Summary of Recurring Displays

Maternal & Child Health Nursing

Care of the Childbearing and Childrearing Family

Maternal & Child Health Nursing

Care of the Childbearing and Childrearing Family

SECOND EDITION

Adele Pillitteri, PhD, RN, PNP

Assistant Professor, School of Nursing
Director, Neonatal Nurse Practitioner Program
State University of New York at Buffalo
Buffalo, New York

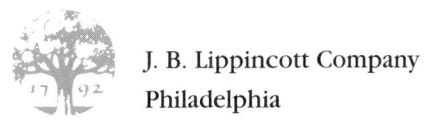 J. B. Lippincott Company
Philadelphia

Sponsoring Editor: Jennifer E. Brogan
Developmental Editor: Marian A. Bellus
Coordinating Editorial Assistant: Danielle DiPalma
Project Editor: Tom Gibbons
Indexer: Maria Coughlin
Senior Design Coordinator: Kathy Kelley-Luedtke
Interior Designer: Anne O'Donnell
Cover Designer: Louis Fuiano
Production Manager: Helen Ewan
Production Coordinator: Nannette Winski
Compositor: Circle Graphics
Printer/Binder: Courier Book Company/Westford
Cover Printer: Lehigh

⊗ This Paper Meets the Requirements of ANSI/NISO Z39.48-1992
(Permanence of Paper).

Photographs opening Units III, IV, VI, and IX © Kathy Sloane.

Color Plates 1 through 6: © R. Gould/Custom Medical Stock Photo
Color Plate 7: © 1991 SIU/Custom Medical Stock Photo
Color Plate 8: © J. Siebert, PhD/Custom Medical Stock Photo
Color Plates 9 and 10: © 1991 M. Fisher/Custom Medical Stock Photo
Color Plate 11: © 1992 J. Barabe/Custom Medical Stock Photo
Color Plates 12 and 17: © 1993 NMSB/Custom Medical Stock Photo
Color Plate 13: © 1994 SIU/Custom Medical Stock Photo
Color Plates 14 and 16: © 1991 NMSB/Custom Medical Stock Photo
Color Plate 15 © 1994 SPL/Custom Medical Stock Photo
Color Plate 18: © 1992 SPL/Custom Medical Stock Photo
Color Plates 19 and 20: © 1990 NMSB/Custom Medical Stock Photo

6 5 4 3 2 1

Library of Congress Cataloging in Publications Data

Pillitteri, Adele.
    Maternal and child health nursing : care of the childbearing and childrearing family / Adele Pillitteri.—2nd ed.
        p. cm.
    Includes bibliographical references and index.
    ISBN 0-397-55113-4
    1. Maternity nursing. 2. Pediatric nursing. 3. Family nursing.
I. Title.
    [DNLM: 1. Maternal–Child Nursing. 2. Family Health.]
RG951.P637 1995
610.73′678—dc20
DNLM/DLC
for Library of Congress   94–16338
                                                                CIP

Any procedure or practice described in this book should be applied by the healthcare practitioner under appropriate supervision in accordance with professional standards of care used with regard to the unique circumstances that apply in each practice situation. Care has been taken to confirm the accuracy of information presented and to describe generally accepted practices. However, the authors, editors, and publisher cannot accept any responsibility for errors or omissions or for any consequences from application of the information in this book and make no warranty express or implied, with respect to the contents of the book.

Every effort has been made to ensure drug selections and dosages are in accord with current recommendations and practice. Because of ongoing research, changes in government regulations and the constant flow of information on drug therapy, reactions and interactions, the reader is cautioned to check the package insert for each drug for indications, dosages, warnings and precautions, particularly if the drug is new or infrequently used.

To my family: Joseph, Rusty, Dawn, Bill, Heather, J.J., and Lynn

with love

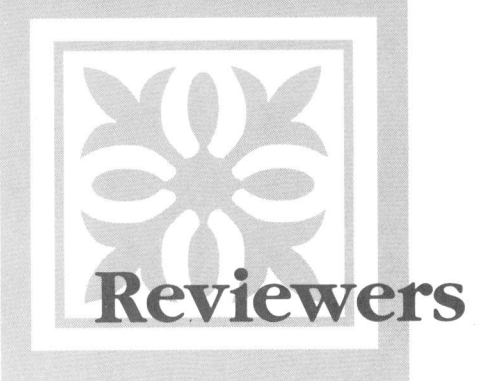

Reviewers

Nina Keller Baker, RNC, MSN
Instructor
Walsh University
Uniontown, Ohio

Patricia Collier, OGNP, MS, ACCE
Clinical Assistant Professor
School of Nursing, Health Sciences Center
State University of New York at Stony Brook
Stony Brook, New York

Lynne Hutnik Conrad, RNC, BSN, MSN
Perinatal Clinical Nurse Specialist
Albert Einstein Medical Center
Philadelphia, Pennsylvania

Edna Boyd Davis, RN, MN
Nursing Instructor
Tuskegee University
Atlanta, Georgia

D'Ann Dennis, RN, MS
Nursing Instructor
Crowder College
Neosho, Missouri

Susan Fowler-Kerry, RN, BA, BSN, MN
Associate Professor
University of Saskatchewan
Saskatoon, Saskatchewan
Canada

Elizabeth I. Hagell, RN, BN, MEd
Nursing Instructor
Red Deer College
Red Deer, Alberta
Canada

Patricia C. Isaacs, RN, PNP, EdD
Professor of Nursing
College of Nursing
Brigham Young University
Provo, Utah

Carol J. Korman, RN, MSN
Nursing Education Specialist
Aultman Hospital School of Nursing
Canton, Ohio

Kris Lishner, DNS, RN
Nursing Instructor
Intercollegiate Center for Nursing Education
Spokane, Washington

Heather McGregor, RegN, BA
Teaching Master
Lambton College
Sarnia, Ontario
Canada

Deborah Scott, DSN, RN
Associate Professor
University of Louisville School of Nursing
Louisville, Kentucky

Jo Trilling, RNC, MS
Nursing Instructor
Intercollegiate Center for Nursing Education
Spokane, Washington

Betty J. Witt, RN, MA
Professor of Nursing Education
San Diego City College
San Diego, California

Helen Zurlo, RN, MS, CNS, CAGS
Associate Professor
Adirondack Community College
Queensbury, New York

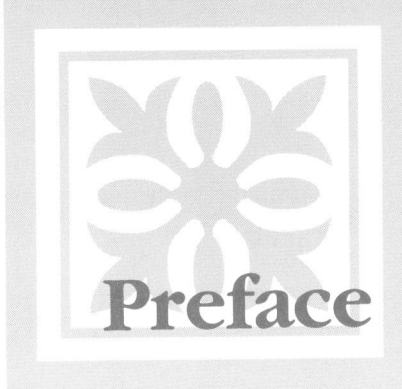

Preface

Maternal–newborn and child health nursing are expanding areas of nursing as a result of the broadening scope of practice within the nursing profession and the recognized need for better preventive and restorative care in these areas. The importance of this need is reflected in the fact that many of the year 2000 health goals for the nation focus on these areas of nursing.

At the same time that the information in these areas of nursing is increasing, less time is available in nursing programs to cover it. Students experience difficulty reading all of the material contained in two separate textbooks.

Maternal and Child Health Nursing: Care of the Childbearing and Childrearing Family, Second Edition, is written with this challenge in mind. It views maternal–newborn and child health care not as two separate disciplines but as a continuum of knowledge. It is designed to present the content of the two disciplines comprehensively but not redundantly. It is based on a philosophy of nursing care that respects clients as individuals yet views them as part of families and the society.

The book is designed for undergraduate student use for a combined course in maternal–newborn and child health, for use in separate maternity and child health courses, or for a curriculum in which concepts of care are integrated throughout the program. It provides a comprehensive, in-depth discussion of the many facets of maternal and child health nursing, while promoting a sensitive, holistic outlook on nursing practice. As such, the book will also be useful for graduate students who are interested in reviewing or expanding their knowledge in these areas.

Basic themes that are integrated into this text include the experience of wellness and illness as family-centered events, the perception of pregnancy and childbirth as periods of wellness in the life of a woman, and the importance of knowledge in the area of child development in the planning of nursing care. Themes reflective of changes in healthcare delivery and settings in a culturally diverse population are discussed in the paragraphs that follow.

The Changing Healthcare Scene

What will ultimately flow from healthcare reform in terms of the kinds of care settings, the cost of care, the roles of healthcare workers, and the educational changes that will have to keep pace with reform has yet to be determined, but it is clear that change is already being effected in each of these areas. In North America an increasingly multicultural population will continue to be reflected among both healthcare workers and their clients, necessitating fine tuning of culturally sensitive care.

New nursing curricula that are in keeping with this spirit of change emphasize outcomes, as reflected in greater emphasis on communication, therapeutic interventions, critical thinking, and nursing process.

Nursing issues that grow out of the current climate of change include the following:

- **The importance of health teaching with families as a cornerstone of nursing responsibilities:** The teaching role of the nurse has greater significance in the new health care milieu as the emphasis on preventive care and short stays in the acute care setting creates the need for families to be better educated in their own care. Focus on Family Teaching displays throughout the text address this issue.

- **An emphasis on National Health Goals:** As a way to focus care and research, National Health Goals have gained wider attention at a time when there is a greater need than ever to be wise in the choice of how healthcare dollars are spent. Students can familiarize themselves with these goals by referring to the Focus on National Health Goals that appear at the beginning of each chapter.

- **The importance of individualizing care according to sociocultural uniqueness:** This is a reflection of both greater cultural sensitivity and an increasingly diverse population of caregivers and care recipients. Greater emphasis is being placed on the implications of multiple sociocultural factors in terms of how they affect the patient's response. Focus on Cultural Awareness displays throughout the text show how cultural factors can be given greater consideration in the planning of care.

- **Changing areas of practice:** The variety of new care settings as well as the diversity of roles in which healthcare workers can practice is reflected both in the proliferation of community-based nursing facilities and in the increase in the numbers of nurse-midwives and pediatric and neonatal nurse practitioners. This new edition places even greater emphasis on the kinds of care settings in which patients find themselves today by including a chapter on the Woman Requiring Home Care, in addition to the chapter on Nursing Care of Children and Their Families in the Home.

Organization of the Text

Maternal and Child Health Nursing follows the family from the pregnancy period, through labor, delivery, and the postpartal period; it then follows the child in the family from birth through adolescence. Coverage includes ambulatory and in-patient care and focuses on primary as well as secondary and tertiary care.

The book is organized in nine units:

Unit I provides an introduction to maternal and child health nursing. A framework for practice is presented, as well as current trends and the importance of considering childbearing and childrearing within a family context.

Unit II examines the nursing role in preparing families for childbearing and childrearing. Reproductive and sexual health, reproductive life planning, and the concerns of the infertile family are discussed.

Unit III presents the nursing role in caring for the pregnant family. Care of the woman during pregnancy and of the growing fetus is discussed. Separate chapters address the role of the nurse when the woman has a preexisting illness, develops a complication of pregnancy, has a special need, or will be cared for at home during pregnancy. Additional chapters detail the role of the nurse as a genetic counselor and an advoate for fetal health.

Unit IV addresses the nursing role in caring for the family during labor and birth. Separate chapters detail the labor process, the role of the nurse in providing comfort during labor, the nursing role when a woman develops a complication of labor and birth, and cesarean birth.

Unit V describes the nursing role in caring for the family during the postpartal period. Separate chapters treat the care of the woman and her family, the newborn, and the changing role when a complication for either the woman or the newborn develops.

Unit VI discusses the nursing role in health promotion during childhood. The chapters in this unit cover principles of growth and development and care of the child from infancy through adolescence, including nutritional needs and child health assessment.

Unit VII presents the nursing role in supporting the health of ill children and their families. The effects of hospitalization on children and their families, health teaching with children, and nursing care of the child and family both in the hospital and in the home are addressed.

Unit VIII examines the nursing role in restoring and maintaining the health of children and families when illness occurs. Disorders are presented according to body systems so that students have a ready orientation for locating content.

Unit IX discusses the nursing role in restoring and maintaining the mental health of children and families. Separate chapters treat the role of the nurse with child abuse and when mental, long-term, or fatal illness is present.

Pedagogic Features

Each chapter in the text is organized to provide a complete learning experience for the student. Numerous pedagogic features help the student understand and increase retention. Important elements include the following.

- **Chapter Objectives:** Learning objectives are included at the beginning of each chapter to identify the outcomes expected after the material in the chapter has been mastered.
- **Chapter Outline:** This feature enables the student to get an overview of the contents of the chapter and to focus on the location of a particular topic when reviewing material.
- **Key Terms:** Terms that would be new to the student are listed at the beginning of each chapter in a ready reference list. The terms first appear in boldface type to draw the student's attention to them and are defined as they are used. They are defined in the glossary as well.
- **Nursing Procedures:** Techniques of procedures specific to maternal and child health care are boxed and presented in a two-column format.
- **Tables and Displays:** Numerous tables and displays summarize important information and provide detail on some topics so that the student has a ready reference.
- **Key Points:** A review of important points is highlighted at the end of the chapter in a list, to help the student monitor his or her comprehension of each chapter.
- **Critical Thinking Exercises:** To involve the student in the decision-making realities of the clinical

setting, several questions are posed at the end of each chapter. They can also serve to form a basis for conference or class discussion.

- **References and Suggested Readings:** These provide the student with the information needed to do more in-depth reading of the sources noted in the text, as well as other relevant articles on the topics included in the chapter.
- **Glossary:** A ready reference-at-hand for the student to clarify the terminology used in the text is included at the end of the book.
- **Appendices:** Ten appendices provide another quick reference to nursing diagnoses, laboratory values, growth charts, vital sign parameters, and drugs safe for use during pregnany and lactation.

Nursing Process

Nursing care plans provide an overview of nursing care in selected situations and show how the nursing process is applied to clinical situations.

- **Nursing Process Overview:** Each chapter begins with a review of nursing process in which specific suggestions, such as examples of nursing diagnoses and outcome criteria helpful to modifying care in the area under discussion, are given. These reviews improve students' preparation in clinical areas to focus their care planning and apply principles to practice.
- **Nursing Interventions:** A consistent format highlights the nursing diagnoses and related interventions throughout the text. A special heading draws the student's attention to these sections where individual nursing diagnoses, goals, and outcome criteria are detailed for the major conditions and disorders discussed.
- **Nursing Care Plans:** Nursing care plans are written for specific clients, not as general summaries, to stress the importance of individualized care planning. Revised and redesigned in a two-column format for this edition, the care plans are written with an emphasis on aiding the student to apply theory to practice and to make use of critical thinking skills.

Recurring Displays

Boxed displays throughout the text help the student focus on important information or provide additional insights.

- **Focus on Nursing Care:** Material that is necessary for quick reference is boxed to give it special emphasis. They focus on key nursing care situations.
- **Focus on Nursing Research:** These displays summarize research carried out by nurses on topics related to maternal and child health nursing. They appear throughout the text to accentuate the use of research as the basis for nursing care.
- **Focus on Family Teaching:** Questions that families frequently ask during the childbearing and childrearing years are presented, followed by a list of detailed and practical information for the family, emphasizing that health teaching should be included as an intrinsic part of nursing care.
- **Focus on Cultural Awareness:** These displays serve to broaden the student's perspective on the many specific cultural influences that can affect the nursing goals and interventions that nurses provide in the maternal and child health setting. They stress the need for nursing care to be modified to meet individualized needs.
- **Focus on National Health Goals:** To emphasize the nursing role in accomplishing the health care goals for our nation, these displays state specific ways in which maternal and child health nursing can provide better outcomes for both mother and child. They help the student to appreciate the importance of national health planning and the influence that nurses can have in creating a healthier nation.

New to the Second Edition

This edition of *Maternal and Child Health Nursing* includes several new features:

- **Two new chapters**
  Sociocultural Aspects of Maternal and Child Health Nursing
  Home Care of the Pregnant Client
- **Key Points**
- **Critical Thinking Exercises**
- **Four new displays**
  Focus on Cultural Awareness
  Focus on Family Teaching
  Focus on National Health Goals
  Focus on Nursing Assessment
- **FREE interactive self-study computer disk**

Ancillary Package

A complete learning and teaching package includes the following:

- **FREE Interactive Self-Study Computer Disk:** Stored on the inside back cover of each book. Two hundred multiple-choice NCLEX-style questions challenge the student's comprehension and application of important material. Feedback is provided for each answer.

- **Instructor's Manual:** The perfect complement to classroom teaching strategies, this resource contains useful media resource lists, case studies, and critical thinking exercises.
- **Computerized Test Bank:** One thousand multiple-choice NCLEX style questions.
- **Overhead Transparencies:** Fifty two-color acetate transparencies illustrating important material enhance student understanding and facilitate classroom discussion.
- **Study Guide:** This companion to the text challenges the student's retention of key concepts and encourages critical thinking and application of information to real nursing situations.
- **Pocket Guide:** The ideal quick reference guide to take along to the clinical area. Essential clinical information, conditions, and problems are organized in an easy-access, alphabetical-outline format. Also includes comprehensive maternity and pediatric content overviews that are excellent for assisting study and review.

Adele Pillitteri, PhD, RN, PNP

Acknowledgments

I would like to express my sincere appreciation to Brian S. Smistek and Timothy R. Palaszewski, Department of Medical Photography, Children's Hospital of Buffalo, Buffalo, New York, for their photographic skill; Marcia Williams for her excellent illustrations; Ann West for her work in the developmental editing of the project; Jennifer Brogan and Marian Bellus, editors at J.B. Lippincott; Tom Gibbons, Project Editor, and all the members of the Production Services Group involved with this text for their assistance and guidance throughout the project; and the countless nursing reviewers who generously added their expertise to this new edition.

A.P.

Contents in Brief

Contents

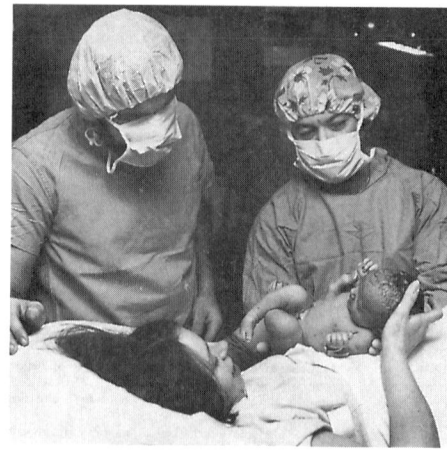

Unit 2
The Nursing Role in Preparing Families for Childbearing and Childrearing   57

Unit 3
The Nursing Role in Caring for the Pregnant Family 137

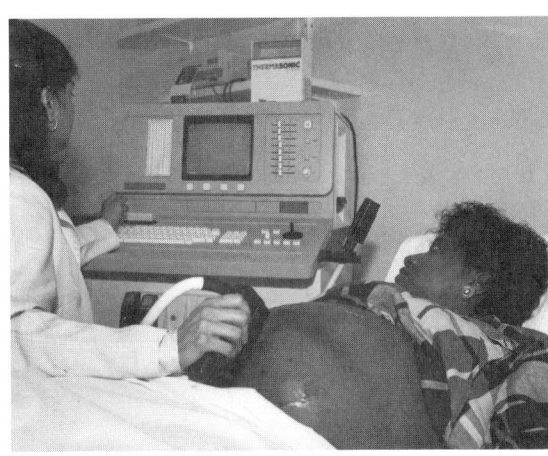

CHAPTER 11
Promoting Fetal and Maternal Health   251

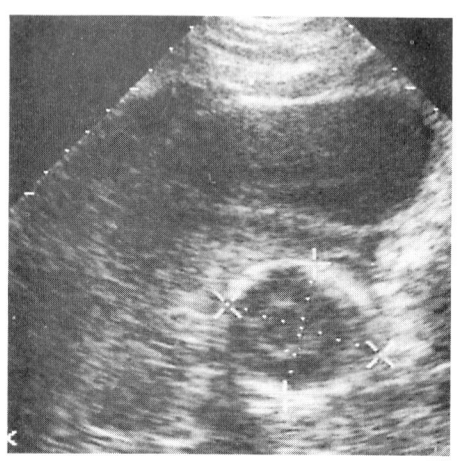

CHAPTER 12
Promoting Nutritional Health During Pregnancy   279

CHAPTER 13
Preparation for Childbirth and Parenting   303

CHAPTER 19
Providing Comfort During Labor and Birth 526

CHAPTER 20
Cesarean Birth 544

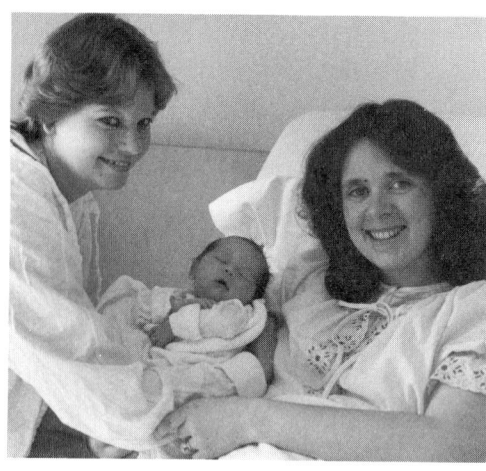

Unit **5**
**The Nursing Role in Caring
for the Family During
the Postpartal Period   601**

CHAPTER 26
**Nursing Care of the High-Risk Newborn
and Family   728**

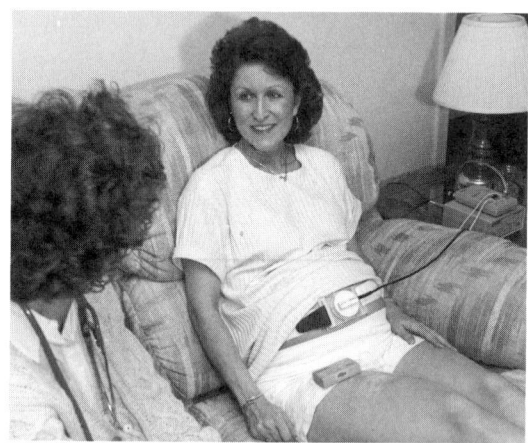

Unit **6**
**The Nursing Role in Health
Promotion for the Childrearing
Family   777**

CHAPTER 27
**Principles of Growth
and Development   778**

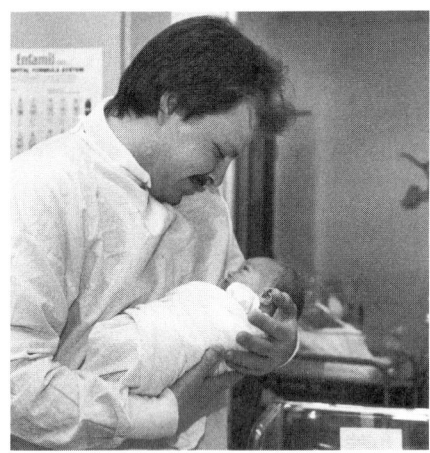

CHAPTER 34

**Nutritional Needs Through Childhood
and Adolescence   980**

Unit **7**

**The Nursing Role in Supporting
the Health of Ill Children
and Their Families   1011**

CHAPTER 35

**The Effects of Hospitalization on Children
and Their Families   1012**

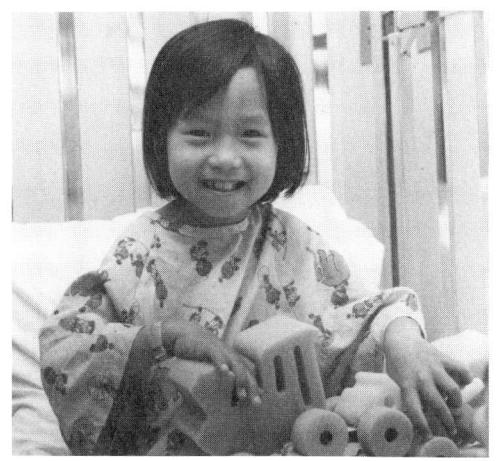

CHAPTER 36

Health Teaching With Children   1041

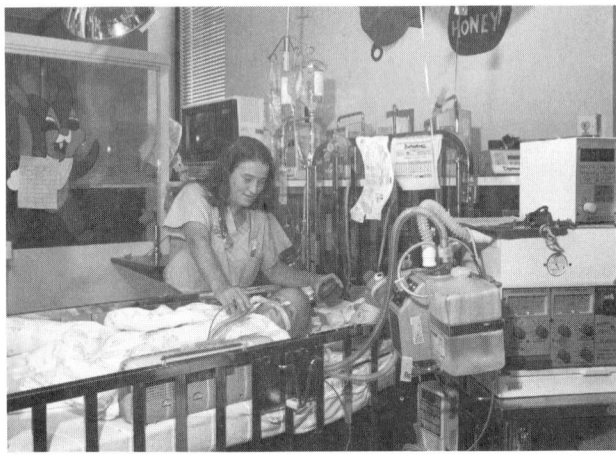

CHAPTER 37
Nursing Care of the Hospitalized Child and Family: Diagnostic and Therapeutic Techniques   1057

CHAPTER 38
Nursing Care of Children and Their Families in the Home   1104

Unit **8**
The Nursing Role in Restoring and Maintaining the Health of Children and Families With Physiologic Disorders   1119

CHAPTER 42
Nursing Care of the Child With an Immune Disorder   1267

NURSING PROCESS OVERVIEW
for the Child With an Immune Disorder   1268

CHAPTER 43
Nursing Care of the Child With an Infectious Disorder   1301

NURSING PROCESS OVERVIEW
for the Child With an Infectious Disorder   1303

CHAPTER 44
Nursing Care of the Child With a Blood Disorder   1341

CHAPTER 45
Nursing Care of the Child With a Gastrointestinal Disorder   1373

CHAPTER 49
Nursing Care of the Child With a Neurologic Disorder   1517

NURSING PROCESS OVERVIEW
for Care of the Child With a Neurologic System Disorder   1518

CHAPTER 50
Nursing Care of the Child With a Disorder of the Eyes or Ears   1562

NURSING PROCESS OVERVIEW
for Health Promotion of Vision and Hearing   1563

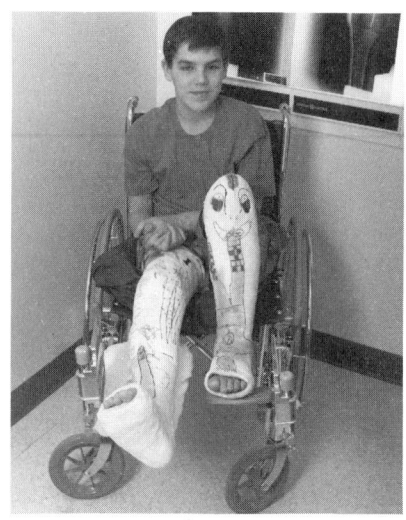

CHAPTER 53
Nursing Care of the Child With Cancer   1675

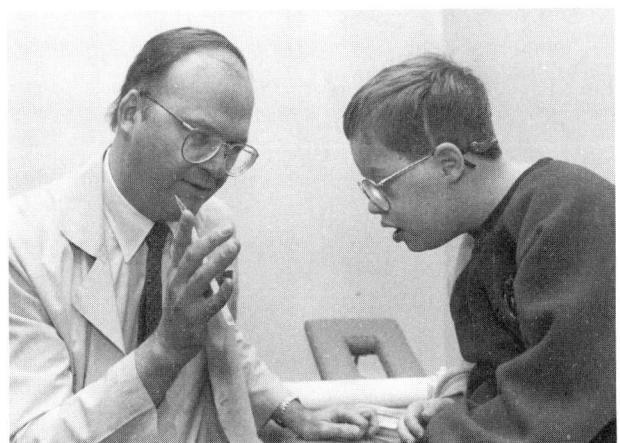

Unit **9**
The Nursing Role in Restoring and Maintaining the Health of Children and Families With Mental Health Disorders   1717

CHAPTER 54
Nursing Care of the Child With a Cognitive or Mental Health Disorder   1718

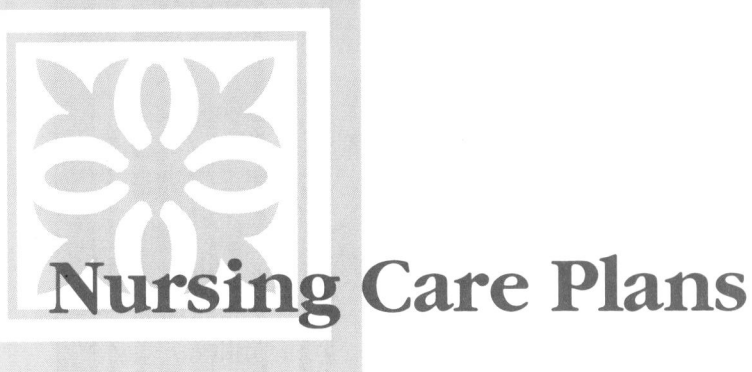

Nursing Care Plans

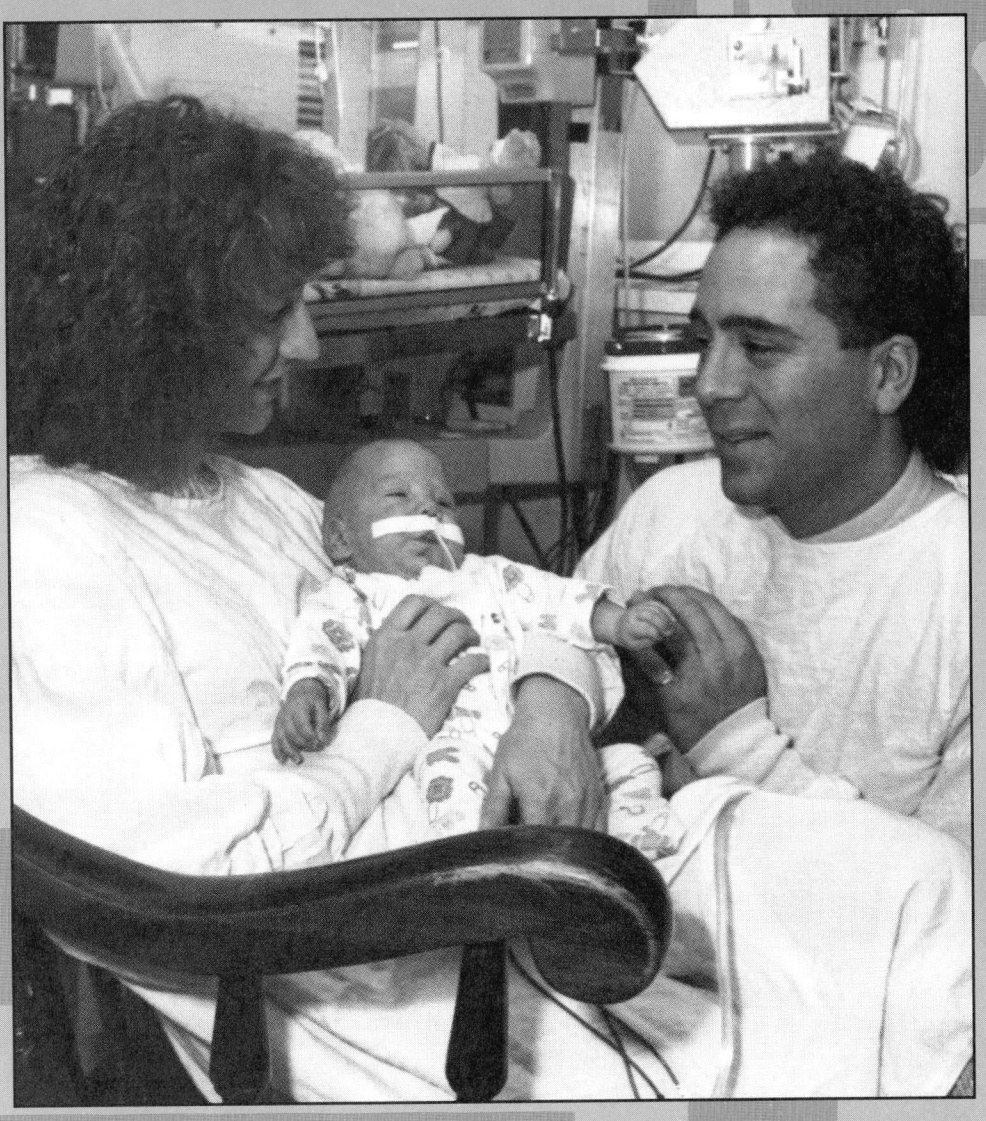

Maternal and Child Health Nursing Practice

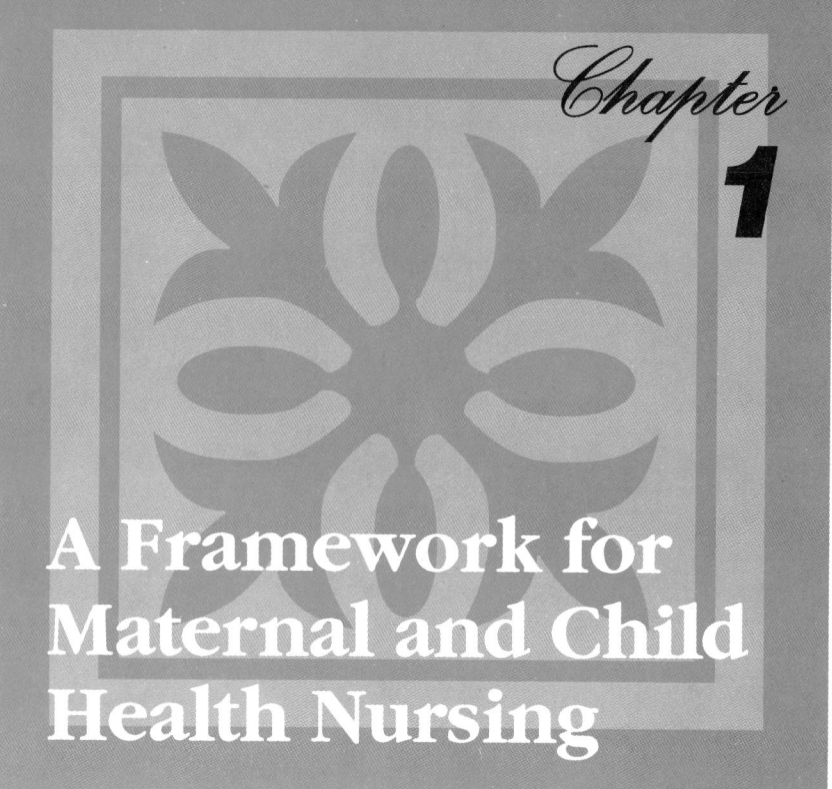

A Framework for Maternal and Child Health Nursing

Chapter 1

Key Terms

- child health nursing
- clinical nurse specialist
- family-centered nursing
- family nurse practitioner
- fertility rate
- maternal and child health nursing
- maternal-newborn nursing
- mortality
- neonatal nurse practitioner
- neonate
- nurse-midwife
- nursing research
- pediatric nurse practitioner
- puerperium

Objectives

After mastering the contents of this chapter, you should be able to:

1. Identify the goals and philosophy of maternal and child health nursing.
2. Describe the evolution, scope, and professional roles of maternal and child health nursing.
3. Define common statistical terms used in the field, such as infant and maternal mortality.
4. Discuss common standards of maternal and child health nursing and the health goals for the nation in terms of their implications for maternal and child health nursing.
5. Discuss the interplay of nursing process, nursing research, and nursing theory as they relate to the future of maternal and child health nursing practice.
6. Use critical thinking to identify areas of care that could benefit from additional nursing research.
7. Synthesize knowledge of trends in maternal and child health care with the nursing process to achieve an understanding of quality maternal and child health nursing care.

Adele Pillitteri: MATERNAL AND CHILD HEALTH NURSING, 2nd Edition. © 1995 Adele Pillitteri.

Care of childbearing and childrearing families has become a major focus of nursing practice today. To have healthy children, it is important to promote the health of the childbearing woman and her family from the time before children are born until they reach adulthood. Prenatal care and guidance is essential to the health of the woman and fetus and to the emotional preparation of a family for childrearing. As children grow, the family needs continued health supervision and support. As children reach maturity, a new cycle begins and new support becomes necessary. The nurse's role in all these phases focuses on promoting healthy growth and development of the child and family in health and in illness.

Although the field of nursing typically divides its concerns for families during childbearing and childrearing into two separate entities—maternity and child health—the full scope of nursing practice in this area is not two separate entities, but one: **maternal and child health nursing**. The nursing role includes the range of responsibilities and concerns involved in care of the woman and family throughout pregnancy and childbirth and the special needs of newborns (**maternal-newborn nursing**) and the health promotion and ill-

ness care for children and families (**child health nursing**).

Goals and Philosophies of Maternal and Child Health Nursing

The primary goal of maternal and child health nursing care can be stated simply as the promotion and maintenance of optimal family health to ensure cycles of optimal childbearing and childrearing. Major philosophical assumptions about maternal and child health nursing are listed in Box 1-1.

Maternal and child health nursing is always **family centered**, which means that the family is considered as the primary unit of care (Figure 1-1). Not only does viewing the family this way provide a context for understanding an individual, but the health of individuals and the ability to function strongly influences the health of family members and overall family functioning. This relationship works both ways. If the family's level of functioning is low, the emotional, physical, and social health and potential of individuals in that family can be ad-

3

1. Maternal and child health nursing is family centered; assessment data must include family as well as individual assessment.
2. Maternal and child health nursing is community centered; the health of families both depends on and influences the health of communities.
3. Maternal and child health nursing is research oriented because research is the means whereby critical knowledge increases.
4. Nursing theory provides a basis for nursing care.
5. A maternal and child health nurse serves as an advocate to protect the rights of all family members including the fetus.
6. Maternal and child health nursing uses a high degree of independent nursing functions because teaching and counseling are so frequently required.
7. Promoting health is an important nursing role because this protects the health of the next generation.
8. Pregnancy or childhood illness are stressful because they are crises. They alter family life in both subtle and extensive ways.
9. Personal, cultural, and religious attitudes and beliefs influence the meaning of illness and its impact on the family. Circumstances such as illness or pregnancy are meaningful only in the context of a total life.
10. Maternal and child health nursing is a challenging role for the nurse and is a major factor in promoting high-level wellness in families.

versely affected. A healthy family, on the other hand, establishes an environment conducive to growth and health-promoting behaviors that sustain family members during crises.

The goals of maternal and child health nursing care are necessarily broad because the scope of practice itself is so broad. Practice ranges from the health care that begins before conception to the care of women during three trimesters of pregnancy and the **puerperium** (the 6 weeks following childbirth, sometimes termed the fourth trimester of pregnancy); to the care of children prenatally, through the neonatal period (the 28 days following birth), and from infancy through adolescence; to the care in settings as varied as the birthing room, the intensive care nursery, and the home. In all of these settings and types of care, keeping the family at the center

of care delivery is essential. Box 1-2 provides a summary of key measures for the delivery of family-centered child health care.

Standards of Maternal and Child Health Nursing Practice

The importance that a society places on caring can best be measured by the concern it places on its vulnerable members or its elderly, disadvantaged, and young citizens. Specialty organizations develop standards of care to promote consistency and ensure quality nursing care in their areas of nursing practice. In maternal child health, standards developed by the Division of Maternal Child Health Nursing Practice of the American Nurses' Association provide important guidelines for planning care and devising outcome criteria for the evaluation of nursing care (ANA, 1986). These standards are summarized in Box 1-3.

Several other specialty groups have developed guidelines for practice and education in this area. The Association of Women's Health, Obstetric, and Neonatal Nurses, or AWHONN (formerly the Nurses' Association of the American College of Obstetricians and Gynecologists, or NAACOG), has developed standards for the nursing care of women and newborns, which are summarized in Box 1-4.

A Framework for Maternal and Child Health Nursing Care

Maternal and child health nursing can be visualized within a framework in which nursing, using nursing process, nursing theory, and nursing research, acts to care for families during childbearing and childrearing years through four phases of health care: health promotion, health maintenance, health restoration, and health rehabilitation. Examples of these phases of health care as they relate to maternal and child health are shown in Table 1-1.

The Nursing Process

Nursing care must be designed and implemented in a thorough manner, using an organized series of steps, to ensure quality and consistency of care. The nursing process, a proven form of problem-solving based on the scientific method, serves as the basis for assessing, plan-

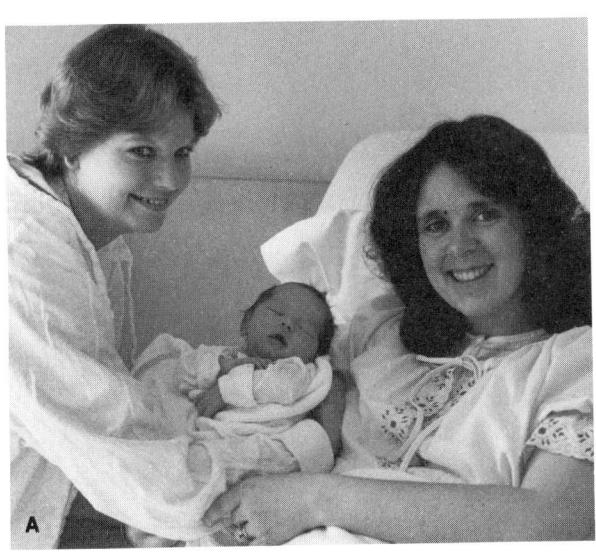
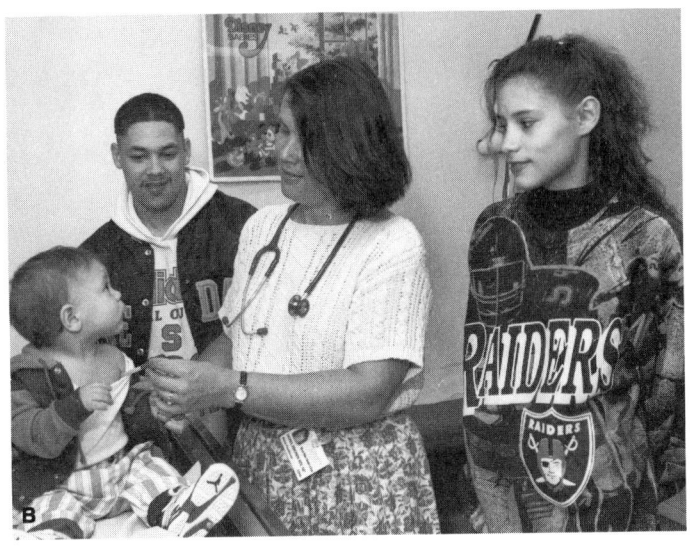

FIGURE 1-1
*Maternal and child health nursing encompasses both childbearing and childrearing aspects.
(**A**) A nurse and mother both show pride in a newborn. (**B**) A nurse takes a child's temperature in an
ambulatory clinic. (Courtesy Department of Medical Photography, Children's Hospital, Buffalo, NY.)*

ning, and organizing care (Henrikson et al., 1992). That the nursing process is applicable to all health care settings from the prenatal clinic to the pediatric intensive care unit is proof that the method is broad enough to serve as the basis for all of nursing care (Carpenito, 1992).

The nursing process according to the NCLEX-RN format (NCSBN, 1987) consists of five steps: (1) assessment, (2) nursing diagnosis, (3) planning, (4) implementation, and (5) evaluation. All subsequent chapters in this book begin with a Nursing Process Overview that summarizes the major nursing concerns in each step of the process for the content of that particular chapter.

Nursing care plans throughout demonstrate the use of the nursing process for a selected client, provide examples of critical thinking in nursing, and clarify nursing care for specific client needs.

Nursing Research

Research is the controlled investigation of a problem using a scientific method. Bodies of professional knowledge grow and expand to the extent that people in that profession plan and carry out research. **Nursing research** is the controlled investigation of problems that have implications for nursing practice. It is the method

---

Box 1-2
Common Measures to Ensure Family-Centered Maternal and Child Health Care

Principle	Nursing Interventions
1. The family is the basic unit of society.	Encourage rooming-in in both maternal and child health hospital settings.
	Participate in early discharge programs to reunite families as soon as possible.
	Encourage family and sibling visiting to promote family contacts.
2. Families represent racial, ethnic, cultural and socioeconomic diversity.	Assess families for strengths and specific needs.
	Respect diversity in families as a special richness of that family.
3. Children grow both individually and as part of a family.	Include developmental stimulation in care.
	Encourage families to give care to a newborn or ill child.
	Share or initiate information on health planning with family members so care is family oriented.

Box 1-3
Standards of Maternal and Child Health Nursing Practice

Standard I

The nurse helps children and parents attain and maintain optimum health.

Standard II

The nurse assists families to achieve and maintain a balance between the personal growth needs of individual family members and optimum family functioning.

Standard III

The nurse intervenes with vulnerable clients and families at risk to prevent potential developmental and health problems.

Standard IV

The nurse promotes an environment free of hazards to reproduction, growth and development, wellness, and recovery from illness.

Standard V

The nurse detects changes in health status and deviations from optimum development.

Standard VI

The nurse carries out appropriate interventions and treatment to facilitate survival and recovery from illness.

Standard VII

The nurse assists clients and families to understand and cope with developmental and traumatic situations during illness, childbearing, childrearing, and childhood.

Standard VIII

The nurse actively pursues strategies to enhance access to and use of adequate health care services.

Standard IX

The nurse improves maternal and child health nursing practice through evaluation of practice, education, and research.

Reprinted from American Nurses' Association. *1986 standards of maternal child health nursing practice.* Kansas City: ANA.

---

by which the foundation of nursing grows, expands, and improves.

The classic example of how the results of nursing research can influence nursing practice is the application of the research carried out by Rubin (1963) on a mother's approach to her newborn. Before this published study, nurses assumed that a woman who did not immediately hold and cuddle her infant at birth was a "cold" or unfeeling mother. Rubin concluded that attachment is not a spontaneous procedure, but more commonly begins with only fingertip touching. Armed with Rubin's finding, nurses became much better able to differentiate healthy from unhealthy bonding behavior in postpartum women and their newborns. Women following this step-by-step pattern of attachment are no longer recognized as unfeeling, but normal; with normal parameters documented, those women who do not follow such a pattern can be identified and helped to gain a stronger attachment to their new infant. Additional nursing research in this area (discussed in Chapter 22) has proved the worth of this original investigation.

Some current examples of questions that warrant nursing investigation in the area of maternal and child health nursing are: What is the best stimulus to encourage women to come for prenatal care or parents to bring children for health maintenance care? What nursing actions are most effective in helping a child adjust to a hospital environment? What are the special needs of women discharged from a hospital or birthing center within 24 hours after childbirth? How much self-care should a preschooler be expected (or encouraged) to provide during illness? What active measures can nurses take to reduce the incidence of child abuse? What are the effects of being in an intensive care unit (ICU) on parents' or children's mental health? How is high self-esteem maintained in couples who are infertile or in disabled children?

Focus on Nursing Research boxes found in chapters throughout this text contain summaries of current maternal and child health nursing research. It is hoped that the content of these boxes will assist students in developing a questioning attitude regarding current nursing practice and in thinking of ways to incorporate research findings into care.

Nursing Theory

One of the requirements of a profession (together with other critical determinants, such as member self-set standards, monitoring of practice quality, and participation in research) is that the concentration of a discipline's knowledge flows from a base of established theory.

Nursing theorists offer helpful ways to view clients and nurses so that nursing activities can best meet client

Standard I

Comprehensive nursing care of women and newborns focuses on helping individuals, families, and communities achieve their optimum health potential. This is best achieved within the framework of the nursing process.

Standard II

Health education for the individual, family, and community is an integral part of comprehensive nursing care. Such education encourages participation in, and shared responsibility for, health promotion, maintenance, and restoration.

Standard III

Written policies, procedures, and protocols clarify the scope of nursing practice and delineate the qualifications of personnel authorized to provide care to women and newborns within the health-care setting.

Standard IV

Comprehensive nursing care for women and newborns is provided by nurses who are clinically competent and accountable for professional actions and legal responsibilities inherent in the nursing role.

Standard V

Nursing care for women and newborns is conducted in practice settings that have qualified nursing staff in sufficient numbers to meet patient-care needs

Standard VI

Ethical principles guide the process of decision-making for nurses caring for women and newborns at all times and especially when personal or professional values conflict with those of the patient, family, colleagues, or practice setting.

Standard VII

Nurses caring for women and newborns utilize research findings, conduct nursing research, and evaluate nursing practice to improve the outcomes of care.

Standard VIII

Quality and appropriateness of patient care are evaluated through a planned assessment program using specific, identified clinical indicators.

From Association of Women's Health, Obstetric, and Neonatal Nurses. (1991). *Standards for the nursing care of women and newborns* (4th ed.). Washington, D.C.: Author.

needs; for example, by seeing the client not simply as a physical form but as a dynamic force with important psychosocial needs. In maternal and child health nursing, it is vital to view clients as extensions or active members of a family as well as holistic beings. Only with this broad focus can nurses appreciate the significant effect of a child's illness or of the introduction of a new member on a family (Gilliss, 1992).

Another issue most nursing theorists address is how nurses should be viewed. At one time, the goal of nurs-

Table 1-1. *Definitions and Examples of Phases of Health Care*

Term	Definition	Examples
Health promotion	Educating clients to be aware of good health through teaching and role modeling	Teaching women the importance of having rubella immunization before pregnancy; teaching children the importance of practices such as thorough tooth brushing or safer sex practices
Health maintenance	Intervening to maintain health when risk of illness is present	Encouraging women to come for prenatal care; teaching parents the importance of safeguarding their home by childproofing it against poisoning
Health restoration	Prompt diagnosis and treatment of illness using interventions that will return client to wellness most rapidly	Caring for a woman during a complication of pregnancy or a child during a respiratory illness
Health rehabilitation	Preventing further complications from an illness; bringing ill client back to optimal state of wellness or helping client to accept inevitable death	Helping a woman with trophoblastic disease to continue therapy or a child with chronic renal disease to continue to attend school

ing could have been stated as providing care and comfort to injured and ill people; currently, most nurses would perceive this view as a limited one, because they are equipped to do much more. Extensive changes in the scope of maternal and child health nursing have occurred as health promotion gains new respect and as new treatment methods become available.

A third issue addressed by nurse theorists concerns the activities of nursing care; as goals become broader, so do activities. For example, when the primary goal of nursing was considered to be caring for ill people, nursing actions were limited to bathing, feeding, and providing comfort. Currently, with the promotion of health as a major nursing goal, teaching, counseling, supporting, and advocacy are also common roles. Because care of women during pregnancy and children during their developing years helps protect not only current health but health of the next generation, maternal child health nurses fill these expanded roles to a unique and special degree.

Table 1-2 summarizes the tenets of a number of common nursing theorists and suggests ways these could be applied to maternal child health care through the situation of one child. The third column of the table ("Emphasis of Care") demonstrates that, although the theoretical bases of these theories differ, the result of any one of them is to provide a higher level of care. These different theories, therefore, are not contradictory, but rather complement each other in the planning and implementation of holistic nursing care.

Maternal and Child Health Nursing Today

The scope of maternal and child health nursing has changed dramatically since the beginning of this century. At that time, research on the benefits of early prenatal care led to the first major national effort to provide prenatal care to all pregnant women through prenatal nursing services (home visits) and clinics. Today, thanks to these and other community health measures (such as the improvement of milk and water supplies and efforts to encourage breast-feeding) as well as many medical advances, the infant mortality rate, or number of infant deaths per 1000 births, has fallen from 100 in 1915 to 8.3 in 1993 (National Center for Health Statistics, 1993b).

Medical technology has contributed to a number of other important advances in maternal and child health: many common childhood illnesses are now largely preventable through immunizations; specific genetic markers and genes responsible for many inherited diseases have been identified and will revolutionize medical therapy in the coming years; and the ability to delay preterm birth and improve life for early born infants has grown substantially. In addition, a growing trend toward health care consumerism, or self-care, has made many child-

bearing and childrearing families active participants in their own health monitoring and care.

But there is still much more to be done. National health care goals established in 1990 for the year 2000 continue to stress the importance of maternal and child health to overall community health (DHHS, 1991) and while health care may be more advanced, it is still not accessible to everyone. These and other social changes and trends have expanded the roles of nurses in maternal and child health care, and at the same time have made the delivery of quality maternal and child health nursing care a continuing challenge.

National Health Goals

In 1979, the United States Public Health Service initiated the formulation of health care objectives to be achieved by 1990. Many of these objectives directly involved maternal and child health care, because improving the health of this young age group has long-term effects. Many of these goals were not met by 1990 due to the limited time period available for problem-solving. Health care goals were reestablished, therefore, in 1990 for the year 2000 (DHHS, 1991). Goals specific for each content area are shown in following chapters. Maternal and child health nurses will play a vital role in helping the nation achieve these objectives and better health.

Trends in the Maternal and Child Health Nursing Population

The maternal and child population is constantly changing along with changes in social structure, variations in family lifestyle, increased health care costs, improvements in medical technology, and changing patterns of illness. Table 1-3 summarizes some of the social changes that have occurred over the last 20 to 30 years that have altered health care priorities for maternal and child health nurses.

What is the best way to measure the health of this population? Health is certainly more complicated than just the absence of illness. For example, some children with chronic but controllable asthma think of themselves as well; others with the same degree of involvement consider themselves ill. Although pregnancy is generally considered a well state, some women think of themselves as ill during this period. A more objective view of health is provided by national health statistics.

Measuring Maternal and Child Health

A number of statistical terms are used internationally to express the outcome of pregnancies and births and describe child health (Box 1-5). The statistics that these terms encompass require accurate collection and analysis in order to provide a descriptive picture of the nation's health. Such a description is useful for comparison and planning of future health care needs.

Table 1-2. *Summary of Nursing Theories*

Terry is a 7-year-old girl who is hospitalized because her right arm was severely injured in an auto-mobile accident. There is a high probability she will never have full use of the arm again. Terry's mother is concerned because Terry showed promise in art. Previously happy and active in Girl Scouts, Terry has spent most of every day since the accident sitting in her hospital bed silently watching television.

Theorist	Major Concepts of Theory	Emphasis of Care
Faye Abdellah	The role of the nurse is to identify and to correct needs according to 21 identified areas; needs may be overt (apparent) or covert (hidden or unknown to the client).	Assess Terry's health care needs according to the 21 areas of concern; care is incomplete until all needs are met.
Dorothy Johnson	A person comprises subsystems that must remain on balance for optimal functioning. Any actual or potential threat to this system balance is a nursing concern.	Assess the effect of lack of arm function on Terry as a whole; modify care to maintain function in all systems, not just musculoskeletal.
Imogene King	Nursing is a process of action, reaction, interaction, and transaction; needs are identified based on client's social system, perceptions, and health; the role of the nurse is to help the client achieve goal attainment.	Discuss with Terry the way she views herself and illness. She views herself as a well child, active in Girl Scouts and school; structure care to help her meet these perceptions.
Florence Nightingale	The role of the nurse is viewed as changing or structuring elements of the environment such as ventilation, temperature, odors, noise, and light to put the client into the best opportunity for recovery.	Turn Terry's bed into the sunlight; provide adequate covers for warmth; leave her comfortable and with electronic games to occupy her time.
Betty Neuman	A person is an open system that interacts with the environment; nursing is aimed at reducing stressors through primary, secondary, and tertiary prevention.	Assess for stressors such as loss of self esteem and derive ways to prevent further loss such as praising her for combing her own hair.
Dorothea Orem	The focus of nursing is on the individual; clients are assessed in terms of ability to complete self-care. Care given may be wholly compensatory (client has no role); partly compensatory (client participates in care); or supportive-educational (client performs own care).	Arrange overbed table so Terry can feed herself; urge her to participate in care by doing as much for herself as she can.
Ida Jean Orlando	The focus of the nurse is interaction with the client; effectiveness of care depends on client behavior, nurse's reaction to behavior, and the nursing action appropriate to client needs. Client should define own needs.	Ask Terry what she feels is her main need. Terry says that returning to school is what she wants most. Stress activities that allow her to maintain contact with school such as doing homework or telephoning friends.
Hildegard Peplau	The promotion of health is viewed as the forward movement of the personality; this is accomplished through an interpersonal process including orientation, identification, exploitation, and resolution.	Plan care together with Terry. Encourage her to speak of school and accomplishments in Girl Scouts to retain self-esteem.
Martha Rogers	The purpose of nursing is to move the client toward optimal health; the nurse should view the client as whole and constantly changing, and help people to interact in the best way possible with the environment.	Help Terry to make use of her left side as much as possible so that she returns to school and previous level of functioning as soon as possible.
Sister Callistra Roy	The role of the nurse is to aid clients to adapt to the change caused by illness; levels of adaptation depend on the degree of environmental change and state of coping ability; full adaptation includes physiological factors, self-concept, role function, and interdependence.	Assess Terry's ability to use her left hand to replace her right-hand functions, which are now lost; direct nursing care toward replacing deficit with other skills.

Birth Rate

The birth rate in the United States has increased slightly over the past few years, from a record low of 14.8 per 1000 population in 1976 to the current rate of 15.5 (NCHS, 1994) (Figure 1-2). This is primarily due to an increased number of women at childbearing age, increased births to unmarried women, and a higher birth rate for older women. Currently, the average U.S. family has 1.2 children. Boys are born more often than girls, at a rate of 1053 boys to every 1000 girls (Wegman, 1993).

Table 1-3. *Trends in Maternal and Child Health Care and Implications for Nurses*

Trend	Implications for Nursing
Families are smaller in size than in previous decades.	Fewer family members are present as support in a time of crisis. Nurses must fulfill this role more than ever before.
Single parents are increasing in number.	A single parent may have fewer financial resources; more likely if the parent is a woman. Nurses need to inform parents of care options and to serve as a "backup" opinion when needed.
An increasing number of mothers work outside the home.	Health care must be scheduled at times a working parent can bring a child for care. Problems of latch-key children and the selection of child care centers need to be discussed.
Families are more mobile than previously.	Good interviewing is necessary with mobile families so a health data base can be established; education for health monitoring is important.
Abuse is more common than ever before.	Screening for the possibility of child or spouse abuse should be included in family contacts. Be aware of the legal responsibilities for reporting abuse.
Families are more health-conscious than previously.	Families are "ripe" for health education; providing this can be a major nursing role.

Fertility Rate

The term **fertility rate** reflects what proportion of women who could have babies are having them. The fertility rate for 1993 was 69%, which demonstrates a healthy reproductive rate for a country (NCHS, 1993a).

Box 1-5

Statistical Terms Used to Report Maternal and Child Health

Birth rate: The number of births per 1000 population.

Fertility rate: The number of pregnancies per 1000 women of childbearing age.

Fetal death rate: The number of fetal deaths (over 500 g) per 1000 live births.

Neonatal death rate: The number of deaths per 1000 live births occurring at birth or in the first 28 days of life.

Perinatal death rate: The number of deaths of fetuses more than 500 g and in the first 28 days of life per 1000 live births.

Maternal mortality: The number of maternal deaths per 100,000 live births that occur as a direct result of the reproductive process.

Infant mortality: The number of deaths per 1000 live births occurring at birth or in the first 12 months of life.

Fetal Death Rate

A fetal death is defined as the death in utero of a child (fetus) weighing 500 g or more, roughly the weight of a fetus of 20 weeks or more gestation. Fetal deaths may occur because of maternal factors (e.g., maternal disease, incompetent cervix, or maternal malnutrition) or fetal factors (e.g., fetal disease, chromosome abnormality, or poor placental attachment). A large number of fetal deaths occur for reasons yet unknown. The fetal death rate of a nation is important in evaluating health care because it reflects the overall quality of maternal health and prenatal care.

Neonatal Death Rate

The first 28 days of life are known as the *neonatal period*. The child during this time is known as a **neonate**. The neonatal death rate reflects not only the quality of care available to women during pregnancy and childbirth but also the quality of care available to infants during the first month of life.

The leading causes of infant mortality during the first 4 weeks of life are prematurity (early gestational age), low birth weight (a weight below 2500 g), and congenital anomalies. Approximately 80% of infants who die within 48 hours of birth weigh less than 2500 g (5.5 lb).

Perinatal Death Rate

The perinatal period is the time beginning when the fetus reaches 500 g (about week 20 of pregnancy) and ending about 4 weeks after birth. The perinatal death rate is the sum of the fetal and neonatal rates.

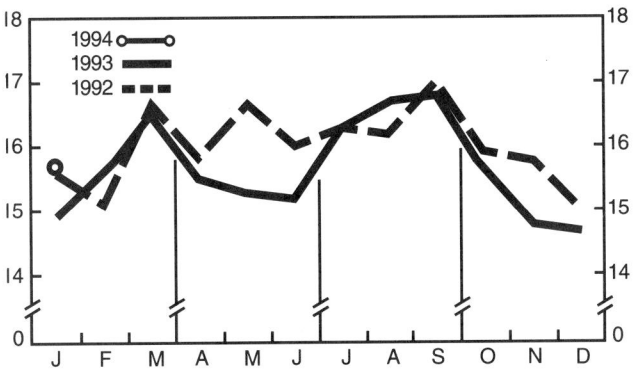

FIGURE 1-2
Monthly birth rates per 1000 population in the United States, 1992–1994. (From National Center for Health Statistics [1994]. Monthly Vital Statistics Report [Vol. 43, p. 2]. Hyattsville, MD: U.S. Public Health Service.)

Maternal Mortality

Mortality rate is the rate of deaths from a specific cause. Early in the 20th century, the maternal mortality (death from childbirth) rate reached levels as high as 600 per 100,000 live births. Currently, the maternal mortality rate has declined to a low of 6.5 per 100,000 live births (NCHS, 1994; Figure 1-3). This dramatic decrease can be attributed to improved prenatal and obstetric care, such as the improved ability to control complications associ-

ated with hypertension of pregnancy and improved anesthetic techniques (Scott et al., 1990).

For most of the 20th century, uterine hemorrhage was the leading cause of death during pregnancy. This has changed owing to the increased ability to prevent or control hemorrhage, so that pulmonary embolism currently is the leading cause of death in childbirth (Lagrew, 1990). Pregnancy-induced hypertension, a condition peculiar to pregnancy, and hemorrhage and infection are other important causes. These conditions are largely preventable, and nurses who are alert to their signs and symptoms are invaluable guardians of the health of pregnant and postpartum women.

Infant Mortality

The infant mortality rate of a country is an index of the general health of the country. This rate is the traditional standard used to compare national health care to previous years and to that of other countries.

Thanks to medical advances and improvements in child care, the infant mortality rate in the United States has been steadily declining in recent years; it reached a record low in 1993 of 8.2 per 1000 population (NCHS, 1994). Unfortunately, infant mortality is not equal for all people. Black infants have a mortality rate of 18.9. This difference in black and white infant deaths is thought to be related to the high proportion of births to young

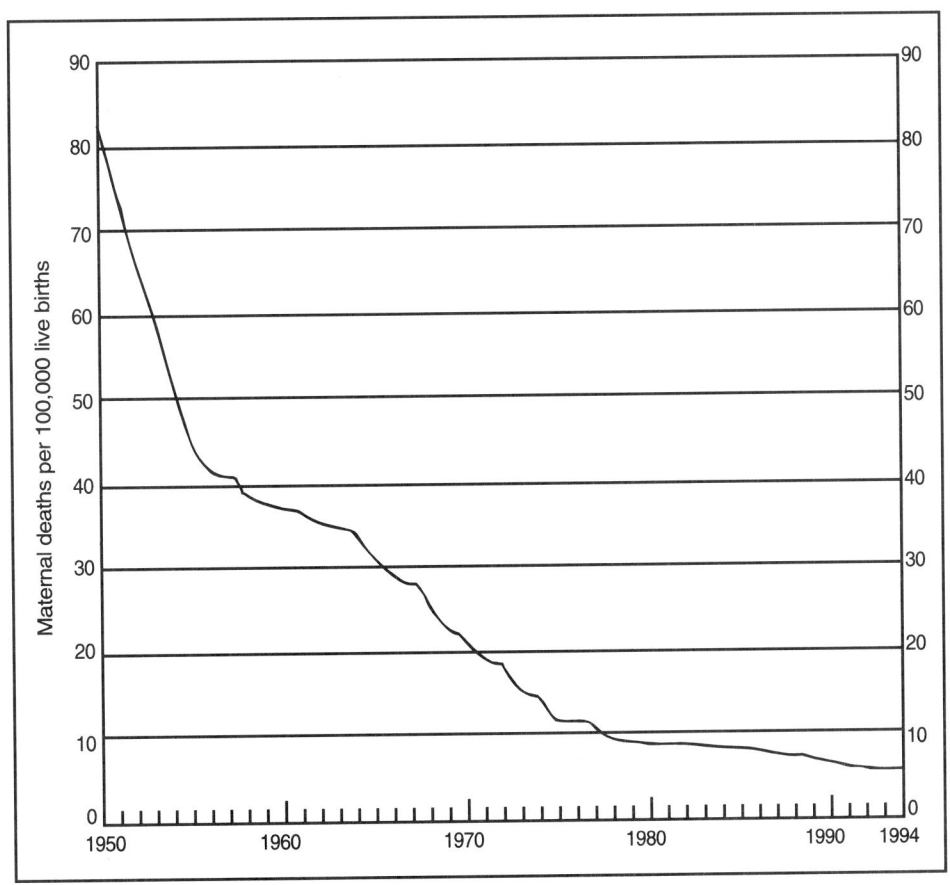

FIGURE 1-3
Maternal mortality rates, 1950–1994. (From National Center for Health Statistics [1994]. Monthly Vital Statistics Report [Vol. 43, p. 4]. Hyattsville, MD: U.S. Public Health Service.)

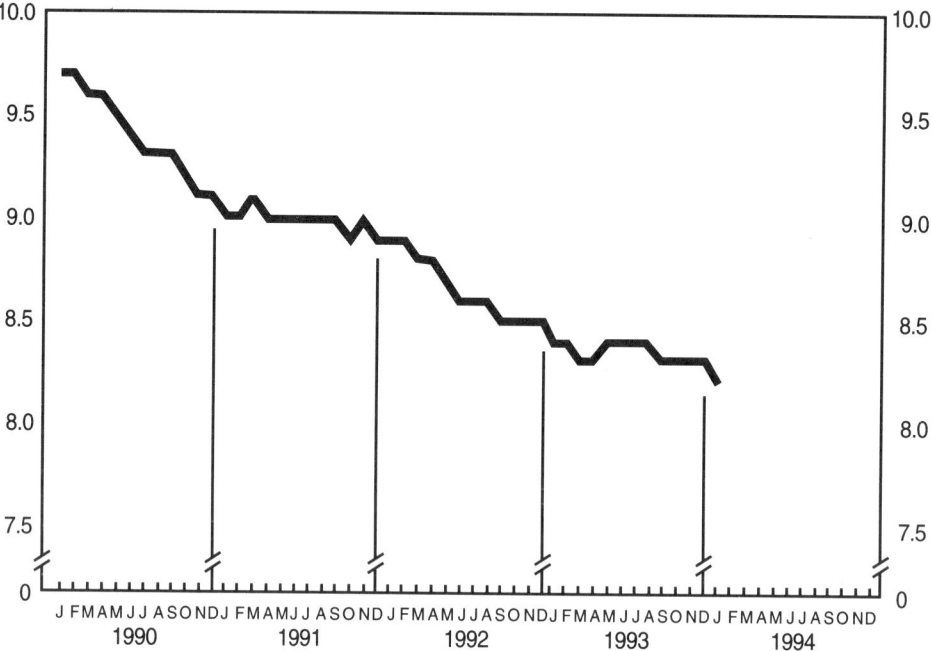

FIGURE 1-4

Infant mortality rates (per 1000 live births), 1990–1994. (From National Center for Health Statistics [1994]. Monthly Vital Statistics Report [Vol. 43, p. 5]. Hyattsville, MD: U.S. Public Health Service.)

black mothers, unequal provision of health care, and the higher percentage of low birth weight babies born to black women—12% as compared to 5% for white and Asian women (Wegman, 1993). Despite this negative trend, the overall steady drop in total infant mortality is encouraging (Figure 1-4).

The infant mortality rate varies greatly from state to state within the United States (Table 1-4). For example, in the District of Columbia, the area with the questionable distinction of having the highest infant mortality, infant mortality is more than four times that in New Hampshire, the state with the lowest infant mortality.

Table 1-5 shows the relative ranking of the United States compared with other developed countries. One would expect that a country such as the United States, which has one of the highest gross national products in the world and is known for its technologic capabilities, would have the lowest infant mortality. Yet, in 1990, the U.S. infant mortality rate was higher than that of 20 other countries (Wegman, 1993).

One factor that may contribute to national differences in infant mortality is the type of health care available. In Sweden, for example, a comprehensive health care program provides free maternal and child health care to all residents. Women who attend prenatal clinics early in pregnancy receive a monetary award for early attendance; this almost guarantees that all women will come for prenatal care. Many people believe that a guaranteed health care system would lead to lower infant mortality in the United States.

Many women in the United States do not begin prenatal care in the first trimester of pregnancy (only 78% do). In addition, 5% of white mothers and 11% of black

Table 1-4. *Infant Mortality per 1000 Live Births by State, 1993*

State	Rate	State	Rate
New Hampshire	4.9	Idaho	8.7
North Dakota	6.1	Pennsylvania	8.7
Vermont	6.2	Kentucky	8.9
Nevada	6.3	Florida	8.9
Iowa	6.5	New York	8.9
Massachusetts	6.6	Missouri	9.1
Hawaii	6.7	Oklahoma	9.3
Maine	6.7	Rhode Island	9.3
Utah	6.7	Arkansas	9.3
California	6.8	Tennessee	9.5
Nebraska	7.1	Louisiana	9.7
Texas	7.2	Virginia	9.7
Minnesota	7.2	West Virginia	9.8
New Mexico	7.3	Indiana	9.8
Washington	7.4	Delaware	9.9
Wisconsin	7.4	Michigan	9.9
Colorado	7.5	Illinois	9.9
Montana	7.5	South Carolina	10.0
Oregon	7.5	Georgia	10.1
Connecticut	7.7	Wyoming	10.2
Alaska	7.8	Alabama	10.3
New Jersey	7.9	South Dakota	10.3
Maryland	8.0	North Carolina	10.5
Arizona	8.2	Mississippi	11.9
Kansas	8.2	District of Columbia	17.4
Ohio	8.3		

From: National Center for Health Statistics. (1993). *Monthly Vital Statistics Report, 42,* 14.

Table 1-5. Infant Mortality Rates per 1000 Live Births for Selected Countries, 1990

Country	Birth Rate	Infant Mortality
Japan	9.9	4.6
Singapore	17.8	5.5
Sweden	14.3	5.6
Finland	13.2	6.1
Switzerland	12.6	6.8
Canada	14.9	6.8
Netherlands	13.2	7.1
France	13.3	7.3
Hong Kong	11.7	7.4
Germany	11.2	7.5
Denmark	12.4	7.5
Spain	10.2	7.7
Austria	12.0	7.7
Norway	14.2	7.8
United Kingdom	13.9	7.9
Belgium	12.6	7.9
Ireland	14.9	8.2
Australia	15.4	8.2
New Zealand	17.8	8.3
Italy	9.8	8.5
United States	16.7	9.1

From: United Nations. (1992). *Population and vital statistics report.* New York: United Nations.

mothers receive no care or only attend prenatal care in the last trimester of pregnancy. This allows complications of pregnancy to become extreme before they are resolved rather than allowing preventive strategies to reduce their intensity. The United States also differs from other countries in the increased number of infants born

to adolescent mothers (about one in four live births are to teenage mothers; Burnhill, 1994).

The main causes of early infant death in the United States are problems occurring at birth or shortly thereafter. Prematurity, low birth weight, respiratory distress syndrome, intrauterine hypoxia, birth asphyxia, and congenital anomalies are major causes (NCHS, 1993a).

Before antibiotics and formula sterilization practices, gastrointestinal disease was a leading cause of infant death. By advocating breast-feeding and teaching mothers strict adherence to good sanitary practices health care practitioners can help ensure that gastrointestinal infection does not again become a major factor in infant mortality.

Childhood Mortality

The risk of death in the first year of life is higher than that in any other year under age 55 (Wegman, 1992). Children in the prepubescent period (age 5 to 14 years) have the lowest mortality of any child age group.

The most frequent causes of childhood death are shown in Table 1-6. Notice that motor vehicle accidents are the leading cause of death in adolescents, and yet many accidents are largely preventable through education on the value of seat belt use, the dangers of drinking and driving, and the hazards of drug abuse.

In addition, there is a high incidence of suicide in the 15- to 24-year-old age group. Many adolescents come to health care facilities for the common physical problems of their age—obesity, acne, and menstrual irregularities. Although an adolescent may not voice feelings of depression or anger during a health care visit, such underlying feelings may actually be a primary concern. The high incidence of homicide and an increase in the number of HIV-positive adolescents are also growing concerns.

Table 1-6. Major Causes of Death in Childhood

Cause	1–4 yrs	Rank Order	5–14 yrs	Rank Order	15–24 yrs	Rank Order
Accidents (other than MV)	11.6	1	4.6	2	9.9	4
Motor vehicle (MV) accidents	5.9	2	5.6	1	32.0	1
Congenital anomalies	5.7	3	1.4	4	1.2	8
Malignant neoplasms	3.5	4	3.1	3	5.0	5
Homicide	2.8	5	1.4	5	22.4	2
Diseases of the heart	2.2	6	0.8	6	2.7	6
Pneumonia and influenza	1.4	7	0.4	8	0.7	9
Human immunodeficiency virus	1.0	8	0.3	9	1.7	7
Suicide	0.0	9	0.7	7	13.1	3

From: National Center for Health Statistics. (1993). Deaths and death rates for the 10 leading causes of death in specific age groups. *Monthly Vital Statistics Report, 42,* 21.

Incidence of Infectious Diseases

As more immunizations become available, fewer children in the United States are affected by common childhood diseases. For instance, the incidence of poliomyelitis (once a major killer of children) is now extremely low (almost extinct), because nearly all children in the United States are immunized against it. In contrast, measles, once considered a disease that would also become extinct because of immunization, flared in incidence in the early 1990s. Measles encephalitis can be as destructive and lethal as poliomyelitis, which underscores the importance of continued health education on measles immunization. Continued education about the benefits of immunization against rubella (German measles) is also needed. If women contract this form of measles during pregnancy, their infants can be born with severe congenital anomalies.

Although the decline in the overall incidence of preventable childhood diseases is encouraging, as many as 50% of children under 4 years in some communities are still not fully immunized (NCHS, 1993b). Childhood infectious diseases will increase again if immunization is not maintained as a high national priority.

The advent of human immunodeficiency virus (HIV) has changed care considerations in all areas of nursing, but it has particular implications for maternal and child health nursing: childbearing women and sexually active teenagers are at risk for becoming infected with the human immunodeficiency virus through sexual contact or parenteral exposure to blood and blood products; infected women may transmit the virus to a fetus during pregnancy through placental exchange (Meadows et al., 1993). To help prevent the spread of HIV, adolescents and young adults must be educated against unsafe sexual practices. Universal precautions must be strictly followed in maternal and child health nursing as in other areas of nursing practice to safeguard health care providers and other clients (Greenbaum, 1993).

Other infectious diseases growing in incidence include syphilis, genital herpes, hepatitis A and B, and tuberculosis. The rise in syphilis and genital herpes probably stems from an increase in premarital or non-monogamous sexual relationships. The increase in hepatitis B is due largely to drug abuse and infected injection equipment. One reason for an increase in hepatitis A is shared diaper-changing facilities in day care centers. Tuberculosis, which was once considered close to eradication, has experienced a resurgence, occurring today at approximately the same rate as measles in young adults. One form, occurring as an opportunistic disease in individuals who are HIV positive, is particularly resistant to the usual therapy (Schurmann et al., 1993).

Health Care Settings

The settings of maternal and child health care are changing to better meet the needs of this increasingly well informed and vocal population.

Alternative Settings and Styles for Childbirth

This century has seen several major shifts in maternity care. At the turn of the century, most births took place in the home with only the very poor or very ill delivering in "lying-in" hospitals. By 1940, about 40% of live births occurred in hospitals and by 1990, the figure had risen to 99%. Today, a less dramatic but no less important trend is occurring as an increasing number of families are once more choosing childbirth at home or in alternative birth settings rather than hospitals. These alternative settings provide families with increased control in the birth experience and options for birth surroundings unavailable in hospitals. One strength of this movement is its encouragement of family involvement in birth. It also increases nursing responsibility for assessment and professional judgment and provides expanded roles for nurse practitioners, such as the nurse-midwife. Of all U.S. births, 3% currently are attended by midwives rather than physicians (Wegman, 1993).

Hospitals have responded to consumer demand for a more natural childbirth environment by refitting labor and delivery suites as birthing rooms often called LDR (labor-delivery-recovery) or LDRP (labor-delivery-recovery-postpartum) rooms. These rooms are designed to make labor and delivery more homelike and relaxing (Figure 1-5). This appeals to many families who might otherwise have opted to give birth at home. Keeping childbirth as natural as a family desires within the hospital or birthing center where experienced nurse-midwives or physicians can provide professional care should contribute to the goal of continued lowering of infant mortality rates.

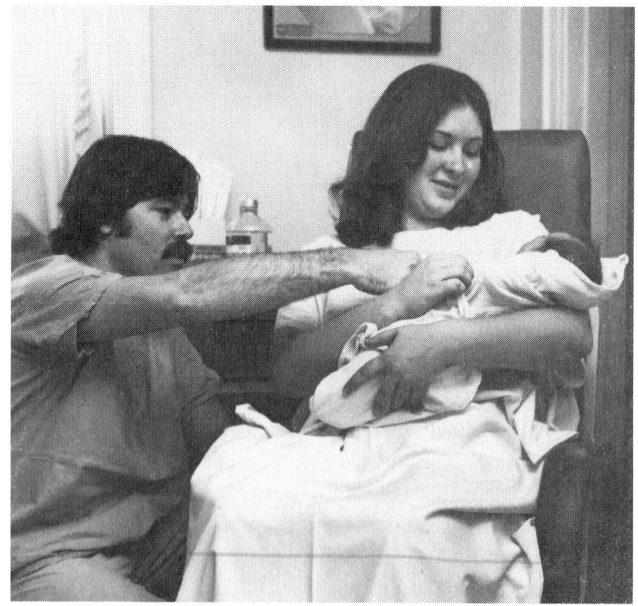

FIGURE 1-5
Mother and father share a close moment in a birthing room. (Courtesy Department of Medical Photography, Children's Hospital, Buffalo, NY.)

Strengthening of the Ambulatory Care System

The ambulatory care system has broadened its base so that more and more people who might have been admitted to a hospital are now being cared for in ambulatory clinics or at home. This option has proved especially important in the care of sick children and women who are experiencing a pregnancy complication or who want early discharge following childbirth (Williams & Cooper, 1993). Separation of a child from his or her family during an illness has been shown to be potentially harmful to the child's development, so any effort to reduce the incidence of separation should have a positive effect (see Chapter 35). Avoiding long hospitalizations for women during pregnancy is also a preferable method of care because it helps to maintain family contact.

Shortening of Hospital Stays

Many hospitals perform children's surgery such as tonsillectomy or umbilical or inguinal hernia repair without requiring an overnight stay. Early in the morning of surgery, the parent and child arrive at the hospital and the child receives a preoperative physical and medication. After surgery, the child is sent to a recovery room and then to a short-term "observation" unit. If the child is doing well and showing no complications by about 4 hours after surgery, the child can be discharged. Similarly, women who have begun preterm labor stay in the hospital while labor is halted, and then are allowed to return home on medication with continued monitoring. Routine hospitalization for mothers and newborns after an uncomplicated delivery is now 2 days or less.

Short-term hospitalization often requires intensive health teaching by the nursing staff. A child's parent must be taught to watch for danger signs in the child without being frightened. A woman with a complication of pregnancy must be taught to watch for signs that warrant immediate attention. A new mother and father must be taught about their newborn's nutritional needs, umbilical cord care, bathing, and safety considerations—all before the euphoria/fatigue of birth has begun to wear off. This is a difficult type of teaching that not only includes imparting the facts of self-care but also includes providing support and reassurance that the client or client's parents are capable of this level of care.

Inclusion of the Family in the Health Care Setting

Many hospitals have developed policies that minimize the effects of separation from parents when children must be admitted for extended stays. Open visiting hours allow parents to visit as much as possible and sleep overnight in a bed next to their child. Parents are allowed to do as much for the child as they wish during a hospital stay, such as feeding and bathing the child or administrating oral medicine. Most of a parent's time, however, should be spent in simply being close by to provide a comfortable, secure influence on the child in order to maintain normal growth and development. For the same reasons, parents on a maternity unit are encouraged to room in and give total care to their well newborn.

Because parents will play such a vital role in their child's hospitalization, they should be considered admitted along with the child. Thus, the nurse's client care load will be not just four children, for example, but four children plus four sets of parents; not just a single newborn, but his or her two parents as well.

Increase in the Number of Intensive Care Nurseries

Over the past 20 years, care of infants and children has become more intensive. It is generally assumed that newborns with a term birth weight (more than 2500 g or 5.5 lb) will thrive at birth. A number of infants are born each year, however, with birth weights lower than 2500 g or who are ill at birth and do not thrive. Such infants are regularly transferred to a neonatal intensive care unit (NICU) or intensive care nursery (ICN). Intensive care at this early point in life is one of the most costly types of hospitalization. Expenses of $1000 a day or $20,000 to $100,000 for a total hospitalization are not rare for care during a high-risk pregnancy and care for a high-risk infant. As the number of these settings increases, the opportunities for advanced practice nursing also increases.

Regionalization of Intensive Care

To avoid duplication of care sites, it is accepted practice for a community to establish one high-risk nursery (Level III) to serve the needs of the entire health system; ill newborns are transported to this central nursery when necessary. Likewise, regions are limited to the number of intensive care units for high-risk women and children that can be opened. Through such planning, there is always one site that is properly staffed and equipped for every potential problem. However, when a newborn is hospitalized in a regional center, the mother who has been left behind in a community hospital needs a great deal of support. She will feel she has "lost" her infant the same as if the child had died, unless health care personnel help her keep abreast of her infant's progress through phone calls and snapshots, and encourage her to visit the baby as soon as she is able.

An important argument against regionalization for pediatric care is that children will feel homesick in strange settings, overwhelmed by the number of sick children they see, and frightened because they are miles from home. These are definitely important considerations. Because nurses more than any other health care group set the tone for hospitals, it is their responsibility to see that children and parents feel as welcome in the regional centers as they would have been in a small hospital, and that staffing is adequate, allowing sufficient time for nurses to comfort frightened children and prepare them for new experiences.

Transportation to Regional Centers. When regionalization concepts of newborn care first became accepted, transporting the ill or premature newborn to the regional care facility was the method of choice (Figure 1-6). Currently, however, health care providers are reconsidering the subject. When it is known in advance that a child may be born with a life-threatening condition, it may be safer to transport the mother to the regional center during pregnancy, because the uterus has advantages as a transport incubator that far exceed any commercial incubator yet designed (Strobino et al., 1993).

Such transportation creates several problems, however. Removing a woman from her community places a great deal of stress on her family; it also limits her own doctor's participation in her care. Women who are transported long distances for perinatal care need strong support from nursing personnel, or else they can feel "lost" in the system.

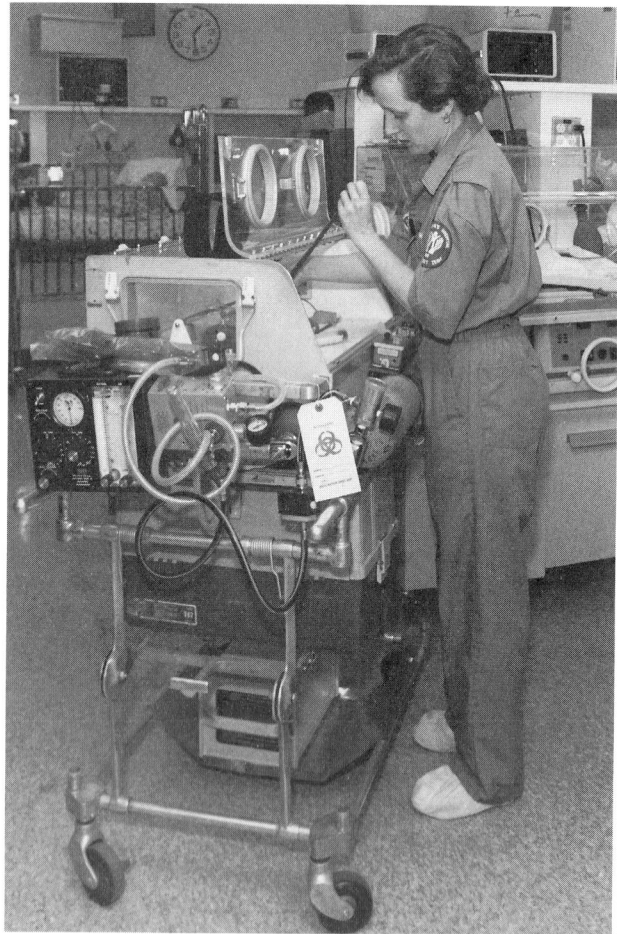

FIGURE 1-6

An infant transport incubator is prepared to move a premature infant to a regional hospital. Helping with safe movement of pregnant women and ill newborns to regional centers is an important nursing responsibility. (Courtesy Department of Medical Photography, Children's Hospital, Buffalo, NY.)

Increased Reliance on Comprehensive Care Settings

Comprehensive health care is designed to be capable of meeting all of a child's needs in one setting. In the past, care of children tended to be specialized. For example, a child with a congenital anomaly such as myelomeningocele or cerebral palsy might have been followed by a team of specialists for each facet of the problem. Such a team might include a neurologist, a physical therapist, an occupational therapist, a psychologist for intelligence quotient testing, speech therapist, orthopedic surgeon, and finally, a special education teacher. The parents might need to find a special dentist who would accept multihandicapped clients. Each specialist would look only at one area of the child's needs rather than the whole child's development. Without extra guidance, parents would find themselves lost in a maze of visits to different health care personnel. If they were not receiving financial support for their child's care, they might not have been able to afford all the necessary services at one time. It might have been difficult to decide which of the child's problems needed to be treated immediately and which could be left untreated, without worsening and developing into permanent disability. Many health care experts now urge that, while specialists are still important to a child's care, a trusted primary care provider to help parents in the coordination of a child's specialized services is also essential.

Throughout the health care system, major attempts are being made to centralize or at least combine care so that one caregiver serves as the primary care provider and follows the child through all phases of care even though specialists are still used. Nurses can be helpful in seeing that children have all their needs met by a primary health care provider (who could be a nurse practitioner) in this way. The family must become empowered to seek out conditions that will be best for their health. Use of a health maintenance organization or family practice often allows all needs to be met in a family-centered setting.

Increased Use of Alternative Treatment Modalities

There is a growing tendency for families to consult providers of alternative forms of therapy such as acupuncture or therapeutic touch in addition to, or instead of, traditional health care providers (Zagorsky, 1993). One study estimated that as frequently as one in every three persons in the United States adult population used some form of unconventional therapy in 1990 (Eisenberg et al., 1993). Nurses have an increasing obligation to be aware of alternative therapies, which have the potential to enhance or detract from the effectiveness of traditional therapy (see Focus on Cultural Awareness box).

In addition, the health care team who is unaware of the existence of some alternative forms of therapy may

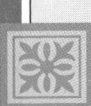

FOCUS ON CULTURAL AWARENESS

The term "alternative health care practices" refers to therapy such as acupuncture, homeopathy, therapeutic touch, herbalism, and chiropractic care (Zagorsky, 1993). Other sources for health care needs include tribal medicine or *yerberos* or *curanderos* (Hanley, 1991; Adams, et al., 1992). Some people seek out these types of therapy prior to consulting a traditional health care provider; others consult them following what they perceive to be inadequate care by a traditional provider.

Respecting these forms of care can be instrumental in showing families that their sociocultural traditions and needs are important to the nurse. The nurse should also assess what nontraditional measures are being used, since the action can interfere with prescribed medications. For instance, the consumption of traditional ethnic remedies such as Jin Bu Huan, a Chinese herbal medicine to relieve pain, has caused adverse effects such as life-threatening bradycardia and respiratory depression (DHHS, 1993a). Lead poisoning has resulted from ingestion of "greta," a traditional Mexican remedy employed as a laxative (DHHS, 1993b).

lose an important opportunity to capitalize on the positive features of that particular therapy. For instance, it would be important for the nurse to know that a child about to undergo a painful procedure was experienced at meditation. The nurse might ask the child if she wanted to meditate before the procedure to help her relax. Not only could this decrease the child's discomfort, but it could also offer the child a feeling of control over a difficult situation.

Increased Reliance on Home Care

Early hospital discharge has resulted in many women and children returning home before they are fully ready to care for themselves. Ill children and women with complications of pregnancy may choose to remain at home for care rather than be hospitalized. This has created a "second system" of care and requires many additional care providers. Nurses are instrumental in devising and modifying procedures for home care, as well as sustaining the client's morale and interest in her own health in situations such as home monitoring to prevent premature labor (Adkins et al., 1993). Because home care is a unique and expanding area in maternal and child health nursing, it is discussed in relation to maternal care in Chapter 16; in relation to children in Chapter 38.

Health Care Concerns and Attitudes

The 1980s brought about considerable change in the health care system and particularly in maternal and child health. As we approach the year 2000, there are likely to be even more changes as the United States actively works toward effective health goals and guaranteed health care for all citizens.

Increasing Concern Regarding Health Care Costs

The cost of health care has increased in recent years to such an extent that, without health insurance programs, the average American is unable to pay for hospital care without a great sacrifice to family needs. This situation has direct implications for maternal and child health nursing because early prenatal care is the single most important determinant of neonatal health (Harvey et al., 1993). Lack of financial ability to pay for the service is a major reason that women do not obtain prenatal care (Braveman et al., 1993).

Increasing Emphasis on Preventive Care

A generally accepted theory is that it is better to keep individuals well than to restore health after they have become ill. Counseling parents on ways to keep their homes safe for children is an important form of illness prevention in maternal and child health nursing. The facts that accidents are still a major cause of death in children and that women still do not receive prenatal care are testaments to the need for much more anticipatory guidance in this area (Wegman, 1993).

Increasing Emphasis on Family-Centered Care

Health promotion with families during pregnancy or childrearing is a family-centered event, because teaching health awareness and good health habits is accomplished chiefly by role modeling. Illness in a child is automatically a family-centered event, because parents have to adjust work schedules to allow one of them to stay with the ill child; siblings may have to sacrifice an activity such as a birthday party or having a parent watch their school play; family finances may have to be readjusted to pay for hospital and medical bills. When a mother is pregnant, family roles or activities may have to change to safeguard her health. A family may feel itself drawn together by the fright and concern of an acute illness; unfortunately, when an illness becomes chronic, it may pull a family apart or destroy it.

Nurses can be instrumental in including family members in events from which they were once totally excluded, such as an unplanned cesarean birth. They can help child health care to be family centered by consulting with family members about a plan of care and providing clear health teaching so family members can monitor their own care (Figure 1-7). Nurses play an active role in both health promotion teaching and sustain-

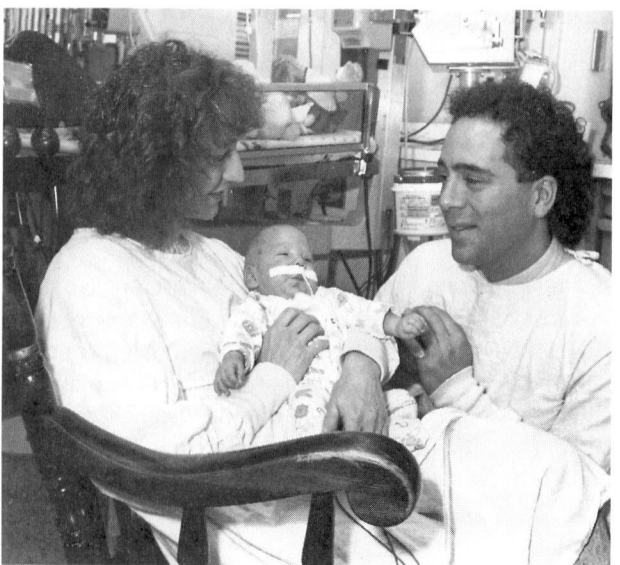

FIGURE 1-7
Childbearing and childrearing families require nursing care that addresses the special needs of their particular stage of development. (Courtesy Department of Medical Photography, Children's Hospital, Buffalo, NY.)

ing families through a child's illness. A nurse is often the person best able to recognize illness as a family problem rather than the illness of a single child.

Increasing Concern for the Quality of Life

In the past, health care of women and children was centered on maintaining physical health. More recently, however, a growing awareness that the quality of life is as important as physical health has expanded the scope of health care to include the assessment of psychosocial facets of life in such areas as self-esteem and independence. Good interviewing skills are necessary to elicit this information at health care visits. Nurses can be instrumental not only in assessing for such information but also in planning ways to improve the quality of life in the areas the client considers most important.

One way in which the quality of life is being improved for children with chronic illness is the national mandate to allow them to attend regular school; they are guaranteed entrance despite severe illness or use of medical equipment such as a ventilator (Public Law 99-452). Nurses, serving as school nurses or consultants to schools, play important roles in making these efforts possible.

Increasing Awareness of the Individuality of Clients

Women having children today do not fit readily into any set category; some are younger than ever before and an increasing number of women are experiencing their first pregnancies after the age of 35. Many women are having children outside of marriage (Campen, 1992). Many families who have come from foreign countries enter the

United States health care system for the first time during a pregnancy or with a sick child. This requires a greater sensitivity in the health care provider to the sociocultural aspects of care (Doucet et al, 1992). Lesbian couples are also beginning to raise families together, conceiving children through artificial insemination or adoption. As a result of advancements in research and treatments, women who were once unable to have children, such as those with cystic fibrosis, are now able to manage a full-term pregnancy (Kotloff et al., 1992). Individuals with mental and physical disabilities are also establishing families and rearing children (Accardo et al., 1990; Sauer & Harvey, 1993). As the level of violence in the world increases, the incidence of abused children and pregnant women is also increasing (Bohn, 1990). All of these concerns require increased nursing concern.

Empowerment of Health Care Consumers

In recent years, individuals and families have begun to take increased responsibility for their own health. For some families this means following a more nutritious diet and planning regular exercise; for others it can mean an entire change in lifestyle. When a family member is ill, empowerment means participation in the treatment plan. Women are very interested in participating in decision-making regarding their childbearing options. Parents want to accompany their ill children into the hospital for overnight stays. They are eager for information about their child's health and want to contribute to the decision-making process. They may question treatments or care plans that they feel are not in their child's best interest. When health care providers do not provide answers to a client's questions or are insensitive to needs, many health care consumers are willing to take their business to another health care setting. Nurses can be instrumental in promoting empowerment of parents and children by respecting views and concerns, addressing clients by name, and by regarding parents as important participants in their child's health—keeping them informed and helping them to make decisions about their child's care. Although the nurse may have seen 25 clients already in a particular day, he or she can make each client feel as important as the first by showing a warm manner and keen interest.

Advanced Practice Roles for Nurses in Maternal and Child Health

As trends in maternal and child health care change, so do the roles of maternal and child health nurses. All maternal and child health nurses function in a variety of settings as caregivers, client advocates, researchers, case managers, and educators. There are also many advanced practice roles (O'Connor, 1994).

Women's Health Care Nurse Practitioner

A women's health care nurse practitioner is a nurse with advanced study in the promotion of health and prevention of illness in women. Such a nurse plays a vital role in educating women about their bodies and sharing with them methods to prevent illness; they care for women with illnesses such as sexually transmitted diseases and counsel them about and offer information regarding reproductive life planning. They play a large role in helping women remain well so that they can enter a pregnancy in good health and maintain their health during the years until their child reaches adulthood.

Maternity or Family Nurse Practitioner

A maternity nurse or **family nurse practitioner** (FNP) in conjunction with a physician provides prenatal care for the woman with an uncomplicated pregnancy. He or she may see the client on an alternate basis with the physician throughout the woman's pregnancy evaluating the progress of the pregnancy, managing minor health care problems including prescribing medication, and providing information and counseling. The nurse practitioner takes the health and pregnancy history, performs physical and obstetric examinations, orders appropriate diagnostic and laboratory tests, and plans continued care through pregnancy and for the family afterward. FNPs follow the family indefinitely to promote health and optimal family functioning.

Neonatal Nurse Practitioner

The **neonatal nurse practitioner** (NNP) is skilled in the care of the newborn, both well and ill. Neonatal nurse practitioners may work in level I, II or III newborn nurseries, neonatal intensive care units, neonatal follow-up clinics, physician groups, or in transporting the ill infant (Zukowsky & Coburn, 1991). The NNP's responsibilities include managing patient care in an intensive care unit, conducting normal newborn assessments and physical examinations, and providing high-risk follow-up discharge planning (see the Focus on Nursing Research box).

Pediatric Nurse Practitioner

Either a **pediatric nurse practitioner** (PNP) or a family nurse practitioner (FNP) is a nurse prepared with extensive skills in physical assessment, interviewing, and well-child counseling and care. In this role, a nurse interviews parents as part of an extensive health history and performs a physical assessment of the child. If the nurse's diagnosis is that the child is well, he or she discusses with the parents any childrearing problems

FOCUS ON NURSING RESEARCH

Can Nurses Make a Direct Impact on Infant Well-being?

Very-low-birth-weight infants benefit from periods of sustained sleep. In order to see if decreasing the noise in an intensive care unit would help these infants coordinate sleep states, Strauch et al. (1993) designated a Quiet Hour for the last hour of every nursing shift. Both noise and procedures were reduced to a minimum during these times. For the study, noise levels and sleep states were monitored. The findings indicated that fewer infants cried during the Quiet Hour than control period and more infants achieved sleep states.

This is an important study in that it demonstrates that nurses can have a direct effect on controlling the environment in which they work and can directly improve patient health.

From Strauch, C., Brandt, S., & Edwards-Beckett, J. (1993). Implementation of a quiet hour: effect on noise levels and infant sleep states. *Neonatal Network, 12,* 31.

mentioned in the interview; gives any immunizations needed; offers necessary anticipatory guidance (based on the nursing plan); and arranges a return appointment for the next well-child checkup. The nurse serves as a primary health caregiver or as the sole health care person the parents and child see at all visits (Forbes et al., 1990).

The PNP who determines that a child has a common illness—for example, iron deficiency anemia—orders the necessary laboratory tests and prescribes appropriate drugs for therapy (Figure 1-8). If the PNP determines that the child has a major illness—for example, congenital subluxated hip, kidney disease, or heart disease—he or she consults with an associated pediatrician; together, they decide what further care is necessary. Nurse practitioners also work in inpatient or specialty settings providing continuity of care to hospitalized children.

Nurse-Midwife

Throughout history, **nurse-midwives,** individuals educated in the discipline of nursing and midwifery and licensed according to the requirements of the American College of Nurse-Midwives (ACNM), have played an important role in assisting women with pregnancy and childbearing. Either independently or in association with an obstetrician, the nurse-midwife can assume full responsibility for the care and management of women with uncomplicated pregnancies. Nurse-midwives play a large role in making birth an unforgettable family event

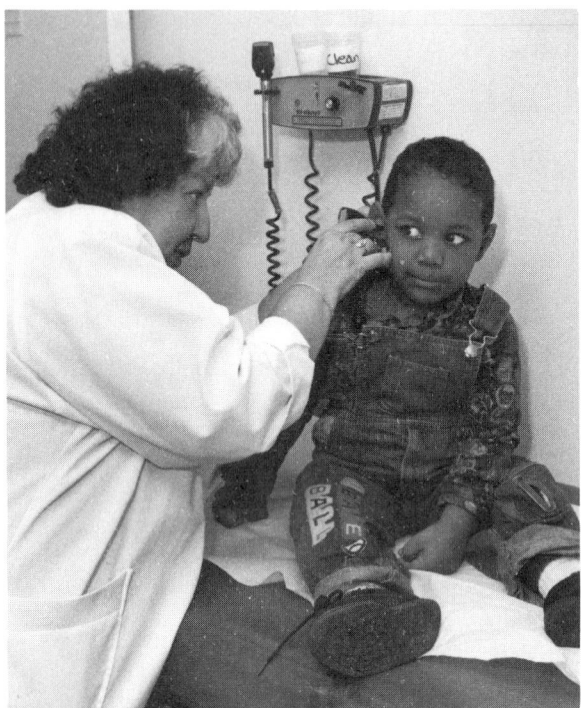

FIGURE 1-8
Pediatric nurse practitioner is an extended role for nurses. (Courtesy Department of Medical Photography, Children's Hospital, Buffalo, NY.)

as well as helping to ensure a healthy outcome for both mother and child (Figure 1-9).

Child Health, Perinatal, and Neonatal Clinical Nurse Specialists

Clinical nurse specialists are nurses prepared at the master's degree level who are capable of acting as a consultant in his or her area of expertise, as well as a role model, researcher, and teacher of quality nursing care (Naylor & Brooten, 1993). Examples of areas of specialization are adolescent health care and lactation consultation for breast-feeding mothers.

Consider, for example how a child health clinician might intervene to help in the care of John, a 4-year-old with diabetes mellitus who has been admitted to the hospital. John's primary nurse determines that John's parents are having difficulty accepting the diagnosis. John is difficult to care for because he is so fearful of hospitalization and so perplexed by his parent's attitudes (he interprets their lack of visits as nonacceptance of him). The primary nurse also notes that nurses are not giving consistent information to the parents. A child health clinician could be instrumental in helping a primary nurse organize care and meeting with the parents to help them accept what is happening. Neonatal clinicians manage infant's care at birth and in intensive care

settings; they provide home follow-up care to ensure the newborn remains well (Zukowsky & Coburn, 1991).

Legal Considerations of Practice

Maternal and child health nursing carries some legal concerns that extend above and beyond other areas of nursing, because care is often given to an "unseen client"—the fetus—or to clients who are not of legal age for giving consent for medical procedures. This concern is long lasting, since children who feel they were wronged by health care personnel can bring a lawsuit at the time they reach legal age. This means that a nursing note written today may need to be defended as many as 20 years in the future. Nurses need to be conscientious about obtaining informed consent for invasive procedures and in determining that pregnant women are aware of any risk of harm to the fetus involved with a procedure or test (Rhodes, 1990). In divorced or blended families (those in which two adults with children from previous relationships now live together), it is important to establish who has the right to give consent for health care.

In a society in which child abuse is of national concern, nurses are becoming increasingly responsible for identifying and reporting each incident of suspected abuse in children (Pillitteri et al., 1993). The exact legal ramifications of procedures or care are discussed in further chapters with procedures or treatment modalities.

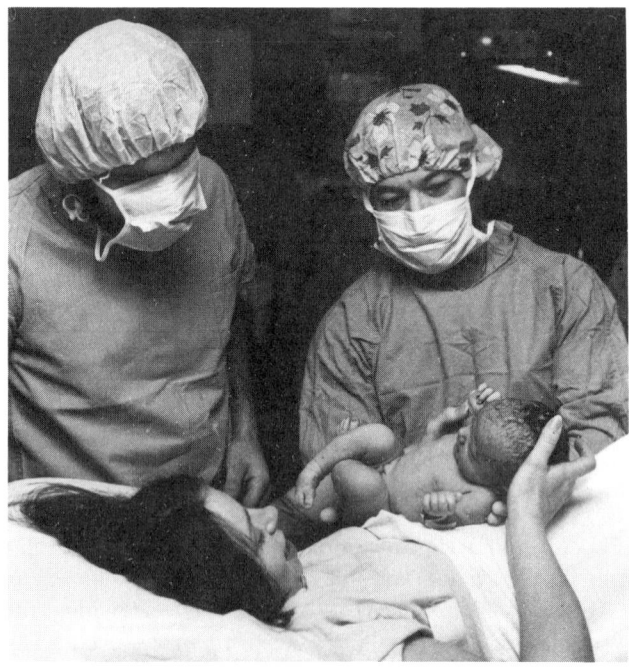

FIGURE 1-9
A nurse-midwife plays an important role in ensuring a safe birth. (Courtesy Department of Medical Photography, Children's Hospital, Buffalo, NY.)

Ethical Considerations of Practice

Some of the most difficult decisions in health care settings must certainly be those that involve children and their families. Just a few of the major potential conflicts include conception issues, especially those related to in vitro fertilization, embryo transfer, and surrogate mothers; abortion; fetal rights versus rights of the mother; the use of fetal tissue for research; resuscitation (how long should it be continued?); how many procedures or how much pain should a child be asked to endure to achieve a degree of better health?; what should be the balance between modern technology and quality of life?

Legal and ethical aspects of issues are often intertwined, which makes the decision-making process complex. Because maternal and child health nursing is so strongly family centered, it is common to encounter some situations in which the interests of one family member are in conflict with those of another. For example, when a pregnancy causes a woman to develop a serious illness, the family must make a decision either to terminate the pregnancy and lose the child or keep the pregnancy and rally to support the mother through the crisis. If the fetus is also at risk from the illness, the decision may be easier to make; however, the circumstances are usually not clear-cut; the decisions that need to be made are difficult. The nurse is certain to discover these and other issues in the course of practice and can do much to aid clients when they reach such decision-making impasses by providing factual information and supportive listening and by aiding the family in clarification of values.

The Pregnant Woman's Bill of Rights and the United Nations Declaration of Rights of the Child (see Appendix A) provide guidelines for determining the rights of clients in health care settings and situations.

Key Points

- Standards of maternal and child health nursing practice have been formulated by the ANA and the Association of Women's Health, Obstetric and Neonatal Nurses (AWHONN) to serve as guides for practice.
- Nursing theory and nursing research are methods by which maternal and child health nursing expands and improves.
- The most significant measure of maternal and child health is the infant mortality rate. It is the number of deaths in infants from birth to 1 year per 1000 live births. This rate is declining steadily but in the United States is still higher than 20 other nations.
- Trends in maternal and child health nursing include changes in the settings of care, increased concern about health care costs, increased preventive care and family centered care.

- Advanced practice roles in maternal and child health nursing include women's health, neonatal, and pediatric nurse practitioners, clinical nurse specialists, and nurse-midwives. All of these expanded roles contribute to making maternal and child health care an important area of nursing and health care.
- Maternal and child health care has both legal and ethical considerations over and above other areas of practice.

Critical Thinking Exercises

1. Canada has a health care delivery system based not on profit but on provision of care for all citizens through a tax-supported program. The infant mortality rate in Canada is lower than in the United States.
   a. What are some reasons that might contribute to this?
   b. How do sociocultural aspects affect infant mortality rate?
2. The age of women having their first baby is advancing. For many women this is 30 years and above.
   a. How do you anticipate this will change care in the future?
   b. Are there special services you can anticipate that should be provided for such women?
   c. How will this trend influence childrearing in the future?

References

Accardo, P. J., et al. (1990). Children of mentally retarded parents. *American Journal of Diseases of Children, 144,* 69.

Adams, R., et al. (1992). Cultural considerations: developing a nursing care delivery system for a Hispanic community. *Nursing Clinics of North America, 27,* 107.

Adkins, R. T., et al. (1993). Prevention of preterm birth: early detection and aggressive treatment with terbutaline. *Southern Medical Journal, 86,* 157.

American Nurses Association. (1986). *Standards of maternal-child health nursing practice.* Kansas City, MO: ANA.

Bohn, D. K. (1990). Domestic violence and pregnancy. *Journal of Nurse-Midwifery, 35,* 86.

Braveman, P., et al. (1993). Access to prenatal care following major Medicaid eligibility expansions. *Journal of the American Medical Association, 269,* 1285.

Burnhill, M.S. (1994). Adolescent pregnancy in the United States. *Contemporary OB/GYN, 39,* 26.

Campen, J. (1992). Statistics corner: a substantial increase in women giving birth outside of marriage. *International Journal of Childbirth Education, 7,* 4.

Carpenito, L. J. (1992). *Nursing diagnosis: Application to clinical practice* (4th ed.). Philadelphia: J. B. Lippincott.

Department of Health & Human Services. (1991). *Healthy people 2000.* Washington, D.C.: Public Health Service.

Department of Health and Human Services. (1993a). Jin bu Huan toxicity in children—Colorado, 1993. *MMWR, 42 (28),* 1.

Department of Health and Human Services. (1993b). Lead poisoning associated with use of traditional ethnic remedies—California, 1991–1992. *MMWR, 42 (27),* 1.

Doucet, H., et al. (1992). Risk of low birthweight and prematurity among foreign born mothers. *Canadian Journal of Public Health, 83,* 192.

Eisenberg, D. M., et al. (1993). Unconventional medicine in the United States. *New England Journal of Medicine, 328,* 246.

Forbes, K. E., et al. (1990). Clinical nurse specialist and nurse practitioner core curriculum survey results. *Nurse Practitioner, 15,* 43.

Gilliss, C. L. (1992). Family nursing research: precepts from paragons and peccadilloes. *Journal of Advanced Nursing, 17,* 28.

Greenbaum, D. M. (1993). History, general overview, and protection of health care workers. *Critical Care Clinics, 9,* 1.

Hanley, C. (1991). Navago Indians. In Giger, J., & Davidhizar, R. *Transcultural Nursing: Assessment and Interventions.* St. Louis: Mosby Year Books.

Harvey, S. M., et al. (1993). Obstacles to prenatal care following implementation of a community-based program to reduce financial barriers. *Family Planning Perspectives, 25,* 32.

Henrikson, M., et al. (1992). Nursing diagnosis and obstetrics, gynecologic, and neonatal nursing: breastfeeding as an example. *Journal of Obstetrics, Gynecologic, and Neonatal Nursing, 21,* 446.

Kotloff, R. M., et al. (1992). Fertility and pregnancy in patients with cystic fibrosis. *Clinics in Chest Medicine, 13,* 623.

Lagrew, D. C. (1990). Strategies for managing emboli in pregnancy. *Contemporary Obstetrics/Gynecology, 20,* 113.

Meadows, J., Catalan, J., & Gazzard, B. (1993). HIV antibody testing in the antenatal clinic. *Midwifery, 9,* 17.

National Center for Health Statistics. (1993a). Trends and current status in childhood mortality. *Vital and Health Statistics, 42,* 1.

National Center for Health Statistics. (1993b). Monitoring maternal mortality. *Vital and Health Statistics, 42,* 5.

National Center for Health Statistics. (1994). Births, marriages, divorces and deaths. *Monthly Vital Statistics Report, 43,* 6.

National Council of State Boards of Nursing. (1987). *Test plan for the national council licensure examination for registered nurses* (NCLEX). Chicago, IL: Author.

Naylor, M. C., & Brooten, D. (1993). The roles and functions of clinical nurse specialists. *Image, 25,* 73.

O'Connor, K. S. (1994). Advanced practice nurses in an environment of health care reform. *MCN: American Journal of Maternal Child Nursing, 19,* 65.

Pillitteri, A., et al. (1993). Parent gender, victim gender and family socioeconomic influences on the reporting of child abuse by nurses. *Issues in Comprehensive Pediatric Nursing, 16,* 287.

Rhodes, A. M. (1990). Maternal liability for fetal injury? *MCN: American Journal of Maternal Child Nursing, 15,* 41.

Rubin, R. (1963). Maternal touch. *Nursing Outlook, 11,* 828.

Sauer, P. M., & Harvey, C. J. (1993). Spinal cord injury and pregnancy. *Journal of Perinatal and Neonatal Nursing, 7,* 22.

Schurmann, E., et al. (1993). Acute and long term efficacy of anti-tuberculous treatment in HIV-seropositive patients with tuberculosis: a study of 36 cases. *Journal of Infection, 26,* 45.

Scott, J. R., et al. (1990). *Danforth's obstetrics and gynecology* (6th ed.). Philadelphia: J.B. Lippincott, p. 124.

Strobino, D. M., et al. (1993). Development of an index of maternal transport. *Medical Decision Making, 13,* 64.

Wegman, M. E. (1993). Annual summary of vital statistics. *Pediatrics, 92,* 743.

Williams, L. R., & Cooper, M. K. (1993). Nurse-managed postpartum home care. *Journal of Obstetrical, Gynecologic and Neonatal Nursing, 22,* 25.

Zagorsky, E. S. (1993). Caring for families who follow alternative health care practices. *Pediatric Nursing, 19,* 71.

Zukowsky, K. S., & Coburn, C. E. (1991). Neonatal nurse practitioners: who are they? *Journal of Obstetric, Gynecologic, and Neonatal Nursing, 20,* 128.

Suggested Readings

Austin, J. K. (1990). Assessment of coping mechanisms used by parents and children with chronic illness. *MCN: American Journal of Maternal Child Nursing, 15,* 98.

Curry, J. (1993). Pediatric nursing; preserving a national treasure. *American Journal of Nursing, 93,* 83.

Davidhizar, R., et al. (1992). Understanding the physical and psychosocial stressors of the child who is homeless. *Pediatric Nursing, 18,* 559.

Evans, M. I, et al. (1993). Fetal therapy: the next generation. *Western Journal of Medicine, 159,* 325.

Gatford, A. (1992). Keeping the sick child out of hospital. *Professional Care of Mother and Child, 2,* 84.

Gilchrist, V. J. (1991). Preventive health care for the adolescent. *American Family Physician, 43,* 719.

Gleeson, R. M., et al. (1990). Advanced practice nursing: a model of collaborative care. *MCN: American Journal of Maternal Child Nursing, 15,* 9.

Hempel, S. (1994). Teenage pregnancy. *Community Outlook, 4,* 26.

Katz, K. S. (1993). Project headed home: intervention in the pediatric intensive care unit for infants and their families. *Infant and Young Child, 5,* 67.

Kuhni, C. Q. (1990). When cultures clash at the bedside. *RN, 53,* 23.

Liu, D. T. Y., et al. (1992). Antenatal care towards the year 2000. *Midwives Chronicle, 105,* 388.

Nesbitt, T. S., et al. (1990). Access to obstetric care in rural areas: effect on birth outcomes. *American Journal of Public Health, 80,* 814.

Newman, B. S., & Muzzonigro, P. G. (1993). The effects of traditional family values on the coming out process of gay male adolescents. *Adolescence, 28,* 213.

Porcher, F. K. (1992). HIV-infected pregnant women and their infants; primary health care implications. *Nurse Practitioners, 17,* 46.

Ranjan, V. (1993). Obstetrics and the fear of litigation. *Professional Care of Mother and Child, 3,* 10.

Styles, M. (1990). Challenges for nursing in the new decade. *MCN: American Journal of Maternal Child Nursing, 15,* 347.

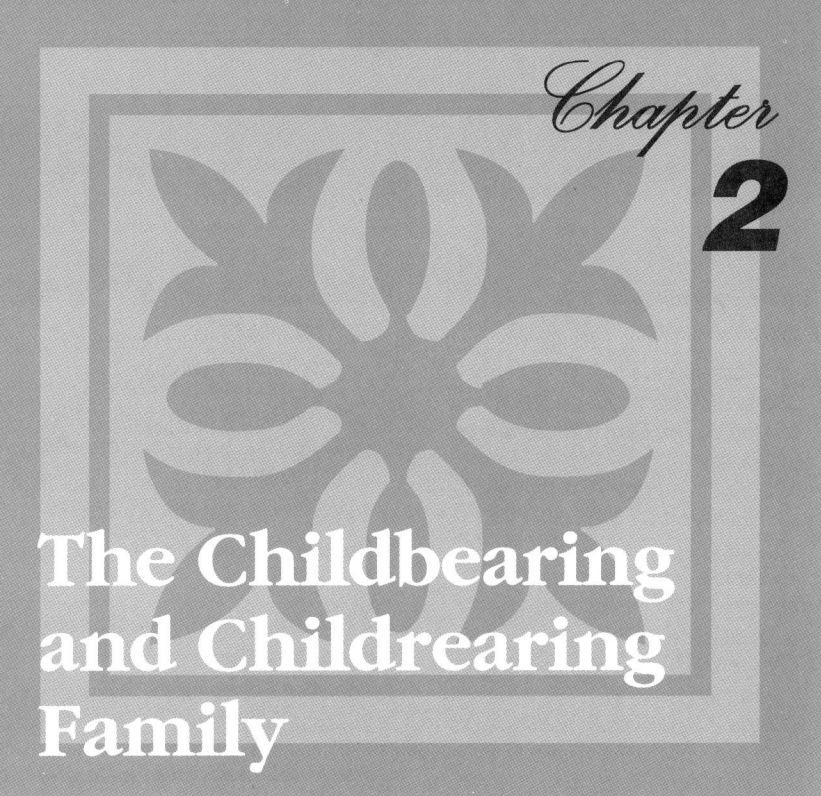

Chapter 2

The Childbearing and Childrearing Family

Key Terms

- *community*
- *community ecomap*
- *family*
- *family nursing*
- *family of orientation*
- *family of procreation*
- *family sculpture*
- *family theory*
- *genogram*

Objectives

After mastering the contents of this chapter, you should be able to:

1. Describe family structure, function, and family roles.

2. Assess a family for structure and health.

3. Formulate nursing diagnoses related to family health.

4. Plan nursing care, such as helping a family modify its lifestyle to accommodate an ill child.

5. Implement nursing care, such as teaching a family more effective wellness behaviors.

6. Evaluate outcome criteria established for care to be certain that goals have been achieved.

7. Identify National Health Goals related to the family and specific ways that nurses can help the nation achieve these goals.

8. Identify areas of care related to family nursing that could benefit from additional nursing research.

9. Use critical thinking to analyze additional ways that nursing care can be family centered or that client care can better include family members.

10. Synthesize knowledge of family nursing with nursing process to achieve quality maternal and child health nursing care.

Adele Pillitteri: MATERNAL AND CHILD
HEALTH NURSING, 2nd Edition. © 1995
Adele Pillitteri.

Outside of one's family, no other social group has the potential to provide the same level of support and long-lasting emotional ties. Maintaining healthy family life is so important that a number of National Health Goals speak directly to maintaining healthy family life (see the Focus on National Health Goals box). Because of the importance of the family to the individual, family-centered care has become a focus of modern nursing practice. **Family nursing,** a distinct specialty area that sees the family rather than the individual as its client, is based on concepts about family behavior (Gilliss & Davis, 1992). **Family theory** is a set of perspectives *from the family's point of view* that helps the nurse address the important health issues of the childbearing and childrearing family. For instance, in order for a family to adjust to a new family member, it is important that family structures and roles be flexible enough to adjust to the changes that pregnancy and the introduction of a newborn will bring. The strain on a family can be tremendous when a child is ill or passing through a difficult developmental period such as adolescence. The roles individuals assume in the family and the general family structure can also influence a couple's perception of a pregnancy or their child's illness, as well as their ability to adjust to these situations and positively influence their outcome.

FOCUS ON
National Health Goals

A number of National Health Goals speak directly to achieving healthy family and community life. The following goals are representative:

- Lower the current baseline of 25.2 children per 1000 who are younger than age 18 who are maltreated.

- Reduce physical abuse directed at women by male partners to no more than 27 per 1000 couples from a current baseline of 30 per 1000.

- Reduce the prevalence of blood lead levels exceeding 15 μg/dL in children aged 6 months to 5 years to no more than 500,000 from a current baseline of 3,000,000 (DHHS, 1991).

Nurses can be instrumental in helping to see that goals such as these for more healthy family living are met by assessing families and their environment in order to identify families at risk, assisting with counseling or further testing, and maintaining contact with families to ensure long-term measures for care can be instituted. Family violence is further discussed in Chapters 14 and 55; lead poisoning from excessive lead in the environment in Chapter 52.

For all these reasons, family-centered maternal and child health nursing considers the strengths, vulnerabilities, and patterns of family functioning in order to support families through the passages of childbirth and childrearing and to encourage healthy coping mechanisms within families facing a crisis. This means that health assessment and intervention planning should include consideration of social, emotional, spiritual, and financial resources, as well as the physical condition of the home and the community environment.

This chapter defines the concept of family and describes family types, family functions, and variations that affect family life. With these elements in mind, it then addresses family assessment and the family's place as part of the community.

NURSING PROCESS OVERVIEW for Promotion of Family Health

ASSESSMENT

Family assessment provides information on the meaning of a current health situation to family members and the emotional support that can be expected to be offered to an individual from the family. It is vital to understanding what a pregnancy or childhood illness means to the family. Family structure and function are both considered.

NURSING DIAGNOSIS

Nursing diagnoses used in connection with families generally relate to the family's ability to handle stress and to provide a positive environment for individual growth and development. Examples include:

- Parental role conflict related to prolonged separation from child during a long hospitalization
- Altered family processes related to emergency hospital admission of oldest child
- Altered parenting related to unplanned pregnancy
- Ineffective family coping related to inability to adjust to child's illness
- Family coping: Potential for growth related to improved perceptions of child's capabilities
- Potential for enhanced parenting
- Health-seeking behaviors related to birth of first child

Altered parenting and Parental role conflict are diagnoses that suggest that parents need additional help with the parenting role. The first coping diagnosis (Ineffective family coping) indicates that a family is not functioning at an optimum level; the second (Potential for growth) is used for a well family or one that is exhibiting enhanced growth with regard to a specific event, such as the sudden diagnosis of illness in a child or an unplanned pregnancy. Potential for enhanced parenting and Health-seeking behaviors are diagnoses that apply to families actively investigating more effective ways to manage stress and improve family functioning.

PLANNING

Planning for nursing care must include a design that is appropriate and desired by the majority of family members. It must also consider community environment; for example, it is not helpful to suggest that a family take regular walks together to improve their relating skills if their neighborhood is unsafe; a regular outing at the local YWCA in a family gym class might be more practical. Urging family members to plan together not only encourages shared decisions but promotes improved family communication.

IMPLEMENTATION

A plan for improving family health can be implemented easily if family members have agreed on it out of support for one another. It may be necessary in some instances to encourage family members to agree on a plan or to abide by a chosen plan; otherwise, they may expend needless energy carrying out an activity that is counterproductive or in direct opposition to the major goal.

EVALUATION

Evaluation should reveal not only that a goal was achieved but that the family feels more cohesive after working together toward the goal. If evaluation does not reveal these two factors, reassessment is needed to determine whether further interventions are still required. Examples of outcome criteria that might be established are:

- Family members state they are adapting well to the presence of a newborn.
- Mother states she feels prepared to manage home care.
- Father states he has arranged the family financial resources to accommodate health care expenses for the family.

The Family

How well a family works together and meets any crisis depends on its structure (family composition) and function (activities or roles family members carry out). Infants born to dysfunctional families, for example, have lower birth weights than those born to functional families (Abell et al., 1991). Children from homeless families (an example of an unstructured type of family) score less well on Denver Developmental Screening Tests than do other children (Bassuk & Rosenberg, 1990) and may have increased depression (Smart & Walsh, 1993).

Defining the Concept of Family

A **family** is defined by the U.S. Census Bureau as "a group of people related by blood, marriage, or adoption living together" (U.S. Bureau of the Census, 1990). This definition is workable for gathering comparative statistics but is necessarily limited when assessing a family for health concerns or support people available because, in reality, families can and do occur between unmarried couples. Spradley (1990, p. 100) defines the family in a much broader context as "two or more people who live in the same household (usually), share a common emotional bond, and perform certain interrelated social tasks." This is a better definition for health care providers because it addresses the broad range of types of families health care providers encounter. Families, like individuals, manifest wellness behaviors under times of lessened stress and illness behaviors under periods of stress. Box 2-1 lists generally accepted characteristics of a "well" or functioning family. Assessing families for these characteristics is helpful in establishing the extent of wellness or illness behavior.

Family Types

Many types of families exist, and a family will change over time as it is affected by birth, work, death, divorce, and the growth of family members. For the purposes of description of family in maternal and child health nursing, two basic family structures can be described: (1) a **family of orientation** (the family one is born into; or oneself, mother, father, and siblings, if any) and (2) a **family of procreation** (a family one establishes; or oneself, spouse, and children). More specific descriptions vary greatly depending on family roles, generational issues, means of family support, and sociocultural influences (see the Focus on Cultural Awareness box). The last United States census revealed some interesting statistics about the American family. While the traditional household of a married couple with children made up 78% of the total families of children, this number represented a decline compared to previous years. Increasing

in incidence is the single-headed family (an increase from 10% of all families in 1960 to nearly 16% in 1990).

The Nuclear Family

The traditional nuclear family structure is composed of a husband, wife, and children. As young people move away from their parents when they marry or establish independent housekeeping, more and more families today are nuclear in structure (no grandparents, aunts, or uncles live in the home). An advantage of a nuclear family is its ability to provide support to family members because interests are common; although a person receives strong support from such a family structure, the nuclear family may offer limited support in time of illness or other crisis (there are fewer family members to share the burden and offer support).

The Extended (Multigenerational) Family

The extended family includes not only the nuclear family but other family members such as grandmothers, grandfathers, aunts, uncles, cousins, and grandchildren. An advantage of such a family is that it offers more people to serve as resources during crises and provides more role models for behavior and learning values. A

Box 2-1
Twelve Behaviors Indicating a Well Family

1. The ability to provide for the physical, emotional, and spiritual needs of family members.
2. The ability to be sensitive to the needs of family members.
3. The ability to communicate thoughts and feelings effectively.
4. The ability to provide support, security, and encouragement.
5. The ability to initiate and maintain growth-producing relationships.
6. The capacity to maintain and create constructive and responsible community relationships.
7. The ability to grow with and through children.
8. The ability to perform family roles flexibly.
9. The ability to help oneself and to accept help when appropriate.
10. The capacity for mutual respect for the individuality of family members.
11. The ability to use a crisis experience as a means of growth.
12. A concern for family unity, loyalty, and interfamily cooperation.

(Reprinted from Otto, H. [1963]. Criteria for assessing family strengths. *Family Process, 2,* 329, with permission.)

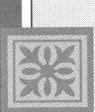

FOCUS ON CULTURAL AWARENESS

Families tend to display characteristics of their culture and community. Knowing some of the basic norms and taboos of different cultural groups is an important part of the nurse's knowledge base. This basic knowledge of a family's cultural background helps the nurse to understand the family's value system and the degree of support family members have available.

The types of families that live in communities tend to be culturally determined: some cultures enjoy extended families; others consist of single-parent families. Some cultures respect elderly family members and depend on them for advice; others are more oriented in the present. Whether families are headed by males or females is also culturally determined.

Remember that poverty is a major problem for many nondominant ethnic groups. Characteristic responses that are sometimes described as cultural limitations are actually the consequences of poverty, for example, parents seeking medical care for their child late in the course of an illness or late in pregnancy. Solving some problems may be a question of locating adequate financial resources rather than overcoming cultural influences.

their own role in the family (they must be the father and the breadwinner but must also provide child care). Trying to fulfill several central roles is not only time consuming but mentally and physically exhausting, and, in many instances, dissatisfying. Such a parent may have low self-esteem (if a spouse left or if the other parent refuses to help with child support). This interferes with decision making and can impede effective daily functioning (Figure 2-1).

A single-parent family has the advantage of offering a child a special parent-child relationship and increased opportunities for self-reliance and independence. If there has been a divorce, one parent may have been given legal custody of the children or both parents may have joint custody. Either way, both parents often participate in decision making. At a time of illness, both may be active in visiting a hospitalized child and anxious to receive reports of the child's progress. Identifying who is the custodial parent is important when consent forms for care are signed.

The Blended Family

In a blended family or "remarriage" or "reconstituted family," a divorced or widowed person with children marries someone who also has children of his or her own. Advantages of blended families are increased secu-

possible disadvantage of an extended family is that family resources must be stretched to accommodate all members. In an extended family, a person's strongest support person or a child's primary caregiver may not be the mother or father. The grandmother or an aunt, for example, may provide the largest amount of child care, for example, even though the child's mother is also present every day.

The Single-Parent Family

In as many as 60% to 70% of families with school-age children today, only one parent lives in the home. This increase in single-parent families is due both to the high rate of divorce and to the increasingly common practice in the United States of women raising children outside marriage (Wegman, 1992). A health problem in a single-parent family is almost always compounded, because if the parent is ill there is no back-up person for child care. If a child is ill, there is no close support person to give reassurance or a second opinion on whether the child's health is improving.

Low income is often an additional problem encountered by single-parent families, because the parent is most often a woman (nationally, women's incomes are lower than men's by about 40%). Single parents also may have difficulty with role modeling or identifying

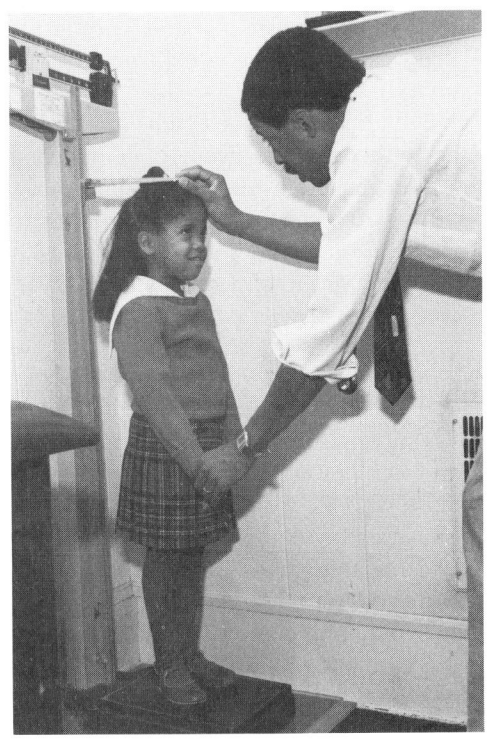

FIGURE 2-1
Many families today are headed by a single parent. A single-parent relationship can create a special bond between parent and child. Here a father measures his daughter's height. (Courtesy Department of Medical Photography, Children's Hospital, Buffalo, NY.)

rity and resources, especially for the female partner. Childrearing problems may arise in this type of family from rivalry among the children for the attention of a parent; grandparents or godparents may compete for the attention of the children. In addition, each spouse may encounter difficulties helping to rear the other's children. Young children often worry about having a stepparent because of the bad reputations stepmothers and stepfathers have in fairy tales. They may also become distressed at seeing their other biologic parent move into another home and become a stepparent to other children.

Moreover, financial difficulties can be severe if a parent pays child support for children from a previous marriage. Nurses can be instrumental in offering emotional support to members of a remarriage family until the adjustments for mutual living have been made.

The Communal Family

Communes comprise groups of people who have chosen to live together as an extended family group; their relationship to each other is social-value or interest motivated rather than kinship. The values of commune members are often religiously based and may be more freedom and free-choice oriented than those of a traditional family structure; because of the number of people present, members may have few set traditional family roles. People with this philosophy may have difficulty conforming with health care regimens (health care itself may be seen as an established system that they are rejecting).

On the other hand, people who reject traditional values may be the most creative people in a community and the most interested in participating in their own care and thus may have the best outcomes from therapy. Some commune communities are described as cults, or are composed of a group of people who follow a charismatic leader.

The Cohabitation Family

Cohabitation families comprise heterosexual couples who are living together but remain unmarried. Such people can offer as much psychologic comfort to each other as those who are formally married. Although such a relationship may be temporary, it may also be as long-lasting and as meaningful as a more traditional alliance. With pressure today to adhere to a monogamous relationship to avoid contracting HIV (human immunodeficiency virus) or other sexually transmitted diseases, these types of long-term cohabitation alliances are growing in number.

The Single Alliance Family

Many single young adults live together in shared apartments or dormitories or homes for companionship and financial security while completing school or beginning their careers. Although these relationships are often temporary, they have the same characteristics as cohabitation families.

The Gay or Lesbian Family

In homosexual unions, individuals of the same sex live together as married partners for companionship and sexual fulfillment. Such a relationship offers support in times of crisis comparable with that offered by a traditional nuclear or a cohabitation family. Some lesbian and gay families include children because of previous heterosexual marriages or through the use of artificial insemination or adoption.

The Foster Family

Children whose parents are unable to care for them may be placed in a foster or substitute home by a child protection agency (Martin, et al., 1992). Foster parents receive remuneration for their care. They may or may not have children of their own or other foster children. Foster home placement is theoretically temporary until children can be returned to their own parents. If return is impossible or is not imminent, children may be raised to adulthood in foster care. Such children may feel insecure in such settings, concerned that soon they will have to move again. They may have some emotional difficulties related to the reason they were removed from their original home.

When caring for children from foster homes, it is important to ascertain who has legal responsibility to sign for health care for the child (a foster parent may or may not have this responsibility). Most foster parents are as concerned with health care as biologic parents and can be depended on to follow health care instructions conscientiously.

Family Function and Roles

A family is a small community group, and as a group it must designate certain people to complete certain tasks. Otherwise, work is duplicated or never completed. The majority of roles that people view as appropriate are the roles they saw their own parents fulfilling. Each new generation takes on the values of the previous generation, passing traditions and culture from generation to generation.

An important part of family assessment is to identify the roles that family members assume. Most families can identify an individual who serves as a financial manager, a problem-solver, a decision-maker, a nurturer, a health manager, and a gate-keeper who allows information into and out of the family. Knowing who fulfills these roles in a family helps you to work effectively with the family. If a hospitalized child will need continued care after he or she returns home, for example, then it would be important to identify and contact the nurturing member of the family because it will probably be this person who will supervise or give the needed care at home. Take care not to make assumptions about role fulfillment based on gender or stereotyping, since every family operates differently. For example, although nurturing has typically been thought of as a female characteristic, many men are just as nurturing as women and in some families fulfill this role.

If a pregnancy will cause a major change in lifestyle for the family, it would be good to identify and contact the person in the family who is the decision-maker or the person who is the problem-solver (not necessarily the same). If the child's illness will involve increased family expense, then identifying and contacting the wage earner for the family would be important.

Knowledge of who is a family's safety and health officer is important before contacting a family for discharge planning. The gate-keeper for a family is the person who allows information into the family and releases information from it. It is important to identify this family member before attempting to introduce a change such as a new pattern of nutrition into a family. Identifying the family's emotional support person helps evaluate the family's ability to cope with stress, such as the care of an ill family member (Baker, 1994).

Family Tasks

Duvall and Miller (1990) have identified eight tasks that are essential for a family to perform to survive as a unit. These tasks differ in degree from family to family and depend on the growth stage of the family, but are usually present to some extent in all families.

1. *Physical maintenance.* A healthy family provides food, shelter, clothing, and health care for its members. Being certain that a family has ample resources to provide for a new member is important in maternal and child health nursing.
2. *Socialization of family members.* This task involves preparation of children to live in the community and interact with people outside the family. A family that is located in a community with a culture or values different from its own may find this a very difficult task (Campanella et al., 1993).
3. *Allocation of resources.* Determining which family needs will be met and their order of priority is called allocation of resources. In healthy families there is justification, consistency, and fairness in the distribution. Resources include not only financial wealth but material goods, affection, and space. In some families, resources are limited, so no one has new shoes. A danger sign would be a family in which one child has one-hundred-dollar sneakers while others are barefoot.
4. *Maintenance of order.* This task includes opening

an effective means of communication between family members, establishing family values, and enforcing common regulations for all family members (see the Focus on Family Teaching box). Determining the place of a new infant and what rules he or she will need to follow may be an important task for a developing family. In healthy families, members know the family rules and respect and follow them without difficulty.

5. *Division of labor.* The issue here is who will fulfill certain roles such as family provider, who will be the children's caregiver, and who will be the home manager. Pregnancy or an illness of a child may change this familial arrangement and cause the family to have to rethink this task.
6. *Reproduction, recruitment, and release of family members.* Often not a great deal of thought is given to this task: who lives in a family often happens more by changing circumstances than by true choice. Having to accept a new infant into an already crowded household may make a pregnancy a less-than-welcome event or cause reworking of this task.
7. *Placement of members into the larger society.* This task consists of selecting community activities, such as school, religious affiliation, or a political group, that correlates with the family's beliefs and values.

FOCUS ON FAMILY TEACHING

Q. Everyone in our family has different school or work schedules. How can we keep our family intact in light of this?

A. Traditionally, families gathered for an evening meal and this allowed for a set time period each day for interaction and problem-solving while the problems were still small enough to be solvable. If this isn't possible, suggestions for better communication might be:

- A bulletin board or chalk board family members check each day for messages.
- Telephone answering or tape or cam recorders used to leave messages.
- An earlier wake-up time so all family members can have breakfast together every morning.
- One night a week that is reserved as "family night" when the family plans a special activity to do together.
- Joining in other's activities (if one is playing in a ball game, all come and watch).

Selecting a birth setting or choosing a hospital or hospice setting is part of this task.

8. *Maintenance of motivation and morale.* A sense of pride in the family group, when created, helps members serve as support people to each other during crises. Assessing to see that this feeling is present or not, helps in care planning.

Family Life Cycles

Families, like individuals, pass through predictable developmental stages (Duvall & Miller, 1990). To be able to predict the likelihood of a family using health promotion activities, therefore, it is helpful to assess its developmental stage. Figure 2-2 shows the relative amount of time a traditional family spends in each of these stages. Because families are delaying the age at which they have a first child and parents are living longer, the length of stages 1, 7, and 8 is growing.

Stage 1: Marriage and the Family

Although Duvall referred to this stage as marriage, what occurs during it is applicable to couples forming cohabitation, lesbian, gay, or single alliances when formal marriage does not occur. During this first stage of family development, members work to achieve three separate identifiable tasks: (1) establish a mutually satisfying relationship, (2) learn to relate well to their families of orientation, and, if applicable, (3) engage in reproductive life planning. Establishing a mutually satisfying relationship includes merging a couple's values brought into the relationship from the families of orientation. This means not only adjusting to each other in terms of routines (e.g., sleeping, eating, or housecleaning) but also sexual and economic aspects. This first stage of family development is a tenuous one, as evidenced by the high rate of divorce or separation of roommates at this stage. Illness

of a member or an unplanned pregnancy at this stage may be enough to destroy the still lightly formed bonds of partners if the partners do not receive support from their former family members or from alert health care providers.

Stage 2: The Early Childbearing Family

The birth or adoption of a first baby is a stress to a family because of the economic and social role changes that are required (Daiges-Pelish, 1993). An important nursing role during this period is health education concerning well-child care and how to integrate a new member into a family (see the Focus on Nursing Research box). It is a further developmental step to change from being able to care for a well baby to caring for an ill baby. One way of determining whether a parent has made this change is to ask what the new parent has tried to do to solve a child-rearing or health problem. Even if what the person answers is not therapeutic or the best solution to the problem, as long as it is sensible (not "I don't do anything when the baby's sick; I just take her right to my mother" but "I've been trying to give her a little water and keep her warm"), it probably means the parent has mastered this developmental step. Parents who have difficulty with this step need a great deal of support and counseling from health care providers to be able to care for an ill child at home or to give care to the child during a hospitalization.

Stage 3: The Family With Preschool Children

A family with preschool children is a busy family because children at this age demand a great deal of time related to growth and developmental needs and safety considerations as accidents become a major health concern (Lee et al., 1990). If a child is hospitalized because of an accident, parents may have difficulty facing the injury because they feel they should have done more to

FIGURE 2-2

Duvall's family life stages: Size of wedge reflects relative percent of total life cycle spent in each stage. Stage 1, marriage; stage 2, early childbearing; stage 3, families with preschool children; stage 4, families with school-age children; stage 5, families with adolescent children; stage 6, launching center families; stage 7, families of middle years; stage 8, families in retirement or old age. (From Spradley, B.W. [1990]. Community health nursing [3rd ed.]. Philadelphia: J.B. Lippincott.)

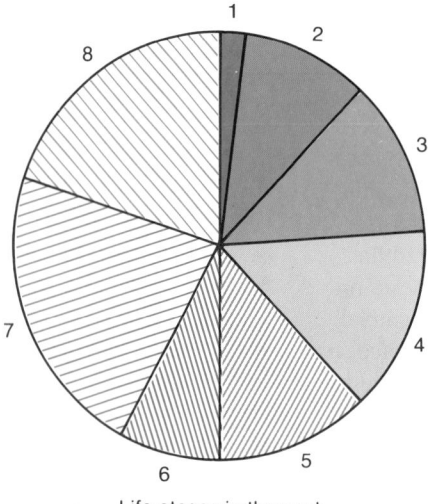

Life stages in the past

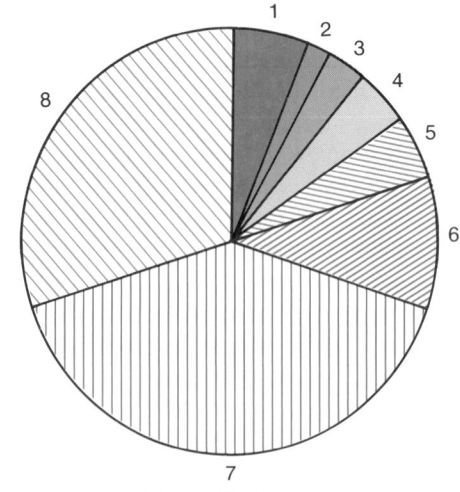

Modern life stages

**FOCUS ON
NURSING RESEARCH**

What Are Stressors for Mothers During the First Years of Their Child's Life?

To answer this question, Coffman et al. interviewed 43 women at the time their child was 1 month old and then again when the child was 13 months old. Frequent concerns mothers noted were not getting enough rest or sleep, not having enough time to do things they wanted to do, having too many responsibilities, concerns about physical appearance and weight gain, and owing money. At the 1-month stage, 69% of this sample named their husband as their closest relation; by 13 months, only 58% named him. More women named their mother as their closest support person at the second interview than the first.

This study has implications for nurses working with young families because it documents that many stressors for new families are not major happenings but everyday issues. It should also alert health care providers not to assume a husband is a woman's chief support person.

From Coffman, S., Levitt, M. J., & Guacci-Franco, N. (1993). Mothers' stress and close relationships: correlates with infant health status. *Pediatric Nursing, 19,*135.

prevent the accident. It may be difficult for parents to visit the hospital because they must care for other young children at home. If the child returns home for further care, a family in this stage may need continued support and help from a community health nurse to provide necessary health care for the ill member.

Stage 4: The Family With School-Age Children
Parents of school-age children have the important responsibility of preparing their children to be able to function in a complex world while at the same time maintaining their own satisfying marriage relationship. For many families, this is a trying time. Illness imposed at this stage adds to the burdens already present and may be enough to dissolve the marriage. Support systems within a family may be deceptive in that family members may be physically present but provide little or no emotional support, if internal tension exists. Many families during this period will need to turn to a tertiary level (e.g., friends, church organizations, or counseling) for adequate support.

Important nursing concerns during this family stage are monitoring children's health in terms of immunization, dental care, and health care assessments; monitoring child safety related to electrical or automobile accidents; and encouraging a meaningful school experience that will make learning a lifetime concern, not to be abandoned after a mere 12 years.

Stage 5: The Family With Adolescent Children
The primary goal for a family with teenagers differs considerably from the goal of the family in previous stages, which was to strengthen family ties and maintain family unity. Now the family must loosen family ties to allow adolescents more freedom and prepare them for life on their own. As technology advances at a rapid rate, the gap between generations increases; life when the parents were young was different from what it is for their teenagers. This makes stage five a trying stage for both children and adults.

Violence—accidents, homicide, and suicide—is the major cause of death in adolescents. The incidence of deaths from HIV infection is growing (DHHS, 1993). The nurse working with families at this stage, therefore, needs to spend time counseling members on safety (driving defensively and not under the influence of alcohol); proper care and respect for firearms; the dangers of drug abuse; and safer sex practices. If a generation gap exists between parents and children, children are unable to talk to parents about these problems, particularly those of a controversial nature such as sexual responsibility. A community health nurse is a neutral person who can assist families at this stage when communication difficulties exist.

Stage 6: The Launching Center Family
For many families, the stage at which children leave to establish their own households is the most difficult stage, because it appears to represent the breaking up of the family. Parental roles change from those of mother or father to once-removed support people or *guideposts.* The stage may represent a loss of self-esteem for parents, who feel themselves being replaced by other people in their children's lives. They may feel old for the first time and less able to cope with responsibilities. Illness imposed on a family at this stage may be detrimental to the family structure, breaking up an already disorganized and noncohesive group.

A nurse, again, serves as a counselor to such a family. He or she can help the parents gain a better perspective to see that what their children are doing is what they have spent a long time preparing them to do, or that leaving home is a positive, not a negative, step.

Stage 7: The Family of Middle Years
When a family returns to a two-partner nuclear unit, as it was before childbearing, the partners may view this stage either as the prime time of their lives (with opportunity to travel, economic independence, or time to spend on hobbies) or as a period of gradual decline (lacking the constant activity and stimulation of children in the home, finding life boring without them, or experiencing an "empty nest" syndrome). Because the family has returned to a two-partner union, support people

may not be as plentiful as they were before. Having a baby at this point in life may be viewed as exciting or worrisome, depending on individual circumstances.

Stage 8: The Family in Retirement or Older Age

The number of families of retirement age is approximately 15% to 20% of the population. As a group, family members in retirement or older age are more apt to suffer from chronic and disabling conditions than members in younger age groups. Although families at this stage are not having children, they remain an important family type in reference to maternal and child health nursing because they often offer a great deal of support to the young adult who is just beginning a family and needs child care advice; many grandparents are full-time child care providers for grandchildren while the parents are at work.

Changing Patterns of Family Life

Family life has changed significantly in the United States over the last 50 years. This is due to many complex and interrelated factors, such as increased mobility, the increase in the number of two wage-earner families, and an increase in the number of one-parent families. Understanding the impact these changes have on family structures and family life can help the nurse create plans of care which are realistic and better meet the needs of today's families.

Mobility Patterns

Population movement has an important influence on the quality of family life. During the 20th century, vast numbers of rural families have moved to urban communities; many urban families have moved to the suburbs. This pattern of mobility is expected to continue in the future. This means that an area with many child health care facilities may find itself with few children to use them; areas with many children may have few facilities specific for their care. Parents will travel a great distance to obtain health care for an ill child, but they are less apt to do so for health maintenance or health promotion care. Thus, if this circumstance goes unrecognized, goals such as routine immunization may be neglected. Families need to be asked if convenient health care is available.

Families of migrant farm workers are a particular group who have difficulty finding consistent health care because of their constant movement (Mobed et al., 1992). Children from these families have been identified as being at high risk for intestinal parasites and low socioeconomic status.

New immigrant families have the problem of adjusting not only to a new country but also to a different health care system. Ensuring their access to health care may require a great deal of education and community outreach. Nurses can be instrumental in seeing that health care organizations consider these issues and institute innovative measures such as providing transportation to facilities, changing locales or services so facilities and needs remain balanced, or setting up outreach and translator programs so that non–English speaking residents can receive adequate health care.

Poverty

Although the United States is a large and wealthy country, extreme poverty still exists and, in some areas, seems to be growing. According to the U.S. Census Bureau (1990), 20% of all children and 10.7% of families have incomes that fall below the poverty line. Poverty places children and families at risk for a variety of health care problems. The pregnant woman living in poverty, for example, is less likely to receive essential prenatal care; her diet may be inadequate for her increasing nutritional needs (Braveman et al., 1993).

A family who, in a given week, must choose between groceries and a child's immunizations will obviously buy groceries; the child's immunizations must wait until another time. If the family is forced to make this same choice week after week, the child could grow up without protection against a number of potentially lethal diseases.

Nurses can be instrumental in helping families to secure benefits such as food stamps or funding from Women, Infants, and Children Special Supplemental Food Program (WIC) and referring them to free or scaled payment health care programs so a healthy environment and health care can be provided despite limited financial resources. Some families who ordinarily would not qualify for Medicaid funding will qualify if the mother is pregnant.

The Homeless Family

It is estimated that more than 3 million people in the United States today are homeless (Berne et al., 1990). Although there is diversity in homeless families as in all others, they share a number of common characteristics. Many homeless families are headed by a female and an increasing number are headed by pregnant and parenting adolescents (Rich, 1992). Such families do not use health care providers or community agencies as effectively as other families. Many mothers of homeless families have a childhood history of physical abuse and of battering as an adult. The frequency of drug, alcohol, and severe psychiatric problems is greater in these families than in non-homeless families.

Half of homeless children are under 5 years of age (Kemsley & Hunter, 1993). Such children tend to perform less well than others on standard screening tests such as the Denver Developmental Screening Test. This is probably due to decreased environmental stimulation and lack of exposure to normal play activities. They have more physical illnesses, such as anemia, pneumonia, and dental problems. They may have inadequate growth (Taylor & Koblinsky, 1993).

When caring for homeless families, it is important to remember that they lack support people. This means they may need a health care provider to serve in this capacity during times of stress or illness (Velsor-Friedrich, 1993).

Increasing Number of One-Parent Families

One-parent families are increasing in number because of the high divorce rate and the number of women having children outside marriage. An increasing number of children are being raised by a male single parent.

Nurses can be instrumental in helping single parents to strengthen parenting skills and to be available to provide a second opinion on a course of action or care. In a study (Duffy et al., 1990) to identify the personal goals of recently divorced women, the most frequently listed goal was independence, followed by employment and education. Assessing a broad range of possible needs in women who have recently divorced can help nurses to direct these women to the appropriate resources.

Increasing Divorce

Divorce is rarely easy for the people involved. Because they are so emotionally involved and their perceptions of their roles are changing so drastically, parents may be unable to give their children the support they need during a divorce (Fishel & Samsa, 1993). For children, the loss of a parent through divorce may be little different from loss of a parent through death. Severing ties with grandparents is also difficult.

Children may manifest grief with physical symptoms such as nausea or fatigue as a response to divorce. Their performance in school may suffer (Neighbors, Forehand, & Armistead, 1992). Boys have been identified as generally having more emotional trauma from divorce than girls, probably because they lose their gender role model if the mother becomes the parent with custody.

Although divorce is a stressful time for children, a redeeming feature may be that the period following a divorce may be less stressful to children than living in a home where there is a high level of conflict between parents. Children need an explanation of why the divorce has occurred and assurance that the divorce was not their fault. The parent who will now be raising them may need help in not assuming the role of the injured party and portraying the other partner as dishonorable. Although a person was not a good marriage partner, he or she may have been a good parent and may be well loved by the children.

Children may have difficulty thinking of themselves as good people if they believe that one of their parents is bad. They may need time to discuss how they feel about their parents so that they do not think of one parent as kind and loving and the other one as selfish and unreliable.

Decreasing Family Size

The birth rate in the United States declined steadily from 1900 to 1990. It is now increasing slightly, although it remains at a point of below-zero population growth, that is, fewer infants are being born in a year than people are dying (Wegman, 1992). The average American family has 1.7 children. Although small families have fewer child care requirements for parents, they also limit parent experience in childrearing; thus, the amount of counseling time per parent may increase.

Dual-Parent Employment

As many as 62% of women of childbearing age work at a full-time job outside their home today; as many as 90% work at least part time. The implication of this trend for health care providers is that health care facilities must schedule times when parents are free to bring children to the facilities (parents will choose to miss work for an ill care visit but not necessarily for a health maintenance one or a routine prenatal visit). It means that a nurse must give health instructions such as medicine administration not only as "three times a day" but at times when a parent will be home to supervise medicine administration (e.g., before breakfast, after a parent returns from work, and at bedtime). Dual parent employment has increased the number of children in day care centers or after school programs. This may complicate child care, since there is an increased incidence of infection such as acute diarrhea in children in day care (Reves, et al., 1993). Nurses can be helpful in aiding parents to choose a quality care center which takes the necessary precautions against infection (see Chapter 31). School-age children often return home from school before parents return from work. Helping parents prevent loneliness in these "latch-key" children and helping children make good use of their time is a nursing responsibility (see Chapter 32).

Increased Family Responsibility for Health Monitoring

In the past, parents relied on health care providers to be the monitors of their child's health. They accepted health care advice with few questions or expressed opinions. Today, the majority of parents expect to take (and should be encouraged to take) an active role in monitoring their child's health and being participants in planning and goal setting.

This increased consumer awareness puts increased responsibility on nurses to include parents and children in health care decisions. Using nursing process for planning helps to accomplish this because the goal setting encourages parent participation. Health teaching such as reducing smoking in the home or increasing the fiber content in diets becomes an important aspect with interested learners. The severity of upper respiratory illnesses and inflammatory bowel disease in children is reduced in the home when parents do not smoke (Lashner, et al., 1993; Murray & Morrison, 1993).

Increased Abuse in Families

An alarming statistic in relation to family nursing is that the number of instances of reported child abuse in families is increasing yearly. This is apparently related to an increased stress level in the population as a whole as well as better reporting of abuse. Detecting child abuse begins with the awareness that it does occur; careful screening for the possibility at child care contacts is essential (Pillitteri, et al., 1993; see Chapter 55).

Unique Concerns of the Adopting Family

Adoption brings a number of challenges to the adopting parents and the adopted child, as well as to other children in the family, if any (Sherrod, 1992). It is helpful if parents of an adopted child visit a health care facility shortly after the child is placed in their home, so that a base of health information can be obtained, potential problems discussed, and possible solutions explored. Like all children, adopted children need good health maintenance and thorough health assessment during the years of childhood. If the birth mother of an adopted child was in socioeconomic circumstances that resulted in an inadequate diet and little prenatal care, the adopted child may be at higher risk for abnormal neurologic development. Children from countries that are war-torn have a greater risk of having illnesses such as hepatitis B and intestinal parasites and growth retardation, because health supervision has not been adequate (Johnson et al., 1992).

It is important when assessing a family with a newly adopted child to ascertain the stage of parenting the parents have reached. The average parent has 9 months to prepare physically and emotionally for a coming baby. Usually it takes the full 9 months for parents to accept the pregnancy and to begin to think of themselves as parents. Although adoptive parents may have been planning on a baby for much longer than 9 months, the actual appearance of a child can occur quite suddenly. The parents are called to say that "their child" has been born; they go to the hospital 2 days later to bring the child home. Children who are adopted from developing countries or who have disabilities and are waiting for adoption also arrive in a short time frame. In a few days' time, adoptive parents are asked to make the mental steps toward parenthood that biologic parents make over 9 months.

Because adoptive parents may be older than nonadoptive parents at the time they have a first child (the average couple conceives a child within 2 years of marriage; the average adopting couple waits 2 years, then undergoes fertility tests for an additional year, then waits for agency adoption up to 5 years), they may be less resilient or less able to adjust their lives to the presence of a child in the home. They may need a great deal of "talk time" at health care visits to explore their feelings about this change in their life and their feelings about being parents (adoptive parents may have low self-esteem because they were unable to conceive or have married a partner who is unable to conceive). To bolster this, they may need frequent assurance that they are functioning well as parents.

It is generally accepted that adopted children should be told early that they are adopted. Knowing from early childhood that they are adopted is not nearly as stressful as growing up not knowing it and then stumbling onto the information because of the carelessness of a neighbor or a relative when they are school-age or adolescent. By age 3 years, children are old enough to understand the story of their adoption: they grew inside the tummy of another woman, but because the woman could not care for them after birth, the woman gave them to the adopting parents to raise and love. It is important for parents not to criticize the birth mother (e.g., by saying she did not love the child or was a bad woman and so gave the child away) as part of the explanation. Children need to know for their own self-esteem that their birth mothers were good people and that they were capable of being loved by them.

By the time children are 6 years old, they are definitely ready to be told about adoption. When children are first told about their adoption they may exhibit "honeymoon behavior" or may try to behave absolutely perfectly for fear of being given away again. Following this "honeymoon," children may deliberately do things that are annoying to parents, testing them to see whether, despite their behavior, parents will still keep them. A child may say things such as "I don't have to listen to you—you're not my real mother" or "My real mother would have let me do that." It helps parents put these comments in perspective if they are reminded that it may happen and that nonadoptive children use the same ploys ("Daddy lets me do it" to mother; "Grandmother lets me do that" to father).

As adopted children enter puberty and begin to think about having children of their own, they may need some talk time to express their feelings about being adopted. Some adopted children of this age have difficulty establishing a sense of identity because they do not know who their birth parents were. It is common for them to spend time tracing records and trying to locate their birth parents. Counsel adopting parents that this is not a rejection of them, but a normal consequence of being adopted. Children seek out their birth parents not because they do not love their adoptive parents, but because they need that information to know where they fit into the eternal scheme of the world.

If the adoptive parents have a child of their own born after the adoption, they may wish to discuss their feelings about the two children. Siblings of an adopted child may sometimes feel inferior to the adopted child, because they were just born, not "chosen from all the babies in the hospital nursery" (a common explanation of how an adopted child came to live in a family). Others feel superior and need talk time to voice their feelings about having an adopted child as a sibling.

Counseling an adopted child or forming a relationship with one as a health care provider carries an additional responsibility, that of making certain that the relationship is not ended abruptly or thoughtlessly. If the health care provider is leaving an agency, he or she should ensure that an adopted child is introduced to the person who will continue health supervision, so that he or she doesn't feel abandoned. When hospitalized, all preschoolers worry about being abandoned and left in the hospital. Preschoolers who have just been told that they are adopted, that they were chosen by their adoptive parents "from all the babies in the hospital nursery," may be terribly afraid that they are now being returned to the hospital to be given back. Parents of an adopted child may need help in preparing the child for this experience and also encouragement to stay with the child in the hospital as much as possible to reduce fear.

Assessment of Family Structure and Function

Assessment of family health can be carried out on a variety of levels and in varying degrees of detail. There are many different ways to collect data on the family; the method chosen should match the way in which the assessment data will be used.

General characteristics of family type and functioning can be assessed using observation and general history questions (Table 2-1). When more detailed information about family environment and roles is required, using an assessment tool specifically developed for that purpose is most effective.

The Well Family

Assessment of psychosocial family wellness requires measurement of how the family relates and interacts as a unit, including communication patterns, bonding, roles and role relationships, division of tasks and activities, governance of the family structure, decision-making and problem-solving, and leadership within the family unit. Assessment also looks at how the family relates to the outside community.

The Family APGAR (Smilkstein, 1978) is a screening tool of the family environment (Figure 2-3). A family APGAR form is administered to each family member, and their scores are compared. The tool can be a helpful adjunct to complement history taking.

Table 2-1. *Family Assessment*

Area of Assessment	Questions to Ask
Type of family	Who lives in the home? Is the family nuclear, extended, or other?
Family finances	Are finances adequate? Is money divided evenly among family members?
Safety	Is the home safe from fire or accidents?
Health	Does the family eat a nutritious diet? Do they receive adequate sleep? Are immunizations current? Is there a balance between work and recreation? Can they cope with problems adequately?
Emotional support	
Within family	Do members eat together or spend an equal amount of time with each other daily? Do they band together to defend each other from outsiders?
Outside family	Is the family active in community organizations or activities? Do they visit (or are they visited by) friends and relatives? Can the family name one outside person they can always rely on for help in a time of crisis?
Family roles	
Nurturing figure	Who is the primary caregiver to children or any disabled member?
Provider	Who is the main family provider?
Decision-maker	Who makes decisions, particularly in the area of finances and leisure time?
Problem-solver	Who does the family depend on to provide the solution for problems?
Health manager	Who ensures that family members keep return health appointments, immunizations are kept current, and preventive care such as a mammogram for the mother is scheduled?
Gatekeeper	Who determines what information will be released from the family or what new information can be introduced?

The **genogram**, a diagram which details family structure, provides information about a family's history and roles of various family members over time, usually through several generations (Figure 2-4). The genogram provides both the nurse and the family with a basis for discussion and analysis of family interactions (Friedman, 1992).

Family sculpture is a more dynamic tool that engages the family in creating a live portrait of themselves. Individual family members act in turn as sculptor, molding other members into postures and spatial relationships that represent to that person the family dynamics and feelings toward one another and their relationship to the outside environment. This exercise serves as the starting point for a discussion about family interactions and can help in planning nursing care (Spradley, 1990).

The Family APGAR Questionnaire

	Almost always	Some of the time	Hardly ever
I am satisfied with the help that I receive from my family* when something is troubling me.	_____	_____	_____
I am satisfied with the way my family discusses items of common interest and shares problem solving with me.	_____	_____	_____
I find that my family accepts my wishes to take on new activities or make changes in my lifestyle.	_____	_____	_____
I am satisfied with the way my family expresses affection and responds to my feelings such as anger, sorrow, and love.	_____	_____	_____
I am satisfied with the way my family and I spend time together.	_____	_____	_____

SCORING

Scoring: The patient checks one of three choices, which are scored as follows: 2 points for "Almost always," 1 point for "Some of the time," and 0 for "Hardly ever." The scores for each of the five questions are then totaled. A score of 7 to 10 suggests a highly functional family. A score of 4 to 6 suggests a moderately dysfunctional family. A score of 0 to 3 suggests a severely dysfunctional family.

WHAT IS MEASURED

Adaptation — How resources are shared, or the member's satisfaction with the assistance received when family resources are needed.

Partnership — How decisions are shared, or the member's satisfaction with mutuality in family communication and problem solving.

Growth — How nurturing is shared, or the member's satisfaction with the freedom available within the family to change roles and attain physical and emotional growth or maturation.

Affection — How emotional experiences are shared, or the member's satisfaction with the intimacy and emotional interaction within the family.

Resolve — How time* is shared, or the member's satisfaction with the time commitment that has been made to the family by its members.

*Besides sharing time, family members usually have a commitment to share space and money. Becuase of its primacy, time was the only item included in the Family APGAR; however, the nurse who is concerned with family function will enlarge understanding of the family's resolve by inquiring about family member's satisfaction with shared space and money.

FIGURE 2-3
The Family APGAR Questionnaire. (From Smilkstein, G. [1978]. The Family APGAR. Journal of Family Practice, 6, 1231.)

The Family in Crisis

Nursing assessment of the family often occurs when the family is in crisis. The way that families react to a crisis situation depends largely on the particular crisis affecting them, their past experiences with problem-solving, their perception of the event (whether they can clearly see what is the problem), and the resources that are available to them to help with problem-solving. McCubbin and Patterson (1983) have suggested that assessing these factors is vital to predicting the probable extent of the crisis for the family. The effect of a crisis on a family changes perceptions and resources available. Renewed assessment is therefore necessary in light of a crisis to see if the family is weathering the impact (a double ABCX model of assessment; Figure 2-5). To use this

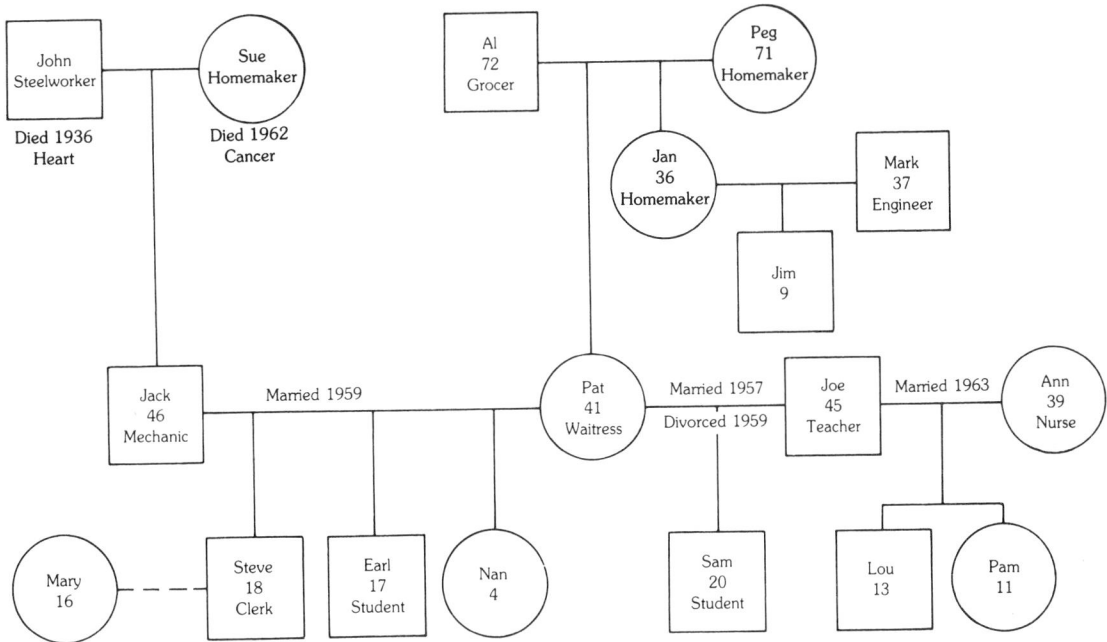

FIGURE 2-4
A family genogram showing three generations. Males are depicted by squares, females by circles. Each family member's name, age, and occupation is supplied. (From Spradley, B. [1990]. Community health nursing: Concepts and practice *[3rd. ed.]. Philadelphia: J.B. Lippincott, with permission.)*

DOUBLE ABCX MODEL
FAMILY ADAPTATION MODEL

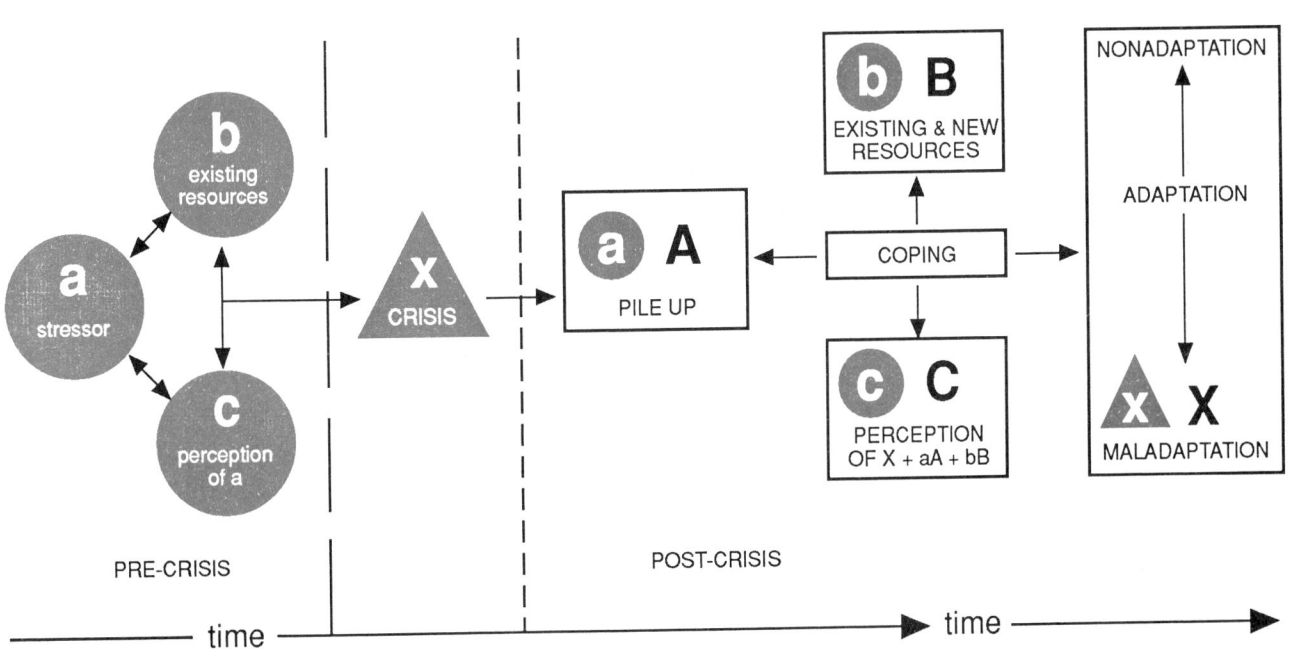

FIGURE 2-5
The ABCX System for Family Assessment. (McCubbin, H.I., & Patterson, J. [1983]. Family stress adaptation to crises: a double ABCX model of family behavior. In McCubbin, H., Sussman, M., & Patterson, J. [eds.]. Social stresses and the family: Advances and developments in family stress theory and research. *New York: Haworth Press.)*

model, first assess what is the stressor, the family's perception of the stressor, and the resources available to evaluate the extent of the crisis on the family. The presence of a crisis leads to added stress, additional coping actions, and identification of new resources, all of which lead to new perceptions of the event. These combined forces determine whether the outcome will be "bonadaptation" or "maladaptation" (McCubbin & McCubbin, 1993).

Listing a family's strengths and coping abilities as well as its areas of vulnerability not only aids in planning care but also the actual process of identifying strengths by and with the family members themselves strengthens the family (see the Focus on Nursing Research box). Family assessment carried out with the family together in this way will bring out these sorts of insights and better prepare family members to cope with the current level of stress and difficult decision-making that may be

ahead for them. Box 2-2 lists practical suggestions to help families enduring a crisis to deal with stress.

The Family as Part of a Community

Community is a term that can be defined in many ways, but it is generally accepted to refer to a limited geographic area in which the residents relate to and interact among themselves (Bullough & Bullough, 1990). When asked what community they are from, therefore, people may mention an entire city; a school district; a geographic district ("the east side"); a street name ("Pine Street area"); or a natural marking ("the lower creek area").

Because the health of individuals is influenced by the health of their community, it is important to become acquainted with the community in which you practice. If

---

Box 2-2
Methods to Help Families Deal With Stress

1. Help people to recognize their individual stress level, a level that differs from person to person. Because a person works next to someone who is not upset by some condition does not mean that the person will not be annoyed or upset. On the other hand, if a situation does not annoy a person, that person should not feel that he or she has to react to it just because a friend does.

2. Help people to learn to change those things they cannot accept and to learn to accept those things they cannot change. Trial and error is often required to determine the difference between the two categories.

3. Often a total change is unnecessary; a modification will be ample to make the difference.

4. Encourage people to verbalize personal reactions to stress. Almost nothing limits the extent of a threat more than being able to accurately describe it.

5. Encourage people to reach out for support. People under stress are often so involved in their problems that they do not realize that people around them want to help. Sometimes the people closest to the person feeling stress are under a similar threat and so are no longer able to offer support. When this happens, the person must then call on second- or third-level support persons (family or community people) for help.

6. Help people to develop a habit of reaching out to give support when others are in threat (to network). Survival is a collaborative function of social groups; a favor offered now can be called in when the person is in need at a later date.

7. Help people to face a situation as honestly as possible. As a rule, knowing the exact nature of a threat is less stressful than a "shadow-haunting, something-is-out-there" feeling. On the other hand, people should not be urged to face intense threats, such as a serious complication of pregnancy or a fatal illness in a child until they have had time to mobilize their defenses, or they may be overwhelmed.

8. Help people not to rush decisions or make final adaptive outcomes to a stress situation. As a rule, major decisions should be delayed at least 6 weeks after an event; 6 months is an even better time interval.

9. Help people anticipate life events and plan for them to the extent possible. Anticipatory guidance this way will not totally prepare clients for a coming event but will at least serve notice that distress over the situation is normal.

10. Alert people that accidents increase when people are under stress. A person worrying about a complication of pregnancy, for example, is more apt to have an automobile accident than a person who is stress free. Children are more apt to poison themselves when the family is under stress than during a nonstress time.

11. Action feels good during stress because doing something brings a sense of control over feelings of helplessness and disorganization. Action often is so satisfying that people do things such as write threatening letters or make harmful remarks that they later regret. Help people to channel energy into therapeutic action (such as going for a long walk) instead.

you are caring for a client from a community unknown to you, then assess that community to see if there are aspects about it that contributed to an illness (and therefore need to be corrected) and to determine whether the person will be able to return to such a community without extra help and counseling from a nurse or some other health care provider (Figure 2-6).

Community assessment consists of examining the various systems that are present in almost all communities to see if they are functioning adequately. Knowing the individual aspects of families or community may help you understand why some children reach the illness level they do before parents bring them in for health care. In addition, such knowledge can set the stage for care (e.g., a woman living alone in a city has no transportation available to her until her husband comes home from work, so she cannot come for prenatal care; a 5-year-old child develops measles because there are no free immunization services in the community). It is easier for the nurse to prepare a woman or child for return to a community after childbirth or a hospitalization if, for example, he or she knows the specific features of the community where the family lives. (Does the Pine Street area have well or city water? How many flights of stairs does someone from the Stevens Plaza area have to walk to reach an apartment? Is there public transportation so the mother can return for her 2-week and 6-week visits with the baby?) Table 2-2 summarizes areas of community assessment to use in discharge planning.

Table 2-2. Community Assessment

Area of Assessment	Questions
Age span	Is the family within the usual age span of the community and thereby assured of support people?
Education	If the person is school age, is there provision for schooling? Is there a public library for self-education? Is there easy access to such places if the person is disabled? If a special program such as diet counseling is needed, does it exist?
Environment	Are there environmental risks present such as air pollution? Busy high ways? Train yards? Pools or water where frequent drownings occur? Will hypothermia be a problem?
Finances, occupation	Is there a high rate of unemployment in the community? What is the average occupation? Will this family have adequate finances to manage comfortably? Are there supplemental aid programs available?
Health care delivery	Is there a health care agency the family can use for comprehensive care? Is it convenient in terms of finances and time?
Housing	Are houses mainly privately owned or apartments? Are homes close enough together to afford easy contact? Are they in good repair? Is upkeep such as constant repair or extensive lawn mowing a problem?
Political	Is the community active politically? Can adults reach a local polling place to vote or do they know how to apply for absentee ballots?
Recreational	Are there recreational activities available of interest? Are they economically feasible?
Religion	Is there a facility where the family can worship as they choose? Is there easy transportation to it?
Safety, protection	Is there adequate protection so that family members can feel safe to leave home or remain home alone? Do they know about available "hot lines" and local police and fire department numbers? Is the home safe from fire?
Sociocultural	What is the dominant culture in the community? Does the family fit into this environment? Are foods that are culturally significant available?
Transportation	Is there public transportation? Will family members have access to it if they are disabled?

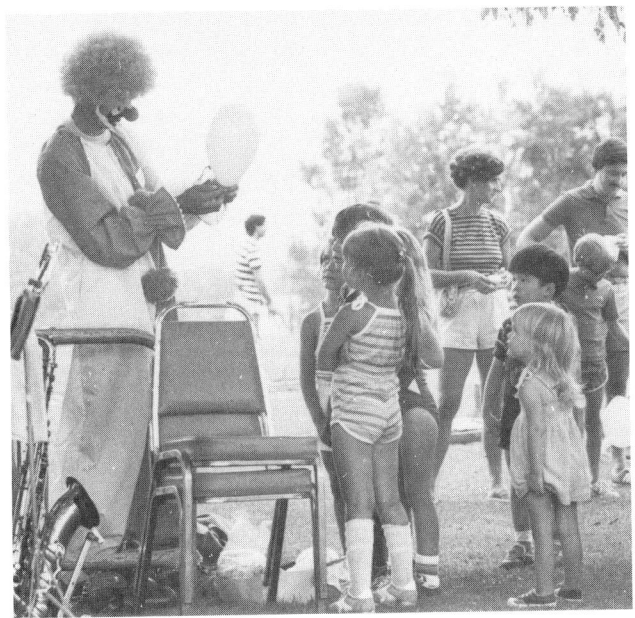

FIGURE 2-6

Community experiences can be a rich source of learning for children. Here a clown attracts a crowd at a summer picnic. (Courtesy Department of Medical Photography, Children's Hospital, Buffalo, NY.)

A second aspect of community assessment is determining the relationship of the family to the community. This is done by means of an **ecomap**, a diagram of family and community relationships (Figure 2-7). Such a "map" helps to assess the emotional support available to

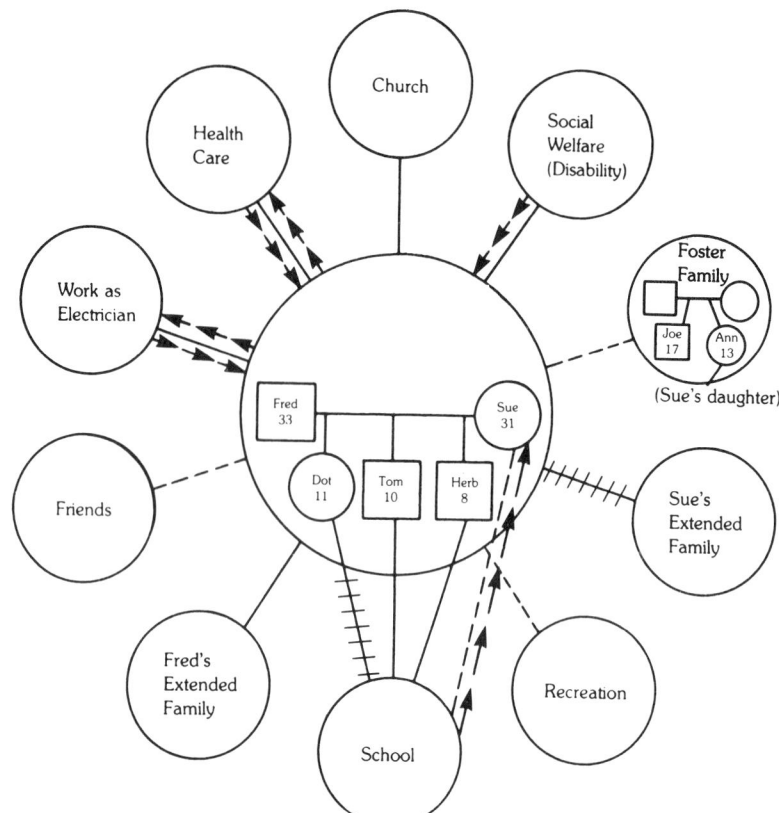

FIGURE 2-7

Ecomap of a family's relationship to its environment. The family members and their ages are shown in the center circle; the outer circles show community contacts. Lines indicate types of connections: solid line, strong; dotted line, tenuous; line with cross bars, stressful. Arrows signify energy or resource flow, and absence of lines indicates no connection. (From Spradley, B. [1990]. Community health nursing: Concepts and practice [3rd. ed.]. Philadelphia: J.B. Lippincott, with permission.)

a family from the community. A family whom you assess as having few connecting lines between its members and community contacts may need increased nursing contact and support in order to remain a well family. The Nursing Care Plan demonstrates both family and community assessment.

Key Points

- A family is a group of people who share a common emotional bond and perform certain interrelated social tasks.
- Common types of families encountered are nuclear, extended, single-parent, blended, cohabitation, single alliance, gay, lesbian, and foster families.
- Common family tasks are physical maintenance, socialization of family members, allocation of resources, maintenance of order, division of labor, reproduction, recruitment and release of members, placement of members into the larger society, and maintenance of motivation and morale.
- Common life stages of families are marriage, early childbearing, families with preschool, school-age, and adolescent children, launching center and middle-years families, and the family in retirement.
- Changes in patterns of family life that are occurring are increased mobility, one-parent families, and dual-

parent employment, divorce, social problems such as abuse and decreased socioeconomic level, and family size.
- Considering a family as a unit (a single client) helps the nurse to plan nursing care that meets the family's total needs.
- Families exist within communities; assessment of the community and the family's place within the community yields further information on family functioning.
- Families are not always functioning at their highest level during periods of crisis; reassessing them during a period of stability may reveal a stronger family than on first assessment.
- Because families work as a unit, unmet needs of any member can spread to become unmet needs of all family members.

Critical Thinking Exercises

Marlo Hanavan is a 32-year-old bookkeeper who is pregnant with her second child. Her first child, 2-year-old Amy, has just been diagnosed by their family practitioner as having cerebral palsy. She needs long-term physical therapy and attends a special school. Mr. Hanavan is unemployed because of an accident at work. He has some income from selling woodworking products at craft shows. Mrs. Hanavan states that on many weeks

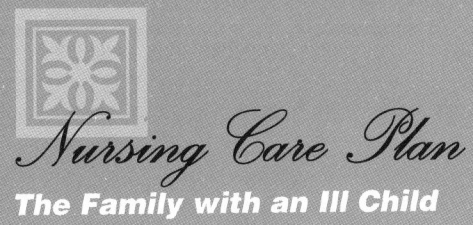

Nursing Care Plan
The Family with an Ill Child

Kevin is a 12-year-old boy with asthma. He is being seen in a child development clinic because he consistently neglects prescribed daily chest exercises and is a behavior problem in school. The following is a nursing care plan you might devise for his family.

Family Assessment:

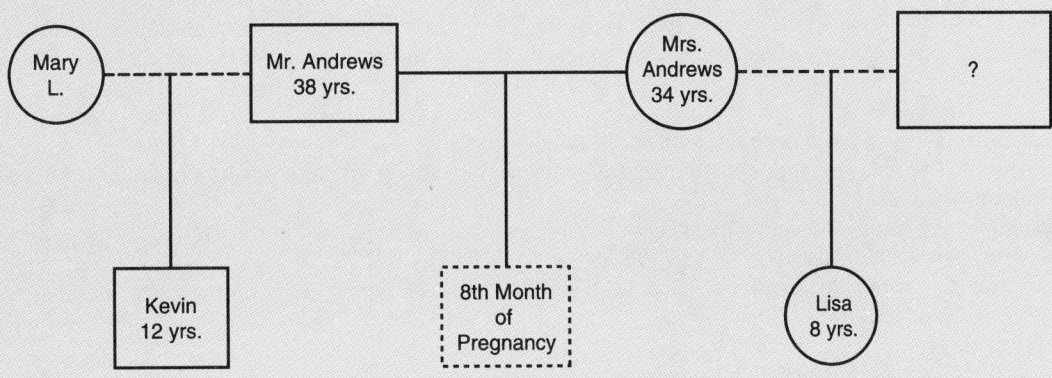

Type of family: Blended
Stage of family: Stage 4 or family with school-age children
Family functions

Ability to provide for physical, emotional and spiritual needs: Client states that mother wishes the family had more money, although father already works two jobs; mother has returned to college for a business degree so she can help earn more. Will interrupt education for one semester because of expected newborn. Schooling often makes her "too busy" to cook favorite foods or help with school projects. Kevin worries that new baby will take even more of mother's time.

Ability to be sensitive to needs: Client states that no one appreciates what it's like to be the one in the family who is always sick. Sister is active in Girl Scouts and wins many awards; parents are involved with work or school. Everyone but Kevin swims at health spa weekly; Kevin does not participate because he dislikes swimming. Kevin is alone a lot after school. He is worried when he is the only one home that he will have difficulty breathing.

Ability to communicate thoughts and feelings effectively: Client states he wishes the family would talk together more. Members used to talk at dinner but now father leaves for second job before dinner. Would like parents to discuss the potential impact of new baby on family.

Ability to provide support, security, and encouragement: Client states he would do breathing exercises if only one other family member would do them with him, but everyone is too busy.

Ability to initiate growth-producing relationships: Both parents encourage children to be independent and think for themselves; very upset over Kevin's disruptive school behavior.

Capacity to maintain community relationships: Father attends church on Sunday with children; mother is "too busy." Mother attends meetings of local Republican women's club once weekly. All of family but Kevin attends health club weekly. Kevin states he wishes the family would do more together but has no suggestions as to what these activities could be.

Ability to grow with and through children: Client states that mother studies with him in the evening. Although school is difficult for her, Kevin is worried she is "growing ahead" of father who is not attending school.

Ability to perform family roles flexibly: Conflict arises over evening dishes. Mother says she is too busy; father says they are not his job; sister is too young, so job is left to Kevin. He resents this.

Ability to accept help when appropriate: Mother accepted financial aid to return to school, although father states this is "demeaning" to his earning capacity. Family has spoken to school psychologist but sees this as help for Kevin, not entire family. Mother refused offer from pastor to discuss family problems.

Capacity for mutual respect for individuality: Client states that no one respects things he wants to do. He is expected to spend time caring for his sister rather than things he wants to do.

(continued)

Ability to use a crisis as a means of growth: Client states he thinks his mother's returning to school has ruined family life. Is afraid that a new baby will do even more damage.

Concern for unity, loyalty, and cooperation: Kevin says everyone is too busy doing their own thing to have time for anyone else.

Community Assessment

Housing: Family lives in a three-bedroom ranch home. Has adequate heat, hot water, and furnishings, indoor plumbing. No furniture or provisions have been purchased for new baby as yet. Kevin aware that if it is a boy, he will have to share room.

Support people: Although family is not emotionally close to any neighbors, they could call on those on either side of house for emergencies; house has a functioning telephone.

Occupation: The majority of people in community are employed. Postal clerk position of father provides a middle-class income.

Transportation: Family owns two cars; client rides school bus to centralized middle school. Most community activities are within walking distance.

Recreation: Community has an active Boy's Club and Boy Scouts Kevin could join. There is a county golf course and health spa nearby for adults.

Safety: Client states he feels safe in his home and on streets near his home.

Religion: There is a church of their denomination nearby.

Health care: Family uses an HMO as a primary health care site; has a pediatrician to provide care to children; mother sees a nurse-midwife for pregnancy care.

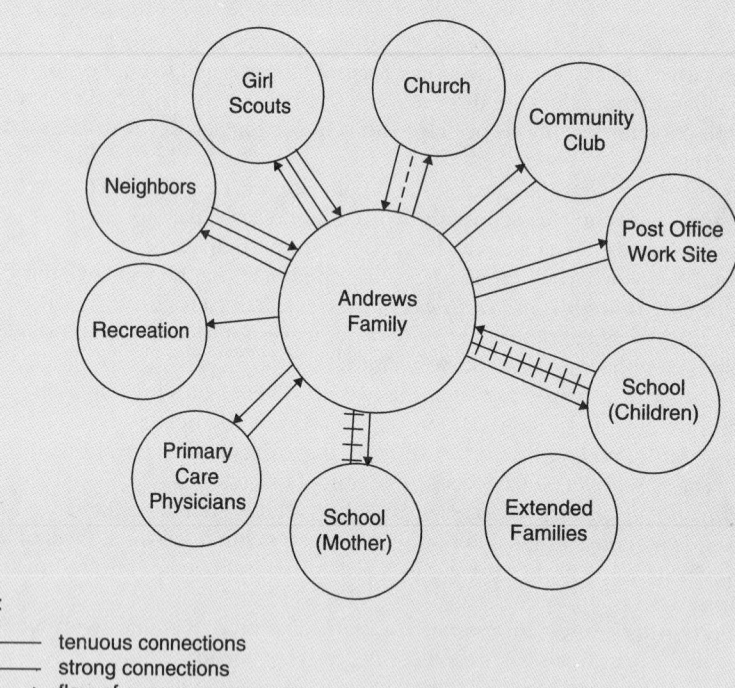

Key:

——————— tenuous connections
——————— strong connections
———————▶ flow of energy or resources
++++++ stressful connections
[absence of lines] no connection

(continued)

Nursing Diagnosis: Ineffective family coping, compromised, related to recent increased stresses on family.

Defining Characteristic: Family member expresses dissatisfaction with the way the family works.

Goal: Family will demonstrate increased support to client by 6 months' time.

Outcome Criteria: Kevin voices feelings of increased support from family; family is participating in at least one shared activity weekly.

Nursing Orders	Rationale
1. Meet with Kevin to help delineate areas of support he feels he needs. Encourage Kevin to express needs in a positive way.	1. Kevin has voiced that he feels a need for increased support. Positive expression of feelings may help reduce behavior problems in school.
2. Meet with mother and father to discuss Kevin's needs, particularly concern over being home alone and insecurity about new baby.	2. Mother is decision-maker; father is economic support person.
3. Assess if there are more support resources the family could call on.	3. Ecogram shows that more energy lines flow out than in.
4. Encourage Kevin to participate in family activities so he is a full family member.	4. Kevin does not participate in the one family activity (swimming) that the family enjoys.
5. Explore relationship with father and whether this could be strengthened.	5. This relationship appears to be the richest relationship for Kevin and could be Kevin's passage back into the family group.

Nursing Diagnosis: Social isolation related to family's busy schedule and disinterest in scheduled family activities.

Defining Characteristic: Family interacts little with community.

Goal: Family will increase community contacts by 3 months.

Outcome Criteria: Family is able to describe at least three interactions with community contacts in last month.

Nursing Orders	Rationale
1. Secure sources of community activities for family information.	1. Family is unaware of community activities.
2. Assess with family if there are community activities they would enjoy participating in as a family.	2. Community activities could both strengthen the family and their potential resources.

she doesn't have enough money to pay bills; she is forced to choose between medical care and groceries.

1. What family stage according to Duvall have the Hanavans reached? What would a genogram of their family look like? An ecogram?
2. Why is this a particularly unfortunate time for the Hanavans to have to choose between medical care and groceries?
3. How would the Hanavans' needs change if they were an extended family? A single-parent family? A cohabitation family?

References

Abell, T. O., et al. (1991). The effects of family functioning on infant birth weight. *Journal of Family Practice, 32,* 37.

Baker, N. A. (1994). Avoiding collisions with challenging families. *MCN: American Journal of Maternal Child Nursing, 19,* 97.

Bassuk, E. L., & Rosenberg, L. (1990). Psychosocial characteristics of homeless children and children with homes. *Pediatrics, 85,* 257.

Berne, S. S., et al. (1990). A nursing model for addressing the health needs of homeless families. *Image, 22,* 8.

Braveman, P., et al. (1993). Access to prenatal care following major Medicaid eligibility expansions. *Journal of the American Medical Association, 269,* 1285.

Bullough, B., & Bullough, V. (1990). *Community health across the age cycle.* St. Louis: C. V. Mosby.

Campanella, K., Korbin, J. E., & Acheson, L. (1993). Pregnancy and childbirth among the Amish. *Social Science Medicine, 35,* 333.

Daiges-Pelish, P. L. (1993). The impact of the first child on marital happiness. *Journal of Advanced Nursing, 18,* 437.

Department of Health and Human Services. (1991). *Healthy people 2000.* Washington, DC: Public Health Service.

Department of Health and Human Services. (1993). Measuring the health of children. In *Vital statistics report, 42,* 8. Hyattsville, MD: U.S. Public Health Service.

Duffy, M. E., et al. (1990). Personal goals of recently divorced women. *Image, 22,* 14.

Duvall, E. M., & Miller, B. (1990). *Marriage and family development.* Philadelphia: J.B. Lippincott.

Fishel, A. H., & Samsa, G. P. (1993). Role perceptions of divorcing parents. *Health Care for Women International, 14,* 87.

Friedman, M. (1992). *Family nursing: Theory and practice* (3rd ed.). Norwalk, CT: Appleton & Lange.

Gilliss, C., & Davis, L. L. (1992). Family nursing research: precepts from paragons and peccadilloes. *Journal of Advanced Nursing, 17,* 28.

Johnson, D. E., et al. (1992). The health of children adopted from Romania. *Journal of the American Medical Association, 268,* 3446.

Kemsley, M., & Hunter, J. K. (1993). Homeless children and families: clinical and research issues. *Issues in Comprehensive Pediatric Nursing, 16,* 99.

Lashner, B. A., et al. (1993). Passive smoking is associated with an increased risk of developing inflammatory bowel disease in children. *American Journal of Gastroenterology, 88,* 356.

Lee, E. J., et al. (1990). Survey of accidents in a university day-care center. *Journal of Pediatric Health Care, 4,* 18.

Martin, E. D., et al. (1992). Improving resources for foster care. *Clinical Pediatrics, 31,* 400.

McCubbin, M.A., & McCubbin, H.I. (1993). Family coping with health crises: the resiliency model of family stress, adjustment and adaptation. In Danielson, C., Hamel-Bissil, B., & Winstead-Fry, P. (eds.). *Families, health and illness.* New York: Mosby.

McCubbin, H.I., & Patterson, J. (1983). Family stress adaptation to crises: a double ABCX model of family behavior. In McCubbin, H., Sussman, M., & Patterson, J. (eds.). *Social stresses and the family: Advances and developments in family stress theory and research.* New York: Haworth Press.

Mobed, K., Gold, E. B., & Schenker, M. B. (1992). Occupational health problems among migrant and seasonal farm workers. *Western Journal of Medicine, 157,* 367.

Murray, A. B., & Morrison, B. J. (1993). The decrease in severity of asthma in children of parents who smoke since the parents have been exposing them to less cigarette smoke. *Journal of Allergy and Clinical Immunology, 91,* 102.

Neighbors, B., Forehand, R., & Armistead, L. (1992). Is parental divorce a critical stressor for young adolescents? Grade point average as a case in point. *Adolescence, 27,* 639.

Pillitteri, A., et al. (1993). Parent gender, victim gender and family socio-economic influences on the reporting of child abuse by nurses. *Issues in Comprehensive Nursing 16,* 287.

Reves, R. R., et al. (1993). Child day care increases the risk of clinic visits for acute diarrhea and diarrhea due to rotavirus. *American Journal of Epidemiology, 137,* 97.

Rich, O. J. (1992). Vulnerability of homeless pregnant and parenting adolescents. *Journal of Perinatology/Neonatal Nursing, 6,* 37.

Sherrod, R. A. (1992). Helping infertile couples explore the option of adoption. *Journal of Obstetric, Gynecologic, and Neonatal Nursing, 21,* 465.

Smart, R. G., & Walsh, G. W. (1993). Predictors of depression in street youth. *Adolescence, 28,* 41.

Smilkstein, G. (1978). The Family APGAR. *Journal of Family Practice, 6,* 1231.

Spradley, B. W. (1990). *Community health nursing* (3rd ed.). Philadelphia: J.B. Lippincott.

Taylor, M. L., & Koblinsky, S. A. (1993). Dietary intake and growth status of young homeless children. *Journal of the American Dietary Association, 93,* 464.

United States Census (1990). *Statistical abstract of the U.S.* Washington, DC: U.S. Department of Commerce.

Velsor-Friedrich, R. (1993). Homeless children and their families. *Journal of Pediatric Nursing, 8,* 122.

Wegman, M. E. (1992). Annual summary of vital statistics—1991. *Pediatrics, 90,* 835.

Suggested Readings

Aldous, J. (1990). Family development and the life course: two perspectives on family change. *Journal of Marriage and Family, 52,* 571.

Arditti, J. (1992). Differences between fathers with joint custody and noncustodial fathers. *American Journal of Orthopsychiatry, 62,* 186.

Arnold, L., & Brecht, M. (1990). Legislative issues affecting parenting; an overview of current policies. *Journal of Perinatology/Neonatal Nursing, 4,* 24.

Brazelton, T. B. (1993). Putting a child in day care; issues for working parents. *Pediatrics, 91,* 271.

Frankowski, B. L., et al. (1993). Advising parents to stop smoking: pediatricians' and parents' attitudes. *Pediatrics, 91,* 296.

Koepke, J., et al. (1991). Becoming parents: feelings of adoptive mothers. *Pediatric Nursing, 17,* 333.

Leventhal-Belfer, L., Cowan, P., & Cowan, C. (1992). Satisfaction with child care arrangements: effects on adaptation to parenthood. *American Journal of Orthopsychiatry, 62,* 165.

Melnyk, B. (1991). Changes in parent-child relationships following divorce. *Pediatric Nursing, 17,* 337.

Portes, P. R., et al. (1992). Family functions and children's postdivorce adjustment. *American Journal of Orthopsychiatry, 52,* 613.

Pridham, K. F. (1993). Anticipatory guidance of parents of new infants: potential contribution of the internal working model construct. *Image, 25,* 49.

Slater, S., & Mencher, J. (1991). The lesbian family life cycle: a contextual approach. *American Journal of Orthopsychiatry, 61,* 372.

Stainton, M. C. (1994). Supporting family functioning during a high-risk pregnancy. *MCN: American Journal of Maternal Child Nursing, 19,* 24.

Tschann, J., et al. (1990). Family process and children's functioning during divorce. *Journal of Marriage and Family, 51,* 431.

Wallace, P., & Gotlib, I. (1990). Marital adjustment during the transition to parenthood: stability and predictors of change. *Journal of Marriage and Family, 52,* 21.

Wineberg, H. (1990). Childbearing after remarriage. *Journal of Marriage and Family, 52,* 31.

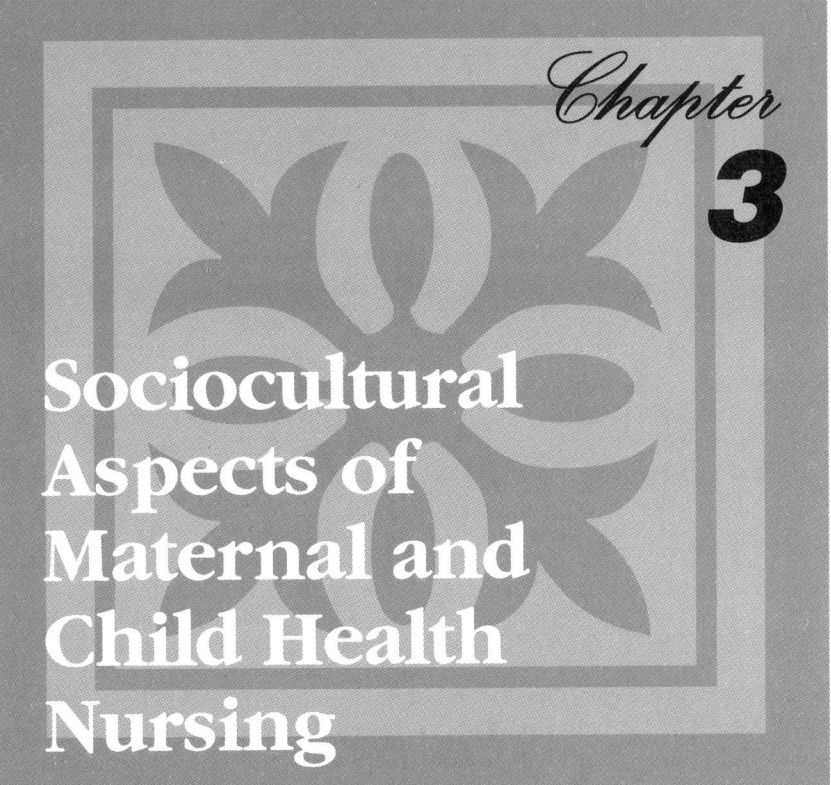

Chapter 3

Sociocultural Aspects of Maternal and Child Health Nursing

Objectives

After mastering the contents of this chapter, you should be able to:

1. *Describe ways that sociocultural influences affect maternal and child nursing care.*

2. *Assess a family for sociocultural influences that might influence the way it responds to childbearing and childrearing.*

3. *Formulate nursing diagnoses that relate to culturally appropriate aspects of nursing care.*

4. *Plan and implement nursing care that respects sociocultural needs and wishes of families.*

5. *Evaluate outcome criteria to be certain that goals of care related to sociocultural aspects have been achieved.*

6. *Identify National Health Goals related to sociocultural considerations that nurses could be instrumental in helping the nation to achieve.*

7. *Identify areas of care related to sociocultural considerations that could benefit from additional nursing research.*

8. *Use critical thinking to analyze how the sociocultural aspects of care affect family functioning and develop ways to make nursing care more family centered.*

9. *Synthesize sociocultural aspects of care with nursing process to achieve quality maternal and child health nursing care.*

Adele Pillitteri: MATERNAL AND CHILD HEALTH NURSING, 2nd Edition. © 1995 Adele Pillitteri.

---

*I*n order to understand why people respond the way they do to preventive health measures or illness, it is necessary to assess their socioeconomic status and their cultural beliefs, as these factors can strongly influence their responses.

Culture is a view of the world and a set of traditions that a specific social group uses and transmits to the next generation. **Cultural values** are preferred ways of acting based on those traditions. In order to understand why people react to health care in differing ways, it is important to understand their cultural values (Spector, 1991).

Cultural values often arise from environmental conditions (in a country where water is scarce, daily bathing is not practiced; in a country where meat is scarce, ethnic recipes use little meat). Such values influence people's view of themselves and their approach or lack of approach to situations such as health care. The usual values of a group are termed **mores** or **norms**. Expecting women to come for prenatal care and for parents to bring children for immunizations are examples of norms. Actions that are not acceptable to a culture are called **taboos**. Three taboos that are almost universal are murder, incest, and cannibalism. Issues such as abortion and child abuse are controversial because these are taboos only to some, not all people.

It is important to be aware of individual and cultural values as these influence the manner in which people plan for child birth, carry out child rearing, and respond to health and illness (Starn, 1991). Nurses need to be certain to include all cultural groups in nursing research samples so more is learned about cultural preferences in relation to nursing interventions (Betz, 1992). In a culture in which the male is the authority figure, for example, it might be expected that the father rather than the mother answers questions about an ill child; if you are from a culture in which females are expected to provide all child care, you might find it annoying to hear a man taking over the responses at a health interview. A nurse

who has been culturally influenced to believe that stoic behavior is the "proper" response to pain may be impatient with a woman who has been influenced to believe that expressing discomfort in childbirth is "proper."

Cultural differences occur across not only different ethnic backgrounds but also different lifestyles. Adolescents, urban city youth, the hearing-impaired, and gays or lesbians also have separate cultures. A parent who has been deaf since birth, for example, expects her deaf culture to be respected by having health care professionals attempt to communicate with her in her language.

The United States is a country of varied cultural groups and socioeconomic conditions, and under any given circumstance you are likely to see a wide range of behaviors exhibited (Figure 3-1). Given the wide range of the cultural mix, almost any behavior can be considered appropriate for some individuals at some time and place. Nursing with cultural aspects as a guide to care is termed **transcultural nursing** (Leininger, 1990).

Stereotyping consists of expecting people to act in characteristic manners without regard to individual characteristics; it is generally derogatory in nature. Statements such as "Men never diaper babies well" or "Japanese women are never assertive" are examples of stereotyping. Stereotyping occurs largely because of lack of exposure to enough people in a particular group and, consequently, a lack of understanding of the wide range of differences among people. In the above examples, the first speaker, having seen one man change diapers poorly, assumes that this represents the entire male population. The second example demonstrates lack of knowledge of a changing culture. If the person who believes that all Japanese females are nonassertive were exposed to more Japanese females, she or he certainly would find that the statement is not true. Using such stereotypes, you could plan health care that would be both inappropriate and resisted.

On the other hand, it is important to be aware of cultural characteristics because most people are proud

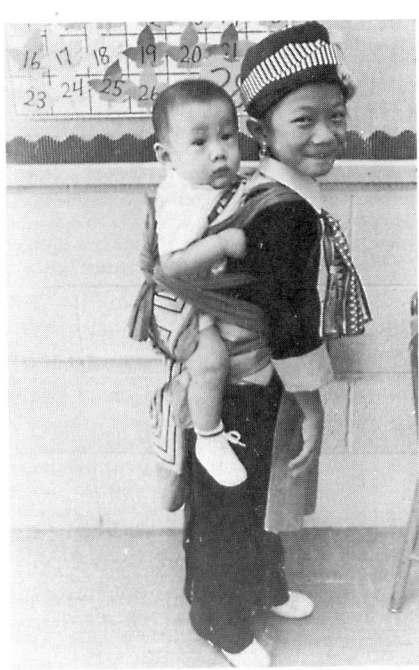

FIGURE 3-1
Cultural preferences vary even in the manner that parents carry children. Learning about different ways is important in care planning. (Schuster, C.S., & Ashburn, S.S. [1992]. The process of human development: A holistic life-span approach [3rd ed.]. Philadelphia: J.B. Lippincott. ©1992 by Clara Shaw Schuster and Shirly Smith Ashburn.)

of their cultural heritage. Making a statement such as "Hispanic women tend to be caring mothers" does not stereotype as much as it supports a characteristic of which the members of the culture are proud (Kulpers, 1991). Nurses should try to meet as many people from different cultures as possible in order to avoid stereotyping. Assess each person you meet as an individual, not merely as one of a group. A number of National Health Goals have been established in reference to sociocultural aspects of care. These are shown in the Focus on National Health Goals display.

 NURSING PROCESS OVERVIEW
That Respects Sociocultural Aspects of Care

ASSESSMENT

Assessment of sociocultural factors is important to be certain that care is not planned based on predetermined assumptions but on actual preferences of the family. Learn as much as you can about different cultures by reading about or talking to as many different ethnic

groups as possible. Specific areas to assess along with important findings in these areas are discussed in the chapter.

NURSING DIAGNOSIS

A number of nursing diagnoses speak to the consequences that occur when cultural preferences are not respected in care. Examples are:

- Powerlessness related to expectations of care not being respected
- Powerlessness related to sociocultural isolation
- Impaired verbal communication related to English not being primary language
- Nutrition, less than body requirements related to cultural preferences
- Anxiety related to a cultural preference for not bathing while ill
- Fear related to inability to buy food related to poor economic status

---

FOCUS ON
National Health Goals

A number of National Health Goals are concerned with health practices that may be influenced by cultural factors. These are:

- Increase to at least 90% the proportion of all pregnant women who receive prenatal care in the first trimester of pregnancy from a baseline of 76%.

- Increase to at least 90% the proportion of babies aged 18 months and younger who receive primary care services at the appropriate intervals.

- Increase to at least 75% the proportion of mothers who breast-feed their babies in the early postpartal period and to at least 50% the proportion who continue to breast-feed until their babies are 5 to 6 months of age from baselines of 54% and 21% (DHHS, 1991).

Nurses can be instrumental in helping the nation achieve these goals by designing prenatal and child care services that take into account the cultural diversity in our country and by promoting the nutrition and immunologic advantages of breast-feeding in a culturally sensitive manner. Additional nursing research on ways that prenatal care and child health services can be made more appealing to culturally diverse populations and education methods to best reach non–English-speaking clients is needed.

PLANNING

Planning needs to be very specific for the family and circumstances involved as sociocultural preferences tend to be very personal. Care may begin with in-service education for health care providers who are unfamiliar with a particular cultural practice and its importance to the specific family involved. It may include arranging for variations in policy, such as the length of family visiting hours, types of food served, or kind of child care. Such planning is beneficial because it can not only make health care more acceptable to a child or woman but also motivate providers to examine policies and question the rationale behind them (see the Focus on Nursing Research box).

IMPLEMENTATION

Appreciate that cultural values are ingrained and usually very difficult to change (in yourself and in others). An example of implementing care might be making arrangements for a Native American woman in labor to be able to take home the placenta if that was important to her or planning home care for a Chinese American

FOCUS ON NURSING RESEARCH

Do Cultural Preferences Influence Attendance at Prenatal Care?

Sculpholme, Robertson, & Kamons conducted a study to determine if ethnicity was a factor in why women from a low socioeconomic background were not making use of prenatal care services in their urban community. Two hundred twenty-seven women who had received no prenatal care during their pregnancies were interviewed in the immediate postpartum period as to why they had not received care. Findings of the study demonstrated that the main barriers to care the women identified were that the location of the clinic and the hours that care was offered were inconvenient, and transportation to the clinic was not available. Only 57 women stated that financial considerations were the main problem. Surprisingly, 29 stated they were turned away from care because they sought care too late in pregnancy. As could be expected, these women had a higher percentage of low-birth-weight infants than comparable women who did receive prenatal care, especially those who were single and African-American.

This study is important for nurses because although it was designed to reveal insights into the culture of the study population, it may have ultimately revealed more about the cultural orientations and beliefs of health care providers.

Sculpholme A., Robertson, E. G., & Kamons, A. S. (1991). Barriers to prenatal care in a multiethnic, urban sample. *Journal of Nurse Midwifery, 36*, 111.

child whose family believes in herbal medicine. It might be establishing a network of interpreters from health care agency personnel or eliciting assistance of personnel from a nearby university or foreign importing firm. It might be educating a child, family, or community as to the reason for a hospital practice. Do not feel that you and the health care agency are always the ones that must adapt; a particular situation may call for both sides to adjust (cultural negotiation).

EVALUATION

Evaluation by assessing if goal outcomes have been met should reveal that a family's sociocultural preferences were considered and respected during care. If this was not achieved, procedures may need to be modified further until this can be realized. Examples of outcome criteria that might be established are:

- Parents list three different ways they are attempting to initiate cultural preservation in their children.
- Child states he or she no longer feels socially isolated because of cultural differences.
- Family members state they have learned to substitute easily purchased foods for traditional foods unavailable in local stores in order to maintain adequate nutrition.
- Child with severe hearing impairment writes that he or she feels communication with ambulatory care staff has been adequate.

Sociocultural Differences and Their Implications for Maternal and Child Health Nursing

People's **ethnicity** refers to the cultural group into which they were born, although the term is sometimes used in a narrower context to mean only race. All people who move into a new community trade some of their ethnic traditions for those of the dominant culture through the processes of **assimilation** or **acculturation**. Both these terms mean that cultural expression is lost by taking on the customs of the dominant culture (Spector, 1991). The more different are the two cultures, the less likely there will be a high degree of assimilation or acculturation. Mutual culture assimilation often occurs. For example, when many Italians moved into American communities in the early 1900s, the average Italian family learned to speak English; the average American family learned to cook spaghetti with Italian sauce.

Ethnocentrism is a belief that one's own culture is superior to all others. Ethnocentrism became a strong component of United States life when, in the 1800s, it was actively stressed that the American way (which actually was the northern European way) was the "best" way. You cannot begin to understand how other people feel about situations or appreciate why they think the way they do unless you accept a philosophy that the world is large enough to accommodate a diversity of ideas and behaviors and that there is probably no "best" way.

Sociocultural Assessment

When assessing families as to whether socioeconomic or cultural influences are present that will make special considerations of care necessary, a number of categories of information related to structure (the composition of the family) and function (the roles and actions of the family) need to be examined.

Communication Patterns

Communication patterns (not only what people say, but how they say it) are determined by culture (Bushy, 1993); it is important to assess these patterns before teaching or giving information (Krauss-Mars & Lachman, 1994). People who ordinarily associate only with members of their own culture speaking their native language may have great difficulty detailing a health history in English to a health care provider. Language barriers can be particularly significant if the health history is given at a time when they or their child is ill, because their ability to cope and to express themselves in English may be at a low point. Even if people are able to converse well in English at work or in stores, they may not be able to recall the English words for symptoms such as nausea or dizziness when under stress. If so, such a person might omit mentioning the symptom rather than try to pantomime it or describe it in a different way.

Children who are embarrassed or bashful about speaking may simply not talk; therefore their needs may go unmet. If a child is frequently asked to interpret for parents, he or she may be forced to miss days of school in order to do this. Translating also can place a child in situations that unfairly require adult judgment; in some cultures it might be unacceptable for a younger person to serve as an interpreter for an older adult.

The term *Hispanic* refers to people who use Spanish as their primary language. There are about 12 million documented persons of Mexican, Puerto Rican, Cuban, or other Spanish-speaking origin in the United States. When added to the number of Hispanics who are undocumented or living illegally in the country, the total size of this group is close to 19 million, or about 9 percent of the total U.S. population.

Communication problems arise not only from foreign languages but also from dialects within a country. Something as simple as a New Englander adding an *r* sound to the end of words ending in *a* ("idear" instead of "idea") may make an explanation difficult to follow;

the slow cadence of a person from the Deep South may seem strange to someone accustomed to the rapid speech pattern of residents of New York City. Inner-city African-Americans often speak a dialect unique to them. In order to care for such clients, it is important to learn their dialect's cadence and common words without attempting to use them yourself, unless that is your own dialect. Trying to speak in a dialect not your own could be misinterpreted as mockery (Box 3-1).

Touch is a form of communication. Whether people greet one another with hugs and kisses or omit touching one another is culturally determined. Not all people like to be touched or even to shake hands (Hanley, 1991). For instance, some Vietnamese-Americans feel that rumpling the hair or palpating fontanels is an intrusive gesture because they believe that the head is the seat of the body's spirit and should not be touched.

Whether people look at one another when talking is also culturally determined. Chinese-Americans, for example, may not make eye contact during a conversation, a social custom that shows respect for the position of the health care professional—a compliment, not avoidance of the issues (Chang, 1991).

Use of Conversational Space

People of different cultures use the space around them differently. In the Western world, examinations of children or of childbearing women are, by necessity, conducted in a very tight (intimate) space because palpation is a part of the examination. Conversation, on the other

---

Box 3-1

Methods to Improve Health Care When Clients Do Not Speak English as Their Primary Language

1. If English is not the client's primary language, reading material may be difficult. Assess the reading level and rewrite information at an easier reading level.
2. Ask an interpreter to translate and rewrite material into other languages.
3. Be certain that rooms such as bathrooms are labeled with international symbols, not just the English words *male* or *female*.
4. Learn a few phrases such as "Good morning" or "This won't hurt" from other languages and use them in interactions with clients.
5. Don't be reluctant to use hand gestures or draw a figure to communicate better.
6. When using an interpreter, be certain not to ignore the primary person seeking health care in preference to the interpreter.

hand, is usually held at a distance of between 18 inches and 4 feet; business is most often conducted at a 4-foot distance. People from Eastern cultures may not be comfortable in this same space (Chang, 1991). Being aware that use of space is culturally determined helps you to respect the use of space for clients.

Time Orientation

The cultural pattern in the United States is geared toward punctuality regarding appointments; "time is money" is an often-quoted axiom. Other cultures do not have this concern for time. They may have instead a concept that time is to be enjoyed; for such a person there is no such thing as wasted time. In some South Asian cultures being late for appointments is not only a proper but a necessary sign of respect (giving the person you are meeting time to organize and be well prepared for your coming). Women who do not have a strict time orientation may view the hospital compulsion of feeding infants at staged times (e.g., 10 AM, 2 PM) as strange. People who are not accustomed to adhering to schedules this way may have difficulty following a strict medical regimen. If they are told, for example, to give a child a medication at 8 AM, 12 noon, and 6 PM daily and to return for another appointment at 2 PM in a week's time, you may have to stress that the important points are that the medication be taken three times a day (not the specific times) and that returning for a checkup at a set time is important (because the physician who will see them is in the health care facility only at that time).

Another way that time orientation differs is in whether a culture concentrates on the past, the present, or the future.

The dominant U.S. culture is present-future oriented; people are expected not only to take care of themselves at the present moment but also to make plans for the future. Other cultures are past oriented: they carefully preserve past traditions, allowing only the slightest change or variations in practices. Still others are present oriented. Saving money for college (a future-oriented action) may not be a high priority in these cultures. If a family's orientation is for the present or the past, members may have difficulty accepting a long-term rehabilitation plan (e.g., by 6 months a brain-injured boy will be crutch walking, and it will be a full year before he will be fully ambulatory again); they may need to be motivated by present indications of progress (e.g., this afternoon the child will be allowed to sit up for the first time; this evening he can begin to have periods of time without oxygen). The Amish are an example of a past-oriented culture in that they adhere to time-honored traditions and do not accept modern technological advances such as immunizations (Palmer, 1992). Some Native Americans hold a time-past orientation (Hanley, 1991). People from lower socioeconomic groups tend to be more present oriented than those from middle or higher socioeconomic groups because of the struggle to get through each day. People with strong religious convictions may be future oriented (looking forward to a future existence better than their present one) (Giger & Davidhizar, 1991).

Work Orientation

The predominant culture in the United States stresses that everyone should be employed productively (called the Protestant work ethic) and that work should be a pleasure and valued in itself (as important as the product of the work). Other cultures do not value work in itself but see it as a means to an end (you work to get money or food). A woman with this latter orientation might be more distressed to learn that bedrest during pregnancy will interfere with her ability to continue a hobby (going to baseball games) than with her occupation (teaching). Do not interpret this behavior as "lazy" or unproductive; it is merely a cultural or individual variation.

Family Orientation

The family structure most common in middle-class communities in the United States is that of the nuclear family (mother, father, and children). Some other cultures more typically form extended families (nuclear family plus grandparents, aunts, uncles, and cousins); such extended families offer many more potential support people in crisis situations and so have many positive attributes (Stauffer, 1991). The roles of family members are also culturally determined. When caring for children from extended families, be certain to identify the child's primary caregiver before giving health care instructions, as the child's natural mother may not be filling this role. Identifying the family decision maker is also important in large families. Family traditions may be well protected in extended families because there are so many people to maintain them. Information about the family may be carefully guarded and not given freely at health care visits as a way of keeping the family intact and unique (and as a reflection of mistrust for health care providers). Most families are interested in preserving their cultural heritage as a way of providing a sense of security and continuity for their children (see the Focus on Family Teaching box).

Male-Female Roles

In most cultures the male is the dominant figure. In such a culture, if approval for hospitalization or therapy must be gained, it would be the man who would give this approval. In a culture where the man is very dominant and the woman is extremely passive, she may be unable to offer an opinion of her own health or be embarrassed to submit to a physical examination. Orthodox Jewish women may be reluctant to remain in an examining

FOCUS ON FAMILY TEACHING

Q. Our family has a different cultural heritage than most of the people in our neighborhood. How can I encourage knowledge and respect for our native culture in my children?

A. Preserving cultural heritage when living in another culture calls for creative planning. Some suggestions for doing this are:

- Plan an "ethnic night" once a week when you serve only ethnic food. Encourage your children to invite friends for the meal and discuss the traditions behind the various foods served.

- If a foreign language is part of your tradition, reserve one night a week when family members speak only the native language.

- Choose books for your children to read that are written by authors from your ethnic origin or that advantageously describe the culture.

- Monitor television for specials or travel or educational programs that focus on your culture and plan to have your children watch them.

- Talk to your children about your childhood and the traditions and values that may have differed from those of other families you knew.

- Celebrate holidays in your traditional manner. Including cultural influences in holiday celebrations adds a very rich ingredient to these occasions.

room with a male physician unless a nurse is also present (Feldman, 1992). In an extremely male-dominated family, a woman may be pregnant not from a mutually planned pregnancy but from sexual relations she felt she could not refuse.

In contrast, in some cultures, such as Native American, the woman may be the dominant person in the family (Spector, 1991). The oldest woman in the home or tribe is the counselor; she would be the person who would give consent for treatment or hospitalization. It is important to evaluate male-female roles, because knowing the dominant person in the household helps you to understand the impact of the illness and/or loss to the family. If a woman is a family's dominant person and can no longer make her usual decisions because she is ill during a pregnancy, for example, the entire family may be thrown into confusion; if the woman is a nondominant member, you may have to act as an advocate for her rights with a more dominant person.

In most hospitals today, the father of the child is expected to play an active role in labor. This may be so different a role expectation or custom than the one the man is used to that he is thrown into confusion. Awareness that male roles differ from country to country helps nurses to find a middle ground for male participation in labor.

Religion

Religion is culturally determined, although there are wide variations in what religion people practice. Because religion guides people's overall life philosophy, it influences how they feel about health and illness.

Knowing what religion a family subscribes to helps you locate a support person when needed, as this differs according to religion. It helps you in planning care, as many nutrition practices, such as whether the family eats pork, are dictated by religious beliefs.

Health Beliefs

Health beliefs are not universal. Most people are familiar with the current controversy about whether male circumcision is necessary or not, for example. More surprising to most people is a belief that female circumcision (amputation of the clitoris and perhaps a portion of the vulva) is thought to be necessary in some cultures (Kluge, 1993).

It is generally assumed in the United States that illness is caused by documented factors such as bacteria, viruses, or trauma. In other cultures illness may be viewed primarily as a punishment from God, an evil spirit, or the work of a person who wishes harm on the sick person. An example of this is a belief among Hispanics that an evil eye (*mal ojo*) can cause illness (Adams et al., 1992). People who believe that their own action (being sinful) caused an illness may not be highly motivated to take medication or other measures to get well again (such a woman when ill during a pregnancy does not believe that a spoonful of penicillin will cure her). People from some cultures may receive more comfort from a spiritualist or witch doctor than from their physician; they may feel that it is necessary to suffer pain in order to be rid of the illness. Adolescents with this belief might be reluctant to ask for medication to make the illness easier for themselves. Understanding

Mary Jo is a 6-year-old Native American admitted to the hospital for a 24-hour admission for a tonsillectomy. The following is a nursing care plan you might devise to safeguard her cultural preferences.

Assessment: Child's father requests that three tribal customs be respected during her hospitalization: she be allowed to wear a charm filled with snake oil around her neck; her bed be placed so it faces north so the power of the North Star can act on her; and corn meal be sprinkled around her bed to ward off evil spirits.

Nursing Diagnosis: Parental fear related to concern that cultural beliefs will not be respected.

Defining Characteristic: Father has voiced concern that cultural beliefs will not be respected.

Goal: Family will voice satisfaction at hospital discharge that health care beliefs were respected.

Outcome Criteria: Family states that nursing staff respected cultural preferences during hospitalization.

Nursing Orders	Rationale
1. Discuss importance of customs with nursing staff.	1. Gains cooperation of all personnel.
2. Admit to room 8.	2. Bed in room 8 faces north yet is readily visible from doorway.
3. Place sign by bed not to remove charm from neck.	3. Alerts nursing personnel of cultural preference.
4. Discuss significance of corn meal with housekeeping staff.	4. Gains cooperation for a short (24-hour) admission.
5. Ask family to provide throw rug at door of room.	5. Allows personnel to wipe feet to prevent spread of corn meal and also encourages family to be an active participant in care.

different beliefs allows you to respect cultural differences and to work out mutual goal setting, even when a patient's views are not the same as you would choose for yourself or a member of your family (see the Nursing Care Plan).

Women's concepts of whether pregnancy is a time of wellness or illness differs in various cultures (Mullahy, 1992). Many American women visit physicians early in pregnancy, follow prenatal directives, and at birth allow a physician to be in charge. In other cultures, pregnancy and childbearing are considered such natural processes that a physician is considered unnecessary. The woman knows the special rules and taboos that she must follow in order to ensure a safe birth and healthy child and she is an active participant in labor and birth. She may plan to breast-feed until the next child is born, or as long as 1 to 5 years. Unless these differences are respected, it is difficult to plan prenatal care that meets women's needs (Mattson et al., 1992; Alcalay, Ghee, & Scrimshaw, 1993).

Choosing a physician as a primary care provider is not well accepted by all people. The health care delivery system in Mexico, for example, is a less structured one

than in the United States; there are few physicians for the total population. Many drugs are available without prescriptions; therefore, a local pharmacist, rather than a physician, may serve as the main health care resource for many Mexicans. Families may first seek help for illness from a trusted family member. Such a family member is termed *el que sabe* (he that knows). During an illness this person's approval of therapy is crucial; if it is not given, the ill person cannot comply with therapy. Outside the family structure are *yerbero* (herbalists) who grow and instruct people in the use of herbs or cures; another advice source is healers, known as *curandero*, who heal by the use of herbs or diet. Other healers are *expiritualistos* who can treat supernaturally caused illnesses and *brujos* who can not only revoke evil spells but turn them around onto others. *Parteras* are midwives who care for women during pregnancy and birth. For many people, turning to a *yerbero* or *curandero* is preferable to professional health care because these people do not charge a fee but only accept donations or an exchange of goods or services. Also, relating health problems to them is not difficult because there is no language problem (Spector, 1991).

Nutrition Practices

Foods and their methods of preparation are strongly culturally related. In many instances hospitalized children cannot find on the menu any foods that appeal to them because of cultural preferences. A Japanese diet, for example, includes many vegetables like bean sprouts, broccoli, mushrooms, water chestnuts, and alfalfa. Children with this preference would probably tire very quickly of the corn and peas common to a middle-class American diet. Fortunately, in most instances, a child's family can provide food that is appealing culturally and is still within a prescribed dietary limitation.

In counseling for good nutrition during pregnancy, remember that respect for culturally preferred food is important. Mexican-American women tend not to eat a large amount of meat compared with other cultures; adequate protein can be ingested, however, by mixing sources of incomplete protein (beans and rice, for example). Some women may omit various foods during pregnancy because they believe a particular food will mark a baby (strawberries cause birth marks, raisins cause brown spots) or because of a necessity to eat hot or cold foods to ensure fetal growth. Pregnancy is considered a hot condition; pork is considered a "hot" food. It may be difficult for a woman who believes in this balance to agree to increase her intake of meat, including pork, during pregnancy (Spector, 1991). Asian women may believe in a similar pattern of required balances (yin and yang beliefs). Be aware of what is locally available in food stores. Women who cannot secure the foods you recommend in their own neighborhood may not eat well because of the inconvenience of shopping elsewhere.

Changing Cultural Concepts

In the 1800s when there were a large number of immigrants from many different countries coming into the United States, the United States was viewed as a giant cultural "melting pot" or "salad bowl," where all new arrivals gave up their native country's traditions and values and became "Americans." Any behavior that was not like that of middle-class Americans was viewed as strange and inferior and a mark that one was a new immigrant.

Today the idea that America ever was a melting pot is being questioned; in addition, it is being stressed that retaining cultural values and traditions is not only acceptable but preferred. Retaining ethnic traditions strengthens and enriches family life; it provides security to younger family members to realize that they are one of a continuing line of people (who have a past and will have a future) (Figure 3-2).

When planning nursing care, it is important not only to respect people's cultural differences but also to help people share their cultural beliefs with health care

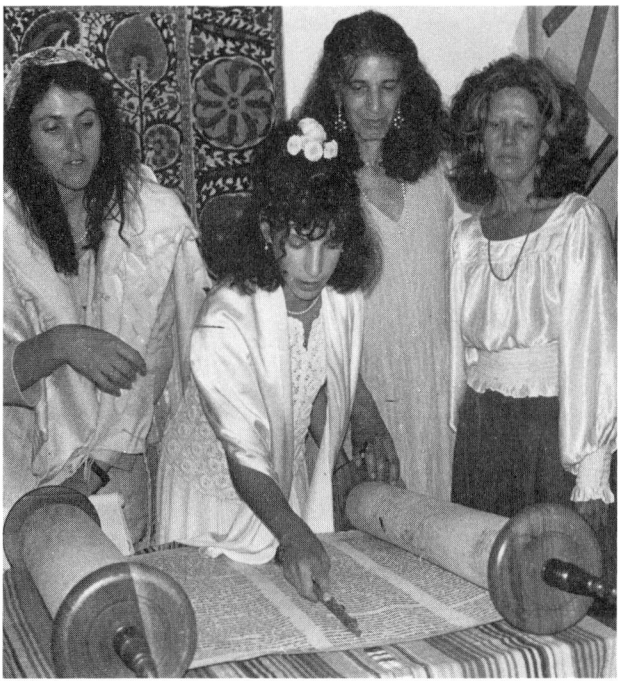

FIGURE 3-2
Cultural traditions offer a sense of security to children. (© Kathy Sloane, 1993.)

providers so that their beliefs can be considered and respected. As a nurse, you will have the opportunity to meet many people who hold cultural values different from your own. Throughout this text, Cultural Awareness boxes feature specific cultural preferences as they relate to health care or nursing. Respecting sociocultural differences is as important in giving holistic care as respecting individual traits or characteristics. Therefore, it is vitally important to include such considerations in care.

Key Points

- Culture is an organized structure that guides behavior into acceptable ways for that group. Usual customs are termed mores or norms. Actions that are not acceptable to a culture are taboos.
- Each culture differs to some degree from every other; most people are proud of these differences or cultural traits.
- Culture is transmitted by both formal and informal ways from generation to generation.
- Although cultural ideas adapt from time to time, they tend to remain constant.
- Cultural practices arise from environmental conditions.
- There is wide variation within a culture concerning values and actions because individuals make up the group and individually express their cultural heritage.

- People bring cultural values and beliefs to nursing interactions and these affect nursing care.
- Cultural aspects that are important to assess are communication patterns; use of conversational space; time, work and family orientation; and social organization, including nutrition, family roles, and health beliefs.

Critical Thinking Exercises

1. Anna Rodriques is a 12-year-old who is hospitalized for surgical repair of a broken tibia. She has a cast on her right leg and will be on bedrest for three days, then gradually be allowed to learn crutch walking.

   In planning care for her, you assume that because her culture is Hispanic, her family orientation will be male-dominated, her time focus will be on the present rather than the future, and nutrition preferences will be Mexican-American. Based on this, you concentrate on talking mainly about her current problem (bedrest) rather than future care at home. You speak to the dietitian about avoiding milk as lactase deficiency is present in many Mexican-Americans. You consult with Anna's father regarding the major aspects of her care.

   You are surprised to hear Anna complain on the second day of her hospitalization that she feels like a second-class person because her father has been asked for more input about her care than she has. She says she is particularly concerned that bone healing will not take place because she has had little milk to drink.
   a. What went wrong with Anna's care? If you had actually planned care in this way what would you have been guilty of?
   b. What would have been a better approach for determining Anna's family's cultural preferences? Supposing it is true that Anna is present oriented, how would you approach discussions of a long-term rehabilitation program for her?
2. Miss Crawford is a woman who is 30 weeks pregnant who has not been coming regularly for prenatal care. When you visit her in her home to see why, she states that before coming to the clinic for another appointment she wants to visit a voodoo doctor who will both predict her child's sex and guarantee a safe birth.
   a. What would be a plan of care that best respects this cultural value?
   b. Would recommending that Miss Crawford have a sonogram evaluation (which also could predict the fetal sex) be likely to be as satisfying for her?

References

Adams, R., et al. (1992). Cultural considerations: Developing a nursing care delivery system for a Hispanic community. *Nursing Clinics of North America, 27*, 107.

Alcalay, R., Ghee, A., & Scrimshaw, S. (1993). Designing prenatal care messages for low-income Mexican women. *Public Health Reports, 108*, 354.

Betz, C. L. (1992). A culturally biased perspective. *Journal of Pediatric Nursing, 7*, 229.

Bushy, S. (1993). Rural women: Lifestyle and health status. *Nursing Clinics of North America, 28*, 187.

Chang, K. (1991). Chinese Americans. In J. Giger & R. Davidhizar (Eds.), *Transcultural nursing: Assessment and intervention*. St. Louis: Mosby Year Book.

Department of Health and Human Services. (1991). *Healthy people 2000*. Washington, DC: Public Health Service.

Feldman, P. (1992). Sexuality, birth control and childbirth in orthodox Jewish tradition. *Canadian Medical Association Journal, 146*, 29.

Giger, J., & Davidhizar, R., eds. (1991). *Transcultural nursing: Assessment and intervention*. St. Louis: Mosby Year Book.

Hanley, C. (1991). Navajo Indians. In J. Giger & R. Davidhizar (Eds.), *Transcultural nursing: Assessment and intervention*. St. Louis: Mosby Year Book.

Kluge, E. T. (1993). Female circumcision: When medical ethics confronts cultural values. *Canadian Medical Association Journal, 148*, 288.

Krauss-Mars, A. H., & Lachman, P. (1994). Breaking bad news to parents of disabled children: a cross-cultural approach. *Child: Care, Health and Development, 20*, 101.

Kulpers, J. (1991). Mexican Americans. In J. Giger & R. Davidhizar (Eds.), *Transcultural nursing: Assessment and intervention*. St. Louis: Mosby Year Book.

Leininger, M. (1990). The significance of cultural concepts in nursing. *Journal of Transcultural Nursing, 2*, 52.

Mattson, S., et al. (1992). Culturally sensitive prenatal care for Southeast Asians. *Journal of Obstetric, Gynecologic and Neonatal Nursing, 21*, 48.

Mullahy, C. (1992). Cultural concerns add complexity to case of high-risk pregnancy. *Case Management Advisor, 3*, 54.

Palmer, C. V. (1992). The health beliefs and practices of an Old Order Amish family. *Journal of American Academy of Nurse Practitioners, 4*, 117.

Sculpholme, A., Robertson, E. G., & Kamons, A. S. (1991). Barriers to prenatal care in a multiethnic, urban sample. *Journal of Nurse Midwifery, 36*, 111.

Spector, R. (1991). *Cultural diversity in health and illness* (3rd ed.). Norwalk, CT: Appleton & Lang.

Starn, J. R. (1991). Cultural childbearing: Beliefs and practices. *International Journal of Childbirth Education, 6*, 38.

Stauffer, R. (1991). Vietnamese Americans. In J. Giger & R. Davidhizar (Eds.), *Transcultural nursing: Assessment and intervention*. St. Louis: Mosby Year Book.

Suggested Readings

Ahumada, L. S. (1991). Multicultural perinatal health care. *Maternal and Child Health Educational Resources, 6*, 1.

Buehler, J. (1993). Nursing in rural Native American communities. *Nursing Clinics of North America, 28*, 211.

Campinha-Bacote, J., et al. (1991). Cultural considerations in childrearing practices: A transcultural perspective. *Journal of National Black Nurses Association, 5,* 11.

Corrine, L., et al. (1992). The unheard voices of women: Spiritual interventions in maternal-child health. *MCN: American Journal of Maternal Child Nursing, 17,* 141.

D'Avanzo, C. E. (1992). Bridging the cultural gap with Southeast Asians. *MCN: American Journal of Maternal Child Nursing, 17,* 204.

Elfert, H., et al. (1991). Parents' perceptions of children with chronic illness: A study of immigrant Chinese families. *Journal of Pediatric Nursing, 6,* 114.

Forsythe, H. E., & Gage, B. (1994). Use of a multicultural food-frequency questionnaire with pregnant and lactating women. *American Journal of Clinical Nutrition, 59,* 2035.

Horn, B. (1990). Cultural concepts and postpartal care. *Journal of Transcultural Nursing, 2,* 48.

Kulig, J., et al. (1992). Prenatal classes for new Canadians. *Canadian Nurse, 88,* 25.

Lefever, D., & Davidhizar, R. (1991). American Eskimos. In J. Giger & R. Davidhizar (Eds.), *Transcultural nursing: Assessment and intervention.* St. Louis: Mosby Year Book.

Miller, S. W., & Supersad Nerala, J. (1991). East Hindu Americans. In J. Giger & R. Davidhizar (Eds.), *Transcultural nursing: Assessment and intervention.* St. Louis: Mosby Year Book.

Norbeck, J., & Anderson, N. (1991). Psychosocial predictors of pregnant outcomes in low-income black, Hispanic and white women. *Nursing Research, 38,* 204.

Phillips, S., & Lobar, S. (1990). Literature summary of some Navajo child health beliefs and rearing practices within a transcultural nursing framework. *Journal of Transcultural Nursing, 1,* 13.

Rairdan, B., et al. (1992). When your patient is a Hmong refugee. *American Journal of Nursing, 92,* 52.

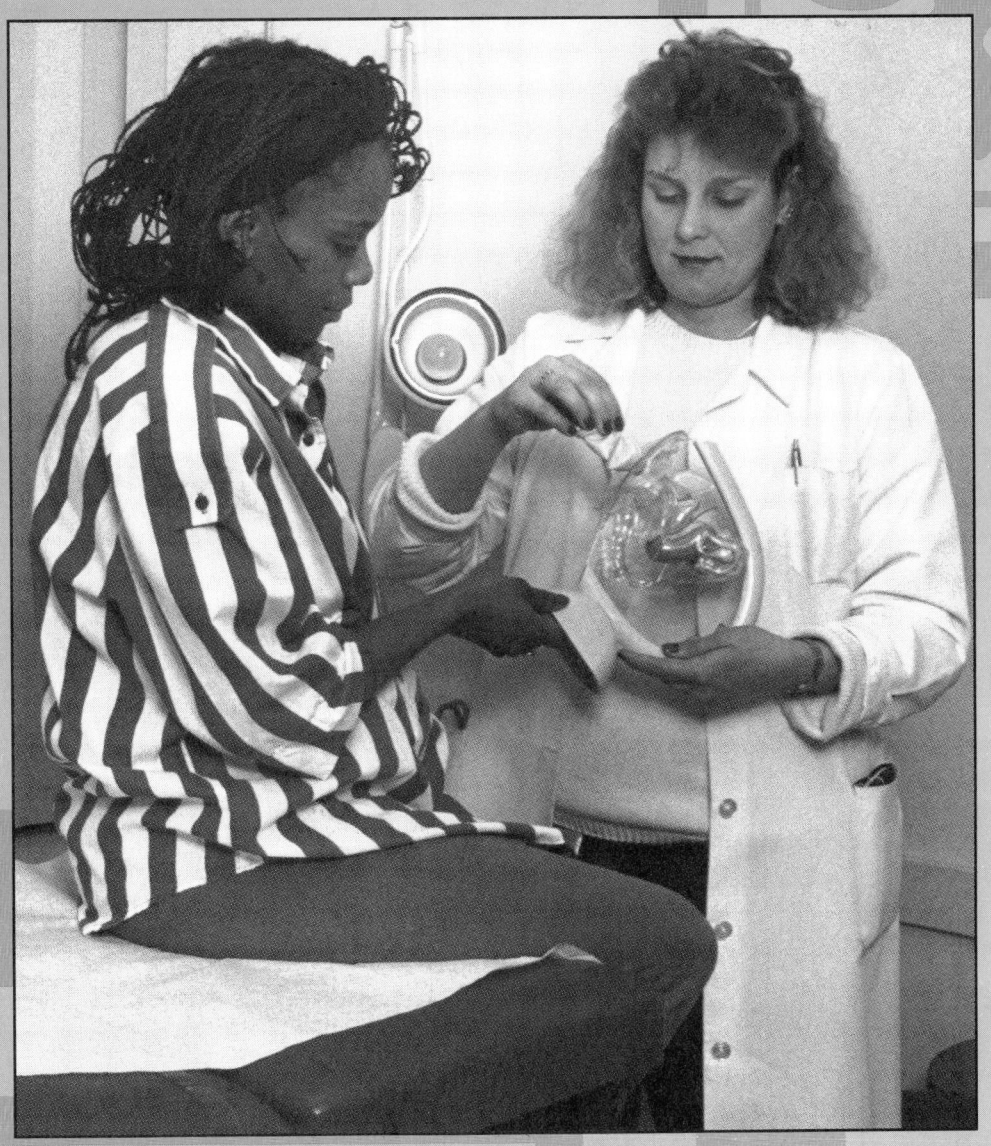

Unit 2

The Nursing Role in Preparing Families for Childbearing and Childrearing

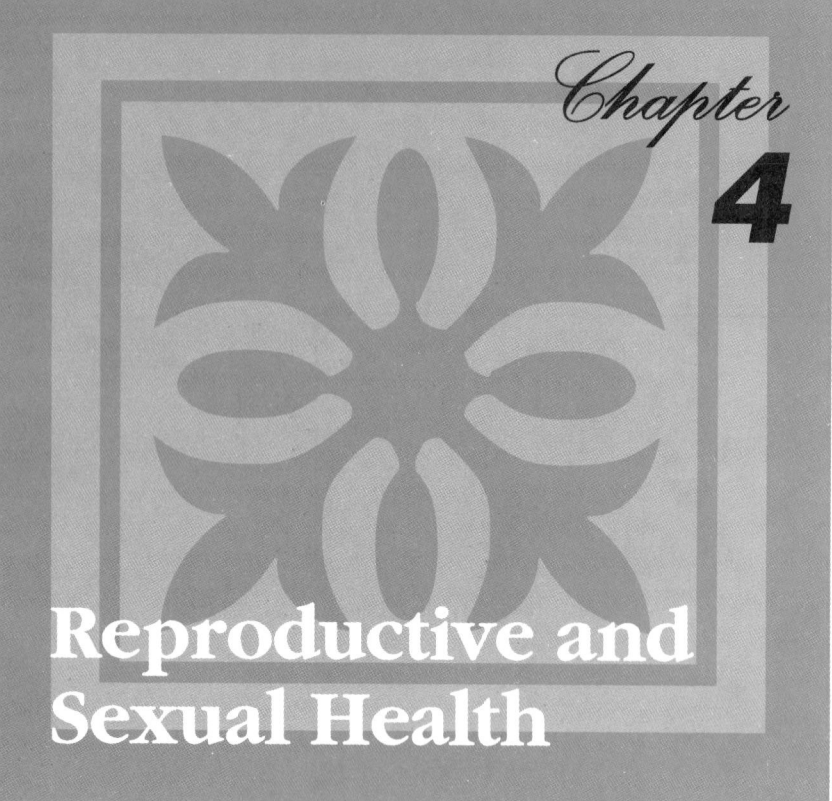

Chapter 4

Reproductive and Sexual Health

Objectives

After mastering the contents of this chapter, you should be able to:

1. Describe anatomy and physiology necessary for reproductive and sexual health.

2. Assess a couple for anatomic and physiologic readiness for childbearing, biologic gender, gender role, and gender identity.

3. Formulate nursing diagnoses related to reproductive or sexual health.

4. Plan nursing care related to anatomic and physiologic readiness for childbearing or sexual health, such as helping adults discuss concerns in these areas.

5. Implement nursing care related to reproductive health, such as educating for menstruation.

6. Evaluate goals and outcome criteria established for care to be certain they have been achieved.

7. Identify National Health Goals related to reproductive health and sexuality and specific ways that nurses can help the nation achieve these goals.

8. Identify areas of care in relation to reproductive and sexual health that could benefit from additional nursing research.

9. Use critical thinking to analyze ways that clients' reproductive and sexual health can be improved for healthier childbearing and adult health.

10. Synthesize knowledge of reproductive health and sexuality with nursing process to achieve quality maternal and child health nursing care.

Key Terms

- adrenarche
- andrology
- anteflexion
- anteversion
- aspermia
- bicornuate uterus
- culdoscopy
- cystocele
- dyspareunia
- endocervix
- endometrium
- erectile dysfunction
- gonad
- gonadostat
- gynecology
- gynecomastia
- homologue
- homosexual
- laparoscopy
- lesbian
- menarche
- mesonephric (wolffian) duct
- myometrium
- oligospermia
- oocytes
- paramesonephric (müllerian) duct
- perimetrium
- premature ejaculation
- rectocele
- retroflexion
- retroversion
- sadomasochism
- thelarche
- transsexual
- transvestite
- vaginismus
- voyeurism

Adele Pillitteri: MATERNAL AND CHILD HEALTH NURSING, 2nd Edition. © 1995 Adele Pillitteri.

Whether planning for childbearing or not, everyone should be familiar with reproductive anatomy and physiology and his or her own body's reproductive and sexual capacity. Women and their partners who are planning for childbearing may be especially curious about reproductive physiology and the changes the pregnant woman will undergo, so this is an opportune time for the nurse to educate both partners about reproductive and gynecologic health. Although the general public is becoming increasingly sophisticated about their bodies, misunderstandings about conception (preventing or promoting), sexuality, and childbearing still abound. Nurses who can clearly explain the phases of menstruation to the adolescent, the physiologic changes of pregnancy to a young adult couple, or the cause of menopause to a middle-aged woman provide much needed health teaching information. A number of National Health Goals that speak directly to improving reproductive or sexual health have been formulated. These are shown in the Focus on National Health Goals box.

Sexuality, in particular, is a major area of concern for adolescents and families of childbearing age. The nurse who cares for childbearing or childrearing families will be asked a variety of detailed questions about sexuality. For instance, many young adults want to know what is considered a "normal" sexual response or the "normal" expected frequency for sexual relations. A general rule of thumb in answering this question is that normal sexual behavior includes any act mutually satisfying to both sexual partners. Actual frequency and type of sexual activity varies widely. One of the biggest contributions nurses can make may be to make it clear that questions about sexual and reproductive functioning are best asked. With this attitude, problems of sexuality and reproduction are brought out into the open and made as resolvable as other health concerns or problems.

NURSING PROCESS OVERVIEW
for Promotion of Reproductive and Sexual Health

The primary role of the nurse concerning reproductive anatomy and physiology is education. Both female and male clients may feel more comfortable asking questions of the nurse than of the doctor, so it is important for a nurse to have this information readily available.

ASSESSMENT

Problems of sexuality may not be evident on first meeting a client, because it may be difficult for that person to bring up the topic until he or she feels more secure with the nurse. Good follow-through and planning is important because a person may find the courage to discuss a problem once but then will be unable to do so again. If the problem is ignored or forgotten through a change in caregivers, it may never be addressed again.

Any change in physical appearance (such as adolescent development or pregnancy) can intensify or create a sexual problem. The person with excessive weight loss or gain, a disfiguring scar from surgery or accident, hair loss such as occurs with chemotherapy, surgery on reproductive organs, inflammation or infection of reproductive organs, chronic fatigue or pain, spinal cord in-

jury, or the presence of a retention catheter need to be assessed for problems regarding sexual role as well as other important areas of functioning.

Sexual assessment is not a routine part of every health assessment. However, it should be included when appropriate, such as before providing reproductive life planning information, during pregnancy, or following childbirth. At other times, it is wise to listen for verbal or nonverbal clues that suggest a person wants to discuss a sexual concern. These clues are often subtle—"I guess marriage isn't for everybody"; "I'm not the woman I used to be"; "Are there ever funny effects from this medicine I'm taking?" Telling a seemingly inappropriate sexual joke may be another clue. Nonverbal clues may include extreme modesty or obvious embarrassment in response to a question about voiding or perineal pain or stitches.

Interviewing to obtain a sexual history takes practice and the conviction that exploring sexual health is as important as exploring less emotionally involved areas such as dietary intake or activity level. Frank admission by the nurse that he or she does not understand words that a person is using, if that is so, helps communication; the nurse's admitting that he or she is not always at his or her best when exploring this facet of a person's life (if that is true) also aids communication because it lets the person know that difficulty explaining it is a common reaction. Specific questions to include in a sexual history are shown in Box 4-1.

On physical examination, observe for normal distribution of body hair (i.e., hair on arms, axilla, and

---

Box 4-1
Specific Questions to Include in a Sexual History

Are you sexually active?

Are you satisfied with your sex life? If not, why not?

Do you have any concerns about your sex life? If so, what are they?

Do you practice "safe sex"?

Have you ever contracted a sexually transmitted disease or been worried that you have one?

Have you ever experienced a problem such as erectile dysfunction, failure to achieve orgasm, or pain during intercourse?

Are you using a contraceptive?

Are you satisfied with your current contraceptive method or do you have any questions about it?

---

triangle-shaped pubic hair in women; diamond-shaped pubic hair in men). Observe for normal genital and breast development (see "Tanner Stages," Chapter 33, for documentation of a stage of development).

Assessment in the area of reproductive health begins with interviewing clients to determine what they know about the reproductive process and any concerns they might have about their own reproductive functioning. The 14-year-old who is not yet menstruating, for instance, may be quite anxious about that fact but may be reluctant to say so unless asked directly. A statement such as the following invites discussion: "Although many of your friends at school may be menstruating already, it's not at all uncommon for some girls not to begin their periods until age 15 or 16. Is this something you find troubling?" This combination of providing information and questioning may encourage the girl to discuss not only her concern about delayed menarche (if she is indeed concerned), but other areas that will show her knowledge or lack of knowledge about reproductive health.

NURSING DIAGNOSIS

Common nursing diagnoses used in regard to reproductive health are:

- Health-seeking behaviors related to reproductive functioning
- Anxiety related to inability to conceive after 6 months without birth control
- Pain related to menstrual discomfort
- Disturbance in body image related to advanced development of secondary sex characteristics

Diagnoses relevant to sexuality include:

- Sexual dysfunction related to as yet unknown cause
- Altered sexuality patterns related to chronic illness
- Self-esteem disturbance related to recent surgery
- Altered sexuality patterns related to pregnant couple's fear of harming the fetus
- Anxiety related to fear of contracting sexually transmitted disease
- Health-seeking behaviors related to responsible sexual practices

PLANNING AND IMPLEMENTATION

A major part of planning in this area is to help a woman begin to see that she has some control over her body—she can do something about a symptom such as menstrual discomfort or a lack of energy related to excessive blood loss with menstruation. Empowering the woman with knowledge about her reproductive system and providing specific information about ways to alleviate discomfort will go far in helping that person understand re-

productive functioning throughout her life. Specific teaching instances might include explaining menstruation to a young girl, teaching a woman what is normal and abnormal in relation to menstrual function, and explaining reproductive physiology to the couple who wishes to become pregnant. Teaching is often enhanced by the use of illustrations from books or journals and models of internal and external reproductive systems. Nursing interventions in this area, however, include much more than education. Often, simply taking seriously a woman's concern of increased tension before menstruation will validate her concern. Role modeling, too, can be a valuable intervention, particularly for young clients. Discussing the subject of reproduction in a matter-of-fact way, or treating menstruation as a positive sign of growth as a woman, rather than as a burden, may help clients assume a positive attitude about these subjects from the start.

Planning for strengthening a person's gender identity or role behavior may involve interventions that strengthen an individual's sense of maleness or femaleness. A woman who feels that a woman's role is to be assertive needs to have built into her care plan opportunities for decision-making and self-care; a hospitalized adolescent who views a woman's role as being a person who is well groomed and has her hair washed every day needs time structured for these activities at the same priority level as other measures of self-care. Planning for these activities must be carefully structured, because they are activities that are easy for a busy health care provider to omit.

Clients who reveal homosexuality to health care providers usually do so not because they are interested in changing their lifestyle, but because they need help dealing with friends or family who refuse to accept their homosexuality. Nurses can be instrumental in designing care that demonstrates acceptance of all lifestyles equally (e.g., including anal and oral-genital sex practices in a discussion of safer sex practices). A helpful referral organization is National Federation of Parents and Friends of Lesbians and Gays, Inc., 8020 Eastern Avenue, NW, Washington, D.C. 20012.

EVALUATION

Evaluation in the area of reproductive health must be ongoing as health education needs change with circumstances and maturity.

How people feel about themselves sexually has a great deal to do with how quickly they recover from an illness, how quickly they are ready to begin self-care following pregnancy, or even how well motivated they are as adolescents to do those things necessary to remain well. Evaluating whether goals related to sexuality have been achieved is important in being certain that the person will be able to accomplish activities in other life phases that depend on being sure of sexuality or gender role. Examples of outcome criteria might be:

- Client states she is no longer fearful of contracting a sexually transmitted disease.
- Couple state they have achieved a mutually satisfying sexual relationship.

Reproductive Development

Physiologic readiness for childbearing begins as early as in intrauterine life; full function is initiated at puberty when the hypothalamus synthesizes and releases gonadotropin-releasing factor stimulator (GnRf), which in turn triggers the anterior pituitary to form and begin to release follicle stimulating hormone (FSH) and luteinizing hormone (LH). FSH and LH initiate the production of androgen and estrogen, which in turn initiate visible signs of maturity or secondary sex characteristics.

Intrauterine Development

The sex of an individual is determined at the moment of conception by the chromosome information of the particular ovum and sperm that joined to create the new life. A **gonad** is a body organ that produces sex cells (the ovary in females and the testis in males). At approximately week 5 of intrauterine life, primitive gonadal tissue is already formed. In both sexes, two undifferentiated ducts, the **mesonephric** (wolffian) and **paramesonephric** (müllerian) ducts are present. By week 7 or 8, in chromosomal males, this early gonadal tissue differentiates into primitive testes and begins formation of testosterone. Under the influence of testosterone, the mesonephric duct begins to develop or the male reproductive organs are formed and the paramesonephric duct regresses. If testosterone is not present by week 10, the gonadal tissue differentiates into ovaries and the paramesonephric duct develops into female reproductive organs. All the **oocytes** (cells that will develop into eggs throughout the woman's mature years) are already formed in this early structure (Scott et al., 1990).

At around week 12, under the influence of testosterone, penile tissue elongates and the urogenital fold on the ventral surface of the penis closes to form the urethra; in females, with no testosterone present, the urogenital fold remains open to form the labia minora; what would be formed as scrotal tissue in the male becomes the labia majora in the female. If, for some reason, testosterone secretion is halted *in utero,* a chromosomal male could be born with female-appearing genitalia. If a woman should be prescribed a form of testosterone during pregnancy or if the woman, because of a metabolic abnormality, produces a high level of

testosterone, a chromosomal female could be born with male-appearing genitalia. Examples of male and female reproductive **homologues**, that is, organs derived from the same embryonic origin, are summarized in Table 4-1.

Pubertal Development

Puberty is the stage of life at which secondary sex changes begin (Behrman et al., 1992). Girls begin dramatic development and maturation of reproductive organs at approximately age 12 to 13 years; for boys, 13 to 14 years. Although the mechanism that initiates this dramatic change in appearance is not well understood, the hypothalamus under the direction of the central nervous system may serve as a **gonadostat** or regulation mechanism set to "turn on" gonad functioning at this age. One theory is that a girl must reach a critical weight of approximately 95 lb (43 kg) before the hypothalamus is "triggered" to send initial stimulation to the anterior pituitary gland to begin gonadotropic hormone formation. The phenomenon of why puberty occurs is even less well understood in boys and the weight theory is often disputed today as not accurate (Goldsmith & Weiss, 1990).

The Role of Androgen

Androgenic hormones are the hormones responsible for muscular development, physical growth, and an increase in sebaceous gland secretions causing typical acne in both boys and girls. In males, androgenic hormones are produced by the adrenal cortex and the testes; in the female, by the adrenal cortex and the ovaries.

The primary androgenic hormone, *testosterone,* is low in males until puberty (approximately age 13 to 14 years). At that time, it rises to influence the development of testes, scrotum, penis, prostate, and seminal vesicles; the appearance of male pubic, axillary, and facial hair; laryngeal enlargement and its accompanying voice change; maturation of spermatozoa; and closure of growth in long bones.

In girls, testosterone influences enlargement of the labia majora and clitoris and formation of axillary and pubic hair. This development of pubic and axillary hair

Table 4-1. *Female and Male Reproductive System Homologues*

Female	Male
Clitoral glans	Penile glans
Clitoral shaft	Penile shaft
Labia majora	Scrotum
Ovaries	Testes
Skene's glands	Prostate
Bartholin's glands	Cowper's glands

due to androgen stimulation is termed **adrenarche** (Behrman et al., 1992).

The Role of Estrogen

When triggered at puberty, ovarian follicles in females begin to secrete a high level of the hormone estrogen. This hormone is actually not one substance but three compounds (estrone [E1], estradiol [E2], and estriol [E3]). It can be considered a single substance, however, in terms of action.

The increase in estrogen level in the female at puberty influences the development of the uterus, fallopian tubes, and vagina, typical female fat distribution and hair patterns, breast development, and an end to growth as it closes epiphyseal lines of long bones. The beginning of breast development is termed **thelarche**.

Secondary Sex Characteristics

Adolescent sexual development has been categorized into stages (Tanner, 1990). There is wide variation in the times that adolescents move through these developmental stages; however, the sequential order is fairly constant. In girls, pubertal changes typically occur in the order of (1) growth spurt, (2) increase in the transverse diameter of the pelvis, (3) breast development, (4) growth of pubic and axillary hair, and (5) vaginal secretions (Behrman et al., 1992). Menstruation usually begins between the time a girl develops pubic hair and the time she develops axillary hair. The average age at which **menarche** (the first menstrual period) occurs is 12.8 years. This may occur as early as age 9 or as late as age 17 years, however, and still be within a normal age range. Irregular menstrual periods are the rule rather than the exception for the first year. Menstrual periods do not become regular until ovulation consistently occurs with them (menstruation is not dependent on ovulation) and this does not tend to happen until 1 to 2 years after menarche. This is one reason that estrogen-based oral contraceptives are not commonly recommended until a girl's menstrual periods have become stabilized or are ovulatory (to prevent administration of a medication to halt ovulation before it is firmly established).

Production of spermatozoa does not begin in intrauterine life as does the production of ova, nor are spermatozoa produced in a cyclic pattern as are ova, but rather in a continuous process. Sperm production continues from puberty throughout the male's lifespan in contrast to production of mature ova, which stops at menopause.

Secondary sex characteristics of boys usually occur in the order of (1) increase in weight, (2) growth of testes, (3) growth of face, axillary, and pubic hair, (4) voice changes, (5) penile growth, (6) increase in height, and (7) spermatogenesis (Behrman et al., 1992).

Anatomy and Physiology of the Reproductive System

Although the structures of the female and male reproductive systems differ greatly in both appearance and function, they are homologues, that is, they come from the same embryonic origin (see Table 4-1). The study of the female reproductive organs is called **gynecology. Andrology** is the study of the male reproductive organs (Guyton, 1991).

The Male Reproductive System

Understanding the male reproductive system is necessary in order to appreciate the process of conception and human sexuality.

Male External Structures

External genital organs of the male include the penis, the scrotum, and the testes (which are encased in the scrotal sac). Spermatozoa are produced in the testes and begin existence, surrounded by semen, in the external structures. Semen is derived from the prostate gland (60%), the seminal vesicles (30%), the epididymis (5%), and the bulbourethral glands (5%). It is alkaline in nature and contains a basic sugar and mucin (protein) (Scott et al., 1990). Figure 4-1 illustrates external and internal male reproductive anatomy.

Penis. The penis is composed of three cylindrical masses of erectile tissue, two termed *corpus cavernosa,* and a third, the *corpus spongiosum,* contained in the shaft. The urethra passes through these layers of erectile tissue and serves as the outlet for both the urinary and the reproductive tracts in men. With sexual excitement, contraction of the ischiocavernosus muscle at the penis base occurs. This causes venous congestion in the three sections of erectile tissue, leading to distention and erection of the penis. At the distal end of the organ is a bulging sensitive ridge of tissue, the *glans.* A retractable casing of skin or *prepuce* protects the nerve-sensitive glans at birth. Many infants in the United States undergo *circumcision,* or surgical removal of the prepuce at birth (Figure 4-2).

The penile artery, a branch of the pudendal artery, provides the blood supply for the penis. Penile erection is stimulated by parasympathetic nerve innervation.

Scrotum. The *scrotum* is a rugated skin-covered muscular pouch suspended from the perineum. It contains the testes, epididymis, and the lower portion of the spermatic cord.

Testes. The *testes* are two ovoid glands 2 to 3 cm wide that lie in the scrotum. Each testis is encased by a

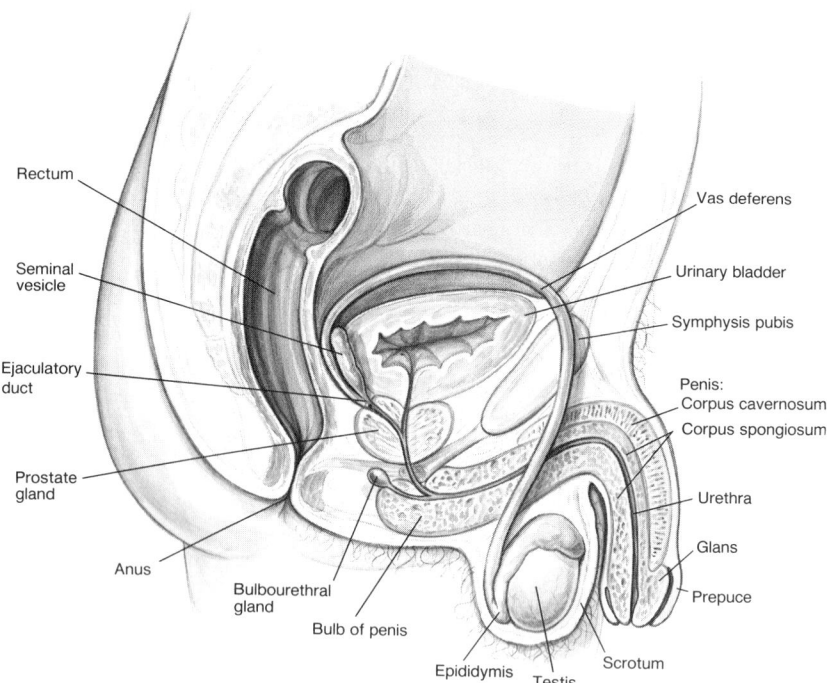

FIGURE 4-1
Male internal and external reproductive organs.

protective white fibrous capsule and is composed of a number of lobules, each lobule containing interstitial cells (*Leydig's cells*) and a seminiferous tubule. Seminiferous tubules produce spermatozoa. Leydig's cells are responsible for the production of testosterone. Testosterone, in turn, is responsible for male characteristics such as hair distribution. The level of testosterone in blood influences the production of spermatozoa indirectly, because if testosterone is low in amount, this stimulates the production of gonadotropic hormones (FSH and LH) by the pituitary gland; when testosterone increases in amount it causes a decrease in production of gonadotropic hormones. The presence of gonadotropic hormones is what stimulates seminiferous tubules to produce spermatozoa (Guyton, 1991).

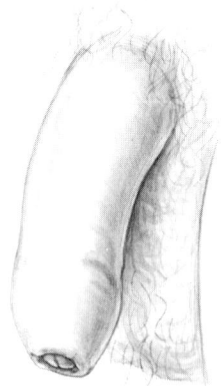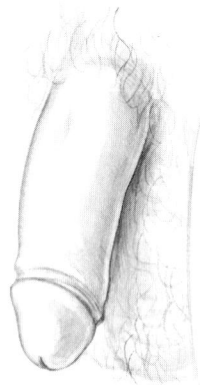

FIGURE 4-2
Uncircumcised and circumcised penis.

In most males, one testis is slightly larger than the other and is suspended slightly lower in the scrotum than the other (usually the left one). Because of this, testes tend to slide past each other more readily on sitting or muscular activity and there is less possibility of trauma to them. Most body structures of importance are more protected than are the testes (the heart, kidneys, and lungs are surrounded by ribs of hard bone, for example). Because spermatozoa do not survive at body temperature, however, the testes are suspended outside the body where the temperature is approximately 1°F lower than body temperature and sperm survival can be ensured.

In very cold weather, the scrotal muscle contracts to bring the testes closer to the body; in very hot weather, or in the presence of fever, the muscle relaxes, allowing the testes to fall away from the body. In this way, the temperature of the testes can remain as even as possible to promote the production and viability of sperm.

Male Internal Structures

The male internal reproductive organs are the epididymis, the vas deferens, the seminal vesicles, the ejaculatory ducts, the prostate gland, the urethra, and the bulbourethral glands (see Figure 4-1).

Epididymis. The seminiferous tubule of each testis leads to a tightly coiled tube, the *epididymis*. Because each epididymis is so tightly coiled, its length is extremely deceptive. It actually totals approximately 20 ft. The epididymis is responsible for conduction of sperm from the testis to the vas deferens, the next step in the passage to the outside. Some sperm are stored in the epididymis, and a part of the fluid that surrounds sperm (*semen,* or seminal fluid) is produced by the cells lining the epididymis. Because the epididymis is so extremely narrow in diameter along its entire length, infection (epididymitis) can lead to easy scarring of the lumen and prohibit passage of sperm beyond the scarred point (Kaler, 1990).

Sperm are immobile and incapable of fertilization as they pass or are stored at the epididymis level. It takes at least 12 to 20 days for sperm to travel the length of the epididymis, and a total of 64 days for sperm to reach maturity. This is one reason that **aspermia** (absence of sperm) or **oligospermia** (fewer than 20 million sperm per milliliter) are problems that do not appear to respond immediately to therapy but rather only after 2 months.

Vas Deferens (Ductus Deferens). The *vas deferens* is an additional hollow tube surrounded by arteries and veins and protected by a thick fibrous coating. It carries sperm from the epididymis through the inguinal canal into the abdominal cavity. The blood vessels and vas deferens together are referred to as the *spermatic cord.* The vas deferens ends at the seminal vesicles and the ejaculatory ducts. Sperm mature in their passage through the vas deferens. They are not mobile at this point, however, probably due to the fairly acidic medium of the semen produced at this level. A *varicocele* or a varicosity of the internal spermatic vein can contribute to male infertility by causing congestion in the testes (Mordel et al., 1990). *Vasectomy,* or severing of the vas deferens, is a popular means of male birth control.

Seminal Vesicles. The *seminal vesicles* are two convoluted pouches that lie along the lower portion of the posterior surface of the bladder and empty into the urethra by way of the *ejaculatory ducts.* These glands secrete a viscous portion of the semen, which has a high content of a basic sugar and protein and is alkaline in *p*H. Sperm become increasingly motile with this added fluid because it surrounds them with nutrients and a more favorable *p*H.

Ejaculatory Ducts. The two ejaculatory ducts pass through the prostate gland. They join the seminal vesicles with the urethra.

Prostate Gland. The prostate gland lies just below the bladder. The urethra passes through the center of it, like the hole in a doughnut. The prostate gland secretes a thin alkaline fluid that, when added to the secretion from the seminal vesicles and that already accompanying sperm from the epididymis, further protects sperm from being immobilized by the naturally low *p*H level of

the urethra due to the passage of urine through the same lumen.

Urethra. The *urethra* is a hollow tube leading from the base of the bladder that, after passing through the prostate gland, continues to the outside through the shaft and glans of the penis. It is approximately 8 in long. It is lined with mucous membrane the same as other urinary tract structures.

Bulbourethral Glands. Two *bulbourethral,* or *Cowper's glands,* lie beside the prostate gland and by short ducts empty into the urethra. Like the prostate gland and seminal vesicles, they secrete an alkaline fluid that helps counteract the acid secretion of the urethra and ensures the safe passage of spermatozoa.

The Female Reproductive System

The female reproductive system, like the male system, has both external and internal components.

Female External Structures

The structures that form the female external genitalia are termed the *vulva* (from the Latin word for covering) and are illustrated in Figure 4-3.

Mons Veneris. The *mons veneris* is a pad of adipose tissue located over the *symphysis pubis,* the pubic bone joint. It is covered by coarse curly hairs. In females, pubic hair appears in a triangular distribution (in males, the pubic hair pattern is more diamond shaped). The purpose of the mons veneris is to protect the junction of the pubic bone from trauma.

Labia Minora. Just posterior to the mons veneris spread two folds of connective tissue, the labia minora. Before menarche, these folds are fairly small; by childbearing age they have become firm and full; after menopause, they atrophy and again become much smaller. Normally, the folds of the labia minora are pink; the internal surface is covered with mucous membrane, the external surface with skin. The area is abundant with sebaceous glands so localized sebaceous cysts may occur here.

Labia Majora. The labia majora are two folds of adipose tissue covered by loose connective tissue and epithelium; they are positioned lateral to the labia minora. Covered by pubic hair, the labia majora serve as protection for the external genitalia, the urethra, and the distal vagina. They are fused anteriorly but separated posteriorly. Trauma to the area such as occurs from childbirth or rape can lead to extensive edema formation in the area because of the looseness of the connective tissue base.

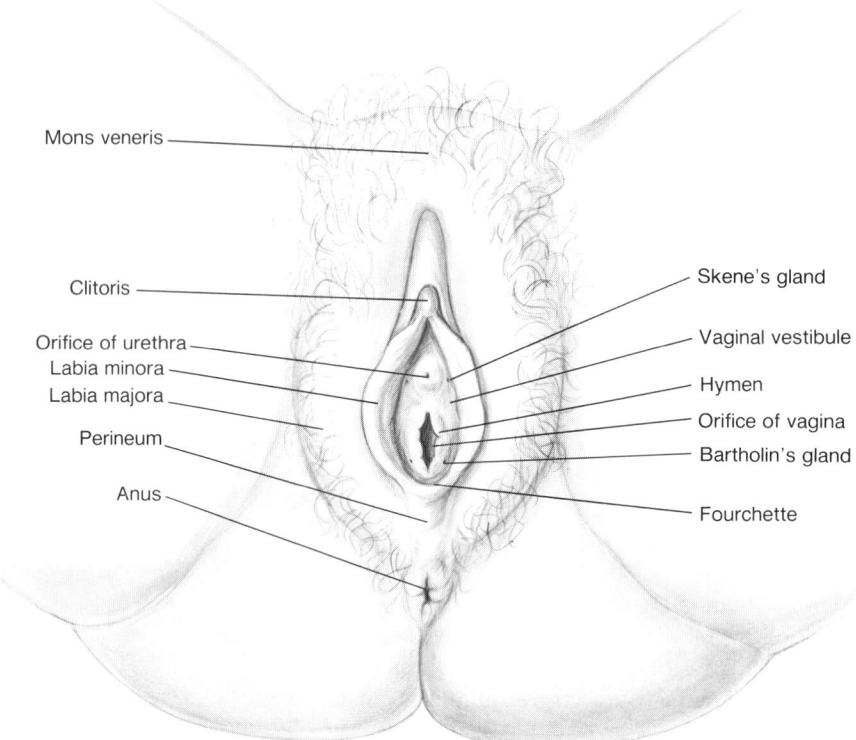

Mons veneris

Clitoris

Orifice of urethra
Labia minora
Labia majora

Perineum

Anus

Skene's gland

Vaginal vestibule

Hymen

Orifice of vagina

Bartholin's gland

Fourchette

FIGURE 4-3
Female external genitalia.

Other External Organs. The *vestibule* is the flattened, smooth surface inside the labia. The opening to the bladder (the urethra) and the uterus (the vagina) both arise from the vestibule. The *clitoris* is a small (approximately 1 to 2 cm) rounded organ of erectile tissue at the forward junction of the labia minora. It is covered by a fold of skin, the *prepuce.* The clitoris is sensitive to touch and temperature and is the center of sexual arousal and orgasm in the female (clitoris is the Greek word for "key"). Arterial blood supply for the clitoris is plentiful. When the ischiocavernosus muscle surrounding it contracts with sexual arousal, the venous outflow for the clitoris is blocked. Venous congestion from this blockage is what leads to clitoral erection.

Two *Skene's glands* (paraurethral glands) are located just lateral to the urinary meatus, one on each side. The ducts open into the urethra. Secretions from them help to lubricate the external genitalia during coitus. *Bartholin's glands* (vulvovaginal glands) are located just lateral to the vaginal opening on both sides. Their ducts open into the distal vagina. These glands lubricate the external vulva during coitus. The alkaline *p*H of their secretion helps to improve sperm survival in the vagina. Both Skene's glands and Bartholin's glands may become infected and produce a discharge and local pain (DiSaia & Woodruff, 1990).

The *fourchette* is the ridge of tissue formed by the posterior joining of the two labia minora and the labia majora. This is the structure that is sometimes cut (epi-

siotomy) before birth of a child to enlarge the vaginal opening.

Posterior to the fourchette is the perineal muscle or the *perineal body.* Because this is a muscular area, it is easily stretched during childbirth to allow for enlargement of the vagina and passage of the fetal head. Many exercises (Kegel's) suggested for pregnancy are aimed at making the perineal muscle more relaxed and more expandable to allow easy expansion during birth without the tearing of this tissue.

The *hymen* is a tough but elastic semicircle of tissue that covers the opening to the vagina in childhood. Due to the use of tampons and active sports participation, even many virginal girls do not have intact hymens at the time of their first pelvic examination. Occasionally, a girl will have an imperforate hymen, or a hymen so complete it does not allow passage of menstrual blood from the vagina or allow for sexual relations until it is surgically incised.

Vulvar Blood Supply. The blood supply of the external genitalia is mainly from the pudendal artery and a portion of the inferior rectus artery. Venous return is through the pudendal vein. Pressure on this vein by the fetal head may cause extensive back pressure and development of varicosities (distended veins) in the labia majora. Because of the rich blood supply, trauma to the area such as occurs from pressure during childbirth can cause the development of large hematomas. This ready blood supply also fortunately contributes to rapid healing of any lesions in the area following childbirth.

Vulvar Nerve Supply. The anterior portion of the vulva derives its nerve supply from the ilioinguinal and genitofemoral nerves (L-1 level). The posterior portions of the vulva and vagina are supplied by the pudendal nerve (S-3 level). Such a rich nerve supply makes the area extremely sensitive to touch, pressure, pain, and temperature. One form of anesthesia for childbirth may be administered locally to block the pudendal nerve to eliminate pain sensation at the perineum during birth. Normal stretching of the perineum with childbirth causes temporary loss of sensation in the area.

Female Internal Structures

Female internal reproductive organs, as shown in Figure 4-4, are the ovaries, the fallopian tubes, the uterus, and the vagina.

Ovaries. The function of the two ovaries (the female gonads) is to produce, mature, and discharge ova (the egg cells). In the process, the ovaries produce estrogen and progesterone and initiate and regulate menstrual cycles. If ovaries are removed before puberty (or are nonfunctional), the resulting absence of estrogen will prevent breasts from maturing at puberty; in addition, pubic hair distribution will assume a more male pattern than normal. After *menopause,* or cessation of ovarian function, the uterus, breasts, and ovaries themselves undergo atrophy or a reduction in size because of a lack of estrogen. Ovarian function, therefore, is necessary for maturation and maintenance of secondary sex characteristics in females. The estrogen secreted by ovaries is further important to prevent *osteoporosis* or faulty withdrawal of calcium from bones. This frequently occurs to women after menopause, making them prone to serious vertebra, hip, and wrist fractures. Estrogen may be prescribed for women at this age to help prevent osteoporosis. Because cholesterol is incorporated in estrogen, the production of estrogen is thought to keep cholesterol levels reduced and so limit the effects of atherosclerosis (artery disease) in women (Youngkin, 1990).

The ovaries are approximately 4 cm long by 2 cm in diameter and approximately 1.5 cm thick, or the size and shape of almonds. They are grayish white in color and appear pitted or with minute indentations on the surface. An unruptured, glistening, clear, fluid-filled *graafian follicle* (an ova about to be discharged) or a miniature yellow *corpus luteum* (the structure left after the ovum has been discharged) often can be observed on the surface.

Ovaries are located close to and on both sides of the uterus in the lower abdomen. It is difficult to locate them by abdominal palpation because they are located so low. If an abnormality is present, such as an enlarging ovarian cyst, however, the tenderness this causes may be evident on lower left or lower right abdominal palpation.

Ovaries are held in suspended positions and kept in close contact with the ends of the fallopian tubes by three strong supporting ligaments attached to the uterus or the pelvic wall. They are unique among pelvic structures in that they are not covered by a layer of peritoneum. Because they are not encased this way, ova can escape from them and enter the uterus by way of the fallopian tubes. Because they are suspended in position

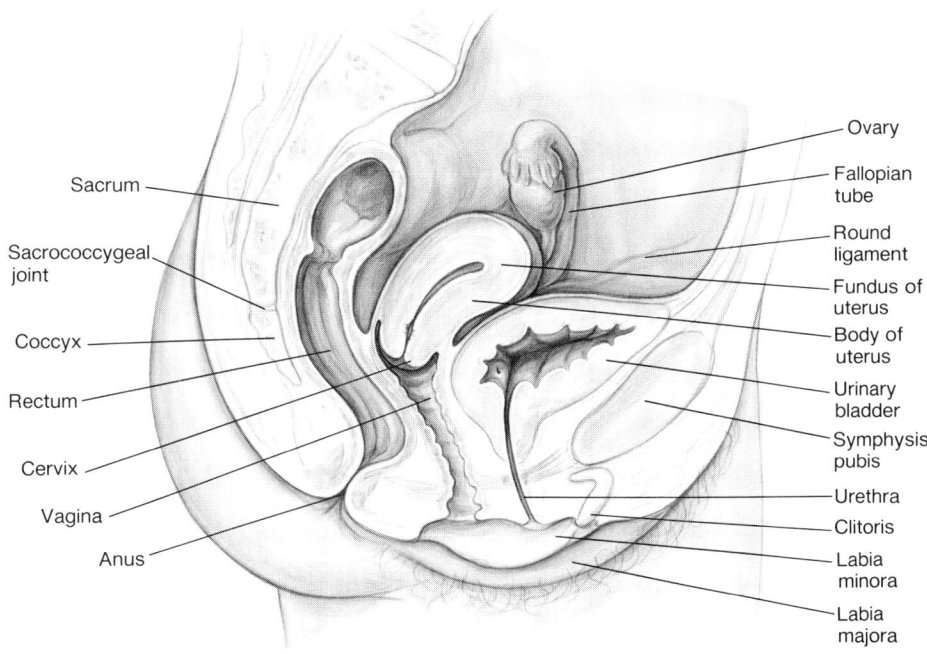

FIGURE 4-4
Female internal reproductive organs.

rather than being firmly fixed in place, an abnormal tumor or cyst growing on them can enlarge to a size easily twice that of the organ before pressure on surrounding organs or the ovarian blood supply leads to symptoms of compression. This is the reason that ovarian cancer continues to be one of the leading causes of death from cancer in women (the tumor grows without symptoms for such an extended period) (DiSaia, 1990a).

Ovaries are formed with three principal divisions: (1) a layer of surface epithelium, (2) inside that, a *cortex* area filled with connective tissue, and (3) a central area termed the *medulla*. It is in the cortex that immature (primordial) follicles that will mature into ova and produce large amounts of estrogen and progesterone important for the physiology of menstrual cycles develop.

Fallopian Tubes. The fallopian tubes arise from each upper corner of the uterine body and extend outward and backward until each opens at the distal end next to an ovary. Fallopian tubes are approximately 10 cm in length in a mature woman. Their function is to convey the ova from the ovaries to the uterus and to provide a place for fertilization of the ova by sperm.

Although a fallopian tube is one smooth hollow tunnel, it is anatomically divided into four separate parts (Figure 4-5). The most proximal division, the *interstitial* portion, is that part of the tube that lies within the uterine wall. This portion is only approximately 1 cm in length; the lumen of the tube is only 1 mm in diameter

at this point. The *isthmus* is the next distal portion. It is, like the interstitial tube, extremely narrow. The segment is approximately 2 cm in length. It is the portion of the tube that is cut or sealed in a tubal ligation or tubal sterilization procedure. The *ampulla* is the third and also the longest portion of the tube. It is approximately 5 cm in length. It is in this ampullar portion that fertilization of an ovum usually occurs. The *infundibular* portion is the fourth most distal segment of the tube. It is approximately 2 cm long and is funnel shaped. The rim of the funnel is covered by fimbria (small hairs) that help to guide the ova into the fallopian tube.

The lining of the entire fallopian tube is comprised of mucous membrane, which contains both mucus-secreting and ciliated (hair-covered) cells. Beneath the mucous lining is connective tissue and a circular muscle layer. The muscle layer of the tube produces peristaltic motions that conduct the ova the length of the tube. This migration of the ova is further aided by the action of the ciliated lining and the mucus, which acts as a lubricant. The mucus produced may also act as a source of nourishment for the fertilized egg because it contains protein, water, and salts.

Because the fallopian tubes are open at the distal end, they provide a connection between the outside of the body (vagina to uterus to tube) and the peritoneum. This pathway makes conception possible. It, unfortunately, can also lead to infection of the peritoneum (peritonitis) if disease spreads from the external genital

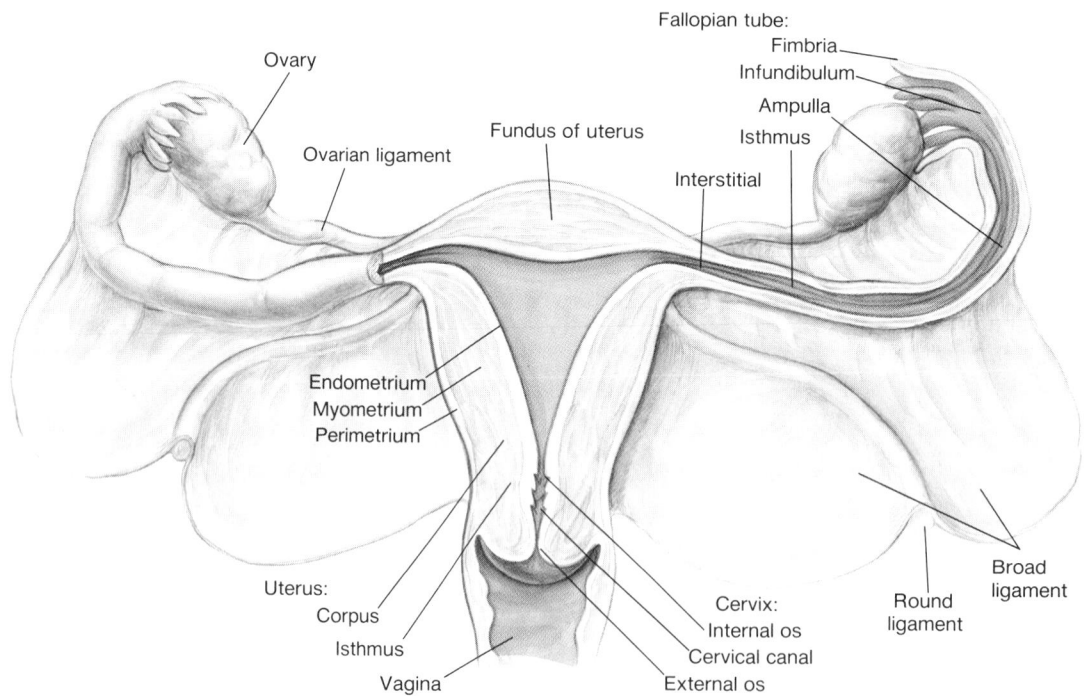

FIGURE 4-5

Anterior view of female reproductive organs showing relationship of fallopian tubes and body of the uterus.

organs through the vagina and uterus to the tubes and the peritoneum. For this reason, careful, clean technique must be used during pelvic examination or treatment. Vaginal examinations done during labor and birth are done with sterile technique to assure that no organisms can enter.

Uterus. The uterus is a hollow, muscular, pear-shaped organ located in the lower pelvis, posterior to the bladder and anterior to the rectum. During childhood, it is approximately the size of an olive, and its proportions are reversed from what they are later on, the cervix being the largest portion of the organ. At approximately age 8 years, an increase in the size of the uterus begins. The maximum increase in size occurs by approximately age 17 years, a fact that probably helps to account for the low-birth-weight babies typically born to adolescents younger than this age.

With maturity, a uterus is approximately 5 to 7 cm long, 5 cm wide, and in its widest upper part 2.5 cm deep. In a nonpregnant state a uterus weighs approximately 60 g. The function of the uterus is to receive the ova from the fallopian tube; provide a place for implantation and nourishment during fetal growth; furnish protection to a growing fetus; and at maturity of the fetus, expel it from the woman's body.

Following a pregnancy, the uterus never returns to quite the small diameters of its nonpregnant size. Therefore, in the woman who has born a child, uterine dimensions are closer to 9 cm long, 6 cm wide, 3 cm thick, and 80 g in weight. Anatomically, the uterus consists of three divisions: (1) the body or *corpus,* (2) the *isthmus,* and (3) the *cervix* (see Figure 4-5). The body of the uterus is the uppermost part and forms the bulk of the uterus. The lining of the cavity is continuous with that of the fallopian tubes, which fuse at its upper aspects (the *cornua*). The portion of the uterus between the points of attachment of the fallopian tubes is the *fundus.* During pregnancy, the body of the uterus is the portion of the structure that expands to contain the growing fetus. The fundus is the portion that can be palpated abdominally to determine the amount of uterine growth occurring during pregnancy, the force of uterine contractions during labor, and to assess that the uterus is returning to its nonpregnant state following childbirth.

The isthmus of the uterus is a short segment between the body and the cervix. In the nonpregnant uterus, it is only 1 to 2 mm in length. During pregnancy, this portion also enlarges greatly to aid in accommodating the growing fetus. It is the portion of the uterus that is cut when a fetus is delivered by a cesarean birth.

The cervix is the lowest portion of the uterus. It represents approximately one third of the total uterus size, or is approximately 2 to 5 cm long. Approximately half of it lies above the vagina; half extends into the vagina. The cavity is termed the *cervical canal.* The junction of the canal at the isthmus is the *internal cervical os;* the distal opening to the vagina is the *external cervical os.* The level of the external os is at the level of the ischial spines (an important relationship in estimating the level of the fetus in the birth canal before birth).

Uterine and Cervical Coats. The uterine wall comprises three separate coats or layers of tissue: (1) an inner one of mucous membrane (the **endometrium**), (2) a middle one of muscle fibers (the **myometrium**), and (3) an outer one of connective tissue (the **perimetrium**). The mucous membrane lining the cervix is termed the **endocervix.**

The endometrial layer of the uterus is important in terms of menstrual function and childbearing. It is not a single structure, but comprises two layers of cells. The layer closest to the uterine wall, or the *basal* layer, is not much influenced by hormones. An inner second glandular layer is greatly influenced by both estrogen and progesterone. This is the layer that grows and becomes so thick and responsive each month under the influence of estrogen and progesterone that it is capable of supporting a pregnancy. If pregnancy does not occur, it is this layer that is shed as the menstrual flow. The endocervix, continuous with the endometrium, is also affected by hormones, but changes are manifested in a more subtle way. The cells of the cervical lining secrete mucus to provide a lubricated surface so that spermatozoa can readily pass through the cervix; the efficiency of this lubrication increases or wanes depending on hormone stimulation. At the point in the menstrual cycle when estrogen production is at its peak, as much as 700 mL of mucus per day are produced; at the point that estrogen is very low, only a few milliliters are produced. Because mucus is alkaline, it helps to decrease the acidity of the upper vagina, aiding sperm survival. During pregnancy, the endocervix becomes plugged with mucus, forming a seal to keep out ascending infections.

The lower surface of the cervix and the lower third of the cervical canal are lined, not with mucous membrane, but with stratified squamous epithelium similar to that lining the vagina. Locating this point at which the tissue changes from epithelium to mucous membrane is important when helping with a Papanicolaou smear (a test for cervical cancer), because this tissue interface is the most frequent place for cervical cancer to originate (DiSaia, 1990b).

The *myometrium,* or muscle layer of the uterus, is composed of three interwoven layers of smooth muscle, the fibers of which are arranged in longitudinal, transverse, and oblique directions—a network that offers extreme strength to the organ. When the uterus contracts at the end of pregnancy to expel the fetus, equal pressure is exerted at all points throughout the cavity because of this unique arrangement of muscle fibers. Following childbirth, this interlacing network of fibers is able to constrict blood vessels coursing through the layers and thus limit loss of blood or hemorrhage in the woman. In addition, the middle muscle layer serves the important function of constricting the tubal junctions and preventing regurgitation of menstrual blood into the tubes. It also holds the internal cervical os closed during pregnancy to prevent a preterm birth. It is the layer from which myomas or benign uterine tumors arise (Merrill & Creasman, 1990). The *perimetrium* or the outermost layer of the uterus offers added strength and support to the structure.

Uterine Supports. The uterus is suspended in the pelvic cavity by a number of ligaments and supported by a combination of fascia and muscle (Nichols, 1990). If these supports become overstretched during pregnancy, they may not support the bladder well afterward and the bladder can then herniate into the anterior vagina (a **cystocele**). A **rectocele** may develop in the same way if the rectum pouches toward the vaginal wall (Figure 4-6).

A fold of peritoneum behind the uterus is the *posterior* ligament. This forms a pouch (Douglas' cul-de-sac) between the rectum and uterus. Because this is the lowest point of the pelvis, any fluid such as blood in the pelvis tends to collect in this space. The space can be examined for the presence of fluid by insertion of a culdoscope through the posterior vaginal wall (**culdoscopy**) or a laparoscope through the abdominal wall (**laparoscopy**).

The *broad* ligaments are two folds of peritoneum that cover the uterus front and back and extend to the pelvic sides. The *round* ligaments are two fibrous muscular cords that pass from the body of the uterus near the attachments of the fallopian tubes through the broad ligaments into the inguinal canal and insert into the fascia of the vulva. The round ligaments act as "stays" to steady the uterus. If a pregnant woman moves quickly, she may pull one of these ligaments and feel a quick, sharp pain that is frightening in its intensity in one of her lower abdominal quadrants.

A uterus is a suspended, not a fixed, organ, which is important in childbearing. Because it is not fixed in one position, this makes the uterus free to enlarge without discomfort during pregnancy (Coulam, 1990).

Uterine Blood Supply. The large descending abdominal aorta divides to form two iliac arteries; main divisions of the iliac arteries are the hypogastric arteries. These further divide to form the uterine arteries and supply the uterus. Because the uterine blood supply is not far removed from the aorta, it is copious and adequate to supply the growing needs of a fetus. As an additional safeguard, after supplying the ovary with blood, the ovarian artery (a direct subdivision of the aorta) joins with the uterine artery as a fail-safe system to ensure that the uterus will have an adequate blood supply. The blood vessels that supply the cells and lining of the uterus are tortuous in appearance against the sides of the uterine body in nonpregnant women. As a uterus enlarges with pregnancy, the vessels "unwind" and so can stretch to maintain an adequate blood supply as the organ enlarges. The uterine veins follow the same twisting course as the arteries; they empty into the internal iliac veins.

An important organ relationship to be aware of is the association of uterine vessels and the ureters. The ureters from the kidneys pass directly in back of the ovarian vessels near the fallopian tubes; as shown in Figure 4-7, they cross just beneath the uterine vessels before they enter the bladder. This close anatomic relationship has implications in surgery such as tubal liga-

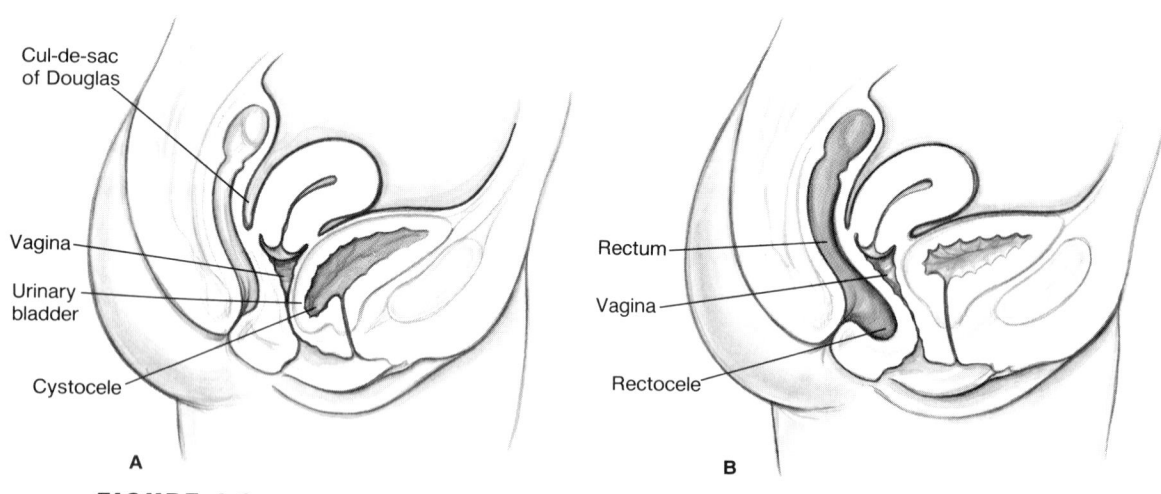

Cul-de-sac of Douglas

Vagina

Urinary bladder

Cystocele

A

Rectum

Vagina

Rectocele

B

FIGURE 4-6

(**A**) *Cystocele. The bladder has herniated into the anterior wall of the vagina.* (**B**) *Rectocele. The posterior wall of the vagina is herniated.*

above this at the T-5 to T-10 level). This is the principle of epidural anesthesia (see Chapter 19).

Uterine Deviations. A number of uterine deviations relating to shape and position may interfere with fertility or pregnancy. In the female fetus, the uterus first forms with a septum or a fibrous division, longitudinally separating it into two portions. As the fetus matures, this septum dissolves, so that typically at birth no remnant of the division remains. In some women, the septum never atrophies, and so the uterus remains as two separate compartments. In others, half of the septum is still present. Still other women have oddly shaped "horns" at the junction of the fallopian tubes, termed a **bicornuate** uterus. All these malformations may decrease the ability to conceive or to carry a pregnancy to term. Some variations of uterine formation are shown in Figure 4-8. The specific effects of these deviations on fertility and pregnancy are discussed in later chapters.

Ordinarily, the body of the uterus is tipped slightly forward. **Anteversion** is a condition in which the fundus is tipped very far forward. **Retroversion** means that the fundus is tipped back. **Anteflexion** means that the body of the uterus is bent sharply forward at the junction with the cervix. **Retroflexion** means that the body is bent sharply back. Minor variations of these generally cause no reproductive problems. Extreme abnormal flexion or version positions may interfere with fertility, because they may block the deposition or migration of sperm. Examples of these abnormal uterine positions are shown in Figure 4-9.

Vagina. The vagina is a hollow musculomembranous canal located posterior to the bladder and anterior to the rectum. It extends from the cervix of the uterus to the external vulva. Its function is to act as the organ of intercourse and to convey sperm to the cervix so sperm can meet with the ovum in the fallopian tube. With childbirth, it expands to serve as the birth canal.

When a woman is lying on her back as she does for a pelvic examination, the course of the vagina is inward and downward. Because of this downward slant and the insertion of the uterine cervix into the distal portion, the length of the anterior wall of the vagina is approximately 6 to 7 cm long and the posterior wall, 8 to 9 cm. At the uterine end of the structure, there are recesses on all sides of the cervix termed *fornices.* Behind the cervix is the *posterior fornix;* at the front, the *anterior fornix;* and at the sides, the *lateral fornices.* The posterior fornix serves as a place for the pooling of semen following coitus; this allows a large number of sperm to remain close to the cervix and encourages sperm migration into the cervix.

The vaginal wall is so thin at the fornices that the bladder can be palpated through the anterior fornix, the

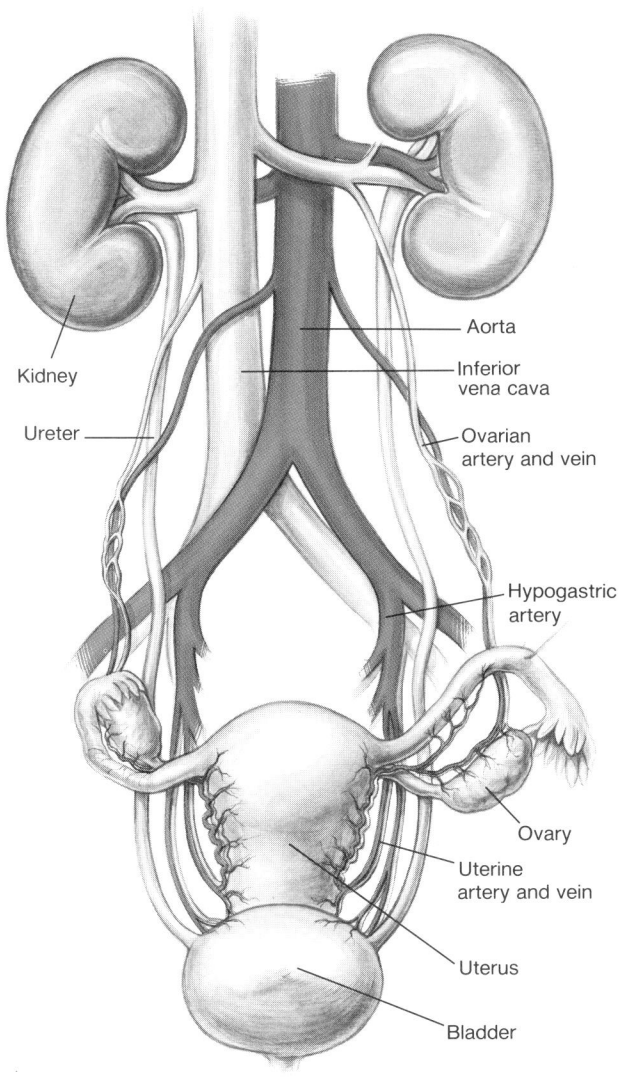

FIGURE 4-7
Blood supply to the uterus.

Kidney

Ureter

Aorta

Inferior vena cava

Ovarian artery and vein

Hypogastric artery

Ovary

Uterine artery and vein

Uterus

Bladder

tion, cesarean birth, and hysterectomy (removal of the uterus), because the ureter may be injured by a clamp if bleeding is controlled by clamping the uterine or ovarian vessels. This is one reason why observing women for urine output following uterine or fallopian tube surgery is always a critical assessment.

Uterine Nerve Supply. The uterus is supplied by both afferent (sensory) and efferent (motor) nerves. The efferent nerves arise from T-5 through T-10 spinal ganglia. The afferent nerves join the hypogastric plexus and enter the spinal column at T-11 and T-12. The fact that sensory innervation from the uterus registers lower in the spinal column than does motor control has implications in controlling pain in labor. An anesthetic solution can be injected near the spinal column and stop the pain of uterine contractions at the T-11 and T-12 levels without stopping motor control or contractions (registered

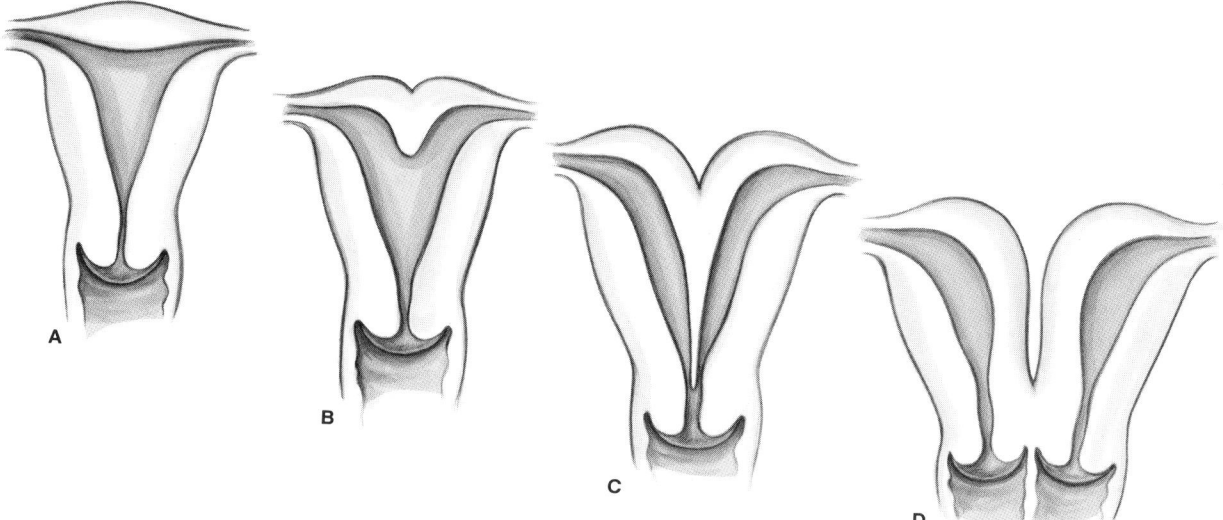

FIGURE 4-8
(**A**) *Normal uterus.* (**B**) *Bicornuate uterus.* (**C**) *Septum dividing uterus.* (**D**) *Double uterus. Abnormal shapes of uterus allow less placenta implantation space.*

ovaries through the lateral ones, and the rectum through the posterior fornix.

The vagina is lined with stratified squamous epithelium similar to that covering the cervix. It has a middle connective tissue layer and a strong muscular wall. Normally, the walls contain many folds or rugae and lie in close approximation to each other. These folds make the vagina very elastic and able to expand at the end of pregnancy to allow a full-term baby to pass through without tearing. A circular muscle, the *bulbocavernosus*, at the external opening to the vagina acts as a voluntary sphincter.

Women preparing for childbirth are advised to relax and tense this external vaginal sphincter muscle a set

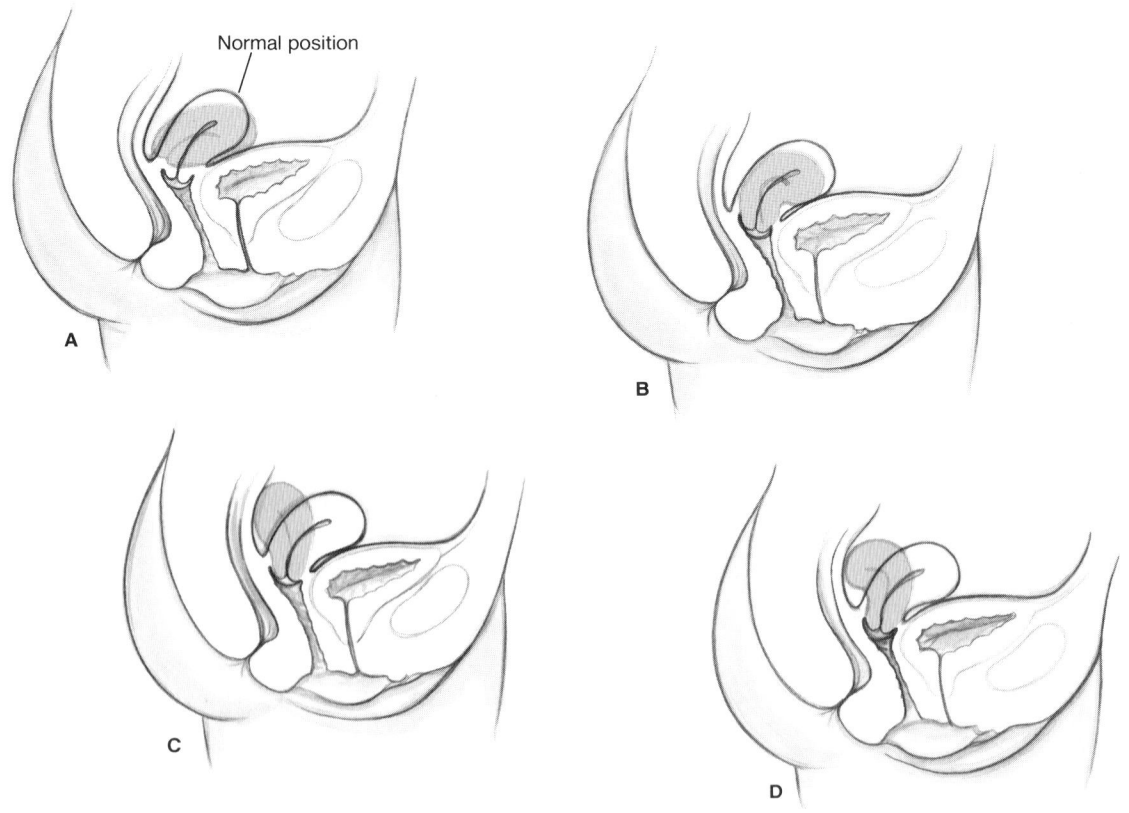

FIGURE 4-9
Uterine flexion and version. (**A**) *Anteversion.* (**B**) *Anteflexion.* (**C**) *Retroversion.* (**D**) *Retroflexion.*

number of times each day to make it more supple for birth and to help maintain tone after birth (Kegel's exercises).

The blood supply to the vagina is furnished by the vaginal artery, a branch of the internal iliac artery. Vaginal tears at childbirth tend to bleed profusely because of this rich blood supply. This rich blood supply is also, however, the reason that healing of any vaginal trauma at birth occurs rapidly.

The vagina has both sympathetic and parasympathetic nerve innervations originating at the S-1 to S-3 levels. It is not an extremely sensitive organ, however. Sexual excitement, often attributed to vaginal stimulation, is influenced mainly by clitoral stimulation.

The mucus produced by the vaginal lining has a rich glycogen content. When this glycogen is broken down by lactose-fermenting bacteria (Döderlein's bacillus) that frequent the vagina, lactic acid is formed. This makes the usual *p*H of the vagina acid, a condition detrimental to the growth of pathologic bacteria, so that even though the vagina connects directly to the external surface, infection is not usually present. Under normal circumstances, use of vaginal douches or sprays should not be a daily hygiene measure or this natural acid medium can be cleaned away, inviting vaginal infections. Following menopause, the *p*H of the vagina becomes closer to 7.5 or slightly alkaline, a reason that vulvovaginitis infections occur more frequently in women in this age group.

Breasts

The *mammary glands* or breasts arise from ectodermic tissue early *in utero*. They remain, however, in a halted stage of development until a rise in estrogen at puberty produces a marked increase in size from increased connective tissue and deposition of fat in girls and a transient increase in boys. Increase in male breast size is termed **gynecomastia**. If boys are not prepared that this is a normal change of puberty, they can be concerned that they are developing abnormally. Gynecomastia is most evident in obese boys. The glandular tissue of the breasts, necessary for successful breast-feeding, remains undeveloped until a first pregnancy begins.

Breasts are located anterior to the pectoral muscle (Figure 4-10). In many women, breast tissue extends well into the axilla, a reason that this region must always be included in self–breast examination or some breast tissue will be missed. Milk glands of breasts are divided by connective tissue partitions into approximately 20 lobes. All the glands in each lobe produce milk by acini cells and deliver it to the nipple by a *lactiferous duct*. The nipple has approximately 20 small openings through which milk is secreted. An ampulla portion of the duct just posterior to the nipple serves as a reservoir for milk before breast-feeding.

A nipple comprises smooth muscle that is capable of erection on manual or sucking stimulation. On stimulation, it transmits sensations to the posterior pituitary gland to release oxytocin. Oxytocin acts to constrict milk gland cells and push milk forward into the ducts that lead to the nipple. The nipple is surrounded by a darkly pigmented area of epithelium approximately 4 cm in diameter termed the *areola;* the areola is rough appearing on the surface owing to the many sebaceous glands called *Montgomery's tubercles.*

The blood supply to the breasts is profuse, being comprised of the thoracic branches of the axillary, internal mammary, and intercostal arteries. This effective blood supply is important in bringing nutrients to the

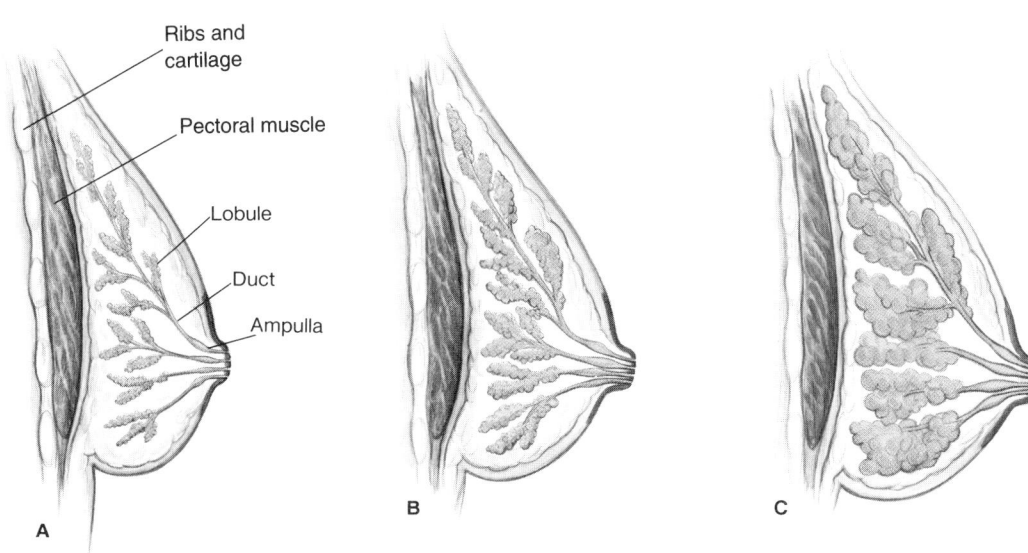

FIGURE 4-10
*Anatomy of the breast. (**A**) Nonpregnant. (**B**) Pregnant. (**C**) During lactation.*

milk glands and makes possible a plentiful supply of milk for breast-feeding. It also unfortunately aids in the metastasis of breast cancer if not discovered early by self–breast examination (Marchant, 1990).

Pelvis

For a baby to be delivered vaginally, he or she must be able to pass through the ring of pelvic bone. The pelvic opening must be sufficient, therefore, or the infant will be too large to be born except by cesarean birth. This is not a problem for the average woman; it may be a problem for the young adolescent girl who has not yet achieved full pelvic growth (girls younger than age 14 years are most prone to this difficulty) or a woman who has had a pelvic injury such as from an automobile accident.

The pelvis serves to both support and protect the reproductive and other pelvic organs. It is a bony ring formed by four united bones: the two *innominate* (flaring hip) bones that form the anterior and lateral portion of the ring, and the coccyx and sacrum, which compose the posterior aspect (Figure 4-11).

Each innominate bone is divided into three parts: (1) the ilium, (2) the ischium, and (3) the pubis. The *ilium* forms the upper and lateral portion. The flaring superior border of this bone is what forms the prominence of the hip (the crest of the ilium). The *ischium* is the inferior portion. At the lowest portion of the ischium are two projections: the *ischial tuberosities*. This is the portion of bone on which a person sits. These projections are important markers used to determine lower pelvic width. The *pubis* is the anterior portion of the in-

nominate bone. The *symphysis pubis* is the junction of the innominate bones at the front of the pelvis.

The *sacrum* forms the upper posterior portion of the pelvic ring. There is a marked anterior projection (the sacral prominence) of this bone at the point where it touches the lower lumbar vertebrae. This landmark must be identified when securing pelvic measurements.

The *coccyx,* just below the sacrum, is composed of five very small bones fused together. Although it is stiff, there is a degree of movement possible in the joint between the sacrum and the coccyx (the *sacrococcygeal* joint). This is important because this movement permits the coccyx to be pressed backward, allowing more room for the fetal head as it passes through the bony pelvic ring at birth.

For obstetric purposes, the pelvis is further divided into the false pelvis (the superior half) and the true pelvis (the inferior half; Figure 4-12). The *false pelvis* supports the uterus during the late months of pregnancy and aids in directing the fetus into the *true pelvis* for birth. The false pelvis is divided from the true pelvis only by an imaginary line: the *linea terminalis.* This imaginary line is drawn from the sacral prominence at the back to the superior aspect of the symphysis pubis at the front of the pelvis. Above the line is the false pelvis; below it, the true pelvis.

Other important terms in relation to the pelvis are the inlet, the pelvic cavity, and the outlet. The *inlet* is the entrance to the true pelvis or the upper ring of bone through which the fetus must first pass to be born vaginally. It is at the level of the linea terminalis or is marked by the sacral prominence in the back, the ilium on the sides, and the superior aspect of the symphysis pubis in

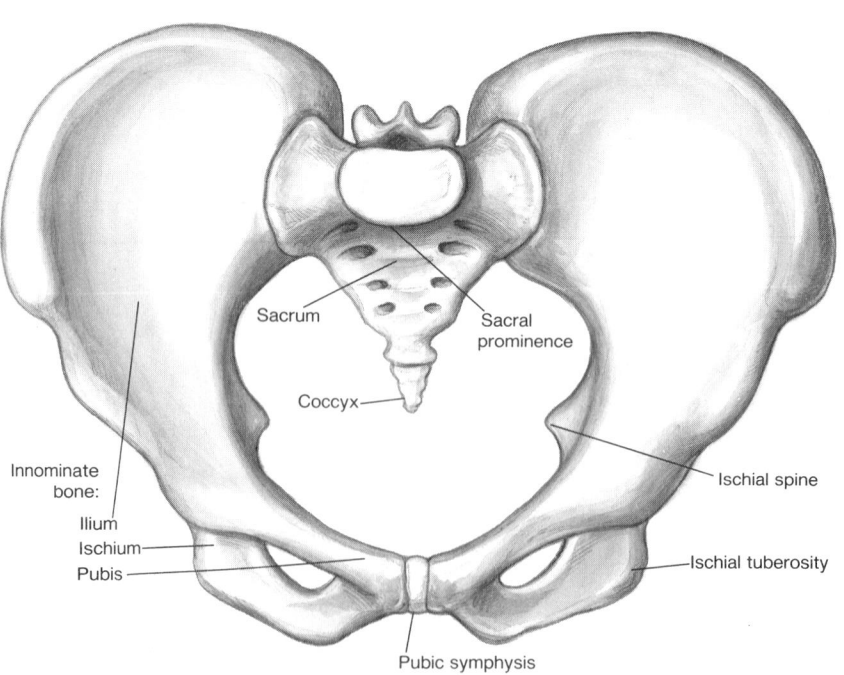

FIGURE 4-11
Structure of the pelvis.

Sacrum

Sacral prominence

Coccyx

Innominate bone:

Ilium
Ischium
Pubis

Ischial spine

Ischial tuberosity

Pubic symphysis

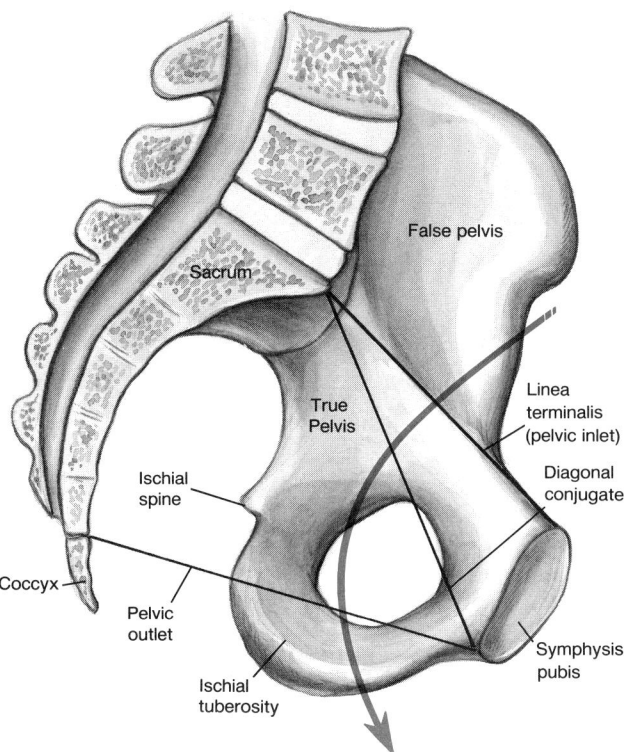

FIGURE 4-12
True and false pelvis. Portion above linea terminalis is false pelvis; portion below is true pelvis. Arrow shows "stovepipe" curve that the fetus must follow to deliver.

the front. If looking down the pelvic inlet, the passageway at this point appears heart-shaped because of the jutting sacral prominence. It is wider transversely (sideways) than in the anteroposterior dimension.

The *outlet* is the inferior portion of the pelvis, or that portion bounded in the back by the coccyx, on the sides by the ischial tuberosities, and in the front by the inferior aspect of the symphysis pubis. In contrast to the inlet of the pelvis, the greatest diameter of the outlet is its anteroposterior diameter.

The *pelvic cavity* is the space between the inlet and the outlet. This space is not a straight passage but is curved like a stovepipe from an old-fashioned wood stove. There are physiologic reasons for this design. The curve slows and controls the speed of birth and therefore reduces sudden pressure changes on the fetal head, which might rupture cerebral arteries. The snugness of the cavity compresses the chest of the fetus as he or she passes through, helping to expel lung fluid and mucus and thereby better prepare the lungs for good aeration at birth. The level of the ischial spines marks the *midplane* or midpoint of the pelvis. This marker is used to assess the level to which the fetus has descended into the birth canal during labor. Different pelvic types and an assessment of pelvic size are discussed in detail in Chapter 10.

Menstruation

A *menstrual cycle* (also termed a female reproductive cycle) can be defined as periodic uterine bleeding in response to cyclic hormonal changes. It is the process that allows for conception and implantation of a new life.

Menarche is the term applied to the first menstruation period in girls. It occurs typically at age 12 to 13 years, but it may occur as early as age 9 or as late as age 17 and still be within normal limits (Goldsmith & Weiss, 1990). Because menarche may occur as early as age 9 years, nurses should include health teaching information on menstruation to both girls and their parents as early as the fourth-grade level as part of routine care. It is a poor introduction to sexuality and womanhood for a girl to begin menstruation unwarned and unprepared for the important internal function it represents.

Menopause is the cessation of menstrual cycles. The *postmenopausal* period is the time of life following menopause. *Perimenopausal* is a term used to denote the period during which menopausal changes are occurring. The age range at which menopause occurs is wide, between 40 and 55 years. Both the age of menarche and the age of menopause tend to be familial (if menarche occurred early in a mother, it will probably occur early in her daughter; if menopause began early in a mother, it may begin early in her daughter). The earlier the age of menarche, the earlier menopause tends to occur. Women need as much health teaching to learn the normal parameters of menopause as they do of menarche to enable them to continue to monitor their own health during this time. Women often call this time of life "change of life" because it marks the end of the ability to bear children, which for some women may mark a big change in their life. An important health teaching measure is helping women to appreciate that loss of uterine function may make almost no change in their life and, for the woman with dysmenorrhea (painful menstruation) or with no desire for more children, may even be a welcome change.

The purpose of a menstrual cycle is to bring an ovum to maturity and renew a uterine tissue bed that will be responsive to its growth should it be fertilized. The length of menstrual cycles differs from woman to woman, but the accepted average length is 28 days (from the beginning of one menstrual flow to the beginning of the next). However, it is not unusual for cycles to be as short as 23 days or as long as 35 days.

The length of the average menstrual flow (termed *menses*) is 2 to 7 days, although women may have periods as short as 1 day or as long as 9 days. Because there is such variation in the times that menarche and menopause occur and such variation in length, frequency, and amount of menstrual flow, many women have questions about what is considered normal. Contact with health care personnel during a yearly health examination or prenatal visit is often the first opportunity some women have to ask questions they have had for some time. Table 4-2 summarizes the normal characteristics of menstruation for quick reference.

Physiology of Menstruation

Four body structures are involved in the physiology of the menstrual cycle: (1) the hypothalamus, (2) the pituitary gland, (3) the ovaries, and (4) the uterus. For a menstrual cycle to be complete, all four structures must contribute their part; inactivity from any part will result in an incomplete or ineffective cycle (Figure 4-13).

The Hypothalamus

The release of a hormone by the hypothalamus initiates the menstrual cycle; the presence of estrogen represses it. During childhood, the hypothalamus is apparently so sensitive to the small amount of estrogen produced by the adrenal glands that release of the hormone is suppressed. Beginning with puberty it becomes less sensitive to estrogen feedback; this causes the initiation every month in females of a luteinizing hormone-releasing hormone (LHRH, sometimes abbreviated GnRH for gonadotropin-releasing hormone). This is transmitted from the hypothalamus to the anterior pituitary gland and signals the anterior pituitary gland to begin production of gonadotropic hormones.

Diseases of the hypothalamus causing deficiency of this releasing factor result in delayed puberty. Diseases causing early activation of the releasing factor lead to abnormally early sexual development or precocious puberty (see Chapter 47). When hormones secreted by the ovary such as estrogen and progesterone rise in amount

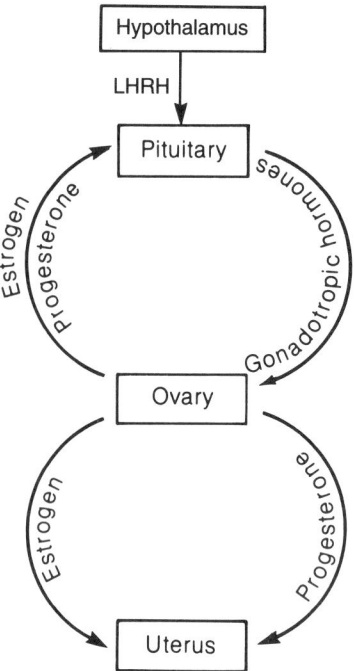

FIGURE 4-13
The interaction of pituitary-uterine-ovarian functions in a menstrual cycle.

each month, they create an inhibitory feedback mechanism, which halts production of the releasing factor for the remainder of the month. This also occurs when high levels of pituitary-based hormones such as prolactin, follicle-stimulating hormone (FSH), or luteinizing hormone (LH) are present.

Because production of LHRH is cyclical, menstrual periods also cycle.

The Pituitary Gland

Under the influence of LHRH, the anterior lobe of the pituitary gland (the adenohypophysis) produces two hormones that act on the ovaries to further influence the menstrual cycle: (1) FSH, a hormone that is active early in the cycle and is responsible for maturation of the ovum, and (2) LH, a hormone that becomes most active at the midpoint of the cycle and is responsible for ovulation or release of the mature egg cell from the ovary and growth of the uterine lining during the second half of the menstrual cycle (Figure 4-14).

The Ovary

Under the influence of FSH and LH—called gonadotropic hormones because they cause growth (trophy) in the gonads (ovaries)—one ovum matures in one or the other ovary and is discharged from it each month.

Division of Reproductive Cells (Gametes). At birth, each ovary contains approximately 2 million immature ova (oocytes), which were formed during the first

Table 4-2. Characteristics of Normal Menstrual Cycles

Term	Description
Beginning (menarche)	Average age of onset: 12 or 13 years; average range of age: 9–17 years
Interval between cycles	Average 28 days; cycles of 23 to 35 days not unusual
Duration of menstrual flow	Average flow: 2–7 days; ranges of 1–9 days not abnormal
Amount of menstrual flow	Difficult to estimate; average 30 to 80 mL per menstrual period; saturating a pad or tampon in less than an hour is heavy bleeding
Color of menstrual flow	Dark red; a combination of blood, mucus, and endometrial cells
Odor of menstrual flow	Odor of marigolds

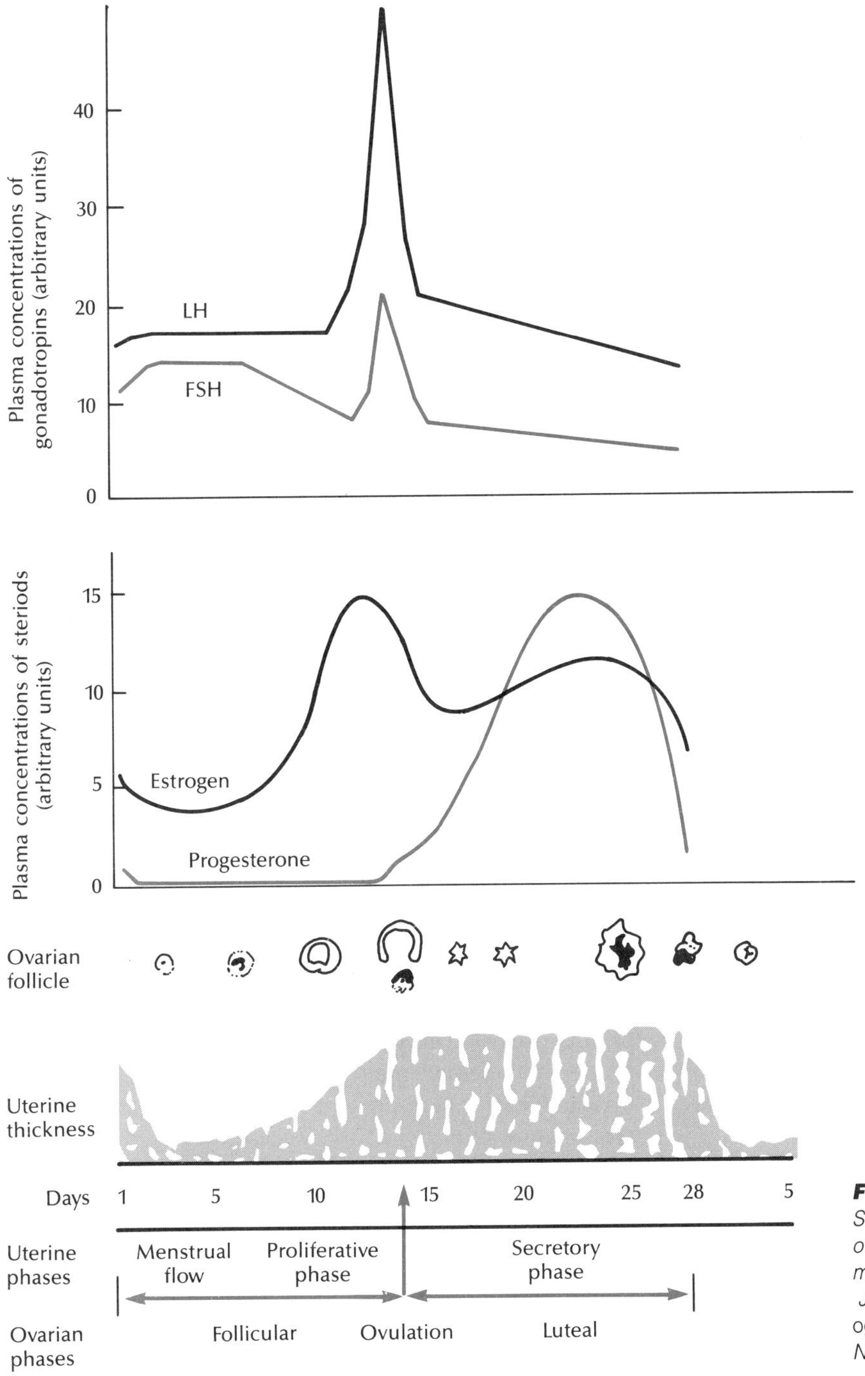

FIGURE 4-14

Summary of plasma hormone concentrations, ovarian events, and uterine changes during the menstrual cycle. (From Vander, A. J., Sherman, J. H., & Luciano, D. S. [1985]. Human physiology: The mechanisms of body function *[4th ed.]. New York: McGraw-Hill, with permission.)*

5 months of intrauterine life. Although these cells have the unique ability to produce a new individual, they basically contain usual cell components: a cell membrane, an area of clear cytoplasm, and a nucleus containing chromosomes.

The oocytes differ from all other body cells in the number of chromosomes they contain in the nucleus. The nucleus of all other human body cells contains 46 chromosomes, consisting of 22 pairs of autosomes (paired matching chromosomes) and one pair of sex chromosomes—two X sex chromosomes in the female

and an X and a Y sex chromosome in the male. Reproductive cells (ova and spermatozoa) have only half the usual number of chromosomes so that when they combine (fertilization), the new individual formed from them will have the normal number of 46 chromosomes. If both ova or spermatozoa carried the full complement of chromosomes, a new individual formed out of them would have twice the normal amount of chromosome material. There is a difference in the way reproductive cells divide that causes this change in chromosome number.

Cells in the body, such as skin cells, undergo cell division by *mitosis,* or daughter cell division. In this type of division, all the chromosomes are reduplicated in each new cell just before cell division, giving every new cell the same number of chromosomes as the original parent cell. Oocytes divide in intrauterine life by *mitotic* division. Division activity then appears to halt until at least puberty, when a second type of cell division, *meiosis* (cell reduction division), occurs. In the male, this reduction division occurs just before the spermatozoa mature. In the female, it occurs just before ovulation. Following this division, ova have 22 autosomes and an X sex chromosome; a spermatozoon has 22 autosomes and either an X or a Y sex chromosome. A new individual formed from the union of an ova and an X-carrying spermatozoa will be female (an XX chromosome pattern); an individual formed from the union of an ova and a Y-carrying spermatozoa will be male (an XY chromosome pattern).

Maturation of Oocytes. Each oocyte lies in the ovary surrounded by a protective sac, or thin layer of cells, called a *follicle.* The structure in this underdeveloped state is called a *primordial follicle.* Originally when these are first formed in utero, there are 5 to 7 million of them present. The maturation of these primitive follicles appears to stop approximately at month 5 of intrauterine life. The majority never develop beyond the primitive state and actually atrophy, so that by birth there are only 2 million present; by age 7 years, only approximately 500,000 are present in each ovary; by 22 years, there are approximately 300,000; by menopause, or the end of the fertile period in females, none are left (all have either matured or atrophied). "The point at which no functioning oocytes remain in the ovaries" is one definition of menopause.

Ovulation. During the fertile period of a woman's life (from menarche to menopause) every month, one of the primordial follicles is activated by FSH from the anterior pituitary and begins to grow and mature. Its cells produce a clear fluid (follicular fluid) containing a high content of estrogen (mainly estradiol) and some progesterone. The structure grows in size, propelling itself toward the surface of the ovary as it develops. At maturity, it is visible on the surface of the ovary as a clear water blister approximately ¼ to ½ inches across. At this stage of maturation, the small ovum (barely visible to the naked eye, approximately the size of a printed period) with its surrounding follicle membrane and fluid is termed a *graafian follicle.*

By day 14 before the end of a menstrual cycle (the midpoint of a typical 28-day cycle), the ovum has divided by mitotic division into two separate bodies: a primary oocyte, which contains the bulk of the cytoplasm, and a secondary oocyte, which contains so little cyto-

plasm it is not functional. The structure also has accomplished its meiotic division or has reduced its number of chromosomes to its *haploid* (having only one member of a pair) number of 23.

Following an upsurge of LH from the pituitary, prostaglandins are released and the graafian follicle ruptures. The ovum is set free from the surface of the ovary, a process termed *ovulation.* It is swept into the open end of a fallopian tube. It is important to teach women that ovulation occurs on the fourteenth day *before the onset of the next cycle.* Because ovulation happens at the midpoint of a 28-day cycle, many women think incorrectly that the midpoint of their cycle will be the time of ovulation. If the cycle is only 20 days long, however, their day of ovulation would be day 6, not the tenth or middle day. If a cycle is 44 days long, ovulation would occur on day 31, not day 22.

After the ovum and the follicular fluid have been discharged from the ovary, the cells of the follicle remain in the form of a hollow, empty pit. The FSH has done its work at this point and now decreases in amount. The second pituitary hormone, LH, continues to rise in amount and acts on the follicle cells of the ovary, causing them to produce instead of follicular fluid, which was high in estrogen with some progesterone, a bright yellow fluid known as *lutein,* which is high in progesterone with some estrogen. This yellow fluid fills the empty follicle, which is then termed a *corpus luteum* (yellow body).

The basal body temperature of a woman drops slightly (1°F) just before the day of ovulation, because of the extremely low level of progesterone present at that time. It rises at least 1°F the day following ovulation, because of the concentration of progesterone (which is thermogenic) that is present at that time. The woman's temperature remains at this increased level until approximately day 24 of the menstrual cycle, when progesterone level again decreases.

If conception (fertilization by a spermatozoon) occurs as the ovum proceeds down a fallopian tube, and the fertilized ovum implants on the endometrium of the uterus, the corpus luteum will remain throughout the major portion of the pregnancy (approximately 16 to 20 weeks). If conception does not occur, the unfertilized ovum atrophies after 4 or 5 days, and the corpus luteum (called a "false" corpus luteum) will then remain for only approximately 8 to 10 days. As the corpus luteum regresses, it is gradually replaced by white fibrous tissue, and the resulting structure is termed a *corpus albicans* (white body). Figure 4-14 shows the times when ovarian hormones are secreted at peak levels during a typical 28-day menstrual cycle.

The Uterus

Stimulation from the hormones produced by the ovaries causes specific monthly effects on the uterus.

First Phase of Menstrual Cycle (Proliferative). Immediately following a menstrual flow (occurring the first 4 or 5 days of a cycle), the endometrium, or lining of the uterus, is very thin, only approximately one cell layer in depth. As the ovary begins to form estrogen (in the follicular fluid, under the direction of the pituitary FSH), the endometrium begins to proliferate, or grow very rapidly, increasing in thickness approximately eightfold. This increase continues for the first half of the menstrual cycle (from approximately day 5 to day 14). This half of a menstrual cycle is termed interchangeably the proliferative, estrogenic, follicular, or postmenstrual phase.

Second Phase of Menstrual Cycle (Secretory). Following ovulation, the formation of progesterone in the corpus luteum (under the direction of LH) causes the glands of the uterine endometrium to become corkscrew or twisted in appearance and dilated with quantities of glycogen and mucin, an elementary sugar and protein. The capillaries of the endometrium increase in amount until the lining takes on the appearance of rich, spongy velvet. This second phase of the menstrual cycle is termed the progestational, luteal, premenstrual, or secretory phase.

Third Phase of Menstrual Cycle (Ischemic). What occurs next in a menstrual cycle depends on whether the released ovum meets and is fertilized by a spermatozoon. If fertilization does not occur, the corpus luteum in the ovary begins to regress after 8 to 10 days. As it regresses, the production of progesterone and estrogen decreases. With the withdrawal of progesterone stimulation, the endometrium of the uterus begins to degenerate (at approximately day 24 or day 25 of the cycle). The capillaries rupture, with minute hemorrhages, and the endometrium sloughs off.

Menses: Final Phase of a Menstrual Cycle. Blood from the ruptured capillaries, along with mucin from the glands, fragments of endometrial tissue, and the microscopic, atrophied, and unfertilized ovum, are discharged from the uterus as the menstrual flow or *menses*. This is actually the end of an arbitrarily defined menstrual cycle, but because it is the only external marker of the cycle, the first day of menstrual flow is used to mark the beginning day of a new menstrual cycle.

Contrary to common belief, a menstrual flow contains only approximately 30 to 80 ml of blood; it seems more because of the accompanying mucus and endometrial shreds. Menstrual blood dries, but it does not clot, because when the capillaries of the endometrium first ruptured, the blood clotted almost immediately and then was liquefied by fibrinolytic activity. Once blood has clotted and liquefied, it will not clot again. The iron loss in a menstrual flow is approximately 11 mg, enough loss that many women need to take a daily iron supplement to prevent iron depletion during their menstruating years.

In women who are going through menopause, menses may typically be a few days of spotting before a heavy flow or heavy flow followed by a few days of spotting, because progesterone withdrawal is more sluggish or tends to "staircase" rather than withdraw smoothly.

The Cervix

The mucus of the uterine cervix as well as the uterine body lining changes each month during the menstrual cycle. During the first half of the cycle, when hormone secretion from the ovary is low, cervical mucus is thick and scant. Sperm survival in this type of mucus is poor. At the time of ovulation when estrogen level is high, cervical mucus becomes thin and copious. Sperm penetration and survival at the time of ovulation in this thin mucus is excellent. As progesterone becomes the major influencing hormone during the second half of the cycle, cervical mucus again becomes thick. Sperm survival is again poor.

Additional changes in cervical mucus are described in Chapter 6, because changes in cervical mucus are helpful in establishing fertility. The awareness that such changes occur with ovulation allows women to plan sexual coitus so that it coincides with ovulation, ensuring that pregnancy will occur, or to avoid sexual coitus at the time of ovulation to prevent pregnancy (see Chapter 5).

Education Regarding Menstruation

Many myths about menstruation still exist (Cumming et al., 1991). Early preparation for menstruation is important preparation for future childbearing and for a girl's concept of herself as a woman, because it teaches her to trust her body or think of menstruation as a mark of pride or growing up. Education regarding menstruation is equally important for boys so they can appreciate the cyclic process that a woman's reproductive system activates and can be active participants in helping plan or prevent the conception of children.

Girls who are well prepared for menstruation and view it as a positive happening are more likely to cope with menstrual discomforts and pain more effectively, thus missing fewer school days than those who view menstruation as an ill time. Important teaching points for girls at menarche regarding menstruation are summarized in Table 4-3. Menstrual disorders including dysmenorrhea (painful menstruation) and premenstrual syndrome are discussed in Chapter 47 with other reproductive tract disorders.

Table 4-3. *Teaching about Menstrual Health*

Area of Concern	Teaching Points
Exercise	It is good to continue moderate exercise during menses because it increases abdominal tone. Excessive exercise can cause amenorrhea.
Sexual relations	Not contraindicated during menses (the male should wear a condom to prevent exposure to blood). Heightened or decreased sexual arousal may be noticed during menses. Orgasm may increase menstrual flow.
Activities of daily living	Nothing is contraindicated (many people believe incorrectly that washing hair or having a permanent is harmful).
Pain relief	Any mild analgesic is helpful. Prostaglandin inhibitors such as ibuprofen (Motrin) are specific for menstrual pain.
Rest	More rest may be helpful if dysmenorrhea interferes with sleep at night.
Nutrition	Many women need iron supplementation to replace iron lost in menses. Eating pickles or cold food does not cause dysmenorrhea.

Sexuality and Sexual Identity

Sexuality is a multidimensional phenomenon that includes feelings, attitudes, and actions. It has both biologic and cultural components. It encompasses and gives direction to a person's physical, emotional, social, and intellectual responses throughout life. Born a sexual being, a child's gender identity and gender role behavior evolve from and usually conform to the societal expectations within that child's culture (see the Focus on Cultural Awareness box). Nurses can play a major role in promoting sexual health through education and discussion (Few, 1994).

FOCUS ON CULTURAL AWARENESS

The way that people manifest maleness and femaleness can be culturally determined. A Mexican-American man, for example, may maintain an air of "machismo" or a distance while his partner is in labor rather than move closer to her and be more comforting. Being aware of cultural differences in this way helps you to view people as individuals and better understand their actions in situations.

Biologic gender is the term used to denote chromosomal sexual development: male (XY) or female (XX). *Gender* or *sexual identity* is the inner sense a person has of being male or female, which may be the same as or different from biologic gender. *Gender role* is the behavior a person conveys about being male or female, which again, may or may not be the same as biologic gender or gender identity.

Development of Gender Identity

Whether gender identity arises from primarily a biologic or psychosocial focus is currently controversial. The amount of testosterone secreted in utero (a process termed "sex typing") may affect this characteristic. How appealing parents or other adult role models portray their gender roles may influence how a child envisions himself or herself. For example, both sons and daughters often relate better to whichever parent is kinder and more caring. This may result in a son assuming characteristics often regarded as feminine or daughters developing interests typically regarded as masculine.

Gender role is also culturally influenced. In Western society, women have in the past been viewed as kind and nurturing, with sole responsibility for childrearing and homemaking. Men were viewed as being expected to provide financial support for the family. Fortunately, gender roles today are more interchangeable than they once were: women pursue all kinds of jobs and careers without loss of femininity; men participate (some as primary homemakers) with childrearing and household duties without loss of masculinity.

An individual's sense of gender identity develops throughout an entire lifespan, and the stage is set by expectations even before a child is born. Although parents usually respond to the question, "Do you want a boy or a girl?" with the answer, "It doesn't matter as long as it's healthy," many parents actually have strong preferences for a male or female child. Although some parents may be disappointed if the child is not the gender they hoped for, most adapt quite quickly and will say later that they always wanted that sex child.

Infancy

From the day of birth, female and male babies are treated differently by their parents (Calhoun & Light, 1993). People generally bring girls dainty rattles and dresses with ruffles; on the whole they are treated more gently by parents and held and rocked more than male babies. People tend to buy boys bigger rattles and sports-related jogging suits. Admonitions given babies can be different. A girl might be told, "Don't cry. You don't look pretty when you cry." A boy might be told, "You've got to learn to be tougher than that if you're ever going to make it in this world." By the end of the first year, differences in play are usually strongly evident.

Girls play for longer periods with quiet soft toys, checking back with the parent frequently; boys spend more time in gross motor activity, staying away from the parent for longer periods than girls.

The Preschool Period

Children can distinguish between men and women as early as age 2 years. By age 3 or 4 years, they know what sex they are, and they have absorbed cultural expectations of that sex role. Often, boys will play rough and tumble games with other boys, and girls will play more quietly with each other, although the two frequently mix at this age. Comments such as, "What kind of mommy are you going to be, treating a doll that way?" or "Is that the way a lady sits?" from parents and well-meaning friends help to govern their choice of actions. Common sayings such as "all boy" or "boys will be boys" are representative of the differences expected between the two sexes.

Sex role modeling also comes from watching programs on television. Based on these sources of information, preschool children's actions are strengthened and maintained as right for them or discarded in favor of actions that will bring approval (Figure 4-15). If the child lives in a home where both mother and father are kind, loving people, sex role identification progresses

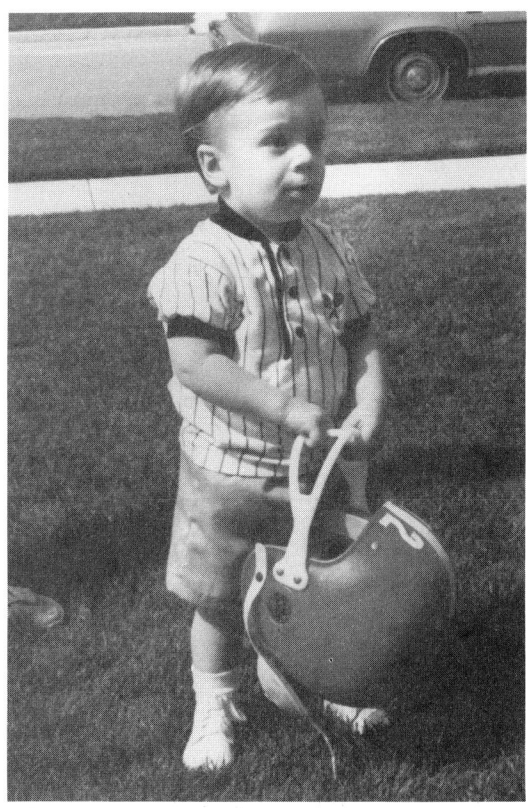

FIGURE 4-15
Children learn gender roles by imitation. Here an 18-month-old already imitates a male sports role.

FOCUS ON FAMILY TEACHING

Sexuality and reproductive function can be an area of care that families have many questions about yet are hesitant to ask. Helping parents to feel comfortable asking this type of question is a major point in health teaching. Here are two commonly asked questions:

Q. Is it all right to call body parts by nicknames such as "peter" or should we use the anatomic name?

A. Although this is strictly up to parents, using anatomic names is usually advised. This prevents children from thinking of one part of the body as so different from others (and perhaps dirty or suspect) that it can't be called by its name.

Q. Is it important to give our children unisex toys? Can't girls play with dolls and boys with trucks?

A. Developing a sense of gender is more involved than what toys children play with. If parents are concerned with instituting unisex roles in children, they need to begin by monitoring their own perspective on what they believe are female and male roles. Once they project a feeling that roles are interchangeable, no one action, but rather the general home milieu will teach this to children in their family.

---

smoothly; it is easy to want to be like someone who treats you well and with whom you feel secure (see the Focus on Family Teaching box). If one parent does not have a high nurturing capacity, however, it may be hard for the child of the same sex to identify with that person, or the identification may occur, but because the adult is not a good role model, the child perpetuates the poor role.

Although the development of an *Oedipus complex*—the strong emotional attachment of a preschool boy for his mother or a preschool girl for her father—may have been overstated by Freud as a result of sexual bias, many children manifest indications that such a phenomenon is occurring (Robinson, 1993). The preschool boy begins to show signs of competing with his father for his mother's love and attention; the preschool girl begins to compete with the mother for the father's attention and love. Parents may need reassurance that this phenomenon of competition and romance in preschoolers is normal and is one step in the development of their child's gender role identity.

The School-Age Child

Early school-age children typically spend play time imitating adult roles as a way of learning gender roles (Figure 4-16). Where once schools promoted differences in

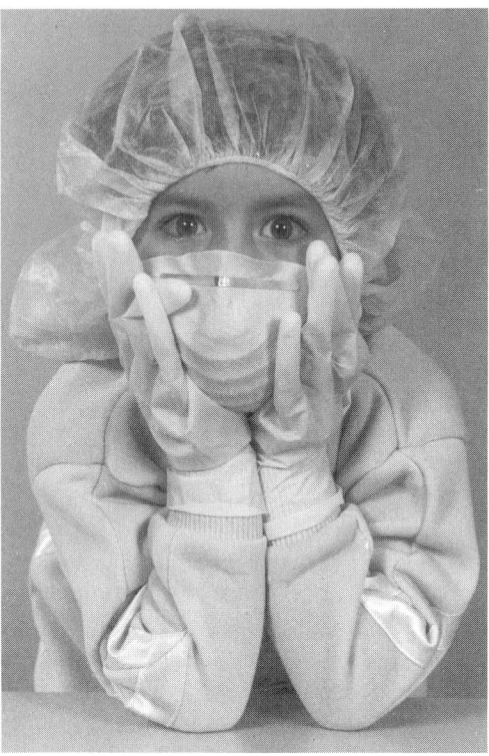

FIGURE 4-16
Early school-age children imitate adult roles to learn more about them. Here a girl "tries on" what being a doctor will feel like.

boys and girls by separating activities and through such beliefs as expecting boys to be poorer readers, to write less neatly, and to act rougher in the school hallways, grade schools have become much more attuned to unisex activities.

Girls may participate in activities that were once male-dominated such as Little League or shop and auto repair courses; boys can take cooking courses or ballet lessons, formerly the province of girls.

The Adolescent

At puberty, as the adolescent begins the process of establishing a sense of identity, the problem of final gender role identification surfaces again. Most early adolescents maintain strong ties to their gender group; boys with boys, girls with girls. The advent of menstruation may provide a common bond for girls at this stage. Some adolescents choose a child of their own gender a few years older than themselves to use as their model of gender role behavior. This is a way that adolescents can be certain that they understand and feel comfortable with their own sex before they are ready to reach out and interact with members of the opposite sex. Interviewing adolescents for a sexual history needs to be done tactfully, since this is a new and sensitive area for them.

More adolescents are sexually active than ever before. As many as 50% of ninth grade boys and 30% of ninth grade girls are already sexually active (CDC, 1992). Guidelines for safer sex are shown in Box 4-2 (see also the Focus on Nursing Research box). Including such instructions in sexual counseling should help to reduce the incidence of sexually transmitted diseases as well as empower clients with better self-care skills. One of the reasons that preventive measures for HIV have not been as successful as first predicted may be that adolescents' total lifestyle and interpretation of sexuality were not at first considered (Smith & Lathrop, 1993).

The Young Adult

When young adults move away from home to attend college or establish their own home, they choose the way they will express their sexuality along with other life patterns. Many young adults marry with a commitment to one sexual partner. Others establish relationships (cohabitation) less binding by legal definitions but perhaps equally binding in concern and support. Young adults may view cohabitation as a means of learning more about a possible marriage partner on a day-to-day basis in the hope that a future marriage will then be stronger and more lasting. Figures are imprecise, but an estimated 50% to 80% of young adults engage in sexual activities outside marriage. Homosexuality or bisexuality may be overtly expressed for the first time during this period (Zeidenstein, 1990).

Gender Identity and Parenting. Gender identity influences many aspects of life such as health perceptions (Anson, et al., 1993). It can affect parenting, since individuals tend to parent as their parents parented. Those who come from intact homes often have rather firmly fixed notions by the age of parenthood about what their gender roles will be in the care of children. They may believe, for example, that fathers should play with babies—toss them in the air, play patty-cake with them—but should not be expected to change diapers; or that fathers should be in charge of discipline; mothers in charge of nutrition, manners, and proper grammar.

Individuals raised in single-parent homes may have more difficulty with parenting than those who had constant role models or they may, because they did not have a firm example of one of the parenting roles, be more flexible and therefore more able to adapt to the expectations of their marriage partner. A son who saw his father only on weekends, making each experience with the father something special, may have trouble being enthusiastic enough every day with his own children and feel that he is failing in his role. Trying to live up to television role models for parenting (the house is always neat, the children are always well behaved, and all problems can be solved by clever one-liners) is also very difficult.

Conflicts in parenting can occur if parents-to-be do not take time to discuss some of the views they have on

---

Box 4-2
Guidelines for Safer Sex Practices

1. Be selective in choosing sexual partners. When you have sex, you are exposing yourself to the infections of everyone with whom your partner has ever had sex. The more partners you have relations with, the greater your danger of contracting a sexually transmitted disease.

2. Don't be reluctant to ask a sexual partner about his or her sexual lifestyle before engaging in sexual relations. If a partner has a history of casual contacts, bisexual or unprotected sex, there is a greater hazard of infection for you than if your partner is also choosy about partners.

3. Avoid sexual relations with IV drug users or prostitutes (male or female) or sexual partners who have had sexual relations with such people, because such people have a greater than usual chance of carrying HIV and hepatitis B infections.

4. Inspect your sexual partner for any lesions or abnormal drainage in the genital area. Do not engage in sexual relations with anyone who exhibits these signs.

5. The use of a condom is the best protection against infection. Condoms should be latex; the chance of the condom tearing is less if it is a prelubricated brand. Those coated with the spermicide nonoxynol-9 appear to be effective in destroying HIV, herpes, gonorrhea, and chlamydia. Use water-based lubricants such as KY Jelly on condoms, because oil-based lubricants can weaken the rubber. Spermicidal cream or jelly or sponges impregnated with nonoxynol-9 not only provide lubrication but also some additional protection against infectious agents.

6. Condoms should be protected from excessive heat to avoid rubber deterioration and should be inspected to be certain they are intact before use.

Do not inflate condoms before use to test for intactness because this weakens the rubber.

7. Condoms should be fitted over the erect penis with a small space left at the end to accept semen. The condom should be held against the sides of the penis while the penis is withdrawn to prevent spillage of semen.

8. Voiding immediately after sexual relations may aid in washing away contaminants on the vulva or in the urinary tract.

9. Anal intercourse carries a high risk for HIV and hepatitis B infection as well as infection from intestinal organisms. Wearing two condoms provides extra protection in case one tears. Use lubricants for anal penetration to keep bleeding and condom resistance to a minimum.

10. Do not engage in oral-penile sex unless the male wears a condom, because even preejaculatory fluid may contain viruses and bacteria. For safer oral-vaginal sex, a condom split in two or a plastic dental dam like that used for pediatric dentistry and covering the mouth should be used to protect against the exchange of body fluids.

11. Hand-to-genital contact may be hazardous if open cuts are present on hands. Use a latex glove or finger cots for protection.

12. To decrease the possibility of transferring germs, do not share sexual aids such as vibrators.

13. If you think you have contracted a sexually transmitted disease, do not engage in sexual relations until you have contacted a health care provider and are again disease free. Alert any recent sexual partners that you might have an infection so they also can receive treatment.

---

parenting and see whether they agree on male and female roles and their relationship with their children. A single parent may be concerned about how he or she can fulfill both roles. Conflicts in the role parents have chosen often come to light for the first time during pregnancy as they worry about what type of parent they are going to be or if they are adequately prepared to be a parent. Being able to talk to health care personnel about the gender role they have adopted in life can be a major step in resolving feelings of inadequacy and preparing themselves to parent. One sad finding that has emerged from studying gender role identification in relation to parenting involves child abuse: Children who are battered by their parents frequently grow up to imitate that role model and become battering parents themselves (Kempe & Helfer, 1980). They assume the role of their

parents even though they can say their parents were not good role models, that their childhood was not a happy one, and that they would have liked it otherwise.

The Middle-Aged Adult

For many women and men in midlife, sexuality has achieved a degree of stability. A sense of masculinity or femininity and comfortable patterns of behavior have been established. Adults in midlife have resolved earlier conflicts with mates and have the freedom to satisfy their sexual needs, including the freedom to remain with a partner or return to a single state.

Following menopause, reproductive functioning alters but sexual functioning does not. Although a woman's response to the physiologic and emotional components of menopause is to a degree culturally determined

**FOCUS ON
NURSING RESEARCH**

*What Type of Safer Sex Information
Is Needed by Men in the United States?*

For this study, 3000 men, ages 20 to 39 years, were asked about their sexual practices. Ninety-five percent of them responded that they had had vaginal intercourse; among these, 23% had had 20 or more vaginal sex partners in their lifetime. Twenty percent of men stated they had engaged in anal intercourse. Seventy-five percent had performed oral sex; 79% had received oral sex. Only 2% of this sample had had any same-gender sexual activity, and only 1% reported being exclusively homosexual.

A nursing implication of this study is that teaching safer sex practices must include much more than teaching the use of condoms. Men need to know protective measures for oral and anal sex as well.

From Billy, J. O., Tanfer, K., Grady, W. R., & Klepinger, D. H. (1993). The sexual behavior of men in the United States. *Family Planning Perspectives, 25,* 52.

and includes anticipation of its effects, generally, a woman engaged in a productive, satisfying lifestyle is more likely to progress through this natural biologic stage without problems.

In men, neither reproductive nor sexual functioning alters at midlife. Midlife is, however, often reported to be the most difficult period of adjustment in a man's life, bringing a need for ego enhancement and reassurance of sexual adequacy. He may find he has sexual dysfunction, such as premature ejaculation, particularly if he has extreme work or family pressure. The increased incidence of sexual encounters with younger women at this age is seen by many as the man's way of reassuring himself of his attractiveness and virility and denying the fear of aging.

Certain medications such as antihypertensives, antianxiety agents, and narcotics may diminish sexual response in both men and women. Being aware of this is important not only for clients, so they can understand that it is an expected response, but also for their partners. A woman who undergoes surgery on her reproductive organs, such as a hysterectomy (removal of the uterus), needs sensitive nurses to listen to her concerns about the meaning of the experience to her. For some women, the loss of a uterus can be synonymous with the loss of femininity. If both ovaries are also removed (oophorectomy), an immediate surgical menopause occurs. The hormonal changes occurring with the removal of both ovaries must be dealt with openly. Limited hormonal replacement is often a means of simulat-

ing the naturally decreasing hormone levels of natural menopause.

Be alert that the individual who comments about the need to maintain a reduced activity level at work or a reduced social schedule may also be seeking information and direction in other important areas of life such as sexual relations.

The Older-Aged Adult
Both male and female older adults can enjoy active sexual relationships (Booth, 1990). Some men experience less erectile firmness or ejaculatory force than when they were younger, but others discover that they are able to maintain an erection longer. Because males remain fertile throughout life they must continue to be responsible sex partners in terms of reproductive planning for life.

Older women may have less vaginal secretions because they have less estrogen after menopause. Using a lubricant before sexual intercourse may enhance their comfort and enjoyment. An estrogen supplement also often corrects this (Youngkin, 1990).

The Individual With a Physical Disability
Individuals with physical disabilities have sexual desires and needs the same as others. They may have difficulty with sexual identity or sexual enjoyment due to the effects of their condition. Males with upper spinal cord injury may have difficulty with erection and ejaculation, because these actions are governed at the spinal level. Manual stimulation of the penis or psychologic stimulation achieves erection in most men with spinal cord lesions, allowing the man a satisfying sexual relationship with his partner. Women with most spinal cord injuries are unable to experience orgasm but are able to conceive and have children.

Those who interpret a procedure such as a colostomy as disfiguring may be reluctant to participate in sexual activities, fearing that the sight of an apparatus will diminish their partner's satisfaction or enjoyment. Individuals with urinary catheters may be concerned about their ability to enjoy coitus with the catheter in place. For women, a retention catheter should not interfere with coitus. Males may be taught how to replace their own catheter so they can remove it for sexual relations. In all instances in which one sexual partner is disabled in some way, the response of a loving partner does much to enhance the body image and feelings and adequacy of a mate.

Sexuality is a facet of rehabilitation that has not always received attention. If a person could accomplish activities of daily living such as eating, elimination, and mobility, then that person was considered to be leading a normal or near-normal life. Today, establishment of a satisfying sexual relationship is considered an activity of daily living and should be included as such in assessment of clients and in rehabilitation programs (Welner, 1993).

Human Sexual Response

Sexuality has always been a part of human life, but it is only in the past few decades that it has been studied scientifically by experts in the field of sex research. One common finding of researchers has been that feelings and attitudes about sex vary widely—the sexual experience is unique to each individual, but sexual *physiology,* that is, how the body responds to sexual arousal, has common features.

Sexual Response Cycle

Two of the earliest researchers of sexual response were Masters and Johnson. In 1966, they published the results of a major study of sexual physiology based on more than 10,000 episodes of sexual activity among more than 300 men and 300 women (Masters et al., 1993). In the study, they described the human sexual response as a cycle with four discrete stages: (1) excitement, (2) plateau, (3) orgasm, and (4) resolution.

Excitement. *Excitement* occurs with physical and psychologic (i.e., sight, sound, emotion, or thought) stimulation that causes parasympathetic nerve stimulation. This leads to arterial dilation and venous constriction in the genital area; the blood supply to this area increases, with resulting vasocongestion and increasing muscular tension. In women, this vasocongestion causes the clitoris to increase in size and mucoid fluid to appear on vaginal walls as lubrication. The vagina widens in diameter and increases in length. The breast nipples become erect. In men, erection occurs; there is scrotal thickening and elevation of the testes. In both sexes, there is an increase in heart and respiratory rates and blood pressure.

Plateau. The *plateau* stage is reached just before orgasm. In the woman, the clitoris is drawn forward and retracts under the clitoral prepuce; the lower part of the vagina becomes extremely congested (formation of the orgasmic platform), and there is increased nipple engorgement.

In men, the vasocongestion leads to full distention of the penis. Heart rate increases to 100 to 175 beats per minute and respiratory rate to approximately 40 respirations per minute.

Orgasm. *Orgasm* occurs when stimulation proceeds through the plateau stage to a point at which the body suddenly discharges accumulated sexual tension (Masters et al., 1993). A vigorous contraction of muscles

in the pelvic area expels or dissipates blood and fluid from the area of congestion. The average number of contractions for the woman is from 8 to 15 contractions at intervals of one every 0.8 sec. In men, muscle contractions surrounding the seminal vessels and prostate project semen into the proximal urethra. These contractions are followed immediately by three to seven propulsive ejaculatory contractions, occurring at the same time interval as in the woman, which force semen from the penis.

As the shortest stage in the sexual response cycle, orgasm is usually experienced as intense pleasure affecting the whole body, not just the pelvic area. It is also a highly personal experience; descriptions of orgasm vary greatly from person to person.

Resolution. *Resolution* is the period during which the external and internal genital organs return to an unaroused state. For the male, a refractory period during which further orgasm is impossible occurs first. Women do not go through this refractory period, so it is possible for women who are interested and properly stimulated to have additional orgasms immediately after the first. The resolution period generally takes 30 minutes for both men and women.

Controversies About Female Orgasm

The female orgasm has been a topic of much controversy over the years, beginning with Freud who posited that there were two types of female orgasms, clitoral and vaginal. He believed that clitoral orgasms (originating from masturbation or other noncoital acts) represented sexual immaturity and that only vaginal orgasms were the authentic, mature form of sexual behavior in women. Accordingly, he considered women to be neurotic if they did not achieve orgasm through intercourse (Robinson, 1993).

Masters and colleagues (1993) showed that there is no physiologic difference between an orgasm achieved through intercourse and one achieved by stimulating the clitoris directly. Women have reported a difference in intensity and character between orgasms achieved through coitus and through other means, and some prefer one to the other, but there is no physiologic difference between them.

Another topic of debate surrounding female orgasm relates to the question of whether all women are capable of experiencing orgasm from intercourse alone. In Sherry Hite's (1977) controversial survey of female sexuality, only 30% of women reported regularly experiencing orgasm from vaginal intercourse alone. Approximately 90% of the women in the study reported being capable of achieving orgasm if manual or direct clitoral stimulation was used in conjunction with coitus. Some researchers such as Helen Kaplan believe that this inability to experience a vaginal orgasm without any other stimulation is just another variant of female sexuality; others feel that lack of coital orgasm is due to psychologic factors such as poor communication or unexpressed anger between partners, anxiety, or low self-esteem (Masters et al., 1993).

Although recent studies have demonstrated that most women are capable of achieving orgasm through vaginal stimulation alone, there appears to be little convincing evidence of the existence of yet another subject of controversy regarding female sexuality—"the G spot." First described in 1950 by the German physician Grafenberg, the G spot, presumably located on the inner portion of the vaginal wall, halfway between the pubic bone and the cervix, has been recently touted as an area of heightened erotic sensitivity. Several studies carried out in the past 10 years have not been able to verify the existence of this particular anatomic site, although some women do claim to possess such an erotic trigger (Masters et al., 1993).

Today, many sex researchers and clinicians are focusing on inhibited sexual desire and orgasm, problems that some studies have found to be common among women. Much of the research and therapy in this area seems to be directed away from a strictly physiologic analysis of sexual behavior in favor of a view of sexuality that stresses the importance of integrating both mind and body for sexual pleasure, a trend that seems both productive and healthy.

Influence of the Menstrual Cycle on Sexual Response

During the second half of the menstrual cycle—the luteal phase—there is increased fluid retention and vasocongestion in the woman's lower pelvis. Because some vasocongestion is already present at the beginning of the excitement stage of sexual response, women appear to reach the plateau stage more quickly and achieve orgasm more readily during this time. Women also seem to be more interested in initiating sexual relations at this time.

Influence of Pregnancy on Sexual Response

Pregnancy is another time in life when, because of the rapidly growing fetus in the lower pelvic area, vasocongestion of the area occurs. Some women experience their first orgasm during their first pregnancy due to this phenomenon. Following a pregnancy, many women experience increased sexual interest as the new growth of blood vessels during pregnancy lasts for some time and continues to facilitate pelvic vasocongestion. This is why discussing sexual relationships is an important part of health teaching during pregnancy. At a time when a woman may want sexual contact very much, she needs to be free of myths and misconceptions such as orgasm will cause a spontaneous abortion (see Nursing Care Plan). Although the level of oxytocin does appear to rise in women following orgasm, it is not enough to cause concern in the average woman without a poor obstetric history.

For some women, the increased breast engorgement that accompanies pregnancy may result in extreme breast sensitivity during coitus. Foreplay that includes sucking or massaging breasts is not contraindicated unless the woman has a history of premature labor.

Types of Sexual Orientation

Sexual gratification is experienced in a number of ways. One's culture determines acceptable forms of sexual expression; what is considered normal varies greatly among cultures, although general components of accepted sexual activity is that privacy, consent, and lack of force are included. Most individual value systems are closely aligned to the cultural norm.

Heterosexuality

A *heterosexual* is one who finds sexual fulfillment with a member of the opposite gender. Because sexual relationships may begin as early as the beginning of puberty (age 10 to 12 years), health care providers need to provide information on "safer sex practices" as early as this for the knowledge to be most helpful.

Homosexuality

A **homosexual** is a person who finds sexual fulfillment with a member of his or her own sex. Many homosexual men prefer to use the term "gay." **Lesbian** refers to homosexual women.

Why homosexual gender identity develops is unknown, although evidence that this is genetically determined is increasing (Pool, 1993). Even before puberty, most individuals who are homosexual report a realization that they are "different" in that they are not interested in opposite sex classmates. It is probably during adolescence in seeking a sense of identity that they realize the reason they feel "different" is because they are homosexual. This can be a frightening time because a homosexual identity is not usually easily revealed to family or friends. Some people refuse to associate with homosexuals to such an extent a fear termed "homophobia" is said to exist.

Young adulthood is the time most persons begin to assume a homosexual lifestyle. Many young adults are worried about the stigma of being labeled a homosexual and so keep their identity secret from heterosexual acquaintances (Smith & McClaugherty, 1993). Others "commit" or "come out" or are able to reveal to friends and family that they are homosexual.

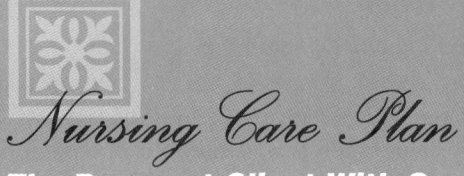

Nursing Care Plan

The Pregnant Client With Concerns Regarding Sexual Activity

Mary Fastfox is a 23-year-old woman you care for in a prenatal setting. She is 12 weeks pregnant. She had a spontaneous abortion 2 years ago followed by 1 year of apparent infertility.

Assessment: Client states that she is concerned because her husband is refusing to have sexual relations with her since she became pregnant. Before pregnancy, couple mutually enjoyed coitus about two times weekly.

Nursing Diagnosis: Altered sexuality pattern related to refusal of husband to engage in sexual relations.

Defining Characteristic: Client voices that frequency of sexual relations is no longer satisfying to her.

Goal: Client and husband will renew satisfactory sexual relationship in 1 month.

Outcome Criteria: Couple states that pattern of sexual relations is again mutually satisfying.

Nursing Orders	Rationale
1. Discuss necessity for client to ask husband for reason for his change in their sexual relation pattern.	1. Change in husband may be positive response to wanting her to complete pregnancy without spontaneous abortion this time. If this is a reaction to pregnancy it may be a positive protective action, although misinformed regarding sexual relations during pregnancy.
2. Discuss more positive means of approaching problem solving than client currently uses (withdrawing from solution) such as actively addressing issue.	2. Parenting will produce many situations when good problem-solving is needed.
3. Discuss modifications of positions for sexual intercourse to use during pregnancy to help ensure enjoyment, for example, side by side or female dominant.	3. Husband may find using alternate positions relieves concern about miscarriage.
4. Reassess at next prenatal visit to be certain that problem has been resolved.	4. Problem may not be a simple one to resolve if it is not directly related to pregnancy.

Because the period of identity confusion during adolescence can be so traumatic to a homosexual youth, it is important for health care providers to be sensitive to their needs in the area of identity formation. In a sample of gay and lesbian youths, Remafedi (1990) found that as many as 34% had attempted suicide, 48% had run away from home, 58% had abused substances, and 72% had consulted mental health professionals. Gay youths may need additional counseling to help them avoid acquiring HIV and other sexually transmitted diseases, since they are at high risk for this. Lesbians, by contrast, are at less risk because they do not have heterosexual relations (Zeidenstein, 1990). Securing a sexual history and providing information on the prevention of sexually transmitted diseases as well as providing their signs and symptoms are important responsibilities for the nurse caring for gay and lesbian, as well as heterosexual, youths. With children being raised by homosexual and lesbian couples today, an important part of health guid-ance is allowing the couples to discuss their concerns and wishes for their children (Javaid, 1993).

Bisexuality

People are *bisexual* if they achieve sexual satisfaction from both homosexual and heterosexual relationships.

Celibacy

Celibacy is abstinence from sexual activity. Celibacy is the avowed state of certain religious orders. It is also a way of life for many adults and one becoming fashionable among a growing number of young adults. The theoretic advantage of celibacy is the ability to concentrate on the means of giving and receiving love other than through sexual expression.

Transsexuality

A **transsexual** is an individual who, although of one biologic gender, feels as if he or she should be of the opposite gender. Such people may have sex change operations so they appear cosmetically as the sex they envision themselves to be. Such operations do not change the person's chromosomal structure, however, so although capable of sexual relations in this new role (a synthetic vagina or penis is created), the person is incapable of reproduction. The incidence of sex change operations has decreased in recent years because of potential disappointment following the surgery—despite a new outward appearance, the person realizes that he or she is still not totally the person he or she wished or envisioned.

Transvestism

A **transvestite** is an individual who desires to take on the role or wear the clothes of the opposite sex. Most transvestites are heterosexual and married (Bullough & Bullough, 1990). They may be under a great deal of strain to keep their lifestyle a secret from friends and neighbors.

Types of Sexual Expression

Masturbation

Masturbation is self-stimulation for erotic pleasure; it can also be a mutually enjoyable activity for sexual partners. It offers sexual release, which may be interpreted by the person as overall tension or anxiety relief. Masters and coauthors (1993) report that women may find masturbation to orgasm the most satisfying sexual expression and use it more commonly than men. Children between ages 2 and 3 years discover masturbation as an enjoyable activity as they explore their body. A child under a high level of tension may become accustomed to using masturbation as a means of falling asleep at night or at naptime. They do this without any attempt at concealment because they have not yet been affected by society's view that such activity is private.

School-age children continue to use masturbation for enjoyment or to relieve tension but limit such activity to privacy. In a hospital setting, a school-age child may assume that he or she has more privacy than actually exists, and thus may be discovered masturbating if the nurse walks unannounced into the room.

Following reproductive tract surgery or childbirth, many adult men and women are concerned with how soon they will be able to have sexual relations again without feeling pain. They may masturbate to orgasm to "test" whether everything in their body is still functional, much as the preschooler does.

Erotic Stimulation

Erotic stimulation is the use of visual materials such as magazines or photographs for sexual arousal. Although this is thought of as mostly a male phenomenon because of the number of "girlie" magazines on newsstands, there is increasing interest in centerfold photographs in magazines marketed primarily to women. Some parents of adolescents may need to be assured that an interest in this type of material is normal. Respect this type of reading material when straightening patient rooms in a health care facility.

Fetishism

Fetishism is sexual arousal by the use of certain objects or situations. Leather and rubber are materials frequently perceived to have erotic qualities. Unpacking a suitcase on hospital admission or helping pack for a return home might be times when a wardrobe of unusual articles of clothing or photographs of the fetishist's sexual arousal object are revealed.

Voyeurism

Voyeurism is sexual arousal by looking at another's body. Almost all children and adolescents pass through a stage when voyeurism is appealing; this passes with more active sexual expressions. That some voyeurism exists in almost everyone is illustrated by the large number of R-rated movies shown on television and in movie theaters and by the erotic descriptions in modern novels. Voyeurism may be practiced to the exclusion of other sexual experiences, but such an extreme probably reflects great insecurity or the inability to feel confident enough to relate to others on more personal levels.

Sadomasochism

Sadomasochism involves inflicting pain (sadism) or receiving pain (masochism) to achieve sexual satisfaction. It is a practice generally considered to be within the limits of normal sexual expression as long as the pain involved is minimal and the experience is mutually satisfying to both sexual partners.

Disorders of Sexual Functioning

Disorders involving sexual functioning can have either a psychogenic origin (produced by psychic factors rather than organic factors) or a biogenic origin (produced by biologic processes) or both. They are also categorized as primary, that is, occurring as a lifelong condition, or secondary, occurring after the person has experienced a period of normal functioning.

Primary Sexual Dysfunction

Several types of primary sexual dysfunction are described in this section. Careful assessment can help to clarify whether the cause is related to physical factors or psychologic factors or a combination of both.

***Erectile Dysfunction.* Erectile dysfunction** is the inability to produce or maintain an erection long enough for vaginal penetration or partner satisfaction. Some reasons why this occurs are physical, such as a debilitating disease or drug dependence. In many instances, the problem appears to be psychologic: related to stress, depression, and anxiety. Doubts about ability to perform or overall masculinity might be the cause. The treatment of erectile dysfunction depends on the factors involved. Surgical implants to aid erection are possible. If the cause is psychologic, sexual counseling is helpful.

***Premature Ejaculation.* Premature ejaculation** is ejaculation before penile-vaginal contact. The term is often used to mean ejaculation before the sexual partner's satisfaction as well. Premature ejaculation is actually unsatisfactory for both partners: for the woman, because she cannot achieve orgasm without the man's erection, and for the man, because he has failed to help her achieve orgasm.

The cause of premature ejaculation, like that of erectile dysfunction, appears to be most often psychologically based. Masturbating to orgasm (in which orgasm is achieved quickly owing to lack of time) may play a role. Other reasons suggested are doubt about masculinity and fear of impregnating. Sexual counseling to help the female partner put less pressure on the male (and the male on himself) to achieve may be helpful in alleviating the problem.

Failure to Achieve Orgasm. The failure of a woman to achieve orgasm can be due to poor sexual technique, concentrating too hard on achievement, or possible negative attitudes toward sexual relationships. Treatment is aimed at relieving the underlying cause. It may include instruction and counseling about sexual feelings and needs.

***Vaginismus.* Vaginismus** is involuntary contraction of the muscles at the outlet of the vagina when coitus is attempted. This muscle contraction prohibits penile penetration.

Vaginismus may occur in women who have been raped. It can also be the result of early learning patterns, in which sexual relations were viewed as bad or sinful. As with other sexual problems, sexual or psychologic counseling to reduce this response may be necessary.

***Dyspareunia.* Dyspareunia** is pain during coitus. It can be due to endometriosis, vaginal infection, or hormonal changes such as those that occur with menopause. It can be psychologic. Treatment is aimed at the underlying cause.

Inhibited Sexual Desire. Lack of a desire for sexual relations may be a concern of young or middle-aged adults. Health teaching can reassure such clients that it is normal in circumstances such as following the death of a family member, divorce, or a stressful job change. Support of a caring sexual partner or relief of the tension causing the stress allows a return of sexual interest.

Secondary Sexual Dysfunction

Chronic diseases, such as peptic ulcers or chronic pulmonary disorders that cause frequent pain or discomfort may interfere with a man or woman's overall well-being and interest in sexual activity (Katzin, 1990). Obese men and women may have difficulty achieving deep penetration because of the bulk of their abdomen. An individual with a sexually transmitted disease such as genital herpes may forgo sexual relations rather than inform a partner of the disease. Encouraging open communication between sexual partners is a nursing intervention that proves useful in all these situations.

Key Points

- The reproductive and sexual organs form early in intrauterine life; full functioning becomes possible at puberty.
- The female internal organs of reproduction include the ovaries, fallopian tubes, uterus, and vagina.
- The female external organs of reproduction include the mons veneris, labia minora and majora, vestibule, clitoris, fourchette, perineal body, hymen, Skene's and Bartholin's glands.
- The male external reproductive structures are the penis, scrotum, and testes. Internal organs are the epididymis, vas deferens, seminal vesicles, ejaculatory ducts, prostate gland, urethra, and bulbourethral glands.
- A menstrual cycle is periodic uterine bleeding in response to cyclic release of hormones. Menarche is the first menstrual period. Menstrual cycles are possible because of the interplay between the hypothalamus, pituitary, ovaries, and uterus.
- Biologic gender is determined by chromosomal content (XX or XY), which is set at conception. Gender identity is a person's concept of being male or female. This develops over a lifetime.
- Masters and Johnson have identified a sexual response cycle consisting of excitement, plateau, orgasm, and resolution stages. Disorders of sexual dysfunction include premature ejaculation, failure to achieve orgasm, vaginismus, dyspareunia, inhibited sexual desire, and erectile dysfunction.

- Educating people about reproductive function is an important primary prevention measure because it teaches them to better monitor their own health through breast and vulvar or testicular self-examination.
- Adolescents should be taught that with sexual maturity comes sexual responsibility. The best protection against either a sexually transmitted disease or an unintentional pregnancy is the practice of safer sex or abstinence.

Critical Thinking Exercises

1. Joel is a 15-year-old whom you see in your role as a school nurse. He is concerned because a number of his friends have sexually transmitted diseases. What would you advise him regarding safer sex practices?
2. Mrs. Desmond is concerned because her daughter, age 7, seems to be a "tom boy." She asks you how she can convince her daughter to be more of a "lady." What advice would you give her? Suppose her daughter was 17? Would your advice be different? Suppose Mrs. Desmond was concerned because a son was not "boy" enough? Would your answer be any different?

References

Anson, O., et al. (1993). Gender differences in health perceptions and their predictors. *Social Science Medicine, 36,* 419.

Behrman, R., et al. (1992). *Nelson's textbook of pediatrics.* Philadelphia: W. B. Saunders.

Booth, B. (1990). Does it really matter at that age? Sexuality and the older person. *Nursing Times, 86,* 50.

Bullough, B., & Bullough, V. (1990). *Nursing in the community.* St. Louis: C. V. Mosby.

Calhoun, C., & Light, D. (1993). *Sociology* (6th ed.). New York: McGraw-Hill.

Centers for Disease Control. (1992). Sexual behavior among high school students, United States, 1990. *Monthly Mortality and World Report, 40,* 1.

Coulam, C. B. (1990). Neuroendocrinology and ovarian function. In Scott, J. R. *Danforth's obstetrics and gynecology.* Philadelphia: J.B. Lippincott.

Cumming, D. C., et al. (1991). Menstrual mythology and sources of information about menstruation. *American Journal of Obstetrics and Gynecology, 164,* 472.

Department of Health and Human Services. (1991). *Healthy people 2000.* Washington, D.C.: Public Health Service.

DiSaia, P. J. (1990a). Ovarian disorders. In Scott, J. R. *Danforth's obstetrics and gynecology.* Philadelphia: J.B. Lippincott.

DiSaia, P. J. (1990b). Malignant lesions of the uterine cervix. In Scott, J. R. *Danforth's obstetrics and gynecology.* Philadelphia: J.B. Lippincott.

DiSaia, P. J., & Woodruff, J. D. (1990). Disorders of the vulva and vagina. In Scott, J. R. *Danforth's obstetrics and gynecology.* Philadelphia: J.B. Lippincott.

Few, C. (1994). Promoting sexual health. *Community Outlook, 4,* 29.

Goldsmith, L. T., & Weiss, G. (1990). Puberty, menarche and the clinical aspects of normal menstruation. In Scott, J. R. *Danforth's obstetrics and gynecology.* Philadelphia: J.B. Lippincott.

Guyton, A. C. (1991). *Textbook of medical physiology* (8th ed.). Philadelphia: W. B. Saunders.

Hite, S. (1977). *The Hite report.* New York: Dell Press.

Javaid, G. A. (1993). The children of homosexual and heterosexual single mothers. *Child Psychiatry & Human Development, 23,* 235.

Kaler, S. R. (1990). Epididymitis in the young adult male. *Nurse Practitioner, 15,* 10.

Katzin, L. (1990). Chronic illness and sexuality. *American Journal of Nursing, 90,* 54.

Kempe, C. H., & Helfer, R. E. (Eds.). (1980). *The battered child* (3rd ed.). Chicago: University of Chicago Press.

Marchant, D. J. (1990). The breast. In Scott, J. R. *Danforth's obstetrics and gynecology.* Philadelphia: J.B. Lippincott.

Masters, W. H., et al. (1993). *Biological foundations of human sexuality.* New York: Harper College.

Merrill, J. A., & Creasman, W. T. (1990). Disorders of the uterine corpus. In Scott, J. R. *Danforth's obstetrics and gynecology.* Philadelphia: J.B. Lippincott.

Mordel, N., et al. (1990). Spermatic vein ligation as treatment for male infertility. *Journal of Reproductive Medicine, 35,* 123.

Nichols, D. H. (1990). Relaxation of pelvic supports. In Scott, J. R. *Danforth's obstetrics and gynecology.* Philadelphia: J.B. Lippincott.

Pool, R. (1993). Evidence for homosexuality gene. *Science, 261,* 291.

Remafedi, G. (1990). Fundamental issues in the care of homosexual youth. *Medical Clinics of North America, 74,* 1169.

Robinson, P. (1993). *Freud and his critics.* Berkeley: University of California Press.

Scott, J. R., et al. (1990). *Danforth's obstetrics and gynecology* (6th ed.). Philadelphia: J. B. Lippincott.

Smith, L.L., & Lathrop, L. M. (1993). AIDS and human sexuality. *Canadian Journal of Public Health, 84,* 514.

Smith, S., & McClaugherty, L. O. (1993). Adolescent homosexuality: a primary care perspective. *American Family Physician, 48,* 33.

Tanner, J. M. (1990). Fetus into man. *Physical growth from conception to maturity* (2nd ed.) Cambridge, MA: Harvard University Press.

Welner, S. L. (1993). Gynecologic care of the disabled woman. *Contemporary OB/GYN, 38,* 55.

Youngkin, E. Q. (1990). Estrogen replacement therapy and the estraderm transdermal system. *Nurse Practitioner, 15,* 19.

Zeidenstein, L. (1990). Gynecological and childbearing needs of lesbians. *Journal of Nurse Midwifery, 35,* 10.

Suggested Readings

Brooks, T. R. (1994). Sexuality in the aging woman. *Female Patient, 19,* 63.

Cook, R. J. (1993). International human rights and women's reproductive health. *Studies in Family Planning, 24,* 73.

Nettina, S. L., & Kauffman, F. H. (1990). Diagnosis and management of sexually transmitted genital lesions. *Nurse Practitioner, 15,* 20.

Netting, N. S. (1992). Sexuality in youth culture: identity and change. *Adolescence, 27,* 961.

Olsen, J., et al. (1992). Student evaluation of sex education programs advocating abstinence. *Adolescence, 27,* 369.

Petrosa, R., & Jackson, R. (1991). Using the health belief model to predict safer sex intentions among adolescents. *Health Education Quarterly, 18,* 463.

Pittman, K. J., et al. (1992). Making sexuality education and prevention programs relevant for African-American youth. *Journal of School Health, 62,* 339.

Rosenfield, A. (1993). Women's reproductive health. *American Journal of Obstetrics & Gynecology, 169,* 128.

Sciarra, J. J. (1993). Reproductive health: a global perspective. *American Journal of Obstetrics & Gynecology, 168,* 1649.

Taylor, B. A., & Remafedi, G. (1993). Youth coping with sexual orientation issues. *Journal of School Nursing, 9,* 26.

Wall-Haas, C. L. (1991). Nurses' attitudes toward sexuality in adolescent patients. *Pediatric Nursing, 17,* 549.

Wolf, P. H., et al. (1991). Reduction of cardiovascular disease: related mortality among postmenopausal women who use hormones. *American Journal of Obstetrics and Gynecology, 164,* 489.

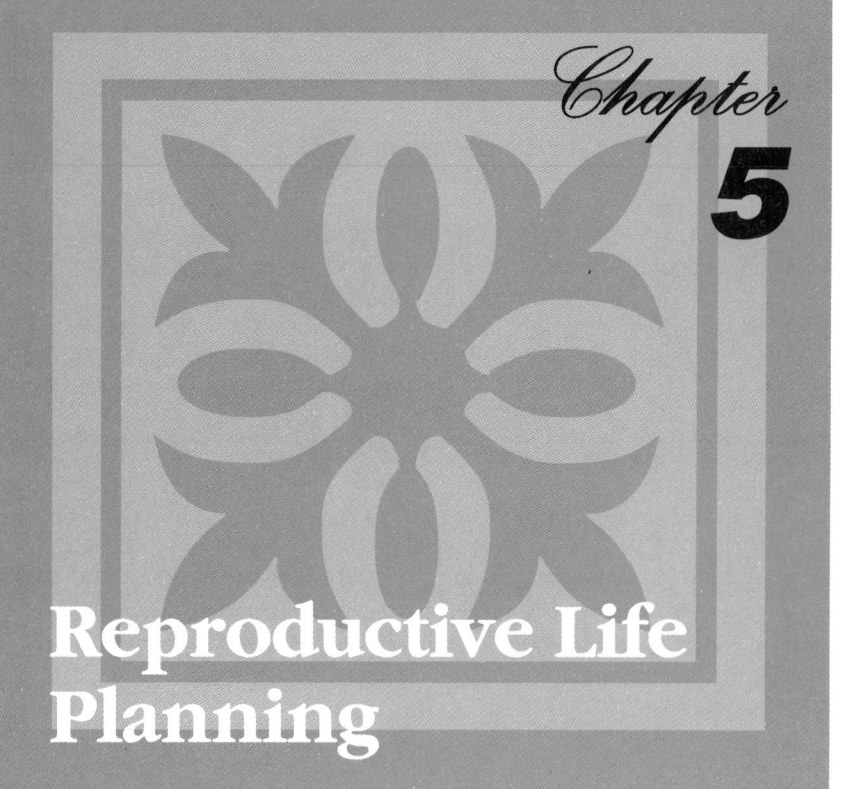

Chapter 5

Reproductive Life Planning

Adele Pillitteri: MATERNAL AND CHILD HEALTH NURSING, 2nd Edition. © 1995 Adele Pillitteri.

Key Terms

- abstinence
- barrier method
- basal body temperature method
- calendar method
- cervical cap
- coitus interruptus
- condom
- contraceptive
- diaphragm
- elective termination of pregnancy
- fertility awareness
- intrauterine device
- laparoscopy
- natural family planning
- reproductive life planning
- tubal ligation
- vasectomy

Objectives

After mastering the contents of this chapter, you should be able to:

1. Describe common methods for reproductive life planning.
2. Assess clients for reproductive life planning needs.
3. Formulate nursing diagnoses related to reproductive life planning concerns.
4. Plan nursing care related to reproductive life planning, such as helping a client select a suitable family planning measure.
5. Implement nursing care related to reproductive life planning such as educating adolescents about the use of condoms to promote safe sex practices as well as prevent unwanted pregnancy.
6. Evaluate goals and outcome criteria established for care to be certain they have been achieved.
7. Identify National Health Goals related to reproductive life planning that nurses can be instrumental in helping the nation achieve.
8. Identify areas related to reproductive life planning that could benefit from additional nursing research.
9. Use critical thinking to analyze methods that could be used to promote reproductive health.
10. Synthesize aspects of reproductive life planning with nursing process to achieve quality maternal and child health nursing care.

Reproductive life planning includes all the decisions an individual or couple make about if and when to have children, how many children are desired in a family, and how they are spaced. Not so long ago, **contraceptive** products (products to prevent pregnancy) were not all that reliable or could not be easily purchased. Today, however, technologic advances, especially development of the birth control pill and hormonal injections and implants, have created numerous contraceptive choices. Reproductive health has become so important that a number of National Health Goals speak directly to this area of care (see the Focus on National Health Goals box). Nurses can be instrumental both in informing couples about the choices available and helping them choose a method that best suits their needs to help the nation meet these goals.

A woman or a couple's choice of contraceptive method, if any, should be made carefully with complete knowledge about the advantages, disadvantages, and side-effects of the various options. It is a choice based on personal values, knowledge of the reliability of each method, and how the chosen method will affect sexual enjoyment. A couple will also weigh financial factors, the status of their relationship, prior experiences, and future plans.

Nursing responsibilities related to reproductive life planning include helping couples who are having difficulty conceiving children to explore infertility programs, helping couples who wish to space children to do so, and helping individuals and couples who do not want to have children to avoid conception. It may include counseling a couple whose contraceptive has failed and who now wish to know about abortion or adoption options.

The widespread use of contraceptives and the increased number of elective abortions in recent years point to both an increased awareness of the responsibility and the options available for controlling reproduction and family size. Understanding how various methods of contraception work and how they compare in terms of benefits and disadvantages is necessary for successful counseling. It is also important to be able to answer questions about elective termination of pregnancy with accurate, up-to-date knowledge and objectivity. With information and the ability to discuss specific concerns couples can better clarify their values so that they are better prepared to make the decisions that are right for them.

⊠ **NURSING PROCESS OVERVIEW**
for Reproductive Health

ASSESSMENT

As a result of changing social values and lifestyles, many people are able to talk more easily about reproductive life planning today than people were 20 years ago. Remember, however, that others still are uncomfortable with this topic and may not voice their interest in the subject independently. Many women in the immediate postpartal period may believe that they cannot conceive immediately (especially if they are breast-feeding). As many as two thirds of pregnancies to teenagers are unintended, as if adolescents do not believe that preg-nancy can happen to them (DHHS, 1992a). At health assessments people need to be asked if they want more information or need any help with reproductive life planning.

NURSING DIAGNOSIS

Nursing diagnoses applicable to reproductive life plan-ning include:

- Health-seeking behaviors regarding contraception options related to desire to prevent pregnancy
- Knowledge deficit related to use of diaphragm
- Decisional conflict regarding choice of birth control because of health concern
- Decisional conflict related to unwanted pregnancy
- Powerlessness related to failure of chosen repro-ductive life planning method

- Altered sexuality patterns related to fear of getting pregnant

PLANNING AND IMPLEMENTATION

When establishing goals for care in this area, be certain that they are realistic for that person. If the person has a history of poor drug compliance, for instance, it may not be realistic for her to plan to take an oral contraceptive every day. It is important, too, to be sensitive to a cou-ple's religious or cultural beliefs when suggesting possi-ble methods (see the Focus on Cultural Awareness box).

Some couples are unable to make realistic plans about reproductive life planning because they are unin-formed or misinformed about the available options. Ed-ucation is an important nursing role. An organization helpful for referral for reproductive life planning is Planned Parenthood, 810 7th Avenue, New York, NY 10019. When counseling, be certain to emphasize "safer sex" measures as well as contraceptive ones (see Guide-lines for Safer Sex Practices, Box 4-2, Chapter 4). This, for instance, means that although a woman may feel confident her oral contraceptive, barrier method, or a natural family planning method is offering her protec-tion against conception, her partner should still wear a condom to protect her against sexually transmitted dis-eases if the relationship is not a monogamous one.

EVALUATION

Evaluation is important in reproductive life planning because anything that causes a woman or couple to discontinue or misuse a particular method will leave them without the protection needed. It is important to reassess early (within 1 to 3 weeks) after a woman begins a new method of birth control in order to prevent such an occurrence. Evaluation is much broader than simply assuring that no unwanted conception occurs. The satisfaction of a woman and her sexual partner with the method chosen is also important. Examples of outcome criteria include:

- Client uses chosen method of family planning without pregnancy for next year.
- Couple state they are no longer afraid of pregnancy because of better information on birth control by next visit.
- Couple voices satisfaction with natural family planning at follow-up visit.

Abstinence

Obviously, the most effective way to protect against conception is to abstain from sexual intercourse (**abstinence**). This has a 0% failure rate. Although this seems obvious, it is not as obvious to people in everyday life situations. An adolescent, for example, may not have adequate self-confidence to be able to say no. In a moment of irresponsibility or passion, many otherwise responsible people may fail to consider this as an option. Abstinence is also the most effective way to prevent sexually transmitted diseases. Unless it is mentioned for adolescents among contraceptive options, they may overlook the importance of considering this option (see the Nursing Care Plan: The Adolescent Seeking Contraceptive Information).

Contraceptives

As many as 38 million women in the United States use some form of reproductive life planning measure, a figure that represents three fourths of women of childbearing age (Hatcher et al., 1993). To be ideal as a method of reproductive life planning, a contraceptive should be completely safe, 100% effective, totally free of side-effects, easily obtainable, easily affordable, acceptable to the user and sexual partner, and have no effect on future pregnancies. The effectiveness of various contraceptive measures is contrasted in Table 5-1. This table gives failure rates for each method in the first year of use. The failure rate represents the number of pregnancies that occur among couples who use the method consistently and correctly.

Oral Contraception

Oral contraceptives, commonly known as *the pill* or OCs, are composed of synthetic estrogen combined with a small amount of synthetic progesterone. The estrogen content acts to suppress follicle-stimulating hormone and luteinizing hormone, the gonadotropic hormones of the pituitary, thereby halting ovulation. The progesterone action complements that of estrogen by causing a decrease in the permeability of cervical mucus, thereby limiting sperm motility and access to ova. Progesterone also interferes with endometrial proliferation to such a degree that implantation becomes unlikely.

Oral contraceptives must be prescribed by a physician, nurse practitioner, or nurse-midwife following a pelvic examination and a Papanicolaou (Pap) smear. When used correctly, they are nearly 100% effective in preventing conception. Because women occasionally forget to take them and there are individual differences in women's physiology, the typical failure rate is around 3%.

In addition to the high rate of effectiveness, the pill has some other positive benefits. For example, women who use ovulation suppressants rarely experience dysmenorrhea because ovulation does not occur; premenstrual syndrome is also lessened because of the increased progesterone levels. The use of oral contraceptives reduces the amount of menstrual flow, making iron deficiency anemia not as great a problem as in nonpill users. The incidence of acute pelvic inflammatory disease (PID) with tubal scarring is also reduced in women who use the pill.

In addition, there are some positive long-term effects. The rates of endometrial cancer and ovarian cancer appear to be reduced by as much as 50% in pill users; the risk of developing osteoporosis may also be reduced (Mastroianni & Robinson, 1994). Although there has been a fair amount of publicity about the increased risk of breast cancer in pill users, only one of a number of studies conducted has shown any link between OC use and breast cancer.

The instructions for taking oral contraceptives are roughly similar for all brands. They are packaged 21 pills to a container. It is generally recommended that the first pill be taken on a Sunday (the first Sunday following the beginning of a menstrual flow). If following childbirth, a woman should start the contraceptive on the Sunday closest to 2 weeks postdelivery; if postabortion, then on the first Sunday following the procedure. As pills are not effective for the first 7 days, she is advised to use a second form of contraception during the initial 7 days she takes pills. The woman takes a pill at the same time every day for 21 days. Pill taking by this regimen will end on a Saturday. The woman would then not take any pills for 1 week. She would restart a new month's supply of pills on the Sunday 1 week after she stopped. A men-

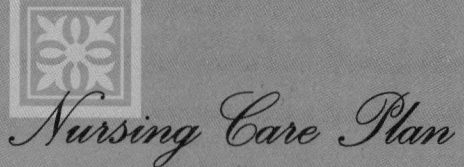

Nursing Care Plan

The Adolescent Seeking Contraceptive Information

> Christine McFadden is a 15-year-old girl whom you see in a reproductive life planning clinic. The following is a nursing care plan devised for her related to this area of care.

Assessment: 15-year-old female seen for advice on contraception. Has been sexually active for 3 months; has not been using any form of contraception. Menarche at 12 years, usual menstrual cycle is 28 to 35 days duration, flow is moderately heavy, cramping is enough to keep her home from school 1 day/month. Last menstrual flow 1 week ago. No history of STD, vaginal infections, pelvic inflammatory disease, or uterine malformation. Height: 5′2″; development: mature (Tanner 4). States she "has to do something about birth control" but doesn't know what.

Nursing Diagnosis: Health-seeking behaviors related to preventing pregnancy

Defining Characteristic: Client states she is concerned about becoming pregnant.

Goal: Client will choose and be using a method of reproductive life planning by one month's time; will not engage in sex before a choice is made and implemented.

Outcome Criteria: Client voices contraceptive options available and her preference; client explains how to correctly use the method of her choice; client explains any following care necessary for method chosen.

Nursing Orders	***Rationale***
1. Review options for birth control with client.	1. Poor compliance by adolescents leaves some methods in doubt.
2. Provide routine VDRL test, gonorrhea plate, chlamydia culture, and Pap test with pelvic examination.	2. It is important to use this opportunity to carry out assessment and related interventions.
3. Discuss ability to say "no" to sexual relations she does not want and to insist partner use a condom.	3. The adolescent may need some support in learning how to practice safer sex.
4. Discuss necessity for pelvic examinations every year.	4. Yearly pelvic examinations are recommended for sexually active women.

Nursing Diagnosis: Knowledge deficit related to potential for contracting STDs through unprotected sexual activity

Defining Characteristic: Client reveals no concern about the possibility of acquiring an STD through sexual activity.

Goal: Client will describe process of transmission of common STDs and ways to prevent contracting such diseases.

Outcome Criteria: Client states realistic possibility of contracting an STD during sexual activity; client correctly explains how she can effectively prevent contracting disease; client correctly describes symptoms of commonly occurring STDs and states intention to return to health care provider if any of these occur.

Nursing Orders	***Rationale***
1. Discuss importance of instituting measures for safe sex as accompaniment to all sexual activity.	1. A knowledge base of safer sex practices will empower the client to protect herself from STDs.
2. Discuss symptoms of commonly occurring STDs and importance of notifying health care provider if any of these occur.	2. A knowledge base of STDs will empower the client to monitor her own health.

Table 5-1. Contraceptive Failure Rates

Contraceptive	Failure Rate (%)*	Advantages	Disadvantages
Chance	85	No motivation necessary	Highly unreliable
Spermicides	21	No major health risks; no prescription necessary	Unaesthetic to some; must be properly inserted
Periodic abstinence	20	No cost; acceptable to Roman Catholic Church	Requires high motivation and periods of abstinence
Withdrawal	18	No cost	Requires motivation
Cervical cap	18	Can wear for several days if desired	May be difficult to insert; may irritate cervix
Sponge	23	Simple to use; effective with several acts of intercourse	Aesthetic objections; needs water to activate
Diaphragm	18	No major health risks; easy to use	Aesthetic objections
Male condom	12	Protects against STDs; male responsibility; no prescription necessary	Unaesthetic to some; requires interruption of sexual activity
Female condom	15	Protection against STDs	Insertion may be difficult
IUD	3	No memory or motivation needed	Cramping, bleeding, expulsion may occur. Possible risk of PID
Pill	3	Coitus independent	Possible side-effects; daily use; continual cost
Injectable progestogen	0.3	Coitus independent	Continual cost; continued injections
Implanted progestogen	.04	Very dependable	Initial cost; appearance on arm
Female sterilization	0.4	Permanent and highly reliable	Initial cost; irreversible
Male sterilization	0.1	Permanent and highly reliable	Initial cost; irreversible

*Number of pregnancies that occur among couples who use the method consistently and correctly during a year's time.
Modified from Trussell, L., Hatcher, R., Cates, W., et al. (1990). Contraceptive failure in the United States: An update. *Studies in Family Planning, 1,* 52; and Hatcher, R.A., et al. (1990). *Contraceptive technology* (15th ed.). New York: Irvington.

strual flow begins about 4 days after the woman finishes a cycle.

A pattern of this kind (always starting on a Sunday) helps in remembering when it is time to start a new dispenser. Sunday, however, may not be a good day for some women to begin new cycles because it is such an atypical day. They may choose to start on another day, because then they can schedule the time of a menstrual period to some extent by the day a new cycle is started (if she starts taking pills on a Sunday, she will begin her period 4 days after she ends a 3-week cycle, or on a Tuesday or Wednesday; if she starts her 3-week cycle on a Friday, she will begin her menstrual flow on a Monday (thus avoiding having menstrual flows on weekends if that is important to her).

Oral contraceptives are packaged in convenient dispensers (Figure 5-1). To help women remember the pattern of pill taking (and to eliminate having to count days between pill cycles) certain brands of oral contraceptives are packaged with 28 pills in the circular dial dispenser. With this type, the woman begins to take pills on the first day of her menstrual period. The first 7 pills are placebos; the next 21 are the real pills. She starts a second dispenser of pills the day after finishing the first

dispenser. There is no need to skip days because, again, the first 7 pills of the new dispenser are placebo tablets.

For ovulation suppressants to be effective, they must be taken consistently and conscientiously. Some women leave them in plain sight on the bathroom

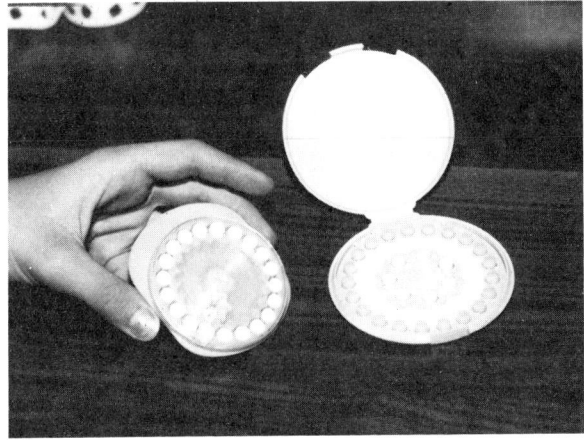

FIGURE 5-1
Oral contraceptives are supplied in a circular monthly dispenser of 21 or 28 pills.

counter or kitchen counter so they are easily reminded to take them. Women with young children in the house need to be cautioned that this is a dangerous practice. Poisoning (increased blood clotting from the high estrogen content) could result if a small child ingested them accidentally. Women who have difficulty remembering to take a contraceptive in the morning may find it easier to remember to take a pill a day if they do it at bedtime. It makes no difference what time of day the pill is taken; the key word is the same time *daily.*

If the woman forgets to take one pill, she should take it as soon as she remembers and then continue the following day with her usual schedule. This might mean she is taking two pills on one day if she doesn't remember until the second day. Missing one pill this way should not initiate ovulation.

If the woman misses two consecutive pills, she should take two pills on the day she remembers and two pills the following day and then continue the following day with the usual schedule. However, missing two pills may be enough to allow ovulation to occur, so an added protection, such as a spermicidal cream, should be used for the next 7 days. She may experience some breakthrough bleeding (vaginal spotting) with two forgotten pills. She needs to be cautioned not to mistake this bleeding for her menstrual flow. If three or more pills are missed in a row, the woman should throw out the rest of the pack and start a new pack of pills the following Sunday. She might not have a period because of this routine and should use extra protection for the first 7 days starting a new pack of pills (Williams-Dean & Potter, 1993).

Side-Effects and Contraindications

Modern oral contraceptives contain only one fifth the amount of estrogen and only one eighth the amount of progesterone that was used in the earliest OC compounds. This means they produce fewer side-effects and are safer than the earlier pills. The main side-effects of oral contraceptives are nausea, weight gain, headache, breast tenderness, breakthrough bleeding (spotting outside the menstrual period), monilial vaginal infections, mild hypertension, and perhaps depression.

Early studies found that breast-fed infants had lower weight gains when the mother was on an oral contraceptive containing a high level of estrogen during lactation, because the estrogen content decreased the woman's milk supply. Although there is less estrogen in today's preparations, it is rarely recommended that women who are breast-feeding take estrogen-based oral contraceptives until their milk supply is well established (Saarikoski, 1993). Women may take progesterone-only (mini-pills) during breast-feeding (see below) (Brenner & Mishell, 1990).

Although it is no longer believed that the use of oral contraceptives leads to an increased risk of myocardial infarction, women with a history of thromboembolic disease or a family history of cerebral or cardiovascular accident are not routinely placed on the pill because of the increased tendency toward clotting in the presence of estrogen. Women who smoke; are older than age 40 years; are obese; have high blood pressure, high serum cholesterol levels, or pulmonary disease may also be poor candidates for pill use (Hatcher et al., 1993).

Oral contraceptives cause some interference with glucose metabolism. Women with diabetes mellitus or a history of liver disease, therefore, including hepatitis, should also be considered individually before being placed on birth control pills. Other instances in which oral contraceptives may be contraindicated are breast or reproductive tract malignancy, undiagnosed vaginal bleeding, migraine headache, epilepsy, or sickle cell disease (Yuzpe, 1991).

The cost of oral contraceptives and the woman's ability to follow instructions faithfully must both be considered before oral contraceptives are prescribed. The woman on oral contraceptives should return for a follow up visit in 3 months, 6 months, and 1 year, then yearly for a pelvic examination and breast examination as long as she remains on this form of reproductive life planning.

Effect on Sexual Enjoyment

For the most part, not having to worry about pregnancy because the contraceptive being used is reliable makes sexual relations more enjoyable for couples.

Some women appear to lose interest in coitus after taking the pill for about 18 months, possibly because of the long-term effect of altered hormones in their body. Sexual interest increases again after they change to another form of contraception. Some women find the nausea they experience with the pill interferes with sexual enjoyment as well as with other activities. If they are having side effects with one brand they might be able to take another brand involving a different strength of estrogen without problems. Taking pills at bedtime rather than in the morning may eliminate nausea.

Discontinuing Use

After a woman discontinues an oral contraceptive, she should expect that she may not become pregnant for 1 or 2 months, and probably 6 to 8 months because the pituitary gland requires a recovery period to begin cyclic gonadotropin stimulation again. If ovulation does not return spontaneously following discontinuation of the pill, it can be stimulated by clomiphene citrate (Clomid) therapy.

If the woman taking an oral contraceptive suspects that she has become pregnant, she should discontinue taking the pill if she intends to continue the pregnancy.

High levels of estrogen or progesterone might be teratogenic to a growing fetus (although this is not as great a concern now that birth control pills contain low doses of hormones in contrast to the high doses of estrogen they once contained) (Hatcher et al., 1993).

Use by the Adolescent

It is usually recommended that adolescent girls have well-established menstrual cycles of at least 2 years' duration before beginning oral contraceptives. This reduces the chance that the oral contraceptive will cause permanent suppression of pituitary-regulating activity. Estrogen has the side-effect of causing epiphyseal lines of long bones to close and growth to halt; therefore, waiting at least 2 years will also ensure that the preadolescent growth spurt will not be halted. Because adolescent compliance to any form of medicine taking is low, adolescent girls may not take pills reliably enough to make them effective (Wilson, 1994). In addition, the cost of a continuing supply of pills may make this a prohibitive method of birth control for the girl who has a limited money supply. Oral contraceptives have a side-benefit of improving facial acne in some girls, because of the increased estrogen-androgen ratio created, and of decreasing dysmenorrhea, a problem of many adolescents. In some girls, the pill may be prescribed for dysmenorrhea especially if endometriosis is present (see Chapter 47).

Mini-pills

Oral contraceptives containing only progesterone are popularly called *mini-pills.* Without the estrogen, ovulation occurs, but because the uterine lining has not developed fully, implantation will not take place. Such a pill has advantages for the woman who cannot take an estrogen-based pill and wants high-level contraception assurance. This type of pill is taken every day even through the menstrual flow, which minimizes the planning involved in taking the pills.

Postcoital Contraception

Oral contraceptives may also be used to prevent pregnancy after unprotected sexual intercourse, particularly after a sexual assault has occurred. This one-time contraception consisting of high doses of estrogen and progesterone must be started no later than 24 hours after the unprotected coitus. The high level of estrogen interferes with the production of progesterone and therefore prohibits good implantation. It is a helpful method of preventing pregnancy for victims of rape. The method should always be used cautiously, because high levels of estrogen are associated with congenital anomalies if the pregnancy is not prevented. RU486 (mifepristone) (discussed below) may be prescribed in the future for emergency postcoital contraception (Glasier, et al, 1992).

Subcutaneous Implants

Norplant, a subdermal hormonal implant, is a form of contraception which received FDA approval in 1991. Six Silastic implants about the width of a pencil lead and filled with levonorgestrel (a synthetic progesterone) are embedded just under the skin on the inside of the upper arm (Figure 5-2). Once embedded, the implants appear only as irregular lines on the skin, simulating small veins. The implants slowly release the hormone, suppressing ovulation and stimulating thick cervical mucus for a 5-year period.

The implants are inserted using a local anesthetic during the menses or no later than the seventh day of the menstrual cycle to be certain that the woman is not pregnant at the time of insertion. They can be inserted immediately following an abortion or 6 weeks after delivery of a baby. They can be used during breast-feeding with no effect on milk production. In 20 years of experimental use, the failure rate increased to 4% by the fifth year of use, which is close to the failure rate of OCs (Sharts-Engel, 1991).

A disadvantage of the implants is the cost (about $150) and side-effects such as weight gain, headaches, irregular periods, and an increased incidence of ovarian cysts and possibly depression (Kaunitz, 1990). The major advantage is that they eliminate the responsibility for taking an oral contraceptive daily. They can be used safely with adolescents (Berenson & Wiemann, 1993). When a woman wishes to have a child, the implants can be removed under local anesthesia. Fertility returns in about 3 months (Flattum-Reimers, 1991).

Subcutaneous Injections

Injection of medroxyprogesterone acetate (DMPA or Depo-Provera) has recently been approved for contraceptive use in the United States (Kaunitz, 1993). A single injection is given every 3 months. Side-effects are similar to those of subcutaneous implants: menstrual spotting, headache, and weight gain. Depo-Provera may impair glucose tolerance in women at risk for diabetes. There also may be a slight increase in the development of breast cancer and osteoporosis. Women should be advised to ingest a high amount of calcium and exercise

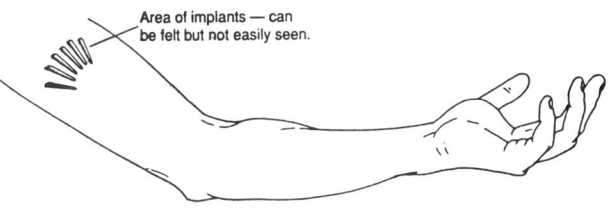

Area of implants — can be felt but not easily seen.

FIGURE 5-2
Norplant implants are placed under the skin.

daily to minimize the osteoporosis risk (Sharts-Hopko, 1993). An advantage of subcutaneous injections over implants is that there is no visible sign that a birth control measure is being used. A disadvantage is that the woman must return to a health care provider for a new injection every 3 months for the method to remain reliable.

Intrauterine Devices

The **intrauterine device** (IUD) is a small, plastic object inserted into the uterus through the vagina where it remains in place. IUDs became popular as a method of birth control 20 years ago, but few women use them now because few manufacturers continue to provide them for the U.S. market. For many the legal liability became too great, in association with the increased incidence of pelvic inflammatory disease (PID, infection of the pelvic organs) in women using one particular brand.

Although this method of contraception was used in camels during the time of Christ (a stone was inserted into the camel's uterus), the mechanism of action is still not fully understood. The presence of a foreign substance in the uterus apparently interferes with the ability of an ovum to develop as it traverses the fallopian tube. Another possibility is that the endometrium of the uterus forms cytotoxins that attack and destroy a growing ovum. A local sterile inflammatory action may result that prevents implantation. Copper added to the device appears to affect sperm mobility, decreasing the possibility of sperm being able to traverse the uterine space.

An intrauterine device must be fitted by a physician, nurse practitioner, or nurse-midwife who first performs a pelvic examination and takes a smear for a Pap test. The device is inserted either during the menstrual flow or before the client has had coitus following the menstrual flow. The health care provider is thus assured that the woman is not pregnant at the time of insertion, and insertion is easiest because the cervical canal os is slightly dilated during menses. Insertion may be made immediately following childbirth or before the cervical os closes again. An IUD inserted this closely after childbirth does not affect uterine involution or return to a pre-pregnant uterine size (Chi, 1993).

The insertion procedure may be performed in an ambulatory setting such as a physician's office or a reproductive planning clinic. The woman may feel a sharp cramp as the device is passed through the internal cervical os but will not feel it after it is in place. It is inserted in a collapsed position, then enlarged to its final shape in the uterus when the inserter is withdrawn. Properly fitted, such devices are contained wholly within the uterus, although the string attached protrudes through the cervix into the vagina.

The two types of IUDs currently approved for use in the United States are the *Progestasert*, a T-shape of permeable plastic with a drug reservoir of progesterone in

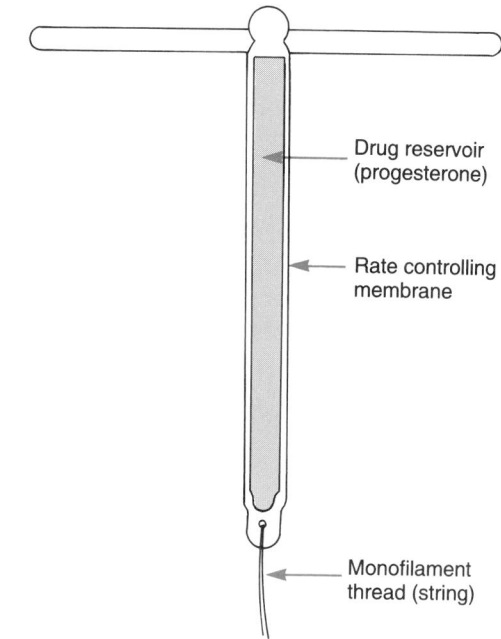

FIGURE 5-3
Intrauterine device (Progestasert IUD, ALZA Corporation, Palo Alto, CA).

the stem (Figure 5-3). and the *Copper T380*, a T-shaped plastic device wound with copper. The progesterone in the drug reservoir of *Progestasert* gradually diffuses into the uterus through the plastic and prevents endometrium proliferation. This type of IUD must be changed yearly or the progesterone supply will become depleted. It has a 2% failure rate. The *Copper T380* or *ParaGard* has a failure rate less than 1 per 100. In the United States, it is approved for only 4 years of use, after which time it should be removed and replaced with a new IUD (Hatcher, et al., 1993).

IUDs have several advantages over other contraceptives. Only one insertion is necessary and no further attention is needed except for yearly pelvic examinations. Thus, although the initial insertion involves the cost of a health care agency visit, there is only one yearly cost, not a continual expense.

Side-Effects and Contraindications

A woman with an IUD in place has a higher than usual risk for pelvic inflammatory disease, although the new copper devices may actually have a lower risk. There is also a higher risk of ectopic (tubal) pregnancy. She may notice some spotting or uterine cramping the first 2 or 3 weeks after insertion; as long as this is present, she should use an additional form of contraception such as vaginal foam. Some women have a heavier than usual menstrual flow for 2 or 3 months accompanied by dysmenorrhea. Ibuprofen, a prostaglandin inhibitor, is helpful in relieving this problem. Occasionally, a woman continues to have cramping and spotting and is likely, in these instances, to expel the device spontaneously. After each menstrual flow, the woman should examine with a finger the string attached to the IUD to make certain that the device is still in place. Women with IUDs in place should take active steps to avoid toxic shock syndrome (*Staphylococcus* infection from the vaginal insertion of tampons), because infection might travel by the IUD string into the uterus to cause uterine infection. They also need to know the most common symptoms of pelvic inflammatory disease (fever, lower abdominal tenderness, and dyspareunia; see Chapter 47).

An IUD is not recommended for women who have not been pregnant (their small uterus could be punctured with insertion), who have multiple sexual partners, or who have a past history of having had PID (Toivonen, 1993). If PID is suspected, the device should be removed and the woman should receive antibiotic therapy.

IUDs are also contraindicated in women whose uterus is known to be distorted in shape (the device might perforate an abnormally shaped uterus). They are not advised for women with dysmenorrhea, menorrhagia, or a history of ectopic (tubal) pregnancy, because their use may increase the symptoms or incidence. Women with valvular heart disease may be advised against the use of an IUD because the increased risk of PID may lead to accompanying valvular involvement (bacterial endocarditis). Because IUDs cause a heavier than usual menstrual flow, a woman with anemia is generally not considered to be a good candidate for IUD use.

Effect on Sexual Enjoyment

A woman should not feel an IUD once it is in place, thus it should not interfere with sexual enjoyment. If a woman with an IUD in place suspects she is pregnant, she should call her health care provider. Although the IUD may be left in place during the pregnancy, it is usually removed vaginally to prevent the introduction of infection during the pregnancy. The woman should receive an early sonogram to rule out ectopic pregnancy.

Use by the Adolescent

IUDs are rarely prescribed for adolescents because at that age they tend to have variable sexual partners and no prior child, which are criteria contradictory to IUD insertion.

Barrier Methods

Barrier methods of birth control work by the physical placement of a barrier between the cervix and sperm so that sperm cannot enter the uterus and fallopian tubes.

Vaginally Inserted Spermicidal Products

Spermicidal jellies or creams, when inserted into the vagina, cause the death of spermatozoa before they can enter the cervix. These jellies are not only actively spermicidal but change the vaginal *p*H to a strong acid level, a condition not conducive to sperm survival. Nonoxynol 9, the preferred ingredient, apparently also helps prevent sexually transmitted disease. Because no prescription is necessary for the purchase of spermicidal creams or jellies, these products offer an independent method of birth control.

With an applicator supplied with each product, the woman inserts the jelly or cream into the vagina before coitus (Figure 5-4). She should do this no more than 1 hour before coitus for the most effective results. She should not douche for 6 hours following coitus to ensure that the cream or jelly has completed its spermicidal action.

Another form of spermicidal protection is a film of glycerin impregnated with nonoxynol 9 that is folded and inserted vaginally. On contact with vaginal secretions or precoital penile emissions, the film dissolves and a carbon dioxide foam that protects the cervix against invading spermatozoa forms. Also available is a foam-impregnated sponge that is moistened with water and then inserted vaginally. Moisture, again, creates an internal foaming action and contraception protection. An advantage of the sponge is that it can be left in the vagina for 24 hours and will continue to be effective during this time. A disadvantage is that water is necessary to activate it. Still other vaginal products are cocoabutter and glycerin-based vaginal suppositories filled with nonoxynol 9. Inserted vaginally, these dissolve and free the spermicidal ingredients. Because it may take about 15 minutes for a suppository to dissolve, it must be inserted 15 minutes before coitus.

Side-Effects and Contraindications. Vaginally inserted spermicidal products are contraindicated in

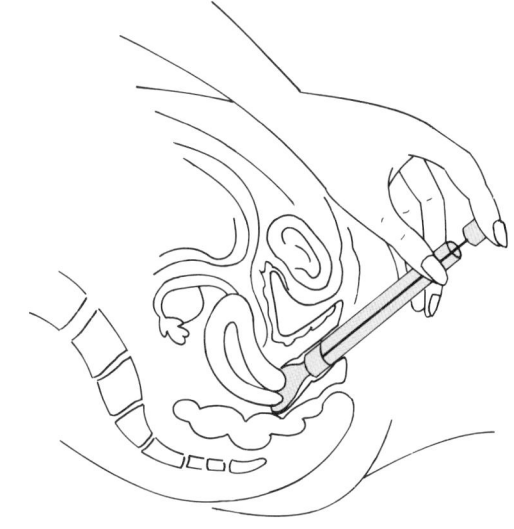

FIGURE 5-4
Vaginal insertion of a spermicidal agent.

women with acute cervicitis because they might further irritate the cervix. They are generally inappropriate for couples who *must* prevent conception (perhaps the woman is taking a drug that is teratogenic or the couple absolutely does not want the responsibility of children), because the overall failure rate of all forms of these products is about 20%, compared with the much lower failure rate of diaphragms, IUDs, and oral contraceptives. Women nearing menopause should be advised not to use a type of contraceptive that depends on vaginal moisture to be activated because they tend to have less vaginal moisture at this time of life than they did previously. Some women find the vaginal "leakage" after use of these products bothersome. Vaginal suppositories, because of the cocoa butter or glycerin base, are the most bothersome; the sponge is the least so. Women should be cautioned not to leave sponges in place over 24 hours or these may be associated with toxic shock syndrome (Brenner & Mishell, 1990).

Effect on Sexual Enjoyment. Although spermicidal products must be inserted fairly close to the time of coitus, they also are so easily purchased (no prescription and no physician appointment necessary) that many couples find the inconvenience of insertion only a minor problem. If a couple is concerned that the method does not offer enough protection, worry about becoming pregnant may interfere with sexual enjoyment. Some couples find the foam or moisture irritating to vaginal and penile tissue during coitus.

If conception should occur, there is no reason to think that the fetus will be affected by the spermicide. Some women worry that a sperm that survived the cream or foam must have been weakened by migrating through it and will produce a defective child. They can be assured that conception occurred most likely because the product did not completely cover the cervical os; the sperm that reached the uterus was free of the product and unharmed.

Use by the Adolescent. Many adolescents use vaginal products as their method of birth control. There is little money involved because a physician appointment is not needed and no parental permission is involved. Adolescents should be cautioned that this method has a high failure rate (20%). All women need to be cautioned that preparations labeled "feminine hygiene" products are for vaginal cleanliness and are not spermicidal: they are not birth control products.

Because of the nontraditional settings in which adolescents may engage in coitus (e.g., in cars or on couches), some girls find having to insert the product awkward and consequently do not use it, even though they have purchased it and intended to be more cautious.

Diaphragms

A **diaphragm** is a circular rubber disk that fits over the cervix and forms a barricade against the entrance of spermatozoa. Although newer studies demonstrate that a spermicide may not be required, using a spermicidal jelly with a diaphragm combines a barrier and a chemical method of contraception. A diaphragm is prescribed and fitted initially by a physician, nurse practitioner, or nurse-midwife to ensure a correct fit. Because the shape of the cervix changes with pregnancy, miscarriage, cervical surgery (dilatation and curettage, or D&C), or therapeutic abortion, a woman must return for a fitting after any of these occurrences. Gaining or losing more than 15 pounds in weight may change pelvic and vaginal contours to such an extent that having the diaphragm competency checked after weight gain or loss is also advisable.

Before coitus, the woman coats the rim of the diaphragm with a contraceptive jelly, and using either a squatting position, a position with one leg elevated on a chair, or lying supine, she inserts the diaphragm into the vagina, sliding it along the posterior wall and pressing it up against the cervix so it is held in place by the vaginal fornices. After insertion, she should always check that it is secure against the cervix by palpating the cervical os through the diaphragm (Figure 5-5). Spermatozoa remain viable in the vagina for 6 hours. Thus, a diaphragm should remain in place for at least 6 hours following coitus, and it may be left in place for as long as 24 hours. If it is left in the vagina longer than this, the stasis of fluid may cause cervical inflammation (erosion). A diaphragm is removed by inserting a finger vaginally and

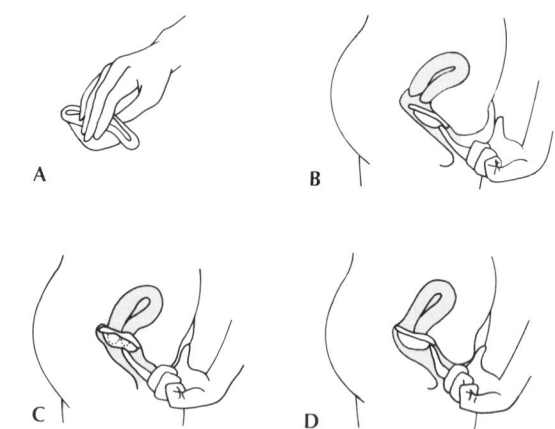

FIGURE 5-5
*Proper insertion of a diaphragm. (**A**) After spermicidal jelly or cream is applied to the rim, the diaphragm is pinched between the fingers and thumb. (**B**) The folded diaphragm is gently inserted into the vagina and pushed backward as far as it will go. (**C**) To check for proper positioning, the woman should feel the cervix to be certain it is completely covered by the soft rubber dome of the diaphragm. (**D**) A finger is hooked under the forward rim to remove the diaphragm. (Reprinted from Masters, W.H., & Johnson, V.E. [1990]. Human sexuality [4th ed.]. Philadelphia: Harper.)*

loosening it by pressing against the anterior rim, and withdrawing it again vaginally.

If the woman washes the diaphragm in mild soap and water, dries it gently and stores it in its protective case, it will last for 2 to 3 years. If she inspects the diaphragm periodically to see that the rubber is not deteriorating, uses it with a spermicidal jelly, and checks it with a finger after insertion to be certain it is fitted well up over the cervix, its failure rate may be as low as 5% to 6% (Trussell, Strickler, & Vaughan, 1993).

Side-Effects and Contraindications. Users of diaphragms may experience a higher number of urinary tract infections than nonusers probably because of pressure on the urethra (Brenner & Mishell, 1990). Diaphragms may not be competent if the uterus is prolapsed, retroflexed, or anteflexed to such a degree that the cervix is also displaced in relation to the vagina. Intrusion on the vagina by a cystocele or rectocele (walls of the vagina are displaced by bladder or bowel) may make inserting a diaphragm difficult. Diaphragms should not be used in the presence of acute cervicitis, because the close contact of the rubber may cause additional irritation.

Effect on Sexual Enjoyment. Some women dislike using diaphragms because they must insert them before coitus (although they may be inserted up to 2 hours beforehand, minimizing this problem). Use of a vibrator as a part of foreplay, frequent penile insertion, or the woman superior during coitus may dislodge the diaphragm, so it may not be the contraceptive of choice for some couples. If coitus is repeated before 6 hours, the diaphragm should not be removed and replaced, but more spermicidal jelly should be added. Some couples may find this precaution restricting. An advantage of the diaphragm is that it allows sexual relations during the menstrual flow without the flow of menstrual blood interfering with enjoyment. If a woman should become pregnant while using a diaphragm, there is no risk of harm to the fetus.

Use by the Adolescent. Adolescents may be fitted for diaphragms, although because an adolescent's vagina will vary in size as she matures and starts sexual relations, the device may not remain as effective as with older women. Adolescents may need to be reminded that diaphragms must be individually fitted; otherwise, they may borrow a friend's, or a group of girls will pool their money to pay for one to share. A young girl usually needs to be shown an anatomic diagram of what is meant by her cervix. Being shown the appearance of her cervix during a pelvic examination by use of a mirror helps her to visualize what she is feeling when she checks for diaphragm placement.

Cervical Caps

A **cervical cap** is yet another barrier method of contraception. Caps have been available in Europe for years but have only recently been approved for use in the United States. A cervical cap is made of soft rubber and shaped like a thimble, and fits snugly over the uterine cervix (Figure 5-6). As with the diaphragm, it is filled just before insertion with a spermicidal jelly (Weiss et al., 1991). The lowest reported failure rate of the cervical cap is 8%, although the typical rate of failure is estimated to be as high as 18% (Hatcher et al., 1993).

Many women are unable to use cervical caps because their cervix is too short for the cap to fit properly. Also, the cap tends to dislodge more readily than a diaphragm during coitus. One advantage it has over the diaphragm is that it can be left in place longer than a diaphragm (48 hours). Although a cervical cap may increase the risk of cervical irritation, unlike the diaphragm it does not put pressure on the vaginal walls or urethra, which could possibly interfere with vaginal blood supply or urine flow. Cervical caps, like diaphragms, must be fitted individually by a health care provider.

Condoms

A **condom** is a latex rubber or synthetic sheath (similar to a finger cot but larger in diameter) that is placed over the erect penis before coitus (Figure 5-7). It prevents pregnancy because spermatozoa are deposited not in

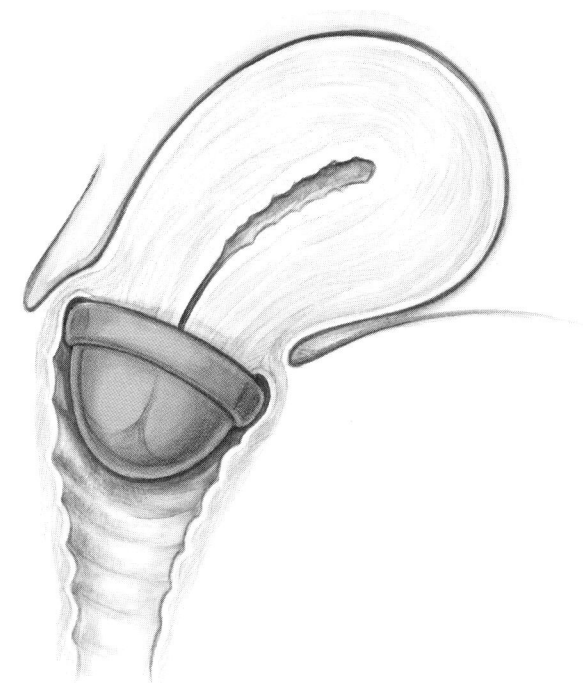

FIGURE 5-6
Cervical caps are used with a spermicidal jelly the same as with a diaphragm.

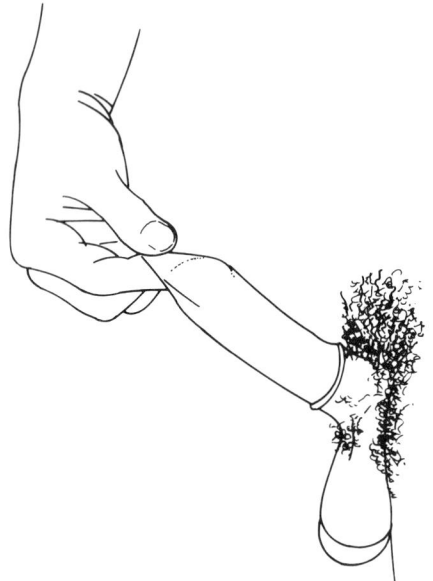

FIGURE 5-7
Male condom. Being certain that space is left at the tip helps to ensure the condom will not break with ejaculation.

the vagina but in the tip of the condom. The use of condoms has an ideal failure rate of 2% and a typical failure rate of about 12%. This is one of the few "male-responsibility" birth control measures available, and no health care visit or prescription is needed. Condoms have the additional potential of preventing the spread of sexually transmitted diseases—their use has become a major part of the fight against human immunodeficiency virus (HIV) infection; it is recommended that they always be worn during coitus between partners who do not maintain a monogamous relationship (DHHS, 1993a) (see the Focus on Nursing Research box).

Side-Effects and Contraindications. There are no contraindications to the use of condoms except for a rare sensitivity to rubber.

Effect on Sexual Enjoyment. To be effective, condoms must be applied before any penile-vulvar contact, because even preejaculation fluid may contain some sperm. The condom should be positioned so it is loose enough at the penis tip to collect the ejaculate without undue pressure on the condom. Before the penis begins to become flaccid after ejaculation, the penis (with the condom held carefully in place) must be withdrawn. If it is not withdrawn at this time, sperm may leak from the now loosely fitting sheath into the vagina. Some men find that condoms dull their enjoyment of coitus; some women resent that men must withdraw promptly following ejaculation.

Use by the Adolescent. One study of male adolescents showed the incidence of condom use in the age

group to have increased to about 50% (DHHS, 1992b). Adolescent boys who have infrequent coitus may use condoms that they have owned and stored for a long time. The effectiveness of these old condoms, especially if they are carried in a warm pocket, should be questioned. Adolescents may need to be cautioned that condoms should never be reused, because even a pinpoint hole can allow thousands of sperm to escape. For many adolescent couples, use of a vaginally inserted preparation by the girl and a condom by her partner is the preferred method of birth control. Effectiveness of these two methods of birth control used in conjunction becomes about 95%. With the exception of abstinence, condoms are the best method of preventing sexually transmitted diseases and their use should be encouraged (Kirkman & Chantler, 1993).

Female Condoms

Condoms for females have received provisional approval by the Federal Drug Administration. These latex sheaths are made of polyurethane, lubricated with nonoxynol 9, and cover the vulva as well as line the vagina and cervix. The sheath may be inserted any time before sexual activity and must be removed after ejaculation occurs. Like male condoms, they are intended for one-time use and offer protection against both conception and sexually transmitted disease (Soper et al., 1993) (Figure 5-8). Although still being tested, the failure rate in preliminary studies was somewhat greater than the

FOCUS ON NURSING RESEARCH

Who Are the Adolescents Most Apt to Use Contraception?

To answer this question, a nationally representative sample of 1880 young men ages 15 to 19 years were asked about their use of contraceptives. In this sample, young men who lived in poor neighborhoods were more likely to feel pleased about an unplanned pregnancy than those who had better living conditions (12% vs 2%) and also more likely to view impregnating a woman as enhancing their masculinity (8% vs 3%). Sexually active black men and Hispanic men were more likely than white men to have discussed contraception with their last sexual partner; black men were more likely to have used a condom at last intercourse.

An implication for nursing is that young men are assuming responsibility for contraception more than previously. Encouraging this trend can be a nursing responsibility.

From Marsiglio, W. (1993). Adolescent males' orientation toward paternity and contraception. *Family Planning Perspectives, 25,* 22.

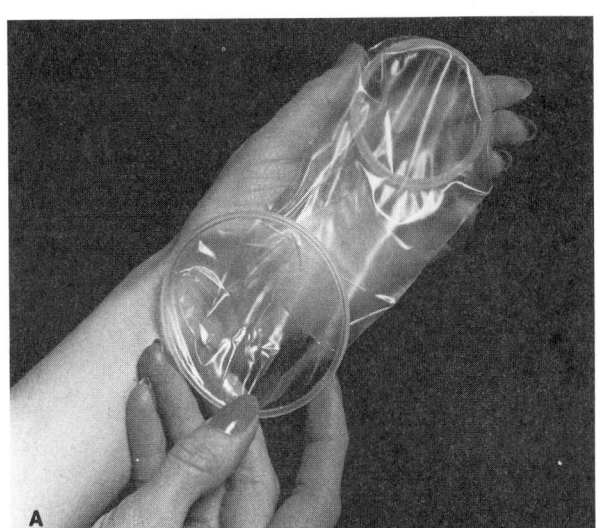

Insertion of the REALITY™ Vaginal Pouch

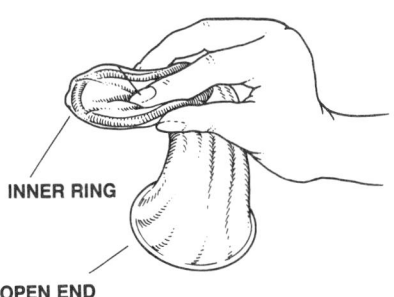

INNER RING

OPEN END

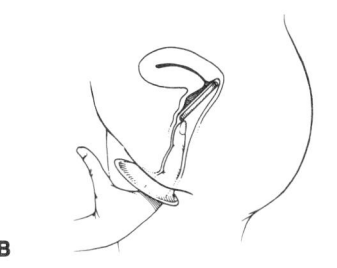

B

FIGURE 5-8
Female condom. Women have a way to protect themselves against both STDs and pregnancy with the female condom. (A) The REALITY (WP-333) female condom. (B) Insertion technique. (Courtesy of Wisconsin Pharmaceutical Company, Inc.)

failure rate for male condoms, about 15%. Most of these pregnancies occurred because of incorrect or inconsistent use (Hatcher et al., 1993).

Natural Family Planning (Periodic Abstinence or Fertility Awareness)

Natural family planning or **fertility awareness** methods rely on periods of temporary abstinence or temporary contraceptive use and require an understanding of the changes that occur in the woman's ovulatory cycle. With fertility awareness, couples determine fertile days and abstain from sex or use a birth control method during these days. They are then free to go without contraception during the rest of the month (Hatcher et al., 1993). As described below, there are a variety of ways to determine a fertile period. Couples may do this by calculating the period based on a set formula, body temperature, or cervical mucus, or they may use an over-the-counter test kit. These tests detect the midcycle surge of luteinizing hormone that occurs 12 to 24 hours before ovulation.

Many people hold religious beliefs that rule out the use of birth control pills or devices; others believe that a "natural" way of planning pregnancies is best for them. These people are candidates for natural family planning methods. No expense is involved in these methods and no foreign materials are used. They are methods approved by the Roman Catholic Church and Orthodox Judaism. The effectiveness of these methods varies greatly, depending mainly on the couple's ability to observe sexual abstinence on fertile days. Failure rates

range from 10% to 20% (Hatcher et al., 1993). If unwanted pregnancy should occur with these methods, there is no risk to the fetus except the obvious one: a child so conceived might be unwanted.

Calendar (Rhythm) and Basal Body Temperature Methods

The **calendar method** requires a couple to abstain from coitus on the days of a menstrual cycle when the woman is most apt to conceive (3 to 4 days before and after ovulation). To plan for this, a woman should keep a diary of six menstrual cycles. To calculate "safe" days, she subtracts 18 from the shortest cycle documented. This number represents her *first* fertile day. She subtracts 11 from her longest cycle. This is her *last* fertile day. If she had six menstrual cycles ranging from 25 to 29 days, her fertile period would be from the 7th day (25−18) to the 18th day (29−11). To avoid pregnancy, she would avoid coitus during these days (Figure 5-9*A*).

The basis of the **basal body temperature method** is that just before the day of ovulation, a woman's basal body temperature falls about half a degree. At the time of ovulation, her temperature rises a full degree because of the influence of progesterone. This higher level will be maintained for the rest of the menstrual cycle.

To use this method, the woman should take and chart her temperature each morning immediately after waking, before she undertakes any activity. This is her basal body temperature. As soon as she notices a slight dip in temperature followed by an increase, she knows that she has ovulated. She maintains abstinence from this point until after the third day of the sustained high

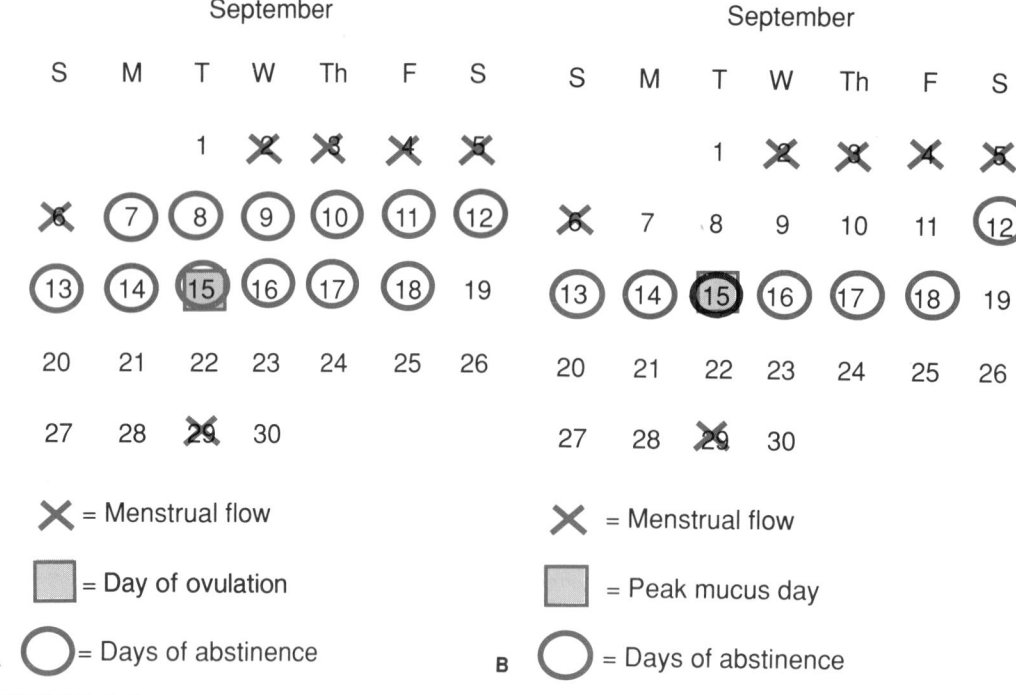

FIGURE 5-9

(**A**) A month using the calendar method as a natural family planning method. (**B**) A month using the cervical mucus method of natural family planning. Unmarked days are those safe for sexual relations.

temperature (the combined life of ova and sperm). For more information on basal body temperature and fertility, see Chapter 6 and Figure 6-2.

A problem with this method is that a temperature rise from illness could be mistaken as the signal of ovulation. If this happens, a woman can mistake a fertile day for a safe one.

The Symptothermal (Cervical Mucus) Method

Another method to predict ovulation is to use the changes in cervical mucus that occur naturally with ovulation (Roth, 1993). Before ovulation each month, cervical mucus is thick and does not stretch when pulled between the thumb and finger (the property of *spinnbarkeit*). Just before ovulation, mucus secretion becomes copious. With ovulation (the peak day) the mucus becomes thin, watery, and transparent, feels slippery, and stretches a distance of at least 1 inch before the strand breaks. In addition, breast tenderness and an anterior tilt to the cervix occur. All the days the mucus is copious and the 3 days after the peak day are considered to be fertile days, or days the woman should maintain sexual abstinence to avoid conception.

The woman using this method must be conscientious about assessing vaginal secretions daily or she will miss the phenomenon of changing cervical secretions. The feel of vaginal secretions following sexual relations is unreliable, because seminal fluid (the fluid containing sperm from the male) has a watery, postovulatory consistency and can be confused with ovulatory mucus. Figure 5-9B shows a hypothetical month using this method.

Ovulation Awareness

Yet another method used to predict ovulation is to use an over-the-counter ovulation detection kit. These tests detect the midcycle surge of luteinizing hormone that occurs 12 to 24 hours before ovulation (Demystifying ovulation and pregnancy kits for your patients, 1993). Using such a kit in place of cervical mucus secretion testing makes this form of natural family planning more attractive to many women.

Effect on Sexual Enjoyment. Once a couple is certain of nonfertile days using one of the natural planning methods, more spontaneity in sexual relations is possible than with methods that involve vaginal insertion products. On the other hand, the required days of abstinence may make a natural planning method unsatisfactory and unenjoyable for a couple.

Use by the Adolescent. Natural methods of family planning (with the exception of abstinence) are usually not the contraceptive method of choice for adolescents (see the Focus on Family Teaching box). Girls tend to have occasional anovulatory menstrual cycles for several years after menarche and they do not always experience

FOCUS ON FAMILY TEACHING

Reproductive life planning can be a subject that adolescents want to learn more about at health care visits. Here are some common questions they may have:

Q. If a method prevents pregnancy, does it automatically also prevent sexually transmitted disease?

A. No. Only condoms (both male and female) and spermicidal agents with nonoxynol 9 are effective against STDs.

Q. I want to use abstinence as my contraceptive method. What measures could I take to let my partner know I mean no when I say it?

A. Discuss with your partner in advance what sexual activities you will permit and what you will not. Try and avoid high pressure situations (a party with excessive alcohol consumption and no adult supervision). If pressured, say no as if you mean it. Be certain your partner understands that you consider being forced into relations against your wishes the same as rape, not simply irresponsible conduct.

definite cervical changes or an elevated body temperature. Also, these methods require girls to be able to say no to sexual relations on fertile days, a difficult task to do under peer pressure.

Ovulation Suppression by Lactation

As long as a woman is breast-feeding an infant, there is some natural suppression of ovulation. Use of lactation as a birth control method is not highly reliable. Because women may ovulate but not menstruate while breast-feeding, the fact they have not had a menstrual period following childbirth does not ensure that they are not fertile.

Coitus Interruptus

Coitus interruptus is one of the oldest known and least effective methods of contraception (Lethbridge, 1991). The couple proceeds with coitus until the moment of ejaculation. Then the man withdraws and spermatozoa are emitted outside the vagina. Unfortunately, ejaculation may occur before withdrawal is complete and, despite the care used, some spermatozoa may be deposited in the vagina. Because there may be a few spermatozoa in preejaculation fluid, even though withdrawal seems controlled, fertilization may occur. For these reasons, coitus interruptus offers little protection against conception. In particular, adolescent boys often lack the control or experience to use the method.

Permanent Methods of Reproductive Life Planning

Permanent methods of reproductive life planning include sterilization (a **tubal ligation** procedure for women and **vasectomy** for men). Sterilization is the most frequently used method of contraception in the United States. About 14% of all women in the United States of childbearing age choose sterilization to prevent unwanted pregnancy. Vasectomy is the contraceptive method of choice for about 10% of men (Brenner & Mishell, 1990). So many people choose a permanent method because it is the most effective method of contraception. Because it is permanent, it should not be chosen without great thought and care. Although procedures for the reversal of both male and female sterilization do exist, such techniques are much more complicated than the sterilization itself, and success rates vary greatly. Before anyone of childbearing age undergoes a sterilization procedure, he or she should understand that it is permanent. Counseling should be especially intensive for men and women under the age of 25. Couples should consider the possibilities of divorce, death of a partner, loss of a child, or remarriage before considering this option. In addition, sterilization is not recommended for individuals whose fertility is important to their self-esteem. Candidates for sterilization can be apprised that these procedures have no effect on sexuality (Shain et al., 1991).

Vasectomy

In vasectomy, a small incision is made in each side of the scrotum. The vas deferens at that point is then cut and tied or cauterized or plugged, blocking the passage of spermatozoa (Figure 5-10). Vasectomy can be done under local anesthesia in an ambulatory setting such as a physician's office or a reproductive life planning clinic. The man experiences a small amount of local pain afterward that can be managed by taking a mild analgesic and applying ice to the site. Vasectomy is 100% effective, although spermatozoa that were present in the vas deferens at the time of surgery may remain viable for as long as 6 months. Although the man can resume sexual coitus within 1 week, an additional birth control method should be used until two negative sperm reports have been examined (proof that all sperm in the vas deferens have been eliminated). The man should think of vasectomy as irreversible, although the newer techniques of silicone plugs and microsurgery can make it reversible to a limited extent.

Some men resist the concept of vasectomy because they are not sufficiently aware of their anatomy to know exactly what the procedure involves. It does not interfere with the production of sperm; the testes continue to produce sperm as always; the sperm simply do not pass beyond the severed vas deferens but are absorbed at

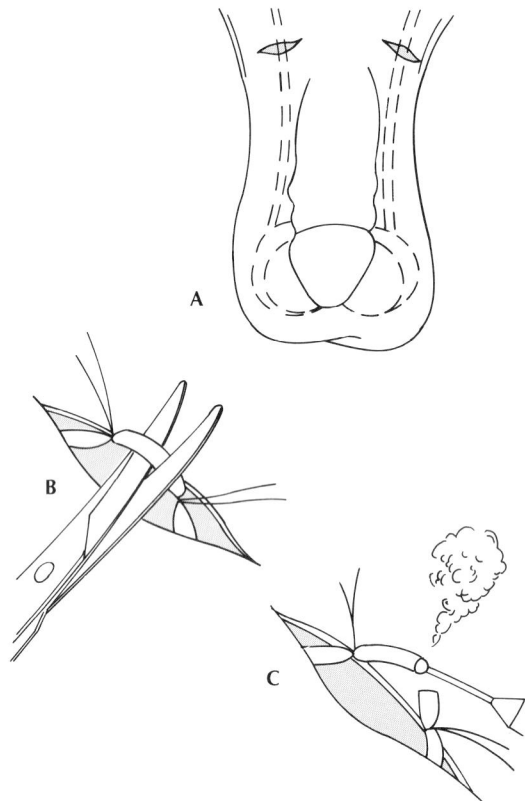

FIGURE 5-10

*Vasectomy. (**A**) Site of vasectomy sutures. (**B**) The vas deferens being cut with surgical scissors. (**C**) Cut ends of the vas deferens are cauterized to completely ensure blockage of the passage of sperm.*

that point. The man will still have full erection and ejaculation capacity. Because he also continues to form seminal fluid, he will ejaculate seminal fluid, only it will not contain sperm.

There are very few complications associated with vasectomy (Giovannucci et al., 1992). Hematomas may occur in up to 5% of men undergoing the procedure, but these may be prevented by carefully securing hemostasis during the procedure (Brenner & Mishell, 1990). Six percent to 7% of men in the U.S. who have had a vasectomy seek medical reversal. The success rate for reanastomosis is 45% to 60% (Brenner & Mishell, 1990). Some men develop autoimmunity or form antibodies against sperm, so that even if reconstruction of the vas deferens is successful at a later date, the sperm they produce do not have good mobility and are incapable of fertilization (Hatcher et al., 1993). The possibility that vasectomy may be associated with development of prostate cancer has been raised. The data as to whether this occurs or not, however, are unclear (Klitsch, 1993).

Tubal Ligation

Sterilization of women could include removal of the uterus (*hysterectomy*), but it generally refers to a minor

surgical procedure, such as tubal ligation, that occludes the fallopian tubes by cautery, crushing, clamping, or blocking the tube and thereby preventing passage of the sperm into the tube to meet the ova. If a silicone gel is instilled into the tubes as a blocking agent, this can be removed at a later date to reverse the procedure. Even this technique, however, as with vasectomy, should not be undertaken unless the woman does view it as a permanent, irreversible procedure. Not only is it difficult to reconstruct fallopian tubes after they have been cauterized, but there is a possibility that afterwards the anastomosis site, because of its irregular surface, could be host to an ectopic (tubal) pregnancy.

The most common operation to achieve tubal ligation is **laparoscopy**. Following a menstrual flow and before ovulation, an incision as small as 1 cm is made just under the woman's umbilicus with the woman under general or local anesthesia (Lipscomb, 1993). A lighted laparoscope is inserted through the incision. Carbon dioxide is then pumped into the incision to lift the abdominal wall upward out of the line of vision. The surgeon locates the fallopian tubes by viewing the field through the laparoscope. An electrical current is then passed through the instrument for about 3 to 5 seconds. This coagulates the tissue of the tube and seals it (Figure 5-11). The woman is either kept in the hospital overnight or discharged in a few hours. She may notice abdominal bloating after the procedure for the first 24 hours until the carbon dioxide that was infused at the beginning of the procedure is absorbed. She may notice sharp diaphragmatic or shoulder pain if some of the carbon dioxide escapes under the diaphragm.

Women need to be certain that they have no unprotected coitus before the procedure (sperm trapped in the tube could fertilize an ovum there and cause an ectopic pregnancy). They need to be informed before the procedure that laparoscopy, unlike a hysterectomy, will not affect the menstrual cycle, so they will still have a monthly menstrual flow. Complications include the risk of bowel perforation, hemorrhage, and the risks of general anesthesia with the procedure. A woman may return to coitus as soon as 2 to 3 days after the procedure.

Tubal ligation can be done as soon as 1 day after delivery (usually not sooner to allow good uterine contraction) of a child, although the abdominal distention at this time may make locating the tubes difficult. The procedure can also be done by *culdoscopy* (a tube inserted through the posterior fornix of the vagina) and *colpotomy* (incision through the vagina), but the incidence of pelvic infection is higher with these procedures and visualization is less.

Contraindications to laparoscopy are an umbilical hernia, because bowel perforation might result, and extensive obesity, which would probably require a full laparotomy to allow adequate visualization. A number of women develop vaginal spotting, intermittent vaginal

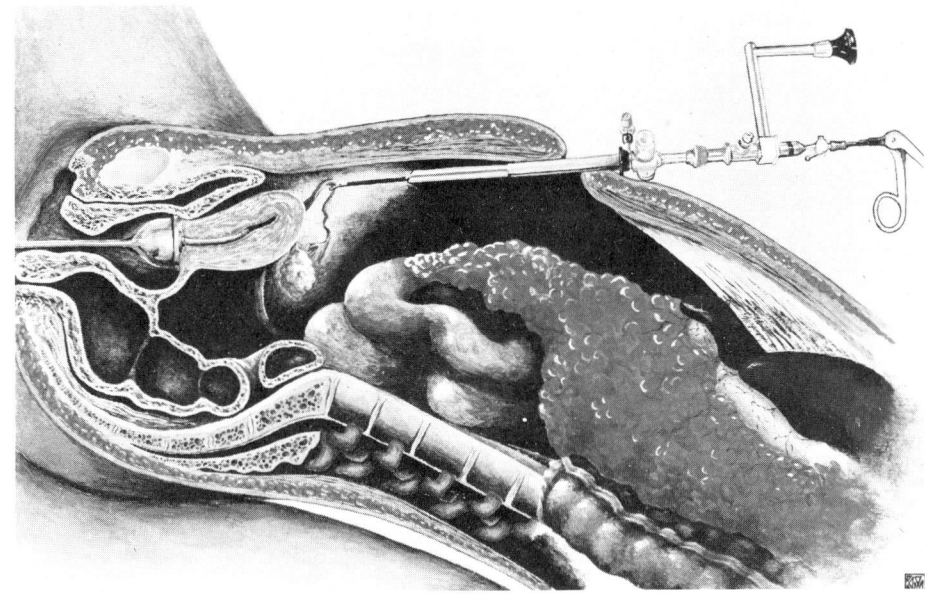

FIGURE 5-11
Laparoscopy for tubal sterilization. (From Richard Wolf Medical Instruments Corporation, with permission).

bleeding, and severe lower abdominal cramping after tubal ligation (post–tubal ligation syndrome) (Townsend et al., 1993). Removing the fallopian tubes appears to relieve the symptoms.

A *minilaparotomy* is used post childbirth or post abortion. Many such procedures are done in the ambulatory surgery department. A local anesthetic can be used. An incision is made 2 to 3 cm transversely just above the pubic hair. The fallopian tubes are pulled to the surface and lifted out of the incision to be visualized. Metal or plastic clips or rubber rings are then used to seal the tubes. Clips obscure tubes by causing necrosis at that point. The woman may notice a day or two of abdominal discomfort caused by the local necrosis at the clip site. A *fimbriectomy,* or removal of the fimbria at the distal end of the tubes, is possible.

Effect on Sexual Enjoyment. Both tubal ligation and vasectomy may lead to increased sexual enjoyment because they completely eliminate the possibility of pregnancy. If either partner changes his or her mind about having children or additional children, however, the surgery may become an issue between them that interferes not only with sexual enjoyment but with other aspects of their relationship as well.

Use by the Adolescent. Sterilization is not advised for adolescents, since their future goals may change so drastically that what they want at age 16 or 18 may not be what they want at all at age 30. Adolescents should be counseled to use more temporary forms of birth control. Later, if they still feel vasectomy or tubal ligation is the method of reproductive life planning for them, the option is still open (Figure 5-12).

The Disabled Couple

A couple with a disability should be asked at health care visits if reproductive life planning is a concern (Welner, 1993). A man, for example, who has unsteady coordination, might not have adequate hand coordination to place a condom effectively. A female, likewise, might have difficulty inserting a diaphragm; a woman with mental retardation might not appreciate the necessity for

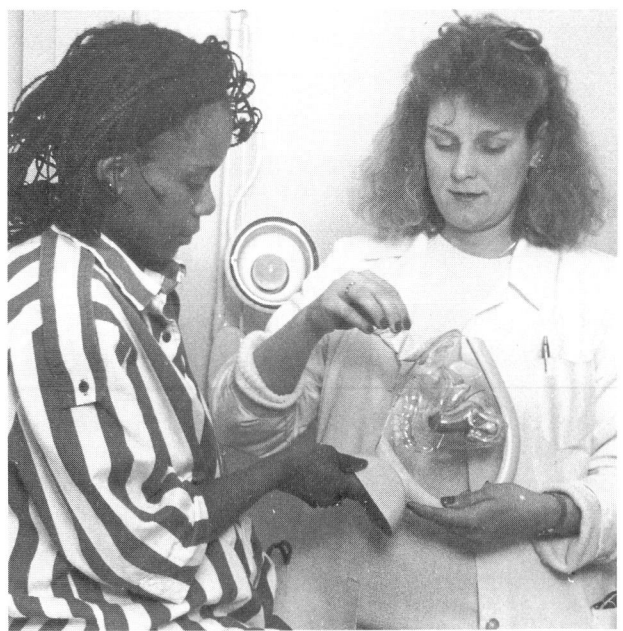

FIGURE 5-12
Counseling adolescents regarding reproductive life planning is an important health promotion measure that can also prevent sexually transmitted disease. (Courtesy Department of Medical Photography, Children's Hospital, Buffalo, NY.)

taking birth control pills daily and so not use them effectively. For these reasons, subcutaneous implants and injections may prove to be the ideal contraceptives for many persons with a disability.

Future Trends in Contraception

Because estrogen is responsible for most of the side-effects associated with oral contraceptives, studies are being made of even lower dose estrogen pills. A progesterone-filled vaginal ring is a possibility (Mishell, 1993). A progesterone-impregnated diaphragm may be used in the future. A birth control vaccine consisting of antibodies against human chorionic gonadotropin hormone and linked to a tetanus or diphtheria toxoid as a carrier is being investigated (Talwar et al., 1993). Even a male contraceptive of synthetic androgen is being developed (Sundaram et al., 1993). Until some method satisfies all the criteria for an ideal contraceptive—that is, completely safe, no side-effects, low cost, easy availability, easy reversibility, and user acceptability—research in the field will continue.

Elective Termination of Pregnancy

An **elective termination of pregnancy** is a procedure performed to deliberately end a pregnancy before fetal viability. Such procedures are also referred to as *therapeutic, medical,* or *induced* abortions. Nurses employed in a health care agency where induced abortions are performed or who work for physicians or clinics who perform them are asked to assist with the procedures as a part of their duties.

Induced abortions are done for a number of reasons: to end a pregnancy which threatens a woman's life (e.g., pregnancy in a woman with class IV heart disease) or which involves a fetus found on amniocentesis to have a chromosomal defect; to end a pregnancy that is unwanted because it is the result of rape or incest; or to terminate the pregnancy of a woman who chooses not to have a child at this time in her life. The majority of induced abortions are done for the last reason.

In 1973, the U.S. Supreme Court ruled that induced abortions must be offered in all states as long as the pregnancy is under 12 weeks. It is left up to the individual state to determine whether induced abortions may be performed after the first trimester and to mandate additional regulations regarding the procedure, such as requiring a 24-hour waiting period from counseling until the procedure can be done or requiring parental approval for minors. The July 1992 ruling of the Supreme court in *Casey v Planned Parenthood of Pennsylvania* confirmed the right to abortion and the right of states to

make these kinds of restrictions. Whether a particular institution provides abortion services depends on the policy and choice of that institution.

About 28 in every 1000 U.S. women have an induced abortion in their lifetime. The majority of these are done when the pregnancy is less than 12 weeks in length. The maternal mortality of abortion is 0.6 per 100,000 abortions performed (Henshaw, 1990). This makes abortion about 11 times safer for women than childbirth, for which the mortality rate is 6 per 100,000 births.

Choosing an abortion is a decision that a woman can make on her own. The consent of the father is unnecessary. Most midtrimester abortions occur in hospitals; a hospital may require that the permission of the husband be obtained before the procedure is performed, but this is hospital policy only. Although the law is being debated and is subject to changes in state laws, in most instances, minors may consent to abortion without knowledge or consent of their parents (although the average adolescent tells a parent before the procedure; Henshaw & Kost, 1992).

Abortion Procedures

Women having surgically induced abortions have laboratory studies performed before the procedure, including a pregnancy test, complete blood count, blood typing (including Rh factor), gonococcal smear, a serologic test for syphilis, urinalysis, and a Pap smear.

Elective abortions involve a number of techniques, depending on the gestation age at the time the abortion is performed.

Menstrual Extraction
Menstrual extraction is the simplest type of abortion procedure. It may be performed on an out-patient basis at 5 to 7 weeks after the last menstrual period (often before pregnancy tests are reliable enough to prove that a pregnancy exists). The woman voids and her perineum is washed with an antiseptic (shaving is unnecessary). A speculum is then introduced vaginally, the cervix is stabilized by a tenaculum, and then a narrow polyethylene catheter is introduced through the vagina into the cervix and uterus (Figure 5-13A). The lining of the uterus that would be shed with a normal menstrual flow is then suctioned and removed by means of the vacuum pressure of a syringe. Menstrual extraction is an ambulatory procedure, completed quickly and with a minimum of discomfort (some abdominal cramping may occur as the tenaculum grasps the cervix and as the last of the endometrium is suctioned away). The woman should remain supine for about 15 minutes after the procedure until uterine cramping quiets and to prevent hypoten-

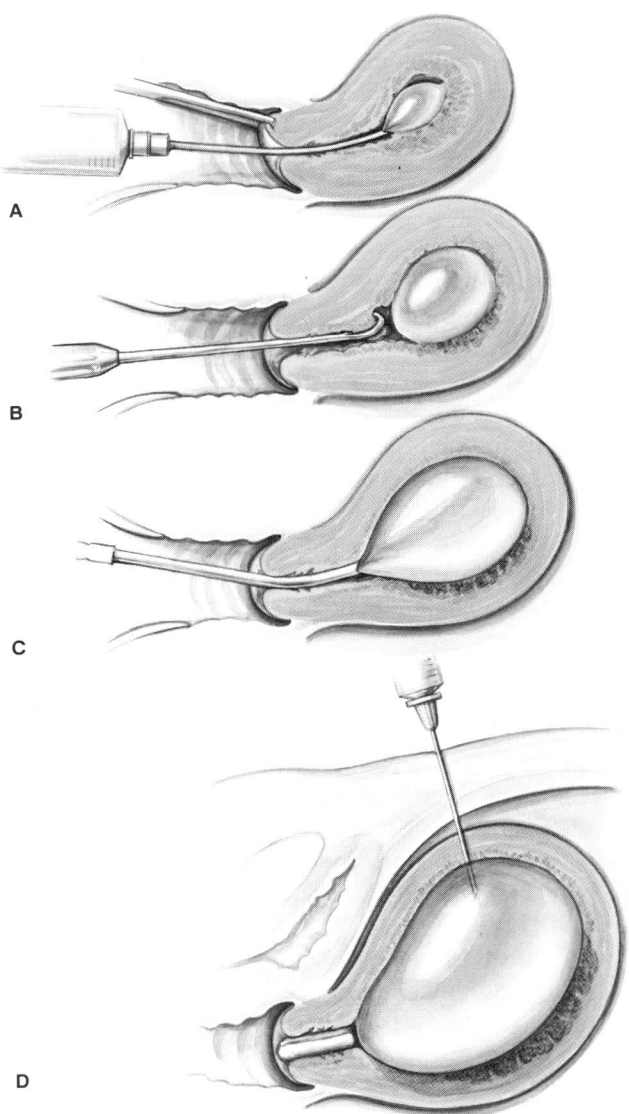

FIGURE 5-13
*Techniques of elective termination of pregnancy. (**A**) Vacuum extraction. (**B**) Dilatation and curettage (D&C). (**C**) Dilatation and vacuum extraction (D&E). (**D**) Saline induction.*

sion on standing. She may be given an oral oxytocin to ensure full uterine contraction following the procedure.

She can expect to have vaginal bleeding similar to her normal menstrual flow for a week following the procedure; she may have occasional spotting up to 2 weeks. She should not douche, use tampons, or resume coitus until 1 week after the procedure. She should return in 2 weeks for a pelvic examination and pregnancy test to be certain that the procedure was successful and her pregnancy was effectively terminated.

Menstrual extraction carries with it the same possibility of hemorrhage and infection as other abortion procedures. Because a pliable catheter is used, however, the possibility of uterine puncture is greatly reduced.

The woman needs to know danger signs to watch for following an abortion and who to telephone if any of these should be apparent (Table 5-2). She should be asked if she wants contraceptive counseling for better reproductive life planning.

Dilatation and Curettage

If the gestation age of the pregnancy is under 13 weeks, a dilatation and curettage (D&C) may be used as the procedure. For this, the woman is admitted to a hospital or clinic. If in the hospital, she may receive a general anesthetic, although a regional anesthetic such as a paracervical block works well for pain relief and is used in ambulatory settings. The use of a paracervical block does not completely obliterate pain but limits what the woman experiences to cramping and a feeling of pressure at her cervix.

After voiding, cleaning of the perineum, and the anesthetic block, the cervix is dilated by graduated dilators until a uterine sound and a curette can be inserted through the cervical os. The uterus is then scraped clean with the curette, removing the zygote and trophoblast cells (Figure 5-13*B*). Following the procedure, the woman should remain in the hospital or clinic for an hour or, preferably, 4 hours. She is given the same careful assessment of vital signs and perineal care as a woman following childbirth receives. She is given an oxytocin medication to ensure firm uterine contraction and minimize bleeding. If there are no complications, she may return home after approximately 4 hours and after being told of the danger signs of abortion (see Table 5-2) and pertinent contraceptive counseling.

D&C has the potential risks over menstrual extraction of uterine puncture from the instruments used, and increased danger of uterine infection because of greater cervical dilatation.

Dilatation and Vacuum Extraction

Most second-trimester abortions (those between 12 and 16 weeks) are done by dilatation and vacuum extraction (D&E), which can be either an inpatient or ambulatory

Table 5-2. *Danger Signs Following Elective Termination of Pregnancy*	
Sign	**Possible Meaning**
Heavy vaginal bleeding (more than two pads saturated in 1 hour)	Hemorrhage
Passing of clots	Hemorrhage
Abdominal pain or tenderness	Infection (endometritis)
Fever over 100.4°F	Infection (endometritis)
Severe depression	Inadequate coping ability

procedure. With this, as with D&C, the woman must void before the procedure; as with other uterine procedures, the perineum is washed; a paracervical block is carried out and the cervix is dilated. In some centers, dilatation of the cervix is accomplished by having the woman come into the center the day before the procedure; a laminaria "tent" is inserted into the cervix under sterile conditions. *Laminaria* is seaweed that has been dried and sterilized. In a moist body part such as the cervix, it begins to absorb fluid and swell in size. Over a 24-hour period, gradually, painlessly, and without trauma, it dilates the cervix enough for a vacuum extraction tip to be inserted. There is some concern that frequent dilatation of the cervix can lead to an incompetent cervix, or one that dilates so easily that it will not remain contracted during pregnancy. Laminaria dilatation is often chosen for adolescent girls, therefore, who may have more than one abortion in their life-time, to try to safeguard their bodies for later childbearing. Antibiotic prophylaxis may begin at the time of the laminaria insertion to protect against infection. The woman is cautioned not to have sexual relations until the abortion is complete to reduce the possibility of infection.

After either *Laminaria* dilatation or dilatation by traditional dilators, a narrow suction tip specially designed for the incompletely dilated cervix is introduced into the cervix (Figure 5-13*C*). The negative pressure of a suction pump or vacuum container then gently evacuates the uterine contents over a 15-minute period. The woman will feel pain as the cervical dilatation is performed and some pressure and cramps similar to menstrual cramps during suction, but it is not a markedly painful procedure.

After the procedure, the woman lies flat for at least 15 minutes. She remains in the hospital or clinic for about 4 hours. She is given the same careful assessment of vital signs and perineal care as a woman following childbirth receives. She usually receives an oxytocin medication to ensure firm uterine contraction and minimize bleeding. If there are no complications, she may return home after 4 hours after receiving appropriate contraceptive counseling. She can expect to have bleeding comparable to a menstrual flow for the first week afterward, and spotting up to 2 or 3 weeks afterward. Cramping may continue for up to 24 to 48 hours; she may be advised to take a mild analgesic such as acetaminophen (Tylenol) for discomfort. She should not douche, use tampons, or resume coitus until she returns 2 weeks later for an examination; be certain she knows the danger signals shown in Table 5-2. If none of these signals is present, she can resume normal activities within 24 hours after the procedure.

D&E has a potential for uterine puncture, because a rigid cannula is used for the procedure. Moreover, because the cervix was dilated, there is a potential for post-procedure infection.

Saline Induction

Saline induction is a method used if a pregnancy is between 16 and 24 weeks (Figure 5-13*D*). It is based on the principle that hypertonic (20%) saline causes fluid shifts and placenta and endometrium sloughing. It is an inpatient procedure.

The woman is admitted to the hospital and has laminaria cervical suppositories inserted to help prepare the cervix for dilatation. Four hours later, she voids to reduce the size of her bladder so that it will not be accidentally punctured by the saline injection. Her abdominal wall is then prepared with an antiseptic solution and a local anesthetic. A sterile spinal needle is inserted into the uterus through the abdominal wall, and 100 to 200 mL of amniotic fluid is removed by a sterile syringe with amniocentesis technique (see Chapter 9). A 20% hypertonic saline solution of up to 200 mL is then injected through the same needle through the abdominal wall into the amniotic fluid. The needle is withdrawn. Within 12 to 36 hours following the injection, labor contractions begin. The labor (which takes an additional 12 to 36 hours) may be shortened by administration of a dilute oxytocin intravenous solution. The woman is cared for the same as any woman in labor: she needs frequent explanations of what is happening; she needs medication for discomfort; she may find breathing exercises helpful to minimize discomfort; and she needs to have her family or a support person and health care personnel close at hand.

In most hospitals, women undergoing saline induction complete the abortion in a labor room and are not transferred to the delivery room. Because the products of conception are small, the actual delivery causes only a momentary stinging pain as the perineum is stretched.

A serious potential complication of saline abortion is *hypernatremia* from accidental injection of the hypertonic saline solution into a blood vessel within the uterine cavity. The presence of such a concentrated salt solution in the bloodstream could cause body fluid to shift into the blood vessels in an attempt to equalize osmotic pressure. Serious dehydration of tissue could result. If an intravenous puncture should occur, there is an intense reaction that occurs at the moment of injection that is manifested by increased pulse rate, flushed face, and severe headache. The injection must be stopped immediately in the event of such a reaction and an intravenous solution such as 5% dextrose begun to restore fluid balance.

If large amounts of oxytocin are necessary to induce labor with a saline abortion, the woman must be observed closely for signs of *water intoxication,* or body fluid accumulating in body tissue, a side-effect of oxytocin administration. Signs of water intoxication are severe headache, confusion, drowsiness, edema, and decreased urinary output. These symptoms occur subtly at first, then grow in severity. Stopping the oxytocin drip is necessary. Water intoxication will then decrease as body fluid shifts back to normal compartments. Always infuse oxytocin in a piggy-back method during an abortion procedure, the same as with a woman in labor, so as to be able to stop the infusion of oxytocin quickly yet maintain a fluid line for emergency drugs or fluid.

After delivery of the products of conception, it is important that the tissue be examined to determine whether the entire conceptus has been delivered. The woman should be carefully observed for hemorrhage, just as if the fetus had been born at term. If the delivery was unusually prolonged, the woman is prone to the development of disseminated intravascular coagulation (see Chapter 15); if this occurs, she is very susceptible to hemorrhage. If she wishes to see the fetus, swaddle it as if it were a full-term infant and allow her to see it.

All women should be asked if they want contraceptive counseling following saline induction. A follow-up examination 2 to 4 weeks after the abortion should be scheduled so that it can be assessed that the organs of reproduction have returned to their pre-pregnant state. Sexual relations and douching are generally contraindicated until the time of the postabortion checkup or for 2 weeks. The woman can expect to have spotting for as long as 2 weeks and a menstrual flow 2 to 8 weeks after the procedure.

Hysterotomy

If the gestation age for a pregnancy is more than 16 to 18 weeks, a *hysterotomy*, or removal of the fetus by surgical intervention, may be performed. Surgery is necessary because the uterus becomes resistant to the effect of oxytocin as it reaches this phase of pregnancy and may not respond to saline induction even with an oxytocin assist. Further, the chance is great at this gestational age that the uterus will not respond and contract afterward, leading to hemorrhage after a vaginal delivery. The technique for hysterotomy is the same as that for cesarean birth (see Chapter 20). Because this is so late in pregnancy, less than 1% of abortions are done using this technique (Henshaw, 1990).

Orally Induced Abortion

RU 486 (mifepristone) is a compound that blocks the effect of progesterone (a progesterone antagonist) and is currently used in France as a commonly prescribed drug for abortions (Glasier et al., 1992). The compound has a 95% effectiveness rate when it is administered with a prostaglandin within 49 days of the last menstrual period; 90% if it is used without a prostaglandin.

The complications of the compound are incomplete abortion and the possibility of prolonged bleeding. Advantages are the decreased risk of damage to the uterus and use of anesthesia necessary for surgically performed abortions (Henshaw, 1990).

RU 486 may in the future have additional applications such as regression of uterine leiomyomas (Murphy et al., 1993), labor induction (Frydman et al., 1992), and detoxification in cocaine overdose (Sharma et al., 1993).

Isoimmunization

Whenever a placenta is dislodged, either by spontaneous delivery or surgical intervention at any point in pregnancy, blood from the placental villi (the fetal blood) may enter the maternal circulation. This has implications for the Rh-negative woman. Enough Rh-positive blood may enter her circulation to cause *isoimmunization*: the production by her immunologic system of antibodies against Rh-positive blood. If her next child should have Rh-positive blood, these antibodies would attempt to destroy the red blood cells of the infant during the months in utero.

After either an orally induced or surgically induced abortion, because the blood type of the conceptus is unknown, all women with Rh-negative blood should receive $Rh_o(D)$ immune globulin (RhoGAM or RHIG) to prevent the buildup of antibodies in the event the conceptus was Rh-positive.

Psychological Aspects of Elective Termination of Pregnancy

Women of all ages, married or unmarried, with or without children, request induced abortions. The usual profile of a woman who is having an abortion is young, white, unmarried, no previous live births and undergoing the procedure for the first time. She is having the procedure done to end an unwanted pregnancy (DHHS, 1993b).

Women having induced abortion need the same kind of explanations that women in labor receive (often more, because women do not share abortion experiences with each other as they share labor experiences, so they usually have received little advance preparation).

Most women feel anxious when they appear at the hospital or clinic for an abortion. Some of the anxiety comes from having made a difficult decision to reach this step; some comes from having to face the unknown; some may come from feelings of loss or shame and sadness that they had to make a decision with which they are not totally comfortable. Remembering that this is not a decision taken lightly helps to plan nursing care aimed at making an abortion as untraumatic as possible.

Key Points

- Reproductive life planning involves personal decisions based on an individual's background, experiences, and sociocultural beliefs and thorough planning, so that any contraceptive method chosen is acceptable and can be maintained effectively.

- Oral contraceptives are combinations of estrogen and progesterone that provide one of the most reliable forms of contraception outside of abstinence. Women older than age 40 years who smoke are not candidates for oral contraceptive use because of the danger of cardiovascular complications. Counsel them to find a form of contraception that is reliable and allows them to remain sexually active.

- Subcutaneous implants (renewed every 5 years) and subcutaneous injections (renewed every 3 months) are new methods of contraception. These are 100% effective.

- Intrauterine devices are mechanical methods that prevent fertilization and implantation by placement in the uterus. Women with IUDs need to be aware that they are at greater risk for pelvic inflammatory disease (PID) than others. Counsel them to limit the number of sexual partners and be aware of the signs of PID as practical measures to help avoid serious illness.

- Barrier methods include the diaphragm, cervical cap, vaginal spermicides, sponge, and condom (male and female). Such methods are low in cost but are not as effective as ovulation suppressant methods.

- Natural family planning (periodic abstinence) methods are varied but involve determining the fertile period each month and then avoiding sexual relations during that time.

- Permanent methods of contraception are tubal ligation in women and vasectomy in men. Counsel individuals who wish to undergo these procedures that they are largely irreversible.

- Elective termination of pregnancy is accomplished by menstrual extraction, dilatation and curettage, saline induction, or hysterotomy. Counsel women not to think of elective termination of pregnancy as a contraceptive method. It is a recourse to be used only when preventive measures fail. Women who are Rh negative need to receive $Rh_0(D)$ immune globulin after these procedures.

- When counseling clients about reproductive life planning, nurses have a responsibility to counsel them regarding safer sex practices, such as using a condom during sexual intercourse.

Critical Thinking Exercises

1. Judy is a 16-year-old you care for in a family planning clinic. Would your interview differ if Judy were 39 rather than 16? Would your recommendations for a method of birth control differ?

2. John is a young adult male who is interested in having an active role in reproductive life planning and avoiding contracting a sexually transmitted dis-

ease. He has no regular sexual partner at present. What recommendations would you make to John? Would this be different if he had a monogamous relationship?

3. Betty Jo is a 16-year-old who has been admitted to the hospital for saline induction of elective termination of pregnancy. Her doctor tells you to give her only a minimum of analgesia so Betty remembers the experience as painful and, therefore, won't get pregnant again. Do you agree with this philosophy? Are there other measures you could take to help ensure that she doesn't become pregnant irresponsibly again?

References

Berenson, A. B., & Wiemann, C. M. (1993). Patient satisfaction and side effects with levonorgestrel implant use in adolescents 18 years of age or younger. *Pediatrics, 92,* 257.

Brenner, P. F., & Mishell, D. R. (1990). Control of hormone reproduction, contraception, sterilization and pregnancy termination In Scott, J. R. *Danforth's obstetrics and gynecology.* Philadelphia: J.B. Lippincott.

Chi, I. (1993). What we have learned from recent IUD studies: a researcher's perspective. *Contraception, 48,* 81.

Demystifying ovulation and pregnancy kits for your patients. *Contemporary OB/GYN, 38,* 67.

Department of Health and Human Services. (1991). *Healthy people 2000.* Washington, DC: Public Health Service.

Department of Health and Human Services. (1992a). Sexual behavior among high school students, United States, 1990. *Morbidity and Mortality Weekly Report, 40,* 1.

Department of Health and Human Services. (1992b). Unintended childbearing: pregnancy risk assessment monitoring system. *Morbidity and Mortality Weekly Report, 41,* 1.

Department of Health and Human Services. (1993a). Update: barrier protection against HIV infection and other sexually transmitted diseases. *Morbidity and Mortality Weekly Report, 42,* 589.

Department of Health and Human Services. (1993b). Abortion surveillance. *Morbidity and Mortality Weekly Report, 42,* 11.

Flattum-Reimers, J. (1991). Norplant: a new contraceptive. *American Family Physician, 44,* 103.

Frydman, R. (1992). Labor induction in women at term with mifepristone (RU 486). *Obstetrics and Gynecology, 80,* 972.

Glasier, A., et al. (1992). Mifepristone (RU 486) compared with high-dose estrogen and progestogen for emergency postcoital contraception. *New England Journal of Medicine, 327,* 1041.

Giovannucci, E., et al. (1992). Vasectomy and its effects on life-span. *New England Journal of Medicine, 326,* 1392.

Hatcher, R. A., et al. (1993). *Family planning at your fingertips.* New York: Irvington.

Henshaw, S. K. (1990). Induced abortion: A world review. *Family Planning Perspectives, 22,* 76.

Henshaw, S. K., & Kost, K. (1992). Parental involvement in minors' abortion decisions. *Family Planning Perspectives, 24,* 196.

Kaunitz, A. M. (1990). Long-acting progestin contraceptives. *Contemporary OB/GYN, 35,* 59S.

Kaunitz, A. M. (1993). DMPA: a new contraception option. *Contemporary OB/GYN, 38,* 19.

Kirkman, R., & Chantler, E. (1993). Contraception and the prevention of sexually transmitted diseases. *British Medical Bulletin, 49,* 171.

Klitsch, M. (1993). Vasectomy and prostate cancer; more questions than answers. *Family Planning Perspectives, 25,* 133.

Lethbridge, D. J. (1991). Coitus interruptus: considerations as a method of birth control. *Journal of Obstetric, Gynecologic, & Neonatal Nursing, 20,* 80.

Lipscomb, G. H. (1993). Laparoscopic sterilization under local anesthesia. *The Female Patient, 18,* 67.

Mastroianni, L., & Robinson, J. C. (1994). Contraception in the 1990s. *Patient Care, 28,* 107.

Mishell, D. R. (1993). Vaginal contraceptive rings. *Annals of Medicine, 25,* 191.

Murphy, A. A., et al. (1993). Regression of uterine leiomyomata in response to the antiprogesterone RU 486. *Journal of Clinical Endocrine Metabolism, 76,* 513.

Roth, B. (1993). Fertility awareness as a component of sexuality education. *Nurse Practitioner, 18,* 40.

Saarikoski, S. (1993). Contraception during lactation. *Annals of Medicine, 25,* 181.

Shain, R. N., et al. (1991). Impact of tubal sterilization and vasectomy on female marital sexuality. *American Journal of Obstetrics and Gynecology, 164,* 763.

Sharma, A., et al. (1993). Progesterone antagonist mifepristone (RU 486) decreases cardiotoxicity of cocaine. *Proceedings of the Society for Experimental Biology and Medicine, 202,* 279.

Sharts-Engel, N. (1991). Levonorgestrel subdermal implants (Norplant) for long term contraception. *MCN: American Journal of Maternal Child Nursing, 16,* 232.

Sharts-Hopko, N. C. (1993). Depo-Provera. *MCN: American Journal of Maternal Child Nursing, 18,* 128.

Soper, D. E., et al. (1993). Prevention of vaginal trichomoniasis by compliant use of the female condom. *Sexually Transmitted Diseases, 20,* 137.

Sundaram, K., et al. (1993). 7-a-methyl-notestosterone (MENT): the optimal androgen for male contraception. *Annals of Medicine, 25,* 199.

Talwar, G. P., et al. (1993). A birth control vaccine is on the horizon for family planning. *Annals of Medicine, 25,* 207.

Toivonen, J. (1993). Intrauterine contraceptive devices and pelvic inflammatory disease. *Annals of Medicine, 25,* 171.

Townsend, D.E., et al. (1993). Post-ablation-tubal sterilization syndrome. *Obstetrics & Gynecology, 82,* 422.

Trussell, J., Strickler, J., & Vaughan, B. (1993). Contraceptive efficacy of the diaphragm, the sponge and the cervical cap. *Family Planning Perspectives, 25,* 100.

Weiss, B. D., et al. (1991). The cervical cap. *American Family Physician, 43,* 517.

Welner, S. L. (1993). Gynecologic care of the disabled woman. *Contemporary OB/GYN, 38,* 55.

Williams-Dean, M., & Potter, L. (1993). Standardizing the instructions for oral contraceptive use. *The Female Patient, 18,* 77.

Wilson, M. D. (1994). Adolescent pregnancy and contraception. In Oski, F. A., et al. *Principles and practice of pediatrics.* Philadelphia: J. B. Lippincott.

Yuzpe, A. (1991). Current status of OCs. *Contemporary OB/GYN, 36,* 77.

Suggested Readings

Bullough, B., et al. (1991). Contraceptives for teenagers. *Journal of Pediatric Health Care, 5,* 237.

Croxatto, H. B. (1993). Norplant: levonorgestrel-releasing contraceptive implant. *Annals of Medicine, 25,* 155.

Emerling, J. M., et al. (1993). Subdermal contraceptive implants in nurse-midwifery practice. *Journal of Nurse Midwifery, 38,* 80S.

Fehring, R. V. (1991). New technology in natural family planning. *Journal of Obstetrical, Gynecologic and Neonatal Nursing, 20,* 199.

Goldstein, M. (1993). Vasectomy reversal. *Comprehensive Therapy, 19,* 37.

Howard, M., & McCabe, J. (1990). Helping teenagers postpone sexual involvement. *Family Planning Perspectives, 22,* 21.

Jarrett, M. E., & Lethbridge, D. J. (1990). The contraceptive needs of midlife women. *Nurse Practitioner, 15,* 34.

Orr, D. P., et al. (1992). Factors associated with condom use among sexually active female adolescents. *Journal of Pediatrics, 120,* 311.

Parazzini, F., et al. (1994). Contraceptive methods and risk of pelvic endometriosis. *Contraception, 49,* 199.

Poindexter, A. N. (1990). Laparoscopic tubal sterilization under local anesthesia. *Obstetrics and Gynecology, 75,* 5.

Root, W. B. (1992). Contraception for midlife women. *NAACOGS Clinical Issues in Perinatal & Women's Health Nursing, 3,* 227.

Trussell, J., & Grummer-Strawn, L. (1990). Contraceptive failure of the method of periodic abstinence. *Family Planning Perspectives, 22,* 65.

Weiss, B., et al. (1991). The cervical cap. *American Family Practice, 43,* 517.

Wells, C. B. (1993) Speaking of sex. *American Journal of Nursing, 93,* 93.

Wendell, E., et al. (1992). Youth at risk: sex, drugs and human immunodeficiency virus. *American Journal of Diseases of Children, 146,* 76.

Winter, L., & Breckenmaker, L. C. (1991). Tailoring family planning services to the special needs of adolescents. *Family Planning Perspectives, 23,* 24.

The Infertile Family

Chapter 6

Key Terms

- anovulation
- cryptorchidism
- endometriosis
- failure to achieve ejaculation
- infertility
- mumps orchitis
- primary infertility
- secondary infertility
- sperm count
- sperm motility
- spermatogenesis

Objectives

After mastering the contents of this chapter, you should be able to:

1. Describe common causes of infertility in men and women.

2. Describe common assessments necessary to detect infertility.

3. Formulate nursing diagnoses related to infertility.

4. Plan nursing care specific to relieving or coping with a diagnosis of infertility.

5. Assist with implementations involved in a diagnostic fertility study or assist a couple to achieve further fertility, such as health teaching about the time of ovulation.

6. Evaluate outcome criteria to be certain that nursing goals were achieved.

7. Identify National Health Goals related to infertility that nurses can participate in helping the nation to achieve.

8. Identify areas of nursing care related to fertility that could benefit from additional nursing research.

9. Use critical thinking to analyze nursing strategies that can be used to support a couple through a fertility assessment.

10. Synthesize concern for problems of infertility with nursing process to achieve quality maternal and child health nursing care.

Adele Pillitteri: MATERNAL AND CHILD
HEALTH NURSING, 2nd Edition. © 1995
Adele Pillitteri.

Infertility, or the inability to conceive a child or sustain a pregnancy to childbirth, affects as many as 10% to 15% of couples who desire children (Bernhardt, 1990). When a couple comes to a health care agency for fertility counseling, they often arrive with a set of fears and anxieties not only about the inability to conceive but what this condition means to themselves and their family. Without information about the cause of their infertility, each may blame himself or herself or carry unexpressed anger toward his or her partner. In addition, the couple may strongly desire a child but also feel the normal anxieties associated with impending parenthood—loss of independence and an established lifestyle. Infertility screening and counseling in itself can be an emotionally difficult and physically demanding process, often creating much strain on a couple's relationship.

A number of National Health Goals aimed at reducing infertility are shown in the Focus on National Health Goals box. Nurses are vital members of fertility health care teams and often assume responsibility for health assessment and client education and counseling (Marshak, 1993). The nurse will work with clients and other members of the health care team to determine the cause of infertility; help clients solidify their feelings about the desire to have children and how far they are willing to go in terms of testing and procedures to achieve this de-

sire; educate clients about the available procedures (many of which are complex and demand knowledgeable, ongoing participation); and participate in the planning and implementation of treatment strategies. When pregnancy cannot be achieved, nurses can counsel clients about the available alternatives.

 ## NURSING PROCESS OVERVIEW
for Families With Infertility

ASSESSMENT

Infertility is a problem that strikes at the core of a couple's self-image and self-esteem. Nursing assessment will often reveal that one or both partners feels inadequate or angry and frustrated. It may be possible to detect such feelings while gathering information for the history. Questions such as, "How do you feel about this problem?" or "How do you think your wife [husband] feels about not being able to conceive thus far?" may be enough to encourage partners to express their concerns. Talking with both the man and woman together may be advantageous because they may feel more comfortable speaking about their problem together. On the other hand, it is important to spend some time alone with each client in case there is anything a partner wishes to discuss privately. This might be the only opportunity one of them has to ask that one "silly" question or voice a fear that they feel is too foolish to ask or bring up in front of their partner.

NURSING DIAGNOSIS

Nursing diagnoses related to problems of infertility are likely to focus on psychosocial issues associated with the inability to conceive and the long, arduous process of fertility testing and management. Possible diagnoses include:

- Fear related to outcome of infertility studies
- Decreased self-esteem related to the inability to conceive
- Anxiety related to the heavy schedule of planned testing
- Grieving related to failed conception or failed pregnancy

If a specific problem is revealed in this area or if testing and therapy become so overwhelming for a couple that their relationship (including sexual patterns) begins to unravel, Sexual dysfunction related to "command performance" of infertility therapy might be applicable. Powerlessness related to repeated unsuccessful attempts at achieving conception and Hopelessness related to no viable alternatives to usual conception being perceived may also be relevant.

PLANNING AND IMPLEMENTATION

In setting goals with a couple for fertility testing, attempt to ensure that the couple realizes that because testing takes a long time, results will not be instantaneous. A couple may need to change or modify their goals if tests begin to show that what they first wanted—to have a child without medical intervention—is impossible.

Some health insurance programs do not provide money for fertility testing, although coverage of surgery such as that to relieve endometriosis would be covered. Because of this, couples need specific estimates of the cost of testing or therapy and may need help budgeting and planning their resources accordingly.

Suggesting that a couple begin a new activity together such as taking a night school course, planting a garden, or learning a new sport or hobby at the same time they begin fertility testing is a way of helping them reduce the feeling that their entire existence is revolving around the testing procedures. This also gives them hours of shared experiences and intimacy that helps to compensate for any decreased enjoyment that comes from "scheduled" sexual relations.

Depending on their motivations, a couple's reaction to study results may vary from relief to stoic acceptance to grief for children never to be born. Each partner may wonder whether the other will be able to accept marriage if he or she turns out to be the "infertile" one. Couples need the support of health care personnel throughout the course of infertility studies, so that in the event of bad news, they have people who have stood by them from the first day they braced themselves to ask, "Exactly why are we childless?"

Participation in a support group may be helpful to allow a couple to work through the stress this places on their lives (Marshak, 1993). Resolve (1310 Broadway, Somerville, MA 02144-1731) is a national support group for couples with infertility that can be helpful in offering referral sources and support that a couple can use to aid in planning. Another organization is the American Fertility Society, 2140 11th Avenue, Suite 200, Birmingham, AL 35205-2800.

EVALUATION

Examples of goal outcomes in this area might be:

- Client rearranges work plans in order to manage heavy schedule of testing by one month.
- Couple demonstrates a high level of self-esteem following fertility studies, even in the face of disappointing study outcomes.

Evaluation should be ongoing with a couple who has a problem of infertility, because as circumstances around them change, so may their goals and desires. Until they can accept an alternative method of having children, such as adoption or artificial insemination, for-

---

FOCUS ON
National Health Goals

One of the year 2000 National Health Goals directly addresses the problem of infertility. This is:

- Reduce the prevalence of infertility to no more than 6.5% from a baseline of 7.9% (DHHS, 1991).

To meet this health goal, nurses will need to be active in teaching safer sex practices (see Chapter 4) in order to help reduce the incidence of sexually transmitted diseases and pelvic inflammatory disease that can contribute to infertility. Nursing research to investigate such areas as how to help women better recognize the symptoms of pelvic inflammatory disease is also necessary.

mer plans have been crushed. It is not unusual to see a couple move through steps of denial, anger, bargaining, and depression before they reach a level of acceptance that they are different in this one area of life from others, but not limited in their ability to achieve in other areas. With acceptance, they are able to make adjustments in their wants or plans to feel fulfilled.

Future evaluation is also important, because a couple who decides at age 20 that they want to choose childfree living may change their mind at a later date. A couple who chooses artificial insemination may decide after a number of unsuccessful attempts that they are no longer interested in this method of conception. Keeping evaluation an ongoing process allows such a plan to be modified as necessary. Couples seen for fertility testing can be encouraged to telephone or visit every 6 months to 1 year to inquire about new discoveries in the field of fertility and how these apply to their situation.

Infertility

Infertility is said to exist when a pregnancy has not occurred after at least 1 year of unprotected coitus (Hughes & Hammond, 1990). In **primary infertility**, there have been no previous conceptions; in **secondary infertility**, there has been a previous viable pregnancy but the couple is unable to conceive at present. *Sterility* refers to the inability to conceive because of a known condition, such as the absence of a uterus; about one in five to six couples is infertile. In about 40% of couples with an infertility problem, the cause of infertility is multifactorial; in about 30% of couples, it is the man who is infertile; 20% to 30% of couples experience ovulatory failure; and 20% to 40% experience tubal, vaginal, or uterine problems as the cause of their infertility. In as many as 15% of couples, no known cause for the infertility can be discovered despite all the diagnostic tests currently available (Richard-Davis & Moghissi, 1993).

Some couples (unaware of the average length of time it takes to achieve a pregnancy) may worry that they are infertile when they are not. When engaging in coitus an average of four times per week, 50% of couples take 6 months to conceive; after 12 months, 85% of couples will conceive. These periods are longer if sexual relations are less frequent.

Couples who engage in coitus daily, hoping to cause early impregnation, may actually have more difficulty conceiving than those who delay coitus to every other day, because too frequent coitus can lower a man's spermatozoa count to a level below optimal fertility. Couples who focus their sexual relations on trying to increase sperm-ova exposure may also find their lives governed by temperature charts and "good days" and "bad days" to such an extent that their relationship suffers.

The chance of infertility increases with age. Because of this gradual decline in fertility, about one third of women who defer pregnancy to their mid- to late thirties will have an infertility problem (Maroulis, 1993). Women who have been taking oral contraceptives, using Depo-Provera or Norplant (levonorgestrel) should know that they may have difficulty becoming pregnant for several months after discontinuing the medication (anywhere between 2 to 7 months on average), because it takes this long to restore normal body functioning.

Male Infertility Factors

A number of factors may lead to male infertility: a disturbance in **spermatogenesis** (the production of sperm cells); an obstruction in the seminiferous tubules, ducts, or vessels that prevents movement of spermatozoa; qualitative or quantitative changes in the seminal fluid that prevents **sperm motility** (movement of sperm); autoimmunity that immobilizes sperm; or a problem in ejaculation or deposition that prevents spermatozoa from being placed close enough to the woman's cervix to penetrate it and fertilize the ovum.

Inadequate Sperm Count

A **sperm count** is a count of the number of sperm in a single ejaculation or milliliter of semen. The minimum sperm count considered normal is 20 million per milliliter of seminal fluid, or a total of 50 million per ejaculation. At least 60% of sperm should be motile, and 60% should be normal in shape and form. Spermatozoa must be produced and maintained at a temperature slightly lower than body temperature to become normal and fully motile. The testes, in which sperm are produced and stored, are suspended in the scrotal sac away from body heat. Men who work at desk jobs or who drive a great deal every day, such as salesmen or motorcyclists (actions which increase scrotal heat), may have lower sperm counts than men whose occupations allow them to be ambulatory at least part of each day. Frequent use of hot tubs or saunas may also lower sperm counts appreciably. Yet another reason for an inadequate sperm count is a chronic infection such as tuberculosis or recurrent sinusitis because of the elevated temperature that may accompany an infection.

Many other conditions can impair spermatogenesis. Congenital abnormalities such as **cryptorchidism** (undescended testes) may lead to lowered sperm production if surgical repair of this problem was not completed until after puberty, or if the spermatic cord became twisted following the surgery (Thompson, 1993). Sons of women who took diethylstilbestrol during pregnancy have an increased chance of producing abnormal sperm.

Other conditions that may inhibit sperm production include trauma to the testes; surgery on or near the testicles that results in impaired testicular circulation; the presence of varicocele (varicosity of the spermatic vein);

and endocrine imbalances, particularly in the thyroid, pancreas, and pituitary glands. Drug or alcohol abuse and environmental factors such as excessive exposure to x-rays or radioactive substances have been found to negatively affect spermatogenesis (Bernhardt, 1990). Men exposed to radioactive substances on the job should have adequate protection of the testes. When undergoing pelvic x-rays men should always be furnished with a protective lead shield.

Obstruction or Impaired Sperm Motility

Obstruction may occur at any point in the pathway that spermatozoa must travel to reach the outside: the seminiferous tubules, the epididymis, the vas deferens, the ejaculatory duct, and the urethra (see Chapter 4, Figure 4-1). Diseases such as *mumps orchitis* (testicular inflammation and scarring) and *epididymitis* (inflammation of the epididymis) may impair transport of sperm through the seminiferous tubules (Kaler, 1990). Tubal infection such as occurs with gonorrhea or ascending urethral infection may result in adhesions and occlusions; congenital stricture of a spermatic duct is sometimes seen. Hypertrophy of the prostate gland occurs in many men beginning at about age 50 years. Pressure from this on the vas deferens may interfere with sperm transport. Infection of the prostate gland through which the seminal fluid passes or infection of the seminal vesicles (spread from urinary tract infections) can change the composition of the seminal fluid enough to reduce sperm motility.

It has been shown that men who have vasectomies may develop an autoimmune reaction or may form antibodies that immobilize their own sperm. It is conceivable that men with obstruction in the vas deferens from other causes could also develop a reaction that is immobilizing sperm (Alexander, 1990).

Anomalies of the penis, such as *hypospadias* (urethral opening on the ventral surface of the penis) or *epispadias* (urethral opening on the dorsal surface) may cause deposition of spermatozoa too far from the cervix to allow for cervical penetration. Extreme obesity may also interfere with penetration.

Ejaculation Problems

Psychologic problems and debilitating diseases may result in **failure to achieve ejaculation** (formerly called impotence). This is *primary* if the man has never been able to achieve erection and ejaculation, *secondary* if the man has been able to achieve ejaculation in the past. Failure to achieve ejaculation may be a relatively easily solved problem if it is associated with stress. If the failure of ejaculation is caused by a deep-seated psychologic issue (*psychogenic infertility*), a solution to the problem will include psychologic or sexual counseling and may involve long-term care (Ackerman et al., 1994). Premature ejaculation (ejaculation before penetra-

tion) is yet another problem often attributed to psychologic causes. This may affect the proper deposition of sperm (Stine & Collins, 1990).

Female Infertility Factors

The factors that cause infertility in women are analogous to those causing infertility in men: **anovulation** (faulty or inadequate production of ova); problems of ova transport through the fallopian tubes to the uterus; uterine factors such as tumors or poor endometrial development; and cervical and vaginal factors that immobilize spermatozoa.

Anovulation

Anovulation is the most common cause of infertility in women. Anovulation may occur from a genetic abnormality such as Turner's syndrome (*hypogonadism*) in which there are no ovaries to produce ova. It may also occur not as a primary ovarian problem but as an imbalance of hypothalamus-pituitary-ovarian interplay caused by a condition such as hypothyroidism. Ovarian tumors may produce anovulation due to feedback stimulation on the pituitary. Chronic or excessive exposure to x-rays or radioactive substances may be involved. General ill health, poor diet, or stress may all contribute to poor ovarian function. Stress affects the ovaries by reducing hypothalamus GnRH secretion, which then lowers luteinizing hormone (LH) and follicle-stimulating hormone (FSH) production (Berga, 1993). Decreased body weight, or a body-fat ratio of less than 10%, such as develops in female athletes (such as runners) or in women who are excessively lean or anorexic, can reduce pituitary hormones and halt ovulation.

In addition, ovulatory patterns vary greatly among women; some women may only ovulate a few times a year. Sometimes this can be determined by looking at the menstrual history, but even if a woman experiences regular monthly menstruation, it does not necessarily indicate that she is also ovulating on a regular basis.

Tubal Transport Problems

Difficulty with tubal transport usually occurs because of scarring in the fallopian tubes. This usually occurs from chronic salpingitis (chronic pelvic inflammatory disease or PID; Benrubi, 1990). It can result from a ruptured appendix or abdominal surgery in which infection was involved and adhesions formed.

Pelvic Inflammatory Disease. Pelvic inflammatory disease (PID) is infection of the pelvic organs: the uterus, fallopian tubes, ovaries, and their supporting structures. The infection can extend to cause pelvic peritonitis. Many organisms can cause PID, but gonorrhea and chlamydia are the most frequent offenders (Romanowski, 1993). The rate of PID among 15- to 24-year-olds has risen dramatically in recent years, primarily due to the prevalence of sexually transmitted infections (Eschenbach, 1990). Although sexual transmittal accounts for about 75% of all PID, infections from other causes such as *Escherichia coli* and *Streptococcus* are beginning to be recognized and may be as severe. There is also a higher incidence of PID in women using IUDs, a compelling reason for not recommending IUDs to women with multiple sexual partners (Farley et al., 1992).

PID begins with a cervical infection that spreads by surface invasion along the uterine endometrium and then out to the fallopian tubes and ovaries. Bacterial invasion is most apt to occur at the end of a menstrual period, because menstrual blood provides an excellent growth medium and there is loss of the normal cervical mucous barrier at this time. When left unrecognized and untreated, pelvic inflammatory disease enters a chronic phase, which can result in the scarring that can lead to stricture of the fallopian tubes and resulting fertility problems. The number of episodes of PID increases the risk of infertility. As many as 25% of women with PID are hospitalized; of these, 25% will need major surgery and 20% will be left with significant tube blockage that will reduce fertility (Eschenbach, 1990).

Uterine Problems

Inadequate endometrium formation resulting from poor secretion of estrogen or progesterone from the ovary is the main cause of infertility from a uterine factor (the primary factor here is actually ovarian). Tumors such as fi-

bromas (leiomyomas) may be a cause of infertility in that they block the entrance to fallopian tubes into the uterus or limit the space available for effective implantation; many women with huge fibromas, however, do become pregnant. A congenitally deformed uterine cavity may limit implantation sites, but this is a rare occurrence.

Endometriosis. **Endometriosis** is the implantation of uterine endometrium, or nodules, which have spread from the uterus to locations outside the uterus (Younger, 1993). The most common sites of endometrium spread are Douglas's cul-de-sac, the ovaries, the uterine ligaments, and the outer surface of the uterus and bowel (Figure 6-1).

Endometriosis occurs in as many as 25% of women (Berger, 1993). The spread of endometrium this way is probably due to regurgitation through the fallopian tubes at the time of menstruation. Viable particles of endometrium regurgitated this way begin to proliferate and grow at the new sites. When fallopian tube implants occur, they may cause tube obstruction; the presence of peritoneal macrophages drawn to the abnormal tissue can destroy sperm; adhesions that form from these growths may displace fallopian tubes away from the ovaries and so prevent ova from entering tubes. The occurrence of endometriosis may indicate an endometrium that has different or more friable qualities than the normal endometrium (perhaps due to a luteal phase defect); such an endometrium also may not support implantation as well (see Chapter 47 for the treatment of endometriosis).

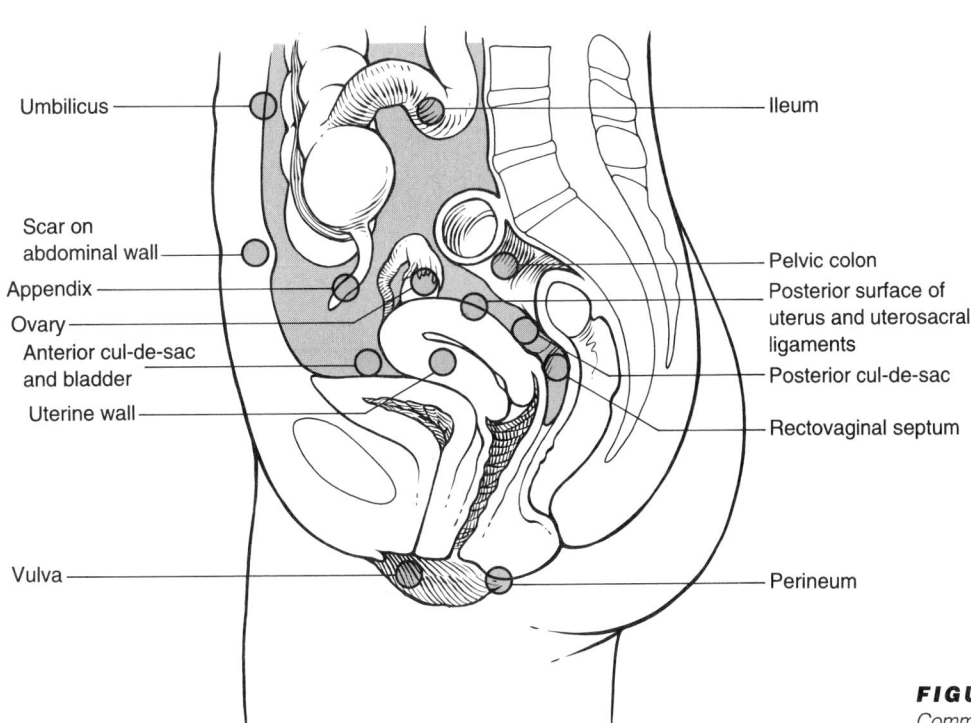

Umbilicus

Scar on abdominal wall

Appendix

Ovary

Anterior cul-de-sac and bladder

Uterine wall

Vulva

Ileum

Pelvic colon

Posterior surface of uterus and uterosacral ligaments

Posterior cul-de-sac

Rectovaginal septum

Perineum

FIGURE 6-1
Common sites of endometriosis formation.

Cervical Problems

At the time of ovulation, cervical mucus becomes thin and watery and can be easily penetrated by spermatozoa for a period of 12 to 72 hours. If coitus is not synchronized with this time period, spermatozoa may not be able to penetrate the cervix. Infection or inflammation of the cervix (erosion) may cause so much thickening in cervical mucus that spermatozoa cannot penetrate it easily or survive in it. A tight cervical os or obstruction of the os by a polyp may compound infertility but is rarely enough of a problem to be the sole cause of it. The woman who has undergone dilatation and curettage (D&C) procedures several times or cervical conization (cervical surgery) should be evaluated in light of the possibility that scar tissue and tightening of the cervical os could have occurred. A woman who has undergone several D&C procedures or has had vacuum extractions for abortions performed may develop a cervix that does not close completely (an incompetent cervix). This is not as much a problem of conception, however, as it is of maintaining a pregnancy (see Chapter 15).

Vaginal Problems

Infection of the vagina may cause the *p*H of the vaginal secretions to become acidotic, limiting or destroying the motility of spermatozoa (Shesser, 1990). Some women appear to have sperm-immobilizing or sperm-agglutinating antibodies in the blood plasma that act to destroy sperm cells in the vagina (Alexander, 1990). Both or either of these problems can limit the ability of sperm to enter the uterus.

Unexplained Infertility

In about 10% of couples, no known cause for infertility can be discovered. Possibly the problems of either partner alone are not significant, but when combined they become enough to create infertility. It is obviously discouraging for couples to complete a fertility series and be told that no reason for their inability to conceive can be explained. Such couples need support from health care providers to help them find alternative solutions, such as continuing to try to conceive, choosing to adopt, or agreeing to a childfree life.

Fertility Assessment

Not all couples who desire fertility testing want children. Some want to know for their own peace of mind that they are fertile, but do not plan on having children at the present time; others want to know that they are indeed infertile so that they can discontinue contraceptive measures.

The age of the couple and the degree of apprehension they feel make a difference in determining when

they should be referred for fertility evaluation. As a rule of thumb, if the woman is younger than age 30 years, she should be referred after 1 year of infertility; if older than age 30 years, after 6 months of infertility. Studies are more quickly undertaken with older women, because adoption, artificial insemination, and embryo transfer (ET)—the alternatives to natural childbearing (besides childfree living, which must not be discounted)—are limited by age. It would be doubly unfortunate if a couple delayed fertility testing past the point of being able to conceive, and also to a point at which an adoption agency would consider them "too old" to be prospective parents. If the couple is extremely apprehensive over their apparent infertility, studies should never be delayed, regardless of the couple's age.

Because infertility may be a problem of either partner, fertility studies must involve both partners (see the Focus on Nursing Research box).

History

Nurses often assume the responsibility for initial history taking with the infertile couple. Because of the wide variety of factors potentially responsible for causing infertility, it is important that the history be as thorough as possible. The history for the man should cover general health, nutrition, alcohol, drug or tobacco use; congenital health problems such as hypospadias or crypt-

FOCUS ON NURSING RESEARCH

Are There Differences in the Ways That Men and Women React to Infertility?

To answer this question, Phipps asked a sample of 8 white, middle-class couples about the meaning of being infertile. The males ranged in age from 26 to 40; all were college graduates, held white collar jobs, and had yearly incomes of $35,000/year or more. The wive's ages were 23 to 41; all had completed or attended college.

Feelings associated with infertility by men were sorrow, isolation, hope, urgency, guilt, powerlessness, and anger. Women identified sorrow, isolation, urgency, guilt, powerlessness, and loss of control. Methods of coping that men employed to deal with infertility were cognitive processes, avoidance, and faith in God; in addition to these, women identified verbal expression and humor.

The researcher concluded that infertility is a frustrating experience for both men and women. Nurses could be therapeutic by helping couples identify their coping strategies and supporting them with these.

From Phipps, S. A. (1993). A phenomenological study of couples' infertility: gender influence. *Holistic Nursing Practice, 7,* 44.

orchidism; illnesses such as mumps orchitis, urinary tract infection, or sexually transmitted disease; operations such as surgical repair of a hernia, which could have resulted in a blood compromise to the testes; and current illnesses, particularly endocrine illnesses. The man's occupation and work habits now and in the past (e.g., Does his job involve sitting at a desk all day or exposure to x-rays or other forms of radiation?) are also important.

It is important to document the frequency of coitus and masturbation, the occurrence of failure to achieve ejaculation or premature ejaculation, the coital positions used, whether lubricants are used, what contraceptive measures have been used, and whether the man has ever produced children in a previous marriage or relationship. Cultural or religious values should also be elicited (see the Focus on Cultural Awareness box).

For the woman, a menstrual history should be obtained, including the age of menarche, the length and frequency of menstrual periods, the amount of flow, and any difficulties she experiences such as pain or premenstrual syndrome. The woman should be asked about current or past reproductive tract infections; her overall health, emphasizing endocrine problems; and any abdominal or pelvic operations she might have had. Ask also: How often does she use douches or intravaginal medication or sprays? (These may interfere with vaginal

pH.) Is she exposed to occupational hazards such as x-rays or toxic substances? It is also important to obtain a history of previous pregnancies or abortions and to ask questions about her use of contraceptives.

In addition to history taking, take time with each partner individually, as well as a couple, to encourage questions and to discuss overall attitudes toward sexual relations, pregnancy, and parenting. A frank discussion centered on resolving the couple's fears and clearing up any longstanding confusion or misinformation will set a positive tone for future interactions, establish a feeling of trust, and increase self-esteem. When talking together with both partners, this process can also help them clarify their own feelings about infertility and why they are seeking help in this area (see the Nursing Care Plan: The Family Seeking a Fertility Evaluation).

Physical Assessment

Following a thorough history, both men and women need a complete physical examination. Of particular importance in men is the observation of secondary sexual characteristics and genital abnormalities, such as the absence of a vas deferens or the presence of undescended testes. The presence of a *varicocele* (enlargement of a testicular vein) is associated with infertility probably due to venous congestion and scrotal warmth. The presence of a *hydrocele* (collection of fluid in the tunica vaginalis of the scrotum) is indirectly associated with infertility but should be documented if present.

For the woman, a thorough physical assessment is also necessary to rule out current illness. Of particular importance are secondary sex characteristics, which indicate maturity and pituitary function. A complete pelvic examination (see Chapter 10) is needed to rule out gross anatomic defects and infection (Willms & Newman, 1994).

Laboratory Tests

To rule out poor health as a causative factor for infertility, the following laboratory tests are usually included in the male studies: urinalysis; complete blood count; blood typing, including Rh factor; serologic test for syphilis; sometimes a sedimentation rate (increased rate indicates inflammation); protein-bound iodine (test for thyroid function); cholesterol level; gonadotropin; prolactin; and testosterone level. A sonogram or x-ray study of the excretory portion of the genital tract using a contrast medium might be indicated (Werner & Lipshultz, 1993). Semen analysis (see below) is done.

To determine the woman's general state of health, laboratory tests similar to those done on the man will be ordered: urinalysis and complete blood count, and possibly a sedimentation rate, a serologic test for syphilis,

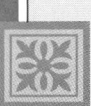

FOCUS ON CULTURAL AWARENESS

Many marriage customs such as throwing rice are rituals to promote fertility. That such rituals commonly exist is evidence of how important having children is to the average couple and to society as a whole. If an infertility problem arises it can, therefore, cause an extreme hardship for a family and can result in dissolution of marriages or relationships. If infertility does occur, it is automatically assigned to be the woman's fault in most societies. Many women, even after careful explanation that the problem is their male partner's and not theirs, continue to show low self-esteem as if the fault rests with them.

How often couples engage in sexual relations can affect fertility. This can be influenced by culture and religion. According to Orthodox Jewish law, for example, a couple may not engage in sexual relations for 7 days following menstruation (the "nida" period). This can result in fertility problems if the woman ovulates within the 7-day period.

Being aware that cultural differences can influence how a couple reacts to a diagnosis of infertility helps you to appreciate the meaning of this diagnosis to an individual couple.

Susan Mercer is a 23-year-old woman you care for in a health care setting for a fertility evaluation. The following is a nursing care plan designed for her.

Assessment: Client is unable to conceive after 2 years of unprotected coitus. Sexual relations about 2 times a week. Keeps temperature chart daily; is aware of concept of fertile and infertile periods. Has temperature increase, suggesting ovulation on 17th day of cycle as a rule. Menstrual cycle 30–32 days, 5 days' duration, heavy flow with painful cramping. No history of STD; normal activity level, although she has a scanty diet pattern. Had abdominal surgery for appendicitis as 12-year-old. No gynecologic surgery. Sometimes has dyspareunia. Has slight vaginal frothy discharge now; some pruritus. Hemoglobin: 12 mg; normal urinalysis; vaginal culture positive for *Trichomonas*.

Nursing Diagnosis: Fear related to apparent infertility

Defining Characteristic: Client expresses fear that she will be unable to conceive children.

Goal: Client will demonstrate understanding of the process of fertility testing and how it helps pinpoint problems that are often, although not always, correctable.

Outcome Criteria: Client states realistic future plans related to outcomes of fertility testing.

Nursing Orders	*Rationale*
1. Explain and schedule fertility testing pattern as determined by physician.	1. A year of no pregnancy with unprotected coitus is the definition of infertility. Understanding the assessment plan can decrease fear and frustration.
2. Discuss husband-wife relationship and coping ability; frustrations and disappointment;	2. Fertility testing can be frustrating and disappointing if length of testing period is prolonged.

Nursing Diagnosis: Knowledge deficit related to symptoms of *Trichomonas*

Defining Characteristic: Client is unable to associate current symptoms with infection.

Goal: Client will describe symptoms of vaginal infection and necessity for therapy by next clinic visit.

Outcome Criteria: Vaginal culture is negative for organisms at next clinic visit; client describes vaginal discharge as symptom of infection.

Nursing Orders	*Rationale*
1. Discuss importance of taking drug metronidazole (Flagyl) as prescribed by physician for vaginal infection.	1. Flagyl is the drug of choice for *Trichomonas*.
2. Discuss importance of husband reporting to clinic for a culture and using a condom for next week.	2. Ensure that husband does not reinfect the client.
3. Discuss importance of not continuing to take Flagyl if she should suspect she is pregnant.	3. The drug may be teratogenic in early pregnancy.

and a T_3 and T_4 uptake determination. A basal metabolic rate may be taken. If the woman has a history of menstrual irregularities, blood will be assayed for follicle-stimulating hormone (FSH); estrogen; luteinizing hormone (LH); and progesterone levels. A pelvic sonogram may reveal ovarian, tubal, or uterine structural disorders.

Semen Analysis

For a semen analysis, after 3 or 4 days of sexual abstinence, the man ejaculates by masturbation into a clean, dry specimen jar, and the spermatozoa are examined under a microscope before 2 hours. If the man brings in the specimen to the health care facility, he must be certain that it is not exposed to extreme cold or heat in transport, which destroys sperm mobility. For the analysis, the number of spermatozoa in the specimen are counted, and their appearance and motility are noted. An average ejaculation should produce 2.5 to 5.0 mL of semen. Moreover, it should contain a minimum of 20 million spermatozoa per milliliter of fluid, or a total of 50 million per ejaculation (the average normal sperm count is 50 to 200 million per milliliter). Two hours after ejaculation, 60% to 70% of sperm cells should still be vigorously active.

Ovulation Determination by Basal Body Temperature

Basal body temperature is a test for ovulation; it documents the slight temperature increase (from .5 to 1°F) that normally occurs with the release of progesterone following ovulation. To determine this, the woman takes her temperature before getting out of bed each morning or engaging in any activity or eating or drinking. She plots this daily temperature on a monthly graph, noticing conditions that might affect her temperature (colds, other infections, or sleeplessness). At the time of ovulation, the basal temperature can be seen to dip slightly (about .5°), then rise to a degree higher than normal body temperature and stay at that level until 3 or 4 days before the next menstrual flow. The increase in basal body temperature marks the time of ovulation (actually the beginning of the luteal phase of the menstrual cycle, which only could have occurred if ovulation occurred). A temperature rise should last 10 days; if not, there is a luteal phase defect present (progesterone production begins but is not sustained). Graphs of basal body temperature are shown in Figure 6-2.

Ovulation Determination by Test Strip

Various brands of commercial kits are available for assessing the upsurge of LH that occurs just before ovulation. The woman dips a test strip into a midmorning urine specimen and then compares it with the kit instructions for a color change. Such kits are easy to use and have the advantage of marking the point just before ovulation occurs rather than after ovulation, as is the case with basal body temperature (Demystifying ovulation and pregnancy kits for your patients, 1993).

Ovulation Determination by Cervical Mucus Assessment

At the height of estrogen stimulation, cervical mucus is copious in amount, thin in consistency, and has a low viscosity and cellularity. It "ferns" or forms a distinct pattern when allowed to dry. It can be graded according to Table 6-1.

Fern Test. When high levels of estrogen are present in the body, as they are just before ovulation, the cervical mucus forms fernlike patterns when it is smeared

Basal body temperature

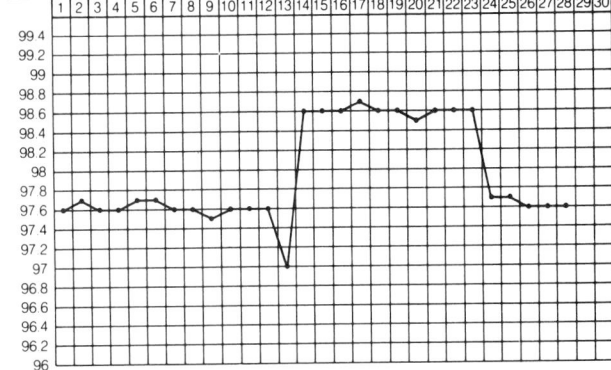

A   Ovulation without conception

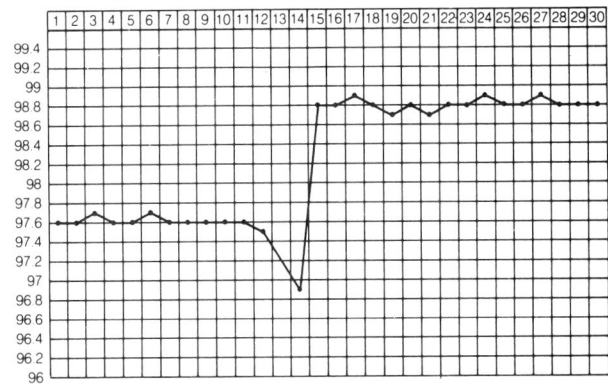

B   Ovulation with conception

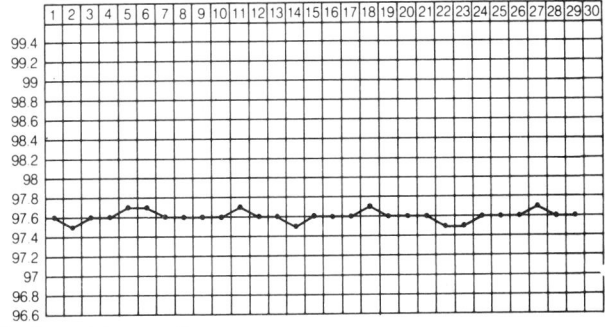

C   Anovulatory cycle

FIGURE 6-2
*Basal body temperature graph. (**A**) The woman's temperature dips slightly at midpoint in the menstrual cycle, then rises sharply, an indication of ovulation. Toward the end of the cycle (the 24th day), her temperature begins to decline, indicating that progesterone levels are falling and that she did not conceive. (**B**) The woman's temperature rises at the midpoint in the cycle and remains at that elevated level past the time of her normal menstrual flow, suggesting that pregnancy has occurred. (**C**) There is no preovulatory dip, and no rise of temperature anywhere during the cycle. This is the typical pattern of a woman who does not ovulate.*

Table 6-1. *Cervical Mucus Scoring**

Assessment Factor	Conditions	Score
Amount	None	0
	0.1 mL	1
	0.2 mL	2
	0.3 mL or greater	3
Spinnbarkeit	None	0
	1–4 cm	1
	5–8 cm	2
	9 cm or greater	3
Ferning	None	0
	Atypical (1+)	1
	2+	2
	3+ or 4+	3
Viscosity	4+	0
	3+	1
	2+	3
	1+	3
Cellularity	11 or greater	0
	6–10	1
	1–5	2
	Occasional	3

*Maximum score is 15; scores less than 10 represent unfavorable mucus, and scores less than 5 represent hostile cervical secretion.
(Richard-Davis, G., & Moghissi, K.S. [1993]. Basic evaluation of the infertile couple. *The Female Patient, 18,* 71.)

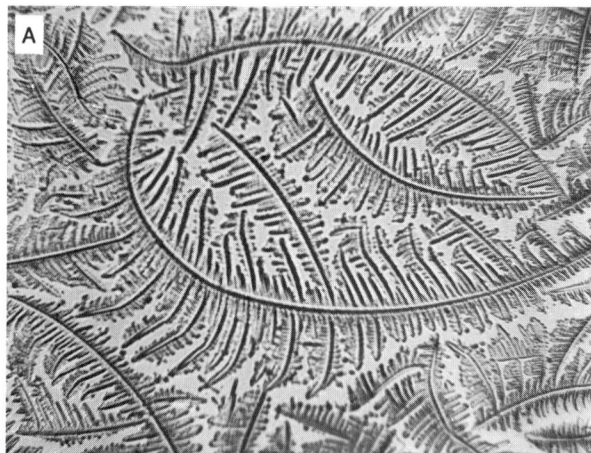

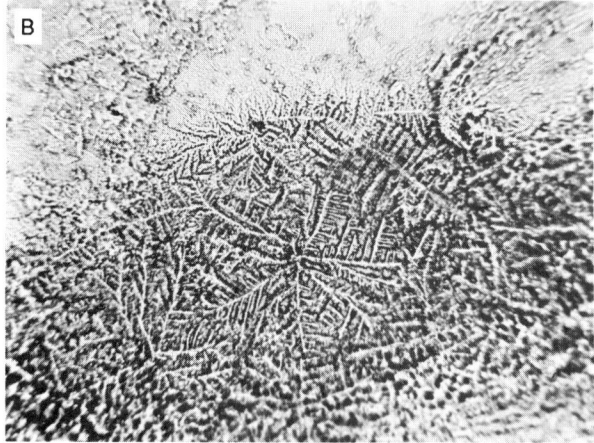

FIGURE 6-3
(**A**) *A ferning pattern of cervical mucus occurs with high estrogen levels.* (**B**) *Incomplete ferning during secretory phase of cycle.* (From Scott, J. R. [1990]. Danforth's obstetrics and gynecology [6th ed.]. Philadelphia: J.B. Lippincott, with permission.)

and dried on a glass slide. The patterns are due to crystallization of sodium chloride on mucus fibers, and this is known as *arborization,* or *ferning* (Figure 6-3). When progesterone is the dominant hormone, as it is just after ovulation when the luteal phase of the menstrual cycle is beginning, a fern pattern is no longer discernible. Fern tests are usually done at midcycle and again before menstruation, so that both patterns can be demonstrated. Women who do not ovulate continue to show the fern pattern throughout the menstrual cycle (progesterone levels never become dominant), or they never demonstrate it because their estrogen levels never rise.

Spinnbarkeit Test. At the height of estrogen secretion, the cervical mucus becomes thin and watery and can be stretched into long strands. This stretchability (to a distance of 13 cm to 15 cm) is in contrast to its thick, viscous state when progesterone is the dominant hormone. Taking spinnbarkeit patterns at a midpoint and a late point in the menstrual cycle can demonstrate that progesterone is being produced and, by implication, that ovulation has occurred. A woman can do this herself by stretching the sample between thumb and finger; or it can be tested in an examining room by smearing a cervical mucus specimen on a slide and stretching the mucus between the slide and cover slip (Figure 6-4).

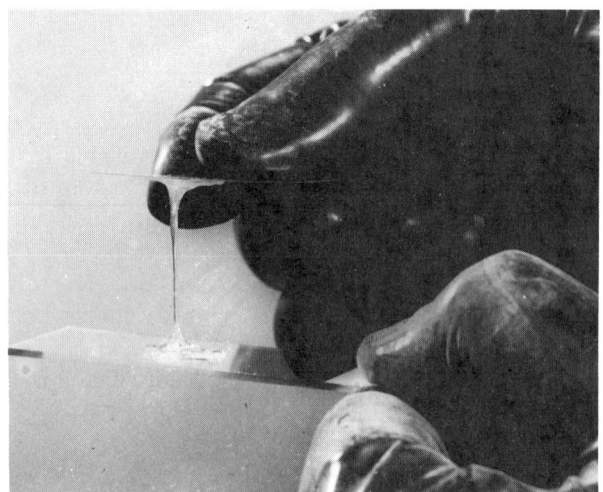

FIGURE 6-4
Spinnbarkeit is the property of cervical mucus to stretch a distance of 13 to 15 cm before breaking. (From Scott, J.R. [1990]. Danforth's obstetrics and gynecology [6th ed.]. Philadelphia: J.B. Lippincott, with permission.)

Postcoital Test

In a postcoital test, the time of ovulation is predicted from the woman's basal body temperature chart or a commercial ovulation predictor kit. The couple has coitus at this time and then the woman reports to the health care facility within 2 to 8 hours. With the woman in a lithotomy position, a specimen of cervical mucus is removed and examined microscopically for ferning and cell count and for viable spermatozoa. The postcoital test demonstrates how sperm interact with the woman's vaginal and cervical environment. A good result would show abundant, elastic mucus with a high number of motile sperm. If sperm are found to be clumped and immobile or if the mucus is very thick, this may indicate a problem with timing or could point to a sperm antibody problem. A finding of no sperm could indicate azoospermia. Once a mainstay of infertility testing, postcoital tests currently are not used as much as formerly because their scheduling is difficult and they may yield little more information than a single sperm or cervical mucus analysis reveals.

Surgical Testing

Uterine Endometrial Biopsy

Uterine endometrial biopsy may be used as a test for ovulation or to reveal an endometrial problem such as a luteal phase defect (Mashburn, 1993). If a corkscrew-like appearance of the endometrium (a typical progesterone-dominated endometrium) is found on examination, it suggests that ovulation has occurred.

The biopsy is usually done 2 or 3 days before an expected menstrual flow (day 25 or 26 of a typical menstrual cycle) by introducing a thin probe and biopsy forceps through the cervix. It involves slight discomfort from the maneuvering of the instruments, and there is a moment of sharp pain as the biopsy specimen is taken from the anterior or posterior uterus. The risks of the procedure are pain, excessive bleeding, infection, or uterine perforation. It is contraindicated if pregnancy is suspected, although the chance it would interfere with a pregnancy is probably under 10%. It is also contraindicated if an infection such as acute PID or cervicitis is present. The woman should be cautioned to expect a small amount of spotting following the procedure, but she should call back if she develops a temperature of more than 101°F, has a large amount of bleeding, or passes clots. It is important for the woman to telephone the health care agency when she has her next menstrual flow to help "date" the endometrium.

Laparoscopy

Laparoscopy is the introduction of a thin, hollow, lighted tube (a fiberoptic telescope or *laparoscope*) through a small incision in the abdomen just under the umbilicus to examine the position and state of the fallopian tubes and ovaries. It is scheduled during the follicular phase of a menstrual period and done under general anesthesia to allow for good relaxation and a steep Trendelenburg position (which brings the reproductive organs down out of the pelvis). Carbon dioxide is introduced into the abdomen to cause the abdominal wall to move outward and offer better visualization. Women may feel a bloating of their abdomen after such a procedure; if some carbon dioxide escapes under the diaphragm, they may feel extremely sharp shoulder pain.

Laparoscopy technique is shown in Figure 5-11. It may be used to view the proximity of the ovaries to the fallopian tubes (if the distance is too great, the discharged ovum cannot enter the tube). Dye can be injected into the uterus during the procedure by a polyethylene cannula placed in the cervix and tubal patency assessed by observing if the dye appears in the abdominal cavity (tubal lavage). Inspection of the fallopian tubes reveals whether fimbria are present or not. If fimbria have been destroyed owing to pelvic inflammatory disease, the chance for normal conception is in doubt, because ovum seem unable to enter the tube without the fimbrial currents present.

Hysterosalpingography

Hysterosalpingography (uterosalpingography) is roentgenography of the fallopian tubes using a radiopaque medium. It is done immediately following the menstrual flow to avoid unintentional irradiation of a growing zygote. It is contraindicated if infection of the vagina, cervix, or uterus is present (infectious organisms might be forced into the pelvic cavity). For the procedure, radiopaque material is introduced into the cervix under pressure (Figure 6-5). This outlines the uterus and both tubes, provided the tubes are patent. Because the medium is thick, it distends the uterus and tubes slightly, causing uterine cramping that is momentarily painful. Following the study, the contrast medium will drain out through the vagina. The instillation of radiopaque material may be therapeutic as well as diagnostic. The pressure of the solution may actually break up adhesions as it passes through the fallopian tubes, thereby increasing their patency. The procedure carries a degree of risk of infection; allergic reaction to the contrast medium (it is iodine based); and embolism from dye entering a uterine blood vessel.

Hysteroscopy

Hysteroscopy is visual inspection of the uterus through the insertion of a hysteroscope through the cervix. This is helpful if uterine adhesions or other abnormalities were discovered on hysterosalpingogram.

Ultrasonography and Magnetic Resonance Imaging

Both ultrasound and magnetic resonance imaging are yet other methods that can be used to determine pa-

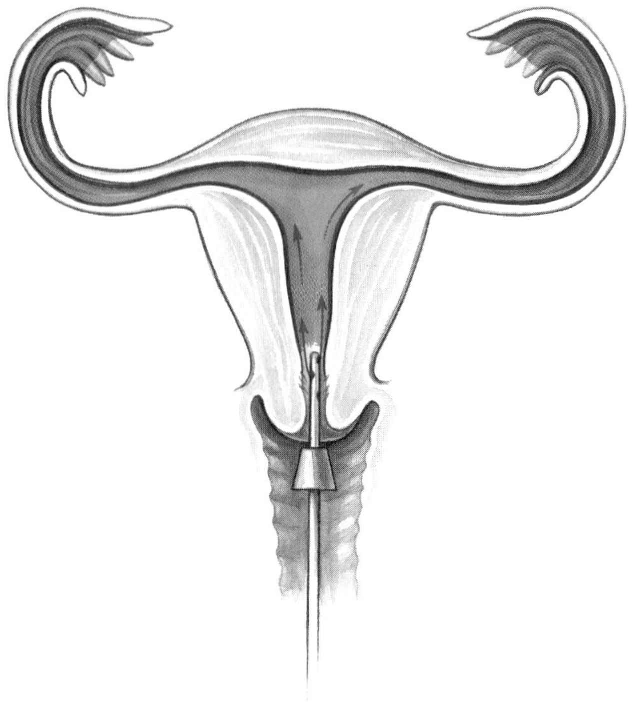

FIGURE 6-5
Insertion of a dye for a hysterosalpingogram. The contrast dye will outline the uterus and fallopian tubes on x-ray to show that they are patent.

tency of fallopian tubes and assess the depth and consistency of the endometrial lining (Allahbadia, 1993; Woodward et al., 1993).

Infertility Management

The overall management of infertility involves treating the underlying cause of the infertility, such as chronic disease or current infection. If that is impossible, infertility management will focus on achieving conception with the help of a sperm donation or other medical intervention.

Correction of the Underlying Problem

When it is possible to determine a specific cause of infertility, management will focus on correction of the underlying problem. In the meantime, whether the cause is known or not, all couples may benefit from some practical information on how to increase the chances of achieving conception on their own. Some suggestions to discuss with a couple are included in the Focus on Family Teaching box.

Increasing Sperm Count and Motility

Administration of clomiphene citrate (Clomid) may be successful in increasing an inadequate sperm count, as

may injections of testosterone and human chorionic gonadotropin.

If the vas deferens is obstructed, the obstruction is unfortunately usually extensive and difficult or impossible to relieve by surgery. If spermatozoa are present but the total count is low, a man might be advised to abstain from coitus for 7 to 10 days at a time to increase the count. If the underlying cause cannot be corrected, which unfortunately often happens (e.g., a prior infection that has left extensive scarring), artificial insemination by a donor is a possible solution. Ligation of a varicocele if this is present and advising changes in lifestyle such as suggesting wearing looser clothing and not taking prolonged hot baths may be helpful to reduce scrotal heat and increase a sperm count.

If spermatozoa appear to be destroyed by vaginal secretions due to an immunologic factor, the response may be reduced by abstinence or condom use for about 6 months. The administration of corticosteroids to the woman may have some effect. Direct insemination of the sperm into the cervix may be a solution (Alexander, 1990).

Reducing the Presence of Infection

If a vaginal infection is present, the infection will be treated according to the causative organism (see Chapter 14). Vaginal infections such as *Trichomonas* and *Monilia* are obstinate and tend to recur, requiring close supervision and follow-up (Shesser, 1990). The possibility that the sexual partner is reinfecting the woman needs to be considered. Women who are prescribed metronidazole (Flagyl) for a *Trichomonas* infection should be warned that it is teratogenic early in pregnancy and should not be continued if a pregnancy is suspected.

If there are white blood cells in the cervical mucus, an endocervical or endometrial infection may be present. Culturing the specimen will reveal the specific organism present and allow for appropriate antibiotic therapy. *Chlamydia trachomatis* infections are becoming more and more common and are one of the bacteria responsible for pelvic inflammatory disease. The treatment for chlamydia infection is oral erythromycin or doxycycline.

Hormone Therapy

If the problem appears to be a disturbance of ovulation, endocrine therapy may be necessary. In some instances, therapy with estrogen and progesterone is sufficient. Clomiphene citrate (Clomid), an estrogen antagonist, may also be used to stimulate ovulation. In other women, this can be stimulated by the administration of human menopausal gonadotropins (Pergonal) followed by administration of human chorionic gonadotropin (HCG). Human menopausal gonadotropins (derived from postmenopausal urine) are combinations of FSH and LH. If prolactin levels are increased, bromocriptine

FOCUS ON FAMILY TEACHING

Q. My husband and I want to start our family as soon as possible. Are there practical suggestions to help us conceive quickly?

A. A number of suggestions are generally helpful:

- Couples can determine the time of ovulation through the use of a basal body temperature, analysis of cervical secretions, or a commercial ovulation determination kit. Planning sexual relations for every other day around the time of ovulation is ideal.

- Although frequent intercourse may stimulate sperm production, males need sperm recovery time following ejaculation to maintain an adequate sperm count. This is why coitus every other day, rather than every day, during the fertile period will probably yield faster results.

- The male superior position is the best position for intercourse to achieve conception because it places sperm closest to the cervical opening.

- The male should try for deep penetration so ejaculation places sperm as close as possible to the cervix. Elevating the woman's hips on a small pillow is another way to facilitate sperm collection near the opening to the cervix.

- The woman should remain on her back with knees drawn up for at least 20 minutes after ejaculation to help sperm remain near the cervix.

- No artificial lubricants should be used because they may interfere with sperm motility.

- No douching should be used before or after intercourse so that vaginal *p*H is unaltered.

(Parlodel) is added to the medicine regime to reduce these levels and allow for rise of gonadotropin stimulation. Either the administration of clomiphene citrate or human menopausal gonadotropins may overstimulate the ovary, and multiple births may result. Women who are administered these compounds should be counseled that this is a possibility. If the problem is that spermatozoa do not appear to survive in the vaginal secretions because secretions are too scant or tenacious, the woman may be placed on low-dose estrogen to increase mucus production during day 5 to 10 of her cycle. Conjugated estrogen (Premarin) is a type of estrogen used for this purpose.

If the problem appears to be a luteal phase defect, this may be corrected by progesterone vaginal suppositories begun on the third day of the temperature rise and continued for the next 6 weeks if pregnancy occurs or until the menstrual flow resumes. Oral progesterone is not prescribed because it may cause fetal reproductive tract abnormalities if pregnancy occurs.

Surgery

If the cause of infertility is a *myoma* (fibroid tumor), then *myomectomy,* or removal of the tumor by surgery, may be necessary. Myomectomy may be done with a hysteroscope if the growth is small. For problems such as abnormal uterine formation, which may result in a septal uterus, surgery is also available. Septal defects, however, are generally related to early pregnancy loss, not infertility. Uterine adhesions may be lysed by hysteroscopy. Following this procedure, an intrauterine device (IUD) may be placed for 3 months and estrogen administered to prevent adhesions from reforming. This treatment may be difficult for the woman to accept, because preventing pregnancy (using an IUD) is exactly what she does not want to do.

If the problem is tubal insufficiency, diathermy or steroid administration may be helpful in reducing adhesions. A hysterosalpingography may be repeated to see whether it has a therapeutic effect. Canalization of fallopian tubes and plastic surgical repair (microsurgery) are possible treatments (Moore et al., 1991). If peritoneal adhesions or nodules of endometriosis are holding the tubes fixed and away from the ovaries, these can be removed by laparoscopy or laser surgery. Additional therapy for endometriosis is discussed in Chapter 47.

Artificial Insemination

Artificial insemination is the instillation of sperm into the uterus to aid conception. It can either be accomplished by the introduction of the husband's sperm (*AIH*—artificial insemination by husband) or by introduction of donor sperm (*AID*—artificial insemination by donor). It is a technique that may be used when the man has an inadequate sperm count or the woman has a vaginal or cervical factor interfering with sperm motility. It is useful for men who, feeling their family is complete, undergo vasectomy, and then later wish to have additional children (Humphrey & Humphrey, 1993). In the past, men who underwent chemotherapy or radiation for testicular cancer were not able to produce sperm afterward. Today, such men can have their sperm reserved in a sperm bank before undergoing therapy, so that it is available for insemination afterward (Sanger et al., 1992).

To prepare for artificial insemination, the woman

must take basal body temperature, assess cervical mucus, or use an ovulation predictor kit to be able to predict her day of ovulation. Just before, on and 2 days after the day of ovulation, the physician takes the seminal fluid of the husband or donor's ejaculate and, using a syringe, places it at the opening to the cervix (Figure 6-6). The woman rests in a supine position for approximately 20 minutes to allow the spermatozoa ample opportunity to enter the cervix. A cervical cap may be fitted to ensure that the sperm remain in contact with the cervix.

Donors for artificial insemination are volunteers who have no history of disease and no family history of possible heritable disorders. The blood type, or at least the Rh factor, can be matched with the mother's to prevent Rh incompatibility. Sperm banks, supplying frozen spermatozoa, are now available. Sperm from these sources can be selected according to desired physical characteristics and from donors screened for human immunodeficiency virus.

One disadvantage of using frozen sperm is that it tends to have slower motility than unfrozen specimens. However, although the rate of conception may be lower from this source, there appears to be no increase in incidence of congenital anomalies in children conceived by this method (Subak et al., 1992).

A man who has a low sperm count may pool and freeze ejaculations for 1 week or more, forming a pooled specimen that can be used in insemination. This technique may not be as effective as hoped, however, because of poor sperm motility from individuals with low sperm counts and the added insult of freezing. Thus, conception may not be improved under these circumstances.

Legal considerations must also be considered, because some states have specific laws regarding inheritance and child support and responsibility. Some couples have religious or ethical beliefs that prohibit them from using artificial insemination.

Because the process takes an average of 6 months to achieve conception, artificial insemination may be a discouraging process to some couples. The 6 months are long and filled with the tension of having pregnancy so near and yet so elusive.

In Vitro Fertilization and Embryo Transfer

In vitro fertilization (*IVF*) refers to fertilization of a mature oocyte recovered from the woman's ovary by laparoscopy by exposing it to sperm under laboratory conditions outside the woman's body (Beaudoin et al., 1993). *Embryo transfer* (also called ova transfer) refers to the insertion of laboratory-grown ova into the woman's uterus approximately 40 hours after fertilization, where ideally one or more will implant and grow.

IVF is most often used for couples who have not been able to conceive because the woman has blocked or damaged fallopian tubes. It is also used when the man has oligospermia or a low sperm count, because the controlled concentrated conditions require fewer sperm (perhaps as few as 50,000 whereas nearly 50 million are normally required). IVF may be helpful to couples when an absence of cervical mucus prevents sperm from traveling to or entering the cervix or antisperm antibodies cause immobilization of sperm. In addition, couples with unexplained infertility of long duration may be helped by IVF. A donor ova may be used for the woman who does not ovulate or who carries a sex-linked disease, which she does not want to pass on to her children.

Before the procedure, the woman is administered an ovulation agent such as clomiphene citrate (Clomid) or human menopausal gonadotropin (Pergonal). The woman is monitored closely for increasing serum estrogen as a sign of follicular growth. Beginning about the 10th day of the menstrual cycle, ovaries are examined daily by sonography to see the number and size of developing follicles. When a follicle appears to be mature, the woman is administered an injection of HCG hormone. This creates an LH effect and causes ovulation in 38 to 42 hours.

A needle is then introduced abdominally or intravaginally guided by ultrasound to aspirate the oocyte with a needle and sterile tubing from its follicle. Often, many oocytes ripen at once, and perhaps as many as 3 to 12 can be removed, impregnated, and reimplanted (Massey, 1991). Following aspiration and removal, the oocytes are incubated for at least 8 hours to be certain they are apparently viable. In the meantime, the husband or donor supplies a fresh semen specimen and this is prepared by a procedure called *sperm washing*, which separates sperm cells from seminal fluid by centrifuge. The sperm cells and oocytes are then mixed and allowed

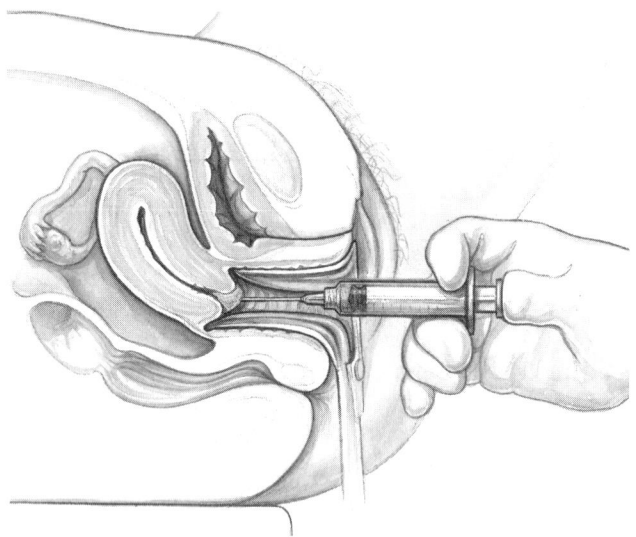

FIGURE 6-6
Artificial insemination. Donor sperm are deposited next to the cervix.

to incubate in a growth medium. If fertilization occurs, the zygotes formed will almost immediately begin to divide and grow. By 40 hours post fertilization, they will have undergone their first cell division. The fertilized eggs are examined and, if normal, a chosen number are transferred back to the uterine cavity through the cervix by a thin catheter (Figure 6-7). If the couple desires, any eggs not used can be frozen for use at a later time.

Progesterone may be given to the woman if it is felt that she will not produce enough to support implantation. A lack of progesterone can occur if the corpus luteum was injured by the aspiration of the follicle. Proof that the zygote has implanted can be demonstrated by a routine pregnancy test as early as 11 days after transfer.

The overall results of IVF vary from site to site. The recovery rate for harvesting ripened eggs is high (about 90%), as is the ability to fertilize eggs by sperm in vitro. However, the overall pregnancy rate is as low as 11% per treatment cycle in some centers (Hatcher et al., 1990). Although IVF programs do not result in an increase in birth defects, about 25% of pregnancies will end in spontaneous abortion (the same rate as for natural pregnancies). Once a pregnancy has been successfully implanted, the woman's prenatal care is the same as for any pregnancy. If a sonogram reveals that a multiple pregnancy of more than two zygotes has been achieved, selective termination of gestational sacs until only two are remaining may be recommended. This is done by the intraabdominal injection of potassium chloride into the gestational sacs chosen to be eliminated. Reducing the number of growing embryos in this way to a number a woman could carry to term helps to ensure the success of the pregnancy.

IVF–embryo transfer is expensive and only available at specialized centers. In addition, waiting to be accepted by a center's program and waiting for the time to obtain the oocyte, laboratory growth, and pregnancy success is a psychologic strain. There is a risk that if bacteria are introduced at any point in the transfer, maternal infection could occur.

Gamete Intrafallopian Transfer

In gamete intrafallopian transfer (GIFT), ova are obtained from ovaries exactly as in IVF procedures (Nelson et al., 1993). Instead of waiting for fertilization to occur, however, both ova and sperm are instilled within a matter of hours into the open end of a fallopian tube by laparotomy. This procedure has a pregnancy rate slightly higher than IVF–embryo transfer. The procedure is contraindicated if the woman's fallopian tubes are blocked, because this could lead to ectopic (tubal) pregnancy.

Direct Intraperitoneal Insemination

Yet another technique for aiding sperm and ova fertilization is direct intraperitoneal insemination (DIPI). DIPI is most effective for couples whose fertility problem is related to the male's low sperm count. Following ovulation stimulation, sperm, under ultrasound visualization, are injected through the posterior wall of the vagina into Douglas's cul-de-sac. They are placed into the pool of follicular fluid that accumulates following ovulation (Figure 6-8). In a preliminary study using this technique, 42% of patients became pregnant (Melnick & Ruzhnikov, 1990). DIPI is both less invasive and less costly than IVF or GIFT.

Sex Preselection

Approximately 200 genetic diseases such as hemophilia are known to be sex-linked or transmitted to male offspring on the X chromosome. These illnesses could be prevented from occurring if a woman who carried the X-linked gene had only girls as offspring. The thought that people can preselect the sex of their children (have

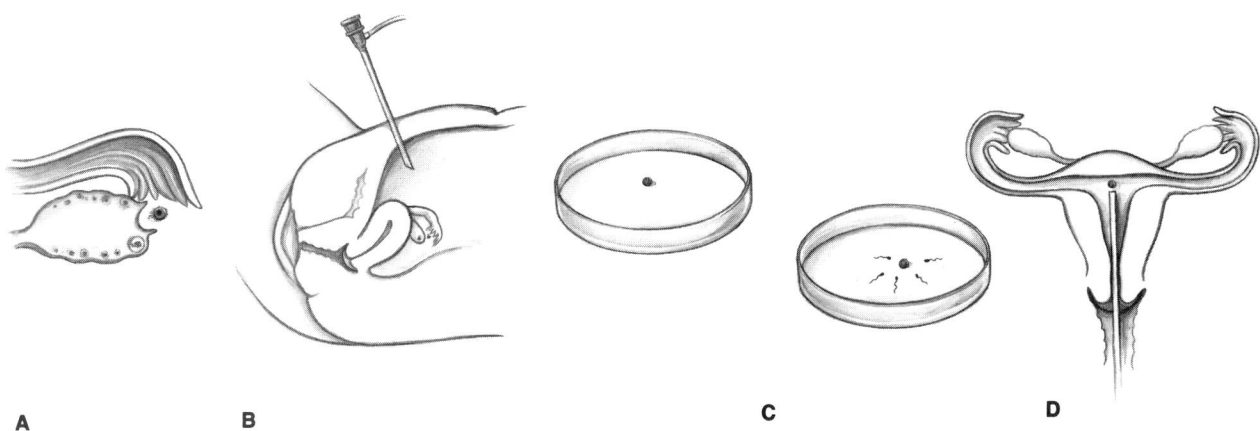

A   B   C   D

FIGURE 6-7
*Steps involved in in vitro fertilization. (**A**) Ovulation. (**B**) Capture of ova. (**C**) Fertilization of ova and growth in Petri dish. (**D**) Insertion of fertilized ova into uterus. (Reprinted from Masters, W.H., Johnson, V.E, and Kolodny, R.C. [1990]. Human sexuality [4th ed.]. Philadelphia: J.B. Lippincott, with permission.)*

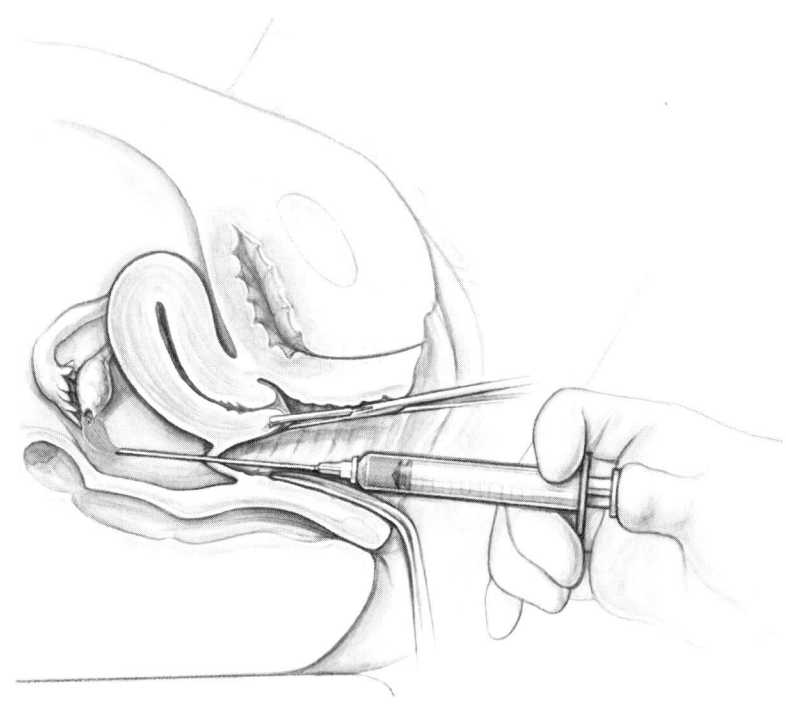

FIGURE 6-8
Direct intraperitoneal insemination. Sperm are deposited in the cul-de-sac of Douglas through a posterior vaginal injection.

only boys or only girls) has been appealing to people not only for this reason but for simple preference.

A number of methods to differentiate X-carrying and Y-carrying sperm have been identified (Beernink et al., 1993). Couples participating in intrauterine transfer and artificial insemination can have sex predetermined to some extent using these methods. Such techniques can be useful because popular methods to influence the sex of a child (such as douching with a baking soda mixture before coitus to have a boy or with a vinegar solution to have a girl) have proven to be more folklore than scientific fact.

Normally the ratio of male to female births is 105: 100. What would happen to this ratio if parents were able to preselect their children's sex? Walker & Conner (1993) in a survey of what sex pregnant women in their second trimester wished their baby to be, showed that males and females were desired equally. If a first child was a male, a female was wanted for the second child and vice versa. This would seem to be reassuring, that the average couple in the United States desires both a boy and a girl, implying that at the point that reliable preselection methods are devised, a significant change in this natural female/male ratio is not apt to occur.

Alternatives to Childbirth

For some couples, treatment for infertility will be unsuccessful. These couples need to consider other life options.

Surrogate Mothers

A *surrogate mother* is a woman who agrees to be impregnated by a man's sperm and then to carry a fetus to term for him and his partner. Surrogate mothers are often a friend or family member who take the role out of friendship or compassion, or they can be someone who is interested in the arrangement for monetary gain.

The infertile couple can enjoy the pregnancy as they watch it progress in the surrogate. However, a number of ethical and legal problems may arise with surrogate motherhood if the surrogate mother decides at the end of pregnancy that she wants to keep the baby despite the pre-pregnancy agreement she signed. Another potential problem occurs if the child is imperfect and the infertile couple no longer wants it (Lawrence, 1992). Who should be responsible? For these reasons, couples and the surrogate mother should be certain they have given adequate thought to the process before attempting it.

Adoption

Adoption, once a ready alternative for infertile couples, is still a viable alternative, although there are fewer children available for adoption and it often takes longer to find a child than it once did. And like other alternatives, adoption may not be right for every couple.

Agency Adoption

In traditional agency adoption, a couple usually contacts an agency by first attending an informational meeting. If they decide to apply to the agency, they are then put on a waiting list for processing; extensive interviewing and a home visit by an agency social worker determines if the couple can be relied on to provide a safe and nurturing environment for an adopted child. This investigation may consist of a single visit or several lengthy home interviews. Once approved by the agency, the couple is placed on a second waiting list. The agency calls the couple when a baby has been located for them. Depending on the area of the country, this may take anywhere from less than a year to 5 or 6 years. There is little or no communication between the woman placing the baby for adoption and the adopting couple. In the past this was seen as an advantage, since the birth mother could then not interfere in the new couple's lives. Today, the disadvantage of this for the child is being realized. Should a child want to learn his or her birth family's name or medical history or location, this information may not be available.

There are a number of alternatives to the traditional agency adoption. Some of these include international adoption, adoption of children with special needs, and private adoption. International adoptions can often provide a baby in less time than a traditional agency adoption, but there may be unanswered questions about prenatal health care or the birth family's background. In addition, countries willing to permit abandoned or orphaned children to be adopted internationally are often war or strife torn. They may allow children to be released from the country one day but refuse to do so the next. Thus, couples who are waiting for an international adoption must be ready at a moment's notice either to travel to a foreign country or the airport to pick up their child or to give up the adoption because new political reforms have stopped the release of children.

A home visit from a local agency as well as a significant amount of paperwork and communication with the international agency are usually required before a family can be approved for this type of adoption. International adoptions have been very successful for some families. However, it is important that the parents think through beforehand how they will feel about having a child who does not necessarily look like them and the ways they can respect the child's natural heritage. Local support groups consisting of other families who have gone through international adoption can be very helpful to couples who are considering this option. It may be difficult for internationally adopted children to learn about or locate their natural parents in years to come, since records of their birth may have been destroyed in their native countries during war or political turmoil.

There are children in every state who are waiting for adoption and can be placed almost immediately into adopting homes. Many of these children are older and have lived with many foster families or have gone back and forth between the homes of their birth parents and foster care. Many others have special health care needs or learning disabilities. Although this is not an option that is appealing for every couple, adoption of such children can be a very rewarding experience for the right couple.

Private Adoption

For families who have exhausted other options, or who can't wait for the traditional agency adoption process, private adoption is a possible alternative. Some pregnant women prefer to place their child for adoption directly with a couple this way rather than through an agency, so that they can be assured of approving of the couple and so they can maintain contact with the child.

Usually a lawyer serves as the go-between to make certain that all the legal ramifications of adoption have been considered by each party. The adopting parents usually agree to pay a certain amount of money, part of which presumably goes toward the birth mother's prenatal and medical expenses. Sometimes strict anonymity is maintained between the two parties, but in other instances the adopting couple and birth mother come to know each other quite well. The adopting parents might even attend the child's birth if the birth mother wishes. Close familiarity between the two parties can create difficulties later on. The birth mother may find it difficult to lose contact not only with the baby she has carried for 9 months but also with her new friends, who may have been extremely supportive of her during the pregnancy. Some couples may want to have the birth mother play a continued role in their lives, but others don't, and it is essential that these issues be worked out legally well in advance of the child's birth. Once she has received support during a pregnancy, it is possible for a birth mother, once delivered, to change her mind about giving the baby up before the adoption is settled. There is nothing that an adopting couple can do in this circumstance. At any point that a birth mother changes her mind about adoption, the courts have ruled in favor of returning an adopted child to the birth mother.

Childfree Living

Childfree living is an alternative lifestyle available to both fertile and infertile couples alike. However, for many infertile couples who have been through the rigors and frustrations of infertility testing and unsuccessful treatment regimens, childfree living may emerge as the option they finally wish to pursue. A couple in the midst of fertility testing may begin to reexamine their motives for pursuing the pregnancy in the first place and decide that the pregnancy and parenting is not worth the emotional or financial cost of future treatments; they may decide that the additional stress of going through an adoption is not for them; or a couple may simply decide that children are not necessary for them to fulfill their family unit. For these couples, childfree living is a positive choice.

Childfree living has advantages for a couple in that it allows time for both to pursue careers. They can travel more or have more time to pursue hobbies or continue their education. If a couple still wishes to include children in their lives in some way, there are many opportunities to do this: either through family connections (most parents welcome offers from siblings or other family members to share in childrearing) or through volunteer organizations (such as Big Brother or Big Sister programs) or through local schools and town recreational programs. Childfree living can be as equally fulfilling as having children because it allows a couple more time to help other people and to contribute to society through personal accomplishment. Many couples today who feel that overpopulation is a major concern are choosing childfree living, even when a problem of infertility is not present.

Key Points

- Infertility is said to exist when a pregnancy has not occurred after 1 year of unprotected coitus. Sterility refers to the inability to conceive because of a known condition.
- About 1 in 10 couples experience infertility. The incidence increases with the age of the couple.
- Male factors that contribute to infertility are inadequate sperm count, obstruction or impaired sperm motility, and problems with ejaculation.
- Female factors that cause infertility are problems with ovulation, tubal transport, impaired implantation, or interference with sperm motility.
- Infertility assessment procedures consist of a health history, physical examination, laboratory tests to document general health, and specific tests for semen analysis, ovulation, tubal patency, and hormone assessment.
- Measures to induce fertility are aimed at improving sperm number and transport, decreasing infections, and regulating hormones.
- Artificial insemination, in vitro fertilization, adoption, surrogate motherhood, and childfree living may all be suggested as solutions for infertility.
- Infertility testing is an intense psychologic stress period for couples. Support from health care personnel is necessary during this time not only to help couples through the experience on an individual basis but also to help them maintain their relationship as a couple.
- Couples who are told that an infertility problem has been discovered are apt to suffer a great loss of self-esteem. The nursing role includes offering support to help them look at other aspects of their lives where they do achieve to help them feel that they are productive healthy people in many ways.

Critical Thinking Exercises

1. Joanne Bigwan is a 30-year-old woman who has just been married; she wants to have a child as soon as possible. What advice would you give her to help increase her chances of conceiving quickly?
2. When Joanne doesn't conceive within a year, she is scheduled for a hysterosalpingogram and an endometrial biopsy. How would you prepare her for these procedures? What should she expect when the procedures are over?
3. Joanne states that she feels fertility testing is extremely stressful. What are measures you could take to make the process easier for her?

References

Ackerman, M., et al. (1994). Impotence: help for erectile dysfunction. *Patient Care, 28*, 22.

Alexander, N. J. (1990). Treatment of antisperm antibodies: Voodoo or victory? *Fertility and Sterility, 53*, 602.

Allahbadia, G. N. (1993). Fallopian tube patency using color Doppler. *International Journal of Gynaecology & Obstetrics, 40*, 241.

Beaudoin, D., et al. (1993). Motherhood at any price. *Canadian Nurse, 89*, 41.

Beernink, F. J., et al. (1993). Sex preselection through albumin separation of sperm. *Fertility and Sterility, 59*, 382.

Benrubi, G. L. (1990). Pelvic inflammatory disease. *The Female Patient, 15*, 50.

Berga, S. L. (1993). How stress can affect ovarian function. *Contemporary OB/GYN, 38*, 87.

Berger, G. S. (1993). How many women are affected by endometriosis? *Contemporary OB/GYN, 38*, 47.

Bernhardt, J. H. (1990). Potential workplace hazards to reproductive health. *Journal of Obstetric, Gynecologic, and Neonatal Nursing, 19*, 53.

Demystifying ovulation and pregnancy kits for your patients. (1993). *Contemporary OB/GYN, 38*, 67.

Department of Health and Human Services. (1991). *Healthy people 2000.* Washington, D.C.: U.S. Public Health Service.

Eschenbach, D. A. (1990). Pelvic infections and sexually transmitted diseases. In Scott, J. R., et al. (Eds.) *Danforth's obstetrics and gynecology* (6th ed.) Philadelphia: J. B. Lippincott.

Farley, T. M., et al. (1992). Intrauterine devices and pelvic inflammatory disease: an international perspective. *Lancet, 339*, 785.

Hatcher, R. A., et al. (1990). *Contraceptive technology: 1990-1992* (15th ed.). New York: Irvington Publishers.

Hughes, C. L., & Hammond, C. B. (1990) Infertility. In Scott, J. R. et al. (Eds.) *Danforth's obstetrics and gynecology* (6th ed.). Philadelphia: J.B. Lippincott.

Humphrey, M., & Humphrey, H. (1993). Vasectomy as a reason for donor insemination. *Social Science & Medicine, 37*, 263.

Kaler, S. R. (1990). Epididymitis in the young adult male. *Nurse Practitioner, 15*, 10.

Lawrence, R. A. (1992). The medico-legal, social and ethical implications of surrogate parenthood. *Medicine & Law, 11*, 661.

Maroulis, G. B. (1993). Fertility, pregnancy and the older woman. *Contemporary OB/GYN, 38*, 101.

Marshak, L. S. (1993). The role of the female doctorally prepared nurse in caring for infertile women. *Clinical Nurse Specialist, 7*, 8.

Mashburn, J. (1993). Endometrial biopsy in the office setting. *Journal of Nurse-Midwifery, 38,* 31S.

Massey, J. B., et al. (1991). In vitro fertilization: recent improvements in technology. *The Female Patient, 16,* 63.

Melnick, H. D., & Ruzhnikov, L. (1990). Direct intraperitoneal insemination: An alternative treatment for infertility. *The Female Patient, 15,* 21.

Moore, D. E., et al. (1991). Selective fallopian tube canalization. *American Family Physician, 43,* 889.

Nelson, J. R., et al. (1993. Predicting success of gamete intrafallopian transfer. *Fertility and Sterility, 60,* 116.

Richard-Davis, G., & Moghissi, K. S. (1993). Basic evaluation of the infertile couple. *The Female Patient, 18,* 71.

Romanowski, B. (1993). Pelvic inflammatory disease: current approaches. *Canadian Family Physician, 39,* 346.

Sanger, W. G., et al. (1992). Semen cryobanking for men with cancer. *Fertility and Sterility, 58,* 1024.

Shesser, R. (1990). Common vaginal infections. *The Female Patient, 15,* 53.

Stine, C. C., & Collins, M. (1990). Male sexual dysfunction. *Primary Care, 16,* 1031.

Subak, L. L., et al. (1992). Therapeutic donor insemination: a prospective randomized trial of fresh versus frozen sperm. *American Journal of Obstetrics & Gynecology, 166,* 1597.

Thompson, S. T. (1993). Preventable causes of male infertility. *World Journal of Urology, 11,* 111.

Walker, M. K., & Conner, G. K. (1993). Fetal sex preference of second-trimester gravidas. *Journal of Nurse-Midwifery, 38,* 110.

Werner, M. A., & Lipshultz, L. I. (1993). How practical are male infertility technologies? *Contemporary OB/GYN, 38,* 76.

Willms, J. L., & Newman, L. (1994). The pelvic examination in primary practice. *Consultant, 34,* 175.

Woodward, P. J., et al. (1993). MR imaging in the evaluation of female infertility. *Radiographics, 13,* 293.

Younger, J. B. (1993). Endometriosis. *Current Opinion in Obstetrics & Gynecology, 5,* 333.

Suggested Readings

Adamson, G. D. (1991). Management of endometriosis. *Female Patient, 16,* 35.

Bernstein, J., et al. (1992). Coping with infertility: a new nursing perspective. *NAACOGS Clinical Issues in Perinatal & Women's Health Nursing, 3,* 335.

Damewood, M. D. (1993). Pathophysiology and management of endometriosis. *Journal of Family Practice, 37,* 68.

Domar, A. D., Seibel, M. M., & Benson, H. (1990). The mind body program for infertility—a new behavioral treatment approach for women with infertility. *Fertility and Sterility, 53,* 246.

Gibson, M. (1990). Chronic sequelae of salpingitis. *Contemporary OB/GYN, 35,* 13.

Hajal, F. & Rosenberg, D. (1991). The family life cycle in adoptive families. *American Journal of Orthopsychiatry, 61,* 78.

James, C. A. (1992). The nursing role in assisted reproductive technologies. *NAACOGS Clinical Issues in Perinatal & Women's Health Nursing, 3,* 328.

Nachtigall, R. D. (1993). Secrecy: an unresolved issue in the practice of donor insemination. *American Journal of Obstetrics & Gynecology, 168,* 1846.

Paulson, R. J., et al. (1990). Embryo implantation after human in vitro fertilization: Importance of endometrial receptivity. *Fertility and Sterility, 53,* 870.

Reame, N. E. (1991). The surrogate mother as a high-risk obstetric patient. *Women's Health Issues, 1,* 151.

Sherrod, R. A. (1992). Helping infertile couples explore the option of adoption. *Journal of Obstetrical, Gynecologic and Neonatal Nursing, 21,* 465.

Update: New guidelines for STD management. (1994). *Consultant, 34,* 182.

White, G. B. (1992). Understanding the ethical issues in infertility nursing practice. *NAACOGS Clinical Issues in Perinatal & Women's Health Nursing, 3,* 347.

Witt, M. A., & Grantmyre, J. E. (1993). Ejaculatory failure. *World Journal of Urology, 11,* 89.

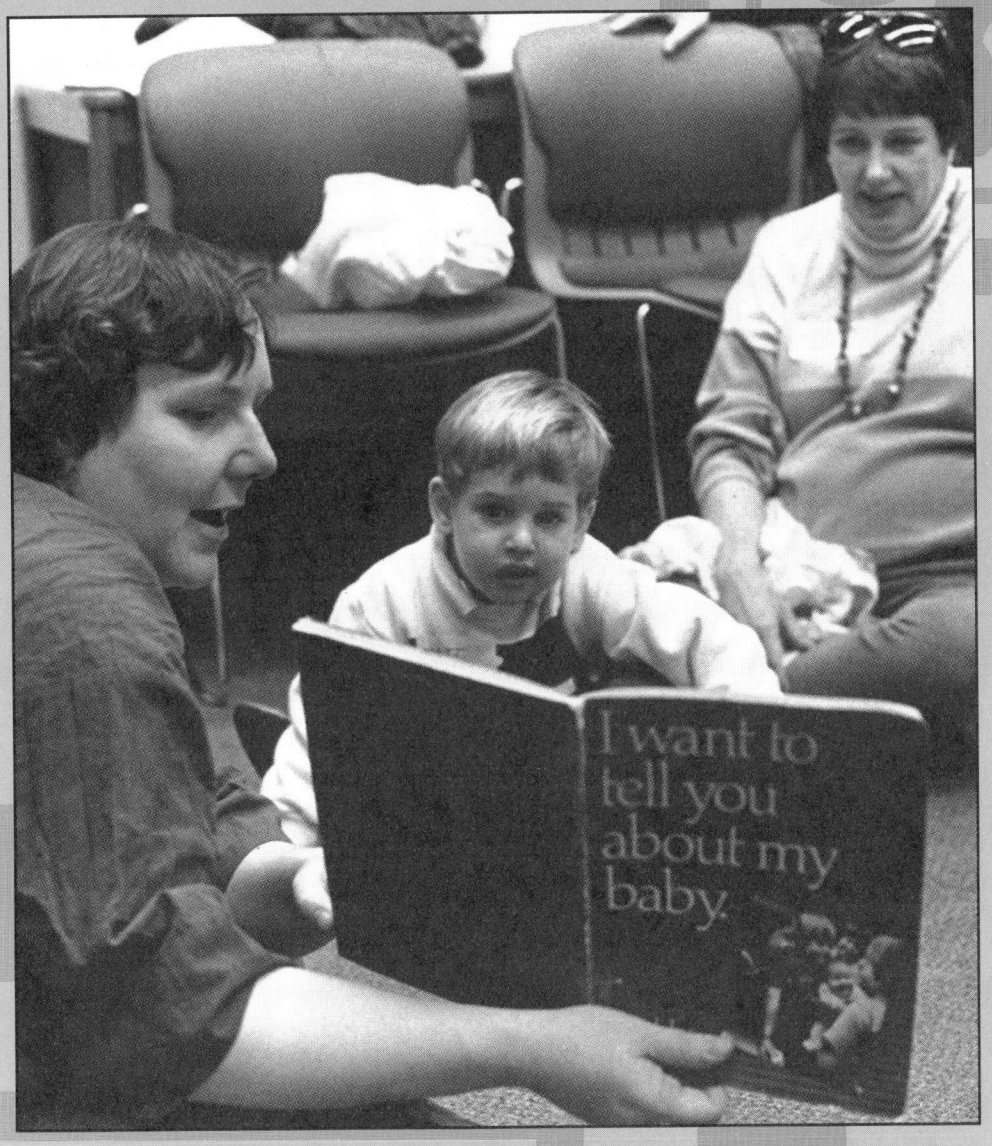

Unit
3

The Nursing Role
in Caring for
the Pregnant Family

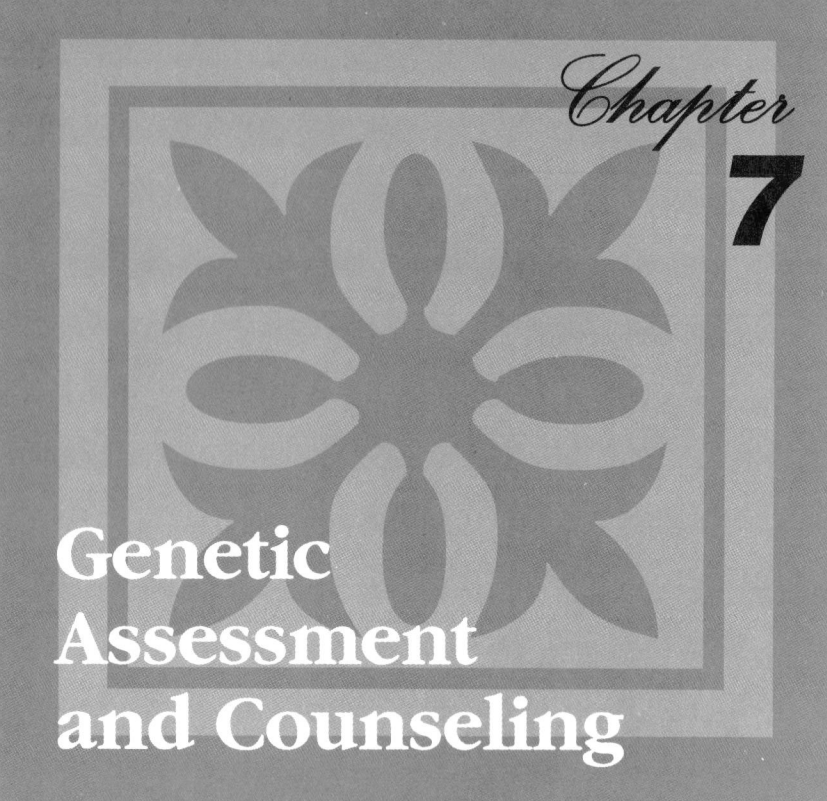

Chapter 7

Genetic Assessment and Counseling

Objectives

After mastering the contents of this chapter, you should be able to:

1. Describe the nature of inheritance, patterns of recessive and dominant mendelian inheritance, and common chromosomal aberrations such as nondisjunction syndromes.

2. Assess a family for the probability of inheriting a genetic disorder.

3. Formulate nursing diagnoses related to genetic disorders.

4. Plan nursing care related to an alteration in genetic health, such as assisting with an amniocentesis.

5. Implement nursing care related to identification of or counseling for a genetic disorder.

6. Evaluate goals and outcome criteria established for care to be certain they were achieved.

7. Identify National Health Goals and specific measures that nurses can take to help the nation achieve these goals.

8. Identify areas related to genetic assessment that could benefit from additional nursing research.

9. Use critical thinking to analyze ways that nurses can contribute to health education and counseling as genetic counselors.

10. Synthesize knowledge of genetic inheritance with nursing process to achieve quality maternal and child health nursing care.

Key Terms

- acrocentric chromosome
- alleles
- centromere
- chromosomes
- dermatoglyphics
- dominant gene
- genes
- genetics
- genome
- genotype
- heterozygous trait
- homozygous trait
- imprinting
- karyotype
- meiosis
- metrocentric chromosome
- nondisjunction
- phenotype
- recessive gene
- submetrocentric chromosome

Adele Pillitteri: MATERNAL AND CHILD HEALTH NURSING, 2nd Edition. © 1995 Adele Pillitteri.

The possibility of genetic illness crosses the minds of most pregnant women and their partners at some point in a pregnancy, whether or not there is any family history of genetic illness. Many pregnant couples will ask health care providers about their chances of having a child with a genetic disorder. Advances in genetic screening techniques over the last decade have made genetic testing a common feature of prenatal care. For instance, women 35 years of age and over are routinely asked if they want to be tested by alpha-fetoprotein serum screening for Down syndrome, a genetic disorder that increases in incidence as maternal age increases. Couples who already know of the existence of genetic disease in their family or those who have had a previous child born with a congenital anomaly often require even more testing; following a positive test for a genetic disease they will almost certainly undergo an emotional period of decision-making. Informative and sensitive genetic counseling by health care providers educated in the specialty of genetics is essential for these couples.

This chapter reviews the basic principles by which illness is inherited and provides guidelines of care for couples considering or undergoing genetic counseling. National Health Goals include several aimed at improved screening for genetic disorders (see the Focus on National Health Goals box). Nurses can be instrumental in helping to see that these goals are achieved.

 NURSING PROCESS OVERVIEW
for Genetic Counseling

ASSESSMENT

Assessment is a crucial step in any nursing intervention, but it plays an especially vital role in genetic counseling. Assessment measures include a detailed family history, physical examination, and an ever-growing series of laboratory assays of blood, chorionic villi, and amniotic fluid that demand equally varied techniques for obtaining maternal, fetal, and cell samples for analysis.

NURSING DIAGNOSIS

Typical nursing diagnoses related to the area of genetic disorders are:

- Decisional conflict related to testing for an untreatable genetic disorder
- Fear related to outcome of genetic screening tests
- Situational low self-esteem related to identified chromosomal abnormality
- Knowledge deficit related to inheritance pattern of Down syndrome
- Health-seeking behaviors related to potential for genetic transmission of disease
- Altered sexuality pattern related to fear of conceiving a child with a genetic disorder

PLANNING AND IMPLEMENTATION

Planning care and outcome criteria for families following genetic assessment differs according to the assessment results. It may include helping couples to arrange for further assessment measures during a pregnancy. Setting realistic goals that are consistent with the individual's or couple's lifestyle is important.

Parents' reactions to the birth of a child with a genetically inherited disorder are apt to be the same as those of parents whose child dies at birth: grief. They must work through stages of shock and denial ("This cannot be true"), anger ("It's not fair this happened to us"), bargaining ("If only this would go away"), to reorganization and acceptance ("It has happened to us and it is all right"). Planning with parents may be difficult in the newborn period before they have finished working through these stages of grief (Simpson, 1990).

As a rule, it is beneficial to concentrate on short-term goals in these instances. Will the baby need to be hospitalized for immediate surgical correction of accompanying congenital anomalies? Will the parents take the baby home or will he or she be placed temporarily in foster care?

Identifying support people who can be helpful to the parents during the time of disorganization and shock is also important. These may be the usual family resource people, such as grandparents or other family members; in some families, these people are as disturbed by the diagnosis as the parents and so cannot offer their usual support. Secondary support sources that may be helpful include organizations such as the March of Dimes Birth Defects Foundation (1275 Mamaroneck Avenue, White Plains, NY 10605), Klinefelter Syndrome and Associates (P.O. Box 119, Roseville, CA 95678-0119), the Fragile X Foundation (1441 York Street, Suite 215, Denver, CO 80206), Association for Children with Down Syndrome (2616 Martin Avenue, Bellmore, NY 11710), and the Turner's Syndrome Society (15500 Wayzata Boulevard, Wayzata, MN 55391). Not all parents are ready to talk to members of such organizations at the time of diagnosis (to join the organization makes the diagnosis "real" or moves them out of denial before they are ready to do that).

Identifying health care personnel with whom the parents will need to maintain contact during the next few months offers additional support. At some point there will be care decisions concerning schooling, surgical procedures, behavior problems, or future development. Do not leave parents without health care providers they know they can turn to when they are moving out of denial; become ready to deal with the problem at that time yourself.

EVALUATION

Examples of outcome criteria for the family with a known genetic disorder might be:

- Couple states they feel capable of coping no matter what the outcome of genetic testing.
- Client accurately states the chances of Down syndrome occurring in her next child.
- Couple states they have resolved their feelings of low self-esteem related to birth of child with trisomy 13.

It is important to remember that a couple's decisions about genetic testing and childbearing may change over time. A decision made at age 25 not to have children because of a potential genetic disorder may be difficult to maintain as the couple, now age 30, sees many of their friends with growing families. Provide individuals and couples who have asked for genetic counseling with the phone number of a genetic counselor and urge them to call periodically for news of recent advances in genetic screening techniques or disease treatments.

FOCUS ON
National Health Goals

Two National Health Goals speak directly to genetic disease and screening. These are:

- Increase to at least 90% the proportion of women enrolled in prenatal care who are offered screening and counseling for prenatal detection of fetal abnormalities.

- Increase to at least 95% the proportion of newborns screened by state-sponsored programs for genetic disorders and other disabling conditions and to 90% the proportion of newborns testing positive for disease who receive appropriate treatment (DHHS, 1991).

Nurses can be instrumental in helping these goals to be achieved by being sensitive to the need for genetic screening and counseling in prenatal and birth settings. Nursing research asking such questions as when are people most responsive to genetic counseling or what is the effect on bonding of learning alpha-fetoprotein level during pregnancy can also help meet these goals.

Genetic Disorders

Inherited or *genetic disorders* are disorders that can be passed from one generation to the next. They result from some disorder in gene or chromosome structure. **Genetics** is the study of the way such disorders occur.

Genetic abnormalities can occur at the moment of ova and sperm fusion or even earlier, in the meiotic division phase of the gametes (ova and sperm). Some genetic abnormalities are so severe that normal fetal growth cannot continue, and many early, spontaneous abortions apparently are the result. Genetic disorders are so common that as many as 50% of first trimester spontaneous abortions involve chromosomal abnormalities (Simpson, 1990). Other genetic disorders do not affect life in utero; only after birth or at the time of fetal testing will the result of the disorder become apparent. In the near future it will be possible to not only identify aberrant genes for illnesses but to insert healthy genes in place of diseased genes to treat disorders such as inborn errors of metabolism. Gene replacement therapy has already been used with some success in the treatment of blood and immunodeficiency syndromes.

The Nature of Inheritance

Deoxyribonucleic acid (DNA), the material of heredity, is woven into strands in the nucleus of all body cells to form **chromosomes**. **Genes** are designated points along the chromosomes that are responsible for specific body characteristics, traits, or illness. Chromosomes are like structures in that they are all composed of four "arms" joined at a point termed the **centromere**. A chromosome is said to be **metrocentric** if the centromere is located so all four arms are the same length. It is **submetrocentric** if the location results in two long upper arms; **acrocentric** if it results in two short upper arms.

In order for cell formation to remain constant, DNA always remains guarded in the cell nucleus. The genetic information in the DNA is copied onto ribonucleic acid (RNA) strands. RNA is a separate protein component that passes out of the nucleus into the cell cytoplasm and guides cell function and reproduction of new cells. A wrong communication by an RNA molecule can lead to severe genetic abnormalities in the formation of a new cell.

In humans, each cell, with the exception of the sperm and ova, contains 46 chromosomes (44 autosomes and 2 sex chromosomes). The spermatozoa and ova are exceptions to this in that they each carry only half of the chromosome number, or 23 chromosomes. For each chromosome in the sperm cell, there is a like chromosome of similar size and shape and function (autosomes, or homologous chromosomes) in the ovum. As genes are always located at fixed positions on chromosomes, two like genes (**alleles**) for every trait are represented in the ovum and sperm on autosomes. The one chromosome in which this does not occur is the chromosome that determines sex. The female sex chromosome is medium size, with arms of equal length (metrocentric); the male sex chromosome is small and has an off-center midpoint (acrocentric). If the sex chromosomes are both X in the zygote formed from the union of a sperm and ovum, the individual is female (Figure 7-1*A*); if one sex chromosome is an X and one a Y (the small, acrocentric type), the individual is a male (Figure 7-1*B*).

A person's **phenotype** refers to his or her outward appearance or the expression of the genes. A person's **genotype** refers to his or her actual gene composition. A person's **genome** is the complete set of genes present. A normal genome is abbreviated as 46XX or 46XY (designation of the total number of chromosomes plus a graphic description of the sex chromosomes present). If a chromosomal aberration exists, it is listed after the sex chromosome pattern. In such abbreviations, the letter *p* stands for short arm defects and *q* stands for the long arm of chromosomes. The abbreviation 46XX5p−, for example, is the abbreviation for a female with 46 total chromosomes but with the short arm of chromosome 5 missing (Cri-du-chat syndrome). In Down syndrome the person has an extra chromosome 21, which is abbreviated as 47XX21+ or 47XY21+.

Mendelian Inheritance: Dominant and Recessive Patterns

The principles of genetic inheritance of disease are the same as those that govern genetic inheritance of other physical characteristics, such as eye or hair color. These principles were discovered and described by Gregor Mendel, an Austrian naturalist, and are known as *mendelian laws*.

A person who has two like genes for a trait—for blue eyes, for example (one from the mother and one from the father)—on two homologous chromosomes is said to be **homozygous** for that trait. If the genes differ (a gene for blue eyes from the mother and a gene for brown eyes from the father, or vice versa), the person is said to be **heterozygous** for that trait (Campbell, 1992). Many genes are **dominant** in their action over others; that is, when paired with other genes, dominant genes are always expressed in preference to the other genes. For example, brown eye color is dominant over blue, so a person with a heterozygous pattern would appear to have brown eyes. An individual with two homozygous genes for a dominant trait is said to be *homozygous dominant;* the individual with two genes for a recessive trait is *homozygous recessive.*

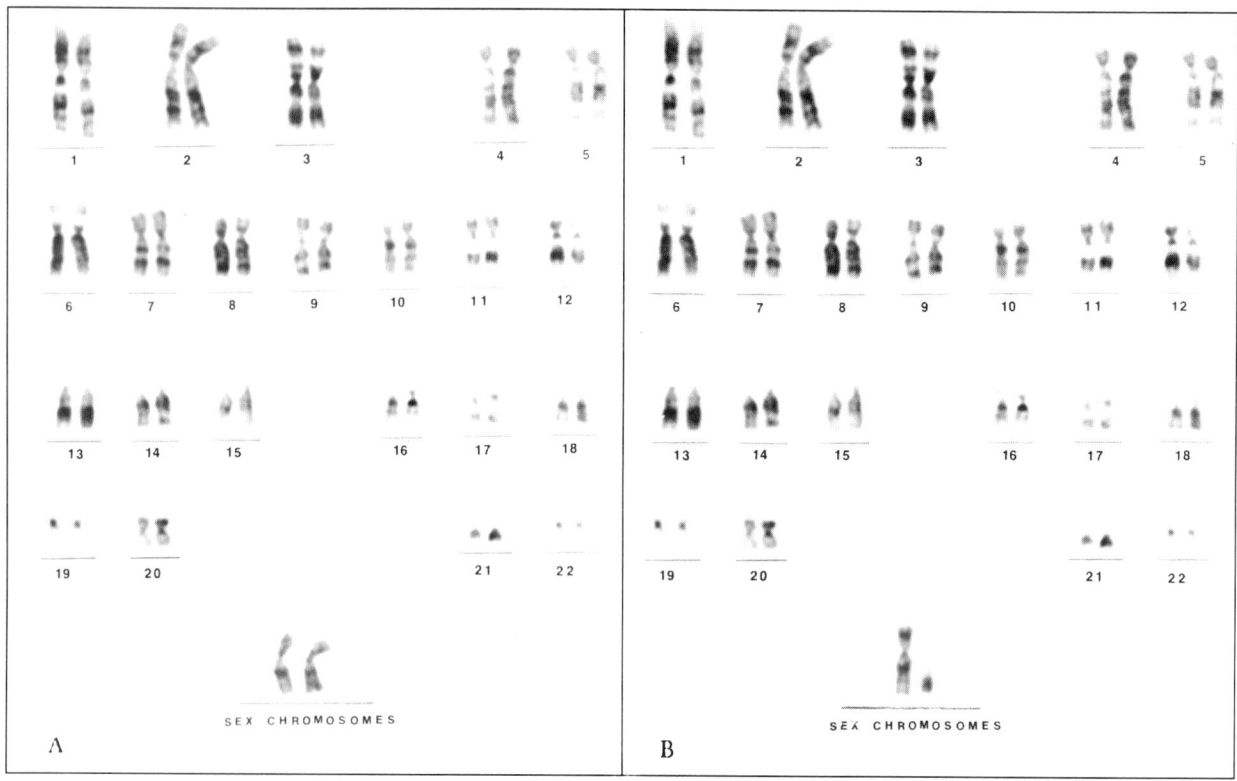

FIGURE 7-1

Photomicrographs of human chromosomes (karyotypes). If a blood sample is taken from a child or adult and the white blood cells are examined at the mitotic division phase of reproduction, transferred to slides, and photographed under high-power magnification, the individual chromosomes can be cut from the photograph and arranged according to size and shape. (A) Normal female karyotype. (B) Normal male karyotype.

Mendelian laws permit the prediction of inheritance of traits, such as eye color, or the chance that a child born to parents with a certain genotype will be born with a disease. Inheritance patterns for eye color provide a useful example of these principles. If the father is homozygous dominant (has two dominant genes for brown eye color) and the mother is homozygous recessive (has two genes for blue eye color), it can be predicted that their children have a 100% chance of being heterozygous for the trait (Figure 7-2*A*); they will appear brown eyed (the phenotype), but will carry a recessive gene for blue eyes (the genotype). If the father, however, is heterozygous (has one dominant gene and one recessive gene), a child born to this couple will now have an equal chance of being brown eyed or blue eyed (Figure 7-2*B*).

Suppose the mother is heterozygous instead of homozygous recessive and the father is homozygous dominant. As can be seen in Figure 7-2*C*, when this pairing occurs, the chances are equal that their child will be homozygous dominant like the father or heterozygous like the mother. All the children's phenotypes will be brown eyes.

Suppose both parents are heterozygous. As can be seen in Figure 7-2*D*, there is a 25% chance of their children being homozygous recessive (appear blue eyed); a 50% chance of their being heterozygous (appear brown eyed); and a 25% chance of their being homozygous dominant (appear brown eyed). This is how two brown-eyed parents can produce a blue-eyed child, or two brunette parents can produce a blonde child. It is impossible to predict a person's genotype from the phenotype, or outward appearance.

Inheritance of Disease

The same principles governing inheritance are applicable to predicting inherited diseases. Diseases may be transmitted as either dominant or recessive traits. A list of single-gene disorders seen in children is shown in Table 7-1.

FIGURE 7-2

Possibilities of inheritance. (A–D) Eye color. (E–F) Autosomal dominant inheritance. (G–K) Autosomal recessive inheritance. (L) Sex-linked dominant inheritance. (M–N) Sex-linked recessive inheritance. ➤

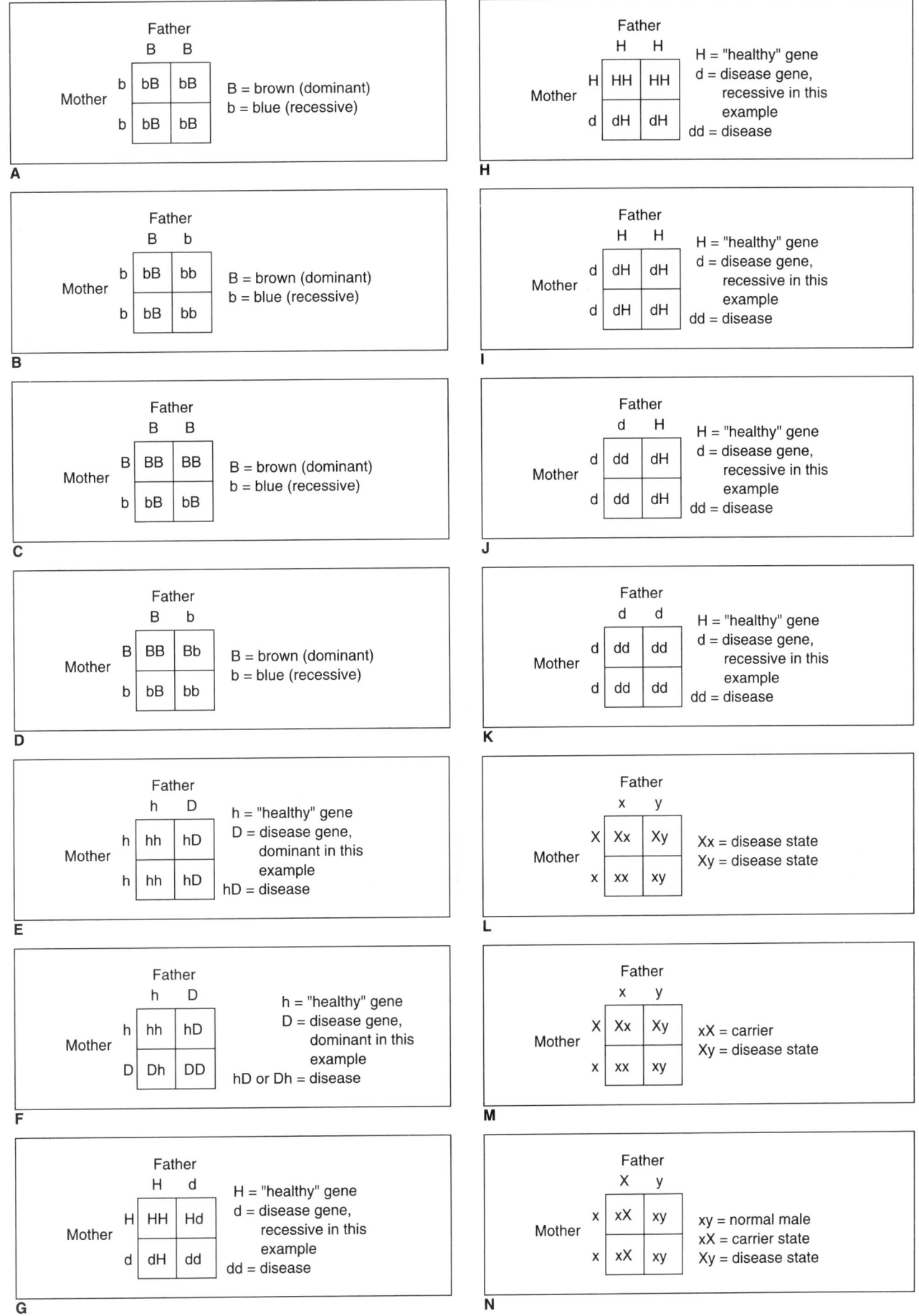

A

Father
B   B

Mother
b | bB | bB
b | bB | bB

B = brown (dominant)
b = blue (recessive)

B

Father
B   b

Mother
b | bB | bb
b | bB | bb

B = brown (dominant)
b = blue (recessive)

C

Father
B   B

Mother
B | BB | BB
b | bB | bB

B = brown (dominant)
b = blue (recessive)

D

Father
B   b

Mother
B | BB | Bb
b | bB | bb

B = brown (dominant)
b = blue (recessive)

E

Father
h   D

Mother
h | hh | hD
h | hh | hD

h = "healthy" gene
D = disease gene,
   dominant in this
   example
hD = disease

F

Father
h   D

Mother
h | hh | hD
D | Dh | DD

h = "healthy" gene
D = disease gene,
   dominant in this
   example
hD or Dh = disease

G

Father
H   d

Mother
H | HH | Hd
d | dH | dd

H = "healthy" gene
d = disease gene,
   recessive in this
   example
dd = disease

H

Father
H   H

Mother
H | HH | HH
d | dH | dH

H = "healthy" gene
d = disease gene,
   recessive in this
   example
dd = disease

I

Father
H   H

Mother
d | dH | dH
d | dH | dH

H = "healthy" gene
d = disease gene,
   recessive in this
   example
dd = disease

J

Father
d   H

Mother
d | dd | dH
d | dd | dH

H = "healthy" gene
d = disease gene,
   recessive in this
   example
dd = disease

K

Father
d   d

Mother
d | dd | dd
d | dd | dd

H = "healthy" gene
d = disease gene,
   recessive in this
   example
dd = disease

L

Father
x   y

Mother
X | Xx | Xy
x | xx | xy

Xx = disease state
Xy = disease state

M

Father
x   y

Mother
X | Xx | Xy
x | xx | xy

xX = carrier
Xy = disease state

N

Father
X   y

Mother
x | xX | xy
x | xX | xy

xy = normal male
xX = carrier state
Xy = disease state

Table 7-1. *Selected Examples of Single-Gene Disorders*

Disorder	Occurrence	Brief Description
Autosomal Dominant Inheritance		
Familial hypercholesterolemia (type II)	1:200–1:500	Deficiency in cell receptors for low density lipo-proteins, hypercholesterolemia, xanthomas, coronary heart disease
Huntington's disease	1:18,000–1:25,000 (United States)	Progressive neurologic disease, involuntary muscle movements, mental deterioration with memory loss, personality changes
Neurofibromatosis	1:3000–1:3300	Disorder of neural crest–derived cells with skin and central and peripheral nervous system manifestations; café au lait spots, neurofibromas, and malignant progression are common; variable expression of manifestations
Tay-Sachs disease	1:3600 (Ashkenazi Jews)	Lipid storage disease; progressive mental and motor retardation with onset at about age 6 months, deafness, blindness, convulsions; death by age 3–4 years
X-Linked Dominant Inheritance		
Pseudohypoparathyroidism (Albright hereditary osteodystrophy)	Rare	Short stature, delayed dentition, hypocalcemia, hyperphosphatemia, mineralization of skeleton, round facies
Vitamin D–resistant rickets (familial hypophosphatemia)	1:25,000	Disorder of renal tubular phosphate transport; low serum phosphate, rickets, short stature
Polydactyly	1:100–1:300 (blacks) 1:630–1:3300 (Caucasian)	Extra (supernumerary) digit on hands or feet
Polycystic renal disease (adult)	1:250–1:1250	Enlarged kidneys with cysts, hematuria, proteinuria, abdominal mass; may be associated with hypertension, hepatic cysts
Autosomal Recessive Inheritance		
Albinism (tyrosinase negative)	1:15,000–1:40,000 1:85–1:650 (American Indians)	Melanin lacking in skin, hair, and eyes; nystagmus; photophobia; increased susceptibility to neoplasia
Cystic fibrosis	1:2000–1:2500 (Caucasians) 1:16,000 (American blacks)	Abnormal exocrine gland function with pancreatic insufficiency and malabsorption, chronic pulmonary disease, excessive salt in sweat
Cystinuria	1:10,000	Defect in transport of cystine, lysine, arginine, and ornithine in intestines and renal tubules; tendency toward renal calculi
Familial dysautonomia (Riley-Day syndrome)	1:10,000–1:20,000 (Ashkenazi Jews)	Dysfunction of autonomic nervous system, sensory abnormalities, small stature, poor coordination, scoliosis, lack of tears leading to corneal ulcers
Hurler syndrome	1–2:100,000	Mucopolysaccharide disorder; mental retardation, coarse facies, skeletal and joint deformities, deafness, dwarfism, corneal clouding, onset age 6–12 months, fatal in childhood
Phenylketonuria (PKU)	1:15,000 (United States) 1:5000 (Scotland)	Deficiency in phenylalanine by hydroxylase causing excess phenylalanine in blood and urine, mental retardation if untreated, normal development and lifespan with low phenylamine diet
Sickle cell disease	1:400–1:600 (American blacks)	Hemoglobinopathy with chronic hemolytic anemia, growth retardation, susceptibility to infection, painful crises, leg ulcers, dactylitis

(continued)

Table 7-1. (continued)		

X-Linked Recessive Inheritance

Color blindness (red-green deuteranopia)	8:100 (Caucasian males) 4–5:100 (Caucasian females) 2–4:100 (black males)	Normal visual acuity, defective color vision with red-green confusion
Duchenne's muscular dystrophy	1:3000–1:5000 males	Progressive muscle weakness, atrophy contractures, eventual respiratory insufficiency and death
G6PD (glucose-6-phosphate dehydrogenase) deficiency	1:10 black American males 1:50 black American females	Enzyme abnormality with subtypes; manifestations involve RBC since it cannot replace unstable enzyme; usually asymptomatic unless person is under stress or exposed to certain drugs or infection, which increase need for chemical-reducing power generated by action of G6PD; decreased reducing power eventually results in denaturation of hemoglobin and hemolysis
Hemophilia A	1:2500–1:4000 male births	Coagulation disorder due to deficiency of factor VIII
Hemophilia B	1:4000–1:7000 male births	Coagulation disorder due to deficiency of factor IX
X-linked ichthyosis	1:5000–1:6000 males	May be born with sheets of scales (collodion babies), dry scaling skin, corneal opacities, steroid sulfatase deficiency

(Adapted from Cohen, F. *Clinical genetics in nursing practice.* Philadelphia: J.B. Lippincott, 1984. pp. 78, 81, 84, 87, 91. Additional material from Connor, J.M., & Ferguson Smith, M.A. *Essential medical genetics.* Oxford. Blackwell Scientific, 1984, pp. 185, 186, 198.)

Autosomal Dominant Inheritance

Although there are over 1000 autosomal disease disorders known, only a few are commonly seen. A person with a dominant gene for a disease is usually heterozygous, that is, has a corresponding healthy recessive gene for the trait. Huntington's disease, a progressive neurologic disorder characterized by loss of motor control and intellectual deterioration, is an example of a dominantly inherited disease. The onset of Huntington's disease is usually between the ages of 35 to 45 years. It is now possible to detect those people who will develop this disease by analyzing for a specific gene on chromosome 4. Unfortunately, there is as yet no cure for the disease, which means potentially affected individuals must make a difficult choice in deciding to undergo the analysis when they can do nothing but worry if the result is positive.

Other examples of dominantly inherited diseases include facioscapulohumeral muscular dystrophy, a form of *osteogenesis imperfecta* (a disorder in which bones are exceedingly brittle), and Marfan syndrome (a disorder of connective tissue in which the child is abnormally thinner and taller than normal and has associated heart defects). If a person with a dominant disease trait such as facioscapulohumeral muscular dystrophy mates with a person who does not have the trait, as shown in Figure 7-2E, the chances are even (50%) that a child would be born with the disease or be both disease and carrier free.

Two persons with a dominantly inherited disease are unlikely to choose each other as reproductive partners. If they do, however, their chances of having disease-free children decline (Figure 7-2F). Now there is only a 25% chance of a child being disease and carrier free; a 50% chance the child would have the disease like themselves, and a 25% chance that a child would be homozygous dominant (have two dominant disease genes), a condition that is probably incompatible with life.

In assessing family pedigrees for the incidence of inherited disease, a number of common findings are usually discovered when a dominantly inherited pattern is present in the family:

1. One of the parents of a child with the disorder also will have the disorder.
2. The sex of the affected individual is unimportant in terms of inheritance.
3. There is usually a history of the disease in other family members.

Figure 7-3 shows a typical pedigree of a family with a dominantly inherited autosomal disorder.

Autosomal Recessive Inheritance

Most heritable diseases are inherited not as dominant but as recessive traits. Such diseases do not occur unless two genes for the disease are present, that is, a homozygous recessive pattern. Many inborn errors of metabolism are recessively inherited (Strobel & Keller, 1993). Examples are cystic fibrosis, adrenogenital syndrome, albinism, Tay-Sachs disease, galactosemia, phenylketonuria, limb-girdle muscular dystrophy, and Rh-factor incompatibility problems that arise with pregnancy.

An example of autosomal recessive inheritance is shown in Figure 7-2G, in which both parents are disease free. Both are heterozygous in genotype, however, and thus carry a recessive gene for cystic fibrosis. As can be

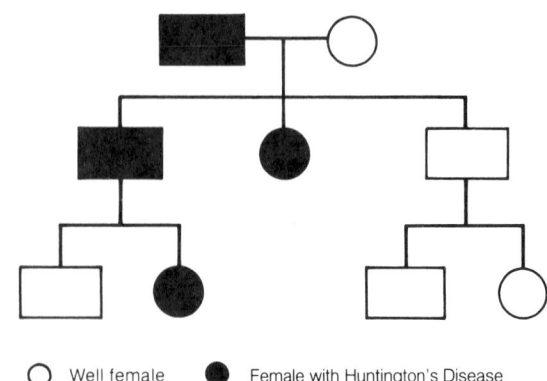

○ Well female   ● Female with Huntington's Disease
▢ Well male   ◼ Male with Huntington's Disease

FIGURE 7-3
Family pedigree: autosomal-dominant inheritance.

seen, there is a 25% chance of a child born to them being disease and carrier free (homozygous dominant for healthy genes); a 50% chance of a child being, like themselves, free of disease but carrying the unexpressed disease gene (heterozygous); and a 25% chance of a child having the disease (being homozygous recessive).

Suppose the woman with the heterozygous genotype shown in Figure 7-2*G* mates with a male who has no trait for cystic fibrosis. The chances are even that a child born to them will be completely disease and carrier free or heterozygous like the mother, as shown in Figure 7-2*H*. There is no chance in this case of a child having the disease. The child should be aware, however, that his or her children may manifest the disease if he or she carries the trait and if a sexual partner also has a recessive gene for the trait (see Figure 7-2*G*).

Ten or twenty years ago, most children with cystic fibrosis died in early childhood and so never reached childbearing age. Today, with good management, some do live to have children of their own (Fernbach & Thomson, 1992). If a person with cystic fibrosis should choose a sexual partner without the trait, all their children would be free of the disease. They all would carry a recessive gene, however, as shown in Figure 7-2*I*.

If the person with cystic fibrosis mated with a person with an unexpressed gene for the disease, the chances are equal that a child would have the disease or would carry a recessive gene for the disease (see Figure 7-2*J*). If a person with the disease should mate with a person who also has the disease, as shown in Figure 7-2*K*, the chances are 100% that a child would have the disease.

When family pedigrees are assessed for incidence of inherited disease, situations commonly discovered when a recessively inherited disease is present in the family include the following:

1. Both parents of a child with the disorder are clinically free of the disorder.

2. The sex of the affected individual is unimportant in terms of inheritance.
3. The family history for the disorder is negative (no one can identify anyone else who had it).
4. A known common ancestor between the parents sometimes exists. This is how both male and female have come to possess a like gene for the disorder.

Figure 7-4 shows a typical pedigree of a family with an autosomal recessive inherited disorder.

X-Linked Dominant Inheritance

Some genes for disease are located on, and therefore transmitted only by, the female sex chromosome (the X chromosome). This is called *X-linked inheritance*. When the gene is dominant it need be present on only one of the X chromosomes for symptoms of the disorder to be manifested (Figure 7-2*L*). Family characteristics seen with this type inheritance are:

1. All individuals with the gene are affected.
2. Female children of affected males are all affected; male children of affected males are unaffected.
3. It appears in every generation.
4. All children of homozygous affected females are affected. Fifty percent of heterozygous affected females are affected (Figure 7-5). An example of a disease in this group is hypophosphatemia.

X-Linked Recessive Inheritance

The majority of X-linked inherited diseases are recessive. With this, the mother will be the carrier for the disorder. Any time a normal gene also is present, as in her female children, the expression of the disease will be blocked, but if the gene is not paired, as in her male children, the disease will be manifested.

Hemophilia A, Christmas disease (a blood-factor deficiency), color blindness, Duchenne (pseudohyper-

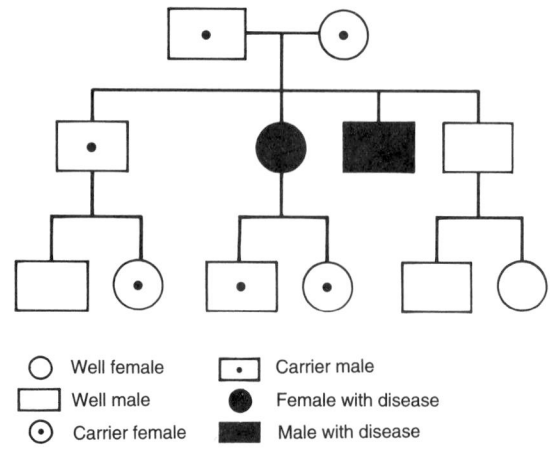

○ Well female   ▢• Carrier male
▢ Well male   ● Female with disease
⊙ Carrier female   ◼ Male with disease

FIGURE 7-4
Family pedigree: autosomal recessive inheritance.

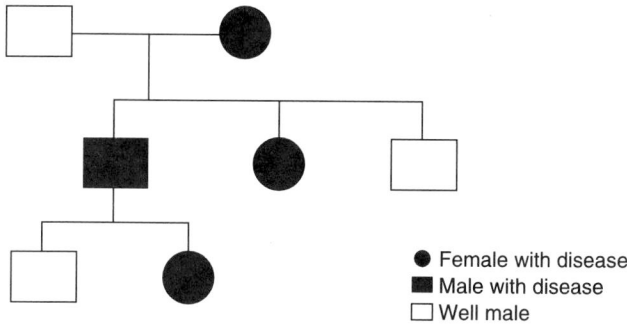

● Female with disease
■ Male with disease
□ Well male

FIGURE 7-5
Family pedigree: X-linked dominant inheritance.

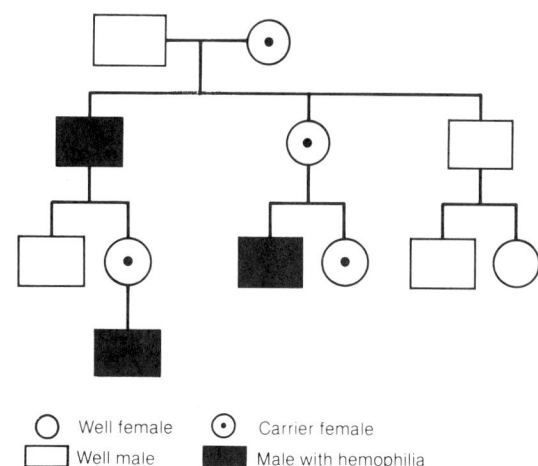

○ Well female   ⊙ Carrier female
□ Well male   ■ Male with hemophilia

FIGURE 7-6
Family pedigree: X-linked recessive inheritance.

trophic) muscular dystrophy, and fragile X syndrome are examples of this type of inheritance (Giannopoulou & Turk, 1992). Such a pattern is shown in Figure 7-2*M,* in which the mother has the affected gene on one of her X chromosomes and the father is disease free. The chances are 50% that a male child will manifest the disease and 50% that a female child will carry the disease gene. If the father has the disease and chooses a sexual partner who is free of the disease gene, the chances are 100% that a daughter will have the sex-linked recessive gene. There is no chance a son will have the disease. This is shown in Figure 7-2*N.*

When family pedigrees are assessed for inherited disorders, the following findings usually are apparent if an X-linked recessive inheritance disorder is present in the family:

1. Only males in the family will have the disorder.
2. A history of females dying at birth for unknown reasons often exists (females who had the affected gene on both X chromosomes, a condition incompatible with life).
3. Sons of an affected male are unaffected.
4. The parents of affected children do not have the disorder.

Figure 7-6 shows a typical family pedigree in which there is an X-linked recessive inheritance pattern.

Multifactorial (Polygenic) Inheritance

Many congenital disorders (disorders present at birth) such as heart disease, pyloric stenosis, cleft lip and palate, neural tube disorders, hypertension, and mental illness tend to have a higher-than-usual incidence in some families. Diabetes is an example of this type of disorder that has been studied closely. Children inherit human lymphocyte antigens (HLAs) from both parents. Certain HLA genes appear to play a role in genetic susceptibility to diabetes mellitus. Children who will develop diabetes mellitus can be shown to have an increased frequency of HLA B8, B15, DR3, and DR4 on chromosome 6. They lack DR2, an HLA that appears to

be protective against diabetes mellitus. Those diseases caused by multifactorial reasons do not follow the mendelian laws of inheritance probably because more than a single gene or HLA is involved. Environmental influences may be instrumental in determining whether the disorder is expressed or not. It is difficult to counsel parents regarding these disorders because their occurrence is so unpredictable. A family history, for instance, reveals no set pattern. Some of these conditions have a predisposition to occur more frequently in one sex (e.g., cleft palate occurs more often in females), but they can occur in either sex.

Imprinting

Imprinting refers to the differential expression of genetic material and allows researchers to identify whether the chromosomal material has come from the male or female parent (Hall, 1990). In some instances, such as hydatidiform mole (see Chapter 15), it can be shown that no maternal contribution is made to a fertilized ovum. In Prader-Willis syndrome, a mental retardation syndrome involving chromosome 15, no paternal contribution is present.

Genetic Markers

A *genetic marker* is a specific point on a chromosome that, if present, marks the location of a missing or abnormal gene. Chromosomal markers can be identified in varying types of pediatric illnesses, such as leukemias and lymphomas, or suggest that a genetic basis exists for some of these illnesses. Cystic fibrosis can now be detected prenatally because of a gene marker on chromosome 7 (Rosenstein, 1994). It is hoped that more markers can be identified, and, with recombinant DNA processing techniques, a healthy gene can be reimplanted at these sites as a means of curing inherited diseases.

Chromosomal Abnormalities

In some instances of genetic disease, the abnormality occurs not because of dominant or recessive gene patterns but through a fault in the number or structure of chromosomes.

Nondisjunction Abnormalities

Meiosis is a type of cell division in which the number of chromosomes in the cell are reduced to the haploid (half) number for reproduction (23 rather than 46 chromosomes). All sperm and ova initially undergo a *meiosis* cell division early in formation. During this, half of the chromosomes are attracted to one pole of the cell and half to the other pole. The cell then divides cleanly, with 23 chromosomes in the first new cell and 23 chromosomes in the second new cell. Chromosomal abnormalities occur when the division is uneven (nondisjunction). The result may be that one new sperm cell or ovum has 24 chromosomes and the second only 22 (Figure 7-7). If one of these defective spermatozoon or ovum fuses with a normal spermatozoon or ovum, the zygote (sperm and ova combined) will have 47 or 45 chromosomes, not the normal 46. The presence of 45 chromosomes does not appear to be compatible with life, and the embryo or

fetus probably will be aborted. Down syndrome (trisomy 21) (47XX21+ or 47XY21+) is an example of a disease in which the individual has 47 chromosomes: there are three rather than two of chromosome 21 (Figure 7-8).

The incidence of Down syndrome is highest if the mother is over 35 years of age and the father is over 45, so aging seems to present an obstacle to clean cell division. The incidence is 1:150 in women over 45, compared to 1:2500 in women under 20 (Tunnessen, 1994). Other examples of cell nondisjunction are trisomy 13 (Figure 7-9) and trisomy 18 (mental retardation syndromes).

When nondisjunction occurs in the sex chromosomes, as opposed to the autosomes, other types of abnormalities occur. Turner's and Klinefelter's syndromes are the most common of this type of chromosomal abnormality. In Turner's syndrome (45XO), marked by webbed neck, short stature, sterility, and possible mental retardation, the individual, although female, has only one X chromosome or has two X chromosomes but one is defective. She appears to be female (female phenotype) because of the one X chromosome. In Klinefelter's syndrome (marked by sterility and possibly mental retardation), the individual has male genitals but his sex chromosomal pattern is 47XXY.

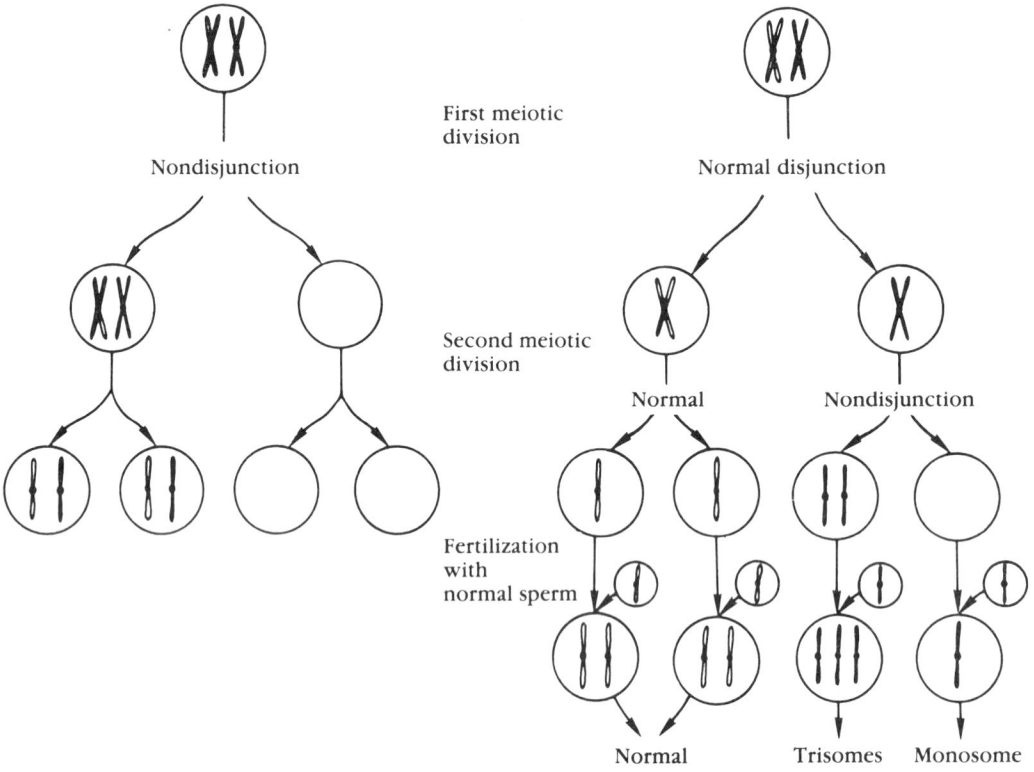

FIGURE 7-7

Process of nondisjunction at the first and second meiotic divisions of the ovum and fertilization with normal sperm. (From Bullock, B. L., & Rosendahl, P. P. [1992]. Pathophysiology: Adaptations and alterations in function *[2nd ed.]. Philadelphia: J.B. Lippincott, with permission.)*

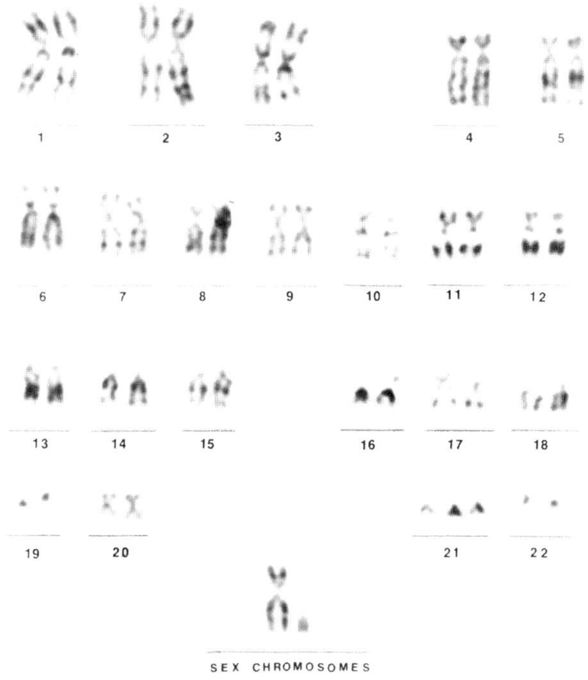

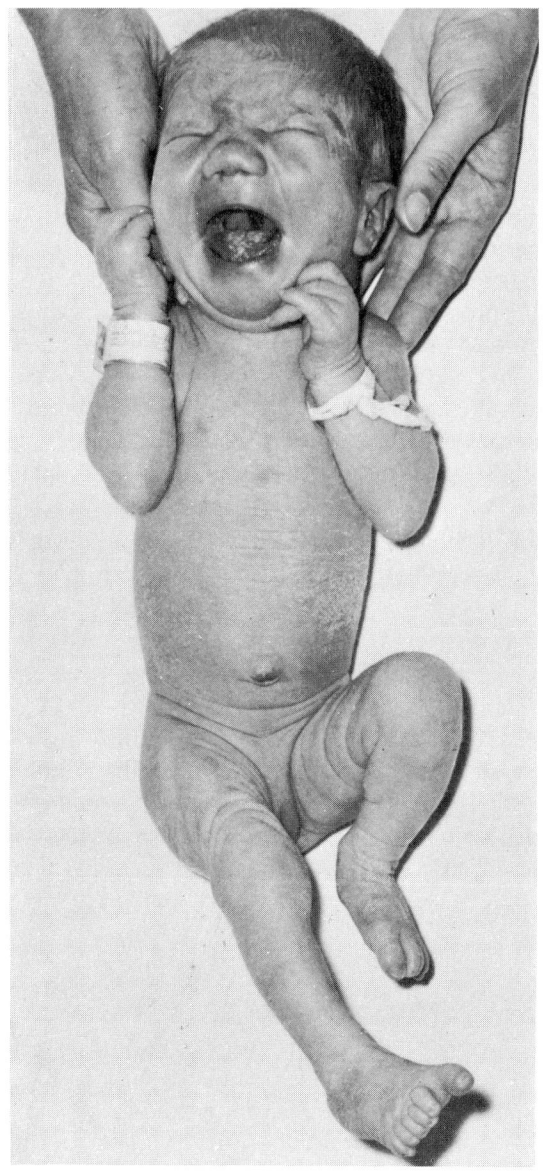

FIGURE 7-8
Karyotype of trisomy 21.

Deletion Abnormalities

Deletion abnormalities are a form of chromosome disorder in which part of a chromosome breaks during cell division, causing an affected person to have the normal number of chromosomes plus or minus an extra portion of a chromosome, such as 45 and ¾ chromosomes or 47 and ½.

In Cri-du-chat (cat's cry) syndrome (46XY5q−), a mental retardation syndrome named for the child's cat-like cry, one portion of chromosome 5 is missing. Deletion of the long arm of chromosome 18 (46XX18q−) results in a syndrome marked by hypotonus, mental retardation, seizures, heart defects, and hyperplastic genitalia.

Translocation Abnormalities

Translocation abnormalities are perplexing situations in which a child gains an additional chromosome through another route. A form of Down syndrome occurs as a translocation abnormality. In this instance, one parent of the child has the correct number of chromosomes (46), but chromosome 21 is misplaced and abnormally attached to chromosome 14. The parent's appearance and functioning are normal, because the total chromosome count is a normal 46; he or she is termed a *balanced translocation carrier.*

If with meiosis, however, this abnormal chromosome 14 (carrying the extra 21 chromosome) plus the normal chromosome 21 are both included in one sperm or ova, the resulting child will have a total of 47 chromosomes, including the extra number 21. The child

FIGURE 7-9
An infant with trisomy 13. The child has a cleft palate and polydactyly (7 toes). (From Barnett, H. Pediatrics [15th ed.]. New York: Appleton-Century-Crofts. Courtesy of Drs. J. Lindsten and P. Zetterquist.)

has an *unbalanced translocation syndrome.* The phenotype (appearance) of the child will be indistinguishable from the form of Down syndrome that occurs from nondisjunction.

About 2% to 5% of children with Down syndrome have this type of chromosome pattern. It is important to identify parents who are translocation carriers, because their chance of having a child born with Down syndrome is higher than normal. If the father is the carrier, this risk is about 2%; if the mother is the carrier, the risk is about 10% (Simpson, 1990). As many as 15% of couples who have frequent early spontaneous abortions may have this type of chromosomal aberration.

Mosaicism

Normally, a nondisjunction abnormality occurs during the meiosis stage of cell division when sperm and ova halve their number of chromosomes. *Mosaicism* is an abnormal condition that is present when the nondisjunction disorder occurs after fertilization of the ovum as the structure begins *mitotic* (daughter-cell) division. When this occurs, different cells in the body will have different chromosome counts. The extent of the disorder depends on the proportion of tissue with normal chromosome structure to tissue with an abnormal chromosome constitution. Children with Down syndrome who have near-normal intelligence may have this type of pattern. The occurrence of such a phenomenon at this stage of development suggests that a teratogenic (harmful to the fetus) condition, such as x-ray or drug exposure, existed at that point to disturb normal cell division. This genetic pattern in a female would be abbreviated as 46XX/47XX21+.

Isochromosomes

If a chromosome accidentally divides not by a vertical separation but a horizontal one, a new chromosome with mismatched long and short arms can result. This is an *isochromosome*. It has much the same effect as a translocation abnormality when an entire extra chromosome exists. Some instances of Turner's syndrome (45XO) may occur because of isochromosome formation.

Genetic Counseling

Any person who is concerned about the possibility of transmitting a disease to his or her children should have access to genetic counseling for advice on the inheritance of disease.

Such counseling can serve to:

Reassure people who are concerned about their children inheriting a particular disorder that their fears are groundless (if what they are concerned about is not an inherited disorder, for example).

Allow people who are affected by inherited disorders to make informed choices about future reproduction.

Educate people about inherited disorders and the process of inheritance.

Offer support by skilled health care professionals to people who are affected by genetic illness.

Confidentiality of information revealed in genetic screening must be guarded closely; in the wrong hands, such information could be used to damage a person's reputation or harm a future career or relationship. A woman with a history of mental illness, for example, might seek genetic counseling to determine the likelihood that her children will have the same illness. This information could be detrimental to her if inadvertently given to an employer or used by a political adversary. Often, an entire family is advised of a condition that affects it to allow all members to make equally informed responsible choices.

Confidentiality, however, prevents the health care provider from alerting other family members unless the member requesting genetic assessment has given consent. In some instances, a history reveals new information, such as that a child has been adopted or is the result of artificial insemination, or that the child's father is not the current husband. The member of the family seeking counseling has the right to decide whether he or she wants this information imparted to other family members.

The timing of genetic counseling is important, because counseling given after the fact is useless and counseling given before a couple is ready to accept it will be ignored. The ideal time for genetic counseling is before the first pregnancy. Some couples take this step before committing themselves to marriage, offering out of compassion for the partner to not involve him or her in a marriage commitment if children of the marriage would be subject to an inherited disorder. Other couples first become aware of a need for genetic counseling after the birth of a child with a disorder. Couples who seek counseling after a first affected child is born need counseling before a second pregnancy occurs. They are not ready for this, however, until the initial shock of their first child's condition and the grief reaction that may accompany it has run its course. Only then are they ready for information and future decision-making. (See the Focus on Family Teaching box for common questions about genetic counseling or procedures.)

Even if a couple decides not to have any more children, it is important for them to know that genetic counseling is available if they change their minds in the future. They also should be aware that as their children reach reproductive age, they, too, may benefit from genetic counseling.

Specific examples of couples who might benefit from a referral for genetic counseling would be:

A couple who have a child with a congenital abnormality or an inborn error of metabolism. Many congenital abnormalities occur because of teratogenic invasion during pregnancy that is often unrecognized. More important perhaps for the couple is learning that the abnormality occurred by chance rather than inheritance, so that they do not have to spend the remainder of their childbearing years in fear that another of their children may be born this way (although a chance circumstance could occur again). If a definite teratogenic agent, such as a

FOCUS ON FAMILY TEACHING

Families often have questions about genetic diagnostic procedures. A number of these are:

Q. Why do I have to wait so late in pregnancy for genetic studies by amniocentesis?

A. Genetic analysis is done on skin cells obtained from amniotic fluid. The test cannot be scheduled until enough amniotic fluid is present for analysis. Fortunately this now can be done as early as the 12th week of pregnancy.

Q. Why do laboratories take so long to return karyotyping results?

A. Karyotyping has traditionally (and by necessity) been done on cells at the metaphase (center phase) of division. This means the laboratory has to delay testing until the cells grow to reach this phase. New techniques now allow analysis to be done immediately so that results are available much sooner.

Q. There are no inherited diseases that we know of in our family, but should my husband and I have a karyotype done "just to be sure" before we have our first baby?

A. Most people don't recommend that a genetic analysis be done routinely, only if there is evidence or suspicion of disease in the family. Remember that karyotyping only reveals diseases that are present on chromosomes. A "perfect" karyotype doesn't guarantee that a newborn will not be ill in a noninherited way.

---

drug the woman took during pregnancy, can be identified, the couple can be advised about preventing this in a future pregnancy.

A couple whose close relatives have a child with a genetic disorder, including those with a child who has a congenital abnormality or inborn error of metabolism (see the Nursing Care Plan). Many conditions are caused by multifactorial inheritance. It is difficult to predict the expected occurrence of these "familial" or multifactorial disorders because they are caused by multiple gene disorders. Counseling should be aimed, therefore, at helping the couple learn as much as possible about the disorder, what treatment is available, and the prognosis or outcome. Based on this information, the couple can make an informed reproductive choice.

Any individual who is a known balanced translocation carrier. A balanced translocation carrier needs to understand his or her own chromosome structure and the process by which future children could be affected. Based on this information, the individual can make a choice to not reproduce or can be alerted to the probable wisdom of fetal karyotyping during any future pregnancy.

Any individual who has an inborn error of metabolism or chromosomal disorder. Any person with a disease should know the inheritance pattern of the disease, and like those who are balanced translocation carriers, be alerted to the wisdom

of prenatal diagnosis, if possible, for their particular disorder.

A couple that is consanguineous (closely related). The more closely related two people are, the more genes they share in common, so the more likely a recessively inherited disease will be expressed. A brother and sister for example, have about 50% of their genes in common; first cousins have about 12% of their genes in common.

Any woman over 35 years of age and any man over 45. This is directly related to the association between advanced maternal age and the occurrence of Down syndrome.

Couples of ethnic backgrounds in which specific illnesses are known to occur (see the Focus on Cultural Awareness box).

Genetic counseling may result in making individuals feel "well" or free of guilt for the first time in their lives; they may discover that the disorder they were worried about was not an inherited one but rather a chance occurrence.

In other instances, counseling results in informing individuals that they are carriers of a trait that is responsible for a child's condition. Even when people understand that they have no control over this, knowledge about passing along a genetic abnormality can cause guilt and self-blame. Marriages and relationships can suffer unless both partners are given adequate support (Weil, 1991).

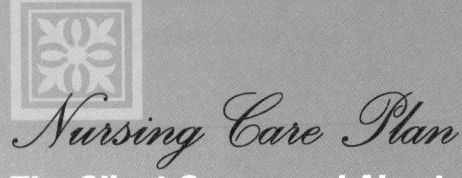

Nursing Care Plan

The Client Concerned About a Genetic Disorder in Future Offspring

Edna Harrison is a 26-year-old woman who is 2 months pregnant and in a prenatal clinic. Her twin sister has Down syndrome. Edna has been afraid until now to have a child because of the chance the child would also have Down syndrome.

Assessment: Client states, "My family has always been so ashamed that a genetic defect could happen in our family; I've always felt like something must be wrong with me, too." She states she wants chorionic villi testing done during all pregnancies to prevent a child of hers being born that way.

Medical chart obtained from her home hospital reveals that her twin sister's karyotype is 47XX21+; they were born when their mother was 42 years old. Her twin's characteristic features include mental retardation, epicanthal folds, bilateral simian palm creases, an endocushion heart defect (repaired), and hypertelorism (widespaced eyes). Client's karyotype is normal (46XX) as is her husband's (46XY). Client's parents have refused to have karyotyping done, stating they do not want to know who "caused" their daughter's retardation.

Nursing Diagnosis: Health seeking behaviors related to knowledge regarding probability of genetic abnormality in children.

Defining Characteristic: Client states she is concerned about having a child with a genetic abnormality.

Goal: Client will demonstrate increased understanding of nature of chromosomal disorders by 1 week.

Outcome Criteria: Client voices that she is not apt to have a genetically abnormal child except by routine chance.

Nursing Orders	Rationale
Schedule appointment with couple to discuss: 1. Pattern of nondisjunction and maternal age as the probable inheritance pattern involved in sister's syndrome. 2. The cause of twinning; she and her sister must be fraternal twins and therefore they do not carry like genes.	1. Down syndrome increases in incidence with maternal age. 2. Client needs to know that she and her sister do not share chromosome genomes.

Nursing Diagnosis: Self-esteem disturbance related to lack of knowledge about cause of sister's illness.

Defining Characteristic: Client states family is "ashamed" of sister; she feels something is wrong with her.

Goal: Client will express increasing ability to deal with forces in her life such as inheritance by 6 months' time.

Outcome Criteria: Client states that because she now understands the basis for genetic disease, she no longer feels as if she is imperfect.

Nursing Orders	Rationale
1. Discuss with client that feelings of shame in regard to genetic abnormalities of offspring were common reactions before the causes of many disorders were known. Now that much more is known about the causes of genetic disorders, including the fact that they are not caused by anything the parent may have done or not done, shame is an outmoded concept. 2. Discuss the risk-benefit of having CVS performed during a pregnancy when chromosomal abnormality is unlikely to occur except by chance.	1. Client's continued feelings of shame about her sister are preventing her from being objective and positive about her own future children. 2. Client needs to know that CVS has a pregnancy loss incidence of about 5%; alpha-fetoprotein would be a safer assessment.

Responsibilities of the Nurse

Nurses play important roles in assessing for genetic disorders, in offering support to individuals who seek genetic counseling, and in helping with reproductive genetic testing procedures (Thomson, 1993). Nurses can be instrumental in alerting a couple to what procedures they can expect to undergo; explaining how different genetic screening tests are done and when they are usually offered; supporting a couple during the wait for test results; and assisting couples in values clarification, planning, and decision-making based on test results. A great deal of time may need to be spent offering support for a grieving couple who realize for the first time how tragically the laws of inheritance affect their lives.

Genetic counseling, however, is a role for nurses only if they are adequately prepared in the study of genetics. Without this background, genetic counseling can be as dangerous and destructive as parlor psychology.

Whether acting as a generalist member of a genetic counseling team or as a genetics counselor, some common principles apply. First, be certain to make sure that the individual or couple being counseled has a clear understanding of the information provided. People may listen to the statistics of their situation ("Your child has a 25% chance of having this disease") and misinterpret what they hear. They can construe a "25% chance" to mean that, if they have one child with the disease, they can then have three normal children without any worry. A 25% chance, however, means that with each pregnancy, there is a 25% chance the child will have the disease (chance has no memory of what already happened). It is as if the couple has four cards, all aces, with the ace of spades representing the disease. When a card is drawn from the set of four, the chance of its being the ace of spades is 1 in 4 (25%). And so it is for the first pregnancy. When the couple is ready to have a second child, it is as if the card drawn during the first round is returned to the set. The chance of drawing the ace

of spades in the second draw is exactly the same as in the first draw. Similarly, the couple's chances of having a child with the disease remain 1 in 4 in the second pregnancy.

Second, be certain never to impose your own values or opinion on others. Individuals with known inherited diseases in their family have to face difficult decisions, such as how much genetic testing to undergo or whether to terminate a pregnancy that will result in a child with a specific genetic disease. Couples should be made aware of all the options available to them, but then they need to think about the options and make their own decisions. It may be difficult to avoid making your opinion known, but couples always should understand that nobody is judging their decision, because it must be one *they* can live with.

Assessment for the Presence of Genetic Disorders

Genetic counseling begins with careful assessment of the pattern of inheritance in the family by history, physical examination of family members, and laboratory analysis, such as karyotyping (see later discussion), in order to define the extent of the problem and the chance of inheritance.

History

A detailed family history is obtained to see if any disorders are present in family members. The mother's age is important to obtain, since some disorders increase in incidence with age. Ethnic background is important, because certain disorders occur more commonly in some ethnic groups than others. If the couple seeking counseling is unfamiliar with the family history, ask them to talk to senior family members about grandparents, aunts, uncles, and so forth before they come for an interview. Ask specifically for instances of spontaneous abortion or children in the family who died at birth. In many instances, these children died of unknown chromosomal disorders or were spontaneously aborted because of one of the 70 or more known chromosomal abnormalities inconsistent with life.

An extensive prenatal history of any affected person should be obtained to see whether environmental conditions could account for the condition. A family pedigree is drawn (see Figure 7-4) to attempt to diagnose the trend of inheritance. Such a diagram not only identifies the possibility of a chromosomal disorder occurring in a couple's children but also helps to identify other family members who would benefit from genetic counseling.

Taking a health history for a genetic pedigree determination is often difficult because facts must be detailed that may evoke uncomfortable emotions such as sorrow, guilt, or inadequacy. Many people may have only sketchy information about their families, such as, "The baby had some kind of nervous disease," or "Her heart didn't work right." You may obtain more information by asking the couple to describe the appearance or activities of the affected individual or asking for permission to obtain health records.

When a child is born dead, parents are currently advised to have a chromosomal analysis and autopsy performed on the infant. If at some future date they wish genetic counseling, this would allow their genetic counselor to have accurate medical information available.

Physical Assessment

A careful physical assessment of any family member with a disorder, that child's siblings, and the couple seeking counseling needs to be made. This is because genetic disorders often occur in various degrees of expression. It might be possible for an individual to have a minimal expression of a disorder and have been undiagnosed up to that point. Important body parts to inspect are the space between the eyes; the height, contour and shape of ears; and the number of fingers and toes and whether webbing exists between them. **Dermatoglyphics** (the study of surface markings of the skin) should also be done, noting any abnormal fingerprints or palmar creases, which appear with some disorders. Abnormal hair whorls or coloring can also be present.

Careful inspection of newborns is often sufficient to identify a child with a potential chromosomal disorder. Infants with multiple congenital anomalies, those born at less than 35 weeks' gestation, and those whose parents have had previous children with chromosomal disorders need extremely critical assessment. Table 7-2 lists the physical characteristics that are suggestive of common inherited syndromes.

Laboratory Analysis

For genetic counseling to be effective, the exact type of genetic disorder being considered must be identified as accurately as possible. There are many laboratory tests which provide important clues into possible disorders. Karyotyping of both parents and those of an already affected child provides a picture of that person's chromosome pattern that can be used to make predictions about future children. When a couple is already pregnant, several other laboratory tests may be performed to help in the prenatal diagnosis of a genetic disorder. These include alpha-fetoprotein analysis, chorionic villi sampling (CVS), amniocentesis, percutaneous umbilical blood sampling (PUBS), sonography, and fetoscopy.

Karyotyping

A **karyotype** is a visual presentation of the chromosome pattern of an individual. For karyotyping, a sample of peripheral venous blood or a scraping of cells from the buccal membrane is taken. Cells are allowed to grow until they reach a stage of metaphase or are at their most easily observed phase. They are then stained, placed

Table 7-2. *Common Physical Characteristics of Children With Chromosomal Syndromes*

Characteristic	Probable Syndrome
Late closure of fontanelles	Down syndrome
Bossing (prominent forehead)	Fragile X syndrome
Microcephaly	Trisomy 18, trisomy 13
Low-set ears	Trisomy 18, trisomy 13
Slant of eyes	Down syndrome
Epicanthal fold	Down syndrome
Abnormal iris color	Down syndrome
Large tongue	Down syndrome
Prominent jaw	Fragile X syndrome
Low-set hair line	Turner's syndrome
Multiple hair whorls	Trisomy 18, trisomy 13
Webbed neck	Turner's syndrome
Wide-set nipples	Trisomy 13
Heart abnormalities	Many syndromes
Large hands	Fragile X syndrome
Clinodactyly	Down syndrome
Overriding of fingers	Trisomy 18
Rocker-bottom feet	Trisomy 13
Abnormal dermatoglyphics	Down syndrome
Simian crease on palm	Down syndrome
Absence of secondary sex characteristics	Klinefelter's and Turner's syndromes

under a microscope, and photographed through the microscope. Chromosomes are identified according to size and shape and stain, cut from the photograph, and arranged as in Figure 7-1. Additional, lacking, or abnormal chromosomes can be visualized by this method.

A new method allows karyotyping to be done immediately, rather than waiting for the cells to reach metaphase. *Fluorescence in situ hybridization (FISH)* staining can be done in interphase as well. This makes it possible for a report to be obtained in a day's time (Shapiro & Wilmot, 1993).

Barr Body Determination

If a child is born with ambiguous genitalia (it is difficult to determine if the child is male or female from outward appearance), a quick test to determine whether the child has two X chromosomes (female) is a Barr body determination. For this, cells are scraped from the buccal membrane of the inner surface of the child's cheek; these are then stained and magnified. Only one X chromosome is functional in females; the nondominant one appears to be uninvolved in cell metabolism. After staining, the presence of this nondominant X chromosome will appear as a black dot on the edge of the nucleus. It is called a *Barr body*. The presence of a Barr body confirms that the child is chromosomally female. Following this rapid procedure, the child will need further chromosomal investigation, including a complete karyotype, to reveal his or her complete chromosomal pattern. In order for the laboratory technician performing a Barr body test to be certain the cell stain was adequately absorbed, a known female's buccal membrane scraping is examined as well. Technicians may ask a female nurse assisting with the buccal scraping procedure to serve as the test control.

Chorionic Villi Sampling

Chorionic villi sampling (CVS) is retrieval and analysis of chorionic villi for chromosome analysis. Although this procedure may be done as early as the fifth week of pregnancy (Brambati et al., 1990), it is more commonly done at 8 to 10 weeks (Stringer, Librizzi, & Weiner, 1991). With this technique, the chorion cells are located by ultrasound. A thin catheter is then inserted vaginally or a biopsy needle is inserted abdominally or intravaginally, and a number of chorionic cells are removed for analysis (Figure 7-10). CVS carries a small risk (about 2% to 4%) of causing labor contractions and excessive bleeding, and parents should be counseled about this risk prior to the procedure (Rosenfield & Fathalla, 1990). There have been some instances of children born with missing limbs following the procedure (limb reduction syndrome), but the risk of this is apparently small (Shulman et al., 1994). Following CVS, women need to be instructed to report chills or fever suggestive of infection or symptoms of abortion (uterine contractions or vaginal bleeding). Women with an Rh-negative blood type need Rh immune globulin administration to guard against isoimmunization in the fetus.

The cells removed by chorionic villi sampling are karyotyped or submitted for DNA analysis to reveal whether or not the fetus has a genetic disorder. Because chorionic villi cells are dividing rapidly, results are available rapidly, perhaps as soon as the following day. If a twin or multiple pregnancy is present, with two or more separate placentas, it is important that cells be removed separately from each placenta. Because fraternal twins are derived from separate ova, one twin could have a chromosomal abnormality while the other is normal.

It is important for parents to understand that not all inherited diseases can be detected by CVS (only those which involve abnormal chromosomes or whose gene location or specific DNA disorder is known). Table 7-3 shows common chromosomal dysjunction disorders that can be diagnosed prenatally through karyotyping. Other conditions, such as cystic fibrosis, muscular dystrophy, and Huntington's chorea are identified by gene markers on individual chromosomes.

Whether or not to have CVS is a major decision for a couple because, as a rule, they are not making a decision simply for CVS; if the CVS reveals that their child is abnormal, they will be asked to make a decision about aborting the pregnancy.

Making an abortion decision during a pregnancy is rarely easy. The couple may need a great deal of support to carry through with their decision; they also will

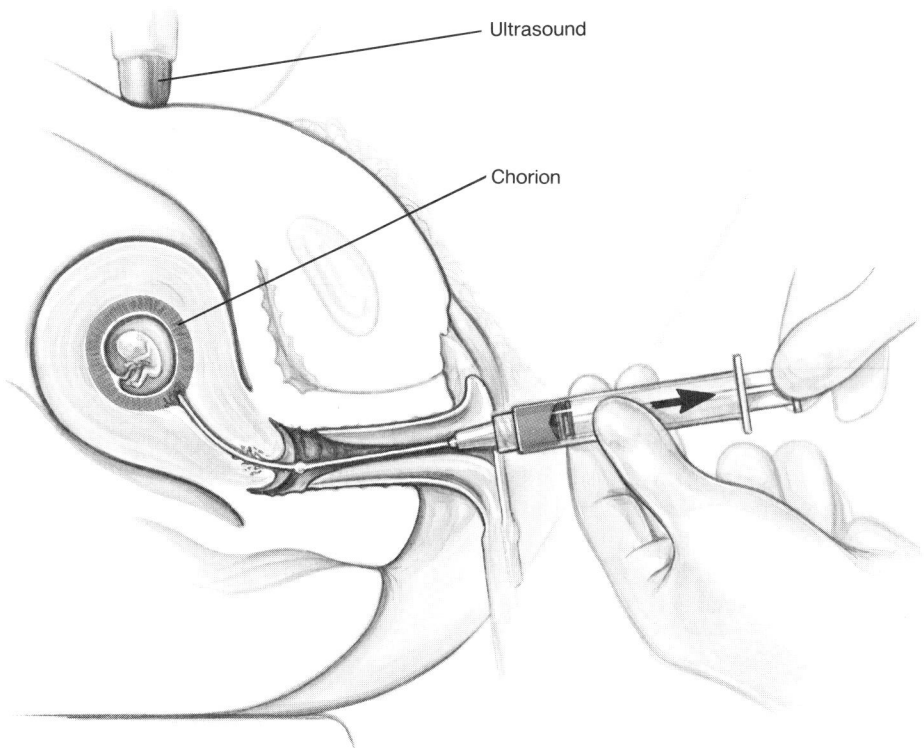

FIGURE 7-10

Chorionic villi sampling. Since the villi arise from trophoblast cells, their chromosome structure is the same as the fetus's.

Table 7-3. *Chromosomally Determined Diseases That Can Be Detected by Amniocentesis or CVS*

Syndrome	Chromosomal Characteristics	Clinical Signs
Down syndrome	Extra chromosome 21	Mental retardation; protruding tongue; epicanthal folds; hypotonia
Translocation Down syndrome	Translocation of a chromosome, perhaps 14/21	Same clinical signs as trisomy 21
Trisomy 18	Extra chromosome 18	Mental retardation; congenital malformations
Trisomy 13	Extra chromosome 13	Mental retardation; multiple congenital malformations; eye agenesis
Cri-du-chat syndrome	Deletion of short arm of chromosome 5	Mental retardation; facial structure anomalies; peculiar, cat-like cry
Fragile X syndrome	Distortion of the X chromosome	Mental retardation
Philadelphia chromosome	Deletion of one arm of chromosome 21	Chronic granulocytic leukemia
Turner's syndrome	XO	Short stature; streak gonads; infertility; webbing of the neck
Klinefelter's syndrome	XXY	Small testes; gynecomastia; infertility

need support during the remainder of the pregnancy and in the days following birth if they decide not to end the pregnancy. It may be hard for a couple to believe that what the test showed is real. Only when they inspect the baby and see that the test was accurate—that the child does have Down syndrome, for example—do they realize the truth. The result may be a long-lasting depression.

Because CVS is not without risk, some physicians are reluctant to perform the procedure for chromosomal analysis unless the couple agrees that they will consent to an abortion if an abnormality is detected. Parents do not need to feel bound to this prior agreement, however; they can decide against abortion even after learning of the chromosomal disorder. The consent they sign before the CVS cannot be considered "informed" consent and therefore would not be binding.

Alpha-fetoprotein Analysis

Alpha-fetoprotein is a glycoprotein produced by the fetal liver. The level of alpha-fetoprotein present in amniotic fluid (AFAFP) or maternal serum (MSAFP) will change from normal if a chromosomal or a spinal cord disorder is present. The test is done at the 15th week of pregnancy. The level is elevated in spinal cord disease (twice the value of the mean for that gestational age). It will be decreased in a chromosomal disorder such as trisomy 21 (Palomaki, 1990).

Amniocentesis

Amniocentesis is the withdrawal of amniotic fluid through the abdominal wall for analysis at the 14th to 16th week of a pregnancy. Analysis may include the karyotyping of skin cells obtained or analysis of alpha-fetoprotein or acetylcholinesterase. Assessing for acetylcholinesterase helps to reduce false-positive results. It is a substance present in blood. If the acetylcholinesterase result is negative it shows that an elevated alpha-fetoprotein level is truly elevated and is not a false-positive reading from blood in the fluid obtained. Some disorders such as Tay-Sachs disease can be identified by the presence of a specific enzyme in amniotic fluid. Since amniocentesis is also a common assessment for fetal maturity, it is discussed further in Chapter 9 (see Figure 9-16).

New techniques of amniocentesis allow it to be done as early as the 12th week of pregnancy (Shulman, 1994). Although not as much amniotic fluid can be removed at this time (only about 2 mL compared to 5 mL later), this will yield enough fluid for genetic testing. For the procedure, a pocket of amniotic fluid is located by sonogram; a needle is inserted abdominally and fluid aspirated. Skin cells in the fluid are karyotyped for chromosomal number and structure. The level of alpha-fetoprotein is analyzed. Amniocentesis has the advantage over CVS of carrying only a 0.5% risk of labor occurring from the procedure (Rosenfield & Fathalla, 1990). Unfortunately, it is usually not done until the 14th to 16th week of pregnancy, which is a time when the woman is beginning to accept her pregnancy and perhaps to "nest build." Women with an Rh-negative blood type need Rh immune globulin administration after the procedure to protect against isoimmunization in the fetus. All women need to be monitored for about 30 minutes afterward to be certain that labor contractions are not beginning.

Percutaneous Umbilical Blood Sampling

Percutaneous umbilical blood sampling (PUBS) is the removal of blood from the umbilical cord using an amniocentesis technique (Figure 7-11). This allows for more rapid karyotyping than is possible when only skin cells are removed. PUBS is discussed further in Chapter 9.

Sonography

Sonography is a diagnostic tool that is helpful in assessing a fetus for general size and structural disorders of internal organs, spine, and limbs. Sonography may be used concurrently with amniocentesis, because it causes no apparent risk to the fetus (Rottem & Chervenak, 1990).

Fetoscopy

Fetoscopy is the insertion into the uterus and membranes of a fiberoptic fetoscope through a small incision in the mother's abdomen to inspect the fetus for gross abnormalities. It could be used to confirm a sonography finding or remove skin cells for DNA analysis.

Preimplantation Diagnosis

It is not recommended at present, but in the future it may be possible for a fertilized embryo to be removed

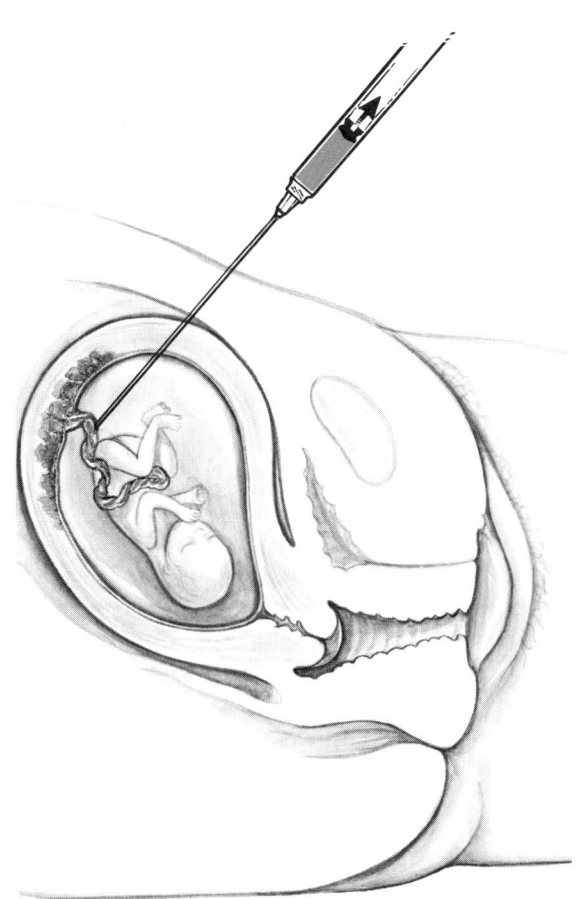

FIGURE 7-11
Percutaneous umbilical blood sampling. Blood is withdrawn from the cord using amniocentesis technique.

from the uterus by lavage before implantation, with cells from the zona pellucida removed and biopsied for DNA or cell analysis. The ova would then be reinserted or not, depending on the findings and the parent's wishes (Simpson, 1990). This would provide genetic information extremely early in a pregnancy. It may also one day allow healthy genes to be inserted to correct underlying disorders very early in pregnancy.

Reproductive Alternatives

Some couples are reluctant to seek genetic counseling because they are afraid they will be told it would be unwise to have children. Helping them to realize that viable alternatives for having a family exist for them allows them to seek the help they need.

Artificial insemination by donor (AID) is an option for couples in whom the genetic disorder is one inherited by the male partner or is a recessively inherited disorder carried by both partners. AID is available in all major communities and permits the couple to experience the satisfaction and enjoyment of a normal pregnancy.

If the inherited problem is one caused by the female partner, use of a surrogate mother (a woman who agrees to be artificially inseminated by the male partner's sperm and bear a child for the couple) is a possibility. Donor embryo transfer (an ovum is taken from a donor, fertilized in the laboratory by the husband's sperm, and then implanted in the wife's uterus) is a procedure that is performed in major centers. Like AID, donor embryo transfer offers the couple a chance to experience a normal pregnancy. All these procedures are expensive and, depending on the individual circumstances, may have disappointing success rates. They are discussed in more detail in Chapter 6.

Pregnancy interruption or therapeutic abortion of any pregnancy that reveals a chromosomal or metabolic abnormality is yet another option. Diagnosis of a disorder during pregnancy and prompt treatment at birth to minimize the prognosis and outcome of the disorder is another possibility.

Adoption is an alternative many couples find rewarding (see Chapters 2 and 6). Also, choosing to remain childfree should not be discounted as a viable option. Many couples who have every reason to think they would have normal children choose this alternative because they believe their existence is full and rewarding without the presence of children.

Couples need support from health care personnel to decide on the alternative that is correct for them. It is most important for a couple to select the option that is right for them, not one that they sense a counselor feels would be best. They may need to consider the ethical philosophy or beliefs of other family members when making their decision, although ultimately they must do what they feel is best.

Legal and Ethical Aspects of Genetic Screening and Counseling

Nurses can be instrumental in seeing that couples who seek genetic counseling receive results in a timely manner and with compassion as to what the results may mean to future childbearing (Aylsworth, 1992). When participating in genetic screening or counseling, there are a number of legal responsibilities to keep in mind. These are shown in Box 7-1. Failure to heed these guidelines could result in charges of invasion of privacy, breach of confidentiality, or psychologic injury caused by "labeling" someone or imparting unwarranted fear and worry about the significance of a disease or carrier state. All couples who seek counseling and are identified as being at risk for having a child with a genetic disorder must be informed of the risk and offered appropriate diagnostic procedures such as amniocentesis. "Wrongful birth" lawsuits have been initiated against health care providers for not making this information available to them.

Genetic screening and counseling can raise serious ethical questions for a couple, particularly when they choose to abort a pregnancy based on CVS or amniocentesis findings. Some people argue that a decision to abort a child just because he or she will be mentally or physically handicapped is unethical. The problem becomes thornier when a disorder that affects only male or only female offspring is present. For instance, a woman who carries the gene for an X-linked disorder for which there is no prenatal screening test might choose to abort all male fetuses, even though each will have a 50% chance of not inheriting the disease. Another dilemma can occur if it is discovered that a twin pregnancy includes one normal and one affected child. Is it ethical to attempt to abort the diseased child when the procedure also might endanger the child without the disorder?

It is important to remember that the choice to be made is the couple's, not the counselor's. A useful place to start counseling might be with values clarification, to be certain the couple understands what is most important to them.

Common Chromosomal Disorders Resulting in Physical or Cognitive Developmental Disorders

A number of chromosomal disorders may be detected at birth on physical examination. The most common chromosome disorders revealed this way are nondisjunction syndromes. All have the potential for causing mental retardation. Care of the child with mental retardation is discussed in Chapter 54.

Trisomy 13 Syndrome

Trisomy 13 syndrome (Patau's syndrome) is a syndrome in which children have an extra chromosome 13. Children with this disorder are grossly mentally retarded. The incidence is low, approximately 0.45 per 1000 live births. Midline body disorders are present and common findings are microcephaly with abnormalities of the forebrain and forehead; eyes that are smaller than normal (*microphthalmia*) or absent; cleft lip and palate; low-set ears; heart defects, particularly ventricular septal defects; and abnormal genitalia. Most of these children do not survive past early childhood.

Trisomy 18 Syndrome

Children with *trisomy 18 syndrome* have three number-18 chromosomes. They are severely mentally retarded. The incidence is approximately 0.23 per 1000 live births. These children tend to be small for gestational age at birth. They have markedly low-set ears, a small jaw, congenital heart defects, and misshapen fingers and toes (the index finger tends to deviate or cross over other fingers). Also, the soles of their feet are often rounded instead of flat (rocker-bottom feet). Most of these children do not survive beyond early infancy.

Cri du Chat Syndrome

Cri du Chat syndrome (46XX5q−) is the result of a short arm on chromosome 5. In addition to an abnormal cry, which is much more like the sound of a cat's than a

---

Box 7-1
Focus on Nursing Care

Legal Guidelines for Genetic Screening

Participation in genetic screening programs must be elective, not mandatory.

People desiring genetic screening should sign an informed consent form for the procedure.

Results must be interpreted carefully and relayed to individuals as promptly as possible.

The results must not be withheld from individuals.

The results must not be given to persons other than those directly involved.

After genetic counseling, persons must not be coerced to undergo procedures such as abortion or sterilization. This should be a free, individually dictated choice.

human infant's, children with cri du chat syndrome tend to have a small head, wide-set eyes, and a downward slant to the palpebral fissure of the eye. They are severely mentally retarded.

Turner's Syndrome

The child with *Turner's syndrome* (gonadal dysgenesis; 45X0) has only one functional X chromosome (Lippe, 1991). The child is short in stature. The hairline at the nape of the neck is low-set, and the neck may appear to be webbed and short. The newborn may have appreciable edema of the hands and feet and a number of congenital anomalies, most frequently *coarctation* (stricture) of the aorta and kidney disorders. The child has only *streak* (small and nonfunctional) gonads, so that, with the exception of pubic hair, secondary sex characteristics do not develop at puberty. Lack of ovarian function results in sterility. The incidence is approximately 1 per 10,000 live births (Williams, 1992). With Barr body determination, the child is shown to have only one X chromosome (no Barr body present).

Although children with Turner's syndrome may have mental retardation, more commonly they have learning disabilities that interfere with learning ability (see the Focus on Nursing Research box). Socioemotional adjustment problems often accompany the syndrome as well.

If treatment with estrogen is begun at approximately age 13 years, secondary sex characteristics will appear. If females continue taking estrogen for 3 out of every 4 weeks, they will have withdrawal bleeding that results in a menstrual flow. This flow, however, does not correct the problem of sterility; the gonadal tissue is scant and inadequate for ovulation because of the basic chromosomal aberration. Growth hormone may help children with Turner's syndrome to achieve additional height.

Klinefelter's Syndrome

Infants with Klinefelter's syndrome are males with an XXY chromosome pattern (47XXY). Characteristics of the syndrome may not be noticeable at birth. At puberty, the child has poorly developed secondary sex characteristics and small testes that produce ineffective sperm (Mandoki & Sumner, 1991). They tend to develop gynecomastia (increased breast size). The incidence is about 1 per 1000 live births. A Barr body test can be used to reveal the additional X chromosome present.

Fragile X Syndrome

Fragile X Syndrome is an X-linked pattern of inheritance in which one long arm of an X chromosome is weakened. The incidence is about 1 in 1000 live births. It

FOCUS ON NURSING RESEARCH

Do Children with Turner's Syndrome Benefit from Instruction in Problem-Solving?

Children with Turner's syndrome typically exhibit learning difficulties that can interfere with progress in school. Although many teaching strategies have been designed to increase the attention span and learning ability of children with nonverbal learning disabilities, it was unknown if the learning disabilities that occur in association with Turner's syndrome were similar enough to these that children with Turner's syndrome could benefit from the same teaching strategies.

For this study, two control groups of children ages 7 to 13 years with learning disabilities were matched against an experimental group of like age children with Turner's syndrome. All groups were pretested by five tests of memory and attention. Children were then taught a problem-solving strategy.

The results of the study showed that following the problem-solving sessions, all children improved significantly. There were not significant differences in overall scores of the groups, or children with Turner's syndrome appeared to have the same difficulties with learning as the others. Children with Turner's syndrome are therefore likely to benefit from educational strategies designed for the nonverbal learning difficulties population.

Williams, J. K. (1992). School-aged children and Turner's syndrome. *Journal of Pediatric Nursing, 7,* 14.

is the commonest cause of mental retardation in boys (Giannopoulou & Turk, 1992).

Before puberty, boys with fragile X syndrome typically have maladaptive behaviors such as hyperactivity and autism. They have reduced intellectual functioning with marked deficits in speech and arithmetic. They may be identified by the presence of a large head, a long face with a high forehead, a prominent lower jaw, and large protruding ears. Hyperextensive joints and cardiac disorders may also be present. After puberty, enlarged testicles may become evident. Affected individuals are fertile and can reproduce (Caskey et al., 1994).

Carrier females may show some evidence of the physical and cognitive characteristics. Although intellectual function from the syndrome cannot be improved, both folic acid and phenothiazide administration may improve symptoms of poor concentration and impulsivity.

Down Syndrome (Trisomy 21)

Trisomy 21, the most frequent chromosomal abnormality, occurs as frequently as 1 in 800 live births. Formerly called mongolism because an upward slant of the eyes makes the child look Asian, the syndrome occurs most frequently in the pregnancies of women who are over 35 years of age (the incidence is as high as 1 in 100 live births for these women). Paternal age (over 55) may also contribute to the increased incidence in this age group (Cooley & Graham, 1991).

The physical features of children with Down syndrome are so marked that fetal diagnosis is possible by sonogram in utero. The nose is broad and flat; the eyelids have an extra fold of tissue at the inner canthus (an epicanthal fold); and the palpebral fissure (opening between the eyelids) tends to slant laterally upward. The iris of the eye may have white specks in it called Brushfield's spots (Tunnessen, 1990). Even in the newborn, the tongue may protrude from the mouth because the oral cavity is smaller than normal. The back of the head is flat; the neck is short, and an extra pad of fat at the base of the head causes the skin there to be so loose it can be lifted up (like a puppy's neck). The ears may be low-set. Muscle tone is poor, giving the baby a rag-doll appearance; this can be so lax, the child's toe can be touched against the nose (not possible in the average mature newborn). The fingers of many children with Down syndrome are short and thick, and the little finger is often curved inward. There may be a wide space between the first and second toes and first and second fingers. The palm of the hand shows a peculiar crease (a simian line) or a horizontal palm crease rather than the normal three creases in the palm (Figure 7-12).

Children with Down syndrome usually have some degree of mental retardation, but the retardation can range from that of an educable child (intelligence quotient [IQ] of 50 to 70) to one requiring institutionalization (IQ less than 20). The extent of retardation is not evident at birth. Educable children may represent mosaic chromosomal patterns. The fact that the brain is not developing well is shown by a head size that is generally under the 10th or 20th percentile at well child visits.

These children appear to have altered immune function; they are prone to upper respiratory infections. Congenital heart disease, especially atrioventricular defects, are common (Walker, 1991). Stenosis or atresia of the duodenum and strabismus and cataract disorders are also common. For unknown reasons, acute lymphocytic leukemia occurs approximately 20 times more frequently in children with Down syndrome than in the healthy population. Even if children are born without an accompanying disorder such as heart disease, their lifespan generally is only 40 to 50 years and aging seems to occur faster than normal.

Children with Down syndrome need to be exposed to early educational and play opportunities (see Chapter 54). Because they are prone to infections, sensible precautions such as using good handwashing technique should always be taken when caring for them. The enlarged tongue may interfere with swallowing and cause choking unless the child is fed slowly.

As with all newborns, they need physical examination at birth in order that the genetic disorder can be detected and counseling and support for parents can begin.

Key Points

- Genetic disorders are ones that result from malstructure or number of genes or chromosomes. Genetics is the study of how and why such disorders occur.

- A phenotype is a person's outward appearance. Genotype refers to actual gene composition. A person's genome is the complete set of genes present. A karyotype is a graphic representation of chromosomes present.

- A person is homozygous if he or she has two like genes for a trait; heterozygous if he or she has two unlike genes for a trait.

- Mendelian laws can predict the likely incidence of recessive or dominant diseases in offspring. Division disorders including nondisjunction abnormalities, deletion, translocation, and mosaicism also create genetic disorders.

- Genetic counseling can be a role for nurses if they are well versed in genetics. Assessment of genetic disorders consists of a health history, physical examination, and laboratory studies such as chorionic villi sampling, amniocentesis, and buccal smears.

- Some karyotyping tests such as chorionic villi sampling and amniocentesis introduce a risk of initiating labor. Be certain that women undergoing these tests remain in the health care facility for at least 30 minutes after a procedure to be certain that a complication such as vaginal bleeding or labor contractions are not beginning.

- Women with an Rh-negative blood type need

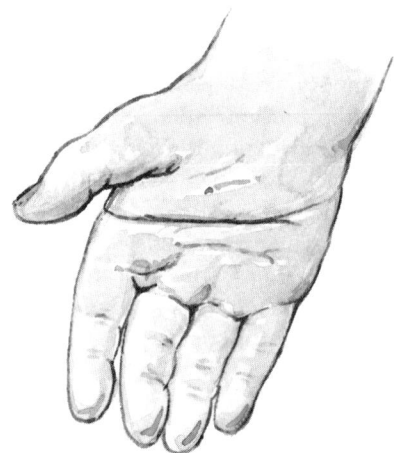

FIGURE 7-12
A simian line, a horizontal palm crease seen in children with Down syndrome.

Rh immune globulin administration after these procedures.

- An important aspect of genetic counseling is respecting a couple's right to privacy. Be certain that information is not given indiscriminately to other family members.
- People who are told that a genetic abnormality does exist in their family may suffer a loss of self-esteem. Offering support to help them deal with the feelings they experience is an important nursing intervention.
- Common nondisjunction genetic disorders are Down syndrome (trisomy 21), trisomy 13, trisomy 18, Turner's syndrome, and Klinefelter's syndrome. Most of these syndromes include mental retardation, which is discussed in Chapter 54.

Critical Thinking Exercises

Edna Harrison, the woman described in the nursing care plan in this chapter, is a 26-year-old woman seen in a prenatal clinic. Her twin sister has Down syndrome. Edna has been afraid until now to have a child because of the chance her child will also have the syndrome. She states, "My family has always been so ashamed that a genetic defect could happen in our family."

1. Why would a genetic syndrome appear in one twin and not the other this way?
2. What does the client's statement about her family feeling ashamed reveal about her knowledge of genetic disorders?
3. Would it be realistic to assure Edna that her child will not have Down syndrome?
4. What genetic tests would you anticipate Edna will have ordered during pregnancy in order that Down syndrome in her child can be detected?
5. Suppose Edna is so worried that her child has the syndrome that she decides to abort her fetus and remain childless rather than undergo genetic testing? Is this her right? What would be her fetus's rights?

References

Aylsworth, A. S. (1992). Genetic counseling for patients with birth defects. *Pediatric Clinics of North America, 39,* 229.

Brambati, B., et al. (1990). Transabdominal and transcervical chorionic villus sampling. *American Journal of Medical Genetics, 35,* 160.

Campbell, J. (1992). Making sense of the principles of genetics. *Nursing Times, 88,* 36.

Caskey, C. T., et al. (1994). Human genes: The map takes shape. *Patient Care, 28,* 28.

Cooley, W. C., & Graham, J. M. (1991). Down syndrome: An update and review. *Clinical Pediatrics, 30,* 233.

Department of Health and Human Services. (1991). *Healthy people 2000.* Washington, DC: Public Health Service.

Fernbach, S. D., & Thomson, E. J. (1992). Molecular genetic technology in cystic fibrosis: implications for nursing practice. *Journal of Pediatric Nursing, 7,* 20.

Giannopoulou, I., & Turk, J. (1992). Clues to the detection of fragile X syndrome. *Health Visitor, 65,* 113.

Hall, J. (1990). Genomic imprinting: Review and relevance to human diseases. *American Journal of Human Genetics, 46,* 857.

Lippe, B. (1991). Turner syndrome. *Endocrinology and Metabolic Clinics of North America, 20,* 121.

Mandoki, M., & Sumner, G. (1991). Klinefelter syndrome; the need for early identification and treatment. *Clinical Pediatrics, 30,* 161.

Palomaki, G. E., et al. (1990). Maternal serum alphafetoprotein screening for fetal Down syndrome in the United States: Results of a survey. *American Journal of Obstetrics and Gynecology, 162,* 317.

Rosenfield, A., & Fathalla, M. F. (1990). *The F.I.G.O. manual of human reproduction.* Park Ridge, NJ: Parthenon.

Rosenstein, B. J. (1994). Cystic fibrosis. In Oski, F. A., et al. *Principles and practice of pediatrics.* Philadelphia: J. B. Lippincott, pp. 1362–1372.

Rottem, S., & Chervenak, F. A. (1990). Ultrasound diagnosis of fetal anomalies. *Obstetrics and Gynecology Clinics of North America, 17,* 17.

Shapiro, L. R., & Wilmot, P. L. (1993). Cytogenetic diagnosis of genetic diseases. *Pediatric Annals, 22,* 298.

Shulman, L. P., et al. (1994). Amniocentesis performed at 14 weeks' gestation or earlier: comparison with first-trimester transabdominal chorionic villus sampling. *Obstetrics and Gynecology, 83,* 543.

Simpson, J. L. (1990). Genetic factors in obstetrics and gynecology. In Scott, J. R. *Danforth's obstetrics and gynecology* (6th ed.). Philadelphia: J. B. Lippincott.

Spector, R. E. (1991). *Cultural diversity in health and illness* (3rd. ed.). Norwalk, CT: Appleton & Lange.

Stringer, M., Librizzi, R., & Weiner, S. (1991). Establishing a prenatal genetic diagnosis: the nurse's role. *MCN: American Journal of Maternal Child Nursing, 16,* 152.

Strobel, S. E., & Keller, C. S. (1993). Metabolic screening in the NICU population: proposal for change. *Pediatric Nursing, 19,* 113.

Thomson, E. J. (1993). Reproductive genetic testing: implications for nursing education. *Fetal Diagnosis & Therapy, 1,* 232S.

Tunnessen, W. W. (1994). Common syndromes with morphologic abnormalities. In Oski, F. A., et al. *Principles and practice of pediatrics.* Philadelphia: J. B. Lippincott.

Walker, C. (1991). Down's syndrome and congenital heart defects: anatomical and functional anomalies: prognosis and treatment. *Intensive Care Nursing, 7,* 94.

Weil, J. (1991). Mothers' postcounseling beliefs about the causes of their children's genetic disorders. *American Journal of Human Genetics, 48,* 145.

Williams, J. K. (1992). School-aged children and Turner's syndrome. *Journal of Pediatric Nursing, 7,* 14.

Suggested Readings

Beaudet, A. L. (1992). Genetic testing for cystic fibrosis. *Pediatric Clinics of North America, 39,* 213.

Buist, N. R., & Tuerck, J. M. (1992). The practitioner's role in newborn screening. *Pediatric Clinics of North America, 39,* 199.

Collins, J. E. (1994). Fetal surgery: Changing the outcome before birth. *Journal of Obstetrics, Gynecologic, and Neonatal Nursing, 23,* 166.

George, J. B. (1992). Genetics: challenges for nursing education. *Journal of Pediatric Nursing, 7,* 5.

Kenner, C., et al. (1990). Nursing in genetics: current and energizing issues for practice and education. *Journal of Pediatric Nursing, 5,* 370.

MacGregor, E. (1991). Dilemmas in genetic screening. *Nursing (London), 4,* 13.

Monsen, R. B. (1992). Endpaper: a national agenda for nursing and genetics. *Journal of Pediatric Nursing, 7,* 63.

Moskowitz, C. B. (1991). The primary dystonias of childhood. *Journal of Neuroscience Nursing, 23,* 175.

Oehler, J. M., et al. (1993). How to target infants at highest risk for developmental delay. *MCN: American Journal of Maternal Child Nursing, 18,* 20.

Prows, C. A. (1992). Utilization of genetic knowledge in pediatric nursing practice. *Journal of Pediatric Nursing, 7,* 58.

Rowley, P. T., et al. (1991). Prenatal screening for hemoglobinopathies: applicability of the health belief model. *American Journal of Human Genetics, 48,* 447.

Van Dyke, D. L., et al. (1991). Mental retardation in Turner syndrome. *Journal of Pediatrics, 118,* 415.

Walker, C. (1991). Down's syndrome and congenital heart defects: an extended care plan. *Intensive Care Nursing, 7,* 148.

Wright, L., et al. (1992). Newborn screening; the miracle and the challenge. *Journal of Pediatric Nursing, 7,* 26.

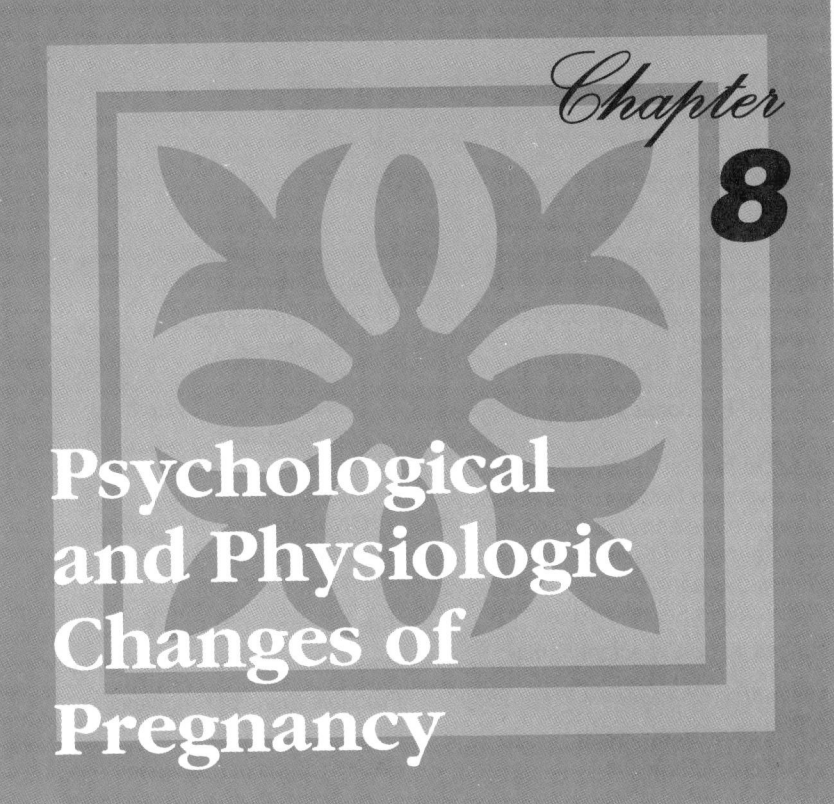

Psychological and Physiologic Changes of Pregnancy

Objectives

After mastering the contents of this chapter, you should be able to:

1. Describe the psychological and physiologic changes that occur with pregnancy, the underlying principles for these changes, and the relationship of the changes to pregnancy diagnosis.

2. Assess a woman for the psychological and physiologic changes that occur with pregnancy through health history and physical examination.

3. Formulate nursing diagnoses related to psychological and physiologic changes of pregnancy.

4. Plan nursing care related to the changes and diagnosis of pregnancy, such as helping women plan to get adequate rest.

5. Implement nursing care, such as health teaching related to the expected changes of pregnancy.

6. Evaluate outcome criteria to be certain that nursing goals established for care were achieved.

7. Identify National Health Goals that nurses could be instrumental in helping the nation achieve.

8. Identify areas of nursing care related to the psychological and physiologic changes of pregnancy that could benefit from additional nursing research.

9. Use critical thinking to analyze how the physical and psychological changes of pregnancy affect family functioning and develop ways to make nursing care more family centered.

10. Synthesize knowledge of psychological and physiologic changes in pregnancy with nursing process to achieve quality maternal and child health nursing care.

Key Terms

- ballottement
- Braxton Hicks contractions
- couvade syndrome
- diastasis
- Goodell's sign
- Hegar's sign
- hyperptyalism
- lightening
- melasma
- multipara
- operculum
- polyuria
- positive signs of pregnancy
- presumptive signs of pregnancy
- primigravida
- probable signs of pregnancy
- pseudoanemia

Adele Pillitteri: MATERNAL AND CHILD
HEALTH NURSING, 2nd Edition. © 1995
Adele Pillitteri.

Pregnancy brings both psychological and physical changes to the woman and her partner.

The physiologic changes of pregnancy occur gradually but eventually affect all organ systems of the woman's body. Psychological changes occur in response not only to the physiologic alterations that are occurring but also to the increased responsibility associated with welcoming a new and completely dependent person to the family. Although physiologic changes that occur with pregnancy are extensive, they are also temporary; when pregnancy ends, the woman's body returns virtually to its pre-pregnant state. The changes occur in order for the woman to provide oxygen and nutrients for the growing fetus as well as extra nutrients for her own increased metabolism during the pregnancy. They ready her body for labor and birth and for lactation if she chooses to breast-feed once the baby is born. Despite the magnitude of some of these changes, it cannot be stressed enough that they are extensions of *normal physiology*. This means that pregnancy represents *wellness*, not illness. Because of this, the major responsibility of the nurse caring for the pregnant woman and family is to help the family maintain a state of wellness throughout the pregnancy and into early parenthood. A National Health Goal relevant to this issue is shown in the Focus on National Health Goals box.

⊠ **NURSING PROCESS OVERVIEW**
for Healthy Adaptation to Pregnancy

ASSESSMENT

Women are interested in the changes pregnancy brings, because these changes verify the reality and mark the progress of a pregnancy. Physical findings are gained through health history, physical assessment, and laboratory tests. Assessment in psychological areas is obtained primarily through interviewing. Be certain that you establish a trusting relationship with a woman early in her pregnancy so that she will see you as a person who is capable of counseling her and helping her solve problems and in whom she is willing to confide necessary information.

NURSING DIAGNOSIS

Nursing diagnoses involving the changes that occur with pregnancy include:

- Anxiety related to unexpected pregnancy
- Ineffective breathing pattern related to respiratory system changes of pregnancy
- Body image disturbance related to weight gain with pregnancy

PLANNING

Even though a woman may have read pamphlets or talked to her friends about the physiologic changes of pregnancy, she is often surprised to see these changes occurring in herself. She may say, "I knew I'd be tired, but I never guessed it would be this bad," or "I've read about a brown line forming on my abdomen, but is it normal for it to be this dark? Will this go away?"

Planning nursing care in connection with physiologic and psychological changes of pregnancy should involve a plan to review this type of concern with women as well as a plan to ask about individual responses they are experiencing.

IMPLEMENTATION

The changes of pregnancy may appear insignificant if taken one by one, but together they add up to major changes.

Most women of childbearing age have a mental picture of themselves. A woman may have a good idea how she will look in a dress before she tries it on in a store. She participates in sports or other activities that conform to her self-image. Then, in 9 months, she gains 25 to 30 lb and her figure changes so drastically that none of her pre-pregnancy clothes fit. At the beginning of pregnancy, she may feel constantly nauseated. To-

ward the end of pregnancy, the extra weight and the strain of waiting may make her feel tired and short of breath. Endocrine changes make her moody and, perhaps, quick to cry. She may never have been concerned with her health before, and now, every month (and toward the end of pregnancy, every week), she must report for a prenatal checkup. She may worry that she will never lose all the weight she has gained, that the stretch marks on her abdomen will remain forever, and that she will always be as tired or as nauseated as she feels during various stages of her pregnancy.

At prenatal visits, women need help in voicing their concerns about these physiologic changes of pregnancy. The worry brought on by these changes may compound an already stressful situation if the woman is not forewarned that the changes are a normal but transitory part of pregnancy.

EVALUATION

Evaluation should determine if a woman has really "heard" your teaching. Remember that people under stress do not always comprehend well, and pregnancy is a 9-month stress period. It is not unusual for a woman to pocket away information, thinking, "I'll concentrate on what that means when it happens to me, not now." Then, when a particular change has happened, she realizes that she has forgotten what you said. Evaluation that reveals learning did not take place confirms that pregnancy is a period of stress more often than it reflects the quality of teaching. Examples of outcome criteria you might strive for are:

- Client states that she is able to continue usual lifestyle through pregnancy.
- Family members describe ways they have adjusted lifestyle to accommodate mother's fatigue.
- Couple states they accept physiologic changes of pregnancy as normal happenings.

Psychological Changes of Pregnancy

A woman's attitude toward a pregnancy depends a great deal on the environment in which she was raised, the messages about pregnancy her family communicated to her as a child, and the society and culture in which she lives as an adult.

Social Influences

Until recently, the heavy emphasis on medical management for women during pregnancy conveyed the idea that pregnancy was a 9-month-long illness. The preg-

FOCUS ON
National Health Goals

At least one National Health Goal speaks directly to the physiologic and psychologic changes of pregnancy:

- Increase to at least 60% the proportion of primary care providers who provide age-appropriate preconception care and counseling (DHHS, 1991).

Nurses can be instrumental in helping the nation achieve this objective by being certain that adolescents receive counseling in nutrition and safe sex practices so they can enter intended pregnancies in good health. Nursing research to identify the best way to reach mature women with preconception counseling is also important.

nant woman went alone to a physician's office for care; at the time of birth, she was separated from her family and admitted to a health care facility. She was hospitalized in seclusion from visitors and even from the new baby for a week afterward.

In the last decade, our society has come to view pregnancy more in terms of health. Nurses have played an important role in helping to convince the medical establishment that certain longstanding protocols are no longer appropriate. As a result, women are being encouraged to participate in all aspects of the experience. Instead of coming alone for prenatal care, they now bring their families. Instead of being given general anesthetics so they can "sleep through" labor and birth, women now are never denied the opportunity to participate actively in childbirth. Many alternatives to the traditional in-hospital labor and birth experience now exist, both inside and outside many hospitals. The addition of birthing rooms and an emphasis on family-centered care have helped involve families, not just the women, in childbirth. These new measures help to make pregnancy to be a well, not an ill, time.

How the pregnant woman and her partner feel about pregnancy and childbirth may be just as affected by their cultural background, their personal experiences and those of friends and relatives as by the current public philosophy of childbirth. By informing women about their options and continuing to work with other health care providers for "demedicalization" of childbirth, nurses can improve the chances for their clients and families of being able to enjoy pregnancy and childbirth.

Cultural Influences

A woman's cultural background may strongly influence how active a role she wants to take in her pregnancy. Certain beliefs and taboos may place restrictions on her behavior and activities (Boyle & Andrews, 1990). The Focus on Cultural Awareness box lists some common cultural beliefs that exist about activities considered appropriate during pregnancy. It is important to keep in mind that these beliefs may not be held by all members of a particular group, but they are held by many. Supporting these activities is important and shows respect for the individuality of the woman.

Family Influences

The home in which a woman was raised can be as influential to her beliefs about pregnancy as her cultural environment. If she was raised in a family in which children were loved and viewed as the pleasant outcome of a happy marriage, she is more likely to have a positive attitude toward her pregnancy than if she were reared in a home in which children were felt to be intruders or were blamed for the breakup of a marriage. No matter how often a woman is told that pregnancy is natural and

simple, she will not be overjoyed to find herself pregnant if all she has heard are stories about excruciating pain and endless suffering in labor. If her mother has constantly reminded her, "If you hadn't come along, I could have gone to college," or "I could have had a career," the daughter may view pregnancy as disastrous in her life.

That "people love as they have been loved" is said so often it has become a cliché. It is highly relevant, however, to whether pregnancy and childbirth will be viewed in a positive or a negative light. If a woman has had difficulty loving others because of a lack of receiving love, she may have difficulty loving and accepting an unseen fetus growing within her. To mother her baby well, she should be able to feel a pleasurable anticipation at the prospect of rearing a child; becoming a mother is a second adjustment above and beyond being pregnant. The woman who views mothering as a positive activity is more likely to be pleased when she becomes pregnant than one who devalues mothering.

Individual Influences

A woman's ability to cope with or adapt to stress plays a major role in how she will resolve conflict and adapt to new life contingencies. This ability to adapt—to being a mother without needing mothering, to loving a child as well as a husband, to becoming a mother of each new child—depends, in part, on the woman's basic temperament, on whether she adapts to new situations quickly or slowly, faces them with intensity or maintains a low-key approach, and whether she has had experiences coping with change and stress.

The extent to which a woman feels secure in her relationship with the people around her, especially the father of her child, is usually important to her acceptance of a pregnancy. Acceptance will be easier if she has confidence in the solidity of her relationship with the child's father and knows that he will be there to give her emotional support. On the other hand, she may be uneasy to find herself pregnant if she has a partner who may disappear shortly, leaving her alone to raise the child.

A woman who thinks of brides as young but mothers as old may believe that pregnancy will rob her of her youth. If she thinks children are sticky-fingered and time-consuming, she may view the pregnancy as taking away her freedom. If she has heard that pregnancy will permanently stretch her abdomen and breasts, her concern may be that she will lose her looks. She may feel that pregnancy will rob her financially and ruin her chances of job promotion. These are real feelings and must be taken seriously when counseling pregnant women. Such concerns cannot be shrugged off with simple clichés ("One door closes, another one opens") or with repression ("You shouldn't think that way, you'll love having a baby in the house"). The

FOCUS ON CULTURAL AWARENESS

Beliefs about the proper activities to undertake during pregnancy are often culturally determined. Some examples are:

Prescriptive Beliefs

- Remain active during pregnancy to aid the baby's circulation (Crow Indian)
- Remain happy to bring the baby joy and good fortune (Pueblo and Navajo Indians, Mexican, Japanese)
- Sleep flat on your back to protect the baby (Mexican)
- Keep active during pregnancy to ensure a small baby and an easy delivery (Mexican)
- Continue sexual intercourse to lubricate the birth canal and prevent dry labor (Haitian, Mexican)
- Continue daily baths and frequent shampoos during pregnancy to produce a clean baby (Filipino)

Restrictive Beliefs

- Avoid cold air during pregnancy (Mexican, Haitian, Asian)
- Do not reach over your head or the cord will wrap around the baby's neck (Black, Hispanic, White, Asian)
- Avoid weddings and funerals or you will bring bad fortune to the baby (Vietnamese)

- Do not continue sexual intercourse or harm will come to you and the baby (Vietnamese, Filipino, Samoan)
- Do not tie knots or braid or allow the baby's father to do so as it will cause difficult labor (Navajo Indian)
- Do not sew (Pueblo Indian, Asian)

Taboos

- Avoid lunar eclipses and moonlight or the baby may be born with a deformity (Mexican)
- Don't walk on the streets at noon or five o'clock as this may make the spirits angry (Vietnamese)
- Don't join in traditional ceremonies like Yei or Squaw dances or spirits will harm the baby (Navajo Indian)
- Don't get involved with persons who cast spells or the baby will be eaten in the womb (Haitian)
- Don't say the baby's name before the naming ceremony or harm might come to the baby (Orthodox Jewish)
- Don't have your picture taken because it might cause stillbirth (Black)

Boyle, J., & Andrews, M. (1990). *Transcultural concepts in nursing care.* Glenview, IL: Scott, Foresman, with permission.

woman needs an opportunity to express these feelings and become aware of their intensity in order to work at resolving them.

Whether or not the father is able to accept the pregnancy and the coming child depends on the same factors that affect the woman—cultural background, past experience, and relationship with family members. If he was raised to believe that men should not show their emotions, he may not be able to say easily, "I want this baby" or "I'm glad," when his partner tells him of the positive diagnosis. He may not be able to say such things as, "It's great to feel it kick."

Even though he might be inarticulate, however, he may be able to convey such emotions by a touch or a caress, one reason his presence is always desirable at a prenatal visit and certainly in a birthing room. His wife will know that his hand on hers is as meaningful an expression of emotion as a spoken word.

The Psychological Tasks of Pregnancy

During the 9 months of pregnancy, a woman runs a gamut of emotions, from surprise at finding herself pregnant (or wishing she were not) to pleasure and accep-

tance of the fact as she feels the child stir, to fear for herself and the child, to boredom with the process and wishing to get it all over with so that she can get on with the next step of childrearing near the end of pregnancy. Once the child is born, she may feel surprised again that it really happened and she has really given birth.

From a physiologic standpoint, it is fortunate that a pregnancy is 9 months long, because this gives the fetus time to mature and be prepared for life outside the protective uterine environment. From a psychological standpoint, the 9-month period is fortunate for the family, giving it time to prepare emotionally as well.

First Trimester: Accepting the Pregnancy

Most cultures structure celebrations around important life events. Christenings, coming of age, marriages, birthdays, and deaths all have rituals to help individuals take a step forward or accept the coming change in their lives. A diagnosis of pregnancy is a similar rite of passage. This aura of initiation into one of the large mysteries of life gives special meaning to the health care visit in which the diagnosis of pregnancy is confirmed, making it more than an ordinary visit to a health care facility.

Today's availability of family planning measures and home pregnancy test kits would, in theory, seem to prevent the diagnosis of pregnancy from being a surprise. In reality, as many as 50% of pregnancies are unintended (DHHS, 1991). Every pregnancy is a surprise to some extent, either because the woman had not planned on becoming pregnant or had been looking forward to being pregnant but cannot believe it has happened so quickly. No woman is absolutely confident in advance that she will be able to conceive until it happens. If pregnancy announced itself with more reliable signs than a (possibly) skipped period, slight breast tenderness, or vague nausea and tiredness, women could become more certain how they feel about being pregnant sooner. Home pregnancy test kits have helped women in this regard by confirming pregnancy early on. Until it is verified by a home test or health care visit, however, the uncertainty of symptoms makes pregnancy a vague theoretical possibility and leaves room for denial. It is strange that such an important life event is heralded by the cessation of a bodily function (menstruation) rather than by the addition of one.

Some women who are surprised to find themselves pregnant immediately experience something less than pleasure and closer to disappointment or anxiety at the news. Fortunately, most women are able to change their attitude toward the pregnancy by the time they feel the child move inside them.

FOCUS ON NURSING RESEARCH

Do Women Have a Fetal Sex Preference During Pregnancy?

If asked conversationally, most women during pregnancy deny they have a sex preference for their fetus. To determine if this is actually true, Walker and Conner asked 300 women who had had an amniocentesis for fetal chromosome studies what was their sex preference for their fetus. A total of 243 woman, age 18 to 43 years, supplied an answer. Of these women, 39% said they desired a male; 41% wanted a female. Seven percent of the sample reported trying to conceive a child of a specific sex. The gender of previous children influenced their preferences. If women had a previous male, 58% wanted their fetus to be a female; if the woman had a previous female child, the same percent wanted a male.

The researchers suggest that most women have strong preferences as to gender of a fetus, and the birth of a child of the undesired gender could be a cause of postpartal depression or distress.

Walker, M. K., & Conner, G. K. (1993). Fetal sex preference of second-trimester gravidas. *Journal of Nurse-Midwifery, 38,* 110.

Second Trimester: Accepting the Baby

A second turning point in pregnancy is often *quickening,* or the first moment the woman feels fetal movement. Until a woman experiences for herself this proof of the child's existence, she may think of the life inside her as an integral part of herself rather than as a separate entity. She knows it is there; she eats to meet its needs and takes special vitamins to help it grow, but it seems just another part of her body. With quickening, however, she is able to give the child an identity. She begins to imagine how she will feel at the birth when the physician or midwife announces, "It's a boy!" or "It's a girl!" (See the Focus on Nursing Research box for a study on sex preferences in pregnancy.) She begins to imagine herself as a mother, perhaps teaching her child the alphabet or how to ride a bicycle. This anticipatory role playing is an important task for the pregnant woman. It leads her to a larger concept of her condition. It helps her realize that not only is she pregnant but there is a *child* inside her.

It would be easy to suppose that a woman who uses the term *it* for the fetus inside her has not yet accepted the pregnancy or still considers the baby an inanimate object. This is not necessarily true. Although they might deny being superstitious, some women feel that referring to the child as "she" or "he" will be bad luck as this will surely cause the child to be the opposite sex. From a practical standpoint, it makes sense to avoid disap-

pointment by not becoming attached to a mental image of a child as "he" or "she" but rather to keep an open mind, especially if one sex is desired more than the other. Many women today have sonograms, which reveal the sex of the child and let the woman know about this early in pregnancy.

Most women can pinpoint a moment during each pregnancy when they knew definitely that they wanted the child. For a woman who carefully planned the pregnancy, this moment of awareness occurs as soon as she recovers from the surprise of learning she has actually conceived. For others, it may come when she announces the news to her parents and hears them express their joy or when she sees a look of pride on her partner's face. It might be the moment of quickening, when she realizes that the fetus inside her is not passive but an active being. Shopping for baby clothes for the first time, setting up the crib, seeing a blurry outline on a sonogram screen—any of these small actions may suddenly make the coming baby seem real and desired.

On the other hand, accepting the baby as a welcome family addition might not come until labor has begun or after several hours of labor. It might even be the moment the woman first hears the baby's cry or first touches or feeds the newborn. It could take several weeks after the baby is born for the woman to accept her new reality. Unfortunately, some women have great difficulty coming to terms with motherhood, especially if they have a complication of pregnancy, are having financial difficulty, or lack emotional support (Burger et al., 1992). The tremendous emotional and physical upheaval brought about by the hormonal changes of pregnancy and impending childbirth can lead to postpartum depression or, in rare instances, even psychosis.

A good way to measure the level of a woman's acceptance of the coming baby is to measure how well she follows prenatal instructions (Figure 8-1). Until a woman views the growing structure inside her as something desired, it may be difficult for her to discipline herself to follow a proper diet. If she wants very much to be pregnant but is not yet convinced that she is, she may have difficulty eliminating her favorite high-carbohydrate, low-protein food from her diet. After all, gaining weight may be the most certain proof she has of being pregnant.

Third Trimester: Preparing for Parenthood

During the third trimester, the woman usually begins "nest-building" activities, such as planning the infant's sleeping arrangements, buying clothes, choosing names for the infant, and "ensuring safe passage" by learning about birth.

Women at this point are interested in attending prenatal classes or preparation for childbirth classes. It is

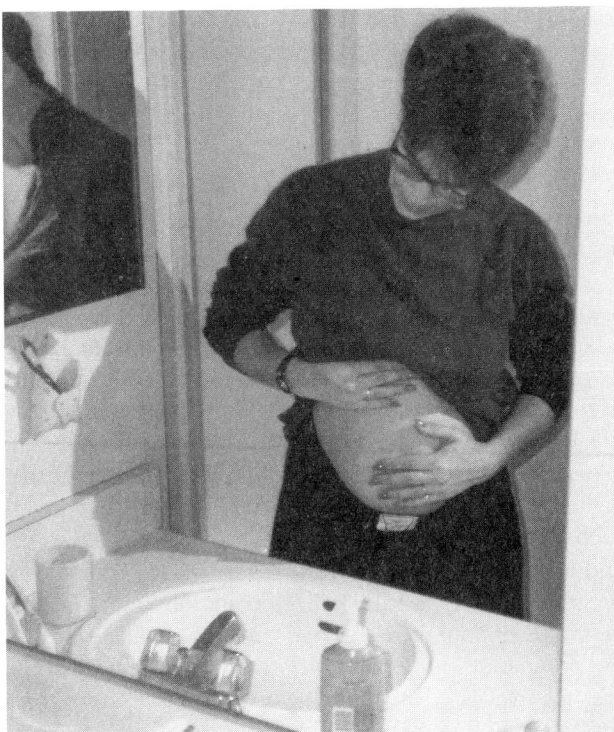

FIGURE 8-1
How well women follow prenatal instructions is an indication of how pleased they are at being pregnant. This woman admires her growing abdomen.

helpful to ask women what specifically they are doing to get ready for birth to document how prepared they will be for a baby's arrival.

A number of external life contingencies may interfere with a woman developing a relationship with her child or becoming a mother by slowing down the process of the mental work of pregnancy. Common occurrences in this area are listed in Box 8-1.

During prenatal visits, the type of question that will reveal a woman's external difficulties might be "How does your partner feel about your being pregnant?" or "Has anything changed in your home life since you last came to clinic?" It is unrealistic to believe that one health care professional has all the solutions to the problems that women can develop during pregnancy. Referral is often necessary to help solve some of these multifaceted problems.

Pregnancy Tasks

In order to be ready to parent, there are a number of specific tasks a couple must complete. These steps, discussed in the following sections, are important with each pregnancy, not just the first one. Whereas once the father used to be the forgotten person in the childbearing process, today he has an important role. This means that as the woman adapts to pregnancy, her partner may go through some of the same psychological changes.

Fathers-to-be may not voice their concerns well because they think they ought to already know about certain things and do not want to compound their partner's anxieties by appearing anxious themselves. Many men obtained their sex education in boyhood from other boys and grew up misinformed, sometimes not even knowing for certain where the fetus grows in the woman's body. A man might believe, for example, that breast-feeding will make his wife's breasts pendulous and no longer attractive and will advise against it. He may believe that childbirth will stretch his wife's vagina so much that sexual relations will no longer be enjoyable and will advocate for a cesarean birth. Such a man needs factual education to correct misinformation.

Reworking Developmental Tasks

One of the tasks of pregnancy is working through previous life experiences. Needs and wishes that have been repressed for years may surface, to be studied and reworked to such an extent that were the woman not pregnant, her behavior might be called pathologic.

Primary among these life experiences is the woman's relationship with her parents, particularly with her mother. For the first time in her life, she finds she can empathize with her mother and the way she used to worry when she came home later than expected from high school activities. The pregnant woman has already begun to worry about her child, to the point that she

Box 8-1
Possible LIfe Events That Could Contribute to Difficulty Accepting a Pregnancy

1. Learning that a pregnancy is going to be a multiple pregnancy
2. A pregnancy occurring within 10 to 12 months of a previous one
3. Relocating moves during pregnancy that involve a need to find new support people
4. Moving away from a family group or back to the group for economic reasons during pregnancy
5. Unexpected loss of security to family or the pregnant woman because of job loss
6. Marital infidelity discovered in prenatal period
7. Illness in self, husband, or relative who must be cared for during pregnancy
8. A role reversal: a previously supporting person who becomes dependent or vice versa
9. Conception and course of pregnancy associated with loss of a person with whom there was a deeply significant tie, especially the husband or the infant's father
10. History of previous abortions, sterility problems, traumatic past births
11. Pregnancy health complications
12. Experience of close friends or relatives who have had children born with a health disorder
13. A series of devaluing experiences such as failure in school or loss of a boyfriend, occurring with pregnancy

wonders if something is wrong when she feels no movement for a few hours, even though she is only 5 months into the pregnancy.

Fear of dying is a common childhood fear that can be revived during pregnancy. Although the likelihood of this happening is remote, it is not entirely unrealistic; without proper health supervision, women may indeed die in childbirth.

For the woman to work through past fears and conflicts of this kind, she needs to think about them when she is alone as well as to discuss them with others. She may "throw out comments" to her husband or to health care personnel to test their reactions to these thoughts. A typical opening statement is, "I really hated my mother when I was a kid." If she is responded to in a therapeutic way, with an open-ended response, (e.g., "You hated her?") the woman may feel able to reveal the intensity of her conflict with her mother and how she cannot bear to think of the child inside her feeling that way about *her*. Unless these feelings are resolved, they may continue to negatively influence her view of becoming a mother.

Other cues that signal a woman's distress about pregnancy and childbirth itself may be more subtle, such as, "Am I ever going to make it through this?" This expression might mean simply that she is tired of her backache, but it also might be a plea for reassurance that she will survive this event in her life.

A woman needs to have confidence in those who provide health care for her during pregnancy so that she can express some of these disturbing thoughts and work through them to resolution.

A pregnant woman's partner needs to do the same reworking of old values and forgotten developmental tasks, such as rethinking his relationship with his father, to understand better what kind of father he is going to be.

For generations, the unwed father was dismissed as a person who had no interest in pregnancy or further concern about the mother's or infant's health. Statements such as, "It's always the woman who pays" or, "Love 'em and leave 'em" reflect these societal beliefs. Today, with pregnancy out of wedlock more common, unmarried fathers are encouraged to have an emotional interest in the pregnancy. Some men who want to have a child but are not interested in marriage may even arrange for a surrogate mother to have a child for them.

Role Playing

The second step in preparing for motherhood is role playing. Just as a preschooler learns what to do by following her mother as she sets a table or balances her checkbook, the pregnant woman begins to spend time with other pregnant women or mothers of young children to learn how to mother. She may spend more time talking to her own mother, perhaps for the first time since the conflicts of adolescence set up a barrier between them. A pregnant woman will offer to babysit for a neighbor or relative so she can "practice" caring for a new baby. Role playing and fantasies about being a mother may be hard for a young, unmarried woman who has not fully made the transition to adulthood and is still so obviously a daughter.

As part of the woman's need for role playing during pregnancy, she is drawn into a world of talk about babies. It is helpful for most couples to attend childbirth education classes or classes on preparing for parenthood. Attending these classes will help the couple accept the pregnancy, expose them to other parents as role models, and provide practical information about pregnancy and child care. The typical material covered in these classes is discussed in Chapter 13.

The father also has role playing and grief work to do during pregnancy before he becomes a father. He has to imagine himself as the father of a boy and as the father of a girl. If he already is a father, he has to cast aside a "father of one" identity to accept a "father of two" image, and so forth. If this is his first time as a father, he may have to relinquish the image of being "one of the boys" or a "carefree bachelor." These freedoms may not seem so precious if he examines them truthfully, but giving them up may be difficult. Just as people do not feel thirsty until you deny them water, men may not mind giving up a well-ordered, uncluttered life until compelled to do so by their partner's pregnancy.

Fantasy

During this step, the woman performs much the same work as she did in initially accepting the pregnancy. She fantasizes about what it will be like to be the mother of a boy, then to be the mother of a girl, and, ideally, finds either fantasy a comfortable "fit." Unless she is informed of the sex of her child in advance, she has no way of knowing which role she will be called on to assume.

This step is an important one in helping the adolescent girl to become a mother. If the only role models she has are other girls her age, who typically are not interested in the commitment to mothering, or if the role model is her own mother who might be unable to cope with problems such as poverty, too many children, or an ineffectual husband, then the young girl will probably assume the same role. She needs exposure to good role models—in mothers' classes, at the health care agency, in a social agency—to be able to find a maternal role that will be worth copying and integrating into her own behavior.

As a part of this process, women's dreams tend to change with pregnancy to being about pregnancy. The frequency of this type of dream increases with advancing gestational age and may include disturbing images (Blake & Reimann, 1993).

Emotional Responses to Pregnancy

Pregnancy is an intrusive process. A separate individual is growing inside the woman's body and she cannot ignore its presence any more than she can ignore a stranger who walks into her home and sits for 9 months at her dining room table. On some days, she might try to pretend no one was there or forget he was there when out of the house. Sometimes, if he conversed with her or told her amusing stories, she might be grateful he was there. But it would be impossible not to have some feelings about his presence.

Much of a woman's reaction to pregnancy resembles the woman's reaction in the example above, that is, it is ambivalent. She wants to be pregnant and yet she is not enjoying it. Ambivalence does not mean that the positive feelings counteract the negative feelings so that the woman is left feeling almost nothing toward her pregnancy, thereby making pregnancy a calm, neutral period. No matter how neutral she wants to be, sooner or later she will have to walk into the dining room and confront the stranger waiting for her. She has to experience some reaction to his being there. *Ambivalence to pregnancy,* therefore, refers to the fact that the feelings of wanting and not wanting always exist at high levels; they are interwoven.

For the father of the child, accepting the pregnancy means not only accepting the certainty of the pregnancy and the reality of the child to come but also accepting the woman in her changed state. It is helpful to caution men of the changes they can expect. Otherwise, they might interpret the woman's mood swings, decreased sexual interest, introversion, or narcissism not as changes of pregnancy but as loss of interest in their relationship.

A man should try to give the woman emotional support while she is learning to accept the reality of pregnancy, and she should reciprocate when he begins to go through the process. It is not unusual for a father to feel somewhat jealous of the growing baby, who, although not yet physically apparent, seems to be taking up a great deal of his partner's time and thought. He may feel as if he has been left standing in the wings, waiting to be asked to take part in the event. To compensate for this feeling, a man may become overly absorbed in his work, striving to produce something concrete on the job or to earn enough money to buy the house they need, to demonstrate that he, too, is capable of creating something. This preoccupation with work may limit the amount of time he spends with the family, just when his partner most needs his emotional support.

Many men experience physical symptoms, such as

nausea, vomiting, and backache, to the same degree or even more intensely than their partners experience them. This is common enough that it has been given a name—**couvade syndrome**. The more involved the father is, attuned to the changes of his partner's pregnancy, the more symptoms he may experience. As the woman's abdomen begins to grow, taking up more body space, men may perceive themselves as growing larger, too, as if they were the ones who were pregnant. This change is most noticeable at about the 8th month of pregnancy and may extend for as long as the 12th postpartum month (Fawcett, 1989). These are healthy happenings and are a measure of the man's interest in and acceptance of the pregnancy.

An unwed father may have a great deal of difficulty accepting a pregnancy, unless he is actively involved in prenatal care. He tries to picture himself as a father, then realizes that if he does not marry his partner, he may never play a full father role to this child; the image disappears again. Because the unwed father can relate to the fact that he fathered the child, however, he may feel a deep sense of loss if the woman decides to have an abortion or if the baby is born less than perfect. In addition, he may not have anyone to turn to for support because no one recognizes his loss, and so he must suffer the loss alone.

Grief

The thought that grief could be associated with such a positive process as childbirth seems at first out of place. But before a woman can take on a mothering role, she has to "give up" present roles. She cannot be the mother of two and the mother of three at the same time; the "mother-of-two" image will have to go. She cannot be a child herself if she is to be an effective mother. The daughter image she has of herself will have to go.

Narcissism

A woman's reaction to the intrusion of pregnancy can be manifested in many ways. Self-centeredness is generally an early reaction to pregnancy. A woman who previously was barely conscious of her body, who dressed in the morning with little thought about what to wear, who was unconcerned about her posture or her weight, suddenly begins to concentrate on these aspects of her life. She dresses so that her pregnancy will or will not show, and dressing becomes a time-consuming, mirror-studying procedure. She makes a ceremony out of fixing her meals. She may lose interest in her job, because the work seems alien to the events taking place in her body, which constantly remind her that a new round of life is beginning.

A woman sometimes manifests narcissism by a change in her activities. She may stop playing tennis, even though her physician tells her it will do no harm in moderation. She criticizes her husband's driving when it never bothered her before. She does these things to unconsciously "protect" her body and thus her baby. She may be so unaware of what she is doing that she rationalizes her behavior. Tennis becomes "too tiring" or "boring." She describes her husband's driving as "reckless." What she means in both instances is that she feels threatened.

When caring for the pregnant woman, it is important to remember that she may feel a need to protect her body in this way, that her *own self* is important. This means she may regard unnecessary nudity as a threat to her body (as her nurse, be sure to drape properly for pelvic and abdominal examinations). She may resent casual remarks, such as, "Oh my, you've gained weight" (a threat to appearance) or, "You don't like milk?" (a threat to judgment).

There is a tendency to organize health instruction during pregnancy around the baby. "Be sure and keep this appointment. You want to have a healthy baby." "You really ought to drink more milk for the baby's sake." This approach may be particularly inappropriate early in pregnancy, before the fetus stirs and before the woman is convinced not only that she is pregnant but that there is a baby inside her who is going to be born. At this stage a woman may be much more interested in doing things for herself, because it is her body, her tiredness, and her well-being that will be directly affected.

Introversion Versus Extroversion

Introversion, or turning inward to concentrate on oneself and one's body, is a common finding during pregnancy. Some women, however, react in an entirely opposite fashion and become more extroverted. They become more active, appear healthier than ever before, and are more outgoing. This tends to occur in women who are finding unexpected fulfillment in pregnancy, perhaps who had seriously doubted they would be lucky enough or fertile enough to conceive. Such a woman regards her expanding abdomen as proof that she is equal to her sisters. Although such a woman may become more varied in her interests during pregnancy, she may surprise those around her who previously regarded her as quiet and self-contained.

Body Image and Boundary

Body image (the way your body appears to yourself) and body boundary (a zone of separation you perceive between yourself and objects or other people) (Fawcett, 1989) change during pregnancy as the woman begins to envision herself as a mother in addition to being a daughter and/or wife. This change in body image is part of the basis for the woman becoming narcissistic and introverted. Changes in the body boundary concept lead to a firmer distinction between objects, yet at the same time the boundary is perceived as extremely vulnerable, as if the body were delicate and easily harmed. This change in boundary perception is so startling that pregnant women may walk far away from an object such as a table in order to avoid it. Fathers who are involved with a pregnancy demonstrate this same enlarged body image.

Decreased Decision-Making

A common effect of stress is decreased decision-making ability. As pregnancy is a period of stress, this may be noticeable, therefore, in pregnant women. People who were dependent on a woman before pregnancy may feel hurt, because now that she is pregnant she seems to have strength only for herself.

It helps families to keep their perspective to remind them that a decrease in responsibility taking is a reaction to the stress of pregnancy, not the pregnancy itself. Nonpregnant women and many men function at work under just as much stress due to marital discord or a loved one's illness or death and have just as much difficulty with decision-making in these circumstances. Pregnancy may actually be less stressful than these situations because of its predictable 9-month outcome.

A woman with few support people around her almost automatically has more difficulty adjusting to and accepting a pregnancy and a new child than if she had more support. During pregnancy, she may feel acute loneliness, which brings with it depression, and a common symptom of depression is further inability to function or make decisions.

Determining whether the twinges she feels in her back are beginning labor contractions or just backache, and whether she should telephone her primary care provider or not, are difficult decisions to make for someone who is depressed. A woman who begins a pregnancy with a strong support person and then loses that person through trauma or illness, separation or divorce, needs special attention in regard to loneliness. She should be evaluated carefully and given extra support, because her loneliness is likely to be extremely acute. A loss of this kind has the potential to interfere not only with her concern about her own health but also with parent-child bonding.

Emotional Lability

Mood changes occur frequently in a pregnant woman, partly as a manifestation of narcissism (her feelings are easily hurt by remarks that would have been laughed off before) and partly because of hormonal changes, particularly the sustained increase in estrogen and progesterone. Mood swings are so common they may make a woman's reaction to her family and to health care routines unpredictable. What she finds acceptable one week she may find intolerable the next. She may cry over her children's bad table manners at one meal and find the situation amusing and even charming the next. Women need to be cautioned that such mood swings occur, beginning with early pregnancy, so that they can accept them as part of pregnancy (see the Focus on Family Teaching box).

Changes in Sexual Desire

Most women report that their sexual desire changes, at least to some degree, during pregnancy. For women who were worried about becoming pregnant, sex during pregnancy may be truly enjoyed for the first time. Others may feel a loss of desire due to the estrogen increase or may unconsciously view sexual relations as a threat to the fetus they must protect. Some may be frightened that sexual relations may bring on early labor.

When a couple knows early in pregnancy that such changes may occur, they can be interpreted in the correct light, that is, as a difference, not as loss of interest in the sexual partner.

Changes in the Expectant Family

Most parents today are aware that their older children need some preparation when a new baby is on the way; however, knowing that such preparation is called for and being able to give it are two different things. For this reason, some couples appreciate suggestions from health care personnel as to how this task can be best accomplished.

Preparing a child for the birth of a sibling is discussed in Chapters 13 and 31. Both preschool and school-age children need to be reassured periodically during pregnancy that a new baby is *adding* to a family and will not replace anyone in either parent's affection.

Physiologic Changes of Pregnancy

Physiologic changes that occur during pregnancy can be categorized as *local* (confined to the reproductive organs) or *systemic* (affecting the entire body). Both the symptoms (subjective findings) and signs (objective findings) of the physiologic changes of pregnancy are used to diagnose and mark the progress of pregnancy. Table 8-1 summarizes the physiologic changes that occur during a typical 40-week pregnancy. In order that they can be used as diagnostic criteria, changes are rated as **presumptive** (slightly predictive), **probable** (moderately predictive), or **positive** (definitely predictive). These terms are discussed later in the chapter, in the Diagnosis of Pregnancy section.

Reproductive Tract Changes

Reproductive tract changes are those involving the uterus, ovaries, vagina, and breasts.

Uterine Changes

The most obvious alteration in the woman's body during pregnancy is the increase in the size of the uterus that occurs to accommodate the growing fetus. Over the 10 lunar months of pregnancy, the uterus increases in length from approximately 6.5 cm to 32 cm; in depth,

FOCUS ON FAMILY TEACHING

Q. My back often hurts at the end of the day since I've been pregnant. How can I evaluate if this is serious or not?

A. Backache is a common symptom or pregnancy owing to the strain on lower vertebrae from carrying extra weight. It may be serious if:

- It is experienced as waves of pain (could be preterm labor).
- There are accompanying urinary symptoms such as frequency and pain on urination (could be a urinary tract infection).
- The backs feels tender at the point of backache (could be pylonephritis or a kidney infection).
- Rest doesn't relieve it (could be a muscle strain).

Q. Since I've been pregnant, I "fly off the handle" easily. How can I prevent this?

A. Mood swings tend to happen with pregnancy probably because of changing hormones. Some tips for reducing the effect of this are:

- Try to avoid fatigue, since this is when your normal defenses are most apt to be down (ask yourself if everything you're doing really needs to be done).
- Try to reduce your level of stress by setting priorities.
- Don't let little problems grow into big ones; attack them when they first occur.
- Try to see situations from other persons' perspective (they're not as involved in your pregnancy as you). Things that don't seem important to you may be important to them.
- Let others know you're aware you're having trouble with emotions since you became pregnant. Your family and friends will be more than willing to help you through this time if they realize it is of concern to you.

---

from 2.5 to 22 cm; and in width, from 4 to 24 cm. Its weight increases from 50 to 1000 g. At the beginning of pregnancy the uterine wall is about 1-cm thick, and its cavity is barely large enough to hold a 2-mL bulk. As pregnancy begins, the wall first hypertrophies and thickens to about 2 cm. Then it begins to thin, so that by the end of pregnancy it is quite supple and only about 0.5 cm thick (so thin that the fetus can be easily palpated through it). By term, the increase in size of the uterus is so extensive that the uterus can hold a 7-lb (3175 g) fetus plus 1000 mL of amniotic fluid, or a total of about 4000 g.

This great uterine growth is due partly to formation of a few new muscle fibers in the uterine myometrium, but principally to the stretching of existing muscle fibers (by the end of pregnancy, muscle fibers in the uterus are two to seven times longer than they were pregestationally). The uterus is able to withstand this stretching of its muscle fibers because of the formation of extra fibroelastic tissue between fibers, which binds them closely together. Because uterine fibers only stretch during pregnancy and are not newly built, the uterus is able to return to its pre-pregnant state at the end of the pregnancy with little difficulty and almost no destruction of

tissue (which explains why the postpartal period is a period of wellness, not illness).

The woman becomes aware of the growing uterus early in pregnancy; by the end of the 12th week of pregnancy, it is large enough to be palpated as a firm spheroid under the abdominal wall just above the symphysis pubis. An important factor to assess regarding uterine growth is its *constant, steady, predictable* increase in size. By the 20th or 22nd week of pregnancy, for example, it should reach the level of the umbilicus. By the 36th week, it should touch the xyphoid process and can make breathing difficult. About 2 weeks before term (the 38th week for a **primigravida**, a woman in her first pregnancy), the fetal head settles into the pelvis to prepare for birth, and the uterus returns to the height it was at 36 weeks. This is termed **lightening**, because the better lung expansion and easier breathing pattern this allows seem to lighten the woman's load. When lightening will occur is not predictable in **multiparas** (women who have had one or more children). In these women, it may not be experienced until the morning of birth.

The fundus of the uterus usually remains in the midline during pregnancy, although it may be pushed slightly to the right side because of the larger bulk of the

Table 8-1. *Timetable for Physiologic Changes of Pregnancy*

Location of Change	1st Trimester	2nd Trimester	3rd Trimester
		Body Occurrence	
Cardiovascular	Blood volume increasing		
	Pseudoanemia	Blood pressure slightly decreased	Blood pressure returns to pre-pregnancy levels
	Clotting factors increasing ———————————————————————————————➤		
Ovarian	Corpus luteum active —— Corpus luteum fading		
Uterine	Increased growth —————————————————————————————————————➤		
		Placenta forming estrogen and progesterone ——————————➤	
Cervix	Softening progressive ————————————————————————————————➤ "ripe"		
Vaginal	White discharge present ———————————————————————— increasing ➤		
Musculoskeletal		Progressive cartilage softening —————————————————————➤	
		Lordosis increasing ——————————————————————————————➤	
Pigmentation		Progressively increasing ——————————————————————————➤	
Kidney	GFR increasing ——————————————————————————————————➤		
		Glycosuria ————————————————————————————————————➤	
	Aldosterone increased, increasing sodium and fluid ————————➤		
Gastrointestinal		Slowed peristalsis ——————————————————————————————➤	
Thyroid	Increased metabolic rate —————————————————————————————➤		

sigmoid colon on the left. Changes in fundal height during pregnancy are shown in Figure 8-2. Uterine height is measured from the top of the symphysis pubis over the top of the fundus (Engstrom et al., 1993; see the Focus on Nursing Research box in Chapter 9 for problems in measurement). As a uterine tumor could mimic this steady growth, uterine growth is only a presumptive sign of pregnancy.

As the uterus increases in size, it pushes the intestines to the sides of the abdomen and elevates the diaphragm at term. The slender woman may worry that there will not be enough room inside her abdomen for the increase in size. She can be assured that the abdominal contents shift readily to accommodate uterine enlargement (Figure 8-3).

Uterine blood flow increases during pregnancy as the placenta grows and requires more and more blood volume for perfusion. Before pregnancy, uterine blood flow is at the rate of 15 to 20 mL/min. By the end of pregnancy, it is as much as 500 to 750 mL/min, with 75% of that volume going to the placenta. One method for measuring and monitoring uterine blood velocity during pregnancy is Doppler ultrasound. One sixth of the total body blood supply is circulating through the uterus at any given time; thus, uterine bleeding in pregnancy is always potentially serious, because it could result in a major blood loss.

A bimanual examination (one finger of the examiner placed in the vagina, the other hand on the abdomen) demonstrates that, with pregnancy, the uterus is more anteflexed, larger, and softer to the touch than usual. At about the 6th week of pregnancy (at the time of the second missed menstrual period), the lower uterine seg-

ment just above the cervix becomes so soft that when it is compressed between the examining fingers by bimanual examination, the wall cannot be felt or feels as thin as tissue paper. This extreme softening of the lower uterine segment is known as **Hegar's sign** (Figure 8-4).

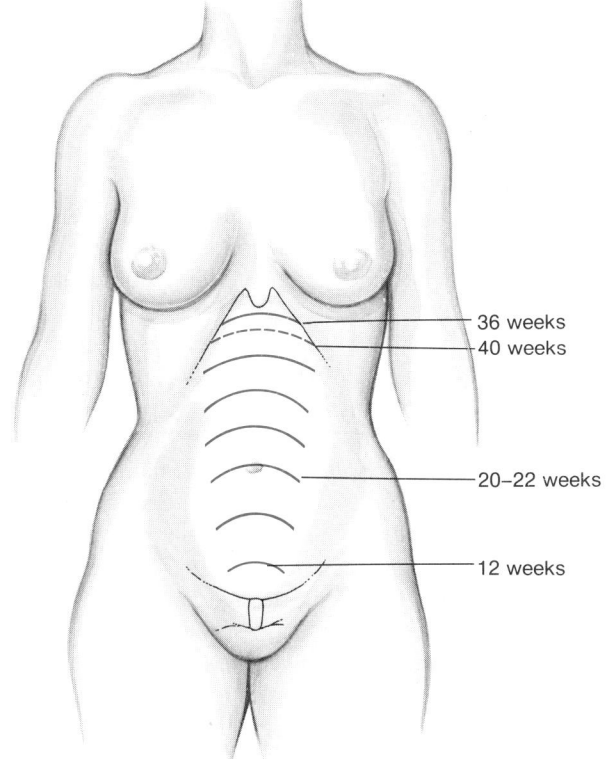

FIGURE 8-2
Fundus height at various weeks of pregnancy.

36 weeks
40 weeks
20–22 weeks
12 weeks

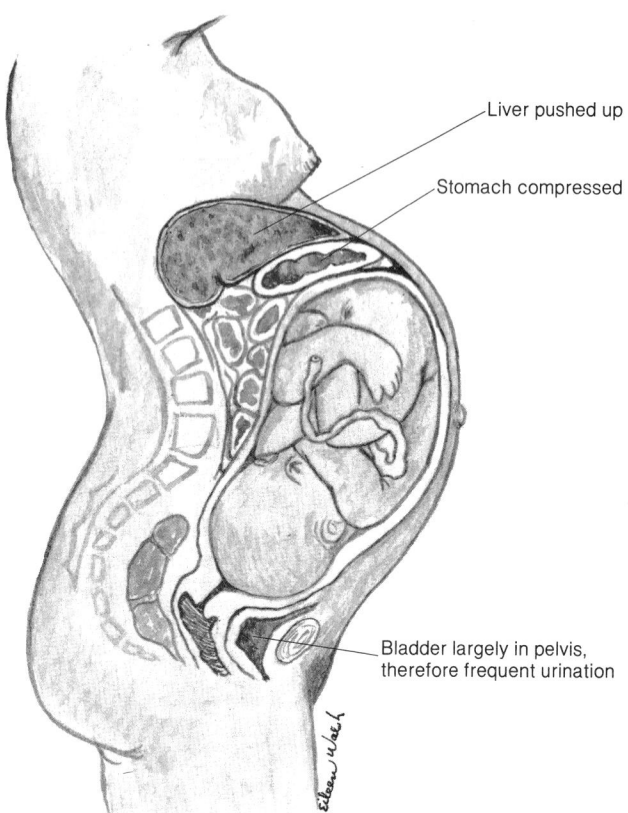

Liver pushed up

Stomach compressed

Bladder largely in pelvis, therefore frequent urination

FIGURE 8-3
Crowding of abdominal contents late in pregnancy.

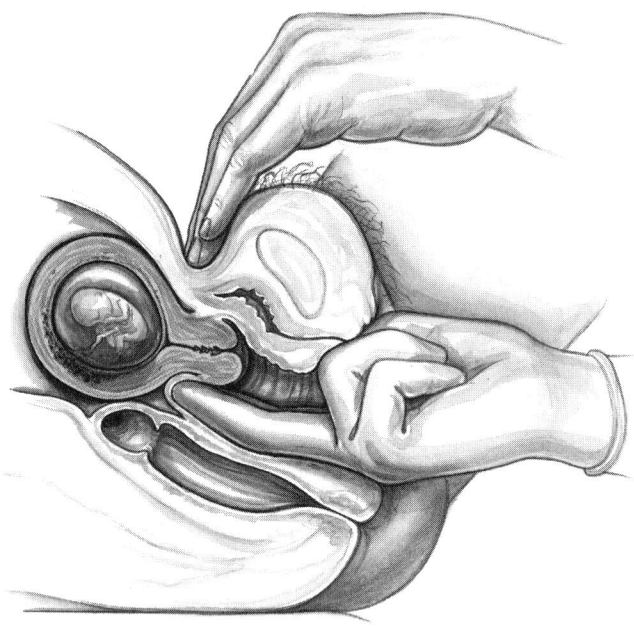

FIGURE 8-4
Examining for Hegar's sign. If the sign is present, the wall of the uterus is softer than normal.

During the 16th to 20th week of pregnancy, when the fetus is still small in relation to the amount of amniotic fluid present, **ballottement** (from the French word *balloter,* meaning "to toss about") may be demonstrated. On bimanual examination, if the lower uterine segment is tapped sharply by the lower hand, the fetus can be felt to bounce or rise in the amniotic fluid up against the top examining hand. This phenomenon is interesting; again, however, it may be simulated by a uterine tumor, so it is no more than a probable sign of pregnancy.

Between the 20th and 24th week of pregnancy, the uterine wall has become thinned to such a degree that a fetal outline within the uterus may be palpated by a skilled examiner. Because a tumor with calcium deposits could simulate a fetal outline, palpation of a uterine mass does not constitute a positive confirmation of pregnancy.

Uterine contractions begin early in pregnancy, at least by the 12th week, and are present throughout the rest of pregnancy, becoming stronger and harder as the pregnancy advances. They may be felt by a woman as waves of hardness or tightening across her abdomen. An examining hand may be able to feel a contraction as well, and an electronic monitor will be able to measure the frequency and length of such contractions.

These "practice" contractions are termed **Braxton Hicks contractions**. They serve as warm-up exercises for labor and increase placental perfusion. They may become so strong and noticeable in the last month of pregnancy that they are mistaken for labor contractions (false labor). They can be differentiated from true labor contractions on internal examination because they do not cause cervical dilation. Although these contractions are always present with pregnancy, they also could accompany any growing uterine mass and so, like ballottement, they are no more than a probable sign of pregnancy.

Amenorrhea

Amenorrhea (absence of menstruation) occurs with pregnancy because of the suppression of follicle-stimulating hormone. In a healthy woman who has menstruated previously, the absence of menstruation strongly suggests that impregnation has occurred. Amenorrhea, however, also heralds the onset of menopause or could result from delayed menstruation due to unrelated reasons, such as uterine infection, climate change, worry (perhaps over becoming pregnant), chronic illness such as severe anemia, or stress. It occurs in athletes who train strenuously and especially in long-distance runners whose percentage of body fat drops below a critical point. Amenorrhea is therefore only a presumptive sign of pregnancy.

Cervical Changes

In response to the increased level of circulating estrogen from the placenta during pregnancy, the cervix of the uterus becomes more vascular and edematous. Increased fluid between cells causes the cervix to soften in consistency and increased vascularity causes it to darken from a pale pink to a violet hue. The glands of the endocervix undergo both hypertrophy and hyperplasia as they increase in number and distend with mucus. A tenacious coating of mucus fills the cervical canal. This mucous plug, called the **operculum**, will act to seal out bacteria during pregnancy and so help prevent infection in the fetus and membranes.

Softening of the cervix in pregnancy (**Goodell's sign**) is so extensive that, although the consistency of a nonpregnant cervix may be compared with that of the nose, the consistency of a pregnant cervix more closely resembles that of an earlobe. This softening is so marked it is rated as a probable diagnostic sign of pregnancy. Just before the onset of labor, when the cervix becomes so soft that it takes on the consistency of butter, it is said to be "ripe" for birth.

Vaginal Changes

Under the influence of estrogen, the vaginal epithelium and underlying tissue become hypertrophic and enriched with glycogen; they loosen from their connective tissue attachment in preparation for great distention at birth. This increase in the activity of the epithelial cells results in a white vaginal discharge throughout pregnancy.

An increase in the vascularity of the vagina, beginning early in pregnancy, parallels the vascular changes in the uterus. The resulting increase in circulation to the vagina changes the color of the vaginal walls from the normal light pink color to a deep violet (Chadwick's sign).

Vaginal secretions during pregnancy fall from a *p*H of over 7 (an alkaline *p*H) to 4 or 5 (an acidotic *p*H). This occurs owing to the action of *Lactobacillus acidophilus,* a bacteria which grows freely in the increased glycogen environment and by so doing increases the lactic acid content of secretions. This changing acid content makes the vagina resistant to bacterial invasion for the length of the pregnancy. This change in *p*H also, unfortunately, favors the growth of *Candida albicans,* a species of yeastlike fungi. A candidal infection is manifested by an itching, burning sensation in addition to a cream cheese–like discharge. A nonpregnant woman needs medication for such an infection to relieve discomfort. A pregnant woman needs medication not only to relieve discomfort but also to prevent transmission of the infection to the infant as it passes through the birth canal at term. Candidal infection in the newborn is termed thrush or oral monilia.

Ovarian Changes

Ovulation stops with pregnancy because of the active feedback mechanism of estrogen-progesterone produced by the corpus luteum early in pregnancy and the placenta later in pregnancy. This feedback causes the pituitary gland to halt production of follicle-stimulating

hormone and luteinizing hormone. Without stimulation from these, ovulation will not occur.

The corpus luteum that was created following the ovulation that lead to the pregnancy continues to increase in size on the surface of the ovary until about the 12th week of pregnancy. At that time, the placenta begins to take over as the chief provider of progesterone and estrogen. The corpus luteum, no longer essential for the continuation of the pregnancy, begins to regress in size (Hume & Killam, 1990).

Integumentary Changes

A number of integumentary changes occur with pregnancy. As the uterus increases in size, the abdominal wall must stretch to accommodate it. This stretching (plus possibly increased adrenal cortex activity) can cause rupture and atrophy of small segments of the connective layer of the skin. This leads to pink or reddish streaks (striae gravidarum) appearing on the sides of the abdominal wall and sometimes on the thighs (Figure 8-5). In the weeks following birth, striae gravi-

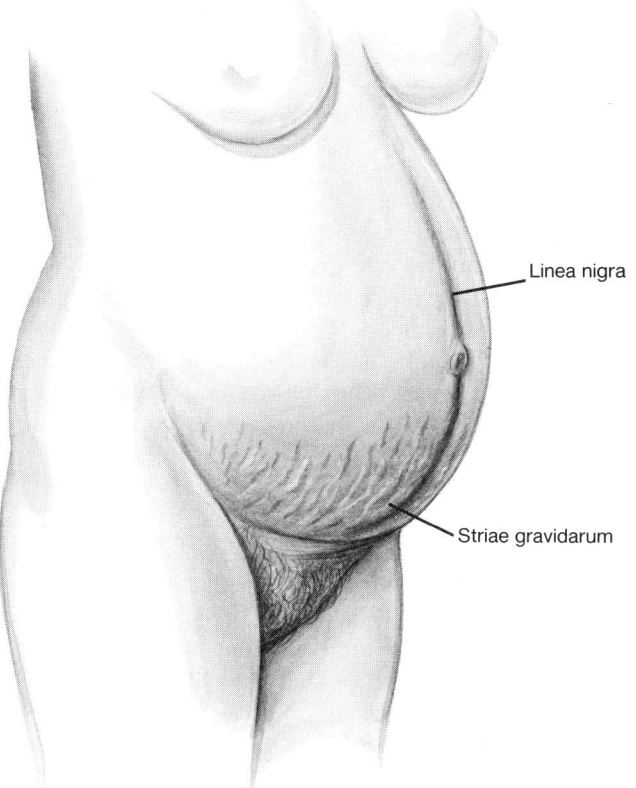

Linea nigra

Striae gravidarum

FIGURE 8-5

Skin changes in pregnancy. In the later months of pregnancy, reddish, slightly depressed streaks called striae gravidarum often develop in the skin of the abdomen and, sometimes, the breasts and thighs. Following pregnancy, these fade to glistening, silvery lines. In many pregnancies, the abdominal skin at the midline becomes markedly pigmented, assuming a brownish-black color, referred to as a linea nigra.

darum lighten to a silvery-white color (striae albicantes or atrophicae) and, although permanent, become barely noticeable.

Occasionally, the abdominal wall has difficulty stretching enough to accommodate the growing fetus, causing the rectus muscles to actually separate, a condition known as **diastasis**. If this happens, it will appear after pregnancy as a bluish groove at the site of separation.

The umbilicus is stretched by pregnancy to such an extent that by the 28th week, its depression becomes obliterated and smooth because it has been pushed so far outward. In most women it may appear as if it has turned inside out, protruding as a round bump at the center of the abdominal wall.

Extra pigmentation generally appears on the abdominal wall. A brown line (linea nigra) may be present, running from the umbilicus to the symphysis pubis and separating the abdomen into a right and left hemisphere (see Figure 8-5). Darkened areas may appear on the face, particularly on the cheeks and across the nose as well. This is known as **melasma** (chloasma), or the "mask of pregnancy." These increases in pigmentation are due to melanocyte-stimulating hormone secreted by the pituitary. With the decrease in the level of the hormone after pregnancy, these areas lighten and again disappear.

Vascular spiders (small, fiery-red branching spots) are sometimes seen on the skin of pregnant women, particularly on the thighs. These probably result from the increased level of estrogen in the body. These may fade but not completely disappear again after pregnancy.

The activity of sweat glands increases throughout the body during pregnancy. This is manifested as an increase in perspiration. Palmar erythema (redness and itching) may occur on the hands from the increased estrogen level. Fewer hairs on the head enter a resting phase so scalp hair growth is increased (Hume & Killam, 1990).

Changes in the Breasts

Subtle changes in the breasts that occur as a result of the effect of estrogen-progesterone production may be one of the first physiologic changes of pregnancy the woman notices (at about 6 weeks). She may experience a feeling of fullness, tingling, or tenderness in breasts because of the increased stimulation of breast tissue by the high estrogen level in the body. As pregnancy progresses, breast size increases, because of hyperplasia of the mammary alveoli and fat deposits. The areola of the nipple darkens in color, and its diameter increases from about 3.5 cm to 5 or 7.5 cm (1.5 in to 2–3 in). There is additional darkening of the skin surrounding the areola in some women, forming a secondary areola. As vascularity of the breasts increases, blue veins may become prominent over the surface of the breasts. The seba-

ceous glands of the areola (Montgomery's tubercles) enlarge and become protuberant. The secretions from these glands keep the nipple supple and help to prevent the nipples from cracking and drying during lactation.

Early in pregnancy, the breasts begin readying themselves for the secretion of milk. By the 16th week, *colostrum,* the thin, watery, high-protein fluid that is the precursor of breast milk, can be expelled from the nipples.

Systemic Changes

Although the most interesting physiologic changes first noticed by a woman are apt to be those of the reproductive system and breasts, changes do occur in almost all body systems.

Respiratory System

The change in CO_2 level and the compensating mechanisms can be described as a chronic respiratory alkalosis fully compensated by a chronic metabolic acidosis.

As the uterus enlarges during pregnancy, a great deal of pressure is put on the diaphragm and, ultimately, on the lungs. The diaphragm may be displaced by as much as 4 cm upward. This crowding of the chest cavity causes an acute sensation of shortness of breath late in pregnancy, until lightening (see discussion above) relieves the pressure.

Even with all this crowding, vital capacity (the maximum volume exhaled following a maximum inspiration) of the woman does not decrease during pregnancy. Although lungs are crowded in the vertical dimension, they can expand horizontally. Residual volume (the amount of air remaining in the lungs following expiration) is decreased up to 20% by the pressure of the diaphragm. Tidal volume (the volume of air inspired) is increased up to 40% as the woman draws in extra volume to increase the effectiveness of air exchange. Total oxygen consumption increases by as much as 20%.

The increased level of progesterone during pregnancy appears to set a new level in the hypothalamus for acceptable blood carbon dioxide levels (PCO_2), since during pregnancy a woman's body tends to maintain a PCO_2 at closer to 32 mm Hg than the normal 40 mm Hg.

This low PCO_2 level causes a favorable CO_2 gradient at the placenta (the fetal CO_2 level is higher than that in the mother, allowing CO_2 to cross readily from the fetus to the mother).

To keep the mother's *p*H level from becoming acidotic from the load of CO_2 being shifted to her by the fetus, increased ventilation (mild hyperventilation) to blow off excess CO_2 begins early in pregnancy. At full term, a woman's total ventilation capacity may have risen by as much as 40%. This increased ventilation may

Table 8-2. Respiratory Changes During Pregnancy

Variable	Change
Vital capacity	No change
Tidal volume	Increased
Respiratory rate	Increased
Residual volume	Decreased
Plasma P_{CO_2}	Decreased
Plasma pH	Increased
Plasma P_{O_2}	Increased
Respiratory minute volume	Increased
Expiratory reserve	Decreased

become so extreme that the woman develops a respiratory alkalosis. To compensate for this, plasma bicarbonate is excreted by the kidneys in larger than normal amounts. With greater urine output, additional sodium is lost and, therefore, additional water. The effect is **polyuria**, an early sign of pregnancy.

The slight increase in pH in serum due to the increased expiratory effort is advantageous because it slightly increases the binding capacity of maternal hemoglobin and thereby raises the oxygen content of maternal blood (the level of PO_2) from a normal level of about 92 mm Hg to a level of 106 mm Hg early in pregnancy. This is advantageous to fetal growth by allowing good placental exchange.

The cumulative effect of these respiratory changes is often experienced by the woman as chronic shortness of breath. She will need a clear explanation that, while her breathing rate is more rapid than normal (18 to 20 breaths per minute), it is part of pregnancy, and so she should not be alarmed.

A local change that often occurs in the respiratory system is marked congestion, or "stuffiness," of the nasopharynx, a response to increased estrogen levels. Women may worry that this stuffiness indicates an al-

lergy or a cold. Some women, unfortunately, may take over-the-counter cold medications or antihistamines to try to relieve the congestion, not realizing that it is happening because they are pregnant. Some continue to take the medication after pregnancy is confirmed, not mentioning it to their physician because they think the stuffiness is a separate problem and not pregnancy related. Asking a woman at prenatal visits if she is taking any kind of medicine or if she has noticed nasal stuffiness is an important nursing responsibility.

Changes in respiratory function during pregnancy are summarized in Table 8-2.

Temperature

Early in pregnancy, body temperature increases slightly because of the secretion of progesterone from the corpus luteum (the temperature, which elevated at ovulation, remains elevated). As the placenta takes over the function of the corpus luteum at about 16 weeks, the temperature generally decreases to normal.

Some women may mistakenly assume this slight rise in temperature (99.6°F orally), associated with pregnancy-related nasal congestion, is a sure sign of a cold, and may think they need medication. It is important to explain the reason for these changes to allow the woman to accept them without worrying.

Circulatory System

Changes in the cardiovascular system are extremely significant to the health of the fetus because they are important for adequate placental and fetal circulation. Table 8-3 summarizes the changes that are described in the following sections.

Blood Volume. To provide for an adequate exchange of nutrients in the placenta and to provide adequate blood to compensate for blood loss at birth, the circulatory blood volume of the woman's body increases at least 30% (and possibly as much as 50%) during pregnancy. Blood loss for a normal vaginal birth is about 300

Table 8-3. Changes in the Cardiovascular System During Pregnancy

Assessment Factor	Pre-pregnancy	Pregnancy
Cardiac output		25% to 50% increase
Heart rate	70–80	80–90
Plasma volume (mL)	2600	3600
Blood volume (mL)	4000	5250
Red blood cell mass (mm³)	4,200,000	4,650,000
Leukocytes (mm³)	7000	20,500
Total protein (g/dL)	7.0	5.5–6.0
Fibrinogen (mg/dL)	300	450
Blood pressure		Decreases in 2nd trimester, at pre-pregnancy level in 3rd trimester

to 400 mL, whereas blood loss from a cesarean birth is much higher, about 800 to 1000 mL. The increase in blood volume occurs gradually near the end of the first trimester. It reaches its peak at about the 28th to the 32nd week and continues at this high level through the third trimester. As the plasma volume first increases, the concentration of hemoglobin and erythrocytes may decline, giving the woman a **pseudoanemia**. The woman's body compensates for this change by producing more red blood cells, creating nearly normal levels of red blood cells again (Blackburn & Loper, 1992).

Almost all women need some iron supplementation during pregnancy owing to a variety of factors. They usually have comparatively low iron stores (less than 500 mg) because of their monthly menstrual loss. The fetus requires about 350 to 400 mg of iron to grow. The increases in the mother's circulatory red blood cell mass require an additional 400 mg of iron. This is a total increased need of about 800 mg. As the average woman's store of iron is less than this (about 500 mg), and iron absorption may be impaired during pregnancy as a result of decreased gastric acidity (iron is absorbed best from an acid medium), additional iron is often prescribed during pregnancy to prevent a true anemia.

Either a hemoglobin concentration of less than 11.5 g/100 mL or a hematocrit value below 30% is generally considered true anemia, for which iron therapy above normal supplementation is advocated. (See Chapter 14 for additional information on anemia in pregnancy.) The need for folic acid also increases during pregnancy, or else megalohemoglobinemia (large, nonfunctioning red blood cells) will result. Prenatal vitamins include added folic acid to supply this need (Loeb, 1993).

To handle the increase in blood volume in the circulatory system, a woman's cardiac output increases significantly by 25% to 50%; the heart rate increases by 10 beats per minute. Like the circulating volume increase, the bulk of the cardiac work increase occurs during the second trimester, with a small increase in the third trimester. This rise in circulating load has implications for the woman with cardiac disease. Although the average woman's heart is able to adjust to these changes readily, a woman whose heart has difficulty handling her normal circulating load may be overwhelmed by the requirements placed on it when she is pregnant (Syverson et al., 1991). For the average woman, significant changes related to her circulatory system are occurring inside her, yet she is not even aware of them.

Because the diaphragm is elevated by the growing uterus late in pregnancy, the heart is shifted to a more transverse position in the chest cavity and may appear enlarged on x-ray examination. Some women have audible functional (innocent) heart murmurs during pregnancy, probably because of the altered heart position.

During the third trimester, blood flow to the lower extremities is impaired by the pressure of the expanding uterus on veins and arteries, which slows circulation. This decrease in blood flow in the venous system leads to edema and varicosities of the vulva, rectum, and legs.

Palpitations. Palpitations of the heart are not uncommon during pregnancy, particularly on quick motion. A woman should be cautioned that if palpitations do occur, not to be frightened. Palpitations in the early months of pregnancy are probably caused by sympathetic nervous system stimulation; in later months, they may result from increased thoracic pressure caused by the pressure of the uterus against the diaphragm.

Blood Pressure. Average blood pressures for adult women are shown in Appendix G. Despite the hypervolemia of pregnancy, the blood pressure does not normally rise, since the increased heart action takes care of the greater amount of circulating blood.

In most women, blood pressure actually decreases slightly during the second trimester because of the lowered peripheral resistance to circulation as the placenta expands rapidly. If this occurs, during the third trimester, the blood pressure rises again to first-trimester levels (Figure 8-6).

Supine Hypotension Syndrome. When a pregnant woman lies supine, the weight of the growing uterus presses the vena cava against the vertebrae, obstructing blood flow from the lower extremities. This causes a de-

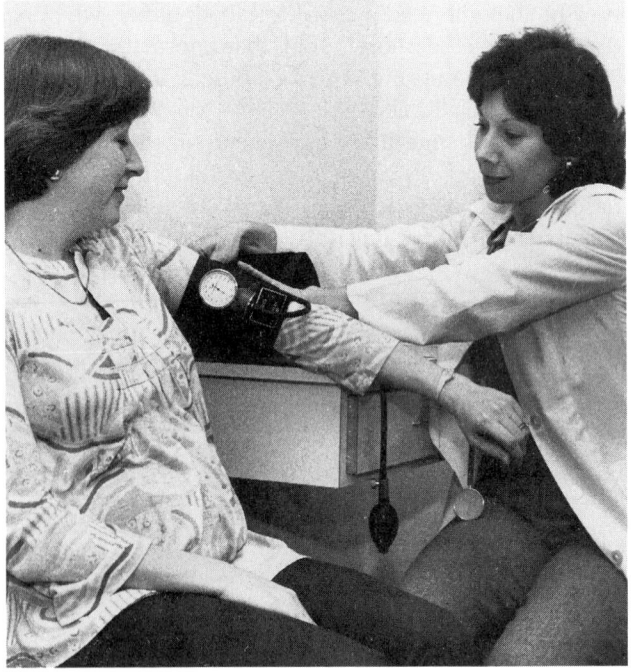

FIGURE 8-6
Blood pressure determination is an important assessment during pregnancy; normally, this does not elevate during pregnancy.

crease in blood return to the heart and, consequently, immediate decreased cardiac output and hypotension (Figure 8-7). The woman experiences this as lightheadedness, faintness, and palpitations. Supine hypotension syndrome can be corrected easily by having the woman turn onto her side (preferably the left side) to free blood flow through the vena cava. To lessen the possibility of this phenomenon, women have an increase in collateral blood circulation during pregnancy. Teach women to always rest on their left side rather than their back because, even with additional collateral circulation, a supine position tends to lead to hypotension.

Blood Constitution. The level of circulating fibrinogen, a constituent of the blood necessary for clotting, increases as much as 50% during pregnancy, probably because of the increased level of estrogen. Other clotting factors, such as VII, VIII, IX, and X, and the platelet count also increase. This increase is a safeguard against major bleeding should the placenta be dislodged and the uterine arteries or veins are opened. Total white blood cell count rises slightly as both a protective mechanism and a reflection of the woman's total blood volume (up to about 20,000/mm^3). The total protein level of blood decreases, perhaps indicating the amount of protein needed by the fetus. Because the circulating system has a lowered total protein load and hypervolemia, fluid readily leaves the intravascular spaces in order to equalize osmotic and hydrostatic pressure. This causes the common ankle and foot edema of pregnancy (not to be confused with nondependent edema, which is a symptom of pregnancy-induced hypertension).

Overall, blood lipids increase by one third; cholesterol serum level increases 90% to 100%. These increases provide a ready supply of available energy for the fetus.

Gastrointestinal System

As the uterus increases in size, it tends to displace the stomach and intestines toward the back and sides of the abdomen. At about the midpoint of pregnancy, the pressure may be sufficient to slow intestinal peristalsis and the emptying time of the stomach, leading to heartburn, constipation, and flatulence. Relaxin, a hormone produced by the ovary, may contribute to decreased gastric motility; this may cause a decrease in blood supply to the gastrointestinal tract (blood is drawn to the uterus). Progesterone also has an effect on smooth muscle, such as that in the intestine, making it less active.

At least 50% of women experience some nausea and vomiting early in pregnancy. This is one of the first sensations the woman may experience with pregnancy (sometimes noticed even before the first missed menstrual period). It is most apparent early in the morning on rising or if she becomes fatigued during the day. Known as *morning sickness,* nausea and vomiting begin to be noticed at the time human chorionic gonadotropin and progesterone begin to rise. It may occur as a systemic reaction to increased estrogen levels and decreased glucose levels, or glucose being utilized in great quantities by the growing fetus. Common interventions to decrease nausea and vomiting are discussed in Chapter 12.

This common feeling of nausea usually subsides after the first 3 months, after which the woman may acquire a voracious appetite. Although the acidity of stomach secretions decreases during pregnancy, heartburn may result from the reflux of stomach content into the esophagus as a result of upward displacement of the stomach and the relaxed cardioesophageal sphincter. Interventions for heartburn are also discussed in Chapter 12.

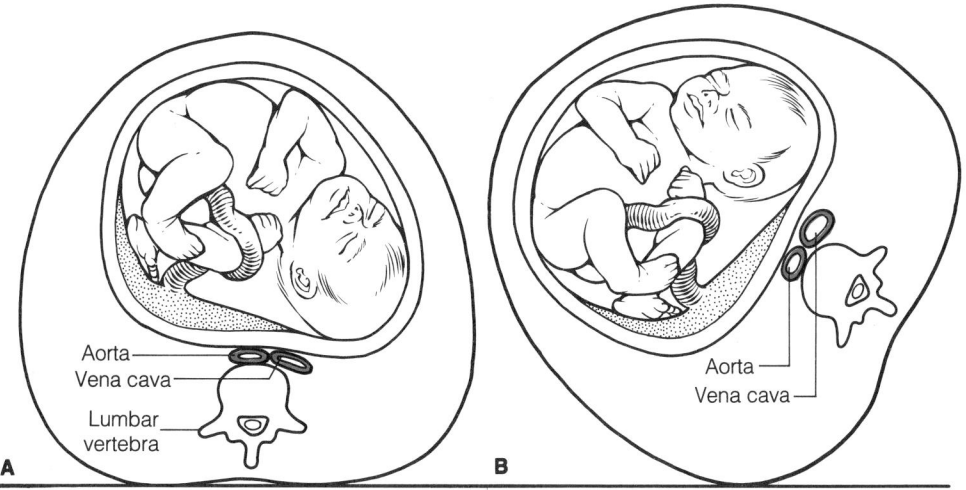

FIGURE 8-7
*Supine hypotension can occur if a pregnant woman lies on her back. (**A**) The weight of the uterus compresses the vena cava, trapping blood in the lower extremities. (**B**) If a woman turns on her side, pressure is lifted off of the vena cava.*

Due to the gradual slowing of the gastrointestinal tract, decreased emptying of bile from the gallbladder may result. This can lead to reabsorption of bilirubin into the maternal bloodstream, giving rise to the symptom of generalized itching (subclinical jaundice). A woman who has had previous gallstone formation may have an increased tendency to stone formation during pregnancy as a result of the increased plasma cholesterol level and additional cholesterol incorporated in bile. Women with peptic ulcer generally find their condition improved during pregnancy, because the acidity of the stomach is decreased.

Some women notice hypertrophy at their gumlines and bleeding of gingival tissue when they brush their teeth. There may be increased saliva formation (**hyperptyalism**), probably as a local response to increased levels of estrogen. It is an annoying but not serious problem. A lower than normal *p*H of saliva may lead to increased tooth decay if toothbrushing is not continued conscientiously.

Urinary System

During pregnancy, the kidneys must excrete not only the waste products of the woman's body but those of the growing fetus as well. Thus, urinary output gradually increases (about 60% to 80%) and the specific gravity of urine decreases.

In order to provide sufficient fluid volume for effective placental exchange, total body water increases to 7.5 L; this requires the body to increase its sodium reabsorption in the tubules in order to maintain osmolarity. Under the influence of progesterone, there is an increased response of the angiotensin-renin system in the kidney, which leads to an increase in aldosterone production. Aldosterone aids sodium reabsorption. Progesterone appears to be potassium sparing, so that even with an increased urine output, potassium levels remain adequate.

Water is retained during pregnancy to aid the increase in blood volume and to serve as a ready source of nutrients to the fetus. As nutrients can only pass to the fetus when dissolved in or carried by fluid, this ready fluid supply is a fetal safeguard (Theunissen & Parer, 1994).

At one time, pregnant women were administered diuretics to help clear this excess fluid from their system. Today it is recognized that this practice is potentially harmful, because the fluid has physiologic benefits for the fetus. In addition, the excess fluid can serve to replenish the mother's own blood volume should hemorrhage occur.

Occasionally, a trace of albumin will remain in urine, because of congestion in renal capillaries. Glomerular filtration rate (GFR) and renal plasma flow are both most effective (they temporarily increase as much as 50%) when a person lies in a lateral recumbent position (on the side). Women should be advised to rest and sleep in this position during pregnancy to prevent cardiovascular problems, such as supine hypotension, as well as to assist the kidneys to function at maximum efficiency.

Both the GFR and the renal plasma flow must (and do) increase by 30% to 50% to meet the increased needs of the circulatory system. This rise is consistent with that of the circulatory system increase, peaking at about 24 weeks. This efficient GFR level leads to a lowered blood urea nitrogen (BUN) and low creatinine levels in maternal plasma. A BUN of 15 mg/100 mL or higher and a serum creatinine over 1 mg/100 mL are considered abnormal and reflect kidney difficulty in handling the increased blood load. The higher GFR leads to increased filtration of glucose into the renal tubules. Because reabsorption of glucose by the tubule cells occurs at a fixed rate, this means there will be some accidental spilling of glucose into urine during pregnancy. Lactose, the sugar of breast milk (which is being produced by the mammary glands but is not used during pregnancy), will also be spilled into the urine. Although minimal spilling of glucose may occur by this route, the finding of more than a trace of glucose in a routine sample of urine from a pregnant woman is considered abnormal until proven otherwise, since it can be an indication of gestational diabetes (see Chapter 14).

To differentiate the types of sugar spilling into the urine, a test material for urine analysis specific for glucose (Tes-Tape) must be used. A urine test method that is positive for all sugars (Benedict's solution) will give false-positive results, because it reports the presence of the harmless lactose as well.

Other changes that the increased level of progesterone produces are an increase in diameter of the ureters and an increase in bladder capacity to about 1500 mL. The uterus tends to rise on the right side of the abdomen, because it is pushed slightly in that direction by the greater bulk of the sigmoid colon. As a result, pressure on the right ureter may lead to urinary stasis and pyelonephritis if not relieved.

The woman may notice an increase in urinary frequency during the first 3 months of pregnancy until the uterus rises out of the pelvis and relieves pressure on the bladder. Frequency of urination may return at the end of pregnancy as lightening occurs and the fetal head exerts renewed pressure on the bladder.

Changes in the urinary tract during pregnancy are summarized in Table 8-4. Creatinine clearance has become the standard test for renal function during pregnancy, as creatinine is cleared from the body at a steady rate in relation to GFR. A normal pregnancy value is 90 to 180 mL/min. This is analyzed from a 24-hour urine sample.

Table 8-4. Urinary Tract Changes During Pregnancy	
Variable	*Change*
Glomerular filtration rate	Increased
Renal plasma flow	Increased
Blood urea nitrogen	Decreased
Plasma creatinine level	Decreased
Renal threshold for sugar	Decreased
Bladder capacity	Increased
Diameter of ureters	Increased
Frequency of urination	Increased 1st trimester, last 2 weeks of pregnancy

Skeletal System

Calcium and phosphorus needs are increased during pregnancy because the fetal skeleton must be built. As pregnancy advances, there is a gradual softening of the pelvic ligaments and joints to create pliability and to facilitate passage of the baby through the pelvis at the time of birth. This softening is probably due to the influence of the ovarian hormone *relaxin* and placental progesterone. Excessive mobility of the joints may cause discomfort, and a wide separation of the symphysis pubis, as much as 3 to 4 mm by 32 weeks of pregnancy, may occur.

To change her center of gravity and make ambulation easier, the pregnant woman tends to stand straighter and taller than usual. This stance is sometimes referred to as the *pride of pregnancy*. Standing this way, unfortunately, with the shoulders back and the abdomen forward, creates a *lordosis* (forward curve of the lumbar spine), which may lead to backache (see the Focus on Family Teaching box).

Endocrine System

The most striking change in the endocrine system during pregnancy is the addition of the placenta as an endocrine organ in its role of producing large amounts of both estrogen and progesterone. Many women experience palmar erythema during early pregnancy as a response to the high circulating estrogen levels.

The pituitary gland is affected by pregnancy because there is a halt in the production of follicle-stimulating hormone and luteinizing hormone brought on by the high estrogen and progesterone levels of the placenta. There is increased production of growth hormone and melanocyte-stimulating hormone (causing skin pigment changes). Late in pregnancy, the posterior pituitary begins to produce oxytocin that will be needed to aid labor. Prolactin production is also begun late in pregnancy as the breasts prepare for lactation following birth.

The thyroid gland is altered significantly. The gland enlarges in early pregnancy to such an extent that the basal body metabolic rate increases by about 20%. Levels of protein-bound iodine, butanol-extractable iodine, and thyroxine are all elevated in blood serum. If a sufficient supply of iodine is not present during pregnancy, goiter (thyroid hypertrophy) can occur as the gland intensifies its productive effort.

These thyroid changes, along with emotional lability, tachycardia, palpitations, and increased perspiration, may lead to a mistaken diagnosis of hyperthyroidism if pregnancy has not been determined.

The parathyroid glands, which are necessary for the metabolism of calcium, also increase in size during pregnancy. Because calcium is an important ingredient of fetal growth, the hypertrophy is probably necessary to satisfy the increased regulation of calcium.

Glucocorticoid levels increase in pregnancy, perhaps because of increased plasma binding rather than increased production by the adrenal glands. Although the pancreas increases production of insulin in response to the higher glucocorticoid levels, the insulin is less effective than normal because of increased estrogen, progesterone, and human chorionic somatomammotropin. Thus, a woman who is diabetic and taking insulin before pregnancy will need more insulin during pregnancy. A woman who is prediabetic may develop overt diabetes for the first time during pregnancy.

Carbohydrate Metabolism

The glucose level of a fetus is about 30 mg/100 mL below that of the maternal glucose level. To prevent fetal hypoglycemia, with resultant cell destruction or lack of fetal growth, a maternal glucose level is maintained at a higher than normal level during pregnancy. A number of fail-safe physiologic measures are effected to achieve this.

As mentioned, although the pancreas secretes an increased level of insulin throughout pregnancy, it appears to be not as effective. This is because of the human chorionic somatomammotropin hormone secreted by the placenta, cortisol secreted by the adrenal gland, and possibly the high levels of estrogen and progesterone now present. With insulin that is less effective, fat stores of the woman are utilized as well as available glucose. This maintains maternal glucose levels at a fairly steady level despite long intervals between meals or days of increased activity. To ensure against hypoglycemia, a pregnant woman should be conscientious of keeping her diet high in calories and of never going longer than 12 hours between meals. Because the rapidly developing fetus uses so much glucose in early pregnancy, a fasting blood glucose level at this time is generally slightly low (80 to 85 mg/100 mL).

Adrenal Glands

Adrenal gland activity increases in pregnancy as elevated levels of corticosteroids and aldosterone are produced. The function of corticosteroids is generally unknown, but it is assumed that this increased level aids in suppressing an inflammatory reaction or helps to reduce the possibility of the woman's body rejecting the foreign protein of the fetus, the same as it would automatically do for a foreign-tissue transplant. It also helps to regulate glucose metabolism in the woman. The increased level of aldosterone aids in promoting sodium reabsorption and maintaining osmolarity in the amount of fluid retained. This indirectly helps to safeguard the blood volume and provide adequate perfusion pressure across the placenta.

Immune System

Immunologic competency during pregnancy apparently decreases, probably to prevent the woman's body from rejecting the fetus as if it were a transplanted organ. IgG production is particularly decreased; this may make the woman more prone to infection during pregnancy. A simultaneous increase in white blood cell count may help to counteract the decrease in IgG response.

The Diagnosis of Pregnancy

Diagnosis of pregnancy marks a major life milestone. If a pregnancy was planned, diagnosis produces a feeling of intense fulfillment and achievement; or, if it was not planned or not desired, can result in an equally extreme crisis state. Medical diagnosis of pregnancy serves to date the expected birth and help predict the existence of a high-risk status (see the Nursing Care Plan: A Woman Seeking Pregnancy Confirmation).

When a sexually active woman is scheduled for diagnostic testing that includes a pelvic x-ray such as an intravenous pyelogram, you might suggest that she first have a rapid serum pregnancy test to rule out pregnancy as a possibility, to avoid exposing a fetus to radiation.

Most women who come to a health care facility for a diagnosis of pregnancy have already "hunched" that they are pregnant based on a multitude of presumptive signs. Often, they have already done a home pregnancy test to see if they are pregnant.

Pregnancy is officially diagnosed on the basis of the symptoms reported by the woman and signs elicited by a health care provider. These signs and symptoms are traditionally divided into three classifications: presumptive, probable, and positive (Table 8-5).

Presumptive Signs of Pregnancy

Presumptive signs of pregnancy are those that are least indicative of pregnancy; taken as single entities, they could easily indicate other conditions. These findings are largely subjective in that they are experienced by the woman but cannot be documented by the examiner.

Probable Signs of Pregnancy

In contrast to presumptive signs, *probable signs of pregnancy* can be documented by the examiner. Although they are more reliable than the presumptive signs of pregnancy, they still are not positive or true diagnostic findings.

Laboratory Tests

The commonly used laboratory tests for pregnancy are based on determining the presence of human chorionic gonadotropin (HCG), a hormone created by the chorionic villi, in the urine or serum of the pregnant woman. Because all laboratory tests for pregnancy are inaccurate to some degree, positive results from these tests are considered probable rather than positive signs.

For pregnancy testing, HCG is measured in international units. In the nonpregnant woman, no units will be detectable, because there are no trophoblast cells producing HCG. In the pregnant woman, trace amounts of HCG appear in the serum as early as 24 to 48 hours following implantation. They reach a measurable level of 50 to 100 mIU/mL on common immunologic serum tests by the 30th day after the last menstrual period (Kochenour, 1990). HCG levels peak at about 100 mIU/mL between the 60th and 80th day of gestation. After this point, the level declines again so that at term it is barely detectable in serum or urine.

Urine, formerly used extensively for pregnancy testing, is now used only rarely in health care settings, because blood serum tests give earlier results. Urine tests still form the basis of home pregnancy tests. Any woman who thinks she might be pregnant but gets a negative result from a pregnancy test should be advised to have a repeat test 1 week later if she is still experiencing amenorrhea. If she is not pregnant, she might have a condition such as an ovarian tumor causing the amenorrhea and need appropriate therapy.

Home Pregnancy Tests. Several brand name kits for pregnancy testing based on immunologic reactions are available over the counter (Demystifying ovulation and pregnancy kits for your patients, 1993). These tests have a high degree of accuracy (about 97%) if the instructions are followed exactly. They are convenient for women, because waiting for a physician's appointment to have a pregnancy diagnosed is an anxious, stressful time for many women. For this type of testing, the woman dips a reagent strip into her stream of urine. A color change on the strip denotes pregnancy. Home tests are able to detect as little as 50 to 150 mIU/mL of HCG.

In the past, one of the chief reasons women sought early prenatal care was to obtain an official diagnosis of pregnancy and not so much for reasons of health. Now

Table 8-5. *Presumptive and Probable Signs of Pregnancy*

Time from Implantation (weeks)	Presumptive Finding	Probable Finding	Positive Finding	Description
1		Serum laboratory tests		Tests of blood serum reveal the presence of human chorionic gonadotropin hormone.
2	Breast changes			Feeling of tenderness, fullness, or tingling; enlargement and darkening of areola
2	Amenorrhea			Absence of menstruation
3	Frequent micturition			Sense of having to void frequently
6		Chadwick's sign		Color change of the vagina from pink to violet
6		Goodell's sign		Softening of the cervix
6		Hegar's sign		Softening of the lower uterine segment
6		Sonographic evidence of gestational sac		A characteristic ring is evident.
8			Sonograph evidence of fetal outline	A fetal outline can be seen and measured by sonogram.
10			Fetal heart audible	Doppler ultrasound reveals heart beat.
12	Fatigue			General feeling of tiredness
12	Uterine enlargement			Uterus can be palpated over symphysis pubis.
16		Ballottement		When lower uterine segment is tapped on a bimanual examination, the fetus can be felt to rise against abdominal wall.
16		Fetal outline		A fetal outline can be felt through abdominal wall.
18	Quickening			Fetal movement felt by woman
20			Fetal movement felt by examiner	Fetal movement can be palpated through abdomen.
20		Braxton Hicks sign		Periodic uterine tightening occurs.
20		Fetal outline felt by examiner		Fetal outline can be palpated through abdomen.
24	Linea nigra			Line of dark pigment on the abdomen
24	Melasma			Dark pigment on face
24	Striae gravidarum			Red streaks on abdomen

that women can diagnose their pregnancies at home by means of a test kit, they may not seek prenatal care until something seems to be wrong with the pregnancy or until they are far along and feel they should do something about arranging medical coverage for the birth. Caution women that early and regular prenatal care is important to safeguard the pregnancy outcome and that after a positive pregnancy test, their next step should be to arrange for prenatal care.

Women who are taking psychotropic drugs (antianxiety agents) may have false-positive results on pregnancy tests. Women on oral contraceptives also may have false-positive results; for such a test to be accurate, oral contraceptives should have been discontinued 5 days before the test. Women who have proteinuria, are postmenopausal, or have hyperthyroid disease also may show false-positive results.

Positive Signs of Pregnancy

There are only three *positive signs of pregnancy:* demonstration of a fetal heart separate from that of the mother's, fetal movements felt by the examiner, and visualization of the fetus by ultrasound.

Nursing Care Plan

A Woman Seeking Pregnancy Confirmation

Mary Kraft is a 25-year-old woman you meet in an obstetrician's office at a confirmation of pregnancy visit. The following is a nursing care plan designed for her at this first prenatal visit.

Assessment: Client has been married 4 years; gravida 2, para 0; last spontaneous menstrual period 9 weeks ago. Last pregnancy ended in spontaneous abortion at 2½ months. She asked, "How do I know that won't happen again?" and appears nervous discussing possibility of another early pregnancy loss. States she has only minimal nausea. States biggest problem is with backache; hurts when climbing ladder at work. This pregnancy was planned after surgery for endometriosis 4 months ago. Reaction to pregnancy confirmation: "Unbelievably happy." Husband attends night school so "some nights are lonely." Client works as a public librarian, family lives out of town; she has few close friends, "one at work." They are only black family in condominium so sometimes feels "out of place." Appeared nervous at discussing lack of friends.

Nursing Diagnosis: Social isolation related to lifestyle.

Defining Characteristic: Client states she has few support people.

Goal: Client will increase social contacts during pregnancy.

Outcome Criteria: Client establishes a satisfying relationship with at least one neighbor or new acquaintance outside work; client demonstrates ability to use health care personnel as her support people until outside sources are established.

Nursing Orders	*Rationale*
1. Urge client to communicate with family out of town by letter, telephone.	1. Pregnancy is a situational crisis and support people are important in times of crisis.
2. Urge client to have husband accompany her for at least one prenatal visit.	2. Involving the husband in prenatal care helps to family center the event.
3. Discuss ways to fill in free time to counteract feelings of loneliness.	3. Feelings of loneliness could interfere with the psychologic work of pregnancy.
4. Discuss ways of meeting more people to establish her own network of friends outside husband's acquaintances.	4. Establishing a network of friends could serve to not only alleviate loneliness now but also build a network of support in the future.

Nursing Diagnosis: Fear about pregnancy outcome related to previous miscarriage.

Defining Characteristic: Client voices concern about early pregnancy loss.

Goal: Client will experience decreased anxiety about pregnancy outcome by next clinic visit.

Outcome Criteria: Client voices decreased anxiety about pregnancy outcome; Client voices she is able to view herself as a mother by end of pregnancy.

(continued)

Demonstration of a Fetal Heart Separate from the Mother's

Presence of a fetal heart can be demonstrated by hearing its sound (auscultation) or seeing it beating by an ultrasound examination. Although the fetal heart has been beating since the 24th day after conception, it is audible by auscultation of the abdomen with an ordinary stethoscope only at about 18 to 20 weeks of pregnancy. Fetal heart sounds are difficult to hear when abdomens have a great deal of subcutaneous fat or there is a greater-

Nursing Orders	Rationale
1. Discuss the frequency of miscarriages and the fact that having one does not necessarily predispose a person to another.	1. Factual information can help reduce her anxiety.
2. Assure client that pregnancy is going well (as appropriate) at visits.	2. Promote parent-child bonding, which may be threatened owing to previous pregnancy loss.
3. Schedule appointments so consistent health care personnel are present.	3. Health care personnel can serve as important support people to this client who has few support people of her own close by.
4. Encourage client to express concerns at prenatal visits.	4. Voicing concerns can be the beginning of self–problem solving. It can also alert health care personnel to anxiety-related problems they can help solve.

Nursing Diagnosis: Pain related to lumbar lordosis accompanying pregnancy.

Defining Characteristic: Client voices she has discomfort.

Goal: Client will experience increased comfort by next prenatal visit.

Outcome Criteria: Client voices she has less discomfort concerning back and leg pain; is able to continue working.

Nursing Orders	Rationale
1. Review with client that backache can accompany pregnancy because of lordosis; the necessity of good posture during pregnancy.	1. Good posture can help reduce strain on back ligaments.
2. Give client pamphlet *Your Baby Inside You,* and review photos of correct posture.	2. Improve health teaching with visual example.
3. Discuss wardrobe during pregnancy and possibility of limiting amount of time spent each day wearing high heels.	3. High heels can increase a lordosis.
4. Help client plan ways to rest daily with feet elevated; caution about ladder climbing as pregnancy progresses.	4. Increasing abdominal size can interfere with balance.
5. Teach client pelvic rocking exercise.	5. Pelvic rocking can reduce back discomfort.

than-normal amount of amniotic fluid present (hydramnios). They are heard best when the position of the fetus is determined by palpation and the stethoscope is placed over the area of the fetus's back. A fetal heart rate usually ranges between 120 and 160 beats per minute.

Ultrasonic monitoring systems that convert ultrasonic frequencies to audible frequencies (Doppler technique) are extremely helpful in detecting fetal heart sounds. Fetal heart sounds may be heard as early as the 10th to 12th week of gestation by this method. Echocardiography can demonstrate a heart beat as early as 5 weeks (Kochenour, 1990).

Fetal Movements Felt by the Examiner

Movements of the fetus perceived by the woman may be felt as early as 16 to 20 weeks of pregnancy. Those felt by an objective examiner are considered much more reliable and constitute a positive sign of pregnancy. Such movements may be felt by the 20th to 24th week of pregnancy unless the woman is extremely obese.

Visualization of Fetus by Ultrasound

High-frequency sound waves projected toward a woman's abdomen are useful in diagnosing pregnancy. In the event of pregnancy, a characteristic ring, indicating the gestational sac, will be revealed on the oscilloscope as early as the 5th to 6th week of pregnancy. This method of determination also gives information about the site of implantation and whether a multiple pregnancy exists. By the 8th week, a fetal outline can be seen so clearly within the sac that the crown to rump length can be measured to establish the gestational age of the pregnancy (Kochenour, 1990). By using a "real-time" technique of ultrasound, fetal heart movement may be demonstrated as early as the 6th week by the use of transvaginal sonography, the 7th week by transabdominal sonography.

Seeing or hearing a fetal heart beat is not only positive proof for a health care provider that a pregnancy exists, but for many women as well. It can be an important step in initiating bonding.

Key Points

- The ability of a woman to accept a pregnancy depends on social, cultural, family, and individual influences.
- The psychological tasks of pregnancy are centered on ensuring safe passage for the fetus. These consist of, first trimester: accepting the pregnancy; second trimester: accepting the baby; and third trimester: preparing for parenthood. Fathers undergo the same steps.
- Common emotional responses that occur with pregnancy can be grief, narcissism, introversion or extroversion, decreased decision-making ability, body image and boundary confusion, emotional lability, and changes in sexual desire.
- Physiologic changes that occur with pregnancy are both local (uterine, ovarian, and vaginal) and systemic changes (changes in respiratory, cardiovascular, urinary, and skin changes).
- The diagnosis of pregnancy is based on three types of findings: presumptive, probable, and positive.
- The positive signs of pregnancy are demonstration of a fetal heart separate from the mother's, fetal

movement felt by an examiner, and visualization of the fetus by ultrasound.
- Women may have read about the expected psychological and physiologic changes of pregnancy, but once these changes are actually being experienced, they may find them more intense than anticipated.
- Although a woman may be in a physician's office or prenatal clinic for only an hour, if her pregnancy was confirmed at that visit, she invariably feels "more pregnant" when she leaves. From that day, most women try to eat a proper diet and give up cigarette smoking, alcohol ingestion, and stop taking over-the-counter medication. Because a woman may not take these measures before confirmation of her pregnancy, early diagnosis is important. If the woman does not wish to continue the pregnancy, early diagnosis is imperative; elective termination of pregnancy always should be carried out at the earliest stage possible for the safest outcome.

Critical Thinking Exercises

1. Molly is a young adult woman you care for in a prenatal setting. She tells you that she "hates" her parents and "would die" if she thought she might be the same type of parent they were. Has Molly completed the psychological development tasks of pregnancy? Are there suggestions you could make to her to help her be a better parent?

2. Teresa is a 15-year-old adolescent you know who is 4 months pregnant. She tells you she has had almost constant heartburn and nausea since she became pregnant. How would you explain why these symptoms happen with pregnancy?

3. Teresa used a home test kit to determine that she is pregnant and has not been to a health care setting, because she says the most important reason for going would be to learn whether she is pregnant or not and she already knows that. What argument could you use to convince her that prenatal care is important for more than pregnancy diagnosis?

References

Blackburn, S., & Loper, D. (1992). *Maternal, fetal and neonatal physiology: A clinical perspective.* Philadelphia: W. B. Saunders.

Blake, R. L., & Reimann, J. (1993). The pregnancy-related dreams of pregnant women. *Journal of the American Board of Family Practice, 6,* 117.

Boyle, J., & Andrews, M. (1990). *Transcultural concepts in nursing care.* Glenview, IL: Scott, Foresman.

Burger, J., et al. (1993). Psychological sequelae of medical complications during pregnancy. *Pediatrics, 9,* 566.

Demystifying ovulation and pregnancy kits for your patients. (1993). *Contemporary OB/GYN, 38,* 67.

Department of Health and Human Services. (1991). *Healthy people 2000.* Washington, D.C.: Public Health Service.

Engstrom, J. L., McFarlin, B., & Sittler, C. P. (1993). Fundal height measurement: three measurement techniques. *Journal of Nurse-Midwifery, 38*, 17.

Fawcett, J. (1989). Spouses' experiences during pregnancy and the postpartum. *Image, 21,* 149.

Hume, R. F., & Killam, A. P. (1990). Maternal physiology. In Scott, J. R., et al. *Danforth's obstetrics and gynecology.* Philadelphia: J. B. Lippincott.

Kochenour, N. K. (1990). Normal pregnancy and prenatal care. In Scott, J. R., et al. *Danforth's obstetrics and gynecology.* Philadelphia: J. B. Lippincott.

Loeb, S. (1993). *Nurses' handbook of drug therapy.* Springhouse, PA: Springhouse.

Syverson, C. J., et al. (1991). Pregnancy-related mortality in New York City. *American Journal of Obstetrics and Gynecology, 164,* 603.

Theunissen, I. M., & Parer, J. T. (1994). Fluid and electrolytes in pregnancy. *Clinical Obstetrics and Gynecology, 37,* 3.

Walker, M. K., & Conner, G. K. (1993). Fetal sex preference of second-trimester gravidas. *Journal of Nurse-Midwifery, 38,* 110.

Suggested Readings

Brown, D. (1992). All pregnant women need prenatal care. *RN, 55,* 88.

Cerrato, P. L. (1992). Improving the odds of a healthy birth. *RN, 55,* 71.

Culpepper, L., & Jack. B. (1993). Psychosocial issues in pregnancy. *Primary Care, 20,* 599.

Flagler, S., & Nicoll, L. (1990). A framework for the psychological aspects of pregnancy. *NAACOGS Clinical Issues in Perinatal & Women's Health Nursing, 1,* 267.

Fogel, C. I. (1993). Pregnant inmates: risk factors and pregnancy outcomes. *Journal of Obstetric, Gynecologic and Neonatal Nursing, 22,* 33.

Hofmeyr, G., Marcos, E., & Butchart, A. (1991). Pregnant women's perceptions of themselves: a survey. *Birth, 17,* 205.

Kenney, J., & Tash, D. (1992). Lesbian childbearing couples' dilemmas and decisions. *Health Care of Women International, 13,* 209.

May, K. M. (1992) Social networks and help seeking experiences of pregnant teens. *Journal of Obstetric, Gynecologic and Neonatal Nursing, 21,* 497.

Mercer, R. T., & Ferketich, S. L. (1994). Predictors of maternal role competence by risk status. *Nursing Research, 43,* 38.

Muller, M. (1992). A critical review of prenatal attachment research. *Scholarly Inquiry in Nursing Practice, 6,* 5.

O'Connor, A. M., et al. (1992). Effectiveness of a pregnancy smoking cessation program. *Journal of Obstetric, Gynecologic and Neonatal Nursing, 21,* 385.

Tulman, I., et al. (1991). The inventory of functional status—antepartal period. *Journal of Nurse-Midwifery, 36,* 117.

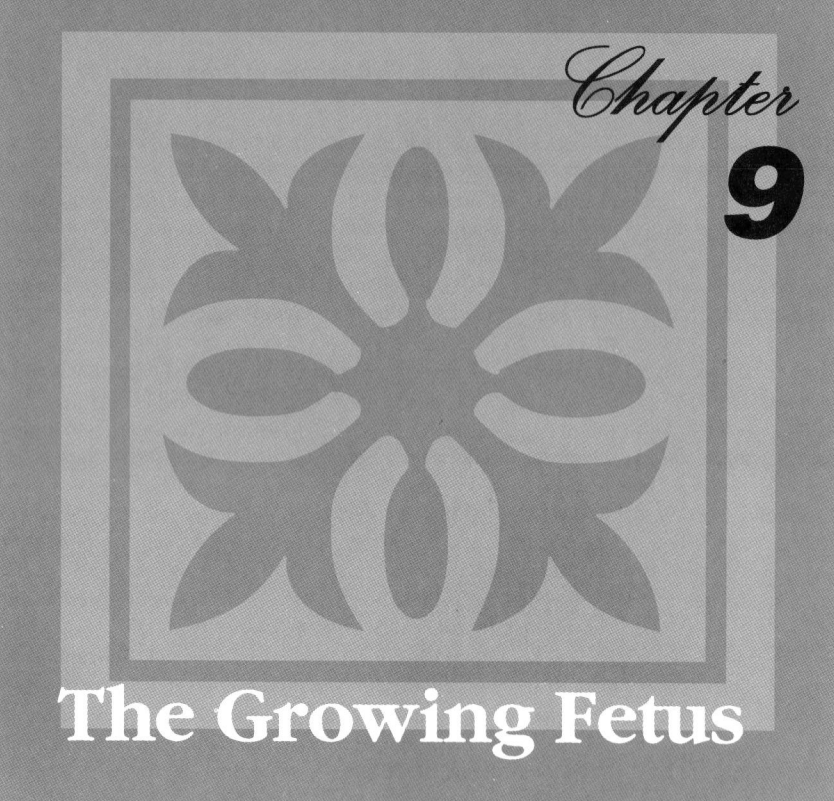

Chapter 9

The Growing Fetus

Objectives

After mastering the contents of this chapter, you should be able to:

1. Describe the growth and development of the fetus by gestational week.

2. Assess fetal growth and development through maternal and pregnancy landmarks.

3. Formulate nursing diagnoses related to the needs of the pregnant woman and developing baby.

4. Plan nursing care that promotes healthy fetal growth.

5. Implement nursing care to help ensure a safe pregnancy outcome and a safe fetal environment.

6. Evaluate outcome criteria established in relation to fetal growth to be certain that nursing goals have been achieved.

7. Identify National Health Goals related to fetal growth that nurses can help the nation to achieve.

8. Identify areas of fetal health that could benefit from additional nursing research.

9. Use critical thinking to analyze ways to promote fetal growth and development appropriate for individual families.

10. Synthesize knowledge of growth and development of the fetus with nursing process to achieve quality maternal and child health nursing care.

Key Terms

- amniocentesis
- amniotic cavity
- amniotic membrane
- blastocyst
- cephalocaudal
- chorionic membrane
- chorionic villi
- coelocentesis
- corona radiata
- cotyledons
- decidua basalis
- decidua capsularis
- decidua vera
- ductus arteriosus
- ductus venosus
- ectoderm
- embryo
- entoderm
- expected date of birth
- fertilization
- fetoscopy
- fetus
- foramen ovale
- hydramnios
- implantation
- lightening
- McDonald's rule
- mesoderm
- morula
- neural plate
- nonstress test
- oligohydramnios
- quickening
- surfactant
- trophoblast
- umbilical cord
- Wharton's jelly
- yolk sac
- zona pellucida
- zygote

Adele Pillitteri: MATERNAL AND CHILD HEALTH NURSING, 2nd Edition. © 1995 Adele Pillitteri.

*T*hroughout history, different societies have held a variety of beliefs and superstitions about the way the **fetus** (the infant during intrauterine life) grows. Medieval artists depicted the child in utero completely formed as a miniature man. Leonardo da Vinci, in his notebooks of 1510 to 1512, made several sketches of unborn infants that indicated he believed the fetus was immobile and essentially a part of the mother, sharing her blood and internal organs. During the 17th and 18th centuries, a baby was thought to form to a miniature size in the mother's ovaries; when male cells were introduced, the baby expanded to birth size. A second theory was that the child existed in the head of the sperm cell as a fully formed being, the uterus being used only as an incubator in which it grew. It was not until 1759 that Kaspar Wolff proposed that both parents contribute equally to the structure of the baby (De Lia, 1990). Thanks to the work of modern medical researchers and photographers like Lennart Nielsson, who have been able to capture the process of fertilization and fetal development through the use of enhanced, high-tech photography, we now have a clear idea of what the fetus looks like from the moment of conception until birth.

A number of National Health Goals have been devised specifically to increase the health of fetuses during pregnancy. These goals are shown in the Focus on National Health Goals box.

⊞ **NURSING PROCESS OVERVIEW**
for Teaching Families About Fetal Growth and Development

ASSESSMENT

The predictable stages of fetal development provide a guide for determining the well being of an individual fetus. Health care providers can also use these stages as guidelines to predict the expected date of birth of the fetus more accurately. For the expectant family, knowledge about fetal growth and development can provide an important frame of reference, helping the mother to understand some of the changes going on in her body and allowing all family members to begin thinking about and accepting the newest member of their family before the baby actually arrives. Conveying findings gained from fetal assessment in as much detail as parents request is an important nursing role.

191

NURSING DIAGNOSIS

Common nursing diagnoses related to growth and development of the fetus focus on the mother and family as well as the fetus. Examples include:

- Health-seeking behaviors related to knowledge of normal fetal development
- Anxiety related to lack of fetal movement
- Potential for enhanced parenting related to need for good prenatal care for healthy fetal development

PLANNING

Goals and outcome criteria established for teaching about fetal growth should be realistic in light of the parents' knowledge base and desire for information. When additional assessment measures are necessary, it is important that new teaching material is readied that explains why further assessment is necessary and what results are to be expected.

IMPLEMENTATION

Teaching women about fetal growth and development helps them to visualize the fetus at each stage of development, which, in turn, helps them to understand the

---

FOCUS ON
National Health Goals

A number of National Health Goals address fetal growth. These are:

- Reduce the fetal death rate (death below 20 or more weeks of gestation) to no more than 5 per 1000 live births from a baseline of 7.6/1000.

- Reduce low birth weight to an incidence of no more than 5% of live births and very low birth-weight to no more than 1% of live births from baselines of 6.9 and 1.2% (DHHS, 1991).

Nurses can be instrumental in helping the nation achieve these goals by urging women to preplan pregnancies so they can enter a pregnancy in good health. Educating women about the importance of attending prenatal care is another vital role. Nursing research in such areas as why women avoid prenatal care or how soon women change a lifestyle during pregnancy to more healthy actions could lead to increased success for these national health goals.

---

importance of eating well and avoiding substances that may be dangerous to the fetus. Viewing sonograms helps to begin parent-infant bonding. Chapters 10 and 11 discuss specific health-maintenance teaching measures that are vital to fetal health and well being.

EVALUATION

Evaluation of outcome criteria in regard to fetal growth and development usually focuses on determining whether the mother or family is demonstrating any necessary changes in lifestyle to ensure fetal growth and whether or not the mother voices that she feels confident that the baby inside her is healthy and growing normally. Examples are:

- Parents describe smoke-free living at next prenatal visit.
- Client records number of movements of fetus for 1 hour daily.
- Couple attends prenatal care regularly.

Stages of Fetal Development

In just 38 weeks, a fertilized egg is able to mature from a single cell carrying all the necessary genetic material to a fully developed fetus ready to be born. Table 9-1 lists common terms used to describe the fetus at various stages in this growth.

Fertilization: The Beginning of Pregnancy

Fertilization is the union of the ovum and a spermatozoon. Other terms used to describe this phenomenon are *conception, impregnation,* or *fecundation.*

Following ovulation, as the ovum is extruded from the graafian follicle, it is surrounded by a ring of mucopolysaccharide fluid (the **zona pellucida**) and a circle of cells (the **corona radiata**). These structures increase the bulk of the ovum, facilitating its migration to the uterus, and probably also serve as a protection from injury. The ovum and surrounding cells are propelled into the near fallopian tube by currents initiated by the *fimbriae,* the fine, hair-like structures that line the openings of the fallopian tubes. The ovum is propelled the length of the tube by peristaltic action of the tube and movement of the tube cilia. Fertilization must occur fairly quickly after release of the ovum because an ovum is capable of fertilization for only 24 hours (48 hours at the most). After that time, it atrophies and becomes nonfunctional.

Table 9-1. Terms Used to Denote Fetal Growth

Name	Time Period
Ovum	From ovulation to fertilization
Zygote	From fertilization to implantation
Embryo	From implantation to 5–8 weeks
Fetus	From 5–8 weeks until term
Conceptus	Developing embryo or fetus and placental structures throughout pregnancy

Although only one ovum reaches maturity each month, a normal ejaculation of semen averages 2.5 mL of fluid containing 50 to 200 million spermatozoa per milliliter, or an average of 400 million per ejaculation. To promote the possibility of a sperm reaching the ovum, there is a reduction in the viscosity (thickness) of cervical mucus at the time of ovulation, making it easier for spermatozoa to penetrate it. Sperm transport is so efficient close to ovulation that spermatozoa deposited in the vagina during intercourse generally reach the cervix of the uterus within 90 seconds after deposition and the outer end of a fallopian tube in 5 minutes (one reason why douching is not an effective contraceptive measure). Spermatozoa move by means of their *flagella* (tails) and uterine contractions through the cervix, the body of the uterus, and into the fallopian tubes toward the waiting ovum. The mechanism whereby spermatozoa are drawn toward an ovum is probably a species-specific reaction, similar to an antibody-antigen reaction. *Capacitation* is a final process that sperm must undergo to be ready for fertilization. This process consists of changes in the plasma membrane of the sperm head which reveals the sperm-binding receptor sites (Flood & Hodgen, 1990).

Fertilization usually occurs in the outer third of a fallopian tube, the ampullar portion. The functional life of a spermatozoa is about 48 hours (maybe as long as 72 hours), so sexual coitus as long as this time interval before ovulation may result in fertilization. That makes the total critical fertilization timespan during which fertilization may occur about 72 hours (48 hours preceding ovulation plus 24 hours afterward).

All the spermatozoa that achieve capacitation reach the ovum and cluster around the protective layer of corona cells. Hyaluronidase (a proteolytic enzyme) is apparently released by the spermatozoa and acts to dissolve the layer of cells protecting the ovum. The reason that an ejaculation contains so many sperm although only one is necessary for fertilization is probably to provide enough enzymes to dissolve the corona cells. Once one spermatozoon effectively penetrates the zona pellucida, a reaction sweeps through the layer that makes it difficult for other spermatozoa to penetrate it. Under or-

dinary circumstances, only one spermatozoon is able to penetrate the cell membrane of the ovum. After it has done so, the cell membrane becomes impervious to other spermatozoa. An exception to this is the formation of hydatidiform mole in which multisperm enter; this leads to abnormal growth (see Chapter 15).

Immediately after penetration of the ovum, the chromosomal material of the ovum and spermatozoon fuse. The resulting structure is called a **zygote**. Because the spermatozoon and ovum each carried 23 chromosomes (22 autosomes and 1 sex chromosome), a fertilized ovum has 46 chromosomes. If an X-carrying spermatozoon enters the ovum, the resulting child will have two X chromosomes and will be female (XX). If a Y-carrying spermatozoon fertilizes the ovum, the resulting child will have an X and a Y chromosome and will be male (XY).

Fertilization is never a certain occurrence because it depends on at least three separate factors: (1) maturation of both sperm and ovum, (2) ability of sperm to reach the ovum, and (3) ability of the sperm to penetrate the zona pellucida and cell membrane and achieve fertilization.

Out of the fertilized ovum (the zygote) will form not only the future child but also the accessory structures the child needs for support during intrauterine life: the placenta, the fetal membranes, the amniotic fluid, and the umbilical cord.

Implantation

Implantation or contact between the blastocyst and the uterine endothelium occurs approximately 8–10 days after fertilization. Once fertilization is complete, the zygote migrates toward the body of the uterus, aided by the currents initiated by the muscular contractions of the fallopian tubes. It takes 3 or 4 days for the zygote to reach the body of the uterus. During this time, mitotic cell division, or *cleavage,* begins at a rapid rate. The first cleavage occurs at about 24 hours; cleavage divisions continue to occur at a rate of one about every 22 hours. By the time the zygote reaches the body of the uterus, it consists of 16 to 50 cells. At this stage, because of its bumpy outward appearance, it is termed a **morula** (from the Latin word *morus,* meaning "mulberry").

The morula continues to multiply as it floats free in the uterine cavity for 3 or 4 more days. Large cells tend to mass at the periphery of the ball, leaving a fluid space surrounding an inner cell mass. At this stage, the structure is termed a **blastocyst**. The cells in the outer ring are known as **trophoblast** cells. They are the part of the structure that will later form the placenta and membranes. The inner cell mass (embryoblast cells) is the portion of the structure that will later form the embryo.

After the 3rd or 4th day of free floating (about 8

days from ovulation), the last residues of the corona and zona pellucida are shed by the growing structure. The blastocyst brushes against the rich uterine endometrium (in the second [secretory] phase of the menstrual cycle), a process termed *apposition*. It attaches to the surface of the endometrium (*adhesion*) and settles down into its soft folds (*invasion*). Stages to this point are depicted in Figure 9-1.

The blastocyst is able to invade the endometrium because as the trophoblast cells on the outside of the structure touch the endometrium, they produce proteolytic enzymes that dissolve the tissue they touch. This action allows the blastocyst not only to burrow deeply into the endometrium but to receive some basic nourishment of glycogen and mucoprotein from the endometrial glands. As invasion continues, the structure establishes an effective communication network with the blood system of the endometrium. The touching or implantation point is usually high in the uterus and on the posterior surface. If the point of implantation is low in the uterus, the growing placenta may occlude the cervix and make delivery of the child at term difficult (*placenta previa*).

Implantation is an important step in pregnancy because as many as 50% of zygotes never achieve it. In these instances, a pregnancy ends as early as 8 to 10 days after conception, often before the woman is even aware it had begun. Occasionally, a small amount of vaginal spotting appears with implantation because capillaries are ruptured by the implanting trophoblast cells. A woman who normally has a particularly scant menstrual flow may mistake implantation bleeding for her menstrual period. If this happens, the predicted date of birth of her baby (based on the time of her last menstrual period) will then be calculated 4 weeks late. Once implanted, the zygote is an **embryo**.

The Decidua

Following conception, the corpus luteum in the ovary continues to function rather than to atrophy because of the influence of human chorionic gonadotropin (HCG) hormone secreted by the trophoblast cells; thus, the endometrium of the uterus, instead of sloughing off as in a normal menstrual cycle, continues to grow in thickness and vascularity. The endometrium is now termed **decidua** (the Latin word for "falling off"), because it will be discarded following the birth of the child. The decidua has three separate areas: (1) the **decidua basalis** or the part of the endometrium lying directly under the embryo (or the portion where the trophoblast cells are establishing communication with maternal blood vessels); (2) the **decidua capsularis**, or the portion of the endometrium that stretches or encapsulates the surface of the trophoblast; and (3) the **decidua vera**, or the remaining portion of the uterine lining (Figure 9-2).

As the embryo continues to grow, it pushes the decidua capsularis before it like a blanket. Eventually, enlargement brings the structure into contact with the opposite uterine wall. Here, the decidua capsularis fuses with the endometrium of the opposite wall. This is why, at delivery, the entire inner surface of the uterus is stripped away, leaving the organ highly susceptible to hemorrhage and infection.

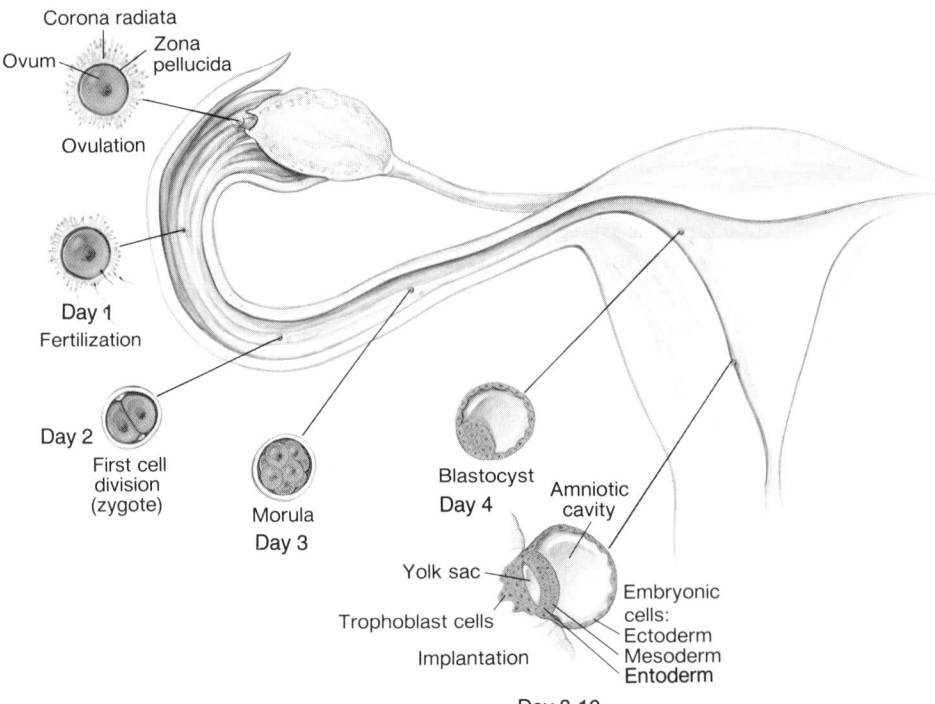

FIGURE 9-1
Schema of ovulation, fertilization, and implantation. At the time of implantation, the blastocyst is already differentiated into germ layers (ectoderm, mesoderm, and entoderm). Cells at the periphery of the structure are trophoblast cells that mature into the placenta.

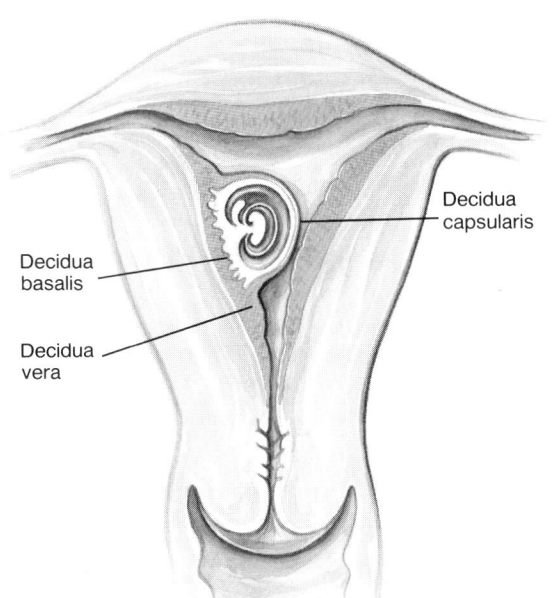

FIGURE 9-2
Division of uterine decidua into three areas.

Labels: Decidua capsularis; Decidua basalis; Decidua vera

Chorionic Villi

Once implantation is achieved, the trophoblastic layer of cells of the blastocyst begins to mature rapidly. As early as the 11th or 12th day, miniature villi, or probing "fingers," reach out from the single layer of cells into the uterine endometrium; these are termed **chorionic villi**. At term, nearly 200 such villi will have formed.

Chorionic villi have a central core of loose connective tissue surrounded by a double layer of trophoblast cells. The central core of connective tissue contains fetal capillaries. The outer of the two covering layers is termed the *syncytiotrophoblast,* or the *syncytial layer.* This layer of cells is instrumental in the production of various placental hormones, such as HCG, somatomammotropin (human placental lactogen), estrogen, and progesterone. The inner layer, known as the *cytotrophoblast* or *Langhans'* layer, is present as early as 12 days' gestation and appears to be functional early in pregnancy but then disappears between the 20th and 24th week. This layer of cells protects the growing embryo and fetus from certain infectious organisms such as the spirochete of syphilis. This is why syphilis is considered to have high potential for fetal damage late in pregnancy, when cytotrophoblast cells are not functioning. Unfortunately, the layer appears to offer little protection against viral invasion.

The Placenta

The placenta arises out of trophoblast tissue. It serves as the fetal lungs, kidneys, and gastrointestinal tract and as a separate endocrine organ throughout pregnancy. Its growth is as phenomenal as that of the fetus, growing from a few identifiable cells at the beginning of pregnancy to an organ 15 to 20 cm in diameter and 2 to 3 cm in depth at term. It covers about half the surface area of the internal uterus. The word placenta is Latin for "pancake," which is descriptive of its size and appearance at term.

Circulation

Placental circulation is depicted in Figure 9-3. As early as the 12th day of pregnancy, maternal blood begins to collect in spaces (intervillous spaces) of the uterine endometrium surrounding the chorionic villi. By the 3rd week, oxygen and other nutrients, such as glucose, amino acids, fatty acids, minerals, vitamins, and water, diffuse from the maternal blood through the cell layers of the chorionic villi to the villi capillaries. From there, nutrients are transported back to the developing embryo.

For practical purposes, there is no direct exchange of blood between the embryo and the mother during pregnancy; the exchange is carried out only by selective osmosis through the chorionic villi. In actuality, because the layer of exchange is only one cell thick, miniature breaks in the chorionic villi do allow occasional cells to cross. Placenta osmosis is so effective that all but a few substances are able to cross the placenta into fetal circulation (Ward, 1992). For this reason, it is important that a woman take no drugs (including caffeine, alcohol, and nicotine) other than those prescribed for her during pregnancy because almost all drugs are able to cross into fetal circulation (Rurak, 1992). Table 9-2 describes the specific mechanisms by which nutrients cross the placenta. All these processes are affected by blood pressure and *p*H of the fetal and maternal plasma. Specific transport of nutrients is discussed in Chapter 12.

As the number of chorionic villi increases with pregnancy, the villi form a network of communication with the maternal blood that becomes more and more complex. Intervillous spaces grow larger and larger and become separated by a series of partitions or septa. In a mature placenta there are as many as 30 separate segments, called **cotyledons**. These compartments are what make the maternal side of the placenta at term look rough and uneven.

About 100 maternal uterine arteries supply the mature placenta. To provide enough blood for exchange, the rate of uteroplacental blood flow in pregnancy increases from about 50 mL/min at 10 weeks to 500 to 600 mL/min at term. No additional maternal arteries appear after the first 3 months of pregnancy, but to accommodate the increased blood flow, the arteries increase in size. Systemically, the mother's heart rate, total cardiac output, and blood volume all increase to supply the placenta.

In the intervillous spaces, maternal blood jets from the coiled or spiral arteries in streams or spurts. It is propelled from compartment to compartment by the cur-

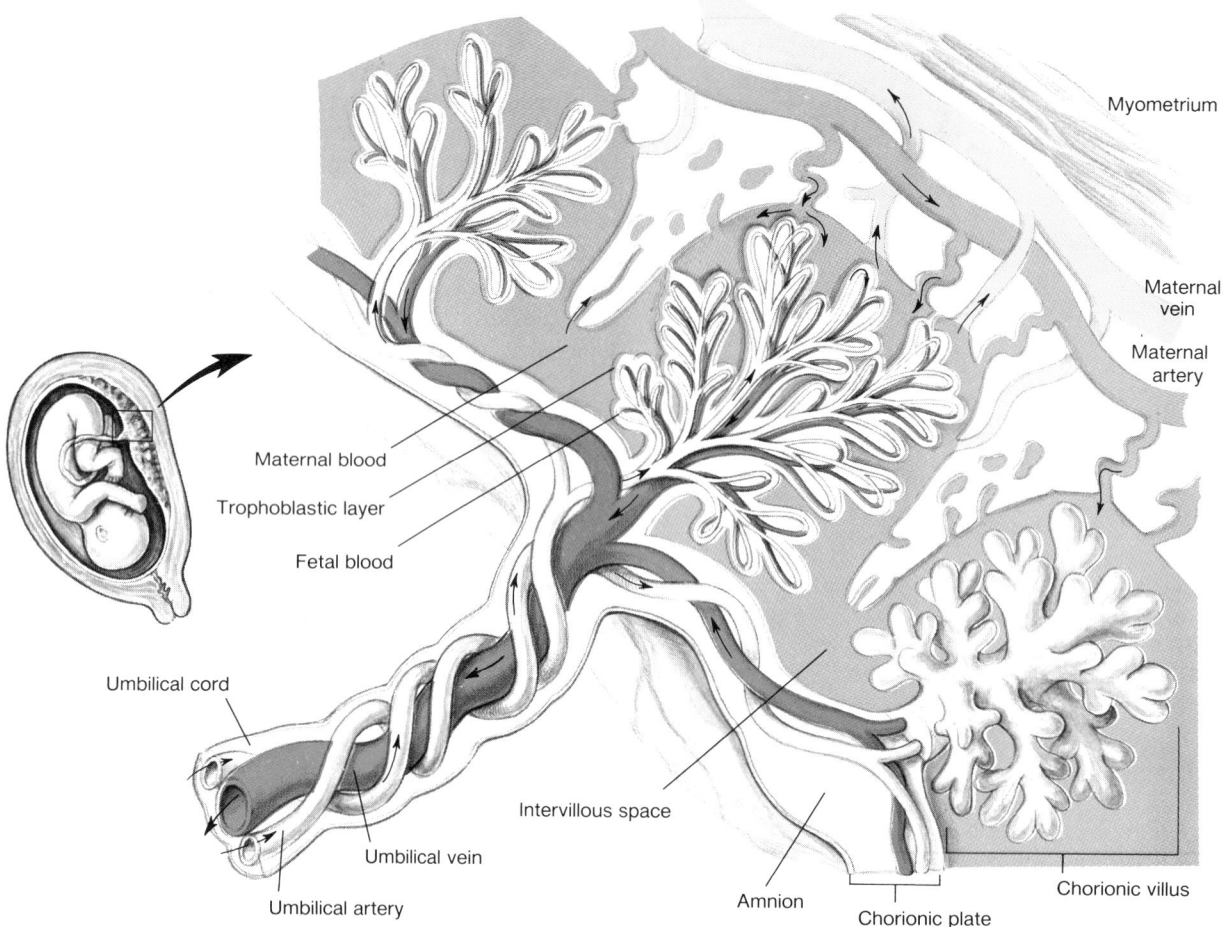

FIGURE 9-3
Placental circulation.

rents initiated and not through definite anatomic channels. Thus, the movement of maternal blood appears to be controlled physiologically rather than anatomically. As the blood circulates around the villi and nutrients osmose from it, it gradually loses its momentum and is crowded toward the placental floor. From there, it enters the orifices of maternal veins and is returned to the maternal circulation. Braxton Hicks contractions, the barely noticeable uterine contractions that are present from about the 12th week of pregnancy, aid in maintaining pressure in the intervillous spaces by closing off the uterine vessels momentarily with each contraction.

Uterine perfusion is most efficient when the mother lies on her left side. This position lifts the uterus away from the inferior vena cava and so prevents blood from being trapped in the lower extremities and unable to circulate. Placental circulation can be sharply reduced if the mother lies on her back and the weight of the uterus compresses the vena cava.

At term, the placental circulatory network is so extensive that a placenta weighs 400 to 600 g (1 lb) and is one-sixth the weight of the baby. If a placenta is smaller than this, it suggests that circulation to the fetus

may have been inadequate. Interestingly, a placenta of greater weight than this also may indicate that circulation to the fetus was in threat because the placenta was forced to spread out in an unusual manner to organize a sufficient blood supply. A fetus of a woman with diabetes may develop a larger-than-usual placenta, probably from excess fluid collected between cells.

Endocrine Function

Aside from serving as the source of oxygen and nutrients for the fetus, the syncytial (outer) layer of the chorionic villi develops into a separate, important hormone-producing system.

Human Chorionic Gonadotropin. The first hormone to be produced is HCG. The presence of this hormone can be demonstrated in maternal blood serum and urine as early as the time of the first missed menstrual period (shortly after implantation has occurred) through about the 100th day of pregnancy. Before or after this period, a false-negative result from a pregnancy test may be reported. The mother's serum will be completely negative for HCG within 1 to 2 weeks after delivery. Testing for

Table 9-2. *Mechanisms by Which Nutrients Cross the Placenta*

Mechanism	Description
Diffusion	When there is a greater concentration of a substance on one side of a semipermeable membrane than on the other, substances of correct molecular weight cross the membrane from the area of higher concentration to the area of lower concentration. Oxygen and carbon dioxide cross the placenta by simple diffusion.
Facilitated diffusion	In order that the fetus receives enough concentrations of necessary growth substances, some substances cross the placenta more rapidly or more easily than would occur if only simple diffusion were operating. Glucose is an example of a substance that crosses by this process.
Active transport	This process requires that an enzyme act to facilitate transport. Essential amino acids and water-soluble vitamins cross the placenta against the pressure gradient or from an area of lower molecular concentration to an area of greater molecular concentration. Amino acid concentrations in the fetal plasma are twice what they are in the mother, a situation that must occur to provide building substances for active fetal growth.
Pinocytosis	Absorption by the cellular membrane of microdroplets of plasma and dissolved substances. Gamma globulin, lipoproteins, phospholipids, and other molecular structures that are too large for diffusion and that cannot participate in active transport cross in this manner. Unfortunately, viruses that then infect the fetus may also cross in this manner.

HCG following delivery can be used as proof that all the placental tissue has been delivered.

The purpose of HCG is to act as a fail-safe measure to ensure that the corpus luteum of the ovary continues to produce progesterone and estrogen. If the corpus luteum should fail, falling levels of progesterone would cause endometrial sloughing, with loss of the pregnancy followed by a rise of pituitary gonadotropins to induce a new menstrual cycle. HCG also may play a role in suppressing the maternal immunologic response so placental invasion is not rejected. Because the structure of HCG is similar to luteinizing hormone of the pituitary gland, if the fetus is male, it exerts an effect on the fetal testes to begin testosterone production. The presence of testosterone causes the maturation of the male reproductive tract in contrast to the female reproductive tract of the fetus.

At about the 8th week of pregnancy in humans, the outer layer of cells of the developing placenta begins to produce progesterone. At this point, the corpus luteum is no longer needed so the production of HCG which sustained it begins to decrease.

Estrogen. Estrogen (primarily estriol) is produced as a second product of the syncytial cells of the placenta. Estrogen contributes to the mother's mammary gland development in preparation for lactation and stimulates the uterus to grow to accommodate the developing fetus. Assessing the amount of estriol in maternal serum can be used as a test of fetal welfare because the immediate precursor of estrogen synthesis by the placenta is a compound produced by the fetal adrenal gland and liver. When a fetus is stressed, the production of this fetal compound is decreased; estrogen, therefore, cannot be synthesized, and the level of estriol in maternal serum will then decrease. After the 32nd week of pregnancy, a level less than 14 ng/mL suggests that fetal well being is in jeopardy.

Progesterone. Estrogen is often referred to as the "hormone of women," progesterone as the "hormone of mothers." Progesterone is indisputably necessary to maintain the endometrial lining of the uterus during pregnancy. It is present in serum as early as the 4th week of pregnancy as a result of the continuation of the corpus luteum. When placental synthesis begins (at around the 12th week), the level rises progressively during the remainder of the pregnancy. A second function of this hormone appears to be to reduce the contractility of the uterine musculature during pregnancy, which prevents premature labor. Such reduced contractility is probably produced by a change in electrolytes (notably, potassium and calcium), which decreases the contraction potential of the uterus.

Human Placental Lactogen (Chorionic Somatomammotropin). Human placental lactogen (HPL) is a hormone with both growth-promoting and lactogenic (milk-producing) properties. It is produced by the placenta beginning as early as the 6th week of pregnancy. It then increases in amount to a peak level at term. It can be assayed in both maternal serum and urine. It functions to promote mammary gland (breast) growth in preparation for lactation in the mother (accounting for its name). It also serves the important role of regulating maternal glucose, protein, and fat levels so that adequate amounts of these are always available to the fetus.

The Umbilical Cord

As chorionic villi form and begin to function, initiating circulatory communication with maternal blood, they join together to form larger and larger veins and arteries, until they form the **umbilical cord**. The function of the cord is to transport oxygen and nutrients to the fetus from the placenta and to return waste products from the fetus to the placenta. The umbilical cord is about 53 cm (21 in) in length at term. It is about 2 cm (¾ in) in thickness. It contains one vein (carrying blood from the placental villi to the fetus) and two arteries (carrying blood from the fetus back to the placental villi). The remnant of the yolk sac may be found in the fetal end of the cord as a white fibrous streak at term. The bulk of the cord is a gelatinous mucopolysaccharide called **Wharton's jelly**, which gives the cord body and prevents pressure on the vein and arteries. The outer surface is covered with amniotic membrane.

The number of veins and arteries in the cord is always assessed at birth: about 1% of all infants are born with a cord that contains only a single vein and artery. About 15% of these infants are found to have accompanying congenital anomalies, particularly of the kidney and heart (Barness, 1994).

The rate of blood flow through an umbilical cord is rapid (350 mL/min at term). Whether an adequate blood flow (blood velocity) is present in the cord can be determined by ultrasound. Both systolic and diastolic pressure can be determined by this method. Rapid blood flow through the cord makes it unlikely that a cord will twist or knot enough to interfere with the fetal oxygen supply. Blood can be withdrawn from the umbilical vein or transfused into the vein during intrauterine life for fetal assessment or treatment (termed percutaneous umbilical blood sampling) (Davis, 1993). In about 20% of all deliveries, a loose loop of cord is found around the fetal neck (a *nuchal* cord). If this loop of cord is removed before the newborn's shoulders are extruded, so that there is no traction on it, the oxygen supply to the fetus remains unimpaired. Smooth muscle is abundant in the arteries of the cord; the constriction of these circular muscles after birth contributes to hemostasis and helps prevent hemorrhage of the newborn through the cord. Because the umbilical cord contains no nerve supply, it can be cut at birth without discomfort to the child or mother.

The Membranes and Amniotic Fluid

The chorionic villi on the medial surface of the trophoblast (those that are not involved in implantation because they do not touch the endometrium) gradually thin and leave the medial surface of the structure smooth (the *chorion laeve,* or *smooth chorion*). The smooth chorion eventually becomes the **chorionic membrane**, the outermost fetal membrane. Once it smooths, its purpose for the remainder of pregnancy is to offer support to the sac that contains the amniotic fluid. A second membrane lining the chorionic membrane, the **amniotic membrane** or amnion, forms beneath the chorion (Figure 9-4). Early in pregnancy, these membranes become so adherent that they seem as one at term. These membranes cover the fetal surface of the placenta and are what give the placenta its typical shiny appearance. Like the umbilical cord, they have no nerve supply. Thus, when they rupture at term, neither mother nor child experiences any sensation.

Unlike the chorionic membrane, the amnion membrane not only offers support to amniotic fluid but actually produces the fluid. In addition, it produces a phospholipid that initiates the formation of prostaglandins. Prostaglandins cause uterine contractions and may be the "trigger" that initiates labor.

Amniotic fluid is constantly being newly formed and reabsorbed, so it is never stagnant within the membranes (Smith & Weiner, 1990). Reabsorption occurs because the fetus continually swallows the fluid, and it is absorbed across the fetal intestine into the fetal blood stream; from there, the umbilical arteries exchange it across the placenta. Some fluid is probably absorbed in direct contact with the fetal surface of the placenta. At term, the average amount of fluid present is 1000 mL; the range is about 800 to 1200 mL. If, for any reason, the

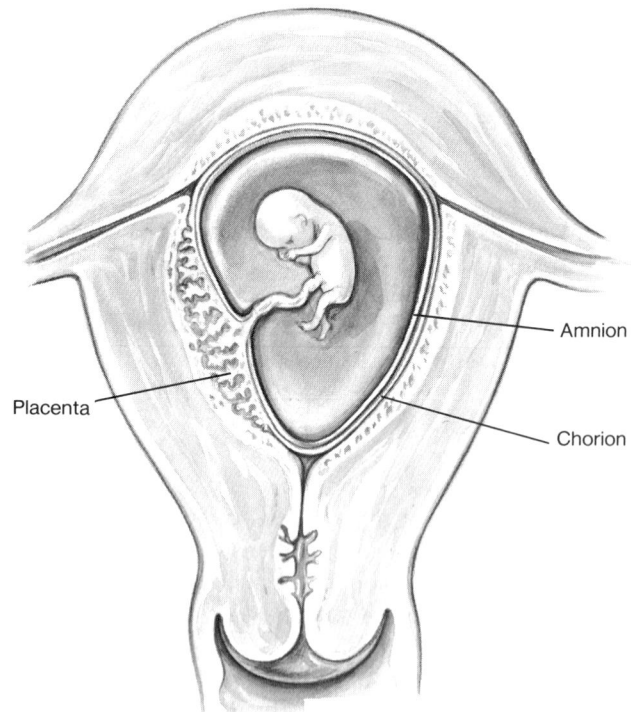

FIGURE 9-4
Membranes, with embryo lying within amniotic sac.

Placenta

Amnion

Chorion

fetus is unable to swallow (esophageal atresia or anencephaly are the two most common reasons), **hydramnios**, or excessive amniotic fluid (more than 2000 mL total or pockets of fluid larger than 8 cm on ultrasound), will result. Early in fetal life, as soon as the fetal kidneys become active, fetal urine adds to the quantity of the amniotic fluid. A disturbance of kidney function may cause **oligohydramnios**, or a reduction in the amount of amniotic fluid (under 300 mL total or no pocket on ultrasound larger than 1 cm) (Smith & Weiner, 1990).

Amniotic fluid is an important protective mechanism for the fetus: (1) it shields against pressure or a blow to the mother's abdomen; (2) it protects the fetus from changes in temperature, because liquid changes temperature more slowly than air; (3) it probably aids muscular development, because it allows the fetus freedom to move; and (4) it protects the umbilical cord from pressure, protecting fetal oxygenation.

Even if the membranes rupture before birth and the bulk of the amniotic fluid is lost, some will always surround the fetus in utero because of the constant new formation of fluid. Amniotic fluid is slightly alkaline with a *p*H of about 7.2. This might be important at the time of rupture in differentiating it from urine, which is acidic (*p*H 5.0 to 5.5). The specific gravity of amniotic fluid is only slightly heavier than that of water—1.005 to 1.025.

Origin and Development of Organ Systems

From the beginning of fetal growth, development proceeds in a **cephalocaudal** (head-to-tail) direction, that is, head development occurs first and is followed by development of the middle and, finally, lower body parts. This pattern of development continues after birth: newborns can lift up their head approximately a year before they can walk.

Primary Germ Layers

At the time of implantation, the blastocyst already has differentiated to a point at which two separate cavities appear in the inner structure: (1) a large one, the **amniotic cavity**, which is lined with a distinctive layer of cells, the **ectoderm** and (2) a smaller cavity, the **yolk sac**, which is lined with **entoderm** cells (see Figure 9-1).

In chicks, the yolk sac serves as a supply of nourishment for the embryo throughout its development. In humans, the yolk sac appears to supply nourishment only until implantation. After that, it provides a source of red blood cells until the embryo's hematopoietic system is mature enough to perform this function (at about the 12th week of intrauterine life). The yolk sac atrophies after the hematopoietic function is complete and remains only as a thin white streak discernible in the cord at birth.

Between the amniotic cavity and the yolk sac forms a third layer of primary cells, the **mesoderm**. The embryo will begin to develop (form an *embryonic shield*) at the point where the three cell layers (ectoderm, entoderm, mesoderm) meet. Each germ layer of primary tissue develops into specific body systems (Table 9-3). It is helpful to know which structures rise from each germ layer because coexisting congenital defects found in newborns usually arise from the same layer. For example, a tracheoesophageal fistula (both organs arising from the entoderm) is a common birth anomaly. Heart and kidney defects (both organs arising from the mesoderm) are also commonly seen together. It is rare, however, to see a newborn with a heart malformation (arises from the mesoderm) and a lower urinary malformation (bladder and urethra arise from the entoderm). One reason rubella infection is always serious in pregnancy is because this virus is capable of affecting all the germ layers and thereby causing congenital anomalies in a myriad of body systems, irrespective of their primary origin.

Knowing the origins of body structures helps you to understand why certain screening procedures are ordered for newborns with congenital malformations. A kidney x-ray examination, for example, may be ordered for a child born with a heart defect. A child with a malformation of the urinary tract is often investigated for reproductive abnormalities as well.

All organ systems are complete, at least in a rudimentary form, at 8 weeks' gestation (the end of the embryonic period). It is during this early time of organogenesis (organ formation) that the growing structure is most vulnerable to invasion by teratogens (any factor that affects the fertilized ovum, embryo, or fetus adversely; see the Focus on Family Teaching box) (Ward, 1992). Figure 9-5 illustrates critical periods of fetal growth. Teratogens are discussed in Chapter 11.

Cardiovascular System

The cardiovascular system is one of the first systems to become functional in intrauterine life. Its development is a progression from simple blood cells joined to the walls of the yolk sac, to a network of blood vessels, to a sin-

Table 9-3. *Origin of Body Tissue*

Tissue Layer	Body Portions Formed
Mesoderm	Supporting structures of the body (connective tissue, bones, cartilage, muscle, and tendons); upper portion of the urinary system (kidneys and ureters); reproductive system; heart; circulatory system; and blood cells
Entoderm	Lining of the gastrointestinal tract, respiratory tract, tonsils, parathyroid, thyroid, thymus glands; and lower urinary system (bladder and urethra)
Ectoderm	The nervous system; skin, hair, and nails; sense organs; and mucous membranes of the anus and mouth

FOCUS ON FAMILY TEACHING

Q. I want to continue to work during pregnancy. How can I guard against fetal teratogens at work?

A. Some preconceptual planning may be necessary to do this. Some sugggestions are:

- Avoid rooms where smokers gather, such as coffee rooms.
- Alcohol is a frequent accompaniment to work lunches or social functions; make sure that non-alcoholic drinks are available.
- Headaches can occur at work from eye strain. Stock some acetaminophen so you won't be tempted to borrow aspirin.
- Ask your employer for a statement on hazardous substances at your work site; discuss your need to avoid these during pregnancy.

gle heart tube that begins to form as early as the 16th day of life and to beat as early as the 24th day. The heart beat is governed by the sinoatrial node and spreads to the ventricles by the atrioventricular node the same as in adults. The septum that divides the heart into chambers develops during the 6th or 7th week, and the heart valves begin to develop in the 7th week. With a Doppler system, the heart beat may be heard by an examiner as early as the 10th to 12th week of pregnancy. An electrocardiogram (ECG) may be recorded on a fetus as early as the 11th week, although the accuracy of such ECGs is in doubt until about the 20th week of pregnancy when neuro conduction is more regulated.

The heart rate of a fetus is affected by fetal oxygen level, body activity, and circulating blood volume just as in adult life. After the 28th week of pregnancy, when the sympathetic nervous system has matured, the heart rate will begin to show a baseline variability of about 5 beats per minute on a fetal heart rate rhythm strip.

Fetal Circulation. As early as the 3rd week of intrauterine life, fetal blood has begun to exchange nutrients with the maternal circulation across the chorionic villi. Fetal circulation (Figure 9-6) differs from extrauterine circulation in several respects. During intrauterine life, the fetus derives its oxygen and excretes carbon dioxide not from oxygen exchange in the lungs but from the placenta. Blood does enter lung vessels while the child is in utero, but this blood flow is to supply the cells of the lungs themselves, not for oxygen exchange.

Blood arriving at the fetus from the placenta (blood

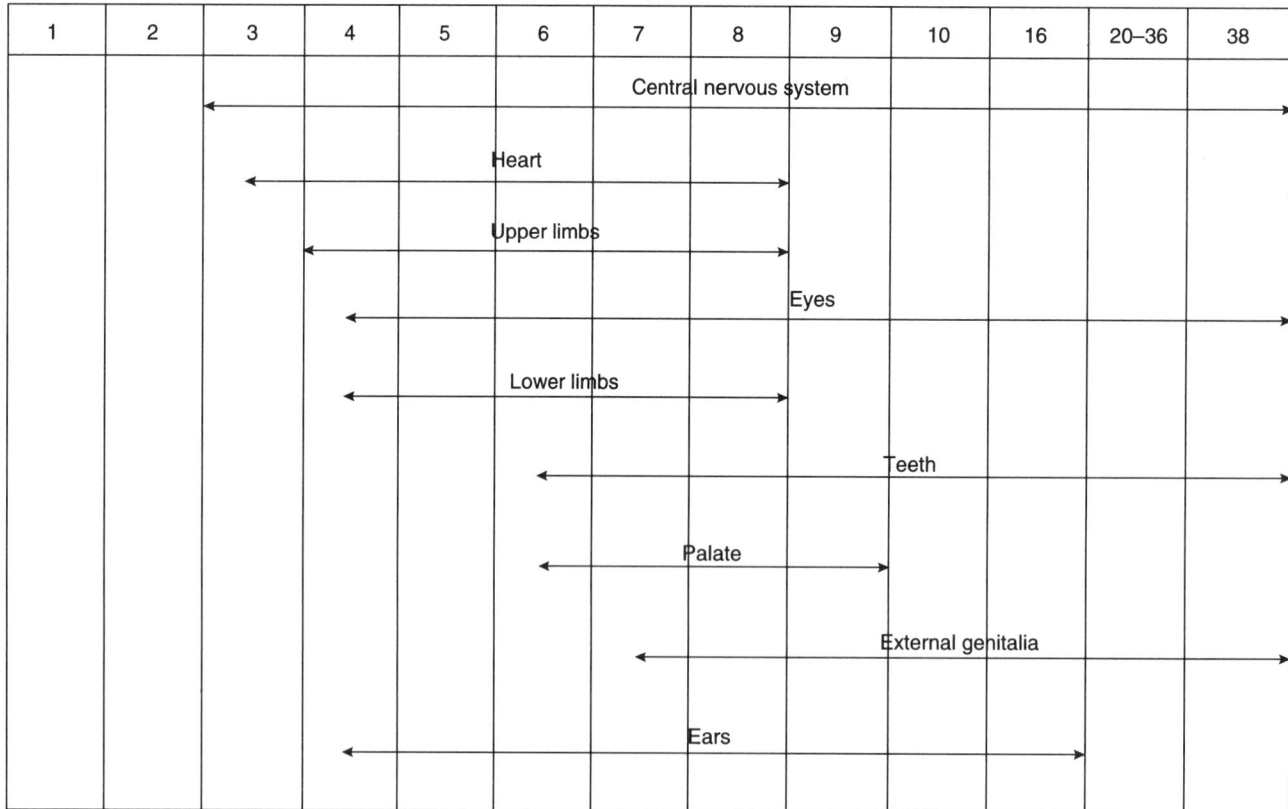

FIGURE 9-5
Critical periods of fetal growth.

with a high oxygen content) enters the fetus through the umbilical vein (called a vein even though it carries oxygenated blood, because the direction of the blood is toward the fetal heart) and into an accessory vein, the **ductus venosus**. The ductus venosus supplies blood to the fetal liver and then empties into the inferior vena cava, through which blood flows to the right side of the heart. As the blood enters the right atrium, the bulk of it is shunted into the left atrium through an opening in the atrial septum, the **foramen ovale**. From the left atrium it follows the course of normal circulation into the left ventricle and into the aorta.

Blood returning from the superior vena cava enters the right atrium and leaves it by the normal circulatory route, that is, through the tricuspid valve into the right ventricle. This blood leaves the right ventricle through the pulmonary artery in the normal manner. A small portion of this blood flow services the lung tissue; the larger portion is shunted away from the lungs, through an additional vessel, the **ductus arteriosus**, directly into the aorta.

Two umbilical arteries (called arteries because they carry blood away from the fetal heart, even though they are now transporting unoxygenated blood) transport most of the blood flow from the descending aorta back through the umbilical cord to the placental villi, where new oxygen exchange takes place.

The shunts of fetal circulation are necessary to supply the most important organs of the fetus: the brain, liver, heart, and kidneys. The ductus venosus supplies the liver, and the foramen ovale allows oxygenated blood to move directly to the left side of the heart and

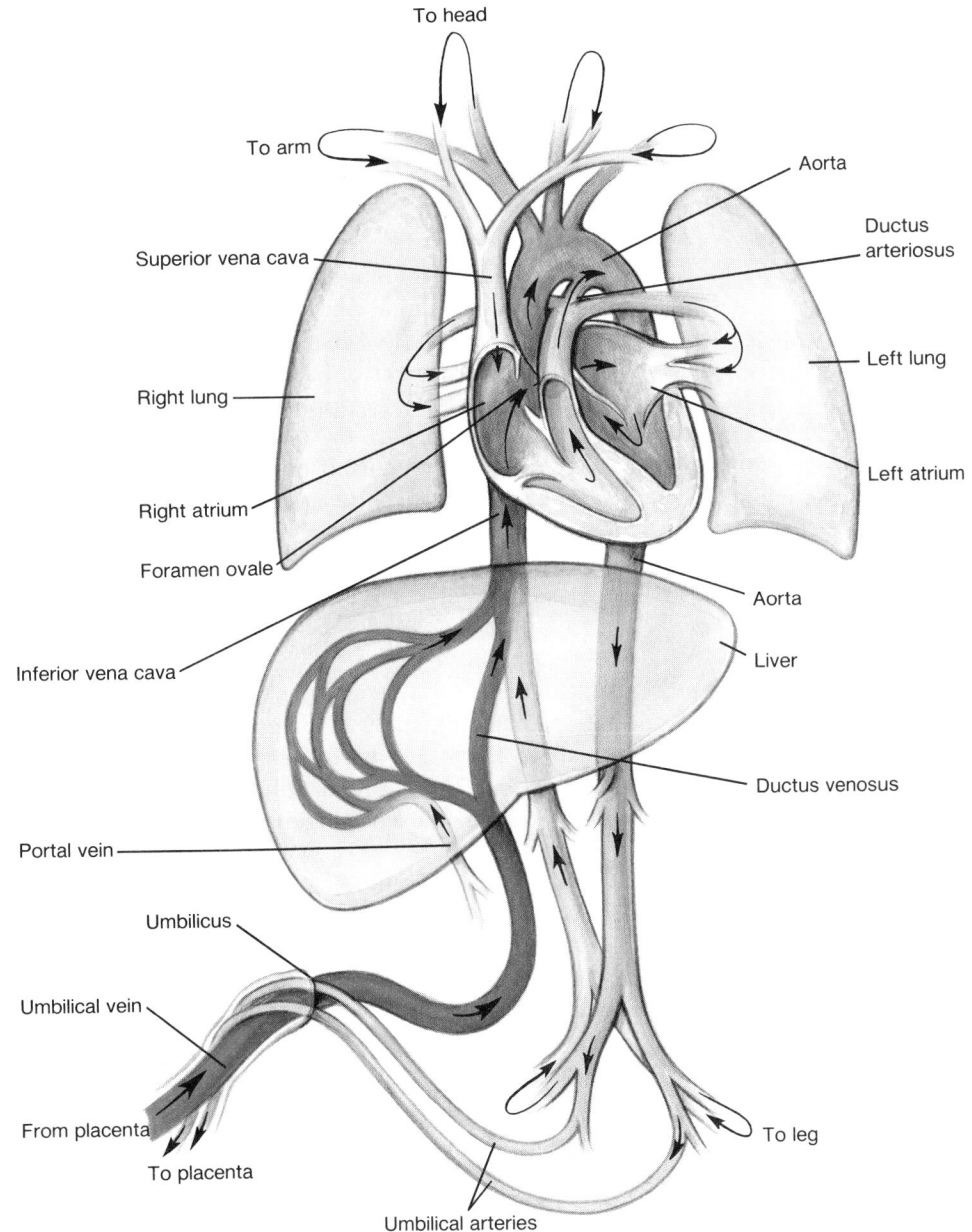

FIGURE 9-6
Fetal circulation.

the aorta, the vessel from which the arteries arise that supply the brain, heart, and kidneys.

The fetus exists at a blood oxygen saturation level of about 80% of the newborn's saturation level. The rapid rate of the fetal heart beat during pregnancy (120 to 160 beats per minute) is necessary to supply oxygen to cells when red blood cells are never fully saturated. Fortunately, a fetus has a high hemoglobin concentration (about 50% greater than the mother). In addition, fetal hemoglobin has a greater affinity for oxygen (about 20% to 30% higher) and a higher disassociation level than adult hemoglobin so that the movement and release of oxygen are facilitated. Despite a low blood oxygen saturation level, carbon dioxide does not accumulate in the fetal system because of rapid diffusion into maternal blood across a favorable placental pressure gradient.

Fetal Hemoglobin. Fetal hemoglobin differs from adult hemoglobin in several ways. It has a different composition (two alpha and two gamma chains as compared with two alpha and two beta chains of adult hemoglobin). As mentioned above, it has a greater oxygen affinity, which means it is more efficient. It is more concentrated (at birth, a newborn's hemoglobin level is about 17.1 g/100 mL compared with an adult's normal level of 11 g/100 mL; a newborn's hematocrit is about 53% compared with an adult's normal level of 45%). These same changes occur in people who live at high altitudes, where the atmosphere has a reduced oxygen content. The change from fetal to adult hemoglobin levels begins before birth and accelerates following birth. The major blood dyscrasias, such as sickle cell anemia, are defects of the beta hemoglobin chain, so clinical symptoms do not become apparent until the bulk of fetal hemoglobin has matured to adult hemoglobin composition at about 6 months of age.

Respiratory System

At the 3rd week of life, the respiratory and digestive tracts exist as a single tube. Like all body tubes this is at first a solid structure which then canalizes (hollows out). By the end of the 4th week, a septum begins to divide the esophagus from the trachea. At the same time, lung buds appear on the trachea.

Until the 7th week of life the diaphragm does not completely divide the thoracic cavity from the abdomen. During the 6th week of life, lung buds may extend down into the abdomen, reentering the chest only as the chest's longitudinal dimension increases and the diaphragm becomes complete (at the end of the 7th week). If the diaphragm fails to close completely, the stomach, spleen, liver, or intestines may enter the thoracic cavity. The child then will be born with a diaphragmatic hernia, compromising the lungs and perhaps displacing the heart.

Alveoli and capillaries begin to form between the 24th and 28th weeks. Both capillary and alveoli development must be complete before gas exchange can occur in the fetal lungs. This is why 24 weeks is a practical lower limit of prematurity or the earliest gestation age at which a fetus can survive in an air-filled extrauterine environment.

As early as during the first 3 months of pregnancy, the fetus begins to make spontaneous respiratory movements. These movements continue throughout pregnancy and can be demonstrated on sonogram. Although babies are born with fluid in their lungs, it is not amniotic fluid but a specific lung fluid that has a low surface tension and low viscosity and is capable of being rapidly absorbed after birth. The presence of this fluid aids in the expansion of the alveoli at birth.

At about the 24th week of pregnancy, alveolar cells begin to excrete **surfactant**, a phospholipid substance that decreases alveolar surface tension on expiration. This prevents alveoli from collapsing on expiration and so greatly adds to the infant's ability to maintain respirations in the outside environment. Surfactant has two components: *lecithin* and *sphingomyelin*. Early in the formation of surfactant, sphingomyelin is the chief component; at about 35 weeks, there is a surge in the production of lecithin, and this then becomes the chief component by a ratio of 2:1. As surfactant is mixed with amniotic fluid due to lung movements, it becomes present in amniotic fluid. Analysis of the lecithin/sphingomyelin (L/S) ratio by an amniocentesis technique is one of the primary tests of fetal maturity. Lack of surfactant is a factor in the development of respiratory distress syndrome (see Chapter 26). Any interference with the blood supply to the fetus as might occur with placental insufficiency from hypertension appears to hurry lung development. This type of stress probably increases steroid levels in the fetus; increased steroid levels are associated with alveoli maturation.

Nervous System

Like the circulatory system, the nervous system begins to develop extremely early in pregnancy. During the 3rd and 4th weeks of life, when the woman may not even realize yet that she is pregnant, active formation of the nervous system and sense organs has already begun.

By the 3rd week of gestation, a **neural plate** (a thickened portion of the ectoderm) is apparent in the developing embryo. The top portion of the neural plate differentiates into the neural tube, which will form the central nervous system (brain and spinal cord), and the neural crest, which will develop into the peripheral nervous system. Brain waves can be detected on electroencephalogram by the 8th week.

Although all parts of the brain (cerebrum, cerebellum, pons, and medulla oblongata) form in utero, the brain is not mature at birth. It continues rapid growth during the 1st year; growth continues at high levels until

5 or 6 years of age. Thus, the newborn infant still has many findings of neurologic immaturity, such as a positive Babinski sign (toes flare on stroking of the bottom of the foot).

The eye and inner ear both develop as projections of the original neural tube. The ear is so developed by 24 weeks that the fetus can respond to sound. The neurologic system seems particularly prone to insult during the early weeks of the embryonic period. All during pregnancy and at birth, the system is vulnerable to damage from anoxia.

Endocrine System

As soon as endocrine organs mature in intrauterine life, function begins. The fetal adrenal glands play a direct role in placental estrogen production, as they supply a precursor of estrogen synthesis. (One theory of why labor begins is that the uterus senses from estrogen production that the fetus is mature and ready to be born.) The fetal pancreas produces the insulin needed by the fetus. (Insulin is one of the few known compounds that does not cross the placenta from the mother to the fetus.) The thyroid and parathyroid glands play vital roles in metabolic function and calcium balance.

Digestive System

Once the digestive tract is separated from the respiratory tract (at about the 4th week), the intestinal tract grows extremely rapidly. At first, tubes are solid; they canalize to become hollow. Later, the endothelial cells of the gastrointestinal tract proliferate so extensively that the lumen is once more closed. Atresia or stenosis can develop if either the first or second canalization does not occur. The proliferation of cells which are shed in the second recanalization forms the basis for meconium (see below).

During the 6th week of intrauterine life, the abdomen becomes too small to contain the intestine, and a portion of the intestine, guided by the vitelline membrane, a part of the yolk sac, enters the base of the umbilical cord. Intestine remains in the base of the cord until about the 10th week, a time when the fetal trunk has extended and enlarged the abdominal cavity so much it can finally accommodate all the intestinal mass. As the intestine returns to the abdominal cavity, it must make a rotation of 180 degrees. Failure to do so can result in inadequate mesentery attachments which can lead to volvulus of the intestine. If any intestinal coils remain outside the abdomen, in the base of the cord, a congenital anomaly, *omphalocele*, develops. A similar defect, gastroschisis, occurs when the original midline fusion is incomplete.

If the vitelline duct does not atrophy following return of the intestines, a Meckel's diverticulum (a pouch of intestinal tissue) or an opening between the intestine and the umbilicus can result. *Meconium* forms in the intestines as early as the 16th week. It consists of cellular wastes, bile, fats, mucoproteins, mucopolysaccharides, and portions of the vernix caseosa, the lubricating substance that forms on the fetal skin. Meconium is black or dark green and it is sticky in texture. It derives its dark color from bile pigments.

The gastrointestinal tract is sterile before birth. Because vitamin K is synthesized by the action of bacteria in the intestines, vitamin K levels may be low in the newborn infant.

Sucking and swallowing reflexes are not mature until the fetus is about 32 weeks or weighs 1500 g. That this function, so necessary for survival outside the uterus, develops so late in pregnancy has implications for nursing care of the fetus born before this time.

Ability of the gastrointestinal tract to secrete enzymes essential to carbohydrate and protein digestion is mature at 36 weeks. *Amylase,* an enzyme found in saliva and necessary for digestion of complex starches, is not mature until 3 months after birth. Many newborns have not yet developed *lipase,* an enzyme needed for fat digestion. This fact also has implications for newborn nutrition (see Chapter 24).

The liver is active throughout gestation, functioning as a screen between the incoming blood and the fetal circulation and a deposit for fetal stores such as iron and glycogen. It is still immature at birth, however. Two of the most serious problems of infants in the first 24 hours after birth are hypoglycemia and hyperbilirubinemia, both related to immature liver function.

Musculoskeletal System

The fetus can be seen to move on ultrasound as early as the 11th week, although the mother usually does not feel this movement (**quickening**) until nearly 20 weeks. In the first 2 weeks of fetal life, cartilage prototypes provide position and support. Ossification of bone tissue begins about the 12th week. The ossification process continues all through fetal life and actually until adulthood. Carpals, tarsals, and sternal bones generally do not ossify until birth is imminent.

Reproductive System

Whether the child will be male or female is determined at the moment of conception by a spermatozoon carrying an X or a Y chromosome. At about the 6th week of life, the gonads (ovaries or testes) form. If testes form, testosterone secretion from them apparently influences the sexually neutral genital duct to form other male organs (maturity of the wolffian, or mesonephric, duct). In the absence of testosterone secretion, female organs will form (maturation of the müllerian, or paramesonephric, duct). This is an important phenomenon, because if the mother should be prescribed an androgen or an androgen-like substance during this stage of pregnancy, the child, although chromosomally female, would appear more male than female at birth because clitoral growth would be stimulated. If deficient testosterone is secreted by the testes, both the müllerian (female) duct and the male (wolffian) duct could develop (pseudohermaphroditism).

Masculinization in female infants also may occur with adrenogenital syndrome, a genetic disease in which there is deficient cortisol production and excess androgen production by the adrenal gland. These female infants are born with a clitoris that resembles a penis, and if close inspection is not carried out at birth, they may be assumed to be males with cryptorchidism (undescended testes). Males with this syndrome are born with abnormally enlarged genitalia.

Testes in a normal male tend to descend from the pelvic cavity, where they first form into the scrotal sac late in intrauterine life, at the 34th to 38th week. Thus, many male low-birth-weight infants are born with undescended testes. These children should be followed closely to see that the testes descend when the child reaches what would have been the 34th to 38th week of gestational age, because testicular descent does not occur as readily in extrauterine life as it would in utero. The gender of a fetus can be determined by chromosome analysis of the chorionic villi as early as 8 weeks of the pregnancy; it can be detected by sonogram late in pregnancy if the penis is evident on the screen. Most women have a preference for gender although they may not voice this (see the Focus on Nursing Research box in Chapter 8).

Urinary System

Although rudimentary kidneys are present as early as the end of the 4th week, they do not appear to be essential for life before birth. Urine is formed by the 12th week and is excreted into the amniotic fluid by the 16th week of gestation. At term, fetal urine is being excreted at the rate of 500 mL/day. An amount of amniotic fluid that is less than normal (oligohydramnios) suggests that fetal kidneys are not secreting adequate urine. The complex structure of the kidneys is gradually developed during pregnancy and for months afterward. The loop of Henle, for example, is not fully differentiated until the child is born. Glomerular filtration and concentration of urine in the newborn are not efficient because the kidneys are not fully mature at birth.

Early in the embryonic stage of urinary system development, the bladder extends to the umbilical region. On rare occasions, an open lumen between the urinary bladder and the umbilicus fails to close. This is a *patent urachus* and is discovered at birth by the persistent drainage of a clear, acid-*p*H fluid (urine) from the umbilicus.

Integumentary System

The skin of a fetus appears thin and almost translucent until subcutaneous fat begins to be deposited at about 36 weeks. Skin is covered by soft downy hairs (lanugo) and a cream-cheese-like substance, vernix caseosa, that is important for lubrication and keeping skin from macerating.

Immune System

Maternal antibodies of the IgG class of immunoglobulins cross the placenta into the fetus primarily during the third trimester of pregnancy. These will give a fetus temporary passive immunity against diseases for which the mother has antibodies, which often include poliomyelitis, rubella (German measles), rubeola (regular measles), diphtheria, tetanus, infectious parotitis (mumps), and pertussis (whooping cough). Little or no immunity to varicella (chicken pox) or the herpes virus (the virus of cold sores and genital herpes) is transferred to the fetus; thus, the average newborn is potentially susceptible to these diseases.

The level of passive IgG immunoglobulins peaks at birth and then decreases over the next 9 months while infants begin to build up their own stores of IgG as well as IgA and IgM. Because the passive immunity received by the newborn has already declined substantially by about 2 months, immunization against diphtheria, tetanus, pertussis, and poliomyelitis is typically begun at this age. Passive antibodies to measles have been demonstrated to last over a year; consequently, the immunization for measles is not given until 15 months' extrauterine age.

It has been shown that a fetus is capable of active antibody production late in a pregnancy. The fetus is generally not called on to use this ability, however, because antibodies are manufactured only when stimulated by an invading antigen, and antigens rarely invade the intrauterine space. This is possible, though, because babies whose mothers had an infection such as rubella during pregnancy typically have IgM antibodies to rubella in their blood serum at birth. IgA and IgM antibodies cannot cross the placenta (IgG does, however), so their presence in a newborn is proof that the fetus has been challenged by disease invasion and has produced active antibodies.

Milestones of Fetal Growth and Development

During pregnancy, couples ask many questions about their baby's appearance and age. To answer these questions effectively and to plan care that safeguards the growth of the new child, it is helpful to be able to describe the developmental milestones by weeks of intrauterine life.

This can be confusing because the life of the fetus is generally measured from the time of ovulation or fertilization (ovulation age), but the length of the pregnancy is generally measured from the first day of the last menstrual period (gestation age). Because ovulation and fertilization take place about 2 weeks after the last menstrual period, the ovulation age of the fetus is always 2 weeks less than the length of the pregnancy or the gestation age. The relationship of ovulation age to gestation age is shown in Figure 9-7.

Both ovulation and gestation age are also sometimes measured in lunar months (4-week periods) or in trimesters (3-month periods) rather than in weeks. In lunar months, a pregnancy is 10 months (or 40 weeks) long; a fetus grows in utero 9½ lunar months or three full trimesters (38 weeks).

The following discussion of fetal developmental milestones is based on gestation weeks (Figure 9-7) because it is helpful when talking to expectant parents to be able to correlate fetal development to the way they measure pregnancy: from the first day of the last menstrual period. Figures 9-8 and 9-9 illustrate the comparative size and appearance of human embryos and fetuses at different stages.

End of 4 Gestation Weeks

At the end of the 4th week of gestation, the human embryo is a rapidly growing formation of cells but does not resemble a human being as yet. The spinal cord has formed and fused at the midpoint. Lateral wings have

folded forward to fuse at the midline. Shortly, the head will fold forward and become prominent, comprising about one-third of the entire structure. The back is bent so that the head almost touches the tip of the tail (yes, a human embryo does have a tail at this point). The heart (still rudimentary) appears as a prominent bulge on the anterior surface. The arms and legs are bud-like structures. Rudimentary eyes, ears, and nose are discernible. Length is 0.75 cm to 1 cm. Weight is 400 mg.

End of 8 Gestation Weeks

Length is 2.5 cm (1 in). Weight is 20 g. Organogenesis is complete. The heart has a septum and valves and is beating rhythmically. The facial features are definitely discernible. Legs, arms, fingers, toes, elbows, and knees have developed. Although the external genitalia are present, male and female are not distinguishable by simple observation. The primitive tail is undergoing retrogression. The abdomen appears large as the fetal intestine is growing rapidly. A sonogram taken at this time demonstrates a gestational sac and is diagnostic of pregnancy (Figure 9-10).

End of 12 Gestation Weeks (First Trimester)

Length is 7 to 9 cm. Weight is 45 g. Nail beds are forming on fingers and toes. The fetus is capable of sponta-

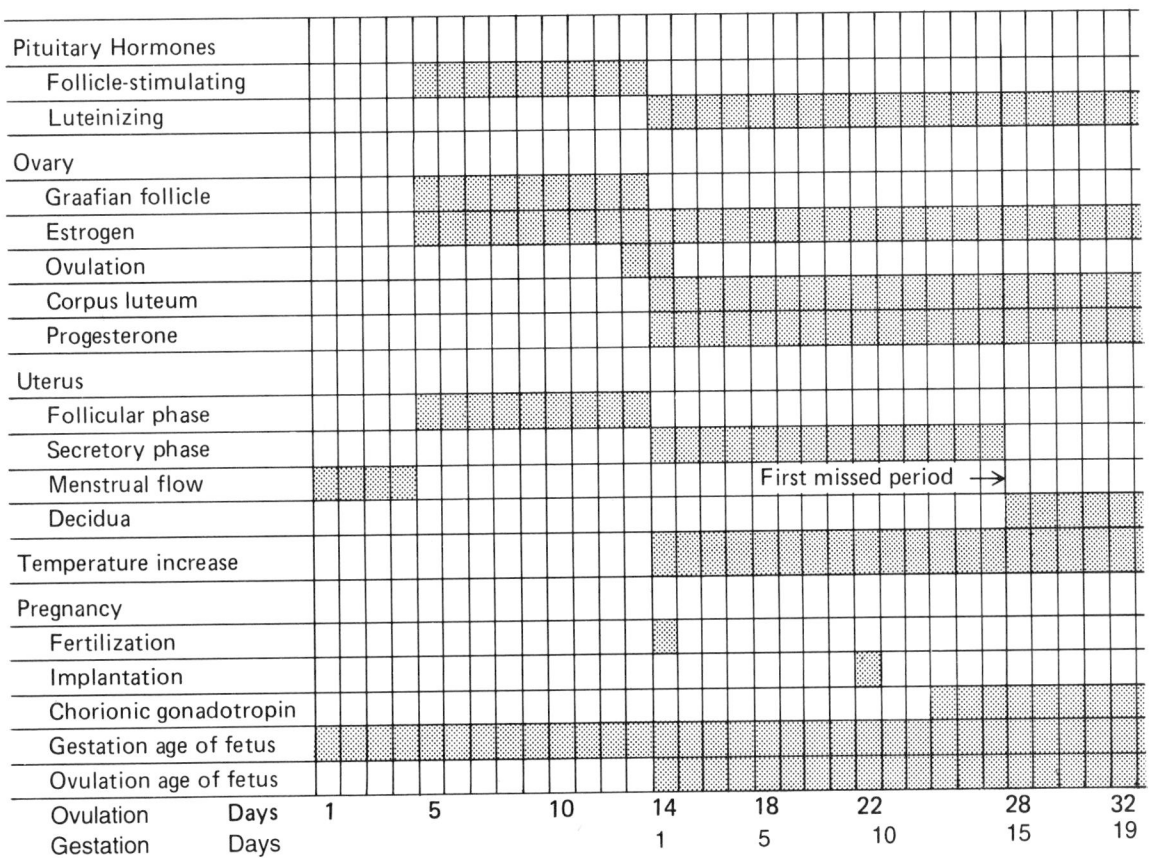

FIGURE 9-7
Ovulation age and timing of pituitary, ovarian, and uterine functions as they affect gestation age.

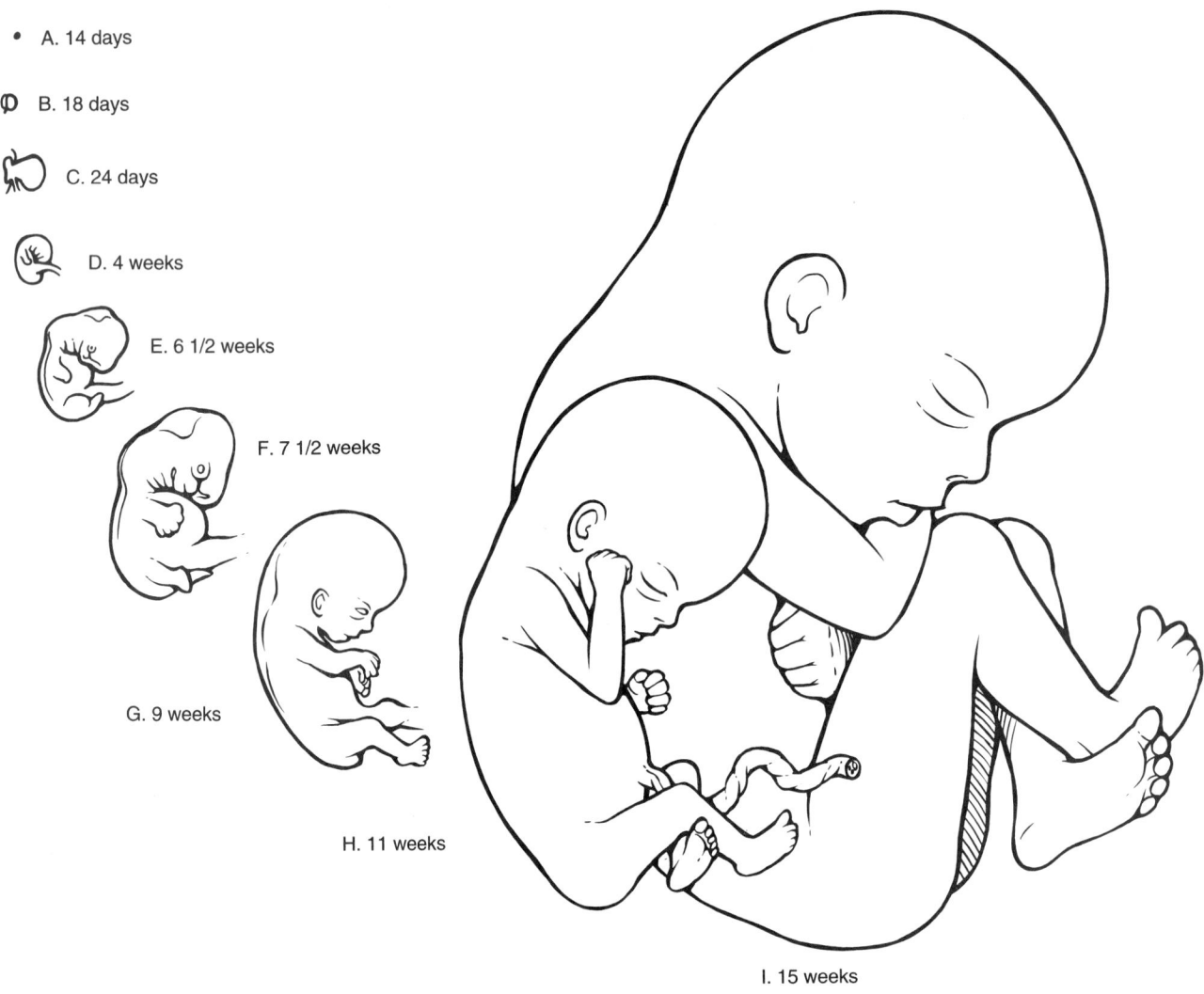

- A. 14 days
- B. 18 days
- C. 24 days
- D. 4 weeks
- E. 6 1/2 weeks
- F. 7 1/2 weeks
- G. 9 weeks
- H. 11 weeks
- I. 15 weeks

FIGURE 9-8
Comparative sizes of the human embryo at nine different ages. (Arey, L. [1965]. Developmental anatomy *[7th ed.]. Philadelphia: W.B. Saunders, with permission.)*

neous movements, although they are usually too faint to be felt by the mother. Some reflexes are present, notably the Babinski reflex. Ossification centers are forming in bones, and tooth buds are present. Male and female fetuses are distinguishable by outward appearance. Kidney secretion has begun, although urine may not yet be evident in amniotic fluid. The heart beat is audible by a

Doppler instrument, allowing the mother and father to hear the beat.

End of 16 Gestation Weeks

Length is 10 to 17 cm. Weight is 55 to 120 g. It may be possible to hear fetal heart sounds through an ordinary stethoscope. The formation of *lanugo* (the fine, downy

FIGURE 9-9
*Human embryos at different stages of development. (**A**) Surface view of a human implantation on the uterus 7 to 8 days after conception. The openings of the uterine glands of the epithelium appear as dark spots surrounded by light circles. (**B**) Embryo at 32 days. Notice the primitive tail. The heart fills a large portion of the upper torso. (**C**) Embryo at 37 days. The abdominal contents are beginning to grow rapidly. (**D**) Embryo at 41 days. Arms and legs are becoming clearly defined. The tail is regressing. (**E**) Embryo at 48 days. Fingers and toes are formed. The bulk of fetal intestine is protruded into the umbilical cord. (**F**) Embryo at 48 days, surrounded by amniotic membrane and fluid, the opened chorion, and the projecting chorionic villi. (**G**) Embryo at 57 days (8 weeks). Organogenesis is complete. (Courtesy of the Department of Embryology, Davis Division, Carnegie Institution of Washington, D.C.)*

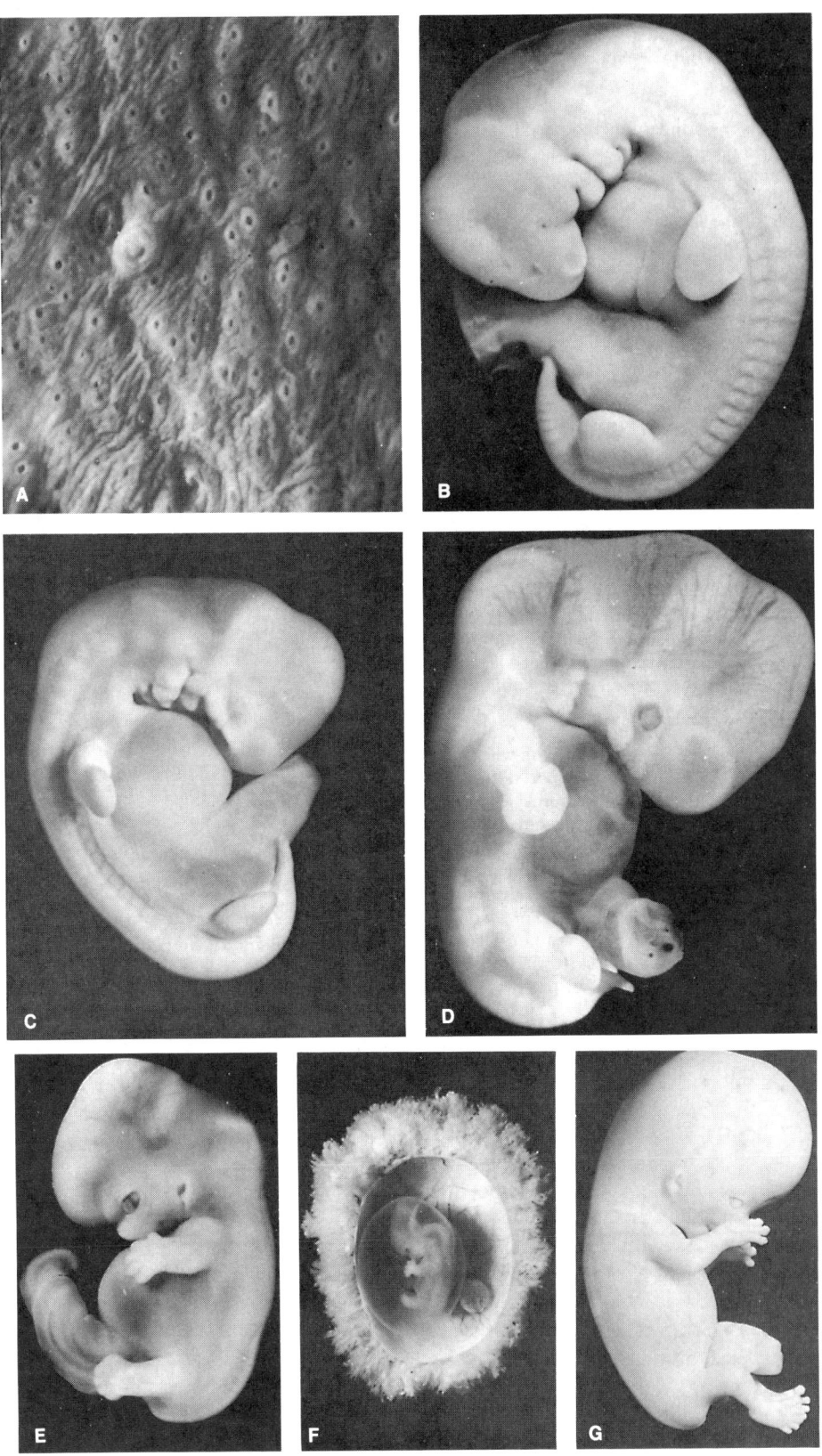

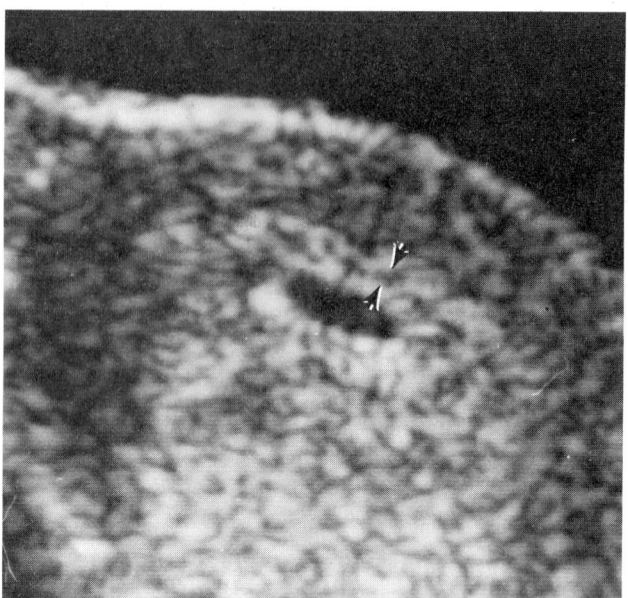

FIGURE 9-10
Sonogram showing the characteristic circle diagnostic of pregnancy (the gestational sac). (Benson, C. B., et al. [1988]. Atlas of obstetrical ultrasound. Philadelphia: J.B. Lippincott, with permission.)

hair on the back and arms of newborns, apparently serving as a source of insulation for body heat) is well formed. The liver and pancreas are functioning. At this time, the fetus actively swallows amniotic fluid, demonstrating an intact swallowing reflex.

End of 20 Gestation Weeks

Length is 25 cm. Weight is 223 g. The spontaneous movements of the fetus have become strong enough for the mother to feel. The sensation is like the fluttering of wings or fluid moving rapidly through the bowels. This event is termed *quickening*. It is a major milestone in pregnancy. For many women it is the first time the pregnancy seems real to them. It is such an exciting event in a first pregnancy that most mothers can remember for the rest of their lives not only at what month in pregnancy quickening occurred but exactly where they were when it happened.

A 20-week-old fetus is capable of antibody production. Hair formation extends to include eyebrows and hair on the head. Meconium is present in the upper intestine. Brown fat, a special fat that will aid in temperature regulation at birth, begins to be formed behind the kidneys, sternum, and posterior neck. The fetal heart beat is strong enough to be heard readily through the abdomen with an ordinary stethoscope. Definite sleeping and activity patterns are distinguishable; at this point in pregnancy, the fetus has developed biorhythms that will guide sleep/wake patterns throughout life.

End of 24 Gestation Weeks (Second Trimester)

Length is 28 to 36 cm. Weight is 550 g. Passive antibody transfer from mother to fetus probably begins as early as the 20th week of gestation, certainly by the 24th week of gestation. Infants born before antibody transfer has taken place have no natural immunity and need more than the usual protection against infectious disease in the newborn period until the infant's own store of immunoglobulins can build up.

Vernix caseosa, a cream cheese–like substance produced by the sebaceous glands that serves as a protective skin covering during intrauterine life, begins to form following the 20th week. Meconium is present as far as the rectum. Active production of lung surfactant begins, and features as detailed as eyebrows and eyelashes are well defined. The eyelids of the fetus have been fused since the 12th week. Now the membrane that had fused them dissolves, the eyes can open, and the pupils are capable of reacting to light.

When fetuses reach 24 weeks, or 601 g, they have achieved a practical low-end age of viability if they are cared for after birth in a modern intensive care facility.

End of 28 Gestation Weeks

Length is 35 to 38 cm. Weight is 1200 g. The lung alveoli begin to mature, and surfactant can be demonstrated in amniotic fluid. In the male fetus, the testes begin to descend into the scrotal sac from the lower abdominal cavity.

The blood vessels of the retina are extremely susceptible to damage from high oxygen concentrations (an important consideration when caring for low-birth-weight infants who need oxygen).

End of 32 Gestation Weeks

Length is 38 to 43 cm. Weight is 1600 g. Subcutaneous fat begins to be deposited in the fetus during this month, and the former stringy, "little-old-man" appearance is lost. The fetus is aware of sounds outside the mother's body, has an active Moro reflex, and in some cases, has already assumed delivery position (vertex or breech). Iron stores to provide iron for the time during which he or she will ingest only milk following birth begin to be laid. Fingernails grow to reach the end of fingertips.

End of 36 Gestation Weeks

Length is 42 to 49 cm. Weight is 1900 to 2700 g (5 to 6 lb). In the last 2 months of intrauterine life, body stores of glycogen, iron, carbohydrate, and calcium are augmented and additional amounts of subcutaneous fat are deposited. At this time, the sole of the foot has only one or two crisscross creases compared with the full crisscross pattern that will be evident at term. The amount of lanugo present begins to diminish.

Many babies turn in utero into a vertex or head-down presentation during this month.

End of 40 Gestation Weeks (Third Trimester)

Length, crown to heel, is 48 to 52 cm. Weight is 3000 g (7 to 7½ lb).

The fetus kicks actively during these weeks, hard enough to cause the mother considerable discomfort. Fetal hemoglobin begins its conversion to adult hemoglobin. The conversion is so rapid that, at birth, about 20% of hemoglobin will be adult in character.

Vernix caseosa is fully formed. Fingernails extend over the tips of fingers. Creases on the soles of the feet cover at least two-thirds of their surface.

In primiparas (women having their first babies), the fetus often sinks into the birth canal during these last 2 weeks, giving the mother a feeling that her load is being lightened. This event is termed **lightening**. It is a fetal announcement that the third trimester of pregnancy has ended and birth is at hand.

Determination of Estimated Birth Date

It is impossible to predict the day of birth of a child with a high degree of accuracy. Traditionally, this date has been referred to as the EDC, for expected date of confinement. As women are no longer confined following childbirth, EDB **(expected date of birth)** or EDD (expected date of delivery) are more commonly used today.

As mentioned, the average length of a pregnancy from ovulation is 9½ lunar months, or 38 weeks, or 266 days; from the last menstrual period, a pregnancy is 10 lunar months, or 40 weeks, or 280 days. In fact, however, fewer than 5% of pregnancies end exactly 280 days from the last menstrual period; fewer than half end within 1 week of the 280th day (Zlatnik, 1990). Nagele's Rule, the standard method used to predict the length of a pregnancy, is shown in Box 9-1.

If fertilization occurs early in a menstrual cycle, the pregnancy will probably end "early"; if ovulation and fertilization occur later in the cycle, the pregnancy will

---

Box 9-1
Nagele's Rule

To calculate the date of birth by this rule, count backward 3 calender months from the first day of the last menstrual period and add 7 days. For example, if the last menstrual period began May 15, you would count back 3 months (April 15, March 15, February 15) and add 7 days, to arrive at a date of birth of February 22.

---

end "late." Because of these normal variations, a pregnancy ending 2 weeks before or 2 weeks after the calculated date of birth is considered well within the normal limit (a pregnancy of 38 to 42 weeks in length).

Assessment of Fetal Growth and Development

Much information about the size and health of the unborn child can be gathered through a variety of assessment techniques (see the Nursing Care Plan). Nursing responsibility for these assessment procedures includes seeing that consent is obtained as needed; scheduling the procedure; explaining the procedure to the woman and her support person; preparing the woman physically and psychologically; providing support during the procedure; assessing both fetal and maternal responses to it; and providing after care to the woman, equipment, and specimens.

Additional consent to perform a procedure must be obtained if the procedure carries any risk that would not be present if it were not performed. For a woman to sign a consent form, she must be informed what the procedure consists of and what risk (to herself and/or the fetus) is present by having or not having the procedure performed.

Estimating Fetal Growth

McDonald's rule is a method of determining that the fetus is growing in utero by measuring fundal (uterine) height. The rule is the fundus to symphysis distance in cms is equal to the week of gestation between the 20th to 31st weeks of pregnancy (Kochenour, 1990). The measurement is made from the notch of the woman's symphysis pubis to over the top of the uterine fundus as the woman lies supine (Figure 9-11) (Engstrom & Sittler, 1993). McDonald's rule becomes inaccurate during the third trimester of pregnancy as the fetus is growing more in weight than height during this time. Until then, a fundal height much greater than this standard suggests multiple pregnancy, miscalculated due date, a large-for-gestation-age infant, hydramnios (increased amniotic fluid volume), or hydatidiform mole (see Chapter 15). A fundal measurement much less than this suggests that either the fetus is failing to thrive (small for gestational age), the pregnancy length is miscalculated, or an anomaly, such as anencephaly, is developing (see the Focus on Nursing Research box for problems in measurement).

Recording that the fundus reaches typical milestone measurements, such as over the symphysis pubis at 12 weeks, at the umbilicus at 20 weeks, and at the xyphoid process at 36 weeks, is also a helpful determination.

Nursing Care Plan

A Growing Fetus

Mary Colton is an 18-year-old client you care for at a prenatal clinic. The following is the part of her nursing care plan designed to help her safeguard fetal growth and development.

Assessment: Client states that she feels ugly since becoming pregnant; asks if she should quit school. Unsure of date of last menstrual period (about 16 weeks ago). Is worried that she might have hurt fetus because she is a member of high school swimming team and had two "wrong dives" from high board, hitting abdomen hard against water in last 2 weeks. Client smokes "occasionally"; drinks beer "sometimes on Saturday night." No intravenous drug use or cocaine. Was evasive about use of marijuana. Nutrition: eats two meals at home daily, one at school. States, "My Mom is a good cook. I eat okay." Uterine height 4 cm above symphysis. Fetal heart tones by Doppler at 150.

Nursing Diagnosis: Health-seeking behaviors concerning fetal growth and development related to first pregnancy experience and young age.

Defining Characteristic: Client states she is interested in protecting the fetus throughout remainder of pregnancy.

Goal: Client will describe and demonstrate behaviors that safeguard fetal health for pregnancy duration.

Outcome Criteria: Client takes actions, such as discontinuing alcohol and cigarette smoking, and keeps sports activities to sensible level for duration of pregnancy.

Nursing Orders	Rationale
1. Schedule for sonogram per nurse-midwife.	1. Establishes pregnancy length (last menstrual period not known).
2. Educate about importance of discontinuing drug and alcohol use during pregnancy.	2. Drug and alcohol use can be teratogenic to fetal growth.
3. Caution client to discontinue high school diving; to telephone clinic for advice if in doubt about what is appropriate sports activity during pregnancy.	3. Severe blow to abdomen could cause rupture of membranes and loss of amniotic fluid.

Nursing Diagnosis: Body image disturbance related to change in appearance from pregnancy.

Defining Characteristic: Client states she feels "ugly."

Goal: Client will voice improved body image by next prenatal visit.

Outcome Criteria: Client uses positive terms to describe self rather than a term such as "ugly"; speaks of growing fetus in positive terms.

Nursing Orders	Rationale
1. Discuss with client the body changes she can expect to occur with pregnancy and the stage of fetal growth.	1. Knowledge of change tends to make it easier to accept; acceptance can help with mother-child bonding.
2. Discuss with client activities she can continue during pregnancy to ensure contact with friends.	2. Help client to view pregnancy as a positive time in her life.
3. Encourage client to remain in school.	3. Help her to feel a sense of self worth from her accomplishment.

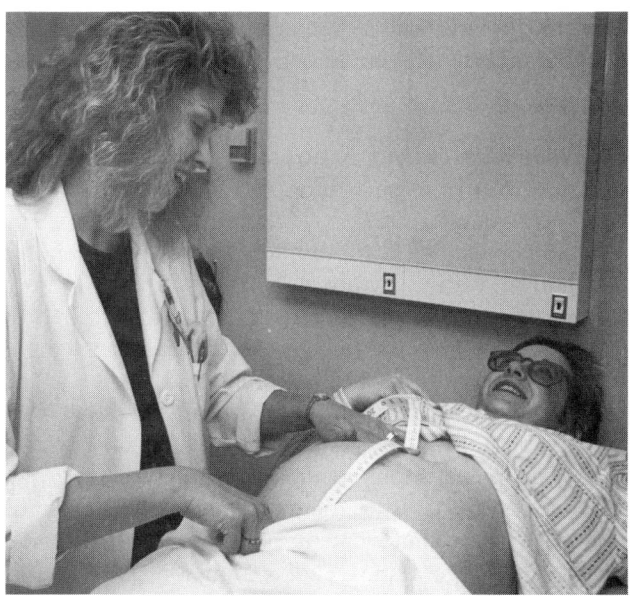

FIGURE 9-11
Measuring fundal height from the superior aspect of the pubis to the fundal crest. (Courtesy of the Department of Medical Photography, Children's Hospital, Buffalo, NY.)

Assessing Fetal Well Being

Fetal Movement

Fetal movement that can be felt by the mother (quickening) begins at 18 to 20 weeks of pregnancy and reaches a peak at 29 to 38 weeks. A healthy fetus moves with a degree of consistency, but a fetus affected by placental insufficiency will greatly decrease its movements. Asking the mother to observe and record the number of movements the fetus makes daily offers a gross assessment of fetal well being (Marnoch, 1992).

One popular way to approach this assessment is to ask the mother to lie in a left recumbent position after a meal and record how many fetal movements she feels over the next hour. A fetus normally moves a minimum of two times every 10 minutes or an average of 10 to 12 times an hour. The mother is instructed to telephone her health care provider if she has felt fewer than five (half the normal number) during the chosen hour. Another protocol is "Count-to-Ten." For this the mother records the time interval it takes for her to feel ten fetal movements. This usually occurs within 20 minutes so is a shortened version (Smith, Davis, & Rayburn, 1992). It is important to realize that, because of variations in movements among normal, healthy fetuses as well as variations in different health care providers' level of confidence in the techniques, a variety of protocols have been developed by different institutions. There is great variety, too, in what is accepted as normal in different areas of the country.

Before being asked to be responsible for this type of observation, women must be taught that fetal move-

ments do vary, especially in relation to sleep cycles of the fetus and their activity during the observation time. Otherwise, the strain of waiting for the fetus to move may become unbearable even though the fetus may be doing well. Although this assessment is easy and inexpensive, the false positive rate (not detecting movements although the fetus is healthy) is extremely high (McCaul & Morrison, 1990). Busy women may have difficulty finding an uninterrupted hour in their day to complete the assessment.

Fetal Heart Rate

Fetal heart rate should be 120 to 160 beats per minute throughout pregnancy. Fetal heart sounds can be heard and counted as early as the 11th week of pregnancy by the use of an ultrasonic Doppler technique (Figure 9-12).

Rhythm Strip Testing. The term *rhythm strip testing* has come to mean assessment of the fetal heart rate in terms of baseline and long- and short-term variability.

FOCUS ON NURSING RESEARCH

When Different People Measure Fundal Height, Are There Differences in the Measurements?

Most women attending prenatal care have a fundal height measurement taken at each visit. In many health care settings, personnel are so numerous these measurements may be made each month by a different health care provider. If these measurements differ, it is assumed that is because the fetus has grown. It would be unfortunate if differences in measurements due to different techniques or equipment made it seem as if a fetus has not grown or vice versa.

To see if differences do exist among examiners, Engstrom, McFarlin, and Sittler compared the fundal measurements made by three examiners on 60 pregnant women. The findings revealed that differences among the three examiner's measurements were always greater than differences among any single examiner's measurements on different occasions. Interexaminer differences were smaller when the tape was placed over the curve of the abdomen rather than held straight with an attempt made to judge the top of the fundus; it was even less when calipers were used instead of a tape measure. To ensure maximal reliability of measurements, the researchers suggest that fundal height measurements be obtained by the use of calipers and by the same clinician throughout pregnancy.

Engstrom, J. L., McFarlin, B. L., & Sittler, C. P. (1993). Fundal height measurement: Intra- and interexaminer reliability of three measurement techniques. *Journal of Nurse-Midwifery, 38,* 17.

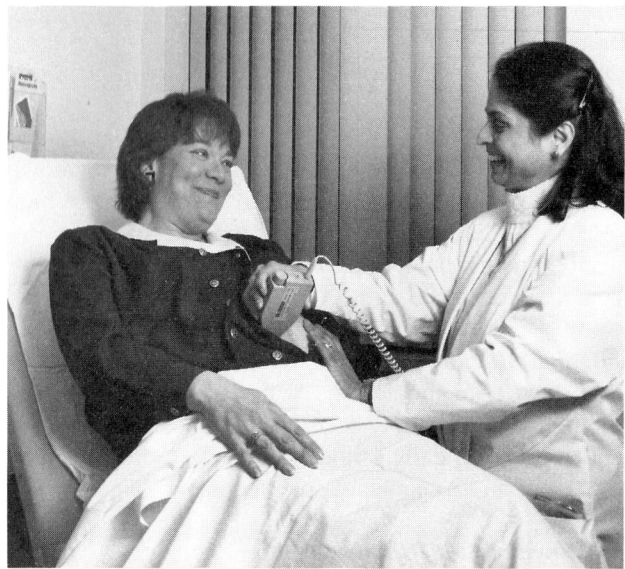

FIGURE 9-12
Measuring fetal heart rate with a Doppler. A Doppler detects and broadcasts the fetal heart rate so the parents-to-be as well as you can hear it. (Courtesy of the Department of Medical Photography, Children's Hospital, Buffalo, NY.)

For the test, the woman is placed in a semi-Fowler's position (either in a comfortable lounge chair or on an examining table or bed with an elevated back rest) to prevent supine hypotension syndrome during the test. An external fetal heart rate monitor is attached abdominally (Figure 9-13*A*) and allowed to record the fetal heart rate for 20 minutes.

The *baseline reading* refers to the average rate of the fetal heart beat per minute. *Short-term variability* (also called beat-to-beat variability) denotes the small changes in rate that occur from second to second if the fetal parasympathetic nervous system is receiving adequate oxygen and nutrients. In the rhythm strip in Figure 9-13*B,* for example, the baseline (average) of the fetal heart beat would be 140 beats per minute. Beat-to-beat variability is present.

Long-term variability denotes the differences in heart rate that occur over the 20-minute time period. Note in Figure 9-13*B* how the heart rate varies from 160 to 110. As the average fetus moves about two times every 10 minutes, and movement causes the heart rate to increase, there will typically be two or more instances of fetal heart rate acceleration in a 20-minute rhythm strip. Long-term variability this way reflects the state of the fetal sympathetic nervous system.

Rhythm-strip testing requires the mother to remain in a fairly fixed position for 20 minutes so the ultrasound scanner does not lose the fetal heart. If she lies supine, she should turn to the left side to prevent vena cava compression. It is important with this and other tests of fetal health to keep the mother well informed of the pur-

pose of the test, how it is interpreted, and the meaning of results. The more she understands about the process, the better she can cooperate to make it successful.

Nonstress Testing. A **nonstress test** adds another measure to a simple rhythm strip: the response of the fetal heart rate to fetal movement (Devoe, 1990). The woman is positioned, and the fetal heart rate monitor is attached as with a rhythm strip. The woman pushes a button attached to the monitor (similar to a call bell) whenever she feels the fetus move. The paper tracing is marked by a dark line at these points.

When a fetus moves, the fetal heart rate should increase about 15 beats per minute and remain elevated for 15 seconds. It should decrease again as the fetus quiets (Figure 9-13*C*). If no increase in beats per minute is noticeable on fetal movement, poor oxygen perfusion of the fetus is suggested (McCaul & Morrison, 1990).

A nonstress test is done for 10 to 20 minutes. The test is *reactive* if two accelerations of fetal heart rate (15 beats or more) lasting for 15 seconds occur following movement within the chosen time period. The test is *nonreactive* if no accelerations occur with the fetal movements. The results also can be interpreted as nonreactive if no fetal movement occurs or there is low short-term fetal heart rate variability (less than 6 beats per minute) throughout the testing period.

If a 20-minute period passes without any fetal movement, it may mean only that the fetus is sleeping. If the mother is given an oral carbohydrate snack, such as orange juice, her blood glucose level may increase enough to cause fetal movement. Because both rhythm strip and nonstress testing are not invasive procedures and cause no risk to either mother or fetus, they can be done at home daily as part of a home monitoring program for the mother with a complication of pregnancy (see Chapter 16).

If a nonstress test is nonreactive, additional fetal assessment, such as a contraction stress test or biophysical profile test, will be scheduled.

Vibroacoustic Stimulation. Acoustic stimulation is the application of an instrument to produce a sharp sound to the mother's abdomen to startle and wake the fetus (Kisilevsky, Kilpatrick, & Low, 1993). Two such instruments used are an artificial larynx and a fetal acoustic stimulator specifically designed for this. These devices emit sound levels of approximately 80 dB at a frequency of 80 Hz (Clark, 1990).

During a standard nonstress test, if a spontaneous acceleration has not occurred within 5 minutes, a single 1- to 2-second sound stimulation is applied to the lower abdomen. This could be repeated again at the end of 10 minutes if no further spontaneous movement occurs, so two movements within the 10-minute window can be evaluated.

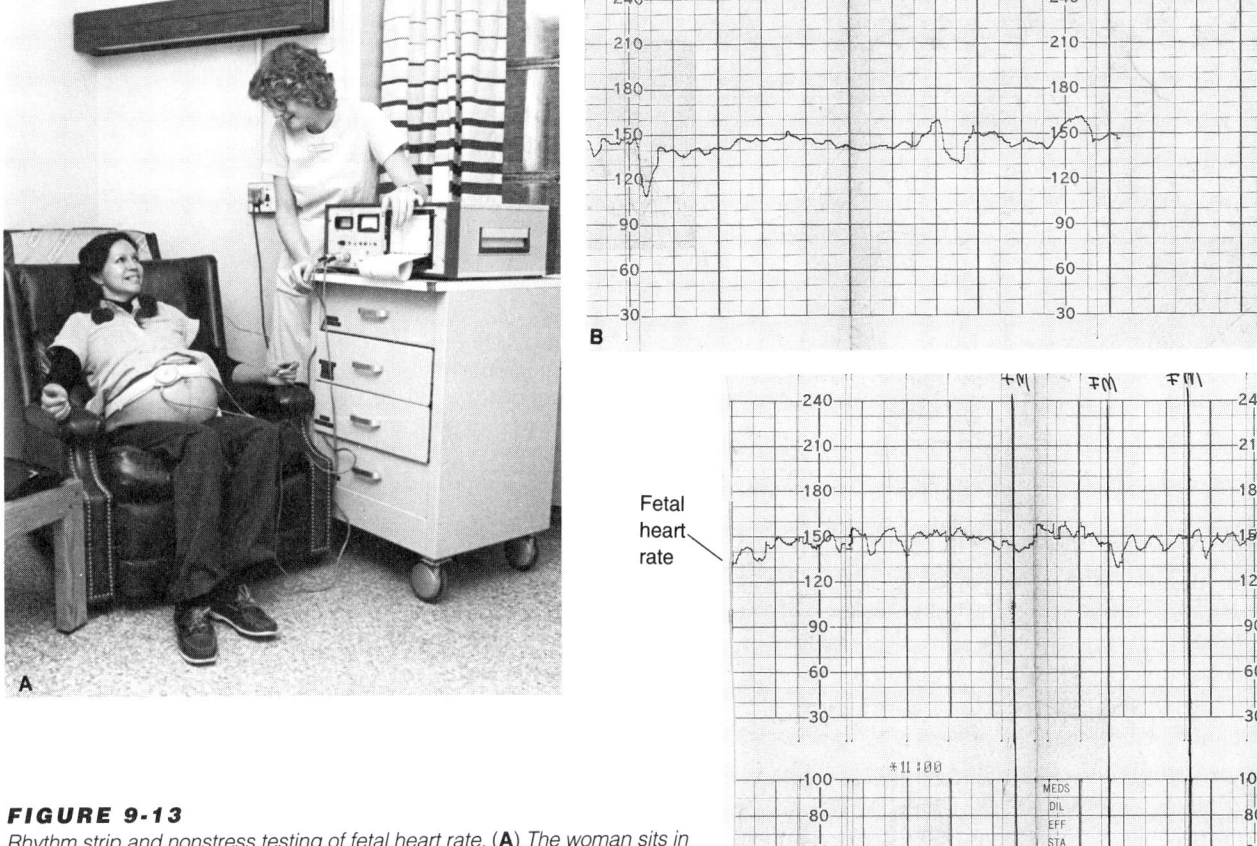

FIGURE 9-13
*Rhythm strip and nonstress testing of fetal heart rate. (**A**) The woman sits in a comfortable chair to avoid supine hypotension. Both a uterine contraction and fetal heart rate monitor are in place on her abdomen. (Courtesy of the Department of Medical Photography, Children's Hospital, Buffalo, NY.) (**B**) A rhythm strip. Fetal baseline is 140 beats/min. (**C**) Nonstress test rhythm strip. Following the three marked fetal movements (FM), the heart rate increases 15 beats/min and stays elevated for 15 sec.*

Fetal heart rate

Uterine monitor

Contraction Stress Testing

With contraction stress testing (CST), fetal heart rate is analyzed in reference to contractions (Pircon & Freeman, 1990). When this test was first developed, contractions were initiated by the intravenous infusion of oxytocin. The technique had innate difficulties as once started, contractions begun this way may be difficult to stop and lead to preterm labor. For this reason, contraction stress testing is currently most often done by nipple stimulation. Gentle stimulation of the nipples releases oxytocin in the same way as with breast-feeding.

Following identification of the baseline fetal heart rate, the mother rolls a nipple between her finger and thumb until uterine contractions begin. These are recorded by a uterine monitor. Three contractions with a duration of 40 seconds or more must be present in a 10-minute window before the test can be interpreted (McCaul & Morrison, 1990). The test is negative (normal) when no fetal heart rate decelerations are present with contractions. It is positive (abnormal) when 50% or more of contractions cause a late deceleration (a dip in fetal heart rate that occurs toward the end of a contrac-

tion and continues after the contraction). See Chapter 18 for further discussion of fetal heart rate monitoring with labor contractions.

Nonstress tests and contraction stress tests are compared in Table 9-4. Following a CST, encourage women to remain in the health care facility for about 30 minutes to be certain that contractions have quieted and labor is not a risk.

Ultrasound

Ultrasound, or the response of sound waves against objects, is a well-used tool in modern obstetrics although the recommendations for its use may change because of unproven benefits in the face of added expense. It most likely is used in fetal assessment at least once during a normal pregnancy. It can be used to diagnose pregnancy as early as 6 weeks' gestation age and later to confirm the presence, size, and location of the placenta and to establish that the fetus is increasing in size and has no gross defects, such as hydrocephalus, anencephaly, or spinal cord, heart, kidney, and bladder defects. Ultrasound may be used at term to establish the

Table 9-4. *Comparison of Nonstress and Contraction Tests*

Assessment	Nonstress	Contraction
What is measured	Response of fetal heart rate in relation to fetal movements.	Response of fetal heart rate in relation to uterine contractions, which are nipple or oxytocin stimulated
Normal findings	Two or more accelerations of FHR of 15 beats/min lasting 15 sec or more following fetal movements in a 20-min period.	No late decelerations with contractions
Safety considerations	Woman should not lie supine to prevent supine hypotension syndrome.	In addition to supine hypotension syndrome, observe woman for 30 min afterward to see that contractions are quiet and preterm labor does not begin.

presentation and position of the fetus, to predict maturity by measurement of the biparietal diameter (see later discussion), and during the early stages of labor to determine the presence of any abnormality, such as placenta previa.

Ultrasound is also used to discover complications of pregnancy, such as the presence of an intrauterine device, hydramnios or oligohydramnios, ectopic pregnancy, missed abortion, abdominal pregnancy, placental previa, premature separation of the placenta, coexisting uterine tumors, or multiple pregnancy. Fetal death can be revealed by a lack of heart beat and respiratory movement. Following birth, sonogram may be used to detect a retained placenta or poor uterine involution.

With ultrasound, intermittent sound waves of high frequency (above the audible range) are projected toward the uterus by a transducer. The sound frequencies that bounce back can be displayed on an oscilloscope screen as a visual image; the frequencies returning from tissues of various thicknesses and properties present distinct appearances. A permanent record can be made by Polaroid photography.

The intricacy of the image obtained depends on the type or mode of process used. *B-mode* scanning is the process most frequently used and generally what people refer to as a sonogram. This mode allows patterns to merge and form a picture similar to a black-and-white television picture (called *gray-scale imaging*). *Real-time* mode involves the use of multiple waves that allow the screen picture to be two dimensional or actually to move. This technique is termed *echocardiography* when it is used to study heart movements. On this type of sonogram, the fetal heart can be seen actually to move, and even movement of extremities, such as the fetus bringing a hand to the mouth to suck a thumb, can be seen. A parent who is in doubt that her fetus is well or whole cannot help but be assured by viewing a real-time sonogram image.

Prior to an ultrasound study, the woman needs to be given a good explanation of what will happen and assured that the process does not involve x-ray. This means it is also safe for the father of the child to remain in the room during the test. Comparing it with the process by which sonar detects submarines may be helpful (it is the same). For the sound waves to reflect best and the uterus to be held stable, it is helpful if the mother has a full bladder at the time of the procedure. To ensure this, she should drink a full glass of water every 15 minutes beginning an hour and a half before the procedure and then be certain not to void before the procedure. For the actual procedure, the mother lies on an examining table and is draped for privacy but with her abdomen exposed. (To prevent supine hypotension syndrome, place a towel under her right buttock to tip her body slightly so the uterus will roll away from the vena cava.) A contact gel is applied to her abdomen to improve the contact of the transducer. (Be certain the gel is room temperature or even slightly warmer or you can cause uncomfortable uterine cramping.) The transducer is then applied to her abdomen and moved both horizontally and vertically until the uterus and its contents are fully scanned (Figure 9-14). Ultrasound also may be done by an intravaginal technique.

Although the long-term effects of ultrasound are not yet known, the technique appears to be safe for both mother and fetus. It involves no discomfort for the fetus, and the only discomfort for the mother is that she might interpret the contact lubricant which must be applied to her abdomen at the beginning of the scan as messy. She may experience a strong desire to void before the scan is completed. If Polaroid photos are taken of the sonogram image, ask if the mother can have one for her baby book. Having a photo this way can enhance bonding as it is proof that the pregnancy exists and the fetus appears well.

Biparietal Diameter. Ultrasound may be used to predict the maturity of the fetus by measuring the biparietal

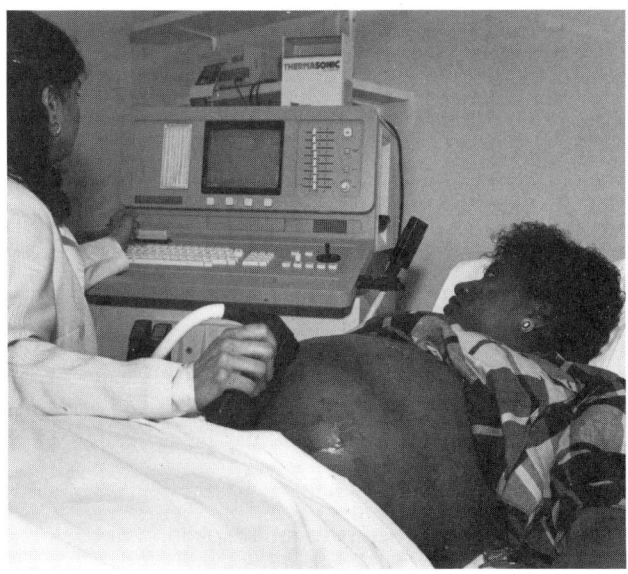

FIGURE 9-14
A sonogram being recorded. Notice the mother's interest in being able to see her baby's first picture. (Courtesy of the Department of Medical Photography, Children's Hospital, Buffalo, NY.)

diameter (side to side measurement) of the fetal head on the permanent record. When the biparietal diameter of the fetal head is 8.5 cm or more, in 90% of pregnancies the infant will weigh more than 2500 g (5½ lb). A biparietal diameter of 9.5 cm indicates a fetus of 40 weeks. Figure 9-15 is a sonogram showing the biparietal diameter of a fetus at 24 weeks.

Two other measurements commonly made by sonogram are head circumference (34.5 cm is a 40-week fetus) and femoral length.

Doppler Umbilical Velocimetry. Doppler ultrasonography measures the velocity at which red blood cells in the uterine and fetal vessels are traveling. The velocity at which they are moving is proportional to the blood pressure in vessels and inversely proportional to vascular resistance (Trudinger, 1993).

As early as 20 weeks' gestation, transabdominal ultrasound can locate the umbilical artery. On a monitor screen a waveform with a triangular shape should be present at this time. The top of the waveform represents the systolic blood pressure; the lowest point before the wave rises represents the diastolic pressure. As the placenta matures, the systolic/diastolic ratio of the waveform should fall to less than 3. If this does not happen by 30 weeks, intrauterine growth retardation from the poor blood flow can be predicted (Farmakides & Coury, 1990).

Assessment of the uterine blood vessels in this way is helpful in determining the vascular resistance present in women with diabetes or hypertension of pregnancy (Trudinger, 1993).

Placental Grading. Based on changes, particularly the amount of calcium deposits present in the base of the placenta, placentas can be graded as 0 (a placenta 12 to 24 weeks), 1 (30–32 weeks), 2 (36 weeks), and 3 (38 weeks). As fetal lungs are apt to be mature at 38 weeks, a grade 3 placenta suggests that the fetus is mature.

Amniotic Fluid Volume Assessment. The amount of amniotic fluid present is an important fetal assessment measure because a portion of the fluid is formed by fetal kidney output. If a fetus is becoming stressed in utero so that circulatory and kidney functions are failing, urine output and, consequently, the volume of amniotic fluid also will decrease. A decrease in amniotic fluid volume puts the fetus at risk for compression of the umbilical cord and interference with nutrition.

Amniotic fluid volume is measured by placing an ultrasound scanner against the side of the abdomen. For gestations of less than 20 weeks, the uterus is hypothetically divided along the linea nigra into two vertical halves. The vertical diameter of the largest pocket of amniotic fluid present is measured in centimeters on each side. The amniotic volume index (total) is the sum of the two measurements. For gestations of 20 weeks or more, the uterus is divided into four quadrants, using the linea nigra again as the vertical dividing line and the level of the umbilicus as the horizontal dividing line. The vertical diameter of the largest pocket of fluid in each quadrant is obtained, and the four values are then added to produce the amniotic fluid index (AFI). The average AFI is approximately 15 cm between 28 and 40 weeks. An AFI

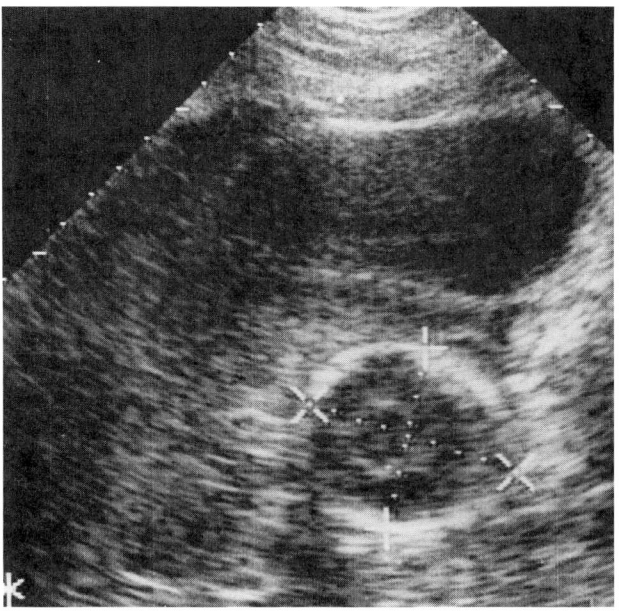

FIGURE 9-15
A sonogram at 24 weeks' gestation showing measurement of the head circumference. (Courtesy of the Department of Medical Photography, Children's Hospital, Buffalo, NY.)

greater than 20 to 24 cm indicates hydramnios (excessive fluid, perhaps caused by inability of the fetus to swallow); an AFI less than 5 to 6 cm indicates oligohydramnios (decreased amniotic fluid, perhaps caused by poor perfusion and kidney failure) (Smith & Weiner, 1990).

Electrocardiography
Fetal ECGs may be recorded as early as the 11th week of pregnancy. The ECG is inaccurate before the 20th week, however, because until this time the fetal cardiac electrical signal is so weak that it is easily masked by the mother's. The art of monitoring fetal ECGs as an additional measure of fetal assessment is being investigated. In the future, evaluation of the ECG during labor may become preferred over Doppler studies (Hess et al., 1990).

Magnetic Resonance Imaging
Magnetic resonance imaging (MRI) uses a computerized axial tomography scanner with a magnetic field activated by radio waves substituted for the x-ray tube (Barton et al., 1993). For an MRI examination, the woman lies on a moving pallet that is pushed into the core of the machine (see Chapter 37, Figure 37-3B). When the magnetic field is turned on, it causes tissue atoms to line up in a parallel fashion. This unique alignment is sensed and converted into a visual display on a computer screen. The technique has the potential to offer a much more striking gray matter-white matter contrast than ultrasound. As the technique apparently causes no harmful effects to the fetus or mother (although extensive long-term testing is not yet available), MRI has the potential to replace or complement ultrasound as a fetal assessment technique. It may be most helpful in diagnosing ectopic pregnancy or trophoblastic disease (see Chapter 15).

Assay of Maternal Serum
Maternal serum may be used to determine the levels of various hormones as assessments of fetal well being. Diamine oxidase, oxytocinase, progesterone, alkaline phosphatase, and human placental lactogen are all chemical substances that rise in the blood serum of a pregnant woman if the fetus is growing well. These are rarely assayed, however, as information on the fetus can be derived more directly from a single study such as serum alpha fetoprotein or a triple screen (see below).

Alpha Fetoprotein. Alpha fetoprotein (a substance produced by the fetal liver) will be abnormally high in the maternal serum (MSAFP) if the fetus has an open spinal or abdominal defect and low if the fetus has a chromosomal defect, such as Down syndrome (Keenan et al., 1991). Alpha fetoprotein begins to rise at 11 weeks' gestation, then steadily increases until term. Tra-

ditionally assessed at the 15th week of pregnancy, due to new analysis techniques it is now feasible to analyse this as early as the 11th week of pregnancy (Crandall et al., 1993). "Triple screening," or analysis of three indicators (maternal serum for alpha fetoprotein, estriol, and human chorionic gonadotropin), may be performed in place of only alpha fetoprotein in order to yield more reliable results.

Chorionic Villi Sampling (CVS)
Chorionic villi sampling is biopsy and analysis of chorionic villi for chromosome analysis done at 5 to 10 weeks of pregnancy. As this is used almost exclusively for chromosome analysis, it is discussed in Chapter 8.

Coelocentesis
Coelocentesis is the transvaginal aspiration of coelomic fluid at the 6th to 10th week of pregnancy for analysis. Coelomic fluid collects in the extraembryonic cavity early in pregnancy and may be a safer source of cells for analysis than chorionic villi (Jurkovic et al., 1993).

Amniocentesis
Amniocentesis (from the Greek *amnion* for sac and *kentesis* for puncture) is aspiration of amniotic fluid from the pregnant uterus for examination. The procedure can be done in a physician's office or an ambulatory clinic as early as the 12th to 13th week of pregnancy (Shulman, 1992). Formerly, the procedure was delayed until the 14th to 16th week to allow for a generous amount of amniotic fluid to form. Refined analysis requires only 1 mL of fluid for analysis so earlier intervention is possible. Amniocentesis is used late in pregnancy to test for fetal maturity (Table 9-5.)

Although amniocentesis is a technically easy procedure, it may be frightening to a woman and it is not totally without risk to the fetus because it involves penetrating the integrity of the amniotic sac. It can lead to complications in rare instances (under 1% of procedures), such as hemorrhage from penetration of the placenta, infection of the amniotic fluid, puncture of the fetus, and irritation of the uterus, leading to premature labor (Rosenfield & Fathalla, 1990).

To prepare for amniocentesis, the woman is asked to void (to reduce the size of the bladder so that it is out

Table 9-5. *Timing of Amniocentesis Procedures*

Reason for Procedure	Timing (Weeks)
Chromosomal determination	14–16
Rh isoimmunization	20–28
Maturity determination	34–42
Assessment of fetal well being	34–42

of the field). She lies in a supine position on the examining table and is draped for privacy but with her abdomen exposed. (Place a folded towel under her right buttock to tip her body slightly to the left and move the uterus off the vena cava to prevent supine hypotension syndrome.) Take the maternal blood pressure and the fetal heart rate for baseline levels. The position of the fetus, a pocket of amniotic fluid, and the placenta are all located by sonogram. The woman's abdomen is then washed with an antiseptic solution, and the skin is infiltrated with a local anesthetic, causing momentary pain because abdominal skin is tender. This is the extent of the pain the woman will experience; she may feel a sensation of pressure as the needle used for aspiration is introduced. Do *not* suggest that the woman take a deep breath and hold it as a distraction against pressure; this lowers the diaphragm against the uterus and shifts intrauterine contents.

The needle used is a 3- or 4-in 20- to 22-gauge spinal needle. This is inserted into the abdomen and into the amniotic cavity over the pool of amniotic fluid, carefully avoiding the fetus and placenta (Figure 9-16). A syringe is attached to the needle, and a chosen amount of

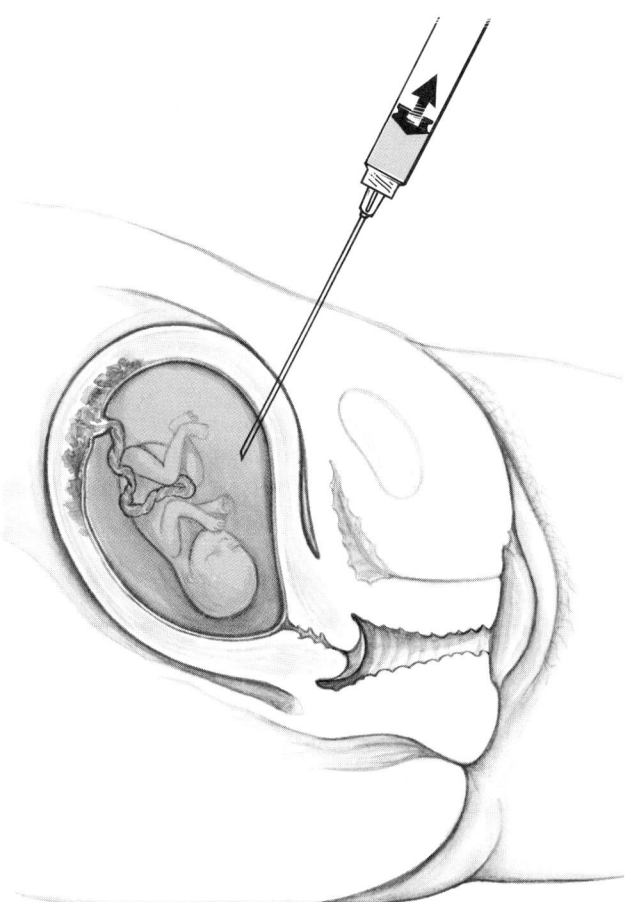

FIGURE 9-16
Amniocentesis. A pocket of amniotic fluid is located by sonogram. A small amount of fluid is removed by aspiration.

fluid is withdrawn. The needle is then removed, and the woman rests quietly for a short period. A fetal heart monitor and uterine contraction monitor are put in place and assessed for about 30 minutes to be certain that the fetal heart rate remains normal and no uterine contractions are occurring. If the woman has Rh negative blood, Rho (D) immune globulin (RhIG) (RhoGAM) may be administered following the procedure to prevent fetal isoimmunization. This is to ensure that maternal antibodies will not form against any placental red blood cells that accidentally were released during the procedure. Amniocentesis can reveal information in a number of areas.

Color. Normal amniotic fluid is the color of water; late in pregnancy it may have a slightly yellow tinge. A strong yellow color suggests a blood incompatibility (the yellow results from the presence of bilirubin released with the hemolysis of red blood cells). A green color suggests meconium staining, a phenomenon associated with fetal distress.

Lecithin/Sphingomyelin Ratio. Lecithin and sphingomyelin are the protein components of the lung enzyme surfactant that the alveoli begin to form about the 22nd to 24th weeks of pregnancy. Following amniocentesis, the L/S ratio may be determined quickly by a shake or bubble test or sent for laboratory analysis.

To do a shake test, amniotic fluid is placed in a test tube and diluted with saline; ethanol alcohol is then added and the mixture is shaken. If stable bubbles appear, the L/S ratio is greater than 2:1 and the fetal pulmonary system is sufficiently mature for birth. If the bubbles are unstable, the L/S ratio is below 2:1—that is, not enough lecithin is present to ensure lung function if the fetus should be delivered at this time.

More accurate information on lecithin production is accomplished by laboratory analysis. As mentioned previously, infants of mothers with severe diabetes may have false-mature readings of lecithin because the stress to the infant in utero tends to mature lecithin pathways early. Fetal values must be considered in light of the presence of maternal diabetes, or the infants may be delivered with mature lung function but be immature overall (fragile giants) and so not do well in postnatal life. Some laboratories interpret an L/S ratio of 2.5:1 or 3:1 as a mature indicator in these infants.

Phosphatidyl Glycerol and Desaturated Phosphatidylcholine. Phosphatidyl glycerol and desaturated phosphatidylcholine phospholipid are compounds in addition to lecithin and sphingomyelin found in surfactant. Pathways for these compounds mature at 35 to 36 weeks. Because they are present only with mature lung function, when they are present, it can be predicted that respiratory distress syndrome will not occur.

Bilirubin Determination. Determining the presence of bilirubin is important when a blood incompatibility is suspected. When bilirubin is being analyzed, the specimen must be blood free or a false-positive reading will occur.

Chromosome Analysis. A few fetal skin cells are always present in amniotic fluid. These cells may be cultured and stained for chromosomal analysis (karyotyping). The chromosomal diseases that can be detected by prenatal amniocentesis and their significance to health are discussed in Chapter 7.

Inborn Errors of Metabolism. Some inherited diseases caused by inborn errors of metabolism can be detected by amniocentesis. For a condition to be identified this way, the enzyme defect must be present in the amniotic fluid as early as the time of the procedure. Examples of illnesses that can be detected this way are cystinosis and maple syrup urine disease (amino acid disorders).

Alpha Fetoprotein. If the fetus has an open body defect, such as anencephaly, myelomeningocele, or omphalocele, alpha fetoprotein will be present at increased levels in the amniotic fluid because of leakage of alpha fetoprotein into the amniotic fluid. The level will be decreased in the fluid of fetuses with chromosomal defects such as Down syndrome. Acetylcholinesterase is a similar compound obtained from amniotic fluid in high levels if a neural tube defect is present.

Percutaneous Umbilical Blood Sampling (PUBS)

Percutaneous umbilical blood sampling (also called *cordocentesis* or *funicentesis*) is aspiration of blood from the umbilical vein for analysis (Davis, 1993). For the procedure, the umbilical cord is localized by sonogram. A thin needle is then inserted by amniocentesis technique into the uterus; it is guided by ultrasound until it pierces the umbilical vein. A sample of blood is removed for blood studies, such as a complete blood count, direct Coombs, blood gases, and karyotyping. Blood obtained is determined to be fetal blood by a Kleihauer-Betke test. If a fetus is found to be anemic, blood may be transfused by this same technique. Because the umbilical vein continues to ooze for a moment following the procedure, fetal blood could enter the maternal circulation, so RhIG is given to Rh negative women to prevent sensitization. The fetus is monitored by a nonstress test before and after the procedure to be certain that uterine contractions are not present and by ultrasound to see that no bleeding is evident. Cordocentesis carries little additional risk to the fetus or mother over amniocentesis and can yield information not available by any other means, especially about blood dyscrasias (Bell & Weiner, 1993).

Amnioscopy

Amnioscopy is visual inspection of the amniotic fluid through the cervix and membranes with an amnioscope (a small fetoscope). The main use of the technique is to detect meconium staining. It carries some risk of membrane rupture.

Fetoscopy

Fetoscopy, or actually visualizing the fetus by inspection through a fetoscope (an extremely narrow, hollow tube inserted by amniocentesis technique), is helpful in assessing fetal well being in some instances (Copel et al., 1990). A Polaroid photo can be taken through the fetoscope as assurance for the parents that their infant is well and perfectly formed. Intactness of the spinal column can be confirmed by this method. Biopsies of fetal tissue and fetal blood samples can be removed through a fetoscope for analysis. Elemental surgery, such as inserting a polyethylene shunt into the fetal ventricles to relieve hydrocephalus or anteriorly into the fetal bladder to relieve a stenosed urethra, can be accomplished (Collins, 1994).

The 16th or 17th week of pregnancy is about the earliest time in pregnancy that fetoscopy can be performed. For the procedure, the mother is prepared and draped as for amniocentesis (see earlier discussion). A local anesthetic is injected into the abdominal skin. The fetoscope is then inserted following a minor scalpel incision. If the fetus is very active, meperidine (Demerol) may be administered to the mother to avoid fetal injury by the scope and to provide for better observation. This drug crosses the placenta and sedates the fetus.

Fetoscopy carries a small risk of premature labor. *Amnionitis* (infection of the amniotic fluid) may occur. To avoid this, the mother may be placed on 10 days of antibiotic therapy following the procedure. The number of procedures performed by fetoscopy is limited because of the manipulation involved and the ethical quandary of the mother's autonomy being compromised by the fetal needs (asking the mother to undergo a general anesthesia so the fetus can have surgery).

Biophysical Profile

A biophysical profile combines four to six parameters—(1) fetal breathing movements, (2) fetal movement, (3) fetal tone, (4) amniotic fluid volume, (5) fetal heart reactivity, and (6) placental grade—into one assessment. The scoring for a profile is shown in Table 9-6. By this system, each item has the potential for scoring a 2, so 12 would be the highest score possible. If only four parameters are used, 8 is a perfect score; if five parameters are used, 10 is the perfect score. A biophysical profile is more accurate in predicting fetal well being than any single assessment (Manning, 1990). As the scoring sys-

Table 9-6. *Biophysical Profile Scoring*

Assessment	Instrument Used	Criteria for a Score of 2
Fetal breathing	Sonogram	At least one episode of 30 sec of sustained fetal breathing movements within 30 min of observation
Fetal movement	Sonogram	At least three separate episodes of fetal limb or trunk movement within a 30-min observation
Fetal tone	Sonogram	The fetus must extend and then flex the extremities or spine at least once in 30 min
Amniotic fluid volume	Sonogram	A pocket of amniotic fluid measuring more than 1 cm in vertical diameter must be present
Placental grade	Sonogram	Placenta is grade 3. Grading is based on structure and amount of calcium present
Fetal heart reactivity	Nonstress test	Two or more fetal heart-rate accelerations of at least 15 beats/min above baseline and of 15 sec duration occur with fetal movement over 20 min

(From Gebauer, C. L., & Lowe, N. K. [1993]. The biophysical profile: Antepartal assessment of fetal well-being. *Journal of Obstetric, Gynecologic and Neonatal Nursing, 22*, 115.)

tem is so much like the Apgar score determined at birth on infants, it is popularly called a *fetal Apgar.*

Biophysical profiles may be done as often as daily during a high-risk pregnancy. If a fetus scores 8 to 12, the fetus is considered to be doing well. A score of 4 to 6 denotes a fetus in jeopardy. Nurses play a large role in obtaining the information for a biophysical profile by obtaining either the nonstress test or sonogram readings (Gebauer & Lowe, 1993).

Key Points

- The union of a single sperm and egg (fertilization) signals the beginning of pregnancy. The fertilized ovum (a zygote) travels by way of a fallopian tube to the uterus where implantation takes place in about 8 days. From implantation to 5 to 8 weeks, the growing structure is called an embryo. The period following this until birth is the fetal period.
- Growth of the umbilical cord, amniotic fluid, and amniotic membranes proceeds in concert with fetal growth. The placenta produces a number of important hormones: estrogen, progesterone, chorionic somatomammotropin, and human chorionic gonadotropin as it grows.
- Various methods to assess fetal growth and development are fundal height, fetal movement, fetal heart tones, ultrasound, magnetic resonance imaging, alpha fetoprotein analysis, amniocentesis, percutaneous umbilical blood sampling, amnioscopy, and fetoscopy. A biophysical profile is a combination of fetal assessments that better predicts fetal well being than single parameters.

- A fetus needs protection from teratogens such as drugs in order to develop normally. Nicotine and alcohol should be avoided.
- Although fetal growth can be demonstrated by x-ray, it is not assessed this way to avoid exposing the fetus to x-ray. Women need to tell health care providers that they are pregnant before they have an x-ray for any reason so they can be furnished with a lead apron for the procedure to protect the fetus.

Critical Thinking Exercises

1. Jessica Ayers is a woman who is 6 weeks pregnant. She asks you how big her fetus is at this point. What would be the best way to illustrate this for her?
2. Jessica is scheduled for an ultrasound at 20 weeks gestation to assess fetal growth. She states she does not want to know her fetus' sex if it is revealed by the test. Why do you think some women want to know the sex of a fetus and some do not? Is there an advantage to knowing or not knowing?
3. Late in pregnancy, Jessica is scheduled for a number of nonstress and contraction stress tests. She states she hates to have these done because they are time consuming and boring. What are ways you could make such tests more appealing and so increase compliance?

References

Barness, L. A. (1994). The pediatric history and physical examination. In F. A. Oski et al. *Principles and practice of pediatrics* (pp. 28–43). Philadelphia: J.B. Lippincott.

Barton, J. W., et al. (1993). Pelvic MR imaging findings in gestational trophoblastic disease, incomplete abortion and ectopic pregnancy; are they specific? *Radiology, 186,* 163.

Bell, J. G., & Weiner, S. (1993). Has percutaneous umbilical blood sampling improved the outcomes of high-risk pregnancies? *Clinics in Perinatology, 20,* 61.

Clark, S. L. (1990). How a modified NST improves fetal surveillance. *Contemporary Obstetrics and Gynecology, 35,* 45.

Collins, J. E. (1994). Fetal surgery: Changing the outcome before birth. *Journal of Obstetric, Gynecologic and Neonatal Nursing, 23,* 166.

Copel, J. A., et al. (1990). Invasive fetal assessment in the antepartum period. *Obstetrics and Gynecology Clinics of North America, 17,* 201.

Crandall, B. F., et al. (1993). Maternal serum screening for alphafetoprotein, unconjugated estriol, and human chorionic gonadotropin between 11 and 15 weeks of pregnancy to detect fetal chromosome abnormalities. *American Journal of Obstetrics and Gynecology, 168,* 1864.

Davis, J. G. (1993). Reproductive technologies for prenatal diagnosis. *Fetal Diagnosis & Therapy, 1,* 28S.

De Lia, J. E. (1990). Placental and fetal development. In Scott, J. R., et al. *Danforth's obstetrics and gynecology.* Philadelphia: J.B. Lippincott.

Department of Health and Human Services. (1991). *Healthy people 2000.* Washington, DC: Public Health Service.

Devoe, L. D. (1990). The nonstress test. *Obstetrics and Gynecology Clinics of North America, 17,* 111.

Engstrom, J. L., & Sittler, C. P. (1993). Fundal height measurement: Techniques for measuring fundal height. *Journal of Nurse-Midwifery, 38,* 5.

Farmakides, G., & Coury, A. (1990). Pregnancy surveillance with Doppler velocimetry. *Female Patient, 15,* 49.

Flood, J. T., & Hodgen, G. D. (1990). Physiology of fertilization, implantation and early human development. In Scott, J. R., et al. *Danforth's obstetrics and gynecology.* Philadelphia: J. B. Lippincott.

Gebauer, C. L., & Lowe, N. K. (1993). The biophysical profile: Antepartal assessment of fetal well-being. *Journal of Obstetric, Gynecologic and Neonatal Nursing, 22,* 115.

Hess, L. W., et al. (1990). Fetal echocardiography. *Obstetrics and Gynecology Clinics of North America, 17,* 41.

Jurkovic, D., et al. (1993). Coelocentesis: A new technique for early prenatal diagnosis. *Lancet, 341,* 1623.

Keenan, K. L., et al. (1991). Low level of maternal serum alphafetoprotein: Its associated anxiety and the effects of counseling. *American Journal of Obstetrics and Gynecology, 164,* 54.

Kisilevsky, B. S., Kilpatrick, K. L., & Low, J. A. (1993). Vibroacoustic induced fetal movement: Two stimuli and two methods of scoring. *Obstetrics & Gynecology, 81,* 174.

Kochenour, N. K. (1990). Normal pregnancy and prenatal care. In Scott, J. R., et al. *Danforth's obstetrics and gynecology.* Philadelphia: J. B. Lippincott.

Manning, F. A. (1990). The fetal biophysical profile score: Current status. *Obstetrics and Gynecology Clinics of North America, 17,* 147.

Marnoch, A. (1992). An evaluation of the importance of formal, maternal fetal movement counting as a measure of fetal well-being. *Midwifery, 8,* 54.

McCaul, J. F., & Morrison, J. C. (1990). Antenatal fetal assessment: An overview. *Obstetrics and Gynecology Clinics of North America, 17,* 1.

Pircon, R., & Freeman, R. K. (1990). The contraction stress test. *Obstetrics and Gynecology Clinics of North America, 17,* 129.

Rosenfield, A., & Fathalla, M. F. (1990). *The F.I.G.O. manual of human reproduction.* Park Ridge, N.J.: Parthenon Publishing.

Rurak, D. W. (1992). Fetal behavioral states: Pathological alterations with drug/alcohol abuse. *Seminars in Perinatology, 16,* 239.

Shulman, L. P. (1992). Early amniocentesis: How feasible? *Contemporary Obstetrics and Gynecology, 37,* 29.

Smith, C. S., & Weiner, S. (1990). Amniotic fluid volume: Importance and assessment. *Female Patient, 15,* 85.

Smith, C. V., Davis, S. A., & Rayburn, W. F. (1992). Patients' acceptance of monitoring fetal movement. *Journal of Reproductive Medicine, 37,* 144.

Trudinger, B. J. (1993). How Doppler ultrasound assesses fetal condition. *Contemporary Obstetrics and Gynecology, 38,* 54.

Ward, R. M. (1992). Maternal drug therapy for fetal disorders. *Seminars in Perinatology, 16,* 12.

Zlatnik, F. J. (1990). Normal labor and delivery and its conduct. In Scott, J. R., et al. *Danforth's obstetrics and gynecology* (6th ed.). Philadelphia: J.B. Lippincott.

Suggested Readings

Burton, B. K., et al. (1992). Limb anomalies associated with chorionic villus sampling. *Obstetrics and Gynecology, 79,* 726.

Chervenak, F. A., & McCullough, L. B. (1992). Fetus as patient: An ethical concept. *Contemporary Obstetrics and Gynecology, 37,* 11.

Eganhouse, D. J. (1992). Fetal monitoring of twins. *Journal of Obstetric, Gynecologic, and Neonatal Nursing, 21,* 17.

Inglis, S. R., et al. (1993). The use of vibroacoustic stimulation during the abnormal or equivocal biophysical profile. *Obstetrics & Gynecology, 82,* 371.

Luke, B. (1994). Maternal-fetal nutrition. *Clinical Obstetrics and Gynecology, 37,* 93.

Martin, J. N., & Cowan, B. D. (1990). Biochemical assessment and prediction of gestational well-being. *Obstetrics and Gynecology Clinics of North America, 17,* 81.

Meyers, C. M., & Blitzer, M. G. (1993). Managing unexplained elevated MSAFP with ultrasound and amniocentesis. *Contemporary Obstetrics and Gynecology, 38,* 10.

Miller-Slade, D., et al. (1991). Acoustic stimulation-induced fetal response compared to traditional nonstress testing. *Journal of Obstetric, Gynecologic and Neonatal Nursing, 20,* 160.

Petrikovsky, B. M., & Kalan, G. (1992). Assessment of fetal behavior. *Female Patient, 17,* 32.

Rapp, R. (1993). Sociocultural differences in the impact of amniocentesis. An anthropological research report. *Fetal Diagnosis & Therapy, 1,* 90S.

Rhodes, A. M. (1990). Maternal liability for fetal injury? *MCN: American Journal of Maternal Child Nursing, 15,* 41.

Rottem, S., & Chervenak, F. A. (1990). Ultrasound diagnosis of fetal anomalies. *Obstetrics and Gynecology Clinics of North America, 17,* 17.

Roussis, P., et al. (1991). Fetal Assessment: The biophysical profile. *Female Patient, 16,* 70.

Shaw, K. J., & Paul, R. H. (1990). Fetal responses to external stimuli. *Obstetrics and Gynecology Clinics of North America, 17,* 235.

Smith, C. V. (1990). Amniotic fluid assessment. *Obstetrics and Gynecology Clinics of North America, 17,* 187.

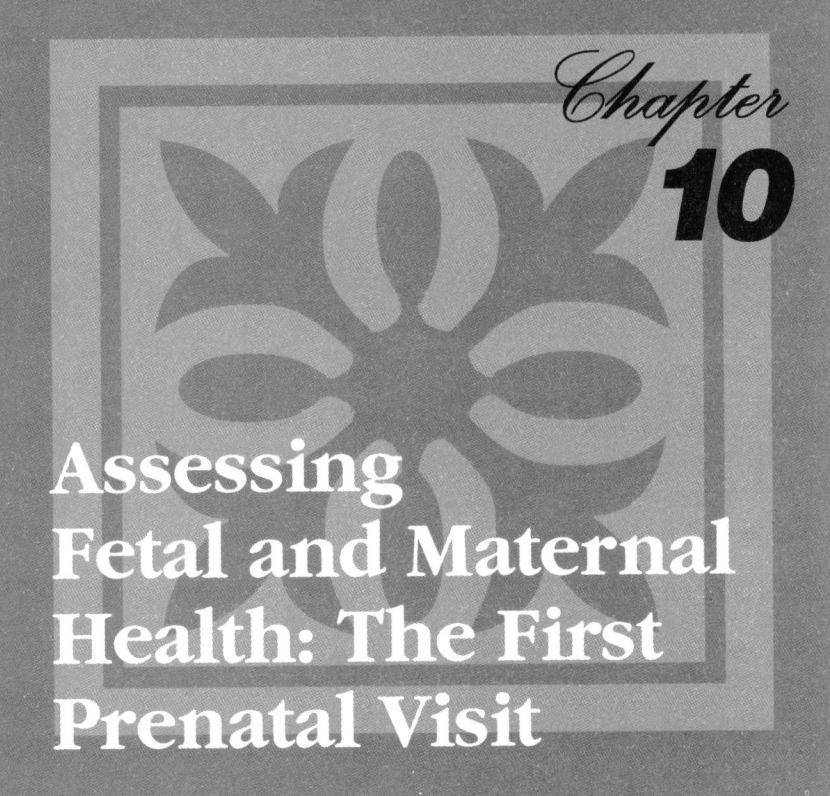

Chapter 10

Assessing Fetal and Maternal Health: The First Prenatal Visit

Objectives

After mastering the contents of this chapter, you should be able to:

1. Describe health assessment measures commonly included in a first prenatal visit.

2. Assess a pregnant woman for optimal health status by such actions as obtaining a health history.

3. Formulate nursing diagnoses related to health status of pregnancy.

4. Plan nursing care such as preparing a woman for a pelvic examination or a fundal measurement.

5. Implement nursing care such as establishing a risk score for pregnancy.

6. Evaluate outcome criteria related to fetal or maternal health to be certain goals of care were achieved.

7. Identify National Health Goals that nurses can be instrumental in helping the nation to achieve.

8. Identify areas of prenatal care that could benefit from additional nursing research.

9. Use critical thinking to analyze ways that the family can be included in prenatal care to keep care family centered.

10. Synthesize knowledge of pregnancy health assessment with nursing process to achieve quality maternal and child health care.

Adele Pillitteri: MATERNAL AND CHILD HEALTH NURSING, 2nd Edition. © 1995 Adele Pillitteri.

Prenatal care is essential for assuring the overall health of babies and their mothers and is a major strategy for helping to reduce the number of low-birth-weight babies born yearly. It is seen as so important a number of National Health Goals speak directly to it (see Focus on National Health Goals box). Ideally, prenatal care begins in the mother's childhood. It includes a good calcium and vitamin D intake during infancy and childhood, so that the woman does not develop rickets (which can distort pelvic size); adequate immunizations against contagious diseases so that, when pregnant, she will be protected against viral diseases such as rubella; and a healthy daily diet, so that both she and her sexual partner enter pregnancy in the best state of health possible.

Promotion of prenatal health also includes the development of positive attitudes about sexuality, womanhood, and childbearing so that the woman enters pregnancy in good psychological health. Once a woman becomes sexually active, preparation for a successful pregnancy includes practicing safer sex, regular pelvic examinations, and prompt treatment of any sexually transmitted disease to prevent complications that could lead to infertility. Acquisition and use of reproductive planning information help to assure that each pregnancy is planned and the child desired. Women who have maintained this type of healthy lifestyle come to a first prenatal visit prepared to follow health promotion

strategies for a healthy pregnancy. For many women, the first prenatal visit represents the first time they have been to a health care facility since the routine health maintenance visits of childhood. It may be the first time she has had an appointment that focuses more on health

---

FOCUS ON
National Health Goals

A number of National Health Goals speak directly to the importance of prenatal care. These are:

- Increase to at least 60% the proportion of primary care providers who provide age-appropriate preconception care and counseling.

- Increase to at least 90% the proportion of all pregnant women who receive prenatal care in the first trimester of pregnancy from a baseline of 76% (DHHS, 1991).

Nurses can be instrumental in helping the nation to achieve these goals by educating women and their families about the importance of prenatal care and by making sites of prenatal care receptive to women and families. Additional nursing research to investigate ways to promote prenatal care or to enlarge the scope of nursing involvement in prenatal care would be important to help the nation meet these goals.

promotion than on the diagnosis of disease. A woman may have a specific reason for coming to the first prenatal visit, e.g., to confirm the diagnosis of pregnancy (her agenda), which makes the visit an ideal time to impress on her that this is only the first of many health promotion visits necessary during pregnancy (your agenda). Hopefully, her motivation will allow you not only to provide the information, counseling, and care necessary during pregnancy but also to establish a positive pattern of health promotion behaviors in the woman and her family to use throughout their lives.

▨ NURSING PROCESS OVERVIEW
for the First Prenatal Visit

ASSESSMENT

The first prenatal visit is a time to establish a baseline of assessment data that will be relevant to planning health promotion information at the first and every subsequent visit. Explaining why specific assessment data are relevant to the pregnancy may be the first step in this process. For instance, when weighing the woman, discussing what routine weight gain is to be expected in the next couple of months supplies important information while demonstrating that weight measurement is an important routine procedure. Relating assessment measures and health promotion activities throughout the pregnancy this way keeps the woman and her family well informed and eager to comply with further health care recommendations. An important assessment measure for the first and subsequent visits is obtaining a health history to screen for the presence of teratogens and any problems the woman may be experiencing early in her pregnancy. Chapter 11 discusses assessment measures used later in pregnancy.

NURSING DIAGNOSIS

Nursing diagnoses appropriate to early pregnancy include:

- Health-seeking behaviors related to guidelines for nutrition or activity during pregnancy
- Knowledge deficit regarding the danger of alcohol ingestion during pregnancy related to youth and lifestyle
- High risk for injury to fetus related to current lifestyle

In addition, as the first prenatal visit serves to confirm pregnancy, nursing diagnoses may focus on the response of the woman and her family to that information, e.g.:

- Decisional conflict related to desire to be pregnant
- High risk for ineffective family coping related to confirmation of unwanted pregnancy

PLANNING

It is important that sufficient time be reserved for a first prenatal visit so the visit can be a thorough one, allowing for sufficient time to set realistic goals and outcome criteria with both the woman and the baby's father, if he desires. It is important to make sure that a woman leaving an initial prenatal visit schedules an appointment for a following visit. This may not occur to a woman whose mind is full of all the new things that are happening to her and her family, but establishing a pattern of regular appointments is crucial to providing adequate prenatal care. During a normal pregnancy, return appointments are usually scheduled every 4 weeks through the 32nd week of pregnancy, every 2 weeks through the 36th week, and then every week until birth. Women who are categorized as high risk are followed more closely.

IMPLEMENTATION

The purposes of prenatal care are to establish a baseline of present health, determine gestation age of the fetus, monitor fetal development, identify the woman at risk for complications, minimize the risk of possible complications by anticipating and preventing problems before they occur, and provide time for education about pregnancy and possible dangers (Kochenour, 1990).

Much time in a first visit is spent on client teaching regarding prenatal care. It may be helpful, in addition, to give the woman and her partner pamphlets or books that cover the same topics. After their initial surprise wears off, they may be better able to grasp the material and will enjoy reading it. Be sure you have read all the printed material you give families, to be certain the advice it contains is consistent with what you have already said and with the views of their primary care physician or nurse-midwife. A beautiful picture on the cover of a pamphlet does not ensure the quality of the advice inside. In addition, assure the woman that she may call the health care setting if she has any problems or questions during the coming month. Some women may feel reluctant to "bother" a health care provider outside of scheduled visits and will worry about a problem without calling unless you indicate beforehand that they are welcome to do this. Suggesting that women attend prenatal classes is another way that teaching can be effectively accomplished during pregnancy.

EVALUATION

Evaluation during the first prenatal visit should concentrate on the woman's initial progress toward understanding goals of care for pregnancy and assessing outcome criteria established for specific diagnoses. Examples of outcome criteria might be:

- Client states she feels well informed about the common discomforts of pregnancy.
- Client lists the dangers of alcohol consumption during pregnancy and states her intention not to consume any more alcohol during pregnancy.
- Couple telephones to indicate they have reached a decision about maintaining or discontinuing the pregnancy.

Health Promotion During Pregnancy

The Preconceptual Visit

Some women may have scheduled examinations with a physician or nurse-midwife before becoming pregnant to obtain authoritative reproductive life planning information, receive reassurance about fertility (as much as can be given based on a health history and a routine physical examination), and detect any problems that need correction. Many women choose to do this before getting married. At this visit, hemoglobin level and blood type (including Rh factor) can be determined; minor vaginal infections such as those arising from *Candida* can be corrected to help ensure fertility; and the woman can be counseled on the importance of a good protein diet and early prenatal care in the event she does become pregnant. More often, however, women arriving for their first prenatal visit will not have had a recent health care appointment oriented toward reproduction. Thus, the first prenatal visit usually must cover a wide range of assessment criteria.

Choosing a Health Care Provider for Pregnancy and Childbirth

Once a woman is or suspects that she may be pregnant, she chooses a primary health care provider to see her through the pregnancy and birth. Various options are a prenatal clinic; her HMO health care provider; or a nurse-midwife, obstetrician, or family practitioner in private practice. The important thing is that a woman initiates prenatal care early in pregnancy and continues with care throughout pregnancy (see the Focus on Nursing Research box).

Nursing can contribute a great deal to the success of prenatal care as listening, counseling, and teaching, three areas of nursing expertise, are important to successful prenatal care (Brown, 1992). Many clinics and

FOCUS ON NURSING RESEARCH

Why Do Women Delay Prenatal Care?

In the United States, as many as 5% of pregnant women wait until the third trimester of pregnancy to come for prenatal health care or else receive no prenatal care. As many as 25% of women of reproductive age have no health insurance for maternity care. Such women are more likely to obtain late care or to receive no prenatal care. To determine if there are other than financial reasons for delaying prenatal care, researchers in this study interviewed 144 women who came to a prenatal clinic for care only in their last trimester. Women's reasons for seeking care this late in pregnancy according to age group are shown below. As indicated from these results, need to conceal the pregnancy or social isolation are important factors that contribute to late seeking of prenatal care.

	Age <20 yr (N=64)	Age >20 yr (N=80)
1. Acceptance of pregnancy		
Didn't realize was pregnant	21.9	25.8
Had considered an abortion	7.8	11.3
Wanted to conceal pregnancy	26.6	1.3
Unwanted pregnancy	7.8	12.5
Psychological problems (depression, anger, anxiety related to pregnancy)	0.0	11.5
2. Utilization of prenatal care		
Afraid of hospitals/doctors	7.8	5.0
Motivation problem obtaining care (making and keeping appointments)	26.6	13.8
Didn't feel need for care	10.9	12.5
3. Financial issues		
Financial problem obtaining private care	10.9	12.5
Unaware of free prenatal care	7.8	6.3
4. Family responsibilities		
Conflict with father of baby	3.1	12.5
Babysitting problems	0.0	8.8
Other family crises	1.6	12.5
Geographic move	4.7	7.5

Young, C., McMahon, J., Bowman, V., & Thompson, D. (1990). Maternal reasons for delayed prenatal care. *Nursing Research, 38*, 243; with permission.

group practices provide an initial educational seminar for women in the early stages of their pregnancy, which is often led by a nurse or nurse practitioner. Box 10-1 summarizes ways to improve and individualize prenatal care.

1. Women should be seen within a week after they first call the health care setting. This initial contact can be done through a group orientation session, individually by a health team member, or, if risk status warrants, by a physician. Try and schedule further appointments at times convenient for support people as well as the client to encourage attendance.

2. Make waiting time at a visit educational time by providing educational materials such as pamphlets or videotapes in the waiting room.

3. Provide privacy for assessments such as blood pressure, weight, and urine checks rather than doing these in a public waiting room.

4. Women should feel responsible for their health record. If a woman's first language is not English, provision should be made to record pregnancy information so she can read it.

5. Be certain that pregnant women meet health care providers while fully clothed and upright, not naked and in a lithotomy position on an examining table.

6. Encourage family members and friends to come for prenatal care. Allow them to enter the examination room and participate in all aspects of care to the extent they and the client desire.

7. Schedule appointments to provide continuity of care. Be certain that women have a specific person's name as a phone contact for pregnancy-related questions. Without this, they tend not to call.

8. Educate pregnant women about care options and encourage them to participate in decision making about their care.

Health Assessment During the First Prenatal Visit

The major causes of death in childbirth today are ectopic pregnancy, embolism, intrapartum cardiac arrest, and hypertension (Syverson et al., 1991). An important focus of all prenatal visits, therefore, is to screen for indications that bleeding or circulatory impairment, infection, or hypertension of pregnancy (a unique phenomenon of pregnancy) are not occurring. The symptoms of these conditions, summarized in Table 10-1, are considered danger signs of pregnancy.

At the first visit, an extensive health history, a complete physical examination, including a pelvic examination, and blood and urine specimens for laboratory work are obtained. Although pelvic measurements may be obtained by a combination of x-ray pelvimetry and fetal ultrasound later in pregnancy, manual pelvic measurements can be taken to determine pelvic adequacy (Morgan & Thurnau, 1992).

Danger Signs

Assure the pregnant woman that you have no reason to think she is going to experience any serious problems, that you have every reason to believe she is going to have a normal, uncomplicated pregnancy (assuming that is true), but that, if any of the things described below should occur, she should inform a health care provider by telephone immediately. Be certain you give her an alternate telephone number to call if the health care facility is closed. Emphasize that if one of these danger signs should occur, it does not mean something bad has happened to her or her baby; they serve merely to alert all of you to the possibility that something may happen. It is important for her to report them immediately, so

Table 10-1. Danger Signs of Pregnancy

Sign	Possible Importance
Vaginal bleeding	Low implanted placenta, premature separation of placenta, premature birth
Persistent vomiting	Systemic infection, hyperemesis of pregnancy
Chills, fever	Intrauterine infection
Sudden escape of fluid from vagina	Premature rupture of membranes
Abdominal or chest pain	Ectopic pregnancy, premature separation of placenta, uterine rupture, pulmonary embolus
Swelling of face or fingers	Hypertension of pregnancy
Vision changes, flashes of light, diplopia, dimness or blurring of vision	Hypertension of pregnancy
Severe, continuous headache	Hypertension of pregnancy
Increase or decrease in intensity or frequency of fetal movements	Fetal distress

that they can be dealt with before something harmful occurs.

Vaginal Bleeding

A woman should report vaginal bleeding, no matter how slight, as some of the serious bleeding complications of pregnancy begin with *slight* spotting. If you are talking to the woman on the telephone, ask her how she discovered the spotting. If she discovered it on toilet paper following a bowel movement, she may be reporting spotting from hemorrhoids. When a woman has spotting, she needs referral to a physician or nurse-midwife for further evaluation. This clinician will either see her or offer her advice on the telephone, depending on the length of her pregnancy and the individual circumstances.

Persistent Vomiting

Once- or twice-daily vomiting is not uncommon during the first trimester of pregnancy. Persistent vomiting that occurs more often than this is not normal; vomiting that continues past the 12th week of pregnancy is also extended vomiting. Persistent or extended vomiting depletes the nutritional supply available to the fetus, and for this reason it is a danger to the fetus.

Chills and Fever

Chills and fever may be evidence of an intrauterine infection, which is a serious complication for both the woman and the fetus. They also may be symptoms of a relatively benign gastroenteritis. The woman herself, however, is not capable of making a definite determination as to the cause.

Sudden Escape of Fluid From the Vagina

When fluid is discharged suddenly from the vagina, it is evident that the membranes have ruptured: the fluid is amniotic fluid. Although this may be one of the first signs of labor, mother and fetus are now both threatened, because the uterine cavity is no longer sealed against infection. If the fetus is small and the head does not fit snugly into the cervix, the umbilical cord may prolapse with the membrane rupture and the fetal head may be compressed against the cord, creating an immediate and grave danger. Alerting you to any sudden escape of fluid is crucial so that a safe and controlled birth can be planned. Occasionally, a woman confuses stress incontinence (involuntary loss of urine on coughing or sneezing or lifting a heavy object) for this. Vaginal examination will reveal that the membranes are still intact.

Abdominal or Chest Pain

Abdominal pain at any time is a signal that something abnormal is occurring. Some women may think that it is normal in pregnancy because of the growing uterus, which is deflecting their other organs from the usual alignment. They are wrong: the uterus expands painlessly. Abdominal pain is announcing something else: a tubal (ectopic) pregnancy; a separation of the placenta; preterm labor; or something unrelated to the pregnancy but perhaps equally serious, such as appendicitis, ulcer, or pancreatitis. Chest pain may indicate a pulmonary embolus, a complication that follows thrombophlebitis.

Pregnancy-Induced Hypertension (PIH)

A number of symptoms signal developing pregnancy-induced hypertension:

1. Rapid weight gain (over 2 lb/wk in second trimester, 1 lb/wk in third trimester)
2. Swelling of the face or fingers
3. Flashes of light or dots before the eyes
4. Dimness or blurring of vision
5. Severe, continuous headache
6. Decrease in urine output

Some edema of the ankles during pregnancy is normal, particularly if it occurs after the woman has been on her feet for a long period of time. Swelling of the hands (ask if she has noticed that her rings are tight) or face (difficulty opening eyes in the morning due to edema of the eyelids) indicates edema too extensive to be normal. Visual disturbance or continuous headache may be a sign that cerebral edema is present or that hypertension is becoming acute. Be certain the woman is not reporting symptoms she had before she became pregnant. If she had the same visual difficulties and headaches before pregnancy as she is reporting now, she may need to see an ophthalmologist rather than her obstetrician for help with the problem. (See Chapter 15 for more on pregnancy-induced hypertension.)

Increase or Decrease in Fetal Movements

Since a fetus normally moves more or less the same amount every day, an unusual increase or decrease in movement suggests that the fetus is responding to oxygen want. Tests of fetal movement are discussed in Chapter 9.

The Initial Interview

Interviewing expectant women often elicits a welter of contradictions. Women are likely to want to talk about their past health and current pregnancy, so interviewing them should go smoothly and be productive. On the other hand, pregnancy symptoms are subtle, so a woman may not regard certain information as important and answer questions about these areas vaguely; perhaps she is unaware that she is the only person who knows the answers to a number of vital questions ("How do you feel about being pregnant?" or "What have you been taking for your morning nausea?"). Outside pressures, such as older children coming home from school or having to report for work may take a toll on interview effectiveness. Later in pregnancy, a woman may feel uncomfortable sitting for a long time.

Interviewing is best accomplished in a private, quiet setting. Trying to talk to a woman in a crowded hallway or a waiting room full of other patients is rarely effective; pregnancy is too private an affair to be discussed under these circumstances (Figure 10-1).

It is helpful if the receptionist in the clinic or office—or you, if you make the appointment—cautions a patient that the first visit will necessarily be a long one. This caution prevents the woman from trying to sandwich the visit in between other errands or from having to terminate the interview because of another appointment.

Be certain to determine what name a woman wants you to use when addressing her in a prenatal setting. If you are a student or a new graduate and the woman is older than you are, you should probably not call her by her first name. On the other hand, if the woman is close to your age, ask if she would like you to call her by her first name. This personal, concerned touch is appreciated by most women.

Make certain that a woman knows *your* name and understands your role correctly. If she views you as a secretary, she will be willing to discuss superficial facts (name, address, phone number, and the like) but will resist discussing more intimate things (her feelings toward this pregnancy, the difficulty she has reworking old fears, how scared she is about birth).

Because initial health history taking is time consuming, the use of forms the patient fills in herself is often advocated. Pregnancy is such a personal experience, however, that it seems callous to depersonalize it in this way. A better solution to the time problem is for nurses to practice good interviewing technique so they can se-

cure thorough and meaningful health histories within a time constraint. The rapport that is established by face-to-face interviewing gives a woman the feeling that she is more than just a file card. It may be as important in bringing her back to a health care setting as her desire to be assured that her pregnancy is progressing normally.

Components of the Health History

An initial interview has several purposes: to establish rapport, to gain information about the woman's physical and psychosocial health, and to obtain a basis for anticipatory guidance for the pregnancy. It is a good idea to establish a baseline health picture at the initial pregnancy visit: if on subsequent visits a symptom is mentioned, you can then check your records to see whether it is truly a new symptom. It may be that the woman is just becoming more aware of it. General interviewing techniques are discussed in Chapter 28. Included in the following section are those elements that are pertinent to a pregnancy history (see the Nursing Care Plan).

Demographic Data
Demographic data usually obtained are name, age, address, telephone number, religion, and health insurance information.

Chief Concern
The chief concern in a history is the reason the woman has come to the health care setting—in this instance, the fact she is or thinks she is pregnant. To explore the chief concern, you need to know whether or not a pregnancy was planned. "All pregnancies are a bit of a surprise. Is that how it was with this one?" is the kind of statement that will give you this information if you feel uncomfortable asking it directly. Other ways to word such a question would be, "Some couples plan on having children right away, some plan on waiting. How was it with you?"

Ask the date of the last menstrual period and whether the woman has had a pregnancy test or used a home test kit as yet. Ask if signs of early pregnancy, such as nausea, vomiting, breast changes, or fatigue are present. Are any discomforts of pregnancy, such as constipation, backache, or frequent urination present? Has she been exposed to any contagious diseases? Has she taken any medicine that might be harmful to fetal growth? Ask as well about danger signs of pregnancy, such as bleeding, continuous headache, visual disturbances, or swelling of the hands and face. If the woman said the pregnancy was not planned, explore far enough to learn if she has reached a point in pregnancy where she can say she wants this child growing inside her. A question such as, "Some women change their mind about wanting a baby once they realize they are pregnant; some don't. How has it been for you?" is the type of question that is effective for obtaining this type of in-

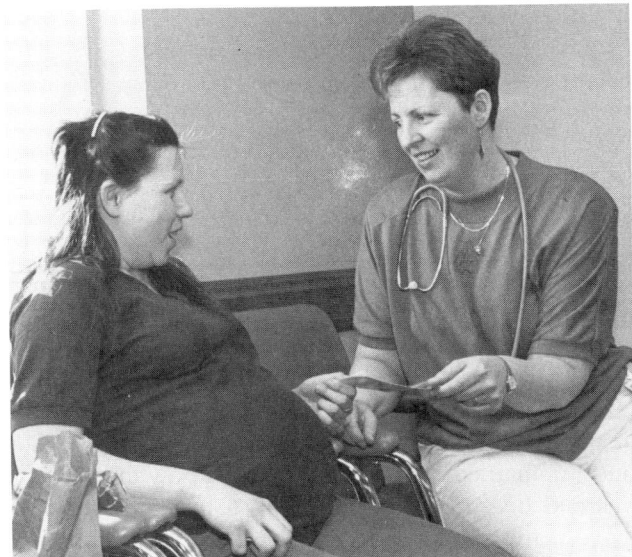

FIGURE 10-1
Interviewing at prenatal visits begins with establishing rapport, as the relationship will extend over months. (Courtesy of the Department of Medical Photography, Children's Hospital, Buffalo, NY.)

Jessine Wardall is a 22-year-old gravida 2, para 0 you see in a prenatal setting. She is 13 weeks pregnant. The following is a nursing care plan devised for her.

Health History

Chief Concern: "I think I'm pregnant."

History of Present Illness: Has had nausea and constipation for last 2 weeks. Last menstrual period 6 weeks ago. Feels "constantly fatigued."

Family Profile: Lives in apartment with husband (married 4 years). Works as part-time Spanish teacher for grade school children; husband is an accountant and also goes to night school for an M.B.A. Client states she has no regular exercise program. Smokes 2 packs cigarettes/day. No longer drinks alcohol since realizing she might be pregnant. States she can't imagine totally quitting smoking during pregnancy. Client states her husband could be free on Tuesdays for prenatal visits; would like appointments scheduled for then so he can come. Client wants to take her own blood pressure; states testing urine is "not her thing." Husband present at this visit and appears supportive. Learned blood pressure taking today.

Past Health History: Had mumps at 10 years; fell and dislocated knee at 16 years (in cast for 6 weeks). No apparent sequelae. No major illnesses; had surgery 4 months ago for endometriosis. Negative for sickle cell trait and disease.

Gynecologic History: Menarche at 10 years; duration of menstrual cycles: 30 days; flow for 5 days. Has a "lot of cramping" with menstrual flow.

Obstetric History: Had one previous pregnancy, ending in spontaneous abortion (no known cause) 2 years ago. Risk assessment by Goodwin scale is 2 (Para 0 = 1; spontaneous abortion = 1).

Family Medical History: No kidney, heart, lung disease, or cancer reported.

ROS: Negative except for symptoms of chief concern.

Physical Examination

General Appearance: Well appearing, slightly obese, black adult female.

Mental Status: Alert appearing; nervous mannerism of wringing hands.

Head and Neck: Normocephalic. Neck supple; full range of motion. One "shotty" lymph node present in anterior cervical chain.

Eyes: Red reflex present; extraocular muscles grossly intact. Conjunctivae pale.

Nose: Midline septum; mucus membrane slightly swollen and soft.

Mouth: One cavity present in left lower molar; gingiva slightly hypertrophied; pink and moist.

Chest: Lungs clear to auscultation and percussion; respiratory rate: 20/min. Heart rate: 80/min. No adventitious sounds heard.

Breasts: Tender to touch; no masses or nipple discharge present. Montgomery's tubercles prominent.

Abdomen: 8 cm-long surgical scar present on lower abdomen; some keloid growth present. Abdomen soft; liver palpated at 1 cm below costal margin. Femoral pulses equal bilaterally. Uterine height, not palpable above symphysis. Fetal heart rate by Doppler at 154/min.

(continued)

formation as it says either option is possible; you just want her to tell you which is happening.

Family Profile

In the past, the social history or family setting history (family profile) was left until the end of a health interview. It is now more often obtained at the beginning following the chief concern. Placing this early in the interview helps you to know the woman earlier and helps shape the nature and kind of later questions such as whether she is married. This is one of the hardest and sometimes most awkward questions to ask. You might simply ask, "Who else lives at home with you?" The married woman answers, "My husband and my 4-year-old son." The single woman answers, "No one," "My parents and my brothers and sisters," or "My boyfriend." If this method of discovering marital status makes you more comfortable than a direct question, use it. As a rule, most unmarried women want you to know they are unmarried because this can alert you that they may not have ready support people available. If a woman lives alone, whom does she approach for emotional support, advice, or help with problems?

It is good to know the size of the apartment or

Physical Examination (continued)

Genitalia: Pubic hair female distribution; slight white vaginal discharge present. Pelvic exam performed by nurse-midwife. Reported cervix as clean and slightly soft, uterus enlarged and soft, vagina purple-hued. Culture taken for gonorrhea and chlamydia; Pap smear obtained.

Extremities: Full range of motion; no varicosities present.

Back: No tenderness of joints; vertebrae midline and straight.

Neurologic: Biceps, triceps, patellar, and Achilles reflexes 2+.

Nursing Diagnosis: Health-seeking behaviors related to prenatal care.

Defining Characteristic: Client voices she intends to continue prenatal care.

Goal: Client will participate in family-centered prenatal care for duration of pregnancy.

Outcome Criteria: Client and husband both attend all prenatal care appointments.

Nursing Orders	**Rationale**
1. Mark chart for Tuesday appointments.	1. Scheduling appointments for a day preferred by client should increase compliance.
2. Husband to attend all prenatal visits as support person.	2. Support people are important in a crisis situation.
3. Mark for self-participation at visits.	3. Greater participation in prenatal care can offer a greater sense of control.
4. Blood drawn for hemoglobin, hematocrit, rubella titer, HBsAg, and serum human chorionic gonadotropin (HCG) analysis.	4. These tests confirm general health and confirm pregnancy.
5. Urine obtained by clean-catch for routine urinalysis. Negative for protein and glucose.	5. These tests are performed to rule out potential problems: urinary tract infection can lead to spontaneous abortion; protein in urine could signify hypertension of pregnancy; glucose could signify gestational diabetes.
6. Inform client to telephone tomorrow to ask about HCG report. If test is positive, schedule for return visit for pregnancy instruction and counseling.	6. Early diagnosis can lead to improved lifestyle and opportunities for health education.
7. If pregnancy test is negative, advise as indicated according to nurse-midwife's further instructions.	7. Client wants to be pregnant so this would be a disappointing event for her.

house in which a woman lives. If she is expecting a baby, you are going to be talking to her in the coming months about a bedroom or space for the baby's bed. It is important to know whether the essential rooms are on the ground floor or upstairs in case she is restricted from climbing stairs more than once or twice a day during the last part of pregnancy or following birth.

Before you can begin to offer a woman any more than stereotyped health care instruction, it is important to know her and her husband's or sexual partner's age (additional testing such as genetic screening may be necessary if her age is over 35), their educational levels (of-

fers an estimation of how well they will be able to understand teaching), and occupation (does the woman's involve heavy lifting, long hours of standing in one position, handling of a toxic substance?) (Bernhardt, 1990).

Situations such as changing status from independence to dependence because of stopping work, chronic illness at home, the death of a significant person during pregnancy, the infidelity of a husband, geographical moves, financial hardship, or lack of support people are representative of situations that can be injurious to a woman's ability to accept her pregnancy and child. No one in the health care setting will be aware of these potentially harmful situations if you do not ask the questions about family profile that expose them.

Past Medical History

Questions about the past medical history are an important part of an interview because a past condition may become active during or immediately following pregnancy. Representative diseases which can pose potential difficulty during pregnancy are kidney disease, heart disease (coarctation of the aorta and rheumatic fever cause problems most often), hypertension, sexually transmitted disease (including hepatitis B and HIV), diabetes, thyroid disease, recurrent convulsions, gallbladder disease, urinary tract infections, varicosities, phenylketonuria, tuberculosis, and asthma. It is vital to find out whether a woman had childhood diseases, such as mumps (epidemic parotitis), measles (rubeola), German measles (rubella), or poliomyelitis. From this information you can reach an estimate of the antibody protection she has against these diseases if she is exposed to them during her pregnancy. If pregnant, she can be immunized against poliomyelitis by the Salk (killed virus) vaccine. She *cannot* be immunized against the others, because the vaccines contain live viruses, as does the oral Sabin poliomyelitis vaccine. Live virus vaccines could be harmful to the fetus ("Immunization During Pregnancy," 1993).

Ask as well about any allergies including any drug sensitivities, so that a prescription that might harm her can be avoided during pregnancy. As a rule, women with allergies of any magnitude should probably breastfeed rather than bottle-feed their infants in order to avoid possible milk allergy in the infant. This choice is the woman's, not yours to make; however, you will need the information to counsel her appropriately.

Any past surgical procedures are also important as adhesions resulting from past abdominal surgery could cause difficulty with the growth of the uterus.

Family History

A family history documents illnesses that occur frequently in the family and helps to identify potential problems in the mother during pregnancy or in the infant at birth. Ask specifically about cardiovascular and renal disease, mental retardation, blood disorders, or any known inherited disease or congenital anomalies.

Social Profile

A social profile provides information on the woman's lifestyle. Ask how much she exercises weekly to see if her routine pattern will be consistent with a recommended pregnancy level. Ask if she hikes or camps to determine exposure to Lyme disease (Williams & Strobino, 1990). Ask about hobbies; working with lead-based glazes and ceramics, for example, might not be wise during pregnancy.

Because of the known deleterious effect of smoking on the growth of a fetus, a woman's smoking history (if any) should be obtained. Excessive alcohol intake may lead to poor nutrition or be directly responsible for fetal alcohol syndrome in the baby, so ask about alcohol consumption. If a woman answers vaguely, "I drink socially," or "I only smoke occasionally," ask her *exactly* what she means so you can judge accurately the frequency of these events.

Pregnant women are vulnerable to spouse abuse (Campbell et al., 1992). Ask if this is a potential or a real problem. Ask whether a woman takes any medication, prescribed or over the counter, as the effect of these on a growing fetus will have to be evaluated. Even seemingly innocent medications for simple conditions can be detrimental during pregnancy. Isotretinoin (Acutane), a vitamin A preparation taken for acne, for example, is associated with spontaneous abortion and congenital anomalies. Include as well the use of recreational drugs, such as marijuana or cocaine, as these also can be deleterious to fetal growth. Include intravenous drug use to investigate the possibility of exposure to HIV or hepatitis B, which can be spread this way. Although this is a type of information not readily revealed by people, most women will answer these questions honestly during pregnancy because they are concerned about protecting the health of the fetus.

Gynecologic History

Table 10-2 lists common gynecologic illnesses and their possible significance in pregnancy. When most women had children early in their childbearing years, the number of reproductive tract or women's health problems, such as breast disease, that they had experienced before pregnancy were few. Today, when women often delay conception of their first child past 30 years of age, it is not unusual to discover a woman who has had a problem with her reproductive tract or breast health.

A woman's past experience with her reproductive system may have some influence on how well she accepts a pregnancy. For a history, you need to know her age of menarche (first menstrual period) and how well she was prepared for it as a normal part of being a mature woman. Ask the interval, duration, and amount of menstrual flow. Does she have discomfort? If she describes menstrual cramps as "horrible" and wonders how she "lives through them some months," imagine what her concept of labor, which is usually described as worse than these, must be like. If this is so, she may need more counseling than average as pregnancy progresses to be prepared for labor. Some women who have extreme dysmenorrhea are looking forward to pregnancy as 9 months without discomfort; they may need counseling in the postpartal period about active ways to relieve menstrual discomfort (see Chapter 47).

Ask if the woman does a monthly breast and/or perineum examination (see Chapter 28 for these techniques). Be certain to ask about past surgery. If a

Table 10-2. *Gynecologic Disorders*

Disorder	Possible Symptoms	Significance and Suggested Therapy
Vulva		
Cysts of Skene's or Bartholin's glands	Asymptomatic swelling at the sides of the urinary meatus or vestibule	Such cysts are surgically incised to prevent blockage and infection of the gland.
Condylomata acuminata	Cauliflower-like lesion on vulva	Tends to occur in women with chronic vaginitis. Caused by the epidermatrophic virus that causes common warts. Removed by cryocautery or knife excision.
Lichen sclerosus	Whitish papules on the vulva; asymptomatic	No need for removal; the area is biopsied because leukoplakia, a potentially cancerous condition, has an almost identical appearance.
Leukoplakia	Thick, gray, patchy epithelium that cracks and infects easily, accompanied by itching and pain	Possibly a premalignant state. Therapy involves systemic antibiotics and frequent return visits to health care personnel (every 6 months) for observation to detect any changes suggestive of carcinoma.
Carcinoma of the vulva	A shallow vulvar ulcer that does not heal	Occurs most often in postmenopausal women; represents only 3% to 4% of all reproductive tract cancer in women. Therapy is vulvectomy—vagina is left intact, and sexual relations and pregnancy with cesarean birth to prevent tearing of fibrotic vulvar tissue may be possible.
Vagina and Cervix		
Adenosis	Asymptomatic vaginal cysts	Caused by diethylstilbestrol (DES) administration while in utero. Columnar rather than squamous epithelium is present on vaginal walls. Has the potential for becoming malignant (clear cell adenocarcinoma). If adenosis is present, an examination 2 or 3 times a year with a Pap test and Lugol's staining is necessary and the woman should not use estrogen sources such as oral contraceptives. If adenocarcinoma occurs, local destruction of atypical cells can be achieved by excision, cautery, or cryosurgery.
Cervical polyp	Red, vascular, protruding pedunculated tissue that bleeds readily with trauma	A polyp may be discovered because of vaginal spotting on coitus, tampon insertion, or vaginal examination. Removed vaginally by excision. Often associated with chronic cervical inflammation.
Cervicitis (erosion)	Reddened cervical tissue with a whitish exudate	Douching with a vinegar solution aids healing. May be treated with cryosurgery if extensive.
Nabothian cyst	Clear shining circles on cervix from blocked ducts of glands	No therapy necessary.
Cervical carcinoma	Postcoital spotting, unexplained vaginal discharge, or vaginal spotting between menstrual periods	Most frequent type of reproductive tract malignancy. High-risk factors are coitus with multiple partners or uncircumcised males, herpes type II infections, or DES during pregnancy. Diagnosed by Pap test or colposcopy. Therapy is conization, radiation, or surgical excision. Pregnancy is possible following cervical carcinoma; cesarean birth may be necessary because of fibrotic cervical tissue.
Ovaries		
Endometrial cyst	Chocolate-brown colored cyst on tender enlarged ovary; may cause acute pain if rupture occurs	Caused by endometriosis; occurs in women aged 20 to 40 years. Therapy is surgical excision; ovary may or may not be removed depending on extent of cyst.
Follicular cyst	Amenorrhea and possibly dyspareunia; ovary is tender and enlarged	Follicular cysts regress after 1–2 months, a low-dose oral contraceptive may be prescribed for 6–12 weeks to suppress ovarian activity; estrogen may be continued for 6 months.
Polycystic disease	Multiple follicular cysts of both ovaries are present	There is excess adrenal supply of estrogen leading to inhibition of follicle-stimulating hormone and anovulation. Clomiphene citrate therapy to induce ovulation or wedge resection of the ovaries is used as therapy.
Corpus luteum cyst	Delayed menstrual flow followed by prolonged bleeding; ovary is enlarged and tender	A corpus luteum has persisted rather than atrophied. Most regress in about 2 months; a low-dose oral contraceptive may be prescribed for 6 weeks to suppress ovarian activity.

(continued)

Table 10-2. *(Continued)*

Disorder	Possible Symptoms	Significance and Suggested Therapy
Dermoid cyst	Asymptomatic; ovary is enlarged on examination	Arises from embryonic tissue; may contain hair, cartilage, and fat. Most common ovarian tumor of childhood; also occurs at 30–50 years. Therapy is surgical resection.
Serous cystadenoma	Occurs bilaterally; asymptomatic except for signs of pelvic pressure	Most common type of benign ovarian cyst; malignancy rate is high: 20% to 30%. Therapy is surgical resection.
Carcinoma	Asymptomatic	Arises from epithelial tissue most often in women over 50 years of age. Tendency may be inherited; environmental contamination may play a role in development. Therapy is hysterectomy and salpingo-oophorectomy.
Uterus		
Endometrial polyp	Intermenstrual bleeding	Removed by dilatation and curettage.
Leiomyomas (fibroids)	Asymptomatic or with increased menstrual flow	Formed of muscle and fibrous connective tissue in response to estrogen stimulation. May increase in size during pregnancy; may cause interference with cervical dilatation and result in postpartal hemorrhage. Stress to the myometrium by uterine contractions may be the original cause of formation. Therapy is surgical resection (myomectomy) or hysterectomy if childbearing is complete.
Endometrial carcinoma	Vaginal bleeding between menstrual periods	Diagnosis is by endometrial washing, not Pap test. Therapy is hysterectomy.
Uterine prolapse	Vaginal pressure and low back pain	The uterus has descended into the vagina due to overstretching of uterine supports and trauma to the levator ani muscle. Occurs most often in women who had insufficient prenatal care, birth of a large infant, a prolonged second stage of labor, bearing-down efforts or extraction of a baby before full dilatation, instrument delivery, and poor healing of perineal tissue postpartally. Therapy is surgery to repair uterine supports or placement of a pessary, a plastic uterine support. Women with pessaries in place need to return for a pelvic examination every 3 months to have the pessary removed, cleaned, and replaced and the vagina inspected; otherwise, vaginal infection or erosion of the vaginal walls can result.

woman has had a tubal operation, such as surgery for an ectopic pregnancy, the risk of another tubal pregnancy statistically becomes higher. If she has had uterine surgery, her child may have to be delivered by cesarean birth rather than vaginally because her uterus may not be able to stand the strain of labor contractions. If she has had frequent dilatation and curettage of the uterus, her cervix may be incompetent or unable to remain closed for 9 months; this could lead to premature birth unless she has a surgical procedure (cerclage) for this (see Chapter 15). Ask what reproductive planning methods, if any, the woman has been using. Occasionally, a woman becomes pregnant with an intrauterine device in place. It will have to be removed to prevent infection during pregnancy. If the woman did not realize she was pregnant, she may have continued to take an oral contraceptive for some time into the pregnancy. Document if this occurred. Be certain to include a sexual history (number of sexual partners and whether or not she adheres to "safer sex" practices).

A problem that should also be included as part of a woman's gynecologic history is stress incontinence, which is incontinence of urine on laughing, coughing, deep inspiration, jogging, or running (the diaphragm descends with these actions, increasing abdominal pressure, which increases bladder tension and causes emptying). This problem happens so often in some women that they must continually wear a sanitary pad or plastic-lined underpants. If the problem occurs often, the woman's vulva may be chronically irritated and inflamed. Stress incontinence can be intensified during pregnancy from the increasing abdominal pressure.

Stress incontinence occurs from lack of strength in the perineal muscles and bladder supports. It is associated with difficult births, the birth of large infants, grand multiparity, and instrument deliveries. Some women accept stress incontinence as a normal consequence of childbearing and so do not report it at health care assessments unless asked.

Stress incontinence may be prevented and relieved to some degree by strengthening perineal muscles with the use of Kegel exercises (periodic tightening of the perineal muscles; see Chapter 11). Surgical correction can be performed to fix the urethra to the fascia of the rectus muscle of the abdomen following a pregnancy. This offers support to the neck of the bladder and decreases the tendency for easy emptying on abdominal pressure.

Obstetric History

Do not assume that the current pregnancy is the first pregnancy simply because a woman is very young or says she has only recently been married. Ask. Be certain not only to obtain the facts such as date and sex of the child of past pregnancies but to elicit the woman's subjective feelings about these pregnancies as well. Document the child's sex and place and date of birth for each previous pregnancy. It is good to review the pregnancy briefly. Was it planned? Did she have any complications, such as spotting, swelling of her hands or feet, falls, or surgery? Did she take any medication? Did she receive prenatal care? What was the duration of gestation? What was the duration of labor? Was labor what she expected? Worse? Better? What was the type of birth? What was the type of anesthetic used (if any)? What was the infant's birth weight? What was the condition of the infant at birth? Did the infant cry right away? Some mothers know the infant's Apgar score and can tell you this. Also inquire about the need for special equipment, whether the baby was discharged from the health care setting with her, and the child's present state of health. What was the outcome of the pregnancy for her? Did she have stitches following birth? Did she have any complications, such as excess bleeding or infection?

Ask about any previous miscarriages or abortions. Did she have any complications during or following them? **Abortion** is the medical term for any pregnancy terminated before the age of viability. The **age of viability** is the earliest age at which fetuses could survive if they were born at that time, generally accepted as 20 to 24 weeks, or fetuses weighing more than 400 g. Although you chart both induced and spontaneous pregnancy terminations in the same way, women appreciate your separating them into *miscarriage* (a spontaneous abortion) and *abortion* (used in its more limited meaning of induced, therapeutic, or planned termination of pregnancy) when you are talking to them. If the woman's blood type is Rh negative, ask if she received RhIG (RhoGAM) after miscarriages or abortions or previous births so you will know whether Rh sensitization could have occurred. Ask if she had a blood transfusion to establish possible risk of hepatitis B or HIV exposure or Rh sensitization.

After a history of previous pregnancies is obtained, determine a woman's status with respect to the number of times she has been pregnant, including the present pregnancy (**gravida**), and the number of children above the age of viability she has previously delivered (**para**).

Table 10-3 provides an explanation of these terms. For example, a woman who has had two previous pregnancies, has delivered two term children, and is again pregnant is gravida III, para 2. A woman who has had two abortions at 12 weeks (under the age of viability) and is again pregnant is a gravida III, para 0.

A more comprehensive system for classifying pregnancy status (GTPAL or GTPALM) provides greater detail on the pregnancy history. By this system the gravida classification remains the same, but para is broken down into:

T: The number of full-term infants born (infants born at 37 weeks or after).

P: The number of preterm infants born (infants born before 37 weeks).

A: The number of spontaneous or induced abortions.

L: The number of living children.

M: Multiple pregnancies.

Using this system, the woman in the first example above would be gravida 3, para 20020 (320020).

A pregnant woman who had the following past history—a boy born at 39 weeks gestation, now alive and well; a girl born at 40 weeks gestation, now alive and well; a girl born at 33 weeks gestation, now alive and well—would have her pregnancy information summarized as follows: gravida 4; para 21030 (421030).

Day History

Information about a woman's current nutrition, elimination, sleep, recreation, and interpersonal interactions can be elicited best not by direct questions but by asking the woman to describe a typical day of her life. If any of this information is not reported spontaneously as a woman describes her day, ask for additional details. A "24-hour recall" this way is especially helpful in obtaining accurate

Table 10-3. *Terms Related to Pregnancy Status*

Term	Definition
Para	A baby born past a point of viability
Gravida	A pregnant woman
Primigravida	A woman who is pregnant for the 1st time.
Primipara	A woman who has delivered 1 child past age of viability. In common usage, this is used to mean a woman who is pregnant for the 1st time.
Multigravida	A woman who has been pregnant previously
Multipara	A woman who has delivered 1 or more children previously
Nulligravida	A woman who has never been pregnant

nutrition information as the woman tells you what she actually ate, not what she knows she should have eaten.

Review of Systems

A review of systems takes about 10 minutes to obtain and completes subjective information. You will be amazed at the results obtained, however, by telling a woman you are going to start at the top of her head and go through to her toes, asking about body parts or systems and any diseases she has had. This method causes her to recall diseases she forgot to mention earlier, diseases that are important to your history taking.

The following body systems and conditions should constitute the minimum covered in a review of systems for a first prenatal visit:

1. *Head:* Headache? Head injury? Seizures? Dizziness? Syncope?
2. *Eyes:* Vision? Glasses needed? Diplopia? Infection? Glaucoma? Cataract? Pain? Recent changes?
3. *Ears:* Infection? Discharge? Earache? Hearing loss? Tinnitus? Vertigo?
4. *Nose:* Epistaxis (nose bleeding)? Discharge? How many colds a year? Allergy? Postnasal drainage? Sinus pain?
5. *Mouth and pharynx:* Dentures? Condition of teeth? Toothaches? Any bleeding of gums? Hoarseness? Difficulty in swallowing? Tonsillectomy?
6. *Neck:* Stiffness? Masses?
7. *Breasts:* Lumps? Secretion? Pain? Tenderness? Does she know how to do a breast self-examination? Does she do this monthly?
8. *Respiratory system:* Cough? Wheezing? Asthma? Shortness of breath? Pain? Serious chest illness, such as tuberculosis or pneumonia?
9. *Cardiovascular system:* History of heart murmur? Rheumatic fever or Kawasaki Disease? Hypertension? Any pain? Palpitations? Any heart disease? Anemia? Does she know her blood pressure? What was her prepregnancy weight? Has she ever had a blood transfusion?
10. *Gastrointestinal system:* Vomiting? Diarrhea? Constipation? Change in bowel habits? Rectal pruritus? Hemorrhoids? Pain? Ulcer? Gallbladder disease? Hepatitis? Appendicitis?
11. *Genitourinary system:* Infection? Hematuria? Frequent urination? Sexually transmitted disease? Pelvic inflammatory disease? Hepatitis B? HIV?
12. *Extremities:* Varicose veins? Pain or stiffness of joints? Any fractures or dislocations?
13. *Skin:* Any rashes? Acne? Psoriasis?

Conclusion

End an interview by asking if there is something you have not covered that the woman wants to discuss. This gives her one more chance to verbalize any questions she has about this new life experience.

The Father's or Support Person's Role

More and more fathers accompany women for prenatal care today. Young children may accompany their mothers on these visits as well. If family members are present, should they be included in an initial interview? As a whole, interviewing is most effective if it is a one-to-one interaction. A woman may be unwilling to mention certain of her concerns with her family present for fear of worrying them. A husband may not be the father of her child, and she may be unable to voice her concern over this fact or alert you to the possibility she is worried about blood incompatibility because another man is the father.

If childbearing is a family affair, however, it is just as important to determine the father's degree of acceptance of the pregnancy and of being a father as it is to establish how far the woman has come in the process of acceptance. Including siblings in a prenatal visit is an opportune way to involve them with the pregnancy planning and coming baby. Interviewing the woman alone and then inviting the support person and family to join her while you talk about pregnancy symptoms with them as a couple is a good solution (Figure 10-2). Providing some private interview time with a husband allows him to express worries he is reluctant to voice in front of his wife for fear of concerning or hurting her. The main areas you should investigate with the father are his current health, his feelings and concerns about the pregnancy, and his knowledge of pregnancy and childbirth. If the woman wishes, he can accompany her for the physical examination, and following the confirmation of pregnancy, he should be present when health care information is given (see the Focus on Family Teaching box).

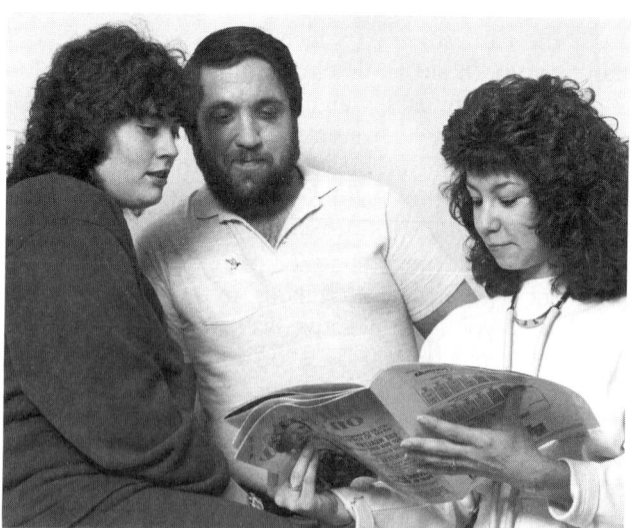

FIGURE 10-2

Include support people in a prenatal visit when appropriate or desired so that visits are family centered. Here a husband and wife both listen to a description of fetal growth. (Courtesy of the Department of Medical Photography, Children's Hospital, Buffalo, NY.)

Q. I had a normal pregnancy with my first child. Why do I need close prenatal supervision for a second pregnancy? Won't this one be normal as well?

A. Although you have every reason to believe a second pregnancy will also be normal, prenatal care is still important as it will detect any problem when it is still small enough to be solved. Infant mortality is significantly reduced in women who attend prenatal care.

Q. I want my husband to come for prenatal visits with me. How can he participate more so he's more interested in doing this?

A. Prenatal care is best if it's a shared event. Some suggestions for doing this are:

- Ask for appointments to be scheduled at a time that is convenient for both of you.

- A prenatal visit can be lengthy. Be certain he reserves enough time so the visit doesn't become more of an inconvenience than an enjoyable event.

- Ask him to accompany you into the examining room at visits so he can share progress or decisions.

- Be certain he listens to the fetal heart at visits as soon as this can be heard.

- If a sonogram is scheduled, ask him to view this with you (it's an exciting moment to see your fetus moving).

Physical Examination

Following the health history, the woman will be given a physical examination. She should undress, put on a gown, and empty her bladder. Emptying the bladder will make the pelvic examination more comfortable for her, allow for easier identification of pelvic organs, and provide urine for laboratory testing. This urine should be obtained by a clean-catch technique so it can be examined for bacteriuria. Procedure 10-1 reviews instructions for women on how to do this. The urine is immediately tested for glucose, protein, and ketones by a dipstick.

A physical examination at a first prenatal visit should include inspection of body systems, with particular emphasis on changes that occur with pregnancy or could signal a developing pregnancy problem. General techniques of physical examination are discussed in Chapter 28.

Baseline Height/Weight and Vital Sign Measurement

The woman is weighed and her height is measured at a first prenatal visit to establish a baseline for future comparison. When weighing, be certain to convey an air of "accuracy is what counts," instead of "minimal weight gain is important," so the woman feels free to gain 25 to 30 lb during pregnancy. Record this assessment with her prepregnancy weight to determine how much weight she has already gained or lost (Figure 10-3).

Blood pressure, respiration rate, and pulse rate should also be measured for baseline information. A sudden increase in blood pressure, like a sudden weight gain, is a danger sign of hypertension of pregnancy; a sudden increase in pulse or respirations may suggest

---

NURSING PROCEDURE 10-1
Instructions to Help a Woman Obtain a Clean-Catch Urine Specimen

Plan	*Principle*
1. Wash your hands	1. Prevent spread of microorganisms.
2. From the commercial clean-catch urine specimen kit, moisten 3 cotton balls in antiseptic solution. Cleanse your urinary meatus with the cotton balls (washing front to back, using each cotton ball for only 1 stroke, then discarding it).	2. Cleansing front to back prevents bringing rectal contamination forward.
3. Begin to void, and dip the sterile specimen container into the urine stream to obtain a midstream urine specimen. After 10–20 mL is obtained in specimen cup, finish voiding in toilet.	3. The flow of urine washes away bacteria from urinary meatus.
4. Avoid touching inside of container or cap.	4. Prevents contamination.
5. Cap the specimen container and bring to nursing desk. If you have any pain on urination, mention this to the nurse.	5. Pain on urination is a symptom of urinary tract infection.

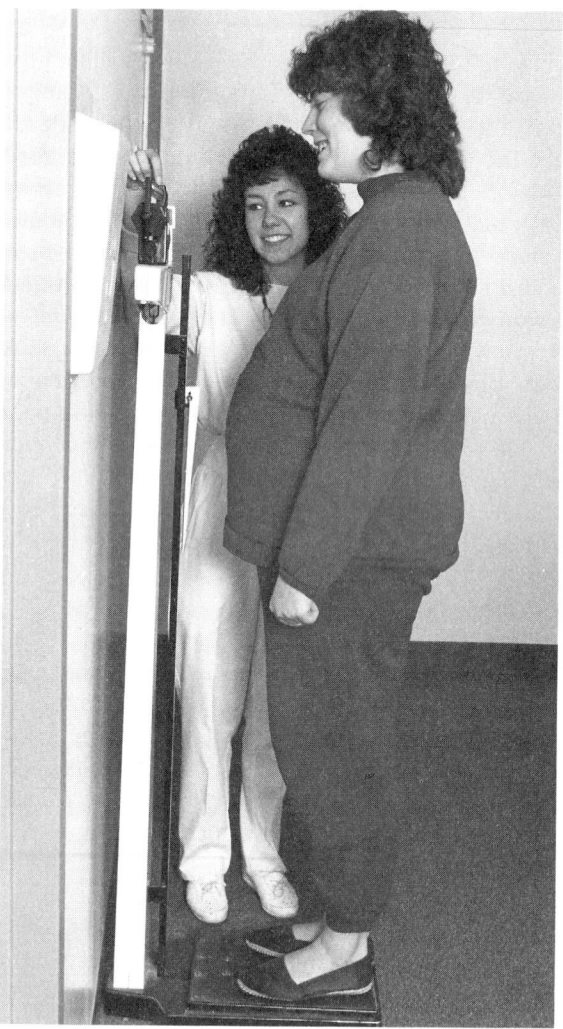

FIGURE 10-3
A woman helps to weigh herself at a prenatal visit. (Courtesy of the Department of Medical Photography, Children's Hospital, Buffalo, NY.)

bleeding, which is equally serious. A support person or the woman herself can be taught the technique of blood pressure recording if close monitoring will be warranted during pregnancy.

Assessment of Systems

General Appearance and Mental Status. Physical examination always begins with inspection of general appearance to form a general impression of the woman's health and well being. General appearance is an important assessment because people suggest how they feel about themselves by the manner in which they dress, the way they speak, and the body posture they assume. Inspect especially for signs that suggest fatigue or depression (careless hygiene, unwashed hair, inappropriate or soiled clothing, sad facial expression).

Remove and replace, as necessary, any bandages and other dressings a woman has in place that could

hide important findings. A growing problem—or perhaps one receiving increased recognition—is that of the battered woman. Ask how any skin abnormality, such as an ecchymotic area, occurred. Most marks from battering occur on the face, the ulnar surfaces of the forearms (from a woman raising her arms to defend herself), the abdomen or buttocks (from being kicked), or the upper arms (from being grabbed and held forcefully) (Noel & Yam, 1992).

Head and Scalp. Examine the head for symmetry, normal contour, and tenderness; the hair for presence, distribution, thickness, excessive dryness or oiliness, or the use of hair dye (hair dye may be carcinogenic over an extended period of time). Hair growth speeds up during pregnancy as a result of the overall increased metabolic rate. Dryness or sparseness of hair suggests poor nutrition; excessive oiliness suggests fatigue to the extent that the woman has not felt well enough to wash it recently. Urge women during pregnancy to let some other task go and save energy for self-care so they can continue to feel good about themselves. Dandruff shampoos may be used during pregnancy as they are not absorbed. Look for chloasma (extra pigment on the face) which can accompany pregnancy.

Eyes. Hypertension of pregnancy may be manifested by eye symptoms of edema in the eyelids, spots before the eyes, or diplopia (double vision). If an ophthalmoscopic examination is done, the optic disc will be swollen from edema in the presence of hypertension. Help pregnant women to recognize symptoms of poor vision as danger signs of pregnancy that they should not delay reporting rather than as symptoms unrelated to pregnancy. Caution them if they do close desk work to take a break every hour so sensations of eyestrain are not confused with actual danger signs.

Nose. The high level of estrogen that occurs with pregnancy causes nasal congestion or the appearance of swollen nasal membranes. Teach pregnant women that even topical medicine such as nose drops are absorbed to some degree; a woman should avoid taking even these during pregnancy without her physician's or nurse-midwife's knowledge and consent.

Ears. The nasal stuffiness that accompanies pregnancy may lead to blocked eustachian tubes and therefore a feeling of "fullness" or dampening of sound during early pregnancy. This disappears as the body better adjusts to the new estrogen level. Normal hearing level and normal tympanic landmarks should be present.

Sinuses. Sinuses should feel nontender. Establishing that tenderness over sinuses does not exist helps to evaluate headache during pregnancy (a danger sign until ruled otherwise).

Mouth, Teeth, and Throat. The pregnant woman is prone to vitamin deficiency because of the rapid growth of the fetus; assess carefully for cracked corners of the mouth that would reveal this. Assess carefully for pinpoint lesions with an erythematous base on the lips; these suggest a herpes infection (a herpes lesion on the gumline is more often a shallow ulcer). Because newborns are susceptible to herpes infection, lesions present at birth may necessitate limit in her contact with the newborn. Gingiva (gums) may be hypertrophied due to estrogen stimulation during pregnancy. They should not appear reddened, only swollen, and may be slightly tender to touch.

Teach all women not to neglect good dental hygiene or yearly dental supervision visits. Pregnant women should maintain thorough toothbrushing at least once a day (some stop thorough brushing because they notice slight blood-tinged mucus due to gingiva hypertrophy).

If many dental caries are obvious, the woman should be referred to a dentist or dental clinic. Carious teeth are a source of infection and should be treated before abscesses develop and cause more serious problems. Contrary to what many women believe, dental x-rays *can* be taken during pregnancy as long as the woman reminds her dentist that she is pregnant and needs a lead apron. No extensive dental work should be done during pregnancy without approval from the woman's primary care provider.

Neck. Slight thyroid hypertrophy may occur with pregnancy as the overall metabolic rate is increased. Encourage a woman to continue to use iodine salt during pregnancy and to eat seafood at least once weekly to supply enough iodine for thyroxine production with this increased rate. Without this precaution, some women will view iodine as an unnecessary additive and discontinue using it during pregnancy.

Lymph Nodes. No palpable lymph nodes should be present. Pregnant women may develop an increased number of upper respiratory infections because of reduced immunologic resistance and this could result in enlarged cervical lymph nodes. If they develop a tooth abscess from bacterial growth under hypertrophied gingival tissue this could lead to palpable submaxillary lymph nodes.

Breasts. As pregnancy begins, the breast areola darkens, Montgomery's tubercles become prominent, size increases, and the tone firms. A secondary areola may develop surrounding the natural one; blue streaking of veins becomes prominent. Colostrum may be expelled from the nipples as early as the 16th week of pregnancy. If a supernumerary nipple is present, this also may become darker, and the woman may need assurance that this is not a growing mole but a normal pregnancy change. All women should be instructed on monthly breast self-examination. The day after the end of each monthly menstrual flow is a good marking point for the nonpregnant woman to use; this is also a time when hormonal influences on breast tissue are at a low ebb, so breast tissue is normally not swollen or tender and does not cause discomfort. A pregnant woman should specify a certain day each month (the first day, the last day) for breast self-examination (see Figure 28-20, Chapter 28). Alert women that 90% of breast lesions are not breast cancer, so if they do discover a lesion on self-examination, they will report it promptly (Simpson, 1992). Otherwise, they might become so fearful of cancer that they are "frozen" into immobility. Benign breast lesions that might be discovered on physical examination are discussed in Chapter 47.

Heart. Heart rate should be 70 to 80 beats per minute; no accessory sounds should be present. It may be difficult to hear the heart beat during pregnancy because of the increase in breast size. An occasional woman will develop an innocent (functional) heart murmur during pregnancy because of the excess amount of blood her heart processes. If this occurs, she needs referral for further investigation to be certain only a physiologic change of pregnancy and not a previously undetected heart condition is involved. Many women notice palpitation (their heart skipping a beat) during pregnancy, especially when lying supine. Teach pregnant women always to rest or sleep on their side (left side is best) to help avoid this problem.

Lungs. Assess respiratory rate and rhythm. Although lung tissue assumes a more horizontal position during pregnancy, vital capacity is not reduced. Late in pregnancy, diaphragmatic excursion (diaphragm movement) is lessened because the diaphragm cannot push as low as a result of the distended uterus.

Back. Assess the spine for any abnormal curve that would suggest scoliosis. Young women with scoliosis may need a referral to their orthopedist during pregnancy to be certain that their condition is not worsening. The lumbar curve in many pregnant women is accentuated on standing so that they can maintain body posture in the face of increasing abdominal size. This response may cause back pain during pregnancy.

Rectum. Assess the rectum closely for hemorrhoidal tissue, which is apt to occur in a pregnant woman from pelvic pressure preventing venous return. This can be very uncomfortable for women and worrisome if they are not assured that it is a normal accompaniment to pregnancy.

Extremities and Skin. Many women develop palmar erythema and itching early in pregnancy from a high estrogen level and perhaps subclinical jaundice. Assess the lower extremities of pregnant women carefully for varicosities, filling time of the toenails (should be under 5 seconds), and the presence of edema; pelvic pressure may be preventing venous return from the lower extremities. Any edema more than ankle swelling may be a danger sign of pregnancy.

Assess the gait of pregnant women to see that they are keeping their pelvis tucked under the weight of their abdomen. This position prevents them from developing muscle strains from abnormal tension on abdominal muscles. Many pregnant women have a "waddling" gait late in pregnancy from relaxation of the symphysis pubis. This development can cause pain if the cartilage is actually so unstable that it moves on walking.

Measurement of Fundal Height and Fetal Heart Sounds

At about 12 to 14 weeks of pregnancy, the uterus is palpable over the symphysis pubis as a firm globular sphere; it reaches the umbilicus at 20 to 22 weeks, the xyphoid process at 36 weeks, and then often returns to about 4 cm below the xyphoid due to "lightening" at 40 weeks. Palpate fundus location, measure fundal height (from the notch above the symphysis pubis to the superior aspect of the uterine fundus), and plot height on a graph such as the one shown in Figure 10-4. If this is not currently done by the prenatal care providers in your setting, it can be done as an independent nursing action. Plotting uterine growth at each visit in this way can

make apparent any variations in fetal growth (Engstrom & Work, 1992). If an abnormality is detected, further investigation with ultrasound can be made to determine the cause of the increase or decrease in growth. See the Focus on Nursing Research box in Chapter 9 for a discussion of the problems of measurement.

Auscultate for fetal heart sounds (120 to 160 beats per minute). These can be heard at 18 to 20 weeks of pregnancy (10 to 12 weeks if a Doppler technique is used). Palpate for fetal outline and position after the 28th week.

Pelvic Examination

A pelvic examination reveals information on the health of both internal and external reproductive organs (Willms & Newman, 1994). It requires the following equipment: a **speculum** (a metal or plastic instrument with movable flat blades; see Figure 10-6), a spatula for cervical scraping, a clean examining glove, lubricant, a glass slide for plating the Papanicolaou (Pap) smear, a culture tube, and two or three sterile cotton-tipped applicators for obtaining cervical cultures. A good examining light and a stool of correct sitting height are also necessary.

For a pelvic examination, the woman should void and then lie in a **lithotomy position** (on her back with her thighs flexed and her feet resting in the examining table stirrups (Figure 10-5). Her buttocks should extend slightly beyond the end of the examining table. Her abdominal muscles will be more relaxed if she has a pillow under her head.

She should be properly draped with a draw sheet over the abdomen and extending over the legs. It is helpful if the foot of the examining table does not face the examining room door to prevent the woman from

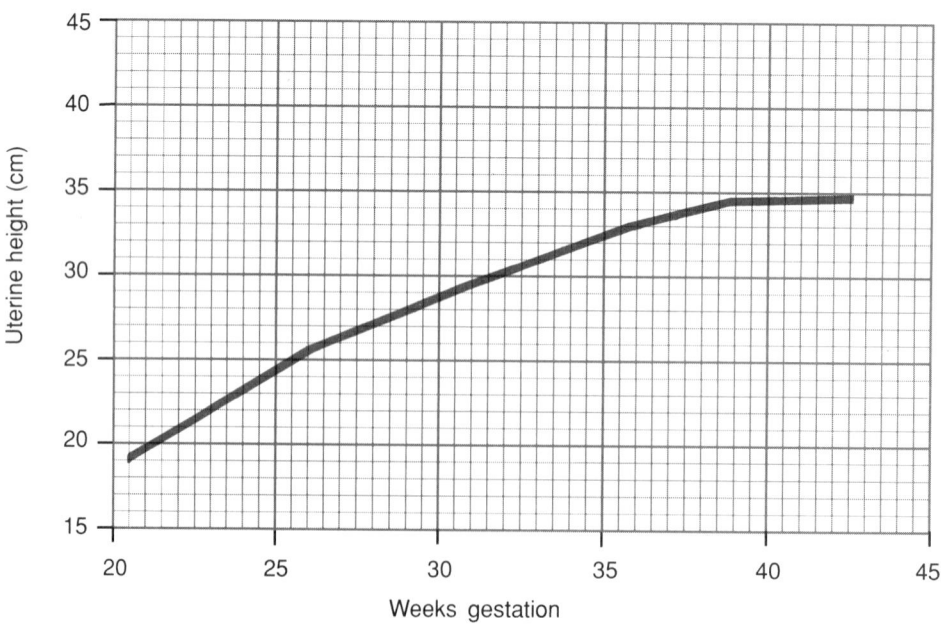

FIGURE 10-4

Plotting uterine height on such a graph at prenatal visits helps to monitor whether fundal growth is adequate.

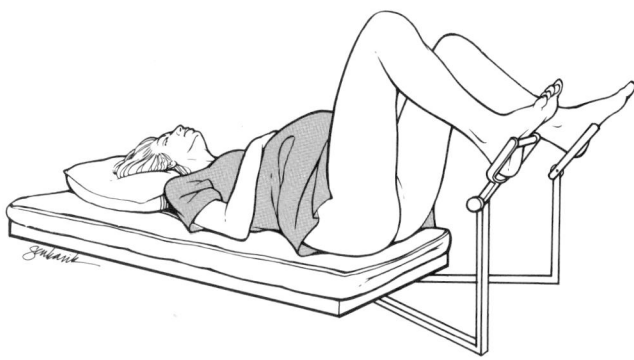

FIGURE 10-5
A lithotomy position used for a pelvic examination. Help position the woman with her buttocks just over the edge of the table for the actual examination. Drape appropriately for modesty.

feeling exposed should someone walk in unexpectedly. She should have an opportunity to talk with the person performing the examination while she is sitting, before she is placed in a lithotomy position, for the sake of her self-esteem and sense of control.

Many women want their support person to remain with them at the head of the table during the exam. In addition, it is customary, especially on an initial visit, for a nurse to be in the room with the woman for the pelvic examination to order to offer additional support. This is true whether the examiner is male or female. This is because if this is a first pregnancy, it may well be the first time the woman has had a pelvic examination. There are so many stories about how painful these examinations are that a woman may tense just thinking about it. When pelvic muscles are tight and tense, not only does the examination become painful, but the examiner has difficulty assessing the status of the pelvic organs.

Helping a woman relax during the examination reduces pain, and having someone with her whom she knows is supportive. Being with her at the head of the table enables you to touch her hand or cheek if she needs the support of physical contact. Explanations of what is happening or what the examiner is doing also are an aid to relaxation. Meaningful conversation with the woman may be helpful, but conversation with the examiner over her head is *not*. Suggesting that the woman breathe in and out (not hold her breath as she is likely to do) may help her relax. Holding her breath pushes the diaphragm down and makes pelvic organs tense and unyielding.

External Genitalia. A pelvic examination begins with inspection of external genitalia. Any signs of inflammation, irritation, or infection, such as redness, ulcerations, or vaginal discharge, are noted (Nattina et al., 1990). A woman may view a pelvic examination if she likes by an overhead mirror or a mirror held by herself or the examiner. Seeing vaginal cervical pathology this way helps

her to understand any kind of problem that is present and the interventions she must continue to improve it. If not already doing it women should be told how to do a monthly perineal examination (holding a mirror) just as they do a monthly breast self-examination (see Chapter 28) (Lawhead, 1990).

If a herpes simplex II virus infection is present, it appears as clustered, pinpoint vesicles on an erythematous (reddened) base on the vulva. These are painful when touched or irritated by underclothing. The presence of herpes lesions on the vulva or vagina at the time of birth will necessitate cesarean birth to prevent exposing the fetus to the virus during passage through the birth canal. As there may be an association between cervical cancer and herpes simplex II virus infections, the presence of a herpes infection should be noted clearly in the woman's record so she can be followed in the future by cytologic (Pap) smears for cervical cancer.

To check whether Skene's glands are infected, insert a sterile gloved finger into the woman's vagina and press it against the anterior vaginal wall to see if any pus can be extruded from the openings to the glands at the urethral opening. To check for possible infection of Bartholin's glands, the sites of Bartholin's glands (5 and 7 o'clock position) are palpated between the vaginal finger and the thumb of the same hand. If a discharge is produced from any of these gland ducts (Skene's or Bartholin's), a culture is obtained by touching the drainage with a sterile applicator tip. Infection here could be caused by something as simple as streptococci; often it is gonorrhea.

To assess whether either a rectocele (a forward pouching of the rectum and posterior vaginal wall due to loss of posterior vaginal muscular support) or a cystocele (an inward pouching of the bladder and anterior vaginal wall due to loss of vaginal muscular support) is present, ask the woman to bear down as if she were moving her bowels while the labia are gently separated to allow a view of the vaginal walls.

Internal Genitalia. To view the uterine cervix, the vagina must be opened with a speculum. No lubricant other than warm water should be used over the speculum blades as a lubricant might interfere with the interpretation of the Pap smear that will be taken. Warm water rather than cold water should be used so that the woman does not contract her vaginal muscles when she feels the cold instrument.

A speculum is introduced with the blades in a closed position and directed toward the posterior rather than the anterior vaginal wall because the posterior wall is less sensitive (Figure 10-6*A*). A speculum enters most readily if it is inserted at an oblique angle (the crease of the blades directed to 4 or 8 o'clock), then rotated to a horizontal position when fully inserted (the crease of the blades pointing to a 3 or 9 o'clock position) (Figure

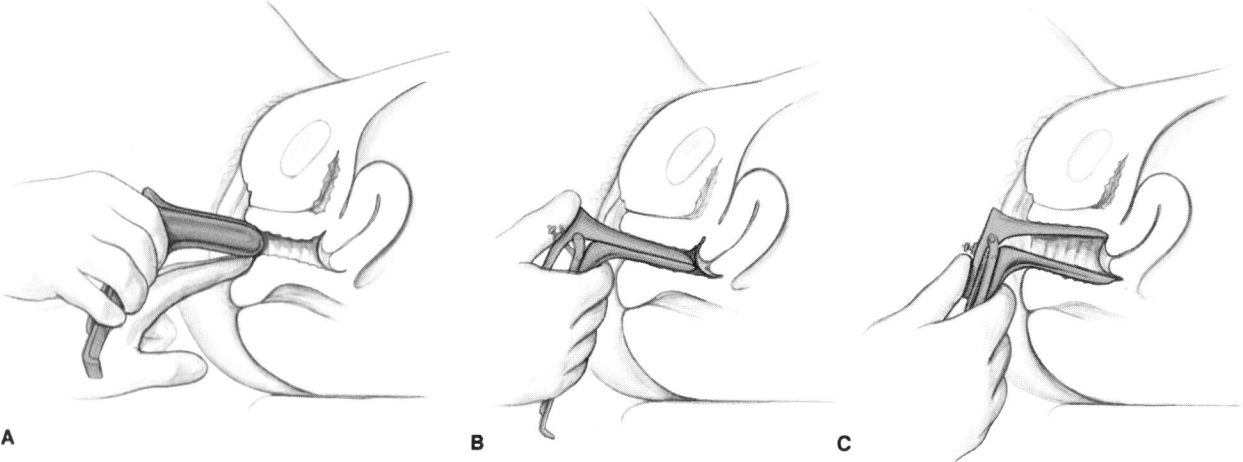

FIGURE 10-6

*Insertion of a vaginal speculum. (**A**) Blades held obliquely on entering the vagina. (**B**) Blades rotated to horizontal position as they pass the introitus. (**C**) Blades separated by depressing thumbpiece and elevating handle.*

10-6*B*). When fully inserted and rotated to a horizontal position, the blades are opened so the cervix is visible and are secured in the open position by tightening the thumb screw at the side (Figure 10-6*C*).

With the speculum in place, the cervix can be inspected for its position (a retroverted uterus has a cervix positioned anteriorly; an anteverted uterus has its cervix positioned posteriorly), its color (a nonpregnant cervix is light pink; in pregnancy it changes to almost purple), and any lesions, ulcerations, discharge, or otherwise abnormal appearance (Bates, 1991).

In a **nulligravida**, a woman who has never been pregnant, the cervical os is round and small. In a woman who has had a previous pregnancy with a vaginal birth, the cervical os has much more of a slit-like appearance (Figure 10-7*A*). If the woman had a cervical tear during a previous birth, the cervical os may appear as a transverse crease the width of the cervix or a typical star-like (stellate) formation. If a cervical infection is present, a mucus discharge may be present. With infection, the epithelium of the cervical canal often enlarges and spreads onto the area surrounding the os, giving the cervix a reddened appearance (called **erosion**; Figure 10-7*B*). This area bleeds readily if it is touched.

Trichomoniasis, a protozoal infection, generally gives signs of redness, a profuse whitish bubbly discharge, and petechial spots on the vaginal walls (Heine & McGregor, 1993). Candidal (*Monilia*) infection typically presents with thick, white vaginal patches that may bleed if scraped away. A gonorrhea infection typically presents with a thick, greenish-yellow discharge and extreme inflammation. *Chlamydia* infection, in contrast, shows few symptoms (Carroll, 1993).

Carcinoma of the cervix appears as an irregular, granular growth at the os. Cervical polyps (red, soft,

pedunculated protrusions) also may occasionally be seen at the os.

Papanicolaou Smear. Although only an endocervical smear may be taken to be plated for a Pap test in some centers, in others three separate specimens, one from the endocervix, one from the cervical os, and one from the vaginal pool, are obtained. In addition, a cervicogram (a photograph of the cervix) may be taken. Cervicograms serve as complements to Pap smears as yet another weapon for detecting cervical cancer (Ferris et al., 1993).

To obtain a first specimen for a Pap smear, take a sterile cotton applicator or cervical brush, wet it with saline, and insert it through the speculum into the os of the cervix. Gently rotate it, first clockwise, then counter-

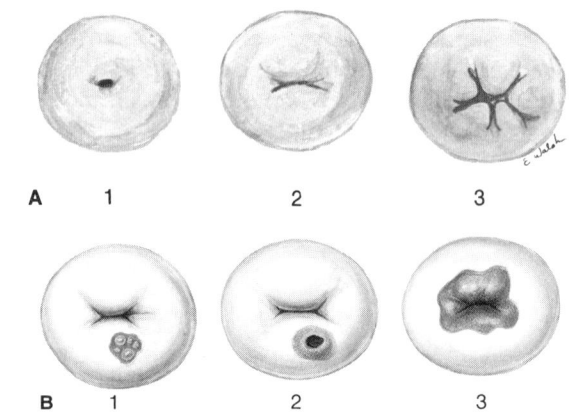

FIGURE 10-7

*(**A**) Appearances of the cervix in nulliparous and multiparous women. (1) Nulliparous cervix. (2) Cervix after childbirth. (3) "Stellate" cervix seen after mild cervical tearing. (**B**) Possible cervical lesions. (1) Herpes II. (2) Chancre of syphilis. (3) Erosion or infection.*

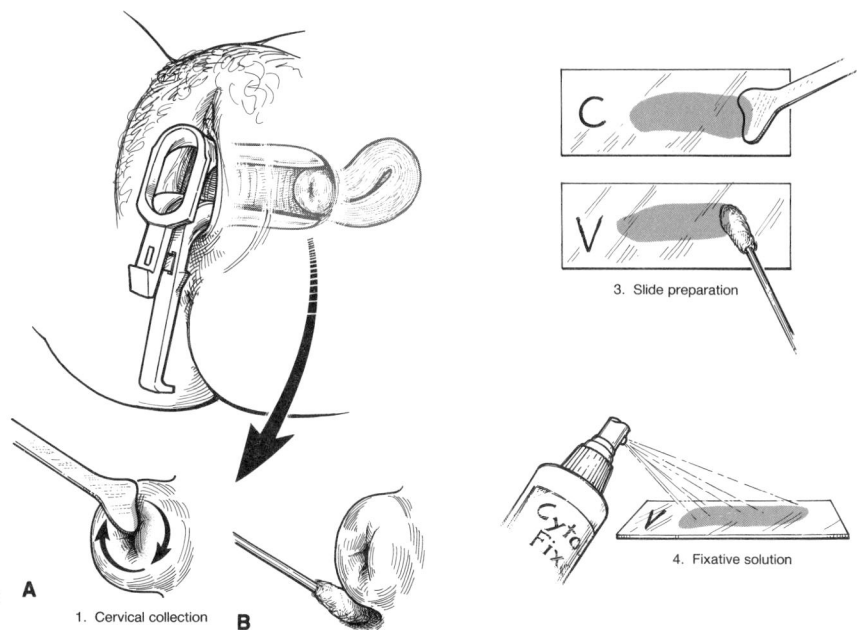

3. Slide preparation

4. Fixative solution

FIGURE 10-8
*Obtaining a Pap smear. (**A**) A specimen taken from the cervix. (**B**) A specimen taken from vaginal pool.*

A 1. Cervical collection

B 2. Vaginal pool collection

clockwise. Remove it without touching the sides of the vagina, and paint a glass slide using a gentle touch so as not to destroy cells. Spray the slide with a fixative to preserve the cells.

To take the cervical specimen, press the uneven end of the spatula supplied for the test on the os of the cervix; rotate it to scrape cells in a circle around the os (Figure 10-8). Smear the scraper onto a slide and spray the slide with fixative.

For the third specimen, place a cotton-tipped applicator or the opposite spatula blade at the posterior fornix just below the cervix (the vaginal pool); roll it gently to pick up secretions collecting there. Remove it carefully and prepare a third slide as described for the first two specimens.

The classification of Pap smears is constantly being revised as the meaning of abnormal cells is further defined (Boyce & Fruchter, 1993). Three methods of classification are shown in Table 10-4. Be certain when discussing these reports with women that they do not overinterpret the classifications. Class I means only normal cells were found. Class II means that cells are inflamed because infection is present (the woman needs to be treated and reexamined in about 3 months). Cervical intraepithelial neoplasia (CIN) levels require a colposcopy exam for further evaluation. Class IV identifies carcinoma in situ or precancerous cells that are present. Class V is indicative of squamous cell carcinoma.

Many women ask how often repeat Pap smears are necessary because the recommendations have changed

Table 10-4. *Classification of Papanicolaou Smears*

Bethesda System	Classic System	Class
Within normal limits	Normal	I
Infection (specify organism)	Inflammatory cells	II
Reactive and reparative changes		
Squamous cell abnormalities		
Atypical squamous cells of undetermined significance	Squamous atypia of uncertain significance	IIR
Low-grade squamous intraepithelial lesion	HPV atypia mild dysplasia	
High-grade squamous intraepithelial lesion	Moderate dysplasia Severe dysplasia	III
	Carcinoma in situ	IV
Squamous cell carcinoma significance	Squamous cell carcinoma	V

(From Boyce, J.C., & Fruchter, R.G. [1993]. Lengthening the interval between Pap smears. *Contemporary Obstetrics and Gynecology, 37,* 82.)

and are confusing. The American Cancer Society recommends a Pap smear as infrequently as every 3 years in women who have had two consecutive negative tests a year apart. Women who should have them more frequently are those who were exposed to diethylstilbestrol (DES) in utero, who have multiple sexual partners, who have a history of human papillomavirus (HPV), who smoke cigarettes, or who were active sexually before age 21. Screening as infrequently as every 3 years could miss pathology in these women (Boyce & Fruchter, 1993).

Vaginal Inspection. Before the speculum is removed, a culture for gonorrhea, chlamydia, or group B streptococcus may be taken. These cultures are done by gentle swabs of the cervix using cotton-tipped applicators; the specimens obtained are then plated onto a medium to allow for their growth. All these organisms can cause disease in the newborn so it is best if they can be eradicated during pregnancy (Coleman, Sherer, & Maniscalco, 1992).

A speculum must be unlocked to be removed because the excessive stretching that would occur if it were removed in an open position would be painful. If the speculum is kept partially open as it is removed, it should not cause any pain, and the sides of the vagina can be inspected as it is withdrawn. Such a vaginal inspection is critical, especially for a woman whose mother took DES during her pregnancy: Female children of mothers who took DES are prone to develop adenosis, or overgrowth of cervical endothelium (which is possibly associated with vaginal cancer). In a nonpregnant woman, vaginal walls are light pink; pregnancy turns them dark blue to purple. Any areas of inflammation, ulceration, lesions, or discharge are noted.

Examination of Pelvic Organs. Following the speculum examination, it is necessary to perform a bimanual (two-handed) examination to assess the position, contour, consistency, and tenderness of pelvic organs (Figure 10-9). The index and middle fingers of one gloved hand are lubricated and inserted into the vagina and the walls of the vagina are palpated for abnormalities. The other hand is then placed on the woman's abdomen and pressed downward toward the hand still in the vagina until the uterus can be felt between the two hands. If a uterus is extremely retroverted, it may not be palpable abdominally. Next, the right and left ovaries are identified by the same method. Ovaries are normally slightly tender, so the pressure caused by palpation may cause the woman some discomfort.

Abnormalities that can be noted by bimanual examination are ovarian cysts, enlarged fallopian tubes (perhaps from pelvic inflammatory disease), and an enlarged uterus. An early sign of pregnancy (Hegar's sign) is elicited on bimanual examination (see Figure 8-4). Table

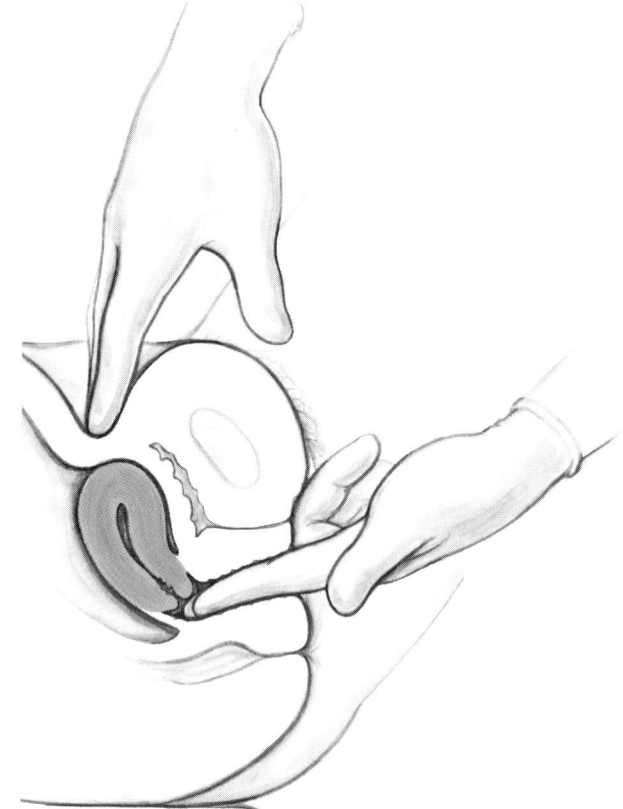

FIGURE 10-9
A bimanual examination to determine uterine size.

10-2 summarizes gynecologic disorders that might be present and their symptoms.

Rectovaginal Examination. Following a bimanual pelvic examination, the hand is withdrawn from the vagina and reinserted with only the index finger in the vagina and the middle finger in the rectum. By palpating the tissue between the examining fingers in this way, it is possible to assess the strength and irregularity of the posterior vaginal wall. This maneuver may be slightly uncomfortable for the woman because of the rectal pressure involved. Some examiners use a clean pair of gloves before they perform a vaginal-rectal examination so that they will not spread an infection from the vagina to the rectum. Following the rectal examination, if it is necessary to reexamine the vagina for any reason, the glove must be changed to avoid contaminating the vagina with fecal material.

After completing the examination, wipe away excess lubricant from the vaginal and rectal openings. It is important to wipe front to back so as not to carry rectal contamination forward to the vaginal introitus.

Estimating Pelvic Size

It is impossible to predict from the outward appearance of a woman whether or not her pelvis is adequate for the passage of a fetus through its center. Some women look as if they have a wide pelvis but, in reality, only have wide iliac crests and a normal or even smaller-than-normal internal ring. Other women appear as if their pelvis will be small because the iliac crests are non-flaring but the internal pelvis, the part that must be sufficiently large for childbirth, is of average size, and they will give birth vaginally without difficulty. Differences in pelvic contour and development occur mainly because of hereditary factors, but disease (e.g., rickets, now rarely seen in the United States, which may cause contraction of the pelvis) or injury (inadequate repair following an accident) also may play a role.

If, on this initial visit, the primary care provider establishes that the woman is pregnant, and if she has never given birth vaginally before, pelvic measurements may be taken.

Some care providers prefer to take these measurements later in pregnancy, when the woman's pelvic muscles are more relaxed, making measurement easier. If a routine sonogram will be prescribed, estimations may be made by a combination of pelvic pelvimetry and fetal sonogram. Estimation of pelvic adequacy must be done at least by the 24th week of pregnancy, because

by this time there is danger that the fetal head will reach a size that will interfere with safe passage and birth if the pelvic measurements are small.

Once a woman has given vaginal birth, her pelvis has been proved adequate, and it is not necessary to take her pelvic measurements again unless she has had an intervening history of pelvic accident.

Types of Pelves. The types of pelves found in women can be categorized into four groups (Figure 10-10):

1. *Gynecoid* pelvis. This is the "normal" female pelvis. The inlet of this type is well rounded forward and backward, and the pubic arch is wide. This pelvic type is ideal for childbirth.
2. *Anthropoid* pelvis. In this pelvis (an ape-like one), the transverse diameter is narrow and the antero-posterior diameter of the inlet is larger than normal. This does not accommodate a fetal head as well as a gynecoid pelvis.
3. *Platypelloid* pelvis. In this pelvis (a flattened one), the inlet is an oval, smoothly curved, but the an-teroposterior diameter is shallow. A fetal head

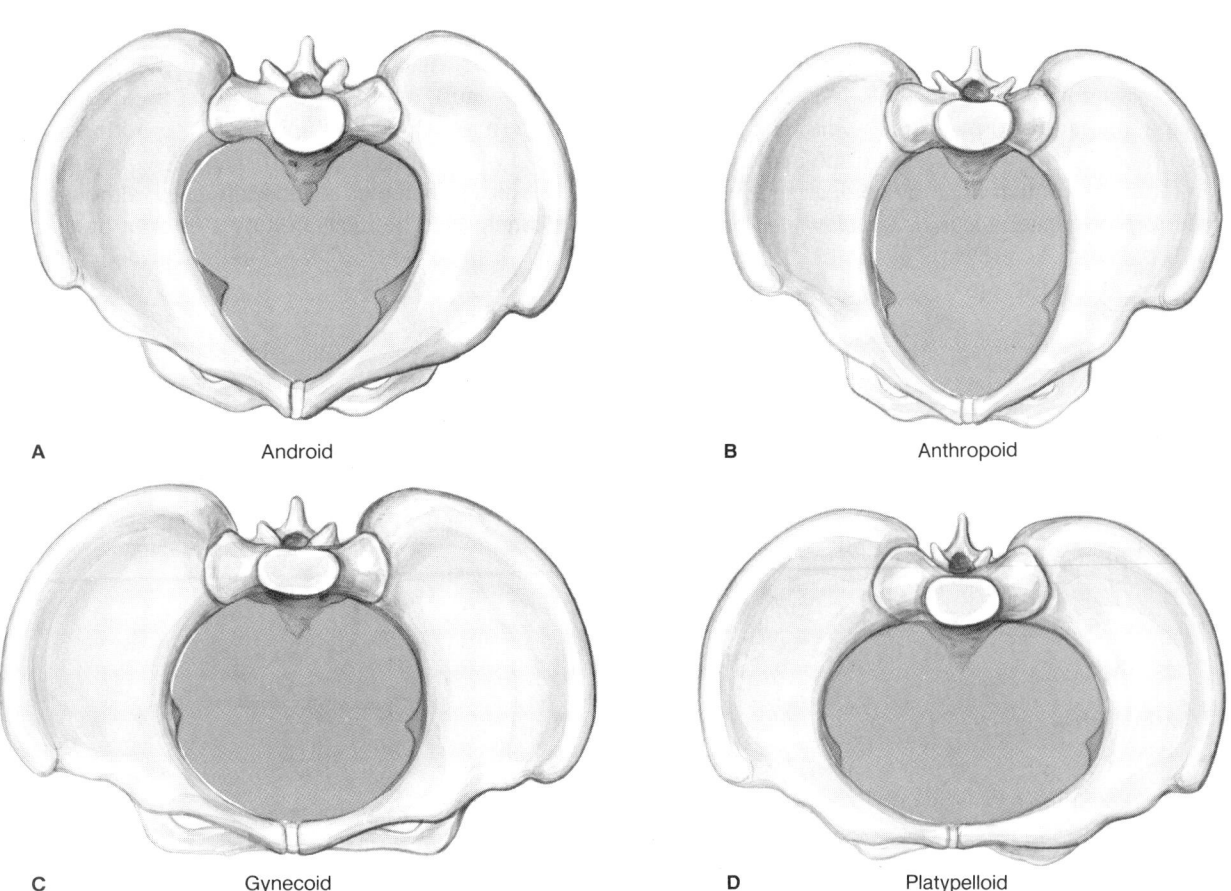

A   Android

B   Anthropoid

C   Gynecoid

D   Platypelloid

FIGURE 10-10
Types of pelves. (**A**) *Android.* (**B**) *Anthropoid.* (**C**) *Gynecoid.* (**D**) *Platypelloid.*

might not be able to rotate to match the curves of the pelvic cavity in this type of pelvis.

4. *Android* pelvis, or "male" pelvis. The pubic arch in this pelvis type forms an acute angle, making the lower dimensions of the pelvis extremely narrow. A fetus may have difficulty exiting from this type of pelvis.

Internal Measurements. Internal measurements give the actual diameters of the inlet and outlet through which the fetus must pass. The following measurements are made most commonly:

1. The **diagonal conjugate**. This is the distance between the anterior surface of the sacral prominence and the anterior surface of the inferior margin of the symphysis pubis (see Chapter 4, Figure 4-11). It is the most useful measurement for estimation of pelvic size, as it suggests the anteroposterior diameter of the pelvic inlet (the narrower diameter at that level, or the one that is most apt to cause a misfit with the fetal head).

   The diagonal conjugate is measured while the woman lies in a lithotomy position. To measure it, introduce two fingers vaginally and press inward and upward until your middle finger touches the sacral prominence. With your other hand, mark the part of your examining hand where it touches the symphysis pubis (Figure 10-11*A*). Withdraw your examining hand and measure the distance between the tip of your middle finger and the marked point on the glove on that hand by comparing it with a ruler or, for greater accuracy, a *pelvimeter.* The

measurement is slightly painful; the woman will feel the pressure of the examining finger as it stretches to touch the sacral prominence. If your hand is small with short fingers, you may not be able to assess pelvic measurements manually because your fingers may not reach the sacral prominence. If the measurement obtained is more than 12.5 cm, the pelvic inlet is rated as adequate for childbirth (the diameter of the fetal head that must pass that point averages 9 cm in diameter).

2. The **true conjugate**, or **conjugate vera**, is the measurement between the anterior surface of the sacral prominence and the posterior surface of the inferior margin of the symphysis pubis. This measurement cannot be made directly, but it can be estimated from the measurement you made of the diagonal conjugate. To do this, subtract the usual depth of the symphysis pubis (assumed to be 1.2 to 2 cm) from the diagonal conjugate measurement. The distance remaining will be the true conjugate, or the actual diameter of the pelvic inlet through which the fetal head must pass. The average true conjugate diameter is, therefore, 12.5 cm minus 1.5 or 2 cm, or 10.5 to 11 cm.

3. The **ischial tuberosity** diameter. This measurement is the distance between the ischial tuberosities, or the transverse diameter of the outlet (the narrowest diameter at that level or the one most apt to cause a misfit). It is made at the medial and lowermost aspect of the ischial tuberosities at the level of the anus (Figure 10-11*B*). A Williams or Thomas pelvimeter is generally used, although the diameter can be measured by a ruler or by compar-

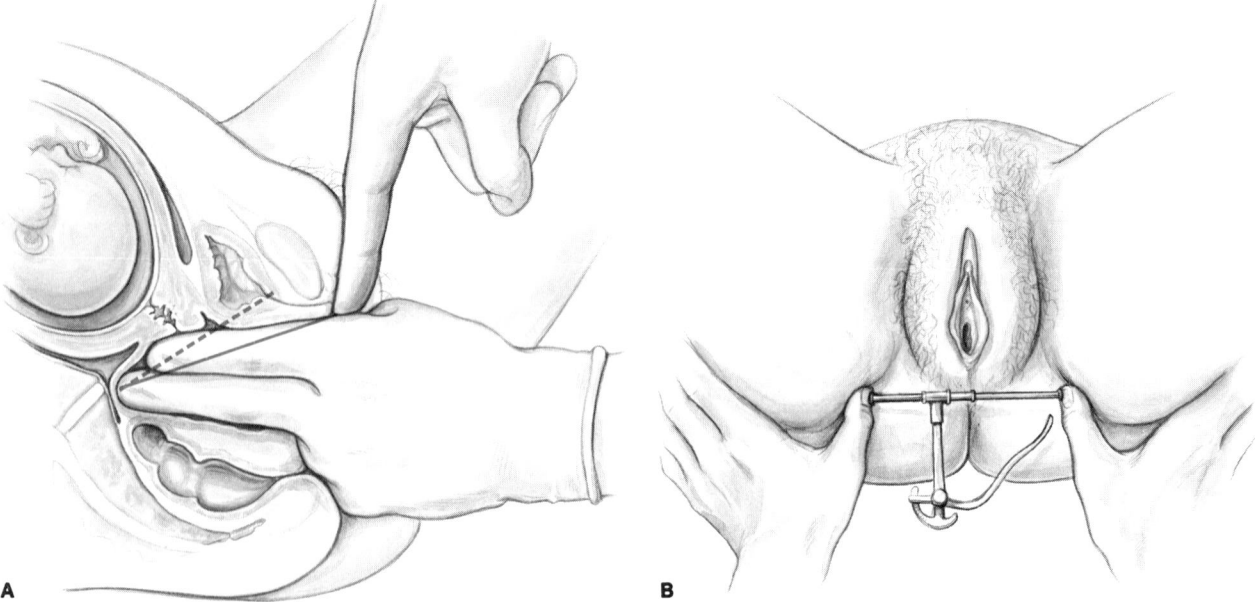

A **B**

FIGURE 10-11
(**A**) *Measurement of diagonal conjugate diameter.* Straight line = *diagonal conjugate;* dotted line = *true conjugate.* (**B**) *Measurement of ischial tuberosity diameter.*

ing it with a known hand span or clenched fist measurement. A diameter of 11 cm is considered adequate because it will allow the widest diameter of the fetal head, or 9 cm, to pass freely through the outlet.

Laboratory Assessment

A number of laboratory studies are included in assessment measures at a first prenatal visit to confirm general health and rule out sexually transmitted diseases that could injure the growing fetus (Wendel & Gilstrap, 1990). Normal levels for these studies are shown in Appendix F.

Blood Studies

The following blood studies are usually done at the first prenatal visit:

1. A complete blood count, including hemoglobin or hematocrit and red cell index to determine the presence of anemia, a white blood cell count to determine infection, and a platelet count to estimate clotting ability. A hematocrit is a simple test that may be done in minutes in the office by a technician or nurse skilled in the technique. African-American women have a blood sample taken to be tested for sickle cell trait or disease and possibly glucose-6-phosphate dehydrogenase if they have not had this done before.

2. A serologic test for syphilis (VDRL or rapid plasma reagin test). Syphilis must be treated early in pregnancy before fetal damage occurs so it is important that this is done at the first visit (Tillman, 1992). A blood sample for a serologic test for gonorrhea may be drawn on women suspected of having the disease.

3. Blood typing (including Rh factor). Blood may have to be made available if the woman has bleeding early in her pregnancy.

4. Maternal serum for alpha fetoprotein (MSAFP). MSAFP will be elevated if a neural tube or abdominal defect is present in the fetus; it may be decreased if a chromosomal anomaly is present in the fetus. It is done at 16 to 18 weeks of pregnancy. A normal value is 2.5 measures of the mean (MOM). If this is elevated, a sonogram will be ordered to assess for a fetal disorder.

5. An indirect Coombs' test (determination if antibodies to the Rh factor are present). This test is generally repeated at 28 weeks of pregnancy. If the titers are not elevated, the woman will receive RhIG (RhoGAM) at 28 weeks of pregnancy and following any procedure that might cause placental bleeding, such as amniocentesis or external version (Scott, 1990).

6. Antibody titers for rubella and hepatitis B (HBsAg). These tests determine whether or not the woman is protected against rubella if exposure should occur during pregnancy and whether a newborn will have the chance of developing hepatitis B (Moyer, 1992). HBsAg may be repeated at about 36 weeks.

7. Human immunodeficiency virus (HIV) screening. Women who are high risk for contracting acquired immunodeficiency syndrome (AIDS) should be asked if they want to be screened for the disease early in pregnancy. This is done by an enzyme-linked immunosorbent assay (also known as *ELISA*) on a blood sample. If this is positive, the finding is confirmed by a second test (a Western Blot).

   Testing women for HIV early in pregnancy allows a woman who is found to be antibody positive for the syndrome the option of choosing to terminate her pregnancy to avoid giving birth to an infant who has a high risk of developing the disease (Lindsay, 1993). It also allows her to begin therapy with AZT, which may decrease the risk of the infant developing the disease.

   General recommendations as to who is high risk for the disease and should be asked if they would like the screening test are women who (1) have used or are using intravenous drugs; (2) have engaged in prostitution; (3) have had sexual partners who are infected or are at risk because they are bisexual, IV drug abusers, or hemophiliacs; or (4) have received a transfusion between 1977 and 1985.

   Because HIV is a fatal disease, some women choose not to have a blood titer taken as they would rather not know that they have the illness. This is their option; screening cannot be mandatory in prenatal settings. Health care providers need to be certain that test results given to clients are accurate (a high blood antibody titer means the person has been exposed to the disease, not that they necessarily have the syndrome) and are presented with tact and compassion with respect for the meaning of the results to the client (Meadows, Catalan, & Gazzard, 1993).

8. If the woman has a history of previously unexplained fetal loss, has a family history of diabetes, has had babies that were large for gestation age (9 lb or more at term), is obese, or has glycosuria, she will need to be scheduled for a 50 gm oral 1-hour glucose loading or tolerance test toward the end of the first trimester of pregnancy to rule out gestational diabetes. If not, she will have this done routinely at the 24th to 28th week visit to evaluate insulin-antagonistic effects of placental hormones, which can register a noticeable effect at this time. The plasma glucose should not be above 135 mg/dL if the woman was fasting and 140 mg/dL if she was not fasting (see Chapter 15 for a discussion of diabetes in pregnancy).

Urinalysis

As mentioned, a urinalysis is performed to test for albuminuria, glycosuria, and pyuria. All three of these can be done by means of test strips and microscopic examination of the urine.

Tuberculosis Screening

Tuberculosis is a disease that is on the rise, an increase related to the HIV epidemic: more people with lowered immune system resistance (ie, those with HIV infection) are contracting tuberculosis and then spreading it to others in the population (May, 1993). In light of this, the physician or nurse-midwife may order a tuberculin skin test to screen for tuberculosis. Any woman who has a positive reaction would then require a chest x-ray for further diagnosis.

If the woman has a history of tuberculosis, she should not be given a tuberculin skin test because the reaction would be extreme. To assess her current disease status, she might receive a chest x-ray. A woman is often reluctant to have this done because she knows that radiation is harmful to a growing fetus. She needs to be assured that she will be provided a lead apron to cover her abdomen to protect the fetus and that only her chest will be exposed to radiation.

It is important to screen for tuberculosis early in pregnancy because it is a chronic and debilitating disease that increases the risk of abortion. Further, the change in the shape of the lung tissue as the growing uterus presses on the lung may reactivate old lesions.

Ultrasonography

If the date of the last menstrual period is unknown, the woman will be scheduled for a sonogram to confirm the pregnancy length or document healthy fetal growth.

Risk Assessment

Table 10-5 summarizes necessary data assessment for a first prenatal visit. Following this assessment, findings are analyzed to determine whether this pregnancy is apt to continue with a good outcome or there is some risk that it will end before term or with an unfavorable fetal or maternal outcome (a high-risk pregnancy).

Many factors enter into the categorization of high risk. The Goodwin Scale, a scale commonly used for risk assessment, is shown in Table 10-6. A score of more than 3 by this scale identifies a fetus as being at high risk. For example, the baby of a woman more than 35 years of age (score 1) in her first pregnancy (score 1)

Table 10-5. *Assessments for a First Pregnancy Visit*

Health History

Demographic data:	Name, address, age, telephone number, health insurance
Chief concern:	Was pregnancy planned? When was last menstrual period? Any exposure to infectious diseases or ingestion of drugs since she thinks she has been pregnant?
Family and social profile:	What is family composition? Who is her chief support person? What is her occupation? Source of income? Level of exercise? Hobbies? Recreational drug use? Living conditions? Nutrition? Sleep pattern?
Past medical history:	Any abdominal surgery, kidney, heart, hypertension, sexually transmitted diseases, diabetes, allergies?
Gynecologic history:	When was menarche? What is length and duration of menstrual cycle?
Obstetric history:	Any previous pregnancies? When? Type and outcome of birth?
Review of systems:	Brief review of all body systems

Physical Examination

Baseline data:	Height, weight, vital signs, fundal height measurements, fetal heart sounds
System assessment:	Full physical exam to confirm general health
Pelvic examination:	General assessment, Pap smear, cultures for chlamydia, gonorrhea, group B streptococcus, pelvic measurements

Laboratory Assessment

Blood assessment:	Complete blood count, serologic test for syphilis, blood type and Rh, alpha fetoprotein, indirect Coombs for antibody titer against Rh, hepatitis B, and HIV
Urinalysis:	Clean catch for glucose, protein, ketones and culture
Tuberculosis:	Tine or PPD
Ultrasound:	To date pregnancy or confirm fetal health

Table 10-6. *Antepartum Fetal Risk Score*

Category I

Baseline Data (Prepregnancy)

Age		*Reproductive History*	
15 or under	1	Abortion, spontaneous	
35+	1	Abortion, therapeutic	
40+	2	Pelvic infection, postabortal or postpartum	
Para		Fetal death	
0	1	Neonatal death	
5+	2	Surviving premature infant	
Interval <2 years	1	Surviving infant, low birth weight for date	
Isolation: 50+ miles from medical care	2	Antepartum hemorrhage	
Weight		Toxemia	
<100 lb (45 kg)	1	Difficult midforceps	
>200 lb (90 kg)	2	Cesarean section	
Diabetes		Hysterotomy	
Class A	1	Myomectomy	
Class B, C, D	2	Major congenital anomaly	
Class F, R	3	Cervical incompetence	
Chronic renal disease	1	Large infant: >10 lb (4.5 kg)	
Chronic renal disease with diminished renal function	3	Malpresentation	
Pre-existing hypertension			
140+/90+	1	One instance of above	1
160+/110+	2	Two or more instances of the above	2
Interpregnancy cardiac failure	2	(in one or more pregnancies)	
Rh-isoimmunized mother (1:8 AHG+)			
With homozygous husband	2		
With previously affected infant (regardless of outcome)	3		

Score (circle one)		0 1 2 3

Category II

Present Pregnancy

Bleeding early (<20 wk)		No antepartum care	2
Alone	1	Less than 3 visits	1
With pain	2	Heart disease: AHA functional	
Bleeding late (>20 wk)		Class III or IV	2
Ceased	1	Anemia	
Continues	2	10 g or less	1
With pain	3	10 g after 36 wk	2
With hypotension	3	8 g or less	2
Spontaneous premature rupture of membranes	1	Megaloblastic anemia	2
With latent period 24 h	2	Specific infections	
Asymptomatic bacteriuria	1	Untreated syphilis	2
Toxemia		Toxoplasmosis	2
Grade I	1	Hepatitis	1
Grade II	3	Vaccination during pregnancy	1
Eclampsia	3	Rubella titer rising significantly	
Hydramnios (single fetus)	3	6 wk	3
Multiple pregnancy	2	9 wk	2
Gestational diabetes		12 wk	1
Diagnosis before 36 wk	1	Inhalation anesthesia (emergency)	1
Diagnosis after 36 wk	2	Abdominal operation	2
Decreasing insulin requirement		Cervical suture (cerclage)	3
(50% + reduction in 48 h)	3	Pelvic irradiation diagnostic 12 wk	1

(continued)

Table 10-6. (Continued)						
Category II						
Present Pregnancy						
Maternal acidosis	3					
Maternal pyrexia (39°C or over)	1					
Maternal pyrexia + fetal heart rate >160	2					
Rising Rh antibody titer (2 tube+)	2					
Score (circle one)			0	1	2	3
Category III						
Gestation Age Achieved						
28 weeks or under	4					
32 weeks or under	3					
35 weeks or under	2					
37 weeks or under	1					
42 weeks or over	1					
43 weeks or over	2					
Score (circle one)			0	1	2	3
Total Score (0–10) =						

(From Goodwin, J. W., & Hewlett, P. T. [1973]. The strategy of fetal risk management. *Canadian Family Physician, 19*[4], 54; with permission.)

who had anemia of 10 g or less (score 1) would, by this scale, be at high risk. The woman needs close observation during pregnancy to see that the pregnancy is progressing well; the infant born of this woman would need close observation in the neonatal period until it was confirmed that no anomalies exist. Category III is scored only after the baby is born.

The failure to identify risk potential in pregnancy leads to increased perinatal mortality. Identifying fetuses at risk by using a standard scoring system such as Goodwin's can be an independent nursing function that can do much to increase the health of newborns and prevent unwanted fetal loss.

Risk assessment should be updated at each pregnancy visit (Andolsek, 1993). See Chapters 14 to 17 for a more detailed discussion of high-risk pregnancy and its management.

Key Points

- Prenatal care has the potential to reduce congenital anomalies and the infant mortality rate. The purposes of prenatal care are to establish a baseline of present health, determine gestation age of the fetus, monitor fetal development, identify the woman at risk for complications, minimize the risk of possible complications by anticipating and preventing problems before they occur, and provide time for education about pregnancy and possible dangers.

- A first visit for prenatal care not only confirms a pregnancy but provides a time to assess client needs and to educate about pregnancy. Assessments consist of a health history, physical examination, and laboratory tests. The physical exam could include measurement of fundal height and assessment of fetal heart sounds, a pelvic examination (including a Pap test), and perhaps estimation of pelvic size.

- Common types of pelves are gynecoid (well rounded with wide pubic arch), anthropoid (narrow), platypelloid (flattened), and android (male or with a sharp pubic arch). A gynecoid pelvis is ideal for childbearing.

- The true conjugate (conjugate vera) is the measurement between the anterior surface of the sacral prominence and the posterior surface of the inferior margin of the symphysis pubis (the anterior-posterior diameter of the pelvic inlet). The average is 10.5 to 11 cm. The ischial tuberosity diameter is the distance between the ischial tuberosities or the transverse diameter of the outlet. The average is 11 cm.

- A first prenatal visit sets the tone for visits to follow. Maintaining a supportive manner is helpful in establishing rapport and allowing the woman to feel comfortable to return for future care.

- Remember that a family, not a woman alone, is having a baby and include family members in procedures and health teaching as desired.

- Pregnant women have decreased balance. For safety,

help them to positions on examining tables as needed. Pregnant women should remain in a lithotomy position for as short a time as possible to help prevent thromboembolism and supine hypotension.

Critical Thinking Exercises

1. It is important to ask enough questions during a health history to be able to estimate health risks. The client, Jessine Wardall, described in the Nursing Care Plan works as a Spanish teacher for grade school students. Are there any special risks you can think of associated with this? Is there a greater opportunity than normal for her to develop upper respiratory infections, for example? Is this a job that probably keeps her on her feet for long periods or not? Is she apt to be exposed to toxic substances at work?

2. Some women do not come early in pregnancy for prenatal care because they know a first visit includes a pelvic examination. What are techniques you can use to help women better accept this procedure?

3. What are things about Jessine Wardall's lifestyle you would like to see her change during a pregnancy that you would stress in pregnancy education for her? Are there factors to make you believe she will comply with instructions well? Are there reasons to think she might not comply?

References

Andolsek, K. M. (1993). Obstetric risk assessment. *Primary Care, 20,* 551.

Bates, B. (1991). *A guide to physical examination* (5th ed.). Philadelphia: J.B. Lippincott.

Bernhardt, J. H. (1990). Potential workplace hazards to reproductive health: Information for primary prevention. *Journal of Obstetric, Gynecologic, and Neonatal Nursing, 19,* 53.

Boyce, J. G., & Fruchter, R. G. (1993). Lengthening the interval between Pap smears. *Contemporary Obstetrics and Gynecology, 37,* 82.

Brown, D. (1992). All pregnant women need prenatal care. *RN, 55,* 88.

Campbell, J. C., et al. (1992). Correlates of battering during pregnancy. *Research in Nursing and Health 15,* 219.

Carroll, J. C. (1993). Chlamydia trachomatis during pregnancy; to screen or not to screen? *Canadian Family Physician, 39,* 97.

Coleman, R., Sherer, D., & Maniscalco, W. (1992). Prevention of neonatal group B streptococcal infections: advances in maternal vaccine development. *Obstetrics and Gynecology, 80,* 301.

Department of Health and Human Services. (1991). *Healthy people 2000.* Washington, DC: Public Health Service.

Engstrom, J. L., & Work, B. A. (1992). Prenatal prediction of small- and large-for-gestational age neonates. *Journal of Obstetric, Gynecologic, and Neonatal Nursing, 21,* 486.

Ferris, D. G., et al. (1993). Cervicography: Adjunctive cervical cancer screening by primary care clinicians. *Journal of Family Practice, 37,* 158.

Heine, P., & McGregor, J. A. (1993). Trichomonas vaginalis: A reemerging pathogen. *Clinical Obstetrics and Gynecology, 36,* 137.

Immunization during pregnancy. (1993). *International Journal of Gynaecology & Obstetrics, 40,* 69.

Kochenour, N. K. (1990). Normal pregnancy and prenatal care. In Scott, J. R., et al. *Danforth's obstetrics and gynecology.* Philadelphia: J. B. Lippincott.

Lawhead, R. A. (1990). Vulvar self-examination: What your patient should know. *Female Patient, 15,* 33.

Lindsay, M. K. (1993). A protocol for routine voluntary antepartum human immunodeficiency virus antibody screening. *American Journal of Obstetrics and Gynecology, 168,* 476.

May, M. (1993). Tuberculosis: A comprehensive review for the certified nurse-midwife. *Journal of Nurse-Midwifery, 38,* 132.

Meadows, J., Catalan, J., & Gazzard, B. (1993). HIV antibody testing in the antenatal clinic: The views of the consumers. *Midwifery, 9,* 63.

Morgan, M. A., & Thurnau, G. R. (1992). Efficacy of the fetal-pelvic index in nulliparous women at high risk for fetal-pelvic disproportion. *American Journal of Obstetrics and Gynecology, 166,* 810.

Moyer, V. A. (1992). Hepatitis B screening in pregnancy: Practical aspects. *Texas Medicine, 88,* 62.

Nattina, S. L., et al. (1990). Diagnosis and management of sexually transmitted genital lesions. *Nurse Practitioner, 15,* 20.

Noel, N., & Yam, M. (1992). Domestic violence: The pregnant battered woman. *Nursing Clinics of North America, 27,* 871.

Scott, J. R. (1990). Immunologic disorders in pregnancy. In Scott, J. R., et al. *Danforth's obstetrics and gynecology.* Philadelphia: J. B. Lippincott.

Simpson, J. F. (1992). Benign conditions affecting the breast. *Contemporary Obstetrics and Gynecology, 37,* 11.

Syverson, C. J., et al. (1991). Pregnancy related mortality in New York City, 1980–1984: Causes of death and other factors. *American Journal of Obstetrics and Gynecology, 164,* 603.

Tillman, J. (1992). Syphilis: An old disease, a contemporary perinatal problem. *Journal of Obstetric, Gynecologic, and Neonatal Nursing, 21,* 209.

Wendel, G. D., & Gilstrap, L. C. (1990). Syphilis rise calls for accurate diagnosis. *Contemporary Obstetrics and Gynecology, 35,* 37.

Williams, C. L., & Strobino, B. A. (1990). Lyme disease transmission during pregnancy. *Contemporary Obstetrics and Gynecology, 35,* 48.

Willms, J. L., & Newman, L. (1994). The pelvic examination in primary practice. *Consultant, 34,* 182.

Suggested Readings

Affonso, D., et al. (1992). Adaptation themes for prenatal care delivered by public health nurses. *Public Health Nursing, 9,* 172.

Dascal, A., et al. (1990). Laboratory tests for the diagnosis of viral disease in pregnancy. *Clinical Obstetrics and Gynecology, 33,* 218.

Davison, C F., et al. (1993). Screening for HIV infection in pregnancy. *AIDS Care, 5,* 135.

Dewey, K. G., & McCrory, M. A. (1994). Effects of dieting and physical activity on pregnancy and lactation. *American Journal of Clinical Nutrition, 59,* 4465.

Dowling, P. T. (1991). The return of tuberculosis: screening and preventive therapy. *American Family Physician, 43,* 457.

Legg, J. J. (1993). Women and HIV. *Journal of the American Board of Family Practice, 6,* 367.

Levy, M., & Koren, G. (1991). Hepatitis B vaccine in pregnancy: maternal and fetal safety. *American Journal of Perinatology, 8,* 227.

Libbus, M., & Sable, M. (1991). Prenatal education in a high risk population: the effect on birth outcomes. *Birth, 18,* 78.

Machala, M., & Winer, M. (1991). Piecing together the crazy quilt of prenatal care. *Public Health Reports, 106,* 353.

McClanahan, P. (1992). Improving access to and use of prenatal care. *Journal of Obstetric, Gynecologic, and Neonatal Nursing, 21,* 280.

Metersky, M. L., & Catanzaro, A. (1993). A rapid tuberculosis screening program for new mothers who have had no prenatal care. *Chest, 103,* 364.

Pettitti, D., et al. (1991). An outcome evaluation of content and quality of prenatal care. *Birth, 18,* 21.

Scupholme, A., et al. (1991). Barriers to prenatal care in a multi-ethnic urban sample. *Journal of Nurse Midwifery, 36,* 111.

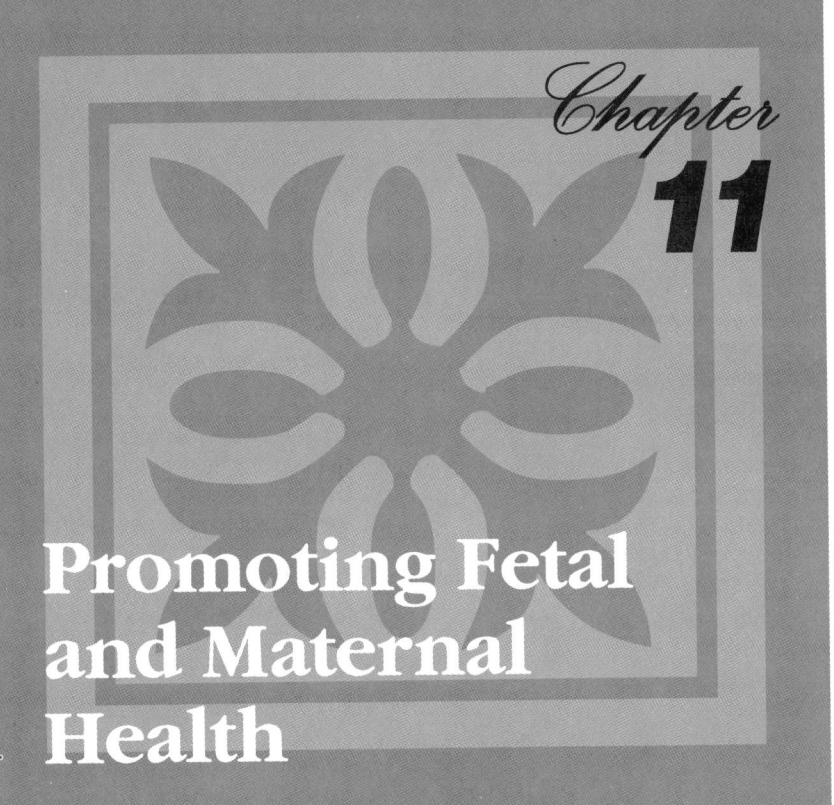

Chapter 11

Promoting Fetal and Maternal Health

Key Terms

- Braxton Hicks contractions
- cytomegalovirus
- fetal alcohol syndrome
- leukorrhea
- organogenesis period
- Sims' position
- teratogen
- teratogenicity
- toxoplasmosis

Objectives

After mastering the contents of this chapter, you should be able to:

1. Describe health practices important for a positive pregnancy outcome.

2. Assess a woman during pregnancy for health practices and concerns.

3. Formulate nursing diagnoses related to health promotion during pregnancy.

4. Plan pregnancy health promotion measures such as ways to limit exposure to teratogens or reduce the minor symptoms of pregnancy.

5. Implement care to promote positive health practices during pregnancy.

6. Evaluate outcome criteria related to health promotion goals to be certain that goals of care were achieved.

7. Identify National Health Goals related to pregnancy care that nurses can help the nation to achieve.

8. Identify areas of prenatal care that could benefit from additional nursing research.

9. Use critical thinking to analyze ways that prenatal care can be made individualized and more family centered to achieve maximum effectiveness.

10. Synthesize knowledge of health promotion measures with the nursing process to achieve quality maternal and child health nursing care.

Adele Pillitteri: MATERNAL AND CHILD HEALTH NURSING, 2nd Edition. © 1995 Adele Pillitteri.

The health of the fetus and mother are inextricably linked. Generally, a woman who eats well and takes care of her own health will provide a healthy environment for the fetus to develop and grow. She may need instructions, however, on what exactly constitutes a healthy lifestyle for herself and her baby. She is apt to have questions regarding how much extra rest she needs, what type of exercise she can continue, and whether all the changes going on in her body, some of which bring her daily discomfort, are normal. As a result, a major role in promoting maternal and fetal health is education. Providing sound and sympathetic advice on ways to alleviate the minor discomforts of pregnancy, alerting the woman to the danger signs of a problem in pregnancy, and keeping abreast of the latest scientific studies done on maternal exposure to teratogens are all part of this role. National Health Goals set to increase the number of women receiving prenatal care are shown in the Focus on National Health Goals box.

⊠ **NURSING PROCESS OVERVIEW**
for Health Promotion of the Fetus
and Mother

ASSESSMENT

A thorough health history, physical evaluation, and initial laboratory data gathering are completed at a first prenatal visit. Continuing assessment concentrates on screening for the presence of teratogens in the pregnant woman's environment and any abnormalities in physical or emotional health that might be occurring with the pregnancy. It is important to encourage the pregnant woman to discuss whatever concerns she has at visits: some of these may represent minor common discomforts associated with normal pregnancy, but others may be early indicators of potential problems with the pregnancy or fetus. In either instance, it is important for you to know what is going on as soon as possible—first, so that you can provide information and guidance on ways to alleviate the discomforts of pregnancy; and, second, so that you can alert the woman's physician or nurse-midwife of your findings early in the pregnancy. The dangers of hypertension and pregnancy-induced diabetes are reduced, for instance, if these conditions are detected early and monitored regularly. Many women do not mention concerns or discomforts they are experiencing unless specifically asked because they are reluctant to use a busy health care provider's time for these things. Unless problems are brought to the health care provider's attention early, however, women may not learn to take the precautions they need to prevent further discomfort during or after the pregnancy. For example, women experiencing constipation may not take care of the problem early or well enough to prevent the occurrence of hemorrhoids, which then become a long-term problem not only throughout the pregnancy but afterward as well.

NURSING DIAGNOSIS

Examples of nursing diagnoses related to health promotion of the pregnant woman and fetus include:

- Health-seeking behaviors related to interest in maintaining optimal health during pregnancy
- Anxiety related to minor symptoms of pregnancy

- High risk for fluid volume deficit related to nausea of pregnancy
- Constipation related to reduced peristalsis during pregnancy
- Disturbance in body image related to change of appearance with pregnancy
- High risk for altered sexual patterns related to fear of harming fetus during pregnancy
- Altered sleep pattern related to frequent need to empty bladder during night
- Fatigue related to metabolic changes of pregnancy
- High risk for fetal injury related to maternal cigarette smoking

PLANNING

When establishing goals and outcome criteria for evaluation of care, be certain that the plans are realistic for the woman's situation and family lifestyle (see Focus on Cultural Awareness box). Try to turn long-term goals into more manageable, short-term ones. Goals to *reduce* smoking in pregnancy or to stop smoking just for the

FOCUS ON
National Health Goals

A number of National Health Goals speak to the importance of prenatal care. These are:

- Increase to at least 60% the proportion of primary care providers who provide age-appropriate preconception care and counseling.
- Increase to at least 90% the proportion of all pregnant women who receive prenatal care in the first trimester of pregnancy from a baseline of 76% (DHHS, 1991).

As nurses are important members of prenatal health care teams, they play a significant role in seeing that services include preconceptual care and that women are aware that early pregnancy care is important. Nursing research to answer such questions as what aspects of preconceptual care are most important in reducing pregnancy complications, and what are effective incentives to make women come early for prenatal care, is important to help the nation meet these goals.

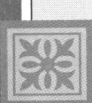

FOCUS ON CULTURAL AWARENESS

Southeast Asians, largely from Cambodia, Laos, and Vietnam, represent a growing population in the United States. Many women from these countries have suffered years of deprivation before emigrating. They may enter the United States with health problems such as parasites, anemia, malnutrition, and tuberculosis. They are at high risk for hepatitis B and genetic blood disorders such as α-thalassemia.

As many of these women do not speak English, providing prenatal care that is meaningful to them can be challenging. Many do not seek care as they do not see pregnancy as a time when medical intervention is necessary. They are often extremely modest and so find pelvic examinations difficult. They may rely on herbs and folk remedies rather than prescribed medicines. A belief that blood is not replaceable prevents them from easily agreeing to pregnancy blood assessment.

Planning prenatal care to meet the needs of Southeast Asians includes furnishing interpreters, providing classes in prenatal health, and maintaining an attitude of advocacy to help adjustment to a formal health care system (Mattson & Lew, 1992).

duration of the pregnancy, for example, may be more realistic than a goal to *stop* smoking altogether. Eliminating the pressure of making a major permanent lifestyle change may help the woman concentrate her efforts on the next several months. Hopefully, she will decide not to smoke again after the baby is born to continue to provide a smoke-free environment for her child. Similarly, you cannot set a goal for a woman to be free of the nausea of early pregnancy; the best you can expect to accomplish is to maintain good nutrition in light of it. Nor can you do much about the frequency of urination, backache, or fatigue that occur with pregnancy, except to help the woman adapt her lifestyle to these symptoms (eg, drink more liquids during the day and less in the early evening; schedule regular rest periods, if possible).

Helping a woman plan to avoid teratogens is often difficult because it may involve a total change in lifestyle (not smoking, not drinking alcohol, changing a work environment, and so on). It is amazing, however, how much a woman will sacrifice to complete a pregnancy satisfactorily. With this level of motivation, planning then becomes the task of determining what will be the best route to achieve a goal rather than education for the need of goal attainment.

When planning teaching strategies, it is important to discover how receptive to instruction a woman will be. No matter how excited and pleased a woman is to be pregnant, she can assimilate only so much information at one particular time. You will need, therefore, to select from all the available health information those points that seem most relevant to the individual woman. The priority for discussing varicosity prevention, for example, would seem higher for a woman who has had varicosities in a former pregnancy than for one who is pregnant for the first time and is an avid sportswoman. The health measures you are teaching must be maintained for an extended time: 40 weeks. To be certain that a woman follows these measures throughout this period, choose priorities and give meaningful, individualized health advice. This kind of advice is much more likely to be followed than that given in a standardized lecture that the woman will recognize is given to everyone.

Remember that a basic tenet of teaching-learning is that people learn best information that has *direct* application to them. Plan to space health promotion and maintenance information in pregnancy according to early and late pregnancy so those measures that are immediately applicable are taught first; those that have relevance only toward the end of pregnancy are taught then.

IMPLEMENTATION

The major interventions for nursing diagnoses associated with health promotion during pregnancy involve teaching. Although the average woman is aware that discom-

forts occur with pregnancy, they will seem different when they are happening to *her*. A woman who knows that it is normal for breast tenderness to occur during pregnancy may not be sure that the *amount* of breast tenderness she is having is normal; a woman who had a mental image of herself as someone who would not gain much weight during pregnancy may be very concerned that she is, in fact, gaining a great deal of weight. Adolescent girls often are uninformed about common discomforts of pregnancy because they lack a set of peers with pregnancy experience, so they may need more teaching and review in this area. Be certain all women understand that they should double check with their primary care practitioner about the safety in pregnancy of any medicine they take.

Other important interventions include good role modeling, such as not smoking in prenatal settings, and evidencing a healthy lifestyle in terms of nutrition or exercise.

EVALUATION

Evaluation of health promotion goals is an ongoing process aided by the regularity of health care visits. Desired outcomes that are developed with the woman at one prenatal visit need to be assessed at the next. Examples of goal outcomes would be:

- The client has stopped smoking.
- The client walks the length of a block daily.

Health Promotion During Pregnancy

Self-Care Needs

Because pregnancy is not an illness, there are few required special care measures other than to use common sense regarding self-care. Many women, however, have heard different warnings about what they should or should not do during pregnancy. Thus, the average woman needs some help separating fact from fiction so she can enjoy her pregnancy unhampered by unnecessary restrictions. It is important to know the common misunderstandings of pregnancy so you can appreciate why so much health teaching is necessary. In no other area of nursing, other than infant feeding, does there seem to be as many misconceptions or inappropriate information available to women.

Bathing

At one time, bathing was restricted during pregnancy because it was feared that bath water would enter the vagina and cervix and contaminate the uterine contents. Further, it was believed that hot water touching the abdomen might bring on labor. Because the vagina normally is in a closed position, however, the danger that water will enter the cervix is minimal. The water temperature has no documented effect on initiating labor. Sweating tends to increase with pregnancy because the woman excretes waste products not only for herself but for the child within her, and she has an abundant vaginal discharge, so daily bathing has now moved from a high place on the *don't* list to a high place on the *do* list.

As pregnancy advances, a woman may have difficulty maintaining her balance when getting in and out of a bathtub. If so, she can shower or take sponge baths instead. If membranes rupture or vaginal bleeding is present, bathing *is* contraindicated because then there would be a danger of contamination of uterine contents. During the last month of pregnancy, when cervical dilatation may be beginning, some physicians restrict tub bathing for the same reason.

Breast Care

All women should observe a few precautions during pregnancy to prevent loss of breast tone, which can result in painful, pendulous breasts later in life. A general rule is to wear a firm, supportive bra. Wide straps spread weight across the shoulders better than narrow ones. The woman may have to buy a larger-sized bra halfway through pregnancy to accommodate increased breast growth.

At about the 16th week of pregnancy, colostrum secretion begins in the breasts. The sensation of a fluid discharge from the breasts can be frightening unless the woman is forewarned that it is likely to happen at about this time. Instruct her to wash her breasts with clear water (no soap) daily to wash the colostrum away and minimize the risk of infection from organisms growing in this medium.

If colostrum secretion is profuse, she may need to place gauze squares or breast pads inside her bra and change them frequently to maintain dryness; otherwise, constant moisture next to the breast nipple may cause nipple excoriation, pain, and fissuring.

Dental Care

It is important for women to continue good toothbrushing habits throughout pregnancy. Gingival tissue tends to hypertrophy during pregnancy; unless the pregnant woman brushes well, pockets of plaque may form readily between the enlarged gumline and teeth (Figure 11-1).

Tooth decay occurs from the action of bacteria on sugar. This action lowers the *p*H of the mouth, and it is the acid medium created that leads to etching of teeth. To keep levels of sugar in the mouth to a minimum, and if she can't give up candy completely, eating snacks that dissolve easily (like a chocolate bar) are preferable to those (like chewy candy) that remain in the mouth a long time. Of course, snacking on foods such as apples

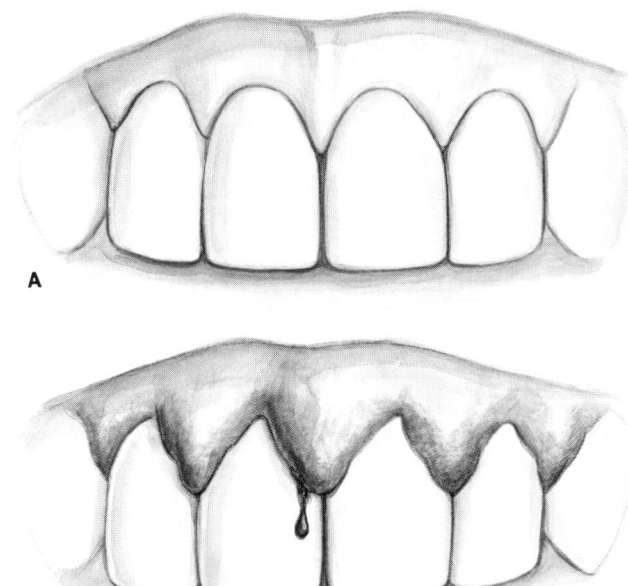

A

B

FIGURE 11-1

*Hypertrophy of the gumline can occur during pregnancy. (**A**) Normal gingiva. (**B**) Swollen gingiva, which makes it difficult to remove plaque from teeth.*

and carrots that are not empty-calorie foods is an even better recommendation for dental care.

Perineal Hygiene

Although women have increased vaginal discharge during pregnancy, douching as a means of vaginal cleansing is contraindicated during pregnancy. The force of the irrigating fluid could possibly enter the cervix and cause infection.

Dressing

The day when a woman had to purchase a completely new maternity wardrobe has disappeared. This has an economic advantage because maternity clothing is expensive, but it may be disappointing to a woman who wants to announce her pregnancy early by wearing maternity clothing.

Early in pregnancy, women may wear an abdominal support such as a light girdle if they wish (for *support*, not to compress and constrict the abdomen). They should avoid garters and extremely firm girdles with panty legs because these impede lower-extremity circulation. A woman may need to purchase a larger-sized bra as her breasts enlarge. If she plans on breast-feeding her newborn, she might choose to buy bras suitable for breast-feeding so she can continue to use these after the baby's birth. She will have less backache if she limits her shoes to those with a low heel. Otherwise, the rules are common sense and comfort.

Sexual Activity

Some women are reluctant to ask questions about sexual relations during pregnancy. Most women are concerned about whether intercourse should be restricted, however, and many need information to refute some of the myths about sexual relations in pregnancy that still exist. Myths such as "coitus on the date her period would have been expected will initiate labor"; "orgasm will initiate labor, but relations without orgasm will not;" "coitus during the fertile days of a cycle will cause a second pregnancy or twins"; and "coitus might cause rupture of the membranes" abound, but none of these is true. If a woman has such concerns, however, she needs to voice them. The fears then can be dispelled and she will not refrain from coitus when she desires it or worry needlessly that coitus is harming her child.

Women who have a history of repeated abortion may be advised to avoid coitus during the time of the pregnancy when the previous abortions occurred. Women whose membranes have ruptured or who have vaginal spotting should be advised against coitus until they are examined in order to prevent infection. Otherwise, there are no sexual restrictions during pregnancy.

Early in pregnancy a woman may notice a decrease in her desire for coitus due to the increased level of estrogen in her body. Breast tenderness may limit a usual pattern of sexual arousal. As pelvic congestion occurs as a result of the additional uterine blood supply, most women may notice increased clitoral sensation; some women experience orgasm for the first time during pregnancy because of the increased pelvic congestion. As pregnancy advances and the woman's abdomen increases in size, she and her sexual partner may need to use new positions for intercourse. A side-by-side position, or the woman in a superior position, may be more comfortable. As vaginal secretions change, the woman may find a lubricant helpful. If she begins to experience discomfort from penile penetration, mutual masturbation or female oral-male genital relations might be satisfying to both partners. Caution women with non-monogamous sexual partners to make sure their partner uses a condom to avoid contracting a sexually transmitted disease during pregnancy. Advise caution about male oral-female genital contact, because accidental air embolism has been reported from this act during pregnancy (Nagey, 1989).

Exercise

Women need exercise during pregnancy to prevent circulatory stasis (Fishbein et al., 1990); it can have the additional positive effect of increased fetal growth, apparently from increased circulation (Hatch et al., 1993). For many women, teaching about exercise is centered on helping them realize the need for exercise and urging them to get enough. Others may need to be cautioned to restrict exercise or participation in contact sports.

The American College of Obstetricians and Gynecologists (ACOG) recommends that both the average nonpregnant and average pregnant woman exercise 3 to 5 times a week for 15 to 60 consecutive minutes (Retts, 1993). An exercise program should consist of 5 to 10 minutes of warm-up exercises, an active "stimulus" phase, and then 5 to 10 minutes of cool-down exercises. The type of activity chosen depends on the woman's interests but those which exercise large muscle groups rhythmically are best. How intense exercise should be depends on the woman's cardiopulmonary fitness. If any complication of pregnancy should occur such as bleeding or hypertension of pregnancy, the woman should discontinue an exercise program.

Both pregnant and nonpregnant women should exercise at 70% to 85% of their maximum heart rate. The easiest way to calculate maximum heart rate is to subtract a woman's age from 220. The target heart rate range for exercise such a woman should aim for is 70% to 85% of this number. A woman 23 years old, therefore, would have a target pulse range of 137 to 167 ($220 - 23 \times 70\%$ and 85%). For a woman of 35, this target range would be 129 to 157.

A quick assessment as to whether a woman is exercising too strenuously is to assess if she is able to continue talking while exercising. If she is too short of breath to be able to do this, she is exercising beyond her target heart rate.

The benefits of a planned exercise program are lowered cholesterol, reduced risk of osteoporosis, increased energy level, maintenance of healthy body weight, decreased risk of heart disease, and increased self-esteem and well being (Retts, 1993). As a rule, a woman can continue any sport she participated in before pregnancy unless it was one that involved body contact. If a woman is a competent horsewoman, for example, there is little reason for her to discontinue riding until it becomes uncomfortable (as long as she does not have a history of early abortion). Pregnancy is no time to learn to ride, however, because a beginning rider is in more danger of being thrown than an experienced one. The same principles apply to skiing and bicycling. An accomplished skier or bicycler may continue activity in moderation until balance becomes a problem; pregnancy is not the time to learn to ski or ride a bicycle, however, because the lack of skill may result in many falls. Swimming is a good activity for pregnant women and, like bathing, is not contraindicated as long as the membranes are intact. Long-distance swimming or any other activity carried out to a point of extreme fatigue is difficult to justify. A program of low-impact aerobics is healthy; high-impact aerobics is strenuous to both pelvic and knee joints and may lead to hyperthermia (although the average healthy woman is able to maintain thermal balance for 20 minutes of exercise; McMurray et al., 1993). Use of hot tubs and saunas following workouts is contraindicated because these could raise internal fetal temperature; hyperthermia may be related to congenital anomalies.

Walking is the best exercise during pregnancy, and women should be encouraged to take a walk daily unless many levels of stairs or an unsafe neighborhood are contraindications. Jogging, in contrast, is questioned because of the strain the extra weight of pregnancy places on the knees. Late in pregnancy, jogging can be painful from relaxed symphysis pubis movement. Guidelines for exercise during pregnancy are given in Box 11-1.

Sleep

The optimal condition for body growth occurs when growth hormone is secreted at its highest level, during sleep. This fact appears to be the physiologic reason for pregnant women needing an increased amount of sleep or at least rest to build new body cells during a pregnancy.

Pregnant women rarely have difficulty falling asleep at night because they have such a physiologic need for sleep. If the woman does have trouble falling asleep, drinking a glass of warm milk is a good sleep inducer. Total relaxation exercises (lying quietly, systematically relaxing neck muscles, shoulder muscles, arm muscles, and so on) can be helpful.

Late in pregnancy, a woman often finds herself awakened from sleep at short, frequent intervals by the activity of the fetus. She may wake with dyspnea if she doesn't sleep with two pillows (sleeping on a couch with an arm rest may be best for her). Because frequent waking leads to loss of REM (rapid-eye-movement sleep), a woman can be left with a feeling of anxiety or not being well rested although she has slept as many hours as usual. To gain enough sleep and rest during pregnancy, most pregnant women need a rest period during the afternoon as well as a full night of sleep. A good resting or

---

Box 11-1
Guidelines for Exercise in Pregnancy

1. Regular exercise (at least 3 times per wk) is preferable to intermittent activity. Competitive activities should be discouraged.
2. Vigorous exercise should not be performed in hot, humid weather or during a period of febrile illness.
3. Ballistic movements (jerky, bouncy motions) should be avoided. Exercise should be done on a wooden floor or a tightly carpeted surface to reduce shock and provide a sure footing.
4. Deep flexion or extension of joints should be avoided because of connective tissue laxity. Activities that require jumping, jarring motions, or rapid changes in direction should be avoided because of joint instability.
5. Vigorous exercise should be preceded by a 5-min period of muscle warm-up. This can be accomplished by slow walking or stationary cycling with low resistance.
6. Vigorous exercise should be followed by a period of gradually declining activity that includes gentle, stationary stretching. Because connective-tissue laxity increases the risk of joint injury, stretches should not be taken to the point of maximum resistance.
7. Heart rate should be measured at times of peak activity. Target heart rate and limits established in consultation with the primary care giver should not be exceeded.
8. Care should be taken to rise gradually from the floor to avoid orthostatic hypotension. Some form of activity involving the legs should be continued for a brief period.
9. Liquids should be taken liberally before and after exercise to prevent dehydration. If necessary, activity should be interrupted to replenish fluids.
10. Women who have sedentary lifestyles should begin with physical activity of very low intensity and advance activity levels very gradually.
11. Activity should be stopped and the primary care giver consulted if any unusual symptoms appear.
12. Maternal heart rate should not exceed 140 beats per minute.
13. Strenuous activities should not exceed 15 minutes in duration.
14. No exercise should be performed in the supine position after the 4th month of gestation is completed; avoid toe pointing to prevent leg cramps.
15. Exercises that employ the Valsalva maneuver should be avoided.
16. Caloric intake should be adequate to meet not only the extra energy needs of pregnancy but also of the exercise performed.
17. Maternal core temperature should not exceed 38°C (100.4°F).

American College of Obstetricians and Gynecologists. *Exercise during pregnancy and the postnatal period.* Washington, DC: ACOG, with permission; Retts, V. S. (1993). Women and exercise, *The Female Patient, 18,* 59.

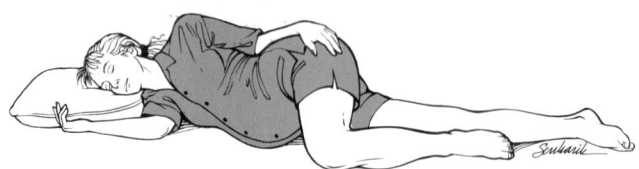

FIGURE 11-2
Modified Sims' position as a rest position during pregnancy. The knees and elbows should be slightly bent, the muscles limp, and the breathing slow and regular. Notice that the weight of the fetus is resting on the floor.

sleeping position is a modified **Sims' position,** with the top leg forward (Figure 11-2). This puts the weight of the fetus on the bed, not on the woman, and allows good circulation in the lower extremities.

Be certain women know not to rest in a supine position or they can develop supine hypotension syndrome (faintness and hypotension from the presence of the expanding uterus on the inferior vena cava). Be certain they know not to rest with their knees bent, as this adds greatly to pooling of blood in the venous system and potential thrombophlebitis.

Work

Unless women's jobs involve exposure to toxic substances, lifting heavy objects, other kinds of excessive physical strain, long periods of standing, or having to maintain body balance, there are few reasons they cannot continue to be employed throughout pregnancy. To protect women from loss of employment benefits during pregnancy, Congress passed an employment rights law in 1978 (Public Law 95-555) (Box 11-2). The only women not covered by this law are those who work for companies with fewer than 15 employees.

Some occupations are more hazardous because they bring women into contact with harmful substances. For example, nurses working with anesthetic gases in operating room suites or dental offices are reported to have a higher incidence of spontaneous abortion and, possibly, congenital anomalies in children than nurses working in other locales (Shepard, 1992). This finding suggests that breathing even a low dose of anesthetic gases such as nitrous oxide can be a serious occupational hazard for these nurses (Bernhardt, 1990). Nurses working with chemotherapy agents should wear gloves to protect themselves from exposure to these drugs, which are possibly teratogenic. Ribavirin, an antibiotic used to treat respiratory syncytial infections, is also apparently teratogenic if inhaled by health care providers (Corey & Clore, 1991).

A number of studies suggest that spontaneous abortion may occur more frequently in women who work outside the home than in those who do not, regardless of occupation, and the longer a woman works beyond 28 weeks of pregnancy, the lower her baby's birth

---

Box 11-2
Employment Rights of Pregnant Women

An employer *cannot:*

1. Deprive women of seniority rights, in pay or promotion, because they take a maternity leave.
2. Treat women returning from maternity leave as new hires, starting over on the eligibility period for pension and other benefits.
3. Force pregnant women to leave if they are able to and want to continue working.
4. Refuse to hire women just because they are pregnant or fire them for the same reason.
5. Refuse to cover employees' normal pregnancy and delivery expenses in the company health plan or pay less for pregnancy then for other medical conditions.
6. Refuse to pay sick leave or disability benefits to women whose difficult pregnancies keep them off the job.

Source: Public law 95-555, United States Congress, 1978.

---

weight may be (Bernhardt, 1990). Other problems that can possibly occur with employment include interferences in adequate rest and nutrition. Based on these findings, the American Medical Association suggests that women employed in jobs that require standing or walking or excess physical exertion stop or reduce their work load 2 to 4 weeks before the expected date of birth (Bernhardt, 1990). Urge the woman who works outside her home to put her feet up to rest when performing tasks that can be done in that position. Review what she eats at fast food restaurants or packs for herself to be certain she understands this type of lunch can be as nutritious as if she were eating at home if she takes the time to plan ahead.

Remember that few women work for the sheer joy of working; most work to augment or supply the family income. Even those who could afford to leave their jobs may not be willing to sacrifice the collegial relationships and sense of fulfillment derived from work, nor the lifestyle their income has allowed them to enjoy. More effective than counseling women to resign from their jobs during pregnancy to get more rest, then, is counseling them to reserve periods during the day for rest and urging them to eat a proper diet (see the Focus on Family Teaching box).

Travel

Most women have questions about travel during pregnancy. Early in a normal pregnancy, there are literally no restrictions except that those who are susceptible to motion sickness should take no medication that is not

FOCUS ON FAMILY TEACHING

Q. What are sensible guidelines I can use to avoid overdoing at work during pregnancy?

A. A good question. Some common-sense guidelines for women working during pregnancy are:

- Use your rest periods for resting, not running errands, etc.

- Try and use at least part of your lunch hour to rest. Lie on your left side in a break room if possible.

- If your job involves long periods of standing, think of times you could stop and elevate your legs (working in a low file drawer, reading time in a classroom, etc.).

- Walk around periodically to avoid periods of long standing in one position if possible; stretch your back periodically to try and avoid backache.

- Wear support hose to improve venous return to lower extremities.

- Avoid excessive overtime or working longer than 8-hour shifts.

- Empty your bladder every 2 hours as a measure to try and prevent bladder infection.

- Get extra rest on weekends or days off.

- Take great caution around equipment that requires sure balance. Avoid ladders or climbing late in pregnancy when balance is a problem.

- Learn your target heart rate for exercise. If your job involves strenuous exercise, stop and rest at the point your target heart rate is exceeded.

- Stop or reduce work 2–4 weeks before your EDB.

---

specifically prescribed or approved by their physician or nurse-midwife. Late in pregnancy, travel plans should take into consideration the possibility of early labor, requiring delivery at a strange setting where the woman's obstetric history is unknown.

If the woman plans to spend her vacation at a remote location, such as a campsite, be certain that no matter what month of pregnancy she is in, she knows of a health care facility near the location should an unexpected complication occur. If she is going to be away from home for an extended vacation, she will need to make arrangements to visit a health care provider in her vacation area at the times her regular prenatal visits would be scheduled. Ask her to make these plans far enough ahead of time to allow her office or clinic records to be copied for her to carry with her or to be forwarded to the health care provider she will see (you need her written permission to send records). She should be certain to pack enough of her prescribed vitamin supplement plus adequate prescriptions for refills as necessary.

Advise a woman who is taking a long trip by automobile to plan frequent rest or stretch periods. Every 100 miles, or at least every 200 miles, she should get out of the car and walk a short distance. This practice will relieve stiffness and muscle ache and improve lower-extremity circulation, helping to prevent varicosities and hemorrhoids.

Women may drive as long as they fit comfortably behind the steering wheel. While pregnant, they should use seat belts like everyone else. Occasionally, uterine rupture has been reported from seat belt use, but, overall, the evidence suggests that seat belts reduce maternal mortality in car accidents. Both shoulder harnesses and lap belts should be used (Hammond, 1990). The lap belt should be worn as snugly as comfortable, so that it fits under the abdomen across the pelvic bones. The shoulder harness should be worn above the uterus and across the shoulder to avoid chafing the woman's neck. It should also be as snug as comfortable.

Pregnancy is also a time for a family to think about safety for the newborn. Purchasing a car seat is an investment that may require some advance planning. Women need to plan during pregnancy because they will need an infant seat in order to take the baby home from the hospital. Families who cannot afford to purchase an infant car seat may want to inquire among friends or relatives about the possibility of borrowing an infant seat that is no longer needed. Many hospitals also provide infant seats on a rental or loan basis for families who may find it difficult to obtain one in other ways.

Traveling by plane shortens traveling time and is not contraindicated as long as the plane has a well-pressurized cabin (true of commercial airlines but not of all small private planes). Some airlines do not permit women who are more than seven months pregnant on board; others require written permission from the woman's primary caregiver. The woman will have to investigate these restrictions herself by calling the airline or a travel agency.

Women who are traveling abroad may need extra vaccination protection for entry into certain countries to safeguard their health. Some vaccines are contraindicated during pregnancy, however, and must not be administered unless the risk of the disease outweighs the risk to the pregnancy. Before any immunization, women should ask their primary caregiver to verify it will be safe during pregnancy (Bia, 1992).

Discomforts of Early Pregnancy: The First Trimester

The symptoms of early pregnancy tend to cause more discomfort than they provide evidence to the woman that she is carrying a child. As such, they can become frustrating to a woman who expected her pregnancy to be a time of glowing good health. Providing sympathetic and sound advice for measures to relieve these discomforts does much to promote the overall health and well being of a pregnant client. Although the symptoms discussed below are classified as minor, they may not seem minor to the woman who wakes up each morning feeling nauseous and despairs of ever feeling herself again. What's more, each of these symptoms has the potential to lead to problems that are more serious.

Nursing Diagnoses

Listening, observing carefully, and developing nursing diagnoses based on assessment data are important steps in prenatal care. Examples of nursing diagnoses that might be developed for women experiencing the symptoms of early pregnancy are listed below. It is important to keep in mind that although many women will have many of these symptoms, each woman will experience them uniquely. Nursing diagnoses must be developed according to each woman's individual needs. Examples are:

- Health-seeking behaviors related to interest in relieving discomforts of pregnancy
- Altered comfort related to breast tenderness during pregnancy
- Body-image disturbance related to breast and abdominal enlargement in pregnancy
- Constipation related to reduced peristalsis in pregnancy
- Fatigue related to increased physiologic need for sleep and rest during pregnancy
- Pain related to frequent muscle cramps secondary to physiologic changes of pregnancy
- Altered sleep pattern related to frequent need to empty bladder during night

Breast Tenderness

Breast tenderness is often one of the first symptoms noticed in early pregnancy; it may be most noticeable on exposure to cold air. For most women, the tenderness is minimal and transient, something they are aware of but not unduly distressed by. If the tenderness is enough to cause discomfort, encourage the woman to wear a bra with a wide shoulder strap for support and to dress warmly to avoid cold drafts if cold increases symp-

toms. If actual pain exists, the presence of conditions such as nipple fissure or other explanations for the pain should be ruled out.

Palmar Erythema

Palmar erythema, or palmar pruritus, occurs in early pregnancy and is probably caused by increased estrogen levels. Constant redness or itching of the palms may make the woman think she is allergic to something. She needs an explanation that this is normal before she spends time and effort trying different soaps or detergents or attempting to implicate certain foods she has eaten. Calamine lotion may be soothing for this condition. As soon as the woman's body adjusts to the increased level of estrogen, the erythema and pruritus disappear.

Constipation

Constipation tends to occur in pregnancy as the pressure of the growing uterus presses against the bowel and slows peristalsis. If you discuss preventive measures with the woman early in pregnancy, she may be able to avoid this problem. Encourage her to evacuate her bowels regularly (many women neglect this first simple rule); to increase the amount of roughage in her diet by eating raw fruits, bran, and vegetables; and to drink extra amounts of water daily.

Some women find that an oral iron supplement leads to constipation. Help the woman to find a method to relieve or prevent constipation through other measures than avoiding taking the iron supplement as she needs this supplement to build iron stores in the fetus.

The woman should not use "home" medications to prevent constipation; she should especially avoid mineral oil. Mineral oil interferes with the absorption of fat-soluble vitamins (A, D, K, and E), which are needed for good fetal growth and maternal health.

Enemas also should be avoided as their action might initiate labor. Over-the-counter laxatives are contraindicated, as are *all* drugs during pregnancy unless specifically prescribed or sanctioned by her physician or nurse-midwife (Cunningham et al., 1993). Stool softeners, mild laxatives, and evacuation suppositories may be prescribed. Some women have extensive flatulence accompanying constipation. Avoiding gas-forming foods, such as cabbage or beans, will help to control this problem.

Nausea, Vomiting, and Pyrosis

At least half of pregnant women experience enough gastrointestinal symptoms to cause discomfort in pregnancy. As these symptoms also interfere with nutrition, they are discussed in Chapter 12.

Fatigue

Fatigue is extremely common in early pregnancy. It is probably due to increased metabolic requirements, and

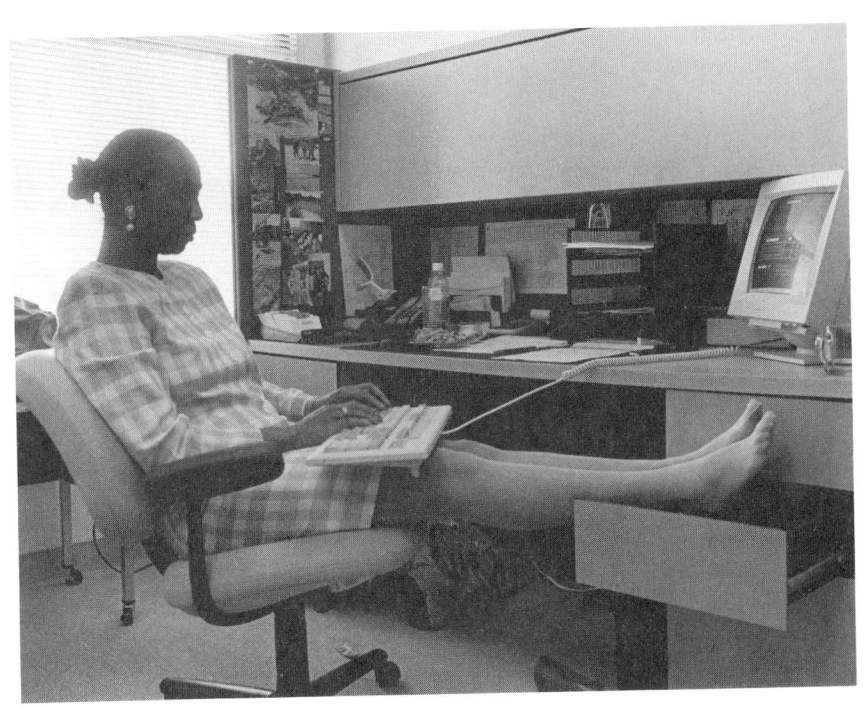

FIGURE 11-3
If at all possible, women who are employed need to arrange a "feet-up" period during their workday.

much of it can be relieved by increasing the amount of rest and sleep. Some women are reluctant to take time out of their day for rest; they know that pregnancy is not an illness, and so they proceed as if nothing is happening to them. Rarely is there justification during a normal pregnancy for women to take extra days off from work because of their condition, but it is also unrealistic to proceed as if nothing is happening. Fatigue can increase morning sickness, so if a woman becomes too tired, she does not eat properly. If she remains on her feet without at least one break during the day, the tendency for varicosities to develop increases as does the danger of thromboembolitic complications.

Ask women at prenatal visits whether or not they manage to have at least *one* short rest period every day. A good resting position is a modified Sims' position, with the top leg forward (See Figure 11-2). This puts the weight of the fetus on the bed, not on the woman, and allows good circulation in the lower extremities.

A woman who works outside her home might use part of her lunch hour to sit with her feet elevated on an adjoining chair (Figure 11-3). After she returns home from work in the evening, she may need to modify a customary routine from cooking dinner, doing the dishes, straightening up the house, and so on, to *resting,* then cooking dinner and so on; or *resting* while her husband cooks the dinner and cleans the dishes (part of "we are having a baby at our house" for a husband who does not usually share in household chores).

Muscle Cramps

Decreased serum calcium, increased serum phosphorus, and, possibly, interference with circulation commonly cause muscle cramps of the lower extremities during pregnancy. These circulation problems are best relieved by the woman lying on her back and extending the involved leg while keeping her knee straight and dorsiflexing the foot (Figure 11-4).

If the woman is having frequent leg cramps, she may need a prescription of aluminum hydroxide gel (Amphojel), which binds phosphorus in the intestinal tract and thereby lowers its circulating level. Lowering milk intake to only a pint daily may also help to reduce the phosphorus level. Elevating the lower extremities frequently during the day to improve circulation and never stretching the legs to full extension with the toes pointed may be of benefit. Muscle cramps are a minor symptom of pregnancy, but the pain may be extreme

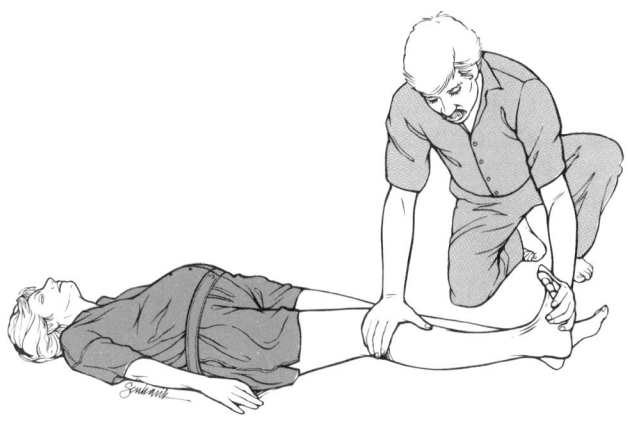

FIGURE 11-4
Relieving a leg cramp in pregnancy. Pressing down on the knee and pressing the toes backward (dorsiflexion) relieves most cramps. A husband assists here.

and the intensity of the contraction can be frightening. Always ask at prenatal visits if this is a problem; otherwise, women may not realize that cramping is pregnancy-related and may not mention the problem spontaneously.

Hypotension

Supine hypotension is a symptom that occurs when a woman lies on her back and the uterus presses on the vena cava, impairing blood return to the heart. Relieving the problem is simple: if the woman turns or is turned on her side, pressure is removed from the vena cava, blood flow is restored, and the symptoms quickly fade.

If a woman rises suddenly from a lying or sitting position or stands for an extended time in a warm or crowded area, she may faint from the same phenomenon (blood pooling in the pelvic area or lower extremities). Rising slowly and avoiding extended periods of standing prevent this problem. If the woman should feel faint, sitting with her head lowered—the same action for any person who feels faint—will alleviate the problem.

Varicosities

Varicosities are common in pregnancy because the weight of the distended uterus puts pressure on the veins returning blood from the lower extremities. This causes a pooling of blood in the vessels. The veins become engorged, inflamed, and painful. Varicosities usually are found in the lower extremities; they may extend to the vulva. They occur most frequently in women with a family history of varicose veins and those who have a large fetus or a multiple pregnancy (Kochenour, 1990). Urge such women to prevent varicosities early in pregnancy; if left until the second trimester, the best you can accomplish is relief of their pain from already formed varicosities.

Resting in a Sims' position or on the back with the legs raised against the wall or elevated on a footstool for 15 to 20 minutes twice a day is a good precaution (Figure 11-5). Be certain that the woman doesn't sit with her legs crossed or her knees bent. She should not wear knee-high hose.

Some women may need the support of elastic stockings or an ace bandage for relief of varicosities. The stocking or bandage should be applied to the leg so that it reaches an area above the point of distention. The woman should apply the support before she arises in the morning; once she is on her feet, the pooling of blood has already begun, and the stockings or bandages will not be as effective. If a woman is going to buy stockings, be certain she understands they are to be medical support hose. Many panty hose manufacturers advertise their stockings as giving "firm support," and the woman may assume erroneously that this is sufficient for her.

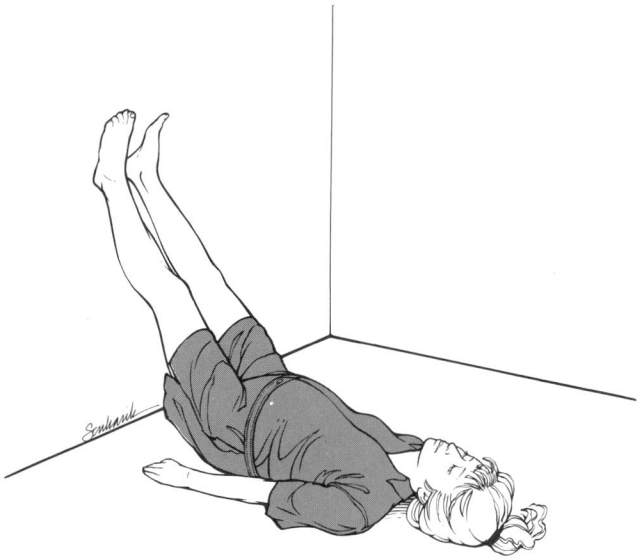

FIGURE 11-5
Position to relieve varicosities. The mother keeps a pad under her right hip to prevent supine hypotensive syndrome.

Exercise is as effective as rest periods in alleviating varicosities, because it stimulates venous return. Most women state that they do not need set exercise periods during pregnancy because they work hard cleaning the house or working on the job. If they analyze the type of work they do, however, they will realize that a great deal of housework and office or factory work leads to stasis of lower-extremity circulation. Women stand in one position to wash dishes, make beds, cook dinner, file, run a duplicating machine, process a part on an assembly line, or teach a class. They need to break up these long periods of standing with a "walk break" at least twice a day, and their families would benefit by accompanying them. Husbands may discover that they, too, walk very little during their workday.

Vitamin C may be helpful in reducing the size of varicosities as it is apparently involved in the formation of blood vessel collagen and endothelium. Ask at prenatal visits whether fresh fruit is included in the woman's diet.

Hemorrhoids

Hemorrhoids are varicosities of the rectal veins that occur commonly in pregnancy because of pressure on these veins from the bulk of the growing uterus. Preventive measures early in pregnancy may be effective in reducing their severity. Daily bowel evacuation not only helps to relieve constipation but also helps to prevent the formation of hemorrhoids. Resting in a modified Sims' position daily is helpful. At day's end, assuming a knee-chest position (Figure 11-6) for 10 to 15 minutes is an excellent way to reduce the pressure on rectal veins. A knee-chest position tends to make a woman feel light-

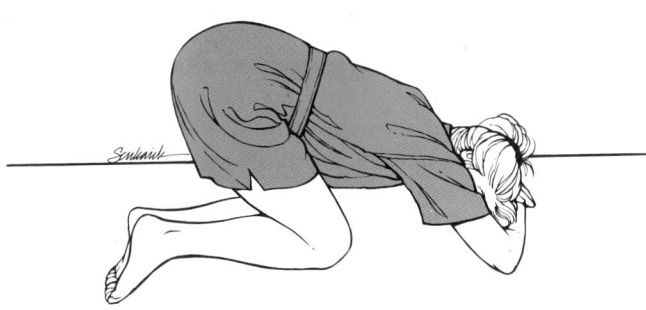

FIGURE 11-6
Knee-chest position. This position allows for free flow of urine from the kidneys (preventing urinary tract stasis and infection) and better circulation in the rectal area (preventing hemorrhoids), because the weight of the uterus is shifted forward.

headed; thus, at first, she should remain in this position for a few minutes only, gradually increasing the time until she can maintain the position comfortably for about 15 minutes. Stool softeners may be recommended for the woman who already has hemorrhoids. Applying witch hazel may help relieve pain. As with varicosities, think *prevent,* not just provide help for already established hemorrhoids.

Heart Palpitations

On sudden movement, such as turning over in bed, a pregnant woman may experience a bounding palpitation of the heart. This is probably due to the circulatory adjustments necessary to accommodate her increased blood supply during pregnancy. Although only momentary, the sensation is frightening because the heart seems to have skipped a beat. Slower movements will prevent its happening so frequently. It is reassuring for women

to know that palpitations are normal and to be expected on occasion.

Frequency of Urination

Frequency of urination occurs in early pregnancy due to the pressure of the growing uterus on the anterior bladder. It may last for about 3 months, sometimes beginning as early as the first or second missed period, disappear in midpregnancy when the uterus rises above the bladder; and return again in late pregnancy as the fetal head presses against the bladder (Figure 11-7).

When a woman describes frequency of urination, be certain this is the only urinary symptom that she has. Ask whether she has burning on urination or whether she has noticed any blood in her urine (signs of urinary tract infection).

There are no solutions for decreasing frequency of urination; the important intervention is to be certain the woman understands that voiding more frequently is a normal phenomenon. Unless a woman is cautioned that the sensation of frequency returns after lightening (the settling of the fetal head into the inlet of the pelvis at pregnancy's end), she may think she has a urinary tract infection. This is less noticeable to women who have practiced Kegel exercises (alternately contracting and relaxing perineal muscles; Box 11-3) as preparation for delivery.

Occasionally, a woman notices stress incontinence (involuntary loss of urine on coughing or sneezing) during pregnancy. Doing Kegel exercises helps to strengthen urinary control and directly strengthen perineal muscles for birth and decreases the possibility that stress incontinence will occur.

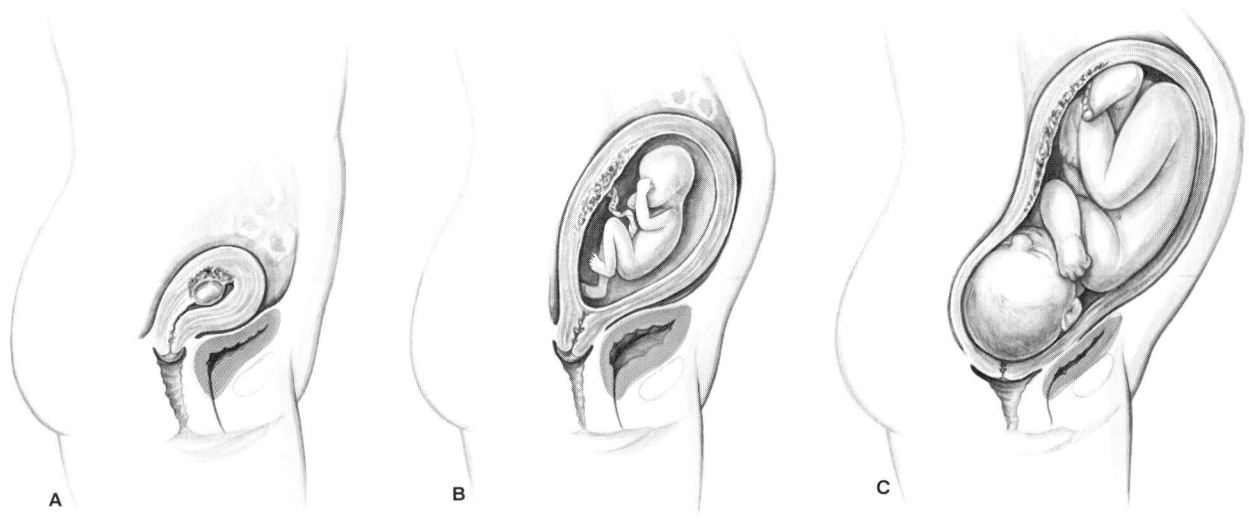

A   B   C

FIGURE 11-7
*Bladder changes during pregnancy. (**A**) Early pregnancy: the uterus presses against the bladder causing frequency of urination. (**B**) Middle pregnancy: urinary frequency is relieved. (**C**) Late pregnancy: the uterus is again pressing on the bladder.*

Box 11-3
Kegel Exercises

Kegel exercises are exercises designed to strengthen the pubococcygeal muscles. They should be done about 3 times a day. Exercises are as follows:

1. Squeeze the muscles surrounding the vagina as if stopping the flow of urine. Hold for 3 seconds. Relax. Repeat 10 times.
2. Contract and relax the muscles surrounding the vagina as rapidly as possible 10 to 25 times.
3. Imagine that you are sitting in a bathtub of water and squeeze muscles as if sucking water into the vagina. Hold for 3 seconds. Relax. Repeat 10 times.
4. Push out with the vagina as if expelling something from it. Hold for 3 seconds. Relax. Repeat 10 times.

It may take as long as 6 weeks of exercise before pubococcygeal muscles are strengthened. In addition to preventing stress incontinence, exercises can lead to increased sexual enjoyment because of the tightened vaginal muscles.

Abdominal Discomfort

Some women experience uncomfortable feelings of abdominal pressure early in pregnancy. Women with a multiple pregnancy may notice this throughout pregnancy. Women learn to relieve the feeling by putting gentle pressure on the uterine fundus. Pregnant women typically stand with their arms crossed in front, as the weight of their arms resting on their abdomens relieves this discomfort.

When women stand up quickly, they may experience a pulling pain in the right or left lower abdomen from tension on the round ligaments. The pain is sharp and frightening. They can prevent this type of pain by always rising slowly from a lying to a sitting, or from a sitting to a standing, position. Because round ligament pain may simulate the abrupt pain that occurs with ruptured ectopic pregnancy, the description of the pain needs to be evaluated carefully.

Leukorrhea

Leukorrhea is a whitish, viscous vaginal discharge or an increase in the amount of normal vaginal secretions. It occurs in response to the high estrogen levels present and the increased blood supply to the vaginal epithelium and cervix in pregnancy. A daily bath or shower to wash away accumulated secretions and prevent vulvar excoriation should be enough to control this problem. The woman should *not* douche. Some women may wear perineal pads to control the discharge. Women

should be cautioned *not* to use tampons, however, because this could lead to stasis of secretions and subsequent infection. Wearing cotton, not synthetic, underpants and sleeping at night without underwear are also helpful measures in reducing moisture and possible vulvar excoriation. Advise women to contact their physician or nurse-midwife if there is a change in the color, odor, or character of this discharge, as this suggests infection.

A woman with vulvar pruritus needs to be seen by a health care provider because this strongly indicates infection. Be certain that when she is describing pruritus-like symptoms she is not really describing burning on urination, a sign of a beginning bladder infection (which also needs therapy, but of a different type). Common vaginal infections that present with pruritus are discussed in Chapter 47.

Avoiding tight underpants and panty hose may help prevent yeast infections. Although over-the-counter medications for yeast infections are available, caution women not to treat vaginal infections by themselves during pregnancy. Some medications (metronidazole [Flagyl], in particular) prescribed for trichomonas are not recommended during early pregnancy due to possible **teratogenicity** (fetal harm) (Reed & Eyler, 1993).

A woman who is uncomfortable about discussing this part of her body or who associates vaginal infections with poor hygiene or sexually transmitted disease may be reluctant to mention an irritating vaginal discharge. It is helpful, therefore, to ask each woman specifically at prenatal visits whether she has this problem.

Discomforts of Middle to Late Pregnancy

At the midpoint of pregnancy (the 20th to 24th weeks) the woman is usually ready for further health teaching that relates to the new developments in the latter half of pregnancy. She should be informed of the signs and symptoms of beginning labor. As she starts to view the child within her as a separate person, she becomes interested in discussing and making plans for labor, birth, and the infant's care. At the midpoint of a pregnancy, it is good to review the precautions she should take to prevent constipation, varicosities, and hemorrhoids and to describe the new minor symptoms that may now be expected.

Nursing Diagnoses

Possible nursing diagnoses associated with the discomforts of middle to late pregnancy include the following:

- Health-seeking behaviors related to discomforts of middle to late pregnancy
- Pain related to postural changes in pregnancy
- Anxiety related to lack of information about shortness of breath secondary to pressure on diaphragm from the expanding uterus

- Altered comfort related to minor ankle edema
- Fear related to occurrence of Braxton Hicks contractions in late pregnancy

Backache

As pregnancy advances, a lumbar lordosis occurs and postural changes necessary to maintain balance will cause backache. Wearing shoes with a moderate-height heel reduces the amount of spinal curvature necessary to maintain an upright posture. Encouraging the woman to walk with her pelvis tilted forward (putting pelvic support under the weight of the fetus) is also helpful. Too often, women are observed at a prenatal visit only lying in a lithotomy position on an examining table. Make it a nursing responsibility to assess the manner in which the woman walks and what type of shoes she is wearing as she moves from the waiting room to the examining room. This assessment can reveal a lot about the cause of her backache. Advising women to squat and not to bend over to pick up objects and to always lift objects by holding them close to the body also may help. Some women may need a firmer mattress during pregnancy than before; sliding a board under the mattress serves the same purpose and is cheaper than buying a new mattress. Pelvic rocking or tilting, an exercise described in Chapter 13, also helps to prevent and relieve backache.

Women who begin preterm labor have a higher frequency of backache than others (Iams et al., 1990). It can also be an initial sign of bladder or kidney infection. Thus, you need a detailed account of a woman's symptoms to make certain she is describing only backache. Caution women not to take muscle relaxants or analgesia (or any other medication) for back pain without first consulting their physician or nurse-midwife. Generally, acetaminophen (Tylenol) is considered to be safe and effective for relieving this type of pain during pregnancy.

Headache

A number of women experience headache during pregnancy apparently from the expanding blood volume which puts pressure on cerebral arteries (Feller & Franko-Filiposic, 1993). Women should try to reduce any situation which normally causes headaches for them, such as eye strain or tension, to try and lessen the number of headaches they experience. Resting with cold towels on their forehead and taking usual adult doses of acetaminophen usually furnishes adequate relief. Although a few women who have migraine headaches find these worsen during pregnancy, most women notice considerable improvement with this type of headache (see Chapter 49). Caution women that if a headache is *unusually intense* or *continuous,* they should report it to their primary care provider as this type of headache may be a danger sign of pregnancy (see Danger Signs of Pregnancy, Chapter 10).

Dyspnea

Shortness of breath occurs in pregnancy as the expanding uterus puts pressure on the diaphragm and causes some lung compression. A woman may notice this mostly at night, when she lies flat, and she will definitely notice it on exertion. Sitting upright, allowing the weight of the uterus to fall away from the diaphragm, will relieve the problem. As pregnancy progresses, she may require two or more pillows to sleep at night. Caution her to limit her activities *before* she becomes short of breath. Remember that anxiety adds to the sensation of breathlessness. Worry over dyspnea may make her more dyspneic, which is one reason this is an important minor symptom to review. Distraction from the discomfort by a support person is helpful and a good way for a support person who plans to help the woman through labor and birth to practice distraction techniques.

Ankle Edema

Most women experience some swelling of the ankles and feet during late pregnancy, most noticeably at the end of the day. Women are often conscious of this first when they kick off their shoes at a restaurant or party and then are unable to put them on again comfortably.

Ankle edema of this nature, as long as proteinuria and hypertension do not accompany it, is a normal occurrence of pregnancy. It is probably caused by reduced blood circulation in the lower extremities due to uterine pressure and general fluid retention. This simple edema can be relieved best by resting in a side-lying position as this increases kidney glomerular flow rate. Sitting for half an hour in the afternoon and again in the evening with the legs elevated is also helpful. Women should avoid constricting panty girdles or knee-high stockings, as these impede lower-extremity circulation and venous return.

Women need reassurance that ankle edema is normal during pregnancy. Otherwise, they worry that it is a beginning sign of pregnancy-induced hypertension. On the other hand, do not dismiss a report of lower-extremity edema lightly until you are certain that the woman does not evidence any signs (proteinuria; edema of other, nondependent parts; sudden increase in weight) that might indicate pregnancy-induced hypertension.

Braxton Hicks Contractions

Beginning as early as the 12th week of pregnancy, the uterus periodically contracts and then relaxes again. Early in pregnancy, these contractions, termed **Braxton Hicks contractions,** are not noticeable. In middle and late pregnancy, the contractions become stronger, and the woman who tenses at the sensation may even experience some minimal pain similar to a hard menstrual cramp. Women need reassurance that the contractions are normal and that they are not a sign of beginning labor. Equally important, be certain they understand that a rhythmic pattern of contractions is probably labor and should not be mistaken for Braxton Hicks contractions. Table 11-1 summarizes common discomforts of pregnancy and steps to take to relieve them.

Preparation for Labor

At about the midpoint of pregnancy, it is time to review the events that signal the beginning of labor so women will not be surprised by these happenings or dismiss them as something other than what they are.

Table 11-1. Common Discomforts of Pregnancy

Discomfort	Possible Solutions
Ankle edema	Rest with feet elevated Avoid standing for long periods Avoid constrictive lower extremity garments
Backache	Avoid periods of long standing Apply local heat Stoop, don't bend to lift objects Take acetaminophen in regular adult doses
Breast tenderness	Wear a support bra
Constipation	Increase fiber in diet Save regular time for defecation Drink additional fluid
Fatigue	Try for full night's sleep Schedule a rest time daily Maintain good nutrition
Headache	Avoid eye strain Rest with cold cloth on forehead Take acetaminophen in regular adult doses
Hemorrhoids	Rest and sleep in Sims' position Avoid constipation Apply witch hazel and replace hemorrhoids gently Take sitz baths
Leg cramps	Reduce milk intake Straighten leg and dorsiflex ankle Avoid pointing toes
Round ligament pain	Rise from a standing position slowly Bend forward to relieve pain Avoid twisting motions
Urinary frequency	Void as necessary Avoid caffeine Practice Kegel exercises
Vaginal discharge	Wear cotton underwear Avoid tight-fitting pantyhose Bathe daily
Varicosities	Walk regularly Rest with feet elevated daily Avoid standing for long periods Avoid crossing legs; avoid knee-high stockings Wear support stockings

Lightening

Lightening is the settling of the fetal head into the inlet of the true pelvis. It occurs approximately 2 weeks before labor in primiparas but at unpredictable times in multiparas. The woman notices that she is not as short of breath as she was; her abdominal contour is definitely changed; and on standing she may experience frequency of urination or sciatic pain (pain across her buttock radiating down her leg) from the lowered fetal position.

Show

Show is the common term for the release of the cervical plug (operculum) that formed during pregnancy. It consists of a mucous, often blood-streaked vaginal discharge and indicates that cervical dilatation is beginning.

Rupture of the Membranes

A sudden gush of clear fluid (amniotic fluid) from the vagina indicates rupture of the membranes. The woman should telephone the clinic or office at once if labor begins this way. Following rupture of the membranes, there is danger of cord prolapse and uterine infection.

Excess Energy

Feeling extremely energetic is a sign of labor that is important for women to recognize. It occurs as part of the body's physiologic preparation for labor. If the woman does not recognize the sensation for what it is, she may use this burst of energy to clean or finish paperwork at the office and exhaust herself before labor begins. If she can recognize this symptom as an initial sign of labor, she can conserve the energy for the purpose for which nature intended it.

Uterine Contractions

For most women, labor begins with contractions. True labor contractions usually start in the back and sweep forward across the abdomen like the tightening of a band. They gradually increase in frequency and intensity. Advise a woman to telephone the health care facility when contractions begin, in order to alert the health care personnel that she is in labor. Inform her at what point in labor her physician or nurse-midwife wants her to come to a health care facility (such as when contractions are five minutes apart) but be certain she knows this is not a hard-and-fast rule. If she should become exceptionally anxious, be home alone, or have a long drive, she should be given the option of arriving ahead of time.

Prevention of Fetal Exposure to Teratogens

A **teratogen** is any factor, chemical or physical, that adversely affects the fertilized ovum, embryo, or fetus. In order to reach maturity in optimal health, a fetus needs not only sound genes (see Chapter 7) but also a healthy intrauterine environment that protects from the influence of teratogens.

At one time it was assumed that a fetus in utero was protected from chemical or physical injury by the presence of the amniotic fluid and by the absence of any direct exchange between mother and fetus at the placenta. When infants were born with disorders, it was often attributed to the influence of "fate," "bad luck," or, in some cultures, "evil spirits." Today it is acknowledged that a fetus is extremely vulnerable to environmental injury; although many anomalies occurring in utero are still unknown, many teratogenic factors can now be isolated.

Effects of Teratogens on the Fetus

Several factors influence the amount of damage a teratogen can cause. Strength of the teratogen is obviously one. For example, radiation is a known teratogen, but in small amounts (everyone is exposed to some radiation every day) it causes no damage. In large doses, however (e.g., the amount of radiation necessary to treat cancer of the cervix), serious fetal defects or death can occur.

The timing of the teratogenic insult is another factor that makes a significant difference. If a teratogen is introduced before implantation, either the zygote is destroyed or appears unaffected. If the insult occurs when the main body systems are being formed (in the 2nd to 8th weeks of embryonic life), the fetus is very vulnerable to injury. During the last trimester, the potential for harm again decreases as all the organs of the fetus are formed and are merely maturing (Dickinson & Gonik, 1990). The times when different anatomic areas of the fetus are most likely to be affected by teratogens are shown in Chapter 9, Figure 9-5.

Two known exceptions to the rule that deformities usually occur in early embryonic life are the effects caused by the organisms of syphilis and toxoplasmosis. These two infections can cause abnormalities in organs that were originally formed normally.

A third factor determining the effects of a teratogen is that each teratogen generally has an affinity for specific tissue. Lead, for instance, attacks and disables nervous tissue. Thalidomide causes limb defects. Tetracycline causes tooth enamel deficiencies and, possibly, longbone deformities. The rubella virus, on the other hand, can affect many organs: the eyes, ears, heart, and brain are the four most commonly attacked (Dickinson & Gonik, 1990).

Nursing Diagnoses

Nurses who care for women during pregnancy should be familiar with the various categories of teratogens described in the following sections, as much of the health history information obtained at prenatal visits is gathered to determine whether or not the woman has been exposed to a teratogen since the last visit.

Possible nursing diagnoses associated with maternal exposure to teratogens include the following:

- Health-seeking behavior related to mother's interest in avoiding exposure to substances that would be harmful to the fetus during pregnancy
- High risk for fetal injury related to lack of knowledge about teratogenicity of alcohol, drugs, and cigarettes
- High risk for infection transmission to fetus related to possible maternal exposure to genital herpes

Women seeking prenatal care need to be educated regarding the teratogenicity of alcohol and chemical substances as well as environmental teratogens and possible exposure to a variety of infections.

Teratogenic Maternal Infections

Teratogenic maternal infections have been described collectively under the umbrella term TORCH, which is an abbreviation for toxoplasmosis, rubella, cytomegalovirus, and herpes simplex virus. (Some sources identify the "O" with "other infections," which could include syphilis, hepatitis B virus [HBV], and HIV.) These are all infections known to cross the placenta and affect the fetus during pregnancy. The TORCH screen was developed as an immunologic survey to determine whether these infections exist in either the pregnant woman (to identify fetal risk factors) or the newborn (to detect if antibodies against the common infectious teratogens are present). Although it is now known that many more than the original four or five maternal infections can harm the embryo or fetus, the TORCH screen still provides a quick way to assess the potential risk of teratogenic infection in pregnant women and newborns.

Teratogenic infections can be viral, bacterial, or protozoan. Most cause relatively mild, flu-like symptoms in the woman, yet can have much more serious effects on the fetus or newborn. Preventing and predicting fetal injury from infection is complicated, because a disease may be subclinical (without symptoms in the mother) and yet injure the fetus. The most common teratogenic infections are described in more detail below.

Rubella

The rubella virus usually causes only mild systemic illness in the mother, but the teratogenic effects on the fetus can be devastating. Fetal damage from maternal infection with rubella (German measles) includes deafness, mental and motor retardation, cataracts, cardiac defects (patent ductus arteriosus and pulmonary stenosis being the most common), retarded intrauterine growth (small for gestation age), thrombocytopenic purpura, and dental and facial clefts, such as cleft lip and palate.

The greatest risk to the embryo from rubella virus is during the **organogenesis period** in early pregnancy. The frequency of defects is about 80% if infection occurs in the first 12 weeks of pregnancy, 54% at 13 to 14 weeks, and 25% after the second trimester. In addition, there is about a 30% chance of spontaneous abortion or stillbirth if the infection occurs in the first trimester.

All women of childbearing age should be immunized against rubella so that this teratogen can be eradicated. About 10% of women are still unimmunized (Eisele, 1993). A woman who is not immunized before pregnancy cannot be immunized during pregnancy because the vaccine uses a live virus that would have effects similar to those occurring with a subclinical case of rubella. Following a rubella immunization, a woman is not advised to become pregnant for three months. Immediately following a pregnancy, all women who have low rubella titers should be immunized so that they will have the needed protection against rubella during their next pregnancy. Helping to screen postpartum women to discover those with low or unknown titers is a responsibility of the nurse on a postpartum unit.

An increasing concern is women who demonstrate antibodies against rubella, yet become reinfected during pregnancy (Weber et al., 1993). Because of this, pregnant women should avoid contact with children with rashes. Infants who are born to mothers who had rubella during pregnancy may be capable of transmitting the disease for up to 8 months after birth (Dickinson & Gonik, 1990). The infant should be isolated from other newborns during the newborn period, and the mother should be made aware of the possibility that her infant might infect others, including pregnant women. Nurses with low rubella titers should avoid caring for these infants (and should act to have their serum titer elevated by immunization). Titer analysis is traditionally done by a hemagglutination inhibition assay. A titer greater than 1:8 suggests immunity to rubella. A titer of less than 1:8 suggests that the woman is susceptible to invasion of the virus. A titer that is increased greatly over a previous reading or is initially extremely high suggests that a recent infection has occurred (Dascal et al., 1990).

Cytomegalovirus (CMV)

The **cytomegalovirus** (CMV), a member of the herpes family, is another teratogen that can cause extensive damage to a fetus. It is transmitted by droplet infection from person to person. It is estimated that over 50% of women are infected with CMV before pregnancy. If a woman acquires a primary CMV infection during a pregnancy, transplacental transmission of the virus may re-

sult in congenital CMV infection (Adler, 1992). The mother has almost no symptoms and so is not aware that she has contracted an infection, yet the infant may be born with severe brain damage (hydrocephalus, microcephaly, spasticity), eye damage (optic atrophy, chorioretinitis), deafness, or chronic liver disease. The child's skin may be covered with large petechiae ("blueberry-muffin" lesions). Diagnosis in the mother or infant can be established by the isolation of CMV antibodies in serum. Unfortunately, no treatment for the infection exists even if it presents with enough symptoms to allow it to be detected in the mother. Because there is no treatment or vaccine for the disease, routine screening for CMV during pregnancy is not recommended (Dascal et al., 1990). Like herpes simplex, a primary CMV infection may become latent and then reactive periodically. These recurrences are not thought to have a teratogenic effect on the fetus, but they can cause infection of the newborn during birth from genital secretions, or postpartum from exposure to CMV-infected breast milk (Landers & Sweet, 1990). CMV infection contracted at birth is not associated with serious adverse effects except in babies of very low birth weight (1200 g) (Landers & Sweet, 1990).

Herpes Simplex Virus (Genital Herpes Infection)

A primary, first-episode genital herpes infection in a pregnant woman poses a substantial risk to the fetus. The first time a woman contracts a genital herpes infection, there is systemic involvement so the virus spreads into the bloodstream (viremia) and crosses the placenta to the fetus (McIntosh & Isaacs, 1992).

If the infection takes place in the first trimester, severe congenital anomalies or spontaneous abortion may occur. If the infection occurs during the second or third trimester, there is a high incidence of premature birth, intrauterine growth retardation, and continuing infection of the newborn at birth. The fetal mortality and morbidity rate is as high as 40% (Baker, 1990).

If the woman has had herpes simplex virus type 1 infections prior to the genital herpes invasion or if the genital herpes (type 2) infection is a recurrence, antibodies to the virus in her system prevent spread of the virus to the fetus across the placenta. If genital lesions are present at the time of birth, however, the fetus may contract the virus during birth, so this is still serious. For women with a history of genital herpes and existing genital lesions when labor or rupture of membranes occurs, cesarean delivery is often performed in order to reduce the risk of neonatal infection (Landers & Sweet, 1990).

This awareness of the placental spread of herpes simplex virus has increased the importance of asking women at prenatal visits if they are aware of their own exposure to genital herpes or have any painful perineal or vaginal lesions that might be symptoms of this viral infection.

Although not yet approved during pregnancy, the use of intravenous or oral acyclovir to prevent harm to the fetus exposed in utero is being investigated. The chief fetal protection at the moment is prevention of the disease. Women with multiple sexual partners should ask their partners to use condoms to lessen their exposure to this and other sexually transmitted diseases.

Other Viral Diseases

So far it has been difficult to demonstrate other viral teratogens, but rubeola (measles), coxsackievirus, mumps, varicella (chicken pox), poliomyelitis, influenza, and viral hepatitis all may be teratogenic (Dickinson & Gonik, 1990). Parvovirus B19 is the causative agent of erythema infectiosum (also called *fifth disease*). If a pregnant woman contracts this infection, the virus can cross the placenta and attack the red blood cells of the fetus. Infection during early pregnancy is associated with fetal death; if the infection occurs late in pregnancy, the infant may be born with severe anemia and congenital heart disease (Berry et al., 1992).

Syphilis

Syphilis, a sexually transmitted infection, has been on the rise in the United States in recent years, and it is of great concern for the maternal/fetal population in spite of the availability of accurate screening tests and proven medical treatment (Wendel & Gilstrap, 1990). In the United States in 1987, 37,231 cases of primary and secondary syphilis were reported; this rose to 49,000 in 1990 (Landers & Sweet, 1990; Tillman, 1992). A syphilis infection during pregnancy can place the fetus at risk for congenital syphilis. The spirochete *Treponema pallidum*, which causes syphilis, can do extensive damage to a fetus after the 16th to 18th week of intrauterine life, when the cytotrophoblastic layer of the placental villi has atrophied and no longer protects against it. If detected and treated before this time, the fetus is rarely affected (Tillman, 1992). However, if left untreated beyond the 18th week of gestation, deafness, mental retardation, osteochondritis, and fetal death are possible results (Evans & Frenkel, 1994).

Prevention of maternal syphilis and early detection and immediate treatment with antibiotics are the best ways to prevent congenital syphilis. Benzathine penicillin is a drug often used since it may be given safely during pregnancy. Serologic screening (either a VDRL or a rapid plasma reagin) should be done at the first prenatal visit; the test may then be repeated again close to term (the 8th month). Even when a woman has been treated with appropriate antibiotics, the serum titer remains high for more than 200 days; an increasing titer, however, suggests an additional infection has occurred. In an infant born to the woman with syphilis, the serologic test for syphilis (fluorescent treponemal antibody absorption test) may remain positive for up to 3 months even though the disease was treated therapeutically during pregnancy.

The newborn with congenital syphilis may have congenital anomalies, extreme rhinitis (snuffles), and a characteristic syphilitic rash, which identify the baby as high-risk at birth. Medical care and nursing treatment for the newborn with congenital syphilis are discussed in Chapter 26.

Lyme Disease

Lyme disease is a multisystem disease caused by the spirochete *Borrelia burgdorferi* and spread by the bite of a deer tick. The highest incidence occurs in the summer and early fall; the largest outbreaks of the disease are found on the east coast of the United States.

Following the tick bite, a typical skin rash, *erythema chronicum migrans* (large, macular lesions with a clear center), develops. Pain in large body joints such as the knee may be present. Infection in pregnancy results in spontaneous abortion or severe congenital anomalies (Williams & Strobino, 1990).

Women anticipating becoming pregnant or who are pregnant should avoid areas where they are apt to be bitten by ticks (woods and tall grass). If hiking in these areas, a woman should wear long, light-colored slacks tucked into her socks to prevent her legs from being exposed. She should avoid the use of tick repellents containing diethyltoluamide as this ingredient is teratogenic. After returning home from an outing, she should inspect her body carefully and immediately remove any ticks she finds. To spread the spirochete, the tick must be present on the body possibly as long as 24 hours. If the woman has any symptoms that suggest Lyme disease or knows she has been bitten, she should contact her primary health care provider. Treatment of Lyme disease for pregnant women must be different than that for nonpregnant women because the drugs used for nonpregnant adults (tetracycline and doxycycline) cannot be used during pregnancy, as they cause tooth discoloration and, possibly, long-bone malformation in the fetus (Kalish, 1993). A course of penicillin may be prescribed to reduce symptoms.

Because the symptoms of Lyme disease are chronic but not dramatic (a migratory rash and joint pain), women may not report them at a prenatal visit unless they are educated about their importance and are asked at prenatal visits if such symptoms are present.

Toxoplasmosis

Toxoplasmosis, a protozoan infection, may be contracted by eating undercooked meat, although the organism is spread most commonly through contact with cat stool in soil or cat litter (Peckham & Logan, 1993). The woman may experience almost no symptoms of the disease except a few days of malaise and posterior cervical lymphadenopathy. Following placental transfer of the infection, however, the infant may be born with central nervous system damage, hydrocephalus, microcephaly, intracerebral calcification, and retinal deformities. Presence of the disease in the woman may be established by serum analysis. A course of sulfonamides may be begun during pregnancy if toxoplasmosis is identified, although the prevention of fetal deformities is unreliable (and sulfa may lead to increased bilirubin in the newborn).

It is not necessary to remove a cat from the home during pregnancy as long as the cat is healthy; on the other hand, taking in a new cat is not wise. Pregnant women should be careful not to change a cat litter box or work in soil in an area where cats may defecate. They should be cautioned to avoid undercooked meat. Prepregnancy serum analysis can be done to identify women susceptible (about 50% of women) who would need to be more careful than those who are not susceptible.

Infections That Cause Illness at Birth

A number of infections are not teratogenic to the fetus during pregnancy but are harmful if they are present at the time of birth. Gonorrhea, candidiasis, chlamydia, and hepatitis B infections are examples of these. Chapter 26 discusses the effects of these infections on maternal, fetal, and neonatal health.

Potential Teratogenicity of Vaccines

Live virus vaccines, such as measles, mumps, rubella, and poliomyelitis (Sabin type), are contraindicated during pregnancy because they may transmit the virus infection to the fetus. Care must be taken in routine immunization programs to make sure that adolescents about to be vaccinated are not pregnant or do not become pregnant until three months afterward (Landers & Sweet, 1990). Women who work in biologic laboratories where vaccines are manufactured are well advised not to work with live virus products during pregnancy (Bernhardt, 1990).

Teratogenicity of Drugs

Many women assume that the rule of being cautious with drugs during pregnancy applies only to prescription drugs and take over-the-counter drugs freely. Not all drugs cross the placenta (for example, heparin does not because of its large molecular size), but most do.

To identify drugs that are unsafe for ingestion during pregnancy, the Food and Drug Administration has established five categories of safety (Table 11-2). In addition to understanding this classification, it is important to recognize two principles related to drug intake during pregnancy. First, any drug, under certain circumstances, may be detrimental to fetal welfare; therefore, during pregnancy, the woman should not take any drug not specifically prescribed or approved by her physician or nurse-midwife. Second, a woman of childbearing age and ability should take no drugs other than those prescribed by a physician or nurse-midwife because a fetus is as endangered at the beginning of a pregnancy as he or she is when the pregnancy is further along.

The classic teratogenic drug is thalidomide, which was once liberally prescribed for morning sickness in Europe. Never approved for use in the United States, thalidomide caused *amelia* or *phocomelia* (total or partial absence of extremities) in 100% of instances when it was taken between the 34th and 45th day of pregnancy. Isotretinoin (Accutane), a drug commonly prescribed for adolescent acne, is an example of a teratogenic drug still in use today (Kizer et al., 1990). Other examples of drugs capable of being teratogenic are shown in Table 11-3.

Table 11-2. *Pregnancy Risk Categories of Drugs*

Category	Description	Example
A	Adequate studies in pregnant women have failed to show a risk to the fetus in the first trimester of pregnancy; there is no evidence of risk in later trimesters.	Thyroid hormone
B	Animal studies have not shown an adverse effect on the fetus but there are no adequate clinical studies in pregnant women.	Magnesium sulfate
C	Animal studies have shown an adverse effect on the fetus, but there are no adequate studies on humans, or there are no adequate studies in animals or humans. Pregnancy risk is unknown.	Docusate sodium (Colace)
D	There is evidence of risk to the human fetus, but the potential benefits of use in pregnant women may be acceptable despite potential risks.	Lithium citrate
X	Studies in animals or humans show fetal abnormalities or adverse reaction reports indicate evidence of fetal risk. The risks involved clearly outweigh potential benefits.	Isotretinoin (Accutane)

(From Loeb, S., et al. [1993]. *Nurses' handbook of drug therapy.* Springhouse, PA: Springhouse Corporation.)

Table 11-3. Some Potentially or Positively Teratogenic Drugs

Drug	Teratism
Accutane (isotretinoin)	Use is associated with congenital anomalies.
Alcohol	Regular use during pregnancy is associated with fetal alcohol syndrome and withdrawal syndromes at birth.
Androgens	Prolonged therapy with high doses during first 12 wk causes masculinization of the female fetus.
Antiepileptics	Phenytoin (Dilantin) may cause cleft palate and congenital heart anomalies. Teratogenicity has also been reported for phenobarbital, trimethadione, and primidone. Risk of teratogenicity has to be weighed against risk to fetus if mother has a seizure during pregnancy. Antiepileptics also cause vitamin K deficiency in fetus.
Antimicrobials	Tetracyclines compete with calcium in the developing fetal skeleton. They should not be used from the middle to the end of pregnancy. Ototoxic antimicrobials, such as gentamicin, streptomycin, and kanamycin, cross the placenta and may damage the fetal labyrinth. The fetal liver cannot metabolize chloramphenicol, and therefore its use in the mother can cause a "gray-baby syndrome." Sulfonamides given near term may cause jaundice in the neonate, but when given earlier in pregnancy, the fetus is protected from this effect by placental metabolism of bilirubin. Other teratogenic antimicrobials include isoniazid, novobiocin, quinine, chloroquine, and nitrofurantoin.
Antineoplastics	Methotrexate, mercaptopurine, cytosine arabinoside, and others have been noted to cause teratogenic effects, most frequently when used during the 1st trimester.
Antithyroid drugs	Hypothyroidism in fetus.
Anxiolytics	No teratogenicity was found in a large study, but there have been isolated reports. FDA requires warning that use of anxiolytics (meprobamate and benzodiazepines) during the 1st trimester of pregnancy may increase risk of congenital malformations.
Digitoxin	Harmful late in pregnancy.
Estrogens	Female offspring have higher risk of adenocarcinoma if exposed to estrogens in utero.
Glucocorticoids	Fetal abnormalities when given in large doses during pregnancy.
Iodide 131	Can destroy thyroid of fetus.
Magnesium sulfate	This drug, often used in pre-eclampsia, causes respiratory depression if used close to time of delivery.
Narcotics	Addiction in mother causes a withdrawal syndrome in the infant at birth. Use near the time of delivery causes difficulty in initiating neonatal respiration that can be alleviated by administering a narcotic antagonist to the infant.
Oral anticoagulants	Coumarins cross the placenta freely and may cause bleeding in the fetus. Coumarins given during the 1st trimester have been associated with fetal anomalies. Heparin can be used safely.
Oral hypoglycemic	Can cause profound hypoglycemia in the baby. Should not be used during pregnancy. Insulin can be used instead because it does not cross the placenta.
Oxidant drugs	May cause hemolysis if fetus has G6PD* deficiency. Oxidant drugs include primaquine, nitrofurantoin, naphthalene, sulfonamides, chloramphenicol, and vitamin K.
Phenothiazines	Accumulate in the eye of the fetus and cause retinopathy.
Piperazine antihistamines	Meclizine and cyclizine are teratogenic at least in animal studies.
Progesterone	Use by the mother during the first 12 wk may be associated with congenital anomalies or masculinization of the female genitalia.
Reserpine	Causes norepinephrine depletion, leading to respiratory distress, lethargy, bradycardia, and nasal stuffiness.
Ribavirin	Inhalation of vapor is associated with congenital anomalies.
Salicylates	Given late in pregnancy, salicylates may cause hypoprothrombinemia and fetal or neonatal hemorrhage. Salicylates compete with bilirubin for protein binding sites and may cause kernicterus.
Thiazide diuretics	Unknown risks. Thiazides cross the placenta and are not recommended for routine use in pregnancy.
Tobacco	Use during pregnancy is associated with decreased birthweight and increased spontaneous abortions.
Vaccines	Live vaccines should be avoided during pregnancy because fetal infection may occur.
Vitamin C	Megadose may cause withdrawal scurvy in the infant at birth.

*G6PD = glucose-6-phosphate dehydrogenase.
(From Swonger, A., & Matejski, N. [1991]. *Nursing pharmacology: An integrated approach to drug therapy and nursing practice* [2nd ed.]. Philadelphia: J.B. Lippincott; with permission.)

Recreational Drug Use

The use of recreational drugs during pregnancy puts a fetus at risk in two ways: (1) the drug itself may have a direct teratogenic effect; and (2) intravenous drug use also risks exposure to diseases such as HIV and hepatitis B (Tinkle et al., 1992).

Narcotics such as meperidine (Demerol) and heroin have long been implicated as causing intrauterine growth retardation. The use of marijuana alone apparently does not (Witter & Neibyl, 1990). Cocaine is particularly harmful to the fetus as it causes vasoconstriction in the mother. This compromises the blood supply to the placenta or cuts off the fetal nutrient supply. Its use is associated with spontaneous abortion, preterm labor, meconium staining, and intrauterine growth retardation (Plessinger & Woods, 1993). Limb defects may occur from loss of blood supply (Viscarello et al., 1992). When pregnant women use crack, a particularly strong form of cocaine that is smoked by pipe, their newborns show symptoms of irritability and tremulousness. Children of cocaine users may suffer long-term effects, such as learning disorders or poor attention span. See Chapter 17 for more information on the hazards of cocaine use during pregnancy.

Teratogenicity of Alcohol

It has been known for years that when women consume a large quantity of alcohol during pregnancy, their babies may show a high incidence of congenital deformities and mental retardation. It was assumed that these defects were the result of the mother's poor nutritional status (drinking alcohol rather than eating food), not necessarily the direct result of the alcohol.

Alcohol, by itself, has now been isolated as a teratogen (Dedam, McFarlane, & Hennessy, 1993). This occurs because fetuses cannot remove the breakdown products of alcohol from their body. The large buildup of these leads to vitamin B6 deficiency and accompanying neurologic damage.

An infant born with **fetal alcohol syndrome** is small for gestational age, mentally retarded, and has a characteristic craniofacial deformity (short palpebral fissures, thin upper lip, and upturned nose). Because of individual variations in metabolism, it is impossible to define a safe level of alcohol consumption (Kochenour, 1990). Women are best advised, therefore, to abstain from alcohol completely or at least limit their intake to less than 1 oz a day. Limiting alcohol consumption is difficult for women who are used to social drinking or who may be addicted to alcohol. Women with alcohol problems should be referred to an alcohol treatment program as early in pregnancy as possible to help them reduce their intake (see the Nursing Care Plan).

Teratogenicity of Cigarettes

Cigarette smoking by a pregnant woman has been shown to have teratogenic effects on the fetus, especially growth retardation. These children continue to be underweight during their early years (Floyd et al., 1993). Low birth weight in infants of smoking mothers results from vasoconstriction of the uterine vessels, limiting the blood supply to the fetus. Part of the influence of cigarettes may be related to inhaled carbon monoxide. If this is true, then inhaling the smoke of another person's cigarettes may be as harmful as actually smoking the cigarettes. All prenatal health care settings should be posted with "No Smoking" signs for both personnel and patients for this reason.

If a woman cannot stop smoking during pregnancy (and, realistically, many women cannot), reducing the number of cigarettes smoked per day should help diminish any adverse effects on the fetus.

Another sound reason women should at least limit the number of cigarettes smoked per day is to protect their own health. A child needs a well mother while growing up. Losing a mother to lung cancer is as deleterious to a child's psychological health as second-hand smoke is to physical health.

The best approach to urge women to discontinue smoking is to educate them about the risks to themselves and their fetus at the first prenatal visit (see the Focus on Nursing Research box). It may be effective to encourage them to sign a contract with a health care provider to try and stop or to join a smoking cessation program. Be certain pregnant women know that they shouldn't enter a stop-smoking program that uses drug

FOCUS ON NURSING RESEARCH

How Effective Are Smoking Cessation Programs With Pregnant Women?

To answer this question, women in a prenatal clinic who were fewer than 31 weeks gestation were asked about their smoking habits. They were then given either a referral to an evening 2-hour cessation program or a 20-minute discussion during the prenatal appointment. Findings revealed that none of the women referred to the evening program ever attended. The group receiving the immediate intervention reduced smoking 2 to 3 times that of the referral group. The researchers recommend that women be given immediate counseling regarding smoking at their first prenatal visit.

O'Connor, A. M., et al. (1992). Effectiveness of a pregnancy smoking cessation program. *Journal of Obstetrics, Gynecologic, and Neonatal Nursing, 21,* 385.

Nursing Care Plan

A Pregnant Woman with Threats to Fetal Health

Margaret McCormack is a 19-year-old woman you see at a prenatal clinic. The following is a nursing care plan devised for her in regard to guarding fetal growth.

Assessment: Gravida 1, para 0. Unsure of date of last menstrual period (about 16 weeks). Heavy smoker—2 packs/day. Alcohol: 1–2 beers/week. Takes Sudafed 60 mg daily for "sinus headache." Evasive about use of marijuana. Complains of severe nausea in morning; occasional vomiting. Says someone told her that "smoking pot would help her nausea go away." Uterine height 4 cm above symphysis. Fetal heart tones by Doppler at 150/min.

Nursing Diagnosis: High risk for fetal injury related to lack of knowledge about potential dangers of maternal cigarette, alcohol, and drug use.

Defining Characteristic: Client states she has used alcohol and smoked cigarettes during pregnancy.

Goal: Client will safeguard fetal health for pregnancy duration.

Outcome Criteria: Client decreases smoking to less than 10 cigarettes daily; client omits all alcohol consumption during pregnancy; client omits all marijuana use during pregnancy; client takes no medication during pregnancy without Women's Health Clinic personnel approval; fetal growth is within normal parameters during pregnancy.

Nursing Orders	Rationale
1. Refer to physician for evaluation of safety of sinus medication during pregnancy.	1. Medications must be assessed to be sure they are not teratogenic.
2. Educate about dangers of drug use (including non-prescription medication) and alcohol during pregnancy.	2. Educating the woman can help her avoid these substances throughout pregnancy.
3. Urge to quit smoking or decrease number of cigarettes smoked per day to less than 10; no marijuana use.	3. Cigarette use during pregnancy can lead to fetal growth retardation.
4. Urge to decrease alcohol consumption completely (substitute caffeine-free beverages).	4. Alcohol consumption during pregnancy can lead to fetal alcohol syndrome.
5. Ask physician if sonogram should be scheduled for fetal growth evaluation.	5. Heavy cigarette smoking may have led to fetal growth retardation.

Nursing Diagnosis: High risk for fluid volume deficit related to nausea and vomiting every morning.

Defining Characteristic: Client states she has nausea or vomiting almost every morning.

Goal: Client will not demonstrate fluid volume deficit during pregnancy.

Outcome Criteria: Nausea and vomiting end at 14 weeks of pregnancy; specific gravity of urine remains below 1.030; client maintains a consistent weight gain during pregnancy; client states she is ingesting a minimum of 1800 calories daily despite nausea and vomiting; client states she is no longer using home remedy to counteract nausea but is using dry crackers before arising and delaying eating instead.

Nursing Orders	Rationale
1. Educate client about importance of maintaining good hydration and nutrition during pregnancy.	1. Good hydration and nutrition are important to fetal growth.
2. Brainstorm with client ways to reduce nausea, such as eating dry crackers after awakening.	2. Including the client in planning may increase feeling of control and improve compliance with health recommendations.

therapy because the substitute drug may be as harmful to their fetus as the original smoking.

Environmental Teratogens

Teratogens from environmental sources can be as lethal to the fetus as those that are directly or deliberately ingested.

Metal and Chemical Hazards

The effects of pesticides and carbon monoxide (from automobile exhaust) are examples of chemical teratogens that are harmful and should be avoided. Chemicals in a variety of work environments also can be quite dangerous (Table 11-4). Lead poisoning generally is considered a problem of early childhood, but it is also a fetal hazard because lead is teratogenic if consumed by a woman during pregnancy (Bernhardt, 1990). Pre-school children ingest lead by eating paint chips or wall plaster; women may ingest it by drinking water that travels through old pipes that are leaching lead or by "sniffing" gasoline. Lead ingestion during pregnancy causes mental retardation and central nervous system damage in the fetus.

Radiation

Rapidly growing cells are extremely vulnerable to destruction by radiation (which is why radiation is used as a cancer therapy) (Oakley, 1990). Radiation has been proved to be a potent teratogen to unborn children because of the high proportion of rapidly growing cells present. Radiation produces a range of malformations, depending on the stage of development of the embryo or fetus and on the strength and length of exposure. If the exposure occurs before implantation, the growing zygote apparently is killed. If the zygote is not killed, it survives apparently unharmed. The most damaging time is from implantation to 6 weeks after conception (when many women are not yet aware that they are pregnant). The nervous system, brain, and the retinal innervation are most affected.

As a rule, therefore, all women of childbearing age should be exposed to pelvic x-rays only in the first 10 days of a menstrual cycle (a time when pregnancy is unlikely because ovulation has not yet occurred), except, of course, in emergency situations. A rapid serum assay pregnancy test can be done on all women who have reason to believe they might be pregnant before diagnostic tests involving x-ray are performed.

Radiation of the pelvis should be avoided during pregnancy if at all possible; it should be undertaken at term in pregnancy only if the data the x-ray will reveal cannot be obtained by any other means and will be important for birth. Sonography or magnetic resonance imaging has replaced x-ray examination for confirmation of situations such as multiple pregnancy because these do not appear to be teratogenic.

If the woman needs nonpelvic radiation during pregnancy (e.g., dental x-rays, limb x-ray after a fall), her pelvis should be shielded by a lead apron during the procedure. Even fluoroscopy, which uses lower radiation doses than regular x-ray photography, can cause deformation of the fetus and should be avoided during pregnancy—again, except in an emergency. Although apparently safe, the effect of long-term use of even slight radiation sources, such as a word processor or computer, is now being questioned.

Evidence exists that, in addition to immediate fetal damage, x-rays have long-lasting effects on the health of the child. There appears to be an increased risk of cancer in children exposed to x-rays while in utero (Fry & Fry, 1990). Exposure of the fetal gonads possibly could lead to a genetic mutation that will not be evident until the next generation.

These restrictions in x-ray use have special meaning for nurses. If you are asked to assist with a client in an x-ray room, you have a right to insist on lead shielding as pelvic protection. Do not be persuaded when x-ray technicians say, "It's just one time," or "It's the buildup of radiation that counts." Protection that is suggested for people in general should be demanded by nurses.

Hyperthermia and Hypothermia

Hyperthermia to the fetus may be detrimental to growth (Fishbein et al., 1990). Hyperthermia can occur from the use of saunas, hot tubs, or tanning beds, or from a work environment next to a furnace, such as in welding or steel making. Maternal fever early in pregnancy (4 to 6 weeks) may cause abnormal fetal brain development and, possibly, seizure disorders, hypotonia, and skeletal deformities.

The effect of hypothermia on pregnancy is not well known. Because the uterus is an internal organ, the woman's body temperature would have to be lowered significantly before a great deal of fetal change would result.

Teratogenicity of Maternal Stress

Many myths exist about the "marking" of infants in utero: "if a woman sees a mouse during pregnancy, her child will be born with a furry or mole-like birthmark"; "eating strawberries causes strawberry birthmarks"; "looking at a handicapped child while pregnant will cause a child in utero to be handicapped the same way." Common sense and awareness of fetal-maternal physiology have dispelled these superstitions. There is growing evidence, however, that an emotionally disturbed pregnancy, one filled with anxiety and worry beyond the usual amount associated with pregnancy, may have

Table 11-4. *Selected Real or Suspected Chemical Hazards to Reproductive Health and Where They May Be Found in the Workplace*

Chemical	Occupational Exposure
Agent Orange (50/50 mixture of 2,4-D and 2,4,5-T)	Herbicide. Exposure during manufacturing and application.
Anesthetic gases and liquids	Used by health care workers, dentists, laboratory personnel, and veterinarians. Examples are nitrous oxide, halothane, enflurane, cyclopropane, and methoxyflurane.
Arsenic	Occurs as a by-product of copper and lead smelting. Used in pesticides, glass, ceramics, paints, dyes, wood preservatives, and leather processing.
Boron	Used to weatherproof woods and fireproof fabrics. Used in manufacture of cement, crockery, porcelain, enamels, glass, leather, carpets, hats, soaps, and artificial gems.
1,3-butadiene*	Used in manufacture of rubber, resins, and latexes.
Cadmium	Used in batteries, pigments, paints, soldering liquids, semiconductors, photo cells, insecticides, and fungicides. Is set free during welding.
Carbaryl*	Broad-spectrum insecticide. Exposure during manufacturing and application.
Chloroprene*	Used as chemical intermediate in rubber manufacturing.
2,4-D	Herbicide. Exposure during manufacturing and application (banned†).
DDT	Pesticide. Exposure during manufacturing and application (banned†).
Dibromochloropropane (DBCP)	Nematocide. Exposure during manufacturing and application (banned†).
Dioxin (TCDD)	Unwanted contaminant in manufacture of several agricultural chemicals.
Epichlorohydrin*	Used as intermediate in the manufacture of a broad range of chemicals, including agricultural chemicals, coatings, adhesives, plasticizers, textile chemicals, and pharmaceuticals.
Ethylene dibromide (EDB)	Used as an antiknock additive in leaded gasoline, as a pesticide, as an intermediate in synthesis of dyes and pharmaceuticals, and as a solvent for resins, gums, and waxes.
Ethylene oxide (EtO)*	Used in production of ethylene glycol for antifreeze, polyester fibers and films, and detergents. Used in sterilizing equipment and supplies in health-care facilities and as a fumigant in the manufacture of medical products, foodstuffs, and in libraries and museums.
Ethylene thiourea*	Used in manufacturing rubber.
Formaldehyde	Used in more than 60 different industrial and laboratory applications. Examples are paper manufacturing; leather tanning; manufacture of film and photographic paper; textile processing; manufacture of particle board, plywood, and foam insulation; and as a biologic preservative.
Kepone (chlordane)	Insecticide: Exposure in manufacturing and application (banned†).
Lead	Found in metallurgic and smelting industries. Used by battery manufacturers, painters, typesetters, and stained glass artists. Used in manufacture of paint, ink, ceramics, pottery, ammunition, and textiles.
Manganese	Used in manufacture of steel, dry cell batteries, glass, inks, ceramics, paints, rubber, and wood preservatives.
Mercury	Used in manufacture of electrical apparatus, mercury vapor lamps, paint, thermometers, and in mining.
Organic solvents	Widely used in manufacturing and in chemical industry as well as in electronics manufacturing. Examples are carbon disulfide,* carbon tetrachloride, styrene, xylene, toluene, and benzene.
Polybrominated biphenyls (PBB)	Used as a flame retardant for thermoplastic products (banned†).
Polychlorinated biphenyls (PCB)*	Used as a collant fluid in electrical transformers; lubricant; plasticizer; and in manufacture of coatings and solvents (banned†).
Polyvinylchloride (PVC)	Used in manufacture of plastics and resins. Occurs in many products such as clothing, flooring, upholstery, wire insulation, phonograph records, and food containers.
Synthetic hormones	Used as a supplement in animal feeds and pharmaceuticals. Exposure during manufacturing.
2,4,5-T	Herbicide. Exposure in manufacturing and application (restricted use).

*Chemicals identified by National Institute for Occupational Safety and Health (NIOSH) as reproductive hazards. NIOSH also includes dinitrotoluene, glycidyl ethers, glycol ethers, and monohalomethanes.
†Although banned, the chemical is important because of its similarities to chemicals still in use, its persistence in the environment, and/or its potential long-term effects on workers previously exposed.
(From Bernhardt, J.H. [1990]. Potential workplace hazards to reproductive health. *Journal of Obstetric, Gynecologic, and Neonatal Nursing, 19,* 53; with permission.)

some effect on the unborn child or at least may lead to preterm labor (Anderson & Merkatz, 1990). Anxiety produces physiologic changes through its effect on the sympathetic division of the autonomic nervous system. The main changes are an increase in heart rate, constriction of the peripheral blood vessels, a decrease in gastrointestinal motility, and dilation of coronary vessels. This effect is called the *fight or flight syndrome.* If the anxiety is prolonged, the constriction of uterine vessels could possibly interfere with the blood supply to the fetus.

These phenomena are characteristic only of long-term, extreme stress, not of the normal anxiety of pregnancy. Illness or death of one's partner, difficulty with relatives, marital discord, and illness or death of another child are examples of stressful situations that might provoke excessive anxiety.

Helping a woman resolve these complex problems during pregnancy is not easy. If maternal stress is severe, however, securing counseling for the woman during pregnancy is as important as ensuring good physical care.

Key Points

- The more women know about measures they should take during pregnancy to safeguard their health, the more likely they will avoid substances or activities harmful to fetal growth. This makes prenatal education an important part of prenatal care.
- Discussion and health teaching periods during pregnancy should cover such topics as bathing, sexual activity, sleep, and exercise.
- Women who work outside of their homes need to make provisions for rest periods during their day and to be aware of any potential teratogens at their work site such as radiation or heavy metals. Women who travel should plan for break periods to avoid congestion in the lower extremities; they should use seatbelts when traveling by car.
- Common discomforts of early pregnancy include breast tenderness, constipation, palmar erythema, nausea and vomiting, fatigue, muscle cramps, pain from varicosities or hemorrhoids, heart palpitations, frequency of urination, vulvar pruritus, and leukorrhea. If women know that these symptoms occur they will not interpret them as complications.
- Minor discomforts of middle or late pregnancy may include backache, dyspnea, ankle edema, and uterine contractions.
- Beginning signs of labor that women should be made aware of are lightening, show, rupture of membranes, and uterine contractions.
- Women should be aware of the danger to the fetus of infectious diseases such as rubella, HIV, cytomegalovirus, herpes simplex virus, syphilis, Lyme disease, and toxoplasmosis during pregnancy and how to avoid these illnesses.
- All women should also be counseled about the necessity to avoid the use of any drugs not specifically approved by their physician or nurse-midwife, as well as alcohol and cigarettes, during pregnancy.
- Urge women to find the best way for them to modify their lifestyle for pregnancy. Pregnancy is 9 months long, so modifications must be agreeable to a woman or she will not maintain them over such a long time span.
- It is almost impossible for a woman to modify a lifestyle, such as stopping smoking, if her support person does not agree to the change (and usually change also). Including the family in care is an important way of helping support persons understand the necessity for the modification and increase cooperation.

Critical Thinking Exercises

1. Jackie is a 19-year-old college student you see in a prenatal clinic. She is unmarried and lives in a college dormitory. She admits she has not been taking her prenatal vitamins and describes a day to you that involves long periods of sitting with almost no exercise.
   a. What would be some recommendations you could make to help Jackie increase her exercise level?
   b. What suggestions could you make to improve her medication compliance?
   c. Jackie mentioned no support person that she relies on for advice during pregnancy. Would you make any recommendations for who she might consult on a college campus for this?

2. Mel and Harriet are a young couple you see in an obstetrician's office. They report that Harriet's pregnancy has been "terrible—one ache or pain or problem after another." Harriet's record shows that the only symptoms she reported to the doctor were mild nausea, some constipation, and occasional backache that the physician considered all within normal parameters. Why do you think this discrepancy in the perceived seriousness of Harriet's concerns has occurred? Are there measures that could have been employed to make Harriet's pregnancy a better experience for her?

References

Adler, S. P. (1992). Cytomegalovirus and pregnancy. *Current Opinion in Obstetrics & Gynecology, 4,* 670.

Anderson, H. F., & Merkatz, I. R. (1990). Preterm labor. In Scott, J. R., et al. *Danforth's obstetrics and gynecology.* Philadelphia: J.B. Lippincott.

Baker, D. A. (1990). Herpes and pregnancy: New management. *Clinical Obstetrics and Gynecology, 33,* 253.

Bernhardt, J. H. (1990). Potential workplace hazards to reproductive health. *Journal of Obstetric, Gynecologic, and Neonatal Nursing, 19,* 53.

Berry, P. J., et al. (1992). Parvovirus infection of the human fetus and newborn. *Seminars in Diagnostic Pathology, 9,* 40.

Bia, F. J. (1992). Medical considerations for the pregnant traveler. *Infectious Disease Clinics of North America, 6,* 371.

Corey, M. A., & Clore, E. R. (1991). Management of the infant with respiratory synctial virus. *Journal of Pediatric Nursing, 8,* 93.

Cunningham, F. G., et al. (1993). *Williams obstetrics* (19th ed.). Norwalk, CT: Appleton & Lange.

Dascal, A., et al. (1990). Laboratory tests for the diagnosis of viral disease in pregnancy. *Clinical Obstetrics and Gynecology, 33,* 218.

Dedam, R., McFarlane, C., & Hennessy, K. (1993). A dangerous lack of understanding. *Canadian Nurse, 89,* 29.

Department of Health and Human Services. (1991). *Healthy people 2000.* Washington, DC: Public Health Service.

Dickinson J., & Gonik, B. (1990). Teratogenic viral infections. *Clinical Obstetrics and Gynecology, 33,* 242.

Eisele, C. J. (1993). Rubella susceptibility in women of childbearing age. *Journal of Obstetric, Gynecologic, and Neonatal Nursing, 22,* 260.

Evans, H. E., & Frenkel, L. D. (1994). Congenital syphilis. *Clinics in Perinatology, 21,* 149.

Feller, C. M., & Franko-Filiposic, K. J. (1993). Headache during pregnancy: Diagnosis and treatment. *Journal of Perinatal and Neonatal Nursing, 7,* 1.

Fishbein, E. G., et al. (1990). How safe is exercise during pregnancy? *Journal of Obstetric, Gynecologic, and Neonatal Nursing, 19,* 45.

Floyd, R. L., et al. (1993). A review of smoking in pregnancy: Effects on pregnancy outcome and cessation efforts. *Annual Review of Public Health, 14,* 379.

Fry, R. J., & Fry, S. A. (1990). Health effects of ionizing radiation. *Medical Clinics of North America, 74,* 475.

Hammond, T. L., et al. (1990). The use of automobile safety restraint systems during pregnancy. *Journal of Obstetric, Gynecologic, and Neonatal Nursing, 19,* 339.

Hatch, M. C., et al. (1993). Maternal exercise during pregnancy, physical fitness, and fetal growth. *American Journal of Epidemiology, 137,* 1105.

Iams, J. D., et al. (1990). Symptoms that precede preterm labor and preterm premature rupture of the membranes. *American Journal of Obstetrics and Gynecology, 162,* 486.

Kalish, R. (1993). Lyme disease. *Rheumatic Diseases Clinics of North America, 19,* 399.

Kizer, K. W., et al. (1990). Vitamin A—a pregnancy hazard alert. *Western Journal of Medicine, 152,* 78.

Kochenour, N. K. (1990). Normal pregnancy and prenatal care. In Scott, J. R., et al. *Danforth's obstetrics and gynecology.* Philadelphia: J.B. Lippincott.

Landers, D. V., & Sweet, R. L. (1990). Perinatal infections. In Scott, J. R., et al. *Danforth's obstetrics and gynecology.* Philadelphia: J.B. Lippincott.

Mattson, S. & Lew, L. (1992). Culturally sensitive prenatal care for southeast Asians. *Journal of Obstetrics, Gynecologic, and Neonatal Nursing, 21,* 48.

McIntosh, D., & Isaacs, D. (1992). Herpes simplex virus infection in pregnancy. *Archives of Disease in Childhood, 67,* 1137.

McMurray, R. G., et al. (1993). Thermoregulation of pregnant women during aerobic exercise on land and in the water. *American Journal of Perinatology, 10,* 178.

Nagey, D. A. (1989). The content of prenatal care. *Obstetrics and Gynecology, 74,* 516.

Oakley, K. (1990). Making sense of x-ray precautions. *Nursing Times, 86,* 50.

O'Connor, A. M., et al. (1992). Effectiveness of a pregnancy smoking cessation program. *Journal of Obstetrics, Gynecologic, and Neonatal Nursing, 21,* 385.

Peckham, C. S., & Logan, S. (1993). Screening for toxoplasmosis during pregnancy. *Archives of Disease in Childhood, 68,* 3.

Plessinger, M. A. & Woods, J. R. (1993). Maternal placental and fetal pathophysiology of cocaine exposure during pregnancy. *Clinical Obstetrics & Gynecology, 36,* 267.

Reed, B. D., & Eyler, A. (1993). Vaginal infections: Diagnosis and management. *Infectious Disease Clinics of North America, 6,* 371.

Retts, V. S. (1993). Women and exercise. *Female Patient, 18,* 59.

Shepard, T. H. (1992). *Catalog of teratogenic agents.* Baltimore: Johns Hopkins University Press.

Tillman, J. (1992). Syphilis: An old disease, a contemporary perinatal problem. *Journal of Obstetric, Gynecologic, and Neonatal Nursing, 21,* 209.

Tinkle, M. B., Alvarez, A. M., & Tamayo, O. W. (1992). HIV disease and pregnancy. *Journal of Obstetrics, Gynecologic, and Neonatal Nursing, 21,* 86.

Viscarello, R. R., et al. (1992). Limb-body wall complex associated with cocaine abuse: Further evidence of cocaine's teratogenicity. *Obstetrics and Gynecology, 80,* 523.

Weber, B., et al. (1993). Congenital rubella syndrome after maternal infection. *Infection, 21,* 118.

Wendel, G. D., & Gilstrap, L. C. (1990). Syphilis rise calls for accurate diagnosis. *Contemporary Obstetrics and Gynecology, 35,* 37.

Williams, D. L., & Strobino, B. A. (1990). Lyme disease transmission during pregnancy. *Contemporary Obstetrics and Gynecology, 35,* 48.

Witter, F. R., & Niebyl, J. R. (1990). Marijuana use in pregnancy and pregnancy outcome. *American Journal of Perinatology, 7,* 36.

Suggested Readings

Ausman, L. F. (1993). Toxoplasmosis and pregnancy. *Canadian Nurse, 89,* 31.

Buekens, P., et al. (1993). A comparison of prenatal care use in the United States and Europe. *American Journal of Public Health, 83,* 31.

Fogel, C. I. (1993). Pregnant inmates: Risk factors and pregnancy outcomes. *Journal of Obstetrics, Gynecologic, and Neonatal Nursing, 22,* 33.

Heine, P., & McGregor, J. A. (1993). Trichomonas vaginalis: A reemerging pathogen. *Clinical Obstetrics and Gynecology, 36,* 137.

Lippman, A., et al. (1992). The role of the telephone in providing prenatal care. *American Journal of Preventive Medicine, 8,* 373.

McClanahan, P. (1992). Improving access to and use of prenatal care. *Journal of Obstetrics, Gynecologic, and Neonatal Nursing, 21,* 280.

Mercer, R. T., & Ferketich, S. L. (1994). Predictors of maternal role competence by risk status. *Nursing Research, 43,* 38.

Merlin, R. (1992). Understanding bulimia and its implications in pregnancy. *Journal of Obstetrics, Gynecologic, and Neonatal Nursing, 21,* 199.

Peoples-Sheps, M. D., et al. (1991). Prenatal records: A national study of content. *American Journal of Obstetrics and Gynecology, 164,* 514.

Progress toward achieving the 1990 objectives for the nation for sexually transmitted diseases. (1990). *Mortality/Morbidity World Report, 39,* 53.

Remkes, T. (1993). Saying no—completely. *Canadian Nurse, 89,* 25.

Rhodes, A. M. (1990). Maternal liability for fetal injury? *MCN: American Journal of Maternal Child Nursing, 15,* 41.

Rosen, M. G., et al. (1991). Caring for our future: A report by the expert panel on the content of prenatal care. *Obstetrics and Gynecology, 77,* 82.

Shaw, N. (1990). Common surgical problems in the newborn. *Journal of Perinatal and Neonatal Nursing, 3,* 50.

Vandenter, M. C. (1991). Ptyalism in pregnant women. *Journal of Obstetrics, Gynecologic, and Neonatal Nursing, 20,* 206.

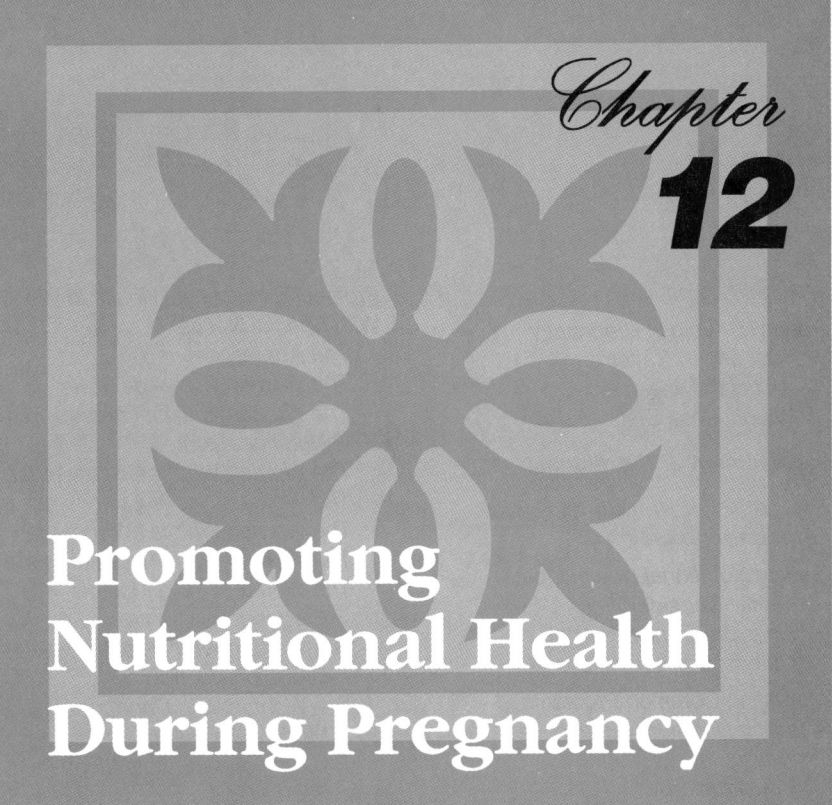

Chapter 12

Promoting Nutritional Health During Pregnancy

Objectives

After mastering the contents of this chapter, you should be able to:

1. Describe the requirements of healthy pregnancy nutrition.

2. Assess a woman's nutritional intake during pregnancy.

3. Formulate nursing diagnoses related to nutritional concerns during pregnancy.

4. Plan health teaching for nutritional intake during pregnancy, including ways a woman can increase her iron and calcium intake.

5. Implement nursing care that encourages healthy nutritional practices during pregnancy such as eating a high-protein diet.

6. Evaluate outcome criteria related to nutritional care goals to be certain that goals were achieved.

7. Identify National Health Goals related to nutrition and pregnancy that nurses can be instrumental in helping the nation achieve.

8. Identify areas related to nutrition and pregnancy that could benefit from additional nursing research.

9. Use critical thinking to analyze the effects of different life situations on nutrition patterns and ways nutritional health can be improved.

10. Synthesize nutrition knowledge with nursing process to achieve quality maternal and child health nursing care.

Adele Pillitteri: MATERNAL AND CHILD HEALTH NURSING, 2nd Edition. © 1995 Adele Pillitteri.

A good diet cannot guarantee a good pregnancy outcome, but it certainly makes an important contribution (Giotta, 1993). Both the nutritional state that a woman brings into pregnancy and her nutrition during pregnancy have direct bearing on her health as well as on fetal growth and development.

Early in pregnancy, fetal growth occurs largely by an increase in the number of cells formed (**hyperplasia**); late in pregnancy it occurs mainly by enlargement of existing cells (**hypertrophy**). A fetus who is deprived of adequate nutrition early in pregnancy, then, will be small for gestational age because of too few cells in the fetus's body; later on, retarded growth is due to a normal number but smaller than usual size cells. To be certain that early pregnancy deficiencies do not occur, women of childbearing age should be especially encouraged to follow a balanced diet; otherwise, in the time before they recognize that they are pregnant (about 6 weeks), their poor diet and lack of important nutrient stores could seriously impair fetal growth. Good nutrition is so important in pregnancy that the subject is addressed in National Health Goals (see the Focus on National Health Goals box).

☒ **NURSING PROCESS OVERVIEW**
for Promoting Nutritional Health
in the Pregnant Woman

ASSESSMENT

A thorough assessment of nutritional health patterns is crucial before any nutritional planning can begin. Determining not only whether the client is eating a "balanced" diet but what cultural, environmental, and social lifestyle factors affect eating habits is also important. Using a 24-hour recall history can help the woman appreciate that she needs some help with nutrition or can provide confirmation that she is eating well.

NURSING DIAGNOSIS

Nursing diagnoses related to nutritional status of the pregnant woman must consider the desired health and growth of both the fetus and the mother. Common nursing diagnoses are:

- Altered nutrition, less than body requirements, related to nausea every morning
- Health-seeking behaviors related to determining best food choices in pregnancy

- Altered nutrition, more than body requirements, related to chronic poor eating habits

These are serious diagnoses, because they mean that the woman may not be taking in enough nutrients to sustain fetal growth or is taking in so many high-calorie foods that the fetus could weigh more than usual (be large for gestational age, or LGA). Taking in less nutrition than desirable can occur equally to the woman who is eating a great deal of nutritionally inferior food and the woman who has a problem eating because of nausea and vomiting or fatigue. Being sensitive to a client's concern about maintaining her own appearance in light of her need to gain sufficient weight helps her keep a healthy perspective on "eating for two."

PLANNING

In large health centers, nutritionists are available to meet with women prenatally and help them plan pregnancy nutrition. In other settings, a nutritionist may be available only for women with special needs. When helping a woman set goals for improving nutritional patterns, be certain to consider all the cultural and lifestyle factors that give different meanings to food. Because food is an expensive commodity, financial resources must also be considered. It is important to teach women about long-term goals such as rebuilding iron stores or muscle mass. Eating an improved diet for a week will probably not make a radical change; however, continuing a healthy eating pattern throughout the pregnancy (and maintaining it throughout life) will bring about important changes. At the same time, some goals need to be short-term and specific. For instance, some goals might include the following:

- Client will plan weekly menu that includes three main meals and two snacks per day.
- By next prenatal visit, client will demonstrate knowledge of meat and non-meat sources of protein by relaying that meals during the last week included fish, eggs, beans, and peanut butter.

IMPLEMENTATION

Changing a dietary pattern can be a lonely and seemingly unrewarding endeavor. Women often need support through a telephone conversation or person-to-person contact to eat a different lunch than others around them are eating; to be motivated enough to get up 15 minutes earlier in the morning to prepare breakfast rather than just dashing to work without anything more than coffee; or to resist a soft drink with their fast-food dinner and drink orange juice instead. Asking women to list what foods they eat daily and to bring in the chart to show the nurse at a health maintenance visit is an effective motivating technique for many people. In research studies, this is called a **Hawthorne effect**, in which people who are being watched do better than those who are not. With this system, the average person will eat better than normally so her list looks better when she presents it. As soon as she understands that better eating patterns make her feel better, it is hoped that she will continue them indefinitely.

Be careful with statements such as "Eat high-protein foods." Such statements are meaningless for many women because food, after all, does not come from the supermarket labeled "high-protein food." Women need advice given in more specific terms—for example, "Eat three servings of some type of meat every day."

The word *diet* has come to mean a form of unpleas-

FOCUS ON
National Health Goals

A number of National Health Goals speak to nutrition in pregnancy. These are:

- Increase calcium intake so at least 50% of pregnant and lactating women consume three or more servings daily of foods rich in calcium from a baseline of 24%.

- Reduce iron deficiency to less than 3% among women of childbearing age from a baseline of 5%.

- Increase to at least 85% the proportion of women who achieve the minimum recommended weight gain during their pregnancies from a baseline of 67% (DHHS, 1991).

Nurses can be instrumental in helping the nation achieve these goals by stressing the importance of a balanced diet for all people so women enter pregnancy with adequate nutritional stores. They can help pregnant women plan ways to ingest three servings of calcium daily and to remember to take their prenatal vitamin (which contains an iron supplement) daily. Nursing research on such problems as what are effective methods to help people remember to take daily medications, how can women who cannot drink milk obtain adequate calcium, and in what ways can women be helped to gain weight in pregnancy by eating high protein, not empty carbohydrate foods could add important information in this area of care.

ant food denial. Rather than a "pregnancy diet," it is better to talk about the "foods that are best for you during pregnancy" or "pregnancy nutrition." These statements have a positive sound and refer more closely to foods the nurse is encouraging the woman to eat. A list of prenatal instructions listing appropriate foods is good to distribute to women as long as it is short and clear. Complicated lists of foods or a list of *don'ts* will land in the wastepaper basket rather than being followed.

Because some supplementation of vitamins and minerals is encouraged during pregnancy, a woman may think that consuming many vitamins is even better for her. Caution women against taking vitamin preparations indiscriminately, just as she avoids any medication during pregnancy that is not specifically prescribed or approved by her health care provider (Kizer et al., 1990). The woman should take the supplement her primary health care provider recommends and no others.

EVALUATION

When evaluating whether an improved nutrition pattern has been successful, rely on the most important assessments: weight, energy level, general appearance, bowel function, and, when accessible, hemoglobin and urinalysis findings.

Urge women to be honest about whether they are actually following a new nutrition pattern. If they are not, it probably means that the nursing plan did not fit their lifestyle or degree of motivation, and they need additional modifications for it to be successful. Examples of outcome criteria that might be used are:

- Client states that she is able to make up for meals missed because of nausea later each day.
- Client's food lists for 1 week include three sources of calcium per day.
- Client describes pattern she is using to increase fluid intake to six glasses daily.

People always have some degree of "back-sliding" at holidays and special events. Respect this as a fact of human nature. If it is vital that this not occur on the next holiday, help the woman make definite, concrete plans to avoid back-sliding, or the next evaluation will reveal the same problem. Be certain to comment on the things the woman is doing correctly. This is an elemental rule of teaching that almost every teacher forgets in his or her zeal to create a perfect student.

Relationship of Maternal Diet to Infant Health

Women must eat adequately during pregnancy in order to supply enough nutrients to the fetus so the fetus can grow. In addition, adequate protein intake may help prevent complications of pregnancy such as pregnancy-induced hypertension or preterm birth (Newman & Fullerton, 1990). Deficiencies or overuse of vitamins may contribute to birth defects such as neural tube abnormalities (Olson, 1994). Good nutrition plays a role in preventing preterm birth (Scholl et al., 1993).

Recommended Weight Gain During Pregnancy

A weight gain of 12 to 14 kg (25 to 35 lb) is currently recommended as an average weight gain in pregnancy (Kochenour, 1990). If a woman is high-risk for nutritional deficits, a more precise estimation of adequate weight gain can be calculated. This is done by computing **body mass index** (BMI), which is the ratio of weight to height. The formula for calculating BMI is weight (in kilograms) divided by height (in meters^2). Women who are high or low weight for height (BMI below 19.8 or above 26.1) will have weight gain goals adjusted in light of this. Figure 12-1 summarizes the reasons for weight gain in pregnancy. Figure 12-2 shows projected adequate weight gains for average-weight women.

Weight gain during pregnancy occurs as roughly 0.4 kg (1 lb) per month during the first trimester and then 0.4 kg (1 lb) per week during the last two trimesters (a trimester pattern of 3-12-12) (see Figure 12-2). Weight gain is excessive if it is more than 3 kg a month during the second and third trimesters; it is less than normal if it is under 1 kg per month during the second and third trimesters (Kochenour, 1990). Women can be assured that most of the gain in weight that occurs with pregnancy will be lost afterward (Parham, Astrom, & King, 1990).

Women who are underweight coming into pregnancy should gain more weight than the average woman during pregnancy (0.5 kg per month or week rather than 0.4). An obese woman may gain less than average (0.3 kg). As a rule, women should not diet to lose weight during pregnancy to be certain the fetus receives adequate nutrition. Weight gain should be higher for a multiple pregnancy than for a single pregnancy. Sudden increases in weight that suggest fluid retention or a loss of weight that suggests illness should be carefully evaluated at prenatal visits.

Components of Healthy Nutrition for the Pregnant Woman

The old saying that a pregnant woman must "eat for two" is not just a myth—it is a scientific fact. This does not mean that the woman needs to eat enough for *two adults,* but she does need to increase intake to provide enough nutrients for the growing fetus. Many women will not have to increase by much the *quantity* of food

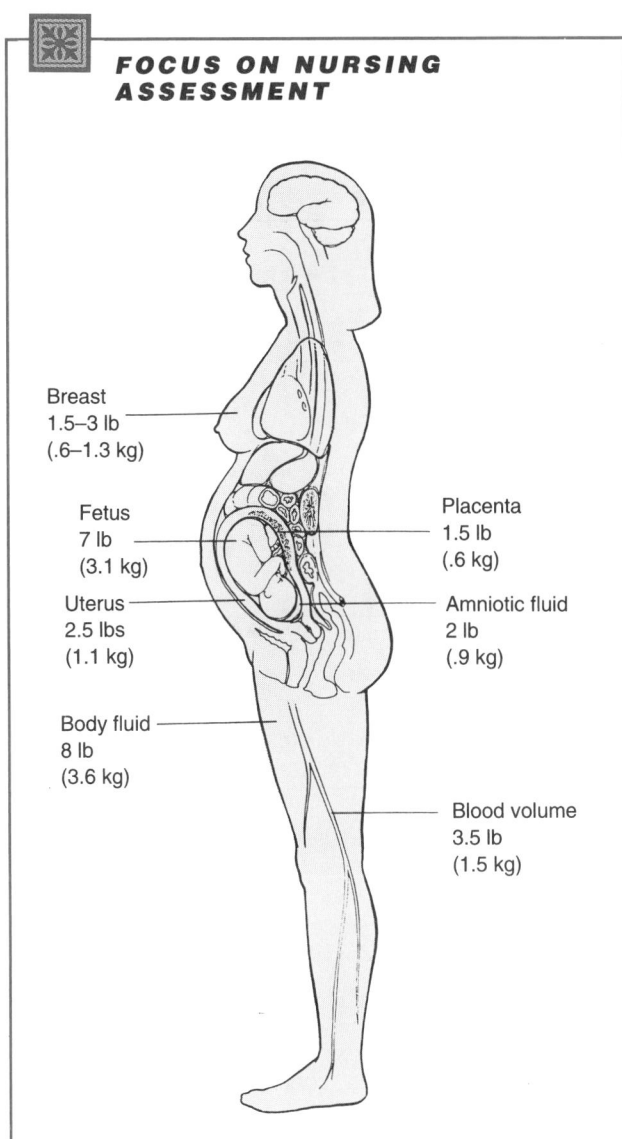

FOCUS ON NURSING ASSESSMENT

Breast
1.5–3 lb
(.6–1.3 kg)

Fetus
7 lb
(3.1 kg)

Uterus
2.5 lbs
(1.1 kg)

Body fluid
8 lb
(3.6 kg)

Placenta
1.5 lb
(.6 kg)

Amniotic fluid
2 lb
(.9 kg)

Blood volume
3.5 lb
(1.5 kg)

FIGURE 12-1
Weight gain in pregnancy occurs from both growth of the fetus and accumulation of maternal stores.

eaten but they will have to increase the *quality* of their intake (Chez, 1991).

The recommended daily dietary allowances (RDA) for girls and women and the requirements for pregnancy were revised in 1989 (Table 12-1). Foods eaten should represent all food groups in a food pyramid (Figure 12-3 and Table 12-2). Be sure to discuss nutrition in terms of servings of food rather than milligrams or percentages to better increase comprehension (Herron, 1991).

Calorie Needs

The RDA of calories for women of childbearing age is 2200. As can be seen in Table 12-1, an additional 300 calories, or a total caloric intake of 2500 calories, is recommended to meet the increased needs of pregnancy.

In addition to supplying energy for the fetus and placenta, this increase provides for an elevated metabolic rate from increased thyroid function and an increased work load from the extra weight she must carry. The use of sugar substitutes is not recommended, because the woman needs the sugar to maintain carbohydrate levels. A danger of not taking in adequate calories is that her body will use protein for energy, depriving the fetus of essential protein. Even in obese women, a pregnancy diet should never contain fewer than 1500 calories.

In helping a woman plan an increased caloric intake, be certain that she is planning on adding calories by eating foods rich in protein, iron, and other essential nutrients, rather than eating empty-calorie foods such as pretzels and doughnuts. Effective advice often is for her to prepare snacks such as carrot sticks or cheese and crackers early in the day when she is not tired and keep them readily available in the refrigerator. Otherwise, later in the day when she is tired, she will snack on empty-calorie food simply because it takes no preparation.

Protein Needs

The RDA for protein in women is 46 to 50 g. During pregnancy, the intake of protein should be increased to 60 g daily (an increase of 10 g). If protein needs are met in this way, overall nutritional needs are likely to be met (with the possible exceptions of ascorbic acid, vitamin A, and

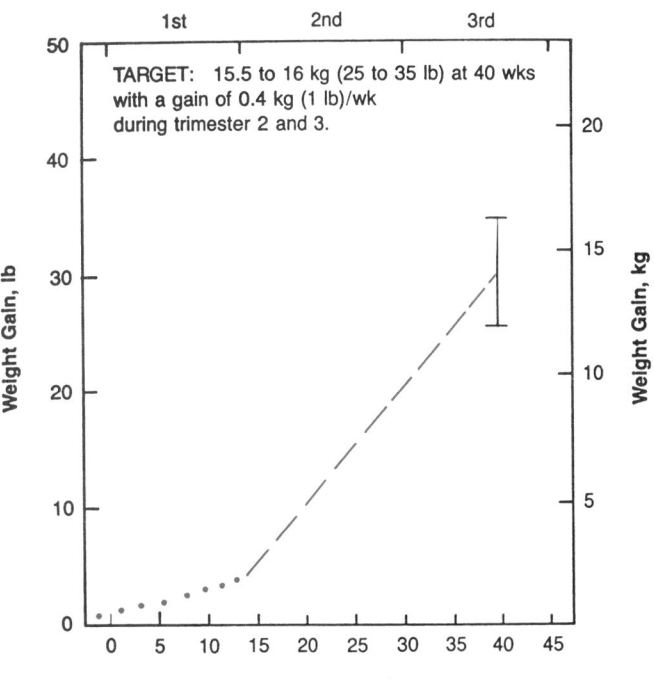

FIGURE 12-2
Provisional weight gain graph for normal weight women with BMI of 19.8 to 26.0 (metric). (Assumes a 1.6-kg [3.5-lb] gain in first trimester and the remaining gain at a rate of 0.44 kg [0.97 lb] per week.) (Dudek, S.G. [1993]. Nutrition handbook for nursing practice [2nd ed.]. Philadelphia: J.B. Lippincott.)

Table 12-1. *Recommended Daily Dietary Allowances for Pregnant and Nonpregnant Women*

	Nonpregnant Women				
	Age 11–14	Age 15–18	Age 19–24	Age 25–50	Pregnant Women
Calories (kcal)	2200	2200	2200	2200	2500
Protein (gm)	46	44	46	50	60
Fat Soluble Vitamins					
Vitamin A (μg)	800	800	800	800	800
Vitamin D (μg)	10	10	10	5	10
Vitamin E (mg)	8	8	8	8	10
Water Soluble Vitamins					
Ascorbic acid (mg) Vitamin C	50	60	60	60	70
Folic acid (μg)	150	180	180	180	400
Niacin (mg)	15	15	15	15	17
Riboflavin (mg)	1.3	1.3	1.3	1.3	1.6
Thiamine (mg)(B$_1$)	1.1	1.1	1.1	1.1	1.5
Vitamin B$_{12}$ (μg)	2.0	2.0	2.0	2.0	2.2
Vitamin B$_6$ (mg)	1.4	1.5	1.6	1.6	2.2
Minerals					
Calcium (mg)	1200	1200	1200	800	1200
Phosphorus (mg)	1200	1200	1200	800	1200
Iodine (μg)	150	150	150	150	175
Iron (mg)	15	15	15	15	30
Magnesium (mg)	280	300	280	280	320
Zinc (mg)	12	12	12	12	15

(National Academy of Sciences. [1989]. *Recommended daily dietary allowances* (10th ed.). Washington, DC: National Academy Press.)

vitamin D) because of the high incorporation of other nutrients with protein foods. If protein is inadequate in the diet, iron, B vitamins, calcium, and phosphorus also will undoubtedly be inadequate. Vitamin B$_{12}$ is found almost exclusively in animal protein so is apt to be insufficient if animal protein is totally excluded from the diet.

Extra protein is best supplied by meat, poultry, fish, yogurt, eggs, and milk because the protein in these forms contains all eight essential amino acids, or is a **complete** protein. The protein in nonanimal sources does not contain all eight essential amino acids (and thus is **incomplete**). It is possible by choosing nonanimal proteins carefully to provide all amino acids in the diet. Proteins that when cooked together provide all eight essential amino acids are termed *complementary proteins*. Examples are beans and rice, legumes and rice, or beans and wheat.

A woman who comes from a family with a tendency to high cholesterol levels (**hypercholesterolemia**) probably should not eat more than one egg per week because of the high cholesterol content of eggs. Encourage such women to eat lean meat, cook with vegetable oil instead of lard or butter, and remove the skin from poultry to reduce its fat content. Lunch meats (e.g., bologna or salami) should not be included as staples in the diet because their protein content may not be high and their salt content is invariably exceptionally high.

Milk is a rich source of protein but some women resist drinking it because it is high in calories and fat. Some cannot drink it because of lactose intolerance. Skim milk, either liquid or dry, supplies the same protein as regular milk but half the calories and is very low in fat. Some women find it difficult to drink a quart of milk a day because they simply do not like its taste. Buttermilk can be substituted, or chocolate or another flavoring can be added to make milk palatable (buttermilk has the disadvantage of having a high salt content). Yogurt or cheese may also be substituted for milk, or milk may be incorporated into custards, eggnogs, or cream soups. Women who are lactose intolerant can add lactase, which predigests the milk and makes it palatable.

Fat Needs

Only one fatty oil—linoleic acid, an essential fatty acid necessary for new cell growth—cannot be manufactured in the body from other sources. Thus, women must be

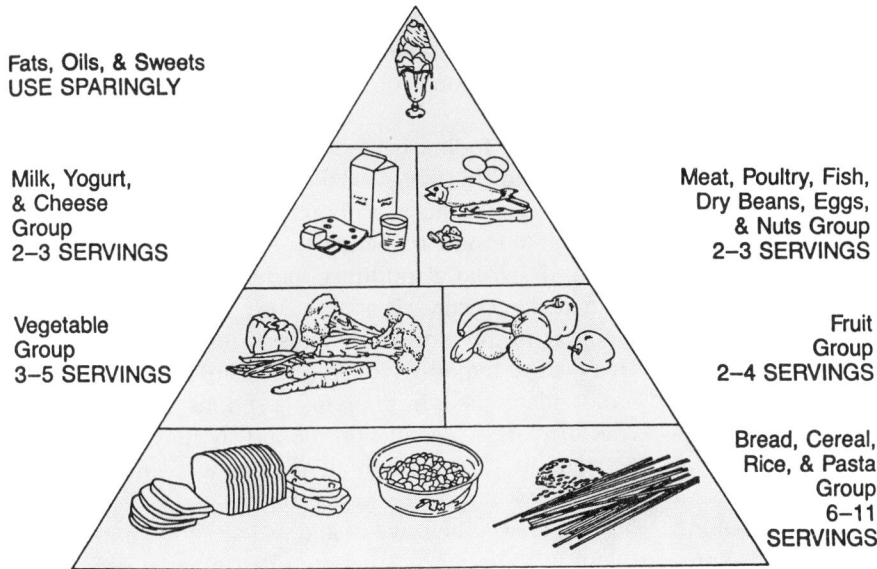

Fats, Oils, & Sweets
USE SPARINGLY

Milk, Yogurt,
& Cheese
Group
2–3 SERVINGS

Meat, Poultry, Fish,
Dry Beans, Eggs,
& Nuts Group
2–3 SERVINGS

Vegetable
Group
3–5 SERVINGS

Fruit
Group
2–4 SERVINGS

Bread, Cereal,
Rice, & Pasta
Group
6–11
SERVINGS

FIGURE 12-3
The food pyramid. (Dudek, S.G. [1993].
Nutrition handbook for nursing practice
[2nd ed.]. Philadelphia: J.B. Lippincott.)

concerned about consuming it during pregnancy. Using vegetable oils (e.g., safflower, corn, peanut, and cottonseed) rather than animal oils (lard) that have low cholesterol content is recommended for all adults as a means of preventing cholesterolemia and atherosclerosis. Vegetable oils serve the additional advantage of containing linoleic acid.

Vitamin Needs

The intake of vitamins as a daily dietary supplement has become so common that their importance may be underestimated by some women. Vitamin requirements of both fat-soluble and water-soluble vitamins increase during pregnancy to support the growth of new fetal cells (see Table 12-1). Vitamin deficiency can result in several problems. Severe folate deficiency can lead to megaloblastic anemia; it has also been associated with fetal neural tube defects (see below). A lack of vitamin D, which is essential to calcium absorption, can begin to diminish maternal mineral bone density; studies have also shown a direct correlation between maternal cal-

cium intake during gestation and neonatal bone density (Kochenour, 1990).

Even though vitamin needs do increase during pregnancy, most of the vitamin intake requirements (with the exception of folic acid) can be met by eating a healthy, varied diet with plenty of fruits and vegetables. Women who were on oral contraceptives before they became pregnant should be certain to include good sources of vitamins A and B_6 and folic acid in their early pregnancy diets, since OCs may deplete stores of these vitamins. Women should also be counseled not to use mineral oil as a laxative, since it can prevent absorption of fat-soluble vitamins from the gastrointestinal tract, thus hindering their availability to the body.

Women should, however, avoid taking megadoses of vitamins. The fat-soluble vitamins are stored in the body rather than excreted and thus can reach toxic levels. Some animal studies have found an association between excessive vitamin intake and fetal malformation (Kochenour, 1990). The intake of excessive vitamin A as isotretinoin (Accutane), a medication prescribed for

---

Table 12-2. *Quantities of Food Suggested During Pregnancy*

Food Group	Nonpregnant Woman	Pregnant Woman
Meat, poultry, fish, dry beans, eggs, and nut group	2–3 servings (only 2–3 eggs per week)	2–3 servings (only 2–3 eggs per week)
Vegetable group	3–5 servings	3–5 servings
Fruit group	2–4 servings	2–4 servings
Bread, cereal, rice and pasta group	6–11 servings	6–11 servings
Milk, yogurt, and cheese group	2–3 servings	3–4 servings
Additional fluid	As desired	At least 2 glasses

acne, is documented as causing congenital anomalies in humans (Loeb, 1993). In addition, the mechanism of placental transfer of water-soluble vitamins makes fetal blood levels regularly higher than maternal blood levels; maternal overdosage can thus potentially cause fetal toxicity (Kochenour, 1990). Megadoses of vitamin C may cause withdrawal scurvy in the infant at birth (Swonger & Matejski, 1991).

Folic Acid. Although folic acid (folacin) belongs to the B vitamin group, its importance during pregnancy warrants separate discussion. Folic acid is necessary for red blood cell formation. It is found predominantly in fresh fruits and vegetables. As the woman's blood volume doubles during pregnancy, her folic acid needs increase substantially. Without adequate folic acid, a megaloblastic anemia (large but ineffective red blood cells) may develop. If the woman manifests such symptoms at the time of birth, the infant may be affected as well. In addition, low levels of folic acid in the woman have been associated with premature separation of the placenta, spontaneous abortion, and neural tube defects (Murphy, 1992).

For these reasons, women should eat foods high in folic acid such as vegetables and fruit, and are prescribed prenatal vitamins which contain a folic acid supplement of 0.4 to 1.0 mg.

Mineral Needs

Minerals are necessary for new cell building in the fetus. Because they are found in so many foods and because mineral absorption improves during pregnancy, mineral deficiency, with the exceptions of calcium, iodine, and iron, is rare.

Calcium and Phosphorus. The skeleton and teeth constitute a major portion of the fetus (tooth formation begins as early as 8 weeks and bones begin to calcify at 12 weeks in utero). To supply adequate calcium and phosphorus for bone formation, pregnant women need to ingest a diet high in calcium and vitamin D (necessary for calcium to enter bones). Milk is the best source of calcium. If a woman cannot drink milk or eat milk products such as cheese, she can be prescribed a daily calcium supplement.

Before nutrition counseling in pregnancy became as common as it is today, women expected to lose "a tooth a child"; that is, they believed the fetus, as he or she grew, would drain calcium from their teeth. Although it is unlikely that a woman will lose a tooth with pregnancy nowadays, the concern reflected in this myth about the fetus taking calcium from the mother is well-founded. However, the calcium in teeth is not as readily absorbed as that of bone, so it is more likely that inadequate calcium intake will result in diminished maternal bone density rather than weakened teeth. With a good calcium intake during pregnancy, the fetus will receive as much calcium as needed for growth and mineralization of the fetal skeleton without taking any away from the maternal bones or teeth.

Iodine. Iodine is essential for the formation of thyroxine and therefore for the proper functioning of the thyroid gland. It is important that a woman ingest enough during pregnancy to supply the needs of increased thyroid gland function during this time. If iodine deficiency occurs, it may cause thyroid enlargement (goiter) in the woman or fetus; in extreme instances, it may cause hypothyroidism (cretinism) in the fetus. Thyroid enlargement in the fetus is serious at birth because the increased pressure on the airway may lead to early respiratory distress; hypothyroidism leads to mental retardation if not discovered at birth.

In areas where water and soil are known to be deficient in iodine, it is suggested that women use iodized salt and include a serving of seafood in their diet at least once a week.

Iron. A fetus at term has a hemoglobin level of 17 to 21 g per 100 mL of blood. This high hemoglobin level is necessary to oxygenate the blood during intrauterine life, because with fetal circulation, venous and arterial blood are so mixed that 100% oxygenation of red blood cells is not attained. In addition to needing iron to build this high level of hemoglobin, after week 20 of pregnancy, the fetus begins to store iron in the liver to last him or her through the first 3 months of life, when intake will consist mainly of milk, which is low in iron. In addition to fetal needs, the woman needs iron to build an increased red cell volume for herself and to replace iron lost in blood at delivery.

The RDA of iron for pregnant women is 30 mg per day. An average diet supplies about 6 mg of iron per 1000 calories. If the woman eats a 2500-calorie diet daily, she therefore takes in about 15 mg of iron daily. Because only 10% to 20% of dietary iron is absorbed, however, she is actually taking in less than this amount (closer to 1.5 mg to 3 mg). Therefore, a prenatal diet should be supplemented with 15 mg of iron per day to ensure that adequate iron is ingested and absorbed. It is important for women to understand that iron supplementation is intended as a supplement to, not a replacement for, an iron-rich diet.

Women in low-income groups may find it difficult to include adequate iron in their diets, because the foods richest in iron (e.g., organ meats; eggs; green, leafy vegetables; whole grain; enriched breads; or dried fruits) are also the most expensive foods. Iron is better absorbed from the stomach in an acid environment than an alkaline one, so taking an iron supplement with orange juice may increase absorption. Oral iron compounds turn stools black and tend to cause constipation in some women. Women should not stop taking the iron compound because constipation occurs. Increasing fluid intake or fiber in the diet is a better way to relieve the constipation. Some women may need a prescribed stool softener to be comfortable. Stool softeners such as docusate sodium (Colace) are not associated with teratogenic action and so can be taken safely during pregnancy.

Fluoride. Because fluoride aids in the formation of sound teeth, a pregnant woman should drink fluoridated water. In an area where water is not fluoridated either naturally or artificially, supplemental fluoride may be recommended. Fluoride in large amounts causes brown-stained teeth, so the woman must not take the supplement more often than prescribed or if tap water in her area is already fluoridated.

Sodium. Sodium is the major electrolyte that acts to maintain fluid balance in the body, because when sodium is retained rather than excreted by the kidney tubules, an equal or balancing amount of fluid is also retained. It is important that enough fluid be retained in the maternal circulation during pregnancy to cause a pressure gradient across the placenta for optimal exchange to occur.

Unless the woman is hypertensive or has heart disease when she enters pregnancy and has previously been on a salt-restricted diet, she should continue to season foods as usual during pregnancy. She should, however, avoid foods that are extremely salty, such as lunch meats, potato chips, and monosodium glutamate. Too much salt could result in retention of excessive amounts of fluid, putting a strain on the heart as blood volume doubles.

Zinc. Zinc is necessary for synthesis of DNA and RNA and so is important for fetal growth. A deficiency of zinc has been associated with preterm birth (Scholl et al., 1993). The RDA of zinc during pregnancy is 15 mg per day, or an increase of 3 mg over prepregnancy need. Most people who take in adequate protein also take in adequate zinc as zinc is contained in foods such as meat, liver, eggs, and seafood. It is a component of pregnancy vitamins.

Fluid Needs

Extra amounts of water are needed during pregnancy for good kidney function, because the woman must excrete waste products for two. Two glasses of fluid daily over and above a daily quart of milk are recommended.

Fiber Needs

Constipation occurs readily in pregnancy from the pressure of the uterus on the intestine. Eating fiber-rich foods daily is a natural way of preventing constipation, because the bulk of the fiber in the intestine aids evacuation. Fiber also has the advantage of lowering cholesterol levels and may remove carcinogenic contaminants

from the intestine. A food has a high fiber content when it consists of parts of the plant cell wall that are resistant to normal digestive enzymes of the small intestine (such as broccoli and asparagus). Crude fiber content refers to how much fiber is left after intestinal breakdown.

Foods to Avoid in Pregnancy

As discussed in Chapter 11, alcoholic beverages should not be ingested by the pregnant woman because of their potentially teratogenic effects on the fetus. Other foods to be avoided are those that contain food additives.

Foods With Caffeine

Caffeine is thought of by many women as just an incidental ingredient in beverages. It is much more than this, however, because it is a central nervous system stimulant capable of increasing heart rate, urine production in the kidney, and secretion of acid in the stomach.

Caffeine is related in chemical structure to uric acid. In animals, the administration of caffeine is associated with infertility and the development of structural anomalies such as cleft palate. In humans, a daily intake of caffeine of more than 300 mg (comparable to four cups of coffee) has been associated with low birth weight (McDonald et al., 1992). For this reason, the Food and Drug Administration (FDA) has issued a formal warning to women to limit their caffeine intake during pregnancy. A moderate intake apparently carries little risk (Mills et al., 1993).

To limit their caffeine intake, women should not only limit the amount of coffee they drink but also other sources of caffeine as well, such as chocolate, soft drinks, and tea. If a woman has difficulty omitting these common foods from her diet, she can still reduce the amount of caffeine she ingests by modifying their preparation. Instant coffee, for example, as a rule, has less caffeine than brewed coffee; percolated coffee has less caffeine than dripped coffee. Decaffeinated coffee, as the name implies, contains almost no caffeine.

Tea, like coffee, varies in caffeine content, depending on the type and time of brewing. The longer tea brews, the more the caffeine content increases. Green tea has less caffeine than black tea. Both herbal teas and decaffeinated tea are available in most communities.

The cocoa bean that is used to make chocolate and cocoa is yet another natural source of caffeine. Chocolate sources tend to be low in caffeine, however, compared with coffee. Whereas a cup of coffee contains approximately 120 mg of caffeine, a cup of hot chocolate contains only 10 mg. Baking chocolate, used for cake frostings and glazes, is proportionately higher, containing about 35 mg of caffeine per ounce.

Soft drinks do not naturally contain caffeine; it is added to them to improve their appeal. To limit the amount of caffeine consumed, pregnant women should choose caffeine-free brands.

Artificial Sweeteners

Artificial sweeteners are used to improve the taste and limit the caloric content of foods and are a common component of many popular foods. Federal controls regulate the use of these ingredients, but it is probably safest for pregnant women to reduce intake of these substances. For instance, although the sweetener Aspartame has been approved by the FDA for consumption and is apparently safe during pregnancy, large amounts of the compound should be avoided by pregnant women until its safety is completely confirmed (Niebyl, 1990). The use of saccharine is not recommended during pregnancy because it is eliminated slowly from the fetal bloodstream. In any event, pregnant women need carbohydrate furnished by sugar rather than artificial substances.

Weight Loss Diets

Every year new diets to help people lose weight painlessly are introduced. As a rule, pregnant women should not be on reducing diets. If women have been following such diets before becoming pregnant, they may have few nutritional stores, and additional vitamin supplementation may be appropriate.

Assessment of Nutritional Health

Nutritional risk factors during pregnancy are summarized in Table 12-3. The best method for assessing nutritional intake is to ask for a "typical day" history or a 24-hour dietary recall. Ask first if yesterday was a typical day. If it was, ask the woman to list all the food she ate within the past 24 hours. Be certain she includes all the snack foods she ate as well as sit-down meals. This method of history-taking yields much more accurate information about actual intake than if the woman is asked how often during the week she eats citrus fruit, or how much milk she drinks every day. A woman who knows how much milk she ought to drink a day will probably say she drinks a quart a day during pregnancy. However, if asked to list the foods she ate the day before, she may report that she drank only one glass of milk all day.

After obtaining the day's list of food, compare the types and amounts on the list with those shown in Table 12-2 to see if all food groups and adequate amounts are included. Comparing foods from the person's 24-hour recall against such a table is a helpful way of showing clients that what they thought was a "perfect" intake is imperfect or what they thought was a "little" problem actually involves the loss of an entire food group. Once a woman sees that an actual defect exists, she is more apt to be ready to set goals to improve nutrition. Such a picture also offers an instant reward for the woman who is ingesting an adequate diet.

In addition to actual food intake, ask the woman if she thinks she has any problem with nutrition (such as cravings) and assess circumstances of eating, such as cultural preferences, who prepares food in the family, and how many meals are eaten outside the home weekly. Table 12-4 summarizes this type of additional information.

To strengthen history findings, assess the woman's prepregnancy weight and calculate her body mass index. People with poor nutrition are over or underweight and demonstrate typical physical signs. Table 12-5 lists

Table 12-3. *Nutritional Risk Factors During Pregnancy*

Risk	Rationale
Adolescent (less than 18 years old at LMP)	An adolescent already has increased nutritional needs.
Short intervals between pregnancies	The woman's body has not had time to replace nutritional stores depleted during previous pregnancy(ies).
Low income	Family may not have resources to purchase adequate foods to meet pregnancy nutritional needs.
Follows food fads	Foods eaten may not be those adequate for pregnancy. (Some diets may be lacking in essential nutrients.)
Drug use (including cigarettes and alcohol)	Drugs may be ingested in preference to healthy foods.
Existence of a chronic illness requiring a special diet	Intake may be low in an essential substance such as carbohydrate or protein.
Underweight or overweight	Underweight and overweight status may indicate chronic inadequate dietary patterns.
Multiple pregnancy	The woman must supply enough nutrition for multiple fetal development.
Anemic at conception	The woman has no iron stores for fetal growth.
Lactose intolerance	The woman may not be ingesting adequate calcium for fetal skeletal growth.

Table 12-4. *Areas to Be Assessed for a Total Nutrition History*

Area of Assessment	Pertinent Questions
Food preparation	Who does the cooking?
	How many people does the woman cook for?
	How are foods usually prepared (fried or baked)?
	What spices or condiments are commonly used?
	What type oil is used for frying (saturated or unsaturated)?
Food pattern	How many meals are eaten a day?
	Which is the biggest meal?
	How many snacks are eaten a day?
	What are they?
	How many meals are eaten outside the home?
	Where are they eaten? Cafeteria? Fast-food store? Restaurant? Bagged lunch?
Financial concerns	Is there enough money for food?
	Would the woman eat differently if more money were available?
	Is any supplementary financial program used?
Activity level	Is she normally active or sedentary?
	(Could increase calorie need.)
Health	Does she know of any allergies to food?
	Does she have any trouble with chewing or digestion?
	What is bowel movement frequency?
	Was she taking oral contraceptives before pregnancy?
	Does she take supplemental vitamins? What type? How many?
	Does she drink alcohol? What type? How much?
	Does she smoke cigarettes?
	What is her stress level? Does this affect her appetite?
Personal food preferences	Are there any foods she particularly enjoys or dislikes?
	Are there any foods she feels are harmful or particularly beneficial to her?
	Are there any cultural or religious preferences?
Family dietary patterns	Does anyone in the family eat a special diet?
	Is anyone obviously overweight or underweight?
	Does the family eat meals together?
	Is mealtime a social time?

important physical examination assessments that suggest a good nutritional intake or evidence of poor nutrition.

Hemoglobin or hematocrit determinations are also important assessments of good nutrition (see Table 12-5). Women have these measured early in pregnancy and then usually repeated close to term and again at birth. A urinalysis can also be important because a finding such as elevated specific gravity of urine suggests a disturbed fluid balance.

Promotion of Nutritional Health During Pregnancy

Setting Nutritional Health Goals

Plans made for improving nutrition patterns must be within the woman's lifestyle, family preferences, financial resources, customs, and cultural desires for a family

to follow them for 9 months (Figure 12-4; see also the Nursing Care Plan).

Family Considerations

Meal planning must involve the entire family. Even if a woman is receptive to changing her eating habits, she may have difficulty carrying out recommendations if her family resists such changes. With an adolescent, it is important to speak to her mother or whoever prepares the meals at home to effect a change. In families in which a member needs a special diet, cooking is more difficult than in others; thus, change may be even more difficult.

Financial Considerations

Food is costly. To provide the extra servings required during pregnancy, a woman is being asked to spend more on food for herself per week than she is used to spending. Women generally view this increased expense

Table 12-5. *Physical Signs and Symptoms of Adequate Pregnancy Nutrition*

Assessment Area	Signs of Good Nutrition	Signs of Malnutrition
Hair	Shiny; strong with good body	Hair dull and lifeless.
Eyes	Good eyesight, particularly at night; conjunctiva moist and pink	Pale and dry conjunctiva; difficulty with night vision.
Mouth	No cavities in teeth; no swollen or inflamed gingiva; no cracks or fissures at corners of mouth; mucous membrane moist and pink; tongue smooth and nontender	Fissures at corners of mouth; tongue rough and tender; mucous membrane pale.
Neck	Normal contour of thyroid gland	Thyroid gland enlarged.
Skin	Smooth, with normal color and turgor; no ecchymotic or petechial areas present	Rough texture; poor turgor.
Extremities	Normal muscle mass and circumference; normal strength and mobility; edema limited to slight ankle involvement; normal reflexes	Poor muscle tone; diminished reflexes.
Finger and toenails	Smooth; pink; normal contour	Pale; break easily; little growth.
Weight	Within normal limits of ideal weight chart before pregnancy; following normal pattern of pregnancy weight gain	Over or underweight; unusually slow or rapid weight gain.
Blood pressure	Within normal limits for length of pregnancy	Decreased from anemia; increased from hypertension.

as an investment in their child's health and do not regard it as a burden. However, the family on a marginal income, though willing to shoulder the additional cost, may have trouble actually doing so. The woman with this problem needs to review her diet to be certain she is not buying only starchy foods because they are more filling and cheaper than buying protein foods. She may need help in securing any financial assistance that is available, such as food stamps or nutrition aid programs such as Women, Infants and Children Special Supplemental Food Program (WIC) (Kahler et al., 1992). The WIC program is a federal program that provides nutritional support for low-income women and children. Established in 1972 as a pilot program, WIC is funded by the Food and Nutrition Service of the U.S. Department of Agriculture. The program supplies supplemental foods and nutrition education not only to pregnant women but also to postpartal women up to 6 months, nursing mothers up to 1 year, and children from birth to age 5 (see Chapter 34 for a discussion of WIC supplements for children).

Eligibility for the program is based on income level, geographic area, and nutritional risk. Each state defines the income eligibility level. To receive food, clients must live in an area that has been designated a funding area. The nurse or nutritionist in the health care facility determines nutritional need. Factors that are considered to put pregnant women at nutritional risk include age (adolescent or woman over 40); poor obstetric history such as previous spontaneous abortion, a short period between pregnancies, previous low-birth-weight infant or gestational diabetes; anemia; poor weight gain; or inadequate consumption of food by diet history.

Typical foods offered by the program to pregnant women are those with high-quality protein, iron, calcium, and vitamins A and C, such as fruit juice, eggs, milk, and cheese. WIC clients are reevaluated at predetermined intervals to see if the program supplements are still necessary. WIC has been successful in increasing nutrition during pregnancy not only because it supplies additional food to recipients but because the periodic evaluations provide time for nutrition counseling. WIC supplementation not only reduces the risk of low birth weight but reduces medical costs by preventing costly newborn care (Buescher et al., 1993).

Cultural Considerations

Women during pregnancy may not want to change from familiar patterns of food preparation. Many women prepare food for their families as well as for themselves, and asking them to change to different foods involves changing the food patterns of other family members as well. Common cultural differences that are important to be aware of in nutrition counseling are shown in the Focus on Cultural Awareness box.

Managing Common Problems Affecting Nutritional Health

Specific nutrition problems in pregnancy may result from a number of factors or circumstances.

Nausea and Vomiting

As many as 50% of pregnant women report nausea and vomiting. No definite cause has been established for this

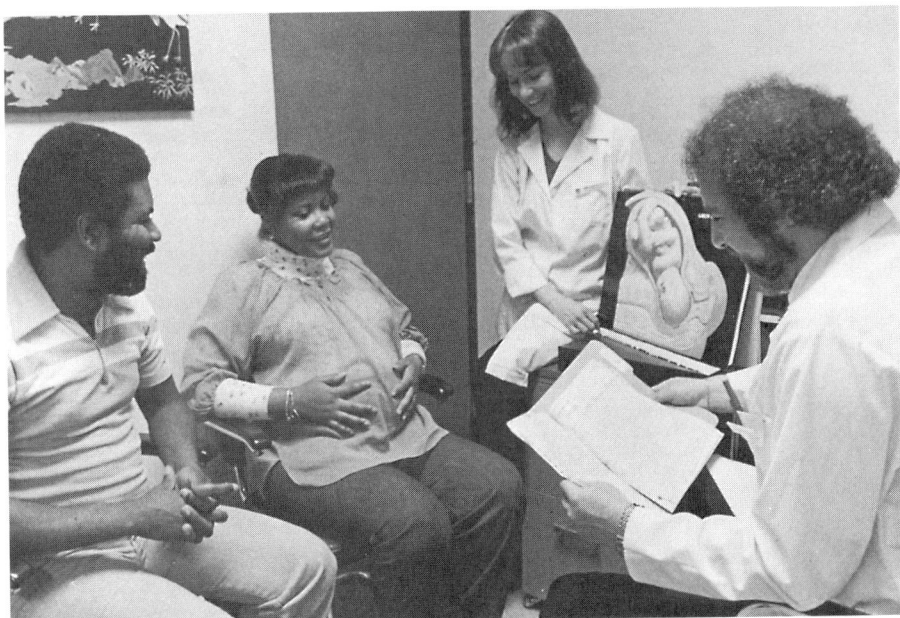

FIGURE 12-4

Encourage pregnant women to eat a varied diet with a high iron and protein content. This may be difficult early in pregnancy because of nausea, late in pregnancy because of fatigue. (Courtesy of Harvard Community Health Plan, Boston, MA.)

almost universal symptom of early pregnancy. It may be due to sensitivity to the high chorionic gonadotropin hormone levels produced by the trophoblast; to high estrogen or progesterone levels; to lowered maternal blood sugar caused by the needs of the developing embryo; to lack of pyridoxine (vitamin B$_6$); or to diminished gastric motility. It is known that nausea is aggravated by fatigue and may be aggravated by emotional disturbance (Newman, Fullerton, & Anderson, 1993).

Most women notice the sensation as early as the first missed menstrual period; it lasts the first 3 months of pregnancy. The sensation is usually most intense on arising but may occur while the woman is preparing meals and smelling food. Vomiting at least once a day is not uncommon. Women who work nights and sleep days often experience "evening sickness," because that is when they arise (see the Focus on Nursing Research box).

Methods such as acupressure have been tried with good success (DeAloysio & Penacchioni, 1993). Women may find that antimotion sickness wrist bands give some relief. Ginger may be effective. Increasing glucose intake seems to relieve nausea better than any other remedy. The traditional solution is for women to keep dry crackers or potato chips by the bedside and eat a few before rising; sourball candy may serve the same purpose. The woman can then eat a light breakfast or delay breakfast until 10 AM or 11 AM, past the time her nausea seems to persist. It is essential for her to maintain a good food intake during pregnancy, so she must compensate for missed meals later in the day. If preparing food for others makes her feel queasy, she should try to give these responsibilities to another family member, at least

through the worst phase of this symptom. Preparing meals ahead of time, perhaps at night when the nausea is less bothersome, may also help.

It is a good rule not to go longer than 12 hours between meals during pregnancy to prevent hypoglycemia, so a woman may need to include a late evening snack in her meals. Fruit and raw vegetables may be tolerated during the morning before other food; urge her to experiment with soups or vegetable drinks that she may not usually think of as breakfast foods but will give her early morning calories.

Women should be cautioned against taking home remedies for nausea, including antacids. Preparations of antacids containing sodium bicarbonate may cause fluid retention because of the sodium content. It is a sound rule that a woman should take *no* medication during pregnancy unless her physician or nurse-midwife agrees to its use.

Nausea in pregnancy was formerly treated with antiemetics (Bendectin, a drug similar to those used for motion sickness, was commonly prescribed). A number of drugs in this classification are now being investigated for teratogenic effects and so are no longer routinely prescribed. Advise women that natural measures of controlling early morning nausea, such as eating food high in carbohydrates on arising and delaying breakfast, are safer methods (see the Focus on Family Teaching box).

Fortunately, nausea usually disappears spontaneously as the woman enters her fourth month of pregnancy. If it persists beyond this month or is so extreme in early pregnancy that it interferes with nutrition, it may indicate the development of hyperemesis gravidarum, a complication of pregnancy (see Chapter 15).

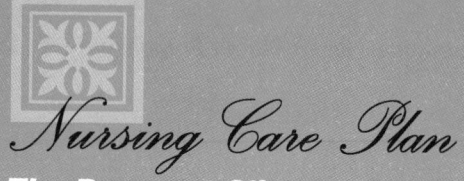

Nursing Care Plan

The Pregnant Client With an Inadequate Nutritional Pattern

Trisha Morane is a 26-year-old woman you see at a prenatal care visit. The following is a nursing care plan designed for her that addresses the nutritional requirements of pregnancy.

Assessment: Thin-appearing client who works as buyer for department store. Cooks for self and husband; reports she is "not a good cook." Often cooks just for herself because husband travels 3 days a week. Culture: African-American. Finances "adequate." Had a weight problem in high school that she now keeps under control by "eating almost nothing," especially when husband is away. Concerned with constipation since beginning of pregnancy. Twenty-four hour dietary history is:

Breakfast: 1 cup black coffee
Lunch: none
Dinner: 1 serving macaroni and cheese; 1 serving green peas, 1 cup coffee
Snacks: 1 glass milk, 1 candy bar, 1 cup coffee

Height: 5'6"; prepregnancy weight: 110 lb (10 lb under desirable weight for height; BMI: 14. Weight today (last menstrual period 9 weeks ago): 111 lb.

Nursing Diagnosis: Altered nutrition, less than body requirements, related to inadequate food intake.

Defining Characteristic: Client describes a daily intake with low total calories, low protein, no fruit, high caffeine; is underweight by BMI criteria.

Goal: Client will ingest adequate nutrition daily throughout pregnancy.

Outcome Criteria:
1. Pregnancy weight gain totals 35–40 lbs.
2. Hemoglobin remains above 11 g/100 mL.
3. Client describes adequate pregnancy nutrition at visits.
4. Client takes daily prenatal vitamin.

Nursing Orders	Rationale
1. Diet to be 3000 calories daily; one prenatal vitamin (Stuartnatal 1+1) prescribed by M.D.	1. 500 additional calories added to increase weight.
2. Counsel regarding pregnancy nutrition and the need to increase intake.	2. Client needs to increase intake to add additional calories.
3. Return in 1 week for nurse appointment for further nutrition review and suggestions.	3. Changing nutritional habits is difficult without follow-up.
4. Client to bring suggestions that might make cooking for herself in evening or packing a lunch easier or more fun.	4. Active participation should help compliance.

(continued)

Constipation

Many women experience constipation during pregnancy. This is related to the reduced activity of the gastrointestinal tract from pressure of the growing uterus, effects of the placental hormone relaxin, or possibly progesterone levels. Constipation leads to a feeling of bloating or fullness and lack of appetite. Including an adequate intake of fiber-rich foods in the diet should create enough intestinal bulk to promote peristalsis. Preventing constipation by nutritional intervention this way is preferable to treating constipation with laxatives or enemas.

Cravings

Cravings for food during pregnancy are so common that they are considered a normal part of pregnancy. It was formerly considered that these strange desires for food reflected a woman's need to call attention to the pregnancy or were a reaction to her imposed dependent state. However, cravings are actually more likely the re-

Nursing Diagnosis: Potential for injury to fetus related to excessive caffeine ingestion.

Goal: Client will reduce caffeine use by next prenatal visit.

Outcome Criteria: Client lists only 1 cup of coffee on 24-hour recall dietary history by 1 month.

Nursing Orders	Rationale
1. Educate regarding possible teratogenic effect of excessive caffeine.	1. Awareness of problem can be the beginning of action.
2. Plan with client beverages she would enjoy other than coffee such as herbal tea.	2. Maintaining high fluid intake is important for kidney and bowel function.
3. Plan a schedule with client to reduce caffeine intake by half each day until she reaches 1 cup daily.	3. Help prevent headache from caffeine withdrawal.

Nursing Diagnosis: Constipation related to physiologic changes of pregnancy.

Goal: Client will use self-care measures to prevent constipation for the remainder of pregnancy.

Outcome Criteria: Client states she has a bowel movement at least every other day.

Nursing Orders	Rationale
1. Counsel client regarding causes of constipation with pregnancy such as pressure on bowel and slowed bowel motility.	1. Understanding can be the basis for action.
2. Remind client of importance of a regular time for bowel evacuation.	2. Bowel evacuation is stimulated by habit.
3. Help client plan a way to include more roughage in meals such as additional fruits, vegetables, and legumes.	3. Roughage can aid bowel evacuation.
4. Help client plan on ways to increase fluid in diet.	4. Additional fluid can help relieve constipation.

sult of a physiologic need for more carbohydrates or particular vitamins and minerals.

Now that the recommended pregnancy diet allows for more calories, and a greater pregnancy weight gain is encouraged, cravings are seen less often than before. When taking a nutritional history, ask if the woman notices any particular cravings. Planning nutrition to include the food or foods that she craves will prevent her from cheating on her diet to include this item. This is a more positive approach to nutrition counseling than leaving her feeling guilty because she is eating her favorite foods and enjoying her pregnancy.

Pica. Some women report an abnormal craving for nonfood substances during pregnancy (termed **pica** from the Latin magpie, a bird that is an indiscriminate eater). The most common form of pica in the past was a craving for laundry starch; now that this is rarely present in homes, pica may be revealed by a craving for clay, dirt, corn starch, or ice cubes. Although some of these

FOCUS ON CULTURAL AWARENESS

Culture	Influences on Nutrition	Possible Nutritional Problems
Asian	Diet rich in vegetables (bean sprouts, broccoli, bamboo shoots, or mushrooms) that are stir-fried quickly so that their vitamins are retained. Meat served with vegetables; portions may be small. Rice is dietary staple. Milk not consumed much because many people tend to have lactase deficiency and cannot digest the lactose in milk.	Lack of protein due to small meat servings. Because bean curd, soybeans, and green leafy vegetables supply calcium, calcium deficiency is not a problem despite lack of milk. Rice used should be enriched or thiamine deficiency can occur.
Puerto Rican	Meat often cooked in stews, so portions may be small. Beans and rice cooked together for complementary protein sources. Little milk consumed due to lactase deficiency.	Lack of protein due to small meat servings; lack of folic acid in diet
Mexican-American	Corn often used as basic grain. Meat generally mixed with beans and sauce so portions may be small. Milk use limited.	Lack of vitamin A and folic acid: small meat portions may lead to protein deficiency.
European	Wide range of dietary patterns. English tend to overcook vegetables, thus losing water-soluble vitamins; Italians tend to eat a large amount of pasta (leading to obesity). Fresh fruit not used extensively.	Deficiency of vitamin C
Jewish	Level of dietary practices varies according to whether the family is Orthodox (follows restrictions firmly); Reformed; or Conservative (follows rules at individual level). For Orthodox family, food must be *kosher* (clean): Meat is soaked in salt water to remove blood; only four-footed animals that are cloven-hooved and chew a cud allowed (eg, beef and lamb). Pork and fish without scales (shellfish) prohibited. Milk and meat cannot be combined.	People may develop increased cholesterol level owing to high level of saturated fat used in cooking.
African-American	Meat consumed is often pork; vegetables cooked with salt pork for long periods. Little milk consumed owing to lactose intolerance. Popular broadleaf vegetables (e.g., collard greens or beet greens) are good sources of calcium.	Iron and protein deficiency may occur; high level of dietary salt may contribute to chronic hypertension in adults.
Vegetarian	A person who is a vegan (i.e., all animal foods, dairy products, and eggs are prohibited) by religion or culture eats only vegetables and fruit. A lacto-vegetarian eats vegetables, fruits, milk, and cheese. A lacto-ovo vegetarian eats vegetables, fruits, milk, cheese, and eggs. These diets are nutritious and can be well balanced with careful meal planning.	It is easy to develop deficiencies unless person is knowledgeable about complementary protein. Vitamin B_{12} (present almost entirely in animal sources) and vitamin D (supplied in normal diets by fortified milk and exposure to sunlight) may be deficient without a supplement.

things can do no harm in themselves, the ingestion of large quantities may leave the woman deficient in protein, iron, and calcium, nutrients essential for a healthy pregnancy outcome (Horner, 1991).

Pica is a symptom that often accompanies iron deficiency anemia. Always ask women at prenatal visits if

any form of pica is present. Most women do not supply this information unless asked directly because they worry that you will find their behavior odd and because they may not realize their habit is pregnancy-related as much as being a nervous habit.

Encouraging a woman to stop eating the nonfood

substance may not be effective because the habit may be deeply ingrained. Correcting iron deficiency anemia with an iron supplement will generally automatically correct the pica. At subsequent visits, however, be certain to assess the woman for this and ask her if she notices any difference in her cravings.

Pyrosis

Pyrosis (heartburn) is a burning sensation along the esophagus caused by regurgitation of gastric contents. In pregnancy, it may accompany nausea, but it may persist beyond the resolution of nausea and even increase in severity as pregnancy advances.

Pyrosis is probably caused by decreased gastric motility. It may be relieved by eating small meals frequently and by not lying down immediately after eating, to help prevent reflux. Aluminum hydroxide (Amphojel) or a combination of aluminum and magnesium hydroxide (Maalox) may be prescribed for relief. Be certain a woman understands that this "chest" pain is from her gastrointestinal tract and that, although it is called heartburn, it has nothing to do with her heart.

Flatulence

Flatulence may occur with pregnancy owing to decreased gastrointestinal motility and delayed emptying of the bowel. Remedies for this are to avoid gas-forming foods such as cabbage or beans and to maintain normal bowel habits.

Hypercholesterolemia

Women who have an inherited tendency towards hypercholesterolemia may enter pregnancy with an elevated cholesterol level. During pregnancy, increasing progesterone levels cause a further elevation of cholesterol, which can result in an increased tendency to form gallstones (cholelithiasis) and an increased risk of cardiovascular disease. Preventing these complications during pregnancy is important. An attack of gallstones causes extremely sharp pain, and surgery to remove them during pregnancy can be a threat to the fetus because of the necessary anesthesia (Scott, 1992). A woman who has had difficulty with hypercholesterolemia before pregnancy may need to continue to reduce her intake of fat during pregnancy to prevent any increase in cholesterol. Exercising daily, broiling meat rather than frying it, using a minimum of salad oils, and substituting margarine for butter are good ways to keep down cholesterol levels. Women should check with their health care provider about the wisdom of continuing cholesterol-lowering drugs during pregnancy, as these may be teratogenic. A low-cholesterol diet will automatically be lower in calories than the average diet, because oils and fats add many calories. Assess these women carefully for adequate weight gain during pregnancy. Make sure that a woman does include *some* oil daily (perhaps as salad

FOCUS ON NURSING RESEARCH

What Is the Usual Pattern and Intensity of Nausea With Pregnancy?

To answer this question, Dilorio, van Lier, and Manteuffel asked 19 pregnant women to record in a daily diary for 1 week the pattern and intensity of the nausea they were experiencing. All the women in the study were less than 14 weeks pregnant; all but one were employed. Their ages ranged from 23 to 38 years. Findings from the diaries revealed four patterns of nausea: morning only, evening only, morning and evening, and continuous. The periods when it was most apt to occur were 3 P.M. to 6 P.M. and 7 A.M. to 10 A.M. The researchers suggest that using the term "morning sickness" to describe nausea of pregnancy could be confusing to women who experience it continuously or at times of the day other than morning.

Dilorio, C., van Lier, D., & Manteuffel, B. (1992). Patterns of nausea during first trimester of pregnancy. *Clinical Nursing Research, 1,* 127.

oil) so that she has included a source of linoleic acid in her daily intake.

Promoting Nutritional Health in Women With Special Needs

The Adolescent

Good nutrition is apt to be a problem with pregnant teenagers because of the dual demands of pregnancy and adolescence (Scholl & Hediger, 1993). The girl must be certain to consume enough food to provide not only for fetal growth but for her own continuing growth. Often involved in adolescents' search for identity is an avoidance of foods that their parents see as important for them (e.g., milk, warm cereal, vegetables, or fruit). Teenagers may indulge themselves instead in foods of which their parents usually disapprove such as pizza, soft drinks, potato chips, and french fries. To help the adolescent plan a diet for pregnancy, respect her right to reject traditional foods as long as her diet includes sufficient nutrients. A cheese and sausage pizza, a glass of milk, and an apple is a lunch that provides all basic food groups (meat: sausage; bread: pizza crust; vegetable: tomato sauce; dairy: cheese and milk; and fruit: apple). A hamburger "with everything" plus a tangerine and milk provides the same nutrition.

Many adolescents snack frequently during the day. Toward the end of pregnancy when a girl is tired, she may begin to eat more and more "junk food" because preparing nutritious snacks takes more effort. Advise her to prepare some nutritious snacks such as carrot sticks or cheese bites early each day when she has energy so

---

Q. I'm really uncomfortable in the morning with nausea since I've been pregnant. What are some practical suggestions I can use to relieve this?

A. Medications are rarely prescribed to relieve nausea with pregnancy because they may have an effect on the fetus. Some measures you can take to reduce nausea are:

- Be aware that at least 50% of women experience nausea during pregnancy, so what you are experiencing is normal.
- Eat a few dry crackers, potato chips, toast, or a sour ball before you get out of bed in the morning.
- Eat small but frequent meals rather than large infrequent ones.
- Avoid greasy or highly seasoned food.
- Delay breakfast until nausea passes (dinner if it is evening nausea).
- Make up missed meals at some other time of the day to maintain nutrition.
- Avoid sudden movements and fatigue as these may increase or cause nausea.
- Eat a snack before bedtime so delaying breakfast won't cause you to go a long time between meals.

- If adventurous, try a wrist acupressure band (purchased in travel stores for motion sickness).

If nausea is present:

- Try sipping a carbonated beverage, water, or an herbal noncafffeinated tea.
- Try a walk outside in the fresh air.

Q. How do I judge if the amount of nausea I'm having is beyond the usual amount?

A. Nausea would be greater than normal if:

- If you are losing weight rather than gaining it.
- You have not gained the projected amount of weight for your week of pregnancy.
- You are unable to make up for lost meals some other time of the day.
- You have signs of dehydration such as little urine output.
- Nausea has lasted past 12 weeks of pregnancy.
- You vomit more than once daily.

---

that eating a nutritious snack later in the day when she is tired will not involve much effort.

Counseling adolescents may be difficult because they often are not responsible for cooking the food they eat. You may need to speak to parents about certain foods to prepare before you can alter an adolescent's diet pattern.

The pregnant adolescent needs a high caloric intake (2500 calories) to supply energy for her high level of activity and growth. The nutrients most often lacking from a typical adolescent diet tend to be calcium, iron, vitamin A, and total calories. Look for sources of these when analyzing teenage pregnancy intake. Advise a girl to drink fruit or vegetable drinks and decaffeinated soft drinks instead of the caffeine-rich kinds.

The Woman Over Age 35

In light of a growing tendency today for women to delay childbearing, many women are older than 35 by the time they have their first child. Many more are older than 35 years when they have their second or third child. The nutritional needs of women in this age group are poorly studied, but these women should maintain the same careful pregnancy nutrition as younger women. Because women in this age group have slightly decreased kidney function, they need to maintain a high fluid intake to re-

move waste products for themselves and for the fetus. Many women have delayed childbearing to establish a career and thus depend on packed or fast-food lunches for at least part of their nutrition each week. Nutrition counseling should focus on maintaining adequate nutrition during pregnancy, based on this lifestyle.

The Woman With Decreased Nutritional Stores

A woman with high parity or a short interval between pregnancies or who has been dieting rigorously to lose weight before pregnancy may have depleted her nutritional reserves to such an extent that she has little to draw on during the first part of pregnancy when she may not be able to eat well because of the normal nausea and vomiting of pregnancy. As many as 30% of women in low-income families enter pregnancy with anemia (DHHS, 1991). Women who used diuretics for a dieting program may be potassium deficient. Women who have been on oral contraceptives may have decreased folate stores. Women who were using intrauterine devices or who have menorrhagia may be iron deficient from excessive blood loss with menstrual flows. Women who drink alcohol excessively may be thiamine deficient. A woman who is a frequent or recent blood donor could be anemic.

Women with these decreased nutritional stores need

to be identified early in pregnancy through history taking so that specific nutrition counseling can be begun early. They may need additional supplements during pregnancy to restore a particular nutrient.

The Woman Who Is Underweight

Fashion's concentration on slim female figures makes it easy to overlook the health problem of the woman who is underweight. A woman who enters a pregnancy underweight, however, needs dietary counseling just as much as the overweight woman or the one who eats nonfood substances.

Underweight in pregnancy is defined as a state in which a woman's weight is 10% to 15% less than ideal weight for height, or she has a body mass index of less than 19.8 (Suitor et al., 1993). Being underweight usually occurs because of a long-standing poor nutritional pattern, or it may signify underlying disease. Most women who are underweight have an accompanying iron deficiency anemia, reduced resistance to disease, and tire easily. They have a higher than usual incidence of low-birth-weight infants (Kim et al., 1992).

Being underweight can occur because of poverty and the inability to buy adequate food, although many poor women are obese, not underweight, because high-starch foods are cheaper to purchase than those that have a higher protein content such as meat and eggs. Being underweight may occur due to excessive worry or stress, emotions that can lead to a loss of appetite. It may be due to depression that causes a chronic loss of appetite. It may be present as a symptom of anorexia nervosa or bulimia, conditions in which the woman has developed a revulsion to food (see Chapter 54). The major reason for being underweight, however, is insufficient intake of food due to chronic poor nutrition habits.

Nutrition counseling with underweight women, therefore, may not be easy because the woman is being asked to change lifelong eating habits. Counseling produces an extreme challenge during the first trimester of pregnancy, when fetal need is greatest; at a time when she has nausea and vomiting and has lost all desire to eat, it is crucial that a woman does eat.

Begin counseling by asking the woman for a 24-hour dietary recall. If only asked if she eats well, she will usually say that she does (it seems adequate to her because it is her usual pattern).

Total daily caloric intake for the underweight woman may need to be 3500 calories (500 to 1000 calories more than the usual specified daily amount). Working out well-planned meals rather than depending on quick take-out foods is generally helpful in accomplishing this. Additional calories might be added in the form of a concentrated formula such as an instant liquid breakfast drink. Be certain the woman understands this should not be a high-protein drink devised for high-protein dieting regimes. Such diet drinks deliver a con-

centrated solute load (breakdown products of protein) to the kidney (already working to capacity because of the pregnancy) and provide so little carbohydrate in proportion to protein that they encourage the breakdown of protein for body energy, a process that results in acidosis. High-protein diets of this nature are not recommended for long-term use by any individual; they should be totally avoided by women during pregnancy.

A 500-calorie increase over normal calorie requirements should result in a weight gain of an additional pound per week. Be certain when the total weight gain during pregnancy is calculated at each office visit that this additional pound per week is planned for, or the total weight gain of the woman may seem excessive when it is actually healthy.

If being underweight is making the woman feel tired, she needs to be urged to schedule adequate rest periods daily so that she can feel sufficiently energetic to prepare nutritious meals. She should be assessed for iron deficiency anemia and treated if necessary. She may need additional nutrition counseling in the postpartal period so that she can maintain better nutrition throughout her life and can enter a subsequent pregnancy (if there is one) in a state of nutritional health. Even when underweight women gain excessive weight during pregnancy, they still tend to have a higher than usual incidence of low-birth-weight infants, probably because of depleted nutrient stores at the pregnancy's beginning. This is one reason that preconceptual health care visits are important.

The Woman Who Is Overweight

A woman is considered **overweight** during pregnancy if she is 20% above ideal weight or has a body mass index over 26.1 (Suitor et al., 1993). She is considered **obese** if her weight is more than 200 pounds, she is 50% above ideal body weight for height, or her BMI is above 29. Although obesity may occur from hypothyroidism, it most often occurs as a result of excessive caloric intake and decreased energy expenditure.

Obesity is a serious problem among women in the United States (approximately 10% of pregnant women are overweight). Women with less education and who live in poverty tend to be more overweight than others because they may not be so aware of the comparative levels of carbohydrates in foods and because many starchy foods (e.g., macaroni or spaghetti) are cheaper than less caloric but more nutritious foods such as meat and cheese. Native Americans have an exceptionally high ratio of obesity (Botash et al., 1992).

Obesity becomes a problem during pregnancy because as the woman's circulatory volume increases 20% to 50% and her metabolism increases to meet the demands of the pregnancy, this can put additional stress on a possibly already overworked body. The incidence of gestational diabetes is increased in such women; they are also at high risk to develop hypertension of pregnancy. It is often difficult to hear fetal heart tones in an obese woman; palpating for position and size of the fetus is difficult. Obese women are also more apt to have infants with *macrosomia* (large for gestational age), which increases the incidence of cesarean births in this population (Larsen et al., 1990). Yet another problem in obese women is that their pregnancies are more apt to be prolonged, leading to postmature infants. If a cesarean birth is needed at delivery, it is difficult to perform because of the excessive adipose tissue that must be cut to reach the uterus. Ambulating during pregnancy and immediately afterward is more difficult because of the increased energy expenditure necessary; thus, thrombophlebitis and complications such as pneumonia tend to occur more frequently.

Nutrition counseling with obese women during pregnancy may be difficult because overeating has many causes. For some women, overeating is a coping mechanism for stress; whenever they feel tense or worried, they have something "comforting" to eat. Because pregnancy is stressful, it may be difficult for a woman to change food intake patterns at this time. Other women overeat because their parents did and they were raised to consume a diet overly rich in calories. Changing this pattern means changing a lifelong habit. If the woman's family also enjoys an excessive intake of calories, then the entire family may have to change their eating patterns to effect a change in the woman's intake.

Dieting to reduce weight is not recommended during pregnancy, however, because if carbohydrates are reduced too much, the body will use protein and fat for energy. This can deprive the fetus of protein and can lead to ketoacidosis in the woman. Although the long-term effects of mild ketoacidosis are not well studied (Rizzo et al., 1990), it can be avoided if the pregnancy diet, even in the most obese women, does not go below 1500 to 1800 calories.

Overweight women tend to exercise less than women of normal weight (exercising is more awkward and more tiring, and they may feel self-conscious dressed in sports clothing). Try to encourage them to engage in at least a minimum activity program such as walking around the block once a day in addition to a high-protein diet.

Helping a woman look at her diet in terms of empty-calorie versus nutritious-calorie foods may help her to eat more sensibly. Early in pregnancy when she is eager to appear pregnant, she may be resistant to any limitation of intake. She needs to understand that a fetus grows best on nutritious foods, not necessarily those with the most calories. She may need additional nutrition counseling in the postpartal period so she can prepare more nutritious meals in the future for herself and her growing family and so she will not enter another pregnancy severely overweight.

The Woman Who Is a Vegetarian

Most women who practice vegetarianism are knowledgeable about their diets and able to discuss what foods are high in various nutrients and how they incorporate such foods in their diet. They can be a helpful source of nutrition information. There are many different types of vegetarian diets (see Chapter 34). Special concerns for a pregnant woman on this diet include lack of vitamin B_{12} (meat is the chief source of B_{12}), and an inadequate intake of calcium (recommend dark green vegetables as sources) and vitamin D (fortified milk and sunlight are the main sources of vitamin D).

The Woman With Phenylketonuria

Phenylketonuria (PKU) is an inherited disorder in which a person is unable to convert the essential amino acid phenylalanine into tyrosine, the form in which it is used for cell growth. Without this conversion, the raw phenylalanine builds up in the person's serum and eventually leaves the bloodstream to invade body cells. When it invades brain cells, it leaves severe mental retardation and accompanying neurologic damage such as recurrent seizures (see Chapter 48).

Children with PKU stay on a restricted phenylalanine diet until they are past adolescence. A woman with PKU (named because the breakdown product of phenylalanine is excreted in the urine in this form) should consult her internist when she is planning on becoming pregnant and plan to return to a low phenylalanine diet for at least 3 months before she becomes pregnant. Foods low in phenylalanine include orange juice, bananas, squash, spinach, and peas. The woman follows this diet until she becomes pregnant and during the pregnancy; if she should breast-feed, then she follows this diet during this time also (Peng, 1993).

The woman with PKU needs support during pregnancy to follow such a restrictive diet. It is particularly disappointing for her if she does not become pregnant immediately after starting the diet, because each month that she is "prepregnant" extends the period she must follow the diet. A woman with PKU is usually well informed about her dietary needs. She is aware that phenylalanine is destructive to developing brain cells and that not following her prescribed diet could leave her future child mentally retarded.

The Woman With a Multiple Pregnancy

The woman carrying twins gains more weight overall (an average of 32.1 pounds in the twin pregnancy versus 24.5 pounds in the single pregnancy) and with greater speed than the woman carrying a single child (Garcia & Gall, 1990). Despite this increased weight gain, the energy and protein intake for the woman with a multiple pregnancy is the same as that for the single pregnancy. However, an increased burden is placed on maternal iron and folic acid stores. It is important that multiple pregnancy be recognized early and dietary supplements be added as needed.

The Woman Who Smokes or Uses Drugs or Alcohol

The specific effects of alcohol, cigarette smoking, and drug use on fetal growth are discussed in Chapter 11. In addition to specific teratogenic fetal effects, these substances can lead to general nutrition problems because the woman is ingesting these substances rather than nutritious foods (Armstrong et al., 1992).

The Woman With Concurrent Medical Problems

Any medical condition that requires rigid salt, protein, or carbohydrate restriction poses a potential fetal nourishment problem during pregnancy. Women who have medical problems such as kidney disease, diabetes, tuberculosis, bulimia, or anorexia nervosa need special dietary considerations during pregnancy because of the specific metabolic disorders that can occur with these diseases. Nursing interventions and nutrition concerns for women with medical problems such as these are discussed in Chapters 15 and 17.

The Woman Who Eats Many Fast-Food Meals

As many as 80% of women of childbearing age work at least part-time outside their homes (Calhoun & Light, 1993). This means that nutrition counseling must involve helping the woman who relies on a packed lunch or fast food to maintain adequate pregnancy nutrition. The difficulty with using fast-food restaurants is the limited choice of food available (the woman may grow tired of the same thing and thus eat little) and, unless there is a salad bar, there is apt to be a limited menu of fruits and vegetables. Fast-food restaurants have also been associated with outbreaks of infection due to undercooked hamburger. This could lead to severe gastrointestinal symptoms such as vomiting and diarrhea and possible electrolyte imbalance.

A packed lunch lends few problems in pregnancy as long as the woman uses some degree of creativity in preparation so she does not grow so tired of packed lunches that she reduces her noon intake. Packing a lunch at bedtime rather than in the morning when she possibly feels nauseous (and therefore packs little because nothing looks good) is a good recommendation early in pregnancy. Late in pregnancy, a woman may feel too tired at bedtime to do this and should change to preparing it in the morning when she has more energy. Including a thermos with a cream soup is a good way to add milk and calcium to the diet. A woman should avoid using lunch meat daily because it tends to be high in salt. Packing carrot sticks or sliced cucumbers, tomatoes, or apples not only makes the lunch nutritious but provides for midmorning or midafternoon snacks as well, so that the woman does not go long stretches of time without eating.

The Woman With Lactose Intolerance

The sugar in milk is lactose. In the intestine, lactose is broken down into glucose and galactose by the enzyme **lactase**. In most of the world's population, lactase is present in infants but disappears by school age. After this point, many people have difficulty digesting lactose or are *lactose intolerant*. African Americans, Native Americans, and Asians tend to have the highest percentage of lactose intolerance (approximately 70% of African American adults cannot drink milk). Those most able to tolerate milk are North Europeans and their descendants.

When people who are lactose intolerant drink milk, they report symptoms of nausea, diarrhea, cramps, gas, and a general feeling of bloatedness. Some express these symptoms as simply, "I don't like milk."

Women who cannot drink milk may be able to eat cheese because the processing of cheese changes the lactose content; yogurt may also be tolerable. Fortified soy milk can also be substituted. Women can be prescribed lactase tablets to chew before ingesting milk products. Even with this, they may need a calcium supplement (1200 mg daily) and a vitamin D supplement (400 IU) because the amount of cheese or yogurt that would need to be eaten to replace the calcium of milk would be too great to be practical. Because milk is a good source of protein, it is important to take a thorough diet history to assess whether, without milk, the woman is also taking in enough protein.

Many baby magazines, television advertisements, and government pamphlets on pregnancy mention repeatedly that it is important to drink milk during pregnancy, so it may be necessary to spend time reassuring women who cannot drink milk that it really is unnecessary as long as they ingest the same nutrients from other foods.

The Woman With Hyperemesis Gravidarum

Hyperemesis gravidarum (sometimes called pernicious vomiting) is nausea and vomiting of pregnancy that is prolonged past week 12 of pregnancy or is so severe that dehydration, ketonuria, and significant weight loss occur within the first 12 weeks. Women with the disorder tend to have increased thyroid function due to thyroid-stimulating properties of HCG hormone (Lazarus, 1993). It occurs at an incidence of 1 in 200 to 300 women (Varner, 1990).

Assessment. A woman with normal nausea and vomiting of pregnancy usually notices nausea for only part of the day, so is able to maintain nutrition even without therapy such as an antiemetic.

With hyperemesis gravidarum, the woman's symptoms are so severe that she is unable to maintain nutrition. She may show an elevated hematocrit concentration at her monthly prenatal visit, not because her hemoglobin level is so high, but because her inability to retain fluid has resulted in hemoconcentration. Concentrations of sodium, potassium, and chloride may be reduced, and hypokalemic alkalosis may result if vomiting is severe during the day or persists for an extended period. In some women, polyneuritis, due to a deficiency of vitamin B, develops. She may be losing weight. Her urine may test positive for ketones, evidence that her body is breaking down stored fat and protein for cell growth. The condition is not associated with spontaneous abortion but is associated with intrauterine growth retardation.

Ask women at prenatal visits whether they are having nausea and vomiting. Determine exactly how much. Ask a woman to describe the events of the day before if she says it was a typical day. How late into the day did the nausea last? How many times did she vomit? What was the total amount of food she ate?

The biggest danger with pernicious vomiting is that the woman will become dehydrated and no longer be able to provide the fetus with essential nutrients for growth. Prolonged hospitalization with this disorder may result in social isolation.

Therapeutic Management. The woman usually needs to be hospitalized so that her intake, output, and blood chemistries can be monitored and dehydration prevented.

During the first 24 hours of the hospital admission, no food and fluid are allowed by mouth. The woman should receive approximately 3000 mL of an intravenous solution such as Ringer's lactate with added vitamin B. A sedative such as phenobarbital may be ordered to encourage rest, and an antiemetic may be prescribed such as chlorpromazine. Measure intake and output, including the amount of vomitus.

Visitors may be excluded for the first 24 hours or until the vomiting has ceased. If there is no vomiting after this time, small amounts of clear fluid may be begun. If this is tolerated, small quantities of dry toast, crackers, or cereal are given every 2 or 3 hours. If no vomiting occurs, the woman is gradually advanced to a soft diet, then to a normal diet. If these measures are ineffective, total parenteral nutrition (hyperalimentation) may be attempted (Charlin et al., 1993). Women can be discharged home on this therapy.

Nursing Diagnoses and Related Interventions

If stress is a possible factor in the development of hyperemesis gravidarum, a relevant nursing diagnosis may be "Ineffective individual coping related to stress of pregnancy or concurrent life events." Be certain that goals established are realistic in relation to the basic problem. It may not be possible to stop vomiting completely, but enough supplemental fluid to counteract the loss of fluid with vomiting can be supplied.

Nursing Diagnosis: High risk for fluid volume deficit related to vomiting secondary to hyperemesis gravidarum.

Goal: Client will regain adequate hydration for her own and the baby's needs.

Outcome Criteria: Client demonstrates no signs and symptoms of dehydration (i.e., poor skin turgor or dry skin or mucous membranes). Urine output is greater than 30 mL/h; SG is 1.003–1.030.

Like the normal nausea and vomiting of pregnancy, hyperemesis gravidarum is precipitated by fatigue and the smell of cooking. The portions of food served should be small, so that the amount does not appear overwhelming. Food should be prepared attractively. Hot foods should be hot and cold foods cold.

Although an emesis basin is an important piece of equipment for the womann who is vomiting, put it out of sight and not on the bedside table so that she is not constantly reminded of vomiting. Be sure that food carts smelling of food such as fish, bacon, or coffee are not parked outside her door at mealtimes.

Nursing Diagnosis: Altered nutrition, less than body requirements, related to prolonged vomiting.

Goal: Client will ingest orally or intravenously enough nutrients to sustain herself and growing fetus for remainder of pregnancy.

Outcome Criteria: Client takes in at least 2500 calories daily.

A number of women have such extreme symptoms that vomiting recurs with the introduction of food. To maintain adequate nutrition to support fetal growth, the woman may need to be maintained on total parenteral nutrition or enteral feedings. Women may remain on home care during this time. They should assess a urine sample twice daily for glucose and ketones. If there is glucose in the urine, this suggests that the infusion solution contains more glucose than the body's metabolism can use. Ketones in the urine mean that the body is not receiving enough nutrients and it is breaking down cells.

A woman with hyperemesis gravidarum needs the

opportunity to express how she feels about the strange thing that is happening to her. She needs to talk about how it feels to be pregnant and to live with the ever-present nausea. In some women, so many psychosocial factors are involved that counseling is required to help them decide whether to terminate the pregnancy or allow it to go to completion.

Key Points

- Pregnant women should increase intake of calories, protein, and certain vitamins and minerals during pregnancy to help ensure fetal growth.
- Nutrition during pregnancy should be high in calories to provide for protein sparing and high in protein for fetal growth requirements.
- Important minerals necessary for pregnancy are iron, iodine, calcium, fluoride, sodium, and zinc. Most women need to take an iron supplement to supply enough of this mineral to prevent iron deficiency anemia.
- Women should reduce caffeine and artificial sweeteners during pregnancy.
- Assessment of nutritional health consists of a health history (24-hour recall) as well as a physical examination.
- Women who are at high risk for nutrition problems are those who are adolescent or over age 35; have decreased nutrition stores; are carrying a multiple pregnancy; are lactose intolerant; are underweight or overweight; are on a special diet; use drugs, including alcohol or cigarettes; or develop hyperemesis gravidarum (extreme nausea and vomiting).
- Hyperemesis gravidarum is nausea and vomiting of pregnancy that extends past 12 weeks of pregnancy or is too extreme to allow for adequate nutrition. Women with this condition may need nutrition supplemented by total parenteral nutrition or enteral feedings.
- Common nutrition concerns associated with pregnancy are nausea and vomiting, constipation, cravings (including pica), and pyrosis.
- Advise women during pregnancy not to go longer than 12 hours between meals, to avoid hypoglycemia.
- Pregnancy vitamins contain additional folic acid supplements and iron, so these should be used instead of regular vitamins during pregnancy. The vitamins should be kept from the reach of small children, as excess ingestion of these additives could result in acute poisoning. Be certain that women regard pregnancy vitamins as medication and follow the medication rule: take nothing other than medications specifically recommended by the primary care provider, or else toxicity could result.

Critical Thinking Exercises

1. Mary is a 30-year-old woman who is 2 months pregnant. She works as a cashier at a supermarket from 6 AM to 2 PM daily. She states she is too nauseous in the morning to eat before she leaves for work; she is too tired of seeing food go by her to prepare a good meal after work. Prepare a care plan for Mary that will help her increase her food intake.
2. Anita is a 21-year-old who rarely eats vegetables. When she does she fries them in butter. How would you use a food pyramid to explain better pregnancy nutrition to Anita?
3. Chris is a 19-year-old college student. The food plan she subscribes to provides for only lunch and dinner and these must be obtained from the college cafeteria. What suggestions could you make to Chris to be certain she obtains adequate nutrition during pregnancy?

References

Armstrong, B. G., et al. (1992). Cigarette, alcohol and coffee consumption and spontaneous abortion. *American Journal of Public Health, 82,* 85.

Botash, A. S., et al. (1992). Cardiovascular risk factors in Native American children. *New York State Journal of Medicine, 92,* 378.

Buescher, P. A. (1993). Prenatal WIC participation can reduce low birth weight and newborn medical costs. *Journal of the American Dietetic Association, 93,* 163.

Calhoun, C., & Light, D. (1993). *Sociology* (6th ed.). New York: McGraw.

Charlin, V., et al. (1993). Parenteral nutrition in hyperemesis gravidarum. *Nutrition, 9,* 29.

Chez, R. A. (1991). Advising pregnant women about nutrition. *Contemporary Obstetrics and Gynecology, 36,* 80.

DeAloysio, D. & Penacchioni, P. (1993). Morning sickness control in early pregnancy by Neiguan point acupressure. *Obstetrics & Gynecology, 80,* 852.

Department of Health and Human Services. (1991). *Healthy people 2000.* Washington, DC: Public Health Service.

DiIorio, C., van Lier, D., & Manteuffel, B. (1992). Patterns of nausea during first trimester of pregnancy. *Clinical Nursing Research, 1,* 127.

Garcia, P. M., & Gall, S. A. (1990). Multiple pregnancy. In J. R. Scott et al., *Danforth's obstetrics and gynecology.* Philadelphia: J.B. Lippincott.

Giotta, M. P. (1993). Nutrition during pregnancy: Reducing obstetric risk. *Journal of Perinatology and Neonatal Nursing, 6,* 1.

Herron, D. G. (1991). Strategies for promoting a healthy dietary intake. *Nursing Clinics of North America, 26,* 875.

Horner, R. D., et al. (1991). Pica practices of pregnant women. *Journal of the American Dietetic Association, 91,* 34.

Kahler, L. R., et al. (1992). Factors associated with rates of participation in WIC by eligible pregnant women. *Public Health Report, 107,* 60.

Kim, I., et al. (1992). Pregnancy nutrition surveillance system. *Mortality & Morbidity Weekly Report, 41,* 25.

Kizer, K. W., et al. (1990). Vitamin A—a pregnancy hazard alert. *Western Journal of Medicine, 152,* 78.

Kochenour, N. K. (1990). Normal pregnancy and prenatal care. In J.R. Scott et al., *Danforth's obstetrics and gynecology.* Philadelphia: J.B. Lippincott.

Larsen, C. E., et al. (1990). Macrosomia: Influence of maternal overweight among a low-income population. *American Journal of Obstetrics and Gynecology, 162,* 490.

Lazarus, J. H. (1993). Treatment of hyper and hypothyroidism in pregnancy. *Journal of Endocrinological Investigation, 16,* 391.

Loeb, S. (1993). *Nurse's handbook of drug therapy.* Springhouse, PA: Springhouse.

McDonald, A. D., et al. (1992). Cigarette, alcohol and coffee consumption and prematurity. *American Journal of Public Health, 82,* 87.

Millis, J. L., et al. (1993). Moderate caffeine use and the risk of spontaneous abortion and intrauterine growth retardation. *Journal of the American Medical Association, 269,* 593.

Murphy, P. A. (1992). Periconceptional supplementation with folic acid: Does it prevent neural tube defects? *Journal of Nurse Midwifery, 37,* 25.

Newman, V., & Fullerton, J. T. (1990). Role of nutrition in the prevention of preeclampsia: Review of the literature. *Journal of Nurse Midwifery, 35,* 282.

Newman, V., Fullerton, J. T., & Anderson, P. O. (1993). Clinical advances in the management of severe nausea and vomiting during pregnancy. *Journal of Obstetric, Gynecologic, and Neonatal Nursing, 22,* 483.

Niebyl, J. (1990). Teratology and drugs in pregnancy and lactation. In J. R. Scott, et al. *Danforth's obstetrics and gynecology.* Philadelphia: J. B. Lippincott.

Olson, C. M. (1994). Promoting positive nutritional practices during pregnancy and lactation. *American Journal of Clinical Nutrition, 59,* 525S.

Parham, E. S., Astrom, M. F., & King, S. H. (1990). The association of pregnancy weight gain with the mother's postpartum weight. *Journal of the American Dietetic Association, 90,* 550.

Peng, T. C. (1993). Maternal disease and injury in pregnancy. *Current Opinion in Obstetrics & Gynecology, 5,* 3.

Rizzo, T., et al. (1990). Correlations between antepartum maternal metabolism and newborn behavior. *American Journal of Obstetrics and Gynecology, 163,* 1458.

Scholl, T. O., et al. (1993). Low zinc intake during pregnancy: Its association with preterm and very preterm delivery. *American Journal of Epidemiology, 127,* 1115.

Scholl, T. O., & Hediger, M. L. (1993). A review of the epidemiology of nutrition and adolescent pregnancy: Maternal growth during pregnancy and its effect on the fetus. *Journal of the American College of Nutrition, 12,* 101.

Scott, L. D. (1992). Gallstone disease and pancreatitis in pregnancy. *Gastroenterology Clinics of North America, 21,* 803.

Suitor, C. W., et al. (1993). Nutrition care during pregnancy and lactation: New guidelines from the Institute of Medicine. *Journal of the American Dietetic Association, 93,* 478.

Swonger, A. K., & Matejski, M. P. (1991). *Nursing pharmacology: An integrated approach to drug therapy and nursing practice.* Philadelphia: J.B. Lippincott.

Varner, M. (1990). General medical and surgical diseases in pregnancy. In J. R. Scott et al., *Danforth's obstetrics and gynecology.* Philadelphia: J.B. Lippincott.

Suggested Readings

Brown, D. (1992). All pregnant women need prenatal care. *RN, 55,* 88.

Carruth, B. R., & Skinner, J. D. (1991). Practitioners beware: Regional differences in beliefs about nutrition during pregnancy. *Journal of the American Dietetic Association, 91,* 435.

Clark, N. (1992). Shower your baby with good nutrition. *Physician and Sportsmedicine, 20,* 39.

Forsythe, H. E., & Gage, B. (1994). Use of a multicultural food-frequency questionnaire with pregnant and lactating women. *American Journal of Clinical Nutrition, 59,* 203S.

Heins, H. C., et al. (1990). A randomized trial of nurse-midwifery prenatal care to reduce low birth weight. *Obstetrics and Gynecology, 75,* 341.

Koch, R., et al. (1993). The effect of nutrient intake on pregnancy outcome in maternal phenylketonuria. *Annals of the New York Academy of Sciences, 678,* 348.

Lacey, E. P. (1990). Broadening the perspective of pica: Literature review. *Public Health Report, 105,* 29.

McElroy, D. (1992). Nutritional and medical concerns: Bizarre food cravings and aversions. *International Journal of Childbirth Education, 7,* 7.

Pietz, C. L. (1991). Weight gain and nutritional supplement during pregnancy; An updated view. *International Journal of Childbirth Education, 6,* 7.

Schneck, M. E., et al. (1990). Low-income pregnant adolescents and their infants: Dietary findings and health outcomes. *Journal of American Dietetic Association, 90,* 555.

Thompson, J. (1993). Nutrition in pregnancy. *Nursing Times, 89,* 38.

Vogt, C. (1991). Iron requirements of pregnancy. *NAACOG's Clinical Issues in Perinatal and Women's Health Nursing, 2,* 364.

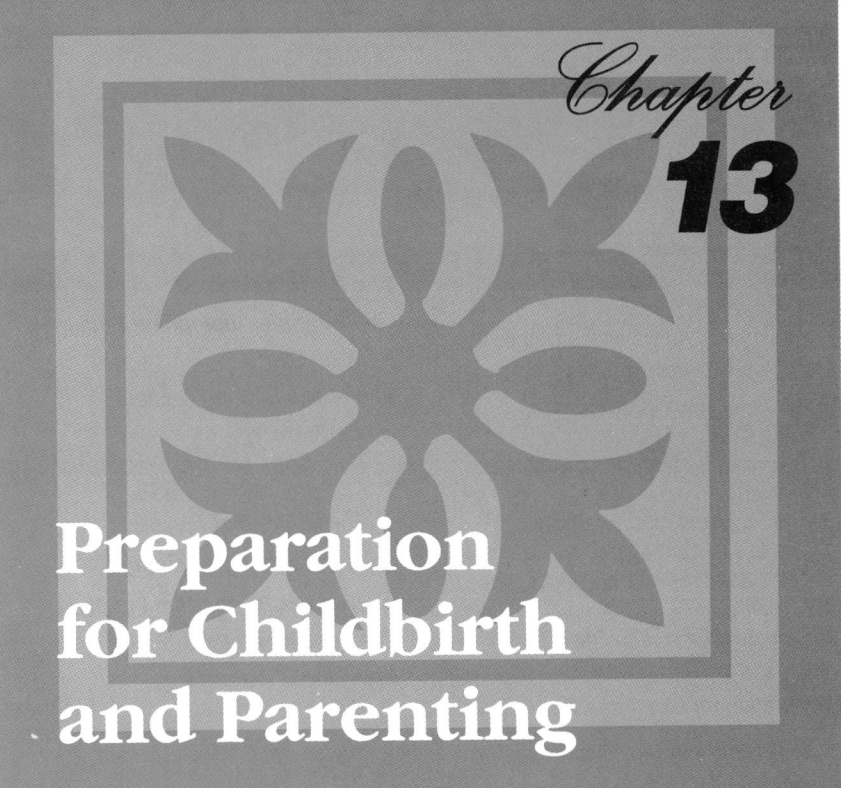

Chapter 13

Preparation for Childbirth and Parenting

Objectives

After mastering the contents of this chapter, you should be able to:

1. Describe common alternative settings for birth and preparation necessary for childbirth and parenting.

2. Assess a couple for readiness for childbirth in regard to choice of birth attendant, preparation for labor, and setting.

3. Formulate nursing diagnoses related to preparation for childbirth.

4. Plan nursing care such as teaching exercises that are effective for strengthening abdominal and perineal muscles for childbirth.

5. Implement nursing care such as supporting a woman during labor by the Lamaze (psychoprophylactic) method of prepared childbirth or helping a couple select and prepare for an alternative birth setting such as the home.

6. Evaluate outcome criteria to be certain that goals of nursing care were achieved.

7. Identify National Health Goals related to preparation for parenthood that nurses could be instrumental in helping the nation to achieve.

8. Identify areas related to preparation for childbirth that could benefit from additional nursing research.

9. Use critical thinking to analyze ways that birth can be made more family centered through the use of expectant parents' prepared childbirth classes and alternative birth settings.

10. Synthesize the principles of prepared childbirth with nursing process to achieve quality maternal and child health nursing care.

Adele Pillitteri: MATERNAL AND CHILD HEALTH NURSING, 2nd Edition. © 1995 Adele Pillitteri.

As active consumers of health care, expectant families are faced with a wide array of choices about a childbirth experience and preparation for parenting. Two of the most important decisions they need to make involve choice of birth attendant and setting. Families may choose, for example, to have a nurse-midwife present for an at-home delivery, or they may elect to have their baby born in a hospital setting with their family doctor, obstetrician, or nurse-midwife attending. Birthing centers and birthing rooms within hospitals provide environments for families who desire a childbirth experience that is also relaxed and "family centered." These options within hospitals appeal to many expectant families because they offer some of the "homeyness" of a nontechnical setting with all the medical resources a hospital can offer should any complication arise during the birth or early postpartal period.

No matter what setting a woman or couple chooses, expectant parents need to be prepared for childbirth itself. Childbirth preparation courses help prepare expectant couples for the physical and emotional rigors of childbirth and teach nonmedication methods of pain relief during labor. Courses are individualized to meet parents' needs and may be divided into classes for women with special needs such as adolescents or women over 35 (Predmore, 1992; Raymond, 1992). Also available are classes to help prepare siblings and classes for grandparents to learn more about their role. Women having a **vaginal birth after a cesarean birth** (VBAC) or women who know they will need a cesarean birth also can attend specially designed classes (Tighe et al., 1990; Crawford, 1992). In some communities, classes are offered at work sites (MacLachian & Merkel, 1990). Classes offered at work sites benefit the employer as much as the employee because prenatal care and guidance is correlated with healthier pregnancy outcome and fewer lost work days. Women hospitalized for high risk pregnancy care and disabled women are special groups who can benefit from childbirth preparation classes. Classes for adolescents can be offered in schools (Wood, 1992).

Although parenting is unarguably the most important of occupations, it is one of the few that requires no formal education, no examination to test a person's ability to take on such a role, and no refresher course to ensure that a parent is following healthy standards of child-rearing. Encouraging preparation is a nursing role because educating families about both childbirth and parenting is important in making childbirth a satisfying experience, helping a family bond to its new member, and promoting wellness behaviors that could last throughout the family's life cycle. National Health Goals related to preparation for parenting are shown in the Focus on National Health Goals box.

 ### NURSING PROCESS OVERVIEW
for Childbirth and Parenting Education

ASSESSMENT

Some couples have a clear idea of where and how they wish their child's birth to occur. Others may not even be able to think about the actual birth until they are better adjusted to the idea of pregnancy. Assessing each woman or couple's readiness for decision making as well as providing information early in the process helps the woman or couple make this kind of decision. For couples who have chosen what may be considered an "alternative birthing option" such as home delivery, it is important that they understand both the physical and emotional requirements of such a choice. In addition, it is important to ask each pregnant client whether she is primipara or grand multipara, and whether she would be interested in participating in a course aimed at preparing her and her support person for childbirth or parenting, so she can gain access to this information as needed.

 ### FOCUS ON
National Health Goals

Preparation for childbirth classes supply information not only on how to prepare for childbirth but also on how to parent. A number of National Health Goals speak to the importance of monitoring health in young children:

- Increase to at least 90% the proportion of babies aged 18 months and younger who receive recommended primary care services at the appropriate intervals.

- Increase to at least 75% the proportion of mothers who breastfeed their babies in the early postpartum period.

- Reduce to no more than 20% the proportion of children aged 6 and younger who are regularly exposed to tobacco smoke at home (DHHS, 1991).

Nurses actively participate as instructors in preparation for childbirth and parenting classes and teach these measures. Nursing research that addresses such issues as how best to teach parents the importance of breastfeeding and early immunization and the importance of stopping smoking is needed in order for the nation to reach these goals.

NURSING DIAGNOSIS

A typical nursing diagnosis for this area of nursing care is:

- Health-seeking behaviors related to a lack of information about childbirth and newborn care

If there is a lack of support people, diagnoses that would apply are:

- Ineffective coping related to lack of support people
- Anxiety related to absence of significant others

For the couple who cannot make a decision about childbirth setting, an appropriate diagnosis would be:

- Decisional conflict related to lack of information regarding advantages and disadvantages of childbirth settings

If there are older children in the family, a nursing diagnosis might be:

- Anxiety related to role in pending birth event, and ability to welcome a sibling

PLANNING

Be certain when planning with couples for labor and birth that the goals they set are realistic and flexible. Not all women want to go through labor without any analgesia, but most would like to participate as fully as possible. Some women may be reluctant to attend a childbirth preparation course because they fear that would mean committing themselves to a medication-free birth. They can be assured that learning about "natural childbirth" methods does not preclude also learning about what medications are available for pain relief and using those medications if desired. At the same time a couple is planning goals for childbirth, it is best to encourage them to be flexible in expectations for themselves. A woman who has decided ahead of time that she absolutely will not take any medication during labor and birth may find the intensity or duration of labor to be so severe that she will need an analgesic or epidural block to make the experience tolerable. If she and her support person have made the goal of medication-free labor too strict, this may make them feel they have failed when medication becomes necessary.

Finally, it is important to establish with the woman or couple that the ultimate goal of childbirth is a healthy baby and healthy parents. This will prevent them from concentrating on limited goals such as not having fetal monitoring or a particular birthing position and concentrate instead on doing whatever is required to make the birth safest for both them and the baby.

The following organizations are helpful referral sources for couples:

Maternity Center Association
48 E. 92nd Street
New York, NY 10128

American Society for Psychoprophylaxis
in Obstetrics (ASPO)
1101 Connecticut Avenue, NW, Suite 700
Washington, DC 20036

National Association of Parents and Professionals
for Safe Alternatives in Childbirth (NAPSAC)
Route #1, Box 646
Marble Hill, MD 63764-9725

La Leche League International
9616 Minneapolis Avenue
P.O. Box 1209
Franklin Park, IL 60131

IMPLEMENTATION

Nurses play vital roles in preparing parents for childbirth. It is important to provide a woman and her partner with information on the benefits and drawbacks of birth setting options, without influencing them in a particular direction. With referral to a childbirth preparation course, many questions about different settings can be answered in a sympathetic group setting, where feelings and anxieties can be shared as well. Being familiar with the content of courses in the community helps the nurse be certain that the courses advocated present adequate and accurate information.

Be certain to review the arrangements the woman needs to make for labor and birth at a midpoint in pregnancy. No matter how calm a woman seems when discussing these details, many women have some fear that at the last minute they will forget what they need to do when labor begins. In addition, the woman should be encouraged to work out arrangements for transportation to the hospital or birthing center and to arrange for child care if she has other children at home. The woman who anticipates a home birth must organize her home and purchase supplies well in advance of her expected due date.

EVALUATION

Evaluation of whether goals for childbirth education have been achieved should be carried out during the last few prenatal visits. By the last trimester, the woman or couple should know where the baby will be born, and should have worked out transportation and child-care details. Women who will be coached through childbirth by their husbands or another support person

should be encouraged to continue practicing breathing and relaxation techniques together up to the time of birth so they do not lose these skills.

Examples of outcome criteria related to this are:

- Couple states they feel prepared for childbirth.
- Client states she feels confident she can use breathing exercises to get through contractions as long as 70 seconds.
- Sibling states she is ready to welcome a new brother or sister into family.

The Childbirth Plan

Key among the decisions a couple must make during pregnancy is choice of setting and birth attendant. The expectant woman and her partner should also think about other issues such as the extent of family participation they wish during labor, specific labor procedures, birthing positions, medication options, plans for the immediate postbirth and baby care, and the postpartum stay and family visitation. Examples of some suggestions for a woman and her partner to ask in planning these specific childbirth details are shown in the Focus on Family Teaching box.

Birth planning is usually part of the curriculum for childbirth education classes. The group setting may be the best way for couples to sort out their questions and feelings about how best to plan for a healthy and enjoyable birth. It is important for couples to make decisions concerning these issues before the day of birth, or else decisions could be determined by agency policy or the circumstances of the moment, without the couple's input. If the expectant family has a strong desire in a certain area, planning ahead will allow them to communicate this so their particular wish can be accommodated if possible. Be certain all couples understand, however, that in the event of a complication of labor or birth, a certain preference may have to be modified in the interest of the mother's or baby's safety.

Childbirth Education

The overall goals of childbirth education are to prepare expectant parents emotionally and physically for childbirth while promoting wellness behaviors that can be used by parents and their families for life. Specific goals of preparation for childbirth classes are to prepare the expectant mother and her support person for the childbirth experience, make them knowledgeable consumers of obstetric care, help them reduce and manage pain with as little pharmacologic intervention as possible, and help increase their overall enjoyment of and satisfaction with the childbirth experience.

FOCUS ON FAMILY TEACHING

Q. What questions should I ask to explore whether a birth setting will be right for me?

A. Choosing a birth setting is a personal decision. Some questions you might want to ask are:

- What type of care giver will supervise my prenatal care and labor and birth? Nurse-midwife? Family doctor? Obstetrician?

- Will the same person be present at prenatal visits as for birth? Does the setting offer preparation for childbirth or childrearing classes?

- What setting can I choose from? A birthing room? An alternative birthing center? My home?

- Will I be allowed to choose a birth position? Will I have input into the amount of anesthesia used? Will administration of ophthalmic ointment for the baby be delayed? Can I begin breastfeeding immediately? Will there be nurses who are supportive and informed about breastfeeding available?

- Will the setting allow my partner to participate? Will he or she be allowed to be with me through labor and birth? Could he or she cut the cord or help deliver the baby? Can older children participate? Can I record the birth on video tape or by photograph?

- Is early discharge available? Will a follow-up home visit be included in care?

- If I should have a complication during labor or birth are there adequate supplies and personnel available for emergency care? If the baby should have a complication, is there provision for immediate emergency care or transport to a high-risk facility?

Childbirth Educators and Methods of Teaching

Childbirth educators teach expectant parents about the physical and emotional aspects of pregnancy, childbirth, and early parenthood, and present coping skills and labor support techniques. Although childbirth education is an interdisciplinary field, it has historically been associated with nursing, and nurses play a major role in designing, planning curriculum for, and teaching childbirth education courses (see the Focus on Nursing Research box). Childbirth educators usually have a professional degree in the helping professions as well as a certificate from a course specifically on childbirth education. Classes are taught in a group format; most incorporate a variety of teaching techniques such as videotapes and slides, lecture, and demonstration (especially for content on relaxation and breathing techniques). One of the most important aspects of these courses, however, is group interaction. Women and their partners enjoy the opportunity to share their fears and hopes about their pregnancy and upcoming birth with others as they learn together.

Efficacy of Childbirth Education Courses

Many studies have been done to determine just how effective childbirth courses are in reducing the pain of childbirth, shortening the length of labor, decreasing the amount of medication used, and increasing overall enjoyment of the experience. Because of the variability in courses offered, however, it is often difficult to compare

FOCUS ON NURSING RESEARCH

What Content Do Women Want Taught in Childbirth Education Classes?

For this study, 71 pregnant women (34 primiparas and 37 multiparas), 25 to 38 years of age, were asked to identify their major needs during pregnancy.

Women in their first trimester of pregnancy expressed interest in learning more about fetal development, positive and negative influences of nutrition and teratogens, and physical and psychologic changes they would experience during pregnancy. Second trimester women were more interested in labor and birth, nutrition and exercise, how to care for themselves afterward, how to combine motherhood with a career, and infant feeding and care. Third trimester women were most interested in nutrition, physical preparation, and analgesia for labor and birth, labor and birth complications, successful parenting, and how to manage infant feeding and care.

An unexpected finding of the study was that 78% of multiparous women said they did not plan to attend a childbirth education or preparation for childbirth class.

Important implications of this study are that women like information paced through pregnancy, and nurses cannot necessarily depend on childbirth education classes to be sources of information for multiparas, as the majority of these women in this study did not plan on attending childbirth education classes.

Sullivan, P. (1993). Felt learning needs of pregnant women. *Canadian Nurse, 89,* 42.

results of attending childbirth classes versus not attending classes. Each course has a different set of goals depending on the instructor and participants. In addition, it has been found that participants already have a high degree of positive motivation, which may also skew the results. Despite these difficulties with measurements, it is generally accepted that preparation courses can lead to an increase in satisfaction, reduced amount of reported pain, and increased feeling of control (MacKey, 1990).

Perineal and Abdominal Exercise

In childbirth preparation classes, women learn exercises to strengthen pelvic and abdominal muscles and make them more supple, as well as exercises to help manage discomfort in labor. Supple perineal muscles allow for ready stretching for birth; strengthened muscles more quickly revert to their normal condition and function quickly and efficiently following childbirth.

A woman may begin exercises as early in pregnancy as she likes; however, women enrolled in Lamaze prepared programs generally do not begin until the last 6 weeks of pregnancy. This time frame allows for learning the conditioned responses necessary for prepared labor closer to the time they will be used, but it limits the total amount of time directed to perineal exercises. If labor begins early, the woman may have had little or no practice with the perineal exercises.

Women should not participate in a formal exercise program without their physician's or nurse-midwife's approval. They should not attempt exercise if any of the danger signs of pregnancy appear, and they should never exercise to a point of fatigue. Common safety precautions for preparation for childbirth exercise in pregnancy are summarized in Box 13-1.

Many of these exercises described below can be incorporated into daily activities so they take little time from a woman's day. It is best, however, for the woman to set aside a specific time each day for the task; otherwise, participation is apt to be sporadic. Initially, women should do each exercise only a few times, gradually increasing the number at each session.

Tailor Sitting

All kindergarten children know how to tailor sit. Many women have to be retaught. To do this correctly, so the perineum stretches and blood supply to the lower legs is not occluded, the woman should not put one ankle on top of the other but should place one leg in front of the other (Figure 13-1). As she sits in this position, she should gently push on her knees (pushing them toward the floor) until she feels her perineum "stretch." This is a good position to use to watch television, to read, or to talk to friends. It is good to plan on sitting in this position for at least 15 minutes every day. By the end of pregnancy, the woman's perineum should be so supple

---

Box 13-1

Safety Precautions for Exercises During Pregnancy

- Never exercise to a point of fatigue.
- Always rise from the floor slowly to prevent orthostatic hypotension.
- To rise from the floor, roll over to the side first and then push up to avoid strain on the abdominal muscles.
- For leg exercises, to prevent leg cramps, never point the toes (extend the heel).
- Do not attempt exercises that hyperextend the lower back to prevent muscle strain.
- Do not hold your breath while exercising because this increases intraabdominal and intrauterine pressure.
- Do not continue with exercises if any danger signal of pregnancy occurs.
- Do not practice second-stage pushing. Pushing increases intrauterine pressure and could rupture membranes.

---

that when she tailor sits her knees will almost touch the floor if pushed to that position.

Squatting

Squatting (Figure 13-2) also stretches the perineal muscles, so a woman should also practice this position for about 15 minutes a day. Women in nonindustrial cul-

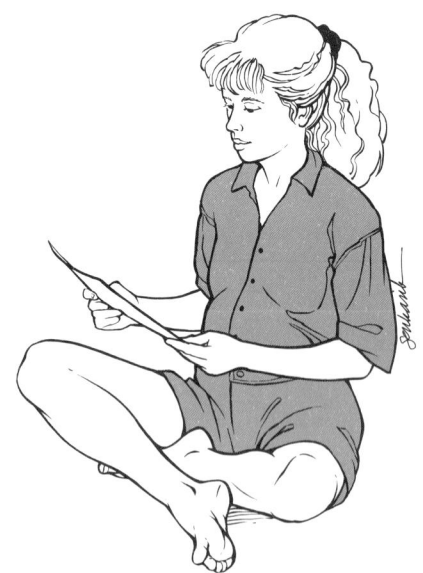

FIGURE 13-1

Tailor sitting strengthens the thighs and stretches perineal muscles. Notice that the legs are parallel so that one does not compress the other. A woman could use this position for television watching, telephone conversations, or playing with an older child.

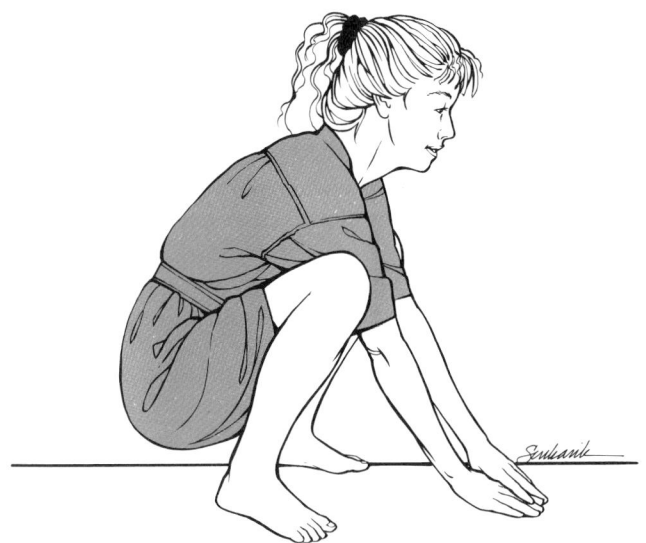

FIGURE 13-2
Squatting helps to stretch the muscles of the pelvic floor. Notice that the feet are flat on the floor for optimum stretching.

tures squat many times a day—to tend a fire, to pick up a child, to wash vegetables—but women in the United States rarely squat. Most women need a demonstration of effective squatting. Otherwise, they have a tendency to squat on tiptoes. For the pelvic muscles to stretch, the woman must keep her feet flat on the floor. Incorporating squatting into daily activities such as picking up toys from the floor reduces the amount of time a woman has to devote to daily exercises.

Pelvic Floor Contractions (Kegel Exercises)

Pelvic floor contractions can be done during the course of daily activities as well. While sitting at her desk or working around the house, the woman can tighten the muscles of the perineum by doing Kegel exercises (see Chapter 11, Box 11-3). Such perineal muscle-strengthening exercises are helpful in the postpartum period as well to promote perineal healing, to increase sexual responsiveness, and to help prevent stress incontinence.

Abdominal Muscle Contractions

Abdominal muscle contractions help strengthen abdominal muscles during pregnancy and therefore help restore abdominal tone following pregnancy. Strong abdominal muscles can also contribute to effective second-stage pushing during labor and help to prevent constipation. Abdominal contractions can be done in a standing or lying position along with pelvic floor contractions. The woman merely tightens her abdominal muscles, then relaxes, and she can repeat the exercise as often as she wishes during the day.

Another way to do the same thing is to practice "blowing out a candle." The woman takes a fairly deep inspiration, then exhales normally; then holding her fin-

ger about 6 inches in front of herself, as if it were a candle, exhales forcibly, pushing out residual air from her lungs. She can feel her abdominal muscles contract as she reaches the end of her forcible exhalation.

Pelvic Rocking

Pelvic rocking (Figure 13-3) helps relieve backache during pregnancy and early labor by making the lumbar spine more flexible. It can be done in a variety of positions: on hands and knees, lying down, sitting, or standing. The woman arches her back, trying to lengthen or stretch her spine. She holds the position for one minute, then hollows her back. A woman can do this at the end of the day about five times to relieve back pain and make herself more comfortable for the night.

Methods for Pain Management

Beginning in the late 1950s, many specific methods for nonmedication pain reduction for labor were developed. These included the Lamaze, Dick-Read, and Bradley methods, all named after the professionals who developed them. More recently, however, childbirth education has been moving away from the method approach to a more eclectic one. Much research is currently being done to verify the effectiveness of each of these many techniques, and in practice, many educators are using a variety of approaches in their courses (see the Focus on Cultural Awareness box).

Most of the methods advocated are based on three premises. The first is that discomfort during labor can be minimized if the woman comes into labor informed about what is happening and prepared with breathing exercises to use during contractions. In classes, therefore, the woman learns about what will be her body's response in labor, the mechanisms involved in childbirth, and breathing exercises she can use during labor. The second premise is that discomfort during labor can be minimized if the woman's abdomen is relaxed and the uterus is allowed to rise freely against the abdominal

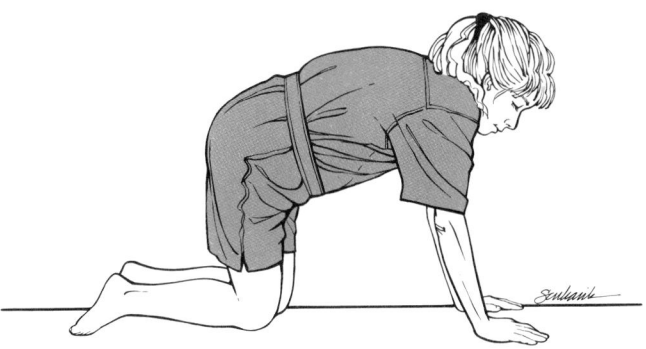

FIGURE 13-3
Pelvic rocking is helpful in relieving backache during pregnancy and labor. The woman hollows her back and then arches it.

wall with contractions. Childbirth methods differ only in the manner by which they achieve this relaxation. The third premise is that pain perception can be altered by distraction techniques or by a "gate control" theory of pain perception.

Gate Control Mechanisms

According to the gate control theory of why people experience pain, as soon as the endings of small peripheral nerve fibers detect a stimulus, they transmit it to cells in the dorsal horn of the spinal cord. Impulses pass through a dense, interfacing network of cells in the spinal cord (the substantia gelatinosa) and, immediately, a synapse occurs that returns the transmission to the peripheral site through a motor nerve (a person touches a candle flame; the impulse travels to the spinal cord and back, and the person jerks his or her hand away from the flame). Following this short-circuit synapse, the impulse then continues in the spinal cord to reach the hypothalamus and cortex of the brain. There, the impulse is interpreted (the candle is hot) and perceived as pain. Gate control mechanisms in the substantia gelatinosa are capable of halting an impulse at the level of the spinal cord so the impulse is never perceived at the brain level as pain, or a process similar to closing a gate occurs. This is the **gating theory of pain control**. Three techniques to assist gating mechanisms are: (1) cutaneous stimulation, (2) distraction, and (3) reduction of anxiety.

Cutaneous Stimulation. If large peripheral nerves next to an injury site are stimulated, the ability of the small nerve fibers at the injury site to transmit pain impulses appears to decrease. Therefore, rubbing an injured part or applying heat or cold to the site (**cuta-**

neous stimulation) are effective maneuvers to suppress pain. **Effleurage**, or light massage used in the Lamaze method, accomplishes this.

Distraction. If the cells of the brain stem that register an impulse as pain are preoccupied with other stimuli, a pain impulse cannot register. **Distraction** or imagery (having a person focus on some pattern or action) accomplishes this. Different preparation-for-childbirth classes use different breathing techniques or focusing to accomplish this.

Reduction of Anxiety. Pain impulses are perceived more quickly if anxiety is also present. Thus, the third technique of gating is to reduce patient anxiety as much as possible. Teaching a woman what to expect during labor is a means of achieving this.

The Bradley (Husband Coached) Method

The Bradley method of childbirth, originated by Robert Bradley, M.D. (1981), is based on the premise that childbirth is a joyful natural process and stresses the important role of the husband during pregnancy, labor, and the early newborn period. During pregnancy, the woman performs muscle-toning exercises and limits or omits foods that contain preservatives, animal fat, or a high salt content. Pain is reduced in labor by abdominal breathing. In addition, the woman is encouraged to walk during labor and to use an internal focus point as a disassociation technique. The Bradley method is used widely in some areas of the United States and at specific centers.

The Psychosexual Method

The psychosexual method of childbirth was developed by Sheila Kitzinger (1990) in England during the 1950s. The method stresses that pregnancy, labor and birth, and the early newborn period are important continuing points in the woman's life cycle. It includes a program of conscientious relaxation and levels of progressive breathing that encourages the woman to "flow with" rather than struggle against contractions of labor.

The Dick-Read Method

The Dick-Read (1987) method is based on the approach proposed by Grantly Dick-Read, an English physician. The premise of the method is that fear leads to tension, which leads to pain. If one can prevent this chain of events from occurring, or break the chain between fear-tension or tension-pain, then one can reduce the pain of childbirth contractions. The woman achieves relaxation and reduced pain in labor by using abdominal breathing during contractions.

The Lamaze (Psychoprophylactic) Method

The Lamaze method of prepared childbirth is the method most often taught in the United States today. It is based on the theory that through stimulus-response conditioning women can learn to use controlled breathing and therefore reduce pain sensation during labor. The method was developed in Russia based on Pavlov's conditioning studies but was popularized by a French physician, Ferdinand Lamaze. Formal classes are organized by the American Society for Psychoprophylaxis in Obstetrics or the International Childbirth Education Association, and many other classes teach variations on the Lamaze method. A popular book on the subject—*Thank you, Dr. Lamaze*—was written by Marjorie Karmel (1965) who had personally used the method. The word **psychoprophylaxis** is a combination of what is attempted by the method: preventing pain in labor (prophylaxis) by use of the mind (psyche).

Three main premises are taught in the prenatal period related to the gate control method of pain relief: (1) with relaxation, pain does not have to occur with contractions, (2) sensations such as uterine contractions can be inhibited from reaching the brain cortex and registering as pain, and (3) conditioned reflexes are a positive action to use to displace pain sensations in labor. Much time in class is spent reviewing or teaching reproductive anatomy and physiology and the process of labor and birth. Thus, the couple is familiar with what will happen to the woman in labor and with the nature of contractions and so enters labor without a great deal of unnecessary tension.

To use the second premise in labor—that sensations coming into the brain can be inhibited from registering—the woman is taught to concentrate on breathing patterns and use imagery or focusing (concentration on an alternative thought) on a specified object, blocking out other phenomena. The effectiveness of focusing can be observed in athletes who hurt themselves in basketball or football games but do not feel the pain until after the game because of their concentration on winning. A mother running to scoop her child away from danger will manifest the same inhibition phenomenon, not even aware that she has wrenched her ankle in the process of rescuing her child until the child is safe. In the past, breathing patterns taught tended to be complex; today the emphasis is on simpler patterns that can be more easily learned and practiced (Janke, 1992).

Time in class is also spent on learning **conditioned reflexes**, or reflexes which automatically occur in response to a stimulus. While conducting studies of salivation in dogs, Pavlov noticed that every time he put out food for his dogs, the dogs salivated at the mere sight of it. To learn more about this phenomenon, he tried ringing a bell each time he presented food and found that after a time the dogs salivated at the sound of the bell even when food was not offered. This is called a conditioned response. The same training technique is applied to the birth process in the Lamaze method. The woman is conditioned to relax automatically on hearing a command ("contraction beginning") or on the feel of a contraction beginning.

To use the Lamaze method, the responses to contractions must be recently conditioned to be effective (because conditioned responses fade if not reinforced). It is generally recommended, therefore, that women not begin classes in this method before week 26 of pregnancy. They then continue the classes to the end of pregnancy. Such timing corresponds nicely to that of the psychologic nestbuilding that occurs at about the same time.

A woman is required to bring a support person who will act as her coach in labor with her to class. Classes are kept small so there is time for individual instruction attention with each couple (Figure 13-4). Breathing exercises taught vary from teacher to teacher, especially

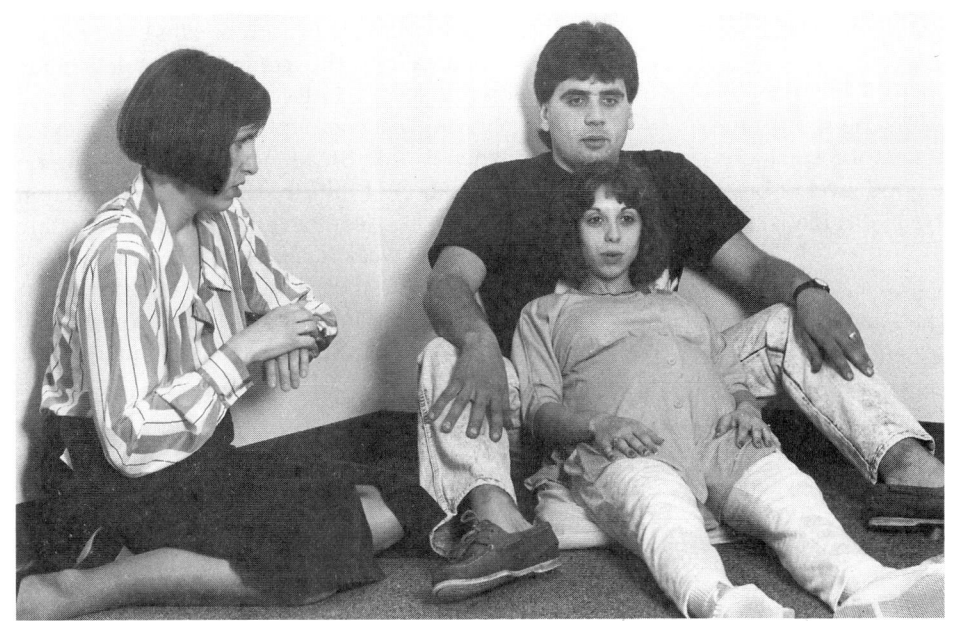

FIGURE 13-4
Every woman needs to be well prepared for birth. Here a couple practices breathing patterns in a preparation-for-childbirth class. (Courtesy of the Department of Medical Photography, Children's Hospital, Buffalo, NY.)

in terms of complexity, but have common features shown below.

Conscious Relaxation.
Conscious relaxation is learning to relax body portions deliberately so, unknowingly, the woman does not remain tense and cause unnecessary muscle strain and fatigue during labor. She practices relaxation during pregnancy by deliberately relaxing one set of muscles, then another, and another until her body is completely relaxed. A support person concentrates on noticing symptoms of tension such as a wrinkled brow, clenched fists, or a stiffly held arm. By either placing a comforting hand on the tense body area or telling the woman to relax that area, the support person helps her to achieve relaxation.

The Cleansing Breath.
To begin all breathing exercises, the woman breathes in deeply and then exhales deeply (a "**cleansing breath**"). To end each exercise, she repeats this step. It is an important step to take because it limits the possibility of hyperventilation with rapid breathing patterns; it helps ensure an adequate fetal oxygen supply.

Consciously Controlled Breathing.
Using **consciously controlled breathing**, or set breathing patterns at specific rates, prevents the diaphragm from descending fully and therefore prevents it from putting pressure on the expanding uterus. To practice, the woman inhales comfortably but fully, then exhales, with her exhalation a little stronger than her inhalation. She practices breathing in this manner at a controlled pace, depending on the intensity of contractions. Various levels of breathing are:

Level 1. Slow chest breathing at this level consists of comfortable but full respirations at a rate of 6 to 12 breaths per minute. The level is used for early contractions.

Level 2. For this level, breathing is lighter than level 1. The rib cage should expand but be so light the diaphragm barely moves. The rate of respirations is up to 40 per minute. This is a good level of breathing for contractions when cervical dilation is between 4 cm and 6 cm.

Level 3. Breathing at this level is even more shallow, mostly at the sternum. The rate is 50 to 70 breaths per minute. As the respirations become faster, the exhalation must be a little stronger than the inhalation for good air exchange and to prevent hyperventilation. If the woman practices saying "out" with each exhalation, she almost inevitably will make exhalation stronger than inhalation. The woman uses this level for transition contractions. Keeping the tip of her tongue against the roof of her mouth helps prevent oral mucosa from drying out during such rapid breathing.

Level 4. At this level, the woman uses a "pant-blow" pattern, such as taking three or four quick breaths (in and out), then a forceful exhalation. Because this type of breathing sounds like an imitation of a train (breath-breath-breath-huff), it is sometimes referred to as "choo-choo" breathing or "hee-hee-hee-hoo" breathing.

Level 5. The woman pants at this level. Chest panting is continuous, very shallow panting at about 60 breaths per minute. It can be used during strong contractions or during the second stage of labor to prevent the woman from pushing before full dilatation.

Some courses stop teaching at the point a woman has mastered the levels of breathing; others have her learn to shift from one level to the other on command, or at the point she feels a need for more pain relief. To do this, at the sound of "contraction beginning," she breathes at 12 breaths a minute; at the sound of "contraction getting harder," 40 breaths a minute; "harder still," 70 breaths a minute; and so on, imitating basic shifts she will use in labor.

A woman who can successfully perform various levels of breathing and change from one to the other on command is prepared to handle all labor contractions up to the pelvic division of labor.

Figure 13-5 illustrates the use of levels of breathing. An early labor contraction is mild. When the contraction begins, the coach says, "contraction beginning." The woman breathes at level 1; she feels no bite from the contraction and so does not need to change to a more involved breathing pattern. Later in labor, the contraction is stronger and longer. Now, at the sound of "contraction beginning," the woman begins level 1 breathing (3 breaths); shifts to level 2 (4 to 6 breaths); then shifts to level 3 (10 breaths). The contraction is lessening. She shifts down to level 2 (4 to 6 breaths), then to level 1 (3 to 4 breaths). The contraction is gone. Her coach can tell her when to shift breathing levels depending on the coach's estimation of the strength of the contraction with words such as, "contraction beginning, getting stronger, now getting weaker, almost gone, gone." In the time before transition to the second stage of labor, when contractions are longest and strongest, the woman may need to use her level 4 breathing or continuous light panting as well.

Effleurage.
One additional technique to displace pain sensation in the Lamaze method is *effleurage,* which is light abdominal massage, done with just enough pressure to avoid tickling. To ensure that she is maintaining a steady rhythm for massage, the woman

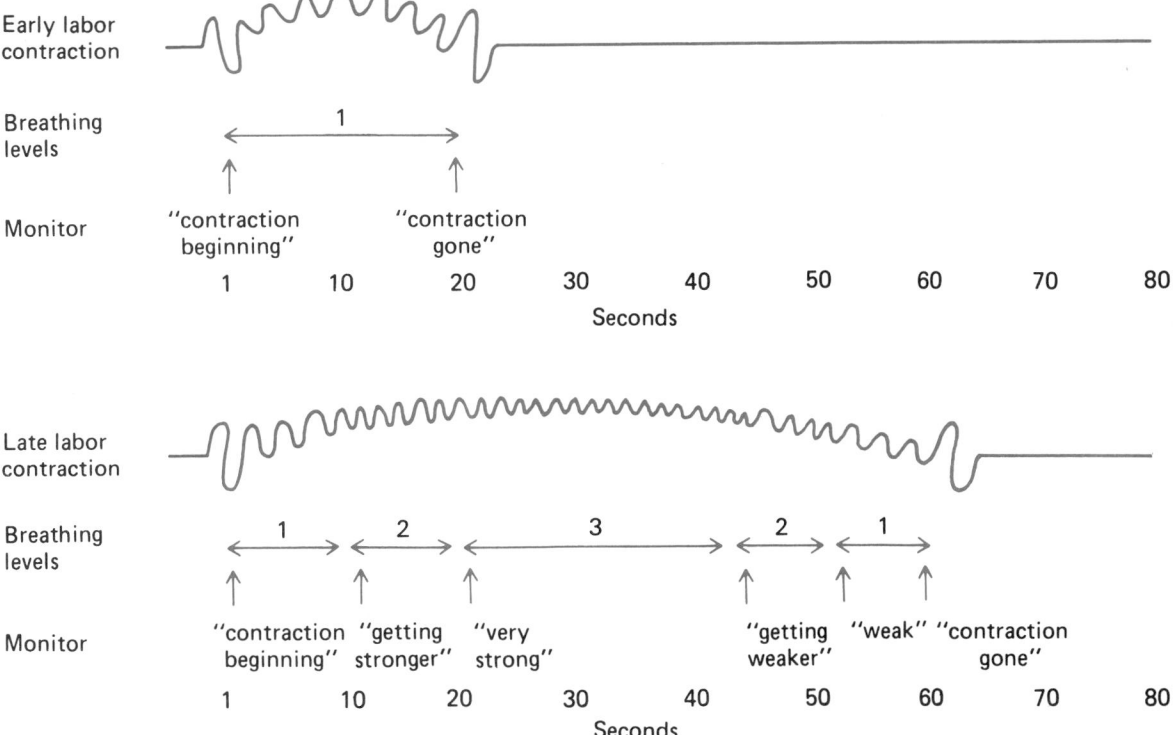

FIGURE 13-5
Example of differing Lamaze breathing patterns during a single contraction. 1, 2, and 3 are levels of breathing.

should trace a pattern on her abdomen with her fingertips such as the one shown in Figure 13-6. The rate of effleurage should remain constant, even though breathing rates change. Effleurage decreases sensory stimuli transmission from the abdominal wall and so helps limit local discomfort.

Focusing or Imaging. Focusing intently on an object (sometimes called "sensate focus") is another method of keeping sensory input from reaching the cortex of the brain. The woman brings with her into labor a photograph of her partner or children, a graphic design, or just something that appeals to her (Figure 13-7). She concentrates on it during contractions. Be careful not to step in the woman's line of vision during a contraction and break her concentration. Other women use imaging by mentally concentrating on an image such as watching waves rolling onto a beach or relaxing on a porch swing. Do not ask questions or talk to women using this technique because you will break their concentration.

Second Stage Breathing. During the second stage of labor when the baby is actually pushed down the birth canal, what type of breathing is best to use is controversial. In the past, women were told to hold their breath while they pushed. Now it is believed that holding the breath impairs blood return from the vena cava (a Val-

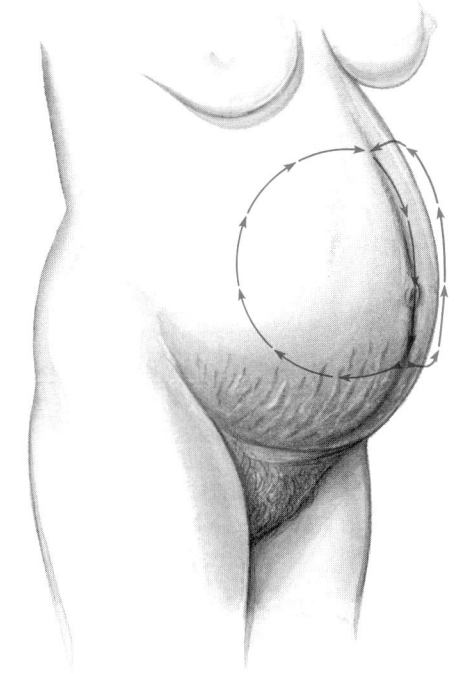

FIGURE 13-6
Effleurage patterns. Effleurage is light massage, performed with only enough pressure to avoid tickling. It desensitizes the abdominal skin, in turn relaxing the underlying muscles. During uterine contractions, a woman traces the pattern on her bare abdomen with her fingers.

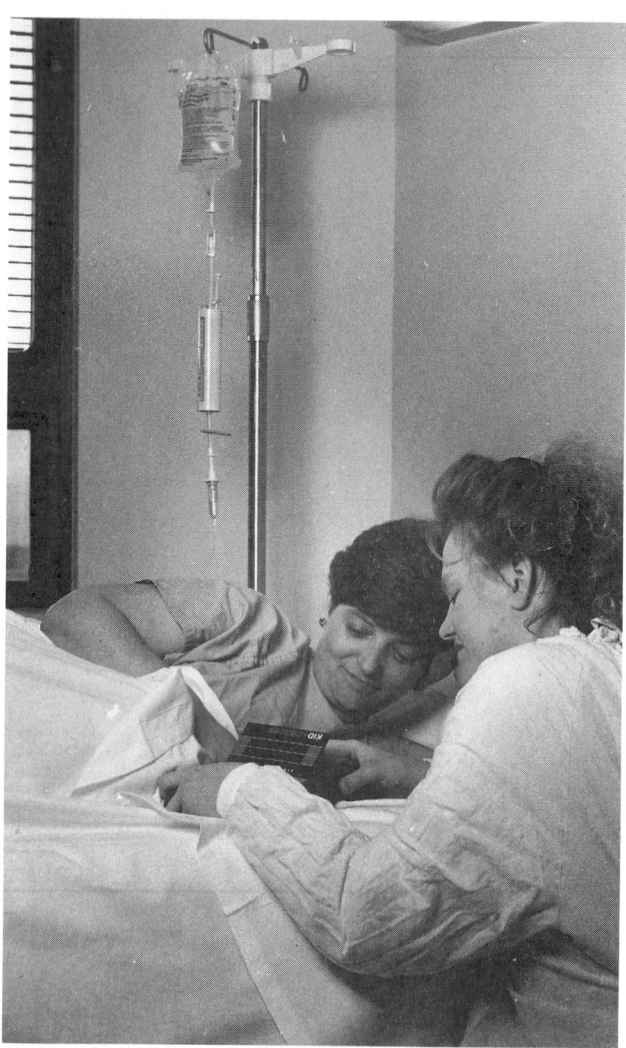

FIGURE 13-7
A woman chooses what object she wishes to focus on during labor. Here, a woman and nurse listen to the taped music the woman will focus on during contractions. (Courtesy of the Department of Medical Photography, Children's Hospital, Buffalo, NY.)

salva maneuver) so this is now discouraged. Teaching women to breathe out while pushing may be helpful. Other instructors suggest women breath any way that is natural for them, except holding the breath.

Women should not practice breathing and pushing. The possibility that they would rupture membranes by doing this is too great. Furthermore, in labor, the urge to push is uncontrollable so practice at this technique is not necessary.

Sample Curriculum Based on Lamaze

The following outlines the typical content of a series of preparation for childbirth classes.

Class One. The first class generally begins with an introduction of couples to each other and a review of the course objectives by the instructor. Stressed is the concept that the goal of classes is to make childbirth a satisfying experience and that there is no such thing as failure in prepared childbirth. Anatomy and physiology of the reproductive system and the process of pregnancy from fertilization to term are reviewed. Common discomforts of pregnancy such as constipation, backache, and urinary frequency are reviewed and tips on avoiding the problems suggested. Good nutrition for pregnancy is reviewed and suggestions for improving it are offered.

Exercises to improve posture, decrease fatigue, and strengthen the muscles used in labor such as Kegel exercises, pelvic rocking, and tailor sitting are discussed, demonstrated, and redemonstrated. A number of neuromuscular control exercises to introduce the concept of concentration-relaxation may be introduced, demonstrated, and practiced. A major goal is to increase the woman's ability to respond to verbal commands and to establish a feeling of close communication between her and her support person who will coach her in labor.

Class Two. Exercises for body strengthening and neuromuscular control are reviewed and the woman and her support person are moved a step further by a presentation of the stages of labor. Following this, a breathing technique (slow chest breathing) to be used in the first stage of labor and the technique of effleurage are introduced, demonstrated, and practiced.

Class Three. For a third class, stages of labor and the principles of breathing with contractions using effleurage are reviewed. Other breathing patterns that allow the woman to accelerate and decelerate breathing and panting to use during birth are demonstrated and practiced. Variations of labor such as back labor and how to avoid and correct hyperventilation are stressed. A list of labor supplies that the woman or couple might pack in advance to bring with them to the hospital is discussed. Such a list is shown in Table 13-1.

Class Four. Class four begins with the usual review of past material. More variations of breathing such as pant-blow are taught. Pushing without holding the breath is taught as are effective measures to decrease the length of the second stage of labor such as maintaining a semi-Fowler's position or squatting. Women should not practice pushing during pregnancy or increased abdominal pressure can cause enough increased intrauterine pressure possibly to rupture membranes. The importance of not holding the breath while pushing is stressed.

Class Five. For the fifth class, past material is reviewed and questions answered; new material concerning analgesia and anesthesia and other variations such as malpresentation, forceps birth, cesarean birth, and the role of fetal and uterine monitoring is introduced. Use of

Table 13-1. Supplies to Prepare for Labor	
Item	*Purpose*
Lip balm	To prevent dry lips
Mouthwash	For rinsing dry mouth
Toothbrush and toothpaste	To prevent dry mouth
Warm socks	Comfort
Small rolling pin covered with soft cloth	Back massage
Focal point	To increase concentration
Busy work (e.g., knitting or magazines)	To pass time
Paper bag	To prevent hyperventilation
Extra pillow	For semi-Fowler's position in labor
Watch	For timing contractions
Baby powder	For reducing friction of effleurage
Lollipops	For energy and dry mouth
Snacks (e.g., apples or potato chips)	For coach's comfort
Tapes or compact discs and player	To increase relaxation

a uterine monitor can be helpful for the prepared woman in labor because it can help to alert her or her coach when a contraction is beginning (a monitor registers uterine tightening before she feels the sensation).

Class Six. For a final class, a complete run-through of a simulated labor and birth is staged. Events that will occur in the postpartal period are discussed. The role of breast-feeding in the immediate postpartal period and uterine involution are included.

Preparation for Cesarean Birth

The fact that cesarean birth may be necessary to ensure a safe birth is covered in most preparation for childbirth classes. The woman who knows that she is to have a cesarean birth due to a pelvic abnormality or because she is a candidate for a repeat cesarean birth needs specific preparation (Fawcett, 1993). This is discussed in Chapter 20.

Expectant Parenting Classes

A number of other types of courses are offered to expectant parents that focus on concepts other than preparing for the actual labor and birth. Hospitals, health maintenance organizations, and community health services may provide classes for women and their families that focus on family health. These include sibling prepa-

ration classes, refresher classes for "repeat parents or grandparents," classes for expectant adoptive parents, preparation for parenting specially geared toward adolescents, breast-feeding classes, and many others. The most common of these courses is the expectant parenting class, which generally covers the normal stages of pregnancy and newborn care.

Most preparation-for-parenthood programs are planned to cover 4 to 8 hours of content spaced over a 4- to 8-week period. Both women and their support people are included. The curriculum should be individualized for the group and that group's particular needs (Ancheta, 1992). If all the women in the group already have children, for example, they may not feel a need for a tour of a maternity unit as part of the program; instead, they may want a review of what is new in baby food or child care. If all the women are teenagers, they may be most interested in what is going to happen to their bodies during pregnancy, or what sports are safe to continue during pregnancy. They may also need more information on what to expect when their baby is born. They probably will want a tour of the maternity unit (Figure 13-8). If all the women in the class work at least part-time, discussion of "brown bag nutrition" and how to include rest periods during work might be useful. A typical course plan for 8 weeks is shown in Box 13-2.

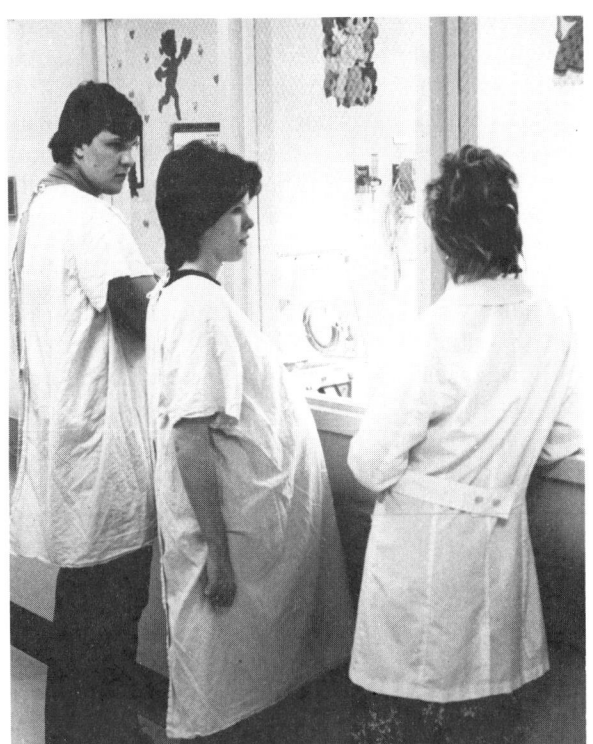

FIGURE 13-8

An enjoyable part of a preparation-for-parenthood class is touring a maternity service. Here, parents-to-be view a newborn nursery. (Courtesy of the Department of Medical Photography, Millard Filmore Hospital, Buffalo, NY.)

Lesson 1 Review of Physiological Changes of Pregnancy and Fetal Growth
Lesson 2 Personal Care During Pregnancy
   Nutrition
   Hygiene
   Exercise
   Rest
Lesson 3 Emotional Changes During Pregnancy
Lesson 4 Labor and Delivery
   The Process of Birth
   Exercises and Breathing Techniques
   Medication in Labor
Lesson 5 The Postpartum Period
Lesson 6 Infant Care
   Nutrition
   Hygiene
Lesson 7 Plans for Birth
   Birth Settings Available
   Supplies to Take to Birth Settings
   Tour or Film of a Typical Setting
Lesson 8 Reproductive Life Planning

Sibling Education Classes

Sibling classes are organized to acquaint older brothers and sisters with what happens during birth and what they can expect a newborn to be like. Where babies grow and things children can do to help their mother during a pregnancy such as not leaving toys on the floor that need to be picked up and helping her eat healthy foods during pregnancy are reviewed.

If the classes are held at a hospital, a tour of a newborn nursery is included so children can see how small their new sibling will be. A hospital room like the one their mother will occupy may be visited. Sibling classes can be helpful in allowing older children to feel a part of family planning for a new baby.

The Birth Setting

The setting for birth that a couple chooses depends on the woman's health and that of the fetus as well as the couple's preferences on how much supervision they desire at the birth. Although hospitals are the usual site for birth today, that has not always been the case. Up until the late 1800s, childbirth was conducted in the home. Analgesia or anesthesia for childbirth was unpopular until Queen Victoria delivered Prince Leopold under chloroform in 1853. Unfortunately, this extensive level

of anesthesia for childbirth led to additional interventions, because under anesthesia women were no longer able to push effectively during the pelvic division of labor. It became necessary to use a lithotomy position and an episiotomy and forceps for birth as well.

Part of the reason for so much anesthesia during birth can be attributed to physicians misinterpreting the types of pain in childbirth. It was assumed that the moment of birth was the major time of discomfort. As a result, women were allowed to labor without any pain medication and then given anesthesia or analgesia right before the baby was born. In reality, although the pain felt during the last stage of labor is intense, women may not be as uncomfortable during that time as early in labor because it is also the most fulfilling and even most exhilarating time, and it is directly followed by the birth of the baby.

Fortunately, birthing practices have changed to incorporate women's needs based on their descriptions of the pain of childbirth. There is also an economic incentive for change. If women choose physicians or hospitals who subscribe to more progressive birth practices over the services of more traditional facilities, the overall standard of care in communities leans toward the more progressive settings. The addition of birthing rooms to hospitals in the past 10 years is an example of this change. Nurses are in a strong position to advocate for making childbirth a "natural" process in the least restrictive setting possible. At the same time, nurses have a strong responsibility to encourage parents to maintain enough restrictions that birth remains safe.

Choosing the Appropriate Setting

Women choose hospitals, birthing centers, or their homes as settings for birth. Women with high-risk pregnancies have little choice; most nurse-midwives and physicians who deliver babies at home insist that women with any potential complication deliver at a hospital rather than at home.

Hospital Birth

Advantages and disadvantages of hospital birth are summarized in Box 13-3. A hospital has the advantage of having ready supplies and expert personnel if the mother or fetus or newborn should have a complication of birth.

In evaluating studies that compare the complications of birthing centers or home births to hospitals, be sure to consider that high-risk mothers deliver their children at hospitals; thus, the number of complications in hospital settings is bound to be higher than in other settings.

A woman usually comes to the hospital when her contractions are approximately 5 minutes apart and reg

Advantages

- The woman is encouraged to be prepared to control the discomfort of labor through nonmedication measures such as controlled breathing.
- The woman is encouraged to be knowledgeable about the labor process and make decisions about procedures performed.
- The woman is encouraged to consider breastfeeding to aide uterine contraction and infant bonding.
- Labor, birth, and immediate postpartal care can all be scheduled in a single room.
- The woman is attended by skilled professionals during labor and birth and the postpartal period.
- Emergency care and extended high-risk care are immediately available.

Disadvantages

- Separation of the family for at least one night.
- Mother does not feel as much in control of the childbirth experience as she may wish.
- Care may be fragmented, particularly if the woman's physician is not present during the entire labor and birth, or if labor nurses change shifts in the middle of labor. (Many nurse-midwives and physicians make it a point, however, to remain with their client throughout the entire childbirth experience.)

ular in pattern. If she has preregistered at the hospital, she is admitted to a **birthing room** without any separation time from her support person. A birthing room is sometimes called an LDR for **labor-delivery-recovery** or an LDRP, for **labor-delivery-recovery-postpartum room**. It is often decorated in a home-like atmosphere; the bed can be used as a labor bed until birth, when it converts into a birthing bed or a lithotomy position (Figure 13-9). A woman is expected to use a prepared method of childbirth with a minimum of analgesia and anesthesia (although an advantage of a hospital birth is that anesthesia such as an epidural is readily available for her if she needs it). Her support person can stay with her for the entire birth experience. (In the 1950s, maternity services had small waiting rooms for fathers because they were unwelcome. In the 1960s, they created large waiting rooms to show they were welcome. In the 1970s, they converted back to small waiting rooms because the support person is rarely separated from the woman.) Couples can bring favorite music or reading materials with them to use during labor.

Most hospitals screen women in early labor with an external monitor for both fetal heart rate and uterine contractions. If the fetal heart rate is good, such a monitor can usually be removed and used again only for periodic screening as labor progresses. The woman may have intravenous fluid started as a prophylactic measure. If this is done, it can be inserted in a dorsal surface vein so that it causes little discomfort and inconvenience for her.

At the time of birth, additional cupboards in the

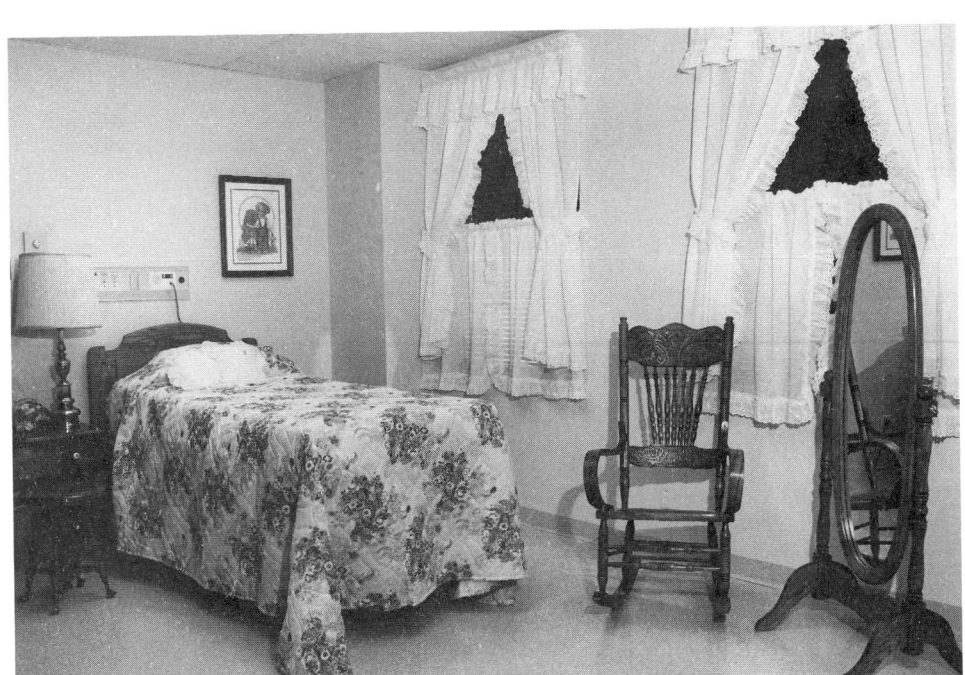

FIGURE 13-9
A birthing (labor-birth-recovery) room designed to maintain a home-like atmosphere in a hospital setting. (Courtesy of the Department of Medical Photography, Children's Hospital, Buffalo, NY.)

room are opened and converted into a space for baby care. A support person remains with the woman during birth and in some settings can cut the umbilical cord if desired. Women can choose a birthing position: lithotomy, supine recumbent, or side-lying.

Postpartal Care. Following birth, eye care for the infant can be delayed until the parents and infant have had a chance to become acquainted. Women giving birth.in LDRPs remain there with their families for the rest of the hospital stay (anywhere from 4 hours to 2 nights). Women giving birth in birthing rooms may be transferred to the postpartal unit almost immediately following birth, and remain there for a stay of 12 to 36 hours depending on preferences and insurance provisions. Both LDRPs and postpartal units generally advocate "rooming-in," in which the infant remains in the mother's room for the majority of the day. Breast-feeding on demand for infants should be the rule. There should be no restrictions on visiting for the primary support person; in many institutions a roll-away bed is provided so this person can remain constantly. Siblings of the newborn should be allowed to visit at least once and touch and become acquainted with the newborn. Because hospital stays are so short, the more women know about the experience and infant care, the more teaching can be accomplished (McGregor, 1994).

Alternative Birthing Centers

Alternative birthing centers (ABCs) are wellness-oriented childbirth facilities designed to bring childbirth out of acute care hospital settings yet provide enough medical resources for emergency care should a complication of labor and birth arise. Such a setting is established within or nearby a hospital or at least in easy transport distance of one. Because it is located outside an acute care setting where infections abound, the risk of nosocomial infection to the mother is thought to be reduced, an advantage of these settings. The birth attendants tend to be nurse-midwives. Women who deliver in ABCs are screened for complications before being admitted. Because women are carefully screened, the mortality rate of mothers and infants is no higher in these out-of-hospital settings than in hospital settings.

ABCs have LDRP rooms where a woman and her support person can invite friends and siblings to participate in the birth. In some centers, a central play area for siblings and cooking facilities are also available. ABCs also encourage the woman to express her own needs and wishes during the labor process. A minimum of analgesia and anesthesia is provided, and she can choose a birth position. She can bring her own music or distraction objects and the partner can perform such tasks as cutting the umbilical cord if he or she chooses.

Advantages and disadvantages of ABCs are summarized in Box 13-4.

Women remain in an ABC from 4 to 24 hours following birth. Because a minimum of analgesia or anesthesia is used, a woman recovers quickly following birth and is prepared to be discharged this early.

Home Birth

Home birth is the usual mode of birth in developing countries. Under the supervision of nurse-midwives, it is a popular choice for birth in Europe but only about 1% of women in the United States choose this method (DHHS, 1992). The Frontier Nursing Service of Kentucky is an example of an organization in the United States that maintains an active and well-accepted program of home birth. Home birth may be supervised by a physician, but nurse-midwives are the more likely choice as birth attendants in this setting. The nurse-midwife works in consultation with a physician and refers any woman who develops a complication during pregnancy. Such a woman is no longer a candidate for home birth. With conscientious selection of candidates, home birth with a nurse-midwife in attendance is as safe as hospital birth (Duran, 1992).

Most women who choose home birth in the United

Box 13-4
Advantages and Disadvantages of ABCs

Advantages

- The woman is encouraged to be prepared to control the discomfort of labor through nonmedication measures such as controlled breathing.
- The woman is encouraged to be knowledgeable about the labor process and help care-providers with decision making.
- The woman is encouraged to breastfeed to aide uterine contraction and infant bonding.
- Family integrity can be maintained because family members may accompany her to the birthing center.
- The woman is attended by skilled professionals during labor and delivery.
- Emergency care is immediately available. Extended high-risk care is easily arranged.

Disadvantages

- Extended high-risk care is not immediately available.
- The woman may be fatigued following birth because of early discharge.
- She must independently monitor her postpartal status because of early discharge.

States are well-educated and from middle-income families (O'Connor, 1993). They choose home birth in order to have the baby close by after birth, to have more control over the childbirth experience, to give birth in familiar surroundings, and to avoid a nosocomial infection (Anderson & Greener, 1991).

The main advantage of a home birth is that it allows for family integrity—the woman and her family are not separated. On the other hand, it puts the responsibility on the woman to prepare her home for the birth (difficult if she is exhausted toward the end of pregnancy) and to take care of the infant at birth and assess his or her wellness. Many women passing through a "taking-in" phase postpartally may be happier maintaining a dependent passive role than taking responsibility for the infant's actual care. Home birth also requires adequate support people. Unfortunately, some people, however willing, may be unable to take on this role in a crisis situation such as childbirth. Advantages and disadvantages of home birth are summarized in Box 13-5.

Requirements and Preparation

To be a candidate for a home birth, a woman must be in good health and have an adequate system of support people who will sustain her during labor and assist her for the first few days of the postpartal period. She needs a home that has basic necessities such as running water, adequate heat, and cooking and sewer facilities. The windows should have screens so that a multitude of flies

or other vectors are not present. A personal characteristic needed is the ability to adjust to changing circumstances (see the Nursing Care Plan).

The couple is responsible for providing necessary supplies other than those the birth attendant will bring, such as sterile gloves and scissors. Examples of supplies and equipment they need to organize are shown in Box 13-6.

In preparation for a home birth, parents should be-

Box 13-5
Advantages and Disadvantages of Home Birth

Advantages
- The woman is encouraged to become knowledgeable about the birth process and be an active participant in independently reducing the discomfort of labor.
- The woman has the greatest freedom for expressing her individuality.
- There is no separation of the family at birth.

Disadvantages
- Adequate equipment other than first-line emergency equipment is unavailable.
- An abrupt change of goals is necessary if hospitalization is required.
- Exhaustion of the woman and support person may occur because of the responsibility placed on them.
- Interference with the "taking-in phase" may occur postpartally because the woman must "take hold."
- The woman must independently monitor her postpartal status.

Box 13-6
Supplies Necessary for a Home Birth

For the Mother
Birth suface; this could be a bed or the floor. If a bed is used, it should be firm. Placing a wooden door or piece of plywood under a mattress can make it firmer.
Plastic protection for bed during the birth such as a shower curtain or plastic tablecloth
Clean towel and wash cloths
2 dozen disposable plastic pads to use as buttock pads
2 dozen sterile 4 × 4s
A bowl for the placenta
1 Fleets enema
A flashlight with new batteries for an examining light
2 pillows (to prop against for pushing)
Newspaper (to protect the floor and to wrap placenta for disposal)
A trash receptable with plastic bag
Paper towels and hand soap for handwashing
Antiseptic solution for handwashing
A telephone to call for emergency help (if this will be a public telephone, correct change for the call)
A mirror (dresser, standing, or hand-held) so the woman can view the birth
Warmed olive oil (to lubricate perineum)
Honey or sugar cubes (to promote energy)

For the Infant
A rubber bulb syringe to suction mouth at birth
Alcohol and cotton balls for cord care
A tape measure
Six receiving blankets
Diapers
A baby gown

For Postpartal Care
Vitamin A and D ointment for breast care
1 box sanitary pads (unopened)
1 nursing bra
Extra gauze squares or pieces of cotton for bra pads

Nursing Care Plan

The Family Who Desires a Home Birth

Carla is a 26-year-old primigravida, 24 weeks gestation, who with Bob, her 28-year-old support person, has decided on a home birth. They have a 4-year-old son, Zak, who was born under general anesthesia because of a sudden fetal bradycardia. The following is a nursing care plan designed to assist them with a home birth.

Assessment: Client is committed to home birth "to avoid a hospital admission like last time." She also wants her son to view birth. Support person is interested in home birth from a financial standpoint (they do not have hospital insurance). Client states she has bed supplies readied; having some difficulty purchasing other supplies because of limited finances. Bathroom sink is inoperable; home has no telephone.

Client follows vegetarian diet. Diet reviewed by nutritionist and found to be adequate except for iron content. Client has prenatal vitamins she takes "not very regularly." Has attended no preparation for childbirth classes. Has read on subject and feels this will be adequate. Birth attendant will be nurse-midwife.

Nursing Diagnosis: Knowledge deficit regarding true advantages and disadvantages of home birth related to inexperience.

Defining Characteristic: Couple voices financial concerns and avoidance of medication as primary motivations.

Goal: Couple will reexamine motivation for home birth in 3 weeks.

Outcome Criteria: Couple expresses a healthy mother and healthy child as their goal for birth and can elaborate on plans to fulfill this through home birth.

Nursing Orders	Rationale
1. Urge couple to discuss plans with each other.	1. Assures that couple shares same goals and plans for achieving them.
2. Ask mother to locate a caretaker for Zak during birth.	2. A caretaker is essential in order to make experience enjoyable for older child.
3. Sign contract to stipulate financial arrangements and agree to allow emergency hospital care if necessary.	3. Safeguard well being in case of unexpected circumstances.

(continued)

come familiar with the birth process. Stress should be placed on the events of early labor such as when and how the woman should telephone the birth attendant team (preferably as early as she realizes that she is in labor); how to time contractions; and danger signs she should watch for before the birth attendant arrives, such as rupture of membranes, vaginal bleeding, or no relaxation between contractions. The couple will be relying on their own judgment during this time, thus it is crucial that they be well informed. They should also be aware of emergency birth procedure in case traffic or other delays prevent the birth attendants from arriving or the labor is precipitous. They should have the telephone number of the community emergency service posted conspicuously by a telephone; if the house has no telephone, the couple needs to have a car (with a full gas tank) available for emergency transport.

Children and Home Birth

An advantage of home birth is that it allows other children to view the birth. If older children will be present, a person separate from the mother's main support person needs to be designated to care for them. This person will need to plan to provide entertainment (timing contractions for more than 10 minutes is not interesting), explanations, food, and sleep. It is particularly important that the mother not be expected to provide such supervision during labor when she becomes introverted and has concern only for herself. A child who is without supervision during this time can remember the experi-

Nursing Diagnosis: Health-seeking behaviors regarding healthy fetal outcome related to first childbirth experience.

Defining Characteristic: Client voices that she is interested in learning more about health during pregnancy and at birth.

Goal: Client and support person will both demonstrate increased knowledge about and participation in preparing for safe home birth.

Outcome Criteria: Client describes normal pattern of labor and birth and means used to control pain of labor; client completes formal preparation course for labor and birth and readies adequate supplies by week 38 of pregnancy.

Nursing Orders	Rationale
1. Urge couple to make bed more firm for childbirth (take kitchen door off hinges and use as a bedboard) and begin to save money weekly for purchasing supplies.	1. Assures that physical environment and couple will be ready when labor begins.
2. Ask couple to buy a gallon of distilled water for handwashing and damp-dust floor with wet cloth attached to broom daily beginning in week 38 of pregnancy.	2. Provides safe alternative for maintaining asepsis, as bathroom sink is not operable.
3. Ask couple to arrange to have neighbor provide a key to her apartment or remain home during labor (if realistic), to give access to emergency telephone.	3. Assures access to emergency telephone, as client has no telephone in apartment.
4. Urge couple to keep car more than half-filled with gasoline after week 38 of pregnancy.	4. Assures that there will be emergency transportation as needed.

ence as a time of rejection rather than an exciting, happy experience.

Women need to ask themselves if the birth experience would be enjoyable for an older child or whether the sight of her undressed and in pain would be so different from usual that it would be shocking or bewildering. Allowing a child to witness the birth of kittens or puppies in this instance might be a more appropriate way to expose a child to birth.

The Day of Birth

Beginning with week 38 of pregnancy, the woman must be certain that the room that will be used for the birth is clean and prepared for the birth. Encourage damp dusting in the room and vacuuming or damp mopping every day to keep the microorganism count low. When the woman realizes that she is in labor, she needs to make the final preparations for a labor bed. To do this, she spreads out a plastic sheet or shower curtain or table cloth and covers that with a freshly washed clean sheet. The top sheet will become badly stained and probably never wash completely free of blood stains again so using an old one is more practical.

The woman then notifies the birth attendant team that she is in labor and reports her contraction pattern. She is encouraged to continue with daily activities as much as possible (but to stop short of fatigue) to make the time of labor seem shorter, the same instructions given to women who are planning on giving birth at a birthing center or hospital. When labor contractions become moderate in intensity and have a regular pattern, she or her support person should notify the birth attendant team that they are needed.

Sterile technique is just as important for a home birth as in an agency setting. Because most women will not be having an anesthetic, they can drink carbohydrate-rich fluids such as orange juice or eat easily digested foods such as yogurt early in labor. Fetal heart rate should be assessed every 15 minutes during active labor and every 5 minutes closer to birth, as no electronic monitors will be used.

The temperature of the room should be raised slightly close to birth so the infant will not be born into a cool climate. Baby blankets can be warmed for 5 minutes in a 150°F oven or for about 20 seconds in a microwave oven.

Because the woman will not be receiving any oxytocin to contract her uterus, there is a much greater possibility of uterine atony and massive hemorrhage following birth than in an alternative birth center or hospital setting.

For safety, someone should keep their hand on the fundus of the uterus and apply gentle but firm pressure for the next full hour. The woman herself should not do this as she may fall soundly asleep from exhaustion following birth. Take maternal pulse and blood pressure every 15 minutes for the first hour as another gauge of hemostasis.

The infant should be encouraged to breast-feed immediately after birth because this action releases maternal oxytocin, which will assist uterine contractions. Make certain the woman realizes that this action is for her health, not solely for infant nutrition.

Eye prophylaxis is mandatory for the infant at home births (as in a hospital setting). If the infant does not receive vitamin K, he or she must be observed closely in the next 3 days for ecchymotic bleeding (which can lead to extreme jaundice as the blood is absorbed).

Women must take the responsibility for assessing their own uterine contraction for the next week; they are usually advised to take their temperature daily and report a temperature over 100.4°F, as this could indicate a postpartal infection.

At present, home birth is chosen by only a small segment of the population and, despite predictions that the rate will increase, it does not appear to be gaining in popularity. The changes that hospitals have made in providing attractive welcoming rooms for birth are probably a major reason for this.

Alternative Methods of Birth

In addition to setting, there are a number of different methods of childbirth that have become popular in the past 10 to 15 years. These include using a birthing chair (which saw renewed popularity only to become somewhat neglected again) and some alternative birth methods such as the LeBoyer method and birth under water.

Birthing Chairs and Birthing Beds

Birthing chairs (Figure 13-10) are comfortable reclining chairs with a slide-away seat that allow a woman a comfortable position during labor and also furnish perineal exposure so a birth attendant can assist with the infant's birth. Many hospitals and alternative birth centers have birthing chairs available for a woman to use if she should choose to do so. They have the advantage of maintaining the woman in a semi-Fowler's position, a position that, because it acts with gravity, appears to speed the second stage of labor.

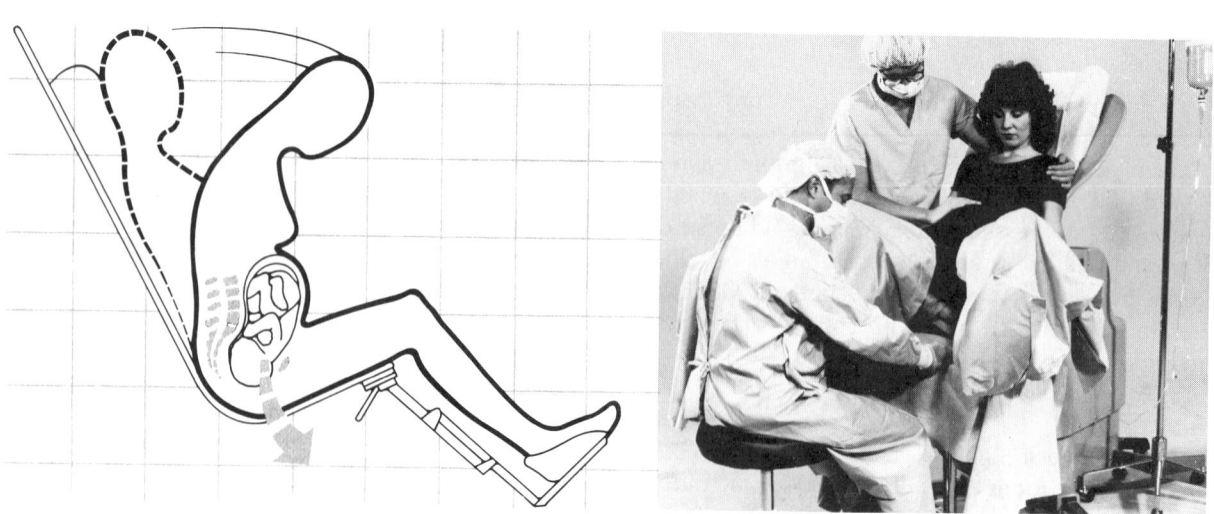

FIGURE 13-10

A birthing chair. (Reprinted by permission of the Century Manufacturing Company.)

If a woman chooses to use a supine recumbent position (on her back with knees flexed) rather than a lithotomy position (legs elevated into stirrups) for birth, she can use a **birthing bed**. Such a position reduces tension on the perineum and may result in fewer perineal tears than in the lithotomy position (Olson et al., 1990).

The Leboyer Method

Frederick Leboyer (1975) is a French obstetrician who proposed that moving from a warm, fluid-filled intrauterine environment to a noisy, air-filled, brightly lighted birth room is a major shock to a newborn. With the **Leboyer method**, the birthing room is darkened so there is no sudden contrast in light; it should be pleasantly warm, not chilled. There should be soft music playing, or at least no harsh noises in the room. The infant should be handled gently—the cord cut later and the infant placed immediately after birth into a warm water bath.

These principles have received a great amount of publicity in the press as being new and different. In reality, the concept that infants should be handled gently at birth is always practiced. Some neonatologists question the wisdom of a warm bath because it may reduce spontaneous respirations and allow a high level of acidosis to occur. Late cutting of a cord may lead to excess blood viscosity to the newborn (Nelle et al., 1993). Certainly, soft music, gentle handling, and a welcome atmosphere are important ingredients for all birth attendants to try to incorporate into birth. Providing dim lights (or at least not bright, glaring ones) could be given more consideration in most institutions.

Birth Under Water

Reclining or sitting in warm water during labor can be soothing; the feeling of weightlessness that occurs under water as well as the relaxation from the warm water both can contribute to reduce discomfort in labor. Using this principle, a number of birthing centers allow women to labor in tubs of warm water. The baby is born under water and then immediately brought to the surface for a first breath. Some potential difficulties with underwater birth are contamination of the bath water with feces expelled with pushing efforts during the second stage of labor that could lead to uterine infection, aspiration of bath water by the fetus, and maternal chilling when she leaves the water. A number of unfortunate newborn deaths have occurred using the method. Until the safety of this method has been fully established, women should be advised not to choose underwater birth over more tested methods (Zimmerman et al., 1993).

Key Points

- Couples should be encouraged to make a childbirth plan early in pregnancy which includes birth attendant and setting.
- Common exercises taught in pregnancy to strengthen perineal muscles are tailor sitting, squatting, and Kegel exercises. Abdominal muscle contraction and pelvic rocking exercises strengthen abdominal muscles and help relieve backache.
- Types of childbirth preparation include the Bradley (husband-coached), psychosexual (Kitzinger), Dick-Read, and Lamaze (psychoprophylactic) methods. Lamaze is the most-used method in the United States.
- Commonly used nonmedication techniques for pain relief in labor are conscious relaxation, consciously controlled breathing, effleurage, focusing, and imaging.
- Expectant parents' classes provide information on pregnancy, birth, and child care.
- Common sites for childbirth include hospitals, alternative birthing centers, and home.

Critical Thinking Exercises

1. Avery is a 19-year-old expecting her first baby, who tells you she does not intend to attend a preparation for labor class because she wants to have epidural anesthesia as soon as she is admitted to the hospital in labor. Would you advise her to attend a class or not?
2. Bob and Rae are a couple having their third child. They ask you if they should allow their oldest child to view the birth. How would you advise them? What further information would you need before you could give informed advice?
3. Susan is a 23-year-old who tells you that the father of her baby will not be with her during labor. She asks you if it is really important or not to have someone with her. She intends to use Lamaze breathing patterns and hopes to use no medication. How would you advise her?

References

Ancheta, R. (1992). Using a skit to teach question-asking skills. *International Journal of Childbirth Education, 7,* 29.

Anderson, R., & Greener, D. (1991). A descriptive analysis of home births attended by CNMs in two nurse midwifery services. *Journal of Nurse Midwifery, 36,* 95.

Bradley, R. (1981). *Husband-coached childbirth* (3rd ed.). New York: Harper Collins.

Crawford, K. (1992). Childbirth education for VBAC. . . vaginal birth after a cesarean. *International Journal of Childbirth Education, 7,* 20.

Department of Health & Human Services. (1991). *Healthy people 2000.* Washington, DC: Public Health Service.

Department of Health & Human Services. (1992). Surveillance of birth practices. *Morbidity & Mortality Weekly Reports, 41,* 33.

Dick-Read, G. (1987). *Childbirth without fear: The original approach to natural childbirth* (5th ed.). New York: Harper Collins.

Duran, A. M. (1992). The safety of home birth: The farm study. *American Journal of Public Health, 82,* 450.

Fawcett, J., et al. (1993). Effects of information on adaptation to cesarean birth. *Nursing Research, 42,* 49.

Geissler, E. M. (1994). *Pocket guide to cultural assessment.* St. Louis: C. V. Mosby.

Janke, J. (1992). Teaching breathing techniques in the '90s. *International Journal of Childbirth Education, 7,* 33.

Karmel, M. (1965). *Thank you, Dr. Lamaze.* New York: Doubleday.

Kitzinger, S. (1990). *The experience of childbirth.* New York: Viking Penguin.

Leboyer, F. (1975). *Birth without violence.* New York: Alfred A. Knopf.

MacKey, M. C. (1990). Women's preparation for the childbirth experience. *Maternal-Child Nursing Journal, 19,* 143.

MacLachian, D. J., & Merkel, S. F. (1990). Prenatal education and family centered health promotion at the worksite. *American Association of Occupational Health Nurses Journal, 38,* 114.

McGregor, L. A. (1994). Short, shorter, shortest: Improving the hospitalized stay of mothers and newborns. *MCN: American Journal of Maternal Child Nursing, 19,* 91.

Nelle, M., et al. (1993). The effect of Leboyer delivery on blood viscosity and other hemorrheologic parameters in term neonates. *American Journal of Obstetrics and Gynecology, 169,* 189.

O'Connor, B. B. (1993). The home birth movement in the United States. *Journal of Medicine and Philosophy, 18,* 147.

Olson, R., et al. (1990). Maternal birthing positions and perineal injury. *Journal of Family Practice, 30,* 553.

Predmore, P. (1992). A new outreach population? The "thirty-something" crowd. *International Journal of Childbirth Education, 7,* 31.

Raymond, T. (1992). Moms younger than eighteen and older than thirty-five: Should they have their own classes? *International Journal of Childbirth Education, 7,* 37.

Sullivan, P. (1993). Felt learning needs of pregnant women. *Canadian Nurse, 89,* 42.

Tighe, D., et al. (1990). The perioperative experience of cesarean birth preparation: Considerations and complications. *Journal of Perinatal and Neonatal Nursing, 3,* 14.

Wood, D. (1992). TAPP: A school-based pregnancy program that shines. *International Journal of Childbirth Education, 7,* 19.

Zimmerman, R., et al. (1993). Water birth—is it safe? *Journal of Perinatal Medicine, 21,* 5.

Suggested Readings

Begley, C. M. (1991). Postpartum haemorrhage. *Midwives' Chronicle, 104,* 102.

Biasella, S. (1993). A comprehensive perinatal education program. *AWHONNS Clinical Issues in Perinatal and Women's Health Nursing, 4,* 5.

Coleman, C. (1992). Marketing your childbirth classes: The strategic planning process. *International Journal of Childbirth Education, 7,* 7.

Duffin, C. (1992). Teaching 1st stage: What's new and what's being taught. *International Journal of Childbirth Education, 7,* 31.

Hotelling, B. A. (1992). What can these babies possibly learn about having babies? *International Journal of Childbirth Education, 7,* 10.

Janke, S. (1992). Pregnancy over 35. *International Journal of Childbirth Education, 7,* 35.

Jeffers, D. (1992). Outreach childbirth education classes for low income families: A strategy for program development. *International Journal of Childbirth Education, 7,* 17.

Lauer, E. L. (1992). Relaxation: Back to basics. *International Journal of Childbirth Education, 7,* 31.

Luke, B. (1994). Maternal-fetal nutrition. *Clinical Obstetrics and Gynecology, 37,* 93.

O'Brien, M. P. (1992). Expanding your childbirth education practice. *International Journal of Childbirth Education, 7,* 40.

Perrin, K. M. (1992). The 4Ms of teen pregnancy: Managing, mending, mentoring and modeling. *International Journal of Childbirth Education, 7,* 29.

Waldenstrom, U., & Nilsson, C. A. (1993). Women's satisfaction with birth center care: A randomized, controlled study. *Birth, 20,* 3.

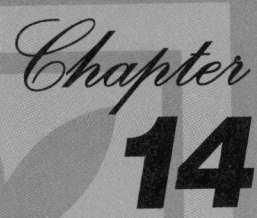

Chapter 14

High-Risk Pregnancy: The Woman With a Preexisting or Newly Acquired Illness

Objectives

After mastering the contents of this chapter, you should be able to:

1. Define high-risk pregnancy and identify factors that can make a pregnancy high risk.

2. Describe common illnesses such as heart disease, diabetes mellitus, or renal and blood disorders that can result in complications when they exist with pregnancy.

3. Assess the woman with an illness during pregnancy for changes occurring because of the pregnancy.

4. State nursing diagnoses related to the effect of a preexisting or newly acquired illness on pregnancy.

5. Plan interventions that will contribute to a safe pregnancy outcome when illness occurs with pregnancy (e.g., planning ways a woman can secure more rest).

6. Implement a plan of care for the woman with an illness during pregnancy (eg, teaching insulin administration to a woman newly diagnosed with diabetes).

7. Evaluate outcome criteria to be certain nursing goals related to care for the high-risk pregnant woman have been achieved.

8. Identify National Health Goals related to complications of pregnancy that nurses can be instrumental in helping the nation achieve.

9. Identify areas related to illness and pregnancy that could benefit from additional nursing research.

10. Use critical thinking to analyze ways that nursing care can remain family centered when a preexisting or newly acquired illness develops.

11. Synthesize knowledge of high-risk pregnancy and nursing process to achieve quality maternal and child health nursing care.

Adele Pillitteri: MATERNAL AND CHILD HEALTH NURSING, 2nd Edition. © 1995 Adele Pillitteri.

When a woman enters pregnancy with a chronic condition such as heart disease or kidney disease, both she and the pregnancy are at risk for complications. The course of a normal pregnancy can complicate the disease, and the disease can cause complications that may affect the baby or leave the woman less equipped to function as a mother or undergo a future pregnancy. Nursing care for the woman with a preexisting illness focuses on close observation of maternal health and fetal well being, education of the woman and her family about danger signs to watch for during pregnancy, and actions to keep complications to a minimum whenever possible.

In addition to preexisting illnesses, the pregnant woman, like any other person, may develop non–pregnancy-related illnesses or suffer from trauma during a pregnancy. When this occurs, the illness or injury can have adverse effects not only on the woman but on the unborn child as well. Nursing care for the well, pregnant woman focuses on preventing illness and trauma by promoting an especially healthy lifestyle. When accidents and illness occur despite these safeguards, nursing care must focus on preventing such disorders from affecting the health of the fetus as well as helping the mother regain her health as quickly as possible so that she can continue a healthy pregnancy and prepare herself psychologically and physically for labor and birth and the arrival of her newborn.

Conditions that cause severe symptoms such as a marked change in fluid and electrolyte balance, altered cardiovascular or respiratory function, or severe blood loss, are especially dangerous to a fetus. Some infections, notably toxoplasmosis (as discussed in Chapter 11) and some of the sexually transmitted infections, are devastating for the unborn child and need to be ad-

dressed as soon as they are discovered. National Health Goals related to complications of pregnancy are shown in the Focus on National Health Goals box.

Although pregnancy is a stressful time, women generally do experience overall good health during their pregnancies, perhaps in part because of their extra care and concern in keeping healthy for two. This extra motivation also encourages the woman with a high-risk pregnancy to follow carefully the therapeutic regimen established to keep her and her developing fetus safe.

NURSING PROCESS OVERVIEW
for Care of the Woman With Preexisting or Newly Acquired Illness

ASSESSMENT

Accurate prenatal assessment of the woman with a preexisting or newly acquired illness requires a thorough understanding of the signs and symptoms of illnesses, such as cardiac disease and diabetes mellitus, that can strike women of childbearing age, in addition to an understanding of the course of a normal pregnancy. Assessment techniques include objective measures such as fetal heart monitoring and observation of more subjective factors such as the extent of edema or exhaustion. Such assessment is best made by health care personnel who care for the woman consistently throughout the pregnancy so that subtle changes in data can be best recognized. In the absence of a consistent care provider, teach the woman to assess her health in relation to objective parameters. Teach her to report exhaustion, for example, in relation to daily activity (e.g., "Two weeks ago, I could walk a block without being short of breath. Today, I could walk only half a block"; "The last time I was in for a checkup, edema didn't occur until bedtime. Now I notice it every afternoon by the time my child comes home from school").

NURSING DIAGNOSIS

Nursing diagnoses developed for the woman with a high-risk pregnancy address the specific, disease-related conditions as well as the therapeutic restrictions such conditions might require, such as:

- High risk for altered tissue perfusion related to mitral valve prolapse during pregnancy
- Pain related to pyelonephritis during 4th month of pregnancy

- Social isolation related to prescribed bedrest during pregnancy secondary to concurrent illness
- Ineffective individual coping related to increasing level of daily restrictions secondary to chronic illness and pregnancy
- Knowledge deficit related to normal changes of pregnancy versus illness complications
- Fear regarding pregnancy outcome related to chronic illness
- Health seeking behaviors related to the increasing knowledge of the effects of illness on pregnancy
- Self-identity disturbance related to diagnosis of HIV infection

PLANNING

Be certain that outcome criteria and goals established are realistic in light of the mother's health and the restrictions placed on her by her health. One family member with illness affects all family members; goals should relate to the entire family's health.

Planning with the woman with a preexisting medical condition must be done based on the pattern of her life before the pregnancy (Figure 14-1). Planning adequate rest during pregnancy, for example, usually means planning for two rest periods a day. For a woman with

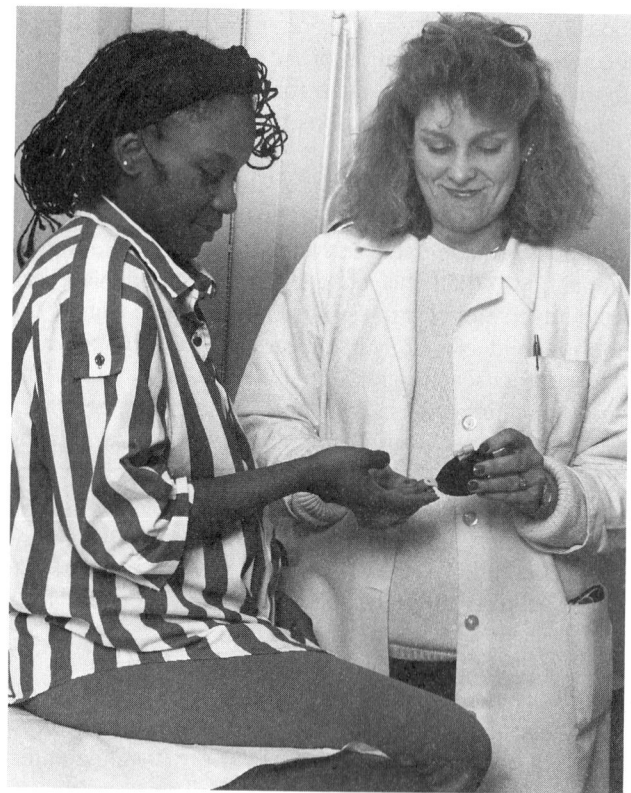

FIGURE 14-1
Planning with women with a preexisting illness should consider both the impact of the illness and the pregnancy. (Courtesy of the Department of Medical Photography, Children's Hospital, Buffalo, NY.)

cardiac disease who took two rest periods a day before pregnancy, however, this would be ineffective planning. Remember that the additional medical supervision needed during pregnancy may involve increased expenses for the family; the family may need to develop new ways to meet expenses. A major goal for a woman with a severe chronic condition might be to maintain the woman's health during pregnancy so that she can remain at home as long as possible and hospitalization can be kept to a minimum.

Planning following trauma may be difficult for the client because of the shock of the accident. Be careful, however, not to make plans completely for her (e.g., "Your best plan would be to allow the doctor to put a cast in place"). Instead, give the woman the available alternatives (e.g., "As the doctor explained, there are two separate therapies for a dislocated knee; let me review with you the advantages and disadvantages of each therapy"). Allowing the woman to choose among alternatives helps her to participate in planning care.

Most women who sustain a form of trauma during pregnancy need time to talk about the event after the emergency care is complete. They may feel guilty they were not more careful. In some instances, the woman's support person caused the injury (e.g., by driving carelessly) and she may feel both anger at that person's carelessness and yet relief that he or she was not injured and is there to offer support.

A woman and her partner can work through these emotions satisfactorily if the pregnancy progresses normally after this point and the fetus was uninjured. If the fetus was injured or the pregnancy disrupted, the event may be too great for the relationship to survive without counseling.

IMPLEMENTATION

Nursing interventions for the pregnant woman with an illness unrelated to her pregnancy may focus on teaching her new or additional measures to maintain health. Imaginative solutions to problems must be created or, after a time, the woman may be unable to adjust adequately to the changes she must make.

EVALUATION

If evaluation of goals at health care visits reveals that a goal is not being met, new assessment, analysis, and planning need to be done. In some instances, a goal is not met because the woman did not appreciate the need for an added pregnancy measure (she is so used to adjusting and compensating for her illness, she feels as if she can sense when she needs further restrictions). Evaluation may reveal that the woman needs more psychological support to continue to follow a pregnancy routine consistently. Nine months is a long time not to know whether restrictions or following a new regimen is

going to be successful. Examples of outcome criteria that might be established are:

- Client states she rests for 1 hour morning and afternoon; dependent edema has not increased from 1+ at next prenatal visit.
- Family state they are all participating in exercise program since mother developed gestational diabetes.
- Client reports no increase in frequency of urination or burning at next prenatal visit.

Identifying the High-Risk Pregnancy

A **high-risk pregnancy** is one in which some maternal or fetal factor, either psychosocial or physiologic, is apt to result in the birth of a high-risk infant or in some way harm the woman herself.

Some women enter pregnancy with a chronic illness that, superimposed on the pregnancy, makes it high risk. Other women enter pregnancy in good health but then develop a complication of pregnancy that causes it to become high risk. In some instances, particular circumstances—poverty, lack of support people, poor coping mechanisms, genetic inheritance, or past history of pregnancy complications—can cause a pregnancy to be categorized as high risk.

In most instances, more than one factor will contribute to the classification of a pregnancy as high risk (see the Focus on Cultural Awareness box). The preg-

FOCUS ON CULTURAL AWARENESS

An illness during pregnancy can complicate not only a pregnancy but also a woman's entire lifestyle and family. Women who think of pregnancy as a time of wellness may have a great deal of difficulty accepting a medical regimen such as daily blood glucose monitoring as this is contradictory to their primary belief. Women in extended families may have an easier time accepting hospitalization during pregnancy than those from nuclear families because there are more people available to take over their role at home. On the other hand, women in extended families may have more difficulty with hospitalization because there are more people depending on them to be home.

Assessing all families individually and asking about the effect of an illness during pregnancy on the entire family helps to identify problems and lead to timely problem-solving.

nancy of a woman who is diabetic, for example, is automatically termed one with greater than normal risk. The fetus growing in an environment in which **hyperglycemia** (increased serum glucose) is the rule runs increased danger. During the pregnancy, the woman, worrying that something will happen to her baby, fails to begin the "pregnancy work" that she must do so that bonding can take place. At birth, the child is in double jeopardy. Not only may the baby be born with an illness, but he or she is at high risk for poor maternal-child attachment as well.

The preterm infant born to a teenage girl, likewise, has a double problem. Not only is the infant immature (and at risk for all the complications that accompany immaturity), but he or she has an immature mother as well (see Chapter 17 for discussion of the special needs of the pregnant adolescent).

Box 14-1 lists common psychological, social, and physical areas that, when present, can cause the pregnancy to be categorized as high risk. Categorizing the risks as minimal, moderate, or extensive differs with each woman because of her individual coping mechanisms and level of support. A woman living in extreme poverty, for example, isolated on a mountain, would be extremely high risk for poor nutritional intake during pregnancy; a woman with a similar income who could depend on a nutritional assistance program such as WIC and counseling from a community health nurse might be only at minimal risk.

Remembering that the term "high risk" rarely refers to just one causative factor helps in the planning of holistic and, ultimately, effective nursing care.

A high-risk classification system such as Goodwin's Antepartum Fetal Risk Score (see Table 10-6) should be used routinely with all pregnant women to attempt to identify high-risk status as early as possible in pregnancy. Preexisting or newly acquired maternal illnesses that can make a pregnancy high-risk are covered in this chapter. Chapters 15 and 16 discuss pregnancy-related conditions and illnesses that make the pregnancy high risk for mother or child. Chapter 17 covers populations that are high risk due to age (younger than 18 years or older than 35 years), the presence of a disability, or drug abuse.

Sexually Transmitted Diseases and Pregnancy

Sexually transmitted diseases (STDs) are those spread by coitus. A number of STDs produce only local effects during pregnancy; thus, women do not always report them unless asked about specific symptoms. Almost all STDs have some effect on the fetus, though, and so they need to be identified. This chapter provides a brief overview of those STDs most important to identify during pregnancy because of their potential effect on the pregnancy or newborn. Chapter 26 discusses specific effects on the fetus.

All STDs can be prevented to some extent by the use of "safer sex practices" (see Chapter 4), including use of a condom and a spermicide containing nonoxynol 9 for sexual relations. Little disease immunity is developed against an STD once it has been contracted, so it is possible to become reinfected if prevention measures are not followed. In most instances, the male partner should also be treated or the disease will recur from cross infection.

Treatment of most STDs begins with determining the causative organism so that the appropriate antibiotic or antifungal medication can be prescribed. The woman can reduce discomfort of vulvar or vaginal irritation by following guidelines discussed in Chapter 47.

Nursing Diagnoses and Related Interventions

Nursing Diagnosis: Pain related to vulvar irritation secondary to existence of STD.

Goal: Client will be free of symptoms of infection and will take measures to prevent contracting this or other STDs in the future.

Outcome Criteria: No vaginal discharge or pruritus is present by history or examination. Client reports she is using safer sex practices.

The Woman With Candidiasis

Candidiasis causes a vaginal infection spread by the fungus *Candida*. The woman notices a thick, cream cheese–like vaginal discharge and extreme pruritus. The vagina appears red and irritated. Candidiasis occurs more frequently during pregnancy than normally because of the increased estrogen level present during pregnancy. In the pregnant population, it occurs most frequently in women being treated with an antibiotic for another infection, in women with gestational diabetes, and in women with human immunodeficiency virus (HIV) infection. Women with repeated infections should have urine tested for glucose to detect if gestational diabetes is present.

The disease is diagnosed by microscopic analysis of a wet slide. It is treated by the local application of an antifungal agent such as nystatin suppositories or miconazole. It may be necessary to continue therapy longer during pregnancy than usual (6–14 days) (Ernest, 1992). It is important that the infection is treated during pregnancy, not only because it is uncomfortable for the woman, but also because, if infection is present in the vagina at the time of childbirth, it may cause a candidal

Box 14-1
Factors that Categorize a Pregnancy as High Risk

Psychological

Prepregnancy

History of drug dependence (including alcohol)

History of abusive behavior

History of tolerating battering

Cigarette smoker

History of mental illness

History of poor coping mechanisms

Mental retardation

Social

Occupation involving handling of toxic substances (including radiation and anesthesia gases)

Environmental contaminants at home

Isolated

Lower economic level

Poor access to transporation for emergency care

High altitude

Highly mobile lifestyle

Poor housing

Lack of support people

Physical

Visual or hearing impaired

Pelvic inadequacy or malshape

Uterine incompetency, position, or structure

Secondary major illness (heart disease, diabetes mellitus, kidney disease, hypertension, chronic infection such as tuberculosis, hemopoietic or blood disorder, malignancy)

Poor gynecologic or obstetric history

History of previous poor pregnancy outcome (spontaneous abortion; stillbirth)

History of child with congenital anomalies

Obesity

Pelvic inflammatory disease (PID)

History of inherited disorder

Small stature

Potential of blood incompatibility

Younger than age 18 years or older than 35 years

Pregnancy Period

Loss of support person

Illness in a family member

Decrease in self-esteem

Drug abuse (including alcohol and cigarette smoking)

Poor acceptance of pregnancy

Refusal of or neglected prenatal care

Exposure to environmental teratogens

Disruptive family incident

Decreased economic support

Subject to trauma

Fluid or electrolyte imbalance

Intake of teratogen such as a drug

Multiple gestation

A bleeding disruption

Poor placental formation or position

Gestational diabetes

Nutritional deficiency of iron, folic acid, or protein

Poor weight gain

Pregnancy-induced hypertension

Infection

Amniotic fluid abnormality

Postmaturity

Conception under 1 year from last pregnancy

(continued)

Box 14-1 (continued)

Labor and Delivery Period

Severely frightened by labor and delivery experience

Lack of participation due to anesthesia

Separation of infant at birth

Lack of preparation for labor

Delivery of infant who is disappointing in some way (e.g., sex, appearance, or congenital anomalies)

Illness in newborn

Lack of support person

Inadequate home for infant care

Unplanned cesarean birth

Lack of access to continued health care

Lack of access to emergency personnel or equipment

Hemorrhage

Infection

Fluid and electrolyte imbalance

Dystocia

Precipitous delivery

Lacerations of cervix or vagina

Celphalopelvic disproportion

Induced labor

Internal fetal monitoring

Anesthesia, analgesia

Forceps delivery (other than outlet)

Retained placenta

Cesarean birth

---

infection, or thrush, in the newborn (see Chapter 43). A number of over-the-counter preparations are available for candidiasis. Caution pregnant women to telephone their primary health care provider before using one of these products to be certain the product will be safe during pregnancy and so the primary care provider can know that vaginal infections are occurring.

The Woman With Trichomoniasis

Trichomonas vaginalis is a single-cell protozoan spread by coitus. The woman notices a yellow-gray frothy vaginal discharge (Heine & McGregor, 1993). It is diagnosed by appearance on a wet slide which has been treated with potassium hydroxide (KOH). It is important that trichomoniasis infections are identified because they are possibly associated with preterm labor, preterm premature rupture of membranes, and postcesarean infection.

The drug of choice for the disorder, metronidazole (Flagyl), is possibly teratogenic during the first trimester of pregnancy. Thus, the disorder is usually not treated until the second trimester.

The Woman With Bacterial Vaginosis (Gardnerella Infection)

Bacterial vaginosis is local infection of the vagina by the invasion, most commonly, of *Gardnerella* or *mobilumus curtsii* organisms (Hill, 1993). The associated discharge is gray and has a fish-like odor. Pruritus may be intense. The treatment for nonpregnant women is metronidazole (Flagyl). Because this is not recommended during the first trimester of pregnancy, women are usually treated with ampicillin or amoxicillin during this time. Assure

women that these are safe drugs to take during pregnancy so that they will finish the full prescription. Untreated bacterial infections are associated with amniotic fluid infections and, perhaps, preterm labor.

The Woman With Chlamydia Trachomatis

A *chlamydia* infection is the most common vaginal infection seen during pregnancy (Blackburn, 1992). All women are usually screened for this by a vaginal culture at their first prenatal visit and, if they are from a high-risk population (i.e., have had multiple sexual partners), they are screened again in the third trimester. The infection causes a heavy, gray-white vaginal discharge. Diagnosis is made by culture of the organism. Therapy for nonpregnant women is tetracycline. This is contraindicated in pregnancy because of possible long bone deformities; erythromycin or amoxicillin are used instead. There is a high association between gonorrhea and chlamydia; therefore, if a chlamydia infection is documented, women are usually cultured for gonorrhea as well.

Chlamydia infections are associated with premature rupture of the membranes, preterm labor, and endometritis in the postpartal period. An infant who is born while a chlamydia infection is present in the vagina can suffer from conjunctivitis or pneumonia following birth (see Chapter 40).

The Woman With Syphilis

Syphilis is a systemic disease caused by the spirochete *Treponema pallidum* that, unlike most diseases, is currently increasing in frequency in the United States (Berry & Dajani, 1992). The first stage of syphilis results in a painless ulcer (chancre) on the vulva or vagina. Early in pregnancy (before week 18), the placenta appears impervious to the disease organism. Following this, however, the spirochete crosses the placenta freely and may be responsible for preterm labor, stillbirth, or congenital anomalies in the newborn (Donders et al., 1993) (see Chapter 26). All pregnant women are screened for syphilis at the first prenatal visit by a VDRL, RPR, or FTA-ABS antibody reaction test, and those who have a lifestyle that includes multiple sexual partners are tested again at about week 36 of pregnancy. In most institutions, women are screened once again at the beginning of labor. In some institutions newborns are also screened for congenital syphilis by a cord blood sample. One injection of benzathine penicillin G is the drug of choice for the treatment of syphilis. This drug is safely administered during pregnancy.

Following therapy, the woman may experience a sudden episode of hypotension, fever, tachycardia, and muscle aches. This is called a Jarisch-Herxheimer reaction and is caused by the sudden destruction of spirochetes. The reaction lasts about 24 hours and then fades (Eschenbach, 1990).

The Woman With a Herpes (Herpes Simplex Virus Type 2) Infection

Genital herpes infection (HSV) is a sexually transmitted disease caused by the herpes simplex virus type 2. The woman develops painful, small, pinpoint vesicles surrounded by erythema on the vulva or in the vagina 3 to 7 days following exposure. There may be a genetic susceptibility to the herpes virus, so some women are more prone to infection than others (Shornick, 1993).

Herpes can be transmitted across the placenta to cause congenital infection in the newborn or it can be transmitted at birth if lesions are present at that time in the vagina or on the vulva (Jenkins & Kohl, 1992). Congenital herpes in the newborn results in a severe systemic infection that is often fatal (see Chapter 26). To avoid this second form of transmission, women with active lesions are scheduled for a cesarean birth.

Diagnosis is made by the appearance of the lesions, Pap smear, and enzyme linked immunosorbent assay (ELISA). The drug of choice for the treatment of herpes infection, acyclovir (Zovirax), is contraindicated during pregnancy because its effects on fetal growth are not yet documented (Loeb, 1993); it may be prescribed on an experimental basis. Women can reduce the pain of the infection by sitz baths. Because herpes simplex virus type 2 infections are associated with the development of cervical cancer, women who have had one episode of infection should be conscientious about having yearly Pap tests for the remainder of their life.

The Woman With Gonorrhea

Gonorrhea is a sexually transmitted disease caused by the gram-negative coccus *Neisseria gonorrhoeae*. It may not produce symptoms in women or a yellow-green vaginal discharge may be present. The male partner usually has severe symptoms of pain on urination and a purulent penile discharge. It is presently being spread at an epidemic rate among young adults.

Gonorrhea is associated with spontaneous abortion, preterm birth, and endometritis in the postpartal period (Gabbe et al., 1991). It is a cause of pelvic infectious disease (PID) and infertility. Diagnosis is made by culture of the organism from the vagina, rectum, or urethra. Although gonorrhea has traditionally been treated with amoxicillin and probenecid, the incidence of penicillinase-producing strains has made this traditional therapy ineffective. Ceftriaxone IM is therefore now the drug of choice (Cunningham et al., 1993) and can be administered during pregnancy (pregnancy risk category B). A sexual partner should be treated as well to prevent reinfection.

It is important that gonorrhea be identified and treated during pregnancy because if the infection is present at the time of birth, it can cause a severe eye infection that can lead to blindness in the newborn (ophthalmia neonatorum; see Chapter 26).

The Woman With Human Papilloma Virus Infection

The human papilloma virus (HPV) causes fibrous tissue overgrowth on the external vulva (condyloma acuminatum). It tends to occur in about 1% of women and most often in women who have chronic vaginitis and long-term vulvar irritation. It is spread by sexual contact (Nettina & Kauffman, 1990). At first, lesions appear as discrete papillary structures, which then spread, enlarge, and coalesce to form large, cauliflower-like lesions. These tend to increase in size during pregnancy because of the high vascular flow in the pelvic area. They may become secondarily ulcerated and infected; when this occurs a foul vulvar odor may develop.

Therapy for such lesions is aimed at dissolving the lesions and also ending any secondary infection present. Podophyllum applied directly to lesions is the drug of choice for nonpregnant women but is contraindicated during pregnancy because of fetal toxic effects. Trichloroacetic acid applied to the lesions three times weekly may be effective and can be applied during pregnancy. Large lesions may be removed by laser therapy, cryocautery, or knife excision. With cryocautery, edema at the site is evident immediately; lesions become gangrenous and sloughing occurs in 7 days. Healing will be complete in 4 to 6 weeks with only slight depigmentation at the site. Sitz baths and a lidocaine cream may be soothing during the healing period. Unless they are bothersome, lesions may be left in place during pregnancy and removed during the postpartal period.

The presence of vulvar lesions appears to have no effect on the fetus during pregnancy but if they are present at the time of birth, a cesarean may be performed to avoid exposure of the fetus to the virus in the birth canal. An exposed infant can develop lesions in the throat and trachea, possibly causing respiratory obstruction (Smith et al., 1991). Lesions may physically interfere with vaginal birth if they obstruct the vaginal orifice; they may also interfere with episiotomy. Human papilloma virus infections are serious infections because they are associated with the development of cervical cancer later in life. Women who have had one episode of infection should be conscientious about having yearly Pap tests for the rest of their lives.

The Woman With a Group B Streptococci Infection

Although a less publicized disease than STDs such as herpes type 2 or gonorrhea, streptococcus B infection perhaps occurs at a higher incidence during pregnancy than those diseases or in as high as 10% to 30% of pregnant women (Dinsmoor, 1990). When the infection develops, the mother usually experiences no symptoms. Consequences can be urinary tract infection, intraamniotic infection, and postpartal endometritis. Approximately 40% to 70% of neonates whose mothers have an active infection will become infected from placental transferral or from direct contact with the organisms at birth. Infected neonates develop severe pneumonia or meningitis (see Chapter 26).

Women who are at high risk (i.e., who have had multiple sex partners or previous infection) may be screened for the infection at 38 weeks of pregnancy by a vaginal culture and treated with a broad spectrum penicillin.

The Woman With Human Immunodeficiency Virus (HIV) Infection

HIV, which leads to acquired immunodeficiency syndrome (AIDS), is the most serious of the STDs as it may be fatal to both mother and child. Women are contracting this at much faster rates than formerly and in many areas they are the fastest growing category of HIV-infected persons. About 1.5 out of every 1000 women giving birth is HIV positive (ACOG, 1992).

The disease is caused by a retrovirus that infects T-lymphocytes. This disables the body's ability to fight infection through either T-cell or B-cell activity (see Chapter 42). It may be contracted through sexual inter-

course, by exposure to infected blood, by vertical transmission across the placenta to the fetus at birth, or by breast milk to the newborn. Women at greatest risk are those who have multiple sexual partners or a sexual partner who has multiple partners, use intravenous drugs, have a sexual partner who is a drug user, or engage in prostitution (Smith & Lathrop, 1993).

Assessment

Unlike other STDs, HIV rarely begins with reproductive tract irritation. Instead, early symptoms are more subtle and often difficult to differentiate from other diseases or even from the symptoms of early pregnancy (e.g., fatigue, anemia, diarrhea, and weight loss) (De Ferrari et al., 1993) (see the Nursing Care Plan: A Woman Who Is HIV Positive).

HIV infection progresses through various stages from the initial invasion of the virus (perhaps accompanied by mild, flu-like symptoms); seroconversion (the woman converts from HIV serum negative to HIV serum positive 6–12 weeks after exposure); an asymptomatic latency period in which the woman appears to be disease free except for symptoms such as weight loss and fatigue (a wasting syndrome); and finally a symptomatic period in which the woman develops opportunistic infections and malignancies (such as toxoplasmosis, oral and vaginal candidiasis, gastrointestinal illness, herpes simplex, pneumocystis carinii pneumonia, candida esophagitis, Kaposi's sarcoma, and HIV-associated dementia). Ordinarily, toxoplasmosis presents with few symptoms; in the HIV positive woman, it may invade cerebral spinal fluid and cause extreme neurologic involvement. Cervical dysplasia and the incidence of cervical cancer increases (Cohn, 1993). There is no clear evidence that pregnancy accelerates the progression of HIV (De Ferrari et al., 1993).

Although women are not as yet routinely screened for this infection during pregnancy (as a rule, no screening program is initiated for any disease until there is a cure for the disease), women who practice high-risk behaviors are usually asked if they want to be screened. The woman with HIV may also have contracted other STDs such as syphilis, gonorrhea, chlamydia, and hepatitis B, and so should be screened for these as well. Because women are also high risk for the development of toxoplasmosis and cytomegalovirus infections, a history should include questions on cat ownership and mild, flu-like symptoms (see Chapter 9). Tuberculosis occurs at a higher rate in people with HIV than others, and may grow worse during pregnancy; thus, a test for this should also be included.

Testing for HIV is done by an ELISA antibody reaction; for confirmation, a Western blot analysis is required. If women are found to be HIV positive (have been exposed to the virus), the issues of safer sex practices, testing of sexual contacts, and continuation or termination of the pregnancy need to be addressed. HIV is associated with low-birth-weight and preterm birth. Preliminary statistics indicate that from 20% to 50% of infants born to HIV-positive women develop AIDS in the 1st year of life. The more serious the mother's disease symptoms, the more apt placental transmission is to occur (De Ferreri, 1993). Therapy with AZT may reduce the possibility of placental transmission (Luzuriaga & Sullivan, 1994).

A CD4 cell count is the laboratory test for functioning lymphocytes. CD4 molecules are found on the surface of T-helper and B cell lymphocytes. The number of CD4 sites present should normally equal the number of functioning lymphocytes present. CD4 molecules are necessary for the HIV virus to bind to and gain entry to cells. Inside the cell, the virus lies dormant for years. When proliferation does begin, the cell can no longer function and dies, leaving fewer CD4 sites present in the blood stream. Normally the CD4 levels fall during pregnancy, possibly as a natural protection against placental rejection. A count less than 300 cells/mm^3 suggests severe immunological compromise or HIV infection.

Therapeutic Management

Women who are identified as HIV positive are usually advised not to become pregnant until more is learned about how to prevent transmission to the fetus. Often, however, the existence of HIV is only discovered after pregnancy is already present. Because the woman does not have the usual response to antibiotics as a result of low lymphocyte levels, infections must be treated with stronger than usual antibiotics. The antiviral agent zidovudine (AZT), the drug of choice for the primary disorder, may be teratogenic (it is associated with polydactyly), but it is administered if a woman's CD4 count is below 200 mm^3 to prevent opportunistic infections, especially pneumocystis carinii pneumonia. AZT has side effects of thrombocytopenia and granulocytopenia from suppression of bone marrow. Some women may need a blood transfusion to help restore these levels (Tinkle et al., 1992). At birth, the infant needs to be assessed for this same suppression.

If pneumocystis carinii pneumonia (PCP) develops, the woman is treated with trimethoprim with sulfamethoxazole. Trimethoprim may be teratogenic in early pregnancy; sulfamethoxazole may lead to increased bilirubin in the newborn if administered late in pregnancy. Pentamidine, the drug of choice for PCP pneumonia in nonpregnant women, may be administered by aerosol.

Kaposi's sarcoma, a rare malignancy that tends to occur with AIDS, is normally treated with chemotherapy. Chemotherapy is contraindicated during early pregnancy because of the potential for fetal injury but is used later in pregnancy to halt these malignant growths.

Thrombocytopenia (lowered platelet count) may be present as a part of the disease pathology or as a response to AZT therapy. This may make the woman a poor candidate for an epidural injection for anesthesia during labor or episiotomy. She may need a platelet transfusion to restore coagulation ability.

Nursing Diagnoses and Related Interventions

Nursing Diagnosis: High risk for opportunistic infections and spread of illness to others through sexual relations or body fluids related to dysfunction of the immune system secondary to invasion of HIV

Goal: Client will not develop a severe opportunistic infection during the remainder of pregnancy; she will not knowingly be responsible for infection in another.

Outcome Criteria: CD4 counts remain above 500 mm^3; no symptoms of lung, vaginal, esophageal, or CNS infections are present. Client states she is using safer sex practices.

Women who are HIV positive need to be aware of the danger that they can spread this illness to others through unprotected sexual relations or unintentional contamination by blood.

Health care providers must take care to use universal infection control precautions (see Chapter 43) to protect against the spread of HIV. This includes the use of gloves when there is a possibility of contact with body secretions; cover gowns if clothing will be exposed to secretions; and at birth, when there may be splashing of amniotic fluid, goggles. The newborn should not be handled without the use of gloves until all maternal blood has been removed by a first bath.

Women who have CD4 counts below 200 mm^3 are usually administered drugs to help prevent opportunistic infections. Such drugs include acyclovir for herpes simplex, clotimazote troches for oral thrush, pyrimethamine and sulfadizone for toxoplasmosis, and trimethoprim with sulfamethoxazole for pneumocystis carinii pneumonia. They may be immunized against pneumonia, influenza, and hepatitis B.

During pregnancy and at birth, active interactions must be made to reduce the possibility that the fetus may be exposed to maternal blood. Amniocentesis presents a risk of this, so fetal age is determined by sonogram if possible, not amniocentesis. During labor, internal fetal monitors, scalp blood sampling, forceps, and vacuum extraction are avoided to prevent an open lesion on the fetal scalp.

The woman is at increased risk for infection if membranes rupture early, so these are usually not ruptured

Bonnie is a 19-year-old woman you care for in a prenatal clinic. She first came to the clinic last week at 30 weeks of pregnancy. Because she had frequent upper respiratory and vaginal infections for the past 3 months, she asked to be screened for HIV and was found to be HIV positive. She returned today to learn results of tests and for confirmation of pregnancy.

Assessment: Last menstrual period "about March 15th." Had bad nausea during April. Has had an episode of white, pruritic vaginal discharge almost every month since March. Has taken over-the-counter Monistat-7 with good relief each time. Has had frequent "colds" with sore throats and cough since about February. No pregnancy care because "I had other things to contend with."

Patient's parents were divorced when she was 8. Her mother remarried when she was 10. New father "didn't like her" so she ran away from home at age 13 years. Has lived "anywhere it's warm" and earned money by prostitution since then. Has used intravenous drugs since age 15. Current boyfriend (also an intravenous drug user) was tested last month and found to be HIV negative; but positive for syphilis. He received treatment for this; Bonnie has not.

Presently lives with boyfriend and one cat in two-room apartment. Boyfriend does not work because of post-traumatic stress disorder. Patient cried when told that the ELISA and Western blot antibody assays were positive for HIV and CD4 level was at $400/mm^3$. VDRL for syphilis is positive. Stated it was unfair her HIV result was positive if boyfriend's was negative. Stated, "He's no better than I am."

On physical exam, client has a white vaginal discharge and numerous herpes-like lesions on the vulva; mild cervical dysplasia is present.

Nursing Diagnosis: Anticipatory grieving related to positive result of HIV antibody titer.

Defining Characteristic: Client cried and was obviously sad at diagnosis of HIV.

Goal: Client will express grief and share feelings with others over coming weeks.

Outcome Criteria: Client expresses fears and feelings about HIV to nurse; states she is able to function effectively and maintain prenatal care even in face of grief.

Nursing Orders	*Rationale*
1. Client advised of HIV-positive status in meeting with clinic social worker, nurse, and physician.	1. Client asked to be informed of diagnosis.
2. Client was offered spiritual support through agency clergy service but this was declined. Client was encouraged to express her feelings about the diagnosis and what it means to her; continue to encourage this at future visits.	2. Expressing feelings can help her use adaptive coping mechanisms during a period of crisis.
3. Phases of usual grief response explained (denial, anger, depression).	3. Prevent client from feeling surprised by usual feelings of grief.

(continued)

artificially. If the woman is too fatigued to be able to push with the second stage of labor or if fetal distress occurs, a cesarean birth will be planned. There appears to be no increased incidence in the development of HIV in the newborn with cesarean over vaginal birth.

Postpartally, the woman needs to be assessed carefully for endometritis because she is at risk for contracting any type of infection; she is also at risk for developing anemia.

Breast milk may transmit HIV, so the woman is ad-

Nursing Orders	**Rationale**
4. Client urged to reveal diagnosis to boyfriend.	4. Boyfriend has a right to be informed of risk to himself.
5. Client supplied with health care facility and social worker's telephone number.	5. Providing a continuing source of information and support is important to care during pregnancy.

Nursing Diagnosis: High risk for opportunistic infections related to lowered resistance to disease secondary to CD4 level of 400/mm^3.

Defining Characteristic: Client is documented as HIV positive with low CD4 count and positive for syphilis by VDRL.

Goal: Client's number of opportunistic infections will be kept to a minimum during pregnancy.

Outcome Criteria: Client tests negative for syphilis and *Candida* infection at next prenatal visit; no additional symptoms of infections are present.

Nursing Orders	**Rationale**
1. Administer benzathine penicillin G 2.4 million units intramuscularly per protocol as syphilis therapy.	1. Therapy for eradication of syphilis.
2. Teach client regarding insertion of miconazole nitrate (Monistat) vaginal suppositories two times daily for 10 days to help prevent vaginal yeast infections.	2. Therapy for candidiasis.
3. Suggest oral acetaminophen and warm sitz baths to promote comfort and healing of herpes lesions; given prescription for acyclovir.	3. Therapy and pain relief for herpes lesions.
4. Refer client to department of medicine for medical consult to evaluate illness fully.	4. Client needs HIV status fully evaluated.
5. Provide information on safer-sex practices such as necessity for boyfriend to use condom for coitus.	5. Client is HIV positive and sexual partner is HIV negative.
6. Discuss legal and ethical necessity of no longer engaging in prostitution. Referral made to social services to secure an additional source of finances in place of this.	6. Continuing prostitution exposes clients to the virus.
7. Advise client to attempt to avoid people with obvious infections in everyday contacts.	7. Client will be more prone than usual to contracting any infection.
8. Advise client not to change cat litter.	8. Client is now at high risk for toxoplasmosis.
9. Advise client to telephone health care agency at first sign of fever, cough, or other suggestions of infection.	9. Client can secure prompt therapy.
10. Teach client symptoms of ruptured membranes and encourage her to notify health care agency promptly if this should occur.	10. Ruptured membranes will put her at high risk for amnionitis.

vised not to breast-feed her infant (Porcher, 1992). Breast-feeding could also be exhausting for a debilitated woman.

Caring for the woman who is HIV positive during pregnancy and childbirth calls for great sensitivity to re-spect the woman as a patient with a baffling yet fatal disease yet encourage her to continue with prenatal care in the hope that prenatal transmission to the fetus will not occur. In most states, the confidentiality of persons with the disease must be preserved. Sexual contacts of a woman cannot be notified they may have been exposed without permission of the woman.

Hematologic Disorders and Pregnancy

Hematologic disorders during pregnancy involve either blood formation or coagulation disorders.

Anemia and Pregnancy

Because the blood volume expands during pregnancy slightly ahead of the red cell count, most women have a pseudoanemia of early pregnancy. This is normal and should not be confused with the true anemia that can occur as a complication of pregnancy.

Nursing Diagnoses and Related Interventions

> ***Nursing Diagnosis:*** High risk for altered tissue perfusion related to maternal anemia during pregnancy
>
> ***Goal:*** Client will take adequate measures to guard against anemia during pregnancy and experience adequate tissue perfusion during pregnancy.
>
> ***Outcome Criteria:*** Client takes prenatal supplement daily; hemoglobin is above 11 mg/dL; fetal heart rate is 120 to 160 bpm.

The Woman With Iron Deficiency Anemia

Iron deficiency anemia complicates as many as 15% to 25% of all pregnancies; it occurs in as many as 40% of pregnant African American women (Cruikshank, 1990). Many women enter pregnancy with an iron deficiency anemia which has resulted from poor diet, heavy menstrual periods, or unwise weight-reducing programs. As a rule, the average woman needs to depend on iron stores to supply enough iron for pregnancy. Iron stores are apt to be low if there was a short period (under 2 years) between pregnancies. Low iron stores and iron deficiency anemia are both strongly correlated with poverty (DHHS, 1992). When the hemoglobin level is below 11 mg/dL (hematocrit under 33%), iron deficiency is suspected.

Iron is made available to the body by absorption from the duodenum into the blood stream where it is bound to transferrin for transport to the liver, spleen, and bone marrow. At these sites it is incorporated into hemoglobin or stored as ferritin.

Iron deficiency anemia is characteristically a *microcytic* (small-sized red blood cell), *hypochromic* (less hemoglobin than the average red cell) anemia, because when an adequate supply of iron is not ingested, iron is unavailable for incorporation into red blood cells and so cells are not as large or as rich in hemoglobin as normally (Hoffman, 1993). Both hematocrit and hemoglobin will be reduced (under 33% and 11 g/dL, respec-

tively). Serum ferritin will be under 10 *ug*/L, transferrin saturation level will be under 16%, serum iron will be under 30 *ug*/dL, and mean corpuscular hemoglobin concentration (MCHC) will be under 30; iron-binding capacity, in contrast, will be increased (over 400 *ug*/dL). Iron deficiency anemia is associated with low fetal birth weight and preterm birth. Because the body recognizes it needs increased nutrients, some women develop pica or the eating of substances such as ice or starch. The woman experiences extreme fatigue and poor exercise tolerance.

All women should take prenatal vitamins that contain an iron supplement of 60 mg of elemental iron as prophylactic therapy against iron deficiency anemia during pregnancy; those with iron deficiency anemia will be prescribed therapeutic levels of medication (120 to 180 mg of elemental iron/day). This is usually prescribed as ferrous sulfate 325 mg orally T.I.D. with vitamin C 500 mg orally once a day. Iron is best absorbed in an acid medium so women should take iron supplements with orange juice. In addition, they need to maintain a high iron and vitamin intake. If they are not already enrolled in a WIC program and are eligible, a referral should be made. If women are taking a prescribed iron supplement, new red blood cells should begin to increase in proportion or a reticulocyte count should rise from a normal of between 0.5% and 1.5% to between 3% and 4% by 2 weeks' time.

If iron deficiency anemia is severe and a woman is noncompliant with oral iron therapy, this can be administered as iron-dextran IM or IV (Cruikshank, 1990).

The Woman With Folic Acid Deficiency Anemia

Folic acid deficiency anemia is seen in 1% to 5% of pregnancies. It occurs most often in multiple pregnancies because of the increased fetal demand; in those with a secondary hemolytic illness in which there is rapid destruction and production of red blood cells; and in women who are taking hydantoin, a drug that interferes with folate absorption. This is a **megaloblastic anemia** (enlarged red blood cells). The mean corpuscular volume (MCV) will be elevated, in contrast to the lowered level seen with iron deficiency anemia. Folic acid deficiency is apparently responsible for neural tube defects (Repke, 1992) and may be responsible for early abortion or abruptio placentae (premature separation of the placenta). The deficiency may take a number of weeks to develop so often becomes most apparent during the second trimester of pregnancy.

Over-the-counter multivitamin preparations generally do not contain adequate folic acid for pregnancy, whereas vitamins specifically designed for pregnancy, such as Natalins or Stuart-Natels, do. Ask at prenatal visits whether a woman is taking her prescribed vitamin source. To save money, women may not have a prescription filled and may be using over-the-counter, less expensive types, not aware of the difference.

The Woman With Sickle Cell Anemia

Sickle cell anemia is a recessively inherited hemolytic anemia caused by an abnormal amino acid in the beta chain of hemoglobin. If there is a substitution in place of the amino acid valine, sickle hemoglobin (HbS) results; if lysine is substituted, nonsickling hemoglobin (HbC) results. An individual who is heterozygous (has only one gene in which the abnormal substitution has occurred) has the sickle cell trait (HbAS). If the person is homozygous (has two genes in which the substitution has occurred), sickle cell disease (HbSS) results.

Approximately 1 in every 10 African-Americans has the sickle cell *trait*—that is, carries a recessive gene for S hemoglobin but is asymptomatic; 1 in every 400 African-American women theoretically has the disease. The sickle cell trait does not appear to influence the course of pregnancy in terms of pregnancy-induced hypertension, prematurity, abortion, or perinatal mortality. Women with the trait do seem to have an increased incidence of asymptomatic bacteriuria, however, resulting in an increased incidence of pyelonephritis. They should be certain to take the regular iron and folic acid supplement during pregnancy to build new red blood cells. Clean-catch urine should be collected periodically during pregnancy to attempt to detect developing bacteriuria while it is still asymptomatic.

Pregnancy can be a severe complication for the woman with sickle cell *disease* (Perry & Morrison, 1990). With the disease, the majority of red blood cells are irregular or sickle shaped. They can not carry as much hemoglobin as normally shaped red blood cells. When oxygen tension is reduced, as happens at high altitudes, or blood becomes more viscid than usual (dehydration), the cells tend to clump because of the irregular shape. This clumping results in blockage of vessels and infarcts of organs. The cells will then hemolyze. At any time in life, sickle cell anemia is a threat to life if vital blood vessels such as those to the liver, kidneys, heart, lungs, or brain are blocked. In pregnancy, blockage to the placental circulation can lead to direct fetal compromise with low birth weight and possibly death.

Early in pregnancy when the woman may be nauseated, her fluid intake may decrease and dehydration then becomes a real possibility. Pooling of blood in the lower extremities because of uterine pressure may take place as pregnancy advances, leading to red cell destruction. If the woman develops an infection that raises her temperature and causes her to perspire more than normally (creates dehydration) or contracts a respiratory infection that compromises air exchange so that her PO_2 is lowered, she will be hospitalized for observation until it is established that she is not beginning a sickle cell crisis and hemolysis of crowded cells has not begun. All during pregnancy, the woman with sickle cell anemia should be asked how well she is eating (she must include enough fluid—at least eight glasses daily) and whether she is standing for long periods during the day.

She needs always to rest with her legs elevated when sitting in a chair; lying on her side in a modified Sims' position is even better because it encourages venous return from the lower extremities.

Assessment. A woman with sickle cell disease may normally have a hemoglobin level of 6 to 8 mg per 100 mL, a level she will maintain during pregnancy unless it is corrected. Hemolysis in a sickle cell crisis may occur so rapidly that her hemoglobin level can fall to 5 to 6 mg per 100 mL in a few hours. There is an accompanying rise in her indirect bilirubin level because she cannot conjugate the bilirubin released from red blood cells so quickly destroyed. She is 4 to 6 times more susceptible to preeclampsia and urinary tract infection than others so needs urine tested for protein and organisms at all prenatal visits.

Fetal health will be monitored during pregnancy by an ultrasound exam at 16 to 24 weeks to assess for intrauterine growth retardation and weekly nonstress or ultrasound exams beginning at 30 weeks. Blood flow through the uterus and placenta may be measured by blood flow velocity. If blood flow velocity is reduced, the chance of intrauterine growth retardation is increased (Billett et al., 1993).

Therapeutic Management. Interventions to prevent sickle cell crisis can include replacing sickle cells with normal cells by exchange transfusion periodically throughout pregnancy. An exchange transfusion serves a secondary purpose of removing a quantity of the increased bilirubin level as well as restoring hemoglobin level. If a crisis occurs, controlling pain, administering oxygen as needed, and increasing the fluid volume of the circulatory system to lower viscosity are important interventions (see Chapter 44 for further discussion of therapy of sickle cell anemia). Fluid administered is often hypotonic (0.45 saline) to keep plasma tension low because of the difficulty the woman has concentrating urine to remove large amounts. Women with sickle cell disease are not given an iron supplement during pregnancy as a rule. The cells cannot incorporate iron as can normal cells, and therefore an excessive iron buildup may result. Women do need a folic acid supplement to keep new cells produced from being megaloblastic.

When the fetus is mature, birth must be individualized. The woman must be kept well hydrated in labor. If an operative birth is necessary, she generally receives nerve block anesthesia rather than a general anesthetic to avoid anoxia.

Women generally are interested in determining at birth whether the child has inherited the disease. Because the disorder is recessively inherited, with one of the parents having the disease and the other free of the trait, the chances that the child will inherit the disease are zero. If one parent has the disease and the partner has the trait, the chances that the child will be born with the disease are 50% (see Chapter 7).

Symptoms of sickle cell disease do not become clinically apparent until the child's hemoglobin converts to a largely adult pattern (in 3 to 6 months). Fetal hemoglobin comprises two alpha and two gamma chains; adult hemoglobin comprises two alpha and two beta chains. Because the sickle cell trait is carried on the beta chain, it will not be manifested clinically until this chain appears. Electrophoresis of red blood cells during fetal life by percutaneous umbilical blood sampling or amniocentesis and at birth will reveal the manifestation of the disease on the few beta chains present (infants have approximately 15% adult hemoglobin at birth). Nursing care of the child with sickle cell disease is discussed in . Chapter 44.

Coagulation Disorders and Pregnancy

Most coagulation disorders are sex linked, or only occur in males. Von Willebrand's disease is a coagulation disorder that does occur in women as it is inherited as an autosomal dominant trait. The woman has symptoms of menorrhagia and frequent episodes of epistaxis. If the symptoms are not severe, a woman may be undiagnosed until pregnancy when she experiences a spontaneous abortion or else experiences postpartal hemorrhage.

Women with the disorder have normal platelet counts but bleeding time is prolonged. Factor VIII related antigen (VIII-R) and factor VIII coagulation activity (VIII-C) are both reduced. Replacement of these factors by infusion of cryoprecipitate or fresh frozen plasma may be necessary before labor to prevent excessive bleeding.

Hemophilia B (Christmas disease, factor IX deficiency) is a sex-linked disorder, so the actual disease occurs only in males. Female carriers may have such a reduced level of factor IX (only 33% of normal), however, that hemorrhage with labor or with a spontaneous abortion can be a serious complication. Carriers of the disorder need to be identified prior to pregnancy. Restoration of factor IX levels can be done by infusion of factor IX concentrate or fresh frozen plasma.

With these disorders, whether a male fetus has the disease can be detected by percutaneous umbilical blood sampling (Shipley & Nelson, 1993). Before an internal fetal heart rate monitor or fetal scalp blood sampling is done during labor, the child's status needs to be determined. Otherwise the procedures could result in extensive fetal blood loss.

Renal and Urinary Disorders and Pregnancy

Adequate kidney function is important to successful pregnancy outcome; any condition that interferes with kidney or urinary function is potentially serious.

The Woman With a Urinary Tract Infection

As many as 4% to 10% of nonpregnant women have asymptomatic bacteriuria (organisms are present without symptoms of infection). Symptomatic urinary tract infections occur in as many as 10% to 15% of pregnancies (Cruikshank, 1990). In the pregnant woman, because of the dilated ureters from the effect of progesterone, stasis of urine occurs and asymptomatic infections can flame into pyelonephritis (infection of the pelvis of the kidney). The minimal glucosuria that occurs with pregnancy contributes to the growth of organisms. Women with known vesicoureteral reflux often develop a UTI or pyelonephritis more often than others. An increased incidence of preterm labor; preterm, premature rupture of membranes; and fetal loss may be associated with pyelonephritis. The organism most commonly responsible for urinary tract infection is *Escherichia coli* from an ascending infection (Johnson, 1990). A urinary tract infection can also occur as a descending infection or begin in the kidneys from the filtration of organisms present from other body infections. If the infectious organism is determined to be streptococcus B, vaginal cultures should be obtained as streptococcal B infection is associated with pneumonia in newborns.

Assessment

With pyelonephritis, the woman notices pain in the lumbar region (usually on the right side) that radiates downward. The area is tender to palpation. She may have accompanying nausea and vomiting, malaise, pain, and frequency of urination. Her temperature may be elevated only slightly or may be as high as 103°F to 104°F (39°C to 40°C). The infection usually occurs on the right side because the uterus is pushed to that side by the large bulk of the intestine on the left side. This greater compression on the right ureter creates greater stasis on that side. A urine culture will reveal over 100,000 organisms per mL of urine.

Therapeutic Management

A clean-catch urine should be obtained for culture and sensitivity (see Nursing Procedure 10-1). Many health care agencies ask women for clean-catch urine specimens at intervals during pregnancy (tested by a rapid dip-stick method) to detect infection before it becomes symptomatic. A sensitivity test following a culture will determine which antibiotic will be prescribed. Amoxicillin, ampicillin, and cephalosporins are effective against most organisms causing urinary tract infection and are safe antibiotics for pregnancy. The sulfonamides are used early in pregnancy but not near term because they interfere with protein binding of bilirubin, which could lead to hyperbilirubinemia in the newborn. Tetracyclines are contraindicated in pregnancy; they cause retardation of bone growth and staining of the fetal teeth (Loeb, 1993).

Nursing Diagnoses and Related Interventions

Nursing Diagnosis: High risk for infection related to stasis of urine with pregnancy

Goal: Client will demonstrate no signs of infection during pregnancy.

Outcome Criteria: Oral temperature is below 38°C and a clean-catch urine specimen has a bacteria count below 100,000 colonies per mL.

All women during pregnancy can be reminded of common measures to prevent UTIs, such as voiding frequently; wiping front to back after bowel movements; wearing cotton, not synthetic fiber underwear; and voiding following sexual intercourse. The pregnant woman with a urinary tract infection needs to take some measures in addition to this such as drinking additional fluid to flush out the infection from the kidney. Do not merely tell her to "push fluids" or "drink lots of water." Give her a specific amount to drink every day (up to 3 to 4 L per 24 h), to make certain that her fluid intake will be sufficiently increased.

A woman can promote urine drainage by assuming a knee-chest position for 15 minutes morning and evening. In this position, the weight of the uterus is shifted forward, freeing the ureter for drainage.

If the woman has one urinary tract infection during pregnancy, the chance that she will develop another late in pregnancy is high. She may therefore be kept on prophylactic antibiotics throughout the remainder of the pregnancy. Ask at prenatal visits whether she is continuing to take this type of prophylactic medicine. When women have pain and symptoms of urinary frequency, they take medication well. When they no longer have any clinical evidence that they are sick, their compliance rate begins to fall dramatically. A woman may need to post a chart on her refrigerator door or in her bathroom to remind herself to take this kind of medication. Leaving the medicine on a counter to remind herself to take it is not a good habit to develop. Shortly, she will have a new baby in the house. Encourage her to keep medicine out of sight and reach to get into the habit of "childproofing" at this early stage. The woman who develops pyelonephritis will be hospitalized and treated with intravenous antibiotics. Following this acute episode, she may be maintained on oral nitrofurantoin for the remainder of the pregnancy. Acidifying urine by the use of ascorbic acid, which is often recommended in nonpregnant women, is not recommended during pregnancy as the newborn can develop scurvy in the immediate neonatal period from withdrawal. Following birth, the woman who developed more than one urinary tract infection may have an intravenous pyelogram scheduled to help detect any urinary tract abnormality that might be present to help prevent future infections.

The Woman With Chronic Renal Disease

In the past, children with chronic renal disease did not reach childbearing age or were advised not to have children because of the high risk for them during pregnancy. Today, women with chronic renal disease are having children as pregnancy does not appear to cause progressive deterioration of kidney lesions. Children even have been born to women who have had renal transplants.

Pregnancy increases the workload on the kidneys because the woman's kidneys must excrete waste products not only for herself but for the fetus for 40 weeks. Many women with renal disease take a corticosteroid (prednisone) at a maintenance level, and they should continue to do so throughout pregnancy. Although reports of animal studies have demonstrated an increased incidence of cleft palate from the taking of corticosteroids during pregnancy, this does not appear to happen in humans. The infant may be hyperglycemic at birth because of the suppression of insulin activity by corticosteroids. Infants of women with chronic renal disease tend to have intrauterine growth retardation from lessened placental perfusion. Women may develop severe anemia because of lack of erythropoietin by their diseased kidneys. Fortunately, synthetic erythropoietin is now available and can be administered safety to pregnant women (Hou et al., 1993).

It is difficult to interpret kidney function during pregnancy based on nonpregnant values (Figure 14-2). Many women spill a trace of glucose and protein during pregnancy because of increased glomerular permeability. If the woman is told about this possibility, she will understand that it is an expected change of pregnancy, not a forecast of changing kidney function. Many women with renal disease have elevated blood pressure; the woman's blood pressure level during pregnancy must therefore be compared with prepregnancy levels as well as the normal level to be meaningful (Ferris, 1990). Proteinuria must also be compared to a prepregnancy level to be meaningful.

Because the glomerular filtration rate normally increases during pregnancy, a woman is able to clear waste products for both herself and the fetus from her body with such efficiency that her serum creatinine level is actually slightly below normal during pregnancy. Normal serum creatinine is 0.7 mg per 100 mL; during pregnancy, it falls to about 0.5 mg per 100 mL. Women with kidney disease who normally have an elevated serum creatinine level more than 2.0 mg/dL probably should not undertake a pregnancy or the increased strain on already damaged kidneys may lead to kidney failure (Reveille, 1990).

Women with kidney transplants should be considered individually to determine whether they will be able to carry a pregnancy to term before a pregnancy is initiated. Criteria that should be evaluated are the woman's general health and the time since the transplant (prefer-

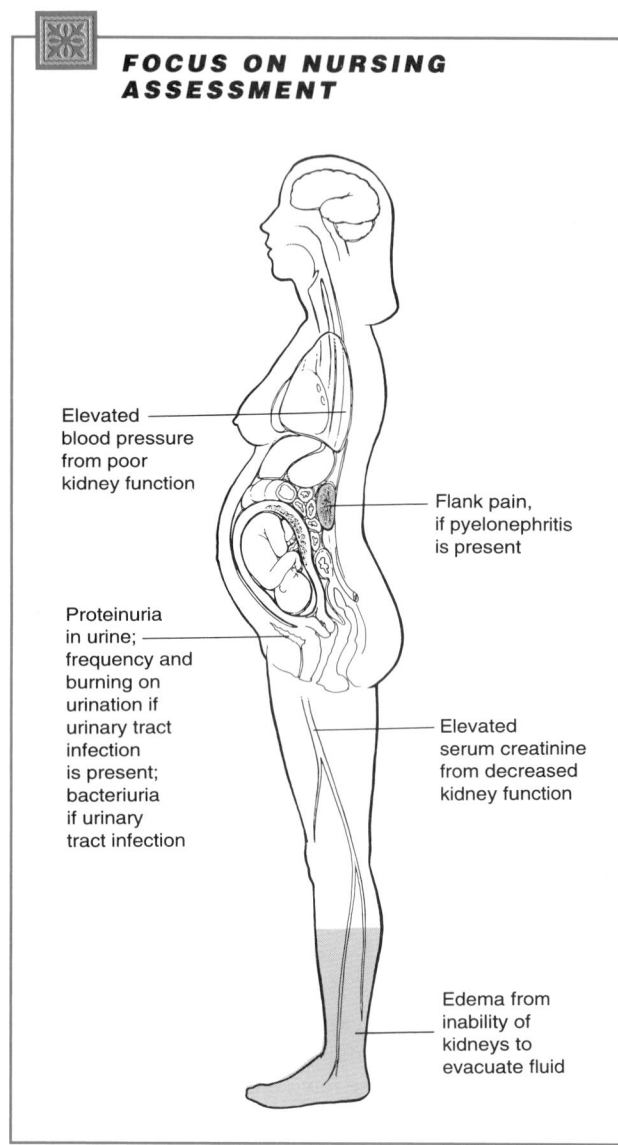

FOCUS ON NURSING ASSESSMENT

Elevated blood pressure from poor kidney function

Flank pain, if pyelonephritis is present

Proteinuria in urine; frequency and burning on urination if urinary tract infection is present; bacteriuria if urinary tract infection

Elevated serum creatinine from decreased kidney function

Edema from inability of kidneys to evacuate fluid

FIGURE 14-2
Symptoms of renal disease in pregnancy.

ably more than 2 years); whether she has proteinuria, signs of graft rejection, or hypertension; her level of serum creatinine; and whether she is taking medication to reduce graft rejection. If the drugs she is taking are limited to prednisone and azathioprine (an antimetabolite, but with no reports of fetal compromise from its use), pregnancy may be possible. Women with severe renal disease may require dialysis to aid kidney function during pregnancy. This is associated with a risk of preterm labor, perhaps because progesterone is removed with the dialysis. To prevent this complication, women may be administered IM progesterone before dialysis. If hemodialysis is used, it should be scheduled frequently and for short durations to avoid acute fluid shifts. The heparin administered in connection with hemodialysis is safe during pregnancy as it does not cross the placenta. Peritoneal dialysis is actually preferred because it normally causes less drastic fluid shifts. This can

be accomplished on an ambulatory basis (continuous ambulatory peritoneal dialysis) throughout pregnancy (Lew & Watson, 1992).

Women with renal disease need a great deal of support during pregnancy. They are aware that kidneys are vital for life and that the stress of pregnancy on damaged kidneys may cause them to fail. They are aware that they are risking not only the life of the child growing inside them but their own. They may need extra time with their infant at birth for bonding because they may have been too concerned during pregnancy to begin bonding. They may need extra assurance that the baby is well.

Respiratory Disorders and Pregnancy

Respiratory diseases range from the mild, such as the common cold, to the severe, such as active tuberculosis. Chronic respiratory conditions may worsen in pregnancy because the rising uterus compresses lung space just when increased lung function is needed to provide adequate oxygen exchange for the fetus and mother. Any respiratory disorder can pose serious hazards to the fetus if allowed to progress to the point where the mother's oxygen-carbon dioxide exchange is altered.

Nursing Diagnoses and Related Interventions

> ***Nursing Diagnosis:*** High risk for ineffective breathing pattern related to respiratory disorder during pregnancy
>
> ***Goal:*** Client will not experience a significantly altered breathing pattern during pregnancy.
>
> ***Outcome Criteria:*** Respiratory rate is between 16 and 20 per minute, PO_2 above 80 mm Hg, PCO_2 below 40 mm Hg, and fetal heart rate at 120 to 160 bpm with good variability.

The Woman With Acute Nasopharyngitis

Acute nasopharyngitis (common cold) tends to be more severe during pregnancy than otherwise. With pregnancy, there is normally some degree of nasal congestion due to estrogen stimulation. With even a minor cold, therefore, the woman finds it difficult to breathe. Women should be cautioned that, unless they have a fever with the cold, taking acetaminophen (Tylenol) is unnecessary. Aspirin should be avoided during pregnancy because of a possible interference with blood clotting and prolonged pregnancy at term. Because common colds are invariably caused by a virus, antibiotic therapy is unnecessary except to prevent a secondary infection. Women should check with their health care provider before taking any over-the-counter medication for a cold.

The Woman With Influenza

Influenza is caused by a virus that is identified as type A, B, or C. Type A causes most infections. The disease spreads in epidemic form and is accompanied by high fever, extreme prostration, aching pains in the back and extremities, and generally a sore, raw throat. There is no clear correlation between influenza outbreaks and congenital anomalies in children, although during the famous Asian flu epidemic of the 1950s (caused by a variant of type A virus), preterm labor and abortion rates increased. Influenza is treated with an antipyretic to control fever and perhaps a prophylactic antibiotic to prevent a secondary infection. As the influenza vaccines are made from killed virus, women may be immunized safely during pregnancy if an epidemic is present.

The Woman With Pneumonia

Pneumonia is the bacterial or viral invasion of lung tissue. Following the invasion, an acute inflammatory response occurs with exudate of red blood cells, fibrin, and polymorphonuclear leukocytes into the alveoli. This process confines the bacteria or virus within segments of the lobes of the lungs. Pneumonia poses a serious complication of pregnancy because fluid collects in alveolar spaces causing limited oxygen-carbon dioxide exchange in the lungs. If collection of fluid is extreme, it will limit the oxygen available to the fetus. For therapy, the woman will be placed on an appropriate antibiotic and perhaps oxygen administration. With severe disease, ventilation support may be necessary. There is a tendency for women with pneumonia late in pregnancy to begin preterm labor. During labor, oxygen should be administered so that the fetus has adequate oxygen resources during contractions.

The Woman With Asthma

Asthma is paroxysmal wheezing and dyspnea in response to an inhaled allergen. It complicates about 1% of pregnancies (Varner, 1990). Most people who are susceptible to allergens in this way are said to be *atopic* individuals or have a predisposition to allergy over and above others. With inhalation of the allergen, there is an immediate histamine release from IgE immunoglobulin interaction. This results in constriction of the bronchial smooth muscle, marked mucosal swelling, and the production of thick bronchial secretions. These three processes reduce the lumen of air passages markedly. The woman has difficulty with air exchange; on exhalation, she makes a high pitched whistling sound (bronchial wheezing) from air being pushed past the bronchial secretions. Asthma has the potential of reducing the oxygen supply to the fetus if a major attack should occur during pregnancy. Women with asthma have a higher rate of preterm birth than others (Doucette & Bracken, 1993). Many women find that their asthma is improved during pregnancy by the high circulating levels of corticosteroids that are present during pregnancy (D'Alonzo, 1990). A woman should check with her physician about the safety of the medications she routinely takes for this disorder *before pregnancy* to be certain it will be safe to continue them during pregnancy and during breast-feeding.

Beta-adrenergic agonists such as terbutaline and albuterol are the drugs of choice for asthma. If these are ineffective, then theophylline, a corticosteroid such as prednisone, or cromolyn sodium may be added to the regimen. All these drugs are safe during pregnancy; serum levels of theophylline must be monitored closely to avoid toxicity. Beta-adrenergic agonists have the potential to reduce labor contractions so are tapered close to term if possible (Loeb, 1993). Women who have been taking a corticosteroid during pregnancy may need parenteral administration of hydrocortisone during labor because of the added stress during this time.

The Woman With Tuberculosis

Tuberculosis is a disease that should have been eradicated in view of the effective treatment available. However, in some highly populated areas, the incidence has increased and is at epidemic proportions. Worldwide, it is still one of the leading causes of death.

With tuberculosis, lung tissue is invaded by the *mycobacterium tuberculosis,* an acid-fast bacillus. Macrophages and T-lymphocytes surround the bacillus, but rather than actually killing it, they merely surround the invasion site. Fibrosis, calcification, and a final ring of collagenous scar tissue develop, effectively sealing off the organisms from the body and any further invasion or spread. Antibodies developed will thereafter cause a positive tine or purified protein derivative (PPD) test in the individual.

Assessment

In high-risk areas for tuberculosis, women should be skin tested with a tine or PPD test at their first prenatal visit. A chest x-ray can then be taken of women who show positive reactions to skin testing. Women need to be cautioned that a positive reaction does not necessarily mean that they have the disease; it can mean that they have at some time been exposed to tuberculosis and so have antibodies in their system. A chest x-ray confirms the diagnosis and this can be taken safely in pregnancy if the abdomen is shielded. A woman with tuberculosis shows symptoms of a chronic cough, weight loss, hemoptysis, night sweats, a low-grade fever, and chronic fatigue.

Therapeutic Management

Women with active tuberculosis should be treated during pregnancy (Mays, 1993). Isoniazid (INH) and ethambutol hydrochloride, drugs of choice for tuberculosis, may be given without apparent teratogenic effects. INH may result in a peripheral neuritis if the woman does not take supplemental pyridoxine as well. Ethambutol may cause optic nerve involvement (optic atrophy and loss of green color recognition) in the mother. To detect this, the woman should be tested monthly using a Snellen (eye test) chart.

A woman who has had tuberculosis is usually advised to wait 1 year, perhaps 2 years, before attempting to conceive after tuberculosis becomes inactive, because tuberculosis lesions never actually disappear but are only "closed off" and made inactive. The woman who has active tuberculosis, or has had it recently, must be especially careful to maintain an adequate level of calcium during pregnancy to ensure that tuberculosis pockets form or are not broken down. Recent inactive tuberculosis can become active during pregnancy, because pressure on the diaphragm from below changes the shape of the lung, and a sealed pocket may be broken in this process. Pushing during labor may increase intrapulmonary pressure and cause the same phenomenon. Recent inactive tuberculosis may become active during the postpartal period, as the lung suddenly returns to its more vertical prepregnant position and breaks open calcium deposits.

Although tuberculosis can be spread by the placenta to the fetus, it usually is spread to the infant after birth. A woman with a recent history of tuberculosis should have at least three negative sputum cultures before she holds or cares for her infant. If these are negative, there is no need to isolate the infant from the mother; she can even breast-feed. If there is active tuberculosis in the home, the infant is generally discharged on prophylactic INH to prevent infection and is skin tested at 3-month intervals. If the infant is to be placed on INH, a mother also taking INH should not breast-feed or the combined dosage the infant receives (INH is found in breast milk) might be toxic.

The Woman With Cystic Fibrosis

Cystic fibrosis is a recessively inherited disease in which there is generalized dysfunction of the exocrine glands. This dysfunction leads to mucus secretions, particularly in the pancreas and lungs, becoming so viscid that normal secretion is blocked.

The cause of the disorder is unknown, but DNA markers have been used to localize the gene mutation to the seventh chromosome (Harrington & Fujimura, 1992). Whether a fetus has cystic fibrosis may be identified by chorionic villi sampling or amniocentesis and identification of the gene marker (a technique called restriction fragment length polymorphism) (Simpson, 1990). As

many as 98% of men with cystic fibrosis are sterile from reduced semen (Rosenstein, 1994). Women with the disorder may have lessened fertility from inability of sperm to migrate through viscid cervical mucus. Artificial insemination may be necessary so sperm is not obstructed by cervical mucus.

Persons with the disease typically develop symptoms of chronic respiratory infection and overinflation of their lungs as well as an inability to digest fat and protein because the pancreas cannot release amylase. Because of poor pulmonary function that results in inadequate oxygen supply to the fetus, there is an increased risk for preterm labor and perinatal death (Cunningham et al., 1993).

Therapy for the illness consists of taking pancrelipase (Pancrease) to supplement pancreatic enzymes and a bronchodilator or antibiotic to reduce pulmonary symptoms. Pancrelipase is a pregnancy risk category C drug (teratogenic effects are unknown) but does not appear to affect the fetus. In addition to pharmacologic measures, women with cystic fibrosis must perform postural drainage daily.

Modifications for Pregnancy

During pregnancy, the woman is at high risk for anemia because pancrelipase interferes with iron absorption. She needs to conscientiously add an iron supplement to her diet. Persons with cystic fibrosis have a higher-than-usual incidence of developing diabetes mellitus due to pancreas involvement; therefore, they need to be monitored for serum glucose levels at prenatal visits to detect whether gestational diabetes is developing.

Postural drainage becomes difficult late in pregnancy as the process itself is exhausting. Moving to new positions is difficult, and lying prone, a position used frequently in postural drainage, is contraindicated in late pregnancy. The woman may need to plan more frequent and shorter sessions in modified positions to prevent exhaustion. Fetal health will be monitored by ultrasound and nonstress tests to identify intrauterine growth retardation.

The Postpartal Period

It is usually not recommended that women with cystic fibrosis breast-feed as their breast milk contains more fatty acid than usual and it is tiring for the mother (Luder et al., 1990). Help the woman plan how to conserve her energy for infant care in the immediate postpartal period so she does not become exhausted and can enjoy her newborn.

Rheumatic Disorders and Pregnancy

A number of rheumatic disorders occur in young adult women and thus are seen during pregnancy. Because most of these illnesses result in discomfort, potential or actual pain related to disease pathology is the primary nursing diagnosis used. Women may not achieve a pain-free outcome because of the nature of these illnesses, but outcome criteria should center on the woman stating that her pain level is tolerable.

Nursing Diagnoses and Related Interventions

Nursing Diagnosis: Pain related to rheumatic disorder during pregnancy

Goal: Client will not experience an intolerable level of pain during pregnancy.

Outcome Criteria: Client states that she is moderately comfortable and is able to maintain level of daily activity.

The Woman With Juvenile Rheumatoid Arthritis

Juvenile rheumatoid arthritis, a disease of connective tissue with joint inflammation and contracture, occurs for unknown reasons but is probably the result of an autoimmune response.

The disease pathology is synovial membrane destruction. Inflammation with effusion, swelling, erythema, and painful motion of the joints occurs. Over time, formation of granulation tissue can fill the joint space, resulting in permanent disfigurement and loss of joint motion.

Symptoms of the disease may improve during pregnancy because of the naturally increased circulating level of corticosteroids in the maternal bloodstream during pregnancy (Ostensen, 1992). During the postpartal period, when the woman's corticosteroid levels fall to normal again, arthritis symptoms will probably recur. Women with juvenile rheumatoid arthritis frequently take corticosteroids and salicylate therapy to prevent joint pain and loss of mobility (Scott, 1990).

Although they continue to take these medications during pregnancy, a danger of large amounts of salicylates is prolonged pregnancy (salicylate interferes with prostaglandin synthesis, so labor contractions are not initiated). The infant may have a bleeding defect due to the high salicylate level as well as premature closure of the ductus arteriosus. For this reason, the woman is asked to decrease her intake of salicylates approximately 2 weeks before term. Women should be considered individually in the postpartal period as to whether it is safe for them to breast-feed based on the medication they will be taking; those on a nonsteroidal antiinflammatory agent such as ibuprofen can breast-feed; those on indomethacin or acetosalicylic acid probably should not because of the danger of early patent arteriosus closure and increased bleeding.

The Woman With Systemic Lupus Erythematosus

Systemic lupus erythematosus (SLE) is a multisystem chronic disease of connective tissue that can occur in women of childbearing age: its highest incidence is in women ages 20 to 40 years. With onset of the illness, widespread degeneration of connective tissue, especially of the heart, the kidneys, the blood vessels, spleen, skin, and retroperitoneal tissue, occurs (Reveille, 1990). The most marked skin change is a characteristic erythematous "butterfly-shaped" rash on the face. Most serious of the kidney changes are fibrin deposits that plug and block the glomeruli, leading to necrosis and scarring. The thickening of collagen tissue in the blood vessels causes vessel obstruction. This could be life-threatening to the woman if blood flow to vital organs becomes compromised and to the fetus if blood flow to the placenta is obstructed. The woman may be taking corticosteroid, nonsteroidal antiinflammatory agents, and salicylate therapy to reduce symptoms of joint pain and inflammation. A number of women with SLE have antiphospholipid antibodies, which increase the tendency to thrombi formation.

The increased circulation of corticosteroids during pregnancy may lessen symptoms in some women. In others, the chief complication of the disorders—acute nephritis with glomeruli destruction—may occur for the first time during pregnancy.

With nephritis, the woman's blood pressure will rise. She will develop hematuria and decreased urine output. Proteinuria and edema may begin. It is difficult to differentiate these symptoms from the symptoms of pregnancy-induced hypertension, except that with pregnancy-induced hypertension, there is no hematuria. Women will be followed during pregnancy by frequent serum creatinine levels to assess kidney function. If this value is over 1.5 mg/dL and proteinuria and a decreased creatinine clearance value are also present, the fetus is seriously threatened. Dialysis or plasmapheresis may be necessary.

Women are asked to decrease salicylate use close to birth to reduce the possibility of bleeding in the newborn. Infants of women with SLE tend to be small for gestational age due to the decreased blood flow to the placenta. The incidence of abortion and preterm birth rises (Julkunen et al., 1993). Intravenous hydrocortisone is generally administered during labor to help the woman adjust to the stress at this time. During the postpartal period, there may be an acute exacerbation of symptoms in the woman as corticosteroid levels again fall to normal. Infants may be born with a lupus-like rash, anemia, and thrombocytopenia (low platelet count). This lasts about 6 months and then fades. Congenital heart block for which a pacemaker may be necessary may occur in the newborn (Scott, 1990). Screening for the exact type of autoantibodies present may be helpful in predicting which newborns are susceptible to this.

Gastrointestinal Disorders and Pregnancy

Although minor gastrointestinal discomfort (e.g., nausea, heartburn, constipation) is common during pregnancy, acute abdominal pain or protracted vomiting are causes for concern. Pregnancy complications such as abruptio placentae or ectopic pregnancy often manifest with acute abdominal pain, so differentiating the cause of abdominal pain can be difficult. In some instances, abdominal pain is associated with a condition completely unrelated to the pregnancy such as ulcerative colitis, viral hepatitis, hiatal hernia, or cholecystitis. These conditions may be known to the woman before she becomes pregnant, or they may develop or be discovered during her pregnancy. Women who have colostomies complete pregnancy without difficulty. Even a previous liver transplant is not a contraindication to pregnancy (Scantlebury et al., 1990).

Nursing Diagnoses and Related Interventions

> ***Nursing Diagnosis:*** High risk for altered nutrition, less than body requirements related to a gastrointestinal disorder during pregnancy
>
> ***Goal:*** Client will ingest adequate nutrition during pregnancy.
>
> ***Outcome Criteria:*** Client's weight gain is 25 to 30 lb for pregnancy; hemoglobin is above 11 mg/dL; specific gravity of urine is below 1.030.

The Woman With Appendicitis

Appendicitis is inflammation of the appendix. It has a high incidence in young adults so occurs at an incidence of about 1 in 1500 to 2000 pregnancies (Varner, 1990).

Assessment

History-taking is important. Appendicitis usually begins with a few hours of nausea (e.g., the woman reports she skipped lunch because she just did not feel hungry). An hour or two of generalized abdominal discomfort follows. The woman may have vomiting during this time. Then comes the typical sharp, peristaltic, lower-right-quadrant pain of acute appendicitis.

This is different from the pain of an overstretched round ligament that may cause lower quadrant pain during pregnancy. Pain from the round ligament occurs with sudden motion, and is only transient. Appendicitis pain is also different from that of ectopic pregnancy; with ectopic pregnancy there is no nausea and vomiting.

In the nonpregnant woman, the sharp localized pain of appendicitis appears at McBurney's point (a point halfway between the umbilicus and the iliac crest on the lower right abdomen). If one presses at that point, it is not so tender while pressing; releasing one's hand abruptly, however, causes the abdominal contents to jiggle, and the jiggling of the inflamed appendix brings sharp pain (rebound tenderness). In the pregnant woman, the appendix is often displaced upward in the abdomen, and the localized pain may be so high it resembles the pain of gallbladder disease. Blood work will reveal leukocytosis. Because pregnant women have an elevated white blood cell count, this increased finding is not so helpful in pregnancy as it might be otherwise. Her temperature may be elevated. There are typically ketones in the urine. A sonogram will reveal the inflamed appendix (Lim et al., 1992).

The woman should not take food, liquid, or laxatives while she is waiting to be seen by a physician, because increasing peristalsis tends to cause an inflamed appendix to rupture.

Therapeutic Management

If the woman is near term (past 36 weeks) and there is reason to believe that the fetus is mature, a cesarean birth may be done to deliver the baby and then remove the inflamed appendix. If appendicitis occurs early in pregnancy, an abdominal incision to remove the inflamed appendix can usually be made without disturbing the pregnancy (a midline rather than a right-sided one is done). As long as the anesthesiologist is aware that the woman is pregnant and carefully controls oxygen levels during anesthesia administration, the outcome of the pregnancy will be good (Mahmoodian, 1992).

If the appendix ruptures before surgery, the risk to both mother and fetus increases dramatically. This is because with rupture, infected material is free in the peritoneum. It can spread by the fallopian tubes to the fetus. Generalized peritonitis is such an overwhelming infection it is difficult for the woman's body to combat it effectively and maintain the pregnancy too. Women who have a ruptured appendix may develop extreme peritoneal adhesions, which later result in infertility due to changes in the placement of fallopian tubes.

The Woman With a Hiatal Hernia

Hiatal hernia is a condition in which a portion of the stomach extends and protrudes up through the diaphragm into the chest cavity. Although the condition can be constantly present, symptoms are most often present only sporadically following increased peristaltic action. Hiatal hernia may generate symptoms during pregnancy as the uterus pushes the stomach against the diaphragm and increases the hernia. With a hiatal hernia, the symptoms the woman notices are "heartburn," gastric regurgitation, indigestion, and dysphagia (difficulty swallow-ing); heartburn is particularly extreme if she lies supine following a full meal. The woman may lose weight be-cause of her inability to eat. If the problem is extreme, she may have hematemesis (vomiting of blood).

That a hiatal hernia is present is usually diagnosed by direct endoscopy or sonogram during pregnancy to avoid x-rays. She can be prescribed antacids to relieve pain; sleeping so her head is elevated also helps. Fol-lowing pregnancy, as the uterine pressure is decreased, the symptoms generally become less noticeable or disappear.

The Woman With Cholecystitis and Cholelithiasis

Cholecystitis (gallbladder inflammation) and cholelithia-sis (gallstone formation) are most frequently associated with women older than 40 years, obesity, multiparity, and ingestion of a high fat diet. Gallstones are formed from cholesterol. It is debated whether the hypercholes-terolemia that naturally occurs during pregnancy leads to increased cholecystitis or cholelithiasis (Cunningham et al., 1993). Symptoms of cholecystitis (constant aching and pressure in the right epigastrium, perhaps accompa-nied by jaundice) typically occur following a meal rich in fat. Medical therapy is to lower fat intake. A woman can eat a low-fat but not a fat-free diet during pregnancy be-cause of the importance of linoleic acid for fetal growth. Cholecystitis can be diagnosed by sonogram. If acute episodes occur during pregnancy, they can generally be managed by IV fluid, nasogastric suction, and analgesics.

Surgery for gallbladder removal by laparoscopy technique may be done during pregnancy if the wom-an's symptoms cannot be controlled by conservative management (Elerding, 1993).

The Woman With Viral Hepatitis

Hepatitis is liver disease that may occur from invasion of either the A, B, C, or D virus. Hepatitis A is spread mainly by contact with another person who has the in-fection or by ingestion of fecally contaminated water or shellfish after an incubation period of 2 to 6 weeks. Women exposed to hepatitis A may be given prophylac-tic gamma globulin while pregnant to try and abort the disease after exposure. This form follows a rather benign course and is not known to be transmitted to the fetus.

Hepatitis B (serum hepatitis) is spread by transfu-sion of contaminated blood or blood products; it can be spread by semen and thus is considered a sexually trans-mitted disease (STD). Hepatitis C and D are apparently spread by the same methods as hepatitis B but are rarely seen in pregnant women. Hepatitis B has an incubation period of 6 weeks to 6 months. It occurs in both an acute and chronic form leading to liver cell necrosis with scarring and inability to convert indirect to direct biliru-bin or excrete direct bilirubin. Urine will be dark yellow from excretion of bilirubin by this alternate route; stools will be light colored from lack of bilirubin.

With both hepatitis A or B, the woman may notice symptoms of nausea and vomiting. Her liver area may feel tender to palpation. Jaundice is a late symptom. On physical examination, her liver is found to be enlarged. Her bilirubin level will be elevated. Liver enzymes such as transaminase will be increased. Specific antibodies against the virus can be detected in the blood serum. If a liver biopsy is necessary for diagnosis, this can be per-formed safely during pregnancy.

The woman is usually prescribed bedrest and en-couraged to eat a high-calorie diet as her liver has diffi-culty converting stored glycogen into glucose in a dis-eased state. Enteric precautions (i.e., a cover gown, washing hands well on entering and leaving the room, and wearing gloves to handle articles contaminated with fecal material) are followed. If the woman has hepatitis B infection (i.e., is HB Ag-positive), precautions with blood samples or blood drawing equipment should be used as well.

The danger of hepatitis during pregnancy is that a high incidence of abortion or preterm labor can result. Approximately 85% of infants whose mothers are HB Ag-positive will develop chronic hepatitis B (Cunning-ham et al., 1993). The later in pregnancy the mother contracts the infection, the greater the risk the infant will be affected. This is a serious consequence in newborns because a proportion of HB Ag-positive infants will de-velop liver cirrhosis or carcinoma later in life. If the mother has anti-HB antibodies present (antibodies to-ward a virus subgroup), the incidence of this occurring appears to be less. Following birth, the infant should be washed well to remove any maternal blood, and hepati-tis B immune globulin (HBIG) and immunization against hepatitis B will be administered. The infant needs to be observed carefully for symptoms of infection over the first few months of life. The mother will be advised not to breast-feed because HB Ag antigens can be recovered from breast milk.

The Woman With Inflammatory Bowel Disease

Crohn's disease (inflammation of the terminal ileus) and ulcerative colitis (inflammation of the distal colon) occur most often in young adults between ages 12 and 30 years (childbearing years). The cause of these diseases is unknown, but an autoimmune process may be responsi-ble. In both diseases, the bowel develops shallow ulcers. The woman experiences chronic diarrhea, weight loss, occult blood in stool, and nausea and vomiting. If extreme, obstruction and fistula formation with peritoni-tis can occur. With Crohn's disease, malabsorption, particularly of vitamin B_{12} (a substance whose absorption occurs almost entirely in the ilium) occurs.

These diseases obviously have the potential for interfering with fetal growth if malabsorption occurs (Korelitz, 1992). Therapy for the disorders is total rest for the gastrointestinal tract by administration of total parenteral nutrition. Although it is possible to sustain a pregnancy by this route, it is obviously not a desirable nutrition pattern. Sulfasalazine, an antiinflammatory and a mainstay of therapy, may be continued during pregnancy without fetal injury. Close to birth, the dosage of sulfasalazine is reduced as it may interfere with bilirubin binding sites and cause neonatal jaundice.

Neurologic Disorders and Pregnancy

Neurologic illness is not a common affliction of women of childbearing age. However, any neurologic disease with symptoms of seizures must be carefully managed during pregnancy because the anoxia caused by severe seizures could also deprive the fetus of oxygen, with serious outcomes.

The Woman With a Seizure Disorder

Recurrent seizures have a number of causes, such as head trauma or meningitis. The causes of most instances of recurrent seizures, however, are unknown (*idiopathic*).

Recurrent seizures were at one time so incapacitating that women who suffered them were generally advised not to have children. Today, however, there is no contraindication to such a woman having children as long as she is aware that the medications she must take to control seizures may increase the chance of anomalies in her infant.

Therapeutic Management

In the early months of pregnancy, women with recurrent seizures need to be cautioned to continue taking their seizure control medications despite nausea or vomiting of pregnancy. Be certain they understand that the rule "Do not take medication during pregnancy" does not apply to their seizure control medications.

Phenytoin sodium (Dilantin), a drug frequently prescribed for the control of seizures, appears to be teratogenic, resulting in a Dilantin syndrome (i.e., mental retardation and a peculiar facial proportion, not unlike that of the fetal alcohol syndrome). This may occur because of competition for folic acid binding sites (Loeb, 1993). Trimethadione is associated with mental retardation and physical deformities; valproic acid is associated with neural tube defects; carbamazepine (Tegretol) is a pregnancy risk category C drug, or unproven during pregnancy. Ethosuximide, a drug often used to control

absence seizures, is untested during pregnancy. The woman is in a "catch-22" position of having to take drugs to safeguard her own health, but by taking them she may not be safeguarding the health of the fetus.

Women who have been taking Dilantin may have chronic hypertension. For these women, a baseline blood pressure should be established early in pregnancy so that later changes can be interpreted in terms of this already elevated pressure. All women should have serum evaluations of drug level before pregnancy or early in pregnancy. As the blood volume increases with pregnancy, some women may need their dosage increased.

Infants of woman taking seizure medications are prone to hemorrhagic disease of the newborn because of decreased vitamin K coagulation factors at birth. To counteract this, women may be prescribed vitamin K during labor. Some infants may have an increased danger of neural tube disorders and childhood malignancies as a result of folic acid displacement during intrauterine life (Varner, 1990).

Nursing Diagnoses and Related Interventions

Nursing Diagnosis: High risk for altered placental perfusion related to anoxia resulting from maternal seizure

Goal: Client will take prescribed anticonvulsant therapy during pregnancy; will be prepared for emergency management of seizures. Adequate fetal oxygenation will be maintained throughout pregnancy.

Outcome Criteria: Client informs health care personnel about history of seizures; states importance of immediate care and oxygen therapy should she begin a seizure. Fetal Apgar score at birth is between 7 and 10 and no birth anomalies are apparent.

Many women wonder what a seizure during pregnancy might do to the unborn child. Seizures in people vary so that it is difficult to predict an individual effect. Absence seizures (i.e., often just a rapid fluttering of the eyelids or a moment's staring into space) will have no effect on the fetus. Tonic-clonic seizures (sustained, full-body involvement) could conceivably affect the fetus because of the anoxia that can occur from the spasm of chest muscles.

If a seizure should occur, the woman must be evaluated to be certain that the seizure occurred from her underlying disease, not from beginning hypertension of pregnancy. Nonpregnant people having tonic-clonic seizures do not need oxygen administered to them during a seizure. In pregnancy, administering oxygen by mask is good prophylaxis to ensure adequate fetal oxygenation.

It is also important that a woman be advised to alert hospital personnel at the time of labor that she has recurrent seizures and to report the type of medication she is taking. She should continue to take the medication during labor. If a general anesthetic should be necessary, the anesthesiologist needs to know about her condition before administering anesthesia; otherwise, during the excitement phase of anesthesia induction, a seizure may occur if the anesthesiologist is not forewarned to prevent it.

Nursing Diagnosis: High risk for altered parenting related to maternal feelings of low self-esteem and fear that her child will inherit seizure disorder

Goal: Client will be informed about the low statistical possibility that her child will have inherited her disorder and will demonstrate confidence in her ability to care for the infant by hospital discharge.

Outcome Criteria: Client states accurately the nature of her disorder (acquired or idiopathic) and the statistical chances of her child inheriting the disorder. After child is born, client identifies sudden jerking movements in her newborn (such as Moro reflex) as healthy newborn characteristics.

Some women with recurrent seizures suffer from low self-esteem because of the inability to control their body. Feelings of low self-worth or powerlessness can contribute to delayed or ineffective bonding once the baby is born. All through pregnancy, women require encouragement and support for the things that they are doing right.

In addition, a woman may worry that her child will have seizures as the child grows older. If the woman's seizures are the result of an acquired disorder—that is, infection, such as meningitis or head trauma—the woman can be assured that her child will have no more tendency toward seizures than any other child. If the etiology of her seizures is unknown, the chance that her child will have them too is slightly higher than in the normal population. This prediction is only theoretical, however, and cannot be made without a thorough review of the onset and nature of the woman's disorder (Cunningham et al., 1993). Be certain the woman has her newborn with her for long periods so she can become acquainted with sudden jerking motions such as occur when a newborn is startled (Moro reflex) or quivering of the jaw with prolonged crying so she does not interpret these as seizure activity.

The Woman With Myasthenia Gravis

Myasthenia gravis is an autoimmune disorder characterized by the presence of an IgG antibody against acetylcholine receptors in striated muscle. This causes failure of the striated muscles to contract, particularly those of the oropharyngeal, facial, and extra ocular groups.

Myasthenia gravis is treated by the administration of anticholinesterase drugs such as pyridostigmine or neostigmine and possibly prednisone. These medications may be continued during pregnancy. Plasmapheresis to remove immune complexes from the bloodstream may be prescribed to reduce symptoms further. Plasmapheresis must be carried out gradually so there is no danger of fluid overload or hypotension. As smooth muscle is not affected by the disease, labor should occur as normally. Magnesium sulfate and procaine anesthetics should be avoided (Varner, 1990).

An infant born of a woman with the disease may demonstrate disease symptoms at birth from transfer of antibodies (Tzartos et al., 1990). This is further discussed in Chapter 51.

The Woman With Multiple Sclerosis

Multiple sclerosis (MS) occurs predominantly in woman between 20 and 40 years of age, so it is seen in women of childbearing age. With MS, nerve fibers become demyelinated and therefore lose function. Women develop symptoms of fatigue, numbness, blurriness of vision, and loss of coordination. Woman are commonly administered ACTH or a corticosteroid to strengthen nerve conduction. These are safe for administration during pregnancy. Cyclosporine, azathioprine, and cyclophosphamide, drugs also frequently administered, are not. Interferon is untested as to pregnancy safety. Women may continue with plasmapheresis (withdrawal and replacement of plasma) during pregnancy as long as the volume is well controlled. Women with this disorder grow increasingly fatigued as pregnancy progresses. Urinary tract infections tend to occur as a poorly defined consequence of the illness.

A danger at term is that a painless precipitous birth will occur if quadriplegia is present. Women may be prone to autonomic dysreflexia caused by the pain of labor. This leads to severe hypertension, headache, diaphoresis, and bradycardia. Administration of an epidural anesthetic may decrease the risk of this.

Women may notice a decrease of symptoms during pregnancy because of the naturally occurring elevated level of corticosteroids during pregnancy (Davis & Maslow, 1992). In the postpartal period, symptoms return; some women experience a level of symptoms worse than their prepregnancy level.

Musculoskeletal Disorders and Pregnancy

Women of childbearing age have few common musculoskeletal disorders. One that may be seen is scoliosis.

The Woman With Scoliosis

Scoliosis is lateral curvature of the spine; it occurs most often in females approximately 12 years of age; if not corrected at this time, it continues to grow progressively worse until it causes cosmetic deformity and even interferes with respiration and heart action because of chest compression. Pelvic distortion can interfere with childbirth, especially at the inlet (Sokol & Brindley, 1990). Spinal or epidural anesthesia may be more difficult to place for analgesia with labor if the woman's spine is extremely curved.

Girls with scoliosis may wear a Milwaukee brace during their adolescent years to maintain an erect posture. Obviously, such a brace cannot be continued during the last half of pregnancy. Other girls have stainless steel rods (Harrington rods) implanted on both sides of their spinal vertebrae to strengthen and straighten their spine. Such rod implantations do not interfere with pregnancy; the woman will notice some back pain as does the average woman from tension on back muscles. If the woman's pelvis is distorted, a cesarean birth may need to be anticipated for a safe birth. If a vaginal birth is permitted, plot the course of labor on a Friedman graft so an unusually long first stage of labor suggesting cephalopelvic disproportion can be recognized. Chapter 51 discusses the nursing care of adolescents with scoliosis in detail.

Cardiovascular Disorders and Pregnancy

The number of women of childbearing age who have heart disease is diminishing as more and more congenital heart anomalies (discussed in Chapter 41) are corrected in early infancy and rheumatic fever is being more actively prevented and treated so that cardiac damage from the disorder is reduced. Heart disease is still a problem in pregnancy, however, because improved management of women with heart disease has enabled women who might never have risked pregnancy in the past to do so now (Jackson et al., 1993). Cardiac disease complicates about one percent of all pregnancies (Cunningham et al., 1993).

The majority of cardiovascular problems that cause difficulty with pregnancy are congenital anomalies such as atrial septal defect or uncorrected coarctation of the aorta. Valve damage caused by rheumatic fever or Kawasaki disease can also cause difficulty. Because women are becoming pregnant at older ages than previously, the incidence of primary myocardial infarction or ischemic cardiac disease during pregnancy is increasing (Sala, 1992). Heart disease that occurs specifically with the pregnancy (*peripartal heart disease)* can rarely occur. A woman with heart disease needs a team approach to care during pregnancy, combining the talents of an internist, obstetrician, and nurse. Ideally, the woman should visit her obstetrician or family physician before conception, so that a health care team can become familiar with her state of health when she is not pregnant and establish baseline evaluations of her heart function. The woman should begin prenatal care as soon as she suspects she is pregnant (1 week after the first missed menstrual period), so that close assessment of her general condition and circulatory system can be maintained.

Pregnancy taxes the circulatory system of every woman, even without cardiac disease, because both the blood volume and cardiac output increase approximately 30% (perhaps as much as 50%). Most of this increase occurs in the first 28 weeks of pregnancy, and then this greater blood volume continues to be maintained for the remainder of pregnancy.

Because of the increased blood flow past valves, heart murmurs are heard in many women during pregnancy. These are functional (innocent) murmurs, are transient, and will disappear following the pregnancy. Heart palpitations on sudden exertion are also normal in pregnancy. Neither of these symptoms is a sign of heart disease, but merely of the normal physiologic adjustment to pregnancy.

The danger of pregnancy in a woman with heart disease occurs mainly because of the increased circulatory volume. The most dangerous time for her is in weeks 28 to 32, just after the blood volume reaches its peak, although if heart disease is severe, symptoms can occur almost immediately. The woman's heart may become so overwhelmed by increased blood volume that her cardiac output falls to the point that vital organs (including the placenta) are no longer perfused adequately. When this happens, the oxygen and nutrition requirements of cells are not met.

The determination of whether a woman with heart disease can complete a pregnancy successfully depends on the type and extent of her disease. As a rule, a woman with artificial but well-functioning heart valves can be expected to complete a pregnancy without difficulty as long as she has consistent prenatal and postpartal care. The occasional woman with a pacemaker implant can also expect to complete pregnancy successfully. To predict pregnancy outcome, heart disease is divided into four categories based on the criteria originated by the New York State Heart Association (Table 14-1). The woman with class I or II heart disease can expect to experience a normal pregnancy and birth. Women with class III can complete a pregnancy if they abide by almost complete bedrest. Women with class IV heart disease are poor candidates for pregnancy because they are in cardiac failure even at rest and when they are not pregnant; they are usually advised to avoid pregnancy. Table 14-2 shows the predicted mortality of women with various heart diseases in pregnancy.

Table 14-1. *Classification of Heart Disease*

Class	Description
I	Uncompromised. Women have no limitation of physical activity. Ordinary physical activity causes no discomfort. They have no symptoms of cardiac insufficiency and no anginal pain.
II	Slightly compromised. Women have slight limitation of physical activity. Ordinary physical activity causes excessive fatigue, palpitation, and dyspnea or anginal pain.
III	Markedly compromised. Women have a moderate to marked limitation of physical activity. During less than ordinary activity they experience excessive fatigue, palpitations, dyspnea, or anginal pain.
IV	Severely compromised. Women are unable to carry out any physical activity without experiencing discomfort. Even at rest they experience symptoms of cardiac insufficiency or anginal pain.

(From Criteria Committee of the New York State Heart Association. [1979]. *Nomenclature and criteria for diagnosis of disease of the heart and blood vessels* [8th ed.]. Boston: Little, Brown, with permission.)

The Woman With Left Sided Heart Failure

Left sided heart failure occurs with conditions such as mitral stenosis and mitral insufficiency (the most common cardiac sequelae of rheumatic heart disease and Marfan syndrome, a congenital connective tissue disorder) and aortic coarctation.

Left sided heart failure occurs when the left ventricle is unable to move forward the volume of blood received by the left atrium from the pulmonary circulation. The reason for the failure is often at the level of the mitral valve. The normal physiologic tachycardia of pregnancy

Table 14-2. *Risks for Maternal Mortality by Various Heart Diseases*

Mortality 0–1%

Atrial septal defect
Ventricular septal defect
Patent ductus arteriosus
Pulmonic or tricuspid disease
Tetralogy of Fallot, corrected
Bioprosthetic valve
Mitral stenosis, NYHA class I and II

Mortality 5–15%

Mitral stenosis, NYHA class III and IV
Aortic stenosis
Aortic coarctation without valve involvement
Tetralogy of Fallot, uncorrected
Previous myocardial infarction
Marfan syndrome, normal aorta
Mitral stenosis with atrial fibrillation
Artificial valve

Mortality 25–50%

Pulmonary hypertension
Aortic coarctation with valve involvement
Marfan syndrome with aortic involvement

(From American College of Obstetricians and Gynecologists. [1992]. *Mortality of congenital heart disease.* New York: ACOG.)

shortens diastole (atrial contraction) and decreases the time available for blood to flow across this valve. The inability of the mitral valve to push blood forward causes back pressure on the pulmonary circulation, causing this to become distended; systemic blood pressure falls in the face of lowered cardiac output and pulmonary hypertension occurs. When pressure in the pulmonary vein reaches a point of about 25 mm Hg, fluid begins to pass from the pulmonary capillary membranes into the interstitial spaces surrounding the alveoli and then into the alveoli themselves (pulmonary edema). The normal decrease in serum albumen that occurs with pregnancy can cause pulmonary edema to form at even lower capillary pressure than usual. Pulmonary edema interferes with oxygen-carbon dioxide exchange as the fluid coats the exchange space. If pulmonary capillaries rupture under the pressure, small amounts of blood will leak into the alveoli. This will be manifested by a productive cough of blood-speckled sputum. Women with pulmonary hypertension are extremely high risk for spontaneous abortion, preterm labor, and maternal death during pregnancy (Jackson et al., 1993).

As the oxygen saturation of the blood decreases from dysfunction of the alveoli, chemoreceptors stimulate the respiratory center to increase the respiratory rate. At first this is noticeable only on exertion, then finally with rest also. Body cells receive little oxygen and the woman experiences increased fatigue, weakness, and dizziness (specifically from lack of oxygen in brain cells). As the systemic fall in blood pressure registers on the pressoreceptors in the aorta, the woman's heart rate increases and peripheral vasoconstriction occurs in attempts to increase the systemic blood pressure. As the fall in blood pressure is registered with the renal angiotensin system, both sodium and water retention occur.

As pulmonary edema becomes severe, the woman will be unable to sleep in any position but one with her chest and head elevated (**orthopnea**). Elevating her chest allows edema to settle to the bottom of her lungs and frees up exchange space. She may also notice **paroxysmal nocturnal dyspnea**—suddenly waking at night short of breath. This occurs because heart action is more effective when she is at rest. With the more effective heart action, interstitial fluid is returned to the circulation. This overburdens the circulation, causing increased left side failure and increased pulmonary edema. The end result of severe heart failure is poor placental perfusion with intrauterine growth retardation.

If mitral stenosis is present, it is so difficult for blood to leave the left atrium that a secondary problem of thrombus formation can occur (Kirkland, 1990). If coarctation of the aorta is causing the difficulty, both dissection of the aorta and thrombus formation can be secondary problems. The woman may be prescribed antihypertensives in order to control upper body blood pressure and may be prescribed beta blockers to decrease the force of myocardial contractions. If blood flow to the uterus is impaired by the aortic constriction, fetal mortality will be high. The woman needs serial ultrasound and nonstress tests done after weeks 30 to 32 of pregnancy to monitor fetal health.

The Woman With Right Sided Heart Failure

Congenital heart defects such as pulmonary valve stenosis and atrial and ventricular septal defects may result in right sided heart failure. Right sided failure occurs when the output of the right ventricle is less than the blood volume the heart receives at the right atrium from the vena cava or venous circulation. Back pressure from this results in congestion of the systemic venous circulation and decreases cardiac output to the lungs. Blood pressure falls in the aorta because less blood is reaching it; pressure is high in the vena cava; both jugular venous distention and increased portal circulation occur. Both the liver and spleen become distended. Distention of abdominal vessels can lead to exudate of fluid from the vessels into the peritoneal cavity (ascites). Fluid moves from the systemic circulation into interstitial spaces (peripheral edema). Liver enlargement can cause extreme dyspnea and pain in a pregnant woman because the enlarged liver, as it is pressed upward by the enlarged uterus, will put extreme pressure on the diaphragm.

The congenital anomaly which is most apt to cause right sided failure in women of reproductive age is Eisenmenger's syndrome (a right to left atrial or ventricular septal defect with an accompanying pulmonary stenosis). Women who have an uncorrected anomaly of this type have a 50% risk of dying during pregnancy (Weiss & Atanassoff, 1993). They can be expected to be hospitalized during pregnancy. They need oxygen administration and frequent arterial blood gases to ensure fetal growth. During labor they may need a Swan-Ganz

catheter inserted for monitoring pulmonary pressure. They need extremely close monitoring following epidural anesthesia to be certain that hypotension does not occur.

The Woman With Peripartal Heart Disease

An extremely rare condition, **peripartal cardiomyopathy**, can originate late in pregnancy in women with no previous history of heart disease. It is apparently due to the effect of the pregnancy on the circulatory system. The cause is unknown although in many instances it may occur from previously undetected heart disease; it occurs most often in African-American multiparas (Cunningham et al., 1993). It often occurs in conjunction with hypertension of pregnancy. Late in pregnancy, the woman develops signs of myocardial failure (i.e., shortness of breath, chest pain, and edema). Her heart begins to increase in size (cardiomegaly). If this occurs, activity must be sharply reduced. Many women need diuretic and digitalis therapy. Low-dose heparin may be administered to decrease the risk of thromboembolism. Immunosuppressive therapy may improve the prognosis.

If the cardiomegaly persists past the postpartal period, it is generally suggested that the woman not attempt any further pregnancies as the condition tends to repeat in future pregnancies. Oral contraceptives are contraindicated to prevent further pregnancies because of the danger of thromboembolism with these.

Fetal Effects

Cardiac failure will affect fetal growth at the point maternal blood pressure is insufficient to provide an adequate supply of blood to the placenta. The infants of women with severe heart disease tend to have low birth weights because not enough nutrients are available due to poor placental perfusion. This poor perfusion level may lead to severe fetal distress if blood flow is inadequate for carbon dioxide exchange and the environment of the fetus becomes acidotic (Cunningham et al., 1993). Preterm labor may occur. This exposes the infant to the hazards of immaturity as well as low birth weight at birth. The infant may not respond well to labor (evidenced by late deceleration patterns on a fetal heart monitor) if cardiac decompensation has reached a point of placental incompetency.

Assessment

Nurses play a major role in the care of the pregnant woman with heart disease. Continuous assessment of the woman's health status, health education, and health promotion activities are essential. Assessment of the woman with heart disease begins with a thorough health history so her prepregnancy heart status can be documented (Figure 14-3). Ask about her level of exercise performance (what level can she do before growing short of

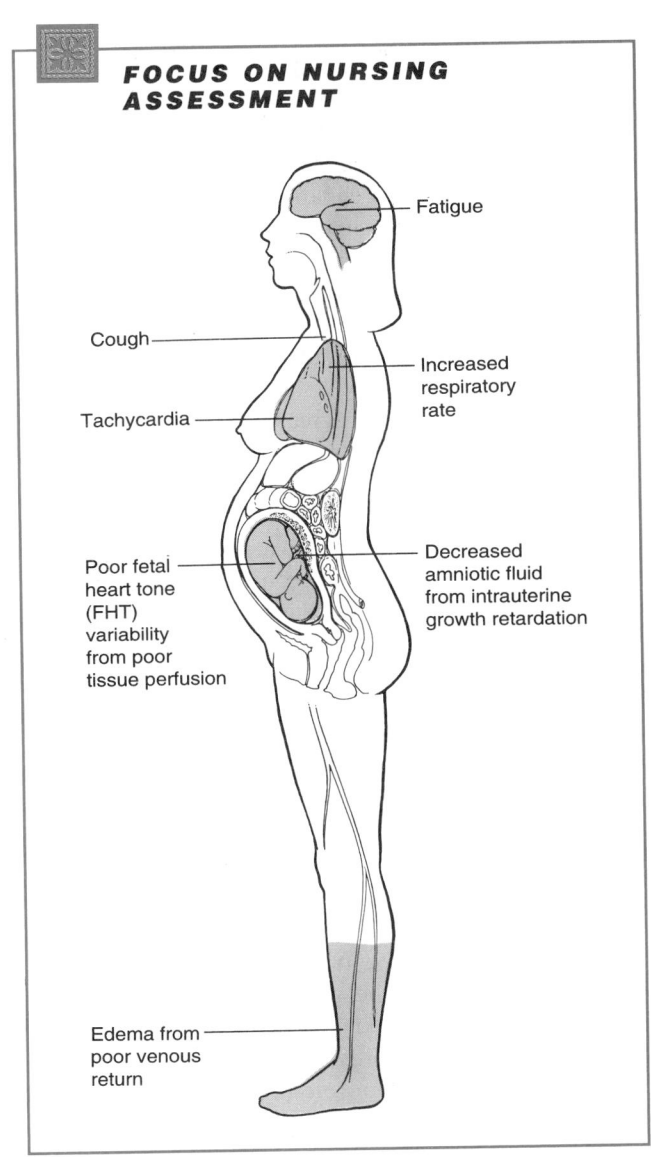

FOCUS ON NURSING ASSESSMENT

Fatigue

Cough

Tachycardia

Increased respiratory rate

Poor fetal heart tone (FHT) variability from poor tissue perfusion

Decreased amniotic fluid from intrauterine growth retardation

Edema from poor venous return

FIGURE 14-3
Symptoms of heart disease in pregnancy.

gins after week 20. If the edema is a sign of heart failure, it can begin at any time and other symptoms will probably also be present: irregular pulse, rapid or difficult respirations, and perhaps chest pain on exertion. Be certain to record a baseline blood pressure, pulse rate, and respiratory rate in either a sitting or lying position; then, at future health visits, always take these in the same position for a most accurate comparison. Assessing for nailbed filling (should be under 5 seconds) and jugular venous distention are helpful comparison assessments throughout pregnancy. If a woman's heart disease involves right sided heart failure, assessment of liver size at visits is helpful. Liver assessment becomes difficult and probably inaccurate late in pregnancy because the enlarged uterus presses the liver upward.

For additional cardiac status assessment, the woman may have an ECG, chest x-ray, or echocardiogram done at periodic points in pregnancy. Assure her that an ECG merely measures cardiac electrical discharge and thus does not harm the fetus in any way. Echocardiography uses sonography and thus will not harm the fetus. Chest x-ray is safe as long as the woman's abdomen is covered by a lead apron during the exposure. An ECG may become inaccurate late in pregnancy (demonstrates left axis deviation) as the enlarged uterus presses upward on the diaphragm and displaces the heart laterally.

Nursing Diagnoses and Related Interventions

> **Nursing Diagnosis:** Knowledge deficit regarding potential for altered tissue perfusion in fetus or self related to maternal cardiovascular disease
>
> **Goal:** Client will demonstrate understanding of danger signs that indicate inadequate tissue perfusion and when she should contact physician.
>
> **Outcome Criteria:** Client identifies danger signs and steps to take when they occur; maternal blood pressure is maintained above 100/60 mm Hg and fetal heart rate between 120 and 160 bpm.

Be certain that goals and outcome criteria established are realistic to the situation. Not all women with heart disease will be able to complete a pregnancy; some infants of women with severe involvement will be born with the effects of placental insufficiency such as neurologic involvement or mental retardation. There are positive actions the woman with heart disease can take, however, to reduce or eliminate complications during pregnancy. These include measures to rest and strengthen heart action. Nursing interventions are concerned with helping her to achieve these measures.

Promote Rest. A woman with heart disease needs more rest during pregnancy than the average woman to

breath and what physical symptoms she experiences, such as cyanosis of the lips or nailbeds). Ask if she normally has a cough and edema. Every woman with heart disease should report coughing during pregnancy and should be seen even if she assumes it is just a simple upper respiratory infection, because pulmonary edema from heart failure may first be manifested as a cough.

Evaluation of edema in women with heart disease must never be taken lightly. A decision must be made as to whether the edema is the normal edema of pregnancy (innocent); the beginning of pregnancy-induced hypertension (serious); or the edema of heart failure (serious). The normal edema of pregnancy involves only the feet and ankles. Edema of either pregnancy-induced hypertension or heart failure may *begin* as ankle edema. Edema of pregnancy-induced hypertension usually be-

lessen the strain of the increased burden of the pregnancy on her heart. Remember that at the point that cardiac output is not enough to meet systemic body demands, peripheral vasoconstriction occurs. Because the uterus is a peripheral organ, this causes uterine/placental constriction. A rest program must be carefully designed, therefore, so a woman stops exercising before this point is reached. Exactly how much rest she is to have should be carefully detailed for her. She may need to discontinue work early in pregnancy rather than work until midpregnancy or the end of pregnancy as the average woman usually plans to do. Exactly how much she will be allowed to do should be detailed as well. Allowing "normally heavy" housework may mean nothing more strenuous than dusting to some women. To others, it may mean washing windows, turning mattresses, and shoveling snow. Make certain that the woman's definition of "heavy work" is the same as yours and her physician's.

Many women need two rest periods a day (fully resting, not getting up frequently to answer the door or telephone) and a full night's sleep at night (not tossing and turning because of excess noise or heat in the room) in order to obtain adequate rest. Rest should be in the left lateral recumbent position to prevent hypotension and increase heart effort.

Many physicians prefer that women with heart disease remain on complete bedrest after week 30 of pregnancy. The purpose of this is to ensure that the pregnancy will be carried to term, or at least past week 36 so that fetal maturity can be assured.

Promote Healthy Nutrition. The woman with heart disease may need closer supervision of nutrition during pregnancy than does the average woman. She must gain enough weight to ensure a healthy pregnancy and a healthy baby. However, she must not gain so much excess weight that she has to supply additional cells with nutrients as this could overburden her heart and circulatory system.

Be certain that she is taking her prenatal vitamins as these contain an iron supplement to help prevent anemia. Anemia requires the body to circulate blood more vigorously to distribute oxygen to all body cells; if her heart is already taxed, she cannot do this. If the woman was following a sodium restricted diet before pregnancy, this may be continued during pregnancy. Because sodium is necessary for fluid volume, however, and allowing the woman's body to retain enough blood volume to supply blood to the placenta is important, the woman's sodium intake is usually limited, not severely restricted during pregnancy.

Educate Regarding Medication. Women who were taking cardiac medication before pregnancy may need to increase their maintenance dose because of the ex-

panded blood volume during pregnancy (Hess et al., 1992). A woman who needed digitalis for heart action before pregnancy will continue to require it during pregnancy (and can take it safely). A woman who was not digitalis-dependent before pregnancy may need such therapy prescribed as pregnancy advances and her cardiac output has to be increased or strengthened (the action of a digitalis preparation is to slow and strengthen myocardial contraction). In order to help the woman to continue thinking of herself as a fully functioning person, help her to understand that this does not mean her heart function is weakening, but rather that it is being stressed further by the increased circulatory load of pregnancy. Digitalis is sometimes administered to a woman during pregnancy if tachycardia is present in the fetus to slow the fetal heart. Propranolol, a beta-adrenergic blocker frequently used for cardiac arrhythmias, is a class C drug (unstudied in pregnancy), but apparently does not cause fetal abnormalities. Nitroglycerin, a compound often prescribed for angina, is also a category C drug but apparently safe.

A woman who was taking penicillin prophylactically following rheumatic fever to prevent a recurrence (often taken for 10 years following the occurrence of rheumatic fever or at least until age 18 years) should continue to take this drug during pregnancy because penicillin is not known to be a fetal teratogen (a category B drug). Close to the anticipated day of birth, some physicians begin women with valvular or congenital heart disease on a course of an antibiotic such as penicillin. This is because the postpartal period always involves some mild invasion of bacteria from the denuded placental site on the uterus (why lochia is always considered potentially contaminated). Because this invading bacteria may be streptococci, the bacteria often responsible for subacute bacterial endocarditis, a course of ampicillin, gentamicin, or amoxicillin at this time offers women needed protection.

It is often difficult to keep healthy women from taking over-the-counter medicines during pregnancy; conversely, it can be just as difficult to encourage women to take the medicine they need during pregnancy. Help them understand that there are valid exceptions to the rule of "no medicine during pregnancy."

Educate Regarding Avoidance of Infection. A systemic infection almost automatically increases body temperature, causing a woman to have to expend more energy and increase her cardiac output. This insult may be too much for the woman with heart disease to withstand. Caution the client to avoid visiting or being visited by people with infection. She should alert health care personnel at the first indication of an upper respiratory tract or urinary tract infection (be certain she knows the symptoms of this; Box 14-2) so that, if warranted, antibiotic therapy can be begun early in the course of the

Box 14-2
Signs and Symptoms of Urinary Tract Infection

Pain on urination
Frequency of urination
Hematuria
Bacterial count of more than 100,000 colonies per mL in a clean-catch specimen

infection. Monthly screening with clean catch urines for bacteriuria may be recommended.

Promote Reduction of Psychological Stress. Reducing psychological stress in a high-risk pregnancy is a worthy goal but often an unattainable one if the reason for the worry and stress is the pregnancy. Stress outside the pregnancy, however, such as financial responsibilities or lack of support people, should be reduced as much as possible. Provide extra time at prenatal visits for discussing any problems the woman may have. Be certain the woman understands that the purpose of any fetal assessment test made, such as a nonstress test, is prophylactic so she does not worry unnecessarily. Reinforce teaching points and positive aspects of the pregnancy for support people so they do not share unwarranted concerns and worries with the woman.

Women worry not only for the fetus but also, realistically, for themselves. In many instances, a well-meaning physician or family member or friend has told a woman long ago that she would never be able to have children. Much as she would like to believe the obstetrician who is telling her now that she can, she cannot forget the earlier prediction. If she feels that the pregnancy will never reach a safe conclusion, it is hard for her to follow instructions; everything seems more or less in vain. This can interfere with infant bonding. It helps some women to look at the pregnancy one day at a time rather than at the entire pregnancy. "Today, everything is going well. Let's do everything that is necessary today. Tomorrow we will think about what needs to be done then."

Nursing Interventions During Labor and Birth

The anesthetic of choice for labor in women with heart disease is often an epidural as this can make both labor and birth effort-free as well as pain-free. Many women with heart disease should not push with contractions; pushing requires more effort than they should expend. If an epidural anesthetic is used, low forceps will be used for birth. A woman may be disappointed that her birth is not more "natural"; help her to remember that her ultimate goals are a healthy newborn and a mother

able to care for her new baby, and these are the measures that can achieve such goals.

Fetal heart beat and uterine contractions should be closely monitored during labor on all women with heart disease. The mother's blood pressure, pulse, and respirations are assessed frequently. Rapidly increasing pulse rate (more than 100 bpm) is an indication that her heart is pumping ineffectively and therefore has increased its rate in an effort to compensate. She should remain in a side-lying position to reduce the possibility of supine hypotension syndrome. If she has some pulmonary edema, it may be necessary for her to have her chest and head elevated (semi-Fowler's position) to breathe adequately. Remember that fatigue is a symptom of heart decompensation. If this occurs in labor, evaluate carefully whether it is heart or labor related.

A major problem that can occur in women with atrial or ventricular heart defects during labor or birth is that a shunt reversal can occur if the systemic circulatory pressure falls from hypovolemia or the effect of epidural anesthesia. If this happens, there will be severe underperfusion of the lungs as blood shunts right to left across the heart septum. The woman will become cyanotic and dyspneic. To prevent this, women should be well hydrated before epidural administration, blood loss should be kept to a minimum, and the supine position must be avoided.

Postpartal Nursing Interventions

The period immediately following birth may be the most critical time for the woman with heart disease (Cunningham et al., 1993). This is because with delivery of the placenta, the blood that supplied the placenta is now released into the general circulation, and the blood volume increases between 20% to 40%. During pregnancy, the rise in blood volume occurred over a 6-month period, so the heart had time to adjust to this change gradually. Following birth, the rise in pressure takes place within 5 minutes, so the heart must make a rapid and major adjustment.

If the woman is in severe congestive failure following birth, she needs a program of decreased activity and possibly anticoagulant and digitalis therapy until her circulation stabilizes. As soon as possible, she should be ambulated to avoid the formation of emboli; she may need to wear elastic stockings to increase venous return. If she was not already begun on prophylactic antibiotics previously, she will be started on them immediately postpartally to discourage subacute bacterial endocarditis caused by introduction of microorganisms from the denuded uterus.

A woman with heart disease is often interested in close inspection of her baby immediately following birth because she wants to know that her infant does not have a heart defect. Be sure to point out that acrocyanosis is normal in newborns, so that she does not interpret her baby's severe peripheral cyanosis as cardiac inadequacy.

In the postpartal period, compounds to encourage uterine involution such as methylergonovine maleate (Methergine) must be used with caution because they tend to increase blood pressure and this necessitates increased heart action. The woman with heart disease can breast-feed without difficulty as a rule, although she needs to be individually assessed. Postpartal exercises to improve abdominal tone should not be undertaken until her physician approves them. Kegel's exercises are acceptable for perineal strengthening. Suggest a stool softener if it has not been prescribed to prevent her from straining with bowel movements.

The woman may require a longer than usual hospital stay so that her cardiac condition can be stabilized. Be certain she has thought through what help she will need at home so she can continue periods of adequate rest. Be certain she schedules a return appointment for a postpartal checkup for both her gynecologic health and cardiac status.

The Woman With an Artificial Valve Prosthesis

Once women with a heart valve prosthesis were advised not to become pregnant. Today, caring for a woman with a valve prosthesis during pregnancy would not be unusual. A problem that arises is that many women with valve prostheses take oral anticoagulants such as Coumarin derivatives to prevent the formation of clots at the valve site. Unfortunately, these medications may increase the risk of congenital anomalies in infants (pregnancy risk category D). Women, therefore, are usually placed on heparin therapy before becoming pregnant to reduce this risk. Heparin does not cross the placenta so does not interfere with fetal development or fetal coagulation (category C). Subclinical bleeding from the anticoagulant in the mother may cause placental dislodgment, so the woman must be observed closely for signs of premature separation of the placenta during pregnancy and labor (Cosico et al., 1992). If coagulation therapy other than heparin is continued, it may be discontinued about 2 weeks before birth to reduce the level in the fetus at birth and prevent the fetus's being born with a coagulation defect (Cosico, et al, 1992).

The Woman With Chronic Hypertensive Vascular Disease

Women with chronic hypertensive disease come into pregnancy with an elevated blood pressure (140/90 or above). Hypertension of this kind is usually associated with arteriosclerosis or renal disease. It tends to be a problem of the older pregnant woman. Retinal changes

may be apparent on physical examination from the chronic hypertension in retinal vessels. Deterioration of the renal glomeruli may have occurred, resulting in chronic **proteinuria** (excretion of protein in urine). Chronic hypertension produces a high-risk status as fetal well being may be compromised by poor placental perfusion during the pregnancy.

Usually, the woman who enters pregnancy with slight hypertension will have an additional elevation of blood pressure with pregnancy; she is prone to the development of edema and proteinuria. It is difficult to differentiate this increased blood pressure and proteinuria from developing preeclampsia if the woman comes to the health care facility late in pregnancy for her first prenatal visit (see Chapter 15 for a discussion of pregnancy-induced hypertension).

Women with chronic hypertensive vascular disease should be followed by an internist during pregnancy, as well as by an obstetrician. They will likely be scheduled for an ultrasound exam at 16 to 24 weeks to document adequate fetal growth. Baseline renal function studies such as creatinine clearance and a 24-hour protein will be scheduled early in pregnancy and repeated about every 8 weeks throughout pregnancy. Nonpregnant women with hypertension are frequently prescribed diuretics, so a woman may be taking one of these at the beginning of pregnancy. The thiazides are pregnancy risk category D; ethacrynic acid is category D; furosemide is category C. Methyldopa (Aldomet), a commonly used antihypertensive, is a category B, so many women are changed to this at the beginning of a pregnancy. Calcium channel blockers are usually avoided as they may decrease uterine blood flow. If blood pressure becomes extremely elevated as pregnancy progresses, complete bedrest on the left side to promote diuresis may be necessary (Zuspan, 1991). In some women, pregnancy may have to be terminated to prevent a cerebral vascular accident. The infants of women with chronic hypertension tend to have retarded fetal growth or can be stillborn or register fetal distress during labor due to poor placental perfusion. Abruptio placenta may occur during pregnancy because the increased vascular tension leads to rupture of capillaries supplying the placenta, with placenta infarcts developing. Because women with hypertension are advised not to take birth control pills, other methods of contraception will need to be discussed.

The Woman With Venous Thromboembolic Disease

The incidence of venous thromboembolic disease increases during pregnancy due to a combination of stasis of blood in the lower extremities from uterine pressure and hypercoagulability (the effect of increased estrogen; Figure 14-4) (Skudder & Farrington, 1993). When pres-

cough with hemoptysis, tachycardia or missed beats, and severe dizziness or fainting from lowered blood pressure. Pulmonary embolism is an emergency situation. Care measures for this are discussed in Chapter 15.

The risk of thrombus formation can be prevented or reduced through common-sense measures such as avoiding the use of constrictive knee-high stockings, not sitting with legs crossed at the knee, and avoiding standing in one position for a long period. If a thrombus does occur during pregnancy, the woman will be treated with bedrest and intravenous administration of heparin for 24 to 48 hours. Following this, she may be prescribed subcutaneous heparin for the duration of the pregnancy. It is generally recommended that the lower abdomen be used for rotating sites for subcutaneous heparin administration. With pregnancy, this site of choice is usually avoided and the injection sites limited to arms and thighs. Heparin dosage is regulated by frequent partial thromboplastin time (PTT) determinations. Additional measures of care for the woman with deep vein thrombosis (DVT) such as heat, elevation, and bedrest are discussed in Chapter 25 because the highest incidence of this occurs in the postpartal period.

A particular group of women has been identified as being more susceptible than normal to thrombi formation, spontaneous abortion, fetal death, and hypertension of pregnancy: women with antiphospholipid antibodies (aPLA) (Aoki et al., 1993). It is unknown why aPLA occurs in some clients but not in others, but these antibodies probably represent an autoimmune process. Women who are identified as aPLA-positive may be started on a prophylactic program of aspirin or subcutaneous heparin during pregnancy, continued postpartally to reduce the possibility of DVT. Administration of a corticosteroid helps to reduce the formation of additional antibodies and, thus, may also be prescribed. Following pregnancy, such women should not begin an oral contraceptive, which can increase blood coagulation and the possibility of thrombi formation.

Women taking heparin during pregnancy should not take any additional injections once labor begins to help reduce the possibility of hemorrhage at birth; they are not routine candidates for episiotomy or epidural anesthesiology for this same reason. Heparin administration with close PTT monitoring is resumed following birth.

Endocrine Disorders and Pregnancy

As a normal effect of pregnancy, the thyroid gland enlarges (hypertrophies) slightly as a result of increased vascularity due to the increased metabolic rate necessary to supply nutrients to both the maternal and fetal systems. The woman with preexisting thyroid problems may have difficulty making this pregnancy transition.

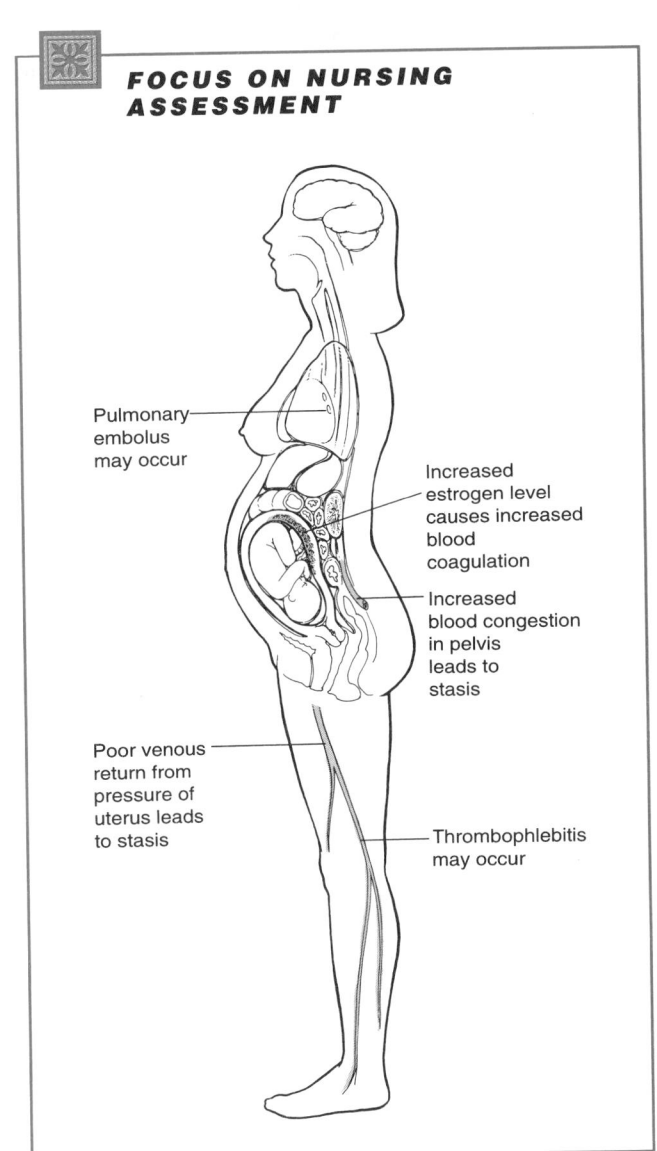

FOCUS ON NURSING ASSESSMENT

Pulmonary embolus may occur

Increased estrogen level causes increased blood coagulation

Increased blood congestion in pelvis leads to stasis

Poor venous return from pressure of uterus leads to stasis

Thrombophlebitis may occur

FIGURE 14-4
Symptoms of venous thromboembolic disease in pregnancy.

sure of the fetal head at birth puts additional pressure on lower extremity veins, actual damage can occur to the walls of vessels. When this triad of effects is in place (i.e., stasis, vessel damage, and hypercoagulation), the stage is set for thrombus formation in the lower extremities (Sipes & Weiner, 1990). As more women delay childbearing until after age 30 years, the likelihood of **deep vein thrombosis** (DVT) leading to pulmonary emboli increases as increased age is yet another risk factor for thrombosis formation. With hemorrhage and infection of pregnancy reduced in amount because of better therapy for these complications of pregnancy, pulmonary emboli has become a major cause of death in childbirth (Lagrew, 1990). Symptoms of pulmonary embolism are chest pain, sudden onset of dyspnea,

Nursing Diagnoses and Related Interventions

Nursing Diagnosis: High risk for altered placental perfusion related to imbalance of hormones secondary to preexisting endocrine disorder during pregnancy

Goal: Fetus will suffer no adverse effects from maternal hormonal imbalance.

Outcome Criteria: No congenital anomalies are present in infant at birth; Apgar score is 7 to 10.

The Woman With Hypothyroidism

Hypothyroidism is a rare condition in young adults; those women with symptoms of untreated hypothyroidism are often unable to conceive because they are anovulatory. Because their thyroid cannot increase function to maintain even normal limits (and, thus, cannot increase to a pregnancy level), the woman often has a history of early spontaneous abortion. A woman with hypothyroidism fatigues easily and tends to be obese; her skin is dry (myxedema) and she has little tolerance for cold. Most women with hypothyroidism take thyroxine to supplement what their body cannot produce. A woman who is taking thyroxine for therapy for hypothyroidism needs to consult with her obstetrician and internist when she is planning on becoming pregnant. She needs to come for early diagnosis and close follow-up as soon as she suspects she is pregnant (1 week past her missed menstrual period). As a rule, her dose of thyroxine will be increased for the duration of the pregnancy to simulate the effect that would normally occur in pregnancy. Be certain that the woman realizes the importance of this increased dose.

Hypothyroidism is associated with extreme nausea and vomiting during pregnancy (hyperemesis gravidarum) so she may be more prone to this than normally. Following the pregnancy, the dose of thyroxine prescribed for pregnancy must be gradually tapered back to the prepregnancy level. Be certain the woman does not continue to take her pregnancy dose (trying to be economical and use up her higher dose pills) or she will pass the line between normal thyroid function and develop hyperthyroidism.

The Woman With Hyperthyroidism

Hyperthyroidism causes symptoms of rapid heart rate; exophthalmos (protruding eyeball); heat intolerance; nervousness; heart palpitation; and weight loss. Hyperthyroidism is more apt to be seen in pregnancy than hypothyroidism. If undiagnosed, the woman may develop heart failure during pregnancy because her rapid heart rate cannot adjust to the increasing serum volume occurring with pregnancy. She is more prone to symptoms of hypertension of pregnancy and preterm labor than the average woman. Hyperthyroidism is normally diagnosed by a radioactive uptake of ^{131}I subtype. This diagnostic procedure should not be used during pregnancy because the fetal thyroid will also incorporate this drug; this could result in destruction of the fetal thyroid.

Treatment for hyperthyroidism is with thioamides (methimazole or propylthiouracil) to reduce thyroid activity. These drugs are unfortunately teratogens in that they cross the placenta and lead to congenital hypothyroidism and consequent enlarged thyroid gland (a goiter) in the fetus. If this abnormal neck growth enlarges enough, it can obstruct the airway and make resuscitation difficult for the infant at birth. These drugs also increase the potential for bleeding during birth (Loeb, 1993). The woman should be regulated on the lowest dose possible and cautioned to keep a careful record of doses taken so she does not forget or accidentally duplicate a dose. Surgical treatment to reduce the functioning of the maternal thyroid gland can be accomplished but this is generally not the treatment of choice due to the need for general anesthesia during pregnancy. Following a pregnancy, if the woman desires other children, the procedure might be possible as an interpregnancy procedure.

If the woman's thyroid function was not regulated during pregnancy, infants may be born with symptoms of hyperthyroidism because of the excess stimulation they receive in utero. An assay of fetal cord blood will reveal the level of T4 and TSH and if therapy is needed. The infant appears jittery; tachypnea and tachycardia may be present. Women on antithyroid drugs are advised not to breast-feed their babies, because these drugs are excreted in breast milk (Loeb, 1993).

The Woman With Diabetes Mellitus

Diabetes mellitus is an endocrine disorder in which the pancreas is unable to produce adequate insulin to regulate body glucose. The incidence of the disorder affects 1% to 5% of women during pregnancy (Dickinson & Palmer, 1990). Before insulin was produced synthetically in 1921, women with diabetes either failed to survive to reach childbearing age, were infertile, or had spontaneous abortions early in pregnancy. Now that diabetes can be well controlled, three new problems have developed: (1) how to bring a woman with diabetes through a pregnancy with good glucose-insulin control; (2) how to protect her infant in utero from the adverse effects of the diabetes; and (3) how to care for the infant in the first 24-hour period after birth until the infant's insulin-glucose regulatory mechanism stabilizes.

Reproductive planning may be a fourth concern for a diabetic woman. Many women with diabetes cannot take birth control pills because progesterone interferes with insulin activity and therefore increases blood glucose levels. The estrogen in contraceptives has the potential for increasing lipids, cholesterol levels, and blood clotting. In the woman with a potential for vessel complications, taking such a substance is a questionable practice. Intrauterine devices lead to a high incidence of PID; because women with diabetes have difficulty fighting infections, these are not usually advised either. Norplant, subcutaneous implanted progestin, may be an ideal choice (see Chapter 5).

Pathophysiology and Clinical Manifestations

The possible etiology and pathology of diabetes mellitus is discussed in detail in Chapter 48. The primary problem of any woman with the disorder is control of the balance between insulin and blood glucose to prevent acidosis. Acidosis is dangerous during pregnancy because it is a threat to the fetus.

If insulin amount is insufficient, glucose cannot be used by body cells. The cells register their glucose want and the liver quickly converts stored glycogen to glucose to increase the blood glucose level. Because of the insulin insufficiency, however, the body cells still cannot use the glucose, and the serum glucose levels continue to rise (hyperglycemia). When the level of blood sugar of the woman rises to 150 mg per 100 mL (normal is 80 to 120 mg/dL), the kidneys begin to excrete quantities of glucose in the urine in an attempt to lower the level (**glycosuria**). During pregnancy the point at which this happens may be even lower than 150 mg per 100 mL. Because of osmotic action, the increased amount of glucose in the urine reduces fluid absorption in the kidney, and large quantities of fluid are lost in urine (polyuria).

Dehydration begins to occur; the blood serum becomes concentrated and the blood volume may fall. With the reduced blood flow, cells do not receive adequate oxygen, and anaerobic metabolic reactions cause large stores of lactic acid to pour out of muscle into the bloodstream. Fat is mobilized from fat stores and metabolized for energy, and large amounts of ketone bodies are poured into the bloodstream. Ketone bodies are acidic (the best example is acetone). These two acid sources affect the *p*H of the blood. The woman has developed a metabolic acidosis.

Protein stores are next tapped by the body as it attempts to find a source of energy for body cells. Protein catabolism reduces the supply of protein to body cells. Cell catabolism also results in the loss of potassium and sodium from the body. Long-term effects of diabetes mellitus are vascular narrowing, leading to kidney and retinal dysfunction and increasing blood pressure.

Diabetes During Pregnancy

Even a woman who has successful regulation of glucose-insulin metabolism before pregnancy is apt to develop less than optimum control during pregnancy because all women experience a number of changes in the glucose-insulin regulatory system as pregnancy progresses (Figure 14-5). Glomerular filtration of glucose is increased (the glomerular excretion threshold is lowered), causing slight glycosuria. The rate of insulin secretion is increased, and the fasting blood sugar is lowered. All women appear to develop an insulin resistance as pregnancy progresses (i.e., insulin does not seem normally effective during pregnancy), a phenomenon that is probably caused by the presence of the hormone human placental lactogen (chorionic somatomammotropin) and high levels of cortisol, estrogen, progesterone, and catecholamines. Placental insulinase may cause increased breakdown or degradation of insulin. This resistance to or destruction of insulin is helpful in a normal pregnancy because it prevents the blood glucose from falling to dangerous limits, despite the increased insulin

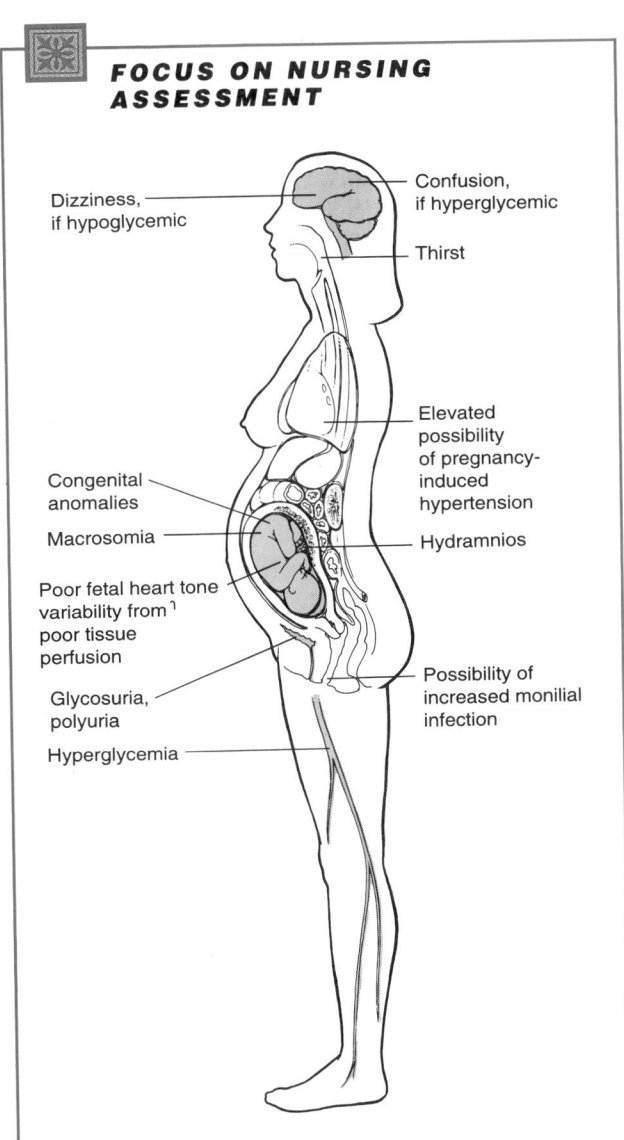

FOCUS ON NURSING ASSESSMENT

Dizziness, if hypoglycemic

Confusion, if hyperglycemic

Thirst

Elevated possibility of pregnancy-induced hypertension

Congenital anomalies

Macrosomia

Hydramnios

Poor fetal heart tone variability from poor tissue perfusion

Glycosuria, polyuria

Hyperglycemia

Possibility of increased monilial infection

FIGURE 14-5
Symptoms of diabetes during pregnancy.

secretion that occurs. It causes difficulty for a diabetic pregnant woman in that she must increase her insulin dosage beginning at about week 24 of pregnancy to prevent hyperglycemia.

At the same time, the continued use of glucose by the fetus may lead to **hypoglycemia** (lowered serum glucose levels) for the mother between meals; this is apt to occur overnight. A low maternal level of glucogenic amino acids (used by the liver to produce glucose) add to this. She may become ketoacidic from breakdown of stored fat between meals. This is particularly likely to happen during the second and third trimester of pregnancy. If the woman has preexisting kidney disease (revealed by proteinuria, decreased creatinine clearance, and hypertension), the risk of fetal growth retardation, asphyxia, stillbirth, and maternal pregnancy-induced hypertension rise markedly (Cunningham et al., 1993).

When glucose regulation is poor, the woman is more prone to pregnancy-induced hypertension and infection (particularly monilial infection) than other women. Infants of poorly controlled diabetic women tend to be large (more than 10 lb) because the increased insulin the fetus must produce to counteract the overload of glucose he or she receives acts as a growth stimulant. The increased glucose adds subcutaneous fat deposits. A large-size infant may create delivery problems at the end of the pregnancy due to cephalopelvic disproportion (Sacks, 1993). There is a high incidence of congenital anomaly, abortion, and stillbirth in infants of women with diabetes, and at birth they are more prone to hypoglycemia, respiratory distress syndrome, hypocalcemia, and hyperbilirubinemia. The first trimester of pregnancy is the most critical time for fetal development; if the woman's serum glucose level can be kept from becoming hyperglycemic during this time, the chances of congenital anomaly are greatly lessened (Cunningham et al., 1993).

Hydramnios occurs in at least 25% of diabetic women, probably due to hyperglycemia in the fetus that causes a fluid shift of amniotic fluid. Amniocentesis may be done to decrease the level of amniotic fluid. This unfortunately submits the woman to potential infection and preterm labor and is only a temporary measure because amniotic fluid is continually produced.

The Woman With Gestational Diabetes

Approximately 2% to 3% of all women who do not begin a pregnancy with diabetes become diabetic during the pregnancy, usually at the midpoint of pregnancy when insulin resistance becomes most noticeable. This is termed gestational diabetes. The symptoms will fade again at the completion of pregnancy, but the woman with gestational diabetes may have as high a risk as 50% of developing diabetes later in life (Cunningham et al., 1993). It is unknown whether this disease results from inadequate insulin response to carbohydrate or from ex-

cessive resistance to insulin; a combination of both may occur. Women who are particularly prone to this are those who are obese, over age 30, or have a history of large babies (10 lb or more); unexplained fetal loss; congenital anomalies in previous pregnancies; unexplained natal or neonatal loss; or a family history of diabetes (one close relative or two distant ones).

Classification of Diabetes Mellitus

White (1978) has divided diabetes into various categories to predict pregnancy outcome (Table 14-3). The pregnancy outcome becomes less successful with more diabetic involvement in the mother. In class A, fetal survival is high. Infants of mothers in classes D and E may have a perinatal mortality as high as 25%. Class F and class R women may have a perinatal mortality close to 100%. Women with diabetes mellitus this severe are generally advised not to become pregnant. Women in class T (kidney transplant) can complete a pregnancy successfully.

Assessment

All women should be screened during pregnancy for diabetes. This is usually done using a 50-g oral glucose screening test at weeks 24 to 28 of pregnancy. Women who have a history of large babies (10 lbs or more), unexplained fetal loss, or congenital anomalies in previous pregnancies, who are obese, or who have a family history of diabetes should be screened early in pregnancy because they represent a high-risk group for developing diabetes.

Glucose Screening Test. Fasting is not necessary for a 1-hour glucose screening test. Following the oral 50-g glucose load a venous blood sample is taken for glucose determination 60 minutes later. If the serum glucose at 1 hour is more than 140 mg/dL, diabetes is said to be present (Dickinson & Palmer, 1990). If a 1-hour screening test is positive, women are then scheduled for a 100-g, 3-hour fasting **glucose tolerance test**. The values that confirm diabetes with this are shown in Table 14-4.

Monitoring the Woman With Diabetes. The woman with overt diabetes should come to her obstetrician for care before she becomes pregnant; during this waiting period, her condition can be well regulated so she has no hyperglycemia during the early weeks of pregnancy when the tendency for congenital anomalies is highest. The woman should use a basal body temperature graph or a home test kit to determine she is pregnant at the earliest possible time. The best insulin control program for her during pregnancy can then be determined. The measurement of **glycosylated hemoglobin** is used to detect the degree of hyperglycemia present. This is a measure of the amount of glucose attached to hemoglobin. As glucose circulates in the bloodstream, it binds to a portion of the total hemoglobin in the blood. The

Table 14-3. *Classification of Diabetes Mellitus*

Class	Description
Class A	Pregnant women whose glucose tolerance test is only slightly abnormal; dietary regulation is minimal; no insulin is required (gestational diabetes is included)
Class B	Pregnant women whose diabetes is of less than 10 years' duration or whose disease began at age 20 years or older; there is no vascular involvement
Class C	Pregnant women whose diabetes began between ages 10 and 19 years or whose disease has lasted from 10 to 19 years; there is minimal vascular involvement
Class D	Pregnant women whose diabetes has lasted 20 years or more or whose disease began before age 10 years; there is greater vascular involvement than in class C D1 = Under age 10 years at onset D2 = More than 20 years' duration D3 = Beginning retinopathy is present D4 = Calcified vessels of legs are present D5 = Hypertension is present
Class E	Pregnant women in whom calcification of the pelvic arteries has been demonstrated on x-ray; technique is not done during pregnancy because of teratogenic effect of x-ray
Class F	Pregnant women whose diabetes has caused nephropathy
Class H	Cardiopathy is present
Class R	Pregnant women with active retinitis proliferans
Class T	Women who have had kidney transplants

(From White, P. [1978]. Classification of obstetric diabetes. *American Journal of Obstetrics and Gynecology, 50*, 229, with permission.)

amount of glucose that attaches to hemoglobin in this way will be high if the hemoglobin has been exposed to a greater level of glucose than normally. Measuring glycosylated hemoglobin (HbA$_1$ or HbA$_{1c}$) reflects the average blood glucose level over the past 4 to 6 weeks (the time the red blood cells were picking up the glucose). The upper normal level of HbA$_{1c}$ is 6% of total hemoglobin. Yet another monitoring measure is the use of serum fructosamine. Fructosamine levels vary, like glycosylated hemoglobin, according to recent ingestion of glucose.

The glucose level in urine is not indicative of the actual blood sugar because, due to the decreased renal threshold, glucose may be spilled at unusually low glucose serum levels. Monitoring the woman's serum glucose by blood monitoring is much more accurate. Women can be taught to do this themselves.

Table 14-4. *Oral Glucose Tolerance Test Values (Plasma Values)**

Test Type	Pregnant mg/dL Glucose
Fasting	105
1 h	190
2 h	165
3 h	145

*Following a 100 g glucose load. Rate is abnormal if two values are exceeded. (From Fischbach, F. [1992]. *A manual of laboratory and diagnostic tests.* Philadelphia: J.B. Lippincott, p. 305.)

Ophthalmic examination should be done once during pregnancy for gestational diabetes and with each trimester for known diabetics because background retinal changes, such as increased exudate (Figure 14-6), dot hemorrhage, and macular edema, progress or originate during pregnancy. If proliferation retinopathy was present before pregnancy, this also progresses and can

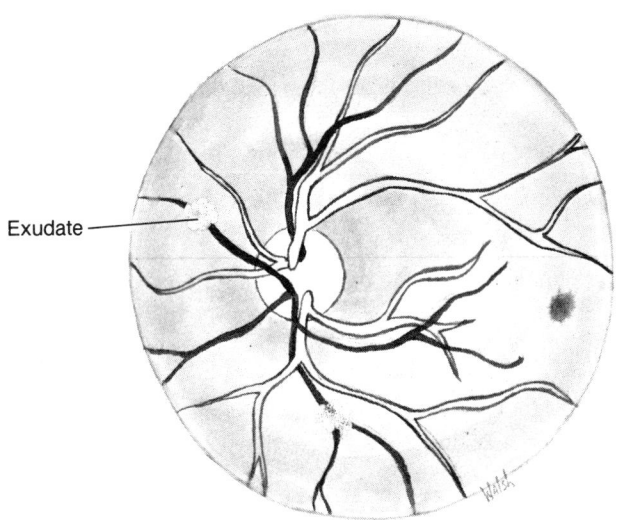

Exudate

FIGURE 14-6
Increased exudate in the retina can occur with progressing diabetes during pregnancy. It appears as a "cloud-like" finding obscuring a retinal vessel.

lead to blindness. Laser therapy to halt these changes can be done during pregnancy without risk to the fetus. A urine culture may also be done each trimester to detect asymptomatic urinary tract infection.

Nursing Diagnoses and Related Interventions

Because diabetes is such a complex disorder, associated nursing diagnoses are many and varied. They include but are not limited to

- High risk for altered tissue perfusion related to reduced vascular flow
- Altered nutrition, less than body requirements, related to inability to use glucose
- High risk for ineffective individual coping related to required change in lifestyle
- High risk for infection related to impaired healing accompanying condition
- Fluid volume deficit related to polyuria accompanying disorder
- Knowledge deficit related to voiced misconceptions of illness
- Health-seeking behaviors related to voiced need to learn home glucose monitoring

The following nursing diagnosis and related interventions illustrate one of the most important facets of the nursing role in caring for the diabetic pregnant client: health teaching.

> **Nursing Diagnosis:** Health-seeking behaviors related to diabetic therapeutic regimen changes during pregnancy
>
> **Goal:** Client will demonstrate knowledge about effects of pregnancy on diabetic condition and vice versa by 1 month.
>
> **Outcome Criteria:** Woman states importance of careful attention to diet, exercise, and home monitoring of glucose levels during pregnancy; describes diet and exercise program; states intention to keep diet and exercise constant.

Nurses are instrumental in teaching women with diabetes how to change a therapeutic regimen during pregnancy (or begin one if newly diagnosed). Important topics include diet, exercise, insulin administration, blood glucose monitoring, and explanation of the various fetal assessment tests that will be done.

Education Regarding Diet During Pregnancy. Many women who are of childbearing age and who have had diabetes since early childhood do not follow a strict diabetic diet but eat sensibly and then cover any excess food eaten with additional insulin. This type of regimen

is apt to require excessive insulin during pregnancy. A woman is well advised, therefore, to alert her health care providers that she is anticipating a pregnancy and begin to subscribe to a stricter diabetic diet regimen that includes exchange lists before she becomes pregnant. She should wait to become pregnant until she has good disease control. Women who develop gestational diabetes begin a diet as soon as they are diagnosed (ADA, 1990).

Dietary control or maintaining an adequate glucose intake so that hypoglycemia does not occur may be extremely difficult early in pregnancy because of nausea and vomiting. An 1800- to 2200-calorie diet (or one calculated at 35 Kcal per kg of ideal weight), divided into three meals and three snacks, is a usual regimen for a woman with diabetes during pregnancy. Keeping calories evenly distributed this way during the day helps to keep the blood glucose constant. If a woman cannot eat due to vomiting or nausea early in pregnancy or heartburn in later pregnancy, she must notify the health care agency. She may need temporary intravenous fluid supplemented. Women are extremely vulnerable to hypoglycemia at night during pregnancy due to the continuous fetal use of glucose during the time they sleep. Urge the woman to make her final snack of the day one of protein and complex carbohydrate so this is slowly digested during the night.

The diet should include a reduced amount of saturated fats and cholesterol and an increased amount of dietary fiber. Increased fiber decreases postprandial hyperglycemia and thus lowers insulin requirements. Of dietary calories, 20% should be from protein, 50% from carbohydrate, and 30% from fat.

Even though a woman is overweight, she should not reduce her intake to below 1800 calories during pregnancy. A diet this low in carbohydrate causes breakdown of fat, which produces acidosis. In the woman with diabetes, the weight of the infant is directly correlated with what the woman gains in pregnancy (which directly correlates with her disease control). She thus must be extremely nutrition conscious to maintain good control and keep her weight gain to a suitable amount (approximately 25 lb), in the hope of limiting the size of her infant and making a vaginal birth possible.

Education Regarding Exercise During Pregnancy. Exercise is another mechanism that lowers serum glucose and thereby the need for insulin. If a woman begins to exercise during pregnancy, she may notice excessive glucose fluctuations at first. The woman is urged, therefore, to begin her pregnancy exercise program before pregnancy, when glucose fluctuation can be evaluated and food and snacks adjusted accordingly before a fetus is involved.

When the woman exercises, she lowers her blood glucose level because of uptake of glucose by the muscle. This effect lasts for at least 12 hours following exercise. If the arm in which she injected insulin is actively exercised, the effect will be greatly increased. To avoid this phenomenon, the woman should eat a snack of protein or complex carbohydrate before exercise and she should maintain a consistent exercise program (not doing aerobic exercises one day and then none the next but rather 30 minutes of walking every day). In the woman who is in poor diabetic control, extreme exercise will cause hyperglycemia and ketoacidosis as the liver both releases glucose and breaks down fatty acids in an attempt to supply enough energy for the exercise (yet the body cannot use them because of inadequate insulin).

Therapeutic Management

Both women with gestational diabetes and those with overt diabetes need more frequent prenatal visits than the average woman. Women with gestational diabetes are usually briefly hospitalized early in pregnancy to determine whether insulin will be necessary or whether diet management will be enough. Then they are monitored every week or two during pregnancy. Women with known diabetes may be admitted to the hospital early in pregnancy for insulin adjustment and then monitored weekly (preferably in a high-risk diabetic center where an internist, an obstetrician, a nurse, a diabetic educator, and a nutritionist work in combination).

Insulin. Because of the change in body metabolism, the woman who was diabetic before pregnancy may need to increase her insulin dose during pregnancy. If she has been taking one particular kind of insulin and a specified dosage for a long time before the pregnancy, changing the type and dosage may be unnerving for her. She can be informed that reregulation is a necessity for pregnancy because of the changes in her metabolism. Women with gestational diabetes will be started on insulin therapy if diet alone is unsuccessful in regulating glucose values.

Early in pregnancy a woman may need less insulin because the fetus is taking so much glucose in rapid cell growth. Later in pregnancy she will need an increased amount because of increased metabolic need.

The dosage and type of insulin will be specific for each woman. The insulin chosen is usually a short-acting insulin (regular) combined with an intermediate type (NPH). Two-thirds of the total amount of the day's insulin is given in the morning; the other one-third in the evening. This is self administered in combination 30 minutes before breakfast in a ratio of 2:1 (NPH to regular) and again just before dinner in the evening in a ratio of 1:1 (Gabbe, 1990).

Oral hypoglycemia agents (aside from being controversial at present for any client) are not used for regulation because, unlike insulin, they cross the placenta and

are potentially teratogenic. Humulin insulin is generally recommended because it has the potential for provoking a lesser antibody response than beef or pork insulins. Remind women of the time interval their insulin takes to reach its peak. An intermediate insulin given prebreakfast reaches its peak after lunch or late in the afternoon just before dinner. Regular insulin given prebreakfast reaches its peak just after breakfast. An intermediate insulin given in the evening reaches peak into the next day before breakfast; the evening regular insulin injection peaks after dinner or at bedtime. Knowing when insulin reaches its peak level makes blood glucose monitoring meaningful and alerts women to the time of the day when they are most apt to be hypoglycemic.

Be certain that women are using an injection technique of stretching the skin taut and injecting at a 90° angle. Although this is normally intramuscular injection technique, insulin syringes have such short needles (⅝ in) that this places the insulin in the subcutaneous tissue. Because insulin is absorbed more slowly from the thigh than the upper arm, the woman should maintain a consistent rotating injection routine (either all sites in one limb before using another or rotating limbs) in order to maintain as consistent a level of absorption as possible. Insulin is adjusted to keep a fasting blood sugar below 100 mg/dL range and a 1-hour postprandial level below 120 mg/dL.

Insulin Pump Therapy (continuous subcutaneous insulin infusion). Because a woman will have some periods of relative hyperglycemia and hypoglycemia no matter how carefully she maintains her diet and balances her exercise level, the best solution to keep serum glucose constant that can be devised is to administer insulin by a continuous pump during pregnancy.

When **insulin pump therapy** (administration of insulin by an automatic infusion devise) is begun, the woman is usually hospitalized for at least 3 days to assure that she is familiar with the equipment and that the proposed insulin coverage is indeed adequate for her. An insulin pump is an automatic pump about the size of a transistor radio. A syringe of regular insulin is placed in the pump chamber; a thin polyethylene tubing leads to the woman's abdomen where it is implanted into the subcutaneous tissue of her abdomen by a small gauge needle (Figure 14-7). Throughout the day at a continuous rate of about 1 u per hour, the pump edges the syringe barrel forward, infusing insulin continually into the subcutaneous tissue. Before a snack and before a meal, the woman manually presses on the syringe barrel and forces a bolus of insulin forward to increase her insulin amount for these large carbohydrate times. The site of the pump insertion is cleaned daily and covered with sterile gauze; the site is changed every 24 to 48 hours to ensure absorption is still optimum.

Restrictions with pump therapy are that the pump

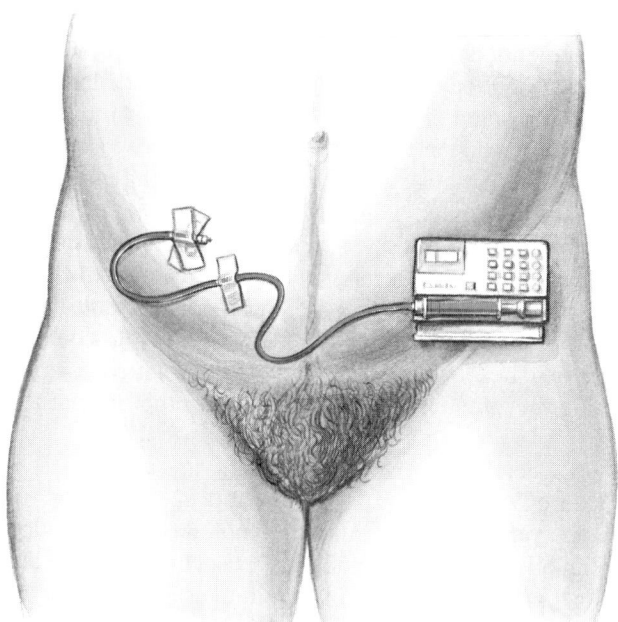

FIGURE 14-7
Using an insulin pump during pregnancy is the best assurance that insulin levels will remain constant.

must not be allowed to become wet; a woman must remove the pump (not the syringe and tubing) while showering. She removes the needle and pump to bathe or swim (caution her not to leave it disconnected for more than 1 hour). She might prefer to wear clothing that hides the pump's outline (it can either be held against her abdomen by an over-the shoulder sling or hung from a belt around her waist). To assess that the pump is delivering insulin at the designated rate, the woman must do blood glucose determinations four times throughout the day (fasting and 1 hour after each meal). When pump therapy first begins, she must wake at night and do a 2 AM blood glucose as this is a vulnerable time for hypoglycemia.

Blood Glucose Monitoring. All women with diabetes can be taught to do blood glucose monitoring to determine if hyperglycemia or hypoglycemia exists. For this, a woman uses a Dextrostix technique using one of her fingertips as the site of lancet puncture. If she uses a glucose meter with a digital readout, it is easier for her to assess the level than if she merely compares the color of the test strip to a color-coded chart. A fasting plasma glucose level below 100 mg/dL and a postprandial level below 120 mg/dL are well-adjusted values. Because home monitors are based on whole blood values, which are 14% to 15% higher than plasma values, levels of 115 mg/dL fasting and 138 mg/dL are levels the woman should strive to maintain.

When a woman discovers hypoglycemia is present, she treats this by drinking a glass of milk and eating some crackers. Taking a less concentrated fluid such as

milk rather than orange juice and including a complex carbohydrate helps prevent a rebound phenomenon in which high glucose is created that then becomes even more pronounced hypoglycemia.

If the woman discovers an elevated blood glucose, she should assess urine for acetone. The finding of acetone in two separate specimens should be reported to a health care provider. Acidosis during pregnancy must be prevented because maternal acidosis leads to fetal anoxia due to fetal inability to use oxygen when body cells are acidotic. The most frequent time during pregnancy for insulin coma (hyperinsulinism) is the 2nd and 3rd month, before insulin resistance peaks; for diabetic coma (hypoinsulinism) it is the 6th month, or the time insulin resistance is becoming most pronounced.

Tests for Placental Function and Fetal Well Being. Because women with diabetes tend to have infants with a higher incidence of birth anomalies than normal, the woman may have a serum for alpha-fetoprotein done at 15 to 17 weeks to assess for a neural tube defect and an ultrasound examination done at approximately 18 to 20 weeks gestation for inspection of gross abnormalities. A creatinine clearance test may be ordered each trimester. A normal creatinine clearance suggests that the woman's vascular system is intact and uterine perfusion is probably adequate.

Placental functioning may also be established by means of a weekly nonstress test or biophysical profile (see Chapter 9) if the woman is in good control or a daily nonstress test if her regulation is poor. Fetal stress tests are difficult procedures for the woman. Having to wait during each weekly test to hear how the fetus is doing is like having to take a final examination every week. The woman may feel that it is somehow her fault, her doing, her failure (it is, after all, her diabetes) if the monitor equipment shows fetal distress. The failure may be absolute, because if the distress is acute, the fetus can no longer live in utero. If the gestation age is below 34 weeks, the infant is exposed to the serious consequences of immaturity.

The woman's partner is often unable to come to the hospital and be with the woman once or twice a week while she is having these tests. (It may be difficult enough for her to schedule this time.) The woman needs health care personnel with her who can help her to minimize the feeling that she is all alone. Sufficient emotional support during pregnancy is correlated with increased compliance in women with diabetes (Ruggiero et al., 1990).

A woman may be asked to self-monitor fetal well being by recording how many movements occur an hour. Be certain she knows that fetal activity varies depending on her activity and meal patterns so she is not alarmed at discovering this herself. The healthy fetus has approximately 10 movements per hour (see Chapter 9).

Sonography to determine fetal growth, amniotic fluid volume, placental location, and biparietal diameter may be taken at week 28 and then again at weeks 36 to 38 of pregnancy. With fetal growth retardation, there is often accompanying oligohydramnios. With poor disease control, there is hydramnios formation in as many as 25% of pregnancies (probably due to hyperglycemia in the fetus which causes a fluid shift to amniotic fluid). Lecithin–sphingomyelin ratio by amniocentesis is undertaken by week 36 of pregnancy to assess fetal maturity. The L/S ratio in pregnancies complicated by diabetes tends not to show maturity as early as in other pregnancies because the synthesis of phosphatidyl glycerol, the compound that stabilizes surfactant, is delayed in a diabetes-complicated pregnancy.

As lung surfactant does not appear to form as early in these fetuses as others (due to the decreased level of cortisone present because of high serum glucose levels) most people accept 3:1 rather than 2:1 for a mature L/S ratio. The presence of phosphatidyl glycerol indicates lung maturity. Although it is known that administering corticosteroids to the mother during the last week of pregnancy can hurry lung maturity, corticosteroids may also impair fetal insulin release and perhaps fetal islet development. Therefore, with a fetus who already has a risk at birth from poor glucose control, this is not usually attempted.

Timing for Birth. Before women were managed with maximum control during pregnancy, the timing of the birth was a chief concern. One of the most hazardous times for the infant are weeks 36 to 40 of pregnancy (the fetus is drawing large stores of maternal nutrients because of its large size). In the past, many pregnancies were terminated early enough to prevent fetal loss from placental insufficiency due to poor perfusion during these susceptible weeks; hopefully this was not so early that immaturity of the child posed further complications.

For many years, cesarean birth was almost routinely performed in pregnant diabetic women at approximately 37 weeks gestation. Cesarean birth was chosen because it is difficult to induce labor this early in pregnancy as the cervix is not yet ripe or responsive to labor contractions. Furthermore, babies of diabetic women may be large, making vaginal delivery difficult. Moreover, a fetus suffering placental dysfunction or insufficiency, which may occur with maternal diabetes, will not do well in labor and may actually die. Early cesarean deliveries, however, often resulted in immature infants who died in the neonatal period because of respiratory distress syndrome (infants of diabetic women may be more prone to this than usual even without a cesarean birth).

Today, when accurate assessment of fetal age is available and the pregnancy can be maintained within safe limits by use of nonstress testing for a longer period, the last weeks of pregnancy are not as haz-ardous as before and the timing of birth is much more individualized. A woman may be hospitalized from week 34 or 37 until birth, however, so close monitoring can be accomplished.

Birth should be vaginal if this seems at all a possibility. Cesarean birth always presents a higher risk than vaginal birth for the fetus, and because of the difficulty of glucose-level regulation, the fetus of a diabetic mother is already under enough stress. Labor is induced by rupture of the membranes or an oxytocin infusion. Both maternal labor contractions and fetal heart sounds should be monitored continuously during labor so that placental dysfunction can be detected if it does occur. An internal fetal monitor may be used with scalp *p*H recordings. The woman's glucose level is regulated during labor by an intravenous infusion of regular insulin, with blood glucose assay every hour. Regulating the glucose level carefully during labor reduces the possibility of rebound hypoglycemia in the newborn (see Chapter 26 for care of the infant of a diabetic woman at birth).

If the woman will be given an epidural anesthetic, be certain that an intravenous glucose solution is not used for a plasma volume expander (or its presence is accounted for by additional insulin administration).

Postpartal Adjustment. During the postpartal period, a woman with diabetes has to undergo another readjustment to insulin regulation. With insulin resistance gone, often she needs no insulin during the immediate postpartal period; she will then return to her prepregnant insulin requirements. Blood glucose will be regulated in correlation with 1- or 2-hour postprandial blood glucose determinations. The woman with gestational diabetes will usually demonstrate normal glucose values by 24 hours after birth and need no further diet or insulin therapy. Urine or plasma should be assessed at health maintenance visits throughout life to detect if diabetes is developing in the woman. Women with diabetes may breast-feed, because insulin is one of the few substances that does not pass into breast milk from the bloodstream. The woman requires careful observation during the immediate postpartal period because if hydramnios was present during pregnancy, she is at risk of hemorrhage from poor uterine contraction.

Be certain the woman has contraceptive information as appropriate. Remind her that before she plans a second pregnancy, she will first need to be certain that her disease is stabilized and in good control (the first trimester of pregnancy is crucial fetal developmental time).

Cancer and Pregnancy

Malignancies seen with pregnancy are those that reach peak incidence during childbearing years: cervical, breast, ovarian, and thyroid tumors plus leukemia, melanoma, and lymphomas. As women delay the age at which they are having their first child, the incidence of malignancy during pregnancy is expected to rise.

Although women's immunologic mechanism is altered during pregnancy, there is no proof that pregnant women are more prone to cancer than others or that pregnancy changes the course of an existing disease. If a woman is in the first trimester when the malignancy is diagnosed, she and her partner are asked to make a difficult decision: delay treatment to avoid teratogenic risks to a fetus (possibly increasing the woman's risk); abort the pregnancy to allow for chemotherapy treatment; or choose chemotherapy or radiation treatment with the almost certain knowledge that they will cause birth anomalies in the fetus.

As a rule, women can receive chemotherapy in the second and third trimesters of pregnancy without untoward fetal effects. Radiation therapy, in contrast, another modality that is a mainstay of cancer therapy, puts the fetus at risk throughout pregnancy if the fetus is directly exposed.

Surgery to remove a tumor can be successfully completed during pregnancy with the understanding that there is a risk the fetus may suffer anoxia during anesthesia administration. The woman is at more than usual risk of thrombus formation postoperatively due to the increased coagulation process accompanying pregnancy. Cervical conization has a particularly high fetal risk because the surgery may directly disrupt the pregnancy (Giuntoli, 1990; Duggan, 1993).

A cancer present in the woman does not appear to metastasize to the fetus during pregnancy (Scott, 1990). This is because the placenta serves as an effective barrier against this spread and also because the fetus may be capable of resisting the invasion of the foreign cells.

Mental Illness and Pregnancy

Psychiatric illnesses affect all age groups, including women of childbearing age. Depression is the most common mental illness seen. Schizophrenia tends to occur in adolescence and thus may occur in pregnant women.

Mental illness may precede or occur with pregnancy. Stress makes it more difficult to use coping mechanisms, and pregnancy or childbirth may be the stress that reveals mental illness for the first time. It is important that any psychotropic medication being taken by a pregnant woman be evaluated for possible fetal harm. For example, lithium, a mainstay of therapy for bipolar disorders such as manic depression, is a known teratogen. The woman with a psychiatric disorder should be cared for by both a psychiatric care team and a prenatal care group to assure that the stress of pregnancy is not increasing mental illness and distorted perceptions or depression from mental illness is not causing complications of pregnancy (Forcier, 1990).

Mental illness may also occur in the postpartal period (postpartal psychosis; see Chapter 25).

Trauma and Pregnancy

Trauma (injury by force) is a phenomenon that seems remote from pregnancy because the pregnant woman usually takes extra safety precautions to protect her body from harm. However, trauma in women occurs at a high incidence during the childbearing years because, for this age group, automobile accidents, homicide, and suicide are among the three leading causes of death. During pregnancy, the incidence of trauma is between 6% and 7% (as many as 250,000 pregnant women experience trauma per year), with the highest incidence during the last trimester due to clumsiness, fainting, and hyperventilation. Orthopedic injuries such as broken wrists or sprained ankles occur because the pregnant woman's sense of balance is altered. In an automobile accident, a pregnant woman is often the front seat passenger and this is the passenger who often receives the most severe injury in an accident. Other women seen in emergency rooms have suffered physical abuse.

Preventing Accidents

Accidents occur more frequently in people under stress than in those with little stress in their lives. Because pregnancy is a life event that may cause some stress in a family's life, a woman and her family should take sensible precautions for safety. Pregnancy counseling should include education about ways to avoid accidents and trauma (see the Focus on Family Teaching box).

Physiologic Changes in Pregnancy That Affect Trauma Care

In an emergency situation, the physiologic changes that normally occur with pregnancy must be considered in order for physical assessment to be meaningful. A primary rule to remember is that following a traumatic injury, a woman's body will maintain her own homeostasis at the expense of the fetus. To maintain blood pressure in the face of hemorrhage, for example, the woman's body will use peripheral vasoconstriction. The uterus is a peripheral organ in a shock response, so blood supply to the uterus will be greatly diminished and nutrient supply to the fetus greatly compromised when this happens (Figure 14-8).

The woman's total plasma volume increases during pregnancy from approximately 2600 mL to 4000 mL at term. This increase serves as a safeguard to the woman if trauma with bleeding should occur because the woman can lose more blood than normally (up to 30% of her blood volume) before hypovolemia is clinically evident (Dudley & Cruikshank, 1990). It also means,

Q. How can I reduce the chance I'll have an accident such as a fall during pregnancy?

A. This is a good question because during the latter half of pregnancy, accidents are more prone to happen from poor balance. Some preventive measures are:

- Don't stand on stepstools or step ladders (difficult to maintain balance on a narrow base).
- Keep small items such as toys out of pathways (a pregnant woman has difficulty seeing her feet).
- Avoid throw rugs without a nonskid backing.
- Use caution stepping in and out of a bathtub.
- Do not overload electrical circuits (it is difficult for a pregnant woman to escape a fire because of poor mobility).
- Do not smoke so falling asleep with a cigarette will not be a problem.
- Do not take medicine in the dark so an error is not apt to occur.
- Avoid handling toxic substances at work.
- Avoid working to a point of fatigue because this lowers judgment.
- Avoid long periods of standing because this can lead to orthostatic hypotension and fainting.
- Use a seat belt when driving at all times.
- Refuse to ride with anyone who has been drinking alcohol or whose judgment might be impaired.

mal. It is important to remember that this elevated rate is normal so a rapid pulse rate is not interpreted as a sign of hemorrhage. The heart is displaced by the elevated diaphragm so interpretation of an ECG will show a left axis deviation.

Peripheral venous pressure in the pregnant woman is unchanged, although it tends to be higher in lower extremities because of compression of the vena cava and back pressure. This causes lacerations of the legs or perineum to bleed much more profusely than usual. Peripheral blood flow in general is increased due to decreased peripheral vascular resistance (the effect of estrogen and decreased sympathetic activity all through pregnancy). This means that the pregnant women can be in severe shock and her extremities will still not feel cold and clammy.

During pregnancy, the leukocyte count rises (to 20,000 at term), so it is difficult to use this determination

however, that fluid replacement volume will undoubtedly have to be high because the woman needs more fluid than the nonpregnant woman to restore fully her circulatory volume. The central venous pressure (normal is 0 to 5 cm H_2O in a nonpregnant state) is increased to 2 to 7 cm H_2O. Although a woman needs a large amount of replacement fluid, this means her circulation can also be overwhelmed more easily than normal by intravenous fluid infusion.

To accommodate the increased vascular load of pregnancy, cardiac output increases in pregnancy from 1 L/min early in pregnancy to 6 to 7 L/min in the second trimester. This volume circulates through the placenta at such a rapid rate, approximately one-sixth total blood volume is present in the placenta at all times. If a uterine laceration occurs, this is always serious because up to one-sixth of blood volume would be immediately lost.

To move this increased blood volume adequately through the circulation, the heart rate increases 15 to 20 beats above normal, so a pulse rate of 80 to 95 is nor-

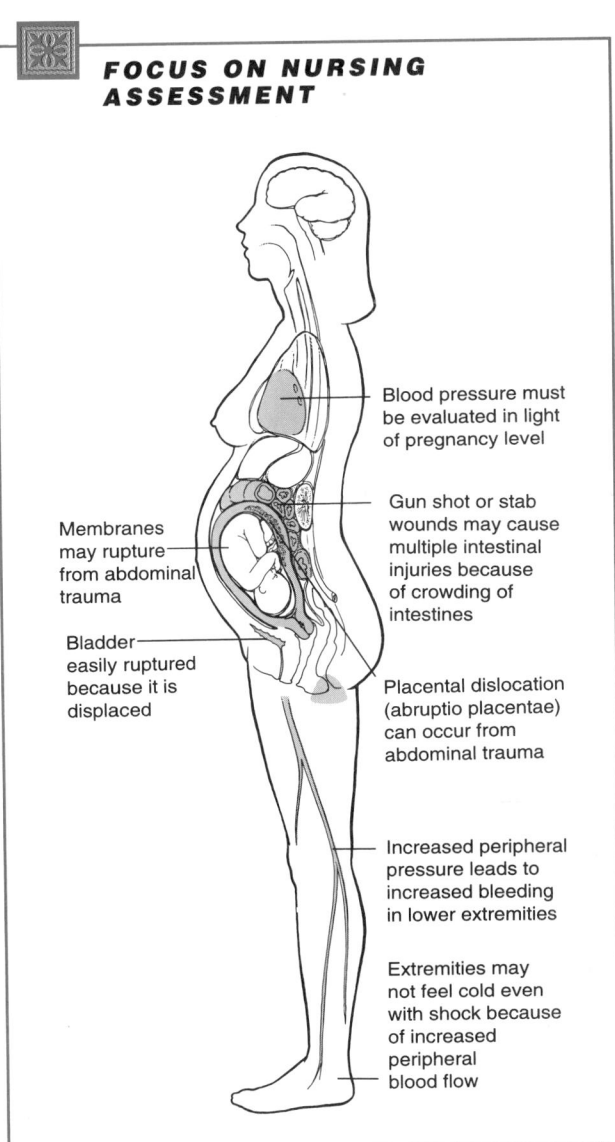

FOCUS ON NURSING ASSESSMENT

Blood pressure must be evaluated in light of pregnancy level

Gun shot or stab wounds may cause multiple intestinal injuries because of crowding of intestines

Membranes may rupture from abdominal trauma

Bladder easily ruptured because it is displaced

Placental dislocation (abruptio placentae) can occur from abdominal trauma

Increased peripheral pressure leads to increased bleeding in lower extremities

Extremities may not feel cold even with shock because of increased peripheral blood flow

FIGURE 14-8
Effects of trauma on pregnancy.

as a sign of infection following an open wound. Serum albumin level decreases during pregnancy, making the large loss that normally occurs with burns a more serious than usual response. Serum liver enzyme levels (i.e., serum glutamic-oxaloacetic transaminase, serum glutamate pyruvate transaminase, and lactate dehydrogenase) remain the same during pregnancy, so if these are elevated following trauma, liver trauma can be detected. Alkaline phosphatase, a substance also usually helpful in detecting liver trauma, is three to four times greater in the pregnant woman at term than normally (from placental origin), so this marker loses its importance. Pancreatic amylase is the same as normal during pregnancy so the pancreas can be evaluated normally.

Abdominal pain is difficult to localize during pregnancy because organs are pushed aside by the growing uterus. The abdomen always feels tense during pregnancy so guarding and rigidity of the abdominal wall are lost as important findings. Bleeding into the abdominal cavity with an abdominal injury is apt to be forceful and extreme because of the increased pressure in the pelvic vessels. A procedure such as a needle paracentesis to assess for bleeding into the abdominal cavity is dangerous because the bowel, dislocated from its usual position, can be easily punctured. *Culdocentesis* or needle aspiration through the posterior vaginal fornix into the peritoneal cavity may be done. Peritoneal lavage, or inserting a peritoneal dialysis catheter into the abdominal cavity, adding a liter of an isotonic solution, aspirating it again, and analyzing it for blood or urine, may reveal bleeding best.

The bladder of pregnant women is susceptible to rupture because it is the most anterior organ and is elevated abnormally. Following abdominal trauma, an indwelling bladder catheter is often inserted to assess for blood in urine.

Emotional Considerations

When a pregnant woman is seen at a health care facility because of an accident, she is both apprehensive and frightened, not only for herself but for the health of the fetus. She is worried not only about what has happened but also about what could have happened (if the knife had slipped an inch farther, if the automobile accident had been worse, if she had fallen from farther up the stepladder) and about what medical care will be required (does she need an x-ray; if she does, will this be safe for the fetus?). She may feel guilty about her carelessness (if she were really a good mother she would have had her seatbelt fastened or not tried to stand on a stepladder to hang drapes alone). A feeling of guilt lowers self-esteem and increases the level of stress. Remember that people under stress do not process well and so may not perceive correctly the information given to them. Always try to review information with a woman at

a later date to be certain that she does have the facts of her injury and she is accurate in her knowledge of follow-up care needed.

Assessment

Assessment of the injured woman must be done quickly yet thoroughly and include both the woman's psychologic as well as her physical status. A pregnant woman may be so concerned with her fetus's health that she does not appreciate she is injured. Another woman might not even consider the possibility that her fetus could be injured until someone asks if she has felt the fetus move since the accident (not realizing that a loss of blood from her leg would affect uterine blood flow). Assessment should be done concurrently with reassurance ("Your blood pressure is low but the fetal heart beat sounds good") to try and relieve fear of fetal health. Use a Doppler method of assessing fetal heart tones if possible to demonstrate to the woman as well as yourself that the fetus still appears to be well. External monitoring of fetal heart rate and uterine contractions best rules out fetal distress and preterm labor.

In an emergency situation, a woman needs her support people around her. Locate them as necessary and also assess their reaction to the trauma.

Health History

In an emergency situation, a few minutes spent attempting to calm the woman and move her past her initial fright is time well spent unless symptoms of major body system disturbances require that immediate efforts are directed elsewhere. Reducing the woman's level of anxiety will help her to better cooperate with history giving and physical assessment procedures.

Take a brief pregnancy history as well as a trauma history (i.e., length of pregnancy or any complications). Ask specifically if fetal heart tones have been heard by an examiner during the pregnancy, if she has felt the fetus move since the accident, if she has any sensation of tightening or pain in her abdomen that could be uterine contractions, and if she knows what her prepregnancy and pregnancy blood pressures have been to help evaluate the extent of blood loss from the trauma.

Document the circumstances of the trauma: what happened, the time that has passed since the injury, signs and symptoms of injury the woman is experiencing, and actions she has taken to counteract these.

If the woman fell, for example, how far did she fall? (A fall from the top of a stepladder is more likely to be serious than a fall from a low rung.) What body part did she land on? (Landing on her abdomen may be very serious, although she may be in less pain than if she injured a wrist in the fall.) For an automobile accident, ask how fast the car was traveling, if she was thrown from the car, or if the windshield broke (generally in automobile accidents, windshields are broken from the impact of a head striking the windshield; thus, the woman needs to be assessed for a head injury).

As a final measure, assess whether the woman's degree of injury is in proportion to the history. Injuries out of proportion to the history (a woman states that all that happened is that she tripped on her front steps but you notice that all her extremities are ecchymotic and her jaw is broken) suggest abuse (battering) rather than a simple accident. Analyze also whether the woman seemed to be using a sensible degree of caution for the circumstances. If not, assess whether she might have wanted the pregnancy to end. A naive adolescent, for example, may attempt to end a pregnancy by a deliberate fall or poisoning, which she then reports as an accident.

Physical Examination

Accidents become fatal when lung, heart, kidney, or brain function becomes inadequate; fetal health is in jeopardy when uterine function is impaired. It is important that these body systems be evaluated first, therefore. Table 14-5 lists signs and symptoms to assess to evaluate function of these major body organs.

With multiple trauma, a nasogastric tube is usually passed to empty the stomach. A Foley catheter is passed to assess for urine output and to rule out a ruptured bladder (blood would return or urine would be blood tinged if bleeding were occurring).

To prevent supine hypotension syndrome, be certain that the woman does not lie supine for an examination. If it is necessary for her to lie on her back, manually displace the uterus from the vena cava by placing rolled towels or a blanket under her right side to tip her body approximately 15 degrees to the side. If surgery is necessary, an operating room table can be tipped to achieve this same effect or a uterine displacement bar, a metal bar attached to the table that presses the uterus away from the vena cava, can be used.

Nursing Diagnoses and Related Interventions

Nursing care during the initial phase of an emergency focuses on stabilizing the woman and protecting the fetus. Examples of nursing diagnoses that would be appropriate are:

- Fear related to threat of injury to the fetus
- High risk for fetal injury related to apparent suicide attempt
- Altered tissue perfusion related to severed artery
- Altered respiratory function related to gun shot

Once the immediate emergency phase is passed, nursing diagnoses will focus on prevention of more severe injury and alleviation of emotional distress, and will depend on the type of injury received. Examples are:

Table 14-5. *Initial Assessments Following Trauma During Pregnancy*

Body System	Assessment
Respiratory System	Quality of respirations (labored or even?)
	Rate of respirations
	Sounds of obstruction (wheezing, retractions, coughing?)
	Color (cyanotic?)
	Oxygen hunger (inability to lie flat, nasal flaring?)
Cardiovascular System	Color (pallor from hemorrhage?)
	Gross bleeding?
	Pulse rate (increases with hemorrhage)
	Blood pressure (decreases with hemorrhage)
	Feeling of apprehension from altered vascular pressure?
Nervous System	Level of consciousness (woman answers questions coherently?)
	Pupils (equal and reacting to light?)
	Bruises or raised bump on head or spinal column?
	Loss of motion or sensory function in a body part?
Renal System	Bruising on anterior abdominal wall over bladder or on back over kidneys?
	Blood in urine?
Uterine-Fetal System	Bradycardia, tachycardia, or absence of fetal heart tones or loss of variability on fetal monitor?
	Vaginal bleeding?
	Clear (amniotic) fluid leaking from vagina?
	Bruising on abdomen over uterus?

- High risk for infection related to loss of skin integrity or wound contamination
- Situational low self-esteem related to occurrence of accident
- Powerlessness related to seriousness of the injury sustained or inability to prevent accident from occurring

Nursing Diagnosis: High risk for altered tissue perfusion related to blood loss from trauma

Goal: Client will maintain adequate tissue perfusion throughout remainder of pregnancy.

Outcome Criteria: Client's blood pressure is above 100/60 mm Hg; pulse below 100 bpm; no signs of labor are present; fetal heart rate is 120 to 160 bpm; non-stress test shows good variability.

Therapeutic Management

Planning in an emergency always involves two phases: planning for immediate care to stabilize the client and planning for continuing care once the emergency has passed.

Implementations in emergency situations must be done quickly yet always remembering that the woman's primary health condition is that she is pregnant.

If respirations are not present or are ineffective, cardiopulmonary resuscitation (CPR) should begin the same as with any person following trauma (Table 14-6). To be certain a woman has not just fainted, try to rouse her by calling her name or shaking her shoulders. If this is unsuccessful, assess whether her airway is obstructed by holding your cheek next to her nostrils and assessing for air exchange; look in her mouth for a foreign object; if she is not breathing, pull her chin forward and using a resuscitation bag administer 2 breaths. Although an enlarged uterus puts considerable pressure on the diaphragm and consequently the lungs, unusual pressure is unnecessary to fully inflate lungs in a resuscitation attempt. Assess cardiovascular function by palpating the carotid pulse. If this is not palpable or the pupils are fixed, heart function must also be supplemented. Begin external heart massage at a rate of two breaths to every 15 heart compressions (one rescuer) or one breath to five cardiac beats for two rescuers (the same as for all adults). Cardiac massage may be awkward late in pregnancy because of the size of the uterus, but undue pressure should not be necessary to create heart action. Cardioversion can be done successfully (Neufeld, 1993).

Following assessment of the level of consciousness and cardiovascular and respiratory status, if there has been blood loss, a central venous pressure line is often inserted and lactated Ringer's or another isotonic solution infused to restore fluid volume or provide an open line for emergency medication.

If hypotension is present, it must be corrected quickly to maintain a pressure gradient across the placenta. Any antihypotensive agent, however, that achieves an increased blood pressure by causing peripheral vasoconstriction is contraindicated. Ephedrine is the drug of choice with a pregnant woman to restore blood pressure because it has a minimal peripheral vasoconstriction effect. Dopamine in low doses is a second drug that can be used. Following emergency implementations, care will depend on the specific injury or trauma present.

Table 14-6. CPR During Pregnancy

Action	Technique
1. Shake and shout	Shake shoulders and attempt to rouse her to be certain woman has not fainted.
2. Position the airway	Lift the chin to straighten airway.
3. Establish lack of respirations	Assess if exhalations are occurring by placing your face next to woman's mouth; if none is present, go to step 4.
4. Begin rescue breathing	Deliver 2 breaths to woman's mouth and lungs.
5. Assess cardiovascular system	Assess for presence of carotid pulse; if present, continue to breathe at 10–12 b/min. If none is present, go to step 6.
6. Begin heart massage	With one rescuer, place both hands on the lower sternum just above xyphoid process and deliver 15 chest compressions followed by 2 rescue breaths until cardiopulmonary function returns; with two rescuers, deliver 5 chest compressions followed by 1 breath.
7. Prevent supine hypotension syndrome	To prevent the uterus from compressing the vena cava, place a folded towel under one hip.

(From American Heart Association. [1992]. Adult basic life support. *Journal of the American Medical Association, 268,* 2184.)

Open Wounds

A number of types of wounds occur with trauma.

Lacerations. A laceration is a jagged cut. It may involve only the skin layer or penetrate to deeper subcutaneous tissue or tendons. Lacerations generally bleed profusely. Bleeding should be halted by pressure on the edge of the laceration (remember: this is difficult to achieve in lower extremities because venous pressure is so great in the lower extremities during pregnancy). Following cleaning, the area is sutured through each layer of tissue involved to approximate edges. For sutures to be used, a local anesthetic such as Xylocaine is necessary. Because this has only a local effect, it is safe during pregnancy. If the laceration is superficial and the woman is nervous about the use of an anesthetic, the edges can be approximated by use of a "butterfly" strip made from a commercial adhesive strip. This may allow it to heal with a slightly more noticeable scar, however. Antishock trousers should be used with caution to halt lower extremity bleeding as the top of these may put pressure on the uterus and press it against the vena cava causing a supine hypotension syndrome (Neufeld, 1993).

Again, the white blood count is normally elevated during pregnancy and thus is a poor indicator of the presence or extent of infection in wounds.

Puncture Wounds. A puncture wound results from penetration of a sharp object such as a nail, splinter, nail file or knife. Puncture wounds bleed little—an advantage in terms of minimizing blood loss but not in terms of wound cleaning. A puncture wound is usually not sutured so that a sealed unoxygenated cavity is not created below the sutures and a space where tetanus bacilli can grow is not created. If the woman has had a tetanus immunization within the past 10 years, tetanus toxoid is administered. If the woman did not have a tetanus immunization within 10 years (the usual condition) tetanus toxoid plus immune tetanus globulin is administered.

Puncture wounds are frightening because the average woman knows that they can have severe consequences from tetanus and they also usually occur in association with a degree of violence.

Knife wounds cause deep penetration and are often directed into the abdomen. They may easily reach the depth of the uterus so they may directly injure the fetus. Most stab wounds of the abdomen, however, occur in the upper quadrants of the abdomen above the height of the uterus. To determine the depth and extent of the wound, a fistulogram may be done. This involves insertion of a thin catheter into the wound; the wound is then filled with radiopaque solution. An x-ray of the area the solution fills will reveal the extent of the puncture. If the peritoneal cavity was perforated, dye will outline the intestines. If there is suspicion that there is bleeding in the abdominal cavity, a *celiotomy* or an exploratory surgical procedure into the abdominal cavity may be performed. Surgery this close to the uterus usually does not result in preterm birth (Dudley & Cruikshank, 1990). If the diaphragm was cut, intestine may herniate into the chest cavity (diaphragmatic hernia) due to the increased abdominal pressure from the enlarged uterus. Following surgical repair of an injured diaphragm, cesarean birth may be planned to avoid strain on a newly repaired diaphragm during labor. The uterus appears to have a natural resistance to infection so even if punctured, infection in the uterus rarely occurs.

Animal Bites. Pregnant women are rarely bitten by any animal but a dog. Animal bites are a form of puncture wound, so if the rabies immunization status of the dog is known, the wound is washed and treated as a puncture wound. If the dog cannot be located or is proved to be rabid after 48 hours of observation, the woman must be administered rabies immune globulin and vaccine. Pregnancy is not a contraindication to rabies immunization since contracting the disease would be very serious (Wilson, 1994).

Pregnant women should be advised to use caution not to pet unfamiliar dogs or, if camping in a remote location, for example, not to try to feed wild animals such as squirrels and raccoons.

Blunt Abdominal Trauma

Blunt trauma occurs generally from automobile accidents when the woman's abdomen strikes the steering wheel or dashboard or from someone deliberately kicking or punching her abdomen. No visible break is present in the skin. Following the injury, the underlying tissue becomes edematous; broken underlying blood vessels may ooze and form ecchymosis or a hematoma at the site. To assess if there is abdominal bleeding, a diagnostic peritoneal lavage may be done by introducing a small amount of normal saline by a syringe and then withdrawing it to see if blood is evident.

Careful assessment that the pregnancy has not been harmed must be made because a traumatic blow to the abdomen could cause dislodgement of the placenta (abruptio placenta) or, if uterine bleeding is occurring, may cause preterm labor. The uterus should be palpated for any abnormal contours that would suggest edema or internal bleeding. Fetal heart tones should be counted. Using a Doppler instrument is helpful to assure the woman that her fetus is unharmed. Real time sonogram may also be helpful in showing that the uterus and placenta are not torn. A pelvic examination is usually performed to assess for vaginal bleeding or seepage of clear fluid that would suggest the amniotic membranes were ruptured from the force of an abdominal blow and amniotic fluid is not continuously leaking vaginally. If the woman reports uterine contractions, a uterine and fetal monitor should be placed to estimate the strength and effect on the fetal heart rate of these and the possibility that preterm labor has begun. Magnesium sulfate is usually selected to halt preterm labor following trauma because it has fewer hemodynamic effects than beta-mimetic drugs (see Chapter 16 for a full discussion of these drugs).

The possibility that placental blood will enter the maternal circulation with uterine trauma is a threat to the Rh-negative woman. Rh-negative women are therefore typically administered Rh immune globulin (RHIG). The presence of fetal blood cells in the maternal bloodstream can be documented by a Kleihauer-Betke test (on staining, maternal cells remain colorless; fetal cells turn purple-pink).

Gunshot Wounds

A woman may receive a gunshot wound as an intended victim or innocent bystander; occasionally a woman attempts suicide by a gunshot wound. Assessment of the wound includes inspection not only for the point where the bullet entered the woman's body but also the point where the bullet exited (the entry wound is small but the exit wound is large because as a bullet slows, it begins to tumble, enlarging the space it occupies). The uterine wall is so thick during pregnancy that it may trap a bullet; thus, there is no exit point from her body if the uterus was punctured. If the bullet entered high in the woman's abdomen, intestine will surely be injured; because so much is compressed above the uterus, intestine may sustain many tears from the one bullet.

Gunshot wounds are surgically cleaned and debrided and the woman is treated with a high concentration of antibiotics. Ampicillin is frequently ordered for this; fortunately, ampicillin is safe during pregnancy. Gunshots wounds to the uterus have a high incidence of fetal mortality. Following emergency therapy for the injury, it is important to investigate carefully the circumstances of the injury. Gunshot wounds must be reported to the police. Stay with the woman as necessary while she recounts her history of the accident again for law enforcement officers.

Poisoning

Pregnant women are not apt to swallow a poison, although this can occur accidentally during pregnancy, especially if a woman wakes at night and attempts to take medicine in the dark. It can occur as a suicide attempt. Poisoning in the pregnant woman should be managed the same as in any individual. The woman should telephone the local poison control center, state what she accidentally swallowed, and follow the specific recommendation of personnel at the poison control center. Syrup of ipecac (15 mL) taken followed by a glass of water is the best emetic to cause vomiting and discharge

of the poison from her body and is safe for use during pregnancy. However, no ipecac should be taken until the woman has checked with her poison control center. Some poisons can be more harmful if vomited than if allowed to remain in the body.

After the woman has been treated and the emergency of the poisoning is over, investigate carefully the circumstances of the poisoning to help the woman learn safer habits of medicine taking or to discover if there was a possibility she intentionally took a poison.

Choking

If a pregnant woman chokes on a piece of meat or any foreign object blocks the airway, it is difficult to dislodge it by a sudden upward thrust to the upper abdomen (a Heimlich maneuver) in the same way it would be done to the average adult. This difficulty is because of a lack of space between the uterus and the end of the sternum and because a person cannot reach from the rear around the woman's enlarged abdomen. Late in pregnancy, therefore, a rescuer must use successive chest thrusts instead. The instructions for this are to (1) stand behind the woman and encircle her chest with your arms; (2) place the thumb side of your fist on the middle of the woman's sternum; and (3) grab the fist with the other hand and perform backward thrusts until the foreign body is expelled (American Heart Association, 1992). This could be done with the woman lying down. The hand position for the application of chest thrusts in this position is the same as that for external heart compressions (heel of the hand on the lower sternum; Figure 14-9).

Orthopedic Injuries

Because a woman has poor balance late in pregnancy, she may trip more readily than usual; when she falls, she automatically reaches out a hand to cushion the fall and prevent landing on her abdomen. Ordinarily, if a young adult falls this way, his or her wrist is uninjured; the extra weight the pregnant woman carries, however, puts a greater proportion of weight on the wrist, so more serious injuries can occur. Applying ice to the area decreases swelling as an immediate first-aid measure. An x-ray may be necessary to determine whether a fracture is present. Assure the woman that an x-ray of an extremity is safe for her during pregnancy as long as her abdomen is shielded during the radiation exposure. Accompany the woman to the x-ray department and remain with her (outside the actual x-ray room) to both assure that lead protection will be offered her and to be available if signs of preterm labor should suddenly develop as a result of a yet undetected injury.

Because women of childbearing age are usually healthy, healing of fractures or torn ligaments generally occurs quickly and without complications. Be certain she can identify good calcium sources if she has a frac-

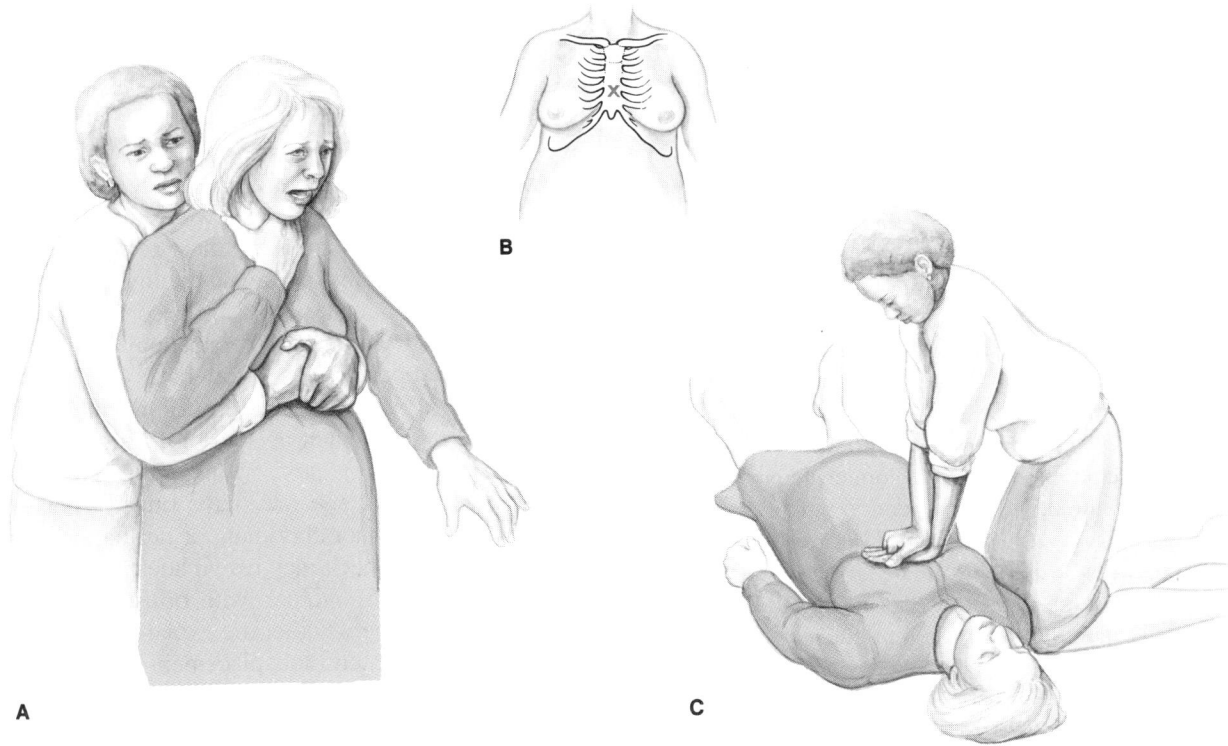

FIGURE 14-9
*Choking. Chest thrust administered for foreign body airway obstruction in advanced stages of pregnancy. (**A**) Conscious victim (standing). (**B**) Correct position for hand on sternum. (**C**) Unconscious victim (lying).*

ture so both she and the fetus can have adequate calcium for new bone growth.

Because many more adolescent girls and young adult women participate in sports today than ever before, there is an increasing number of women of childbearing age who have a weakened knee cartilage from having dislocated a knee joint during active sports play (formerly thought of only as a football injury). During pregnancy, when all body cartilage softens, combined with the excessive abdominal weight the woman carries, the woman may dislocate her knee again.

Any woman who has had a previous knee injury of this type should have it reevaluated early in pregnancy and may need to wear a knee support such as a knee immobilizer for the last 3 months of pregnancy to prevent the knee joint from dislocating again. Discuss with her the advantage of prevention because if the knee cartilage should not be able to sustain her added weight and dislocates again, she will surely fall. In addition, she will then need to wear an immobilizer for approximately 6 weeks for therapy. Preventing the dislocation prevents possible injury due to a fall and will allow her to be fully mobile at the time she has a new child to care for. She can be assured that a knee immobilizer in place at the time of birth will not interfere with birth; if a lithotomy position and stirrups for birth are necessary, a modified stirrups position can be devised for her.

The laxness of body cartilage may also cause separation of the symphysis pubis if a woman falls with her legs outspread. This is painful on walking or turning. To avoid pain and allow the cartilage to heal, she needs to remain on bedrest for 4 to 6 weeks. If separation of the symphysis pubis is present at the time of birth, this may cause labor to be painful, especially the pelvic division as the fetus is pushed through the pelvic ring.

Burns

Burns are dangerous to the pregnant woman not only because of the actual thermal injury that occurs but also because the woman can inhale carbon monoxide gases from the fire. Such inhalation can lead to extreme fetal anoxia as carbon monoxide crosses the placenta in place of oxygen. Smoke is irritating to lung tissue and can result in extensive lung edema; this can cause anoxia from the lack of oxygen-carbon dioxide exchange space. Because the fluid and electrolyte loss is great with burns, hypotension from hypovolemia or an electrolyte imbalance can occur. A body response to a harsh trauma such as a burn is the production of prostaglandins, which may cause preterm labor (Jain & Garg, 1993). Both maternal and fetal prognoses are poor if burns cover more than 50% of body surface area. Fortunately, few women in the childbearing age group experience this degree of burn in the United States.

Interestingly, burn tissue heals more quickly than normal during pregnancy. This is probably related to the generally increased metabolism and possibly to the increased corticosteroid serum level that keeps inflammation and damage to tissue from the pressure of edema from occurring.

Postmortem Cesarean Birth

If a pregnant woman does not survive serious trauma, it may still be possible for her child to be born safely by a postmortem cesarean birth. This is usually attempted if the fetus is past 24 weeks and fewer than 20 minutes have passed since the mother expired. Infant survival is best in these circumstances if no longer than 5 minutes has passed (Neufeld, 1993). By general practice, no consent is necessary for this procedure because the fetus is assumed to want to live but cannot give consent. A classic cesarean incision is used. Personnel should be available to resuscitate the newborn immediately.

The Battered Woman

As many as 25% of women seen in emergency departments are there because they have been abused by a spouse. Abused women may be pregnant because they were unable to resist sexual advances from their abusive partner. Beatings may increase during pregnancy because stress is often a "trigger" to beatings, and pregnancy, with all that an expected new child entails (another mouth to feed, body to clothe, or dependent to protect), increases stress (Campbell, Oliver, & Bullock, 1993). The woman may desire the pregnancy very much because she thinks that having a child will change the partner and make him a better person. She may be grateful thinking that she will have an infant to love her.

Assessment

A battered woman may come for care late in pregnancy because of lack of transportation (her partner controls the use of the car) or because she has tried to pretend that the pregnancy did not exist to reduce stress. Keeping the stress level down is her best defense against violence. She may be noticeable in a prenatal setting in that she purchases no clothing especially for the pregnancy (she has no funds for herself and asking for money may incite violence). She may not be able to go for laboratory tests if going involves transportation or money.

The battered woman may have difficulty following recommended pregnancy nutrition (she must cook what her partner wants or she will be beaten). She may leave before the nurse-midwife or physician sees her at a prenatal setting, or she may grow anxious if her prenatal appointment is running late (she must be home to cook dinner or risk a beating).

She may call and cancel appointments frequently (or simply not keep appointments) because she has an obvious black eye or a bleeding facial laceration she does not want to reveal.

She may be anxious to listen to the baby's heartbeat at prenatal visits because her partner recently punched or kicked her abdomen and she is worried that the fetus has been hurt. A sonogram is the most accurate method of assessing fetal health following trauma. Fetal heart tones and fundal height should be recorded. Minimal placental infarcts from blunt abdominal trauma may lead to poor placental perfusion and low birth weight.

She may dress inappropriately for warm weather, wearing long-sleeved, tight-necked blouses to cover up bruises on her neck or arms. When undressed for a physical examination, she may have bruises or lacerations on her breasts, her abdomen, or her back that she cannot explain. Her neck may reveal linear bruises from strangulation. Ask any woman with bruises to account for them. Listen to see whether the explanation seems to correlate with the extent and placement of a bruise or laceration.

Nursing Diagnoses and Related Interventions

Nursing diagnoses for the battered woman may pertain to physical injuries sustained but they should also address the emotional manifestations of abuse. Some examples include:

- Powerlessness related to perception that it is impossible to break away from abusing partner
- Fear related to constant threat of beatings
- Social isolation related to client's need to hide evidence of her abuse
- Ineffective denial related to inability to face the fact that spouse is abusive
- Ineffective family coping: Compromised, related to poor communication between client and abusive spouse.

Goals should address ways to keep the woman safe from further abuse. Outcome criteria should be specific tasks the woman could accomplish to meet the goals, such as:

- Client carries phone number for Home for Abused Women with her.
- Client states she has filed restraining order.
- Client states she feels secure living in Safe House.

Nursing Diagnosis: Chronic low self-esteem related to continuing physical and mental abuse

Goal: Client will express realistic positive aspects about self and situation she is in by 3 months time.

Outcome Criteria: Client identifies positive traits about self; begins to discuss possible reasons that explain why she has remained in abusive situation; makes concrete, realistic plans for future; states that she feels able, with continuing help and outside resources, to protect herself in future.

It may be difficult to work with battered women because it is hard to understand why they stay in their situation. A common finding is that they may be immobilized and unable to leave by fear of the abusive person (if they leave, he may find them and kill them) and the guilt and low self-esteem they feel (he has told them so many times that this is their fault and they deserve to be treated this way that they believe it). In order to free them from this emotional paralysis, they need outside help. To compound the problem, their low self-esteem and depression leads them to believe that no one would be interested in helping them (Bohn, 1990).

The battered woman may need support to make simple decisions. Support any ability to make constructive decisions that she has left. Be familiar with safe shelters for battered women in the community; discuss with her how she can call the police at any time and they will take her to the shelter. Help her obtain a restraining order to keep the abusive person from coming near her again if this is necessary.

After the birth of the child, assuming the woman moved away from the abuser, a woman may be depressed because she is lonely. She may have unreal expectations of the child, trying to make the infant smile at her and interact with her more than a newborn is capable of doing in order to have someone to love her. Try to caution her that her newborn does love her but she has to give the child time to grow. Show the mother all the things her child can do, such as attend to the sound of her voice or cuddle against her. Otherwise her unreal expectations may lead to disappointment and an interference with her mothering. Do not leave a battered woman without a support system after birth of the child. If she was depending on prenatal personnel during pregnancy, the gap with another support system must be filled. This could be a social agency that deals specifically with battered women in the community; it could be a community health nurse who will be visiting when she returns home. If she is left without a support person, her low self-esteem may not allow her to reach out and seek help. She may decide suicide or returning to the person who abused her is her best recourse.

Battered women need to be identified during pregnancy not only so they can be helped but to help the mental health of the child (see the Focus on Nursing Research box). A child raised in a home where the mother is battered will learn that this is acceptable conduct, and the battering may extend to yet another generation (see Chapter 55).

FOCUS ON NURSING RESEARCH

Why Are Pregnant Women Subject to Battering by Their Spouses?

Three nursing researchers, Campbell, Oliver, and Bullock, attempted to answer this question by interviewing 79 battered women whom they recruited by newspaper or bulletin board advertisement. Twenty-seven women who were beaten during pregnancy were compared to 24 women who were not beaten while pregnant. Answers to why they thought abuse occurred during pregnancy were jealousy or anger toward the unborn child, pregnancy-specific violence not directed toward the unborn child, and "business as usual." Women who were beaten during pregnancy overall had a relationship in which they were more frequently and severely beaten than those who were not beaten during pregnancy. The researchers stress the importance of nurses identifying battered women at prenatal visits so appropriate advice and help can be offered them to decrease injury to themselves and their fetus.

Campbell, J. C., Oliver, C, & Bullock, L. (1993). Why battering during pregnancy? *AWHONNS Clinical Issues in Perinatal & Women's Health Nursing, 4,* 343.

Key Points

- A high-risk pregnancy is one in which some maternal or fetal factor, either psychological or physiologic, may result in the birth of a high-risk infant or in some way cause harm to the woman herself.
- Pregnancy is a stress to any family because it involves financial expenses plus changes in family roles. If a complication of pregnancy develops, this stress is almost automatically intensified. Families need support during this time to be able to cope with the increased burden.
- When women with a preexisting disease become pregnant, it is important that a thorough history and physical examination is done at their first prenatal visit to establish a baseline of information on their condition and vital signs such as blood pressure. Documentation of any medication being taken for a secondary condition is also necessary to protect against adverse drug interactions and the possibility of teratogenic action on the fetus.
- Teaching is an important nursing concern because the woman with a preexisting illness must make modifications in her usual therapy to adjust to pregnancy. Pregnancy often stimulates women to learn more about their primary disease as well.
- Women who have a complication early in pregnancy may continue to worry about the health of their fetus all during pregnancy. They need to be assured

(appropriately) that the episode was temporary and that with continued monitoring, the fetus should not suffer harm. After giving birth, they may need additional time to spend with their newborn to convince themselves that the infant is healthy so bonding can begin.

- Because blood volume increases by as much as 50% during pregnancy, cardiac function may become inadequate if cardiovascular disease is present. Illnesses that cause difficulty can be either acquired disorders such as Kawasaki disease and rheumatic fever or congenital disorders such as mitral valve prolapse and coarctation of the aorta.
- Various forms of anemia can cause complications of pregnancy; iron deficiency, sickle cell, and folic acid deficiency are examples. All these anemias can result in fetal distress because of inadequate oxygen transport.
- Urinary tract disorders can lead to pregnancy complications because pregnancy increases the workload of kidneys. Urinary tract infection and chronic renal disease are two disorders that may lead to early pregnancy loss.
- Acute nasopharyngitis, asthma, pneumonia, influenza, and tuberculosis are respiratory disorders seen in pregnancy. Because tuberculosis is on the increase, it needs special assessment and care.
- Juvenile rheumatoid arthritis and systemic lupus erythematosus are examples of rheumatic disorders seen in pregnancy. These disorders generally require large doses of salicylate and nonsteroidal antiinflammatory agents for therapy; women are usually advised to discontinue NSAID agents during pregnancy. They are advised to decrease use of salicylates 2 weeks before birth to avoid bleeding disorders in the newborn.
- Some gastrointestinal illnesses that occur with pregnancy are hiatal hernia, cholecystitis, viral hepatitis, inflammatory bowel disease, and appendicitis. If surgery is necessary for conditions such as cholecystitis or appendicitis, this can be scheduled during pregnancy but may result in preterm labor.
- Recurrent seizure is the most frequently seen neurologic condition during pregnancy. Many drugs used to control seizures are teratogenic; women need to have their medical regimen evaluated prior to pregnancy to be certain that they are regulated on the lowest number of medications possible.
- The major endocrine disorder seen during pregnancy is diabetes mellitus. Gestational diabetes is diabetes that occurs during pregnancy and fades following it.
- Sexually transmitted diseases such as candidiasis, trichomoniasis, chlamydia, syphilis, herpes type 2, gonorrhea, papilloma, and HIV may occur during pregnancy. These illnesses need prompt treatment

when they occur. Women need to follow safer sex practices to help prevent these diseases.
- Trauma in pregnancy includes automobile accidents and falls. Women with traumatic injuries need to be carefully assessed to determine if spouse abuse was the cause of the trauma.

Critical Thinking Exercises

1. Mary G. is a 23-year-old you care for who has gestational diabetes. Mary is resistant to teaching about her condition because she knows that the condition is only temporary and will fade at the end of pregnancy. What type of teaching plan would you devise to help Mary learn in the face of this attitude?

2. In the past many women with heart disease were advised not to attempt pregnancy. What has changed to make this advice different in most instances today? Describe the modifications an average women with heart disease would have to make in her lifestyle if she were required to rest at least 4 hours every day. How difficult do you anticipate this is for the average woman?

3. One of the most devastating medical diagnoses today is that of acquired immune deficiency syndrome (HIV). How is this illness a threat to the newborn as well as the mother? Summarize measures nurses can use to help prevent the spread of this disorder. Are there changes a prenatal clinic would have to make to care for an HIV positive woman?

References

ACOG. (1992). *HIV in pregnancy.* ACOG Technical Bulletin. Washington, DC: ACOG.

American Diabetic Association. (1990). Clinical practice recommendations: Gestational diabetes mellitus. *Diabetes Care, 13,* 1.

American Heart Association. (1992). Adult basic life support. *Journal of the American Medical Association, 268,* 2184.

Aoki, K., et al. (1993). Specific antiphospholipid antibodies as a predictive variable in patients with recurrent pregnancy loss. *American Journal of Reproductive Immunology, 29,* 82.

Berry, M. C., & Dajani, A. S. (1992). Resurgence of congenital syphilis. *Infectious Disease Clinics of North America, 6,* 19.

Billett, H. H. (1993). Doppler velosimetry in pregnant patients with sickle cell anemia. *American Journal of Hematology, 42,* 305.

Blackburn, L. S. (1992). Effective treatment of chlamydia trachomatis infection during pregnancy to prevent perinatal and infant complications. *Nurse Practitioner, 17,* 56.

Bohn, D. C. (1990). Domestic violence and pregnancy: Implications for practice. *Journal of Nurse Midwifery, 35,* 86.

Campbell, J. C., Oliver, C., & Bullock, L. (1993). Why battering during pregnancy? *AWHONNS Clinical Issues in Perinatal & Women's Health Nursing, 4,* 343.

Cohn, J. A. (1993). Human immunodeficiency virus and AIDS—1993 update. *Journal of Nurse Midwifery, 38,* 65.

Cosico, J. N., et al. (1992). Indications, management and patient education: Anticoagulation therapy during pregnancy. *MCN: American Journal of Maternal Child Nursing, 17,* 130.

Criteria Committee of the New York State Heart Association. (1979). *Nomenclature and criteria for diagnosis of diseases of the heart and blood vessels* (8th ed.). Boston: Little, Brown.

Cruikshank, D. P. (1990). Cardiovascular, pulmonary, renal and hematologic diseases in pregnancy. In J.R. Scott et al., *Danforth's obstetrics and gynecology.* Philadelphia: J.B. Lippincott.

Cunningham, F. G., et al. (1993). *Williams obstetrics* (19th ed.). Norwalk, CT: Appleton and Lange.

D'Alonzo, G. E. (1990). The pregnant asthmatic patient. *Seminars in Perinatology, 14,* 119.

Davis, R. K., & Maslow, A. S. (1992). Multiple sclerosis in pregnancy: A review. *Obstetrical & Gynecological Survey, 47,* 290.

De Ferrari, E., et al. (1993). Nurse-midwifery management of women with human immunodeficiency virus disease. *Journal of Nurse-Midwifery, 38,* 86.

Department of Health and Human Services. (1991). *Healthy people 2000.* Washington, DC: Public Health Service.

Department of Health and Human Services. (1992). Nutrition surveillance—United States. *MMWR: Morbidity and Mortality Weekly Report, 42,* 1.

Dickinson, J. E., & Palmer, S. M. (1990). Gestational diabetes: Pathophysiology and diagnosis. *Seminars in Perinatology, 14,* 2.

Dinsmoor, M. J. (1990). Group B streptococcus still poses a challenge. *Contemporary Obstetrics and Gynecology, 35,* 93.

Donders, G. G., et al. (1993). The association of gonorrhea and syphilis with premature birth and low birthweight. *Genitourinary Medicine, 69,* 98.

Doucette, J. T., & Bracken, M. B. (1993). Possible role of asthma in the risk of preterm labor and delivery. *Epidemiology, 4,* 143.

Dudley, D. J., & Cruikshank, D. P. (1990). Trauma and acute surgical emergencies in pregnancy. *Seminars in Perinatology, 14,* 42.

Duggan, B., et al. (1993). Cervical cancer in pregnancy: Reporting on planned delay in therapy. *Obstetrics & Gynecology, 82,* 598.

Elerding, S. C. (1993). Laparoscopic cholecystectomy in pregnancy. *American Journal of Surgery, 165,* 625.

Ernest, J. M. (1992). Topical antifungal agents. *Obstetrics & Gynecology Clinics of North America, 19,* 587.

Eschenbach, D. A. (1990). Pelvic infections and sexually transmitted diseases. In J.R. Scott et al., *Danforth's obstetrics and gynecology.* Philadelphia: J.B. Lippincott.

Ferris, T. F. (1990). Pregnancy complicated by hypertension and renal disease. *Advances in Internal Medicine, 35,* 269.

Forcier, K. I. (1990). Management and care of pregnant psychiatric patients. *Journal of Psychosocial Nursing and Mental Health Services, 28,* 11.

Gabbe, S. G. (1990). Diabetes mellitus: Individualizing care. *Contemporary Obstetrics and Gynecology, 35,* 68.

Gabbe, S., et al. (1991). *Obstetrics: Normal and problem pregnancies.* New York: Churchill Livingstone.

Giuntoli, R. L. (1990). Management of an atypical Pap smear in the pregnant patient. *Female Patient, 15,* 59.

Harrington, D. S., & Fujimura, F. K. (1992). A guide to genetic testing for cystic fibrosis. *Female Patient, 17,* 22C.

Heine, P., & McGregor, J. A. (1993). Trichomonas vaginalis: A reemerging pathogen. *Clinical Obstetrics & Gynecology, 36,* 137.

Hess, D. B., et al. (1992). Management of cardiovascular disease in pregnancy. *Obstetric and Gynecologic Clinics of North America, 19,* 679.

Hill, G. B. (1993). The microbiology of bacterial vaginosis. *American Journal of Obstetrics & Gynecology, 169,* 450.

Hoffman, J. A. (1993). Iron deficiency anemia: An update. *Journal of Perinatal and Neonatal Nursing, 6,* 13.

Hou, S., et al. (1993). Pregnancy in women with end-stage renal disease: Treatment of anemia and premature labor. *American Journal of Kidney Diseases, 21,* 16.

Jackson, G. M., et al. (1993). Severe pulmonary hypertension in pregnancy following successful repair of ventricular septal defects in childhood. *Obstetrics & Gynecology, 82,* 680.

Jain, M. L., & Garg, A. K. (1993). Burns with pregnancy: A review. *Burns, 19,* 166.

Jenkins, M., & Kohl, S. (1992). New aspects of neonatal herpes. *Infectious Disease Clinics of North America, 6,* 57.

Johnson, M. A. (1990). Urinary tract infections in women. *American Family Physician, 41,* 565.

Julkunen, H., et al. (1993). Fetal outcome in lupus pregnancy: A retrospective case control study of 242 pregnancies in 112 patients. *Lupus, 2,* 125.

Kirkland, C. J. (1990). Mitral stenosis in pregnancy: The nursing challenge. *NAACOGS Clinical Issues in Perinatal and Women's Health Nursing, 3,* 429.

Korelitz, B. I. (1992). Inflammatory bowel disease in pregnancy. *Gastroenterology Clinics of North America, 21,* 827.

Lagrew, D. C. (1990). Strategies for managing emboli in pregnancy. *Contemporary Obstetrics and Gynecology, 35,* 113.

Lew, S. Q., & Watson, J. P. (1992). Urea and creatinine generation and removal in a pregnant patient receiving peritoneal dialysis. *Advances in Peritoneal Dialysis, 8,* 131.

Lim, H. K., et al. (1992). Diagnosis of acute appendicitis in pregnant women: Value of sonography. *American Journal of Roentgenology, 159,* 539.

Loeb, S. (1993). *Nurse's handbook of drug therapy.* Springhouse, PA: Springhouse.

Luder, E., et al. (1990). Current recommendations for breastfeeding in cystic fibrosis centers. *American Journal of Diseases of Children, 144,* 1153.

Luzuriaga, K., & Sullivan, J. L. (1994). Pathogenesis of vertical HIV-1 infection: Implications for interventions and management. *Pediatric Annals, 23,* 159.

Mahmoodian, S. (1992). Appendicitis complicating pregnancy. *Southern Medical Journal, 85,* 19.

Mays, M. (1993). Tuberculosis: A comprehensive review for the certified nurse-midwife. *Journal of Nurse-Midwifery, 38,* 132.

Nettina, S. L., & Kauffman, F. H. (1990). Diagnosis and management of sexually transmitted genital lesions. *Nurse Practitioner, 15,* 20.

Neufeld, J. D. (1993). Trauma in pregnancy, what if . . .? *Emergency Medical Clinics of North America, 11,* 207.

Ostensen, M. (1992). The effect of pregnancy on ankylosing spondylitis, psoriatic arthritis and juvenile rheumatoid arthritis. *American Journal of Reproductive Immunology, 28,* 235.

Perry, K. G., & Morrison, J. C. (1990). The diagnosis and management of hemoglobinopathies during pregnancy. *Seminars in Perinatology, 14,* 90.

Porcher, R. (1992). HIV-infected pregnant women and their infants: Primary health care implications. *Nurse Practitioner, 17,* 49.

Repke, J. J. (1992). Drug supplementation in pregnancy. *Current Opinion in Obstetrics & Gynecology, 4,* 802.

Reveille, J. D. (1990). Systemic lupus erythematosus: Issues in long-term management and pregnancy. *Female Patient, 15,* 21.

Rosenstein, B. J. (1994). Cystic fibrosis. In F. A. Oski et al., *Principles and practice of pediatrics.* Philadelphia: J.B. Lippincott.

Ruggiero, L., et al. (1990). Impact of social support and stress on compliance in women with gestational diabetes. *Diabetes Care, 13,* 441.

Sacks, D. A. (1993). Fetal macrosomia and gestational diabetes: What's the problem? *Obstetrics & Gynecology, 81,* 775.

Sala, D. J. (1992). Myocardial infarction. *NAACOGS Clinical Issues in Perinatal and Women's Health Nursing, 3,* 443.

Scantlebury, V., et al. (1990). Childbearing after liver transplantation. *Transplantation, 49,* 317.

Scott, J. R. (1990). Immunological disorders in pregnancy. In J. R. Scott et al., *Danforth's obstetrics and gynecology.* Philadelphia: J.B. Lippincott.

Shipley, C. F., & Nelson, G. H. (1993). Chorionic villus sampling in a patient who is an unusual carrier of hemophilia B. *American Journal of Obstetrics & Gynecology, 169,* 70.

Shornick, J. K. (1993). Herpes gestationis. *Dermatologic Clinics, 11,* 527.

Simpson, J. L. (1990). Genetic factors in obstetrics and gynecology. In J. R. Scott et al., *Danforth's obstetrics and gynecology.* Philadelphia: J.B. Lippincott.

Sipes, S. L., & Weiner, C. P. (1990). Venous thromboembolic disease in pregnancy. *Seminars in Perinatology, 14,* 103.

Skudder, P. A., & Farrington, D. T. (1993). Venous conditions associated with pregnancy. *Seminars in Dermatology, 12,* 72.

Smith, E., et al. (1991). Perinatal vertical transmission of human papillomavirus and subsequent development of respiratory tract papillomatosis. *Annals of Otology, Rhinology & Laryngology, 100,* 479.

Smith, L. L., & Lathrop, L. M. (1993). AIDS and sexuality. *Canadian Journal of Public Health, 84,* S14.

Sokol, R. J., & Brindley, B. A. (1990). Practical diagnosis and management of abnormal labor. In J. R. Scott et al., *Danforth's obstetrics and gynecology.* Philadelphia: J.B. Lippincott.

Tinkle, M., et al. (1992). HIV disease and pregnancy: Epidemiology, pathogenesis and natural history. *Journal of Obstetric, Gynecologic and Neonatal Nursing, 21,* 86.

Tzartos, S., et al. (1990). Neonatal myasthenia gravis: Antigenic specificities of antibodies in sera from mothers and their infants. *Clinical Experiments in Immunology, 80,* 376.

Varner, M. (1990). General medical and surgical diseases in pregnancy. In J.R. Scott et al., *Danforth's obstetrics and gynecology.* Philadelphia: J.B. Lippincott.

Weiss, B. M., & Atanassoff, P. G. (1993). Cyanotic congenital heart disease in pregnancy: Natural selection, pulmonary hypertension, and anesthesia. *Journal of Clinical Anesthesia, 5,* 332.

White, P. (1978). Classification of obstetric diabetes. *American Journal of Obstetrics and Gynecology, 50,* 229.

Wilson, M. H. (1994). Immunization. In F. A. Oski et al., *Principles and practice of pediatrics.* Philadelphia: J.B. Lippincott.

Zuspan, F. P. (1991). Dealing with chronic hypertension. *Contemporary Obstetrics and Gynecology, 36,* 31.

Suggested Readings

Bushnell, F. K. (1992). A guide to primary care of iron deficiency anemia. *Nurse Practitioner, 17,* 68.

de Swiet, M. (1992). Medical disorders in pregnancy. *Current Opinion in Obstetrics & Gynecology, 4,* 28.

Donders, G. G., et al. (1993). The association of gonorrhoea and syphilis with premature birth and low birth weight. *Genitourinary Medicine, 69,* 98.

Drummond, S. B. (1992). Cardiac disease in pregnancy: Intrapartum considerations. *Critical Care Nursing Clinics of North America, 4,* 659.

Goodwin, T. M., & Breen, M. T. (1990). Pregnancy outcome and fetomaternal hemorrhage after noncatastrophic trauma. *American Journal of Obstetrics and Gynecology, 162,* 665.

Hanshaw, J. B. (1994). Congenital cytomegalovirus infection. *Pediatric Annals, 23,* 159.

Heine, P., & McGregor, J. A. (1993). Trichomonas vaginalis: A reemerging pathogen. *Clinical Obstetrics & Gynecology, 36,* 137.

Helman, N. S. (1990). Sickle cell disease and pregnancy. *NAACOGS Clinical Issues in Perinatal and Women's Health Nursing, 1,* 194.

Hess, D. B., & Hess, L. W. (1992). Management of cardiovascular disease in pregnancy. *Obstetric & Gynecology Clinics of North America, 19,* 679.

Lindheimer, M. D., & Katz, A. I. (1991). OB renal problems. *Contemporary Obstetrics and Gynecology, 36,* 76.

Niebyl, J. R. (1991). Drugs with potential fetal toxicity. *Contemporary Obstetrics and Gynecology, 36,* 68.

Paavonen, J. (1991). Chlamydial disease during pregnancy. *Contemporary Obstetrics and Gynecology, 36,* 91.

Packham, D. K. (1993). Aspects of renal disease and pregnancy. *Kidney International, 42* S64.

Schenk, S. (1992). Anticoagulation during pregnancy. *Nurse Practitioner Forum, 3,* 114.

Scott, L. D. (1992). Gallstone disease and pancreatitis in pregnancy. *Gastroenterology Clinics of North America, 21,* 803.

Sharts-Hopko, N. C. (1993). Coping with multidrug resistant tuberculosis. *MCN: American Journal of Maternal Child Nursing, 18,* 184.

Torres, S. (1993). Nursing care of low-income battered Hispanic pregnant women. *AWHONNS Clinical Issues in Perinatal & Women's Health Nursing, 4,* 416.

Williams, M., & Wheby, M. (1992). Anemias in pregnancy. *Medical Clinics of North America, 76,* 631.

Chapter 15

High-Risk Pregnancy: The Woman Who Develops a Complication of Pregnancy

Objectives

After mastering the contents of this chapter, you should be able to:

1. Describe complications of pregnancy such as bleeding, hypertension of pregnancy, and Rh incompatibility.

2. Assess the woman with a complication of pregnancy.

3. Formulate nursing diagnoses that address the needs of the woman with a complication of pregnancy as well as the needs of her family.

4. Plan nursing interventions that address both short-term and long-term goals and that allow the woman to feel a measure of control in her daily life.

5. Implement nursing actions specific to the complications of pregnancy (e.g., begin intravenous fluid, prepare for an emergency cesarean birth).

6. Evaluate outcome criteria to be certain that nursing goals established for care were achieved.

7. Identify National Health Goals related to complications of pregnancy and specific measures nurses can take to help the nation achieve these goals.

8. Identify areas of nursing care related to high risk pregnancy that could benefit from additional nursing research.

9. Use critical thinking to analyze ways that nurses can help prevent complications of pregnancy through health teaching and risk assessment as well as keep nursing care family centered in the midst of a pregnancy complication.

10. Synthesize knowledge of complications of pregnancy with nursing process to achieve quality maternal and child health nursing care.

Key Terms

- abortion
- abruptio placentae
- cervical cerclage
- cervical ripening
- complete abortion
- couvelaire uterus
- ectopic pregnancy
- eclampsia
- erythroblastosis fetalis
- gestational trophoblastic disease
- HELLP syndrome
- hemolytic disease of the newborn
- hydatidiform mole
- hydramnios
- imminent abortion
- incompetent cervix
- incomplete abortion
- isoimmunization
- missed abortion
- placenta previa
- post-term pregnancy
- preeclampsia
- premature separation of the placenta
- pseudocyesis
- Rh incompatibility
- spontaneous abortion
- threatened abortion

Adele Pillitteri: MATERNAL AND CHILD HEALTH NURSING, 2nd Edition. © 1995 Adele Pillitteri.

*T*he leading causes of maternal death during pregnancy are thromboembolism, hemorrhage, infection, hypertension of pregnancy, anesthesia complications, ectopic pregnancy, and heart disease. When a complication of this kind occurs, it has the potential to threaten the life of the mother and the fetus directly and, indirectly, the health of the family.

Most women enter pregnancy in apparent good health and achieve a normal pregnancy and birth without complications. In a few women, however, for reasons that usually are unclear, unexpected deviations from the course of normal pregnancy occur. National Health Goals designed to reduce complications of pregnancy are shown in the Focus on National Health Goals box. A complication of pregnancy can place a severe burden on the woman and her family. Any woman benefits from the support and the skill of a professional nurse who helps her work through the tasks of pregnancy, accept it, and prepare to become a mother. The support and skill of a professional nurse are essential to a woman who, in addition to the usual tasks of pregnancy, must take special care to ensure the continuation of the pregnancy and who may be very concerned that she will not carry the baby to term.

NURSING PROCESS OVERVIEW
*for Care of the Woman Who Develops
a Complication of Pregnancy*

ASSESSMENT

Nurses are often the first to discover a complication of pregnancy. Enough time should be provided for a thorough health history during prenatal visits so that problems such as headache, blurred vision, or vaginal spotting can be uncovered.

It is important to ask women at prenatal visits for symptoms of potential complications so that they can recognize potential problems and telephone the health care center if problems occur. Assure women when giving this information that they are free to call; otherwise, they may wait until their symptoms are acute rather than call when they first notice them.

NURSING DIAGNOSIS

Many nursing diagnoses pertain to the woman with a pregnancy complication. They include:

- Anxiety related to guarded pregnancy outcome
- Fluid volume deficit related to third-trimester bleeding
- High risk for infection related to incomplete abortion
- Altered tissue perfusion related to hypertension of pregnancy
- Grieving related to intrauterine fetal death

PLANNING

In an emergency situation, goals established for care must reflect the short time frame involved. Be certain they address fetal as well as maternal welfare; often they may also reflect family welfare. Protocols for action related to bleeding, premature labor, and hypertension of pregnancy, once established, should be regularly updated and maintained so they remain current. Be certain that they reflect a current nursing management level so nurses are free to act rather than wait for a physician to arrive to begin actions such as routine intravenous fluid or monitoring or typing and crossmatching of blood.

Many women who develop a pregnancy complication will spend a few days (or weeks) in the hospital for therapy and monitoring. It is hard enough waiting for a pregnancy to come to term, but it is even harder for a woman to wait in a hospital, especially when some complication has occurred that might threaten the pregnancy

outcome. Planning must consider the many feelings this experience will cause.

IMPLEMENTATION

Interventions with a complication of pregnancy not only include measures to maintain the physiologic functioning of the pregnancy but the woman's and family's psychological acceptance and maintenance of the pregnancy as well. So that the woman does not begin "anticipatory grieving" for the fetus and halt the growth of bonding, maintain an optimistic attitude of fetal progress. If the complication can be sufficiently contained and the pregnancy continue uninterrupted, this will help protect the mental health of the family. If the pregnancy cannot be continued, be available to offer support to the family who grieves for the loss of the unborn child and, in rare instances, loss of future childbearing potential or the woman herself.

Following a pregnancy with complications, the mother has reason to be especially worried about the infant's health at the time of birth. Be certain she spends enough time with the child to be able to see that, although perhaps born prematurely, the infant is well and healthy. It is helpful to assess the infant in her presence for such things as ability to follow a finger and respond to a voice to demonstrate that the infant is well.

 FOCUS ON
National Health Goals

Preventing complications of pregnancy are viewed as so important by the majority of people that they are included in National Health Goals. Two of these are:

- Increase to at least 90% the proportion of pregnant women and infants who receive risk-appropriate care.
- Reduce severe complications of pregnancy to no more than 15 per 100 deliveries from a baseline of 22 per 100 (DHHS, 1991).

Nurses working in prenatal settings can be helpful in seeing that women are well informed about the normal course of pregnancy so they can recognize and alert health care providers when a complication is occurring; nurses actively participate in risk assessment at prenatal visits. Nursing research is needed in areas such as what is the best way to determine each woman's individual needs so prenatal instructions can be specifically planned, or does increasing the number of prenatal visits for high-risk women reduce complications during pregnancy.

EVALUATION

Established goals should be evaluated throughout the pregnancy (although the success or failure of some nursing interventions cannot be fully evaluated until the child is born or even into the postnatal period). Be aware that following a complication of early pregnancy, a woman cannot help but continue to worry during the remainder of the pregnancy that the complication will recur or that the original insult to the fetus was severe enough to cause long-term damage. Evaluate a woman's psychological attitude as well as her physical status at each continuing health care visit to be certain that she is coping with the fear and strain she lives under until the child is born.

Some fetal outcomes will not be optimal, however, so evaluation will then include the ability of the family to adjust to care of an ill infant. Examples of outcome criteria might be:

- Client's blood pressure is maintained above 100/60 mm Hg.
- Couple state they feel able to cope with anxiety about medical diagnosis of placenta previa.
- Client's temperature remains below 100.4°F; vaginal discharge has no unusual odor.

Bleeding During Pregnancy

Vaginal bleeding is a deviation from the normal that may occur at any time during pregnancy. It is never normal, and it is always frightening. It may or may not be serious, but it must always be carefully investigated, because if it occurs in sufficient amount or for sufficient cause it can impair both the outcome of the pregnancy and the woman's life or future health. The primary causes of bleeding during pregnancy are summarized in Table 15-1.

Bleeding and the Development of Shock

Any degree of vaginal bleeding during pregnancy is potentially serious. This is because the amount that is able to be visualized may be only a fraction of the blood lost because an undilated cervix and intact membranes can be effective at containing blood within the uterus. A woman with any degree of bleeding, therefore, needs to be evaluated for hypovolemic shock.

The process of shock due to blood loss is shown in Figure 15-1. Note that because the uterus is a nonessential body organ, danger to the fetal blood supply occurs not as a last physiologic step but at the point the woman's body begins to decrease blood flow to peripheral organs (although the increased blood volume of pregnancy allows more than normal blood loss before hypovolemic shock occurs) (Clark, 1990). Signs of hypovolemic shock (Table 15-2) will occur when 10% of blood volume or approximately two units of blood have been lost; fetal distress occurs when 25% is lost (Figure 15-2). It is important to know a baseline blood pressure for a pregnant woman to evaluate shock because "normal" varies from woman to woman. Women should be informed of their blood pressure at prenatal visits (e.g., "Your blood pressure is 110 over 70—that's normal," not just "Your pressure is normal"). Then if blood loss should occur, the woman can be helpful in offering her baseline pressure.

Therapeutic Management

Therapy for hypovolemic shock is aimed at both restoring blood volume and halting the source of hemorrhage. These steps are summarized in Table 15-3. A woman suspected of serious bleeding should have an intravenous fluid line begun with a large angiocath (16 or 18) for rapid fluid expansion with a solution such as Ringer's lactate. A blood transfusion can be administered through the same site as soon as blood is available. Hemoglobin and hematocrit levels and typing or crossmatching for blood are essential. The woman may have a central venous pressure (CVP) or a capillary wedge pressure catheter inserted (see Chapter 41). During pregnancy, these values differ from the average so they should be evaluated in light of the pregnancy. A CVP during pregnancy is 2 to 7 mm Hg; pulmonary capillary wedge pressure is 6 to 10 mm Hg (Clark, 1990). Urge the woman not to lie flat on her back but in a lateral position or, if on her back, with a wedge under one hip so that there is minimal uterine pressure on the vena cava and as little blood as possible is trapped in the lower extremities. If respirations are rapid, oxygen by mask should be administered and blood gases drawn. Frequent assessments of vital signs and continuous fetal monitoring by an external monitoring device should be started.

Nursing Diagnosis and Related Interventions

Nursing Diagnosis: High risk for fluid volume deficit related to bleeding during pregnancy.

Goal: Client will not experience significant fluid volume deficit during pregnancy.

Outcome Criteria: Client's blood pressure is more than 100/60 mm Hg; pulse, less than 100 beats per minute; minimal bleeding is apparent; fetal heart rate (FHR) is 120 to 160 bpm, with adequate short-term and long-term variability.

A number of women need blood transfusions during pregnancy or at delivery to restore their normal cir-

Table 15-1. *Summary of Causes of Bleeding During Pregnancy*

Time	Type	Cause	Assessment	Cautions
First trimester	Threatened abortion (early—under 16 wk) (late—16 to 24 wk)	Unknown; possibly chromosomal, uterine abnormalities	Vaginal spotting perhaps slight cramping	
	Imminent (inevitable) abortion		Vaginal spotting, cramping, cervical dilatation	
	Missed abortion		Vaginal spotting, perhaps slight cramping; no apparent loss of pregnancy	Disseminated intravascular coagulation associated with missed abortion
	Incomplete abortion		Vaginal spotting, cramping, cervical dilatation, but incomplete expulsion of uterine contents	
	Complete abortion		Vaginal spotting, cramping, cervical dilatation, and complete expulsion of uterine contents	
	Ectopic (tubal) pregnancy	Implantation of zygote at site other than in uterus; tubal constricture, adhesions associated	Sudden unilateral lower-abdominal-quadrant pain; minimal vaginal bleeding, possible signs of shock or hemorrhage	May have repeat ectopic pregnancy in future if tubal scarring is bilateral
Second trimester	Hydatidiform mole (gestational trophoblastic disease)	Abnormal proliferation of trophoblast tissue; fertilization or division defect	Overgrowth of uterus; highly positive human chorionic gonadotropin (HCG) test; no fetus present on sonogram; bleeding from vagina of old or fresh blood accompanied by cyst formation	Retained trophoblast tissue may become malignant (choriocarcinoma); follow for 1 year with HCG testing
	Incompetent cervix	Cervix begins to dilate and pregnancy is lost at about 20 wk; unknown cause, but cervical trauma from dilatation and curettage (D & C) may be associated	Painless bleeding leading to expulsion of fetus	Can have cervical sutures placed to ensure a second pregnancy
Third trimester	Placenta previa	Low implantation of placenta possibly due to uterine abnormality	Painless bleeding at beginning of cervical dilatation	No vaginal exams to minimize placental trauma
	Premature separation of the placenta (abruptio placentae)	Unknown cause; associated with hypertension	Sharp abdominal pain followed by uterine tenderness; vaginal bleeding; signs of maternal shock, fetal distress	Disseminated intravascular coagulation associated with condition
	Premature labor	Unknown cause; increased chance in multiple gestation, maternal illness	Show—pink-stained vaginal discharge accompanied by uterine contractions becoming regular and effective	Premature labor may possibly be halted if the cervix is less than 4 cm dilated and the membranes are intact

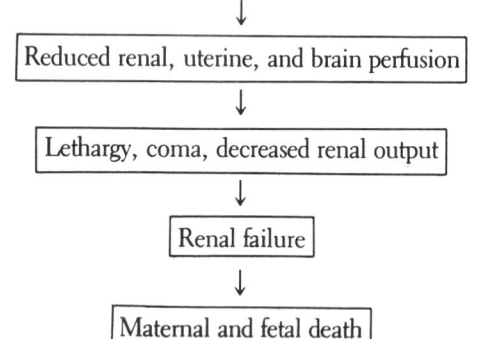

```
Blood loss
   ↓
Decreased intravascular volume
   ↓
Decreased venous return, decreased cardiac output,
and lowered blood pressure
   ↓
Body compensating by increasing heart rate to
circulate the decreased volume faster;
vasoconstriction of peripheral vessels (to save blood
for vital organs). Increased respiratory rate and a
feeling of apprehension at body changes also occur
   ↓
Cold, clammy skin, decreased uterine perfusion. In
the face of continued blood loss, although the body
shifts fluid from interstitial spaces into intravascular
spaces, blood pressure will continue to fall
   ↓
Reduced renal, uterine, and brain perfusion
   ↓
Lethargy, coma, decreased renal output
   ↓
Renal failure
   ↓
Maternal and fetal death
```

FIGURE 15-1
The process of shock due to blood loss (hypovolemia).

Table 15-2. *Signs and Symptoms of Hypovolemic Shock*

Assessment	Significance
Increased pulse rate	Heart attempting to circulate decreased blood volume
Decreased blood pressure	Less peripheral resistance because of decreased blood volume
Increased respiratory rate	Increased gas exchange to better oxygenate decreased red blood cell volume
Cold, clammy skin	Vasoconstriction occurs to maintain blood volume in central body core
Decreased urine output	Inadequate blood is entering kidney due to decreased blood volume
Dizziness or decreased level of consciousness	Inadequate blood is reaching cerebrum due to decreased blood volume
Decreased CVP	Decreased blood is returning to heart due to reduced blood volume

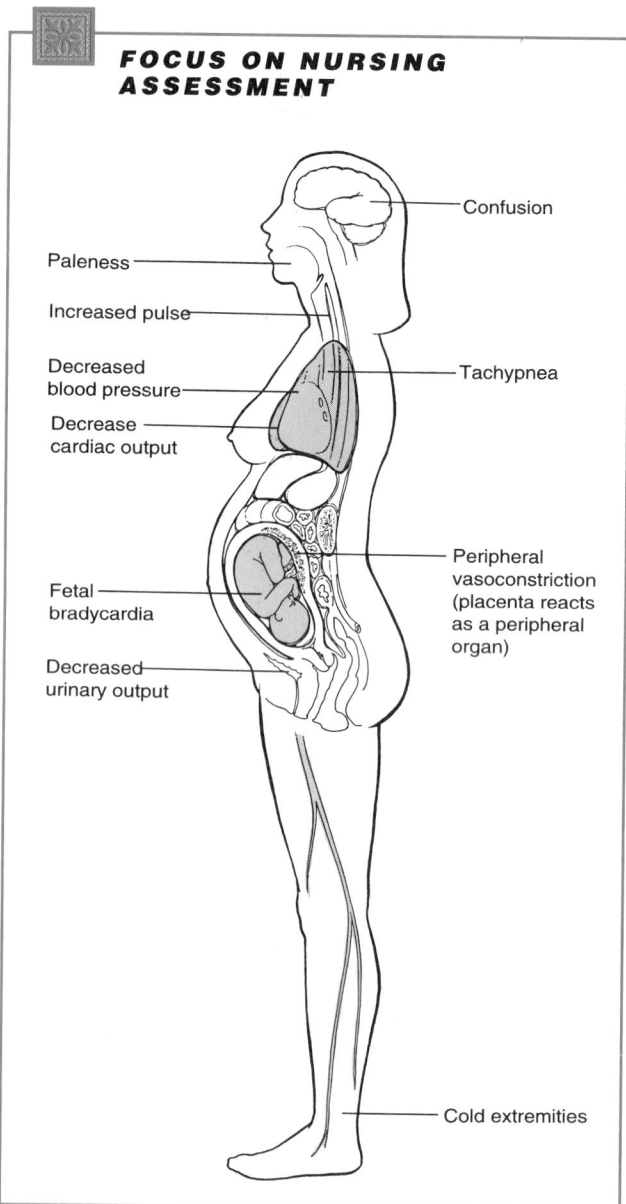

FOCUS ON NURSING ASSESSMENT

Confusion

Paleness

Increased pulse

Decreased blood pressure

Decrease cardiac output

Tachypnea

Fetal bradycardia

Peripheral vasoconstriction (placenta reacts as a peripheral organ)

Decreased urinary output

Cold extremities

FIGURE 15-2
Signs of hypovolemic shock.

culating blood volume following a blood loss. To avoid the risk of receiving blood contaminated by a viral disease, women may donate a unit of blood before pregnancy or early in pregnancy and then receive this blood as a transfusion following the bleeding episode (autologous blood transfusion) (Droste et al., 1992). Donating blood during pregnancy this way does not appear to be detrimental to fetal growth and may be a wise anticipatory measure for the woman who has a placenta previa where substantial blood loss can be anticipated (Cohen, 1991). It is recommended that women donate more than 2 weeks before their EDB so there is time to restore full blood volume before birth (Bottoms & Scott, 1990).

Table 15-3. *Emergency Implementations for Bleeding in Pregnancy*

Implementation	Rationale
Alert health care team of emergency situation	Provides maximum coordination of care
Place woman flat in bed on her side	Maintains optimal placental and renal function
Begin intravenous fluid such as lactated Ringer's with a 16 or 18 angiocath	Replaces intravascular fluid volume; intravenous line is established if blood replacement will be needed.
Adminsiter oxygen as necessary at 6–10 L/min by face mask	Provides adequate fetal oxygenation despite lowered maternal circulating blood volume
Monitor uterine contractions and fetal heart rate by external monitor	Assesses whether labor is present and fetal status; external system avoids cervical trauma
Omit vaginal examination	Prevents tearing of placenta if placenta previa is cause of bleeding
Withhold oral fluid	Anticipates need for emergency surgery
Order type and crossmatch of two units whole blood	Preparation for restoring circulating maternal blood volume
Measure intake and output	Enables assessment of renal function (will decrease to under 30 mL/h with massive circulating volume loss)
Assess vital signs (pulse, respirations, and blood pressure every 15 min; apply pulse oximeter and automatic BP cuff as necessary)	Provides baseline data on maternal response to blood loss
Assist with placement of CVP or pulmonary wedge catheter and blood determinations	Provides more accurate data on maternal hemodynamic state
Measure maternal blood loss by weighing perineal pads; save any tissue passed	Saturating a sanitary pad in less than 1 hour is heavy blood loss; tissue may be abnormal trophoblast tissue
Set aside 5 mL of blood drawn intravenously in a clean test tube; observe in 5 min for clot formation	Tests for possible blood coagulation problem (disseminated intravascular coagulation; suspect this if no clot forms within time limit)
Assist with ultrasound examination	Supplies information on placental and fetal well being
Maintain a positive attitude toward fetal outcome	Supports mother–child bonding
Support woman's self-esteem	Supports problem solving as this is lessened by poor self-esteem

Conditions Associated With First-Trimester Bleeding

The time during pregnancy at which bleeding occurs helps to identify its cause. The two most common causes of bleeding during the first trimester of pregnancy are spontaneous abortion and ectopic pregnancy.

Spontaneous Abortion

An **abortion** is defined as any interruption of a pregnancy before the fetus is viable (a stage of development that will enable the fetus to survive outside the uterus if born at that time). A nonviable fetus is usually defined as a fetus of 20 to 24 weeks gestation age or weighing 500 g. A fetus born at this point would be considered a premature or immature birth (Scott, 1990a). **Spontaneous abortion**, also called miscarriage, happens in 15% to 30% of all pregnancies and occurs from natural causes. *Elective abortion,* which is discussed in Chapter 5, is planned, medical termination of a pregnancy.

A spontaneous abortion is an *early* abortion if it occurs before week 16 of pregnancy and a *late* abortion if it occurs between weeks 16 and 24. For the first 6 weeks of pregnancy, the developing placenta is tentatively attached to the decidua of the uterus; during weeks 6 to 12, a moderate degree of attachment to the myometrium is accomplished. After week 12, the attachment is penetrating and deep into the uterine myometrium. Because of the degrees of attachment achieved at different weeks of pregnancy, it is important to try and establish the week of the pregnancy at which bleeding has become apparent. Bleeding before week 6 is rarely severe; bleeding after week 12 can be great in amount. Fortunately, at this time, with such deep placental implantation, the fetus is expelled as in natural childbirth before the placenta separates. Uterine contraction then helps to control placental bleeding as it does postpartally. For some women, then, the stage of attachment between weeks 6 and 12 can lead to the most severe bleeding and threat to their life (the placenta delivers before the fetus; uterine contraction does not occur readily and bleeding continues).

Causes of Spontaneous Abortion

The most frequent cause of abortion in the first trimester of pregnancy is abnormal fetal formation, due either to a teratogenic factor or to a chromosomal aberration. Approximately 60% of fetuses aborted early have structural abnormalities: 40% have grossly observable pathologic conditions. In other abortions, immunologic factors may be present or "rejection" of the embryo may occur. Sonogram examination during early pregnancy may demonstrate hematomas on the placenta of pregnancies that then abort. Women with maternal lupus anti-coagulant factors have both more abortions and preterm births than other women (Rosove et al., 1990). Administering heparin to these women may decrease the tendency toward early pregnancy loss.

Another common cause of early abortion is implantation abnormalities (approximately 50% of zygotes are never implanted). With inadequate implantation, the placental circulation will not be well established, and fetal formation will be inadequate. Poor implantation may result from inadequate endometrial formation or from an inappropriate site of implantation.

Abortion may also occur if the corpus luteum fails to produce enough progesterone to maintain the decidua basalis. Progesterone therapy may be attempted to prevent this if this cause is documented.

Abortion may occur following trauma, such as a blow to the woman's abdomen in an automobile accident. The reason for the abortion in this instance is probably hemorrhage in the decidua basalis, resulting in placental detachment. It is always amazing, however, to discover how many women have accidents or falls during pregnancy without abortion. Such pregnancy histories provide good justification for the presence of the amniotic fluid: it truly serves as a buffer against fetal trauma.

Infection in the woman may be yet another cause of abortion. Rubella and poliomyelitis viruses cross the placenta readily and may cause fetal death. Cytomegalovirus and toxoplasmosis infections are both implicated in early abortion. Urinary tract infections also increase the incidence. With failure of growth in the fetus, estrogen and progesterone production by the placenta falls; this leads to endometrial sloughing. With the sloughing,

prostaglandins are released and uterine contraction and cervical dilatation and expulsion of the products of conception begin. Ingestion of a teratogenic drug is yet another cause. Isotretinoin (Accutane) is an example of a drug that if taken early in pregnancy, can lead to abortion or fetal abnormality (Loeb, 1993). Because abortion can occur from so many causes it can be difficult for a couple to understand why it happened to them (see the Focus on Family Teaching box).

Assessment

The presenting symptom of spontaneous abortion is almost always vaginal spotting, which is why this is one of the danger signs of pregnancy. At the first indication of vaginal spotting, a woman should telephone her health care provider and describe what is happening. Because a nurse often takes this initial call, nurses should be aware of guidelines to assess vaginal bleeding quickly during pregnancy (Table 15-4).

The history of the episode is important in helping the physician or nurse-midwife form a diagnosis of the cause. Knowledge of the woman's actions is important to ensure she did not attempt to self-abort. She may prefer not to mention such an attempt, but usually will if asked directly. Ask what she has done about the bleeding to be sure she has not inserted a tampon to stop bleeding and actually has an unknown amount of blood loss, although reporting only slight spotting.

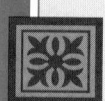

FOCUS ON FAMILY TEACHING

Q. Why did my doctor keep referring to my miscarriage as an abortion? She made me feel as if she thought I did something to cause it.

A. Abortion is the medical term for any pregnancy loss before the fetus could have lived outside the uterus. Think of the word as interchangeable with miscarriage.

Q. Are there special things I should do with a second pregnancy to keep an early abortion from happening again?

A. Early abortion is largely unpreventable because it is caused by such things as abnormal chromosome formation or poor uterine implantation—things over which you have no control. Following sensible guidelines such as eating a nutritious diet so you enter a pregnancy in good health and avoiding cigarette smoking or drinking alcohol are sensible recommendations. If you had extensive blood loss with your miscarriage, you might want to be certain to eat iron-rich foods (meat, green vegetables) to help restore red blood cells for a second pregnancy.

Table 15-4. *Immediate Assessment of Vaginal Bleeding During Pregnancy*

Assessment Factor	Specific Questions to Ask
Confirmation of pregnancy	Does the woman know for certain that she is pregnant (positive pregnancy test or physician/nurse-midwife confirmation)? A woman who has been pregnant before and states that she is sure she is pregnant is probably right even if she has not yet had this confirmed.
Pregnancy length	What is the length of the pregnancy in weeks?
Duration	How long did the bleeding episode last? Is it continuing?
Intensity	How much bleeding occurred? (Ask the woman to compare it to a common measure [e.g., a tablespoonful, a cup].)
Description	Was it mixed with amniotic fluid or mucus? Was it bright red (fresh blood) or dark (old blood)? Was it accompanied by tissue fragments? Was it odorous?
Frequency	Steady spotting? A single episode?
Associated symptoms	Cramping? Sharp pain? Dull pain? Has she ever had cervical surgery?
Action	Did anything happen that may have started the bleeding? What has she done (if anything) to control bleeding?
Blood type	Does she know this? (Rh negative women will need Rh immune globulin to prevent Rh isoimmunization.)

Therapeutic Management

Depending on the symptoms and the description of the bleeding or spotting the woman gives, the physician or nurse-midwife will decide whether the woman should be seen in an ambulatory setting or the hospital for care.

Threatened Abortion

Threatened abortion is manifested by vaginal bleeding, usually bright red in color and moderate in amount. There are no associated symptoms such as cramping and no cervical dilatation present on vaginal examination. The woman may be asked to come to the clinic or office to have a sonogram done to confirm a pregnancy. Blood for human chorionic gonadotrophin hormone may be drawn at the start of bleeding and again in 48 hours (if the placenta is still intact, the level of this in the bloodstream should double in this time [Cowan, 1993]). Serum progesterone may also be assessed (a diminishing level suggests pregnancy disruption). The only therapy usually advised for threatened abortion is to limit activities for 24 to 48 hours; complete bed rest is unnecessary. Complete bed rest will stop the vaginal bleeding

but this occurs only because blood is pooling vaginally; when the woman does ambulate again, bleeding will reoccur. The woman is apt to be extremely worried at the sight of bleeding and perhaps watching a pregnancy end, so needs some time to talk with a sympathetic support person about how distressed she is.

It is important to convey concerned reassurance that abortions happen spontaneously, not because of anything the woman did (see the Focus on Nursing Research box). Women with threatened abortions look for reasons as to why they could have happened and never fail to find some, such as running up a flight of stairs, forgetting to take an iron pill, or getting angry with an older child. Being told that none of these events causes abortions helps to free women of guilt for the abortion.

Although human chorionic gonadotrophin hormone may be prescribed on an experimental basis (Harrison, 1993), most women are disappointed to learn that there is no cure to "hold the pregnancy." In the past, estrogen or progesterone were prescribed for this purpose, but there is no sure evidence that this helps. Nearly 20 to 30 years ago, diethylstilbestrol (DES) was routinely administered to women at the time of threatened abortion; although this drug never proved to be effective, daughters born of the DES-aided pregnancies are now in danger of developing vaginal cancer following adenosis from their intrauterine exposure to DES (Faber et al., 1990); male children from such pregnancies are more susceptible to cystic testicular development.

FOCUS ON NURSING RESEARCH

What Are Women's Reactions to Miscarriage in Early Pregnancy?

Two researchers attempted to answer this question by interviewing ten women 2 to 4 months after a miscarriage. The miscarriages had occurred within the first 15 weeks of a pregnancy. Findings of the interviews revealed that the "hush" surrounding miscarriage was not helpful to women and contributed to the inadequate support they perceived they had received. Women wanted (and benefited) from unconditional acceptance of their feelings, not to be told how to feel. It was not uncommon for women to feel responsible for their miscarriage; several experienced enough pain and bleeding that they perceived this as a life-threatening event. It was so serious an event in several women's lives that they grieved over their loss as they would have mourned the deaths of other family members. All women emerged from the experience with changed perspectives on their lives.

Bansen, S. S., & Stevens, H. A. (1992). Women's experiences of miscarriage in early pregnancy. *Journal of Nurse-Midwifery, 37,* 84.

If the spotting with threatened abortion is going to stop, it usually does so within 24 to 48 hours of the time the woman begins to reduce her activity. After that, she can gradually resume normal activities. Coitus is usually restricted for 2 weeks following the bleeding episode to prevent the possibility of infection and to avoid possibly inducing further bleeding.

As many as 90% of women with threatened abortion continue the pregnancy; for the other 10%, unfortunately, the threatened abortion changes to imminent or inevitable abortion.

Imminent (Inevitable) Abortion

A threatened abortion becomes an **imminent** or **inevitable abortion** if uterine contractions and cervical dilatation occur. With cervical dilation, the loss of the product of conception cannot be halted. A woman who reports cramping or uterine contractions is usually asked to come to the hospital, where she is examined (Figure 15-3). She should save and bring to the hospital with her any tissue fragments that she has passed. In the hospital,

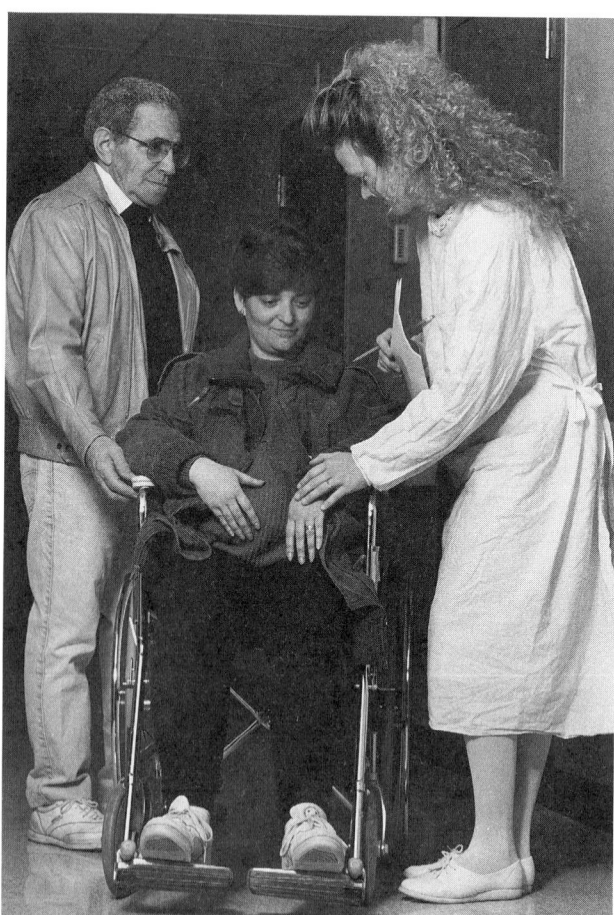

FIGURE 15-3

Hospital admission for a spontaneous abortion is a serious and frightening experience. It requires compassionate nursing care. (Courtesy of the Department of Medical Photography, Children's Hospital, Buffalo, NY.)

if no fetal heart sounds are detected, the woman's physician may perform a D & C to ensure that all the products of conception are removed. Be certain the woman has an explanation that the pregnancy was already lost at hospital admission and all procedures such as a suction curettage are to clean and ready the uterus for another pregnancy (forward moving steps) not actually causing the pregnancy loss. Any tissue fragments passed in the labor room should be saved, so that they can be examined for an abnormality such as gestational trophoblastic disease (**hydatidiform mole**) (see below) or for assurance that all the products of conception have been removed from the uterus. Weighing perineal pads before and after use and subtracting the difference is a good way to accurately determine how much vaginal blood loss is occurring.

Complete Abortion

In a **complete abortion**, the entire contents of conception (fetus, membranes, and placenta) are expelled spontaneously without any assistance. There is minimal, self-limiting bleeding.

Incomplete Abortion

In an **incomplete abortion**, part of the conceptus (usually the fetus) is expelled, but the membranes or placenta are retained in the uterus. Incomplete can be a confusing term for women. They may interpret it as indicating that because the abortion is only partial, the pregnancy can continue. Be careful not to encourage false hopes by also misinterpreting this term.

In an incomplete abortion, there is a danger of maternal hemorrhage as long as part of the conceptus is retained in the uterus, as the uterus cannot contract in this state. The woman's physician will usually perform a D & C or suction curettage to evacuate the remainder of the pregnancy from the uterus. Be certain that the woman is informed what is happening—that she knows the pregnancy is already lost and that the procedure is being done only to protect her from hemorrhage and infection, not to end the pregnancy.

Missed Abortion

In a **missed abortion**, the fetus dies in utero but is not expelled. Women may also find this term misleading. A missed abortion is usually discovered at a prenatal examination when the fundal height is measured and no increase in size can be demonstrated, or when previously heard fetal heart sounds cannot be heard. The woman may have had symptoms of a threatened abortion (painless vaginal bleeding); she may have had no prior clinical symptoms before this time.

A sonogram can establish that the fetus is dead; following this, the pregnancy will be ended by one of the same techniques used with induced abortion, such as dilatation and evacuation or PGE_2 vaginal suppositories (see Chapter 5). If symptoms of fetal death are not detected within 2 weeks, abortion usually spontaneously occurs at this time. There is a danger of allowing this normal course to happen, however, because disseminated intravascular coagulation, a coagulation defect, may develop if the dead (and possibly toxic) fetus remains too long in utero. Disseminated intravascular coagulation is a potential complication of other bleeding disorders in pregnancy as well (Drummond, 1992).

Most women hope until the moment the abortion is induced that the sonogram was mistaken, that their baby is alive. They need support in accepting the reality of the situation. They may need counseling to accept a future pregnancy because of fears that whatever "force" struck silently and strangely in one pregnancy might strike again.

Recurrent Abortion

In the past, women who had three spontaneous abortions that occurred at the same gestation age in three pregnancies were called "habitual aborters." They were often advised that they were apparently too "nervous" or that something was so wrong with their hormones that childbearing was not for them. Today, the term *recurrent abortion* is used to describe this abortion pattern and a thorough investigation is done to discover the cause of the loss and help ensure the outcome of a future pregnancy (Kutteh, 1993). Recurrent abortion occurs in about 1 in 200 women (Scott, 1990a). There are a number of causes of recurrent abortion.

Defective Spermatozoa or Ova. A careful family history of such women may reveal a familial tendency to produce children with defects. If a woman has had more than one aborted fetus, a pathologic report and chromosomal karyotype on the fetus should be carried out to reveal a possible inherited chromosomal abnormality. A chromosomal investigation of both parents will then be done to see whether aberrant chromosomes can be detected in either the husband or the wife's karyotype. (Chromosome abnormalities are discussed in Chapter 7.) If such a chromosomal aberration is discovered, artificial insemination using donor sperm or donor embryo transfer can be suggested.

Endocrine Factors. Ordinarily during pregnancy, the protein-bound iodine (PBI), butanol-extractable iodine (BEI), and globulin-bound iodine (GBI) levels are elevated; the outcome of this is an increased basal metabolism rate. In women with recurrent abortions, these values may be lowered. Thyroid function is assessed by T3 and T4 serum levels. Poor thyroid function can be a cause of infertility as well as of abortion. Thus, if the tests indicate poor thyroid function, the woman may be started on therapy to aid in conception as well as to help carry the next pregnancy to term.

Ovarian dysfunction such as a luteal phase defect that leads to poor progesterone production may also be a cause. An endometrial biopsy will be scheduled to detect this. Therapy with progesterone suppositories or clomiphene (Clomid) may be prescribed to correct this (Bopp & Shoupe, 1993).

Deviations of the Uterus. In the female fetus, the uterus first forms as an organ with a midseptum (see Chapter 4). As the organ matures, the septum atrophies and disappears. Occasionally, a woman reaches adulthood with a uterine septum still intact. The blood supply to the septum is ordinarily not as good as that to the endometrium covering the normal walls of the uterus. Placental implantation on the septum, therefore, may result in an inadequate nutrient supply to the fetus and consequent abortion. In addition, the uterus may be only half the normal size because of the dividing septum; this can cause a pregnancy to end prematurely.

A bicornuate uterus is one with sharp poles (horns). This abnormal shape may lead to early pregnancy loss, although most women with a bicornuate uterus carry pregnancies to term (Fedrizzi & Cothren, 1993). Although many women with leiomyomas (fibroid tumors) also carry a fetus to term, extensive tumors can block out implantation space and lead to abortion (Exacoustos & Rosati, 1993). Women with these disorders will be scheduled for abdominal metroplasty (reconstructive surgery) or vaginal hysteroscopy to correct the problems.

Infection. Any infection of the developing embryo could lead to abortion. *Listeriosis*, an infection caused by the gram-positive rod *Listeria monocytogenes* is an example of an organism which can cause this (Lallemand et al., 1992). Listeriosis is transmitted in contaminated food such as coleslaw or cheese, and so it may cause several episodes of abortion in a community at the same time. The organism is susceptible to penicillin G, ampicillin, or erythromycin.

Autoimmune Disorders. Women who have autoimmune diseases may have a tendency to early pregnancy loss (Mishell, 1993). The presence of lupus anticoagulant and anticardiolipin antibodies are most associated with this phenomenon. With these antibodies present, women have an increased tendency for embolic formation. This can lead to decidual and placental insufficiency from infarcts forming under the placenta. Administration of prednisone, heparin, or aspirin may be helpful in reducing the reaction. A program of immunotherapy to reduce rejection of the fetus may be attempted.

Complications of Abortion

As with full-term childbirth, hemorrhage and infection are two of the most likely complications following abortion. Isoimmunization and the woman's psychological state both need to be considered.

Hemorrhage. With a complete spontaneous abortion, serious or fatal hemorrhage is rare. With incomplete abortion or in the woman who develops an accompanying coagulation defect (usually disseminated intravascular coagulation), major hemorrhage is a possibility. If excessive vaginal bleeding is occurring, for an immediate measure, keep the woman flat and massage the uterine fundus to try and achieve contraction. The woman may need a D & C to empty the uterus of the material that is preventing it from contracting and achieving hemostasis. She may need a transfusion to replace blood, and she may require direct replacement of fibrinogen to aid coagulation.

The woman who is being managed at home after a self-limiting complete abortion should have clear instructions on how much bleeding is abnormal (a rule of thumb is more than one sanitary pad per hour); what color changes she should expect in bleeding (gradually changing to a dark color and then to the color of serous fluid as it does with the postpartal woman); and that any unusual odor or passing of large clots is also abnormal. If the physician has prescribed an oral medication such as methylergonovine maleate (Methergine) to aid with contraction, check to see that she is aware of its importance. Some women want to forget the experience as quickly as possible; repression helps them to handle their anger or grief at the loss of the pregnancy most effectively. Be careful that in repressing the experience the woman does not also repress the memory of her medication and leave herself open to hemorrhage. If the woman is hospitalized following an abortion, the same observations, in addition to careful recording of vital signs, are carried out.

Infection. Infection is a minimal possibility when pregnancy loss occurs over a short period, bleeding is self-limiting, and instrumentation is limited.

Women should still be observed closely for signs of infection following abortion, however, including fever, local tenderness, and a foul vaginal discharge. Some women have a transient fever with abortion that is probably due to a period of lowered fluid intake that preceded abortion in some instances. In other instances, the fever may be a systemic reaction to the abortion process. All fevers of more than 100.4°F should be evaluated carefully, however, so that the woman who is contracting an infection will not be overlooked.

Infection tends to occur in women who have lost appreciable amounts of blood due to the debilitating effect of blood loss. Such women need especially careful observation to rule out this second, possibly fatal, complication.

The organism responsible for infection following abortion is usually *Escherichia coli* (spread from the rectum forward into the vagina). The woman should be cautioned to wipe the perineal area from front to back after voiding and particularly after defecation, to prevent the spread of bacteria from the rectal area. Caution her not to use tampons to control vaginal discharge, because stasis of any body fluid increases the risk of infection. Be careful about statements such as, "You'll have some vaginal flow now almost exactly like a menstrual flow," so the woman does not treat it as a menstrual flow and use tampons.

Endometritis (infection of the uterine lining) is the infection that usually occurs following abortion. It may be more extensive, however, and parametritis, peritonitis, thrombophlebitis, and septicemia can occur. The management of these infections is the same as if they were occurring postpartum, after the safe delivery of a child (see Chapter 25).

Septic Abortion. A septic abortion is an abortion that is complicated by infection (Stabile, 1992). Infection can happen following a spontaneous abortion but more frequently occurs in women who have tried to self abort using a nonsterile instrument such as a knitting needle.

As the uterus is a warm, moist, dark cavity, once introduced, infectious organisms grow rapidly in this environment, particularly if there are still products of conception present such as necrotic membranes.

The woman has symptoms of fever and crampy abdominal pain and her uterus feels tender to palpation. Left untreated, such an infection can lead to toxic shock syndrome, septicemia, kidney failure, and death.

In order for her life to be saved, the woman needs immediate, intensive assessment including a complete blood count, electrolytes, creatinine, and type and cross match of blood. Cultures will be taken of the cervix, vagina, and urine. She will have a foley catheter inserted to monitor urine output; she will be begun on intravenous fluid both to restore fluid volume and provide a route for high dose broad spectrum antibiotic therapy. Penicillin (gram positive coverage), tobramycin (gram negative coverage), and clindamycin (gram negative anaerobic coverage) are common antibiotics used.

A CVP or Swan-Ganz catheter to monitor left atrial filling pressure may be put in place. The removal of all infected or necrotic tissue from the uterus is important, so a D & C will be performed. Tetanus toxoid SQ or tetanus immune globulin IM will be administered for prophylaxis against tetanus.

The woman is usually admitted to an intensive care setting for continuing care. Dopamine and digitalis may be necessary to maintain sufficient cardiac output. Oxygen and perhaps ventilatory support may be necessary to maintain respiratory function.

Assuming the woman recovers from the intense episode, septic abortion may lead to future infertility due to uterine scarring or fibrotic scarring of the fallopian tubes. If the woman caused the infection by trying to self-abort she needs to be counseled following the acute episode to seek better problem solving methods in the future.

Isoimmunization. Whenever a placenta is dislodged, either by spontaneous birth or by D & C at any point in pregnancy, some blood from the placental villi (the fetal blood) may enter the maternal circulation. This has implications for the Rh-negative woman. Enough Rh-positive fetal blood may enter her circulation to cause **isoimmunization**—that is, the production by her immunologic system of antibodies against Rh-positive blood. If her next child should have Rh-positive blood, these antibodies would attempt to destroy the red blood cells of the next infant during the months the infant is in utero.

Following an abortion, because the blood type of the conceptus is unknown, all women with Rh-negative blood should receive Rh$_o$ (D antigen) immune globulin (RHIG) to prevent the buildup of antibodies in the event the conceptus was Rh-positive.

Grieving. As with pregnancy loss for any reason, women need to be assessed as to how they are adjusting to a spontaneous abortion. A feeling of sadness over the loss is to be expected. Spontaneous abortion can be particularly heartbreaking for the woman who waits until almost 40 to have her first child, as she realizes that her window of childbearing is limited.

Ectopic Pregnancy

An **ectopic pregnancy** is one in which implantation occurs outside the uterine cavity (Sepulveda et al., 1993). The implantation may occur on the surface of the ovary or in the cervix, but the most usual site (in approximately 95% of such pregnancies) is in the fallopian tube (Figure 15-4). Of these fallopian tube sites, approximately 60% occur in the ampullar portion, 25% in the isthmus, and 5% are interstitial. Approximately 1 in every 200 pregnancies is ectopic; ectopic pregnancy is the second most frequent cause of bleeding early in pregnancy (Cunningham, 1993).

With ectopic pregnancy, fertilization occurs normally in the distal third of the fallopian tube, and immediately after the union of ovum and spermatozoon, the zygote that is formed begins to divide and increase in size normally. Unfortunately, if an obstruction is present, such as an adhesion of the fallopian tube from previous infection (chronic salpingitis or pelvic inflammatory disease), congenital malformations, scars from tubal surgery, or a uterine tumor pressing on the proximal end of the tube, the zygote is unable to traverse the length of the tube and lodges at a strictured site along the tube; it

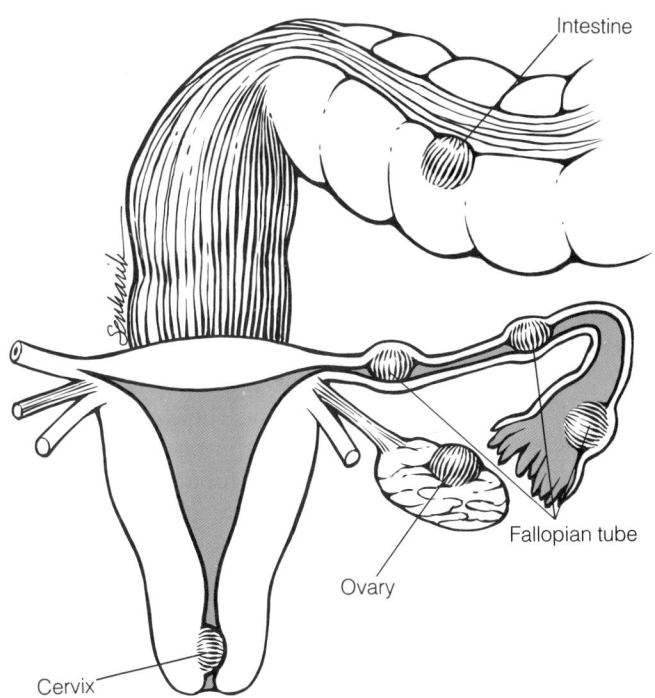

FIGURE 15-4
Sites at which an ectopic pregnancy may occur.

implants there instead of in the uterus. There is some evidence that intrauterine devices (IUDs) used for contraception may slow the transport of the zygote and lead to tubal or ovarian implantation as these are also associated with pelvic inflammatory disease. Progestin-only oral contraceptives, postconceptual estrogen, or ovarian induction drugs may also be causes of ectopic pregnancy. Women who have one ectopic pregnancy have a 10% to 20% chance that a subsequent pregnancy will also be ectopic (Scott, 1990b). This is because salpingitis that leaves scarring is usually bilateral. Congenital anomalies such as webbing may also be bilateral.

Assessment

With ectopic pregnancy, there are no unusual symptoms at the time of implantation. The corpus luteum of the ovary continues to function as if the implantation were in the uterus. No menstrual flow occurs, the woman may experience the nausea and vomiting of early pregnancy, and a pregnancy test for HCG will be positive.

At week 6 to 12 of pregnancy (4 to 10 weeks following a missed menstrual period), the growing zygote ruptures the slender tube, or the trophoblast cells break through the narrow base of the fallopian tube, with resultant invasion and destruction of the blood vessels in the tube. The extent of the bleeding that occurs depends on the number and size of the ruptured vessels. If implantation is in the interstitial portion of the tube (where the tube joins the uterus), rupture will cause severe intraperitoneal bleeding. Fortunately, the incidence of tubal pregnancies is highest in the ampullar area (the distal third), where the blood vessels are smaller and profuse hemorrhage is less likely. However, the continued bleeding from this area may in time result in as great a loss of blood. The bottom line is ruptured ectopic pregnancy is serious, no matter what the site of implantation.

The amount of bleeding evident with ruptured ectopic pregnancy is often deceptive. This is because the products of conception from the ruptured tube and the accompanying blood may be expelled into the pelvic cavity rather than into the uterus and so blood does not reach the vagina to become evident. The woman usually experiences a sharp, stabbing pain in one of the lower abdominal quadrants at the time of rupture followed by a little vaginal spotting. (With placental dislodgment, progesterone secretion stops and the uterine decidua begins to slough, causing this bleeding.) She may experience light-headedness and rapid pulse, signs of shock.

The possibility of ectopic pregnancy is the reason it is important when women call a health care agency in the first trimester of pregnancy reporting vaginal spotting to ask whether there is any associated pain. Any woman with sharp pain and vaginal spotting must be seen so that ectopic pregnancy can be ruled out. Occasionally, a woman will move suddenly and pull one of the round ligaments, the anterior uterine supports. This can cause a sharp, momentary, innocent lower-quadrant pain. However, it would be rare for this phenomenon to be reported in connection with vaginal spotting.

By the time the woman with a ruptured ectopic pregnancy arrives at the hospital or physician's office, she may be in deep shock, with a rapid, thready pulse, rapid respirations, and falling blood pressure. Leukocytosis may be present, not from infection, but from the trauma. Temperature is usually normal. A sonogram will demonstrate the ruptured tube and collecting pelvic fluid. If the diagnosis of ectopic pregnancy is in doubt, the physician may, under sterile conditions, insert a needle through the postvaginal fornix into the cul-de-sac to see whether blood that has collected there from internal bleeding can be aspirated. Either laparoscopy or culdoscopy can be used to visualize the fallopian tube if the symptoms alone do not reveal a clear-cut picture of what has happened.

Gradually, the woman's abdomen becomes rigid from peritoneal irritation. If blood is slowly seeping into the peritoneal cavity, the umbilicus may develop a bluish tinge (Cullen's sign). The woman may have continuing extensive or dull vaginal and abdominal pain; movement of the cervix on pelvic examination may cause excruciating pain. There may be pain in her shoulders from blood in the peritoneal cavity causing irritation to the phrenic nerve. A tender mass is usually palpable in Douglas's cul-de-sac on vaginal examination.

Therapeutic Management

Because ruptured ectopic pregnancy is an emergency situation, the woman's condition must be evaluated quickly, the amount of blood *evident* being a poor estimate of her actual blood loss. Blood is drawn immediately for hemoglobin value, typing, and cross matching, and possibly progesterone or human chorionic gonadotropin (HCG) level for immediate pregnancy testing if pregnancy has not been confirmed. Intravenous fluid to restore intravascular volume is begun (use a large size angiocath so blood can be administered when available through the same site).

The therapy for ruptured ectopic pregnancy is laparotomy to ligate the bleeding vessels and to remove or repair the damaged fallopian tube. A rough suture line on a fallopian tube may lead to another tubal pregnancy, so suturing on the tube must be done with microsurgery technique.

If a tube is removed, the woman is theoretically only 50% fertile, because every other month, when she ovulates from the ovary next to the removed tube, sperm cannot reach the ovum on that side. This cannot be counted on as a contraceptive measure, however. It has been shown in rabbits that translocation of ova can occur—that is, an ovum released from the right ovary can pass through the pelvic cavity to the opposite (left) fallopian tube, and vice versa.

As with abortion, women with Rh-negative blood should receive Rh_o (D) immune globulin (RHIG) following an ectopic pregnancy for isoimmunization protection in future childbearing.

If ectopic pregnancy can be diagnosed by a routine sonogram before the tube has ruptured, it can be treated medically by the oral administration of methotrexate ("Local methotrexate," 1990) followed by leucovorin. Methotrexate is a chemotherapeutic agent that attacks and destroys fast-growing cells. Because trophoblast and zygote growth is rapid, the drug is drawn to the site of the ectopic pregnancy (see Chapter 53 for a general discussion of chemotherapy agents). Methotrexate is also effective in cervical pregnancies (Punch, 1992). Clients are treated until a negative HCG titer is achieved. A hysterosalpingogram is usually performed following chemotherapy to assess whether the tube is fully patent. RU486, a medication used in Europe as an abortion agent, is also effective at causing sloughing of the tubal implantation site (Pansky et al., 1991). The advantage of these therapies is that the tube is left intact with no surgical scarring.

Nursing Diagnoses and Related Interventions

Nursing Diagnosis: Grieving related to early loss of pregnancy secondary to ectopic pregnancy

Goal: Client will satisfactorily complete grief reaction by six months.

Outcome Criteria: Client states she feels sad at pregnancy loss but is able to deal with situation; has returned to work and has forward thinking plans.

A woman who has an ectopic pregnancy not only has grief stages to work through (she has lost a child) but may have problems of diminished self-image to resolve as well if surgery included removal of a fallopian tube. She may believe that she is now half a woman if she equated childbearing with being a woman. She needs to verbalize concerns about this and future childbearing. The process of working through grief and role images takes weeks to months. It should begin in the hospital, however, where the woman has professional people to help her through the first days and estimate whether she will need counseling.

Abdominal Pregnancy

Very rarely after ectopic pregnancy rupture—so rarely that the instances are difficult to document—the product of conception is expelled into the pelvic cavity with a minimum of bleeding. The placenta continues to grow in the fallopian tube, spreading perhaps into the uterus for a better blood supply; or it may escape into the pelvic cavity and successfully implant on an organ such as an intestine (Costa, Presley, & Bastert, 1991). The fetus will grow in the pelvic cavity (an abdominal pregnancy).

In an abdominal pregnancy, the fetal outline is not easily palpable. The woman may not be as aware of movements as she would be normally or she may experience painful fetal movements and abdominal cramping with fetal movements.

Past history of the woman may include previous uterine surgery or the sudden pain of ectopic pregnancy earlier in the pregnancy. A sonogram or magnetic resonance imaging is used to reveal the fetus outside the uterus.

The danger of abdominal pregnancy is that the placenta will infiltrate and erode a major blood vessel in the abdomen, leading to hemorrhage. If implanted on the intestine, it may erode so deeply that it causes bowel perforation and a peritonitis. The risk to the fetus is also high because without a good uterine blood supply, nutrients may not adequately reach the fetus. Survival in an abdominal pregnancy is only approximately 20% because of poor nutrient supply. In those infants who do survive, there is an increased incidence of fetal deformity.

At term, the infant must be born by laparotomy. The placenta is often difficult to remove following birth if it is implanted on an abdominal organ such as the intestine. It may be left in place and allowed to be absorbed spontaneously in 2 or 3 months (a follow-up sonogram can be used to detect this has occurred) or the woman can be treated with methotrexate, which will destroy the placenta cells.

Conditions Associated With Second-Trimester Bleeding

There are two main causes of bleeding during the second trimester: gestational trophoblastic disease and incompetent cervix.

Gestational Trophoblastic Disease (Hydatidiform Mole)

Gestational trophoblastic disease is proliferation and degeneration of the trophoblast villi. As the cells degenerate, they become filled with fluid, appearing as fluid-filled, grape-sized vesicles; in this condition, the embryo fails to develop beyond a primitive start. Such structures must be identified as they are associated with choriocarcinoma, a rapidly metastasizing malignancy (Figure 15-5) (Lewis, 1993).

The incidence of gestational trophoblastic disease is approximately 1 in every 2000 pregnancies. The condition tends to occur most often in women from low socioeconomic groups who have a low protein intake, in young women (under age 18 years), in women older than age 35 years, and in women of Asian heritage (Deicas et al., 1991).

Two types of mole growth can be identified by chromosome analysis. With a *complete mole,* all trophoblastic villi swell and become cystic. If an embryo forms it dies early at only 1 to 2 mm in size; no fetal blood is present in the villi. On chromosomal analysis, although

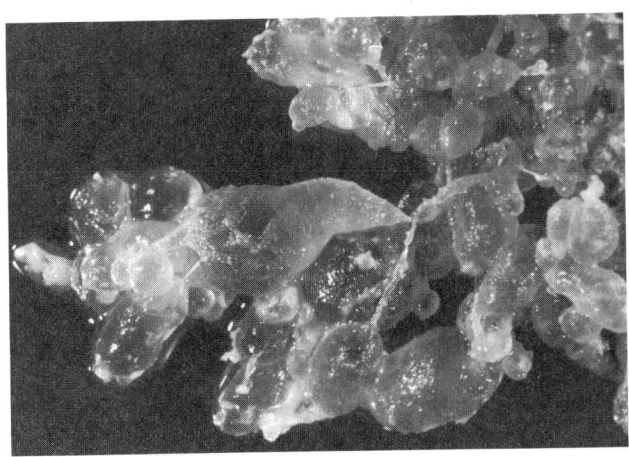

FIGURE 15-5
Gestational trophoblastic disease. (Courtesy of Bryan Smistek.)

the karyotype of the growth is a normal 46XX or 46XY, this chromosome component was contributed only by the paternal material or an "empty ovum" was fertilized and the chromosome material duplicated (Figure 15-6*A*).

With a *partial mole,* some of the villi form normally; the syncytiotrophoblast layer of villi, however, is swollen and misshaped. Even though no embryo is present, fetal blood may be present in villi. A macerated embryo of approximately 9 weeks gestation may be present. A partial mole has 69 chromosomes (a triploid formation in which there are three chromosomes instead of two for every pair, one set supplied by an ova that apparently was fertilized by two sperm or an ova fertilized by one sperm in which meiosis or reduction division did not occur). This could also occur if one set of 23 chromosomes was supplied by one sperm and an ova that did not undergo reduction division supplied 46 (Figure 15-6*B*).

In contrast to complete moles, partial moles rarely lead to choriocarcinoma. Although still above average, HCG titers are lower in partial than complete moles; they return to normal faster after mole evacuation.

Assessment

Because the proliferation of the trophoblast cells occurs so rapidly with this condition, the uterus expands faster than normally. This causes the uterus to reach its landmarks (just over the symphysis brim at 12 weeks, at the umbilicus at 20 to 24 weeks) before the usual time. This rapid development is also diagnostic of multiple preg-

nancy or miscalculated due date, however, so this finding must be evaluated carefully. No fetal heart sounds will be heard because there is no viable fetus. A blood or urine test of HCG for pregnancy will be strongly positive (1 to 2 million IU compared with a normal pregnancy level of 400,000 IU) because HCG is produced by the trophoblast cells and this is what is overgrowing.

Results continue to be strongly positive after day 100 of pregnancy, when the level of HCG normally would begin to decline. This fact must be evaluated carefully also, because highly positive test results can be characteristic of multiple pregnancies with more than one placenta. The nausea and vomiting of early pregnancy is usually marked, probably due to the high HCG level present. Symptoms of hypertension of pregnancy (i.e., hypertension, edema, and proteinuria) are ordinarily not present before week 20 of pregnancy; with gestational trophoblastic disease, they may appear before this time. A sonogram will show dense growth (typically a "snowflake pattern") but no fetal growth in the uterus.

At approximately week 16 of pregnancy, if the structure was not identified earlier by sonogram, it will identify itself with vaginal bleeding. This may begin as vaginal spotting of dark brown blood or as a profuse fresh flow. As the bleeding progresses, it is accompanied by discharge of the clear-fluid–filled vesicles. This is one reason women who begin to abort at home should bring to the hospital with them any clots or tissue they have passed. The presence of clear-fluid–filled cysts changes the diagnosis to gestational trophoblastic disease.

If bleeding is heavy with the discharge of the mole, a great deal of blood loss can occur. In addition, gestational trophoblastic disease can cause extreme psychological distress because the woman realizes she is not only not pregnant as she thought but that a "tumor-like" structure has been growing inside her.

Therapeutic Management

Therapy for gestational trophoblastic disease is suction curettage to evacuate the mole. Although HCG levels are usually negative within 1 week following a normal pregnancy, the level remains high following gestational trophoblastic disease. One-half of women will still have a positive reading at 3 weeks; one-fourth will still have a positive test result at 40 days.

Every woman who has had gestational trophoblastic disease should have a blood serum test for HCG every 2 to 4 weeks along with a chest x-ray until HCG levels are again normal, then every month for a full year. If the HCG titer is gradually declining, it suggests no complication is developing. If it plateaus for 3 times or increases in amount, it suggests malignant transformation has occurred. The woman should use a reliable contraceptive method during the year, so that a positive pregnancy test (the presence of HCG) resulting from a new pregnancy

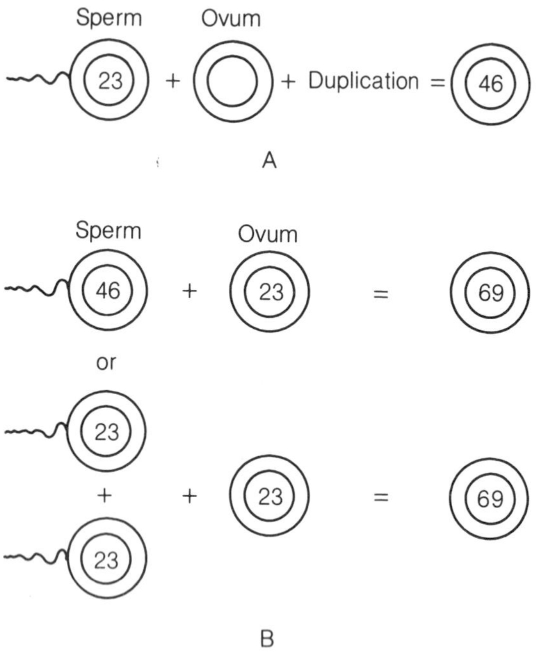

FIGURE 15-6
Formation of gestational trophoblastic disease. (**A**) *Complete mole.* (**B**) *Partial mole.*

will not be confused with developing malignancy. Some physicians give women who have had gestational trophoblastic disease a prophylactic course of methotrexate, the drug of choice for choriocarcinoma. Because the drug has side effects that interfere with blood formation (leukopenia), however, the wisdom of prophylaxis must be weighed carefully. If malignancy should occur, it can be treated effectively in most instances with methotrexate (Lewis, 1993).

After 1 year, if pregnancy test results are still negative, the woman is theoretically free of the risk of a malignancy developing; she could plan a second pregnancy at this time. Although the development of gestational trophoblastic disease means that a pregnancy never materialized, that a fetus never formed, the woman may experience the same feeling of loss following its evacuation that she would have experienced following the loss of a true pregnancy. She did, after all, believe that she was pregnant. On top of losing the pregnancy, she has the added anxiety of being aware that a malignancy may develop. She also must delay her childbearing plans for a full year. If she has already put off having a child for some time, the 1 year may seem the longest one of her life.

Women need the opportunity to express their anger and sense of unfairness at this type of event. They may feel inadequate because something went wrong with the pregnancy. They may wonder whether it will happen again, whether they will ever be able to have children. Unfortunately, women who have one incidence of gestational trophoblastic disease have a 4 to 5 times increased risk of a second molar pregnancy. They need early screening with ultrasound during a second pregnancy to be certain this is not happening again (Soper & Hammond, 1990).

Incompetent Cervix

An **incompetent cervix** is a cervix that dilates prematurely and therefore cannot hold a fetus until term. The dilation is usually painless. The first symptom is show (a pink-stained vaginal discharge), which is followed by rupture of the membranes and discharge of the amniotic fluid. Uterine contractions begin, and after a short labor the fetus is born, but unfortunately at approximately week 20 of pregnancy when the fetus is too immature to survive.

It is often difficult to explain in a particular instance what has caused incompetent cervix. It is associated with increased maternal age (Williams & Mittendorf, 1993). Congenital development factors or endocrine factors may be responsible. Trauma to the cervix such as might have occurred with a D & C or traumatic delivery is probably often the cause.

Therapeutic Management

Following the loss of one child due to an incompetent cervix, a surgical operation termed **cervical cerclage** can be performed to prevent this from happening again (Marks et al., 1992). As soon as it is confirmed by sonogram that the fetus is healthy, at approximately weeks 12 to 14 of a new pregnancy, under regional anesthesia, purse-string sutures are placed in the cervix by a vaginal route. This is called a McDonald or a Shirodkar procedure after the surgeons who perfected it. The sutures serve to strengthen the cervix and prevent it from dilating (Figure 15-7). With these procedures, the suture may be removed at weeks 38 to 39 of pregnancy so that the fetus may deliver vaginally, or sutures may be left in place and the woman delivered by cesarean birth.

It is important with these procedures that the suture be removed before vaginal birth is attempted or the cervix will be torn. Be certain to ask women who are reporting painless bleeding (the symptoms of spontaneous abortion also) whether they have had past cervical operations.

Still newer techniques allow the purse-string sutures to be set before the woman is pregnant. This gives her the added assurance that she will not begin aborting before week 14 of pregnancy. Women who are discovered to have cervical dilatation but with membranes still intact at a prenatal visit may have "emergent cerclage" sutures placed in the cervix even at this late point (Barth et al., 1990).

Women with an incompetent cervix were formerly included in the category of habitual aborters and told to accept their fate. Their cervix was thought simply not strong enough to support a pregnancy. Currently, women are followed by ultrasound examinations during pregnancy; the prognosis for a successful pregnancy is favorable (Carson, 1991). The success rate with both types of cerclage techniques is between 80% and 90%.

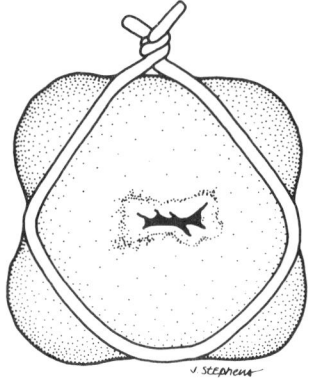

FIGURE 15-7
Cervical cerclage. (Courtesy of Childbirth Graphics, Rochester, NY.)

Conditions Associated With Third-Trimester Bleeding

Bleeding during late pregnancy occurs because of either placenta previa, premature separation of the placenta, or premature labor, all of which are serious conditions. Slight spotting late in pregnancy can be caused also by trauma from a pelvic examination or coitus, innocent findings.

Placenta Previa

Placenta previa (Figure 15-8) is low implantation of the placenta. It occurs in four degrees: (1) implantation in the lower rather than in the upper portion of the uterus (low-lying placenta); (2) marginal implantation (the placenta edge approaches that of the cervical os); (3) implantation that occludes a portion of the cervical os (partial placenta previa); and (4) implantation that totally obstructs the cervical os (total placenta previa) (Timor-Tritsch & Monteagudo, 1993). The degree to which the placenta covers the internal cervical os is generally estimated in percentages: 100%, 75%, 30%, and so forth.

Increased parity, the number of past cesarean births, the number of past uterine curettages, smoking, residence at high altitude, a male fetus, and multiple gestation are all associated with placenta previa (Lockwood, 1990). It is thought to occur whenever the placenta is forced to spread to find an adequate exchange surface. The incidence is approximately 3 to 6 per 1000 pregnancies. An increase in congenital anomalies in the fetus may occur if the low implantation does not allow for optimal fetal nutrition or oxygenation.

Assessment

Because routine sonograms are performed so frequently during pregnancy, many placenta previas are diagnosed today before any symptoms occur. In these instances, the condition is explained to the woman and she is cau-

tioned to avoid coitus, try and get adequate rest, and telephone her health care agency at any sign of vaginal bleeding. Bleeding with placenta previa occurs when the lower uterine segment begins to differentiate from the upper segment late in pregnancy (approximately week 30) and the cervix begins to dilate. The bleeding results from the placenta's inability to stretch to accommodate the differing shape of the lower uterine segment or the cervix. The bleeding that occurs is usually abrupt and painless and bright red; it is not associated with increased activity. It may stop as abruptly as it began, so that by the time the woman is seen at the hospital she is no longer bleeding, or it may slacken after the initial hemorrhage but continue as continuous spotting. The bleeding is usually acute and sudden enough to frighten the woman thoroughly. She telephones her physician or nurse-midwife, who instructs her to come to a hospital. She may arrive by ambulance. In any event, she is frightened for herself and for her baby.

Therapeutic Management

Immediate Care Measures. The bleeding of placenta previa, like that of ectopic pregnancy, is an emergency situation. The bleeding is from the uterine decidua (maternal blood), so the mother is in danger of hemorrhage. Because the placenta is loosened, the fetal oxygen supply may be compromised so the fetus may be in threat also. With the placenta loosening, premature labor may begin (another threat to the fetus). Once more it is difficult to evaluate how much blood has been lost or whether bleeding is still occurring, because the blood may pool at the base of the uterus above the placenta and not be apparent.

The woman requires immediate bed rest in a side-lying position. Assess the following: the time the bleeding began; the woman's estimation of the amount of blood—ask her to estimate in terms of cupfuls or tablespoonfuls (a cup is 240 mL; a tablespoon is 15 mL); whether there was accompanying pain; the color of the

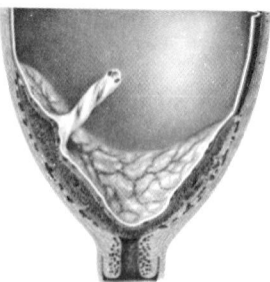

Total Placenta
Previa

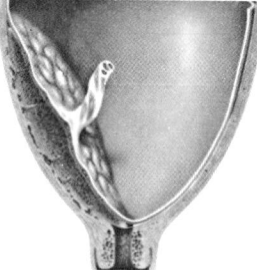

Partial Placenta
Previa

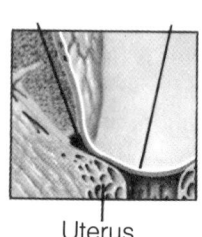

Uterus

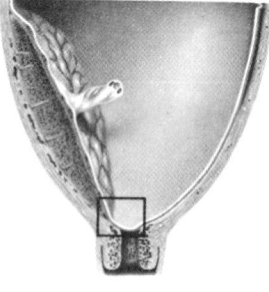

Low
Implantation

FIGURE 15-8

Degrees of placenta previa. (Used with permission of Ross Products Division, Abbott Laboratories, Columbus OH 43216 from Clinical Education Aid No. 12. © 1963 Ross Products Division, Abbott Laboratories.)

blood (the redder the blood, the fresher it is); what she has done for the bleeding (it is important to know that she did not insert a tampon to halt the bleeding, so that there may be hidden bleeding); whether there were prior episodes of bleeding during the pregnancy; and whether she had prior cervical surgery for an incompetent cervix. To help determine management, it is also important to know the duration of the pregnancy.

In the birthing room, check the woman's perineum for bleeding. Estimate the present rate of blood loss. Weighing perineal pads before and after use and subtracting the difference is a good method to determine vaginal blood loss. An Apt or Kleihauer-Betke test is used to detect whether blood is of fetal or maternal origin. *Never attempt a pelvic or rectal examination with painless bleeding late in pregnancy as any agitation of the cervix when there is a placenta previa may initiate massive hemorrhage, fatal to both mother and child.* Take vital signs to determine whether symptoms of shock are present and continue this assessment every 15 minutes. Measuring the specific gravity of urine is another way of assessing fluid volume adequacy. Attach an external fetal monitor and begin recording fetal heart sounds and uterine contractions. Obviously, an internal monitor that requires invasion of the cervix is completely contraindicated. Hemoglobin, hematocrit, prothrombin, partial thromboplastin, fibrinogen, platelet count, and type and cross-match should be assessed to establish baselines, detect a possible clotting disorder, and ready blood for replacement if necessary. Vaginal birth is always safest for an infant. Therefore, it is essential to locate the placenta as accurately as possible in the hope that its position will make vaginal birth feasible.

On abdominal examination, the fetal head may be discovered to be nonengaged because of the interfering placenta. However, this finding gives little indication of how much of the placenta is obscuring the os and thus preventing the head from engaging. A sonogram will be ordered to detect this.

The woman's physician may attempt careful speculum examination of the vagina and cervix to rule out a source of bleeding such as ruptured varices or cervical trauma and to establish the percentage of placenta covering the os. If this is under 30%, it may be possible for the fetus to be born past it. If over 30%, and the fetus is mature, the safest birth method for both mother and baby will be a cesarean delivery.

Vaginal examinations (actual investigation of dilation) to determine whether placenta previa exists are done in an operating room or a fully equipped birthing room so that if hemorrhage does occur with the manipulation, the woman may be immediately sectioned to remove the child and the bleeding placenta, contract the uterus, and save both the child and the woman.

Oxygen equipment should be available in case the fetal heart sounds indicate fetal distress (bradycardia or tachycardia; late deceleration or variable deceleration dips if the woman is in labor). An intravenous fluid line for emergency intravascular volume replacement should be begun.

Continuing Care Measures. Once a tentative diagnosis of placenta previa has been made, the age of the gestation will largely dictate the management. If labor has begun, or bleeding is continuing, or the fetus is being compromised (measured by the response of FHR to contractions) birth must be accomplished irrespective of gestation age. If the bleeding has stopped, the fetal heart sounds are of good quality, maternal vital signs are good, and the fetus is not yet 36 weeks of age, the woman is usually managed by expectant watching. As many as half of all women with bleeding from placenta previa will be managed this way.

The woman remains in the hospital on bed rest for close observation. Careful assessment of fetal heart sounds is carried out, and daily determination of hemoglobin or hematocrit is necessary for detection of hidden bleeding. The woman is administered betamethasone to encourage maturity of fetal lungs.

Nursing Diagnoses and Related Interventions

The medical diagnosis of placenta previa is an emergency situation. All goals should reflect the emergency condition and a short time frame for goal resolution.

Nursing Diagnosis: Fear related to outcome of pregnancy following episode of placenta previa bleeding

Goal: Client will be able to express her fears about the baby openly and continue to think about the baby in a positive manner.

Outcome Criteria: Client discusses concerns with nurse and other health care providers; states that hearing fetal heart beat helps to reassure her about baby's health.

It is difficult for the woman who has experienced bleeding late in a pregnancy to wait for the baby to come to term. She cannot stop wondering whether her infant is all right. She cannot help but wonder if the next bleeding she experiences may kill her, or her infant, or both. Listening to fetal heart sounds and being reassured that they are in a healthy range is helpful. She also needs to be able to talk to someone about her fears. If not, she may become so worried about the safety of her child that she begins to think of the baby as already dead. She might begin to neglect her diet or her supplementary vitamins because "it doesn't matter anymore." No matter what her outward appearance is at this time, she is bound to be under severe emotional stress.

Birth

As soon as the fetus reaches 37 weeks of age (2500 g), an amniocentesis analysis for lung maturity shows a positive result (a favorable L/S ratio), bleeding occurs again, labor begins, or the fetus shows symptoms of distress, the fetus will be delivered. The woman should be told during her weeks or days of waiting that birth will probably be cesarean because of the low implantation of the placenta. If the pregnancy is not yet at term, her baby will have a low birth weight.

On the chosen day of birth, a woman needs a great deal of support. It is one thing to talk about being ready for surgery; it is another to be truly ready. She may be as frightened as she was the evening her bleeding first began. If, at the time of the initial bleeding, the pregnancy is past 36 weeks, a birth decision will generally be made immediately. If the placenta previa is found to be total, delivery through the placenta is impossible, and the baby must be delivered by cesarean birth. If the placenta previa is partial, the amount of the blood loss, the condition of the fetus, and the woman's parity will influence the birth decision. When a cesarean birth is used in placenta previa, although the skin incision is still a transverse (bikini) one, because the uterine cut must be made high, it may be made longitudinally above the low implantation site of the placenta. If a sonogram clearly reveals the placental location, a transverse incision may be possible.

Following delivery, whether by vaginal or cesarean birth, the mother inspects her child carefully, looking for defects. If the placenta was implanted wrongly, she thinks, there might possibly be something wrong with her child as well. During the postpartal period, she needs long visiting periods with her child to make certain that he or she is all right.

Any woman who has had a placenta previa is more prone than normal to postpartal hemorrhage because the placental site is in the lower uterine segment, which does not contract as efficiently as the upper segment. Also, because the uterine blood supply is less in the lower segment, the placenta tends to grow larger than it would normally, leaving a larger denuded surface area when it is removed. As a second complication, the woman is more likely to develop endometritis, too, because the placental site is close to the cervix, the portal of entry for pathogens.

Premature Separation of the Placenta (Abruptio Placentae)

Unlike placenta previa, in **premature separation of the placenta** (also called **abruptio placentae**) (Figure 15-9), the placenta appears to have been implanted correctly. Suddenly, however, it begins to separate and bleeding results. By definition, this occurs after week 20 to 24 of pregnancy; separation occurring earlier would be considered a spontaneous abortion. Although this generally occurs late in pregnancy, it may occur as late as during the first or second stage of labor. Because premature separation of the placenta may occur during an otherwise normal labor, it is important always to be alert to the amount and kind of vaginal discharge a woman is having in labor. Listen to her description of the kind of pain she is having to detect this grave complication.

The primary cause of premature separation is unknown, but certain predisposing factors contribute to it: high parity, chronic hypertensive disease, hypertension of pregnancy, direct trauma as from an automobile accident, and vasoconstriction from cocaine use (Richardson et al., 1993). Pressure on the vena cava from the enlarging uterus may contribute to the problem because this puts tension on the uterus from back pressure.

Premature separation may follow a rapid decrease in uterine volume, as occurs with sudden release of am-

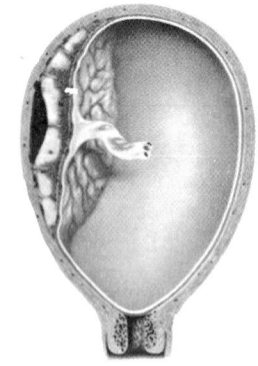

Partial Separation
(Concealed Hemorrhage)

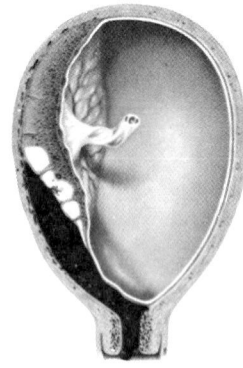

Partial Separation
(Apparent Hemorrhage)

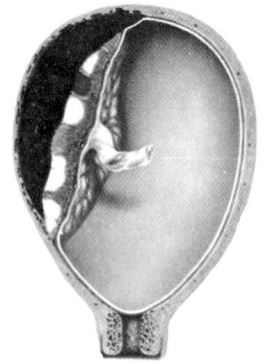

Complete Separation
(Concealed Hemorrhage)

FIGURE 15-9

Premature separation of the placenta. (Used with permission of Ross Products Division, Abbott Laboratories, Columbus OH 43216 from Clinical Education Aid No. 12. © 1963 Ross Products Division, Abbott Laboratories.)

niotic fluid. Because the fetal head is usually so low in the pelvis that it prevents loss of the total volume of the amniotic fluid at one time, a rapid reduction in amniotic fluid this way does not occur normally.

Assessment

A woman may experience a sharp stabbing pain high in the uterine fundus as the initial separation occurs. If labor begins with the separation, each contraction will be accompanied by pain over and above the pain of the contraction. In some women, the pain is not evident with contractions but tenderness is felt on uterine palpation.

Heavy bleeding usually accompanies premature separation of the placenta, although it may not be readily apparent. There will only be external bleeding if the placenta separates first at the edges and blood escapes freely from the cervix. If the center of the placenta separates first, however, blood will pool under the placenta and be hidden from view. Blood may infiltrate the uterine musculature (**couvelaire uterus** or utero-placental apoplexy), forming a hard, board-like uterus with no apparent, or minimally apparent, bleeding present. Signs of shock usually follow quickly because of the blood loss, and the uterus becomes tense and rigid to the touch.

If bleeding is extensive, the woman's reserve of blood fibrinogen may be used up in her body's attempt to accomplish effective clot formation, and disseminated intravascular coagulation (DIC) syndrome occurs (see below).

If the woman is being admitted to the hospital after experiencing symptoms at home, assess the time the bleeding began, whether pain accompanied it, the amount and kind of bleeding, and the woman's actions. Initial blood work should include not only hemoglobin level, typing, and cross matching but a fibrinogen level and fibrin breakdown products (FBP) test to detect the occurrence of DIC. For a quick assessment of blood clotting ability, draw 5 mL and place it in a clean, dry test tube. Stand it aside untouched for 5 minutes. At the end of this time, if a clot has not formed, an interference with blood coagulation can be suspected.

Therapeutic Management

On her admission to the hospital, the woman needs oxygen by mask to limit fetal anoxia. Fetal heart sounds should be monitored by an external monitor and maternal vital signs recorded to establish baselines and observe progress. The baseline fibrinogen determination is followed by additional determinations up to the time of delivery. Keep the woman in a lateral, not supine, position to prevent pressure on the vena cava and additional compromising of fetal circulation. It is important not to disturb the injured placenta any further; therefore, do not perform any vaginal or pelvic examination or give an enema to the woman with a diagnosed or suspected placental separation.

For better prediction of fetal and maternal outcome, the degrees of placental separation are graded, as shown in Table 15-5. Unless the separation is minimal (grades 0 and 1) the pregnancy must be terminated as the fetus cannot obtain adequate oxygen and nutrients. If the premature separation occurs during active labor, rupturing the membranes or assisting labor with intravenous oxytocin may be the method of choice to speed birth. Rupturing membranes keeps so much blood from being trapped in the myometrium of the uterus wall that the accumulating blood prevents contraction of the uterus. It may also help to prevent DIC by preventing pressure of placenta blood into the mother's venous circulation. Because membranes are ruptured with just a pinprick opening to allow a slow, steady escape of amniotic fluid, a sudden change in uterine pressure does not encourage more separation. If delivery does not seem imminent, cesarean birth is the delivery method of choice.

If the woman has developed DIC, surgery may be a grave risk for her because of the possibility that she will hemorrhage from the surgical incision. Her fibrinogen level must be elevated by the intravenous administration of fibrinogen or cryoprecipitate (which contains fibrinogen) or one of the other forms of therapy for DIC.

Fetal prognosis depends on the extent of the placental separation and the degree of fetal hypoxia. Maternal prognosis depends on how promptly treatment is instituted. Death can occur from massive hemorrhage leading to shock and circulatory collapse or renal failure from the circulatory collapse.

Any woman who has had bleeding before delivery is more prone to infection following delivery than the average woman. A woman with a history of premature separation of the placenta, therefore, needs to be ob-

---

Table 15-5. *Premature Separation of the Placenta: Degrees of Separation*

Grade	Criteria
0	No symptoms of separation were apparent from maternal or fetal signs; the diagnosis that a slight separation did occur is made after delivery when the placenta is examined and a segment of the placenta shows a recent adherent clot on the maternal surface.
1	This is minimal separation, but enough to cause vaginal bleeding and changes in the maternal vital signs; no fetal distress or hemorrhagic shock occurs, however.
2	This is moderate separation; there is evidence of fetal distress; the uterus is tense and painful on palpation.
3	This is extreme separation; without immediate interventions, maternal shock and fetal death will result.

served closely for the development of infection in the postpartal period.

Other Causes of Bleeding During Pregnancy

In addition to the major causes of bleeding during pregnancy already discussed, a few other causes exist.

Premature Labor

Premature labor can begin with vaginal spotting. This is discussed in Chapter 16 as it is an example of a pregnancy condition managed by home care.

Coexisting Disease

Cervical or vaginal polyps, vaginal varicosities, carcinoma of the cervix, or blood dyscrasias such as leukemia or decreased platelet levels may cause bleeding during any phase of pregnancy. These are not complications of pregnancy, however, but the reverse: pregnancy is a complication of the disease entity.

Cervical Ripening

Following a pelvic examination late in pregnancy, a woman may notice some slight vaginal spotting due to the manipulation of the cervix as **cervical ripening** (preparation for labor) is occurring. The bleeding should be slight and of short duration if this is the only cause.

Disseminated Intravascular Coagulation

DIC is an acquired disorder of blood clotting that results from excessive trauma or some similar underlying stimulus. Examples of situations associated with childbirth that may cause it are premature separation of the placenta, hypertension of pregnancy, amniotic fluid embolism, placental retention, septic abortion, retention of a dead fetus, and saline abortion. In a normal clotting sequence, platelets quickly form a seal over the point of bleeding to prevent further loss of blood. This plug is strengthened by fibrin threads into a firm, fixed structure. To prevent too much clotting from occurring, at the same time the clot is being formed, fibrinolysin, a proteolytic enzyme, begins to digest excess fibrin threads. This lysis results in the release of fibrin degradation products (FDPs). DIC occurs when there is extreme bleeding and so many platelets and fibrin from the general circulation are used that there are not enough left for clotting. This results in a paradox: at one point in the circulatory system, the person has increased coagulation; throughout the rest of the system, a bleeding defect exists. DIC is an emergency situation; goals must reflect the presence of the emergency (Harding & Keegan, 1992).

Therapeutic Management

To stop the process of DIC, the underlying insult that began the phenomenon must be halted. When the insult was a complication of pregnancy, ending the pregnancy by delivering the fetus and placenta is part of the answer. Next, the marked coagulation must be stopped so that coagulation factors are available elsewhere in the bloodstream. This is accomplished by the intravenous administration of heparin. Heparin must be given with caution close to delivery or postpartal hemorrhage can occur following delivery of the placenta. Although blood transfusion will be necessary to replace blood loss if bleeding during pregnancy is the beginning stimulus, blood administration may be delayed until after heparin has been administered so that the new blood factors are not also consumed by the coagulation process. Fresh frozen plasma, fibrinogen, or cryoprecipitate (which contains fibrinogen) may all be administered. If neither fibrinogen nor cryoprecipitate (cryoprecipitate is the blood product administered to persons with hemophilia and therefore may be unavailable in hospitals that do not routinely treat a large number of persons with hemophilia) is at hand, then fresh frozen plasma or platelets will aid in restoring clotting function.

It is bewildering to a patient with a disorder such as premature separation of the placenta to have the physician tell her one minute that bleeding is what he or she is worried about and the next minute hear heparin ordered (or watch a nurse add heparin to her intravenous line). If the woman understands the action of heparin—to discourage blood coagulation—it seems as if the physician has ordered exactly the wrong medication (or the nurse is adding exactly the wrong one). Be certain that the woman and her support person have a full explanation of what is happening—the woman has an increased risk of hemorrhaging because part of her system has tied up coagulation factors; by releasing them, you can aid coagulation throughout the rest of her body—so that confidence in her caregivers is maintained.

Evaluation is aimed at determining whether the woman's blood coagulation studies are returning to normal and if any destruction has occurred, particularly in renal or brain cells from occluded coagulated capillaries. Obviously, fetal assessment and, following birth, newborn assessment is important to determine that placental circulation remained sufficient. Because heparin does not cross the placenta, the infant does not need assessment for blood coagulation ability at birth.

Pregnancy-Induced Hypertension

Pregnancy-induced hypertension (PIH) is a condition unique to pregnancy that occurs in 5% to 10% of pregnancies in the United States. Despite years of research, the cause of the disorder is still unknown. Originally it was called *toxemia* because researchers pictured a toxin of some kind being released by the woman in response to the foreign protein of the growing fetus, the toxin leading to typical symptoms of hypertension, proteinuria, and edema. Although this may be so, no toxin has ever been identified (Khong et al., 1992).

Pregnancy-induced hypertension tends to occur more frequently in primiparas younger than age 20 years or older than 40 years; women from a low socioeconomic background (perhaps because of poor nutrition); women who have had five or more pregnancies; women of color; women with multiple pregnancy; women with hydramnios; and women with underlying disease such as heart disease, diabetes with vessel or renal involvement, and essential hypertension. The condition may be associated with poor calcium or magnesium intake.

Causes

PIH is a systemic disorder with effects to almost all organs. A basic cause of the three symptoms that mark the disorder (hypertension, proteinuria, and edema) is peripheral vascular spasm, but why this vascular spasm occurs is difficult to establish. It may be caused by the action of prostaglandins (notably decreased prostacyclin and increased thromboxane) (Gilstrap & Gant, 1990). Increased cardiac output may cause injury to endothelial cells of the arteries, leading to spasm. Normally, blood vessels during pregnancy are resistant to the effects of pressor substances such as angiotension and norepinephrine so blood pressure remains normal during pregnancy. With hypertension of pregnancy, this reduced responsiveness to blood pressure changes appears to be lost, vasoconstriction occurs, and blood pressure increases dramatically.

The cardiac system is strained as the heart is forced to pump against rising peripheral resistance. This reduces the blood supply to organs. This effect is most marked in the kidney, pancreas, liver, brain, and placenta. Tissue hypoxia may follow in the maternal vital organs; poor placental perfusion may reduce the fetal nutrient and oxygen supply. Ischemia in the pancreas may result in epigastric pain and an elevated amylase/creatinine ratio. Spasm of the arteries in the retina leads to vision changes; if hemorrhages occur in the retina, blindness can result.

Vasospasm in the kidney increases blood flow resistance. Degenerative changes develop in kidney glomeruli because of the back pressure; this leads to increased permeability of the glomerular membrane allowing the serum proteins albumin and globulin to escape into the urine (proteinuria). The degenerative changes also result in decreased glomerular filtration so there is lowered urine output and clearance of creatinine. Increased tubular reabsorption of sodium occurs; as sodium retains fluid, edema results. Edema is further increased because as more protein is lost, the osmotic pressure of the

circulating blood falls, and fluid diffuses from the circulatory system into the denser interstitial spaces to equalize the pressure (edema) (Figures 15-10 and 15-11). Extreme edema can lead to brain edema and convulsions (eclampsia).

The arterial spasm causes the bulk of the blood volume in the maternal circulation to be pooled in the venous circulation so the woman has a deceptively low arterial intravascular volume. Additionally, thrombocytopenia or a lowered platelet count occurs as platelets cluster at the sites of endothelial damage. Measuring hematocrit levels helps to assess the extent of plasma loss to interstitial space or the extent of the edema (the higher the hematocrit, the more is being lost). An HCT above 40% suggests significant fluid loss.

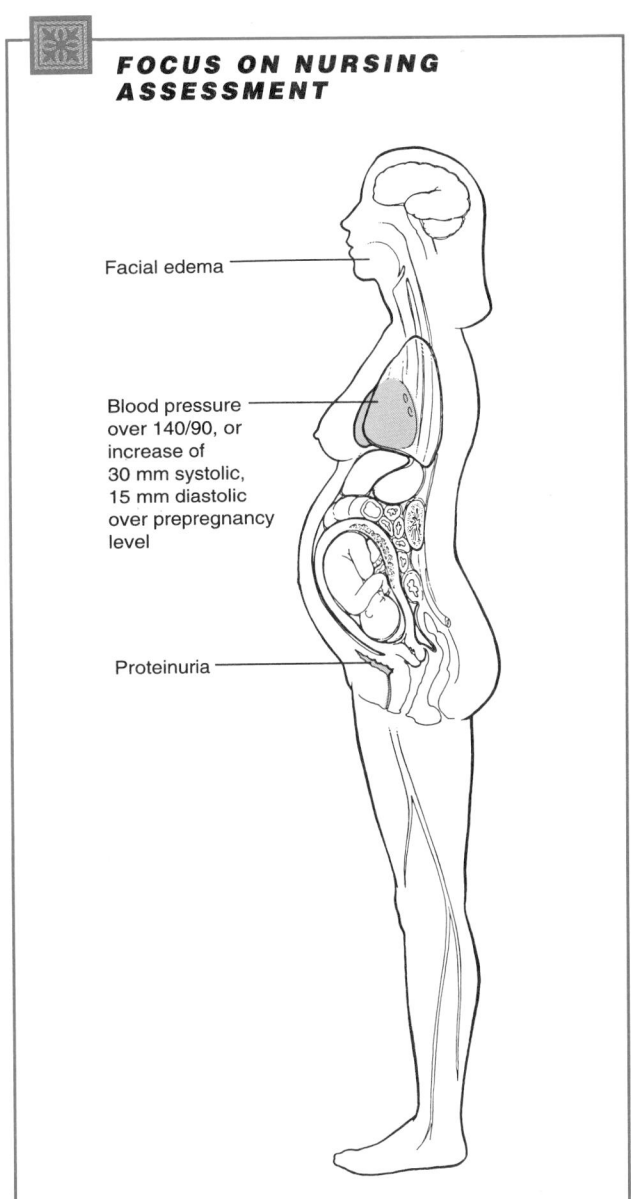

FOCUS ON NURSING ASSESSMENT

Facial edema

Blood pressure over 140/90, or increase of 30 mm systolic, 15 mm diastolic over prepregnancy level

Proteinuria

FIGURE 15-10
Major manifestations of hypertension of pregnancy.

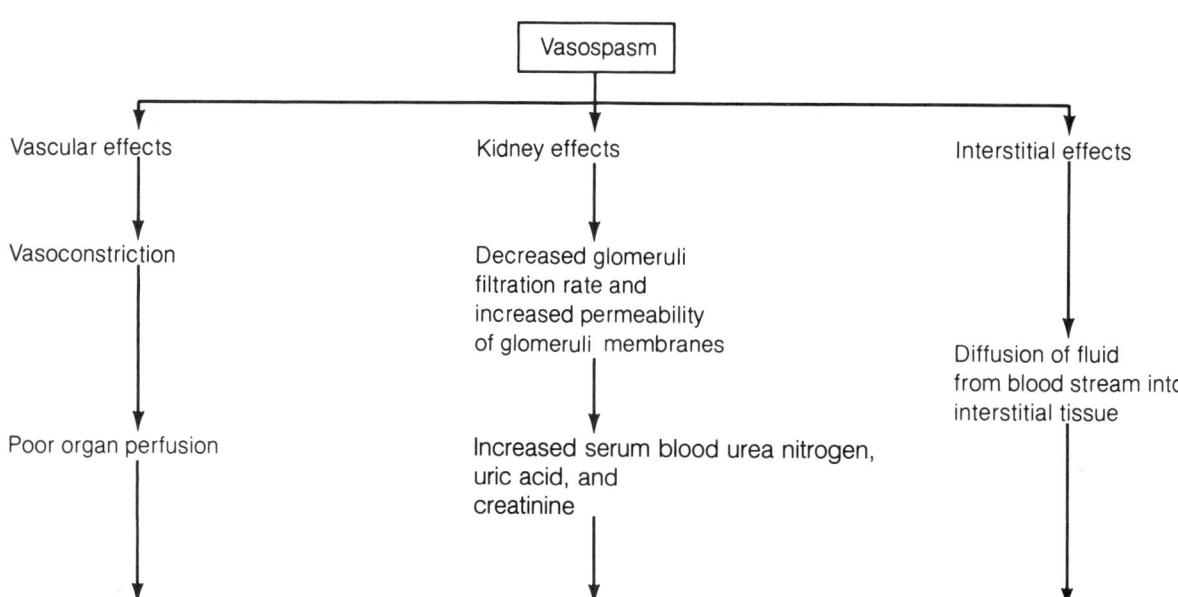

FIGURE 15-11
Physiologic changes with pregnancy-induced hypertension.

Assessment

Symptoms of the levels of pregnancy-induced hypertension are summarized in Table 15-6. Any woman who falls into one of the high-risk categories for pregnancy-induced hypertension should be observed especially carefully for symptoms at prenatal visits. She must know the symptoms herself to watch for so that she can call and alert prenatal personnel if additional symptoms occur between visits. Symptoms rarely occur before 20 weeks of pregnancy.

Gestational Hypertension. A woman is said to have gestational hypertension when she develops an elevated blood pressure but has no proteinuria. Perinatal mortality is not increased with simple gestational hypertension. Chronic hypertension may develop in these women later in life, however.

Mild Preeclampsia. If a convulsion from hypertension of pregnancy occurs, the woman has **eclampsia**. Any status before this point is **preeclampsia**. A woman is said to be mildly preeclamptic when her blood pressure rises 30 mm Hg or more systolic or 15 mm Hg or more diastolic above her prepregnancy level, taken on two occasions at least 6 hours apart. The diastolic value of blood pressure is extremely important to note because it is this pressure that best indicates the degree of peripheral arterial spasm present.

At one time if a woman developed a blood pressure of 140/90 or over, she was considered to have preeclampsia. This general rule is obviously less meaningful than the comparison of an individual woman's blood pressure against her early pregnancy baseline. This value is still a useful "cutoff" point, however, and should be used when there are no baseline data available, such as when a woman seeks prenatal care late in pregnancy.

Average blood pressures in American females are shown in Appendix G. An examination of the average pressure for young Caucasian women reveals that a

Table 15-6. *Symptoms of Pregnancy-Induced Hypertension*

Hypertension Type	Symptom
Gestational hypertension	Blood pressure 140/90 or systolic pressure elevated 30 mm Hg or diastolic pressure elevated 15 mm Hg above prepregnancy level; no proteinuria
Mild preeclampsia	Blood pressure 140/90 or systolic pressure elevated 30 mm Hg or diastolic pressure elevated 15 mm Hg above prepregnancy level; proteinuria of 1–2+ on a random sample; weight gain over 2 lb per wk in second trimester and 1 lb per wk, third trimester; mild edema in upper extremities or face
Severe preeclampsia	Blood pressure of 160/110 mm Hg; proteinuria 3–4+ on a random sample and 5 g on a 24-hour sample; oliguria (500 mL or under in 24 h); cerebral or visual disturbances (headache, blurred vision); pulmonary edema; extensive peripheral edema; hepatic dysfunction; thrombocytopenia; epigastric pain
Eclampsia	A tonic-clonic convulsion occurs

woman in the younger-than-age-20-years category could have a blood pressure of 98/61 and still be within normal limits. If her blood pressure were elevated 30 mm Hg systolic and 15 mm Hg diastolic, it would be only 128/76. This is well beneath the traditional warning point of 140/90 yet would be hypertension for her.

With mild preeclampsia, in addition to the hypertension, the woman has proteinuria (1+ or 2+ on a reagent test strip on a random sample). Many women show a trace of protein during pregnancy. Actual proteinuria is said to exist when it registers as at least 1+ or more (this represents a loss of 1 g/L).

Occasionally, women have orthostatic proteinuria (on long periods of standing, they excrete protein; at bed rest they do not). If a woman has no other signs of hypertension of pregnancy (no hypertension and no edema) and the urine she offers for testing is not her first morning one but one she has voided in the health care facility, asking her to bring in a first morning urine may reveal that this is the problem, not preeclampsia.

Edema will also be present. This develops, as mentioned, because of the protein loss, sodium retention, and a lowered glomerular filtration rate. Edema begins to accumulate in the upper part of the body, rather than just the normal ankle edema of pregnancy. A gain in weight of more than 2 lb/wk in the second trimester or 1 lb/wk in the third trimester usually indicates abnormal tissue fluid retention. This is likely to be the first symptom to appear and is discovered when the woman is weighed at a prenatal visit. Noticeable edema may or may not be present when this sudden increase in weight first occurs.

Severe Preeclampsia. A woman has passed from mild to severe preeclampsia when her blood pressure has risen to 160 mm Hg systolic and 110 mm Hg diastolic or above on at least two occasions 6 hours apart at bed rest (the position in which blood pressure is lowest) or her diastolic pressure is 30 mm Hg above prepregnancy level. Marked proteinuria and extensive edema are also present. Marked proteinuria is a reading of 3+ or 4+ on a random urine sample or more than 5 g in a 24-hour sample.

With severe preeclampsia, the extreme edema will be noticeable in the woman's face and hands as "puffiness." It is most readily palpated over bony surfaces, where the sponginess of fluid-filled tissue can be palpated best. Palpating or pressing over the tibia on the anterior leg, the ulnar surface of the forearm, and the cheekbones is a good way to detect edema. Edema is nonpitting if there is swelling or puffiness at these points to a palpating finger but the swelling cannot be indented with finger pressure. If the tissue can be indented slightly, this is 1+ edema; moderate indentation is 2+; deep indentation is 3+; and indentation so deep it remains as a pit after removal of the finger is 4+ pitting edema. Further assess edema by asking the woman if she

has been aware of any. Most women at the end of pregnancy have edema of the feet at the end of the day. They report this as difficulty fitting into their bedroom slippers or kicking off their shoes at dinnertime and then not being able to put them back on again. This is normal edema. Edema that has progressed to upper extremities or the face is abnormal. Women report upper-extremity edema as "rings are so tight that I can't get them off" and facial edema as "when I wake in the morning, my eyes are swollen shut," or "I'm unable to talk until I walk around awhile."

Some women have severe epigastric pain and nausea and vomiting possibly due to abdominal edema or ischemia to the pancreas and liver. Pulmonary edema may cause them to feel short of breath. Cerebral edema will cause visual disturbances such as blurred vision or seeing spots before their eyes. Cerebral edema also produces symptoms of severe headache and marked hyperreflexia and perhaps muscle clonus. This accumulating edema will reduce their urine output to approximately 400 to 600 mL per 24 hours.

Eclampsia. This is the most severe classification of hypertension of pregnancy. A woman has passed into this third stage when cerebral edema is so acute that a convulsion occurs. With eclampsia, maternal mortality is as high as 15%.

Eclampsia can result in death of the mother from cerebral hemorrhage, circulatory collapse, or renal failure. Fetal prognosis in eclampsia is poor because of hypoxia and consequent fetal acidosis. If premature separation of the placenta from vasospasm occurs, the prognosis is even graver. If the fetus must be delivered before term, all the risks of the immature infant will be faced. In preeclampsia, fetal mortality is approximately 10%. If eclampsia develops, the mortality increases to as high as 25%.

Nursing Diagnoses and Related Interventions

The nursing diagnoses used with hypertension of pregnancy are numerous because the disease has such wide-ranging effects.

- Altered tissue perfusion related to vasoconstriction of blood vessels
- Fluid volume deficit related to fluid loss to subcutaneous tissue
- High risk for fetal injury related to reduced placental perfusion secondary to vasospasm
- Social isolation related to prescribed bed rest

Nursing Diagnosis: High risk for altered tissue perfusion related to arterial vasospasm

Goal: Client will not experience reduced tissue perfusion during pregnancy.

Outcome Criteria: FHR is 120–160 bpm; maternal blood pressure is below 140/90 mm Hg; maternal urine output is above 30 mL/hr.

Nursing Interventions for the Woman With Mild Hypertension of Pregnancy

Promote Bed Rest. When the human body is in a recumbent position, sodium tends to be excreted at a more rapid rate than during activity. Bed rest, therefore, is the best method of aiding increased evacuation of sodium and encouraging diuresis.

Rest should always be in a left lateral recumbent position to avoid uterine pressure on the vena cava and prevent supine hypotension syndrome. If the woman is able to rest at home, she can remain at home. If there is a question as to her compliance, she may be hospitalized even at this early date. Water immersion may possibly reduce blood pressure (Katz et al., 1990). The woman may have baths, with water up to her chin, prescribed twice a day for this therapeutic effect.

Promote Good Nutrition. Because the woman is losing protein in the urine, she needs a high-protein diet. At one time stringent restriction of salt was advised to reduce edema. This is no longer true as stringent sodium restriction may activate the angiotensin system and result in increased blood pressure, compounding the problem.

Provide Emotional Support. It is difficult for a woman to appreciate the potential seriousness of symptoms at this point because they are still so vague. Neither high blood pressure nor protein in urine are things that she can see or feel. She is aware that edema is present, but it seems unrelated to the pregnancy; it is her hands that are swollen, not a body area near her growing child. Many women, therefore, take instructions such as getting rest at this time rather lightly.

Women are also used to having severe disorders treated with some form of medication, and their physician has given them none here. How can this be really serious? In addition, it is not always easy to comply with an instruction such as get additional rest during the day. Of women of childbearing age, 90% work outside their home. Approximately half the women with pregnancy-induced hypertension, therefore, are being asked to stop work to rest more. The contribution of most working women today goes not for luxuries but for a good part of the mortgage or rent or car payments. If a woman is not married, her income is probably her sole support. Thus, asking her to stop work on the basis of a few vague symptoms—a little swelling or a little headache—when she may be evicted or have a car or house loan foreclosed on because of missed payments is asking a great deal.

Health care providers cannot solve all of people's financial problems, but be certain to ask enough questions at health care visits so that a problem of financial need can be documented. A question such as "What will it mean to your family if you have to quit work?" brings concerns out into the open.

People can make arrangements with loan companies or banks to make partial payments or delayed payments during periods of hardship. The couple may have savings they were planning to use for the baby that can carry them over during this time (and is still being used for the baby). Perhaps they can borrow money or change their living arrangements.

A woman with children must usually make changes to get additional rest. The mother who spends considerable time chauffeuring school-age children to activities may have to investigate car pooling as an alternative. A mother may have to drop being a volunteer leader or ask her family for more help in cleaning or cooking. Ask "What will it mean to your other children or your husband if you have to rest?" to allow her to face this problem.

Women with beginning signs of hypertension will be seen approximately every 2 weeks for the remainder of pregnancy. Be certain the woman understands that if symptoms worsen before 2 weeks she should not wait for the scheduled visit but call for an earlier appointment. There is little cure for eclampsia of pregnancy. Prevention at the early stage is what is important.

Nursing Interventions for the Woman With Severe Hypertension of Pregnancy

If the preeclampsia is severe (i.e., systolic blood pressure of more than 160 mm Hg, diastolic blood pressure of more than 110 mm Hg, or both on two occasions 6 hours apart after the woman has been on bed rest; extensive edema; marked proteinuria—3+ to 4+; cerebral or visual disturbances; marked hyperreflexia; or oliguria—500 mL per 24 hours or less), hospitalization is strongly recommended. If the pregnancy is 36 weeks or more in length, or fetal maturity can be confirmed by amniocentesis, induction of labor may be undertaken. If the pregnancy is less than 36 weeks, or the amniocentesis reveals immature lung function, interventions will be instituted to attempt to alleviate the symptoms and allow the fetus to come to term (see the Nursing Care Plan).

Support Bed Rest. With hospitalization, bed rest can be enforced, and the woman can be observed closely. The woman with severe preeclampsia should be admitted to a private room so she can rest undisturbed by a roommate. She should lie in a left lateral recumbent position as much as possible. She should be away from the sound of women in labor or the crying of infants on a postpartal unit. A loud noise such as a crying baby or a dropped tray of equipment may be sufficient to trigger a convulsion, initiating eclampsia.

The room should be darkened; a bright light can also trigger convulsions. However, the room should not be so dark that caregivers need to use a flashlight to make assessments. Having to shine a flashlight beam into the woman's eyes is the kind of stimulus to avoid. Visitors are usually restricted to support people (e.g., husband, father of the child, mother, or older children).

Monitor Maternal Well Being. The woman's blood pressure should be taken at least every 4 hours to detect any increase, which is a warning that her condition is worsening. If blood pressure is fluctuating, it may need to be assessed hourly. Blood studies (i.e., complete blood count, platelet count, liver function, blood urea nitrogen, and creatine and fibrin degradation products) may be taken daily to assess for renal and liver function and the development of DIC which often accompanies severe vasospasm. She may have a type and cross match for blood drawn because she is high risk for premature separation of the placenta and resulting hemorrhage.

A daily hematocrit level is determined to monitor blood concentration (the level will rise if increased fluid is leaving the blood stream for interstitial tissue). Plasma estriol and electrolyte levels will also be measured frequently. The woman's optic fundus is assessed daily for signs of arterial spasm, edema, or hemorrhage.

A urinary catheter is usually inserted to allow accurate recording of output and comparison with intake. Urinary output should be more than 600 mL per 24 hours (more than 30 mL/h); an output lower than this means that oliguria is present. Urinary proteins and specific gravity should be measured and recorded with voidings or hourly by catheter. Urine should be saved for 24-hour protein and creatinine clearance determinations to evaluate kidney function. A woman with mild preeclampsia spills between 0.5 g to 1 g of protein every 24 hours (1+ on a random sample); a woman with severe preeclampsia spills approximately 5 g per 24 hours (3+ to 4+ on an individual specimen).

Weight should be measured daily at the same time each day for evaluation of tissue fluid retention. Ask the woman to bring a light duster or bathrobe to the hospital with her to wear at every weighing, so that any change in weight does not merely reflect a change in the weight of her clothing.

Monitor Fetal Well Being. FHR may be assessed by continuous fetal external monitor, but generally single Doppler auscultation at approximately 4-hour intervals is sufficient at this stage of management. The woman may have a nonstress test or biophysical profile done daily to assess placental uterine sufficiency (see Chapter 9). Oxygen administration to the mother may be necessary to maintain adequate fetal oxygenation and prevent bradycardia.

Provide a Safe Environment. The siderails on the woman's bed should be raised to keep her from falling should she have a convulsion. She needs to be told that the side rails have been raised not to imprison her but for her safety and the safety of her unborn child. With this explanation, a side rail rule is not difficult to enforce, and protection is provided when no nurse is present.

Support High-Protein Diet. The woman needs a high-protein, moderate-sodium diet to compensate for the protein she is losing in the urine.

Administer Medications to Prevent Eclampsia. A fluid line to serve as an emergency route for drug administration and to reduce hemoconcentration and hypovolemia should be initiated and maintained. It is important that the insertion site be observed carefully for infiltration because if the woman is heavily sedated she may be unaware that the site is swelling and irritation from an infiltrated intravenous site is the sort of irritation that can trigger a convulsion in a severely preeclamptic woman.

A hypotensive drug such as hydralazine (Apresoline) may be prescribed to reduce the hypertension. Hydralazine acts to lower blood pressure by peripheral dilatation and thus causes no interference with placental circulation. Hydralazine may cause tachycardia; thus, not only blood pressure but pulse as well should be assessed following its administration. Diazoxide (Hyperstat) may be used for its ability to produce a rapid decrease in blood pressure. If vasopressors of this nature are used, diastolic pressure should not be lowered below 80 to 90 mm Hg or inadequate placental perfusion may occur. A low dosage of aspirin of 60 mg 4 times a day may be prescribed (Walsh, 1990). This acts to decrease prostaglandins, which results in vasodilation. Other drugs which may reduce the development of symptoms are calcium and magnesium.

Despite these new drugs suggested for the treatment of hypertension of pregnancy, magnesium sulfate is still the drug of choice once symptoms are present (Box 15-1). The drug is classified as a cathartic. It is able to reduce edema by causing a shift in fluid from the extracellular spaces into the intestine. It also has a CNS depressant action (it blocks peripheral neuromuscular transmissions) that lessens the possibility of convulsions.

To achieve immediate reduction of the blood pressure, magnesium sulfate is first given intravenously in a loading or bolus dose (4 g in 100 mL of 5% dextrose in water). Given intravenously over 15 to 20 minutes, the drug begins to act almost immediately but the effect lasts only 30 to 60 minutes.

Following the initial reduction of blood pressure, magnesium sulfate is then continued by slow intravenous infusion (1 to 2 g/h). This is usually mixed as

(text continues on page 408)

Hannah Rawling is a 28-year-old G3P2 woman admitted to the obstetrics unit for severe preeclampsia. She is 27 weeks pregnant.

Health History: Obese-appearing pregnant black woman, height: 5′5″; prepregnant weight: 172 (BMI = 29); present weight: 192 lbs (gained 3 lbs in last week); BP: 146/92 mm Hg. Edema present around eyes. Client states, "My legs are so swollen I can't wear no shoes." First noticed swelling in legs shortly after last prenatal visit 2 weeks ago. Swelling has grown worse every day. Is unable to wear wedding ring because of swelling in hands. Has headache "all the time," which she thinks is "sinusitis" (the reason she agreed to hospitalization). Two episodes of blurriness of vision; no diplopia. Experienced no increased blood pressure with previous pregnancies. Has attended prenatal care with this pregnancy since 4th month of pregnancy. Had sonogram at 4 months; no intrauterine growth retardation noted.

Client is not married; works behind counter at fast food store. Boyfriend is student in community college. Concerned because she has no one to watch children while boyfriend is in school. Has no hospital insurance; finances are "a disaster." Lives in a two-room apartment; has "left-over" clothes for baby but nothing new because of finances.

Laboratory Results: Urine positive for protein (3+) and ketones by dipstick. S.G. = 1.020. Hemoglobin: 10.6 mg/dL; hematocrit: 33%.

Nursing Diagnosis: Anxiety regarding hospitalization related to family responsibilities.

Defining Characteristic: Client states she is anxious over hospitalization because of lack of child care.

Goal: Client will demonstrate acceptance of hospitalization by 4 h.

Outcome Criteria: Client complies with bedrest and therapy for hypertension of pregnancy.

Nursing Orders	*Rationale*
1. Encourage client to voice feelings about difficulties with hospitalization.	1. Expressing concerns could be the beginning of problem solving.
2. Encourage boyfriend to visit for emotional support.	2. Emotional support can reduce stress.
3. Help client plan ways to adjust to hospitalization so she can maintain bedrest.	3. Bedrest is helpful in alleviating symptoms of PIH; stress over hospitalization can interfere with bedrest.

Nursing Diagnosis: High risk for fluid volume deficit related to loss of fluid into interstitial space.

Defining Characteristic: Edema is present in both upper and lower extremities and face.

Goal: Client will not experience continued increase in edema during remainder of pregnancy.

Outcome Criteria: Edema remains at 2+ in face and hands; proteinuria is not above 2+; urine output is over 30 mL/h.

(continued)

Nursing Orders	***Rationale***
1. Admit to room 204.	1. A quiet, dark, private room is best to help prevent eclampsia.
2. Enforce total bedrest in left side-lying position.	2. A left lying position helps increase kidney glomerular function and urine output.
3. Restrict visitors to boyfriend.	3. Rest is essential to care.
4. No radio, alarm clock, or telephone in room. Do not use intercom in room.	4. Loud noises can cause convulsions in the preeclamptic woman.
5. Insert indwelling urinary catheter to gravity drainage.	5. Provide an effective means of measuring urinary output.
6. Measure intake and output; assess urine sample every 4 h for protein. Save total for daily 24 h urine for protein and creatinine clearance, report output less than 30 mL/h.	6. Kidney failure is evidenced by increased protein-uria, a decreased creatinine clearance value, and decreased urine output.
7. Begin intravenous therapy of Ringer's lactate at 120 mL/h per physician's order.	7. Magnesium sulfate therapy will need a solution for "piggyback" infusion.
8. Loading dose of magnesium sulfate (4 g) to be administered intravenously followed by maintenance dose of 2 g/h.	8. Magnesium sulfate therapy acts to reduce the possibility of seizures.
9. Assess patellar reflex (2+ or better); urine output (more than 30 mL/hour); and respiration (more than 12/min) every hour.	9. A weak patellar reflex, urine output below 30 mL/hr, and respiratory rate below 12/min indicates unsafe serum levels of magnesium sulfate which could lead to respiratory failure.
10. Hematocrit daily; weight daily. Maintain intake and output.	10. An increasing hematocrit level indicates hemoconcentration is occurring or fluid is leaving the blood stream. An increasing weight and intake and output contrast can reveal fluid retention.

Nursing Diagnosis: High risk for fetal injury related to poor placental perfusion secondary to hypertension.

Defining Characteristic: Increased BP (146/92) indicates peripheral vascular resistance is increased.

Goal: Fetus will continue to demonstrate well being for remainder of pregnancy.

Outcome Criteria: Nonstress test is reactive; FHR is between 120 and 160 bpm with good variability.

Nursing Orders	***Rationale***
1. Monitor with nonstress test daily using external uterine and fetal monitors.	1. A nonstress test is a good indicator of fetal well being, especially if used as part of a complete biophysical fetal profile; external monitors are necessary as membranes are not ruptured and cervix is not dilated.
2. Assess fetal heart rate every 4 h; report tachycardia or bradycardia.	2. Increased or decreased heart rate are signs of poor placental perfusion.
3. Remind client to maintain a side lying position.	3. A side lying position improves placental perfusion because it takes pressure off the vena cava.

Box 15-1

Drugs Used in Pregnancy-Induced Hypertension

Drug	Indication	Dosage	Comments
Magnesium sulfate Pregnancy Risk Category B	Muscle relaxant; prevents seizures	Loading dose 4–6 g Maintenance dose 1–2 g/h IV	Loading dose is infused slowly over 15–30 min. Always administer as a "piggyback" infusion. Assess respiratory rate, urine output, deep tendon reflexes, and clonus q hour. Urine output should be over 30 mL/h and respiratory rate over 12/min. Serum magnesium level should remain below 7.5 mEq/L. Observe for depression and hypotonia in infant at birth.
Hydralazine (Apresoline) Pregnancy Risk Category C	Antihypertensive (peripheral vasodilator); used for increasing hypertension	5–10 mg/IV	Administer slowly to avoid sudden fall in BP. Maintain diastolic pressure over 90 mm Hg to ensure adequate placental filling.
Diazoxide (Hyperstat) Pregnancy Risk Category C	Peripheral vasodilator; used for severe hypertension	1–3 mg/kg	Assess BP every 1–2 min until stable then q 15–30 min as precipitous drop may occur. Maintain diastolic pressure over 90 mm Hg to ensure adequate placental filling.
Diazepam (Valium) Pregnancy Risk Category D	Halt seizures	5–10 mg/IV	Administer slowly. Dose may be repeated q 5–10 min (up to 30 mg/hour). Observe for depression or hypotension in mother; depression and hypotonia in infant at birth.
Calcium gluconate Pregnancy Risk Category C	Antidote for magnesium intoxication	1 gm/IV (10 mL of a 10% solution)	Have prepared at bedside when administering magnesium sulfate. Administer at 5 mL/min.

Loeb, S. (1993). *Nurse's handbook of drug therapy.* Springhouse, PA: Springhouse.

40 g MgSO₄ in 1000 mL lactated Ringer's solution to yield 2 g MgSO₄ per 50 mL. The drug should be given "piggybacked" to a main infusion line so it can be discontinued immediately without interfering with the main intravenous line; it should be administered with an automatic pump to ensure safe and controlled administration (Mandeville & Troiano, 1992).

For magnesium sulfate to act as an anticonvulsant, blood serum levels are maintained at 4 to 7 mg/100 mL. If a blood serum level above this occurs, respiratory depression, cardiac arrhythmias, and cardiac arrest can occur. These serum levels are shown in Table 15-7.

The most evident symptoms of overdose from magnesium sulfate administration are decreased urine output, depression of respirations, reduced consciousness, and decreased deep tendon reflexes. It is important that urine output remains adequate because magnesium is excreted from the body almost entirely through the urine. If severe oliguria should occur (less than 100 mL in 4 hours), excessively high serum levels of magnesium can result. Before further magnesium sulfate is administered, urine output should be above 25 to 30 mL/h (specific gravity 1.010 or lower). Respirations should be above 12 per minute, the woman should be able to answer questions asked of her, ankle clonus should be minimal, and deep tendon reflexes should be present. These assessments should be made every hour if a continuous intravenous infusion is being used (Figure 15-12).

The easiest deep tendon reflex to assess is the patellar reflex (knee jerk). Instructions for initiating this reflex and ankle clonus are shown in Box 15-2. If an epidural block has been given for labor anesthesia, assess a biceps or triceps reflex (see Chapter 28).

In addition to making the above assessments when magnesium sulfate is being given, a solution of 10 mL of a 10% calcium gluconate solution (1 g) should be kept ready nearby for immediate intravenous administration. Calcium is the specific antidote for magnesium toxicity. Severe oliguria may be treated by intravenous infusion of salt-poor abdomen. This high colloid solution will "call" fluid into the intravascular space by osmotic pressure; the kidneys will then excrete the extra fluid along with magnesium sulfate levels.

On the day of birth, the anesthesiologist must be alerted to the fact that the woman has been receiving magnesium sulfate. If magnesium sulfate is given intravenously within 2 hours of delivery, the baby may be born depressed because the drug crosses the placenta. A fetus may show loss of variability of heartbeat immediately following magnesium therapy, and sonogram may reveal reduced fetal breathing movements. Observe carefully for other signs of fetal effects such as late deceleration with labor contractions. Magnesium sulfate is continued for 12 to 24 hours following birth to prevent

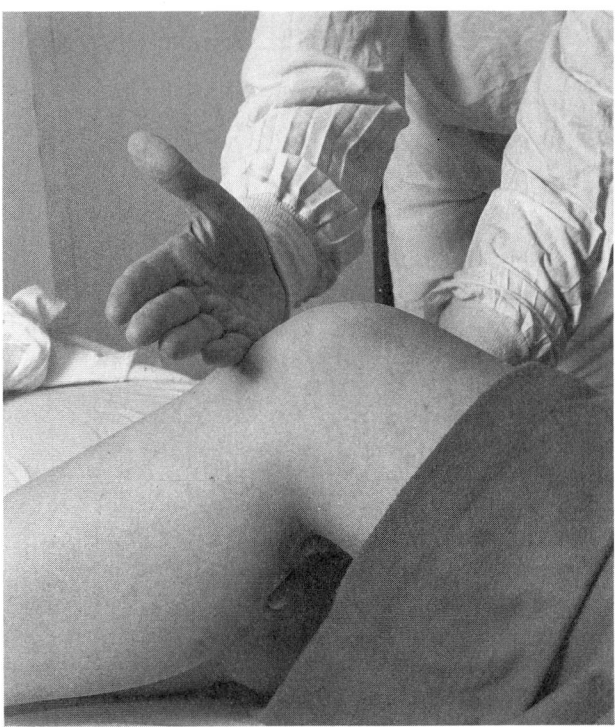

FIGURE 15-12
Eliciting a patellar reflex is an important assessment before administration of magnesium sulfate. The patellar tendon is struck sharply. (Courtesy of the Department of Medical Photography, Children's Hospital, Buffalo, NY.)

eclampsia from occurring during this period. The dose is then tapered and discontinued; the woman should delay breast-feeding until the medication is discontinued.

Promote Relaxation. A woman hospitalized with severe hypertension needs almost constant nursing observation. Stress is a stimulus capable of increasing blood pressure and possibly evoking convulsions in the woman with severe preeclampsia so plans must be made to avoid this. Be certain she receives clear explanations of what is happening and what is planned for her. If she understands the importance of complete bed rest, she will tend not to "cheat" and get out of bed. She will accept the fact that, in the interest of maximal rest and minimal stimulation, visitors must be restricted to just a few people of her choice. She must have opportunities to express how she feels about what is happening or how bewildered she is because the few simple symptoms she noticed 2 weeks ago (increase in weight or increasing edema) have now developed into a syndrome that may be lethal to her baby and possibly to her. She needs to talk about the things she did during pregnancy that she believes may have brought on her condition. Perhaps the night before her symptoms first became apparent she ate a half box of potato chips. Could that have set off this event? The first 3 months of the preg-

Table 15-7. *Effects of Increasing Magnesium Sulfate Serum Levels*	
Medication Range	*Serum Level*
Therapeutic range	4–7 mg/100 mL
Patellar reflex disappears	8–10 mg/100 mL
Respiratory depression occurs	10–12 mg/100 mL
Cardiac conduction defects occur	More than 15 mg/100 mL

Box 15-2
Eliciting a Patellar Reflex and Ankle Clonus

Patellar Reflex

With the woman in a supine position, ask her to bend her knee slightly. Place your hand under her knee to support the leg. Locate the patellar tendon in the midline just below the knee cap. Strike it firmly and quickly with a reflex hammer or the side of your hand. If the leg and foot move, a patellar reflex is present. The reflex is scored as:

0 = No response; hypoactive; abnormal
1+ = Somewhat diminished response but not abnormal
2+ = Average response
3+ = Brisker than average but not abnormal
4+ = Hyperactive; very brisk; abnormal

Ankle Clonus

To elicit ankle clonus, dorsiflex the woman's foot 3 times in rapid succession. As you take your hand away, observe the foot. If no further motion is present, no ankle clonus is present. If the foot continues to move involuntarily, clonus is present. Although usually just rated as present or absent, it can be rated as:

Mild (2 movements)
Moderate (3 to 5 movements)
Severe (over 6 movements)

nancy she wished she were not pregnant. Could that have been responsible?

The woman may want to discuss the financial and stress-related impact of the hospitalization. She planned to work until the end of pregnancy. She planned on delivering her child at an alternative birthing center, and now she may be hospitalized for 1 month. Where is the money for all this to come from?

A woman with severe pregnancy-induced hypertension should not have a telephone in her room, because a ringing phone is a sudden, sharp stimulus and all such stimuli are to be avoided. She can be encouraged to write short notes to her family to maintain contact unless she is too heavily sedated to do so. Older children should be encouraged to send her notes or school drawings.

If the woman cannot be freed of these worries even with help, it is a fallacy to think that she could be waiting calmly for her pregnancy to come to term.

Nursing Interventions for the Woman With Eclampsia

Degeneration of the woman's condition from severe preeclampsia to eclampsia occurs when cerebral irrita-

tion from increasing cerebral edema becomes so acute that a convulsion occurs. This usually occurs late in pregnancy but can happen up to 48 hours after childbirth. Immediately prior to a convulsion, the woman's blood pressure may rise suddenly from additional vasospasm. Her temperature may rise sharply to 39.4°C or 40°C (103°F to 104°F) from increased cerebral pressure. She may notice blurring of vision or severe headache (from the increased cerebral edema). She may have hyperactive reflexes. She may have a premonition that "something is happening." There may be epigastric pain and nausea as a result of vascular congestion of the liver or pancreas. Urinary output may slacken abruptly, to less than 30 mL/h. Eclampsia has actually occurred, however, only when the woman convulses.

Tonic-Clonic Convulsions. An eclamptic convulsion is a tonic-clonic convulsion that occurs in stages. Following the preliminary signals, all the muscles of the woman's body contract. Her back arches, her arms and legs stiffen, and her jaw closes abruptly. She may bite her tongue from the rapid closing of her jaw. Respirations will be halted, because her thoracic muscles are held in contraction. This phase of the convulsion, called the tonic phase, lasts approximately 20 seconds. It may seem longer because the woman may grow slightly cyanotic from the cessation of respirations.

Oxygen administered by face mask may be needed to protect the fetus during this time interval; attach a pulse oximeter to assess oxygen saturation. The woman should be turned on her side; or, even though she is almost at term, she can be placed on her abdomen to allow secretions to drain from her mouth to prevent aspiration. An external fetal heart monitor should be attached if it is not already in place to follow the condition of the fetus. Inserting a tongue blade between the woman's teeth to prevent her from biting her tongue is not recommended. The convulsion occurs suddenly, and thus the action that causes the jaw to clench shut has occurred before anyone can put a tongue blade between her teeth. Attempting to do so after the contraction has occurred rarely has any therapeutic effect and leads to broken teeth, scraped gums, bitten fingers, or broken tongue blades.

Following the tonic phase of the convulsion, all the muscles of the woman's body begin to contract and relax, contract and relax, causing the woman's extremities to flail wildly (the *clonic* phase). She inhales and exhales irregularly as her thoracic muscles contract and relax. She may aspirate the saliva that collected in her mouth during the tonic phase if she was not placed on her side or abdomen during this time. Blowing air through the collected saliva, and any blood that is present in her mouth, may cause the "foaming at the mouth" sometimes associated with convulsions. Her bladder and bowel muscles contract and relax; incontinence of urine and feces may occur. Although she begins to breathe during this stage, the breathing is not entirely effective. Her color may remain cyanotic and she may need continued oxygen therapy, not for herself but for the fetus. The clonic stage of a convulsion lasts up to 1 minute. Magnesium sulfate or diazepam (Valium) may be administered intravenously as an emergency measure at this time.

The third stage of the convulsion is a *postictal* state. During this stage, the woman is semicomatose and cannot be roused except by painful stimuli for at least 1 hour and sometimes up to 4 hours. Extremely close observation is as necessary during the postictal stage as it is during the first two stages. If the convulsion caused premature separation of the placenta, labor may begin during this period, and because the woman is unconscious, she will be unable to report the sensation of contractions. Also, the painful stimuli of contractions may initiate another convulsion. Fetal heart sounds and uterine contractions should be continuously monitored. Check for vaginal bleeding every 15 minutes. Evidence that placental separation may have occurred will appear first on the fetal heart sound record; vaginal bleeding will strengthen the presumption. The woman should be regarded as and treated like any comatose patient. She should remain on her side, so that secretions can drain from her mouth. She should be given nothing to eat or drink. Remember that in coma hearing is the last sense lost and the first one regained. Be aware that when talking at the woman's bedside, she may be able to hear even though she does not respond.

Birth. If the gestational age of the pregnancy is more than 24 weeks, a delivery decision will be made as soon as the woman's condition stabilizes, which is usually 12 to 24 hours after the convulsion. There is some evidence that the fetus does not continue to grow after eclampsia occurs. Thus, terminating the pregnancy at this point is appropriate for both mother and child. For an unexplained reason, fetal lung maturity appears to advance rapidly with hypertension of pregnancy (possibly from the intrauterine stress), so even though the fetus is younger than 36 weeks, the lecithin-sphingomyelin ratio of amniotic fluid may be mature.

Cesarean birth is always more hazardous for the fetus because of the association of retained lung fluid (see Chapter 26). Further, the woman with eclampsia is not a good candidate for general anesthesia and surgery. Because the vascular system is low in volume, the woman may become hypotensive with regional anesthesia such as an epidural block. The preferred method for birth, therefore, is vaginal. If labor does not begin spontaneously, rupture of the membranes or induction of labor by intravenous oxytocin may be instituted. If this is ineffective and the fetus appears to be in imminent danger, the infant will be delivered by cesarean birth.

Postpartal Hypertension. Pregnancy-induced hypertension may occur up to 10 to 14 days after birth, although most postpartal hypertension occurs in the first 48 hours following birth. Women need blood pressure monitored in the postpartal period to detect residual hypertensive or renal disease. Women who had an elevation of blood pressure during pregnancy need to be certain to return for a postpartal checkup to have their postpregnancy blood pressure evaluated to be certain it is again normal and chronic hypertension has not occurred.

HELLP Syndrome

HELLP syndrome is a variation of hypertension of pregnancy named for the common symptoms that occur: *h*emolysis, *e*levated *l*iver enzymes, and *l*ow *p*latelets (Sauer & Harvey, 1992). HELLP syndrome occurs in 4% to 12% of patients with hypertension of pregnancy or affects approximately 1 in every 150 births. It is a serious syndrome because it results in a maternal mortality rate as high as 20% (Sauer & Harvey, 1992).

Why the syndrome occurs is unknown; it occurs in both primigravidas and multigravidas. It may accompany either mild or severe preeclampsia. It occurs either late in pregnancy or immediately following birth.

The first symptoms to be present are usually nausea, epigastric pain, general malaise, and right upper quadrant tenderness. Laboratory studies reveal hemolysis of red blood cells (they appear fragmented on a peripheral blood smear), thrombocytopenia (below $100,000/mm^3$), and the elevated liver enzyme tests alanine-aminotransferase (ALT) and serum aspartate aminotransferase (AST). The liver enzymes are elevated from hemorrhage and necrosis of the liver.

Complications associated with the syndrome are subcapsular liver hematoma, hyponatremia, and hypoglycemia. Severe hemorrhage may occur at birth because of the poor clotting ability present. Epidural anesthesia may not be possible because of the low platelet count and the high possibility of bleeding at the epidural site (Sauer & Harvey, 1992). Therapy for the condition is to improve the platelet count by transfusion of fresh frozen plasma or platelets. If hypoglycemia is present, this is corrected by an intravenous dextrose infusion. The infant is delivered as soon as feasible by either vaginal or cesarean birth.

Multiple Pregnancy

Multiple gestation is considered a complication of pregnancy because the woman's body must adjust to the effects of more than one fetus. Although multiple birth occurs in only 1% of pregnancies, it accounts for 11%

of neonatal deaths (Garcia & Gall, 1990). The rate of twinning in the United States is 1 in 84 births; triplets, 1 in 6400.

Identical (monozygotic) twins begin with a single ovum and spermatozoon. In the process of fusion, or in one of the first cell divisions, the zygote divides into two identical individuals. Single-ovum twins usually have one placenta, one chorion, two amnions, and two umbilical cords. The twins are always of the same sex. Fraternal (dizygotic, nonidentical) twins are the result of the fertilization of two separate ova by two separate spermatozoa (possibly not from the same sexual partner). These twins are actually siblings growing at the same time in utero. Double-ova twins have two placentas, two chorions, two amnions, and two umbilical cords. The twins may be of the same or different sex (Figure 15-13). Two-thirds of twins are dizygotic.

It is sometimes difficult to determine by sonogram or at delivery whether twins are identical or fraternal because the two fraternal placentas may fuse and appear as one large placenta.

Multiple pregnancies of three, four, five, or six children may be single-ovum conceptions, multiple-ova conceptions, or a combination of the two types. Multiple pregnancies are more frequent in nonwhites than in whites. They often occur as a side effect of ovulation stimulation by clomiphene (Clomid); with in vitro fertilization, several fertilized ova are introduced into the uterus resulting in a high possibility of multiple birth.

The higher a woman's parity and age, the more likely she is to have a multiple gestation. Inheritance appears to play a role in dizygotic twinning; this has a familial maternal pattern of occurrence (see the Focus on Cultural Awareness box).

Assessment

Multiple gestation is suspected early in pregnancy when the uterus begins to increase in size at a rate faster than usual. A sonogram will reveal multiple gestation sacs. In some instances early ultrasound examinations reveal double amniotic sacs but then later in pregnancy, only one remains (a vanishing twin syndrome). Alpha-fetoprotein levels will be elevated (Johnson et al., 1990). At the time of quickening, the woman may report flurries of action at different portions of her abdomen rather than at one consistent spot (where the feet are located). On auscultation of the abdomen, two sets of fetal heart sounds may be heard, but if one twin has his or her back positioned toward the woman's back, only one set may be heard. On occasion, twinning is not discovered until after the birth of the first child when it is found that the uterus is not empty.

Therapeutic Management

Women with a multiple gestation are more susceptible than women carrying one fetus to complications of pregnancy such as pregnancy-induced hypertension, hydramnios, placenta previa, and anemia, and they are more prone to postpartal bleeding because of the additional uterine stretching. Because a multiple pregnancy usually ends before the normal term, immaturity of the newborns is a crisis superimposed at birth. It is impor-

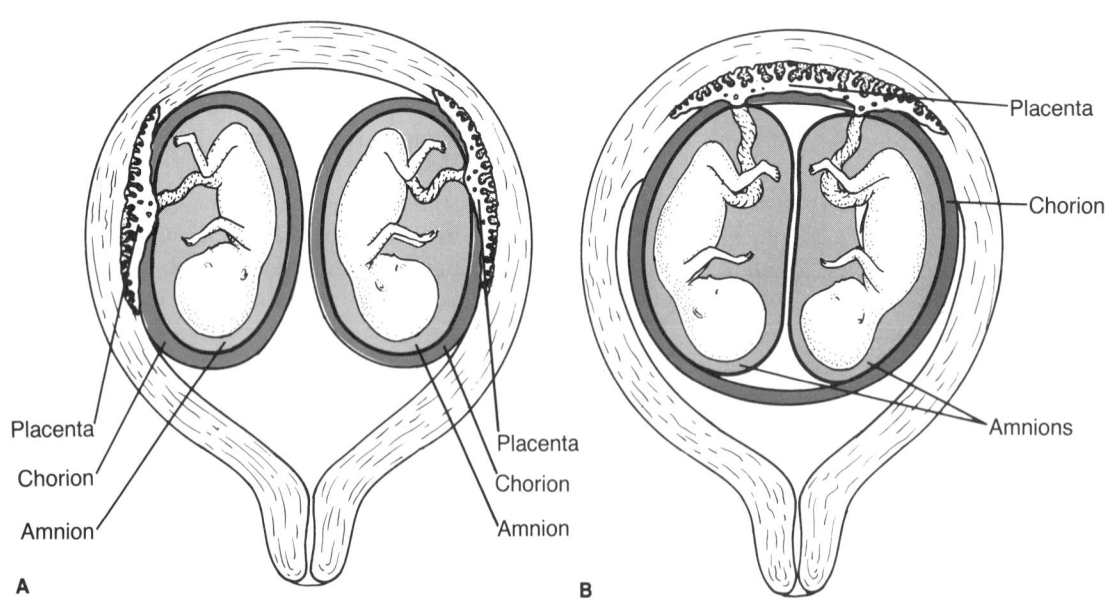

FIGURE 15-13

Multiple gestations. (**A**) *Dizygotic twins showing two placentas, two chorions, and two amnions.* (**B**) *Monozygotic twins with one placenta, one chorion, and two amnions. (From Reeder, S., et al. [1992].* Maternity nursing *[17th ed.]. Philadelphia: J. B. Lippincott, with permission.)*

FOCUS ON CULTURAL AWARENESS

Ethnic origin can influence the incidence of multiple pregnancy. Dizygotic twinning is an inherited tendency. It is most likely to occur in African-Americans, and least likely to occur in Asians.

tant that women with a multiple gestation do not smoke so that they do not add to this risk. There is a higher risk of congenital anomalies in twins such as spinal cord defect than with single births. There is a higher incidence of velamatous cord insertion (the cord inserted into the fetal membranes) with twins than with single births so bleeding at the time of delivery from a torn cord is increased. A complication of monozygotic twins is that the fetuses can share vascular communication. This can lead to overgrowth of one fetus and undergrowth of the second (a twin-to-twin transfusion). If a single amnion is present, there can be knotting and twisting of umbilical cords causing fetal distress or difficulty with birth. The woman will need closer prenatal supervision than the woman with a single gestation to detect these problems as early as possible (Yeast, 1990).

Spend time at health care visits reviewing with the woman her need for extra rest and "shoes off" times during the day, to increase tissue perfusion. Most people are aware that a twin pregnancy will require special precautions so are willing to offer them to her as soon as she makes it known that two heart beats have been heard.

Nursing Diagnoses and Related Interventions

Nursing Diagnosis: Fatigue related to increased stress on body functioning secondary to multiple gestation

Goal: Client will understand cause of fatigue and establish regular rest periods to counteract exhaustion for remainder of pregnancy.

Outcome Criteria: Client states that she is tired but identifies steps she has taken to minimize fatigue.

Because the woman is carrying a double weight during pregnancy, she may notice extreme fatigue and backache. She may have more difficulty resting or sleeping than the average woman because of greater discomfort and increased fetal activity. As the growing uterus compresses her stomach, she may find her appetite decreasing and her intake falling. In order to compensate and maintain nutrition, she may need to eat six small meals a day rather than three large ones. She

must take her iron, folic acid, and vitamin supplement (Keith, 1992).

Toward the end of pregnancy, the woman may have extreme difficulty ambulating because of fatigue and backache. Her abdomen may become so stretched that she feels as if she were going to burst.

Many women with a multiple pregnancy are prescribed bed rest during the last 2 or 3 months of pregnancy in the hope of minimizing the number of falls and accidents that occur from body imbalance and increase the possibility that the pregnancy will come to term, or at least pass week 34, when the chances for survival of the fetuses rises markedly (Elliott & Radin, 1992). The woman is usually urged to refrain from coitus during the last 2 or 3 months of pregnancy because the cervix may be dilating prematurely due to early onset of beginning labor. She is asked to come to a health care facility for monthly ultrasound examinations or weekly nonstress tests to document normal fetal growth beginning with the 28th week of pregnancy. Be certain that these appointments are scheduled to conserve her energy as much as possible.

Nursing Diagnosis: Parental role conflict related to recent discovery of multiple (as opposed to single) pregnancy

Goal: Client will demonstrate positive attitude about event of twins and be able to form close bonds with both infants.

Outcome Criteria: Client states that she is looking forward to two infants (may express concern about her ability to manage their arrival); client identifies changes she is making in preparation now that two babies are expected. *

The woman with a multiple pregnancy has to work through two role changes during pregnancy rather than one. First, she is surprised to find out that she is pregnant (pregnancy is almost always a surprise to every woman) and must begin to work through to acceptance of being pregnant. Suddenly, at a routine office visit, two gestational sacs are seen on ultrasound or two sets of heart sounds are heard. She is told that she has a twin pregnancy. Now she has to work through a second role change: becoming a mother of two, not of one, or a mother of five, not of four. This role change may be difficult to complete, especially if the pregnancy ends early at 32 to 34 weeks. The woman may need some extra help postpartally to form a close mother-child relationship with her newborns.

Nursing Diagnosis: Fear concerning her own and the babies' health related to risks of multiple pregnancy

Goal: Client will express her fears and is able to

manage them well enough to keep positive outlook on pregnancy.

Outcome Criteria: Client accurately states risks of multiple pregnancy; expresses confidence in health care team's ability to care for her and her babies through pregnancy and birth.

In addition to having to rework a role change, the woman with a multiple pregnancy has more reason to fear for her life and the life of her babies than does the average woman. Most women worry at some time during a twin or multiple pregnancy that the infants will be born joined. The chances of this event with twin pregnancy are so small that they can be discounted (and would show on ultrasound if this were so). Every woman has also heard stories about twins being born so prematurely that they did not survive, and about the special danger for the second twin at birth. If she has not already heard these stories, she will surely hear them before her due date. Unfortunately, all these risks cannot simply be filed away under the heading of untrue stories. Both prematurity and high risk to the second twin during birth are real hazards in multiple gestation. Help the woman deal with her fears as positively as possible. It is helpful to tell her that there is no indication so far that her babies are in any danger; that right now it is best to continue doing the things that have to be done. If any problems should arise, the health care team and the woman's family will be there to support her.

Sometimes a woman is so fearful that one or both of her twins will not survive that she makes no preparations for the infants or buys clothes and a crib only for one. This is an indication not so much that she does not accept the second child as that she lacks confidence in herself. She cannot imagine that she will be lucky enough or "good" enough to be able to carry a twin pregnancy to completion. She needs assurance during pregnancy that she is managing well and that she is following instructions well, so that her self-esteem is maintained at as high a level as possible. When her babies are born and both are healthy, the proof she needs that she "deserved" this or was "capable" of it will be present in her arms. Then she will be free to begin interaction with the second child.

Nursing care at the birth of multiple infants is discussed in Chapter 21.

Hydramnios

Hydramnios is excessive amniotic fluid formation. Amniotic fluid is usually 500 to 1000 mL in amount at term. An amount of more than 2000 mL or an amniotic fluid index above 24 cm is considered hydramnios (Chauhan et al., 1993). Hydramnios can cause fetal mal-

presentation because of the extra uterine space it provides. It can lead to premature rupture of the membranes and premature labor because of the increased intrauterine pressure. Premature rupture of the membranes adds the additional risks of both infection and prolapsed cord (see Chapter 16).

Assessment

The first sign of hydramnios may be an unusually rapid enlargement of the uterus. The small parts of the fetus are difficult to palpate because the uterus is unusually tense. Auscultating FHR is difficult because of the increased amount of fluid surrounding the fetus.

The woman will begin to notice extreme shortness of breath as the overly distended uterus pushes up against her diaphragm. She may develop lower-extremity varicosities and hemorrhoids because of poor venous return from the extensive uterine pressure. She will have an increased weight gain. Sonography will generally be ordered to attempt to document the presence of hydramnios and to discover a reason for the excessive amount of fluid (Browne, 1993). Amniotic fluid is formed by the cells of the amniotic membrane and from fetal urine. It is swallowed by the fetus, absorbed across the intestinal membrane into the fetal blood stream, and transferred across the placenta. Accumulation of amniotic fluid suggests difficulty with the fetus's ability to swallow or absorb or excessive urine production. Inability to swallow occurs in infants who are anencephalic or who have tracheoesophageal fistula with stenosis or intestinal obstruction. Excessive urine output occurs in the fetuses of diabetic women (hyperglycemia in the fetus causes increased production).

Therapeutic Management

Women with severe hydramnios are admitted to the hospital for bed rest and further evaluation of their condition. Maintaining bed rest helps to increase uteroplacental circulation and reduces pressure on the cervix which may help prevent preterm labor. Educate the woman to report any sign of ruptured membranes or uterine contractions. Help her avoid constipation by eating a high-fiber diet (although not common, there is a possibility that straining to defecate could increase uterine pressure and cause rupture of membranes). Suggest that a stool softener be prescribed if diet alone is ineffective.

Assess vital signs and lower extremity edema every 4 hours because the extremely tense uterus puts unusual pressure on the diaphragm and vessels of the pelvis.

It is possible for an amniocentesis to be performed to remove some of the extra fluid to give the woman some relief from the increasing pressure. Because amniotic fluid is replaced rapidly, however, this is only a temporary measure unless it is repeated daily. A nonsteroidal anti-inflammatory agent such as indomethacin therapy may be effective in reducing the amount of fluid formed (Mamopoulus et al., 1990). Tocolysis with magnesium sulfate may be begun to try and prevent or halt premature labor.

In most instances of hydramnios, there is premature rupture of the membranes due to excessive pressure, followed by premature labor. In order to prevent the sudden loss of fluid and an accompanying prolapsed cord, membranes can be "needled" (a thin needle is inserted vaginally to pierce them) to allow for slow, controlled release of fluid. Following birth, the infant must be assessed carefully for factors that made him or her unable to swallow in utero.

Post-term Pregnancy

A term pregnancy is 38 to 42 weeks long. A pregnancy that exceeds these limits is prolonged (**post-term**, *postmature,* or *postdate*). The infant of such a pregnancy is considered postgestational, postmature, or dysmature.

Post-term pregnancy occurs in approximately 10% of all pregnancies. Included in this group are some pregnancies that appear to extend beyond the due date set for them because of a faulty due date. Women who have long menstrual cycles (40 to 45 days) do not ovulate on day 14 as in a typical menstrual cycle; they ovulate 14 days from the end of their cycle, or on day 26 or 31. Thus their child will be "late" by 12 to 17 days.

In other instances the pregnancy is truly overdue. For some reason, the "trigger" that initiates labor did not work. Prolonged pregnancy can occur in a woman on a high dose of salicylates (for severe sinus headaches or rheumatoid arthritis) because salicylate interferes with the synthesis of prostaglandins and prostaglandins may be responsible for the initiation of labor. It is also associated with myometrial quiescence or a uterus that does not respond to normal labor stimulation (Smith, 1990).

It is dangerous for a fetus to remain in utero more than 2 weeks beyond term. If the fetus continues to grow, macrosomia will create a delivery problem. The usual effect that occurs, though, is lack of growth. A placenta seems to have a growth potential for only 40 to 42 weeks. After that time it acquires calcium deposits (becomes a Grade III) and is unable to function adequately. A fetus still in utero will be forced to live with decreased blood perfusion. Oligohydramnios leading to variable decelerations may occur. The fetus may suffer from a lack of oxygen, fluid, and nutrients. The amniotic fluid is often stained with meconium at birth (Tongsong & Srisomboon, 1993).

If labor has not begun by 41 weeks, a nonstress test or a biophysical profile may be done (Smith, 1990). If these findings are normal and the physical examination suggests an infant smaller than a normal-term infant,

checked by sonogram, the due date is recalculated. If the tests are abnormal or the physical examination or biparietal diameter measured on sonogram suggests that the fetus is term size, the infant will be delivered by inducing labor. Prostaglandin gel may be applied to the cervix to initiate ripening and labor (Harris et al., 1991). FHR must be monitored closely during labor to be certain that placental insufficiency is not occurring from aging of the placenta. Amnioinfusion may be necessary (Macri et al., 1992). If oxytocin is ineffective, cesarean birth will be necessary. Amnioinfusion is discussed in Chapter 18. Nursing care for the post-term infant at birth is discussed in Chapter 26.

Pseudocyesis

In **pseudocyesis** (false pregnancy), nausea and vomiting, amenorrhea, and enlargement of the abdomen occur in a nonpregnant woman; this is also seen in men (Shutty & Leadbetter, 1993). There are a number of theories as to why the phenomenon occurs: wish-fulfillment theory suggests that the woman's desire to be pregnant actually causes physiologic changes to occur; conflict theory suggests that a desire for or fear of pregnancy creates an internal conflict leading to changes; depression theory attributes the cause to major depression (Paulman & Sadat, 1990). The woman's body responds to her needs with physiologic symptoms. In some women, the abdomen is so enlarged that they appear to be 7 or 8 months pregnant. On physical examination, it is obvious the woman is not pregnant. Sonographic imaging rules out pregnancy.

Both men and women with the disorder need psychologic counseling to learn how to handle better their needs or conflicts.

Rh Incompatibility (Isoimmunization)

Approximately 15% of Caucasians and 10% of African-Americans in the United States are missing the Rh (D) factor in their blood or have an Rh-negative blood type. Although a blood incompatibility problem of this nature is basically a problem that affects the fetus, it causes such concern and apprehension in the woman during pregnancy that it becomes a maternal problem as well.

Rh incompatibility during pregnancy can be predicted when an Rh-negative mother (one negative for a D antigen or one with a dd genotype) is carrying a fetus with an Rh-positive blood type (DD or Dd genotype). For such a situation to occur, the father of the child must either be homozygous (DD) or heterozygous (Dd) Rh-positive. If the father of the child is homozygous (DD) for the factor, 100% of the couple's children will be Rh positive (Dd). If the father is heterozygous for the trait, 50% of their children can be expected to be Rh positive (Dd).

It is easiest to understand how the Rh factor can endanger the fetus if one thinks of it as an antigen (which it is). People who have Rh-positive blood have a protein factor (the D antigen) that Rh-negative people do not. When an Rh-positive fetus begins to grow inside an Rh-negative mother, it is as though her body is being invaded by a foreign agent, or antigen. Her body reacts in the same manner it would if the invading factor were a foreign substance such as measles or mumps virus: her body begins to form antibodies against the invading substance. The Rh factor exists as a portion of the red blood cell. In the case of Rh invasion, therefore, to destroy the antigen, the entire red cell must be destroyed. The maternal antibodies formed cross the placenta and cause red blood cell destruction (hemolysis) of fetal red blood cells (Figure 15-14). The fetus becomes so deficient in red blood cells that sufficient oxygen transport to body cells cannot be maintained. This condition is termed **hemolytic disease of the newborn** or **erythroblastosis fetalis**. Management of the infant born with this condition is discussed in Chapter 26.

Theoretically, there is no connection between fetal blood and maternal blood during pregnancy so the mother should not be exposed to fetal blood. In fact, an occasional villus ruptures, allowing a drop or two of fetal blood to enter the maternal circulation; procedures such as amniocentesis or percutaneous umbilical blood sampling (PUBS) can also cause this. As the placenta separates following delivery of the child, there is an active exchange of fetal and maternal blood from damaged villi. Therefore, most of the maternal antibodies formed against the Rh-positive blood are formed by the Rh-negative woman in the first 72 hours after delivery.

The woman with Rh-negative blood whose sexual partner is Rh-positive used to be advised that she could have no more than three children. This advice was based on the fact that during a first pregnancy, little sensitivity to the foreign Rh antigen developed. However, as described, following delivery of the first child, a large number of antibodies formed and were in the maternal circulation when a second pregnancy began. Many antibodies were formed at the end of the second pregnancy when the fetal-maternal exchange occurred. Thus, an even greater number—in many women, a lethal number—of antibodies were present when the third pregnancy began. Today, the number of children Rh-negative women can have is unlimited because of passive antibody immunization during pregnancy and following birth (see below).

Assessment

All women with Rh-negative blood should have an anti-D antibody titer done at a first pregnancy visit. If the results of this are normal or the titer is minimal (normal is 0; a ratio below 1:8 is minimal), the test will be repeated at week 28 of pregnancy.

If the woman's anti-D antibody titer is elevated at a first assessment, showing Rh sensitization, the titer will be monitored approximately every 2 weeks during the remainder of the pregnancy. The well being of the fetus in this potentially toxic environment will be monitored every 2 weeks (or more often) by amniocentesis (see Chapter 9). Spectrophotometer readings are made of the amniotic fluid obtained by this technique to reveal the fluid density. If the readings (at 450 μm optical density) are plotted on a graph and correlated with gestation age, the extent of involvement and the amount of bilirubin present can be judged.

If the fluid density remains low, the fetus either is in

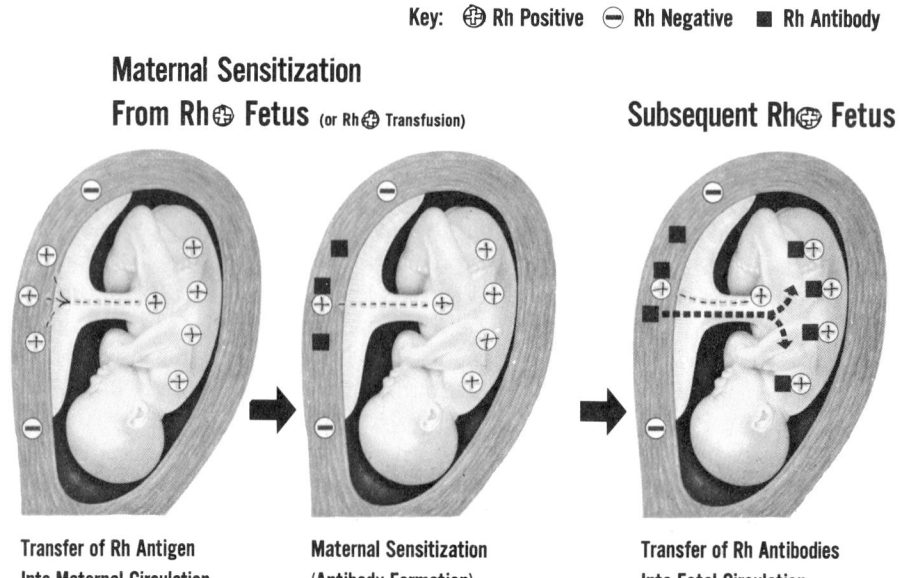

Key: ⊕ Rh Positive ⊖ Rh Negative ■ Rh Antibody

Maternal Sensitization From Rh⊕ Fetus (or Rh⊕ Transfusion)

Subsequent Rh⊕ Fetus

FIGURE 15-14
Maternal antibody formation preceding sensitization of the fetus to Rh antigen. (Used with permission of Ross Products Division, Abbott Laboratories, Columbus OH 43216 from Clinical Education Aid No. 9. © 1962 Ross Products Division, Abbott Laboratories.)

Transfer of Rh Antigen Into Maternal Circulation

Maternal Sensitization (Antibody Formation)

Transfer of Rh Antibodies Into Fetal Circulation

no distress or, more likely, is an Rh-negative fetus. If the spectrophotometer reading is moderate, preterm delivery by induction of labor at fetal maturity is indicated. If the reading is high, the fetus is in imminent danger, and immediate delivery will be carried out or intrauterine transfusion begun. An antibody-D titer in the mother of more than 1:64 is also a critical point at which intrauterine transfusion may be initiated.

Therapeutic Management

Today, with the discovery of Rh_o (D) immune globulin (RHIG), the problem of maternal isoimmunization to an Rh-positive fetus should be eliminated. RHIG is a commercial preparation of passive antibodies against the Rh factor. RHIG is administered to women at 28 weeks of pregnancy. RHIG does not cross the placenta late in pregnancy and destroy fetal red blood cells because the antibodies are not the IgG class, the only type that crosses the placenta. If this is given again by injection to the mother in the first 72 hours following delivery of an Rh-positive child, the mother forms no natural antibodies. Because RHIG is passive antibody protection, it is transient, and in 2 weeks to 2 months, the passive antibodies are destroyed. Only those few antibodies that were formed during pregnancy are left. Thus, every pregnancy is like a first pregnancy in terms of the number of antibodies present, assuring a safe intrauterine environment for as many pregnancies as the woman wishes to have.

If there was no change in the woman's antibody-D titer at week 28 of pregnancy, no special therapy except injection of RHIG needs to be undertaken. Following delivery, the infant's blood type will be determined from a sample of the cord blood. If it is Rh positive—Coombs' negative, indicating that a large number of antibodies are not present in the mother—the mother will receive an RHIG injection. If the newborn's blood type is Rh negative, no antibodies have been formed in the mother's circulation during pregnancy and none will form. Thus, passive antibody injection is unnecessary.

Although in future years the problem of Rh sensitization will be greatly reduced, it currently remains a complication of pregnancy. This is because some women of childbearing age began childbearing before RHIG was available and so have high Rh antibody titers in their blood. Some women do not receive RHIG injections following abortions, ectopic pregnancy, or amniocentesis as they should, and so antibody formation begins.

Intrauterine Transfusion. Formerly, although it was evident that the antibody titer was rising in pregnancy and fetal well being was being threatened, nothing could be done until the fetus became mature enough to be delivered. Some infants were so affected by red cell destruction that they were stillborn; some died in the

neonatal period of heart failure (erythroblastosis fetalis). Others suffered permanent brain damage with resulting motor and mental retardation from high bilirubin levels (kernicterus). The one measure that helps to combat the red cell destruction, exchange blood transfusion to remove the hemolyzed cells and replace them with healthy cells, could be done only after the infant was delivered. Currently, blood transfusion, although not exchange transfusion, can be performed in utero. This can be done by injecting red blood cells directly into a vessel in the fetal cord or depositing them in the fetal abdomen using amniocentesis technique.

Blood used for transfusion in utero is either the fetus's own type (determined by percutaneous blood sampling) or group O negative if the fetal blood type is unknown. From 75 to 150 mL of washed red cells will be used, depending on the age of the fetus. Following deposition of the blood in the cord, the cannula is withdrawn, and the woman is urged to rest for approximately 30 minutes while fetal heart sounds and uterine activity are monitored. The woman is discharged to her home to resume her usual routine.

Obviously, intrauterine transfusion is not without risk. A cord blood vessel may be lacerated by the needle or the uterus may be so irritated by the invasive procedure that labor contractions begin. For the fetus who is becoming severely affected by isoimmunization, however, such a risk is no greater than that of leaving the fetus untreated in the intrauterine environment. The mother receives an RHIG injection following the transfusion to help reduce increased sensitization from the amniocentesis (Vomund & Witter, 1994).

To reduce the possibility of the fetus receiving virus-contaminated blood, women can donate blood themselves for the transfusions (Droste et al., 1992). Women restore their blood volume promptly following blood donation, so there is no fetal or maternal injury from this. Transfusion is sometimes done only once during pregnancy or it may be repeated every 2 weeks for five or six times. As soon as fetal maturity is reached as shown by a mature lecithin sphingomyelin ratio, delivery will be induced.

A woman in whom a high-antibody titer is developing needs a great deal of support to help her reach the end of her pregnancy. She may feel that this is somehow her fault, that she is responsible for literally destroying her child's blood. Often, a day-by-day approach is most helpful in managing such anxiety: "Today, everything seems to be going all right; let's worry about tomorrow when it comes."

Following birth, the infant may require an exchange transfusion to remove hemolyzed red blood cells and replace them with healthy blood cells (see Chapter 26). The woman needs to discuss her plans for further childbearing and to be provided with contraceptive information if she feels that the strain of this pregnancy, the constant feeling of wishing that everything was all right but never being certain that it was, is more than she wants to endure again.

Fetal Death

Obviously the most severe complication of pregnancy that can occur is fetal death. The most likely causes of this are chromosomal abnormalities, congenital malformations, infections such as hepatitis B, immunologic causes, and complications of maternal disease (Chervenak, 1990). If fetal death happens before the time of quickening, the woman will not be aware that the fetus has died because she was not able to feel fetal movements. This type of fetal death may be discovered at a routine prenatal visit when no fetal heart beat can be heard; a real-time sonogram will reveal that no fetal heart beat is present. Following fetal death, delivery will occur naturally, but this may not occur for 4 to 5 weeks after the death. A dead fetus in utero this long can initiate DIC. To prevent this, once it is established by sonogram that the fetus is definitely dead, terminating the pregnancy by oxytocin infusion prevents this complication (Maurer, 1993).

That a fetus has died early in intrauterine life may first be revealed by the natural abortion that occurs. The woman begins painless spotting; this is gradually accompanied by uterine contractions with cervical effacement and dilatation. No fetal heart beat can be heard on assessment. The fetus is born lifeless and emaciated. Observe carefully all women who deliver a dead fetus because if the fetus is dead in utero for any length of time, the risk of developing DIC is present.

If a fetus dies in utero past the point of quickening, the woman becomes aware that fetal movements are suddenly absent. She may lie down or sit in a position that she knows usually causes fetal movement; unable to believe that something could have happened, she may attribute the lack of movement as due to "sleeping" or "saving enough strength to be born." Because she is denying what is happening, it may be a full 24 hours before she telephones the health care facility to report the apparent lack of fetal movement. On assessment, no fetal heart beat can be heard; a sonogram will reveal no fetal heart beat.

If labor does not begin spontaneously, it will be induced through a combination of prostaglandin gel application to the cervix to effect ripening and oxytocin administration to begin uterine contractions. Blood for coagulation studies to detect DIC should be drawn.

Nursing Diagnoses and Related Interventions

Nursing Diagnosis: Grieving related to fetal death
Goal: Client and family will express and share grief among themselves and with significant others.

Outcome Criteria: Client and support person express meaning of pregnancy loss to them; identify other support people/family with whom they can share grief.

Going through labor knowing that the fetus is dead is difficult. The woman grieves for both her dead child and her inability to carry a pregnancy to completion. She cannot help but think she did something to cause this (e.g., forgot an iron supplement or painted a crib) or that she is basically not as good a woman as others. Give her opportunities to express how she feels about this loss. A statement such as "This must be a very difficult day for you" is the kind of statement that opens up the topic for discussion. If there are older children, it might be a help to explore how the woman plans to explain the fetal death to them.

Encourage a support person to remain with the woman during labor. Although this is a difficult time, it makes the birth real, ends the pregnancy, and allows the couple to begin active grieving (Maurer, 1993).

Labor will simulate term live labor because a live fetus is basically a passive participant during labor. It is difficult for the woman to use controlled breathing exercises, although encouraging her to use them is helpful in making the experience one of controllable pain. If the woman wishes a high level of analgesia, she may have it because there is no fetus to protect from narcotic effects, although too much may lead to poor uterine involution in the postpartal period.

Ask if the parents wish to see the child. If they do, wash away obvious blood, swaddle the baby as if he or she were a well newborn, and bring the baby to them. Point out particularly endearing features of the child that may provide a focus for memories. Some parents want to keep a lock of the child's hair. Others want the hospital identification bracelet or to take a photograph. All of these measures are helpful in making the death real to parents and letting them begin the healthy process of grieving.

If the child has a congenital anomaly that led to the death, prepare them for this before bringing the child to them and explain how the anomaly affected the child. Explain hospital procedures such as when the body will be released or what additional permission for autopsy is needed. Different communities have different laws concerning whether burial for an immature fetus is necessary. Consult local health department regulations so you can serve as a resource person for parents concerning this.

The woman need only remain for a short stay in the hospital, assuming there were no complications with labor. Many couples ask if it will be safe for them to have another child. They need to consult with their obstetrician or nurse-midwife about why this fetal death occurred to learn that answer. Some ask if it would be best if they have another baby right away. For some couples, this is a good recommendation providing no physical health problem intervenes. For others, waiting for an interval of time (perhaps 6 months) may be necessary so they can work through their grief before starting a new pregnancy. This helps prevent the new baby from becoming a "replacement" baby or someone to take the place of the dead infant rather than a unique individual in his or her own right. This is important because replacement children are rarely able to live up to the image of what the dead baby would have been if only she or he had lived.

Prepare the couple for the possibility that they may feel sad on the day the infant would have been born if the pregnancy had been carried to term or they visit a friend's child of the age their child would have been. Be certain before the woman is discharged that she has a support person she can rely on during the following week or month when the full impact of the fetal loss registers. Be certain she has a return appointment for a gynecologic checkup so both her physiologic and psychological health can be evaluated at that time.

Key Points

- As the uterus is such a vascular organ during pregnancy, a major complication that can occur all during pregnancy is bleeding. First trimester causes of this are abortion (the spontaneous loss of a pregnancy) and ectopic pregnancy (pregnancy outside the uterus).
- The bleeding evident with bleeding disorders of pregnancy is invariably not indicative of the actual amount of bleeding occurring because so much internal bleeding is also happening. As a rule, women with bleeding of pregnancy should be positioned flat on their left side to help improve placenta circulation.
- Vaginal bleeding during pregnancy is always serious until ruled otherwise as it has the potential to diminish the blood supply of both the mother and fetus. The most usual causes of bleeding during the first trimester are spontaneous abortion and ectopic pregnancy.
- Spontaneous abortion is the loss of a pregnancy before viability of the fetus (20 to 24 weeks). The majority of these early pregnancy losses are attributed to chromosomal abnormality. Abortions are classified as threatened, inevitable, complete, incomplete, missed, or recurrent. Women who have a spontaneous abortion at home should bring any tissue passed with them to the hospital for an analysis for gestational trophoblastic disease.
- Ectopic pregnancy is pregnancy implantation outside the uterus, usually in a fallopian tube. If discovered before the tube ruptures, this can be treated with methotrexate. If not discovered early, it produces sharp lower quadrant pain at about 6 to 12 weeks as the tube ruptures. Surgery is removal or repair of the tube to halt bleeding.
- Common causes of bleeding in the second trimester are gestational trophoblastic disease (abnormal growth of trophoblastic tissue) and incompetent cervix (cervical dilatation before fetal maturity).
- Gestational trophoblastic disease is abnormal growth of the trophoblast tissue. If not discovered by sonogram before this, bleeding will occur at about the 16th week of pregnancy. Women need close follow-up following this as it can lead to choriocarcinoma, a malignancy.
- An incompetent cervix is a cervix that dilates early in pregnancy before viability of the fetus. Sutures (cervical cerclage) can be placed to prevent the cervix from dilating prematurely in a second pregnancy.
- Common causes of third trimester bleeding are placenta previa (low implantation of the placenta) and premature separation of the placenta.
- Placenta previa is low implantation of the placenta so it crosses the cervical os. If not discovered before labor, cervical dilatation may cause the placenta to tear and result in extreme blood loss. Women who have symptoms of placenta previa (painless vaginal bleeding in the third trimester) should not have routine vaginal examinations done to avoid tearing the low-implanted placenta.
- Premature separation of the placenta (abruptio placentae) usually occurs late in pregnancy and means the placenta has separated from the uterus before the fetus is born. This separation immediately cuts off blood supply to the fetus. Women over age 35, those with previous uterine surgery, and those who use cocaine are at highest risk for this. It is manifested by sudden sharp fundal pain, then a continuing dull pain and vaginal bleeding.
- Pregnancy-induced hypertension is a unique disorder that occurs with pregnancy. The three classic symptoms are hypertension, edema, and proteinuria. A sudden increase in weight (more than 1 lb per week) or facial or finger edema are the first symptoms a woman usually reports. It is categorized as preeclampsia or eclampsia. If mild (blood pressure not over 140/90), treatment is bed rest. If severe (BP over 160/110), bed rest plus administration of magnesium sulfate is necessary. If a convulsion occurs the condition is eclampsia. The mortality of the fetus is high following eclampsia. Helping prevent disease progress to this stage is an important nursing responsibility.
- The HELLP syndrome is a unique form of preeclampsia marked by *h*emolysis of red blood cells, *e*levated *l*iver enzymes, and *l*ow *p*latelet count.
- Multiple gestation puts an additional strain on a woman's physical resources and may lead to birth complications or immaturity of the infant. Helping a

woman obtain adequate nutrition and rest during pregnancy are nursing responsibilities.

- Post-term pregnancy is pregnancy that extends beyond 42 weeks. As the placenta is a timed organ, the fetus may receive decreased nutrients post-term.
- Hydramnios is overproduction of amniotic fluid (above 2000 mL). This can lead to premature labor from ruptured membranes because of increased intrauterine pressure. Newborns must be assessed carefully to be certain a swallowing defect was not the cause of the hydramnios.
- Disseminated intravascular coagulation is a blood disorder that can occur with any degree of trauma. It can accompany premature separation of the placenta and pregnancy-induced hypertension. Blood coagulation is so extreme at one point in the circulatory system that clotting factors are used up and absent in the remainder of the system. Beginning symptoms of this are easy bruising, petechiae, and oozing from intravenous sites. A woman with DIC can bleed profusely. Therapy is treatment with heparin to stop the coagulation and free up clotting factors for systemic use.
- Rh incompatibility is a possibility when the woman is Rh negative and the fetus is Rh positive. When this happens, maternal antibodies form that can actually destroy fetal red blood cells, leading to anemia, edema, and jaundice in the newborn. Being certain that women are screened for blood type early in pregnancy is a nursing responsibility.

Critical Thinking Exercises

1. Mrs. Graver is a 30-year-old G1P0 admitted to the labor service with a probable diagnosis of placenta previa. Everyone else on the unit is at lunch so you are alone. You know you should not do a pelvic exam with a placenta previa. How would you estimate her amount of blood loss? How would you determine that blood loss was not affecting the fetus?

2. Alu Wu is a college student who has just been diagnosed as having gestational trophoblastic disease. She tells you she thinks the sonogram she had in early pregnancy caused this. How would you explain gestational trophoblastic disease to her? Was the sonogram responsible for this?

3. Berta is a 30-year-old woman with signs of pregnancy-induced hypertension. Her doctor asks you to explain the necessity for bed rest to her as she insists that she has to continue her job as a lawyer or she will be passed over for promotion to a full partner in her firm. How would you explain this to her? If Berta is prescribed bed rest, what suggestions would you give her so she could achieve this?

Does Berta have an ethical obligation to rest? What about a legal obligation?

4. Jessica is a 25-year-old who is pregnant for the second time. A first pregnancy ended in an early spontaneous abortion 2 years ago. Because she felt well following the abortion, she did not see a health care provider at the time. Looking at Jessica's prenatal record, you realize that she is Rh negative. Is she high risk for Rh incompatibility with this pregnancy?

References

Barth, W. H., et al. (1990). Emergent cerclage. *Surgical Gynecology and Obstetrics, 170*, 323.

Bopp, B., & Shoupe, D. (1993). Luteal phase defects. *Journal of Reproductive Medicine, 38*, 348.

Bottoms, S. F., & Scott, J. R. (1990). Transfusions and shock. In Scott, J. R., et al. *Danforth's obstetrics and gynecology.* Philadelphia: J.B. Lippincott.

Browne, P. C. (1993). Polyhydramnios: Diagnosis, implications and management. *Female Patient, 18*, 19.

Carson, S. A. (1991). Nongenetic causes of recurrent fetal loss. *Contemporary Obstetrics and Gynecology, 36*, 14.

Chauhan, S. P., et al. (1993). Intrapartum hydramnios at term and perinatal outcome. *Journal of Perinatology, 13*, 186.

Chervenak, J. (1990). Ask the expert. *Female Patient, 15*, 100.

Clark, S. L. (1990). Shock in the pregnant patient. *Seminars in Perinatology, 14*, 52.

Cohen, A. W. (1991). Prenatal care, screening and complications. *Current Opinion in Obstetrics & Gynecology, 3*, 759.

Costa, S. D., Presley, J. & Bastert, D. (1991). Advanced abdominal pregnancy. *Obstetrical & Gynecological Survey, 46*, 515.

Cowan, B. D. (1993). Ectopic pregnancy. *Current Opinion in Obstetrics & Gynecology, 5*, 328.

Cunningham, F. G., et al. (1993). *Williams obstetrics* (19th ed.). Norwalk, CT: Appleton and Lange.

Deicas, R. E., et al. (1991). The role of contraception in the development of postmolar gestational trophoblastic tumor. *Obstetrics & Gynecology, 78*, 221.

Department of Health & Human Services. (1991). *Healthy people 2000.* Washington, DC: Public Health Service.

Droste, S., et al. (1992). Maternal and fetal hemodynamic effects of autologous blood donation during pregnancy. *American Journal of Obstetrics and Gynecology, 167*, 89.

Drummond, S. B. (1992). Disseminated intravascular coagulation. *NAACOGS Clinical Issues in Perinatal and Women's Health Nursing, 3*, 530.

Elliott, J. P., & Radin, T. G. (1992). Quadruplet pregnancy: Contemporary management and outcome. *Obstetrics and Gynecology, 80*, 421.

Exacoustos, C., & Rosati, P. (1993). Ultrasound diagnosis of uterine myomas and complications in pregnancy. *Obstetrics and Gynecology, 82*, 97.

Faber, K., et al. (1990). Invasive squamous cell carcinoma of the vagina in a diethylstilbestrol-exposed woman. *Gynecologic Oncology, 37*, 125.

Fedrizzi, R. P., & Cothren, J. D. (1993). Rudimentory uterine horn pregnancy. *Female Patient, 18*, 21.

Garcia, P. M., & Gall, S. A. (1990). Multiple pregnancy. In Scott, J. R., et al. *Danforth's obstetrics and gynecology*. Philadelphia: J.B. Lippincott.

Gilstrap, L. C., & Gant, N. F. (1990). Pathophysiology of preeclampsia. *Seminars in Perinatology, 14,* 147.

Harding, J. A., & Keegan, K. (1992). Coagulation disorders in pregnancy. *Female Patient, 17,* 59.

Harris, B., et al. (1991). Prolonged pregnancy: Monitoring and interventions. *Female Patient, 16, 47.*

Harrison, R. F. (1993). A comparison study of human chorionic gonadotropin, placebo and bedrest for women with early threatened abortion. *International Journal of Fertility and Menopausal Studies, 38,* 160.

Johnson, J. M., et al. (1990). Maternal serum alpha-fetoprotein in twin pregnancy. *American Journal of Obstetrics and Gynecology, 162,* 1020.

Katz, V. L., et al. (1990). A comparison of bed rest and immersion for treating the edema of pregnancy. *Obstetrics and Gynecology, 75,* 147.

Keith, L. G. (1992). Management of twin pregnancy. *Female Patient, 17,* 65.

Khong, T., et al. (1992). An immunohistologic study of endothelialization of uteroplacental vessels in human pregnancy. *American Journal of Obstetrics and Gynecology, 167,* 751.

Kutteh, W. H. (1993). Diagnosis and management of recurrent pregnancy loss. *Female Patient, 18,* 85.

Lallemand, A. V., et al. (1992). Fetal listeriosis during the second trimester of gestation. *Pediatric Pathology, 12,* 665.

Lewis, J. L. (1993). Diagnosis and management of gestational trophoblastic disease. *Cancer, 71,* 1639.

Local methotrexate used for tubal pregnancy. (1990). *Nurses Drug Alert, 14,* 23.

Lockwood, C. J. (1990). Placenta previa related disorders. *Contemporary Obstetrics and Gynecology, 35,* 47.

Loeb, S. (1993). *Nurse's handbook of drug therapy*. Springhouse, PA: Springhouse.

Macri, C. J., et al. (1992). Prophylactic amnioinfusion improves outcome of pregnancy complicated by thick meconium and oligohydramnios. *American Journal of Obstetrics & Gynecology, 167,* 117.

Mamopoulus, M., et al. (1990). Maternal indomethacin therapy in the treatment of polyhydramnios. *American Journal of Obstetrics and Gynecology, 162,* 1225.

Mandeville, L. K., & Troiano, N. H. (1992). *High-risk intrapartum nursing*. Philadelphia: J.B. Lippincott.

Marks, F., et al. (1992). Surgical treatment of incompetent cervix. *American Journal of Perinatology, 9,* 481.

Maurer, M. C. (1993). Intrauterine fetal death: Medical, nursing and psychosocial considerations for the childbearing patient. *Journal of Perinatology, 13,* 36.

Mishell, D. R. (1993). Recurrent abortion. *Journal of Reproductive Medicine, 38,* 250.

Pansky, M., et al. (1991). Nonsurgical management of tubal pregnancy. *American Journal of Obstetrics and Gynecology, 164,* 888.

Paulman, P. M., & Sadat, A. (1990). Pseudocyesis. *Journal of Family Practice, 30,* 575.

Punch, M. R. (1992). Cervical pregnancy. *Female Patient, 17,* 21.

Richardson, G. A., et al. (1993). The impact of prenatal marijuana and cocaine use on the infant and child. *Clinical Obstetrics and Gynecology, 36,* 302.

Rosove, M. H., et al. (1990). Heparin therapy for pregnant women with lupus anticoagulant or anticardiolipin antibodies. *Obstetrics and Gynecology, 75,* 630.

Sauer, P. M., & Harvey, C. J. (1992). Pregnancy-induced hypertension: Understanding severe preeclampsia and the HELLP syndrome. *Critical Care Nursing Clinics of North America, 4,* 703.

Scott, J. R. (1990a). Spontaneous abortion. In Scott, J. R., et al. *Danforth's obstetrics and gynecology*. Philadelphia: J.B. Lippincott.

Scott, J. R. (1990b). Ectopic pregnancy. In Scott, J. R., et al. *Danforth's obstetrics and gynecology*. Philadelphia: J.B. Lippincott.

Sepulveda, W. H., et al. (1993). Cervical pregnancy: A case report. *Archives of Gynecology & Obstetrics, 252,* 155.

Shutty, M. S., & Leadbetter, R. A. (1993). Recurrent pseudocyesis in a male patient with psychosis, intermittent hyponatremia, and polydipsia. *Psychosomatic Medicine, 55,* 146.

Smith, C. I. (1990). Postterm pregnancy: Monitoring vs intervention. *Female Patient, 15,* 19.

Soper, J. T., & Hammond, C. B. (1990). Gestational trophoblastic neoplasms. In Scott, J. R., et al. *Danforth's obstetrics and gynecology*. Philadelphia: J.B. Lippincott.

Stabile, I. (1992). Spontaneous abortion: A clinical perspective. *Female Patient, 17,* 14.

Timor-Tritsch, I. E., & Monteagudo, A. (1993). Diagnosis of placenta previa by transvaginal sonography. *Annals of Medicine, 25,* 279.

Tongsong, T., & Srisomboon, J. (1993). Amniotic fluid volume as a predictor of fetal distress in postterm pregnancy. *International Journal of Obstetrics & Gynecology, 40,* 213.

Vomund, S. L., & Witter, S. E. (1994). Advanced techniques for the treatment of severe isoimmunization. *MCN: American Journal of Maternal Child Nursing, 19,* 18.

Walsh, S. W. (1990). Physiology of low-dose aspirin therapy for the prevention of preeclampsia. *Seminars in Perinatology, 14,* 152.

Williams, M. A., & Mittendorf, R. (1993). Increasing maternal age as a determinant of placenta previa. *Journal of Reproductive Medicine, 38,* 425.

Yeast, J. D. (1990). Maternal physiologic adaptation to twin gestation. *Clinical Obstetrics and Gynecology, 33,* 10.

Suggested Readings

Alto, W. A. (1990). Abdominal pregnancy. *American Family Physician, 41,* 209.

Alvarez, M., & Berkowitz, R. (1990). Multifetal gestation. *Clinical Obstetrics and Gynecology, 33,* 79.

Cox, S. M., & Klein, V. R. (1993). Partial molar pregnancy associated with severe pregnancy-induced hypertension. *Journal of Perinatology, 13,* 103.

Edozien, L. C. (1992). The incomplete cervix—a review. *British Journal of Clinical Practice, 46,* 264.

Elliott, B., et al. (1990). Maternal gonococcal infection as a preventable risk factor for low birth weight. *Journal of Infectious Disease, 161,* 531.

Freda, M. C., et al. (1990). Lifestyle modification as an intervention for inner city women at high risk for preterm birth. *Journal of Advanced Nursing, 15,* 364.

Hennessy, M. B., & Polk-Walker, G. C. (1990). Case study analysis of pseudocyesis: Consideration of the diagnosis of child sexual abuse. *Nurse Practitioner, 15,* 31.

Kreutner, A. K. (1992). Postabortal infections. *Contemporary Obstetrics and Gynecology, 37,* 13.

Nageotte, M. P. (1990). Prevention and treatment of preterm labor in twin gestation. *Clinical Obstetrics and Gynecology, 33,* 61.

Oppenheimer, L. W., et al. (1991). What is a low-lying placenta? *American Journal of Obstetrics and Gynecology, 165,* 1036.

Phelan, J. P., & Easter, T. (1990). HELLP syndrome: The great masquerader. *Female Patient, 15,* 79.

Queenan, J. T. (1992). Reducing the threat of ectopic pregnancy. *Contemporary Obstetrics and Gynecology, 37,* 6.

Reveille, J. D. (1990). Systemic lupus erythematosus. *Female Patient, 15,* 21.

Schroder, W., & Heyl, W. (1993). HELLP syndrome. *Clinical & Experimental Obstetrics & Gynecology, 20,* 88.

Smith, D., et al. (1993). Current approaches to diagnosis and treatment of gestational trophoblastic disease. *Current Opinion in Obstetrics and Gynecology, 5,* 84.

Stainton, M. C. (1994). Supporting family functioning during a high-risk pregnancy. *MCN: American Journal of Maternal Child Nursing, 19,* 24.

Thomas, S. R. (1992). Cervical pregnancy. *Female Patient, 17,* 24.

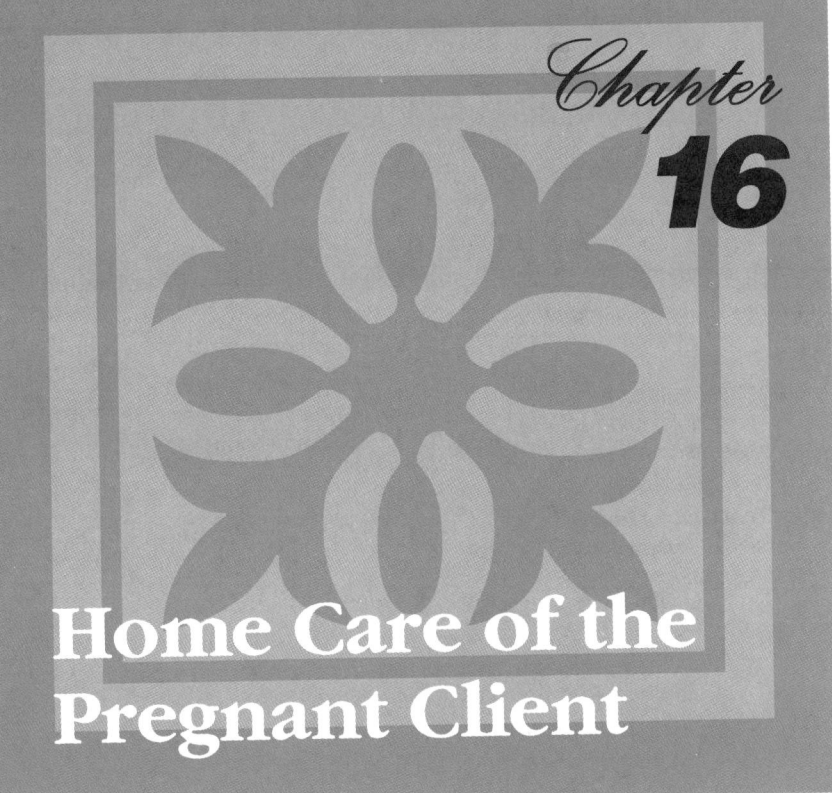

Chapter 16

Home Care of the Pregnant Client

Objectives

After mastering the contents of this chapter, you should be able to:

1. Describe the usual health concerns that require home care nursing during pregnancy.

2. Assess the pregnant woman who is being cared for at home for both physical and psychosocial aspects of care.

3. Formulate nursing diagnoses related to care of the pregnant client at home.

4. Plan home nursing care interventions such as teaching a woman the signs of preterm labor.

5. Implement nursing care such as attaching and using a home uterine monitor to detect uterine contractions.

6. Evaluate outcome criteria to be certain that home care is a satisfying and effective experience for the woman and her family.

7. Identify National Health Goals related to home care during pregnancy that nurses can be instrumental in helping the nation to achieve.

8. Identify areas of home care nursing that could benefit from additional nursing research.

9. Use critical thinking to analyze how home care influences family functioning and develop ways to make nursing care more family centered.

10. Synthesize knowledge of home care with nursing process to achieve quality maternal and child health nursing care.

Adele Pillitteri: MATERNAL AND CHILD HEALTH NURSING, 2nd Edition. © 1995 Adele Pillitteri.

Home care for women during pregnancy means that women who have a complication of pregnancy are cared for in their homes rather than in a hospital setting. This is a method of care that is increasing in frequency. When complications of pregnancy such as preterm labor, hyperemesis gravidarum, preterm premature rupture of membranes, multiple gestation, hydramnios, and hypertension of pregnancy occurred in the past, women were required to spend weeks or even months in the hospital so their condition could be closely monitored. Today, such women are able to remain at home with periodic (perhaps daily) supervision visits by a community or home care nurse. The advantages of home care are numerous. It prevents extensive disruption of the family unit; it can increase self confidence of women because it allows them to have more control of their circumstances; and it can reduce the cost of health care.

Possible disadvantages are that it can actually increase costs to an individual family if their insurance coverage is not geared for home care. It can cause increased anxiety because of the added decision making required. Nurses have an important responsibility to orient families to home care, make home visits, and evaluate whether home care remains appropriate during the remainder of a pregnancy. National Health Goals related to preterm birth are shown in the Focus on National Health Goals box.

■ NURSING PROCESS OVERVIEW
for the Pregnant Woman on Home Care

ASSESSMENT

Most women on home care are first admitted to a hospital for initial fetal monitoring and stabilization and then discharged to a home care program. They are taught self assessment before they leave the hospital so that they can monitor their own condition. This means the nurse who prepares them for home care must spend time with them to teach them the importance of various assessments. The nurse who visits in the home not only continues this health teaching but also carries out the assessments. Women on home care frequently self assess such measures as blood pressure, pulse, temperature, proteinuria, fundal height, and uterine contractions.

NURSING DIAGNOSIS

Nursing diagnoses may speak to the physiologic reason for the supervised home care or the effect of the experience on the family such as:

- High risk for infection related to preterm premature rupture of membranes
- Altered family processes related to necessity for home care
- Altered role performance related to bedrest at home
- Social isolation related to need for home care
- Anxiety related to possibility of pregnancy loss

PLANNING

Planning for home care requires close collaboration between health care providers at a health care agency and those providing care through a home care agency. A major portion of planning for home care is reviewing with the woman and her family exactly what will be expected of them and what they can expect of you. If this is not carefully done, some women, for example, will assume that staying at home is all that is required of them, when what is actually required is complete bedrest. "Walking through a day" with them helps them to determine at what points during the day they will need assistance to be able to remain in bed at home.

IMPLEMENTATION

Women on home care have the advantage of being with their families but the disadvantage of not being constantly supervised by health care personnel. An important aspect of home visits is to reassure the woman and family following assessment that her condition has not changed and it is safe for her to remain at home on the present program or, based on changes, to introduce new interventions. Interventions range from teaching and counseling to hands-on care.

EVALUATION

Evaluation of a home care program not only includes whether the woman is remaining well in her home but whether she feels comfortable and secure with the arrangements. Although the exact requirements necessary for a home care program are yet to be determined (Villar et al., 1992), for many women, successful home care can mean the difference between early birth and a successful pregnancy outcome (Starn, 1992).

Examples of outcome criteria that might be devised are:

- Client's white blood count remains less than 18,000/mm^3.
- Family members state they have adjusted to home care of mother.
- Client states she is able to maintain contact with work setting and family in spite of home care for preterm labor.

Home Visiting

A number of steps of planning are necessary for a home visit to be successful (see the Focus on Cultural Awareness box).

Making a Home Visit

Before making a home visit, be certain to obtain a copy of the client's hospital discharge plan so you are familiar with what her hospital care consisted of and what is the plan for home care. Telephone in advance to arrange a time for the visit so it will be convenient for the family. Confirm this as necessary on the day of the visit and obtain necessary instructions to reach the home. Try not to visit at mealtime unless observing what the woman is eating for a typical meal is necessary for assessment, in order not to disrupt family routines.

Remember that patient confidentiality must be maintained despite the informality of the setting. When transporting a chart or notes on a client, be certain to maintain confidentiality of these.

FOCUS ON
National Health Goals

One National Health Goal speaks directly to the necessity to prevent preterm birth:

- Reduce low birth weight (infants born weighing less than 2500 g) to an incidence of no more than 5% of live births from a baseline of 6.9% and very low birth weight (infants weighing less than 1500 g) to no more than 1% of live births from a baseline of 1.2% (DHHS, 1991).

Low birth weight occurs in newborns because preterm labor cannot be halted. Nurses can be instrumental in seeing that women seek prenatal care, as this is important in preventing preterm birth. Educating women about the signs and symptoms of preterm labor so they can recognize it as soon as it begins—a point at which it possibly can be halted—is important. Areas of nursing research that would be helpful are determining effective ways to alert women to the danger of cocaine use in pregnancy; identifying reasons why many women with preterm labor ignore the initial symptoms until it is too late to halt birth; and determining whether home care, although cost effective, is more effective at preventing preterm labor than hospital care.

FOCUS ON CULTURAL AWARENESS

Because the structure of families is culturally determined, home care of a woman during pregnancy will be easier for some than for others. If the family is extended, for example, the woman may be so involved in the care of other family members that she is unable to rest adequately at home. On the other hand, in such a family, there may be many people to offer care and so rest at home is ideal. Assess each family individually to determine what family members are present and how home care will affect that family.

In some settings it may be necessary to take some precautions to avoid getting flea bites or ingesting questionable food. Good judgment should be used in regard to parking the car safely or carrying a large sum of money.

Wash your hands before touching the client, as you would in a health care setting, so as to prevent spread of infection between clients (ask permission to use the kitchen sink to wash; carry a liquid soap and paper towels with you). If a home situation should become unsafe while you are visiting (a fist fight breaks out, a dog is menacing), leave. If both the client and you are in danger, call the community emergency number for help.

Client Assessment

Women on home care are usually anxious to have a nurse confirm that the self assessments they have been making are accurate. Be certain to provide privacy for both health histories and physical examinations in the home. Some homes are too cool early in the morning for physical assessment because the heat has been turned down during the night. Arranging for a visit later in the day may alleviate this problem. If a home has few rooms, finding a private location can be difficult. Be certain to include assessment not only of physical aspects but of mental or psychosocial ones as well. If the woman is on bedrest, ask how she occupies her time. A woman cannot rest if she is concerned about her family or the family's finances or is caring for older children. She also may find it difficult to rest if she is bored. Be certain that the woman has a means of obtaining refills on prescriptions and measures to take if her condition should worsen (telephone 911? telephone the hospital? her doctor's office?). Be certain that she knows it is important to keep health care appointments in addition to home care visits and also that she has transportation for these appointments.

Environmental Assessment

Observe that the house is safe for home care. Ask if there is adequate water, heat, and refrigeration. Are there any drafts or broken windows? Are there rodents or insects in the house? If the woman is on bedrest, do the arrangements seem adequate or is it likely that she is getting up every few minutes to care for small children (Figure 16-1)?

Preterm Labor

Preterm labor is labor that occurs before the end of week 37 of gestation (Travis & McCullough, 1993). It occurs in approximately 9% of all pregnancies (Anderson & Merkatz, 1990). A woman is considered to be in pre-

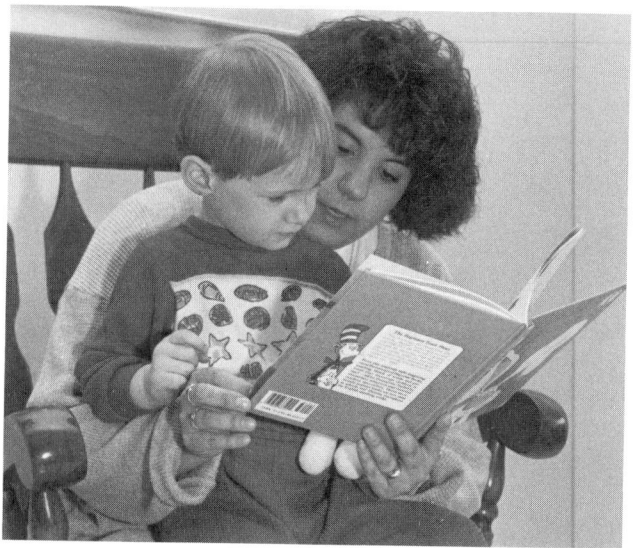

FIGURE 16-1

Assess that women on bedrest at home are truly resting and not maintaining a usual household routine. Activities such as caring for older children can interfere with this.

term labor if she is having uterine contractions that cause cervical effacement and dilatation. Any woman having a pattern of labor for more than an hour with contractions lasting 30 seconds and occurring as frequently as every 10 minutes apart should be considered to be in labor. Preterm labor is always serious because if it results in the infant's birth, the infant will be premature. Preterm births are responsible for almost two thirds of all infant deaths in the neonatal period (Papke, 1993).

Why labor begins before the fetus is mature is unclear in most instances. During pregnancy, those women who will deliver prematurely may have more painless contractions, more backache, and more vaginal discharge than others (Iams et al., 1990). Preterm labor occurs at a higher rate in African Americans than in others; it is frequently associated with dehydration, urinary tract infection, and **chorioamnionitis** (infection of the fetal membranes and fluid). A scale that can be used to score the likelihood of preterm birth based on socioeconomic factors is shown in Table 16-1. Such a scale should be used at the initial prenatal visit and again at 26 to 28 weeks gestation. The higher the score, the more likely the woman is to have a preterm birth. Zero to 5 denotes low risk; 6 to 9, moderate risk; 10 or over, high risk. Box 16-1 lists common symptoms of early preterm labor. Any woman who has these symptoms or feels she is in preterm labor for any reason needs to be carefully evaluated because symptoms of labor are subtle and best recognized by the woman herself (Kragt & Keirse, 1990). Women who continue to work strenuous jobs during pregnancy or work shift work that leads to extreme fatigue may have a higher incidence than others (Infante-Rivard et al., 1993).

Table 16-1. *Preterm Labor Risk Assessment Scale*

Score	Socioeconomic	Past History	Daily Habits	Current Pregnancy
1	2 children at home Low socioeconomic status	1 abortion Less than 1 year since last birth	Work outside home	Unusual fatigue
2	Under 20 years old Over 40 years old Single parent	2 abortions	More than 10 cigarettes/day	Albuminuria Hypertension Bacteriuria
3	Very low socioeconomic status Under 5 ft tall Under 100 lb	3 abortions	Heavy work; long, tiring trips	Breech at 32 weeks Weight loss of 5 pounds Head engaged Febrile illness
4	Under 18 years old	Pyelonephritis		Metrorrhagia after 12 weeks Effacement; dilatation; uterine irritability
5		2nd trimester abortion		Uterine anomaly; placenta previa; polyhydramnios
10		DES exposure Preterm birth Repeated second trimester abortion		Uterine myoma Twins Abdominal surgery

(From Creasy, R., & Merkatz I. [1990]. Prevention of preterm birth: Clinical opinion. *Obstetrics and Gynecology, 76,* 2S.)

Therapeutic Management

It is not possible to definitely predict which pregnancies will end early with preterm labor, although a number of diagnostic tests are being evaluated. In the future, it may be possible to analyze changes in vaginal mucus, such as the presence of fibronectin, a protein produced by trophoblast cells, to predict this (Creasy, 1991). Until recent years, there were no measures available to halt preterm labor. Currently, medical attempts can be made to stop labor if fetal membranes are intact; fetal heart sounds are good; there is no evidence that bleeding is occurring that will affect maternal or fetal welfare; the cervix is not dilated more than 3 to 4 cm; and effacement is not more than 50%.

Box 16-1

Symptoms of Preterm Labor That Women Can Self Assess

Persistent, dull, low backache
Vaginal spotting
Feeling of pelvic pressure or abdominal tightening
Menstrual-like cramps
Increase in vaginal discharge
Uterine contractions
Intestinal cramping

A woman who is in preterm labor is usually first admitted to the hospital and placed on bedrest to relieve pressure of the fetus on the cervix. Hydration may also have an influence on stopping contractions so intravenous fluid therapy to keep the woman well hydrated is begun. This effect of hydration is probably related to the fact that oxytocin is secreted by the pituitary gland. The pituitary gland also secretes antidiuretic hormone. If the woman is dehydrated, the gland is activated to secrete antidiuretic hormone and this may also release oxytocin. By keeping her well hydrated, the release of oxytocin may be minimized.

Vaginal and cervical cultures and a clean catch urine for culture are obtained to rule out infection. Assuring the woman that everything that can be done is being done is important. Following stabilization, the woman is discharged to home care. Women in preterm labor can be safely cared for at home as long as they can dependably remain on almost complete bedrest, drink enough fluid to remain well hydrated, and take an oral tocolytic such as oral terbutaline (Dineen, 1992; Poland et al., 1992). It is important that women also maintain adequate nutrition and do not smoke cigarettes (poor nutrition and smoking cigarettes are activities that put them at high risk for preterm birth; see the Nursing Care Plan).

Drug Administration

For reasons not clearly understood, the administration of a corticosteroid to the fetus appears to accelerate the formation of lung surfactant. During the time labor is being

Cecelia Armitage is a 23-year-old woman (G2P1) at week 32 of pregnancy who began preterm labor. She was admitted to the labor and delivery service of the hospital with contractions 40 sec long and 7 min apart. She was placed on tocolytic therapy and now is home on uterine monitoring. The following is a nursing care plan you might design for her.

Nursing Diagnosis: High risk for fetal injury related to preterm labor.

Defining Characteristic: Client had labor contractions at 32 weeks gestation; at 32 weeks, the fetus has limited lung capacity to function well if born.

Goal: Preterm labor will be deterred by tocolytic therapy and home monitoring.

Outcome Criteria: Labor contractions do not resume before 38 weeks' gestation; fetal heart rate is 120 to 160 bpm by external monitor with good variability; infant Apgar score at birth is 7 to 10.

Nursing Orders	Rationale
1. Review medication therapy and necessity to follow schedule exactly with client.	1. Tocolytic therapy must maintain blood levels in order to be effective.
2. Review importance of a high fluid intake (1 quart every 4 hours).	2. Hydration can help allay preterm birth.

Nursing Diagnosis: Fear related to threatened pregnancy loss.

Defining Characteristic: Client voices she is afraid fetal outcome will be poor.

Goal: Client will demonstrate adequate ability to deal with fear during crisis period.

Outcome Criteria: Client cooperates with instructions and participates actively in home care.

Nursing Orders	Rationale
1. Maintain an optimistic attitude at home visits.	1. Preterm labor is preventable by tocolytic therapy and home monitoring.
2. Review technique of home monitoring and instructions client should follow if contractions resume.	2. Knowledge can aid self-confidence and ability to manage stress.
3. Encourage couple to verbalize their fears.	3. Verbalizing problems is a means of helping people begin problem solving.

chemically halted, therefore, the woman may be given a steroid (betamethasone) to attempt to hasten fetal lung maturity (Crowley, 1990). It takes about 48 hours for betamethasone to have an effect so it is important that labor be halted for at least this long.

A drug that is able to halt labor is a **tocolytic agent** (Box 16-2). Calcium channel blockers such as nifedipine (Procardia) may also be effective. A prostaglandin antagonist such as indomethacin (Indocin) can be used as a tocolytic; however, the danger this will lead to premature closure of the fetal ductus arteriosus and cause

fetal pulmonary hypertension limits its use (Anderson & Merkatz, 1990).

Beta-sympathomimetic drugs are the most frequently used tocolytic agents today. Beta-1 receptor sites are found in adipose tissue, heart, liver, pancreatic islet cells, and gastrointestinal smooth muscle. Beta-2 receptor sites are found in uterine smooth muscle, bronchial smooth muscle, and blood vessels. Beta-adrenergic drugs act to halt contractions by coupling with adrenergic receptors on the outer surface of the membrane of myometrial cells. This releases adrenylcyclase, which triggers the

Box 16-2
Tocolytic Therapy

Drug: Magnesium Sulfate

Action: Central nervous system (CNS) depressant that acts by decreasing acetylcholine level, thereby blocking neuromuscular transmission. Antidote is calcium gluconate.

  Pregnancy risk category: B

  Dosage: Loading dose of 4 g IV infused over 15–30 min, then 1–4 g/h until contractions halt. Following this, it may be administered orally (500 mg every 4 h).

  Maternal side effects: hypotension, diarrhea, depressed deep tendon reflexes, depressed respirations, oliguria, vasodilatation producing feeling of warmth.

  Fetal effects: depressed biophysical profile; possibly bone abnormalities with long-term administration.

  Nursing responsibilities: Assess every hour, woman's respirations are more than 12/min; urine output is more than 30 mL/h and patellar reflex is present.

Drug: Ritodrine Hydrochloride (Yutopar)

Action: Beta-receptor agonist that stimulates the Beta-2 adrenergic receptors in uterine smooth muscle, inhibiting contractions.

  Pregnancy risk category: B

  Dosage: A loading dose of 0.05–0.1 mg/min. Dosage may be increased if no effect by 10-min increments of 0.05 mg/min per increment to a maximum of 0.35 mg/min until contractions halt. Following this, the drug is continued for 24 h, then oral administration (10 mg every 4 to 6 h up to 120 mg/24 h) may be begun. The first oral dose should be administered 30 min before discontinuation of the intravenous solution to ensure continual serum levels.

  Maternal side effects: Tachycardia, chest pain, hypotension, drowsiness, nausea, vomiting, hyperglycemia, hypokalemia, pulmonary edema.

  Fetal effects: Tachycardia, hypoglycemia at birth.

  Nursing responsibilities: Pulse and respirations should be assessed hourly with intravenous infusion.

Notify physician if pulse is more than 120 bpm before continuing drug. Auscultate chest for rales and rhonchi daily. Fasting and 2 h postprandial blood glucose levels may be ordered to assess for hyperglycemia.

Drug: Terbutaline (Brethine)

Action: Beta-adrenergic agonist that stimulates the Beta-2 adrenergic receptors in uterine smooth muscle, inhibiting contractions.

  Pregnancy risk category: B

  Dosage: 0.01 mg/min IV infusion is begun; this is then increased by 0.005 mg/min every 10 min up to 0.08 mg/min until contractions halt. Following this, it may be administered orally at 2.5 to 5 mg every 4–6 h. The first oral dose should be started 30 min before the intravenous infusion is discontinued to ensure continual serum drug level. Also may be administered subcutaneously at 0.25–0.5 mg every 2–4 h.

  Maternal side effects: Hypokalemia, hyperglycemia, pulmonary edema, hypertension.

  Fetal effects: Possibly hypoglycemia in newborn.

  Nursing responsibilities: Assess if maternal pulse is more than 120/min before administering next oral dose, every 1 h with intravenous infusion.

Drug: Nifedipine (Procardia)

Action: Calcium channel blocker.

  Pregnancy risk category: C

  Dosage: Sublingual using gelatin capsule or orally 10 mg every 6 h.

  Maternal side effects: Palpitations, hypotension, headache, heartburn, nausea, muscle cramps.

  Fetal effects: Few documented; possibly tachycardia.

  Nursing responsibilities: Maternal vital signs should be taken every 4 h.

(From Loeb, S. [1993]. *Nurse's handbook of drug therapy.* Springhouse, PA: Springhouse.)

conversion of adenosine triphosphate into cyclic adenosine monophosphate. This substance is responsible for reducing the intracellular concentration of calcium through protein binding. With a lowered intracellular calcium concentration, muscle contraction is ineffective and uterine contractions halt. An ideal tocolytic drug is one that acts entirely on beta-2 receptor sites and does not cause any heart or gastrointestinal symptoms.

Magnesium sulfate is often the first drug used to halt contractions. It is administered with a loading dose followed by continuous intravenous administration. The same safeguards of safe administration as for hypertension of pregnancy (assessment of urinary output and

respiratory rate) should be followed (see Chapter 15). Following this initial therapy, oral magnesium oxalate can be begun.

Ritodrine hydrochloride (Yutopar) and terbutaline (Brethine) are two drugs that are also used often. These drugs act almost entirely on beta-2 receptor sites, and thus have only a mild hypotensive and tachycardiac effect. As beta-2 receptors, however, blood vessels and bronchi relax along with the uterine muscle. As a result, the heart rate increases to move blood more effectively. Hypocalcemia may occur from a shift of potassium into cells, and blood glucose and accompanying plasma insulin levels may increase. Pulmonary edema may also occur (Cowan, 1993). Headache, due to the dilatation of cerebral blood vessels, is a common side effect; nausea and emesis also may occur. Headache, nausea, and vomiting are side effects to be observed for but are not reasons in themselves to discontinue therapy. Both drugs should be used cautiously with clients with diabetes mellitus and thyroid dysfunction. In a woman who is predisposed to developing gestational diabetes, terbutaline can raise her blood sugar levels and cause her to become overtly diabetic. This adds further complications to her pregnancy.

Before a tocolytic drug is administered, baseline blood data (hematocrit, serum glucose, potassium, sodium chloride, carbon dioxide) and an electrocardiogram (perhaps) are recorded. An external uterine and fetal monitor should be in place. Be certain that the woman meets the criteria for labor (contractions 10 seconds in length, every 10 minutes for more than 1 hour). Be certain the woman falls within the safe criteria for tocolytic administration: no vaginal bleeding, no elevated temperature, and no cervical dilatation of more than 4 cm or effacement of more than 50%.

If ritodrine is being used, 150 mg of ritodrine is added to 500 mL Ringer's lactate (Ringer's lactate is used rather than a dextrose solution to prevent any unnecessary hyperglycemia). The drug should be administered by a "piggy-back" method, connected to a mainline intravenous solution, so it can be stopped immediately if effects such as tachycardia or arrhythmias occur. A microdrip and an automatic infusion pump should be used to ensure a constant infusion.

An initial flow rate is calculated and begun; this initial flow rate may be increased every 10 minutes until uterine activity halts, a rate of .35 mg/min (the maximum dosage) is reached, or side effects become extreme. Pulse and blood pressure should be assessed every 15 minutes during the time the flow rate is being increased; thereafter, every 30 minutes until contractions halt. Assess also for chest pain and dyspnea. Auscultate the lungs for rales to detect signs of pulmonary edema. Report promptly a pulse rate of more than 120 bpm, blood pressure below 90/60, chest pain, dyspnea, rales, or cardiac arrhythmias. Hematocrit and electrolytes may be drawn every 4 hours during administration. Observe the fetal heart rate closely for tachycardia (heart rate over 160 bpm), late decelerations, or variable decelerations that suggest possible uterine bleeding or the need for emergency delivery of the fetus rather than continuation of the pregnancy.

During administration, propranolol (Inderal) may be administered to counteract the decreased diastolic blood pressure in the mother and allow ritodrine infusion to continue. Weigh the woman daily because an increasing daily weight suggests retention of fluid or accumulation of edema.

Assess the total parenteral intake. If this exceeds 100 mL/h, the woman may develop a fluid overload and pulmonary edema. Measure intake and output every hour and then every 4 hours following the infusion.

Following the halt of contractions, the infusion is continued for 12 to 24 hours, then oral administration of ritodrine or terbutaline is begun. The first oral dose to be administered is given 30 minutes before the intravenous infusion is discontinued to be certain no drop in serum concentration occurs. Following this initial stabilization, the woman continues to take an oral tocolytic until 37 weeks gestation or fetal lung maturity is established by amniocentesis. Safe rules for home administration of medicine are shown Chapter 38, Box 38-1. Teach the woman to take her pulse before each dose and to call for further advice if the pulse is more than 120 bpm or if she experiences cardiac palpitation or extreme nervousness.

If terbutaline is used as the primary tocolytic, it may be begun with a similar, but subcutaneous, protocol. Terbutaline may also be administered by pump subcutaneously while on home care (Allbert et al., 1992).

The disadvantage of oral terbutaline is that a large dose (30 to 40 mg daily) is required to maintain uterine inactivity. Such a high dose can lead to tachycardia in both the woman and the fetus; it can also desensitize beta-2 receptor sites and allow uterine contractions to "break through." Women on large oral doses of terbutaline need to assess their radial pulse daily and keep a permanent record of this. Alert them to report a pulse rate of more than 120 bpm or a feeling of their heart "pounding" or "jumping" that might suggest an arrhythmia.

Oral tocolytics must be taken every 4 to 6 hours to maintain uterine inactivity. This means women must set their alarm clocks so that they wake during the night, or by morning their serum level of medication will be too low to be effective. Caution them that if they forget a dose, they must take a pill as soon as they remember and then space their doses accordingly from that time. They should not double the dose to make up for the missed pill because of the extreme tachycardia this could cause.

The terbutaline pump provides another method of home drug administration that uses lower doses of medicine with better results. Oral terbutaline therapy has the potential of prolonging labor an average of 2 weeks; with subcutaneous pump infusions, labor can be delayed an average of 8 to 9 weeks.

Similar to an insulin pump (see Figure 14-7), a terbutaline pump is filled with a syringe of the drug. A small polyethylene catheter leads from the pump to a subcutaneous needle. When the needle is inserted into the subcutaneous tissue of the abdomen or the thigh, the pump automatically injects a continuous low dose of medication subcutaneously. The pump can be set to "bolus" an injection of the drug at the time of day when contractions tend to occur the most; a woman could manually trigger the pump to inject extra medicine (within set limits) if she should begin to feel contractions. The pump can be carried in a sash around the waist or kept in a pocket of her clothing (Sala & Moise, 1990).

Pumps should never get wet, so the syringe should be removed from the pump while the woman showers. For tub bathing, she should remove both the pump and needle and replace it immediately afterward.

Fetal Assessment

In addition to tocolytic therapy, it is important to assess fetal welfare daily in the woman trying to delay preterm labor. Women may be instructed to use a "Daily Fetal Movement Count" or "Count to Ten" test (Smith, Davis, & Rayburn, 1992). The typical fetus moves 10 times in an hour. To evaluate fetal movement, the woman lies down on her left side and times the number of minutes it takes for her to feel 10 fetal movements (about an hour) or counts the number of fetal movements she feels in 1 hour (10 to 12). If the time it takes to feel 10 fetal movements is twice what it was the day before or she feels fewer than five movements during an hour (half of what she should feel), she monitors again for a second hour. If at the end of this second hour, fetal activity has not increased, she should telephone her primary care provider for consultation. Because of the variation of movements among normal, healthy fetuses, different perinatal centers use different protocols for counting fetal movements. What standard is accepted as normal also varies.

A rhythm strip or nonstress test can be conducted and evaluated by use of a portable monitor approximately the size of a transistor radio. The woman straps this to her abdomen for 20 to 30 minutes at a set time every day or at any time she feels contractions or is concerned about the lack of fetal movement (Figure 16-2). Both uterine contractions and FHR are monitored. At the conclusion of the monitoring period, the monitor is held next to a telephone and the tracing is transmitted to a central center for evaluation. If a woman is asked to take fundal height measurements, be certain she demonstrates the correct technique to you, as this measurement varies greatly depending on where a tape measure is placed (Engstrom & Sittler, 1993).

Bedrest and Hydration

Be certain that women with threatened preterm labor are maintaining bedrest while at home. Arranging for a homemaker service to care for children or an aging parent may allow the woman to rest completely. Restricting activity in the mother puts additional responsibility on the father (May, 1994). Assess how he is coping as well.

Women on home care should drink at least eight full glasses of fluid a day to obtain adequate fluid intake.

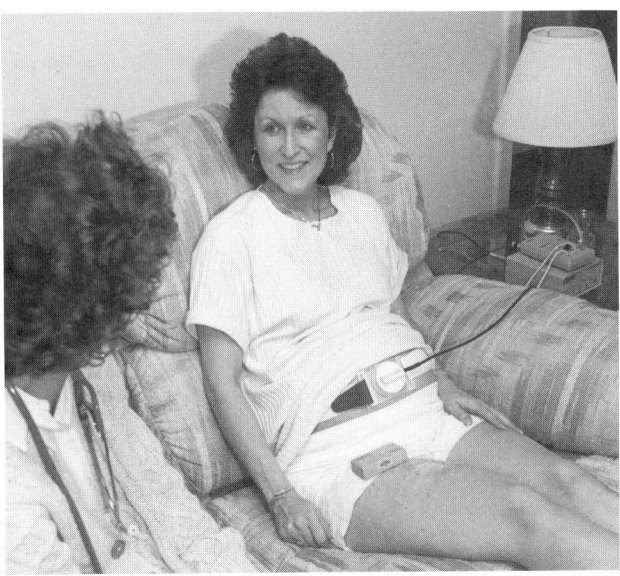

FIGURE 16-2
Uterine and fetal monitoring can be conducted safely at home under the guidance of a community or home health care nurse. (Courtesy of the Department of Medical Photography, Children's Hospital, Buffalo, NY.)

Common instructions for home care and actions for the woman to take if she should detect uterine contractions are beginning again are shown in the Focus on Family Teaching box.

Labor That Cannot Be Halted

In some women, preterm labor will be too far advanced when they are first seen in a health care facility for it to be halted. Preterm labor may begin with rupture of the membranes or show from cervical dilatation, the same as term labor. Because the mucus plug that seals the cervix, ("show") is often blood tinged, initially the woman may report this as bleeding in pregnancy.

If membranes have ruptured or the cervix is more than 50% effaced and 3 to 4 cm dilated, it is unlikely that labor can be halted. The rupturing of membranes, especially, can be thought of as a point of no return in stopping or delaying labor because of the risk of infection that begins with ruptured membranes.

Some women wait, unwilling to face the fact that labor contractions have started. Some diagnose their contractions as nothing more than extremely hard Braxton Hicks contractions and do not seek help until membranes rupture. Currently, when labor can be delayed until the fetus reaches a level of maturity that will allow him or her to survive in the outside environment, evaluation and the institution of therapy before membranes rupture is vitally important (Hill & Lambertz, 1990).

If the fetus is very immature at the time labor cannot be halted, a cesarean birth may be planned to reduce

FOCUS ON FAMILY TEACHING

Q. My preterm labor has been effectively halted and now I'm home on bedrest. What are actions I can take to help prevent contractions from starting again?

A. No one can guarantee that preterm labor won't recur. Measures you can take hopefully to postpone a recurrence are:

- Remain on bedrest except to use the bathroom (use a bed or feet up on a couch or lounge).
- Drink eight to ten glasses of fluids daily (keep a pitcher by your bed so you don't have to get up to get some).
- Be certain to take your prescribed tocolytic medication on time to maintain a constant blood level. Set an alarm clock as necessary, especially at night.
- Monitor fetal heart rate and uterine contractions daily.
- Keep mentally active by reading or working on a project to prevent boredom.
- Avoid activities that could stimulate labor such as nipple stimulation.
- Consult your primary care provider as to whether sexual relations should be restricted.
- Immediately report signs of ruptured membranes (sudden gush of vaginal fluid) or vaginal bleeding.
- Report signs of urinary tract or vaginal infection (burning on and frequency of urination; vaginal itching or pain).
- Report symptoms of pulmonary congestion (cough and difficulty breathing unless upright), which can be effects of tocolytic drugs.
- Keep appointments for prenatal care.

If uterine contractions recur:

- Empty your bladder to relieve pressure on the uterus.
- Lie down on your left or right side to encourage blood return to the uterus.
- Attach the fetal and uterine contraction monitor.
- Drink two to three glasses of fluid to increase hydration.
- Telephone your health care provider to report incident and ask for further care measures.

---

pressure on the fetal head and hopefully reduce the possibility of subdural or intraventricular hemorrhage.

Most women assume that if they are going to have a vaginal birth, labor will be shorter than normal labor because the infant is so small. This is not necessarily the case. The first stage of labor, the longest stage, proceeds exactly as it would with a term pregnancy. The second stage of labor *may* be shorter, because a small infant can be pushed through the dilated cervix and the birth canal much more easily than one of normal size. Because the second stage takes at most 1 hour, the difference will be not more than approximately 30 minutes to 1 hour. Unless a woman is given this explanation, she may worry not only that her labor is preterm but also that something is going wrong because it is taking so long (see the Focus on Nursing Research box for other concerns of women in preterm labor).

Artificial rupture of the membranes is not done as a rule in preterm labor until the fetal head is firmly engaged because there is such a potential for prolapse of the cord around the small head. Delaying rupture of the membranes may prolong the first stage of labor.

Analgesic agents are administered with caution during preterm labor. The immature infant will have enough difficulty breathing on his or her own at birth without the additional burden of being born sedated. If the woman wants anesthesia relief, an epidural anesthetic is preferable rather than a general anesthetic because this does not further compromise the infant's ability to initiate respirations at birth. Again, the woman needs to know why a particular method of anesthesia is chosen. She will bear a great deal of pain in the interest of her child's welfare. She will tolerate very little if she feels it is for the convenience of the hospital staff.

Uterine contractions and fetal heart sounds should be continuously monitored during labor (Eganhouse et al., 1992). The woman can feel reassured by the evidence of the monitor screen or graph or the projected sound that, although her infant is likely to be small, his or her heart tones seem to be of good quality and the infant is reacting well to labor.

Most women assume that because the infant's head will be small, an episiotomy will be unnecessary for delivery, and they will therefore escape the discomfort of postpartal stitches. Although the head of a preterm infant is smaller than that of a mature infant, it is also more fragile. Excessive pressure might result in a subdural or intraventricular hemorrhage that could be fatal. The woman may therefore need an episiotomy incision larger than usual. Forceps may also be used at delivery to reduce pressure on the fetal head.

The cord of the preterm infant is usually clamped immediately rather than waiting for the pulsating to halt. This is because an immature infant has a difficult time excreting the large amount of bilirubin that will be formed if this extra blood is added to the circulation. The extra amount of blood may also overburden the circulatory system.

FOCUS ON NURSING RESEARCH

What Are the Needs of Women in Preterm Labor?

To answer this question, nurse researchers asked 14 postpartum women who had experienced preterm labor what they perceived as their greatest needs. Findings revealed the 10 most important needs of these women were:

• To be asked opinions and preferences regarding type of delivery

• To be informed of how my baby is tolerating the labor process

• To have the father of my baby stay during labor

• To have questions answered honestly

• To be assured of a safe outcome for my baby

• To have explanations given in simple terms

• To be told about other patients and/or hospital personnel who can discuss care of my children at home

• To have the physician who specializes in preterm babies discuss what the baby will look like, how big the baby will be, and what support measures the baby will need, before the baby is born

• To know why labor began prematurely

• To feel that hospital personnel care about me

Lynam, L. E., & Miller, M. A. (1992). Mothers' and nurses' perceptions of the needs of women experiencing preterm labor. *Journal of Obstetric, Gynecologic and Neonatal Nursing, 21,* 126.

Nursing Diagnoses and Related Interventions

Primary nursing diagnoses for the woman with preterm labor that cannot be halted are:

• Fear related to uncertain outcome of pregnancy
• Pain related to labor contractions
• Self-esteem disturbance related to inability to carry pregnancy to term
• High risk for fetal injury related to preterm birth
• Anger related to early onset of labor

Be certain that goals established for care are realistic; although there are many measures available to help the preterm baby adjust to birth, the baby born preterm will be at risk for a variety of medical problems (see Chapter 26).

Nursing Diagnosis: Self-esteem disturbance related to feelings of responsibility for preterm labor

Goal: Client will demonstrate understanding of areas of pregnancy over which she does and does not have control (i.e., labor beginning); will express positive hopes for future.

Outcome Criteria: Client expresses feelings and worries to nurse and states that it is unknown why labor begins but that she knows she is not responsible for her labor beginning prematurely.

A woman in preterm labor is undergoing an extreme crisis situation. She cannot help asking herself, "What did I do to cause this?" People who are looking for reasons find them. She may believe that the large meal she ate the night before is responsible because it "crowded out" the fetus. She may worry that sexual relations the night before precipitated the preterm labor. She needs to be assured that in no way is preterm labor her fault. Why labor begins at all is still a mystery (see Chapter 18). Why it sometimes begins prematurely is even more mysterious.

Provide Opportunity for Open Discussion. Time spent taking the initial history or timing contractions presents an opportunity to bring the concern out in the open: "Did Dr. Smith explain to you that labor sometimes begins early this way without any reason?" "Some women worry that they did something to bring on preterm labor. Have you had any thoughts like that?"

Most women in preterm labor are anxious to talk to someone who gives them any opening to express this concern. Help the woman to be able to say to herself afterward, "I'm sorry this happened. I'd give anything to stop it from happening. I didn't mean for it to happen. *But it was not my fault.*"

Be careful at the same time not to give either false reassurances about the health or weight of the child or be overly pessimistic in an effort to relieve any guilt. If the woman is going to establish a good mother–infant relationship, she needs to perceive her child as viable. At the point that labor cannot be stopped, find a middle ground. "The baby's heartbeat is good. Labor is going well. Let's face one thing at a time."

Provide Support and Reassurance. A woman in preterm labor that cannot be halted needs a support person with her because she is apt to be more concerned than the average person about being alone in labor. She needs frequent assurance during labor that she is breathing well with contractions or just that she is "doing well." She may not be mentally prepared for labor because it has come unexpectedly. During the postpartal period a woman may need continued reassurance. Helping rebuild self-esteem this way can better prepare her to be ready to be a mother to her preterm infant.

Preterm Premature Rupture of Membranes

Preterm premature rupture of membranes (PPROM) is rupture of fetal membranes with loss of amniotic fluid before labor begins either at term or earlier in pregnancy. The cause of preterm premature rupture is unknown but it is associated with infection of the membranes (chorioamnionitis) before rupture. If this occurs early in pregnancy, it poses a major threat to the fetus, because, following rupture, the seal to the fetus is lost and uterine and fetal infection may occur. Preterm labor may follow rupture, posing the additional risk of immature birth to the fetus. Inhibition of labor is rarely used following rupture of membranes because it may effectively halt labor, but if this results in infection, fetal welfare will not be substantially benefitted.

A second complication that can occur with premature membrane rupture is increased pressure on the umbilical cord or prolapse (extension of the cord out of the uterine cavity into the vagina), particularly if rupture happens when the fetal head is still too small to fit the cervix firmly. An additional risk to the fetus of remaining in a non–fluid-filled environment is the development of a Potter-like syndrome of distorted facial features and pulmonary hypoplasia (Garite, 1990).

Assessment

Rupture of the membranes is suggested by the history. A woman will usually describe a sudden gush of clear fluid from the vagina, with continued minimal leakage. Occasionally, a woman will mistake urinary incontinence caused by exertion for rupture of the membranes. Amniotic fluid cannot be differentiated from urine by appearance, so a sterile vaginal speculum exam is done

to observe for vaginal pooling of fluid. A strip of nitrazine test paper is dipped into this; amniotic fluid will cause an alkaline reaction on the paper (appears blue) and urine an acidic reaction (remains yellow). Another test used is ferning. A swab taken from the vagina is spread on a slide, allowed to dry, and observed under a microscope: amniotic fluid has a high estrogen content so shows a ferning pattern; urine will not (Rosemond et al., 1990). Because preterm premature rupture of membranes is associated with vaginal infection, cultures for *Neisseria gonorrhoeae*, beta-streptococcus, and chlamydia are usually taken following rupture. If there is a question as to whether membranes have ruptured, a sonogram may be ordered to assess amniotic fluid index. Avoid doing a vaginal examination as the risk of infection rises significantly when digital examinations are performed after premature rupture of membranes (Lewis et al., 1992).

If the fetus is estimated to be mature enough to survive in an extrauterine environment at the time of rupture and labor does not begin within 24 hours, labor contractions are usually induced at the end of that time period by intravenous administration of oxytocin to prevent infection.

Therapeutic Management

If labor does not begin and the fetus is too young to survive outside the uterus, the woman will be placed on bedrest either in the hospital or at home. The time between rupture and birth of the infant is called the latency period. Although prophylactic administration of antibiotics during this period seems attractive, there is little evidence that such administration delays the onset of labor. It is usually not necessary to administer a corticosteroid to accelerate fetal lung maturity following rupture of membranes as the lack of amniotic fluid causes early maturation of lung tissue by itself. In addition to not being necessary, administration of a corticosteroid may increase the possibility of maternal infection (Anderson & Merkatz, 1990).

If home, a woman is instructed to take her temperature twice a day and to report a fever (a temperature greater than 100.4°F), uterine tenderness, or odorous vaginal discharge. She should refrain from tub bathing, coitus, and douching because of the danger of introducing infection. White cell count will need to be assessed daily: a count of more than 18,000/mm^3 to 20,000/mm^3 suggests infection is present.

Nursing Diagnoses and Related Interventions

Nursing Diagnosis: High risk for infection related to preterm premature rupture of membranes without accompanying labor

Goal: No infection will develop during the period between membrane rupture and birth of the baby.

Outcome Criteria: Maternal white blood cell count is less than 18,000/mm^3; maternal temperature is less than 100.4°F.

An infection can be dangerous for both the mother and the fetus. After the initial observation period and before the woman is discharged to home care, be certain that she knows how to read a thermometer (have her demonstrate her knowledge); that she has specific instructions (i.e., what degree of temperature to report and when she should report to her physician for her first check-up); and that she understands that bedrest should be strictly followed. Help her make arrangements for the daily white blood cell count (through a laboratory service or home care nurse). Be certain she knows that as soon as the fetus is mature, she will be delivered by labor induction.

There are many misconceptions about the agony of labor following preterm premature rupture of the membranes (dry labor). Every day the woman hopes that the fetus is ready to be born, ending the long wait, yet she is also afraid to begin labor. She needs a great deal of support for the remainder of the pregnancy and reassurance that because amniotic fluid is always being formed, there is no such thing as a "dry" labor. Intrauterine amnioinfusion may be used to supply additional uterine fluid and help protect the umbilical cord from compression and the fetus from compression deformities or pulmonary hypoplasia (see Chapter 18).

Key Points

- Home care is more cost effective than hospital care. Women with preterm labor or preterm premature rupture of the membranes can be monitored on bedrest at home.
- Home care requires careful planning and a combined effort between home care and hospital personnel so there is collaboration and continuity between the two types of care.
- Labor is preterm if it occurs after 20 weeks and before the end of the 37th week of pregnancy. A woman is said to be in preterm labor when she has had uterine contractions every 10 minutes for 1 hour.
- Tocolytics are drugs that can halt labor. The most frequent ones used are magnesium sulfate and β-adrenergic agents such as ritodrine (Yutopar) and terbutaline (Brethine). All these drugs have toxic effects. Magnesium sulfate should not be administered unless the maternal respiratory rate is more than 12/min, urine output is more than 30 mL/h, and a patellar reflex is present. Beta-adrenergic drugs (rito-

drine and terbutaline) should not be administered if the maternal pulse is more than 120 bpm.
- Once preterm labor is halted, women can be discharged to home care. They need instructions in uterine monitoring and the importance of taking their tocolytic consistently and on time.
- Preterm premature rupture of the membranes is tearing of the fetal membranes with loss of amniotic fluid before the pregnancy is at term. Preterm premature rupture is a serious complication because following rupture, there is a high risk of fetal and uterine infection (chorioamnionitis).
- If a fetus is not yet at a point of viability, following preterm premature rupture of the membranes the woman may be discharged to home care. Important aspects of care are bedrest and assessment of maternal temperature, white blood count, and fetal well being.

Critical Thinking Exercises

1. Amy is an 18-year-old on bedrest at home following preterm premature rupture of membranes at 32 weeks of pregnancy. Amy belonged to a competitive synchronized swimming team before she became pregnant. She is concerned that she will miss too much school to be able to graduate and will be so weak from lack of exercise by the time she delivers that she won't be able to take care of a newborn.
   a. Identify areas for assessment that will help you to assure that Amy is not developing chorioamnionitis. What questions would you want to ask to be certain that she is maintaining bedrest?
   b. Outline patient teaching points that address her concerns about lack of exercise.
   c. Amy is home alone most of the day because her parents work. Her boyfriend visits between 9 AM and 10 AM and school friends visit in the afternoon. What time of the day would be best to schedule a home visit for Amy? What signs and symptoms of preterm labor would you want her to know?
2. Mary Beth is a woman who has started preterm labor at 32 weeks of pregnancy.
   a. Summarize conditions you would want to assess before Mary Beth is begun on a tocolytic to halt labor.
   b. What if Mary Beth states that she doesn't want the baby? How would this influence care?
   c. Mary Beth's contractions are effectively halted and she is being cared for at home. Identify measures you would instruct her to take if she should start to feel contractions.

References

Allbert, J. R., et al. (1992). Subcutaneous tocolytic infusion therapy for patients at very high risk for preterm birth. *Journal of Perinatology, 12,* 28.

Anderson, H. F., & Merkatz, I. R. (1990). Preterm labor. In J. R. Scott et al., *Danforth's obstetrics and gynecology* (6th ed.). Philadelphia: J.B. Lippincott.

Cowan, M. (1993). Home care of the pregnant woman using terbutaline. *MCN: American Journal of Maternal Child Nursing, 18,* 86.

Creasy, R. K., & Merkatz, I. R. (1990). Prevention of preterm birth: Clinical opinion. *Obstetrics and Gynecology, 76,* 2S.

Creasy, R. K. (1991). Preventing preterm birth. *New England Journal of Medicine, 325,* 727.

Crowley, P., et al. (1990). The effects of corticosteroid administration before preterm delivery: An overview of the evidence from controlled trials. *British Journal of Obstetrics and Gynaecology, 97,* 11.

Department of Health and Human Services. (1991). *Healthy people 2000.* Washington, D. C.: Public Health Service.

Dineen, K., et al. (1992). Antepartum home-care services of high-risk women. *Journal of Obstetric, Gynecologic and Neonatal Nursing, 21,* 121.

Eganhouse, D. J., et al. (1992). Nursing assessment and responsibilities in monitoring the preterm pregnancy. *Journal of Obstetric, Gynecologic and Neonatal Nursing, 21,* 355.

Engstrom, J. L., & Sittler, C. P. (1993). Fundal height measurement. *Journal of Nurse Midwifery, 38,* 5.

Garite, T. J. (1990). Premature rupture of membranes. In J. R. Scott et al., *Danforth's obstetrics and gynecology* (6th ed.). Philadelphia: J.B. Lippincott.

Hill, W. C., & Lambertz, E. L. (1990). Let's get rid of the term Braxton Hicks contractions. *Obstetrics and Gynecology, 75,* 709.

Iams, J. D., et al. (1990). Symptoms that precede preterm labor and preterm premature rupture of the membranes. *American Journal of Obstetrics and Gynecology, 162,* 486.

Infante-Rivard, C., et al. (1993). Pregnancy loss and work schedule during pregnancy. *Epidemiology 4,* 1.

Kragt, H., & Keirse, M. J. (1990). How accurate is a woman's diagnosis of threatened preterm delivery? *British Journal of Obstetrics and Gynecology, 97,* 317.

Lewis, D., et al. (1992). Effects of digital vaginal examinations on latency period in preterm premature rupture of membranes. *Obstetrics and Gynecology, 80,* 630.

Lynam, L. E., & Miller, M.A. (1992). Mothers' and nurses' perceptions of the needs of women experiencing preterm labor. *Journal of Obstetric, Gynecologic and Neonatal Nursing, 21,* 126.

May, K. A. (1994). Impact of maternal activity restriction for preterm labor on the expectant father. *Journal of Obstetric, Gynecologic and Neonatal Nursing, 23,* 246.

Papke, K. R. (1993). Management of preterm labor and prevention of premature delivery. *Nursing Clinics of North America, 28,* 279.

Poland, M. L., et al. (1992). Effects of a home visiting program on prenatal care and birthweight: A case comparison study. *Journal of Community Health, 17,* 221.

Rosemond, R. L., et al. (1990). Ferning of amniotic fluid contaminated with blood. *Obstetrics and Gynecology, 75,* 338.

Sala, D. J., & Moise, K. J. (1990). The treatment of preterm labor using a portable subcutaneous terbutaline pump. *Journal of Obstetric, Gynecologic and Neonatal Nursing, 19,* 108.

Smith, C. V., Davis, S. A., & Rayburn, W. F. (1992). Patients' acceptance of monitoring fetal movement. *Journal of Reproductive Medicine, 37,* 144.

Starn, J. R. (1992). Community health nursing visits for at-risk women and infants. *Journal of Community Health Nursing, 9,* 103.

Travis, B.E., & McCullough, J. M. (1993). Pharmacotherapy of preterm labor. *Pharmacotherapy, 13,* 28.

Villar, J., et al. (1992). A randomized trial of psychosocial support during high risk pregnancies. *New England Journal of Medicine, 327,* 1266.

Suggested Readings

Brown, D. (1992). All pregnant women need prenatal care. *RN, 55,* 88.

Fresquez, M. L., et al. (1992). Advancement of the nursing role in antepartum fetal evaluation. *Journal of Perinatology and Neonatal Nursing, 5,* 16.

Gjerdingen, D. K. (1992). Premature labor: Risk assessment, etiologic factors, and diagnosis. *Journal of the American Board of Family Practice, 5,* 495.

Goodwin, L. (1992). Home fetal assessment. *Journal of Perinatology and Neonatal Nursing, 5,* 33.

Gregor, C. L., et al. (1992). Antepartum fetal assessment techniques: An update for today's perinatal nurse. *Journal of Perinatology and Neonatal Nursing, 5,* 1.

Hill, W. C., et al. (1990). Home uterine activity monitoring is associated with a reduction in preterm birth. *Obstetrics and Gynecology, 76,* 13S.

Kosasa, T. S., et al. (1990). Evaluation of the cost-effectiveness of home monitoring of uterine contractions. *Obstetrics and Gynecology, 76,* 71S.

Moss, N., & Carver, K. (1993). Pregnant women at work: Sociodemographic perspectives. *American Journal of Industrial Medicine, 23,* 541.

Murphy, P. M. (1992). Problem pregnancies: Hemorrhagic complications in the third trimester. *Journal of Emergency Medical Services, 17,* 44.

Stainton, M. C. (1994). Supporting family functioning during a high risk pregnancy. *MCN: American Journal of Maternal Child Nursing, 19,* 24.

Update on Yutopar for preterm labor. (1992). *Nurses Drug Alert, 16,* 71.

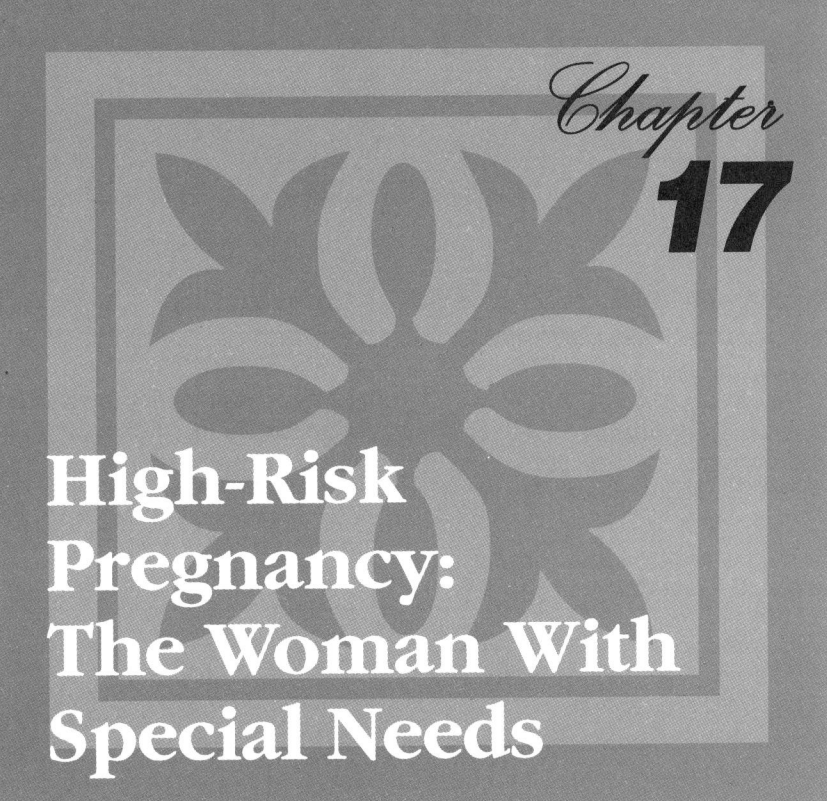

Chapter 17

High-Risk Pregnancy: The Woman With Special Needs

Key Terms

- *autonomic dysreflexia*
- *drug dependence*
- *drug tolerance*
- *elderly primipara*

Objectives

After mastering the contents of this chapter, you should be able to:

1. Describe the risks of pregnancy in the woman with special needs, such as the adolescent, the woman over age 35, the woman with a drug dependency, and the woman with a disability.

2. Assess the woman with special needs for safe health practices during pregnancy.

3. State nursing diagnoses related to pregnancy for the woman with special needs.

4. Plan nursing care to respect the special growth and development needs of the adolescent and the woman over age 35 and the specific strengths and weaknesses of the woman with a physical disability or drug dependency during pregnancy.

5. Implement nursing care that is effective with a woman with special needs, such as education about the importance of exercise or participation in a drug withdrawal program.

6. Evaluate outcome criteria to be certain that goals for care have been achieved.

7. Identify National Health Goals related to the woman with a special need that nurses can be instrumental in helping the nation to achieve.

8. Identify areas related to care of the woman with special needs during pregnancy that would benefit from additional nursing research.

9. Use critical thinking to analyze ways that nursing care of the pregnant woman with a special need can be optimally family centered.

10. Synthesize knowledge of the risks of pregnancy with age extremes, drug use, and disability with nursing process to achieve quality maternal and child health nursing care.

Adele Pillitteri: MATERNAL AND CHILD HEALTH NURSING, 2nd Edition. © 1995 Adele Pillitteri.

Many women seen in a prenatal care setting do not fit the description of the average pregnant woman—a well, young adult who maintains healthy patterns of living. Chapter 14 described high-risk pregnancy for women who are ill when they become pregnant and for those who develop an illness while pregnant. Chapter 15 discussed high-risk pregnancy for women who develop a complication related to the pregnancy itself. This chapter describes high-risk pregnancy for women with other special needs—those who are at the two age extremes (adolescents and "elderly primipara"), those who have a disability, such as a spinal cord injury or hearing impairment, and those who are drug dependent.

The pregnancy rate is increasing among adolescents and women over age 35. Adolescents require special consideration because they are physically and psychosocially immature. Women over age 35 need special consideration because their bodies may have passed a point of optimum childbearing; in addition, psychosocial adjustment to pregnancy (especially a first pregnancy) at this time in life may be difficult.

The pregnancy rate also is increasing among women with mental and physical disabilities, including disabilities that might have precluded pregnancy even a few years ago. These conditions present a challenge to childbearing and childrearing but do not necessarily prevent women from establishing their own families. Supportive nursing care that considers the limitations imposed by a particular disability, while focusing on the normal aspects of childbearing and childrearing, is vital to these women.

The pregnancies of women who are drug dependent also require a great deal of nursing support and care. Ideally, a woman would give up her substance abuse for the health of the fetus, but that may not be possible; every effort must be made to provide enough prenatal care and attention to protect the fetus in other ways. National Health Goals related to women with special needs during pregnancy are shown in the Focus on National Health Goals box.

 NURSING PROCESS OVERVIEW
for Care of the Pregnant Woman
With Special Needs

ASSESSMENT

It is important always to assess the strengths and weaknesses of the individual client to establish accurate nursing diagnoses and realistic goals and to plan effective nursing interventions. When a client has a special need, however, this part of the assessment becomes even more essential. Establishing as thorough a data base as possible early in pregnancy helps to predict the risks a woman will undergo when the risks of pregnancy are increased by age, physical disability, or unhealthy lifestyle.

When caring for the woman with a physically disabling condition, keep in mind that physical disabilities occur in degrees; establish, first, the impact of the disability on the woman's life before offering any care or guidance for care measures during pregnancy. Be certain to assess not only physical limitations and abilities but also psychosocial or emotional strengths. The capacity of the woman with special needs to adapt to pregnancy will depend not only on physical capabilities but on the ability to persevere against odds and overcome what the average woman might think of as unsurmountable obstacles. The woman with a spinal cord injury, for example, is likely to have developed ways of coping in daily life that may never occur to someone who has not experienced that disability.

For the drug-dependent woman, pregnancy may be the avenue by which she can find the strength to break a drug habit. Other women cannot accomplish this. Your main goal should be to encourage her to keep coming for prenatal care. As long as she feels comfortable with you during regular visits, you may be able to establish a trusting relationship that could eventually provide her

with the confidence to try a more healthful pattern of living.

NURSING DIAGNOSIS

Nursing diagnoses established for pregnant women with special needs are different in degree, but not substance, from the nursing diagnoses established for all pregnant women. As with any client, you want to be especially careful to establish goals that are realistic for that person, given her particular condition or situation. The adolescent, for instance, cannot achieve goals that rely on her making decisions independently if her family is still making decisions for her. If a pregnant adolescent is still growing, nutrition is an important problem for her and for the fetus. Examples of diagnoses are:

FOCUS ON
National Health Goals

A number of National Health Goals have been formulated to improve the health of women with special needs during pregnancy. These are:

- Reduce pregnancy among girls aged 17 and younger to no more than 50/1000 adolescents from a baseline of 71/1000.

- Increase the proportion of high school seniors who perceive social disapproval associated with the heavy use of alcohol, occasional use of marijuana, and experimentation with cocaine.

- Increase abstinence from cocaine and marijuana by pregnant women by at least 20% (DHHS, 1991).

Nurses can be instrumental in helping the nation to achieve these goals by teaching adolescents about the dangers of substance abuse and the complications, both psychologically and physically, of teenage pregnancy.

Nurses can add knowledge to this area by being active research investigators. Special topics that could be investigated are what is the most effective way to impress adolescents with the dangers of substance abuse; what would be the ideal birth control measure for adolescents (one that would actually be used); and how does the typical woman over 35 who becomes pregnant integrate the pregnancy into her life? As more and more women over 40 are becoming pregnant, the exact effects of pregnancy on this age group and their adjustment to it also need to be investigated.

- High risk for altered nutrition, less than body requirements, related to combined needs of adolescence and pregnancy
- High risk for fetal injury related to drug and alcohol use
- Impaired mobility related to spinal cord injury
- High risk for injury related to unstable balance
- Impaired verbal communication related to spastic muscle functioning
- Impaired home maintenance management related to hearing loss
- Family coping: Potential for growth, related to commitment to have a child in the face of a disabling condition

PLANNING

Often, the pregnant woman with a special need already has some significant stressors to deal with in her life. For the teenager, adolescence itself is a period of growth and change that can be stressful for her and her family. The physically disabled woman must constantly cope with a condition that must be considered in all activities, even if she has adjusted completely to the limitations such a disability imposes. The drug-dependent woman is held hostage by a life-threatening habit.

Pregnancy brings a new overlay of stressors that can prove overwhelming if the woman has no outside support. Planning for the pregnant woman with a special need often involves identifying support people who can help her adjust to the added burden of pregnancy. This support can consist of family, friends, and health care providers. If the woman is not totally independent in her care, you will have to do some planning with her support person, who may be the person who actually carries out the proposed action. At the same time you are planning, be sure not to ignore the woman and plan around her. Only if she approves of the plan can pregnancy be the enjoyable experience it should be. This principle applies as much to the adolescent as it does to the disabled woman.

A major problem encountered when planning with the pregnant adolescent is that she may have difficulty accepting the reality of the pregnancy and may not be interested in pursuing prenatal care.

Some primiparas older than 35 may have delayed pregnancy to pursue further education or solidify a loving, stable relationship. Remember that the woman who has been submerged in a career instead of the world of babies and homemaking may, like the adolescent, be less informed about normal pregnancy findings or healthful pregnancy practices than the average woman. Be certain that you do not equate a woman's knowledge in one field, such as chemistry or law, with her knowledge of prenatal care.

Plans should include ways to strengthen confidence

and self-esteem, as these are crucial attributes for the mother. These also are areas in which the woman with a special need, especially one who perceives herself as too young or too old or who has experienced physical dysfunction, may not have developed fully. Drug dependence itself may be related to feelings of lowered self-worth, which may have been strengthened if the drug-dependent woman has tried unsuccessfully to limit her drug intake in the past.

Being certain that plans are established in a wide range of areas helps to ensure that planning is comprehensive. Be certain, too, to include safe care of the newborn in plans for all women with special needs. Once the infant is born, it is too late to make these plans in a comprehensive manner.

IMPLEMENTATION

The goal of interventions for the high-risk pregnant woman is to prevent pregnancy complications. A great deal of time is spent teaching and encouraging the woman with any special need to determine how best to manage her pregnancy according to her particular situation.

A high proportion of adolescents unfortunately do not seek prenatal care early in pregnancy because they deny that they are, in fact, pregnant. Others simply may not feel comfortable in a health care facility. The same may be true of the woman with a drug dependency who fears reprisals from health care providers regarding her drug use. A welcoming attitude, with the focus on the pregnancy and the baby, and avoidance of recriminations regarding the woman's youth or circumstances are essential to attracting such women to prenatal care and keeping them coming for regular visits. (They may hear from a friend that the staff members at your clinic are helpful, not judgmental, and then take the first step into your facility.) Allow adolescents as many independent decisions as they are capable of making at prenatal visits, to strengthen their self-esteem.

Some nursing interventions for women who are physically disabled will be modifications of interventions associated with typical pregnancy-related procedures. For example, it may be necessary to modify a pelvic examination when a woman is not able to place her legs in table stirrups. Modifying procedures in this way develops your ability to individualize nursing interventions for all women, improving your nursing care as a whole.

EVALUATION

Evaluation of nursing interventions in the care of the pregnant woman with a special need will often focus on the woman's physical and emotional readiness for childbearing, maintenance of fetal health, and ability of the woman to provide a safe and healthy environment for her newborn. Some examples of outcome criteria might be:

- Client states she will use walker to maintain balance during pregnancy.
- Adolescent lists intake of adequate nutrition even with frequent meals at fast-food restaurants.
- Family members state they have been able to adjust to changing demands of pregnancy in mother with cerebral palsy.

The Pregnant Adolescent

Adolescent pregnancy is not a new phenomenon. In the 18th century, it was common for women to marry at an early age, often by age 16; these young women often found themselves pregnant with their first child by age 17.

In today's society, however, marriage during the teenage years is unusual, and teenage pregnancy without marriage is generally not condoned. Even so, the pregnancy rate is increasing in the adolescent population. Seven percent of births in the United States are to girls under 18 years (DHHS, 1993). A combination of factors has contributed to the rising rate of teenage pregnancy: the earlier age of menarche in girls (many girls begin menstruating at age 10, so are ovulating and able to conceive by age 11) (Cunningham et al., 1993); an increase in the rate of sexual activity among teenagers; and a lack of knowledge (or inability to use) contraceptive information among sexually active teenagers.

The inability of adolescents to obtain adequate knowledge of contraceptive measures is an issue that can be addressed by the health care profession. Providing information, however, does not always resolve the problem entirely because adolescents often lack money to purchase such protection as birth control pills or a diaphragm. In addition, the egocentric phenomenon at adolescence makes the sexually active teenager believe that she just will not become pregnant. On the other hand, some adolescent girls actually plan pregnancy. They feel that being pregnant will free them from an intolerable school or home situation and will give them someone to love. This phenomenon must be recognized because it puts a tremendous responsibility on a newborn baby to furnish love and change a girl's life: child abuse can occur when the newborn cannot meet such expectations.

At one time, pregnant, unmarried girls were sent to a "secret" home or shelter where they would stay through the pregnancy, deliver, place the child for adoption, and return home as if nothing had happened to them. But something did happen, as much as the girl and her family wanted to pretend it did not; the girl was left with the psychological scars of starting to love a kicking stranger inside her and then having to give the newborn away and never mention him or her again. Today, pregnant girls attend prenatal clinics or come to physician's offices just as most older women do. They deliver in birthing rooms at hospitals, and as many as 90% keep their babies. Few deliver in alternative birth centers since adolescent pregnancy is considered high risk. Home birth is not recommended for the same reason.

Developmental Crises of Adolescence

Adolescence is a vulnerable time for pregnancy because the developmental tasks of pregnancy are superimposed on those of adolescence. The developmental tasks of the average adolescent are fourfold: to establish a sense of self-worth and a value system; to establish lasting relationships; to emancipate from parents; and to choose a vocation (Erikson, 1963). A girl who is in the process of separating from her parents may be devastated by the knowledge that in less than a year someone will be dependent on her. She may have decreased ability to separate from her parents when she realizes she is pregnant because she needs their financial help more than ever to obtain prenatal care and buy prenatal vitamins. If she must depend on her parent's health insurance, she may feel virtually trapped into dependence. Helping adolescents at health care visits to make their own health care decisions helps them feel independent in the middle of this forced dependency. Consider, for example, the decision that the adolescent must make about where to hang her medication reminder chart: if it hangs in the kitchen, her mother will monitor it; in her bedroom or in her school locker, she alone will monitor it. An adolescent may not be able to choose when she comes for care (her mother has the car to drive her only on Tuesday afternoons), but during a visit she can do many things to feel independent (weigh herself, hold a mirror to view the pelvic examination, be interviewed apart from her parent).

Parents may have difficulty allowing a daughter to participate in making her own health care decisions. You may need to remind them that a pregnant woman may sign permission for her own care. Soon she will be caring for an infant, so she needs this practice in independence.

Pregnancy may interfere with the development of a healthy sexual relationship and cause difficulty in establishing future intimate relationships if the girl realizes that her present relationship has led to a situation detrimental to her. To prevent this, it is useful to help her view the pregnancy as a growth-producing experience. Most people can point to a day in their life when they "grew up" (perhaps a day a parent became ill or the day they left home for college). This pregnancy can be a "growing-up" revelation or a growth-producing experience for her.

Establishing a value system or sense of identity can be difficult if health care personnel treat a pregnant adolescent as though she were irresponsible. Encouraging her to continue school is crucial to her self-esteem and to her future, as well as to the future of her unborn child.

Prenatal Assessment

Adolescents are considered high-risk clients because they have a high incidence of pregnancy-induced hypertension and iron deficiency anemia. They have a higher incidence of preterm birth, with low-birth-weight infants (Jacono et al., 1992). They tend to give birth to high-risk infants. Early and consistent prenatal care is essential to their health and the health of their baby (Burnhill, 1994).

Unfortunately, many adolescents do not seek prenatal care until late in their pregnancies. This may be partly due to the girl's denial of the pregnancy. Not going for prenatal care is also a way of protecting the pregnancy—if she doesn't tell anyone, no one can suggest that she terminate it. After the 6th month, abortion is no longer a possibility so she can feel free to come for care without being subjected to this pressure.

Other factors contributing to the lack of prenatal care are lack of knowledge of the importance of prenatal care and dependence on others for transportation. The girl may feel awkward in a prenatal setting (an adult setting) and frightened about her first pelvic examination. Ideally, every community should have a facility that is designed especially for adolescents; if this is not possible, all settings should accommodate adolescents' needs so this last reason for poor prenatal care can be eliminated. Lack of adequate facilities for pregnant adolescents is denial of the existence of adolescent pregnancy on the part of health care providers and the community. Adolescents have a difficult time relating to authority figures. A primary nursing or case management approach may be the most effective method for providing care during the prenatal period for adolescents, to minimize the number of health care providers the girl is exposed to.

Health History

A detailed health history should be taken at the first prenatal health care visit. It is best to take this history without the girl's parents present. The girl needs practice in being responsible for her own health, and having to account for her health practices helps her to do this. It also helps prevent her from fabricating an answer to please a parent.

Some adolescents present not with the acknowledgment that they are pregnant but with concerns such as "weight gain" or they feel "tired all the time." They depend on health care providers to think of pregnancy as a possible reason for their symptoms. This is part of denial or pregnancy protection. Think of possible preg-

nancy when an adolescent's symptoms are vague and hard to define. If you miss the importance of what she is saying when she mentions feeling "tired" or "nauseated," she may ask if someone will feel her stomach. If you tell her that this is not necessary for any of the symptoms she has mentioned, she may describe bigger symptoms, such as "terrible stomach pain." Think of possible pregnancy when you hear such a "growing" history.

Many adolescents feel that their world is totally separate from the adult world and, to keep it separate, do not voluntarily share information. Be certain in interviewing adolescents that you press for the responses you need to assess safely and do not accept statements such as "I eat okay" as a nutrition history or "I'm a very active person" as a history of rest and activity.

If the adolescent delayed seeking health care, ask for the reason at her first prenatal visit. Acknowledge that "protecting" the pregnancy is a desirable motive, but a better method of doing that in the future is to continue with prenatal care.

If a parent does accompany the girl, ask the parent separately what, if any, concerns he or she wishes to discuss. A young adolescent is still a daughter, and a parent may be as concerned about her health during this pregnancy as he or she was at health visits when the girl was being seen for a cold or sports injury.

The baby's father may accompany the girl into the clinic or office to have the diagnosis established. Although he may not have a legal right to participate in the girl's decision concerning pregnancy, abortion, or whether the child will be adopted at the pregnancy's end, he may not be devoid of feelings for either the girl or the conceived child. If he is an adolescent, he may feel sorrow that because of his age he cannot provide adequately for the girl and baby. If a complication occurs, he may feel genuine grief. The concept of the boy as one who irresponsibly uses a girl reveals a lack of understanding of human behavior, especially that of adolescents. He will need compassionate understanding as well as education in preventing further pregnancies. Helping him offer support in the present pregnancy helps him to better define his role.

Adolescents have not necessarily been exposed to many pregnant women, so they may need extra teaching to help them become aware of common pregnancy symptoms such as urinary frequency, fatigue, and vaginal discharge. Asking what symptoms an adolescent is having, and reassuring her that they are part of a normal pregnancy, will help prevent her from attempting to treat them with potentially teratogenic over-the-counter medications.

As pregnancy progresses, listen for signs of "nest-building" behavior during a pregnancy history. An adolescent girl may not have the financial resources for buying clothing or a baby bed. She may reveal nest-building feelings by asking an increasing number of questions about newborns. Suggesting that she make one article of clothing for the baby or save her own money for one article is a way of actively involving her in the pregnancy and provides a measure of nest-building potential (the girl who, week after week, spends her money on something else is probably not as involved in the pregnancy as the girl who puts away even 25 cents each week toward a pair of baby shoes).

Some adolescents have difficulty telling their parents about the pregnancy. They need help in knowing how to tell someone what is happening. Role playing or simulated game playing may be an effective technique for this. Most girls report on a second visit that their parents were not nearly as angry as they had anticipated. Some parents react as if they had been waiting to hear this news, having accepted it as inevitable months before.

Family Profile. Adolescents may leave home if their family disapproves of the pregnancy. Others do not leave home but separate themselves emotionally from their family. Trying to manage by themselves leaves young girls with tremendous financial strain and a devastating sense of loneliness. Ask the girl at prenatal visits where she is living, what the source of her income is, and whom she would call if she suddenly became ill.

Asking about home life may reveal a dysfunctional family or an incest relationship as the cause of the pregnancy. If the girl is under legal age, incest is considered child abuse; inform yourself about how your state handles this and make the necessary report.

Because of family relation problems, a girl may need help in making arrangements for the next few months. Will her parents allow her to live at home during the pregnancy? If not, is there a relative she may go to? Is there an institution such as a Salvation Army home for unwed mothers in the community that will shelter her during her pregnancy? What kind of financial support does she need? Family and social support for pregnant adolescents have been shown to be important influences on the maintenance of a healthy pregnancy lifestyle and, thus, prevention of low birth weight in their children.

Ask if the girl is planning to continue with school. Pregnancy is an egocentric time when outside interests do not always seem important. Help her to see that the months of pregnancy will go faster if she is busy. Remaining in and doing well in school is a way of keeping busy as well as preparing for the future.

A high school education is necessary to obtain marketable skills. A girl will have little chance of supporting herself and her baby later if she is not allowed to continue with her education. Once she delivers the baby, returning to school will be difficult because she may have baby sitter problems and because she may feel she is more mature than the other girls (or the other girls may make her feel this way). Any school that obtains

federal money cannot discriminate against students because they have a physical disability. Many states interpret pregnancy as a physically disabling condition, so in those states a girl cannot be forced to leave school (or even asked to go to an alternate school) because of pregnancy. You may need to advocate for the girl with the school committee of the physically disabled for a proper school placement.

Day History. Few adolescents are willing to provide detailed day histories unless the purpose of a day history is well explained. Tell her the purpose of the history is to learn more about her as a whole person, not to discover if she is doing things during the day she should not do. Adolescents are private people; to allow you to walk through their adolescent world for a day is a breach of adolescent philosophy.

Ask in particular about nutritional practices, daily activity, use of drugs, and whether they have friends who can support them through this experience.

Ask if she is taking any medicine. Some adolescents take acne medication that is potentially teratogenic, such as tetracycline or isotretinoin (Accutane). Some take frequent doses of aspirin for tension (studying) headaches. Impress upon her the importance of not taking any medication—even nonprescription medication—without prior approval from her physician or nurse-midwife.

Physical Examination

Physical examination procedures with pertinent adolescent findings are discussed in Chapter 28. A statement such as "Oh, you're starting to have colostrum," a positive finding of pregnancy, may be frightening to an adolescent who does not know what colostrum is.

A better way to phrase a finding might be "Your hair looks healthy and well textured; you must be eating healthy foods; later we'll talk about ways to make sure you're including extra food that's adequate for your body's increased needs." This kind of feedback makes the health examination a learning experience, relieves anxiety for adolescents who tend to be very concerned about body appearance, and provides a way of encouraging healthy behavior patterns.

Adolescents are prone to pregnancy-induced hypertension, so be certain to obtain a baseline blood pressure determination at the first prenatal visit. Few adolescents are told the results of blood pressure determinations at health maintenance visits so they will not know what their typical finding is. Make a point of informing them of their blood pressure reading to encourage future active health care participation. Adolescents are often active in a waiting room—walking to get a magazine, returning it, looking out the window; be certain that the girl has 15 minutes of rest before you take a blood pressure or the recording will be falsely high.

Use a Doppler technique to obtain fetal heart tones,

if possible, as hearing the fetal heart helps the adolescent acknowledge the reality of her pregnancy. For the same reason, make a point of assessing fundal height growth from visit to visit to show that the baby is growing.

Adolescents who use drugs may be reluctant to supply a urine specimen for testing because they are afraid you are secretly looking for evidence. In this instance, you may receive a cupful of water in place of a urine specimen. If in doubt as to the substance you are testing, check the specific gravity. The specific gravity of water is 1.000, whereas urine specific gravity ranges from 1.003 to 1.030.

Many adolescents like to weigh themselves at prenatal visits. Weight gain in early pregnancy is proof that they are pregnant. It is good practice to make a note of what type of clothing the girl is wearing the first time she is weighed (jeans, T-shirt) so later weight determinations can be compared more accurately.

Nursing Diagnoses and Related Interventions

Nursing Diagnosis: Health-seeking behaviors related to special care necessary for healthy adolescent pregnancy

Goal: Client will obtain necessary information on self-care during pregnancy.

Outcome Criteria: Client states she feels confident in her ability to take care of herself and avoid pregnancy complications.

Provide Prenatal Health Teaching. Adolescents often are unwilling to follow health care advice that might make them different in any way from their peers. On the other hand, adolescents often do not have well-established health practices, so they are adaptable to a well-health approach. They need a great deal of health teaching during pregnancy because they do not know many of the common measures of care that the older woman may have learned from experience over the years.

Adolescent girls may respond to health teaching that is directed to their own health more than to that of the fetus inside them: "Eat a high protein diet because protein makes your hair shiny (or prevents split fingernails)" often leads to better compliance than a statement that protein is good for the baby. "Taking the iron supplement should make you feel less tired," is better than "It will help build the baby's blood supply," for the same reason. These are truthful statements that appeal to an adolescent's preoccupation with self. In addition, this type of health teaching is the only form to which the adolescent who is denying her pregnancy can respond.

Be certain to include information on the effects of all drugs, including recreational drugs, on fetal welfare.

Pregnancy could become an important growth experience if it provides the motivation some adolescents need to withdraw from recreational drug use.

Nutrition. Good nutrition is a major problem during adolescent pregnancy, as many enter pregnancy with poor nutritional stores (Gutierrez & King, 1993). There is an association between low-birth-weight babies and girls who are still growing during pregnancy (Scholl et al., 1990). The younger the girl is, the more likely she is to have a low birth-weight infant. The girl's diet must be sufficient not only to maintain her own health and allow for growth of the fetus but also to provide the needs of her own growing body. Protein, iron, folic acid, and vitamin A and C deficiencies may become acute (Chez, 1991). Besides eating larger amounts of food, the pregnant adolescent must eat the proper foods and possibly abandon the adolescent food fads she has been following. Some girls are so peer oriented that they balk at substituting a glass of orange juice for a cola beverage because no one else they know drinks orange juice. The best you may be able to accomplish is to secure her agreement to switch to noncaffeinated soft drinks. agreement to switch to noncaffeinated soft drinks.

Many adolescent girls are willing to eat a nutritious diet during pregnancy; they simply do not know what constitutes a good diet. Some girls have little choice in what foods are prepared at home. To change her dietary pattern, you may have to talk to the person who cooks for her.

Many adolescents eat at least one meal a week at a fast-food restaurant. Remember that if the girl is attending school, she eats at least one meal away from home each day. If she travels by school bus, she may have to leave by 6:00 or 7:00 in the morning, so she needs suggestions on how to construct a quick but healthy breakfast; if she leaves home this early she will have a long wait until lunchtime. Suggest midmorning snacks that are not just empty calories. Be certain that nutrition education includes how to "brown-bag" or buy a nutritious cafeteria lunch (type A school lunches are discussed in Chapter 34).

Adolescents traditionally demonstrate poor compliance to medication. They may need frequent reminders that vitamin and iron supplements during pregnancy not only have to be purchased but also have to be swallowed. Be sure the girl posts a medication reminder chart at home or in her school locker.

Activity and Rest. Adolescents vary greatly in their preferred level of activity. Assess the girl's participation in sports activities and determine which ones (if any) should be discontinued during pregnancy (diving, gymnastics, touch football). Many girls practice sports not for the enjoyment of the sport but for the feeling of "team" or companionship. You may need to suggest alternative activities for her (joining the drama or language club, inviting friends over once a week to watch a movie) or she will suffer from the loss of companionship.

Adolescent girls may not plan enough rest time during pregnancy, especially if they are acting as if nothing is happening to them. It may help to explore their typical day and suggest ways to rest without compromising social relationships.

Pregnancy Information. A young girl may have distorted beliefs about her body. Despite all the health information given to children in school, it still is not uncommon to find an adolescent who thinks that her baby is growing in her stomach. Such a girl is unwilling to eat large meals during pregnancy for fear of suffocating the fetus. All adolescent girls need substantial education on the physiologic changes that occur during pregnancy. In addition, specific information about labor and delivery is essential to counteract all the scare stories they may have heard from their peers. Gaining knowledge is another way that pregnancy can be a growth experience. At the end of the pregnancy, the adolescent will know a great deal more about her body and her ability to monitor her health than her average classmate (see the Nursing Care Plan).

Prepare for Childbirth. Adolescents have a strong need for peer companionship. When they become pregnant, they often are cut off from fellow adolescents. This makes them "ripe," therefore, to join a class of adolescents in preparation for childbirth. They are excellent students because being a student is so age-appropriate for them. They have enough childish magical belief operating that they are not skeptical that prepared childbirth will work for them. In fact, believing that prepared childbirth will work is an important component in a successful prepared childbirth experience, so this becomes a self-fulfilling prophecy.

Birth Decisions. Pelvic measurements should be taken early and carefully in adolescent girls; cephalopelvic disproportion is a real possibility because of the girl's incomplete pelvic growth. Most girls who are told that their baby will have to be delivered by cesarean birth respond well to the news, and many are frankly relieved. Surgery seems controlled and simple compared with the agonies of labor that they imagine are in store. The decision on the method of delivery should be shared with the girl and her parents when it is reached by the health care team. This is part of being honest with the girl. It cannot be stressed enough that adolescents, for the most part, want to know the truth. They tend to regard the withholding of information not as a way of protecting them from worry but as an indication that they are being treated like children.

Plans for the Baby. Adolescents may need additional time at prenatal visits to talk to a good listener concerning their feelings about being pregnant and becoming a mother. Scared? Bewildered? Numb? Happy? Be certain they know all the options available to them: keeping the baby or placing the baby in a temporary foster home or for adoption.

Adolescents should be encouraged to breast-feed. Breast tissue matures with pregnancy, so even the very young adolescent is physically capable of breast-feeding.

Complications of Adolescent Pregnancy

Adolescent pregnancy carries an increased incidence of pregnancy-induced hypertension, iron deficiency anemia, preterm labor, and cephalopelvic disproportion. Cephalopelvic disproportion leads to an increased incidence of cesarean birth (Figure 17-1).

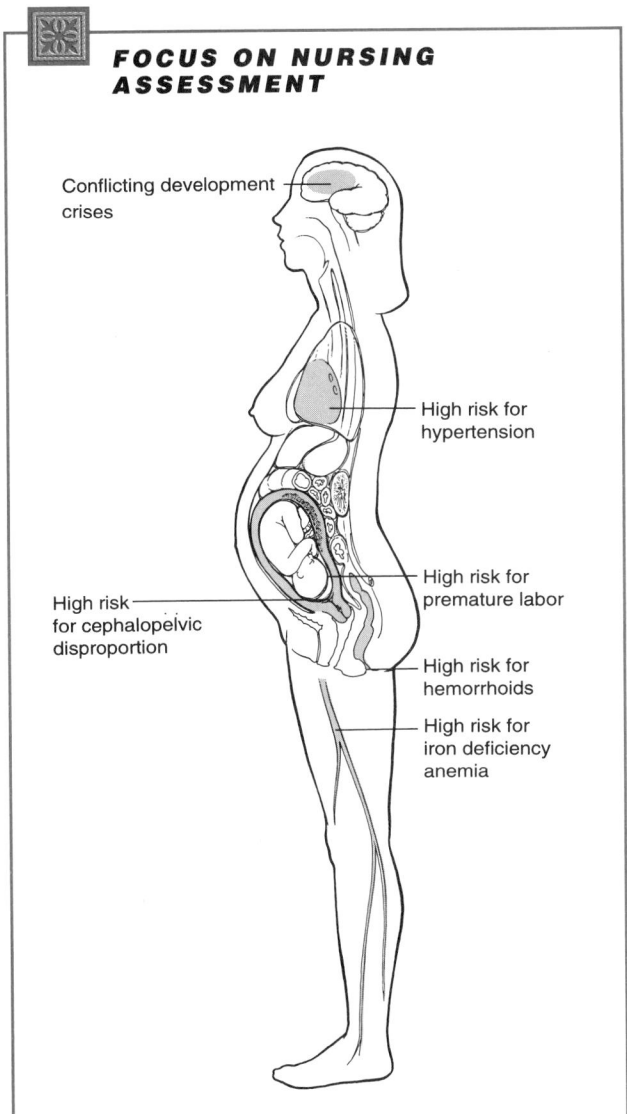

FOCUS ON NURSING ASSESSMENT

Conflicting development crises

High risk for hypertension

High risk for premature labor

High risk for hemorrhoids

High risk for iron deficiency anemia

High risk for cephalopelvic disproportion

FIGURE 17-1

Because of immaturity, the pregnant adolescent is at high risk for various problems.

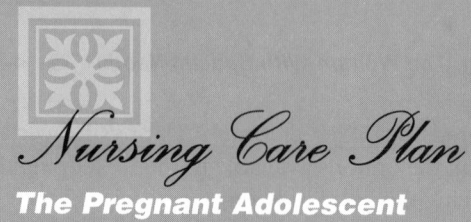

Nursing Care Plan
The Pregnant Adolescent

> Megan Ryan is a 16-year-old G1P0 adolescent you see in a prenatal clinic who has just been diagnosed as being pregnant. The following is a nursing care plan developed for part of her care.

Health History: Pale and tired-appearing adolescent who has noticed intense itching of pubic hair for last 4 days. Voices concern she has "caught" something from boyfriend. Is also concerned because she has not had a menstrual period for 2 months. Has not been using contraception although she has been sexually active for 6 months. Has experienced nausea in early morning for past 2 months. Lives in upstairs flat with parents and 5-year-old sister. Has taken responsibility for sister's care after school since she was 12. Parents own a delicatessen downstairs and both work in it. Has not told either parent or father of baby (a senior in high school) about possibility of pregnancy. States: "My parents will be wild. They'll be so disappointed I'll have to drop out of school."

Nutrition: States "Eating for 2 will be fun. I can't wait." Typical breakfast: none (because of early hour she leaves for school). Lunch: tuna sandwich, 1 banana. Dinner: 1 serving roast beef, 1 serving potatoes, 1 serving lima beans; 1 glass milk. Snack: 1 serving popcorn.

Nursing Diagnosis: High risk for altered growth and development related to potential disruption of peer relationships and interruption of schooling secondary to unplanned pregnancy.

Defining Characteristic: Client states that pregnancy is unplanned and will disrupt lifestyle.

Goal: Client will demonstrate ability to adjust to crisis with family support by 1 month.

Outcome Criteria: Client states specific plans she has developed to continue school and maintain peer contacts; describes workable relationship with parents; clarifies relationship she wants to have with father of child; states safe and healthy practices during pregnancy and intention to follow them.

(continued)

Pregnancy-Induced Hypertension

Adolescents are five times more prone to pregnancy-induced hypertension than the average woman (see Chapter 15). Establishing a baseline blood pressure is important in adolescents because some will not have had their blood pressure measured since a preschool checkup as long as 10 years earlier.

The best intervention for reducing an increasing blood pressure during pregnancy is bedrest, preferably in a left side-lying position. This is difficult for a teenager to do because she easily grows bored on bedrest, and being confined to bed limits her interactions with peers and school activities. Many girls on bedrest at home may rest better if they are lying on the living room couch where they can be aware of household activity than in an upstairs bedroom where they have to get up time and again to see what is happening; it is easier for a parent to enforce bedrest if the girl is within eyesight also. If called too many times to the distant bedroom for small tasks, a parent tends to say, "Get up and get it yourself this time."

Girls on bedrest need activities to keep them busy. This can include homework or listening to music. "Assignments" from the health care agency, such as reading about appropriate toys and games for infants, may provide a way to occupy time. A daily telephone call from the health care facility to the girl not only occupies time but shows concern and offers an opportunity to enforce health teaching points.

If a girl is going to be on bedrest for a significant portion of the pregnancy, she will need to make arrangements for continuing school. If the end of the pregnancy is near, she may be able to have a friend bring her homework assignments. If the bedrest period will be longer than 2 weeks, however, she will need to make arrangements for home tutoring. You may need to advocate for her with the school system for this service (remembering that only rarely can it be denied on the basis of pregnancy).

Be certain that the girl does not interpret being placed on bedrest as being ill. This may cause her to reduce her nutritional intake or to limit body hygiene.

Nursing Orders	*Rationale*
1. Urge client to tell parents about pregnancy. Role playing rehearsal may be helpful to prepare her for this.	1. Client will need both financial and emotional support from her family as the pregnancy progresses.
2. Urge client to tell father of child about pregnancy.	2. Father needs time to define his role.
3. Discuss ways that being pregnant will change her life and possible adaptations she will need to make so she knows more about what to expect. Stress that remaining in school is important.	3. A teenager may already be feeling the pressures of adolescence; she may need extra help in adapting to the additional stress of pregnancy.
4. Later in pregnancy after adaptation has improved, discuss childrearing plans and need for help with baby care.	4. Client will need continued support with childrearing once her child is born.

Nursing Diagnosis: High risk for altered nutrition, less than body requirements, related to adolescent diet pattern.

Defining Characteristic: Client describes a poor dietary intake.

Goal: Client will ingest an adequate pregnancy diet daily.

Outcome Criteria: Client ingests a 2500-kcal, 60-g protein diet daily.

Nursing Orders	*Rationale*
1. Discuss that "eating for two" means eating a healthy diet, not necessarily consuming more food.	1. Client's present diet is inadequate for pregnancy.
2. Plan ways to include adequate nutrition in busy school and activity life style.	2. Adolescents have difficulty adjusting to pregnancy if their adolescent lifestyle cannot be maintained.

If the hypertension continues following a period of bedrest at home (or if the symptoms of pregnancy-induced hypertension are acute when they are first discovered) the girl will be admitted to the hospital so bedrest can be better enforced. Establish a specific routine of bedrest—does it mean being strictly confined to bed or sitting up part of the day in a lounge chair with legs elevated? Could she lie on a stretcher by the desk? Can she take a shower once a day? Use the bathroom? Knowing the exact rules from the beginning helps prevent misunderstandings and hurt feelings.

Iron Deficiency Anemia

Many adolescent girls are iron deficient because their low protein intake cannot balance the amount of iron lost with menstrual flows. Deficiency is revealed by chronic fatigue, pale mucus membranes, and a hemoglobin less than 11 g. As if the girl's body has identified a mineral lack, iron deficiency anemia is associated with pica, or the ingestion of inedible substances. Cravings for ice cubes or candy bars also may develop because of this (Horner et al., 1991).

A pregnancy compounds iron deficiency anemia because the girl must now supply enough iron for fetal growth and her increasing blood volume. All women should take an iron and folic acid supplement (folic acid is important for red blood cell growth and possibly, prevention of neural tube defects) during pregnancy; this is especially important for the adolescent (Schneck et al., 1990).

Help the girl plan a daily time for taking the nutrition supplement. Review with her how much iron-rich food she eats daily; an iron supplement is not a supplement until her dietary intake is already strong in iron-rich foods.

Blood can be drawn in 2 weeks for a reticulocyte count to prove that the iron supplement is being taken (as soon as the body has iron it will begin forming immature red blood cells [reticulocytes] rapidly). If the reticulocyte count is not elevated by 2 weeks, it implies the girl did not take the supplement. Taking a stool

447

swab and assessing it for the black tinge of an iron supplement is another method of assessment for medicine compliance.

Preterm Labor

Review with adolescent girls the signs of labor by the 3rd month of pregnancy. Stress that labor contractions begin as only a sweeping contraction no more intense than menstrual cramps. Stress that any vaginal bleeding is suspicious until ruled otherwise. Adolescent girls have gained much of their knowledge of labor from television (where a woman suddenly announces she is in labor and within 15 minutes delivers a baby). They can therefore dismiss light contractions as simple discomfort, not realizing they might be the start of labor. Adolescents who recognize labor contractions early on can seek care to have premature labor halted.

Hemorrhoids

Many adolescents develop hemorrhoids during pregnancy because the disproportion of their body size to the fetus puts extra pressure on pelvic vessels and causes blood to pool in rectal veins. Measures to reduce this are discussed in Chapter 11. Reassure her that this is a pregnancy-related phenomenon and will resolve when the pregnancy is over.

Striae and Chloasma

Adolescents may develop many striae across the sides of the abdomen because so much stretching of the abdominal skin occurs. They can be assured that because they have such elastic skin, these marks will probably fade following pregnancy. Chloasma, excess pigment deposition on the face and neck, appears at the same rate in adolescents as in older women. Adolescents, however, may be more conscious of this pigment because, overall, they are more conscious and concerned about their facial appearance. Suggesting a cover makeup and offering reassurance that the pigmentation will fade after pregnancy may help.

Complications of Labor, Birth, and the Postpartal Period

Cephalopelvic Disproportion

Adolescent labor does not differ from labor in the older woman if no cephalopelvic disproportion is present. Cephalopelvic disproportion is suggested by lack of engagement at the beginning of labor, a prolonged first stage of labor, and, finally, poor fetal descent. Plotting labor on a Friedman graph is a good way to detect labor that is becoming abnormal at these points (see Chapter 18). Be certain that the adolescent has a support person with her so she can relax during labor and breathe effectively with contractions. If this person is also an adolescent, you may need to serve as the true support person during labor or at least spend considerable time coaching so that he or she can effectively support the girl in labor. It is important that a first labor be a positive experience so the girl does not have to live in dread of a second pregnancy.

Postpartal Hemorrhage

Young adolescents are more prone to postpartal hemorrhage than the average woman because if the girl's uterus is not yet fully developed, it is overdistended by pregnancy. An overdistended uterus does not contract as readily as a normally distended uterus in the postpartal period. The young adult also may have more frequent or deeper perineal and cervical lacerations because of the size of the infant in relation to her body. On the other hand, young adolescents are generally healthy and have supple body tissue that allows for adequate perineal stretching; if a laceration does occur, it will heal readily without complication.

Inability to Adapt Postpartally

The immediate postpartal period may be an almost unreal time for the adolescent. Giving birth is such a stress and a major crisis that all women have difficulty integrating it into their life. It may be particularly difficult for the adolescent. The girl may "block out" the hours of labor as if they didn't happen; if she was particularly frightened by labor, she may have been administered a narcotic so her memory of the labor hours are not clear. Urge her to talk about labor and birth to make the happening real to her. As many as 20% of adolescent mothers have minimal postpartum depression due to the stress of the event (Troutman & Cutrona, 1990).

Lack of Knowledge About Infant Care

Adolescents show the same positive bonding behavior with their infants as their more mature counterparts. They may, however, lack knowledge of infant care (Figure 17-2). Though they may consider themselves to be knowledgeable in child care because they baby-sat for a neighbor's child or a younger sibling, they may be overwhelmed in the postpartal period to realize that when the baby is their own, child care is not as simple as it once seemed. When the child cries, they cannot hand it to someone else; at the end of 4 hours, when they are tired of caring for the baby, they cannot leave it and walk away. Even though you and others may have discussed this with the girl during her pregnancy, these feelings may not arise until the child is actually born. Spend time with the girl observing how she handles the infant; demonstrate bathing and changing the baby as appropriate. Model mothering behaviors whenever possible, by being aware of how you hold and care for the child.

Unfortunately, most adolescent mothers do not

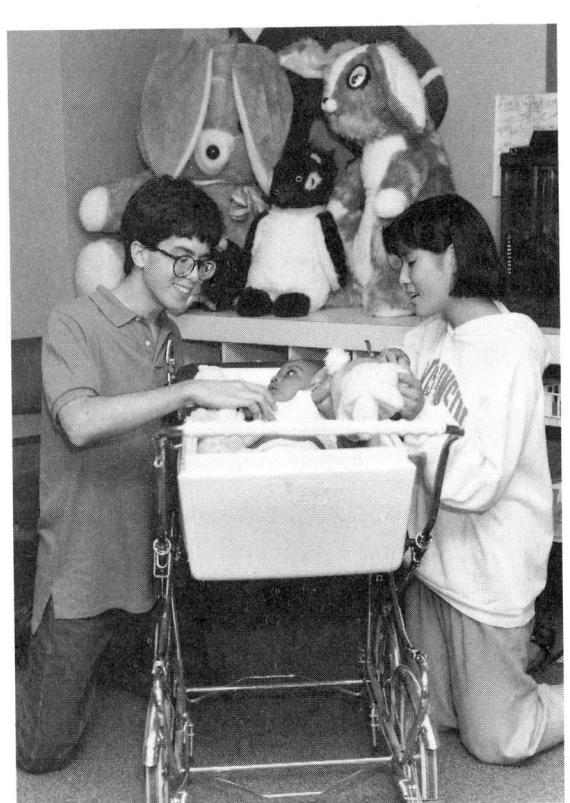

FIGURE 17-2
Adolescents need extra time for health education to be certain they are prepared to be parents. (Courtesy of Department of Medical Photography, Children's Hospital, Buffalo, NY.)

breast-feed. This is related to their perception of breast-feeding as something that will "tie them down" and the reality (in many instances) that they will be returning to a full-time school program soon after birth. Help young mothers who do not choose to breast-feed to find a feeding method that is satisfying to them and safe for the infant.

The Pregnant Woman Over Age 35

The incidence of women delaying their first pregnancy until their late 30s or early 40s is increasing (see the Focus on Cultural Awareness box). Seven percent of births in the United States today are to women over 35; 1% are to women over 40 (DHHS, 1993). No woman over 35 likes to be referred to as elderly, but women over 35 who are pregnant for the first time are traditionally termed **elderly primiparas.** In the past, it was assumed that a woman of this age was past the optimum age for childbearing and was at risk for many complications. With the exception of greater chromosomal abnormality, there is little evidence of increasing complications in women older than 35 as long as prenatal care is begun early in the pregnancy (Berkowitz et al., 1990).

Women of this age, however, are still considered at high risk, for some of the reasons discussed below.

The woman over age 35 is more likely than a younger woman to have a previously diagnosed condition such as hypertension, varicosities, or hemorrhoids; if these conditions increase in severity during pregnancy, complications can arise. In addition, by age 35, a woman usually has a major role change to undertake during pregnancy because she is well established in a career or has an accustomed routine at home or in her community. She needs to think through how this pregnancy and childrearing are going to fit into and change her life. Although she may feel rich in the number of support people she perceives around her, she may discover she has few "pregnancy support" people since she does not have many friends her age who are also having babies—some may be close to becoming grandmothers. The only things these friends remember of pregnancy and labor are their particular highs and lows, and these memories may be dated in terms of what goes on today in the typical birthing room. This may leave her without access to the daily shop talk of other pregnant women, or someone to turn to, to ask questions such as whether the backache she is experiencing or frequent need to urinate is normal. On the other hand, because many women delay childbearing today, she may be one of a sizable group of women in the community experiencing pregnancy at this stage of life.

Childbirth education classes oriented toward the older woman not only provide important information on pregnancy but can bring these women and their support people together. The woman over 35, like any other pregnant woman, needs access to health care personnel who can supply her with factual information during pregnancy. She also needs a sympathetic ear while she works through this role change in her life.

FOCUS ON CULTURAL AWARENESS

What is perceived as the best time in life to have children is culturally influenced. Some people believe that having children young allows parents to grow with children; in other cultures, delaying childbirth until a family is financially secure is thought to be best. What you believe, therefore, may not be the belief of a family for whom you are caring. What may be a catastrophe to you may seem like a blessing to someone else (and vice versa). Assess couples by history and observation to determine if childrearing appears to be timed correctly for them. If not, they may need extra time to accept a pregnancy and adapt to becoming parents.

Developmental Tasks and Pregnancy

The developmental challenge of the over-35 age group is to expand their awareness or develop generativity—that is, a sense of moving away from themselves and becoming involved with the world or community (Erikson, 1963). Some people assume that once they reach adulthood, the way they are is the way they always will be, and they are surprised to see that changes still occur. They are amazed to find that their bodies change (men become bald; women and men both gain weight) and so do their interests. They find themselves joining committees and clubs, coaching Little League teams, or organizing fundraising or community events.

A woman in this age group who is pregnant may begin to feel ambivalent during pregnancy, as she may want to continue with community activities, yet also want to daydream or concentrate on the fetus inside her. You may need to help her balance her life so she can manage crossing two life phases this way.

Many middle-age adults are caring for aging parents. This additional responsibility may make it difficult for women to complete the psychological work of pregnancy. It also may create extra strain on the woman's finances and time.

Prenatal Assessment

The woman over 35 should begin prenatal care early in pregnancy. Fortunately, most women of this age group are well informed about the advisability of early prenatal care and so do seek an early appointment (Rosenfeld, 1990). A few mistakenly believe that their lack of menstruation is the result of early menopause, so they do not seek an early health care consultation.

Health History

Ask women not only about their present symptoms of pregnancy but how they feel about the pregnancy and how it fits into their lifestyle. If the woman did not realize that she was pregnant, she may have self-medicated. Ask if she has been taking any medication to relieve reported symptoms, such as nausea or fatigue. Because a woman is functioning well in a business world does not mean she has a healthy pregnancy lifestyle. Don't accept answers such as "I drink socially" or "I take the usual drugs" without exploring what the phrases mean specifically.

Family Profile. Some women over age 35 who are pregnant for the first time are women who have recently changed their life pattern (married or become involved in a long-term sexual relationship) or have decided to have a child without a marriage partner before they are no longer able to conceive. Whereas the younger woman often waits awhile after marrying to become

pregnant, the over-35-age woman often plans to become pregnant immediately after marriage because she senses her reproductive years are running out. Because of this, she may find herself making many adjustments at once (not only to a new life partner, house or apartment, and perhaps community, but also to a pregnancy).

Identify her source of income (if both she and her partner work, stopping work when her child is born may reduce their income greatly) and how many people are financially or emotionally dependent on her (children from a partner's former marriage, elderly parents, an elderly neighbor, fellow workers that count on her). During pregnancy, when a woman often needs extra emotional support, feeling responsible for so many people may be difficult for her.

Day History. Ask specifically about her job and estimate the amount of walking or back strain this entails. Ask about recent diet or exercise programs; if she belongs to a health club, remind her that saunas are contraindicated during pregnancy because of possible hyperthermia and teratogenic effects of extreme heat on the developing fetus. Identify personal habits, such as cigarette smoking and alcohol consumption. Many women of this age group still smoke cigarettes, and businesswomen may drink alcohol daily as part of their job of entertaining business contacts. Smoking in older women leads to a much greater risk of preterm birth than it does in younger women (Wen et al., 1990).

Physical Examination

The woman over age 35 needs a thorough physical examination at her first prenatal visit to establish her general health and, in particular, to identify any circulatory disturbances. Inspect lower extremities thoroughly for varicosities, as these tend to occur in women over 30. Be certain to test a urine specimen for specific gravity as well as glucose and protein to assess adequate kidney function.

Assess the woman's breasts for any abnormalities and urge her to continue breast self-examination during pregnancy. This is easy for women to neglect as they no longer have menstrual period markers to remind them to do this. Women over 35 are in a higher-risk group for breast cancer than younger women, however, so it is especially important that they continue to self-examine their breasts. Be certain to assess for fetal heart sounds and fetal movement at prenatal visits as hydatidiform mole has a higher than usual incidence in the woman over 35 (see Chapter 15).

Chromosomal Assessment

Women over 35 may be offered the opportunity for chorionic villi sampling at 8 to 10 weeks of pregnancy to detect chromosomal abnormalities. An amniocentesis may be performed in place of this at the 14th to 16th week of pregnancy. A triple-screen (serum alpha-feto-protein, human chorionic gonadotropin, and unconjugated estriol levels) drawn at the 15th week of pregnancy is recommended to detect an open spinal cord or chromosomal defect (Schmidt, 1993). Be certain the woman is well prepared for these studies and receives support during them. Many women of this age group do not begin nest-building until these tests confirm that the child probably will be healthy.

Nursing Diagnoses and Related Interventions

Nursing Diagnosis: Health-seeking behaviors related to special care necessary for healthy pregnancy

Goal: Client will obtain information about healthful care practices.

Outcome Criteria: Client states she feels confident in self-care and ability to decrease complications of pregnancy.

Prenatal teaching needs to be adjusted to fit the woman's lifestyle. If she has not planned on ever being pregnant, she may have isolated herself through the years from "mothering" activities and so, despite her years, knows little about pregnancy and newborn care. Knowledge-wise, she is at the same level as the adolescent. Others have read so extensively that they may know more theoretical information than the woman who has already given birth.

Nutrition. Assess the number of meals the woman eats outside her home each week, including those she packs as a lunch or eats in restaurants. She may need some tips on how to adjust pregnancy nutrition so she can obtain the same nutrition whether she prepares meals at home or eats them at an office or school luncheon. Urge her to substitute a caffeine-free soft drink in place of alcoholic beverages. In some offices, large amounts of coffee are consumed. Urge her to substitute milk or juice. Many women this age normally drink little milk; rather than getting used to milk again, she may appreciate suggestions on other ways to ingest calcium, such as in puddings or yogurt.

Prenatal Classes. Because a pregnant woman over 35 may be unique in her circle of friends, she may feel shut out of her usual group because of the pregnancy. She may be ready, therefore, to join a childbirth preparation class where she is "one of the group."

Be certain the woman plans (or they plan together as a couple) to set aside a specific time every day when she will do breathing exercises. Otherwise, she will never find time to get to these in a busy day and will discover herself unprepared in labor.

Complications of Pregnancy for the Woman Over Age 35

The complications of pregnancy most likely to occur in a woman over age 35 are those related to the phenomenon that her circulatory system may not be as competent as when she was younger or her body tissues may not be as elastic as they once were (hypertension of pregnancy, preterm birth, and cesarean birth). Post-term birth also occurs at a higher rate in this age group than others (Figure 17-3).

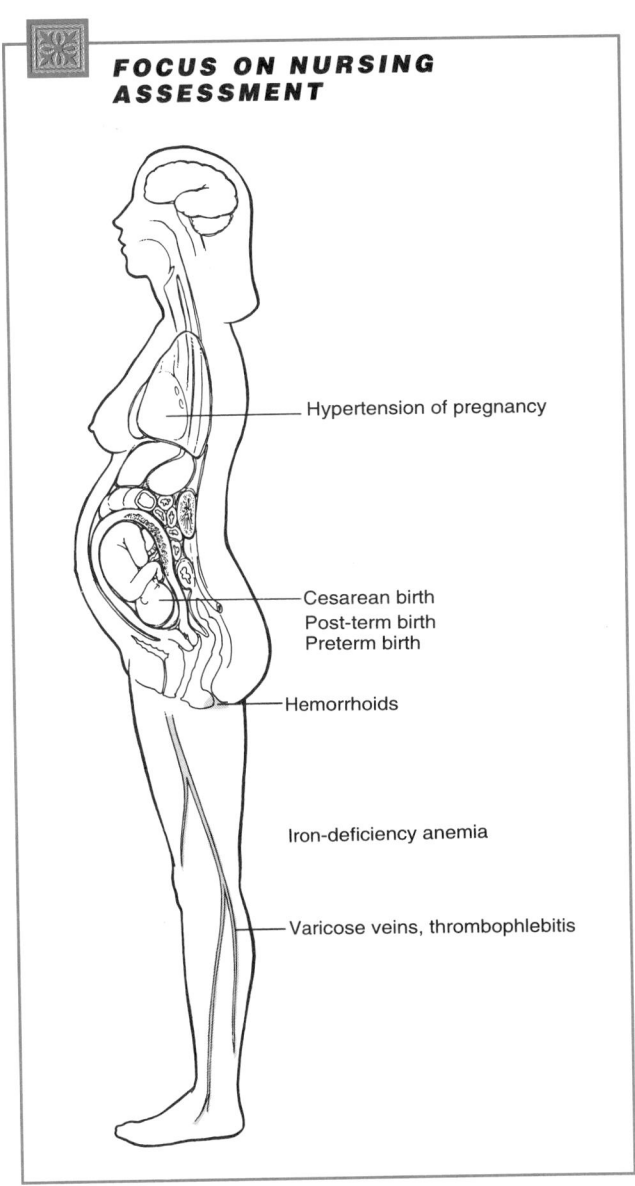

FOCUS ON NURSING ASSESSMENT

- Hypertension of pregnancy
- Cesarean birth
  Post-term birth
  Preterm birth
- Hemorrhoids
- Iron-deficiency anemia
- Varicose veins, thrombophlebitis

FIGURE 17-3
Effects of pregnancy on the woman over 35.

Hemorrhoids

The woman over age 35 is prone to hemorrhoids as she may have some degree of rectal varicosities present at the beginning of pregnancy. Pain from rectal distention may, in fact, be one of the primary symptoms that she reports at a first visit. Measures to reduce these and increase comfort are discussed in Chapter 11.

Varicosities

Varicosities, like hemorrhoids, develop readily in the woman over 35 because she may have some tendency toward them even before the pregnancy. As with hemorrhoids, her best approach during pregnancy is to prevent varicosities rather than to allow them to develop. Measures to prevent varicosities are discussed in Chapter 11 (see also the Focus on Family Teaching box).

Flag the chart of the woman with any degree of varicosity formation during pregnancy so nurses caring for her during the postpartal period can take special precautions to prevent thrombophlebitis. With venous stasis present, the woman is more prone to develop this complication.

Pregnancy-Induced Hypertension

A woman over 35 may have a higher incidence of pregnancy-induced hypertension than a younger woman, possibly related to blood vessel inelasticity. As with any woman, the best way to reduce the symptoms of pregnancy-induced hypertension is for the woman to rest most of each day. If the woman has a job, this may be quite difficult for her, not only because she feels she may miss out on a promotion, receive reduced pay, or risk losing her job altogether, but also because she is used to being productive, not merely lying in bed all day. To allow her to rest effectively, you may need to help her plan activities she can accomplish on bedrest, such as reworking a school course outline, restructuring her office filing system, or working at a hobby, like embroidery, that she has wanted to pursue but never had time for before.

If resting at home is not effective in reducing symptoms, she will be admitted to the hospital where bedrest can be better enforced and antihypertensive therapy begun. Remember that the woman may be a new marriage partner, so this separation may cause a major strain on the marriage. You may need to advocate for increased visiting time for her husband and provision of privacy for them as a couple so they do not feel shut away from each other.

Iron Deficiency Anemia

Iron deficiency anemia is a potential problem for all women, particularly if a woman had an IUD in place for contraception. Be certain the woman hangs a reminder sheet on her refrigerator door, bathroom mirror, or at her office to cue her to take her daily prenatal vitamins and iron supplement. A usually well-organized woman may

FOCUS ON FAMILY TEACHING

Q. I'm 37 and having my first baby. What are some practical measures I can take to prevent varicose veins from developing during this pregnancy?

A. Women over 35 do develop more varicose veins than women who are younger during a pregnancy unless they take some precautions. Some practical suggestions are:

- Find opportunities at work to elevate your legs, such as a coffee or lunch break.
- Be certain your diet includes vitamin C as this is important to strengthen vein walls.
- Rest in a side-lying position with your body tipped slightly forward (Sims' position) as this allows leg veins to drain and empty.
- Avoid long periods of standing in one place by taking "walk breaks"; active muscle contraction helps venous return.
- Avoid sitting with crossed legs.
- Don't wear anything constricting on your lower legs, such as knee-high stockings.
- Support hose are helpful. Be certain to put them on before you get out of bed in the morning, before veins become swollen, for best results.

think she will be able to remember this without help, but pregnancy is a time of stress so it distorts memory, and without a reminder sheet she may easily forget.

Complications of Labor, Birth, and the Postpartal Period

Failure to Progress in Labor

Labor in the elderly primipara may be prolonged, as cervical dilatation may not occur as spontaneously as in the younger woman, probably because of decreased elasticity in cells (Cunningham et al., 1993). Plotting labor on a Friedman graph is a good method of determining when labor is becoming prolonged. A number of women this age will need a cesarean birth if labor becomes overly prolonged, putting the fetus at risk. Urge women to ask for no more than a regional anesthetic if possible so they can be awake for the birth. Urge their support person to be present for the birth.

Difficulty Accepting the Event

Women in the over-age-35 group may begin to have second thoughts about planning a pregnancy this late in life as the reality of a new baby registers with them during the postpartal period. Although they may have read a great deal about babies during pregnancy, they may wish they had read more or were as confident with this phase of their life as they are about their home, office, or schoolroom. Review plans for child care and postpartal rest, with an emphasis on helping women learn to balance their lives. They will particularly need this help if they plan on returning to work soon after the birth.

Postpartal Hemorrhage

Just as the cervix may not dilate as readily during the older woman's labor, it may not contract as readily in the postpartal period; the older woman is, therefore, at higher risk for postpartal hemorrhage. Observe closely for this complication. Because she tends to be an independent woman who is interested in self-care, she may ask for few measures of care that would allow you to assess the amount of lochial flow unless you ask directly.

The Pregnant Woman With a Physical Disability

In the past, women with conditions such as vision or hearing impairment, mental retardation, or spinal cord or orthopedic injuries were sheltered by their families to such an extent that a woman with even a moderate physical disability did not meet potential marriage partners and so did not become (and it was believed should not become) pregnant. Although care of the woman with a physical disability has always been important to nursing, there has been little application of that care to the maternal child health area. Today, women with varying degrees of disability attend public schools, work in offices, join community organizations, establish sexual relationships, marry, and plan pregnancies. Because such women (and in some instances, their support persons also) face special problems related to a physical disability, nursing care during pregnancy must be designed with these special concerns in mind so that it addresses the woman and her family's problems and needs.

Table 17-1 lists general areas of care that are important in planning for the physically disabled woman who is pregnant. Women with a degree of physical disability that makes them more sedentary than usual, such as those with a spinal cord injury, have a special risk during pregnancy of forming thrombi in lower extremity veins. This must be prevented as the development of thrombi can lead to pulmonary emboli, one of the chief causes of death in childbirth today (Lagrew, 1990).

Rights of the Physically Disabled

By federal law, physically disabled persons must have freedom of access to public buildings with ramps or handrails placed so they can enter and leave buildings safely. All health care facilities should be in compliance with these laws not only in terms of physical facilities but in the true spirit of the law (people are psychologi-

Table 17-1. *Areas of Planning With Physically Disabled Women During Pregnancy*

Area	Assessment and Planning Guidelines
Transportation	Ask if the woman has transportation for prenatal care and for emergencies.
Pregnancy counseling	Assess the special modifications of care that will need to be made depending on the woman's special disability. Use additional visual or sound aids to make your teaching points clear.
Support person	Assess who is the woman's support person. In some instances, the woman's condition requires so much assistance during pregnancy that one support person will not be enough. If necessary, contact community agencies to lend second-ring support.
Health	Don't lose track of the fact that the woman has a primary health problem. The woman with cerebral palsy will need to continue an active muscle exercise program during pregnancy for her primary illness, for example.
Work	Assess whether the woman works outside her home and if this is discontinued during pregnancy what she could substitute for a social contact activity. Many women with a disabling condition are lonely because they do not have a wide range of friends or social contacts.
Recreation	Many women with a physically disabling condition lead a rather sedentary life (partly because they do not have many social contacts). Assess whether her level of activity is adequate and make concrete suggestions within her limitations for increasing it.
Self-esteem	Assess the woman's level of self-esteem: it may be low because of repeated failure situations in her life. Give praise at prenatal visits and help her to make pregnancy a growth experience.

cally welcome as well as physically able to reach the inside of the building). By the same law, a hospital cannot deny care to a person with a physical disability even though the disabling condition complicates treatment considerably and may require extra personnel time.

The Woman With a Spinal Cord Injury

Severe spinal injury leaves loss of sensory and motor control distal to the point of injury. Many women who have paraplegia (loss of sensory and motor control of their lower extremities) were born with a congenital spinal cord defect, such as myomeningocele, or were injured in a violent accident during childhood or adolescence (e.g., they were hit by a motor vehicle or thrown from a horse or motorcycle, or they struck their head on the bottom of a shallow swimming pool). Many such women are ambulatory by wheelchair only.

Table 17-2 lists the expected levels of ambulatory function in different types of spinal cord injury.

Modifications for Pregnancy

Explore in a prenatal health history the cause of the woman's physical problem and her general image of herself. Some women who are confined to a wheelchair maintain high self-esteem and so are as able to deal with a pregnancy as any woman. Others have a poor sense of self-esteem that will make this particularly difficult for them. For many women, pregnancy becomes a special event: a 9-month time to show everyone they are capable of completing one of life's miracles.

Be certain to explore with the woman whom she would count on for emergency transportation if a pregnancy emergency should occur. Ask about her ability to reach a telephone if she is home alone. Late in pregnancy, she might want always to rest near a telephone by sleeping on the couch or in a sleeping bag on the kitchen floor so reaching it will not be a problem. Most communities have a telephone contact system that connects physically disabled persons with a paramedic or

Table 17-2. Level of Ambulatory Function Anticipated Following Spinal Injury

Level of Spinal Cord Injury	Functional Abilities
C3–4	Manipulate electric wheelchair using mouthstick
C5–7	Propel wheelchair with handrim on wheels
T1–4	Propel wheelchair without special projections
T5–L2	Use bilateral long leg braces and crutches
L3–4	Use short leg braces with or without crutches
L5–S3	Be ambulatory without aids

hospital emergency service through a specifically designed beeper system. If she has not already, a physically disabled woman might want to invest in this service during pregnancy.

Physical examination may present some difficulties. Many obstetric examining tables are built for the comfort of the examiner and so are too high for a patient to transfer from a wheelchair by simply sliding onto the table. To help a woman move to the examining table, you may have to borrow a ramp from the physical therapy department so the wheelchair can be elevated to the level of the table. The woman may be unable to maintain her legs in a lithotomy position because of either hip flexion contracture or laxness of leg support, so she may need to be in a dorsal recumbent rather than a lithotomy position for a pelvic examination.

Pregnancy Counseling

All women who use wheelchairs are taught to press with their arms against the armrests and lift their buttocks up off the wheelchair seat for 5 seconds every hour. This prevents the formation of decubiti of the buttocks and posterior thighs that would result from continual pressure against these areas. It is important that the woman continues to perform this maneuver during pregnancy, as the increased weight of her abdomen makes her more prone than usual to decubiti formation from compression.

The sharp bend of her hips as she sits in a wheelchair limits venous return from the lower extremities. Raising her buttocks as described above decreases this angle and allows better venous return, another desired goal in pregnancy. For at least 1 hour every morning and afternoon, she should also elevate her feet to decrease the sharp bend at her knees, promoting venous return at that site and helping to prevent varicosities and thrombi formation. For this same reason, she should adjust the footrests so her legs are not sharply bent at the knees at any time.

Women who have no sensation of voiding as a result of lack of bladder innervation have been taught (1) to empty their bladder every 2 hours either by the Credé method (pressing on the upper anterior surface of the bladder to constrict and empty it) or by self-catheterization, or (2) to use a continuous indwelling catheter.

All of these methods may still be used during pregnancy. However, the size of the woman's abdomen may interfere with self-catheterization late in pregnancy (Sauer & Harvery, 1993).

Women with spinal cord injury are at high risk of contracting urinary tract infections during pregnancy, probably because of increased glucose in the urine (Craig, 1990). Urge the woman with an indwelling catheter to continue good perineal care (washing her perineum well with soap and water two times a day and applying an antiseptic ointment, such as povidone-iodine

[Betadine], to the insertion site). Be certain when changing the catheter (some women do this themselves by lying on their back and holding a hand mirror to view the perineum) that she uses optimal sterile technique during pregnancy. Urge her to place a folded towel under one buttock while she does this to displace the uterus off the vena cava so supine hypotension does not occur. She may be unable to continue changing her own catheter late in pregnancy as her abdomen is so large she can no longer visualize her perineum and vulva edema enlarges the labia so much that she needs a "third hand" to displace these to view the urethral opening. Discuss with her what arrangements she wants to make concerning this (a support person can change the catheter, a community health nurse could visit and do this, or it could be done at frequent prenatal visits). Women without full bladder control will be scheduled to have catheterized specimens obtained at intervals during pregnancy to be certain that a urinary tract infection is not occurring, as urinary tract infection is associated with preterm birth.

Planning Child Care

During pregnancy, the woman needs to think through the problems she may face in caring for an infant. Encourage her to breast-feed so she won't have to get up at night and go to the refrigerator for formula (some women worry that their bodies will not allow them to breast-feed, but it shouldn't be a problem). Explain that breast innervation will not be affected by her physical disability and that she should be able to breast-feed successfully and find it a satisfying accomplishment.

Some infant crib rails are lowered by pressure on a foot pedal, others by a waist-high lever. Urge the woman to test different types of cribs to find one that she can manage from her wheelchair (otherwise, she will leave the crib rail down and her infant could suffer a serious fall). Investigate how she anticipates carrying the infant (using an anterior baby backpack is usually effective with a wheelchair).

Childbirth

The woman who has no sensory involvement to her abdomen will not be able to feel uterine contractions. Remember that sensory innervation of the uterus is at the T10 spinal level; the motor innervation is at the T7 level. This means that a woman's uterus may begin to initiate contractions but the woman will not be able to feel them. Late in pregnancy she will need to palpate her abdomen periodically for tightening or the presence of contractions that she cannot otherwise feel. She may be admitted to a hospital at 38 weeks' gestation for continuous monitoring to detect uterine contractions. She may be scheduled for an amniocentesis to determine fetal maturity followed by a cesarean birth if the fetus is mature. If she is unable to control abdominal muscles, she is unable to push with the pelvic stage of labor; therefore, cesarean birth may be necessary in any event (Cross et al., 1992). If she has some abdominal muscle control, it may be possible for the infant to be born vaginally with forceps to help descent and birth. Encourage the woman to attend preparation for childbirth classes because even though her labor and birth may not be typical, she will benefit from the overall knowledge on fetal development and child care offered by such courses.

After giving birth, the woman has a strong need to see the baby and assure herself that he or she is healthy. She undoubtedly wants to observe the baby's back, which means unwrapping the baby from a warm cover. Even in a chilly birthing room the woman should be allowed to do this, as the inspection is so important to her. Point out to the mother how the infant spontaneously brings the knees up under the abdomen when lying prone to prove to her that the infant has full use of the legs.

The Postpartal Period

In a woman who has a high spinal cord injury (cervical or high thoracic), a condition that must be observed for during pregnancy, labor, and the immediate postpartal period is **autonomic dysreflexia.** This is an exaggerated autonomic response to stimuli. Any irritating condition, such as a distended bladder, increasing uterine size, or breast-feeding, may initiate the response; without upper motor neuron control to reverse the symptoms, extreme changes can occur. Severe hypertension (300/160 mm Hg) will occur, and the woman will experience a throbbing headache; flushing of the skin and profuse diaphoresis above the level of the spinal lesion; nausea; and bradycardia. Immediate action is necessary to protect against cerebral vascular accident or intraocular damage. Elevate the woman's head to reduce cerebral pressure, and locate the irritating stimulus (usually a distended bladder or bowel). Remove the bladder pressure by catheterization if an indwelling catheter is not in place. If a catheter is in place, check to see why it is not draining, then encourage it to drain by unkinking or flushing to allow urine to flow freely again. A hypotensive agent may be necessary to alleviate the extreme blood pressure.

As soon as the source of irritation is removed, symptoms fade quickly back to normal. Autonomic dysreflexia is an extremely frightening event for the woman, however, and, as mentioned, can cause severe, additional damage to her neurologic ability.

Be certain the woman carries out conscientious perineal care during the postpartal period (she does not sense pain in the area, so a hematoma or an infection of a perineal suture line could occur without her being aware of it). Assess carefully for bladder filling in the postpartal period as, again, the woman is not aware of bladder filling. She can return to her usual method of bladder emptying following delivery (Credé method, indwelling catheter, or self-catheterization).

Be certain the woman spends enough time with her infant to develop confidence in her ability to lift him or her from a bassinet into the wheelchair and in diapering and feeding. Be certain she has a return appointment for health care for both herself and the infant. Ask if she desires contraceptive information as she is probably aware that two small children close together in age could be more of a challenge than she would like to manage (Figure 17-4).

The Woman With Cerebral Palsy

Cerebral palsy is discussed in detail in Chapter 49. The exact cause of cerebral palsy is unknown, but it is associated with anoxia to brain cells during intrauterine life, during labor, or at birth (Paneth, 1993). It may include mental retardation, depending on the extent of the anoxia effect. With the most common type of cerebral palsy, the woman has spasticity of all body muscles. This causes her to reach past objects and to walk unsteadily as her muscles overcontract on voluntary motion. Her speech may be unclear if her facial and throat

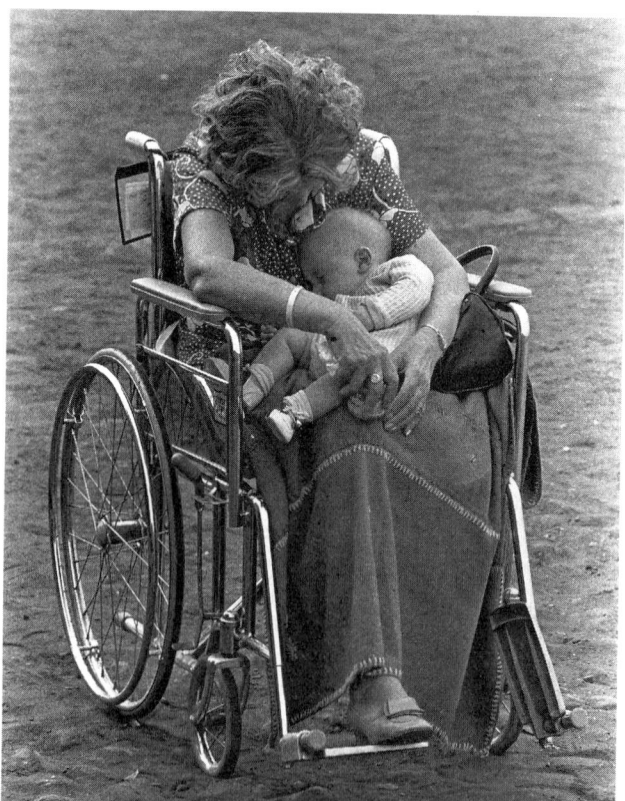

FIGURE 17-4
Being confined to a wheelchair doesn't prevent a woman from providing the love and stimulation her baby needs. (Maje Waldo/Stock Boston.)

muscles also are affected. Cerebral palsy is a condition that has a wide range of involvement, from only slight spasticity (a woman who has difficulty with only fine motor control), to an extreme level where the woman would be limited to a wheelchair for ambulation and have a great deal of difficulty performing even tasks of daily living such as self-feeding. Some women walk with the aid of forearm-supported crutches or may be ambulatory without aids (but with an unsteady gait). Evaluate each woman individually so as not to overestimate or underestimate her special needs during pregnancy.

Modifications for Pregnancy

As pregnancy progresses, a woman with cerebral palsy may need a referral to a physical therapist to evaluate carefully her ability to maintain self-ambulation. The weight of her abdomen may necessitate the use of crutches if she did not use them before or the use of a wheelchair if she was ambulatory with crutches before pregnancy. Appreciate that the woman achieved the degree of ambulation that she first presents with only after years of physical therapy and strengthening of leg and arm muscles. Help her to see that reducing her degree of independence during pregnancy is not a step backward for her but a step forward in that it will allow her to have a safe pregnancy without repeated falls.

To maintain the strength of muscle groups, especially the knees and hips, and to prevent contractures, she may need to perform active range of motion exercises each day and to spend about an hour walking in a physical therapy department with the support of parallel bars. Bringing her to a hospital daily may not be realistic in terms of the time her support person has to do this. If necessary, help her to contact a community support group, such as her church organization or a community organization for the physically disabled, to supply this transportation for her or to arrange a home care service. Otherwise, she may continue to try to be independently ambulatory beyond her capacity and fall or, at the end of pregnancy, discover that she can no longer be ambulatory beyond the limits of a wheelchair because contractures have developed.

If the woman's speech cannot be readily understood, evaluate whether she can use a telephone to call for help if an emergency should occur. When calling the health care agency, ask her to state her name first, "Hello, I'm Mary Smith," and then ask for help. Inform the switchboard operators and department receptionists of her name and her degree of speech impairment, so that staff members can communicate quickly with her in an emergency and keep her from getting so frustrated that she gives up trying to relay her message. Be certain that the woman knows how to summon help (perhaps a community 911 number) when the health care facility is closed.

Women with cerebral palsy may find that lying on

an examining table is uncomfortable because their muscle spasticity limits their ability to conform to a hard surface. They may have enough hip flexion contraction that they are unable to raise their feet comfortably into obstetric stirrups.

An important facet of pregnancy counseling for the woman with cerebral palsy is increasing her self-esteem and ability to see herself as capable of maintaining a pregnancy and caring for a child. Children can be cruel to a person who cannot control muscle motion smoothly, so her years of schooling have probably included experience after experience of hurtful occasions. This pregnancy is her chance to accomplish, to succeed. She makes an eager and excellent student and is ready to learn all that you can teach her about how to make pregnancy successful.

Allow time during prenatal visits for her to ask questions. If her speech is unclear, suggest that she bring her questions already written down before the visit so that all her concerns can be addressed.

Planning Child Care

Help the woman to think through how she will carry a crying, struggling infant if she is unsteady on her feet or uses crutches to ambulate. She might be encouraged to use an infant backpack or a wheelchair with an anterior baby sling (so her hands are free to move the wheels and control the chair). If her home is spacious enough, she might consider using a toy wagon to pull the infant. Some women lie on their back, place the infant on their chest, and slide across the floor by pushing with their feet. Impress on her that the way she chooses to do this is not as important as the fact that it is done safely without danger of her falling with a small infant. Encourage her to breast-feed because this will eliminate her having to walk an extra distance to warm or prepare formula. She may be reluctant to try this because she has little confidence in her body's ability to function correctly. If her spasticity is severe, she may not be successful at breast-feeding as the let-down reflex, which depends on muscle relaxation, may not occur.

Childbirth

Encourage the woman to attend a childbirth preparation class even though she may not be able to use breathing exercises effectively during labor, because the spasticity of her muscles may not allow for a controlled breathing pattern. Gaining general knowledge about labor and birth and participating in a shared experience with her life partner will still be valuable.

Labor may be acutely painful because her abdominal muscles remain tight and the uterus grows tender, raising and pressing against a tense abdomen with each contraction. Because she has poor use of the abdominal muscles, she may not be able to push effectively during the pelvic division of labor, so fetal descent may not

occur and cesarean birth or a forceps delivery may be necessary. If she is unable to assume a lithotomy position because of hip contractures, she will be vaginally delivered from a Sims' or dorsal recumbent position.

The Postpartal Period

Help the woman to begin self-care at the level with which she is capable. Mark her nursing care plan and her chart with a note that states clearly she has a speech impediment so people do not underestimate her intelligence and do wait patiently for her to make her needs clear to them.

Urge her to use infant disposable diapers so she does not employ safety pins because with a quick, uncontrolled hand motion, she could injure the infant. Allow her adequate time to feed and hold the infant to increase her competence.

Be certain that she has a return appointment for health care supervision for herself and the infant. Ask if she desires contraceptive information: she is probably aware that caring for two children born close together might be beyond her capabilities.

The Woman With Mental Retardation

Mental retardation may occur as a result of (1) anoxia suffered during intrauterine life or in birth or (2) a chromosomal retardation syndrome, such as Down syndrome. This does not affect childbearing ability or even, in many instances, childrearing capability (see Chapter 54 for a more detailed discussion of mental retardation).

Some women with mental retardation of childbearing age were raised in an institution and only recently discharged to a half-way home or their own apartment. These women have unusual difficulty making plans for pregnancy or child care because they have never experienced normal family life or seen younger children being cared for. If the woman became pregnant because she was taken advantage of sexually or if she has little understanding of reproductive physiology, she may not realize how she became pregnant. Some women come late in their pregnancy for prenatal care because they do not recognize the changes they may have noticed in their bodies as symptoms of pregnancy.

Women with mental retardation need frequent and consistent prenatal care as they do not have the same judgment as the average woman to determine if they are developing a complication of pregnancy. Because they do not have the same level of common pregnancy knowledge as other women, they will need more teaching to complete the pregnancy safely.

Modifications for Pregnancy

When interviewing a woman with mental retardation, ask her level of education. The number of years in school, however, may not be that helpful in assessment of functional level. Many women report that they finished high school, and although they did attend school for 12 years, their curriculum may have been limited. Be certain while interviewing that you limit your words to ones the woman can easily understand. Keep the interview time brief (10 to 15 minutes) and the environment free of distractions because the average person with mental retardation has a short attention span.

Investigate who lives at home with the woman, whom she would turn to if she had a problem, and what sources of financial support exist. The woman may be eligible for a Social Security assistance program but is not receiving benefits because she was not aware of the paperwork required. Ask if the woman has a telephone at her home and if she understands how to call the health care facility when she needs help.

Many women with mental retardation do not drive. Ask what transportation would be available in an emergency. (Is there a neighbor, family member, or friend who would drive her to the hospital?)

Explain carefully any procedure, such as blood drawing, so the woman understands that this is a helping, not a punishing, procedure. If she has not had a pelvic examination before, she may be reluctant to reveal this portion of her body to a stranger. Offer helpful support during the procedure.

Pregnancy Counseling

Limit instructions to those few items about pregnancy that are crucial for safety (do not drink alcohol; don't take any medicine); use photos or drawings to illustrate your teaching points to increase understanding.

It is usually helpful to allow the woman to visualize (using drawings) how her baby is growing from month to month. Teach her as well what a newborn is like and can do. Without this information, she may expect more of the baby than he or she is capable of (e.g., the baby will answer when spoken to or be able to play games) and so not be prepared to give safe care.

Planning Child Care

Help the woman and her family plan realistically for child care. Encourage the woman to breast-feed to limit the possibility of her misinterpreting instructions about formula preparation. If her attention span is short, however, she may not be a candidate for breast-feeding, as she may be unable to grasp the importance of food for the infant and put him or her down when she is tired of feeding, not when enough milk has been consumed. If she will not actually be the primary caregiver to the child because of severe retardation, she is probably best advised to formula-feed the infant.

If the woman has more than mild retardation, you have a legal obligation to help devise a safe plan of care for the child (e.g., ensure that the woman will move in with a responsible friend) or counsel the woman's mother if she will be raising the child. Even though she is mentally retarded, the woman has full rights to the child so it cannot be taken from her at birth without her full consent. Likewise, she cannot be forced to terminate the pregnancy unless that is her informed decision.

Childbirth

A woman with mental retardation may not be able to benefit from a childbirth preparation class if her attention span is not long enough to enjoy the sessions and learn breathing exercises. If her retardation is not severe, she may benefit greatly from the classes. If she does not work or attend school, she has ample time to practice breathing exercises, and she may become very adept at using such a method to control pain in labor.

Labor may be a confusing time for the woman because even though she has been told that she would have labor contractions, she may not be fully prepared for their degree of severity or length. This is usually overwhelming for every woman. She may need an epidural anesthetic during labor to withstand this strange experience.

Following the birth, she will need time to examine the infant to understand the shift from "being pregnant" to "having a baby." If she is disappointed in the sex or appearance of the child, it would not be unusual for her to ask the nurse to "give her another baby" because she does not fully understand the uniqueness of each child.

The Postpartal Period

During the postpartal period, encourage the woman to spend time with the infant so that she learns safe care. It may be difficult for her to judge how much to feed the baby or that it is not safe to place the baby on a bed alone. You will need to model safe child care as a visual teaching strategy.

Ask if she desires contraceptive information. She may not be interested in prevention of another child at this time because a new baby is cute and "like a doll." As a rule, suggest that a community health nurse visit her within a week to be certain that the child's environment is safe; note on the referral if the woman did not accept contraceptive information as this might be mentioned again by the community health nurse once a working relationship has been established with her.

Be certain that she has a return appointment for both herself and the infant for follow-up care. Do not discharge the infant to her care until you are certain that she will be safe with the baby.

The Woman With Visual Impairment

Visual impairment in women of childbearing age may be the result of a variety of causes—for example, accidental injury in childhood, diabetes mellitus, or congenital anomalies, such as cornea or lens destruction from rubella invasion in utero. Visually impaired women may have suffered retinal damage from the use of oxygen if they were born prematurely. Unlike those who have lost their eyesight because of accidental injury or illness in childhood or young adulthood, women who have been visually impaired since birth tend not to grieve for their lack of vision but instead have a positive "I can do it" attitude about what they can accomplish. This is a positive characteristic to reinforce during pregnancy. It is interesting to help these women complete pregnancy safely and make plans for childrearing.

Degrees of Impairment

A designation of *visual impairment* means that a woman has some loss of vision; however, this could range from loss of peripheral vision to complete lack of eyesight. Each woman needs to be evaluated individually. A woman with loss of peripheral vision will have few special problems during pregnancy because, by turning her head, she can bring objects into her area of central vision. She may not be able to drive, however, and so will be dependent on a support person for transportation. A woman who is legally blind has a visual field not greater than 20 degrees or central distance vision in her better eye that is 20/200 or worse with the use of corrective lenses. A person with loss of central vision has to make some accommodations for pregnancy and child care.

Modifications for Pregnancy

Visually impaired women need to come early and consistently for prenatal care because they may not be able to self-assess for some of the danger signs of pregnancy, such as diplopia, blurring of vision, edema, or vaginal spotting. Because the woman may depend on a support person for transportation to the health care facility, you may need to schedule her appointments according to that person's schedule so that the woman does not miss visits. If a woman brings a guide dog with her, mark the dog's name as well as hers on the chart so you can also greet the dog by name and make yourself familiar to the animal. Although a guide dog's chief function is to offer direction to its owner, natural instincts cause it to become her protector. In this role, the dog may feel threatened by people who try to pet it and may snap at them. Children in the waiting room need to be cautioned about this.

In interviewing or teaching visually impaired women, do not use your hands to illustrate points ("I'll need a urine sample of at least this much urine [measured with your fingers]"). Be careful not to raise your voice to make a point and be certain to look at her, not her support person, as you speak. Do not use colors as descriptions of objects ("put on the blue gown").

It is important to determine the reason for the woman's visual impairment when taking a health history

and to address her worries about the impairment being passed on to her baby. If her lack of eyesight is for congenital reasons, she might benefit from genetic counseling. This is particularly important if the loss of vision is due to retinoblastoma, an inherited malignancy (see Chapter 53). If the cause was rubella, the woman might be advised to be certain her serum titer against rubella is adequate before undertaking a pregnancy to prevent this from occurring in her child.

Ask about a woman's financial resources (all persons legally blind are eligible for financial assistance through Social Security benefits) and whether this amount will be adequate for pregnancy expenses. Ask if someone lives with her and if she has someone to turn to if she has a problem. Investigate how the woman would contact the health care agency if she had an emergency, such as ruptured membranes. If she is visually impaired but has some eyesight, write an emergency telephone number in large letters for her to tape over her telephone. If she has no vision but reads Braille, ask if she has access to a Braille typewriter (she may own one or work in a sheltered workshop that has one). The number can then be written in Braille for her. Ask about whom she could rely on for transportation in an emergency (possibly a neighbor or a friend).

Ask about the woman's education level to help determine what health teaching will be necessary. It is quite possible for a visually impaired woman to have finished college and graduate school. Do not assume that she has received less than the usual amount of schooling or will not be well acquainted with body physiology.

When helping with or performing the physical assessment, make a point that you are closing the door or drawing a curtain to assure her that you are providing privacy. Always alert the woman that you are going to touch her, so as not to startle her. Otherwise, you may find yourself facing a growling guide dog that rises to protect her.

Pregnancy Counseling

If a woman and her support person are both visually impaired, use of pamphlets about pregnancy care is limited. If the woman's support person has vision, offering the pamphlets to him and suggesting he read them to her as a shared activity will not only be helpful to her but make him a more informed support person.

Schedule prenatal visits as needed to cover orally all the information the woman needs to be well informed about her pregnancy. Using three-dimensional models of anatomy or fetal growth is helpful in allowing the woman to appreciate how big her child is month by month (Figure 17-5). Many visually impaired women have tape recorders that are supplied free of charge to them from Recording for the Blind, a national nonprofit, voluntary organization. Telephone the local association

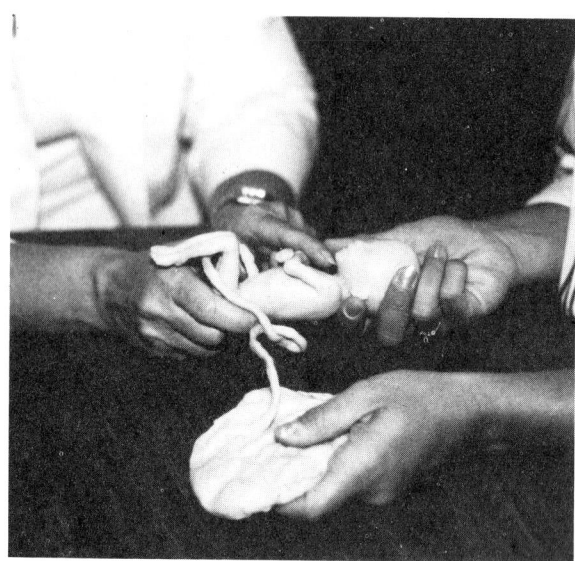

FIGURE 17-5
Health teaching with disabled women is modified to meet their particular needs. Visually impaired women benefit from tactile aids, such as this rubber model of a fetus.

for the visually impaired and ask if they have any material already recorded on pregnancy or breast-feeding that they could supply. If not, make a tape recording of any information you particularly want the woman to remember or she seems concerned about. You could supply the health care facility telephone number at the beginning of the tape for easy access in an emergency, and, perhaps, the date of her next visit.

Discuss her level of activity during pregnancy. If she depends on the sound of a cane against the sidewalk to direct her while she walks, she may not go out on days when there is snow or ice that obscures the sound. Stress that walking is important during pregnancy; if she cannot go outside, walking around her house or apartment 20 to 30 times will help promote venous return from the lower extremities. Women with a visual impairment may have developed a keen sense of hearing and touch. At visits, use a Doppler instrument to listen to fetal heart sounds so they can hear them also. Show her how to assess her ankles and fingers for edema so she will be able to check for this danger sign of pregnancy independently.

As with any pregnant woman, investigate the visually impaired woman's knowledge of good nutrition for pregnancy. Ask who does the cooking in her household. She may prepare breakfast and lunch, for example, meals that do not necessarily require a stove, whereas her support person may prepare a hot evening meal. Nutrition counseling, for two meals daily, therefore, may need to center on foods that can be prepared without cooking. Do not be reluctant to use food names such as "green, leafy vegetables" or "orange" when dis-

cussing food. Although these words are colors, they are also the most common names by which these foods are known.

Planning Child Care

Ask during pregnancy about the woman's plans for child care. Encourage her to breast-feed, as this is easier than preparing formula. If she chooses to use formula, suggest she use the ready-prepared kind that needs no dilution and can be poured into a clean bottle just before feeding, so that she can avoid having to measure amounts. Caution her against propping the baby's bottle, which could cause aspiration.

Explore with her how she will manage to supervise the child as he or she gets older and begins exploring the house. All women should remove harmful items from lower cupboards during pregnancy; then, if a child crawls or walks sooner than anticipated, dangerous substances will already be hidden. Many visually impaired people do not turn on lights because they do not perceive the difference between light and dark. This is particularly true if two visually impaired persons live together. Urge the woman to develop the habit of turning on lights after dinner as the infant will need light to develop vision. Suggest she check with a neighbor monthly to see that light bulbs have not burned out.

Childbirth

Encourage the woman to attend a childbirth preparation class. Explain that a number of films may be used in the introductory sessions concerning childbirth; although she will be unable to view them, the audio portion will still be helpful to her. She will be as able as a sighted woman to use breathing exercises in labor. If her support person is also visually impaired, he cannot time the length of contractions by looking at a watch (most Braille watches do not have second hands), but he can count the contractions in seconds. The most important role of a support person in labor is not counting contractions, in any event, but simply being there as a supporting presence.

Labor can be a confusing time for the visually impaired woman. She is able to function competently by arranging many aspects of her life in a way that allows her to stay in charge of situations; during labor, however, she may feel she is losing this psychologic edge as her body takes charge. Be certain to explain any sound in a labor or birthing room, such as the buzz of a central supply routing system, the fetal monitor, or the client call light system. Hearing sounds and not being able to identify them is frightening. Be certain that everyone who comes into the birthing room introduces themselves (or you interrupt to introduce them) so she is not frightened by strangers' voices speaking to her. Be sure to give the baby to the visually impaired woman as soon as possible so she can reassure herself that the child is perfect. Describe the baby to her (long hair, pretty eyes, 10 fingers, and so forth). Even if she does not voice her fear, she cannot help but worry that the baby is vision impaired. Assess whether the infant has a red reflex and whether he or she follows a moving light, then assure the woman that her infant is indeed able to see. (On the other hand, do not act too excited that the baby has sight. This reaction could be interpreted as belittling the mother herself.) Touching the baby is much more satisfying for the visually impaired mother than hearing your assuring words. If the birthing room is cold, explain to the woman that you want to rewrap the baby to prevent chilling, not because her touching is wrong or because you are trying to hide an imperfection in the baby.

The Postpartal Period

Be certain that a woman has her child with her for long stretches of time so she can become used to such phenomena as the irregular pattern of breathing of a newborn (she may notice this where others do not because of her acute awareness of sound) and she is comfortable with changing diapers and feeding. Suggest disposable diapers to avoid sharp safety pins. As a rule, suggest a community health nurse visit her daily for the first few weeks she is home with the infant unless she has a sighted family member who will be home with her.

Teach her to look at the child when talking to him because making eye contact is important to the child in feeling secure and developing vision. Be certain that she has an appointment for follow-up child health supervision and a return appointment for herself as well. Ask if she desires contraceptive information.

The Woman With a Hearing Impairment

Hearing impairment ranges from having difficulty hearing whispered conversation to being totally deaf. A hearing loss of 30 dB means that a woman has some difficulty hearing normal instructions and questions. A loss of 50 dB or more is a severe hearing loss. This is the decibel level used to conduct normal conversation. Many women with a hearing impairment also have a speech impairment. (The older term *deaf and dumb* is no longer used as it unfairly correlates a hearing impediment with mental retardation or total speechlessness [Armstrong, 1991].)

The average woman of childbearing age with a hearing impairment has been hearing impaired since birth because of an infection such as rubella during intrauterine life, meningitis in early infancy, or a genetically inherited hearing disorder. These types of hearing losses are sensorineural; they can be helped to some degree by a hearing aid, but hearing can never be fully restored.

Explore with the woman the reason for her hearing impairment; as with visual impairment, it may affect her concerns during pregnancy. If her hearing loss is the result of a genetic disorder, she may be concerned that her child will also develop this problem. If it occurred because of an infection while she herself was in utero, ensure that her rubella titer is adequate so that her own child will not be infected.

Modifications for Pregnancy

A woman with a hearing impairment needs to establish a regular pattern of prenatal care. As she may have missed the everyday discussions of pregnancy that other women have listened to or the spot announcements on television about avoiding alcohol or smoking during pregnancy, she may lack "savvy" about pregnancy and need more time at appointments so these areas can be discussed.

Lip-reading is a hard skill to learn so many people with hearing impairments are unable to do this with ease. Even if skilled at this, new words such as *amniotic, gestation,* or *edema* cannot be deciphered. Make a habit of showing the woman the printed word so she can see what your lip motion represents when presenting a new term. Speak slowly but without exaggerated enunciation so she can follow your meaning. Remember that if she is lip reading, she cannot understand your instruction or question if you turn away from her or hold a chart so she cannot see your lips. If she uses sign language, she may bring an interpreter with her to translate. Be certain that you talk to her, the client, not to her interpreter when interviewing.

Many women who have been hearing impaired since birth have difficulty enunciating words clearly because they have never heard the sound they are trying to imitate. The more you listen to the woman, the more adept you can become at understanding her speech pattern. Do not be reluctant to ask her to repeat a question you did not understand. If she repeats a question a second time and you still have difficulty understanding it, ask her to write it down for you.

Assess whether hearing impaired women have support people available and who they would depend on in an emergency. How would they contact the health care facility if an emergency, such as ruptured membranes, occurred? (Most women have a neighbor they could ask to telephone for them or use a specially equipped telephone [a TDD device] that prints out messages for them.) Discuss how she can secure emergency help (perhaps a community 911 number) when the health care agency is not open. Ask about financial resources for pregnancy (most women with hearing impairment qualify for Social Security assistance).

Pregnancy Counseling

Use visual aids liberally to explain the physiologic changes of pregnancy or what care is planned at a health visit (Hall, 1991).

Be certain you have a woman's attention before you touch her to avoid startling her. During a pelvic examination, she may not be able to see the examiner's face, so be aware that any questions or reassurances made during this time will not be noticed and must be repeated.

Planning Child Care

One of the biggest worries of the hearing impaired woman is that she will not be able to hear the baby crying to tell her he or she is hungry and needs her, especially at night. Help her to plan to bring the infant's crib or bassinet close to her bed so she can feel the vibration of the baby's stirring and waking. Suggest she breastfeed so that if she misses the first hungry demands, she can feed the infant immediately without making him or her wait while she prepares a bottle.

Childbirth

Encourage the woman to attend a childbirth preparation class. She may not be able to hear the soundtrack of films used in class, but the visual picture of a birth will be helpful to her. She can learn and use breathing exercises during labor. Since she will be unable to hear a coach say "contraction beginning," plan with her how her coach will alert her to relax (a hand on her forehead or her arm?).

Remember that during labor the hearing-impaired woman cannot hear information on how she is progressing if you are not directly facing her or if your face is hidden (as often happens with pelvic examination). If she needs to communicate with her support person in sign language, act as an advocate for keeping her hands unencumbered by intravenous lines. Remember that she cannot hear the infant cry at birth (which is how the average woman is reassured that her newborn is healthy); be sure she knows the baby is crying and breathing well.

Hearing-impaired women have a strong need to see their infant as soon as possible to assure themselves that the infant is well. Even if they do not voice this fear, they may be concerned that the infant is hearing impaired. You can assess for this disability by showing her how the infant startles at a loud noise, such as clapping your hands. A better way is to show her how the baby quiets at the sound of your voice. This will also encourage her to talk to him or her. If she continues to feel anxious and tests her baby for hearing in the weeks to come, the latter method is much more preferable than making loud noises to startle the baby.

The Postpartal Period

Be certain that a woman's nursing care plan is marked clearly that she is hearing impaired. A woman who is severely hearing impaired may not appreciate the comforting quality that speech has for infants. Some women whose speech is severely affected are reluctant to speak to strangers. Assure her that her infant is not a stranger in this sense and will quiet readily to the sound of her voice. Unfortunately, the child may develop her speech pattern and need speech therapy during preschool years to learn to enunciate words clearly. Having been spoken to and sung to during the first year is important for overall development, however, so this is still preferable to living in a world of silence. If her partner is not hearing impaired, he should be encouraged to talk and sing to the baby to provide a normal pattern of speech. Tapes of songs, stories, and nursery rhymes also can be played.

Be certain that the woman has learned to tell from vibration when her infant is crying. Schedule a follow-up health care appointment for both her and her child. Ask the woman if she desires contraception information about spacing possible future children.

The Woman Who Is Drug Dependent

Drug dependence is a growing health problem in women of childbearing age and, thus, of increasing incidence during pregnancy. As many as 10% to 20% of pregnant women use illegal drugs during pregnancy (Evans, 1991). Cocaine use, in particular, has increased dramatically in recent years. Many women are multiple-drug users (Little et al., 1990). It is both an urban and rural issue (see the Focus on Nursing Research box).

Someone who is **drug dependent** craves a particular drug for psychologic as well as physical well being. Typically, substance-abusing women are in the younger age group. They may have less traditional lifestyles because they spend their money for drugs rather than for domestic needs. Even women who appear settled or "typical homemakers" may be drug dependent, however, so all pregnant women need to be assessed for drug consumption.

A woman with a substance abuse problem may come late for prenatal care and is apt to have difficulty following instructions. Although she means to eat well, she rarely has enough money for both drugs and food, and so her nutrition is apt to be inadequate. Further, she is unlikely to have money for supplemental vitamins or iron preparations.

The substance-abusing woman may be reluctant to come for prenatal care, afraid that she will be "found out" and reported to legal authorities. She may not have money to pay for prenatal services or transportation to and from a clinic because she spends her income on drugs. If she is using a drug that sustains her only for a few hours, she cannot wait long at a health care facility to be seen for an appointment.

Illicit drugs tend to be of small molecular weight, so they cross the placenta readily. As a result, the fetus of an addicted mother has a drug concentration of about

FOCUS ON NURSING RESEARCH

Is Drug Use During Pregnancy Only an Urban Problem?

To see if drug use during pregnancy was a problem in a rural community, two nursing researchers tested urine on a sample of 202 women enrolled for prenatal care to see if residuals of drug use could be detected. The mean age of the sample was 28 years with a range of 16 to 41 years. The mean education level was 14.25 years. Findings of the study revealed the prevalence of perinatal drug use in this population was 3.9%. No instance of ethanol, amphetamines, barbiturates, benzodiazepines, cocaine, or phencyclidine use was detected. Marijuana use was found in 3.5% of specimens and 0.5% were positive for opiates. These findings are significantly lower than the 10% to 11% prevalence level seen in urban communities. Although drug use during pregnancy was revealed to be lower than in urban populations, the researchers stress that because it is present, it should continue to be screened for by interview at prenatal visits.

Matti, L. K., & Caspersen, V. M. (1993). Prevalence of drug use among pregnant women in a rural area. *Journal of Obstetric, Gynecologic and Neonatal Nursing, 22,* 510.

pressure increase dramatically in response to extreme vasoconstriction. Immediate death may result from cardiac failure. Alkaloidal cocaine (crack) is a concentrated mixture and produces an even more rapid and intense "high" when it is inhaled (Niebyl, 1991).

Cocaine has become one of the most frequently abused drugs during pregnancy (Lynch & McKeon, 1990). As many as 21% of women between the ages of 26 and 34 have used it (Savoy-Moore et al., 1992). Cocaine use is exceptionally harmful during pregnancy as the extreme vasoconstriction that occurs can occlude circulation to the placenta. This may cause congenital anomalies in the fetus. It also leads to abruptio placentae, or a tearing loose of the placenta, which can result in preterm labor or fetal death (Figure 17-6). Infants of

50% of that of the mother. Because fetal effects occur, drug use accounts for 4% to 5% of fetal abnormalities. Many drugs cause withdrawal and neurobehavioral effects on the fetus (Dattel, 1990). If a woman uses drugs that she injects, she may develop hepatitis B or human immunodeficiency virus (HIV) unless her injection equipment is clean each time. Because many women addicts become prostitutes to earn money for drugs, they are more likely than the average woman to contract sexually transmitted diseases, posing an additional threat to the fetus.

Women who are drug dependent need nursing support and anticipatory guidance during pregnancy as they may have few effective support people with whom they feel free to discuss their problems or concerns or who can answer their questions about pregnancy. Pregnancy may become a stimulus for drug withdrawal, so this year in their life can become a maturing and health advocacy experience for them. The effects of alcohol, cigarette, and caffeine use are discussed in Chapter 11.

Cocaine

Cocaine is derived from *Erythroxylon coca,* a plant grown almost exclusively in South America. When sniffed into the nose or smoked in a pipe, cocaine is absorbed across the mucous membranes and affects the central nervous system, leading to restlessness and excitement; the respiratory and cardiac rates and blood

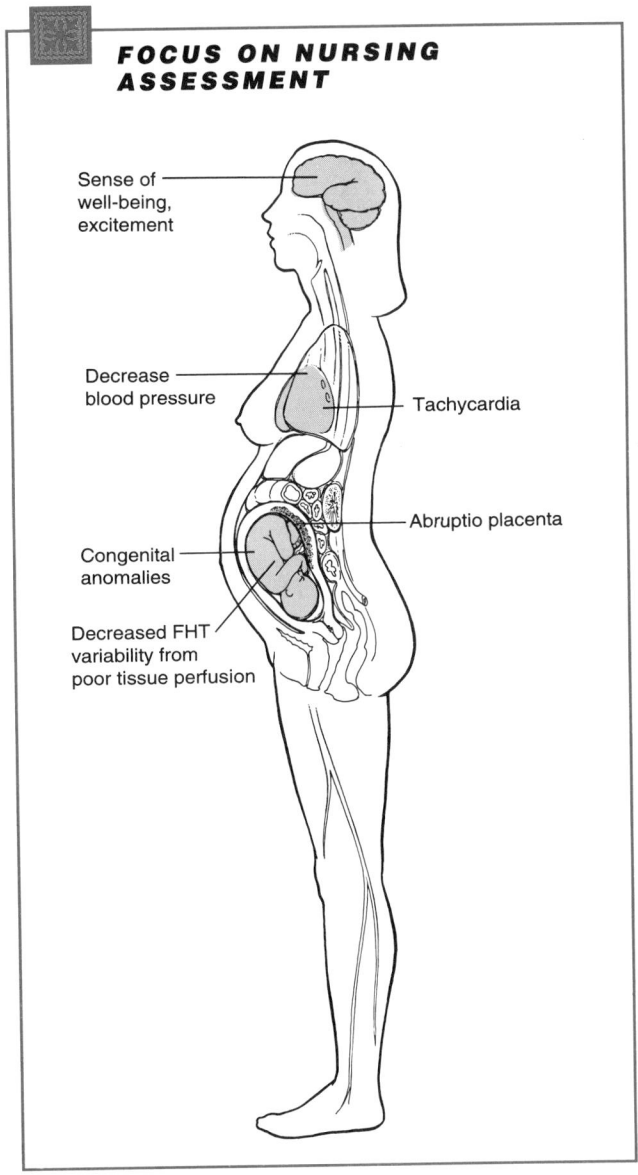

FOCUS ON NURSING ASSESSMENT

Sense of well-being, excitement

Decrease blood pressure

Tachycardia

Abruptio placenta

Congenital anomalies

Decreased FHT variability from poor tissue perfusion

FIGURE 17-6
The effects of cocaine abuse in the pregnant woman.

cocaine-dependent women may suffer intracranial hemorrhage at birth and long-term emotional and learning deficits. Another result is a withdrawal syndrome of tremulousness, irritability, and muscle rigidity.

Women who are at high risk for suspected cocaine use as identified by Dattel (1990) are those who do not attend prenatal care (or only make erratic visits), appear to have a placental abruption, have a history or physical signs of other substance abuse, show bizarre behavior or have a psychiatric history, and have a history of prostitution, other family members abusing drugs, or incarceration.

Cocaine use can be detected by urinalysis. The metabolites of cocaine can be detected in urine up to 1 week after use but, for best results, a urine for drug analysis should be obtained within the first 24 hours. Counseling women to discontinue cocaine use during pregnancy is often disappointing, as the effects of the drug are so dramatic it is difficult for addicted woman to withdraw.

Amphetamines

Methamphetamine (speed) has a pharmacologic effect similar to cocaine. It is usually identified in polydrug abuse. Ice, a rock type of methamphetamine that is smoked, has the potential for causing high concentrations of drug in the maternal circulation. Newborns show signs of jitteriness and poor feeding at birth (Evans, 1991).

Marijuana and Hashish

Both marijuana and hashish are obtained from the hemp plant, cannabis. When smoked, they produce tachycardia as well as a sense of well being. As these drugs are frequently part of polydrug abuse, their singular effects are not well documented. They are associated with loss of short-term memory and increased respiratory infection in adults; newborns may suffer some intelligence reduction if the mother's use is extensive. A frequent user may not be able to breast-feed because of reduced milk production and excretion of the drug in the milk.

Phencyclidine

Phencyclidine (PCP) is an animal tranquilizer that is a frequently used street drug in polydrug abuse (Carroll, 1990). It causes increased cardiac output and a sense of euphoria. PCP tends to leave the maternal circulation and concentrate in fetal cells, so it has the potential to be particularly injurious to the fetus. It has the potential for causing long-term hallucinations (flashback episodes) in the user.

Opiates

Opiates, which are used for the treatment of pain (e.g., morphine or meperidine [Demerol]) and cough suppression (codeine), are also widely abused because of their potent analgesic and euphoric effect. Heroin, a raw opiate, is the main opiate used recreationally to the point of dependence. A short-acting narcotic, heroin is inactive until it crosses the blood-brain barrier (which it does more quickly than morphine). It may be administered intradermally ("skin popping"), through inhalation ("snorting"), or intravenously ("shooting"). It produces an immediate and short-lived feeling of euphoria (high) followed by sedation (nodding).

There is great potential for the development of tolerance in the use of opiates, which eventually leads to drug dependence: both psychologic and physical dependence occur with chronic narcotic abuse (Loeb, 1993). Withdrawal symptoms, which include nausea, vomiting, diarrhea, abdominal pain, hypertension, restlessness, shivering, insomnia, body aches, and muscle jerks, may begin as soon as 6 hours after the last drug dose and can continue for several days. Their severity and duration will depend on the amount of drug used daily and length of the dependence period. Maternal complications include pregnancy-induced hypertension, phlebitis, subacute bacterial endocarditis, and, because narcotics are often injected with shared needles, hepatitis B and HIV.

Heroin abuse in the pregnant woman results in fetal opiate dependence. At one time, fetal morbidity and mortality with maternal opiate dependence were extremely high. With the development of methadone maintenance programs and protocols to manage the drug-dependent newborn, however, the infant's prognosis has improved. The baby born to a heroin-addicted mother is still considered to be at risk for a number of disorders. Infants of opiate-abusing women tend to be small for gestation age and have an increased incidence of fetal distress and meconium aspiration. They will have the same withdrawal symptoms after birth as the mother would if she abruptly stopped taking the drug; they are at higher than usual risk for sudden infant death syndrome.

Because the fetus is exposed to drugs that must be processed by the liver during pregnancy, the fetal liver is forced to mature faster than normal. For this reason, newborns of substance-abusing women seem better able to cope with bilirubin at birth than other babies; hyperbilirubinemia is, therefore, rarely a problem. Fetal lung tissue also appears to mature more rapidly than is normal. Thus, even though the infant is born preterm, the chance that he will develop a condition such as respiratory distress syndrome is less than average.

If at all possible, the opiate-dependent woman should be enrolled in a methadone maintenance program during pregnancy. Infants of women on methadone do not escape withdrawal symptoms (some infants appear to have more severe reactions to methadone withdrawal than to heroin withdrawal), but because the woman is being provided an oral drug legally, the fetus is at least assured better nutrition, better prenatal care, and less exposure to pathogens such as hepatitis B and HIV. A nonstress test is apt to be depressed in variability for 1 to 2 hours following administration of methadone so its results should be evaluated in light of this (Archie et al., 1989). Drug withdrawal symptoms of the newborn are discussed in Chapter 26.

Key Points

- As many as 7% of births in the United States are to teenagers. Adolescent pregnancy is a major problem not only because it occurs at such a high rate but also because it can interfere with the development of both the adolescent and fetus. Nursing care needs to be individualized to meet the prenatal needs of this age group. Helping adolescents to view a pregnancy as a growth experience can help them mature in their ability to parent.
- Women who delay childbearing until age 35 may have some needs during pregnancy that need special consideration by health care providers. They may need additional discussion time at prenatal visits to help them incorporate a pregnancy into their lifestyle. They may need reminding to save time during the day for rest, particularly if they have a degree of hypertension before pregnancy.
- Women who have physical disabilities such as vision and hearing impairment or spinal cord injury are apt to have special needs during pregnancy that must be addressed by health care providers. Providing time for discussion early in pregnancy so these needs can be identified and anticipated is an important role for nurses.
- Women with a physical disability may need help in adjusting their usual medical regimen to pregnancy. Be certain they are aware of how to contact help in an emergency. Assess that all medications they are taking for their primary disorder are safe during pregnancy.
- Women with mental retardation may need help in planning ways to follow prenatal instructions. As with all women with special needs, be certain they have support people around them so you can feel confident the baby will receive safe care.
- The woman who is drug dependent presents a unique challenge during pregnancy. Short-term goals must be directed toward encouraging the woman to decrease or halt her drug intake in order to safeguard the health of the fetus. Long-term goals must

address the need for the woman to decrease drug intake for the reminder of her life so she can be a quality parent for her child.
- The fetus of a woman with drug dependency is at high risk because of the direct effects of the drug and the indirect effects of an unhealthy lifestyle. Women addicted to opiates should be encouraged to join methadone maintenance programs if possible.

Critical Thinking Exercises

1. Mindy is a 14-year-old you meet in a prenatal clinic. She is 20 weeks pregnant. She lives with her mother and two younger sisters. She tells you she is old enough to be a responsible parent so plans on keeping her baby. Describe the specific measures you would want to teach Mindy to help her be ready for parenting. What clues would you look for in Mindy to see if her evaluation of herself is correct?
2. Chelsa is a 40-year-old woman who was recently married and is pregnant following in vitro fertilization. She works out at a health spa daily and flies 3 days every week to out-of-state locations for work. Outline a plan of care for Chelsa to help her avoid complications of pregnancy. Suppose she had a very sedentary life. Would your advice be different?
3. Terry is a 22-year-old who is drug dependent on heroin. You suspect she supports her drug habit by prostitution. She refuses to be seen in clinic if she has to wait over 15 minutes. Describe modifications to Terry's plan of care to assure consistent prenatal care. What specific advice would you want to stress with Terry to avoid complications of pregnancy?

References

Archie, C. L., et al. (1989). The effects of methadone treatment on the reactivity of the nonstress test. *Obstetrics & Gynecology, 74,* 254.

Armstrong, N. T. (1991). Nursing care of the deaf-blind client. *Insight, 16,* 20.

Berkowitz, G. S., et al. (1990). Delayed childbearing and the outcome of pregnancy. *New England Journal of Medicine, 322,* 659.

Burnhill, M. S. (1994). Adolescent pregnancy in the U.S. *Contemporary Obstetrics and Gynecology, 39,* 26.

Carroll, M. E. (1990). PCP and hallucinogens. *Advances in Alcohol and Substance Abuse, 9,* 167.

Chez, R. A. (1991). Advising pregnant women about nutrition. *Contemporary Obstetrics and Gynecology, 36,* 80.

Craig, D. F. (1990). The adaptation to pregnancy of spinal cord injured women. *Rehabilitation Nursing, 15,* 6.

Cross, L. L., et al. (1992). Pregnancy, labor and delivery—postspinal cord injury. *Paraplegia, 30,* 890.

Cunningham, F. G., et al. (1993). *Williams obstetrics* (19th ed.). Norwalk, CT: Appleton and Lange.

Dattel, B. J. (1990). Substance abuse in pregnancy. *Seminars in Perinatology, 14,* 179.

Department of Health & Human Services (1991). *Healthy people 2000.* Washington, D.C.: U.S. Public Health Service.

Department of Health & Human Services (1993). Comparability of the birth certificate and 1988 maternal and infant health survey. *Vital & Health Statistics, 2,* (116)12.

Erikson, E. (1963). *Childhood and society* (3rd ed.). New York: Norton.

Evans, A. (1991). Perinatal chemical use. In K. Niswander & A. Evans (Eds.), *Manual of obstetrics* (4th ed.). Boston: Little, Brown.

Gutierrez, Y. & King, J. C. (1993). Nutrition during teenage pregnancy. *Pediatric Annals, 22,* 99.

Hall, J. (1991). Jane: The care of a deaf woman. *Midwives Chronicle, 104,* 251.

Horner, R. D., et al. (1991). Pica practices of pregnant women. *Journal of the American Dietetic Association, 91,* 34.

Jacono, J. J., et al. (1992). Teenage pregnancy: A reconsideration. *Canadian Journal of Public Health, 83,* 196.

Lagrew, D. C. (1990). Strategies for managing emboli in pregnancy. *Contemporary Obstetrics and Gynecology, 35,* 113.

Little, B. B., et al. (1990). Patterns of multiple substance abuse during pregnancy: Implications for mother and fetus. *Southern Medical Journal, 83,* 507.

Loeb, S. (1993). *Nurses' handbook of drug therapy.* Springhouse, PA: Springhouse.

Lynch, M., & McKeon, V. A. (1990). Cocaine use during pregnancy. *Journal of Obstetric, Gynecologic, and Neonatal Nursing, 19,* 285.

Niebyl, J. R. (1991). Drugs with potential fetal toxicity. *Contemporary Obstetrics and Gynecology, 36,* 68.

Paneth, N. (1993). The causes of cerebral palsy: Recent evidence. *Clinical & Investigative Medicine, 16,* 95.

Rosenfeld, J. A. (1990). Pregnancy in women over 35: Risks for mother and baby. *Postgraduate Medicine, 87,* 167.

Sauer, P. M. & Harvey, C. J. (1993). Spinal cord injury and pregnancy. *Journal of Perinatal & Neonatal Nursing, 7,* 22.

Savoy-Moore, R. T., et al. (1992). Cocaine use and reproductive function. *Female Patient, 17,* 109.

Schmidt, S. (1993). What is a multiple marker (triple screen) test? *AWHONN Voice, 1,* 8.

Schneck, M. E., et al. (1990). Low-income pregnant adolescents and their infants: Dietary findings and health outcomes. *Journal of the American Dietetic Association, 90,* 555.

Scholl, T. O., et al. (1990). Maternal growth during pregnancy and decreased infant birth weight. *American Journal of Clinical Nutrition, 51,* 790.

Troutman, B. R., & Cutrona, C. E. (1990). Nonpsychotic postpartum depression among adolescent mothers. *Journal of Abnormal Psychology, 99,* 69.

Wen, S. W., et al. (1990). Smoking, maternal age, fetal growth, and gestational age at delivery. *American Journal of Obstetrics and Gynecology, 162,* 53.

Suggested Readings

Accardo, P. J., et al. (1990). Children of mentally retarded parents. *American Journal of Diseases of Children, 144,* 69.

Byrne, M. W., et al. (1992). Communicating with addicted women in labor. *MCN: American Journal of Maternal Child Nursing, 17,* 22.

Donovan, C. (1990). Adolescent sexuality. *British Medical Journal, 300,* 1026.

Elster, A. B., et al. (1990). Association between parenthood and problem behavior in a national sample of adolescents. *Pediatrics, 85,* 1044.

Faye, E. E., et al. (1994). Help people with disabilities help themselves. *Patient Care, 28,* 65.

Fingerhut, L., et al. (1990). Smoking before, during and after pregnancy. *American Journal of Public Health, 80,* 541.

Howard, M., & MaCabe, J. B. (1990). Helping teenagers postpone sexual involvement. *Family Planning Perspectives, 22,* 21.

Kelsall, J. (1991). She'll be all right. She can lip read. *Midwives Chronicle, 104,* 254.

Parker, B., et al. (1993). Physical and emotional abuse in pregnancy: A comparison of adult and teenage women. *Nursing Research, 42,* 173.

Peters, H., & Heorell, C. J. (1991). Fetal and neonatal effects of cocaine use. *Journal of Obstetric, Gynecologic, and Neonatal Nursing, 20,* 121.

Scholl, T. O., et al. (1990). Weight gain during pregnancy in adolescence: Predictive ability of early weight gain. *Obstetrics & Gynecology, 75,* 948.

Stevens-Simon, C., et al. (1990). Repeat adolescent pregnancy and low birth weight. *Journal of Adolescent Health Care, 11,* 114.

Tsang, R. C. (1993). Teenage pregnancy is preventable—a challenge to our society. *Pediatric Annals, 22,* 133.

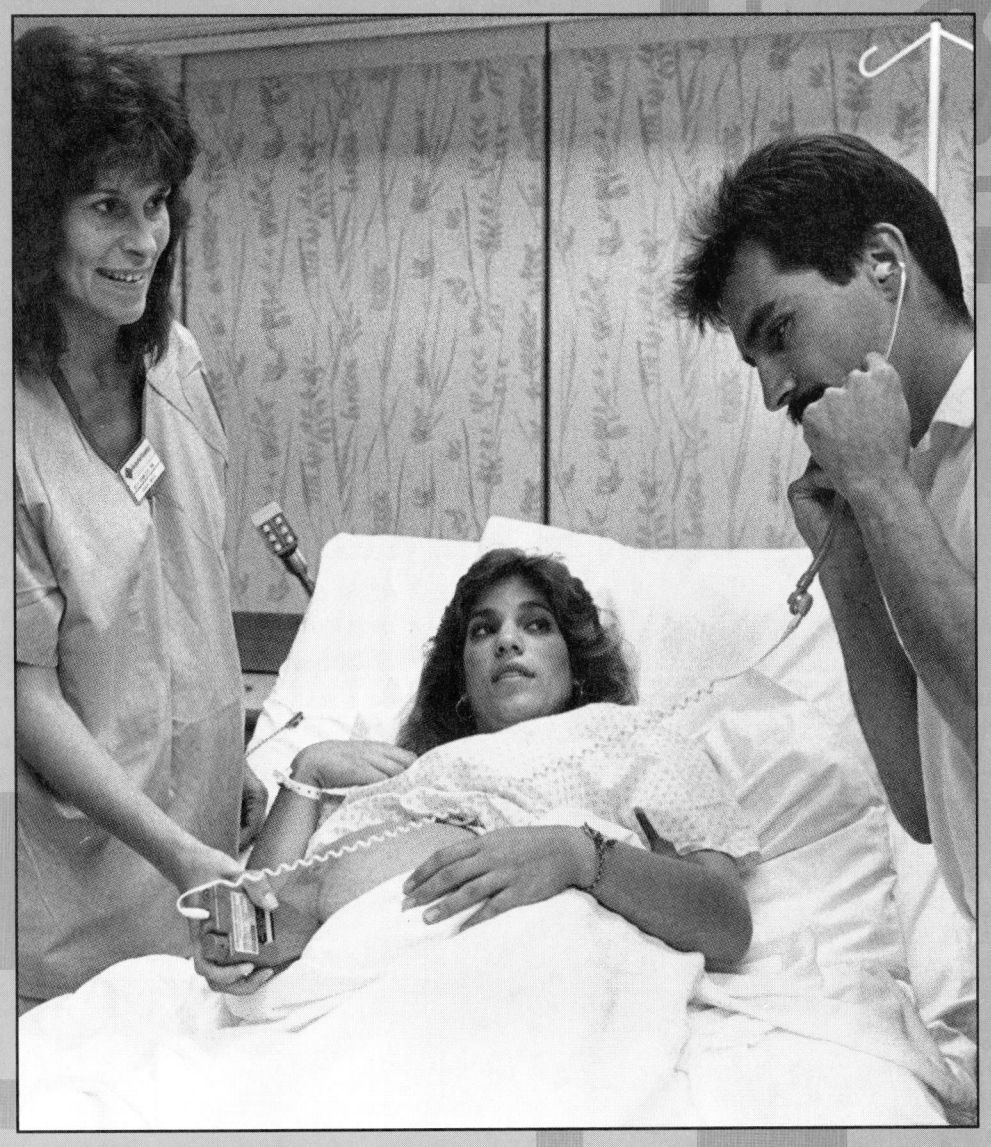

Unit 4

The Nursing Role in Caring for the Family During Labor and Birth

Chapter 18

The Labor Process

Adele Pillitteri: MATERNAL AND CHILD
HEALTH NURSING, 2nd Edition. © 1995
Adele Pillitteri.

Key Terms

- attitude
- breech presentation
- cardinal movements of labor
- cephalic presentation
- crowning
- dilatation
- effacement
- engagement
- episiotomy
- fetal descent
- Leopold's maneuver
- lie
- lightening
- molding
- passage
- passenger
- pathologic retraction ring
- physiologic retraction ring
- position
- ripening
- station
- transition

Objectives

After mastering the contents of this chapter, you should be able to:

1. Describe the common theories explaining the onset and continuation of labor as well as the role of the passenger, the passage, and the force in the labor process.

2. Assess a woman for stages and progress of labor.

3. Formulate nursing diagnoses related to both the physiologic and psychologic aspects of labor.

4. Assist the woman in labor to establish realistic goals and outcome criteria for progress in labor.

5. Implement nursing care for the family during labor, such as providing for comfort, and educating them about the process of labor.

6. Evaluate outcome criteria to be certain that nursing goals for care have been achieved.

7. Identify National Health Goals related to safe labor and birth that nurses can be instrumental in helping the nation to achieve.

8. Identify areas related to labor and birth that could benefit from additional nursing research.

9. Use critical thinking to analyze whether current nursing care measures truly meet the needs of women and their families in labor.

10. Synthesize knowledge of nursing care in labor with nursing process to achieve quality maternal and child health nursing care.

Labor is the series of events by which uterine contractions expel the fetus and placenta from the woman's body. Regular contractions cause progressive dilatation of the cervix and sufficient muscular force to allow the baby to be pushed to the outside. Labor is an apt term for the process because it involves a great deal of work. For the woman, the fetus, and the family, it is a time of change, both an ending and a beginning.

Labor and birth call for all the psychological and physical coping methods that a woman has available to her. No matter how much childbirth preparation she has had, nor how many times she has already gone through the experience, a woman will require nursing care that is efficient and family focused, because childbirth marks the beginning of a new family structure.

Nursing interventions to make labor safe, comfortable, and effective are vital. Any support person should be treated with respect and should be included in all phases of the process, whenever possible. Labor and birth are enormous emotional and physiologic accomplishments for a woman and her support person, and interventions that make the experience more positive and memorable for them will contribute to future family interactions.

National Health Goals related to labor or birth are shown in the Focus on National Health Goals box.

NURSING PROCESS OVERVIEW for the Woman in Labor

ASSESSMENT

Assessment of a woman in labor must be done with a degree of speed but also with gentleness. The woman is keenly aware of words spoken around her and the manner with which procedures are carried out. Due to this sensitivity, she may perceive a venipuncture as an excessively painful experience rather than a simple momentary pain. She may have difficulty relaxing for a vaginal examination if she is worried that pressure on the fetal head will cause her pain. Remember that pain is a subjective symptom. The woman is the only person who can evaluate how much she is having or how much she will be able to endure.

Assess how much discomfort a woman is having in labor not only by what she voices, but also by subtle signs of pain such as facial tenseness, flushing or paleness of face, hands making a fist, rapid breathing, or rapid pulse rate. Knowing the extent of the woman's discomfort is a guide to the choice of medication or intervention she needs in labor.

NURSING DIAGNOSIS

Common nursing diagnoses used during labor include:

- Pain related to labor contractions
- Anxiety related to process of labor and birth
- Health-seeking behaviors related to management of discomfort of labor
- Situational low self-esteem related to inability to use prepared childbirth method

Even though the discomfort of labor is commonly referred to as "contractions" rather than "pain," do not omit the word "pain" from a nursing diagnosis because the term strengthens an understanding of the problem.

PLANNING

When establishing goals with the woman in labor and her partner, be certain that the goals are realistic for the situation. Labor takes place over a relatively short time (an average of 12 hours), so goals must be met within this period. On the other hand, it is important not to project a definite time limit for labor to be completed. The length of labor can vary greatly from person to person and still be within normal limits. It is necessary also to appreciate the magnitude of labor. It is unlikely that all the fear or anxiety during the woman's labor can be alleviated; it is such an unusual and significant experience that the average couple lacks coping resources large enough to resolve all associated stress.

Be certain to incorporate both the woman and her support person in planning so that the experience is a shared one for the couple. Planning may include review and education of the normal labor process; even though a couple may have learned this during pregnancy, the reality of labor may seem much different from what they imagined. Plans for nursing interventions must be flexible so that they can change with the progress of labor. Plans must also be individualized. Modify "standard" nursing care plans or else the significance of the experience for an individual woman may be lost.

A plan addressing the discomforts of labor includes planning for education, validation, and response to the woman's pain to help her maintain realistic perceptions about it. Be certain to include planning for comfort measures such as changing a wet sheet or offering a moisturizing cream for dry lips.

IMPLEMENTATION

Interventions in labor must always be carried out between contractions if possible so the woman is free to use a prepared childbirth technique to limit the discomfort of contractions. This calls for good coordination of care between health care providers and planning with the woman and her support person.

EVALUATION

Evaluation must be included as a continual step of care for the woman in labor to preserve her and her about-to-be born child's safety. Evaluation should reveal that the woman found labor and birth to be not only an endurable experience but one that allowed her self-esteem to grow and the family to grow through a shared experience. It is advantageous to talk to women in the early postpartal period about their labor experience, both as a means of evaluation of nursing care during labor and as a chance for the woman to "work through" this overwhelming experience and incorporate it into her self-image. Examples of outcome criteria that might be established are:

* Client states pain in labor was tolerable because of her advance preparation.
* Family members voice that the labor and birth experience was a growth experience for them, both individually and as a family.

Theories of Labor Onset

Labor normally begins when a fetus is sufficiently mature to cope with extrauterine life, yet not too large to cause mechanical difficulties with birth. The trigger that

---

FOCUS ON
National Health Goals

As labor and birth are both high risk times for the fetus and the mother, a number of National Health Goals speak directly to these times. These goals are:

* Reduce the maternal mortality rate to no more than 3.3/100,000 live births from a baseline of 6.6/100,000.
* Reduce the fetal death rate to no more than 5/1000 live births from a baseline of 7.6/1000 (DHHS, 1991).

Nurses can be instrumental in helping the nation to achieve these goals by close monitoring of women during labor and birth and by teaching women as much as possible about labor so they are able to use as little analgesia and anesthesia as possible. The less anesthesia and analgesia used, the fewer the complications that can result in fetal or maternal death.

Topics that could benefit from additional nursing research in this area are advantages and disadvantages of different birthing settings; the best way to teach unprepared women to learn breathing patterns for labor; how support people can best be prepared for a support role; and advantages and disadvantages of different birthing or labor positions.

---

converts the random, painless Braxton Hicks contractions into strong, coordinated, productive labor contractions, however, is unknown. In some instances, labor begins before the fetus is mature (preterm birth); in others, labor is delayed until the fetus and the placenta have both passed beyond the optimum point for birth (postterm birth).

A number of theories have been proposed to explain why labor begins. These include the *uterine stretch theory* (when an organ is full, it will empty); the *oxytocin theory* (oxytocin released by the posterior pituitary gland initiates labor); and the *progesterone deprivation theory* (when the level of progesterone decreases, contractions are initiated). Currently, however, it is believed that the initiation of labor contractions is caused by an interplay between the adrenal gland of the fetus and the uterus, which results in the production of prostaglandins—the *prostaglandin cascade theory.*

Interestingly, Hippocrates wrote in 400 BC that the fetus initiated labor. Nearly 2000 years later, new research is beginning to suggest that his hunch was accurate. It has been shown that progesterone has a relaxing effect on uterine muscle; estrogen a stimulating one. From early in pregnancy, a precursor from the fetal adrenal gland is conjugated in the placenta into estrogen. As estrogen from this source reaches a high level, glycerophospholipids (A1 prostaglandin precursors) are laid down. At the point that estrogen becomes the dominant hormone, phospholipase A2 begins to convert prostaglandin precursors into prostaglandin. Prostaglandins stimulate the myometrium (smooth muscle) to contract. That prostaglandins can initiate uterine contractions has been established by the usefulness of prostaglandins in initiating labor in postterm pregnancies (Cunningham et al., 1993). This is why inhibitors of prostaglandin synthesis such as aspirin may delay labor in women. The relatively low progesterone level causes the uterine muscle to be sensitive to oxytocin (possibly by blocking calcium sequestration in the muscle fiber) and aids contractions.

Other factors that stimulate the release of phospholipase A2 are damage to fetal membranes, stretching of the uterus, infection, decreased uterine blood flow, heavy smoking, abruptio placentae, and a stressed fetus. Immunologic responses may also contribute (Akin et al., 1990).

Signs of Labor

Preliminary Signs of Labor

Labor begins with subtle signs that women should be taught to recognize.

Lightening

In primiparas, **lightening,** or settling of the fetal presenting part to the level of the ischial spines, occurs approximately 10 to 14 days before labor begins. This changes the woman's abdominal contour as the uterus becomes lower and more anterior. Lightening gives the woman relief from the diaphragmatic pressure and shortness of breath she has been experiencing, and thus "lightens" her load. Lightening probably occurs early in primiparas because of tight abdominal muscles. In multiparas it is not as dramatic and usually occurs on the day of labor or even after labor has begun.

Increase in Level of Activity

A woman may wake on the morning of labor full of energy, in contrast to her feelings the previous month. This increase in activity is due to an increase in epinephrine release that is initiated by a decrease in progesterone produced by the placenta. The secretion of additional epinephrine prepares the woman's body for the work of labor ahead.

Braxton Hicks Contractions

In the last week or days before labor begins, the woman usually notices extremely strong Braxton Hicks contractions, which she may interpret as true labor contractions. Table 18-1 summarizes the ways these contractions can be differentiated from true labor.

Primiparas in particular have great difficulty in distinguishing between the two forms of contractions. A woman may be admitted to the labor unit of a hospital or birthing center because false contractions so closely simulate true labor. It is discouraging for a woman who is having what seem like contractions (and strong Braxton Hicks cause real discomfort) to be told that she is not in true labor and should return home. When this happens, women need sympathetic support. They can be reassured that misinterpreting labor signals is a natural mistake (it happens to many pregnant nurses and physicians, too). They can be reminded that if false contractions have become strong enough to be mistaken for true labor, true labor must not be far away.

Ripening of the Cervix

Ripening of the cervix is an internal sign seen only on pelvic examination. Throughout pregnancy the cervix feels softer than normal, with the consistency of an earlobe (Goodell's sign). At term, the cervix becomes still softer, until it can be described as "butter-soft," and tips forward. This is ripening, an internal announcement that labor is close at hand.

Signs of True Labor

Signs of true labor involve uterine and cervical changes. The more women know about true labor signs, the better, because they will be able to recognize them. This is helpful both in preventing preterm birth and being able to feel secure during labor (Bonovich, 1990).

Uterine Contractions

The surest sign that labor has begun is the initiation of effective, productive, involuntary uterine contractions. Because contractions are involuntary and come without warning, they can be frightening in early labor until the woman realizes that she can predict their pattern and can control the degree of discomfort if she uses the breathing exercises she has learned in preparation-for-labor classes.

Show

As the cervix softens and ripens, the mucus plug that filled the cervical canal during pregnancy is expelled. The exposed cervical capillaries seep blood as a result of pressure exerted by the fetus. The blood, mixed with mucus, takes on a pink tinge and is referred to as "show" or "bloody show."

Rupture of the Membranes

Labor may begin with rupture of the membranes, which the woman experiences as either a sudden gush or scanty, slow seeping of clear fluid from the vagina. Some women may worry when labor begins with rupture of the membranes because they believe labor will then be "dry" and thus be difficult and long. Actually, amniotic fluid continues to be produced until delivery of the membranes after the birth of the fetus, so no labor is ever dry. Early rupture of the membranes can be advantageous if it causes the fetal head to settle snugly into the pelvis, as this can actually shorten labor.

The main risks of ruptured membranes are intrauterine infection and possible prolapse of the cord, which can cut off the oxygen supply to the fetus. If labor has not spontaneously occurred by 24 hours after membrane rupture and the pregnancy is at term, in most instances labor will be induced to help reduce the possibilities of infection and prolapse of the cord.

Table 18-1. *Differentiation Between True and False Labor Contractions*

False Contractions	True Contractions
Begin and remain irregular.	Begin irregularly but become regular and predictable.
Felt first abdominally and remain confined to the abdomen.	Felt first in lower back and sweep around to the abdomen in a wave.
Often disappear with ambulation.	Continue no matter what the woman's level of activity.
Do not increase in duration, frequency, or intensity.	Increase in duration, frequency, and intensity.
Do not achieve cervical dilatation.	Achieve cervical dilatation.

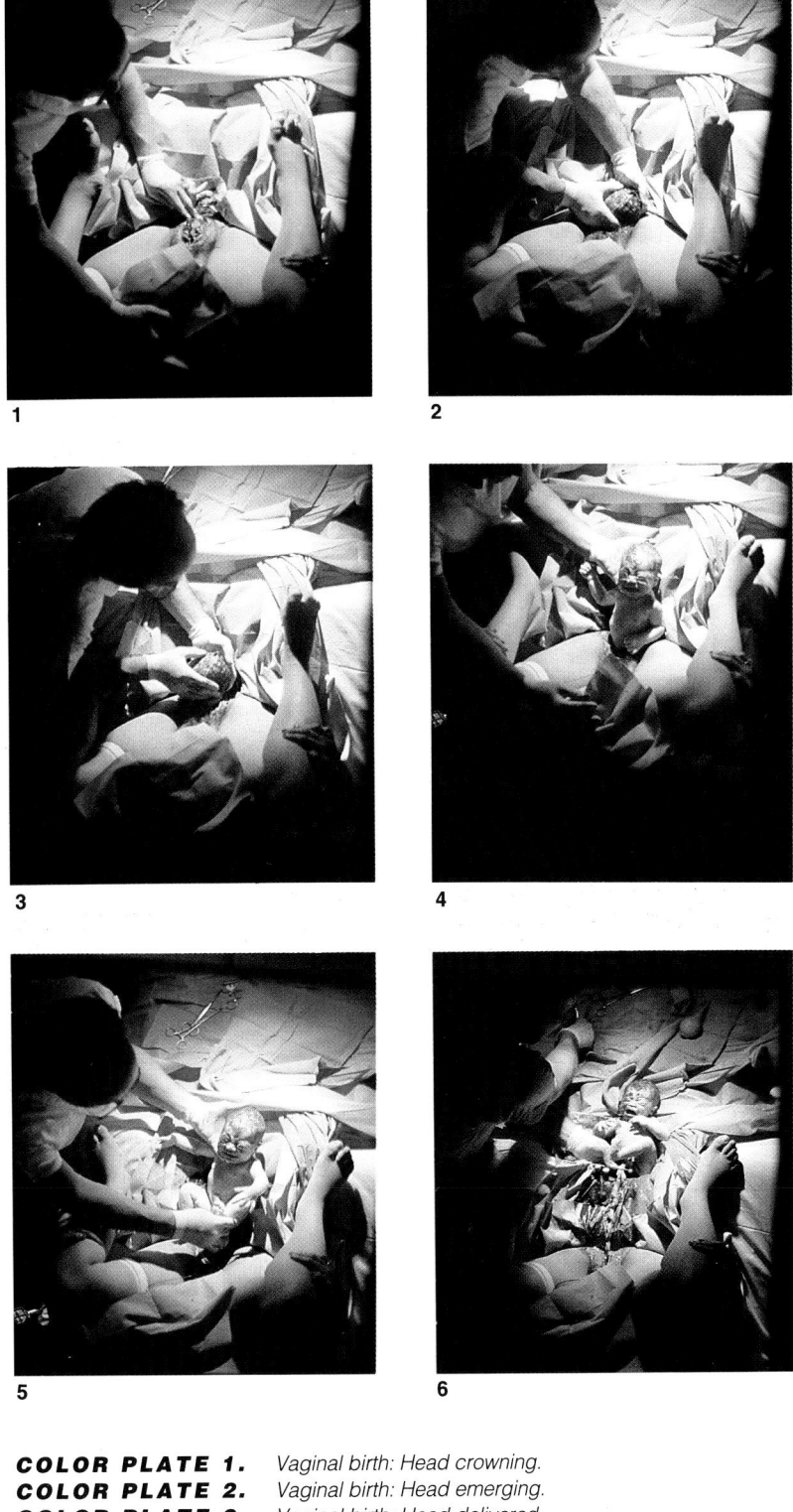

COLOR PLATE 1. *Vaginal birth: Head crowning.*
COLOR PLATE 2. *Vaginal birth: Head emerging.*
COLOR PLATE 3. *Vaginal birth: Head delivered.*
COLOR PLATE 4. *Vaginal birth: Head and torso born.*
COLOR PLATE 5. *Infant several seconds following birth.*
COLOR PLATE 6. *Cutting umbilicus of newborn.*

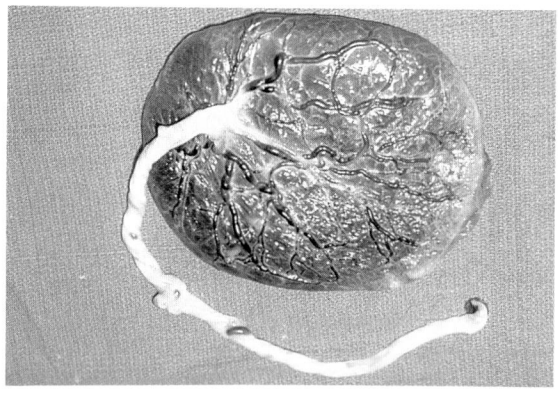

7

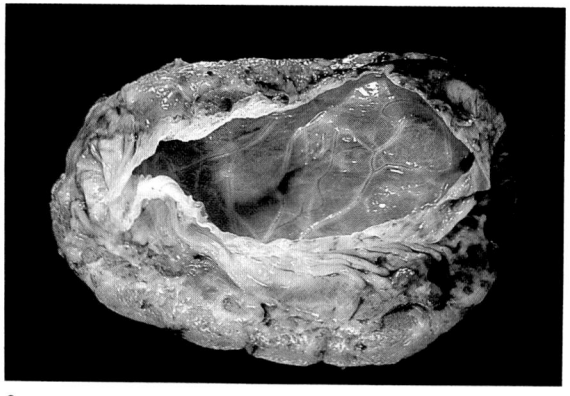

8

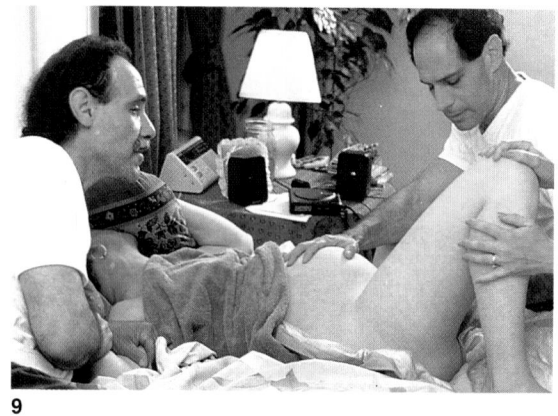

9

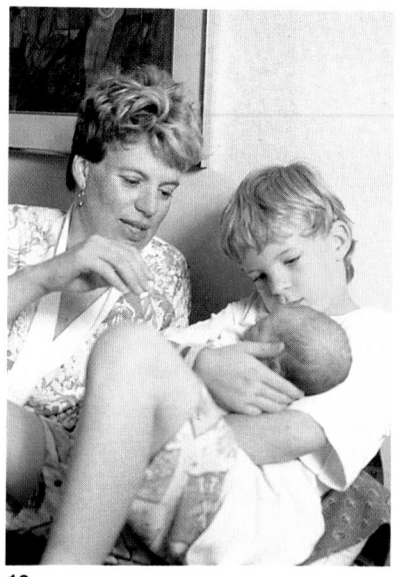

10

COLOR PLATE 7. *Human placenta: fetal side.*
COLOR PLATE 8. *Circumvalate placenta.*
COLOR PLATE 9. *Woman in labor during home birth.*
COLOR PLATE 10. *Mother, infant, and sibling following home birth.*

Components of Labor

A successful labor depends on three integrated concepts: (1) the woman's pelvis (the **passage**) is of adequate size and contour; (2) the **passenger** (the fetus) is of appropriate size and in an advantageous position and presentation; and (3) the powers of labor (uterine factors) are adequate. A fourth concept or "p"—psyche—is sometimes added to reflect the importance of the woman's frame of mind in dealing with the labor experience.

Passage

The passage refers to the route the fetus must travel from the uterus through the cervix and vagina to the external perineum; because these organs are contained inside the pelvis, the fetus must also pass through the pelvic ring. Pelvic anatomy is discussed in Chapter 4 (see especially Figures 4-11 and 4-12). Important pelvic measurements include the diagonal conjugate (the anterior-posterior diameter of the inlet) and the transverse diameter of the outlet (see Figs. 10-10 and 10-11). The narrowest diameter of the pelvis at the inlet is the anteroposterior diameter; at the outlet, the transverse diameter is the narrowest (Figure 18-1).

In most instances in which a disproportion does occur, the pelvis is the structure at fault. When the fetus is causing the problem, it is often because the fetal head is presented to the birth canal at less than its narrowest diameter, not because the head is actually too large. This is important to consider when discussing with parents why an infant cannot be delivered vaginally. When discussing such a situation with the parents, emphasize that the pelvis is too small, not that the head is too big. It is one thing for parents to learn that a child cannot be born vaginally because the mother's pelvis is too small and another to learn that the infant's head is too large. The first fact is merely unfortunate; the second implies that something is seriously wrong with the baby (which is generally not the case). Such a negative thought can lead to tension and fear during the labor process.

Passenger

The fetal head is the body part with the widest diameter and therefore the part least likely to be able to pass through the pelvic ring. Whether a fetal skull can pass depends on both its structure and its alignment with the pelvis. To understand how such a presentation occurs, it is necessary to appreciate the bones, fontanelles, and suture lines of the fetal skull (Figures 18-2 and 18-3).

Structure of the Fetal Skull

The cranium (the uppermost portion of the skull) comprises eight bones. The four superior ones—the frontal bone, the two parietal bones, and the occipital bone—are the important bones in terms of obstetrics. The frontal bone is actually two fused bones; for obstetric purposes, the area over the bone is referred to as the *sinciput*. The area over the occipital bone is referred to as the *occiput*. The other four bones of the skull (i.e., sphenoid bone, ethmoid bone, and two temporal bones) do not play a large part in obstetrics because they lie at the base of the cranium and therefore are never presenting parts. The chin can be a presenting part. For obstetric purposes, it is referred to by its Latin name, *mentum*.

The two parietal bones of the skull are joined by a membranous interspace, the *sagittal suture*. The *coronal suture* is the line of junction of the frontal bones and the two parietal bones. The *lambdoid suture* is the line of junction of the occipital bone and the two parietal bones. The suture lines are important in birth because they allow the cranial bones to move and overlap, thus molding or diminishing the size of the skull so that it can more readily pass through the birth canal.

At the junction of the main suture lines are significant membrane-covered spaces called the fontanelles. The *anterior fontanelle* lies at the junction of the coronal and sagittal sutures. Because the frontal bone consists of two fused bones, four bones (counting the two parietal bones) are actually involved at this junction, making the anterior fontanelle diamond shaped. It measures approximately 3 to 4 cm in its anteroposterior diameter and 2 cm to 3 cm in its transverse diameter. For obstetric purposes, the anterior fontanelle is referred to as the *bregma*.

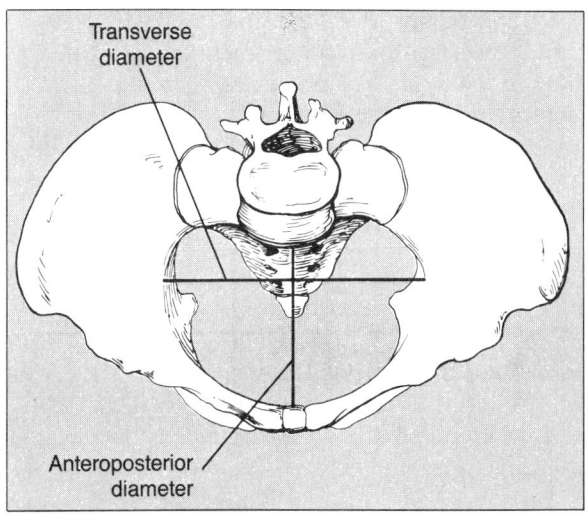

FIGURE 18-1

Inlet of normal female pelvis showing transverse and anteroposterior diameter. The narrowest diameter of the pelvis at the inlet is the anteroposterior diameter; at the outlet, the narrowest diameter is the transverse diameter. (From Reeder, S.J., Martin, L.L., & Koniak, D. [1992]. Maternity nursing: Family, newborn, and women's health care [17th ed.]. Philadelphia: J.B. Lippincott.)

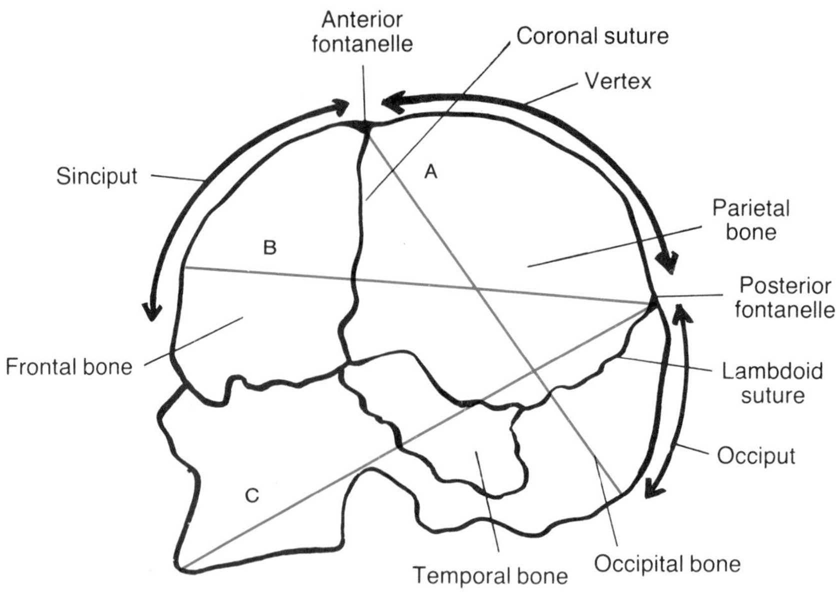

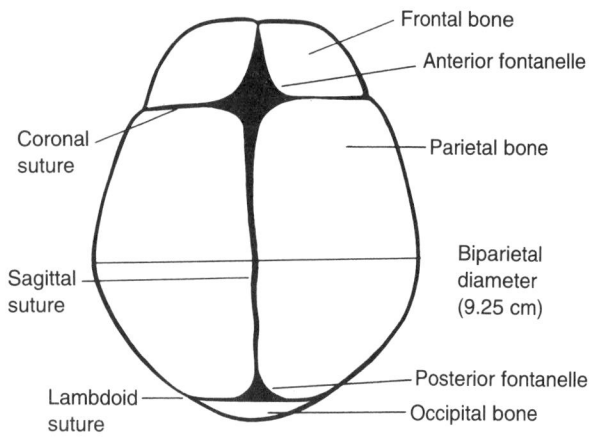

FIGURE 18-2
*The fetal skull (lateral view), showing (**A**) antero-posterior diameter, (**B**) suboccipitobregmatic diameter (9.5 cm), and (**C**) occipitomental diameter (13.5 cm).*

Three bones (the two parietal bones and the occipital bone) are involved at the junction of the lambdoid and sagittal sutures; thus, the *posterior fontanelle* is triangular. It is smaller than the anterior fontanelle, measuring approximately 2 cm across its widest part. Fontanelle spaces compress during birth to aid in molding of the fetal head. Their presence can be assessed on manual examination of the cervix after it has dilated during labor to establish the position of the fetal head and whether it is in a favorable position for birth. The space between the two fontanelles is referred to for obstetric purposes as the *vertex*.

Diameters of the Fetal Skull

The shape of a fetal skull causes it to be wider in its anteroposterior diameter than in its transverse diameter. To fit through the birth canal, the fetus must present the

smaller diameter (the transverse diameter) to the smaller diameter of the maternal pelvis; otherwise, progress will halt and birth cannot be accomplished.

At the pelvic inlet, for example, the fetus must present the narrowest diameter—the biparietal diameter, which is approximately 9.25 cm (see Figure 18-3)—to the anteroposterior diameter of the pelvis, a space approximately 11 cm wide. At the outlet, this narrow diameter must be presented to the transverse diameter, a space approximately 11 cm wide (Figure 18-4). If the anteroposterior diameter of the skull (a measurement wider than the biparietal diameter) is presented to the anteroposterior diameter of the inlet, **engagement**, or the settling of the fetal head into the pelvis, may not occur. If the anteroposterior diameter of the skull is presented to the transverse diameter of the outlet, arrest of progress may occur at that point.

The diameter of the anteroposterior fetal skull depends on where the measurement is taken. The narrowest diameter (approximately 9.5 cm) is from the inferior aspect of the occiput to the center of the anterior fontanelle (the suboccipitobregmatic diameter). The occipitofrontal diameter, measured from the bridge of the nose to the occipital prominence, is approximately 12 cm. The occipitomental diameter, which is the widest anteroposterior diameter (approximately 13.5 cm), is measured from the chin to the posterior fontanelle (see lines *A, B,* and *C* in Figure 18-2).

The degree of flexion of the fetus' head determines which anteroposterior diameter will be presented to the birth canal (Figure 18-5). In full flexion, the head flexes so sharply that the chin rests on the thorax, and the smallest anteroposterior diameter, the suboccipitobregmatic, will be presented to the birth canal. If the head is held in moderate flexion, the occipitofrontal diameter

FIGURE 18-3
The fetal skull (from above) showing biparietal diameter.

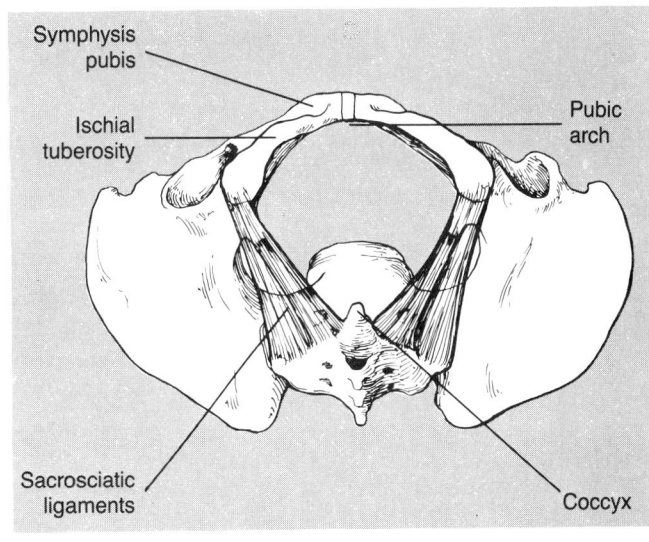

FIGURE 18-4
*Views of the pelvic inlet and outlet with fetal head in place. (**A**) For the largest diameter of the fetal head to pass through the largest diameter of the inlet, the fetal head enters transversely. (**B**) For the largest diameter of the fetal head to pass through the largest diameter of the outlet, the head must rotate 90 degrees and pass through anteroposteriorly. (From Reeder, S.J., Martin, L.L., & Koniak, D. [1992]. Maternity nursing: Family, newborn, and women's health care [17th ed.]. Philadelphia: J.B. Lippincott.)*

will be presented. In poor flexion (the head hyper-extended), the largest diameter—the occipitomental—will be presented.

This anteroposterior diameter must fit through the transverse diameter of the pelvic inlet, a space of approximately 12.4 cm to 13.5 cm; and at the outlet, through the anteroposterior diameter of the pelvis, a space of 9.5 cm to 11.5 cm. It follows that a fetal head presenting a diameter of 9.5 cm will fit through a pelvis much more readily than if the diameter is 12.0 or 13.5

cm. Table 18-2 compares diameters of the fetal skull with maternal pelvic diameters.

Molding

Molding is the change in shape of the fetal skull produced by the force of uterine contractions pressing the vertex against the not-yet-dilated cervix. Because the bones of the fetal skull are not yet completely ossified and therefore do not form a rigid structure, they overlap and cause the head to become narrower but longer,

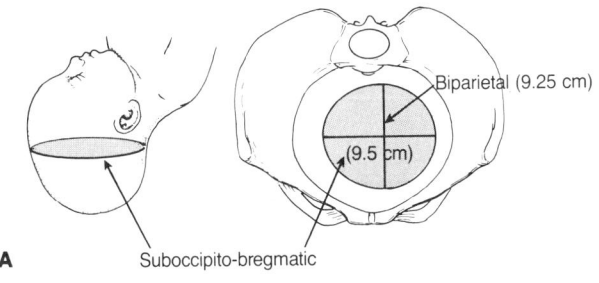

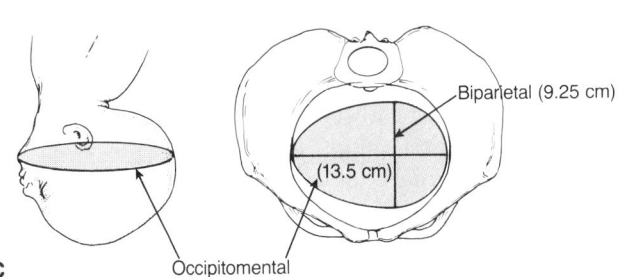

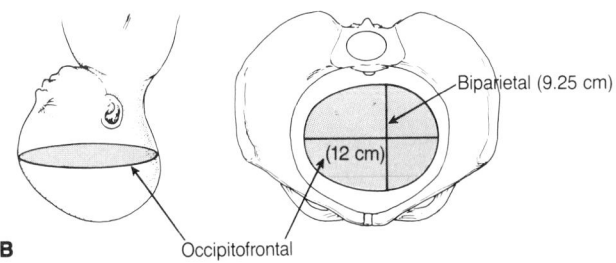

FIGURE 18-5
*(**A**) Complete flexion allows the smallest diameter of the head to enter the pelvis. (**B**) Moderate extension causes the larger diameter to enter the pelvis. (**C**) Marked extension forces the largest diameter against the pelvic brim, but the head is too large to enter the pelvis. (From Reeder, S.J., Martin, L.L., & Koniak, D. [1992]. Maternity nursing: Family, newborn, and women's health care [17th ed.]. Philadelphia: J.B. Lippincott.)*

Table 18-2. *Diameters of Fetal Skull Compared With Maternal Pelvic Diameters*

Diameter	Measurement	Average Diameter (cm)
Anteroposterior Fetal Skull Diameters		
Suboccipitobregmatic	Inferior aspect of occiput to center of anterior fontanelle	9.5
Occipitofrontal	Bridge of nose to occipital prominence	12.0
Occipitomental	Chin to posterior fontanelle	13.5
Transverse Fetal Skull Diameter		
Biparietal	Distance between parietal prominences	9.25
Anteroposterior Pelvic Diameters		
Diagonal conjugate	Inferior margin of symphysis pubis to sacral promontory	12.5
True conjugate	Internal aspect of symphysis pubis to sacral promontory	11.0
Transverse Pelvic Diameter		
Ischial tuberosities	Distance between ischial tuberosities at the level of the anus	11.0

facilitating its passage during birth. Parents can be reassured that molding only lasts a day or two and is not a permanent condition.

At birth, the overlapping of the sagittal suture line and generally the coronal suture line can be easily palpated in the newborn skull. In a brow presentation (described in the following section), there is little molding because frontal bones are fused. Labor will undoubtedly be arrested and the fetus will be unable to pass through the pelvis. In a breech presentation (see below), no skull molding occurs, and the fetal head may present a birth problem.

Fetal Presentation and Position

In addition to being familiar with the parts and diameters of the fetal head, it is necessary to be able to understand and use the terms describing fetal presentation and position.

Attitude. **Attitude** is a term used to describe the degree of flexion the fetus assumes or the relation of the fetal parts to each other (Figure 18-6). A fetus in good attitude is in *complete flexion:* the spinal column is bowed forward, the head is flexed forward so much that the chin touches the sternum, the arms are flexed and folded on the chest, the thighs are flexed onto the abdomen, and the calves of the legs are pressed against the posterior aspect of the thighs (Figure 18-6*A*). This is the normal "fetal position" and is advantageous for birth not only because it helps the fetus present the smallest anteroposterior diameter of the skull to the pelvis but also because it puts the whole body into an ovoid shape, occupying the smallest space possible.

A fetus is in *moderate flexion* if the fetus' chin is not touching his or her chest but is in an alert or "military

position" (Figure 18-6*B*). This position causes the next widest anteroposterior diameter to present to the birth canal, the occipital frontal diameter. A fair number of fetuses assume a military position at the early part of labor. This does not usually interfere with labor because part of the mechanisms of labor (descent and flexion) causes the fetus to flex his or her head fully at that point.

The fetus in *partial extension* presents the "brow" of the head to the birth canal (Figure 18-6*C*). If a fetus is in *poor flexion,* the back is arched, the neck is extended, and the fetus presents the occipitomental diameter of the head to the birth canal (face presentation; Figure 18-6*D*). This is an unusual position; it presents too wide a skull diameter to the birth canal for normal birth. Such a position may occur if there is less than normal amniotic fluid present (oligohydramnios), which does not allow the fetus adequate movement; it may reflect a neurologic abnormality that is causing spasticity.

Engagement. The presenting part of the fetus is said to be engaged when it has settled far enough into the pelvis to be at the level of the ischial spines, a midpoint of the pelvis. Descent to this point means that the widest part of the fetus (the biparietal diameter in a cephalic presentation or the intertrochanteric diameter in a breech presentation) has passed through the pelvis intact or the pelvic inlet is adequate for birth. Engagement is another term for **lightening**. In a primipara, nonengagement of the head at the beginning of labor indicates a possible complication: an abnormal presentation or position, abnormality of the fetal head, or cephalopelvic disproportion. In multiparas, engagement may or may not be present at the beginning of labor. A presenting part that is not engaged is said to be "floating." One that is descending but has not yet reached the iliac spines is

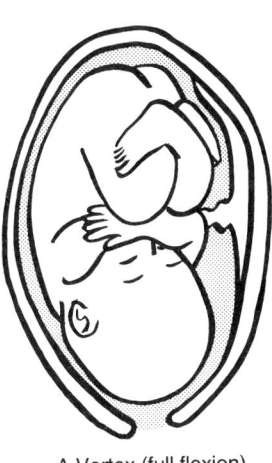

A Vertex (full flexion)

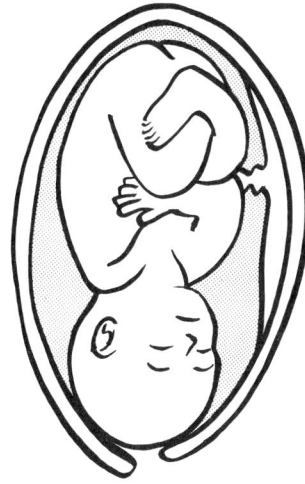

B Sinciput (military attitude)

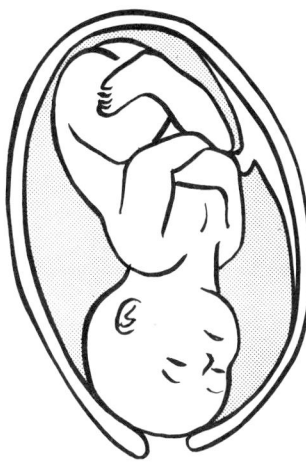

C Brow (partial extension)

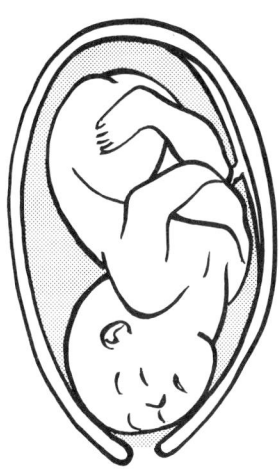

D Face (complete extension)

FIGURE 18-6
*Fetal attitude. (**A**) Fetus in full flexion presents smallest (suboccipitobregmatic) anteroposterior diameter of skull to inlet in this good attitude (vertex presentation). (**B**) Fetus is not as well flexed (military attitude) as in **A** and presents occipitofrontal diameter to inlet (sinciput presentation). (**C**) Fetus in partial extension (brow presentation). (**D**) Fetus in complete extension presents wide (occipitomental) diameter (face presentation).*

said to be "dipping." Engagement is assessed by vaginal and cervical examination.

Station. **Station** refers to the relationship of the presenting part of the fetus to the level of the ischial spines (Figure 18-7). When the presenting part is at the level of the ischial spines, it is at a 0 station (synonymous with engagement). If the presenting part is above the spines, the distance is measured and described as minus stations which range from −1 cm to −4 cm. If the presenting part is below the ischial spines, the distance is stated as plus stations (+1 cm to +4 cm). At a +3 or +4 station, the presenting part is at the perineum and can be seen if the vulva is separated (synonymous with **crowning**). To remember whether a plus or minus station is below the spines, think about what is trying to be accom-

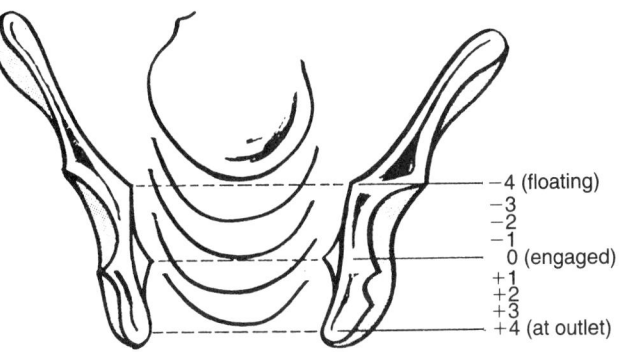

−4 (floating)
−3
−2
−1
0 (engaged)
+1
+2
+3
+4 (at outlet)

FIGURE 18-7
Station (anteroposterior view). Station, or degree of engagement, of the fetal head is designated by centimeters above or below the ischial spines. At −4 station, head is "floating." At 0 station, head is "engaged." At +4 station, head is "at outlet."

plished (moving the fetus from above the pelvic ring to below it). As the fetus passes farther toward the goal of being born (beyond the midpelvis) the stations become plus designations. When describing the terms "engagement" and "station" to parents, reassure them that when their child is passing the ischial spines, these are not the same as vertebrae, but are dull bony protrusions within the pelvis. No parent likes to think of their child traversing through needle-sharp "spines."

Fetal Lie. **Lie** is the relationship between the long (cephalocaudal) axis of the fetal body and the long (cephalocaudal) axis of the woman's body, that is, whether the fetus is lying in a horizontal (transverse) or a vertical (longitudinal) position. Approximately 99% of fetuses assume a longitudinal lie (with their long axis parallel with the long axis of the woman). Longitudinal lies are further classified as *cephalic* (the head is the presenting part, that is, it is the first part to contact the cervix) or *breech* (the breech, or buttocks, is the portion to contact the cervix first).

Types of Fetal Presentation

A fetal presentation denotes the body part that will first contact the cervix or deliver first. This is determined not only by the fetal lie but by the degree of flexion (attitude).

Cephalic Presentations. **Cephalic presentation** is the most frequent type of presentation (presenting as much as 95% of the time). The four types of cephalic presentation—vertex, brow, face, and mentum—are de-

scribed in Table 18-3. The area of the fetal skull that contacts the cervix often becomes edematous during labor due to continual pressure against it (called a *caput succedaneum*). In the newborn infant, the point of presentation can be analyzed from the location of the caput.

Breech Presentations. **Breech presentations** occur in only a small number of births, approximately 3%. They are affected by fetal attitude—a good attitude brings the knees up against the umbilicus; a poor attitude does not. Breech presentations are difficult deliveries; the presenting point influences the degree of difficulty. Three types of breech presentation—complete, frank, and footling—are possible; these are shown in Figure 18-8 and described in Table 18-4.

Shoulder Presentations. In a transverse lie, the fetus is lying horizontally in the pelvis so that its long axis is perpendicular to that of the mother. The presenting part usually becomes one of the shoulders (acromion process); an iliac crest; a hand; or an elbow (Figure 18-9).

Fewer than 1% of fetuses lie transversely. This may be caused by relaxed abdominal walls from grand multiparity that allows the uterus to be unsupported and fall forward. Another cause is pelvic contraction, in which there is more horizontal then vertical space. Placenta previa (the placenta is located low in the uterus, obscuring some of the vertical space) may also limit the fetus' ability to turn, resulting in a transverse lie. The usual contour of the at-term abdomen is distorted or is fuller side to side rather than top to bottom.

Table 18-3. Types of Cephalic Presentations

Type	Lie	Attitude	Description
Vertex	Longitudinal	Good (full flexion)	The head is sharply flexed, making the parietal bones or the space between the fontanelles (the vertex) the presenting part. This is the most common presentation and allows the suboccipitobregmatic diameter to present to the cervix.
Brow	Longitudinal	Moderate (military)	Because the head is only moderately flexed, the brow or sinciput becomes the presenting part.
Face	Longitudinal	Poor	The fetus has extended his or her head to make the face the presenting part. From this position, extreme edema and distortion of the face may occur. The presenting diameter (the occipitomental) is so wide delivery may be impossible.
Mentum	Longitudinal	Very poor	The fetus has completely hyperextended the head to present the chin. The widest diameter (occipitomental) is presenting. As a rule, the fetus cannot enter the pelvis in this presentation.

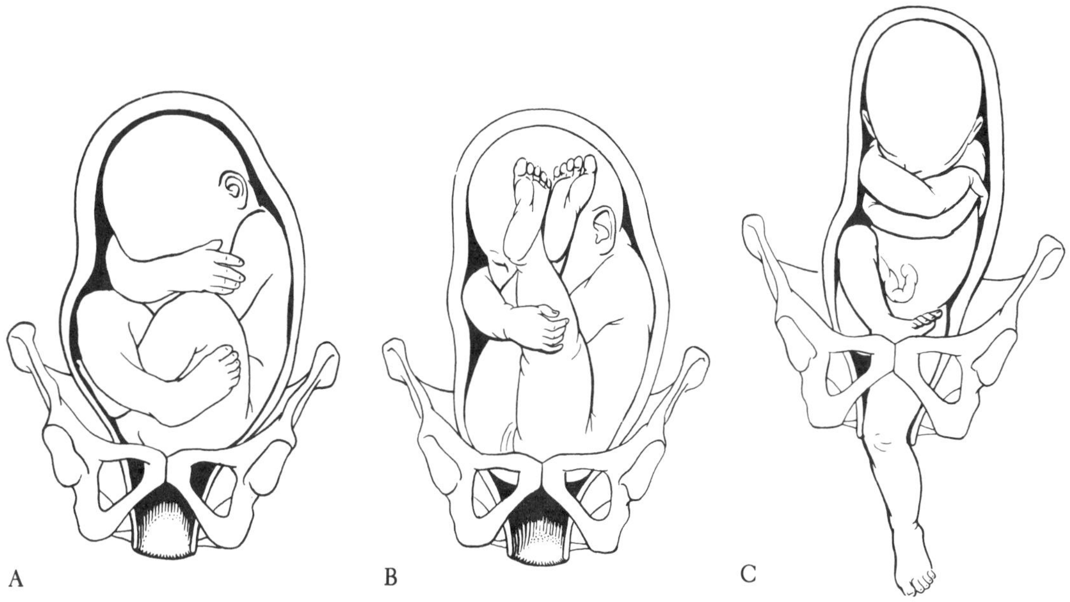

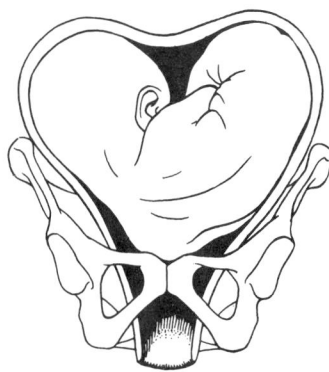

FIGURE 18-8
*Breech presentation. (**A**) Complete breech. (**B**) Frank breech. (**C**) Footling breech. (Used with permission of Ross Products Division, Abbott Laboratories, Columbus, OH 43216. From Clinical Education Aid, No. 18, ©1958 Ross Products Division, Abbott Laboratories.)*

Table 18-4. Types of Breech Presentations			
Type	**Lie**	**Attitude**	**Description**
Complete	Longitudinal	Good (full flexion)	The fetus has thighs tightly flexed on the abdomen; both the buttocks and the tightly flexed feet present to the cervix.
Frank	Longitudinal	Moderate	Attitude is moderate because the hips are flexed but the knees are extended to rest on the chest. The buttocks alone present to the cervix.
Footling	Longitudinal	Poor	Neither the thighs nor lower legs are flexed. If one foot presents, it is a single-footling breech; if both present, it is a double-footling breech.

FIGURE 18-9
Transverse or shoulder presentation. (Used with permission of Ross Products Division, Abbott Laboratories, Columbus, OH 43216. From Clinical Education Aid, No. 18, ©1958 Ross Products Division, Abbott Laboratories.)

Most infants in a transverse lie must be delivered by cesarean birth because they are unable to deliver normally from this "wedged" position. Discovering a shoulder presentation is an important assessment because it almost automatically identifies a birth position that puts both mother and child in jeopardy unless skilled health care personnel are available to deliver the child safely by cesarean birth.

Types of Fetal Position

Position is the relationship of the presenting part to a specific quadrant of the woman's pelvis. For convenience in defining position, the maternal pelvis is divided into four quadrants according to the mother's, rather than the examiner's, right and left: (1) right anterior, (2) left anterior, (3) right posterior, and (4) left posterior.

Four parts of the fetus have been chosen as points of direction to describe the relationship of the presenting part to one of the pelvic quadrants. In a vertex presentation, the occiput is the chosen point; in a face presentation, it is the chin (mentum); in a breech presentation, it is the sacrum; in a shoulder presentation, it is the scapula or the acromion process.

A position is marked by an abbreviation of three letters. The middle letter denotes the fetal landmark (*O* for occiput, *M* for mentum or chin, *Sa* for sacrum, and *A* for acromion process). The first letter defines whether the landmark is pointing to the mother's right (*R*) or left (*L*). The last letter defines whether the landmark points anteriorly (*A*), posteriorly (*P*), or transversely (*T*).

When the occiput of the fetus points to the left anterior quadrant in a vertex position, for example, this is termed *left occipitoanterior* (*LOA*); the fetus is in good attitude in a vertical cephalic lie. When the occiput points to the right posterior quadrant, the position is *right occipitoposterior (ROP)*. LOA is the most common fetal position and right occipitoanterior (ROA) the second most frequent position. Box 18-1 summarizes possible positions. Six common positions in cephalic presentations are depicted in Figure 18-10.

Position is important because it influences the process and efficiency of labor. A fetus delivers fastest from an ROA or LOA position. Labor is considerably extended if the position is posterior; it may be more painful for the mother because the rotation of the fetal head puts pressure on the sacral nerves, causing sharp back pains.

Importance of Determining Fetal Presentation and Position

There are four methods by which the fetal position and presentation and lie are established: (1) combined abdominal inspection and palpation, (2) vaginal examination, (3) auscultation of fetal heart tones, and (4) sonography.

The vertex is the ideal presenting part because the skull bones are capable of molding so effectively to accommodate the cervix; it may actually aid in cervical dilatation; and it prevents complications such as a *prolapsed cord* (cord passing between the presenting part and the cervix and entering the vagina before the fetus). When a body part other than the vertex presents, labor is invariably longer due to ineffective descent of the fetus, ineffective dilatation of the cervix, and irregular and weak uterine contractions.

The less effective labor is, the longer it is, tiring the mother and reducing the excitement of the experience. If an operative birth is necessary, and postoperative complications occur, the mother may have a longer hospitalization and more pain and disability following the birth. If the fetus delivers vaginally after a complicated labor, the mother has a greater chance of having per-

ineal tears or cervical laceration, which may also increase her disability and decrease her chances of having problem-free childbearing in the future. When labor is threatening and unsatisfactory, it can interfere with maternal-child bonding.

The presentation of a body part other than the vertex puts the fetus at a risk because there is apt to be a proportional difference between the fetus and pelvis, making a cesarean birth necessary and the membranes more apt to rupture early, increasing the possibility of infection. The fetus is more apt to suffer anoxia and meconium staining, complications that lead to respiratory distress at birth.

Mechanisms (Cardinal Movements) of Labor

Passage of the fetus through the birth canal involves a number of different position changes to keep the smallest diameter of the fetal head (in cephalic presentations) always presenting to the smallest diameter of the birth

---

Box 18-1
Possible Fetal Positions

Vertex Presentation
LOA, left occipitoanterior
LOP, left occipitoposterior
LOT, left occipitotransverse
ROA, right occipitoanterior
ROP, right occipitoposterior
ROT, right occipitotransverse

Breech Presentation
LSA, left sacroanterior
LSP, left sacroposterior
LST, left sacrotransverse
RSA, right sacroanterior
RSP, right sacroposterior
RST, right sacrotransverse

Face Presentation
LMA, left mentoanterior
LMP, left mentoposterior
LMT, left mentotransverse
RMA, right mentoanterior
RMP, right mentoposterior
RMT, right mentotransverse

Shoulder Presentation
LSCA, left scapuloanterior
LSCP, left scapuloposterior
RSCA, right scapuloanterior
RSCP, right scapuloposterior

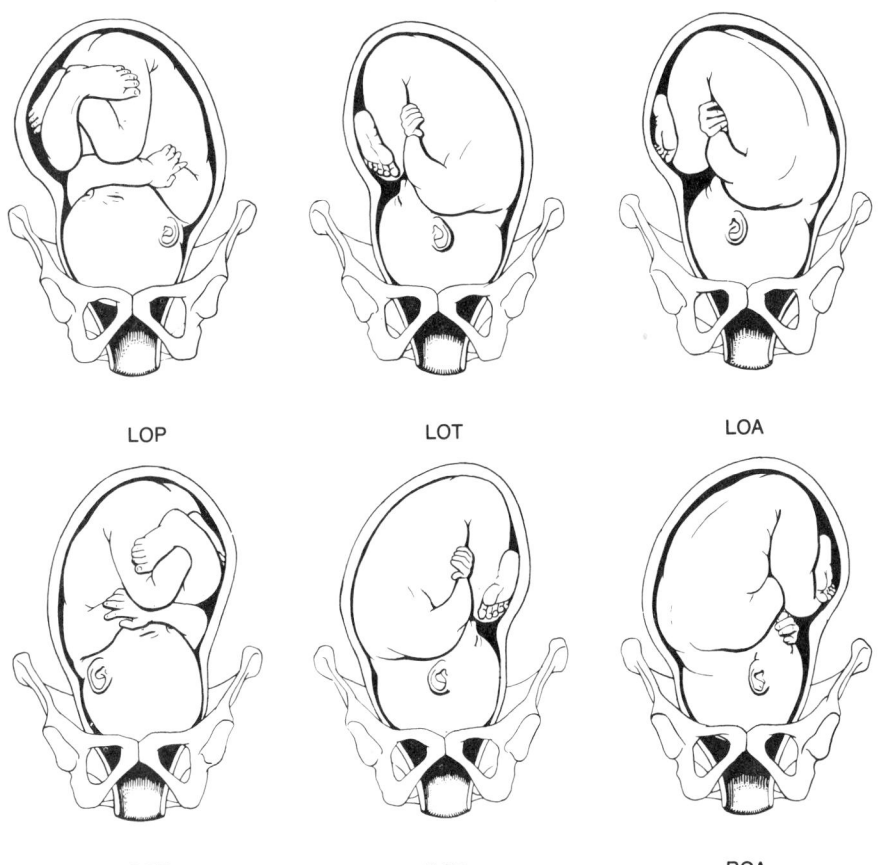

LOP   LOT   LOA

ROP   ROT   ROA

FIGURE 18-10
*Fetal position. All are vertex presentations.
A = anterior; L = left; O = occiput; P =
posterior; R = right; T = transverse. (Used
with permission of Ross Products Division,
Abbott Laboratories, Columbus, OH
43216. From Clinical Education Aid,
No. 18, ©1958 Ross Products Division,
Abbott Laboratories.)*

canal. These position changes are termed the **cardinal movements of labor**. They are descent, flexion, internal rotation, extension, external rotation, and expulsion (Figure 18-11).

Descent. Descent is the downward movement of the biparietal diameter of the fetal head to within the pelvic inlet. Full descent occurs when the fetal head extrudes beyond the dilated cervix and touches the posterior vaginal floor. The pressure of the fetus on the sacral nerves causes the mother to experience a pushing sensation. Descent occurs because of pressure on the fetus by the uterine fundus; full descent may be aided by abdominal muscle contraction.

Flexion. As descent occurs, pressure from the pelvic floor causes the fetal head to bend forward onto the chest. The smallest anteroposterior diameter (the suboccipitobregmatic diameter) is the one presented to the birth canal in this flexed position. Flexion is aided by the abdominal muscle contraction during pushing.

Internal Rotation. During descent, the head enters the pelvis with the fetal anteroposterior head diameter in a diagonal or transverse position. The head flexes as it touches the pelvic floor, and the occiput rotates until it is superior, or just below the symphysis pubis, bring-

ing the head into the best diameter for the outlet of the pelvis (the anteroposterior diameter is now in the anteroposterior plane of the pelvis). This movement brings the shoulders, coming next, into the optimum position to enter the inlet or puts the widest diameter of the shoulders (a transverse one) in line with the wide transverse diameter of the inlet.

Extension. As the occiput is born, the back of the neck stops beneath the pubic arch and acts as a pivot for the rest of the head. The head thus extends, and the foremost parts of the head, the face and chin, are born.

External Rotation. In external rotation, almost immediately after the head of the infant is born, the head rotates (from the anteroposterior position it assumed to enter the outlet) back to the diagonal or transverse position of the early part of labor. The aftercoming shoulders are thus brought into an anteroposterior position, which is best for entering the outlet. The anterior shoulder is delivered first, assisted perhaps by downward flexion of the infant's head.

Expulsion. Once the shoulders are delivered, the rest of the baby is delivered easily and smoothly because of its smaller size. This is expulsion and is the end of the pelvic division of labor.

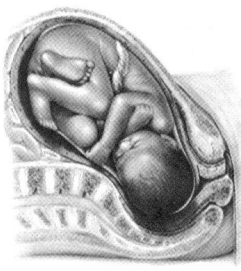
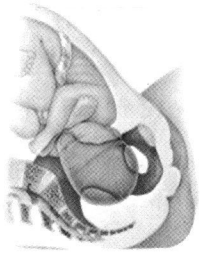
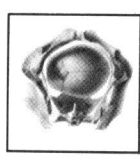

Engagement,
Descent,
Flexion

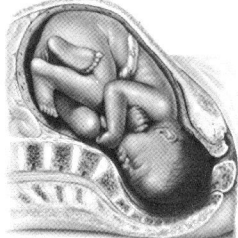
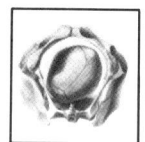

Internal Rotation

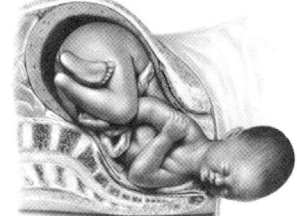
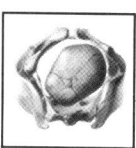

External Rotation (Restitution)

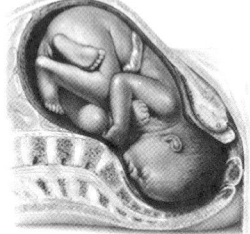
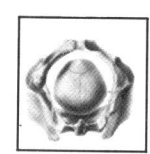

Extension Beginning (Rotation Complete)

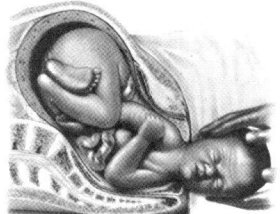
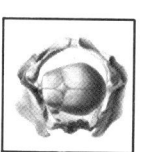

External Rotation (Shoulder Rotation)

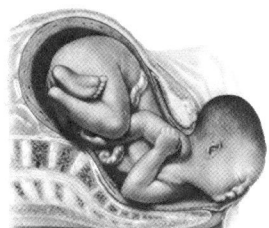
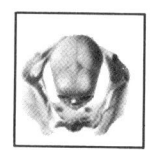

Extension Complete

Expulsion

FIGURE 18-11
Mechanism of normal labor and cardinal positions of the fetus from a left occipitoanterior position. (Used with permission of Ross Products Division, Abbott Laboratories, Columbus, OH 43216. From Clinical Education Aid, No. 13, ©1964 Ross Products Division, Abbott Laboratories.)

For a view of the complete birth sequence see Figure 18-12.

Powers of Labor

The powers of labor are supplied by the fundus of the uterus and implemented by uterine contractions, a process that causes cervical dilatation and then expulsion of the fetus from the uterus. Following full dilatation of the cervix, the primary power is supplemented by the use of the abdominal muscles. It is important for women to understand they should not bear down with their abdominal muscles until the cervix is fully dilated; this will impede the primary force or cause fetal and cervical damage.

FIGURE 18-12
Birth of a baby. (A) Episiotomy. (B) Crowning. (C, D) Extension. (E) External rotation. (F, G) Birth of anterior shoulder. (H, I) Birth of posterior shoulder. (J) Birth of torso. (K, L) Birth of total baby. (From Danforth, D., & Scott, J.R. [Eds.]. [1990]. Danforth's obstetrics and gynecology [5th ed.]. Philadelphia: J. B. Lippincott.)

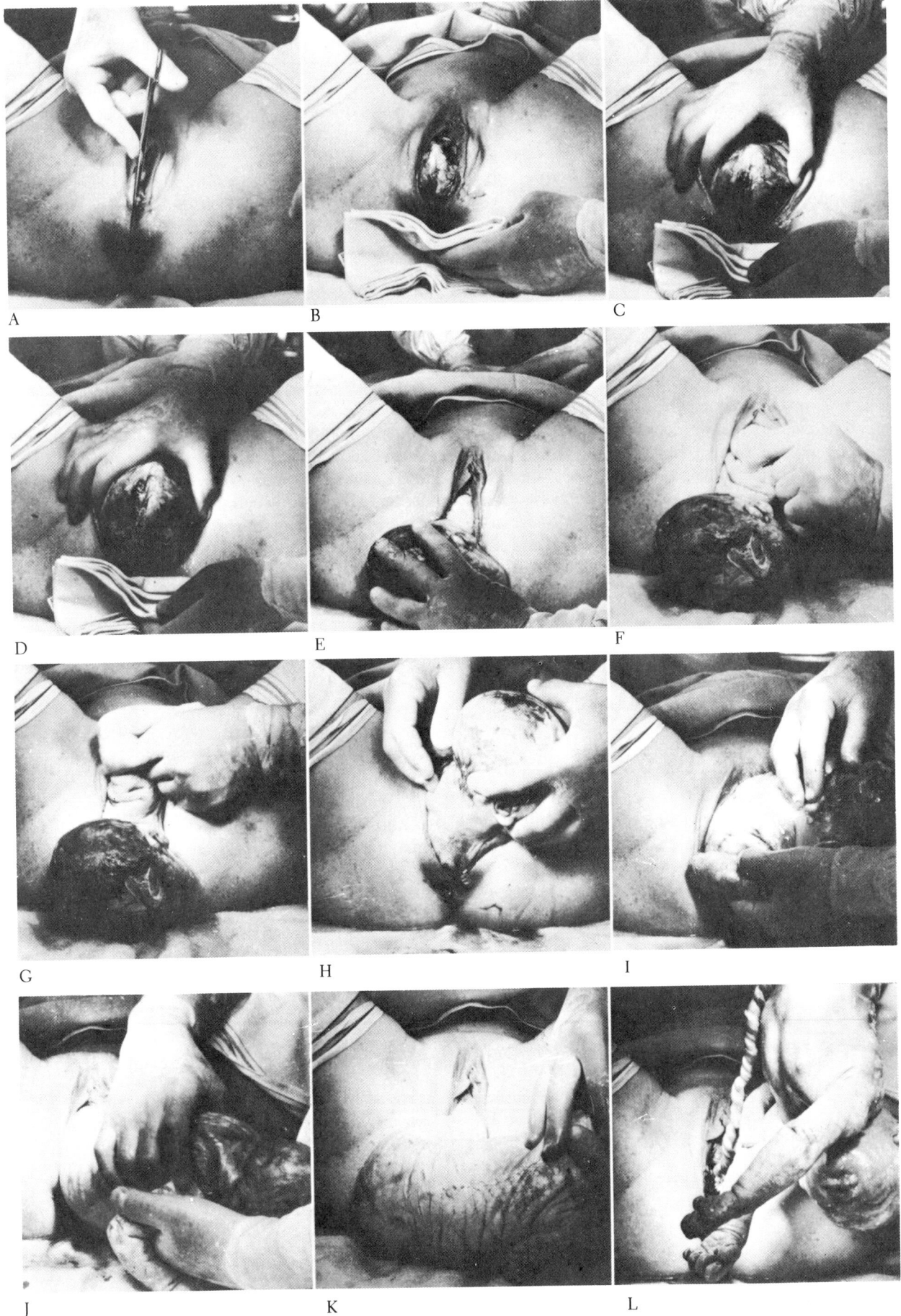

A

B

C

D

E

F

G

H

I

J

K

L

Uterine Contractions

Origins. Like cardiac contractions, labor contractions begin at a "pacemaker" point. This point is located in the myometrium of the uterus near one or the other uterotubal junctions. Each contraction begins at that point and then sweeps down over the uterus as a wave. After a short rest period, another contraction is initiated and the downward wave begins again.

In early labor, the uterotubal pacemakers may not be working in a synchronous manner; this makes contractions sometimes strong, sometimes weak, and irregular. This mild incoordination of early labor improves after a few hours as the pacemakers become more attuned to calcium concentrations in the myometrium and begin to function smoothly.

In some women, contractions appear to originate in the lower uterine segment rather than in the fundus. These are reverse, ineffective contractions, and actually cause tightening rather than dilatation of the cervix. That contractions are being initiated in a reverse pattern is difficult to tell from palpation. It can be suspected if a woman tells you that she feels pain in her lower abdomen before the contraction is readily palpated at the fundus. It is truly revealed only when cervical dilation does not occur.

Some women seem to have additional pacemaker sites in other portions of the uterus, in which case severe incoordination of contractions will occur. Uncoordinated contractions slow labor and may lead to failure to progress in labor and fetal distress because they do not allow for adequate placental filling. Therefore, evaluating the rate, intensity, and pattern of uterine contractions is an important nursing responsibility.

Phases. A contraction consists of three phases: the *increment*, when the intensity of the contraction increases; the *acme*, when the contraction is at its strongest; and the *decrement*, when the intensity decreases (Figure 18-13). Between contractions the uterus relaxes. As labor progresses the relaxation intervals decrease from 10 minutes early in labor to 2 to 3 minutes. The duration of contractions also changes, increasing from 20 to 30 seconds to a range of 60 to 90 seconds.

Contour Changes. As labor contractions progress and become regular and strong, the uterus is gradually differentiated into two distinct portions. The upper portion becomes thicker and active, preparing it to exert the strength necessary to expel the fetus when the expulsion phase of labor is reached. The lower segment becomes thin-walled, supple, and passive, so that the fetus can be pushed out of the uterus easily.

As the lower segment thins and the upper segment thickens, the boundary between the two portions becomes marked by a ridge on the inner uterine surface, the **physiologic retraction ring**.

In addition to this change in the contour of the uterine wall is a change in the contour of the overall uterus. The contour changes from a round ovoid to a structure more markedly elongated in a vertical diameter than horizontally. This lengthening of the uterus body serves to straighten the body of the fetus and place it in better alignment to the cervix and pelvis. Round ligaments move with the uterus as it contracts and keep the fundus forward, again to assist with placing the fetus in good alignment with the cervix. The elongation of the uterus causes it to press against the diaphragm and causes the often expressed sensation that a uterus is "taking control" of the woman's body.

In a difficult labor, particularly in obstructed labor when the fetus is larger than the birth canal, the round ligaments of the uterus become tense during dilatation and expulsion and may be palpable on the abdomen. The normal physiologic retraction ring may become prominent and observable as an abdominal indentation. This is termed a **pathologic retraction ring** or **Bandl's**

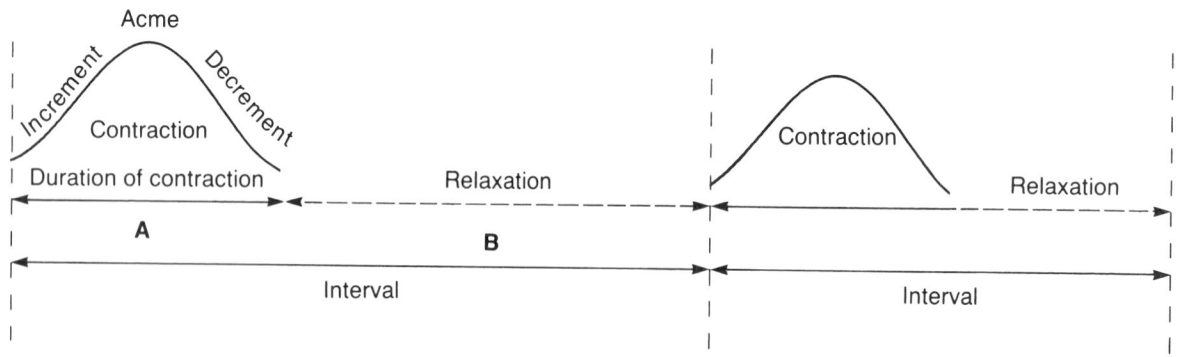

FIGURE 18-13

*The interval and duration of uterine contractions. The frequency of contractions is the interval timed from the beginning of one contraction to the beginning of the next contraction. The interval consists of two parts: (**A**) the duration of the contraction and (**B**) the period of relaxation. The broken line indicates an indeterminate period because the relaxation time (**B**) is usually of longer duration than the actual contraction (**A**). (From Reeder, S.J., Martin, L.L., & Koniak, D. [1992].* Maternity nursing: Family, newborn, and women's health care *[17th ed.]. Philadelphia: J.B. Lippincott.)*

ring. It is a danger sign that signifies impending rupture of the lower uterine segment if the obstruction to labor is not relieved (Cunningham et al., 1993).

Cervical Changes

Even more marked than the changes in the body of the uterus are two changes that occur in the cervix: effacement (thinning) and dilatation (enlargement).

Effacement. Effacement is the shortening and thinning of the cervical canal from its normal length of 1 cm to 2 cm to a structure with paper-thin edges in which no canal distinct from the uterus appears to exist (Figure 18-14). It occurs because of longitudinal traction from the contracting uterine fundus.

In primiparas, effacement is accomplished before dilatation begins. This is important to point out to a woman during her first labor. Otherwise, she can become discouraged if, for example, at noon her physician examines her and reports that she is 2 cm dilated and then examines her again at 4:00 PM and reports that she

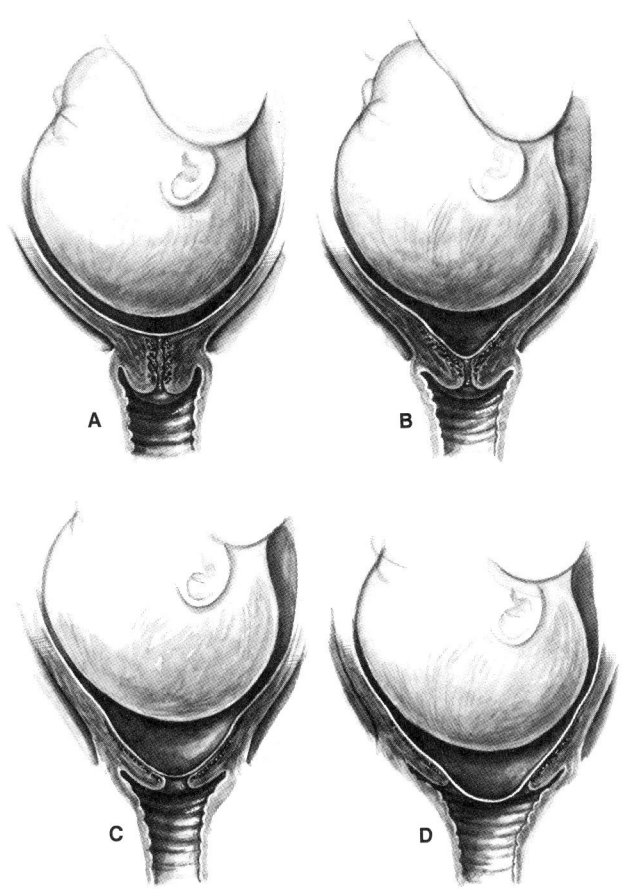

FIGURE 18-14
*Effacement and dilatation of cervix. (**A**) Beginning labor. (**B**) Effacement is beginning; dilation is not apparent yet. (**C**) Effacement is almost complete. (**D**) After complete effacement, dilatation proceeds rapidly.*

is still 2 cm dilated; it will seem to her that absolutely nothing has happened in 4 hours. However, effacement will have been occurring, and when this is complete, dilatation will then progress rapidly.

In multiparas, dilatation may proceed before effacement is complete. Effacement must occur at the end of dilatation, however, before the fetus can be safely pushed through the cervical canal or cervical tearing can result.

Dilatation. Dilatation refers to the enlargement of the cervical canal from an opening a few millimeters wide to one large enough (approximately 10 cm) to permit passage of the fetus (see Figure 18-14).

Dilatation occurs for two reasons. First, uterine contractions gradually increase the diameter of the cervical canal lumen by pulling the cervix up over the presenting part of the fetus and second, the fluid-filled membranes press against the cervix. If the membranes are intact, they push ahead of the fetus and serve as an opening wedge; if they are ruptured, the presenting part will serve this same function.

There is an increase in the amount of vaginal secretions as dilatation begins (termed *show*), because the last of the operculum or the mucus plug in the cervix is dislodged, and minute capillaries in the cervix rupture (Duffin, 1992).

Stages of Labor

Labor has traditionally been divided into three stages: a first stage of dilatation, beginning with true labor contractions and ending when the cervix is fully dilated; a second stage, from the time of full dilatation until the infant is born; and a third or placental stage, from the time the infant is born until following the delivery of the placenta. The first 1 to 4 hours following birth of the placenta are sometimes termed the "fourth stage" to emphasize the importance of the close observation needed at this time. This designation can be helpful in planning nursing interventions as it stresses the importance of interventions to ensure safety of the mother.

The work of Friedman (1978) is often cited in reference to the progress of labor. His studies of laboring women have yielded data that when plotted in graph form are useful in monitoring an individual woman's labor progress (Figure 18-15). Friedman's terms—preparatory division, dilatational division, and pelvic division—correspond to the first and second stages of labor described here. (See Table 18-5 for clinical features of divisions of labor as described by Friedman.)

First Stage

The first stage of labor is divided into three phases: the latent, the active, and the transition phases.

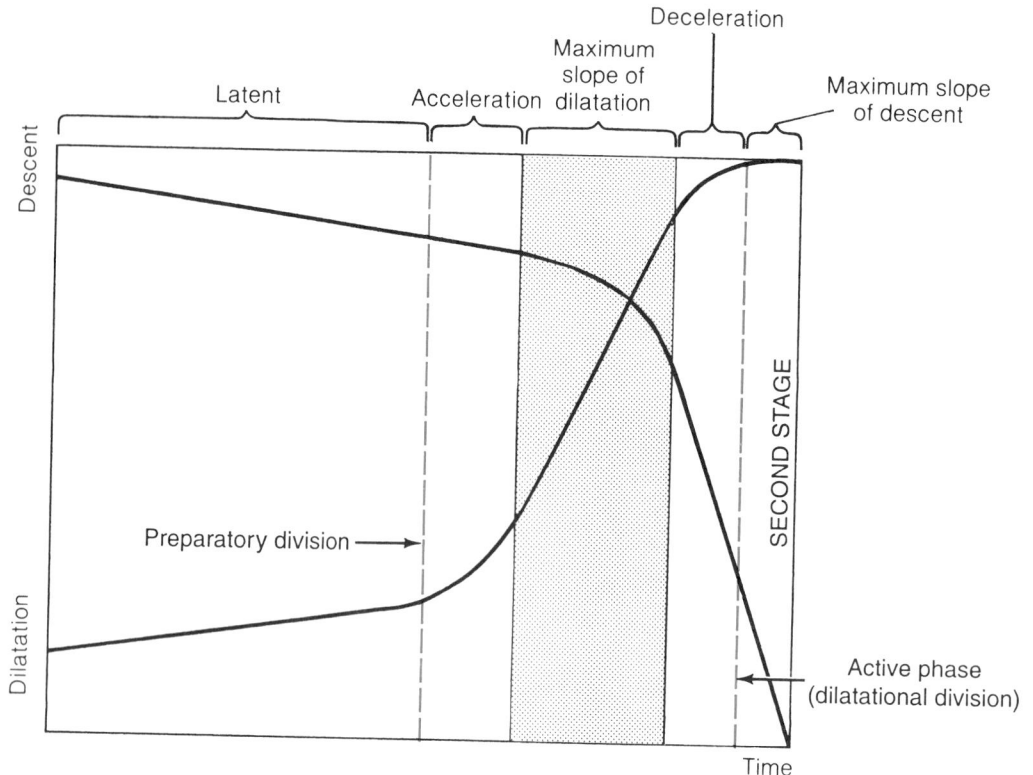

FIGURE 18-15

Divisions of labor. (Friedman, E. [1978]. Labor, clinical evaluation and management *[3rd ed.]. New York: Appleton-Century-Crofts, with permission.)*

Latent Phase

The latent phase begins at the onset of regularly perceived uterine contractions and ends when rapid cervical dilatation begins. Contractions during this phase are mild and short (20 to 30 seconds in length). Cervical effacement occurs and the cervix dilates to 3 or 4 cm. The phase lasts approximately 6 hours in a nullipara and 4.5 hours in a multipara. A woman who enters labor with a "nonripe" cervix will also have a longer than usual latent

phase. Analgesia given too early in labor will also prolong this phase. The latent phase may be prolonged if a cephalopelvic disproportion exists.

In a woman who is psychologically prepared for labor and who does not tense at each tightening sensation in her abdomen, latent phase contractions cause only minimal discomfort. The woman can continue to walk about and make preparations for birth, such as doing last-minute packing for her stay at the hospital or

Table 18-5. *Principal Clinical Features of the Divisions of Labor*

| Feature | First Stage | | Second Stage |
	Preparatory Division	Dilatational Division	Pelvic Division
Functions	Contractions coordinated, cervix prepared	Cervix actively dilating	Pelvis negotiated; mechanisms of labor; fetal descent; delivery
Interval	Latent and acceleration phases	Phase of maximum slope	Deceleration phase and second stage
Measurement	Elapsed duration	Linear rate of dilatation	Linear rate of descent
Diagnosable disorders	Prolonged latent phase	Protracted dilatation; protracted descent	Prolonged deceleration; secondary arrest of dilatation; arrest of descent; failure of descent

(From Friedman, E. [1978]. *Labor, clinical evaluation and management* [2nd ed.]. New York: Appleton-Century-Crofts, p. 54, with permission.)

birthing center, preparing older children for her departure, and giving instructions to the person who will take care of them while she is away.

Active Phase

During the active phase of labor cervical dilatation occurs more rapidly, going from 4 cm to 8 cm, and contractions are stronger (45 to 60 seconds long and 3 to 5 minutes apart). This phase lasts approximately 3 hours in a nullipara and 2 hours in a multipara. Show (increased vaginal secretions) and perhaps spontaneous rupture of the membranes occur. Although this is a difficult time for a woman in labor (contractions begin to cause true discomfort), it is also an exciting time because she realizes that something dramatic is happening. It may also be frightening because she realizes that labor is truly progressing and her life is about to change.

The active phase of labor in Friedman's graph can be subdivided into the following two periods: acceleration (4 to 5 cm) and maximum slope (5 to 9 cm). During the period of maximum slope, cervical dilatation proceeds at its most rapid pace, averaging 3.5 cm per hour in nulliparas and 5 to 9 cm per hour in multiparas. Administration of an analgesic at this point has little effect on the progress of labor.

Transition Phase

During the transition phase, maximum dilatation of 8 to 10 cm occurs, and contractions reach their peak of intensity (every 2 to 3 minutes) and duration (60 to 90 seconds). Dilatation continues at a rapid rate. If the membranes have not previously ruptured or been ruptured by amniotomy, they will rupture as a rule at full dilatation (10 cm). If it has not previously occurred, show will be present as the last of the mucus plug from the cervix is released. By the end of this phase, full dilatation (10 cm) and complete cervical effacement (obliteration of the cervix) has occurred.

The woman at this stage in labor may be experiencing intense discomfort or pain. Because of the intensity and duration of the contractions, she experiences a feeling of loss of control, anxiety, panic, and irritability. This may be accompanied by nausea and vomiting. The sensation in her abdomen is so intense that it may seem as though labor has taken charge of her. A few minutes before, she enjoyed having her forehead wiped with a cool cloth; now she may knock the nurse's hand away. A moment before, she enjoyed having her partner rub her back; now she may resist being touched and push that person away. Her focus is entirely inward on the task of delivering her baby.

The peak of the transition phase can be identified by a slight slowing in the rate of cervical dilatation when 9 cm is reached. As the woman reaches the end of this stage at 10 cm of dilatation, a new sensation—that is, an irresistible urge to push—begins to occur.

Second Stage

The second stage of labor is the period from full dilatation and cervical effacement to birth of the infant. At first there may be a short period during which the intensity, duration, and frequency of contractions may slow somewhat. The urge to bear down also begins to grow stronger at this time as the fetus descends into the lower pelvis.

With retraction of the cervix over the presenting part, **fetal descent** and negotiation of the pelvis occurs rapidly. The woman may experience momentary nausea or vomiting, because pressure is no longer exerted on the stomach after the downward movement of the fetus. Contractions change from the characteristic crescendo-decrescendo pattern she has grown accustomed to, to an overwhelming, uncontrollable urge to push or bear down with contractions as if she were moving her bowels. She pushes with such force that she perspires and the blood vessels in her neck become distended. As the fetus descends in the pelvic ring, being pushed beyond the open cervix, the woman's perineum begins to bulge, the labia part, and the vaginal introitus stretches apart.

The anus of the woman appears everted; stool may be expelled from the pressure exerted on it. As the fetal head touches the internal perineum, the perineum begins to bulge and appear tense. As the fetal head is pushed still tighter against the perineum, the fetal scalp becomes visible at the opening to the vagina. At first this is a slit-like opening, then oval, then circular. The circle enlarges from the size of a dime to that of a quarter to that of a half dollar. This is called **crowning**.

It takes a few contractions of this new type for the woman to realize that everything is still all right, just different, and to appreciate that it feels good, not frightening, to push with contractions. In fact, the need to push becomes so intense that she cannot stop herself. She barely hears the conversation in the room around her. All of her energy, her thoughts, her being are directed toward delivering her child. As she pushes, using her abdominal muscles and the involuntary uterine contractions, the fetus is pushed out of the birth canal.

Graphing Labor Progress

Graphing labor progress can be an independent nursing function. If a health care agency does not have commercial graph forms, simple square-ruled graph paper can be used. Number the left side of the graph 1 to 10 (representing centimeters of cervical dilatation). Number the bottom line to represent hours of labor. Number the right side of the graph −4 to +4 to represent the station of the fetal presenting part.

After each cervical examination, plot the extent of cervical dilatation and the fetal descent on the graph. The pattern of cervical dilatation when graphed in this way is typically an S-shaped curve. The descent pattern

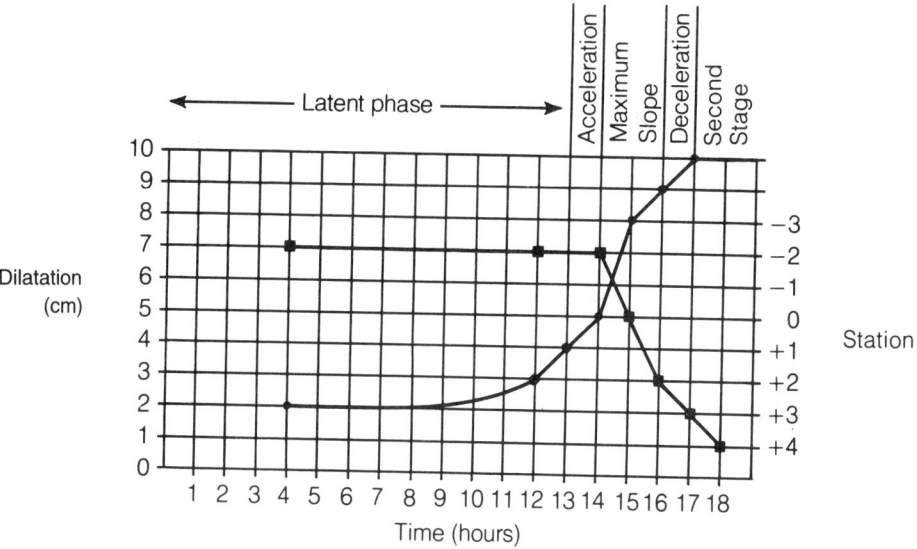

FIGURE 18-16

Normal labor graph. Fetal descent and cervical dilatation are occurring at the same time.

●—cervical dilatation

■—fetal descent

of the fetus typically forms a downward curve. The sharp downward slope of fetal descent should cross the dilatation line at the same time as maximum cervical dilatation occurs (phase of maximum slope). A typical labor graph is shown in Figure 18-16.

Plotting the duration of labor phases offers another indication that something is wrong with labor. Various abnormal patterns that may be detected are shown in Figure 18-17 and defined in Table 18-6.

Third Stage

The third stage of labor, or the *placental stage,* begins with the birth of the infant and ends with the delivery of the placenta. Two separate phases are involved: (1) placental separation, and (2) placental expulsion.

Following the birth of the infant, the uterus can be palpated as a firm, round mass just inferior to the level of the umbilicus. After a few minutes of rest, uterine contractions begin again, and the organ assumes a discoid shape. It retains this new shape until the placenta has separated, approximately 5 minutes after birth of the infant.

Placental Separation

Placental separation occurs automatically as the uterus resumes contractions. As the uterus contracts down on an almost empty interior, there is such a disproportion between the placenta itself and its attachment site that folding and separation of the placenta occur. Active bleeding on the maternal surface of the placenta begins with separation; the bleeding helps to separate the pla-

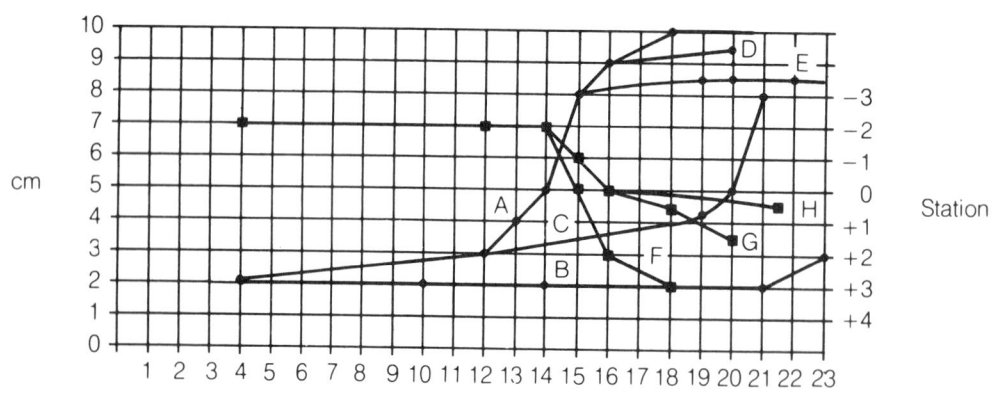

FIGURE 18-17

*Graph showing types of abnormal labor. (**A**) Normal labor curve. (**B**) Prolonged latent phase. (**C**) Protracted active-phase dilatation. (**D**) Prolonged deceleration phase. (**E**) Secondary arrest of dilatation. (**F**) Normal descent. (**G**) Protracted descent. (**H**) Arrest of descent.*

Table 18-6. *Abnormal Phases of Labor Detectable by Graphing*

Phase	Definition
Prolonged Latent Phase	A latent phase that is more than 20 hours in a nullipara and 14 hours in a multipara is a prolonged latent phase.
Protracted Active Dilatation Phase	If the phase of maximum slope occurs at a rate less than 1.2 cm per hour for multiparas and 1.5 cm per hour for nulliparas, it is a protracted or abnormally extended phase.
Prolonged Deceleration Phase	If a deceleration phase is longer than 3 hours in a nullipara and 1 hour in a multipara, the phase is abnormally long or protracted.
Protracted Descent	The slope of fetal descent is normally greater than 1 cm per hour in nulliparas, 2 cm per hour in multiparas. A descent under these limits is considered protracted descent.
Secondary Arrest of Dilatation	This is cessation of progressive dilatation in the active phase before full dilatation.
Arrest of Descent	This is cessation of progressive linear descent occurring in the pelvic division.

centa still further by pushing it away from its attachment site. As separation is completed, the placenta sinks to the posterior aspect of the lower uterine segment or the upper vagina.

The following signs indicate that the placenta has loosened and is ready to deliver: a lengthening of the umbilical cord, a sudden gush of vaginal blood, or a change in the shape of the uterus.

If the placenta separates first at its center and last at its edges, it tends to fold on itself like an umbrella and will present at the vaginal opening with the fetal surface evident (Figure 18-18A). This appears shiny and glistening from the fetal membranes, and is called a *Schultze's placenta.* Approximately 80% of placentas separate and present in this way. If, however, the placenta separates first at its edges, it slides along the uterine surface and presents at the vagina with the maternal surface evident (Figure 18-18B). It looks raw, red, and irregular with the cotyledons showing, and is called a *Duncan placenta.* A simple trick of remembering the presentations is associating "shiny" with Schultze (the fetal membrane surface) and "dirty" with Duncan (the irregular maternal surface) (Figure 18-19).

Bleeding occurs as part of the normal consequence

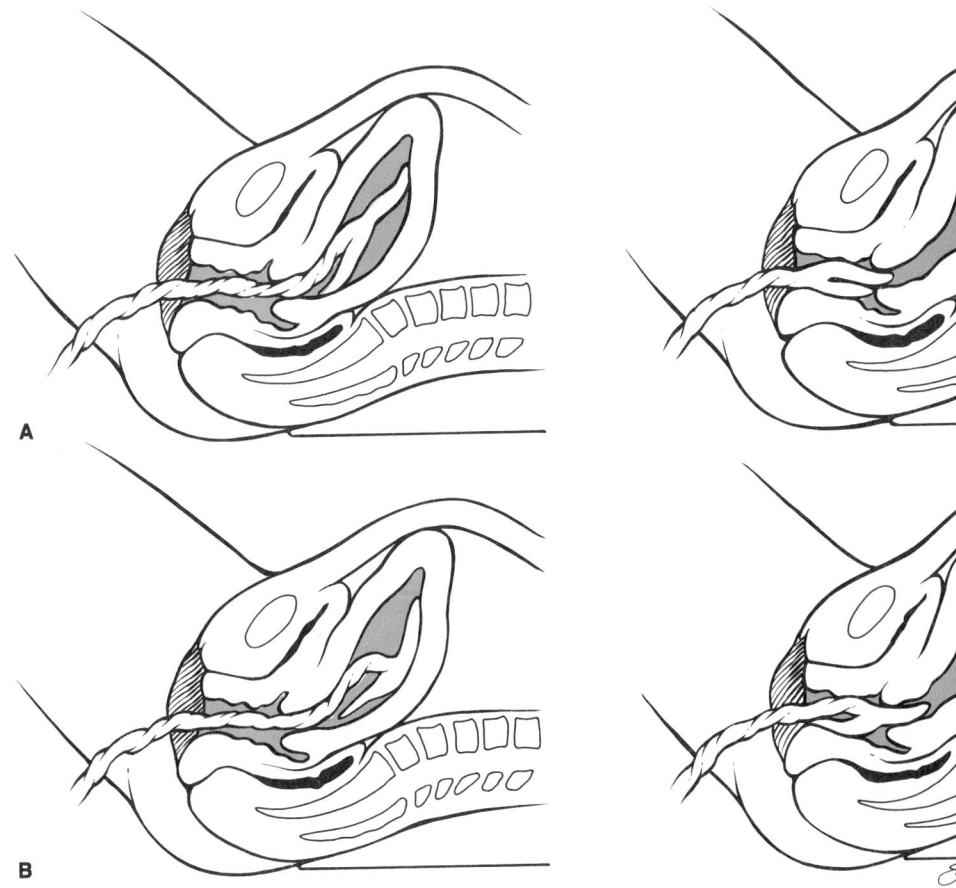

FIGURE 18-18
*Delivery of the placenta. Note the change in contour of the woman's abdomen after separation of placenta. (**A**) Placenta separates first at center and delivers with fetal surface in evidence (Schultze's placenta). (**B**) Placenta separates first at edge and delivers with maternal surface in evidence (Duncan placenta).*

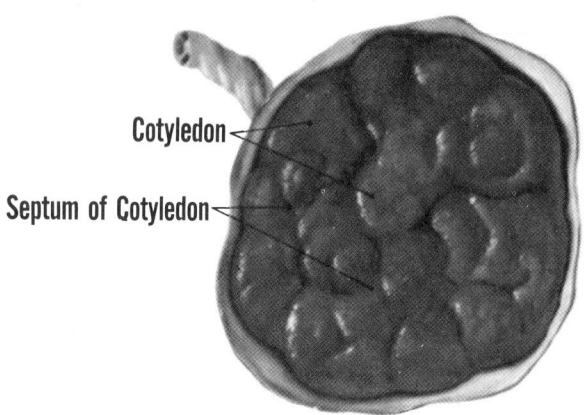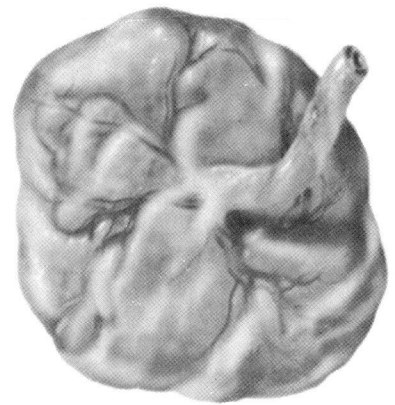

Cotyledon

Septum of Cotyledon

FIGURE 18-19
*Maternal (**left**) and fetal (**right**) surface of the placenta. (Used with permission of Ross Products Division, Abbott Laboratories, Columbus, OH 43216. From Clinical Education Aid, No. 2, ©1960 Ross Products Division, Abbott Laboratories.)*

of placental separation, before the uterus contracts sufficiently to seal maternal sinuses. The normal blood loss is 300 to 500 mL.

Placental Expulsion

The placenta is delivered either by the natural bearing-down effort of the mother or by gentle pressure on the contracted uterine fundus by the physician or nurse-midwife (Credé maneuver). *Pressure must never be applied to a uterus in a noncontracted state or the uterus may evert and hemorrhage.* This is a grave complication of birth, because the maternal blood sinuses are open and gross hemorrhage occurs.

If the placenta does not deliver spontaneously, it can be removed manually. With delivery of the placenta, the third stage of labor is over. In some cultures, the placenta is saved for symbolic rituals or is important to the couple. Parents should be asked if this is important to them before the placenta is destroyed.

Maternal and Fetal Responses to Labor

Physiologic Effects of Labor on the Mother

Although labor is a local process that involves the abdomen and reproductive organs, its intensity also has systemic effects.

Cardiovascular System

Labor is hard effort, causing an increase in cardiac output, blood pressure, and pulse rate.

Cardiac Output. A contraction greatly decreases the blood flow to the uterus. The blood previously supplied to the uterus remains in the general circulation and leads to an increase in peripheral resistance. This in turn leads to an increase in systolic and diastolic blood pressure. An added factor during the second stage is the effect of the woman bearing down while pushing. During the pushing phase, the cardiac output may be increased as much as 40% to 50% above the prelabor level. Immediately after delivery, cardiac output peaks at 80% above prelabor levels as pressure is released from the vena cava. Within the first hour of delivery it will decrease from these high levels by about 50%.

With birth, there is a blood loss averaging 300 to 500 mL. Because the woman's blood volume has increased 30% to 50% during pregnancy, the blood loss during birth is not detrimental to the average woman and actually plays a role in reducing her blood volume to prepregnancy levels. Immediately following birth, with the weight and pressure removed from the pelvis, blood from the peripheral circulation may "flood" into the pelvic vasculature, momentarily dropping the pressure in the vena cava. This is quickly compensated for, and actually a heavy load of blood is then delivered by the vena cava to the heart. These hemodynamic changes have implications for the mother who has a cardiac problem at the time of birth (Cunningham et al., 1993).

Blood Pressure. With increased cardiac output during contractions, the systolic blood pressure rises an average of 15 mm Hg. Blood pressure should be assessed between contractions to monitor any further increase. Higher increases could be a sign of pathology. When the woman is in a supine position and pushes, her blood pressure can drop precipitously, leading to hypotension. An upright or sidelying position during the second stage of labor may help avoid such a problem.

Hemopoietic System

The major change in the blood-forming system that occurs during birth is the development of leukocytosis or a sharp increase in the number of circulating white blood cells, possibly as a result of stress and heavy exertion. At the end of labor, the average woman has a white blood cell count of 25,000/mm³ to 30,000/mm³ cells compared with a normal of 5000/mm³ to 10,000/mm³ cells. Being alert to this rise helps health care providers not to interpret an elevated leukocytosis during this time as a suggestion of infection.

Respiratory System

Whenever there is an increase in cardiovascular parameters, an accompanying increase in respiratory rate to supply additional oxygen for the bloodstream occurs but can result in hyperventilation. Encouraging appropriate breathing patterns will help avoid severe hyperventilation (which can lead to nausea and vomiting) or lengthy breath-holding. Total oxygen consumption increases about 100% during the second stage of labor, comparable with that of a person performing a strenuous exercise such as running.

Temperature Regulation

The increased muscular activity associated with labor has a tendency to elevate the woman's temperature a degree. To prevent excessive temperature increases, diaphoresis occurs with accompanying evaporation to cool and limit warming.

Fluid Balance

Insensible water loss increases during labor because of the increase in rate and depth of respirations (which causes moisture to be lost with each breath) and the presence of diaphoresis. The average woman eats nothing during labor and her fluid intake is reduced to only sips of fluid or ice cubes or hard candy. The combination of increased losses during this time and decreased intake may make supplemental fluid by intravenous therapy necessary as a prophylactic measure. It is important that the woman recognizes the administration of fluid during labor as prophylactic. Otherwise, she may misinterpret fluid administration as an indication that something is wrong when actually it is being used to ensure that everything will go well. Be sure that the woman knows that intravenous therapy does not hurt once the needle is inserted and should not interfere with ambulation or turning.

Urinary System

With the decrease in fluid intake during labor and the increased insensible water loss, kidneys begin to concentrate urine to preserve both fluid and electrolytes (specific gravity will rise to a high normal level of 1.020 to 1.030). It is not unusual for a trace of protein to be evident in urine from the breakdown of protein due to increased muscle activity (trace to 1+). Pressure of the fetal head as it descends in the birth canal against the

anterior bladder reduces bladder tone or the ability of the bladder to sense filling. If the woman is not asked to void approximately every 2 hours during labor, her bladder can overfill and leave her in the postpartal period with lessened bladder tone.

Musculoskeletal System

All during pregnancy, relaxin, an ovarian-released hormone, has acted to soften the cartilage between bones. In the week before labor, considerable additional softening causes the symphysis pubis and sacral/coccyx joints to be even more relaxed and movable, as this allows them to stretch apart to increase the size of the pelvic ring by as much as 2 cm. The woman may notice this increased pubic flexibility as increased back pain or irritating nagging pain at the pubis as she walks or turns in labor.

Gastrointestinal System

The gastrointestinal system becomes fairly inactive during labor, probably due to a shift in blood away from it to more life-sustaining organs and to pressure on the stomach and intestine from the contracting uterus. Digestive and emptying time of the stomach is prolonged, which is why eating during labor is usually restricted. Some women experience a loose bowel movement as contractions grow strong, similar to what may occur with painful menstrual cramps.

Neurologic and Sensory Responses

The neurologic responses that occur during labor are those responses related to pain (increased pulse and respiratory rate). Early in labor, it is the contraction of the uterus and dilatation of the cervix that causes the discomfort. Uterine and cervical nerve plexuses register at the 11th and 12th thoracic nerves. At the moment of birth, the pain is centered on the perineum as it stretches to allow the fetus to move past it. Perineal pain is registered at sacral-2 to sacral-4 nerves.

Psychological Responses of the Woman to Labor

Labor can lead to emotional distress because it represents the beginning of a major life change for the woman and her partner. Even for the most organized woman, pain reduces her ability to cope and may make her quick-tempered and quick to criticize things around her. If, for example, she has done last-minute shopping, dropped off a crying 2-year-old at her parents' house, driven or ridden in the car, and walked into the hospital from a distant parking lot, all the while trying to remember to breathe at a prepared rate through contractions, she will arrive at the labor unit in pain and with a sense of disorganization. Admitting her quickly to a birthing room in an environment free from outside interference will help her begin to control her breathing patterns and reduce the pain of early contractions, as well as begin to organize coping strategies.

Fatigue

By the time a date of birth approaches, a woman is generally tired from the burden of carrying an extra 30 to 35 pounds of weight with her. In addition, most women do not sleep well during the last month of pregnancy because they have backache in a side-lying position; they turn on their back and the fetus kicks and wakens them; they turn to their side and their back aches again, and so on. Sleep hunger from this discomfort makes it difficult for them to perceive situations clearly or to adjust rapidly to new situations. A little deficiency such as a wrinkled draw sheet can appear as a threatening discrepancy in their care. The process of labor can loom as an overwhelming, unendurable experience.

Fear

Women appreciate a review of labor process early in labor because it serves as a reminder that childbirth is not a strange, bewildering experience but a predictable and well-documented one. The labor process includes an explanation that contractions last a certain length and reach a certain firmness and are following the expected course.

Being taken by surprise—labor moving faster or slower than a woman thought it would—can be frightening. It brings to mind any horror stories of labor that a woman has heard. Compounding this, women may begin to worry that their infant may die or be born with an abnormality; they may be afraid they will not meet their own behavior expectations.

Cultural Influences

Cultural factors influence a woman's experience of labor and, as a result, the nurse's plan of care for each woman. Many American women are accustomed to following hospital procedures and the medical model of care. However, every woman in labor responds to cultural cues in some way; these are manifested in her response to pain, her choice of nourishment, her preferred birthing position, the proximity and involvement of a support person, and customs related to the immediate postpartum period.

Good nursing care can be given only by the nurse who is knowledgeable about cultural variations in these areas of human response and who is willing to be adaptable to specific circumstances. When a woman has traditions that run counter to American hospital protocols, the plan of care needs to address these differences and specific arrangements made to accommodate the individual's beliefs or customs (for instance, providing warm food or fluids during labor or saving the placenta for the

mother to take home). Being able to meet these needs may also include arranging for an interpreter if the woman does not speak English or working closely with a family member who can interpret for the nurse.

Fetal Responses to Labor

Although the fetus is basically a passive participant in labor, the effect of pressure and circulatory changes that occur with contractions cause detectable physiologic differences.

Neurologic Changes

Uterine contractions exert pressure on the fetal head that can be detected by a change in fetal cardiac rate during contractions. This causes the fetal heart rate (FHR) to decrease by as much as 5 bpm during a contraction as soon as contraction strength reaches 40 mm Hg. This is the same response that occurs in any instance of increased intracranial pressure; it shows on a fetal heart monitor as an early deceleration pattern.

Cardiovascular Effects

The average fetus has such mature response ability to cardiovascular change that he or she is unaffected by the continual variations of heart rate—a slight slowing and then return to normal (baseline) levels—that occur with labor. During a contraction, the arteries of the uterus that are corkscrew in contour are sharply constricted. Filling of cotyledons therefore almost completely halts during a contraction. The amount of nutrients exchanged during this time is reduced, causing a slight hypoxia. The corresponding increase in blood pressure that occurs from increased intracranial pressure serves to keep circulation from falling below normal during the duration of a contraction.

Integument

The pressure involved in birth is often reflected in minimal petechiae or ecchymotic places on the fetus (particularly the presenting part). There may also be edema of the presenting part (a caput succedaneum).

Musculoskeletal System

The force of uterine contractions tends to push the fetus into a position of full flexion. A fully flexed position is the most advantageous for birth, as it can speed labor.

Respiratory System

The process of labor appears to aid in the maturation of surfactant production by alveoli in the fetal lung. The pressure applied to the chest from contractions and passage through the birth canal clears it of lung fluid so the infant born by vaginal birth tends to be able to establish respirations easier than the fetus born by cesarean birth.

Maternal and Fetal Assessment During Labor

Immediate Assessment of the Woman in Stage One

There are a number of immediate assessment measures that need to be taken to safeguard maternal and fetal health once a woman is admitted to a labor unit. After the woman and her support person are oriented to the unit, admission procedures focus on obtaining this vital assessment data (see the Focus on Family Teaching box).

Initial Interview

Certain information must be obtained on hospital admission so that the extent of the woman's labor, her general physical condition, and her preparedness for labor and birth can be evaluated and comprehensive nursing care planned.

For an initial interview, ask about the woman's expected date of birth so that all health care personnel can be alerted to the possibility of a preterm birth. Document the frequency, duration, and intensity of the woman's contractions, the amount of and character of show, and whether the membranes have ruptured. Ask when the woman last ate to establish risk in case a general anesthetic must be planned. Ask whether she has any known allergies to drugs to determine if there will be a problem with medication administration. Ask her past pregnancy history to establish gravida and para. Ask about the outcome and any complications of labor or birth she may have experienced from previous pregnancies.

This amount of information is scant but helps to establish whether the woman is in active labor and needs intense care or whether she has arrived at the hospital or birthing center in an earlier stage of labor and will benefit from paced interventions.

Determining Maternal and Fetal Well Being

To evaluate a woman's physical well being, assess her temperature, pulse, respiration, and blood pressure, as well as the fetal heartbeat. Next, assess contractions for their duration, intensity, and frequency to establish a firm baseline. Always take the woman's blood pressure between contractions because blood pressure may rise 5 mm Hg to 10 mm Hg during a contraction.

Following initial assessment procedures, a woman is categorized as being at low, moderate, or high risk to have difficulty in labor herself or to deliver a newborn who will need special care at birth. If a risk assessment scale (see Chapter 10) was used during pregnancy, it should be updated at this time and new factors gained from the labor assessment added.

Detailed Assessment During the First Stage

If the woman is not facing imminent delivery, a more extensive history and physical examination can be carried out.

History

If the woman is in active labor, the history taken on arrival may be the only history obtained until after the baby is born. However, most women get to the hospital or birthing center in time for thorough history taking.

The history taken at this point should include a review of the woman's pregnancy, both physical and psychologic events, and a review of past pregnancies, general health, and family medical information to aid in planning nursing care.

Interviewing a woman in labor in detail can be difficult because the woman is constantly interrupted by labor contractions. Be patient. Remember that the longest contraction is rarely more than 60 seconds. A woman may concentrate so intently on a breathing exercise that she completely forgets the question asked just before the contraction. As the contraction subsides, repeat the question as if it had not been asked before, or act as if it is no trouble to ask it again.

Current Pregnancy History. Important information needed for a complete history is documentation of gravida and para; a description of the pregnancy (if it was planned or not, pattern and place of prenatal care,

FOCUS ON FAMILY TEACHING

Q. I'm nervous that admission procedures to a hospital while I'm in labor will be so overwhelming they'll interrupt my breathing exercises. What can I expect on admission?

A. Every agency has specific procedures but generally these would include:

- Orientation to a birthing room
- Temperature, pulse, respirations, and blood pressure assessment
- Nursing and medical history and physical examination
- Assessment of fetal heart rate
- Vaginal examination
- Urine specimen and necessary blood samples obtained
- Explanation of fetal or uterine monitoring equipment to be used; connecting this equipment

whether nutrition was adequate, if any complications such as spotting, falls, hypertension of pregnancy, infection, or alcohol or drug ingestion occurred); plans for labor (does she want medication for pain or not, will she use breathing exercises or not, will she have a support person with her?); and child care (will she breast- or bottle-feed? Has she chosen a pediatrician?).

Past Pregnancy History. Document prior pregnancies (numbers, dates, types of birth, any complications and outcomes, including sex and birth weight of children). What is the current health status of previous children?

Past Health History. Document any previous surgery (surgical adhesions might interfere with free fetal passage); heart disease or diabetes (she will need special precautions during labor and birth); anemia (blood loss at birth may be more important than normally); tuberculosis (tuberculosis lung lesions may be reactivated at birth by changes in lung contour); kidney disease or hypertension (blood pressure will need to be watched even more carefully than normally); or a sexually transmitted disease such as herpes (the infant may be exposed to the disease by vaginal contact if the disease is still active). Ask if her lifestyle is high risk for human immunodeficiency virus exposure: multiple sexual partners, history of intravenous (IV) drug use, or a sexual partner who uses IV drugs or is bisexual.

Family Medical History. Ask if any family member has a heart disease, a blood dyscrasia, diabetes, kidney disease, cancer, allergies, seizures, congenital defects, or mental retardation. Adequate preparation can then be made for a child who might be born with a disease.

Physical Examination

Following history taking, the woman needs a thorough physical examination, including a pelvic examination, to confirm the presentation and position of the fetus and determine the stage of dilatation.

Physical assessment during labor begins, as does all physical assessment, with the woman's overall appearance. Does she appear tired? Pale? Ill? Frightened? Is there obvious edema or dehydration? Are there open lesions anywhere?

Assess by palpation for enlargement of lymph nodes to detect the possibility of infection. Inspect the mucous membrane of the mouth and the conjunctiva of the eyes for color. Does the color (paleness) suggest anemia? What is the condition of her teeth? Are they carious? Do any teeth appear abscessed (such a condition needs to be documented as it might account for a postpartum temperature)? Examine the outer and inner surfaces of her lips carefully. Does she have herpes lesions (pinpoint vesicles on an erythematous base)? Type II (genital) virus can be lethal to newborns. If herpetic lesions

are present anywhere, the woman will probably be isolated from her child until the lesions crust.

Assess lungs to be certain they are clear to auscultation. Listen for normal heart sounds and rhythms. Many pregnant women at term have a grade II to III systolic ejection murmur from the extra volume of blood that must cross heart valves. Inspect and palpate her breasts. Are they free of cysts and lumps? Ask if she inspects her own breasts monthly. Do not try to teach breast self-examination while a woman is in labor; she will be unable to concentrate on the instructions. If she needs education in this area, indicate it on her chart, so that the postpartum nursing staff can provide it before she leaves the hospital or birthing center.

Mark the chart also of a woman who has a palpable mass in her breasts for reexamination following labor and birth. This is probably an enlarged milk gland but needs further evaluation.

Estimate fetal size by fundal height (should be at the level of the xyphoid process at term); assess presentation and position by Leopold's maneuvers (see below). Palpate and percuss the bladder area (over the symphysis pubis) to detect a full bladder. Even though the woman has just voided, she might not have emptied her bladder sufficiently because of pressure of the fetal head. A full bladder is uncomfortable during labor and may impede the descent of the fetus. In addition, an overly distended bladder can be injured in labor from pressure of the fetus; this can cause urinary retention in the postpartum period. Assess for abdominal scars as abdominal or pelvic surgery can leave adhesions. Assess skin turgor for dehydration.

Finally, inspect the lower extremities for edema and varicose veins. Women with large varicosities are prone to thrombophlebitis following birth. Some physicians prefer not to use birth room stirrups if varicosities are prominent during labor, because the stirrups may press against them. Severe edema suggests hypertension of pregnancy, so the extent and intensity of edema must be assessed and correlated with the woman's blood pressure.

Leopold's Maneuvers

Leopold's maneuvers (Figure 18-20) are a systematic method of observation and palpation to determine fetal presentation and position. Begin by observing the woman's abdomen. What is the longest diameter in appearance? Is it horizontal or vertical? If the fetus is active, where is the movement apparent? The long axis is the length of the fetus. The activity probably reflects the position of the feet.

In Leopold's maneuvers, as in any form of palpation, best results are obtained if the palpation is done systematically. The woman should lie in a supine position with her knees flexed slightly so that her abdominal muscles are relaxed. Hands that are warm (by washing them in warm water first if necessary) aid comfort; cold

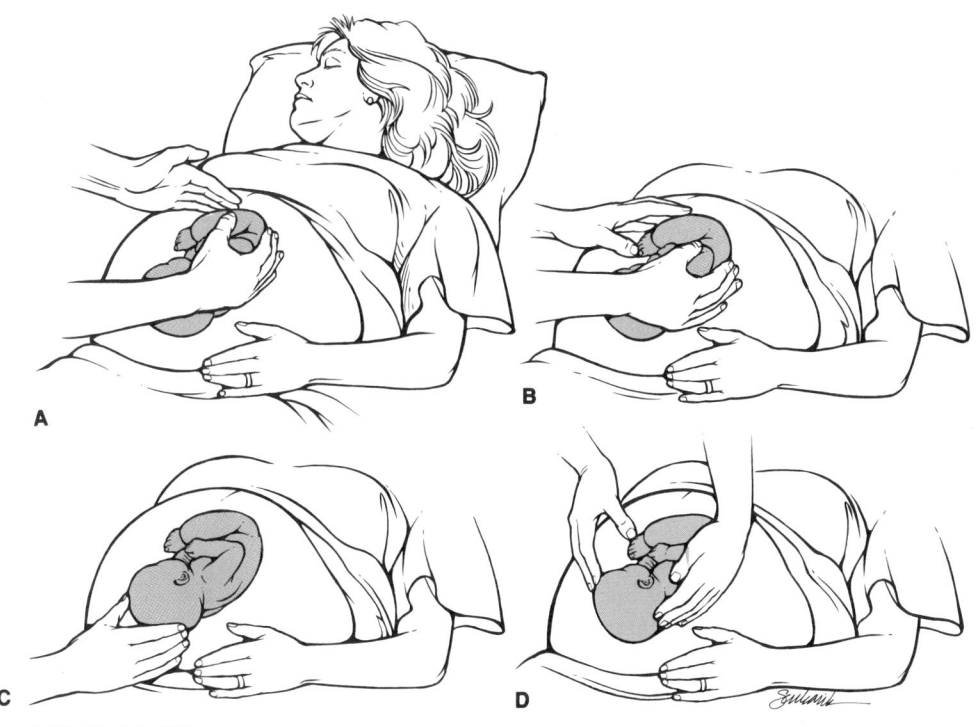

FIGURE 18-20
Leopold's maneuvers. (**A**) *First maneuver.* (**B**) *Second maneuver.* (**C**) *Third maneuver.* (**D**) *Fourth maneuver.*

hands cause abdominal muscles to contract and tighten. Use gentle but firm motions.

If the woman empties her bladder before palpation is begun, she will be more comfortable and the results more productive, because the fetal contours will then not be obscured by a distended anterior bladder.

First Maneuver. Palpate the superior surface of the fundus (Figure 18-20*A*). What is the consistency? A head feels more firm than a breech. What is the shape? A head is round and hard; the breech is less well defined. What is the mobility of the palpated part? A head moves independently of the body; the breech moves only in conjunction with the body. Form an opinion of what portion of the fetus lies in this fundal area.

Second Maneuver. Palpate the sides of the uterus to determine which direction the fetal back is facing (Figure 18-20*B*). This maneuver is accomplished most successfully if the left hand is held stationary on the left side of the uterus while the right hand palpates the opposite side of the uterus from top to bottom. Next, hold the right hand stationary to immobilize the uterus, and palpate top to bottom on the left side. One hand will feel a smooth, hard, resistant surface (the back), while on the opposite side, a number of angular nodulations (the knees and elbows of the fetus) will be felt.

Third Maneuver. Next, palpate to discover what is at the inlet of the pelvis (Figure 18-20*C*). Gently grasp the

lower portion of the abdomen just above the symphysis pubis between the thumb and index finger and try to press the thumb and finger together. If the presenting part moves upward so an examiner's hands can be pressed together, the presenting part is not engaged (not firmly settled into the pelvis). Is it firm (the head)? Or is it soft (the breech)?

Fourth Maneuver. Assuming the fetus has been found to be in a cephalic presentation, the fetal attitude should then be determined (degree of flexion). Place fingers on both sides of the uterus approximately 2 inches above the inguinal ligaments (Figure 18-20*D*). Press downward and inward. The fingers of one hand will slide along the uterine contour and meet no obstruction; this is the back of the fetal neck. The other hand will meet an obstruction an inch or so above the ligament; this is the fetal brow. The position of the fetal brow should correspond to the side of the uterus that contained the elbows and knees of the fetus. If the fetus is in a poor attitude, the examining fingers will meet an obstruction on the same side as the fetal back; that is, the fingers will touch the hyperextended head.

Information about the infant's anteroposterior position may also be gained from this final maneuver. If the brow is very easily palpated (as if it lies just under the skin), the fetus is probably in a posterior position (the occiput is pointing toward the woman's back).

Leopold's maneuvers provide information about the presentation, presenting part, position, and attitude of the fetus, which are all important facts to know to help predict the course of labor. It is difficult to palpate fetal contour in an obese woman or one with hydramnios (excessive amniotic fluid).

Assessing Rupture of Membranes

In as many as 25% of labors, labor begins with spontaneous rupture of the fetal membranes. In most instances with rupture of membranes, there is a sudden gush of amniotic fluid from the vagina. Women are startled by this sensation (it feels as if they have lost bladder control). It may happen while they are shopping or in another public place, and they may be embarrassed before they realize that the warm moist fluid on their perineum and legs is not urine but the announcement that labor is beginning. In other women, rupture of membranes is not a dramatic event but only a slow loss of fluid, and there is a question whether membranes have ruptured.

A simple test with nitrazine paper may help determine if the membranes have ruptured. To obtain vaginal secretions for testing, insert a sterile, cotton-tipped applicator deeply into the vagina and then touch it to a strip of nitrazine paper or a glass slide. Vaginal secretions are acid; amniotic fluid is alkaline. If amniotic fluid has passed through the vagina recently, the *p*H of the vagina will probably be alkaline (with a *p*H greater than 6.5) if tested by nitrazine paper. A false reading may occur in women with intact membranes who have a heavy, bloody show, because blood is also alkaline. An additional test is a fern test. Because of its high estrogen content, amniotic fluid will show a fern pattern when dried and examined under a microscope; urine will not.

Ask the woman whose membranes ruptured at home to describe the color of the amniotic fluid. It should be clear as water. Yellow-staining fluid may indicate a blood incompatibility between mother and fetus (the amniotic fluid is bilirubin-stained from the breakdown of red blood cells). Green-colored fluid indicates meconium staining. Although this is normal in breech deliveries because of buttock compression, which expels meconium into the amniotic fluid, in a vertex presentation, meconium staining may indicate that the fetus has suffered anoxia in utero and the anoxia has led to spontaneous sphincter relaxation (a vagal response), resulting in meconium loss into amniotic fluid. A fetus with meconium staining needs immediate interventions to safeguard his or her well being. The infant will need close assessment following birth because it is possible that he or she will have aspirated some meconium into the trachea or lungs.

Vaginal Examination

Vaginal examination is necessary to determine the extent of cervical effacement and dilatation and to confirm the fetal presentation, position, and degree of descent. If careful technique is used, and vaginal examinations are kept to the few required, they do not increase the incidence of infection. The technique for a vaginal examination in labor is shown in Nursing Procedure 18-1.

Women practitioners usually have an advantage over men in performing vaginal examinations because their fingers, which often are narrower, cause less pressure and less discomfort (Figure 18-21). Fingernails should not extend beyond the edge of the fingertips of the examining fingers so that there is no danger of piercing an examining glove.

Vaginal examinations may be done either between contractions or during contractions. More fetal skull may be palpated during a contraction because the cervix retracts more at that time, but examining during a contraction is more painful and rarely justifies the additional amount of information gained. Palpating membranes during a contraction when they are under pressure may cause them to rupture.

Women are anxious to have frequent progress reports during labor, to assure them that their work is not in vain. Tell the woman immediately after the examination about the progress of dilatation. Most women are aware of dilatation but not the word *effacement*. Just saying "no further dilatation" is a depressing report. "You're not dilated a lot more, but a lot of thinning out is happening and that's just as important" is the same report given in a positive manner.

Vaginal examinations are never done in the presence of fresh bleeding, because this may indicate a placenta previa (implantation of the placenta so low in the uterus that it encroaches on the cervical os). Performing a vaginal examination in this instance might tear the placenta and cause hemorrhage, with resultant danger to both mother and fetus. If in doubt, err on the side of postponing a vaginal examination until a physician or nurse-midwife arrives.

After finishing a vaginal examination, plot the new degree of dilatation and descent of the presenting part on a labor progress graph as described earlier.

Assessment of Pelvic Adequacy

Evaluating pelvic adequacy by means of an internal conjugate and ischial tuberosity diameters is generally done during pregnancy so that by weeks 32 to 36 of pregnancy, the nurse-midwife or physician is alerted to the problem that a cephalic disproportion could occur. Women with this potential problem are cautioned not to attempt a home birth or use a birthing center without nearby hospital facilities.

Pelvic capacity can be reassessed during early labor, although these procedures involve excessive vaginal manipulation and discomfort (and the diameters obtained during pregnancy have not changed), so they do not need to be retaken routinely. Procedures for these estimates are described in Chapter 10. They need to be

NURSING PROCEDURE 18-1
Vaginal Examination in Labor

Purpose
Determine cervical readiness and fetal position and presentation.

Procedure	*Principle*
1. Wash your hands; explain procedure to client. Provide privacy.	1. Prevent spread of microorganisms; ensure client cooperation and compliance.
2. Assess client status; analyze appropriateness of plan; adjust plan to individual client need.	2. Care is always individualized according to a client's needs.
3. Implement plan by assembling equipment: sterile examining gloves, sterile lubricant, antiseptic solution. Ask the woman to turn onto back with knees flexed (a dorsal recumbent position). Pull on sterile examining gloves.	3. Position allows for good visualization of perineum. A sterile glove prevents contamination of birth canal.
4. Discard one drop of clean lubricating solution and drop an ample supply on tips of gloved fingers.	4. To ensure that quantity you use will not be contaminated.
5. Pour antiseptic solution over vulva using nondominant hand.	5. Prevent the spread of organism from perineum to birth canal.
6. Place nondominant hand on the outer edges of the woman's vulva and spread her labia so you can inspect the external genitalia for lesions such as occur with primary syphilis or herpes infections.	6. Allow for good perineal visualization. Look for red, irritated mucous membranes; open, ulcerated sores; clustered, pinpoint vesicles.
7. Look for escaping amniotic fluid or the presence of umbilical cord or bleeding.	7. Amniotic fluid implies membranes have ruptured and umbilical cord may have prolapsed. Bleeding may be a sign of placenta previa. *Do not do a vaginal examination if a possible placenta previa is present.*
8. If there is no bleeding or cord visible, introduce your index and middle fingers of dominant hand gently into the vagina, directing them toward the posterior vaginal wall.	8. The posterior vaginal wall is less sensitive than the anterior wall. Stabilize the uterus by placing your nondominant hand on the woman's abdomen.
9. Touch the cervix with your gloved examining fingers. Palpate for cervical consistency and rate if *firm* or *soft*. Measure the extent of dilatation; palpate for an anterior rim or lip of cervix.	9. The cervix feels like a circular rim of tissue around a center depression. Firm is similar to the tip of a nose; soft is as pliable as an earlobe. The anterior rim is usually the last portion to thin. You should measure the width of your fingertips on a centimeter scale if you are going to do vaginal examination so you know how wide your index and middle fingers are at the tip. An index finger averages about 1 cm; a middle finger about 1½ cm. If they can both enter the cervix, the cervix is dilated 2½ to 3 cm. If there would be room for double the width of your examining fingers in the cervix, the dilatation is about 5 to 6 cm. When the space is four times the width of your fingertips, dilatation is complete—10 cm.
10. Estimate the degree of effacement.	10. Effacement is estimated in percentage. A cervix before labor is 2 to 2½ cm thick. If it is only 1 cm thick now, it is 50% effaced. If it is tissue paper thin, it is 100% effaced. It is difficult to feel for dilatation with a 100% effaced cervix because the

(continued)

NURSING PROCEDURE 18-1 (continued)
Vaginal Examination in Labor

Procedure	Principle
10. Continued.	edges of the cervix are so thin; it is difficult to be certain whether you are touching fetal scalp or brushing against an edge of the paper-thin rim of the cervix. Practice is necessary.
11. Estimate whether membranes are intact.	11. The membranes (with a slight amount of amniotic fluid in front of the presenting part) are the shape of a watch crystal. With a contraction, they bulge forward and become prominent and can be felt much more readily.
12. Locate the ischial spines. Rate the station of the presenting part. Identify the presenting part (confirm what you suspect from having done Leopold's maneuvers).	12. Ischial spines are palpated as notches at the 4 and 8 o'clock positions at the pelvic outlet. Station is the number of centimeters the presenting part is above or below the spines. Differentiating a vertex from a breech may be more difficult than would first appear. A vertex has a hard, smooth surface; buttocks feel softer and give under fingertip pressure. Fetal hair may be palpable but massed together and wet and may be difficult to appreciate through gloves, however. Palpating the two fontanelles, one diamond-shaped and one triangular, helps the identification. You can identify the anus because the sphincter action will "trap" your index finger.
13. Establish the fetal position.	13. The fontanelle you are able to palpate is invariably the posterior one because the fetus maintains a flexed position, presenting the posterior not the anterior fontanelle. In an ROA position, the triangular fontanelle will point toward the right anterior pelvic quadrant. In an LOA position, the posterior fontanelle will point toward the left anterior pelvis. In a breech presentation, the anus can serve as a marker for position. When the anus is pointing toward the left anterior quadrant of the woman's pelvis, the position is LSA.
14. Withdraw your hand. Wipe the perineum front to back to remove secretions or examining solution. Leave client comfortable and turned to side.	14. Use as gentle a technique with withdrawal as insertion. Wipe front to back to avoid moving rectal contamination forward to the vagina. Side-lying is the best position to prevent supine hypotension syndrome in labor.
15. Evaluate effectiveness of procedure. Record procedure and assessment findings.	15. Document nursing care and client status.
16. Inform the woman of labor progress and graph the new findings on a labor graph.	16. Providing knowledge is a prime method of reducing anxiety during labor. Graphing progress is a part of risk assessment.

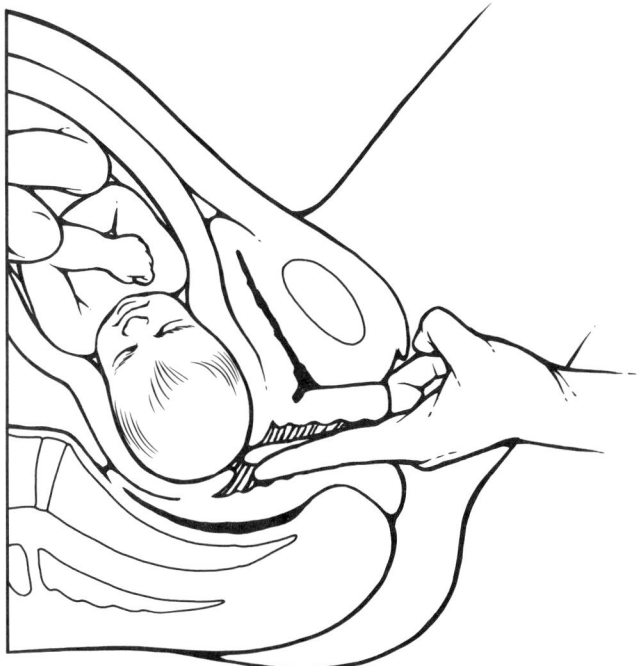

FIGURE 18-21
Technique of vaginal examination during labor.

estimated at this time if the woman did not receive prenatal care.

A further estimation done in early labor may be the degree of the suprapubic angle, since this influences how readily the fetal head will deliver. To estimate this, place the fingers vaginally and press up against the pubic arch. If the fingers cannot be separated in this position, the angle is unusually steep (less than 90 de-

grees). An unusually steep pubic arch may prevent the fetal head from delivering freely and increase the possibility that the perineal tissue may tear during birth as the fetal head is pushed posteriorly.

Sonography

Sonography may be used at term to determine the diameters of the fetal skull and to determine presentation, presenting part, position, flexion, and degree of descent of the fetus. If a woman is going to be transported to another department to have this done, a nurse should accompany her so if labor does become more active, she can be returned quickly to the labor and birth service.

Vital Signs

Vital signs are taken at the beginning of labor and then repeated periodically as summarized in Table 18-7.

Temperature. Temperature should be repeated every 4 hours during labor. A temperature higher than 37.2°C (99°F) should be reported to the attending physician or nurse-midwife because the sign may indicate the development of infection. It is more likely that, unless there are accompanying symptoms, it reflects dehydration in the woman who is taking no fluids by mouth (a different situation but one that still requires some intervention). Following rupture of membranes, temperature should be taken hourly because the possibility for infection increases markedly after this time.

Pulse and Respiration. Pulse and respiration rate should be taken and recorded every hour during labor. A woman's pulse may be rapid on admission because

Table 18-7. *Time Intervals for Nursing Interventions During First Stage of Labor*

		Continued Pregnancy	
Intervention	Admission	Latent Phase	Active Phase
Assess and Record			
Temperature	X	q4h (unless membranes are ruptured, then q1h)	q4h (unless membranes are ruptured, then q1h)
Pulse	X	q1h	q1h
Respirations	X	q1h	q1h
Blood pressure	X	q1h	q1h
Voiding	X	q2–4h	q2–4h
FHR	X	Continuously by monitor or q30min	Continuously by monitor or q15min
Contractions	X	Continuously by monitor or q30min	Continuously by monitor or q15min
Provide			
Ambulation	Until membranes rupture		
Support	X	Continuously	Continuously

she is nervous and anxious. After she has become better acquainted with her surroundings and has been assured that everything is going well, her pulse should be in a range of 70 to 80 bpm. A persistent pulse rate of more than 100 bpm suggests tachycardia from dehydration or hemorrhage. Respiration rate during labor is 18 to 20 bpm. Do not count respirations during contractions, because women tend to breath rapidly from pain. Conversely, if a woman is using controlled breathing to decrease pain in labor, her respirations will be counted as abnormally slow.

Observe for hyperventilation (i.e., rapid, deep respirations). Prolonged hyperventilation will result in "blowing off" carbon dioxide and symptoms of dizziness and tingling of hands and feet. Rebreathing into a paper bag and reassurance to reduce anxiety is necessary to reverse this process.

Blood Pressure. Blood pressure also should be taken and recorded every hour during labor. If a woman receives an analgesic agent that tends to be hypotensive (such as meperidine), check the woman's blood pressure approximately 15 minutes after administration to be certain that the medication's effect is not causing hypotension. Blood pressure should be recorded between contractions, both for the woman's comfort and for best accuracy, because blood pressure tends to rise 5 mm Hg to 10 mm Hg during a contraction. An increase in blood pressure may indicate the development of pregnancy-induced hypertension. A decrease in blood pressure or a decrease in the pulse pressure (the difference between the systolic and diastolic pressures) may indicate hemorrhage.

A blood pressure of more than 140/90 suggests pregnancy-induced hypertension. If a woman knows her prepregnancy blood pressure, a systolic elevation of 30 mm Hg or a diastolic elevation of 15 mm Hg over the prepregnancy level can also be used to screen for pregnancy-induced hypertension.

Laboratory Analysis

Blood. Blood is drawn for hemoglobin and hematocrit, VDRL (serologic test for syphilis), hepatitis B antibodies, and blood typing to assure everyone dealing with the woman that she is in good physical health. It also alerts the laboratory that a woman with a certain blood type is in labor and predicts whether a blood incompatibility is likely to exist in the newborn.

Urine. A urine specimen to be tested immediately for protein and glucose and then sent to the laboratory for a complete urinalysis should be obtained. A woman is able to void most easily if she is allowed to use a bathroom. A bedpan or receptacle placed on the toilet will allow for comfort and also will permit any material

passed by the vagina to be preserved. If the woman describes any symptoms that suggest urinary tract infection (e.g., burning on urination, blood in her urine, extreme frequency, or flank pain), then a clean-catch urine for culture should be obtained. Women who report ruptured membranes should not be ambulated until it is confirmed that the fetal head is engaged so that the umbilical cord cannot slip past the loosely fitting head and prolapse, causing fetal distress.

Assessment of Uterine Contractions

Uterine contractions may be monitored continuously by an internal or external system. Most women are monitored at least for a short period in early labor to screen for fetal well being. Monitoring the duration, strength, and interval between contractions can aid in tracking the progress of labor.

Length of Contractions. To determine the beginning of a contraction, rest a hand on the woman's abdomen at the fundus of the uterus *very gently* to sense the gradual tensing and upward rising of the fundus that accompanies a contraction (Figure 18-22). It is possible to palpate this tensing approximately 5 seconds before the woman is able to feel the contraction. (Contractions are palpable when the intrauterine pressure reaches approximately 20 mm Hg. The pain of a contraction is not felt until pressure reaches approximately 25 mm Hg.) The duration of a contraction is timed from the moment the uterus first tenses until it has relaxed again.

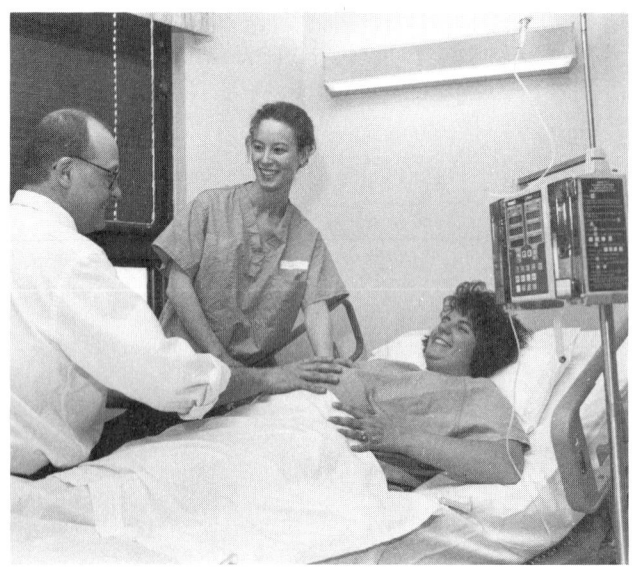

FIGURE 18-22
Contractions can be assessed by very gently placing the hand over the fundus of the uterus. Involving the support person in this activity can enhance the birthing experience.

Intensity of Contractions. In addition to observing duration of contractions, estimate the intensity or the strength of the contraction. Contractions are rated as *mild* (the uterus is contracting but does not become more than minimally tense); *moderate* (the uterus feels firm); or *strong* (the contraction is so intense the uterus feels as hard as wood at the peak of the contraction). The uterus cannot be indented by your fingertips in a strong contraction.

Following estimating the intensity of contractions, check the fundus at the conclusion of the contraction to determine that it does relax and become soft to the touch again. If it does, this demonstrates that the uterus is not in continuous contraction but is providing a relaxation time during which blood vessels can fill to supply the fetus with adequate oxygen.

Frequency of Contractions. Next, time the frequency of contractions. The frequency is timed from the *beginning* of one contraction to the *beginning* of the next. The duration and frequency of contractions are depicted diagrammatically in Figure 18-23.

Use as light a touch as possible on the woman's abdomen while timing contractions or estimating their strength. The fundus of the uterus becomes tender if it has to push against extra weight with each contraction—unnecessary discomfort for a woman in labor.

Initial Fetal Assessment

Fetal assessment must be undertaken along with maternal assessment as soon as the woman is admitted to a labor unit. Though passive in labor, a fetus is subjected to extreme pressure by uterine contractions and passage through the birth canal, as described previously. Compression of the umbilical cord and the placenta by uterine contractions may compromise the fetal blood and oxygen supply during these times. It is important to ascertain that FHR remains within normal limits to ensure that labor is not too strenuous for the fetus.

Auscultation of Fetal Heart Sounds

Fetal heart sounds are transmitted through the convex portion of the fetus, because that is the part lying in close contact with the uterine wall. In a vertex or breech presentation, fetal heart sounds are best heard through the fetal back; in a face presentation, the back becomes concave, and so the sounds are best heard through the

more convex thorax. In breech presentations, fetal heart sounds are heard most clearly high in the uterus at the woman's umbilicus or above. In cephalic presentations, they are heard loudest low in the abdomen. In ROA position, the sounds are heard best in the right lower quadrant; in LOA position, in the left lower quadrant. In posterior positions (LOP or ROP), the heart sounds are loudest at the maternal side. Figure 18-24 shows how to locate heart sounds for different fetal positions.

Hearing the fetal heart sounds in these positions provides confirmatory information about fetal position. Conversely, recognizing the fetal position aids in locating fetal heart sounds.

Fetal heart rate should be counted every 30 minutes during beginning labor, every 15 minutes during active labor, and every 5 minutes during the second stage of labor. This can be done by viewing a fetal heart rate monitoring strip.

Fetoscope. Fetal heart sounds can be auscultated with a stethoscope or a fetoscope, which is a modified stethoscope attached to a headpiece (Figure 18-25). With a fetoscope, sound is conducted through the bones of the head of the person wearing the instrument. Fetal heart tones can be auscultated with the fetoscope during and immediately following a contraction.

Although a fetoscope is a very direct and easy way of assessing fetal heart tones, it has given way in many hospital settings to the portable Doppler.

Portable Doppler or Ultrasound Units. A Doppler unit uses ultrasound waves that bounce off the fetal heart to produce echoes, which are then transformed into clicking noises (Figure 18-26). These clicks reflect the rate of the fetal heart beat. The system is easy to use and less cumbersome and restricting than continuous electronic monitoring devices, but it is limited in the detail it can provide concerning fetal well being.

Electronic Monitoring

In most hospitals, fetal heart rate (FHR) is screened for a short time in early labor by an electronic monitoring system. The monitor is left in place for continuous monitoring on women who are categorized as high risk for any reason or who have oxytocin stimulation.

The use of fetal monitors, however, has provoked

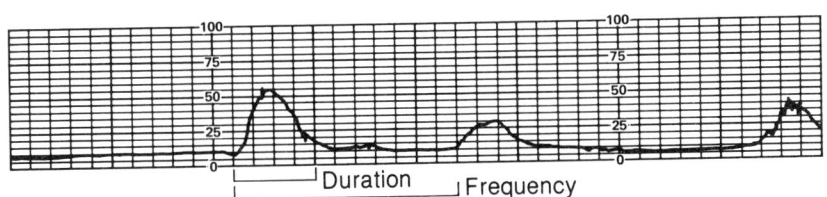

FIGURE 18-23
Duration and frequency of contractions. On this graph, the duration of the first contraction is 40 secs; frequency between the first two contractions is 110 secs (each space is 10 secs).

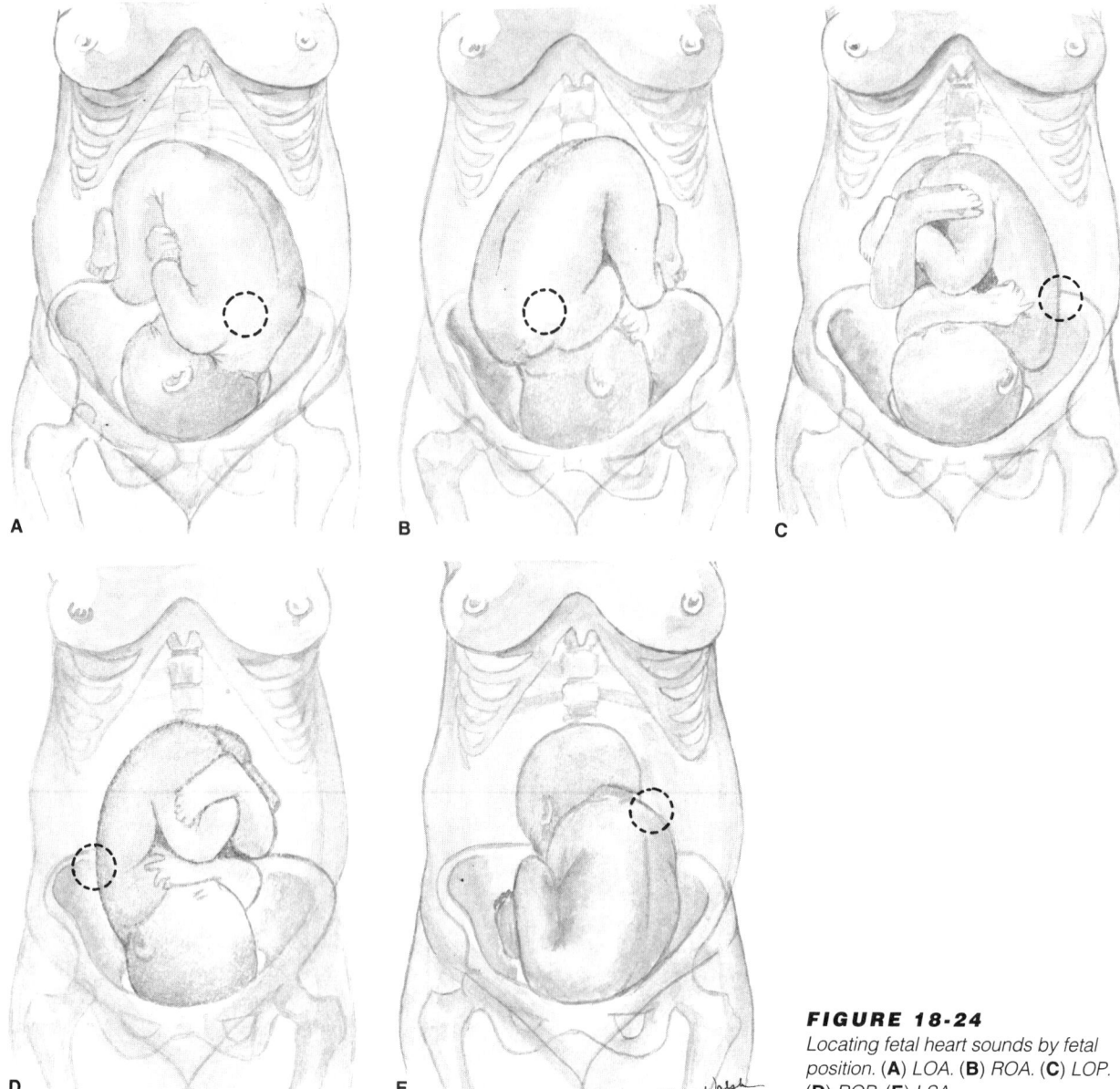

FIGURE 18-24

*Locating fetal heart sounds by fetal position. (**A**) LOA. (**B**) ROA. (**C**) LOP. (**D**) ROP. (**E**) LSA.*

one of the biggest controversies in modern obstetric health care (Lehman, 1990). Monitors were widely adopted in the mid-1970s as a means of immediately detecting variations in FHR that were assumed to be related to a deprivation of oxygen in the fetus. It was felt that if fetal distress could be detected early, forceps or cesarean birth could save the baby's life or prevent brain damage.

However, studies have been unable to confirm that the use of monitors has improved infant survival rates or morbidity. In one review of research addressing the efficacy of monitors, electronic monitoring was not found to be more efficient at saving babies or improving newborn health than frequent checks with a stethoscope or fetoscope (Freeman, 1990). Moreover, monitoring has not been found to be superior to the use of stethoscopes

in the birth of preterm babies at risk for cerebral palsy (Shy et al., 1990). Natural childbirth advocates have long criticized the overuse of monitoring devices, saying they intrude into the childbirth experience, needlessly discomforting and distracting the mother. The medical profession readily admits that monitors have contributed to the growing number of cesarean births, currently estimated at one in five nationwide, over the past 2 decades (Lehman, 1990). Advocates of monitoring would say that the prevention of complications for many babies is worth this increase. However, others believe that monitors often point to a problem where none exists, resulting in unnecessary cesarean births (which carries its own set of risks) and unnecessary frightening of parents (which could adversely affect early parent–infant bonding).

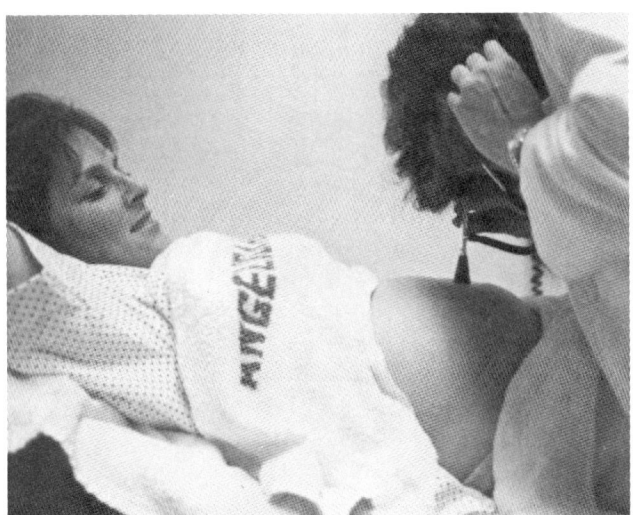

FIGURE 18-25
Auscultation of the fetal heartbeat using the fetoscope. (From Reeder, S.J., Martin, L.L., & Koniak, D. [1992]. Maternity nursing: Family, newborn, and women's health care [17th ed.]. Philadelphia: J.B. Lippincott.)

Monitoring does offer many advantages from a health care provider's standpoint. Observing a fetal heart rate on a monitor is easier than listening by a stethoscope or fetoscope. In addition, most health care providers have grown accustomed to monitors and may feel uncomfortable without them. Few people advocate the return to using stethoscopes for assessment; using monitors for periodic assessment rather than continuous monitoring is a compromise solution.

Parents should know that monitors can provide a valuable early warning of possible fetal distress, but they should also be aware that FHR does vary a great deal during labor, and a normal pattern includes variations. Parents can become so focused on what is happening on the monitor that they lose the ability to concentrate on previously learned relaxation techniques. The monitor is an aid only and should not be the focus of their attention.

External Electronic Monitoring

External electronic monitoring can be used to monitor both uterine contractions and fetal heart rates on a continuous or intermittent basis. The information is obtained from sensors strapped to the woman's abdomen (Figure 18-27).

Contractions are monitored by means of a pressure transducer or tocodynamometer (*toko* is Greek for contraction). The transducer is placed against the abdomen over the uterine fundus and held in place by an adjustable strap (Figure 18-28*A*). The transducer then converts the pressure registered into an electronic signal that is recorded on graph paper. The transducer must be placed over the uterine fundus to register the area of greatest contractility.

The fetal heart rate is monitored through an ultrasonic sensor or monitor (Figure 18-28*A*) also strapped against the woman's abdomen with an adhesive (Velcro) closure. The small Doppler unit converts fetal heart movements into audible beeping sounds and also prints out a permanent graph paper recording.

External monitoring has the advantage of being noninvasive and easily applied, although it can be con-

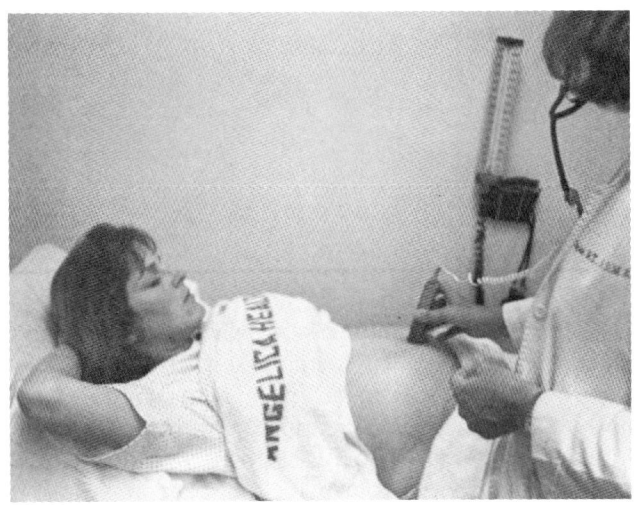

FIGURE 18-26
A Doppler ultrasound device can be used to monitor fetal heart rate intermittently in low-risk labor. (From Reeder, S.J., Martin, L.L., & Koniak, D. [1992]. Maternity nursing: Family, newborn, and women's health care [17th ed.]. Philadelphia: J.B. Lippincott.)

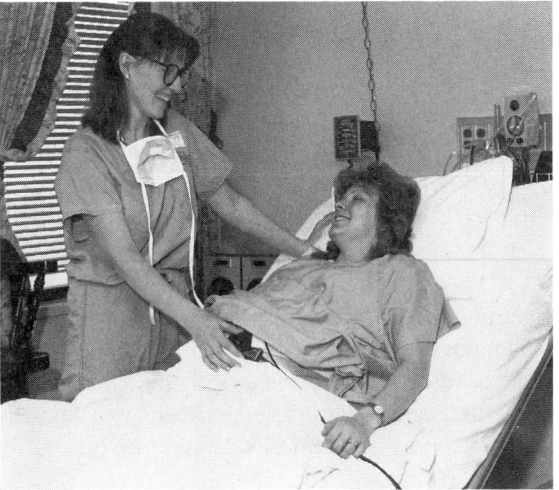

FIGURE 18-27
External electronic monitoring in place. Two devices (a transducer for the uterus and an ultrasound sensor for the fetus) are strapped to the woman's abdomen. (Courtesy of the Department of Medical Photography, Children's Hospital, Buffalo, NY.)

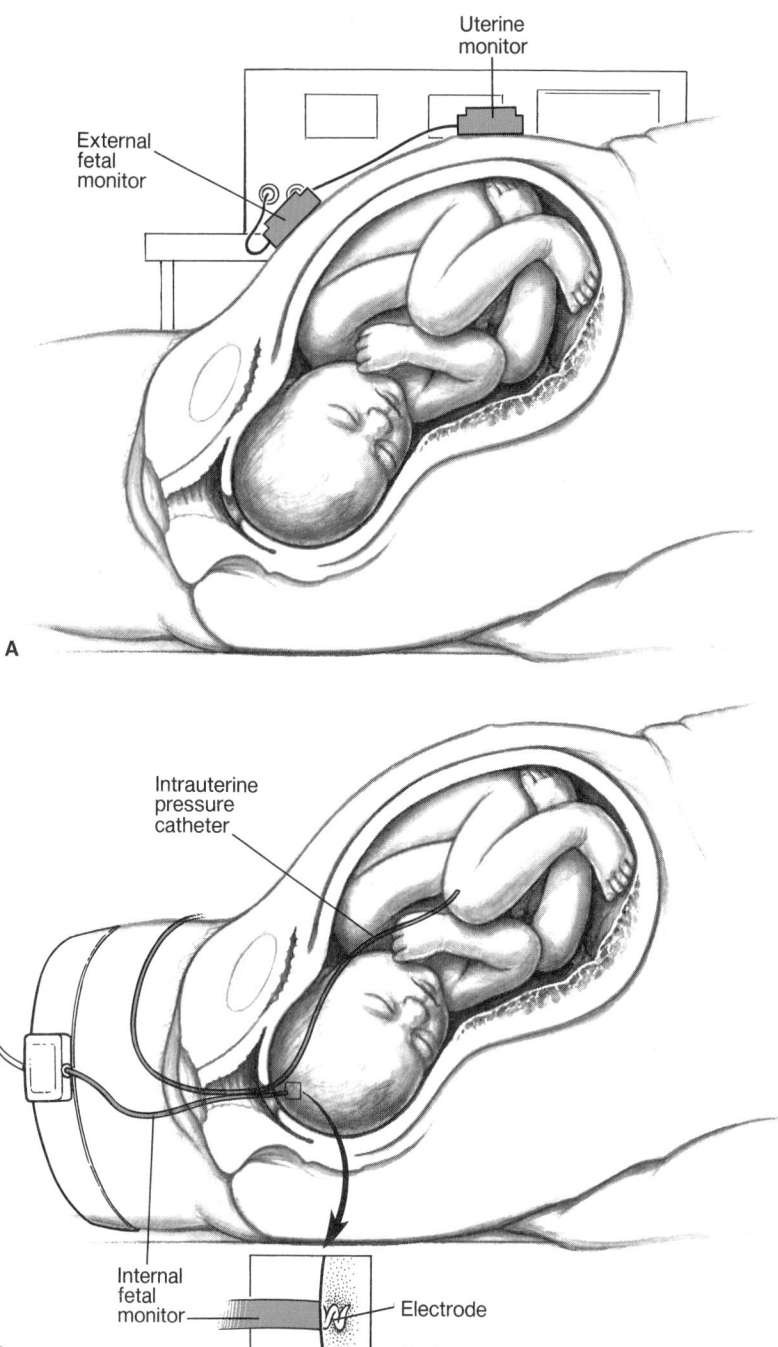

FIGURE 18-28
Placement of electronic monitoring leads.
(A) External leads to monitor for FHR and uterine
contractions. (B) An internal fetal heart rate lead
in place on the fetal scalp. Uterine contractions
are monitored by the intrauterine catheter.

fining and limit the woman's movement. It is not as reliable as internal monitoring in that a change in maternal or fetal position may interfere with the quality of the tracing, but it can be introduced early in labor because it does not depend on cervical dilatation or on the fetus being well descended.

When an external monitoring device is used, it is important to assure both parents that monitoring is a routine procedure and that it provides more accurate information about progress in labor than manual palpation. The woman who is worried that something will

happen to her child during labor will find it reassuring to listen to the regular beeping sound of the undistressed fetal heart from an accompanying fetal heart transducer. Many women ask for a graph tracing to save for their child's baby book.

Occasionally, a woman feels discomfort from the strap holding an external monitoring unit in place, or the snugness of the sensor head limits her ability to breathe deeply. Spreading talcum powder on the abdomen may make the strap more comfortable. Taking off the sensor periodically and allowing for a position change is helpful. If the woman changes her position herself (and she will change position often during labor), repositioning the sensor will be necessary. Remind her that the accompanying fetal heart signal may stop when this happens so that she will not think her baby's heart has stopped when her change of position shifts the beam of the sensor.

Women do not need to lie on their back for monitoring, so it does not increase the likelihood of supine hypotension syndrome. With a monitor attached, be careful not to fall into the habit of nursing the equipment and not the woman or communicating with the monitor and not with the woman and her support person. Monitoring equipment frees nurses from the task of listening to FHRs or timing contractions every 15 to 30 minutes so they can spend more time giving emotional support in labor.

Internal Electronic Monitoring

Internal electronic monitoring is the most precise method for assessing fetal heart rates and uterine contractions. For it to be used, the membranes must have ruptured and the cervix dilated to at least 3 cm. Contractions are monitored via a pressure-sensing catheter that is passed through the vagina, alongside the fetus, into the uterine cavity (Figure 18-28B). The cathether extending from the vagina is attached to a pressure recorder. As each contraction puts pressure on the uterine contents, the pressure exerted on the catheter is recorded. A correlation can then be made between the FHR and uterine pressure from contractions.

The FHR recording is obtained from a fetal scalp electrode. When the fetal head is engaged, the electrode is inserted vaginally and attached to the fetal scalp. A fetal electrocardiograph signal is obtained and amplified and then fed into a cardiotachometer. The output from the cardiotachometer is recorded on permanent graph paper.

When uterine contractions are monitored by an internal pressure gauge, the frequency, duration, baseline strength, and peak strength of contractions can all be

evaluated (Figure 18-29). Strength of contractions is evaluated by the size of the peak of the contraction on the tracing. Equally important to evaluate is the return of the uterine tone to baseline strength between contractions. This ensures placental filling between contractions.

With latent contractions, the baseline level is under 5 mm Hg; with active contractions, it is approximately 12 mm Hg. During the second stage of labor, the baseline may be as high as 20 mm Hg. If baseline readings do not return to 20 mm Hg or below, uterine hypertonia and a compromise of fetal well being are indicated.

This level of feedback cannot be matched by external monitoring, which records only the frequency and duration of contractions. The detail on fetal heartbeats is also clearer with internal monitoring (described in the next section). On the other hand, internal monitoring is intrusive and carries the risk of uterine infection. Thus it is not used as routinely as external monitoring but is reserved for women who are categorized as high risk during labor.

Telemetry

Telemetry allows monitoring of both FHR and uterine contractions to be carried out free of connecting wires that could hamper a woman's movements in labor. For this method, an internal pressure uterine lead is inserted and a fetal scalp electrode is attached; a miniature radio transmitter is placed in the vagina to broadcast the FHR and uterine contraction signals to a distant monitor. The major advantage of telemetry is that it allows the woman to ambulate while being internally monitored. Because it is more expensive than other equipment, not all birth settings use telemetry.

Fetal Heart Rate Patterns

Assessing and interpreting FHR patterns involves evaluating three parameters: the baseline rate, variabilities in the baseline rate (long-term and short-term), and periodic changes in the rate (acceleration and deceleration).

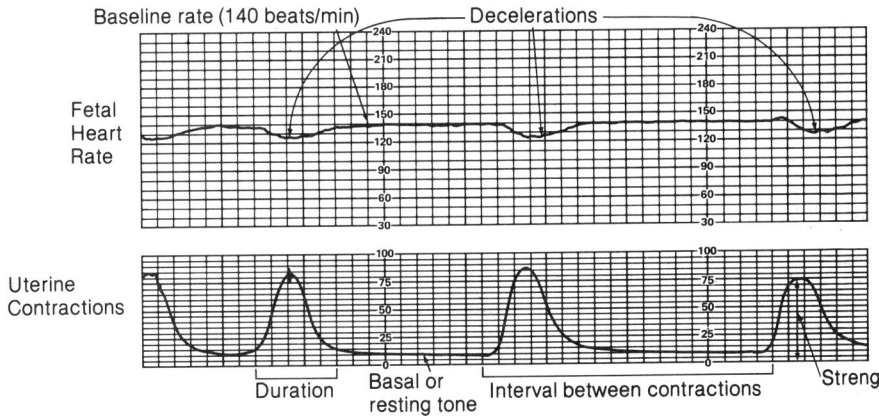

FIGURE 18-29
Common terms used to evaluate monitoring strips.

Baseline FHR

A baseline FHR is determined by analyzing a range of fetal heartbeats recorded on a 10-minute tracing that is obtained between contractions. A normal rate is considered to be between 120 to 160 beats per minute. The rate fluctuates slightly (5 to 15 beats per minute) when the fetus moves or sleeps. If an increase or decrease occurs and is sustained for a 10-minute period, then a new baseline or a baseline change is established. Abnormal patterns in the baseline rate include fetal bradycardia and fetal tachycardia.

Fetal bradycardia occurs when the FHR is below 120 beats per minute for 10 minutes. A moderate bradycardia of 100 to 119 is not considered serious and is probably due to a vagal response elicited by the fetal head being compressed during labor. Marked bradycardia (under 100 beats) is a sign of hypoxia and is considered dangerous.

Fetal tachycardia occurs when the rate is 160 beats per minute (for a 10-minute period). A moderate tachycardia of 161 to 180 beats per minute is a sign of hypoxia. Marked tachycardia is registered at a heart rate of more than 180 beats per minute. A fetus in distress has an increased heart rate of this nature before the heart rate begins to fall. Marked fetal tachycardia may be due to fetal hypoxia, maternal fever, drugs, fetal arrhythmia, or maternal anemia or hyperthyroidism.

Variability

Baseline variability is variation in the heart rate over time and is reflected on the FHR tracing as a slight irregularity or "jitter" to the wave. Baseline variability increases when the fetus is stimulated and slows when the fetus sleeps. If no variability is present, it indicates that the natural pacemaker activity of the fetal heart (effects of sympathetic and parasympathetic nervous system) has been affected. The cause may be a response to narcotics or barbiturates administered to the woman in labor, but the possibility of fetal hypoxia and acidosis must be in-

vestigated. Very immature fetuses will show diminished baseline variability because of a reduced nervous system response to stimulation and immature cardiac node function.

Baseline variability is defined as being long-term or short-term (beat-to-beat) (Figure 18-30). Long-term variability (LTV) is seen on a broad view of the recording and results from fluctuations in FHR of 6 to 10 beats occurring 3 to 10 times per minute. Short-term variability (STV) or beat-to-beat variability refers to the difference between successive heartbeats, usually about 2 to 3 beats per minute. These changes are very subtle and can be picked up only with internal electronic monitoring. Beat-to-beat variability can be rated as "present," "decreased," or "absent." Decreasing variability indicates the development of fetal distress. Absent variability is considered a severe sign, indicating serious fetal compromise.

FHR variability is considered to be one of the most reliable indicators of fetal well-being.

Periodic Changes

Periodic changes in FHR occur in response to contractions and fetal movement and are described in terms of *accelerations* or *decelerations*. Four such responses include acceleration, early deceleration, late deceleration and variable deceleration.

Accelerations. Accelerations are temporary normal increases in FHR due to fetal movement or compression of the umbilical vein during contraction.

Early Decelerations. Early decelerations are periodic decreases in FHR resulting from pressure on the fetal head during contraction. Parasympathetic stimulation in response to vagal nerve compression brings about a slowing of FHR. Early deceleration follows the pattern of the contraction, beginning when the contraction begins

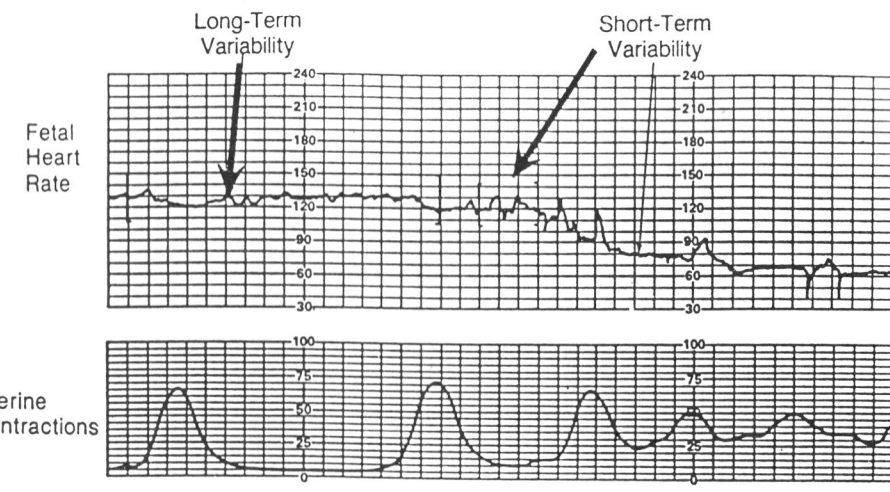

FIGURE 18-30
Fetal monitoring strip showing both long-term and short-term (beat-to-beat) variability. (From Paul, R.H. [1971]. Fetal intensive care. Los Angeles: LAC/USC Medical Center, with permission.)

and ending when the contraction ends. However, the waveform of the FHR change is inverse to the contraction waveform, with the lowest point of the deceleration occurring with the peak of the contraction. The rate rarely falls below 100 beats per minute and returns quickly to between 120 and 160 beats at the end of the contraction.

Early decelerations normally occur late in labor when the head has descended fairly low. As such, they are viewed as a normal pattern. However, if they occur early in labor before the head has fully descended, the head compression causing the waveform change could be the result of cephalopelvic disproportion and is a cause of concern.

Late Decelerations. Late decelerations are those that are delayed until 30 to 40 seconds after the onset of the contraction and continue beyond the end of the contraction (Figure 18-31). This is an ominous pattern in labor because it suggests uteroplacental insufficiency or decreased blood flow through the intervillous spaces of the uterus during uterine contractions. The lowest point of the deceleration (nadir) occurs near the end of the contraction instead of at the peak. This pattern may occur with marked hypotonia or with abnormal uterine tonus caused by the administration of oxytocin. Immediate steps to correct the situation must be initiated. If oxytocin is being used, it should be stopped or the rate of administration slowed. Change the woman's position from supine to lateral (to relieve pressure on the aorta and vena cava and to supply more blood to the uterus). Administer intravenous fluids or oxygen to the woman as prescribed. Prepare for possible prompt delivery of the infant if the occurrence of late decelerations persists and if FHR variability becomes abnormal (absent or decreased).

Variable Decelerations. The variable pattern of deceleration occurs at unpredictable times during contractions and indicates compression of the cord, which is an ominous development in terms of fetal well being (Figure 18-32). However, because the pattern is variable, it can be completely missed if monitoring is not continuous. If this pattern is recognized on the monitor, changing the woman's position from supine to lateral or to a Trendelenburg position is recommended to relieve pressure on the cord. Administering oxygen to the woman may also be helpful. If these measures do not correct the fetal heart pattern, a cesarean birth may have to be performed to save the fetus's life. If accompanying oligohydramnios (a deficiency in aminiotic fluid) is present, uterine amnioinfusion may be attempted to reduce cord pressure.

Amnioinfusion

Variable decelerations present on an FHR monitor suggest cord compression. This may occur because of a prolapsed cord but also may occur because the fetus is lying on the cord; it tends to occur more frequently following rupture of the membranes than when they are intact, or with oligohydramnios (less than a normal amount of amniotic fluid) such as occurs in postterm pregnancy or with intrauterine growth retardation.

If variable decelerations are not relieved by a change in position or hydration and oxygen administration to the mother, enlarging the amount of amniotic fluid present by administration of normal saline intravaginally may be effective (amnioinfusion) (Snell, 1993).

For this, a sterile catheter is introduced through the cervix into the uterus following rupture of the membranes (Figure 18-33). This is attached to intravenous tubing and a solution of warmed normal saline. The solution rate is regulated to allow a large amount (ap-

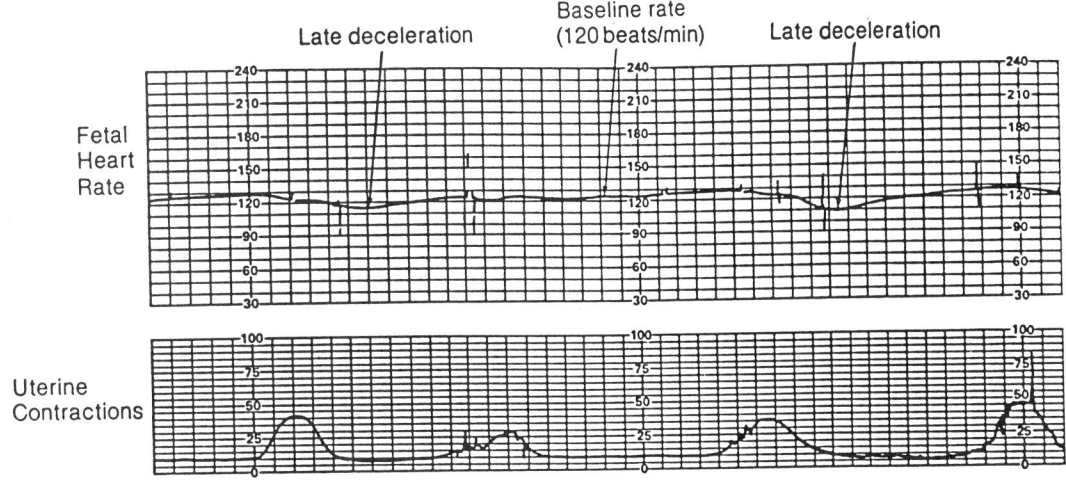

FIGURE 18-31
Late decelerations. Note that the fetal decelerations (arrows) *occur after the uterine contractions. (From Paul, R.H. [1971].* Fetal intensive care. *Los Angeles: LAC/USC Medical Center, with permission.)*

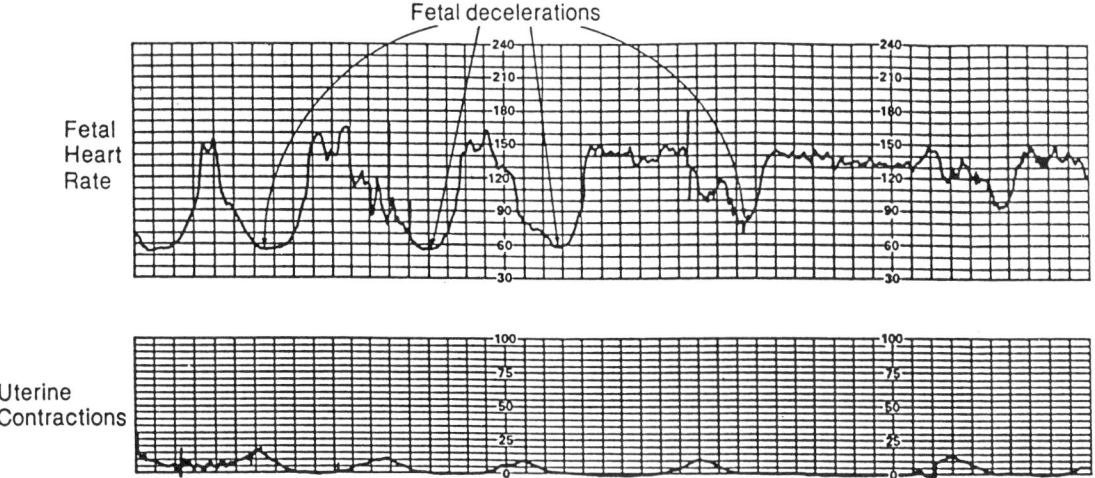

Fetal decelerations

Fetal
Heart
Rate

Uterine
Contractions

FIGURE 18-32

Variable decelerations. Notice that the fetal decelerations (arrows) *occur at unpredictable times in relation to contractions. (From Paul, R.H. [1971]. Fetal intensive care. Los Angeles: LAC/USC Medical Center, with permission.)*

proximately 500 mL) to infuse rapidly. The rate is then adjusted to the least amount necessary to maintain a monitor pattern without variable decelerations.

Strict aseptic precautions must be adhered to while the catheter is inserted. Both the fetal heart rate and uterine contractions should be continuously monitored by internal monitors during the infusion. Maternal temperature should be recorded hourly to detect infection. It is important that the infusing solution is warmed to body temperature before the infusion to prevent chilling of the mother and fetus. This can be done by placing the bag of fluid on a radiant heat warmer before administration.

The mother will have a continuous flow of the infusing solution out of the vagina during the procedure, so her bed must be changed frequently to prevent it

from becoming uncomfortable. This is also a time to assess that constant drainage is occurring. If vaginal leakage should stop, it usually means the fetal head is firmly engaged and all fluid being infused is being held in the uterus. This is dangerous as it will lead to hydramnios (excessive amniotic fluid) and possibly uterine rupture.

Sinusoidal FHR Pattern

In a fetus that is severely anemic or hypoxic, central nervous system control of heart pacing may be so impaired that the FHR pattern resembles a frequently undulating wave. Long-term variability consists of 5 to 15 beats per minute every 3 to 5 minutes, beat-to-beat variability is minimal or absent, and there is a lack of specific responses to contraction. Although the cause of this

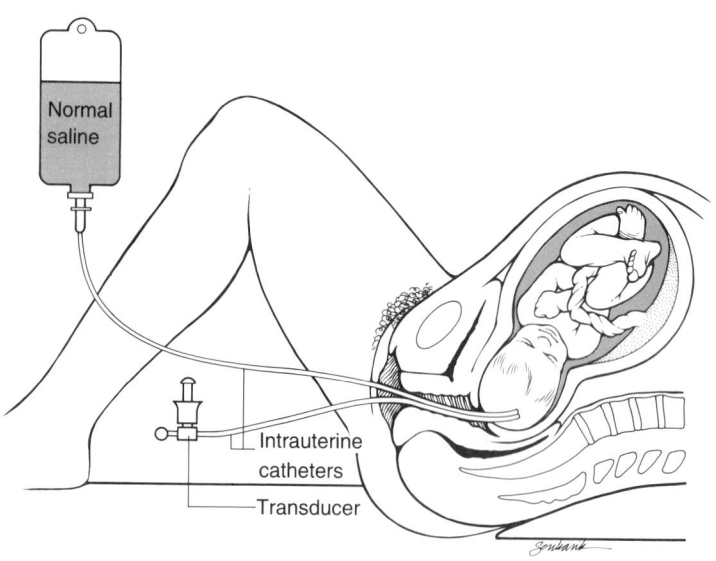

FIGURE 18-33

Amnioinfusion. Increasing the amount of fluid decreases the pressure on the cord.

pattern is poorly understood, it is recognized to be as ominous as a late deceleration or variable deceleration pattern.

Other Assessment Techniques

Fetal Blood Sampling

By monitoring fetal blood composition, hypoxia in the fetus may be determined before it is apparent on an ECG or an external monitoring system. This is because changes in blood composition lead to alterations in FHR. It is unnecessary and impractical to monitor all fetuses by blood sampling during labor. The procedure is therefore reserved for high-risk fetuses.

The oxygen saturation, PO_2, PCO_2, pH, bicarbonate excess, and hematocrit of fetal blood may all be determined during labor if a sample of capillary blood is taken from the fetal scalp as it presents at the dilated cervix. After cervical dilatation of 3 cm to 4 cm and rupture of the membranes, the fetal head is visualized by the use of an *amnioscope,* a small, cone-shaped instrument with a light source at the far end. The scalp is cleaned with povidone-iodine and sprayed with silicon. A small scalpel is introduced vaginally into the cervix and the fetal scalp is nicked. The silicon causes blood to form in beads, which are then caught by a capillary tube. The incision is then compressed until the bleeding has fully stopped. Following the procedure, the mother must be observed after two contractions to be certain that no new scalp bleeding occurs.

Although a blood sample obtained this way may be analyzed for many parameters, usually only the pH results are necessary. If a fetus is hypoxic, the pH will fall (become acidotic). A scalp blood pH below 7.25 is recognized as a level of fetal distress. This technique may be used to verify a heart rate pattern on a monitor that is becoming ominous. It can also be used to verify that no acidosis is occurring, even when a monitor rate is showing decreased variability. Fetal scalp sampling is becoming less popular because it has been found that firm pressure against the fetal head by a finger inserted vaginally will increase monitor strip variability. If the variability increase occurs by this method blood sampling will no longer be necessary.

Fetal blood sampling involves no pain for the mother but may involve an uncomfortable sensation of pressure similar to an examining hand in the vagina. Infants who have had internal scalp blood samples taken should not be delivered by vacuum extraction because this can lead to renewed bleeding at the puncture site. Pulse oximetry that continuously measures oxygen and tissue perfusion in the fetus will be available in the near future (Dildy et al., 1993).

Scalp Stimulation

If fetal heart tone variability is depressed, the welfare of the fetus can be further assessed by scalp stimulation. This is done by applying pressure with fingers to the fetal scalp through the dilated cervix (Figure 18-34). This causes a tactile response in the fetus that will momentarily increase FHR. If the fetus is in distress and becoming acidotic, however, FHR acceleration will not occur. Scalp stimulation, therefore, is an assessment of acid-base balance in the fetus.

Acoustic Stimulation

Acoustic stimulation, or instrumentally producing a sharp sound, is used with nonstress tests during pregnancy to produce FHR acceleration. It can also be used during labor to demonstrate that the fetus is reactive.

Care of the Woman During the First Stage of Labor

Nursing Diagnoses and Related Interventions

Care during the first stage of labor centers on helping the woman feel confident in her ability to control the pain and progress of labor and maintain physiologic stability. At first, it is exciting for the woman to feel labor contractions. They are little more than menstrual cramps and project a "this-is-really-happening" quality. Soon, however, if a woman is not concentrating on controlled breathing exercises, contractions become biting in their intensity. Despite the fact that she is becoming more and more uncomfortable, however, nothing seems to be

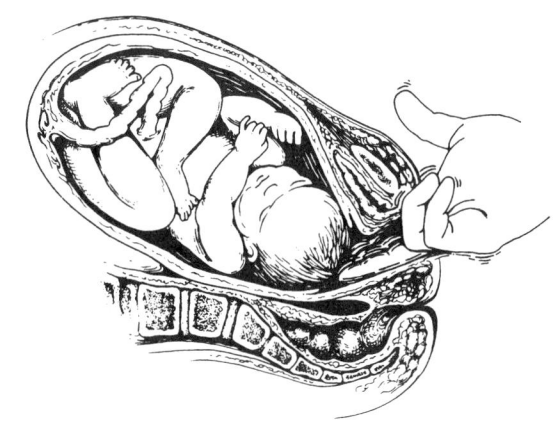

FIGURE 18-34
Technique for scalp stimulation. (Redrawn from Journal of Perinatal and Neonatal Nursing, 1*, 16, with permission from Aspen Publishers, Inc.)*

happening. A couple can begin to worry that something is going wrong and may think that because the 9 months are over victory is near, yet it is eluding them. Couples need to be given progress reports in labor so they do not become discouraged or fearful at this seeming lack of progress.

Powerlessness

> **Nursing Diagnosis:** Powerlessness related to duration of labor.
>
> **Goal:** Client will demonstrate that she feels some control over the labor process after 30 minutes.
>
> **Outcome Criteria:** Client expresses preferences for position and techniques to control pain; asks questions about her progress and states feelings about what is happening.

A woman wants to feel that she has some control over her situation during labor. Most women accomplish this by stating their preferences, breathing with contractions, and changing their position to the one that makes them feel most comfortable. Some women handle the stress of labor by becoming extremely quiet. Others feel most comfortable when they can show their emotions by shouting or cursing. As a rule, then, to help women express their feelings, anything short of hysterical screaming or thrashing is "good" behavior in labor.

Respect Contraction Time. It is important not to interrupt women in the middle of breathing exercises during labor. Once their concentration is disrupted, they feel the bite of the contraction; if they have been successfully using breathing exercises to reduce pain, suddenly feeling the full force of a contraction is frightening. The woman tenses, the pain becomes worse, and she may doubt her ability to breathe constructively in the face of such sharp pain with the next contraction. Allow the woman to finish breathing with her contraction, then ask questions or announce what procedure needs to be done next, or ask the question but wait patiently for the answer. (See Chapter 19 for a discussion of pain management techniques.)

Promote Change of Positions. In early labor, a woman may be out of bed walking or sitting up in bed or in a chair, kneeling, squatting, or in whatever position she prefers. Because a bed is the main piece of furniture in a birthing room, most women assume that they are expected to lie in bed and so must be assured otherwise. A woman whose membranes have ruptured should lie on her side until a fetal monitor shows good baseline variability and no variable decelerations or she has been checked by a physician or nurse-midwife; unless the head of the fetus is well engaged (firmly fitting

into the pelvic inlet), an umbilical cord may prolapse into the vagina if she walks.

Following the administration of medication such as a narcotic, a woman should remain in bed for approximately 20 minutes to avoid a fall if she should become dizzy. As labor becomes advanced, remaining in bed or squatting is her best position so that if birth is precipitous, the infant will not be born while she is walking upright, and suffer an injury. A squatting position is effective in that it helps to align the fetal presenting part with the cervix and also uses the fetal weight to help effect cervical dilation. Remaining in an upright position during labor may also shorten the length of labor.

While women are in bed, they should be encouraged to lie on their side. This position causes the heavy uterus to tip forward away from the vena cava, allowing free blood return from the lower extremities and adequate placental filling and circulation.

Most women are comfortable in this position and adjust to it readily. Check that the chair for the woman's support person is on the side of the bed she faces; otherwise, she will keep turning to her back to talk.

Some women have learned to do breathing exercises in a supine position and may need additional coaching to do them in a side-lying position. If a woman must turn to her back during a contraction to make her breathing exercises effective, help her to remember to return to her side between contractions.

Promote Voiding and Provide Bladder Care. A full bladder or bowel can impede fetal descent. The relationship of a full bladder to descent of the fetus is shown in Figure 18-35. A woman in labor should therefore be encouraged to void spontaneously if possible, but at least every 2 to 4 hours. She may need to be reminded to do this because she may misinterpret the discomfort of a full bladder as part of the sensations of labor. A full bladder can best be discerned by percussion of the bladder area (an empty bladder sounds dull, a full one will sound resonant). If she cannot void and the bladder is distended, she may need to be catheterized. Catheterizing a woman in labor is uncomfortable for her and difficult for the nurse: the vulva is edematous from the pressure of the fetal presenting part, making the urethra difficult to locate and the urethral canal stretched downward. Use a small catheter (No. 12–14F) and insert the catheter between contractions. Use extremely careful aseptic technique to avoid introducing any microorganisms that might result in a urinary tract infection.

Hyperventilation

> **Nursing Diagnosis:** High risk for ineffective breathing pattern (hyperventilation) related to breathing exercises.

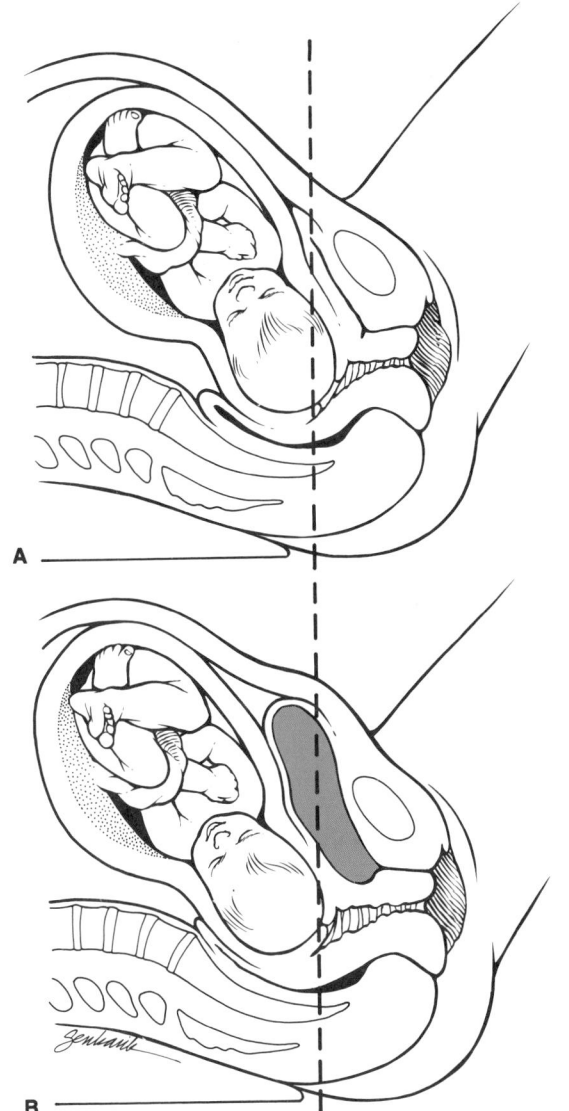

FIGURE 18-35
*Effect of a full bladder versus an empty bladder on ease of fetal descent: (**A**) empty bladder; (**B**) full bladder blocks descent.*

Goal: Client will not experience hyperventilation when using breathing techniques during labor.

Outcome Criteria: Client reports no feelings of lightheadedness or tingling/numbness in extremities.

Hyperventilation is a state of respiratory alkalosis that occurs when a woman exhales more deeply than she inhales ("blows off") extra carbon dioxide. This can occur when a woman is practicing breathing exercises in preparation for labor but is more apt to occur during actual labor. She feels lightheaded and may have tingling or numbness in her toes and fingertips. If allowed to progress to its ultimate end, it can lead to coma.

To halt hyperventilation, teach a woman to keep a paper bag nearby when doing breathing exercises. She can ward off symptoms of hyperventilation by breathing in and out into the paper bag. This causes her to re-breathe the carbon dioxide she exhales and so replace the carbon dioxide lost. If a paper bag is unavailable she can use her cupped hands instead.

The best way to handle hyperventilation is to prevent it from occurring. Be certain that when women are breathing rapidly they are not hyperventilating, and that they end all breathing sessions with a long cleansing breath to help to restore carbon dioxide balance.

Anxiety

> ***Nursing Diagnosis:*** Anxiety related to stress of labor.
>
> ***Goal:*** Client will manage the stress of situation with positive coping mechanisms.
>
> ***Outcome Criteria:*** Client states that she feels somewhat in control of her situation; she and her support person express confidence in themselves and health care personnel.

Labor is such an intense process that it creates a high level of emotional stress for both the woman and her support person. Ability to tolerate stress (to cope adequately) depends on a person's perception of the event, support people available, and past experience in using coping mechanisms. Ways to reduce stress in labor, therefore, center around helping a woman to perceive labor clearly and providing the opportunity for her partner to provide support as well as being personally available to provide support to the woman and her partner throughout the labor process (see the Focus on Nursing Research box).

Offer Support. There is no substitute for personal touch and contact as a way to provide support during labor. Patting a woman's arm while telling her that she is progressing in labor, brushing a wisp of hair off her forehead, wiping her forehead with a cool cloth—these are indispensable methods of conveying concern. This caring attitude has several benefits. First, it may make the difference in helping the woman feel safe and able to continue in control. In addition, a woman who is touched, who experiences the warmth and friendliness of human contact during labor—a time when she is physically dependent—may handle her newborn (who is also physically dependent and undergoing an adjustment not unlike the one she has just gone through) more warmly and affectionately. On the other hand, be aware that not all women care for physical contact during labor (see the Focus on Cultural Awareness box).

Respect and Promote the Support Person's Activities. The expectant husband or father or someone else

FOCUS ON NURSING RESEARCH

What Role Do Fathers See Themselves Fulfilling During Labor and Birth?

To answer this question, 20 couples who gave birth to healthy infants were asked 4 weeks after the birth to identify the role the man fulfilled during labor. Men were aged 25 to 41 years of age with a mean of 33 years.

The three roles men saw themselves as fulfilling most were witness, coach, or teammate. "Witness" was the most common role identified (12 of 20 men). When in a witness role, men viewed themselves as mainly companions with emotional and moral support as their task. They were often observed watching TV, reading a book, sleeping, or leaving the room for long periods. When the father saw himself as a coach, his partner viewed him as critical to her ability to maintain control during labor. When men saw themselves as a teammate, they viewed themselves as assisting their partners throughout the experience by responding to requests for physical or emotional support.

The researcher stresses that it is important for men to adopt a labor role that is a natural part of the couple's pattern of interactions, not necessarily a role that seems ideal to health care providers.

Chapman, L. L. (1992). Expectant fathers' roles during labor and birth. *Journal of Obstetric, Gynecologic and Neonatal Nursing, 21,* 114.

that the woman chooses (such as a sister, mother, or friend) should be admitted to the birthing room with the woman and allowed to remain with her throughout birth. Having someone with her is important to a woman in early labor. Everything is new and she may not be used to the sensation of contractions, so this may be when she will most need a support person. Acquaint the woman and the support person with the unit and point out where supplies such as towels, washcloths, and ice chips (if allowed) are stored so that the support person can get them when necessary. Review procedures for the birthing room so that the support person can be assured early in labor that he or she is welcome there.

Often the support person will be acting as a labor coach. Ask both the woman and the support person if they have been to prepared childbirth classes and whether the support person plans to help the woman with her breathing. Support this person's role. When he or she is hesitant, it is better to review techniques than to take over. Offer praise not only for the woman but for the support person. Relieve the person as necessary so he or she can get something to eat or visit with older children.

Support Woman's Pain Management Efforts. Some women believe that using a prepared childbirth method

will bring them a totally painless labor. When they realize that this is untrue, they can panic and lose the ability to use prepared breathing. Some support people are more nervous than they anticipated and have difficulty being supportive, leaving a woman to manage her anxiety on her own. In these instances, administering an analgesic might be effective in reducing anxiety or taking the edge off of contractions. With this degree of relaxation, the woman is then able to return to effective breathing techniques. Sometimes simply the support of a person such as a nurse, who is confident that breathing can be effective in reducing the discomfort of labor, is all the woman needs to resume her breathing exercises with success.

Fluid Intake

Nursing Diagnosis: High risk for fluid volume deficit related to lack of oral intake and duration of labor.

Goal: Client will not experience fluid volume deficit during labor.

Outcome Criteria: Client voices that she does not feel thirsty; voids every 2 to 4 hours.

How much fluid or food a woman should ingest during labor is controversial. Most hospitals limit the amount of oral fluid or food intake during labor to ice chips or lollipops to prevent aspiration if, in an emer-

FOCUS ON CULTURAL AWARENESS

The person a woman chooses to accompany her during childbirth can be a husband, the father of the child, a sister or parent, or a close friend. Which of these persons a woman chooses is somewhat culturally determined. A Mexican-American woman, for example, might choose a female family member to accompany her instead of her male partner.

It is important for women to be able to understand what is happening to them during labor. If English is not the woman's primary language, arrangements should be made to locate an interpreter. If the woman is hearing impaired, it is the hospital's responsibility to provide an interpreter for her so she can receive adequate explanations of her progress. Remember that whether women enjoy being touched or not during labor is in part culturally determined. Assess early in a woman's labor whether or not she might benefit from such caring measures as having her hand held or her back rubbed.

gency, anesthesia administration should be necessary. Because of this, a woman may have a dry mouth and lips from mouth breathing during labor. Applying a cream to her lips or allowing her to suck on hard candy or ice chips is generally enough to relieve this discomfort. Women in prolonged labor may need additional fluid and caloric intake to prevent secondary uterine inertia (a cessation of labor contractions) as well as generalized dehydration and exhaustion. If all oral fluids are contraindicated by the birth plan, intravenous glucose solutions may be administered to maintain caloric reserve. See the Nursing Care Plan: A Woman in Labor.

Amniotomy

Amniotomy is the artificial rupturing of membranes (Milhan, 1992). Rupturing these if they do not rupture spontaneously allows the fetal head to contact the cervix more directly and may increase the efficiency of contractions. For this, the woman is placed in a dorsal recumbent position; an amniohook (a long thin instrument) or a hemostat is passed vaginally. The membranes are torn and amniotic fluid is allowed to escape. This is a potentially hazardous moment for the fetus as there is a possibility that a loop of cord will escape with the fluid (Strong & Phelan, 1991). Always take FHR immediately following the rupture of membranes to determine that this did not happen.

Care of the Woman During the Second Stage of Labor

Even women who have taken preparation-for-labor classes are surprised at the intensity of the contractions in this phase of labor. Because the feeling of pushing is so strong, many women react by tensing their abdominal muscles and trying to resist, which makes the sensation painful and even more frightening. Some women react to this change of contractions by growing increasingly argumentative and angry, or by crying and screaming.

The next hour will consist of sensations for the woman that are difficult to appreciate unless they are experienced. All the preparations done up to this point may still not be enough to sustain a woman unless she has a support person with her. It will be important later that this person shared this moment with her; in years to come the couple will talk of it often. Birth is such a new phenomenon for most people, however, that most of a support person's effectiveness may be lost.

Women need to have an experienced health care person with them as they enter this stage of labor to reassure them that the change in contractions is normal, and that as soon as they get used to the sensation of pushing, labor from this point on can be exhilarating. Family support people may be inadequate at this point. The woman momentarily wants someone with her to give more knowledgeable support that everything is all right than a family member may be qualified to give.

Fetal heart sounds should be counted at the beginning of the second stage of labor to be certain that the start of the baby's passage in the birth canal is not occluding the cord and interfering with fetal circulation. A timetable for second-stage interventions is shown in Table 18-8.

Preparing the Place of Birth

Birthing Room. A birthing room is converted to a birth room by the addition of sterile packs of supplies on waiting tables; the partition at the end of the room is opened to reveal the "baby island," or newborn care area. The infant equipment available should include a radiant heat warmer, equipment for suction and resusci-

Table 18-8. *Time Intervals for Nursing Interventions During Second Stage of Labor*

Intervention	Beginning of Second Stage	Continued Frequency	After Birth of Infant	After Delivery of Placenta
Assess and Record				
Temperature	X	q2h		X
Pulse	X	q1h	X	X
Respirations	X	q1h	X	X
Blood pressure	Following anesthetic administration	q1h	X	X
FHR	X	Continuously by monitor or q5min		
Contractions	X	Continuously by monitor or q5min		
Provide				
Support	X	Continuously	Continuously	Continuously

Bergin Colton is a 29-year-old woman (gravida 3; para 1; premature 0; abortion 1; stillborn 0; living children 0) you care for in labor. A previous child died shortly after birth from congenital heart disease. An admission care plan you might establish with her might be as follows:

Assessment: Breathing regularly with contractions; likes to turn to supine position to do breathing. Temperature, 99.2°F (37.3°C); pulse, 74; respirations, 20; blood pressure, 110/78. Contractions, 60 sec duration, 2 min frequency, moderate intensity. Labor began 4 h ago. Effacement, 70%; dilatation, 2 cm; station, −1; vertex presentation; position, LOA; FHR baseline, 130. Moderate amount pink-tinged show; membranes ruptured spontaneously just before coming to hospital. Client reported fluid was clear; no blood or meconium staining. Client states, "I didn't remember labor hurting this much." Using slow chest breathing exercises learned in Lamaze class; has husband with her as support person. Baby planned; has clothing, etc. ready for baby. Wants a girl but boy would be "okay." Wants to deliver in delivery, not birthing room, "in case the baby isn't all right." Husband not sure he wants to see birth; says "we'll see when time comes." Did not see previous birth by own choice. Client appears relaxed although bites lip when not actively engaged in conversation.

Nursing Diagnosis: High risk for infection related to early rupture of membranes.

Defining Characteristics: Client states that membranes ruptured 1 h ago.

Goal: Client will not demonstrate signs of infection during labor, birth, or postpartal period.

Outcome Criteria: Client's temperature is below 38.0°C orally.

Nursing Orders	Rationale
1. Notify private physician and house officer of client admission.	1. Ensures continuity of care.
2. Keep client nonambulatory until checked by physician.	2. Cord prolapse may occur if head of fetus is not engaged.
3. Take temperature orally every 2 h during labor. Report temperature of more than 38.0°C.	3. Infection may occur with ruptured membranes.
4. Change bed pad frequently.	4. Provides comfort and helps reduce the possibility of infection.
5. Use strict sterile technique for pelvic exam.	5. Helps reduce the possibility of infection.

(continued)

tation, and supplies for eye care and identification of the newborn. The radiant heat warmer should be turned on well enough in advance so the bottom mattress is pleasantly warm to the touch at the time of birth. If sterile towels and a blanket are placed on the warmer these will also be warm to use to dry and cover the infant.

Drapes and materials used for birth are sterile so no microorganisms are accidentally introduced into the uterus. A table with equipment is set up far enough in advance that preparation does not need to be hurried.

Covered, a table set this way can be left up to 8 hours. Equipment usually provided on an instrument table is listed in Box 18-2. In addition, a sterile gown, gloves, and a sterile towel to dry the hands should be provided for the person who will deliver the infant.

Delivery Room. If a woman is high risk for any reason, a physician may choose to use a delivery room rather than allow the woman to remain in the birthing room. A delivery room table puts the mother in a

Nursing Diagnosis: Fear related to previous poor outcome of pregnancy.

Defining Characteristic: Client states that she is concerned this baby might have congenital heart disease.

Goal: Client will complete her labor within bounds of psychologic well being.

Outcome Criteria: Couple completes labor as a family unit. Couple demonstrates adequate coping behavior during labor.

Nursing Orders	***Rationale***
1. Provide adequate psychologic support; show sonogram report that revealed no obvious heart or valve disorder.	1. Mother needs reassurance and objective evidence (as much as possible) that baby does not have congenital heart disease.
2. Reassure frequently that labor is going well and fetus is doing well (as appropriate).	2. Provides continuous reassurance to relieve anxiety about labor.
3. Assess parent–child relationship in postpartal period.	3. Mother's perception that infant may be ill and "a boy is okay" may lead to poor parent–child relationship.

Nursing Diagnosis: Pain related to labor contractions.

Defining Characteristic: Client states she is having pain with contractions.

Goal: Client will not experience pain above a tolerable level during labor and birth.

Outcome Criteria: Client states that pain is at a tolerable level for her.

Nursing Orders	***Rationale***
1. Admit to birthing room; explain benefits of single care room.	1. Orients client to new environment; promotes relaxation.
2. Place external fetal and uterine monitors and teach her to use these to detect when contractions begin.	2. Knowing how the monitors work will allow client to use them in the most effective way.
3. Encourage client to lie on side, not back, for labor.	3. Side-lying position helps prevent supine hypotension syndrome.
4. Encourage husband to be active support person during labor and birth.	4. Active support can help the woman relax and therefore reduce pain.
5. Assure client that additional measures for pain relief are available if she desires them.	5. Allows client to relax as she knows help is available, if pain becomes unmanageable.

position that makes the birth canal more accessible for surgical procedures, and the room invariably holds more emergency supplies than does a birthing room.

A delivery room's dominant piece of furniture is the delivery table, a stainless steel obstetrics platform. An instrument table stands at its foot and holds the sterile instruments and supplies required during a birth. A second table or stand with basins is also at the foot of the table; one basin will receive used sponges and the other will receive the placenta (Figure 18-36).

If a delivery room is used, the woman must be moved at the beginning of the second stage of labor. This transfer is awkward because she is intensely involved in what is happening inside her at this point. Also, she has grown used to the birthing room surroundings, and being transferred to a sterile-appearing operating room can be intimidating. Her support person may feel powerless and particularly threatened by the strange, obviously surgical surroundings in a delivery room.

It is easiest for the woman to be transferred in her labor room bed rather than on a stretcher, because then she does not have to slide onto a stretcher in the labor room and again onto the delivery table in the delivery room. Once in the delivery room, the woman should be helped to slide over onto the table. Delivery rooms are kept at approximately 68°F to reduce the danger that the gases used for anesthesia in some deliveries might explode. A woman may complain that the room or the sheet on the delivery table seem cold. More often, however, she is too involved in the final climactic moments of labor to notice the change in temperature. Help her make the transfer from the bed or stretcher to the table between contractions, so that it is most comfortable for her. Be certain the bed is held snugly against the delivery table so that she feels secure during the move. Be-

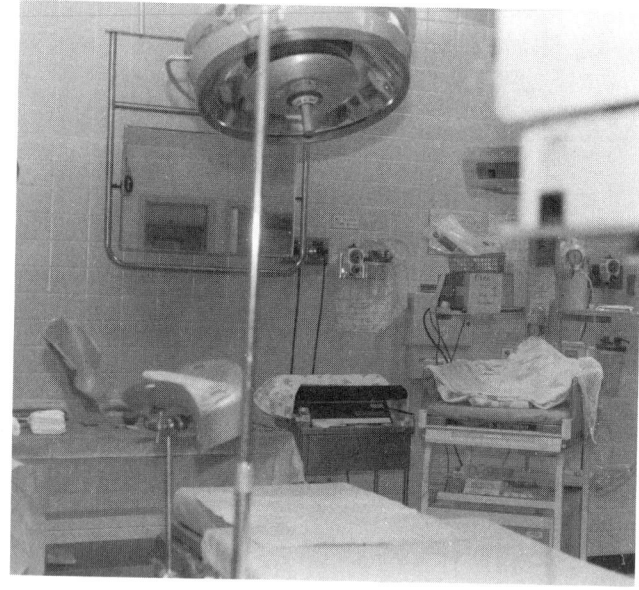

FIGURE 18-36
Delivery room.

cause contractions will now be coming approximately every 1 to 2 minutes, this transition must be done quickly and efficiently yet without seeming to rush.

Positioning for Birth

Alternative Positions. A variety of positions can be used for delivery as shown in Figure 18-37.

At one time the lithotomy position was the major position for birth, but it is no longer the position of choice in birthing rooms or alternative birth centers—although the labor beds in these locales usually have attached stirrups to allow birth in a lithotomy position. Alternative birth positions include the lateral or Sims' position, dorsal recumbent (on the back with knees flexed), semisitting, and squatting, in which a birthing bar may be used (Figure 18-37).

Nurse-midwives tend to favor these alternative birth positions for their clients because less tension seems to be placed on the perineum, resulting in fewer perineal tears. An episiotomy can be made in some alternative positions, although suturing is more difficult than in a lithotomy position.

In the United States, most physicians prefer a lithotomy position for birth. While the physician is scrubbing and donning a sterile mask, gown, and gloves, the woman is positioned into the table stirrups. It is important that both legs be raised at the same time to prevent strain on back and lower abdominal muscles. It is also important that the strap holding the leg in the stirrups is secured snugly but not so tightly that it causes constriction. Stirrups are perceived by women as an unnatural position for birth. They do, however, provide the most

---

Box 18-2
Delivery Equipment and Supplies

For Preparation of Mother
Preparation cup for antiseptic
4 × 4 sponges
Sponge forceps
Buttocks pad
Leg drapes
Towels
Abdominal drape
Towel clips
Needle holder
No. 14 urinary catheter
Basin for urine

Episiotomy and Perineal Repair
Pair episiotomy scissors
Pair suture scissors
Thumb forceps with teeth
Suture material
Kelly clamps
Allis clamps

For Placenta Delivery
Basin for placenta

For Newborn Care
2 bulb syringes
Cord clamp
3 cord blood tubes
Baby blanket

For Safety
Vaginal packing

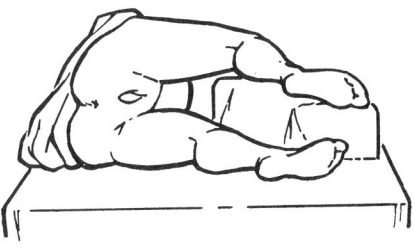

A Left lateral position

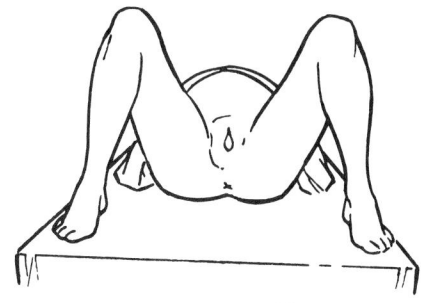

B Dorsal position

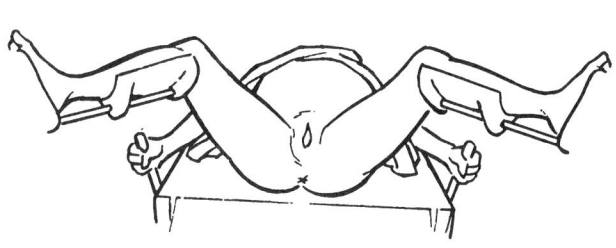

C Lithotomy position

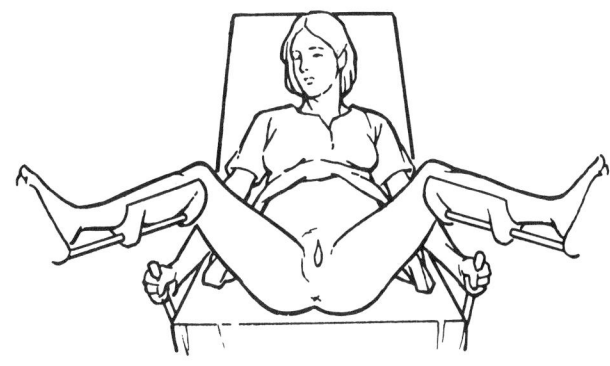

D Back elevated: semisitting position

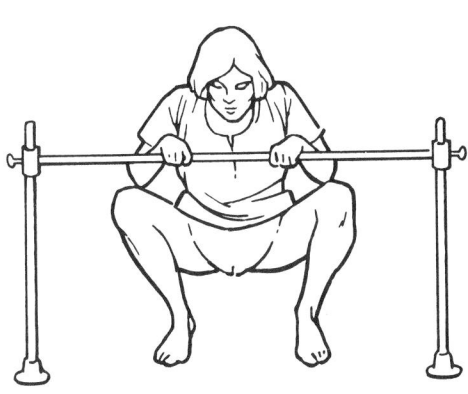

E Squatting position

FIGURE 18-37
*Positions for delivery. (**A**) Left lateral position. (**B**) Dorsal position (with slight left tilt). (**C**) Lithotomy position (with slight left tilt). (**D**) Back elevated: semisitting position. (**E**) Squatting position. (From May, K.A., & Mahlmeister, L.R. [1994]. Maternal and neonatal nursing: Family-centered care [3rd ed.]. Philadelphia: J.B. Lippincott.)*

advantageous position for accomplishing an episiotomy or a forceps-assisted birth, or for viewing the perineum to detect lacerations or other problems at birth, and they are generally not uncomfortable. Pad the stirrups with abdominal pads if a woman has ankle edema; be certain that there is no pressure on the calves of her leg in order to prevent thrombophlebitis.

Because pushing becomes less effective in a lithotomy position, the top portion of the table can be raised to a 30- to 60-degree angle so the woman can continue to push effectively. Lying for longer than 1 hour in a lithotomy position leads to intense pelvic congestion be-

cause blood flow to the lower extremities is impeded. For this reason, legs should be placed in lithotomy position only at the last moment. Pelvic congestion may lead to an increase in thrombophlebitis in the postpartal period. It may also contribute to excessive blood loss with birth and placental loosening.

Once a woman has been placed in a lithotomy position by means of the table stirrups, the table is "broken" (its lower half is folded downward) so that the physician can be in close proximity to the birth outlet. Never step away from the foot of a broken delivery room table until replaced by the birth attendant so that if birth should occur precipitously, the infant will not fall and be injured.

Gowning Procedure

All health care providers who will assist with the birth need to scrub their hands for 3 minutes at a sink and pull on clean gowns, caps, and masks. If anesthesia is going to be used, cloth "boots" may be needed over shoes to prevent static electricity. The support person who is going to stay with the woman for the birth must follow the same gown procedure. If he or she seems intimidated by wearing a mask and gown and unsure about what to do once they are in place, offer help and instruction. Do not feel compelled to keep the support person busy with tasks such as timing contractions during the birth. Sitting on a high stool at the head of the bed where the woman can see him or her, and where the couple can watch the birth in the table mirror, will be the most satisfying position. The support person is there for support, not busy work.

Promoting Effective Second-Stage Pushing

For the most effective pushing during the second stage of labor, the woman must push *with* contractions and rest between them. The best approach to aid women at this stage is to allow them to push when they feel the urge and using the position and technique they feel is best for them (Janke, 1992). Pushing is usually best done from a semi-Fowler's, squatting, or kneeling position rather than lying flat, to allow gravity to aid the effort (Mayberry, 1994). To position a woman in a semi-Fowler's position, place one or two pillows under her head and let her flex her thighs on her abdomen. Most women achieve the best effect if they grasp their legs just below the knees, and as a contraction begins, bear down as if they were starting to move their bowels. The woman can use short pushes or long, sustained ones, whichever is most comfortable for her. Holding her breath during a contraction could cause a Valsalva's maneuver or temporarily impede blood return to the heart because of increased intrathoracic pressure. This could also conceivably interfere with blood supply to the uterus. To prevent her from holding her breath during pushing, urge her to breathe out during a pushing effort.

To keep the second stage of labor from moving too fast in a multipara, it may be necessary to prevent her from pushing. The best way to accomplish this is to have her pant with contractions. Because it is difficult to push effectively when she is using her diaphragm for panting, this limits pushing. Remember that pushing is involuntary. No matter how much a woman wants to cooperate, stopping this overwhelming urge to push is almost beyond her power. Demonstrating "panting like a puppy"

and panting with her may be most effective. Be sure that she is inhaling adequately or she will hypoventilate and become lightheaded while panting. Have her take deep breaths between contractions to prevent this.

For a multipara, the birthing room is converted into a birth room when the cervix reaches 7 to 9 cm dilatation; for a primipara, this may not be done until the baby's head has crowned the size of a quarter or half dollar (full dilatation and descent).

Perineal Cleaning

The perineum is cleaned with an antiseptic and then rinsed with a designated antiseptic solution before birth by the physician, nurse-midwife, or nurse. To do this, use a sterile glove and sterile compresses impregnated with whatever specific cleansing solution is designated by health care agency procedure. Use warm water (set a bottle of sterile water in a warm water basin) because cold water could cause uterine cramping. Cleaning should be done from the vagina outward (so that microorganisms are moved away from the vagina), using a clean compress for each stroke. A wide area including vulva, upper inner thighs, pubis, and anus are included. See Figure 18-38 for a typical pattern for cleaning. Following cleaning, sterile drapes are placed around the perineum as the next step.

Fecal material may be expelled from the rectum due to compression from pressure of the fetal head. This is sponged away by the physician or nurse-midwife to prevent contamination of the birth canal as it occurs.

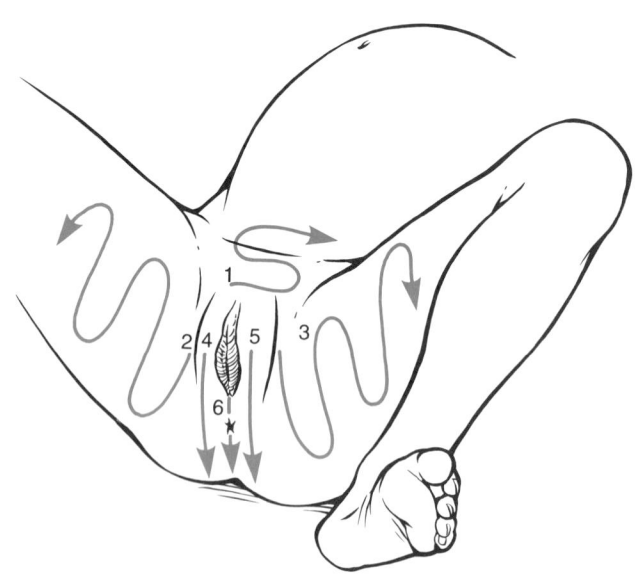

FIGURE 18-38
Pattern for cleaning perineum before birth. Cleaning from the birth canal outward moves bacteria away from, not into, the vagina. Numbers refer to steps of the procedure.

Episiotomy

An **episiotomy** is a surgical incision of the perineum made to prevent tearing of the perineum with birth and to release pressure on the fetal head with birth. An episiotomy incision is made with blunt-tipped scissors in the midline of the perineum (a midline episiotomy) or begun in the midline but directed laterally away from the rectum (a mediolateral episiotomy; see Figure 18-39). Mediolateral episiotomies have the advantage over midline cuts in that, if tearing occurs beyond the incision, it will be away from the rectum with less danger of complication from rectal mucosal tears. However, midline episiotomies appear to heal more easily, cause less blood loss, and result in less discomfort to a woman in the postpartal period.

Obstetrical practice varies as to how often episiotomies are done. They were once done only when tearing seemed imminent, then were considered routine with a normal birth, and now are used less frequently. The advantage of an episiotomy is that it substitutes a clean cut for a ragged tear, minimizes pressure on the fetal head, and shortens the last portion of the second stage of labor (Cunningham et al., 1993).

The pressure of the fetal presenting part against the perineum is so intense that the nerve endings in the perineum are momentarily deadened. Thus, an episiotomy may be done in a woman who has received no anesthesia. However, in some cases a pudendal block is done, whereby lidocaine is injected via a long needle into the vaginal wall near the ischial spine, numbing the lower vaginal area and the perineum.

There is a slight loss of blood at the time of the incision, but the pressure of the presenting part serves to tamp the cut edges and keep bleeding to a minimum. The fetal head generally moves forward considerably once the tension on the perineum is relieved.

Birth

As soon as the head of the fetus is prominent (approximately 8 cm across), the physician or nurse-midwife may place a sterile towel over the rectum and press forward on the fetal chin while the other hand is pressed downward on the occiput (a Ritgen maneuver; Figure 18-40). This helps the fetus achieve extension, so that the head is born with the smallest diameter presenting, and the rate at which the head is born is controlled. Pressure should never be put on the fundus of the uterus to effect birth, as this could rupture the uterus.

The woman is asked to continue pushing until the occiput of the fetal head is firmly at the pubic arch; then the head is actually delivered between contractions to prevent it from being expelled too rapidly and to avoid tearing of the perineum and a rapid pressure change in the infant's head (which could rupture cerebral blood vessels). The woman may be asked to pant deliberately so she does not push during a contraction. She may be asked to push again without a contraction present to deliver the shoulders. She is so involved with the coming birth that instructions often have to be repeated for her. Her support person may be almost as overwhelmed by the birth process as the woman herself, so he or she needs support as well.

The woman who has not had anesthesia experiences the birth of the head as a flash of pain or burning sensa-

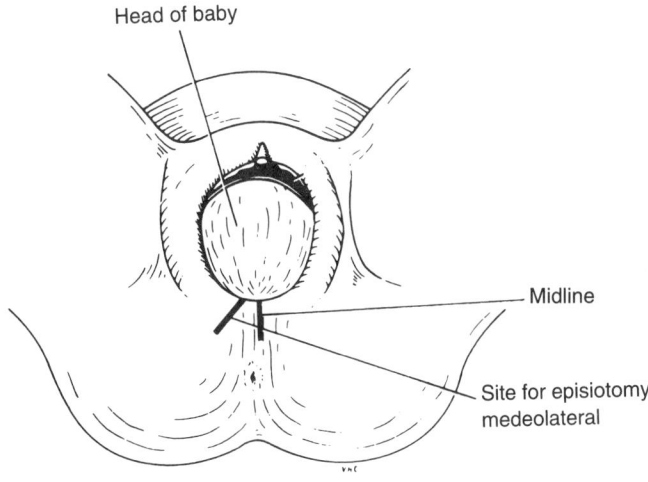

FIGURE 18-39
Position of episiotomy incision in a woman during second stage of labor. Baby's head is presenting to vaginal outlet (crowning).

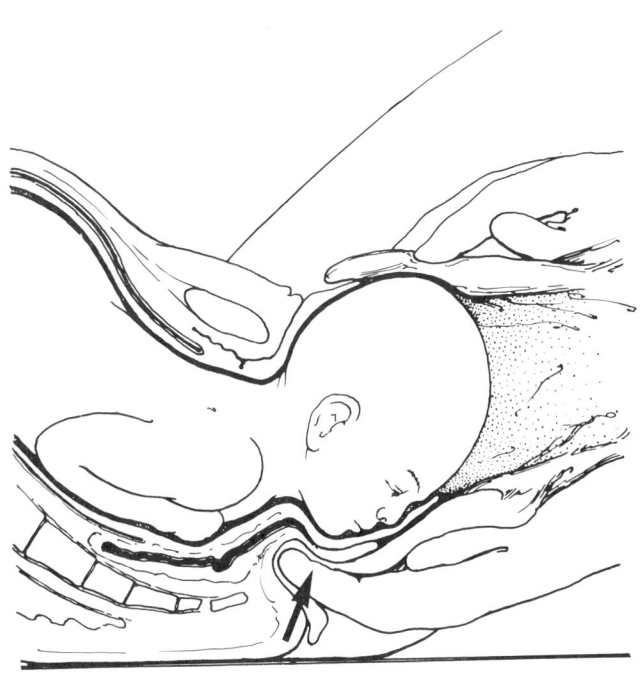

FIGURE 18-40
Ritgen's maneuver as it appears in median section. Arrow shows direction of pressure. (Reeder, S.J., Martin, L.L., & Koniak, D. [1992]. Maternity nursing: Family, newborn, and women's health care [17th ed.]. Philadelphia: J.B. Lippincott.)

tion, as if someone had momentarily poured hot water on her perineum. It is a fleeting sensation and is not particularly uncomfortable. Reassure her that this is normal.

Immediately following birth of the head, the physician or nurse-midwife suctions out the infant's mouth with a bulb syringe and then passes his or her fingers along the occiput to the newborn's neck to determine whether a loop of umbilical cord is encircling the neck. It is not uncommon for a single loop of cord to be positioned this way (termed a *nuchal cord).* If such a loop is felt, it is gently loosened and drawn down over the fetal head. If it is too tightly coiled to allow for this, it must be clamped and cut before the shoulders of the infant are delivered, or else interference with the fetal oxygen supply or tearing of the umbilical cord could result.

Following expulsion of the fetal head, restitution and external rotation occur. The shoulders and the remainder of the newborn must now be delivered to free the chest for the first breath. Gentle pressure is exerted downward on the side of the infant's head, and the anterior shoulder is born. Slight upward pressure on the side of the head allows the anterior shoulder to nestle against the symphysis and the posterior shoulder to be born. The remainder of the body then slides free without any further difficulty.

A child is considered born when the whole body is delivered. This is the time that should be noted and recorded as the time of birth—a nursing responsibility. (Most physicians and nurse-midwives regard it as their responsibility or pleasure to announce the sex of the infant.) With the birth of the infant, the second stage of labor is complete (Figure 18-41).

Cutting and Clamping the Cord

The infant is held with his or her head in a slightly dependent position to allow secretions to drain from the nose and mouth; the mouth may be gently aspirated by a bulb syringe to remove more secretions. The infant is then laid on the abdominal drape of the mother while the cord is cut. The cord will continue to pulsate for a few minutes after birth and then the pulsation ceases. There are a number of theories about the optimum time for cutting the cord and position of the infant. Delaying the cutting until pulsation ceases and maintaining the infant at a uterine level allows as much as 100 mL of blood to pass from the placenta into the fetus. This may help to prevent iron deficiency anemia in infants. On the other hand, late clamping of the cord may cause overinfusion with placental blood and the possibility of polycythemia and hyperbilirubinemia in the infant. This is a particular concern in preterm infants. Raising the infant on the abdomen may modify the amount of blood infused as well as allow the parents a free, unobstructed view of the new child. The timing of cord clamping therefore will vary depending on the individual physician or midwife's preference and the maturity of the infant.

The cord is clamped 8 inches to 10 inches from the infant's umbilicus by two Kelly hemostats and is cut between them; an umbilical clamp is then applied (Figure 18-42). A cord blood sample is taken because this is a ready source of infant blood if blood typing or other emergency measures need to be done. The vessels in the cord are counted to see that three are present. An umbilical cord clamp or tie is then applied.

Clamping the cord is part of the stimulus that initiates a first breath. With this, the infant's most important transition to the outside world, the establishment of independent respirations, has been made.

Introducing the Infant

Following birth, the infant is handed to a nurse who receives him or her in a sterile blanket. Use a firm grip with newborn babies in the first few minutes of life because they are covered with slippery amniotic fluid. Lay

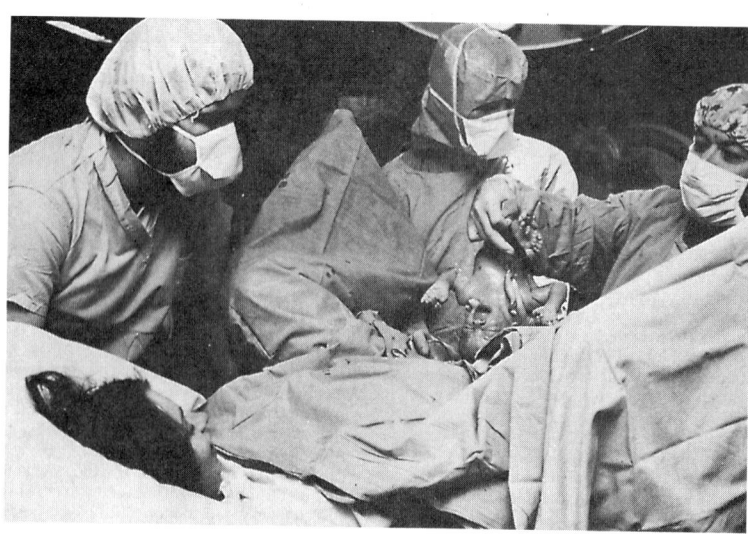

FIGURE 18-41
New parents watch their baby being born. (Courtesy of the Department of Medical Photography, Children's Hospital, Buffalo, NY.)

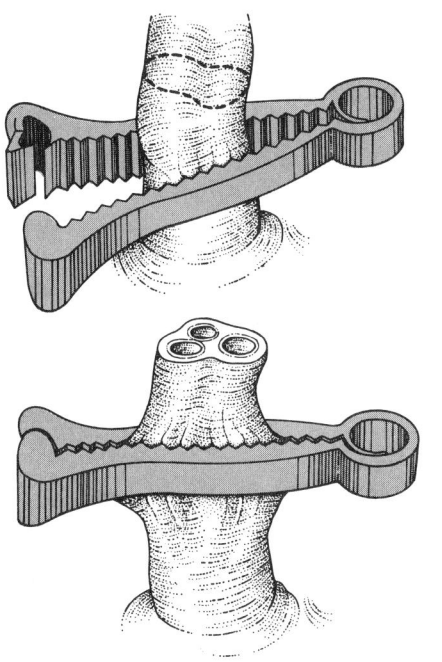

FIGURE 18-42
Umbilical clamp applied to cord. (From Reeder, S.J., Martin, L.L., & Koniak, D. [1992]. Maternity nursing: Family, newborn, and women's health care [17th ed.]. Philadelphia: J.B. Lippincott.)

the infant on the radiant heat warmer and dry him or her well with a warmed towel. Cover the infant's head with a wrapped towel or cap. If the infant was not placed on the mother's abdomen immediately after birth so she could see the baby, wrap the infant snugly now and if the respirations are good, take the infant to the head of the table to show to the mother and father.

Although the theory that parent–infant bonding takes place within a limited time frame is currently being disputed, there is evidence that immediately following birth, the parents are sensitive or "ripe," or most responsive, to beginning attachment or "bonding" with the infant (Klaus & Kennell, 1983).

Both mother and father usually want to see and touch their newborn immediately after birth. This assures them that the baby is well and is important in getting a parent–child relationship off to a good start. For this reason, parents should be encouraged to hold the baby following birth. Prophylactic eye ointment should not be administered to the infant until after parents have had this chance to see their infant (and the infant has had a chance to see them). (See Chapter 23 for infant care after birth.) If a woman wishes to breast-feed, this is an optimal time for her to begin. An infant sucking at the breast stimulates release of endogenous oxytocin. Although it is not well documented that this actually makes a difference, it theoretically aids in uterine contractions and involution, or the return of the uterus to its prepregnant stage.

Use of Forceps

Forceps are metal instruments that may be used during the second stage of labor to extract the fetus from the birth canal. Refer to the section on forceps birth in Chapter 21.

Care of the Woman During the Third Stage and Postpartum

Oxytocics

Once the placenta is delivered, oxytocin is generally administered intramuscularly or intravenously on the physician's or nurse-midwife's order. Such medication increases uterine contractions and therefore minimizes uterine bleeding.

Oxytocin (Pitocin) may be added to an existing intravenous line (4 U as a bolus and 20 to 30 U/L of IV fluid) or given intramuscularly. A complication of bolus injection can be severe hypotension. Methylergonovine maleate (Methergine), a semisynthetic derivative of ergonovine, may also be administered intramuscularly. Methergine produces strong and effective contractions, and its effect lasts several hours. The usual dose is 0.2 mg (1 mL) given intramuscularly (Loeb, 1993).

The administration of these drugs is a nursing responsibility in most health care facilities. Medication should not be given until the birth attendant indicates that it is appropriate, as the birth attendant may want it given as early as when the fetal anterior shoulder is delivered or may want to inspect the placenta first to ensure that it is intact and without gross abnormalities and that none of its cotyledons remains in the uterus. Because oxytocin causes hypertension by vasoconstriction, a baseline blood pressure should be determined before administration. It should not be used with women with elevated blood pressures. Be certain that intramuscular oxytocin administered in the delivery or birthing room is recorded on the maternal record. The next dose of medication to maintain contraction cannot be given closer than 3 or 4 hours to this dose or severe hypertension can occur. Intravenous administration of Pitocin may be continued for up to 8 hours after birth to ensure uterine contraction.

Placental Delivery

If the placenta does not deliver spontaneously, the birth attendant will need to remove it manually by inserting a gloved hand into the uterus. He or she needs fresh sterile gloves for this procedure to avoid introducing pathogens into the uterus. The placenta is inspected following delivery to be certain that it is intact and is normal in appearance and weight (normally a placenta is one sixth the weight of the infant). If unusually large or small, it may be weighed.

Perineal Repair

Following delivery of the placenta, any perineal stitches needed are put in place by the birth attendant. This suturing of the perineum is a long, tedious process from the mother's perspective. She must lie on her back and wait for the procedure to be completed, while attention of others is riveted on the newborn lying in the baby warmer off to one side. This can make the mother feel rejected, perhaps no more important than the discarded packing case in which a new appliance has arrived. It is important that health care personnel be sensitive to this and not appear to be much more interested in trying out the new "appliance"—commenting on its lusty cry, its weight, or its sex—than in seeing to the "carton" that allowed the appliance to arrive safely.

A woman is as vulnerable to hurt feelings in the immediate postpartum period as she was during pregnancy and early labor. Be certain to include her in explanations and appreciate how anticlimactic she may feel. Otherwise, the "postpartum blues" can begin just minutes after birth.

If suturing of an episiotomy is done immediately after the birth of the placenta, a woman who delivered without the aid of an anesthetic will theoretically still have so much natural-pressure anesthesia of the perineum that she will not require an anesthetic. In actual practice, however, by the time the placenta is delivered (approximately 5 minutes), enough sensation has returned to the perineum that the woman will probably need injection of a local anesthetic for comfort during this procedure. Women who received a regional anesthetic during labor, such as a pudendal block, or those who have had epidural anesthesia, do not need additional medication during episiotomy repair.

Immediate Postpartal Assessment and Nursing Care

When the episiotomy repair is complete, remove the drapes covering the woman, ask for help, and with extreme care lower both of the woman's legs from the table stirrups simultaneously to prevent back injury.

Take vital signs (i.e., pulse, respirations, and blood pressure) and palpate the uterus fundus for size, consistency, and position. Pulse and respirations may be fairly rapid (80 to 90 beats per minute and 20 to 24 respirations per minute) and blood pressure slightly elevated due to the excitement of the moment and recent oxytocin administration. Vital signs will be required every 15 minutes for the first hour, and the second set taken is probably a better baseline.

Cleanse the woman's vulva and perineum front to back of any secretions with warmed sterile water and a sterile compress. Dry with a sterile towel and apply a sterile perineal pad held by a sanitary belt to absorb vaginal discharge (lochia).

If the birth was in a birthing room, the birthing bed is returned to its original position. Offer a clean gown and a warmed blanket because a mother often experiences a chill and shaking sensation 10 to 15 minutes after birth. This may be due in part to the low temperature of a delivery room but also may be caused by the sudden release of pressure on pelvic nerves or excess epinephrine production during labor. It is a normal phenomenon but can be frightening to the mother. She may associate the shaking chill with fever or infection and worry that she will be ill at a time when she most wants to be well to care for her new child. Reassure her that this is a normal happening. Fortunately, the sensation is transitory.

Transfer to Recovery Room

If the woman delivered in a delivery room, help her slide to a recovery room bed or stretcher for transfer to the recovery room. This is the beginning of the postpartal period or the fourth stage of labor. It is one of the most hazardous periods of childbirth because the uterus may be so exhausted from labor that it cannot maintain contraction and may hemorrhage. In addition, the woman is so exhausted she generally falls asleep almost immediately and thus loses all ability to assess her own condition. Specific assessments done during this time are continued throughout the postpartal period. These assessments are discussed in Chapter 22 with other aspects of postpartal care.

Danger Signs of Labor

There is wide variation among individuals in the pattern of labor contractions and maternal responses to labor and birth. Certain signs, however, indicate that the course of events is deviating too far from normal. These signs, both fetal and maternal, are described in the following sections. Nursing care of the woman experiencing a complication during labor or birth is addressed in Chapter 21.

Fetal Danger Signs

High or Low Fetal Heart Rate

As a rule, an FHR of more than 160 bpm (fetal tachycardia) or less than 120 bpm (fetal bradycardia) is a sign of possible fetal distress. An equally important sign is a late or variable deceleration pattern on the fetal monitor. The fetal heart may return to a normal range in between these irregular patterns and give a false sense of security if FHR alone is assessed.

Meconium Staining

Although meconium staining of the amniotic fluid is not always a sign of fetal distress, its correlation is high and should be taken seriously. It may indicate that the fetus is experiencing hypoxia, which stimulates the vagal reflex and leads to increased bowel motility. Loss of sphincter control causes escape of meconium into the amniotic fluid. Although meconium staining may be normal in a breech presentation, because pressure on the buttocks can cause meconium loss, it should always be reported to the physician or nurse-midwife, who can then evaluate its meaning and seriousness.

Hyperactivity

Ordinarily, a fetus is quiet and barely moving during labor. Fetal hyperactivity may be a sign that hypoxia is occurring.

Fetal Acidosis

When blood analyses are made on the fetus during labor by use of a scalp capillary technique, the finding of acidosis (blood pH below 7.2) is a certain sign that fetal well being is becoming compromised.

Maternal Danger Signs

Rising or Falling Blood Pressure

Blood pressure in the mother normally rises slightly in the second (pelvic) stage of labor due to her pushing effort. A rule of thumb in labor is to report a systolic pressure of more than 140 mm Hg and a diastolic pressure of more than 90 mm Hg, or an increase in the systolic pressure of more than 30 mm Hg and a diastolic pressure of more than 15 mm Hg (the basic criteria for pregnancy-induced hypertension). A falling blood pressure is just as crucial to report as an increasing one, because it may be the first sign of an occult intrauterine hemorrhage. A falling blood pressure is often associated with other clinical signs of shock such as apprehension, increased pulse rate, and pallor.

Abnormal Pulse

Most pregnant women have an average pulse rate of 70 to 80 bpm. Pulse normally increases slightly during the second stage of labor due to the exertion involved. A maternal pulse of more than 100 bpm during the normal course of labor is unusual and should be reported as a possible indication of hemorrhage.

Inadequate or Prolonged Contractions

Uterine contractions normally become more frequent, intense, and longer as labor progresses. If they become less frequent, less intense, or shorter in duration, this may indicate uterine exhaustion (inertia). This problem must be corrected or else a cesarean birth may have to be performed.

A period of relaxation must be present between contractions so that the intervillous spaces of the uterus can fill and maintain an adequate supply of oxygen and nutrients for the fetus. As a rule, uterine contractions

lasting longer than 70 seconds should be reported because they may begin to compromise fetal well being by not allowing adequate uterine artery filling. The physician or nurse-midwife can then determine whether these long contractions will have an adverse effect on fetal or maternal well being.

Pathologic Retraction Ring

An indentation across the woman's abdomen where the upper and lower segments of the uterus join may be a sign of impending uterine rupture, or at least of extreme uterine stress. For this reason, it is important to observe the contours of the abdomen periodically during labor. If fetal heartbeat is being auscultated by stethoscope, this automatically provides a regular opportunity to assess the woman's abdomen. If an electronic monitor is in place, it is necessary to make this observation deliberately.

Abnormal Lower Abdominal Contour

A full bladder during labor may be manifested as a round bulge on the lower anterior abdomen. This is a danger signal for two reasons: first, the bladder may be injured by the pressure of the fetal head; second, the pressure of the full bladder may not allow the fetal head to descend.

Increasing Apprehension

Warnings of psychological danger during labor are as important to consider in assessing maternal well being as physical signs. A woman who is becoming increasingly apprehensive despite clear explanations of unfolding events may only be approaching the pelvic division of labor. She may, however, not be "hearing" because she has a concern that has not been met. Try an approach such as this: "You seem more and more concerned. Could you tell me what is worrying you?" Increasing apprehension also needs to be investigated for physical reasons. It can be a sign of oxygen deprivation or internal hemorrhage.

Unique Concerns of the Woman in Labor

The Woman Without a Support Person

Some women have chosen to reject or know they must do without the support of the baby's father during labor; some have husbands in the military or who are temporarily not available. Such women may appreciate having a family member or close friend act as their support person. A young girl who did not receive prenatal care may not be aware that she could have asked the father of her child to accompany her, and may appreciate being told that she can telephone him and ask him to join her. If he chooses to include himself in the labor experience, it will reflect his commitment to the mother of his child and his value to her as an important person in her life.

A woman whose acceptance of her pregnancy was slow to develop due to lack of adequate support people may not have completed the psychological tasks by the time she is in labor. This could make her more apprehensive about a new life role and calls for increased assessment of parent–child bonding in the immediate postpartal period.

The Woman Who Will Be Placing Her Baby for Adoption

Even if a woman has decided to place her baby for adoption, she needs to be an active participant in her labor and birth experience. She should watch the baby being born and be allowed to hold it as desired. Legally, she has 4 days (this may vary by state) in which to decide whether to keep the baby. Though the decision may have been easy to make during pregnancy, once she holds the baby in her arms, the prospect of giving it up may be more painful than she realized. She needs support no matter what decision she eventually makes (New England Adoption, 1991).

Vaginal Birth After Cesarean Birth (VBAC)

Women who have had a previous cesarean birth that involved a low transverse uterine incision are often allowed a trial labor with their next pregnancy to see if vaginal birth will be possible. Length of labor in these women is comparable with that of primiparas, not multiparas, because it is their first vaginal birth (Clemenson, 1993). Women should be externally monitored for both fetal heart tones and uterine contractions during VBAC, as they are more prone to uterine rupture than others. Most women are anxious for vaginal birth to be successful so they do not have to undergo surgery. At the same time they may be surprised and dismayed at the length and discomfort of normal labor. They need support to breathe with contractions, push effectively, and accept vaginal birth.

Key Points

- Labor is the series of events by which uterine contractions expel the fetus and placenta from the woman's body.
- The exact reason why labor begins is unknown. It most likely occurs because of an interplay between fetal and uterine factors.
- Effective labor depends on interactions between the passage, the passenger, the power of contractions, and psychological readiness.
- Labor is an almost overwhelming experience because it involves sensations and emotions at such

an intense level. Women need support people with them to help them cope with this experience.

- Fetal presentation (the fetal body part that will initially contact the cervix) and position (the relationship of the fetal presenting part to a specific quadrant of the woman's pelvis) are both important in determining the success of labor.
- The first stage of labor is the time span between beginning dilatation and the time the cervix is fully dilated. The second stage is from the time of full dilatation until the infant is born. A third or placental stage is from the time the infant is born until after the delivery of the placenta. A fourth stage is the first few hours following birth.
- Cervical changes that occur during labor are effacement (shortening and thinning of the cervix) and dilatation (enlargement of the cervical canal from 1 to 2 cm to 8 to 10 cm).
- Important nursing assessments to make in labor are health history, length and intensity of contractions, fetal assessment, and maternal vital signs.
- Monitoring uterine contractions and fetal heart rate are nursing responsibilities. Recognizing fetal bradycardia, tachycardia, and late and variable decelerations are important observations. Interventions to help prevent fetal distress include keeping the woman on her left side and promoting voiding. Offering psychologic support is crucial to maternal well being.
- Pushing during the second stage of labor should be guided by the woman's felt need to push. Urge her to not hold her breath while doing this to prevent a Valsalva maneuver.
- The placental stage follows birth and consists of placental separation and expulsion. Observe for excessive bleeding during this time. Do not pull on the cord to hasten separation as this can lead to uterine inversion.
- Danger signs of labor are abnormal fetal heart rate, meconium staining of amniotic fluid, abnormal maternal pulse or blood pressure, inadequate or prolonged contractions, formation of a pathologic retraction ring, development of an abnormal lower abdomen contour, and increasing apprehension.
- A fetus is in potential danger when membranes rupture because of the possibility of cord prolapse. Always assess FHR at this point to safeguard the fetus.
- A woman is at potential risk all during labor for hemorrhage because of the possibility the placenta could be dislodged. Assess for vaginal bleeding and vital signs to be sure that this is not occurring.

Critical Thinking Exercises

1. Mrs. Travillato is a woman in active labor you admit to a birthing room. She admits she has read nothing during her pregnancy about labor so has

little idea of what to expect. Would it be better to educate her about labor or let her follow her practice of not knowing? If you decide to teach her, what would you tell her early in labor? Midway in labor? Why would a woman enter labor not having read about it?

2. Mrs. Travillato's fetus is in a vertex presentation and an occipitoposterior position and has a military attitude. Explain how this presentation and position might affect the process of labor and what concerns you might anticipate in preparing Mrs. Travillato for delivery.

3. Most women today accept fetal monitoring equipment as an expected part of labor care. How would you care for a woman who states she absolutely does not want this type of monitoring?

References

Akin, J. W., et al. (1990). Increasing quantity of maternal immunoglobulin G in trophoblastic tissue before the onset of normal labor. *American Journal of Obstetrics and Gynecology, 162,* 1154.

Bonovich, L. (1990). Recognizing the onset of labor. *Journal of Obstetric, Gynecologic, and Neonatal Nursing, 19,* 141.

Clemenson, N. (1993). Promoting vaginal birth after cesarean section. *American Family Physician, 47,* 139.

Cunningham, F. G., et al. (1993). *Williams obstetrics* (19th ed.). Norwalk, CT: Appleton & Lange.

Department of Health and Human Services. (1991). *Healthy people 2000.* Washington, DC: Public Health Service.

Dildy, G. A., et al. (1993). Preliminary experience with intrapartum fetal pulse oximetry in humans. *Obstetrics and Gynecoloy, 81,* 630.

Duffin, C. (1992). Teaching 1st stage: What's new and what's being taught. *International Journal of Childbirth Education, 7,* 31.

Freeman, R. (1990). Intrapartum fetal monitoring: A disappointing story. [Editorial]. *New England Journal of Medicine, 322,* 624.

Friedman, E. (1978). *Labor, clinical evaluation and management* (2nd ed.). New York: Appleton-Century-Crofts.

Janke, J. (1992). Teaching breathing techniques in the '90s. *International Journal of Childbirth Education, 7,* 33.

Klaus, M. A., & Kennell, H. (1983). *Bonding: The beginnings of parent-infant attachment.* New York: New American Library.

Lehman, B. (1990, October 8). Doubts growing over fetal monitors. *The Boston Globe,* pp. 59, 61.

Loeb, S. (1993). *Nurse's handbook of drug therapy.* Springhouse, PA: Springhouse.

Mayberry, L. (1994). Intrapartum nursing care: Research into practice. *Journal of Obstetric, Gynecologic and Neonatal Nursing, 23,* 170.

Milhan, D. (1992). The amniotomy. *International Journal of Childbirth Education, 7,* 17.

New England Adoption, Inc. (1991). *Making the adoption decision.* Boston: New England Adoption, Inc.

Shy, K. K., et al. (1990). Effects of electronic fetal-heart rate monitoring as compared with periodic auscultation on the neurologic development of premature infants. *New England Journal of Medicine, 322,* 588.

Snell, B. J. (1993). The use of amnioinfusion in nurse-midwifery practice. *Journal of Nurse Midwifery, 38,* 625.

Strong, T. H., & Phelan, J. P. (1991). Umbilical cord prolapse. *Female Patient, 16,* 19.

Suggested Readings

Abitbol, M. M., et al. (1993). Vaginal birth after cesarean section: The patient's point of view. *American Family Physician, 47,* 129.

Allen, R. E., et al. (1991). Pelvic floor damage and childbirth: A neurophysiological study. *Obstetrical and Gynecological Survey, 46,* 209.

Berg, T. G., & Rayburn, W. F. (1992). Effects of analgesia on labor. *Clinical Obstetrics and Gynecology, 35,* 457.

Cosner, K. R., & deJong, E. (1993). Physiologic second stage labor. *MCN: American Journal of Maternal Child Nursing, 18,* 38.

Guild, S. D. (1994). A comprehensive fetal monitoring program for nursing practice and education. *Journal of Obstetric, Gynecologic and Neonatal Nursing, 23,* 34.

Kruse, J. (1993). The physiology of labor and management of prolonged labor. *Primary Care, 20,* 685.

Lowe, N. K. (1991). Maternal confidence in coping with labor: A self-efficacy concept. *Journal of Obstetric, Gynecologic, and Neonatal Nursing, 20,* 457.

McCurdy, C. M., & Seeds, J. W. (1993). Oligohydramnios: Problems and treatment. *Seminars in Perinatology, 17,* 183.

Smith, M. A., et al. (1993). The rational management of labor. *American Family Physician, 47,* 1471.

Chapter 19

Providing Comfort During Labor and Birth

Objectives

After mastering the contents of this chapter, you should be able to:

1. Describe the physiologic basis of pain in labor and birth and relative theories of pain relief.

2. Compare and contrast the action of local, regional, and general anesthesia as used in labor and birth.

3. Assess the degree and type of discomfort a woman is experiencing and her ability to cope with it effectively during labor and birth.

4. State nursing diagnoses related to the effect of pain in labor.

5. Plan nursing interventions to relieve pain in labor such as teaching breathing techniques or relaxation.

6. Implement common measures used for pain relief in labor and birth, such as administering an analgesic or assisting with local or regional anesthesia.

7. Evaluate outcome criteria to be certain that labor is a satisfying experience for the woman and her family.

8. Identify National Health Goals related to anesthesia and childbirth that nurses can be instrumental in helping the nation to achieve.

9. Identify areas related to comfort in labor that could benefit from additional nursing research.

10. Use critical thinking to analyze ways to maintain family-centered care when analgesia and anesthesia are used in childbirth.

11. Synthesize knowledge of pain relief measures during labor and birth with the nursing process to achieve quality maternal and child health nursing care.

Adele Pillitteri: MATERNAL AND CHILD
HEALTH NURSING, 2nd Edition. © 1995
Adele Pillitteri.

Concerns about the pain involved in labor and birth can sometimes dominate a pregnant woman or couple's thoughts about childbirth, particularly as the baby's due date approaches. Providing information during prenatal visits about natural methods for pain relief as well as the pharmacologic options available in her health care setting can help to allay these fears. As discussed in Chapter 13, prepared childbirth classes can provide couples with an opportunity to learn more about and to practice a variety of pain relief techniques, such as prepared breathing patterns. Often, however, the overwhelming nature of the labor experience is greater than the couple expected. When this occurs, administration of an analgesic or a regional anesthetic can reduce discomfort sufficiently to allow the woman to regain some control over the labor process and the childbirth experience. The result may be an experience that the woman and her partner will remember positively, which ultimately promotes the entire family's health.

A great deal has been written in nursing literature about the benefits of using the neutral term "contractions" instead of "labor pains." The theory is a sound one, not only because the woman is experiencing a *contracting* sensation but also because calling it *pain* magnifies her fear and tension, and tension magnifies pain. Remember, however, that renaming it will not change its basic nature. By any name, discomfort accompanies

labor. Fortunately, many nursing interventions can help reduce pain, so that labor is as fulfilling and rewarding an experience as the woman hopes it will be. National Health Goals related to anesthesia and labor are shown in the Focus on National Health Goals box.

⊠ **NURSING PROCESS OVERVIEW**
for Pain Relief During Childbirth

ASSESSMENT

Pain is any sensation of discomfort. Pain thresholds cause the amount of pain experienced to be unique to each individual. Pain is a subjective symptom, so no one but the woman herself can describe or know the extent of her pain. Assess how much discomfort a woman is having in labor by what she says, but also look for subtle signs of pain such as facial tenseness, flushing, or paleness; hands in a fist; rapid breathing; or rapid pulse rate. Knowing the extent of a woman's discomfort is a guide to whether she needs any additional assistance and to the choice of medication she needs in labor.

NURSING DIAGNOSIS

Although Pain related to labor contractions is the most obvious nursing diagnosis applicable to labor, it is not the only relevant one during this time. Pain can create other problems for the laboring woman that can negatively affect the childbirth experience and, if not resolved, can intensify pain. Some women may become more concerned with their reaction to the pain than to the pain itself. Other nursing diagnoses, therefore, are applicable:

- Powerlessness related to duration and intensity of labor contractions
- Anxiety related to lack of knowledge about "normal" labor process
- Self-esteem disturbance related to ineffectiveness of prepared childbirth breathing exercises
- Decisional conflict related to use of anesthesia during labor

PLANNING

Labor and birth medications may pose risks for both the mother (e.g., hypotension) and the fetus (e.g., bradycardia), so their use must always be weighed against the alternative risk to the mother (enduring a painful labor). The decision may also affect family functioning if the method chosen limits the father's participation in the

---

FOCUS ON
National Health Goals

As both analgesia and anesthesia administration during labor can increase both maternal and fetal mortality, a number of National Health Goals are related to pain relief in labor. For example:

- Reduce the maternal mortality rate to no more than 3.3 per 100,000 live births from a baseline of 6.6 per 100,000.

- Reduce the fetal death rate to no more than 5 per 1000 live births from a baseline of 7.6 per 1000 (DHHS, 1991).

Nurses can be instrumental in helping the nation to achieve these goals by educating women about the advantages of prepared childbirth, helping them to use breathing patterns or other comfort techniques during labor so that they need a minimum of analgesia and anesthesia, and conscientious monitoring of women who receive analgesics and anesthesia during labor and birth.

Among the areas that could benefit from additional nursing research are women's satisfaction with regional anesthesia in labor and their reasons why the prepared childbirth method they anticipated using was not adequate.

---

birth. When planning interventions to manage discomfort, consider the woman's perceptions about childbirth, her past childbirth experiences, if any, and the amount and type of childbirth preparation she and her partner have had.

IMPLEMENTATION

Many interventions to help relieve pain are available to the nurse. Among the most important of these are providing comfort; informing the woman and her support person about the progress of labor—simply knowing that birth is getting even a little closer can make the next few contractions easier to withstand; and supporting and encouraging the woman to use methods of nonpharmacologic pain management such as relaxation. Offering analgesia or assisting with anesthesia administration during labor or birth requires nursing judgment and a caring presence to help one woman accept analgesia when she needs it and to encourage another to experience childbirth without heavy sedation.

EVALUATION

Evaluation is ongoing and generally must occur within a short time frame. Examples of outcome criteria are:

- Client states pain during labor was never above a tolerable level for her.
- Couple report they were not rendered powerless by force or duration of labor.
- Client states she will not feel intimidated by thoughts of pain in labor in the future.

Long-term evaluation should reveal that a woman found labor and birth to be an experience that was not only endurable but allowed her to grow in self-esteem and the family to grow through a shared experience. Asking a woman to describe her labor experience in relation to pain not only aids evaluation but also helps her work through this emotional period of life and integrate it into her previous experience.

Experience of Pain During Childbirth

Etiology of Pain During Labor and Birth

The contractions of the uterus are unique among involuntary muscle contractions in that they cause pain (contractions of the heart, stomach, and intestine also involve involuntary muscles but do not normally cause pain). Several explanations exist as to why pain accompanies uterine contractions in labor. Contractions undoubtedly constrict blood vessels, reducing the blood supply to uterine and cervical cells, resulting in anoxia to muscle fibers. This anoxia can cause pain in the same way that blockage of the cardiac arteries causes the pain of a heart attack. As labor progresses and contractions become longer and harder, the ischemia to cells increases, the anoxia increases, and the pain intensifies.

Another major source of pain is probably the stretching of the cervix and perineum. This phenomenon is the same as that causing intestinal pain when intestines are stretched by gas. At the end of the transitional point in labor, when stretching of the cervix is complete and the woman begins to feel she has to push, pain from the contractions often magically disappears as long as she is pushing, until the fetal presenting part causes the final stretching of the perineum.

Additional discomfort in labor may stem from the pressure of the presenting part of the fetus on tissues, including pressure on surrounding organs: the bladder, the urethra, and the lower colon. Pain at birth is largely from the stretching of the perineal tissue (Whelton, 1990).

Physiology of Pain

Pain is apparently transmitted by small-diameter nerve fibers. These small nerve fibers can be blocked by stimulation of large-diameter nerve fibers lying near them. This is why rubbing the skin (an almost involuntary action after stubbing a toe or bumping a knee) reduces the pain felt. Pain sensation may also be reduced by distracting the woman or by changing its meaning and interpretation for that particular person. The reduction of pain in labor by natural methods based on the Gating theory is described in Chapter 13.

Sensory impulses from the uterus and cervix synapse at the spinal column at the level of T-10, T-11, T-12, and L-1. Pain relief for the first stage of labor, therefore, must be either systemic relief or medication that blocks these upper synapse sites. For the elimination of pain during cesarean birth, T-6 to T-8 level receptors must be blocked.

Sensory impulses from the perineum are carried by the pudendal nerve to join the spinal column at S-2, S-3, and S-4. Pain relief for birth, therefore, when the perineum is initiating the pain, must be provided either systemically or regionally to block these lower receptor sites. This is an important point to remember when talking to women in labor about pain relief. Some interventions relieve pain for both the first *and* second stages of labor; others for first *or* second stage but not for both.

Perception of Pain

The amount of discomfort a woman experiences during contractions differs according to her expectations of and preparation for labor, the length of the labor, the posi-

tion of the fetus, and the availability of support people around her (Figure 19-1). The discomfort a woman experiences becomes compounded when fear and anxiety are also present. Green (1993) asked women during pregnancy how much pain they expected to experience during labor. Eighty-five percent of primiparas reported they anticipated pain to be "quite" to "unbearably" painful; only 2% said it would be "moderately" painful; no one said it would be pain-free.

Pain may be perceived differently by different individuals not only because of psychosocial responses but also because of physiologic responses. (See the Focus on Cultural Awareness box.) When the body experiences pain, it appears to produce opiate-like substances called **endorphins** to reduce that pain. The level of these naturally occurring substances, or the body's ability to produce and maintain them, may influence a person's overall pain threshold and the amount of pain a person perceives at any given time (Guyton, 1990).

Women who come into labor believing the pain will be horrible are usually surprised afterward to realize that the agony they expected never materialized. On the other hand, expectations of pain may make a woman so tense during labor that her pain is worse than it would be if she were relaxed. A woman cannot relax simply because she is instructed to do so by another person, however. Some additional intervention must be used.

Nursing Diagnoses and Related Interventions for Pain Relief During Labor

Nursing Diagnosis: Anxiety related to lack of knowledge about labor experience

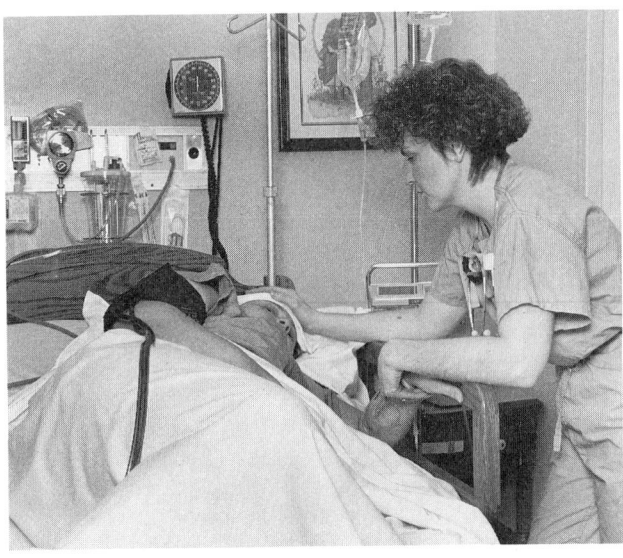

FIGURE 19-1
The discomfort a woman experiences during childbirth may be related to the amount of support she receives from her family or health care providers. (Courtesy, Department of Medical Photography, Children's Hospital, Buffalo, NY.)

Goal: Client will demonstrate good understanding of what is happening during her labor.

Outcome Criteria: Client identifies beginning and ending of contractions; expresses confidence rather than confusion about ongoing process.

In addition to causing local discomfort, pain can evoke a general stress response (a fight-or-flight syndrome). This releases epinephrine, which causes peripheral vasoconstriction. Because the uterus is a peripheral organ, it responds with vasoconstriction during epinephrine release. This may increase the degree of pain experienced as it increases tissue anoxia. Relieving pain, therefore, includes reducing anxiety by helping the woman to relax with planned breathing exercises, or by administration of medication that improves the blood supply to the uterus and reduces vasoconstriction.

Reduce Anxiety
With Explanations of Labor Process

Planning with women as to their options for pain relief during labor should begin prenatally (Fields & Wall, 1993; see the Focus on Family Teaching box). The reduction of pain in labor by natural methods based on

the gating theory is described in Chapter 13. Careful explanation of what is happening or what will happen once a woman begins labor goes a long way toward alleviating anxiety and thereby reducing some discomforts. To a nursing student, the process of explaining everything seems natural and comfortable because it is new to the student as well. However, after having cared for 100 women in labor, a nurse may explain things less and less often. The nurse may begin to assume that everyone knows that the rupturing of membranes is painless, that a pink-stained show is normal, and that contractions change in character during the pelvic division of labor. A woman having her first child, however, *does not know;* a woman having her second child *may not remember* or finds this time so different from the last time (even if it is well within normal limits) that she is frightened. Be certain to give explanations to the woman's husband or support person as well as to her. Otherwise, the support person may start to transmit anxiety back to the woman.

Women in labor relax best if they have a clear understanding that labor contractions are rhythmic in nature and come and go repeatedly, but when each contraction ends, unless the fetus is positioned posteriorly and causing continuous pressure in the woman's back, the woman's discomfort disappears. It seems that the woman should be aware of this since she is experiencing the contractions. She may be feeling so much pain, however, that she is not aware of relief between contractions; she may fear that things will worsen as labor progresses and that the pain will become continuous; she may tense with each contraction, dreading the unknown.

This on-off effect differentiates the pain of labor contractions from that of a toothache or headache, which is continuous. Just knowing that the pain will soon vanish can make even a high level of pain easier to tolerate.

> ***Nursing Diagnosis:*** Ineffective individual coping related to combination of uterine contractions and anxiety
>
> ***Goal:*** Client will be able to cope with labor experience through active participation in labor.
>
> ***Outcome Criteria:*** Client expresses confidence in her ability to maintain active participation during labor (e.g., continues breathing techniques; expresses need to change position) and expresses confidence in labor nurse and other health care providers.

Provide Comfort Measures

Anyone can stand a little discomfort from a backache. Anyone can stand being thirsty and having dry lips for a little while. Anyone can stand having a leg cramp. Few

FOCUS ON CULTURAL AWARENESS

Responses to pain are culturally determined. Based on this, some believe that being stoic and nonverbal is what is expected of them. Others believe that expressing their discomfort by screaming or actively verbalizing their feelings is "correct" behavior. If English is not a woman's primary language, it may be particularly difficult for her to describe her level of distress. Assess each woman individually to determine not only what level of comfort she feels is right for her during labor but also the manner in which she feels most able to express discomfort. Depend on facial expression, body posture and tension, as well as voiced expressions to determine the comfort level of a client.

The amount of analgesia that women desire or will accept is both situational and culturally determined. In a culture in which birth is seen as a "natural" process, less analgesia is generally desired. Kennel et al. (1991) investigated the effect of a continuous support person (a *doula*) on pain perception during labor. In this study, women with such a person present needed less epidural anesthesia for pain relief and had shortened labors. Providing support, therefore, can have a positive influence on pain relief in labor.

FOCUS ON FAMILY TEACHING

Q. I'm having my first baby and am worried I'll need some pharmacologic help with the pain of labor. How do I learn what is available and what are advantages and disadvantages of various methods?

A. One of the advantages of having a baby today is that a number of effective options for pain relief are available. There are several things you can do to learn more:

• Ask your obstetrician or nurse-midwife about options early in pregnancy. The options your care provider suggests may actually influence your decision as to whether this is the optimal care provider for you.

• Attend prepared childbirth classes during pregnancy and conscientiously practice breathing exercises. These measures can be adequate all by themselves; if not, they complement pharmacologic methods of pain relief.

• Late in pregnancy, if you are still concerned, let your primary care provider know. In addition to medication for pain relief during labor, medication to reduce anxiety is available.

• On admission to the hospital, let the medical and nursing staff know that you are concerned. The most commonly used options today are oral, intramuscular, or intravenous administration of narcotics and injection of regional anesthesia by epidural block. Ask questions about any method suggested that you do not understand.

• Be aware that the choice of receiving analgesia or anesthesia is yours to make. On the other hand, if a complication occurs, be ready to compromise in the interest of safety for yourself or your child.

people can tolerate having all of these discomforts simultaneously or feeling even one of them while experiencing labor contractions.

Provide the ordinary comfort measures to a woman in labor that are provided for anyone with pain. The woman will need ice chips to suck on to prevent feeling the additional discomfort of thirst, or perhaps a wet cloth to moisten her lips or moisturizing jelly to apply if her lips are dry during labor. She needs a cool cloth to wipe perspiration from her forehead.

Be aware of what is happening to the woman's bedclothes, which will wrinkle rapidly if she is uncomfortable and moving about a great deal. Her hospital gown also will wrinkle and stick to her skin because she is perspiring. The waterproof pad under her buttocks, soiled with vaginal secretions, will become hot and sticky. To avoid this happening, never apply sanitary pads in labor. Although they absorb vaginal secretions well, they tend to slip out of place and may carry pathogens from the rectal area forward to the vaginal opening. Instead, change the waterproof pad frequently. Halfway through the first stage of labor, change the sheets and give the woman a clean gown, so that she has a fresh, ready-to-go-again feeling. Think of comfort measures for the woman's support person as well. Is the chair by the side of the bed comfortable? Does he or she need to stretch or take a beverage or bathroom break? It

is hard for the support person to comfort the woman if he or she is uncomfortable from hours of sitting still in one position.

Nursing Diagnosis: Pain related to labor contractions

Goal: Client will be able to breathe through contractions or use other techniques (including pain medication) to reduce pain to tolerable level during labor and birth.

Outcome Criteria: Client states that she is able to handle or "work with" contractions; demonstrates ability to listen and respond to questions and instructions from nurse, physician, and support person.

Encourage Comfortable Positioning

An upright position during labor may not only be the most comfortable for the woman in early labor, but also promotes safety and the most efficient contractions. Before membranes have ruptured, therefore, a woman may be most comfortable either sitting in a chair or ambulating. After the membranes have ruptured, and if the fetal head is not engaged, there may be danger in walking about; the cord might prolapse and impede fetal circulation. If this is so, the woman should remain in bed. Urge her not to lie on her back in order to avoid supine hypotension syndrome.

Encouraging a change in position from time to time may well be the most important element of positioning. It is unlikely the woman will not initiate changes on her own, but assisting her to find a satisfying position by moving bedclothes or monitor leads, if any are attached, may help. If she wishes to walk and has no support person, walk with her. Pelvic rocking between contractions may relieve tense back muscles.

Position changes are also essential in the second stage of labor, and, depending on medical protocols and barring any medical contraindications, the woman might prefer to sit, stand, kneel on hands and knees, lie in dorsal recumbent or lateral recumbent positions, or squat. Keep in mind that maintaining these positions often requires assistance from one or two support people.

Assist Women With Prepared Childbirth Exercises

The best analgesia for labor is relaxation. Depending on the type of childbirth preparation the woman and her support person have had, the type of relaxation method used may include breathing exercises, distraction by focusing on an external object, acupressure, therapeutic touch, music therapy, guided imagery, self-hypnosis, or a combination of these methods (see Chapter 13). Biofeedback is not well documented in labor but may be effective. Help the woman who wishes to use prepared breathing patterns to apply them in labor. It is helpful to urge her to begin these early in labor even before contractions become painful. A woman can use less complicated breathing patterns early on, working into the more involved patterns as contractions intensify. It may be necessary to review previously learned breathing techniques with her, because it is easy to forget what was learned in a relaxed, fun setting while in the extreme discomfort and stress of labor. It is not essential for women to use complex breathing patterns in labor; even the woman who has had no prior training in breathing exercises can use a simple breathing pattern to alleviate discomfort with just a little guidance from the nurse. (See the Nursing Care Plan: A Woman Who Desires a Choice of Medication During Labor and Birth.)

Massage is another pain relief method that can be taught to a woman and her support person on the spot. It may be especially useful if the woman is experiencing back pain from labor. Rubbing or massaging the sacral area often alleviates back pain. Firm counterpressure on the lower back, thighs, feet, hands, or shoulders can provide a relaxing distraction from the sensation of internal pressure and pain.

Provide Pharmacologic Pain Relief

Pharmacologic management of pain during labor and birth includes **analgesia**, which reduces or decreases

awareness of pain, and **anesthesia**, which provides for partial or complete loss of sensation. A short-acting narcotic such as fentanyl (Sublimaze) may be administered in combination with a local anesthetic as an additional pain prevention measure. This increases the rate at which action from the anesthetic is achieved. The addition of fentanyl also allows for less local anesthetic to be necessary, and thus can increase the ability of the woman to push effectively during the second stage of labor.

Helping the woman decide if and when medication should be given requires an in-depth understanding of the available drugs, their effects on the mother and the fetus, and their mechanism and duration of action. It also requires sympathetic listening and counseling skills. Many women come into labor wishing to avoid drugs entirely. They may change their minds once in labor but hesitate to say so, especially if their partners also felt that a birth without the use of drugs was ideal. Other women may come into labor asking to receive something immediately to avoid experiencing any pain. In both of these instances, it is important to provide information about the use of drugs and their ultimate effects but also to maintain a supportive presence to help the woman make the best decision for herself and her baby. Some women require analgesia or anesthesia because a complication of labor develops. Helping these women and their support person to understand why the medication is necessary calls for equal care and skill (Figure 19-2).

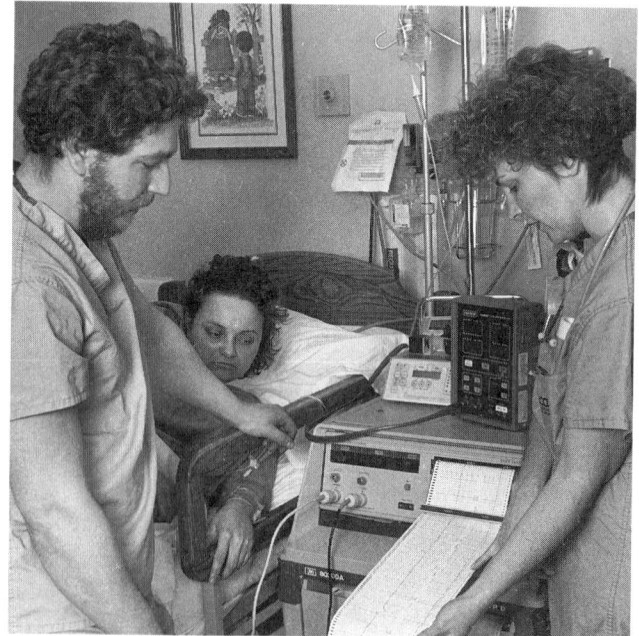

FIGURE 19-2
A support person needs to be oriented to equipment the same as the woman herself to help relieve anxiety. (Courtesy, Department of Medical Photography, Children's Hospital, Buffalo, NY.)

Provide Instructions Regarding Other Available Methods of Pain Relief

Hydrotherapy during early labor may be an effective method of pain relief (Aderhold et al., 1991; see Chapter 13). **Transcutaneous electrical nerve stimulation** (TENS) is yet another method. Two pairs of electrodes are taped to the woman's back to coincide with the T10–L1 nerve pathways. Low-intensity electrical stimulation is given continuously or applied by the woman herself as a contraction begins. This stimulation blocks the afferent fibers, or prevents pain from traveling to the spinal cord synapses from the uterus. As labor progresses and the pelvic division begins, the electrodes are moved to stimulate the S2–4 level. High-intensity stimulation is generally needed to control the pain at this stage.

TENS can be an effective method of pain relief in labor and has no known fetal effects, but because many women object to being "tied down" to monitors, they may object to TENS equipment. Women with extreme back pain during labor may benefit the most from a TENS unit, because this type of pain is difficult to relieve with controlled breathing exercises. TENS is discussed further in Chapter 20.

Medication for Pain Relief During Labor

Virtually all medication given during labor crosses the placenta and has some effect on the fetus. Thus, it is important that a woman receive as little medication as possible during labor. On the other hand, labor should not test a woman to the limit of her endurance. She is in labor to be a mother, not a martyr. Caution women not to take acetylsalicylic acid (aspirin) for pain in labor. Aspirin interferes with blood coagulation and thus can lead to increased bleeding in the newborn or mother.

History of Pain Management in Labor

The pattern of intervention to manage pain in labor has swung from a philosophy of no intervention (none given) to a philosophy of drug intervention as an essential element (too much given) to a modern approach of empowering women and their partners with information so they can decide how to best relieve pain during labor, within the limits of medical safety. For centuries, in Western civilization, offering pain relief in labor was thought to be amoral because, according to the Biblical account, God commanded Eve, "I will greatly multiply thy sorrow and thy conception; in sorrow thou shalt bring forth children . . ." (Genesis 3:16). In the witch-burning period in American history, the concept that childbirth should be painful was so strongly ingrained that women were burned as witches for providing comfort to other women in labor.

With the discovery of ether and chloroform in the 1800s, it became apparent that childbirth could be managed completely pain free. Unfortunately, this goal was achieved by means of complete anesthesia or unconsciousness during labor and birth. In 1847, Sir James Simpson described the first time a woman was delivered under chloroform: "Shortly after her infant was brought in by the nurse from the adjoining room, it was a matter of no small difficulty to convince the astonished mother that labor was entirely over and the child presented to her was really her own living baby" (Lichtiger & Moya, 1978). Aside from the physiologic risk to women from general anesthesia, this inability to accept the event of birth, to change from "being pregnant" to "being a mother" is a major disadvantage of general anesthesia or too much intervention in childbirth.

Goals of Pharmacologic Management of Pain During Labor

Effective medication for use during labor must relax the woman and relieve her discomfort, yet have minimal systemic effects on her uterine contractions, her pushing effort, or the fetus. Whether a drug affects the fetus depends on its ability to cross the placenta. Drugs with a molecular weight of more than 1000 cross poorly; those with a molecular weight of less than 600 cross very readily. Drugs with highly charged molecules or molecules that are strongly bound to protein cross more slowly than others; fat-soluble drugs cross most easily. A preterm fetus, which has an immature liver and is unable to metabolize or inactivate drugs, is generally more affected by drugs than a term fetus. If a drug causes a systemic response such as hypotension in the woman, it can cause a decreased PO_2 gradient across the placenta and fetal hypoxia. If it causes confusion or disorientation in the woman, she may be unable to work effectively with labor and labor may be prolonged. If a medication causes changes in the fetus such as a decreased heart rate or central nervous system (CNS) depression so that it is difficult for the newborn infant to initiate respirations at birth, the infant could be severely compromised in the important first minutes of life.

Once labor is well under way, medication to relieve discomfort can speed its progress because the woman is able to work with, not against, contractions. Medication given too early, however, tends to slow or even stop labor contractions. As a rule, do not give an analgesic to a primipara before she is dilated at least 5 cm; a multipara should be dilated 3 cm before receiving analgesia. Because pain is a subjective sensation, women experience different levels during labor. Some women are most aware of pain early in labor; some report the second stage of labor as the most difficult. The point at

A Woman Who Desires a Choice of Medication During Labor and Birth

Danita Conte is a 23-year-old woman (gravida 2; para 0) you care for in labor. Her cervical dilatation is 2 cm; effacement is 70%.

Assessment: Client states, "I don't want any drugs for labor or delivery." Last ate 2 hours ago (roast beef, potatoes, Jello). Has lollipops with her to suck on during labor. Knowledgeable of Lamaze method for control of discomfort in labor; husband will be support person and coach. Using breathing exercises effectively with contractions. Focuses on photograph at foot of bed for distraction.

Nursing Diagnosis: High risk for pain related to labor contractions.

Defining Characteristic: Labor contractions are likely to cause some degree of discomfort.

Goal: Client will complete labor and birth experiencing tolerable level of discomfort.

Outcome Criteria: Client states pain is at tolerable level; responds to questions and instructions from husband and others.

Nursing Orders	*Rationale*
1. Provide comfort measures such as back massage, change of sheets, etc.	1. Simple comfort measures are helpful in relieving anxiety associated with pain.
2. Support breathing pattern efforts as needed.	2. Interrupting breathing patterns can make them ineffective as a means of controlling pain in labor.
3. Respect necessity to focus during contractions (do not block vision).	3. Interrupting focusing can make the technique ineffective as a means of controlling pain in labor.
4. Reassure client that her wishes for the amount of medication desired will be respected.	4. Client needs to know that she has some control over the childbirth experience and that you respect her decisions.
5. Offer husband relief as desired from role as coach.	5. As labor can be a long process, coaches need periodic relief.

(continued)

which pain medication is needed, therefore, also differs from one individual to another. Unfortunately, there is no perfect analgesic agent for labor or birth that has no effect on labor, the mother, and the fetus.

Preparation for Medication Administration

Medications used during labor vary among different health care agencies and the effectiveness of new drugs is constantly being explored. Thus, it is impractical to memorize a list of drugs that are safe. It is better to remember the criteria that a drug must fulfill to be used in labor and expand the rule of basic medication administration from "Never give any drug unless you know it is safe for your individual client" to "Never give a drug in labor without knowing it is safe for both your clients: the mother and the fetus."

The analgesia and anesthetic preparations frequently used in labor and birth are shown in Table 19-1.

A woman should be well prepared for the type of anesthetic she will receive during labor and birth in terms of how the anesthetic will be administered (e.g., "You'll need to lie on your side") and what she can expect to happen following administration (e.g., "I'll be taking your blood pressure frequently.") Women in labor are under stress. Experiencing surprising body sensations without preparation can be frightening and may defeat an individual's coping abilities. When a person struggles against anesthetic administration because she does not understand what is going on, risks of anesthesia increase.

Narcotic Analgesics

Narcotics are drugs often given in labor because of their potent analgesic effect. As a category, all these drugs cause fetal CNS depression and need to be questioned when ordered for a woman in preterm labor. A preterm

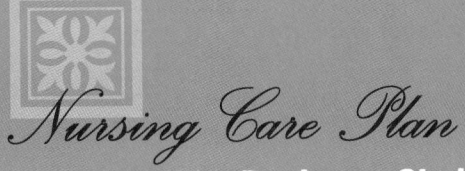

Nursing Care Plan

A Woman Who Desires a Choice of Medication During Labor and Birth (continued)

Interim Assessment: Client asked for epidural block; administered at 3:30 p.m. Client stated afterward, "I don't feel a thing. Is anything still happening?" Client voices fear of baby being "stuck" inside her because she no longer feels contractions. Blood pressure has remained at 124/88 since anesthesia injection. Appears noticeably tense; startles at sound of young girl in next labor room crying.

Nursing Diagnosis: Anxiety related to inability to feel contraction secondary to epidural anesthetic.

Defining Characteristic: Client appears tense and asks why she has no feeling of contractions.

Goal: Client will express confidence with progress of labor.

Outcome Criteria: Client states satisfaction with medication chosen and demonstrates ability to carry out instruction given by nurse, husband, and others.

Nursing Orders	Rationale
1. Assure client that dilation is progressing; help her note uterine contractions on monitor.	1. Client needs to be informed that her contractions are continuing, but she just can't feel them.
2. Support husband as necessary and keep him informed of progress.	2. The client relies on him to remain calm.
3. Assess blood pressure, pulse, and respirations every 15 min per protocol.	3. Hypotension is a side-effect of epidural anesthesia.
4. Encourage client to lie on left side.	4. Reduces possibility of supine hypotensive syndrome.

Interim Assessment: Client had 8 lb, 5 oz male at 5:15 P.M. Client states labor was not "as bad as expected"; happy that she had epidural anesthesia as this let her "enjoy last half."

infant may have extreme difficulty enduring the added insult of respiratory depression.

Narcotic analgesics commonly used are meperidine hydrochloride (Demerol), morphine sulfate, nalbuphine (Nubain), fentanyl (Sublimaze), and butorphanol tartrate (Stadol). Meperidine is advantageous as an analgesic in labor because it has additional sedative and antispasmodic actions. Thus, it is effective in relieving pain and also helps to relax the cervix and give a feeling of euphoria and well-being. Demerol may be given either intramuscularly or intravenously. The dose is 25 mg to 100 mg depending on the woman's weight and route of administration. Action begins in about 30 minutes after intramuscular injection and about 5 minutes after intravenous administration; duration of action is 2 to 3 hours (Loeb, 1993).

Because Demerol crosses the placenta, it may cause depression in the fetus. The drug crosses the placenta minutes after being administered to the mother. The fetal liver takes 2 to 3 hours to activate the drug in the fetal system, however, so the effect will not be registered in the fetus for 2 to 3 hours after administration. For this reason, Demerol is given when the mother is more than 3 hours away from birth (allowing the peak action time of the drug in the fetus to have passed by the time of birth). It may be puzzling to see a sleepy baby delivered to a woman who was given Demerol 2 hours before birth and an alert baby delivered to a woman who had Demerol within 1 hour of birth. In the second instance, the peak action or peak effect has not yet occurred in the infant. This newborn needs careful assessment for the next 4 hours until the drug does peak. Demerol may be self-administered by a patient-controlled analgesic pump for low-dose but frequent administration during labor (see the Focus on Nursing Research box). It may be administered intrathecally (injected into the cerebral spinal fluid), although this method is not successful with all women.

Table 19-1. *Analgesics and Anesthetics Commonly Used in Labor and Birth*

Type	Drug	Usual Dosage/Route	Effect on Mother	Effect on Labor Progress	Effect on Fetus or Newborn
Narcotic analgesic	Meperidine (Demerol)	25 mg IV, 50–100 mg IM q3–4 h; also epidurally	Effective analgesic; feeling of well-being	Relaxation may aid progress during cervical relaxation. Will halt labor contractions if given too early	Should be given 3 h away from delivery to avoid respiratory depression in newborn
	Nalbuphine (Nubain)	10 mg IM q3–6 h, 0.3–3 mg/kg over 10–15 min IV	Slows respiratory rate; effective analgesic	Causes mild maternal sedation	Some respiratory depression may occur
	Pentazocine HCl (Talwin)	30 mg q 3–4 h IM; 50 mg q 3–4 h orally	Do not mix in same syringe with barbiturate		
	Butorphanol (Stadol)	1–2 mg IM or IV q 3–4 h	Causes withdrawal symptoms if woman is opiate-dependent	Will possibly slow labor if given too early	Some respiratory depression
	Morphine sulfate	8–15 mg IM or 1–2 mg IV; also epidurally	Nausea and vomiting, slows respiratory rate; effective analgesia	Will slow labor if given too early	Respiratory depression may occur
	Fentanyl (sublimaze)	50–100 µg IM or 25–50 µg IV; also epidurally	Hypotension; respiratory depression	Will slow labor if given too early	Respiratory depression may occur
Lumbar epidural block	Local anesthetic	Administered for first stage of labor; with continuous block, anesthesia will last through delivery; injected into epidural space at L3–4	Rapid onset in minutes; lasts 60–90 min; loss of pain perception for labor contractions and delivery; possible maternal hypotension	Will slow labor if given too early; obliterates pushing feeling, so that second stage may be prolonged	May be some differences in response in first few days of life
Pudendal block	Local anesthetic	Administered just before delivery for perineal anesthesia; injected through vagina	Rapid anesthesia of perineum	None apparent	None apparent
Local infiltration of perineum	Local anesthetic	Injected just before delivery for episiotomy incision	Anesthesia of perineum almost immediately	None apparent	None apparent
General intravenous anesthetic	Thiopental	Administered IV by anesthesiologist	Rapid anesthesia; also rapid recovery	Forceps required, since abdominal pushing is no longer possible	Infant will be born depressed

(Adapted from Loeb, S. [1993]. *Nurse's handbook of drug therapy.* Springhouse, PA: Springhouse.)

Nalbuphine hydrochloride, butorphanol tartrate, and pentazocine hydrochloride (Talwin) are synthetic narcotic analgesics also used extensively in labor. The action of these is comparable to that of Demerol. Like Demerol, they may also leave a degree of respiratory depression in the newborn.

Whenever a narcotic is given during labor, a narcotic antagonist such as naloxone (Narcan) should be available for administration to the infant at birth. The dose is 0.1 mg/kg administered into the umbilical vein (Cunningham et al., 1993). If severe infant respiratory depression is suspected, Narcan can be given to the mother just before birth. It crosses the placenta readily and may increase the chance for spontaneous respiratory activity, because it interferes with or competes for narcotic binding sites. Observe carefully an infant who receives Narcan in the immediate birth period, because when the Narcan effect wears off, the infant's respirations may become severely depressed again.

Sedative-Hypnotics and Ataractics

Additional drugs such as secobarbital sodium (Seconal) may be administered to encourage rest in a woman who

FOCUS ON NURSING RESEARCH

Does Intramuscular or Intravenous Meperidine Provide Better Pain Relief in Labor?

To answer this question, two nursing researchers designed a study in which a control group of 20 women in labor were offered meperidine intramuscularly and an experimental group of 19 women received meperidine intravenously by a patient-controlled analgesia pump. All women were assessed as being low-risk with singleton, term pregnancies. Women were asked to rate the degree of pain they were experiencing during labor by a 10-point Visual Analogue Scale every 10 minutes during labor.

Results of the study showed that women who received the intravenous meperidine reported significantly less pain in labor. There were no differences in accompanying measures such as length of labor or the Apgar scores of their infants. The researchers recommend that nurses advocate for intravenous meperidine administration for pain relief during labor.

Isenor, L., & Penny-MacGillivray, T. (1993). Intravenous meperidine infusions for obstetric analgesia. *Journal of Obstetric, Gynecologic and Neonatal Nursing, 22,* 349.

is becoming exhausted by labor. An ataractic such as promethazine (Phenergan) may be administered to decrease anxiety and complement the action of a narcotic.

Regional Anesthesia

Regional anesthesia is the injection of a local anesthetic to block specific nerve pathways. It achieves pain relief by blocking sodium and potassium flux in the nerve membrane, thereby stabilizing the nerve in a polarized resting state so it is unable to conduct sensations.

Depending on the region anesthetized, a woman may or may not continue to be aware of contractions following administration of such anesthesia. Injection sites of various regional anesthetic procedures are shown in Figure 19-3. Because women with preeclampsia may have associated bleeding defects, they need to be assessed carefully prior to regional anesthesia (Albright et al., 1991).

Because regional anesthetics are not introduced into the maternal circulation, it was once believed they had no effect on the fetus. However, it has been demonstrated that there is some uptake of these drugs by the fetus (possibly resulting in symptoms of flaccidity, bradycardia, hypotension, and convulsions in the newborn; Loeb, 1993). Effects on the fetus are minimal compared with those of systemic anesthetic agents, however; most important, they allow the woman to be

completely awake and aware of what is happening during birth. Because regional anesthetics do not depress uterine tone, they leave the uterus capable of optimal contraction after birth, which is an important concern in the prevention of postpartal hemorrhage.

It is rare that an infant is born with symptoms of toxicity from a regional anesthetic, but if so, an exchange transfusion at birth will remove the anesthetic from the bloodstream. Gastric lavage will also remove a great deal of anesthetic, because anesthetics have a strong affinity for acid mediums such as stomach acid.

Epidural Anesthesia (Peridural Blocks)

The spinal nerves in the cord are protected by a number of layers of tissue. The *pia mater* is the membrane adhering to the nerve fibers; surrounding this is the *cerebral spinal fluid* (*CSF*); next comes the *arachnoid membrane* and outside that, the *dura mater.* Outside the dura mater is a vacant space (the *epidural space*), and beyond it is the *ligamentum flavum,* yet another protective shield to the vulnerable spinal cord.

An anesthetic agent introduced into the area of the CSF (the subarachnoid space) is called a *spinal* injection or spinal anesthesia. An anesthetic placed just inside the ligamentum flavum in the epidural space is an *epidural anesthesia* (see Figure 19-3). Anesthetic agents placed in the epidural space block not only spinal nerve roots in the space but also the sympathetic nerve fibers that travel with them. Such a block, therefore, provides pain relief for both labor and birth. Such a block may actually increase contraction strength and blood flow to the uterus: because the woman no longer experiences pain, the release of catecholamines (epinephrine) with a beta-blocking effect from a pain response is decreased.

"Spinal headaches" occur rarely after epidural anesthesia, because those headaches are caused by leakage of CSF or the instillation of air into CSF; the CSF space is not entered with this technique.

Advantages. Epidural blocks are commonly used for many women in labor. They are advantageous for women with heart disease, pulmonary disease, diabetes, and sometimes severe pregnancy-induced hypertension, because they make labor virtually pain free and stress from the discomfort of labor is minimal. Because the woman does not feel contractions, her physical energy is preserved. Epidural blocks are acceptable for use in preterm labor because the drug has scant effect on the fetus. They allow for a controlled and gentle birth with less trauma to an immature fetal skull. Because the woman receives no systemic medication, the infant responds more quickly after birth than if narcotic analgesics are used.

Disadvantages. The chief problem with epidural anesthesia is its tendency to induce hypotension in the

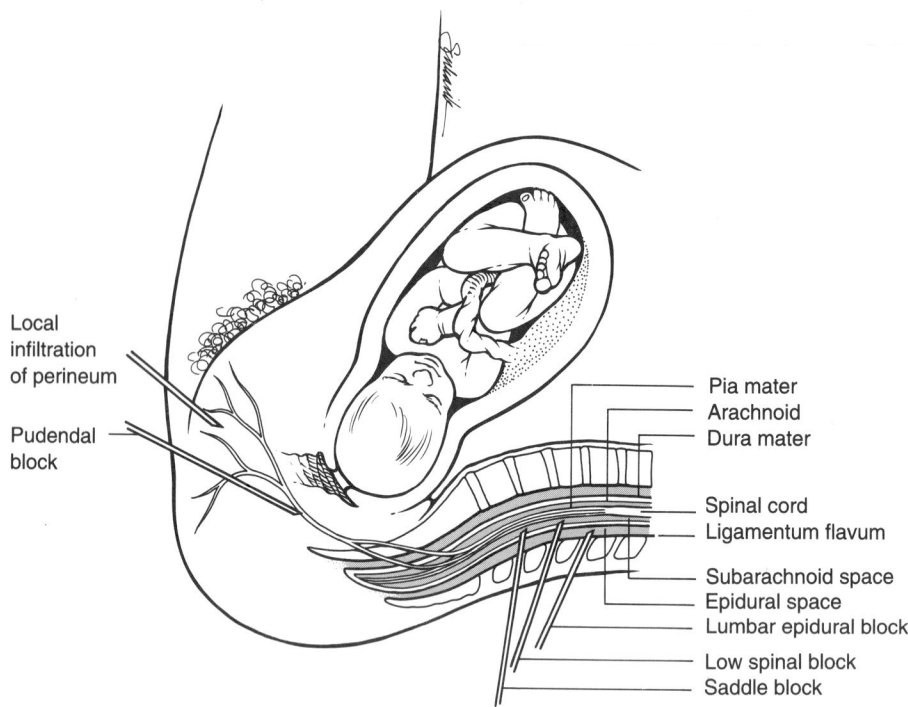

FIGURE 19-3
Anatomy of the spinal canal and sites of injection for regional anesthesia.

woman because of its blocking effect on the sympathetic fibers in the epidural space. This blocking leads to decreased peripheral resistance in the woman's circulatory system; blood flows freely into peripheral vessels and a pseudohypovolemia registering as hypotension occurs. This can be largely prevented by ensuring that the woman is well hydrated before the anesthetic is given (has received 500–1000 mL of intravenous fluid); a goal usually achieved by infusion of a solution such as Ringer's lactate. This is preferable to a glucose solution, because too much maternal glucose can cause hyperglycemia with rebound hypoglycemia in the newborn. Be certain that the woman does not lie supine but remains on her side after an epidural to prevent supine hypotension syndrome.

If hypotension does occur, raising the woman's legs and administering oxygen and intravenous fluid and a drug such as ephedrine to elevate blood pressure may be necessary to stabilize cardiovascular status. If a reaction is so severe that convulsions occur, small amounts of short-acting barbiturates or diazepam (Valium) will control these. Such reactions are rare but should be considered when caring for women in labor who receive large amounts of regional anesthetics.

In addition, the second stage of labor may be prolonged by the use of an epidural block, because the woman, unaware of contractions, does not push with them, which slows descent (e.g., taking 3 hours rather than 2 hours). This leads to a greater need for vacuum

extraction or cesarean birth. Yet another problem is that relaxation of the levator ani muscle may impede internal rotation of the fetal head and further slow labor or make it necessary for forceps to be used to effect rotation (O'Grady & Youngstrom, 1990). This occurs especially if the fetus is in an occiput-posterior position. Allowing an epidural to wear off by the second stage of labor so the woman can push with contractions is an option to try to avoid these problems. Experiencing contractions at this point, however, can be overwhelming for the woman and counteracts the original reason for giving the anesthetic. Oxytocin may be given to shorten labor.

Technique for Administration. Lumbar epidural anesthesia is begun when the cervix is dilated 4 cm to 6 cm. An intravenous infusion and equipment for blood pressure monitoring should be in place (Figure 19-4). The woman is positioned on her side or sitting upright. Her back should not be flexed because this increases the possibility the dura will be punctured and the anesthetic will accidentally be given as spinal, not epidural, anesthesia. The lumbar area of her back is cleaned with an antiseptic solution. A local anesthetic is injected into the skin to form a wheal over the L3–4 vertebra. A special 3-inch to 5-inch needle is then passed through the L3–4 space into the epidural space. After needle placement, a polyethylene catheter is passed through the needle into the space and the needle is then withdrawn, leaving the catheter to be taped in place. A closed system (a syringe

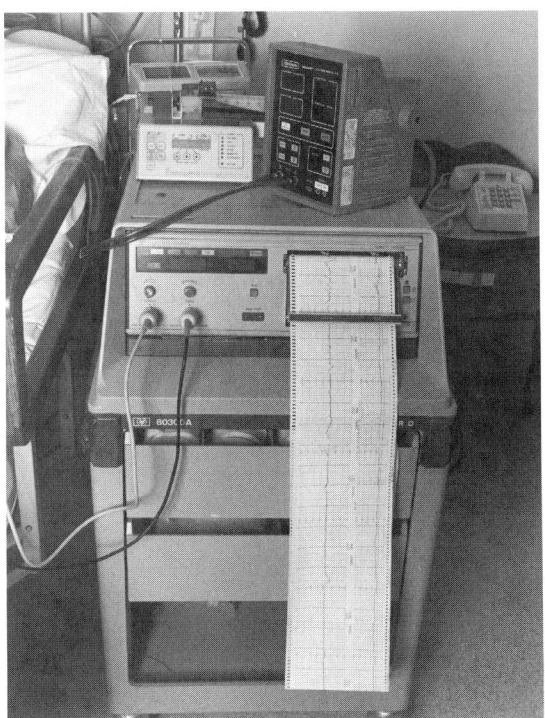

FIGURE 19-4
Equipment necessary for a continuous epidural infusion includes an electronic blood pressure monitor, a Holter pump for the infusion, uterine and fetal heart monitors, and an intravenous infusion. (Courtesy, Department of Medical Photography, Children's Hospital, Buffalo, NY.)

is attached) is established to prevent infection through the catheter.

A small test dose of a local anesthetic solution is injected through the catheter. Five minutes later, the woman's legs are inspected for flushing and warmness, evidence that the anesthetic is in the epidural space (peripheral dilatation is beginning). Assess the woman's pulse and blood pressure. If the anesthetic was accidentally placed in a blood vessel, toxic symptoms of hypotension, nervousness, and rapid pulse would be present. Following assurance that the anesthetic is epidural, an initial dose of anesthetic is then given through the catheter. This produces anesthesia up to the level of the umbilicus in 10 to 15 minutes. The effect of the anesthetic is unfortunately short-lived (40 minutes to 2 hours). Periodically, another dose of anesthetic, termed a "top-up," must be administered or additional anesthetic may be continually infused by an infusion pump to keep the woman free from discomfort (Chestnut et al., 1990; MacDonald, 1992). Self-administration of additional boluses may be effective (Gordon et al., 1994).

Slow absorption of the drug into the maternal circulation may result in toxic reactions of drowsiness, loss of coordination, slurred speech or nervousness, and anxiety. Before an additional top-up dose is administered,

the woman should be asked to both write and say out loud a phrase such as "I can do it" three times. If she is unable to do this (lack of fine motor coordination and slurred speech), the dose needs to be questioned.

Epidural anesthesia may also be given in a "segmented" fashion. With this technique, after the test dose, only a small dose (about 4 mL) is given. This provides anesthesia for uterine contractions but not perineal relaxation. Close to birth, if the woman sits up and an additional dose is given, perineal anesthesia will result. Leaving the lower anesthesia for late in labor this way allows for better internal rotation of the fetal head, because the perineal muscle is not lax and there is less chance that forceps for rotation will be necessary.

A nurse should be in continuous attendance when an epidural anesthetic is given. To detect hypotension, blood pressure should be taken every 2 minutes for the first 20 minutes after each new injection of anesthetic (Figure 19-4). Blood pressure should be monitored throughout the time the anesthetic is in effect to be certain the systolic pressure does not fall below 100 mm Hg or decrease 20 mm Hg in a hypertensive woman. The magnitude of a greater drop than this may be life-threatening to the fetus unless prompt, effective corrective measures such as repositioning and administering an antihypotensive are undertaken. If such measures are instituted quickly, fetal outcome will not be compromised. Epidural anesthesia may cause a temporary elevation in temperature (Vinson et al., 1993), which needs to be kept in mind when the woman's temperature is evaluated.

With an epidural block, the woman loses sensation of her bladder filling. Remind the woman to void every 2 hours, and monitor intake and output carefully and observe and palpate for bladder distention. She cannot walk to the bathroom owing to loss of motor control in her lower extremities. Nursing responsibilities for epidural anesthesia are summarized in Table 19-2.

Medication for Pain Relief During Birth

Pain during birth is caused by stretching of the perineum. The simplest form of pain relief for birth is the natural **pressure anesthesia** that results from the fetal head pressing against the stretched perineum. This natural anesthesia is often adequate to allow an episiotomy to be performed without concern that the woman will feel the cut. The pain she experiences as the fetal head is born, although intense and hot, is not particularly unpleasant, occurs suddenly, and is quickly over. After the hours of hard contractions the woman has come through, this flash of pain may seem almost too easy to be real. For some women, however, additional medication may be needed to reduce the pain of birth.

Table 19-2. *Nursing Responsibilities With Epidural Anesthetic Administration During Labor*

Action	Rationale
Prepare woman for procedure.	Women need to know what the procedure consists of in order to sign for informed consent.
Establish a fluid line and administer a fluid bolus of 500 to 1000 mL of intravenous fluid.	Increasing the fluid volume can help decrease the possibility of hypotension, a frequent complication due to peripheral vasodilatation.
Attach a continuous blood pressure cuff.	Frequent monitoring of blood pressure and pulse is necessary to detect hypotension.
Assist the anesthesiologist with positioning the woman and injection of the local anesthetic, while providing support to the woman as she undergoes a potentially frightening procedure.	Women are positioned side-lying or sitting upright. Fear of medication injection is common.
Assist the anesthesiologist with evaluating whether the catheter is placed appropriately in the epidural space.	A test dose of anesthetic administered into the catheter should produce lower extremity flushing and a feeling of warmth from vasodilatation. If catheter is inadvertently placed below dura, paralysis of lower extremities will occur; if in bloodstream, extreme symptoms of confusion will occur.
Remain with woman to evaluate that pain relief is adequate	Pain relief occurs in 10–15 min. Occasionally, epidural anesthesia fails to have an effect.
Keep woman positioned on left side to prevent supine hypotension syndrome.	Hypotension is a potential problem throughout the procedure.
Help woman to see that labor is progressing despite her loss of pain sensation by teaching about uterine monitor.	Provide active support and education.
Monitor for bladder filling, since woman will have decreased ability to detect bladder filling.	A full bladder can interfere with fetal descent and possibly cause bladder injury.
Help woman with effective second-stage pushing efforts.	This may be difficult due to loss of sensation.
Evaluate whether couple is satisfied with epidural anesthesia as a means of pain relief in labor.	Evaluation helps both consumers and health care providers to advance the number of options for pain relief in labor.

Local Anesthetics

Pudendal Nerve Block

A **pudendal nerve block** (Figure 19-5) is the injection of a local anesthetic into the right and left pudendal nerves at the level of the ischial spine. The injection is made through the vagina with the woman in a lithotomy or dorsal recumbent position. It provides relief of perineal pain during birth. Anesthesia achieved with this method is sufficiently deep to allow the use of low forceps during birth and an episiotomy repair. Although the injection is only a local one, the fetal heart rate and the mother's blood pressure should be checked immediately following the injection in case maternal hypotension occurs. The onset of a pudendal nerve block takes 2 to 10 minutes; the effect lasts for approximately 60 minutes.

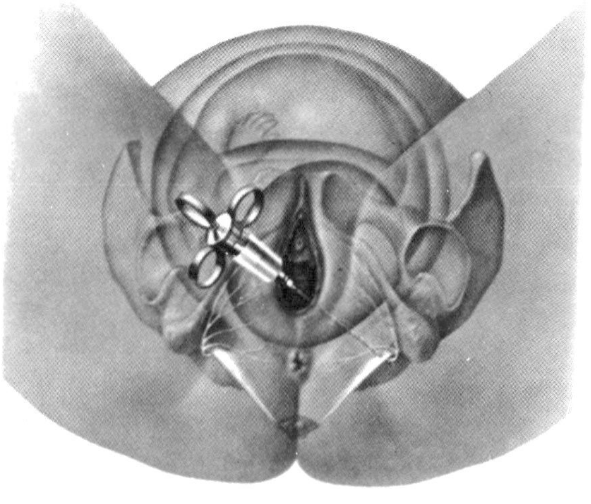

Local Infiltration

Local infiltration is the injection of an anesthetic such as lidocaine (Xylocaine) into the superficial nerves of the perineum by the placement of the anesthetic along the borders of the vulva. Local infiltration is used for episiotomy incision and repair.

Spinal Anesthesia

Spinal anesthesia is rarely used today in preference to lumbar epidural blocks. It may be used, however, in an emergency, since the administration technique is simpler than that of an epidural and can be accomplished more rapidly.

For spinal anesthesia, a local anesthetic agent such as bupivacaine (Marcaine) is injected using lumbar puncture technique into the subarachnoid space (into

FIGURE 19-5
Pudendal nerve block. (From Clinical Education Aid, No. 17, Ross Laboratories, Columbus, OH, with permission.)

the CSF) at the third or fourth lumbar interspace. For administration, the woman is placed in a sitting position on the side of the delivery table. She is asked to bend her head forward so her back curves and the intravertebral spaces open. She needs to be supported in this position, since she is "front-heavy" by her pregnancy and could easily fall forward if not well supported.

The skin over the lumbar vertebrae is cleaned and the skin is then anesthetized. Following this, a spinal needle is inserted through the anesthetized area, a few drops of CSF are allowed to drip from the needle to prove that the needle is in the subarachnoid space, and then the anesthetic is injected. The anesthetic normally reaches the level of T10. Anesthesia up to the umbilicus and including both legs will be achieved.

Spinal anesthetic agents may be "loaded" or "weighted" with glucose to make them heavier than CSF. This helps prevent them from rising too high in the spinal canal and interfering with the motor control of the uterus or with respiratory muscles. Following injection of the anesthetic, the anesthesiologist asks the woman to lie down again. It is important that she does lie down at this time, because if she sits up too long, the anesthetic will not rise high enough in the canal to achieve pain relief. On the other hand, she must not lie down before this time or the anesthetic will rise too high in the canal. Lying with a pillow under her head also helps assure that the anesthesia will be confined to the lower spinal canal.

The major complication with spinal anesthesia that can occur immediately after administration is hypotension from sympathetic blockage in the lower extremities, which leads to vasodilation and a fall in central blood pressure. If hypotension occurs, placental blood perfusion will be compromised. Turn the woman to her left side to reduce vena cava compression. The anesthesiologist will quickly increase the rate of intravenous fluid to increase blood volume; a vasopressor to increase blood pressure and oxygen may be given. Do not place a woman in a Trendelenburg position after spinal anesthesia is given in order to help restore blood pressure; this could make the anesthetic rise high in her spinal column and stop uterine contractions or respiratory function.

In order to guard against hypotension, women are administered intravenous fluid such as lactated Ringer's prior to the injection so they are fully hydrated. Be certain this is flowing well before the anesthesia administration.

A late complication of spinal anesthesia is "spinal headache." This occurs because of leakage of spinal fluid from the needle insertion and possibly from the irritation of a small amount of air that enters at the injection site. The shift in the pressure of CSF on the cerebral meninges initiates pain. The incidence of such headaches is reduced if a small-gauge needle is used for the injection and the woman remains flat in bed for 8 to 12

hours after giving birth (so any air present will not rise to the cerebral meninges), and she drinks a quantity of fluid. A high fluid intake provides fluid for replacement of spinal fluid most rapidly. Be certain the woman understands that she must remain flat, not merely remain in bed (only a flat pillow allowed), and drinking a lot of fluid means drinking about 3000 mL per day.

If a headache occurs, it can be relieved by lying flat again. Administration of an analgesic can be helpful. Some women find a cold cloth to their forehead helpful. If a headache is incapacitating, it can be treated with a blood patch technique. For this, 10 mL of blood is withdrawn from the woman's arm and then immediately injected into the epidural space over the spinal injection site. The blood injected then clots and seals off any further leakage of CSF.

General Anesthesia

General anesthesia administration is never preferred for childbirth, because it carries the dangers of hypoxia and possible inhalation of vomitus during administration (Cunningham et al., 1993). Pregnant women are particularly prone to gastric reflux because of increased stomach pressure from the pressure of the full uterus beneath it. The gastroesophageal valve may be displaced also and so may not be functioning properly. Despite these risks, general anesthesia may be necessary in emergency situations such as an abruptio placenta requiring an immediate cesarean birth.

For complete and rapid anesthesia during childbirth, thiopental sodium (Pentothal), a short-acting barbiturate, is usually the drug of choice. Pentothal causes rapid induction of anesthesia and minimal postpartal bleeding. After induction with Pentothal, the woman is intubated and anesthesia is then generally maintained by nitrous oxide and oxygen. Pentothal crosses the placenta rapidly. Infants born of a woman anesthetized by this method, therefore, may be slow to respond at birth and may need resuscitation. However, in view of the degree of barbiturate intoxication demonstrable in the infant, his or her ability to respond and alertness at birth are always surprising.

All women who receive a general anesthesia must be observed closely in the postpartum period because of the possibility of uterine atony and hemorrhage. Most gases used for general anesthesia cause uterine relaxation, thereby reducing effective contractions and hemostasis postpartum.

Preparation for the Safe Administration of General Anesthesia

A delivery room or birthing room should be checked before every birth to be certain that adequate equipment is available for the safe administration of anesthetic agents.

The anesthesiologist needs a minimum of six drugs

readily available: (1) ephedrine, to use in the event blood pressure falls; (2) atropine sulfate, to dry oral and respiratory secretions to prevent aspiration; (3) thiopental sodium, for rapid induction of a general anesthetic in an emergency; (4) succinylcholine, to achieve laryngeal relaxation for intubation in an emergency; (5) diazepam, to control convulsions, a possible reaction to anesthetics; and (6) isoproterenol, to reduce bronchospasm if aspiration should occur. In addition to these medications, an adult laryngoscope, endotracheal tube, a breathing bag with a source of 100% oxygen, and a suction catheter and suction source should be at hand.

Although the anesthesiologist checks these supplies because they are such important safeguards of the mother's health, particularly the suction and oxygen sources, it is also a nursing responsibility to make sure they are all available.

Aspiration of Vomitus

Anesthesia is the fifth most common cause of death in childbirth (after hemorrhage, infection, pregnancy-induced hypertension, and heart disease). Half the obstetric deaths due to anesthesia are attributed to pneumonia resulting from the aspiration of gastric contents (Cunningham, et al, 1993).

Inhalation of vomitus may be fatal because the woman's airway becomes occluded by foreign matter. Also, stomach contents have an acid pH that can cause chemical pneumonitis and secondary infection of the respiratory tract.

Some anesthesiologists may order cimetidine (Tagamet), ranitidine (Zantac), or an antacid such as sodium citrate or milk of magnesia to be given to the woman before general anesthesia is administered, to reduce the level of acid in stomach contents in case aspiration should occur. Metoclopramide (Reglan) to increase gastric emptying may also be prescribed.

For general anesthesia administration, the woman should be placed on her back with a wedge under her right hip to displace the uterus from the vena cava. To prevent the occurrence of hypotension and to establish a line for emergency medications, intravenous fluid is begun. She is given a rapid induction intravenous agent and is then intubated with a cuffed endotracheal tube. In order to prevent gastric reflux and aspiration before intubation is achieved, cricoid pressure (which seals off the esophagus by compressing it between the cricoid cartilage and the cervical vertebrae) must be applied as soon as the intravenous agent is begun until the cuff on the tube is in place.

The moments of induction of general anesthesia before the endotracheal tube is safely in place are critical ones for the anesthesiologist. Respect his or her necessity to concentrate until the task is achieved. After having general anesthesia, some women may comment that their throat feels raw or sore. This is due to pain from the insertion of the endotracheal tube and is normal. Sipping cold liquids or ice cubes (as soon as this is safe after general anesthesia) relieves the discomfort.

If aspiration of vomitus occurs in the delivery room, prompt attention is essential. The trachea is suctioned by the anesthesiologist to remove as much foreign material as possible; the woman is intubated if she was not previously and given 100% oxygen. She will be given a medication such as isoproterenol intravenously to reduce bronchospasm and a corticosteroid intravenously to reduce an inflammatory reaction. Positive pressure ventilation may be started. Blood gases and a chest x-ray film will be taken to demonstrate the degree of aeration of which she is capable.

The woman will be kept on mechanical ventilation until the chest x-ray films, blood gases, and her overall clinical condition improve. She is critically ill at the time of aspiration and often will be transferred to an intensive care unit for the special care she requires to survive this occurrence.

Key Points

- Pain in labor occurs because of anoxia to uterine cells, stretching of the cervix and perineum, and pressure of the presenting part of the fetus on tissues.
- Pain is perceived differently by each person. Only the woman herself can describe the extent of her pain.
- The better prepared a woman is for childbirth, the less amount of analgesia and anesthesia is necessary. Methods such as reducing anxiety, providing changes in position, increasing knowledge, and supporting prepared childbirth exercises should be used in conjunction with prescribed analgesics.
- Be certain to ask about allergy to medication before administering it in labor. Women under stress may omit mentioning this unless directly asked.
- Record a baseline FHR and maternal blood pressure and pulse before administering medication; reassess 15 minutes later for fetal and maternal safety.
- Women may lose their ability to use controlled breathing after narcotic administration because of a "light-headed" feeling. They may need additional support during this time to be able to continue with a breathing technique until the analgesic begins to have an effect.
- Regional anesthesia such as epidural anesthesia can be extremely effective in relieving labor pain. Be certain the woman is well hydrated with intravenous fluid and that blood pressure is within normal limits prior to administration.
- During regional or general anesthesia administration, if the woman must lie supine, she should have a wedge positioned under her right buttock to help

prevent supine hypotension syndrome. If hypotension should occur after epidural anesthesia administration, elevating the woman's legs is an emergency measure to help relieve hypotension.

- Analgesics or anesthetics may interfere with labor progress if given too early in labor. As a rule of thumb, medication is not given until a primipara is 5 to 6 cm dilated; a multipara, 3 to 4 cm.
- If a narcotic analgesic is used, naloxone (Narcan) must be available for possible newborn resuscitation.
- General anesthesia is rarely administered for an uncomplicated labor, because it has risks for both the mother and infant.

Critical Thinking Exercises

1. Heather is a G1P0 who is admitted to your birthing service. She receives an epidural anesthetic for pain relief and develops hypotension. Formulate the steps you would take to safeguard fetal circulation. Heather asks to have the epidural stopped for another method equally easy and effective. How would you go about describing the other methods available to her?

2. Mrs. Batten is also admitted to your birthing service. She states she wants a general anesthetic for labor or she will leave the hospital. Her physician has said he cannot justify a general anesthetic for uncomplicated labor. What do you consider your role to be in this situation? What criteria do you have for advocating for a general anesthetic?

3. Carla is a woman who seemed well prepared for labor but, after an injection of meperidine early in labor, grows angry with her coach and refuses to use breathing exercises because she feels "light headedness and pain worse than before." How would you help her at this point?

References

Aderhold, K. J., et al. (1991). Jet hydrotherapy for labor and postpartum pain relief. *MCN: American Journal of Maternal Child Nursing, 16,* 97.

Albright, G. A., et al. (1991). Anesthesia for patients with preeclampsia. *Journal of the American Medical Association, 265,* 1587.

Chestnut, D. H., et al. (1990). Continuous epidural infusion of 0.0625% bupivacaine and 0.0002% fentanyl during the second stage of labor. *Anesthesiology, 72,* 613.

Cunningham, G., et al. (1993). *Williams obstetrics* (19th ed.). Philadelphia: W. B. Saunders.

Department of Health and Human Services. (1991). *Healthy people 2000.* Washington, DC: Public Health Service.

Fields, S. A., & Wall, E. M. (1993). Obstetric analgesia and anesthesia. *Primary Care, 20,* 705.

Gordon, S. C., et al. (1994). Self-administered versus nurse-administered epidural analgesia after cesarean section. *Journal of Obstetric, Gynecologic and Neonatal Nursing, 23,* 99.

Green, J. M. (1993). Expectations and experiences of pain in labor. *Birth, 20,* 65.

Guyton, A. C. (1990). *Textbook of medical physiology.* Philadelphia: W. B. Saunders.

Isenor, L., & Penny-Mac Gillivray, T. (1993). Intravenous meperidine infusions for obstetric analgesia. *Journal of Obstetric, Gynecologic and Neonatal Nursing, 22,* 349.

Kennell, J., et al. (1991). Continuous emotional support during labor in a U.S. hospital. *Journal of the American Medical Association, 265,* 2197.

Lichtiger, M., & Moya, F. (1978). *Introduction to the practice of anesthesia* (2nd ed.). New York: Harper & Row.

Loeb, S. (1993). *Nurses' handbook of drug therapy.* Springhouse, PA: Springhouse.

Macdonald, R. (1992). Epidural analgesia for labour. *Midwives Chronicle, 105,* 79.

O'Grady, J. P., & Youngstrom, P. (1990). Must epidurals always imply instrumental delivery? *Contemporary Obstetrics and Gynecology, 36,* 19.

Vinson, D. C., et al. (1993). Association between epidural analgesia during labor and fever. *Journal of Family Practice, 36,* 317.

Whelton, J. (1990). Pain control in labor. *Nursing, 4,* 14.

Suggested Readings

Berg, T. G., & Rayburn, W. F. (1992). Effects of analgesia on labor. *Clinical Obstetrics and Gynecology, 35,* 457.

Budd, S. (1992). Traditional Chinese medicine in obstetrics. *Midwives Chronicle, 105,* 140.

Cassidy, J. (1993). A picture-perfect birth: guided imagery interrupts the pain/anxiety cycle. *RN, 56,* 45.

Holmes, H. S. (1991). Options for painless local anesthesia. *Postgraduate Medicine, 89,* 71.

Kershner, J., et al. (1991). Music therapy assisted childbirth. *International Journal of Childbirth Educators, 6,* 32.

Lea, P. (1992). Delivering women from labor pain. *Canadian Nurse, 88,* 17.

Lowe, N. K. (1991). Maternal confidence in coping with labor: a self-efficacy concept. *Journal of Obstetric, Gynecologic, and Neonatal Nursing, 20,* 457.

Mayberry, L. (1994). Intrapartal nursing care: Research into practice. *Journal of Obstetric, Gynecologic and Neonatal Nursing, 23,* 170.

Radin, T. G., et al. (1993). Nurses' care during labor: its effect on the Cesarean birth rate of healthy, nulliparous women. *Birth, 20,* 14.

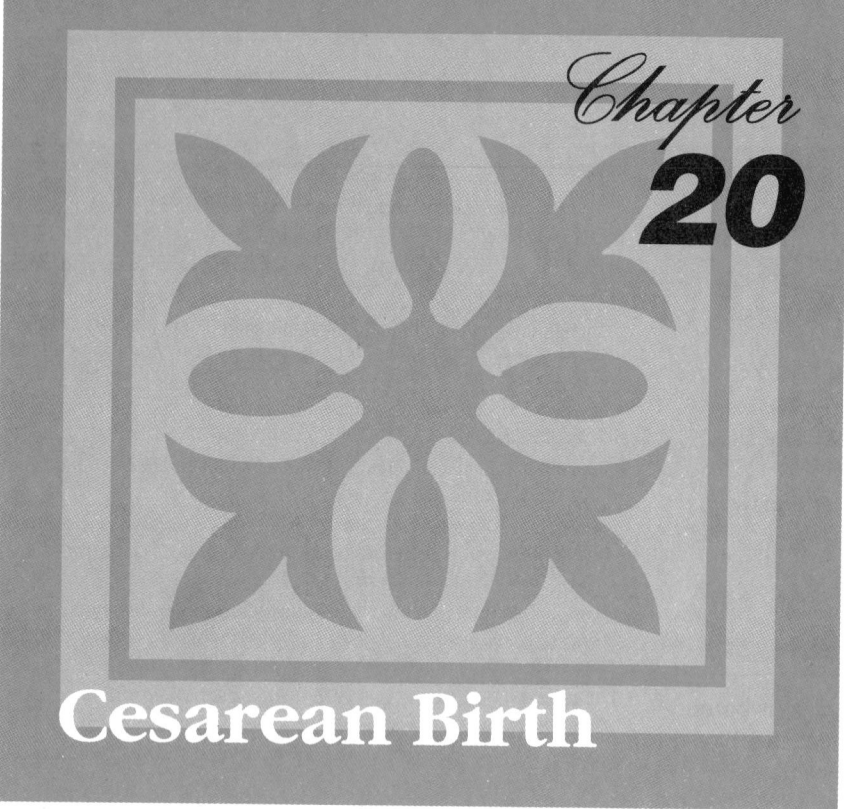

Chapter 20

Cesarean Birth

Key Terms

- cesarean birth
- classic cesarean incision
- low segment incision
- patient-controlled analgesia
- transcutaneous electrical nerve stimulation (TENS)

Objectives

After mastering the contents of this chapter, you should be able to:

1. Describe the indications for cesarean birth.

2. Assess a woman in terms of surgical risk for cesarean birth in order to plan nursing care preoperatively, intraoperatively, and postoperatively.

3. Formulate nursing diagnoses related to cesarean birth.

4. Plan nursing care such as preoperative teaching measures for cesarean birth or ways to maintain family-centered care.

5. Implement common preoperative and postoperative care measures for cesarean birth, such as providing relief for pain.

6. Evaluate outcome criteria to be certain that goals for nursing care were achieved.

7. Identify National Health Goals related to cesarean birth that nurses can be instrumental in helping the nation to achieve.

8. Identify areas related to cesarean birth that could benefit from additional nursing research.

9. Use critical thinking to analyze common complications of cesarean birth and ways they can be prevented.

10. Synthesize knowledge of cesarean birth with nursing process to achieve quality maternal and child health nursing care.

Adele Pillitteri: MATERNAL AND CHILD HEALTH NURSING, 2nd Edition. © 1995 Adele Pillitteri.

Cesarean birth, birth through an abdominal incision into the uterus, is one of the oldest types of surgical procedures known. Although cesarean birth is always more hazardous than vaginal birth, in comparison with other surgical procedures it is one of the safest types of surgery performed.

The word "cesarean" is derived from the Latin *caedore,* which means "to cut." At one time, there was a popular belief that Julius Caesar was delivered by a cesarean birth and that the procedure was named for him. However, because Caesar was born before antibiotics and sterile surgical technique, it seems unlikely that his mother (who is known to have been alive in his adult years) would have survived such a procedure.

Up until the 1800s, cesarean procedures were done only postmortem on women who had died in childbirth as an attempt to save the baby. When it was begun to be used on live women, the operation always involved cesarean hysterectomy, or removal of the uterus with the child. In 1879, Sanger developed the classic cesarean

birth in which the uterus is saved (Cunningham et al., 1993). Currently, cesarean birth is used most often as a prophylactic measure to alleviate problems of birth for conditions such as those listed in Box 20-1. Cesarean birth may be accomplished to deliver a preterm fetus who is not doing well in utero or for multiple births (Dunn, 1990). It is generally contraindicated when there is a documented dead fetus (labor can be induced to avoid a surgical procedure).

A major concern in maternal and child health nursing is the increasing number of cesarean births being performed annually (see the Focus on National Health Goals box). In 1970, only 5.5% of women had infants born by cesarean birth; by 1980, 16.5% of women gave birth by this method. Currently, the incidence is more than 25% (Taffel et al., 1992). This rate is rising owing to a combination of the increasing safety of cesarean birth and the use of fetal monitors, which detect an infant in utero who is not responding well to labor. Its increase may also be related to the phenomenon that physicians,

Box 20-1
Indications for Cesarean Birth

Maternal Factors

Cephalopelvic disproportion

Severe hypertension of pregnancy

Active genital herpes or papilloma

Previous cesarean birth, especially if by classic incision

Disabling conditions that prevent pushing to accomplish the pelvic division of labor

Placenta Factors

Placenta previa

Premature separation of the placenta

Fetal Factors

Transverse fetal lie

Breech presentation

Extreme low birth weight

Fetal distress

Large fetus

FOCUS ON
National Health Goals

One National Health Goal speaks directly to cesarean birth:

- Reduce the cesarean birth rate to no more than 15/100 deliveries from a baseline of 24.4/100 (DHHS, 1991).

Nurses can be instrumental in helping the nation achieve this goal by encouraging women who fulfill the criteria for vaginal birth after cesarean (VBAC) to attempt a vaginal birth with a second child. One study (Radin, et al., 1993) showed that compassionate nursing practice to women in labor can reduce the cesarean birth rate.

Additional nursing research in this area could include additional studies on the effect of nursing practice and the cesarean birth rate, effective pain management for cesarean birth, and measures to help the family adjust smoothly from the hospital to home setting after a cesarean birth.

skilled in doing cesareans, have less experience with other methods that might be used to solve a problem; it may also be related to physician fears of malpractice suits should a fetus be allowed to deliver vaginally and then be discovered to have suffered anoxia. Although the rising incidence of cesarean birth is a concern, this concern must be weighed against the potential of the procedure to reduce the incidence of mental retardation and fetal death. Few parents would insist that giving birth vaginally is more important than ensuring the birth of a healthy baby by cesarean surgery. Cesarean birth is recommended to women when nonstress or oxytocin challenge tests show that a fetus will probably not do well with labor because of poor uteroplacental circulation. A number of legal and ethical issues have arisen in recent years when women have refused to undergo cesarean births in these instances. As women do have a right to decide if they will undergo surgery or not, the right to refuse the procedure is respected. Fortunately, most circumstances do not come to this point of conflict with health care providers. Nurses working in labor and delivery services should be aware of the opinion of their agency's ethics committee on this issue.

NURSING PROCESS OVERVIEW
for the Woman Having a Cesarean Birth

ASSESSMENT

Many women know during pregnancy that they are apt to have a cesarean birth, because they have been shown to have smaller than usual pelvic diameters. Others learn during labor that a cesarean birth will be likely. Assessment as to whether the woman will be a good candidate for surgery, therefore, can in some instances be done over a considerable time period; in others, it is done very quickly as an emergency.

Assessment must include not only whether the woman is physically prepared but psychologically prepared as well.

NURSING DIAGNOSIS

Nursing diagnoses specific to the woman having a cesarean birth are often related to common complications from surgery or client/family concerns about surgical birth. Specific examples include:

- High risk for infection related to a surgical incision
- Fear related to impending surgery
- Pain related to a surgical incision
- Fluid volume deficit related to abdominal surgery

- Powerlessness related to medical need for cesarean birth

PLANNING

The same goal applies to the woman delivering by cesarean birth as the woman delivering vaginally: a healthy mother and child. As cesarean birth decisions are sometimes made suddenly, planning for one may be limited to a few minutes. Whether or not the surgery is anticipated, however, certain presurgery steps will be taken to prepare the woman and her support partner. Helpful referral agencies include the following:

International Cesarean Awareness Network
P.O. Box 152
Syracuse, NY 13210

C/S
22 Forest Road
Framingham, MA 01701

IMPLEMENTATION

Every woman is aware that childbirth carries some risk to her health. Superimposing major surgery on top of this makes it imperative that the woman and her support person have confidence in the health care personnel caring for them, or they could have difficulty coping with the insult of surgery. When giving care to any woman during labor, be certain to establish a helping relationship with both the woman and her support person so they feel they are among friends should the birth method be altered. The nurse who cares for the woman during labor may or may not follow her to surgery, depending on hospital policy.

During surgery, sterile technique is essential. A postpartal infection can be devastating to the woman who already has made many other physical adaptations. Many implementations focus on teaching and support. The more the woman understands about what is happening to her, the more she can accept and cooperate with the procedure. Provide adequate "talk time" after the procedure to allow the woman time to review what happened and fit it in with what she and the father expected.

Another important intervention includes coordination of health care team members (i.e., anesthesiologist, surgeon, pediatrician or neonatologist, and recovery room or nursery personnel). This is particularly important if the surgery will be performed in a hospital surgery department rather than in the labor and delivery suite, or if the infant will be transferred to a careful watch nursery or a distant site for intensive care after the birth.

EVALUATION

Evaluation of outcome criteria is important in the care of a woman after cesarean birth to be certain there are no complications. It is especially important to consider the overall goals of a healthy baby and mother and the development of a positive mother–infant relationship. Specific outcome criteria might include these:

- Client states that she felt well-prepared for cesarean birth even in light of an emergency.
- Couple state that they feel able to cope with newborn care even with mother recovering from surgery.
- Client states that she understands the reason for a cesarean birth.

Cesarean Birth

There are two types of cesarean birth: scheduled and emergency. In the first instance, there is time for thorough preparation for the experience. Some women may have even taken a childbirth preparation class specifically for cesarean birth. With the second type, preparation must be done much more rapidly but with the same concern for fully informing the woman and her support person about what circumstances created the need for a cesarean birth and how the birth will proceed. Cesarean birth is mentioned in most childbirth classes, so that any woman who has taken such classes may at least be familiar with the procedure should one become necessary for her.

Scheduled Cesarean Birth

In the 1950s, cesarean birth became a status symbol when movie actresses asked to have cesarean births to save themselves the strain of labor and in some instances to conveniently schedule the birth between movie contracts. The average woman came to think of cesarean birth as an easy method of painless childbirth. Because the risk of injury from cesarean birth is higher than from vaginal birth, this philosophy put both mothers and fetuses at greater risk than necessary. Scheduling cesarean births this freely also resulted in preterm births. Currently, the practice of truly elective cesarean birth is interesting only as a historic aside. In a reliable health care facility, a physical indication for a cesarean birth such as a transverse presentation, genital herpes, or cephalopelvic disproportion must be documented before a cesarean procedure can be performed. With new surgical techniques, particularly the use of a low cervical incision, "once a cesarean, always a cesarean" no longer applies. Most women who have had a cesarean in the past 10 years are eligible to deliver vaginally in subsequent births if the circumstances otherwise are appropriate for vaginal birth (Rosen et al., 1991).

Emergency Cesarean Birth

Emergency cesarean births are done for reasons such as placenta previa, abruptio placenta, or fetal distress. An emergency cesarean birth carries with it the risk of all emergency surgery: a woman who may not be a prime candidate for anesthesia and who is psychologically unprepared for the experience. In addition, the woman may have a fluid and electrolyte imbalance and be both physically and emotionally exhausted from a long labor.

Effects of Surgery on the Woman

Cesarean birth, like any surgical procedure, has systemic effects.

Stress Response

Whenever the body is subjected to stress, either physical or psychosocial, it responds with measures to preserve the function of major body systems. A stress response results in release of epinephrine and norepinephrine from the adrenal gland medulla. Epinephrine causes an increased heart rate, bronchial dilatation, and elevation of the blood glucose level. Norepinephrine leads to peripheral vasoconstriction, which forces blood to the central circulation and increases blood pressure. These normally positive responses (the person is tensed or ready for action with good heart and lung function and glucose for energy) may contradict anesthetic action, which is aimed at minimizing body activity. In the pregnant woman, such responses may minimize blood supply to her lower extremities. Already prone to thrombophlebitis from stasis of blood flow, these responses compound or increase the risk of thrombophlebitis greatly. Combined with interferences to major body systems, these effects can add to the risk of surgery.

Interference With Body Defenses

The skin serves as the primary line of defense against bacterial invasion. When skin is incised for a surgical procedure, this important line of defense is automatically lost. Strict adherence to aseptic technique during surgery and the days following the procedure must be maintained to compensate for the impaired defense. If cesarean birth is performed after membranes have been ruptured for hours, the woman is doubly at risk for infection due to the surgery.

Interference With Circulatory Function

The cutting of blood vessels is required in even the simplest of surgical procedures. Although incised vessels are immediately clamped and ligated during surgery, there will always be some blood loss. Extensive blood loss leads to hypovolemia and lowered blood pressure. This could lead to ineffective perfusion of all body tissues if the problem is not quickly recognized and corrected. The amount of blood lost in cesarean birth is comparatively high; pelvic vessels are congested with blood needed to supply the placenta, and with pressure on these vessels blood loss occurs freely. During a vagi-

nal birth, a woman loses 300 to 500 mL of blood; this loss increases to 500 to 1000 mL with a cesarean birth.

Interference With Body Organ Function

When any body organ is handled, cut, or repaired in surgery, it may respond with a temporary disruption in function. Pressure of edema or inflammation as fluid moves into the injured area will further impair function of the organ involved and that of surrounding organs. If blood vessels are compressed due to the edema, distant organs may be deprived of blood flow and thus function will be reduced in those organs. After a surgical procedure, therefore, broad observation of not only the one organ involved but of total body function is necessary to assess the total degree of disruption.

During cesarean birth, the uterus is obviously handled and may not contract as well afterward. This may lead to postpartum hemorrhage. To reach the uterus, the bladder must be displaced anteriorly; enough pressure is exerted on the intestine to cause a paralytic ileus or halting of intestinal function. After a cesarean birth, therefore, not only uterine function, but bladder, intestine, and lower circulatory function must be carefully assessed.

Interference With Self-Image or Self-Esteem

Surgery always leaves an incisional scar that will be noticeable to some extent afterward. If the resulting scar from cesarean birth (a horizontal one across the lower abdomen) is noticeable, its appearance may cause the woman to feel self-conscious later. She may feel a loss of self-esteem if she feels that it marks her as a woman unable to give vaginal birth (see the Focus on Cultural Awareness box).

FOCUS ON CULTURAL AWARENESS

In cultures in which birth is viewed as a strictly "natural" process, it is more difficult for women to accept the need for cesarean birth than in a culture which views medical interventions as more acceptable. Establishing rapport with a couple early in labor so they have optimal confidence in health care providers is an effective measure, because if surgery becomes necessary, a couple at least knows that they are with people who have their best interests in mind and will offer support to them. Being certain that women have a support person with them in labor can also help them accept a surgical decision.

Nursing Care of the Woman Anticipating a Cesarean Birth

The woman admitted to the hospital for an anticipated cesarean birth may be more worried about the procedure, because she has more time to worry than the woman who is told during labor that an emergency cesarean is necessary. She needs some time after routine admission to talk about any fears she has; she needs encouragement to do as much as possible for herself preoperatively so she feels in control to reduce her fear. With proper preparation, women who experience cesarean birth can have as positive an outlook about birth as those who deliver vaginally (see the Focus on Nursing Research box).

A woman undergoing surgery cannot begin to relax as long as her support person is nervous and worried. Make a point of including this person in all explanations and admission routines.

Preoperative Interview

Both the physician and anesthesiologist will interview a woman preoperatively to obtain a medical history and make an assessment and decision for safe anesthetic use. In addition, a nursing interview is also essential. Determine whether the woman has had any past surgery, has any secondary illnesses, is currently taking any medication, or has any allergies to foods or drugs to help establish surgical risk. Additional information to be obtained includes the woman's knowledge about the procedure she will undergo, the length of the hospitalization that will be required following surgery, any postsurgical equipment that will be used such as an indwelling catheter and intravenous fluid, and any extra precautions for her infant that will be taken. Cesarean birth is not without extra risk to the newborn. When a fetus is pushed through the birth canal, pressure on the chest helps to rid the lungs of lung fluid, making respirations more likely to be adequate at birth than if the fetus is not subjected to this pressure. Approximately 5% of all infants delivered by cesarean birth have some degree of respiratory difficulty for a day or two after birth because of this omission (Cunningham et al., 1993). (See Chapter 26 for a discussion of this condition, often referred to as transient tachypnea of the newborn).

Establishing Operative Risk

For any surgery to be performed safely, the person must be in the best possible physical and psychological state before surgery. People who are in less than optimal physical or psychological health are at risk for a complicated surgical outcome unless the risk factor is identified and special precautions are taken. The following factors create surgical risk.

Poor Nutritional Status

A woman who is obese is at risk because such a condition interferes with wound healing. Tissue that contains an abundance of fatty cells is difficult to suture, so the incision may take longer to heal; an increased healing period invites infection and rupture of the incision (dehiscence). The person's heart may also have an increased workload; the physiologic shock of surgery may place too much stress on an already overworked organ. In addition, an obese person often has more difficulty moving and turning postoperatively than a person of normal weight and thus has an increased risk for developing respiratory or circulatory complications (pneumonia or thrombophlebitis).

A woman with a protein or vitamin deficiency is also at risk. Protein and vitamins C and D are necessary for new cell formation at the incision site. Vitamin K is necessary for blood clotting to effect hemostasis after surgery. Although most pregnant women do follow sound nutritional practices and take iron supplements, some may still be iron deficient (particularly women

FOCUS ON NURSING RESEARCH

Are Women's Perceptions of Cesarean Birth More Negative Than Perceptions of Vaginal Birth?

For this study, 106 women following unplanned cesarean births, 113 women following planned cesarean births, and 254 women following vaginal birth were interviewed as to their perceptions of birth. The average woman in this study was 30 years of age, had attended college, had a professional occupation, and had a combined household income of over $50,000. Results of the study revealed those women who had had a vaginal birth had more positive perceptions of birth than those who had had an unplanned cesarean birth. There was no significant difference in perception between those who had had planned cesarean and those who had had vaginal births. In general, women who had had a general anesthesia for birth had more negative perceptions than those who had had regional anesthesia.

The results of the study seem to reinforce that good preparation for cesarean birth can make a cesarean experience as enjoyable as vaginal birth.

Fawcett, J., Pollio, N., & Tully, A. (1992). Women's perceptions of cesarean and vaginal delivery: another look. *Research in Nursing and Health, 15,* 439.

with a multiple gestation or women who have not taken supplements), making them high risks in this category.

Age

Age affects surgical risk because it can result in decreased circulatory and renal function. Most pregnant women fall within the young adult age group, making them excellent candidates for surgery. The young adolescent and the woman older than age 35 years both fall into categories of slightly higher risk.

General Health

A person who has a secondary illness (e.g., cardiac disease, diabetes mellitus, anemia, or kidney or liver disease) is at surgical risk depending on the extent of the disease, because the pathology present from the secondary illness may not allow her to make the physiologic adjustments demanded by surgery. Women with a secondary illness may also have an accompanying nutritional or electrolyte imbalance related to their primary illness.

For these reasons, it is important to ask in the preoperative nursing history if the woman has any secondary illnesses. Before surgery, people are under stress and this limits their reasoning ability. It is not unusual for people admitted for any type of surgery to state that they are generally healthy and minutes later request insulin on the day of surgery because they are diabetic.

The woman is asked if she is taking any medication, because some drugs will increase surgical risk by interfering with either the effect of the anesthetic or healing of tissue. A number of drugs that pregnant women might be taking and their potential complications are shown in Table 20-1.

Fluid and Electrolyte Balance

A woman who enters surgery with a lower than normal blood volume will feel the effect of surgical blood loss more than the woman with a normal blood volume. Hypovolemia may result from recent vomiting, diarrhea, or a poor fluid intake before surgery. The woman who began labor and now has been told she is to have a ce-

sarean birth may easily fall into this category, because she may have had nothing to eat or drink for almost 24 hours. To prevent fluid and electrolyte imbalances, many women who are to have a cesarean birth are begun on intravenous fluid therapy preoperatively. Correction is continued postoperatively.

Psychological Condition

Anyone who is frightened when a general anesthesia is administered is at greater risk for cardiac arrest than the person who is calm and relaxed. Women who are extremely worried need a very detailed explanation of the procedure before they can enter surgery without intense fear. Most cesarean births currently are performed under epidural or spinal anesthesia, so they are less frightening in this regard.

In many instances, just helping the woman acknowledge that fear of surgery is normal is beneficial. The procedure does not become any less awesome, but the woman can view her feelings as "normal" and expected.

Preoperative Diagnostic Procedures

For surgery to be performed safely, adequate circulatory and renal function must be documented immediately preoperatively (Kanto et al., 1990).

Vital Signs Determination

Vital signs—temperature, pulse, respiration, blood pressure, and fetal heart rate (FHR)—need to be assessed and recorded. An increased temperature may suggest an upper respiratory infection that might make a general anesthetic inappropriate; an irregular heart beat may suggest a heart evaluation is indicated before surgery. Weight and height are carefully measured to aid in determining the amount and type of preoperative medication or anesthesia necessary.

Urinalysis

All surgical clients have a urinalysis done before surgery to estimate metabolic and kidney function. It would be dangerous, for example, for a person with undetected

Table 20-1. *Drugs That May Result in Complications of Surgery*

Type of Drug	Action
Antibiotics	Specific antibiotics may predispose to renal insufficiency or increase neuromuscular blockage; can lead to opportunistic infections
Anticoagulants	May cause hemorrhage due to lack of hemostasis during surgery
Anticonvulsants	May increase liver action and metabolism of anesthetic agent
Antihypertensives	May result in hypotension following anesthesia
Corticosteroids	May block body's response to shock and lead to lack of adrenal function
Insulin	May lead to hypoglycemia during labor or hyperglycemia if a dextrose solution is administered
Antianxiety agents	May cause hypotension following anesthesia

diabetes to undergo surgery without extra precautions, because intravenous fluid containing glucose could be extremely dangerous to the person during this time. This determination is especially important in pregnant women, because gestational diabetes is a complication of pregnancy. It is equally dangerous for a person with poor kidney function to face the degree of physiologic shock of surgery unless special precautions are taken. Poor kidney function is revealed by the presence of protein and abnormal specific gravity in urine. In addition, the woman should be assessed for a normal voiding pattern and if edema is present, as these suggest renal or bladder impairment.

Blood Studies

Complete Blood Count. A complete blood count is routinely ordered before surgery to document that the woman has adequate blood components so that subsequent blood loss will not reduce her functioning blood components below a safe level. If a woman has a low hemoglobin level preoperatively, a blood loss that appears normal could be fatal. A woman with inadequate blood platelets will not have normal blood clotting ability, so that blood loss will be appreciably more than usual. A person with an inadequate leukocyte count will have a difficult time resisting infection after surgery. A woman during pregnancy, and particularly one who was in prolonged labor, may have an elevated leukocyte count (up to 20,000/mm³), so this finding is not necessarily as helpful with the pregnant woman as with others.

Serum Electrolytes and pH. Normal body electrolytes are necessary to allow the woman to adapt to the shock of surgery. Women who have had nothing by mouth for labor can experience serious electrolyte imbalance. In many hospitals, serum electrolytes are ordered as a single battery of tests (an SMA-12 or SMA-18).

Blood Typing and Cross-Matching. Cesarean birth involves a greater loss of blood than many surgeries. In most health care agencies, blood is drawn to be used for typing and cross-matching before surgery. Women having planned repeat cesareans may donate blood during pregnancy to make it available at the time of surgery.

Sonogram

A sonogram may be done to locate the placenta to be certain it is not lying just under the area where the surgical incision will be made.

Preoperative Teaching

Fear of the unknown is one of the hardest fears to conquer. Preoperative teaching is aimed at acquainting the woman with the procedure and any special equipment used so that she will be as informed about the surgery as possible. Activities to help maintain respiratory and skeletal function to prevent postsurgical complications from stasis of body secretions or circulation are also taught.

Assess first how much the woman already knows about surgery before teaching. The woman who had a cesarean birth for her first child and now is being admitted for a second procedure already knows many details. Even so, she will undoubtedly appreciate having her memory refreshed and recall confirmed. Answer all specific questions and fill in gaps in knowledge. Ensure that all information offered is accurate. It is confusing and potentially frightening for a woman to be told, for instance, that she will not have intravenous fluid after the surgery and then discover the intravenous line in place. Be certain not to use hospital jargon such as "NPO." People under stress do not process new information well. They cannot process at all information they do not understand. Have the woman demonstrate activities such as deep breathing to show that she can do this well.

Teaching Points

Explain preoperative measures that will be necessary such as surgical skin preparation; eating nothing before the time of surgery; premedication (if this will be used); and method of transport to surgery. Review the necessity for an indwelling catheter, intravenous fluid, and early ambulation afterward.

Use visual aids as necessary. Draw pictures or show illustrations of anatomy, if necessary. Do not leave textbooks about cesarean procedure techniques with the client, however, because such books also describe complications. The woman has to know possible complications of the procedure to sign an informed consent, but she may be frightened by reading about complications complete with color illustrations.

Teaching to Prevent Complications

Women who work to maintain good respiratory and circulatory function postoperatively will probably have a postoperative course with fewer respiratory and circulatory complications than those who do not. These preventive measures are best taught during the preoperative period, when the woman is free of pain and can concentrate on the teaching. Such teaching also gives the woman a positive outlook about surgery (a sense of control as well as reassurance that, because the nurse is taking time to teach her postoperative measures, he or she thinks the woman is going to recover safely from surgery). Her obstetrician and anesthesiologist both say to her, "I'll see you in the operating room in a few minutes." By teaching postoperative care, the nurse is saying, "I'll see you and your new child safely back here in your room afterward," a message with a comforting subliminal message for the woman who has serious doubts that there will be an afterward or at least not one with a newborn.

Deep Breathing. Periodic deep breathing exercises fully aerate the lungs and help to prevent stasis of lung mucus (stasis tends to occur because of the long supine period). Because stasis always has the potential for causing infection, it must be prevented as much as possible.

It helps to increase lung function if the woman takes 5 to 10 deep breaths every hour postoperatively. She does this simply by inhaling as deeply as possible, holding her breath for a second or two, and then exhaling as deeply as possible. She must be certain that she inhales and exhales fully or she will feel lightheaded from hyperventilation.

Incentive Spirometry. Another device used postoperatively to encourage deep breathing is the incentive spirometer, a plastic tube with a table tennis (Ping-Pong) ball suspended in the tube. The woman places her lips around the mouthpiece and inhales. The harder she inhales, the farther the ball rises in the hollow tube. Such an exerciser is fun to operate and gives a client a sense of reward for the effort (see Figure 40-18). Women need a good explanation before using an incentive spirometer, because their initial impression is usually that the ball rises as a result of blowing *into* the instrument. Its purpose is to cause the person to take deep breaths and fully aerate lung spaces, however, so most models are triggered by *inhalation,* not exhalation.

Turning. Women do not need to practice turning side to side before surgery because this activity is tiring for them to do while pregnant. However, they should understand that turning is important to prevent both respiratory and circulatory stasis. This will be contraindicated if a spinal anesthetic is used to try and reduce the possibility of a spinal headache.

Leg Exercises. Another means of preventing circulatory stasis postoperatively is ankle, knee, and hip flexion and extension approximately five times every hour. Lifting each foot off the mattress and moving it in a circle (circumduction) is also an effective motion to teach (Figure 20-1). Leg exercises are extremely important following cesarean birth, because the edema of the low pelvic surgery compresses circulation to the lower extremities and makes the woman prone to lower extremity circulatory stasis.

Immediate Preoperative Care Measures

A number of measures must be taken immediately before surgery to ensure a safe outcome.

Obtaining Informed Consent

Obtaining operative consent is the surgeon's responsibility, but seeing that it is obtained is everyone's responsibility. Nurses are often asked to witness the woman's

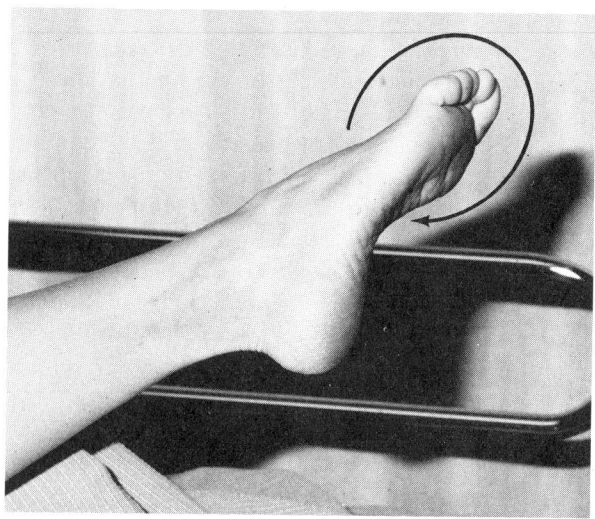

FIGURE 20-1
Leg exercises, such as moving the leg in a circle, help to lessen the possibility of thrombophlebitis postoperatively.

signature on such a form; be certain it was *informed* consent (i.e., the woman was explained the risks and benefits of the procedure in terms that she could understand) before signing as a witness.

The law differs from state to state regarding emancipated minors (girls under legal age but who are pregnant or the previous mother of a child). Emancipated minors can sign their own surgical permission even though they are legally under age.

Overall Hygiene

Most women having repeat cesarean births are admitted on the morning of surgery; they have showered or bathed at home. Provide a clean hospital gown on admission. If the woman's hair is long, encourage her to braid it or put it into a ponytail so that it will more easily fit under the surgical cap she will wear in the operating room (hair contained by a cap is less likely to spread microorganisms). Suggest she not use bobby pins in her hair, because these can lacerate the skin unnoticed while she is unconscious from anesthesia (even women who will be having surgery under an epidural anesthesia need to have these precautions followed, because if a complication should occur during surgery, she may be instantly anesthetized while the emergency is managed). Check the woman's nails for nail polish; if present, ask her to remove it from at least two fingers on each hand to allow determining whether nail bed color is remaining pink during anesthesia administration. Caution the woman not to apply cosmetics following her shower, because extreme paleness or cyanosis from lack of oxygen could be hidden by blush or lipstick. Follow agency regulations on whether jewelry must be removed or not. Some women may have elastic stockings ordered to be applied before surgery to ensure venous return during surgery. Apply these using gentle technique with the woman in a supine position (Figure 20-2).

Gastrointestinal Tract Preparation

A woman may have an enema ordered before surgery to empty her bowel and allow the bowel a few days' rest during the first few days postsurgery when her abdominal muscles are nonfunctional owing to the surgical incision. If this is ordered, be certain to administer an enema to a pregnant woman with gentle, gravity-only pressure. Provide a bed pan for her to expel the enema, or remain with her and accompany her to the bathroom so she does not hurry to reach a bathroom and slip and fall.

Baseline Intake and Output Determinations

To reduce the anterior bladder in size and keep it away from the surgical field, the woman needs to have an indwelling catheter inserted before surgery. Bladder catheterization is reviewed in Nursing Procedure 37-3. Catheterizing a pregnant woman is more difficult than catheterizing a nonpregnant woman, because the pressure of the fetal head puts pressure on the urethra; the vulva may be swollen and distorted in shape from vulval varicosities or edema. Be certain to provide a good light so the perineum is clearly revealed; take special care during the time of skin preparation to locate the urinary meatus. Use a gentle touch to avoid or minimize pain. Be certain after insertion of the catheter that urine is draining, because fetal pressure on the urethra may reduce the flow of urine considerably. Be certain during the transport time to surgery that the drainage bag is kept below the level of the woman's bladder so there is no backflow and so that microorganisms are not introduced into the bladder.

If catheterization cannot be done easily before surgery, do not traumatize the urethra by repeated attempts, because catheterization can be done in the delivery room after the anesthetic for surgery is given. If there is a delay between the catheter insertion time and surgery, mark the drainage bag just before surgery with

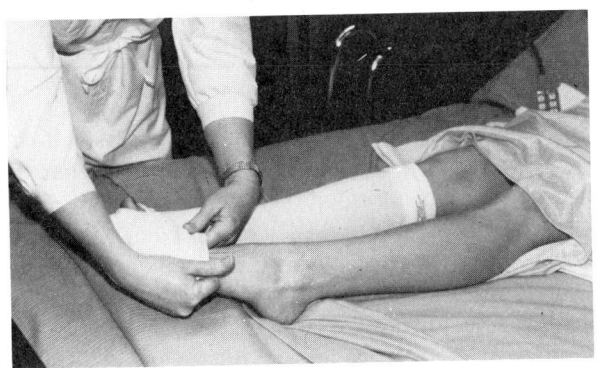

FIGURE 20-2
When applying antiembolitic stockings, be certain the woman is in a supine position, so that veins are not full at the time of application.

the amount in the bag or empty it so that presurgery urine can be differentiated from postsurgery urine. One of the gravest dangers of any surgery procedure is that kidneys may fail under the physiologic stress of surgery or because of lack of blood flow to them due to decreased blood pressure. All reproductive tract surgery puts ureter flow at risk because of edema in the surgery area. Separating presurgical and postsurgical urine drainage allows the nurse to accurately assess urine drainage after the procedure.

Hydration

Most women have an intravenous fluid line begun before surgery so that they are fully hydrated and do not experience hypotension from the blood loss at birth. Be certain this line is started in the woman's nondominant hand to allow her to hold her newborn after surgery without interference. Use a large intercath needle so that replacement blood can be administered through the needle if needed.

Preoperative Medication

A minimum of preoperative medication is used with a woman having a cesarean birth in order not to compromise the fetal blood supply and to assure that the newborn is wide awake at birth and initiates respirations spontaneously.

Intramuscular administration of cimetidine (Tagamet) to decrease stomach secretions or an oral antacid such as sodium citrate (Bicitra) to neutralize the acid of the stomach secretions may be ordered. These precautions are taken also because the woman will be lying on her back during the procedure and esophageal reflux is likely during this time. A gastric emptying agent such as ranitidine or metoclopramide (Reglan) may also be ordered.

Client Chart and Surgery Checklist

Recording of nursing care up to the time the woman leaves the nursing care unit or labor room must be completed before the woman leaves for the delivery room. Many hospitals use an additional preoperative checklist, such as that shown in Figure 20-3, as a reminder of all necessary measures to be taken. Checking and signing such a form indicates that the specific measures are complete.

Transport to Surgery

To transfer the woman to surgery, she may either be taken in her bed or helped to move to a stretcher. It is important to hold the stretcher tightly against the side of the bed for safe transfer, because the woman is awkward in her movements owing to her pregnancy. Urge her to lie on her side to prevent supine hypotension syn-

Patient concerns
   Skin preparation
   Identification in place
   Temperature, pulse, respiration _____
   Blood pressure _____
   Height _____ Weight _____
   Voided _____ Time _____ Amount _____
   NPO after _____
   Hospital gown
   Hairpins removed
   Nail polish removed
   Jewelry removed
   Preoperative medication _____
   Dentures removed _____ In place _____
   Contact lenses removed _____
   Prosthetic devices removed _____

Chart concerns
   Addressograph plate attached
   Operative permit obtained
   Urinalysis
   Hematocrit or CBC
   Blood order of _____

Completed
_____
_____
_____
_____
_____
_____
_____
_____
_____
_____
_____
_____
_____
_____
_____

Signature _____ R.N.

FIGURE 20-3
Preoperative checklist for cesarean birth. Checklists will vary from hospital to hospital.

drome during transport. Use optimal safety features such as having the side rails up and the cart straps secure for transport. Cover her with a blanket as well as a sheet to prevent her from feeling chilled in the cool surgical suite. Her chart with the surgical checklist must accompany her. Check that her identification is secure before she leaves the client unit.

Role of the Support Person

In most instances with cesarean birth, a woman's family can be as involved in the birth as they would be for a vaginal birth. Every couple needs to attend preparation for childbirth classes, because most of the material covered in these classes is on pregnancy and newborn care and this information is the same for her as for others. Many communities have special classes for women who know they will have a cesarean birth. These are especially valuable because they directly address special concerns such as fear of surgery.

With the mother awake for the birth, a support person is allowed to share this with her the same as for a vaginal birth. A support person may need more encouragement to watch a cesarean birth more than a vaginal one, because he or she may visualize the surgery as being much more bloody than it actually is. Helping family members realize that cesarean birth is little different from vaginal birth helps them move on to bonding with the infant and incorporating a new member into the family. It will be necessary to help the support person wash and put on a gown and mask.

Nursing Care of the Woman Having an Emergency Cesarean Birth

Many women who will have a cesarean birth have no warning during pregnancy that this will happen; it becomes necessary during labor when they develop a complication such as prolapsed cord or fetal distress. When surgery is arranged as an emergency this way, only a few minutes of preparation time are available.

The woman who is told during labor that an emergency procedure is necessary may actually be relieved that surgery has been suggested; if she was having a great deal of pain with labor, this will alleviate it. Another woman might feel great disappointment when told that her baby must be born by cesarean birth. In many women, both emotions are present.

Surgical risk in an emergency situation is determined from the baseline history and physical examination information previously obtained on hospital admission at the beginning of labor. Preoperative preparation measures such as vital signs, urinalysis, and blood work have also been previously obtained. Immediate preparation concerns such as informed consent, application of elastic stockings, gastrointestinal tract preparation, bladder catheterization, and establishing an intravenous line will be the same. There is little or no time for postoperative teaching, since the available time must be spent explaining the immediate procedures to the woman: she will be transferred to an operating room; her abdomen will be prepared; she will receive anesthesia; and so on. Mark on the nursing care plan that postpartal teaching was not done so the nurse on the postpartal unit will be aware this will need to be done immediately postpartum.

The Surgical Procedure

Observing or participating in a cesarean birth offers health care providers information about specific areas to explain to women before surgery and complications to watch for after surgery. To observe or participate, one must be free of infection, particularly cutaneous or respiratory infection. Before entering the operating room suite, it is necessary to change to scrub clothing (i.e., cap, mask, gown, and shoe covers) and thoroughly wash hands and arms. This procedure automatically reduces the level of bacteria in the operating room. The head cap should completely cover the hair; the mask covers both mouth and nose and should be pulled snugly against the edges of the face by ties at the back. Shoes should be rubber-soled so they do not conduct sparks, which could cause the explosion of some anesthetic gases; covering them with a cloth or paper impregnated with a conduction strip further reduces their capacity to conduct electricity. If no flammable gases are present, such a precaution may be unnecessary.

In a typical operating room, the operating table is located in the center of the room under a large overhead light. The light is attached to a track so that it can be tilted or focused by means of an overhead handle. The table is built so that it can be tilted in many directions, allowing clients to be positioned with good support for different surgical approaches. Anesthesiology equipment (the portable machine for administering inhalation anesthesia with accompanying oxygen and suction equipment) is placed at the head of the table, and an instrument table at the foot of the table. Additional equipment includes a small over-the-table stand (Mayo) for instruments that will be used first during surgery; a table for surgeon's gloves and gowns; and kickbuckets (stainless steel buckets on wheels) for disposal of used sponges. A newborn care area with a radiant heat warmer stands nearby.

Administration of Anesthesia

The surgical nurse will assist the woman to move from the transport stretcher to the operating room table and remain with her while anesthesia is administered. If the woman has an epidural catheter in place, be careful it is not dislodged while she is moved. If anesthesia administration will be delayed, encourage the woman to remain on her side or insert a pillow under her left hip to keep her body slightly tilted to the side. If she will have a spinal anesthetic, the anesthesiologist will generally ad-

minister this with the woman sitting up. The anesthesiologist may ask a nurse to help the woman curve her back to separate the vertebrae and facilitate entry of the spinal needle. It is difficult for a woman having uterine contractions to remain in this position for long. Talking to her while gently restraining her is the most effective means of helping her maintain this position (Carp, 1990).

Following spinal anesthesia, be certain the woman keeps her head flat or she can develop a post-spinal headache (see discussion of spinal anesthesia in Chapter 19).

Skin Preparation

Reducing the number of bacteria on the skin before surgery automatically reduces the possibility of bacteria entering the incision at the time of surgery. Shaving away abdominal hair and washing the skin area over the incision site accomplishes this.

The skin preparation area for a cesarean birth varies from very extensive in some health care agencies to a limited area in others. A typical pattern is shown in Figure 20-4. Review with the woman that a much wider skin area than the actual incision site is prepared to ensure a wide safe area as free as possible from bacteria. Otherwise she may be alarmed that the procedure planned is more extensive than she had anticipated. Steps in preoperative skin preparation are shown in Nursing Procedure 20-1. To ensure that skin is not irritated or cut, actions that would invite infection, use a generous supply of shaving lather or soap and a sharp razor. Use small, controlled, smooth strokes; shave with the grain of the hair shaft for comfort; use a good light to accurately see that all hair has been removed from the area; use warm water for patient comfort.

Surgical Incision

Following anesthetic administration, the woman is tipped into a slight Trendelenburg position with a towel under her left hip to move abdominal contents up away from the surgical field and to lift her uterus off the vena cava. A metal screen may be placed at the client's shoulder level and covered with a sterile drape to block the flow of bacteria from the woman's respiratory tract to the incision site. The incision area on her abdomen is then scrubbed and appropriate drapes are placed around the area of incision so only a small area of skin is left exposed. Watching a cesarean birth is usually the first surgery the average father or support person has ever witnessed. Because of this, the person is often too overwhelmed by and interested in the procedure to be of optimum support. He or she may become concerned about the amount of manipulation and cutting that occurs before the uterus itself is cut (assuming fetal distress

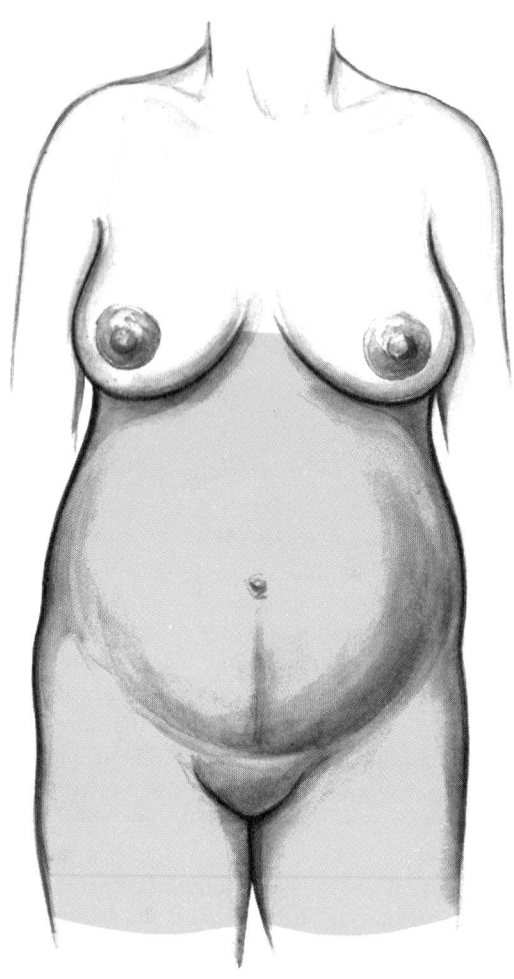

FIGURE 20-4
Skin preparation for a cesarean birth extends from under the breasts and includes pubic hair.

is not extreme). Review with the support person preoperatively that operating incisions are made with careful precautions against excess bleeding so just the skin layer is cut first and the capillaries there that begin to bleed are clamped with hemostats (small metal clamps). The layer of fat beneath the skin is cut and bleeders there are clamped in the same way. The incision is extended deeper through fascia and muscle using the same cut-clamp technique.

Types of Cesarean Incisions

There are two types of cesarean incisions. The type chosen depends on the presentation of the fetus and the speed with which the procedure will be performed (Figure 20-5). In a **classic cesarean incision**, the incision is made vertically through both the abdominal skin and the uterus. The advantage of a classic incision is that it is high on the uterus so it can be used with a placenta previa to avoid cutting the placenta; its disadvantage is that the incision leaves a wide skin scar and runs through the active contractile portion of the uterus. Be-

cause this type of scar could rupture during labor, it is likely that the woman will not be able to have a subsequent vaginal birth.

A **low segment incision** is one made horizontally across the abdomen just over the symphysis pubis and also horizontally across the uterus just over the cervix. This is the most common type of cesarean incision currently made; it is also referred to as a Pfannenstiel incision or a "bikini" incision, because even a low-cut bathing suit would cover it. Because this type of incision is through the nonactive portion of the uterus (the part that contracts minimally), it is less likely to rupture in subsequent labors, making it possible for a woman to deliver vaginally with a future pregnancy. It also results in less blood loss, is easier to suture, decreases postpartal uterine infections, and is less likely to cause postpartal gastrointestinal complications. The major disadvantage of this incision is that it takes longer to perform, possibly making it impractical for an emergency cesarean delivery. In a few instances, a skin incision is made horizontally and then the uterine incision is made vertically, or vice versa. For this reason, you cannot assume during a future pregnancy that just because a woman has a small skin incision, she will have a small uterine incision as well.

Birth of the Infant

Once the surgical incision is complete, retractors (long, metal, curved instruments) are slipped into the incision. Gentle traction on the handles by an assistant keeps the incision spread apart and allows for good visualization of the uterus and the internal incision. Sterile towels may be placed in the incision to separate the uterus from other organs. The uterus itself is then cut and the child's head may be delivered manually or by the application of forceps (Figure 20-6). The mouth and nose of the baby are suctioned by a bulb syringe, the same as in a vaginal birth before the remainder of the child is delivered. Oxytocin is administered intravenously by the anesthesiologist as the child or placenta is delivered, to increase uterine contraction and reduce blood loss. Following full birth, the uterus is pulled forward onto the abdomen and covered with moist gauze; the internal cavity of the uterus is inspected and the membranes and placenta are manually removed. If the woman wishes to have a tubal ligation, this can be done at this time. The uterine, subcutaneous tissue, and skin incisions are then closed (remind the woman and her support person that closing the incision will be a long process and they should not become concerned that something is wrong). Metal staples are usually used on the exterior skin because they leave the least amount of scarring.

Observing the amount of abdominal manipulation that is accomplished during surgery increases understanding of how tender a woman's abdomen will be

NURSING PROCEDURE 20-1
Preoperative Skin Preparation

Purpose
To provide a skin area clear of body hair to reduce chance of infection at a surgical incision site.

Plan	*Principle*
1. Wash your hands; identify client; explain procedure.	1. Prevent spread of microorganisms; ensure client safety and cooperation.
2. Assess client status; analyze appropriateness of procedure; plan modifications as necessary.	2. Nursing care is always individualized according to client needs.
3. Implement care by assembling supplies: safety razor with new blade, shaving soap or lather according to agency policy, waterproof pad, emesis basin, dry gauze sponges, good light source. Determine extent of skin area to be prepared.	3. A good light source is important to be certain that all hair is removed. Check with the surgeon or surgical suite if you are uncertain as to the extent of the preparation.
4. Provide privacy; fanfold covers as necessary to reveal body area to be prepared. Place waterproof pad under area to protect bed. Fill basin with warm water to use to rinse razor.	4. Protect against chilling; protect bed linen.
5. Lather area well with a moistened sponge, using predetermined soap or lather. Stretch skin taut; shave off all hair using short strokes in direction of hair shafts. Be careful not to nick skin.	5. Lather softens hair and reduces friction to skin. Any open area would be an invitation to infection.
6. Wipe away all removed hair; dry area well. Inspect it carefully for additional hair. Evaluate effectiveness, efficiency, cost, comfort, and safety of procedure. Plan health teaching as necessary; for example, inform the patient of the importance of consuming nothing by mouth before surgery.	6. Health teaching is an independent nursing action always included as part of care.
7. Leave client comfortable. Chart area prepared and time of preparation.	7. Document client status and nursing care.

afterward and why a postsurgery client often has an overall "aching" feeling after surgery.

Introduction of the Newborn

Once it is determined that the newborn is breathing spontaneously, he or she is shown to the mother and support person, just as is done after a vaginal birth. The mother may not be able to hold her newborn because she has intravenous fluid infusing into one hand and the surgical drapes are still in place. If the father or support person chooses, he or she may hold the new child. Visiting with the newborn is an effective distraction in making the time of incision closure pass quickly as well as in laying a firm foundation for bonding. Breast-feeding is usually delayed until the woman has been moved to a recovery room, because it initiates uterine contraction and may interfere with suture placement. Breast-feeding also may be awkward with the anesthesia screen in place and because of the lack of privacy.

Postpartal Phase

Women who deliver by cesarean birth have an additional care concern in the immediate postpartal period, because they are not only postpartal clients but postsurgical ones as well. Owing to the strain of the unexpected procedure, they may have increased difficulty bonding with their new infant. As with all postpartal women, the postpartal phase for the woman who delivers by cesarean birth can be divided into an immediate recovery period (the so-called fourth stage of labor) and an extended postpartal period.

Nursing Diagnoses and Related Interventions During the Immediate Postpartal Period

Immediately after surgery is completed, the woman is transferred by stretcher from the operating room table to a recovery or postpartal room. If either epidural or

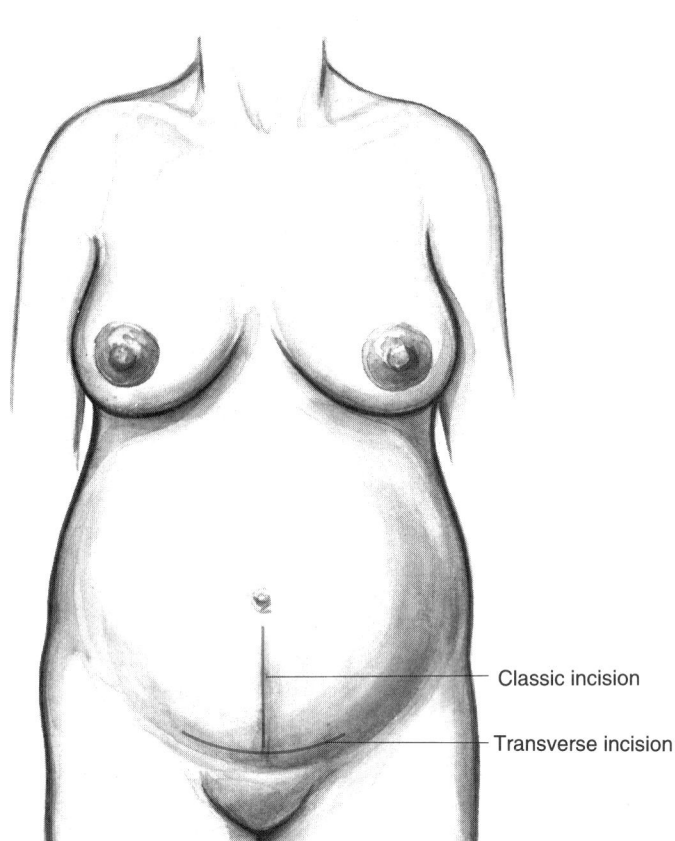

Classic incision

Transverse incision

FIGURE 20-5
Types of cesarean incisions.

spinal anesthesia was used, remember that her legs are fully anesthetized so she will not be able to move them.

> ***Nursing Diagnosis:*** Pain related to surgical incision
>
> ***Goal:*** Client will experience tolerable level of pain during postpartal period.
>
> ***Outcome Criteria:*** Client states that level of pain is tolerable.

A major problem in the woman following cesarean birth is control of pain. Pain is serious in the woman, because it not only may lead to surgical complications such as pneumonia or thrombophlebitis (it prevents her from moving) but also may impair bonding with her newborn if holding him or her is painful. The woman's physician generally orders a narcotic analgesic to be given with a patient-controlled analgesia (PCA) pump for the first 24 to 48 hours after surgery, followed by a less strong analgesic such as acetaminophen (Tylenol) orally. Transcutaneous electrical nerve stimulation (TENS), intranasally administered butorphanol (Stadol), or epidural morphine may also be used. A woman

who is concerned about her infant may experience more pain than the woman who is assured that her infant is doing well, because a tense body posture causes pressure on sutures.

Be certain when administering analgesics following surgery that they are supplemented with other comfort measures, such as change of position or straightening of bed linen. Check for an uncomfortable distended abdomen, which suggests intestinal gas pain rather than incision pain. Always ask the woman what type of pain she is experiencing to be certain that she is describing incisional pain and not pain in a leg or some other body part that would suggest a complication.

Many women who are breast-feeding are reluctant to accept an analgesic especially just before breast-feeding for fear of the analgesic being passed in breast milk to the infant. It is true that most analgesics do pass in breast milk, but the infant takes such a small amount of breast milk (mainly colostrum) during this time that the amount of analgesia received is negligible. Also, without the analgesic, the woman may be so uncomfortable that she is unable to hold the infant comfortably and enjoy having the infant with her. Placing a pillow over her lap will deflect the weight of the infant from the suture line and lessen pain. Some women still have considerable pain on their day of hospital discharge. Advocate for a prescription for her or instruct her to take acetaminophen (Tylenol) every 4 hours for pain. Be certain she understands not to take salicylic acid (aspirin), because this can interfere with blood clotting and healing.

Epidural Analgesia. Women who have cesarean surgery using an epidural anesthetic may have a narcotic such as fentanyl or morphine (Duramorph) added at the beginning of the procedure to aid in anesthesia. If an additional amount is added at the conclusion of surgery, this can provide analgesia for about 24 hours.

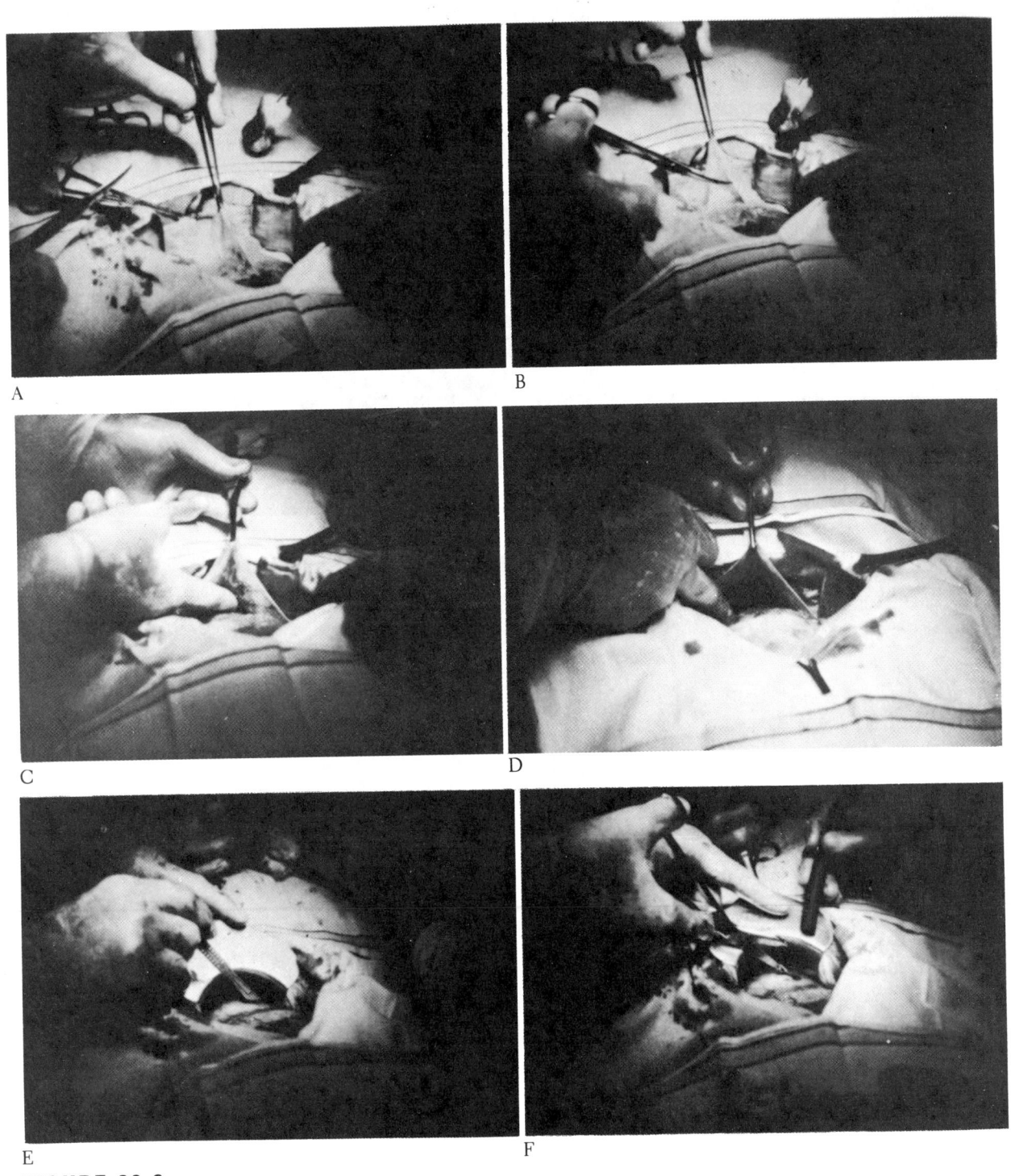

A B C D E F

FIGURE 20-6
(A–L) *Cesarean birth. (From Scott, J.R. (1990).* Danforth's obstetrics and gynecology. *Philadelphia: J.B. Lippincott.)*

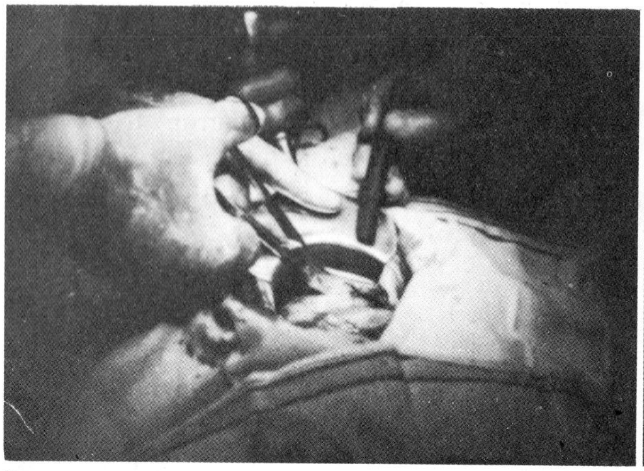

G

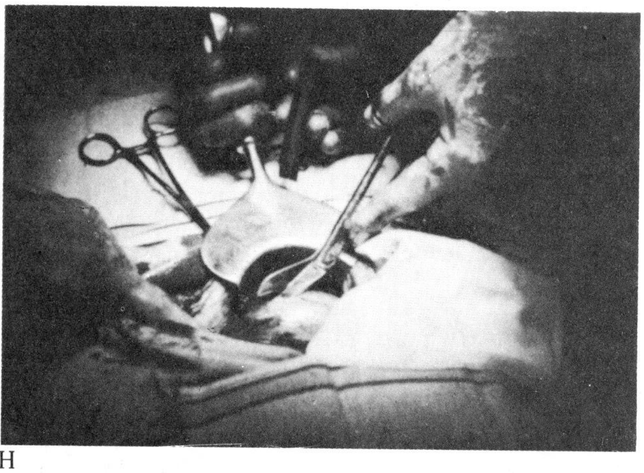

H

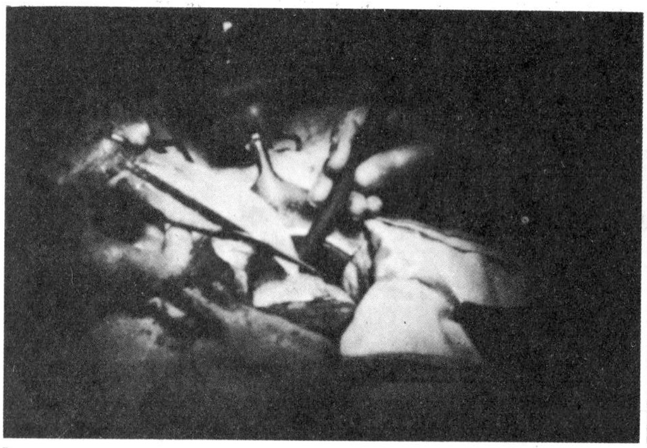

I

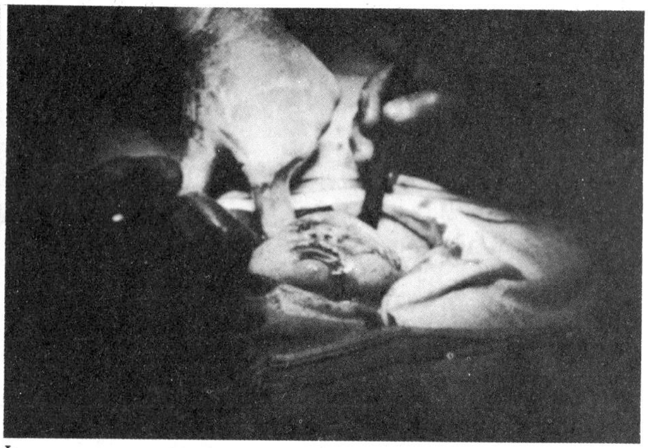

J

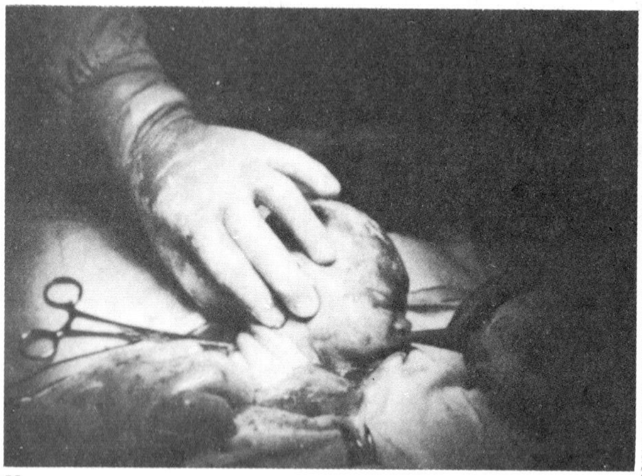

K

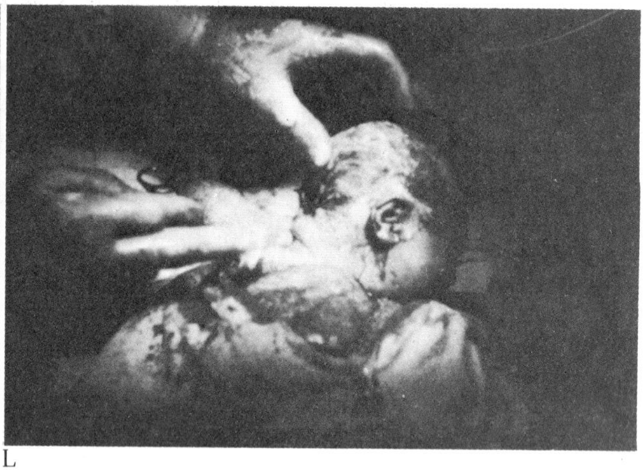

L

FIGURE 20-6 *(Continued)*

Administration of epidural analgesia may result in a depressed respiratory rate from the effect of the opiate. Respirations should be assessed every 15 minutes for the first hour; then every 30 to 60 minutes depending on agency protocol. If respiratory depression should occur (respiratory rate less than 13 breaths per minute), oxygen should be administered and a pulse oximeter attached to measure oxygen saturation. Elevate the head of the bed to facilitate lung expansion. A narcotic antagonist such as naloxone hydrochloride (Narcan) may be administered to counteract the respiratory depression. Narcan's effect lasts only about 30 minutes, so that respiratory depression may occur again at this time. Narcan also counteracts the pain-relieving effect of the narcotic and thus allows the woman to experience pain.

Side-effects of epidural narcotic administration are

intense itching and nausea and vomiting. An antihistamine such as Benadryl may be given to reduce pruritus; an antiemetic such as metoclopramide (Reglan) may be administered to counteract nausea. Despite these annoying side-effects, epidural analgesia can be a very effective means of pain control following cesarean birth. Women can self-administer epidural boluses of drug for pain relief (Gordon et al., 1994).

Patient-Controlled Analgesia. **Patient-controlled analgesia** (PCA) is a method of pain control in which patients administer doses of intravenous narcotic analgesia to themselves as needed. It may be used during labor, although its most frequent use is to control post-surgical pain. An intravenous solution such as Ringer's lactate or 5% dextrose is begun. A PCA pump with a syringe of narcotic (meperidine or morphine) locked inside is attached to the intravenous line at a port close to the client. To receive a dose of analgesia, the client pushes a button similar to a call bell. This alerts the automatic pump to deliver a set amount of narcotic into the intravenous line. The pump has a "lock-out" setting that prevents a client from administering a larger dose than would be safe or doses more frequently than would be safe (e.g., every 8 minutes) (Figure 20-7).

PCA administration corrects most of the problems inherent in intramuscular administration. When injections are given intramuscularly, a high level of narcotic in the bloodstream occurs, but by the end of the 4 hours when another injection is due, the mother may already be experiencing pain once again. With PCA, neither of these phenomena occurs, because a fairly constant level of pain relief can be maintained. The pain and fear of injec-

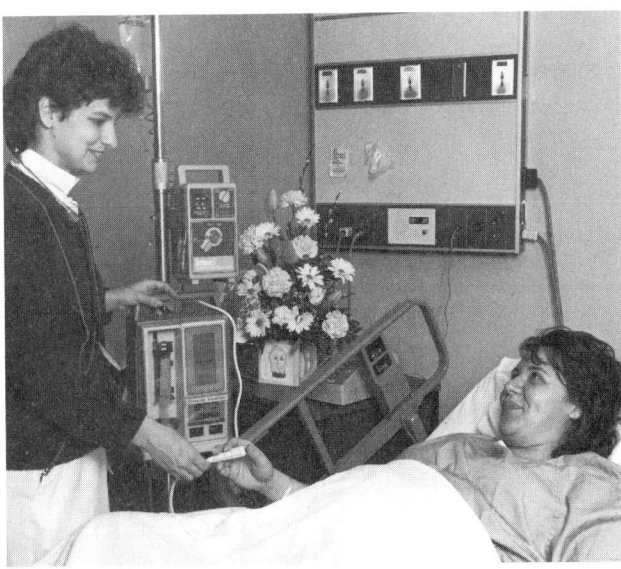

FIGURE 20-7
Patient-controlled analgesia (PCA) pump. By pushing the button, a client delivers a bolus of narcotic to herself. (Courtesy, Department of Medical Photography, Children's Hospital, Buffalo, NY.)

tions are eliminated. Overall, women tend to use a much lower dosage with a PCA system than they would with intramuscular injections. PCA works well with post-cesarean clients because they feel well enough to be interested in self-care and self-administration of analgesia.

Transcutaneous Electrical Nerve Stimulation. **Transcutaneous electrical nerve stimulation (TENS)** is, as the name implies, the transmission of an electrical current across the skin. This is done by the application of electrodes to the surface of the skin. It is an effective method of controlling pain sensation because pain is carried by small affective (sensory) nerve fibers. Irritation or stimulation of the large afferent (sensory) nerve fibers by the electrical stimulation blocks the ability of the cerebral cortex to interpret the incoming small afferent sensation (a gating theory). This is the same phenomenon that rubbing or scratching skin at the point of pain achieves (Welton, 1990).

To begin TENS, two electrodes are positioned one each side of the abdominal surgical incision and taped in place under the surgical dressing in the operating room immediately following surgery. Following surgery, the electrode leads are attached by cords to a monitor about the size of a transistor radio. This can be attached to the side rail of the bed or carried by the client as she ambulates. When the unit is turned on, a mild electrical stimulation is transmitted to the skin. The woman controls the unit herself; stimulation for 30 minutes at a time as infrequently as four times a day is all that is necessary in most women to control pain. Be certain that the activation unit is removed when the woman showers or takes a sitz bath so it is not exposed to water. If placed on the side rail, place it on the opposite side of the bed from the bedside stand and water glass to prevent an accidental spill of water from wetting it. Keep it on the opposite side from an intravenous infusion so that if the intravenous tubing loosens and the bed becomes wet, the unit is not exposed to water. Locating the cord before helping the woman turn in bed and get out of bed will prevent the electrodes from being pulled out. If electrodes should pull free, clean the electrode with an antiseptic solution or use a new sterile one and reattach it by lifting or changing the wound dressing. Do not replace the electrode without cleaning it, because once it has laid in the bed near lochia, it is potentially too contaminated to be replaced near a yet unhealed surgical incision.

TENS therapy has some disadvantages. It may add to the feeling of "unnaturalness" of cesarean birth because of the involvement of an electrical monitor and leads. Disinterest in self-pain control may be apparent during the taking-in period, and the accompanying euphoric effect that accompanies a drug such as meperidine (Demerol) may be helpful to some women with minimal postpartal depression. Many postoperative clients are unable to use TENS because, not only have they had surgery, but they are ill. It appears to have its most appeal with postcesarean clients because, although they are postsurgical, they are not ill and therefore are capable of a high level of self-care.

Nursing Diagnosis: High risk for fluid volume deficit related to blood loss during surgery

Goal: Client will not experience a postsurgical hemorrhage.

Outcome Criteria: Client's blood pressure is 100/60 mm Hg or more; pulse is between 60 and 100 beats/min; no more than scant bleeding on dressing is apparent.

The potential always exists for fluid volume deficit related to blood loss during surgery. The possibility of hemorrhage following surgery exists until all blood vessels cut and ligated during surgery have thrombosed, sclerosed, and permanently sealed closed (Combs et al., 1991). The postpartum woman is at double threat: she may hemorrhage vaginally from an uncontracted uterus as well as internally from "bleeders" or blood vessels that were not securely ligated. The danger of hemorrhage from both forms is most acute in her first hour following surgery; it remains an acute problem for the first 24 hours.

To detect the earliest signs of hemorrhage, blood pressure, pulse, and respiration rate should be taken every 15 minutes for the first hour after surgery, every 30 minutes for the next 2 hours, every hour for the next 4 hours, or as specifically ordered. Signs that hemorrhage is occurring include a falling blood pressure, increased pulse, and rapid respirations. The woman may be restless and feel thirsty. Box 20-2 lists common vital sign "endpoints" to use as points of danger in assessment. The dressing over the surgical incision should be checked for blood staining, the perineal pad observed for lochia flow, and the fundal height palpated every time the vital signs are taken. Lochial discharge may be decreased in a woman after a cesarean birth because the uterus was cleaned during surgery, but some will always be present. The woman who had either a spinal or epidural anesthesia will not experience pain on uterine palpation until the anesthesia has worn off (2 hours to 4 hours), so uterine palpation for measurement will not hurt her. When the anesthetic has worn off, always palpate gently but thoroughly enough to determine uterine consistency. You are not doing the woman a favor if you avoid causing her pain by not palpating her uterus, only to have postpartal hemorrhage occur.

At the same time the uterus is assessed for firmness, assess the remainder of the abdomen for softness, because a hard, "guarded" abdomen is one of the first signs of peritonitis (peritoneal infection), a complication that may occur with any abdominal surgical procedure. Be certain to turn the woman to look under her body for bleeding. Blood oozing from a surgical wound or vaginally can pool considerably under a client before it is visible.

Many physicians order an oxytocin such as Pitocin to be added to the first one or two liters of fluid following surgery to ensure firm uterine contraction. If the rate of fluid administration gets behind, be careful about "catch-up" administration. An oxytocin can elevate blood pressure by causing vasoconstriction. It may be safer to allow the fluid to remain behind for a time, rather than risk dangerously elevating blood pressure. At the point that the oxytocin is discontinued, be aware that the woman is prone to hemorrhage, because this is the first time the uterus is really asked to maintain contraction on its own following the surgical procedure. The woman's physician must be notified of changes in vital signs that might indicate hemorrhage, so that action can be taken to infuse additional fluid to replace loss or to return the client to surgery. Remember that a minimal but continued change in vital signs (pulse steadily increasing, blood pressure steadily declining) is as ominous a sign of hemorrhage as a sudden alteration in these measurements.

Nursing Diagnoses and Related Interventions During the Extended Postpartal Period

The average woman who has delivered her child by cesarean birth will remain in the hospital from 24 hours to 4 days. During this period, a number of interventions are necessary to promote healing and prevent postoperative complications as well as establish bonding with the new child. Common concerns of women are pain, fatigue, interference with gastrointestinal function, and reduced activity level (Miovech et al., 1994).

Nursing Diagnosis: High risk for fluid volume deficit related to postsurgical fluid restriction

Goal: Client will not experience fluid volume deficit following surgery.

Box 20-2
Postoperative Vital Sign Parameters

- Fall in systolic blood pressure more than 20 mm Hg
- Systolic blood pressure less than 80 mm Hg
- Blood pressure dropping 5 to 10 mm Hg over several readings
- Pulse more than 110 beats/min or under 60 beats/min

Outcome Criteria: Client's urine specific gravity is between 1.003 and 1.030; weight loss is not more than 5 to 10 pounds.

Adequate fluid intake is important after surgery to replace blood loss from surgery and to maintain blood pressure and renal function. It must be monitored carefully to prevent giving it at too rapid a rate (which could lead to cardiac overload) or too slow a rate (which could lead to inadequate circulatory compensation). Keep an accurate intake and output record for at least the first 24 hours to ascertain an adequate fluid balance. The handling of the intestine during surgery causes it to halt or slow in function; it takes approximately 24 to 48 hours before full function is restored and oral intake is possible.

The woman will be maintained on intravenous fluid until her gastrointestinal system has recovered and is functioning competently again. Help the woman learn to "guard" the intravenous fluid line, because she needs a high proportion of fluid during this time (all postpartal women undergo diuresis as a physiologic postpartal change). At the same time, do not urge such caution that the woman is afraid to turn or ambulate. She is at high risk for thrombophlebitis so she must turn, do leg exercises, and ambulate early in the postpartal period.

Assess the woman's abdomen once during each nursing shift for bowel sounds, small "pinging" sounds heard on auscultation at a rate of 5 to 10 per minute that denote air and fluid are moving through the intestines. Ask if she is passing flatus as another indication that intestinal function is again active. As soon as these signs are present, the surgeon will order the intravenous fluid to be discontinued and sips of fluid to be begun (begin the fluid and wait 1 hour before removing the intravenous line to be certain that the woman will not have nausea and need the intravenous fluid restarted). Introduce fluid slowly (ice chips for the first hour, then sips of clear fluid such as ginger ale, Jello, tea, or flavored frozen ice) and gradually return the woman to a soft and then regular diet as ordered. Some woman assume that they will not be allowed to eat for a long time following surgery and are surprised (and suspicious) to learn that they can have ice chips only hours after surgery. Ice chips dissolve so slowly that the woman receives little fluid from them; they feel cool, however, and will quickly take away the "cottony" feeling in her mouth caused by lack of fluid.

Note carefully the time of a first bowel movement after surgery. If the woman has had no bowel movement by hospital discharge, the physician may order a stool softener, a suppository, or an enema to facilitate stool evacuation. Assure the woman who is not receiving much food yet that it is normal not to have bowel movements for 3 or 4 days postoperatively, especially if she had an enema administered before surgery.

Nursing Diagnosis: High risk for altered patterns of urinary elimination related to surgical procedure
Goal: Client will have adequate urinary output during postpartal period.
Outcome Criteria: Urinary output is more than 30 mL/h.

Because the bladder was handled and displaced during surgery, its tone may be inadequate to initiate voiding after surgery. The indwelling catheter placed before surgery will usually be left in place for approximately 24 hours to ensure good urine drainage. Assess that the catheter is draining (a postpartal woman has a urine output of 3000 to 5000 mL per 24 hours); bladder distention will occur rapidly if the catheter becomes blocked.

Before the catheter is removed, the physician may order a urine culture to ensure that a urinary infection did not occur. Such cultures are usually taken from the catheter port by a sterile syringe after the port has been cleaned with an antiseptic solution.

Following removal of the catheter, the average woman voids in 4 to 8 hours. Determine whether a bladder is filling by palpation, pressing lightly over the symphysis pubis to assess fullness (Figure 20-8*A*) and by percussion—an empty bladder sounds dull; a full bladder, resonant; and an extended bladder, hyperresonant (Figure 20-8*B*). If a bladder has filled to capacity but cannot empty properly, the woman may have "retention with overflow" or void 30 to 60 mL of urine every 15 to 20 minutes. This voiding pattern is potentially dangerous, because it means that the woman's bladder is held continuously under tension. This can result in permanent bladder damage if the condition goes undetected. In addition, the constantly full bladder may prevent the uterus from contracting and may increase the risk of postpartal hemorrhage.

To help women void, administer an analgesic, which helps to relax abdominal musculature; provide privacy for voiding; help the woman to walk to the bathroom if that is possible; pour warm water over her vulva (measure the amount of water used so that it can be differentiated from urine); and run water from a tap within hearing distance of the woman.

Voiding after surgery not only proves renal competency but also circulatory competency, because the kidneys must have adequate blood flow through them to function.

Nursing Diagnosis: High risk for altered peripheral tissue perfusion related to immobility during and after surgery
Goal: Client will experience no significant cardiovascular effects from surgery.
Outcome Criteria: Homans' sign is negative; fin-

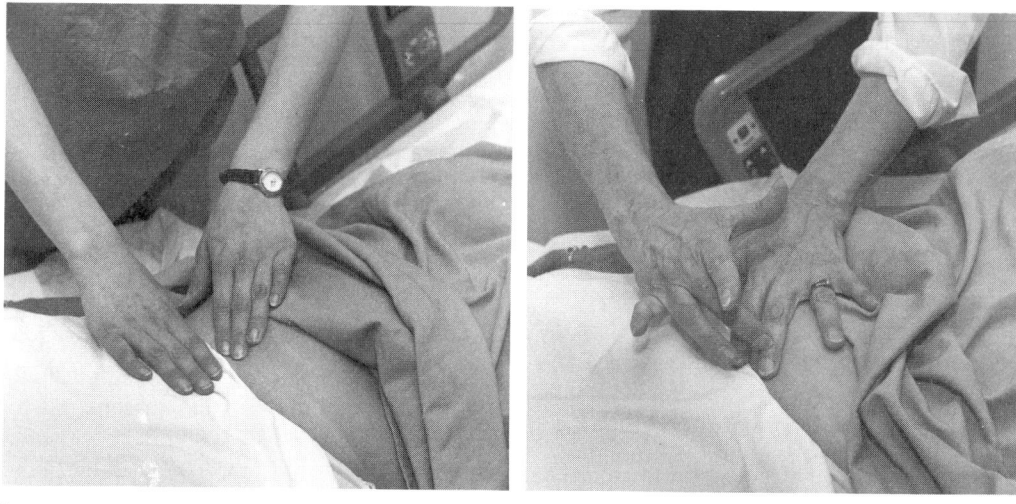

A   **B**

FIGURE 20-8

(**A**) *Assessing bladder filling by palpation.* (**B**) *Assessing bladder filling by percussion.*

gernails and toenails blanch and return to color in less than 5 seconds.

Leg exercises such as flexing and extending the knee and early ambulation are the woman's best safeguards against circulatory problems. She may feel more comfortable turning and sitting up if she supports her abdomen with one hand. Because her abdominal muscles are so lax from having been stretched from pregnancy, abdominal contents tend to shift forward and put pressure on the suture line, causing pain and an uncomfortable feeling often described as "falling apart." Many women will need to have thromboembolitic stockings ordered for them after surgery. These promote venous return. Be certain they are put on with the woman supine when venous distention is minimal. Always allow the woman to sit on the edge of the bed for a few minutes before helping her to a standing position, to prevent orthostatic hypotension. Elicit a Homans' sign (pain in the calf on dorsiflexion of the foot) or pain or redness in the calf to detect if a blood clot is present before ambulation. It would be dangerous to ambulate anyone with this sign, because a thrombus could shift and become an embolus, a potentially lethal situation.

It is difficult for women to appreciate how important it is for them to turn and ambulate as soon as possible after surgery (Figure 20-9). Still in pain and experiencing the "taking in" postpartal phase, a woman may prefer to spend the first days after surgery just resting quietly in bed. Give analgesia as necessary during that time to enable her to move and ambulate with the least amount of pain.

Nursing Diagnosis: High risk for altered parenting related to the emergency nature of birth or discomfort from surgery .

Goal: Parents demonstrate adequate bonding behavior in the postpartal period.

Outcome Criteria: Parents hold and feed child and voice positive comments about him or her.

Many cesarean births are scheduled so quickly that the woman does not have much time preoperatively to think about how she will feel after surgery; most women are surprised to realize how well they feel overall but

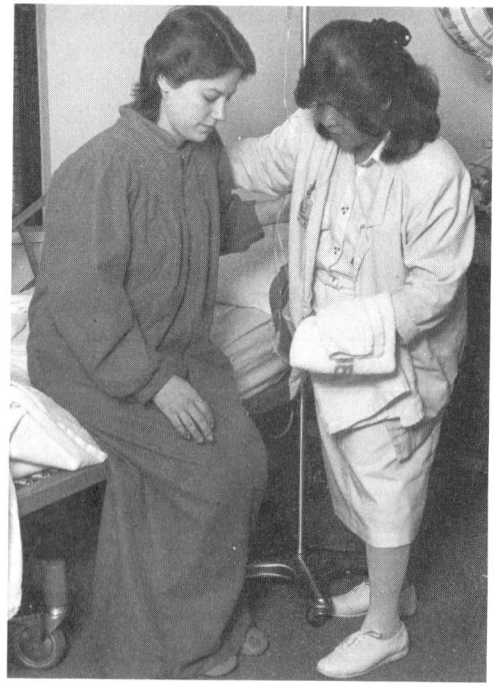

FIGURE 20-9

Encouraging women to walk and to be out of bed to feed their newborns will help prevent thrombophlebitis from venous stasis. (Courtesy, Department of Medical Photography, Children's Hospital, Buffalo, NY.)

also how quickly they become fatigued and how painful a simple surgical incision can be. Being assured that they are recovering well and that surgery is a physiologic shock to their system helps them to accept temporary discomforts.

If the woman's baby was born with a complication or has been transferred to a distant hospital, the postpartal course is difficult because she experiences a sense of loss (depression can slow all body functions and certainly her ability to "take hold" in the postpartal period).

Unless the baby was transferred to another site, be certain that the woman has ample time to hold and feed her child. Most women can breast-feed satisfactorily (Kearney et al., 1990). She may have some reason to think that her baby is not quite perfect—after all, the baby did not deliver "perfectly"—so she may need additional time to inspect the baby and feel comfortable with him or her (Figure 20-10; see also the Nursing Care Plan).

Nursing Diagnosis: Fatigue related to effects of surgery

Goal: Client is able to gradually take over self-care activities in the first 24 hours.

Outcome Criteria: Client voices that she is pleased with level of self-care; ambulates well by 24 hours and sleeps restfully at night.

Although a woman needs active movement after surgery, she also needs adequate rest. Many women attempt to handle their own and their newborn's needs immediately after surgery, because their excitement over their baby and their new role makes them oblivious to

their symptoms of underlying fatigue. Extreme fatigue does not aid healing, however, and it makes the woman prone to postpartal infection. It can eventually interfere with bonding with the child, rather than promote it, if it does lead to postpartal complications. Help the woman plan a day that includes care of her new child and periods of rest for herself as well. Be certain at bedtime that she has adequate analgesic administered to allow her to be pain-free for the night. Provide a time in the middle of the morning and again in the afternoon for uninterrupted rest. Explore her plans for care at home to be certain that her plans seem realistic for a postsurgical-postpartal woman.

Nursing Diagnosis: Altered skin integrity related to surgical incision

Goal: Surgical incision will heal without complication in 7 days.

Outcome Criteria: Incision line is not erythematous; no foul drainage is present; oral temperature is less than 38°C.

Surgical incisions heal by primary intention or by the gradual removal and replacement of dead or damaged cells at the wound site with new cells produced by the surrounding tissue. Some women may receive a course of antibiotics following surgery to help prevent infection (Watts et al., 1991). Assess the surgical incision once during each nursing shift to be certain that the wound edges are approximated and that no signs of infection such as erythema are present. As soon as the woman can walk steadily (usually the second postoperative day), she can take a shower after first removing the dressing. Warm

(*text continues on page 568*)

FIGURE 20-10
To promote bonding, equipment such as for intravenous therapy should not be allowed to interfere with a postpartal woman's interaction with her newborn. (Courtesy, Department of Medical Photography, Children's Hospital, Buffalo, NY.)

FOCUS ON FAMILY TEACHING

Q. I had a cesarean section two years ago for my first child. Now that I'm pregnant again, my doctor has told me he wants me to have this one vaginally. How do I know I'm a good candidate for this?

A. Many women today are having vaginal births after previous cesarean births (called VBACs). The American College of Obstetricians and Gynecologists cites the following criteria for candidates for VBACs:

• No documented cephalopelvic disproportion.

• Previous cesarean incision was low transverse.

• A physician is readily available during a trial labor.

• Emergency surgical facilities are available.

• The fetus is estimated to be less than 4000 g (8 lb, 13 oz).

Christine McFadden is a 15-year-old you care for in a labor-birth-recovery room who has been scheduled for cesarean birth for cephalopelvic disproportion. The following is a nursing care plan designed for her.

Health History: *Chief concern:* "I don't want surgery. I'd rather die!"

History of present problem: Client's obstetrician cautioned her during pregnancy that her pelvic measurements were "borderline" and a cesarean birth might be necessary. Christine was allowed a trial labor. When labor failed to progress, cesarean birth was scheduled. Mother is with client as support person in the labor room, but a degree of mother-adolescent antagonism appears to limit her effectiveness as a support person.

Nursing Diagnosis: Fear related to impending cesarean birth.

Defining Characteristic: Client voices anxiety about procedure.

Goal: Client will state she can accept surgery procedure within 15 minutes.

Outcome Criteria: Client signs informed consent for cesarean birth.

Nursing Orders	*Rationale*
1. Review procedure with client and support person (mother).	1. Knowing the steps of the anticipated procedures can help reduce fear.
2. Review necessity for surgical consent.	2. Knowing purpose of required signature reduces apprehension.
3. Answer questions about procedure.	3. Allowing questions provides a reassuring atmosphere.

Nursing Diagnosis: High risk for injury related to complications of cesarean birth.

Defining Characteristic: All surgical procedures carry risks, such as infection and kidney failure.

Goal: Client will be prepared against common risks of cesarean birth by 20 minutes.

Outcome Criteria: Client has skin preparation, bladder drainage system in place, and states postpartal measures necessary to help prevent circulatory disorders.

Nursing Orders	*Rationale*
1. Administer preoperative medication (sodium citrate).	1. Sodium citrate can reduce lung trauma if aspiration should occur.
2. Insert indwelling catheter to gravity drainage.	2. Provides for assessment of kidney function and ensures emptying of bladder.
3. Maintain nothing-by-mouth status.	3. Reduces possibility of aspiration.
4. Remove nail polish (if any) from two fingers, two toes.	4. Helps ensure safe anesthesia administration.
5. Perform skin preparation from beneath breasts to perineum.	5. Helps protect from infection post surgery.

(continued)

Nursing Orders	**Rationale**
6. Continue FHR monitoring until transfer to operating room; report FHR below 120 or above 160 bpm or decelerations.	6. Help protect safety of fetus.
7. Review deep breathing, leg exercises, and importance of early ambulation for postpartal period.	7. Learning these techniques will help prevent cardiovascular complications in the postpartal period.

Following the cesarean birth of a 6-lb girl, you design the following postpartal plan:

Assessment: Client states, "I hurt all over. I can't breathe, I have so much pain!" Lies holding hands over abdomen, barely moving in bed. Urinary output 100 mL in the past hour. Skin turgor good. Slight lochia rubra vaginal drainage; slight serosanguineous drainage on surgical dressing. Blood pressure: 110/80; respirations: 22; temperature 98.6°F orally. Uterus firm and 1 fingerwidth below umbilicus. Abdomen soft. Client states, "I'm glad I had a girl." Held infant for only a moment in the delivery room. States she feels too tired to feed her now; will "try it later."

Nursing Diagnosis: Pain related to cesarean birth.

Defining Characteristic: Client voices she has pain.

Goal: Client will experience a tolerable level of pain within 20 minutes.

Outcome Criteria: Client voices pain is tolerable; no discernible tension present by facial expression or posture.

Nursing Orders	**Rationale**
1. Teach client about use of PCA pump.	1. Education will help client accept method of pain relief.
2. Set up meperidine (Demerol) by PCA pump, 10 mg bolus q 6 min up to 150 mL q 4 h.	2. PCA pumps are effective to provide analgesia for cesarean birth and promote self-care in the postpartum client.
3. Teach client to support incision when moving.	3. Support to incision can prevent pain on motion.
4. Review that pain is expected postsurgically, but analgesia will be effective in reducing pain.	4. Pain is accentuated by anxiety.

Nursing Diagnosis: High risk for fluid volume deficit related to blood loss.

Defining Characteristic: Blood loss was estimated at 700 mL.

Goal: Client will maintain adequate fluid volume during postpartal period.

Outcome Criteria: Specific gravity of urine is within normal level (1.003 to 1.030); skin turgor is good; lochial or incision drainage is scant.

(continued)

Nursing Orders	Rationale
1. Infuse 3000 mL of Ringer's lactate at 125 mL/h per physician's order.	1. Intravenous fluid will reestablish fluid volume.
2. Add 10 mL of oxytocin (Pitocin) to first 1000 mL of fluid per physician's order.	2. Oxytocin will contract uterus and decrease blood loss.
3. Maintain strict intake and output.	3. Careful record-keeping will document fluid balance and will help the nurse detect potential hemorrhage or bladder retention early.
4. Remove Foley catheter at 12 hours postprocedure following culture of urine. Measure next two voidings for amount and specific gravity.	4. The bladder may not fully function after Foley removal; measuring urine volume documents that the bladder is emptying.
5. Assess for bowel sounds every 8 hours until return.	5. Bowel sounds indicate that the bowel is recovering function following surgery.
6. Begin ice chips when bowel sounds are present.	6. Ice chips allow the client to begin oral fluids slowly and safely.
7. Blood pressure and pulse q 15 min for 1 h, then every 1 h for 4 times, then q 8 h up to 24 h.	7. Vital signs help document amount of blood loss from surgery or can indicate the signs of hemorrhage.
8. Schedule hematocrit and hemoglobin at 4 hours and 24 hours postprocedure.	8. Hematocrit and hemoglobin levels help document amount of blood loss from surgery.

Nursing Diagnosis: High risk for complications of immobility related to painful surgical incision.

Defining Characteristic: Surgical incision is present and this prevents easy motion.

Goal: Client will experience no postpartum immobility complication such as thrombophlebitis.

Outcome Criteria: Homans' sign is negative; client reports no pain in calf of leg.

(continued)

clean water on the incision is healing. Many obstetricians allow the woman to decide if she wants to continue to wear a dressing after this point (lack of a dressing prevents moisture accumulation at the incision site and decreases the possibility of infection). With a cesarean birth, healing will be adequate enough that by day 4 or 5, removable skin sutures or clamps can be removed.

Discharge Planning

The woman being discharged following cesarean birth not only takes home her new baby, but a fair amount of pain and discomfort as well. It is important to discuss home care arrangements to emphasize the need for adequate help with the newborn and other responsibilities at home. Be certain the woman understands that she is going to be extremely tired. She should be aware of any restriction on exercise or activity (as a rule she should not lift any object heavier than 10 pounds for the first

2 weeks) as well as signs of possible complications directly related to the surgery, such as redness at the incision line or frequency or burning on urination. She should also be informed about the normal postpartal concerns such as tender breast tissue and normal lochia flow. She can resume coitus as soon as the act is comfortable for her (as early as 1 more week), and she should have an appointment for a return visit for health assessment and reproductive health planning with her physician (usually in 2 weeks).

The Woman Having a Vaginal Birth After Cesarean Birth (VBAC)

The woman who will be having a vaginal birth after a previous cesarean birth may have a great deal of apprehension and questions about labor (see the Focus on Family Teaching box). If during the previous labor, a complication occurred that necessitated the cesarean,

Nursing Orders	*Rationale*
1. Encourage turning side to side and not crossing legs.	1. Turning encourages venous return in legs.
2. Ambulate at 6 hours.	2. Ambulation also aids venous return.
3. Encourage deep breaths every 2 hours.	3. Deep breathing helps aerate lungs.
4. Use no knee gatch on bed.	4. Bending the knee promotes thrombus formation.
5. Assess for Homans' sign or pain or redness in calf every 8 hours.	5. Homans' sign, redness, and pain are assessments for thrombophlebitis.

Nursing Diagnosis: High risk for altered parenting related to bonding interference secondary to cesarean birth and client's postsurgery exhaustion.

Defining Characteristic: Client states rest is a priority over baby care.

Goal: Client will demonstrate adequate bonding behavior by hospital discharge.

Outcome Criteria: Client holds infant warmly and speaks of her in a positive light.

Nursing Orders	*Rationale*
1. Encourage client to keep infant in room with her for extended periods.	1. Extended contact between mother and infant encourages bonding.
2. Help her to handle and feed infant with support.	2. Support allows the mother to risk trying new holding positions.
3. Review normal growth and development of newborn and point out positive points (long hair, alert expression).	3. Awareness of infant's appearance and actions can prevent surprises; pride in newborn can encourage bonding.
4. Attempt to increase mother's self-esteem by praising her for managing so well during a difficult time in her life.	4. High self-esteem helps clients to manage new situations.

she cannot help but worry that this will happen again. If she has discussed the fact she will be having a vaginal birth this time, she surely is aware that uterine rupture is one of the complications of vaginal birth after cesarean birth.

She needs a support person with her and health care providers who are aware of her possible level of apprehension. Fortunately, the outcome of vaginal birth after cesarean birth is usually without complication. If necessary, oxytocin augmentation (see Chapter 21) can be used to strengthen uterine contractions as with any labor; vacuum extraction and forceps birth can be used as necessary.

Many women are reluctant to try a vaginal birth because they are concerned about the degree of pain involved (Abitbol et al., 1993). Afterward, many are relieved to realize that although they did have more discomfort before birth, they had appreciably less pain afterward.

Key Points

- The term cesarean "birth" is preferred to cesarean "section" because of the focus on the childbirth rather than surgery elements of the procedure.
- Cesarean birth may be either planned or unplanned. Cesarean birth is more hazardous to the infant than vaginal birth and is undertaken only when medically necessary.
- Establishing surgical risk should include assessment of nutritional status, age, general health, fluid and electrolyte balance, and psychological condition.
- Measures prior to surgery should include vital sign determination, urinalysis, blood studies such as complete blood count, electrolytes, blood typing, and cross-matching, and sonography.
- Skin preparation for a cesarean incision is generally from under the breasts to the mid-thigh, including the pubic hair. The skin incision may be vertical

(a classic incision), although it is usually a horizontal one just above the pubic hair. The internal incision into the uterus is also usually a horizontal incision into the lower uterine segment.

- The old saying "Once a cesarean, always a cesarean" is no longer true, providing that cephalopelvic disproportion does not exist and the previous incision was a low transverse one.

- When women have epidural or spinal anesthesia for cesarean birth, a support person can share the experience with them.

- Support people can lose a great deal of their ability to support if they feel intimidated and out of place in an operating room; offer them support as needed to make this a positive experience for them as well.

- Cesarean birth is one of the safest types of surgery performed. To keep the woman safe following the procedure, remember that she is both a surgical and a postpartum client after the surgery. Make assessments to ensure neither postpartum nor postsurgical complications occur.

- Women are physically exhausted after cesarean birth and may be psychologically exhausted because of the emergency nature of the experience. Provide rest time to relieve the physical strain and a chance to verbalize the experience to help relieve the psychological strain.

- A major intervention after cesarean birth is early ambulation. The woman has incisional pain, making this difficult, and will require strong nursing support.

- Patient controlled anesthesia (PCA) is an ideal method for providing pain relief after cesarean birth, because it allows a woman a sense of control as well as effective pain relief.

Critical Thinking Exercises

1. Marjorie is a woman you admit to a birthing room. When she is told that she will need to have a cesarean birth because her fetus is presenting breech, she begins to scream hysterically. What would be your best action?

2. Beth is a woman who has patient-controlled anesthesia ordered after a cesarean birth. She tells you she is not interested in this and would rather have injections for pain. Describe and explain the action you might take. Would you advocate for use of PCA or advocate with her physician for a changed order?

3. Mr. Trevino tells you he cannot possibly stay with his wife in the operating room while she has a cesarean birth. He states he will feel nauseous and probably faint. His wife wants very badly to have him come with her. What would be your action?

References

Abitbol, M. M., et al. (1993). Vaginal birth after cesarean section: the patient's point of view. *American Family Physician, 47,* 129.

Carp, H. (1990). Anesthesia for cesarean delivery. *International Anesthesiology Clinics, 28,* 25.

Combs, C. A., et al. (1991). Factors associated with hemorrhage in cesarean deliveries. *Obstetrics and Gynecology, 77,* 77.

Cunningham, F. G., et al. (1993). *Williams obstetrics* (19th ed.). Norwalk, CT: Appleton and Lange.

Department of Health and Human Services. (1991). *Healthy people 2000.* Washington, DC: Public Health Service.

Dunn, L. J. (1990). Cesarean section and other obstetric operations. In Scott, J. R. *Danforth's obstetrics and gynecology.* Philadelphia: J. B. Lippincott.

Gordon, S. C., et al. (1994). Self-administered versus nurse-administered epidural analgesia after cesarean section. *Journal of Obstetric, Gynecologic and Neonatal Nursing, 23,* 99.

Kanto, J., et al. (1990). Pre-operative preparation. *Nursing Times, 86,* 39.

Kearney, M. H., et al. (1990). Cesarean delivery and breastfeeding outcomes. *Birth 17,* 97

Miovech, S. M., et al. (1994). Major concerns of women after cesarean delivery. *Journal of Obstetric, Gynecologic and Neonatal Nursing, 23,* 53.

Radin, T. G., Harmon, J.S., & Hanson, D. A. (1993). Nurses' care during labor: its effect on the cesarean birth rate of healthy nulliparous women. *Birth, 20,* 14.

Rosen, M. G., et al. (1991). Vaginal birth after cesarean: a meta-analysis of morbidity and mortality. *Obstetrics and Gynecology, 77,* 465.

Taffel, S. M., et al. (1992). U.S. cesarean section rates 1990: an update. *Birth, 19,* 21.

Watts, D. H., et al. (1991). Upper genital tract isolates at delivery as predictors of post-cesarean infections among women receiving antibiotic prophylaxis. *Obstetrics and Gynecology, 77,* 287.

Welton, J. (1990). Pain control in labour. *Nursing, 4,* 14.

Suggested Readings

Berenson, A. B., et al. (1990). Bacteriologic findings of postcesarean endometritis in adolescents. *Obstetrics and Gynecology, 75,* 627.

Clemenson, N. (1993). Promoting vaginal birth after cesarean section. *American Family Physicians, 47,* 139.

Johnson, S. A. (1992). Ethical dilemma: a patient refuses a life-saving cesarean. *MCN: American Journal of Maternal Child Nursing, 17,* 121.

Norman, P., et al. (1993). Elective repeat cesarean sections: how many could be vaginal births? *Canadian Medical Association Journal, 149,* 431.

Pridjian, G., et al. (1991). Cesarean: changing the trends. *Obstetrics and Gynecology, 77,* 195.

Resnick, L. K., & Erlen, J. A. (1990). Vaginal birth after cesarean: issues and implications. *Journal of the American Academy of Nurse Practitioners, 2,* 100.

Shearer, E. (1992). Should the electronic fetal monitor always be used for women in labor who are having vaginal birth after a previous cesarean section? *Birth, 19,* 33.

Stainton, M. C. (1994). Supporting family functioning during a high-risk pregnancy. *MCN: American Journal of Maternal Child Nursing, 19,* 24.

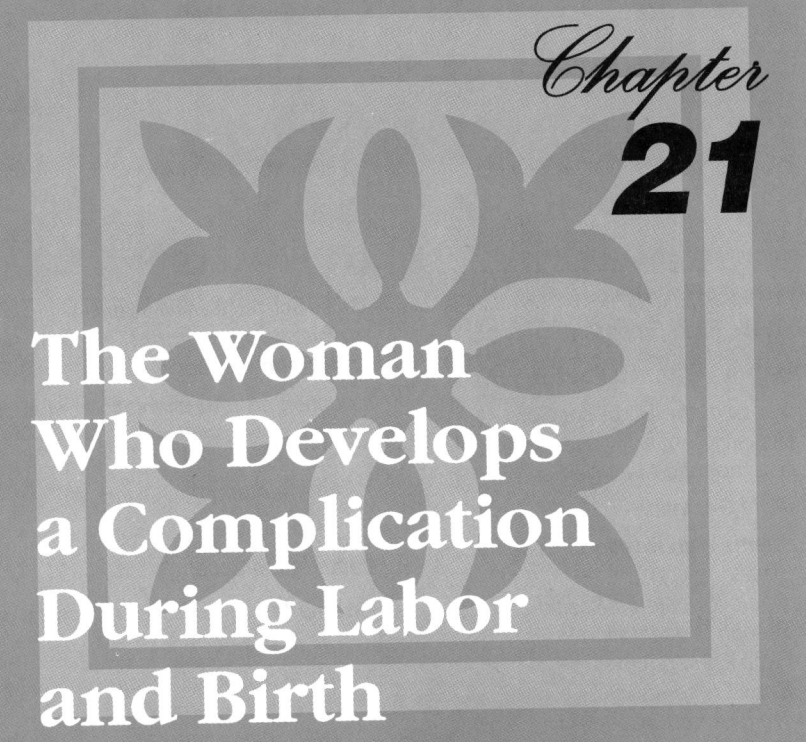

Chapter 21

The Woman Who Develops a Complication During Labor and Birth

Objectives

After mastering the contents of this chapter, you should be able to:

1. Define the general term dystocia and the common deviations in the force of labor, the passage, or passenger that can cause dystocia.

2. Assess the woman in labor and during birth for deviations from the normal labor process.

3. Formulate nursing diagnoses related to deviations from normal in labor and birth.

4. Plan nursing interventions, such as helping a woman prepare for a cesarean birth or augmentation of labor that will help the family meet established goals.

5. Implement care related to potential complications in labor or birth, such as those caused by breech presentation, multiple gestation, fetal distress, and prolapsed cord.

6. Evaluate outcome criteria to ensure that nursing goals related to deviations from the normal in labor and birth were achieved.

7. Identify National Health Goals related to complications of labor that nurses could be instrumental in helping the nation achieve.

8. Identify areas related to complications of labor that could benefit from additional nursing research.

9. Use critical thinking to analyze ways that nursing care can be kept family centered when deviations from the normal in labor and birth occur.

10. Synthesize the knowledge of deviations of normal in labor and birth with nursing process to achieve quality maternal and child health nursing care.

Adele Pillitteri: MATERNAL AND CHILD HEALTH NURSING, 2nd Edition. © 1995 Adele Pillitteri.

Although the usual labor proceeds without a deviation from the normal, a multitude of potential problems exists. Some abnormality is estimated to occur in approximately 8% of all deliveries (Cunningham et al., 1993). A difficult labor—**dystocia**—can arise from any of the three main components of the labor process: (1) the force that propels the fetus (uterine contractions); (2) the passenger (the fetus); or (3) the passageway (the birth canal). In addition, the medical interventions used to prevent or manage certain complications can cause some problems of their own.

Because complications can occur at any point in the process, one of the primary roles of the nurse caring for a woman in labor is continuous monitoring of the mother and fetus. A parallel role, and one that may be just as crucial to the health of the mother and child, is providing emotional support for the laboring woman and her partner. The hours of labor are stressful even when everything is proceeding normally. The laboring woman needs to be assured periodically that everything is going smoothly and that both she and the infant appear to be doing well. When a complication arises, however, and assurances cannot be given as freely, the stress

for the woman and her support person can increase 100-fold (Swinnerton, 1991).

Every woman in labor should have with her a nurse who is highly skilled in both the physical aspects of care and the interpersonal relationships, and who is compassionate as well. The woman who realizes she is having a complication in labor has willed her body to successfully complete the job it started 9 months before; without any idea she would lose control over the final hours before birth, she now needs someone to be with her who understands her fears and feelings of helplessness. National Health Goals related to complications of labor are shown in the Focus on National Health Goals box.

☒ **NURSING PROCESS OVERVIEW**
for the Woman With a Labor Complication

ASSESSMENT

One of the chief assessment measures used to detect deviations from normal labor and birth is fetal and uterine monitoring. Working with such apparatus involves explaining to parents its importance, winning their cooperation, and using judgment in reading the various patterns. Monitoring high-risk women in labor entails problems not found in other high-risk areas such as an intensive care unit (ICU). In an ICU, the person being monitored has been admitted to the unit because he or she is seriously ill; the person, recognizing the seriousness of the illness, accepts almost any monitoring or other procedure without protest. He or she lies still to prevent artifacts on the tracing. A maternity patient, however, may be less compliant because she may be wary of technologic intervention in the course of her labor and birth. She moves because she is in pain. Her movement causes artifacts on tracings and requires frequent adjustment of the equipment to achieve a clear tracing. The nurse needs to accept this problem as inherent in caring for the woman who is otherwise well.

NURSING DIAGNOSIS

Common nursing diagnoses specific to the woman experiencing a complication during labor refer to specific problems present. These include the following:

- Fear related to uncertainty of pregnancy outcome
- Anxiety related to medical procedures and apparatus necessary for ensuring health of mother and fetus

- Fatigue related to loss of glucose stores through work and duration of labor
- High risk for altered tissue perfusion related to excessive loss of blood
- Grief related to death of newborn at birth

PLANNING AND IMPLEMENTATION

Goal-setting during this time is often difficult. One of the ways to be most helpful is to encourage a couple to clarify their priorities. A woman might say early in labor that avoiding monitoring equipment or an episiotomy are her goals in labor. When, for example, the baby is detected to have bradycardia, it becomes apparent that a cesarean birth will be necessary. Reminding the woman that the primary goal is to have a healthy baby will help her accept changes in goals and whatever interventions are necessary to achieve them.

A complication of labor and birth invariably becomes at least a priority action situation, if not an emergency. Planning must be done efficiently based on the individual circumstances, so that when the moment of action occurs, it can be accomplished without hesitation or failure. All actions must safeguard both the woman and the fetus while providing psychological reassurance for the woman and her support person.

EVALUATION

Evaluation of client care goals may be a sad period, because not every woman who experiences a deviation from the normal in labor and birth will be able to deliver a healthy child. Some deviations will be too extreme; some interventions will not be maximally effective owing to individual circumstances. Some infants will die; some women will be left unable to bear future children. Evaluation may lead to new analysis that the couple's chief need at that point is to grieve for the child and a lifestyle that can no longer be theirs. When the outcome is more positive, the couple needs to be evaluated for signs that they are able to begin interaction with the child after a harrowing experience.

Examples of outcome criteria might be:

- Client voices confidence she can cope with fear.
- Client demonstrates adequate energy during course of labor to maintain effective breathing patterns.
- Client's blood pressure remains above 110/60 in spite of excessive blood loss with placenta delivery.
- Client begins grief response because of loss of newborn.

Problems With the Force of Labor

Inertia is a time-honored term to denote that the sluggishness of contractions, or the force of labor, has occurred. The current, commonly used term is **dysfunctional labor**. Dysfunction can occur at any point in labor but is generally classified as *primary* (occurring at the onset of labor) or *secondary* (occurring later in labor). The incidence of postpartal infection and hemorrhage in the woman and mortality in the infant are higher in women who have a prolonged labor than those who do not, making it vital to recognize and prevent dysfunctional labor (Mayberry, 1994).

Prolonged labor appears to result from a number of factors (Box 21-1). Hypotonic, hypertonic, and uncoordinated contractions all play roles in dysfunctional labor.

Ineffective Uterine Force

The contractions of the uterus are the basic force that moves the fetus through the birth canal. As described in Chapter 18, uterine contractions occur because of the interplay of contractile hormones (adenosine triphosphate, estrogen, and progesterone) and the influence of major electrolytes such as calcium, sodium, and potassium, specific contractile proteins (actin and myosin), epinephrine and norepinephrine, oxytocin, and prostaglandins. About 95% of labors are completed with contractions following a predictable, normal course. Three types of abnormal contractions that may occur are (1) hypotonic contractions, (2) hypertonic contractions, and (3) uncoordinated contractions. All of these types of contractions are ineffective, resulting in an ineffective labor.

Hypotonic Contractions

Figure 21-1*A* illustrates the appearance of normal uterine contractions. With **hypotonic uterine contractions** the number of contractions is usually low or infrequent (not increasing beyond two or three in a 10-minute period). The resting tone of the uterus remains below 10 mm Hg and the strength of contractions does not rise above 25 mm Hg (Figure 21-1*B*). Hypotonic contractions are most apt to occur during the active phase of labor. They may occur when analgesia has been administered too early (before cervical dilatation of 3–4 cm) or when bowel or bladder distention is present and prevents descent or firm engagement. They may occur in a uterus overstretched by a multiple gestation, a larger than usual single fetus, hydramnios, or in a lax uterus from grand multiparity. Such contractions are not exceedingly painful, because of the lack of intensity (strength being a subjective symptom, however, some women could interpret contractions as very painful).

Hypotonic contractions increase the length of labor, because so many of them are necessary to achieve cervical dilatation. During the postpartal period, the uterus can be exhausted from a long labor and may not continue to contract as effectively, thus increasing the woman's chance for postpartal hemorrhage. With the cervix dilated for a long period, both the uterus and the fetus are prone to infection.

For these reasons, after it is confirmed by sonogram that a cephalopelvic disproportion does not exist, an infusion of oxytocin to augment labor is usually begun to strengthen contractions and increase their effectiveness. Membranes may be artificially ruptured (amniotomy) in order to speed labor. In the first hour postpartum, the uterus needs to be palpated every 15 minutes and lochia should be assessed carefully to ensure that postpartal contractions are adequate.

Hypertonic Contractions

Hypertonic uterine contractions are marked by an increase in resting tone to more than 15 mm Hg. The intensity may be no stronger than with hypotonic contractions, however; they tend to occur frequently and are most commonly seen in the latent phase of labor. Hypertonic contractions occur because the muscle fibers of the myometrium do not repolarize following a contraction, "wiping it clean" to accept a new pacemaker stimulus, perhaps because more than one pacemaker is stimulating the contractions (Figure 21-1*C*). Hypertonic contractions tend to be painful, because the myometrium becomes tender from constant lack of relaxation and resultant anoxia to uterine cells. The woman may become frustrated or disappointed with her breathing exercises for childbirth, because they are ineffective

---

Box 21-1

Common Causes of Dysfunctional Labor

Inappropriate use of analgesia (excessive or too early administration)

Pelvic bone contraction that has narrowed the pelvic diameter so that the fetus cannot pass, such as might have occurred in a client with rickets

Poor fetal position (posterior rather than anterior position)

Extension rather than flexion of the fetal head

Overdistention of the uterus, as with multiple pregnancy, hydramnios, or an excessively oversized fetus

Cervical rigidity

Presence of a full rectum or urinary bladder that impedes fetal descent

Mother becoming exhausted from labor

Primigravida

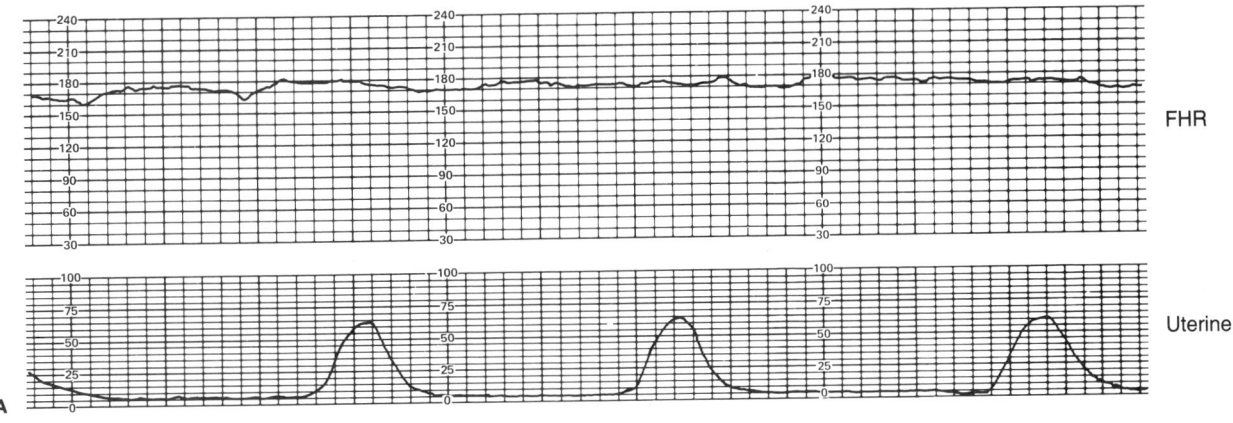
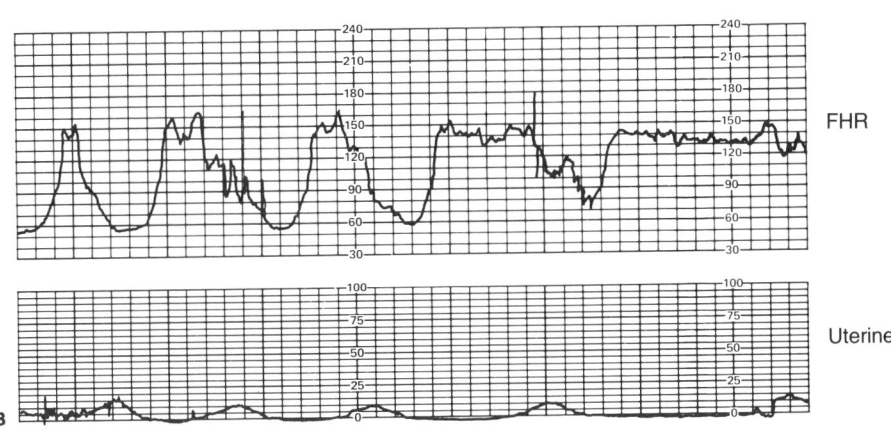
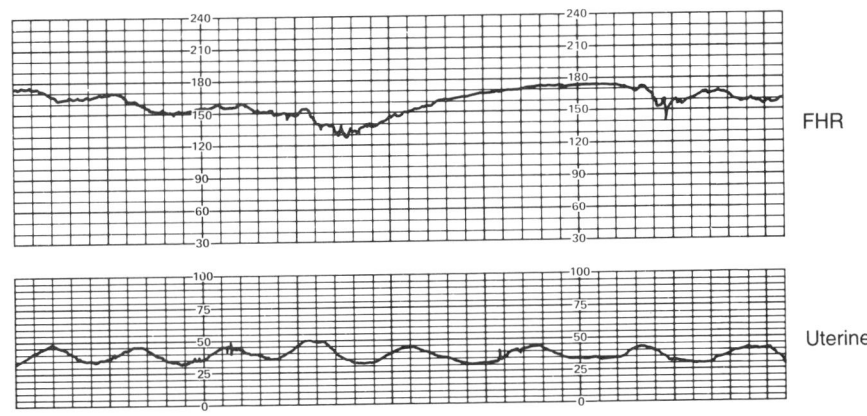

FIGURE 21-1

(**A**) *Normal uterine contractions.* (**B**)*Hypotonic contractions; notice that the fetal heart rate (FHR) on this strip shows late decelerations even with these ineffective contractions of no more than 10 mm Hg pressure.* (**C**) *Hypertonic contractions; notice the high resting pressure (40–50 mm Hg). FHR is rapid (170 beats/min) with variable decelerations.*

in keeping her pain free. Telling her to relax and "breathe with" contractions is ineffective because the problem is reversed: the lack of relaxation makes it impossible for her to breathe effectively.

The lack of relaxation between contractions does not allow optimal uterine artery filling, which may cause

the fetus to begin to suffer anoxia early in the latent phase of labor. Any woman whose pain seems out of proportion to the quality of her contractions should have both a uterine and fetal external monitor applied for at least a 15-minute interval to ensure the resting phase of the contractions is adequate and the fetal pattern is not

Table 21-1. *Comparison of Hypotonic and Hypertonic Contractions*

Criteria	Hypertonic	Hypotonic
Phase of labor	Latent	Active
Symptoms	Painful	Painless
Medication		
Oxytocin	Unfavorable reaction	Favorable reaction
Sedation	Helpful	Little value

(Modified from Cunningham, F. G., et al. [1993]. *Williams obstetrics* [19th ed.]. Norwalk, CT: Appleton & Lange.)

showing late deceleration. Management of hypertonic contractions is rest, analgesia with morphine sulfate, and possibly sedation. Changing the linen and the client's gown, darkening room lights, and decreasing noise and stimulation are also helpful. If deceleration in the fetal heart rate, an abnormally long first stage of labor, or lack of progress with pushing ("second stage arrest") occur, the woman will be scheduled for a cesarean birth. Both the woman and her support person need to understand that, although the contractions are strong, they are in reality ineffective and not achieving cervical dilatation. Hypotonic and hypertonic contractions are compared in Table 21-1.

Uncoordinated Contractions

Normally, all contractions are initiated at one pacemaker point in the uterus. A contraction sweeps down over the uterus, encircling it; repolarization occurs, a low resting tone is achieved, and another pacemaker-activated contraction begins. With uncoordinated contractions, more than one pacemaker may be initiating contractions; or, receptor points in the uterus myometrium are acting independently of the pacemaker. Uncoordinated contractions may occur so closely together that they do not allow good cotyledon filling. They make it difficult for the woman to rest or use breathing exercises between contractions, because they occur so erratically (one on top of another and then a long period without any).

Applying a fetal and uterine external monitor and assessing the rate, pattern, resting tone, and fetal response to contractions for at least a 15-minute interval (a longer time may be necessary to show the disorganized pattern in early labor) reveals the abnormal pattern.

Oxytocin administration may be helpful in uncoordinated labor to stimulate a more effective and consistent pattern of contractions with a better lower resting tone.

Dysfunctional Labor

Dysfunction at the First Stage of Labor

Prolonged Latent Phase. Table 21-2 gives the normal parameters for stages of labor. The major dysfunction that can occur in the first stage of labor is a prolonged latent phase (Friedman, 1985).

A *prolonged latent phase,* defined as a latent phase that is longer than 20 hours in a nullipara and 14 hours in a multipara, may happen if the cervix is not "ripe" at the beginning of labor and time has to be spent getting truly ready for labor (Figure 21-2). It may occur if there is excessive use of an analgesic early in labor. With a prolonged latent phase, the uterus tends to be in a hypertonic state. Relaxation between contractions is inadequate, and the contractions themselves are only mild (less than 15 mm Hg on a monitor printout) and therefore ineffective. One segment of the uterus may contract with more force than another segment.

Management of a prolonged latent phase in labor includes helping the uterus to rest and administering adequate fluid to the woman to prevent dehydration. It may be wise to administer the fluid intravenously to keep the woman's gastrointestinal tract free of fluid in case anesthesia is necessary for birth. Administration of morphine may relax hypertonicity. When the woman awakens from a short sleep, labor usually becomes effective and begins to progress. If it does not, the infant may have to be delivered by cesarean birth or the labor assisted with amniotomy and oxytocin infusion.

Protracted Active Phase. A *protracted active phase* is usually associated with cephalopelvic disproportion (CPD) or fetal malposition, although it may reflect inef-

Table 21-2. *Lengths of Phases of Stages of Normal Labor in Hours*

Phase	Nullipara		Multipara	
	Average	Upper Normal	Average	Upper Normal
Latent phase	8.6	20.0	5.3	14.0
Active phase	5.8	12.0	2.5	6.0
Second stage	1	1.5	.25	1

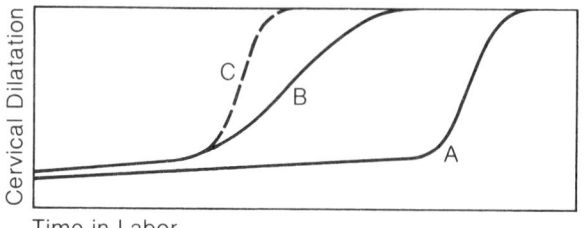

FIGURE 21-2
Labor patterns. (**A**) *Prolonged latent phase.* (**B**) *Prolonged active phase.* (**C**) *Normal labor pattern.*

fective myometrial activity. This phase is prolonged if cervical dilatation does not occur at a rate of 1.2 cm/h or more in a nullipara or 1.5 cm/h or more in a multipara or if the active phase lasts over 12 hours in a primigravida, 6 hours in a multigravida. If the cause of the delay in dilatation is fetal malposition or CPD, cesarean birth may have to be initiated to effect birth. Dysfunctional labor during the dilatational division tends to be hypotonic in contrast to the hypertonic action at the beginning of labor (see Figure 21-2). Oxytocin may be prescribed to augment labor.

Prolonged Deceleration Phase. A deceleration phase has become prolonged when it extends beyond 3 hours in a nullipara and 1 hour in a multipara.

Secondary Arrest of Dilatation. A secondary arrest of dilatation has occurred when there is no progress in cervical dilatation for more than 2 hours.

Prolonged Descent. *Prolonged descent* of the fetus occurs if the rate of descent is less than 1.0 cm/h in a nullipara or less than 2.0 cm/h in a multipara.

With both a prolonged active phase of dilatation and prolonged descent, contractions have been of good quality and proper duration, and effacement and beginning dilatation have occurred; but then the contractions gradually become infrequent and of poor quality, and dilatation stops. If everything except the suddenly faulty contractions is normal (CPD or poor fetal presentation has been ruled out by sonogram), then rest and fluid intake, as advocated for hypertonic contractions, also apply to this situation. If membranes have not ruptured, rupturing them at this point may be helpful. Intravenous oxytocin may be used to induce the uterus to contract effectively. A semi-Fowler's position, squatting, kneeling, or more effective pushing may speed descent.

Whether the dysfunctional labor occurs in the first or second stage of labor, the effect on the woman and her support person will be the same: anxiety, fear, or discouragement. The woman needs a continuous explanation of what is happening: "We're going to take a sonogram to check the baby's position." "This is a drug to urge your uterus into stronger contractions." "I know resting is the last thing you feel like doing, but that is what I want you to try to do."

Dysfunction at the Second Stage of Labor

Arrest of Descent. *Arrest of descent* is when no descent has occurred for 1 hour in a multipara, 2 hours in a nullipara. *Failure of descent* has occurred when expected descent of the fetus does not begin (engagement or movement beyond 0 station has not occurred).

The most likely cause for arrest in labor during the

second stage is CPD. Cesarean birth is generally chosen as the method of birth of the infant. If there is no contraindication to vaginal birth, oxytocin may be used to assist in labor.

Nursing Diagnoses and Related Interventions for Dysfunctional Labor

It is impossible to prevent all dysfunctional labor, just as it is impossible to predict the functioning of anyone's hormone system or individual response to labor. There are a number of nursing interventions, however, that can contribute to the progression of normal labor or re-start a dysfunctional one.

Nursing Diagnosis: High risk for fatigue related to prolonged labor

Goal: Client will maintain adequate energy for continued labor.

Outcome Criteria: Woman states she is able to continue active participation in labor; maintains effective breathing with contractions.

Because labor is such hard work, it can cause a woman to deplete her glucose stores. On a client's admission to a birthing room, assess how likely this is to happen by asking the time of her last meal. If she ate breakfast at 8 AM and then began labor by 2 PM, she is only 6 hours away from a full meal. If, however, she last ate at 5 PM the preceding evening and did not eat breakfast because she awoke with labor this morning, she is 11 hours away from a full meal. The chance that she will deplete glucose stores is three times greater. Alert the physician or nurse-midwife to this possibility, and if the client is still in early labor she may be allowed to drink some high-carbohydrate fluid such as orange juice; an intravenous solution to provide glucose may be started.

Many women react negatively to the suggestion of intravenous fluid during labor. They perceive it as losing control over their bodies, of having the naturalness of labor and birth taken away from them. Introduce the suggestion of intravenous fluid and explain its purpose *before* arriving with the bag of fluid and tubing. Once you have convinced her it is necessary, be certain that the needle is placed in the nondominant hand and only a small "reminder" handboard is used rather than a long one. Assure the woman that she can be out of bed and walking, can turn freely, squat, sit, or use whatever position she prefers; that none of these acts will interfere with the infusion (Figure 21-3). Most physicians and nurse-midwives also allow women to have lollipops or hard candy to suck on during labor to supply additional glucose.

If the woman is neither tense nor frightened during labor, her cervix will dilate more rapidly and therefore

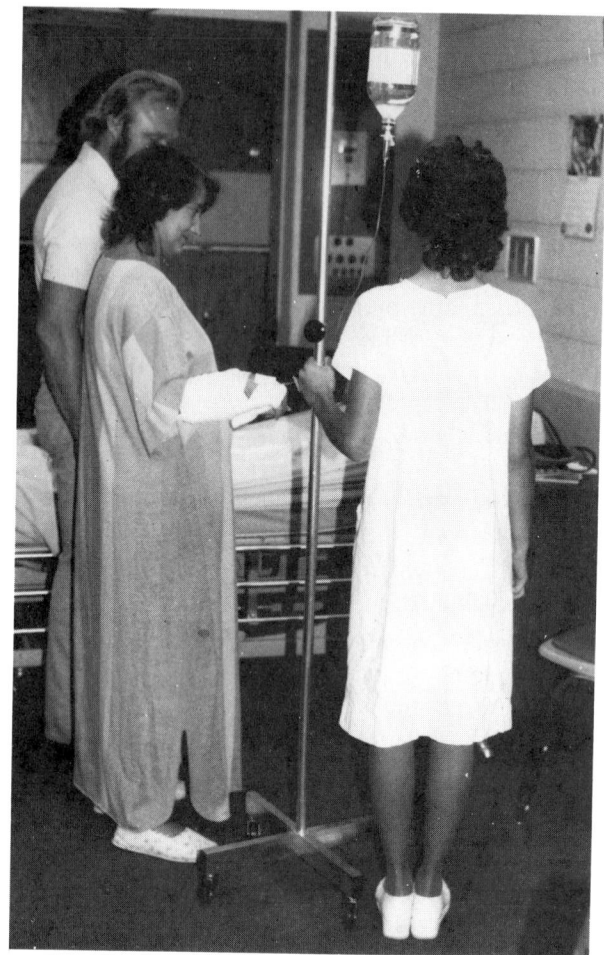

FIGURE 21-3
An intravenous line is becoming a more common piece of equipment for women in labor. However, it does not need to limit mobility.

labor will be shortened. Manage stress by making the transfer from home to health care facility as least traumatic as possible. Ask directly if the woman has any concerns. Offer explanations of all procedures. Make the support person just as welcome and comfortable as the woman herself. A question such as, "Is labor what you thought it would be?" to both the woman and her support person often helps them to express different concerns.

Remember that pain is an exhausting phenomenon. Praise breathing attempts; breathe with the woman, give back rubs, change sheets, use cool washcloths, and so forth. If breathing exercises can be effective, the need for analgesia (which can lead to hypotonic contractions) can be reduced.

To increase the blood supply to the uterus and prevent hypotension, urge the woman to lie on her side so that the uterus is lifted off the vena cava. If a woman insists on lying supine, place a hip roll under one or the

other buttock to cause her pelvis to "tip" and, at least to some extent, move the uterus to the side.

A full bladder prevents descent of the fetus and may impede uterine contractions. Urge the laboring woman to void every 2 hours during labor to keep the bladder empty and to aid progress.

> ***Nursing Diagnosis:*** High risk for fluid volume deficit related to length and work of labor and accompanying (potential) vomiting and diarrhea
>
> ***Goal:*** Client will maintain adequate fluid and electrolyte balance during labor.
>
> ***Outcome Criteria:*** There is no evidence of ketones in urine; specific gravity of urine is between 1.003 and 1.030.

Low levels of serum electrolytes or body fluid can occur in labor for the same reason as a decreased glucose level: a long interval between eating and the end of labor. Electrolyte losses can be increased by vomiting and diarrhea that occasionally accompany labor. Ask if these occurred and the extent of them (e.g., one episode of a small amount of diarrhea or vomiting that lasted on and off for 30 minutes). Profuse diaphoresis and hyperventilation that occur with labor can further increase fluid and electrolyte losses through insensible water loss. Test all voidings during labor for glucose, protein, ketones, and specific gravity (place a urine collector container on the bathroom toilet if the woman is going to use the toilet). Ketones suggest starvation ketosis; a concentrated specific gravity suggests a lack of fluid. Extreme dehydration leads to increased blood viscosity; this may increase the possibility of thrombophlebitis during the postpartal period. Thus, intravenous fluid administration may prevent not only fluid and electrolyte loss but postpartal complications as well.

Contraction Rings

Two types of contraction ring can occur in an abnormal labor. The most common is a **pathologic retraction ring** (Bandl's ring) at the juncture of the upper and lower uterine segments that forms as a warning sign that severe dysfunctional labor is occurring. The ring usually appears during the second stage of labor as a horizontal indentation across the abdomen (Figure 21-4). It is formed by excessive retraction of the upper uterine segment; the uterine myometrium is much thicker above than below the ring.

A second type of ring is a **constriction ring**, which can occur at any point in the myometrium and at any time during labor. With fetal monitors in place, there is a tendency not to observe a woman's abdomen in labor as much as when fetal heart sounds are being auscultated.

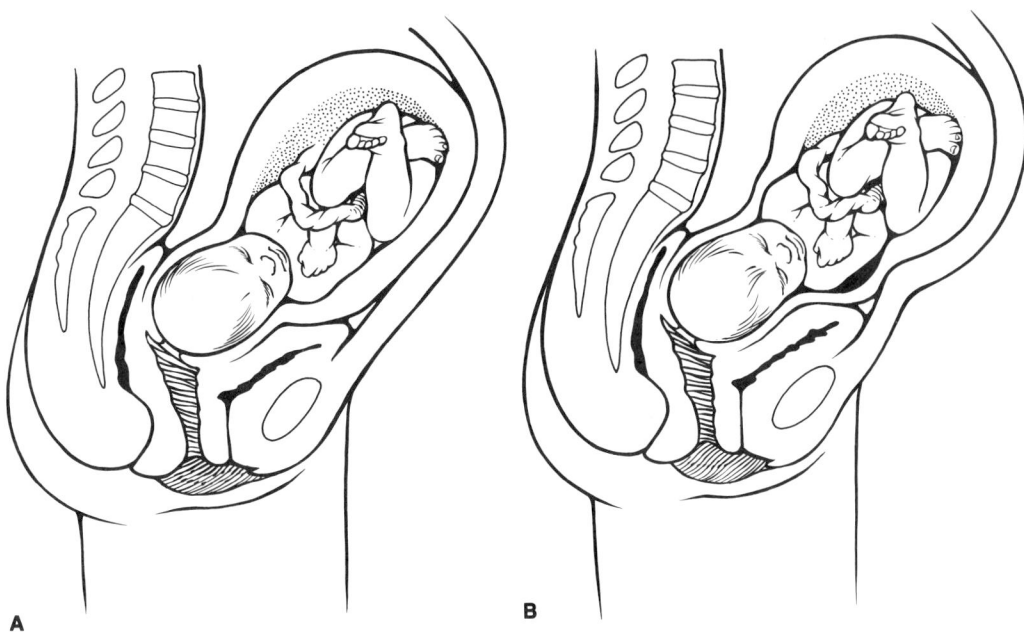

FIGURE 21-4

Pathologic retraction ring. (**A**)*Uterus in the normal second stage of labor. Notice how the upper uterine segment is becoming thicker and the lower uterine segment is thinning. A physiologic retraction ring is normally formed at the division of the upper and lower uterine segments. (**B**) Uterus with a pathologic retraction ring (Bandl's ring). The wall below the ring is thin and the abdomen shows an indentation. This constriction is caused by obstructed labor and is a warning sign that if the obstruction is not relieved, the lower segment may rupture.*

It is important to observe the woman's abdomen, however, in case a pathologic retraction ring appears. When this occurs in early labor, it is usually from uncoordinated contractions; in the pelvic division of labor, it is usually caused by obstetric manipulation or the result of the administration of oxytocin. The fetus is gripped by the retraction ring and cannot advance beyond that point. The undelivered placenta will also be held at that point.

Such a finding is extremely serious and should be reported promptly. Administration of intravenous morphine sulfate or the inhalation of amyl nitrite may relieve the retraction ring. A tocolytic may be administered to halt contractions. If the situation is not relieved, uterine rupture and death of the fetus may occur. In the placental stage, massive maternal hemorrhage may result, because the placenta is loosened but not delivered, which prevents the uterus from contracting.

Cesarean birth will be chosen to ensure safe birth of the fetus. Manual removal of the placenta under general anesthesia may be necessary in the event of placental-stage pathologic retraction rings.

Precipitate Labor

A **precipitate labor** and birth occurs when uterine contractions are so strong that the woman delivers with only a few rapidly occurring contractions. It is often defined as a labor that is completed in fewer than 3 hours (Cunningham et al., 1993). Such rapid labor is likely to occur with multiparity and may follow induction of labor by oxytocin or amniotomy. Rapid labor poses a risk to the fetus, because subdural hemorrhage may result from the sudden release of pressure on the head; the woman may sustain lacerations of the birth canal. Forceful contractions may lead to premature separation of the placenta and both maternal and fetal risk.

A precipitate labor can be predicted from a labor graph if, during the active phase of dilatation, the rate is greater than 5 cm/h (1 cm every 12 minutes) in a nullipara and more than 10 cm/h (1 cm every 6 minutes) in a multipara. If this is occurring, a tocolytic may be administered to reduce the force of contractions.

The woman with multiparity should be told by week 28 of pregnancy that her labor might be shorter than a previous one and that she should make plans for rapid transportation to the hospital or alternative birthing center. Women who had a prior precipitate labor and birth should be alerted that they may well deliver this way again. Both grand multiparas and women with histories of precipitate labor should have the birthing room converted to birth readiness before full dilatation; birth can then be accomplished in controlled surroundings.

Uterine Rupture

Rupture of the uterus during labor is rare, occurring only in about 1 in 1500 births, but is always a possibility. A uterus ruptures when it undergoes more strain than it is capable of sustaining. Rupture occurs most commonly when a vertical scar from a previous cesarean birth, hysterotomy, or plastic repair of the uterus tears. However, other contributing factors are prolonged labor, faulty presentation, multiple gestation, unwise use of oxytocin, obstructed labor, and traumatic maneuvers using forceps or traction. Uterine rupture accounts for as many as 5% of all maternal deaths; 50% of the time, fetal death results.

Impending rupture is suggested by a pathologic retraction ring (an indentation is apparent across the abdomen over the uterus) and strong uterine contractions without any cervical dilatation.

To prevent rupture when these symptoms are present, a cesarean birth will be scheduled immediately. If a uterus should rupture, the woman experiences a sudden, severe pain during a strong labor contraction. She may report a "tearing" sensation. Rupture can be complete, going through endometrium, myometrium, and peritoneum, or incomplete, leaving the peritoneum intact. With rupture, uterine contractions will stop. There is hemorrhage from the torn uterus into the abdominal cavity and possibly into the vagina. Signs of shock begin, including rapid, weak pulse, falling blood pressure, cold and clammy skin, and dilatation of the nostrils from air hunger. The woman's abdomen will change in contour, and two distinct swellings will be visible: the retracted uterus and the extrauterine fetus. Fetal heart sounds fail. If the rupture is incomplete, the signs are less evident than in complete rupture: the woman experiences a localized tenderness and a persistent aching pain over the area of the lower segment; contractions usually cease; and fetal heart sounds and the woman's vital signs will gradually reveal fetal and maternal distress.

Because the uterus at the end of pregnancy is such a vascular organ, uterine rupture is an immediate emergency situation comparable with splenic or hepatic rupture. Emergency fluid replacement must be administered; intravenous oxytocin may be administered to attempt to contract the uterus and minimize bleeding. A laparotomy must be scheduled as an emergency measure to control bleeding and effect a repair. The viability of the fetus will depend on the extent of the rupture and the time that elapses between the rupture and abdominal extraction. The woman's prognosis will depend on the extent of the rupture and blood loss.

It is inadvisable for a woman to conceive again after a rupture of the uterus unless it occurred in the inactive lower segment. The physician, with consent, may sterilize the woman, either by removal of the damaged uterus (hysterectomy) or by tubal ligation at the time of the laparotomy. The woman may have difficulty giving her consent at the moment she is given anesthesia, because it is unknown whether the fetus will live. If blood loss was acute, she may be unconscious from hypotension so that her support person must be the one who gives this consent, relying on the integrity of the operating surgeon to decide whether a functioning uterus can be saved.

Be prepared to offer information to the support person and to inform him or her as soon as possible about the fetal outcome, the extent of the surgery, and the woman's safety. The woman and her support person will probably be intensely grateful initially because her life was saved; however, they may become almost immediately angry that the rupture occurred, especially if the fetus died and the woman will no longer be able to have children. Allow them time to express these justifiable emotions without feeling threatened. They may grieve both for the loss of the child and her fertility.

Inversion of the Uterus

Inversion of the uterus is a rare phenomenon, occurring in about 1 in 15,000 births, in which the uterus is turned inside out. It may occur following the birth of the infant if traction is applied to the umbilical cord to remove the placenta or if pressure is applied to the uterine fundus when the uterus is not contracted. It may also occur when there is insertion of the placenta at the fundus, so that during birth the passage of the fetus pulls the fundus down.

Inversion occurs in various degrees. The inverted fundus may lie within the uterine cavity or the vagina or, in total inversion, protrude from the vagina. When an inversion occurs, there is a large sudden gush of blood from the vagina; the fundus is no longer palpable in the abdomen. If the loss of blood continues unchecked for more than a few minutes, the woman will immediately show signs of blood loss: hypotension, dizziness, paleness, or diaphoresis. The uterus is not contracted in this position and so the bleeding continues unchecked. A woman could exsanguinate within a period as short as 10 minutes.

Never attempt to replace the inversion; without good pelvic relaxation this may only increase bleeding. Never attempt to remove the placenta if it is still attached; this will only create a larger bleeding area. The administration of an oxytocic drug only compounds the inversion. The woman needs to be given general anesthesia or a tocolytic drug intravenously immediately; the delivering physician or nurse-midwife then replaces the fundus manually. An intravenous fluid line needs to be started if one is not already present (if doing this, use a large intercath needle, because blood will need to be replaced); a present fluid line should be opened to achieve optimal flow of fluid to try to restore fluid volume. Administration of an oxytocin at this point helps the uterus to contract into place. Administer oxygen by mask and assess vital signs. Be prepared to perform cardiopulmonary resuscitation (CPR) if her heart should fail from the sudden blood loss. The woman will need antibiotic coverage to prevent infection because the uterine endometrium was exposed.

Amniotic Fluid Embolism

Amniotic fluid embolism occurs when amniotic fluid is forced into an open maternal uterine blood sinus through some defect in the membranes or after membrane rupture or partial premature separation of the placenta. Solid particles (such as skin cells) in the amniotic fluid enter the maternal circulation and reach the lungs as small emboli. They produce a pulmonary embolism the severity of which is out of proportion to the size of the particles. This may occur during labor or in the postpartal period. The incidence of this is no more than 1 in 8000 births. Amniotic fluid embolism is unpreventable, but risk factors are oxytocin administration, placenta abruptio, and polyhydramnios.

The clinical picture is dramatic. The woman, in strong labor, sits up suddenly and grasps her chest because of inability to breathe and sharp pain. She pales and then turns the typical bluish gray associated with pulmonary embolism and lack of blood flow to the lungs. The immediate management is oxygen administration by face mask or cannula. Within minutes the woman will need CPR. This may be ineffective, because these procedures (inflating the lungs and massaging the heart) do not move the emboli so that blood still cannot circulate to the lungs. Death may occur in minutes.

The woman's prognosis depends on the size of the embolism and the skill and speed of the emergency aid available to her. Even if she survives the initial insult, there is a high likelihood of disseminated intravascular coagulation developing from the presence of particles in the bloodstream, further compounding her condition. In this event, she will need continued management that includes intubation and therapy with fibrinogen to counteract disseminated intravascular coagulation. She will be moved to an ICU for this level of care. The prognosis for the fetus is guarded, because reduced placental perfusion results from the severe drop in maternal blood pressure (Sisson, 1992). The fetus must be delivered immediately by cesarean birth or forceps.

Problems With the Passenger

Birth complications may arise if the umbilical cord prolapses, if there is more than one fetus, if the fetus is too large for the birth canal, or if it is malpositioned in the canal.

Prolapse of the Umbilical Cord

In *umbilical cord prolapse,* a loop of the umbilical cord slips down in front of the presenting fetal part (Figure 21-5). Prolapse may occur at any time after the membranes rupture and if the presenting part is not fitted firmly into the cervix. Thus, it tends to occur most often with the conditions shown in Box 21-2. The incidence is 1 in 200 pregnancies.

Assessment

In rare instances, the cord may be felt as the presenting part on vaginal examination or be evident in this position on sonogram. In the event of this presentation, cesarean birth will be necessary before rupture of the membranes occurs; otherwise, with rupture, the cord will be flushed down into the vagina. More often, however, cord prolapse is first discovered when the variable deceleration pattern of cord compression suddenly becomes apparent on a fetal monitor. The cord may then be visible at the vulva.

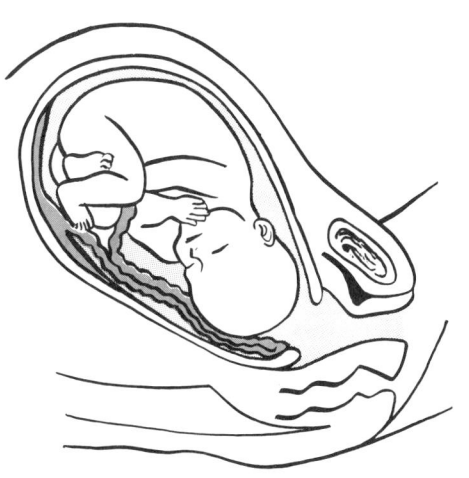

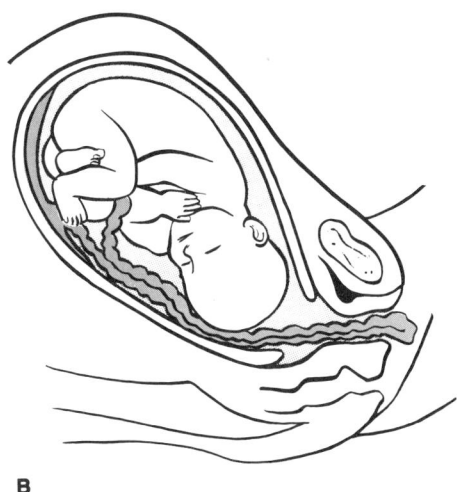

A   **B**

FIGURE 21-5
*Prolapse of the umbilical cord. (**A**) The cord is prolapsed but still within the uterus. (**B**) The cord is visible at the vulva. In both instances the fetal nutrient supply is being compromised, although only a cord such as that shown in **B** would be visible. Both prolapses could be detected by fetal monitoring equipment.*

Premature rupture of the membranes
Fetal position other than cephalic presentations
Placenta previa
Intrauterine tumors that prevent the presenting part from engaging
A small fetus
Cephalopelvic disproportion that prevents firm engagement of the fetus
Polyhydramnios
Multiple gestation

To rule out cord prolapse, fetal heart sounds should always be recorded immediately following rupture of the membranes, whether this occurs spontaneously or by amniotomy.

Therapeutic Management

Cord prolapse automatically leads to cord compression, because the fetal presenting part presses against the cord at the pelvic brim. Management is aimed toward relieving pressure on the cord and thereby relieving the compression and the resulting fetal anoxia. This may be done by placing a hand in the vagina and manually elevating the fetal head off the cord, or by placing the woman in a knee-chest or Trendelenburg position, which causes the fetal head to fall back from the cord. Administering oxygen at 10 L/min by face mask to the mother is also helpful. A tocolytic to reduce uterine activity may be ordered.

If the cord is exposed to room air, drying will begin, leading to atrophy of the umbilical vessels. Do not attempt to push any exposed cord back into the vagina, however, or this may add to the compression by causing knotting or kinking. Instead, cover any exposed portion with a sterile saline compress to prevent drying.

If the cervix is fully dilated at the time of the prolapse, the physician may choose to deliver the infant rapidly, possibly with forceps, to prevent a lengthy period of anoxia. If dilatation is incomplete, the birth method of choice is upward pressure on the presenting part by a practitioner's hand in the woman's vagina until cesarean birth is complete.

Multiple Gestation

Twin gestations occur approximately 1 in every 99 conceptions, triplets 1 in 5000, and quadruplets 1 in 400,000. A woman with a multiple gestation usually causes a flurry of excitement in the labor room. Additional personnel have to be assembled for the birth (two

nurses to attend to possibly immature infants and a pediatrician for immature care). In the middle of all the preparatory activity it is easy to forget that the woman may be more frightened than excited. Be careful that the air of anticipation focuses on her needs and those of the babies, not gratification of the health care team's curiosity about the multiple births. The majority of multiple gestations are delivered by cesarean birth to decrease the risk to the second or more fetus. This is certainly the case in multiple gestations of three or more when there is a high incidence of cord entanglement and premature separation of a placenta.

If a woman with a multiple gestation does deliver vaginally, the first stage of labor will not differ greatly from the first stage of a single gestation labor, except that the woman is usually instructed to come to the hospital early in labor, and it is important to try to monitor each fetal heart rate (FHR) by a separate fetal monitor, if possible. Coming to a hospital this early in labor will make labor seem long; urge the woman to spend the early hours of labor engaged in an activity such as playing cards to make the time pass more quickly.

Because the babies are usually small, firm head engagement may not occur and cord prolapse is an increased possibility after rupture of the membranes. Uterine dysfunction from a long labor, an overstretched uterus, and premature separation of the placenta after the birth of the first child may be more common. Because of the multiple fetuses, abnormal fetal presentation of other than the first infant may occur. Analgesia administration should be conservative, so that it will not add to any respiratory difficulties the infants may have at birth because of their immaturity. To avoid the need for analgesia or anesthesia, support breathing exercises. Multiple pregnancies often end before full term, so the woman may not yet have practiced breathing exercises. The early hours of labor can be used for this. Anemia and hypertension of pregnancy occur at higher than usual incidences during multiple gestations. Be certain to assess her hematocrit level and blood pressure conscientiously during labor.

The first fetus usually presents vertex. After the first infant is born, both ends of the baby's cord will be tied or clamped permanently rather than with cord clamps, which could slip. This will prevent hemorrhage through an open cord end if the placenta has been shared by additional infants. The first infant is identified as *A,* and newborn care will be started for him or her. A product such as methylergonovine (Methergine) to begin uterine involution will not be given to the woman to avoid compromising the circulation of the infants not yet born.

Most twin pregnancies present with both twins vertex, followed in frequency by vertex and breech, breech and vertex, and then breech and breech (Figure 21-6). Multiple gestations of three or more have extremely varied presentations. After the birth of the first child, the

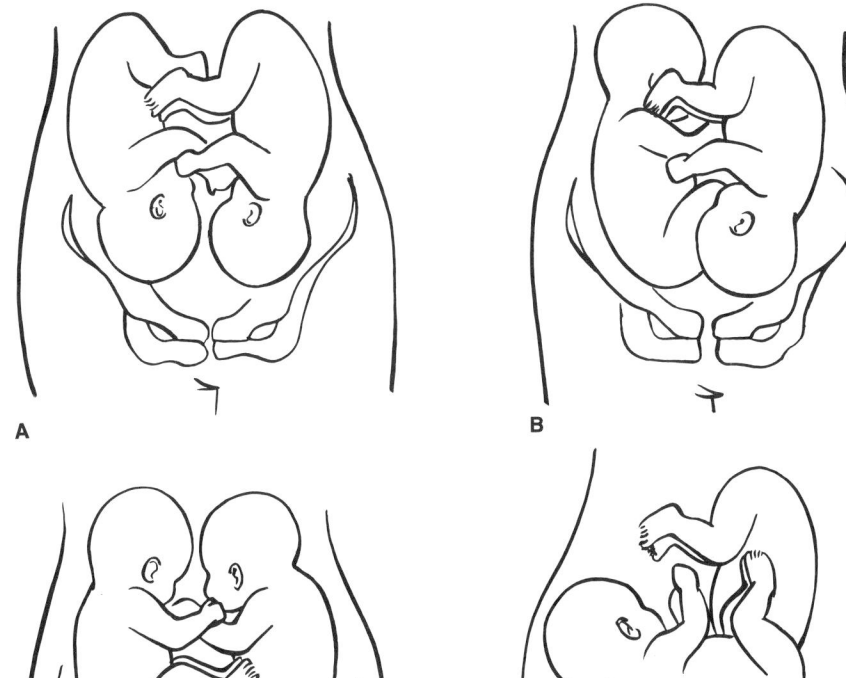

FIGURE 21-6
Four different twin presentations.
*(**A**) Both infants vertex. (**B**) One infant vertex and one breech. (**C**) Both infants breech. (**D**) One infant vertex and one in a transverse lie.*

lie of the second fetus is determined by external abdominal palpation. If the lie is not longitudinal, external version is attempted to make it so. The presentation is confirmed by vaginal examination and ultrasound, and the second set of membranes is ruptured. This action brings down the presenting part of the second infant and may initiate contractions if they are not already active. An oxytocin infusion may be begun at this point to assist uterine contractions in order to shorten the time span between the births.

Occasionally, the placenta of the first infant separates before the second fetus is born, and there is sudden, profuse bleeding at the vagina. This creates a risk for the woman; the uterus cannot contract as it normally would and thereby halt the bleeding because it is still filled with the additional fetus. If the separation of the first placenta caused loosening of the additional placentas, or if a common placenta is involved, the fetal heart sounds of the additional fetuses will immediately register distress, and they will have to be delivered at once if they are to survive. This is the reason that most multiple gestations today are delivered by cesarean birth. In some instances, the first baby is delivered vaginally and the second by cesarean birth because of this complication.

Parents usually want to inspect multiple gestation

infants thoroughly following the birth. The time allowed for this inspection will depend on the infants' weight and condition. Some parents of multiple children worry that the hospital will confuse them through improper identification. Review with them the careful measures that are being taken to ensure correct identification.

Many women who have a multiple birth have difficulty believing that it is real. They need to recount over and over their surprise and to view all their infants together to prove to themselves that it is true. If unable to inspect the infants thoroughly immediately after the birth because of the infants' low birth weight and the danger of chilling, the woman needs the opportunity to do so as soon as possible to dispel any fears she had throughout pregnancy that the babies would be born less than perfect.

The mother needs to be observed carefully in the immediate postpartal period because, overdistended, her uterus may have more difficulty than usual contracting and she is prone to postpartal hemorrhage from uterine atony. She may be more prone to uterine infection if birth was prolonged. The infants need careful assessment to determine their true gestational age and whether a phenomenon such as twin-to-twin transfusion has occurred (see Chapter 26).

Problems With Position, Presentation, or Size

Occipitoposterior Position

In approximately one tenth of all labors, the fetal position is posterior rather than anterior; that is, the occiput (assuming the presentation is vertex) is directed diagonally and posteriorly: right occipitoposterior (ROP) or left occipitoposterior (LOP) (Cunningham et al., 1993). In these positions, in the process of internal rotation, the fetal head must rotate not through a 90-degree arc, which is necessary for the anterior position (Figure 21-7), but through an arc of approximately 135 degrees (Figure 21-8).

Posterior positions tend to occur in women with android, anthropoid, or contracted pelves. A posterior position is suggested by a dysfunctional labor pattern such as a prolonged active phase, arrested descent, or fetal heart sounds heard best at the lateral sides of the abdomen.

The position of the fetus is confirmed on vaginal examination. A posteriorly presenting head does not fit the cervix as snugly as one in an anterior position. Because this increases the risk of prolapse of the umbilical cord, it needs to be assessed for during labor. The majority of in-

fants presenting in these posterior positions, if they are of average size and in good flexion and aided by forceful uterine contractions, will rotate through the large arc, will arrive at a good birth position for the pelvic outlet, and will be delivered satisfactorily with only increased molding and caput formation. Because the arc of rotation is greater, it is usual for the labor to be somewhat prolonged. Because the fetal head rotates against the sacrum, the woman may experience pressure and pain in her lower back from sacral nerve compression during labor, which may be so intense that she asks for medication for relief, not for her contractions but for the intense back pressure and pain she is feeling. Pressure on the sacrum such as that afforded by a back rub or a change of position may be helpful in relieving a portion of the pain (Figure 21-9). Lying on the side opposite the fetal back or maintaining a hands and knee position may help the fetus rotate (see the Focus on Nursing Research box). During a long labor, be certain that the woman voids approximately every 2 hours to keep the bladder empty; a full bladder impedes descent of the fetus. Be aware how long it has been since she last ate; she may need intravenous glucose to ward off uterine dysfunction.

If contractions are ineffective, or the infant is above

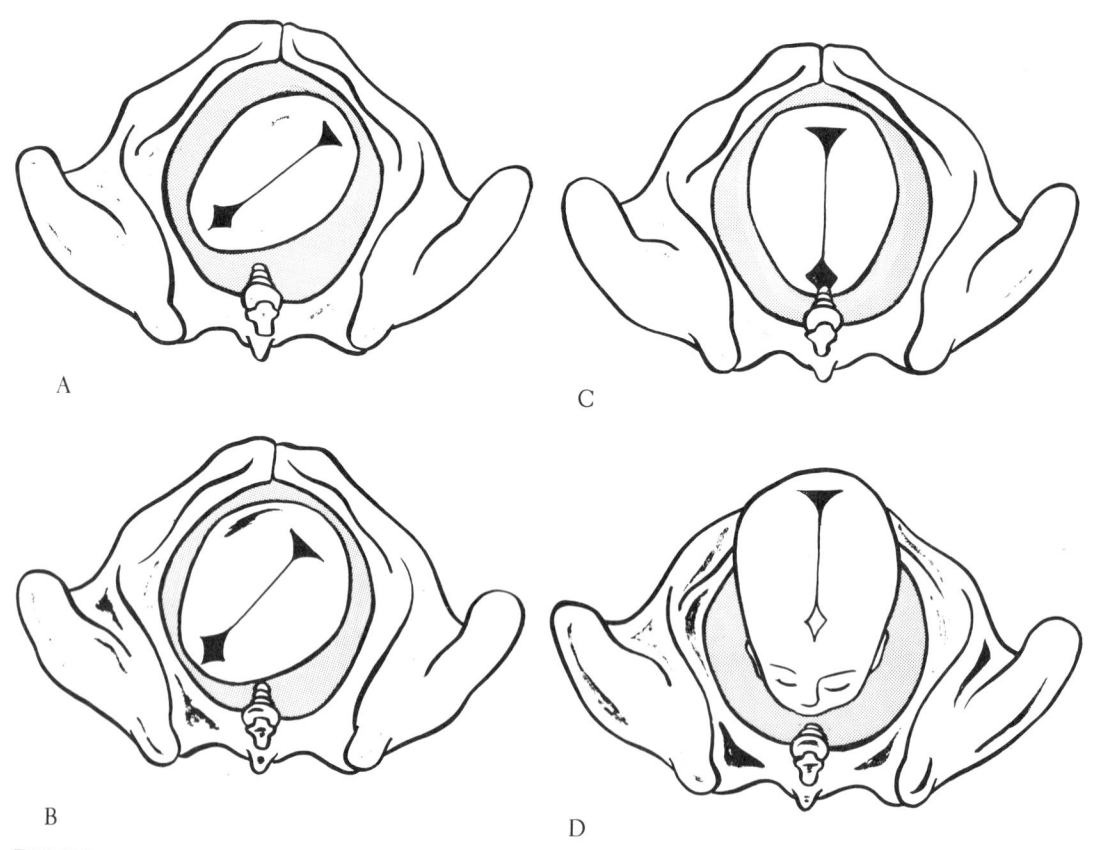

A

B

C

D

FIGURE 21-7

Left occipitoanterior (LOA) rotation. (**A**) *A fetus in a cephalic presentation, LOA position. View is from the outlet. The fetus rotates 90 degrees from this position.* (**B**) *Descent and flexion.* (**C**) *Internal rotation complete.* (**D**) *Extension; the face and chin are born.*

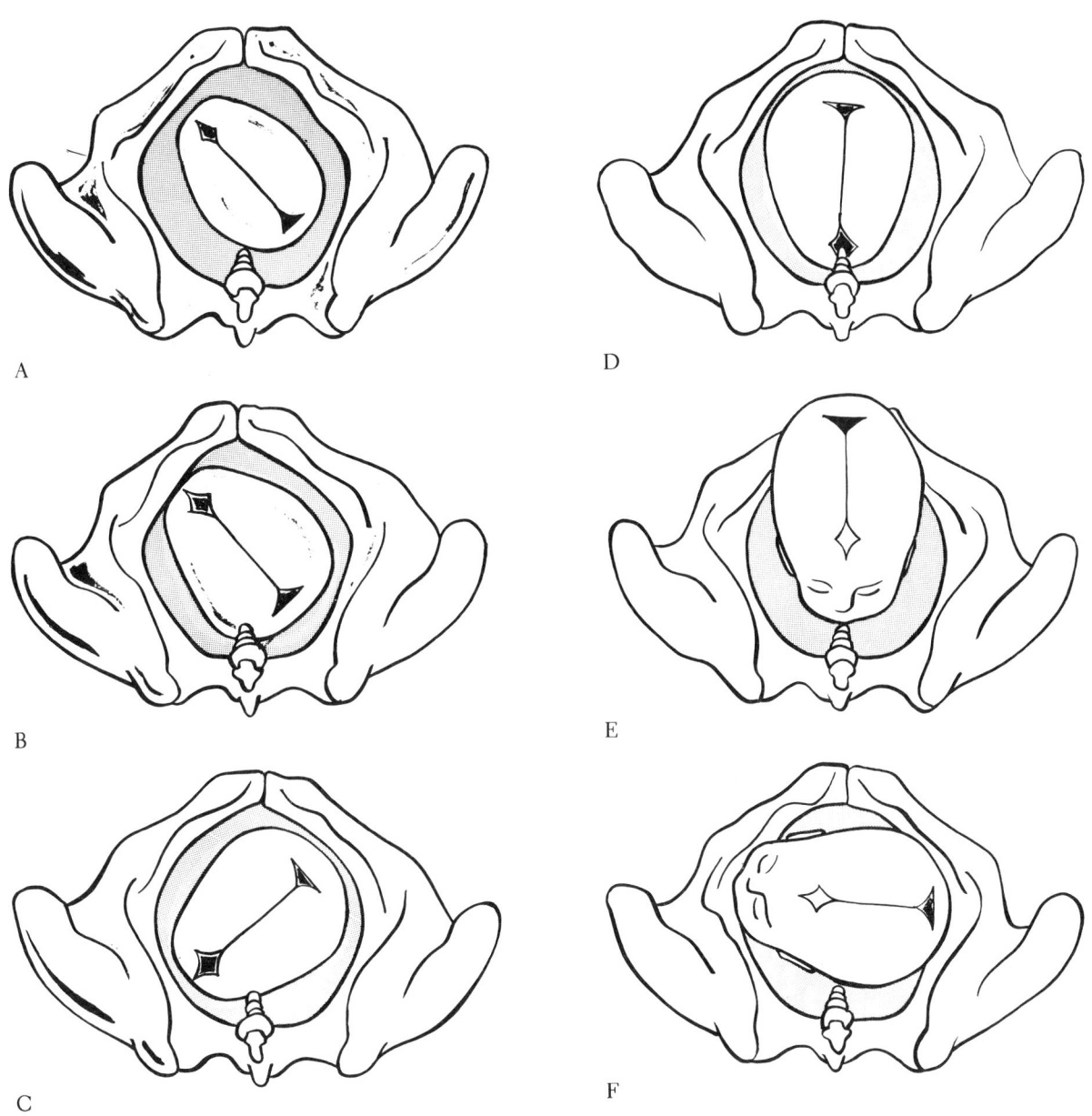

FIGURE 21-8
*Left occipitoposterior (LOP) rotation. (**A**) Fetus in a cephalic presentation, LOP position. View is from outlet. The fetus rotates 135 degrees from this position. (**B**) Descent and flexion. (**C**) Internal rotation beginning. Because of the posterior position, the head will rotate in a longer arc than if it were in an anterior
position. (**D**) Internal rotation complete. (**E**) Extension; the face and chin are born. (**F**) External rotation;
the fetus rotates to place the shoulders in an anteroposterior position.*

average size or not in good flexion, rotation through the
135-degree arc may be impossible. Uterine dysfunction
may result from maternal exhaustion. The head may
arrest in the transverse position (transverse arrest). Rotation may not occur (persistent occipitoposterior position). In both instances, if the fetus has reached the mid-
portion of the pelvis, he or she may be rotated to an
anterior position with forceps and then delivered. Cesarean birth is often elected over rotation and extraction,
because the risk of a midforceps maneuver exceeds the
risk of a cesarean birth.

A woman who has had a long labor is more prone
to postpartal hemorrhage and infection than others. If
forceps were used for birth, the woman is at risk for
reproductive tract lacerations. During labor, she needs a
great deal of support to prevent her from becoming
panicky over the length of the labor, and she needs
practical step-by-step explanations of what is happening. Paradoxically, women who are best prepared for
labor are often most frightened when deviations occur,
because things are not going "by the book"—not happening just as described by the instructor of the course

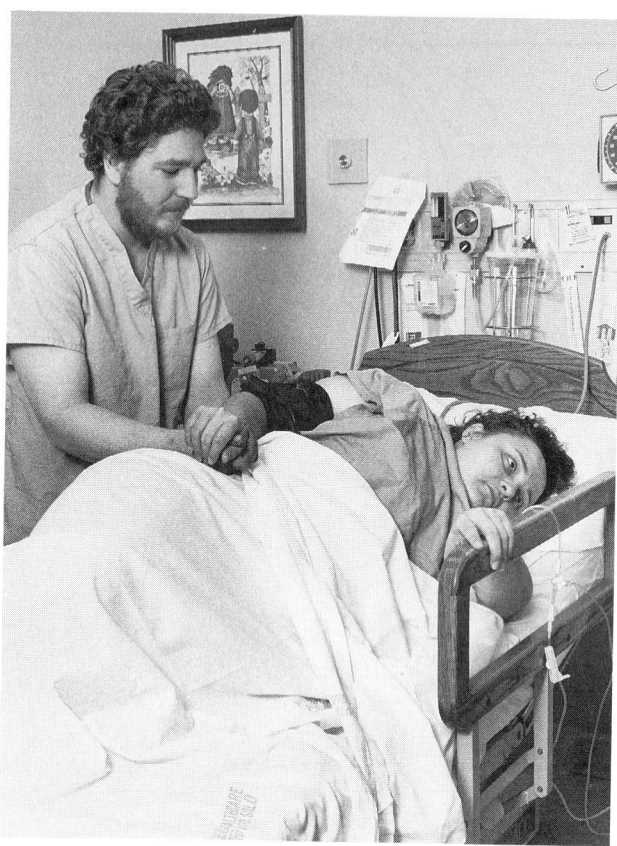

FIGURE 21-9
With a posterior fetal position, the woman may feel extensive back pressure. Pressure on her lower back by her support person may help relieve this problem. (Courtesy of the Department of Medical Photography, Children's Hospital, Buffalo, NY.)

they attended. Such women should have frequent reassurance that, although their pattern of labor is not "textbook," it is still within safe, controlled limits.

Breech Presentation

The majority of fetuses are in a breech presentation early in pregnancy. By week 38 of gestation, however, the fetus normally turns to a cephalic presentation. Although the fetal head is the widest single diameter, the fetus's buttocks (breech), plus the lower extremities, actually takes up more space. The fundus, being the largest part of the uterus, probably accounts for the fact that in approximately 97% of all pregnancies the fetus turns so that the buttocks and lower extremities are in the fundus. If women assume a knee-chest position for approximately 15 minutes three times a day during pregnancy, there is some evidence that breech presentations are less likely to occur.

There are several types of breech presentations. These are shown in Table 21-3. Breech presentation may occur for any of the reasons shown in Box 21-3. Currently, most infants in a breech presentation are turned by external version or delivered by cesarean birth.

Can Nurses Help Shorten Labor When a Fetus Presents in an Occipitoposterior Presentation?

Although this is a difficult area to study because there are so many intervening variables, Biancuzzo (1991) reviewed charts of women whose fetus was in an occipitoposterior position at the beginning of labor to see if positioning, such as placing the woman in a hands and knees position, decreased the length of labor. Findings revealed that this appeared to be so. The researcher suggests that nurses identify fetal position early in labor and take active interventions to aid fetal rotation by making positioning changes.

Biancuzzo, M. (1991). Does the hands and knees position during labor help to rotate the occipitoposterior position? *Birth, 18,* 40.

Breech presentation is more hazardous than a cephalic presentation because there is a higher risk of anoxia from a prolapsed cord; traumatic injury to the aftercoming head (that can result in intracranial hemorrhage or anoxia); or fracture of the spine or arm. Dysfunctional labor may result because the presenting part does not fit the cervix snugly.

Early rupture of the membranes tends to occur because of the poor fit of the presenting part. The inevitable contraction of the buttocks often causes meconium to be extruded before birth. This is not indicative of fetal distress but is expected from the buttock pressure. Such meconium excretion, however, can lead to meconium aspiration if the infant breathes in any amniotic fluid.

Assessment. With a breech presentation, the fetal heart sounds are heard high in the abdomen. Leopold's

Table 21-3. *Classification of Breech Presentations*

Type	Description
Complete	Feet and legs are flexed on thighs; thighs are flexed on abdomen; buttocks and feet are the presenting parts.
Frank	Legs are extended and lie against abdomen and chest; feet are at the level of shoulders; buttocks are presenting part.
Double footling	Legs are unflexed and extended; feet are the presenting part.
Single footling	One leg is unflexed and extended; one foot is the presenting part.

Box 21-3
Causes of Breech Presentation

Gestational age under 40 wk

Abnormality in the fetus, such as anencephaly, hydrocephalus, or meningocele. (In a fetus with hydrocephalus, the widest fetal diameter is the head, and so it retains the most "comfortable" position.)

Hydramnios that allows for free fetal movement, so that the fetus does not have to make a "most comfortable" choice

Congenital anomaly of the uterus such as a midseptum that traps the fetus in a breech position

Any space-occupying mass in the pelvis, such as a fibroid tumor of the uterus or a placenta previa that does not allow the head to present

Pendulous abdomen. If the abdominal muscles are lax, the uterus may fall so far forward that the fetal head comes to lie outside the pelvic brim, causing a breech presentation.

Multiple gestation. The presenting infant cannot turn to a vertex position.

Unknown factors

maneuver, a vaginal examination, and ultrasound will reveal a breech presentation. If the breech is complete and firmly engaged, the tightly stretched gluteal muscles may be mistaken on vaginal examination for a head; the natal cleft may be mistaken for the sagittal suture line. Confirmation of a breech presentation is made by sonography. Such studies also give information on pelvic diameters, fetal skull diameters, and whether a placenta previa exists. Also revealed is any bony fetal abnormality (such as hydrocephalus) that will make vaginal birth impossible.

With every breech presentation, a fetal monitor and uterine contraction monitor should be in place during labor. This will make possible detection of fetal distress from a complication such as a prolapsed cord at the earliest possible moment. In a breech birth, the same stages of flexion, descent, internal rotation, expulsion, and external rotation occur as in a vertex birth (Figure 21-10).

Birth Technique. If the infant will be born vaginally, when full dilatation is reached, the woman is allowed to push, and the breech, trunk, and shoulders are delivered. As the breech spontaneously emerges from the birth canal, it is steadied and supported by a sterile towel held against the infant's inferior surface (Figure 21-10C). The shoulders present to the outlet with their widest diameter anteroposterior. If they do not deliver readily, the arm of the posterior shoulder may be drawn down by passing two fingers over the infant's shoulder and down the arm to the elbow, then sweeping the

flexed arm across the infant's face and chest and out. The other arm is delivered in the same way. External rotation is allowed to occur to bring the head into the best outlet diameter.

Birth of the head is the most hazardous part of the breech birth. The umbilicus precedes the head, and a loop of cord passes down alongside the head. This loop of cord will automatically be compressed by the pressure of the head against the pelvic brim.

A second danger of a breech birth is intracranial hemorrhage. With a cephalic presentation, molding to the confines of the birth canal occurs over hours; with a breech birth, pressure changes occur instantaneously. The result may be tentorial tears, which can cause gross motor and mental incapacity or lethal damage to the fetus. The infant who is delivered suddenly to reduce the amount of time of cord compression may suffer an intracranial hemorrhage; and the infant who is delivered gradually to reduce the possibility of intracranial injury may suffer hypoxia. This makes it obvious that birth of an aftercoming head involves a great deal of judgment and skill.

To aid in delivery of the head, the trunk of the infant is usually straddled over the physician's right forearm (Figure 21-10D). Two fingers of the physician's right hand are placed in the infant's mouth. The left hand is slid into the mother's vagina, palm down, along the infant's back. Pressure is applied to the occiput to flex the head fully. Gentle traction applied to the shoulders (upward and outward) delivers the head. An aftercoming head may also be delivered by the aid of Piper forceps to control the flexion and rate of descent (Figure 21-11).

Parents usually inspect a breech baby after the birth a little more closely than do the average parents. They are looking for the reason that made the presentation breech, as will the person who makes the initial physical assessment of the infant. An infant who was delivered in a frank breech position may tend to keep his or her legs extended and at the level of the face for the first 2 or 3 days of life; the infant who was a footling breech may tend to keep the legs extended in a footling position for the first few days. It is good to point this out to the parents, so that they do not read more than this into the strange posture of the infant.

Face Presentation

Face (chin, or mentum) presentation is rare, but when it does occur, the diameter the fetus presents to the pelvis is often too large for birth to proceed. A face presentation is suggested by a head that feels more prominent than normal and with no engagement apparent on Leopold's maneuvers. It is also suggested when the head and back are both felt on the same side of the uterus on Leopold's maneuvers. The back is difficult to outline in this presentation because it is concave. If the back is extremely concave, fetal heart tones may be transmitted to

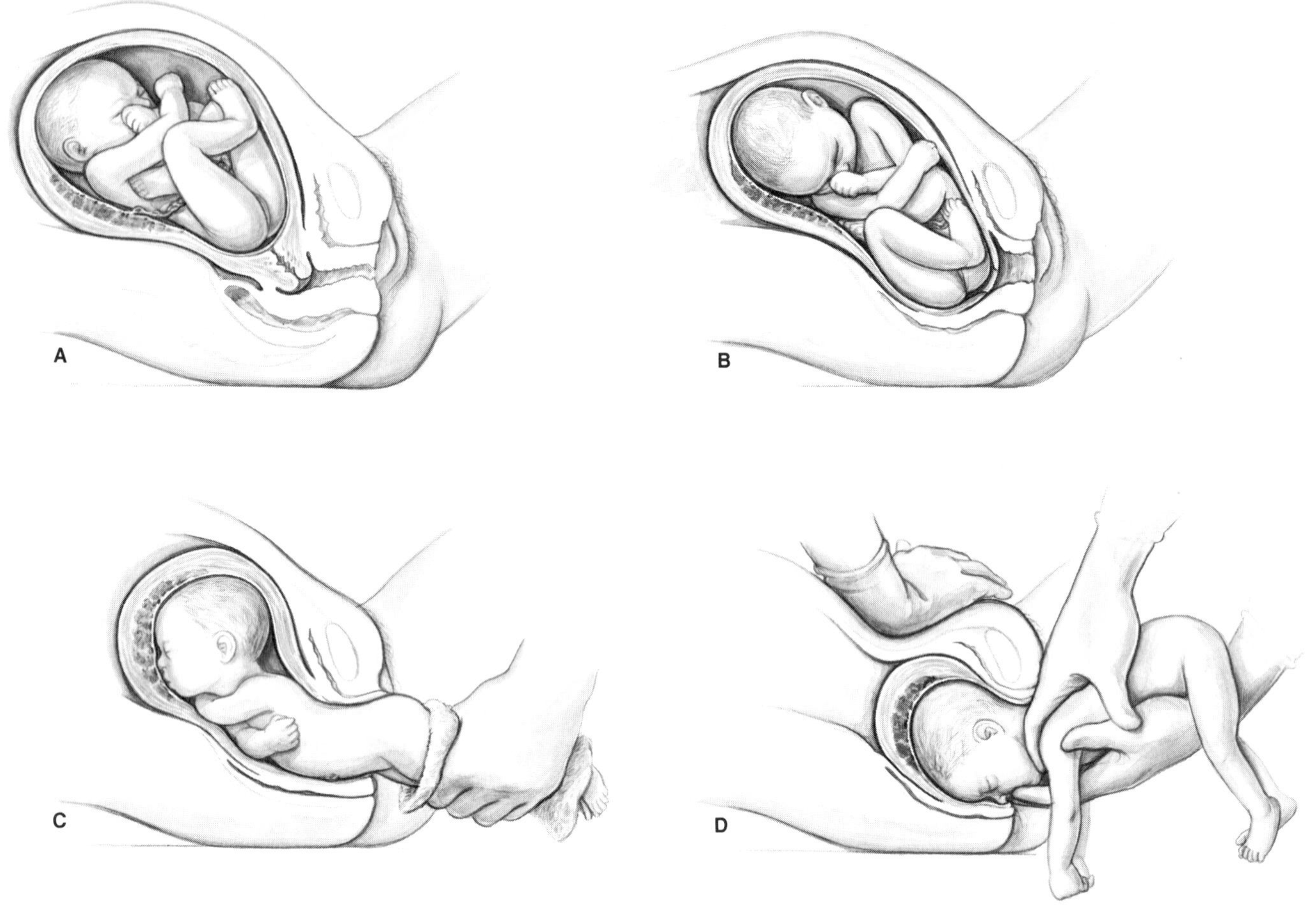

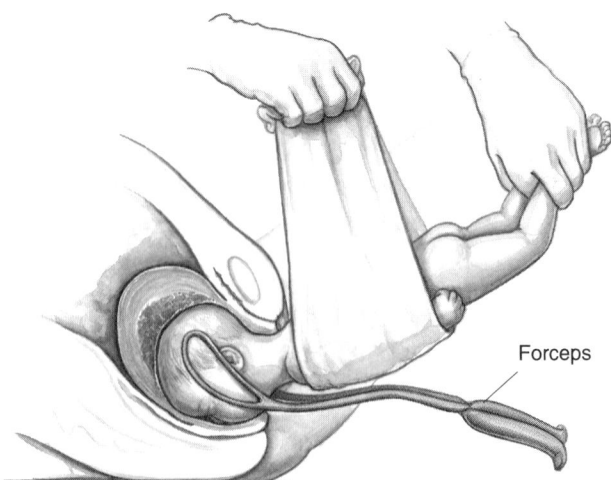

FIGURE 21-10

*Breech birth. (**A**) Position before labor; left sacroposterior. (**B**) Descent and internal rotation. (**C**) Legs being born; the shoulders turn to present to the anteroposterior diameter. (**D**) The head is born. External rotation has put the anteroposterior diameter of the head in line with the anteroposterior diameter of the mother's pelvis. The head is delivered by gentle pressure to flex the head fully and by gentle traction to the shoulders upward and outward. Additional pressure might be applied by an assistant to the abdominal wall to ensure head flexion.*

FIGURE 21-11

With Piper forceps, traction is applied directly to the head, and damage to the infant's neck is avoided.

the forward-thrust chest and heard on the side of the fetus where feet and arms can be palpated. A face presentation is confirmed by vaginal examination when the nose, mouth, or chin can be felt as the presenting part.

A fetus in a posterior position, instead of flexing the head as labor proceeds, may extend the head, resulting in a face (chin) presentation. The usual situation in which this occurs is in a woman with a contracted pelvis or in the presence of a placenta previa. It may occur in the relaxed uterus of a multipara, with prematurity, hydramnios, and fetal malformation. It is a warning signal, in that something abnormal is causing the chin presentation.

When a face presentation is suspected, a sonogram will be done to confirm it and, if indicated, measurements of the pelvic diameters are made. If the chin is anterior and the pelvic diameters are within normal limits, the infant may be delivered without difficulty (perhaps following a long first stage of labor, because the face does not mold well to make a snugly engaging part). If the chin is posterior, cesarean birth will be the choice of birth; otherwise, it would be necessary to wait for a long posterior-to-anterior rotation to occur. Such rotation can result in uterine dysfunction or a transverse arrest.

Babies born following a chin presentation have a great deal of facial edema and may be purple from ecchymotic bruising. Lip edema may be so severe that the infant is unable to suck for a day or two. The infant may have to have gavage feedings to obtain enough fluid until he or she can suck effectively. The infant must be observed closely for a patent airway; thus, the infant usually is transferred for the first 24 hours to a careful watch nursery. The mother needs to be assured that the edema is transient and will disappear in a few days, with no aftermath.

Brow Presentation

A brow presentation is the rarest of the presentations. It occurs with a multipara or with relaxed abdominal muscles. It almost invariably results in obstructed labor, because the head becomes jammed in the brim of the pelvis as the occipitomental diameter presents. Unless the presentation spontaneously corrects, cesarean birth will be necessary to deliver the infant safely. Brow presentations also leave the infant with extreme ecchymotic bruising on the face. Upon seeing this bruising over the same area as the anterior fontanelle or "soft spot," parents may need additional reassurance that the child is well following birth.

Transverse Lie

Transverse lie occurs in women with pendulous abdomens, with uterine masses such as fibroid tumors that obstruct the lower uterine segment, with contraction of the pelvic brim, with congenital abnormalities of the uterus, or with hydramnios. It may occur in infants with hydrocephalus or other gross abnormalities that prevent the head from engaging. It may also occur in prematurity, when the infant has room for free movement; in multiple gestation (particularly in a second twin); or when there is a short umbilical cord.

A transverse lie is usually obvious on inspection, when the ovoid of the uterus is found to be more horizontal than vertical. By means of Leopold's maneuvers the abnormal presentation will be detected. A sonogram may be taken to confirm the abnormal lie and to give information such as pelvic size (Harris, 1990).

A mature fetus cannot be delivered vaginally from this presentation. Often, the membranes rupture at the beginning of labor. Because there is no firm presenting part, the cord prolapses, or an arm may prolapse, or the shoulder obstructs the cervix. Cesarean birth is necessary.

Oversized Fetus (Macrosomia)

Size may become a problem in a fetus who weighs more than 4500 g (10 lb); a weight lower than this is unlikely to cause difficulty. Only 1 in 100 infants weighs this much at birth; weights up to 7800 g (17 lb) have been reported (Cunningham et al., 1993). Babies of this size are most frequently born to women who are diabetic. Large babies may be associated with multiparity, because each infant born to a woman tends to be slightly heavier and larger than the one born just before.

An oversized infant may cause uterine dysfunction during labor or at birth owing to the overstretching of the fibers of the myometrium. The wide shoulders may pose a problem at birth, because they cause cephalopelvic disproportion or even uterine rupture from obstruction. The large size of the fetus may be missed in an obese woman because the fetal contours are difficult to palpate. Because she is obese does not mean that she has a larger than usual pelvis. Pelvimetry or sonography can be used to compare the fetal size with the woman's pelvic capacity. If the infant is so oversized that he or she cannot deliver vaginally, cesarean birth becomes the birth method of choice.

There is a substantial increase in the perinatal mortality of larger infants (15% versus the normal 4%). The large infant who is born vaginally has a higher than normal risk of cervical nerve palsy, diaphragmatic nerve injury, or fractured clavicle because of shoulder dystocia. The mother in the postpartal period has a greater than usual chance of hemorrhage because the overdistended uterus may not contract as readily as normal (Cunningham et al., 1993).

Shoulder Dystocia

Shoulder dystocia is a delivery problem that is increasing in incidence along with the increasing average weight of infants. The problem occurs at the second stage of labor when the fetal head is born but the shoulders are too broad to enter and be delivered through the pelvic outlet. This is a hazard to the mother because it can result in vaginal or cervical tears; it is a hazard to the fetus because the cord is compressed between the fetal body and the bony pelvis; it can result in a fractured clavicle or a brachial plexus injury.

Shoulder dystocia is most apt to occur in women with diabetes, multiparas, and in post-date pregnancies. The problem is often not identified until the head has been born; and then the wide anterior shoulder locks beneath the symphysis pubis. The condition may be suspected earlier if the second stage of labor is prolonged, if there is arrest of descent, or if when the head appears on the perineum (crowning) it retracts instead of protruding with each contraction (a turtle sign; Penny & Perlis, 1992).

Asking the woman to flex her thighs sharply on her

abdomen (McRobert's maneuver) widens the pelvic outlet and may let the anterior shoulder deliver. Applying suprapubic pressure may help the shoulder escape from beneath the symphysis pubis.

Fetal Anomalies

Fetal anomalies of the head such as hydrocephalus (fluid-filled ventricles) or anencephaly (absence of the cranium) can also complicate birth (see Chapter 39).

Problems With the Passage

Another problem that can cause dystocia is a contraction or narrowing of the passageway or birth canal. The pelvis may be contracted (narrow) at the inlet, the midpelvis, or the outlet; this is cephalopelvic disproportion, or a disproportion between the size of the normal fetal head and the pelvic diameters. It causes failure to progress in labor.

Inlet Contraction

Inlet contraction is ordinarily due to rickets in early life or an inherited small pelvis. It is defined as narrowing of the anteroposterior diameter to less than 11 cm, or a maximum transverse diameter of 12 cm or less. In primigravidas, the fetal head normally engages at weeks 36 to 38 of pregnancy. When this event occurs before labor begins, it is proof that the pelvic inlet is adequate. Following the general rule that "what goes in, comes out," a head that engages or proves it fits into the pelvic brim will probably also be able to pass through the midpelvis and through the outlet.

When engagement does not occur in a primigravida, then either a fetal abnormality (larger-than-usual head) or a pelvic abnormality (smaller-than-usual pelvis) is suspect of causing the lack of engagement. As a rule, engagement does not occur in multigravidas until labor begins. This is not a concern because a woman who has delivered a previous full-term infant vaginally without problems has already proved that her birth canal is adequate.

Every primigravida should have pelvic measurements taken and recorded before week 24 of pregnancy so that a birth decision can be made, based on these measurements and on the assumption that the fetus will be of average size.

With CPD, because the fetus does not engage but remains "floating," malposition may occur accompanying an already difficult situation. The possibility of cord prolapse is great with a "floating" head if membranes should rupture.

Outlet Contraction

Outlet contraction is defined as the narrowing of the transverse diameter to less than 11 cm. This is the distance between the ischial tuberosities, a measurement that is easy to make during a prenatal visit and thus can be anticipated before labor begins.

Trial Labor

If a woman has a borderline (just adequate) inlet measurement, and the fetal lie and position are good, her physician may allow her a "trial" labor to see whether labor can progress normally; this is allowed to continue as long as descent of the presenting part and dilatation of the cervix are occurring. Fetal heart sounds and uterine contractions should be monitored during a trial labor. It is especially important that the urinary bladder be kept emptied to allow all the space available to be used by the fetal head (urge the woman to void every 2 hours). Assess FHR carefully after rupture of the membranes, because if the fetal head is high, there is increased danger of prolapsed cord and anoxia in the fetus. If after a definite period (6 to 12 hours) adequate progress in labor cannot be documented, the woman will be scheduled for a cesarean birth.

It is difficult for women to undertake a labor they know they may be unable to complete. Emphasize that it is best for the baby to be born vaginally. However, do not overstress this fact. If the trial labor fails and cesarean birth is scheduled, you will need to explain why a cesarean birth is necessary for the baby.

Some women having a trial labor feel as if they themselves are on trial. When dilatation does not occur, they feel discouraged and inadequate, as if they are somehow at fault. A woman may not even have realized how much she wanted the trial labor to work until she is told that it is not working. The support person may be as frightened and feel as helpless as the woman when a deviation occurs in labor. The couple needs assurance from health care personnel that a cesarean birth is not an inferior method of birth but an alternative method; in this instance, it is the method of choice. A cesarean birth will secure for them the goal they seek: a healthy mother and a healthy child.

External Cephalic Version

External cephalic version is the turning of a fetus from a breech to a cephalic position prior to birth (Clay, Criss, & Jackson, 1993). For the procedure, fetal heart rate and possibly ultrasound should be recorded continuously; the breech and vertex of the fetus are located and grasped transabdominally. Gentle pressure is then exerted to rotate the fetus in a forward direction (Figure

21-12). The use of external version can decrease the number of cesarean births necessary. Contraindications to the procedure are multiple gestation, severe oligo-hydramnios, contraindications to vaginal birth, Rh-iso-immunization, a nuchal cord, and unexplained third trimester bleeding.

Therapeutic Management of Problems or Potential Problems in Labor and Birth

When labor contractions are ineffective, a number of interventions, such as augmentation of labor with oxy-tocin or *amniotomy* (rupture of the membranes), may be initiated to strengthen them. Since amniotomy is also used in normal labor, it is discussed in Chapter 18.

Induction and Augmentation of Labor

Induction of labor means that labor is artificially started; **augmentation** refers to assisting a labor that has started spontaneously to be more effective. It may be necessary to initiate labor before the time when it would have occurred spontaneously because a fetus is in danger or because labor does not occur sponta-neously and the fetus appears to be at term. The primary reasons for inducing labor are the presence of pre-eclampsia, eclampsia, severe hypertension or diabetes, Rh sensitization, prolonged rupture of the membranes, intrauterine growth retardation, and postmaturity (a pregnancy lasting beyond 42 weeks) or situations in which it seems risky for the fetus to remain in utero. Augmentation of labor or assistance to make uterine contractions stronger may be necessary when contrac-tions are too weak or infrequent to be effective.

Before induction of labor is begun, the following conditions must be present:

The fetus is in a longitudinal lie and at a point of extrauterine viability;

The cervix is ripe, or ready for birth;

A presenting part is engaged; and

There is no CPD.

It is a procedure used cautiously with multiple ges-tation, hydramnios, grand parity, maternal age older than 35 years, and the presence of previous uterine scars, since it carries a risk of uterine rupture, a decrease in the fetal blood supply from poor cotyledon filling, and premature separation of the placenta.

A fetal estimation of maturity should be made, such as a lecithin-sphingomyelin ratio or sonogram biparietal diameter, to rule out preterm birth.

Cervical Ripening

Cervical ripening implies a change in the cervical consis-tency from firm to soft. Such softness is necessary for dilatation and coordination of uterine contractions. To determine whether a cervix is ripe, Bishop (1964) de-vised a method of scoring criteria for readiness (Table 21-4). If a woman's total score is 8 or more on this scale, the cervix is considered ready for birth and should re-spond to induction. To "ripen" a cervix, various methods

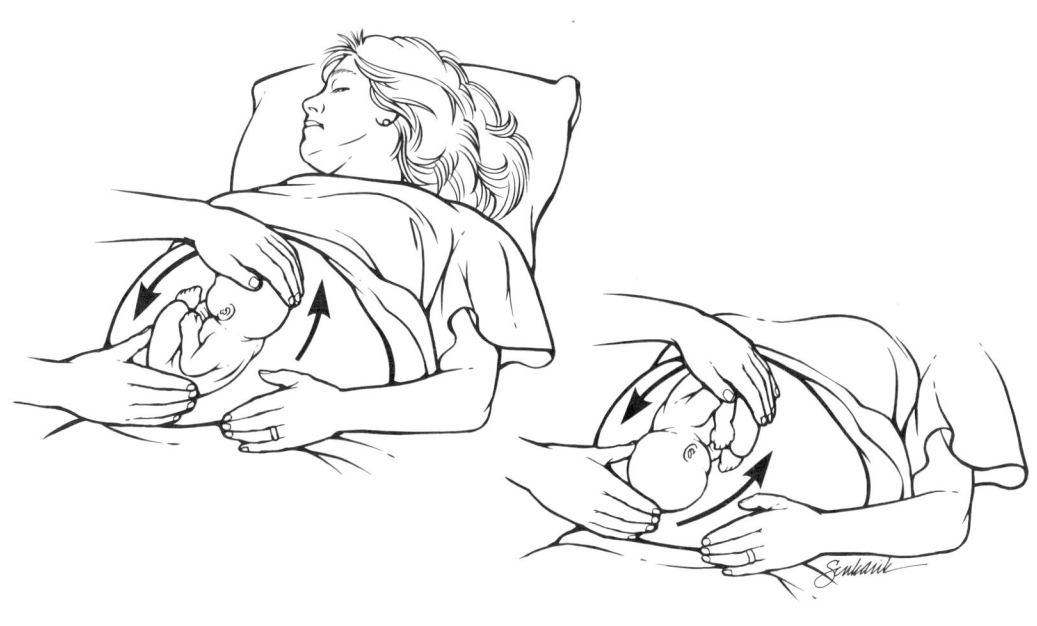

FIGURE 21-12
External cephalic version. The fetus is rotated by external pressure to a cephalic lie.

Table 21-4. Scoring of Cervix for Readiness for Elective Induction

Scoring Factor	Score			
	0	1	2	3
Dilation (cm)	0	1–2	3–4	5–6
Effacement (%)	0–30	40–50	60–70	80
Station	−3	−2	−1–0	+1–+2
Consistency	Firm	Medium	Soft	
Position	Posterior	Mid position	Anterior	

(From Bishop, E. H. [1964]. Pelvic scoring for elective induction. *Obstetrics and Gynecology, 24,* 266, with permission.)

can be instituted. One is "stripping the membranes" or separating the membranes from the lower uterine segment. Possible complications of this mechanical method include bleeding from an undetected low-lying placenta, inadvertent rupture of membranes, and the introduction of infection (Trofatter, 1992). Hygroscopic suppositories (suppositories of seaweed that swell on contact with cervical secretions) can be inserted to gradually and gently urge dilation. These are held in place by gauze sponges that have been saturated with povidone-iodine or an antifungal cream. Documenting how many dilators and sponges were placed during the procedure is important. Yet another method of speeding cervical ripening is application of a prostaglandin gel to the interior surface of the cervix by a catheter or suppository or to the external surface by diaphragm (Day & Snell, 1993).

Induction of Labor by Oxytocin

Administration of **oxytocin**, a synthetic form of the naturally occurring pituitary hormone, initiates contractions in a uterus at pregnancy term (Cardozo & Pearce, 1990). Oxytocin is always administered intravenously (never intramuscularly) so that its effect can be quickly discontinued to avoid hyperstimulation. The half-life of oxytocin is approximately 3 minutes; thus, with intravenous administration, the functioning level will end this quickly. In contrast, if intramuscular administration is used, it might take hours before the serum level decreases.

Induction is begun by the administration of a dilute intravenous form of oxytocin such as Pitocin or Syntocinon. The drug is traditionally mixed in the proportion of 10 IU in 1000 mL of Ringer's lactate. Ten IU of oxytocin is the same as 10,000 milliunits (mU), so each milliliter of this solution will contain 10 mU of oxytocin. An alternative dilution method is to add 15 IU of oxytocin to 250 mL of an intravenous solution. This yields a concentration of 60 mU/1 mL (Table 21-5). Physician's orders for administration of oxytocin for induction generally

designate the number of milliunits to be administered per minute; thus, recognizing the concentration in each milliliter is important. The oxytocin solution must be "piggybacked" with a maintenance intravenous solution such as 5% dextrose and water; then, if the oxytocin needs to be turned off abruptly during the induction, the intravenous line will not be lost. The dose should be piggybacked into a port close to the patient; this way if it is stopped, little remains in the tubing. A constant infusion pump should be used to control the small amount of fluid given and to ensure a uniform infusion rate even when the woman changes position. A physician should be immediately available during the entire procedure to ensure safety (Posiac, 1993).

Infusions are usually begun at a rate of 0.5 mU/min to 1 mU/min. If there is no response from this, the infusion is gradually increased in amount every 15 minutes to 60 minutes by small increments of 1 to 2 mU until contractions begin (ACOG, 1991). Many women respond with as little as 4 mU/min; most women respond at 16 mU/min. An administration rate of more than this will likely cause tetanic contractions. The rate should not be increased more than 20 mU/min without check-

Table 21-5. Solution Concentration of Oxytocin with Various Dilutions

Rate (mU/min)	10 IU Oxytocin/1000 mL (10 mU/mL) mL/Hour	15 IU Oxytocin/250 mL (60 mU/mL) mL/Hour
0.5	3	0.5
1	6	1
2	12	2
3	18	3
4	24	4
5	30	5
6	36	6
7	42	7
8	48	8
9	54	9
10	60	10
11	66	11
12	72	12
13	78	13
14	84	14
15	90	15
16	96	16
17	102	17
18	108	18
19	114	19
20	120	20

(From Posiac, S. [1993]. Induction and augmentation of labor. In Mandeville, L. K., & Troiano, N. H. *High-risk intrapartum nursing.* Philadelphia: J. B. Lippincott.)

ing for further instructions. Aggressive induction (a 6 mU/min increment instead of the usual 1 to 2 mU/min has been suggested as a way to shorten labor and may be used in some research facilities). When cervical dilatation reaches 4 cm, artificial rupture of the membranes will further induce labor and the infusion can be discontinued at that point; for others, it will be continued through full dilatation.

Both fetal heart sounds and uterine contractions should be continuously monitored during the procedure. Oxytocin has the side-effect of causing peripheral vessel dilatation, which may result in extreme hypotension. Excessive stimulation of the uterus by oxytocin may lead to tonic uterine contractions with fetal death or, in extreme instances, rupture of the uterus. The woman's pulse and blood pressure and the FHR should be taken every 15 minutes. Contractions should occur no more than every 2 minutes, should not be stronger than 50 mm Hg pressure, and should last no longer than 70 seconds. The resting pressure between contractions should not exceed 15 mm Hg by monitor (Figure 21-13). If contractions become more frequent or longer in duration than these safe limits or signs of fetal distress occur, stop the intravenous infusion and seek help. Administering oxygen may be necessary. It is better for contractions to slow from a period of inadequate oxytocin administration because the infusion was stopped unnecessarily than for tonic contractions to continue. Because of the short half-life of oxytocin, stopping the flow rate almost immediately stops the oxytocin effect. If this is not effective, a beta-2-adrenergic receptor drug such as terbutaline sulfate (Brethine) to decrease myometrial activity may be ordered.

Oxytocin has an antidiuretic effect, so there will be a decreased urine flow during its administration. This can result in water intoxication in the woman. Water intoxication is first manifested by headache and vomiting. If these danger signs are observed in the woman during induction of labor, they should be reported and the infusion will then be discontinued. Water intoxication in its severest form can lead to convulsions, coma, and

death because it causes a shift in interstitial tissue fluid. Keep an accurate intake and output record and test and record specific gravity of urine to detect discrepancies in the pattern. Limit the amount of intravenous fluid to 150 mL/h by being certain that during a time when the mainline intravenous fluid is flowing that it is doing so at a slow rate (not more than 2.5 mL/min).

Induction of labor with oxytocin may predispose the newborn to hyperbilirubinemia and jaundice. Be sure the infant is observed for this in the first few days of life.

Women may have heard that induced labor is more painful or "so different" from normal labor that breathing exercises are worthless, or that it goes so fast it will be harmful to the fetus (see the Focus on Family Teaching box). Induced labors do tend to have a slightly shorter first stage than the average unassisted labor. This is an advantage to the woman, however, not a disadvantage. Once contractions begin by this method, they are basically normal uterine contractions. The woman can be assured of this so that she does not fight the contractions or become unnecessarily tense, which would prevent her from using her breathing techniques effectively (see the Nursing Care Plan).

Augmentation by Oxytocin

Augmentation of labor is required when labor contractions begin spontaneously but then become so weak, irregular, or ineffective (hypotonic) that assistance is needed to strengthen them.

Precautions regarding oxytocin assist are the same as for primary induction of labor. A uterus may be very responsive to oxytocin when it is used as augmentation. Be certain that the drug is increased in small increments only, and fetal heart sounds are well monitored during the procedure. Nipple stimulation, which releases naturally occurring oxytocin, may be used as augmentation in labor. Unfortunately, because the breasts in most women become tender after only a few minutes, the procedure cannot be continued long enough to be effective.

(text continues on page 596)

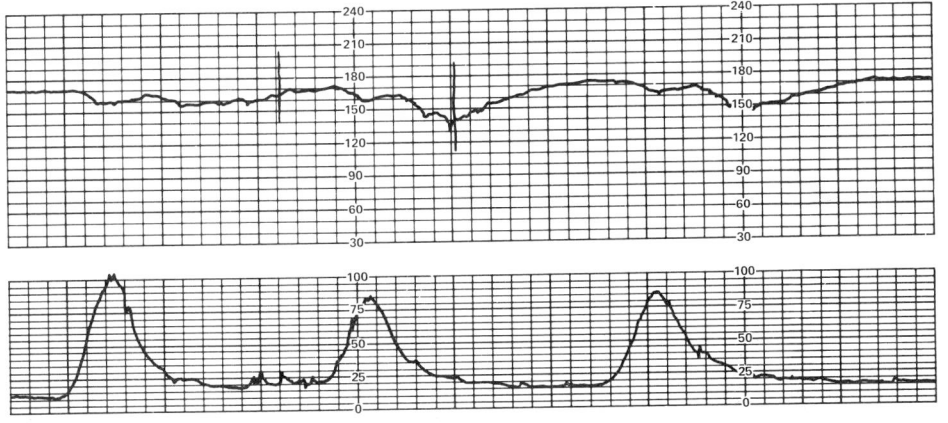

FIGURE 21-13

Hypertonic uterine contractions caused by an oxytocin infusion. Contractions are as high as 100 mm Hg in intensity. Late decelerations and an FHR of 170 bpm baseline are present.

Nursing Care Plan

A Woman Experiencing a Labor Complication

Terry Mavahato is a 33-year-old G5P3 woman in labor. She awoke with labor contractions during the night. Has been in labor now for 12 hours with dilatation at 4 cm; effacement 80%. Husband with her. Urine: negative for protein and glucose; FHR: 130 bpm. Contractions: duration, 30 sec; frequency, 3 min; intensity: moderately strong. Intravenous line of 1000 Ringer's lactate begun in left hand at 150 mL/h.

Nursing Diagnosis: High risk for maternal and/or fetal injury related to prolonged latent stage of labor.

Defining Characteristic: Length of labor is prolonged for a multipara.

Goal: Client will complete labor and delivery within normal parameters without preventable injury to self or fetus.

Outcome Criteria: Fetal heart tones remain within normal limits (120–160 bpm) by monitor; and dilatation continues to increase.

Nursing Orders	Rationale
1. Explain purpose of monitors.	1. Client is scheduled to have external monitor until membranes are ruptured, then internal. She needs to be given this information and told why the monitors are needed so that she sees them as an aid, not an intrusion.
2. Explain purpose of intravenous infusion.	2. Keeping client informed of therapy will help her relax.
3. Maintain client on nothing-by-mouth status.	3. Cesarean birth and anesthesia may be necessary later on.
4. Keep client on left side.	4. Lying on the left side provides for best uterine perfusion.
5. Schedule sonogram per physician's order.	5. Sonogram will reveal cephalopelvic disproportion.

At 2 more hours into labor, you make additional assessments: Client asking if baby is all right. Very apprehensive of any change in sound of fetal monitor. Asking for something to eat "to keep up energy." Internal monitor inserted. FHR baseline: 120–130 bpm, beat-to-beat variability: 5–10 bpm. Contractions still minimal; 30–45 mm Hg by monitor; duration, 30 sec; frequency, 3 min. Continuous intravenous infusion of Ringer's lactate at 150 mL/hr by automatic infuser. Sonogram pelvimetry report: no difficulty with vaginal delivery expected.

Nursing Diagnosis: Fear related to possible pregnancy outcome.

Defining Characteristic: Client states she is fearful of pregnancy outcome.

Goal: Client will demonstrate decreased fear about pregnancy outcome.

Outcome Criteria: Client states she can maintain a positive outlook about pregnancy outcome.

(continued)

Nursing Orders	Rationale
1. Continue to reassure that fetal heart tones are good.	1. Reassures client that fetus is doing well.
2. Continue with explanations of all care given.	2. Reduces anxiety by making client aware of plans.
3. Explain reason for nothing-by-mouth status.	3. Understanding why she must be NPO will help client accept that she must not drink.

After an additional 2 hours, her physician orders an oxytocin infusion to assist with contractions.

Assessment: Both parents seem discouraged with labor progress, happy to hear that oxytocin assist will be started to strengthen contractions. Both parents are observed watching monitor patterns carefully; noticeably apprehensive.

Nursing Diagnosis: High risk for fluid volume excess related to oxytocin infusion.

Defining Characteristic: Water intoxication is a potential risk with an oxytocin assist.

Goal: Client will not develop a fluid volume excess.

Outcome Criteria: Client's blood pressure is below 150/90 mm Hg; client does not evidence confusion or headache.

Nursing Orders	Rationale
1. Explain to both parents all new equipment used.	1. Reduces anxiety to continue to keep client familiar with equipment.
2. Obtain baseline vital signs (blood pressure, pulse, respirations, and FHR).	2. Baseline values allow for better evaluation of infusion.
3. Administer oxytocin (Pitocin) intravenously (10,000 mU in 1000 mL Ringer's lactate) begun at 0.5 mU/min (or 3 mL/h) piggybacked to existing intravenous line.	3. Oxytocin is given piggyback so it can be discontinued abruptly in an emergency.
4. Put internal fetal and uterine monitors in place.	4. Provides for continued monitoring of fetal well-being.
5. Assess FHR, blood pressure, pulse, and respirations every 15 min.	5. It is important to monitor vital signs often during oxytocin infusion in order to detect dangerous side-effects such as maternal hypotension.
6. Assess the duration, frequency, and strength of contractions every 15 min.	6. Allows for early detection of tonic contractions.
7. Advance oxytocin infusion in 2 mU/min increments (up to 16 mU/min) every 30 min until contractions reach duration of 60 sec and frequency of 2 min.	7. Advancing drug dose slowly helps to prevent overdose.
8. Discontinue oxytocin and notify physician if FHR is above 160 bpm or below 120 bpm, or decelerations occur; if contractions are longer than 60 sec, resting pressure of contractions is more than 15 mm Hg, or frequency is less than 2 min; or if general apprehension, confusion, or headache is present.	8. Oxytocin toxicity can lead to fetal injury.

FOCUS ON FAMILY TEACHING

Q. I've heard a lot about augmentation of labor. How will I know if I need this? How would my labor be different?

A. Augmentation of labor is used when labor contractions are ineffective. It has the advantage of shortening labor and avoiding the necessity of cesarean birth. Oxytocin is the drug used; this is a synthetic form of the hormone naturally released by your body during labor. It is administered intravenously. Once labor contractions begin by this method, they are the same as naturally occurring contractions. You will be able to use your prepared breathing exercises with them.

Forceps Birth

Forceps may be necessary to deliver the baby if a woman is unable to push with contractions in the pelvic division of labor, such as after regional anesthesia; if cessation of progress in the second stage of labor occurs; or if the fetus is in an abnormal position. A fetus in distress from a complication such as prolapsed cord can be delivered more quickly by the use of forceps. Forceps are designed to prevent pressure from being exerted on the fetal head. They may be used also, then, to reduce pressure and avoid subdural hemorrhage in the fetus as the fetal head reaches the perineum.

Forceps are steel instruments constructed of two blades that slide together at their shaft to form a handle. Forceps are applied first by one blade being slipped into a woman's vagina next to the fetal head, and then the other side being slipped into place. Next, the shafts of the instrument are brought together in the midline to form the handle. Five commonly used types of forceps are described in Table 21-6.

A **forceps birth** is an outlet procedure when the forceps are applied after the fetal head reaches the perineum. The term **low forceps birth** may be used to indicate the fetal head is at a +2 station. If the fetal head is still at the level of the ischial spines (0 station), this is a **midforceps birth**. Cesarean birth currently involves less risk to the fetus than the use of midforceps, so such a procedure is rarely seen today. Some anesthesia, at least a pudendal block, is necessary for forceps application to achieve pelvic relaxation and reduce pain.

Before forceps are applied, membranes must be ruptured, no CPD must be present, the cervix must be fully dilated, and the woman's bladder must be empty

(Sokol & Brindley, 1990). The FHR should be recorded prior to forceps application; and since a danger of forceps use is that the cord could be compressed between the blade and head, the FHR should be assessed again immediately after application. An episiotomy is usually used to prevent perineal tearing due to pressure on the perineum. The woman's cervix should be assessed after forceps birth to be certain that no laceration occurred. To rule out bladder injury, the first voiding should be recorded (time and amount). The infant should be assessed to be certain that no facial palsy or subdural hematoma exists. Forceps birth may leave a transient erythematous mark on the newborn's cheek. Parents can be assured this will fade in 1 to 2 days' time.

Vacuum Extraction

A fetus positioned far enough down the birth canal may be delivered by means of a vacuum extractor in place of forceps. With the fetal head at the perineum, a disk-shaped cup is pressed against the fetal scalp over the posterior fontanelle. When vacuum pressure is applied, air beneath the cup is sucked out and the cup then adheres so tightly to the fetal scalp that traction on the cord leading to the cup will deliver the fetus (Figure 21-14).

Vacuum extraction has advantages over forceps birth in that little anesthesia is necessary (making the fetus less depressed at birth) and fewer lacerations of the birth canal occur. Its major disadvantage is that it causes a marked caput that may be noticeable as long as 7 days after birth. Tentorial tears from extreme pressure can also occur (Hanigan et al., 1990). A mother may need to be assured that caput swelling will decrease rapidly and is harmless to her infant (Johnson & Pace, 1993). Vacuum extraction should not be used as a method of birth if scalp blood sampling was done, because the suction pressure can cause severe bleeding. Moreover, vacuum extraction is not advantageous for preterm infants because of the softness of the preterm skull.

Table 21-6. *Common Types of Delivery Forceps*

Name	Description
Barton	Forceps with a hinge in the right blade used to rotate the fetal head to a more favorable position such as ROP to ROA
Kielland's	Forceps with short handles and a marked cephalic curve used to rotate the fetal head to a more favorable position such as ROP to ROA
Piper	Used to deliver the head in a breech presentation
Simpson's	Forceps used most commonly as outlet forceps
Tarnier's	Axis traction forceps

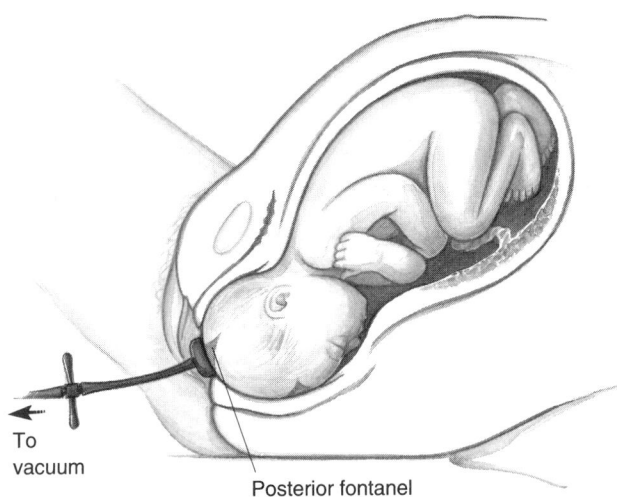

FIGURE 21-14
Vacuum extraction.

To vacuum

Posterior fontanel

Anomalies of the Placenta and Cord

Anomalies of the Placenta

The placenta and cord are always examined for the presence of anomalies after birth. The normal placenta weighs approximately 500 g and is 15 to 20 cm in diameter and 1.5 to 3.0 cm thick. Its weight is approximately one sixth that of the fetus. A placenta may be unusually enlarged in women with diabetes. In certain diseases, such as syphilis or erythroblastosis, the placenta may be so large that it weighs half as much as the fetus. If the uterus has scars or a septum, the placenta may be wide in diameter, because it was forced to spread out to find implantation space.

Placenta Succenturiata

A **succenturiate placenta** (Figure 21-15*A*) has one or more accessory lobes connected to the main placenta by blood vessels. No fetal abnormality is associated with it. However, it is important that it be recognized, because the small lobes may be retained in the uterus at birth, leading to severe maternal hemorrhage. On inspection, the placenta will appear torn at the edge, or torn blood vessels may extend beyond the edge of the placenta. The remaining lobes must be removed from the uterus manually to prevent hemorrhage in the mother from poor uterine contraction.

Placenta Circumvallata

Ordinarily, the chorion membrane begins at the edge of the placenta and spreads to envelop the fetus; no chorion covers the fetal side of the placenta. In **placenta circumvallata**, the fetal side of the placenta is covered to some extent with chorion (Figure 21-15*B*). The umbilical cord enters the placenta at the usual midpoint, and large vessels spread out from there. They end abruptly at the point where the chorion folds back onto the surface, however. (In **placenta marginata**, the fold of chorion reaches just to the edge of the placenta.) Although no abnormalities are associated with this type of placenta, its presence should be noted.

Battledore Placenta

In a **battledore placenta**, the cord is inserted marginally rather than centrally (Figure 21-15*C*). This anomaly is rare and has no known clinical significance.

Velamentous Insertion of the Cord

Velamentous insertion of the cord is a situation in which the cord, instead of entering the placenta directly, separates into small vessels that reach the placenta by spreading across a fold of amnion. This form of cord insertion is most frequently found with multiple pregnancy; it is associated with fetal anomalies (Blackburn & Loper, 1992).

Vasa Previa

The situation in which the umbilical vessels of a velamentous cord insertion cross the cervical os so they would deliver before the fetus is called a **vasa previa**. The vessels may tear with cervical dilatation the same as a placental previa may tear. This would result in sudden fetal blood loss. Before inserting any instrument such as an internal fetal monitor, structures should be identified to prevent accidental tearing of a vasa previa. The infant needs to be delivered by cesarean birth. If sudden painless bleeding occurs with the beginning of cervical dila-

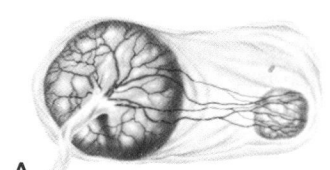
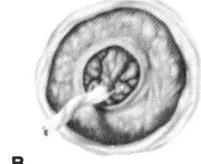
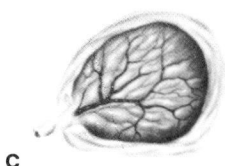

A

B

C

FIGURE 21-15
*Abnormal placental formation. (**A**) Placenta succenturiata. (**B**) Placenta circumvallata. (**C**) Battledore placenta. (From Clinical Education Aid, No. 12, Ross Laboratories, Columbus, OH, with permission.)*

tion, vasa previa should be suspected. Vaginal blood can be differentiated as fetal or maternal blood by an Apt test as described in Box 21-4 (Carlan & Knuppel, 1990).

Placenta Accreta

Placenta accreta is the unusually deep attachment of the placenta to the uterine myometrium. The placenta will not loosen and deliver, and attempts to remove it manually may lead to extreme hemorrhage because of the deep attachment. Hysterectomy may be necessary at this point or the woman may be treated with methotrexate to destroy the still attached tissue.

Anomalies of the Cord

Two-Vessel Cord

A normal cord contains one vein and two arteries. The absence of one of the umbilical arteries is associated with congenital heart and kidney anomalies, because the insult that caused the loss of the vessel probably led to other mesoderm germ layer structures as well (Cochran, 1990). Inspection of a cord must be made immediately at birth before it begins to dry; if drying occurs, the cut surface will then be distorted in appearance. It should be marked prominently on the infant's chart that only two vessels are present. The child needs to be observed carefully for other anomalies during the newborn period.

Unusual Cord Length

An unusually short umbilical cord can result in premature separation of the placenta or an abnormal fetal lie. An unusually long cord can be compromised more eas-

ily because of its tendency to twist or knot more. The length of the umbilical cord rarely varies to these extremes, however. An occasional cord will actually form a knot, but the natural pulsations of the blood through the vessels and the muscle in the vessel walls keep the blood flow adequate. It is not unusual for a cord to wrap once around the fetal neck, but again, with no interference to fetal circulation.

Key Points

- Complications of labor arise from problems with the force of labor, the passage, or the passenger. Hypotonic, hypertonic, and uncoordinated contractions all can occur, resulting in ineffective first or second stages of labor.
- Precipitate labor is delivery that is completed in less than 3 hours. It can be responsible for subdural hemorrhage in the fetus and cervical lacerations in the mother.
- Uterine rupture is a rare occurrence that is suggested by a pathologic retraction or constriction ring (an indentation across the abdomen over the uterus).
- Uterine inversion is a grave complication. If the situation is not immediately corrected, emergency hysterectomy is necessary to save the woman's life. Almost all occurrences of uterine inversion can be avoided by two axioms of care: *Do not put pressure on an uncontracted fundus immediately postpartum* (massage first to cause it to contract); and *do not exert pressure on an umbilical cord to achieve placental delivery*. Patience will achieve the same result in most instances and do it safely.
- Amniotic fluid embolism occurs when amniotic fluid is forced into an open maternal uterine blood sinus. The woman notices chest pain and dyspnea. Administer oxygen and notify the woman's primary care provider of this emergency.
- Prolapse of the umbilical cord is an emergency situation that requires prompt action. Often, the nurse is the person with the woman when this occurs. Position the woman quickly into either a Trendelenburg or knee-chest position to relieve cord compression; apply manual pressure vaginally to lift the head away from the cord; notify the woman's physician of the emergency. With cord prolapse, there are fewer than 5 minutes to institute relief measures to prevent irreparable central nervous system damage to the infant.
- Multiple gestation can complicate delivery. Many infants of multiple gestations are delivered by cesarean birth.
- Abnormal position, presentation, or size of the fetus (e.g., occipitoposterior position, breech, face, or brow presentation, and transverse lie) as well as

---

Box 21-4
Apt Test

An Apt test is a laboratory determination to determine whether a sample of blood is maternal or fetal in origin. The test is used to distinguish whether vaginal blood discovered during labor is from the mother or fetus; it can be used in the newborn period to determine if blood-stained vomitus in the newborn is newborn gastric bleeding or if it is vomited swallowed maternal blood.

For the test, a commercial dipstick may be used or the sample mixed with a 1% solution of sodium hydroxide. If the blood contains fetal hemoglobin (Hgb F), the sample or dipstick will remain pink. If the sample contains maternal hemoglobin (Hgb A), it will turn a yellow-brown.

(Oski, F., et al. [1990]. *Principles and practice of pediatrics.* Philadelphia: J. B. Lippincott, p. 434.)

problems of the passage such as inlet and outlet contraction can lead to labor complications.

- Be certain that a woman meets the criteria for labor induction before preparing an oxytocin solution: no cephalopelvic disproportion is suspected; the fetal head is engaged and the cervix is "ripe." Question an order if the above criteria are not present.
- Always prepare oxytocin as a "piggyback" solution, being extremely careful of the dose used. Both a uterine and FHR monitor should be used continuously during labor induction.

    Observe that contractions occur no more than 2 minutes apart and are no longer than 70 seconds in duration.
- Increase oxytocin flow rate only in increments of 1 to 2 mU to avoid causing hypertonic contractions or uterine tetany. Urge and support the woman to use breathing exercises and to remain on her left side during a labor induction to offer a good blood supply to the uterine muscle.
- If uterine contractions should become too strong or too frequent or fetal bradycardia, tachycardia, or abnormal decelerations should occur, discontinue an oxytocin solution immediately. Do not increase the rate of oxytocin more than 16 mU/min without specific directions to do so, because this high a rate invariably leads to tonic uterine contractions.
- Anomalies of the placenta and cord such as placenta succenturiata, placenta circumvallata, battledore placenta, or a two-vessel cord can lead to delivery complications.
- Vacuum extraction and forceps delivery are methods to assist delivery. Both mother and infant need special observation following these procedures.

Critical Thinking Exercises

1. Josiah and Eva are a young couple having their first child. After rupture of membranes, you notice that the fetal monitor shows variable decelerations. On inspection, you are able to see the cord at the vaginal opening. You are aware that this is a fetal emergency. How would you proceed, in order of priority, to address this situation?
2. Brenda is a 23-year-old having her first child. Her obstetrician has told her that her baby is in a posterior position. She asks you what this means in terms of the length and type of her labor. How would you answer her and why?
3. Mrs. Cranley began labor spontaneously at 10 AM. Mrs. Bellow had an oxytocin infusion for induction of labor at 10 AM because her pregnancy has extended 2 weeks beyond her expected due date. How would you develop a plan of care addressing the following factors: (1) which woman you anticipate will deliver first; (2) whether both women will

be able to use breathing exercises with contractions; and (3) what the priority observations are for each woman?

References

American College of Obstetricians & Gynecologists (ACOG). (1991). *Induction and augmentation of labor.* Washington, DC: ACOG.

Bishop, E. H. (1964). Pelvic scoring for elective induction. *Obstetrics and Gynecology, 24,* 266.

Blackburn, S., & Loper, D. (1992). *Maternal, fetal, and neonatal physiology.* Philadelphia: W. B. Saunders.

Cardozo, L., & Pearce, J. M. (1990). Oxytocin in active-phase abnormalities of labor: A randomized study. *Obstetrics and Gynecology, 75,* 152.

Carlan, S. J., & Knuppel, R. A. (1990). Vasa praevia: Approaches to detection. *The Female Patient, 15,* 37.

Clay, L. S., Criss, K., & Jackson, U. C. (1993). External cephalic version. *Journal of Nurse-Midwifery, 38,* 72S.

Cochran, W. D. (1990). Management of one normal newborn. In Oski, F. A., et al. *Principles and practice of pediatrics.* Philadelphia: J. B. Lippincott.

Cunningham, F. G., et al. (1993). *Williams obstetrics* (19th ed.). Norwalk, CT: Appleton and Lange.

Day, M. L., & Snell, B. J. (1993). Use of prostaglandins for induction of labor. *Journal of Nurse-Midwifery, 38,* 42S.

Department of Health & Human Services. (1991). *Healthy people 2000.* Washington, DC: Public Health Service.

Friedman, E. (1985). Failure to progress in labor. In Queenan, J. (Ed.). *Management of high-risk pregnancy.* Oradell, NJ: Medical Economics Books.

Hanigan, W. C., et al. (1990). Tentorial hemorrhage associated with vacuum extraction. *Pediatrics, 85,* 534.

Harris, B. A. (1990). Shoulder dystocia. *The Female Patient, 15,* 69.

Johnson, P., & Pace, S. (1993). Guide to the use of the vacuum extractor by nurse-midwives. *Journal of Nurse-Midwifery, 38,* 88S.

Mayberry, L. (1994). Intrapartal nursing care: Research into practice. *Journal of Obstetric, Gynecologic and Neonatal Nursing, 23,* 170.

Penny, D., & Perlis, D. (1992). Shoulder dystocia. *MCN: American Journal of Maternal Child Nursing, 17,* 34.

Posiac, S. (1993). Induction and augmentation of labor. In Mandeville, L. K., & Troiano, N. H. *High-risk intrapartum nursing.* Philadelphia: J. B. Lippincott.

Sisson, M. C. (1992). Amniotic fluid embolism. *Critical Care Nursing Clinics of North America, 4,* 667.

Sokol, R. J., & Brindley, B. A. (1990). Practical diagnosis and management of abnormal labor. In Scott, J. R., et al. *Danforth's obstetrics and gynecology.* Philadelphia: J. B. Lippincott.

Swinnerton, T. (1991). Alternative remedies during labor. *Nursing Times, 87,* 64.

Trofatter, K. F. (1992). Cervical ripening. *Clinical Obstetrics & Gynecology, 35,* 476.

Urang, S. (1993). Fetal scalp blood sampling. *Journal of Nurse-Midwifery, 38,* 95S.

Suggested Readings

Brost, L., et al. (1992). Pregnancy after perinatal loss: Prenatal reactions and nursing interventions. *Journal of Obstetric, Gyecologic, and Neonatal Nursing, 21,* 457.

Daddario, J. B. (1992). Fetal surveillance in the ICU: Understanding electronic fetal monitoring. *Critical Care Nursing Clinics of North America, 4,* 711.

Eganhouse, D. J. (1991). Electronic fetal monitoring: Education and quality assurance. *Journal of Obstetric, Gynecologic, and Neonatal Nursing, 20,* 16.

Harvey, M. G. (1992). Promoting parenting: The obstetric patient in an ICU. *Critical Care Nursing Clinics of North America, 4,* 721.

Kruse, J. (1993). The physiology of labor and management of prolonged labor. *Primary Care, 20,* 685.

Porcher, F. K. (1992). HIV-infected pregnant women and their infants. *Nurse Practitioner, 17,* 46.

Rooks, J. P., et al. (1992). The National Birth Center Study: Intrapartum and immediate postpartum and neonatal complications and transfers, postpartum and neonatal care, outcomes and client satisfaction. *Journal of Nurse Midwifery, 37,* 361.

Rosen, M. G., et al. (1992). Abnormal labor and infant brain damage. *Obstetrics and Gynecology, 80,* 961.

Shailer, T. L., et al. (1992). Management of the intrapartum patient in the intensive care unit: preparing for delivery. *Critical Care Nursing Clinics of North America, 4,* 675.

Stainton, M. C. (1994). Supporting family functioning during a high-risk pregnancy. *MCN: American Journal of Maternal Child Nursing, 19,* 24.

Zerbe, M., et al. (1992) Critical hemorrhage during pregnancy. *Critical Care Nursing Clinics of North America, 4,* 729.

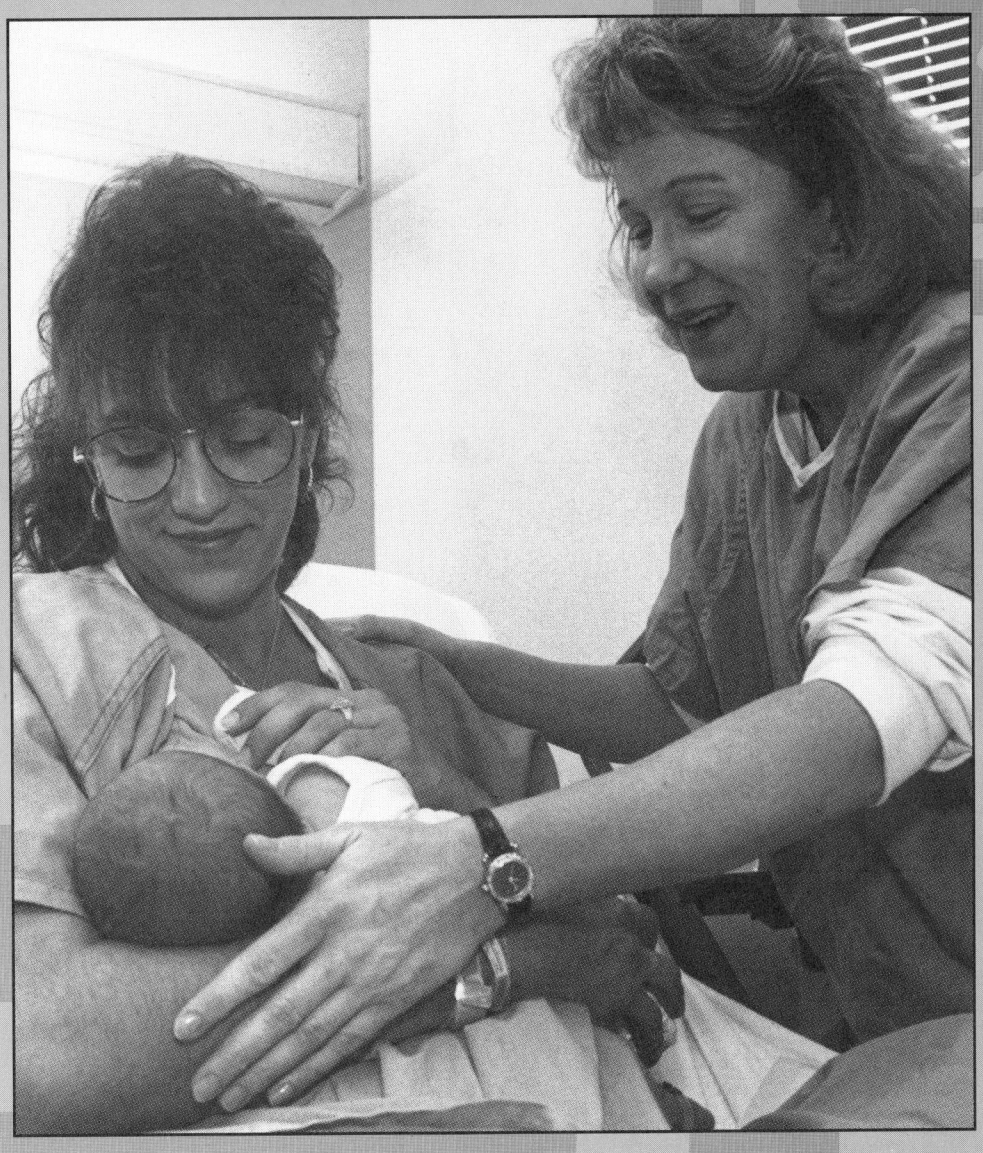

The Nursing Role
in Caring for the Family
During the Postpartal Period

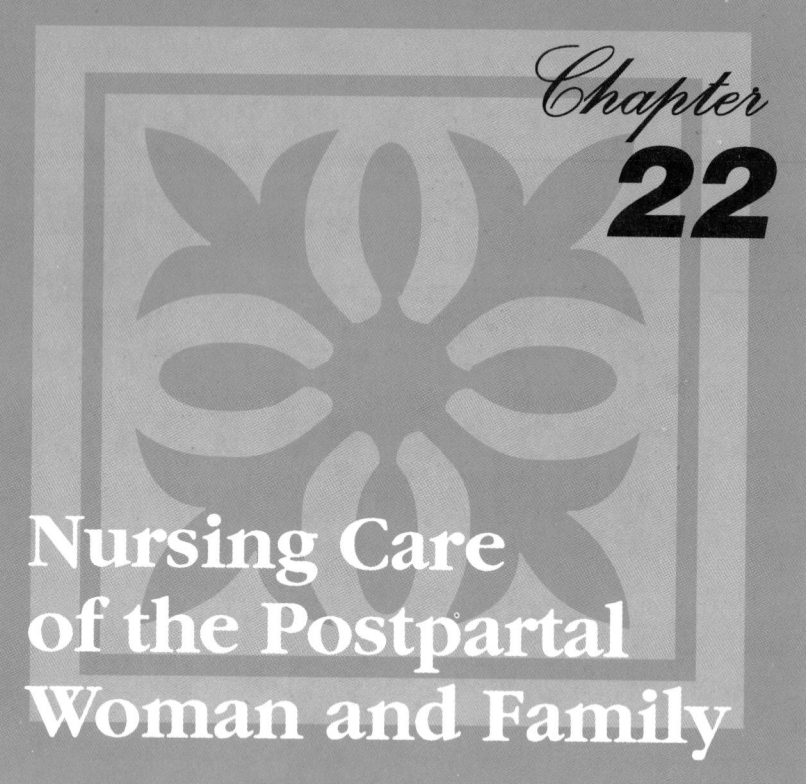

Chapter 22

Nursing Care of the Postpartal Woman and Family

Objectives

After mastering the contents of this chapter, you should be able to:

1. Describe the psychological and physiologic changes that occur in the postpartal woman.

2. Assess a woman and her family for physiologic and psychological changes following childbirth.

3. State nursing diagnoses related to physiologic and psychological changes of the postpartal period.

4. Plan nursing care such as measures to aid uterine involution or encourage bonding.

5. Implement nursing care such as helping aid the progression of physiologic changes or psychological family changes.

6. Evaluate outcome criteria to be certain that goals for nursing care were achieved.

7. Identify National Health Goals related to the postpartal period that nurses can be instrumental in helping the nation to achieve.

8. Identify areas related to care of the postpartal family that could benefit from additional nursing research.

9. Use critical thinking to analyze ways that postpartum nursing care can be more family centered.

10. Synthesize knowledge of the physiologic and psychological changes of the postpartal period with the nursing process to achieve quality maternal and child health nursing care.

Adele Pillitteri: MATERNAL AND CHILD HEALTH NURSING, 2nd Edition. © 1995 Adele Pillitteri.

The postpartal period, or *puerperium* (from the Latin *puer,* "child," and *parere,* "to bring forth"), refers to the 6-week period following childbirth. This is a time of maternal changes that are retrogressive (the involution of the uterus and vagina) and progressive (the production of milk for lactation, the restoration of the normal menstrual cycle, and the beginning of a parenting role). Protecting a woman's health as these changes occur is important for preserving future childbearing function and for ensuring that she is physically well enough to help incorporate her new child into the family. This period is popularly termed the *fourth trimester of pregnancy.*

The postpartal period has unique meaning for each family. Early in the immediate puerperium, a woman wants those people who care for her to share her excitement about her newborn. To a large extent, women base their reactions to their new child on how health care personnel act toward their infants, whether tenderly, compassionately, or routinely, during this time.

The physical postpartal care a woman receives can influence her health for the rest of her life. The emotional support she receives can influence the emotional health of her child and family and so can be felt into the next generation. National health goals related to the postpartal period are shown in the Focus on National Health Goals box.

☒ NURSING PROCESS OVERVIEW
for the Postpartal Woman and Family

ASSESSMENT

Assessment of a woman during the puerperium is done by health interview, physical examination, and analysis of laboratory data. Assessment of a woman's psychological adjustment should begin with her reaction at birth (is she happy the baby is a girl or faintly disappointed? is she happy to be through with the pregnancy or still longing to be back in it?) and continue with every contact with the family in the next few days. Assess the extent and quality of the woman's interaction with the child (does she hold the infant and talk to him or her?),

her overall mood (do you observe her crying? does she have long periods of staring into space or not talking?), and her ability to begin self and infant care. Observe for self care. If a woman feels good about herself, even though she is exhausted from childbirth, she will generally try to look her best. If she is depressed, she probably has little energy to do things such as comb her hair or worry about her appearance.

It is also important to ensure that physical changes, such as uterine involution, are occurring by evaluating uterine size and consistency and lochia flow amount.

NURSING DIAGNOSIS

Nursing diagnoses during the postpartal period usually are concerned with either the family's inability to accept and bond with the new child or physiologic considerations. Examples include:

- High risk for altered parenting related to disappointment in the sex of the child
- Fear related to lack of preparation for child care
- High risk for fluid volume deficit related to postpartal hemorrhage

---

FOCUS ON
National Health Goals

The 1st hour postpartum is an extremely dangerous one for hemorrhage. It is also the optimum period when breast-feeding should first begin. National Health Goals that involve this time period include the following:

- Reduce the maternal mortality rate to no more than 3.3/100,000 live births from a baseline of 6.6/100,000.
- Increase to at least 75% the proportion of mothers who breast-feed their babies in the early postpartum period (DHHS, 1991).

Nurses can be instrumental in helping the nation to achieve these goals by maintaining close observation in the immediate postpartal period to detect maternal hemorrhage and encouraging and supporting women who breast-feed.

Areas that could benefit from additional nursing research include delineating effective means to encourage women to maintain breast-feeding and effective ways to teach women to monitor their own health in the postpartal period, particularly when, because of early discharge, they may be home when uterine hemorrhage occurs.

PLANNING

Be certain that goals established during this time are realistic in light of the woman's changed life pattern. Most postpartum families remain in the hospital for a relatively brief time (often only 12 to 24 hours); the average postpartum stay in an alternative birth center is as short as 4 hours. Goals for care, therefore, must be short-term to be evaluated within the time of the client contact.

When planning care in the postpartal period, try to arrange procedures so there is optimal time for the woman to spend with her child and yet get adequate rest to relieve exhaustion. With exhaustion relieved, coping ability improves and the woman can plan better for self-care. After adequate instruction, women should be able to monitor their own health.

Planning should include ample time for health teaching. An important part of teaching related to care of the newborn should include preparation for the unexpected—flexibility—because parents don't yet know what their new life will be like (whether their child will sleep deeply or fitfully at night, whether their child will become hungry at long or short intervals) or how tired they will become being woken at least twice a night. Brainstorming—practicing to produce at least three different methods of reaching a particular goal—is excellent practice for parenting.

IMPLEMENTATION

All interventions in the postpartal period should be family-centered so that the family will be drawn as close together as possible during this important period of parent–child bonding.

Interventions also are geared toward increasing the woman's self-esteem and allowing her to view herself as a new mother and the infant as part of her family. Do not be as quick to teach new mothers as to explore with them what they already know about child care and what they think would be a sensible solution to a problem. Giving advice only solves an immediate problem; helping the woman to learn good problem-solving techniques enhances her ability to handle effectively the many challenges to come.

EVALUATION

If the woman fails to make an adequate adjustment in the postpartal period, she may have difficulty integrating the infant into the family. The child's mental health, self-esteem, and ability to form a sense of trust will be affected. Follow-up evaluation must be done by telephone or at follow-up home visits and at postpartal and well-child return visits.

Evaluation in the postpartal period involves being certain not only that the woman and her baby are safe but also that the woman knows how to maintain her health after returning home from a health care facility. Examples of outcome criteria include:

- Parents spontaneously make at least one positive comment about child's appearance by hospital discharge.
- Client states she feels she will be able to manage newborn care with support of her mother by 24 hours.
- Client's lochial flow is no more than 50 mL (1 saturated perineal pad) every 3 hours.

Psychological Changes of the Postpartal Period

Phases of the Puerperium

In her classic 1977 work on maternal behavior, Reva Rubin, a nurse, divided the puerperium into three separate phases. She viewed the first of these, called the **taking-in phase,** as encompassing the first 2 or 3 days. The subsequent phases, called **taking-hold** and **letting-go,** are times of renewed action and forward movement and follow the first phase. At the time that phases of the puerperium were identified, women were hospitalized for 5 to 7 days following childbirth. Today, with hospitalization as short as a number of hours, women appear to move through these phases much more quickly (Ament, 1990).

Taking-In Phase

The taking-in phase is a time of reflection for a woman. During this period, she is largely passive. She prefers having a nurse minister to her, to get her a bath towel or a clean nightgown, and make decisions for her rather than doing these things herself. This dependence is due partly to her physical discomfort from possible perineal stitches, afterpains, or hemorrhoids; partly to her uncertainty in caring for a newborn; and partly from the extreme exhaustion that follows childbirth.

As a part of thinking about and pondering her new role, a woman usually wants to talk about her pregnancy, especially about her labor and birth. She holds the child with a sense of wonder. Can this child really be hers? Is birth really over? Could she be this lucky? She needs time for resting to regain her physical strength and for calming and containing her swirling thoughts. Encouraging her to talk about the wonderment of birth helps her do this.

Taking-Hold Phase

Following the time of passive dependence, a woman begins to initiate action herself. She prefers to get her own washcloth and to make her own decisions. Women who give birth without any anesthesia may reach this second phase in a matter of hours following birth.

During the taking-in period, a woman may have expressed little interest in caring for her child. Now, she begins to take a strong interest in caring for her baby. As a rule, therefore, it is always best to give the woman brief demonstrations of baby care and then allow her to care for the child herself—with watchful guidance.

Even though a woman's actions suggest strong independence during this time, she often still feels insecure about her ability to care for her new child. She needs praise for the things she does well: supporting the baby's head, beginning breastfeeding, bubbling the baby correctly, and so on in order to give her confidence before she leaves the hospital or birthing center.

Do not rush a woman through the phase of taking-in or prevent her from taking-hold when she reaches that point. For many young mothers, learning to make decisions about their child's welfare is one of the most difficult phases of motherhood. It helps if the woman has practice in making such decisions in a sheltered setting rather than first taking on that level of responsibility when she is on her own.

Letting-Go Phase

In the third phase, called **letting-go,** the woman finally redefines her new role. She gives up the fantasized image of her child and accepts the real one; she gives up her old role of being childless or the mother of only one or two (or however many children she had before this birth). This process requires some grief work and readjustment of relationships similar to what occurred during pregnancy. It is extended and continues during the child's growing years.

Development of Parental Love and Positive Family Relationships

Almost every woman worries during pregnancy about her ability to be a "good" mother. This concern doesn't evaporate as soon as the baby is born. Some women seem able to recognize a newborn's needs immediately and to give care with confident understanding right from the start. More often, however, a woman enters into a relationship with her newborn tentatively and with qualms and conflicts that she has to address before the relationship can be meaningful. This is because parental love is only partly instinctive. A major portion develops gradually, in stages: planning the pregnancy, hearing the pregnancy confirmed, feeling the child move in utero, birthing, seeing the baby, touching the baby, and, finally, caring for the child. Factors such as a difficult labor or transport and separation from the newborn may interfere with the woman's ability to bond with her baby.

Many women work through these steps slowly and may not experience maternal feelings for their infants until days or even weeks after giving birth. Some fathers admit they have difficulty "claiming" or bonding with an infant (feeling fatherly toward the new child) until as late as 3 months or so after the birth, when the child can smile or coo and interact more directly with them. Both parents' ability to reach out can be strengthened by allowing them to touch and spend time with the new child in the first few hours of life.

Forming a strong bond with a child is not a problem only for first-time parents. Experienced parents can have just as much difficulty—they know they love 4-year-old Johnny and 2-year-old Sue at home, but worry that their heart may not be big enough to love a new child, too.

Because of these mixed feelings, parents may not show genuine warmth the first time they hold their infant. Even though a woman carried an infant inside her for 9 months, she now approaches her newborn as she would a stranger. The first time she holds the infant, she may touch only tentatively. She may hold him or her, so she touches only the blanket and never makes physical contact. If she unfolds the blanket to examine the baby or count the fingers or toes, she may use only her fingertips (Figure 22-1).

Gradually, as a woman holds her child more, she begins to express more warmth. She touches the child with the palm of her hand rather than with her fingertips. She holds her newborn tighter, in a more motherly way. She smoothes the baby's hair, brushes a cheek, plays with toes, and lets the baby's fingers clasp hers, as sweethearts might on a date. Soon, she feels comfortable enough to press her cheek against the baby's or kiss the infant's nose or mouth; she has become a mother tending to her child. This identification process is termed *claiming* or *bonding* (Klaus & Kennell, 1982). A woman looking directly at her newborn's face, with direct eye contact (termed an **en face position**), is a sign that she is beginning effective interaction (Figure 22-2). The length of time parents take to bond with a child depends on the circumstances of the pregnancy and birth, the wellness and ability of the child to meet the parent's expectations, and the opportunities the parents have to interact with the child. An environment free of stringent rules is conducive to the development of good parent-child relationships. To help parents sort out their feelings about being a mother or father and about their new responsibility, provide a supportive presence and be able to offer anticipatory guidance when necessary.

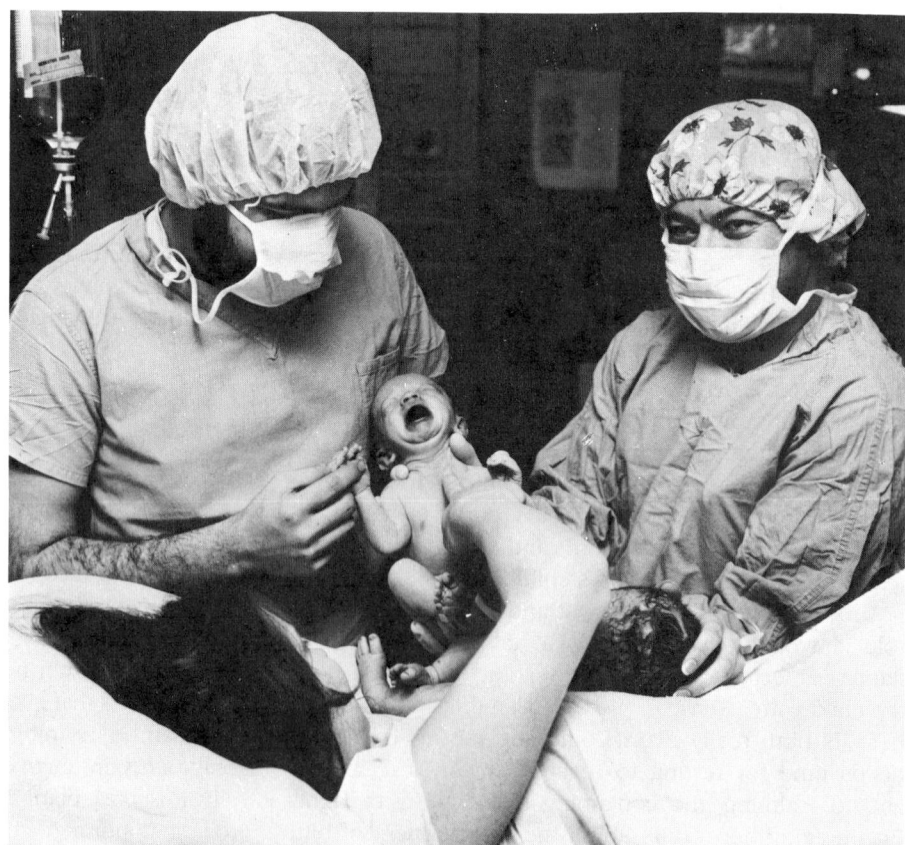

FIGURE 22-1

A mother beginning interaction with her twins immediately after birth. Note the way she touches with only a fingertip. (Courtesy of the Department of Medical Photography, Children's Hospital, Buffalo, NY.)

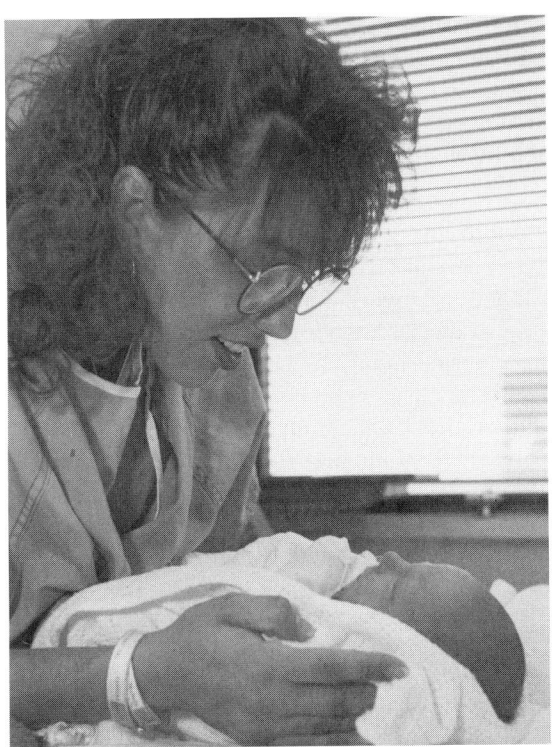

FIGURE 22-2
Mothering a new baby is a responsibility. It takes time and exposure to each other for mother-child interaction to be effective. Notice the healthy "en face" position, however. (Courtesy of the Department of Medical Photography, Children's Hospital, Buffalo, NY.)

Rooming-In

The more time a woman has to spend with her baby, the faster a mother–child relationship is likely to develop. Because the average postpartal hospital stay is not more than 1 or 2 days, a woman today has very little time to become acquainted with her newborn before going home. If the infant stays in the room with her (called **rooming-in**) rather than in a central nursery, she can become better acquainted with her child and begin to feel more confidence in her ability to care for him or her after discharge.

There are two types of rooming-in: *complete,* which implies that the mother and child are together 24 hours a day, and *partial,* in which the infant remains in the woman's room for part of the time, perhaps from 10:00 AM to 9:00 PM, after which he or she is taken to a small nursery near the woman's room or returned to a central nursery for the night. With both complete and partial rooming-in, the father and siblings can also hold and feed the infant. In many settings, the father can stay overnight, or "room-in," as well.

Not only does rooming-in allow mother–child and father–child relationships to develop rapidly, but a couple tends to retain anticipatory guidance and instructions in newborn care better when a nurse demon-

strates bathing, feeding, changing, and so forth on their own child. Fewer parents make anxious phone calls to the hospital after discharge if they have spent more time in the hospital learning how to care for their baby (Figure 22-3).

Sibling Visitation

Whether a child grows up feeling loved partly depends on how older siblings react to having a new family member. Waiting at home separated from their mother and listening only to telephone reports of what a new brother or sister looks like is difficult for children. They may picture the new baby as much older than he or she actually is. "He is eating well" may produce an image of a child sitting at a table using a fork and spoon. "He weighs 8 pounds" can be meaningless information. A chance to visit the hospital and see the new baby and mother reduces feelings that a mother cares more about the new baby than about them.

Children should be free of contagious diseases (upper respiratory illnesses, recent exposure to chickenpox) when they visit. After this is assured, and they have washed their hands, they should be encouraged actually to hold or touch the newborn (Figure 22-4). Some hospitals may require siblings to gown as well.

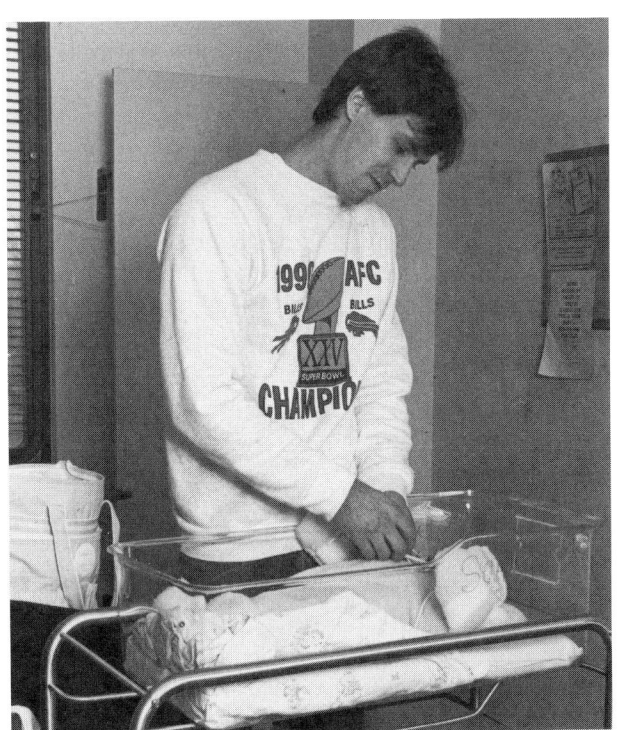

FIGURE 22-3
Fathers should be encouraged to care for their newborns as much as new mothers in order to feel confident in care. (Courtesy of the Department of Medical Photography, Children's Hospital, Buffalo, NY.)

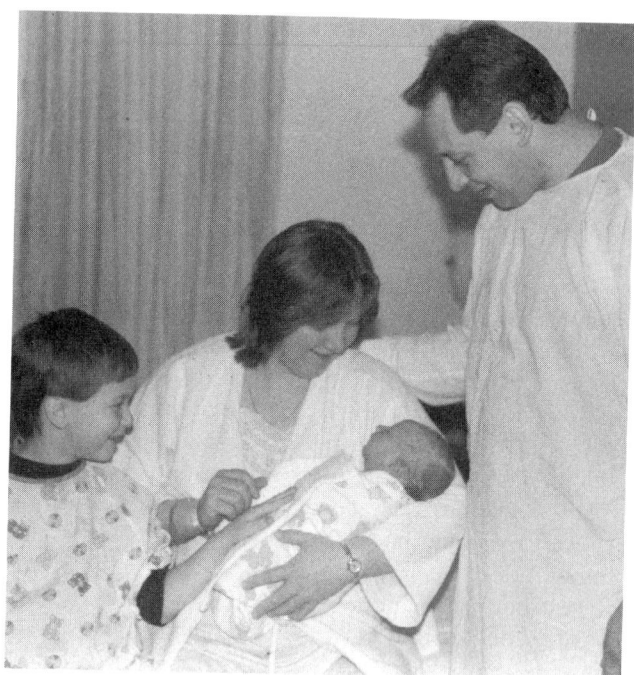

FIGURE 22-4
Sibling visiting is important to bring a family together. Here a brother meets a new sister for the first time. (Courtesy of the Sisters of Charity Hospital, Buffalo, NY.)

Separation from children is often as painful for a mother as for the children. Sibling visitation usually goes a long way toward preventing postpartal depression by relieving some of the impact of separation. You may need to caution a woman that preschoolers' opinions of a new brother or sister may not be complimentary. This baby with little hair is not their idea of a "pretty baby." If they thought the new baby would be big enough to play with, they may not feel he is a "big baby." Seeing the baby, however, even if his or her appearance is not what they expected, is helpful in establishing strong relationships and is a practice to be encouraged in postpartal units.

Maternal Concerns and Feelings in the Postpartal Period

Traditionally, most of a woman's concerns in the postpartal period have been assumed to be with care of the infant. Classes in the postpartal period have centered around teaching how to breastfeed and bathe infants. Although these are concerns for many mothers, they are not necessarily their chief concerns. A woman has come through a tremendous psychological experience during pregnancy and birth of a child. She has made a complete role change. It is only to be expected, then, that some of her attention and interest during this time will be inward-directed as she tries to view herself in this new role.

Major issues identified by postpartum women are often baby feeding or behavior, breast soreness, and regaining their figure; regulating the demands of housework, their partner, and their children; coping with emotional tension and sibling jealousy; and fatigue.

Abandonment

Many mothers, if given the opportunity, admit to feeling abandoned following birth. Only hours before, they were the center of attention. Everyone asked about their health and well being. Now, suddenly, the baby is the chief interest. Everyone asks about the baby, the gifts are all for the baby. Even her obstetrician, who has made her feel so important for the last 9 months, may ask during a visit, "How's that healthy 8-pound boy?" The woman feels confused by a sensation very close to jealousy. How can a good mother be jealous of her own baby?

You can help the woman by verbalizing the problem: "How things have changed! Everyone's asking about the baby today and not about you, aren't they? How strange, even uncomfortable, that must make you feel." These are welcome words for a woman to hear. It is reassuring to know the sensation she is experiencing, while still uncomfortable, is normal.

When a newborn comes home, the father may have much the same feelings. He may become resentful of the time his wife spends with the infant. Perhaps the two used to sit at the table after dinner discussing the day or the future. Now she hurries away to feed the baby. She used to watch the late show with him at night. Now she goes to bed earlier because she knows she will be up again at 2:00 AM.

This is a good subject to discuss with new parents. Both motherhood and fatherhood involve some compromising in favor of the baby's interests. Examination of competitive feelings should start during pregnancy or early in the postpartal period. Making infant care a shared responsibility helps to make both partners feel equally involved in the baby's care and can help alleviate these feelings.

Disappointment

Another common feeling parents may experience is disappointment in the baby. All during pregnancy, they pictured a chubby-cheeked, curly-haired, smiling girl. They have instead a skinny boy, without any hair, who is crying constantly.

It is difficult for partners to feel positive immediately over a child who does not meet their expectations. If the child's sex is not what they desired, the woman may feel she has failed, even though she understands that this is something over which she has no control. If the child looks scrawny and definitely is not as cute as the infant in the next crib, parents may remember their adolescence, when they felt gangly and unattractive, and may experience all over again the inadequacy they felt then.

You can never change the sex or size of a child, but in the short time that you care for a postpartal family, you can hope to change a mother's or father's feelings about the infant's sex and appearance. Handle the child as if you find the infant satisfactory or even special. Comment on the child's good points: long fingers, lovely eyes, good appetite, and so on. During periods of crisis like childbearing, it is possible for a key person such as a nurse to offer support that can tip the scale toward acceptance or at least help the person involved to take a clearer look at his or her situation and begin to cope with the new circumstances.

Postpartal Blues

During the puerperium, as many as 80% of women experience some feelings of overwhelming sadness that they cannot account for (Cunningham et al., 1993). They burst into tears easily and are irritable over trifles. This temporary feeling after birth has long been known as the *baby blues*.

This phenomenon may be due to hormonal changes, particularly the decrease in estrogen and progesterone that occurs with the delivery of the placenta. For some women, it may be a response to dependence caused by exhaustion, being away from home, physical discomfort, and the tension engendered by assuming a new role. The syndrome is evidenced by tearfulness, feelings of inadequacy, mood lability, anorexia, and sleep disturbance.

A woman needs assurance that sudden crying jags are normal; otherwise, she will not understand what is happening to her. Her support person also needs such assurance or he may think that she is unhappy with him or with the baby or is keeping some terrible secret about the baby from him.

Individualized nursing attention, ensuring that a woman is treated as an important client, helps to alleviate postpartal blues. It also is important to give a woman a chance to verbalize her feelings: "I know there's absolutely no reason for me to be crying but I cannot stop." Allowing her to make as many decisions as possible can help give her a sense of control over her life.

Remember, however, that not all women on a postpartal unit cry because they have baby blues. A woman sometimes has other reasons to feel sad during this time. Perhaps problems at home have become overwhelming. Her husband may have been laid off from his job just when they most need the money. Her mother may be ill, or their house may have been damaged in some way. Keeping open lines of communication with postpartal women is important to help you differentiate between problems that can be handled best with discussion and concerned understanding and those that should be re-

ferred to the hospital social service department or a community health agency.

Occasionally, serious depression requiring formal counseling or psychiatric care occurs during the postpartal period (Crisp, 1992). This postpartal psychosis is discussed in Chapter 25.

Physiologic Changes of the Postpartal Period

Retrogressive physiologic changes during the postpartal period include those related specifically to the reproductive system and systemic changes.

Reproductive System Changes

Involution is the process whereby the reproductive organs return to their nonpregnant state. The woman is in danger of hemorrhage from the uterus until involution is complete.

The Uterus

Involution of the uterus involves two main processes. First, the area where the placenta was implanted is sealed off, and bleeding is thus prevented. Second, the organ is reduced to its approximate pregestational size.

The sealing of the placenta site is accomplished by rapid contraction of the uterus immediately following the delivery of the placenta. This contraction pinches the blood vessels entering the 7-cm-wide area left denuded by the placenta and controls bleeding. With time, thrombi form within the uterine sinuses and permanently seal the area. Eventually, endometrial tissue undermines the site and obliterates the organized thrombi, completely covering and healing the area. This process leaves no scar tissue within the uterus, so it does not compromise future implantation sites (Zlatnik, 1990).

The same contraction process reduces the bulk of the uterus. Freed of the placenta and the membranes, the walls of the uterus thicken and contract, reducing the uterus from being a container large enough to hold a full-term fetus to one the size of a grapefruit. Uterine contraction can be compared with a rubber band that has been stretched for many months and now is regaining its normal contour. None of the rubber band is destroyed; the shape is simply altered. A few cells of the uterine wall are broken down by an autolytic process into their protein components, and these components are then absorbed by the bloodstream and excreted by the body in urine. The main mechanism that reduces the bulk of the uterus, however, is contraction. This is the reason the postpartal period, like pregnancy, is not a period of illness, of necrosing cells being evacuated, but primarily a period of healthy change.

With involution, the uterus will never completely return to its prepregnancy state, but its reduction in size is dramatic. Immediately after birth the uterus weighs about 1000 g. At the end of the first week, it weighs 500 g. By the time involution is complete (6 weeks), it will weigh approximately 50 g, its prepregnant weight.

In the first minutes following placenta delivery, as contraction takes place, the fundus of the uterus may be palpated through the abdominal wall halfway between the umbilicus and the symphysis pubis. One hour after birth, it has risen to the level of the umbilicus, where it remains for approximately the next 24 hours. From then on it will decrease a fingerbreadth (1 cm) a day in size. Thus, on the first postpartal day the fundus of the uterus will be palpable 1 fingerbreadth below the umbilicus; on the second, 2 fingerbreadths below the umbilicus; and so on. As a fingerwidth is about 1 cm, this can be recorded as 1 cm below the umbilicus, 2 cm below it, and so forth. The average woman's uterus will have contracted so much by the 9th or 10th day and be so far withdrawn into the pelvis that it can no longer be detected by abdominal palpation (Figure 22-5). Because oxytocin is released with breastfeeding, which leads to uterine contractions, the uterus of the breastfeeding woman may contract even more quickly than this, al-though breastfeeding does not protect against postpartum hemorrhage.

On palpation, the fundus can usually be felt in the midline of the abdomen, although occasionally it is found slightly to the right because the bulk of the sigmoid colon forced it to the right during pregnancy and it tends to remain in that position. Measurements of the height of the fundus should be made shortly after the woman's bladder has been emptied, because a full bladder will keep the uterus from contracting and push it upward due to the laxness of the uterine ligaments, giving a false reading.

Uterine involution may be retarded by a condition such as birth of multiple fetuses, hydramnios, exhaustion from prolonged labor or a difficult birth, grand multiparity, or physiologic effects of excessive analgesia. Contraction may be difficult in the presence of a retained placenta or membranes or a full bladder. Involution will occur most dependably in a woman who is well nourished and who ambulates early following birth (gravity may play a role).

An estimation of the consistency of the postpartal uterus is as important as measurement of its height. A well-contracted fundus feels firm. It can be compared with a grapefruit not only in size but also in tenseness, or consistency. Whenever the fundus feels soft or flabby, it is not as contracted as it should be, despite its position in the abdomen.

The first hour postpartum is potentially the most dangerous time for the newly delivered woman. If the uterus should become relaxed during this time (**uterine atony**), the woman will lose blood very rapidly, because no permanent thrombi have yet formed at the placental site.

In some women, the contraction of the uterus after birth causes cramps similar to those accompanying a menstrual period. These are termed **afterpains**. They occur more frequently in multiparas than primiparas and in mothers who have delivered large babies or had an overdistended uterus for any other reason, as the uterus must contract more forcefully to regain its prepregnancy size. These sensations are noticed most intensely with breastfeeding, as the infant's sucking causes a release of oxytocin from the posterior pituitary, increasing contractions (Acheson & Danner, 1993).

Lochia

The separation of the placenta and membranes occurs in the spongy layer or outer portion of the decidua basalis. By the 2nd day following birth, the layer of decidua remaining under the placental site (an area 7 cm wide) and throughout the uterus differentiates into two distinct layers. The inner layer attached to the muscular wall of the uterus will remain and serve as the foundation from which a new layer of endometrium will be formed. The layer adjacent to the uterine cavity will become necrotic

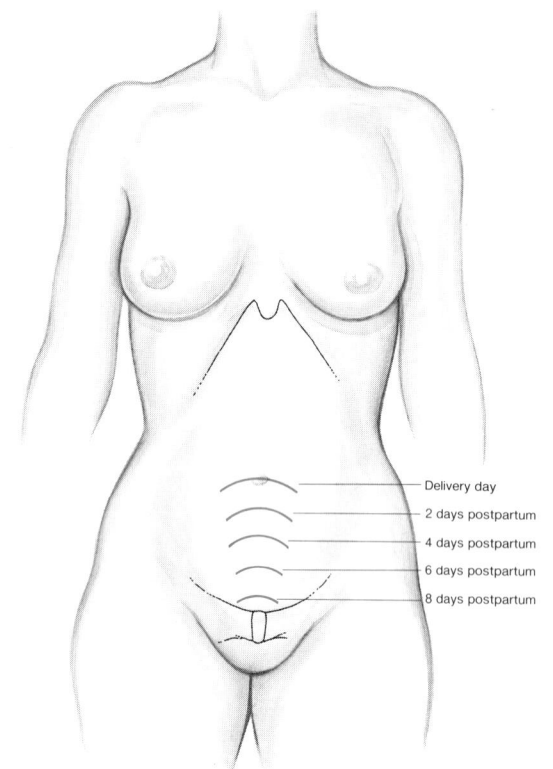

FIGURE 22-5
Uterine involution. The uterus decreases in size at a predictable rate during the postpartal period. After 10 days, it recedes under the pubic bone and is no longer palpable.

Delivery day
2 days postpartum
4 days postpartum
6 days postpartum
8 days postpartum

and will be cast off as a uterine discharge similar to a menstrual flow. This uterine flow, consisting of blood, fragments of decidua, white blood cells, mucus, and some bacteria, is known as *lochia*.

The portion of the uterus where the placenta was not attached will be fully cleansed by this sloughing process and will be in a reproductive state in about 3 weeks. The placental implantation site will take approximately 6 weeks (the entire postpartal period) to be cleansed and healed.

For the first 3 days after birth, a lochia discharge consists almost entirely of blood, with only small particles of decidua and mucus. Because of its red color, it is termed **lochia rubra**. As the amount of blood involved in the cast-off tissue decreases (about the 4th day), and leukocytes begin to invade the area as they do any healing surface, the flow becomes pink or brownish in color (**lochia serosa**). On about the 10th day, the amount of the flow decreases and becomes colorless or white (**lochia alba**). Lochia alba is present in most women until the 3rd week following birth, although it is not unusual for a lochia flow to last the entire 6 weeks of the puerperium. Characteristics of lochia are summarized in Table 22-1. Several rules for judging whether or not lochia flow is normal are summarized in the Focus on Family Teaching box.

The Cervix

Immediately following birth, the cervix is soft and malleable. Both the internal and external os are well open. Like contraction of the fundus of the uterus, contraction of the cervix begins at once. By the end of 7 days, the external os is narrowed to the size of a pencil opening, and the cervix feels firm and nongravid again.

In contrast to the process of involution in the fundus, in which the changes consist primarily of old cells being returned to their former position by contraction, the process in the cervix does involve the formation of new muscle cells. Like the fundus, the cervix does not return exactly to its virginal state. The internal os will close as before, but, assuming that the birth was vaginal,

the external os will usually remain slightly open and appear slitlike or stellate (star shaped) where it was round before. Finding this pattern on pelvic examination suggests that childbearing has taken place.

The Vagina

Following a vaginal birth, the vagina is soft, few rugae are present, and its diameter is considerably greater than normal. The hymen is permanently torn and heals with small separate tags of tissue. It takes the entire postpartal period for the vagina to involute (as in the uterus, by contraction) until it gradually returns approximately to its prepregnant state. Thickening of the walls also appears to depend on renewed estrogen stimulation from the ovaries; a woman who is breastfeeding and in whom ovulation is delayed may continue to have thin-walled or fragile vaginal cells that cause slight vaginal bleeding during sexual intercourse until about 6 weeks' time. Like the cervix, the vaginal outlet will remain slightly more distended than before; if the woman practices Kegel's exercises, the strength and tone of the vagina will increase more rapidly (see "Perineal Exercises"). This may be important for both the woman and her partner's sexual enjoyment.

The Perineum

The perineum is put under a great deal of pressure during birth, to which it responds, after birth, with the development of edema and generalized tenderness. Portions of the perineum may show ecchymosis from the rupture of surface capillaries. The labia majora and labia minora typically remain atrophic and softened in a woman and never return to their prepregnant state. Many women have episiotomy incisions that are extremely painful (Thranov et al., 1990).

Systemic Changes

The same body systems involved in pregnancy are involved in postpartal changes as the body returns to its prepregnant state.

The Hormonal System

Pregnancy hormones begin to decrease as soon as the placenta is no longer present. The level of chorionic gonadotropin in urine is almost negligible by 24 hours. By week 1, progestin, estrone, and estradiol are at prepregnancy levels. Estrol may be elevated for an additional week before it reaches prepregnancy levels (Cunningham et al., 1993).

The Urinary System

During a vaginal birth, the fetal head exerts a great deal of pressure on the bladder and urethra as it passes on the bladder's underside. This pressure may leave the bladder with a transient loss of tone and such edema

Type of Lochia	Color	Duration (day)	Composition
Lochia rubra	Red	1–3	Blood, fragments of decidua, and mucus
Lochia serosa	Pink or brown	3–10	Blood, mucus, and invading leukocytes
Lochia alba	White	10–14 (may last for 6 weeks)	Largely mucus; leukocyte count high

Table 22-1. *Characteristics of Lochia*

FOCUS ON FAMILY TEACHING

Q. How can I judge that the vaginal flow I have after childbirth is normal?

A. A number of guidelines are helpful for evaluating a lochia flow. These are:

Amount	Lochia should approximate a menstrual flow in amount. Like the amount of menstrual flow, this amount will vary from woman to woman. Two women in adjoining beds may be having very different quantities of lochia discharge, yet each may be normal for that woman. Mothers who breast-feed tend to have less lochial discharge than those who do not, because the natural release of oxytocin during breast-feeding strengthens uterine contractions. Conservation of fluid for lactation also may be a factor. Lochial flow increases on exertion, especially the first few times the woman is out of bed, but decreases again with rest. The increase in amount that occurs with ambulation, however, is the result of vaginal discharge of pooled lochia, not a true increase in amount. Lochia amount truly does increase on strenuous exercise, such as lifting a heavy weight or walking up stairs. Saturating a perineal pad in less than an hour is considered an abnormally heavy flow.
Consistency	Lochia should contain no large clots. Clots may indicate that a portion of the placenta has been retained and is preventing closure of the maternal uterine blood sinuses. In any event, clotting denotes poor uterine contraction, which needs to be corrected.
Pattern	Lochia is red for the first 1–2 days (lochia rubra), pinkish-brown from 3–10 days (lochia serosa), and then white (lochia alba) for as long as 6 weeks after birth. The pattern of lochia (rubra to serosa to alba) should not reverse. A red flow after it has turned pink or white may indicate that placental fragments have been retained or that uterine contraction is decreasing and new bleeding is beginning.
Odor	Lochia should not have an offensive odor. Lochia has the same odor as menstrual blood (sometimes compared with the odor of marigolds). An offensive odor usually indicates that the uterus has become infected. Immediate intervention is needed to halt postpartal infection.
Absence	Lochia should never be absent during the first 1 to 3 weeks. Absence of lochia, like presence of an offensive odor, may indicate postpartal infection. Lochia may be scant in amount following cesarean birth, but it is never altogether absent.

surrounding the urethra that voiding is difficult. Thus, even though a bladder fills rapidly and becomes distended, the woman may have no sensation of having to void. The woman who has had an epidural, a spinal, or a general anesthetic for birth can feel no sensation in the bladder area until the anesthetic has worn off.

To prevent permanent damage to the bladder from overdistention, assess the woman's abdomen frequently in the immediate postpartal period to see whether bladder distention is developing. A full bladder is felt as a hard or firm area on palpation just above the symphysis pubis. On percussion (placing one finger flat on the woman's abdomen over the bladder and tapping it with the middle finger of the other hand), a full bladder sounds resonant in contrast to the dull, thudding sound of nonfluid-filled tissue. Pressure on this area may make the woman feel as if she has to void, but she is then unable to do so. As the bladder fills, it displaces the uterus; uterine position is thus a good gauge of whether the bladder is full or empty. If the uterus is becoming uncontracted and flabby and is being pushed to the side, the usual cause is an overfilled bladder. The hydronephrosis or increased size of ureters that occurred during pregnancy remains present for about 4 weeks postpartum. The increased size of these organs increases the possibility of urinary stasis and urine infection in the postpartal period (Stray-Pederson et al., 1990).

During pregnancy, as much as 2000 mL to 3000 mL excess fluid accumulates in the body. An extensive diuresis begins to take place almost immediately following birth to rid the body of the fluid; this increases the daily output of the postpartal woman greatly. Urinary volume may easily rise from a normal level of 1500 mL to as much as 3000 mL during the 2nd to 5th day after birth. This marked increase in urine production causes the bladder to fill rapidly.

In the postpartal period, urine tends to contain more nitrogen than normal. This development is probably due in part to the woman's increased muscle activity during labor and in part to the breakdown of protein in a portion of the uterine muscle that occurs during involution (Cook, 1992). Lactose levels in the urine may be the same as during pregnancy. If any urine testing for sugar is done either during pregnancy or the postpartum period, therefore, agents such as Clinistix or Tes-Tape that test only the glucose, not the lactose, component of sugar should be used for testing.

Diaphoresis (excessive sweating) is another way by which the body rids itself of excess fluid. This is noticeable in women soon after birth.

The Circulatory System

The diuresis evident between the 2nd and 5th days postpartum plus the blood loss at birth act to reduce the added blood volume the woman accumulated during pregnancy. This reduction occurs so rapidly that by the 1st or 2nd week postpartum, the blood volume has returned to its normal prepregnancy level.

Usual blood loss is 300 mL to 500 mL at vaginal birth and 500 mL to 1000 mL with a cesarean birth. A 4-point decrease in hematocrit (proportion of red blood cells to proportion of circulating plasma), and a 1-g decrease in hemoglobin value will occur with each 250 mL of blood lost. If the average woman enters labor with a hematocrit of 37%, therefore, it will be about 33% on the first postpartal day. Hemoglobin will fall from 11 g to 10 g/dL. If the woman was anemic during pregnancy, she can expect to continue to be anemic postpartum. As excess fluid is excreted, the hematocrit will gradually rise from hemoconcentration to be at prepregnancy levels by 6 weeks.

Women generally continue to have the same high level of plasma fibrinogen during the first postpartal weeks as they did during pregnancy. This is a protective measure against hemorrhage but, unfortunately, also increases the risk of thrombophlebitis formation (Gerbasi et al., 1990). There is also an increase in the number of leukocytes in the blood. The white blood cell count may be as high as 30,000 total (mainly granulocytes), particularly if the woman had a long or difficult labor. This, too,

is part of the body's defense system, a defense against infection and an aid to healing.

Varicosities present will recede but rarely will return to a completely prepregnant appearance. Although vascular blemishes, such as spider angina, fade slightly, they also invariably remain.

The Gastrointestinal System

Digestion and absorption begin to be active again in the gastrointestinal system soon after birth. The woman feels almost immediately hungry from the glucose used during labor and thirsty from the long period of restricted fluid plus the beginning diaphoresis. Unless she has the aftereffects of general anesthesia, she can eat without difficulty from nausea or vomiting during this time.

Hemorrhoids (distended rectal veins) that have been pushed out of the rectum due to the effort of pelvic-stage pushing often are present. Bowel sounds are active, but passage of stool through the bowel may be slow because of the still-present effect of relaxin on the bowel; bowel evacuation is difficult due to pain of episiotomy sutures or hemorrhoids.

The Integument

Following birth, the stretch marks on the abdomen (striae gravidarum) still appear reddened and may be even more prominent than during pregnancy, when they were tightly stretched. A white woman can be assured that these will fade to a pale white over the next 3 to 6 months; they will be revealed as only slightly darker pigment in a black woman. Excessive pigment on the face and neck (chloasma) and on the abdomen (linea nigra) will be barely detectable in 6 weeks' time. If **diastasis recti** (overstretching of the abdominal musculature) is present, this will always be present as a slightly indented, bluish-tinged area in the abdominal midline.

The abdominal wall and the ligaments that support the uterus that were obviously stretched during pregnancy usually require the full 6 weeks of the puerperium to return to their former state. If the woman does postpartal exercises, such as head raising or sit-ups, this tone returns more dependably. Otherwise, the muscle will remain protuberant and soft.

Effects of Retrogressive Changes

The overall effects of the postpartal changes discussed above are exhaustion and weight loss.

Exhaustion

As soon as birth is completed, the woman experiences total exhaustion. For the last several months of pregnancy, she has probably not slept soundly. Near the end of pregnancy, she was unable to find a comfortable position in bed because of the fetus's activity or the presence of back or leg pain. All during labor she has eaten nothing and worked very hard, with little or no sleep. Now she has sleep hunger, which makes it difficult for her to cope with new experiences and stressful situations. This sleep starvation probably adds to the development of postpartal depression.

Weight Loss

The rapid diuresis and diaphoresis during the 2nd to 5th day postpartum will ordinarily result in a weight loss of an additional 5 lb (2 kg to 4 kg) over the approximately 12 lb (5.8 kg) that the woman lost at birth. Little loss occurs after 6 weeks. The weight a woman reaches at this time will be her baseline postpartal weight; in many women, this is above their prepregnancy weight (Parham et al., 1990).

Vital Signs

Vital sign changes in the postpartum period reflect the internal adjustments that are occurring as the woman's body begins its return to its prepregnant state.

Temperature

Temperature is always taken orally or at the tympanic membrane during the puerperium because of the danger of vaginal contamination and the discomfort involved in rectal intrusion.

A woman may show a slight increase in temperature during the first 24 hours of the puerperium because of the period of dehydration she underwent during labor. If she receives adequate fluid during the first 24 hours, the temperature will be reduced and should be normal thereafter. As stated, most women are thirsty immediately after birth and so are eager to drink. Drinking a large quantity of fluid is not a problem unless the woman is nauseated from a birth anesthetic.

Any woman whose oral temperature rises above 38°C (100.4°F), excluding the first 24-hour period, is considered by criteria of the Joint Commission on Maternal Welfare to be febrile, and a postpartal infection should be suspected.

Occasionally, on the 3rd or 4th day postpartum, when milk "comes in," the woman's temperature rises for a period of hours because of the increased vascular activity involved in engorgement. If the elevation in temperature lasts more than a few hours, however, infection is a much more likely reason for the fever. Infection is a major cause of postpartal mortality and morbidity, and a major nursing role is detecting signs of infection in a postpartal woman.

Pulse

The pulse rate during the postpartal period is generally slightly slower than normal. The decline is the result of increased stroke volume that occurs because a large amount of venous blood is returning to the heart as it is no longer obstructed by the distended uterus. The pulse rate is reduced to between 60 to 70 bpm. As diuresis diminishes the blood volume and blood pressure falls, the pulse rate increases accordingly. By the end of the first week, the pulse rate has returned to normal.

Pulse rate should be evaluated carefully in the postpartal period as a rapid and thready pulse is a possible sign of hemorrhage. Be certain that you are comparing the woman's pulse rate with the normal range in the postpartal period, not with the normal pulse rates in the general population; otherwise, you may misinterpret the finding.

Blood Pressure

Blood pressure should also be monitored carefully during the postpartal period because of the information it gives in regard to the presence of bleeding. A blood pressure reading should be compared with the woman's prebirth level rather than the standard blood pressures, because this varies with the age of the woman.

A reading above 140 mm Hg systolic or 90 mm Hg diastolic may indicate the development of postpartal pregnancy-induced hypertension, an unusual but serious complication of the puerperium (see Chapter 15). Oxytocics are drugs frequently administered during the postpartal period to achieve uterine contraction. These drugs cause contraction of all smooth muscle including blood vessels and, consequently, increase blood pressure. Always take a blood pressure prior to administration of one of these agents; if it is over 140/90, omit the administration to prevent hypertension and possible cerebrovascular accident. A major complication of acute blood loss is *orthostatic hypotension* or dizziness that occurs on standing because the vascular system does not have enough volume to maintain nourishment of brain cells. To test if a woman will be susceptible to this, assess her blood pressure and pulse with her lying supine. Next, raise the head of the bed fully upright, wait 2 or 3 minutes, and then reassess these values. If pulse rate is increased more than 20 bpm and blood pressure is 15 to 20 mm Hg lower than formerly, the woman will be susceptible to dizziness and possibly falling when she ambulates. Advise her to sit up slowly and "dangle" on the side of her bed before attempting to walk. If she notices obvious dizziness on sitting upright, consult with her physician or nurse-midwife before helping her ambulate to avoid the possibility of her falling. Caution her to not attempt to walk carrying her newborn until her cardiovascular status adjusts better to her blood loss.

Progressive Changes

Two physiologic changes during the puerperium involve progressive changes or the building of new tissue. For this reason, strict dieting that limits cell building ability is contraindicated in the first 6 weeks following childbirth.

Lactation

The formation of breast milk (lactation) is initiated in a woman whether or not she plans to breastfeed.

Early in pregnancy, the increased estrogen level produced by the placenta stimulated the growth of milk glands and growth in breast size from accumulated fluid and extra adipose tissue. For the first 2 days postpartum, the average woman notices little change in her breasts from the way they were during pregnancy. Since midway through pregnancy, she has been secreting colostrum, the thin, watery prelactation secretion. She continues to excrete this fluid the first 2 days postpartum. On the 3rd day, her breasts tend to become full and feel tense or tender as milk forms within breast ducts.

Breast milk forms as a result of the fall in estrogen and progesterone levels that follows delivery of the placenta (which causes an increase in prolactin and stimulates milk production). When the production of milk begins, a great deal of distention occurs in the milk ducts. The woman experiences this distention as a feeling of heat or throbbing breast pain. Breast tissue may appear reddened, its appearance simulating that of an acute inflammatory or infectious process. The distention is not limited to the milk ducts but occurs in the surrounding tissue as well, because blood and lymph enter the area to contribute fluid to the formation of milk. The feeling of tension in the breasts on the 3rd or 4th day postpartum is termed **engorgement** and, although painful, is a welcome sign that breast milk production is starting. Whether milk production continues depends on the infant sucking at the breasts and the ability of milk to come forward in the breasts (a let-down reflex). Care of breasts postpartum and breastfeeding are discussed in Chapter 24.

Return of Menstrual Flow

With the delivery of the placenta, the production of placental estrogen and progesterone is no longer available to the woman; this decrease in hormones causes a rise in the production of follicle-stimulating hormone and, therefore, with only a slight delay, the return of ovulation. This will initiate prepregnancy menstrual cycles.

If the woman is not breastfeeding, she can expect her menstrual flow to return within 6 or 10 weeks after birth. If she is breastfeeding, menstrual flow may not return for 3 or 4 months, or, in some women, for the entire lactation period. The absence of a menstrual flow, however, does not guarantee that a woman will not conceive during this time. She may be ovulating, with the absence of menstruation being the body's way of conserving fluid for lactation.

Nursing Care of the Woman and Family in the First Twenty-Four Hours Postpartum

Women remain in a birthing or recovery room for the 1st hour postpartum for careful assessment. When the hour is up, they are encouraged to shower, are taught perineal care, and then remain in the room as a postpartal patient or are transferred to a postpartal room. The most dangerous hour in childbearing has passed.

A timetable for nursing interventions in the 1st hour postpartum and remaining hours is shown in Table 22-2. A woman's care must be completed with extreme conscientiousness because during the entire first 24 hours after birth, the uterus is prone to hemorrhaging until the myometrial vessels have healed. One of the worries with a couple delivering at home is that they will not appreciate how dangerous a time this is for the mother; with

Table 22-2. *Timetable for Nursing Interventions: Postpartum*

Intervention	1st hour Postpartum	2 to 8 hr Postpartum	1 to 4 days Postpartum
Evaluate fundal height and consistency	q 15 min	q 1 h	q 8 h
Evaluate lochia color and amount	q 15 min	q 1 h	q 8 h
Assess perineum for hematoma or stressed suture line	q 15 min	q 1 h	q 8 h
Take pulse and blood pressure	q 15 min	q 2 h	q 4 h
Assess to see if lactation suppressant is desired	During first h	—	—
Assess bladder distention	At end of h	q 2–4 h	q 4–8 h
Ask woman to void	At end of h	—	—
Take temperature	—	q 4 h	q 4–8 h
Assess breasts for degree of firmness	At end of h	q 8 h	q 8 h
Give bath, first perineal care	At end of h	—	—
Observe mother-child (parent-child) interaction	At each encounter	At each encounter	At each encounter

Abbreviations: q = every; h = hour.

attention focused more on the newborn than the mother, postpartal hemorrhage could occur.

Assessment

Health History

As with all health assessment, assessment during this time begins with history taking. Technical aspects of pregnancy, labor, and birth can be learned from the woman's pregnancy and labor and birth chart. Most of this information is best obtained from the woman herself, however, as this supplies not only information on events of her pregnancy or labor but her emotions and impressions about them. If the nurse previously cared for the woman during labor and birth, it is unnecessary to obtain this information again.

Family Profile. Information you need to know includes age, support persons, other children, type of housing and community setting, occupation, education level, and socioeconomic level. This information is necessary to evaluate the impact of this new child on the woman and her family. It lays a foundation for teaching of self and child care that is specific to her knowledge level and needs.

Pregnancy History. Information you need is para and gravida (and the reason for any discrepancy), expected date of birth, whether the pregnancy was planned, and problems such as spotting or hypertension of pregnancy. This information helps you to know the woman's potential for bonding, as whether the pregnancy was planned and complications during pregnancy may interfere greatly with this.

Labor and Birth History. The length of labor, position of fetus, type of birth, any analgesia and anesthesia used, problems during labor such as fetal distress, supine hypotension syndrome, and perineal sutures are all important information to gather. This information helps you to plan what procedures will be necessary in the postpartal period.

Infant Data. The sex and weight of the infant, any difficulty at birth or during labor, plans to breastfeed or formula feed, and any congenital anomalies present are the major facts needed. This information helps you to plan care for the infant and promote bonding with the parents.

Postpartal Course. Ask about general health; activity level since birth; a description of lochia; presence of perineal, abdominal, or breast pain; success with infant feeding; and response of her support person to parenting. This information helps in planning anticipatory guidance for home care.

Laboratory Data

Women routinely have a hemoglobin and hematocrit level done 12 to 24 hours after birth to determine whether the blood loss at birth left them anemic. If the hemoglobin is below 10 g/100 mL, supplementary iron is usually prescribed. Take note of the laboratory reports on postpartal women and make certain that any abnormal finding, such as low hemoglobin, is brought to the attention of the physician or nurse-midwife. The woman's new responsibility at home will tax her energies enough. She does not need the additional burden of an undetected low hemoglobin level to increase her fatigue. If the woman was catheterized during labor or had a urinary tract infection during pregnancy, a urinalysis or urine culture may be ordered done in the postpartal period. A urine specimen should be obtained during this time with a clean-catch technique using a sterile cotton ball tucked in the vagina introitus. This will prevent lochia from contaminating the specimen and changing the urine's acidity, specific gravity, red blood cell count, and, possibly, bacterial count.

Physical Assessment

During early labor, a woman is given a fairly complete physical examination. During the immediate postpartal period, therefore, she does not need all of this procedure repeated. She does need crucial assessments that examine particular aspects of health, however, such as an estimation of nutrition and fluid state, energy level, presence or absence of pain, breast health, fundal height and consistency, lochia amount and character, perineal integrity, and circulatory adequacy. Be certain to provide privacy for physical assessment during this period. A frequent complaint of women during this time is that they feel as if modesty is a forgotten concept.

General Appearance. A woman's general appearance in the postpartal period reveals a great deal about her energy level, her self-esteem, and whether she is moving into the taking-hold phase of recovery. Before an assessment, ask her to void so she has an empty bladder. Observe how much energy she uses when reaching for her robe or walking to the bathroom—does she struggle or move listlessly, or can she accomplish this task quickly? Observe for a cringing expression or hand pressure against her abdomen that suggests pain on movement. Observe whether she has combed her hair, applied makeup, and has put on her own clothing or an agency gown. Many women choose to sleep in an agency gown to prevent getting lochia stains on their own clothing, but a woman who is pleased with herself, her pregnancy, and her birth experience is usually anxious to wear her own clothing and "fuss" with her appearance within an hour after birth. A woman who is extremely exhausted or depressed probably will not bother with her appearance. Keep in mind, however, that a woman whose labor progressed rapidly and who came to the health care agency as an emergency admission may not have had time to pack a comb or brush or her own clothing. Cultural variations will also affect appearances (see the Focus on Cultural Awareness box).

Hair. Ask the woman to lie supine in bed. Palpate her hair to determine its firmness and strength. A woman who had a good pregnancy diet has firm, crisp hair; when a diet was deficient in nutrients, hair becomes listless and "stringy." Many women begin to lose a quantity of hair in the postpartal period. This occurs because while her metabolism was elevated during pregnancy, hair growth was rapid. She has many hairs reaching maturity at the same time and, as her body returns to a normal metabolism level, this hair is lost. You may need to assure her that this is not a sign of illness but just another aspect of returning to her prepregnant state.

Face. Assess the woman's face for evidence of edema. This is most apparent early in the morning because the woman has had her head level during the night. Edema is manifested as puffy eyelids or a prominent fold of tissue inferior to the lower eyelid. This is normally negligible but will be evident in the woman who had hypertension of pregnancy and so was accumulating excessive fluid. It will become evident in the rare woman who is developing hypertension of pregnancy in the postpartal period.

Eyes. Place your finger on the woman's lower eyelid and gently pull it downward to inspect the color of the inner conjunctiva. Normally this should appear pink and moist. The conjunctiva of the woman who is anemic from poor pregnancy nutrition or excessive blood loss at birth will have a pale-colored conjunctiva. If the woman is dehydrated, the area will appear dry. Make a note to check the hematocrit determination of any woman with pale conjunctivae. Use common sense in assessing extremely fair-skinned or darkly pigmented persons. The conjunctiva always appears lightly shaded in fair-skinned women. Dark-skinned women may have a ruddy conjunctiva appearance in the face of anemia.

Breasts. A woman should wear a bra in the postpartal period to offer support to breast tissue as increased accumulation of fluid preparatory to breastfeeding occurs. This prevents undue stretching of ligaments and the occurrence of pendulous breasts later in life, and it offers a great deal of comfort. Assess whether a bra is in place, and observe that it is an adequate, comfortable size. Properly fitted, the straps should not leave erythemic marks on the shoulders or the bottom part should not be pressing so firmly against the breasts that reddened areas are left there. Breast tissue increases in

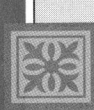

size as breast milk forms, so a bra that was adequate during pregnancy may no longer be adequate by the 2nd or 3rd postpartal day. Advise women to buy a nursing bra for the postpartal period that is one to two sizes larger than her pregnancy size to allow for this size increase.

Ask the woman to remove the bra and cover her breasts with a towel or folded sheet to protect modesty; ask the woman to raise her hand over her head and tuck it under her head as this stretches and thins breast tissue. Observe and then palpate for size, shape, and color.

Breast tissue feels soft on palpation the 1st and 2nd day; on the 3rd day as engorgement occurs, it feels firm and warm (described as *filling*); it may appear flushed. Occasionally, a firm nodule will be detected on palpation. This is usually only a temporarily caked milk duct or milk contained in a gland that is not flowing forward to the nipple. The location of the nodule should be noted, however, reported to the physician or nurse-midwife, and reassessed before discharge. Such caking of breast milk generally is relieved by the infant sucking. Any nodule needs reassessment, however, because a fibrocystic or malignant growth unrelated to the pregnancy could be present. Normal engorgement causes the entire breast to feel warm or appear reddened. If only one portion of a breast is warm or reddened, mastitis or inflammation and, possibly, infection of glands or milk ducts is suggested.

Note whether the nipple is normally erect and not inverted. Assess the nipple for a crack, fissure, or presence of caked milk. Squeezing the nipple is not necessary as it is painful to sensitive nipples, and unnecessary nipple manipulation increases the risk of mastitis.

Uterus. For uterine assessment, be certain the bed is flat so that the height of the uterus is not influenced by an elevated position. Observe the woman's abdomen for contour to detect distention and the appearance of striae or a diastasis. If a diastasis is present (appears as a slightly indented, bluish tinged groove in the midline of the abdomen) measure the width and length by fingerbreadths (a fingerbreadth equals a centimeter). Palpate the fundus of the uterus by placing a hand on the base of the uterus just above the symphysis pubis and the other at the umbilicus. Press in and downward with the hand on the umbilicus until you "bump" against a firm globular mass in the abdomen: the uterine fundus (Figure 22-6). For the 1st hour after birth, the height of the fundus is at the umbilicus or even slightly above it. Assess the fundus for consistency (firm, soft, or boggy), whether it is in the midline, and its height. Measure in fingerbreadths (e.g., 2 F↓ umbilicus, or 2 cm beneath the umbilicus). Although this measurement seems less scientific than a measurement of the height of the uterus from the pubis, it is the most useful measurement because it

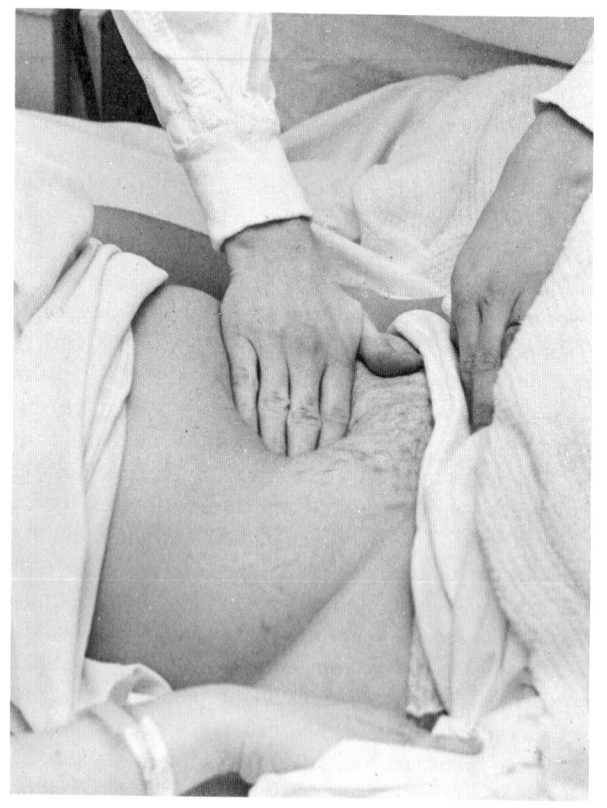

FIGURE 22-6
To palpate the uterus, be certain to place one hand at the base of the uterus. This fundus is about 4 fingerbreadths below the umbilicus. Notice the striae gravidarum marks on the abdomen. (Courtesy of the Department of Medical Photography, Children's Hospital, Buffalo, NY.)

shows the gradual decline in size or distance from the umbilicus.

Never palpate a uterus without supporting the lower segment, as the uterus potentially can invert (and in so doing cause a massive hemorrhage) if not supported this way.

Palpating of a fundus should not cause pain as long as the action is done gently. If the uterus is not firm (the consistency of a grapefruit) on palpating, massage it gently with the examining hand. This generally causes it to contract and become firm immediately. Massage is a gentle rotating motion of the hand. It should never be hard or forceful, lest it be painful to the mother or cause the uterus to expend excess energy. If the fundus does not grow firm with massage, this denotes extreme atony or perhaps retained placenta, or indicates that the woman is experiencing an excess amount of blood loss. The woman's physician or nurse-midwife should be notified or an oxytocin administered if it has been ordered p.r.n. Placing the infant at breast will cause endogenous release of oxytocin and achieve the same effect.

If the woman received no oxytocin agent following birth to help her uterus contract, someone should sit with one hand resting on the woman's abdomen, ready to assist the fundus to contract if it should become soft or relaxed during the important 1st hour. If massage does not seem to be effective in causing the uterus to contract, there may be a clot in the cavity of the uterus. The clot may be expressed from the uterus by gentle pressure on the fundus, but only after the uterus has been massaged. If the uterus is totally relaxed, this type of fundal pressure could cause inversion of the uterus, an extremely serious complication that leads to rapid hemorrhage and could necessitate an emergency hysterectomy to save the woman's life. Another reason that the uterus may not be well contracted is because a rapidly filling bladder is preventing contraction (Begley, 1991). If contraction seems inadequate, a uterine sonogram may be ordered to help detect any abnormalities.

Following the 1st hour after birth, the uterus may be evaluated for height and consistency less frequently: every hour for the next 8 hours, then once each nursing shift. The woman should be taught to make this assessment herself so she can continue it once a day at home. Always stress that she put one hand on the lower uterine segment for support before she massages the fundus. By the 9th or 10th day postpartum, the uterus will have become so small that she will no longer be able to palpate it above the symphysis pubis.

Lochia. A woman can expect to have lochia for 2 to 6 weeks. Characteristics of normal lochia and the change in pattern from red to pink to white are described in Table 22-1.

During the 1st hour postpartum, when the fundus is checked for contraction every 15 minutes, the mother's perineal pad should be removed and the character, amount, color (rubra, serosa, or alba), and presence of any clots evaluated; smell the pad for odor. Be certain the pad is not adherent to perineal stitches before removing.

In the 1st hour, you will see lochia rubra; it may contain small clots. Whether the amount of lochia is normal is evaluated against the amount the woman has during a normal menstrual flow. Ask how often during a normal menstrual flow she changes pads or tampons.

Be certain that when you turn the woman to inspect her perineum, you check under her buttocks so as not to miss bleeding that may be pooling below her. If you observe a constant trickle of vaginal flow or the woman is soaking through a pad every 60 minutes, she is losing more than the average amount of blood. She needs to be checked by a physician or nurse-midwife to be certain that there is no cervical or vaginal tear present.

Women should be encouraged to change perineal pads frequently as they begin self-care. Lochia is an excellent medium for bacterial growth that could spread through the vagina to the uterus, and the presence of constantly wet pads against an episiotomy suture line slows healing. This is not often a problem for the woman while she is at a health care facility, but the woman who is trying to save money at home may try to conserve on the number of pads she uses. Be certain she knows not to use tampons until she returns for her postpartal checkup as she is at high risk for toxic shock syndrome until the uterine lining is healed completely. Be certain that women know the criteria for judging the amount and type of normal lochia (see the Focus on Family Teaching box).

While the woman is at a health care facility, you need to inspect her lochia discharge once every 15 minutes for the first hour, once every hour for the next 8 hours, and then once every 8 hours. Make certain a woman understands that she must wash her hands after handling pads and must use only her own personal care equipment so that she does not contract or spread infection. Demonstrate good role modeling yourself in terms of handwashing and equipment use.

Perineum. At the time that lochia is evaluated, the perineum should be inspected. Ask the woman to turn on her side into a Sims' position with her back toward you. Gently press on the upper buttock to lift it and inspect the perineum. Observe for ecchymosis, hematoma, erythema, edema, intactness, and presence of any drainage or bleeding from any episiotomy stitches. An episiotomy is usually 1 or 2 in long, but if a laceration was involved, stitches may extend from the vagina back to the rectum. Rarely, they extend forward toward the urethra. If a midline episiotomy was performed, which side the mother turns to does not make any difference. If a mideolateral incision is present, turning so the inci-

sion is on the bottom buttock often causes less pain and better visibility. An episiotomy incision is generally fused (edges sealed) by 24 hours following birth; if it is a midline incision, it may be almost invisible as the perineal fold obscures it. A hematoma (blood-filled protruding sphere) is only present if surface capillaries were broken during the pressure of birth. If there is clotted lochia along the incision, the woman probably needs a review of postpartal perineal care so this does not continue to occur. Before discharge, a woman who has perineal stitches can be taught to lie on her back and view her perineum with a hand-held mirror. Once a day while at home, she should inspect for redness, sloughing of sutures, or pus formation at the suture line.

Following perineal assessment, assess the rectal area for the presence of hemorrhoids. Count the number and appearance and note their size in centimeters.

Nursing Diagnoses and Related Interventions

Nursing Diagnosis: High risk for pain related to uterine cramping (afterpains) or perineal sutures

Goal: Client will not experience pain above a tolerable level during postpartal period.

Outcome Criteria: Client states that degree of pain is tolerable.

Provide Pain Relief for Afterpains. Women can be assured that this discomfort is normal and rarely lasts more than 3 days. If necessary, either ibuprofen (Motrin and others), an analgesic specific for relief of afterpains in that it reduces inflammation, or a common analgesic such as acetaminophen (Tylenol) can be taken for relief. As with any abdominal pain, heat should not be placed on the abdomen. This could cause relaxation of the uterus and consequent uterine bleeding.

Relieve Muscular Aches. Many women feel sore and aching after labor and birth because of the excessive energy they used for pushing during the pelvic division of labor. They say they feel as if they have "run for miles," which is indeed comparable to the energy expended. The woman may need a mild analgesic such as Tylenol for the pain. A backrub is effective for relieving aching shoulders or back. Assess carefully the woman who states she has pain on standing. Pain in the calf of the leg on standing (a position that dorsiflexes the foot) is a sign like Homans' that suggests thrombophlebitis (see "Assess Peripheral Circulation").

Give Episiotomy Care. Although episiotomy is becoming a rare procedure, some women will still be given one and will consequently have painful sutures. It is easy to inspect an episiotomy incision and think that because of its minimal size it should not cause much discomfort to the mother. The perineum is an extremely tender area, however, and the muscles of the area are involved in many activities (sitting, walking, stooping, squatting, bending, urinating, defecating). Thus, an incision in this area causes a great deal of discomfort (Wright, 1994).

Women expect the pain of labor to be excruciating and are usually surprised to find that it is not nearly as bad as they feared; however, they usually do not anticipate the pulling pain from perineal stitches in the postpartal period. They may be distracted by it and unable to concentrate on what you are telling them about baby care. This discomfort interferes with their rest and sleep, with eating, and with being able to sit and hold the baby comfortably.

Women can be assured that this discomfort is normal and, fortunately, does not usually last more than 5 or 6 days, because the perineal area heals rapidly. Many physicians and nurse-midwives order a soothing cream or anesthetic spray to be applied to a suture line to reduce discomfort. A cortisone-based cream or sitz bath (see below), which helps to decrease inflammation in the area and therefore to decrease tension, is also helpful. Because of their cooling effect, witch hazel preparations are a mainstay for relief of both perineal and hemorrhoidal discomfort. A woman may worry that she will experience additional discomfort when the episiotomy sutures are removed. Explain to her that these are made of an absorbable material that will not need to be removed, and usually dissolve within 10 days.

Promote Perineal Exercises. Some women find that carrying out a perineal exercise three or four times a day greatly relieves episiotomy discomfort. The exercise consists of contracting and relaxing the muscles of the perineum five times in succession as if trying to stop voiding (Kegel's exercises). This improves circulation to the area and so helps decrease edema. It is only one of a number of postpartal exercises that can help the woman regain her prepregnant muscle tone and form. Others will be discussed later.

Administer Cold and Hot Therapy. Applying an ice-bag or cold pack to a suture line during the 1st hour reduces perineal edema and the possibility of hematoma formation, and therefore reduces pain and promotes healing and comfort. Be certain not to place ice or plastic directly on the perineum, but wrap it first in a towel or disposable pad to decrease the chance of a thermal injury (easy to cause because the perineum has decreased sensation due to edema). Commercial cold packs that are combined with perineal pads are available. An ice pack can be made by partially filling a rubber glove with ice chips.

Ice to the perineum after the first 24 hours is no longer therapeutic, and healing after this time takes place faster if blood is encouraged to enter the area through the use of heat, not cold application. Dry heat in the form of a perineal hot pack or moist heat by a sitz bath is a good way of increasing circulation to the perineum and providing comfort, reducing edema and promoting healing.

Commercial hot packs that grow warm after they are "cracked" and the chemicals in them combined are available. Caution women not to apply these directly to their perineum but with a washcloth or gauze square between the pack and their skin to prevent a possible burn.

Administer Sitz Baths. A **sitz bath** is a small, portable basin that fits on a toilet seat with water constantly swirling in it (Figure 22-7A). The movement of water soothes healing tissue, decreases inflammation by vasodilatation to the area, and therefore effectively reduces discomfort and promotes healing.

Sitz baths may be either cold or warm. Be certain that the water in the sitz bath is not too hot before you help a woman to use it. The woman herself will not be sensitive to the temperature because healing surfaces are not good indicators of heat and cold. This caution applies particularly to the woman who is using an analgesic cream or spray on the perineum or has a great deal of generalized perineal edema. Both these situations make her prone to burns from scalding water unless you act to protect her (see Nursing Procedure 22-1).

A sitz bath should not last more than 20 minutes but may be repeated three or four times a day. Because of the soothing effect of the warm water and the sitting position, the woman may feel extremely tired and unsteady on her feet after using a sitz bath and may need help in getting back to bed.

Administer Medications as Prescribed. Most women who have had an episiotomy require an oral or injected analgesic to relieve their perineal discomfort. Be certain the woman understands how to use any cream or suture-line spray ordered for her. A number of topical medications with xylocaine bases, such as Hurricane Gel or Americaine Spray, are available. These are applied to the incision line with a clean gauze square or sprayed and, because of their anesthetic action, instantly reduce incision line pain. Tucks, a commercial form of soft pads impregnated with witch hazel, which can be tucked between the perineum and a sanitary pad, also are effective in relieving perineal pain. Some women doubt the efficiency of suture-line medications or worry that applying the cream will hurt more than not applying it; they may need extra encouragement to try these helpful aids.

Most physicians and nurse-midwives order a strong analgesic such as propoxyphene/acetaminophen (Darvocet) or codeine for the first 24 hours, then a milder one such as acetaminophen for the remainder of the first

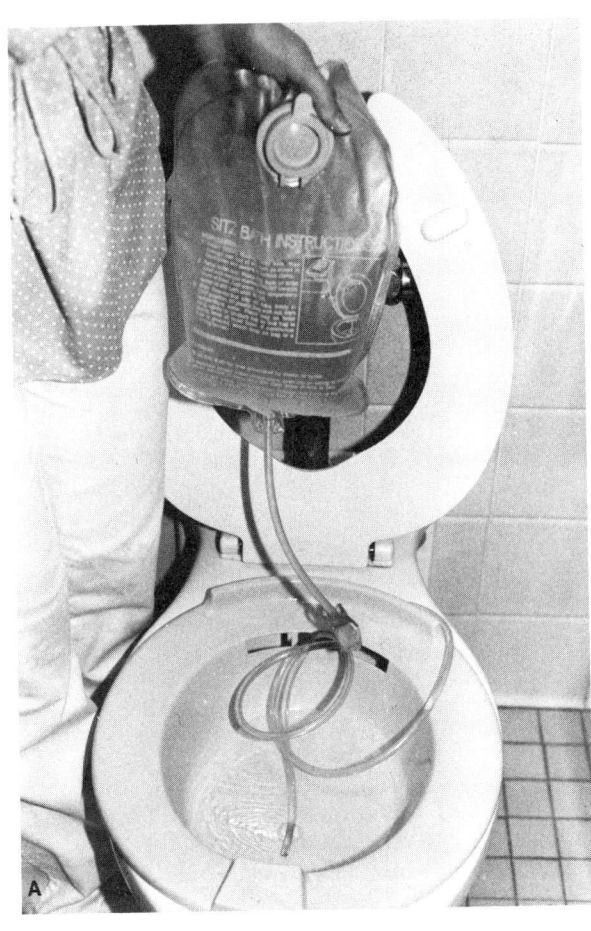

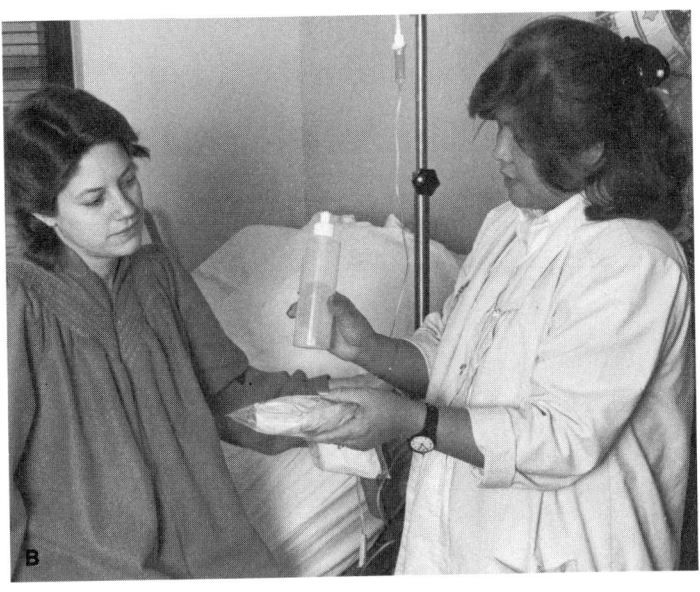

FIGURE 22-7
*Measures to promote perineal hygiene and comfort. (**A**) A sitz bath being set up on a toilet. (**B**) A "peri" bottle used for perineal care.*

week. Aspirin is not used routinely with pain during the postpartal period because it interferes with blood clotting and may make the woman more prone to hemorrhage from the denuded placental site.

    Nursing Diagnosis: High risk for uterine infection related to presence of lochia in vaginal area

    Goal: Client will not demonstrate symptoms of infection during postpartal period.

    Outcome Criteria: Client's temperature is below 100.4°F; no redness or abnormal discharge is present at an episiotomy line.

    Provide Perineal Care. Every woman needs attention to perineal cleanliness in the postpartal period to prevent infection, as lochia allowed to dry and harden on the vulva and perineum furnishes a bed for bacterial growth. Because the vagina lies in close proximity to the rectum, there is also always the danger that bacteria will spread from the rectum to the vagina and cause uterine infection.

    Perineal care should be undertaken as a part of the daily bath and after each voiding or bowel movement. If a woman is on bed rest during the first hour after birth, you will need to provide perineal care for her. As soon as she is ambulatory, she can be instructed to carry it out

herself. Perineal care should be a procedure that is easy to learn and not time-consuming so that the woman can spend most of her time with her new child, not completing a complicated ritual of care.

    Before beginning perineal care, wash your own hands and pull on clean gloves as most postpartal infection is caused and spread by the unclean hands of caregivers. A plastic-covered pad should be placed under the woman's buttocks to protect the bed during the procedure. With the woman lying in a supine position, remove the perineal pad from the front to back; the direction is important in preventing the portion of the pad that has touched the rectal area from sliding forward to the vaginal opening.

    Perineal care is a clean but not a sterile procedure. Agencies differ as to the type of cleansing that is done and the articles and solutions used. If actual washing is to be done, use a clean gauze square or a clean portion of a washcloth with soap and water for each stroke, always washing from front to back, from the pubis toward the rectum. Rinse the area in the same manner and dry.

    A second common method is to spray the perineum with clear tap water from a spray bottle (peri bottle; Figure 22-7*B*). Be certain that none of the solution enters the vagina, because it might be a source of contamination; spray gently to avoid splashing any blood-tinged

NURSING PROCEDURE 22-1
Sitz Baths

Purpose
To aid healing of the perineum through application of moist heat.

Procedure	Principle
1. Wash your hands; identify client; explain procedure.	1. Prevent spread of micro-organisms; ensure client safety and cooperation.
2. Assess client condition; analyze appropriateness of procedure; plan modifications as necessary.	2. A sitz bath can make a woman feel lightheaded; assess whether she is capable of ambulation.
3. Implement procedure by assembling equipment; a sitz bath, clean towel, and clean perineal pad.	3. Organization of equipment increases efficiency of procedure.
4. Place sitz bath on toilet seat; fill collecting bag with warm water, hang overhead so a steady stream of water will flow into basin through tubing.	4. Warm, flowing water increases circulation to perineum and so reduces inflammation and aids healing.
5. Assist woman to walk to bathroom; help her remove perineal pad and sit in bath. Instruct her in use of clamp on tubing to allow water to continue to flow.	5. Swirling water aids in edema reduction.
6. Provide privacy; be certain woman is not chilled; review call bell system for her.	6. Provide for safety and modesty.
7. After 20 minutes, assist woman to pat perineum dry and apply clean pad; assist her to return to room.	7. After 20 minutes, heat is no longer therapeutic as vasoconstriction occurs.
8. Evaluate effectiveness, cost, comfort, and safety of procedure. Plan health teaching such as advantage of continuing sitz baths after return home.	8. Health teaching is an independent nursing action always included in care.
9. Record on chart that sitz bath was taken, condition of perineum, and client condition.	9. Document client care and client status.

solution on yourself (to guard against contacting body secretions). Since the labia normally have a tendency to close and cover the vaginal opening, this will prevent solution from entering the vagina. Do not separate the labia; instead, allow them to perform their protective function. If the solution is to be sprayed with the woman lying on her back, the flow will naturally be from front to back because of gravity.

It may be advantageous to have the woman turn on her side in a Sims' position so that you can fully view an episiotomy area; in some women, better cleaning of the episiotomy area can also be done in this position.

In unwrapping a new perineal pad to apply it, be careful that you do not grasp the portion of the pad that will touch the perineum; hold it by the bottom side or the ends.

Promote Perineal Self-Care. As soon as the woman is allowed to get up to go to the bathroom (if she delivered without an anesthetic, this is within the first hour after birth), she should be instructed in how to carry out her own perineal care.

The bathroom of a birthing room or a postpartal room should have a stand or shelf close to the toilet where the woman can place the equipment she needs for care; the peri bottle, sponges to dry, her clean pad, and so forth. She needs instructions on how to remove the soiled perineal pad and where to dispose of it. She also may need to be reminded of the importance of using any cream or medication that has been prescribed. She should be cautioned not to flush the toilet until she is standing upright; otherwise, the flushing water might spray the perineum.

If women are given a clear explanation as to why perineal care is important, they do it well. Self-care, however, does not free you from your responsibility of checking the woman's perineum and ascertaining whether or not a suture line is healing and the lochia flow is normal as long as she remains in the health care agency. By continuing with these assessments, you remain the woman's first line of defense against postpartal complications such as infection and hemorrhage.

Nursing Diagnosis: High risk for sleep pattern disturbance related to exhaustion from and excitement of childbirth

Goal: Client will receive enough sleep to feel rested during postpartal period.

Outcome Criteria: Client states she feels rested during postpartal period.

After birth, a woman is a paradox. She is excited. She has a baby and she wants to hold and be with this new person in her life. She wants to talk to her support person about the experience, their child, and their future. At the same time, she is exhausted from lack of sleep and increased effort and will fall instantly asleep (Mead-Bennett, 1990).

This first wish of hers, to have time with her expanded family, should be granted in the birthing room immediately after the baby's birth. If the father did not watch the birth for some reason, time should be allowed for mother, father, and baby to be together as soon as possible. Following this, rest should be encouraged.

Promote Rest in the Early Postpartal Period. Following a first get-acquainted meeting with the infant, the woman should be encouraged to sleep to counteract the deficit from sleep lost during labor. All the procedures that must be carried out with her (blood pressures, pulse, checking of fundal height, and perineal inspection) should be done swiftly and gently to allow her as much sleep as possible. If she has discomfort from hemorrhoids, perineal stitches, or afterpains, she needs the cause of the discomfort relieved so that she can sleep.

Some women experience a shaking chill immediately after birth or within a half hour of birth. This is due in part to the pressure changes in the abdomen that occur with reduction in the bulk of the uterus and temperature readjustment following the excessive sweating of labor. It also may result from the exhilaration they are feeling combined with exhaustion. In any event, shaking chills at this point are common, and the woman can be reassured of this or she may attribute them to a developing cold or infection.

Covering the woman with a warm blanket, offering her a warm drink if she is not nauseated from an anesthetic, and assuring her that the occurrence is a normal one is usually enough to make the chill transient and allow her to fall into a sound, much-needed sleep. Most women will then sleep for at least an hour.

Although a woman may choose any position to sleep, she may enjoy being able to sleep on her stomach as she has not been able to do so during pregnancy. Be certain that the woman who had spinal anesthesia (a subarachnoid or saddleblock regional block) remains flat with not more than one pillow for the entire first 8 hours. Sitting up following spinal anesthesia may cause tension on the meninges that could result in an intense spinal headache that may leave her incapacitated for up to a week. Warning her of this possibility should be enough to convince her of the importance of remaining flat during this time.

Promote Rest Throughout the Puerperium. The importance of rest throughout the puerperium cannot be stressed enough. Throughout the woman's agency stay, time for naps (shoes off, feet up) should be provided. Discharge instructions should include a firm statement encouraging the woman to continue to get adequate rest when she is home. This will not be easy for her; she has a newborn who wakes at least twice a night, and relatives and friends who come to see the baby during the day.

Many women do not realize how long it takes to return to their previous level of functioning or that at 6 months, as many of 50% of new mothers still have not achieved this (Tulman, 1990). When families were closely knit and neighborhoods were smaller, a new mother usually had someone in her family or neighborhood to call on to look after the baby while she napped. Today, a young couple is likely to live in an apartment building and may not have family or close friends nearby. If the parents have not thought through this problem before birth, you can help them to look at their situation and see what is available to them. Perhaps the woman's mother, her sister, her partner's mother, or another relative could come and stay with them for the first week. Perhaps the husband could take a week off from work or school to help out at home. If none of these solutions seems appropriate, the couple might appreciate being given the name of a community service agency that supplies homemakers on a short-term basis; or you might make a referral to a community health agency, urging an early home visit.

The woman without support does not have an auspicious start for her new role—being a mother instead of a daughter, a mother as well as a wife, a mother of three, not two—if she is so overcome by sleep hunger that her judgment and sense of balance are blurred.

Nursing Diagnosis: High risk for bathing/hygiene self-care deficit related to exhaustion from childbirth

Goal: Client will meet own self-care hygiene needs during the postpartal period.

Outcome Criteria: Client takes daily responsibility for own hygiene.

Following childbirth women often complain that their hospital or birthing center room is being kept too warm; to prove it, they point out how heavily they are perspiring. Postpartal rooms often are kept warm so newborns will be comfortable in them, but the profuse perspiration the woman is experiencing normally comes more from the body's attempt to regulate fluid than from the heat.

The woman can be reassured that sweating not only is a normal postpartal event but is a help to bring her body back to its prepregnant state. She should be cautioned against becoming chilled during this time and perhaps contracting an upper respiratory infection. If she has soaking sweats, particularly at night, she usually prefers a hospital gown to one of her own. She needs frequent gown changes to be comfortable.

A daily shower is refreshing because of this diaphoresis of the postpartal period. Be certain to accompany a woman for a shower on her first postpartal day as she often is more fatigued than she realizes. Standing under warm water may make her dizzy, which makes it difficult for her to walk safely back to bed.

Formerly, women were not allowed to take tub baths following birth for fear bacteria from the bath water would enter the vagina and cause infection. There appears to be little evidence that this is a real danger, so if the woman wants to bathe instead of shower, she may do so.

Nursing Diagnosis: High risk for altered nutrition, less than body requirements, related to lack of knowledge about postpartal needs

Goal: Client will ingest an adequate diet during the postpartal period for a breastfeeding woman.

Outcome Criteria: Client will ingest a 2700-kcal diet and 6 to 8 glasses of fluid daily.

Postpartal menu planning should include a diet of between 2200 and 2300 calories daily and should be high in protein and the vitamins and minerals needed for good tissue repair. It should have an adequate supply of roughage to help restore the peristaltic action of the bowel. The woman who is breastfeeding needs an additional 500 calories (a 2700-kcal diet) and an additional 500 mL of fluid (these may be from the same source) in her diet to encourage the production of high-quality breast milk. Most mothers are hungry during the immediate postpartal period and consume an adequate diet without urging.

On discharge, the woman needs to be instructed to continue to eat a nutritious diet after she returns home. Some women become too fatigued during their first weeks at home to prepare adequate meals. Thus, neglecting to eat properly leads to more fatigue and so to an even less nutritious diet.

If the woman has any prenatal vitamins or supplementary iron preparations left over from pregnancy, she should, as a rule, continue to take them until her supply is used up. If she needs further supplements, her physician or nurse-midwife will order them for her either on discharge or when she returns for her postpartum checkup.

Promote Adequate Fluid Intake. The rapid diuresis and diaphoresis during the 2nd to 5th day postpartum will ordinarily result in a weight loss of an additional 5 lb over the approximate 12 lb that the woman lost at birth.

The woman often feels thirsty during this period of rapid fluid loss and wants additional fluid. It seems a paradox that while the body is ridding itself of unwanted fluid, it should also demand fluid. Part of this paradox stems from the woman's having had little to drink during a part of her labor. She may say immediately following birth, "I don't think I'll ever get enough to drink again." Part of the need for fluid stems from the increased amount of nitrogen being released from catabolized uterine cells. The woman needs to increase her fluid intake to rid her body of these wastes.

Some women need to be urged to drink adequate fluid in the first few days postpartum because they are restricting fluid themselves in the hope of preventing their breasts from becoming engorged. Other mothers are beginning diets that they hope will bring their bodies more quickly back to their nonpregnant slim state. As mentioned previously, fluid restriction does little to thwart breast engorgement, and unless the woman is extremely obese, this is not a good time for dieting. The postpartal period is a time of rebuilding and readjusting, for which a woman needs both ample nourishment and adequate fluid intake. She should drink three to four 8-oz glasses of fluid a day (6 to 8 if breastfeeding).

Nursing Diagnosis: High risk for altered elimination related to loss of bladder and bowel sensation following childbirth

Goal: Client will not experience difficulty in elimination during the postpartal period.

Outcome Criteria: Client voids over 30 mL/h without urinary retention, beginning the hour after birth, and has a bowel movement by 4 days postpartum.

Promote Urinary Elimination. Because the diuresis of the postpartal period begins almost immediately after birth, the woman's bladder begins filling almost immediately. A full bladder puts pressure on the uterus and may interfere with effective uterine contraction. An overdistended bladder may cause damage to bladder function.

Encourage the woman to walk to the bathroom and void at the end of the 1st hour postpartum. Some women have too much perineal edema to be able to void this early. Women with episiotomies may be reluctant to void because they know that acid urine against the sutures will sting. Many woman will have enough residual effect of epidural, spinal, or pudendal anesthesia at this time so that voiding is painless. You can be of assistance by providing privacy (but remaining in close proximity because the woman may become dizzy if this is her first time out of bed), running water at the sink, or offering the woman a drink of water. Pouring warm tap water over the vulva, if that is consistent with the agency's policy of perineal care, also may help.

If the woman's bladder is distended, she will need to be catheterized if unable to void at the end of the 1st hour. Most women, however, do not have this much filling at this time. They must void within 4 to 8 hours after birth, however, or bladder distention will surely have occurred.

Because the perineum is usually edematous following birth, the vulva in postpartal women appears out of proportion, and it is usually difficult to locate the urinary urethra for catheterization. Be certain that, in catheterization, you do not invade the vagina by mistake and thereby carry contamination to the denuded uterus. Occasionally, because of poor tone, the bladder in some women retains large amounts of residual urine following voidings. This urine harbors bacteria, which may cause bladder infection. Also, permanent loss of bladder tone can result if the distended condition is allowed to persist.

The first voiding after birth should be measured to detect urinary retention (only a small amount of urine was voided). Whether or not the bladder is emptying also may be judged by measuring fundal height and position (a full bladder pushes the fundus up or to the side) or by palpating or percussing bladder prominence in the lower abdomen. If the woman is voiding less than 100 mL at a time or has a displaced uterus or a palpable bladder, the physician may order catheterization for residual urine following a voiding. Be certain you know, before catheterization, how much residual there must be before you leave the catheter in place. As a rule, if the residual urine is over 150 mL, the catheter is left in place for 12 to 24 hours to give the bladder time to regain its normal tone and to begin to function efficiently.

This is an example of why professional judgment is necessary in nursing. A woman may report that she is out of bed and using the bathroom to void. Only a person with knowledge of the extent of the diuresis being accomplished and the amount that should be voided during this time is able to estimate whether bladder function is adequate.

Fortunately, for most women who must be catheterized, the procedure need be done only once following birth. After another 6 to 8 hours have passed and the bladder has filled again, some of the perineal edema has subsided, the bladder has achieved better tone, and the woman is able to void by herself if helped to the bathroom.

Catheterization in the postpartal period should not be used indiscriminately. On the other hand, it should be done before the woman's bladder is injured or the uterus is displaced and uncontracted and bleeding results.

Prevent Constipation. Many women have difficulty moving their bowels during the first week of the puerperium, a condition that can be worrisome and uncomfortable.

Constipation tends to occur because of the relaxed condition of the abdominal wall and the intestine now that it is no longer compressed by the bulky uterus. For a bowel movement, the abdominal wall must exert pressure and, in its relaxed state, the pressure is not strong enough to be effective. Also, if hemorrhoids or perineal stitches are present, the woman may decline to try to move her bowels for fear of pain.

To prevent constipation, many women will have a stool softener prescribed, beginning with the 1st day after birth. If the woman has not moved her bowels by the third day, a mild laxative or cathartic may be ordered for her. There is danger in giving cathartics before the 3rd day; the resulting increase in intestinal activity may also cause uterine irritation and lead to insufficient contraction.

Early ambulation, a good diet with adequate roughage, and an adequate fluid intake all aid in preventing the problem of constipation (see the Nursing Care Plan).

Prevent Development of Hemorrhoids. The pressure of the fetal head on the rectal veins during birth tends to aggravate or produce hemorrhoids (swollen rectal veins). Some women find that the discomfort from distended hemorrhoidal tissue is their chief discomfort in the first few days following birth. The discomfort can be relieved by sitz baths, anesthetic sprays, witch hazel or astringent preparations, or preparations such as hydrocortisone acetate (Proctofoam). Gently, manually replacing hemorrhoidal tissue may be attempted. Assuming a Sims' position several times a day aids in good venous return of the rectal area and also reduces discomfort. Increased fluid and the administration of a stool softener prevents the irritation of hemorrhoids by hard stool.

Nursing Diagnosis: High risk for altered peripheral tissue perfusion related to immobility and increased estrogen level

Goal: Client will experience adequate tissue perfusion during postpartal period.

Outcome Criteria: Homans' sign is negative; there is no evidence of erythema or pain in calves of legs.

Assess Peripheral Circulation. To determine whether peripheral circulation is adequate, assess the thigh for skin turgor by lifting a ridge of tissue and observing whether it falls readily back into place or not. Assess for edema at the ankle and over the tibia on the lower leg by observing for any indication of swelling and pressing into the tissue to detect pitting. Assess for any indication of thrombophlebitis by dorsiflexing the woman's ankle and asking her if she notices any pain in her calf on that motion (**Homans' sign**; Figure 22-8). Assess also for redness in the calf area as thrombophlebitis can be present even with a negative Homans' sign.

If you suspect a thrombophlebitis, *do not* massage the area—that could cause circulatory emboli.

This test should be done once each nursing shift or

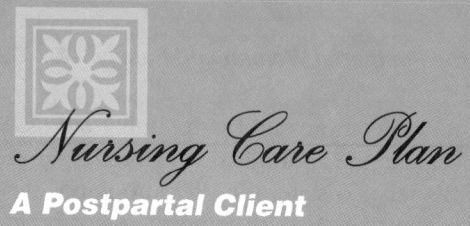

Nursing Care Plan

A Postpartal Client

Margaret Tiegler, 34 years old (para 2, gravida 2), is a client you provide care for on a postpartum unit. The following is a nursing care plan devised for her.

Assessment: Client is day 1 postpartum. Reports acute afterpains "as if my stomach is falling out" when she ambulates; perineal suture line also painful. Suture line intact, no erythema, no separation. Doing own perineal care; dried lochia present on suture line. Voiding in large amount (over 100 mL/h). Abdominal muscles soft. Fundus ½ fingerbreadth under umbilicus and boggy. Large amount of lochia rubra (2 pads every 2½ hours). States she is too tired to hold baby to feed him. Sleeping between procedures or meals. Client has had no bowel movement as yet. Has hemorrhoids that are painful on movement or touch. Client states she understands perineal care; will be discharged at 5 p.m. Her husband will stay home from work for 1 week. Twice during the morning client was observed sitting on side of her bed crying. Stated "I don't know why I'm doing this. I've never been happier." Husband appeared and scolded her for acting so inappropriately.

Nursing Diagnosis: High-risk for fluid-volume deficit related to subinvolution

Defining Characteristic: Client states she has heavy lochia flow; fundus is above standard measurement and soft.

Goal: Client will not experience significant fluid volume deficit during postpartal period.

Outcome Criteria: Client's pulse is between 50 and 70 bpm; blood pressure is above 100/60 mm Hg; lochia slows to moderate amount of flow, equal in amount to menstrual flow, with no large clots; uterus becomes firm and decreases at rate of 1 cm/day; hemoglobin level remains above 11 g/dL.

Nursing Orders	**Rationale**
1. Assess uterine contraction and lochia flow every 2 h.	1. Provides early detection of lochia flow.
2. Assess vital signs every 2 h until lochia flow is lessened.	2. Provides early indication of hypovolemic shock.
3. Administer methylergonovine 0.2 mg every 6 h until bleeding is moderate, as per physician's order.	3. Methylergonovine is an oxytocin that causes uterine contraction. It was ordered because this client's uterus may not be contracting well on its own.
4. Inform physician if above measure is not effective in reducing amount of lochia flow.	4. Lochia flow that persists in presence of an oxytocin warrants further investigation.

Nursing Diagnosis: Pain related to perineal sutures

Defining Characteristic: Client states she has perineal pain.

Goal: Client will not experience pain above a tolerable level during postpartal period.

Outcome Criteria: Client states that pain is not above a tolerable level.

Nursing Orders	**Rationale**
1. Administer appropriate analgesic (acetaminophen 10 grain q4h or ibuprofen 400 mg q4h ordered by physician).	1. Analgesic will relieve afterpains.

every 8 hours during the woman's health care agency stay.

Helping the woman out of bed and assisting her to be ambulatory shortly after birth seems inconsistent in the face of the woman's exhaustion and need for rest. Those who ambulate quickly, however, have fewer bowel and bladder complications and fewer circulatory complications such as thrombophlebitis, and they

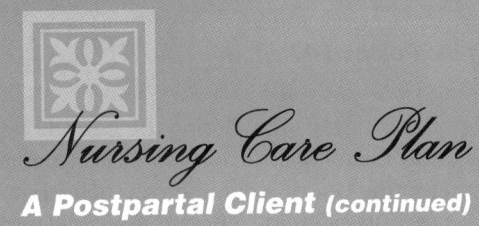

Nursing Orders	**Rationale**
2. Encourage client to do Kegel's exercises q4h.	2. Doing Kegel's exercises may increase circulation in the perineal area, thereby reducing edema.
3. Teach client perineal self-care, including use of benzocaine 20% (Hurricaine) ointment and Tucks pads.	3. These additional measures can aid in pain relief.
4. Encourage client to take a warm sitz bath q8h as prescribed.	4. Warmth improves blood supply and reduces edema, and can provide pain relief.

Nursing Diagnosis: High risk for altered bowel elimination related to lax abdominal tone and hemorrhoids

Defining Characteristic: Client states she is concerned about lack of bowel movement; states hemorrhoids are painful.

Goal: Client will resume normal bowel elimination within 3 days.

Outcome Criteria: Client has daily bowel movements without excessive pain or any bleeding.

Nursing Orders	**Rationale**
1. Encourage oral fluid (at least 1000 mL/day).	1. Fluid can aid in preventing constipation.
2. Encourage ambulation and high fiber diet.	2. Additional measures to prevent constipation.
3. Ask physician for order for stool softener.	3. A stool softener could aid evacuation.
4. Teach chin and leg raising to strengthen abdominal muscles.	4. Good abdominal tone aids effective elimination.

Nursing Diagnosis: Self-esteem disturbance related to lack of knowledge regarding psychological changes during postpartal period

Defining Characteristic: Client states she is having conflicting feelings.

Goal: Client will demonstrate adequate self-esteem despite seemingly inappropriate emotions.

Outcome Criteria: Client voices that she understands conflicting emotions commonly occur during postpartal period and are probably related to the rapid change in hormone levels.

Nursing Orders	**Rationale**
1. Review with client that postpartal sadness is common.	1. Knowledge about her reactions can offer a sense of control.
2. Explore if there are factors that are a concern or worry to her.	2. Investigate if there are additional, but undetected reasons for sadness.
3. Assure her that simple postpartal sadness runs a short, natural course and will pass.	3. Provides client with some relief about expected duration of her sad feelings.

feel stronger and healthier by the end of their 1st week than do those who remain in bed during this time (Figure 22-9).

The first time the woman is out of bed she can expect to feel dizzy and wobbly. Be certain to allow her to dangle her legs on the edge of the bed for a few minutes the first time she is up. Then, assist her as needed for the few steps to a nearby bathroom. Remain with her the

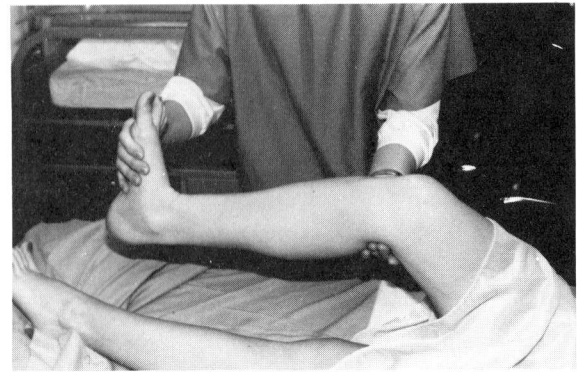

FIGURE 22-8
Evoking Homans' sign (asking if a woman has pain in her calf on dorsiflexion of her foot) is a good test for the presence of thrombophlebitis.

first time she is up; some women are extremely unsteady on their feet and discover that a seemingly easy task like walking across the room becomes overwhelmingly difficult when one is exhausted. Once the woman has been out of bed with your assistance, she may be up on her own as she wishes.

> *Nursing Diagnosis:* High risk for pain related to primary breast engorgement
>
> *Goal:* Client will not experience pain above a tolerable level during postpartal period.
>
> *Outcome Criteria:* Client states pain from breast engorgement is at a tolerable level.

Prevent/Alleviate Breast Engorgement. If the woman is breastfeeding, the sucking of the infant is the main treatment for relief of the tenderness and soreness of primary breast engorgement (breastfeeding is discussed in Chapter 24). In addition, the woman needs a firm, supporting bra to eliminate a tugging sensation and possibly a medication such as synthetic oxytocin (Syntocinon) nasal spray used just prior to breastfeeding. The nasal spray is absorbed across the mucous membrane of the nose and helps bring milk forward in the breast ducts, reducing engorgement. She may find the application of hot or cold compresses or standing under a hot shower beneficial. The woman who is breastfeeding needs reassurance that primary engorgement is a normal finding 3 or 4 days after birth, so that she does not view it as a result of something she is doing wrong with breastfeeding. Engorgement with breastfeeding lasts about 24 hours.

The woman who is not breastfeeding experiences similar discomfort. When little or no milk is removed from the breasts, however, the accumulation of milk inhibits further milk formation, and so engorgement will subside in about 2 days. Cold compresses, applied to the

breasts three or four times a day during the period of engorgement, and/or an oral analgesic provide relief. Wearing a snug-fitting bra or a commercial breast binder may help. Restriction of fluid and pumping milk from the breasts are not effective measures, and are to some degree harmful and so should be avoided. Breastfeeding women need breast support from a bra throughout the period of lactation. As lactation begins, the breasts increase in weight and feel heavy. Good support offers a degree of relief from the resultant pulling sensation and prevents unnecessary strain on the supporting muscles of the breasts, preserving muscle tone. Good support also positions the breasts in good alignment and diminishes the amount of engorgement caused by blocked milk ducts. If the woman has not packed a bra in her suitcase, she can usually arrange to have one brought from home.

Lactation Suppression. If the woman is not planning to breastfeed, some intervention is helpful to stop the formation of breast milk and increase her comfort on

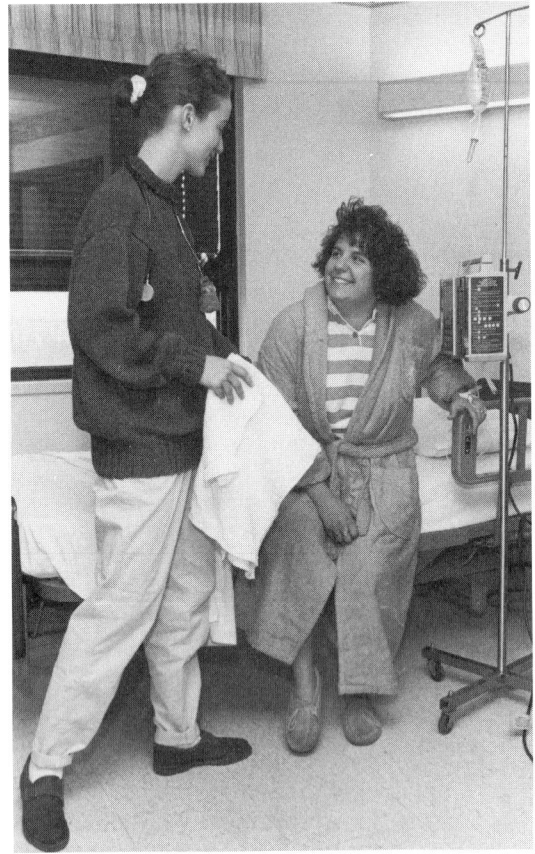

FIGURE 22-9
Ambulating postpartally helps to prevent thrombophlebitis. Encourage this effort even if a woman has equipment such as intravenous therapy. (Courtesy of the Department of Medical Photography, Children's Hospital, Buffalo, NY.)

the 3rd or 4th day postpartum, when engorgement takes place.

Because breast milk forms in mammary glands under stimulation by the pituitary hormone prolactin, administering a drug to decrease prolactin levels effectively prevents breast milk from being formed. Bromocriptine (Parlodel) is a compound given orally to achieve this. One side effect of bromocriptine is gastrointestinal pain, so it should be given with meals to reduce discomfort. Hypertension with CVA has been reported in association with bromocriptine so it is prescribed much less now than it once was (Zlatnik, 1990). Assess blood pressure before administration to be certain it is normal.

Promote Breast Hygiene. Breast care during the postpartal period is directed toward cleanliness and support. These are basically the same whether or not the woman is breastfeeding, although more care may need to be taken by the breastfeeding woman.

The woman should wash her breasts daily at the time of her bath or shower and should not use soap on her breasts, because soap tends to dry and crack nipples. This could lead to fissures and possible breast abscess. It is not necessary for women to wash their breasts more often than this. Excessive washing means unnecessary manipulation, making the process of breastfeeding more complicated than it should be.

A woman who has a considerable discharge of colostrum or milk from her breasts (whether breastfeeding or not) should insert clean gauze squares or commercial pads in her bra to absorb the moisture. These should be changed as often as necessary to keep the nipples dry. If nipples remain wet for any length of time, fissures may form and lead to infection.

Nursing Diagnosis: Health-seeking behaviors related to procedure for breast self-examination

Goal: Woman will demonstrate understanding of importance of regular breast self-examination at time of discharge.

Outcome Criteria: Woman demonstrates procedure for self-examination and states intention to perform it regularly.

All women should know how to examine their breasts so that they can check them routinely for signs of breast carcinoma. This procedure can be taught during pregnancy, but many women are not interested in hearing about cancer prevention measures at that time—the possibility of their developing cancer seems far removed from what they are doing during pregnancy: creating life. In the postpartal period they are conscious that they must remain well to raise this new child to maturity. They are receptive to having you review with them or teach them for the first time the technique of self-examination.

A week after her menstrual period begins is the best time of the month for breast self-examination because during a menstrual period or just prior to it, breasts may be tender and the examination uncomfortable. The woman who is breastfeeding may not have a menstrual flow for 3 or 4 months. During this time, she should pick a day (eg, the 1st day of every month) to do the examination until menstrual flow "markers" return.

The technique of self-breast examination is discussed in Chapter 28. The breastfeeding woman will, of course, have a milk discharge when she squeezes her nipples as part of an examination. She may occasionally discover a distended milk gland that feels very much like a cyst or tumor. She should not worry about such lumps unless they persist beyond two breastfeedings.

Remind women that if they do find a lump or have nipple discharge in a breast on self-examination, they should telephone their doctor about the finding but should not worry. Most lumps found in breasts are benign. Many women do not examine their breasts because they are afraid they will find something; other women find something but are then afraid to tell anyone about it. Breast carcinoma discovered early and treated promptly (often without removal of more than the local lesion) has an excellent cure rate.

Nursing Diagnosis: Health-seeking behaviors related to woman's desire to return to prepregnant weight and appearance

Goal: Woman will demonstrate understanding of what to expect in terms of timetable for returning to prepregnant appearance during postpartal period.

Outcome Criteria: Woman states realistic goals for return to former appearance; is able to demonstrate exercises she plans to use.

Following childbirth, the abdominal wall and the uterine ligaments are stretched. The abdomen pouches forward.

Wearing an abdominal binder or a girdle may make a woman more comfortable during the first few weeks postpartum but does not aid, and may actually hinder, the strengthening of the tone of the abdominal wall. If an abdominal binder is applied for comfort in the postpartal period, it should always be applied from the top down, so that it pushes the uterus down, not up, and uterine contraction is not hampered.

The woman can best help her abdominal wall to return to good tone by proper body mechanics and posture, adequate rest, and prescribed exercises. Exercises to strengthen the abdominal and pelvic muscles may be started with the physician's or nurse-midwife's consent as early as the 1st day after birth. The woman begins with easy exercises and gradually progresses to more difficult ones. She should continue these exercises until the end of the puerperium if she is to derive the maximum benefit from them. Common abdominal and perineal strengthening exercises are shown in Table 22-3 and Figures 22-10 and 22-11.

Teach Methods to Promote Uterine Involution. All during the postpartal period, lying on the abdomen gives support to abdominal muscles and aids involution, because it tips the uterus into its natural forward position. If this puts too much pressure on sore breasts, a small pillow under the stomach usually solves the problem.

A knee-chest position is dangerous for the woman to assume until at least the third week postpartum. In a knee-chest position, the vagina tends to open. Because the cervical os remains open to some extent until the 3rd week, there is a danger that air will enter the vagina and the open cervix, penetrate the open blood sinuses inside the uterus, enter the circulatory system, and cause an air embolism.

It is therefore good practice for a woman to avoid this position until she returns for a postpartal examination and is assured her cervix has closed properly (Cunningham et al., 1993). Women who have used a knee-chest position during pregnancy to relieve the pressure of hemorrhoids need to be instructed that a modified Sims' position, such as they used for a rest position during pregnancy, is better for them now.

Nursing Diagnosis: High risk for altered sexuality patterns related to physiologic changes of postpartal period

Goal: Client will not experience sexual dysfunction following childbirth.

Outcome Criteria: Client states she has a satisfactory sexual relationship with her partner.

At one time, women were cautioned not to resume sexual relations after the birth of a baby until their med-

Table 22-3. *Muscle-Strengthening Exercises*

Exercise	Description
Abdominal breathing	Abdominal breathing may be started on the first day postpartum, because it is a relatively easy exercise. Lying flat on her back, a woman should breathe slowly and deeply in and out 5 times, using her abdominal muscles. Check by watching her abdominal wall rise that she is actually using these muscles.
Chin-to-chest	The chin-to-chest exercise is excellent for the second day. Lying on her back with no pillow, a woman raises her head and bends her chin forward on her chest without moving any other part of her body (Figure 22-10). She should start this gradually, repeating it no more than 5 times the first time and then increasing it to 10–15 times in succession. The exercise can be done 3 or 4 times a day. She will feel the abdominal muscles pull and tighten if she is doing it correctly.
Perineal contraction	If a woman is not already using this exercise as a means of alleviating perineal discomfort, it is a good one to add on the 3rd day. She should tighten and relax her perineal muscles 5 times in succession as if she were trying to stop voiding (Kegel's exercises). She will feel her perineal muscles working if she is doing it correctly.
Arm raising	Arm raising helps both the breasts and the abdomen return to good tone and is a good exercise to add on the 4th day. Lying on her back, arms at her sides, a woman moves arms out from her sides until they are perpendicular to her body. She then raises them over her body until her hands touch and lowers them slowly to her sides. She should rest a moment, then repeat the exercise 5 times.
Leg raising	Leg raising is a good exercise to add next. To do this, the woman lies supine; she raises one leg upward and then, very slowly, lowers it again. She repeats this with the other leg (Figure 22-11). She should feel her abdominal muscles tense as she lowers her leg.
Sit-ups	It is advisable to wait until the 10th or 12th day after delivery before attempting sit-ups. Lying flat on her back, a woman folds her arms across her chest and raises herself to a sitting position, keeping her knees outstretched and unbent. This exercise expends a great deal of effort and tires a postpartal woman easily. She should be cautioned to begin it very gradually and work up slowly to doing it 10 times in a row.

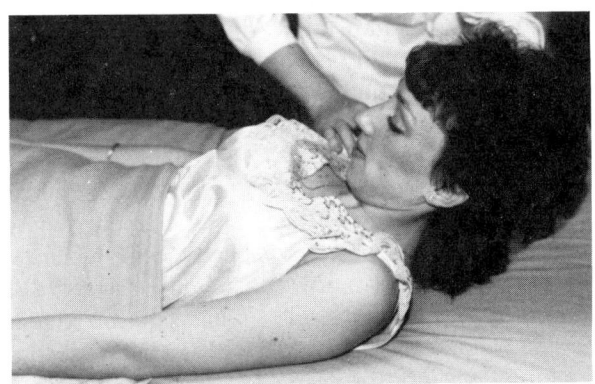

FIGURE 22-10
Chin-to-chest is a good beginning postpartal exercise to strengthen abdominal muscles. From a supine position, a woman raises her chin and touches it to her chest.

ical check-up at 6 weeks. There is no apparent physiologic reason, however, to delay sexual relations this long. For most couples, therefore, coitus may be resumed as soon as lochia serosa has stopped—about 1 to 2 weeks after birth.

Caution women that sex may be painful, however, if begun this early; tissue at an episiotomy site may be sensitive. Because vaginal epithelium is still thin, vaginal tenderness may be noticed; use of a lubricant will help any mucosal dryness. A female-superior position is suggested because it allows a woman to control the depth of penile penetration.

A woman who is breastfeeding will notice that milk is released from her nipples with sexual arousal. Women may already be aware that their degree of exhaustion may make them less receptive to sexual arousal than before.

Nursing Diagnosis: Potential for enhanced parenting related to expected bonding behavior following childbirth

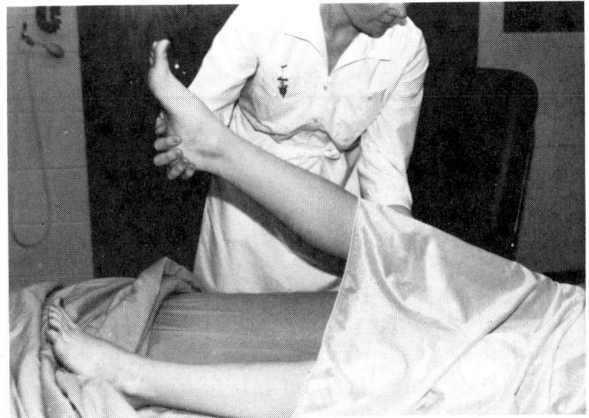

FIGURE 22-11
Leg-raising helps to strengthen abdominal muscles.

Goal: Parents will demonstrate adequate bonding behaviors during the postpartal period.

Outcome Criteria: Parents hold and comfort the infant appropriately and voice positive characteristics of child.

To assess that bonding is occurring, listen to what women say about their newborns in the immediate postpartal period, whether they make positive statements ("I'm glad he's a boy," "She's cute") or negative ones ("I really hoped it would be a girl," "She looks like a circus clown with no hair"). First impressions may not be lasting ones, but unless negative comments are identified so that extra discussion about things such as what it feels like to have four boys can take place, the woman will be discharged from the agency with her needs unmet. At home, away from health care personnel who are attuned to how disappointment can interfere with mother–child interaction, she may have great difficulty adjusting to and relating to this new child. Signs of good parent–child adaptation are shown in Box 22-1.

Nursing Care of the Woman and Family in Preparation for Discharge

The greatest need of the woman preparatory to discharge is education to prepare her to care for herself and her newborn at home. Women must know how to care for themselves to prevent introducing infection to the yet unhealed uterus or suture line before hospital discharge. They must be aware of danger signs to look for and know whom to call if they notice any of these. They must understand safe baby care. Every contact with a woman must include some teaching information, therefore, in order to squeeze everything in during a short period of contact. However, learning does not take place if

---

Box 22-1
Signs of Good Parent–Child Adaptation

Speaks of infant as desirable and attractive
Not upset by vomiting, drooling, etc.
Holds baby warmly
Makes eye contact with infant
Plays with and soothes infant
Talks or sings to baby
Expresses confidence that infant is well
Finds physical or psychological attributes to admire about baby
Is able to discriminate between baby's signs of hunger, sleep, etc.

a learner is overwhelmed and hurried. Common sense is therefore necessary to determine when it is time to teach and when it is time to observe or listen. Observation of mother–child or parent–child interaction and evaluation of the woman's support system at home are the basis for much of the teaching.

Many women attend classes in newborn care during their pregnancies. They remember many points from these classes, but when they actually have a newborn they become worried that they will not remember enough. Many mothers say child care did not seem real during pregnancy. The postpartal period is, therefore, a time for teaching, reteaching, and offering anticipatory guidance to help in the new situations the family can expect to arise when they go home.

During the taking-in phase of the puerperium, the woman may not show much interest in learning; she is more in need of the comfort of being taken care of. As she enters her taking-hold period, she grows increasingly receptive to advice and looks to you for the information she needs. Some nurses assume that multiparas will react negatively to child care suggestions. Multiparas are, after all, veterans of child care. If you listen carefully to a multipara, however, you will discover that a woman of two girls feels insecure about the care of this boy. A woman whose next youngest child is 5 years old admits that in 5 years she has completely forgotten how small newborns are. She yearns to have a nurse who is comfortable with such small human beings reassure her that she is holding her new baby correctly and giving proper care. All mothers, whether primiparas or grand multiparas, therefore, need to be evaluated individually and helped at that point where you find they need guidance.

Group Classes

Providing group classes on bathing infants, preparing formula, breastfeeding techniques, minimizing jealousy in older children, and maintaining health in the newborn can be helpful to mothers and fathers as they can learn from other parents as well as the instructor. Be certain that a time for questions and answers is planned in such classes so that the woman can apply what she is being taught to her individual circumstances. Fathers should be able to attend the classes as well, because many fathers give direct child care for at least part of every day.

Individual Instruction

Every woman needs some individual instruction in how to care for her infant and how to care for herself after discharge. Rooming-in, in which the woman spends at least a portion of the day with her baby, is an ideal setup for letting you observe and work with the woman and her baby. How to bathe and feed the baby, how to care for the infant's cord and circumcision, a review of how much infants sleep during 24 hours, and how to fit a newborn into the family's pattern of living are topics that mothers like to have discussed with them. Teaching in the postpartal unit does not have to be formal. You can teach without lecturing by making a comment such as "Notice how large all newborn's heads seem" while you are showing the woman how to bathe the baby, or "Babies like to be bundled firmly" while you are helping dress the child or "Notice how uneven newborn respirations are?" This kind of instruction saves parents many anxious moments when they are at home. Including the father in teaching is important because the problems that arise with newborn care are, by their nature, family problems, and every effort should be made by nursing personnel to help both parents prepare to deal with them. Home care of the newborn is discussed in Chapter 23.

Discharge Planning

Before the postpartal family is discharged, the woman will be given instructions by her physician or nurse-midwife concerning her care at home. These instructions differ in some aspects among different health care providers but have common points that are summarized in Table 22-4.

Prior to discharge from the health care agency, the woman must be aware that she herself must return for an examination 4 to 6 weeks after birth, and she must make an appointment to take her baby to a pediatrician, family physician, or well-child clinic for an examination at 2 to 4 weeks.

If the woman does not have an adequate rubella antibody titer and anticipates further pregnancies, she may receive a rubella immunization. It is important that discharge instructions be written for the family. The business of getting ready to go home, dressing the baby, seeing him or her in new clothes for the first time, and experiencing the thrill of realizing the baby is really theirs to take home is so exciting that your oral instructions may go unheard. On the other hand, the woman should not simply be handed a list of instructions. They should be reviewed with her to make certain that she understands them.

The health care agency should have on its staff a community liaison person, ideally a nurse, to telephone or make a home visit to mothers within 24 hours of discharge to help them assess their own health and that of the baby and to answer questions from those women who lose their instructions or are unable to interpret them after they have returned home. It is comforting to have a familiar person one trusts this way in the first few days with a new baby at home.

Table 22-4. Postpartal Discharge Instructions	
Area	**Instructions**
Work	All women should avoid heavy work (lifting or straining) for at least the first 3 weeks following birth. Women differ in their concept of heavy work, so it is a good idea to explore with the woman what she considers is heavy work. If she plans to do too much, you can perhaps help her to modify her definition of heavy work. It is usually advised that she doesn't return to an outside job for at least 3 weeks (better 6 weeks) not only for her own health but also for enjoyment of the early weeks with her newborn.
Rest	The woman should plan at least one rest period a day and try to get a good night's sleep. She can rest during the day when her newborn is sleeping unless she has other children or an aged parent to care for. If she has others dependent on her, explore with her the possibility that a neighbor, another family member, or a person from a community health agency will be able to come in to relieve her.
Exercise	The woman should limit the number of stairs she climbs to 1 flight/day for the 1st week at home. Beginning the 2nd week, if her lochial discharge is normal, she may start to expand this activity. This limitation will involve some planning on her part, especially if her washing machine is in the basement and she must wash diapers every day, or if she must go up and down stairs to check on the baby. It is probably better to arrange for a place for the baby to sleep downstairs as well as upstairs, so that he or she has to be taken upstairs only at bedtime. She should continue with muscle-strengthening exercises, such as sit-ups and leg-raising.
Hygiene	The woman may take either tub baths or showers. She should continue to apply any cream or ointment ordered for the perineal area and remember to continue to cleanse her perineum from front to back. Any perineal stitches will be absorbed within 10 days. She should not take vaginal douches until she returns for her postpartal checkup.
Coitus	Coitus is safe as soon as the woman's lochia has turned to alba and if she has an episiotomy, it is healed (about the 3rd week after delivery). Vaginal cells may not be as thick as formerly because prepregnancy hormone balance has not yet completely returned. Use of a contraceptive foam or lubricating jelly will aid comfort. Be certain she knows safe sex precautions (see Box 4-2).
Contraception	The woman should begin a contraception measure with the initiation of coitus (if she desires contraception). If she wishes an IUD, this may be fitted immediately following delivery or at her 1st postpartal checkup. A diaphragm must be refitted at a 6-week checkup. Oral contraceptives are begun about 2–3 weeks after delivery. Until she returns for this checkup, she can use an over-the-counter spermicidal jelly and her sexual partner a condom to provide a high level of protection.
Follow-up	The woman should notify her physician or nurse-midwife if she notices an increase, not a decrease, in lochial discharge, or if lochia serosa or lochia alba becomes lochia rubra. Delayed postpartal hemorrhage can occur in women who become extremely fatigued. Getting adequate rest during her first weeks at home will do much to prevent the possibility of this complication. Four to six weeks after birth, the woman should return to her physician or nurse-midwife for an examination. This visit is important to ensure that involution is complete and reproductive life planning, if desired, can be discussed further.

Making a telephone call to or visiting a woman 24 hours after discharge from a health care facility is a helpful way of evaluating if the woman is able to continue self-evaluation and infant care after discharge and is able to integrate the new infant into the family.

For such a call or visit to be maximally helpful, it is important that it be made fairly close to the day of discharge. After this time, the woman generally solves any problems which she has—for better or worse—and no longer needs a second opinion at that point. Many times, such a call reveals concerns that could not be anticipated before discharge.

Nursing Care of the Woman and Family Following Discharge

Postpartal Home Visits

Early discharge allows the family unit to be interrupted as little as possible; the mother may rest better at home than in a strange hospital setting, and she may eat better if she has cultural preferences for specific foods. The infant can be more quickly exposed to family routines rather than a superficial hospital schedule. Early discharge, unfortunately, has the disadvantage of not allowing a new family to have the ready support of health care personnel if they have questions about the newborn or the woman's condition. In order to be certain that the new family is adjusting well to having a newborn home with them, a home visit may be included as part of an early discharge program. Home visits should always be planned for high risk newborns, including newborns who are preterm, those born with a congenital anomaly, infants of adolescent mothers, or infants of mothers who have abused drugs during pregnancy.

The purposes of a home visit for the well postpartum woman and her newborn are to help the family integrate the infant into the family structure and provide the family with additional information on newborn care they may not have been able to learn during a brief hospital stay. Such a visit also allows for physical examination of the woman and newborn and for phenylketonuria or bilirubin testing to be carried out if this was not done during the hospital stay (Williams et al., 1993).

Because women need to preserve their energy during the postpartal period, a home visit should be arranged at the woman's convenience. Preparation for home visiting is discussed in Chapter 16 with other aspects of home care.

Important assessments to make at a postpartal home visit are:

Pregnancy History: Were there physical factors that could have interfered with pregnancy bonding such as painful varicose veins or gestational diabetes? Were there psychosocial factors such as an unwelcome move or loss of an important support person? Ask the woman to describe her labor and birth at a home visit not only to evaluate if any complications were present but to evaluate her reaction to the event.

Newborn History: Did the baby have a physical exam at birth? Is there anything about the infant the woman is concerned about? What is the baby's current intake? Is the baby sleeping at spaced intervals or constantly fretful?

Postpartal Course: Does the woman have pain? Any concerns about her health? Is she managing to obtain adequate rest? Does she have someone she could call if she had a concern about herself or her child?

Future Plans: Will the woman be returning to work outside her home? If so, what plans has she made for child care? The woman may be unprepared for postpartal depression. Ask if she feels "blue" or extremely fatigued.

Family Assessment: How are other children adapting? Does the client have adequate help with the new baby?

Physical Examination of the Mother: Assess temperature, pulse, and respiratory rate to detect possible infection or excessive blood loss. Assess uterine height and consistency (by the 10th day postpartum, the uterus should no longer be palpable as an abdominal organ). Assess the perineum to be certain there are no signs of infection in episiotomy stitches and that lochia color and odor is normal. Assess breasts to see if engorgement or any sign of infection is present.

Physical Examination of the Child: Assess temperature, heart, respiratory rate, and skin turgor. Assess the abdomen for distention. Inspect for any ecchymotic marks. Assess for full range of motion of extremities and that child follows a moving light. Assess to see that a diaper rash is not present and that the skin around the cord is not reddened. (Assessment of the newborn is discussed further in Chapter 23.)

Follow-Up Information: Be certain that the family has made plans (or knows how to make plans) for continued care for both the infant and the mother. Be certain they have the telephone number of a health care provider they could call if they have a concern before the date of a follow-up appointment.

Visiting a new family a few days following a hospital discharge is an enjoyable type of home visiting, as most families have at least one question about their newborn they are pleased to have answered; they are always pleased to be reassured that they are parenting well.

Postpartal Examination

Every newborn should have a health maintenance visit 2 to 4 weeks following birth (see Chapter 23). Every woman should have a checkup by her physician or nurse-midwife at 4 to 6 weeks following birth (the end of the postpartal period) to assure herself and her health care provider that she is in good health and has no residual problems from childbearing (see the Focus on Nursing Research box).

During this examination, the woman's abdominal

FOCUS ON NURSING RESEARCH

Does a Home Visit Influence Attendance at 6-Week Postpartum Appointments?

Two nurse midwives attempted to answer this question by examining whether 43 clients who did not receive a post-partal home visit came for their 6th-week postpartal health assessment as often as 39 clients who did have such a visit. All subjects in the study had had a vaginal birth of a term, single, living infant without severe congenital anomalies. Content discussed at the home visit included education regarding self and infant care, family planning, and encouragement to attend well child and postpartum checkups.

Findings of the study revealed no significance in attendance at a postpartal health assessment between the women who did not receive a home visit and those who did. Those women who were not home-visited did break and have to reschedule their appointment significantly more times, however, than the visited group or apparently were less attuned to the importance of a health assessment at the end of the postpartal period.

The researchers suggest that home visiting be incorporated as an intrinsic part of routine postpartal care as it provides a way to provide additional postpartal teaching and help ensure or connect the woman with final postpartal health assessment.

Ghilarducci, E., & McCool, W. (1993). The influence of postpartum home visits on clinic attendance. *Journal of Nurse Midwifery, 38,* 152.

wall will be inspected for tone. Her breasts will be inspected to see that they have returned to their nonpregnant state, if she is not breastfeeding, and to see that they are unfissured and free of complications if she is breastfeeding. Most important, a thorough internal examination is performed to see that involution is complete, that the ligaments and the pelvic muscle supports have returned to good functional alignment, and that any lacerations sustained during birth have healed (Table 22-5).

If she has hemorrhoids or varicosities as a result of the pregnancy, her physician or nurse-midwife will discuss with her whether further management of these conditions is necessary. You should discuss breast self-examination with her, as well as the necessity for a Papanicolaou smear and a pelvic examination every year as a means of detecting cervical and uterine cancer. The postpartal examination should also be a time for the woman to discuss with you any problems she had with childbearing and any she now has with childrearing, because these are a continuum. If reproductive life planning was not discussed immediately following birth, this visit is an opportune time for such a discussion. If the woman desires to use a diaphragm or cervical cap, these can be fitted during this examination.

Nursing Care of the Postpartal Woman and Family With Unique Needs

The Woman Who Chooses Not to Keep Her Child

Although the availability of birth control information and the increasing number of abortions that are being performed have reduced the number of unwanted children, some women still may complete a pregnancy and then give up their child for adoption.

The woman may be unmarried or her marriage may be failing and she does not want to raise a child alone. A woman may feel her family is already complete. She may want to finish school before having a child, or she would like to pursue a career.

During pregnancy, most women decide whether or not they will keep their child. During labor, they express confidence in their decision, but with the actual birth of the child, they may find that their resolve wavers. A woman who was certain she was going to surrender her child for adoption may begin to feel she would prefer to change her mind. A woman who was certain she was going to keep her child could become aware for the first time of the responsibility involved and decide that the best course for the child will be adoption. In either event, a woman's feelings become confused.

For a woman who chooses not to keep her child, the long wait in the birthing room for completion of perineal repair and preparations for transfer of the baby to a nursery may seem unusually long. She is usually alone, with no partner or support person with her during this time.

Every woman has a right to see, hold, and feed her child if she wishes. The woman who is not going to keep her child may feel proud that she has produced a healthy baby. The realization that the baby is well may give her a foundation to build a sounder future. It may make her feel truly a whole woman for the first time.

Do not attempt to change a woman's mind about keeping her child or placing her child for adoption during the postpartal period. She is extremely vulnerable to suggestion at this time, and such decisions are too long-range, too important to be made at such an emotional time. Her earlier conclusions may be the sound ones.

During the taking-in phase of the puerperium, be especially careful that you do not influence the woman's decision making. Women enjoy having decisions made for them during this time and may ask you what you think is best. An answer such as "You're the one who

Table 22-5. *Six-Week Physical Assessment*

Area of Assessment	Data Collection
History	Assess chief concern, family profile (support system, bonding, self-esteem, family integrity), interval history, and review of systems (urinary system for pain, frequency, or stress incontinence along with gastrointestinal tract and reproductive tract in particular). Assess maternal intake. Some new mothers are too fatigued to eat well, so they eat mainly carbohydrate snack foods or, at least, not a balanced diet.
Physical Examination	*Expected Findings*
General appearance	Alert; positive mood. If not, woman is probably still extremely fatigued
Weight	Achieved prepregnant weight; if not, this will be her baseline post-pregnant weight
Hair	Healthy, firm hair; excess loss of hair from early postpartal period has halted
Eyes	Pink and moist conjunctiva; if pallor persists, diet may be inadequate due to fatigue
Breasts	
Nursing women	Full and firm to palpation; blue veins prominent under skin; only slightly tender. No palpable nodules or lumps. If erythematous or tender, mastitis may be present. If fissures on nipples are present, the woman may need to expose her nipples to air or to apply additional cream. An occasional filled milk gland may present as a lump; re-examine following breast-feeding
Nonnursing women	Return to prepregnant size; no palpable nodules or lumps
Abdomen	Striae less prominent; linea nigra fading, muscle tone improving. No distended bowel from constipation. No distended bladder from retention. No history of pain, frequency, or blood on urination. (If no abdominal muscle tone is present, women need to increase abdominal exercises. For constipation, increased fluid and fiber. Urinary symptoms probably reflect urinary infection that needs specific treatment.)
Perineum and uterus	No lochia; cervix closed; uterus has returned to prepregnant size. Pap test is normal. Ask woman to bear down during pelvic examination to observe for uterine prolapse, rectocele, or cystocele. If involution is not complete, reason for subinvolution must be investigated
Lower extremities	Varicosities are barely noticeable
Rectum	Hemorrhoids have receded to prepregnant size or are no longer observable
Laboratory Report	
Laboratory values	Hct: 37%; Hb: 11–12 g/100 mL. If these are low, reassess diet; possible iron supplement may be needed
	Rubella antibody titer: 1:8, if low, additional immunization is recommended before a 2nd pregnancy

Abbreviations: Hct = hematocrit; Hb = hemoglobin.

has to make this decision. What are your thoughts about it?" can help her begin to think through the problem.

It is not uncommon for women who surrender their infants for adoption to experience grief reactions like those of women whose children have died. If a woman decides to surrender her child for adoption, refer her to an official adoption agency. An official agency gives the woman the best assurance that the parents chosen for her child will be the right parents. This assurance will

help to relieve any misgivings or guilt the woman has about surrendering the child and should reduce the moments of doubt that can come in future years: Is my child well cared for? Is she getting everything I could have given her?

Some women do not openly voice a wish to give up their child, but they do show you by their actions that they feel little attachment to him or her. The woman who wants to keep her baby has a tentative but eager approach to her newborn; a woman who has doubts is slow to make contact, barely touching the baby even by hospital discharge, and asking few questions about newborn care. She needs tangible help.

The hospital social service department can be of assistance in helping the woman to plan the child's future. A married couple as well as a single woman may place an infant for adoption, although for some couples, family counseling may be their greater need.

It is a fallacy to assume that everything will work out once a woman and infant get home. The number of battered children seen in hospital emergency departments is proof of the harm that can follow when assessment to detect poor parent–child bonding is inadequate in the first few days of life.

The Family Who Is Adopting a Child

A family who is adopting an infant may come into the hospital or birthing center to meet the new infant. Such a couple needs the same introduction to newborn care as biological parents. Additional needs of adopting parents are discussed in Chapter 2.

Key Points

- The postpartal period or the puerperium is the 6-week period following childbirth.
- The postpartal period is an important one for a family as it marks the child's introduction to the family. Women can be seen to move through an initial "taking-in" phase in which they are dependent, a "taking-hold" phase in which they manifest independence, and a "letting-go" phase in which the mother role is finally defined.
- Rooming-in is the preferred health care agency arrangement for postpartal families as it allows the new family the best chance for quality interaction. The more time new parents spend with a newborn, the more likely it is that effective bonding will occur. Help parents to feel comfortable with their newborn by offering anticipatory guidance and role modeling of infant care.
- "Postpartal blues" are a normal accompaniment to childbirth. Women need assurance that this is normal, and supportive care should be given until the emotion passes.
- Uterine involution is the process whereby the uterus returns to its prepregnant state. A uterus decreases in size 1 fingerbreadth a day until it disappears under the pubic bone at about day 10. Lochia is the name of the vaginal flow following childbirth: the flow is lochia rubra (red) for the first 1 to 3 days; lochia serosa (pink to brown) until day 3 to 10; and lochia alba (white) until 2 to 6 weeks.
- A woman is at great risk for hemorrhage in the post-

partal period, so assessments done during this time are some of the most critical assessments made in nursing. Don't discount the importance of these assessments because the overall content of the postpartal period is so focused on wellness.

- Lactation is the production of breast milk. Colostrum is present immediately after birth; milk forms on the 3rd to 4th postpartal day. A feeling of warmth and tension on this day is termed engorgement.
- Women may need various comfort measures to alleviate pain from sutures, uterine pain (afterpains), and breast tenderness. Application of warmth and administration of analgesics are important nursing interventions.
- Women need teaching about self care before health care agency discharge so they can maintain self care at home. Follow-up by a telephone call or home visit is helpful. All women should conscientiously return for a 6-week visit to be certain that their reproductive organs have returned to normal. A menstrual flow should return 6 to 10 weeks following birth in the non-breastfeeding mother; 3 to 4 months in the breastfeeding mother.

Critical Thinking Exercises

1. Liz is a 25-year-old woman 1 day postpartal. She delivered an 8-lb girl without an episiotomy incision. You thought she would have little perineal discomfort because she does not have stitches. Instead, she states her perineal pain is excruciating. You notice she has hemorrhoids. What could you suggest to Liz to make her more comfortable, and why?

2. Marsha Taylor is an 18-year-old woman 1 day postpartal. You hear her telling her husband that he is acting selfishly for paying more attention to their new son than her. You notice that she hands her baby roughly to her husband. How would you evaluate the Taylor family based on your observations? What additional information would you want to know before you reached a firm conclusion regarding this new family's health?

3. Mrs. Acker is a woman you see at a 6-week postpartal checkup. How would you develop an assessment plan to ensure that Mrs. Acker has physically and emotionally adjusted well to childbirth?

References

Acheson, L. S., & Danner, S. C. (1993). Postpartum care and breastfeeding. *Primary Care, 20,* 729.

Ament, L. (1990). Maternal tasks of the puerperium reidentified. *Journal of Obstetrical, Gynecologic, and Neonatal Nursing, 19,* 330.

Begley, C. M. (1991). Postpartum hemorrhage. *Midwives Chronicle, 104,* 102.

Cook, C. (1992). The mystery of the postpartal uterus. *Professional Care of Mothers and Children, 2,* 180.

Crisp, H. (1992). Postnatal depression: Still a neglected illness? *Professional Care of Mothers and Children, 2,* 72.

Cunningham, F. G., et al. (1993). *Williams obstetrics* (19th ed.). Norwalk, CT: Appleton and Lange.

Department of Health and Human Services. (1991). *Healthy people 2000.* Washington, DC: Public Health Service.

Geissler, E. M. (1994). *Pocket guide to cultural assessment.* St. Louis: C. V. Mosby.

Gerbasi, F. R., et al. (1990). Changes in hemostasis activity during delivery and the immediate postpartum period. *American Journal of Obstetrics and Gynecology, 162,* 1158.

Klaus, M. H., & Kennell, J. H. (1982). *Maternal–infant bonding.* St. Louis: C. V. Mosby.

Mead-Bennett, E. (1990). The relationship of primigravid sleep experience and select moods on the first postpartum day. *Journal of Obstetrical, Gynecologic, and Neonatal Nursing, 19,* 146.

Parham, E. S., et al. (1990). The association of pregnancy weight gain with the mother's postpartum weight. *Journal of the American Dietetic Association, 90,* 550.

Rubin, R. (1977). Binding-in in the postpartum period. *Maternal Child Nursing Journal, 6,* 67.

Stray-Pedersen, B., et al. (1990). Bacteriuria in the puerperium. *American Journal of Obstetrics and Gynecology, 162,* 792.

Thranov, I., et al. (1990). Postpartum symptoms: Episiotomy or tear at vaginal delivery. *Acta Obstetricia et Gynecologica Scandinavica, 69,* 11.

Tulman, L., et al. (1990). Changes in functional status after childbirth. *Nursing Research, 39,* 70.

Williams, L. R., et al. (1993). Nurse-managed postpartal home care. *Journal of Obstetrical, Gynecologic, and Neonatal Nursing, 22,* 25.

Wright, A. (1994). Perineal pain after childbirth. *Midwives Chronicle and Nursing Notes, 107,* 22.

Zlatnik, F. J. (1990). The puerperium: Normal and abnormal. In J. R. Scott et al. (Eds.). *Danforth's obstetrics and gynecology.* Philadelphia: J.B. Lippincott.

Suggested Readings

Anderson, R., & Greener, D. (1991). A descriptive analysis of home births attended by CNMs in two nurse midwifery services. *Journal of Nurse Midwifery, 36,* 95.

Duckett, L., et al. (1993). Predicting breastfeeding duration during the postpartal hospitalization. *Western Journal of Nursing Research, 15,* 77.

Garcia, J., et al. (1994). Postnatal home visiting by midwives. *Midwifery, 10,* 40.

Lee, K. A., et al. (1992). Sleep disturbances, vitality and fatigue among a select group of employed childbearing women. *Birth, 19,* 208.

McBride, C. M., et al. (1992). Postpartum relapse to smoking: A prospective study. *Health Education Research, 7,* 381.

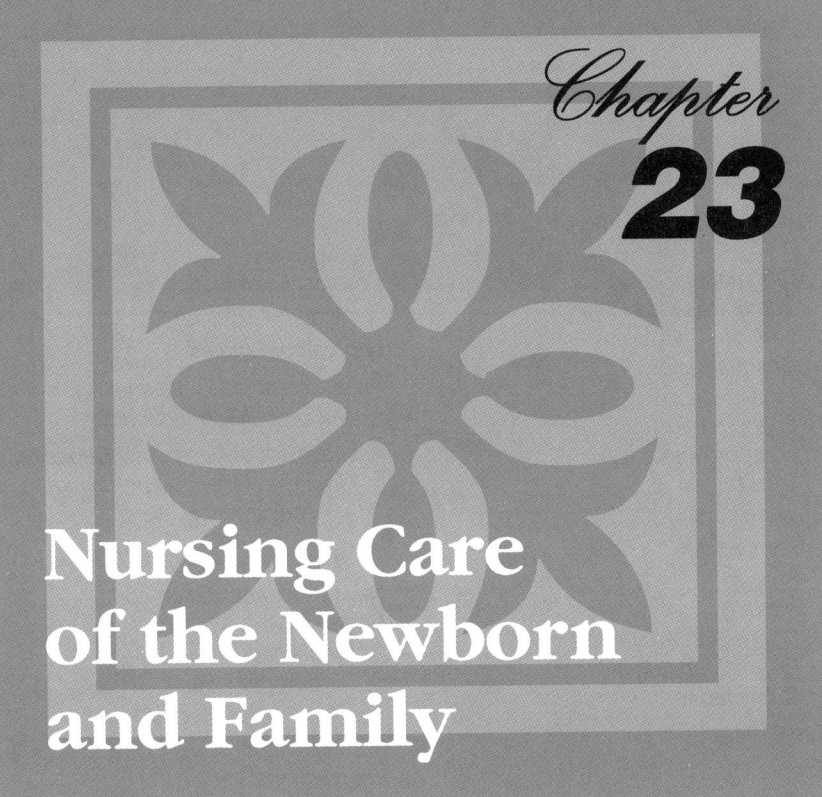

Chapter 23

Nursing Care of the Newborn and Family

Objectives

After mastering the contents of this chapter, you should be able to:

1. Describe the characteristics of the term newborn.
2. Assess a newborn for normal growth and development.
3. Formulate nursing diagnoses related to the newborn and/or family of the newborn.
4. Plan nursing care to enhance normal development of the newborn, such as ways to aid parent-child bonding.
5. Implement nursing care of the normal newborn, such as administering the first bath or instructing parents on how to care for their newborn.
6. Evaluate outcome criteria to be certain that goals of nursing care have been achieved.
7. Identify National Health Goals related to newborns that nurses can be instrumental in helping the nation to achieve.
8. Identify areas related to newborn assessment and care that could benefit from additional nursing research.
9. Use critical thinking to analyze ways that the care of the term newborn can be more family centered.
10. Synthesize knowledge of newborn growth and development and immediate care needs with the nursing process to achieve quality maternal and child health nursing care.

Adele Pillitteri: MATERNAL AND CHILD HEALTH NURSING, 2nd Edition. © 1995 Adele Pillitteri.

Newborns undergo many profound physiologic changes at the moment of birth (and, probably, psychological changes as well), because they have been released from a warm, snug, darkened, liquid-filled environment in which all their basic needs have been met into a chilly, glaring, unbounded, gravity-based, outside world.

Within minutes of being plunged into this strange environment, a newborn's body must initiate respirations and accommodate the circulatory system to extrauterine oxygenation. Within 24 hours, neurologic, renal, endocrine, gastrointestinal, and metabolic functions must be operating competently for life to be sustained.

How well a newborn can achieve these major adjustments will depend on his or her genetic endowment, the competency of the recent intrauterine environment, the care received during the labor and birth period, and the care received during the **neonatal period** (the time from birth through the first 28 days of life). National Health Goals related to the neonatal period are shown in the Focus on National Health Goals display. Nursing has a major contribution to make at all these stages in order to achieve these goals.

Two thirds of all deaths that occur in the first year of life occur in the neonatal period. Over half occur in the first 24 hours after birth—an indication of how hazardous this time is for the infant. Close observation of the neonate for indications of distress is essential during this period (Wegman, 1993).

NURSING PROCESS OVERVIEW
for Health Promotion
of the Term Newborn

ASSESSMENT

Assessment of the **neonate** (a baby in the neonatal period) includes a review of the pregnancy history, physical examination of the infant, analysis of laboratory reports such as hematocrit and blood type, and assess-

ment of the parent-child interaction for the beginning of bonding. Assessment begins immediately after birth and is continued at every contact with the infant during the first few days of life. Teach parents to make assessments concerning their infant's temperature, respiratory rate, and overall health so that they can continue to monitor their infant's health at home.

NURSING DIAGNOSIS

Nursing diagnoses with the newborn often center on the problems of establishing respirations, beginning nutrition, and helping bonding to develop. For example:

- Ineffective airway clearance related to mucus in airway
- Ineffective thermoregulation related to adaptation to extrauterine environment
- Altered nutrition, less than body requirements, related to poor sucking reflex
- Potential for enhanced parenting related to birth of planned infant
- Health-seeking behaviors related to newborn needs. If a minor deviation from the normal is present, a diagnosis such as Parental fear related to hemangioma on left thigh of newborn might be relevant.

PLANNING

Planning nursing care must take into account the mother's need for adequate rest during the postpartal period. Whereas she must learn as much as possible about newborn care, she also must go home from the health setting with enough energy to practice what she has learned. Planning for newborns includes helping them regulate their temperature and grow accustomed to breast- or bottle feeding.

IMPLEMENTATION

A major phase of implementation in the newborn period is role modeling to help new parents grow confident with their newborn. Be aware of how closely parents observe you for guidance in child care. Preserving newborn warmth and energy to prevent hypoglycemia and respiratory distress also is an important consideration in all interventions.

EVALUATION

Evaluation of nursing goals should reveal that parents are able to give beginning newborn care with a certain

---

FOCUS ON
National Health Goals

A number of National Health Goals deal directly with the newborn period. These are:

- Increase to at least 75% the proportion of mothers who breast-feed their babies in the early postpartal period from a base of 54%.

- Increase to at least 50% the proportion of women who continue breast-feeding until their babies are 5 to 6 months old from a base of 21%.

- Increase to at least 75% the proportion of parents and caregivers who use feeding practices that prevent baby bottle tooth decay.

- Reduce the infant mortality rate to no more than 7 per 1000 live births from a base of 10.1 per 1000 live births (DHHS, 1991).

  Nurses can be instrumental in helping the nation achieve these goals not only by encouraging mothers to begin breast-feeding but also by encouraging them to continue it through the first 6 months of life; advising parents on the danger of tooth decay from letting the baby drink from a bottle of milk or juice while falling asleep; and discussing with parents ways to sterilize or provide clean formula to newborns so gastrointestinal illness from contaminated milk does not occur.

  Areas which could benefit from additional nursing research include identifying the reasons why women end breast-feeding shortly after discharge from a health care agency; investigating common methods of encouraging sleep in infants other than by a bottle feeding; and assessing the most effective way to teach formula preparation to new parents.

degree of confidence. Be certain that parents have made arrangements for continued health supervision for their newborn so that evaluation can be continued and the family's long-term health needs met. Examples of outcome criteria might include

- Infant establishes respirations of 30 to 50 per minute.
- Infant maintains temperature at 98.6°F.
- Infant breast-feeds for a minimum of 10 minutes every 3 hours.

Profile of the Newborn

It is not unusual to hear the comment that "all newborns look alike" from people viewing a nursery full of babies. In actuality, every child is born with individual physical and personality characteristics that make him or her unique right from the start (Figure 23-1).

Some neonates are born stocky and short, some large and bony, some thin and rangy. Some have a temperament that causes them to feed greedily, protest procedures loudly, and respond to their parent's inexperienced handling with restlessness and spitting up. Other neonates sleep soundly, make no protest over procedures or diaper changes, and seem to accept passively this new step in life. As you gain experience in working with newborns, it becomes easier to differentiate neonates who are merely demonstrating the extremes of normal neonate characteristics from those whose behavior or appearance indicates a need for more skilled care than is available in normal nursery surroundings.

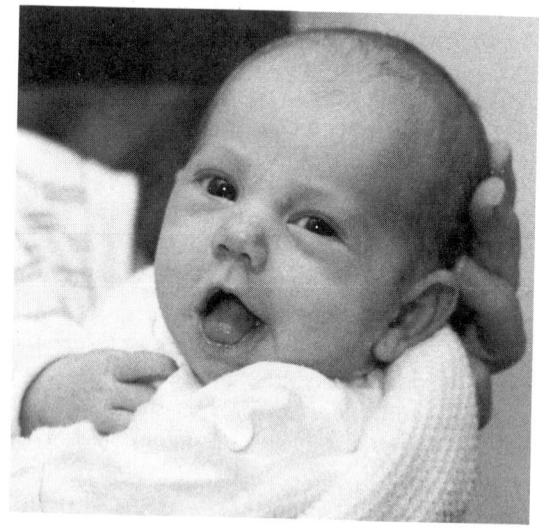

FIGURE 23-1
Personality is apparent in a newborn from the start. Note the alert, searching interest. (Courtesy, Department of Medical Photography, Children's Hospital, Buffalo, NY.)

Vital Statistics

Weight

The birth weight of neonates differs, depending on the racial, nutritional, intrauterine, and genetic factors that were present during conception and pregnancy. The weight in relation to the gestational age should be plotted on a standard neonatal graph such as the one shown in Figure 23-2 (often referred to as a *Lubchenco graph* after its originator), which allows it to be interpreted meaningfully. Plotting in this manner helps to identify neonates at risk because of their small size and to separate those who are small for their gestational age (children who have suffered intrauterine growth retardation) from preterm infants (infants who are small only because they were born early; in other words, weight matches gestational age). These first measurements also serve to establish a baseline for future measurements.

A reason for plotting weight, height, and head circumference is to point out disproportionate measurements (see Appendix E). All three of these measurements should fall close to the same percentile for the same child. A neonate who falls within the 50th percentile for height and weight and whose head circumference is in the 90th percentile, for example, may have abnormal head growth such as occurs from fused suture lines. A neonate who is in the 50th percentile for weight and head circumference but in the 3rd percentile for height may have a growth problem, such as achondroplastic dwarfism.

In the United States, white newborns weigh approximately 0.5 lb more than children of other races (Wegman, 1992). Second-born children generally weigh more than first-borns; weight continues to increase with each succeeding child in a family.

The average birth weight (50th percentile) for a white mature female neonate is 3.4 kg (7.5 lb) and for a white mature male neonate, 3.5 kg (7.7 lb). The arbitrary lower limit of normal is 2.5 kg (5.5 lb). Less than this weight, the child is termed a *low-birth-weight* infant and is given high-risk priority status. Birth weight exceeding 4.7 kg (10 lb) is unusual, but weights as high as 7.7 kg (17 lb) have been documented. When a neonate weighs over 4.7 kg, a maternal illness, such as diabetes mellitus, must be suspected.

The neonate loses 5% to 10% of birth weight (6 to 10 oz) during the first few days after birth. This weight loss occurs because the neonate is no longer under the influence of maternal hormones (which are salt- and fluid-retaining); he or she voids and passes stools; and if breast-fed, intake until about the third day of life is limited by the relatively low caloric content of colostrum, the fluid preceding breast milk. This weight loss also occurs in bottle-fed babies because of the time needed to establish effective sucking.

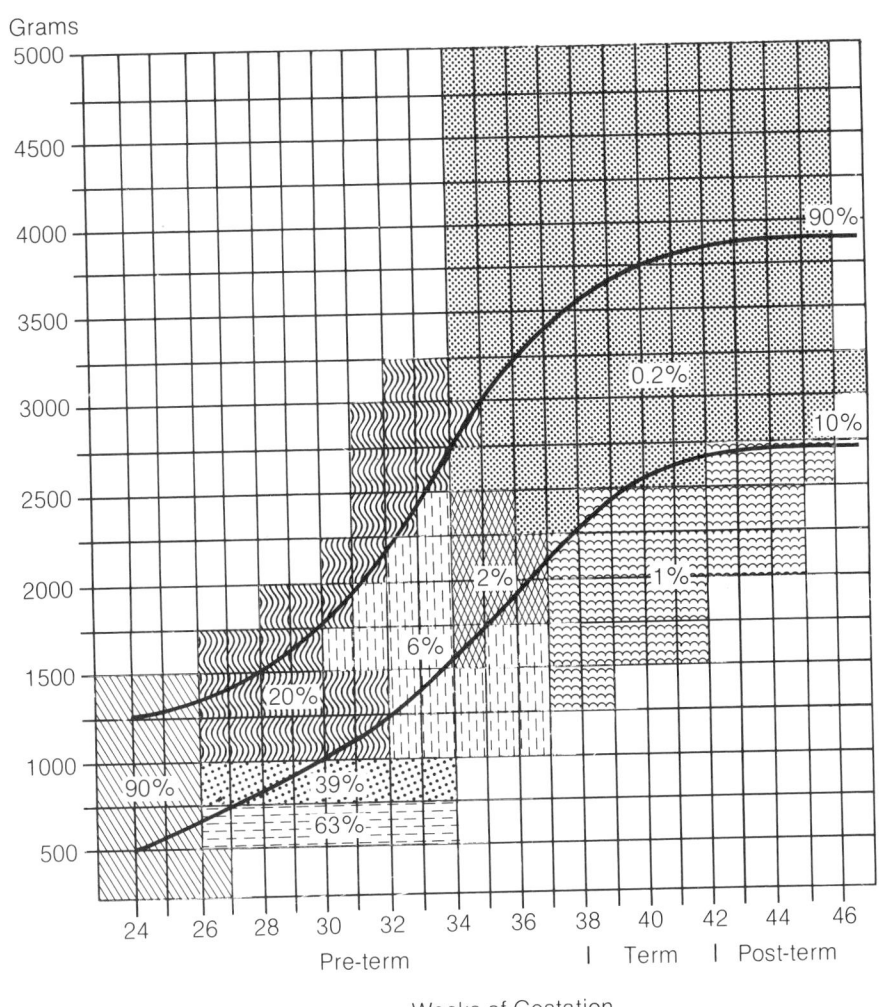

FIGURE 23-2
Classification of newborns by birth weight and gestation age and by neonatal mortality risk. (From Koops, B.L., Morgan, L.J., & Battaglia, F.C. [1982]. Neonatal mortality risk in relation to birth weight and gestational age: An update. Journal of Pediatrics, 101, *969, with permission.)*

Following this initial loss of weight, the neonate has one day of stable weight and then will begin to gain about 2 lb/month (6 to 8 oz/week) for the first 6 months of life.

Length

The average birth length (the 50th percentile) of a white mature neonate female is 53 cm (20.9 in). For white mature males, the average birth length is 54 cm (21.3 in). The lower limit of normal length is arbitrarily set at 46 cm (18 in). Babies with a length as great as 57.5 cm (23 in) have been reported.

Head Circumference

The head circumference is 34 to 35 cm (13.5 to 14 in) in a mature neonate. A mature neonate with a head circumference greater than 37 cm or less than 33 cm (14.8 or 13.2 in, respectively) should be carefully investigated for neurologic involvement, although occasionally a neonate will fall within these limits and still be perfectly normal. Head circumference is measured with a tape measure drawn across the center of the forehead and the most prominent portion of the posterior head (the occiput).

Chest Circumference

The chest circumference in a neonate is about 2 cm (0.75 to 1 in) less than head circumference. It is measured at the level of the nipples. If a large amount of breast tissue or edema of the breasts is present, this measurement will not be accurate until the initial edema has subsided.

Vital Signs

Temperature

The temperature of newborns is about 37.2°C (99°F) at the moment of birth, because they have been confined in an internal body organ. Their temperature falls almost immediately to below normal because of heat loss and immature temperature-regulating mechanisms. The 21° to 22°C (68° to 72°F) temperature of delivery rooms can add to this loss of heat.

Newborns lose heat by four separate mechanisms: convection, conduction, radiation, and evaporation (Figure 23-3).

Convection is the flow of heat from the body surface to cooler surrounding air. The effectiveness of convection depends on the velocity of the flow (a current of air cools faster than nonmoving air). Eliminating drafts from windows or air conditioners reduces convection heat loss.

Conduction is the transfer of body heat to a cooler solid object in contact with the baby. If the baby were laid on a cold counter, for example, or on the cold base of a warming unit, he or she would quickly lose heat to the colder metal surface.

Radiation is the transfer of body heat to a cooler solid object not in contact with the baby. A baby can lose heat by radiation to cold objects, such as a cold window surface.

Evaporation is loss of heat through conversion of a liquid to a vapor. Newborns are wet; they lose a great deal of heat as the amniotic fluid on their skin evaporates. To prevent this rapid loss of heat, they should be dried immediately. Remember to dry their faces

and hair; the head is a large surface area in a newborn. Covering their wet hair with a cap further reduces evaporation cooling.

A neonate not only loses heat easily by the above means but also has difficulty conserving heat under any circumstances. Insulation, an efficient means of conserving heat in adults, is not effective in newborns because they have little subcutaneous fat to provide insulation. Shivering, a means of increasing metabolism and thereby providing heat, is also rarely seen in newborns.

Newborns can conserve heat by constricting blood vessels. *Brown fat,* a special tissue found in mature newborns, apparently helps to conserve or produce body heat by increasing metabolism. Brown fat is found in greatest proportion in the intrascapular region, the thorax, and the perirenal area. It is thought to aid in the control of temperature in the neonate in much the same way it does in the hibernating animal. In later life, it may influence the proportion of body fat retained.

Because newborns have difficulty conserving body heat, exposure to cold can be extremely detrimental. Newborns exposed to cool air will kick and cry to increase their metabolic rate to produce more heat. This reaction, however, also increases their need for oxygen and thus increases their respiratory rate. An immature newborn with poor lung development will have trouble

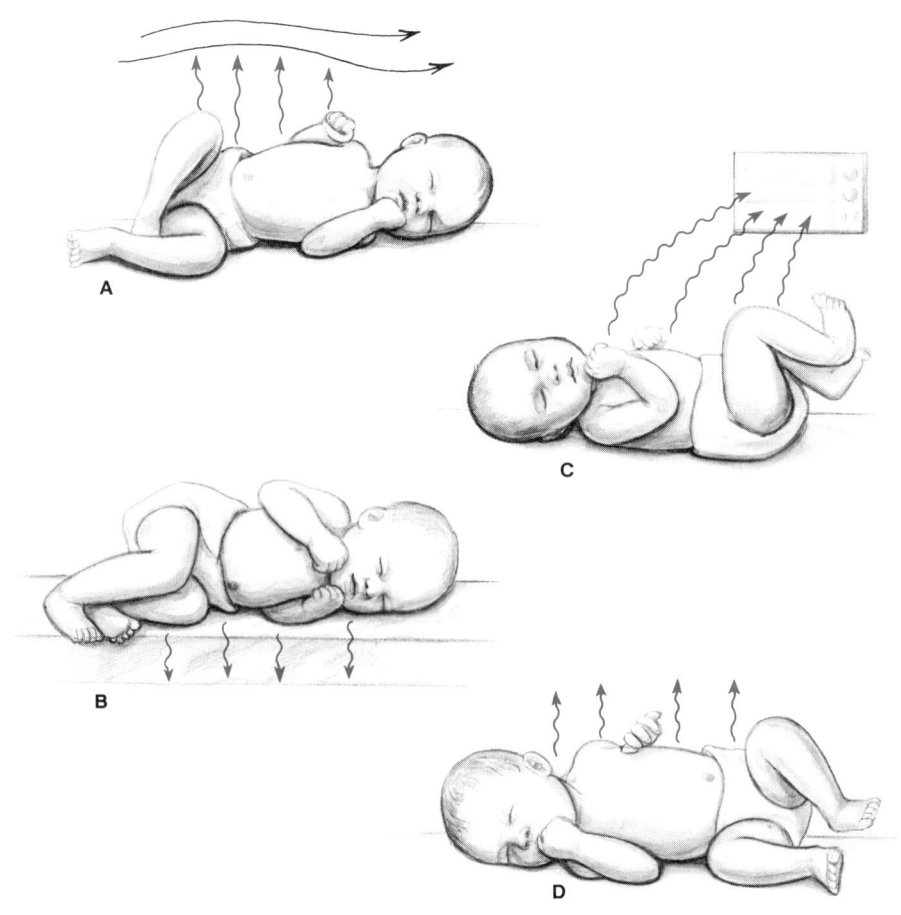

FIGURE 23-3

*Heat loss in the newborn. (**A**) Convection. (**B**) Conduction. (**C**) Radiation. (**D**) Evaporation.*

making such an adjustment. Newborns who cannot increase their respiratory rate in response to increased needs will be unable to deliver sufficient oxygen to their systems. The resultant anaerobic catabolism of body cells releases acid. Every neonate is born slightly acidotic, and any new buildup of acid may lead to severe, life-threatening acidosis. The neonate also becomes fatigued, placing additional strain on an already stressed cardiovascular system.

Drying and wrapping newborns and placing them in warmed cribs or drying them and placing them under a radiant heat source are the best mechanical measures to help conserve heat. All early care should be done speedily to avoid exposing the neonate unnecessarily. Any procedure during which the neonate must be uncovered (e.g., resuscitation, circumcision) should be done under a radiant heat source to prevent damaging heat loss. If chilling is prevented, a neonate's temperature stabilizes at 37°C (98.6°F) within 4 hours after birth.

A neonate who has a bacterial infection may, in contrast to an adult, run a subnormal temperature. Therefore, when a neonate's temperature does not stabilize shortly after birth, the cause must be investigated and corrective measures taken.

Pulse
The heart rate of a fetus in utero averages 120 to 160 beats per minute. Immediately after birth, as a neonate struggles to initiate respirations, the heart rate may be as rapid as 180 beats per minute. Within an hour after birth, as the newborn settles down to sleep, the heart rate falls to an average of 120 to 140 beats per minute, where it stabilizes.

The heart rate of a neonate is often irregular because of immaturity of the cardiac regulatory center in the medulla. Transient murmurs may result from the incomplete closure of fetal circulation shunts. During crying, the rate may rise again to 180 beats per minute.

The femoral pulses can be felt readily in a neonate, but the radial and temporal pulses are more difficult to palpate with any degree of accuracy. Thus, a neonate's heart rate always should be determined by listening for an apical heartbeat for a full minute. It is important that the femoral pulses be palpated, because their absence suggests possible coarctation (narrowing) of the aorta.

Respiration
The respiratory rate of a neonate in the first few minutes of life may be as high as 80 breaths per minute. As respiratory activity is established and maintained, the rate settles to an average of 30 to 60 breaths per minute when the child is at rest. Respiratory depth, rate, and rhythm are likely to be irregular, and short periods of apnea (without cyanosis) sometimes called *periodic respirations* which may occur are normal. Respiration can be observed most easily by watching the movement of the abdomen, because breathing primarily involves the use of the diaphragm and abdominal muscles.

Coughing and sneezing reflexes are present at birth to clear the airway. Neonates are obligate nose-breathers and show signs of acute distress if the nostrils become obstructed. Short periods of crying increase the depth of respirations and aid in aerating deep portions of the lungs and so are beneficial to the neonate. Long periods of crying, however, exhaust the cardiovascular system and serve no purpose. This is an important fact for parents to know.

Blood Pressure
The blood pressure of a neonate is approximately 80/46 mm Hg at birth. By the 10th day it rises to about 100/50 mm Hg. Blood pressure is not routinely measured in newborns unless a cardiac anomaly is suspected, because the blood pressure reading in the neonate is somewhat inaccurate. The cuff width used must be no more than two thirds the length of the upper arm or thigh for any degree of accuracy to be achieved. Blood pressure tends to increase with crying (and a neonate cries when disturbed and manipulated by such procedures as taking blood pressure).

A Doppler method may be used to take blood pressure (see Chapter 37). Hemodynamic monitoring is helpful when continuous assessment is necessary.

Physiologic Function

Cardiovascular System
Changes in the cardiovascular system are necessary at birth because the blood that was formerly oxygenated by the placenta now must be oxygenated by the lungs. When the cord is clamped, a neonate is forced to take in oxygen through the lungs. As the lungs are inflated for the first time, pressure is greatly decreased in the chest in general and in the pulmonary artery in particular (the artery leading to the lungs). The decrease in pressure in the pulmonary artery plays a role in causing the ductus arteriosus to close. As pressure increases in the left side of the heart from increased blood volume, the foramen ovale closes because of the pressure against the lip of the structure (permanent closure does not occur for weeks). With the remaining fetal circulatory structures—the umbilical vein, two umbilical arteries, and the ductus venosus—no longer receiving blood, the blood within them clots, and the vessels atrophy over the next few weeks.

Figure 23-4 shows the respiratory and cardiovascular changes that occur at birth, beginning with the first breath. Table 23-1 shows the timetable for obliteration of fetal structures.

The peripheral circulation of a neonate remains sluggish for at least the first 24 hours. It is not uncommon to observe cyanosis in the feet and hands (**acro-**

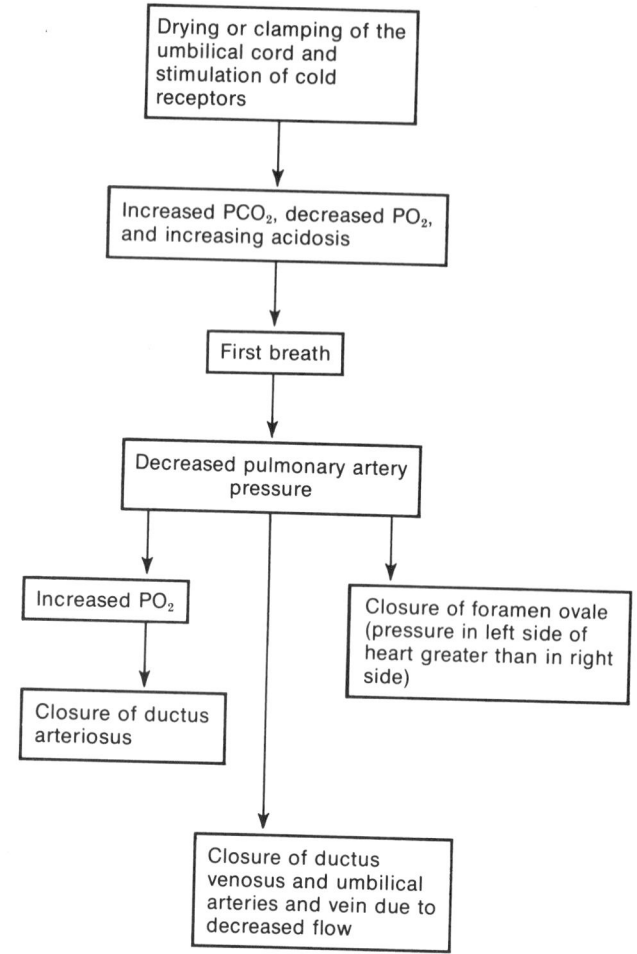

FIGURE 23-4
Circulatory events at birth.

cyanosis) and for the feet to feel cold to the touch for this period of time.

Blood Values. A neonate's blood volume is 80 to 110 mL per kilogram of weight, or about 300 mL. The oxygen dissociation curve of fetal blood is shifted to the left (the quantity of oxygen bound to hemoglobin and partial pressure of oxygen is greater in fetal blood than in the newborn's).

Because of the nature of fetal circulation, a baby is born with a high erythrocyte count, around 6 million per cubic millimeter. A neonate's hemoglobin level averages 17 to 18 g/100 mL of blood. Hematocrit level is between 45% and 50%. Capillary heel pricks may reveal a false high hematocrit or hemoglobin value because of sluggish peripheral circulation. Warming the extremity before the blood drawing improves the accuracy of this value by increasing circulation movement.

Once proper lung oxygenation is established, the need for the high erythrocyte count diminishes. Therefore, within a matter of days, the erythrocyte count begins to fall. An indirect bilirubin level at birth is 1 to 4 mg/100 mL. Any increase over this amount reflects the

release of bilirubin as red blood cells begin their breakdown.

A neonate has an equally high white blood cell count at birth, about 15,000 to 45,000 cells per cubic millimeter. Polymorphonuclear cells (neutrophils) account for a large part of this leukocytosis, but by the end of the first month, lymphocytes become the predominant type. This leukocytosis is a response to the trauma of birth and is nonpathogenic; an increased white blood cell count should not be taken as evidence of infection. On the other hand, although the high white blood cell count makes infection difficult to prove in a neonate, infection must not be dismissed as a possibility if other signs of infection (e.g., pallor, respiratory difficulty, or cyanosis) are present. Blood values in the neonate are summarized in Appendix F.

Blood Coagulation. Most newborns are born with a prolonged coagulation or prothrombin time, because their blood levels of vitamin K are lower than normal. Vitamin K is synthesized through the action of intestinal flora and is necessary for the formation of factor II (prothrombin), factor VII (proconvertin), factor IX (plasma thromboplastin component), and factor X (Stuart-Prower factor). A neonate intestine is sterile at birth unless membranes were ruptured more than 24 hours before birth; therefore, it takes about 24 hours for flora to accumulate and for vitamin K to be synthesized. Because almost all newborns can be predicted to have lessened blood coagulation ability, vitamin K (Aquamephyton) is administered intramuscularly into the lateral anterior thigh, the preferred site for all injections in the newborn (see Chapter 37) immediately after birth.

Respiratory System

The first breath of a neonate is initiated by a combination of cold receptors, a lowered PO_2, (PO_2 falls from 80 mm Hg to as low as 15 mm Hg), and an increased PCO_2

T a b l e 2 3 - 1. *Changes in the Cardiovascular System at Birth*

Structure	Approximate Time of Obliteration	Structure Remaining
Foramen ovale	1 yr	Fossa ovalis
Ductus arteriosus	1 mon	Ligamentum arteriosum
Ductus venosus	2 mon	Ligamentum venosum
Umbilical arteries	2–3 mon	Lateral umbilical ligament
		Interior iliac artery
Umbilical vein	2–3 mon	Ligamentum teres (round ligament of liver)

(Adapted from Moore, M. L. [1972]. *The newborn and the nurse.* Philadelphia: W.B. Saunders; with permission.)

(PCO$_2$ rises as high as 70 mm Hg). A first breath requires a tremendous amount of energy to pull in. A pressure of about 40 to 70 cm H$_2$O is required. The presence of fluid in the lungs eases the pulling apart of alveolar walls during the baby's first breath, allowing the alveoli to inflate more easily than if the lung walls were dry. About a third of this fluid is forced out by the pressure of vaginal birth; additional fluid is quickly absorbed by lung blood vessels and lymphatics following the first breath.

Once the alveoli have initially been inflated, breathing becomes much easier for the baby, requiring only about 6 to 8 cm H$_2$O pressure. Within 10 minutes of birth, a newborn has established a good residual volume. By 10 to 12 hours of age, vital capacity is established at newborn proportions. The heart in a neonate takes up proportionately more space than in an adult, so the amount of lung expansion space available is proportionately limited.

A baby born by cesarean birth does not have as much lung fluid expelled at birth as one born vaginally, and so may have more difficulty with establishing effective respiration (excessive fluid blocks air exchange space). Newborns who are immature and whose alveoli collapse each time they exhale (lack of pulmonary surfactant) have trouble in establishing effective residual capacity and respirations. If the alveoli do not open well, a neonate's cardiac system is compromised, since closure of the foramen ovale and ductus arteriosus depends on free blood flow through the pulmonary artery and good oxygenation of blood. A neonate who has difficulty establishing respirations at birth should be examined closely in the postpartal period for a cardiac murmur or indication that he or she still has patent cardiac structures, especially a patent ductus arteriosus, that did not close.

Gastrointestinal System

Although the gastrointestinal tract is usually sterile at birth, bacteria may be cultured from the intestinal tract in most babies within 5 hours after birth; they can be cultured from all babies at 24 hours of life. Bacteria enter the tract through the newborn's mouth. Some mouth bacteria are airborne; others may come from vaginal secretions at the time of birth, from hospital bedding, and from contact at the breast. Accumulation of bacteria in the gastrointestinal tract is necessary for digestion as well as for the synthesis of vitamin K. Because milk, the infant's main diet for the first year, is low in vitamin K, this intestinal synthesis is necessary for blood coagulation.

Although a neonate's stomach holds about 60 to 90 mL, a neonate has limited ability to digest fat and starch because the pancreatic enzymes, lipase and amylase, are deficient for the first few months of life. The newborn regurgitates easily because of an immature cardiac sphincter between the stomach and esophagus. Immature liver functions may lead to lowered glucose and protein serum levels.

Stools. The first stool of the neonate is usually passed within 24 hours after birth and consists of **meconium**, a sticky, tarlike, blackish-green, odorless material formed from mucus, vernix, lanugo, hormones, and carbohydrates that accumulated during intrauterine life. A newborn who does not pass a meconium stool by 24 hours after birth should be examined for the possibility of meconium ileus, imperforate anus, or bowel obstruction (see Chapter 39).

About the second or third day of life, the neonate stool changes in color and consistency, becoming green and loose. This is termed a **transitional stool**, which may resemble diarrhea to the untrained eye. By the fourth day of life, breast-fed babies pass three or four light yellow stools per day. These are sweet smelling, because breast milk is high in lactic acid, which reduces the amount of putrefactive organisms in the stool. A neonate who receives formula usually passes two or three bright yellow stools a day. These have a slightly more noticeable odor than do breast-fed babies' stools.

A neonate placed under phototherapy lights to be treated for jaundice will have bright green stools because of increased bilirubin excretion. If mucus is mixed with the stool, a milk allergy or some other irritant factor should be suspected. Newborns with obstruction of the bile ducts will have clay-colored (gray) stools, because the bile pigments do not enter the intestinal tract. If the stools remain black or tarry, intestinal bleeding should be suspected. Blood-flecked stools usually indicate an anal fissure. Occasionally, a neonate swallows some maternal blood during birth and will either vomit fresh blood immediately after birth or pass a tarry stool in two or more days. Maternal blood may be differentiated from fetal blood by a dipstick Apt test.

Urinary System

The average neonate voids within 24 hours after birth. A neonate who does not take in much fluid for the first 24 hours may void later than this, but the 24-hour cutoff point is a good rule of thumb. Neonates who do not void within this time should be examined. Possible causes are urethral stenosis or absent kidneys or ureters.

The possibility of obstruction in the urinary tract can be assessed by observing the force of the urinary stream in both male and female infants. Males should void with enough force to produce a small projected arc; females should produce a steady stream, not just continuous dribbling. Urine that is projected farther than normal also may be a sign of urethral obstruction, because it indicates urine is being forced through a narrow channel.

The kidneys of newborns do not concentrate urine well, and thus the urine is usually light in color and odorless. The infant is about 6 weeks of age before much control over reabsorption of fluid in tubules and concentration of urine are evident.

A single voiding in a neonate is only about 15 mL and is easily missed in a thick diaper; specific gravity is

1.008 to 1.010. The daily urinary output for the first 1 or 2 days is about 30 to 60 mL total. By week 1, total daily volume has risen to about 300 mL. A small amount of protein may be normally present in voidings for the first few days of life until kidney glomeruli are more fully mature. The first voiding may be pink or dusky because of uric acid crystals that were formed in the bladder in utero. This is an innocent finding.

Autoimmune System

The neonate has difficulty forming antibodies against invading antigens up to 2 months of age. For this reason immunizations against childhood diseases are not generally given to babies younger than 2 months. The infant at birth, however, has antibodies (IgG) from the mother that crossed the placenta—in most instances, antibodies against poliomyelitis, measles, diphtheria, pertussis, rubella, and tetanus. There is little natural immunity transmitted against varicella (chickenpox) or herpes simplex. Hospital personnel with herpes simplex eruptions (cold sores) should not care for newborns, since herpes simplex II infections can become systemic in the neonate or create a rapidly fatal form of the disease.

Neuromuscular System

Mature newborns demonstrate general neuromuscular function by moving their extremities and attempting to control head movement. Limpness or total absence of a muscular response to manipulation is never normal and suggests narcosis, shock, or cerebral injury. A neonate occasionally makes twitching or flailing movements of extremities in the absence of a stimulus because of the immaturity of the nervous system. A number of reflexes can be tested with consistency by using simple maneuvers.

Blink Reflex. A blink reflex in a neonate serves the same purpose as it does in an adult, that is, to protect the eye from any object coming near it by rapid eyelid closure. It may be elicited by shining a strong light such as a flashlight or otoscope light on the eye. It can rarely be elicited by a sudden movement toward the eye.

Rooting Reflex. If a neonate's cheek is brushed or stroked near the corner of the mouth, the child will turn the head in that direction. This reflex serves to help the baby find food. As the mother holds the child and allows her breast to brush the baby's cheek, the baby will turn toward the breast. The reflex disappears at about the sixth week of life. At about this time, the eyes focus steadily and a food source can be seen. Thus, the reflex is no longer needed.

Sucking Reflex. When a neonate's lips are touched, the baby makes a sucking motion. Thus, as the lips touch the mother's breast or a bottle, the baby sucks and

so takes in food. The sucking reflex begins to diminish at about 6 months of age. It disappears immediately if it is never stimulated—for example, in a neonate with a tracheoesophageal fistula who is not allowed to take oral fluids. It can be maintained in such an infant by offering the child a pacifier after the fistula has been corrected by surgery and until oral feedings can be given.

Swallowing Reflex. The swallowing reflex in the newborn is the same as in the adult. Food that reaches the posterior portion of the tongue is automatically swallowed. Gag, cough, and sneeze reflexes also are present to maintain a clear airway in the event that normal swallowing does not keep the pharynx free of obstructing mucus.

Extrusion Reflex. A newborn will extrude any substance that is placed on the anterior portion of the tongue. This protective reflex prevents the swallowing of inedible substances. It disappears at about 4 months of age. Until then, an infant may seem to be spitting out or refusing solid food placed in the mouth.

Palmar Grasp Reflex. Neonates will grasp an object placed in their palm by closing their fingers on it (Figure 23-5). Mature neonates grasp so strongly that they can actually be raised from a supine position and be suspended momentarily from an examiner's fingers. It is a primitive reflex apparently from a time newborns clung to their mother for safety. The reflex disappears at about age 6 weeks to 3 months. A baby begins to grasp meaningfully at about 3 months of age.

Step (Walk)-in-Place Reflex. Newborns who are held in a vertical position with their feet touching a hard surface will take a few quick, alternating steps (Figure 23-6). This reflex disappears by 3 months of age. By 4

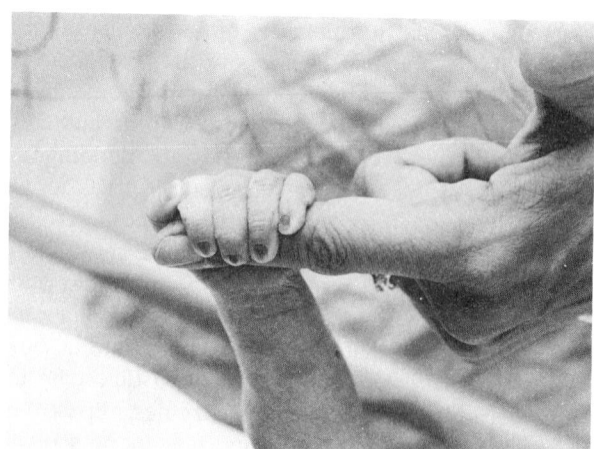

FIGURE 23-5
Palmar grasp reflex. (Courtesy, Department of Medical Photography, Children's Hospital, Buffalo, NY.)

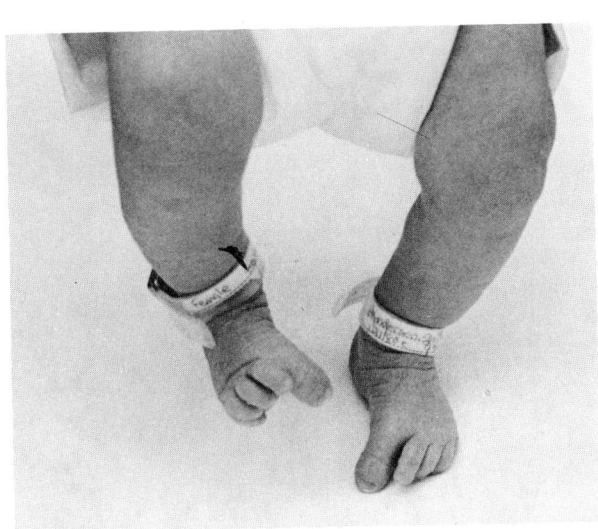

FIGURE 23-6
Step-in-place reflex. (Courtesy, Department of Medical Photography, Children's Hospital, Buffalo, NY.)

months babies can bear a good portion of their weight unhindered by this reflex.

Placing Reflex. The placing reflex is similar to the step-in-place reflex, except it is elicited by touching the anterior surface of a newborn's leg against the edge of a bassinet or table. A newborn will make a few quick lifting motions as if to step onto the table.

Plantar Grasp Reflex. When an object touches the sole of a newborn's foot at the base of the toes, the toes grasp in the same manner as the fingers do. The reflex disappears at about 8 to 9 months of age in preparation for walking, although it may be present in sleep for a longer period of time.

Tonic Neck Reflex. When newborns lie on their backs, their heads usually turn to one side or the other. The arm and the leg on the side to which the head turns extend, and the opposite arm and leg contract (Figure 23-7). If you turn a newborn's head to the opposite side, he or she will often change the extension and contraction of legs and arms accordingly. The movement is most evident in the arms but may be observed in the legs. It is also called a boxer or *fencing reflex*, because the newborn's position simulates that of someone preparing to box or fence. Unlike many other reflexes, the tonic neck reflex does not appear to have a function. It does stimulate eye coordination, however, because the extended arm moves in front of the face. It may signify handedness. The reflex disappears between the second and third months of life.

Moro Reflex. A Moro (startle) reflex (Figure 23-8) can be initiated by startling the newborn by a loud noise

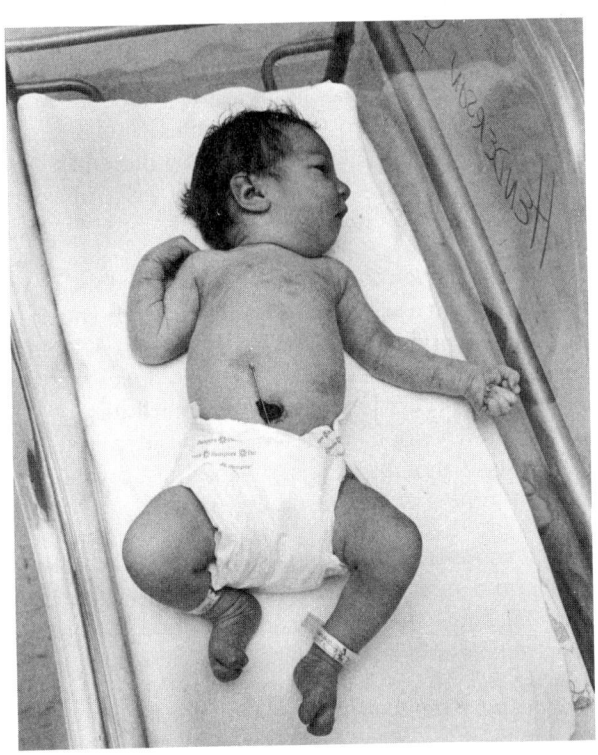

FIGURE 23-7
Tonic neck reflex. (Courtesy, Department of Medical Photography, Children's Hospital, Buffalo, NY.)

or by jarring the bassinet. The most accurate method of eliciting the reflex is to hold newborns in a supine position and allow their heads to drop backward an inch or so. They abduct and extend their arms and legs. Their fingers assume a typical "C" position. They then bring

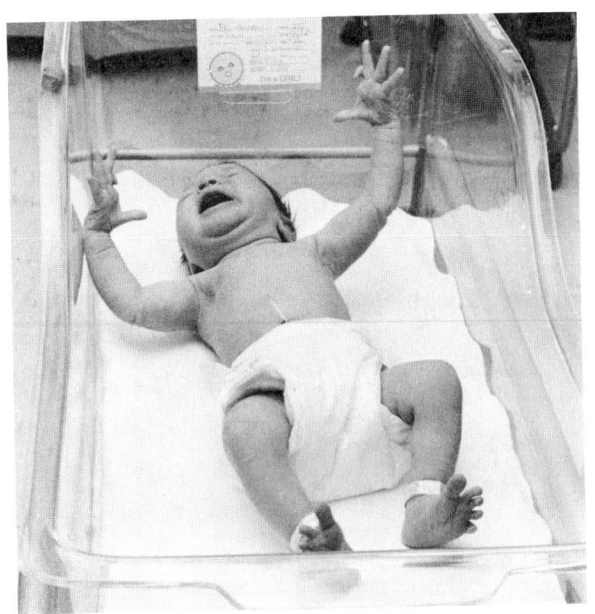

FIGURE 23-8
Moro reflex. (Courtesy, Department of Medical Photography, Children's Hospital, Buffalo, NY.)

their arms into an embrace position and pull up their legs against their abdomen (adduction). The reflex simulates the action of someone trying to ward off an attacker, then covering up to protect himself. It is strong for the first 8 weeks of life and fades by the end of the fourth or fifth month, when the infant can roll away from danger.

Babinski Reflex. When the side of the sole of the foot is stroked in an inverted "J" curve from the heel upward, the newborn fans the toes (positive Babinski sign); this is in contrast to the adult, who flexes the toes. This reaction occurs because of the immaturity of nervous system development. It remains positive (toes fan) until at least 3 months of age, when it is supplanted by the down-turning or flexing adult response.

Magnet Reflex. If pressure is applied to the soles of the feet of a newborn lying in a supine position, she pushes back against the pressure. This and the two following reflexes are tests of spinal cord integrity.

Crossed Extension Reflex. One leg of a neonate lying supine is extended and the sole of that foot is irritated by being rubbed with a sharp object, such as a thumbnail. This causes the newborn to raise the other leg and extend it as if trying to push away the hand irritating the first leg (Figure 23-9).

Trunk Incurvation Reflex. When newborns lie in a prone position and are touched along the paravertebral area by a probing finger, they will flex their trunk and swing their pelvis toward the touch (Figure 23-10).

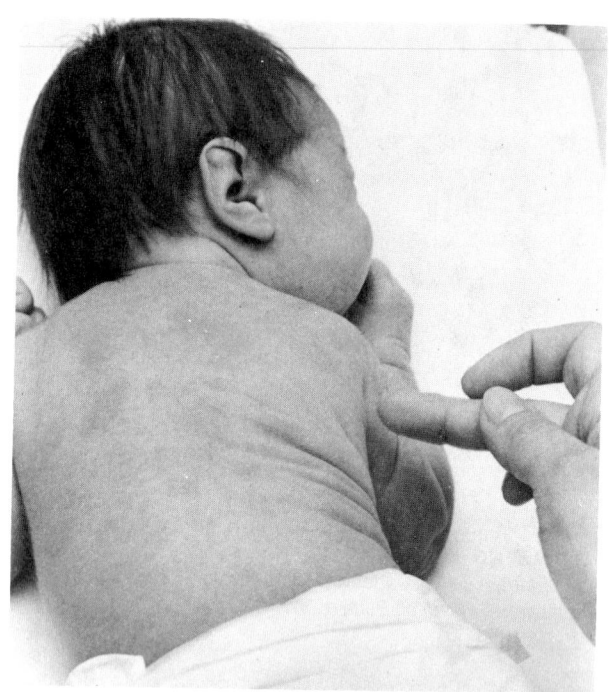

FIGURE 23-10
Trunk incurvation reflex. When the paravertebral area is stroked, the newborn flexes his or her trunk toward the direction of the stimulation. (Courtesy, Department of Medical Photography, Children's Hospital, Buffalo, NY.)

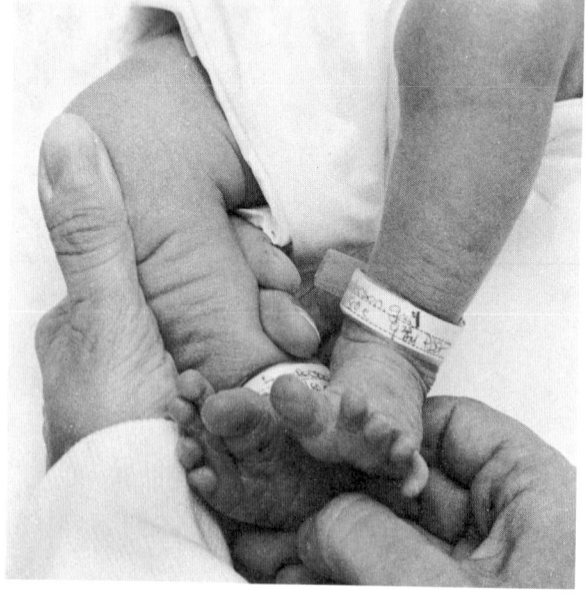

FIGURE 23-9
Crossed extension reflex. When the sole of the foot is stroked, the newborn makes an attempt to push away the irritating object with the other foot. (Courtesy, Department of Medical Photography, Children's Hospital, Buffalo, NY.)

Landau Reflex. A newborn who is held in a prone position with a hand underneath supporting the trunk should demonstrate some muscle tone. Babies may not be able to lift their head or arch their back (as they will at 3 months of age) in this position, but neither should they sag into an inverted "U" position. The latter response indicates extremely poor muscle tone, the cause of which should be investigated.

Deep Tendon Reflexes. A patellar reflex can be elicited in a newborn by tapping the patellar tendon with the tip of the finger; in older children or adults a percussion hammer is needed to demonstrate this reflex. The lower leg will move perceptibly if the infant has a mature reflex. To elicit a biceps reflex, place the thumb of your left hand on the tendon of the biceps muscle on the inner surface of the elbow. Tap the thumb as it rests on the tendon. You are more likely to feel the tendon contract than to observe movement. A biceps reflex is a test for spinal nerves C5 and C6; a patellar reflex is a test for spinal nerves L2 through L4.

The Senses

The senses in newborns appear to be much better developed than previously believed.

Hearing. A fetus is able to hear in utero. As soon as amniotic fluid drains or is absorbed from the middle ear by way of the eustachian tube—within hours after birth—hearing in newborns becomes acute, although they appear to have difficulty locating sound, not turning toward it consistently. Perhaps they must learn to interpret small differences among sounds arriving at their ears at different times. They respond with generalized activity to a sound, such as a bell ringing a short distance from their ear. If they are actively crying at the time the bell is rung, they will stop crying and seem to attend. Similarly, newborns calm in response to a soothing voice and startle at loud noises. They recognize their mother's voice almost immediately as if they have heard it in utero (Damstra-Wijmenga, 1991).

Vision. Newborns see as soon as they are born and possibly have been "seeing" light and dark in utero for the last few months of pregnancy as the uterus and the abdominal wall were stretched thin. Newborns demonstrate sight at birth by blinking at a strong light (blink reflex) or following a bright light or toy a short distance with their eyes. Because they cannot follow past the midline of vision, they lose track of objects easily, so it is sometimes reported that they cannot see. They focus best on black and white objects at a distance of 9 to 12 in. A pupillary reflex is present from birth.

Touch. The sense of touch is well developed at birth. Newborns demonstrate this by quieting at a soothing touch and by the presence of sucking and rooting reflexes, which are elicited by touch. They react to painful stimuli.

Taste. Taste buds are developed and functioning before birth to such an extent that a newborn has dis- criminatory ability. A fetus in utero will swallow amniotic fluid more rapidly than usual if glucose is added to sweeten its taste; the swallowing decreases if a bitter flavor is added. A newborn turns away from a bitter taste such as salt but readily accepts the sweet taste of milk or glucose water.

Smell. The sense of smell is present in newborns as soon as the nose is clear of mucus and amniotic fluid. Neonates turn toward their mothers' breast partly out of recognition of the smell of breast milk and partly as a manifestation of the rooting reflex. Their ability to respond to odors can be used to document alertness and possibly intelligence (Sullivan et al., 1991).

Physiologic Adjustment to Extrauterine Life

All newborns seem to move through a period of irregular adjustment in the first 6 hours of life before their body systems stabilize (Desmond, 1963). The first phase lasts about half an hour. During this time, the baby is alert and exhibits exploring, searching activity, often making sucking sounds. Heart beat and respiratory rate are rapid. This is called the *first period of reactivity*.

Next comes a quiet *resting period*. Heartbeat and respiratory rates slow; the neonate generally sleeps for about 90 minutes. The *second period of reactivity*, between 2 and 6 hours of life, is when the baby wakes again, often gagging and choking on mucus that has accumulated in the mouth. He or she is again alert and responsive and interested in the surroundings.

These three periods are summarized in Table 23-2.

Table 23-2. *Periods of Reactivity: Normal Adjustment to Extrauterine Life*

Assessment	First Period (first 15–30 min)	Resting Period (30–120 min)	Second Period (2–6 h)
Color	Acrocyanosis	Color stabilizing; pink all over	Quick color changes occur with movement or crying
Temperature	Temperature begins to fall from intrauterine temperature of about 100.6° F	Temperature stabilizes at about 99° F	Temperature increases to 99.8° F
Heart rate	Rapid, as much as 180 bpm while crying	Slowing to between 120 and 140 bpm	Wide swings in rate with activity
Respirations	Irregular; 30–90 breaths per min while crying; some nasal flaring, occasional retraction may be present	Slows to 30–50 breaths per min; barreling of chest occurs	Respirations become irregular again with activity
Activity	Alert; watching	Sleeps	Awakes
Ability to respond to stimulation	Reacts vigorously	Difficult to arouse	Becoming responsive again
Mucus	Visible in mouth	Small amount present while sleeping	Mouth full of mucus, causing gagging
Bowel sounds	Able to be heard after first 15 min	Present	Often has first meconium stool

(From Desmond, M. N., et al. [1963]. The clinical behavior of the newly born; the term baby. *Journal of Pediatrics, 62,* 307; with permission.)

Newborns who are ill or who had difficulty at birth may not pass through these typical stages; they may never have periods of alertness or periods of quiet. Their vital signs may not fall and rise again but remain rapid; their temperature may remain subnormal. Exhibition of this typical reactivity pattern, therefore, is an indication that the baby is healthy and adjusting well to extrauterine life.

Appearance of the Newborn

Skin

General inspection of the newborn's skin reveals many characteristic findings.

Color

Most term newborns have a ruddy complexion because of the increased concentration of red blood cells in blood vessels and a decrease in the amount of subcutaneous fat, which makes the blood vessels more visible. This ruddiness fades slightly over the first month.

Cyanosis. The newborn's lips, hands, and feet are likely to appear cyanotic from immature peripheral circulation. Acrocyanosis is so prominent in some newborns that a line seems to be drawn across the wrist or ankle, with pink skin on one side and blue on the other, as if some stricture were cutting off circulation. This is a normal phenomenon in the first 24 to 48 hours after birth.

Generalized mottling of the skin is common. Generalized cyanosis, however, is always a cause for concern, because it usually indicates an underlying disease state.

Mucus obstructing the respiratory tract will cause sudden cyanosis and apnea in a newborn who had previously shown good color. Suctioning the mucus relieves the condition. The mouth may be suctioned if there appears to be a large amount of mucus at the back of the throat, but the nose should be suctioned as well, because in the infant this is the chief conduit for air. Always suction the mouth before the nose, because suctioning the nose first may trigger a reflex gasp, which could lead to aspiration if there is mucus in the posterior throat.

Hyperbilirubinemia. Hyperbilirubinemia leads to **jaundice**, or yellowing of the skin. This occurs on the second or third day in about 50% of all newborns as a result of the breakdown of fetal red blood cells (**physiologic jaundice**). The infant's skin and sclera of the eyes appear noticeably yellow. This occurs as the high red blood cell count built up in utero is destroyed and heme and globin are released. Globin is a protein component that is reused by the body and is not a factor in the developing jaundice. Heme is further broken down into iron (which is also reused and therefore not in-

volved in the jaundice) and protoporphyrin. Protoporphyrin is further broken down into indirect bilirubin. Indirect bilirubin is fat soluble and cannot be excreted by the kidneys in this state. It is instead converted by the liver enzyme glucuronyl transferase into direct bilirubin, which is water soluble and is incorporated into stool and then excreted in feces. Many newborns have such immature liver function that indirect bilirubin cannot be converted to the direct form and, therefore, remains indirect. As long as the bilirubin remains in the circulatory system, the red of the blood cells obscures its color. When the level of this indirect bilirubin rises above 7 mg/100 mL, however, bilirubin permeates the tissue outside the circulatory system and causes the infant to appear jaundiced.

Infants with extensive bruising (large, breech, or immature babies) must be observed carefully for jaundice. Bruising at birth leads to hemorrhage of blood into the subcutaneous tissue or skin. This blood is removed as bruising heals by the breakdown of blood components. As the red blood cells are hemolyzed, indirect bilirubin is released. **Cephalhematoma**, a collection of blood under the periosteum of the skull bone, can lead to the same phenomenon.

Assess for intestinal function also, because if intestinal obstruction is present and stool is not being evacuated, intestinal flora may break down bile into its basic components and release indirect bilirubin into the bloodstream again. Early feeding of newborns promotes intestinal movement and excretion of meconium and helps prevent indirect bilirubin buildup from this source.

The level of jaundice in newborns may be judged grossly by estimating the extent to which it has progressed on the surface of the infant's body, starting in the head and spreading to the rest of the body (Figure 23-11).

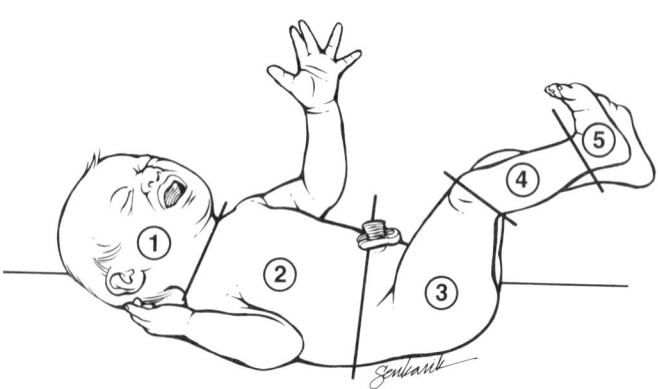

FIGURE 23-11

Jaundice in a newborn. Jaundice may be estimated to some degree by the zone it has reached on the child. The indirect bilirubin level of zone 1 is 8 mg/100 mL; zone 2, 5–12 mg/100 mL; zone 3, 8–16 mg/100 mL; zone 4, 11–18 mg/100 mL; zone 5, 15 mg/100 mL. (Based on data from Kramer, L.I. [1969]. Advancement of dermal icterus in the jaundiced newborn. American Journal of Diseases of Children, 118, 454, with permission.)

Various commercial devices (transcutaneous biliru-binometry devices) are available to aid in estimating jaundice levels (Schumacher, 1990). Although these devices are not yet accurate enough to replace serum measurements, they can be used to identify infants who need serum bilirubin determinations. Serum bilirubin is obtained by heel puncture. The technique for this is shown in Chapter 37.

If the level of indirect bilirubin rises above 10 to 12 mg/100 mL, treatment will be considered. It is important that the level not rise above 20 mg/100 mL. At this point, bilirubin interferes with the chemical synthesis of brain cells and causes permanent cell damage, a condition termed **kernicterus**, which will leave permanent neurologic effects and possibly will cause mental retardation. Treatment for physiologic jaundice in newborns is rarely necessary except for measures such as early feeding (to speed passage of feces through the intestine and prevent reabsorption of bilirubin from the bowel). Phototherapy (exposure of the infant to light to initiate maturation of liver enzymes) may be used (see Chapter 26).

Some breast-fed babies have more difficulty in converting indirect bilirubin to direct bilirubin than formula-fed babies, because breast milk contains pregnanediol (a metabolite of progesterone), which depresses the action of glucuronyl transferase. Rarely does breast-feeding cause enough jaundice to warrant therapy. Stopping nursing in the first week of life must never be a decision taken lightly, as it could interrupt breast-feeding. In rare instances, the mother may be asked to discontinue breast-feeding for 1 or 2 days until the infant's bilirubin level falls again. If the mother expresses her milk manually for the few days that she is not breast-feeding so that her milk supply does not decline, she should be able to breast-feed successfully after the interruption.

Pallor. Pallor in newborns is usually the result of anemia. Anemia may be caused by (1) excessive blood loss at the time the cord was cut; (2) inadequate flow of blood from the cord into the infant at birth; (3) fetal-maternal transfusion; (4) low iron stores caused by poor maternal nutrition during pregnancy; or (5) blood incompatibility in which a large number of red blood cells were hemolyzed in utero. It may be the result of internal bleeding (the baby should be watched closely for signs of blood in stool or vomitus). Infants with central nervous system damage may appear pale as well as cyanotic. A gray color in newborns is generally indicative of infection. Twins may be born with a twin transfusion phenomenon, in which one twin is larger and has good color and the smaller twin has pallor.

Harlequin Sign. Occasionally, because of immature circulation, a neonate who has been lying on his or her side will appear red on the dependent side of the body and pale on the upper side, as if a line had been drawn down the center of the body. This is a transient phenomenon and, although startling, of no clinical significance. The odd coloring fades immediately if the infant's position is changed or the baby kicks or cries vigorously.

Birthmarks
A number of common occurring birthmarks can be identified in newborns. It is important to differentiate the various types of hemangiomas so that you neither give false reassurance to parents nor worry them unnecessarily about these lesions.

Hemangiomas. The hemangiomas are vascular tumors of the skin. Three types are found.

Nevus flammeus (Figure 23-12*A*) is a macular purple or dark red lesion (sometimes called a *port-wine stain* because of its deep color) that is present at birth. These lesions generally appear on the face, although they are often found on the thighs as well. Those above the bridge of the nose tend to fade; the others are less likely to. Because they are level with the skin surface (macular) they can be covered by a cosmetic preparation later in life or can be removed surgically.

Nevus flammeus lesions also occur as lighter, pink patches at the nape of the neck (*stork's beak marks*) (Figure 23-12*B*). These do not fade either, but are covered by the hairline and so are of no consequence. They occur more often in females than in males.

Strawberry hemangiomas are elevated areas formed by immature capillaries and endothelial cells (Figure 23-12*C*). Most are present at birth, although they may appear up to 2 weeks after birth. Formation is associated with the high estrogen levels of pregnancy. They may continue to enlarge from their original size up to 1 year of age. After the first year, they tend to be absorbed and shrink in size. By the time the child is 7 years old, 50% to 75% of these lesions have disappeared. A child may be 10 years old before the absorption is complete. Application of cortisone ointment may speed their disappearance by interfering with the binding of estrogen to its receptor sites.

It is important for parents to understand that the mark may grow; otherwise, they may confuse it with cancer (a skin lesion increasing in size is one of the seven danger signals of cancer). They should also understand that the mark will disappear, so they do not think of their child as imperfect or disfigured. Surgery to remove strawberry hemangiomas may lead to secondary infection, resulting in scarring and permanent disfigurement, and is rarely recommended.

Cavernous hemangiomas (Figure 23-12*D*) are dilated vascular spaces. They are usually raised and resemble a strawberry hemangioma in appearance. They do not disappear with time as do strawberry hemangiomas but can be removed surgically. Cavernous hemangiomas may bleed internally, leading to hyperbilirubinemia or anemia. Children who have a skin lesion

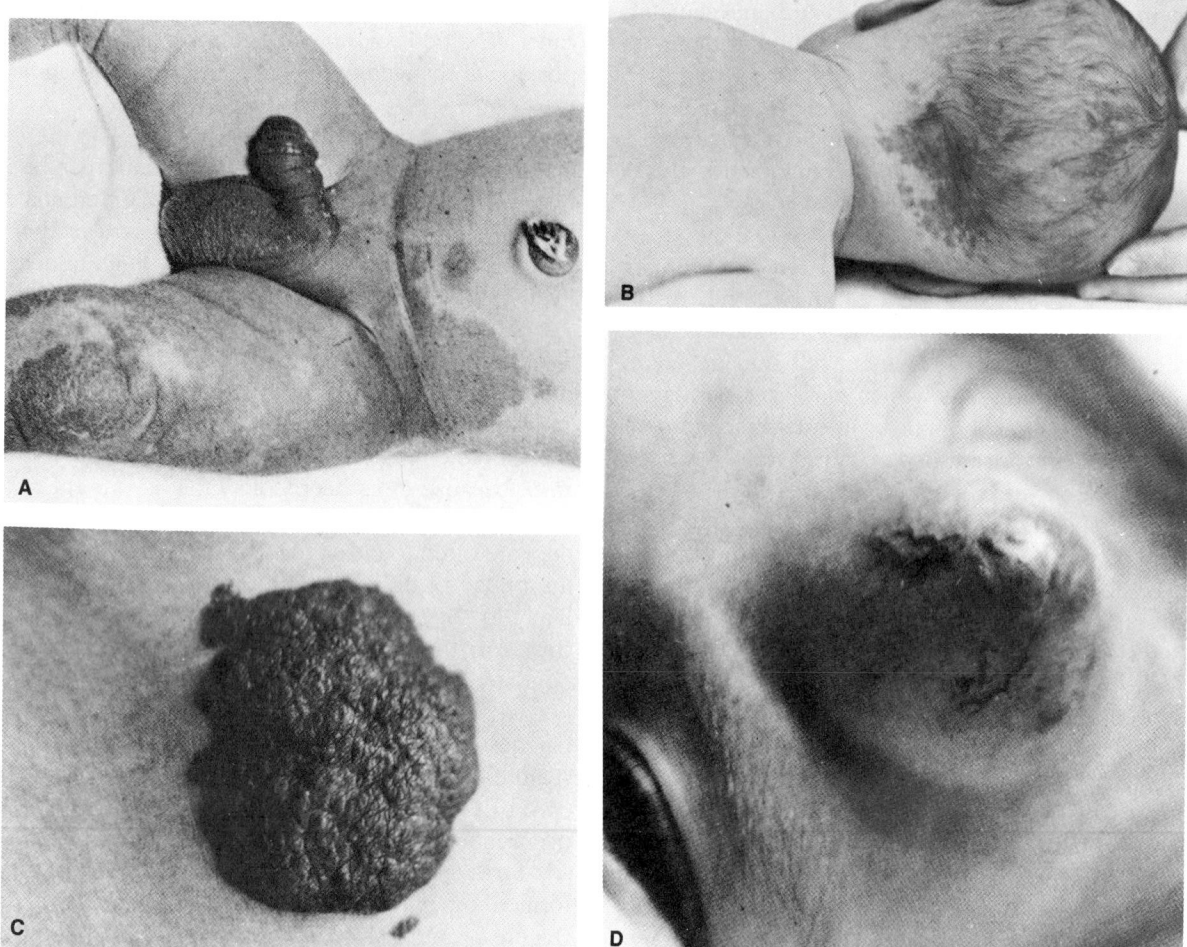

FIGURE 23-12

*Types of hemangiomas found on the newborn. (**A**) Nevus flammeus (port-wine stain) formed of a plexus of newly formed capillaries in the papillary layer of the corium. It is deep red to purple, does not blanch on pressure, and does not fade with age. (**B**) Stork's beak mark, commonly occurring on nape of neck. It blanches on pressure; although it does not fade, it is not noticeable as it becomes covered by hair. (**C**) Strawberry hemangiomas consist of dilated capillaries in entire dermal and subdermal layers. They continue to enlarge after birth but usually disappear by age 10 years. (**D**) Cavernous hemangiomas consist of a communicating network of venules in subcutaneous tissue and do not fade with age. (Courtesy of Mead Johnson & Company, Evansville, IN.)*

may have additional ones on internal organs. Blows to the abdomen, such as those from childhood games, can cause bleeding from internal hemangiomas. Children who have cavernous hemangiomas are usually assessed at health maintenance visits for hematocrit level in order to determine internal blood loss.

Mongolian Spots. Mongolian spots are slate-gray patches across the sacrum or buttocks and consist of a collection of pigment cells (melanocytes). They tend to occur in children of Asian, Southern European, or African extraction. They disappear by school age without treatment. Parents should be assured that they are not bruises, or they may be concerned that the baby has sustained a birth injury.

Vernix Caseosa

Vernix caseosa, a white, cream cheese–like substance that serves as a skin lubricant, is usually noticeable on a newborn's skin, at least in the skin folds, at birth. The color of the vernix should be carefully noted, because it takes on the color of the amniotic fluid. If it is yellow, the amniotic fluid was yellow from bilirubin; if it is green, meconium was present in the amniotic fluid.

Handle newborns with gloves to protect yourself from exposure to body fluids until the first bath when vernix is washed away. Harsh rubbing should never be employed to wash away vernix, because the newborn's skin is tender, and breaks in the skin from too vigorous attempts to remove the vernix may open portals of entry for bacteria.

Lanugo

Lanugo is the fine downy hair that covers a newborn's shoulders, back, and upper arms. It may be found also on the forehead and ears. The newborn of 37 to 39 weeks' gestational age has more lanugo than the 40-week-old infant; postmature infants (over 42 weeks) rarely have lanugo. Lanugo is rubbed away by the friction of bedding and clothes against the newborn's skin. By age 2 weeks, it has disappeared.

Desquamation

Within 24 hours of birth, the skin of most newborns has become extremely dry. The dryness is particularly evident on the palms of the hands and the soles of the feet. It may result in areas of peeling similar to those following a sunburn. This is normal and needs no treatment. If parents wish, they may apply some hand or body lotion to lubricate the dry areas.

Newborns who are postmature and have suffered intrauterine malnutrition have extremely dry skin with a leathery appearance and cracks in the skin folds. This should be differentiated from normal desquamation.

Milia

Newborn sebaceous glands are immature. At least one pinpoint white papule (a plugged or unopened sebaceous gland) can be found on the cheek or across the bridge of the nose of every newborn. Such lesions, termed **milia** (Figure 23-13), disappear by 2 to 4 weeks of age as the sebaceous glands mature and drain.

Erythema Toxicum

In most normal mature infants, a newborn rash called **erythema toxicum** is observed (Figure 23-14). It usually appears in the first to fourth day of life but may appear in neonates up to 2 weeks of age. It begins with a papule, increases in severity to become erythema by the

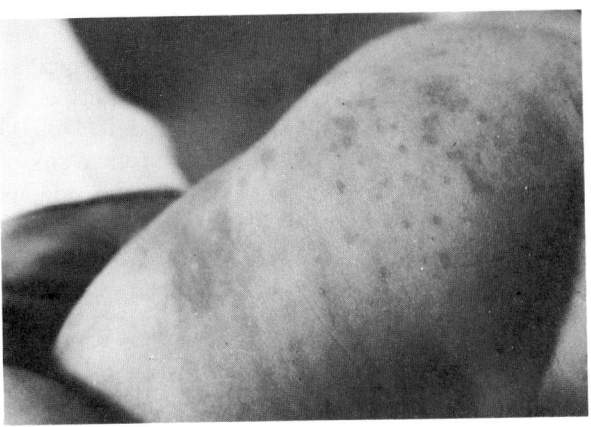

FIGURE 23-14
Erythema toxicum is found on almost all newborns. The reddish rash consists of sporadic pinpoint papules on an erythematous base. It fades spontaneously in a few days. (Courtesy of Mead Johnson & Company, Evansville, IN.)

second day, then disappears by the third day. It is sometimes called a *flea-bite rash* because the lesions are so minuscule. One of the chief characteristics of the rash is its lack of pattern. It occurs sporadically and unpredictably as to time and place on skin surfaces. It may last a matter of hours rather than days. It is probably a response to irritation of the infant's skin by sheets and clothes. It needs no treatment.

Forceps Marks

If forceps were used for birth, there may be a circular or linear contusion matching the rim of the blade of the forceps on the infant's cheek (Figure 23-15). This mark disappears in 1 to 2 days along with the edema that accompanies it. The mark is the result of normal forceps usage and does not denote unskilled or too vigorous application of forceps.

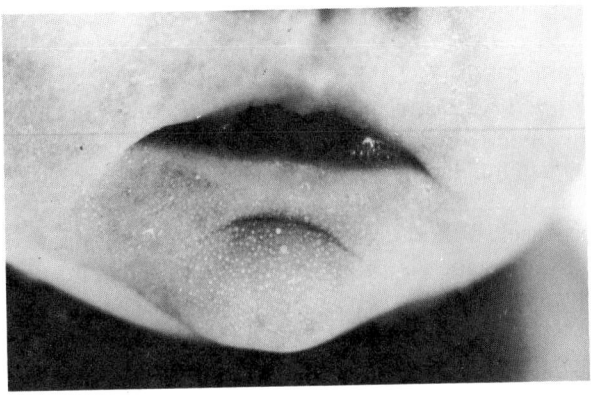

FIGURE 23-13
Milia are unopened sebaceous glands frequently found on the nose, chin, or cheeks of a newborn. They disappear spontaneously in a few weeks' time. (Courtesy of Mead Johnson & Company, Evansville, IN.)

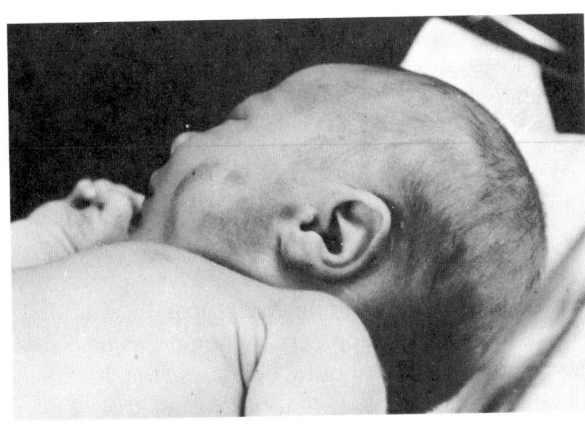

FIGURE 23-15
Forceps marks are commonly found in newborns delivered by forceps. Such marks are transient and disappear in a day or two. (Courtesy of Mead Johnson & Company, Evansville, IN.)

Skin Turgor

Newborn skin should feel resilient if the underlying tissue is well hydrated. If a fold of the skin is grasped between the thumb and fingers, it should feel elastic. When it is released, it should fall back to form a smooth surface. If severe dehydration is present, the skin will not smooth out again but will remain in an elevated ridge. Poor turgor is seen in newborns who suffered malnutrition in utero, who have difficulty sucking at birth, or who have certain metabolic disorders, such as adrenogenital syndrome.

Head

A newborn's head is disproportionately large, about one fourth of the total length; in an adult, the head is one eighth of total height. The forehead of the newborn is large and prominent. The chin appears to be receding, and it quivers easily if the infant is startled or cries. Well-nourished newborns have full-bodied hair; poorly nourished or preterm infants have stringy, lifeless hair.

Fontanelles

The fontanelles are the spaces or openings where the skull bones join. The anterior fontanelle is at the junction of the two parietal bones and the two fused frontal bones. It is diamond shaped and measures 2 to 3 cm (0.8 to 1.2 in) in width and 3 to 4 cm (1.2 to 1.6 in) in length. The posterior fontanelle is at the junction of the parietal bones and the occipital bone. It is triangular and measures about 1 cm (0.4 in) in length.

The anterior fontanelle will be felt as a soft spot. It should not appear indented (a sign of dehydration) or bulging (a sign of increased intracranial pressure). The fontanelle may bulge if the newborn strains to pass a stool or cries vigorously, and with vigorous crying, a pulse may sometimes be seen in the fontanelle. The posterior fontanelle is so small in some newborns that it cannot be palpated readily. The anterior fontanelle normally closes at 12 to 18 months of age. The posterior fontanelle closes by the end of the second month (see Figure 18-2).

Sutures

The skull *sutures,* the separating lines of the skull, may override at birth because of the extreme pressure exerted by passage through the birth canal. Overriding is a normal, transient phenomenon. When the sagittal suture between the parietal bones overrides, the fontanelles will be less perceptible than usual.

Suture lines should never appear separated in newborns. Separation denotes increased intracranial pressure from either abnormal brain formation, abnormal accumulation of cerebrospinal fluid in the cranium (hy-drocephalus), or an accumulation of blood from a birth injury, such as subdural hemorrhage.

Molding

The part of the infant's head (usually the vertex) that engages the cervix is molded to fit the cervix contours and appears prominent and asymmetric; it may be so extreme in the baby of a primiparous woman that it looks like a dunce cap (Figure 23-16). This is a normal finding, although worrisome to new parents. The head will be restored to its normal shape within a few days of birth.

Caput Succedaneum

Caput succedaneum (Figure 23-17*A*) is edema of the scalp at the presenting part of the head. It may involve wide areas of the head or may be the size of a goose egg. The edema will gradually be absorbed and disappear about the third day of life. It needs no treatment.

Cephalhematoma

A *cephalhematoma* is a collection of blood between the periosteum of the skull bone and the bone itself caused by rupture of a periosteum capillary due to the pressure of birth (Figure 23-17*B*). The blood loss is negligible, but the swelling is generally severe and is well outlined as an egg shape. It may be discolored (black and blue) because of the presence of coagulated blood. A caput succedaneum may involve both hemispheres of the head, but a cephalhematoma is confined to an individual bone, so that the associated swelling stops at the bone's suture line.

It takes weeks for a cephalhematoma to be absorbed. It might appear that the blood could be aspirated to relieve the condition. This procedure would introduce the risk of infection, however, and would be an unnecessary intrusion because the condition will subside by itself. As the blood captured in the space is broken down, a great amount of indirect bilirubin may be released, leading to jaundice.

Craniotabes

Craniotabes is a localized softening of the cranial bones. The bone is so soft it can be indented by the pressure of an examining finger. The bone returns to its normal contour when the pressure is removed. The condition corrects itself without treatment after a matter of months.

Craniotabes is probably caused by pressure of the fetal skull against the mother's pelvic bone in utero. It is more common in firstborn infants than in infants born later because of the lower position of the head in the pelvis the last 2 weeks of pregnancy in primiparous women. It is an example of a condition that is normal in a newborn but would be pathologic if found in an older child (probably the result of faulty metabolism or kidney dysfunction).

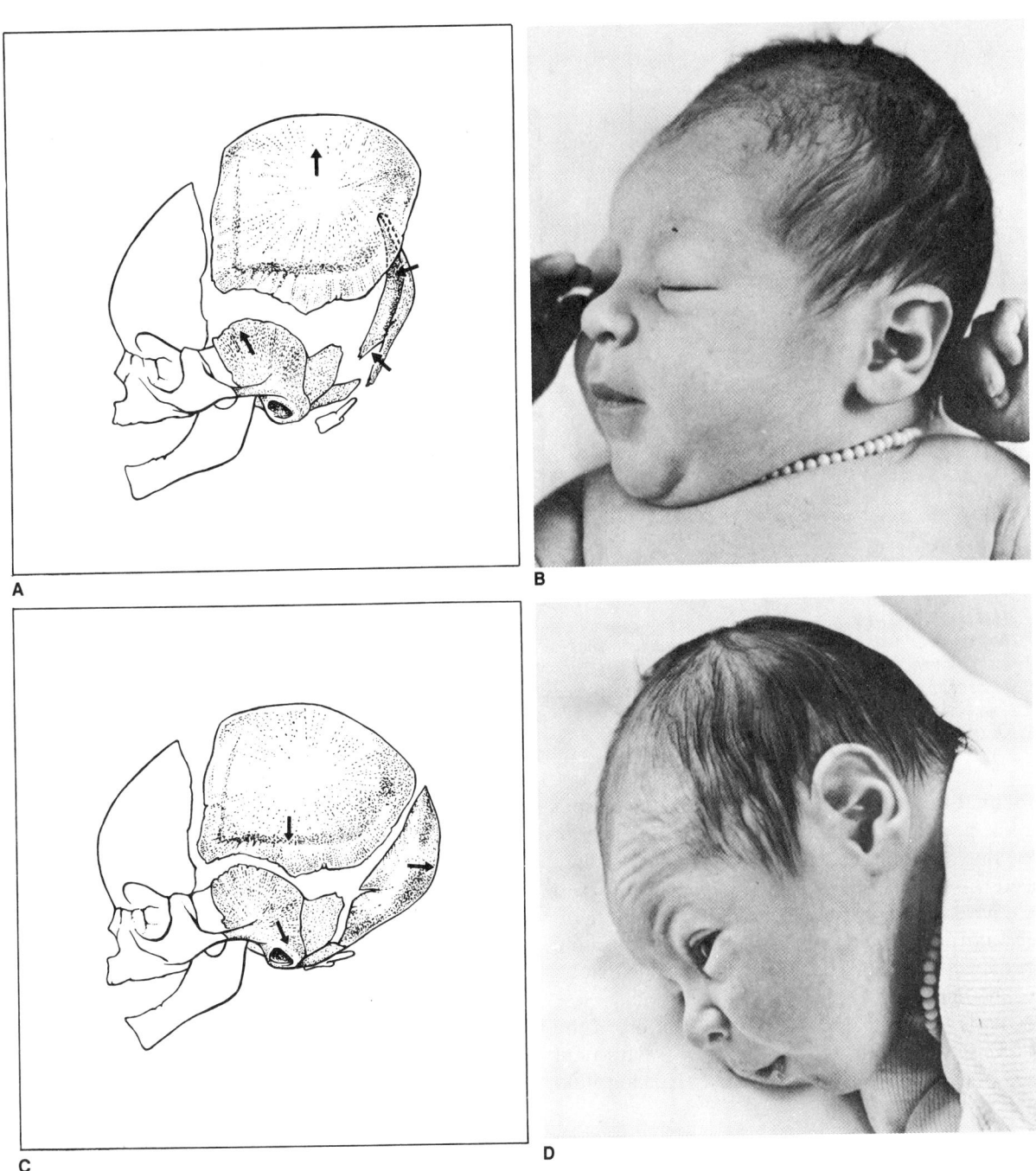

FIGURE 23-16
*Molding. (**A, B**) The infant head molds to fit the birth canal more easily. On palpation, the skull sutures will be felt to be overriding. (**C, D**) The head shape returns to normal within 1 week. (Courtesy of Mead Johnson & Company, Evansville, IN.)*

Eyes

Newborns usually cry tearlessly because the lacrimal ducts are not fully mature at birth. Almost without exception the irises of the eyes of newborns are gray or blue. They do not assume their permanent color until the child is about 3 months of age.

With the infant in a supine position, lift the head. This maneuver usually causes the baby to open the eyes. The eyes should appear clear, without redness or purulent discharge. Occasionally, the administration of antibiotic ointment at birth will cause a purulent discharge for the first 24 hours of life. Antibiotic ointment such as erythromycin is administered to protect against chlamydia infection as well as ophthalmia neonatorum (gonorrheal conjunctivitis).

Pressure during birth sometimes will cause the rupture of a conjunctival capillary, resulting in a small **sub-**

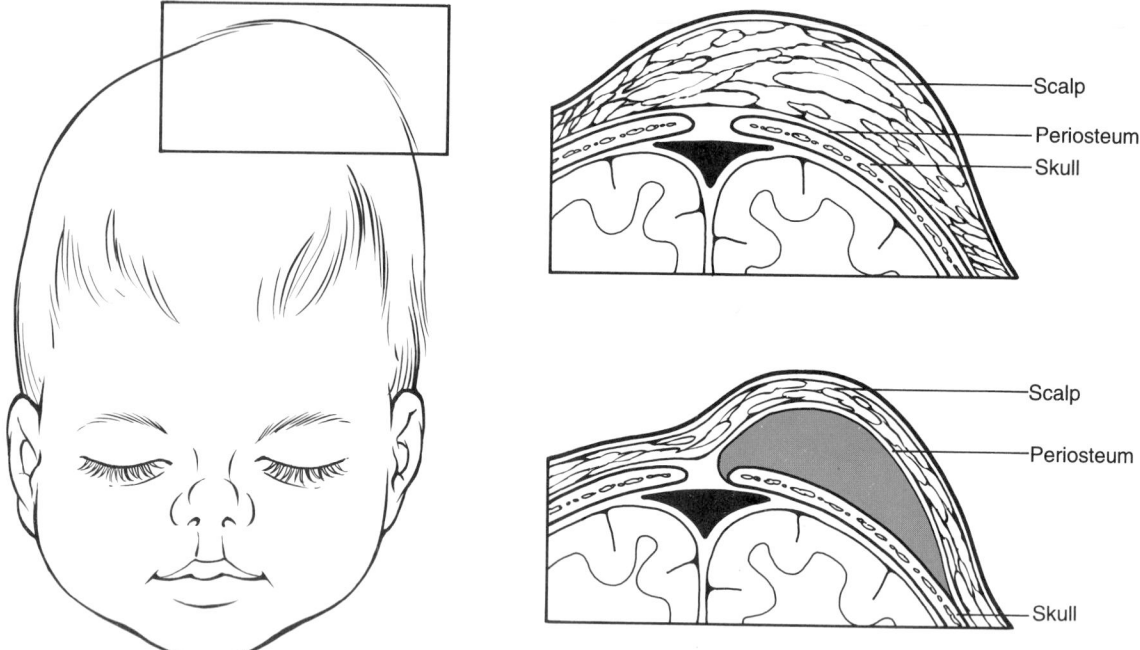

FIGURE 23-17

(**A**) *Caput succedaneum. From pressure of the birth canal, an edematous area is present beneath the scalp. Note how it crosses the midline of the skull.* (**B**) *Cephalhematoma. A small capillary beneath the periosteum of the skull bone has ruptured, and blood has collected under the periosteum of the bone. Note how the swelling now stops at the midline. Because the blood is contained under the periosteum, it is necessarily stopped by a suture line.*

conjunctival hemorrhage. This appears as a red spot on the sclera, usually on the inner aspect of the eye, or as a red ring around the cornea. The bleeding is slight and needs no treatment. It will be completely absorbed in 2 or 3 weeks. Parents can be assured that these hemorrhages are unimportant; otherwise they may assume that the baby is bleeding from within the eye and that vision will be impaired.

Edema is often present around the orbit or on the eyelids. This will remain for the first 2 or 3 days until the newborn's kidneys are capable of evacuating fluid efficiently.

The cornea of the eye should be round and proportionate in size to that of an adult eye. A cornea that is larger than usual may be the result of congenital glaucoma. An irregularly shaped pupil or discolored iris may denote disease (see Chapter 28). The pupil should be dark; a white pupil suggests congenital cataract.

Ears

The newborn's external ear is still not as completely formed as it will be eventually, and the pinna tends to bend easily. When putting an infant on his or her side after a feeding, be sure that you place the ear in good alignment. If you allow a newborn to sleep on an ear in a deformed position, the ear may assume that position permanently.

The level of the top part of the external ear should be on a line drawn from the inner canthus to the outer canthus of the eye and back across the side of the head (see Chapter 28). Ears that are set lower than this are found in infants with certain chromosomal abnormalities, particularly trisomy 18 and 13, syndromes in which low-set ears and other physical defects are coupled with mental retardation (see Chapter 7).

Small tags of skin are sometimes found just in front of the ear. Although these may be associated with chromosomal abnormalities or kidney disease, they generally are isolated findings and are of no consequence. They can be removed by ligation immediately or when the child is a week old. A dermal sinus may be present directly in front of the ear; the area should be inspected for a pinpoint-size opening. The sinus is usually small and can be removed without consequence when a child is near school age.

Visualizing the tympanic membrane in a newborn is difficult and generally is not attempted, because amniotic fluid and flecks of vernix fill the canal and obliterate the drum and its accompanying landmarks.

It is good practice to test the newborn's hearing by ringing a bell held about 6 inches from each ear. If he or she is crying, the infant who can hear will stop momentarily; if quiet, a newborn will blink the eyes, appear to attend to the sound, and may startle. This method of testing is not highly accurate. A negative response should be noted, however, and the child should be retested at a later time. In many health care facilities, all newborns are tested by a standardized response to sound before discharge.

Nose

A newborn's nose may appear large for the face. As the child grows, the rest of the face will grow more than the nose, and the discrepancy will disappear. One or two milia are usually present on the tip or bridge of the nose.

Test for choanal atresia (blockage at the rear of the nose) by closing the newborn's mouth and compressing one naris at a time with your fingers. Note any discomfort or distress.

Mouth

A newborn's mouth should open evenly when the baby cries. If one side of the mouth moves more than the other, cranial nerve injury is suggested. A newborn's tongue appears large and prominent in the mouth. Because the tongue is short, the frenulum membrane is attached close to the tip of the tongue, creating the impression that the infant is "tongue tied." At one time, it was almost routine to snip a newborn's frenulum membrane to lengthen it. Now this procedure is regarded as harmful and unnecessary, because it leaves a portal of entry for infection, risks hemorrhage because of the low level of vitamin K in most newborns, and causes feeding difficulties by making the tongue sore and irritated.

The palate of the newborn should be intact. Occasionally, one or two small round, glistening, well-circumscribed cysts (Epstein's pearls) are present on the palate, a result of the extra load of calcium that is deposited in utero. They are of no significance and need no treatment, because they disappear spontaneously in a week's time. A parent may be concerned about them, mistaking them for *thrush,* a *Candida* infection, which usually appears on the tongue and sides of the cheeks as white or gray patches.

All newborns have some mucus in their mouths. If newborns are placed on their side, the mucus drains from their mouths and gives them no distress. If their mouths are filled with so much mucus that they seem to be blowing bubbles, they may have a tracheoesophageal fistula. This must be determined before a child is fed; otherwise, formula can be aspirated into the lungs from the inadequately formed esophagus.

It is unusual for the newborn to have teeth, but sometimes one or two (called **natal teeth**) will have erupted. Any teeth present must be evaluated for stability. If they are loose, they should be extracted to prevent them from being aspirated during a feeding.

Small, white epithelial pearls (benign inclusion cysts) may be present on the gum margins. No therapy is necessary for these.

Neck

The neck of a newborn is short and often chubby. It is creased with skin folds. The head should rotate freely on it. If there is rigidity of the neck, congenital torticollis from injury to the sternocleidomastoid muscle during birth should be considered (see Chapter 39). In newborns whose membranes were ruptured more than 24 hours prior to birth, nuchal rigidity suggests meningitis.

The neck is not strong enough to support the total weight of the newborn's head, but in a sitting position a newborn should make a momentary effort at head control. When lying prone, newborns can raise their heads slightly, usually enough to lift their nose out of mucus or spit-up formula. If they are pulled into a sitting position from a supine position, their heads will lag behind considerably; however, again, they should make some effort to control and steady their heads as they reach the sitting position.

The trachea may be prominent on the front of the neck. The thymus gland may be enlarged because of the rapid growth of glandular tissue in comparison with other body tissues. The thymus gland triples in size by 3 years of age; it remains at that size until the child is about 10 years old. After that, its size begins to decrease. Although the thymus may appear to be bulging in the newborn, it is rarely a cause of respiratory difficulty as was previously believed.

Chest

The chest in some infants looks small because the infant's head is large in proportion. Not until the child is 2 years of age does the chest measurement exceed that of the head.

In both female and male infants, the breasts may be engorged. Occasionally, the breasts of newborn babies secrete a thin, watery fluid popularly termed *witch's milk.* Engorgement occurs in utero as a result of the influence of the mother's hormones. As soon as these are cleared from the infant's system, the engorgement and any fluid present subsides (about a week). Fluid should never be expressed from infant breasts. The manipulation may introduce bacteria and lead to mastitis.

The chest is as wide in the anteroposterior diameter as it is across. The clavicles should be straight. A lump on one or the other may indicate that a fracture occurred during birth and calcium is now being deposited at that point. Overall, the appearance of the chest should be symmetric. Respirations are normally rapid (30 to 60 breaths per minute) but not distressed. A supernumerary nipple (usually found below and in line with the normal nipples) may be present.

Retraction (the chest wall is drawn in with inspiration) should not be present. A retracting infant is using such strong force to pull air into the respiratory tract that he or she sucks in the anterior chest muscle. Retraction is shown in Figure 23-18.

Because the newborn's alveoli open slowly over the first 24 to 48 hours to full capacity and the baby invariably has mucus in the back of the throat, listening to lung sounds often reveals the sounds of rhonchi, the harsh innocent sound of air passing over mucus. A grunting sound suggests respiratory distress syndrome; a high, crowing sound on inspiration suggests stridor or immature tracheal development (abnormal sounds).

Abdomen

The contour of the newborn abdomen is slightly protuberant. A scaphoid or sunken appearance may be indicative of missing abdominal contents or a diaphragmatic hernia. Bowel sounds should be present within an hour after birth. The edge of the liver is usually palpable at 1 to 2 cm below the right costal margin. The edge of the spleen may be palpable 1 to 2 cm below the left costal margin. Tenderness is difficult to determine in a newborn, but if it is extreme, the infant will cry or possibly thrash about or possibly tense abdominal muscles to protect the abdomen as you palpate it.

For the first hour after birth, the umbilical cord appears as a white, gelatinous structure marked with the red and blue streaks of the umbilical vein and arteries. The one vein and two arteries should be counted when

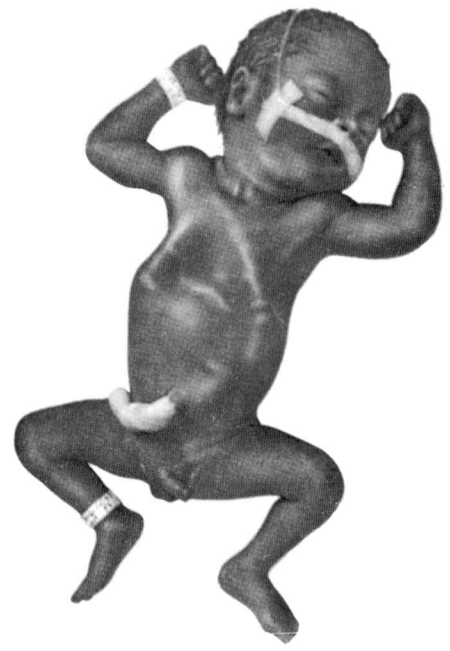

FIGURE 23-18
Sternal retraction in a newborn. Retraction indicates labored and difficult breathing. (Courtesy of Ross Laboratories, Columbus, OH.)

the cord is first cut after birth to be certain they are present. In 0.5% of deliveries (3.5% of twin deliveries), there is only a single umbilical artery, and in a third of such infants, this single artery is associated with a congenital heart anomaly; renal anomalies also may be present. Because the anomaly may not be readily apparent, any child with a single umbilical artery needs close observation and assessment until all anomalies are ruled out (Cochran, 1990).

Inspect the cord clamp to be certain it is secure. After the first hour of life, the cord begins to dry, shrink, and become discolored like the dead end of a vine. By the second or third day, it has turned black. It breaks free by the sixth to tenth day, leaving a granulating area a few centimeters across that heals during the following week.

There should be no bleeding at the cord site. Bleeding suggests that the cord clamp has become loosened or the cord has been tugged loose by the friction of the bedclothes. The base of the cord should appear dry. A moist or odorous cord suggests infection. If present, infection should receive immediate treatment or it may enter the newborn's bloodstream and cause septicemia. Moistness at the base of the cord also may indicate a patent urachus (canal connecting the bladder and the umbilicus), which is draining urine at the cord site.

The base of the cord should also be inspected to be certain there is no defect present in the abdominal wall (umbilical hernia). If there is a fascial (abdominal wall) defect less than 2 cm in size, it will generally close by itself by school age; a defect more than 2 cm wide will probably require surgical correction. Taping or putting buttons or coins on the abdomen are home remedies that do not help such defects to close. Heavy taping may, in fact, worsen the condition by preventing the development of good muscle tone in the abdominal wall. The tape also tends to keep the cord moist and make infection more likely than when the cord is dry (see the Focus on Cultural Awareness box).

You should attempt to verify the presence of kidneys by deep palpation of the right and left abdomen. The right kidney can usually be palpated (at least its lower pole), because it is located lower than the left kidney; the latter is more difficult to locate because the intestine is bulkier on the left side, and the left kidney is higher in the retroperitoneal space. Nonetheless, you should try to locate it; the child's voiding only demonstrates that there is at least one kidney, not that there are two. Placing one hand behind the infant while you palpate offers a firmer base and helps with evaluation of kidney size (newborn kidneys are about the size of a walnut). If a kidney is enlarged, a polycystic kidney or pooling of urine from a urethral obstruction is suggested. Be certain your fingernails are clipped close to your fingertips before you undertake kidney palpation. Otherwise, you will cut the baby's abdominal skin as you press in deeply enough to locate the kidneys.

FOCUS ON CULTURAL AWARENESS

Although it is generally a sound policy to point out the positive aspects of a child to parents to aid parent-child bonding, in some areas of the world, such as traditional Cambodia and Laos, newborns are not given compliments this way, because it is believed to make them vulnerable to evil spirits.

In some African cultures, it is important for newborns to have an amulet (good luck charm) tied around their neck. Oiling the infant's body and placing a belly band over the umbilical cord are also common care procedures. In the traditional Haiti culture, infants are not named immediately, but only after a full month (Geissler, 1994).

Being aware of cultural variations in newborn care such as these helps you plan care that is specific and meaningful to individual parents and that can aid parent-child bonding.

To finish abdominal assessment, elicit an abdominal reflex. Stroking each quadrant of the abdomen will cause the umbilicus to move or "wink" in that direction. This superficial abdominal reflex is a test of spinal nerves T8 through T10. The reflex may not be demonstrable in newborns until the 10th day of life.

Anogenital Area

The anus of the newborn must be inspected to be certain that it is present, patent, and not covered by a membrane (imperforate anus). This condition is best determined by inserting a rectal thermometer into the rectum for the length of the bulb or by inserting the tip of a lubricated, gloved, little finger. The time after birth that the infant first passes meconium should be noted. If a newborn does not do so in the first 24 hours, the suspicion of imperforate anus or meconium ileus is aroused.

Male Genitalia

The scrotum in most male neonates is edematous and rugated. It may be deeply pigmented in black or dark-skinned neonates.

Both testes should be present in the scrotum. Male neonates with one or both undescended testicles (cryptorchidism) need further referral to establish the extent of the problem. It could be due to agenesis (absence of an organ), ectopic testes (the testes cannot enter the scrotum because the opening to the scrotal sac is closed), or undescended testes (the vas deferens or artery is too short to allow them to descend). Neonates with agenesis of the testes are usually referred for inves-

tigation of other anomalies. Because the testes arise from the same germ tissue as the kidney, agenesis of a testes may indicate agenesis of a kidney also. Make a practice of pressing your left hand against the inguinal ring before palpating for the testes, so that they do not slip upward out of the scrotal sac as you palpate (Figure 23-19).

The cremasteric reflex is a reflex elicited by stroking the internal side of the thigh. As the skin is stroked, the testis on that side moves perceptibly upward. This is a test for the integrity of spinal nerves T8 through T10. The response may be absent in newborns less than about 10 days old.

The penis of newborns appears small; it is about 2 cm long. It should be inspected to see that the urethral opening is at the tip of the glans, not on the dorsal surface (epispadias) or the ventral surface (hypospadias).

The prepuce (foreskin) of the penis should be examined to be certain it is not stenosed. In most newborns it slides back poorly from the meatal opening, so this should not be done. Although today most male neonates are circumcised, the necessity for this operation can be questioned. It is rare to find an infant who physically requires it (with a foreskin so constricted that it interferes with voiding or circulation), and surgery this early in life poses the risk of hemorrhage and infection. Circumcision should not be done if hypospadias or epispadias is present, since the plastic surgeon may want to use the foreskin as tissue in the repair of these conditions.

Female Genitalia

The vulva in female newborns may be swollen because of the effect of maternal hormones. Some newborns have a mucous vaginal secretion, which is sometimes

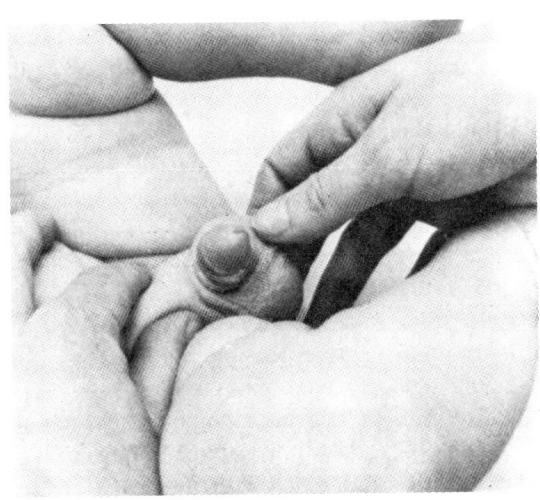

FIGURE 23-19
Technique for blocking the inguinal canal when examining scrotal contents. (From Alexander, M., & Brown, M.S. [1978]. Pediatric physical diagnosis for nurses. *New York: McGraw-Hill: with permission.)*

blood-tinged. Again, this is due to the action of maternal hormones, and the discharge will disappear as soon as the infant's system has cleared the hormones. The discharge should not be mistaken for an infection or taken as an indication that a trauma has occurred.

Back

The spine of a newborn appears flat in the lumbar and sacral areas; the curves seen in the adult appear only when a child is able to sit and walk. The base of the spine should be inspected carefully to be certain there is no pinpoint opening in the skin, which would suggest a dermal sinus.

A newborn normally assumes the position maintained in utero in which, typically, the back is rounded and the arms and legs are flexed on the abdomen and chest. A child who was born in a frank breech position will tend to straighten the legs at the knee and bring them up next to the face. The position of a baby presenting with a face presentation sometimes simulates opisthotonos, because the curve of the back is deeply concave.

Extremities

The arms and legs of a newborn appear short. The hands are plump and clenched into fists. Newborn fingernails are soft and smooth and are usually long enough to extend over the fingertips. Test the upper extremities for muscle tone by unflexing the arms for approximately 5 seconds. When you release an arm, it should return immediately to its flexed position. Hold the arms down by the sides and note their length. The fingertips should cover the proximal thigh. Unusually short arms may signify achondroplastic dwarfism. Observe for unusual curvature of the little finger and inspect the palm for a simian crease (a single palmar crease in contrast to the three creases normally seen in a palm). Both simian creases and inward-curved little fingers are signs of Down syndrome, although curved fingers and simian creases also may occur normally.

The arms and legs should move symmetrically (unless an infant is demonstrating a tonic neck reflex). An arm that hangs limp and unmoving suggests injury to the clavicle or the brachial or cervical plexus or fracture of a long bone, which are possible birth injuries. Assess for webbing (syndactyly), extra toes or fingers (polydactyly), or unusual spacing of toes, particularly between the big toes and the others (a finding in certain chromosomal disorders, although this is also a normal finding in some families). Test to see whether the toenails become blanched and refill after pressure.

The legs are bowed as well as short. The sole of the foot appears to be flat because of an extra pad of fat in the longitudinal arch. In the mature newborn, there are many crisscrossed lines on the sole of the foot. Absence of sole creases usually indicates immaturity.

The feet of many newborns turn in (varus deviation) because of intrauterine position. This simple deviation needs no correction if the feet can be brought into the midline position by easy manipulation; when the infant begins to bear weight, the feet will align themselves. If a foot does not align readily or will not turn to a definite midline position, a talipes deformity (clubfoot) may be present. This condition needs investigation, because congenital problems of this kind are best treated in the newborn period. Put the ankle through a range of motion to evaluate whether the heel cord is unusually tight. Check for ankle clonus by supporting the lower leg in one hand and dorsiflexing the foot sharply two or three times by pressure on the sole of the foot with the other. Following the dorsiflexion, one or two continued movements are normal; rapid alternating contraction and relaxation (clonus) is abnormal (suggests neurologic involvement).

With the newborn in a supine position, both legs can be flexed and abducted to such an extent (180 degrees) that they touch or nearly touch the surface of the bed (Figure 23-20). If the hip joint seems to lock short of this distance (160 to 170 degrees), hip subluxation (a shallow and poorly formed acetabulum) is suggested. If subluxation is present, when the infant's leg is held with the fingers on the greater and lesser trochanters and the hip then abducted, a "clunk" of the femur head striking the shallow acetabulum can be heard (Ortolani's sign). If the hip can be felt to actually slip in the socket, this is Barlow's sign. Subluxated hip may be bilateral but is usually unilateral. It is important that hip subluxation be discovered as early as possible, because correction, as in correction of talipes deformities, is most successful if initiated early.

When lying on the abdomen, newborns are capable

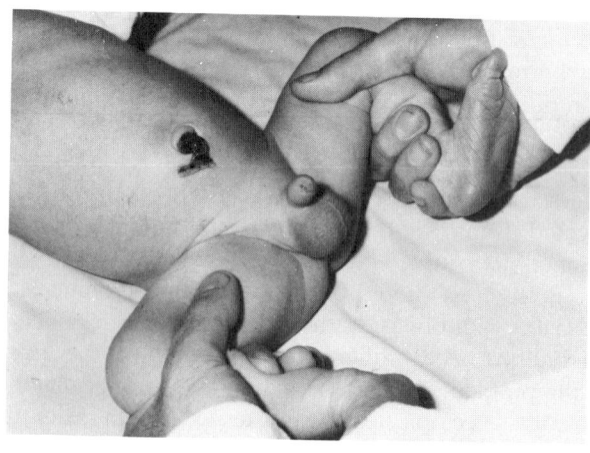

FIGURE 23-20

Hip abduction in a newborn—both hips should abduct so completely they lie almost flat against the mattress (180 degrees). (Courtesy of Mead Johnson & Company, Evansville, IN.)

of bringing their arms and legs underneath them and raising their stomach off the bed enough for a hand to be slipped underneath. This ability helps to prevent pressure or rubbing at the cord site, because in this position the cord site does not actually touch the bedding. The preterm newborn does not have this ability; thus, an infant's ability to do so is an indication of maturity.

Assessment for Well-Being

Apgar Scoring

At 1 minute and 5 minutes after birth, newborns are observed and rated according to an Apgar score (Apgar et al., 1958). As shown in Table 23-3, heart rate, respiratory effort, muscle tone, reflex irritability, and color are rated 0, 1, or 2; all five scores are then added. An infant whose total score is under 4 is in serious danger and needs resuscitation. A score of 4 to 6 means that the condition is guarded and a baby may need clearing of the airway and supplementary oxygen. A score of 7 to 10 is considered good, indicating that the infant scored as high as 70% to 90% of infants at 1 to 5 minutes after birth (10 is the highest score possible).

The Apgar score standardizes infant evaluation and serves as a baseline for future evaluations. There is a high correlation between low 5-minute Apgar scores and mortality and morbidity, particularly neurologic morbidity. The following points should be considered in obtaining an Apgar rating.

Heart Rate. Auscultating the newborn heart with a stethoscope is the best way of determining heart rate; however, heart rate also may be obtained by observing and counting the pulsations of the cord at the abdomen if the cord is still uncut at 1 minute after birth.

Respiratory Effort. A mature newborn usually cries spontaneously at about 30 seconds after birth. By 1 minute he or she is maintaining regular, although rapid, respirations. Difficulty might be anticipated in a newborn whose mother received large amounts of analgesia or a general anesthetic during labor or birth (see Nursing Care Plan: A Term Newborn).

Muscle Tone. Mature newborns hold the extremities tightly flexed, simulating their intrauterine position. They should resist any effort to extend their extremities.

Reflex Irritability. One of two possible cues is used to evaluate reflex irritability: either the newborn's response to a suction catheter in the nostrils or the response to having the soles of the feet slapped. A baby whose mother was heavily sedated will tend to have a low score in this category.

Color. All infants appear cyanotic at the moment of birth. They grow pink with or shortly after the first breath. The color of newborns thus corresponds to how well they are breathing. Acrocyanosis (cyanosis of the hands and feet) is so common in newborns that a score of 1 in this category can be thought of as normal.

Respiration Evaluation

Good respiratory function obviously has the highest priority in newborn care, and thus it is ongoing at every newborn contact. A Silverman and Andersen index

(text continues on page 666)

Table 23-3. *Apgar Scoring Chart*

Sign	Score 0	Score 1	Score 2
Heart rate	Absent	Slow (<100)	>100
Respiratory effort	Absent	Slow, irregular; weak cry	Good; strong cry
Muscle tone	Flaccid	Some flexion of extremities	Well flexed
Reflex irritability			
Response to catheter in nostril	No response	Grimace	Cough or sneeze
or			
Slap to sole of foot	No response	Grimace	Cry and withdrawal of foot
Color	Blue, pale	Body pink, extremities blue	Completely pink

(From Apgar, V., et al. [1958]. Evaluation of the newborn infant: Second report. *Journal of the American Medical Association, 168*, 1985. Copyright 1958, American Medical Association; with permission.)

Nursing Care Plan

A Term Newborn

Robert Bellows is a term newborn. The following is a nursing care plan designed for him.

Physical Examination: Well-proportioned, black male newborn of gravida 1, para 1 single mother. Apgar score: 8 at 1 min; 9 at 5 min. Silverman Index: 0; Ballard score = 40 (40 weeks gestational age).

Weight: 6 lb, 5 oz; 10th percentile (average for gestational age). Height: 19½ inches; 25th percentile.

Head: circumference, 34 cm; 25th percentile; molding at vertex prominent; anterior fontanelle: 3 × 4 cm and soft; posterior fontanelle: pinpoint.

Hair: Mature in thickness and character.

Eyes: Small subconjunctival hemorrhage right eye; extraocular muscles grossly intact; follows both sides to midline; edema on eyelids present; mild inflammatory response in conjunctivae present.

Ears: Normal alignment; apparent patent canal meatus; firm cartilage; no discharge. Pinpoint dermal sinus in front of right ear, not inflamed, no discharge.

Nose: midline septum; no discharge; patent bilaterally.

Mouth: midline uvula; palate intact; no teeth; 2 epithelial cysts on soft palate; gag reflex intact.

Neck: Midline trachea; no dermal sinuses, supple; no nodes palpable; clavicles intact.

Heart: Rate 130 bpm; normal tones; no murmur heard.

Lungs: Air exchange all lobes; rate 70 breaths/min; rhonchi heard in both upper lobes; mild substernal retraction.

Chest: Symmetric; breast tissue palpable 2 cm; no discharge.

Abdomen: soft, no masses; liver palpable 1 cm; spleen not palpable; 2 kidneys palpable; 3-vessel cord.

Genitalia: Urinary meatus present; both testes palpable; scant rugae on scrotum.

Extremities: Full range of motion; hips abduct to 180 degrees.

Back: No dimples; hair tufts visible.

Skin: Slate gray 2 × 3 cm macular area in sacral area; scattered pinpoint papules or erythematous base on abdomen, back arms, and legs.

Neurologic: Moro, grasp, step-in-place, and sucking reflexes tested and present.

Assessment: Mother breast-fed infant in birthing room, but baby didn't suck well because of rapid respirations. Father present at delivery, both concerned with discoloration on back and rash. Birth from left occipito-anterior (LOA) position; breathed at 30 sec after administration of blow-by oxygen. No anesthesia, no forceps used. Catheter inserted through left naris, esophagus, and into stomach; 15 mL stomach contents removed.

Nursing Diagnosis: High risk for ineffective airway clearance related to difficulty establishing respirations.

Defining Characteristic: Respiratory rate is above normal of 30 to 60/min.

Goal: Infant will not experience respiratory difficulty beyond 24 h of age.

Outcome Criteria: Newborn's respiratory rate is between 30 and 60 breaths/min without retractions or expiratory grunting.

Nursing Orders	*Rationale*
1. Infant to remain in birthing room for 1 h postpartum for close observation of respiratory rate. Transfer to rooming-in at end of hour if respiration rate is normal and retractions are no longer present.	1. Provides for safe care.
2. Take respiratory rate every 15 min for 1 h. Note any increase in retractions or expiratory grunting.	2. Assesses for increase in abnormal findings.

(continued)

Nursing Orders

3. Assure parents that some infants have rapid respiratory rates at birth from unabsorbed lung fluid.
4. Encourage mother to hold infant to maintain infant's temperature.
5. Alert high-risk nursery and transfer infant if respiratory rate increases or if retractions or grunting occurs.

Rationale

3. Assurance of health can aid bonding.
4. Hypothermia can add additional stress to respiratory effort.
5. Provide safeguard if rapid respirations are not transitory phenomenon.

Nursing Diagnosis: High risk for altered nutrition, less than body requirement, related to rapid respirations.

Defining Characteristic: Infants with rapid respirations have difficulty coordinating sucking and breathing.

Goal: Infant will ingest adequate oral nutrition during hospital stay.

Outcome Criteria: Infant does not lose more than 10% of birth weight; skin turgor remains good; not crying excessively.

Nursing Orders

1. Review technique of breast-feeding with parents.
2. Stress that infant may need to feed every 2 h for first few days.
3. If infant is moved to high-risk nursery, teach mother to manually express breast milk.

Rationale

1. Mother is breast-feeding for first time.
2. Infants taking small amounts need to eat more frequently.
3. Preserves milk supply and supplies breast milk for infant.

Nursing Diagnosis: Knowledge deficit of parents related to significance of erythema toxicum and mongolian spot.

Defining Characteristic: Parents have voiced concern with these findings.

Goal: Parents will demonstrate increased knowledge of newborn findings by 24 h.

Outcome Criteria: Parents voice they understand these are normal newborn findings; they hold infant warmly as if accepting appearance.

Nursing Orders

1. Discuss mongolian spot and newborn rash with parents and assure them that these are normal findings.
2. Inform parents there is no need for any special skin care.
3. Ask parents if they have any additional concerns.

Rationale

1. Knowing the explanation for observations can aid bonding.
2. Alleviates parents' concern about any special care.
3. Only identified concerns can be met.

(1956) can be used to estimate degrees of respiratory distress in newborns. For this assessment, a newborn is observed and then scored on each of five criteria (Figure 23-21). As shown, each item is given a value of 0, 1, or 2. These values are then added. A total score of 0 indicates no respiratory distress. Scores of 4 to 6 indicate moderate distress. Scores of 7 to 10 indicate severe distress. Note that the scores of this index run opposite to those of the Apgar. In an Apgar score, a value of 7 to 10 indicates a well infant. On a Silverman and Andersen score, a value of 7 to 10 denotes a seriously distressed infant.

Physical Examination

A newborn is given a preliminary physical examination immediately following birth to detect such grossly observable conditions as meningocele, cleft lip and palate, hydrocephalus, birthmarks, imperforate anus, tracheo-esophageal atresia, and bowel obstruction. This assessment may be the responsibility of the delivering physician, the anesthesiologist, a pediatrician, or nurse. This health assessment must be done rapidly, so that the newborn is not exposed for a long period of time, yet it must not be done so swiftly that important findings are overlooked. It is usually performed in the order of heart and respiratory systems first, when the infant is most likely to be quiet.

The immediate birth appraisal should include auscultation of the chest for heart and respiratory sounds (perhaps already done as a part of Apgar scoring). A number of procedures can be performed to rule out the common birth anomalies. Their screening importance is shown in Table 23-4.

In addition to these procedures, a thorough, gener-

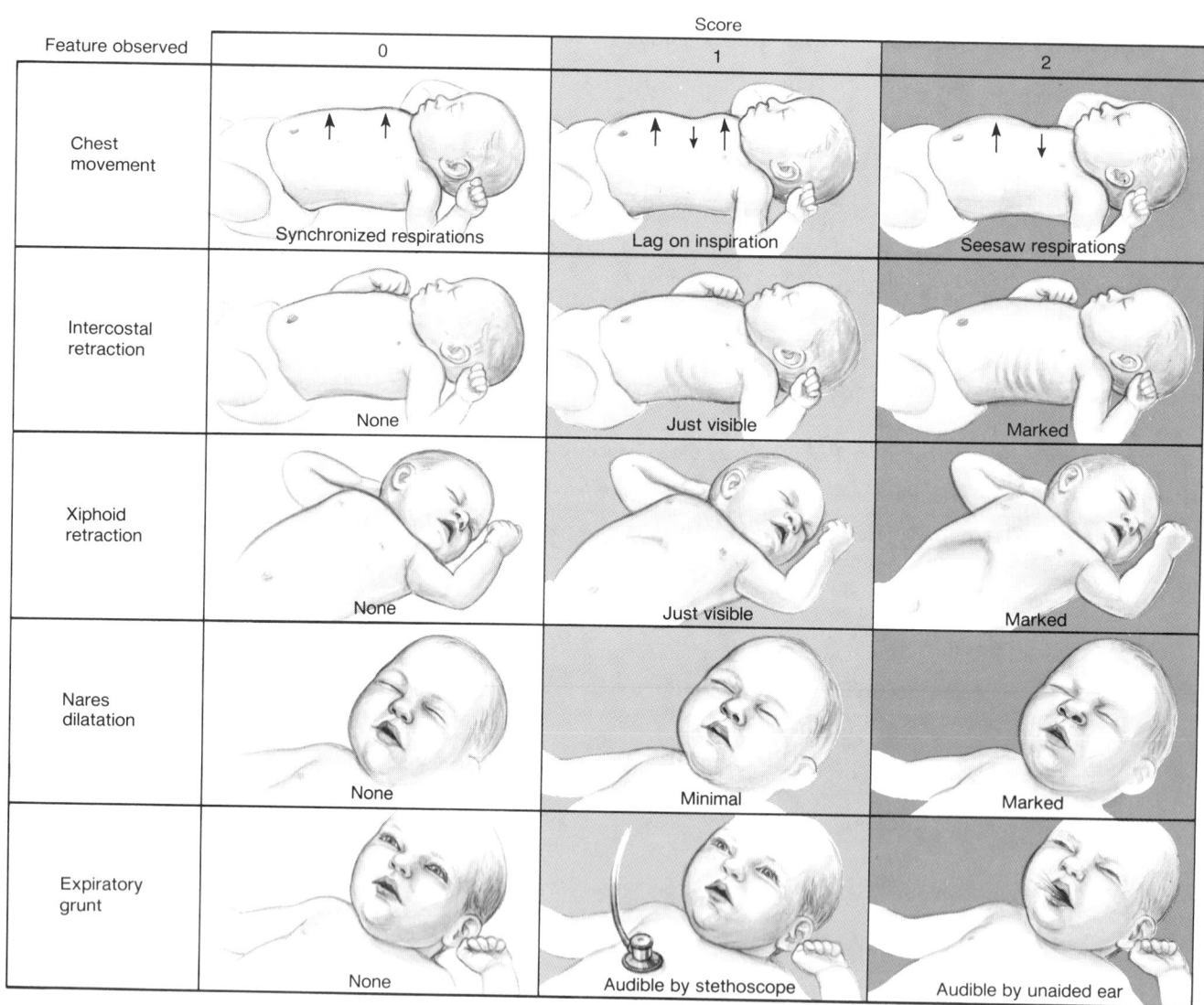

FIGURE 23-21
Grading of neonatal respiratory distress based on Silverman-Andersen index. (Silverman, W. A., & Anderson, D. H. [1956]. A controlled clinical trial of effects of water mist on obstructive respiratory signs, death rate and necroscopy findings among premature infants. Pediatrics, 17, 1.)

Table 23-4. *Congenital Anomaly Appraisal*

Procedure	Abnormalities Considered
Inquire for hydramnios or oligohydramnios	Presence of hydramnios suggests congenital gastrointestinal obstruction. Oligohydramnios suggests genitourinary obstruction or extreme prematurity.
Appearance of abdomen	Distended abdomen suggests ascites or tumor. Empty abdomen suggests diaphragmatic hernia.
Passage of nasogastric tube (No. 8 feeding catheter) through nares into stomach	Failure to pass nasogastric tube through nares on either side establishes choanal atresia. Failure to pass it into the stomach confirms presence of esophageal atresia.
Aspiration of stomach with recording of color and amount of fluid obtained	With excess of 20 mL of fluid, or yellow fluid, duodenal or ileal atresia is suspected.
Insertion of rectal catheter	Failure to obtain meconium suggests imperforate anus or higher obstruction.
Counting of umbilical arteries	The presence of one artery suggests possible congenital urinary or cardiac anomalies or chromosomal trisomy (if other portions of examination are consistent).

(From Van Leeuwen, G., & Glenn, L. [1968]. Screening for hidden congenital anomalies. *Pediatrics, 41,* 147. Copyright American Academy of Pediatrics, 1968; with permission.)

alized inspection and tentative determination of gestational age should be included in the immediate birth appraisal.

Height and Weight

The newborn should be weighed nude and without a blanket in the delivery or birthing room (Figure 23-22). Height and head, chest, and abdominal circumferences can be measured in the newborn or transitional nursery. Doing these measurements while the infant is still damp only exposes a newborn unnecessarily to chilling.

These measurements establish baselines against which all others will be compared. Thereafter, the infant is weighed nude once a day at approximately the same time every day. More frequent weighing subjects the infant to unnecessary manipulation. The weight each day should be compared with that of the preceding day to be certain that the infant is not losing more than the normal physiologic amount (5% to 10% of birth weight).

The first indication that a newborn has an inborn error of metabolism, such as adrenogenital syndrome (salt-dumping type), or is becoming dehydrated may be abnormal loss of weight.

Laboratory Studies

On admission to a nursery or after the first hour of undisturbed rest, newborns have a heel-stick hematocrit or hemoglobin determination and a Dextrostix test for hypoglycemia. Both require a minimum of blood and cause minimal trauma to the baby.

Newborn anemia is difficult to detect by clinical observation. It may be caused by hypovolemia due to bleeding from placenta previa or abruptio placentae or by a cesarean birth that involved incision into the placenta. Another condition as dangerous as anemia is the presence of an excess of red blood cells (polycythemia), probably caused by excessive flow of blood into the infant from the umbilical cord. A heel-stick hematocrit reveals both of these conditions, and treatment then can be instituted. A normal hematocrit at 1 hour of life is about 50% to 55%.

If a Dextrostix reading is less than 45 mg/100 mL of blood, it suggests hypoglycemia. The physician probably will order glucose or infant formula given orally immediately to elevate the infant's blood sugar. It is impor-

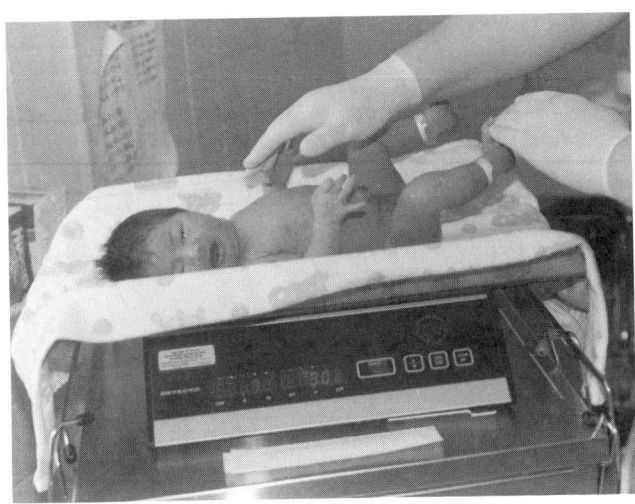

FIGURE 23-22
Weighing a newborn. Notice the protective hand held over the infant. (Courtesy, Sisters of Charity Hospital, Buffalo, NY.)

tant to treat hypoglycemia quickly, because if brain cells become completely depleted of glucose, brain damage can result. If an infant shows symptoms of hypoglycemia (jitteriness, lethargy, convulsions) in addition to the low laboratory report, intravenous glucose probably will be prescribed.

Assessment of Gestational Age

The best way to judge whether a newborn is term or not is not by the due date but by specific findings on physical assessment.

There are many indexes of maturity. Usher (1966) proposed the five criteria given in Table 23-5 as a rapid basis for evaluating gestational maturity. These are easy, quick criteria to use for assessment of all newborns.

Dubowitz Maturity Scale

Dubowitz (1970) has devised a gestational rating scale whereby newborns can be observed, tested, and rated as to maturity level based on much more extensive criteria.

All newborns that appear to be immature by Usher's criteria or who are light in weight at birth or early by dates should be assessed by means of the more definitive criteria. Although completing a Dubowitz assessment takes practice, it is a tool that can yield important results. Alone in a small community hospital nursery, debating whether an infant just born needs immediate high-risk nursery intervention or can wait until morning for transport, the nurse who can complete a Dubowitz examination and report a standardized gestational age report may make the difference in safeguarding the baby's life.

The Dubowitz scale has been modified by Ballard (1977) to an assessment that can be completed in 3 to 4 minutes. The assessment consists of two portions (Figure 23-23). The first is a series of observations about

such things as skin texture, color, lanugo, foot creases, genitalia, ear, and breast maturity. The body part is inspected and given a score of 0 to 5 as described in Figure 23-23A. This observation scoring should be done as soon as possible after birth, because skin assessment becomes much less reliable after 24 hours. Illustrations of mature and immature body parts are shown in Chapter 24 with the discussion of the preterm infant.

To complete the second half of the examination, observe or position the baby as shown in Figure 23-23B. Again, the child is given numerical scores from 0 to 5.

To establish the child's gestational age, the total score obtained (on both sections) is compared with the rating scale in Figure 23-23C. As can be seen by this scale, an infant with a total score of 5 is at 26 weeks' gestational age; a total score of 10 reveals a gestational age of about 28 weeks; a total score of 40 points is found in infants at term or 40 weeks' gestation.

Using such a standard method of rating maturity is helpful in detecting infants who are small-for-gestational age (they are light in weight but the neuromuscular and physical observation scales will be adequate for their weeks in utero) and those who are immature because of a miscalculated due date. An infant who is found to be at a lower gestational age than was predicted by the pregnancy due date needs careful observation in the neonatal period and should not be admitted to routine nursery care.

Assessment of Behavioral Capacity

Term newborns are physically active and emotionally prepared to interact with the people around them. They are people oriented from the beginning—how much so can be demonstrated by the way they immediately attune to human voices or concentrate on their mother's face (Figure 23-24).

Table 23-5. *Clinical Criteria for Gestational Assessment*

	Gestation Age (Weeks)		
Finding	*0–36*	*37–38*	*39 and over*
Sole creases	Anterior transverse crease only	Occasional creases in anterior two thirds	Sole covered with creases
Breast nodule diameter (mm)	2	4	7
Scalp hair	Fine and fuzzy	Fine and fuzzy	Coarse and silky
Ear lobe	Pliable; no cartilage	Some cartilage	Stiffened by thick cartilage
Testes and scrotum	Testes in lower canal; scrotum small; few rugae	Intermediate	Testes pendulous, scrotum full; extensive rugae

(From Usher, R., et al. [1966]. Judgment of fetal age. *Pediatric Clinics of North America, 13*, 835; with permission.)

	0	1	2	3	4	5
SKIN	gelatinous red, transparent	smooth pink, visible veins	superficial peeling &/or rash, few veins	cracking pale area, rare veins	parchment, deep cracking, no vessels	leathery, cracked, wrinkled
LANUGO	none	abundant	thinning	bald areas	mostly bald	
PLANTAR CREASES	no crease	faint red marks	anterior transverse crease only	creases ant. 2/3	creases cover entire sole	
BREAST	barely percept.	flat areola, no bud	stippled areola, 1–2 mm bud	raised areola, 3–4 mm bud	full areola, 5–10 mm bud	
EAR	pinna flat, stays folded	sl. curved pinna, soft with slow recoil	well-curv. pinna, soft but ready recoil	formed & firm with instant recoil	thick cartilage, ear stiff	
GENITALS Male	scrotum empty, no rugae		testes descending, few rugae	testes down, good rugae	testes pendulous, deep rugae	
GENITALS Female	prominent clitoris & labia minora		majora & minora equally prominent	majora large, minora small	clitoris & minora completely covered	

A

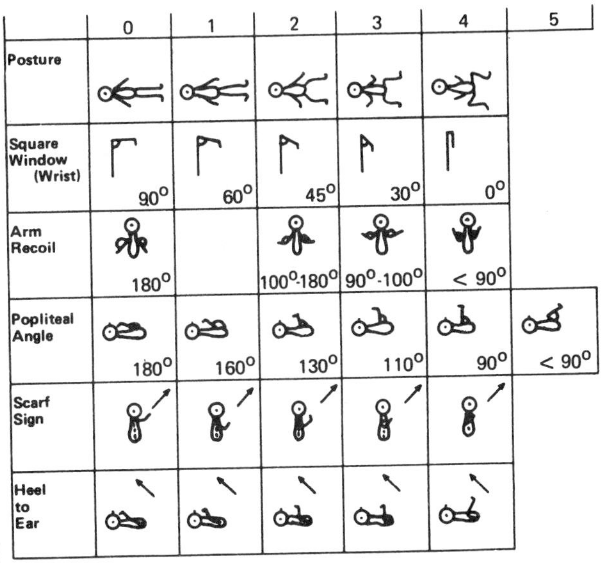

B

Score	Wks
5	26
10	28
15	30
20	32
25	34
30	36
35	38
40	40
45	42
50	44

C

FIGURE 23-23
Ballard's assessment of gestational age criteria. (A) Physical maturity assessment criteria. (B) Neuromuscular maturity assessment criteria. Posture: With infant supine and quiet, score as follows: arms and legs extended = 0; slight or moderate flexion of hips and knees = 2; legs flexed and abducted, arms slightly flexed = 3; full flexion of arms and legs = 4. Square Window: Flex hand at the wrist. Exert pressure sufficient to get as much flexion as possible. The angle between hypothenar eminence and anterior aspect of forearm is measured and scored. Do not rotate wrist. Arm Recoil: With infant supine, fully flex forearm for 5 sec, then fully extend by pulling the hands and release. Score as follows: remain extended or random movements = 0; incomplete or partial flexion = 2; brisk return to full flexion = 4. Popliteal Angle: With infant supine and pelvis flat on examining surface, flex leg on thigh and fully flex thigh with one hand. With the other hand, extend leg and score the angle attained according to the chart. Scarf Sign: With infant supine, draw infant's hand across the neck and as far across the opposite shoulder as possible. Assistance to elbow is permissible by lifting it across the body. Score according to location of the elbow: elbow reaches opposite anterior axillary line = 0; elbow between opposite anterior axillary line and midline of the thorax = 1; elbow at midline of thorax = 2; elbow does not reach midline of thorax = 3; elbow at proximal axillary line = 4. Heel to Ear: With infant supine, hold infant's foot with one hand and move it as near to the head as possible without forcing it. Keep pelvis flat on examining surface. (C) Scoring for a Ballard assessment scale. The point total from assessment is compared to the left column. The matching number in the right column reveals the infant's age in gestation weeks. (From Ballard, J.L., et al. [1977]. A simplified assessment of gestation age. Pediatric Research, 11, 374, with permission.)

Brazelton Neonatal Behavioral Assessment Scale

The *Brazelton Neonatal Behavioral Assessment Scale* is a rating scale devised by Brazelton (1973) to evaluate the newborn's behavioral capacity or ability to respond to set stimuli. Six major categories of behavior—habituation, orientation, motor maturity, variation, self-quieting ability, and social behavior—are assessed. These terms are defined in Table 23-6.

To perform an assessment using the scale requires training in the different techniques to ensure that it is used consistently from one individual to another. There are 27 behavioral items (Box 23-1), which are evaluated on a scale of 1 to 9, and 20 elicited responses or reflexes, which are scored on a 3-point scale. An average baby scores about the midpoint of each scale. Because many infants have uncoordinated behavior for the first 48 hours after birth, it is suggested that the infant be evaluated on the third day of life. Unlike many assessment scales, the infant is scored on best performance rather than on average performance. The total evaluation takes 20 to 30 minutes to complete.

Throughout the testing, the infant's state of consciousness will affect ability to perform. Prior to any stimulation activity, therefore, infants are rated as to their state, as follows:

Sleep States

1. Deep sleep with regular breathing, eyes closed, no spontaneous activity except startles or jerky movements at quiet regular intervals. No eye movements are present.
2. Light sleep with eyes closed; rapid eye movements can be observed under closed lids; low activity level, with random movements and startles or star-

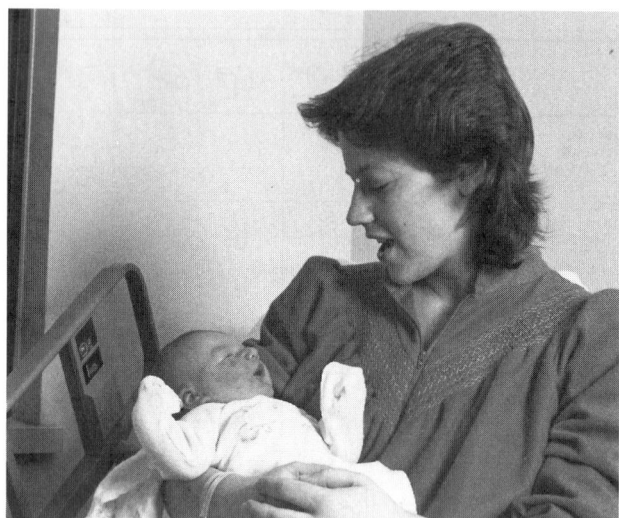

FIGURE 23-24
A newborn recognizes his caregiver's face. (Courtesy, Department of Medical Photography, Children's Hospital, Buffalo, NY.)

tle equivalents. Respirations are irregular, sucking movements occur off and on.

Awake States

1. Drowsy or semidozing; eyes may be open or closed, eyelids fluttering; activity level variable with interspersed, mild startles; reactive to sensory stimuli.
2. Alert, with bright look; seems to focus attention on source of stimulation, such as an object to be sucked or a visual or auditory stimulus. Motor activity is at a minimum.

3. Eyes open; considerable motor activity, with thrusting movement of the extremities, and even a few spontaneous startles; reactive to external stimulation with increase in startles or motor activity.
4. Crying; characterized by intense crying that is difficult to break through with stimulation.

A typical item that is scored in the assessment is the infant's response to being held in the cuddled position against an examiner's chest or shoulder. This typical item (cuddliness) is rated as 1 to 9 based on the following criteria:

1. Actively resists being held, continuously pushing away, thrashing, or stiffening.
2. Resists being held most but not all of the time.
3. Does not resist but does not participate either; lies passively in arms and against shoulder (like a sack of meal).
4. Eventually molds into arms, but after a lot of nestling and cuddling by examiner.
5. Usually molds and relaxes when first held; nestles head in crook of neck or elbow of examiner. Turns toward examiner's body when held horizontally; on shoulder, seems to lean forward.
6. Always molds initially with above activities.
7. Always molds initially with nestling, and turns toward examiner's body and leans forward.
8. In addition to molding and relaxing, baby nestles and turns head, leans forward on shoulder, fits feet into cavity of other arm; all of body participates.
9. Full, active participation; baby grasps hold of the examiner.

Table 23-6. *Categories on Brazelton Neonatal Behavioral Assessment*

Category	Description
Habituation	A newborn is capable of diminishing response to stimuli such as light, sound, and pinprick to the heel. When first stimulated this way, child may startle, respirations become more rapid, blinking becomes rapid. Gradually, a newborn shuts out the stimulus and does not respond to it.
Orientation	A newborn given an auditory or visual stimulus (bell or bright light) looks or turns toward the stimulus or at least indicates by a change of respirations awareness of the new experience being presented.
Motor maturity	The organization of the newborn's motor coordination and the degree of that coordination are assessed throughout the examination by ability to respond to the examiner's interventions.
Variation	Infants have variable degrees of peaks of excitement, general activity, color, and periods of alertness and sleep.
Self-quieting ability	When disturbed, newborns use interventions to console themselves, putting a hand to the mouth, sucking on fist or tongue, etc.
Social behavior	A newborn naturally responds to being held closely by cuddling; despite many unbelievers, a newborn can smile.

(From Brazelton, T. B. [1973]. Neonatal behavioral assessment scale. *Clinics in Developmental Medicine, 50*; 1; with permission.)

1. Response decrement to repeated visual stimuli
2. Response decrement to rattle
3. Response decrement to bell
4. Response decrement to pinprick
5. Orienting response to inanimate visual stimuli
6. Orienting response to inanimate auditory stimuli
7. Orienting response to animate visual stimuli—examiner's face
8. Orienting response to animate auditory stimuli—examiner's voice
9. Orienting responses to animate visual and auditory stimuli
10. Quality and duration of alert periods
11. General muscle tone—in resting and in response to being handled
12. Motor maturity
13. Traction responses as baby is pulled to sit
14. Cuddliness—responses to being cuddled by the examiner
15. Defensive movements—reactions to a cloth over baby's face
16. Consolability with intervention by examiner
17. Peak of excitement and capacity to control self
18. Rapidity of build-up to crying state
19. Irritability during the examination
20. General assessment of kind and degree of activity
21. Tremulousness
22. Amount of startling
23. Lability of skin color
24. Lability of states during entire examination
25. Self-quieting activity—attempts to console self and control state
26. Hand-to-mouth activity
27. Smiling

(Brazelton, T. B. [1973]. Neonatal behavioral assessment scale. *Clinics in Developmental Medicine, 50*; 1 with permission.)

Following the detailed scoring of items using the test form, a descriptive paragraph relating particular characteristics of the infant is written (Brazelton, 1973).

The information supplied by use of this scale provides the concrete evidence that newborns are not passive, nonhearing, unseeing, unresponsive, or even all alike. They can see and hear: they are able to respond to stimuli presented to them and after a time shut out the stimulus so it no longer affects them. They are able to quiet themselves after crying. They respond to the hap-

penings around them. Many of the items tested on the Brazelton assessment scale, such as how infants alert (eyes widen, head held as if listening) or orient to sound (turn toward the direction of the parent's voice or appear to listen to the sound of a voice), how they follow objects (normally, they lose them at the midline), and how they naturally cuddle when held next to their parent, are excellent examples of newborn behavior to point out to parents. If parents perceive a newborn as passive and unresponsive, they are likely to talk or look at him or her very little. If they see that right from the beginning the baby is capable of interacting with them, they are apt to be more responsive. The more they know about their baby, the more they will be able to understand the baby's cues and determine and meet his or her needs.

The descriptive paragraph on each baby is invaluable for helping everyone involved in the infant's care come to know him or her as an individual and be more able to meet newborn needs.

Care of the Newborn at Birth

An island for newborn care should be provided in a delivery or birthing room apart from the equipment needed for the mother's care. Equipment needed includes a radiant heat table or a warmed bassinet, a warm, soft blanket, and equipment for oxygen administration, resuscitation, suction, eye care, identification, and weighing the newborn.

The way babies are cared for at birth may have an effect on the child and family that lasts throughout their lives. The philosophy of caring health care providers has always been that newborns should be handled as gently at birth as they are at any other time. The image of the obstetrician holding a newborn up by the heels and spanking to stimulate breathing has existed only in Hollywood movies. It has long been accepted that holding a baby by the feet and letting the back extend fully is probably painful after the months in a flexed position in utero; a measure such as spanking is not as effective in helping a newborn to breathe as gentle stimulation such as rubbing the back.

Newborn Identification and Registration

Infant identification is important, because there always exists the possibility that a newborn may be kidnapped from a maternity service. The profile of such a kidnapper is a woman who has recently lost a pregnancy or had an infant stillborn and who desires an infant very much (Myrabo, 1993). She often is someone familiar with hospitals; she pretends to be an auxiliary worker and says she needs to take a baby off the maternity service for a procedure or to visit with a parent. Health care agency personnel need to be alert to the potential danger for kidnapping and not only take measures to prevent this from happening but also alert parents to the danger (see the Focus on Family Teaching box).

Identification Band

Some form of identification must be attached to all newborns before they are removed from the delivery or birthing room. One traditional form is a plastic bracelet or bead necklace with permanent locks that need to be cut to be removed (Figure 23-25). A number that corresponds to the mother's hospital number, the mother's full name, and the sex, date, and time of the infant's birth are the information necessary for identification. If an identification band is attached to a newborn's arm or leg, two bands should be used. A newborn's wrist and hand, as well as ankle and foot, are not too different in width, which enables the bands to slide off with little movement.

After the attachment of the identification bands, the

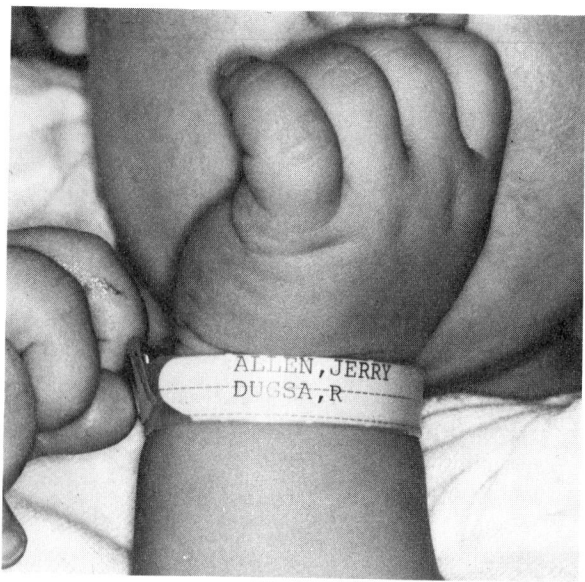

FIGURE 23-25

A newborn identification band in place. Note how the newborn's wrist is almost the size of the hand, which can allow a band to slip off easily.

infant's footprints may be taken (Figure 23-26A) and thereafter kept with the baby's chart for permanent identification. If footprints will be obtained, care should be taken in securing them, since they will be part of the permanent record (Figure 23-26B).

The following procedure will obtain accurate and identifiable prints.

1. Proper equipment must be used, including a disposable footprinter ink plate and high-gloss paper.
2. As soon as the infant is wrapped in a warm blanket, his or her foot should be wiped clean. Vernix caseosa is thus prevented from drying on it and it is easier to clean when the actual footprinting is done.
3. After respiratory and circulatory functions have been established, but before the baby is taken from the delivery or birthing room, the foot should be cleaned gently but thoroughly once more and dried. Flex the baby's knee so that the knee is close to the abdomen, and grasp the ankle between your thumb and middle finger. Next, press your index finger on the upper surface of the foot just behind the newborn's toes to prevent the toes from curling. Press the footprinter gently against the sole of the foot.
4. The footprint paper, attached to a hard surface such as a clipboard, should be pressed gently against the inked foot. The heel should be pressed on the chart first, then the foot "walked" onto the chart with a heel-to-toe motion. The foot should not be rolled back and forth in the hope of making a better print; the result will only be a blurry print.

FOCUS ON FAMILY TEACHING

Q. I'm concerned about the possibility my baby could be kidnapped from my hospital room. What can I do to help prevent this?

A. Kidnapping from a hospital unit is a rare occurrence. Here are a number of steps that can help prevent it:

- Review newborn identification procedure with a nurse so you are familiar with it and can feel comfortable with the safeguards being taken.
- Check that identification bands are in place on your infant as you care for him or her. These can slide off easily over small newborn hands and feet. If a band or necklace is missing, ask a nurse to replace it immediately.
- Don't allow any person without proper hospital identification to remove your baby from your room.
- Don't leave your baby unattended in your room. Either return the baby to the nursery or have the baby accompany you if you are leaving your room to shower, for example.
- Report the presence of any suspicious person in the unit.
- Some hospitals use a microchip system embedded in identification bands which sound an alarm if a baby is removed from the unit (similar to the type tag used to thwart shoplifting in department stores). If this type of band is used, be certain it is removed before hospital discharge or it will set off the alarm.

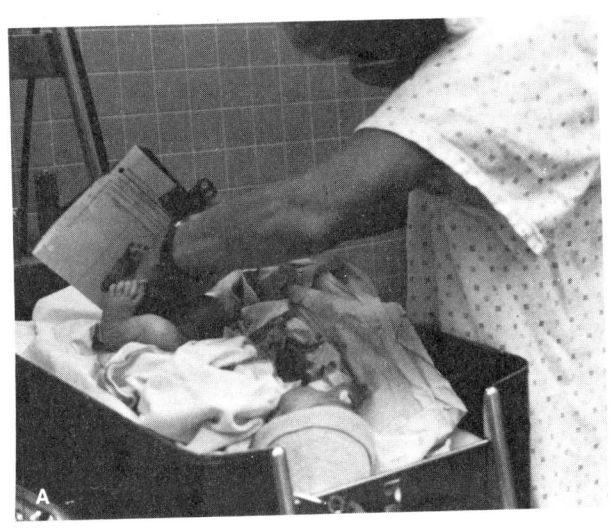

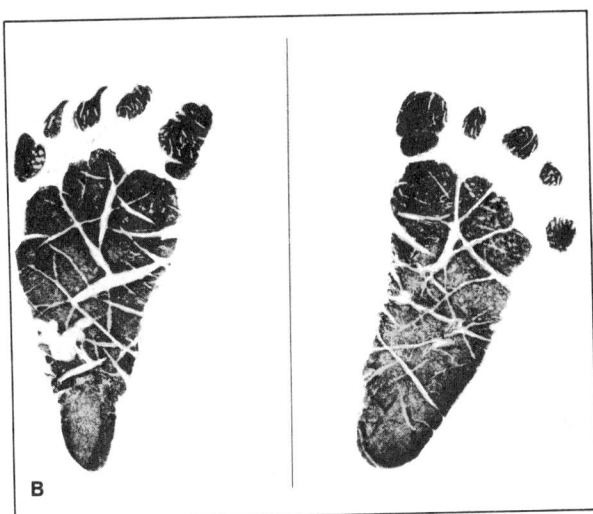

FIGURE 23-26
(**A**) *Footprinting a newborn for identification.* (**B**) *Newborn footprints.*

5. Any excess ink should be wiped from the infant's foot (a new type of carbon paper doesn't leave a black imprint). The baby should then be well swaddled to prevent chilling. The mother's index fingerprint or thumbprint is commonly placed on the same paper, along with the mother's and child's hospital number.

If footprints are required, these should be obtained on babies who are born outside the hospital when they are admitted to the hospital for follow-up care in the same way.

Birth Registration

The physician or nurse-midwife who delivered the infant must be certain a birth registration is filed with the Bureau of Vital Statistics of the state in which the infant was born. The infant's name, the mother's name, the father's name (if the mother chooses to reveal this), and the birth date and place must be recorded. Official birth information is important in proving eligibility for school and later for voting, passports, Social Security benefits, and so on.

Document Birth Record

Be certain the birth record lists the following: the time of birth; the time the infant breathed; whether respirations were spontaneous or aided; the child's Apgar score at 1 and 5 minutes of life; whether eye prophylaxis was given; whether vitamin K was administered; the general condition of the infant; the number of vessels in the umbilical cord; whether cultures were taken (they are taken if at some point sterile delivery technique was broken or the mother has a history of vaginal or uterine infection); and whether the infant (1) voided and (2) passed a stool

(the latter items are helpful if, later on, the diagnosis of bowel obstruction or absence of a kidney is considered). Many nurses indicate a three-vessel cord with the symbol shown in Figure 23-27. Do not mistake this drawing for a "smiling face" and assume it is not important.

Nursing Diagnoses and Related Interventions

In most health care facilities, the delivering physician or nurse-midwife hands the newborn to the nurse moments after birth to begin care. Be certain to don gloves to care for newborns to avoid touching the vernix caseosa as a part of following universal precautions. Holding a warm, sterile blanket, grasp the infant through the blanket by placing one hand under the back and the other around a leg. Newborns are slippery because they are wet from amniotic fluid and the vernix.

> **Nursing Diagnosis:** High risk for ineffective thermoregulation related to newborn's transition to extrauterine environment
>
> **Goal:** Newborn will establish adequate body temperature by 1 hour after birth.
>
> **Outcome Criteria:** Newborn maintains axillary temperature of 37°C.

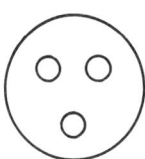

FIGURE 23-27
A chart abbreviation for a three-vessel cord.

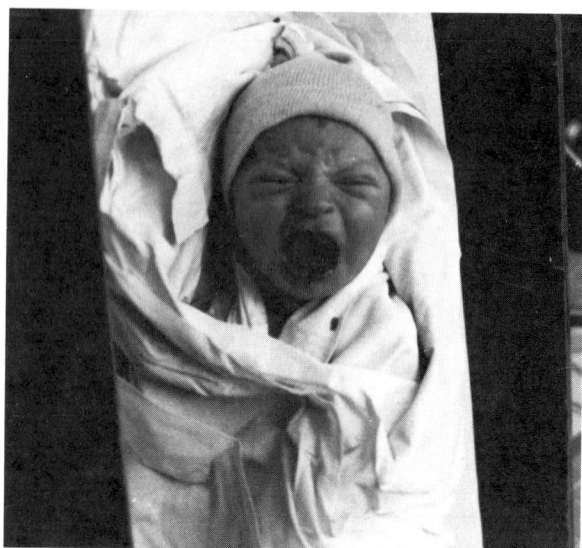

FIGURE 23-28
A newborn wrapped and capped to conserve body heat.

Keep Newborn Warm. Rub infants dry so that little body heat is lost by evaporation. Then swaddle them loosely with the blanket in order that respiratory effort is not compromised, and lay them on their side in a warmed bassinet or unwrapped on a radiant heat table. To help conserve heat, place a cap on the infant's head (Figure 23-28) and be certain all nursing care is accomplished as quickly as possible, with minimal exposure of the newborn to chilling air. Any extensive procedures, such as resuscitation, should be done under a radiant heat source to reduce heat loss.

As soon as it is apparent the infant is breathing well, ask which parent wants to hold the child and place him or her in the parent's arms. This helps conserve heat as well as encourage bonding. The period immediately following birth is an important time for parents to begin interaction. Newborns are alert (first period of activity) and respond well to their parents' first tentative touches or interaction with them. Although the temperature of newborns who are dried and wrapped and then held by their parents immediately after birth apparently falls slightly lower than that of infants placed in heated cribs, their rectal temperature does not fall below safe limits. If a mother wishes to begin breast-feeding immediately after birth, she can be encouraged to do so.

At the end of the first hour of life, reassess a newborn's temperature. Axillary temperatures are recommended for newborns to prevent bowel perforation. If the temperature is subnormal and the baby is in a bassinet, he or she should be placed in an Isolette or under a radiant warmer for additional heat. If the temperature is normal, the newborn can be bathed quickly to remove excess vernix caseosa and blood, then dressed in a shirt and diaper, reswaddled in a snug blanket or sheet (to give the baby a familiar feeling of the tight confines

of the uterus), and placed in a bassinet or returned to the mother's side.

During the first day of life, a newborn's temperature is usually taken every 4 hours. Thereafter, unless it is elevated or subnormal, or the infant appears to be in distress, once a day while in a health care facility is enough.

Nursing Diagnosis: High risk for ineffective airway clearance related to presence of mucus in mouth and nose at birth

Goal: Newborn will establish effective breathing by 5 minutes after birth.

Outcome Criteria: Respiratory rate is 30 to 60 breaths per minute without retraction or grunting sound.

Promote Adequate Breathing Pattern and Prevent Aspiration. Mucus should be suctioned from a newborn's mouth by a bulb syringe as soon as the head is born. As soon as the body is born, he or she should be held for a few seconds with the head slightly lowered for further drainage of secretions. It is important that mucus be removed from the mouth and pharynx before the first breath to prevent aspiration of the secretions. If an infant continues to have an accumulation of mucus in the mouth or nose following these first steps, you may need to suction further when the baby is placed on the warmer (Figure 23-29). Use a bulb syringe or a soft, small (No. 10 or 12) catheter to suction. Vigorous suctioning should never be employed. It irritates the mucous membrane and leaves portals of entry for infection. Brisk suctioning also has been associated with bradycardia in newborns owing to vagal nerve stimulation. If a bulb syringe is used, the bulb should be decompressed before being inserted in the infant's mouth or nose, or the force of decompression will force the secretions back into the pharynx or bronchi rather than remove

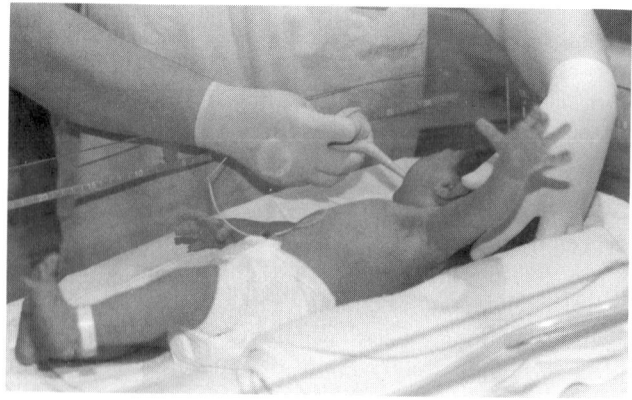

FIGURE 23-29
A newborn is suctioned by means of a bulb syringe to remove mucus from the mouth. The head-down-and-to-the-side position facilitates drainage. Care is given with the infant under a radiant heat source.

them. When an infant is born with meconium-stained amniotic fluid, it is important that the infant be not only suctioned but also intubated so that deep tracheal suction can be accomplished before the first breath. This action prevents meconium, which is very irritating to lung tissue, from being drawn into the lungs with the first breath.

Record the First Cry. A crying infant is a breathing infant, because the sound of crying is made by a current of air passing over the larynx. The more lusty the cry, the more assurance there is that the newborn is breathing deeply and forcefully. Vigorous crying also helps to blow off the extra carbon dioxide that makes all newborns slightly acidotic and thus helps to correct this condition. Although gentleness is necessary to make an infant's transition from intrauterine life to extrauterine life as untraumatic as possible, most people believe you should not be so gentle in handling newborns in the first few minutes of life that you lull them into stopping this initial crying.

It is important to note what time after birth the child first gasped and cried and whether he or she was able to maintain respirations unaided. The newborn who does not breathe spontaneously or who takes a few quick gasping breaths but is unable to maintain respirations needs resuscitation as an emergency measure. An infant with grunting respirations needs careful observation for respiratory distress syndrome (see Chapter 26).

Nursing Diagnosis: High risk for infection related to newly clamped umbilical cord and exposure of eyes to vaginal secretions

Goal: Newborn will show no signs of infection during health care agency stay.

Outcome Criteria: Area around cord is dry and not erythematous. Eyes are not inflamed or draining. Newborn's temperature is not above 38°C axillary.

Inspect and Care for Umbilical Cord. The umbilical cord pulsates for a moment after the infant is born as a last flow of blood passes from the placenta into the infant. Two Kelly clamps are then applied to the cord about 8 in from the infant's abdomen, and the cord is cut between the clamps. Some fathers choose to do this as their responsibility. The infant cord is then clamped again by a cord clamp, such as a Hazeltine or a Kane clamp. The Kelly clamp on the maternal end of the cord should not be released after cord cutting; otherwise, blood still remaining in the placenta will leak out. This loss is not important, because the mother's circulation does not connect to the placenta. It is messy, however, and that is why the clamp is left in place.

Inspect the infant's cord to be certain it is clamped securely. If the clamp loosens before thrombosis obliter-

ates the umbilical vessels, hemorrhage will result. As previously mentioned, the number of cord vessels should be counted and noted immediately after cutting of the cord. Cords begin to dry almost immediately, and by the time of the infant's first thorough physical examination in the nursery, the vessels may be obscured.

Within a few minutes after the cord is cut, assess the cord for possible bleeding; apply antibiotic ointment or triple dye as required by agency policy to help reduce infection. Until the cord falls off, at about the 7th to 10th day of life, the infant should be sponge bathed rather than immersed in a tub of water. Be certain the diaper is folded below the level of the umbilical cord so that when it becomes wet, the cord does not become wet also.

It is important to remind parents to keep the cord dry until it falls off after they return home. The use of creams, lotions, and oils near the cord should be discouraged, because they tend to slow drying of the cord and invite infection. Some health care agencies recommend dabbing rubbing alcohol on the cord once or twice a day to hasten drying; others prefer that the cord be left strictly alone.

After the cord falls off, a small, pink, granulating area about a quarter of an inch in diameter may remain. This should also be left clean and dry until it has healed (about 24 to 48 more hours). If it has remained as long as a week, it may require cautery with silver nitrate to speed healing.

Administer Eye Care. Although the practice may shortly become obsolete (as it is in Europe), every state requires that newborns receive prophylactic treatment against gonorrheal conjunctivitis of the newborn. Such infections are acquired from the mother as the infant passes through the birth canal. Formerly, this procedure was done immediately after birth. Many parents today prefer to visit with the infant before the procedure to be certain the newborn can focus on them without blurry vision from ointment or drops. As long as it is completed before the infant leaves the delivery or birthing room, the exact time the ointment is administered is unimportant. Silver nitrate is the drug that was exclusively used for prophylaxis in the past; today, erythromycin ointment is the drug of choice (Isenberg, 1990). Erythromycin ointment has the advantage of eliminating not only the organism of gonorrhea but that of chlamydia as well.

To instill ointment, the face of the newborn should be dried first with a soft gauze square so that the skin is not slippery. The best procedure to open a newborn's eyes is to shade them from the overhead light and open one eye at a time by pressure on the lower and upper lids. Use an individual tube or package of ointment to avoid transmitting infection from one newborn to another. With one eye open, squeeze a line of ointment along the lower conjunctival sac from the inner canthus outward, then close the eye to allow the ointment to spread across the conjunctiva.

Prophylaxis against gonorrheal conjunctivitis was first proposed by Credé, a German gynecologist, in 1884. For this reason, it is often referred to as the **Credé treatment** and may be listed that way on a health care agency form. Babies born outside hospitals (in taxicabs, for example) must have the prophylactic treatment administered on admission to the hospital. It is also required in babies born at home.

General Infection Precautions

Each infant in a nursery should have his or her own bassinet. Compartments in the bassinet should hold a supply of diapers, shirts, gowns, and individual equipment for bathing and temperature taking. The sharing of equipment leads to the spread of infection.

Personnel, parents, or siblings caring for newborns should wash their hands and arms to the elbows thoroughly with an antiseptic soap before handling infants. Personnel are usually required to wear cover gowns or nursery uniforms.

Personnel with infections (herpes simplex, sore throats, upper respiratory infections, skin lesions, or gastrointestinal upsets) should be excluded from caring for mothers and infants until the condition is completely cleared. Babies should be excluded from the rooms of mothers with infections. A Polaroid photograph can be taken, however, or the baby can be carried to the door of the mother's room and shown to her so that she can follow the baby's progress. If the infant is breast-fed, the mother should manually express milk during the time the infant is excluded to maintain her milk supply and allow for breast-feeding as soon as it is safe.

If central nurseries are used, the number of babies housed together should be limited. Then, if an infection occurs, it will spread to no more than a small number of babies. It is best if nurseries are limited to 6 newborns and are used on a rotating basis, so that each one can be cleaned between each group of 6 babies.

Any baby born outside the hospital or under circumstances conducive to infection (e.g., rupture of the membranes more than 24 h) should be kept in a closed Isolette or separate nursery until negative cultures show that he or she is free of infection. Any newborn in whom symptoms of infection develop (skin lesions, fever, and so forth) should be removed from a central nursery to an isolation nursery or housed in the mother's room to prevent the spread of infection to other babies. There is no reason for parents not to visit a baby housed in isolation care. They may, in fact, have more need to hold a baby who is isolated than the average parents, because they have an extra reason to be worried that something is wrong with the child. To visit in isolation nurseries, parents must use the same isolation techniques as staff members use.

Nursing Care of the Newborn and Family in the Postpartal Period

A newborn should be kept in either a birthing room or a careful watch nursery for optimal safety for the first few hours of life. After this period of careful watch, certain principles of care always apply.

Initial Feeding

A term newborn who is to be breast-fed may be fed immediately after birth. A baby who is to be formula-fed routinely receives a first feeding of about 1 oz of sterile water at 4 to 6 hours of age. This is a test feeding to be certain that the infant can swallow without gagging and aspirating and to rule out the presence of a tracheoesophageal fistula that would cause the infant to aspirate the feeding (see Chapter 39).

After this initial feeding of water, the formula-fed infant is offered formula about every 4 hours. Both formula-fed and breast-fed infants do best on a demand schedule; infants may need to be fed as often as every 2 hours for the first few days of life. Chapter 24 covers the elements of breast-feeding and formula feeding in detail.

Bathing

In most hospitals, newborns receive a complete bath to wash away vernix caseosa within an hour after birth. Thereafter, they are bathed once a day, although the procedure may be limited to washing only the baby's face, diaper area, and skin folds. Wear gloves when handling newborns until a first bath to avoid exposing your hands to body secretions; babies of HIV-positive mothers should be bathed immediately to decrease the possibility of HIV transmission (Luzuriaga & Sullivan, 1994).

Bathing of the infant may be done by the nurse at the mother's bedside or by one of the parents (Figure 23-30). The room should be warm (about 75°F [24°C]) to prevent chilling. Bath water should be around 98° to 100°F (37° to 38°C), a temperature that feels pleasantly warm to the elbow or wrist. If soap is used, it should be mild and without a hexachlorophene base. Bathing should take place prior to, not after, a feeding to prevent spitting up or vomiting and possible aspiration.

The equipment needed consists of a basin of water, soap, washcloth, towel, comb, and clean diaper and shirt. These items should be assembled beforehand, so the baby is not left exposed while the bather goes for more equipment.

Teach parents that when giving a bath, it should proceed from the cleanest to the most soiled areas of the body, that is, from the eyes and face to the trunk and extremities and, last, to the diaper area. Wipe the eyes with clear water from the inner canthus outward, using a clean portion of the washcloth for each eye to prevent

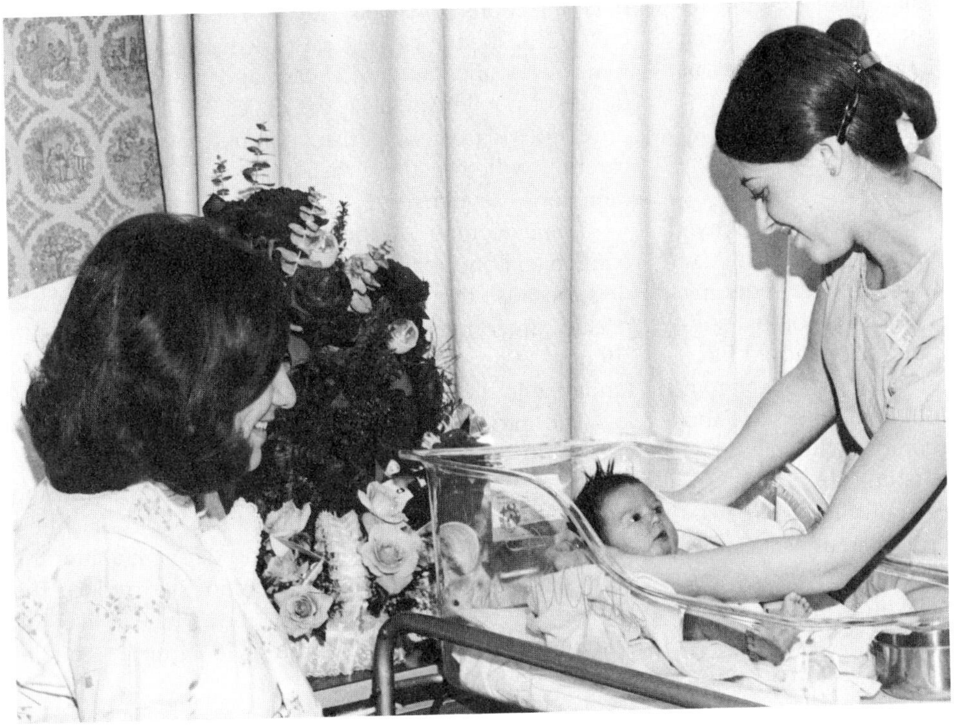

FIGURE 23-30
In a rooming-in unit, a mother has her child with her for a greater part of the day, and mother-child interaction is thus increased. Here, the nurse is demonstrating a newborn bath by the mother's bedside. (Courtesy of the Department of Medical Photography, Children's Hospital, Buffalo, NY.)

spread of infection to the other eye. Wash the face in clear water also to avoid skin irritation by soap, which may be used on the rest of the body.

Teach parents to wash the infant's hair daily with the bath. The easiest way to do this is, first, soap the hair with the baby lying in the bassinet, then hold the infant in one arm over the basin of water as you would a football (Figure 23-31). Splash water from the basin against the head to rinse the hair. Dry the hair well to prevent chilling.

Each area of the baby's body should be washed and rinsed so that no soap is left on the skin (soap is drying and newborns are susceptible to desquamation) and then dried. Wash the skin around the cord, taking care not to soak the cord. A wet cord remains in place longer than a dry one and furnishes a breeding ground for bacteria. Give particular care to the creases of skin, where milk tends to collect if the child spits up after feedings.

In male infants, the foreskin of the uncircumcised penis should not be forced back or constriction of the penis may result. Wash the vulva of female infants, wiping from front to back to prevent contamination of the vagina or urethra by rectal bacteria.

Most health care agencies do not apply powder or lotion to newborns because some infants are allergic to these products. In addition, many adult talcum powders contain zinc stearate, which is irritating to the respiratory tract; these should always be avoided. If the newborn's skin seems extremely dry, and portals for infection are becoming apparent, a lubricant such as Nivea Oil added to the bathwater or applied directly to the baby's skin should relieve the condition.

Diaper Area Care

With each change of diapers, the area should be washed with clear water and dried well. Washing the skin prevents the ammonia in urine from irritating the infant's skin and causing a diaper rash. After the cleaning, an ointment, such as petroleum jelly or A & D ointment, may be applied to the buttocks. The ointment keeps am-

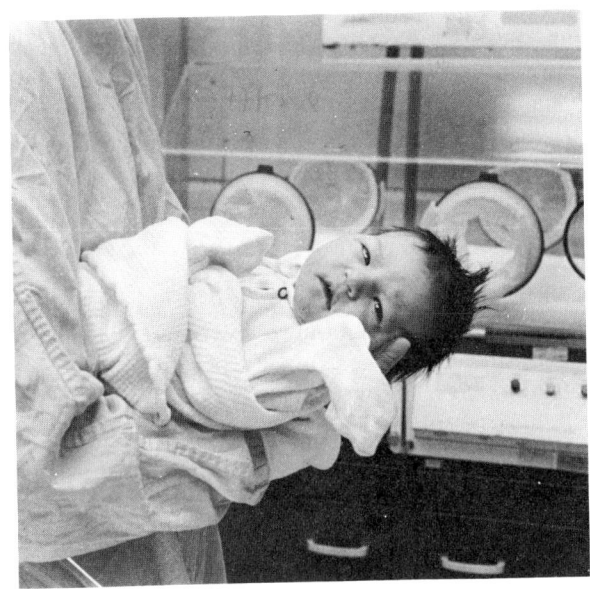

FIGURE 23-31
A football hold. Such a position supports the infant's head and back and leaves the nurse's or mother's other hand free for assembling or using equipment. (Courtesy, Department of Medical Photography, Children's Hospital, Buffalo, NY.)

monia away from the skin and also facilitates the removal of meconium, which is sticky and tarry. Wear gloves for diaper care as part of universal precautions against infection.

Metabolic Screening Tests

By state law, every infant must be screened for phenylketonuria (a disease of defective protein metabolism) by a blood test after birth. This is a simple test requiring three drops of blood from the heel dropped onto a special piece of filter paper. Ideally, the baby should have received formula or breast milk for 2 days (providing an intake of phenylalanine, an essential amino acid found in milk) before the test will be accurate. If the infant has not received adequate milk before taking the blood sample, the results may be falsely negative (a child with phenylketonuria will test as if normal). Many states further require other metabolic tests at birth (e.g., screening for hypothyroidism, galactosemia, and maple syrup urine disease) that also need filter paper blood tests.

If blood testing was not done before discharge, the parents must be made aware this was not done, so that they can return to the hospital or an ambulatory setting in 2 days' time for this. Always assess at first newborn health supervision visits whether parents did bring the baby for this testing. Like any heel prick for blood, sampling of this nature is done best by a spring-activated lancet rather than a regular lancet, so the skin incision is made quickly and painlessly.

Hepatitis B Vaccination

The Centers for Disease Control (1993) have recommended that all newborns receive a first vaccination against hepatitis B within 12 hours after birth. Infants whose mothers are HBsAg+ also receive concurrently hepatitis B immunoglobulin (HBIG). Infants will receive their second vaccination at 1 month and their third one at 6 months.

Circumcision

Circumcision is the surgical removal of the penis foreskin (Gelbaum, 1993). In only a few males, the foreskin is so constricted (phimosis) that it obstructs the urinary meatal opening; otherwise, there is no valid medical indication for circumcision of the newborn male. Circumcision is performed on Jewish males on the 8th day of life as part of a religious requirement, in a ceremony called a *bris*. In the United States, from the 1920s to the 1960s, circumcision became so popular for aesthetic reasons that virtually all male infants were routinely circumcised at birth. The reasons supporting circumcision were easier hygiene, since the foreskin does not have to be retracted during bathing, and possibly fewer urinary

tract infections (Wiswell, 1990). There may be an increased incidence of cervical cancer in the sexual partners of an uncircumcised male and an increased incidence of penile cancer in the male. Because the procedure does carry some risk, parents need to consider carefully whether they wish to have it performed on their sons (Snyder, 1991).

Some contraindications for circumcision include congenital abnormalities such as hypospadias or epispadias, because the prepuce skin may be needed when a plastic surgeon repairs the defect. Another reason not to circumcise an infant would be a history of a bleeding tendency in the family.

The procedure should not be done immediately after birth because the infant's vitamin K level, which would prevent hemorrhage, is at a low point, and the child would be exposed to unnecessary cold. It is best performed during the first or second day of life after the baby has synthesized enough vitamin K to reduce the chance of faulty blood coagulation. Parents may be asked to return the infant to the hospital or an ambulatory setting for the surgery.

For the procedure, the infant is placed in a supine position and restrained either manually or with a commercial swaddling board. The area around the penis is prepared and draped. A specially designed clamp is fitted over the end of the penis, stretching the foreskin taut (Figure 23-32*A*). This inhibits sensory conduction to the foreskin. Under sterile conditions, the prepuce of the penis is separated from the glans and a circle of the prepuce is excised so that the foreskin can be easily retracted and the glans is fully exposed (Figure 23-32 *B,C*).

Although the procedure is traditionally done without anesthesia, many practitioners use a local anesthetic or regional block anesthesia today to reduce the pain as much as possible.

Complications that can occur include hemorrhage, infection, and urethral fistula formation. To keep the risk of these complications to a minimum, infants must be observed closely for about 2 hours after circumcision and checked for hemorrhage. The penis should be wrapped with a strip of petrolatum gauze to keep the diaper from adhering to the denuded glans and also to ensure blood coagulation. The infant should be checked for bleeding every 15 minutes for the first hour. Parents should be taught that when the petrolatum gauze becomes soiled, it can be removed and the penis covered with petrolatum ointment. Circumcision sites appear red but should never have a strong odor or discharge. A film of yellowish mucus often covers the glans (similar to a scab) by the second day after surgery. This should not be washed away. The yellow color is from accumulated serum, an innocent finding, and should not be mistaken for the yellow of a purulent exudate.

Parents should keep the area clean and covered with petrolatum for about 3 days until healing is com-

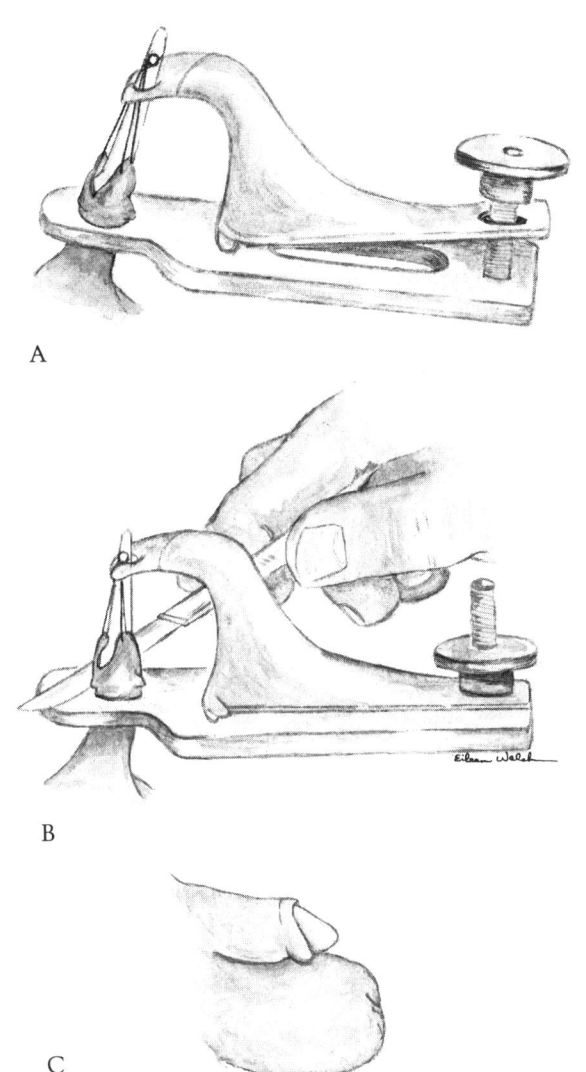

FIGURE 23-32
*Technique for performing circumcision. (**A**) Circumcision clamp in place. (**B**) The foreskin is cut. (**C**) Completed appearance.*

plete. If they see any redness or tenderness or if the baby cries as if in constant pain, they should report it by telephone.

Assessment of Family's Readiness to Care for Newborn at Home

It is important to assess how prepared a family is to care for their newborn at home. They may need to make changes in their usual routine such as shifting their usual dinner time. Sleep schedules are disrupted: infants wake during the night for one or more feedings for about the first 4 months of life.

The physical environment of the home to which a newborn will be discharged is a good subject to explore with parents. Is it an apartment or a house? How many flights of stairs will the mother have to climb when she takes the baby home or when she takes the baby out in a stroller? How many other people live in the home? Will grandparents offer support by visiting or helping with care for the child? Do the parents have anyone to turn to if they have questions about the baby? Will the baby be sleeping alone in a room or with older children? Who will be the primary caregiver?

Is there a bed for the baby? Is there a refrigerator in which formula can be stored? Is there adequate heat? An infant needs a temperature of 70° to 75°F during the day and 60° to 65°F at night. Are the windows draft free? Are they screened to keep out insects? If housing is in poor condition, is there a danger that rats might attack the baby? Is there a danger of lead poisoning? Does the mother or do the parents have a source of income? If not, what sort of referral should be made so that money can be provided to care for this child?

These are not prying questions but are a means of ascertaining whether the home that is to receive the child is adequate and safe. All the good prenatal and postnatal care is wasted if an infant contracts pneumonia the first week home, because no one at the hospital or a birthing center took the time to ask the right questions about the home environment. If a home environment is found to be unsafe, a referral to social services may be necessary before discharge of the infant.

Nursing Diagnoses and Related Interventions

Nursing Diagnosis: Health-seeking behaviors related to needs of a normal newborn following discharge from the health care facility

Goal: Parents will have a general understanding of lifestyle changes made necessary by the addition of a newborn into the family and the principles of newborn care at the time of health facility discharge.

Outcome Criteria: Parents state ways they have already altered their home and lifestyle to accommodate the newborn and indicate they are prepared for other changes; parents voice relative confidence in their ability to care for the newborn and state names of individuals within their family or community who can be resources to them when needed.

Before being discharged from a hospital or birthing center, parents should have thought through how they are going to care for their child at home. Many parents have been mulling over these questions for all 9 months of their pregnancy, but others may not have addressed some or any of the important issues. Young single mothers without family support or mothers who did not seek regular prenatal care in particular may be unprepared for the months ahead. With all parents, try to anticipate problems that may be relevant to them. If there are other children at home, discuss if they are aware that sibling jealousy may occur (see the Focus on Nursing Research box). Discuss with the mother who is not going to breast-feed what she will use to feed the baby until she has had time to buy formula. Most hospitals supply or sell a discharge formula kit to help parents through the first day home. Be sure parents have decided when and where they will take their newborn for health supervision. The child's identification band should be checked against the mother's one final time before discharge. This helps prevent the possibility of infants being confused or kidnapped (Myrabo, 1993).

Daily Care. Neonates thrive on a gentle rhythm of care, a sense of being able to anticipate what is to come next. Parents should decide what is the best daily at-home routine for them and their new child. There are no fixed rules. There is no set time an infant must be bathed or even a rule that requires a bath every day. All infants do not have to be in bed for the night by 8 PM. If the father works evenings, it may be important to have the baby awake at midnight so that he has time to spend with the child.

Your aim in helping a mother and father plan their schedule of care is to arrive at one that (1) offers a degree of consistency (a mother cannot expect an infant to stay awake until midnight five nights a week, then go to sleep at 7 PM the next); (2) appears to satisfy the infant; and (3) gives the parents a sense of well-being and contentment with their child.

Sleep Patterns. Parents may be concerned because they think the baby is sleeping too much or too little. A newborn sleeps an average of 16 hours of every 24 in the first week home and an average of 4 hours at a time. By 4 months of age, the child sleeps an average of 15 hours of every 24 and 8 hours at a time (through the night).

It is exhausting for a parent who is already tired from labor and birth to have to wake at night and feed a newborn. Because of this, parents try various methods to induce a baby to sleep through the night much earlier than 4 months. One approach is to introduce solid food (particularly cereal) in the first weeks of life on the theory that the bulk will fill the infant's stomach for the night, and therefore, he or she will not wake up crying to be fed. Actually, there is no correlation between the age at which solid food is introduced and the baby's capability for sustained sleep. A baby probably wakes every 4, 5, 6, or 8 hours because of physiologic need for fluid. Advise parents that there is no reason to try to eliminate this feeding. Knowing that their baby is not sick, that you are concerned and willing to listen to their questions, and that every other parent of a newborn is also up at night does not solve the difficulty, but it is a help.

Encourage parents to position infants on alternate sides after feedings to keep respiratory secretions or mucus from collecting or pooling in one lung or the other and to prevent flattening of one side of the head.

Crying. Many new parents are not prepared for the amount of time a newborn spends crying. Whenever the mother saw the baby while at the health care agency, the baby was sleeping. She woke the infant for feeding, and immediately he or she went back to sleep. Infants, however, typically cry an average of about 2 hours of every 24 for the first 7 weeks of life. The frequency seems to peak at age 6 or 7 weeks and then tapers off.

Almost all infants have a period during the day when they are wide awake and invariably fussy. New parents need to recognize this as normal and not worry that their child is ill. Parents might use this fussy time for bathing or playing with the infant, arranging their schedules accordingly. The most typical time for wakefulness is between 6 PM and 11 PM, which unfortunately is a time when parents may be tired and least able to tolerate crying.

Parental Concerns Related to Breathing. Some parents report that their newborns have stuffy noses or make snoring noises in their sleep and that they sneeze

FOCUS ON NURSING RESEARCH

What Are Common Reactions of Siblings to Newborns?

To answer this question, two nursing researchers asked 70 married couples expecting their second child to complete a questionnaire before the birth of the second child about what they anticipated their oldest child's reaction to the new baby would be. Parents then completed the questionnaire again after the second baby's birth and the results of the two surveys were compared.

Siblings in this study were aged 15 to 74 months. Findings revealed that siblings were more pleased with the new baby than anticipated, wanted to be involved more with the new baby than expected, and understood better than expected that parents had to care for the new baby instead of play. Making demands on the parents, wanting to play with the baby's toys, drinking from the baby's bottle, and hitting or mistreating the baby were all less than expected.

The researchers suggest that the more parents know about the possibility that sibling jealousy is to be expected, the more prepared they can be for this and the better they can help a first child adjust to a second child in the family.

Gullicks, J. N., & Crase, S. J. [1993]. Sibling behaviors with a newborn: Parents' expectations and observations. *Journal of Obstetrical, Gynecologic and Neonatal Nursing, 22,* 438.

occasionally. Most newborns continue to have some mucus in the upper respiratory tract and posterior pharynx for up to 2 weeks after birth. The snoring noise is a result of this mucus, not a cold. Infants also breathe very irregularly for about the first month. A new parent who did not room with her child at the hospital may wake at night, notice this breathing pattern, and grow alarmed that the child is in respiratory distress. If these are the only symptoms the infant has, this is a normal newborn respiratory pattern. If the child has rhinitis (nasal discharge) or a fever, he or she needs to be seen by a health care provider, since this suggests upper respiratory infection.

Continued Health Maintenance for the Newborn. There is no need for parents to continue to weigh a newborn while at home. This practice only causes worry, because weight fluctuates day by day. Parents should learn to judge an infant's state of health in terms not of increased weight but of overall appearance, eagerness to eat, general activity, and disposition.

Be certain that parents have an appointment for a visit for a first newborn assessment in 4 to 6 weeks. A mother is conscientious throughout pregnancy because she wants to bring a well child into the world. Parents must now begin a health care program that will keep the child well.

Car Safety. Automobile accidents are a safety problem all during childhood (Stewart, 1993). Frequently, infants are injured in car accidents because they are laid on the seat of a car rather than placed in an infant's car seat. If the car stops suddenly, the infant may be thrown onto the floor or, in a collision, thrown out of the car or through the windshield. Many parents do not think initially of a car seat being an essential piece of baby equipment. They envision buying one when the baby sits up. Infant car seats are important from the beginning, however, because in an accident, centrifugal force will cause the infant to exert a force equal to as much as 450 lb, making it impossible for a passenger to hold onto him or her. At only 30 mph, the infant may hit the dashboard with the force equal to a fall from a three-story building. If the adult holding the infant is not wearing a seat belt, the adult can be thrown against the infant and actually kill the child.

In January 1981, a federal safety standard took effect that required infant car seats to meet rigid standards of safety. When purchasing a seat, parents should look at the label to be certain the seat meets these federal guidelines. A local health department or Red Cross chapter should have a list of all the car seats available in a particular area and give details of their comparable features and cost. Some hospitals and Red Cross chapters loan infant car seats for temporary use, such as visiting with grandparents or when first coming home from the hospital.

While an infant is less than 21 lb or 26 inches long, the best type of car seat is an "infant-only" seat that faces the back of the car. It is fairly lightweight and can double as a household seat (Figure 23-33). The ideal model has a five-point harness with broad straps, which help to spread the force of a collision over the chest and hips, and a shield, which cushions the head.

Parents should dress an infant in clothing with pant legs when the infant must be placed in a car seat, because the harness crotch strap must pass between the legs for a snug and correct fit. Advise parents not to use a sack sleeper or papoose bunting, nor should they wrap the baby in a bulky blanket while in the seat. To support the baby's head, parents can use a rolled-up receiving blanket, towel, or diaper on each side of the head. To provide extra warmth, they can cut holes in a blanket for the harness and crotch straps to pass through. Teach parents how to put the blanket in the seat and pull the straps through the blanket holes. Place the baby in the seat, buckle him in, then fold the blanket over him for warmth. Drape a second blanket over the seat if needed.

A parent should keep the seat in a backward-facing position until the child is able to sit up without support

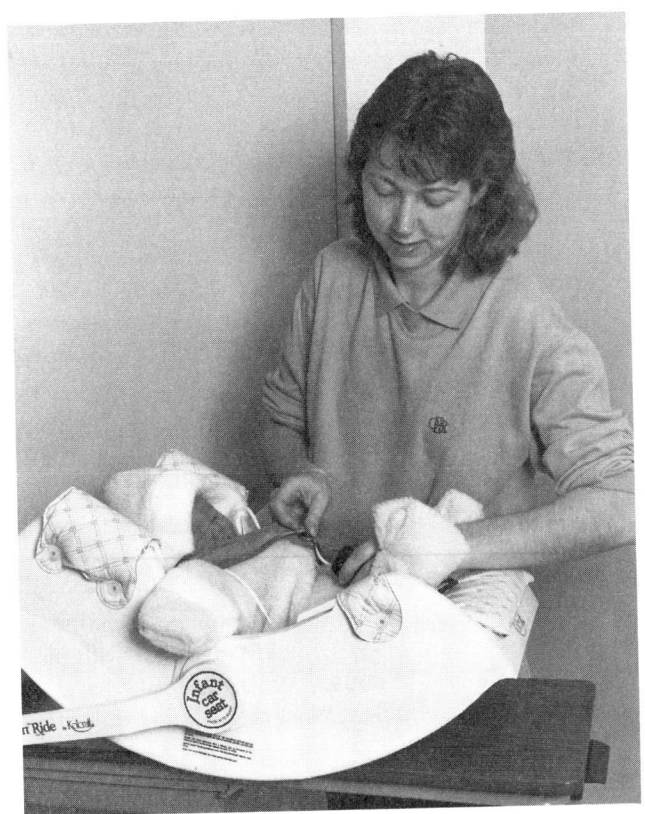

FIGURE 23-33
Most states require infants and children to ride in car seats. It is the nurse's responsibility to make sure that every parent planning to drive a child home from the hospital is properly equipped. (Courtesy, Department of Medical Photography, Children's Hospital, Buffalo, NY.)

or struggles to sit up, usually when the infant weighs about 21 lb. The infant then is old enough for a toddler seat. Caution parents that plastic car seats grow extremely hot in the summer, and they should test the temperature of the surface before placing the infant in it. It should be stressed to parents that it is dangerous to not use the car seat properly, such as not fastening the harness or not securing the seatbelt.

Key Points

- Converting from fetal to adult respiratory function is a major step in adaptation to extrauterine life. Newborns need particularly close observation during the first few hours of life to determine that this adaptation has been made adequately.
- Monitoring body heat is a second major problem of newborns. The temperature of the term baby's environment should be about 75°F (24°C). When procedures that require undressing the infant for an extended period of time are being done (e.g., circumcision), a radiant heat source should be used.
- Newborns may suffer hypoglycemia in the first few hours of life, because they use energy to establish respirations and maintain heat. Signs of jitteriness and a serum glucose under 45 mg by Destrostix help to identify hypoglycemia.
- Identification bands should be attached securely to the infant; careful assessment of these bands should be carried out before hospital discharge. To help prevent the possibility of kidnapping on a newborn unit be certain of the identification of anyone to whom you give a newborn.
- So that parents can feel confident with newborn care, they need to hold and give care to newborns in the hospital. Encouraging them to spend as much time as possible with the newborn and to give care is a major nursing role.
- The best method of care for newborns and their mothers is rooming-in, which allows women to have maximum contact with their new baby.

Critical Thinking Exercises

1. Baby Dowe is a newborn you examine at birth. What newborn reflexes would you assess with him? Suppose it is cold in the room so you only have time to test one reflex. What one would you test? Why?
2. Baby Okasuki is a newborn with a macular purple (port-wine) lesion on her left thigh. Her parents tell you they are not concerned because they know all birthmarks fade by the time children are school-age. Suppose this type of lesion is one that doesn't fade? How would you respond to the parents?
3. The Towers are a family who are getting ready to go home from the hospital with their newborn when you discover that they have no car seat to transport the baby. What would you do? Ask them to stay until they arrange to rent or borrow one? Suppose they insist on putting the baby in the car without a car seat? Do you have a legal obligation to detain them in the health care agency?

References

Apgar, V., et al. (1958). Evaluation of the newborn infant: Second report. *Journal of the American Medical Association, 168,* 1985.

Ballard, J. L., et al. (1977). A simplified assessment of gestational age. *Pediatric Research, 11,* 374.

Brazelton, T. B. (1973). Neonatal behavioral assessment scale. *Clinics in Developmental Medicine, 50,* 1.

Centers for Disease Control. (1993). General recommendations on immunizations. *Morbidity and Mortality Weekly Report, 43,* 9.

Cochran, W. D. (1990). Management of the normal newborn. In Oski, F. A. *Principles and practice of pediatrics.* Philadelphia: J. B. Lippincott.

Damstra-Wijmenga, S. M. (1991). The memory of the newborn. *Midwives Chronicle, 104,* 66.

Department of Health and Human Services. (1991). *Healthy people 2000.* Washington, DC: Public Health Service.

Desmond, M. N., et al. (1963). The clinical behavior of the newly born: The term infant. *Journal of Pediatrics, 62,* 307.

Dubowitz, L., et al. (1970). Clinical assessment of gestational age in the newborn infant. *Journal of Pediatrics, 77,* 1.

Geissler, E. M. (1994). *Pocket guide to cultural assessment.* St. Louis: C. V. Mosby.

Gelbaum, I. (1993). Circumcision: Refining a traditional surgical technique. *Journal of Nurse Midwifery, 38,* 2S.

Isenberg, S. J. (1990). The dilemma of neonatal ophthalmic prophylaxis. *Western Journal of Medicine, 153,* 190.

Luzuriaga, K., & Sullivan, J. L. (1994). Pathogenesis of vertical HIV-1 infection: implications for interventions and management. *Pediatric Annals, 23,* 159.

Myrabo, J. (1993). Neonatal kidnapping. *Journal of Obstetric, Gynecologic and Neonatal Nursing, 22,* 105.

Schumacher, R. E. (1990). Noninvasive measurements of bilirubin in the newborn. *Clinics in Perinatology, 17,* 417.

Silverman, W. A., & Anderson, D. H. (1956). A controlled clinical trial of effects of water mist on obstructive respiratory signs, death rate and necroscopy findings among premature infants. *Pediatrics, 17,* 1.

Snyder, H. M. (1991). To circumcise or not. *Hospital Practice, 26,* 201.

Stewart, D. D. (1993). Child passenger safety: Current technical issues for advocates and professionals. *Family and Community Health, 15,* 12.

Sullivan, R. M., et al. (1991). Olfactory classical conditioning in neonates. *Pediatrics, 87,* 511.

Usher, R., et al. (1966). Judgment of fetal age. *Pediatric Clinics of North America, 13,* 835.

Wegman, M. E. (1992). Annual summary of vital statistics. *Pediatrics, 90,* 1835.

Wegman, M. E. (1993). Annual summary of vital statistics. *Pediatrics, 92,* 743.

Wiswell, T. E. (1990). Routine neonatal circumcision: A reappraisal. *American Family Physician, 41,* 859.

Suggested Readings

Allen, H. D., Golinico, R. J., & Williams, R. G. (1994). Heart murmurs in children: When is a workup needed? *Patient Care, 28,* 123.

Borris, L. C. (1992). Complications of heel pad punctures for blood sampling in the newborn. *Neonatal Intensive Care, 5,* 63.

Kenner, C., et al. (1993). Transition from hospital to home for mothers and babies. *Neonatal Network, 12,* 73.

Lynam, L. E. (1990). An introduction to neonatal pulmonology. *Neonatal Network, 8,* 75.

Mayberry, L. J., et al. (1993). Infant temperament and postpartum depression. *Health Care of Women International, 14,* 201.

Shapiro, C. R. (1993). Nurses' judgments of pain in term and preterm newborns. *Journal of Obstetric, Gynecologic and Neonatal Nursing, 22,* 41.

Symanski, M. E. (1991). Action STAT. Neonatal sepsis. *Nursing, 21,* 33.

Wenger, A. F. (1993). Teaching families from diverse cultural backgrounds. *Neonatal Network, 12,* 69.

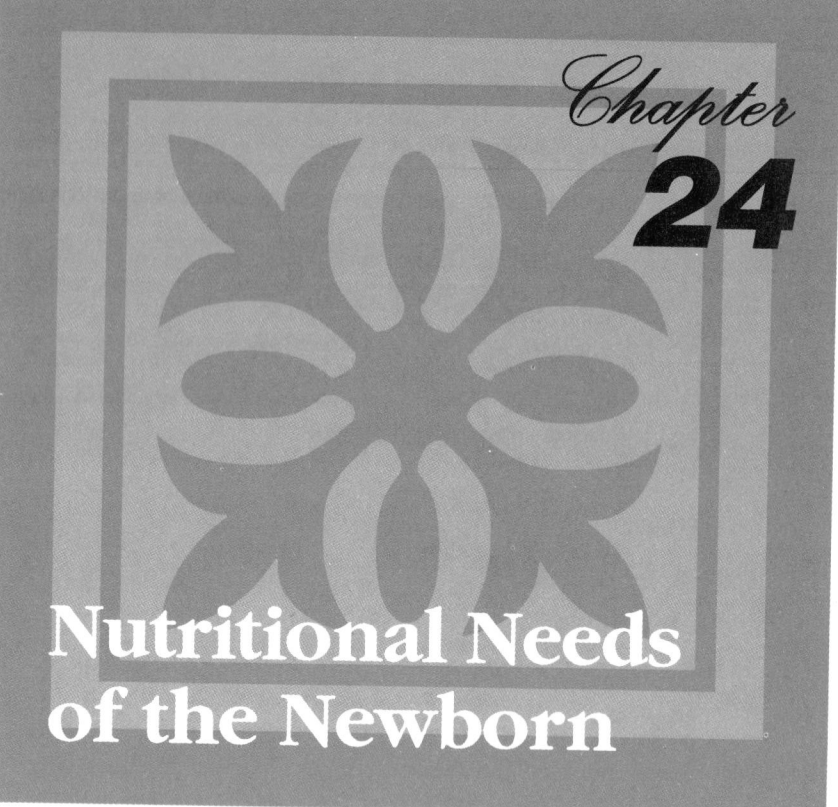

Chapter 24

Nutritional Needs of the Newborn

Objectives

After mastering the contents of this chapter, you should be able to:

1. Describe nutritional requirements of the term newborn.

2. Assess nutritional intake of a newborn to determine if he or she is receiving adequate nutrition.

3. State nursing diagnoses related to newborn nutrition.

4. Plan with a mother a method of infant feeding that will be satisfying for both her and the infant.

5. Implement feeding procedures with newborn infants such as giving a first feeding.

6. Evaluate goal outcomes in relation to nutrition to be certain nursing goals were achieved.

7. Identify National Health Goals related to newborn nutrition that nurses can be instrumental in helping the nation achieve.

8. Identify areas related to nutrition and newborns that could benefit from additional nursing research.

9. Use critical thinking to analyze ways that nurses can help mothers problem-solve feeding difficulties and make newborn nutrition more family centered.

10. Synthesize knowledge of normal newborn nutrition with nursing process to achieve quality maternal and child health nursing care.

Adele Pillitteri: MATERNAL AND CHILD
HEALTH NURSING, 2nd Edition. © 1995
Adele Pillitteri.

Because proper nutrition is essential for optimal growth and development, knowledge of the newborn's nutritional needs is a fundamental requirement for nurses in maternal and child health care. In no other area of nutrition, with the possible exception of weight control or diabetes mellitus, is the nurse asked more questions.

Nutrition is extremely important in the early months of life because brain growth is proceeding at such a rapid rate during this time. Breastfeeding is, for many reasons, the method of choice for providing proper nutrition for human infants. Providing adequate food and nutrition for the newborn extends beyond physiologic need, however. The importance of feeding in terms of the maternal stimulation and love the infant receives in the process cannot be overstated. The parent is close to the infant during feeding time, and the baby will be particularly sensitive to the mother's demonstration of affection or lack of warmth. The infant who does not experience during feedings a warm relationship with the mother or primary caregiver may fail to thrive as surely as the one who is denied sufficient protein or calories. National Health Goals related to newborn nutrition are shown in the Focus on National Health Goals box.

⊞ NURSING PROCESS OVERVIEW for Promotion of Nutritional Health in the Newborn

ASSESSMENT

Assessment of infant nutrition begins in pregnancy with assessment of the mother's (and father's) attitudes and choices about infant feeding. It is well accepted that breastfeeding is the preferred method of newborn nutrition; however, if a particular mother does not choose to breastfeed, she should not be made to feel guilty for her choice. Every person's circumstances are unique. What matters most is that the parents feel comfortable with and confident about the feeding method they have chosen.

Once infant feeding begins, teach a mother to assess whether the amount the infant is receiving is adequate—not by how long the baby takes to empty a breast or a bottle but by whether he or she is growing, voiding, and alert.

NURSING DIAGNOSIS

Assessment of a mother's choice regarding method of feeding and a newborn's nutritional intake and feeding patterns may yield several important nursing diagnoses, although it may be difficult to establish diagnoses during the first part of the newborn period when a mother and infant are still getting used to each other. Examples are:

- Effective breastfeeding related to well-prepared mother and healthy newborn
- High risk for ineffective breastfeeding related to extreme engorgement
- Altered nutrition: less than body requirements related to poor sucking response in newborn
- Altered parenting related to ineffective coping secondary to father feeling resentment because the mother is breastfeeding

PLANNING

Plans made when a woman is still pregnant will focus on providing her with the information she needs to make a knowledgeable choice about breast or bottle feeding. If she makes a decision during pregnancy, that information also can include nutritional needs of the breastfeeding woman. The woman who expects to bottle feed can purchase supplies in advance.

IMPLEMENTATION

A major intervention related to newborn nutrition is supporting a mother's choice of feeding method and helping her to trust her judgment as to when her infant is full and content. Help mothers to make either type of feeding as natural as possible by being certain they are comfortable and relaxed and by removing any unnecessary distractions. A referral to support groups such as La Leche League (9616 Minneapolis Ave., Franklin Park, IL 60131) or International Lactation Consultant Association (201 Brown Avenue, Evanston, IL 60202-3601) might be appropriate. In addition to sponsoring classes on breast-

feeding, a helpful service of La Leche League is its hot-line, through which a breastfeeding woman who is discouraged or is having difficulty can contact a member and ask for advice. *The Womanly Art of Breastfeeding*, published by the League (1991), is a comprehensive and readable book for women. Chapter 34 discusses the addition of solid food for the second half of the first year.

EVALUATION

Evaluation is an important step in this process. Unforeseen circumstances, such as unsuspected milk allergy or mastitis (breast infection) may drastically change goals. Help parents to understand that newborns are adjustable and can adapt to another feeding method if necessary. Examples of outcome criteria related to newborn feeding might be:

- Infant breastfeeds every 3 hours; is content and sleeps between feedings.
- Infant ingests a total of 12 oz formula with iron every 24 hours.
- Mother states she is satisfied with chosen method of infant feeding.

Nutritional Allowances for the Newborn

Calories

Growth in the neonatal period and early infancy is more rapid than at any other period of life. Therefore, the caloric requirements exceed those at any other age. A newborn and an infant up to 2 months of age requires 120 calories per kilogram of body weight (50 to 55 kcal/lb) every 24 hours to provide an adequate amount of food for maintenance and allow for growth as well. After 2 months of age, the amount gradually declines until the requirement at 1 year has decreased to 100 kcal/kg, or 45 kcal/lb/day. In adults, the requirement is 42 kcal/kg, or 20 kcal/lb/day.

The actual caloric requirement, of course, depends on the activity of the baby and the rate of growth. An active infant, one who cries frequently and squirms constantly, will need more calories than one who is more passive and is content to spend long hours playing quietly or just studying the environment.

Many parents tend to feed their babies more formula than babies physiologically need (especially extra quantities of milk), believing that a chubby-cheeked baby is a healthy one. This is not necessarily true. Although the tendency for obesity may be inherited and

FOCUS ON
National Health Goals

Two National Health Goals address nutrition of the newborn. These are:

- Increase to at least 75% from a baseline of 54% the proportion of mothers who breastfeed their babies in the early postpartum period and to at least 50% from a baseline of 21% the proportion who continue breastfeeding until their babies are 5 to 6 months old.
- Increase to at least 75% the proportion of parents and caregivers who use feeding practices that prevent baby bottle tooth decay (DHHS, 1991).

Nurses can be instrumental in helping the nation achieve these goals by educating woman about breastfeeding during pregnancy and supporting the family during the postpartal period while the woman is breastfeeding. Home visits with postpartal families or well child health assessments provide opportunities to advocate for continuing breastfeeding. For the woman who will formula feed her infant, education during pregnancy should include not putting the infant to bed with a bottle of milk or juice to prevent baby bottle tooth decay.

Areas related to this that could benefit from additional nursing research are techniques parents use to initiate sleep without using a bedtime bottle; reasons women discontinue breastfeeding early in the postpartal period; and legislation or education necessary in the workplace to encourage women to continue breastfeeding after they return to work.

thus cannot be controlled, an overweight baby may be more likely to become an overweight adult than one whose weight is within the usual range during the first year of life. This is because when fat cells in the infant increase in size, they remain large, so that such a baby tends to be obese ever afterward.

A formula should contain about 9% to 12% of the calories as protein and 45% to 55% of the calories as lactose carbohydrate. The balance should be fat, of which about 10% (4% of the calories) should be linoleic acid.

Protein

Because of the extremely rapid growth during infancy and because protein is necessary for the formation of new cells and the maturation and maintenance of existing cells, protein requirements are high during the newborn and infancy periods. The nutritional allowance of protein for the first 2 months of life is 2.2 g per kilogram of body weight. Both human milk and cow's milk provide all the essential amino acids. Histidine, an amino acid that appears to be essential for infant growth but is not necessary for adult growth, is found in both forms of milk.

Cow's milk contains about 16% of its calories as protein; human milk, about 8%. Cow's milk creates such a rich solute load (the amount of urea and electrolytes that must be excreted in the urine) that newborn kidneys can be overwhelmed by it. The protein in cow's milk differs from that in human milk in composition as well as in amount. The main protein in human milk is lactalbumin; the main protein in cow's milk is casein. The curd tension in milk is related to the amount of casein present. Thus, the curd in cow's milk is large, tough, and difficult to digest; in human milk, the curd is softer and easier to digest. This is why newborns who are bottle fed need formula, not cow's milk.

Fat

Linoleic acid is an essential fatty acid necessary for growth and skin integrity in infants. It is found in both human and cow's milk, but human milk contains about three times as much. Infants fed on skimmed milk for long periods of time (when other sources of food are not being offered) may become deficient in linoleic acid. Therefore, feeding skimmed milk is not the answer to controlling obesity in young infants. In addition, skimmed milk does not contain sufficient calories (only about half as many as nonskim milk).

Carbohydrate

Lactose, the disaccharide found in human milk, appears to be the most easily digested of the carbohydrates. It also improves calcium absorption and aids in nitrogen retention, both of which are positive factors. When included in a formula, it produces stools in which gram-positive rather than gram-negative bacteria predominate, close to those of a breastfed baby, another positive factor as this decreases the possibility of gastrointestinal illness. It is important that formula contain adequate carbohydrate as this allows protein to be used for building new cells rather than for calories, encouraging normal water balance, and preventing abnormal metabolism of fat.

Cow's milk contains about 29% of its calories as carbohydrate; human milk, 37%. Cow's milk formulas need added carbohydrate to bring their carbohydrate content up to that of human milk.

Fluid

Maintaining a sufficient fluid intake in newborns is important because their metabolic rate is high and metabolism requires water. An adult uses 25 to 30 kcal per kilogram of body weight in 24 hours for metabolism. In the same period, a newborn utilizes 45 to 50 kcal/kg. This high rate of metabolism requires a large amount of water. In addition, the surface area of the newborn is large in relation to body mass. Thus, a baby loses a larger amount of water by evaporation than does an adult.

Water is distributed differently in the newborn than in the adult. In an adult, about 20% of body weight is extracellular fluid; in a newborn, 30% to 35% of body weight is extracellular fluid. Consequently, loss of fluid or inadequate fluid intake, which depletes the extracellular water supply, can affect as much as 35% of the newborn's fluid component. Because the kidneys of a newborn are not yet capable of fully concentrating urine, the newborn cannot conserve body water by this mechanism and must have an adequate fluid intake to prevent dehydration.

The fluid requirement for a newborn is 150 to 200 mL/kg (2.5 to 3.0 oz/lb) per 24 hours.

Minerals

A number of minerals are particularly important to early growth.

Calcium

Calcium is an important mineral because of its contribution to bone growth. Because milk is high in calcium, tetany from a low calcium level seldom occurs in infants who suck well, whether taking human milk or cow's milk formula. Both milks contain more calcium than phosphorus, but the ratio is higher in human milk than in cow's milk (2:1 versus 1.2:1).

Iron

The infant of a mother who had an adequate iron intake during pregnancy will be born with iron stores that, theoretically, will last for the first 3 months of life, until he or she begins to produce adult hemoglobin. Infants are vulnerable to anemia at that time (Mills, 1990). Because not all mothers' diets are iron-rich during pregnancy (and socioeconomic level is not a good criterion for judging the quality of a diet), the American Academy of Pediatrics (1976b) recommends that an iron supplement be included in formula for formula-fed infants for the entire first year of life. It is unnecessary to supplement iron in the breastfed infant.

Fluoride

Fluoride is essential for building sound teeth and for resistance to tooth decay. Because teeth grow into their primary form during pregnancy, it is important for mothers to drink fluoridated water during pregnancy. The lactating mother should continue drinking fluoridated water (although fluoride does not pass in great amounts in breast milk), and formulas should be prepared with fluoridated water. This is an essential point to remember, because a mother may think she is helping her child by using bottled, "natural" water in a formula rather than chlorinated (but fluoridated) water from a tap.

If a mother is breastfeeding and a source of fluoridated water is not available (the family drinks well, spring, or bottled water, or the tap water is not fluoridated), it is recommended that a fluoride supplement, 0.25 mg daily, be given to the infant.

Vitamins

Vitamin additives are necessary for the bottle-fed infant. The American Academy of Pediatrics (1980) recommends supplemental multivitamins (A, C, and D) for the entire first year of life. These vitamins are incorporated into commercially prepared formulas and are not necessary for breastfed infants because of their natural inclusion in breast milk. If the breastfed newborn will not be exposed to sunlight for some reason, four hundred units of vitamin D daily may be prescribed for the mother to increase this level in breast milk, or given to the infant.

Breastfeeding

Breast milk provides numerous health benefits to both the mother and infant and is generally considered to be the superior source of nutrition for infants through the first year of life. Nurses can play a major role in teaching women about the benefits of breastfeeding and providing anticipatory guidance for problems that may occur so increasing numbers of women choose breastfeeding.

Physiology of Breast Milk Production

Breast milk is formed in the acinar or alveolar cells of the mammary glands (see Chapter 4). With the delivery of the placenta, the level of progesterone in the mother's body falls dramatically, stimulating the production of **prolactin**, an anterior pituitary hormone. Prolactin acts on the acinar cells of the mammary glands to stimulate the production of milk. Moreover, when an infant sucks at the breast, nerve impulses travel from the nipple to the hypothalamus to stimulate the production of prolactin-releasing factor. This factor then passes to the pituitary and stimulates further active production of prolactin. Other anterior pituitary hormones, such as adrenocorticosteroid hormone, thyroid-stimulating hormone, and growth hormone, probably also play a role in growth of the mammary glands and their ability to secrete milk.

Milk flows from alveolar cells through small tubules to reservoirs for milk, **lactiferous sinuses**, behind the nipple. This constantly forming milk is called **foremilk**. Its availability depends very little on the infant's sucking at the breast. It is produced in all women 3 to 4 days after birth.

For the first 3 or 4 days after birth, the milk cells produce **colostrum**, a thin, watery, high-protein fluid composed of protein, sugar, fat, water, minerals, vitamins, and maternal antibodies. Colostrum actually is secreted by the acinar cells starting in the fourth month of pregnancy. Because it is high in protein and fairly low in sugar and fat, it is easy to digest. It also provides totally adequate nutrition for the infant until milk begins to flow.

As the infant sucks at the breast, oxytocin is released from the posterior pituitary. Oxytocin causes the collecting sinuses of the mammary glands to contract, forcing milk forward through the nipples and making it available for the baby. This action is the **let-down reflex**. In addition, new milk, called **hind milk**, is formed after the let-down reflex. Hind milk tends to be higher in fat than foremilk and is the milk that makes the breastfed infant grow most rapidly. Oxytocin causes smooth muscle to contract, so when it is produced, the uterus contracts as well. As a result, the woman will feel a small tugging or cramping in her lower pelvis during the first few days of breastfeeding.

Prolonged Jaundice in Breastfed Infants

Physiologic jaundice may occur in as many as nearly 50% of breastfed infants (Brown et al., 1993). This is because pregnanediol (a breakdown product of progesterone) in breast milk depresses the action of glucuronyl transferase, the enzyme that converts indirect bilirubin to the direct form, which is readily excreted. To prevent hyperbilirubinemia in the infant, women should feed frequently in the immediate birth period as colostrum is a natural laxative and helps promote passage of meconium, lowering the potential for jaundice. Breastfeeding rarely results in a serum bilirubin high enough to warrant therapy as pregnanediol remains in breast milk for only 24 to 48 hours (Martinez et al., 1993). If extreme jaundice does occur (bilirubin above 15 or 16 mg/dL), discontinuing breastfeeding for 1 or 2 days usually corrects the problem as by this time, the pregnanediol level in the breast milk will have decreased. The woman should pump her breasts manually during this time to protect her supply of milk.

Advantages of Breastfeeding

Women who are most likely to breastfeed are generally older, well-educated, married, and have participated in prenatal care (Serdula et al., 1991; Hills-Bonczyk et al., 1993). The easiest way for a woman to decide whether or not to breastfeed is to ask herself what would please her most and make her most comfortable. If she is comfortable and pleased with what she is doing, her infant will be comfortable and pleased, will enjoy being fed, and will thrive.

Advantages for the Mother

The woman gains several physiologic benefits from breastfeeding, such as:

1. Breastfeeding may serve as a protective function in preventing breast cancer.
2. The release of oxytocin from the posterior pituitary aids uterine involution (Riordan & Auerbach, 1993).
3. Successful breastfeeding can have an empowering effect (Locklin & Naber, 1993).
4. Breastfed infants appear to have higher scores on intelligence tests than formula-fed infants (Oski, 1993).

Breastfeeding has additional benefits of reducing the cost of feeding and time of preparation of formula. Many woman feel that breastfeeding will give them the best chance of forming a true symbiotic bond with their child. Although this does occur readily with breastfeeding, a woman who holds her baby to bottle feed can form this bond equally well. Some women believe that breastfeeding is a foolproof contraceptive technique; this is incorrect. Among women who breastfeed, 50% resume ovulating by the 4th week postpartum (Gray et al., 1990). Some feel breastfeeding will best help them lose weight gained during pregnancy; this is not true (Potter et al., 1991). Some woman are reluctant to breastfeed because they fear that having to be available to feed the baby every 3 or 4 hours will tie them down. Like mothers who bottle feed, however, they can leave a bottle (with expressed breast milk or formula) with the baby's father or a babysitter if they need to be away from the baby during a feeding. Regardless of feeding method, women should have time away from their babies occasionally.

Advantages for the Baby

Breastfeeding has certain physiologic advantages for the baby. Breast milk contains secretory immunoglobulin A (IgA), which binds large molecules of foreign proteins, including viruses and bacteria, and keeps them from being absorbed through the gastrointestinal tract into the infant. **Lactoferrin** is an iron-binding protein in breast milk that binds iron in such a way that pathogenic bacteria that require protein for growth cannot use it; this decreases the growth of such bacteria. The enzyme **lysozyme** in breast milk apparently actively destroys bacteria by lysing (dissolving) their cell membranes and so it may increase the effectiveness of antibodies. Leukocytes in breast milk provide protection against common respiratory infectious invaders. Macrophages are responsible for producing **interferon**, which interferes with virus growth. The **bifidus factor** is a specific growth-promoting factor that the bacteria *Lactobacillus bifidus* needs to grow. The presence of *L. bifidus* in breast milk interferes with colonization of pathogenic bacteria in the gastrointestinal tract.

In addition to these anti-infection properties, breast milk contains the ideal electrolyte and mineral composition for human infant growth. It is higher than cow's milk in lactose, an easily digested sugar that provides ready glucose for rapid brain growth. The ratio of cysteine to methionine (two amino acids) in breast milk also appears to favor rapid brain growth in early months. Although its protein content is less than that of cow's milk, breast milk is more readily digested and, therefore, the infant actually may receive more. Breast milk contains nitrogen in compounds other than protein so that the infant receives cell-building materials from sources other than just protein. Breast milk contains more linoleic acid, an essential amino acid for skin integrity, than does cow's milk. It contains less sodium, potassium, calcium, and phosphorus than do many formulas. These lower levels are enough to supply infant needs, and they spare the infant's kidneys from having to process a high renal solute load of unused nutrients. Women who have a familial history of allergy are usually encouraged to breastfeed and thus eliminate the possibility of exposing the infant to cow's milk protein, which could be allergenic this early in life. Breast milk also has a better balance of trace elements, such as zinc, than formulas do.

Babies who receive breast milk appear to have less difficulty with regulation of calcium-phosphorus levels than those who are bottle fed. Cow's milk formulas contain a high level of phosphorus. As the phosphorus level in the infant's bloodstream rises, the calcium level falls because of the inverse relationship that always exists between these two minerals. Decreased calcium levels in the newborn may lead to tetany (muscle spasm). The increased concentration of fatty acid in commercial formulas may bind calcium in the gastrointestinal tract and further increase the danger of tetany.

There is a great deal of discussion about the benefits of breastfeeding from the standpoint of the formation of the dental arch. Babies suck differently from a breast than from a bottle (Figure 24-1), pulling their tongue backward as they suck from a breast. They thrust their tongue forward to suck from a rubber nipple, which may lead to malformation of the dental arch.

A disadvantage of breast milk is that it may carry microorganisms such as hepatitis and cytomegalovirus, although the risk to infants is small. Human immunodeficiency virus (HIV) is carried at a high enough level in breast milk that women who are HIV positive are advised not to breastfeed (Burkman, 1993).

Preparing for Breastfeeding

All women should be asked during pregnancy whether they plan to breastfeed or formula feed their newborn. Thinking about feeding in advance allows couples to

make informed choices. Some fathers experience jealousy at the thought of breastfeeding. Early discussion of the problem can help them work through this natural sensation and come to realize that parenting involves more than feeding children (Jordan & Wall, 1993).

Physical preparation such as nipple rolling, advised in the past as a way of making nipples more protuberant, is no longer advised as the oxytocin released by this could lead to the onset of preterm labor. Practicing breast massage to move the milk forward in the milk ducts (manual expression of milk) can be helpful. This allows a woman who may feel hesitant about handling her breasts to grow accustomed to it and will enable her to assist with milk production in the first few days after birth. Manual expression consists of supporting the breast firmly, then placing the thumbs on the areolar margin and first pushing backward toward the chest wall then downward until secretion begins to flow. During the last months of pregnancy and immediately following birth, the fluid obtained will be colostrum. By the 3rd day of infant life, milk will be obtained.

A woman should avoid using any soap on her

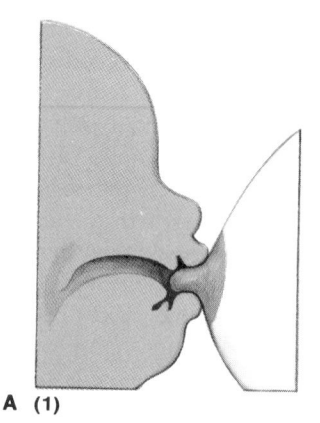
A (1)

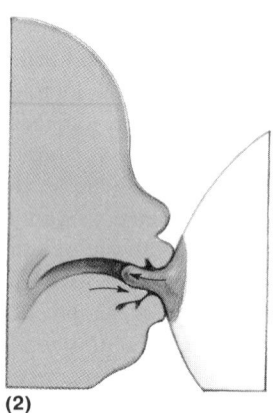
(2)

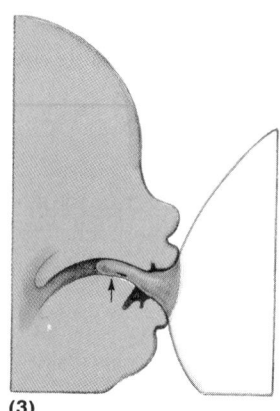
(3)

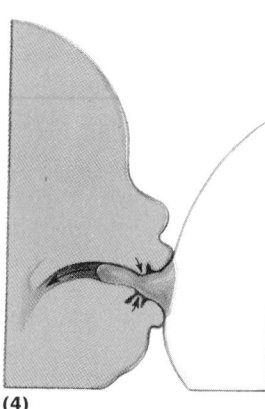
(4)

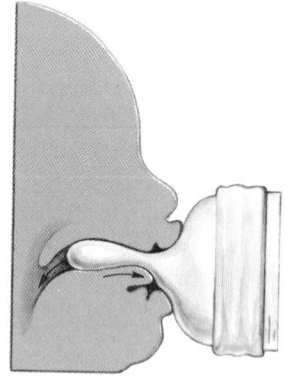
B

FIGURE 24-1

*Differences in sucking mechanism. (**A**) The breast. (**1**) Lips of the infant clamp in a C-shape. The cheek muscles contract. (**2**) The tongue thrusts forward to grasp nipple and areola. (**3**) The nipple is brought against the hard palate as the tongue pulls backward, bringing the areola into the mouth. (**4**) The gums compress the areola, squeezing milk into the back of the throat. (**B**) Bottle-feeding. The large rubber nipple of a bottle strikes the soft palate and interferes with the action of the tongue. The tongue moves forward against the gums to control the overflow of milk into the esophagus.*

breasts during pregnancy because soap tends to dry and crack nipples. The use of creams or lotions other than A & D ointment is not helpful and may lead to nipple fissures and soreness because of too much handling.

Beginning Breastfeeding

Breastfeeding should begin as soon after birth as possible. Ideally, this is while the woman is still in a birthing room and the infant is in the first reactivity period. The release of oxytocin by breastfeeding at this time not only begins the production of milk but also stimulates uterine contraction. If the woman is overly fatigued, however, trying to learn this new skill at this time may only convince her that breastfeeding is not for her (see the Focus on Cultural Awareness box).

It is important that infants grasp the **areola**, or the pigmented circle surrounding the nipple, as well as the nipple itself when they suck. This gives them an effective sucking action and helps to empty the collecting sinuses completely. An infant should be placed first at the breast at which he or she fed last in the previous feeding. Thus each breast is completely emptied at every other feeding.

Milk forms in response to being used. If the breasts are completely emptied, they completely fill again. If half emptied, they only half fill, and after a time, milk production will be insufficient for proper nourishment.

FOCUS ON CULTURAL AWARENESS

Women are the "keepers of the culture" or the main people who transmit customs to the next generation. Chief among these customs is the method for feeding newborns. If a woman comes from a family where no one has ever breastfed, she may be very interested in being a "pioneer" in her family. On the other hand, she may be more interested in following her family's tradition of formula feeding. In a study investigating why women discontinue or continue breastfeeding, Hill and Aldag (1991) found that the mother-in-law's support was important in order for women to continue breastfeeding.

How soon women want to begin breastfeeding after birth is also culturally determined. Although it is the usual practice in hospitals to begin immediately after birth, some women may believe that colostrum is not appropriate for newborns and have a cultural preference not to begin breastfeeding until milk is present, at about 3 days of age. Assessing each family individually is necessary for cultural preferences such as these to be recognized (Geissler, 1994).

Nursing Diagnoses and Related Interventions

In those cultures where breastfeeding is practiced by almost all mothers, the technique is learned early in life by observation. In the United States, they must be helped with beginning the process because they have had few, if any, opportunities to observe breastfeeding. Most hospitals employ a lactation consultant to assist women with breastfeeding. Making a referral to such a person can be extremely helpful.

When a woman begins breastfeeding, one of the first things she must learn to do is relax. If she is tense and anxious, she may have difficulty achieving a good let-down reflex, and her infant will have difficulty obtaining adequate milk. This can lead to the mother's becoming more tense and anxious because her infant does not seem content; the infant will then become hungrier and be left even more unsatisfied, and so on. Receiving support, adequate instruction, and reassurance from health care personnel are important in helping women to feel secure enough to be able to relax (see the Nursing Care Plan).

Nursing Diagnosis: Health-seeking behaviors related to lack of knowledge regarding process of lactation and breastfeeding techniques

Goal: Client will voice understanding of the physiology of breastfeeding and confidence in ability to establish breastfeeding by 24 hours.

Outcome Criteria: Woman states correctly how lactation begins and is maintained in adequate supply; demonstrates effective positioning for baby and herself.

Provide Information Regarding Lactation and Proper Positioning Techniques. Breast milk looks like skimmed milk; it is thin and almost blue-tinged in appearance. Some women may need assurance that the color and consistency are normal. Otherwise, they may think their milk is not nutritious enough.

The woman should wash her hands to be sure they are free of pathogens picked up from handling perineal pads or other sources of germs before breastfeeding. She does not need to wash her breasts unless she notices caked colostrum on the nipples. Lying on her side with a pillow under her head is a good position to assume when she is first attempting to breastfeed (Figure 24-2). This is comfortable for her and allows the infant to rest on the bed. Figure 24-3 shows a sitting position.

If a woman brushes the infant's cheek with her nipple, the baby will turn toward the breast (rooting reflex). Be certain that you do not initiate a rooting reflex by trying to press the baby's face against the mother's breast and cause the child to turn away from the mother towards you.

Joseph Allen Kraft is 1 day old. His mother has planned to breastfeed him as she understands that breast milk has advantages for newborns. She will be returning to a full-time position as a grade-school teacher when he is 6 weeks old.

Assessment: Mother states, "I thought breastfeeding would be difficult. It's easier than it looks." Infant breastfeeding every 2 h; 10 minutes each breast. Doesn't appear totally interested in feedings as yet; needs to be awakened during feedings. Infant content between feedings. Voiding every h; meconium stool x1; skin turgor good, mucous membranes moist. Weight: birth weight minus 2 oz.

Nursing Diagnosis: High risk for altered nutrition less than body requirements related to newborn's immediate sleepiness and return of mother to work in 6 weeks

Defining Characteristic: Sleepiness in a newborn can interfere with breastfeeding; mother states plans to return to work.

Goal: Infant will obtain sufficient nutrition by breastfeeding as entire nutritional pattern for 6 months.

Outcome Criteria: Mother states breastfeeding is an enjoyable activity for her; demonstrates knowledge of technique; infant meets developmental growth milestones.

Nursing Orders	*Rationale*
1. Encourage mother to wake infant prior to feeding.	1. Sleepiness can interfere with effective sucking.
2. Review physiology of engorgement and possible soothing measures (apply warm compresses prior to feeding; encourage infant to suck) with mother.	2. Mother will be home by 3rd day postpartum when this occurs.
3. Review practice of checking with physician before beginning medication while breastfeeding.	3. Almost all medications pass in breast milk.
4. Review need for rest and adequate fluid intake while at home.	4. Mother is planning on returning to work; these measures are necessary for successful breastfeeding.
5. Review availability of hospital lactation consultant for consultation after hospital discharge; provide consultant's name and number.	5. Support is an important aid to successful breastfeeding.
6. Urge mother to extend leave from work as long as possible.	6. Breastfeeding will be most successful if well established before she returns to work.
7. Review techniques for emptying breasts (manual expression of milk or a breast milk pump) for her to use during time she is away from child at work.	7. Manual expression helps to maintain adequate milk supply.

If a woman has large breasts, the infant may have trouble breathing while nursing because breast tissue is pressed against the nose. A woman may prevent this by grasping the areolar margin between her thumb and forefinger, holding the bulk of the breast supported. The nipple is thus made more protuberant as well.

Babies should be fed as often as hungry the first few days of life, because they are receiving only colostrum and need the nutrients and fluid obtained by frequent sucking. Furthermore, the more often breasts are emptied, the more efficiently they will fill and continue to maintain a good supply of milk. A baby may need to be fed as often as every 2 to 3 hours for the first few days (Butte, 1990).

As important as making certain that infants grasp the areola of the breast is helping them to break away from the breast when they are through feeding. This can be done by inserting a finger in the corner of the infant's mouth or by pulling the chin down. Otherwise, the baby may pull too hard on the nipple and cause cracking or soreness (Buchko et al., 1994).

Promote Adequate Sucking. A newborn being breastfed will often drop off to sleep during the first few

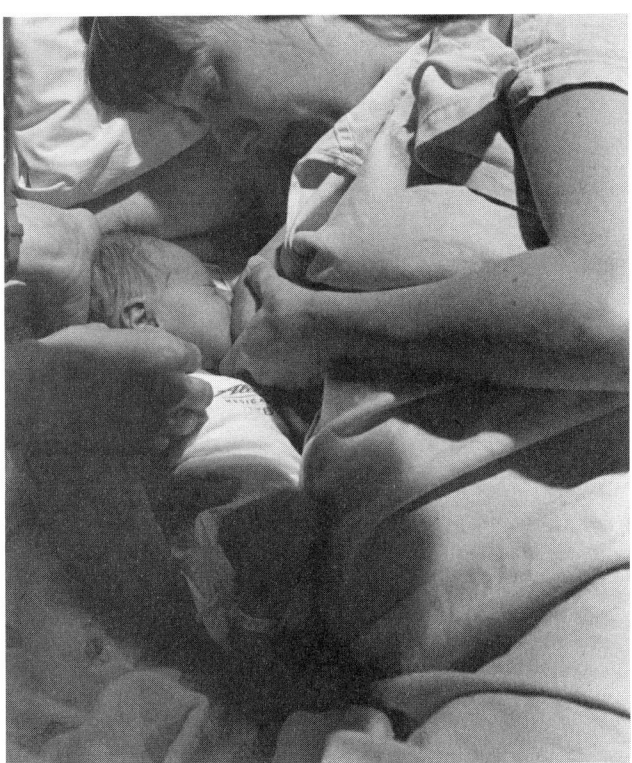

FIGURE 24-2
Side-lying position for breastfeeding. (Photograph © Kathy Sloane.)

wakes him or her up effectively, but many woman are unwilling to cause their newborns discomfort to keep them awake. This attitude may be one of the first signs that the woman is transferring the protectiveness toward her own body she felt during pregnancy to her newborn and is, therefore, a positive reaction.

If an infant is not sucking well, the woman can use breast massage after a feeding to empty her breasts manually (Figure 24-4). This helps to ensure a good milk production for the time when the infant is ready to suck.

Provide Immediate Support When Problems Arise.
The common problems that arise with breastfeeding, if handled intelligently by the health care personnel advising the woman, usually pass and seem unimportant to her. If certain problems are handled wrongly or overemphasized, they may complicate breastfeeding so that a woman becomes discouraged from continuing. It is unfortunate if complications deter a woman from using the most natural and least complicated of all infant feeding methods (see the Focus on Nursing Research box).

Provide Information Regarding Techniques for Burping the Breastfed Baby. Some infants seem to swallow little air when they breastfeed; others swallow a great deal. As a rule, it is helpful to bubble the baby after he

feedings. To stimulate milk production effectively and to ensure adequate fluid intake, the infant should be kept awake and urged to suck. To accomplish this, the woman should be sure to awaken the baby fully before feeding by handling him or her: stroking the baby's back, changing his or her position during feeding, rubbing the arms and chest, or changing the diaper between breasts. Tickling the bottom of a baby's foot

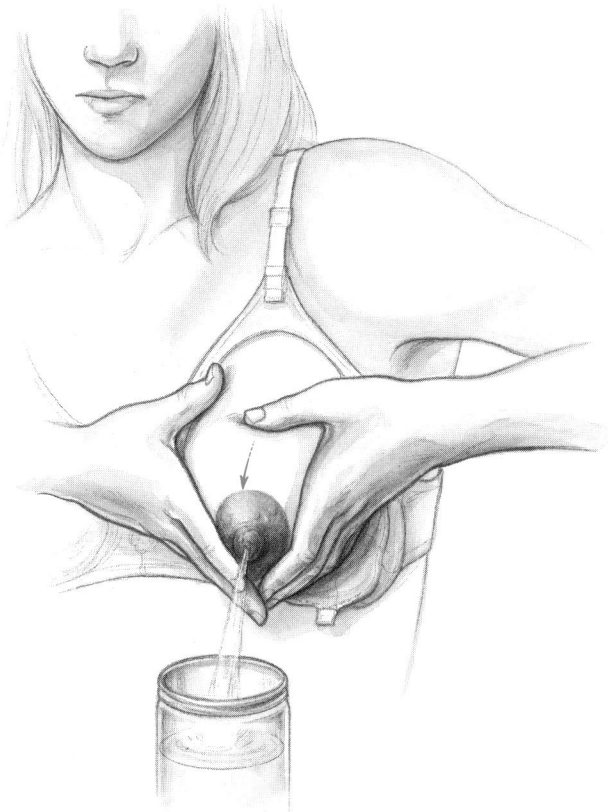

FIGURE 24-4
Manual expression of milk. The breast is supported, and the thumbs are pushed back, then brought forward until breast milk begins to flow.

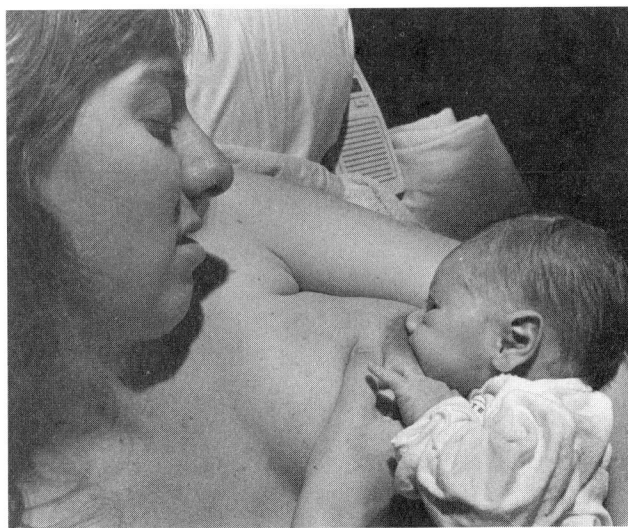

FIGURE 24-3
Sitting position for breastfeeding. (Photograph © Kathy Sloane.)

FOCUS ON NURSING RESEARCH

What Are Common Reactions of Husbands to Breastfeeding?

To examine husbands' experiences of having their wives breastfeed, nursing researchers held in-depth telephone interviews with 14 middle class, urban, Canadian fathers of successfully breastfed infants. Eight of the men were first-time fathers, five had two previous children, and one had three previous children. The men's ages were between 22 and 35 years.

Findings revealed that fathers typically described their major reaction as "postponing" their in-depth relationship with the infant until the infant was weaned. At that point they underwent "catch-up" behavior. A number of men expressed frustration at not being able to comfort their child because he or she would not eat unless breastfed. They typically increased their other caretaking behaviors with the child such as changing diapers, bathing, or putting to bed.

The researchers suggest that nurses should be more aware that breastfeeding influences and possibly changes a father's relationship with a new baby. The more fathers know about breastfeeding, the better able they are to make these adjustments and accept breastfeeding.

Gamble, D., & Morse, J. M. (1993). Fathers of breastfed infants: Postponing and types of involvement. *Journal of Obstetric, Gynecologic, and Neonatal Nursing, 22,* 358.

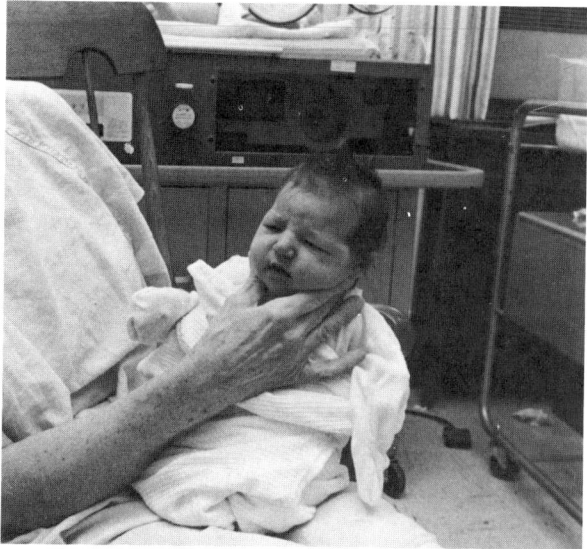

FIGURE 24-5
A sitting position for burping a newborn. The infant's head is supported by the nurse's hand. (Courtesy of the Department of Medical Photography, Children's Hospital, Buffalo, NY.)

minimally inflamed, and she can begin breastfeeding without undue discomfort; infant grasps nipple firmly.

On the 3rd or 4th day, when breast milk forms, some women may notice swelling, hardness, tenderness, and perhaps heat in their breasts. The skin appears red, tense, and shiny. This is called **engorgement** and is caused by vascular and lymphatic congestion arising from an increase in the blood and lymph supply to the breasts. An infant has difficulty sucking on engorged breasts because the areola is too hard to grasp (Figure 24-6). The woman also has difficulty nursing because

or she has emptied the first breast and again after the total feeding.

A parent may place the baby over one shoulder and gently pat or stroke the back. This position is not always satisfactory for a small infant, who has poor head control, and the parent may not be able to support the baby's head and pat the back at the same time. Lying the baby prone across the lap is an alternate position.

Holding the baby in a sitting position on the lap, then leaning the child forward against one hand, with the index finger and thumb supporting the head, is often the best position because it provides head support and yet leaves the other hand free to pat the baby's back (Figure 24-5). Parents usually need to be shown this method. It does not seem as natural as putting the baby against the shoulder.

Nursing Diagnosis: Pain related to breast engorgement or sore nipples

Goal: Client will experience no severe breast discomfort during early breastfeeding period.

Outcome Criteria: Client states that she is experiencing no or reduced discomfort, breasts are only

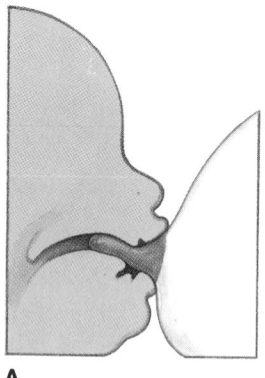
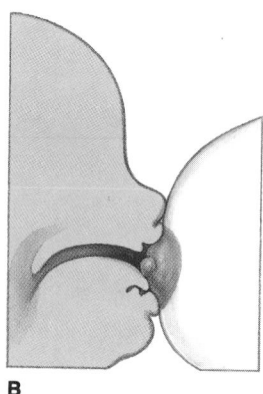

A   **B**

FIGURE 24-6
The problem that breast engorgement causes to breastfeeding. (**A**) *When sucking at a normal breast, the infant's lips compress the areola and fit neatly against the sides of the nipple. The infant also has adequate room to breathe.* (**B**) *When a breast is engorged, the infant has difficulty grasping the nipple. Breathing ability is compromised.*

her breasts are extremely painful, and the baby's sucking accentuates the discomfort.

Prevent or Relieve Engorgement. The primary method for relieving engorgement is emptying the breasts of milk by having the infant suck more often than previously, or at least continuing to suck as much as before. Unfortunately, the breasts are so sore that it is difficult for a mother to continue to breastfeed unless she is given something to alleviate the pain. An analgesic may be necessary, but some mothers find that warm packs applied for about 20 minutes afford the most relief. In addition, good breast support from a firm-fitting bra prevents a pulling feeling.

If an infant cannot grasp the nipple to suck strongly, warm packs applied to both breasts for a few minutes before feeding in combination with massage to begin milk flow (eg, standing under a shower and massaging) will often facilitate drainage and promote softness so that the infant can suck. Manual expression (see Figure 24-4) or the use of a breast pump to complete emptying of the breasts after the baby has nursed can be helpful in maintaining or promoting a good milk supply during the period of engorgement (Figure 24-7).

Fortunately, engorgement is a transient problem. Unfortunately, it occurs just as women are beginning to feel skilled at breastfeeding. Suddenly their breasts are swollen, hot, and painful. They may worry that they have an infection or that the baby will not get enough milk. They can be assured that engorgement is a normal occurrence and actually an important announcement that their breasts are ready to produce milk. They also can be assured that it is only temporary and will begin to subside 24 hours after it first becomes apparent.

Promote Healing of Sore Nipples. Sore nipples result from the strong sucking action of the newborn (Ziemer & Pigeon, 1993). This may be worsened by improper positioning of the infant, that is, from the infant's not grasping the areola as well as the nipple. It can be aggravated by forcefully pulling the infant from the breast, from the infant's sucking too long a time at a breast after it was emptied, or from the nipple remaining wet from leaking milk. Nipples are normally kept supple because of secretions from Montgomery's tubercles. They can become sore when they are excessively dry and so crack or fissure. To help prevent soreness, be certain the mother positions the baby at a reverse angle for feedings to prevent the same area of the areola receiving the main pressure. Exposing the nipples to air by leaving a bra unsnapped for 10 to 15 minutes after feeding is often sufficient to clear up the problem. Some mothers use hair dryers set on low settings. A mother should avoid using the plastic liners that come with nursing bras, so that air is always circulating around her breasts. Applications of vitamin E following air exposure may toughen the nipples and prevent further irritation.

If normal air-drying is not effective, simultaneous exposure to a 20-watt bulb in a gooseneck lamp two or three times a day may be helpful. The light should be 12 to 18 in away from the breasts to prevent burns, and it should be left in place about 10 minutes. If a woman's nipples are so sore that breastfeeding is uncomfortable, she can use a nipple shield to improve comfort. Nipple shields are made of flexible plastic and mold to the contour of the breast covering the nipple. The infant sucks on the plastic rather than the nipple, protecting the nipple from further irritation. Infants must be observed to see that they are obtaining milk and not just achieving

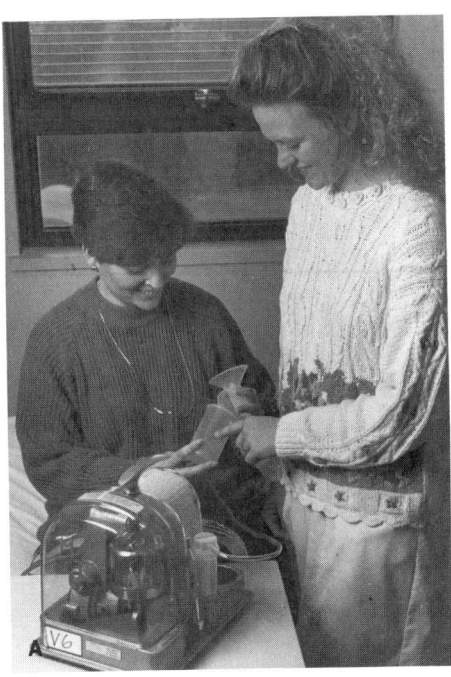
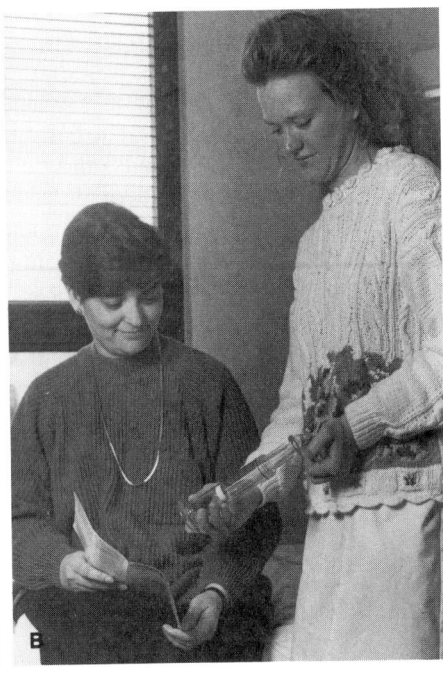

FIGURE 24-7
*A nurse and mother discuss the advantages, disadvantages of (**A**) an electric breast pump and (**B**) a manual pump.*

nonnutritive sucking when a nipple shield is in place. If a woman's nipples are so sore that she cannot nurse even with a breast shield in place, breast milk should be manually expelled and fed to the baby by bottle until the nipples have had a chance to heal. The woman should not use a hand pump with sore nipples, as this may cause fissures to worsen. An electric or battery-operated pump (standard equipment in most maternity or pediatrics hospitals) usually can be used, as these cause less pressure to the nipples.

Sore nipples, like engorgement, are not a contraindication to breastfeeding. If steps to prevent sore nipples are followed, the problem of sore nipples is unlikely to become acute again.

Nursing Diagnosis: Anxiety related to inability to measure amount of food taken by baby

Goal: Client will express confidence that baby is receiving enough milk.

Outcome Criteria: Client states that baby seems satisfied after feeding and voices confidence that baby must be getting enough milk; baby voids 6 to 8 times/day.

Some breastfeeding mothers wonder whether the infant is getting enough to eat. They watch a woman bottle feeding and listen to her report "He took 3 ounces this feeding," and wish they could tell as surely that their infant's intake is adequate. They can be assured that the ultimate test with either breastfeeding or bottle feeding is whether the infant seems content between feedings and is gaining weight, not what was taken at only one feeding. Although the bottle-feeding mother measures the amount of formula as a way of determining this in the early weeks, soon she, too, will be using the alternative criteria: her baby is happy, voids 6 to 8 times a day, and is gaining weight. Helping a woman to use these criteria allows her to develop confidence in her judgment to evaluate her child's health, a role that will be hers for the next 18 or more years.

Nursing Diagnosis: Knowledge deficit related to potential harm to baby of drugs taken by breast-feeding mother

Goal: Client will voice understanding at time of hospital discharge that most drugs pass readily into breast milk.

Outcome Criteria: Client states that almost all drugs she takes will be found in her breast milk; voices importance of consulting physician or nurse practitioner before taking any drug.

For years, people talked about a placental barrier that theoretically protected the fetus from drugs taken by the mother. A similar protection was postulated for breast milk. It has been shown, however, that the fetus is extremely susceptible to drugs ingested by the mother. The same is true of breastfed infants. Almost any drug may cross into the acinar cells and be secreted in breast milk. Drugs that should be avoided by breastfeeding mothers because of their documented harmful effect on infants are shown in Appendix C.

The rule that a woman followed all during pregnancy, that she should take no drug unless prescribed or approved by her physician or nurse practitioner, continues to apply during lactation.

Nursing Diagnosis: Effective breastfeeding related to mother's desire to provide the best nutrition for her child

Goal: Client will voice confidence in ability to breastfeed baby at home.

Outcome Criteria: Client states that she intends to continue breastfeeding at home; voices confidence in her ability to provide adequate milk for infant and names resources for help if needed; infant exhibits adequate weight gain and elimination patterns for age.

Provide Anticipatory Guidance Regarding Potential Problems and Methods for Resolution. Common problems that can arise with breastfeeding are summarized in Table 24-1. Women who do not remember to begin nursing the baby at the breast that the infant finished on the last time may find their milk supply decreasing. It is easy to remember this in the hospital, but the many distractions at home may make the sequence hard to keep in mind. Pinning a safety pin to the bra strap on the correct side to start with at the next time is a useful way to remember.

Another problem after women return home is fatigue. A woman must realize that she cannot expect to feed a baby by any method, attend many social functions, and be a perfect housekeeper and gourmet cook. Adequate rest periods during the day are essential. Sitting relaxed in a comfortable chair with her feet elevated, feeding her baby, and enjoying it is an excellent way to rest.

Adequate fluid intake is also necessary to maintain a milk supply (Morse et al., 1992). In the hospital, fluid intake is supervised by health care personnel. When the woman is at home and involved in other things, she may neglect to drink adequate amounts. Some women deliberately limit fluid intake in the hope of shedding the weight they gained during pregnancy.

Women who are breastfeeding should drink at least four 8-oz glasses of fluid a day; many need to drink six glasses. They need to increase their calorie intake as

Table 24-1. *Common Problems of Breastfeeding*

Problem	Cause	Nursing Interventions
Engorgement	Lymphatic filling as milk production begins	Engorgement subsides best if infant can be encouraged to suck normally; warm packs to breasts before feeding may help soften breast tissue; oxytocin nasal spray before feeding may aid the let-down reflex
Sore nipples	Infant not gripping entire areola Nipple kept wet	Help infant to grasp nipple correctly; expose nipple to air between feedings; aloe vera or vitamin E applied to nipples helps heal tissue
Mother worries about amount of milk being taken	Mother cannot see the amount taken	Assure mother that the best way to judge amount taken is to note if infant is gaining weight and appears content between feedings
Infant does not suck well	Possible effect of anesthesia Infant brought to mother when not hungry Infant exhausted by crying from hunger	Adjust feeding pattern to child's needs; assure mother that effect of anesthesia is temporary
Mother reports infant's stools are loose and thin	Stools normally looser and lighter in color than in formula-fed babies	Examine stools; assure and explain normal stool pattern
Father feels shut out of parent–child relationship	Father does not participate in infant feeding	Suggest father offer a supplemental feeding daily after breastfeeding is established. Show other ways of interacting with infant than through feeding

well (Table 24-2). A daily diet plan for a lactating woman is given in Table 24-3.

At one time, women were given a list of foods not to eat while they were breastfeeding because it was thought they caused diarrhea, constipation, or colic in infants. Today, there are no rules other than to use common sense. A woman can eat anything during lactation that agrees with her and is taken in moderation. She should not eat foods to which she is allergic or that cause gastrointestinal upsets, but then the average woman avoids these foods at all times.

Some women stop breastfeeding after they return home because they have no one to talk to about a problem or to give them support. A nurse who works as a hospital community liaison person or a community health nurse can be a resource for such women. Giving women a complimentary pack of formula on discharge may discourage breastfeeding, so this should be done cautiously (Snell et al., 1992).

Provide Information on the Use of Supplemental Feedings. A breastfeeding woman may leave her child during the day or evening in the care of a babysitter, just as a bottle-feeding woman may. She can express breast milk manually and leave it bottled in the refrigerator or prepare a single bottle of formula for the time she is away. Buying the prepackaged and prepared type of formula is convenient for this; the woman need only

Table 24-2. *Recommended Daily Allowances During Lactation*

	First Six Months	Second Six Months
Calories (kcal)	+500	+500
Protein (g)	65	62
Vitamin A	1300	1200
Vitamin D (μg)	10	10
Vitamin E (mg)	12	11
Vitamin K (μg)	65	65
Vitamin C (mg)	95	90
Folate (μg)	280	260
Niacin (mg)	20	20
Riboflavin (mg)	1.8	1.7
Thiamine (mg)	1.6	1.6
Vitamin B6 (mg)	2.1	2.1
Vitamin B12 (μg)	2.6	2.6
Calcium (mg)	1200	1200
Phosphorus (mg)	1200	1200
Iodine (μg)	200	200
Iron (mg)	15	15
Magnesium (mg)	355	340
Zinc (mg)	19	16

(National Academy of Sciences. [1989]. *Recommended daily dietary allowances* [10th ed.]. Washington: National Academy Press.)

Table 24-3. *Quantities of Food Necessary for Lactating Women*

Food Group	Quantities for Active Nonpregnant Woman	Quantities for Lactating Woman
Meat, fowl, or fish	2 servings daily	3–4 servings daily
Vegetables		
Dark green or deep yellow	1 serving (at least 3 times/ week)	1 serving daily
Other vegetables	2 or more servings daily	2–3 servings daily
Fruits: citrus, melon, strawberry, tomato	1 serving daily	2 or more servings daily
Bread and cereals	4 or more servings daily	4 servings daily
Milk	2 8-oz glasses daily	4–6 8-oz glasses daily
Additional fluid	As desired	At least 2 glasses daily

take a bottle of it down from a shelf, and it is ready. If cost is a problem, using the powdered type of formula is probably the best solution. This can be stored for long periods, and one bottle at a time can be prepared.

Once breastfeeding has been established, after about 6 weeks, missing one feeding will not affect milk production enough to make a difference at the next feeding. Thus, there is no need for her to express milk manually to safeguard a supply, although she may prefer to do so to reduce tension and discomfort and perhaps help prevent mastitis (Auerbach, 1990).

Provide Information for the Mother Who Works Outside Her Home. Many women return to work while continuing to breastfeed by bringing their infant with them to their workplace. Others express breast milk for a caregiver to give by bottle while they work. Some employers have strong feelings about breastfeeding; to avoid difficulties, women should review with an employer the best way for them to continue breastfeeding, perhaps by using a private office or screened area or feeding the baby expressed milk. Problems with expressing milk while at work include maintaining an adequate milk supply and finding a time and place to express the milk (Hills-Bonczyk et al., 1993) (see the Focus on Family Teaching box).

Provide Information on Weaning. Women breastfeed for varying lengths of time. Some do it for 1, 2, or 3 months, then wean the child from breast to bottle. Many continue until the child is 6 to 12 months of age and then wean directly to a small cup or glass. Some continue to breastfeed until the child is preschool age. Lengthy breastfeeding (beyond 1 year), however, may lead to nutritional deficiencies if the child is taking in a large quantity of milk at the expense of other foods (Grummer-Strawn, 1993).

Breastfeeding should be discontinued gradually to prevent engorgement and pain in the mother. To do this, a woman should first omit one breastfeeding a day, sub-stituting a bottle feeding or milk from a glass or cup. Then she should omit two breastfeedings, then three, and so on, until the child is feeding entirely from a bottle, glass, or cup. If the breasts are not emptied by regular feedings, the resulting pressure leads to milk suppression and natural, gradual discontinuance of milk secretion.

Formula Feeding

There is little opposition to the concept that breastfeeding is the best method for feeding human infants—except when a woman cannot or does not want to breastfeed. Women who develop a breast abscess may be advised not to breastfeed. Some women who are uncomfortable with the thought of exposing their breasts may not be able to hold a baby warmly and enjoy feeding an infant at the breast. Others who plan to return to work outside their home or who have older children to care for may choose not to breastfeed. Fortunately, formulas that closely resemble human milk are available for infants who will be bottle-fed.

Preparing for Formula Feeding

Women are advised to use commercial formulas for infant feeding as these so closely mimic human milk.

Commercial Formulas

The contents of commercial formulas are supervised by the Federal Food and Drug Administration and are available in three types: milk-based, soy-based, and elemental (fat, protein, and carbohydrate are modified). Milk-based formulas are used for the average newborn; soy-based formulas are used for infants with lactose intolerance or galactosemia. Elemental formulas are used with infants with protein allergies and fat malnutrition. Both milk and soy-based formulas are designed to simulate breast milk as closely as possible in terms of protein,

FOCUS ON FAMILY TEACHING

Q. I'm going to return to work while breastfeeding. What are some helpful tips for managing this?

A. Continuing breastfeeding while working can be challenging. Some common suggestions are:

- Some women are able to arrange for child care near or at their work site so they can breastfeed at lunch time or during a morning or afternoon break. Discuss with your employer or your immediate work supervisor if this would be a possibility for you.

- Breastfeeding can be done in a public place such as a lounge area without undue exposure if you wear a smock-type or button blouse that you lift or unfasten only as far as necessary; covering any bared breast with a shawl or towel assures modesty.

- If you are not able to breastfeed during work hours, you will need to express milk manually at least once during the day in order to maintain a milk supply. Expressed breast milk can be safely stored in the refrigerator or an iced container for 24 to 48 hours and used by your caregiver to feed the infant the next day.

- Plastic is the best type of storage container for breast milk as antibodies apparently cling to glass and will therefore be lost to the milk.

- Any reminder of a baby while you are breastfeeding may cause leaking of milk from breasts. Wear gauze pads inside your bra to prevent staining your clothing. Pressing against your breasts with the heel of your hands may be helpful in halting leakage.

- Remember to drink a number of glasses of fluid during the day to ensure a high fluid intake.

- Try to avoid fatigue.

- Relax and enjoy your baby during the time you are home.

carbohydrate, fat, mineral, and vitamin content. Those for term newborns contain 20 cal/oz when diluted according to directions. Common brands are shown in Appendix B. Parents should plan on using formula for the first full year of their infant's life (Fomon et al., 1990). Participating in a Supplemental Food Program for Women, Infant, and Children (WIC) helps low-income parents afford formula (see Chapter 34).

Four separate forms of commercial formulas are available: (1) a powder that is combined with water; (2) a condensed liquid that is diluted with an equal amount of water; (3) a ready-to-pour type, which requires no di-

lution; and (4) individually prepackaged and prepared bottles of formula.

The powder is the least expensive and, if a single bottle at a time is prepared, easy to prepare by vigorous shaking. The prepackaged type has the advantage of never needing refrigeration or preparation (take off a bottle cap and it is ready), but is the most expensive type. The ready-to-pour type is also convenient but also expensive. The condensed type is more economical. The cost is as much as 50 cents to $2 a day less than those of ready-to-pour or prepackaged types, which amounts to a savings of $15 to $60 a month. Cost should not be the only basis for a parent to make a choice, however. Tolerance of the formula by the infant and convenience for parents also are important.

Commercial formulas may be purchased with added iron, so separate iron supplementation is not necessary. They also contain added supplemental vitamins.

Calculating a Formula's Adequacy

Calculating the adequacy of a newborn's formula is not complicated. There are only a few rules of thumb to learn, including the following:

1. The total fluid used for 24 hours must be sufficient to meet the child's fluid needs; 75 to 90 mL of fluid per pound of body weight per day (150 to 200 mL/kg) is needed.
2. The protein requirement is 1 g per pound of body weight per day (2.2 g/kg).
3. The number of calories required per day is 50 to 55 per pound of body weight (100 to 120 kcal/kg).

If an infant is taking a commercial formula, total fluid is all that has to be calculated. The 7-lb infant needs 17.5 to 21 oz (7 × 2.5 to 3 oz) per day. As commercial formula contains 20 cal/oz, this supplies 350 to 420 cal/day, which can be divided into six feedings of 3 to 3.5 oz each. A 9-lb infant would need 22.5 to 27 oz of fluid per day, which supplies 450 to 540 cal.

A quick rule of thumb to determine how much an infant usually takes at a feeding is to add 2 or 3 to the infant's age in months. A newborn (0 age) takes 2 to 3 ounces each feeding; a 3-month-old, 5 to 6 ounces; and a 6-month-old, 8 ounces. As infants change from six to five feedings a day (at about 4 months of age), they begin to take more at each one to keep their total intake the same. Knowing the minimum requirements for fluid and calories per day and being able to calculate whether formula is adequate allows you to evaluate the adequacy of an infant's intake.

Nursing Diagnoses and Related Interventions

Nursing Diagnosis: Health-seeking behaviors related to techniques of bottle feeding

Goal: Client will understand techniques of formula feeding by hospital discharge.

Outcome Criteria: Client accurately states what equipment is needed for formula feeding and demonstrates feeding technique with her baby.

Provide Information Regarding Supplies Needed.

Most parents today do not prepare a full day's supply of formula at once but prepare it bottle by bottle, as needed. They can use glass, plastic, or disposable refill bottles. Women who breastfeed and use supplemental bottles can do the same. Caution parents to keep opened cans of liquid formula covered and refrigerated and to use it or discard it within 24 hours.

Nipples for bottles should be firm enough so that the infant sucks vigorously. A soft, flabby nipple allows a baby to suck in milk so rapidly that the need for sucking may not be satisfied. A way to judge a nipple's adequacy is to hold the bottle of milk with nipple attached upside down. The milk should come out at a rate of about one drop a second. While feeding the baby outdoors or anywhere there are flies about, bottle caps to cover the nipples are helpful.

Provide Information Regarding Formula Preparation.

Infant formula of any type must be prepared with careful attention to cleanliness to prevent pathogenic microorganisms from growing in it. The AAP (1976a) states that if a parent uses chlorinated water, a commercial formula, or pasteurized milk, proceeds with clean technique, then refrigerates the prepared formula until it is ready to be used, formula does not need to be sterilized. Sterilization would be necessary, however if any of these conditions were not met—that is, if a parent used unchlorinated well or spring water, unpasteurized milk, or a technique that was not absolutely clean. Women vacationing at rural campsites or living in rural areas may not meet these criteria. Instructions for terminally sterilizing formula for these instances are shown in Box 24-1.

When using presterilized formula, the parent need only do the following to prepare a full day's supply of formula: wash off the top of the can with warm soapy water and rinse; open the can; pour the desired amount of formula and water into each previously cleaned bottle; and put on the nipples, taking care not to handle the nipple projection. Finally, the bottle caps are put on and the bottles refrigerated. To prepare a single bottle, the parent simply combines clean water and liquid or powdered formula, caps the bottle, and shakes it to mix the ingredients.

Provide Information Regarding Feeding Techniques.

To warm or not to warm formula is up to the parents, because studies have shown that infants who are fed cooled formula directly from the refrigerator thrive as well as those who are fed warmed formula. Most par-

---

> ### Box 24-1
> *Terminal Sterilization of Bottles*
>
> Parents who are temporarily away from a chlorinated water supply, such as when they are on a camping trip, should terminally sterilize formula as this eliminates any contamination that may be present in the water. All formula for a day (six bottles) is sterilized at once so the parents must have six bottles. A disadvantage of terminal sterilization is the long cooling period required before the formula can be used (about 2 hours) so parents must sterilize formula at least 2 hours before it is needed. Some brands of disposable or plastic bottles cannot be terminally sterilized or they will melt and leak at the high heat required. For terminal sterilization, use the following steps:
>
> 1. Wash the bottles, nipples, and caps. Prepare the formula as usual and fill bottles. Apply the caps loosely or the pressure inside from the steam as they boil will break the bottles. A good idea is to tighten the caps to the limit and then loosen them a half turn.
>
> 2. Place the bottles in a bottle sterilizer. The rack on the bottom of the sterilizer must be in place; the heat will make the bottles crack if they rest directly on the pan bottom. A high Dutch oven (covered) can be used for sterilizing as long as it is high enough for the bottles to stand upright in it. To protect the bottles from cracking, either a metal pie pan punched with holes (to simulate a rack) or a dishcloth should be placed on the bottom of the pan. Fill the sterilizer or Dutch oven up to the shoulders of the bottles with water, place on the stove to boil, and boil for 25 minutes after boiling starts, determined by listening to the sound of the boiling water and the gentle jiggling of the bottles. The lid should not be lifted to check for boiling or pressure in the bottles from steam will force milk up into the nipples and clog the holes.
>
> 3. After 25 minutes, turn off the stove and move the sterilizer or pan to a cool burner. Do not lift the lid until the sides of the container are cool enough to be touched with bare hands. If the lid is lifted before then, milk will be forced up into the nipples and will clog them. When the pan is cool enough to touch with bare hands, remove the bottles, tighten the caps, and refrigerate until use.

---

ents feel uncomfortable giving cool formula, however, and choose to warm it. To do this, a bottle can be removed from the refrigerator about 1 hour before feeding time and allowed to come up to room temperature gradually. Many parents heat bottles in a microwave oven for about 20 seconds. This can be dangerous because the milk in the center of the bottle becomes hotter than that near the side of the bottle. An infant could burn his tongue from the hot milk at the center. To avoid this, urge parents to shake a bottle well after microwaving it to mix the cool and warm portions and then test the temperature on their wrist before feeding.

A bottle of formula can be put into a pan of hot water or warmed up in a pan of water on the stove. Caution parents to not allow the pan to boil dry or the bottle of milk will burst. They also must be certain to check the temperature of the formula by allowing a drop or two to fall onto the inside of the wrist to make sure that it is not hot enough to burn the baby's mouth.

Disposable bottles with plastic liners should not be heated on the stove; they tend to melt and then leak during feeding. With any type of bottle, once it has been used, any contents remaining should be thrown away; it should never be stored and reused. When sucking, an infant exchanges a small amount of saliva for milk. Because milk is a good growth medium for bacteria and the baby's mouth harbors many bacteria, the bacteria content in reused formula is likely to be high.

Feeding an infant is a skill that, like all skills, has to be learned. A parent needs a comfortable chair (as does a nurse who feeds babies) and adequate time (at least half an hour) to enjoy the process and not rush the baby (Figure 24-8). The baby is held with the head slightly elevated to reduce the danger of aspiration and retention of air bubbles. The parent should be sure that the nipple is filled and the baby is sucking milk, not air. You can tell that a baby is sucking effectively if small bubbles rise in the bottle. Babies in the early weeks should be bubbled after every ounce of fluid taken. The technique is the same as discussed for breastfed infants. Some common problems that can arise with formula feeding are summarized in Table 24-4.

Parents may need to be reminded not to prop up

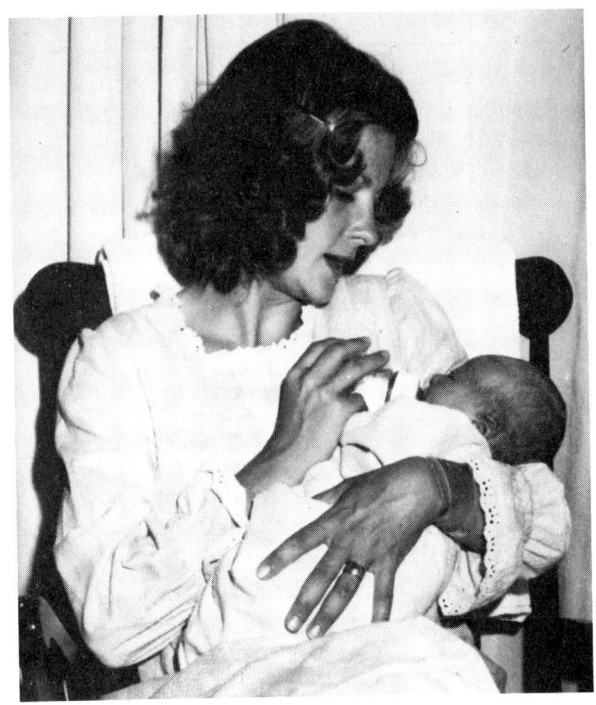

FIGURE 24-8
A newborn receives a bottle feeding from her mother. Notice the en face position. (Courtesy of the Department of Medical Photography, Millard Fillmore Hospital, Buffalo, NY.)

bottles. This is tempting because it frees a busy parent to do something else with the time. Babies are in danger of aspiration if a bottle is propped. It also limits the amount of parent–child interaction that is so important for the health of both the parents and child. Parents also may need to be reminded not to put a baby to bed with a bottle of formula, as this can lead to baby bottle syndrome, or cavities of the lower teeth (see Chapter 29).

Table 24-4. Common Problems in Formula Feeding		
Problem	**Cause**	**Nursing Interventions**
Infant sucks for a few minutes, then stops and cries	Either nipple is blocked and infant is unable to get milk or flow is too fast and baby has choking sensation	Show parent how to test flow of milk from the nipple (hold bottle upside down); milk should flow from nipple at rate of about 1 drop/sec
Infant does not bubble well after feeding	Some infants swallow little air with feeding. Parent may be handling infant too tentatively or not burping effectively	Observe baby feeding and parent's technique of handling; rubbing newborn's back may be more effective than patting it
Parent reports loose stools	Bowel movements from formula-fed infants are not quite as loose as those from breastfed infants but so different from adult stools that parents may be concerned	Examine stools; assure and explain normal stool pattern.

Key Points

- Breastfeeding is the preferred feeding method for newborn infants as it can supply antibodies to the newborn, as well as nutrients. Urge all women at least to try breastfeeding unless they are taking some drug that would interfere with this or there is a potential for spreading a microorganism through breast milk.

- Almost all drugs pass into breast milk. The breastfeeding mother must be certain not to take any medication without contacting her primary care provider for assurance regarding safety with breastfeeding.

- Both breast milk and commercial formulas have 20 kcal/oz. A term newborn requires 120 kcal/kg/day; 160 to 200 mL/kg of fluid.

- Breastfeeding mothers should be encouraged to drink fluoridated water; formula should be prepared using fluoridated water. If a newborn will not have exposure to sunlight, the breastfeeding mother may need to take a supplement of vitamin D.

- If a baby will be bottle fed, be certain the parents understand the potential danger of warming bottles using a microwave oven (the inner core of milk may be very hot).

- Caution parents not to prop bottles. An infant may aspirate from this, and it also deprives him or her of the pleasure of being held for feedings.

- To avoid nursing bottle syndrome (cavitied teeth), infants should not be put to bed with a bottle.

- Linoleic acid is an essential fatty acid necessary for growth and skin integrity that cannot be manufactured by the body. It is supplied by both cow's and human milk but not by skim milk.

Critical Thinking Exercises

1. Jackie is a 1-day-old newborn who is being breastfed. Her mother tells you she is unsure Jackie is receiving enough milk. How could you assure the mother that the baby is receiving enough milk?

2. Mrs. Wheeler has chosen to bottle feed her newborn. Her mother tells you she used to prepare formula using evaporated milk and corn syrup, a form that was cheaper than commercial formula. She asks you why this type of formula isn't recommended today. She also says that at 3 months, babies were changed to skim milk to keep them from gaining too much weight. How would you explain to Mrs. Wheeler the reasons why the formula she described is no longer recommended?

3. Mrs. Curtis is a woman who is breastfeeding and will be returning to work in a busy office. What suggestions for maintaining breastfeeding would you make to her, and why?

References

American Academy of Pediatrics Committee on Nutrition. (1976a). Commentary on breast-feeding and infant formulas. *Pediatrics, 57,* 278.

American Academy of Pediatrics Committee on Nutrition. (1976b). Iron supplementation for infants. *Pediatrics, 58,* 765.

American Academy of Pediatrics Committee on Nutrition. (1978). Breast-feeding. *Pediatrics, 62,* 591.

American Academy of Pediatrics Committee on Nutrition (1980). Vitamin and mineral supplement needs in normal children in the United States. *Pediatrics, 66,* 1015.

Anderson, E., & Geden, E. (1991). Nurses' knowledge of breastfeeding. *Journal of Obstetric, Gynecologic, and Neonatal Nursing, 20,* 58.

Auerbach, K. G. (1990). Assisting the employed breastfeeding mother. *Journal of Nurse Midwifery, 35,* 26.

Berne, R. M., & Levy, M. N. (1993). *Physiology* (3rd ed.). St. Louis: Mosby.

Brown, L. P., et al. (1993). Incidence and pattern of jaundice in healthy breastfed infants during the first month of life. *Nursing Research, 42,* 106.

Buchko, B., et al. (1994). Comfort measures in breastfeeding primiparous women. *Journal of Obstetric, Gynecologic and Neonatal Nursing, 23,* 46.

Burkman, R. T. (1993). Puerperium and breastfeeding. *Current Opinion in Obstetrics and Gynecology, 5,* 683.

Butte, N. F., et al. (1990). Energy utilization of breast fed and formula fed infants. *American Journal of Clinical Nutrition, 51,* 350.

Department of Health and Human Services. (1991). *Healthy people 2000.* Washington, D. C.: Public Health Service.

Fomon, S. J., et al. (1990). Formulas for older infants. *Journal of Pediatrics, 110,* 690.

Geissler, E. M. (1994). *Pocket guide to cultural assessment.* St. Louis: C. V. Mosby.

Gray, R. H., et al. (1990). Risk of ovulation during lactation. *Lancet, 335,* 25.

Grummer-Strawn, L. M. (1993). Does prolonged breast-feeding impair child growth? *Pediatrics, 91,* 766.

Hill, P. D., & Aldag, J. (1991). Potential indicators of insufficient milk supply syndrome. *Research in Nursing and Health, 14,* 11.

Hills-Bonczyk, S. G., et al. (1993). Women's experience with combining breastfeeding and employment. *Journal of Nurse Midwifery, 38,* 257.

Jordan, P. L., & Wall, V. R. (1993). Supporting the father when an infant is breastfed. *Journal of Human Lactation, 9,* 31.

La Leche League International. (1991). *The womanly art of breastfeeding* (35th anniversary ed.). New York: NAL-Dutton.

Locklin, M. P., & Naber, S. J. (1993). Does breastfeeding empower women? *Birth, 20,* 30.

Martinez, J. C., et al. (1993). Hyperbilirubinemia in the breastfed newborn: A controlled trial of four interventions. *Pediatrics, 91,* 470.

Mills, A. F. (1990). Surveillance for anaemia: Risk factors in patterns of milk intake. *Archives of Disease in Childhood, 85,* 420.

Morse, M., et al. (1992). The effect of maternal fluid intake on breast milk supply: A pilot study. *Canadian Journal of Public Health, 83,* 213.

Oski, F. A. (1993). Infant nutrition, physical growth, breastfeeding, and general nutrition. *Pediatrics, 5,* 385.

Potter, S., et al. (1991). Does infant feeding method influence maternal postpartum weight loss? *Journal of the American Dietetic Association, 91,* 441.

Riordan, J., & Auerbach, E. G. (1993). *Breastfeeding and human lactation.* Boston: Jones & Bartlett.

Serdula, M. K., et al. (1991). Correlates of breast-feeding in a low-income population of whites, blacks, and southeast Asians. *Journal of the American Dietetic Association, 91,* 41.

Smith, M. K., et al. (1991). Correlates of breastfeeding in a low-income population of whites, blacks, and southeast Asians. *Journal of the American Dietetic Association, 91,* 41.

Snell, B. J., et al. (1992). The association of formula samples given at hospital discharge with the early discontinuation of breastfeeding. *Journal of Human Lactation, 8,* 67.

Ziemer, M. M., & Pigeon, J. G. (1993). Skin changes and pain in the nipple during the first week of lactation. *Journal of Obstetric, Gynecologic, and Neonatal Nursing, 22,* 247.

Suggested Readings

Coates, M., et al. (1992). Breastfeeding during maternal or infant illness. *NAACOGS Clinical Issues in Perinatal and Women's Health Nursing 3,* 683.

Diflorio, I. (1991). Mothers' comprehension of terminology associated with the care of a newborn baby. *Pediatric Nursing, 17,* 193.

Lethbridge, D. J., et al. (1993). Validation of the nursing diagnosis of ineffective breastfeeding. *Journal of Obstetric, Gynecologic, and Neonatal Nursing, 22,* 57.

Maccagno-Smith, R., et al. (1993). Breastfeeding the sleepy infant. *Canadian Nurse, 89,* 20.

Panetta, I. (1993). Breastfeeding, A to Z. *Canadian Nurse, 89,* 17.

Stashwick, C. A. (1994). Overcoming obstacles to breastfeeding. *Patient Care, 28,* 88.

Taitz, L. (1990). Feeding children in the first year of life. *Midwife, Health Visitor, and Community Nurse, 26,* 81.

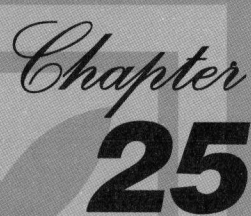

Chapter
25

Nursing Care of the Woman and Family Experiencing a Postpartal Complication

Objectives

After mastering the contents of this chapter, you should be able to:

1. *Describe common deviations from the normal that can occur during the puerperium.*

2. *Assess the woman and her family for deviations from the normal during the puerperium.*

3. *State nursing diagnoses related to deviations from the normal during the puerperium.*

4. *Plan interventions that meet the special needs of the family with a postpartal complication, such as planning for an extended hospitalization.*

5. *Implement nursing care when a postpartal complication such as hemorrhage, infection, hypertension of pregnancy, or postpartal psychosis develops.*

6. *Evaluate outcome criteria to be certain that nursing goals established for care were achieved.*

7. *Identify National Health Goals related to postpartal complications that nurses can be instrumental in helping the nation achieve.*

8. *Identify areas related to care of women with postpartal complications that could benefit from additional nursing research.*

9. *Use critical thinking to analyze ways that nursing care can remain family centered when a postpartal complication occurs.*

10. *Synthesize knowledge of puerperium complications with nursing process to achieve quality maternal and child health nursing care.*

Adele Pillitteri: MATERNAL AND CHILD HEALTH NURSING, 2nd Edition. © 1995 Adele Pillitteri.

Although the puerperium is usually a period of health, complications can occur. When they do, immediate intervention is essential to prevent long-term disability and/or interference with parent–child relationships. The Focus on National Health Goals box describes National Health Goals related to this period.

Most complications of the puerperium are preventable, a fact that is essential to keep in mind when caring for the postpartal woman. A woman with a postpartal complication is at risk from three points of view: her own health, her future childbearing potential, and her ability to bond with her new infant. A complication at this time also invariably causes a family disruption with increased separation of family members due to extended hospitalization. Additional child care that may need to be arranged could cause financial difficulties. Pregnancy and labor and birth, in themselves, create a crisis situation. If the crisis is not resolved but continues, it grows immeasurably in proportion, making it more difficult for the woman and her family to manage.

☒ **NURSING PROCESS OVERVIEW**
for the Woman Experiencing a Postpartal
Complication

ASSESSMENT

Postpartal complications invariably begin with subtle signs such as tenderness in the calf of the leg, slightly increased pain, slightly elevated temperature, and a slightly increased amount of lochia. Because the average woman has no postpartal complications, it is easy to perform postpartal assessments with a degree of "routine." It is important, however, to keep in mind a point at which you will categorize findings as "more than usual" or "more reddened than normal," as these are subjective judgments and it is easy to be misled. Don't rely solely on the mother's report of perineal healing or amount of lochia; be certain to observe the perineum yourself, because the report of "I feel fine" may be deceptive (she expected to have pain and so reports extreme pain as nothing out of the norm; she has no knowledge of "normal" lochia or fundal height against which to compare her own accurately).

An increased temperature exclusive of the first 24 hours following birth is an extremely serious finding. Women may try to "explain away" an increased temperature, because they know that if they have an elevated temperature they may not be allowed to feed their infant. Don't be tempted to rationalize such a finding with explanations such as the woman was smoking a cigarette just before her temperature was recorded, the room was warm, or she just had some coffee. Although these factors may make a slight difference (part of a degree) in temperature level, they do not affect it enough to account for a temperature over 100.4°F.

NURSING DIAGNOSIS

Nursing diagnoses during this time are as varied as the reasons for postpartal complications. Some examples include:

- Fluid volume deficit related to increased lochia flow
- High risk for infection related to microorganism invasion of perineal incision
- Altered peripheral tissue perfusion related to interference with circulation from thrombophlebitis
- Self-esteem disturbance related to postpartal infection and inability to feed infant
- High risk for altered parenting related to extended hospitalization
- Ineffective breast-feeding related to development of mastitis

PLANNING

Setting goals with the woman who has a postpartal complication may be particularly difficult because, although the woman wants to do everything necessary to return to health, she also does not want to allow anything to interfere with her ability to relate with her new child. During the stage of postpartal "taking-in," she may not be interested in doing things for herself; during the second stage of "taking-hold," she may not be interested in having you do procedures for her (see Chapter 22). As a rule, however, never underestimate the degree of pain, inconvenience, or sacrifice that a woman will undergo to prepare herself to care for a new child. That quality is the essence of motherhood.

Be certain in making plans for the postpartal family that you provide for measures that will both restore the woman most quickly to health and promote contact between her and her child, her primary support person,

and full family. Contact with the infant is best if it includes physical contact, such as holding and feeding. If this is not possible, frequent reports of the infant's health and preferences can be supplied by planning for the nursery to contact the mother at least once every nursing shift during the taking-in period and for a telephone call initiated by the mother during the taking-hold phase. Supplying Polaroid photos of the infant who is being cared for in another facility offers the woman something concrete to which to relate. Many mothers respond well to notes written as if they were from the child: "Hi, Mom. Just a note to say hello. I'm drinking well but I miss you and can't wait for you to get better and be allowed to take care of me. Love, Kelsey Marie." Such a note serves to relieve the mother's concern for the child (she is doing well) and also helps increase the mother's self-esteem, which will promote bonding. A number of women develop severe depression and even psychosis following childbirth. One national volunteer support group offers referrals throughout the United States for women who are depressed following childbirth: Depression After Delivery. Call (215) 295-3994 or write in care of P. O. Box 1282, Morrisville, PA 19067.

FOCUS ON
National Health Goals

The postpartal period is a time when women are very susceptible to hemorrhage and women with a complication following childbirth may choose not to breast-feed. Two National Health Goals directly relate to this time period:

- Reduce the maternal mortality rate to no more than 3.3 per 100,000 live births.
- Increase to at least 75% the proportion of mothers who breast-feed their babies in the early postpartal period (DHHS, 1991).

Nurses can be instrumental in helping the nation to achieve these goals by careful monitoring of uterine involution in the postpartal period and by encouraging women to breast-feed even in the face of a postpartal complication.

Areas related to complications of the postpartal period that could benefit from additional nursing research are better identification of risk factors for mastitis and endometritis; identifiable differences in women who stop breast-feeding and those who continue when a complication is present; and health teaching that is effective in preventing mastitis.

IMPLEMENTATION

Interventions for the woman with a complication of the postpartal period must include instruction in child care with (if appropriate) an emphasis on the transitory nature of the complication. Continuing to review well-child care helps the woman to accept the situation as temporary (if it were not, why would you be stressing her ability to return home shortly and care for the child?).

EVALUATION

Evaluation of the woman with a postpartal complication should address both the mother's health and her bonding with the child. Evaluation may suggest that follow-up care by a community health nurse may be necessary for the woman to cope with the responsibility of child care and integrating the child into the family in the face of reduced energy from illness.

Examples of outcome criteria might be:

- Symptoms of infection such as an oral temperature over 100.4°F and foul-smelling lochia are not present.
- Client will not experience fluid volume deficit secondary to hemorrhage as manifested by maintenance of blood pressure over 110/60.
- Client demonstrates warm contact with her child in spite of required bed rest.

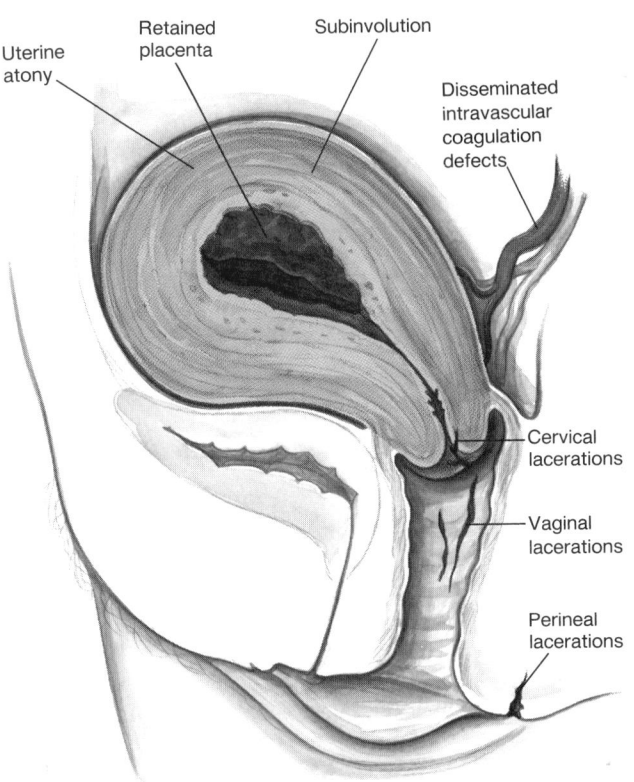

FIGURE 25-1
Common causes of postpartal hemorrhage.

Postpartal Hemorrhage

Hemorrhage, one of the most important causes of maternal mortality associated with childbearing, is a possibility all through pregnancy, but it is a major danger in the immediate postpartal period. With a normal birth, the average blood loss experienced is 300 to 500 mL. Postpartal hemorrhage has been traditionally defined as *any blood loss from the uterus greater than 500 mL within a 24-hour period* (Zahn & Yeomans, 1990). In specific agencies the loss may not be considered hemorrhage until it reaches 1000 mL (Zlatnik, 1990). Hemorrhage may occur either immediately, that is, occurring in the first 24 hours, or late, occurring during the remaining days of the 6-week puerperium (Khong & Khong, 1993). The greatest danger of bleeding is in the first 24 hours because of the grossly denuded and unprotected area left after detachment of the placenta (Cunningham et al., 1993).

There are four main reasons for postpartal hemorrhage: uterine atony, lacerations, retained placental fragments, and disseminated intravascular coagulation (DIC) (Figure 25-1).

Uterine Atony

Uterine atony is the most frequent cause of postpartal hemorrhage (Cunningham et al., 1993). As mentioned in the discussion of involutional changes (see Chapter 22),

the uterus must remain in a contracted state after birth to allow the open vessels at the placental site to seal. Factors that predispose to poor uterine tone and an inability to maintain a contracted state are summarized in Box 25-1. When you are caring for a client in whom any of these conditions are present, be especially cautious in your immediate observations and be on guard for signs of uterine bleeding.

Assessment

If the uterus suddenly relaxes, there will be an abrupt gush of blood from the placental site, with extreme vaginal bleeding and symptoms of shock and blood loss. This may occur immediately following birth or more gradually over the first hour postpartum, as the uterus slowly becomes uncontracted. In this instance, the bleeding that is seen from the vagina is seepage, not a gush of blood. Over a period of hours, however, this seepage results in a condition as lethal as a sudden release of blood.

It is difficult to estimate the amount of blood loss in the postpartal woman, because it is difficult to estimate the amount of blood it takes to saturate a perineal pad (anywhere between 25 and 50 mL.) By counting the perineal pads saturated in given lengths of time, such as half-hour intervals, you can form a rough estimate of blood loss. Five pads saturated in half an hour is obvi-

---

Box 25·1

*Conditions That Make Women at High Risk
for Postpartal Hemorrhage*

**Conditions That Distend the Uterus
Beyond Average Capacity**

Multiple gestation

Hydramnios (excessive amount of amniotic fluid)

Large baby (over 9 lb)

Presence of uterine myomas (fibroid tumors)

**Conditions That Could Have Caused Cervical
or Uterine Tears**

Operative delivery

Rapid delivery

**Conditions With Varied Placental Site
or Attachment**

Placenta previa

Placenta accreta

Premature separation of the placenta

**Conditions That Leave the Uterus Too Exhausted
to Contract Readily**

Deep anesthesia or analgesia

Labor initiated or assisted with an oxytocin agent

Maternal age over 30 years

High parity

Prolonged and difficult labor

Secondary maternal illness such as anemia

Endometritis

**Conditions That Lead to Inadequate Blood
Coagulation**

Fetal death

Disseminated intravascular coagulation

---

postpartal hours to ascertain that the uterus is remaining in a state of contraction is the best preventive measure against immediate hemorrhage. Frequent assessment of lochia and vital signs, particularly pulse and blood pressure, are equally important. If you reach to massage a fundus and are unsure you have located it, the uterus is probably in a state of relaxation. Under normal circumstances, a well-contracted uterus is firm and easily recognized because it feels like no other abdominal structure.

If the woman is losing enough blood to affect systemic circulation, she will develop signs of shock: an increased, thready, and weak pulse; decreased blood pressure; increased and shallow respirations; pale, clammy skin; and increasing anxiety (Lowe, 1990). The woman's circulatory system can compensate for a long time, however; therefore, detecting uterine relaxation should be your first assessment.

Therapeutic Management

The first step in controlling hemorrhage in the event of uterine atony is to attempt uterine massage to encourage contraction (Ritter & deShago, 1994). If the uterus cannot remain contracted, the physician will invariably order an intramuscular injection of methylergonovine (Methergine) or a dilute intravenous infusion of oxytocin to help the uterus maintain tone. Both of these drugs should be kept readily available on a postpartal unit for instant use in the event of postpartal hemorrhage.

Administration of an Oxytocic Agent. Pitocin is the most frequently prescribed intravenous oxytocic; a usual dose is 10 to 40 U per 1000 mL of a 5% dextrose solution. When oxytocin is given intravenously this way, its action is immediate; be aware, however, that oxytocin does not have a sustained action (only about an hour), so that symptoms of uterine atony can occur quickly again after administration of only a single dose. Methylergonovine (Methergine) may be given orally at a dose of 0.2 mg (action begins in 5 to 10 minutes) or intramuscularly at the same dose (action begins in 2 to 5 minutes). The duration of action with methylergonovine is 3 to 4 hours. Both pitocin and methylergonovine have the side-effect of causing hypertension, so they should not be administered if the woman's blood pressure is over 140/90 mm Hg; always assess for this before administration.

Blood Replacement. The number of transfusions given for postpartal bleeding has been reduced owing to the present concern for the safety of the blood supply. If a woman has lost over 500 mL, check if blood should be drawn for cross-matching, so that blood of the woman's specific type can be made available. A number of women donate blood during pregnancy so they can be

ously a different situation from five pads saturated in 8 hours. In either situation, however, the woman will have lost upward of 250 mL of blood; if either rate of flow is allowed to continue untended, the woman will be in grave danger. Be sure you differentiate between *saturated* and *used* when counting pads; *used* in this context is meaningless. Weighing perineal pads before and after use and then subtracting the difference is an accurate way to measure vaginal discharge. In weighing, 1 g (weight) equals 1 mL (volume) of blood, since gram and milliliter are comparable measures. Whether the woman is losing blood rapidly or slowly, always ask her to turn on her side when inspecting for blood loss so you can be certain that large amounts are not pooling undetected underneath her.

Palpating the fundus at frequent intervals in the

autotransfused if hemorrhage should occur (Kruskall, 1990). Be sure that your hands are not tied by hospital policies on ordering blood for replacement. Hemorrhaging women may need replacement, and you should have the authority to request that cross-matching and blood-readying procedures be started. If the necessary forms require a physician's signature, valuable time can be lost waiting for a physician to come to the hospital.

Bimanual Massage. If uterine massage and administration of oxytocin or methylergonovine are not effective in stopping uterine bleeding, the physician or nurse-midwife may attempt the further step of bimanual compression (one hand inserted in the vagina and the other pushing against the fundus through the abdominal wall). It may be necessary to return the woman to a delivery room, so that her uterine cavity can be explored manually for retained placental fragments, which may be preventing good contraction. Uterine packing may be placed to help halt bleeding (Maier, 1993).

Prostaglandin Administration. Prostaglandins promote strong, sustained uterine contractions. Prostaglandin F2a may be injected intramuscularly or intramyometrially to initiate uterine contractions (Oleen & Mariano, 1990). Side-effects to observe for with prostaglandin administration are nausea, diarrhea, tachycardia, and hypertension.

Hysterectomy. The above measures are effective in halting bleeding in all but the extremely atonic uterus. In this rare instance, ligation of the uterine arteries or a hysterectomy may have to be performed (Zelop et al., 1993). Appreciate the fact that this measure is carried out as a last resort only. Despite the emergency conditions, try to comfort and give support to the woman at this time. This is a totally unexpected outcome of childrearing for her and her support person.

Following hysterectomy, the woman will want to talk about what happened, why surgery was necessary, and how she feels now that she can no longer bear children. She needs to discuss her feelings with a person who will listen quietly and help her sort through her "Why me?" feelings. She usually has ambiguous feelings: she wanted to have more children (or at least have the ability to have more), but she also wanted to live. She is grateful to hospital personnel for saving her life, but she may feel resentful that she was not left capable of future childbearing. She may grieve (very genuinely) for children that will not be born. If this child was born outside the hospital and the woman was brought there under emergency circumstances, she has a need to talk about her choice of location for childbirth and perhaps some help with guilt that she did not choose a more controlled place for childbirth.

Open lines of communication between the couple and the hospital staff that allow the family to vent its feelings are most helpful to the couple in this crisis. Grieving for future children that will not be born can interfere with bonding with the present child.

Nursing Interventions

The emergency measure to contract a uterus with atony is to place one hand on the woman's symphysis pubis to give good support to the base of the uterus, grasp the fundus of the uterus with your other hand, and massage gently. Unless the uterus is extremely lacking in tone, this form of massage is usually effective in causing contraction, and, after a few seconds, the uterus will assume its healthy grapefruit-like feel.

The fact that the uterus responds well to massage, however, does not mean that the problem is solved. A few minutes after you remove your hand from the fundus, the uterus may relax and the lethal seepage may begin again. You must therefore remain with the woman following massage to be certain that the uterus is not relaxing again. She needs to be observed closely for the next 4 hours.

A full bladder pushes an uncontracted uterus into an even more uncontracted state. Offer a bedpan at least every 4 hours to keep the woman's bladder empty. To reduce bladder pressure, the physician or nurse-midwife may order insertion of a urinary catheter.

If a woman is experiencing respiratory distress from decreasing blood volume, administer oxygen by face mask. Keep her flat to allow adequate blood flow to her brain and kidneys.

Be certain with uterine atony not only that vital signs are taken frequently during the immediate postpartal period but also that they are interpreted accurately. The pulse rate, for example, may increase only one or two beats at each recording. If you look back at the entire picture, however, you will notice that although the pulse rate is rising slowly, it is rising *continuously,* an ominous pattern. In the event of slow bleeding, there is little change in pulse and blood pressure at first because of circulatory compensation. Suddenly, the system can compensate no more, however, and then the pulse rate rises rapidly. The pulse becomes weak and thready, and the blood pressure drops abruptly. The woman's skin becomes cold and clammy and shows obvious signs of shock. If you are taking frequent vital signs and are carefully monitoring lochia flow, you should be able to detect blood loss before this point is ever reached.

When planning continuing care, remember that any woman is exhausted after birth. If a woman hemorrhages in the immediate postpartal period, she feels even more exhausted. This may make her resent frequent uterine and blood pressure assessment every 15 minutes. Explain that the measures you are taking, although disturbing, are insurance measures. Make vital sign recordings as quickly and gently as possible, so that the woman feels a minimum of discomfort and has time to nap between observations.

The average woman takes the full postpartal period to regain her strength. Women who have a postpartal hemorrhage tend to have a longer than average recovery period because their exhaustion makes it more difficult for them to feel well again. The woman is usually prescribed a course of iron therapy to ensure good hemoglobin formation. She probably will have special orders as to the amount of exertion and postpartal exercise she should undertake. Discuss with her the possibility of having someone stay with her at home at least for the first week to help her with the care of her new baby and to prevent exhaustion from turning childbearing into a less than satisfying event. Extensive blood loss is one of the precursors of postpartal infection because of the general debilitation that results. Any woman who has undergone more than a normal loss of blood should be observed closely for changes in lochia discharge, and her temperature should be monitored closely in the postpartal period to detect the earliest signs of developing infection (see the Focus on Nursing Research box).

Lacerations

Small lacerations or tears of the birth canal are so common they can be considered a normal consequence of childbearing. Large lacerations are complications that occur most often with difficult or precipitate deliveries, in primigravidas, with the birth of a large infant (over 9 lb), and with the use of a lithotomy position and in-

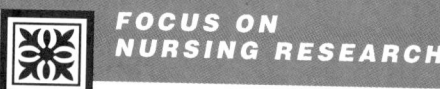

FOCUS ON NURSING RESEARCH

How Soon Do Women Return to Usual Functioning Following Childbirth?

Although the postpartum period is defined as the 6-week period following childbirth, not all women return to full functional status at the end of this time, especially if they have a complication of labor and delivery.

In this study, 97 women were assessed at 3 weeks, 3 months, and 6 months post delivery. At the end of the 6-week postpartal period, although 75% of women reported they were able to give full care to their infant by this time, only 28.9% reported they had assumed full household or social-community responsibilities; only 3.1% reported they had resumed their previous self-care activities.

The researchers stress that the postpartal period is only a theoretically defined period and many women need continued guidance and support beyond this time.

Tulman, L., Fawcett, J., Groblewski, L., & Silverman, L. (1990). Changes in functional status after childbirth. *Nursing Research, 39,* 70.

struments, since these can put added tension on the perineum. Lacerations can occur as either cervical, vaginal, or perineal. Any time the uterus is firm following birth and yet bleeding persists, a laceration of one of these three sites should be suspected.

Cervical Lacerations

Lacerations of the cervix are usually found on the sides of the cervix near the branches of the uterine artery. If the artery is torn, the blood loss will be great. The color of the blood will be brighter red than the venous blood lost with uterine atony because it is arterial bleeding. The force of the blood may be such that it gushes from the vaginal opening. Fortunately, this bleeding ordinarily occurs immediately following delivery of the placenta, when the physician or nurse-midwife is still in attendance.

Repair of a cervical laceration is difficult, because the bleeding is so intense that it can obstruct visualization of the area. Be certain the physician or nurse-midwife has adequate space to work and adequate sponges and suture supplies. The woman is not always aware of what is happening at this point, but she may pick up on the tone in the room that something is seriously wrong. Try to maintain an air of calmness and, if possible, stand beside the woman at the head of the table. She may be worried that the extra activity in the room has something to do with her baby. Assure her that the baby is fine (assuming that it is), but that she will need to stay in the birthing room a little longer than expected while the doctor places additional sutures. Remember that the protective attitude women felt toward their bodies all during pregnancy is now turned toward the baby, so they are generally relieved to learn that it is their problem, not the infant's.

If the laceration appears to be extensive or difficult to repair, it may be necessary for the woman to be given a general anesthetic for relaxation of the uterine muscle and to prevent pain. Be certain the father, assuming he is still present in the room, receives a good explanation as to the need for an anesthetic and the procedures being carried out.

Vaginal Lacerations

Lacerations can also occur in the vagina, although rarely. These are easier to assess because they are easier to view. Because vaginal tissue is friable, however, vaginal lacerations are harder to repair. Some oozing often follows a repair of the vagina, so the vagina may be packed to maintain pressure on the suture line. A Foley catheter may be placed at the same time, because the packing causes pressure on the urethra and can interfere with voiding. If packing is placed, be certain that the woman's chart and the nursing care plan are both marked to show that the packing is in place. Packing usually is removed after 24 to 48 hours and it will be the physician's or nurse-midwife's responsibility to remove it, but by careful recording of the packing's existence and making sure that it is removed, you serve as the woman's first line of defense against infection. Packing left in place too long tends to cause stasis and infection similar to toxic shock syndrome.

Perineal Lacerations

Lacerations of the perineum usually occur when the woman is delivered from a lithotomy position, because this position increases tension on the perineum. Perineal lacerations are classified in four categories, depending on the extent and depth of the tissue involved. These are shown in Table 25-1.

Perineal lacerations are sutured and treated as an episiotomy repair, so much so that it is often difficult to distinguish a repaired perineal laceration from an episiotomy repair on inspection. Lacerations do tend to heal more slowly because the edges of the suture line are ragged. Any woman who has a third- or fourth-degree laceration should not be given an enema or a rectal suppository, and her temperature should not be taken rectally; the sutures include the rectal sphincter, and the hard tips of equipment could open sutures. To prevent constipation and hard stools that could break the sutures, she should have a diet high in fluid and is usually given a stool softener for the first week of the puerperium. Make certain that the degree of the laceration is marked on her nursing care plan; ancillary caregivers such as aides have no appreciation of why these measures are contraindicated unless informed. Unless a secondary complication such as infection occurs, even fourth-degree lacerations should heal without long-term dyspareunia or incontinence (Crawford et al., 1993).

Retained Placental Fragments

Occasionally, the placenta does not deliver in its entirety, but fragments of it separate and are left behind. Because the portion retained keeps the uterus from contracting fully, uterine bleeding occurs. This is most likely to happen with a succenturiate placenta, a placenta with an accessory lobe (see Chapter 21), but it can happen in any instance. A placenta accreta is a placenta that fuses with the myometrium owing to an abnormal decidua basalis layer. Sections of this type of placenta will remain after birth and may need to be surgically incised (Zahn & Yeomans, 1990). To detect the complication of retained placenta, every placenta should be inspected carefully following birth to see if it is complete.

Assessment

If an undetected retained fragment is large, the bleeding will be apparent in the immediate postpartal period, because the uterus cannot contract with it in place. If the fragment is small, bleeding may not be detected until the sixth or tenth day postpartum, when the woman notices an abrupt discharge of a large amount of blood.

On examination, the uterus is usually found to be not fully contracted. If placental tissue is still present in the woman's body, a serum chorionic gonadotropin (HCG) elevation will also be present. Retained placental fragments also may be detected by sonogram.

Therapeutic Management

Removal of the placental fragment is necessary to stop bleeding. The woman will be taken to a delivery room where a dilatation and curettage will be performed to remove the offending placental fragment. In some instances, accreta placentas are so deeply attached they cannot be removed. Therapy with methotrexate may be used to destroy the retained placental tissue. Because the hemorrhage from retained fragments may be delayed until after women are at home, they must be instructed to observe the color of lochia discharge and report any tendency for the discharge to change from lochia alba to rubra.

Disseminated Intravascular Coagulation

Disseminated intravascular coagulation (DIC), a deficiency in clotting ability caused by vascular injury, may occur in any woman in the postpartal period but is usually associated with women who had premature separation of the placenta, missed abortion, or fetal death in utero (Kesteven et al., 1993). It is further discussed in Chapter 15.

Assessment

DIC should be suspected when the usual measures to induce uterine contraction fail to stop vaginal bleeding. Oozing from an intravenous site or a blood-drawing site is also highly suggestive that a level of low fibrinogen exists.

Therapeutic Management

A maternity service should maintain a supply of fibrinogen to be used for treatment of this condition. Increasing the woman's supply of fibrinogen usually decreases

Table 25-1. *Classification of Perineal Lacerations*

Classification	Description
First degree	These involve the vaginal mucous membrane and the skin of the perineum to the fourchette
Second degree	These involve the vagina, perineal skin, fascia, levator ani muscle, and perineal body
Third degree	These involve the entire perineum and reach the external sphincter of the rectum
Fourth degree	These involve the entire perineum, rectal sphincter, and some of the mucous membrane of the rectum

bleeding dramatically if hypofibrinogenemia is the underlying cause (Cunningham et al., 1993). Heparin also may be used as therapy, because it prevents massive clotting and any further lowering of the fibrinogen level.

Subinvolution

Subinvolution is incomplete return of the uterus to its prepregnant size and shape. With subinvolution, at a 4- or 6-week postpartal visit, the uterus is still enlarged and soft and the woman still has a lochial discharge. Subinvolution may result from a small retained placental fragment, a mild endometritis, or an accompanying problem, such as a myoma that is interfering with complete contraction. Oral administration of methylergonovine (0.2 mg four times daily) generally is prescribed to improve uterine tone and complete involution. If the uterus is tender to palpation, suggesting endometritis, an oral antibiotic may be prescribed as well. Be certain that women know at discharge from a health care facility the normal process of involution and lochial discharge. This prevents them from waiting a long interval before seeking health care advice. A chronic loss of blood from subinvolution will result in anemia and lack of energy, conditions that could lead to interference with bonding because of daily exhaustion.

Perineal Hematomas

A perineal hematoma is a collection of blood in the subcutaneous layer of tissue of the perineum. The overlying skin, as a rule, is intact with no noticeable trauma. Such blood collections may be caused by injury to blood vessels in the perineum during birth. They are most likely to occur following rapid spontaneous deliveries and in women who have perineal varicosities. They may occur at an episiotomy or laceration repair site if a vein was pricked during repair. They can cause the woman acute discomfort and concern but, fortunately, they usually represent only minor bleeding.

Assessment
Perineal sutures almost always give the postpartal woman some discomfort. When a woman complains of severe pain in the perineal area or a feeling of pressure between her legs, inspect the perineal area for a hematoma. If one is present, it appears as an area of purplish discoloration and obvious swelling anywhere from 2 cm to as much as 8 cm in diameter (Figure 25-2). The area is tender to palpation; it may at first feel fluctuant, but, as seepage into the area continues and tissue is drawn taut, it palpates as a firm globe.

Therapeutic Management
Report to the physician or nurse-midwife the presence of the hematoma, its size, and the degree of discomfort it is causing the woman. Administer a mild analgesic as ordered for pain relief. Applying an ice pack (covered

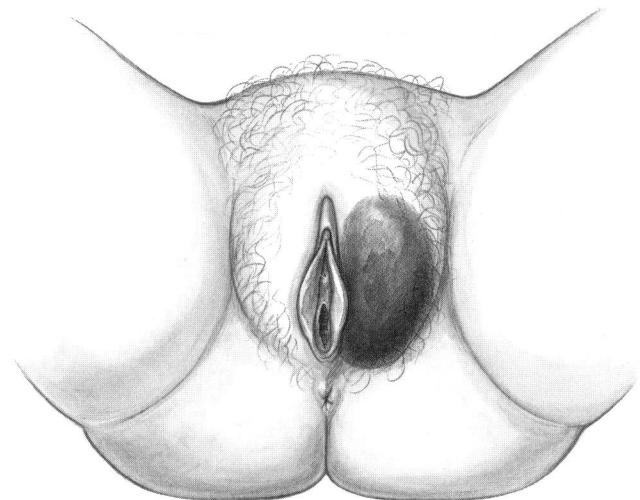

FIGURE 25-2
Appearance of a perineal hematoma from a bleeding subcutaneous vessel.

with a towel to prevent a thermal injury to the skin) may prevent further bleeding; the hematoma is then absorbed over the next 3 or 4 days. If the hematoma is large when discovered or continues to increase in size, the woman may have to be returned to the delivery room to have the site incised and the bleeding vessel ligated (Zahn & Yeomans, 1990). Be certain you assess the size of the collection of blood by measuring it in centimeters each time you inspect the perineum and that this measurement as well as the general appearance is meaningfully recorded. Describing a hematoma as "large" or "small" gives little information to the nurse relieving you about the hematoma's actual size. Describing the lesion as 5 cm across or the size of a quarter or a half dollar is meaningful because it establishes a basis for comparison.

The woman can be reassured that even though the hematoma is causing her considerable discomfort, her hospital stay probably will not be lengthened by its occurrence (unless it is extremely extensive) and the hematoma will absorb over the next 6 weeks, causing no further difficulty. If an episiotomy incision line is opened to drain a hematoma, it may be left open and packed with gauze rather than be resutured. Be certain this packing is recorded on the woman's chart and nursing care plan so you can be certain that it is removed (at about 24 to 48 hours). A suture line opened this way heals by tertiary intention, and thus it will heal slower than a first-degree intention suture line. Be certain the woman has clear instructions before discharge on suture line care she will need to carry out at home.

Postpartal Anterior Pituitary Necrosis

Postpartal anterior pituitary necrosis (also termed **Sheehan's syndrome**) is a rare disorder that may occur in a woman after severe hemorrhage (Gutowksi & Heron,

1993). In these instances, the pituitary gland appears to have been so damaged by the abrupt hypovolemia that it now does not function adequately. This is revealed by signs of decreased or absent lactation, genital and breast atrophy, and loss of pubic and axillary hair; myxedema or symptoms of thyroid dysfunction may result.

The woman needs hormone therapy to replace those hormones that her body now has difficulty producing, most noticeably estrogen, cortisone, and thyroid. Because of decreased stimulation to the ovaries, the woman may be infertile or sterile after this pituitary insult.

Puerperal Infection

Infection of the reproductive tract is another leading cause of maternal mortality. The factors that predispose women to infection in the postpartal period are shown in Box 25-2. When caring for a woman who has any of these circumstances, be extremely aware that postpartal infection is apt to occur.

The uterus is theoretically sterile during pregnancy and until the membranes rupture. It is capable of being invaded by pathogens after that rupture; an even greater risk is present if tissue edema and trauma are present. When infection occurs, the prognosis for complete recovery depends on a multitude of factors: the virulence

Box 25-2
Conditions That Make Women at High Risk for Postpartal Infection

1. Rupture of the membranes over 24 h before delivery (bacteria may have started to invade the uterus while the fetus was still in utero).
2. Placental fragments that have been retained within the uterus (the tissue necroses and serves as an excellent bed for bacterial growth).
3. Postpartal hemorrhage (the woman's general condition is weakened).
4. Pre-existing anemia (the body's defense against infection is lowered).
5. Prolonged and difficult labor, particularly instrument deliveries (trauma to the tissue may leave lacerations or fissures or easy portals of entry for infection).
6. Internal fetal heart monitoring (contamination may have been introduced with the placement of the scalp electrode).
7. Local vaginal infection was present at the time of delivery (direct spread of infection occurred).
8. The uterus was explored following delivery for a retained placenta or abnormal bleeding site (infection was introduced with exploration).

of the invading organism, the general health of the woman, the portal of entry, the degree of uterine involution, and the presence of lacerations in the reproductive tract. A puerperal infection is always serious because, although it usually begins as only a local infection, it can spread to involve the peritoneum (peritonitis) or circulatory system (septicemia), conditions that can be fatal in a woman already stressed from childbirth.

Therapeutic Interventions
Therapy for puerperal infection is prescription of an appropriate antibiotic after culture and isolation of the involved organism. Organisms commonly cultured postpartally are group B streptococci and aerobic gram-negative bacilli such as *Escherichia coli*, although staphylococcal infections are becoming more and more common. Staphylococcal infections are the cause of toxic shock syndrome, an infection not unlike puerperal infection in its ability to cause death and morbidity.

Nursing Diagnoses and Related Interventions

Nursing Diagnosis: High risk for infection related to loss of uterine sterility with childbirth

Goal: The woman will not experience a postpartal infection.

Outcome Criteria: The woman's temperature is below 38°C or 100.4°F orally, excluding the first 24 hours postpartum.

Some bacteria are transferred to the woman as a result of nasopharyngeal infection in hospital personnel. At birth, all persons in a delivery room or birthing room should be masked (nose and mouth). Any article (glove, instruments, and so on) introduced into the birth canal during labor, birth, and the postpartal period should be sterile. The woman must be given good instruction in perineal care, so that she does not bring *E. coli* organisms forward from the rectum. When giving perineal care, nurses should be certain to wash their hands before the procedure and not to open the labia, which would permit contaminated water to enter the vagina. Each maternity patient should have her own bedpan and perineal supplies to prevent transfer of pathogens from one woman to another.

Be certain that antibiotics are administered on time. If women will be continuing a drug at home, stress that they must take the full course to prevent the infection from recurring.

Nursing Diagnosis: High risk for social isolation related to precautions necessary to protect baby and others from exposure to infectious microorganisms

Goal: Woman will demonstrate understanding of the reason for precautions and develop ways to occupy time while in isolation; will demonstrate effective bond with newborn.

Outcome Criteria: The woman describes hospital policy regarding isolation and states plans for diversional activities while in hospital; demonstrates bonding behaviors such as asking about newborn and expressing desire to see infant.

The woman with an infection may be isolated from other clients to reduce the chances that others will contract the infection; she will be administered antibiotics, usually intravenously. Frequently used antibiotics are ampicillin, gentamycin, and first- or second-generation cephalosporins. Be certain to use good handwashing technique after giving care so you do not spread infection to other women or infants.

Whether the woman who has an infection should be allowed to feed and care for her baby is always a concern on postpartal units. Most hospitals have well-defined guidelines in this area (Box 25-3). This is a time in life when the woman is adjusting to a new life role. It is difficult enough to accomplish this when things are going well. When she is segregated from others, frightened by her condition, and denied the pleasure of holding and feeding her baby, the struggle may be more than she is prepared to tolerate. She needs friendly, understanding support from the hospital personnel who give her care.

Endometritis

Endometritis is an infection of the endometrium, the lining of the uterus. Bacteria gain access to the uterus through the vagina and enter the uterus either at the time of birth or during the postpartal period (Monga & Oshiro, 1993).

Assessment

Endometritis usually manifests itself on the third or fourth day of the puerperium, suggesting that a great deal of the invasion occurs during labor or birth.

The white blood cell count of a postpartal woman is normally increased to 20,000 to 30,000/mm^3. Thus, this conventional method of detecting infection is not of great value in the puerperium. An increase in oral temperature above 100.4°F (38°C) for two consecutive 24-hour periods, excluding the first 24-hour period after birth, is defined by the Joint Committee on Maternal Welfare as a febrile condition suggesting infection. All women with temperatures within this range should be suspected of having a postpartal infection until it is proved otherwise.

As a rule, the woman with endometritis demonstrates a rise in temperature well over 38°C. This rise on the third or fourth day postpartum coincides with the time breast engorgement occurs. Do not be led astray by attributing this temperature elevation to breast engorge-

ment. Fever on the third or fourth day postpartum should be considered possible endometritis until proved otherwise.

Depending on the severity of the infection, the woman may have chills, loss of appetite, and general malaise. Most women experience some abdominal tenderness. The uterus is generally not well contracted and is painful to the touch. The woman may feel strong afterpains. Lochia will usually be dark brown in color and have a foul odor. It may be increased in amount because of poor uterine involution, but if the infection is accompanied by high fever, lochia may be scant or absent.

Therapeutic Management

Treatment of endometritis consists of the administration of an appropriate antibiotic determined by a culture of the lochia (take a culture from the vagina by a sterile swab rather than from a perineal pad so you are certain you are culturing the endometrial infectious organism, not an unrelated one from the pad), accompanied by an oxytocic agent to encourage uterine contraction. The woman requires additional fluid to combat the fever. If strong afterpains and abdominal discomfort are present, she needs an analgesic for pain relief.

Fowler's position or ambulating are the best positions for the woman with endometritis, because these positions encourage lochia drainage by gravity and prevent pooling of infected secretions. Both you and the woman must use good handwashing techniques after handling perineal pads, because the pads contain contaminated discharge.

As with any infection, endometritis can be controlled best if it is discovered early in the disease process. If you can interpret the color, quantity, and odor of lochia discharge, and the size, consistency, and tenderness of a postpartal uterus in connection with an increased temperature, you may be the first person to recognize that disease is present.

If the infection is limited to the endometrium, the course of infection is about 7 to 10 days. The woman may have to make arrangements for her baby's discharge prior to her own, because her hospital stay will be extended for a few days. Endometritis can lead to tubal scarring and interference with future fertility. At a future time, if the woman desires more children, she should ask for a fertility assessment (including a hysterosalpingogram) for tubal patency if after a 6- to 12-month period of unprotected coitus she has not conceived. With mild endometritis this is usually not a problem, but the woman should be forewarned that it could occur.

Infection of the Perineum

Assessment

If a woman has a suture line on her perineum from an episiotomy or a laceration repair, there is a ready portal of entry present for bacterial invasion. Infections of the

> ### Box 25-3
> *Common Isolation Guidelines for the Woman With a Postpartal Infection*
>
> 1. As a rule, the baby of a mother with an increased temperature (100.4°F or 38°C) for two consecutive 24-h periods exclusive of the first 24 h is excluded from her room until the cause of the infection is determined. The mother may have an upper respiratory or a gastrointestinal infection unrelated to childbearing but which is transmittable to the newborn.
>
> 2. If the cause of the fever is found to be related to childbirth but involves a closed infection such as thrombophlebitis, when there would be no danger of the baby's contracting the disease, the mother can care for her child as long as she maintains bed rest in the prescribed position while doing so.
>
> 3. If the infection involves drainage (e.g., endometritis, perineal abscess), newborn visiting may be contraindicated. If the mother is allowed to feed her child, she should wash her hands thoroughly before holding the infant. She should never place the baby on the bottom bed sheet, where there may be some infected drainage from her perineal pad (furnish a clean sheet to spread over the covers when you bring in the baby).
>
> 4. Most hospitals are reluctant to return to a central nursery a baby who has visited in a room where there is an infection. The hospital should provide small nurseries that may be used as isolation nurseries for these situations, or the baby can be placed in a closed Isolette in a central nursery or cared for in the mother's room.
>
> 5. If the mother has a high fever, breast milk may be deficient. With modern antimicrobial therapy, puerperal infections are limited, and the period of high fever will be transient. If the mother is too ill to nurse the baby during this time or is receiving an anticoagulant or antibiotic that is passed in breast milk and would be harmful to the baby, the infant should be fed by a supplementary milk formula and the woman's breast milk should be manually expressed to maintain the production of milk so that it will be available when she is again able to nurse. You may need to assist her with this, since she fatigues easily and her energy level may not be enough to support her good intentions. If it appears that the course of the infection will be long, the mother may choose to, or may be advised to, discontinue breastfeeding. In these instances, the physician will usually prescribe a lactation suppressing drug to discourage breast engorgement. Once lactation is well established, however, these drugs are not as effective in suppressing lactation so engorgement may be painful.
>
> 6. If it is necessary for the woman to discontinue breastfeeding, she needs to be assured that she can meet the needs of the child through bottle feeding.
>
> 7. If the woman is going to be hospitalized for a long time, she may have to make arrangements for the discharge and care of the baby. She may be interested in a homemaker service or temporary foster care if she has no close friends or family. If she has older children at home, she needs to keep in close contact with them, calling them on the telephone or writing them short notes if possible. She needs to see a photo of the newborn (a Polaroid camera should be a piece of equipment on every postpartal unit) and hear daily reports of his or her progress and well-being.

perineum generally remain localized and manifest the symptoms of any suture line infection: pain, heat, and a feeling of pressure. The woman may or may not have an elevated temperature, depending on the systemic effect and spread.

Inspection of the suture line reveals the inflammation. One or two stitches may be sloughed away, or an area of the suture line may be open with pus present (Figure 25-3). Notify the woman's physician or nurse-midwife of the localized symptoms and culture the discharge by a sterile cotton-tipped applicator touched to the secretion.

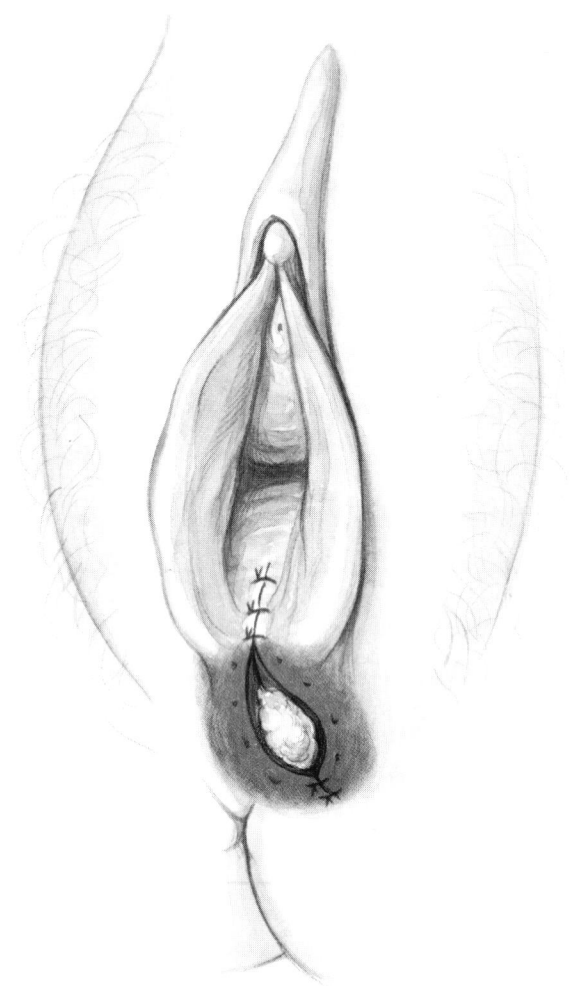

FIGURE 25-3
An infected suture line appears reddened and edematous and often contains infected secretions.

Therapeutic Management

The woman's physician or nurse-midwife may choose to remove the perineal sutures to open the area and allow for drainage. A packing, such as iodoform gauze, may be placed in the open lesion to keep it open and allow it to drain. Be certain the woman is aware that the packing is in place and that she knows not to dislodge the packing as she changes her perineal pad.

An antibiotic will be ordered even before the culture report is returned, and with it an analgesic for discomfort. Sitz baths or warm compresses may be ordered to hasten drainage and cleanse the area. Remind the woman to change perineal pads frequently because they are contaminated by seropurulent drainage. If left in place for a long time, they might cause vaginal contamination or reinfection. The woman should be instructed to also wash her hands (and you want to be certain to do this also) after handling perineal pads. Be certain she wipes front to back after a bowel movement to prevent bringing feces forward onto the healing area.

A local infection of this nature may lengthen the woman's hospital stay by 3 or 4 days, because the incision site, once opened, must then heal by tertiary rather than primary intention. Infections of this nature are annoying and painful to the mother out of proportion to their size. Fortunately, with the use of improved techniques during parturition and the puerperium, perineal infections are now only rarely seen. Because they are localized, there is no need to exclude an infant from the room as long as the woman washes her hands well before holding the newborn. Be certain not to place the infant on the bottom bed sheet where he or she could contact pathogenic bacteria. Be certain that the woman with this type of infection continues to ambulate; the pain from an infected suture line can be severe and she will decrease ambulation unless urged to continue. Assess the mouth of the infant for thrush (oral *Candida*) if a woman is prescribed an antibiotic. A portion of the antibiotic passes into breast milk and can cause an overgrowth of fungal organisms in the infant as well as the woman. Assess the infant for easy bruising; a decrease of microorganisms in the bowel from an antibiotic passed in breast milk may lead to insufficient vitamin K formation and consequently decreased blood-clotting ability.

Thrombophlebitis

Phlebitis is inflammation of the lining of a blood vessel; **thrombophlebitis** is inflammation of the lining of a blood vessel with the formation of blood clots. When thrombophlebitis occurs in the postpartal period, it is usually an extension of an endometrial infection (Magee et al., 1993). It is prone to occur in the postpartal period when blood-clotting ability is high because of (1) increased fibrinogen; (2) dilation of lower extremity veins due to pressure of the fetal head during pregnancy and birth; and (3) the relative inactivity of the period that leads to pooling, stasis, and clotting of blood in the lower extremities (Gerbasi et al., 1990). Women most prone to thrombophlebitis are those with varicose veins, those who are obese, those who had a previous thrombophlebitis, women over 30 years old with increased parity who were in a stirrups position for a long time during birth, or those who have a high incidence of thrombophlebitis in their family.

Prevention of endometritis by use of good aseptic technique helps to prevent thrombophlebitis as well. Early ambulation encourages circulation in the lower extremities and decreases the possibility of clot formation. Women should not remain any longer than an hour in a lithotomy and stirrups position. Be certain that the stirrups of examining and delivery tables are well padded to prevent any sharp pressure against the calf of the legs in this position. If a woman had varicose veins during pregnancy, wearing support stockings for the first 2 weeks postpartum will increase venous circulation and help prevent stasis (Figure 25-4). Be certain the woman puts support stockings on before she rises in the morning; if she waits until she is already up and walking, venous congestion has already occurred and the stockings are less effective. Remove support stockings twice daily and assess skin underneath them for mottling or inflammation that would suggest inflammation of the veins. The Focus on Family Teaching box summarizes these thrombophlebitis prevention measures.

Femoral Thrombophlebitis

With femoral thrombophlebitis, the femoral, saphenous, or popliteal veins are involved. Although the inflammation site in thrombophlebitis is in a vein, an accompanying arterial spasm often diminishes arterial circulation to the leg as well. This decreased circulation, along with edema, gives the leg a white or drained appearance. As the woman's temperature rises because of the infection, her supply of breast milk tends to decrease as the body attempts to save fluid. For these reasons, it was formerly believed that breast milk was going into the leg, giving it its white appearance. The condition was called *milk leg* or *phlegmasia alba dolens* (white inflammation).

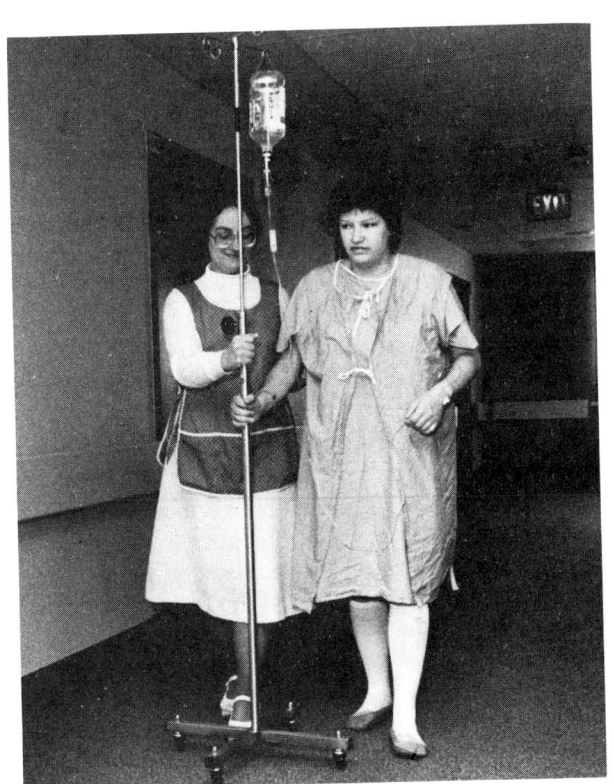

FIGURE 25-4
Ambulation helps to prevent thromboembolism postpartally. Notice the thromboembolitic stockings in place. (Courtesy of the Department of Medical Photography, Children's Hospital, Buffalo, NY.)

FOCUS ON FAMILY TEACHING

Q. I had a mild thrombophlebitis after my first baby. What can I do to help prevent this from happening this time?

A. Thrombophlebitis is directly related to stasis of blood in lower extremity veins and is preventable to a great degree. Common suggestions include the following:

• Ask your primary care provider if you can use a sidelying or supine recumbent position for birth rather than a lithotomy position (lithotomy position can increase the tendency for pooling of blood in lower extremities).

• If you will be using a lithotomy position, ask for padding on the stirrups to prevent sharp calf pressure.

• Early ambulation is the best preventive measure. When resting in bed, wiggle your toes or do leg lifts to improve venous return.

• Ask your primary care provider if he or she recommends support stockings immediately postpartal. Be certain to put these on before ambulating in the morning, before leg veins are full.

Assessment

If femoral thrombophlebitis is present it is revealed on about the tenth day after birth by an elevated temperature, chills, and stiffness, pain, and redness in the affected leg. The leg begins to swell below the lesion, because venous circulation is blocked at that point. The skin becomes stretched to a point of shiny whiteness. Homans' sign (pain in the calf on dorsiflexion of the foot) will be positive (see Figure 22-8). Measure the diameter of the leg at the thigh and calf level and then compare to measurements in the next few days to note any decrease or increase in size.

Therapeutic Management

Treatment consists of bed rest with the affected leg elevated, administration of anticoagulants, and application of heat. Women who have been discharged from the hospital will be cared for at home or may have to return to the hospital so that strict bed rest can be enforced. A cradle is used to keep pressure of the bedclothes off the affected leg, both to decrease the sensitivity of the leg and to improve the circulation (Figure 25-5). A light bulb used with the cradle supplies continual heat to the leg, or heat may be supplied by means of moist, warm compresses.

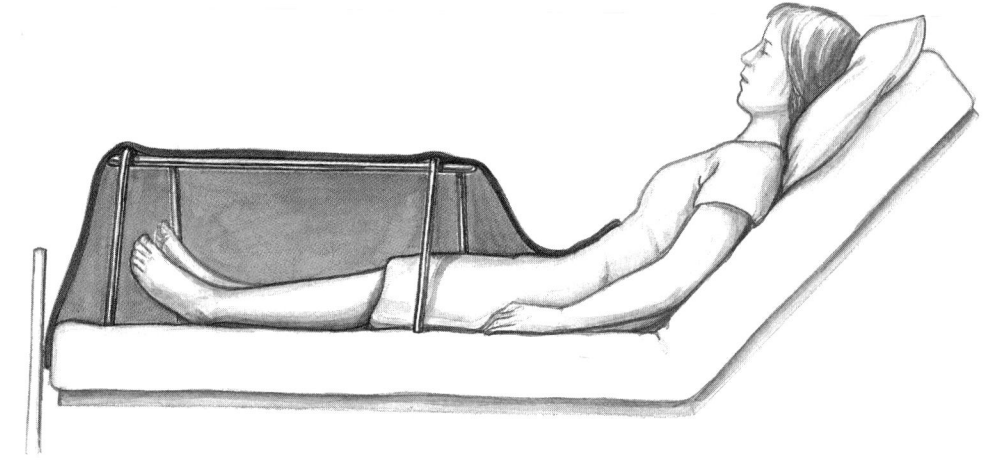

FIGURE 25-5

A bed cradle is used to lift the weight of bedclothes off the legs for the woman with thrombophlebitis.

Warm, wet dressings are one of the most technically difficult treatments to carry out, because dressings invariably dry or become cold after a short time. Compresses and water do not have to be sterile because, with thrombophlebitis, there is no break in the skin. Be certain to test water temperature by dipping your inner wrist in it prior to soaking the dressing to be certain that it is not too warm (sensation in the woman's leg is decreased because of edema so she can be burnt easily). Always cover wet, warm dressings with a plastic pad to hold in heat and moisture. In addition, a K-pad (with circulating heating coils), a Gaymar pump, which consists of a pad that is moistened about every 8 hours and kept warm by a circulating flow of water through an attached pump, or chemical hot packs may be positioned over the plastic to ensure the soaks stay warm. Be certain that the weight of a hot pack or pad does not rest on the leg, obstructing the flow of blood by its weight.

Check the woman's bed frequently when wet compresses are being used to be certain that the bed is not wet from seeping water. For soaks to stay in place, a woman must keep her leg fairly immobile. Be certain she doesn't interpret this as meaning she cannot turn, however. Providing activities for the woman so she doesn't become restless helps to keep dressings in place. Figure 25-6 shows a crossword puzzle relating to newborn care, which is the sort of activity that not only helps a woman maintain bed rest but also educates her about infant care. It could be used as well as a means to assess her health teaching needs. Provide good back, buttocks, and heel care for the woman; check for bed wrinkles so she doesn't develop a secondary problem of a decubitus while remaining this long in bed.

The pain of a thrombophlebitis is usually severe enough to require administration of analgesics. An appropriate antibiotic and often an anticoagulant (dicumarol or heparin) or a thrombolytic agent such as streptokinase to dissolve the clot and prevent further clot formation will be prescribed. The woman will have daily blood coagulation level determinations before administration of the anticoagulant. Lochia will usually increase in amount in the woman who is receiving an anticoagulant. Be sure to keep a meaningful record of the amount of this discharge so it can be estimated. "Lochia serosa with scattered pinpoint clots; three perineal pads saturated in 8 hours" is far more meaningful than "large amount of lochia." Weighing perineal pads before and after use is also effective. Assess also other possible signs of bleeding, such as bleeding gums, ecchymotic spots on the skin, or oozing from an episiotomy suture line.

The dicumarol anticoagulants are passed in breast milk, so the woman will have to discontinue breast-feeding during a course of therapy with these agents. If the infection does not seem to be severe and the woman wants to reinstate breast-feeding after the course of anticoagulant (about 10 days), she should manually express breast milk at the time of normal feedings to maintain a good milk supply. Heparin is one of the few drugs that does not pass into breast milk. If this is the anticoagulant chosen, breast-feeding does not need to be halted. Protamine sulfate is the antagonist for heparin and should be readily available any time heparin is being administered. Check the nursing unit's emergency cart for this. (See the Focus on Cultural Awareness display.)

Heparin can be administered by continuous intravenous infusion or intermittently by subcutaneous injection. If a woman will be discharged on subcutaneous therapy, be certain she has demonstrated good injection technique prior to discharge and understands the importance of required blood work (coagulation time) so that she schedules this appropriately.

Women on anticoagulants are not normally prescribed salicylic acid (aspirin), because salicylic acid acts as a mild anticoagulant. Some women, however, may be prescribed aspirin every 4 hours as their primary anticoagulant. If this is the case, be certain that you do not interpret aspirin used this way as a PRN analgesia order and withhold it depending on the woman's level of pain.

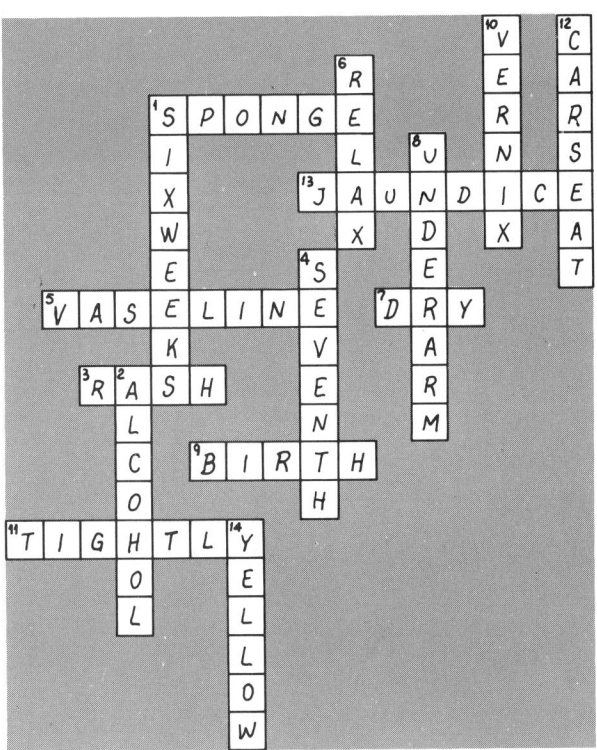

Across

1. Type of bath to give until cord falls off.
3. Consequence of not washing buttocks after bowel movement.
5. Ointment usually applied to circumcision at home.
7. Condition in which to keep umbilical cord.
9. Age at which a newborn sees.
11. Manner in which newborns like to be wrapped.
13. Name of yellow tinge to newborn skin.

Down

1. Age at which infant first smiles.
2. Antiseptic usually applied to cord at home.
4. First day cord can be expected to fall off.
6. Important rule for breastfeeding.
8. Best place to take an infant's temperature.
10. Name of white cream cheese-like substance on newborns.
12. Important piece of safety equipment with newborns.
14. Typical color of infant stool.

FIGURE 25-6
A crossword puzzle can be both a diversional activity and a learning aid for the postpartal woman on bed rest.

With proper treatment, the acute symptoms of femoral thrombophlebitis last only a few days, but the full course of the disease takes 4 to 6 weeks before it is resolved. The affected leg may never return to its former size and may always cause discomfort after long periods of standing (see the Nursing Care Plan: A Woman With Postpartal Thrombophlebitis).

Pelvic Thrombophlebitis

Pelvic thrombophlebitis involves the ovarian, uterine, or hypogastric veins. It occurs later than femoral thrombophlebitis, often around the 14th or 15th day of the puerperium.

Assessment

The woman is suddenly extremely ill, with a high fever, chills, and general malaise. The infection may be so severe that it necroses the vein and results in a pelvic abscess. It can become systemic and result in a lung, kidney, or heart valve abscess.

Therapeutic Management

As with femoral thrombophlebitis, therapy is total bed rest and administration of antibiotics and anticoagulants.

The disease runs a long course of 6 to 8 weeks and, if an abscess forms, may have a fatal outcome (although this can be located and incised by laparotomy, if necessary). An inflammation of this extent may leave tubal scarring and interfere with future fertility.

The woman may need surgery to remove the affected vessel before attempting to become pregnant again. If she should be pregnant in the future, she needs to be careful not to wear constricting clothing on her lower extremities, to rest with feet elevated, and to ambulate daily during pregnancy. She should be cautioned to tell the physician or nurse-midwife at her next birth of the difficulty she experienced this time to ensure that extra precautions are taken to prevent thrombophlebitis.

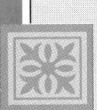

FOCUS ON CULTURAL AWARENESS

The amount of activity that women expect to engage in following childbirth is culturally determined. For this reason, women who assume that they will immediately return to an active lifestyle may see hospitalization for a postpartal complication as more upsetting than women who view the postpartal period as one in which they are expected to rest. The choice to breast-feed or not is also culturally influenced. If there is a postpartal complication that interferes with breast-feeding, the woman who feels that breast-feeding is very important can be expected to react less favorably than the woman from a culture in which formula-feeding is preferred. Assessing each woman individually is necessary to establish the personal impact of a postpartal complication.

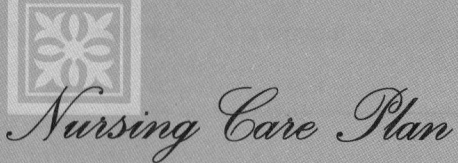

Nursing Care Plan

The Woman With Postpartal Thrombophlebitis

Lynn Barry is a 30-year-old G1P1 woman you care for on her second postpartal day. The following is a nursing care plan devised for her.

Assessment: Client states that her right calf is tender to touch; skin over area is white and shiny. She first noticed symptoms this morning when she awoke (20 minutes ago). Homans' sign positive; right calf larger than left by 2 cm in diameter. Toes blanch equally well in both feet. Temperature is 99.6°F orally.

Nursing Diagnosis: Altered peripheral tissue perfusion related to impaired circulation

Defining Characteristic: Calf painful, skin shiny; positive Homans' sign.

Goal: Client will complete postpartal course without further leg involvement.

Outcome Criteria: Erythema and positive Homans' sign are no longer apparent; client reports pain in leg has resolved.

Nursing Orders	Rationale
1. Complete bed rest with heat cradle and continuous moist warm compresses with Gaymar pump (be certain light bulb of cradle is 15–18 inches away from leg); assess temperature of dressings qh to be certain warmth is maintained.	1. Bed rest may prevent thrombophlebitis from becoming a pulmonary embolus. Warmth from a heated cradle and compresses is comforting and increases circulation to the leg by decreasing edema. Assessing level of warmth helps prevent a burn, since sensation in leg may be decreased because of edema present.
2. Do not rub calf or leg; caution client about doing this.	2. Rubbing could cause clot to move and create a pulmonary embolus.
3. Assess leg for diameter and Homans' sign three times daily.	3. Increased diameter could indicate increased thrombophlebitis formation; Homans' sign indicates inflammation is still present.
4. Encourage good fluid intake (3000–4000 mL daily).	4. Increased fluid decreases blood viscosity.
5. Heparin to be administered subcutaneously daily based on partial thromboplastin time (PTT) report. Schedule PTT daily at 6 A.M. (Do not administer heparin without daily report.)	5. Heparin will decrease tendency for blood clots. Administration of anticoagulant in face of low PTT report could lead to increased bleeding tendency.
6. Assess q4h for excessive amount of lochia (saturating over 1 pad in 1 h); weigh pads if necessary. Assess for bleeding gums, ecchymotic spots, or oozing from episiotomy sutures q4h.	6. Lochia flow could become excessive in light of anticoagulant therapy. Obtain accurate amount of flow and other indications of low clotting level.
7. Position infant bassinet next to bed so client can reach infant easily.	7. Help promote mother–infant bonding.
8. Encourage breastfeeding. Be certain client is comfortable holding infant without pressure on leg.	8. Client may breastfeed safely, because thrombophlebitis is self-contained and not infectious. Careful positioning of infant prevents pressure on thrombophlebitis site.
9. Ask husband to bring in an activity such as a hobby for client.	9. Provides diversion while client remains hospitalized an additional 3 or 4 days.

Pulmonary Embolus

A pulmonary embolus is obstruction of the pulmonary artery with a blood clot, usually seen as a complication of thrombophlebitis. The signs of pulmonary embolus are sudden, sharp chest pain, tachypnea, tachycardia, orthopnea (inability to breathe except in an upright position), and cyanosis (the blood clot is obstructing the pulmonary artery, thus blocking blood flow to the lungs and return to the heart). This is an emergency condition. The woman needs oxygen administered immediately; she almost immediately may need cardiopulmonary resuscitation. Her condition is extremely guarded until the clot is lysed or adheres to the pulmonary artery wall and is reabsorbed. A woman with this degree of postpartal complication is transferred to an intensive care unit for continuing care.

Peritonitis

Peritonitis, or infection of the peritoneal cavity, is usually an extension of endometritis. It is one of the gravest complications of childbearing and accounts for a third of all deaths from puerperal infection (Cunningham et al., 1993). The infection spreads through the lymphatic system or directly through the fallopian tubes or uterine wall to the peritoneal cavity. An abscess may form in the cul-de-sac of Douglas, since this is the lowest point of the peritoneal cavity.

Assessment
The symptoms are the same as those of the surgical patient in whom a peritoneal infection develops: rigid abdomen, abdominal pain, high fever, rapid pulse, vomiting, and the appearance of being acutely ill. It is important when assessing the abdomen of postpartal women that you notice that not only is the uterus well contracted but also it is not tender to touch and the remainder of the abdomen is soft. The occurrence of a rigid abdomen (guarding) is one of the first symptoms of peritonitis.

Therapeutic Management
With peritonitis comes paralytic ileus, which requires a nasogastric tube to be inserted to prevent vomiting; the woman will need intravenous fluid or total parenteral nutrition while she is unable to take food orally because of the intestinal paralysis. She will need analgesics for pain relief. She will be placed on large doses of antibiotics. Her hospital stay will be lengthy, and her prognosis is guarded. A peritonitis may interfere with future fertility, because it leaves scarring and adhesions in the peritoneum. Adhesions formed this way may separate the fallopian tubes from the ovaries so much that ova can no longer easily enter the tubes.

Mastitis

Mastitis (infection of the breast) may occur as early as the seventh postpartal day or may not occur until the baby is weeks or months old (Kaufmann & Foxman, 1991).

The organism causing the infection usually enters through cracked and fissured nipples. Thus, the measures that prevent cracked and fissured nipples also prevent mastitis. These include making certain that the baby is positioned correctly and grasps the nipple properly, including both nipple and areola; releasing the baby's grasp on the nipple before removing the baby from a breast; washing hands between handling perineal pads and breasts; exposing nipples to air for at least part of every day; and using a vitamin E ointment to soften nipples daily. If the woman has one cracked and one well nipple, encourage her to begin breast-feeding (when the infant sucks most forcefully) on the unaffected nipple.

Occasionally, the organism that causes mastitis comes from the nasal-oral cavity of the infant. In these instances, the infant has usually acquired a *Staphylococcus aureus* infection while in the hospital nursery (Olsen et al., 1990). Candidiasis may also be spread this way (Johnstone et al., 1990). Sucking on the nipple, the infant introduces the organisms into the milk ducts, where they proliferate (breast milk is an excellent medium for bacterial growth). This is an epidemic breast abscess; it is usually discovered that several women discharged from the hospital at the same time have similar infections.

Assessment
Mastitis is usually unilateral, although epidemic mastitis (because it originates with the infant) may be bilateral. The affected breast shows localized pain, swelling, and redness. Fever accompanies these first symptoms within a matter of hours, and breast milk becomes scant.

Therapeutic Management
The woman will be placed on a broad-spectrum antibiotic, such as cephalosporin. Breast-feeding is continued, because keeping the breast emptied of milk helps to prevent growth of bacteria. Some women may find an infected breast too painful to allow the infant to suck and may prefer to express milk manually from the affected breast for 2 or 3 days until the antibiotic has taken effect and the mastitis has faded (about 3 days). Ice compresses and good bra support give a great deal of pain relief until the process improves. Warm, wet compresses may be ordered to reduce inflammation and decrease edema.

If therapy is started as soon as symptoms are apparent, the condition runs a short course of about 2 or 3 days. If untreated, a breast infection may become a localized abscess. This may involve a large portion of the breast and rupture through the skin, with thick, purulent drainage. The woman will need incision and drainage of the abscess. If an abscess forms this way, breast-feeding on that breast is discontinued, but the woman is encouraged to continue to pump breast milk until the abscess has resolved in order to preserve breast-feeding. Some women may feel that the breast is too tender to do this; these women can be assured that for this child, formula-feeding is an alternative acceptable feeding method.

Neither mastitis nor breast abscess leaves any permanent breast disease. The woman can be assured that such an incident is not associated with development of breast cancer and does not interfere with future breast-feeding potential.

Urinary System Disorders

Urinary Retention

Urinary retention implies inadequate bladder emptying. It occurs following childbirth because of decreased bladder sensation for voiding due to edema of the bladder from the pressure of birth. Unable to empty, the bladder fills to overdistention. When the woman does void, instead of emptying completely, the bladder only empties a small portion of its contents (retention with overflow). It will quickly, therefore, become overdistended again. Bladder overdistention is potentially serious, because if it is allowed to continue, permanent damage can occur from loss of bladder tone, leading to permanent incontinence (Saultz et al., 1991).

Assessment

In the postpartal woman, urinary retention with overflow is less easy to detect than primary overdistention, because with overdistention, the woman does not void at all. It is easy to detect that a longer-than-usual time (over 8 hours) has passed following birth or between voids than is normal. Assessment by percussion or palpation of the bladder reveals the distention.

With urinary retention and overflow, however, the woman is not only voiding but is voiding very frequently (suggesting that her output must be adequate). It is a good practice to measure the amount of the first voiding after birth by putting a measuring container on the toilet seat in the bathroom. As a rule, if a voiding is less than 50 mL, urinary retention should be suspected.

Urinary retention is proved by catheterizing the woman immediately after a voiding. If the amount of urine left in the bladder after voiding is over 100 mL, the woman has retention above the normal amount. As a rule, a physician or nurse-midwife writes an order to read "Catheterize for residual urine. If this is over 100 mL, leave indwelling catheter in place." Always use a Foley (indwelling) catheter rather than a temporary one (straight catheter) to catheterize for residual urine, and be careful to use absolute aseptic technique so as not to introduce pathogenic bacteria into the sterile urinary tract and cause a urinary tract infection.

Catheterizing a woman during the early postpartal period is often a difficult procedure, because vulvar edema distorts the position and appearance of the urinary meatus. Use a gentle technique, remembering that the woman's perineum is apt to feel tender to touch.

How much urine to remove from an overdistended bladder at one time is controversial. There is a suggestion that removing more than 750 to 1000 mL of urine at any one time will create a great pressure change not only in the bladder but also in the lower abdomen. This decreased pressure in the lower abdomen may cause blood to flow into the area. This could create supine hypotension. There are few actual documented occurrences of this happening, however. Particularly in the postpartal period, when a bladder easily distends and the uterus is larger than normal, this shift in pressure may not be as important. Health care agency policy should be followed in regard to how much urine to remove from a full bladder at catheterization.

If a catheter will be left in place, be certain to explain the principle of it and draw a picture or explain how the balloon is inflated to hold it in place. This prevents the woman from limiting her activity to try and keep it in place and so helps prevent other complications, such as thrombophlebitis. Catheterization is a procedure that has a reputation as being extremely painful. You can assure women that, as a rule, it involves only a momentary sting (like a pin prick) as the catheter is inserted. Since the pain sensation of edematous tissue is decreased, the woman with extreme vulva edema may experience the pain as barely noticeable.

After 24 hours, an indwelling catheter is usually ordered to be removed. Encourage the woman to void by the end of 6 hours after removal of the catheter by offering fluid, administering an analgesic so she can relax, assisting her to the bathroom as necessary, and trying time-honored solutions such as running water at the sink or letting her hold her hand under running water. In most women, bladder and vulvar edema have decreased to such an extent by this time that she is able to void without further difficulty. If she has not voided by 8 hours after catheter removal, the physician or nurse-midwife may suggest another catheter be inserted for an additional 24 hours.

Difficulty with bladder function after childbirth is becoming less of a problem as less anesthesia and fewer forceps are used at birth, lessening bladder and vulvar pressure. When problems do arise, it is difficult for the woman to accept because bladder elimination is a basic step of self-care. It is disappointing and discouraging to a woman who wants not only to be able to care for herself but to care for a new infant as well. Assure women that bladder complications are not that uncommon and invariably are present no longer than 48 hours postpartum. They are not problems that will recur, so that once the difficulty is passed, she does not need to worry about it any longer and can proceed to focus her attention away from her body to her new child.

Urinary Tract Infection

The woman who is catheterized at the time of childbirth or who is catheterized in the postpartal period is prone to developing a urinary tract infection, because bacteria may be introduced into the bladder at the time of catheterization (Stray-Pedersen et al., 1990).

Assessment
When a urinary tract infection develops, the woman notices symptoms of burning on urination, possibly blood in the urine (hematuria), and a feeling of frequency or that she always has to void. The pain is so sharp on voiding that she may resist doing so and thus compound the problem of urinary stasis. She may have a low-grade fever and discomfort from lower abdominal pain.

A clean-catch urine specimen should be obtained for any woman with symptoms of urinary tract infection (see Nursing Procedure 10-1). This can be done as an independent nursing action. So that lochial discharge does not contaminate the specimen, provide a sterile cotton ball for the woman to tuck in her vagina after perineal cleansing. Be certain to ask if the woman removed the vaginal cotton ball after the procedure; otherwise, it could cause stasis of vaginal secretions and increase the possibility of endometritis. Mark the specimen "possibly contaminated by lochia" so any blood in the specimen will not be overly interpreted by the laboratory technician.

Therapeutic Management
The woman will be started on a broad-spectrum antibiotic, such as amoxicillin, to treat the infection. Encourage her to drink large amounts of fluid (a glass every hour) to help flush the infection from her bladder. She may need an analgesic to reduce the pain of urination for the next few times she voids until the antibiotic begins to have an effect and the burning sensation disappears. Otherwise, she may not drink the fluid you suggest, knowing it will increase the number of times she will need to void, and voiding is painful.

Although symptoms of urinary tract infection de-

crease quickly, the woman will need to continue to take the antibiotic for a full 10 days to eradicate the infection completely. Once symptoms have disappeared, people often become noncompliant with medicine, particularly if a person is busy—and a woman at home with a new baby is busy. Make a chart for the woman to post on her refrigerator door as a reminder to continue taking the medication. Otherwise, bacteria in the urine will begin to multiply again, and in another week, symptoms and the active infection will recur. Be certain that the woman is aware of common methods all women should use to prevent urinary tract infections, as shown in the Focus on Family Teaching box in Chapter 46.

If the woman is breast-feeding, she should temporarily discontinue this if her antibiotic is tetracycline or a sulfonamide. Ask her physician if her antibiotic could be changed to one safe for breast-feeding, such as ampicillin. Otherwise, she may decide to breast-feed once she is home and not take the prescribed antibiotic.

Cardiovascular System Disorders

Postpartal Pregnancy-Induced Hypertension

Pregnancy-induced hypertension is discussed in Chapter 15. Mild pre-existing hypertension may increase in severity during the first few hours or days after birth. Rarely, hypertension of pregnancy develops for the first time in a woman who has had no prenatal or intranatal symptoms.

The cardinal symptoms are those of prepartal hypertension of pregnancy, namely, proteinuria, edema, and hypertension.

The treatment measures also will be the same as in prepartal hypertension: bed rest, a quiet atmosphere, and administration of magnesium sulfate or an antihypertensive such as nifedipine (Barton et al., 1990). Antihypertensive therapy can be intense because the fetal risk is no longer present. The woman requires frequent monitoring of her vital signs and urine output. She may be returned to surgery to have a dilatation and curettage to be certain that all placental fragments have been removed from the uterus. After a dilatation and curettage, her blood pressure often falls dramatically to normal.

If convulsions are going to occur with postpartal hypertension of pregnancy, they invariably develop 6 to 24 hours after birth. Convulsions occurring more than 72 hours after birth are probably not due to eclampsia but to some cause unrelated to childbearing.

Women in whom postpartal hypertension develops are bewildered by what is happening to them. If convulsions occur, they are frightened to discover how little control they have over their body. They worry that convulsions will occur after they are home while they are working at a hot stove or holding the baby. The woman should be assured that hypertension of pregnancy, although appearing late, is a condition of pregnancy; now that she is no longer pregnant, it need give her no further cause for concern. Because eclampsia or preeclampsia occurs with one pregnancy, there is no statistical reason to believe it will occur with a future pregnancy (unless chronic hypertension persists).

Reproductive System Disorders

Reproductive Tract Displacement

If the support systems of the uterus are weakened because of pregnancy, the ligaments may no longer be able to maintain the uterus in its usual position or level after pregnancy, and problems of retroflexion, anteflexion, retroversion, and anteversion or prolapse of the uterus may occur (Kvale & Kvale, 1993). These uterine displacement disorders not only may interfere with future childbearing and fertility but also may cause continued pain or a feeling of lower abdominal heaviness or discomfort.

If the walls of the vagina are weakened, a cystocele (outpouching of the bladder into the vaginal wall) or a rectocele (outpouching of the rectum into the vaginal wall) may occur. Stress incontinence (involuntary voiding on exertion) may occur. These problems tend to occur most frequently in women with a high parity and following operative birth, such as forceps birth; they are illustrated in Figure 4-6. Surgery to repair such conditions may be necessary.

Separation of the Symphysis Pubis

During pregnancy, many women feel some discomfort at the symphysis pubis because of relaxation of the joint preparatory to birth. If a fetus is unusually large or fetal position is not optimal, the ligaments of the symphysis pubis may be so stretched by birth that they actually tear (Dhar & Anderton, 1992).

After birth, the woman feels acute pain on turning or walking; her legs tend to rotate externally, giving her a waddling gait. A defect over the symphysis pubis can be palpated; the area is swollen and tender to touch.

Bed rest and the application of a tight pelvic binder to immobilize the joint is necessary to relieve pain and allow healing. As with all ligament injuries, a 4- to 6-week period is necessary for healing to take place. During this time, the woman may need to arrange for some type of child-care help at home and must avoid heavy lifting for an extended time until healing in the ligaments is complete. She may be advised to consider a cesarean birth for any future pregnancy.

Emotional and Psychological Complications of the Puerperium

Any woman who delivers an infant who in any way does not meet her expectations (wrong sex, physically disabled, ill, and so forth) or who is in a stressful situation may have difficulty bonding with the infant. Inability to bond is a postpartal complication with far-reaching implications, affecting the future health of the entire family.

The Woman Whose Child Is Born With an Illness or Disability

Most women say during pregnancy that they do not care about the sex of the child as long as the child is born healthy. How cheated they feel when this one requirement is not met. They are angry, hurt, and disappointed. They may feel a loss of self-esteem: they have given birth to an imperfect child and so they see themselves as imperfect. A woman sometimes responds with a grief reaction, as if the child has died. This is normal, because the image of the "perfect" child she thought she was carrying *has* died.

The average woman has difficulty immediately after birth believing that her child is real. How much greater is the difficulty for the woman of a disabled child. She must not only grasp the fact that the baby has been born but understand that the baby she has delivered is less than what she had wished for.

At one time, the woman of a child born with a disability was put under deep anesthesia at birth, and 24 hours later, when she was "stronger" and "better able to accept the situation," the extent of the disability was explained to her and she was then shown the baby. This method of dealing with the problem seems to have little merit. The woman cannot begin to accept her situation and work through the problem associated with it until she is aware of the situation. Meanwhile, she may imagine a state of affairs much worse than it actually is. The baby may only have a deformed finger, but she may imagine him or her as totally deformed or even dead.

Because of this, parents are now shown the child moments after birth, and the disability is immediately explained to them. This is a shock to couples, but they are not left feeling they have been deceived by the health center staff. Families are not happy over their child's disability, but they can appreciate having honest people who dare to face the problem with them when it first becomes apparent.

The physician or nurse-midwife will usually make it her responsibility to tell the parents of the defect, but you must be prepared to reinforce this information or review the problem. People who are under stress are not good listeners and so may need explanations repeated several times before they completely understand.

It is important for parents to care for the child during the postpartal period if at all possible so they can touch, relate to, and "claim" the infant in as nearly normal a manner as possible. Many women wait until their support person visits, in order that visiting with their newborn is a family activity (Figure 25-7).

Open lines of communication between the parents and the hospital staff that allows for free discussion of feelings and fears will do much to strengthen parent–child relationships and prepare for future hospitalizations or care of the child.

The Woman Whose Child Has Died

The woman whose child dies at birth always has questions about what happened. She is likely to feel bewildered, perhaps bitter, perhaps resentful, that the hospital staff could not save the child. "Why me? Out of all the women here, why did my baby die?" She needs concerned support from health care personnel to help her cope with such a devastating loss (Thomas, 1992).

Many women are interested in seeing the baby; this is generally therapeutic because it helps them begin grieving. Wrap the baby in an infant blanket and bring it into the parents. Remain with them but give them time to handle the child and inspect it as they wish. You should be familiar with the forms the mother or father will have to sign when a baby dies or is born dead, and you should know whether your state requires stillborn infants to be given a name and a funeral.

Other women on the unit tend to stay away from the woman whose child has died as if what has happened to her were contagious. Friends and relatives may be equally unable to talk about the situation. Most women, therefore, want a nurse to approach them and say, "Do you want to talk about what's happened?" or "How do you feel?"

No matter how crowded a maternity service is, a woman whose child has died should never be placed in a room with a woman who has had a healthy child. This is too much to ask her to bear. A private room allows the woman an opportunity to express herself. She does not have to keep up a front for a roommate, and the hospital staff can bend visiting rules for her. She needs her family with her to fill a portion of the void left by her loss.

The process of grieving and support necessary is further discussed in Chapter 56.

Postpartal Depression

Almost every woman notices some immediate **postpartal depression** or a feeling of sadness (postpartal "blues") after childbirth. This probably occurs as a response to the anticlimactic feeling following birth and probably is related to hormonal shifts as estrogen and progesterone levels in her body decline.

In a few women, this postpartal depression continues beyond the one or two days of the immediate postpartal period (Dobie & Walker, 1992). In addition to an overall feeling of sadness, the woman may notice extreme fatigue, an inability to stop crying, increased anxiety about her own or her infant's health, insecurity (unwilling to be left alone or unable to make decisions), and psychosomatic symptoms (nausea and vomiting, diarrhea). Depression that continues beyond a few days may reflect a more serious problem. The woman often has a multitude of related concerns, such as a history of depression, a troubled childhood, stress in the home or work, lack of self-esteem, or lack of effective support people. It is important to recognize women who may be at risk for postpartal depression before birth of their baby so that they can establish good support mechanisms and seek counseling, if necessary. For women who have not been identified as at risk, the discovery of the problem as soon as symptoms develop is a nursing

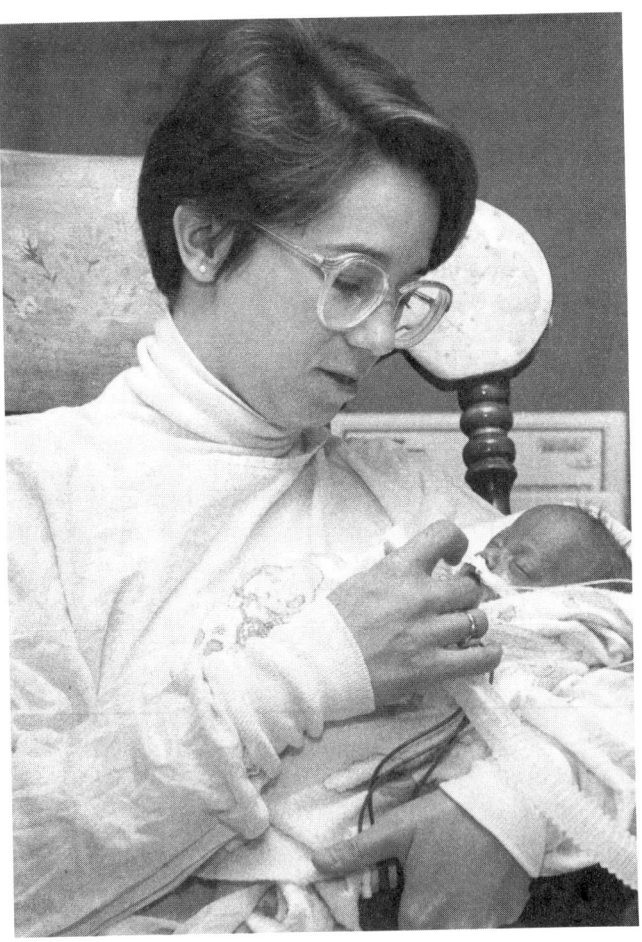

FIGURE 25-7
Be certain that women with a complication of pregnancy or with an ill newborn have adequate care time with their newborns, whenever possible, no matter how much care equipment is involved. (Courtesy of the Department of Medical Photography, Children's Hospital, Buffalo, NY.)

priority (Crisp, 1992). The woman needs counseling to integrate the experience of childbirth into her life. This is crucial to development of a healthy maternal–infant bond, to the health of any other children in the family, and overall family functioning. Ask at postpartal return visits for symptoms that would suggest this depression and suggest an appropriate referral.

Postpartal Psychosis

As many as 1 woman in 500 presents enough symptoms in the year after birth of a child to be considered psychiatrically ill (this statistic represents the current rate of overall mental illness). In about two thirds of these women, the illness develops during the first 6 weeks after birth. Because the illness coincides with the postpartal period, it has been called **postpartal psychosis** (Cunningham et al., 1993). Rather than being a response to the physical aspects of childbearing, however, it is probably a response to the *crisis* of childbearing. Nearly a third of these women will have had symptoms of mental illness prior to the pregnancy. If the pregnancy had not precipitated the illness, a death in the family, the loss of a husband's job, a divorce, or some other major life crisis would probably have precipitated it.

The woman usually appears exceptionally sad. By definition, psychosis exists when a person has lost contact with reality. The woman with a childbearing psychosis may deny that she has had a child and, when the child is brought to her, insist that she was never pregnant. When observation tells you that a woman is not functioning in reality, you cannot improve her concept of reality by a simple measure such as explaining what a correct perception is. Her sensory input is too disturbed to be able to comprehend this, and she may interpret your attempt as threatening. She may respond with anger or become equally threatening. A psychosis is a severe mental illness that requires referral to a professional psychiatric counselor and antipsychotic medication.

While waiting for such a skilled professional to arrive, do not leave the woman alone (distorted perception might lead to her harming herself), nor should you leave her alone with her infant.

Always keep in mind that, although rare, the phenomenon of puerperal psychosis does exist; remembering that childbearing can lead to this degree of mental illness helps you to put childbearing into perspective. For some people, childbearing is such a crisis in their lives that it can trigger mental illness; certainly it cannot be considered an everyday incident in anyone's life.

Key Points

- Establishing a firm family–newborn relationship may be difficult when a woman has a postpartal complication. Investigate ways that will allow the woman to care for her baby or offer necessary support to family members so they can fulfill this role.
- Hemorrhage is a major danger in the immediate postpartal period. It is defined as a loss of blood over 500 mL within a 24-hour period. The most frequent cause of postpartal hemorrhage is uterine atony. Remember that continuous limited blood loss can be as important over time as sudden, intense bleeding. With hemorrhage, administration of an oxytocin may be necessary to initiate uterine tone and halt hemorrhage.
- Other causes of hemorrhage are lacerations (vaginal, cervical, or perineal) and retained placental fragments. Lacerations are most apt to occur with forceps birth or with the birth of a large infant.
- Puerperal infection is a potential complication after any birth until the denuded placental surface has healed. Retained placental fragments and the use of internal fetal heart monitoring leads are potential sources of infection.
- Thrombophlebitis is inflammation of the lining of a blood vessel and is a grave complication of the postpartal period. It occurs most often as an extension of an endometrial infection. Therapy is bed rest with heat applications and anticoagulation administration. Never massage the leg of a woman with a phlebitis or thrombophlebitis; it may cause the clot to move and become a pulmonary embolus, a possibly fatal complication.
- Mastitis is infection of the breast. The symptoms are pain, swelling, and redness in a breast. Antibiotic therapy is necessary.
- A woman whose child is born with a disability needs special consideration following the birth. This is obviously a time of stress for the woman and requires supportive nursing care.
- Postpartal "blues" are a normal accompaniment to birth. Postpartal depression (a feeling of extreme sadness) and postpartal psychosis (an actual separation from reality) are not normal and need accurate assessment so that women can receive adequate therapy for these conditions.

Critical Thinking Exercises

1. Mona is a 29-year-old woman who gave birth to an 8-lb boy yesterday. When you left work yesterday she was rooming-in with the baby and beginning breast-feeding without apparent difficulty. Today, you find her sitting on the side of her hospital bed crying and stating she has to kill her baby because the voices inside her head have told her he is an interplanetary spy. Given the various options available, how would you determine your *first* action? Suppose Mona said she needed to kill herself as well? Would your first action be different?
2. Mary Ann is a 39-year-old who entered her pregnancy with marked varicose veins. One day post-

partum, you notice red streaks on both legs along the course of the veins and she has pain on dorsiflexion of her foot. You are concerned she is developing a thrombophlebitis. How could Mary have reduced the risk of thrombophlebitis during pregnancy? Describe the plan of care that could have reduced this risk during labor and in the immediate postpartal period.

3. Postpartal hemorrhage can lead to extensive hypovolemia if allowed to continue undetected. If you entered a postpartal room and discovered a woman with active vaginal bleeding, how would you determine your *first* action? How would you teach women to assess vaginal bleeding so they can self-assess when they are home?

References

Barton, J. R., et al. (1990). The use of nifedipine during the postpartum period in patients with severe preeclampsia. *American Journal of Obstetrics and Gynecology, 162,* 788.

Crawford, L. A., et al. (1993). Incontinence following rupture of the anal sphincter during delivery. *Obstetrics and Gynecology, 82,* 527.

Crisp, H. (1992). Postnatal depression: still a neglected illness? *Professional Care of Mothers and Children, 2,* 72.

Cunningham, F. G., et al. (1993). *Williams obstetrics* (19th ed.). Norwalk, CT: Appleton and Lange.

Department of Health and Human Services. (1991). *Healthy people 2000.* Washington, DC: Public Health Service.

Dhar, S., & Anderton, J. M. (1992). Rupture of the symphysis pubis during labor. *Clinical Orthopaedics and Related Research, 283,* 252.

Dobie, S. A., & Walker, E. A. (1992). Depression after childbirth. *Journal of the American Board of Family Practice, 5,* 544.

Gerbasi, F. R., et al. (1990). Changes in hemostasis activity during delivery and the immediate postpartum period. *American Journal of Obstetrics and Gynecology, 162,* 1158.

Gutowski, N. J., & Heron, J. R. (1993). Recurrent confusion and hypopituitarism. *Postgraduate Medical Journal, 69,* 392.

Johnstone, H. A., et al. (1990). *Candidiasis* in the breastfeeding mother and infant. *Journal of Obstetric, Gynecologic, and Neonatal Nursing, 19,* 171.

Kaufmann, R., & Foxman, B. (1991). Mastitis among lactating women: occurrence and risk factors. *Social Science and Medicine, 33,* 701.

Kesteven, P., et al. (1993). Disseminated intravascular coagulation. *Care of the Critically Ill, 9,* 22.

Khong, T. Y., & Khong, T. K. (1993). Delayed postpartum hemorrhage. *Obstetrics and Gynecology, 82,* 17.

Kruskall, M. G. (1990). Controversies in transfusion medicine: The safety and utility of autologous donations by pregnant patients: Pro. *Tranfusion, 30,* 169.

Kvale, J. N., & Kvale, J. K. (1993). Common gynecologic problems after age 75. *Postgraduate Medicine, 93,* 263.

Lowe, T. W. (1990). Hypovolemia due to hemorrhage. *Clinical Obstetrics and Gynecology, 33,* 454.

Magee, K. P., et al. (1993). Massive septic pelvic thrombophlebitis. *Obstetrics and Gynecology, 82,* 662.

Maier, R. C. (1993). Control of postpartum hemorrhage with uterine packing. *American Journal of Obstetrics and Gynecology, 169,* 317.

Monga, M., & Oshiro, B. T. (1993). Puerperal infections. *Seminars in Perinatology, 17,* 426.

Oleen, M. A., & Mariano, J. P. (1990). Controlling refractory atonic postpartum hemorrhage with Hemabate sterile solution. *American Journal of Obstetrics and Gynecology, 162,* 205.

Olsen, C. G., et al. (1990). Breast disorders in nursing mothers. *American Family Physician, 41,* 1509.

Ritter, D. C. & de Shago, R. D. (1994). Peripartum complications. *Postgraduate Medicine, 95,* 178.

Saultz, J. W., et al. (1991). Postpartum urinary retention. *Journal of the American Board of Family Practice, 4,* 341.

Stray-Pedersen, B., et al. (1990). Bacteriuria in the puerperium. *American Journal of Obstetrics and Gynecology, 162,* 792.

Thomas, J. (1992). Supporting parents and professionals when a baby dies. *Care of the Critically Ill, 8,* 172.

Tulman, L., et al. (1990). Changes in functional status after childbirth. *Nursing Research, 39,* 70.

Zahn, C. M., & Yeomans, E. R. (1990). Postpartum hemorrhage: Placenta accreta, uterine inversion, and puerperal hematomas. *Clinical Obstetrics and Gynecology, 33,* 422.

Zelop, C. M., et al. (1993). Emergency peripartum hysterectomy. *American Journal of Obstetrics and Gynecology, 168,* 1443.

Zlatnik, F. J. (1990). The puerperium: normal and abnormal. In Scott, J. R., et al. (Eds.). *Danforth's obstetrics and gynecology.* Philadelphia: J. B. Lippincott.

Suggested Readings

Affonso, D. D. (1992). Postpartum depression; a nursing perspective on women's health and behaviors. *Image: The Journal of Nursing Scholarship, 24,* 215.

Chawla, K., et al. (1994). Postpartum ovarian vein thrombosis. *American Journal of Emergency Medicine, 12,* 82.

Fleming, N. (1990). Can the suturing make a difference in postpartum perineal pain? *Journal of Nurse Midwifery, 35,* 19.

Gjerdingen, D. K., et al. (1990). A causal model describing the relationship of women's postpartum health to social support, length of leave, and complications of childbirth. *Women's Health, 16,* 71.

Harrison, L. L. (1990). Patient education in early postpartum discharge programs. *MCN: American Journal of Maternal Child Nursing, 15,* 39.

Littlefield, V. M., et al. (1990). Participation in alternative care: relationship to anxiety, depression, and hostility. *Research in Nursing and Health, 13,* 17.

Mead-Bennett, E. (1990). The relationship of primigravid sleep experience and select moods on the first postpartum day. *Journal of Obstetric, Gynecologic, and Neonatal Nursing, 19,* 146.

Mercer, R. T., & Ferketich, S. L. (1990). Predictors of family functioning eight months following birth. *Nursing Research, 39,* 76.

Potter, S., et al. (1991). Does infant feeding method influence maternal postpartum weight loss? *Journal of the American Dietetic Association, 91,* 441.

Rooks, J. P., et al. (1992). The National Birth Center Study: intrapartum and immediate postpartum and neonatal complications and transfers, postpartum and neonatal care, outcomes and client satisfaction. *Journal of Nurse Midwifery, 37,* 361.

Stanco, L. M., et al. (1993). Emergency peripartum hysterectomy and associated risk factors. *American Journal of Obstetrics and Gynecology, 168,* 879.

Wood, N. J. (1992). The use of vaginal pessaries for uterine prolapse. *Nurse Practitioner, 17,* 31.

Zerbe, M., et al. (1992). Critical hemorrhage during pregnancy. *Critical Care Nursing Clinics of North America, 4,* 729.

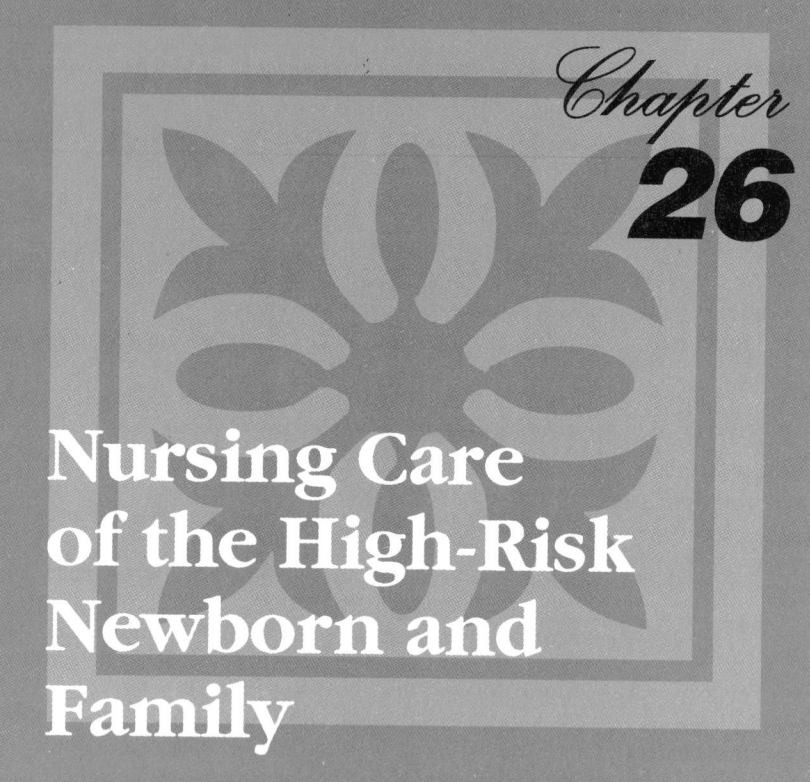

Chapter 26

Nursing Care of the High-Risk Newborn and Family

Objectives

After mastering the contents of this chapter, you should be able to:

1. Define the terms small-for-gestational-age infant, term infant, large-for-gestational-age infant, preterm infant, *and* postterm infant *and describe common illnesses that occur in these high-risk newborns.*

2. Assess a high-risk newborn in the early neonatal period to determine if the infant has completed a safe transition to extrauterine life.

3. List nursing diagnoses concerned with the high-risk newborn.

4. Establish plans for care, respecting priorities of the newborn (i.e., establishing respiratory function, cardiovascular adjustment, temperature regulation, nutrition, bonding, and developmental care) to help a high-risk newborn stabilize body systems.

5. Implement nursing care for the high-risk infant, such as providing an intravenous or gavage-feeding.

6. Evaluate established outcome criteria to be certain that nursing goals for care have been achieved.

7. Identify National Health Goals related to high-risk newborns that nurses could be instrumental in helping the nation to achieve.

8. Identify areas related to the care of high-risk newborns that could benefit from additional nursing research.

9. Use critical thinking to analyze the special crisis imposed on families when alterations of newborn development, length of pregnancy, or neonatal illness occur.

10. Synthesize knowledge of the needs of the high-risk infant with nursing process to achieve quality maternal and child health nursing care.

Adele Pillitteri: MATERNAL AND CHILD HEALTH NURSING, 2nd Edition. © 1995 Adele Pillitteri.

All women should be screened during pregnancy for risk factors that may lead to illness in the newborn (see Table 10-6). As described in Chapters 14 through 17, maternal age (very young or older than average); concurrent disease conditions (e.g., diabetes); pregnancy complications (such as placenta previa); and an unhealthy maternal lifestyle (such as drug abuse) all signify risk potential for the newborn. In addition, the infant who is born with dysmaturity or who is under- or overweight for gestational age is also at risk for complications at birth and in the first few days of life. In addition, not all instances of high risk can be predicted. It is not unusual to discover that an infant of a "perfect" pregnancy is born needing special care or develops a problem over the first few days of life that necessitates special interventions. National Health Goals related to the high-risk newborn are shown in the Focus on National Health Goals box.

Being able to predict that an infant is high-risk makes it possible to arrange for attendance of skilled health care personnel at the child's birth. They may be needed to resuscitate the infant should the infant have difficulty establishing respirations. Immediate, skilled handling of any problems that occur may not only save the infant's life but also prevent future neurologic disorders.

NURSING PROCESS OVERVIEW
for Care of the Family With a Newborn
With High-Risk Status

ASSESSMENT

All infants should be assessed at birth for gross congenital anomalies and **gestational age** (number of weeks they remained in utero); both of these determinations can be done by the nurse who first inspects the infant. Be certain that these assessments are made with the infant under a prewarmed radiant heat warmer to safeguard against heat loss, since the infant who appears to be a term newborn may actually be a large-for-gestational-age preterm infant.

Continuing assessment of high-risk infants involves the use of instrumentation such as cardiac, apnea, and blood pressure monitors. However, no matter how many monitors are in use, they never replace the role of common-sense observation. Carefully evaluate comments from fellow nurses that an infant "isn't himself" or "looks funny." These comments, although not scientific, are the same observations that a parent who knows his or her baby well reports at health visits. A nurse who knows an infant well from having cared for the child consistently over time often senses changes before a monitor or other equipment begins to put a quantitative measurement on the factor.

NURSING DIAGNOSIS

To establish nursing diagnoses for high-risk infants, it is important to be aware of the normal assessment parameters of this population. Nursing diagnosis generally centers on the eight priority areas of care for any newborn; for example,

- Ineffective airway clearance related to presence of mucus or amniotic fluid in airway
- Altered cardiovascular tissue perfusion related to breathing difficulties
- High-risk for fluid volume deficit related to insensible water loss
- Ineffective thermoregulation related to newborn status and stress from illness or prematurity
- High-risk for altered nutrition; less than body requirements related to lack of energy for sucking
- High-risk for infection related to lowered immune response in newborn
- High-risk for altered parenting related to illness in newborn at birth
- Diversional activity deficit (lack of stimulation) related to illness at birth

PLANNING

Be certain that goals established for care are consistent with the infant's potential. A goal that implies complete recovery from a major illness may be unrealistic. An individual care plan that considers the newborn's developmental as well as physiologic strengths, weaknesses, and needs will ensure that parents as well as the health care team have a good understanding of the infant's particular care priorities. Include the parents in plans and interventions. Bathing or feeding their infant in the nursery may be the mechanism that makes the child real to them and helps them begin bonding. Organizations that may be helpful for referral are:

Sudden Infant Death Alliance
10500 Little Patuxent Parkway
Suite 420
Columbia, MD 21044

National SIDS Resource Center
8201 Greensboro Drive, Suite 600
McLean, VA 22102

FOCUS ON
National Health Goals

Preterm birth has the potential for leading to so many complications in newborns that a National Health Goal was written specifically concerning it:

- Reduce low birth weight to an incidence of no more than 5% of live births and very low birth weight to an incidence of no more than 1% of live births from baselines of 6.9% and 1.2%, respectively (DHHS, 1991).

Nurses can be instrumental in helping the nation achieve this goal by teaching women the symptoms of preterm labor so that, hopefully, birth can be delayed until infants are term. They also need to be prepared for resuscitation at birth of preterm infants and to plan development care that can help prevent conditions such as apnea, intraventricular hemorrhage, and periventricular leukomalacia.

Further research is needed as to what materials used to position infants for developmental care best prevent fatigue, what measures can best prevent conditions such as intraventricular hemorrhage, and what measures can make parents feel most comfortable and allow them to interact with their infants best in neonatal intensive care units.

Parent Care (Parents of Premature and High-risk Infants)
9041 Colgate Street
Indianapolis, IN 46268-1210

IMPLEMENTATION

Interventions for any high-risk infant are best carried out by a consistent caregiver (a primary or case-management nursing pattern) and should focus on conserving the baby's energy and providing a thermoneutral environment to prevent exhaustion and chilling. Painful procedures should be kept to a minimum to help the infant achieve a sense of comfort and balance.

EVALUATION

High-risk infants need long-term follow-up so that any consequences of their birth status, such as minimal neurologic injury, can be identified and arrangements for special schooling or counseling can be made for the toddler, preschool, and school years. Examples of outcome criteria are the following:

* Infant tolerates all procedures without accompanying apnea.
* Infant maintains body temperature at 37.0°C in open crib with one added blanket.
* Parents visit at least once and make three telephone calls to neonatal nursery weekly.

Newborn Priorities in First Days of Life

All infants have eight needs that take precedence over all others in the first few days of life: (1) initiation and maintenance of respirations, (2) establishment of extrauterine circulation, (3) control of body temperature, (4) intake of adequate nourishment, (5) establishment of waste elimination, (6) prevention of infection, (7) establishment of an infant–parent relationship, and (8) developmental care that balances rest and stimulation for mental development (see Chapter 23). These are also the eight priority needs of high-risk infants, but with the high-risk infant, fulfilling these needs may require special equipment or care measures. Not all infants will be able to achieve full wellness because of extreme insults to health at birth. Indications that the newborn is having difficulty making the transition from intrauterine life to life outside the uterus may be apparent during the intrapartum period, at birth, or at initial assessment using the Apgar scoring system. (See Chapter 23 for a full explanation of the Apgar score.)

Initiating and Maintaining Respirations

The ultimate prognosis of the high-risk infant depends greatly on how the first moments of life are managed. Most deaths in the first 48 hours after birth are the result of an inability to establish or maintain adequate respirations. An infant who has difficulty accomplishing effective respiratory action in the first hours of life and yet survives may have residual neurologic dysfunction. Extremely thorough care is necessary to make interventions during this time most effective: little victory can be had in a race that ultimately ends in cerebral palsy, recurrent convulsions, or mental retardation.

Most infants are born with some degree of respiratory acidosis, but the spontaneous onset of respirations rapidly corrects this. If respiratory activity does not begin immediately, however, respiratory acidosis will increase. The blood pH and buffer base will fall, and newborn defense mechanisms are inadequate to reverse the process. Therefore, the effort to establish respirations must be begun immediately after birth; by 2 minutes, the development of severe acidosis is already well under way.

Any infant who sustains some degree of asphyxia in utero, which could have occurred from such factors as cord compression, maternal anesthesia, placenta previa, or preterm separation of the placenta, will already be in serious threat from acidosis at birth and have difficulty before the first 2 minutes after birth.

Resuscitation

Factors that commonly make infants high-risk for requiring resuscitation are shown in Box 26-1. If breathing is ineffective, circulatory shunts (particularly the ductus arteriosus) fail to close. Because left side heart pressure is stronger than right side, blood circulates through a patent ductus arteriosus left to right or from the aorta to the pulmonary artery, creating ineffective pump action in the heart. Struggling to breathe and circulate blood, an infant uses available serum glucose quickly and may become hypoglycemic, thus compounding the problem still further.

For all these reasons, resuscitation becomes an important implementation for an infant who fails to take a first breath or has difficulty maintaining adequate respiratory movements on his or her own.

Resuscitation comprises three organized steps: (1) establishing and maintaining an airway, (2) expanding the lungs, and (3) initiating and maintaining effective ventilation. If respiratory depression becomes severe, the heart will fail and resuscitation then must also include cardiac massage.

Establishing an Airway

For the well term newborn, the most care that is needed to help establish the airway is bulb syringe suction, which removes mucus and prevents aspiration of any mucus and amniotic fluid present in the mouth or nose with the first breath (see Chapter 23).

If an infant does not spontaneously draw in a first breath, apply suction to the infant's mouth and nose and rub the back to see if skin stimulation initiates respirations. Be certain the infant is dry, including the hair and head, to prevent chilling. The newborn's attempts to raise his or her temperature will only increase the need for oxygen, which the baby cannot supply because breathing is not yet present. Warmed, blow-by oxygen by face mask or positive pressure mask may be administered.

For deeper suction than is possible by a bulb syringe, place an infant on the back and slide a folded towel or pad under the shoulders to raise them slightly so the head is in a neutral position. Slide a catheter (no. 8F to 12F) over the infant's tongue to the back of the throat (Figure 26-1). Do not suction for longer than 10 seconds at a time (count seconds as you suction) to avoid removing excessive air from an infant's lungs. Use a gentle touch. Bradycardia or cardiac arrhythmias can occur because of vagus stimulation from vigorous suctioning.

The infant who still makes no effort at spontaneous respirations requires immediate laryngoscopy to open the airway. After deep suctioning, an endotracheal tube can be inserted and oxygen can be administered by a positive pressure bag and mask with 100% oxygen at 40 to 60 breaths per minute.

In the first few seconds of life, an infant this severely depressed may take several weak gasps of air and then almost immediately stop; heart rate begins to fall. This period of halted respirations is termed **primary apnea.** Following 1 or 2 minutes of apnea, the infant again tries to initiate respirations with a few strong gasps. The child cannot maintain this effort longer than 4 or 5 minutes, however; following this, the respiratory effort will become weaker again and the heart rate will fall further until the infant stops the gasping effort altogether. The infant then enters a period of **secondary apnea.** Although usually a phenomenon that occurs after birth, both types of apnea may occur in utero.

During the period of the first gasps, resuscitation attempts are generally successful. Once an infant is allowed to enter the secondary apnea period, however, resuscitation measures become difficult and may be ineffective. Resuscitation must always be started as if secondary apnea were occurring, because it is impossible to distinguish between the two periods simply by observation (Phibbs, 1994).

An obstetrician, pediatrician, neonatologist, anesthesiologist, or neonatal nurse practitioner skilled in laryngoscope and endotracheal tube insertion should be present at the birth of all identified high-risk infants. Laryngoscope insertion is easy in theory; in practice, the wide variation in size of infants' posterior pharynx and trachea combined with the emergency conditions always present make it difficult (Figure 26-2).

Laryngoscope blades used with newborns are size 0 or 1. Infants under 1000 g need a size 2.5-mm endotracheal tube; those over 3000 g, a 4.0-mm tube. Be-

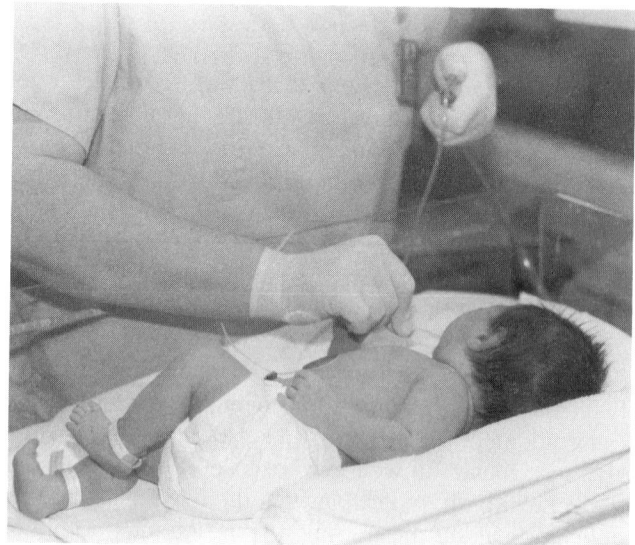

FIGURE 26-1

Suctioning a newborn with mechanical suction controlled by a finger valve. Suction is applied as the catheter is withdrawn. If the catheter is rotated as it is withdrawn, the risk of traumatizing membrane is reduced. (Courtesy of the Sisters of Charity Hospital, Buffalo, NY.)

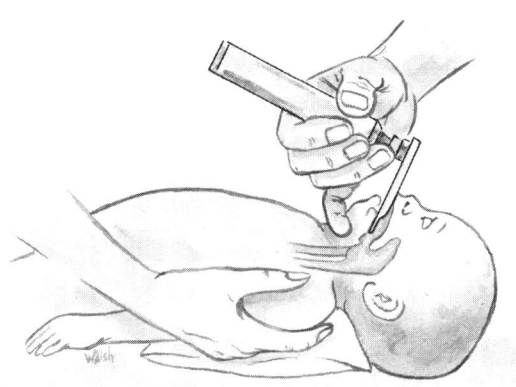

FIGURE 26-2
Intubation. The head should be in a neutral position with a towel under the shoulders. The blade of the laryngoscope is inserted to reveal the vocal cords. An endotracheal tube for ventilation is then passed into the trachea, past the laryngoscope.

cause preterm infants are prone to hemorrhage owing to capillary fragility, extra gentleness must be used in passing an endotracheal tube with these infants.

Expanding the Lungs

Once an airway has been established, an infant needs the lungs expanded. A well infant inflates his or her lungs adequately with the first breath. The sound of a baby crying is proof that lung expansion is good; the vocal sounds are produced by a free flow of air over the vocal cords.

An infant who breathes spontaneously but then is unable to sustain effective respirations may need oxygen by bag and mask to aid lung expansion. An infant mask should cover both the mouth and the nose to be effective. It should not cover the eyes, because it can cause eye injury by mechanical injury or drying of the cornea. Administer 100% oxygen by face mask and pressure bag at a rate of 40 to 60 compressions per minute. To prevent cooling, oxygen should be administered both warmed (between 32°C and 34°C, or 89.6°F and 93.2°F) and humidified (between 60% and 80%), although this is not always possible in an emergency.

Remember that the pressure needed to open lung alveoli for the first time is approximately 40 cm of water pressure. After that, pressures of 15 cm H_2O to 20 cm H_2O are generally adequate to continue inflating alveoli. The pressure from anesthesiology bags is controlled solely by the pressure of a hand; other types of bags such as the AMBU can be set with a "blowoff" valve that limits the pressure in the apparatus.

It is important that no pressure above what is necessary is used, since excessive force can rupture lung alveoli. On the other hand, if adequate insufflation is not achieved, an infant stands little chance of survival. To be certain that oxygen is reaching the lungs, the chest should be auscultated simultaneously with the oxygen administration. In many infants, this degree of resus-

citation will initiate responsive respirations and a strong heartbeat. Color, muscle response, and reflexes will improve.

If an infant's amniotic fluid is meconium stained, do not stimulate the infant to breathe by rubbing or administer air or oxygen under pressure; this could push meconium down into the infant's airway and compromise respirations even further. Give oxygen by mask without pressure and wait for a laryngoscope to be passed and the trachea to be deep-suctioned before oxygen under pressure is given.

The infant who has had an endotracheal tube passed will have oxygen administered by the endotracheal tube. Listen with a stethoscope to both lungs to be certain that both sides are being aerated. If air can be heard on only one side, the endotracheal tube is probably at the bifurcation of the trachea and blocking one of the main stem bronchi. Drawing it back half a centimeter will usually free it and allow oxygen to flow to both lungs.

When oxygen is given under pressure to a newborn, not only the lungs but also the stomach quickly fills with oxygen. If the resuscitation continues for over 2 minutes, inserting an orogastric tube and leaving the distal end open will deflate the stomach and decrease the possibility that vomiting and aspiration of stomach contents will occur.

Drug Therapy

Stimulants have little place in newborn resuscitation unless an infant's respiratory depression appears to be related to the administration of a narcotic such as morphine or meperidine (Demerol) to the mother during labor. In these instances, a narcotic antagonist such as naloxone (Narcan) injected into an umbilical vessel will relieve the depression. The dose of naloxone is determined by institutional policy but is usually 0.1 mg/kg body weight of a 0.4 mg/mL solution (Loeb et al., 1993).

Maintaining Effective Ventilation

To allow a newborn infant to adjust to and maintain cardiovascular changes, effective ventilation (continued respirations) must be maintained. A healthy infant accomplishes this task on his or her own. All infants who had difficulty establishing respirations at birth should be carefully observed in the next few hours to be certain that respirations are maintained.

An increasing respiratory rate in the neonate is often the first sign of obstruction or respiratory compromise. If the respiratory rate is increased, undress the baby's chest and look for retractions (inward sucking of the anterior chest wall on inspiration). Retractions reflect the difficulty the infant is having in drawing in air (tugging so hard to inflate the lungs that the anterior chest muscles are drawn in; see Figure 23-18).

The infant who is having difficulty with breathing

should have the weight of clothing removed from the chest. Positioning the infant with the head of the mattress elevated approximately 15 degrees allows abdominal contents to fall away from the diaphragm, affording optimal breathing space.

Keeping the infant warm remains important. If secretions are accumulating in the respiratory tract, they must be suctioned. "Bagging" an infant for a minute before suction will improve the PO_2 level and prevent it from dropping to dangerous levels during suctioning. The cause of the respiratory distress must be determined and appropriate interventions must be undertaken to correct the difficulty (see Chapter 40).

Establishing Extrauterine Circulation

Although establishing respirations is the usual critical problem at a high-risk infant's birth, lack of cardiac function may be present concurrently or, if respiratory function is not quickly restored, may develop. If there is no audible heart beat, or if the cardiac rate is below 80 bpm, closed chest massage should be started. This technique is accomplished by holding the infant with fingers supporting the back and pressing the thumbs against the sternum or depressing the sternum with two fingers (see Figure 41-32). Depress the sternum approximately 1 or 2 cm, at a rate of 120 times per minute (AHA, 1992). Lung ventilation at a rate of 30 times per minute should be continued interspersed with the cardiac massage at a ratio of 1:3.

Transcutaneous oxygen monitoring or pulse oximetry is used to monitor cardiac efficiency. If pressure and rate of massage are adequate, it should be possible, additionally, to palpate a femoral pulse. If heart sounds are not resumed above 80 bpm after 30 seconds of combined positive pressure ventilation and cardiac compressions, 0.1 to 0.3 mL of epinephrine (1:10,000) may be sprayed into the endotracheal tube to stimulate cardiac function (see Table 26-1). Infants who still have difficulty initiating cardiac function need to be transferred to a transitional or high-risk nursery for continuous cardiac surveillance.

Fluid and Electrolyte Balance

After an initial resuscitation attempt, hypoglycemia (decreased serum glucose) may result from the effort expended; dehydration may result from increased insensible water loss from rapid respiration. Fluid commonly administered to maintain water balance is Ringer's lactate or 5% dextrose in water; electrolytes (particularly sodium and potassium) are added as necessary depending on electrolyte analysis.

The rate of fluid administration must be carefully maintained, because a high fluid intake can lead to patent ductus arteriosus or congestive heart failure. If a radiant warmer is used, more fluid will be required than if a double-walled Isolette is used because of increased water loss from convection and radiation.

Urine output and urine specific gravity must also be carefully monitored; an output less than 2 mL/kg/h or a specific gravity greater than 1.015 to 1.020 suggests dehydration (London, 1993). Elevated specific gravity may also be caused by inappropriate antidiuretic hormone secretion or kidney failure due to a primary illness.

If an infant has hypotension without hypovolemia, a vasopressor such as dopamine may be given to increase blood pressure and improve cell perfusion. If hypovolemia is present, the cause is usually fetal blood loss from a condition such as placenta previa (see Chapter 15) or twin-to-twin transfusion. With hypovolemia, there will be signs of tachypnea, pallor, tachycardia, decreased arterial blood pressure, decreased central venous pressure, and decreased tissue perfusion of peripheral tissue, with a progressively developing metabolic acidosis. The hematocrit may be normal for some time following acute blood loss, because blood cells present are in proportion to plasma. Plasma expanders (whole blood or a protein solution) may be administered to increase blood volume. The rate of these must be controlled carefully to prevent congestive heart failure, patent ductus arteriosus, or intracranial hemorrhage from fluid pressure overload.

Temperature Regulation

Any high-risk infant may have difficulty maintaining a normal temperature, since in addition to stress from an illness or immaturity, the infant's body is often exposed during such procedures as resuscitation and blood drawing.

It is important that infants be kept in a neutral temperature environment, one that is neither too hot nor too cold. At this level of environment, there is less demand on infants to maintain a minimal metabolic rate for effective body functioning. Too hot and they must decrease metabolism to cool their body; too cold and they must increase metabolism to warm body cells. If the infant should become chilled, this requires increased oxygen to raise the metabolic rate; without this oxygen available, body cells become hypoxic. To save oxygen for essential body functions, vasoconstriction of blood vessels occurs. If this process continues for too long, pulmonary vessels become affected and pulmonary perfusion is decreased; the infant's PO_2 level falls and PCO_2 increases; and the decreased PO_2 level may open fetal right-to-left shunts again. Surfactant production may halt, which may further interfere with lung function. To supply glucose to maintain increased metabolism, the infant begins anaerobic glycolysis, which pours acid into the bloodstream. The infant becomes acidotic, and with acidosis comes the increased risk of **kernicterus** (invasion of brain cells with unconjugated bilirubin), as more bilirubin-binding sites are lost and more bilirubin is free to pass out of the bloodstream into brain cells.

To prevent the infant from becoming chilled after birth, the nurse must wipe the infant dry, cover the head with a cap, and place him or her immediately under a prewarmed radiant warmer or in a warmed Isolette. Air, Isolette, or radiant warmer temperatures must be kept regulated to maintain the infant's axillary temperature at 97.8°F (36.5°C).

Be certain that during procedures an infant is not placed directly on cool x-ray plates, scales, or an unheated radiant warmer. In the event of a power failure, wrapping infants with plastic bubble wrap or tin foil is a method to maintain body heat.

Radiant Heat Sources

Radiant heat warmers are open beds that have an overhead radiant heat source. Such units have Servocontrol probes, which when placed on the infant's skin, continually monitor the infant's temperature. Abdominal skin temperature, when measured by a probe this way, should be 35.5° to 36.5°C. If the temperature falls, the unit will alarm. Tape the probe or disk in place on an infant's abdomen between the umbilicus and the xyphoid process. Be sure that it is not over the rib cage where the thin subcutaneous tissue will not allow an accurate reading; it should not be taped under the infant or it will register a falsely high reading. A plastic "bridge" or shield placed over the child will better preserve heat by reducing convection and radiation losses. Plastic wrap can produce this same effect. Sometimes the heads of health care personnel can block the heat from an overhead source and keep it from reaching the baby, so that an additional warming pad placed under the infant may be necessary for very preterm infants or for lengthy procedures.

Isolettes

Following an initial resuscitation attempt, infants may be cared for in Isolettes (square, acrylic-sided incubators). The temperature of Isolettes varies with the amount of time portholes remain open and the temperature of the area in which the Isolette is placed. Direct sunlight or a warm radiator can increase the internal temperature markedly. For this reason, Isolette temperature must be checked at frequent intervals to be certain the temperature level designated is being maintained. Use of an additional acrylic shield inside the Isolette helps prevent radiation heat loss and convection loss when portholes are opened for care.

Some Isolettes have Servocontrol mechanism units that monitor the infant's temperature and automatically change the temperature of the Isolette as needed, just as radiant warmers do. An infant in an incubator should be undressed except for a diaper, so that the flow of air will contact the body surface. Portholes must remain closed to keep the temperature steady.

As the infant's condition improves, weaning from an incubator may be necessary. Dress the infant as if he or she were going to be in a bassinet, then set the incubator about 2°F (1.2°C) below the infant's temperature. Assess after half an hour that the infant is able to maintain body temperature. If so, lower the Isolette temperature another 2° and continue thus until room temperature is reached. If the infant cannot maintain temperature as the incubator temperature level is brought down, he or she is not yet ready for room temperature air, and the weaning process needs to be slowed or stopped until the baby is more mature or better ready to self-regulate temperature.

Kangaroo Care

Kangaroo care is the use of skin-to-skin contact to maintain body heat. The infant is undressed except for a diaper and perhaps a cap. The parent sits in a chair and holds the infant snugly against his or her chest (Ludington-Hoe et al., 1991). This method of care not only supplies heat but also encourages parent and child interaction.

Establishing Adequate Nutritional Intake

An infant who experienced severe asphyxia at birth is maintained on intravenous fluid until it is certain that necrotizing enterocolitis (NEC) is not occurring from the temporary reduction in oxygen to the bowel (see Chapter 45 for a discussion of NEC). After this, if the infant's respiratory rate remains rapid, gavage-feeding may be necessary (Figure 26-3). A mother who wants to breastfeed needs to receive a realistic appraisal of her child's needs. If the infant will have only a brief extended hospital stay, she can manually express breast milk to initiate and continue her milk supply until the infant is mature enough or otherwise ready for breast-feeding. Expressed breast milk may be used in the infant's gavage-feeding. All babies who are gavage-fed need oral stimulation from non-nutritive sucking and should be supplied with a pacifier at feeding times. Exceptions are infants too immature to have a sucking reflex and infants who must not swallow air, such as those with a tracheoesophageal fistula awaiting surgery.

The techniques of gavage-feeding, intravenous feeding, and gastrostomy feeding are all discussed in Chapter 34.

Preventing Infection

Contracting an infection would further complicate a high-risk infant's ability to adjust to extrauterine life. In some instances, such as preterm rupture of the membranes, it is the development of infection (e.g., pneu-

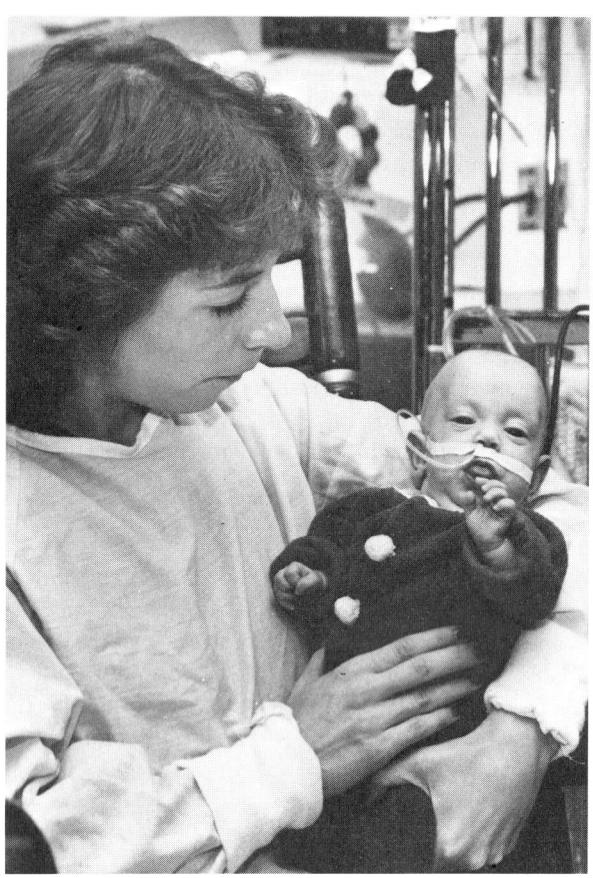

FIGURE 26-3
Infants who are ill at birth often need supplemental feedings by nasogastric or gastrostomy tube. (Courtesy of the Department of Medical Photography, Children's Hospital, Buffalo, NY.)

monia or skin lesions) that places the infant in a high-risk category.

Infections may have prenatal, perinatal, or postnatal causes. The most common viruses to affect infants in utero are the cytomegalovirus and toxoplasmosis viruses. An infant with either of these infections may be born with congenital anomalies (see Chapter 39). The most prevalent perinatal infections are those contracted from the vagina during birth: group B streptococcal septicemia, thrush from *Candida* infection and herpes (see Chapter 39). Postnatal infection is invariably spread to an infant from health care personnel (Cunningham, et al., 1993). All health care personnel caring for infants must observe strict nursery technique to keep the possibility of infection to a minimum. Health care personnel with infections have a professional and moral obligation not to give care to newborn infants.

Establishing Parent–Infant Bonding

During resuscitation at birth, parents of the high-risk newborn should be kept informed of what is happening. They should be able to visit the special nursing unit to which the child is admitted as often as they choose, to wash and gown and hold and touch the child. This makes the child's birth more real to them, and, should the child not survive the illness, will make the death more real. Only when both birth and death seem real can parents begin to work through their feelings and accept these events.

All parents handle newborn babies tentatively until they have "claimed" them or have become better acquainted. It may be months before the parents of a child who has been ill since birth can handle the baby comfortably and confidently. The parents need to spend time with the infant in the intensive care nursery as the infant improves; they also need to have access to health care personnel after discharge, to help them in caring for the child with confidence at home.

If the infant dies, the parents often wish to see him or her. They may never have seen the infant without a great deal of equipment surrounding the child and may need this time to reassure themselves that in every other way except lung function (or whatever the infant's disorder), he or she was a perfect baby. This may give them confidence to plan for other children or simply to continue their lives after such a stressful experience.

Following High-Risk Infants at Home

Each time parents visit in a high-risk nursery, it is important to assess their level of knowledge about their child's condition and development. Some high-risk newborns will return home with extensive care. Referral to a home care agency will be necessary to help parents continue with the level of care that is required (see Chapter 38).

High-Risk Infants and Child Abuse

When a child is born preterm or ill, the expected reaction of the parents would be to protect the child even more than the average child so that no further harm can result. In reality, particularly in reference to preterm children, the opposite may occur. Preterm children are at high-risk for abuse. This is probably due to the separation of the child from the family at birth, which interferes with bonding (Anderson, 1993). Child abuse is discussed in Chapter 55.

Providing Developmental Care

How much rest and how much stimulation preterm infants need for healthy development is unknown. In the 1950s, complete bed rest and minimal handling was advocated for care; in the 1960s, stimulation by rocking or stroking was introduced. Today, *developmental care,* or care designed to meet the specific needs of each infant, is advocated. This type of care can lead to increased weight gain and decreased crying and apnea spells in preterm infants (Blackburn & Vandenberg, 1993).

Nursing care of preterm infants must consider that

their central nervous systems are not mature and their reactions or adjustments to stimuli may be different from those of the term infant; the environment of an intensive care unit is totally different from what the infant would have experienced if he or she had remained in utero until term. Based on these two premises, nursing care must be geared toward making the environment of the infant as untraumatic as possible and helping the infant adjust to new experiences with limited ability.

The usual sound level of nurseries has been documented to be about 40 to 50 dBs; a radio playing raises this to 60 to 65 dBs. The closing of portholes or tapping on the sides of Isolettes raises the sound level inside them to 80 dBs or more. Other abnormal stimuli are bright lights for 24 hours a day, frequent handling, and painful procedures (see the Focus on Nursing Research box).

When a preterm infant is stressed, behaviors such as respiratory pauses, tachypnea, color changes, tremors, sighing, flaccidity, finger splaying, and gaze averting occur. Such behaviors should alert a caregiver that the environment has become too stimulating and needs to

be modified. Activities such as dimming the lights or covering an Isolette, turning the infant to the side and "containing" his body with rolled towels, offering non-nutritive sucking, and maintaining a "quiet hour" to reduce sound are all ways to reduce stimuli.

The Newborn at Risk Because of Altered Gestational Age or Birth Weight

Infants are evaluated as soon as possible after birth to determine their weight and gestational age group classification (Figure 26-4). Classification by growth charts and gestational history is important in determining the immediate health care needs of the newborn and in anticipating any problems that are likely to develop. Birth weight is normally plotted on a growth chart such as the Colorado (Lubchenco) Intrauterine Growth Chart (see Figure 23-2). Infants born after the beginning of week 38 and before week 42 of pregnancy (calculated from the first day of the last menstrual period) are classified as **term infants**. Approximately 93% of all live births are term. Infants born before term (less than the full 37th week of pregnancy) account for approximately 7% of all deliveries and are classified as **preterm infants**. Infants born after the onset of week 43 of pregnancy are classified as **postterm**. Infants who fall below the 10th percentile of weight for their age regardless of gestational age are considered **small-for-gestational-age** infants. Those who fall above the 90th percentile in weight regardless of gestational age are considered **large-for-gestational-age** infants. Preterm infants may be average-for-gestational-age, small-for-gestational-age, or large-for-gestational-age.

Infants who are found to be preterm, postterm, small-for-gestational-age, or large-for-gestational-age have immediate needs that differ from or are more pronounced than the needs of the term newborn. Each of these categories carries its own set of problems and potential risks.

The Small-for-Gestational-Age Infant

An infant is small-for-gestational-age if the birth weight is below the 10th percentile on an intrauterine growth curve for that age (Crouse & Cassady, 1994). The infant may be born preterm (before week 38 of gestation), may be term (weeks 38 to 42) or postterm (past 42 weeks). Infants who are small-for-gestational-age are distinctly different from infants whose weight is low but who are normal for their gestational age.

Causes

The mother's nutrition during pregnancy plays a major role in fetal growth outcome, and lack of adequate nu-

(*text continues on page 740*)

FOCUS ON NURSING RESEARCH

Is It Possible to Detect Pain Responses in Preterm Infants?

To answer this question, three nurse researchers studied the physiologic responses of preterm infants to routine heelsticks. The sample for the study consisted of 40 preterm infants born between 32 and 34 weeks gestational age and not more than 5 postnatal days of age at the time of the study. Infants were observed during 5 phases of the heelstick procedure: just prior to the heelstick, during heel warming, the actual heelstick, heel squeeze, and finally immediately afterward to detect return to baseline responses. Facial expression was videotaped and then analyzed; the infant's cry was converted to spectrographic analysis. The heart rate of these infants rose from a mean of 143 before the procedure, to 146 while the heel was warmed, to 154 during the stick, to 170 while the heel was squeezed. Oxygen saturation fell from 96% to as low as 89% during the squeezing phase; intracranial pressure rose from 7 at the beginning of the procedure to 15 during the actual heelstick.

The researchers stress that painful procedures can cause measurable physiologic responses in preterm infants; nursing actions to calm infants and comfort during and after such procedures are important in helping the infant maintain usual physiologic functioning.

Stevens, B. J., Johnston, C. C., & Horton, L. (1993). Multidimensional pain assessment in premature neonates: a pilot study. *Journal of Obstetrics, Gynecologic and Neonatal Nursing, 22,* 531.

Examination First Hours

WEEKS GESTATION

PHYSICAL FINDINGS		20–25	26–30	31–34	35–37	38–41	42–48
Vernix		Appears	Covers body, thick layer			On back, scalp, in creases (38–39); Scant, in creases (40)	No vernix
Breast tissue and areola		Areola and nipple barely visible; no palpable breast tissue			Areola raised (35)	1–2 mm nodule (36); 3–5 mm (38–39); 5–6 mm (40); 7–10 mm (41)	?12 mm
Ear	Form	Flat, shapeless			Beginning incurving superior (34)	Incurving upper 2/3 pinnae (36); Well-defined incurving to lobe (40)	
	Cartilage	Pinna soft, stays folded		Cartilage scant, returns slowly from folding (32)	Thin cartilage, springs back from folding (34)	Pinna firm, remains erect from head (40)	
Sole creases		Smooth soles without creases		1–2 anterior creases (32)	2–3 anterior creases (35); Creases anterior 2/3 sole (37)	Creases involving heel (38–39)	Deeper creases over entire sole
Skin	Thickness & appearance	Thin, translucent skin, plethoric, venules over abdomen, edema		Smooth, thicker, no edema (32)	Pink (36)	Some desquamation pale pink (40)	Thick, pale, desquamation over entire body
	Nail plates	Appear		Nails to finger tips (32)			Nails extend well beyond finger tips
Hair		Appears on head	Eye brows and lashes (26)	Fine, woolly, bunches out from head (28)	Silky, single strands, lays flat (37)		?Receding hairline or loss of baby hair, short, fine underneath
Lanugo		Appears	Covers entire body	Vanishes from face (34)	Present on shoulders	No lanugo	
Genitalia	Testes		Testes palpable in inguinal canal (28)		In upper scrotum (37)	In lower scrotum (41)	
	Scrotum		Few rugae (28)		Rugae, anterior portion	Rugae cover; Pendulous	
	Labia & clitoris		Prominent clitoris, labia majora small, widely separated (30)		Labia majora larger, nearly cover clitoris		Labia minora and clitoris covered
Skull firmness		Bones are soft	Soft to 1" from anterior fontanelle (28)	Spongy at edges of fontanelle, center firm (35)	Bones hard, sutures easily displaced		Bones hard, cannot be displaced
Posture	Resting	Hypotonic, lateral decubitus	Hypotonic (26)	Beginning flexion, thigh (30); Stronger hip flexion (32); Froglike (34)	Flexion, all limbs (36)	Hypertonic (39)	Very hypertonic
Recoil - leg		No recoil		Partial recoil (32)	Prompt recoil		
	Arm	No recoil		Begin flexion, no recoil (34)	Prompt recoil, may be inhibited	Prompt recoil after 30" inhibition	

FIGURE 26-4

Clinical estimation of gestational age. An approximation based on published data. (From Kempe, C. H., Silver, H. K., & O'Brien, D. O. [1974]. Current pediatric diagnosis and treatment [3rd ed.]. Los Altos, CA: Lange, with permission.)

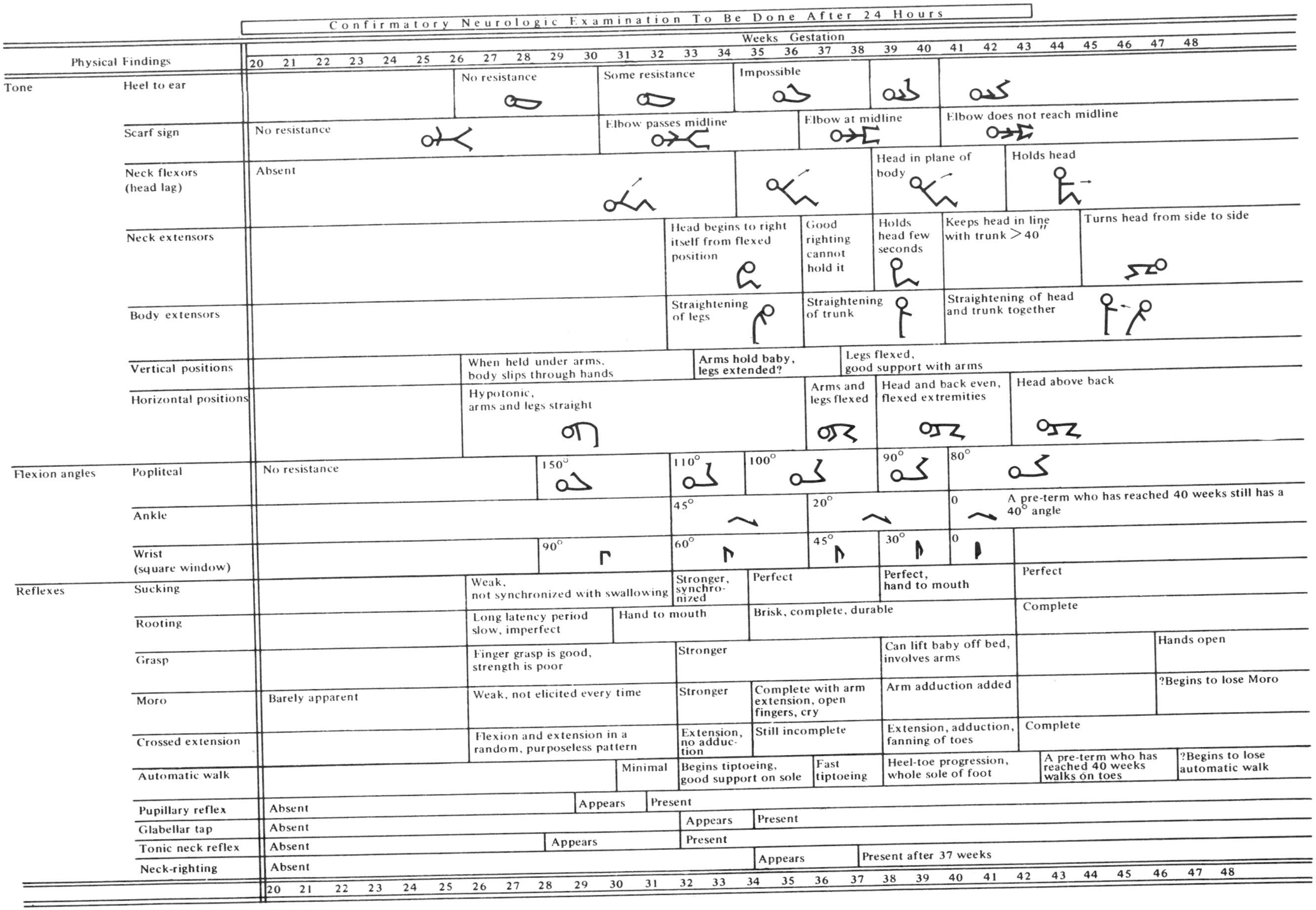

Confirmatory Neurologic Examination To Be Done After 24 Hours
Weeks Gestation
Physical Findings
20 21 22 23 24 25 26 27 28 29 30 31 32 33 34 35 36 37 38 39 40 41 42 43 44 45 46 47 48
Tone
Heel to ear
No resistance
Some resistance
Impossible
Scarf sign
No resistance
Elbow passes midline
Elbow at midline
Elbow does not reach midline
Neck flexors (head lag)
Absent
Head in plane of body
Holds head
Neck extensors
Head begins to right itself from flexed position
Good righting cannot hold it
Holds head few seconds
Keeps head in line with trunk > 40"
Turns head from side to side
Body extensors
Straightening of legs
Straightening of trunk
Straightening of head and trunk together
Vertical positions
When held under arms, body slips through hands
Arms hold baby, legs extended?
Legs flexed, good support with arms
Horizontal positions
Hypotonic, arms and legs straight
Arms and legs flexed
Head and back even, flexed extremities
Head above back
Flexion angles
Popliteal
No resistance
150°
110°
100°
90°
80°
Ankle
45°
20°
0
A pre-term who has reached 40 weeks still has a 40° angle
Wrist (square window)
90°
60°
45°
30°
0
Reflexes
Sucking
Weak, not synchronized with swallowing
Stronger, synchronized
Perfect
Perfect, hand to mouth
Perfect
Rooting
Long latency period slow, imperfect
Hand to mouth
Brisk, complete, durable
Complete
Grasp
Finger grasp is good, strength is poor
Stronger
Can lift baby off bed, involves arms
Hands open
Moro
Barely apparent
Weak, not elicited every time
Stronger
Complete with arm extension, open fingers, cry
Arm adduction added
?Begins to lose Moro
Crossed extension
Flexion and extension in a random, purposeless pattern
Extension, no adduction
Still incomplete
Extension, adduction, fanning of toes
Complete
Automatic walk
Minimal
Begins tiptoeing, good support on sole
Fast tiptoeing
Heel-toe progression, whole sole of foot
A pre-term who has reached 40 weeks walks on toes
?Begins to lose automatic walk
Pupillary reflex
Absent
Appears
Present
Glabellar tap
Absent
Appears
Present
Tonic neck reflex
Absent
Appears
Present
Neck-righting
Absent
Appears
Present after 37 weeks
20 21 22 23 24 25 26 27 28 29 30 31 32 33 34 35 36 37 38 39 40 41 42 43 44 45 46 47 48

FIGURE 26-4

trition may be a major contribution to intrauterine growth retardation. Pregnant adolescents, for example, with poor nutritional habits have a high incidence of small-for-gestational-age infants. However, the most common cause of intrauterine growth retardation is a placental anomaly: either the placenta is unable to obtain sufficient nutrients from the uterine arteries or it is inefficient at transporting nutrients to the fetus. Placental damage, such as partial placental separation with bleeding, limits placental function as the area of placenta that separated becomes infarcted and fibrosed, reducing the placental surface available for exchange. A developmental defect in the placenta can also prevent it from functioning properly. Women with systemic diseases that decrease blood flow to the placenta (e.g., diabetes mellitus or pregnancy-induced hypertension) are at higher risk for delivering small-for-gestational-age babies than others. Mothers who smoke heavily or use narcotics also tend to have small-for-gestational-age infants (Cunningham et al., 1993).

In other instances, the placental supply of nutrients is adequate but the infant is unable to use them. Infants with intrauterine infections such as rubella or toxoplasmosis develop this problem. Babies with chromosomal abnormalities may be small-for-gestational-age in addition.

Assessment

Prenatal Assessment. The small-for-gestational-age infant may be detected in utero when the recorded fundal height during pregnancy becomes progressively less than the expected fundal height. If the woman is unsure of the date of her last menstrual period, this discrepancy can be hard to substantiate. A sonogram can demonstrate the decreased size. A nonstress test can provide additional information on placental function. If poor placental function is apparent from such determinations, it can be predicted that the infant will do poorly during labor; periods of hypoxia could lead to neurologic damage. Cesarean birth is the birth method of choice in such circumstances.

Appearance. The infant who suffers nutritional deprivation early in pregnancy when fetal growth consists primarily of an increase in the number of body cells is generally below average in weight, length, and head circumference. The infant who suffers deprivation late in pregnancy when growth consists primarily in increase of cell size may only have a reduction in weight. Whether deprivation occurs early or late, the infant has an overall wasted appearance. The child may have a small liver, which causes a great deal of difficulty regulating glucose, protein, and bilirubin levels. The infant has poor skin turgor and generally appears to have a large head because the rest of the body is so small from having few fat stores. Skull sutures may be widely separated from

lack of normal bone growth. Hair is dull and lusterless. The abdomen may be sunken. The cord often appears dry and may be stained yellow.

In contrast, because the infant's age is more advanced than the weight implies, the child may have better developed neurologic responses, sole creases, and ear cartilage than expected for a baby of that weight. The skull may be firmer and the infant may seem unusually alert and active for that weight.

The small-for-gestational-age infant needs careful assessment for congenital anomalies that might have occurred as an additional result of the poor nutritional intrauterine environment. Conversely, a congenital anomaly may have caused poor growth by interfering with nutritional use of available substances.

Laboratory Findings. Blood studies at birth on small-for-gestational-age infants usually show a high hematocrit level (less than normal amounts of plasma in proportion to red blood cells) and an increase in the total number of red blood cells (polycythemia). The increase in red blood cells is probably due to a state of anoxia during intrauterine life. The high hematocrit level reflects a lack of plasma due to lack of fluid in utero. The polycythemia causes increased blood viscosity, a condition which puts extra work on the heart, because it is more difficult for the infant to circulate blood effectively. As a consequence, acrocyanosis (blueness of the hands and feet) may be persistent. If the polycythemia is extreme, blocked vessels and thrombus formation can result. If the hematocrit level is more than 65%, an exchange transfusion to dilute the concentration of blood may be necessary.

Because small-for-gestational-age infants have decreased glycogen stores, one of the most common problems in neonatal life is **hypoglycemia** (decreased serum glucose, or a level below 40 mg/dL). Such infants may need intravenous glucose to sustain blood sugar until they are able to suck vigorously enough to take sufficient oral feedings.

Nursing Diagnoses and Related Interventions

Nursing Diagnosis: High risk for altered respiratory function related to underdeveloped body systems at birth

Goal: Newborn will initiate and maintain respirations at birth.

Outcome Criteria: Newborn maintains normal respirations at a rate of 30 to 60 breaths per minute following resuscitation at birth.

Birth asphyxia is a common problem for small-for-gestational-age infants, because they are at risk for developing meconium aspiration syndrome due to anoxia during labor. For this reason, many small-for-gestational-age infants require resuscitation at birth. They should be closely observed for both respiratory rate and character in the first few hours of life, because their chest muscles may be underdeveloped and therefore they are unable to sustain the rapid respiratory rate of a normal newborn.

> ***Nursing Diagnosis:*** High risk for ineffective thermoregulation related to lack of subcutaneous fat
>
> ***Goal:*** Newborn will maintain body temperature within normal limits.
>
> ***Outcome Criteria:*** Infant's temperature is maintained at 36.5°C (97.8°F) axillary.

Small-for-gestational-age infants are less able to control body temperature than the normal newborn because they lack subcutaneous fat. A carefully controlled environment is essential to keep the infant's body temperature in a neutral zone (see Chapter 23).

> ***Nursing Diagnosis:*** High risk for altered parenting related to child's high-risk status and possible cognitive impairment from lack of nutrients in utero
>
> ***Goal:*** Parents will demonstrate beginning bonding with infant while in hospital.
>
> ***Outcome Criteria:*** Parents express interest in infant and ask questions about what will be child's care needs at home.

Although small-for-gestational-age infants may gain weight and appear to thrive in the first few days of life, their mental development may have been impaired because of lack of oxygen and nourishment in utero. Babies who were growing normally in utero but whose gestation was interrupted preterm (true preterm babies) usually gain weight and height so rapidly that by the end of the first year of life they are near the 50th percentile on growth charts. Small-for-gestational-age infants may always be below normal on standard growth charts. This inability to reach normal levels of growth and development may interfere with bonding because the child does not meet the parents' expectations; it can eventually interfere with the child's self-esteem if the child is never able to meet his or her parents' expectations.

One way to promote early parental bonding with the child is to discuss ways parents can promote the infant's development once they are at home. A small-for-gestational-age infant needs adequate stimulation during the infant period to reach normal growth and developmental milestones. Parents need to be encouraged to provide toys that are suitable for their child's chronologic age, *not* physical size. As the infant tires easily in the first few weeks of life, play periods must be spaced

with rest periods or hypoglycemia or apnea can occur (see the Nursing Care Plan: A Preterm Infant).

The Large-for-Gestational-Age Infant

An infant is large-for-gestational-age (also termed **macrosomia**) if the birth weight is above the 90th percentile on an intrauterine growth chart for that gestational age. Such a baby appears deceptively normal at birth because of the weight, but a gestation examination will reveal immature development. It is important that a large-for-gestational-age infant be identified immediately so that the infant is given special care appropriate to his or her gestational age, rather than being treated as a term newborn.

Causes

Infants who are large-for-gestational-age have been subject to an overproduction of growth hormone in utero. This happens most often to mothers with poorly controlled diabetes mellitus. Multiparous women are also prone to delivering large babies, because with each succeeding pregnancy, babies tend to grow larger. Other conditions associated with large-for-gestational-age infants are transposition of the great vessels; Beckwith's syndrome, a rare condition characterized by overgrowth; and congenital anomalies such as omphalocele.

Assessment

A fetus is suspected of being large-for-gestational-age when the size of the uterus measures unusually large for the date of pregnancy. However, because a fetus lies in a flexed fetal position, he or she does not occupy significantly more space at 10 lb than at 7 lb. If a fetus does seem to be growing at an abnormally rapid rate, a sonogram can confirm the suspicion. A nonstress test to assess the placenta's ability to sustain the large fetus during labor may also be performed. The infant's lung maturity may be assessed by amniocentesis. If the infant's large size was not detected during pregnancy, it may be recognized during labor when the baby is unable to descend through the pelvic rim. Cesarean delivery may be necessary because of **cephalopelvic disproportion** (i.e., the biparietal diameter is closer to 10 cm than the usual 9 cm) or **shoulder dystocia** (the wide shoulders are unable to pass through the outlet of the pelvis).

Appearance. Infants who are large-for-gestational-age may show immature reflexes and low scores on gestational age examinations done at birth in relation to their size. The baby may have extensive bruising or a birth injury such as a broken clavicle or Erb-Duchenne paralysis from trauma to the cervical nerves if the infant was delivered vaginally (see Chapter 51). Because the

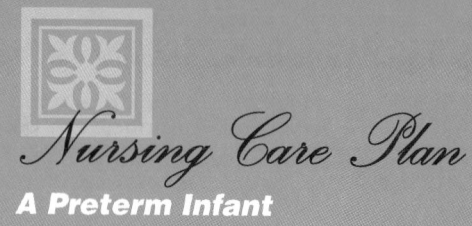

Nursing Care Plan
A Preterm Infant

Baby Harden (the parents have not yet named the infant) is a 34-week gestation, small-for-gestational-age preterm infant (2000 g) in your care. He is 3 days old; the following is a nursing care plan you might design for him.

Assessment: No spontaneous respiratory effort at birth; resuscitated by Ambu respirator and transported to Level III nursery. PO_2 was 40 mm Hg on arrival at Central Nursery. Temperature: 97.6°F axillary with infant in Servocontrol Isolette. No apnea apparent.

Taking 2 mL of breast milk every 3 hours by gavage feeding. No residual aspirated from stomach before feedings. Weight gain; 100 g for past 3 days.

Abraded areas present on elbows and knees from irritation of sheets during transport. Mother has not seen infant because she is still hospitalized at community hospital. Father has visited twice but touched infant only once. He states, "He's not going to make it." Said not to name him, because he doesn't want to "waste" favorite family name on a baby who will die.

Nursing Diagnosis: High risk for ineffective breathing pattern related to lung immaturity

Defining Characteristic: PO_2 was only 40 mm Hg on hospital admission.

Goal: Infant will maintain adequate respiratory function during course of hospital stay.

Outcome Criteria: Infant's PO_2 is maintained between 60 and 100 mm Hg.

Nursing Orders	Rationale
1. Position infant with head and chest elevated.	1. Position allows for maximum lung space.
2. Maintain body temperature in neutral thermal environment; place in oxygen hood.	2. A neutral thermal environment helps prevent an increased metabolic rate and so limits need for oxygen.
3. Observe every 15 min for respiratory rate and sternal retractions.	3. Increased respiratory rate and retractions are signs of respiratory distress.
4. Auscultate for lung sounds every 30 min.	4. Rales and respiratory grunting are signs of respiratory distress syndrome.
5. Suction respiratory tract as necessary.	5. Suctioning maintains airway patency from accumulating mucus.
6. Place pulse oximeter and read every 30 min.	6. Assess for oxygenation saturation of blood.

Nursing Diagnosis: High risk for hypothermia related to immature temperature regulation

Defining Characteristic: Infant's present temperature is maintained only by warmer and servocontrol.

Goal: Infant will maintain temperature at neutral thermal temperature during hospital stay.

Outcome Criteria: Infant's temperature is maintained at 97.6°F (36.5°C) with Servocontrol.

(continued)

head is large it may have been submitted to more than usual pressure during birth, causing a prominent caput succedaneum, cephalhematoma, or molding.

The large-for-gestational-age newborn must be cared for with the same precautions used with a preterm infant. Specific criteria to look for at an initial or continuing assessment are shown in Table 26-1.

Cardiovascular Dysfunction. The heart rate of large-for-gestational-age infants should be carefully observed; cyanosis may be a sign of transposition of the great vessels, a serious heart anomaly (see Chapter 41). Polycythemia, if present, is caused by the infant's sys-tem attempting to fully oxygenate all body tissues. Observe closely for signs of **hyper-**

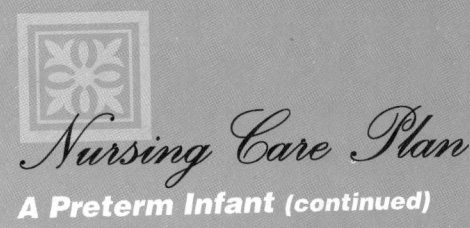

Nursing Orders

1. Place on radiant heat warmer; attach temperature probe to abdomen.
2. Change diapers frequently; keep head covered with cap.
3. Position warmer away from air conditioner or window.
4. Assess and record body temperature every 30 min.
5. Wrap warmly when mother removes him from warmer for feeding or encourage kangaroo care.

Rationale

1. Provides a heat source; assess and maintain neutral body temperature.
2. Prevents chilling from evaporation.

3. Limits radiation cooling.

4. Assess and document body temperature.
5. Prevents cooling by decreasing evaporation or providing a heat source.

Nursing Diagnosis: High risk for altered nutrition, less than body requirements, related to immaturity

Defining Characteristic: Infant is unable to suck for sustained period; presently being gavage-fed.

Goal: Infant will ingest adequate breast milk by gavage or bottle-feeding for calorie and protein needs.

Outcome Criteria: Infant continues weight gain consistent with preterm rate.

Nursing Orders

1. Offer 2 mL breast milk by gavage every 6 h; feed with "preemie" nipple every other feeding.
2. Maintain intravenous fluid of 5% D/W at 3 mL/h.

3. Aspirate stomach contents before gavage-feeding; return amount of aspirate before feeding. Reduce feeding amount by aspirate amount.
4. Bubble well following nipple- or gavage-feeding.

5. Weigh all diapers and test specific gravity of urine. Assess for skin turgor and mucous membrane moisture every 4 hours.
6. Weigh daily.
7. Analyze a serum glucose every 4 hours by heel stick.
8. Record blood loss from blood samples. Assess blood pressure every hour.

Rationale

1. Gavage-feeding prevents fatigue; nipple-feeding provides sucking pleasure.
2. IV solution supplies additional fluid, glucose, and electrolytes to the infant who can not suck effectively.
3. This is assessment for sign of necrotizing enterocolitis; replace fluid to avoid depleting electrolytes.

4. Decrease possibility of retained air in stomach and regurgitation and aspiration.
5. Assessments for hydration.

6. Assessment for continuing growth.
7. Assessment for hypoglycemia.

8. Assessment for anemia and hypovolemia, two sequelae of blood loss.

(continued)

bilirubinemia (increased serum bilirubin) that may result from absorption of blood from bruising and polycythemia.

Hypoglycemia. A large-for-gestational-age infant needs to be carefully assessed also for hypoglycemia in the early hours of life because the infant uses up nutritional stores readily to sustain his or her weight. If the mother is diabetic with poor glucose control, the infant will have an increased blood glucose level in utero, which causes the infant to produce elevated levels of insulin. After birth, these increased insulin levels will continue for the first few hours of life and cause a rebound hypoglycemia.

Nursing Diagnosis: High risk for infection related to immature immune system

Defining Characteristic: The immune system is not mature in preterm infants, so their ability to resist infection is decreased; abrasions or ports of entry are present on skin.

Goal: Infant will remain free of infection during hospital stay.

Outcome Criteria: Infant has negative skin, blood, and urine cultures.

Nursing Orders	**Rationale**
1. Encourage mother to continue to supply breast milk.	1. Breast milk contains antibodies, which may help prevent infection.
2. Apply an emollient (Nivea oil) to dry skin four times daily.	2. Prevent skin from cracking and opening ports of entry for microorganisms.
3. Use clean gavage technique, and sterile bottles to collect breast milk.	3. Prevent spread of infection from equipment.
4. Enforce hand washing before care: use cover gown when holding infant.	4. Prevent spread of infection from health care personnel.
5. Remind parents to wash hands and wear cover gown.	5. Prevent spread of infection from outside environment.
6. Bathe child daily with clear water only.	6. Prevent skin drying from soap; remove surface organisms.
7. Reposition frequently.	7. Prevent any further abraded areas.

Nursing Diagnosis: High risk for altered parenting related to inadequate bonding secondary to separation from child, and anticipatory grief

Defining Characteristic: Father states he feels infant will die.

Goal: Family will develop normal parent–child attachment.

Outcome Criteria: At least one parent visits daily or telephones; both parents express interest in child; parents choose name for child.

(continued)

Nursing Diagnoses and Related Interventions

Nursing Diagnosis: High risk for altered respiratory function related to possible birth trauma in large-for-gestational-age newborn

Goal: Newborn will initiate and maintain respirations at birth.

Outcome Criteria: Newborn initiates breathing at birth; maintains normal newborn respiratory rate of 30 to 60 breaths per minute.

Some large-for-gestational-age infants have difficulty establishing respirations at birth because of birth trauma. Increased intracranial pressure from birth of the larger-than-usual head may lead to pressure on the respiratory center, which causes a decrease in respiratory function. A diaphragmatic paralysis may occur due to cervical nerve trauma as the head is bent laterally to allow for birth of the large shoulders. This prevents active lung motion on the affected side. If the infant had to be delivered by cesarean birth, transient fluid can remain in the lungs and interfere with effective gas exchange.

Nursing Care Plan

A Preterm Infant (continued)

Nursing Orders	Rationale
1. Inform both parents they are allowed to visit any time.	1. Encourage parent–infant bonding by frequent contact.
2. Give snapshot of infant to father to take to mother.	2. Encourage parent–infant bonding by frequent awareness.
3. Urge mother to telephone daily about child's progress. Stress importance of her breast milk for child.	3. Involve parents in care of child to encourage bonding.
4. Encourage father to touch and hold infant at visits.	4. Touching may be instrumental in encouraging bonding.
5. Role model "parenting" at parents visits; encourage verbalization of feelings from parents.	5. Role modeling may aid in teaching parenting behaviors.

Nursing Diagnosis: High risk for altered growth and development related to high-risk status of low-birth-weight infant

Defining Characteristic: Infant is receiving little parent stimulation or interaction because of limited visits this far.

Goal: Infant will demonstrate normal growth and development during hospital stay.

Outcome Criteria: Infant continues to gain weight; shows increased ability to adjust to stress by containment mannerisms.

Nursing Orders	Rationale
1. Observe infant for signs of fatigue and space procedures to avoid this.	1. Preterm infants can develop apnea if fatigue develops.
2. Initiate "containment care" by towel rolls and help to quiet infant with calm environment.	2. Measures to help a preterm infant maintain a midline position and which appear to offer comfort.
3. Maintain "en face" position to speak to infant on warmer.	3. Infants appear to enjoy focusing on human faces.
4. Hang mobile over warmer; stroke back and head for 1 min four times daily.	4. Supply vision and touch stimulation.
5. Encourage parents to touch and hold infant at visits. Describe and demonstrate infant's ability to focus on smiling face and attune to voices.	5. Encourage parents to provide stimulation at visits.

Nursing Diagnosis: High risk for altered nutrition; less than body requirements related to additional nutrients needed to maintain weight and prevent hypoglycemia

Goal: Infant will ingest adequate fluid and nutrients for growth during neonatal period.

Outcome Criteria: Infant's weight follows percentile growth curve; skin turgor is good; specific gravity of urine is 1.003 to 1.030; serum glucose is above 45 mg/dL.

As a rule, the large-for-gestational-age infant needs to be fed early (by 4 hours after birth) to prevent hypoglycemia. The infant may need supplemental glucose water following breast-feeding to supply enough fluid and glucose for the child's larger than normal size.

It is important not to overestimate this infant's ability to feed at birth. The infant may seem as if he or she should do well with breast-feeding because the baby is already the size of a 2-month-old. The infant is an inexperienced newborn, however, so sucking may not be

Table 26-1. Important Assessment Criteria for a Large-for-Gestational-Age Infant	
Assessment	Rationale
Skin color for ecchymosis, jaundice, and erythema	Bruising occurs with vaginal delivery; jaundice may occur from breakdown of ecchymotic collections of blood; polycythemia causes ruddiness of skin.
Motion of extremities on spontaneous movement and in response to a Moro's reflex to detect clavicle fracture (crepitus or swelling may then be palpated at the fracture site) and palsy due to edema of the cervical nerve plexus	Clavicle or cervical nerve injuries may occur due to problem of delivery of wider than normal shoulders.
Asymmetry of the anterior chest or unilateral lack of movement to detect diaphragmatic paralysis from edema of the phrenic nerve	The cervical nerve may be stretched by delivery of wide shoulders.
Eyes for evidence of unresponsive or dilated pupils, vomiting, bulging fontanelles, and a high pitched cry suggestive of increased intracranial pressure	Compression of 3rd, 4th, and 6th cranial nerves by increased pressure limits eye response; other signs of increased intracranial pressure may occur.
Activities such as jitteriness, lethargy, and uncoordinated eye movements that suggest seizure activity	Seizures may be caused by increased intracranial pressure; seizures in newborns often produce only vague symptoms.

effective enough for the infant to obtain an adequate supply of milk.

> ***Nursing Diagnosis:*** High risk for altered parenting related to high-risk status of large-for-gestational-age infant
>
> ***Goal:*** Parents demonstrate adequate bonding behavior during neonatal period.
>
> ***Outcome Criteria:*** Parents hold infant; speak of the child in positive terms; state accurately why the infant needs to be closely observed in postnatal period.

Parents may underestimate this infant's needs because of the child's excessive size. He or she seems so large and healthy the parents may be confused about why the infant needs "careful watch" care. They may read more into the child's condition than is present (he or she must be sick in some way that they are not being told about) and so bonding does not happen as instinctively as it might. If the woman sustained a cervical or perineal tear or had to have a cesarean birth, she needs some time to air any resentment she may feel toward the infant. Otherwise, her perception that the infant is the cause of her additional distress may interfere with her ability to bond with the child.

A large-for-gestational-age infant needs the same developmental care that all other infants need. Singing or talking to the baby, stroking the child's back, and rocking the baby are all important for the large infant's development. Encourage parents to treat their baby as a fragile newborn who needs warm nurturing, not as a tough "big boy or girl" who has grown past that stage.

The Preterm Infant

A preterm infant is usually defined as a live-born infant born before the end of week 37 of gestation; another criterion used is a weight of less than 2500 g (5 lb, 8 oz) at birth. Infants who are born before week 20 to 24 of gestation are generally categorized as products of abortion, not preterm children, because their chances for survival are very slight. Infants born after the 37th week are term. Infants who are born between 30 and 36 weeks gestation (weighing 1500 to 2500 g) are **low-birth-weight** (LBW) infants; those born between 26 and 30 weeks gestation (1000 to 1500 g) are **very-low-birth-weight** (VLBW); those born between 24 and 26 weeks gestation (500 to 1000 g) are **extremely-very-low-birth-weight** (EVLBW) infants. All such infants need level III (neonatal intensive care) care from the moment of birth to give them their best chance of survival without neurologic aftereffects from their being so critically close to the age of viability. A lack of lung surfactant makes them extremely vulnerable to respiratory distress syndrome.

The maturity of a newborn currently is determined by physical findings such as sole creases, skull firmness, ear cartilage, and neurologic findings that reveal gestational age, as well as the mother's report and sonographic estimations of gestational age.

Preterm babies of *every* weight need to be differentiated at birth from small-for-gestational-age babies (who also may have a low birth weight), because the two conditions result from different situations and therefore will have different problems of adjustment to extrauterine life. A preterm infant is immature and small, but well. Unlike the small-for-gestational age infant, this baby appears to have been doing well in utero; for an unexplained reason, the "trigger" that initiates labor was activated too early and birth has resulted even though the baby is immature. Differentiating characteristics of small-for-gestational-age and low-birth-weight infants are compared in Table 26-2.

Incidence

Low birth weight (preterm birth) occurs in approximately 7% of live births of white infants. In black infants, the rate is twice as high—approximately 14%.

If the fact that the infant is preterm is recognized by a gestational-age assessment and health care personnel watch for the specific problems of prematurity such as respiratory distress syndrome, hypoglycemia, and intracranial hemorrhage, LBW infants have a survival rate of 90–95%; VLBW infants, about 80%; EVLBW infants only 40% (Scanlon, 1994).

Causes

With preterm infant death accounting for 80% to 90% of the mortality in the first year of life, infant mortality could be reduced dramatically if the causes of preterm birth could be discovered and corrected and all pregnancies brought to term. The exact cause of early birth, however, is rarely known. There is a high correlation between low socioeconomic level and early termination of pregnancy. In women from the middle and upper socioeconomic groups, only 4% to 8% of pregnancies are terminated early; in women from low socioeconomic levels, 10% to 20% end before term. The major influencing factor in these instances appears to be inadequate nutrition before and during pregnancy, as a result of either lack of money or lack of knowledge of good nutri-

tion. Additional factors that seem to be related to early termination of pregnancy are shown in Box 26-2. It is unfortunate when prematurity results from iatrogenic causes, such as elective cesarean birth and inducement of labor according to dates rather than fetal maturity. Testing fetal maturity by amniocentesis is a current method used to avoid inducing labor prematurely.

Assessment

History. Although a detailed pregnancy history may sometimes point to a potential preterm birth, the pregnancy history is often normal up to the beginning of labor.

When interviewing the mother of a preterm infant, be careful not to convey disapproval of reported pregnancy behaviors such as cigarette smoking or working a 12-hour work shift. The average pregnant woman is not doing these things maliciously, but is likely unaware that they could be detrimental to the fetus. Once the infant is born, she will need a high level of self-esteem and all of her inner resources to sustain her through the crisis. Being overburdened by guilt does not help her in any way and may actually be detrimental to her attempts to bond with her undersized infant. A good answer to her direct inquiries about causes is, "No one really knows what causes prematurity."

In many instances, preterm labor might have been halted had the woman been able to recognize soon enough that she was in true labor, and not having Braxton-Hicks contractions. In a first labor, this can easily occur because the woman does not know what true labor feels like. Television often depicts women in

Table 26-2. Differences Between Small-for-Gestational-Age and Low-Birth-Weight Infants

Characteristic	Small-For-Gestational-Age Infant	Low-Birth-Weight Infant
Gestational age	24–44 wk	Younger than 37 wk
Birth weight	Under 10th percentile	Normal for age
Congenital malformations	Strong possibility	Possibility
Pulmonary problems	Meconium aspiration, pulmonary hemorrhage, pneumothorax	Respiratory distress syndrome
Hyperbilirubinemia	Possibility	Very strong possibility
Hypoglycemia	Very strong possibility	Possibility
Intracranial hemorrhage	Strong possibility	Possibility
Apnea episodes	Possibility	Very strong possibility
Feeding problems	Most likely to be due to accompanying problem such as hypoglycemia	Small stomach capacity; immature sucking reflex
Weight gain in nursery	Rapid	Slow
Future retarded growth	May always be under 10th percentile due to poor organ development	Not likely to be retarded in growth as "catch-up" growth occurs

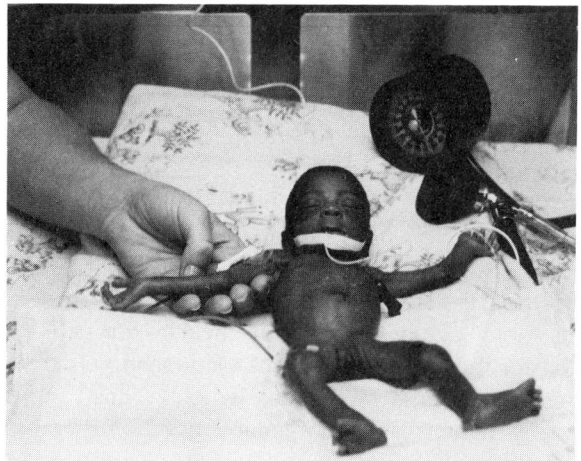

FIGURE 26-5

An immature infant. Notice the frog-leg or lax position due to immature muscle contraction. (Courtesy of the Department of Medical Photography, Children's Hospital, Buffalo, NY.)

labor as having agonizingly painful contractions or, the opposite, simply announcing, "This is it," and then proceeding to deliver within the 30-minute show. The first-time mother does not realize that in real life, labor usually begins with subtle signs and mild contractions, not with a dramatic announcement. Even a multipara may miss the early signs of labor until it is too far advanced to be reversed, because each labor proceeds differently. You can reassure the woman that it is understandable that she did not realize what was happening until cervical dilatation had occurred and labor could not be reversed.

Appearance. On gross inspection, a preterm infant appears small and underdeveloped (Figure 26-5). The head is disproportionately large (3 cm or more greater than chest size). The skin is generally unusually ruddy because the infant has little subcutaneous fat beneath it; veins are easily noticeable, and a high degree of acrocyanosis may be present. The infant has little vernix caseosa, because this is formed late in pregnancy. Lanugo is usually extensive, covering the back, forearms, forehead, and sides of the face, because this is present until late in pregnancy. Both anterior and poste-

rior fontanelles are small. There are few or no creases on the soles of the feet.

Physical findings and reflex tests used to differentiate between term and preterm newborns are illustrated in Figure 26-6. The eyes of most preterm infants appear small. A pupillary reaction is present, although it is difficult to elicit. Ophthalmoscopic examination is extremely difficult and often unrewarding, because the vitreous humor may be hazy. The preterm infant has varying degrees of myopia (near-sightedness) because of lack of eye globe depth.

The cartilage of the ear is immature and allows the pinna to fall forward. The ears appear large in relation to the head. The level of the ears should be carefully inspected to rule out chromosomal abnormalities (Figure 26-6H).

Neurologic function in the preterm child is often difficult to evaluate. The observation of spontaneous movement and provoked movements may yield findings as important as the reflex tests. If tested, reflexes such as sucking and swallowing will be absent if the infant's age is below 33 weeks; deep tendon reflexes such as the Achilles tendon reflex are markedly diminished (Figure 26-6A–E). During an examination, a preterm infant moves far less than a mature infant and rarely cries. If the infant does cry, the cry is weak and high pitched. Assessment charts such as the one shown in Figure 26-4 are helpful in predicting expected neurologic activity in a preterm baby.

Laboratory Findings. Laboratory values for the preterm infant are compared with those of the term infant in Appendix F.

Potential Complications

Anemia of Prematurity. Many preterm infants develop a normochromic, normocytic anemia; blood cells

Full-term Infant

Premature Infant

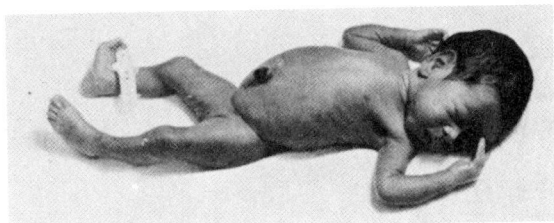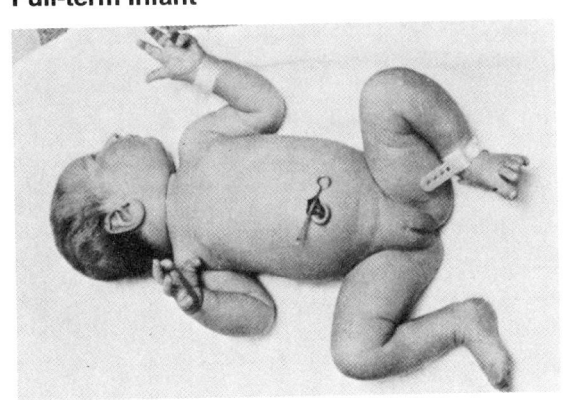

RESTING POSTURE   *The premature infant is characterized by very little, if any, flexion in the upper extremities and only partial flexion of the lower extremities. The full-term infant exhibits flexion in all four extremities.*

A

Premature Infant, 28–32 Weeks

Full-term Infant

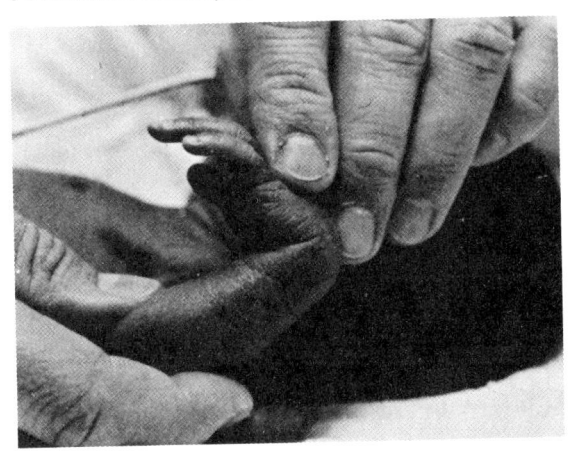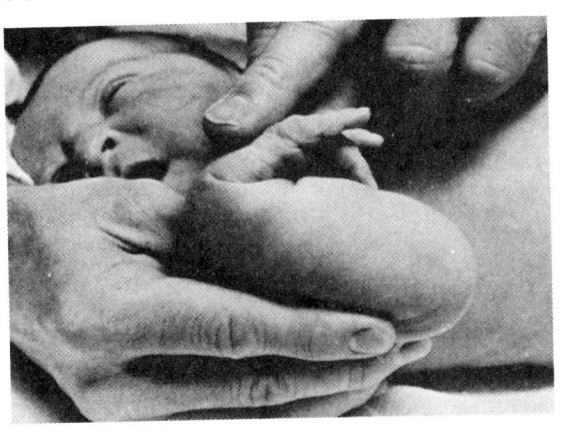

WRIST FLEXION   *The wrist is flexed, applying enough pressure to get the hand as close to the forearm as possible. The angle between the hypothenar eminence and the ventral aspect of the forearm is measured. (Care must be taken not to rotate the infant's wrist.) The premature infant at 28–32 weeks' gestation will exhibit a 90° angle. With the full-term infant it is possible to flex the hand onto the arm.*

B

FIGURE 26-6
*Examples of physical examination findings and reflex tests used to judge gestational age. (**A**) Posture.
(**B**) Wrist flexion. (Figure continues.)*

may be fragmented or irregularly shaped. The reticulocyte count is also low, because the bone marrow appears to have difficulty with the production and maturation of new erythrocytes. The infant will appear pale, may be lethargic and anorectic, and will generally fail to thrive. The fault appears to be immaturity of the hematopoietic system combined with destruction of red blood cells due to low levels of vitamin E. Excessive blood drawing for electrolyte or blood gas analysis can add to the problem. For this reason, records of the amount of blood drawn for analysis must be kept on preterm infants.

Anemia of prematurity will improve with administration of vitamin E (Goetzman & Wennberg, 1991). Red blood cell production can be stimulated by the administration of DNA recombinant erythropoietin. In addition, the infant may need blood transfusions to supply needed red blood cells.

Kernicterus. Kernicterus is destruction of brain cells by invasion of indirect bilirubin (Shaw, 1993). This invasion occurs because of high concentrations of indirect bilirubin in the blood due to excessive breakdown

(*text continues on page 752*)

Flex Extremities and Hold

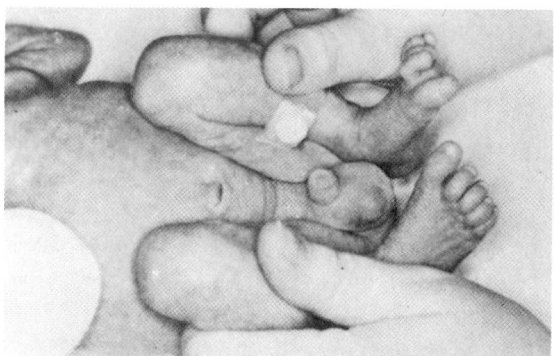

Response in Premature Infant

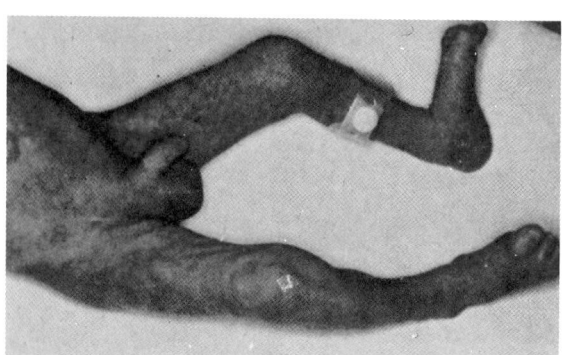

Extend

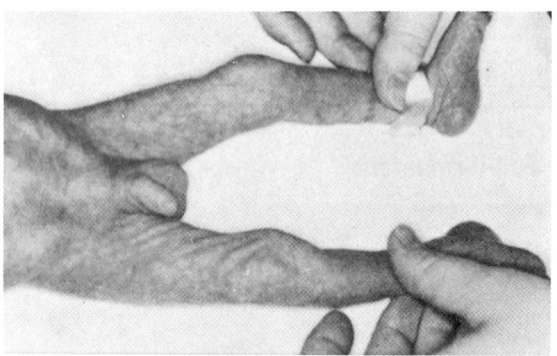

Response in Full-term Infant

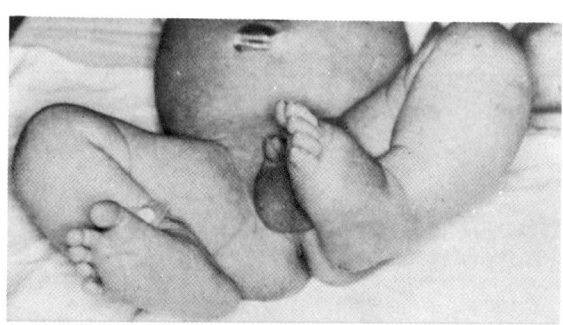

RECOIL OF EXTREMITIES   *Place the infant supine. To test recoil of the legs (1) flex the legs and knees fully and hold for 5 seconds. (2) extend by pulling on the feet, (3) release. To test the arms, flex forearms and follow same procedure. In the premature infant response is minimal or absent; in the full-term infant extremities return briskly to full flexion.*

C

Full-term Infant

Premature Infant

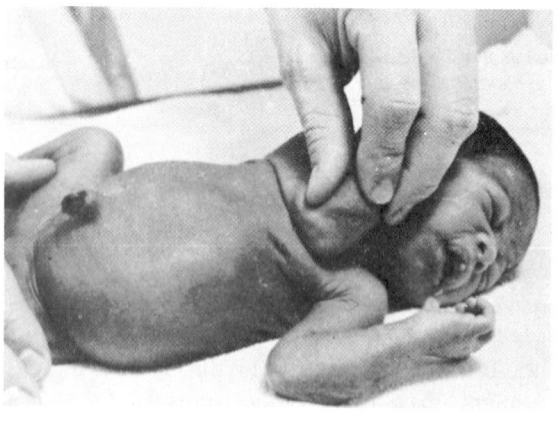

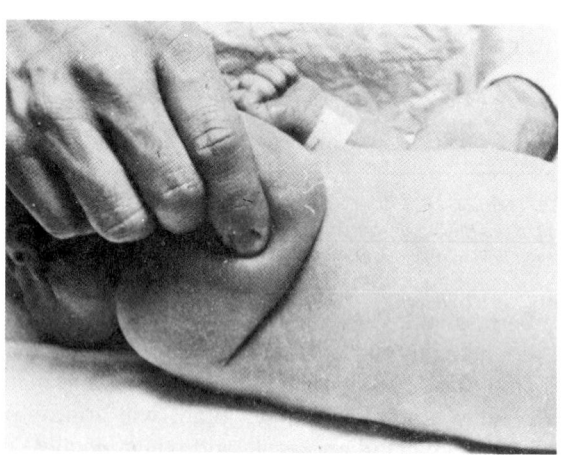

SCARF SIGN   *Hold the baby supine, take the hand, and try to place it around the neck and above the opposite shoulder as far posteriorly as possible. Assist this maneuver by lifting the elbow across the body. See how far across the chest the elbow will go. In the premature infant the elbow will reach near or across the midline. In the full-term infant the elbow will not reach the midline.*

D

FIGURE 26-6 *(Continued)*
(**C**) *Recoil of extremities.* (**D**) *Scarf sign.*

Premature Infant

Full-term Infant

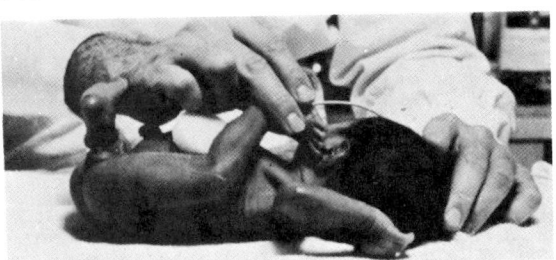
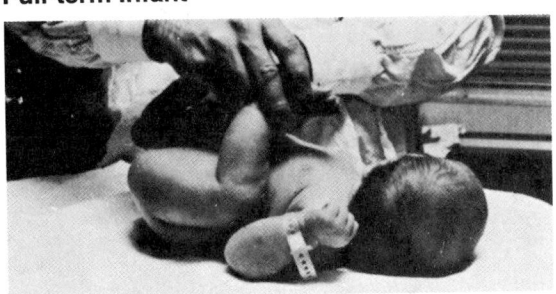

HEEL TO EAR   *With the baby supine and the hips positioned flat on the bed, draw the baby's foot as near to the ear as it will go without forcing it. Observe the distance between the foot and head as well as the degree of extension at the knee. In the premature infant very little resistance will be met. In the full-term infant there will be marked resistance; it will be impossible to draw the baby's foot to the ear.*

E

Premature Infant

Full-term Infant

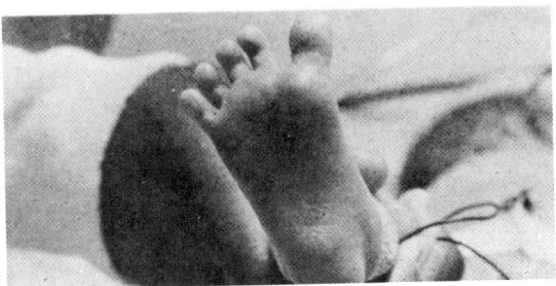
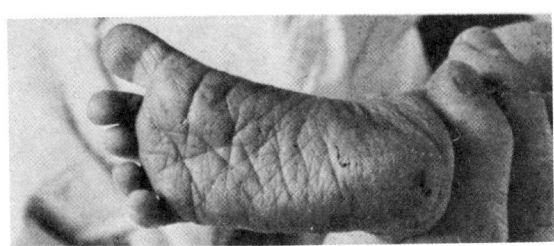

SOLE CREASES   *The sole of the premature infant has very few or no creases. With th increasing gestation age, the number and depth of sole creases multiply, so that the full-term baby has creases involving the heel. (Wrinkles that occur after 24 hours of age can sometimes be confused with true creases.)*

F

Full-term Infant

Premature Infant

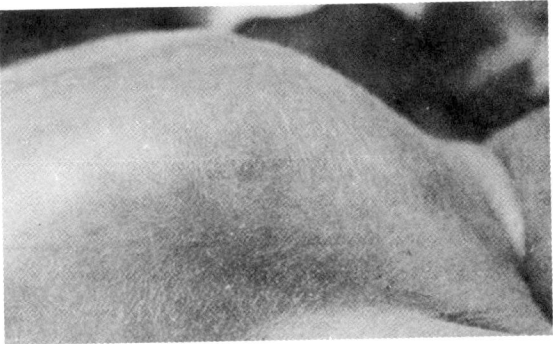
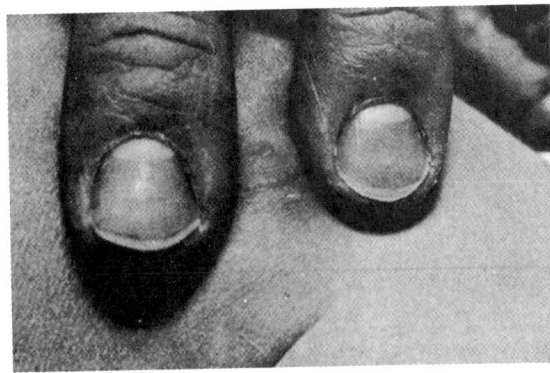

NIPPLES AND BREAST   *In infants younger than 34 weeks' gestation the areola and nipple are barely visible. After 34 weeks the areola becomes raised. Also, the infant of less than 36 weeks' gestation has no breast tissue. Breast tissue arises with increasing gestational age due to maternal hormonal stimulation. Thus, an infant of 39 to 40 weeks will have 5 to 6 mm of breast tissue, and this amount will increase with age.*

G

FIGURE 26-6 *(Continued)*
(**E**) *Heel to ear.* (**F**) *Plantar creases.* (**G**) *Breast tissue.*

Premature Infant, 34–36 Weeks

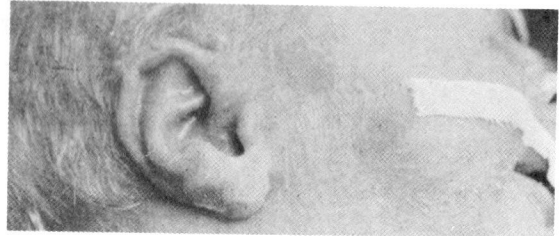

Full-term Infant

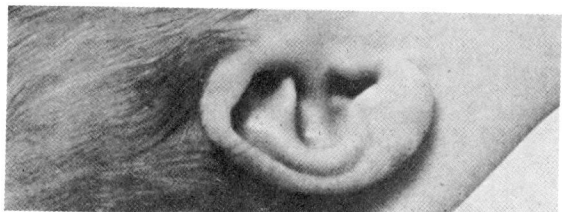

EARS   At fewer than 34 weeks' gestation infants have very flat, relatively shapeless ears. Shape develops over time so that an infant between 34 and 36 weeks has a slight incurving of the superior part of the ear; the term infant is characterized by incurving of two thirds of the pinna; and in an infant older than 39 weeks the incurving continues to the lobe. If the extremely premature infant's ear is folded over, it will stay folded. Cartilage begins to appear at approximately 32 weeks so that the ear returns slowly to its original position. In an infant of more than 40 weeks' gestation, there is enough ear cartilage so that the ear stands erect away from the head and returns quickly when folded. (When folding the ear over during examination be certain that the surrounding area is wiped clean or the ear may adhere to the vernix.)

H

Full-term Male

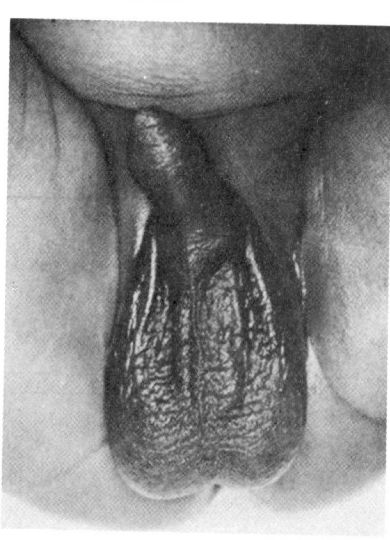

Premature Male

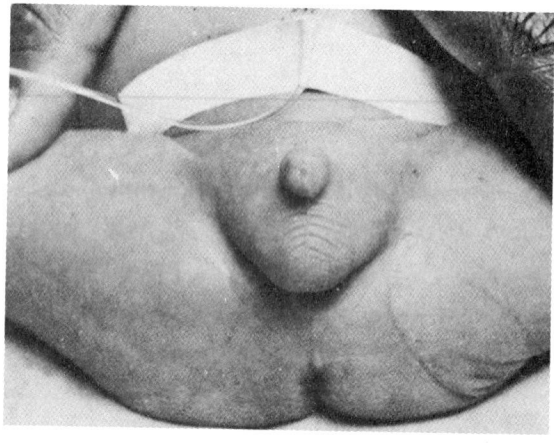

MALE GENITALIA   In the premature male the testes are very high in the inguinal canal and there are very few rugae on the scrotum. The full-term infant's testes are lower in the scrotum and many rugae have developed.

I

FIGURE 26-6 (Continued)
(**H**) Ear. (**I**) Male genitalia.

of red blood cells. Preterm infants are more prone to the condition than term infants, because with acidosis, brain cells are more susceptible to the effect of indirect bilirubin than normally; preterm infants also have less serum albumin to bind indirect bilirubin and therefore inactivate its effect. Because of this, kernicterus may occur at lower levels (as low as 12 mg per 100 mL of indirect bilirubin) in these infants. It is important to monitor indirect bilirubin levels in preterm infants if jaundice occurs, so that phototherapy or exchange transfusion can be started before indirect bilirubin levels become excessive.

Persistent Patent Ductus Arteriosus. Because preterm infants lack surfactant, their lungs are noncompliant and it is more difficult for them to push blood from the pulmonary artery into the lungs. This condition leads to pulmonary artery hypertension, which may interfere with closure of the ductus arteriosus and result in ineffective heart function (see Chapter 41). Intravenous therapy must be administered cautiously to avoid increasing blood pressure and compounding this problem. Indomethacin may be administered to initiate closure of the patent ductus arteriosus.

Premature Female

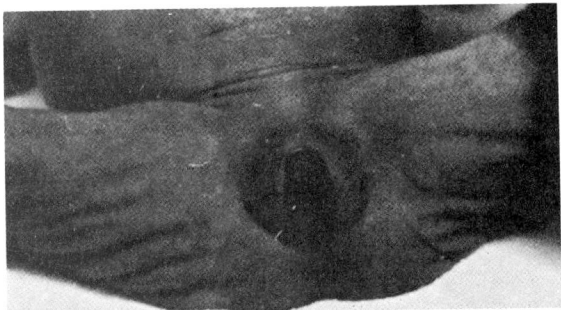

Full-term Female

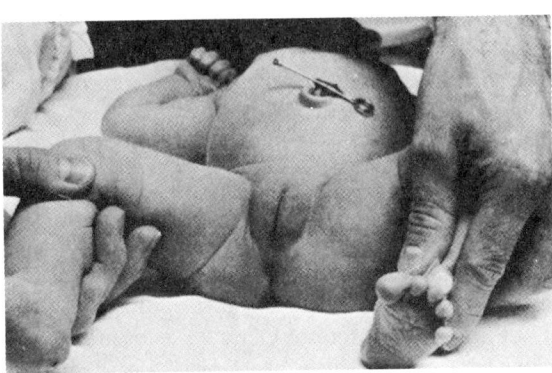

FEMALE GENITALIA *When the premature female is positioned on her back with hips abducted, the clitoris is very prominent and the labia majora are very small and widely separated. The labia minora and the clitoris are covered by the labia majora in the full-term infant.*

J

FIGURE 26-6 *(Continued)*
(J) *Female genitalia. (From Sullivan, R., et al. [1979]. Determining a newborn's gestational age. MCN: American Journal of Maternal Child Nursing, 4, 38. Original source: R. L. Schreiner [Ed.]. [1978]. Care of the newborn. Indianapolis: Indiana University Press, with permission.)*

Periventricular/Intraventricular Hemorrhage. Preterm infants are particularly prone to periventricular hemorrhage (bleeding into the tissue surrounding the ventricles) or intraventricular hemorrhage (bleeding into the ventricles) (Dietch, 1993). These conditions occur in as many as 50% of infants of very low birth weight. Preterm infants are susceptible to this because of fragile capillaries and immature cerebral vascular development. When there is a rapid change in cerebral blood pressure, such as with hypoxia, intravenous infusion, ventilation, and pneumothorax, the capillaries rupture. The infant experiences brain anoxia; hydrocephalus may occur from bleeding into the aqueduct of Sylvius with resulting obstruction of the aqueduct. Preterm infants often have a cranial ultrasound done after the first few days of life to detect if a hemorrhage has occurred. An infant's prognosis is guarded until it can be shown that development in the infant is normal after an intracranial bleed (see Chapter 49).

Other Potential Complications. Preterm infants are particularly susceptible to a number of illnesses in the early postnatal period, including respiratory distress syndrome, apnea, retinopathy of prematurity (discussed later in this chapter), and necrotizing enterocolitis (discussed in Chapter 45).

Nursing Diagnoses and Related Interventions

Because a preterm infant has few body resources, both physiologic and psychological stress must be reduced as much as possible and interventions initiated gently to prevent depletion of resources. Close observation and analysis of findings are essential to managing problems quickly.

Nursing Diagnosis: High risk for altered respiratory function related to immature pulmonary functioning

Goal: Newborn will initiate and maintain respirations following surfactant therapy.

Outcome Criteria: Newborn initiates breathing at birth following resuscitation; maintains normal newborn respirations of 30 to 60 breaths per minute free of assisted ventilation.

Preterm infants have great difficulty initiating respirations at birth because the pulmonary capillary bed has not yet matured. Lung surfactant does not form in adequate amounts until about the 34th to 35th week of pregnancy; it may be inadequate, leading to alveolar collapse with each expiration. This requires the infant to use maximum strength to inflate the alveoli each time. Infants cannot maintain effective expirations under these conditions. Because a fetus usually turns to a vertex presentation late in pregnancy, the preterm infant may still be in a breech position at birth. Breech-born infants are apt to expel meconium into the amniotic fluid. If the fetus aspirates either vaginal secretions or meconium, the respiratory problem is further compromised.

Giving the mother oxygen by mask during the birth will help provide the preterm infant with optimal oxygen saturation at birth. Keeping maternal analgesia and anesthesia to a minimum also offers the infant the best chance of initiating effective respirations. Cesarean birth, although it has the advantage of reducing pressure on the immature head, may lead to additional respiratory complications because of retained lung fluid.

Even term infants are born in temporary respiratory acidosis. Once respirations are established, however, the condition quickly clears. Because the preterm infant is unable to initiate effective respirations as quickly as the mature infant, he or she is prone to irreversible acidosis. To prevent this, the infant must be resuscitated within 2 minutes after birth. The infant must be kept warm during resuscitation procedures so that he or she is not expending extra energy to increase the metabolic rate to maintain body temperature. All procedures must be carried out gently; the preterm infant's tissues are extremely sensitive to trauma and can easily be damaged or bruised by an oxygen mask. When blood from bruising is reabsorbed, this can lead to hyperbilirubinemia, yet another problem.

Giving 100% oxygen to preterm infants during resuscitation or to maintain respirations presents the danger of pulmonary edema and retinopathy of prematurity (blindness of prematurity; see discussion later in chapter). The development of both of these conditions depends on saturation of the blood with oxygen (a PO_2 of more than 100 mm Hg associated with oxygen administered at a concentration over 70%); as long as an infant is cyanotic, the blood saturation level of oxygen is unlikely to be high.

The preterm infant may continue to need oxygen administration after resuscitation, because he or she often has difficulty maintaining respirations. The soft rib cartilage of the preterm infant tends to create respiratory problems because it collapses on expiration. The accessory muscles of respiration may be underdeveloped as well, leaving the preterm infant with no backup muscles to use when he or she becomes fatigued from trying to maintain respirations. Many preterm infants may have higher PO_2 levels when placed prone than when supine, since it increases lung effectiveness.

Many preterm babies, particularly those under 32 weeks of age, have an irregular respiratory pattern (a few quick breaths, a period of 5 seconds to 10 seconds without respiratory effort, a few quick breaths again, and so on). There is no bradycardia with this irregular pattern (sometimes termed **periodic respirations**). Although the pattern is seen in term infants as well, the pattern seems to be intensified by immaturity and uncoordinated respiratory efforts. With true apnea, the pause in respirations is more than 20 seconds and bradycardia does occur. True apnea is discussed in more detail later in the chapter.

Nursing Diagnosis: High risk for fluid volume deficit related to insensible water loss at birth and small stomach capacity

Goal: Newborn will take in adequate fluid and electrolytes to meet body needs.

Outcome Criteria: Plasma glucose is between 40 and 60 mg per 100 mL; specific gravity of urine is maintained at 1.003 to 1.030; urine output is maintained at 1 mL/kg/h.

The preterm newborn has a high insensible water loss due to the large body surface as compared with total body weight. The infant also is unable to concentrate urine well and thus excretes a high proportion of fluid from the body. All these factors make it important that the preterm baby receive 160 to 200 mL of fluid per kilogram of body weight daily (higher than the term infant).

Intravenous fluid administration should begin within hours after birth to fulfill this fluid requirement and provide glucose to prevent hypoglycemia. Intravenous fluid should be given by a continuous infusion pump to ensure a constant infusion rate. A volume control meter and infusion pump must be used to prevent accidental overload. Intravenous sites must be checked conscientiously, because the lack of subcutaneous tissue makes infiltration damaging to tissue. Specially designed no. 27 gauge needles are available to enter small-lumened veins. Many preterm infants have no peripheral veins of a size necessary for even this small a needle; they need to receive intravenous fluid by an umbilical catheter.

The baby's weight, specific gravity and amount of urine, and serum electrolytes all must be monitored to ensure that fluid intake is adequate. Too little fluid and calories leads to dehydration and starvation, acidosis, and weight loss. Overhydration leads to weight gain, pulmonary edema, and heart failure.

A preterm infant should void (and pass meconium) within 24 hours after birth. Urine output should be measured by weighed diapers to limit the number of urine collectors necessary (the constant changing of collectors leads to skin irritation and breakdown). The range of urine output for the first few days of life in preterm babies is high in comparison with that of the term baby—40 to 100 mL per kg per 24 hours, compared with 10 to 20 mL per kg per 24 hours. The specific gravity is low, rarely more than 1.012 (normal term babies may concentrate urine up to 1.030). Dextrostix tests every 4 to 6 hours help to determine hypoglycemia (decreased serum glucose) or **hyperglycemia** (increased serum glucose; the level should be between 40 mg/mL and 60 mg/mL). Be certain to keep a record of all blood drawn so the child does not become hypovolemic from the amount drawn. Conduct a diagnostic test (Hematest Reagent Tablets) for blood in the stools to demonstrate that bleeding from the intestinal tract is not occurring.

Hyperglycemia caused by the glucose infusion may lead to glucose spillage into the urine and an accompanying diuresis. If the glucose being supplied is too low and body cells are using protein for metabolism, ketone bodies will appear in urine. Test urine specimens for glucose and ketones in addition to amount and specific gravity.

Nursing Diagnosis: High risk for altered nutrition; less than body requirements related to additional nutrients needed for maintenance of rapid growth, possible sucking difficulty, and small stomach

Goal: Infant will receive adequate fluid and nutrients for growth during hospitalization.

Outcome Criteria: Infant's weight follows percentile growth curve; skin turgor is good; specific gravity of urine is 1.003 to 1.030; infant has no more than 15% weight loss in first 3 days of life and continues to gain weight after this point.

Nutrition problems arise with the preterm infant because the body is attempting to continue to maintain the rapid rate of intrauterine growth. The infant therefore requires a larger amount of nutrients in the diet than the mature infant, and if not supplied, the infant will develop **hypocalcemia** (decreased serum calcium) or **azotemia** (low protein level in blood). Delayed feeding may also add to hyperbilirubinemia, a problem the infant already is at high-risk of developing when fetal red blood cells begin to be destroyed.

Nutrition problems are compounded by the low-birth-weight infant's immature reflexes, which make swallowing and sucking difficult, and by the small stomach capacity—a distended stomach may cause the infant respiratory distress. Increased activity necessitated by ineffective sucking may increase the metabolic rate and oxygen requirements and require even more calories. An immature cardiac sphincter (between the stomach and esophagus) allows regurgitation to occur readily. The lack of a cough reflex may lead the infant to aspirate regurgitated formula. Digestion and absorption of nutrients in the stomach and intestine may also be immature.

Feeding Schedule. With the early administration of intravenous fluid to prevent hypoglycemia and supply fluid, gastrointestinal feedings may be safely delayed until the infant has stabilized his or her respiratory effort from birth. Preterm infants may be fed by total parenteral nutrition until they are stable enough for other means. Feedings should be begun, however, by gavage or bottle as soon as the infant is able to tolerate them to prevent deterioration of the intestinal villi. If the baby is going to be bottle-fed, there is no need to offer sterile water first, since it is the stomach acid that is harmful if aspirated, not the fluid given; half-strength formula may be used. Most preterm infants have had a chest x-ray prior to a feeding; the presence of air in the stomach shows that the route to the stomach is clear.

The preterm infant needs 115 to 140 cal per kilogram body weight per day, compared with 100 to 110 cal per kilogram body weight per day needed by the term infant. Protein requirements are 3 to 3.5 g per kilogram body weight, compared with 2.0 to 2.5 g per kilo-

gram body weight in a term newborn. Because a preterm infant has a small stomach capacity, he or she cannot take large feedings but must be fed more often than the mature infant (feedings may be as small as 1 or 2 mL every 2 to 3 hours). Both vitamin E and vitamin A supplements may be necessary; iron supplements as soon as the infant reaches term age are recommended (Fletcher, 1994).

Gavage-Feeding. The gag reflex is not intact until an infant is 32 weeks gestation. The ability to coordinate sucking and swallowing is inconsistent until approximately 34 weeks of gestation. Thus, infants born before 32 to 34 weeks of gestation are usually started on gavage-feedings; bottle- or breast-feeding is gradually introduced as they mature (Figure 26-7).

Preterm infants must be observed closely after both oral and gavage-feeding to be certain that the filled stomach is not causing them respiratory distress. As soon as a sucking reflex is present, offering a pacifier will strengthen this reflex and better prepare an infant for bottle-feeding as well as provide oral satisfaction.

As long as the infant is being gavage-fed, stomach secretions are usually aspirated, measured, and replaced before the feeding. An infant who has a stomach content of more than 2 mL just before a feeding is receiving more formula than he or she can digest in the time allowed. Feedings should not be increased but possibly even cut back to ensure better digestion and decrease

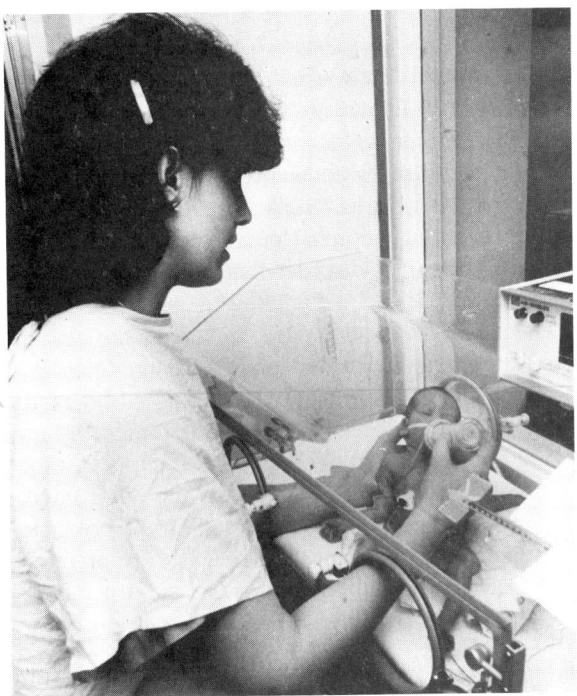

FIGURE 26-7
Feeding a low-birth-weight infant. Notice the small bottle used. (Courtesy of the Department of Medical Photography, Children's Hospital, Buffalo, NY.)

the possibility of regurgitation and aspiration. Inability to digest this way is also a symptom of necrotizing entero-colitis (see Chapter 45).

Formula. The caloric concentration of formulas used for preterm infants is usually 24 cal/oz compared with 20 cal/oz for a term baby (Table 26-3).

Minerals such as calcium and phosphorus and electrolytes such as sodium, potassium, and chloride may have to be supplemented, depending on blood studies. Vitamin K should be administered at birth, same as with a term baby, except that the amount is more often 0.5 mL instead of 1 mL. Vitamin A is important in improving healing and possibly reducing the incidence of lung disease. Vitamin E seems to be important in preventing he-molytic anemia in preterm infants. Iron supplements interfere with the absorption of vitamin E and so are not added to formula until the infant has gained an average birth weight.

The lack of an iron supplement can be confusing to parents, because they have always been told that iron helps to build strong blood. Now they are told that in their particularly vulnerable infant, iron is not being given because it will interfere with blood cell integrity. They need an explanation of the particular blood problem that must be prevented. Iron supplements will be started on discharge from the hospital or at least by age 3 months. Again, parents should have an explanation of what is happening. By the time of discharge, their infant has reached term maturity, and iron deficiency anemia due to low iron stores then becomes the infant's chief health risk.

Breast Milk. There is increasing evidence that, al-though preterm infants need the increased caloric dis-tribution of commercial formulas, the best milk for them as well as for term babies is breast milk. The immuno-logic properties of breast milk apparently play a major role in preventing neonatal necrotizing enterocolitis, a destructive intestinal disorder that often occurs in pre-term babies.

The mother who wants to breast-feed can manually express breast milk for her infant's gavage-feedings. If she cannot bring this in daily, the expressed breast milk can be frozen for safe transport and storage. Whether freezing destroys the antibodies or the factors that make breast milk preferable for sensitive digestive tracts is under investigation. The sodium content of breast milk in mothers whose infant has been born preterm is higher than that of milk at term. It is best if the infant re-ceives his or her own mother's breast milk, in order to receive this high level of sodium, which is necessary for fluid retention in a preterm infant.

Nursing Diagnosis: High risk for hypothermia re-lated to low birth weight

Goal: Infant will maintain temperature within nor-mal limits until term age.

Outcome Criteria: Infant's temperature is 97.6°F (36.5°C) axillary.

A preterm baby has a great deal of difficulty main-taining body heat, because he or she has a relatively large surface area per pound of body weight; in addi-tion, because the infant does not flex the body well but remains in an extended position, rapid cooling from evaporation is more likely to occur (Mayfield et al., 1990).

The preterm infant has little subcutaneous fat for in-sulation, and poor muscular development does not allow the child to move as actively as the older infant to produce body heat. The preterm infant also has a lim-ited amount of **brown fat**, the special tissue present in newborns to maintain body heat. The infant is unable to shiver, which is a useful mechanism to increase body temperature; on the other hand, the child is unable to sweat and thereby reduce body temperature because of an immature central nervous system and hypothalamic control. The infant thus depends on the environmental temperature provided for him or her. The infant must be kept under a radiant heat warmer in a delivery room, because delivery rooms are typically kept at a tempera-ture of 62° to 68°F (16.6° to 20°C). A 1500 g infant ex-posed to this low a temperature loses 1°C of body heat every 3 minutes if left unprotected.

Unless there are obvious abnormalities noted when the child is born, physical assessment of the infant—even weighing—should be delayed until the infant is placed in the warmth of an Isolette or under a radiant warmer with a Servocontrol.

If the infant is going to be transported to a depart-ment within the hospital, such as the x-ray department, or to a regional center for specialized care, he or she must be kept warm during transport. Remember that infants lose heat by radiation. If a warmed Isolette is placed near a cold window or air conditioner, the infant will lose heat to the distant source. Keep this in mind when transporting an infant on a cold day. The ambu-lance must be pulled in close to the hospital door; it, as well as the Isolette, must be prewarmed. An additional heat shield or plastic wrap may be placed over an infant on a radiant warmer to help conserve heat.

Nursing Diagnosis: High risk for infection related to immature immune defenses in preterm infant

Goal: Infant will remain free of infection during hospital stay.

Outcome Criteria: Infant's growth follows per-centile growth curve; temperature is 97.6°F (36.5°C) axillary.

Table 26-3. Formulas Commonly Used with Low-Birth-Weight Infants

Formula	Nutrient Source			Energy Per Oz Nutrients (g/100 mL)					Minerals						Osmolality	
	Protein	Carbo-hydrate	Fat	kcal/oz	Protein	Carbo-hydrate	Fat	Iron (mg/100 mL)	Ca	P	Na (mEq/L)	K	Cl	mos-mol/kg H₂O	Renal Solute Load (mos-mol/L)
Similac 24 LBW (Ross)	Nonfat cow's milk	Lactose, polycose	Soy oil, coconut oil, MCT oil	24	2.2	8.5	4.5	0.3	36	33	16	26	24	290	154
Enfamil Premature (Mead Johnson Nutrition)	Demineralized whey, nonfat cow's milk	Glucose polymers, lactose	Corn oil, MCT oil, coconut oil	24	2.4	8.9	4.1	0.12	48	28	14	23	19	300	220

The skin of the preterm baby is easily traumatized and therefore offers less resistance to infection than the skin and mucous membrane of the mature baby. In addition, the preterm infant has a lowered resistance to infection. The infant has difficulty producing phagocytes to localize infection and has a deficiency of IgM antibodies because of insufficient production.

Linen and equipment used with the preterm infant must be clean to reduce the chances of infection. Staff members must be free of infection, and hand washing and gowning regulations must be strictly enforced.

> ***Nursing Diagnosis:*** High risk for altered parenting related to impaired parent–infant attachment secondary to hospitalization of infant at birth
>
> ***Goal:*** Parents demonstrate adequate bonding behavior by the time of infant's discharge from hospital.
>
> ***Outcome Criteria:*** Parents visit frequently and hold infant; speak of him or her in positive terms.

The first and second periods of reactivity normally observed in newborns at 1 hour and 4 hours of life (see Chapter 23) are delayed in the preterm infant. In some infants, no period of increased activity or tachycardia may appear until 12 to 18 hours of age. If the purpose of a period of reactivity is to stimulate respiratory function, this places the preterm infant in even greater threat of respiratory failure, since respiratory efforts may not be stimulated. A second consequence of a delayed period of reactivity is the loss of an opportunity for interaction between parents and child in the early postpartal period.

At one time, a preterm infant was handled as little as possible by hospital staff to conserve the infant's energy. Parents were strictly isolated from the nursery to prevent the introduction of infection. When the child reached a "magic" weight of 4½ or 5½ lb, the parents were called and told that their child was ready to be discharged. Some nursery personnel offered to allow the mother to feed her infant once under supervision before the day of discharge. In other nurseries, the mother was simply handed the smallest infant she had ever seen and told to take the child home and "mother" this stranger. A child during the preschool years was able to be identified as having been born preterm because of the unusually flat sides to his or her head resulting from lying continually in one position during the first month of life and, sometimes, for behavior problems. A "preterm personality," that of a "spoiled," undisciplined, hard-to-manage child, was defined.

Currently it is recognized that, although it is extremely important to conserve the preterm infant's strength by reducing sensory stimulation as much as possible and handling the infant gently, the child needs as much loving attention as possible. Rocking the infant,

singing and talking to him or her, and gentle holding are measures to help the infant develop a sense of trust in people, which will enable the child to relate satisfactorily to them later on. The parents need to begin interacting with the infant in as normal a manner as possible to promote bonding (see Focus on Family Teaching display).

Before effective bonding can be established, parents may need time to come to terms with their feelings of disappointment and guilt. A nurse can be instrumental in

FOCUS ON FAMILY TEACHING

Q. My son was born at 28 weeks' gestation and will be cared for in a neonatal intensive care nursery for a long time. I feel intimidated by the technology when I visit. What can I do to counteract this feeling?

A. This is a common feeling for parents visiting in such settings. There are several actions you can take:

- Learn the name of your son's primary nurse or care manager and physician. Make a point of talking to them when you visit so the information you receive is consistent and these people can grow to know you.

- Discuss with your son's care manager or primary nurse the time you will usually visit so she or he can reserve this time for you and also schedule your baby's procedures and rest times so this is a good time for you to hold your son and interact with him.

- Ask for explanations of any equipment or medications being used with your son so you understand the plan of care. Insist on being included in care decisions.

- If you cannot visit on any day, feel free to telephone the nursery and ask to talk to your son's primary care nurse or physician. Such telephone calls are not viewed as a bother but are welcomed as the mark of a concerned parent.

- If you planned to breast-feed, ask if you can supply expressed breast milk for your infant as soon as feedings are started; this gives you a feeling of having a greater part in your baby's care.

- Supply a tape recording of your voice so your baby can learn to recognize it and a small toy for your baby's bed; these actions not only supply auditory and visual stimulation for your son but give you a more "normal" feeling toward infant care.

- Use your baby's name when you talk about him (not "the baby") to help you gain a firm feeling that this is your baby, not the nursery's.

- If your child is hospitalized a distance from home, ask if transfer to a local hospital in a less technical environment at a later date will be possible.

helping them air these feelings, and develop a more positive attitude toward their preterm infant.

If the infant cannot be removed from an Isolette or radiant heat warmer, the child can be handled and stroked in the Isolette or warmer. Because parents are not psychologically ready for birth when the preterm baby is born, it may be much harder for them to believe they have a child than if the baby were born at term. Encourage mothers to express breast milk for the infant if the child is too young to nurse. If a woman decides not to breast-feed, she should be encouraged to come into the hospital and hold the baby before and after gavage-feedings or for bottle-feedings. By feeding her baby or expressing milk for the feedings, she is directly participating in the care and taking on responsibility for the infant's welfare.

If the baby is transferred to a regional center, the mother should have an opportunity to see the baby before the transfer. A photograph of the baby for her to keep is helpful in making the birth more real to her. Encourage her to visit as often as possible. Notes that update the baby's condition can be taped to the Isolette or warmer.

On the days they cannot visit, parents can still stay in touch by telephone. By the time the baby is ready for discharge, the parents should be able to feel that they are taking home "their" baby, one that they know and are ready to love.

Parents visiting a high-risk nursery often need a great deal of attention and support from nursing personnel. Remember that, although radiant warmers, Isolettes, ventilators, and monitors are familiar equipment to nurses, they are unusual and frightening equipment to parents. A parent may want very much to touch an infant but be so afraid that touching might set off an alarm that he or she stands back with arms folded instead (Figure 26-8).

Making parents and the baby's siblings welcome in a high-risk nursery is a major role for the nurse of high-risk infants. Because preterm infants are hospitalized for long periods, parents can be baffled by receiving information from a parade of different health care professionals or a different person every time they visit. With primary nursing or case management, one nurse is the consistent caregiver who communicates the baby's nursing needs to the rest of the staff and acts as the liaison with the baby's parents.

> **Nursing Diagnosis:** High risk for diversional activity deficit (lack of stimulation) related to preterm infant's rest needs
>
> **Goal:** Infant will receive adequate stimulation during hospitalization.
>
> **Outcome Criteria:** Infant demonstrates interaction with caregivers by attuning to faces or voices.

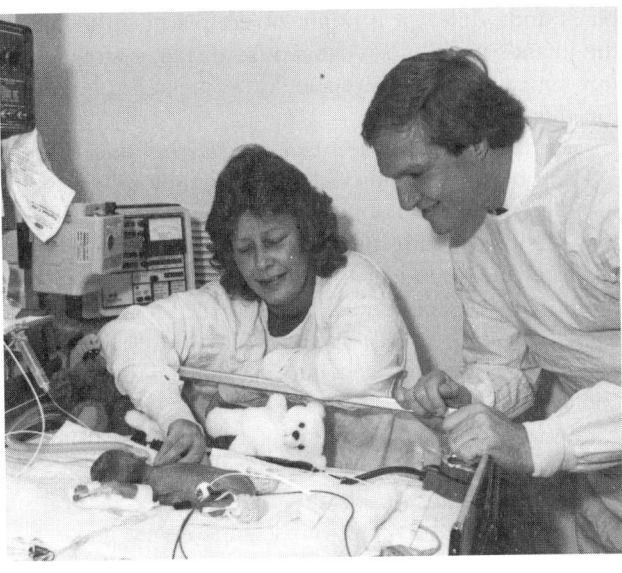

FIGURE 26-8
Parents should be encouraged to visit with immature infants to establish bonding. (Courtesy of the Department of Medical Photography, Children's Hospital, Buffalo, NY.)

Preterm infants need rest to conserve energy for growth and respiratory function, to combat hypoglycemia and infection, to stabilize temperature, and to develop inner balance and attentiveness. Procedures should be organized to maximize the amount of rest available to the infant. If this is not a coordinated effort, the infant may be awakened constantly for procedures. Recent research has shown that preterm infants may have difficulty blocking out stimuli as a result of an immature nervous system; they may react negatively to bright lights, noise, or too strenuous handling with a variety of responses such as gagging, crying, splaying fingers and toes, or going limp. Because these infants have little strength to move away from an unwanted stimulus, it is up to care providers to be sensitive to these cues and move the object or noise away from the infant. Until they are ready to take in stimuli, they may need to be shielded from noise and light as much as possible. They may need handling kept to a minimum to preserve respiratory function (Gorski et al., 1990).

At the same time, the infant needs planned periods of pleasing sensory stimulation. Like all newborns, preterm infants respond best to stimulation that appeals to their senses—sight, sound, and touch. A passive face or picture or decal may be appealing for short periods.

The view from inside an Isolette may be distorted by the acrylic dome. It is most natural for people to view an infant in an Isolette from the side. Thus, the infant's face is rarely in the same line of vision as the adult (an en face position). It is important to look directly at the infant in the straight-forward position so that the infant is provided with the stimulation of a human face. As the infant matures, he or she should have a mobile (perhaps black and white) or a bright object placed in view. As the infant's position is changed from side to stomach to opposite side, the object should be moved in line with the child's vision.

An infant in a closed Isolette may be able to hear nothing but the sound of the Isolette motor. The infant may see people looking or nodding at him or her and may see their mouths moving, but he or she cannot benefit from the sound of their voices because this is obscured by the continuous hum of the motor. Provide some talk time—words spoken softly but clearly to the infant's ear—during each nursing shift to offer normal contact.

Even the infant who cannot be removed from the Isolette should not suffer from lack of touch. Gently stroking the infant's back or smoothing the back of the head should not be tiring. Transcutaneous oxygen determinations allows a nurse to recognize when the infant is comforted by handling and when the child is growing tired. There should be time during every nursing shift for this interaction, particularly if clinical interventions with the infant include hurting procedures such as suctioning or blood drawing. As soon as the infant can be out of the Isolette or removed from the warmer, he or she needs special time to just be rocked and held.

> ***Nursing Diagnosis:*** Parental health-seeking behaviors related to health maintenance needs of preterm infant
>
> ***Goal:*** Parents express confidence in routine health care at time of hospital discharge.
>
> ***Outcome Criteria:*** Parents describe schedule for basic immunizations and health assessments, and state who will provide ongoing health care.

Before discharge from a health care facility, parents of a preterm infant need to learn and practice any special methods of care necessary for their infant and interventions to help maximize their child's development. Some parents have a tendency to overprotect preterm infants (allowing no visitors, not taking the infant outside). Relating to parents that this is often a problem is helpful before discharge. It does not necessarily alleviate the problem but does make the parents feel normal in light of their concern.

Ongoing health maintenance of the preterm infant follows the usual pattern of well child care. Basic immunizations are given according to the age the infant would have been if born at term; the immune system is mature enough to form antibodies upon immunization. In many communities, neonatal intensive care nurseries maintain their own well-child conferences for infants who were hospitalized there; this allows for long-term follow-up studies on the effect of oxygen or drug therapy and continuity of care. Many parents prefer bringing their infant back to such a facility rather than establish-

ing a new network of health care, since they have already established confidence in that health care team. This often also increases their self-esteem because they hear the staff's delight in the progress made by the child. Infants can be followed by any health care provider, however, and if the level III center is a distance away, parents may prefer to change to a facility closer to home.

Remember when plotting height and weight of preterm infants to account for early birth on the growth chart by double charting, that is, plotting the child's weight and height according to the chronologic age (a pattern that probably in the early months places the child below the 10th percentile). Then, in another color, plot the height and weight according to the infant's "set-back" age, or the age the infant would be if he or she had been born at term. A preterm baby typically gains "catch-up" weight in the first 6 months of life, so by age 1 year the baby reaches over the 10th percentile on a growth chart without accounting for a "setback" age.

Evaluate growth and development of the infant by the same manner. A preterm infant can be expected to meet first year milestones not at chronologic age but a "setback" age. Ask at health promotion visits if the parents are beginning to feel more comfortable with the infant. Ask if they are able to allow the child to stay with a babysitter or another family member; ask if the shock of having such a fragile infant has begun to diminish and the infant is beginning to be incorporated normally into their family life.

The Postterm Infant

Most nurse-midwives and obstetricians recommend inducing labor at 2 weeks postterm if it has not begun spontaneously by then. However, when gestational age has been miscalculated, or, if for some other reason, labor is not induced until week 43 of pregnancy or after, the pregnancy may result in a postterm infant.

An infant who stays in utero past week 42 of pregnancy is at special risk, because a placenta appears to be timed to last effectively for 40 weeks. After this time, it seems to lose its ability to function. The postterm infant who remains in utero with a failing placenta may die or develop a **postterm syndrome**.

Postterm infants have many of the characteristics of the small-for-gestational-age infant: dry, cracked, almost leather-like skin from lack of fluid, and absence of vernix. They may be lightweight from a recent weight loss. Fingernails have grown well beyond the end of the fingertips. They may demonstrate an alertness much more like a 2-week-old baby than a newborn. They may be meconium stained, and there may be less amniotic fluid at birth than normal.

When a pregnancy becomes postterm, a sonogram may be obtained to measure the biparietal diameter of the fetus. A nonstress test or complete biophysical profile (see Chapter 9) may be done to establish whether the placenta is still functioning adequately. An amniocentesis will show whether the infant's lungs are mature by detecting the production of surfactant. Some postterm infants must be delivered by cesarean if a nonstress test reveals a placenta that would be extremely compromised during labor because of its failing ability to provide nutrients and oxygen to the fetus.

At birth, the postterm baby is likely to have difficulty establishing respirations. The infant may have meconium aspiration from the effect of anoxia in utero. In the first hours of life, hypoglycemia may develop owing to insufficient stores of glycogen (Beckman, 1990). These stores have been used for nourishment in the last weeks of intrauterine life. Subcutaneous fat levels may also be low, having been used up in utero, so temperature regulation may be difficult. The infant must be protected from chilling at birth or while being transported to a special care center. Polycythemia may be present from decreased oxygenation in the final weeks. The infant's hematocrit may be elevated because of the polycythemia and dehydration, which lowers the circulating plasma level.

Any woman is anxious when she does not deliver on her due date. She becomes extremely anxious and, perhaps, angry when it is found that her baby is postterm. It may seem to her that if the baby stayed so long in utero, he or she should be extra healthy and strong. Why then, is the baby being transferred for special care? She may also feel guilty for not "providing well" for the infant in the last few weeks of pregnancy.

The mother needs to spend time with her newborn to assure herself that, although birth did not occur at the predicted time, the baby is otherwise normal, and with appropriate interventions to control possible hypoglycemia or meconium aspiration, will be a well baby. All postterm infants need follow-up care until at least school age, to track their developmental abilities. The lack of nutrients and oxygen in utero may have left them with neurologic symptoms that will not become apparent until they attempt fine motor tasks.

Illness in the Newborn

Respiratory Distress Syndrome

Respiratory distress syndrome (RDS) of the newborn, formerly termed hyaline membrane disease, most often occurs in preterm infants, infants of diabetic mothers, infants born by cesarean birth, or those who for any reason have decreased blood perfusion of the lungs (Whitsett et al., 1994). The pathologic feature of RDS is a hyaline-like (fibrous) membrane comprised of products formed from an exudate of the infant's blood that lines the terminal bronchioles, alveolar ducts, and alveoli. This membrane prevents exchange of oxygen and car-

bon dioxide at the alveolar–blood interface. The cause of RDS is a low level or absence of surfactant, the phospholipid that lines the alveoli and resists surface tension on expiration to keep alveoli from collapsing on expiration.

As many as 30% of low-birth-weight infants are susceptible to developing RDS; and as many as 50% of very-low-birth-weight infants are susceptible (Whitsett et al., 1994; see Focus on Cultural Awareness display).

Etiology

High pressure is required to fill the lungs with air for the first time and overcome the pressure of lung fluid. It takes a pressure between 40 cm H_2O to 70 cm H_2O to inspire a first breath, but only 6 cm H_2O to 8 cm H_2O to maintain quiet, continued breathing. If alveoli collapse with each expiration, however, it continues to take forceful inspiration to inflate them.

Even very immature infants release a bolus of surfactant at birth into their lungs from the stress of birth. As areas of hypoinflation occur, however, pulmonary blood resistance in the lung is increased. This high tension in the pulmonary artery can cause blood to shunt through the foramen ovale and the ductus arteriosus as it did during fetal life, when passage of blood through the lungs could not be accomplished. With poor lung cell blood perfusion, the production of surfactant decreases even further.

The poor oxygen exchange leads to tissue hypoxia. Tissue hypoxia causes the release of lactic acid. This, combined with an increasing carbon dioxide level resulting from the formation of the hyaline membrane on the alveolar surface, leads to severe acidosis. Acidosis

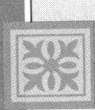

FOCUS ON CULTURAL AWARENESS

The weight of infants at birth is at least partially culturally determined. In the United States, for example, low-birth-weight infants are most apt to be born to unmarried urban black women under age 20 with less than 12 years of schooling who receive late or no prenatal care (Ogata, 1994). This statistic points to the need for the nurse to be aware that the very young mother who is socioeconomically disadvantaged is at higher risk for giving birth to low-birth-weight infants. A number of factors may contribute to this, including lack of knowledge concerning the importance of prenatal care, lack of transportation to prenatal appointments, and poor nutritional status. Assessing the particular needs of these mothers is important in preventing the problems that low-birth-weight infants experience at birth.

causes vasoconstriction, and decreased pulmonary perfusion from vasoconstriction limits surfactant production still further.

With decreased surfactant production, the ability to stop alveoli from collapsing with each expiration becomes impaired. This vicious cycle continues until the oxygen–carbon dioxide exchange in the alveoli is no longer adequate to sustain life without ventilator support.

Assessment

Most infants who will later develop RDS have difficulty initiating respirations at birth, but after resuscitation they appear to have a period of hours or a day when they are free of symptoms because of an initial release of surfactant. During this time, subtle signs such as low body temperature, nasal flaring, sternal and subcostal retractions, and tachypnea (more than 60 respirations per minute) may be present. Within several hours, expiratory grunting, which indicates a prolonged expiratory time, becomes apparent. The sound is a compensatory mechanism that denotes closure of the glottis is occurring. Glottis closure increases the pressure in alveoli on expiration, helps to keep alveoli from collapsing, and makes oxygen exchange more complete. Even with this attempt at better oxygen exchange, however, as the disease progresses infants become cyanotic in room air. On auscultation, there may be fine rales and diminished breath sounds because of poor air entry. As distress increases, the infant shows seesaw respirations (on inspiration, the anterior chest wall retracts and the abdomen protrudes; on expiration, the sternum rises). The infant's heart begins to fail; the urine output decreases; and there may be edema of the extremities from heart failure. The infant's color becomes a pale gray, periods of apnea occur, and bradycardia becomes apparent.

Diagnosis of RDS is made on clinical signs of grunting, cyanosis in room air, tachypnea, nasal flaring, retractions, and shock. A chest x-ray film will reveal a diffuse pattern of radiopaque areas of ground glass (haziness). Blood gas studies (taken from an umbilical vessel catheter) will reveal respiratory acidosis. A beta-hemolytic, group B, streptococcal infection may mimic RDS, because this infection is so severe in newborns that the insult to the lungs is intense enough to stop surfactant production. Cultures of blood and cerebrospinal fluid and skin need to be taken, and antibiotic therapy (penicillin or ampicillin) and an aminoglycoside (gentamicin or kanamycin) may be begun until culture reports are available.

Therapeutic Management

RDS can be largely prevented by the administration of surfactant through an endotracheal tube at birth for the infant at risk because of low gestational age; infants who were not treated at birth can have surfactant administered at the time that symptoms occur (termed surfactant "rescue").

Surfactant Replacement and Rescue. As a preventive measure, synthetic surfactant is sprayed into the lungs by a syringe through an endotracheal tube at birth while the infant is first positioned with the head held upright and then tilted downward (Etherington et al., 1993). It is important that the infant's airway not be suctioned for as long a period as possible after surfactant administration to avoid suctioning the drug away. Although there are almost no unfavorable reactions to surfactant administration, the infant who is receiving surfactant and then is placed on a ventilator needs close observation, since lung expansion can improve rapidly; ventilator settings will then need to be modified to prevent excessive lung pressure.

Oxygen Administration. Administration of oxygen is necessary to maintain correct PO_2 and *p*H levels. Continuous positive airway pressure (CPAP) or assisted ventilation with positive end expiratory pressure (PEEP) will exert pressure on the alveoli at the end of expiration and keep alveoli from collapsing. This greatly improves the oxygen exchange. A possible complication of oxygen therapy in the very immature or very ill infant is retinopathy of prematurity (see later).

Ventilation. Normally, inspiration on a ventilator is shorter than expiration, or an inspiratory/expiratory ratio (I/E ratio) of 1:2. It is difficult to deliver enough oxygen to stiff, noncompliant lungs in the usual ratio without forcing the air into the lungs at such a high pressure and rapid rate that pneumothorax becomes a constant fear. Infant ventilators are available with a reversed I/E ratio (2:1). These are pressure cycled, which controls the force with which air is delivered. High-frequency oscillatory ventilation or "jet" ventilation are other methods of introducing oxygen to infants with noncompliant lungs. These systems maintain a high airway pressure and then intermittently "jet" or oscillate at a rapid rate (up to 600 times a minute) an additional amount of air to inflate alveoli. Complications of any type of ventilation are possible, such as pneumothorax and impairment of cardiac output (decreased flow through the pulmonary artery) from lung pressure. A possible risk of increased intracranial and venous pressure and hemorrhage also exists. Limiting fluid intake may decrease pulmonary artery pressure. The administration of indomethacin will cause closure of the patent ductus arteriosus and make ventilation more efficient. Indomethacin has the side-effects of decreased renal function, decreased platelet count, and gastric irritation. All infants who receive it need careful urine output recorded and should be observed carefully for bleeding, especially at blood puncture sites.

Additional Therapy. Yet another method of increasing pulmonary blood flow is by using muscle relaxants. Pancuronium (Pavulon) is administered intravenously to a point of abolishing spontaneous respiratory action. Doing so allows mechanical ventilation to be accomplished at lower pressures, because there is no normal muscle resistance to overcome. The possibility of pneumothorax is reduced while PO_2 is increased. Obviously an infant who has no spontaneous respiratory function because of drug administration needs critical observation and frequent arterial blood gases, because he or she totally depends on caregivers at this point.

The effects of pancuronium decrease as the life of the drug expires; its effects can be interrupted by the administration of atropine or injectable neostigmine methylsulfate (Prostigmin Methylsulfate Injectable). Some infants will be maintained on extracorporeal membrane oxygenation (ECMO) in order to ensure adequate oxygenation (Short, 1994). Other therapies include liquid ventilation or administration of perfluorocarbons and inhalation of nitric acid (see Chapter 40).

When pancuronium is being administered, both atropine and Prostigmin should be immediately available. The infant's nursing care plan should be specially marked to show that pancuronium therapy is being used, so that in the event of a power failure, manual ventilatory assistance can be begun immediately.

Supportive Care. The infant with RDS needs care in a unit specially designed to meet the needs of such infants. The infant must be kept warm, because cooling increases acidosis in all infants, and may increase it in RDS infants to lethal levels. Keeping the infant warm so that the metabolic rate does not have to increase to maintain an adequate temperature reduces the oxygen need as well. The infant will need intravenous fluid and glucose or gavage-feeding for hydration and nourishment, because the respiratory effort makes the infant too exhausted to suck.

Prevention

RDS rarely occurs in mature infants. Dating a pregnancy by sonogram or the lecithin/sphingomyelin ratio of amniotic fluid are important ways to be certain that an infant born by cesarean or was induced is mature enough that RDS is not apt to occur. (If the level of lecithin in surfactant exceeds that of sphingomyelin by 2:1, the lungs are mature and RDS is not likely to occur).

Preventing labor by using tocolytic agents such as turbutaline helps to prevent preterm infants from being born. It may be possible to further prevent RDS in infants by administering two injections of a glucocorticosteroid (Betamethasone is a common type) to the mother at 12 and 24 hours before birth, since steroids appear to quicken the formation of lecithin production pathways. This is most effective at the 28th to 32nd week of pregnancy. Unfortunately, there is often no warning that preterm birth is imminent until hours before birth, and some labors and births will progress too rapidly for this preventive measure to be effective (the steroid takes effect in 24 to 48 hours).

Transient Tachypnea of the Newborn (TTN)

At birth, a newborn may have a rapid rate of respiration, up to 80 breaths per minute when crying; within 1 hour, however, this rapid rate slows to between 30 and 60 breaths per minute. In about 10 in 1000 live births the respiratory rate remains at a high level, between 80 and 120 breaths per minute. The infant does not appear to be in a great deal of distress, aside from the tiring effort of breathing so rapidly. He or she has mild retractions but not marked cyanosis. Mild hypoxia and hypercapnia may be present. Feeding is difficult for the child because he or she cannot suck and breathe this rapidly at the same time. A chest x-ray film reveals some fluid in the central lung, but aeration is adequate (Haywood et al., 1993).

Transient tachypnea appears to result from slow absorption of lung fluid. It may reflect a slight decrease in production of phosphatidyl glycerol or mature surfactant. These factors limit the amount of alveolar surface available to the infant for oxygen exchange, and the infant must increase the respiratory rate and depth in order to better use the surface available. Transient tachypnea occurs more often in infants who are born by cesarean, in infants whose mothers received extensive fluid administration during labor, and in preterm infants. Infants born by cesarean are probably more prone to develop this form of respiratory distress, because the thoracic cavity is not compressed by the force of vaginal birth and thus less lung fluid is expelled than normally (Haywood et al., 1993).

The major need of the infant is close observation to see that the increased effort is not tiring him or her and to watch for beginning signs of a more serious disorder (a rapid rate of respirations is often the first sign of respiratory obstruction in infants). Oxygen administration may be necessary. Transient tachypnea of the newborn peaks in intensity at approximately 36 hours of life, and then begins to fade, until by 72 hours of life it spontaneously fades as the lung fluid is absorbed and respiratory activity becomes effective (Whitsett, 1994).

Meconium Aspiration Syndrome

Meconium is present in the fetal bowel as early as 10 weeks gestation. An infant who has hypoxia in utero has a vagal reflex relaxation of the rectal sphincter, which releases meconium into the amniotic fluid. Babies born breech may expel meconium into the amniotic fluid from pressure on the buttocks. In both instances, the appearance of the fluid at birth is green to greenish black from the staining. Meconium staining occurs in approximately 10% of all pregnancies; it tends to not occur in extremely-low-birth-weight-infants, since the substance has not passed far enough in the bowel for it to be at the rectum in these infants.

At the time of the initial distress or with the first breath, if the infant inhales any of the fluid, meconium is aspirated. Meconium can cause severe respiratory distress in three ways: (1) It can bring about inflammation of bronchioles because it is a foreign substance; (2) it can block small bronchioles by mechanical plugging; and (3) it can cause a decrease in surfactant production through lung cell trauma. Hypoxemia, carbon dioxide retention, and intrapulmonary and extrapulmonary shunting occur. A secondary infection of injured tissue may lead to pneumonia.

Assessment

Infants with meconium-stained amniotic fluid may have difficulty establishing respirations at birth (those who were not breech born have had a hypoxic episode in utero to cause the meconium to be in the amniotic fluid). The Apgar score is apt to be low. Almost immediately, tachypnea, retractions, and cyanosis occur.

With meconium-stained amniotic fluid, the infant should have the nose and throat suctioned before the first breath is taken to avoid meconium aspiration. The infant should be intubated and meconium suctioned from the trachea and bronchi. It is important that oxygen under pressure (bag and mask) not be administered until the infant has been intubated and suctioned, so that the pressure of the oxygen does not drive small plugs of meconium farther down into the lungs, worsening the irritation and obstruction. After the initiation of respirations, the infant's respiration rate may remain elevated (tachypnea); coarse bronchial sounds may be heard on auscultation. The infant may continue to have retractions; the inflammation of bronchi tends to trap air in alveoli—as in a person with asthma. This may cause the chest to become enlarged in its anteroposterior diameter (barrel chest). Blood gases will reveal the poor exchange of air (a decreased PO_2; an increased PCO_2). A chest x-ray film will show bilateral course infiltrates in the lung, with spaces of hyperaeration (a peculiar honeycomb effect). The diaphragm will be pushed downward.

Therapeutic Management

Infants may be treated with oxygen administration and assisted ventilation as well as an antibiotic to forestall development of pneumonia as a secondary problem. Lung tissue is fairly noncompliant after meconium aspiration, which may necessitate high inspiratory pressure. This can cause pneumothorax or pneumomediastinum. As long as an infant did not undergo a hypoxic incident in utero or during therapy which left him or her with neurologic impairment, the infant can be expected to recover completely in a number of days. Infants must be observed closely for signs of trapping air in alveoli, because alveoli can expand only so far and then will rupture, sending air into the pleural space.

Because of the high pulmonary resistance, the ductus arteriosus may remain open, causing blood to shunt from the pulmonary artery into the aorta, compromising cardiac efficiency and increasing hypoxia. The infant needs to be observed closely for signs of congestive heart failure (e.g., increased heart rate or respiratory distress). The infant must be kept in a thermal neutral environment to prevent the metabolic rate from rising (which would increase the need for oxygen); the infant already has difficulty supplying cells with oxygen because of this unfortunate birth trauma. Amniotransfusion may be used to dilute the amount of meconium in amniotic fluid and reduce the risk of aspiration. Some infants will be maintained on extracorporeal membrane oxygenation (ECMO) in order to ensure adequate oxygenation (Short, 1994).

Postural drainage with clapping and vibration may be helpful to encourage removal of flecks of remaining meconium from the lungs (see Figure 40-12).

Apnea

Apnea is a pause in respirations longer than 20 seconds with accompanying bradycardia and perhaps beginning cyanosis. Many preterm infants have periods of apnea as a result of fatigue or the immaturity of their respiratory mechanisms. Babies with secondary stresses, such as infection, hyperbilirubinemia, hypoglycemia, or hypothermia, tend to have a high incidence of apnea. Gently shaking an infant or flicking the sole of the foot often stimulates the baby to breathe again, almost as if the child needed to be "reminded" to maintain this function. If an infant does not respond to these simple measures, resuscitation by bagging and oxygen administration is necessary. Preterm infants must have extremely close observation to detect these apneic episodes. Apnea monitors that record respiratory movements are invaluable tools to detect failing respiration and sound a warning that an infant needs attention. An infant with frequent or difficult-to-correct episodes will be placed on a ventilator to provide respiratory coordination until he or she is more mature.

To prevent episodes of apnea, maintain thermal neutrality and use gentle handling to avoid excessive fatigue. Always suction gently to minimize nasopharyngeal irritation, which can cause bradycardia due to vagal stimulation. Using indwelling nasogastric tubes rather than intermittent ones can also reduce the amount of vagal stimulation. After feeding, observe an infant carefully, because the full stomach puts pressure on the diaphragm. Careful burping also helps to reduce this effect. Never take rectal temperatures in infants prone to apnea: resulting vagal stimulation can reduce the heart rate (bradycardia), which can lead to apnea. Infants with apnea may be administered theophylline or caffeine sodium benzoate to stimulate respirations (Spitzer & Gibson, 1992). The mechanism by which these drugs reduce the incidence of apneic episodes is unclear, but they appear to increase an infant's sensitivity to carbon dioxide, ensuring better respiratory function. Those infants who have had an apneic episode severe enough to require resuscitation are at high risk for sudden infant death syndrome (SIDS). To prevent SIDS, such infants may be discharged from the health care facility with a monitoring device for apnea for 2 months beyond an apneic episode.

Sudden Infant Death Syndrome

Sudden infant death syndrome (SIDS) occurs in about 4 out of 1000 live births. It tends to occur at a higher than usual rate in the infants of adolescent mothers, infants of closely spaced pregnancies, and underweight male infants. Also prone to SIDS are infants with bronchopulmonary dysplasia as well as preterm infants, twins, siblings of another child with SIDS, Native American infants, Alaskan native infants, economically disadvantaged black infants, and infants of narcotic-dependent mothers.

Although the cause of SIDS is unknown, a number of theories about its cause have been advanced. In addition to prolonged but unexplained apnea, a viral respiratory or botulism infection may occur. Distorted breathing patterns that are familial may be involved. There may be a lack of surfactant in alveoli. Current research has supported studies showing a prevalence in infants who sleep prone rather than on the side or back (Brooks, 1993). The peak ages of incidence are between 2 weeks and 1 year of age.

Affected infants are typically well nourished but have a slight head cold; they have been put to bed at night or for a nap. The infant is found dead a few hours later. Infants who die this way do not appear to make any sound as they die, which indicates that they die with laryngospasm. Although many infants are found with blood-flecked sputum or vomitus in their mouths or on the bedclothes, this seems to occur as the result of death, not as its cause. An autopsy often reveals petechiae in the lungs and mild inflammation and congestion in the respiratory tract, but these symptoms are not severe enough to cause sudden death. It is clear that these children do not suffocate from bedclothes or choke from overfeeding, underfeeding, or crying.

Parents have a difficult time accepting the death of a child when it happens so suddenly this way. In discussing the child, they often use both the past and present tense as if they are not yet aware of the death.

Many parents experience a period of somatic symptoms that occur with acute grief, such as nausea, stomach pain, or vertigo. Parents should be counseled by a nurse or someone else trained in counseling at the time of the infant's death; it helps if they can talk to this same person periodically for however long it takes to resolve their grief. The Sudden Infant Death Syndrome Alliance has chapters in most large cities (see address earlier in this chapter). It offers support to parents and helps them to understand that the feelings they are experiencing are not unique.

The SIDS Alliance suggests that mandatory autopsies be performed on all children who die from SIDS in the hope that the cause of the phenomenon can be identified. Autopsy reports should be given to parents as soon as they are available (if toxicology tests are included in the autopsy, results will not be available for weeks). Reading the report that their child died an unexplained death can be reassuring to them that this was not their fault. They need this assurance if they are to plan for other children. If there are older children in the family, they also need assurance that SIDS is a disease of infants and that the strange phenomenon that invaded their home and killed a younger brother or sister will not also kill them. If they wished the infant dead (as all children wish siblings were dead on some days), they can be assured that their wishes are not that powerful and that they did not cause the baby's death.

When another child is born, the parents can be expected to become extremely frightened at any sign of illness in the child. They need support to see them through the first few months of the second child's life, particularly past the point at which the first child died. Some parents need support to view a second child as an individual child and not as a replacement for the one who died.

Apparent Life-Threatening Event

Some infants have been discovered cyanotic and limp in their beds but have survived after mouth-to-mouth resuscitation by parents. Episodes of this kind are called an **apparent life-threatening event** (ALTE). For these children as well as for preterm infants with a tendency toward apnea or the siblings of a child who died from SIDS, there is a monitoring device that rings when a period of apnea of 20 seconds or more or a decreased heart rate below 80 bpm occurs (Figure 26-9). If parents are going to use an apnea monitor at home, make certain they will be able to hear it in most parts of the house or apartment (usually the alarm is not loud enough to be heard in the basement from an upstairs bedroom). Caution them about household noises that may interfere with hearing the alarm, such as a loud television, radio, vacuum cleaner, hair dryer, and so forth. Be sure they know how to reposition the leads and that they are comfortable enough with the monitor

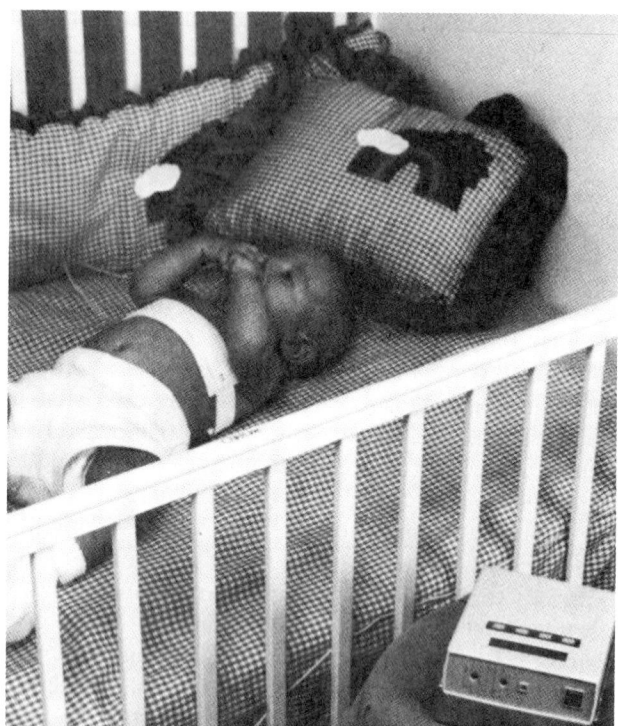

FIGURE 26-9
An apnea monitor for home monitoring. (Courtesy of Life Watch Systems, Inc. 1050 17th St, Suite 900, Denver, CO 80265.)

to see past it to the child. In addition, parents of high-risk infants should be taught cardiopulmonary resuscitation before the infant is discharged from the hospital (Figure 26-10).

Caring for a child on an apnea monitor usually becomes the mother's chief responsibility. This can place severe stress on the mother and on a marriage. Finding a competent babysitter is often described by parents as a major problem. Most parents with a baby on an apnea monitor at home appreciate a community or home care referral, so that they have a second opinion as to how well they are managing as well as a listening ear to discuss the strain of having always to be alert for a sound that means their infant has stopped breathing. They appreciate having someone review with them periodically what steps they should take if the alarm should sound (jiggle the baby, begin mouth-to-mouth resuscitation, call the emergency squad). These parents are under a tremendous strain, accentuated by a lack of sleep at night as a part of them is always listening for an alarm to ring. Because SIDS is a baffling disease, these parents live in fear of it until their child reaches at least 1 year of age.

Periventricular Leukomalacia

Periventricular leukomalacia (PVL) is abnormal formation of the white matter of the brain. It is caused by an ischemic episode, which interferes with circulation to

a portion of the brain. Phagocytes and macrophages invade the area to clear away necrotic tissue, and what is left is an area in the white matter of the brain that is revealed on sonogram as a hollow space. PVL occurs most frequently in preterm infants who experience cerebral ischemia. Once the condition has occurred, there is no therapy for PVL. Infants may die from the original insult; they may be left with long-term effects such as learning disabilities. Any action to reduce environmental stimuli or sudden shifts in cerebral blood flow, such as avoiding rapid fluid infusions, are important to preventing PVL (Blackburn, 1993).

Hemolytic Disease of the Newborn

The term "hemolytic" is Latin for destruction (lysis) of red blood cells. In the past, hemolytic disease of the newborn was most often caused by an Rh blood type incompatibility. Because prevention of Rh antibody formation has been available for more than 20 years, the disorder is now most often caused by an ABO incompatibility. In both instances, the mother builds antibodies against the infant's red blood cells, leading to hemolysis (destruction) of the cells. The destruction of red blood cells causes severe anemia and hyperbilirubinemia. Prevention of the condition begins in pregnancy, as discussed in Chapter 15.

Rh Incompatibility

Theoretically no direct connection exists between the fetal and maternal circulation, and no fetal blood cells

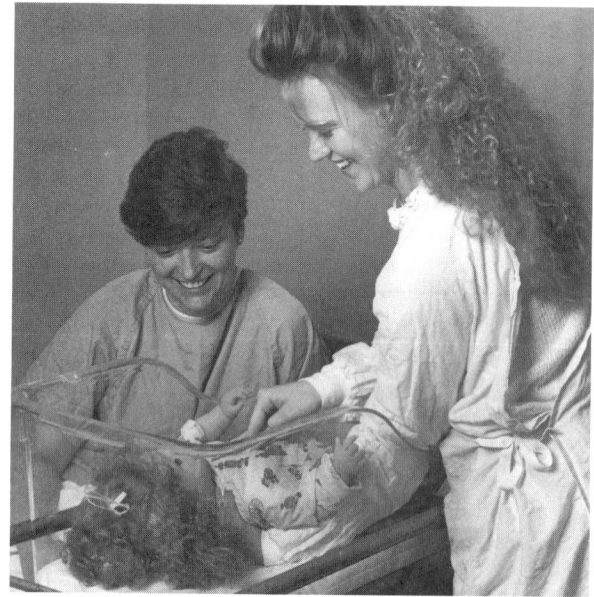

FIGURE 26-10
Parents of infants with respiratory disorders at birth need to learn resuscitation before the infant is discharged from the hospital. Here, a nurse teaches the technique using a doll. (Courtesy of the Department of Medical Photography, Children's Hospital of Buffalo, Buffalo, NY.)

enter the maternal circulation. In actuality, occasional placental villi break and a drop or two of fetal blood does enter maternal circulation. If the mother's blood type is Rh (D) negative and the fetal blood type is Rh positive (contains the D antigen), the introduction of fetal blood causes sensitization to occur, and the mother begins to form antibodies against the D antigen. Few antibodies form this way, however. Most form in the mother's bloodstream in the first 72 hours following birth, because there is an active exchange of fetal–maternal blood as placental villi loosen and the placenta is delivered. After this sensitization, in a second pregnancy, there will be a high level of antibody D circulating in the mother's bloodstream, which acts to destroy the fetal red blood cells early in the pregnancy. By the end of the second pregnancy, the fetus can be severely compromised by the action of these antibodies crossing the placenta and destroying red blood cells. Some infants require intrauterine transfusions to combat red cell destruction. Preterm labor may be induced to remove the fetus from the destructive maternal environment.

ABO Incompatibility

In most instances of ABO incompatibility, the maternal blood type is O and the fetal blood type is A; it may also occur when the fetus has type B or AB blood. A reaction in an infant with type B blood is often the most serious.

Hemolysis can become a problem with a first pregnancy in which there is an ABO incompatibility. The antibodies to A and B cell types are naturally occurring antibodies, which are present from birth in individuals whose red cells lack these antigens. Unlike the antibodies formed against the Rh D factor, these antibodies are large (IgM) class and do not cross the placenta. The infant of an ABO incompatibility, therefore, is not born anemic, as is the Rh-sensitized child. Hemolysis of the blood begins with birth, when blood and antibodies are exchanged during the mixing of maternal and fetal blood as the placenta is loosened.

Assessment

Interestingly, preterm infants do not seem to be affected by ABO incompatibility. This may be because the receptor sites for anti-A or anti-B antibodies do not appear on red cells until late in fetal life. Even in the mature newborn, the direct Coombs' test may only be weakly positive because of the few anti-A or anti-B sites present. The reticulocyte count (immature or newly formed red blood cells) is usually elevated as the infant attempts to replace destroyed cells.

Rh incompatibility of the newborn can be predicted by finding a rising anti-Rh titer or rising level of antibodies (indirect Coombs' test) in the mother during pregnancy. It can be confirmed by detecting antibodies on the fetal erythrocytes in cord blood (positive direct Coombs' test) by percutaneous umbilical blood sampling (see Chapter 9) or at birth. The mother in this situation will always have Rh-negative blood (dd), and the baby will be Rh positive (DD or Dd).

With Rh incompatibility, the infant may not appear pale at birth despite the red cell destruction that has occurred in utero, because the accelerated production of red cells during the last few months in utero compensates for the destruction to some degree. The liver and spleen may be enlarged from an attempt to produce new blood cells. If the number of red cells has decreased, the blood in the vascular circulation may be hypotonic to interstitial fluid; fluid shifts from the lower to higher isotonic pressure by the law of osmosis, causing extreme edema. Finally, the severe anemia results in congestive heart failure.

Hydrops fetalis is an old term for the appearance of a severely involved infant at birth, with *hydrops* referring to the edema and *fetalis* to the lethal state. The infant does not appear jaundiced because the maternal circulation has evacuated the rising indirect bilirubin level. With birth, progressive jaundice, usually occurring within the first 24 hours of life, reveals in both Rh and ABO incompatibility that a hemolytic process is at work. The indirect bilirubin level rises rapidly as red blood cells are destroyed and indirect bilirubin is released. However, indirect bilirubin is fat-soluble and cannot be excreted from the body. Under normal circumstances, the liver enzyme glucuronyl transferase converts indirect bilirubin to direct bilirubin, which is water-soluble, is combined with bile, and is excreted from the body with feces. In preterm infants or those with extreme hemolysis, the liver is unable to convert bilirubin, which is the reason jaundice becomes so extreme.

Normal cord blood has an indirect bilirubin level of 0 to 3 mg/100 mL; the danger of an increasing indirect bilirubin level is that if the level rises above 20 mg/dL in a term or 12 mg/dL in a preterm infant, brain damage from kernicterus can occur. Meanwhile the infant's need to use body stores to maintain metabolism in the presence of anemia causes a progressive hypoglycemia with Rh hemolytic disease in at least 20% of infants to compound their initial problem. A decrease in hemoglobin during the first week of life to a level less than that of cord blood is another indication of blood loss or hemolysis.

Therapeutic Management

Initiation of early feeding, temporary suspension of breast-feeding, use of phototherapy, and exchange transfusion all may be immediate measures necessary to reduce indirect bilirubin levels in the infant affected by ABO or Rh incompatibility. Infants who have severe hemolytic disease of the newborn tend to have a continuing drop in the hemoglobin concentration during the first 6 months of life or their bone marrow fails to increase its production of erythrocytes in response to continuing hemolysis. If this occurs, the infant may need an additional transfusion of blood to correct this late anemia, or therapy with erythropoietin to stimulate red blood cell production is another po sibility.

Initiation of Early Feeding. Bilirubin is removed from the body by being incorporated into feces. Therefore, the sooner bowel elimination begins, the sooner bilirubin removal begins. Early feeding, therefore, stimulates bowel peristalsis and accomplishes this.

Suspension of Breast-Feeding. Pregnanediol, the breakdown product of progesterone, interferes with the conjugation of indirect bilirubin. It is excreted in breast milk until the high levels of progesterone that were present during pregnancy are decreased, usually by 24 to 48 hours. Breast-fed babies, therefore, may evidence more jaundice than bottle-fed babies (Cashore, 1990). Temporary suspension of breast-feeding for 24 hours may be necessary to reduce an accumulating indirect bilirubin level in some infants. If the mother manually expresses breast milk while feeding is halted, her milk supply will be maintained.

Phototherapy. An infant's liver processes little bilirubin in utero because the mother's circulation does this for the infant. With birth, exposure to light apparently "triggers" the liver to assume this function. Additional light appears to speed the conversion potential of the liver. Phototherapy is the light technique that is most often used. In phototherapy, the infant is continuously exposed to three to six fluorescent light tubes with a total strength of 200 to 500 foot-candles. The lights are placed above an Isolette or bassinet and the infant is undressed except for the diaper, so that as much skin surface as possible is exposed to the light (Figure 26-11).

Although no long-term effects have been studied as yet, there appears to be no risk to the infant from phototherapy, provided the infant's eyes remain covered and dehydration from increased insensitive water loss does not occur.

Continuous exposure to bright lights this way may be harmful to the newborn's retina, so the infant's eyes must always be covered while under bilirubin lights. Eye dressings or cotton balls can be firmly secured in place by an additional dressing. The infant must be checked frequently to be certain the dressings have not slipped or are causing corneal irritation.

The stools of an infant under bilirubin lights are often bright green owing to the excessive bilirubin that is excreted as the result of the therapy. They are also frequently loose and may be irritating to skin. Urine may be dark colored from urobilinogen formation. The infant must have his or her skin turgor assessed and intake and output measured to ensure that dehydration is not occurring. Temperature must be monitored to prevent the infant from overheating under the bright lights. An effi-

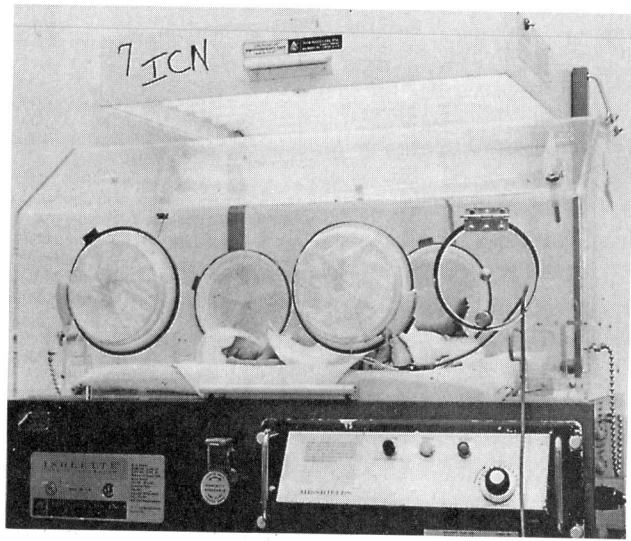

FIGURE 26-11
A newborn receiving phototherapy is undressed except for a diaper so that he receives maximum exposure to the lights. His eyes are covered snugly to protect them from the bright light. (Courtesy of the Department of Medical Photography, Children's Hospital, Buffalo, NY.)

cient way to maintain fluid intake is to offer the infant glucose water every 2 hours.

An infant under phototherapy should be removed for feeding so that he or she continues to have interaction with the mother. The eye patches should be removed during this time to give the infant a period of visual stimulation. To prevent a lengthy hospitalization, infants may be discharged and continue therapy at home (see Chapter 38).

Parents need an explanation of why their infant is being kept under special lights. Isolettes are automatically associated with seriously ill infants. At the same time, the use of lights does not seem scientific (almost a home remedy). Parents can easily be confused by the two interventions, one seemingly serious and the other seemingly not serious at all.

Exchange Transfusion. Phototherapy may take several hours to have an effect. It is not the first method of choice, therefore, if bilirubin levels are rapidly rising. In that instance, the method of clearing indirect bilirubin levels is exchange transfusion. The baby's stomach is aspirated before the procedure so that there is no danger of aspiration caused by the manipulation involved. The umbilical vein is catheterized as the site for transfusion. The procedure involves alternatively withdrawing small amounts (2 to 10 mL) of the infant's blood and then replacing it with equal amounts of donor blood. The blood must be exchanged at this slow rate to prevent alternating hypovolemia and hypervolemia; thus, an exchange transfusion is a lengthy procedure of 1 to 3 hours. An automatic pump is being devised that will perform this exhausting repeated ritual. A hematocrit, bilirubin, electrolytes (especially calcium), glucose determination, and blood culture are taken at the end of the procedure by using the last specimen of blood withdrawn. Exchange transfusion may need to be repeated as additional unconjugated bilirubin from tissue moves into the circulation after the initial exchange.

The therapy can be used for any condition that leads to hyperbilirubinemia or polycythemia. When used as therapy for blood incompatibility, it removes approximately 85% of sensitized red cells. It reduces the serum concentration of indirect bilirubin and often prevents congestive heart failure in infants. Because indirect bilirubin levels rise at relatively predictable levels, exchange transfusion is performed if the indirect bilirubin concentration exceeds 5 mg per 100 mL at birth, 10 mg per 100 mL at age 8 hours, 12 mg per 100 mL at age 16 hours, and 15 mg per 100 mL at 24 hours; or if serum bilirubin is rising more than 0.5 mg/h in infants with Rh incompatibility or 1.0 mg/h in infants with ABO incompatibility.

Infants must be kept warm during the procedure so they do not expend energy on metabolism to warm themselves. The blood being given must be maintained at room temperature, or shock from the cold insult can result. Blood should be warmed only by using a commercial blood warming unit, not hot towels or a radiant heat warmer, which can destroy red cells. Albumin may be administered 1 to 2 hours before the procedure to increase the number of bilirubin binding sites and to increase the efficiency of the transfusion. Be extremely careful to monitor the rate of flow of the albumin transfusion, because rapid flow of such a viscous fluid can quickly overburden the infant heart. The type of blood used for transfusion is O Rh-negative blood, even though the infant's blood type is positive; if Rh-positive or A or B type blood were given, the maternal antibodies that entered the infant's circulation would destroy this blood also, and the transfusion would be ineffective. If the baby is transported to a regional center for the exchange transfusion, a sample of the mother's blood must accompany the infant, so that cross-matching on the mother's serum can be done there.

A baby must be carefully monitored during an exchange transfusion; the heart rate, respirations, and venous pressure all must be observed. The amount of blood given is usually calculated as follows: 85 mL × weight (in kilograms) × 2. The average blood volume of a newborn is 86 mL/kg, but an amount equal to twice the blood volume is used because this quantity will ensure an exchange of erythrocytes that is 85% to 90% effective. Because stored blood for transfusion contains acid-citrate-dextrose (ACD), which is added to blood as an anticoagulant and can lower blood calcium levels and cause acidosis, calcium gluconate is given through the exchange catheter after each 100 mL of blood. If citrate-phosphate-dextrose is used as a preservative, the reaction is less severe than with ACD, but the problem is still present. The infant may become hyperglycemic during the transfusion from the dextrose in the preservative; this is followed by overproduction of insulin and hypoglycemia. If heparinized blood is used, the heparin content may interfere with clotting after the transfusion; and because of its relatively low glucose concentration, it may also lead to hypoglycemia. Administering protamine sulfate aids in the metabolism of heparin and restoration of clotting ability.

After the transfusion, the infant must be observed closely for umbilical vessel bleeding, redness or inflammation of the cord that suggests infection, and changes from normal in vital signs. In addition, the infant needs Dextrostix assessments for about 2 hours and bilirubin levels monitored for 2 or 3 days after the transfusion to ensure that the level of bilirubin is not rising again and that no further transfusion is necessary. Erythropoietin may be administered to increase new blood cell growth and prevent extended anemia (Scaradavou et al., 1993).

Necrotizing enterocolitis may occur as a complication of exchange transfusion. The infant needs to be monitored for signs of this (see Chapter 45).

Hemorrhagic Disease of the Newborn

Hemorrhagic disease of the newborn results from a deficiency of vitamin K. Vitamin K is essential for the formation of prothrombin by the liver, and the lack of it causes decreased prothrombin function and poor blood coagulation. Vitamin K is formed by the action of bacteria in the intestine. Because the intestinal tract of a newborn is sterile at birth, the infant forms minimal amounts of vitamin K until normal intestinal tract flora are established at about 24 hours of age. Babies born to mothers on anticonvulsive medication are at high risk for the condition, because many of these medications interfere with vitamin K formation. Administering vitamin K to these mothers before delivery can help to protect the child.

Newborns with vitamin K deficiency show petechiae from superficial bleeding into the skin. They may have conjunctival, mucous membrane, or retinal hemorrhage. They may vomit fresh blood or pass black, tarry stools because of bleeding into the gastrointestinal tract.

Distinguishing between tarry stools and normal meconium stools is difficult in the first 1 or 2 days of life by simple observation. However, if the infant's stool does not change as it should from greenish black (meconium) to the yellow color of a bottle-fed or breast-fed baby, or if the stool color changes normally, then becomes black again, gastrointestinal bleeding should be suspected. The presence of blood in the stool can be detected by a guaiac or dipstick test.

Such bleeding generally occurs on day 2 to day 5 of life, when the available prothrombin is at its lowest level. The prothrombin time will be prolonged; coagulation time may be normal or prolonged.

Hemorrhagic disease of the newborn can be prevented by the intramuscular administration of 1 mg of vitamin K to all newborns immediately after birth (Blanchette et al., 1994). Make certain that infants who were born in unusual circumstances, such as those born in taxicabs or at home, are administered vitamin K on their admission to the hospital nursery. The same extra double checking must be done in infants whose birth involved an emergency, such as maternal hemorrhaging or failure of the newborn to breathe spontaneously. When there are special duties to be carried out, a routine procedure such as the administration of vitamin K can be forgotten.

The infant who develops hemorrhagic disease of the newborn is treated with vitamin K, given intravenously or intramuscularly. If bleeding is severe, the infant may need a transfusion of fresh, whole blood to increase the prothrombin level immediately.

The infant with this disease should be handled extremely gently (as should all children with bleeding tendencies) to prevent further bleeding, because he or she bruises easily from heavy pressure. Subdural hemorrhage may occur, making hemorrhagic disease a serious and possibly fatal disorder.

Twin-to-Twin Transfusion

Twin-to-twin transfusion is a phenomenon that can occur if twins are monozygotic (identical; share the same placenta) and if abnormal arteriovenous shunts occur that direct more blood to one twin than the other. The process may occur in as many as one third of all identical twin pregnancies, but only enough blood is exchanged to be clinically important in 15% of such pregnancies (Revenis & Johnson, 1994). The result of this shift of blood will lead to anemia in the donor twin and polycythemia in the receiving twin. The anemic twin may also be small-for-gestational-age because of the lack of nutrients or oxygen for growth, and this same small-for-gestational-age twin will be prone to hypoglycemia from lack of glucose stores. He or she will appear pale next to the polycythemic twin, who is prone to hyperbilirubinemia as the excessive red blood cell level is broken down.

Twin-to-twin transfusion can be identified in utero by sonogram (one twin is noticeably larger than the other). All identical twins should have hemoglobin determinations done at birth and the results compared. A difference of more than 5.0 g per 100 mL is enough difference to suggest that a transfusion has occurred. Each twin needs therapy as indicated by the extent of the blood distribution. The donor twin may need a transfu-

sion to establish a functioning blood level; the recipient twin may need an exchange transfusion to reduce the polycythemia and viscosity of the blood (Gardner, 1993).

Necrotizing Enterocolitis

Necrotizing enterocolitis (NEC) is a condition that develops in approximately 5% of all infants in intensive care nurseries. The bowel develops necrotic patches, interfering with digestion and possibly leading to a paralytic ileus. Perforation and peritonitis may follow. This is discussed in Chapter 45.

Retinopathy of Prematurity

Retinopathy of prematurity (ROP) is an acquired ocular disease that leads to partial or total blindness in children due to vasoconstriction of immature retinal blood vessels. It was first recognized as an eye disorder in 1942. It was 10 years, however, before it was established that a high concentration of oxygen is the causative agent. High concentrations of oxygen cause vasoconstriction of immature retinal blood vessels and a secondary proliferation of endothelial cells in the layer of nerve fibers in the periphery of the retina, resulting in detachment of the retina and blindness. Those infants who are most immature and most ill (and consequently receive the most oxygen) are those most susceptible to the condition.

The preterm infant who is receiving oxygen must have blood PO_2 levels monitored by oximeter, or transcutaneous or blood gas monitoring. If PO_2 levels are kept within normal limits, the risk of the condition is lowered. With PO_2 levels of more than 100 mm Hg, the danger of the disease is great. Vitamin E, an antioxidant, may reduce the incidence of ROP because it modifies tissue response to the effect of oxygen, so should be kept within normal serum levels.

Once ROP occurs, there is no reversing it, although the process may be delayed by cryosurgery therapy (Friendly, 1994). A person experienced in recognizing retrolental fibroplasia should examine the eyes of all low-birth-weight newborns and those who have received oxygen therapy at discharge from the nursery and again at age 4 to 6 weeks of age.

The Newborn at Risk Because of Maternal Infection or Illness

Maternal Infection

A newborn who appears ill at birth or becomes ill shortly after birth is usually screened by a TORSCH essay, which tests for the presence of antibodies to *tox*oplasmosis, *r*ubella, *s*yphilis, *c*ytomegalovirus, and *her*-

pes organisms. The effect on the mother from these disorders is discussed in Chapter 15.

Beta-hemolytic, Group B Streptococcal Infection

The major cause of infection in newborn infants currently is the beta-hemolytic, group B streptococcal organism (GBS). This is a gram-positive bacteria and a natural inhabitant of the female genital tract. Between 50 and 300 infants in every 1000 live births display a positive culture for this organism. It may be spread from baby to baby if good hand-washing technique is not used in handling newborns. If a mother is determined to be positive for group B streptococci during late pregnancy, she may be administered ampicillin intravenously during labor to reduce the possibility of newborn exposure.

Colonization by beta-hemolytic, group B streptococci can result in an early onset or a late-onset illness. With the early onset form, symptoms of pneumonia become apparent in the first day of life. Infants will have tachypnea and apnea and symptoms of shock such as decreased urine output, extreme paleness, or hypotonia; a chest x-ray film is almost indistinguishable from that of respiratory distress syndrome. Pneumonia may develop so rapidly that as many as 20% of infants who contract the infection die within 24 hours of birth (Freij & McCracken, 1994).

A late-onset type occurs at 2 to 4 weeks of age; instead of pneumonia being the infection focus, meningitis tends to occur. Infants gradually become lethargic, develop a fever, and lose their appetite. Fontanelles bulge from increased intracranial pressure as meningitis develops. Mortality from the late-onset type is not as high as from the early onset form (15% compared with 20%), but neurologic consequences may occur in up to 50% of infants who survive.

Gentamicin, ampicillin, and penicillin are all effective against beta-hemolytic, group B streptococcal infections. It is difficult for parents to understand how their infant could suddenly become this ill. They may need a great deal of support to care for an infant if he or she does survive the infection but is left neurologically disabled. In the future, immunization of all women of childbearing age against streptococcal B organisms could decrease the incidence of newborns infected at birth.

Congenital Rubella

The rubella virus is capable of causing extensive congenital malformations of the fetus if the mother is infected during the first trimester of pregnancy (Givens et al., 1993). Although childhood immunization programs have greatly decreased the incidence of this infection, in urban areas of the United States, approximately 10% to 20% of women of childbearing age are still susceptible to rubella (Freij & McCracken, 1994). Women can be assessed for this susceptibility by blood sampling

for an antibody titer during pregnancy. A result of less than 1:8 indicates a woman is susceptible.

The greatest risk to an embryo from the rubella virus is during week 2 to week 6 of intrauterine life when body organs are first forming. The frequency of malformations is approximately 50% if the virus invasion is during these early weeks (Taber, 1990).

Assessment. The classic symptoms of the rubella syndrome are thrombocytopenia, cataracts, heart disease, deafness, microcephaly, and motor and mental retardation. The thrombocytopenia is manifested by purpura, which are red-purple macula with a "blueberry muffin" appearance. The diagnosis is confirmed by identifying IgM antibodies against rubella in the infant's serum at birth. IgM antibodies do not cross the placenta, so they cannot have come from the mother; they must have been produced by the fetus in response to invasion by the rubella antigen.

Therapeutic Management. Treatment is symptomatic, depending on the congenital defects present. Live rubella virus may be cultured from nasopharyngeal secretions of affected infants at birth. At age 1 year, approximately 10% of these infants are still shedding live virus. These infants must be isolated in the hospital because this virus is airborne spread; susceptible pregnant women should avoid contact with them. All women in the postpartal period who have low rubella titers should be identified and offered a rubella vaccine to ensure that rubella infection does not occur with a future pregnancy. Women cannot be immunized during pregnancy because the vaccine used contains a live virus.

Ophthalmia Neonatorum

Ophthalmia neonatorum is eye infection at birth or during the first month (O'Hara, 1993). The most common causative organisms of this are *Neisseria gonorrhoeae* or *Chlamydia trachomatis*. The infant contracts the organism during vaginal birth. *N. gonorrhoeae* infection is an extremely serious form of conjunctivitis, because if it is left untreated the infection extends to corneal ulceration and destruction, resulting in opacity of the cornea and severe vision impairment (Patterson, 1990).

Assessment. Ophthalmia neonatorum is generally bilateral. The eye conjunctivae become fiery red, there is thick pus present, and the eyelids are edematous. Although this usually occurs on day 1 to day 4 of life, it should be considered as a possibility when a conjunctivitis occurs in infants younger than 30 days.

Prevention. The prophylactic instillation of erythromycin ointment into the eyes of newborns prevents both gonococcal and chlamydial conjunctivitis. In the past, eye prophylaxis used to be given immediately after birth so was never forgotten. Now it is customary to delay administration of ointment until after the first reactivity period so that the child can see the parents clearly during this important attachment period. It is easy to forget administration, so use a checklist of some sort as a reminder of this important prophylaxis. Infants born in such locations as taxicabs or at home need prophylaxis to prevent ophthalmia neonatorum, the same as infants born in a delivery or birthing room.

Therapeutic Management. Therapy is individualized depending on the organism cultured from the exudate. If gonococci are identified, intravenous ceftriaxone or penicillin are administered. If chlamydia is identified, an ophthalmic solution of erythromycin is used. With a gonococci infection, which is extremely contagious, the newborn must be isolated. In addition to systemic antibiotic therapy, the eyes are washed with saline irrigations to clear the copious discharge. When irrigating eyes, use a sterile medicine dropper or sterile bulb syringe. The solution should be at room temperature and sterile. Direct the stream of the irrigation fluid laterally so that it does not enter and contaminate the other eye. If some fluid should splash into the eyes of the health care providers, they must have antibiotic therapy to avoid contracting the disease.

The mother of the infected infant needs treatment for gonorrhea herself, before fallopian tube sterility or pelvic inflammatory disease results. Sexual contacts of the mother should be treated also, so that the spread of the disease can be halted. With either infection, parents can be assured that with early diagnosis and treatment the prognosis for normal eyesight in the child is good.

Hepatitis B Virus Infection (HBV)

The hepatitis B virus can be transmitted to the newborn infant through contact with infected vaginal blood at birth when the mother is positive for the virus (HBsAg+). Hepatitis B is a destructive illness: 70% to 90% of infected infants become chronic carriers of the virus, and a number of these newborns will develop liver cancer later in life.

To reduce the possibility of HBsAg being spread to newborns in the future, infants are now routinely vaccinated at birth. If the mother is identified as HBsAg+, the infant is also administered immune serum globulin (HBI6) to decrease the possibility of infection. The infant should be bathed as soon as possible after birth to remove HBV-infected blood and secretions. Suctioning should be with gentle technique to avoid possible trauma to the mucous membrane, which could allow HBV invasion. Although the virus is transmitted in breast milk, once immune globulin has been administered, women may breast-feed without risk to the infant. Hepatitis B is further discussed in Chapter 45 as it occurs in older children.

Generalized Herpesvirus Infection

A herpesvirus type 2 (HSV-2) infection can be contracted by a fetus across the placenta if the mother has a primary infection during pregnancy. More often, however, the virus is contracted from the vaginal secretions from the mother who had active herpetic vulvovaginitis at the time of birth. Between 15% and 30% of women of childbearing age demonstrate antibodies to this virus or have the potential to have active lesions during labor. It is most prevalent among women with multiple sexual partners (Freij & Sever, 1994).

Assessment. If the infection was acquired during pregnancy, an infant may be born with vesicles covering the skin; the long-term prognosis of the child is guarded, since severe neurologic damage may have simultaneously occurred. If infants acquire the infection at birth, at approximately day 4 to day 7 of life they show a loss of appetite, perhaps a low-grade fever, and lethargy. *Stomatitis* (ulcers of the mouth) or a few vesicles on the skin appear. Herpes vesicles are always clustered, pinpoint in size, and surrounded by a reddened base. After the vesicles appear, infants become extremely ill. They develop dyspnea, jaundice, purpura, convulsions, and shock. Death may occur within hours or days. Between 25% and 70% of newborns who survive acquired generalized herpesvirus infections may have permanent central nervous system sequelae.

To confirm the diagnosis, cultures are obtained from representative vesicles as well as the nose, throat, anus, and umbilical cord. Blood serum is analyzed for IgM antibodies.

Therapeutic Management. Both acyclovir and vidaribine, drugs that inhibit viral deoxyribonucleic acid synthesis, are effective in combatting this overwhelming infection. Prevention, however, is the newborn's best protection. Women with herpetic vulvar lesions should be delivered by cesarean rather than vaginal birth. Infants with an infection should be isolated from other infants. Women with herpes lesions on their face (herpes simplex or cold sores) should not feed or hold their newborns until lesions are crusted and no longer contagious (although transmission from this source is rare). Health care personnel who have herpes simplex infections must not care for newborn infants. Although herpes simplex lesions are probably caused by herpesvirus type 1, this limitation in contact does not seem excessive in light of the severity of HSV-2 disease. A woman who is isolated from her newborn at birth needs to view the infant from the nursery window and participate in planning care for the infant to aid bonding.

The Infant of a Diabetic Mother

The infant of a diabetic mother (IDM) whose illness was poorly controlled during pregnancy is typically longer and weighs more than other babies (macrosomia). The baby also has a greater chance of having a congenital anomaly such as a cardiac defect than do other infants, as if hyperglycemia were teratogenic to the rapidly growing fetus. Caudal regression syndrome or hypoplasia of the lower extremities is a syndrome that occurs almost exclusively in such infants (Ogata, 1994).

Most such babies have a *cushingoid* (fat and puffy) appearance. They tend to be lethargic or limp in the first days of life, which are effects of hyperglycemia. The macrosomia results from overstimulation of pituitary growth hormone during pregnancy and extra fat deposits created by high levels of glucose during pregnancy. The infant's large size is deceptive, however. Such babies are often immature. Their lungs, especially, may be immature. RDS occurs frequently in these infants because they may be born preterm or possibly because lecithin pathways do not mature as rapidly in them. High insulin secretion during pregnancy by the fetus to counteract the hyperglycemia may interfere with cortisol release; this blocks the formation of lecithin and prevents lung maturity. A term frequently used for these infants is "fragile giant."

An IDM infant loses a greater proportion of weight in the first few days of life than does the average baby, because of the loss of the extra fluid accumulated. The baby needs to be observed closely to be certain that this large weight loss actually represents a loss of extra fluid and that dehydration is not occurring.

Complications

If infants are macrosomic, they may need to be born by cesarean birth to avoid cephalopelvic disproportion. There is greater chance of birth injury, especially shoulder and neck injury. Immediately after birth, the infant tends to be hyperglycemic because the mother was slightly hyperglycemic during pregnancy, which caused excessive glucose to diffuse across the placenta. The fetal pancreas responded to the high glucose level by islet cell hypertrophy, resulting in matching high levels of insulin. After birth, the infant's glucose level begins to fall because the mother's circulation is no longer supplying him or her. The overproduction of insulin causes the development of severe hypoglycemia. Hyperbilirubinemia also tends to occur in these infants, because being immature, they are unable to effectively clear bilirubin from their system. Hypocalcemia also frequently develops because parathyroid hormone is lower in these infants due to hypomagnesemia from excessive renal losses of magnesium (see Chapter 48).

The infant born to a woman with Class D diabetes or beyond will be small for gestational age because of poor placental perfusion. The problems of hypoglycemia, hypocalcemia, and hyperbilirubinemia remain the same.

Therapeutic Management

Hypoglycemia is defined as a serum glucose level of less than 40 mg/dL in a newborn (Gamblien et al., 1993). To avoid the serum glucose level from falling this low, IDM infants are fed early with formula or administered a continuous infusion of glucose. It is important that the child not be given only a bolus of glucose, or else rebound hypoglycemia (accentuating the problem) may occur. Some IDM infants have a small left colon, apparently another effect of intrauterine hyperglycemia, which limits the amount of oral feedings they can take in their first days of life. Signs of a small colon would include vomiting or abdominal distention after the first few feedings.

Infant of a Drug-Dependent Mother

Infants of drug-dependent women tend to be small for gestational age. If the mother is dependent on a narcotic, the infant will show withdrawal symptoms (neonatal abstinence syndrome) shortly after birth. They are usually irritable, with disturbed sleep patterns. They move so constantly that they can cause abrasions on their elbows, knees, or nose. They may have tremors and may sneeze frequently. They may have a shrill high-pitched cry like that of a brain-damaged infant. Hyperreflexia and clonus (neuromuscular irritability) may be present, and convulsions may occur. Tachypnea (rapid respirations) are so severe that hyperventilation and alkalosis develop. Vomiting and diarrhea may begin, leading to large fluid losses and secondary dehydration. These symptoms usually occur in the first 24 hours of life, although they may appear as late as age 7 days in heroin-addicted infants and age 2 weeks in methadone-addicted infants. Methadone-addicted infants tend to have an increased incidence of seizures compared with heroin-addicted infants.

Narcotic metabolites or quinine (heroin is often mixed with quinine) may be obtained from an infant's urine in the first hour after birth. These products are quickly cleared from the body, however, so by the time symptoms become severe, detection of narcotic substances may no longer be possible.

Infants of drug-dependent women usually seem most comfortable when firmly swaddled. They should be kept in an environment free from excessive stimuli (a small isolation nursery, not a large, noisy one). Some quiet best if the room is darkened. Many infants of heroin-addicted women suck vigorously and continuously and seem to find comfort and quiet if given a pacifier. Infants of methadone- and cocaine-addicted women may have extremely poor sucking ability and may have difficulty getting enough fluid intake unless gavage-fed.

Specific therapy for an infant is individualized according to the nature and severity of the symptoms. The infant must have his or her electrolyte and fluid balance maintained; if the infant has vomiting or diarrhea, intravenous administration of fluid may be indicated. The drugs used to counteract withdrawal symptoms include paregoric, phenobarbital, methadone, chlorpromazine (Thorazine), and diazepam (Valium). An infant should not be breast-fed to avoid passing narcotics in breast milk to the child.

Once an infant has been identified as having been exposed to drugs in utero, the mother needs treatment for withdrawal symptoms and follow-up care as much as the infant. In addition, whether an environment that allowed for this much drug abuse will be safe for an infant must be evaluated before the baby is discharged into the parent's care. Infants who are exposed to drugs in utero may have long-term neurologic problems. This is particularly true with cocaine-exposed infants (Mayes et al., 1993).

The Infant With Fetal Alcohol Syndrome (FAS)

Alcohol crosses the placenta in the same concentration as is present in the maternal bloodstream. Fetal alcohol syndrome appears in 2 per 1000 newborns (Ostrea et al., 1994). Because it is unknown if there is a safe threshold of alcohol ingestion during pregnancy, all pregnant women are advised to avoid alcohol intake to prevent any teratogenic effects on their newborn.

The newborn with fetal alcohol syndrome has a number of possible problems at birth (CDC, 1993). Characteristics that mark the syndrome are: pre- and postnatal growth retardation, central nervous system involvement such as mental retardation, microcephaly, and cerebral palsy, and facial features such as short palpebral fissures and a thin upper lip. During the neonatal period, the infant may be tremulous, fidgety, irritable, and demonstrate a weak sucking reflex. Sleep disturbances are common, with the baby either tending to be always awake or always asleep, depending on the mother's alcohol level close to birth.

Native American and socioeconomically deprived black infants are those most apt to be affected. The most serious long-term effect is mental retardation. Behavior problems such as hyperactivity may occur in school-age children. Growth deficiencies may remain through life.

Key Points

- Priorities for infants born with special needs such as the preterm or postterm infant are the same priorities of care as with term infants: initiation and maintenance of respirations, establishment of extrauterine circulation, control of body temperature, intake of adequate nourishment, establishment of waste elimination, establishment of an infant–parent relationship, prevention of infection, and provision of developmental care for mental and social development.
- Many high-risk infants need resuscitation at birth. Prompt action with such measures as suctioning, intubation, oxygen, and warmth are needed.
- A small-for-gestational-age (SGA) infant is one whose birth weight is below the 10th percentile on an intrauterine growth curve for that age infant. The infant could be preterm, term, or postterm.
- Small-for-gestational-age infants have particular difficulty maintaining body warmth because of low fat stores and developing hypoglycemia from low nutritional stores. Common nursing diagnoses identified for them are High risk for altered respiratory function related to underdeveloped body systems at birth, High risk for ineffective thermoregulation related to lack of subcutaneous fat, and High risk for altered parenting related to high-risk status and child's possible cognitive impairment from lack of nutrients in utero.
- A large-for-gestational-age (LGA) infant is one whose birth weight is above the 90th percentile on an intrauterine growth chart for that gestational age. The infant could be born preterm, term, or postterm.
- Large-for-gestational-age infants tend to be infants of diabetic mothers; they are particularly prone to hypoglycemia or birth trauma. Common nursing diagnoses identified for them are High-risk for altered respiratory function related to possible birth trauma, High risk for altered nutrition less than body requirements related to additional nutrients needed to maintain weight or prevent hypoglycemia, and High risk for altered parenting related to infant's high-risk status.
- A preterm infant is one born before 37 weeks of gestation. Preterm birth occurs in as many as 7% of live births. Preterm infants have particular problems of respiratory function, anemia, persistent jaundice, persistent patent ductus arteriosus, and intracranial hemorrhage. Infants who are born between weeks 30 and 36 of gestation (weighing 1500 to 2500 g) are also termed low-birth-weight (LBW) infants; those born between 26 and 30 weeks gestation (1000–1500 g) are very-low-birth-weight (VLBW); those born between 24 and 26 weeks gestation (500 to 1000 g) are extremely-very-low-birth-weight (EVLBW) infants. All such infants need level III (neonatal intensive care) care from the moment of birth to give them their best chance of survival without neurologic aftereffects caused by their being so critically close to the age of viability.
- A postterm infant is one who has remained in utero past week 42 of pregnancy. Postterm infants have particular problems with establishing respirations, meconium aspiration, hypoglycemia, temperature regulation, and polycythemia.
- Respiratory distress syndrome (RDS) occurs in preterm infants from lack of surfactant in alveoli. Without surfactant, alveoli collapse on expiration and require extreme force for reinflation. Primary therapy is synthetic surfactant replacement at birth by endotracheal tube insufflation followed by oxygen and ventilatory support.

- Transient tachypnea of the newborn is a temporary condition caused by slow absorption of lung fluid at birth. Close observation of the infant is necessary until the fluid is absorbed and respirations slow to a normal rate.
- Meconium aspiration syndrome occurs from the infant inhaling meconium-stained amniotic fluid during birth. Meconium is irritating to the airway and may lead to both airway spasm and pneumonia. Infants need oxygen, ventilatory support, and possibly an antibiotic until the effects of the insult to the airway subside. It is important that they are suctioned before oxygen administration under pressure to prevent meconium being forced further into their lungs.
- Apnea is a pause in respirations longer than 20 seconds with accompanying bradycardia. It tends to occur in preterm infants who have secondary stresses such as infection, hyperbilirubinemia, hypoglycemia, or hypothermia. Apnea monitors are used to detect the incidence, and infants who are high risks for this return home on a home monitoring apnea program.
- Sudden infant death syndrome (SIDS) is the sudden unexplained death of an infant. It is associated with infants sleeping on their stomachs (prone) and infants who were born preterm. An important preventive measure may be advising parents to position their infant on the side or back for sleeping.
- Hemolytic disease of the newborn is destruction of red blood cells from Rh or ABO incompatibility. The administration of Rhib (Rh antibodies) to Rh-negative mothers during pregnancy and after the birth of an Rh-positive infant to an Rh-negative mother has greatly reduced the incidence of the condition. Affected infants are jaundiced from release of bilirubin from injured red blood cells. Phototherapy or exchange transfusion is used to prevent kernicterus (the deposition of bilirubin in brain cells causing destruction of the cells).
- Hemorrhagic disease of the newborn is a lack of clotting ability resulting from a deficiency of vitamin K at birth. Prevention is by injection of vitamin K to all infants at birth.
- Retinopathy of prematurity is destruction of the retina due to exposure of immature retinal capillaries to oxygen. Monitoring arterial blood gases is an important preventive measure.
- Severe infections that may be seen in newborns are streptococcal group B pneumonia, hepatitis B infection, gonococcal conjunctivitis and herpesvirus infection. Assessing newborns for symptoms of these infections is an important nursing responsibility.
- Infants of diabetic women and those of drug-abusing women are both examples of infants who are at high risk at birth for further complications. Both need careful assessment for respiratory distress and hypoglycemia.

Critical Thinking Exercises

1. Mrs. Terry is in preterm labor; her child will be at high risk for the development of respiratory distress syndrome. How would you explain to her why her baby will be at high risk for this? Mrs. Terry is asked to make a decision as to whether she wants surfactant administered prophylactically to her baby at birth or to wait and allow the baby to receive it only after (and if) symptoms of respiratory distress begin. Mrs. Terry asks your advice in helping her decide what to do. How would you advise her?

2. Retinopathy of prematurity is an example of a disease that is caused by the therapy given the infant. How can nurses help safeguard infants against this disorder?

3. Infants who are cared for in neonatal nurseries may need either reduced stimulation because they fatigue so easily or increased stimulation because their stay in the nursery will be so extended. How can the nurse demonstrate her understanding of the effects of sensory deprivation and stimulation in this situation?

References

Anderson, C. L. (1993). The parenting profile assessment: screening for child abuse. *Applied Nursing Research, 6,* 31.

American Heart Association. (1992). Neonatal resuscitation. *Journal of the American Medical Association, 268,* 2276.

Beckman, C. A. (1990). Postterm pregnancy: effects on temperature and glucose regulation. *Nursing Research, 39,* 21.

Blackburn, S. T. (1993). Assessment and Management of Neurologic Dysfunction. In Kenner, C., et al. *Comprehensive neonatal nursing*. Philadelphia: W. B. Saunders.

Blackburn, S. T., & Vandenberg, K. A. (1993). Assessment and management of neonatal neurobehavioral development. In Kenner, C., et al. *Comprehensive neonatal nursing*. Philadelphia: W. B. Saunders.

Blanchette, V. et al. (1994). Hematology. In Avery, G., et al. *Neonatology*. Philadelphia: J. B. Lippincott.

Brooks, J. G. (1993). Unraveling the mysteries of sudden infant death syndrome. *Current Opinion in Pediatrics, 5,* 266.

Cashore, W. J. (1990). Neonatal hyperbilirubinemia. In Oski, F. A., et al. *Principles and practice of pediatrics*. Philadelphia: J. B. Lippincott.

Centers for Disease Control. (1993). Fetal alcohol syndrome: United States, 1979–1992. *Morbidity and Mortality Weekly Report, 42,* 339.

Crouse, D. T., & Cassady, G. (1994). The small for gestation age infant. In Avery, G., et al. *Neonatology*. Philadelphia: J. B. Lippincott.

Cunningham, F. G., et al. (1993). *Williams obstetrics*. Norwalk, CT: Appleton & Lange.

Department of Health and Human Services. (1991). *Healthy people 2000*. Washington, DC: Public Health Service.

Dietch, J. S. (1993). Periventricular-intraventricular hemorrhage in the very low-birth-weight infant. *Neonatal Network, 12,* 84.

Etherington, H., et al. (1993). RDS and surfactant replacement: the double-edged sword. *Canadian Nurse, 89,* 14.

Fletcher, A. B. (1994). Nutrition. In Avery, G., et al. *Neonatology.* Philadelphia: J. B. Lippincott.

Freij, B. J., & McCracken, G. H. (1994). Acute infections. In Avery, G., et al. *Neonatology.* Philadelphia: J. B. Lippincott.

Freij, B. J., & Sever, J. L. (1994). Chronic infections. In Avery, G., et al. *Neonatology.* Philadelphia: J. B. Lippincott.

Friendly, D. S. (1994). Eye disorders. In Avery, G., et al. *Neonatology.* Philadelphia: J. B. Lippincott.

Gamblien, V., et al. (1993). Assessment and management of endocrine dysfunction. In Kenner, C., et al. *Comprehensive neonatal nursing.* Philadelphia: W. B. Saunders.

Gardner, K. (1993). Twin transfusion syndrome. *Journal of Obstetric, Gynecologic & Neonatal Nursing, 22,* 64.

Givens, K. T., et al. (1993). Congenital rubella syndrome: ophthalmic manifestations and associated systemic disorders. *British Journal of Ophthalmology, 77,* 358.

Goetzman, B. W., & Wennberg, R. P. (1991). *Neonatal intensive care handbook* (2nd ed.). St. Louis: Mosby Year Book.

Gorski, P. A., et al. (1990). Handling preterm infants in hospitals: stimulating controversy about timing of stimulation. *Clinics in Perinatology, 17,* 103.

Haywood, J. L., et al. (1993). Assessment and management of respiratory dysfunction. In Kenner, C., et al. *Comprehensive neonatal nursing.* Philadelphia: W. B. Saunders.

Loeb, S., et al. (1993). *Nurses' handbook of drug therapy.* Springhouse, PA: Springhouse Corporation.

London, M.L. (1993). Resuscitation and stabilization of the neonate. In Kenner, C., Bruggemeyer, A., & Gunderson, L. P. *Comprehensive neonatal nursing.* Philadelphia: W. B. Saunders.

Ludington-Hoe, S. M., Hadeed, A. J., & Anderson, G.C. (1991). Physiologic responses to skin-to-skin contact in hospitalized preterm infants. *Journal of Perinatology, 11,* 19.

Mayes, L. C., et al. (1993). Neurobehavioral profiles of neonates exposed to cocaine prenatally. *Pediatrics, 91,* 778.

Mayfield, S. R. (1990). The preterm infant. In Oski, F. A., et al. *Principles and practice of pediatrics.* Philadelphia: J. B. Lippincott.

Ogata, E. S. (1994). Carbohydrate homeostasis. In Avery, G., et al. *Neonatology.* Philadelphia: J. B. Lippincott.

O'Hara, M. A. (1993). Ophthalmia neonatorum. *Pediatric Clinics of North America, 40,* 715.

Ostrea, E. M., et al. (1994). The infant of the drug dependent mother. In Avery, G., et al. *Neonatology.* Philadelphia: J. B. Lippincott.

Patterson, L. E. (1990). Gonococcal infections. In Oski, F. A., et al. *Principles and practice of pediatrics.* Philadelphia: J. B. Lippincott.

Phibbs, R. H. (1994). Delivery room management. In Avery, G., et al. *Neonatology.* Philadelphia: J. B. Lippincott.

Revenis, M. E., & Johnson, L. A. (1994). Multiple gestations. In Avery, G., et al. *Neonatology.* Philadelphia: J. B. Lippincott.

Scanlon, J. W. (1994). The very-low-birth-weight infant. In Avery, G., et al. *Neonatology.* Philadelphia: J. B. Lippincott.

Scaradavou, A., et al. (1993). Suppression of erythropoiesis by intrauterine transfusions in hemolytic disease of the newborn: use of erythropoietin to treat the late anemia. *Journal of Pediatrics, 123,* 279.

Shaw, N. (1993). Assessment and management of hematologic dysfunction. In Kenner, C., et al. *Comprehensive neonatal nursing.* Philadelphia: W. B. Saunders.

Short, B. L. (1994). Extracorporeal membrane oxygenation. In Avery, G., et al. *Neonatology.* Philadelphia: J. B. Lippincott.

Spitzer, A. R., & Gibson, E. (1992). Considerations for home monitor management. *Clinics in Perinatology, 19,* 916.

Taber, L. H. (1990). Rubella. In Oski, F. A., et al. *Principles and practice of pediatrics.* Philadelphia: J. B. Lippincott.

Whitsett, J. A., et al. (1994). Acute respiratory disorders. In Avery, G., et al. *Neonatology.* Philadelphia: J. B. Lippincott.

Suggested Readings

Ballard, J. L., et al. (1993). Diabetic fetal macrosomia: significance of disproportionate growth. *Journal of Pediatrics, 122,* 115.

Catlett, A. T., et al. (1990). Environmental stimulation of the acutely ill preterm infant. *Neonatal Network, 8,* 19.

Co, E., & Vidyasagar, D. (1990). Meconium aspiration syndrome. *Comprehensive Therapy, 16,* 34.

Hoffman, H. J., & Hillman, L. S. (1992). Epidemiology of the SIDS syndrome. *Clinics in Perinatology, 19,* 717.

Korner, A. F. (1990). Infant stimulation: issues of theory and research. *Clinics in Perinatology, 17,* 173.

Leonard, C. H., et al. (1990). Effect of medical and social risk factors on outcome of prematurity and very low-birth-weight. *Journal of Pediatrics, 116,* 620.

Levy, M., & Spino, M. (1993). Neonatal withdrawal syndrome: associated drugs and pharmacologic management. *Pharmacotherapy, 13,* 202.

Lindsay, J. K., et al. (1993). Creative caring in the NICU; parent-to-parent support. *Neonatal Network, 12,* 37.

Little, B. B., et al. (1990). Failure to recognize fetal alcohol syndrome in newborn infants. *American Journal of Diseases in Children, 144,* 1142.

Loli, J. G. (1990). Giving surfactant to preterm infants. *American Journal of Nursing, 90,* 59.

Long, C. A., et al. (1992). SIDS and infant parenting: implications for critical care. *Pediatric Nursing, 18,* 524.

McGettigan, M. C., et al. (1994). Psychological aspects of parenting critically ill neonates. *Clinical Pediatrics, 33,* 77.

Moses, S. W. (1990). Pathophysiology and dietary treatment of the glycogen storage diseases. *Journal of Pediatric and Gastroenterology Nutrition, 11,* 155.

Penney, S. (1993). A 24-hour urine collection device for low-birth-weight infants. *Neonatal Network, 12,* 61.

Phelps, D. L. (1993). Retinopathy of prematurity. *Pediatric Clinics of North America, 40,* 705.

Plesko, L. (1992). Nursing implications of surfactant therapy. *Neonatal Intensive Care, 5,* 26.

Schraeder, B. D., et al. (1990). The value of early home assessment in identifying risk in children who were very-low-birth-weight. *Pediatric Nursing, 16,* 268.

Whitby, C. (1990). Infant feeding in adversity: feeding the preterm baby. *Midwives Chronicle, 103,* 12.

Zaichkin, J., et al. (1993). The drug-exposed mother and infant. *Neonatal Network, 12,* 41.

Zwick, M. B. (1993). Decreasing environmental noise in the NICU through staff education. *Neonatal Intensive Care, 6,* 16.

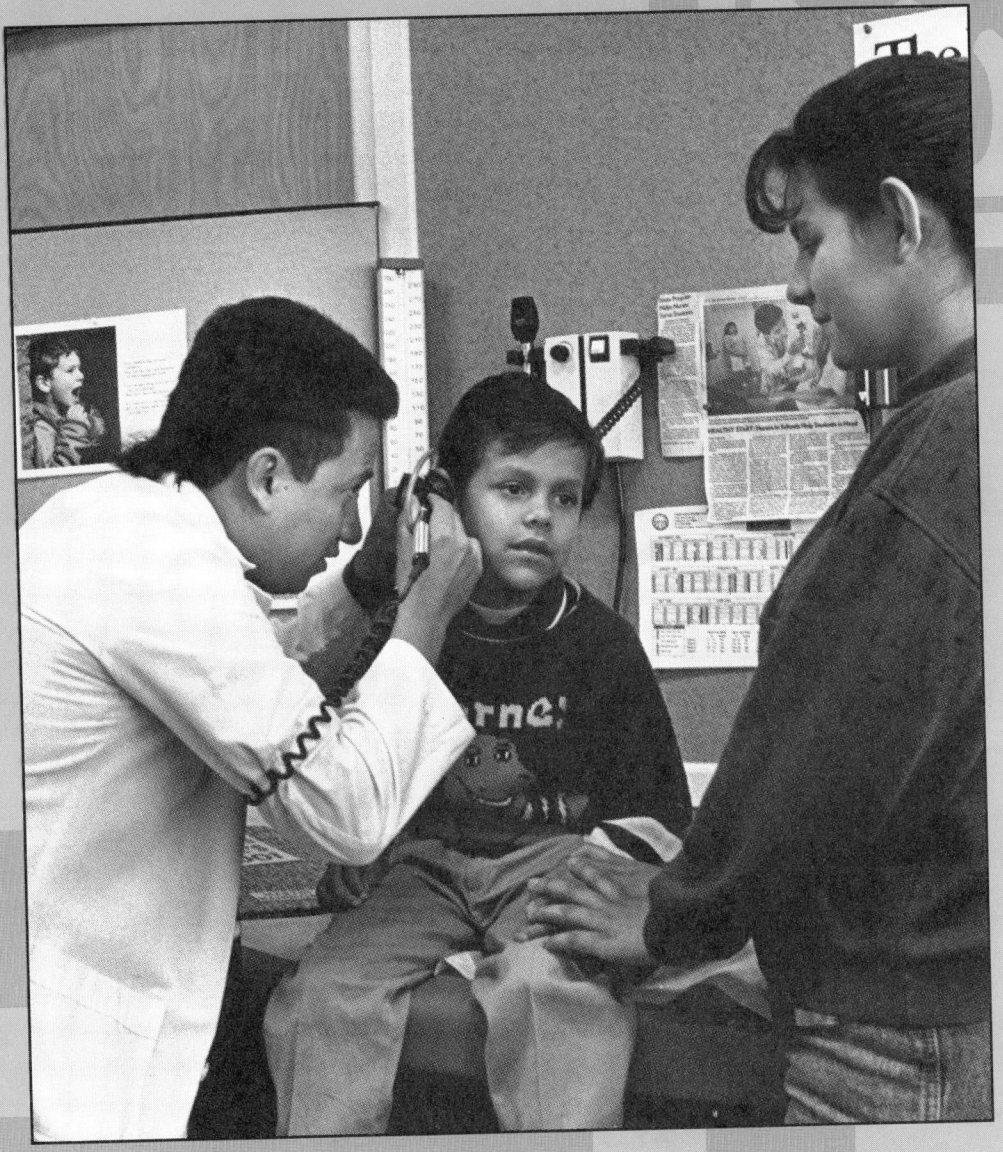

The Nursing Role in Health Promotion for the Childrearing Family

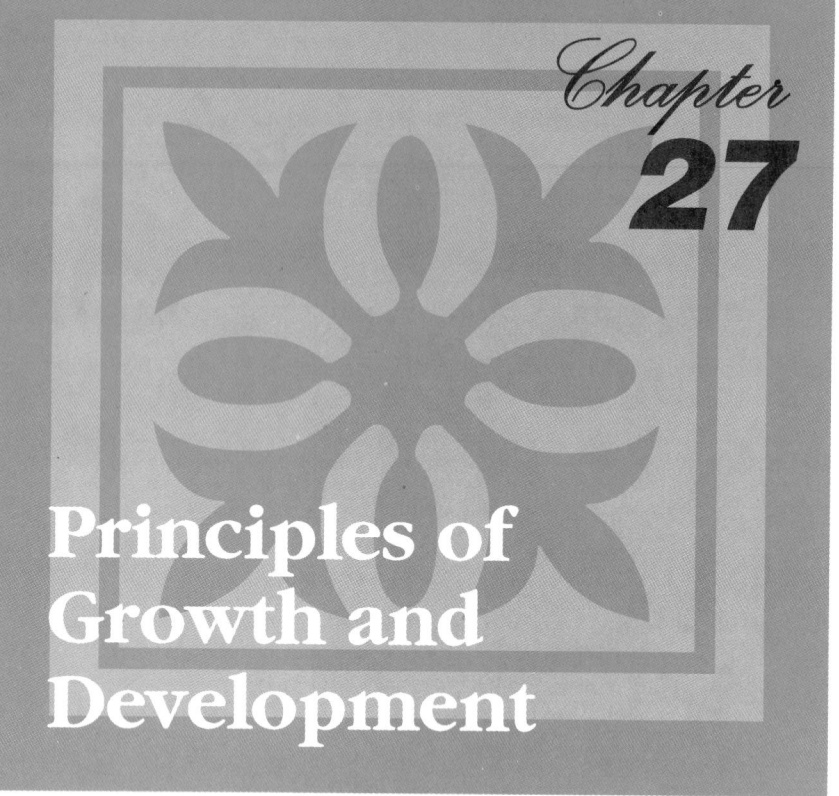

Chapter 27

Principles of Growth and Development

Objectives

After mastering the contents of this chapter, you should be able to:

1. Describe principles of growth and development and developmental stages according to major theorists.

2. Assess a child to determine the stage of development the child has reached.

3. Formulate nursing diagnoses that address both a potential for and an actual delay in growth and development.

4. Plan nursing care to assist a child in achieving and maintaining normal growth and development.

5. Implement nursing care such as providing age-appropriate play materials to support normal growth and development patterns.

6. Evaluate outcome criteria to be certain that nursing goals related to growth and development have been achieved.

7. Identify National Health Goals related to growth and development that nurses can be instrumental in helping the nation to achieve.

8. Identify areas related to growth and development that could benefit from additional nursing research.

9. Use critical thinking to analyze factors that influence growth and development and ways to strengthen paths to achieving a new developmental stage.

10. Synthesize knowledge of growth and development with nursing process to achieve quality maternal and child health nursing care.

Key Terms

- abstract thought
- accommodation
- adaptability
- approach
- assimilation
- attention span
- autonomy versus shame
- cognitive development
- concrete operational thought
- conservation
- conventional development
- development
- developmental milestone
- developmental task
- distractibility
- egocentrism
- formal operational thought
- growth
- identity versus role confusion
- industry versus inferiority
- initiative versus guilt
- intuitive thought
- libido
- maturation
- mood quality
- permanence
- postconventional development
- preoperational thought
- pre-religious stage
- reversibility
- rhythmicity
- role fantasy
- schema
- sensorimotor stage
- temperament
- threshold of response
- trust versus mistrust

Adele Pillitteri: MATERNAL AND CHILD HEALTH NURSING, 2nd Edition. © 1995 Adele Pillitteri.

All children pass through predictable stages of growth and development as they mature. Understanding the stage of development a child has reached is important, because parents often will ask a nurse what to expect from their child regarding developmental progress. Health care visits provide the opportunity to assess present growth and development and to supply anticipatory guidance on the topic. Understanding the psychosocial developmental stage and growth point a child has reached helps in planning care that considers not only age but developmental stage as well.

For these reasons, learning about growth and development is essential to the development of complete and effective nursing care plans for children (Gillis, 1990). This chapter addresses the most important factors to assess for each age group. Later chapters supply detailed descriptions of individual age groups. National Health Goals related to growth and development are shown in the National Health Goals box.

 **NURSING PROCESS OVERVIEW
for Promotion of Normal Growth
and Development**

ASSESSMENT

Height and weight should be measured and plotted on a standard growth chart for children at all health care visits. History-taking and observation should focus on whether **developmental milestones** (major markers of normal development) have been met. Periodic screening tests (i.e., Denver Developmental Screening Test, vision tests, and audiometry screening) should be scheduled at standard times, as discussed in Chapter 28. For the most accurate assessment, be certain to account for sleepiness, fatigue, or "bad days" (a day on which the child did not test well). The developmental stage that a child has reached is assessed through observation and careful listening to how the child describes himself or herself, how the parents describe the child, and what

FOCUS ON
National Health Goals

National Health Goals that address either growth or development of children include the following:

- Reduce to less than 10% the prevalence of mental disorders among children and adolescents from a baseline of 12%.

- Reduce growth retardation among low-income children aged 5 and younger to less than 10% from a baseline of 16%. Growth retardation is defined as height-for-age below the fifth percentile on a standard growth chart (DHHS, 1991).

   Recognizing normal growth and development patterns for children helps in determining if children are following normal development and when referrals are needed. The following are nursing research topics that could shed more information in this area: Are there differences between urban and rural children in the way they approach childhood problems? How do characteristics of temperament effect the way children respond to hospitalization? How does the environment of children influence health?

forced to achieve milestones faster than that child's own timetable will allow. Through anticipatory guidance, a child, however, can be encouraged to reach his or her maximum developmental potential. Nurses can play an important role in offering guidance to both the child and family toward this end.

Planning often includes the child's family even when the child is no longer completely dependent on the family for meeting all of his or her needs. To be able to grow developmentally, a child continues to need emotional support from people who are important to that child, just as he or she needs nutritional support to grow physically. Parents of a developmentally delayed child may use denial as a protective mechanism for a long time; this means that planning may have to be delayed until parents are convinced that a problem truly exists.

IMPLEMENTATION

Interventions to foster growth and development include encouraging age-appropriate self-care in the child and suggesting age-appropriate toys or activities to parents. It may be necessary to help parents accept their child's

activities the child is interested in and can accomplish (Figure 27-1).

NURSING DIAGNOSIS

When assessment is completed, a child profile is devised. Based on this profile, problems and needs can be identified. Nursing diagnoses most frequently used in this area include:

- High risk for altered growth and development related to lack of age-appropriate toys and activities
- Altered growth and development related to prolonged illness
- Family coping: potential for growth related to parent's seeking information about child's growth
- Health-seeking behaviors related to appropriate stimulation for infants

PLANNING

To make care holistic, it is important to consider all aspects of the child's health—physical, emotional, cognitive, and social—and remember that each child's developmental progress is unique. A child cannot be

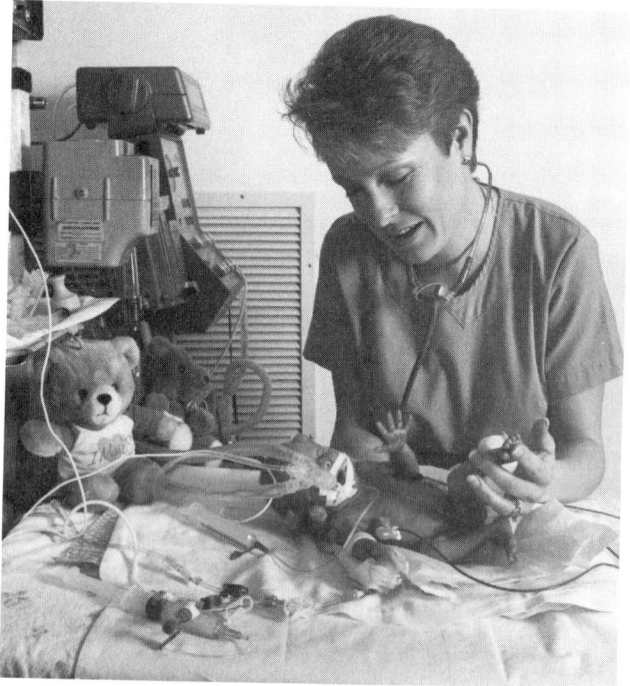

FIGURE 27-1

Growth and development are assessed by both observation and specific testing. (Courtesy of the Department of Medical Photography, Children's Hospital, Buffalo, NY.)

delayed growth or motivate a child to reach his or her upper limits. Role modeling is an important ongoing intervention with children and families. Modeling, for example, can demonstrate that being an adult is an enjoyable life role and that problem-solving is a more effective approach to life's challenges than a temper tantrum.

EVALUATION

Evaluation for growth and developmental milestones (see Chapters 29 through 33) must be ongoing to be accurate and useful, because many children do not test well until school age. If a developmental task involves only gross motor function or sight or hearing development, it may not be apparent that something is wrong until the child is in school and is asked to perform fine motor tasks or listen to and follow detailed instructions. If a child has difficulty achieving one developmental task, he or she may have difficulty with the next as well, another reason for ongoing evaluation. The following are examples of outcome criteria that might be developed:

- Child expresses less negativism by next clinic visit.
- Parents describe at 9-month check-up how they have made a safe space in their home for their infant to crawl so that he is not confined to the playpen.
- Parents list tasks they feel are appropriate for a 6-year-old by next office visit.

Importance of Knowledge About Growth and Development to the Roles of the Nurse

Information about growth and development is important in primary, secondary, and tertiary care settings.

Health Promotion and Illness Prevention

Determining a child's developmental stage is often the primary focus of a health interview. For instance, during her child's 24-month check-up, a mother might ask if it is normal that her child cannot yet pedal a tricycle. This question or any other questions about a child's developmental progress cannot be answered without a full understanding of the average ranges.

In addition to reassurance that their child is doing well, parents also need periodic anticipatory guidance regarding their child's development. For example, it would be important to discuss home safety with a parent when a child is approaching the age for creeping. Parents should be cautioned to think about fencing open

stairways and clearing cleaning compounds out of bottom cupboards. Parents of a child who is almost 2 years old will appreciate being cautioned that the child's appetite may decrease during the coming year. With this caution, they will not see a rejection of food as the beginning of a feeding problem but as a usual step of development. The parent of a child approaching puberty generally welcomes a discussion on how to prepare a child for this growth phase.

It is important that anticipatory guidance be offered at the appropriate time, or it will be useless. Information given too early is forgotten by the time it is needed. If it is given too late, the parents may have already addressed (or ignored) the issues, possibly not in the most growth-enhancing way for the child. In order to be able to supply anticipatory guidance this way at the appropriate time or plan nursing care to meet the needs of children and their families, it is necessary to recognize the predictable stages of growth and development, from newborn to young adult, through which each child passes.

Health Restoration and Maintenance

It is also essential to consider developmental stages when caring for a sick child. It is terribly awkward to prepare a 5-year-old for surgery without being sensitive to how much a 5-year-old can be expected to comprehend. Will the child understand that an anesthetic is a gas? What a surgeon is? What stitches are? Understanding the child's developmental stage helps in choosing the right words. It would be equally frustrating to offer oral medicine to a child to swallow when he or she is too young to coordinate tongue and throat muscles well enough to swallow pills.

Physical growth is another important factor affected by the growth and development stage of a child (see the Focus on Nursing Research display). Disease affects children differently at various stages of growth. A 12-year-old who has fractured a long bone, for example, has a potentially more serious fracture than an 8-year-old who fractures the identical bone. The 8-year-old must metabolize enough calcium to meet two major needs: healing the fracture site and maintaining healthy bone cells. The 12-year-old, who is undergoing a period of rapid growth, must meet three needs: his or her body must supply not only enough calcium for healing and maintaining existing healthy bone cells but also an additional amount for rapid bone growth. If the child does not take in adequate calcium during the healing period to supply the extra amount for growth, the affected limb may be left shorter than its mate. Members of a health care team must recognize this danger and, if necessary, supply extra calcium so that no permanent disability will result.

Principles of Growth and Development

Growing up is a complex phenomenon because of the many interrelated facets involved. Children do not merely grow taller and heavier as they get older. Maturing also involves growth in ability to perform skills, to think, to relate to people, and to trust or have confidence in oneself.

The terms *growth* and *development* are occasionally used interchangeably but they are different. **Growth** is generally used to denote an increase in physical size or a quantitative change. Growth in weight is measured in pounds or kilograms; growth in height is measured in inches or centimeters.

Development is used to denote an increase in skill or the ability to function (a qualitative change). Development can be measured by observing a child's ability to perform specific tasks (e.g., how well the child picks up small objects such as raisins), by recording the parent's description of the child's progress, or by using standardized tests such as the Denver Developmental Screening Test. **Maturation** is a synonym for development.

Cognitive development refers to the ability to learn or understand from experience, to acquire and retain knowledge, to respond to a new situation, and

to solve problems (intelligence; see section on Piaget's Theory of Cognitive Development). It is measured by intelligence tests and by observing the child's ability to function effectively in his or her environment.

Patterns

Neither physical growth nor aspects of maturation occur haphazardly. Several principles govern this process (see the Focus on Family Teaching box). As shown in Figure 27-2, general growth (i.e., growth of respiratory, digestive, renal, musculoskeletal, and circulatory tissue) proceeds fairly smoothly during childhood. Certain body tissues, however, mature more rapidly than others. Neurologic tissue (e.g., spinal cord and brain), for example, grows rapidly the first 2 years so that brain growth has reached mature proportions at 5 years. Lymphoid tissue (e.g., spleen, thymus, lymph nodes, and tonsillar tissue) also grows rapidly during infancy and childhood to provide protection to the child against infection. The spleen is usually a palpable 1 or 2 cm in preschool children, and in 5-year-olds, tonsillar tissue has already reached adult size. On assessment, younger school-age children will appear to have large tonsils and thymus glands because of this early growth of lymphoid tissue (the back of their throat seems to be "all tonsils"). At one time, children's tonsils were routinely removed and their thymus glands were x-rayed to reduce their size, because they were "enlarged." Currently this extreme tissue growth is recognized as being normal. In contrast, the reproductive organs (i.e., genital tissue) show little growth until puberty.

Factors Influencing Growth and Development

Genetic inheritance and environmental influences are the two primary factors in determining a child's pattern of growth and development. For each child, a unique combination of heredity and environment determines how the child grows and matures.

Genetic Influences

From the moment of conception when a sperm and ovum fuse, the basic genetic makeup of an individual is cast. In addition to physical characteristics such as eye color and height potential, inheritance determines other characteristics such as learning style and temperament. The individual may also inherit a genetic defect or defects, which may result in disability or illness at birth or later in life.

Although each child is unique, certain expected gender-related characteristics are important to consider when assessing children for normal growth and devel-

Q. What are general principles of growth and development that I can expect my newborn to follow?

A. No two children are alike, but all do follow general principles of growth and development. Examples of these principles are given in the following table.

Principle	Example
Growth and development are continuous processes from conception until death.	Although there are highs and lows in terms of the rate at which growth and development proceed, at all times a child is growing new cells and learning new skills. An example of how the rate of growth changes is a comparison between that of the first year and later in life. An infant triples birth weight and increases height by 50% during the first year of life. If this tremendous growth rate were to continue, the 5-yr-old child, ready to begin school, would weigh 1600 lb and be 12 ft 6 in tall.
Growth and development proceed in an orderly sequence.	Growth in height occurs in only one sequence—from smaller to larger. Development also proceeds in a predictable order. For example, the majority of children sit before they creep, creep before they stand, stand before they walk, and walk before they run. Occasionally, a child will skip a stage (or pass through it so quickly that the parents do not observe the stage). Occasionally, a child will progress in a different order, but most children follow a predictable sequence of growth and development.
Different children pass through the predictable stages at different rates.	All stages of development have a range of time rather than a certain point at which they are usually accomplished. Two children may pass through the motor sequence at such different rates, for example, that one begins walking at 9 mo, another only at 14 mo. Both are developing normally. They are both following the predictable sequence; they are merely developing at different rates.
All body systems do not develop at the same rate.	Certain body tissues mature more rapidly than others. For example, neurologic tissue experiences its peak growth during the first year of life, whereas genital tissue grows little until puberty.
Development is cephalocaudal.	*Cephalo* is a Greek word meaning "head"; *caudal* means "tail." Development proceeds from head to tail. A newborn can lift only the head off the bed when he or she lies in a prone position. By age 2 mo, the infant can lift the head and chest off the bed; by 4 mo, the head, chest, and part of the abdomen; by 5 mo, the infant has enough control to turn over; by 9 mo, he or she can control the legs enough to crawl; and by 1 yr, the child can stand upright and perhaps walk. Motor development has proceeded in a cephalocaudal order—from the head to the lower extremities.
Development proceeds from proximal to distal body parts.	This principle is closely related to cephalocaudal development. It can best be illustrated by tracing the progress of upper extremity development. A newborn makes little use of the arms or hands. Any movement, except to put a thumb in the mouth, is a flailing motion. By age 3 or 4 mo, the infant has enough arm control to support the upper body weight on the forearms and the infant can coordinate the hand to scoop up objects. By 10 mo, the infant can coordinate the arm and thumb and index finger sufficiently well to use a pincerlike grasp or be able to pick up an object as fine as a piece of breakfast cereal on a high-chair tray.
Development proceeds from gross to refined skills.	This principle parallels the preceding one. Because the child is able to control distal body parts such as fingers, he or she is able to perform fine motor skills (a 3-yr-old colors best with a large crayon; a 12-yr-old can write with a fine pen.)
There is an optimum time for initiation of experiences or learning.	A child cannot learn tasks until his or her nervous system is mature enough to allow that particular learning. A child cannot learn to sit, for example, no matter how much the child's parents have him or her practice, until the nervous system has matured enough to allow back control. Children who are not given the opportunity to learn developmental tasks at the appropriate or "target" times for that task may have more difficulty than the usual child learning the task later on. A child who is confined to a body cast at 12 mo, the time the child would normally learn to walk, may take a long time to learn this skill once free of the cast at, say, age 2 yrs. The child has passed the time of optimal learning for that particular skill.
Neonatal reflexes must be lost before development can proceed.	An infant cannot grasp with skill until the grasp reflex has faded nor stand steadily until the walking reflex has faded.
A great deal of skill and behavior is learned by practice.	An infant practices over and over taking a first step before he or she accomplishes this securely.

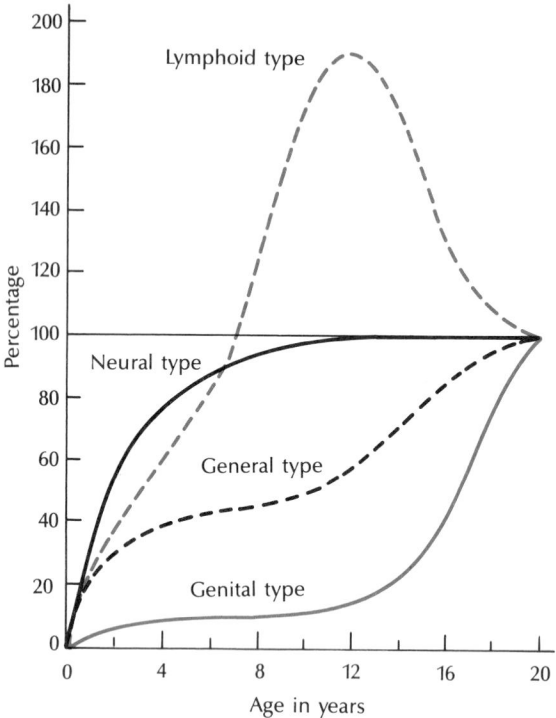

FIGURE 27-2

Main types of postnatal growth of various body tissue types. (From Scammon, R. E. [1930]. The measurement of the body in childhood. In Harris, J. A., et al. [Eds.] The measurement of man, pp. 214–226. Minneapolis: University of Minnesota Press, with permission.)

opment. For instance, on the average, females are born weighing less (by an ounce or two) and measuring less in length (by an inch or two) than males. Boys tend to keep this height and weight advantage until prepuberty, at which time girls surge ahead, because they begin their puberty growth spurt 6 months to 1 year earlier than boys. By the end of puberty (14 to 16 years), males again show a tendency to be taller and heavier than females. This difference in growth patterns is reflected in the different growth charts used for boys and girls (Wegman, 1993; see Appendix E).

Race and cultural influences may also contribute to differences in growth and developmental patterns among children, but it is hard to say whether such differences are genetically or environmentally caused. Although physical differences such as skin color and facial features can be attributed to racial inheritance, any differences in weight, height, and childhood development patterns among different cultural groups may be more closely related to the environment, including the prenatal environment (such as adequate prenatal nutrition) than to any genetic predisposition.

Environmental Influences

Although a child cannot grow taller than his or her genetically programmed height potential allows, the child's adult height may be considerably less than genetic po-

tential if the child's environment hinders growth in some way. For example, the child may receive inadequate nutrition because of low socioeconomic status, inadequate caregiver skills and attention, or chronic illness. Many illnesses lower the child's appetite; others, such as certain endocrine disorders, directly alter the growth rate.

Environmental influences, however, are not always detrimental. For example, a child with phenylketonuria, an inherited metabolic disease, can achieve normal growth and development despite his or her genetic makeup if the child's diet (a part of the environment) is properly regulated. The following environmental influences are most likely to affect growth and development.

Quality of Nutrition

The quality of a child's nutrition during the growing years (including prenatally) has a large influence on eventual health and stature. Poor maternal nutrition may limit the growth and intelligence potential of the child from the moment of birth. Children whose own diets lack essential nutrients show inadequate physical growth. A lack of energy and stamina prevents them from pursuing learning activities at their best intellectual level. Children who eat too many carbohydrates and become obese may develop motor skills more slowly than other children, because physical movement is more tiring for them. Excessively thin or obese children are sometimes taunted by their playmates and may become "loners" or have difficulty relating to their peers.

Socioeconomic Level

Nearly 50% of black children, 40% of Spanish-speaking children, and 16% of white children in the United States live in families with incomes below the poverty line (U.S. Department of Commerce, 1992). Because health care and good nutrition both cost money, the child born into a family of low socioeconomic means may not receive adequate health supervision or good nutrition. Poor health supervision, for instance, could leave a child without immunization against measles or other childhood illnesses and thus vulnerable to diseases that could cause permanent neurologic damage if complications occur. Poor nutrition could leave a child prone to rickets, a disease that affects growth by causing shortening or bowing of long bones.

Parent–Child Relationship

Children who are loved thrive better than those who are not. Either parent or a nonparent caregiver may serve as the primary caregiver or form the primary parent–child love relationship (Levy-Shiff et al., 1990). Loss of love from a primary caregiver, occurring with the death of a parent, or interruption of parental contact through prolonged hospitalizations, divorce, or inadequate parent love, can interfere with the child's desire to eat, improve, and advance. Cultural norms within the family also play a role in determining when a child is expected

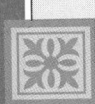

FOCUS ON CULTURAL AWARENESS

Not all nations foster the growth and development of children in the same manner, in part because of cultural variations. In some countries, the predominant theory of child-rearing is protective nurturing. Children are not rushed into new experiences like toilet-training or beginning school. In others, it is customary to treat children in a harsh, strict manner, using shame or corporal punishment for discipline. In Central American nations, toilet training may be begun as early as when the child can sit upright. Praising children for learning a new skill may be viewed as unnecessary or actually harmful, since this could result in a child being subject to an evil eye.

Childhood in the United States covers a relatively long time period; in other countries it is short, because girls are asked to assume domestic responsibilities early in life; outside or farm work is required early for boys. In Cambodia, an infant's personality is thought to depend not so much on genetic or environmental influences but on the year and time of birth (Geissler, 1994).

Recognizing that such cultural variations exist helps in planning care that is specific to a particular child and family.

to achieve particular developmental milestones (see Focus on Cultural Awareness display).

Ordinal Position in the Family

The position of a child in the family, whether a firstborn child, a middle child, the "baby," an only child, or one within a large family, will have some bearing on his or her growth and development. An only child or the oldest child in a family generally excels in language development because conversations are mainly with adults. Children learn by watching other children, however, so that a firstborn or only child, who has no example to watch, may not excel in other skills, such as toilet training at an early age. Parents with large families often say the youngest child "toilet-trained himself or herself" simply by watching the older children.

Health

Diseases that come from environmental sources can have as strong an influence on growth and development as genetically inherited diseases. A child who has a residual heart impairment as a result of rheumatic fever might be limited thereafter in his or her ability to perform active sports, for example. The eventual degree of disability will depend not only on the damage caused by the actual disease but also on the attitudes of the people

around the child—how disabled they feel the child is and how they treat that child. These attitudes are an influence of environment on the child's development. Infants cared for in neonatal intensive care units may have their growth affected by the overstimulation of light and sound, so that their health becomes directly influenced by their environment (Glass, 1994).

Theories of Development

A **developmental task** is a skill or a growth responsibility arising at a particular time in an individual's life, the successful achievement of which will provide a foundation for the accomplishment of future tasks. It is not so much chronologic age as the completion of developmental tasks that defines whether a child has passed from one developmental stage of childhood to another. A child is not a toddler just because he or she is age 1 year plus 1 day old. The child becomes a toddler when that child has passed through the developmental stage of infancy. A child does not leave the adolescent period at age 18 years plus 1 day, but only when that child has completed the developmental tasks of adolescence. For reference, however, childhood is generally divided into the periods shown in Table 27-1.

A number of theories have been proposed to describe how children grow emotionally, psychologically, and intellectually as they pass through these different periods. Some theories deal mainly with negative aspects of childrearing or with events that can cause mental illness in children, either immediately, or later when the child reaches adulthood. Others discuss the positive aspects necessary for normal growth and for development of a mentally healthy and productive adult.

Freud's Psychoanalytic Theory

Sigmund Freud (1856–1939), an Austrian neurologist and founder of psychoanalysis, offered the first real theory of personality development (Robinson, 1993). Freud based his theory of development on his observations of mentally disturbed adults. He described adult behavior as being the result of instinctual drives (**libido**) from within the person and the conflicts that develop be-

Table 27-1. Basic Divisions of Childhood	
Period	*Length*
Neonate	First 28 days of life
Infant	1 mo–1 yr
Toddler	1–3 yr
Preschooler	3–5 yr
School-age child	5–13 yr
Adolescent	13–18 yr

tween these instincts (represented in the individual as the *id*), reality (represented in the individual as the *ego*), and society (represented in the individual as the *super-ego*). He described child development as being a series of psychosexual stages in which the child's interests become focused on a particular body site.

Infant

Freud termed the infant period the *oral phase*, because infants are so interested in oral stimulation or pleasure during this time (Robinson, 1993). According to this theory, infants suck for enjoyment or relief of tension, as well as for nourishment.

Toddler

Freud described the toddler period as the *anal phase*. Toddlers' interests widen and their main focus is on the anal region. Elimination takes on new importance. Children find pleasure in both the retention and defecation of feces. This anal interest is part of toddlers' self-discovery, a way of exerting independence, and thus probably accounts for some of the difficulties parents may experience in toilet-training toddlers.

Preschooler

During the preschool period, children's pleasure zone appears to shift from the anal to the genital area. Freud called this period the *phallic phase*. Children may show exhibitionism, suggesting they hope this will lead to increased knowledge of the two sexes.

School-Age Child

Freud saw the school-age period as being a *latent phase*, a time in which children's libido (energy) appears to be diverted into concrete thinking. No developments as obvious as those in earlier periods appear during this time.

Adolescent

Freudian theory considers the main events of the adolescent period to be the establishment of new sexual aims and the finding of new love objects. Freud's stages of childhood are summarized in Table 27-2.

Erikson's Theory of Psychosocial Development

Erikson (1902–) was trained in psychoanalytic theory but later developed his own theory of psychosocial development that stresses the importance of culture and society in development of the personality (Erikson, 1985). One of the main tenets of his theory, that a person's social view of himself or herself is more important than instinctual drives in determining behavior, allows for a more optimistic view of the possibilities for human growth (Schuster & Ashburn, 1991). Erikson describes

eight developmental stages covering the entire life span. At each stage there is a conflict between two opposing forces. According to Erikson, the successful resolution of each conflict, or accomplishment of the developmental task of that stage, allows the individual to go on to the next phase of development. Table 27-2 shows Erikson's developmental stages through adolescence.

Infant

According to Erikson, the developmental task for infants is learning **trust versus mistrust** (other terms might be *learning confidence* or *learning to love*). Infants whose needs are met when those needs arise, whose discomforts are quickly removed, who are cuddled, fondled, played with, and talked to come to view the world as a safe place and people as helpful and dependable. However, when the care is inconsistent, inadequate, or rejecting, it fosters a basic mistrust—infants become fearful and suspicious of the world and of people. They will carry this attitude through later stages of development. Such children will be "stuck" emotionally at this stage, even though they continue to grow and develop in other ways.

Fortunately, because not all children achieve developmental tasks readily, each task need not be resolved once and for all the first time it arises. The problem of trust versus mistrust, for example, is not resolved forever during the first year of life but arises again at each successive stage of development. Children who enter school with a sense of mistrust may come to trust a teacher who takes the trouble to make himself or herself trustworthy; given this second chance, children overcome early mistrust. On the other hand, children who come through infancy with a vital sense of trust intact may still have a sense of mistrust activated at a later stage if their parents are divorced or separate under unpleasant circumstances.

John, for example, was unable to form a sense of trust. As a 4-year-old, he was seen at an ambulatory care visit because his adoptive parents, who had cared for him for 6 months, now wanted to give him back to the adoption agency. They found John cold and unloving, unable to respond to them. John *was* a cold and apathetic boy, but his background had contributed to this defensive reaction. About 1 year after his birth, he was taken away from his mother, who was not caring for him adequately, and was moved back and forth among several foster homes. Initially, he tried to relate to people in the foster homes, but due to frequent moving, never had a chance to develop relationships. In the end, he gave up trying to initiate bonds with others. The inevitable separations hurt too much.

Like a burned child who avoids fire, emotionally burned children may shun the potential pain of further emotional involvement. John had once trusted his mother but now trusted no one. Similar circumstances

Table 27-2. *Summary of Freud's and Erikson's Theories of Personality Development*

	Freud's Stages of Childhood		Erikson's Stages of Childhood	
	Psychosexual Stage	*Nursing Implications*	*Developmental Task*	*Nursing Implications*
Infant	Oral stage: Child explores the world by using mouth, especially the tongue.	Provide oral stimulation by giving pacifiers; do not discourage thumb-sucking. Breast-feeding may provide more stimulation than formula-feeding because it requires the infant to expend more energy.	Developmental task is to form a sense of trust versus mistrust. Child learns to love and be loved.	Provide a primary care giver. Provide experiences that add to security, such as soft sounds and touch. Provide visual stimulation for active child involvement
Toddler	Anal stage: Child learns to control urination and defecation.	Help children achieve bowel and bladder control without undue emphasis on its importance. If at all possible, continue bowel and bladder training while child is hospitalized.	Developmental task is to form a sense of autonomy versus shame. Child learns to be independent and make decisions for self.	Provide opportunities for decision-making, such as offering choices of clothes to wear or toys to play with. Praise for ability to make decisions rather than judging correctness of any one decision.
Preschooler	Phallic stage: Child learns sexual identity through awareness of genital area.	Accept child's sexual interest, such as fondling his or her own genitals, as a normal area of exploration. Help parents answer child's questions about birth or sexual differences.	Developmental task is to form a sense of initiative versus guilt. Child learns how to do things (basic) problem solving) and that doing things is desirable.	Provide opportunities for exploring new places or activities. Allow play to include activities involving water; clay (for modeling); or finger paint.
School-age child	Latent stage: Child's personality development appears to be nonactive or dormant.	Help the child have positive experiences so his or her self-esteem continues to grow and the child prepares for the conflicts of adolescence.	Developmental task is to form a sense of industry versus inferiority. Child learns how to do things well.	Provide opportunities such as allowing child to assemble supplies for a dressing change (short projects finished completely), so that child feels rewarded for accomplishment.
Adolescent	Genital stage: Adolescent develops sexual maturity and learns to establish satisfactory relationships with the opposite sex.	Provide opportunities for the child to relate with opposite sex; allow child to verbalize feelings about new relationships.	Developmental task is to form a sense of identity versus role confusion. Adolescent learns who he or she is and what kind of person he or she will be by adjusting to a new body image, seeking emancipation from parents, choosing a vocation, and determining a value system.	Provide opportunities for the adolescent to discuss feelings about events important to him or her. Offer support and praise for decision-making.

(Adapted from Erikson, E. H. [1968]. *Childhood and society.* New York: W. W. Norton; and Freud, S. [1962]. *Three essays on the theory of sexuality.* New York: Hearst Corporation, with permission.)

can arise with infants hospitalized for long periods, an important implication for nursing.

Toddler

Erikson defines the development task of the toddler age as learning **autonomy versus shame** or doubt. *Autonomy* (self-government or independence) builds on children's new motor and mental abilities. Children take

pride in new accomplishments and want to do everything independently, whether it is pulling the wrapper off a piece of candy, selecting a vitamin tablet out of the bottle, or flushing the toilet. If parents recognize that toddlers need to do what they are capable of doing, at each child's own pace and in the child's own time, then their children will develop a sense of being able to control muscles and impulses. Toddlers are independent people. When caregivers are impatient and do every-thing for them, however, they enforce a sense of shame and doubt. If children are never allowed to do things they want to do, they will eventually doubt their ability to do them; children stop trying and cannot do them. If children leave this stage with less autonomy than shame or doubt, then they can be disabled in their attempts to achieve independence in adolescence and adulthood (Figure 27-3; see the Nursing Care Plan).

Mary, for example, had difficulty establishing auton-omy. Her mother was a perfect housekeeper who hap-pened to keep many valuable articles at toddler height to maintain her "perfect house" look. As a toddler, Mary could only stand in the middle of rooms, unable to reach out and explore her house. As a school-age child, she still stands apart from an active group. She has no confidence in her ability to achieve. She follows in a quiet, clinging way.

Preschooler

Erikson defines the developmental task of the preschool period as learning **initiative versus guilt**. Learning ini-tiative is learning how to do things. Children can initiate motor activities of various sorts on their own and no longer merely respond to or initiate the actions of other children or their own parents. The same is true for lan-guage and fantasy activities.

Whether children leave this stage with a sense of initiative far outweighing a sense of guilt depends largely on how parents respond to self-initiated activi-ties. When children are given much freedom and oppor-

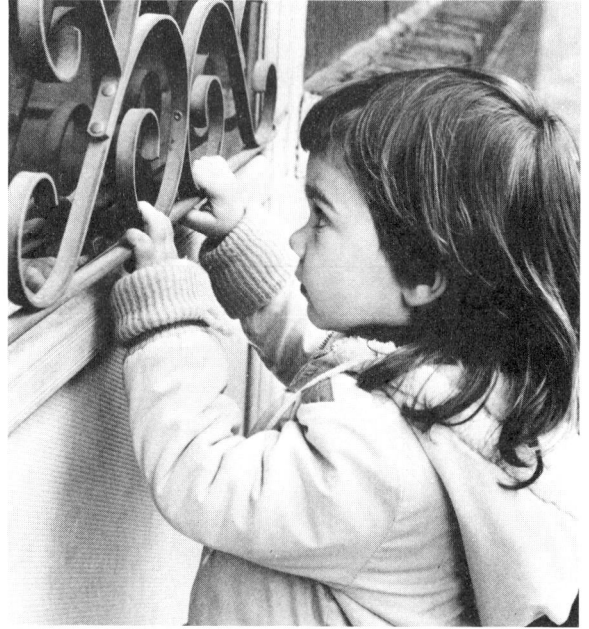

FIGURE 27-3
A toddler enjoys active, independent exploration as part of building a sense of autonomy. (Courtesy of Brian Smistek.)

tunity to initiate motor play such as running, bike riding, sliding, and wrestling or are exposed to such play mate-rials as finger paints, sand, water, and modeling clay, their sense of initiative is reinforced. Initiative is also en-couraged when parents answer their child's questions (intellectual initiative) and do not inhibit fantasy or play activity. If children are made to feel that their motor ac-tivity is bad (perhaps in a small apartment or a hospital), that their questions are a nuisance, and that their play is silly and stupid, they may develop a sense of guilt over self-initiated activities that will persist in later life.

Jill, for example, is a girl with a poor sense of initia-tive. As a preschooler, she was not allowed much exper-imentation because her parents encouraged neatness rather than free play. Now, at high school age, she is unable to "brainstorm" or view more than one way to problem-solve. She waits for clues and guidance from others before acting.

School-Age Child

Erikson states that the developmental task of the school-age period is to develop **industry versus inferiority**, or accomplishment, rather than inferiority. During the preschool period, children were learning initiative—how to do something. Now, children are interested in learning how to do things *well*. When they are absorbed in a project, children's questions are "Am I doing a good job? Am I doing this right?" When children are encour-aged in their efforts to do practical tasks or make practi-cal things and are praised and rewarded for the finished results, their sense of industry grows (Figure 27-4). Par-ents who see their children's efforts at making and doing things as merely "mischief" or who don't show appreci-ation for their children's work may cause them to de-velop a sense of inferiority rather than pride and accom-plishment.

During the years at elementary school, a child's world grows to include the school and community envi-ronment, and success or failure in those settings can have a lasting impact. Children with an intelligence quo-tient of 80 or 90 (slightly below normal), for example, may have a particularly traumatic school experience, even when their sense of industry is rewarded and en-couraged at home. Their learning style may be so differ-ent from the average child's that they cannot compete effectively with children of average ability; they experi-ence repeated failures in their efforts to learn, which re-inforces their sense of inferiority. On the other hand, children whose sense of industry has been destroyed at home may have it revitalized at school through the efforts of a committed teacher. A nurse can also fulfill this role.

Adolescent

Erikson believes that the new interpersonal dimension that emerges during adolescence is a sense of **identity**

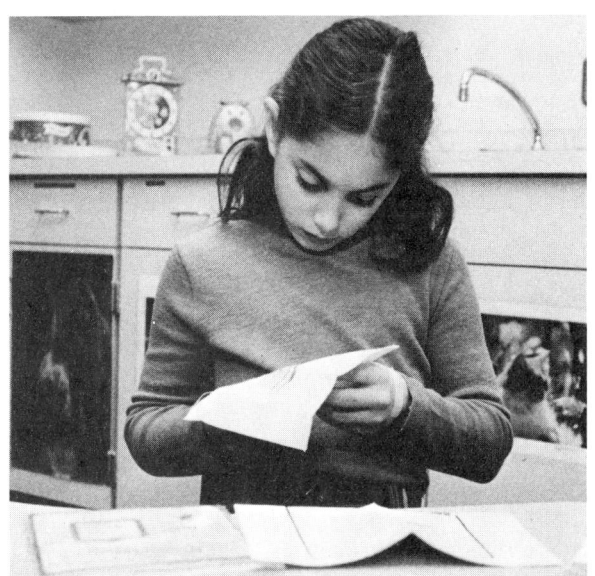

FIGURE 27-4
A school-age child develops her sense of industry by working on projects that result in a feeling of accomplishment. (Courtesy of the Department of Medical Photography, Children's Hospital, Buffalo, NY.)

versus role confusion. To achieve this, adolescents must bring together everything they have learned about themselves as a son or daughter, an athlete, a friend, a drugstore clerk, a student, a scout, and so on, and integrate these different images of themselves into a whole that makes sense. If adolescents are unable to do so, they are left with role confusion—that is, they are unsure what kind of person they are and are uncertain what they can do or what kind of person they can become. Some adolescents seek a negative identity: even being identified as a drug abuser or runaway may be preferable to no identity at all.

Piaget's Theory of Cognitive Development

Piaget (1896–1980), a Swiss psychologist, introduced concepts of cognitive development that are similar to those of both Freud and Erikson and yet separate from each. Piaget defined four stages of cognitive development (Wadsworth, 1989); within each stage are finer units or **schema**. Each period is an advancement over the previous one. To progress from one period to the next, the child reorganizes his or her thinking processes to bring them closer to reality. Piagetian stages of cognitive development are summarized in Table 27-3.

Infant

Piaget refers to the infant stage as the **sensorimotor stage**. Sensorimotor intelligence is practical intelligence, because words and symbols for thinking and problem-solving are not yet available to the child at this age. At the beginning of infancy, babies relate to the world through the senses, using only reflex behavior. As infants progress through this stage (schema of primary and secondary circular reactions and coordination of secondary schema as defined in Table 27-3), they learn the basic theory or concept that people are entities separate from their environment. Piaget uses the term "primary" to refer to activities related to the child's own body, and "circulatory reaction" to demonstrate that repetition of behavior occurs (the infant accidentally brings his or her thumb to the mouth, enjoys the sensation of sucking, and so repeats it).

The term *secondary* refers to activities that are separate from the child's body. An example of *secondary schema* learning is when a baby hits a mobile and notices that this makes it move and so hits it again. During this secondary schema, infants also learn that objects in the environment—bottle, blocks, bed, or even a parent—are permanent and continue to exist even though they are out of sight or changed in some way. For example, infants will search for a block hidden by a blanket, knowing the block still exists. Infants will know that a parent remains the same person whether dressed in a robe and slippers or pants and a T-shirt. Infants learn that they are a separate entity from their playthings. They learn where their body stops and their bed or parent begins. A great deal of the mouthing and handling of objects by infants and the delight of watching a caregiver appear is part of primary and secondary schema and discovering **permanence** (Figure 27-5). The world begins to make sense and the developmental task of achieving trust falls into place when the concept of permanence has been learned (infants know their parents exist and will return to them). Gaining a concept of permanence also contributes to "eighth month anxiety," a stage in which infants continue to cry for their parents because they know their parents still exist even when out of sight.

During the final phase of the infant year (coordination of secondary reactions), infants begin to demonstrate goal-directed behavior. After noticing that hitting a mobile makes it move, infants then reach for and hit a music box nearby, in this way actively seeking new experiences. It is important that infants have enough stimulating objects around for exploring so that experimenting and learning can proceed in this way (Marino, 1991).

Toddler

The toddler period is one of transition as children complete the final stages of the sensorimotor period (defined in Table 27-3 as tertiary circular reaction and invention of new means) and begin to develop some cognitive skills of the preoperative period, such as symbolic thought and egocentric thinking. In the *tertiary circular reaction schema,* children use trial and error to discover new characteristics of objects and events. Toddlers sit-

Bobby is a 2-year-old who is hospitalized for osteomyelitis (infection) of his femur. He will be on bed rest for 2 weeks with continuous intravenous therapy. The following is a nursing care plan that focuses on helping Bobby achieve a sense of autonomy.

Assessment: Child answers "no" to almost all questions. Insists on feeding and dressing himself. Is toilet trained during daytime. Mother will be with him during the day; father to sleep over at night while mother cares for 3-month-old infant at home. Father voices that he is concerned they will become too fatigued with this arrangement, but is unable to think of a better plan.

Nursing Diagnosis: High risk for ineffective family coping, compromised, related to hospitalization and the difficulty for parents to make arrangements to be continually present

Defining Characteristic: Parents state that hospitalization is a stress for the family.

Goal: Family members will demonstrate adequate coping behaviors throughout hospital admission.

Outcome Criteria: Parents state that they are managing adequately with long-term hospitalization.

Nursing Orders	Rationale
1. Encourage parents to continue to discuss child care options with family members to see if there isn't someone who could visit for short periods to relieve one of parents.	1. Helps parents "brainstorm" solutions to their problem.
2. Arrange for primary nursing assignment for child.	2. With primary nursing, Bobby has to adjust to just a few nurses; parents will feel secure leaving their child for short time periods if they are familiar with the nurses.

(continued)

ting in a high chair and dropping objects over the edge of the tray are exploring both permanence and the different actions of toys. During the schema of "invention of new means," children are able to think through actions or mentally project the solution to a problem. If given a box, children will investigate how the top of the box can be removed; if given a second box, even one that varies in shape, children can foresee how the top can be removed. Toddlers following a ball that has rolled under a coffee table no longer have to follow the ball's path to retrieve it but can project where it rolled and walk around the coffee table to find it again.

During the period of **preoperational thought**, children relearn on a conceptual level some of the lessons they mastered as infants at the sensorimotor level, before having language. Now, children are able to use symbols to represent objects. However, they are unable to view one object as necessarily being different from another. On a walk through a department store, for example, children do not know whether they are seeing a succession of toys or if the same ones keep reappearing. They draw conclusions only from obvious facts they see: Daddy is shaving; therefore he must be going to work, because he went to work after he shaved yesterday. This type of faulty reasoning (prelogical reasoning) will lead children to wrong conclusions and will make their judgment faulty as well. How children think has many implications for nursing. If a nurse made John's bed yesterday and then he went to surgery, he may cry at the sight of you approaching with clean sheets today, thinking he will have to go to surgery again.

Preschooler

Piaget sees preschool children as moving on to a substage of preoperational thought termed **intuitive thought**. During this time, neither the properties of **conservation** (the ability to discern truth, even though physical properties change) or **reversibility** (ability to retrace steps) are present. For example, if preschoolers see beads being poured from one glass into another

Nursing Diagnosis: High risk for altered growth and development related to partial immobilization by continuous administration of intravenous therapy

Defining Characteristic: Bed rest is prescribed due to medical condition.

Goal: Child will continue to achieve developmental stage (autonomy) during hospital experience.

Outcome Criteria: Child demonstrates sense of autonomy through attempting dressing self and other self-care measures.

Nursing Orders	Rationale
1. Speak to nutritionist about including finger foods on meal trays for Bobby.	1. Encourages sense of autonomy through self-feeding.
2. Advocate for intravenous line placement in foot or nondominant hand.	2. Allows Bobby use of hands to feed himself and engage in play.
3. Change to training pants in the morning; place potty seat on floor by crib so Bobby can be helped to use it with intravenous line in place.	3. Continuing with toilet training will encourage Bobby's sense of autonomy.
4. Allow Bobby to wear own clothes and dress himself as much as possible within limits of intravenous therapy.	4. Dressing himself will promote independence.
5. Place toys that require action, such as pound-a-peg or toy trucks, within easy reach.	5. Provides age-appropriate stimulation (and distraction from IV line).
6. Allow choices whenever possible; do not offer a choice unless it is truly a choice.	6. Making choices is one of the best ways for any child to demonstrate independence and control.

glass that is taller and thinner, they will usually say that there are now more beads in the second glass (because the level has risen), or that there are fewer beads (because the second glass is narrower), even when told that no beads have been added or removed. When the beads are poured back into the first glass, they still will not understand that the number of beads is unchanged. This immature perception leads children, as it did during the toddler period, to make faulty conclusions. It takes more years of development for children to learn that when thought processes (i.e., they *know* the number of beads did not change) and perceptions conflict, thought processes are more trustworthy.

"Centering" is the tendency to look at an object and see only one of its characteristics (seeing that a banana is yellow but not noticing that it is also long). Centering also contributes to children's faulty conclusion that the number of beads changes when poured from one glass to another (only the characteristic of changing height was noticed). This is noticeable when children are learn-ing about medicine (they observe that it tastes bitter, but cannot understand that it is also good for them).

Preschool thinking is also influenced by **role fantasy**, or how children would like something to turn out. Children use **assimilation** (taking in) information and change it to fit their existing ideas. For example, because a child wants to go outside and play, he or she says that the outside wants him or her to come outside. Children believe that wishes are as real as facts; that dreams are as real as daytime happenings. They perceive animals and even inanimate objects as being capable of movement or thought and feeling (saying that the dog took the doll because the dog was feeling sad). Later, children learn **accommodation,** or change their ideas to fit reality rather than the reverse. **Egocentrism**, or perceiving that one's thoughts and needs are better or more important than those of others, is also strong during this period. Preschoolers are unable to believe that not everyone knows facts they know, and if asked "What is your name?" may reply "Don't you know my name?" Children

Table 27-3. *Piaget's Stages of Cognitive Development*

Stage of Development	Age Span	Nursing Implications
Sensorimotor		
Neonatal reflex	1 mo	Stimuli are assimilated into beginning mental images. Behavior entirely reflexive.
Primary circular reaction	1–4 mo	Hand–mouth and ear–eye coordination develop. Infant spends much time looking at objects and separating self from them. Beginning intention of behavior is present (the infant brings thumb to mouth for a purpose: to suck it). Enjoyable activity for this period: a rattle or tape of parent's voice.
Secondary circular reaction	4–8 mo	Infant learns to initiate, recognize, and repeat pleasurable experiences from environment. Memory traces are present; infant anticipates familiar events (a parent coming near him will pick him up). Good toy for this period: mirror; good game: peek-a-boo.
Coordination of secondary reactions	8–12 mo	Infant can plan activities to attain specific goals. Perceives that others can cause activity and that activities of own body are separate from activity of objects. Can search for and retrieve toy that disappears from view. Recognizes shapes and sizes of familiar objects. Because of increased sense of separateness, infant experiences separation anxiety when primary caregiver leaves. Good toy for this period: nesting toys (i.e., colored boxes).
Tertiary circular reaction	12–18 mo	Child is able to experiment to discover new properties of objects and events. Capable of space perception and time perception as well as permanence. Objects outside self are understood as causes of actions. Good game for this period: throw and retrieve.
Invention of new means through mental combinations	18–24 mo	Transitional phase to the preoperational thought period. Uses memory and imitation to act. Can solve basic problems, foresee maneuvers that will succeed or fail. Good toys for this period: those with several uses, such as blocks, colored plastic rings.
Preoperational Thought	2–7 yr	Thought becomes more symbolic; can arrive at answers mentally instead of through physical attempt. Comprehends simple abstractions but thinking is basically concrete and literal. Child is egocentric (unable to see the viewpoint of another). Displays static thinking (inability to remember what he or she started to talk about so that at the end of a sentence the child is talking about another topic). Concept of time is now and concept of distance is only as far as he or she can see. Centering or focusing on a single aspect of an object causes distorted reasoning. No awareness of reversibility (for every action there is an opposite action) is present. Unable to state cause–effect relationships, categories, or abstractions. Good toy for this period: items that require imagination, such as modeling clay.
Concrete Operational Thought	7–12 yr	Concrete operations includes systematic reasoning. Uses memory to learn broad concepts (fruit) and subgroups of concepts (apples, oranges). Classifications involve sorting objects according to attributes such as color; seriation, in which objects are ordered according to increasing or decreasing measures such as weight; multiplication, in which objects are simultaneously classified and seriated using weight. Child is aware of reversibility, an opposite operation or continuation of reasoning back to a starting point (follows a route through a maze and then reverses steps). Understands conservation, sees constancy despite transformation (mass or quantity remains the same even if it changes shape or position). Good activity for this period: collecting and classifying natural objects such as native plants, sea shells, etc. Expose child to other viewpoints by asking questions such as, "How do you think you'd feel if you were a nurse and had to tell a boy to stay in bed?"
Formal Operational Thought	12 yr	Can solve hypothetical problems with scientific reasoning; understands causality and can deal with the past, present, and future. Adult or mature thought. Good activity for this period: "talk time" to sort through attitudes and opinions.

(From Piaget, J. [1961]. *The growth of logical thinking from childhood to adolescence.* New York: Basic Books, with permission.)

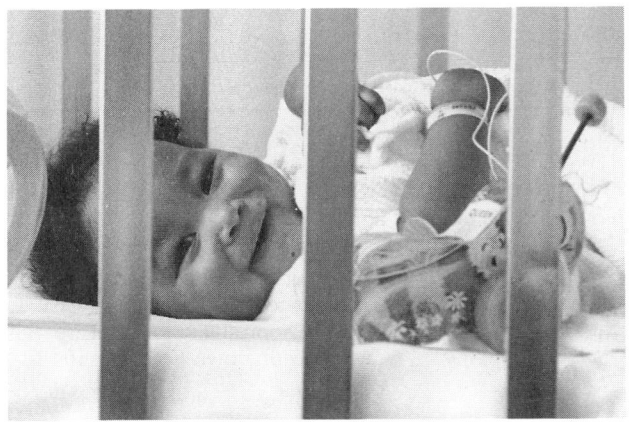

FIGURE 27-5
The infant has discovered permanence when he can tell that objects or people still exist even when out of sight. (Courtesy, Department of Medical Photography, Children's Hospital, Buffalo, NY.)

define objects mainly in relation to themselves, so that a spoon is "what I eat with," not just a curved metal object.

School-Age Child

Piaget viewed school age as a period during which **concrete operational thought** begins. School-age children are able to discover concrete solutions to everyday problems. By understanding that beads do not change in number just because they are poured from one glass to another, children have grasped the concept of conservation. Conservation of numbers is learned as early as age 7 years, of quantity at age 7 or 8 years, of weight at age 9 years, and volume at age 11 years (Wadsworth, 1989). Reasoning during school age tends to be inductive, proceeding from specific to general. Thus, school-age children can reason that a toy they are holding is broken, that the toy is made of plastic, and that all plastic toys break easily.

Adolescent

Piaget sees adolescence as the time when cognition achieves its final form, that of **formal operational thought**. When this stage is reached, adolescents are capable of thinking in terms of possibility—what could be—rather than being limited to thinking about what already is (**abstract thought**). This makes it possible for adolescents to use scientific reasoning.

Moral Development

Children pass through stages of moral development as well as cognitive and psychosocial development. These stages have been described by Kohlberg (1984) and are summarized in Table 27-4. Recognizing these stages can help identify how a child may feel about an illness (e.g., whether or not the child thinks of it as "bad"). Recogniz-

ing moral reasoning also helps in determining whether the child can be depended on to carry out self-care activities such as self-administered medicine, that is, whether the child has internalized standards of conduct so he or she does not "cheat" when away from external control. Moral stages closely approximate cognitive stages of development, because a child must be able to think abstractly (be able to conceptualize an idea without a concrete picture) before being able to understand how rules apply to him or her, even when no one is there to enforce them.

Infant

The infant period is a **prereligious stage**. Infants have little concept of any motivating force beyond that of their parents. Infants learn that when they do certain actions, parents give affection and approval; for other actions, parents scold and label the behavior as "bad." The development of trust is important in moral development, because infants who have developed a sound sense of trust are better able to develop a spiritual orientation in future years and thus be bound by a moral conscience (they can trust in a spiritual being as well as humans around them).

Nursing actions to support this stage of development are to give praise for doing as asked. Appreciate that the average infant is trying hard to please; if he or she falls short of doing this it is probably due to immature development rather than any effort to displease.

Toddler

Toddlers begin to formulate a sense of right and wrong, but their reason for doing right is centered most strongly in "mother or father says so" rather than in any spiritual or societal motivation. Kohlberg refers to this as a punishment obedience orientation (the child is good because a parent says the child must be, not because it is "right" to be good).

Toddlers may not obey a nurse's requests (e.g., "Lie still while I change your dressing"), because they do not view the nurse's authority as being at the same level as their parents' authority. It might be necessary to ask a parent to reinforce instructions to be certain that the toddler will follow them.

Preschooler

Preschoolers tend to do good out of self-interest rather than out of true intent to do good or because of a strong spiritual motivation. When asked why it is wrong to steal from a neighbor, for example, the preschooler will answer, "Because my mother says it's wrong." Children at this age imitate what they see, so if they see less-than-perfect role modeling, they may copy those wrong actions and assume those actions are correct. Preschoolers have great difficulty handling new situations, because they are unable to judge whether a previously learned

T a b l e   2 7 - 4. *Kohlberg's Stages of Moral Development*

Age (Year)	Stage	Description	Nursing Implications
Preconventional (Level I)			
2–3	1	Punishment/obedience orientation ("heteronomous morality"). Child does right because a parent tells him or her to and to avoid punishment.	Child needs help to determine what are right actions. Give clear instructions to avoid confusion.
4–7	2	Individualism. Instrumental purpose and exchange. Carries out actions to satisfy own needs rather than society's. Will do something for another if that person does something for the child.	Child is unable to recognize that like situations require like actions. Unable to take responsibility for self-care, because meeting own needs interferes with this.
Conventional (Level II)			
7–10	3	Orientation to interpersonal relations of mutuality. Child follows rules because of a need to be a "good" person in own eyes and the eyes of others.	Child enjoys helping others because this is "nice" behavior. Allow child to help with bed making and other like activities. Praise for desired behavior such as sharing.
10–12	4	Maintenance of social order, fixed rules and authority. Child finds following rules satisfying. Follows rules of authority figures as well as parents in an effort to keep the "system" working.	Child often asks what are the rules and is something "right." May have difficulty modifying a procedure because one method may not be "right." Follows self-care measures only if someone is there to enforce them.
Postconventional (Level III)			
Older than 12	5	Social contract, utilitarian law-making perspectives. Follows standards of society for the good of all people.	An adolescent can be responsible for self-care because he or she views this as a standard of adult behavior.
	6	Universal ethical principle orientation. Follows internalized standards of conduct.	Many adults do not reach this level of moral development.

(From Kohlberg, L. [1984]. *The psychology of moral development*. New York: Harper & Row, with permission.)

principle of right or wrong can be applied to this new situation. Because of egocentrism, a preschooler will do things for others only in return for things done for him or her. This means it may be necessary to remind the child of actions taken on his or her behalf or trade off actions (e.g., "Lie still now for me while I change your dressing and I'll read you a story when I'm through").

School-Age Child

School-age children enter a stage of moral development termed **conventional development**, the level at which many adults function. Young school-age children adhere to a phase of development termed the "nice girl, nice boy" stage. Children engage in actions that are "nice" rather than necessarily right. Sharing, for example, is "nice." Stealing is not. Young school-age children may lie about their actions to disguise that they have been involved in an action that is not "nice."

When asked why it is wrong to steal from a neighbor, the school-age child most often answers, "Because it's not nice" or "The police will arrest you." School-age children may have difficulty following self-care measures reliably when out of a nurse's or parent's sight, be-

cause they feel it is necessary to obey rules only when the rules can be clearly enforced.

Adolescent

As adolescents become capable of abstract thought, they are capable of internalizing standards of conduct (they do what they think is right regardless of whether they have social rules). This is termed **postconventional development**. In this stage, if asked why it is wrong to steal from a neighbor, the adolescent will answer, "Because it deprives the neighbor of possessions he or she has earned." Adolescents are capable of carrying out self-care measures even when someone else is not present, because they are capable of understanding not only the importance of the measures to themselves but also the principle that certain things should be done simply because they are right. Many adolescents do not enter this phase of development, however, and as adults they continue to act like school-age children, doing right things only when obvious authority or set rules are present. Kohlberg's theory is currently being challenged as being male-oriented because his original research was conducted entirely with boys. Gilligan (1982) suggests that girls do not score well on Kohlberg's scale because, being more concerned with relationships than men, they make moral decisions differently.

Temperament

Temperament can be defined as the usual reaction pattern of an individual or an individual's characteristic manner of thinking, behaving, or reacting to stimuli in the environment (Chess & Thomas, 1985). Unlike cognitive or moral development, temperament is not developed by stages but is an inborn characteristic.

It is important to explore the concept of temperament with parents at child health assessments. Awareness that children are not all alike—some adapt quickly to new situations and others adapt slowly, and some react intensely and some passively—will help parents to better understand their child and therefore to care for the child more constructively (Sheeber & Johnson, 1992).

Reaction Patterns

In assessing the temperament of a child, Chess and Thomas have identified nine separate characteristics that define *reactivity patterns*. Each child's pattern is made up of these individual elements as described below.

Activity Level. The level of activity among children differs widely. Some babies are constantly on the go and rarely quiet. They wiggle and squirm in their crib as early as age 2 weeks. Parents put such children to sleep in one end of a crib and find them in the other end 1 hour later; such children will not stay seated in bathtubs and refuse to be confined in playpens. Other babies, by contrast, move little, stay where they are placed, and appear to take in their environment in a quieter, more docile way. Both patterns are normal; they merely reflect two extremes of motor activity, one characteristic of temperament.

Rhythmicity. A child who has **rhythmicity** manifests a regular rhythm in physiologic functions. Even as infants, such children tend to awake at the same time each morning, are hungry at regular 4-hour periods, nap the same time every day, and have a bowel movement the same time every day. They are predictable and easy to care for in that their parents learn early what to expect from them. On the other end of the scale are infants with an irregular rhythmicity. They rarely awaken at the same time 2 days in a row. They may go a long time without eating one day and the next day appear hungry almost immediately after a feeding. Such children may be difficult to care for because it is not easy to plan a schedule for them, and parents must constantly adapt their own routines to the child's.

Approach. **Approach** refers to a child's response on initial contact with a new stimulus. Some children approach new situations in an unruffled manner. They smile and "talk" to strangers and accept a first feeding or a new food without spitting up or fussing. They explore new toys without apprehension. Other infants demonstrate withdrawal rather than approach to this kind of situation. They cry at the sight of strangers, new toys, and new foods, and the first time they are placed in a bathtub. They are difficult to take on vacation because they react so fearfully to new situations.

Adaptability. **Adaptability** is the ability to change one's reaction to stimuli over time. Infants who are adaptable change their first reaction to situations without exhibiting extreme distress. The first time such children are placed in a bathtub they might protest loudly, for example, but by the third time they sit splashing happily. This is in contrast to infants who cry for months whenever they are put into a bathtub or who cannot seem to accustom themselves to a new bed, new playpen, or new caregiver.

Intensity of Reaction. Some children react to situations with their whole being. They cry loudly, thrash their arms, and begin temper tantrums when their diapers are wet, when they are hungry, and when their parents leave them. Others rarely demonstrate such overt symptoms of anger or have a mild or low-intensity reaction to stress.

Distractability. Children who are easily distracted or have **distractability** can be easily managed. As infants, they are diverted and calmed by a pacifier. If they are crying over the loss of a toy, they can be appeased by the offer of a new one. Others cannot be distracted. Their parents may describe them as stubborn, willful, or unwilling to compromise.

Attention Span and Persistence. **Attention span** is the ability to remain interested in a project or activity, and varies among infants. Some play by themselves with one toy for 1 hour; others spend no more than 1 or 2 minutes with each toy. Degree of persistence also varies. Some infants keep trying to perform an activity even when they fail time after time; others stop trying after one unsuccessful attempt.

Threshold of Response. The **threshold of response** is the intensity level of stimulation that is necessary to evoke a reaction. Children with a low threshold need little stimulation; those with a high threshold need intense stimulation before they demonstrate a change in behavior.

Mood Quality. The child who is always happy and laughing can be said to have a positive **mood quality**. Obviously, mood pattern can make a major difference in the parents' enjoyment of a child. Parents who have fun with their child are bound to spend more time with him or her than parents whose child reacts negatively.

Nursing Implications Regarding Temperament

Children who have a normal activity level and regular rhythmicity, who approach and adapt to new situations easily, who have a long attention span, a high level of persistence, and a positive mood quality are "ideal" or "easy" children to care for, from a parent's point of view. Highly active infants are much more difficult for new parents to learn to care for, especially if they demonstrate irregular physiologic rhythms, withdrawal rather than approach, and little ability to adapt. They require more planning and creative distraction measures.

It is useful to talk to parents about their child's reactivity patterns at health maintenance visits because these patterns tend to persist. The way children will react in the future depends a great deal on their current pattern of behavior. The child who withdraws from rather than approach a first toy may react in the same way to toilet-training or starting day care. The parents of such a child will need to focus on preparing him or her for new activities more than will the parents of a child who approaches new situations easily. Those who are aware that their baby shies away from new experiences such as baths and new foods will be able to take it in stride when the child is slow to adapt to a Head Start program at age 4 years; they will know it is their child's method of coping.

It is good anticipatory guidance to bring these characteristics to parents' attention. Understanding their child is the beginning of acceptance and having respect for the child as an individual and is essential for successful childrearing.

It is important to notice a child's temperamental characteristics when he or she is admitted to a hospital so that the child's reactions to procedures or pain can be anticipated. A child with a mild reactivity pattern, for example, may not show a great deal of response to even acute pain, but a child with an intense pattern may react as strongly to minor discomfort as to major pain, making it difficult to evaluate the true level of pain the child is experiencing. A child who is slow to adapt may need to have a procedure explained repeatedly before being able to accept it.

Carey and McDevitt (1978) developed an Infant Temperament Questionnaire that can be used as a screening tool for temperament in infants; it is described in Chapter 28 with other assessment tools.

Key Points

- Nurses use knowledge of growth and development to promote health and prevent illness through assessment and anticipatory guidance.
- Genetic factors that influence growth and development are gender, race and nationality, intelligence, and health. Environmental influences include quality of nutrition, socioeconomic level, parent–child relationship, ordinal position in the family, and environmental health.
- Common theories of development are Freud's psychoanalytic theory and Erikson's theory of psychosocial development. Both of these theories describe specific tasks, which children which complete at each stage of development in order to mature to a well-adapted adult.
- Piaget's theory of cognitive development describes ways that children learn. Kohlberg has advanced a theory of moral development or how children use moral reasoning to solve problems they face.
- Temperament is a child's characteristic manner of thinking, behaving, or reacting. Chess and Thomas (1985) have described an "easy to care for child" and a "difficult child" based on temperament. Helping parents understand the effect of temperament is a nursing role.
- Although growth and development occur in known patterns, their rate varies from child to child. Caution parents not to be concerned because two siblings are different as long as they both fit within usual parameters.

Critical Thinking Exercises

1. Mrs. Peters is a mother who describes her two children as "totally different." One is shy and quiet and agreeable and one is aggressive and persistent. What characteristic is Mrs. Peters describing? Which child does she probably view as easiest to care for? What anticipatory guidance could you give her to help her better understand these differences in her children?

2. Joey is a 2-year-old from a family whose parents want him to achieve well in life. They ask you what specific steps they should take to foster high achievement in Joey. What advice would you give them?

3. Children who are hospitalized for long periods may fall behind in development. What specific measures could you take to promote developmental growth and encourage a sense of autonomy in a hospitalized 2-year-old? To promote a sense of industry in a hospitalized 10-year-old?

References

Carey, W. B., & McDevitt, S. (1978). Stability and change in individual temperament diagnoses from infancy to early childhood. *American Academy of Child Psychiatry, 17,* 331.

Chess, S., & Thomas, A. (1985). Temperamental differences: A critical concept in child health care. *Pediatric Nursing, 11,* 167.

Department of Health and Human Services. (1991). *Healthy people 2000.* Washington, DC: Public Health Service.

Erikson, E. H. (1985). *Childhood and society.* New York: W. W. Norton.

Geissler, E. M. (1994). *Pocket guide to cultural assessment.* St. Louis: C. V. Mosby.

Gilligan, C. (1982). *In a different voice: Psychological theory and women's development.* Cambridge, MA: Harvard University Press.

Gillis, A. J. (1990). Nurses' knowledge of growth and development principles in meeting psychosocial needs of hospitalized children. *Journal of Pediatric Nursing, 5,* 78.

Glass, P. (1994). The vulnerable neonatal and the neonatal intensive care environment. In Avery, G., et al. *Neonatalogy* (4th ed.). Philadelphia: J. B. Lippincott.

Kohlberg, L. (1984). *The psychology of moral development.* New York: Harper & Row.

Levy-Shiff, R., et al. (1990). Father's hospital visits to their preterm infants as a predictor of father-infant relationship and infant development. *Pediatrics, 86,* 289.

Marino, B. L. (1991). Studying infant and toddler play. *Journal of Pediatric Nursing, 6,* 16.

Robinson, P. (1993). *Freud and his critics.* Berkeley: University of California Press.

Sheeber, L., & Johnson, J. (1992). Child temperament, maternal adjustment, and changes in family life style. *American Journal of Orthopsychiatry, 62,* 178.

Schuster, S., & Ashburn, A. (1991). *The process of human development: A holistic life span approach* (3rd ed.). Philadelphia: J. B. Lippincott.

U. S. Department of Commerce Bureau of the Census (1992). *Poverty in the United States.* Washington, D. C.: Author.

Wadsworth, B. J. (1989). *Piaget's theory of cognitive and affective development* (4th ed.). New York: Longman.

Wegman, M. E. (1993). Annual summary of vital statistics. *Pediatrics, 92,* 743.

Suggested Readings

Canam, C. (1993). Common adaptive tasks facing parents of children with chronic conditions. *Journal of Advanced Nursing, 18,* 46.

Curtis, S. (1992). Promoting health through a developmental analysis of adolescent risk behavior. *Journal of School Health, 62,* 47.

Holaday, B. (1993). Adolescent literature as a means of studying growth and development. *Journal of Nursing Education, 32,* 93.

Kattner, L. (1991). Helpful strategies in working with pre-school children in pediatric practice. *Pediatric Annals, 20,* 120.

Mayfair, A. (1992). Supporting the child with special needs. *Canadian Nurse, 88,* 17.

McConachie, H. (1990). Early language development and severe visual impairment. *Child Care, Health, and Development, 16,* 55.

Prizant, B. M., et al. (1993). Communication and language assessment for young children. *Infants and Young Children, 5,* 20.

Yates, S. R. (1992). The school nurse's role: early intervention with preschool children. *Journal of School Nursing, 8,* 30.

Yoos, H. L. (1994). Children's illness concepts: Old and new paradigms. *Pediatric Nursing, 20,* 134.

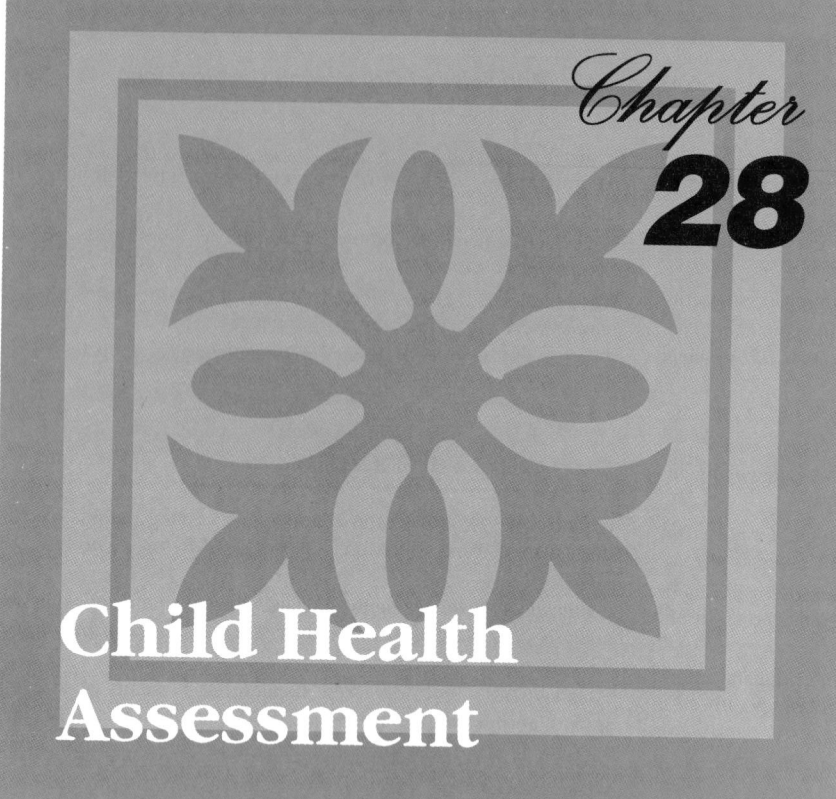

Chapter 28

Child Health Assessment

Objectives

After mastering the contents of this chapter, you should be able to:

1. State the purposes for health assessment in children of all ages.
2. Assess a child and family by health interview, physical examination, and development screening.
3. Formulate nursing diagnoses based on health assessment findings.
4. Plan nursing care based on health assessment findings such as informing parents of health deviations.
5. Implement nursing care such as conducting an age-appropriate health interview or physical examination by modifying techniques based on the child's age.
6. Evaluate outcome criteria to be certain that established goals were achieved.
7. Identify National Health Goals related to health assessment of children that nurses can be instrumental in helping the nation to achieve.
8. Identify areas related to health assessment of children that could benefit from additional nursing research.
9. Use critical thinking to analyze ways that health assessment skills can be incorporated into nursing care procedures.
10. Synthesize nursing process with knowledge of health assessment to achieve quality maternal and child health nursing care.

Key Terms

- audiogram
- auscultation
- bruit
- chief concern
- cognitive learning
- conjunctivitis
- deep tendon reflexes
- diaphragmatic excursion
- epispadias
- esotropia
- exotropia
- fasciculations
- general appearance
- geographic tongue
- gingivae
- hordeolum
- hydrocele
- hypospadias
- inspection
- intelligence
- intercostal spaces
- kwashiorkor
- palpation
- percussion
- physiologic splitting
- point of maximum impulse
- ptosis
- retractions
- review of systems
- sinus arrhythmia
- strabismus
- superficial reflexes
- temperament
- tinea capitis
- turgor
- varicocele

Adele Pillitteri: MATERNAL AND CHILD
HEALTH NURSING, 2nd Edition. © 1995
Adele Pillitteri.

■ **NURSING PROCESS OVERVIEW**
for Health Assessment of the
Child and Family

ASSESSMENT

NURSING DIAGNOSIS

PLANNING

IMPLEMENTATION

EVALUATION

Health History: Establishing a Data Base

Health Interview
Interview Setting
Types of Questions Asked

Conducting a Health Interview
Introduction and Explanation
Chief Concern
Family Profile
Pregnancy History
History of Past Illnesses
Day History
Family Illness History
Review of Systems
Conclusion

Physical Assessment

Purpose and Techniques

Equipment, Setting, and Approach

Variations for Age and Developmental Stage
Newborn
Infant
Toddler and Preschooler
School-Age Child and Adolescent

Components of Physical Examination

Vital Sign Assessment

General Appearance

Mental Status Assessment

Body Measurements
Weight
Height
Head Circumference
Chest and Abdominal Circumference

Skin
Newborn and Infant
Preschool and School-Age Child
Adolescent

Head
Newborn and Infant
Preschool and School-Age Child
Adolescent

Eyes
Newborn and Infant
Preschool and School-Age Child
Adolescent

Nose
Newborn and Infant
Preschool and School-Age Child
Adolescent

Ears
Newborn and Infant
Preschool and School-Age Child

Mouth
Newborn and Infant
Preschool and School-Age Child

Neck
Newborn and Infant
Adolescent

Chest

Breasts
Newborn
School-Age Child and Adolescent

Lungs
Newborn and Infant

Heart
Heart Sounds
Newborn and Infant
School-Age Child and Adolescent

Abdomen
Newborn and Infant
Preschool and School-Age Child

Genitorectal Area
Female Genitalia
Male Genitalia
Inguinal Hernia

Extremities

Back

Neurologic Function
Motor and Sensory Function

Vision Assessment

Vision Screening
Newborn and Infant
Toddler and Preschool Child
School-Age Child and Adolescent

Techniques of Vision Testing
Snellen Chart
Preschool E Chart
National Association of the Prevention of Blindness Home Chart
Allen Cards
Stycar Cards
Titmus Vision Tester
Cover Testing
Color Vision Deficit Testing

Vision Referrals

Hearing Assessment

Auditory Screening
Newborn and Infant
Older Child

Principles of Audiometric Assessment
Frequency
Loudness
Hearing Loss

Acoustic Impedance Testing

Conduction Loss Testing
Rinne Test
Weber's Test

Speech Assessment

Denver Articulation Screening Examination
Administration
Scoring

Developmental Appraisal

Developmental History

Denver Developmental Screening Test
Administration
Scoring
Prescreening Test

Intelligence

Goodenough-Harris Drawing Test

Temperament

Concluding a Health Assessment

Nursing assessment is not only the first step in the nursing process, it is also the fundamental means by which a nurse establishes and maintains contact with a child and family. Child health assessment is especially important as an opportunity to provide families with information about health promotion, signs of health and illness, and expected developmental progress in children. This anticipatory guidance can have a long-lasting positive impact on the health of the child and family.

Assessment for the maternal-child population requires that a nurse first be familiar with health maintenance standards and usual findings. This knowledge is essential to the ability to recognize illness. Most health screening procedures are performed in ambulatory settings (e.g., well-child conferences, physicians' offices, health maintenance organizations, community clinics, and schools), but they can be used to evaluate children in all settings.

Sometimes it is necessary to complete just a partial history or a partial physical examination, as when a child is referred for vision examination. This chapter, however, covers all aspects of the physical examination so that, when necessary, a complete examination can be performed. Procedures specific to a particular illness appear in later chapters with the illness they detect. The Focus on National Health Goals box lists goals related to health assessment.

NURSING PROCESS OVERVIEW
for Health Assessment of the Child and Family

ASSESSMENT

Health assessment of children can be a positive, educational experience for the child and family if time is taken to listen carefully to their concerns and responses to questions. Never rush either an interview or a physical examination: the child needs time to familiarize himself or herself with the environment and equipment that will be used.

NURSING DIAGNOSIS

Health assessment provides the data used to identify potential problems and serves as the basis for the establishment of nursing diagnoses. Be certain not to overlook diagnoses that accentuate the healthy functioning of the child and family, even when diagnoses that address specific problems have been identified. These wellness diagnoses are crucial components of the entire assessment picture and often provide an avenue for ad-

dressing identified problems. For instance, the nursing diagnosis of Impaired social interaction related to lack of self-esteem secondary to disability would be appropriate for a 4-year-old confined to a wheelchair who, according to the parents, feels uncomfortable when around other children. If the parents have difficulty adapting to their child's disability but are eager to accept advice from health care experts on how to provide the most stimulating environment for their child, the diagnosis Potential for enhanced parenting would also be appropriate. Using both these diagnoses allows a care plan to be developed that best takes advantage of this family's strengths.

PLANNING

Nursing diagnoses serve as the basis for planning nursing interventions. Health promotion and illness prevention are vital parts of this process. Help parents plan for their child's next developmental stage; keep them aware of important safety measures and other ways to keep children well. Remind them about immunizations needed in the future and make sure they know when to schedule the next health visit.

IMPLEMENTATION

Health interviewing and physical examination both require a great deal of skill—skill that can only be perfected through practice. To perfect skills and judgment with children of different ages, take advantage of every opportunity to practice interviewing and physical examination techniques.

EVALUATION

Health assessment of children is an ongoing process that does not end when the first data base is obtained. The data must be added to at all future interactions so it remains current and meaningful. Examples of outcome criteria would be:

- Parents state they are satisfied with child's motor development following health exam.
- Child states he or she is aware that his or her vision needs correction following Snellen test.
- Parents state they will continue to assess child's growth by weighing child weekly.

Health History: Establishing a Data Base

The assessment of a young child begins with an interview of the child's parents. An adolescent or preadolescent may choose to be interviewed without parents present, though many preadolescents and adolescents still prefer to have a parent with them as support.

Health Interview

The purpose of a health interview is to gather information that will supplement physical or laboratory examinations to complete a thorough health evaluation (Fred et al., 1994). An extensive interview elicits such facts as parents' problems in childrearing or detecting future health problems (Figure 28-1). Interviewing to obtain a data base is a skill that is learned with practice. A number of important principles of child health interviewing are reviewed below.

Interview Setting

An interview is best conducted in a private room with all parties seated comfortably; if not seated, a health care provider appears rushed. Let parents know that their input and opinions about how their child is developing

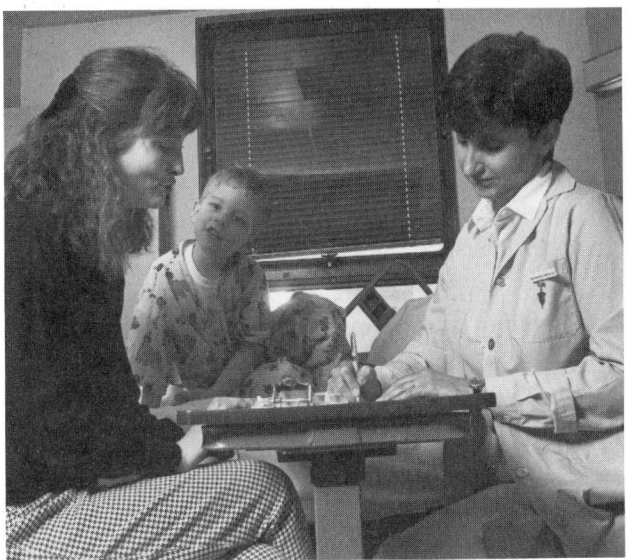

FIGURE 28-1
Health assessment begins with an interview. Allow children as active a part as possible in the assessment process. (Courtesy of the Department of Medical Photography, Children's Hospital, Buffalo, NY.)

are valued by calling them by their names during the interview. A question such as "Does John sit up yet, Mr. Wiser?" is far more personal and a better form than "Does baby sit up yet?"

Types of Questions Asked

The phrasing of questions varies, depending on the type of answer desired. Fact-finding and open-ended questions are two types of effective questions; compound, expansive, and leading questions, on the other hand, are three types to avoid.

Fact-Finding Question. This simplest form of question asks directly for a fact: "Does John walk yet?" "Did you take John's temperature?" This is an effective type of question if a particular point is being sought. It is limited in scope, however, because the response usually will be only a yes or no, with no further elaboration.

Open-Ended Question. An open-ended question allows the parent to elaborate. In contrast to "Did you take John's temperature?" the question "What did you do for John?" is open-ended. The parent answers with a listing of all the things he or she did; the parent took John's temperature, had him lie on the couch, gave him extra fluid, and so on.

Compound Question. Compound questions are confusing and should be avoided because the information they elicit is often inaccurate and must be followed by a clarifying question. An example is, "Did John have nausea and vomiting?" The parent answers yes, but it still is not known whether John had vomiting and nausea, just vomiting, or just nausea.

Expansive Question. This is an open-ended question gone wrong because it is too broad to answer. "What can you tell me about John?" leaves a parent wondering where to start. "How has John been since his last visit?" limits the question and makes it answerable.

Leading Question. A leading question supplies its own answer, and thus should be avoided. "John has had all his immunizations, hasn't he?" implies that John should have had them and that the parent is somehow a poor caregiver if he or she answers that question any way but yes. The penalty for such an exchange could be a child left vulnerable to disease.

Conducting a Health Interview

Data gathering for an initial health assessment can be divided into eight categories: (1) introduction and explanation, (2) chief concern, (3) family profile, (4) pregnancy history, (5) history of past illnesses, (6) day history, (7) family illness history, and (8) review of systems. At return visits, the categories that would be used are generally introduction and explanation, chief concern, family profile, interval history, and day history.

Introduction and Explanation

Parents and the child should be told as a matter of courtesy to whom they are talking and what they will be talking about. A short explanation and introduction such as, "Hello, Ms. Wiser, I'm Janet Dickson, a nurse here in the One Day Surgery Department. I'd like to talk to you about John this morning," is an example of a suitable introduction. Because some families have never had the benefit of in-depth health care, it is helpful to include, as well, a statement about the subjects that will be discussed during the interview, for example, "So that I can get a picture of John's overall health, I'll be asking you questions about why you've brought him here today, your pregnancy with him, concerns you've had in the past, and questions about your typical day with John." The parent begins to concentrate on those areas because he or she realizes that the nurse is interested not just in John's health that particular day, but in his total health (see the Focus on Cultural Awareness box).

Chief Concern

After verifying information about the child's name and age, begin data collection with the reason the parents have brought the child to the health care agency: the **chief concern**. This is what parents are most concerned about, and only after they get this immediate

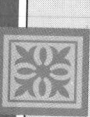

FOCUS ON CULTURAL AWARENESS

Health assessment of children is a skill that is learned with practice. Successful interviewing depends on respecting cultural variations. Whether people establish eye contact with an interviewer, for example, is a characteristic that is culturally determined. In Vietnam, touching the head of a child during physical assessment is thought to be harmful as the head is considered to be the seat of the soul (Geissler, 1994).

Findings and techniques in children also differ depending on racial and ethnic characteristics. Assessing for cyanosis, for example, is more difficult in dark-skinned than in fair-skinned children (mucous membrane is the best place to detect this). As height and weight charts are standardized on middle-class Caucasian children, measurements of children who do not fit this description may not plot well on these charts.

Recognizing that people hold differing cultural expectations and characteristics can help in establishing rapport with children and their families and help make health assessment more meaningful.

concern off their mind will they be ready to talk about other matters. An effective way to elicit this information is to ask an open-ended question such as, "Why did you bring John to the hospital today, Ms. Wiser?" Such an opening allows the parent freedom to answer in a number of areas of concern: physical, emotional, nutritional, and developmental. If asked, "How is John feeling today?" or "Is John ill?" the parent is left to think about only physical aspects and may not voice his or her biggest concern—John's teething difficulty or his frequent temper tantrums.

Once the parent has voiced this chief concern, ask him or her to describe at least six aspects of the problem: (1) duration, (2) intensity, (3) frequency, (4) description, (5) associated symptoms, and (6) actions taken. In discussing duration, it is important to know when the child was last well to determine when he or she became ill. For example, on Saturday morning John began having long crying periods. On Monday night he developed a fever. On Tuesday afternoon he was brought into the clinic for a checkup. The parent states that John vomited three times Monday morning and thinks this was caused by teething. Unless the parent is asked when John was last well, he or she may pinpoint Monday as the beginning of the illness (the vomiting) when actually it was Saturday (the crying).

The intensity of the illness refers in this instance to the kind of vomiting the child is having. Is it drooling, spitting up, or actual vomiting? The description is the amount (a cupful? a mouthful?) and color (whether it contains blood, bile, or mucus). Associated symptoms might include fever, abdominal pain, difficulty eating, or signs of respiratory illness. A good question to obtain this information is "Is John ill in any other way?"

It is important to know the parent's actions for a number of reasons. First, it is important to know whether anything a parent has been doing has been making the illness worse (e.g., offering a great deal of fluid to replace that vomited and, by doing so, causing more vomiting). It also reveals what the parent has previously tried but found ineffective. There is no use telling a parent to give the child 2 grains of acetaminophen (Tylenol) every 4 hours for fever if the parent has already done that and the fever has not improved. This information also reveals the parent's response to caring for an ill child. A parent who says "I tucked him into bed and gave him a little tea to drink" is different from one who replies, "Nothing, I fall all apart when my child is ill." If the child is going to be returned home for the parent to care for, the second parent will need more instructions and support before he or she leaves the health care setting than the first parent.

Obtaining this information about the chief concern puts the parent's observations in proper perspective. In the previous example, the parent is probably not describing teething difficulty (teething does not cause vomiting). More likely, the child has a viral gastroenteritis. Unless the problem is investigated, it is easy to accept the parent's statement at face value as a teething problem and not appreciate its full significance.

After the chief concern is documented, ask another open-ended question to elicit additional ones: "Is there anything else that worries you about John?" Now the parent might want to talk about John's temper tantrums. Unless asked about a second problem, the parent will go home with the first problem cared for well but the second one still not addressed. When the parent arrives home and John begins stomping his feet in the car, unwilling to go into the house, the parent will begin to feel the health care he or she received was less than adequate because the parent did not receive help with this concern.

Do not assume that parents will always reveal their worst fears in the initial minute of an interview: it can be frightening to put these fears into words. As long as a concern is hanging as a nebulous thought in the mind, it is easy to tell oneself that it may not be true. Only when a parent voices the thought ("Do you think that John is retarded?" "Do you think this is leukemia?" "Could this be inherited?") does the fear become real. Before parents dare to speak openly, they must trust health care providers not to treat their statement lightly. For this reason, it is helpful to repeat the question about a second concern at the very end of the interview.

Family Profile

It is helpful before pursuing any further history to learn more about the circumstances in which the child lives by obtaining a family profile. Be certain to make a transition statement before shifting from one part of an interview to another. Without a transition, the parent could be wondering what importance the questions have and may misinterpret their significance. For instance, if a parent has been describing the child's pattern of vomiting and, without a transition statement, is asked about the family's economic status, including hospital insurance, a parent may think that the child needs hospitalization when that is not the intent at all. "Before we talk about any past illnesses or happenings with Jane, let me ask you some questions about your family as a whole" is an example of a good transition statement.

It is important to ascertain socioeconomic level and means of financial support so that it can be determined whether the parent will be able to obtain prescribed care such as medication. Equally important are such questions as "Does Jane have a bed of her own in which to sleep?" "Does she have play space?" "Is there provision for outside play?" "Are there other children?" (If the child has an infectious disease, the siblings will need protection.) "Do you have emotional support in caring for Wendy?" "Do you get away from her sometimes to have a life of your own?" "Do both you and your wife work outside the home?" "How do you manage child care?"

Parents with stressful home situations are usually willing to reveal this to health care personnel. A parent who is unmarried and lives alone with a child in an upstairs apartment with no phone and no hot water wants health care providers to know these facts. Only when they are understood can the difficulties of dealing with the child's illness (and, in all probability, the child's wellness) be appreciated.

Pregnancy History

The health of children is affected by their mother's health during pregnancy. For children under age 5 years, therefore, a pregnancy history is usually obtained. In child health interviewing, document which pregnancy this was for the mother. Were there complications in past pregnancies? Abortions or miscarriages? Stillbirths? Children born prematurely? A history of the pregnancy of the child being assessed can begin with a question such as "How was your pregnancy with John?" This allows the mother to answer in physical and emotional areas. After exploring details she mentions, ask about specific events that are known to occur with pregnancy. Did the mother have the usual discomforts such as morning sickness, backache, or shortness of breath? Did she have any complications such as bleeding, falls, swelling of hands and feet, high blood pressure, or unusual weight gain? Did she take any medication? Were any x-ray films taken? Did she smoke cigarettes or drink alcohol or use recreational drugs?

Because life contingencies such as loss of finances or illness in the family during a pregnancy may affect a parent's ability to form a bond with a child, the emotional experiences of a woman during pregnancy are also important to obtain. Ask if the parents planned the pregnancy. A question such as "A lot of pregnancies come as a sort of surprise. Is that how it was with John?" or "Some unmarried women want to have children and some don't. How was it with you?" lets parents know you accept any answer they give.

Next, review labor and delivery. Were they as the woman expected them to be? How long was labor? Were there complications? Was anesthesia used for delivery? Was the baby born vertex (head first) or breech?

Ask about the health of the child at birth as well. Did the baby cry right away? Did he or she need special procedures or equipment either at birth or in the nursery? Was there cyanosis or jaundice? Did the infant go to a regular nursery? Was he or she discharged from the hospital with the mother? How did the parents feel about having a boy or girl? How did it feel for them to be new parents?

History of Past Illnesses

Ask whether the child ever had any serious illnesses. Parents do not generally think of childhood diseases such as measles, chickenpox, and mumps as serious illnesses; inquire about these separately. Has the child had any accidents? Any surgery? Parents may not think of a tonsillectomy as surgery because there were no stitches; ask for that separately. Did the child ever ingest anything that was inedible? Has the child been hospitalized for any reason? How many times has the child been seen in an emergency room?

The outcome of past illnesses is as important to obtain as the illnesses themselves. If the child had otitis media (middle ear infection) at age 2 years and received an antibiotic and recovered without complications, the parent has every reason to be confident that the child will get better from a present illness also. The parent has confidence in health care personnel. If the child had an allergic reaction to the antibiotic or was left with a hearing difficulty from the previous illness, the parent may distrust the care being given to the child now; he or she may not follow instructions well, thinking that nothing works anyway, or they may need extra support to follow instructions. This is important information for planning care.

Day History

The child's current skills, eating habits, sleep patterns, and interactions with the family can all be elicited by asking the parent to describe a typical day.

Begin by asking "Was yesterday a fairly typical day for John?" (The parent says yes, it was.) "Would you describe for me all that John did yesterday, beginning with his awakening?" Some parents do this with a great deal of detail; with others, it is necessary to backtrack for particular details: "What did he eat for breakfast? Does he use a fork and spoon? Does he sit in a high chair or on your lap?"

Ask the parent to describe the child's play. Is John in a playpen or allowed room to run? Does he play active, chasing games or quiet, pretending kinds? Does the parent play with him or let him play by himself? (This allows for an estimation of the quality of interaction during the day). When the child sleeps, how long does he sleep? Where does he sleep? Does he take a bath in a big tub or in an infant tub? Does he have any irritable periods during the day; if yes, let the parent explain what these are like. What does the parent do when John acts "irritable?" Does John cry as if he's in pain? Can the parent tell the difference among his cries?

These histories are fun to obtain because most parents are eager to describe their day with their child. Information gained this way is surprisingly rich and pertinent, much more so than if parents are just asked how the baby sleeps, eats, or plays.

Family Illness History

Because some diseases are inherited or familial, it is important to know which ones occur in a family. Ask if any family member has heart disease (childhood or adult type); kidney disease; a congenital anomaly; seizures; mental retardation; mental illness; diabetes (insulin dependent or not); tuberculosis; a sexually transmitted disease (STD); or allergies. If a parent reports that someone in the family has allergies, ask about specific symptoms. Some parents believe that their child is allergic to an antibiotic because while the child was taking the drug he or she developed some diarrhea. There is a strong possibility that the diarrhea was associated with the reason for taking the antibiotic, not with the drug itself. Record what the parent says about allergies so that the person who prescribes medication for the child can decide whether a true allergy exists.

Review of Systems

A health interview ends with a summary of body symptoms or a **review of systems.** Once more, make certain to introduce this part of the history with a transition statement, otherwise a parent may think that the local problem (vomiting) he or she has been describing suggests other problems. "I'd like to ask about different parts of John's body, from his head down to his toes, just to be certain I don't miss anything" is such a transition statement.

Although the important items to be covered in a review of systems differ according to the age of the child, a basic list is as follows:

- Neuropsychiatric symptoms: Has the child ever had seizures? Head injury? Has the parent ever had such difficulty rousing the child that the parent believed the child was unconscious?
- Eyes: Has the child had difficulty with crossed eyes? Eye infection? Does the parent have any reason to believe that the child does not see well?
- Ears: Ear infections? Drainage from the ears? Earaches? Reason to believe the child does not hear well?
- Nose: Frequent drainage or cold symptoms? Difficulty breathing? Nosebleeds?
- Mouth: Difficulty with teeth or teething? Mouth infections? Has the child seen a dentist (if older than age 2 years)?
- Throat: Throat infections? Difficulty swallowing?
- Neck: Masses or swelling? Stiffness? Does the child hold his or her head straight? (Torticollis or wry neck will make the child hold his or her head crookedly; children with poor vision also may cock their heads to the side to try to see better.)
- Chest: For adolescent girls, ask about breast self-examination.
- Lungs: Infections? Pneumonia?
- Heart: Has a physician ever said there was difficulty? What exactly was said?
- Gastrointestinal system: Frequent nausea? Vomiting? Ask separately from nausea. (Children with *pyloric stenosis*—obstruction of the pyloric opening of the stomach—have vomiting but no nausea; children with a brain tumor may also have vomiting but no nausea; pregnant teenagers may have nausea but not vomiting.) Diarrhea? Have parents started toilet training? Has it been successful? Any constipation?
- Genitourinary system: Pain or burning on urination? Blood in urine? Does the child have a good urine stream? If a girl is age 10 years or older, has she started menstruation? Any problems with menstruation? If an adolescent, is the child sexually active? Using contraception? Want more information on contraception? Ever had an STD? If an adolescent male, has he begun testicular self-examination?
- Extremities: Painful or swollen joints? Broken bones? Muscle sprains? Is the parent pleased with the child's coordination?
- Skin: Rashes? Lesions such as warts?
- Immunizations: What immunizations has the child received to date?

A review of systems covers a lot of ground, but it generally takes no more than 5 minutes. Do not think of it as just a mop-up operation and ask questions so quickly ("Has John ever had nausea-vomiting-diarrhea-painful joints-broken bones?") that the parent does not have time to answer or begins to feel that this part of the interview is only an exercise and is unimportant. All the questions are important. If the child shows any of the symptoms described, an entirely new area needs to be explored.

Conclusion

A history-taking interview should close with one last open-ended question: "Is there anything more about John that we should know?" or "Is there anything I didn't mention that you want to ask about?" A parent may have been reluctant to bring up something earlier. Asking this final question gives the parent a final opportunity to do this (see the Focus on Nursing Research box).

Physical Assessment

Physical assessment is one of the most frequently practiced skills of a nurse. The scope and extent of pediatric physical assessment varies, like health interviewing, depending on the circumstances of each health visit. Sometimes only a single segment is required to obtain the information needed. For example, if a child has a gastrointestinal disorder, assessment might concentrate on the gastrointestinal system (i.e., mouth, abdomen, and rectum) and assessment of fluid status (i.e., skin turgor, lips, and mucous membranes). At a first health care

---

 **FOCUS ON NURSING RESEARCH**

What Questions About Children Do Parents Most Frequently Ask a Telephone Counseling Service?

To answer this question, nurse researchers tabulated the questions that 3199 parents asked a community telephone counseling service. Such a service uses trained volunteers to answer calls and help parents learn new ways to solve childrearing problems. In this study, mothers were the primary users of the service (93% of calls); mothers of children from birth to 5 years were the most apt to call.

Questions asked varied according to the age of children. Questions about parent-child relationships were asked for all age children. Twenty-nine percent of the calls regarding adolescents from 14 to 18 years concerned this; for early adolescents from 11 to 13 years, this was 23.2%; for school age children, 18.5%; for preschool children, 19.3%; and for infants, 6.9%. Knowing the types of calls which parents ask such a service can help nurses plan parent education programs and sheds light on types of questions to ask at child health assessments.

Jones, L. C., Maestri, B. O., & McCoy, K. (1993). Why parents use the warm line. *MCN: American Journal of Maternal Child Nursing, 18,* 258.

encounter, however, children usually receive a complete physical examination. Mastery of physical examination techniques is essential to being able to incorporate physical assessment data into the assessment step of the nursing process.

Purpose and Techniques

The actual process of physical examination involves four separate techniques: (1) **inspection**, (2) **palpation**, (3) **percussion**, and (4) **auscultation** (Box 28-1). These techniques are carried out in the above order in each area of the body except the abdomen (auscultation should follow inspection and precede palpation of the abdomen, because handling the abdomen may obliterate bowel sounds). Inspection is used to determine whether there is redness or swelling or any break in the skin. Palpation yields information on warmth and edema; percussion helps determine the consistency of tissue beneath the surface area (Figure 28-2) and auscultation reveals the presence of sound. The findings from

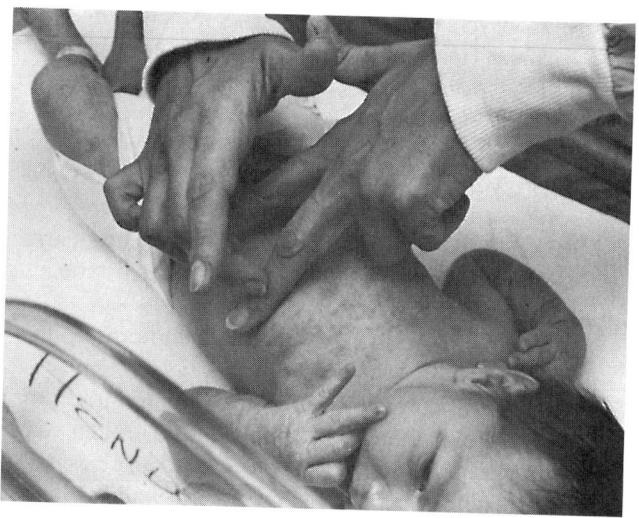

FIGURE 28-2
Percussion. The sound is made by one finger striking a second one. (Courtesy of the Department of Medical Photography, Children's Hospital, Buffalo, NY.)

these techniques strengthen or validate history findings and help determine whether a problem requires immediate action or is secondary to another problem.

Use physical examination to complement the questions asked when a parent describes some symptom a child is experiencing. If a parent says that he or she thinks the child has pain, for example, ask about the duration, intensity, frequency, associated symptoms, and any action or activity that precipitates the pain. Then examine the area for signs of inflammation and palpate for tenderness.

Effective use of physical assessment skills takes practice. Palpating an abdomen, for example, is a simple procedure; recognizing abdominal pathology through palpation is a second, more complicated step. It is difficult to distinguish between normal liver tissue and a distended liver, for example, until both these conditions have been felt many times.

Equipment, Setting, and Approach

A number of items are necessary for complete physical assessment: a thermometer, a stethoscope, a tongue depressor, an ophthalmoscope, an otoscope, a sphygmomanometer, a tape measure, a tuning fork, a reflex (percussion) hammer, rubber gloves, and perhaps a client drape or drawsheet. Nurses who work in community settings or clients' homes must be sure to carry any equipment that may be needed with them.

Examining body parts such as the mouth or an open lesion exposes the hands to body fluids. As part of infection prevention precautions, wear rubber gloves to examine such body parts. During a complete physical examination, every part of the child's body should be

---

> ### Box 28-1
> #### Techniques of Physical Examination
>
> To *inspect* is to examine a child or adolescent initially with your eyes or nose, being alert to visual indications or odors that may point to a health problem.
>
> *Palpation* is examining by touch and can be either light or deep touch. Use light palpation before deep palpation so that the child or adolescent does not tense muscles and make light palpation difficult. The tips of your fingers are most sensitive to texture, vibration, consistency, and contour; the back of your hand is most sensitive to warmth. If a child has a sensitive or painful body part, palpate that area last. Otherwise, the child may be unwilling to allow you to touch other parts for fear he or she will experience additional pain.
>
> *Percussion* is the assessment of a body structure by determining the sound you hear in response to striking the part with an examining finger (Fig. 28-2), and then interpreting the sound. Dense body areas such as bone have a dull flat sound; those filled with air, such as lungs, are resonant. If an organ is stretched (a distended bladder), it has a hyperresonant or low and hollow sound. An organ stretched to an even greater point of distention has a tympanic or extremely hollow, ringing, sound.
>
> *Auscultation* is listening to sounds that are either discernible to the ear (wheezing or heavy breathing) or, as in most cases, made louder by means of a stethoscope. Always listen for four qualities of sound: duration, frequency, intensity (loudness), and pitch (high or low).

exposed for inspection. To protect against chilling and to provide for modesty, do this by exposing body parts individually and only for the amount of time necessary for the examination. Use a client gown or a drawsheet as a drape as necessary.

Be certain that the temperature in an examining room is comfortable. Be certain to provide privacy. Paper table covers should be changed between children to avoid possible spread of illness.

People have the right not to have another person touch their body unless they permit them to do so. It is essential, therefore, to inform children what is happening during a physical examination so that they know when they will be touched (e.g., "Next, let me look at your throat"). If some action will cause discomfort, such as deep palpation of the abdomen, offer fair warning: "You'll feel pressure for a minute." Such actions are also psychologically reassuring because they prevent surprises.

It can be assumed that adolescents will cooperate in placing themselves in whatever position is required to inspect body parts unless they are short of breath or in some other way unable to comply. Small children may not cooperate and so need to be restrained during an examination of body parts such as nose, throat, and ears. This is done not only to enable an examiner to see well but also to ensure that the instrument used will not accidentally injure the child. As a rule, do not ask parents to restrain with any procedure in which the child will be hurt—parents are best used as protectors and comforters. This is not usually a problem with physical examination, which rarely hurts, so parental participation is helpful. Some procedures, such as ear examination, do require a strong restraining hand, and this can be frightening to children. Urge parents to do this with a positive approach such as "Let me help you keep your hand still."

Variations for Age and Developmental Stage

Techniques of physical examination must be tailored to the age and developmental stage of the individual being assessed (Table 28-1) (Wilson et al., 1990). Expected findings also depend on the child's age and developmental stage.

Newborn

All newborns receive a physical examination immediately following birth and again after the first 24 hours of life. When examining newborns, remember that maintaining body temperature is one of the newborn's most difficult tasks. Cover body areas that are not being directly examined. Take axillary temperatures to prevent rupture of rectal mucosa. Take the heart rate apically because peripheral pulses are too faint to be counted accurately. It is important to take femoral pulses in new-

borns to rule out coarctation of the aorta. Include newborn reflexes, head circumference, and an assessment of gestational age (see Chapter 26) as routine parts of the examination. Do not take blood pressure because this value is unreliable in the newborn.

Infant

Infants are usually examined most effectively if a parent holds them during most of the examination. Use an "isn't this fun?" or "this is a game" approach. As a rule, assess heart and lung function first; intrusive procedures such as ear and throat assessment should be done last so the infant does not cry and complicate the remainder of the exam. Blood pressure is not taken routinely. Include newborn reflexes until age 6 months; continue to take heart rate apically and temperature axillary. Include head circumference for a full year.

Toward the end of the first year, children become fearful of strangers. Taking an extra minute to become well acquainted with the infant at the beginning of the examination helps to counteract this problem.

Toddler and Preschool Child

Both toddlers and preschoolers may be afraid of the examining equipment. To alleviate their fears, let them handle items such as stethoscopes, otoscopes, and blood pressure cuffs (Kuttner, 1991) (Figure 28-3). Leave intrusive procedures such as assessment of the genitalia, ears, and throat until last. Give generous praise for cooperation (anything short of hysterical screaming or kicking is good cooperation for intrusive procedures in this age group). The Focus on Family Teaching box describes ways parents can help prepare preschoolers for assessment.

Begin to include blood pressure as part of routine assessment at age 3 years; oral temperature by an electronic thermometer can begin at this age. Before beginning an examination, establish a good rapport with the child's parents, because children this age sense parental trust or suspicion.

School-Age Child and Adolescent

Some children of this age may still be unaware of what a physical examination includes and whether or not it will cause discomfort. Offer good explanations so that they are not frightened by the unknown. Older children may enjoy having a parent with them while they are being examined or they may resent their presence; give them a choice. Adolescents are often worried about some normal physical finding such as a mole or supernumerary (extra) nipple. Make a habit of commenting on such findings—"This is a mole on your hand; that's normal"—as both a means of reassurance and health teaching.

Remember that school-age children and adolescents are modest. Respect this by careful use of gowns or

Table 28-1. *Techniques of Physical Examination Based on Child's Age*

Age	Techniques
Newborn	Undress only the body part being examined or use radiant heat warmer to conserve heat (be certain all body parts are exposed during examination).
	Examine heart and respiratory systems first before infant cries, then follow head-to-toe procedure, performing all manipulative procedures such as throat and eyes last. Examine newborn with parents present, using this assessment time to teach them about normal appearance and development.
Infant	As with newborns, begin examination with heart and respiratory assessment, then follow head-to-toe procedure, performing all manipulative procedures such as throat and ears last.
	Begin examination while parent holds infant in arms or lap to calm the child. Talk to the infant as you proceed; infants calm to sound of your voice or the feeling tone that you radiate as much as they do to what you actually say. Positive feeling tone ("This is like a game") therefore often brings better cooperation than strict, businesslike approach. Infants older than 3 mo like to handle tongue blades. They can be distracted by brightly colored toys while you listen to their heart or lungs. They cooperate best if parent holds them for major portion of examination. Offering a bottle of water or pacifier may be necessary during heart assessment.
Toddler	Allow toddler to handle equipment; include games, such as blowing out otoscope light, to relax child.
	Ask parent to remove clothing or allow child to do it independently.
	Use head-to-toe procedure; leave uncomfortable procedures such as throat and ear examination for last.
Preschooler	Use games such as "Simon Says" to ease child's fright. Ask child to undress; do not remove underpants.
	Preschoolers are extremely threatened by intrusive procedures. Thus, they are frightened of examining instruments. Allow them to handle instruments before use. Assure them that instruments do not hurt. Children up to school age often need to be restrained for ear and throat examinations because they grow fearful about procedures performed on a part of the body they cannot see (ears) or about a throat examination that may be uncomfortable
School-age child	Ask whether child wants parent present or not.
	Proceed with head-to-toe assessment; leave genitalia for last.
	Allow child to undress except for underpants; supply gown.
	Explain equipment and reasons for procedures. Teach whys and hows of procedures.
Adolescent	Ask if the adolescent wants parent present or not.
	Teach adolescent about good health care during examination. Comment on body parts as you examine them: "Your heart sounds good," "Ears look fine." Sometimes an adolescent is so concerned with a part of his or her body (a supernumerary nipple, for example) that he or she is unable to voice this concern. A comment such as, "This is a supernumerary (extra) nipple. Does it ever worry you that you have that?" may help the adolescent to talk about what has indeed been worrying her for years.
	Use head-to-toe procedure; leave genitalia for last.
	Include health teaching on breast and testicular examination.

drapes. Begin to include teaching for self-breast and self-testicular examination by puberty.

Components of Physical Examination

A physical examination may be done in any order, but to ensure thoroughness, develop one system to follow always. Traditionally, this order proceeds from head to toe; examining each body part thoroughly before moving on to the next. With infants and young children, however, it is easiest to begin with the heart and lungs; if the infant cries, findings in these areas become difficult to assess over the sound of crying.

Presented here are the components of a routine or general physical assessment. If abnormalities are discovered during an examination, further assessment would be undertaken. A complete neurologic examination, for example, is not routine so is not included here (see Chapter 49 for details on neurologic examination). It is important to recognize what a "general" physical examination of this nature entails so you can interpret the extent of assessment that a child has received when the parent states, "He had a routine physical."

Vital Sign Assessment

Vital signs refer to temperature, pulse, respiration, and blood pressure or the state of *vital* bodily functions (e.g., heart and lung function or metabolic rate). Because of the important information they provide, measurements of these signs are recorded not only with complete physical examinations but in many other instances of care. Techniques of these measurements and the nursing responsibilities that accompany them, therefore, are discussed in Chapter 37.

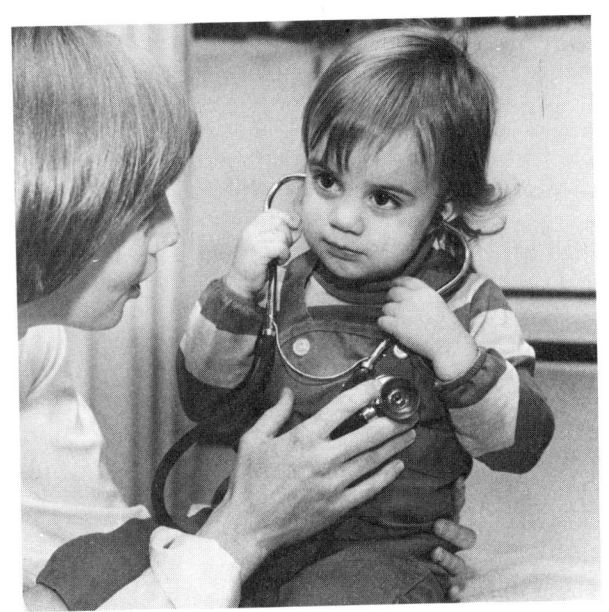

FIGURE 28-3
Children need the opportunity to play with examining equipment to enable them to become more familiar with and less frightened by it. (Courtesy of the Department of Medical Photography, Children's Hospital, Buffalo, NY.)

General Appearance

Physical examination begins with inspection of **general appearance** to form a general impression of the child's health and well-being and to pinpoint specific body areas that will need detailed assessment (Figure 28-4). Assess such areas as: Is the child's height and weight proportional? What is the child's color? Pale? Yellow (jaundiced)? Cyanotic (blue)? Is posture normal? (Children who are in pain sometimes assume an abnormal posture for relief.) Are lesions or symptoms of a specific illness present? Are there any significant body odors (Table 28-2)? Does the child appear relaxed or distressed? Is breathing easy or distressed?

Mental Status Assessment

A mental status assessment is also made early in an examination as a complement to general appearance information. As with general appearance, additional information is gained on mental status throughout the entire exam.

Begin by assessing the child's level of consciousness: Is the child alert? Able to respond to questions easily? Lethargic? Assess *orientation*, or awareness of person, place, and time (awareness of who they are, where they are, and the date). Assess the appropriateness of behavior and mood: hostile, frightened, or relaxed? At some point in the examination of children above preschool age, ask questions that test recent memory and distant memory.

Body Measurements

Body measurements are important determinants of health because with chronic illness the body expends so many nutrients combating the destructive process of the disease that normal height and weight cannot be maintained. Conversely, overweight (obesity) may be the cause of illnesses such as heart and lung disease later in life.

Weight

Until they can stand well, infants are weighed on a sitting or infant scale. Because diapers can be heavy in proportion to total body weight, infants are weighed nude. Always keep a sheltering hand over an infant on an infant scale (hovering but not touching), because infants squirm readily and there is danger of falling (Figure 28-5A). Cover both infant scales and adult scales with scale paper before weighing to prevent spread of illness from one child to another.

Children older than age 2 years are weighed on standing scales, in street clothes (no shoes), or, if in a hospital, in a gown or robe (Figure 28-5B). If children are going to have serial weights (weighed every day or several times a day) taken, it is important that they wear

FOCUS ON FAMILY TEACHING

Q. My 2-year-old son is scheduled for a health assessment next week. What is the best way to prepare him for this?

A. Health assessment always causes some concern with children because it is an unknown and has the threat of possibly causing pain. Some suggestions for preparing a child for a health assessment are:

• Promote the attitude that a health visit will be a positive experience for the child.

• Never threaten a child that if he is not good, a doctor or nurse will punish him.

• Review with the child what he can expect during an assessment (a nurse will ask some questions of his parent; she or he will then look at the child's head, hands, etc.)

• If a child has been taught not to let strangers touch his body (as he should have been taught), a child may need reassurance from a parent that it is all right for a nurse to examine him.

• Dress the child in easy to remove and replace clothing so that you can quickly dress the child after an exam as a way of assuring him that the exam is over.

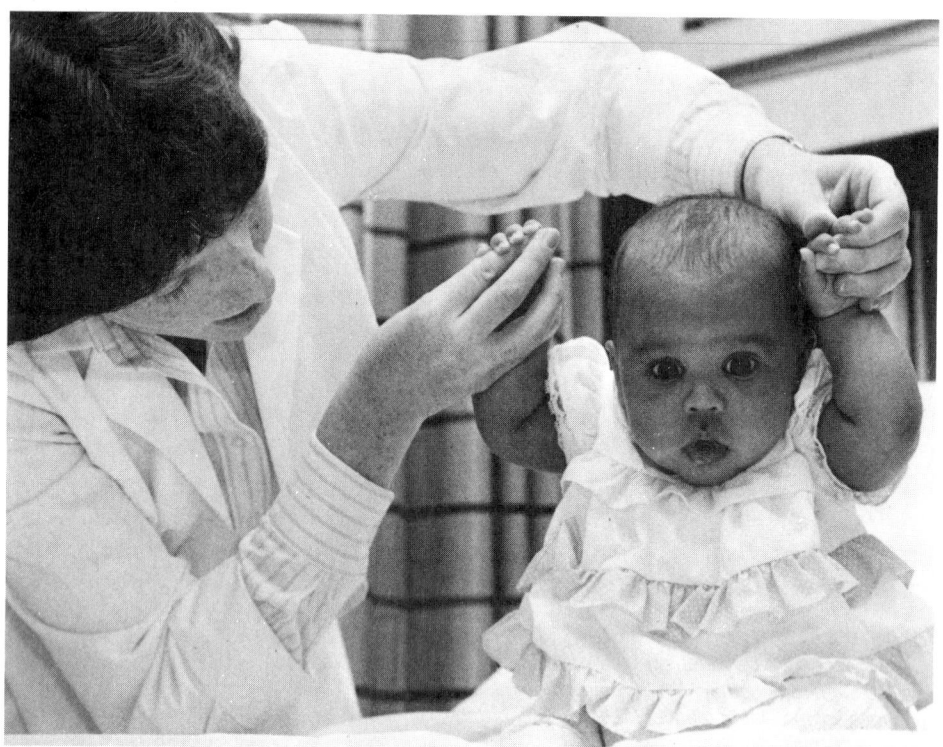

FIGURE 28-4
General appearance assessment reveals that this child is well proportioned and active. (Courtesy Bruce Hill.)

the same clothing every time they are weighed so that any discrepancy in weight is truly a difference in body weight and not a weight change due to more or less clothing. Take the weight at the same time each day (preferably before breakfast) on the same scale for greatest accuracy.

Most children and their parents want to know their weight. To convert from kilograms to pounds, multiply the kilogram amount by 2.2 (50 kg × 2.2 = 110 lb).

To assess whether weight is average for height, compare the child's weight with a standardized height-weight graph. Child and infant values of these are shown in Appendix E for easy reference. In the standardized scale for children, all weights between the 10th and 90th percentiles are considered normal (statistically, a range of weights that includes two standard deviations from the mean or the 50th percentile). As important as the fact that a child's weight falls between the 10th and 90th percentile on a growth chart is that over time the weight follows one of the percentile curves—that they are not at the 80th percentile the first time they are weighed and a month later at the 40th percentile, for example. Although both readings are within the normal range, they reflect a weight loss whose cause needs investigation. Gaining weight in the same way could be equally serious.

Height

In children, height is as good a determinant of health and normal nutrition as weight. Until they can stand securely (at approximately age 2 years), infants are mea-

sured lying down on a measuring frame or an examining table. Align the infant's head snugly against the top bar of the frame and ask an assistant to secure it there. Straighten the infant's body (knees are difficult to straighten in infants because they always keep them flexed); hold the infant's feet in a vertical position; and bring the foot board up snugly against the bottom of the foot (Figure 28-6A). If an examining table is used, mark the spots at the top of the child's head and bottom of feet and then measure between the marks. Parents can help you restrain infants for height measurements because it is a painless procedure.

To measure height in an older child, be certain the child is standing straight with his or her head held level. Align the measuring bar of a standing scale with the top of the head. Placing a flat object such as a clipboard on the child's head in a horizontal position and reading height at the point that it touches a measuring tape on the back of the scale or a flat wall surface is also acceptable technique (Figure 28-6B).

Plot height measurements for children on a standard graph the same as for weight. Height and weight should follow the same percentiles. Remember that height-weight charts have been standardized for "typical" American children, so there will be variations among children of other cultural backgrounds. The important thing to look for is a consistency of measurements over time (always at the same percentile).

A child is defined as having a "failure to thrive" syndrome (medical diagnosis) if height or weight falls below the 3rd percentile on a standardized growth chart.

Table 28-2. *Significant Body Odors*

Source of Odor	Possible Cause
Breath	
Alcohol	Implies recent ingestion (important if coma or neurologic symptoms are present as cause of abnormal functioning)
Camphor	Mothball ingestion
Halitosis (bad breath)	Poor dental hygiene, lung infection; foreign body in respiratory tract
Burnt rope	Marijuana use
Sweet	Acidosis (seen in a child in diabetic coma)
Body	
Stale urine	Incontinence; poor kidney functioning leading to uremia; infrequently changed diapers
Sweat	May imply unusual fatigue recently, or that child has not maintained usual hygiene regimen
"Spoiled fruit"	Wound infection
Sweet	*Pseudomonas* infection
Urine	
Maple syrup	Protein metabolic condition
Musty or mousy	Phenylketonuria or a protein metabolism disorder
Ammonia	Urinary tract infection or poor hydration leading to concentrated urine
Stool	
Putrid	Fat in stool from inadequate absorption

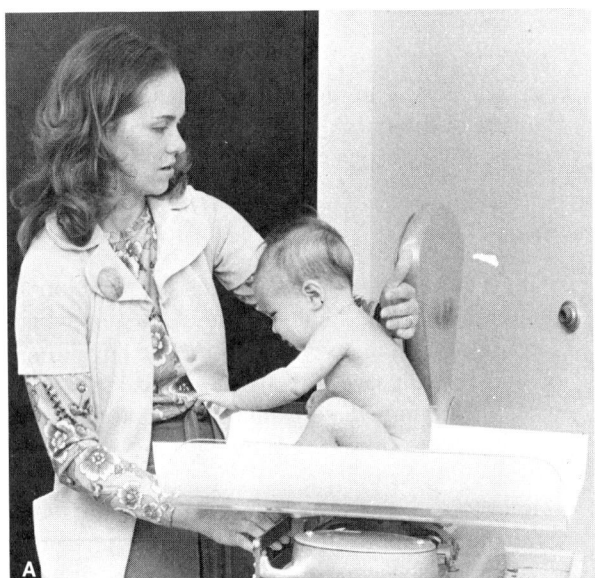
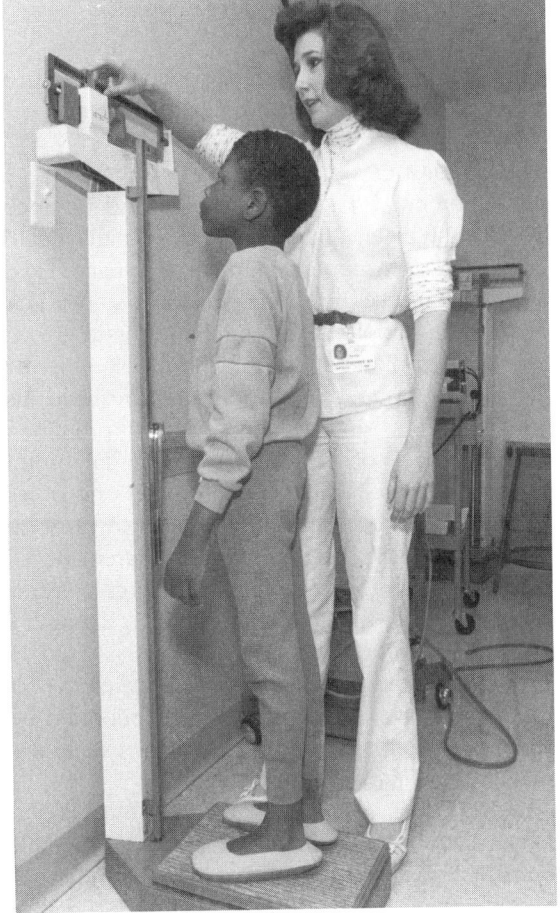

FIGURE 28-5

*Weighing. (**A**) Infants are weighed nude for accuracy. Notice the nurse's hand protecting the infant from falling. (**B**) Weighing an older child. (Courtesy of the Department of Medical Photography, Children's Hospital, Buffalo, NY.)*

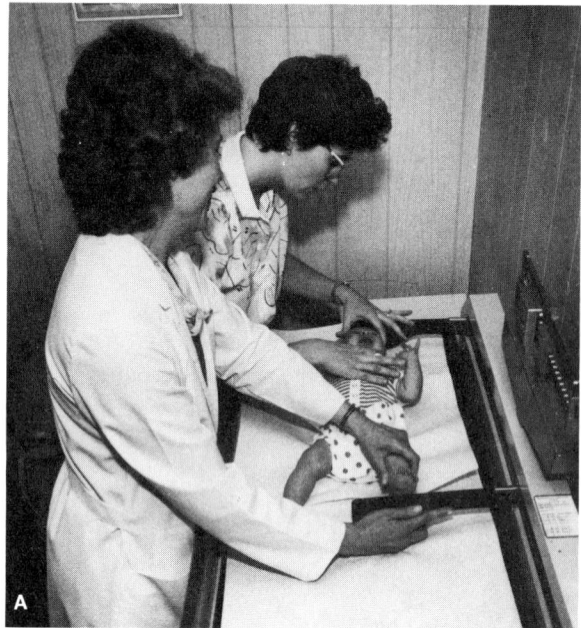

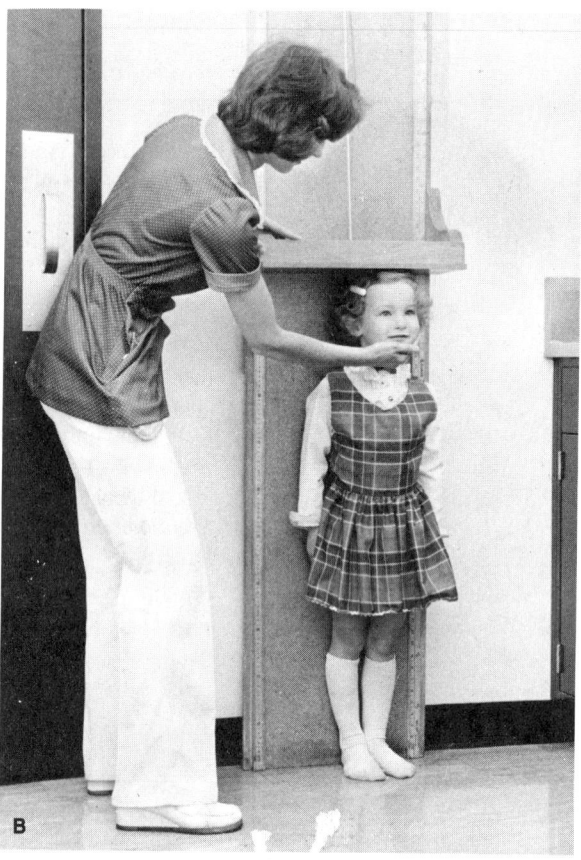

FIGURE 28-6
*Measuring height. (**A**) An infant being measured by a measuring board. The secret is a firmly anchored head and straight legs. (**B**) Measuring an older child. The child must hold his or her head level. (Courtesy of the Department of Medical Photography, Children's Hospital, Buffalo, NY.)*

Any height or weight in this category definitely needs to be reported so that its cause can be investigated.

Head Circumference

Head circumference is measured at birth and routinely on physical assessment until age 1 year (many health care agencies measure routinely until age 2 years). Head growth occurs because the brain is growing, so head circumference is an important determinant of brain growth and potential neurologic function. The measurement is made by placing a tape measure around the head just above the eyebrows and around the most prominent portion of the back of the head, the occipital prominence (Figure 28-7). Babies generally push any object away from their head, so it may be difficult to carry out this otherwise simple procedure. Plot measurements on a standardized graph (Appendix E). Head circumference should correlate with the child's length (e.g., if length is in the 40th percentile, head circumference should be also). If measurements of head circumference plot at different percentiles over time, this should be reported because it implies that brain or skull growth is in some way abnormal and needs investigation.

Chest and Abdominal Circumference

Measurements of chest and abdominal circumference are not done routinely, but only when specific pathol-ogy warrants. The measurement of chest circumference is made at the nipple line; the measurement of abdominal circumference is made at the level of the umbilicus.

Skin

Skin is assessed along with the examination of each body region. Assess color; texture; **turgor**, which is the amount of fluid in body tissue, assessed by lifting a ridge of skin (usually over the abdomen or thigh) and noting whether it immediately falls back into place (Figure 28-8); and the presence of any lesions. Table 28-3 summarizes various other findings that may be detected. Be certain to examine the child's total skin surface at some time during an examination. Remove and replace as necessary adhesive bandages and other dressings that could hide important findings. Good lighting (not just illumination with soft over-the-bed light) is imperative for accurate assessment of the skin, especially when assessing dark-skinned children.

Newborn and Infant

Newborns appear ruddy because their layer of subcutaneous fat is thin and the intense redness of their blood circulation is visible. Birthmarks (hemangiomas, mongolian spots, or nevi) may be present. After the first few days of life, a diaper rash may be present.

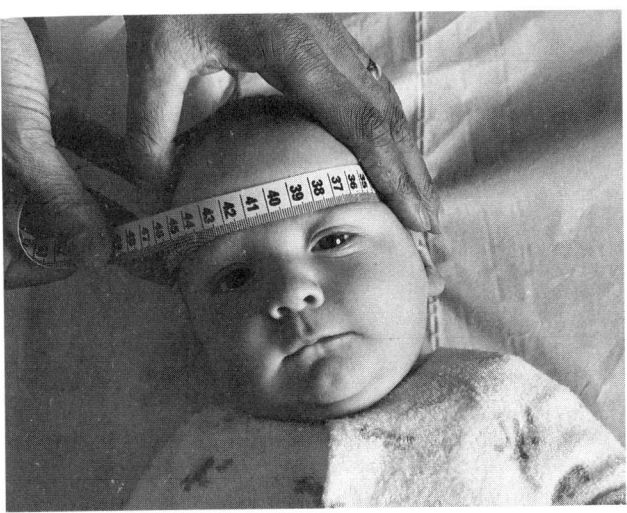

FIGURE 28-7
Measuring head circumference. The measuring tape passes just above the eyebrows and around the prominent posterior aspect of the head. (Courtesy of the Department of Medical Photography, Children's Hospital, Buffalo, NY.)

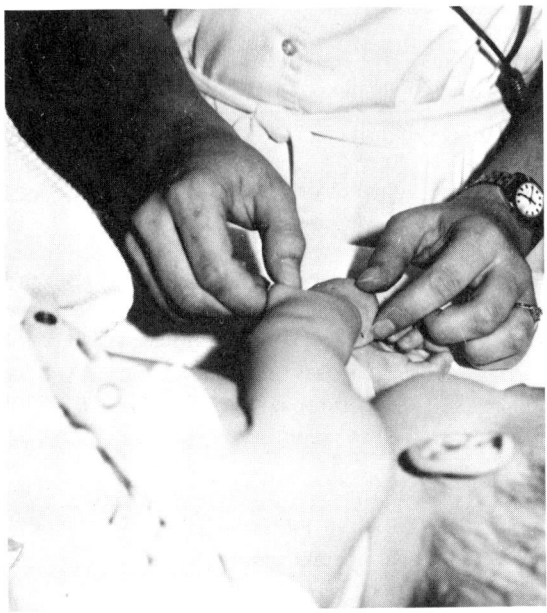

FIGURE 28-8
Assessing skin turgor. If the ridge of tissue does not immediately return to place, the infant is poorly hydrated. (Courtesy Bruce Hill.)

Preschool and School-Age Child

Children this age typically have a number of ecchymotic spots on their lower extremities from bumping into objects during active play. Ecchymotic spots on upper extremities suggest a blood coagulation problem. Be certain in evaluating ecchymotic spots on all age children that the possibility of child abuse is considered (Halverson et al., 1993). Many children also have minor lesions from mosquito bites or from flea bites if they own a pet.

Adolescent

Acne lesions on the face or back are usually present in the adolescent. Lesions or rashes caused by allergies to cosmetics may be apparent.

Head

To examine the head, slide a hand over the skull, assessing for irregular configurations or tenderness. Most children have a prominent occipital outgrowth; do not mistake this natural head contour as an abnormality. Assess the texture and cleanliness of the hair. Children who are well nourished usually have hair of good texture; poorly nourished children tend to have dry, brittle or limp hair. If hair is exceptionally oily, it may mean that a parent or the child has been too fatigued or depressed lately to wash it. If a serious protein deficiency is present such as **kwashiorkor**, the hair becomes striped with dark and light color because dark-colored hair forms during periods of good protein intake and the light color forms during periods of protein deficit. Patches of hair loss (*alopecia*) suggest a fungal infection (*tinea capitis*), child abuse, or a possible drug reaction (chemotherapy will cause total hair loss, not patches).

Newborn and Infant

In the newborn, the head usually shows *molding* (an elongated shape due to pressure against the cervix before delivery). A caput succedaneum or cephalhematoma from the pressure of birth may be present (see Chapter 23). Skull suture lines may be palpable. In both newborns and infants, sit the child upright and palpate the skull for the presence of *fontanelles*—the places where the skull bones fuse. The anterior fontanelle is at the junction of the two parietal bones and the two fused frontal bones. It is diamond shaped and measures 2 cm to 3 cm (0.8 in to 1.2 in) in width and 3 cm to 4 cm (1.2 in to 1.6 in) in length. The posterior fontanelle is at the junction of the parietal bones and the occipital bone. It is triangular and measures approximately 1 cm (0.5 in) in length (see Figure 18-2).

With the infant sitting, fontanelles should be felt as soft spots but should not appear indented (a sign of dehydration) or bulging (a sign of increased intracranial pressure). When an infant cries, cerebral pressure increases, so with crying fontanelles will feel tense, and sometimes even the fluctuation of a pulse is present. The anterior fontanelle normally closes at age 12 to 18 months and the posterior fontanelle by the end of age 2 months, so are not palpable after these times. The closing of fontanelles too early or too late may be an indication of decreased or increased brain or ventricle growth.

A scalp problem commonly encountered in infants is *seborrhea* (scaling, greasy-appearing, salmon-colored patches). This is referred to by parents as "cradle cap." Increasing the frequency of hair washing to once a day will effectively reduce this problem.

Table 28-3. *Skin Findings in Children That Suggest Illness*

Finding	Indication
Bluish color	Cyanosis from decreased respiratory function or cyanotic heart disease
White color	Edema (accumulated subcutaneous fluid is stretching the skin)
Pale color	Anemia or decreased circulation to a body part
Reddened area	Local inflammation or increased systemic temperature
Linear abrasion	Scratch marks from local irritation from an insect bite, or allergic reaction
Ecchymoses (black and blue marks)	Recent injury to skin
Petechiae (pinpoint blood marks)	Blood dyscrasia (poor clotting ability)
Yellow color	Jaundice from increased bilirubin in subcutaneous tissue; carotenemia (excess carotene in skin)
Moistness	Excess perspiration from elevated temperature
Localized cold temperature	Decreased circulation to particular body part
Warm temperature	Local irritation or elevated systemic temperature
Poor turgor	Dehydration
Rash	Infectious childhood illness or excessive heat

Preschool and School-Age Child

Examine the hair of school-age children carefully for small white-yellow sand-sized particles attached to hair strands—the eggs (nits) of *pediculi* (head lice). Nits cling and cannot be readily removed from hair by running fingers the length of the hair. The child may have recent scratch marks on the scalp and generally states that the scalp feels "itchy." Pediculi spread easily in school-age children due to the sharing of combs and towels in school.

Examine the scalp carefully for round circular areas (perhaps weeping in the center, crusting and scaling on the edges) that would suggest **tinea capitis** (ringworm, a fungal infection). Like pediculi, fungal infections are spread readily among school-age children; a prescription medication is necessary to cure the condition (see Chapter 43).

Adolescent

Adolescents may streak their hair with dye or arrange it in a way that requires glue or use of a curling iron. Inspect to see that their scalp and hair is healthy underneath the styling.

Eyes

Observe the eyes for symmetry and signs of frequent blinking, crusting, squinting, or the child's rubbing the eyes. Observe lids and lashes for redness (erythema), which suggests infection. Common infections include **conjunctivitis** (called "pink eye" by parents; an infection of the thin conjunctiva that covers the eye) or a **hordeolum** or sty (an infection of the gland that lubricates an eyelash). Both conditions require an antibiotic for therapy (see Chapter 50).

Assess the location of eyes in relation to the nose (not unusually wide or narrow spaced) and the relationship of the globe to the socket (neither sunken nor protruding from the socket [exophthalmos]). Abnormalities in these areas occur in chromosomal or metabolic illnesses such as hyperthyroidism. Inspect the sclera of the eye for spots of hemorrhage (called *subconjunctival hemorrhage*) or yellowing. Black individuals often have a slight yellowing of the sclera and small black spots on the sclera; do not mistake these for abnormal findings. Note that no sclera shows above the pupil (if it does, this is termed a "sun-set sign," an indication of increased intracranial pressure).

Palpate the eye globe with eyelid closed to assess for tenseness, although the usual cause of this (glaucoma) is rare in children. Determine that, when the child closes the eyes, the eyelids completely cover the eyes (edema or neurologic illnesses may make eyelids too short to do this) and whether, when the child opens the eyes, the lids retract far enough that they do not obscure vision. When a lid obscures vision, a condition termed **ptosis**, it generally denotes neurologic involvement. Be certain not to mistake the normal absence of Eastern palpebral folds for abnormal findings. The difference in Western and Eastern eye creases is shown in Figure 28-9.

Examine the inner lining of the lower eyelid (the conjunctiva) by pulling the lid down slightly with a fingertip. The mucous membrane of this space should appear pink and moist. In children with anemia it often appears pale; with allergy or infection it may appear unusually red and irritated. Do not initiate a blink reflex by touching the cornea with a wisp of cotton, as can be done in adults; this is momentarily painful and frightening to children.

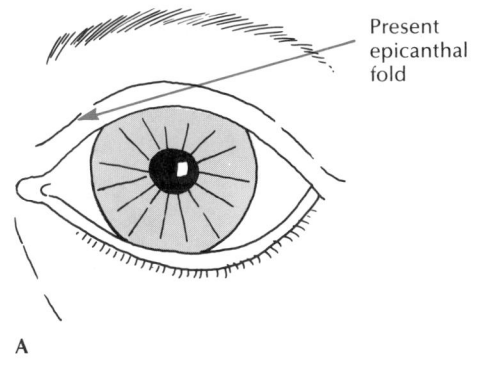

Present epicanthal fold

A

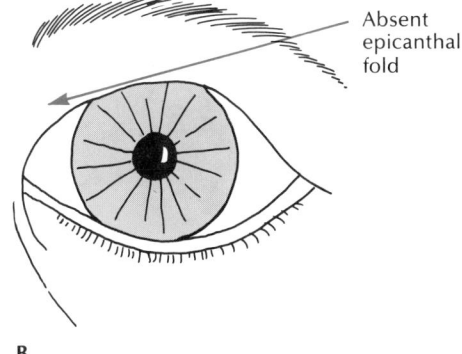

Absent epicanthal fold

B

FIGURE 28-9
*Differences in eye formation. (**A**) Western. (**B**) Eastern. The extra inner fold of tissue is an epicanthal fold.*

In addition, observe whether the eyes appear to be in good alignment. **Strabismus** refers to eyes that are not evenly aligned. If an eye is always turning in, the condition is called **esotropia**; if it always turns out, **exotropia**. Include a cover test as a quick screening procedure to see if eyes are aligned straight (see Figure 28-30) or include a Hirschberg's test—a light should reflect evenly off both pupils if they are in equal alignment (Figure 28-10). Test the eyes for their ability to focus in all fields of vision. To do this, ask the child to follow a moving light (or catch the attention of an infant with a moving light) while holding the child's chin stationary. Move the light out to the side, then up, then down; cross to the opposite side and move it up and down; bring it back to the midline and observe whether the child's eyes converge as the light moves in toward the nose. Remember that infants under age 3 months cannot follow past the midline. Children do not converge well (follow the light to the nose) under school age.

Observe if the pupil constricts (reduces in size) in response to a light, an indication that the third cranial nerve is intact. It is best to approach the child's eye from the forehead so the light suddenly appears on the pupil rather than advancing toward the child slowly. This makes the pupil constrict more dramatically. This should occur in response to a light shining directly on a pupil (direct constriction); when one pupil constricts, this will

also occur in the opposite eye (consensual constriction). Record that pupils are equal in size and react to light as "PERL" (pupils equivalent, react to light). If the pupil converges (moves to follow a light in toward the nose) this is charted as "PEARL" or "PERLA" (pupils equal, react to light, accommodate).

To inspect the inner structures of the eye, use an ophthalmoscope head. For a funduscopic exam, subdue the lights in the room and turn on the light of the ophthalmoscope. Ask the child to look at a point approximately 5 feet in front of himself or herself (name a specific point such as a picture on the wall). The examiner should be positioned so that his or her right eye aligns with the child's left eye; position the ophthalmoscope approximately 15 cm (6 in) in front of the child's eye. Begin with the lens selection of the ophthalmoscope at 0; move forward or backward until the cornea and lens are focused. Observe for opacity. If the cornea, aqueous humor, and vitreous humor are all clear (no cataract, infection, or tumor is present), then there will be an unobstructed view of the retina when shining the ophthalmoscope light directly into the pupil. If the retina is intact, it will appear as a bright red circle in the pupil (a red reflex). (This occasionally appears in colored photographs because the flashbulb initiates the reflex.) If opacity of the lens is present, this will appear as a black dot against the red background of the retina.

Further inspection of the retina is not done routinely in children because retinal disease (arteriosclerosis or diabetic retinopathy) does not occur in a high incidence in children. If further inspection is necessary, move the ophthalmoscope head in closer (to approximately 5 cm, or 1½ to 2 in) and rotate the lens selection dial until a retinal vessel is focused. Veins can be differentiated from arteries by their lighter color and larger size (a ratio of 3:2) (Figure 28-11). Follow a vessel right or left to the optic disc. The optic disc appears as an oval slightly lighter in color than the periphery of the retina. In the center of the disc should be a depressed area that appears even more pale. An optic disc normally measures approximately 1.5 mm in diameter. Observe for swelling of the disc (*papilledema*; a sign of increased intracranial pressure). This makes it larger than normal and the disc borders appear blurry.

The *fovea* is the area of central vision approximately two disc diameters lateral to the disc. It appears darker in color (only slightly so in blondes). The bright light of the ophthalmoscope makes an eye tear when centered on the fovea so the examination of this area must be quick and fleeting to avoid discomfort.

Newborn and Infant
Newborns often have a small bright red spot on the sclera (a subconjunctival hemorrhage) because the pressure of birth has ruptured a small conjunctival blood vessel. This is normal and will fade in 7 days to 10 days as the blood is absorbed.

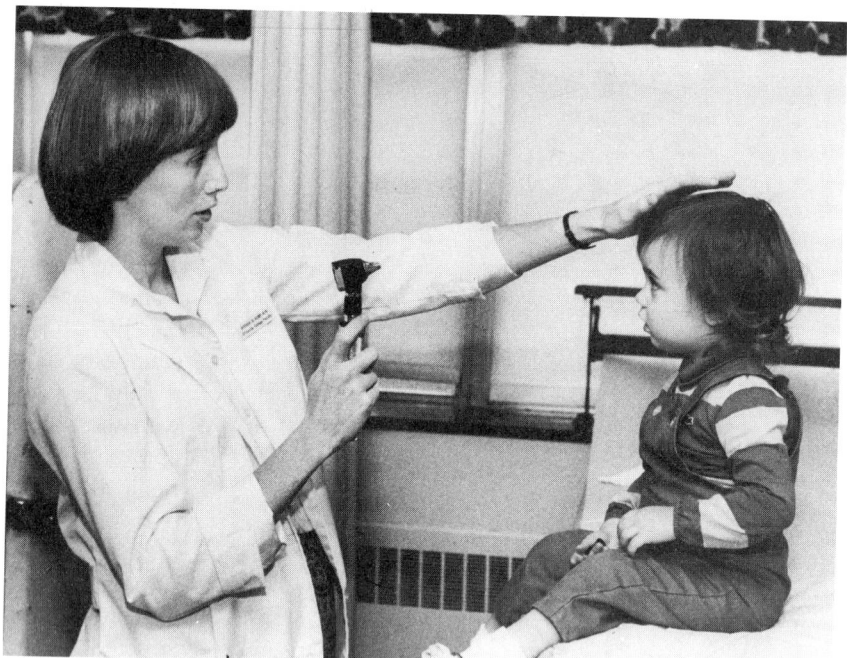

FIGURE 28-10
Testing of good alignment by Hirschberg's test. The child is asked to look directly at the light of the otoscope. The light reflex on the pupils of both eyes will be equal if the eyes are in straight alignment. (Courtesy of the Department of Medical Photography, Children's Hospital, Buffalo, NY.)

Infants can easily be tested for a red reflex, but until they are age 3 months, they cannot follow an object or light across the midline or follow a light into all six positions of gaze. Even a newborn, however, can follow a bright light to the midline.

Preschool and School-Age Child

Many preschoolers are reluctant to let someone look into their eyes. Explaining what will happen during an eye examination is effective in reducing the child's anxiety about this part of the assessment.

Adolescent

Many adolescents wear contact lenses (a red reflex is visible with a contact lens in place); some may be nervous about having their eyes examined because they know they should be wearing prescribed eyeglasses but have omitted wearing them because they do not like their appearance. Observe carefully for pupillary appearance and ability to constrict in adolescents as a sign of drug abuse. Many adolescent girls are anemic and so have pale conjunctiva.

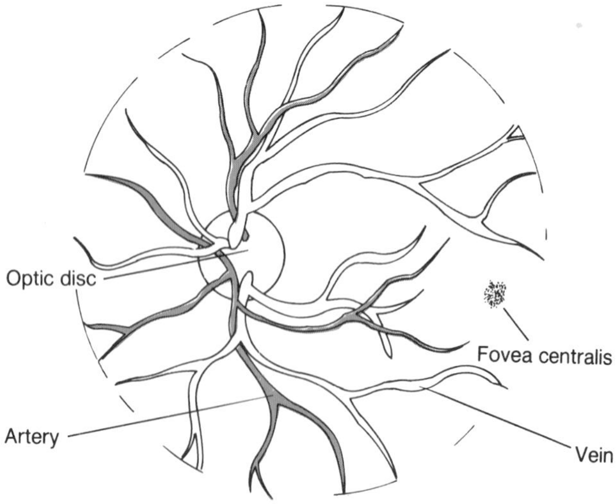

Nose

Observe the nose for flaring of the nostrils (a sign of need for oxygen). Using the otoscope light, observe the mucous membrane of the nose for color (it should be pink; pale suggests allergies, redness suggests infection). Note and describe any discharge. Document that the septum is in the midline (displaced septa such as those that occur after facial injuries can interfere with respiration and make nasal intubation in emergencies difficult). Press one nostril closed with gentle pressure and ask the child to inhale; repeat on the opposite side to assure that both sides of the nose are patent (i.e., that no choanal atresia or no membrane obstructing the posterior nares exists). Palpate the areas over the frontal and maxillary sinuses for tenderness, a symptom of sinus infection in children older than age 6 years. Sense of smell can be assessed in school-age children and adolescents by asking them to identify a familiar odor such as chocolate or an orange.

Optic disc

Fovea centralis

Artery

Vein

FIGURE 28-11
The optic disk and blood vessels of the retina as seen in magnification when viewed by an ophthalmoscope.

Newborn and Infant

Infants are obligate nose breathers. They cannot coordinate mouth breathing, so become disturbed when the nose is temporarily blocked to check for patency; do this only momentarily to avoid discomfort. Most newborns have milia (small white papules) on the surface of the nose.

Preschool and School-Age Child

Many preschool and school-age children have upper respiratory infections that cause nasal mucous membranes to be reddened and also cause a purulent discharge. Children who have frequent nosebleeds from cracked mucosa due to dry air in school buildings may be reluctant to allow inspection of their nose for fear that bleeding will result.

Adolescent

Adolescents who sniff cocaine lose nasal hair and may have abscesses in the mucous membrane.

Ears

Observe ears for proper alignment. In the average child, a line from the inner canthus of the eye to the outer canthus and then to the ear will touch the top of the pinna of the ear (Figure 28-12). Ears set lower than this are associated with chromosomal disorders such as trisomy 13. Observe the opening to the ear canal for any discharge. Touch the pinna and watch for evidence of pain

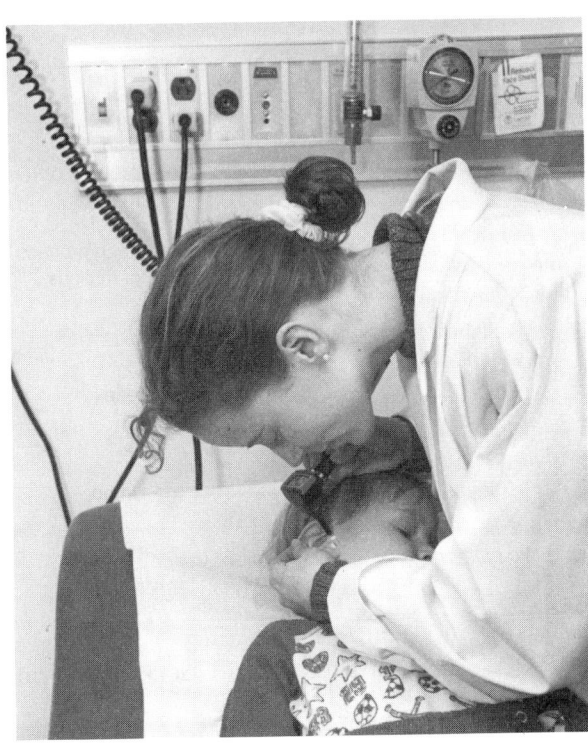

FIGURE 28-13
Otoscopic examination. Note how the nurse's hand rests between the otoscope and the child's head. Should the child move suddenly, no injury to the tympanic membrane will be sustained with this technique because the otoscope will move along with the child's head. (Courtesy of the Department of Medical Photography, Children's Hospital, Buffalo, NY.)

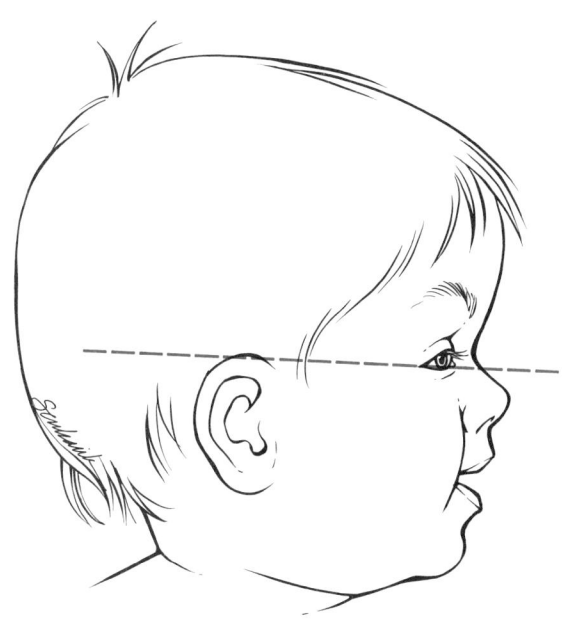

FIGURE 28-12
Normal ear alignment. When a line is drawn from the inner canthus through the outer canthus to the ear, the top of the ear pinna should meet the line. Abnormal ear alignment is associated with certain chromosomal abnormalities.

(a sign of external canal infections). Observe immediately in front of the ear for a dermal sinus or a skin tag (a finding that is usually innocent but may be associated with kidney abnormalities). Observe the ear lobes for redness or drainage from infected pierced earring sites.

To examine the ear canal, the canal must first be straightened. This is done by pulling the pinna gently down and back in the child under age 2 years and up and back in the older child. With the ear canal held straight, insert an otoscope tip into the external canal. Always rest the instrument on a hand, not on the child's head (Figure 28-13). In this position, if the child should move his or her head suddenly, the otoscope will move with the child, avoiding the danger that the plastic tip will scratch the canal. Otoscope tip sizes vary; use the smallest size possible that still gives adequate visibility.

Inspect the sides of the ear canal and locate landmarks on the surface of the tympanic membrane. Landmarks present should be the outline of the malleus of the inner ear through the translucent membrane (Figure 28-14). The color of the membrane itself is pinkish gray; if the tension of the membrane is normal, a cone of light—the light reflex—should be present in one of

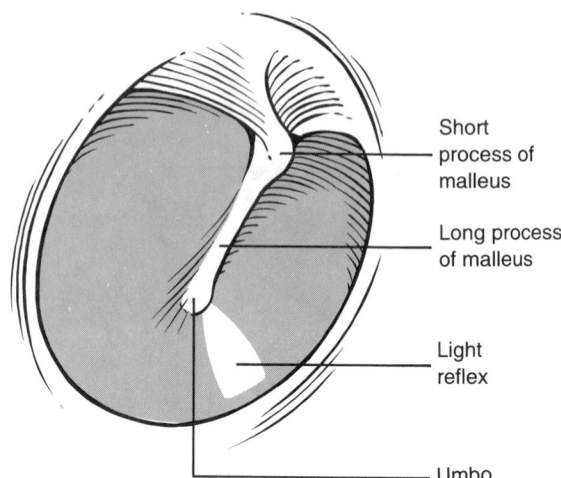

FIGURE 28-14
A tympanic membrane as viewed with an otoscope.

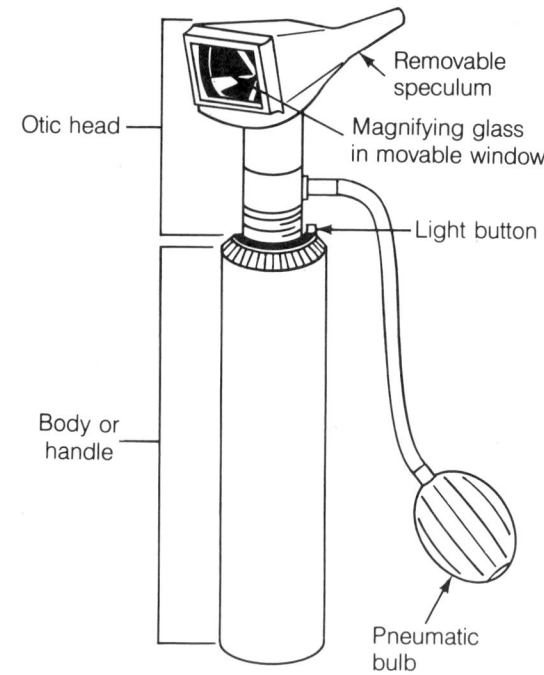

FIGURE 28-15
Otoscope with pneumatic attachment.

the lower corners (at either the 5 o'clock or 7 o'clock position).

Many children have wax (*cerumen*) in their ear canals, appearing as a dark-brown glistening substance, but it is almost always possible to see the tympanic membrane past the wax.

If ear infection is present, the tympanic membrane appears reddened and often bulges forward so that the malleus is no longer able to be discerned, and the cone of light is absent; if there is fluid in the middle ear, it may be possible to see bubbles of air through the membrane. With chronic middle ear disease (serous otitis media), the tympanic membrane may be retracted, the malleus is extremely prominent, and the cone of light is again missing. If the membrane is torn, the jagged edge and opening to the middle ear are discernible from trauma or rupture. In addition to this, inspect for any ulcerated areas that could be a cholesteatoma or an ingrowing tumor.

The mobility of the eardrum can be tested by injecting a column of air into the ear canal against the drum by a pneumatic attachment on the otoscope that looks like the bulb of a blood pressure cuff (Figure 28-15). A normal drum is freely mobile and can be seen to move with pressure on the bulb; one with fluid behind it has decreased mobility. Warn children that this "tickles" before introducing air.

Finally, appraise hearing. Appraisal can be done grossly in an older child by assessing his or her response to questions. Distract an infant with a toy; then make a sound behind the infant's back, out of his or her peripheral vision, and watch for the response. The hearing infant will show some noticeable reaction, although he or she has difficulty looking directly toward or locating the sound until 4 months of age.

Newborn and Infant

Many newborns still have amniotic fluid or vernix caseosa in their ear canal, so inspecting the ear canal is ineffective. Be certain to assess for ear level and normal pinna contour. Assess for hearing by a gross check such as watching the infant startle to a sudden sound or quiet to the calming effect of quiet talking.

Preschool and School-Age Child

Middle ear infection (*otitis media*) is a common childhood illness. This causes the ear to be painful when examined. An external ear infection (often called swimmer's ear) causes any movement of the pinna to be painful. For these reasons and because children are told many times never to put anything into their ears, they usually resist ear examinations. Explaining what is happening helps to allay fear (see the Nursing Care Plan). Preschool and school-age children may have myringotomy tubes (small circular plastic tubes in place on the tympanic membrane) to relieve chronic fluid collected in the middle ear. Inspect that the area surrounding the tube is not inflamed and the tube is not merely lying in the external canal and no longer inserted into the membrane (see Chapter 50).

Mouth

Assess the external appearance of the lips; look for symmetry and color. Ask the child to smile and to frown to evaluate the mobility of facial muscles. Count the num-

Bobby is a 2-month-old infant you care for at a health maintenance setting. The following is a partial nursing care plan designed for him.

Assessment: Mother states that Bobby was well until 3 days ago, then developed mild upper respiratory symptoms (clear rhinitis, slight cough). This morning he woke with a fever (temperature not actually taken but he felt warm). Very sleepy all morning. Refuses to drink (begins to take bottle as if hungry, then stops after sucking 3 or 4 times). No other family members ill. No exposure to communicable disease. General appearance: well-proportioned, irritable-appearing 2-month-old male. Weight: 11 lb (5 kg) = 50th percentile; height: 22 in (56 cm) = 40th percentile; rectal temperature 101°F. Head: normocephalic. Anterior fontanelle open 3 cm × 3 cm. Posterior, closed. Eyes: Red reflex present; extraocular muscles grossly intact. No crusting, erythema, or discharge. Ears: left tympanic membrane pink, good cone of light. Right tympanic membrane erythematous; poor mobility by pneumoscopy. Child observed tugging at right ear. Nose: midline septum. Thick, purulent white discharge present. Mouth and throat: no teeth. Mucous membrane pink and moist. Gag reflex present. Pharynx not erythematous. Mucous discharge from nose present on posterior pharynx. Neck: supple, one shotty anterior chain cervical lymph node present on right. Chest: symmetric. Easy respirations; respiratory rate: 30/min. Heart rate: 120 beats/min., normal heart tones. Lungs: Rhonchi heard in both upper lobes. No rales or wheezing evident. Abdomen: soft, no masses. Liver palpable 1 cm. Genitalia: normal male. Testes down bilaterally. Meatal opening transverse and in good placement. Extremities: full range of motion. No bruising. Good muscle tone. Skin: good turgor. No rashes. Warm and dry to palpation. Neurologic: Moro, tonic neck, grasp reflexes still present. Beginning to support head when pulled to sit.

Nursing Diagnosis: Pain related to inflammation and erythema of tympanic membrane.

Defining Characteristic: Infant refuses to drink; is irritable, observed pulling on ear. Right tympanic membrane erythematous.

Goal: Child will demonstrate relief from pain in 24 hours.

Outcome Criteria: Infant mood is improved with no further pulling at ear.

Nursing Orders	Rationale
1. Amoxicillin prescription given to mother by physician. Instructions and purpose reviewed with her by nurse.	1. Helps ensure compliance.
2. Written instructions on how to administer acetaminophen (Tylenol) to reduce fever reviewed with mother and given to her per protocol. Stress that although Tylenol also relieves pain, pain will be relieved best when inflammation of infection is decreased by antibiotic therapy.	2. Teaches mother how to care for infant now and provides important information for future responses to similar problem.
3. Return to clinic in 2 weeks for follow-up. Mother to call in 24 hours if child's condition has not changed or if she has any further concern.	3. Provides mother with back-up to ease her concerns about child; ensures adequate follow-up care.

ber of teeth present and assess their condition (number missing or cavities present). Inspect the gum line (**gingivae**) for redness, tenderness, and edema, symptoms of periodontal disease. Inspect the buccal membrane and palate for color (pink) and the presence of any lesions. Ask the child to stick out his or her tongue and assess for midline position and no **fasciculations** (trembling). Inspect the area under the tongue for lesions in adolescents who smoke or chew tobacco as this is the most common first site for oral cancer. A child's tongue is normally smooth and moist. With dehydration present, it often appears roughened and dry. **Geographic tongue** is a term for the rough-appearing tongue surface that often accompanies general symptoms of illness such as fever; it may also occur normally. Inspect the uvula to be certain it is in the midline. Use a tongue blade to press down and forward on the back of the tongue (Figure 28-16). The epiglottis can usually be observed with the tongue depressed. Observe for abnormal enlargement, palatine redness, or drainage of tonsils. Tonsillar tissue differs a great deal in size but should not be reddened or have pus in the crypts (indentations). After gagging an infant to view the back of the throat, always turn the infant's head sharply to the side so that he or she does not choke on any saliva that accumulated in the mouth during the throat examination, as an infant is less able to manage this than an adult.

It is important that the tongue of any child who is suspected to have epiglottitis or whose glottis is inflamed not be depressed. Symptoms of this condition are a sore throat, fever, difficulty with respiration, dysphagia, and a barking cough. If a swollen, inflamed epiglottis rises with the pressure of a tongue blade, it can obstruct the respiratory tract so completely that the child is immediately unable to breathe.

Newborn and Infant

Many newborns have considerable mucus in their mouths due to less ability to handle swallowing. If a newborn has teeth, evaluate them carefully for stability; if loose, they need to be removed to prevent aspiration (Nik-Hussein, 1990). Assess carefully for white patches that do not scrape away from the buccal membrane or tongue (thrush), a frequent finding in infants.

Preschool and School-Age Child

Tonsillar tissue in children reaches its maximum growth at early school age, making many preschool children appear to be "all tonsils." As long as the tissue does not appear reddened or tender, it can be assumed to be normal for the age. Many children have irregular pale pink elevated projections on the posterior pharynx as a normal finding. A stream of mucopurulent discharge in the posterior pharynx is not unusual if an upper respiratory infection and a "postnasal" flow of secretions is present. Assess carefully for pinpoint ulcers in the child with teeth braces to be certain that the wires are not causing undue discomfort or infection. Cavities appear as dark brown areas on the tooth enamel. The average school-age child has at least one present.

Neck

Assess the neck for symmetry (the trachea should be in the midline; any deviation suggests lung pathology). Observe the outline of the thyroid gland (barely noticeable below puberty because it is obscured by the sternocleidomastoid muscle) on the anterior neck. Palpate

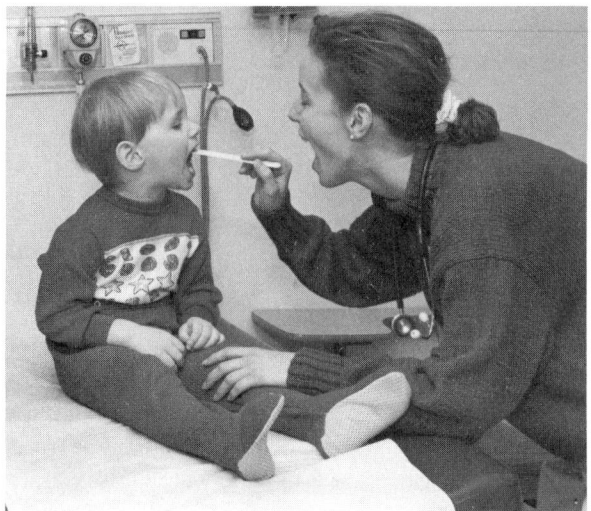

FIGURE 28-16
Inspecting the pharynx in an older child. (Courtesy of the Department of Medical Photography, Children's Hospital, Buffalo, NY.)

the area in front of the ear (location of the parotid gland) and smooth a hand over the location of lymph nodes at the sides of the neck and under the chin to palpate for swelling. Figure 28-17 shows the location of lymph node chains of the head and neck. Because children have so many upper respiratory infections, a few shotty nodes (nodes that are freely movable, about the size of peas) are often present. Preauricular and postauricular nodes may be palpable following ear infections, and postoccipital nodes following a scalp infection. Submental nodes generally denote a tooth abscess. Palpable submaxillary, anterior, and posterior cervical nodes follow throat infections.

Ask the child to move his or her head (or move it for him or her) through flexion (touch chin to chest) and extension (raise chin as high as possible), and turn it right and left (rotation) to see that the child does this easily. Pain on forward flexion is an important sign of neurologic (meningeal) irritation.

Newborn and Infant

With infants, the ability to control the head should be assessed. Lay the infant supine and pull the child to a sitting position. Babies younger than age 4 months will let their heads lag backward as they are pulled up; their heads are righted only as they reach a sitting position. After age 4 months, infants should bring their head up with them (no head lag) if their neuromuscular coordination is adequate for their age. This is a simple but important test in terms of the information it yields on overall neuromuscular control.

Adolescent

In adolescents, palpate the thyroid gland for symmetry and possible nodes. To do this, press on the right side of

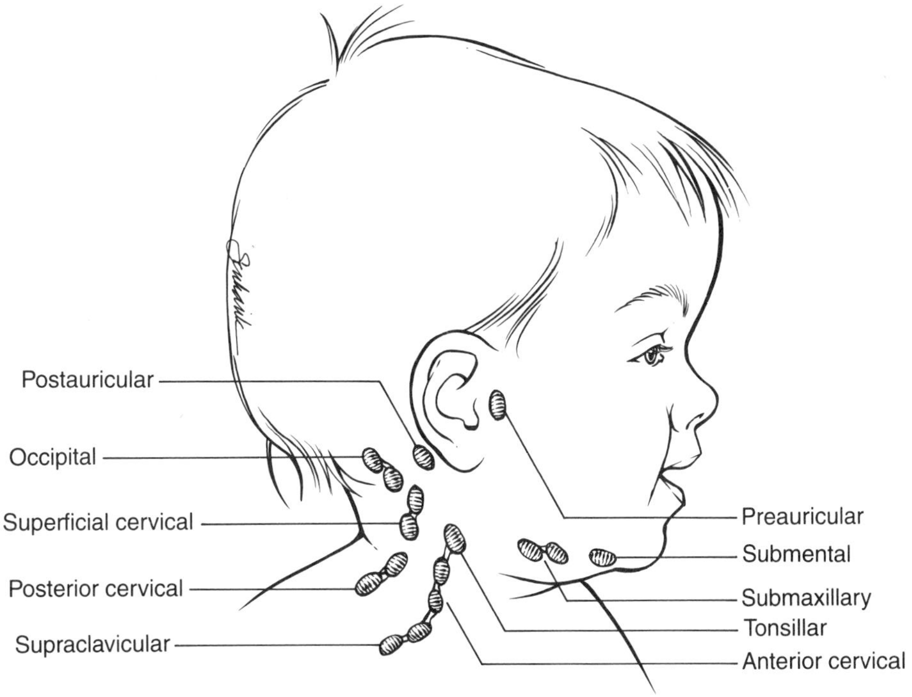

Postauricular

Occipital

Superficial cervical

Posterior cervical

Supraclavicular

Preauricular

Submental

Submaxillary

Tonsillar

Anterior cervical

FIGURE 28-17
Location of lymph node chains in the head and neck.

the gland to cause it to be more prominent on the left side; palpate the left half to discern any irregularities (areas of hardness). Repeat on the right side. A finding of a thyroid node needs to be investigated. It may be only an innocent transient cyst; alternatively, it may be the first indication of thyroid malignancy. Many adolescents have some increase in the size of the thyroid at puberty; this hypertrophy should not be accompanied by any nodes.

Chest

For ease in specifying the location of chest pathology, the chest is divided into sections by imaginary lines drawn through the midclavicle, midmammary, and midsternum points on the front; the midaxilla on the side; and the midscapula on the back. Pathology is described in terms of these lines (e.g., abnormal lung sound heard at left midaxillary line, and so forth). Other helpful means of locating pathology is by the suprasternal notch, the ribs, and the spaces between them (**intercostal spaces**). Intercostal spaces are numbered according to the ribs immediately above them (Figure 28-18).

Inspect both front and back surfaces of the chest for symmetry of appearance and motion. An infant with a diaphragmatic hernia (intestine herniated into the chest cavity) may have a chest enlarged on that side. An infant with an *atelectasis* (collapsed lung) may have a chest that is smaller on that side. If a child has an enlarged heart, the left side of the chest may appear large. Inspect for **retractions** or indentation of intercostal spaces that reflects difficult respirations. Assess the proportion of anteroposterior to lateral diameter (normally 1:2). Chil-

dren with chronic lung disease develop a broad (barrel) chest or one more rounded than normal. This and other chest abnormalities are shown in Figure 28-19.

Breasts

Breast examination should be done on all children past puberty. This is also the time when girls should begin breast self-examination. Inspection of breast tissue is

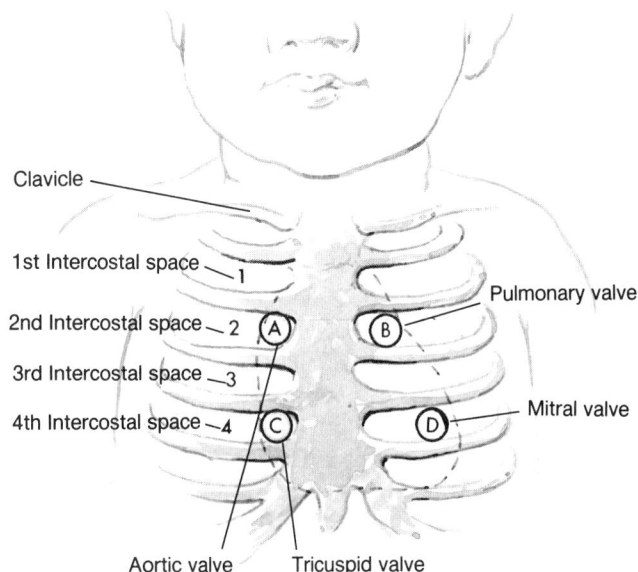

Clavicle

1st Intercostal space — 1

2nd Intercostal space — 2   (A)   (B)   Pulmonary valve

3rd Intercostal space — 3

4th Intercostal space — 4   (C)   (D)   Mitral valve

Aortic valve   Tricuspid valve

FIGURE 28-18
Intercostal (between rib) spaces are numbered according to the ribs immediately above them. The points (A, B, C, and D) to which the sounds of the heart valves radiate and where the sounds can be heard best are the listening posts of the heart.

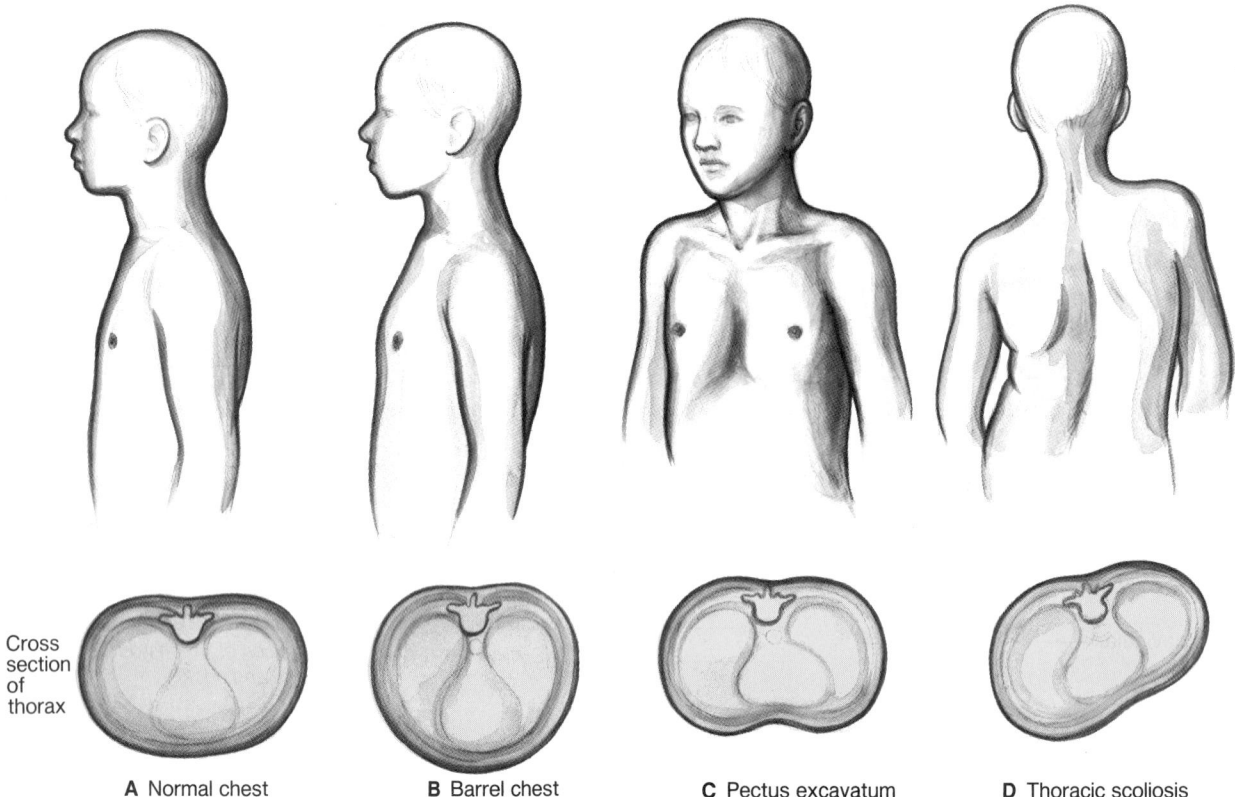

Cross section of thorax

A Normal chest   **B** Barrel chest   **C** Pectus excavatum   **D** Thoracic scoliosis

FIGURE 28-19
*Chest contours that can be assessed by inspection. (**A**) Normal chest. (**B**) Barrel chest. (**C**) Funnel chest (pectus excavatum). (**D**) Thoracic kyphoscoliosis.*

easiest if the child sits on the examining table, arms at the sides, with both breasts exposed. Inspect for symmetry, although it is not unusual (and normal) for a girl to have breasts of slightly unequal size.

Inspect for edema, erythema, wrinkling, retraction, or dimpling of the skin; all suggest that a tumor is growing in deeper layers of the tissue. Erythema occurs from inflammation due to abnormal, rapidly growing tissue; and edema, from the blockage of lymph channels due to tumor pressure. Breast edema makes the skin appear not only swollen but pitted (an orange-peel effect). Note any nipple discharge or "pulled" nipple placement as another way to detect edema.

With the girl's arms at her sides to take pressure off breast tissue, palpate well into each axilla (because breast tissue extends this far), and also palpate to assess axillary lymph nodes. Normally, no nodes should be felt. Ask the girl to lie down; place a folded towel under her near shoulder. Palpate the near breast with the girl lying down with her arm raised and placed under her head because this spreads out breast tissue; begin at the nipple and palpate outward in a circular motion. The lower edge of each breast feels hard; do not mistake this or rib prominences underneath for a tumor. Girls should inspect their own breasts monthly on the day following

the end of their menstrual period. This time not only serves as a marking point but is a time when hormonal influences on breast tissue are at a low ebb and breast tissue is normally not swollen or tender. The American Cancer Society's technique of breast self-examination is shown in Figure 28-20. In the older adolescent, another option might be for a sexual partner to assume this responsibility.

Newborn
Many newborns have breast edema from the influence of maternal hormones. A few drops of clear fluid may even be present from the nipples. This is normal.

School-Age Child and Adolescent
Many preadolescent boys develop hypertrophy of breast tissue due to increased hormonal influences (termed *gynecomastia*); they are generally concerned and need reassurance that it is normal for their age and will fade as soon as androgen becomes their dominant hormone. Adolescent girls may be concerned that breast tissue is inadequate or that breast growth is uneven. They need assurance that not all women have completely symmetric breasts.

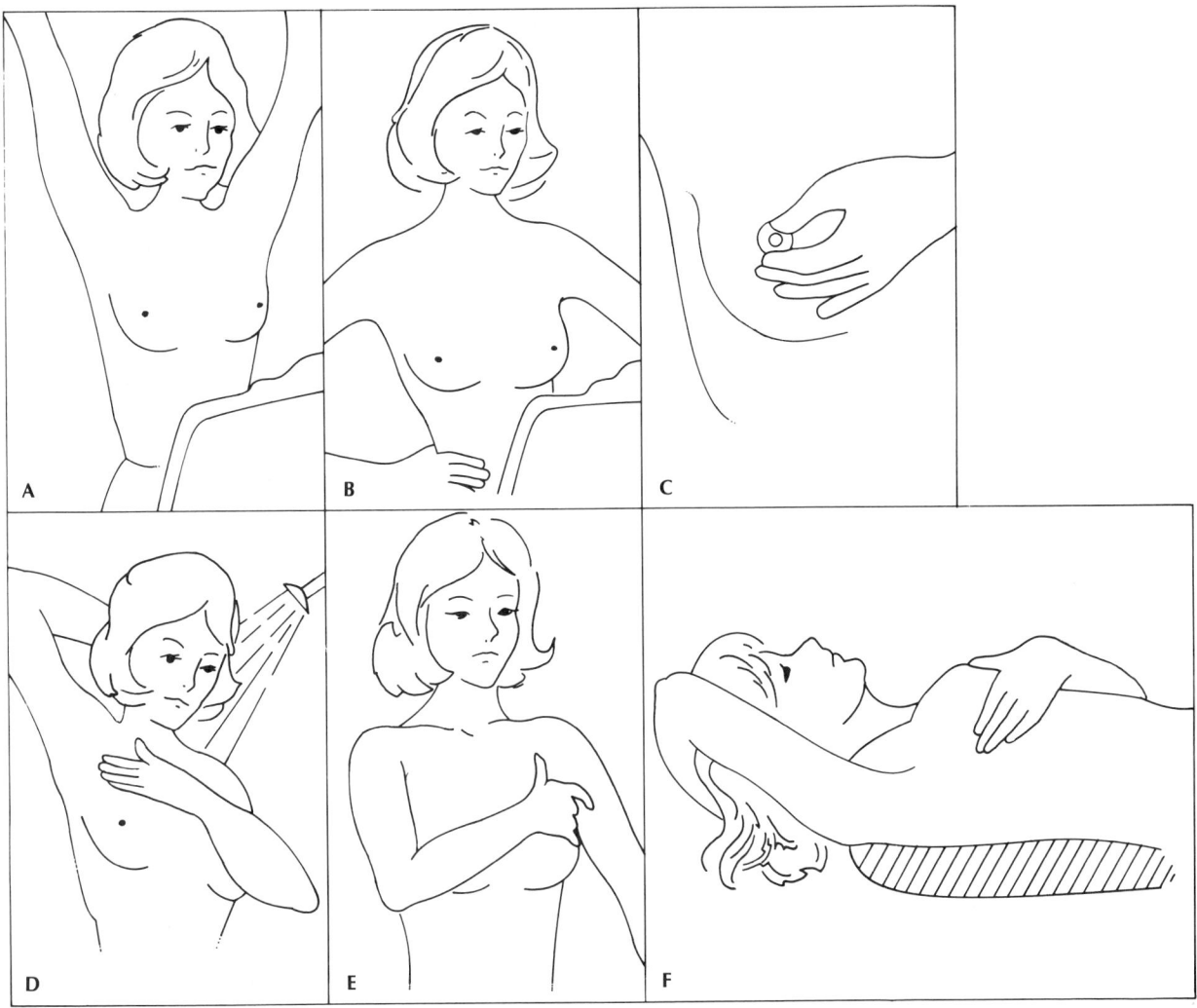

FIGURE 28-20
*Breast self-examination. Step 1. Inspection. (**A**) In front of a mirror, look for any change in the size or shape of the breast, puckering or dimpling of the skin, or changes in the nipple. (**B**) Inspect in three positions: (1) with arms relaxed at sides, (2) with arms held overhead, and (3) with hands on hips, pressing in to contract the chest muscles. Turn from side to side to view all areas. (**C**) Nipple examination. Gently squeeze the nipple of each breast between thumb and index finger to check for discharge. Step 2. Palpation or feeling. (**D**) In shower or bath, fingers will glide over wet soapy skin, making it easier to feel changes in the breast. Check the breast for a lump, knot, tenderness, or change in the consistency of normal tissue. To examine your right breast, put your right hand behind your head. With the pads of your fingers of your left hand held flat and together, gently press on the breast tissue using small circular motions. Imagine the breast as the face of a clock. Beginning at the top (12 o'clock position), make a circle around the outer area of the breast. Move in one finger width; continue in smaller and smaller circles until you have reached the nipple. Cover all areas including the breast tissue leading to the axilla. Reverse the procedure for the left breast. At the lower border of each breast, a ridge of firm tissue may be felt. This is normal. (**E**) Underarm examination. Examine the left underarm area with your arm held loosely at your side. Cup the fingers of the opposite hand and insert them high into the underarm area. Draw fingers down slowly, pressing in a circular pattern, covering all areas. Reverse the procedure for the right underarm. (**F**) Lying down. While lying flat, place a small pillow or folded towel under the right shoulder. Examine the right breast using the same circular motion as was used in the shower. Cover all areas. Repeat this procedure for the left breast. Press firmly but gently while examining your breast, rolling the tissue between your fingers and the chest wall. (Courtesy of the American Cancer Society, New York State Division, Inc. East Syracuse, New York, 1979.)*

Lungs

Assess the rate of respirations and whether respirations are easy and relaxed or if accessory muscles are necessary for effective ventilation. Palpate over lung areas for vibrations caused by difficult respirations.

On the anterior chest, lung tissue extends from above the clavicles to the 6th or 8th rib. On the posterior chest lung tissue is as low as the 10th to 12th thoracic vertebra. The right lung has three lobes; the left, only two. It is important when assessing lung tissue to attempt to evaluate all five lobes because lung disease can be specific for a lobe or involve the entire lung.

Next, percuss over lung tissue. Normal lung sounds are resonant, overexpanded lungs sound hyperresonant, and lungs filled with fluid sound dull. The lower anterior lobe of the right lung will sound dull, as liver covers it on the anterior surface below the fourth or fifth intercostal space. The space over the heart will also sound dull.

Diaphragmatic expanse (the distance the diaphragm descends with inhalation) is an estimate of lung volume. Establish this by asking the child to take in a deep breath and hold it; percuss downward to locate the bottom of the lungs (the percussion note changes from resonant to flat at this point). Next, ask the child to expire fully and momentarily hold that position. Percuss upward to locate the expired or empty lung position (the percussion note changes from flat to resonant). The difference between these two points is the **diaphragmatic excursion.**

Auscultate breath sounds by listening with the diaphragm of a stethoscope over each lung lobe while the child inhales and exhales (preferably with his or her mouth open). Listen both anteriorly and posteriorly; compare left side with right side for equal findings. Normal breath sounds are slightly longer on inspiration than expiration. Consider whether there are any abnormal sounds. Table 28-4 describes normal breath sounds as well as adventitious sounds that if heard might reflect illness.

Newborns and Infant

Infants cannot breathe in and out on request. Try to listen to breath sounds early in an examination, since the breath sounds are difficult to hear clearly over the sound of crying.

Heart

Heart assessment begins with visual inspection to see if there is a point on the chest where the heart beat can be observed. This point represents the location of the left ventricle or the point where the apical heartbeat can be heard best. In children younger than age 4 years, this point is generally lateral to the nipple line and at the fourth intercostal space; it is at the nipple line or just medial to it and at the fourth or fifth intercostal space in children older than age 4 years. This point is termed the **point of maximum impulse** and is observable in approximately 50% of children.

Percuss the left side of the chest to discern the left side of the heart. Percussing in from the axillary, the sound will become dull as the heart is identified. If the heart is farther to the left than usual, it suggests an enlarged heart. Normally the percussion note changes from resonant (percussing over lung) to flat (percussing over heart) midway between the midaxillary and midmammary line.

Heart Sounds

To hear heart sounds, auscultate at four main points. Although these are not the anatomic locations of heart valves, they are the listening points to which the sounds of the valves radiate and can be heard best (see Figure 28-18). The mitral valve is heard best at the fourth or

---

Table 28-4. *Breath Sounds Heard on Auscultation*

Sound	Characteristics
Vesicular	Soft, low-pitched, heard over periphery of lungs, inspiration longer than expiration. Normal.
Bronchovesicular	Soft, medium-pitched, heard over major bronchi; inspiration equals expiration. Normal.
Bronchial	Loud, high-pitched, heard over trachea; expiration longer than inspiration. Normal.
Rhonchi	Snoring sound made by air moving through mucus in bronchi. Normal.
Rales	Crackle (like cellophane) made by air moving through fluid in alveoli. Abnormal; denotes pneumonia, which is fluid in alveoli.
Wheezing	Whistling on expiration made by air being pushed through narrowed bronchi. Abnormal; seen in children with asthma or foreign-body obstruction.
Stridor	Crowing or roosterlike sound made by air being pulled through a constricted larynx. Abnormal; seen in infants with respiratory obstruction.

fifth left intercostal space at the nipple line; the tricuspid near the base of the sternum (fourth or fifth right intercostal space); the pulmonary valve at the second left intercostal space; and the aortic valve at the second right intercostal space. Table 28-5 describes normal and abnormal hearts sounds that may be heard on auscultation. Abnormal sounds are heard best if first the diaphragm and then the bell of the stethoscope is used.

To understand heart sounds, recall heart physiology. The first sound heard (S_1) is that of the mitral and tricuspid valves closing and the ventricles contracting (described as a "lub" sound). The second sound (described as a "dub" and termed S_2) is made by the closure of the aortic and pulmonary valves and atrial contraction. The first sound is generally longer and lower pitched than the second sound. It is louder than the second sound over the heart ventricles; otherwise, it is slightly quieter. Listen for the rhythm of the heart sounds. Rhythm should be regular. **Sinus arrhythmia** is a phenomenon that most school-age children demonstrate; it sounds abnormal but is not. In sinus arrhythmia, there is a marked heart rate increase as the child inspires, a marked decrease as the child expires; ask the child to hold his or her breath, and the rhythm of heart remains the same.

With inspiration and the normal resulting increase of pressure in the lungs, the pulmonary valve tends to close slightly later than the aortic valve. This is termed **physiologic splitting** and is heard as "lub d-dub." As long as this is associated with inspiration, it is a normal finding. Fixed splitting implies that there is always difficulty with the pulmonary valve closing and suggests pathology.

At times, a distinct third heart sound (S_3) may be heard due to rapid filling of the ventricles. This sound should be investigated but it is not necessarily a serious finding. The presence of a fourth heart sound (S_4) generally signifies heart pathology because this sound (a gallop rhythm) is caused by abnormal filling of the ventricles.

Listen to the heart rate in all areas; assess rate and compare this to the child's age to determine if it is a normal rate (Figure 28-21). A *heart murmur* is caused by

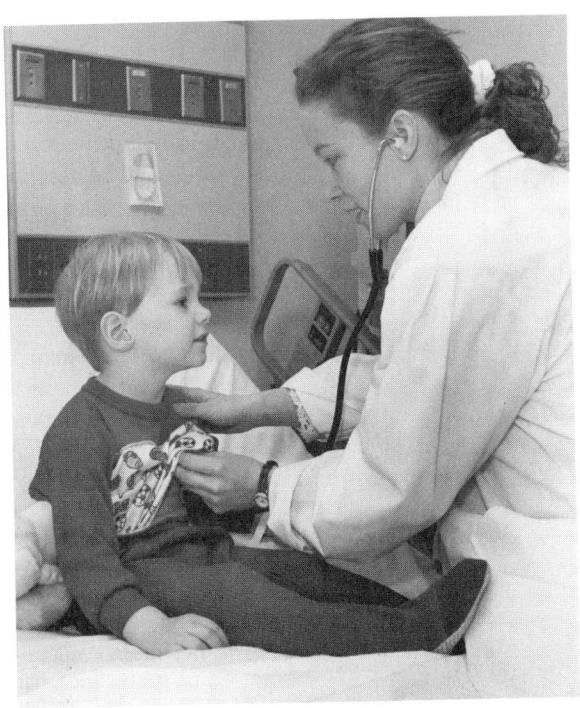

FIGURE 28-21
Auscultating heart sounds. (Courtesy of the Department of Medical Photography, Children's Hospital, Buffalo, NY.)

the sound of blood flowing with difficulty or in a different pathway within the heart (sounds like a swishing sound more than a murmur) and can be either innocent (functional) or pathogenic (organic). If a heart is pumping with abnormal force, there may be a palpable vibration termed a *thrill* on the chest wall. Palpate the precordium (area over the heart) for evidence of this (feels like the sensation of a cat purring) or a *heave* (a definite outward chest movement), which also denotes a struggling heart. Upon hearing or palpating any accessory heart sounds or movements, try to describe them with reference to Table 28-6.

All unusual heart sounds need further identification and investigation of their cause. The skills of listening to and identifying normal and abnormal heart sounds require considerable practice. Determining the cause of an abnormal heart sound requires a cardiac specialist. Determining that an abnormal sound exists, however, and securing proper referral is an important nursing role.

Newborn and Infant

Listen to heart sounds in newborns and infants early in an examination, before the child begins to cry, as it is almost impossible to evaluate heart sounds over the sound of crying. Allowing a parent to hold a child while doing this helps reduce fear.

Table 28-5. *Heart Sounds Heard on Auscultation*

Sound	Cause
S_1 (first heart sound)	Closure of tricuspid and mitral valves with beginning of ventricular contraction (systole)
S_2 (second heart sound)	Closure of pulmonary and aortic valves with beginning of atrial contraction (diastole)
S_3 (third heart sound)	Rapid ventricular filling
S_4 (fourth heart sound)	Abnormal filling of ventricles

Table 28-6. *Description of Accessory Heart Sounds*

Assessment	Information to Be Gathered
Location	At which listening post is the sound most distinct?
Quality	Can sound be described as blowing, rubbing, rasping, musical?
Intensity	*Murmurs* are graded according to the following criteria:
	Grade 6: So loud it can be heard with stethoscope not touching the chest wall; has a thrill (palpable vibration).
	Grade 5: Very loud but must touch stethoscope to chest to hear; has a thrill.
	Grade 4: Loud; may or may not have a thrill.
	Grade 3: Moderately loud; no thrill.
	Grade 2: Quiet but easily discernible.
	Grade 1: Very quiet; difficult to hear.
Timing	When in relation to S_1 and S_2 did you hear it? A sound superimposed between S_1 and S_2 is a *systolic murmur*; one between S_2 and the next S_1 is a *diastolic murmur*. Innocent murmurs (functional, denoting no pathology) are usually systolic, although there are exceptions to this; pathologic murmurs are more likely to be diastolic.
Pitch	Can the sound be described as high- or low-pitched?
Radiation and thrills	Is there an accompanying thrill? Does sound radiate so that it can be heard at another location, such as back of chest?

School-Age Child and Adolescent

Listen carefully for sounds of murmurs in children of school age and older. Refer them to a physician for further evaluation if any abnormalities are detected. Parents are always frightened by an unusual heart sound; unless the child has other symptoms, they can be assured that most murmurs are generally innocent (functional) and caused only by the normal flow of blood across valves.

Abdomen

The abdomen is divided anatomically into four quadrants. The quadrants and the organs that lie within them are shown in Figure 28-22. To assess the abdomen, first inspect the surface for symmetry and contour. It will be slightly protuberant in infants and scaphoid in older children. Note any skin lesions or scars.

Auscultate the abdomen for bowel sounds before palpating, because palpating may alter bowel movement (peristalsis) and therefore disturb bowel sounds. Bowel sounds can normally be heard in all quadrants of the abdomen. They are high "pinging" sounds that occur normally at time intervals of approximately 5 to 10 seconds and are heard best through the bell of a stethoscope. If a bowel is distended, the sounds occur more frequently; if the bowel is blocked so that there is no movement of contents, the sounds will be absent below the obstruction. Listen for 3 to 5 minutes before concluding that no bowel sounds are present.

Listen along the middle of the abdomen over the aorta for irregular sounds. A **bruit** is a swishing or blowing sound that occurs if there is an outpouching of the

aorta (an aneurysm), a condition that can be congenital, although it usually occurs with aging.

Palpate the abdomen in a systematic order to include all four quadrants such as right lower quadrant, right upper quadrant, left lower quadrant, and left upper quadrant. Palpate first lightly, then deeply. If the child has indicated that any portion of his or her abdomen is tender, begin assessment at the farthest point and work toward the tender area. If no tenderness is present, the

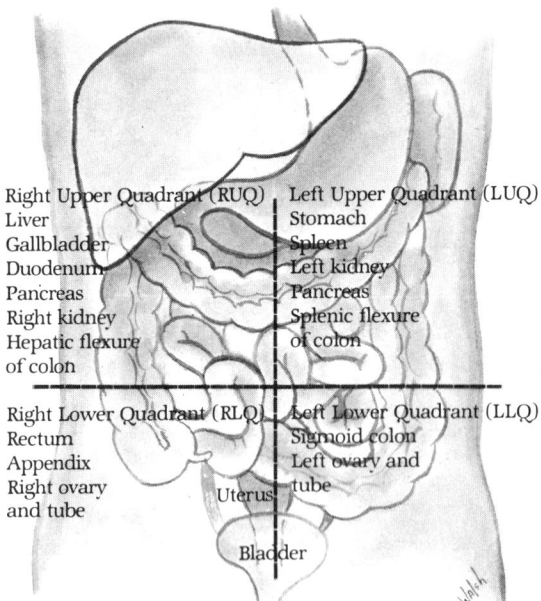

Right Upper Quadrant (RUQ)
Liver
Gallbladder
Duodenum
Pancreas
Right kidney
Hepatic flexure
of colon

Left Upper Quadrant (LUQ)
Stomach
Spleen
Left kidney
Pancreas
Splenic flexure
of colon

Right Lower Quadrant (RLQ)
Rectum
Appendix
Right ovary
and tube

Left Lower Quadrant (LLQ)
Sigmoid colon
Left ovary and
tube

Uterus

Bladder

FIGURE 28-22
Quadrants of the abdomen and underlying structures.

order of palpation is unimportant as long as it is thorough. Ascertain whether any area is tender by watching the child's face while palpating; observe for "guarding" or the child tensing the abdominal muscles to keep anyone from pressing deeply at that point. Note any hard areas or masses.

By palpating from the right lower quadrant to the right upper quadrant, the hand will "bump" against the lower edge of the liver 1 cm to 2 cm below the right ribs (Figure 28-23). On the left side, the lower edge of the spleen may be discernible in the same way. A liver or spleen larger than this is suggestive of disease. Palpate the umbilicus to try to identify the presence of an umbilical hernia. A fascial ring at the umbilicus of more than 2 cm in diameter in an infant denotes a ring of fascia larger than will normally close spontaneously; when this is present, the child will generally need surgery to reduce the umbilical hernia. Liver, spleen, and bladder size can all be documented further by percussion.

Newborn and Infant

Kidneys may be located by deep abdominal palpation in newborns and infants. To do this, place a hand under the infant's back just below the 12th rib; press upward. Place the other hand on that side of the abdomen just below the umbilicus. Press deeply. A kidney can be palpated as a firm mass approximately the size of a walnut between the hands. The right kidney is slightly lower than the left so is easiest to locate.

Preschool and School-Age Child

Children's abdomens at this age are often "ticklish" and children may tense or "guard" their abdominal muscles when touched, making it difficult to palpate. Distract the child by asking him or her a question about home or school or let the child put his or her hand over the examiner's to help relax.

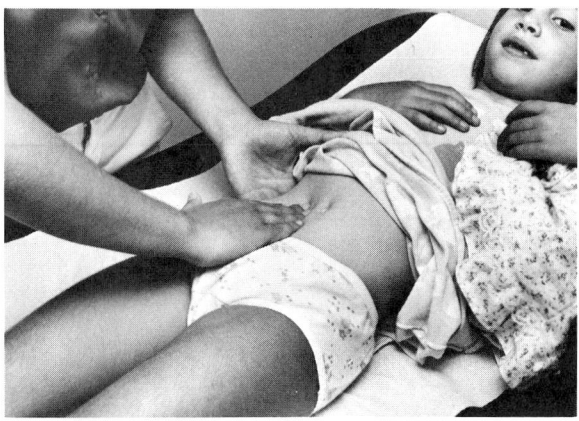

FIGURE 28-23
Deep palpation of the abdomen to locate the lower edge of the liver. (Courtesy of the Department of Medical Photography, Children's Hospital, Buffalo, NY.)

Genitorectal Area

In both sexes, the rectum should be inspected for any protruding hemorrhoidal tissue (rare in children) or fissures.

Female Genitalia

Inspection of external female genitalia and assessment of femoral nodes is included in every complete health assessment. An external examination consists of inspecting for hair growth and configuration (an inverted triangle) and inspection of external genitalia (i.e., clitoris, labia majora, and labia minora) for normal contours. Look for signs of discharge or irritation. A vaginal discharge or fourchette tear in a young child may suggest child abuse (Frasier et al., 1992). Internal pelvic examination is discussed in Chapter 10.

Male Genitalia

Inspection of male genitalia consists of observing the distribution of hair (male pubic hair has a diamond-shaped distribution); lesions of the penis; appearance and placement of the urethral opening (should be slit-like—children with repeated urinary tract infections develop scarring of the meatal opening, making it small and round—and centered at the penis tip); and ability of the foreskin to retract if the boy is uncircumcised. *Phimosis* exists when the foreskin is too tight to retract. **Hypospadias** is a term for a urethral opening located on the inferior or ventral (under) surface of the penis; **epispadias** denotes a urethral opening on the superior or dorsal (upper) surface. Both these conditions need to be identified. If more than a slight deviation is present, repair is usually initiated before school age as such a urethral placement may interfere with fertility and self-image if not corrected.

Inspect the scrotum for size and the presence of testes. In most boys, the left testis is slightly lower than the right, so the scrotum does not appear truly symmetric. Palpate to check that testes are both present by placing one hand over the top of the scrotum at the inguinal ring and then palpating the testis on that side (Figure 28-24). This hand position prevents the testis from slipping up into the inguinal ring and appearing to be absent on palpation. Any swelling or mass in the scrotum needs to be identified. The most likely cause of such a condition is a **hydrocele**, or a fluid-filled sac; it could represent a serious finding such as testicular cancer in adolescents. Hydroceles can be transilluminated: when a flashlight is held in back of the scrotum, the fluid-filled cyst "glows." A **varicocele** (enlarged veins of the epididymis) may be palpated. These are not important findings in young boys; they may interfere with fertility in later life.

Assess the urethral meatus for any discharge that could reveal an STD such as gonorrhea or any lesions

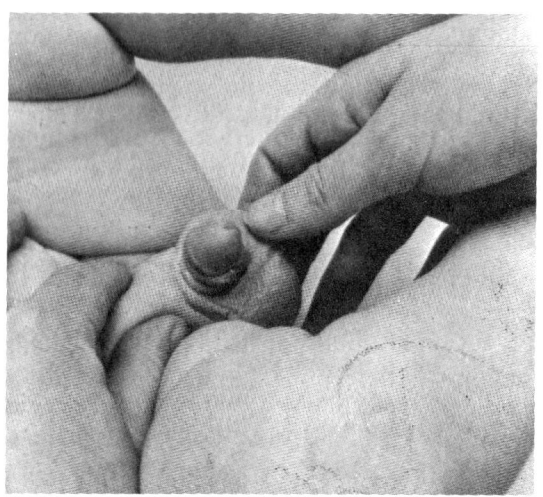

FIGURE 28-24
Assessing for descended testes. The left hand prevents the testes from sliding upward during examination. (Alexander, M., & Brown, M. S. [1978]. Pediatric physical diagnosis for nurses. *New York: McGraw-Hill, with permission.)*

that would suggest herpes II infection or syphilis (see Chapter 47). Beginning at puberty, boys should be taught to do testicular palpation every month. The technique for this is shown in Box 28-2.

Inguinal Hernia

To assess for the presence of an inguinal hernia in an infant, simply observe the groin areas for any bulging (especially while the infant is crying). In a school-age child or adolescent, with the child standing, place a fingertip against the inguinal ring in the groin area and ask the child to cough. If the tendency for a hernia is present, coughing tightens abdominal muscles and forces abdominal contents to bulge against the finger. Palpate femoral nodes (located in the groin and on the inner surface of the upper thigh) for any swelling, which suggests infection.

Extremities

Observe upper extremities for good color and warmth. Inspect fingernails for color, contour, and shape. Normally, nails are pink, smooth, and convex in shape. They should feel hard to touch and not brittle so they do not break readily. Signs of bitten fingernails in the school-age child may reflect a high level of stress. Black children's nails are more deeply pigmented. A blue or purple tinge denotes cyanosis; a yellowed tinge is jaundice. Children who have decreased respiratory function or cyanotic heart disease develop "clubbed" fingers (Figure 28-25); children with endocarditis often have characteristic linear hemorrhages under nails. Iron deficiency anemia may cause extremely concave surfaces

(spoon shaped). Press against a fingernail, release the pressure, and time the refilling interval (should be under 5 seconds). Count the fingers and check for webbing between fingers. Examine for the pattern of fingerprints. Distinctive dermatoglyphics are present on fingertips from the third month of intrauterine life; these are unique to every person but show patterns of circular grooves. Abnormal fingerprints may occur with chromosomal anomalies. Check for normal palmar creases. Children with chromosomal abnormalities often have one central palm crease (a simian line) rather than the nor-

---

Box 28-2
Testicular Self-Examination

Adolescent males should begin testicular self-examination with the same conscientiousness as girls do breast self-examination. Suggest that they select a certain day each month (first day, last day, and so forth) and do it in or immediately after a shower, because that is when scrotal skin is most relaxed. The adolescent should roll each testis gently between thumb and fingers to assess for hard lumps or nodules, change in consistency, or difference in size, any of which he should report. He should know that in most males one testis is slightly larger than the other and hangs a little lower in the scrotal sac, so that he does not think these findings are abnormal. The epididymis, at the rear of the testes, feels like a strong cord; he should be familiar with its feel and recognize it as normal.

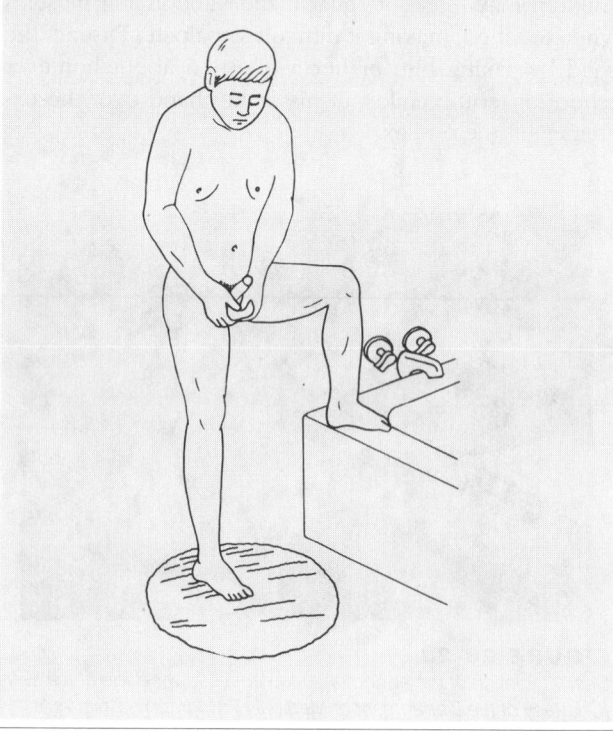

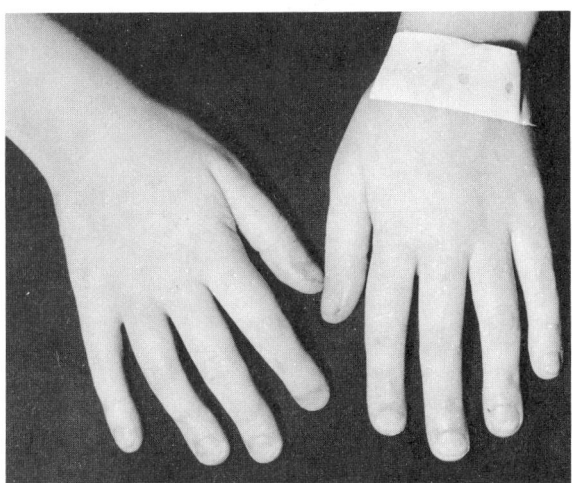

FIGURE 28-25
Clubbed fingers are a sign of cyanosis from congenital heart disease. (Courtesy of the Department of Medical Photography, Children's Hospital, Buffalo, NY.)

mal three. Check the wrist, elbow, and shoulder joints for movement and normal range of motion; palpate joints for swelling or warmth. Palpate to be certain that no lymph nodes are present in the antecubital space; palpate to check that the radial pulse is present.

Inspect the lower extremities for color and warmth. Count the toes and check for webbing between toes. Check the ankle, knee, and hip joints for normal range of motion. Check for subluxated hip in infants by attempting to abduct fully the hip (see Figure 23-20). Palpate to be certain that no lymph nodes are present in the groin or popliteal areas. Palpate that femoral pulses are present and equal bilaterally. Ask the older child to walk and observe for ease of gait, limping, or any foot displacement such as toeing in or out. Toddlers typically walk with a wide-based gait; they walk best if allowed to walk toward their parent (a safe action) rather than away. Many adolescents are self-conscious and slouch or "amble" rather than presenting their true, natural gait.

Back

Inspect the back for symmetry and the spinal column for any deviation. Inspect the base of the spine for a *dermal sinus* (a pinpoint opening) or for a tuft of hair that might reveal a *spina bifida* (a defect of the bony structure of the canal). Inspect also for any dimpling that might denote a dermal cyst (*pilonidal cyst*). This is an innocent finding unless it becomes infected or connects to deeper tissue layers. Assess for tenderness along the spinal column by palpating each vertebra. Have a school-age child bend over; check the straightness of the spine in this position (scoliosis or spinal curvature will be magnified in this position and be more prominent than in a standing position; see Chapter 51).

Neurologic Function

A full neurologic examination takes at least 20 minutes to complete. This is not included in a routine physical examination, therefore. However, it is important to assess for **deep tendon reflexes**, such as triceps, biceps, patellar, and Achilles reflexes, and to test for motor and sensory function. Techniques for eliciting deep tendon reflexes are shown in Figure 28-26. Grade reflexes according to the scale in Table 28-7. The biceps reflex tests 5th and 6th cervical nerves; the triceps reflex, the 7th and 8th cervical nerves; the patellar, the 2nd, 3rd, and 4th lumbar; and the Achilles, the 1st and 2nd sacral. Test the sole of the foot for a *Babinski reflex* (Figure 28-27). This will demonstrate a fanning of the toes in an infant younger than age 3 months and a downward reflex of the toes beyond age 3 months. (Some normal infants demonstrate a flaring Babinski reflex until age 2 years; in the absence of other neurologic findings, this is not significant.)

Test for **superficial reflexes**: abdominal reflexes in both sexes, cremasteric reflex in males. An abdominal reflex is elicited by lightly stroking each quadrant of the abdomen. Normally, the umbilicus moves perceptibly toward the stroke. Presence of the reflex indicates integrity of the 10th thoracic nerve and the 1st lumbar nerve of the spinal cord. A *cremasteric reflex* is elicited by stroking the medial aspect of the thigh in boys. The testes move perceptibly upward in a normal male. The presence of this reflex indicates integrity of the 1st and 2nd lumbar nerves.

Motor and Sensory Function

Test cranial nerve function generally by asking the child to make a face. The child's ability to grasp with his or her hands and push against a surface with his or her feet establishes general motor ability. Recall whether gait was adequate when the child was observed walking.

To test sensory function, ask the child to close his or her eyes and identify the location when he is touched at six points (at least) on different body parts.

Vision Assessment

More than 3 million people in the United States are vision impaired (Tielsch et al., 1990). Assessing vision, therefore, is an important part of physical assessment. The extent of testing depends on the age of the child.

Any child with congenital anomalies, low birth weight, or fetal alcohol syndrome is at high risk for eye abnormalities, as is a child who received oxygen at birth. Because the average parent is careful of a child's eyes, an unreported injury or infection or signs of neglected vision that are noticed during assessment may be indicative of child neglect.

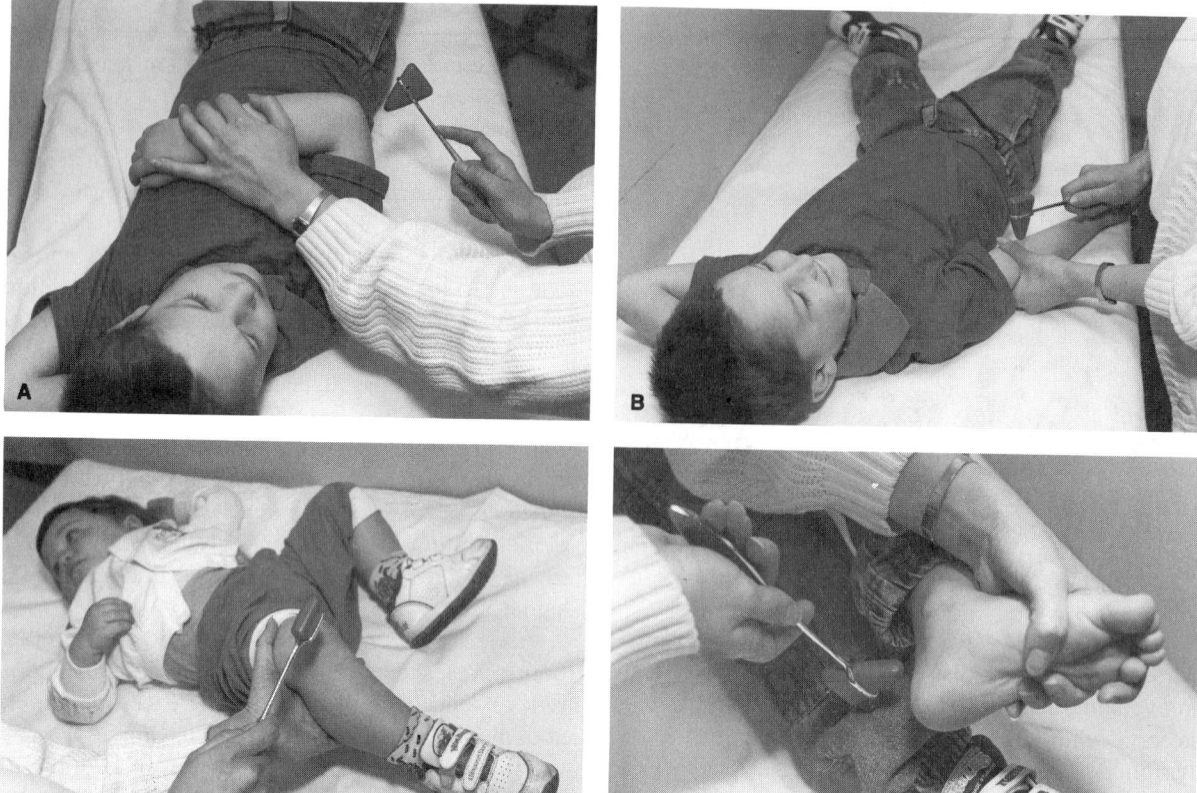

FIGURE 28-26

*Deep tendon reflexes. (**A**) Triceps reflex. The triceps tendon is struck. The forearm will move perceptibly if the reflex is elicited. (**B**) Biceps reflex. The examiner's thumb is placed over the biceps tendon. The reflex hammer actually strikes the examiner's thumb. The examiner will feel the child's forearm move when the reflex is elicited. (**C**) Patellar reflex. The patellar tendon is tapped briskly. The reflex is most obvious when the child's leg is relaxed. (**D**) Achilles reflex. The Achilles tendon is struck. The foot will move if the reflex is elicited. (Courtesy of the Department of Medical Photography, Children's Hospital, Buffalo, NY.)*

Vision Screening

Common vision screening indicators and techniques for children of different ages are summarized in Table 28-8. Parents can provide important clues to possible problems: listen carefully any time a parent expresses concern about or questions a child's ability to see properly.

Table 28-7. *Grading of Deep Tendon Reflexes*

Grade	Interpretation
4+	Hyperactive; extremely marked reaction; abnormal
3+	Stronger than average but within normal range
2+	Average response
1+	Less than average response but within normal range
0	No response; abnormal

Newborn and Infant

A parent's description of a child's activity may give clues to vision problems. Ask the parents if the infant's eyes follow them as they move around the room. Does the infant return their smile? Do the parents have any reason to think the child has difficulty seeing?

Newborns should be able to focus on a moving object such as a finger and follow it to the midline. Infants see black and white objects better than they do colored objects. They seem to see objects most clearly at a distance of 19 cm (8 in to 10 in).

Toddler and Preschooler

Ask the parents of older infants, toddlers, or preschoolers if children rub their eyes, blink frequently, squint, or frown. Cover one eye to look at objects? Tilt their heads to see things better? Stumble over objects in their path? Hold books and toys extremely close or extremely far away? Asking whether children sit close to a television set is meaningless because almost all children do that if allowed.

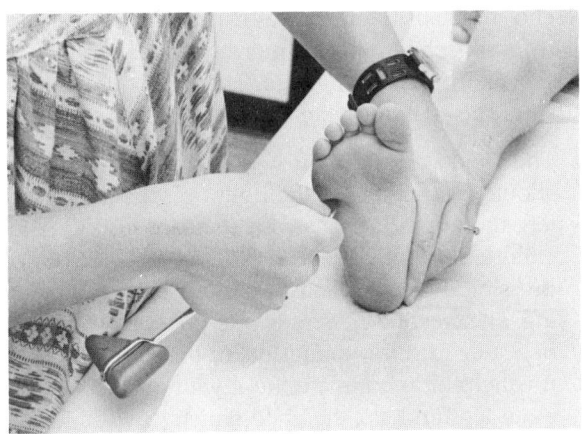

FIGURE 28-27
Babinski reflex. The handle of the reflex hammer is brought along the outside surface in a J-pattern. In newborns, the toes flare; in older children, they plantar flex. (Courtesy of the Department of Medical Photography, Children's Hospital, Buffalo, NY.)

School-Age Child and Adolescent

Ask the parents of school-age children if children state they have frequent headaches. How are children doing with classwork? Do they avoid sports that require long-distance vision, such as baseball or softball? Do they avoid watching movies? Do they skip over words when reading aloud? Have blurriness or double vision? Have reddened conjunctivae or drainage from the eyes? Do they blink at bright light?

Techniques of Vision Testing

Vision is tested by asking the child to read an eye chart. All children need good orientation to such testing. It should be stressed with them that this is not a "test" in

the usual sense of the word, and that "failing" the test will not result in a bad grade.

Snellen Chart

As soon as children can identify letters of the alphabet (early school age), their vision can be tested at a health checkup by using a Snellen eye chart (Figure 28-28). This chart is standardized, so set procedures must be followed when using it to test vision:

1. Hang the chart so that the 20-ft line is at the child's eye level. The child who has to look up or down must look farther than the child who is looking straight across at the chart. A possible solution to avoid moving the chart is to have smaller children stand and taller children sit. To accommodate children in wheelchairs, the chart needs to be lowered (or else have all children sit for the test).

2. Provide a good light for the chart and place it so there is no glare. A light intensity of 20 foot-candles is recommended.

3. Measure a distance of 20 ft from the chart. Mark the floor at this point with a piece of masking tape or other similar mark. For younger children, it is helpful to cut out paper footprints and paste them to the floor with the *heels* of the footprints touching the 20-ft line. If the child sits in a chair, the back legs of the chair should touch the 20-ft line.

4. Provide an individual with a 3″ × 5″ card (to cover the eye not being tested) for each child who is examined.

5. If the child wears glasses, screen the child while he or she is wearing the glasses. Do not screen the child first without glasses and then with them, because this forces the child to strain to read the

Table 28-8. *Common Vision Screening Indicators and Procedures*

Age	Common Test
Newborn	General appearance*
	Ability to follow moving object to midline; focus steadily on an object at 10–12 in.
Infant and toddler	General appearance*
	Ability to follow light past midline
3 yr–school age	General appearance*
	Random dot E for stereopsis (depth perception)
	Allen cards or preschool E chart for visual acuity
	Ishihara's plates for color awareness
School-age–adult	General appearance*
	Snellen's test for visual acuity

* Note redness, blinking, squinting, crusting, and so forth.

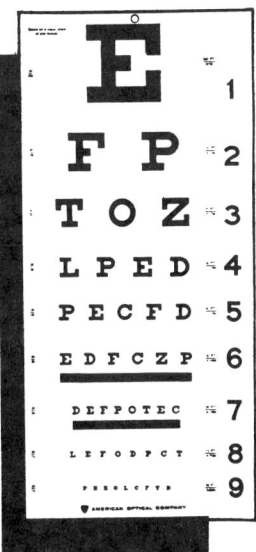

FIGURE 28-28
Snellen vision testing chart. (From the American Optical Corporation, with permission.)

chart. After squinting, a child may have difficulty readjusting to reading with glasses and this makes the prescription appear too weak or too strong. If a child has forgotten his or her glasses, defer the screening until the child can bring the glasses.

6. To begin testing, tell the child to stand with his or her shoes on the footprints (heels against the line); keep both eyes open; and cover the *left* eye with the occluding card. Be certain the child does not press the card against the eye (instead, the edge of the card should rest across the child's nose), because pressure will cause blurred vision when the child removes the card to test that eye.

7. Begin at the 40-ft line of the chart and, using a pointer or pencil, point to each symbol on the line from left to right (the order in which children are taught to read). If the child reads a majority of symbols in a line, he or she sees the line satisfactorily.

8. If the child "passes" the 40-ft line, have the child read the 30- and 20-ft lines or the last line the child can read. Record the last line read. If the child fails to read the 40-ft line satisfactorily, then begin at the top of the chart and move downward to identify the last line the child can read. Record this reading. Because the 200-ft, 100-ft, and 70-ft lines have so few symbols, the child must read all the symbols on them to have read satisfactorily.

9. Visual acuity is always stated as a fraction. The top number is the distance in feet the child stands from the chart (always 20). The bottom of the fraction represents the last line the child read correctly. The adult with good (average) vision can read the 20-ft line from 20 ft away and thus is said to have 20/20 vision.

10. It is important to test the eyes separately, then together. For example, Tony reads all the symbols on the 40-ft line with his right eye; he misses three out of four on the 30-ft line. His visual acuity for his right eye is 20 (the distance from the chart) over 40 (the last line he read correctly). With his left eye, Tony reads the 40-ft, 30-ft, and 20-ft lines correctly. His vision in that eye is 20/20. With both eyes, Tony reads the 40-ft, 30-ft, and 20-ft lines correctly. His visual acuity for both eyes is 20/20. If only this last reading were taken, the right eye weakness (a symptom of *amblyopia* or "lazy eye") would be missed.

11. Observe the child for straining or squinting as he or she reads the chart. By squinting and changing the shape of the eyeball, a child can improve his or her vision and will score higher. The child will appear to see better than he or she actually does in everyday situations.

Preschool E Chart

Between age 3 years and the age they can read the alphabet, children can have vision tested by using a preschool E chart (Figure 28-29). This chart is also helpful in testing children with mental retardation or those who speak a foreign language. The procedure is similar to that of the standard Snellen chart:

1. The child stands 20 ft from the chart. The child should read first with the right eye, then with the left, then both eyes, as with standard testing. Young children do not understand the importance of not pressing the card against their eye or of not peeking, so a second person is often needed to hold the occluder card for youngsters of this age.

2. It is helpful to compare the *E* with a table with three legs and ask the child which way the legs of the table point. Children age 3 years are familiar with tables, but *E*s are strange symbols. Tell the child to point with the entire arm and hand in the direction the legs point so that you do not confuse his or her motion.

3. Begin at the 40-ft line, as with the standard Snellen chart, and work downward until the child passes all lines or cannot read the majority of symbols on a line.

National Association for the Prevention of Blindness Home Test

A home eye test is available from the National Association for the Prevention of Blindness for parents to use to test children age 3 years to 6 years at home. It is similar to the preschool E chart except smaller; the child stands only 10 ft away. The test can help alert parents that a child needs a professional eye examination; it can be given or suggested to parents whose child is tired or for some other reason has not tested well in a health care facility.

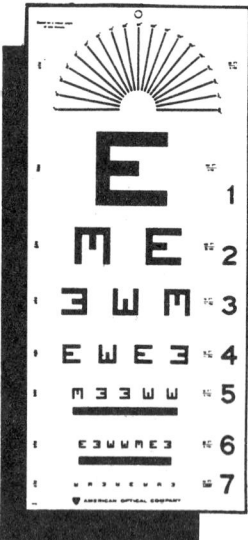

FIGURE 28-29
Astigmatic and preschool E chart. (From the American Optical Corporation, with permission.)

Allen Cards

Preschool children may be tested with Allen cards on which are pictures of common objects such as a horse and rider, car, house, and birthday cake. These are shown to the child at a 15-ft distance, and the child is asked to identify the pictures (proof that the child sees them). Be certain the child has time to examine the cards before the test so that he or she knows the names of the objects (Mayer & Gross, 1990).

Stycar Cards

For this test, the child is given cards with nine letters: *H, C, O, L, U, T, X, V,* and *A.* The child holds up the card that matches the one pointed to on a chart.

Titmus Vision Tester

Another useful method for testing the vision of children is the Titmus Vision Tester. This is the same instrument used by many motor vehicle license offices. As the child looks into the eyepieces of the machine, alphabet letters or preschool *E*s are projected onto a well-lighted screen for the child to identify. Closed vision testers such as the Titmus have an advantage over wall charts in that the child is less easily distracted during testing. Also, because the child cannot see the vision chart beforehand, he or she cannot memorize letters to enable passing the test.

Cover Testing

A cover test is used to detect **strabismus** (misalignment of the eyes).

To perform a cover test (Figure 28-30), have the child fix his or her vision on an attractive object, such as an examining light or a toy, approximately 4 ft in front of the child. Hold a 3″ × 5″ card over the left eye for a count of five. If any degree of strabismus is present, the eye will wander to its misaligned position while covered. Remove the card and observe the eye for movement. As the child again fixes his or her vision on the specified object in front, the child's eye will move to come into line again. This movement reveals the misalignment. Repeat the process with the right eye.

Some children, particularly preschoolers who have wide epicanthic folds, may appear, at a quick glance, to show misalignment. A cover test is helpful in these children. There is no eye movement after removal of the card because there is no misalignment present, only the temporary appearance of misalignment. Reasons for true misalignment are discussed in Chapter 50.

Color Vision Deficit Testing

Color vision deficit is a sex-linked recessive characteristic that tends to occur in males rather than in females, although females carry the gene for the disorder. All male children should be screened once for the disorder during their early school years.

This can be tested by asking the child to identify the

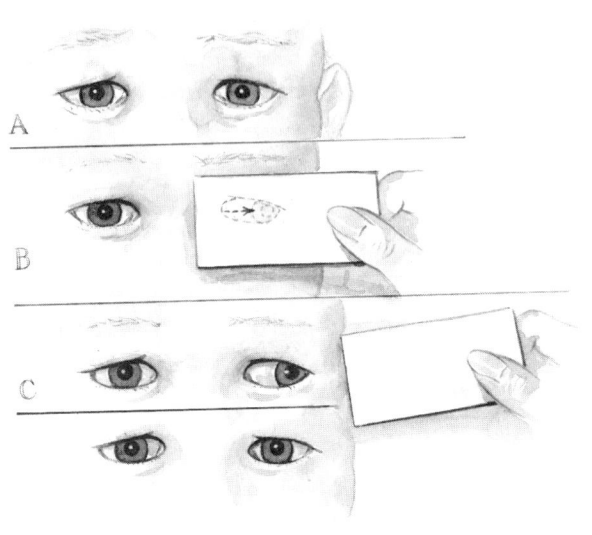

FIGURE 28-30
Cover test. (**A**) *The child's eyes appear to be in good alignment.* (**B**) *The left eye is covered for 5 seconds.* (**C**) *When the card is removed, the left eye is seen to move perceptibly back to good alignment. This movement indicates that it "drifted" into a deviant position while covered, that is, that an exophoria (misalignment) is present. (Courtesy of the Department of Medical Illustration, State University of New York at Buffalo.)*

colored stripes at the top of a Snellen eye chart. This type of screening can also be done by showing the child a series of colored diagrams (Ishihara's plates) in which a person with color vision can see hidden figures, but people with red-green or yellow-blue color vision deficits cannot. Detecting color vision deficit in children is important because many educational materials depend on the ability to identify color, and certain occupations are closed to people who cannot identify colors. Even such a simple childhood pleasure as riding a bicycle safely on city streets depends on being able to distinguish colors, for example, red from green on a traffic light.

Vision Referrals

Children should be screened twice before being referred to a physician for corrective eye care, as some children do not perform well on eye tests because they are easily distracted or do not know their alphabet as well as they pretend. For example, they may say that they do not see a letter when they really mean they do not know or remember its name. Testing twice helps eliminate or identify this type of misleading result.

Following a second screening, the following children should be referred:

- Preschool children who have 20/50 vision in one or both eyes
- Children in kindergarten or later who have 20/40 vision or worse in one or both eyes

- Any child with a two-line difference between the eyes, which might be the beginning of amblyopia
- Any child who states or shows symptoms of visual disturbance

Hearing Assessment

A thorough health assessment should include an evaluation of hearing, including both history and observation, because good hearing is necessary for the development of age-appropriate skills. When taking an auditory history, be certain to ask the accompanying adult or parent an overall question such as, "Have you had any reason to believe Lucy doesn't hear as she should?" Parents and grandparents are usually attuned to hearing difficulty in children and may be suspicious of it in advance of its official detection.

Auditory Screening

Screening for adequate hearing levels requires knowledge of the technique and use of an audiometer. Testing requires a quiet, undistracting setting and consequently is usually not done at routine health appraisals, but only when symptoms suggest ear disease or hearing impairment is present. Screening will vary according to age and developmental stage.

Newborn and Infant

In the past, all newborns at birth were screened for congenital hearing loss. These mass screening programs, however, detected few afflicted infants. Currently, the American Academy of Pediatrics (1983) recommends that mass screening is unnecessary but that certain infants who are high risk should be screened between ages 3 months and 6 months. These may include any of the following conditions:

- History of childhood hearing impairment in the family
- Perinatal infection, such as cytomegalovirus, rubella, herpes, toxoplasmosis, or syphilis
- Anatomic malformations involving the head or neck
- Birth weight less than 1500 g
- Hyperbilirubinemia at a level exceeding indication for exchange transfusion
- Bacterial meningitis, especially when caused by *Hemophilus influenzae*
- Severe birth asphyxia: infants with an Apgar score of 0 to 3, those who failed to breathe spontaneously within 10 minutes of birth, or those with hypotonia persisting to age 2 hours

If a newborn's hearing is assessed, it usually is done through simple response testing (observing whether an infant stirs or responds to a sound made or delivered to the child with a commercial device). It can also be done by auditory-evoked brain stem screening (Figure 28-31). For this method, an earphone is placed on the infant and an electrode is attached to the scalp. When sound is transmitted to the child's ear through the earphone, the electrical potential created as the sound is processed by the brain stem is read by the scalp electrode, processed by a microcomputer, and plotted on a graph such as the one in Figure 28-31. This type of testing may be used at any age and is even successful for comatose or anesthetized persons. Smaller units using otoacoustic emissions are also available. With these, a click stimulus delivered to a normal ear produces an echo from the cochlea. This can be detected by a miniature microphone to reveal even minor hearing loss.

Older Child

Older children who are at high risk for hearing loss are those who have been exposed to loud noises, were of low birth weight, have congenital anomalies, have a repaired cleft palate, or have had repeated ear infections. During history taking, ask children if they ever worry that they have difficulty hearing. Ask them how they are doing in school. Some children with a minimum hearing impairment are considered to have behavioral problems in school because they do not follow directions or appear not to be following the teacher's discussion. In fact,

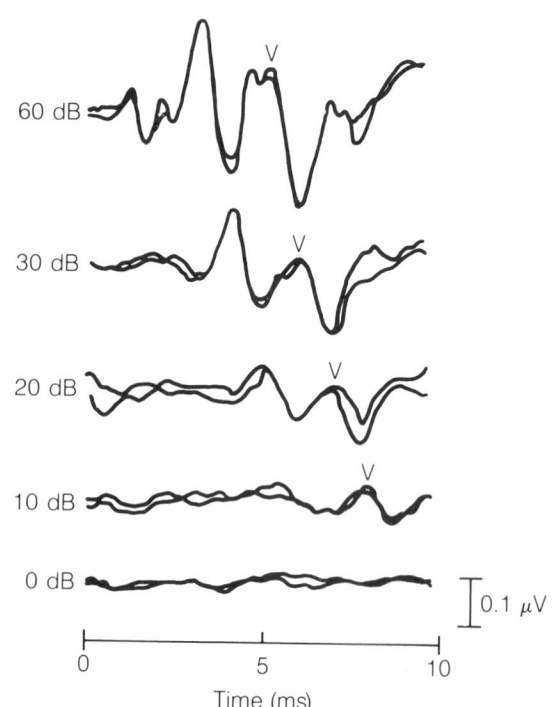

FIGURE 28-31

Wave pattern produced by auditory-evoked brain stem responses. (Stool, S. E. [1984]. Current methods of screening for hearing impairment. Consultant, 24, 131, with permission.)

they may be unable to hear what is being said. Be certain not to confuse difficulty hearing with shyness or recalcitrance in answering. At the age that children can indicate clearly whether they can hear a sound presented to them (at approximately age 3 years), they are judged old enough for audiometric assessment. Children with an ear infection (otitis media) should not be tested because their hearing is temporarily affected by this.

Principles of Audiometric Assessment

Frequency

Sound is the result of vibration; frequency is the number of vibrations a sound creates per second. When frequency is increased, the pitch of the sound increases. For audiometric testing, frequency is measured in Hertz units. Normal speech sounds fall into a narrow range, 500 Hz to 2000 Hz. To function adequately and speak effectively, a child must be able to hear in this range. Children are tested for a wider frequency range than this, from 500 Hz to 6000 Hz, on a routine screening assessment.

Loudness

Decibels are an expression of the intensity of loudness of a sound (or vigor of the vibrations). A decibel level of 0 dB is the softest sound that can be heard. Normal conversation is approximately 50 dB to 60 dB. The sound level at which inner ear damage can occur is about 90 dB. Sound levels of 140 dB are so intense they actually cause pain. Screening audiometry is done at 25 dB.

Hearing Loss

Table 28-9 lists levels of hearing impairment. A hearing loss of 30 dB means the child has some difficulty hearing normal instructions and questions. A loss of 50 dB or more is severe: the child misses most normal conversation and cannot hope to achieve in a regular classroom environment. The child's speech will be impaired because he or she does not hear normal speech sounds.

If a child can hear all frequencies at the 25 dB level, he or she has passed an audiometric screening check. If the child fails to hear two or more frequencies at 25 dB, in either or both ears, the child has failed a screening audiometry test and should be referred to a physician or an otologist (Figure 28-32) shows an **audiogram**, a record of audiometric testing, of a child with normal hearing in the right ear (the child heard all frequencies at the 20 dB level) but a loss of 45 dB in the left ear at frequencies of 1000 Hz, 2000 Hz, and 4000 Hz.

Acoustic Impedance Testing

Acoustic impedance testing is based on the principle that sound entering the ear canal meets resistance at the tympanic membrane. If the middle ear is function-

Table 28-9. Levels of Hearing Impairment

dB Level	Hearing Level Present
Slight (less than 30)	Unable to hear whispered words or faint speech
	No speech impairment present
	May not be aware of hearing difficulty
	Achieves well in school and home, compensating by leaning forward, speaking loudly
Mild (30–50)	Beginning speech impairment may be present
	Difficulty hearing if not facing speaker; some difficulty with normal conversation
Moderate (55–70)	Speech impairment present. May require speech therapy.
	Difficulty with normal conversation
Severe (70–90)	Difficulty with any but nearby loud voice
	Hears vowels easier than consonants
	Requires speech therapy for clear speech. May still hear loud sounds such as jets or whistle of train.
Profound (more than 90)	Hears almost no sound

ing normally, there will be a symmetric pattern of resistance on a tympanogram printout. If the middle ear is functioning abnormally, the level of resistance will be greater or less than normal, so the pattern will be abnormal.

Acoustic impedance testing is performed by audiologists. For the assessment, the child's ear to be tested is plugged with a rubber disc. Sound is then administered to the ear through the center of the disc. The resistance met at the eardrum is registered and recorded as a graph. Tympanograms are inaccurate in children younger than age 7 months because the tympanic membrane is too compliant under that age to register normal impedance.

Conduction Loss Testing

Although not very accurate, both the Rinne and the Weber tests can be used to help determine the cause of hearing loss in older children.

Rinne Test

Strike a 500-Hz tuning fork and hold the stem of it against the child's mastoid bone. Ask the child to say when he or she no longer hears the tuning fork ringing. When the child says it is no longer audible, move the

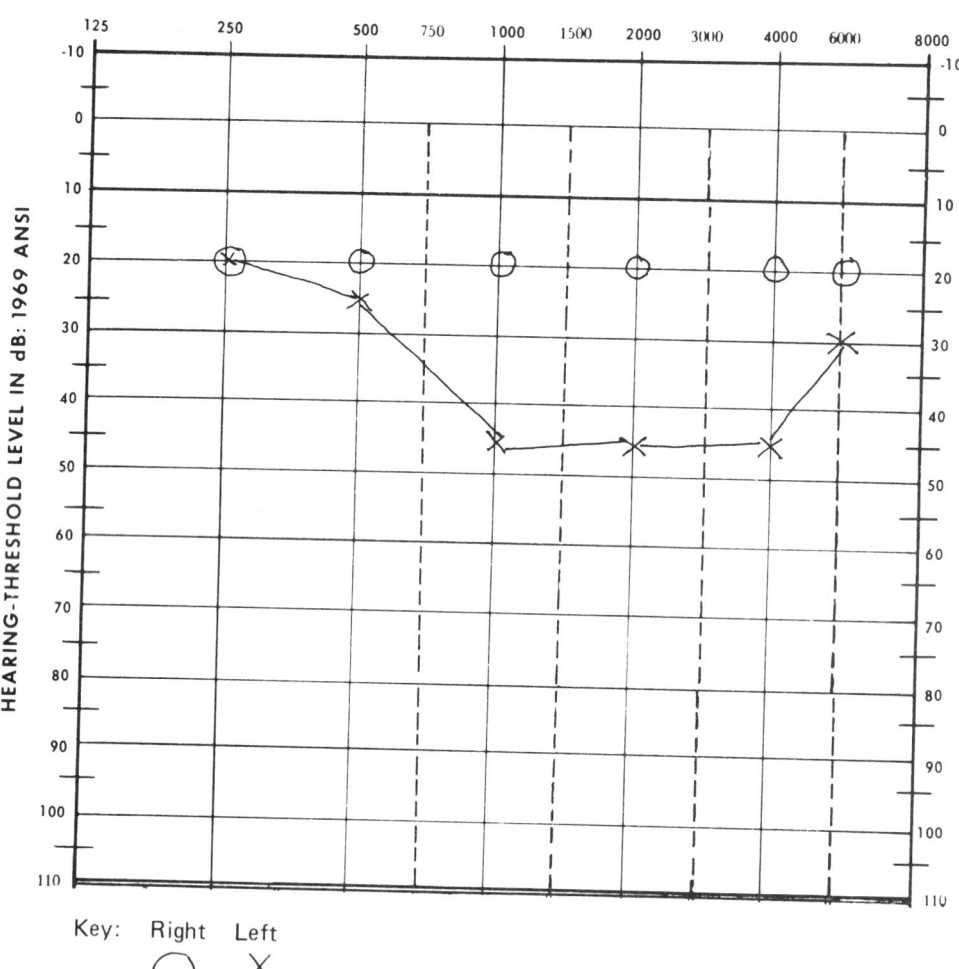

PURE TONE AUDIOGRAM
FREQUENCY IN HERTZ

FIGURE 28-32

An audiogram done as a screening procedure. Notice that hearing is normal in the right ear (all frequencies are heard at the 20-dB level). In the left ear there is hearing loss (the frequencies 1000, 2000, and 4000 Hz are heard only at the 45-dB level). (Courtesy of Dr. H. Schill, Speech Pathology and Audiology Department, Boston University.)

fork forward so that it is at the auditory meatus. Because air conduction is normally better than bone conduction, the child should hear it when it is held in front of the meatus, although he or she no longer heard it when it was held against the bone (Figure 28-33). If the child does not hear it when it is brought forward, then the child's air conduction is probably reduced.

Weber's Test

Strike a 500-Hz tuning fork and hold the stem of it against the center of the child's forehead. The child with normal hearing in both ears will hear the sound equally well with both ears. If the child has an air conduction loss in one ear, the child will hear the sound better in that ear than in the good ear (Figure 28-34). The test must be used in conjunction with other evaluation tools because, if the sound is intensified in one ear, it may mean that there is no hearing perception (there is nerve loss) in the opposite ear.

Speech Assessment

Speech screening is directly related to hearing assessment: the child who does not hear will make preliminary babbling sounds but then will not develop intelligible speech because he or she is unable to hear and repeat sounds. Speech screening is also related to motor development (the child cannot control tongue and facial muscles well enough to form proper words) and intelligence (the child of low intelligence does not grasp the concept of speech or word use until later than normal, or possibly not at all).

Denver Articulation Screening Examination

Assessing for language development is double assessment in that it assesses for both cognitive and hearing ability (Prizant et al., 1993). The Denver Articulation Screening Examination (DASE) is designed to detect sig-

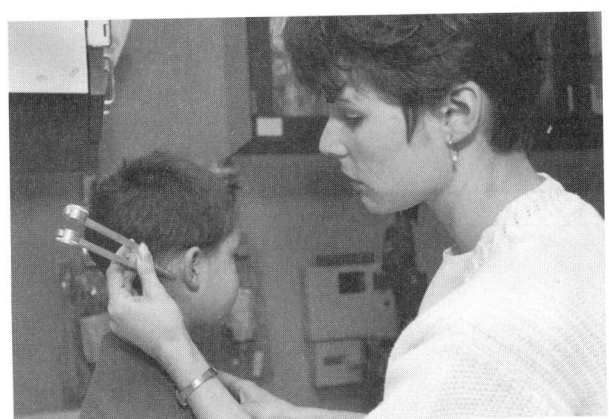

FIGURE 28-33
Rinne's test. The sound of the tuning fork is normally heard longer when the fork is held in front of the ear than when it touches the bony process behind the ear (air conduction is normally better than bone conduction). (Courtesy of the Department of Medical Photography, Children's Hospital, Buffalo, NY.)

nificant developmental delays and normal variations in the acquisition of speech sounds. Because it is a standardized test, its directions must be followed carefully. The test is only useful with English-speaking children.

Administration

For the test, explain that the child will need to repeat some words he or she hears. Give enough examples so that the child will understand what he or she is to do: "When I say 'boat,' then you say 'boat.' " When certain that the child understands the directions, say each of the 22 words shown on the DASE form (Figure 28-35*A*). Convey the impression that there are no right or wrong answers. Give the child approval for responding and fol-

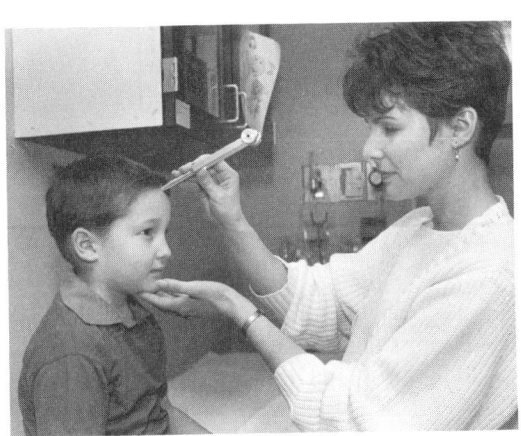

FIGURE 28-34
Weber's test. When the child has an air conduction hearing loss, he or she will hear the sound of the tuning fork better in the affected ear than in the normal ear. (Courtesy of the Department of Medical Photography, Children's Hospital, Buffalo, NY.)

lowing directions correctly, no matter how inaccurately the child repeats the word.

Scoring

The DASE is designed for use with children between ages 2½ years and 6 years. In scoring, consider the child's age to be the closest previous age shown on the percentile rank chart (Figure 28-37*B*). Score the child's pronunciation of the underlined sounds or blends in each word on the test form. A perfect raw score is 30 correctly articulated sounds.

Match this raw score on the percentile rank chart with the column representing the child's age. The number at which the raw score line and the age column meet is the percentile rank of the child (how the child compares with other children of that age). Percentiles shown above the heavy line are abnormal; those below the line are normal. For example, a 3-year-old who says only 12 sounds correctly ranks in the 9th percentile (abnormal ranking); the 3-year-old who scores 20 sounds correctly ranks in the 58th percentile (normal ranking).

In addition to determining the percentile ranking, rate the child's spontaneous speech in terms of intelligibility as 1, easy to understand; 2, understandable half the time; 3, not understandable; or 4, cannot evaluate (eg, the child does not speak in sentences or phrases during the contact with the child). Score intelligibility according to the chart in Figure 28-37*B*. For a final score, rate the child's total test result (normal or abnormal on the DASE or intelligibility).

Children who score abnormally on this screening test should be retested in 2 weeks. If they still score abnormally, they should be referred for complete speech evaluation.

Developmental Appraisal

It would be ideal if children demonstrated all the developmental skills of which they are capable every time they are asked to demonstrate them. Rarely, however, do they accomplish this feat. Infants may become hungry, sleepy, or upset during testing. Older children may become shy. A portion of developmental information on almost all health assessments, therefore, must be elicited by history taking. All previous developmental milestones must be obtained this way.

Developmental History

Many parents keep careful records of their first child's development, a less careful record of their second, a scanty record of the third, and so on. Most of this information must therefore be obtained by recall.

```
┌─────────────────────────────────────────────┬──────────────────────┐
│   DENVER ARTICULATION SCREENING EXAM         │                      │
│   for children 2 1/2 to 6 years of age       │ NAME                 │
│                                              │                      │
│ Instructions: Have child repeat each word    │ HOSP. NO.            │
│ after you. Circle the underlined sounds       │                      │
│ that he pro-nounces correctly. Total correct │ ADDRESS              │
│ sounds is the Raw Score. Use charts on       │                      │
│ reverse side to score results.               │                      │
└─────────────────────────────────────────────┴──────────────────────┘
```

Date: _____ Child's Age: _____ Examiner: _____ Raw Score: _____
Percentile: _____ Intelligibility: _____ Result: _____

1. table	6. zipper	11. sock	16. wagon	21. leaf
2. shirt	7. grapes	12. vacuum	17. gum	22. carrot
3. door	8. flag	13. yarn	18. house	
4. trunk	9. thumb	14. mother	19. pencil	
5. jumping	10. toothbrush	15. twinkle	20. fish	

Intelligibility: (circle one)   1. Easy to understand   3. Not understandable
                                2. Understandable 1/2   4. Can't evaluate
                                   the time.

Comments:

Date: _____ Child's Age: _____ Examiner: _____ Raw Score _____
Percentile: _____ Intelligibility: _____ Result: _____

1. table	6. zipper	11. sock	16. wagon	21. leaf
2. shirt	7. grapes	12. vacuum	17. gum	22. carrot
3. door	8. flag	13. yarn	18. house	
4. trunk	9. thumb	14. mother	19. pencil	
5. jumping	10. toothbrush	15. twinkle	20. fish	

Intelligibility: (circle one)   1. Easy to understand   3. Not understandable
                                2. Understandable 1/2   4. Can't evaluate
                                   the time.

Comments:

Date: _____ Child's Age: _____ Examiner: _____ Raw Score _____
Percentile: _____ Intelligibility: _____ Result: _____

1. table	6. zipper	11. sock	16. wagon	21. leaf
2. shirt	7. grapes	12. vacuum	17. gum	22. carrot
3. door	8. flag	13. yarn	18. house	
4. trunk	9. thumb	14. mother	19. pencil	
5. jumping	10. toothbrush	15. twinkle	20. fish	

Intelligibility: (circle one)   1. Easy to understand   3. Not understandable
                                2. Understandable 1/2   4. Can't evaluate
                                   the time.

Comments:

A

FIGURE 28-35
Denver Articulation Screening Exam (DASE). (**A**) Test form.

Parents may not be able to recall the month during which a skill was first demonstrated. It is often helpful to ask them to try to remember in terms of holidays or seasons. For example, they may not know at which month the infant first used a *pincer grasp* (grasped cleanly with index finger and thumb) but do recall the way the child pinched the ear of the family dog at a summer picnic.

If parents seem to have no recall at all of develop-mental milestones that are important for the child's present evaluation, suggest that they ask other family members or look through family photographs to jog their memories and then call with as much information as they can gather.

In addition to getting the parents' description of the skills a child has mastered, it is often helpful to watch the child perform skills and rate the child according to standard criteria.

To score DASE words: Note Raw Score for child's performance. Match raw score line (extreme left of chart) with column representing child's age (to the closest _previous_ age group). Where raw score line and age column meet number in that square denotes percentile rank of child's performance when compared to other children that age. Percentiles above heavy line are ABNORMAL percentiles, below heavy line are NORMAL.

PERCENTILE RANK

Raw Score	2.5 yr.	3.0	3.5	4.0	4.5	5.0	5.5	6 years
2	1							
3	2							
4	5							
5	9							
6	16							
7	23							
8	31	2						
9	37	4	1					
10	42	6	2					
11	48	7	4					
12	54	9	6	1	1	1	1	
13	58	12	9	2	3	1	2	
14	62	17	11	5	4	2	2	
15	68	23	15	9	5	3	2	
16	75	31	19	12	5	4	3	
17	79	38	25	15	6	6	4	
18	83	46	31	19	8	7	4	
19	86	51	38	24	10	9	5	1
20	89	58	45	30	12	11	7	3
21	92	65	52	36	15	15	9	4
22	94	72	58	43	18	19	12	5
23	96	77	63	50	22	24	15	7
24	97	82	70	58	29	29	20	15
25	99	87	78	66	36	34	26	17
26	99	91	84	75	46	43	34	24
27		94	89	82	57	54	44	34
28		96	94	88	70	68	59	47
29		98	98	94	84	84	77	68
30		100	100	100	100	100	100	100

To Score intelligibility:

	NORMAL	ABNORMAL
2 1/2 years	Understandable 1/2 the time, or, "easy"	Not Understandable
3 years and older	Easy to understand	Understandable 1/2 time Not understandable

Test Result: 1. NORMAL on Dase and Intelligibility = NORMAL

2. ABNORMAL on Dase and/or Intelligibility = ABNORMAL

* If abnormal on initial screening rescreen within 2 weeks. If abnormal again child should be referred for complete speech evaluation.

B

FIGURE 28-35 *(Continued)*
(B) *Percentile rank form. (Reprinted by permission. Copyright 1971 by Amelia F. Drumwright, University of Colorado Medical Center, Denver, CO.)*

Denver Developmental Screening Test

The Denver Developmental Screening Test (Denver II) is the most widely used tool to assess development and has been recently revised (Frankenburg et al., 1992) (Figure 28-36). The DDST detects developmental delays during infancy and preschool years. Four main categories of development are rated: (1) personal-social, (2) fine motor-adaptive, (3) language, and (4) gross motor skills.

Administration

The materials to administer the test must be purchased as a kit. They include a skein of red wool, a box of

(text continues on page 842)

Denver II

Examiner:
Date:

Name:
Birthdate:
ID No.:

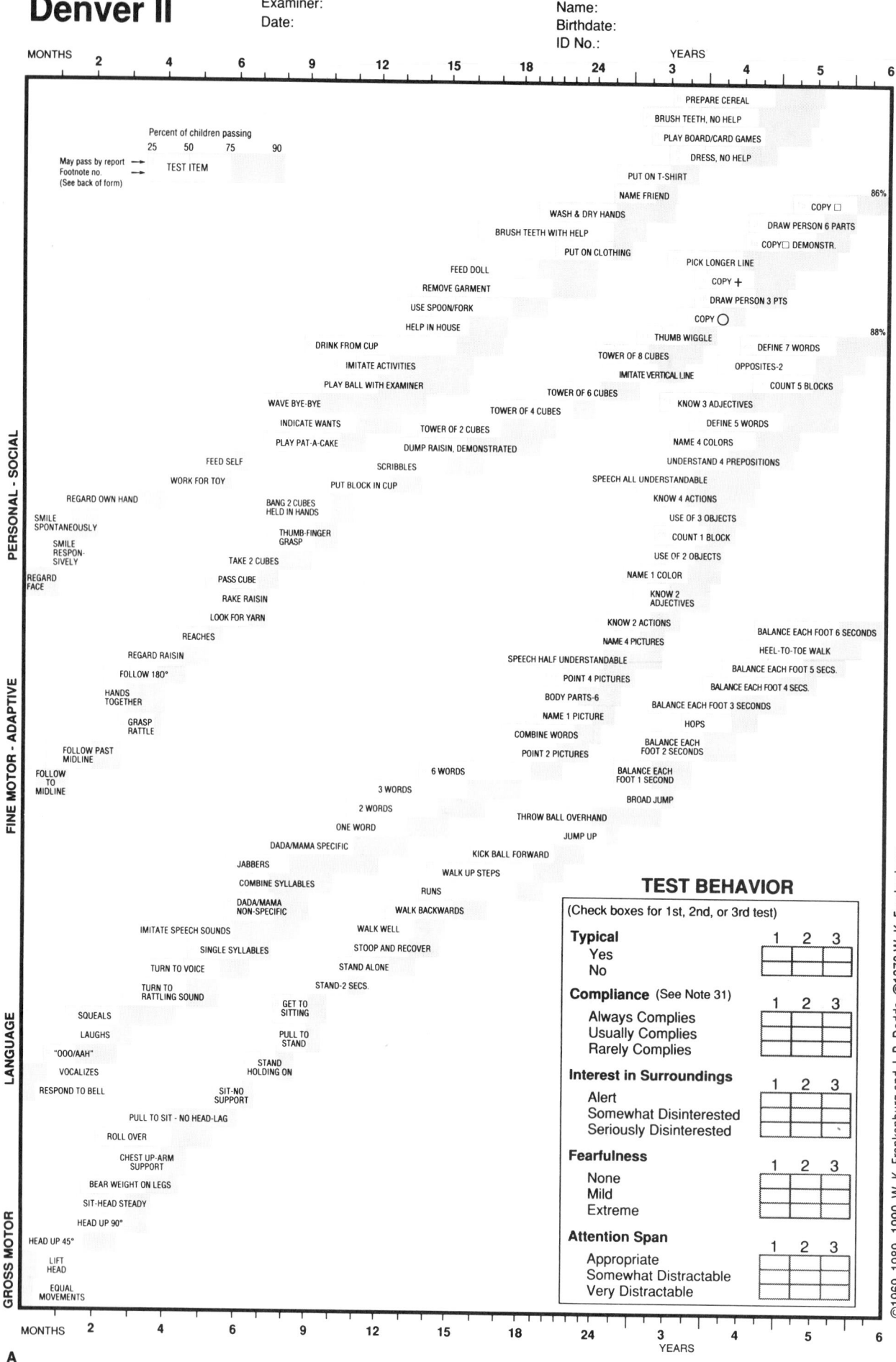

MONTHS 2 4 6 9 12 15 18 24 YEARS 3 4 5 6

Percent of children passing
25 50 75 90

May pass by report →
Footnote no. →
(See back of form) →

TEST ITEM

PERSONAL - SOCIAL

PREPARE CEREAL
BRUSH TEETH, NO HELP
PLAY BOARD/CARD GAMES
DRESS, NO HELP
PUT ON T-SHIRT
NAME FRIEND   86%
WASH & DRY HANDS   COPY □
BRUSH TEETH WITH HELP   DRAW PERSON 6 PARTS
PUT ON CLOTHING   COPY □ DEMONSTR.
FEED DOLL   PICK LONGER LINE
REMOVE GARMENT   COPY +
USE SPOON/FORK   DRAW PERSON 3 PTS
HELP IN HOUSE   COPY ○
DRINK FROM CUP   THUMB WIGGLE   88%
IMITATE ACTIVITIES   TOWER OF 8 CUBES   DEFINE 7 WORDS
PLAY BALL WITH EXAMINER   IMITATE VERTICAL LINE OPPOSITES-2
WAVE BYE-BYE   TOWER OF 6 CUBES   COUNT 5 BLOCKS
INDICATE WANTS   TOWER OF 4 CUBES KNOW 3 ADJECTIVES
PLAY PAT-A-CAKE   TOWER OF 2 CUBES DEFINE 5 WORDS
FEED SELF   DUMP RAISIN, DEMONSTRATED NAME 4 COLORS
WORK FOR TOY   SCRIBBLES   UNDERSTAND 4 PREPOSITIONS
REGARD OWN HAND   PUT BLOCK IN CUP SPEECH ALL UNDERSTANDABLE
SMILE   BANG 2 CUBES   KNOW 4 ACTIONS
SPONTANEOUSLY   HELD IN HANDS   USE OF 3 OBJECTS
SMILE   THUMB-FINGER   COUNT 1 BLOCK
RESPON-   GRASP   USE OF 2 OBJECTS
SIVELY   TAKE 2 CUBES   NAME 1 COLOR
REGARD   PASS CUBE   KNOW 2
FACE   RAKE RAISIN   ADJECTIVES
                  LOOK FOR YARN

FINE MOTOR - ADAPTIVE

REACHES   KNOW 2 ACTIONS   BALANCE EACH FOOT 6 SECONDS
REGARD RAISIN   NAME 4 PICTURES   HEEL-TO-TOE WALK
FOLLOW 180°   SPEECH HALF UNDERSTANDABLE   BALANCE EACH FOOT 5 SECS.
HANDS   POINT 4 PICTURES   BALANCE EACH FOOT 4 SECS.
TOGETHER   BODY PARTS-6   BALANCE EACH FOOT 3 SECONDS
GRASP   NAME 1 PICTURE   HOPS
RATTLE   COMBINE WORDS   BALANCE EACH
FOLLOW PAST   POINT 2 PICTURES   FOOT 2 SECONDS
MIDLINE   6 WORDS   BALANCE EACH
FOLLOW   FOOT 1 SECOND
TO   3 WORDS   BROAD JUMP
MIDLINE   2 WORDS
                  ONE WORD   THROW BALL OVERHAND
                  DADA/MAMA SPECIFIC JUMP UP

LANGUAGE

JABBERS   KICK BALL FORWARD
COMBINE SYLLABLES   WALK UP STEPS
DADA/MAMA   RUNS
NON-SPECIFIC   WALK BACKWARDS
IMITATE SPEECH SOUNDS   WALK WELL
SINGLE SYLLABLES   STOOP AND RECOVER
TURN TO VOICE   STAND ALONE
TURN TO   STAND-2 SECS.
RATTLING SOUND   GET TO
SQUEALS   SITTING
LAUGHS   PULL TO
"OOO/AAH"   STAND
VOCALIZES   STAND
RESPOND TO BELL   HOLDING ON
                         SIT-NO
                         SUPPORT

GROSS MOTOR

PULL TO SIT - NO HEAD-LAG
ROLL OVER
CHEST UP-ARM
SUPPORT
BEAR WEIGHT ON LEGS
SIT-HEAD STEADY
HEAD UP 90°
HEAD UP 45°
LIFT
HEAD
EQUAL
MOVEMENTS

TEST BEHAVIOR

(Check boxes for 1st, 2nd, or 3rd test)

Typical   1 2 3
  Yes
  No

Compliance (See Note 31)   1 2 3
  Always Complies
  Usually Complies
  Rarely Complies

Interest in Surroundings   1 2 3
  Alert
  Somewhat Disinterested
  Seriously Disinterested

Fearfulness   1 2 3
  None
  Mild
  Extreme

Attention Span   1 2 3
  Appropriate
  Somewhat Distractable
  Very Distractable

MONTHS 2 4 6 9 12 15 18 24 YEARS 3 4 5 6

A

DIRECTIONS FOR ADMINISTRATION

1. Try to get child to smile by smiling, talking or waving. Do not touch him/her.
2. Child must stare at hand several seconds.
3. Parent may help guide toothbrush and put toothpaste on brush.
4. Child does not have to be able to tie shoes or button/zip in the back.
5. Move yarn slowly in an arc from one side to the other, about 8" above child's face.
6. Pass if child grasps rattle when it is touched to the backs or tips of fingers.
7. Pass if child tries to see where yarn went. Yarn should be dropped quickly from sight from tester's hand without arm movement.
8. Child must transfer cube from hand to hand without help of body, mouth, or table.
9. Pass if child picks up raisin with any part of thumb and finger.
10. Line can vary only 30 degrees or less from tester's line.⟋
11. Make a fist with thumb pointing upward and wiggle only the thumb. Pass if child imitates and does not move any fingers other than the thumb.

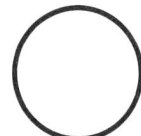

12. Pass any enclosed form. Fail continuous round motions.

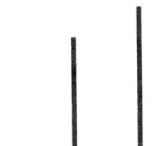

13. Which line is longer? (Not bigger.) Turn paper upside down and repeat. (pass 3 of 3 or 5 of 6)

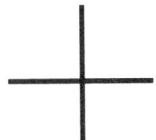

14. Pass any lines crossing near midpoint.

15. Have child copy first. If failed, demonstrate.

When giving items 12, 14, and 15, do not name the forms. Do not demonstrate 12 and 14.

16. When scoring, each pair (2 arms, 2 legs, etc.) counts as one part.
17. Place one cube in cup and shake gently near child's ear, but out of sight. Repeat for other ear.
18. Point to picture and have child name it. (No credit is given for sounds only.)
    If less than 4 pictures are named correctly, have child point to picture as each is named by tester.

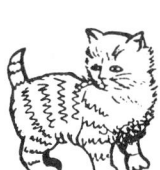 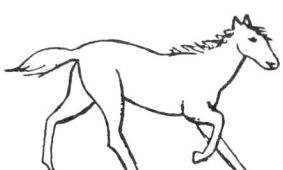 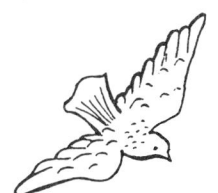 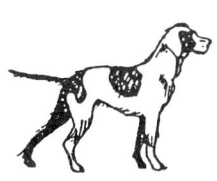 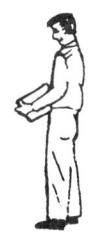

19. Using doll, tell child: Show me the nose, eyes, ears, mouth, hands, feet, tummy, hair. Pass 6 of 8.
20. Using pictures, ask child: Which one flies?... says meow?... talks?... barks?... gallops? Pass 2 of 5, 4 of 5.
21. Ask child: What do you do when you are cold?... tired?... hungry? Pass 2 of 3, 3 of 3.
22. Ask child: What do you do with a cup? What is a chair used for? What is a pencil used for?
    Action words must be included in answers.
23. Pass if child correctly places <u>and</u> says how many blocks are on paper. (1, 5).
24. Tell child: Put block **on** table; **under** table; **in front of** me, **behind** me. Pass 4 of 4.
    (Do not help child by pointing, moving head or eyes.)
25. Ask child: What is a ball?... lake?... desk?... house?... banana?... curtain?... fence?... ceiling? Pass if defined in terms of use, shape, what it is made of, or general category (such as banana is fruit, not just yellow). Pass 5 of 8, 7 of 8.
26. Ask child: If a horse is big, a mouse is __? If fire is hot, ice is __? If the sun shines during the day, the moon shines during the __? Pass 2 of 3.
27. Child may use wall or rail only, not person. May not crawl.
28. Child must throw ball overhand 3 feet to within arm's reach of tester.
29. Child must perform standing broad jump over width of test sheet (8 1/2 inches).
30. Tell child to walk forward, ⟞⟞⟞⟞⟞➤ heel within 1 inch of toe. Tester may demonstrate.
    Child must walk 4 consecutive steps.
31. In the second year, half of normal children are non-compliant.

OBSERVATIONS:

B

FIGURE 28-36
Denver Developmental Screening test. (A) Test form. (B) Instructions for administering specified items. (Reprinted by permission of Dr. W. Frankenburg, University of Colorado Medical Center, Denver, CO.)

raisins, a small bottle, a bell, a rattle with a narrow handle, a tennis ball, 10 1-in brightly colored blocks, a small plastic doll, a toy baby bottle, a plastic cup, and a pencil.*

Although administration of the Denver II is not difficult, it should not be attempted except by health care providers trained specifically in its procedures and interpretation. This precaution is necessary to ensure the validity of its developmental norms. Periodic retraining and proficiency testing are recommended to sustain a high degree of accuracy in administration. Items used on previous forms that were not sensitive to sociocultural influences have been removed (Wade, 1992).

The parent should be told before administration that this is not a test of intelligence but of the child's level of development. The child's inability to perform a task that most children of the same age can accomplish indicates a delay in that area. Further evaluation is then needed to determine the reason for this delay.

Scoring

The child is scored *P* (passed), *F* (failed), *R* (refused), or *N.O.* (no opportunity) on each item by reference to guidelines in the instruction manual. Each item is represented on the test form (see Figure 28-36*A*) by a bar showing the ages by which 25%, 50%, 75%, and 90% of children normally have mastered that item. The left end of the bar is the 25% mark; the tick mark at the top of the bar, 50%; the left end of the colored (gray) area, 75%; and the right end of the bar, 90%. Looking at the form, notice, for example, the item "plays pat-a-cake" in the area of personal-social development. With this item, 25% of children show the trait at age 7 months, 50% between ages 9 months and 10 months, 75% between ages 10 months and 11 months, and 90% by ages 11 months to 12 months.

The Denver II ideally should be presented when the child is approximately ages 3 months or 4 months, again at age 10 months, and again at age 3 years. It is a supplement to the developmental evaluation by history that should be a part of every well-child assessment. Interpretation of performance is detailed in the manual.

Prescreening Test

A Denver Prescreening Developmental Questionnaire (R-PDQ) is available in addition to the Denver II (Frankenburg et al., 1987). The PDQ is designed to identify the child who requires further testing with a full Denver II. It is a questionnaire of 10 developmental items that the parent completes. A child who scores 8 out of 10 or fewer should be retested in approximately 2 weeks. If the initial score is under 6 or the retest score is 8 or below, the child should have a full DDST.

---

* DDST materials may be purchased from Denver Developmental Materials, Inc., P. O. Box 6919, Denver, CO 80205-0919; phone: 303-355-4729.

Intelligence

Children must learn many important concepts or ideas such as near, far, here, there, number sequences, how to judge time intervals, how to reason and solve problems, and how to judge weight before they can function effectively in the world.

This type of learning—gaining concepts—is called **cognitive learning**. It is measured by intelligence tests. **Intelligence** can be defined as an ability to think abstractly, to adjust to new situations, and to profit from experience. Almost everyone has had his or her intelligence quotient (IQ) rated at some point in a school career. Although intelligence tests are not part of routine health appraisals, it is helpful to be familiar with those that are used for childhood measurements because these findings are helpful in evaluating children's development.

The *intelligence quotient* is the ratio of mental age as measured by an intelligence test to chronologic age. The formula is as follows:

$$\frac{\text{Mental age}}{\text{Chronological age}} \times 100 = \text{IQ}$$

A child aged 9 years old (chronologic age) who passes all the items on an intelligence test that an average 9-year-old passes would be scored as follows:

$$\frac{9 \text{ (mental age)}}{9 \text{ (chronologic age)}} \times 100 = 100 \text{ (the child's IQ)}$$

If a child passes no more items than the average 5-year-old would, the IQ would be scored as:

$$\frac{5 \text{ (mental age)}}{9 \text{ (chronologic age)}} \times 100 = 55$$

If a child passed all the items that a 12-year-old normally passes, the IQ would be scored as:

$$\frac{12 \text{ (mental age)}}{9 \text{ (chronologic age)}} \times 100 = 133$$

Children may score poorly on intelligence tests because of test anxiety. Cultural bias and past experience can also affect how they score. Therefore, labeling children by IQ and classifying them into divisions is often unfair and must be done with considerable thought and study.

It is difficult to test young children with any degree of accuracy because they lack the ability to complete tasks in the areas used for scoring intelligence tests: comprehension, imagination, reasoning, memory, and vocabulary. The most common tests used with infants are the Cattell Infant Intelligence Scale, the Bayley Mental Scale, and the Gesell Developmental Schedule. These tests rely heavily on perceptual and motor skills as rating devices.

The two most frequently used tests for older children are the Wechsler Intelligence Scale for Children and the Stanford-Binet test. All school children take one of these tests during the primary school grades. The results are made available to child health teams if they can demonstrate to school officials that such information is necessary for total health care or planning. If the information is unavailable, the child can be referred to a psychologist or a psychological testing clinic for assessment.

Goodenough-Harris Drawing Test

A child's drawing can reveal information on developmental or emotional problems (Wilson & Ratekin, 1990). A Goodenough-Harris Drawing test is a quick intelligence measurement that can be administered without special training (Goodenough, 1926). Give a child between ages 3 years and 10 years a pencil and paper and ask the child to draw a person. Urge the child to draw it carefully in the best way he or she knows how and to take enough time to do it well (Box 28-3).

The child receives one point for each of the items in the drawing listed in Box 28-3. For each four points scored, 1 year is added to a base age of 3 years to get the child's mental age. The picture shown in Box 28-2 was drawn by a 4½-year-old child: it received eight points. The child's IQ level is

$$\frac{5.0}{4.5} \times 100 = 111$$

Scores on the test are reasonably reliable, correlating well with a Stanford-Binet test, although results may not be as reliable with children who are mentally ill. A child who scores significantly lower than his or her chronologic age (after allowing for fatigue, illness, strange surroundings, nervousness, physical ability to use a pencil, and previous practice using a pencil and paper) should be referred for more refined testing.

Temperament

Temperament refers to a child's innate behavioral characteristics such as activity level, rhythmicity, tendency to approach or withdraw, and adaptability to situations (see Chapter 27). A child with an "easy" temperament is generally adaptable and easy to care for; a child with a "difficult" temperament, in contrast, will almost automatically create childrearing concerns (Frankel & Bates, 1990). Helping parents to assess their children's temperament helps them in turn to recognize their children's uniqueness and to anticipate and ideally prevent personality conflicts as a child grows older and expresses identified reactions to situations. If a behavior or parent-child interaction problem is already present, a nursing assessment can be useful to determine whether temperament is a factor in the problem and assist parents with constructive solutions (Thomas & Chess, 1977).

One instrument that is helpful in evaluating temperament is the Carey-McDevitt Infant Temperament Questionnaire (Carey & McDevitt, 1978). This consists of 95 responses and can be answered by a parent in approximately 25 minutes. General categories center on the child's responses to feeding, sleeping, soiling and wetting, dressing, bathing, and diapering, as well as to people and new situations.

The questionnaire should be given to parents when their infant is between ages 4 and 8 months (before this, temperament is not developed enough to be evident). The parent reads each behavioral description and then selects the option that most accurately describes the child. If an item does not apply at all, the parent crosses it out. Finally, the parent is asked to describe general impressions of the child's temperament, activity level, positive and negative moods, and distractibility.

When scored, a child can be categorized into one of 4 groups: (1) difficult (arrhythmic, withdrawing, low in adaptability, intense, and negative in mood); (2) slow to warm up (inactive, low in approach and adaptability, and negative in mood); (3) intermediate (some characteristics of both groups); or (4) easy (rhythmic, approaching, adaptable, mild, and positive in mood).

Concluding a Health Assessment

At every health maintenance visit, the parents and the child, if the child is old enough to understand, should be informed of any available results of screening procedures performed. After learning the results, some parents may require counseling to assist them with health or behavior concerns.

Parents should be asked whether questions remain. If some findings were positive and follow-up procedures are planned, the reason for the upcoming tests should be made clear. Parents should also be encouraged to telephone after they return home from a health assessment so that questions that may occur to them after they leave the facility can be answered.

Key Points

- A health history is an important part of a health assessment. The purpose is to gather information that will supplement physical or laboratory examinations to complete a more thorough health evaluation.
- The parts of a complete health history consist of introduction, chief concern, family profile, pregnancy history, history of past illnesses, day history, family illness history, and review of systems.
- Physical examination consists of 4 techniques: inspection, palpation, percussion, and auscultation. Techniques and approaches must be varied according to the child's age.

Box 28-3
Goodenough–Harris Drawing Test

Score one point for each characteristic listed below that is present on drawing. For every four points, 1 year is added to a base mental age of 3 years.

1. Head present
2. Legs present
3. Arms present
4a. Trunk present
   b. Length of trunk greater than breadth
   c. Shoulders indicated
5a. Both arms and legs attached to trunk
   b. Legs attached to trunk; arms attached to trunk at correct point
6a. Neck present
   b. Neck outline continuous with head, trunk, or both
7a. Eyes present
   b. Nose present
   c. Mouth present
   d. Nose and mouth in two dimensions, two lips shown
   e. Nostrils indicated
8a. Hair shown
   b. Hair nontransparent, over more than circumference
9a. Clothing present
   b. Two articles of clothing nontransparent
   c. No transparencies, both sleeves and trousers shown
   d. Four or more articles of clothing definitely indicated
   e. Costume complete, without incongruities.
10a. Fingers shown
   b. Correct number of fingers shown
   c. Fingers in two dimensions, length greater than breadth, angle less than 180 degrees
   d. Opposition of thumb shown
   e. Hand shown distinct from fingers or arms
11a. Arm joint shown, either elbow, shoulder, or both
   b. Leg joint shown, either knee, hip, or both

12a. Head in proportion
   b. Arms in proportion
   c. Legs in proportion
   d. Feet in proportion
   e. Both arms and legs in two dimensions
13. Heel shown
14a. Firm lines without overlapping at junctions
   b. Firm lines with correct joining
   c. Head outline more than circle
   d. Trunk outline more than circle
   e. Outline of arms and legs without narrowing at point of junction with body
   f. Features symmetric, correct position
15a. Ears present
   b. Ears in correct position and proportion
16a. Eye detail: brow and lashes shown
   b. Eye detail: pupil shown
   c. Eye detail: proportion correct
   d. Eye detail: glance directed to front in profile drawing
17a. Both chin and forehead present
   b. Projection of chin shown

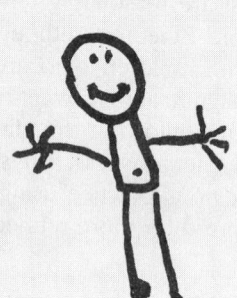

A person drawn by a 4-1/2-year-old.

(From Goodenough, F. L. [1926]. *Measurement of intelligence by drawings*. New York: World Book Company, with permission.)

• The components of a physical examination are vital sign assessment; general appearance; mental status assessment; body measurements; and assessment of head, eyes, nose, ears, mouth, neck, chest, breasts, lungs, heart, abdomen, genitorectal area, extremities, back, and neurologic function.
• Adolescent girls can be taught breast self-examination and boys testicular self-examination at the time of a health appraisal.

• Vision assessment consists of asking children to read a standardized chart such as a Snellen Chart, cover testing, and color awareness assessment.
• Hearing assessment consists of such assessments as audiometric testing and a Rinne and Weber test.
• Development is an important part of total assessment. The Denver Developmental Screening Test and the Denver Articulation Screening examination are specific development tests.

- The Goodenough-Harris Drawing test correlates well with intelligence quotient (IQ) and is an easy test to administer to children between the ages of 3 and 10 years.
- Temperament refers to a child's innate behavioral characteristics such as activity level, rhythmicity, and tendency to approach or withdraw and adapt to situations. Assessing this can help parents to understand behavior in their child better.
- Health assessment always causes some degree of apprehension because parents worry that illness will be detected. Giving reassurance of wellness during examinations helps to alleviate this worry.
- Be certain to use examining instruments safely (supporting an otoscope base so if the child moves, the otoscope moves with the child). Be certain that young children are not left unsupervised on an examining table or a fall could result.

Critical Thinking Exercises

1. Mary is a 2-year-old seen in a health maintenance clinic for well child care. She is very resistant to being examined. How would you determine which techniques you could use to help Mary adjust better to a physical examination?
2. Children may cheat on vision and hearing tests because they do not understand the importance of them. What are techniques to use to keep children from doing this with these assessments?
3. Children should be completely undressed for physical examinations and all body surfaces inspected. What would be your response if a parent said she did not want to undress a child? What if she could not account for multiple bruises on the child?

References

American Academy of Pediatrics, Committee on Hearing Screening. Testing hearing in neonates. (1983). *Pediatrics, 73,* 702.

Carey, W. B., & McDevitt, S. C. (1978). Revision of the infant temperament questionnaire. *Pediatrics, 61,* 735.

Department of Health & Human Services. (1991). *Healthy people 2000.* Washington, D. C.: Public Health Service.

Frankel, K. A., & Bates, J. E. (1990). Mother-toddler problem solving: Antecedents in attachment, home behavior and temperament. *Child Development, 61,* 810.

Frankenburg, W. K., et al. (1992). The Denver II: A major revision and restandardization of the Denver Developmental Screening Test. *Pediatrics 89,* 91.

Frankenburg, W. K., et al. (1987). Revision of Denver Pre-screening Developmental Questionnaire. *Journal of Pediatrics, 110,* 653.

Frasier, L. D., et al. (1992). Physical and behavioral signs of sexual abuse in infants and toddlers. *Infants and Young Children, 5,* 1.

Fred, H. L., et al. (1994). Diagnostic pearls for 10 common problems. *Patient Care, 28,* 70.

Geissler, E. M. (1994). *Pocket guide to cultural assessment.* St. Louis: C. V. Mosby.

Goodenough, F. L. (1926). *Measurement of intelligence by drawings.* New York: World Book Co.

Halverson, K. C., et al. (1993). Treatment of child abuse. *Primary Care, 20,* 355.

Jones, L. C., Maestri, B. O., & McCoy, K. (1993). Why parents use the warm line. *MCN: American Journal of Maternal Child Nursing, 18,* 258.

Kuttner, L. (1991). Helpful strategies in working with pre-school children in pediatric practice. *Pediatric Annals, 20,* 120.

Mayer, D. L., & Gross, R. D. (1990). Modified Allen Pictures to assess amblyopia in young children. *Ophthalmology, 97,* 827.

Nik-Hussein, N. N. (1990). Natal and neonatal teeth. *Journal of Pedodontics, 14,* 110.

Prizant, B. M., et al. (1993). Communication and language assessment for young children. *Infants and Young Children, 5,* 20.

Tielsch, J. M., et al. (1990). Vision deficit and visual impairment in an American urban population. *Archives of Ophthalmology, 108,* 285.

Thomas, A., & Chess, S. (1977). *Temperament and development.* New York: Brunner/Mazel.

Wade, G. H. (1992). Update on the Denver II. *Pediatric Nursing, 18,* 140.

Wilson, C. J., et al. (1990). Preparation for routine physical examination. *Children's Health Care, 19,* 178.

Wilson, D., & Ratekin, C. (1990). An introduction to using children's drawings as an assessment tool. *Nurse Practitioner, 15,* 23.

Suggested Readings

Antwerp, C. V., & Spaniolo, A. M. (1991). Checking out children's life style. *MCN: American Journal of Maternal Child Nursing, 16,* 144.

Black, M., et al. (1994). Sexual abuse: Developmental differences in children's behavior and self-perception. *Child Abuse & Neglect, 18,* 85.

Diefendorf, A. O., et al. (1992). The Joint Committee on Infant Hearing 1990 Position Statement: A close look. *Infants and Young Children, 5,* 5.

Fewell, R. R., et al. (1993). Observing play: An appropriate process for learning and assessment. *Infants and Young Children, 5,* 35.

Johnson, C. F. (1990). Inflicted injury versus accidental injury. *Pediatric Clinics of North America, 37,* 791.

McClowry, S. G. (1992). Temperament theory and research. *Image, 24,* 319.

Paradise, J. E. (1990). The medical evaluation of the sexually abused child. *Pediatric Clinics of North America, 37,* 839.

Silverstein, H., et al. (1992). Diagnosis and management of hearing loss. *Clinical Symposium, 44,* 2.

Tanji, J. L. (1990). The preparticipation physical examination for sports. *American Family Physician, 42,* 397.

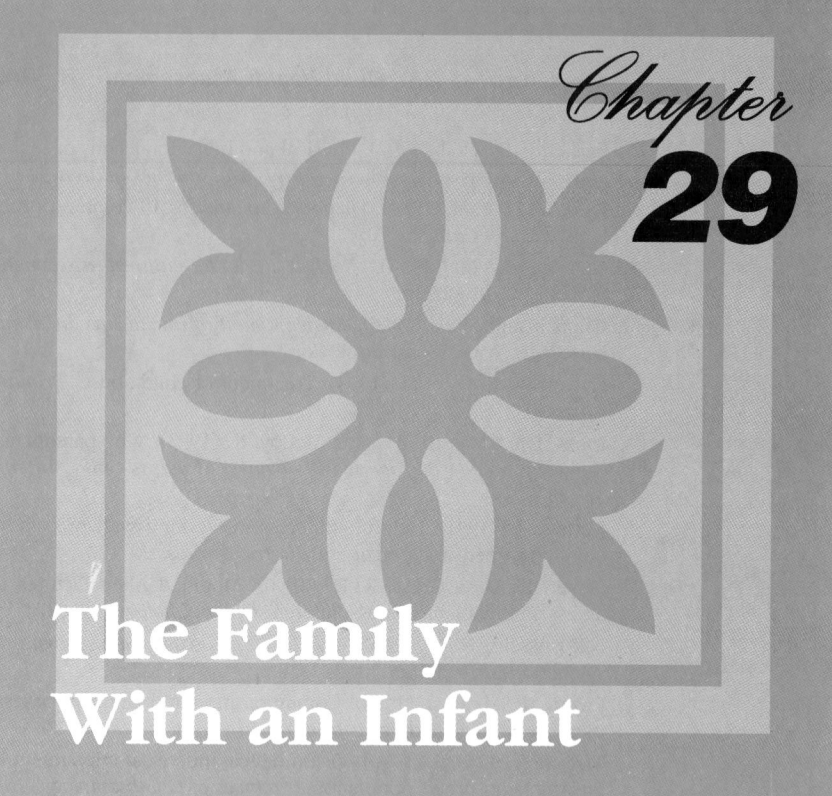

Chapter 29

The Family With an Infant

Adele Pillitteri: MATERNAL AND CHILD
HEALTH NURSING, 2nd Edition. © 1995
Adele Pillitteri.

Objectives

After mastering the contents of this chapter, you should be able to:

1. Describe normal infant growth and development and associated parental concerns.
2. Assess an infant for normal growth and development milestones.
3. Formulate nursing diagnoses related to infant growth and development and associated parental concerns.
4. Plan nursing care to meet the infant's growth and development needs, such as planning anticipatory guidance to prevent problems such as diaper rash and sleep disturbances.
5. Implement nursing care related to normal growth and development of the infant such as helping parents plan stimulating activities.
6. Evaluate goal outcomes established for care to be certain goals associated with growth and development have been achieved.
7. Identify National Health Goals related to infant growth and development that nurses can be instrumental in helping the nation achieve.
8. Identify areas related to nursing care of the infant which could benefit from additional nursing research.
9. Use critical thinking to analyze methods of care for the infant to be certain care is family centered.
10. Synthesize knowledge of infant growth and development with nursing process to achieve quality maternal and child health nursing care.

Key Terms

- baby-bottle syndrome
- binocular vision
- coordination of secondary schema
- deciduous teeth
- eighth-month anxiety
- extrusion reflex
- fine motor development
- gross motor development
- hand regard
- Landau reflex
- natal teeth
- neck-righting reflex
- neonatal teeth
- object permanence
- parachute reaction
- pincer grasp
- prehensile ability
- primary circular reaction
- seborrhea
- secondary circular reaction
- separation anxiety
- social smile
- thumb opposition
- ventral suspension

Infancy is traditionally designated as the period from 1 month to 1 year of age. This year is one of rapid growth and development, with the infant tripling birth weight and increasing length by 50%. In these important months, the infant undergoes such rapid development that parents sometimes feel their baby looks different and demonstrates new abilities each day. During this period, the baby's senses sharpen and, with the process of attachment to primary caregivers, forms his or her first social relationships. Because of the growth and learning potential, this first year is a crucial one. Without proper nutrition, the baby will not grow and physically thrive, and without the proper stimulation and nurturing care by consistent caregivers, the infant may not develop a healthy interest in life or a feeling of security so essential to future development. The Focus on National Health Goals box lists National Health Goals related to the infant year.

Infants are usually seen at health care facilities for health maintenance at least six times during the first year. A standard schedule is for 2-week, 2-month, 4-month, 6-month, 9-month, and 12-month visits, and these visits are as important for the parents as they are for the infants themselves. They provide an opportunity for parents to ask questions about their child's growth pattern and developmental progress and for the nurse to assess for potential problems. Anticipatory guidance offered at these visits can help parents prepare for the rapid changes that mark the first year of life. When appropriate, encouraging parents to join clubs or networking groups helps to increase their knowledge base and confidence level as parents. Table 29-1 details usual procedures at infant maintenance visits. First year immunizations and any risks associated with these are discussed in Chapter 43.

NURSING PROCESS OVERVIEW
for Healthy Development of the Infant

ASSESSMENT

Nursing assessment of the infant should begin by interviewing the primary caregiver. Important areas to discuss are nutrition, growth patterns, and development. The infant's height, weight, and head circumference are important indicators of growth and should be plotted on standard growth charts. These charts represent average growth and are used to see if that individual baby's growth is falling within the same relative percentile with each health check-up.

Physical assessment of the infant must be done quickly yet thoroughly because the baby can tire or become hungry, making it difficult to judge overall behavior and temperament. The primary caregiver should be present to make the child comfortable and thus yield the best results. Using a calm, unhurried approach helps the infant feel safe enough to accept your interventions.

NURSING DIAGNOSIS

Much of your assessment of the infant and family will focus on basic needs such as sleep, nutrition, activity, and parents' adjustment to their new role. Possible nursing diagnoses might be:

- Ineffective breastfeeding related to maternal fatigue
- Maternal sleep pattern disturbance related to baby's need to nurse every 2 hours
- Maternal social isolation related to stress of caring for infant and lack of adequate social support
- Health-seeking behaviors related to adjusting to parenthood
- High risk for impaired verbal communication related to documented hearing impairment
- Altered growth and development related to lack of stimulating environment
- High risk for altered parenting related to long hospitalization of infant
- Family coping: potential for growth related to financial support
- Altered role performance related to new responsibilities within the family

PLANNING

It is important to establish goals for infant care that are realistic. Parents of infants, especially first-time parents, must do a lot of adjusting, and this takes time. Try to suggest activities that can be easily incorporated into the family's lifestyle. If your assessment data indicate that a child needs more exposure to language and you know that both parents work during the day, for example, you might suggest that the parents ask their child's care provider to increase vocalization around the child. Parents could be encouraged to spend a certain amount of time each evening reading or reciting nursery rhymes to their baby.

IMPLEMENTATION

One of the most important interventions of the infant period is teaching new parents about normal growth and development milestones such as the age range for rolling over or reaching for objects. Whenever possible, this information should be anticipatory, so that parents are prepared for changes and developments *before* they occur.

FOCUS ON
National Health Goals

A number of National Health Goals focus on promotion of health during the infant year. These are:

- Increase to at least 75% the proportion of parents and caregivers who use feeding practices that prevent baby bottle tooth decay. Special target population: parents and caregivers with less than high school educations.

- Reduce drowning deaths to no more than 2.3/100,000 for children aged 4 years and younger from a baseline of 4.2/100,000.

- Increase the use of occupant protection systems, such as child automotive safety seats, to 95% from a baseline of 84%.

- Reduce the prevalence of blood lead levels exceeding 15 µg/dL among children aged 6 months through 5 years to no more than 500,000 (DHHS, 1991).

Nurses can be instrumental in helping the nation to achieve these goals by educating parents about the importance of not putting an infant to bed with a bottle of milk or juice, the use of infant car seats, and using lead free paint. A number of areas related to these topics that could benefit from additional nursing research are effective ways that mothers are able to comfort infants while in car seats without removing the infants from the seats; characteristics of programs that were successful for community lead removal; and effective ways to teach cardiopulmonary techniques to parents to prevent fatal outcomes from childhood drownings.

Table 29-1. Health Maintenance Schedule, Infant Period

Area of Focus	Methods	Frequency
Assessment		
Developmental milestones	History, observation	Every visit
	Formal Denver Developmental Screening Test (DDST II)	At 3 months and 1 year
Growth milestones	Height, weight, head circumference plotted on standard growth chart; physical examination	Every visit
Nutritional problems	History, observation; height/weight information	Every visit
Parent–child relationship	History, observation	Every visit
Vision and hearing defects	Grossly, by observation and history	Every visit
Dental health	History, physical examination	Every visit after teeth erupt
Anemia	Hematocrit	9th month visit
Lead screening	Erythrocyte protoporphyrin	9th month visit
Tuberculosis screening	Tine test	12th month visit
Immunizations		
Diphtheria, pertussis, and tetanus (DPT) and *Haemophilus influenzae* type B (HiB)	Check history and past records; inform caregiver about any risks and side effects; administer immunization in accordance with health care agency policies	2nd, 4th, and 6th month visits / 2nd, 4th, and 6th month visits
Trivalent oral poliomyelitis		2nd and 4th month visits Optional 6th month visit
Hepatitis B		1st month visit; 6th month visit
Anticipatory Guidance		
Infant care	Active listening and health teaching	Every visit
Expected growth before next visit		Every visit
Expected developmental milestones before next visit		Every visit
Problem Solving		
Any problems expressed by caregiver during the course of the visit	Active listening and health teaching	Every visit

EVALUATION

Goals established for care should be evaluated at each health supervision visit to detect changes in growth and development. Help parents understand that the total developmental profile, not a single individual element, provides the most important description of their child. Variation is the rule rather than the exception, and a 2-month variation from the average during the infant year is considered normal. Many 4-month-old infants, for example, have mastered most of the 4-month skills and some of the 5-month skills, yet they may still be at a 3-month level on one or two criteria.

Examples of outcome criteria that might be established are:

- Mother states she feels fatigued but able to cope with sleep disturbance from night waking.
- Parents state 5 actions they are taking daily to encourage bonding.
- Father states both he and spouse are adjusting to new role of parent.

Growth and Development of the Infant

Physical Growth

The physiologic changes that occur in the infant year reflect the increasing maturity and growth of body organs.

Weight

As a rule, infants double their weight at 4 to 6 months of age; they triple it by 1 year. This is about 1 lb/month or 6 to 8 oz/week (454 g, or 170 to 277 g/week) for the first 6 months; weight gain is slightly less than this for the next 6 months. The average 1-year-old male weighs 10 kg (22 lb); the average female weighs 9.5 kg (21 lb). The infant's weight, however, is relevant only when plotted on a standard growth chart and compared to that child's own growth curve (see Appendix E). (See Chapter 34 for a discussion of the nutritional needs of the infant.)

Height

The infant increases in height during the first year by 50%, or grows from the average birth length of 20 in to about 30 in (50.8 cm to 76.2 cm). Height, like weight, is best assessed if it is plotted on a standard growth chart. Infant growth is most apparent in the child's trunk during the early months. During the second half of the first year, it becomes more apparent as lengthening of the legs. At the end of the first year, the child's legs may still appear disproportionately short, however, and perhaps bowed. For accuracy, an infant should be measured lying supine on a measuring board (see Figure 28-6A).

Head Circumference

Head circumference increases rapidly during the infant period as a reflection of rapid brain growth. By the end of the first year, the brain has already reached two thirds of adult size.

Some infants have asymmetry of the head until the second half of the first year from always being placed in one sleeping position, causing the skull bones to flatten on that side. This distortion gradually corrects itself as the child sleeps less and spends more time with the head in an erect position. Persistence of asymmetry may suggest that the infant is not receiving enough stimulation.

Body Proportion

Body proportion changes during the first year from newborn to a more typically infant appearance. The mandible becomes more prominent as bone grows. By the end of the infant period, the lower jaw is definitely prominent and remains that way throughout life.

The circumference of the chest is generally less than that of the head at birth by about 2 cm; it is even with the head circumference in some infants as early as 6 months and in most by 12 months. The abdomen remains protuberant until the child has been walking well for some time, generally well into the toddler period. Cervical, thoracic, and lumbar vertebral curves develop as infants hold up their head, sit, and walk.

Lengthening of the lower extremities during the last 6 months of infancy readies the child for walking and often changes the appearance from "baby-like" to "toddler-like."

Body Systems

In the cardiovascular system, heart rate slows from 120 to 160 beats/min to 100 to 120 beats/min by the end of the first year; the heart continues to occupy a little over one half the width of the chest. Pulse rate may begin to slow with inhalation (sinus arrhythmia), but this does not become marked until preschool age. That the heart is becoming more efficient is shown by the decreasing pulse rate and a slightly elevated blood pressure (from an average of 80/40 to 100/60 mm Hg).

Infants are prone to develop a physiologic anemia at 2 to 3 months of age, although this can be prevented by early introduction of oral iron. Anemia occurs because this is the time when many fetal red blood cells are destroyed (the life of a red cell is 3 months) and new cells are not yet being produced in adequate replacement numbers. Hemoglobin in an infant becomes totally converted from fetal to adult hemoglobin at 5 to 6 months of age; infants experience a second decrease in serum iron levels at 6 to 9 months as the last of iron stores established in utero are used.

The respiratory rate of the infant slows from 30 to 60 breaths/min to 20 to 30 breaths/min by the end of the first year. Because the lumen (tubal cavity) of the respiratory tract remains small, and mucous production by the tract is still inefficient, upper respiratory infections occur readily and tend to be potentially more severe in infants than in adults.

At birth, the gastrointestinal tract is immature in both ability to digest food and mechanical action; these functions mature gradually during the infant year. Although the ability to digest protein is present and effective at birth, the amount of amylase, which is necessary for the digestion of complex carbohydrate, is deficient until approximately the third month; lipase, which is necessary for digestion of saturated fat, is decreased in amount during the entire first year.

The liver of the infant remains immature, possibly causing inadequate conjugation of drugs (if a drug should be necessary for treatment of illness) and inefficient formation of carbohydrate, protein, and vitamins for storage. Although a sucking reflex is present at birth, swallowing coordination does not develop effectively until about 6 months. Until age 3 or 4 months an **extrusion reflex** (food placed on the infant's tongue is thrust forward and out of the mouth) prevents some infants from eating effectively. Drinking from a cup rather than from the breast or bottle becomes possible by age 8 or 10 months.

The immune system becomes functional by at least 2 months of age; the infant is able to produce both IgG and IgM antibodies by 1 year of age. The levels of other immunoglobulins (IgA, IgE, and IgD) are not plentiful until preschool age, which is the reason that infants must be protected from infection.

The ability to adjust to cold is mature by age 6 months. By this age, an infant can shiver in response to cold (which increases muscle activity and provides warmth) and has developed additional adipose tissue that serves as insulation. Brown fat, which protected the newborn from cold, decreases in amount during the first year.

The kidneys remain immature and not as efficient at eliminating body wastes as in the adult. The endocrine system remains particularly immature in response to pituitary stimulation, such as adrenocorticotropic hormone, or insulin production from the pancreas. Without these hormones functioning effectively, an infant is unable to react to stress with adequate efficiency.

Although the fluid in body compartments shifts to some extent, extracellular fluid is 35% of body weight and intracellular is 40% at the end of the first year, in contrast to adult proportions of 20% and 40%, respectively. The effect of this proportional difference is to make the infant susceptible to dehydration from illnesses, such as diarrhea, in which body fluid is lost.

Teeth

The first baby tooth usually erupts at age 6 months, followed by a new one monthly. Teething patterns can vary greatly among children, however. Figure 29-1 illustrates the approximate ages of baby tooth eruption by tooth type.

Some newborns may be born with teeth (called **natal teeth**) or have teeth erupt in the first 4 weeks of life (called **neonatal teeth**). This early tooth growth occurs in about 1 of 2000 infants. The mandibular central incisors (see Figure 29-1) are the most frequent teeth involved in this early growth. In some children, natal or neonatal teeth are **deciduous**. They are fixed firmly and should not be removed as no other teeth will grow to replace them until the permanent teeth erupt at age 6 or 7. Deciduous teeth are also essential for protecting the growth of the dental arch. Natal and neonatal teeth may also be supernumerary (extra) teeth, in which case they will be loosely attached; these teeth must be removed before they loosen spontaneously and are aspirated by the infant (Nik-Hussein, 1990).

Motor Development

The average infant progresses through systematic motor growth during the first year that reflects strongly the principles of cephalocaudal development and gross to fine motor development. Control proceeds from head to trunk to lower extremities in progressive, predictable sequence.

To assess motor development, the infant should be evaluated in two major areas. The first is **gross motor development** (ability to accomplish large body movements), in which the infant is observed in four positions: ventral suspension, prone, sitting, and standing. The second is **fine motor development**, which is measured by observing or testing **prehensile ability** (ability to coordinate hand movements).

Gross Motor Development

Ventral Suspension Position. **Ventral suspension** refers to the infant's appearance when held in midair on a horizontal plane, supported by a hand under the abdomen (Figure 29-2*A*). In this position, the newborn allows the head to hang down with little effort at control. A 1-month-old lifts the head momentarily, then drops it again. He or she may flex the elbows, extend the hips, and flex the knees. Two-month-olds hold their head in the same plane as the rest of their body, a major advance in muscle control. The 3-month-old lifts and maintains the head well above the plane of the rest of the body in ventral suspension.

A **Landau reflex** is one that develops at 3 months. When held in ventral suspension, the infant's head, legs, and spine extend. When the head is depressed, the hips, knees, and elbows flex. This reflex continues to be present in most infants during the second 6 months of life, then it becomes increasingly difficult to demonstrate. A child with motor weakness, cerebral palsy, or other neuromuscular defect will not be able to demonstrate the reflex.

At 6 to 9 months, an infant demonstrates a **parachute reaction** from a ventral suspension position. When infants are suddenly lowered toward an examining table from ventral suspension, the arms extend as

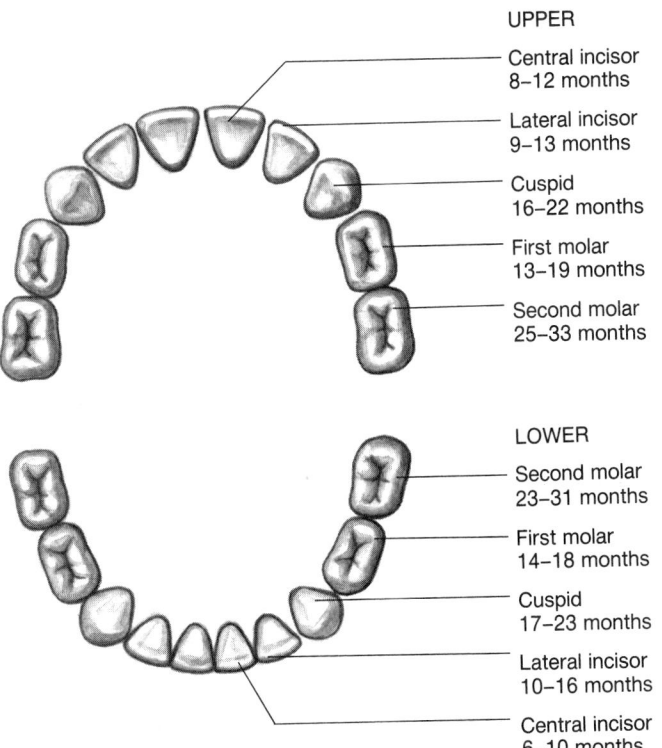

UPPER

Central incisor
8–12 months

Lateral incisor
9–13 months

Cuspid
16–22 months

First molar
13–19 months

Second molar
25–33 months

LOWER

Second molar
23–31 months

First molar
14–18 months

Cuspid
17–23 months

Lateral incisor
10–16 months

Central incisor
6–10 months

FIGURE 29-1
Eruption pattern of deciduous teeth.

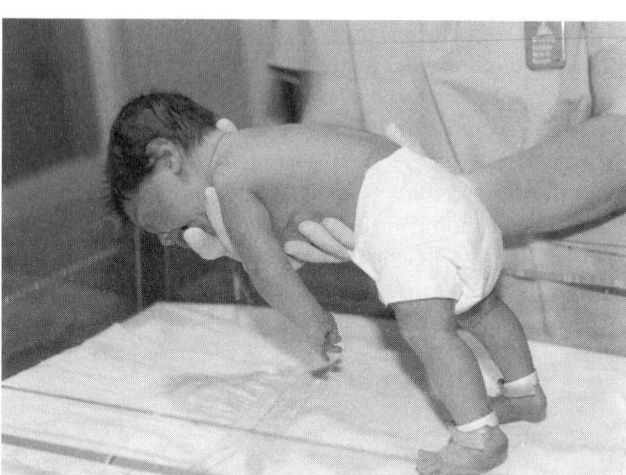
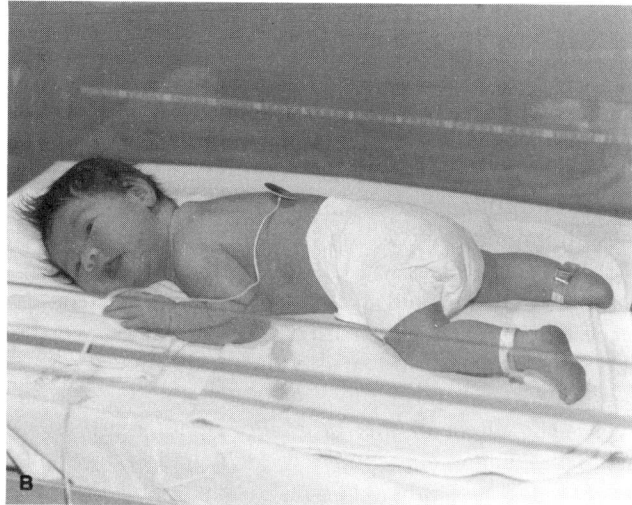

FIGURE 29-2
(**A**) *Ventral suspension position.* (**B**) *Prone position.*

if to protect themselves from falling. In children with hemiplegia, the response is noticeable only on the unaffected side. Children with cerebral palsy do not demonstrate this response because, when in this position, they have extreme flexion activity.

Prone Position. When lying on their stomach, newborns can turn their head to move it out of a position where breathing is impaired, but they cannot hold it raised (Figure 29-2*B*). At age 1 month, infants lift their head and turn it easily to the side. They still tend to keep the knees tucked under the abdomen as they did as a newborn. Two-month-old infants can raise their head and maintain the position, but they cannot raise their chest far enough to look around yet. Their head is still held facing downward.

The 3-month-old lifts the head and shoulders well off the table and looks around when prone. The pelvis is flat on the table, no longer elevated. Some children can turn from a prone to a side-lying position at this age.

Four-month-olds lift the chest off the bed and look around actively, turning the head from side to side. They are able to turn from front to back. The first time, this tends to occur as an extension of lifting the chest combined with the **neck righting reflex** which begins at this age. When the infant turns the head to the side, shoulders, trunk, and pelvis turn in that direction, too. This reflex causes the baby to lose his or her balance and roll sideways when lifting the head up. The baby is frightened by the sudden feeling of rolling free and probably cries. After this happens a few more times, however, the baby begins to delight in this new accomplishment. Most babies turn front to back first and then, 1 month later, back to front. When taking a health history, ask which way the child turned first; those with spasticity *may* turn first in the opposite direction. This is

not necessarily an indication of spasticity, however, because some healthy babies turn back to front first.

A 5-month-old rests his or her weight on the forearms when prone. The infant can turn completely over, front to back and back to front. At 6 months, infants rest their weight on their hands with extended arms. They can raise not only their chest, but also the upper part of their abdomen off the table.

By 9 months, the child can creep from the prone position. Creeping is a new skill, advanced from the crab crawling or hitching he or she has been doing. Creeping means the child has the abdomen off the floor and moves one hand and one leg and then the other hand and leg, using the knees on the floor to locomote (Figure 29-3).

Sitting Position. When placed on his or her back and then pulled to a sitting position, the 1-month-old has gross head lag as in the first days of life (Figure 29-4). In a sitting position, the back is rounded and the infant demonstrates only momentary head control. The 2-month-old can hold his or her head fairly steady when sitting up, although it does tend to bob forward. The infant at this age still has head lag when pulled to a sitting position.

The 3-month-old has only slight head lag when pulled to a sitting position. A 4-month-old reaches an important milestone by no longer demonstrating head lag when pulled to a sitting position.

A 5-month-old can be seen to straighten his or her back when held or propped in a sitting position. By 6 months, children sit momentarily without support. They anticipate being picked up and reach up with their hands from this position. Some parents expect a child this age to sit securely and are worried because the sitting posture is still extremely shaky. It is more normal for the 6-month-old to have only limited ability, how-

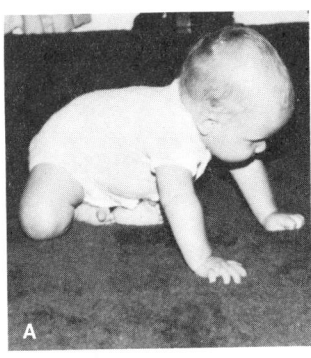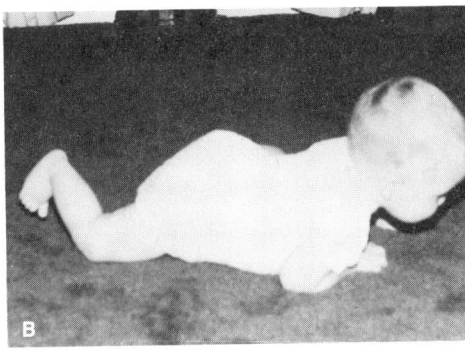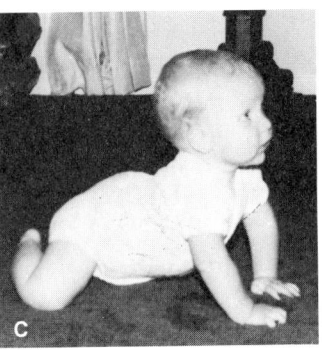

FIGURE 29-3
*Different means of locomotion. (**A**) Hitching. The baby moves backward in a modified sitting position by using the arms and hands to push. (**B**) Crawling. While prone with the abdomen touching the floor and the head and shoulders supported with weight borne on the elbows, the baby pulls the body and drags the legs as the arms move. (**C**) Creeping. The torso is carried above the floor and parallel to it. (Schuster, C. S., & Ashburn, S. S. [1992]. The process of human development (3rd ed.). Philadelphia: J.B. Lippincott, with permission.)*

ever, to sit independently (Figure 29-5). Six-month-olds often sit with their legs spread and their arms stiffened between them, hands on the floor, as a prop. Infants are capable of movement by hitching or sliding backward from this position. It is important that parents be made aware that an infant this young is capable of moving from one spot to another in this way, so that they are prepared for this and can prevent accidents.

A 7-month-old sits alone, but only when the hands are held forward for balance. An 8-month-old is able to sit securely without additional support (Figure 29-6). This is a major milestone in development that should always be considered in assessment. Children with delayed mental or motor development may not accomplish this step at this time.

At 9 months, infants sit so steadily that they can lean forward and regain their balance. They may still lose their balance if they lean sideways for another month.

Standing Position. A stepping reflex can still be demonstrated at 1 month of age. In a standing position, the infant's knees and hips flex rather than support more than momentary weight. A 2-month-old, when held in a standing position, holds his or her head up with the same show of support as in a sitting position. The stepping reflex is still present. At 3 months, infants begin to try to support part of their weight. The stepping reflex begins to fade.

At 4 months, infants make an attempt to sustain their weight actively on their legs. They are successful at doing this because the step-in-place reflex has faded.

The 5-month-old continues the ability to sustain a portion of his or her weight. The tonic neck reflex should be extinguished, and the Moro reflex is fading. By 6 months, infants support nearly their full weight when in a standing position. A 7-month-old bounces with enjoyment in a standing position.

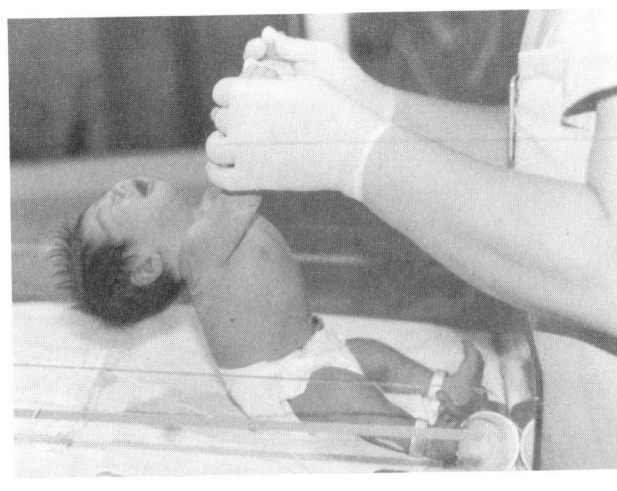

FIGURE 29-4
An infant is pulled to a sitting position to demonstrate head lag. Notice how evident this is in the very young infant.

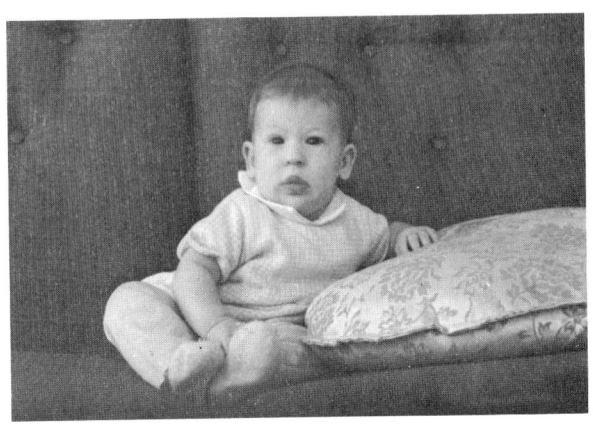

FIGURE 29-5
A 6-month-old infant sitting. Notice how she props herself with her hand to maintain the position.

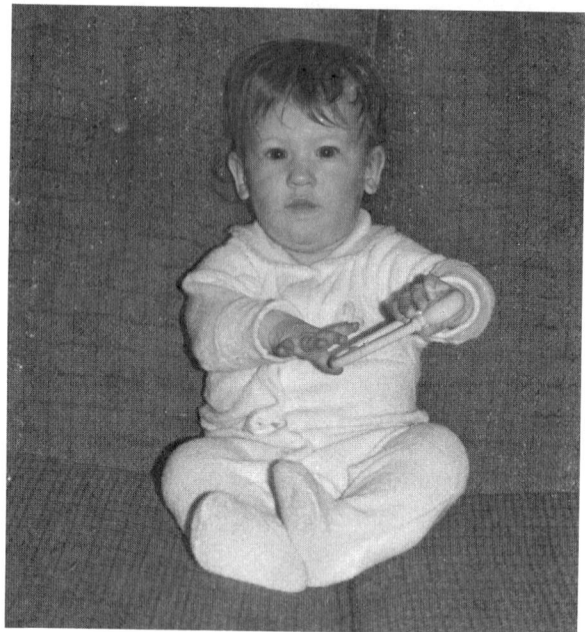

FIGURE 29-6
At 8 months, the same infant shown in Figure 29–5 is able to sit securely.

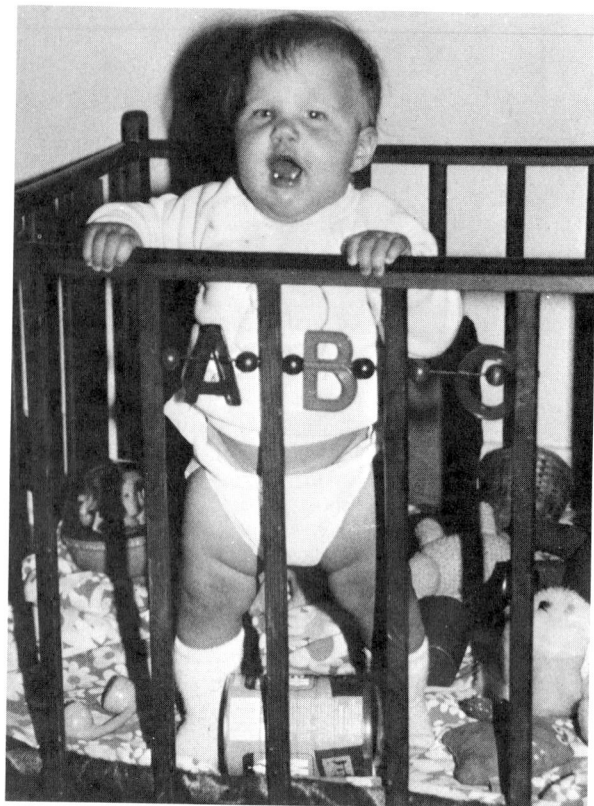

FIGURE 29-7
An 11-month-old child cruising along a crib rail. Further childproofing of the house will be necessary to keep the infant safe.

The 9-month-old can stand holding onto the coffee table if he or she is placed in that position. Some 9-month-olds can pull up to that position. The 10-month-old can pull herself to a standing position by holding onto the side of a playpen or a low table; she cannot let herself down again as yet.

At around 11 months, the child learns to "cruise" or move about the room by holding onto objects such as chairs and low tables (Figure 29-7). At 12 months, a child stands alone at least momentarily. Some parents expect their child to walk at this time and are disappointed to see him or her not moving but merely standing. A child has until about 22 months of age to walk and still be within the normal limit, however (Figure 29-8).

Fine Motor Development

One-month-old infants still hold their hands in fists so tightly it is difficult to extend the fingers. The grasp reflex is very strong. As the grasp reflex begins to fade, the 2-month-old will hold an object for a few minutes before dropping it; the hands are often held open, not fisted.

At 3 months, infants reach for attractive objects in front of them. Their grasp is unpracticed, however, so they usually miss them. It is important for parents to know that this is part of normal development or else they may think the child is nearsighted or farsighted, or has poor coordination.

By 4 months, infants bring their hands together and pull at their clothes. They will shake a rattle placed in their hand for a long time. **Thumb opposition** (ability

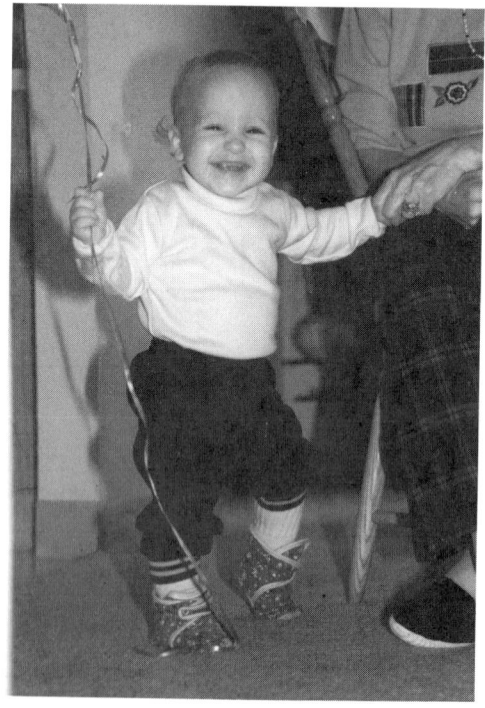

FIGURE 29-8
There is a wide variation in the age at which walking is first accomplished. Here a child has mastered it by 1 year. (Courtesy of Michael Wesniewski.)

to bring the thumb and fingers together) is beginning, but the motion is a scooping, not a picking-up one, and is not very accurate. The infant is limited to handling large objects (Figure 29-9). Palmar and plantar grasp reflexes have disappeared.

The 5-month-old can accept an object that is handed to him or her and grasp it with the whole hand. He or she can reach and pick up an object without its being offered and often plays with his or her toes as objects. Fisting that persists beyond 5 months suggests a delay in motor development. Unilateral fisting suggests hemiparesis or paralysis on that side.

By 6 months, grasping has advanced to a point where the child can hold objects in both hands. Infants at this age will drop one toy when a second one is offered for the same hand. They can hold a spoon and start to feed themselves (with much spilling). Moro, palmar grasp, and the tonic neck reflex have completely faded. A moro reflex that persists beyond this point should arouse grave suspicion of neurologic disease.

The 7-month-old can transfer a toy from one hand to the other. He or she holds a first object when a second one is offered. By 8 months, random reaching and ineffective grasping have disappeared as a result of advanced eye-hand coordination.

A major milestone of 10 months is the ability to bring the thumb and first finger together in a **pincer grasp** (Figure 29-10). This enables the child to pick up objects as small as crumbs, and he or she spends a lot of time picking up such small items as pieces of cereal from the breakfast tray. The infant points with one finger to objects; he or she offers toys to people but then cannot release them.

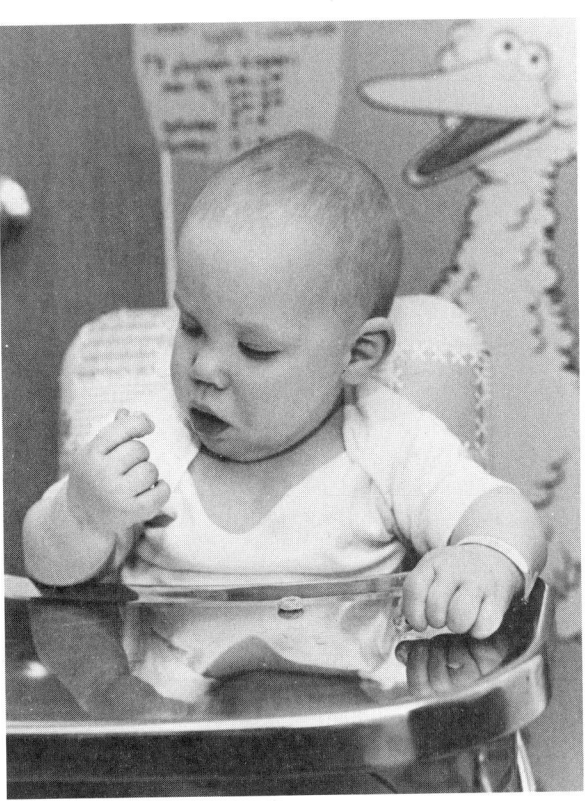

FIGURE 29-10
An infant demonstrating a pincer grasp. (Courtesy of the Department of Medical Photography, Children's Hospital, Buffalo, NY.)

At 12 months, infants can draw a semistraight line with a crayon. They enjoy putting objects such as small blocks in containers and taking them out again. They can hold a cup and spoon to feed themselves fairly well (if they have been allowed to practice) and can take off socks and push their hands into sleeves (again, if they have been allowed to practice). They can offer toys and release them.

Developmental Milestones

In addition to gross and fine motor skills that are developing at this time, language and play behavior also mark major milestones in the first year of life (Curry & Duby, 1994). Motor and cognitive development and play throughout this year are summarized in Table 29-2.

Language Development

A child begins to make small, cooing (dovelike) sounds by the end of the first month. The 2-month-old differentiates a cry. This means caregivers can distinguish a cry that means hungry from one that means wet, from one that means lonely, and so on. This is an important milestone in development for an infant and in marking how far a parent has progressed in the task of learning the infant's cues. A first-time parent has more difficulty mak-

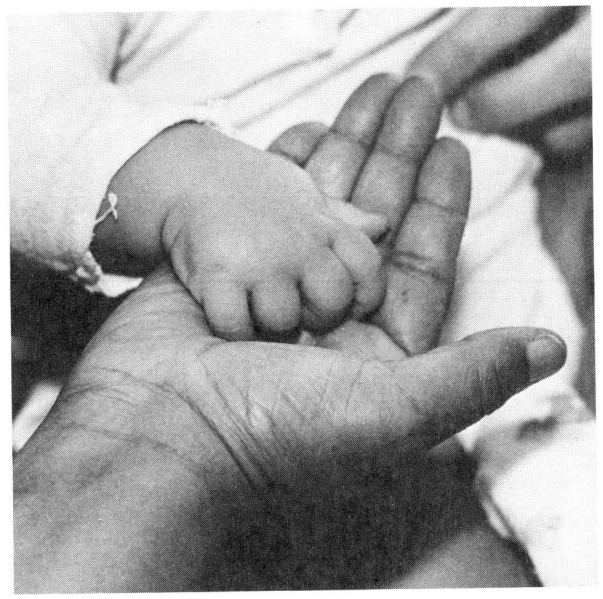

FIGURE 29-9
Hand development. By age 4 months, the infant picks up objects by raking.

Table 29-2. *Summary of Infant Growth and Development*

Month	Motor Development	Fine Motor Development	Socialization and Language	Play
0–1	Largely reflex	Keeps hands fisted; able to follow object to midline		Enjoys watching face of primary caregiver, listening to soothing sounds
2	Holds head up when prone	Has social smile	Makes cooing sounds; differentiates his cry	Enjoys bright-colored mobiles
3	Holds head and chest up when prone. Reflexes: grasp, stepping, tonic neck are fading	Follows object past midline	Laughs out loud	Spends time looking at hands or uses them as toy during the month (hand regard)
4	Turns front to back; no longer has head lag when pulled upright; bears partial weight on feet when held upright			Needs space to turn
5	Turns both ways; Moro reflex fading			Handles rattles well
6	Reaches out in anticipation of being picked up; first tooth (central incisor) erupts; sits unsteadily (still needs support)	Uses palmar grasp	May say vowel sounds (*oh-oh*)	Enjoys bathtub toys, rubber ring for teething
7		Transfers objects hand to hand	Beginning fear of strangers	Likes objects that are good size for transferring
8	Sits securely without support		Fear of strangers (ability to tell known from unknown people) reaches peak	Enjoys manipulation, rattles and toys of different textures
9	Creeps or crawls (abdomen off floor)		Says first word (*da-da*)	Needs space for creeping
10	Pulls self to standing	Uses pincer grasp (thumb and finger) to pick up small objects		Plays games like patty-cake and peek-a-boo
11	"Cruises" (walks with support)			"Cruises"
12	Stands alone; some infants take first step	Holds cup and spoon well; helps to dress (pushes arm into sleeve)	Says two words plus *ma-ma* and *da-da*	Likes toys that fit inside each other (pots and pans); nursery rhymes; will like pull-toys as soon as walking

ing the distinction in crying than a practiced one. The infant's ability to make throaty, gurgling, or cooing sounds also increases at this time.

In response to a nodding, smiling face or a friendly tone of voice, the 3-month-old will squeal with pleasure. This is an important step in development because the baby becomes even more fun to be with. Parents spend increased time with the infant not just to care for him or her but because they enjoy his or her company.

By 4 months, an infant is very "talkative," cooing and gurgling when spoken to. He or she definitely laughs out loud.

By 5 months, the infant says some simple vowel sounds, for example, *goo-goo* and *gah-gah.*

At 6 months, infants learn the art of imitating. They

may imitate a parent's cough, for example, or say "Oh!" as a way of attracting attention.

The amount of talking infants do increases at 7 months. They can imitate vowel sounds well, for example, *oh-oh, ah-ah,* and *oo-oo.* By 9 months, the infant usually speaks a first word: *da-da* or *ba-ba.* Occasionally a mother may need reassurance that *da-da* for daddy is an easier syllable to pronounce than *ma-ma* for mother. German mothers report that the first word their babies say is *da,* which means "here" in German. By 10 months, the infant masters another word such as *bye-bye* or *no.*

At 12 months, infants can generally say two words besides *ma-ma* and *da-da;* they use those two words with meaning.

Play

Because they can fix their eyes on an object, 1-month-olds are interested in watching a mobile over their crib or playpen. Mobiles should be black and white or brightly colored and light enough in weight so that they move when someone walks by them. They should face down towards the infant, not sideways towards the adults standing beside the crib. Musical mobiles provide extra stimulation. One-month-olds spend a great deal of time watching the parent's face and appear to enjoy this activity so much that the face may become their favorite "toy." Help parents to appreciate this fact and not worry that they are spoiling their baby by sitting and holding him or her for long periods of time. They will enjoy recalling such calm moments later, when they are stacking blocks, winding up toys, or playing table games with their growing child.

Hearing is a second sense that is a source of pleasure for the child in early infancy. Even a newborn "listens" to the sound of a music box or a musical rattle. He or she stirs and seems apprehensive at the sound of a raucous rattle.

A 2-month-old will hold a light, small rattle for a short period of time. He or she is very attuned to mobiles or a cradle gym strung across the crib. The infant continues to spend a great deal of time just watching the people around him or her.

Three-month-olds may be more interested in studying their hands than in handling toys (termed **hand regard**). They can handle small blocks or small rattles. Four-month-olds need a playpen or a sheet spread on the floor so they have an opportunity to exercise their new skill of rolling over. Rolling over is so intriguing it may serve as a "toy" for the entire month.

A 5-month-old is ready for a variety of objects to handle: plastic rings, blocks, squeeze toys, clothespins, rattles, plastic keys. All these should be small enough so that the infant can lift them with one hand, yet big enough so that he or she cannot possibly swallow them.

A 6-month-old can sit steadily enough to be ready for bathtub toys such as rubber ducks or plastic boats. Because they are starting to teethe, infants enjoy a teething ring to chew on at this time.

Because 7-month-olds can transfer toys, they are interested in items small enough to do this: blocks, rattles, plastic keys. As their mobility increases, they begin to be more interested in brightly colored balls or toys that previously rolled out of reach.

Eight-month-olds are sensitive to differences in texture. They enjoy having toys that have different feels to them: velvet, fur, fuzzy, smooth, rough.

The 9-month-old needs the experience of creeping. This means time out of a playpen so he or she has room to maneuver. Many 9-month-olds begin to enjoy toys that go inside one another, such as a nest of blocks or rings of assorted sizes that fit on a center post. Some are more interested in pots and pans than toys.

At 10 months, infants are ready for peek-a-boo and will spend a long time playing the game with their hands or with a cloth over their head that they can reach and remove. They can clap and so are also ready to play patty-cake. These games have a positive value just as laughing out loud did for the 3-month-old. They make the baby feel an active part of the household. A family feeling begins to grow as the baby is able to participate in active games.

The 11-month-old has learned to cruise. They often finds this so absorbing that they spend little time doing anything else during the month.

The 12-month-old enjoys putting things in and taking things out of containers. They like little boxes that fit inside one another or dropping objects such as blocks into a cardboard box. As soon as they are able to walk, they will be interested in pull-toys. A lot of time may be spent listening to someone saying nursery rhymes or listening to records of them.

Development of Senses

Vision

A 1-month-old regards an object in the midline of vision (directly in front of himself or herself) as it is brought into close proximity, about 18 in (46 cm) away. The infant follows it a short distance, but not across the midline as yet. He or she studies or regards a human face with a fixed stare. The 2-month-old focuses well (from about age 6 weeks) and follows objects with the eyes (although still not past the midline). This ability is a major milestone in development, indicating that the infant has achieved **binocular vision**, or the ability to fuse two images into one (Figure 29-11).

Three-month-olds typically hold their hands in front of their face and study their fingers for long periods of time (hand regard) (Figure 29-12). Blind children also demonstrate this phenomenon, however, so it may not be so much a test of vision as of cognitive or exploratory development.

A 4-month-old recognizes familiar objects, such as a frequently seen rattle or toy animal. They follow their parents' movements with their eyes eagerly. At 6 months, infants are capable of organized depth perception. This allows them to reach much more accurately for objects as they begin to perceive their distances accurately. Up until 6 months of age, the newborn may experience normal difficulty in establishing eye coordination. After this age, however, an infant whose eyes still "cross" should be examined by a physician.

Seven-month-olds pat their image in a mirror. They have developed such depth perception that they can perform such tasks as transferring toys from hand to hand. By 10 months, the infant looks under a towel or around a corner for a concealed object (beginning of **object permanence**).

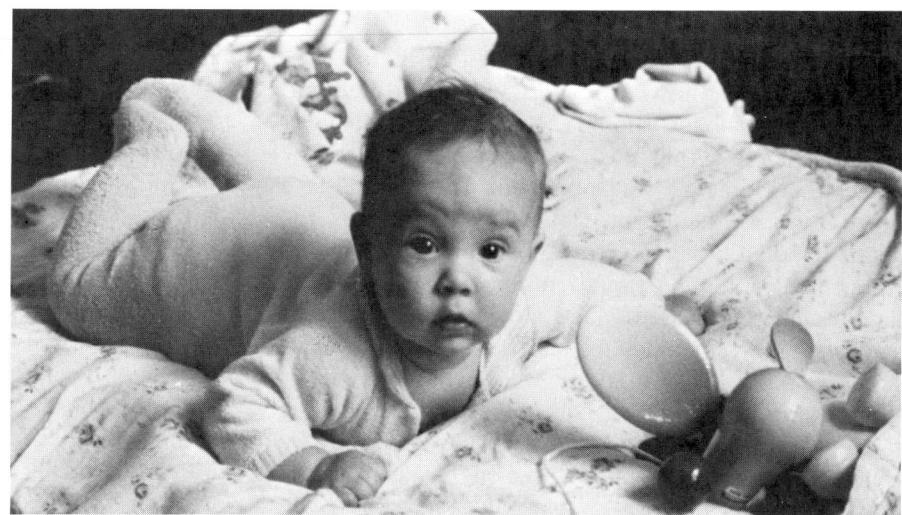

FIGURE 29-11
The 2-month-old infant focuses steadily and lifts her head up while prone. Note her obvious awareness of the photographer. (Courtesy of Brian Smistek.)

Hearing

Hearing is demonstrated in the 1-month-old who quiets momentarily at a distinctive sound such as a bell or a squeaky rubber toy. Hearing awareness becomes so acute by 2 months of age that the infant will listen or stop an activity at the sound of spoken words. Many 3-month-olds will turn their heads to attempt to locate a sound. When the 4-month-old hears a distinctive sound, he or she will turn toward the sound and look in that direction.

At 5 months of age, the infant demonstrates that he or she can localize a sound downward and to the side, by turning the head and looking down. A 6-month-old has progressed to being able to locate a sound made above him or her. By 10 months, the infant can recognize his or her name and listen acutely when spoken to. By 12 months, the infant can easily locate a sound in any direction and turn toward it. A vocabulary of two words

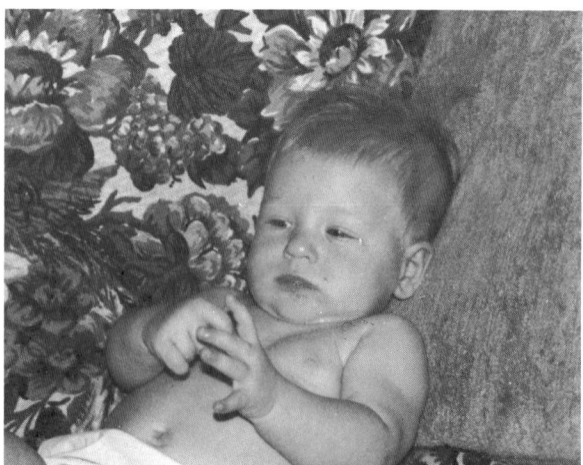

FIGURE 29-12
Three-month-old infants spend time studying their hands. This is a part of cognitive recognition of the self as separate from the environment.

plus *ma-ma* and *da-da* also demonstrates that he or she can hear.

Emotional Development

Developmental Task: Trust Versus Mistrust

Erikson (1986) proposed that the developmental task of the infant period is to form a sense of trust. When the infant is hungry, a parent feeds and makes him comfortable again; she is wet, and the father changes her and makes her dry; he is cold, and the mother holds and warms him. By this process, an infant learns to trust that when he or she has a need or is in distress, a person will come to meet that need.

A synonym for *trust* in this connotation is *love*. By the way that infants are handled, fed, talked to, and held, they learn to love and be loved. Infants who have numerous caregivers, who may be fed one day on a rigid schedule and the next only when they are hungry, who sometimes are treated roughly and sometimes gently, can have difficulty learning to trust anyone. If infants cannot trust, they cannot enjoy deeply satisfying interactions with others and can have difficulty trusting themselves or experiencing high self-esteem. They may have difficulty establishing close relationships as adults.

Socialization

Socialization, or learning how to interact with others, is an extended phenomenon. The 1-month-old shows he or she can differentiate between a face and other objects by studying a face or the picture of a face longer than other objects. They quiet best and eat best for the person who has been their primary caregiver.

When an interested person nods and smiles at a 2-month-old, he or she smiles in return. This is a **social smile** and is a definite response to the interaction, not the faint, quick "smile" that younger infants, even newborns, demonstrate. It is a major milestone for assessing a number of areas, most notably vision, motor control, and intelligence. Mentally disabled children or children with spasticity may not demonstrate a social smile until much later.

At 3 months, the infant demonstrates increased social awareness by readily smiling at the sight of a parent's face. Some 3-month-olds laugh out loud at the sight of a funny face.

By 4 months, when a person who has been playing with and entertaining an infant leaves, the infant is likely to cry to show he or she enjoyed the interaction. Infants at this age recognize their primary caregiver and prefer that person's presence to others. By 5 months, a baby may show displeasure when an object is taken away from him or her. This is a step beyond showing displeasure when a person leaves. The baby can be counted on to laugh at seeing a funny face.

At 6 months, infants are increasingly aware of the difference between people who regularly care for them and strangers. They may begin to draw back from unfamiliar people.

Seven-month-olds show obvious fear of strangers. They may cry when taken from their parent, attempt to cling to him or her, and reach out to be taken back. Parents may view this as a bad trait or a regression in socialization. It is actually a big step forward, for it shows the infant is able to differentiate persons, to know the difference between those he or she trusts and those he or she does not know.

Fear of strangers appears to reach its height during the eighth month, so much so that this phenomenon is often termed **eighth-month anxiety**, or **separation anxiety**. An infant at the height of this phase will not go willingly from a parent's arms to a nurse's. Taking a few minutes to talk to the child and parent first is time well spent.

The 9-month-old is very aware of changes in tone of voice. They will cry when scolded, not so much because they understand what is being said, but because they sense their parent's displeasure.

By 12 months, most children have overcome their fear of strangers and are alert and responsive again when approached. They like to play nursery rhymes and rhythm games, and "dance" with others. They like being at the table for meals and joining in family activities.

Cognitive Development

In the first month of life, an infant uses mainly simple reflex activity. There is little evidence that infants at this age see themselves as separate from their environment. This does not mean that they are not able to respond actively or interact with people, however; they are very people-oriented from within moments after birth.

Primary Circular Reaction

By the third month of life, the child enters a stage identified by Piaget (1966) as **primary circular reaction**. During this time, he or she explores objects by grasping them with his or her hands or by mouthing them (Figure 29-13). The infant at this stage does not appear to be aware of what actions he or she can cause or what actions occur independently of him or her. For example, if an infant's hand should accidentally strike a mobile across the crib, the infant appears to enjoy watching the brightly colored birds move in front of him or her, but makes no attempt to hit the mobile again, not realizing that his or her hand caused the movement.

Secondary Circular Reaction

At about 6 months of age (cognitive development has wide variation), the child passes into a stage that Piaget (1966) called **secondary circular reaction**. During this time, the infant is able to realize that his or her actions can initiate pleasurable sensations. The infant reaches for a mobile above the crib, hits it, watches it move, realizes that his or her hand initiated the motion, and so hits it again.

The infant is still unaware of the permanence of objects; for example, if an object is hidden from vision (a baby drops it from her hand or it is hidden by a blanket), the infant will not search for it. Gone is gone. If any part of the object is exposed, the infant is able to visualize the whole object and will reach to obtain it.

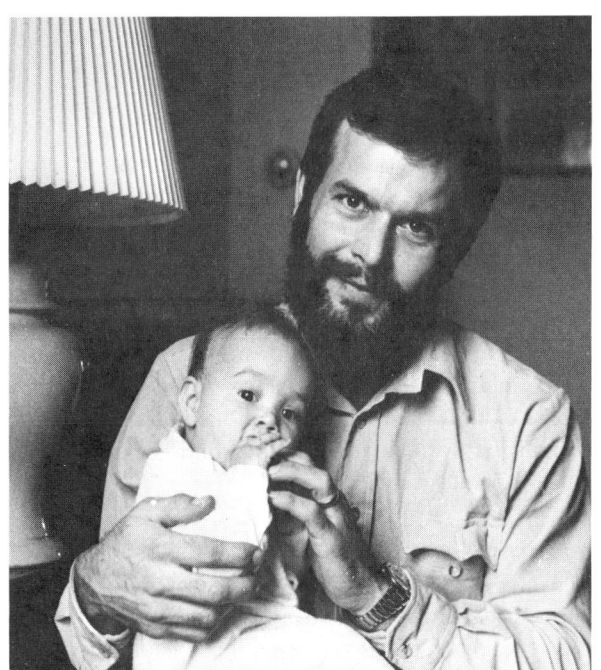

FIGURE 29-13
Mouthing of objects or fingers is a method by which an infant explores the world. This also helps the infant to separate self from environment. (Courtesy of Brian Smistek.)

Coordination of Secondary Schema

An infant of 10 months discovers object permanence, searching for an object that has fallen out of sight. Infants are ready for peek-a-boo once they have gained the concept of permanence, as they know their parent still exists even when hiding behind a hand or blanket. Waiting for the parent to reappear is exciting. If a baby drops a piece of breakfast cereal or a spoon from her highchair tray, she knows it still exists even though it is out of sight and will reach for it. Piaget (1966) called this stage of cognitive development **coordination of secondary schema**.

As infants reach 1 year of age, they are not only capable of reproducing interesting events (she accidentally hits a mobile once; it moves; she hits it again) but are capable of producing new events. She drops objects from a high chair or playpen and watches where they fall or roll. This is a frustrating activity for caregivers because it involves a great deal of reaching and picking up. It is an important activity for infants, however, because it contributes to their awareness of the permanence of objects and how they are able to control events in their world.

The Nursing Role in Health Promotion of the Infant and Family

The nursing role with infants is wide-ranging because infants are so dependent on their caregivers for safety, learning, and emotional development.

Promoting Infant Safety

Accidents are a leading cause of death from 1 month through 24 years of age and are second only to acute infections as a cause of acute morbidity and visits to the physician throughout this time.

Most accidents in infancy occur because parents either underestimate or overestimate the child's ability. Nursing interventions that help parents become sensitive to their infant's developmental progress not only help establish sound parent-child relationships but also provide anticipatory guidance for the child's safety (see the Focus on Family Teaching box).

Preventing Aspiration

The accident that leads to the greatest number of infant deaths is aspiration. Round and cylindrical objects are more dangerous than square or flexible objects in this regard. A 1¼ in (3.2 cm) cylinder, such as a carrot or hotdog, is particularly dangerous because it can totally obstruct the infant's airway. Parents who feed an infant formula should be advised not to prop bottles. By propping bottles, they are overestimating their infant's ability

to push away the bottle, sit up, turn the head to the side, cough, and clear an airway if milk should flow too rapidly into the mouth and the infant begins to aspirate. If an infant bites into an inflated balloon, the balloon can be sucked back into their mouth and obstruct their airway in the same way (Halida, 1993).

Other incidents of aspiration occur because parents underestimate the baby's ability to grasp and place objects in the mouth. Newborns' grasp and sucking reflexes cause them to react this way automatically so from day one, parents must be certain that nothing comes within the child's reach that would not be safe to put into the mouth. Parents should buy clothing without decorative buttons, and check toys and rattles to be certain that they have no small parts that will snap off or fall out. Even a newborn can wiggle to a new position to reach an attractive object such as a teddy bear with small button eyes. When solid foods are introduced, parents must be careful to offer small pieces of hotdogs or grapes, not large chunks. Children under about 5 years should not be offered popcorn because of the danger of aspiration.

As the infant becomes more adept at handling toys, they must be checked for loose pieces or parts such as button eyes on stuffed toys that could be grasped and pulled off. If parents are going to offer an infant a pacifier, they should be certain that it is a one-piece construction and has a flange large enough to keep the object from completely entering the child's mouth (Figure 29-14).

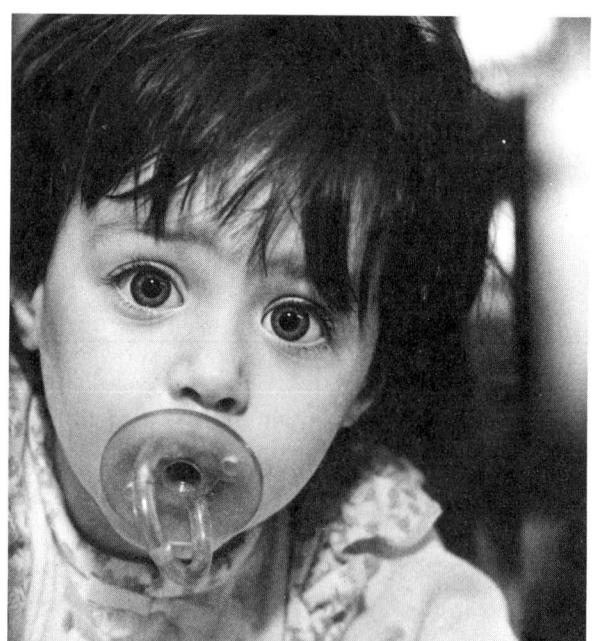

FIGURE 29-14
Many infants enjoy sucking on a pacifier to help them fall asleep. Note the one-piece construction of the pacifier, which prevents the object from completely entering the child's mouth. (Courtesy of Brian Smistek.)

FOCUS ON FAMILY TEACHING

Q. What measures should I take to prevent an accident with my infant?

A. Accident prevention is necessary in a variety of areas.

Potential Accident	Prevention Measure
Aspiration	Be certain any object that an infant can grasp and bring to the mouth is either safe to eat or too big to fit in the mouth. Do not feed an infant popcorn, peanuts, etc., as these are easily aspirated. Store baby products such as powder out of infant's reach; powder is high risk for aspiration.
	Inspect toys and pacifiers for small parts that could be aspirated if broken off; don't make homemade pacifiers.
Falls	Never leave the infant on an unprotected surface, such as a bed or couch, even if the child is in an infant seat.
	Place a gate at the top and bottom of stairways; do not allow an infant to walk with a sharp object in the hands or mouth (it could pierce the throat in a fall).
	Raise crib rails and make sure they are locked before walking away from crib.
	Do not leave a child unattended in a highchair; do not use an infant walker.
Motor vehicle	Never transport unless the infant is buckled into a rear-facing infant seat; question the safety of a passenger side air bag with an infant seat.
	Do not be distracted by an infant while driving.
	Do not leave unattended in a parked car (can become dehydrated from excess heat, move gear shift, or be abducted).
Suffocation	Allow no plastic bags near infant's reach.
	Do not use pillows in a crib.
	Do not allow an infant to sleep in bed with adults.
	Unused appliances such as refrigerators or stoves should be stored with the doors removed.
	Buy a crib that is approved for safety (spacing of rails is not over 2⅜ in [6 cm] apart.)
	Remove constricting clothing such as a bib from neck at bedtime.
Drowning	Do not leave infants alone in a bathtub or unsupervised near water (even buckets of cleaning water).
Animal bites	Do not allow the infant to approach a strange dog; supervise play with family pets.
Poisoning	Never present medication as a candy.
	Buy medications in containers with safety caps; put away immediately after use.
	Never take medication in front of infants.
	Place all medication and poisons in locked cabinets or overhead shelves.
	Never leave medication in a pocket or handbag.
	Use no lead-based paint in any area of the home.
	Hang plants or set on high surfaces.
	Post telephone number of the poison control center by the telephone.
	Provide syrup of ipecac with proper instructions for first-aid supply boxes.
Burns	Test warmth of formula and food before feeding (use extra precaution with microwave warming).
	Do not smoke or drink hot liquids while holding or caring for infant.
	Buy flame-retardant clothing for infants.

(continued)

Potential Accident	Prevention Measure
General	Use a sunshield cream on a child when out in direct sunlight; limit the child's sun exposure to less than ½ h at a time.
	Turn handles of pans toward back of stove.
	Use a cool-mist, not a hot-mist, vaporizer; remain in room to monitor so child cannot reach vaporizer.
	Keep a screen in front of a fireplace or heater.
	Monitor infants carefully near candles.
	Do not leave infants unsupervised near hot-water faucets.
	Do not allow infants to blow out matches (don't teach children that fire is fun).
	Keep electric wires and cords out of reach; cover electrical outlets with a safety plug.
	Know the whereabouts of infants at all times.
	Be aware that the frequency of accidents is increased when parents are under stress.
	Special precautions need to be taken at these times.
	Parents should choose baby sitters carefully and explain and enforce all precautions when sitters are in charge.

Preventing Falls

Falls are a second major cause of infant accidents. No infant, beginning with the newborn, should be left unattended on a raised surface. Normal wiggling can bring a baby to the edge of a bed, couch, or table top and result in a fall.

Parents should be prepared for their infant to roll over by 2 months of age; by that time they must be more careful than ever not to leave a baby unattended on a changing table or counter. If the child sleeps in a crib, the mattress should be lowered to its bottom position so the height of the side rails increases; rails should be 2⅜ inches apart, narrow enough so that the child cannot put his or her head between them. Two months is about the maximum length of time infants can safely sleep in a bassinet. They need the protection of a crib and high side rails *before* they can turn over.

All of the above safety precautions apply to the hospital environment as well as to the home. Be sure that crib sides are raised and secure before you walk away from a crib, even for just a moment. Be certain there is not a wide space between the mattress and head board where the child's head could be trapped. Be certain no cords from nursing call bells or safety pins are within reach.

Car Safety

Teaching car safety for infants (as well as for the whole family) is a vital preventive health measure. The use of car seats with newborns is discussed in Chapter 23. Car seats should continue to be used without interruption through toddlerhood. If parents are firm about keeping their infant in a car seat even when he or she gets fussy or impatient, the child will eventually become more comfortable in the seat than outside it. Rear-facing infant seats should not be used in the front seat of cars with passenger-side air bags as the inflating bag may tip the seat and suffocate the infant ("Health Alert," 1992).

Siblings

As infants become more fun to play with at about 3 months, older brothers and sisters grow more interested in interacting with them. Parents with older children may need to be reminded that children under 5 years of age, as a group, are not responsible enough or knowledgeable enough about infants to be left unattended with them. They might introduce an unsafe toy or engage in play that is too rough for the infant. In addition, some preschoolers are so jealous of a new baby that they will physically harm the infant if left alone.

Bathing and Swimming

As babies begin to develop good back support, many parents move their baths into an adult tub. Be certain parents know that they must not leave an infant unattended in a tub, even when propped up out of the water: normal wiggling may easily cause the baby to slip down below the surface. This applies to the hospital setting as well.

Many communities offer infant swim programs for babies as young as 3 months. If their child is enrolled in one of these programs, parents may become overconfident of the infant's ability to operate safely in water. Because a child can dog-paddle momentarily in a swimming pool, it does not mean he or she can sustain that position for any length of time in a bathtub or pool. Also, the child may lose his or her instinctive fear of water and thus be in more danger when around water than the child who is naturally more cautious. Such programs may also spread microorganisms, such as hepatitis A, because infants this age are not yet toilet trained (AAP, 1987).

Childproofing

When the infant begins teething at 5 to 6 months, there comes a desire to chew on any object within reach. Remind parents to check for sources of lead paint, for example, painted cribs, playpen rails, and windowsills. Paints safe for baby furniture should be marked "Safe for use on surfaces that might be chewed by children." If the infant is going to be allowed to play on the floor, parents should move furniture in front of electrical fixtures or buy protective caps for the outlets, as infants are especially fascinated by the holes and will probe them with (often wet) fingers. Gates should be installed at the top and bottom of stairways.

Parents must move all poisonous substances from bottom cupboards and store them well out of the infant's reach. Infants of any age should not be left unattended in carriages, highchairs, grocery shopping carts, or strollers. Baby walkers are extremely dangerous because infants maneuver them near stairways (AMA, 1991).

When infants begin creeping, it is time for parents to recheck bottom cupboards and stairways for safety. Some 9-month-olds walk. At home, higher areas, such as coffee tables, should be cleared of dangerous items. In a hospital setting, assess low counter areas for dangerous objects. Be certain not to leave possibly dangerous supplies in an infant's room.

By 10 months, the baby's pincer grasp makes him or her able to pick up very small objects. Parents need to check play areas as well as areas such as table tops for pins or other sharp objects that could be swallowed (Figure 29-15). A number of the child's toys are now also 10 months old and need to be rechecked to be certain they are still intact and safe.

The child who can walk securely is likely to walk into streets or into swimming pools if not carefully supervised. Although she seems very independent and able to take care of herself, her judgment about what is dangerous is immature. In a hospital setting, be aware that a 12-month-old can wander onto an elevator, out of

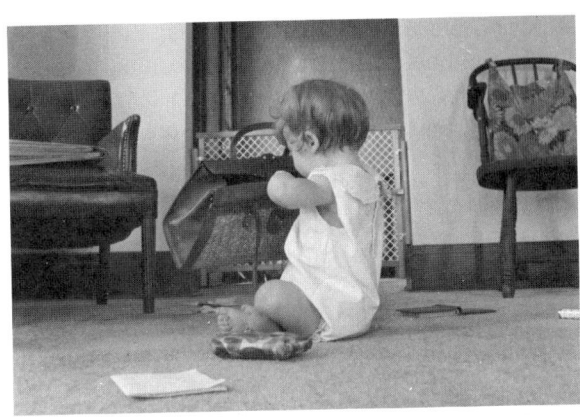

FIGURE 29-15
Once locomotion begins, the extended range of activities brings the infant in contact with potentially dangerous places or objects unless the house is childproofed. A mother's purse is an important object to childproof.

the hospital, or into a laboratory area, or fall down a flight of stairs.

Promoting Emotional Development

The Development of Trust

It is important for people to establish the ability to love, or trust, early in life because development is sequential. If the first developmental step is inadequate, this inadequacy can pervade all future steps. The end result can be an adult who is unable to form deep relationships with others. Such adults may be unable to instill a sense of trust in their own children, and thus the inadequacy is perpetuated from generation to generation.

How do parents (or a nurse) encourage a sense of trust in an infant? Trust arises primarily from a sense of confidence that one knows what is coming next. This does not mean that parents should set up a rigid schedule of care for the child. It does imply that they should establish *some* schedule, for example, breakfast, bath, playtime, nap, lunch, walk outside, quiet playtime, dinner, story, and bedtime. This gentle rhythm of care gives the infant a sense of being able to predict what is going to happen and feel that life has some consistency. All little children thrive on routine: the same story read over and over again; the same bedtime rituals; the same spoon every day for lunch. Infancy is not too early for children to learn family traditions that will help them feel secure in the world as they grow. Some parents have difficulty accepting routine as important to a child. They are so tired of the work treadmill that they want to raise their children as free spirits. Do not discourage this philosophy altogether; however, it may be helpful to suggest a few modifications so as to instill some order into infants' lives.

As important to an infant as the rhythm of care is that the care be given largely by one person (Figure

29-16). This person can be the mother, father, grandparent, conscientious baby sitter, foster parent, or anyone who can give consistent care. For infants ill at birth who are hospitalized for months, this person is often a primary nurse or case manager. Women who work outside their home during the first year of a baby's life (at least 90% of women work at least part-time today) should try to arrange for one person to care for the child while they are away from home or choose a day-care center that will provide a consistent caregiver. They should discuss their methods of child care with alternate caregivers so as not to disrupt the infant's routine. When a child is admitted to a hospital, you must ask for, document, and utilize this information.

Helping parents choose safe child care is discussed in Chapter 31. Parents should assess that the person who will give alternate care will actively interact with the child to provide a sense of trust. Passively caring for infants, not talking to them or touching or stroking them while feeding or changing them, amounts to not being with them. Caregivers may have to be encouraged not to feel self-conscious talking to a baby who does not talk back. Pointing out the importance of such interactions and role modeling them while caring for children helps them to include this type of stimulation as they care for the baby's physical needs. Nursing actions designed to help the ill infant develop a sense of trust are detailed in Table 29-3.

Promoting Sensory Stimulation

Vision

Teach parents that they should make a point of initiating eye-to-eye contact with newborns right from the beginning as a method of stimulating vision as well as promoting socialization.

Most parents are aware that infants enjoy mobiles and also a crib mirror. Occasionally they may overdo the amount of visual stimulation, overwhelming their infant with too many patterns and objects dangling above the crib. Ask parents to consider how all these trappings appear from the infant's view (Figure 29-17).

In a hospital environment, assess that an infant is receiving visual stimulation. Add or reduce objects as appropriate. If the child's movement is restricted in any way, move the position of the mobile from time to time. Photos of family members brought from home or pictures drawn by older brothers or sisters can be posted near the infant's crib. Ask the parents if there are any items from home that the infant would normally see during the course of the day while being fed, changed, or bathed; it may be possible to bring these in to the hospital as well.

Hearing

Infants appear to enjoy soft, musical sounds or soft, cooing voices; they are startled by harsh, raucous rattles or loud bangs. Be certain parents know that they should choose for the infant's first toys ones that make these types of welcoming sounds. For the hospitalized infant, an audiotape of family voices might be a soothing reminder of their presence when they are not around. Tape recordings of maternal heart sounds can be soothing to very young infants.

Touch

An infant needs to be touched so he or she experiences skin-to-skin contact. Clothes should feel comfortable and soft rather than rough; diapers dry rather than wet. Teach parents to handle infants with assurance and gentleness. Some are rough in an ill-timed attempt to "toughen them up so they won't be sissies." Remind such parents that right now their children are babies;

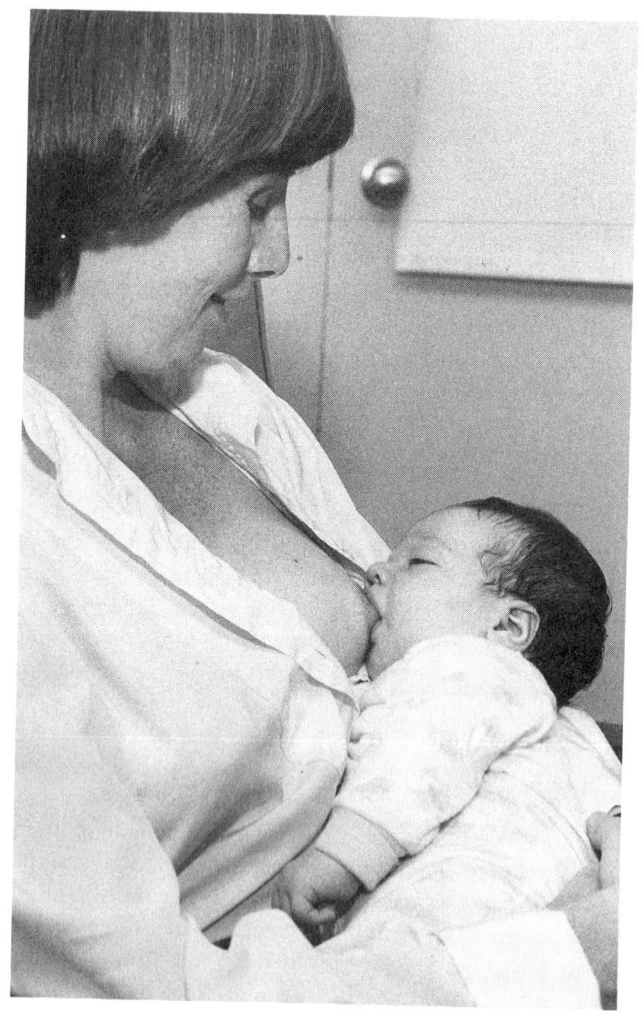

FIGURE 29-16

An infant's sense of trust develops through warm interpersonal relationships. (Courtesy of the Department of Medical Photography, Children's Hospital, Buffalo, NY.)

Table 29-3. *Ways for Nurses to Help Develop a Sense of Trust in an Ill Infant*

Area of Care	Nursing Action
Nutrition	Encourage mothers to breast-feed if possible; provide privacy and support as necessary. Hold the infant no matter what feeding method is used (gavage, total parenteral, oral, enteral). If this is not possible, hold the child for a time after or between feedings so that he or she receives holding equal to that he or she would ordinarily receive. If infant feeding is not oral, provide a pacifier (medical condition considered) five or six times daily for sucking pleasure. Vomiting is not noticeably disturbing to infants, but hold and comfort after an episode.
Dressing change	Try to use nonallergic tape to avoid irritation while applied and pain when removing it. Use a minimum of tape so that the least amount has to be pulled free from sensitive skin (consider using rolled gauze or Kling gauze to hold a bandage in place rather than tape).
	To prevent chilling, be certain irrigation solutions are warm. Try to expose the child minimally during dressing changes to conserve warmth.
	Restrain only those body parts necessary for security.
	Hearing an explanation of what you are doing is comforting to the infant, not for the meaning of the words but for the nonthreatening tone of your voice.
Medicine administration	Flavor oral medicine to disguise disagreeable taste (being careful not to increase the amount to beyond what the child will take readily). Offer a drink of flavorful fluid afterward to counter medicinal taste. Never administer medicine in an infant's formula to prevent changing the formula's taste. Comfort the infant after injections or intravenous insertion by holding and rocking, or give immediately to a parent for this. Check intravenous sites frequently (every 30 min) for swelling to help prevent infiltration and pain. Hold and play with infants despite tubing and restraints.
Rest	Infants sleep in a parent's arms as soundly as they do in bed; therefore, allow parents to sit and hold infants. Rock infants to sleep if this is comforting. If contagion is not a problem, bring the crib to the nursing desk where the infant can see you until he or she falls asleep. Always wake infants gently, because it is frightening (for anyone) to be awakened by a stranger. If bedrest is necessary, check for irritated elbows, heels, and knees from the infant's skin rubbing against sheets; protect with long sleeves or pants.
Hygiene	Check the temperature of bath water for comfort and to prevent chilling. Change diapers frequently to reduce discomfort from irritation. To avoid caries and prevent pain, begin toothbrushing with first tooth.
Pain	Hold and comfort an infant in pain. Do not ask parents to hold a child during a painful procedure; it is difficult for them to see their child in pain. Allow them to comfort the child afterward. Reduce painful procedures to a minimum; combine blood drawing so that only one puncture is necessary for many tests, etc.
Stimulation	Infants focus longest on a human face; talk to them while you care for them so that they come to know you. Provide a crib mirror or a mobile, as visual stimulation is satisfying to an infant. If no mobile is available, create one from a wire coat hanger, string, or strips of adhesive tape and objects that will suspend easily and are light enough to move from motion of the crib or an air current (colored paper, cotton balls, colored tongue blades, inflated rubber gloves). For safety, hang the mobile high enough for the infant to see but not reach.
	During the second half of the 1st year, infants need to try to crawl. Put a pad or sheet on the floor and encourage the infant to come to you or to explore on his or her own while you stand by to offer reassurance (this is almost impossible to accomplish in a crib).

they will have time enough to become strong men or women later.

Because premature infants need to be kept warm while being held, parents may be advised to cuddle an infant next to their bare chest (a kangaroo hold). This is also effective with term infants as a way of promoting close physical contact (see the Focus on Cultural Awareness display).

Taste

Infants demonstrate that they have an acute sense of taste by turning away from or spitting out a taste they do not enjoy. Urge parents to make mealtime a time for fostering trust as well as supplying nutrition. Feedings should be at the infant's pace, and the amount should fit the child's needs and not the parent's idea of how much should be eaten. New foods should be introduced one at a time so that the child can become accustomed to one new taste before another is tried. This also lets parents detect adverse reactions, such as allergy to a new food.

Smell

Infants can smell accurately within 1 or 2 hours after birth. They respond to an irritating smell by drawing back from it. They appear to enjoy pleasant odors and learn early in life to identify the familiar smell of breast

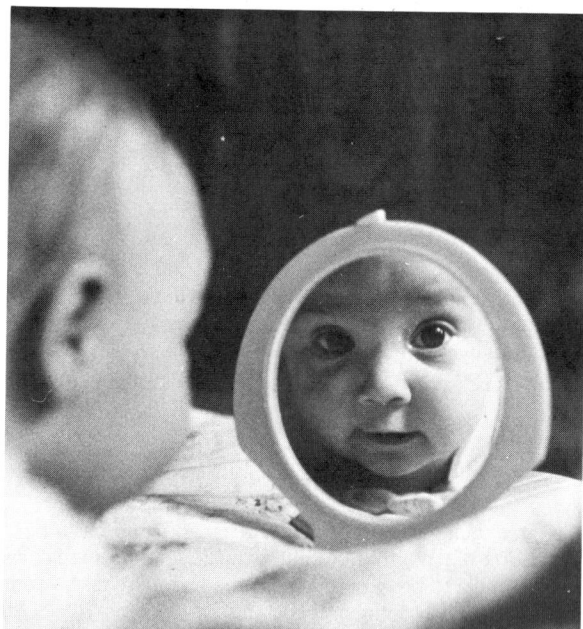

FIGURE 29-17
A 2-month-old infant enjoys her reflection in a crib mirror. (Courtesy of Brian Smistek.)

milk. Teach parents to be alert to substances that cause sneezing when sprayed into the air, such as room deodorizers or cleaning compounds, and to keep irritating odors from the child's environment.

Promoting Infant Development in Daily Activities

In the first year, caring for the infant—feeding, bathing, dressing, and so forth—occupies what may seem like nearly all of parents' waking hours. Worrying about their infant's sleep patterns may take up the rest of their time, often because the parents are not getting enough sleep themselves. But all of these basic care-related activities provide important opportunities for caregivers and infants to get to know one another and to become used to each others' personalities and patterns. Nutritional needs and feeding patterns are paramount during this time; Chapter 34 covers these issues in detail. The other activities of daily living are addressed below.

Bathing

Except in very hot weather, an infant does not need a bath every day. If a parent is tired and would not enjoy bath time or if some days are just too rushed, a complete bath can be omitted, with only the infant's face, hands, and diaper area washed. Some infants do need their head and scalp washed frequently (every day or every other day), however, to prevent **seborrhea**, a scaly scalp condition often called cradle cap. Seborrhea lesions adhere to the scalp in yellow, crusty patches. The

skin beneath them may be slightly erythematous. The patches can be softened by oiling the scalp with mineral oil or petroleum jelly and leaving it on overnight. The crusts can then be removed by shampooing the hair the next morning. A soft toothbrush or fine-toothed comb can be used to help remove crusts.

Bath time should be fun and serves many more functions than just the obvious one of cleanliness (Figure 29-18). Especially during the second half of the first year, a child enjoys poking at soap bubbles and the surface of the water and playing with bath toys. Bathtime also helps an infant learn different textures and sensations and provides an opportunity to exercise and kick. It is a good opportunity for a parent to spend time talking, touching, and communicating with the child.

Diaper-Area Care

The most effective means of promoting good diaper-area hygiene is not to allow an infant to wear soiled diapers for a lengthy period of time. During the day when the child is awake, diapers should be changed frequently (about every 2 to 4 hours). However, it is rarely good practice to interrupt the child's sleep to change diapers. If an infant has such sensitive skin that sleeping in wet diapers constantly causes a rash, sleeping without a diaper at night may be a solution.

At the time of each diaper change, the skin should be washed in clear water or with a commercial diaper wipe and patted or allowed to dry. Routinely using an ointment such as petroleum jelly or A & D ointment to

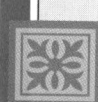

FOCUS ON CULTURAL AWARENESS

Childrearing practices during the first year vary from country to country. One difference is in the way that mothers carry their infants. Many mothers tend to carry infants in their arms and put the infant down to work. Native American mothers, in contrast, may use a papoose board; South American women may carry the infant in a shoulder sling or on their hip. These positions allow the woman to continue to work while holding the infant close.

The amount of infant bathing that is done is also inconsistent across cultures. In the United States, most infants are bathed daily. In colder climates or countries where clean water is not readily available, however, infant bathing is very limited. The use of diapers varies also. In hot climates, infants are often not diapered (Geissler, 1994). Being aware of these cultural differences leads to better understanding of the reasons for an individual woman's particular method of child rearing.

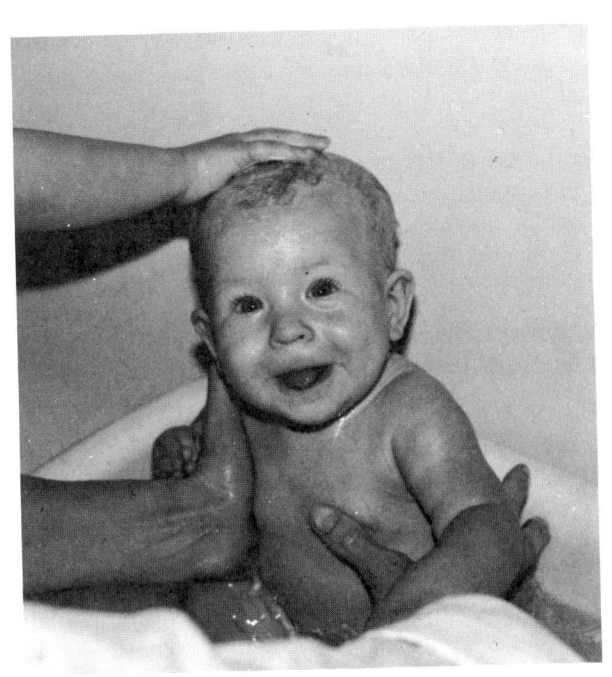

FIGURE 29-18
Infants can have a bath in a tub or sink as soon as they are able to sit securely. Obviously, a parent needs to remain with them for safety.

keep urine and feces away from the infant's skin is good prophylaxis. Parents do not need to use baby powder; if they choose to, it should be used sparingly to reduce the possibility of harmful aspiration. The can should be placed out of the infant's reach afterward.

The benefits and environmental costs of disposable diapers versus cloth diapers have been hotly debated. Some people feel that disposable diapers are environmentally unsound and have contributed greatly to the country's waste disposal problem. Others believe that the water and other energy sources required for the washing of cloth diapers is just as environmentally wasteful. The debate may never be completely resolved, but the nurse can help parents choose what's best for their family by making sure they consider cost, convenience, environmental concerns, and, above all, their baby's comfort. For instance, the cost of laundering diapers or using a diaper service is often less than the cost of buying disposables. However, cloth diapers, if not changed frequently, can be very irritating to the baby's skin. Sometimes home-washed diapers irritate the skin simply because of soap or bleach residue; this can be resolved by giving the diapers an extra rinse after laundering. Parents who live in areas where water must be conserved (or where water is very costly) may prefer disposables for environmental or financial reasons.

Care of Teeth

It is well accepted that exposing developing teeth to fluoride is one of the most effective ways to promote healthy tooth formation and prevent tooth decay. The most important time for children to receive fluoride is between birth and 12 years of age, and the most critical period during this time is the first 3 years of life. A water level of 1 ppm fluoride is recommended as the level that protects tooth enamel. In communities where the water supply does not provide enough fluoride, an oral fluoride supplement before tooth eruption, and using fluoride toothpaste or rinses after eruption, is essential.

Teach parents to inquire about the presence of fluoride in drinking water in their community and help them to determine what, if any, supplementation is necessary. Breastfed infants do not receive a great deal of fluoride from breast milk, so it may be recommended that they receive fluoride drops once a day. Teach parents to begin "brushing" even before teeth erupt by rubbing a piece of gauze over the gum pads. This eliminates plaque and reduces the presence of bacteria, creating a clean environment for the arrival of the first teeth. Once teeth erupt, all surfaces of teeth should be brushed with a soft brush or washcloth once or twice a day. Children lack the coordination to brush effectively until they are school aged, so parents must be responsible for this activity well past infancy. Toothpaste is not necessary for the infant, because it is the scrubbing that removes the plaque, but some health care providers recommend the use of a *slight* amount of fluoridated toothpaste to increase the child's exposure to fluoride.

The initial dental check-up should be made by 2 years of age and continue at 6-month intervals throughout childhood.

Dressing

Clothing for infants should be easy to launder and simply constructed, so that dressing and undressing the child is not a struggle. Infants enjoy kicking and making gross body movements, so their clothing should not be binding. When they begin to creep, they will need long pants to protect their knees. Until they begin to walk, they will need only soft-soled shoes or merely socks or booties to keep their feet warm. Even when they begin walking, their shoes' soles need only be firm enough to protect their feet against rough surfaces; extremely hard soles and high ankle sides are unnecessary (Staheli, 1993).

Sleep

Sleep needs and habits vary greatly among infants, but most require from 10 to 12 hours of sleep at night and one or several naps during the day. If a newborn has been sleeping in a bassinet or in the parents' bed, parents may need some advice on ways to make the adjustment to a crib. Most people advise parents to let the baby sleep in a separate space so that parents do not awaken at every toss and squeak, and so that the baby learns to quiet himself or herself back to sleep should he or she awaken briefly. Caution parents not to place pillows in any kind of infant bed to avoid the possibility of suffocation.

Exercise

The infant benefits from outings in a carriage or stroller, as sunlight provides a natural source of vitamin D. In hot weather, it is important to protect the infant from sunburn by exposing him or her to the sun for only very short periods, beginning with 3 to 5 minutes the first day, a little more the next day, and so on. The sun is most intense between 11:00 AM and 3:00 PM, so early mornings and late afternoons are the best times for the infant to be outside.

Toward the end of the first year, the infant needs space to crawl and then to walk, which can be arranged in an enclosed outdoor play space. In addition to providing fresh air, going for leisurely walks while pointing out the sights of the world—trees, birds, dogs, houses, neighbors—helps the child develop language.

Parents can judge how much outdoor clothing to put on an infant by how much they themselves need. If the adult needs a winter coat, the infant will need a snowsuit; sweaters may be adequate for both; if the adult needs no outer clothing, the infant probably doesn't either.

It is not necessary to enroll infants in formal exercise programs for them to secure adequate exercise, and such programs may put unusual strain on muscles and tendons. Infants using infant walkers must be closely supervised, since they can result in injury if the infant maneuvers the walker too near a stairway.

Promoting Healthy Family Functioning

A primary task of parents during the infant year is to learn to interpret their baby's cues to decipher his or her needs. It is helpful if they can learn early on to perceive the infant as a separate individual with his or her own needs, not a passive being who will accept whatever they offer. This becomes an easier task by 2 months, when infants can indicate by their particular cry whether they are feeling cold, hungry, wet, or lonely. Parents spend a great deal of time with the infant in these first months, which gives them the opportunity to learn and recognize nonverbal cues and to become aware of their baby's needs.

Parental Concerns and Problems Related to Normal Infant Development

Some of the difficulties that parents have in evaluating the health of infants are shown in Table 29-4. New parents may need reassurance and answers to questions about child-care procedures or health during the infant period because they have not yet learned their child's cues. You may find, however, that the need for reassurance is just as great in experienced parents. The unique characteristics of each child require some adjustment from parents.

Teething

Most infants have little difficulty with teething; some, however, appear very distressed. Generally, the gums are sore and tender before a new tooth breaks the surface. As soon as the tooth is through, the tenderness passes.

Because of this pain, the baby might be resistant to chewing for a day or two and be slightly cranky, possibly because he or she is a little hungry from not eating as much as usual. A breastfed baby may refuse the breast because of teething pain. High fever, convulsions, vomiting or diarrhea, and earache, however, are *never* normal signs of teething. An infant with any of these symptoms has an underlying infection or disease and needs to be examined by a physician.

Many over-the-counter medicines are sold for teething pain. As a rule, their use should be discouraged

---

Table 29-4. *Common Difficulties Parents Experience in Evaluating the Health of Infants*

Difficulty	Suggestions for Improving Assessment
Evaluating pain	Infants manifest pain by fussiness. They can reveal arm and leg pain by immobility of the body part; ear pain by brushing or tugging at the ear; stomach pain by pulling up the legs against the abdomen
Evaluating degree of reduced activity	Lack of interest in smiling or interaction is an important observation. Increased sleeping or lying supine with legs nonflexed (frog-legged) as if exhausted is important.
Evaluating infant temperature	All parents should learn how to take an axillary temperature so that they can report a specific degree of fever rather than a subjective finding, such as "feels hot."
Evaluating amount of vomiting or diarrhea	Knowing the number of times vomiting and/or diarrhea has occurred is important. Estimating amount in comparisons with what the child has eaten is helpful as well as estimating an amount (a cupful, etc.). Knowing whether diapers are "soaked" or "stained" with stools is important in estimating amount.

because many contain benzocaine, a topical anesthetic, and, if applied too far back in the throat, could interfere with the gag reflex. Acetaminophen (Tylenol), 1 g per year of age every 4 hours, up to four times a day, is the best suggestion for this discomfort. Teething rings that can be placed in the refrigerator provide soothing coolness against the tender gums. *Caution: an infant who is teething will place almost any object in the mouth; parents must screen articles within the baby's reach to be sure they are edible or safe to chew on.*

Thumb Sucking

Sucking is a surprisingly strong need; sonograms demonstrate fetal thumb sucking in utero. The need is so intense that many infants begin to suck a thumb or finger at about 3 months of age and continue the habit through the first few years of life. It reaches a peak level at about 18 months.

Parents can be assured that thumb sucking is normal and does not deform the jaw line as long as it stops by school age. Also, it does not cause "baby talk" or any of the other symptoms sometimes attributed to it. The parent's best approach is to be certain the infant has adequate sucking pleasure and then to ignore thumb sucking. Making an issue of it rarely causes the child to stop the habit and, if anything, usually intensifies and prolongs it.

Use of Pacifiers

Whether to use pacifiers is a question that parents have to settle for themselves, depending on how they feel about them and their infant's needs. It is rare that infants have such a need for sucking that they must have a pacifier in their mouth constantly. Discussing a few pros and cons with parents clarifies the subject.

An infant who completes a feeding and still seems restless and discontent, who actively searches for something to put into the mouth, and who sucks on hands and clothes may need a pacifier. A baby who has colic craves sucking and enjoys pacifiers because his or her abdomen hurts and he or she interprets this as a hunger sensation. If the child is formula-fed, parents should check the nipples to be certain that the holes are small and the rubber is sturdy, so that the infant can suck hard enough to derive pleasure. If the nipples are satisfactory, parents could offer a pacifier after feeding for more sucking. Theoretically, the child whose sucking needs are met in infancy will not crave as much oral stimulation later in life and is less likely to become a pencil chewer, cigarette smoker, nail biter, or the like.

The major drawback of pacifiers is the problem of cleanliness. They tend to fall on the floor or sidewalk and are then put back into the infant's mouth. If not well constructed, they may come apart and be aspirated. Caution parents not to make pacifiers from a nipple stuffed with cotton. If these come apart, the infant can aspirate the cotton. Wearing the pacifier on a string around the infant's neck could cause strangulation.

Parents should make an attempt to wean a child from a pacifier any time after 3 months of age and certainly during the time that the sucking reflex is fading at 6 to 9 months. Weaning after this age is difficult because the pacifier becomes a well-loved comforter like the warm blanket or fuzzy toy to which a child may cling.

Head Banging

Some infants rhythmically bang their heads against the bars of a crib for a period of time before falling asleep. Such infant head banging is distressing behavior for parents. Besides fearing that children will hurt themselves, some parents may have heard that blind children or those with mental illness do this and will worry that their child is ill in some way.

Head banging in this limited fashion—beginning during the second half of the first year of life and continuing through to the preschool period, associated with nap or bedtime, and lasting for less than an hour at a time—can be considered normal. Children use this measure to relax and fall asleep. Investigating stress factors operating in the house may be helpful. If some of them can be relieved (parents' overestimation of the child's development, marital discord, illness in another family member), the head banging may decrease, or it may have already become such a strong habit that it will persist for months or even years.

Advise parents to pad the rails of cribs so infants cannot hurt themselves and reassure them that this is a normal mechanism for relief of tension in a child of this age. No therapy should be necessary. Excessive head banging done to the exclusion of normal development or activity, or head banging past the pre-school period, suggests a pathologic basis. Such children need a referral for counseling and further evaluation.

Sleep Problems

Sleep problems develop in early infancy because of colic or because an otherwise healthy infant takes longer than usual to adjust to sleeping through the night. Breastfed babies tend to wake more often than those who are formula-fed because breast milk is more easily digested (Adair et al., 1992). When infants wake at night, parents rapidly become fatigued. This is an increasing concern because more and more families today consist of two wage-earning parents. There is no time for parents to nap during the day to make up for sleep lost at night. In late infancy, the problem of waking at night and remaining awake for an hour or more becomes common (Scott & Richards, 1990). Although the infant may be content and not cry during this time, parents are reluctant to sleep while the child is awake and thus may become extremely fatigued again. Suggestions for eliminating or at least coping with night waking are (1) delay bedtime by 1 hour; (2) shorten an afternoon sleep period; (3) do not respond immediately to the child at night so that he or she possibly has time to fall back to sleep on his or her own; and (4) provide soft toys or music and allow the child to play quietly alone during this wakeful time. Reassuring parents that infants take varying lengths of time to adjust to night sleeping is helpful in that it assures them their child is normal. Suggesting parents make use of the time they are awake at night (think through a problem at work, plan a shopping list, and so on) may help them view the situation not as a problem time but as a constructive one.

Constipation

Breastfed infants are rarely constipated because their stools tend to be loose. Constipation may occur in formula-fed infants if the diet is too high in protein (if formula consists of undiluted cow's milk), too high in fat (if it is not diluted properly), or is deficient in fluid. This can be corrected by modifying the diet with the addition of more fluid or carbohydrate. Generally, it is necessary only to clarify the error in formula preparation.

Some parents misinterpret the normal pushing movements of a newborn to be constipation. When defecating, infants' faces do turn red, and they grimace and grunt. As long as stools are not hard and contain no evidence of fresh blood (as might occur with a rectal fissure), this is not constipation but rather normal infant behavior.

If the difficulty persists beyond 5 or 6 months of age, adding foods with bulk, such as fruits or vegetables, and increasing fluid intake generally relieves the problem. Apple juice (3 or 4 oz) or prune juice (0.5 to 1 oz daily) may be given as a temporary measure. It is best not to maintain this therapy over a long period of time, however, because too much apple or prune juice can cause the opposite problem—diarrhea.

All infants with a history of constipation for more than 1 week should be examined for an anal fissure or tight anal sphincter. Softening stools and thereby relieving the pain of defecation often solves the problem and helps the fissure to heal. If an unusually tight anal sphincter exists, parents will be given instructions to manually dilate the sphincter two or three times daily until it dilates sufficiently. Hirschsprung's disease (aganglionic megacolon or lack of nerve innervation to a portion of the colon) may be manifested early in life as constipation. If no stool is present in the rectum of a constipated infant on rectal examination, the possibility of this disease is suggested. A careful history must then be taken to assess whether the infant manifests other symptoms of Hirschsprung's disease: ribbon-like stools, bouts of diarrhea, and a distended abdomen (see Chapter 45).

Chronic constipation also may occur in children with congenital hypothyroidism (decreased functioning of the thyroid gland). An infant with constipation therefore also should be carefully observed for characteristic symptoms of hypothyroidism, such as lethargy, protruding tongue, and failure to meet developmental milestones (see Chapter 48). Infants with either Hirschsprung's disease or hypothyroidism need therapy to correct the disorder.

Loose Stools

Many first-time parents are unfamiliar with the loose consistency or color of normal newborn stools. It is important for parents to care for their newborns before discharge from a hospital or alternative birth center long enough to become familiar with characteristics of the newborn's stools before they take him or her home.

Stools of breastfed infants are generally softer than those of formula-fed infants. Also, if the mother takes a laxative while breastfeeding, its effect may be demonstrated as loose stools in the infant. The infant who is formula-fed may have loose stools if the formula is not mixed properly. It is relatively simple to clear up this form of diarrhea by diluting the infant's formula correctly.

Occasionally, loose stools may begin with the introduction of solid food, such as fruit. Malabsorption syndrome (celiac disease), or inability to digest fat, may manifest itself first by loose stools as well as a distended abdomen and deficiency of fat soluble vitamins (see Chapter 45).

When talking to a parent about this problem, inquire about the duration of the loose stools, the number of stools per day, their color and consistency, and whether there is any mucus or blood in them. Is there associated fever, cramping, or vomiting? Does the infant continue to eat well? Appear well? Seem to be thriving?

Infants with associated symptoms such as fever, cramping, vomiting, loss of appetite, and weight loss should be examined by a physician as this implies an infectious process. Dehydration occurs rapidly in a small infant who is not eating and is losing body fluid through loose stools.

Colic

Colic is paroxysmal abdominal pain that generally occurs in infants under 3 months of age (Pinyerd, 1992b). The discomfort begins abruptly. The infant cries loudly and pulls the legs up against the abdomen. The infant's face becomes red and flushed, the fists clench, and the abdomen is tense. If offered a bottle, the infant will suck vigorously for a few minutes as if starved, then stop as another wave of intestinal pain occurs.

The cause of colic is unclear. It may occur in susceptible infants from overfeeding, from swallowing too much air while feeding, or from a formula too high in carbohydrate. Formula-fed babies are more likely to have colic than breastfed babies.

Although infants continue to thrive despite colic, the condition should not be dismissed as unimportant. It is a distressing and frightening problem for parents because the infant not only appears to be in acute pain, but the distress persists for hours, usually in the middle of the night so that no one in the family gets adequate rest. This is a difficult beginning to a parent-child relationship, which needs to be strong and binding for the parents to enjoy parenting and for the infant to thrive in their care (see the Focus on Nursing Research box).

Take a thorough history of infants with colic symptoms, because intestinal obstruction or infection may mimic an attack of colic and be misinterpreted by the casual interviewer. Ask parents about the duration of the problem and its frequency—it usually lasts up to 3 hours a day and occurs at least 3 days every week. Ask for a description of what happens just prior to the attack (e.g., if it occurs after feeding) and a description of the attack itself and associated symptoms. The number and type of bowel movements is important to document, because bowel movements are not abnormal with colic. Constipation; narrow, ribbon-like stools; and the presence of blood or mucus in the stool suggest other complicating problems. A family medical history is important to obtain because allergy to milk may simulate colic.

Determine the baby's feeding pattern: breast- or bottle-fed; if bottle-fed, type of formula and how it is prepared. Explore with parents how they are feeding the baby and whether they are burping the infant adequately after feeding. Are they holding the baby firmly upright so that air bubbles can rise? For the breastfed baby, a change in maternal diet (e.g., avoiding onions or "gassy" foods) can reduce or limit colicky periods. It may be helpful to recommend that both breast- and formula-fed infants receive small, frequent feedings to prevent distention and discomfort. Offering a pacifier may be comforting.

Many babies with colic are more comfortable sleeping on their abdomens than on their sides or backs after feeding. A towel rolled under the infant's abdomen for a little extra pressure is often helpful.

Some persons recommend placing a hot-water bottle under the infant's stomach, but this should be discouraged. A basic rule for any abdominal discomfort is to avoid heat in case appendicitis is developing. This is highly unlikely in so young an infant, but parents will remember they once used heat and may use it again when the child is older. Hot-water bottles and heating pads should also not be used because they might burn the delicate skin of infants.

If the infant appears to have a great deal of associated intestinal gas, inserting the bulb of a rectal thermometer into the rectum often dramatically relieves the discomfort. Caution parents to be extremely gentle when doing this so that they do not cause rectal fissures or puncture the rectal mucosa. Changing the formula bottle to the type with disposable bags that collapse as the baby sucks may be helpful as these allow less air to be swallowed. Taking the infant for a ride in the car is often reported as being helpful in soothing colicky babies. Commercial manufacturers produce music boxes that simulate the sound of a heart beat, which may be helpful (Hardsell, 1990).

Occasionally, sedation or an antiflatulent, such as simethicone, is required to alleviate attacks and give both the parents and the child some rest. It is important to think of colic as a family problem or else a vicious circle may gradually begin: the infant cries and the parents become tense and unsure of themselves; the infant senses the tension and develops more colic.

In most infants, colic disappears almost magically at 3 months of age, probably because it becomes easier to digest food and the infant maintains a more upright position by this time, which allows less gas to form (see the Nursing Care Plan).

Spitting Up

Almost all infants spit up, although formula-fed babies appear to do it more than breastfed babies. Parents who did not handle their infant much in the health care facility where the child was born may discover that an infant spits up only after they take the baby home. They may

(text continues on page 874)

FOCUS ON NURSING RESEARCH

How Does Persistent Colic Affect the Mental Health of Mothers?

A nurse researcher attempted to answer this question by interviewing 12 mothers who had infants with colic and comparing their responses to those of 12 mothers who had infants without colic. For the purpose of the study, colic was defined as high-pitched infant fussing or crying for at least 2 hours a day for at least 5 out of 7 days plus a maternal report of infant inconsolability. Findings of the study revealed that the mothers of infants with colic had more symptoms of psychological distress, such as more reports of bodily dysfunction, fears, disordered thinking, depression, anxiety, fatigue, hostility, and impulsive thoughts and actions, than the control group. Mothers whose infants had colic also had stronger feelings of personal inadequacy or inferiority than the others. The researcher stresses that colic creates a potentially stressful situation for parents and that parents of infants with colic require concerned support from health care providers.

Pinyerd, B. J. (1992a). Infant colic and maternal mental health: nursing research and practice concerns. *Issues in Comprehensive Pediatric Nursing, 15,* 155.

Nursing Care Plan

Health Maintenance Visit for an Infant

Stuart is a 2-month-old infant brought in by his mother for a routine check-up. The following is a nursing care plan designed for him.

Assessment: Two-month-old, well-proportioned male infant. Chief concerns: "diaper rash" and "always crying." Height and weight both at 50th percentile on growth chart. Taking 4 oz Similac every 4 h. Has erythematous macular diaper area. Mother using no special brand of diapers: "Whatever is on sale." Only occasionally uses baby powder, no ointment. Admits to "stretching" diaper changes to save money. Urine specific gravity: 1.020. Mother attends cosmetology school full-time and works part-time at a grocery store. Father works at garage as a mechanic. Child is at day-care center during morning. Every night infant cries from 6:00 P.M. to about 2:00 A.M. Face gets red. Pulls up legs against abdomen as if abdomen hurts. Has two soft, yellow bowel movements daily. Mother walks with infant to quiet him but she is exhausted; states she is "at end of her rope with crying." Father followed neighbor's suggestion to give infant whiskey, but this didn't help.

Nursing Diagnosis: Impaired skin integrity related to inadequate diaper area care

Defining Characteristic: Child has red macular rash on buttocks.

Goal: Child's diaper rash will be reduced in intensity by 1 week.

Outcome Criteria: Child's diaper area skin is clear of erythema or lesions.

Nursing Orders	Rationale
1. Suggest frequent diaper changes (immediately after each voiding or bowel movement), washing skin, and applying Desitin ointment at diaper changes.	1. Reduces amount of contact of ammonia with skin.
2. "Brainstorm" with mother to identify another way to save money rather than on diapers.	2. Acknowledges family's need to economize while emphasizing that frequent diaper changes are essential to child's health.
3. Discuss with mother the importance of knowing the routines at a day-care center such as how often diapers are changed.	3. Helps mother assess whether day-care center is providing adequate child care.

Nursing Diagnosis: Ineffective family coping, compromised, related to inability to cope with constant crying

Defining Characteristic: Parent states she is at the "end of her rope."

Goal: Parent will demonstrate increased coping behavior by 1 week.

Outcome Criteria: Parent states she feels more in control of situation; states that she and her husband have worked out a plan to relieve stress over baby crying.

(continued)

Nursing Orders

1. Educate mother on common characteristics of colic: duration, timing and intensity of crying, bottle feeding as possible factor, yet presence of normal bowel movements, normal weight gain.
2. Reassure mother that she and her husband are not responsible for their child's discomfort.

3. Caution parents that crying in infants produces great frustration in adults; parents must plan constructive ways to deal with the problem.

4. Help plan parental respite (time away during period the infant is likely to cry most).
5. Caution against actions such as shaking infant. Explain why offering whiskey was not the best approach.
6. Assure mother that she can call the health care facility for suggestions if she or her husband need further help. Explain that colic generally resolves by 3 months, so is a time-limited problem.

Rationale

1. Better understanding of the problem can aid coping.

2. Parents may feel guilty if they can't soothe their baby. Reassurance that the colic is not their fault will help the parents approach the problem more objectively.
3. Acknowledging their frustration will let the mother know these feelings are normal but not necessarily healthy. A plan of action may help them regain some feeling of control over the situation.
4. Time away can help relieve tension.

5. Shaking can be harmful to cerebral vessels or vertebrae of neck. Alcohol, too, can be harmful to infants, and does not relieve the symptoms.
6. Support from health care professionals can aid coping. Knowing that colic generally resolves in time will provide some relief while it is still going on.

Nursing Diagnosis: Health-seeking behaviors related to appropriate actions to take for colic

Defining Characteristic: Mother asked for help to relieve child's symptoms of abdominal pain.

Goal: Mother will voice she feels more confident in caring for child by 1 week's time.

Outcome Criteria: Mother states that child appears playful after feeding; sleeps at least some time between 6 P.M. and 1 A.M. feeding.

Nursing Orders

1. Support parents in attempts to allow infant to cry for short time (5 to 15 min) before comforting.
2. Suggest parents burp child well after feeding; suggest trying a bottle with a disposable bag.
3. Suggest a quiet, soothing atmosphere for feeding away from television.
4. Suggest parents place infant in infant seat for ½ h after feeding, then lay infant on stomach with a folded towel under the abdomen. Other suggestions: rock or jiggle crib; rub infant's back or abdomen; take for drive in car; insert rectal thermometer the length of the bulb.
5. Have parents offer glucose water or a pacifier.

Rationale

1. Infant can be encouraged to comfort self.

2. These measures may help prevent the development of intestinal gas.
3. A quiet time and place may prevent child from being stimulated to drink too rapidly
4. These measures may help relieve intestinal gas.

5. These measures may increase peristalsis and move intestinal gas through intestines to relieve pain.

interpret this as vomiting or think the infant is developing an infection. Ask them to describe carefully what they mean by "spitting up." How long has the baby been doing it? How frequently? What is the appearance of the spit-up milk?

Almost all milk that is spit up smells at least faintly sour, but it should not contain blood or bile. What is the intensity of the spitting? Does the baby spit out forcefully, or are the parents just describing a mouthful of milk rolling down the chin? What have they tried as a remedy? What has been effective?

The baby who spits up a mouthful of milk (rolling down the chin) two or three times a day (or sometimes after every meal) is experiencing normal, early-infancy spitting up. If the parents describe associated symptoms such as diarrhea, abdominal cramps, fever, cough, cold, or loss of activity, the child should be examined by a physician, as these are symptoms of illness. If the infant is spitting up so forcefully that the milk is projected 3 or 4 feet away, it may be beginning pyloric stenosis (an abnormally tight valve between the stomach and duodenum) that requires surgical intervention. If the spitting up is a large amount with each feeding, they may be describing chalasia (gastroesophageal reflux) in which a lax cardiac sphincter and esophagus allow regurgitation of gastric contents into the esophagus. This also requires medical attention (see Chapter 45).

Burping the baby thoroughly following a feeding often helps limit spitting up. Parents may try sitting the infant in an infant chair for half an hour after feeding. Changing formulas generally is of little value or effectiveness. Reassure parents that spitting up decreases in amount as the baby becomes better at coordinating swallowing and digestive processes (the cardiac sphincter matures). In the meantime, a bib can protect the baby's clothing and the parent. After a few months, the child will naturally stay in an upright position longer and gravity will help to correct the problem.

Diaper Dermatitis

Some infants have such sensitive skin that diaper dermatitis (diaper rash) is a problem from the first few days of life (Lane et al., 1990). It occurs for a number of reasons.

When parents do not change their children's diapers frequently, feces is left in contact with skin and a dermatitis may result in the perianal area. More frequent changing of diapers and protecting the skin from fecal material with an ointment, such as petroleum jelly or A & D ointment, are the time-proven solutions to this problem.

Urine that is left in diapers too long breaks down into ammonia, a chemical that is extremely irritating to infant skin. Ammonia dermatitis is generally a problem in the second half of the first year of life when the infant is producing a larger quantity of urine than before, but, for some infants, it is a problem from the first week.

Frequent diaper changing, applying petroleum jelly or A & D or Desitin ointment, and exposing the diaper area to air may relieve the problem. Some infants may have to sleep without diapers at night to control the problem.

Whenever the entire diaper area is erythematous and irritated so that the outline of the diaper on the skin can be identified, one must suspect an allergy to the material in the diaper or to laundry products if a commercially washed or home washed diaper is being used. Changing the brand or type of diaper or washing solution usually alleviates the problem.

If a diaper area is covered with lesions that are bright red and oozing, a fungus (monilial or candidiasis) infection is suggested. This is discussed in Chapter 43.

Miliaria

Miliaria, or prickly heat rash, occurs most often in warm weather or when babies are overdressed or sleep in overheated rooms. The symptoms are clusters of pinpoint, reddened papules with occasional vesicles and pustules surrounded by erythema. They usually appear on the neck first and may spread upward to around the ear and onto the face or down onto the trunk.

Bathing the infant twice a day during hot weather, particularly if a small amount of baking soda is added to the bathwater, may improve the rash. Eliminating sweating by reducing the amount of clothing on the infant or lowering the room temperature should bring about almost immediate improvement and prevent further eruption.

Baby-Bottle Syndrome

Putting an infant to bed with a bottle can result in aspiration or decay of all the upper teeth and the lower posterior teeth (Schwartz et al., 1993) (Figure 29-19). Decay occurs because while the infant sleeps, liquid from the propped bottle continuously soaks the upper front teeth and lower back teeth (the lower front teeth are protected by the tongue). The problem, called **baby-bottle**

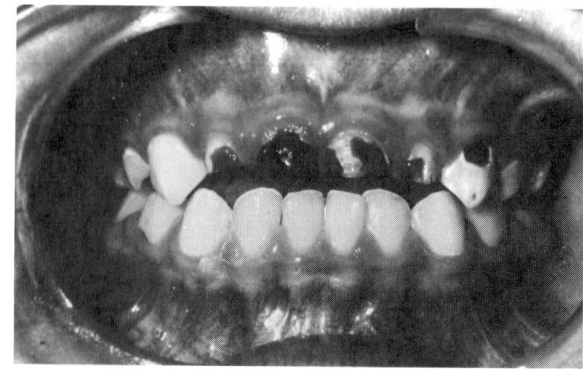

FIGURE 29-19
Baby-bottle syndrome. Notice the extensive decay in the upper teeth. (Nowak, A. J. [1985]. Infant dental health. Public Health Currents, *25, 1. Copyright 1985 Ross Laboratories, with permission.)*

syndrome, is most serious when the bottle is filled with sugar water, formula, milk, or fruit juice, as the carbohydrate in these solutions is fermented to organic acids that demineralize the tooth enamel until it decays.

To prevent this problem, parents should be advised never to put their baby to bed with a bottle. If parents insist that the bottle is necessary, encourage them to fill it with water and use a nipple with a smaller hole to prevent the baby from receiving a large amount of fluid. If the baby refuses to drink anything but milk, the parents might dilute the milk with water more and more each night until the bottle is down to water only.

Unique Concerns of the Family With a Disabled or Chronically Ill Infant

A child who is born with an illness or disability is usually hospitalized immediately after birth for diagnosis and treatment. This can cause bonding to be delayed because the child is separated from the parents during this time. If such an infant is hospitalized, encourage parents to visit regularly to help in forming a strong parent-child attachment. If parents cannot visit, make certain that they know they can telephone the hospital to inquire about their child's well-being. In addition, encourage nurses to supply instant photographs of the infant for parents to take home with them.

Many of the developmental events of the infant year (social smile, laughing out loud, reaching for an object, uttering the first word, sitting, talking) are activities that encourage parent-child interaction as they make an infant fun to be with and naturally make a parent want to spend a great deal of time with the child. The child who is mentally disabled may not reach these milestones. A child with physical limitations may be unable to meet them as well if he or she is unable to reach up and pat a mother's face, or hold out arms to be picked up by a father. If the child cannot interact with the parents in these ways, the parents may find themselves equally unable to interact with the child. If an infant leaves the hospital with a cast or other equipment such as a ventilator for care, parents may be so concerned with these items that they are unable to initiate the normal everyday singing and playing activities with their child.

To encourage parents' relationship with a child, point out the positive things the infant can do. Perhaps the child's facial expression says, "Pick me up," even though he doesn't reach up with his hands; perhaps his eyes follow his mother's actions even though he can't yet call to her.

Helping parents to interact more fully with their infants helps to build a sense of trust in the infant. Without a sense of trust, children have difficulty expressing themselves to others; they do not believe that they are lovable or that people would want to interact with them. Physically disabled individuals—no matter what their ages—need people around them to give them help at whatever point they are unable to meet their own needs. It is unfortunate when a physically disabled child is unable to reach out for help because of not having developed the requisite sense of trust.

It is important to remember also that disabled or chronically ill infants experience the same health and growth problems as other infants. Parents may be reluctant to bring up these concerns, however, as they feel such problems pale in comparison to the child's primary disease or disability. When taking the health histories of children with chronic or longstanding medical problems, be sure to ask the parents about secondary concerns. "What about everyday things? Any problems there?" Treat these concerns seriously, so that parents can feel confident about bringing them to your attention. Also be sure to mention that they are part of normal infant development so that parents can begin to view their child apart from his or her illness or disability.

Teething pain, discomfort from diaper rash, and colic are all potential problems in infancy and may occur even more frequently in babies with other illnesses. For instance, parents may not want to "bother" an ill infant with physical care as often as they would a well child (e.g., before homes were well-heated, bathing an ill infant could cause extensive chilling, and many people still believe that bathing is not appropriate for ill children). Colic may occur because parents are reluctant to tire ill infants by burping them after a feeding. Parents' attention may be so focused on the primary health problem rather than on everyday concerns, such as diaper care, that diaper dermatitis occurs. The bowel movements of physically disabled or chronically ill children may be looser than normal because of a liquid diet or medicine. Their urine may be more concentrated because of reduced intake. These conditions may lead to diaper rashes. Offering anticipatory guidance to parents can go a long way towards helping parents meet the needs of infants with unique needs.

Key Points

- The infant period is from 1 month to 12 months. Children double their weight at 4 to 6 months and triple it at 1 year.
- Infants develop their first tooth at about 6 months; by 12 months they have 6 to 8 teeth.
- Important gross motor milestones during the infant year are lifting chest off bed at 2 months; sitting at 6 to 8 months; creeping at 9 months; "cruising" at 10 to 11 months; and walking at 12 months.
- Important fine motor accomplishments are ability to pass on object from one hand to the other (7 months) and a pincer grasp (10 months).
- Important milestones of language development during the first year are differentiating a cry (2 months); making simple vowel sounds (5 to 6 months); and

saying two words besides ma-ma and da-da (12 months). The more infants are spoken to, the easier language is to acquire.

- Providing infants with proper toys for play helps development. All infant toys need to be checked to be sure that they are not small enough to be aspirated.
- Important milestones of vision development are ability to follow a moving object past the midline (3 months); and ability to focus securely without eyes crossing (6 months).
- The developmental task of the infant year according to Erikson is the development of a sense of trust versus mistrust.
- Infants must be protected from aspiration of small objects and falls. Be aware that a skill an infant cannot accomplish one day, such as crawling, may be accomplished the next.
- Remember that parent-infant attachment is critical to mental health. Urge parents to continue to give as much care as possible to sick infants to maintain this important relationship.
- Common concerns related to infant development are teething, thumb sucking, use of pacifiers, sleep problems, constipation, colic, and diaper dermatitis. Baby-bottle syndrome is a syndrome of decayed teeth from infants sucking on a bottle of formula while they sleep. Nurses can help prevent this by advising against this practice.

Critical Thinking Exercises

1. Katie is a 3-month-old who will be hospitalized for several months in a hospital out of state because of severe burns. As Katie's nurse, what steps could you take to foster a sense of trust in her in light of this extensive parental separation?
2. Marty is a 10-month-old whose mother tells you is "into everything." At a well child assessment, formulate specific questions you would want to ask in order to feel confident that Marty's house is safe for him.
3. Pattie is a 1-month-old who is going to be followed in your health maintenance setting. Describe the immunization schedule you would discuss with her father as recommended for the first year.

References

Adair, R., et al. (1992). Reduced night waking in infancy: A primary care intervention. *Pediatrics 89,* 585.

American Academy of Pediatrics Committee on Accident and Poison Prevention (1987). *Injury control for children and youth.* Elk Grove, IL: Author.

American Medical Association (1991). Use of infant walkers. *American Journal of Diseases of Children, 145,* 933.

Curry, D. M., & Duby, J. C. (1994). Developmental surveillance by pediatric nurses. *Pediatric Nursing, 20,* 40.

Department of Health and Human Services. (1991). *Healthy people 2000.* Washington, DC: Public Health Service.

Erikson, E. (1986). *Childhood and society* (3rd ed.). New York: W. W. Norton.

Geissler, E. M. (1994). *Pocket guide to cultural assessment.* St. Louis: C. V. Mosby.

Halida, D. L. (1993). Latex baloons: They can take your breath away. *Pediatric Nursing, 19,* 39.

Hardsell, M. B. (1990). New products: Sleeptight infant soother and colic. *Journal of Pediatric Nursing, 5,* 59.

Health alert: Car seat and air bag warning. (1992). *American Academy News, 8,* 26.

Lane, A. T., et al. (1990). Evaluations of diapers containing absorbent gelling material with conventional disposable diapers in newborn infants. *American Journal of Diseases of Children, 144,* 315.

Nik-Hussein, N. N. (1990). Natal and neonatal teeth. *Journal of Pedodontics, 14,* 110.

Piaget, J. (1966). *The origins of intelligence in children.* New York: International Universities Press.

Pinyerd, B. J. (1992a). Infant colic and maternal mental health: Nursing research and practice concerns. *Issues in Comprehensive Pediatric Nursing, 15,* 155.

Pinyerd, B. J. (1992b). Strategies for consoling the infant with colic: Fact or fiction? *Journal of Pediatric Nursing, 7,* 403.

Schwartz, S. S., et al. (1993). A child's sleeping habit as a cause of nursing caries. *Journal of Dentistry for Children, 60,* 22.

Scott, G., & Richards, M. P. (1990). Nightwaking in 1-year-old children in England. *Child Care, Health and Development, 16,* 283.

Staheli, L. T. (1993). *Fundamentals of pediatric orthopedics.* New York: Raven Press.

Suggested Readings

Ahmann, E. (1994). Family-centered care: the time has come. *Pediatric Nursing, 20,* 59.

Balsmeyer, B. (1990). Sleep disturbances of the infant and toddler. *Pediatric Nursing, 16,* 447.

Davis, P. B., & May, J. E. (1991). Involving fathers in early intervention and family support programs: Issues and strategies. *Children's Health Care, 20,* 87.

Feldman, K. W., et al. (1993). When is childhood drowning neglect? *Child Abuse & Neglect, 17,* 329.

Gunn, W. J., et al. (1992). Injuries and poisonings in out-of-home child care and home care. *American Journal of Diseases of Children, 145,* 779.

Kenner, C., et al. (1993). Transition from hospital to home for mothers and babies. *Neonatal Network, 12,* 73.

Marino, B. L. (1991). Studying infant and toddler play. *Journal of Pediatric Nursing, 6,* 16.

Wallach, H. R., et al. (1992). College women's expectations about pregnancy, childbirth and infant care: A prospective study. *Birth, 19,* 202.

Woodham, C. (1990). The mystery behind colic. *Community Outlook,* p. 19.

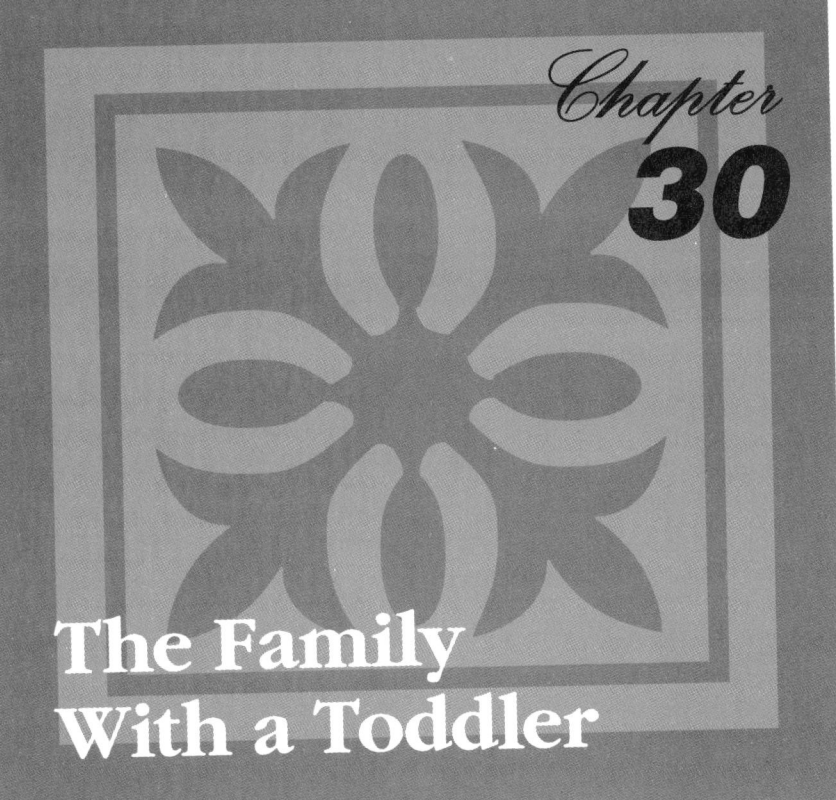

Chapter 30

The Family With a Toddler

Key Terms

- assimilation
- autonomy
- deferred imitation
- discipline
- lordosis
- parallel play
- preoperational thought
- punishment
- tertiary circular reaction stage

Objectives

After mastering the contents of this chapter, you should be able to:

1. Describe normal growth and development of the toddler period and common parental concerns.

2. Assess a toddler for normal growth and development milestones.

3. Formulate nursing diagnoses related to toddler growth and development or parental concerns regarding development.

4. Plan nursing care to meet the toddler's growth and development needs such as anticipatory guidance to prevent problems such as sleep disturbances, temper tantrums, or inappropriate toilet training practices.

5. Implement nursing care to promote normal growth and development of the toddler such as discussing toddler developmental milestones with parents.

6. Evaluate goal outcomes established for care to be certain nursing goals associated with growth and development have been achieved.

7. Identify National Health Goals related to the toddler age group that nurses can be instrumental in helping the nation to achieve.

8. Identify areas related to care of the toddler that could benefit from additional nursing research.

9. Use critical thinking to analyze methods of care for the toddler to be certain care is family centered.

10. Synthesize knowledge of toddler growth and development with nursing process to achieve quality maternal and child health nursing care.

Adele Pillitteri: MATERNAL AND CHILD HEALTH NURSING, 2nd Edition. © 1995 Adele Pillitteri.

The toddler period, usually considered the age from 1 to 3 years, is a period in which enormous changes take place in the child and, consequently, in the family as well. During the toddler period, the child accomplishes a wide array of developmental tasks. He or she changes from a largely immobile and preverbal infant, dependent on caregivers for providing for most needs, to a walking, talking child with a growing sense of autonomy and independence. Parents must also grow during this period. Their task is to support their child's growing independence with patience and sensitivity and to learn methods for handling the child's frustrations that arise from the quest for autonomy. This chapter provides an overview of normal growth and development of the child and family through the toddler period, covering, in particular, those areas to assess at routine health maintenance visits. Because healthy children and families are constantly being challenged by the very process of normal development, parents often have questions about how to guide their children in different situations. This chapter, then, also provides guidelines useful in helping parents cope with special needs and concerns relevant to this age. National Health Goals related to the toddler age group are shown in the Focus on National Health Goals box.

FOCUS ON
National Health Goals

A number of National Health Goals relate specifically to safety during the toddler years. These are:

- Reduce deaths caused by motor vehicle crashes to less than 5.5/100,000 in children under 14 years of age from a baseline of 6.2/100,000.

- Reduce nonfatal poisoning to no more than 520/100,000 emergency department treatments among children aged 4 and younger from a baseline of 650/100,000 (DHHS, 1991).

Nurses can be instrumental in helping the nation to achieve these goals by continuing to educate parents about the importance of using car seats and childproofing their homes against poisoning.

Areas that could benefit from additional nursing research are exploring methods parents use to keep their toddlers entertained while in automobiles, and identifying specific home situations in which poisoning is apt to occur.

NURSING PROCESS OVERVIEW
for Healthy Development of the Toddler

ASSESSMENT

Whether a child is seen for a routine check-up or has come to a health care center because of a specific health concern, assessment begins with taking a careful health history. Asking parents about the toddler's ability to carry out activities of daily living not only offers assessment information on the child's developmental progress but important clues about the child-parent relationship as well.

Careful observation is another crucial element of nursing assessment of the toddler. This is because parents may become so emotionally involved in a health concern that they may not describe it with complete objectivity. On the other hand, parents see their children daily and so are the best source of information and opinion on when a child seems to be acting "out-of-sorts" or different (a typical sign that the child may not be feeling well). Table 30-1 provides some guidelines to help parents evaluate illness at this age.

NURSING DIAGNOSIS

Nursing diagnoses related to normal growth and development of toddlers usually focus on the parents' eager-

---

Table 30-1. *Parental Difficulties in Evaluating Illness in Toddlers*

Problem	Guidelines for Parents
Evaluating seriousness of illness	Toddlers typically answer "No" to almost all questions. A question such as "Does your arm hurt?" may bring a "No" response even if the arm does hurt. Observing children for indications of illness (holding an arm stiffly, rubbing abdomen, crying when they void) is more helpful. Many toddlers do not know the words to describe a feeling of nausea or a sore throat. They reveal these symptoms by not eating. If the child is normally a light eater, as many are, it is difficult for a parent to appreciate these signs.
Differentiating tiredness from illness	Toddlers tend to whine or sleep when they are either tired or ill. Reviewing the child's day and activity often helps to evaluate what is happening. If the child has had no activity all day so is probably not tired, crying and whining or temper tantrums suggest illness.
Evaluating nutritional intake	Toddlers are normally fussy eaters compared to infants. Evaluating children as to whether they are active and growing is better than assessing any one day's food intake (see Chapter 34)
Age-specific diseases to be aware of	The toddler period is an important age to assess speech development; children should be further evaluated if they cannot use simple sentences composed of a noun and verb ("me go") by 2 years of age.
	As children begin to walk they should be observed for abnormal gait. Osteomyelitis (bone infection) occurs with a high frequency in toddlers; symptoms of limping, swollen joints, or arm or leg pain should be regarded as serious until ruled otherwise.
	Toddlers contract 10–12 mild upper respiratory infections a year. Otitis media (middle ear infection) may occur as a complication of these. The child with an upper respiratory infection who suddenly develops a high fever and pulls or manipulates ears should be seen by a physician.
	Children who attend day care programs have a high incidence of hepatitis A, *Giardia* and *Shigella* infections. Teach parents to report jaundice or diarrhea promptly to a health care provider to detect these infections.

ness to learn more about the parameters of normal growth and development or issues of safety or care. Examples are:

- Health-seeking behaviors related to normal toddler development
- Knowledge deficit related to method of toilet training
- High risk for injury related to impulsiveness of toddler
- Altered family process related to need for close supervision of 2-year-old
- Family coping: potential for growth related to parents' ability to adjust to new needs of child
- Potential for enhanced parenting related to increased awareness for poison prevention
- Sleep pattern disturbance related to lack of bedtime routine

PLANNING AND IMPLEMENTATION

The planning necessary to help parents resolve a concern during the toddler period involves not only teaching them how to approach a current problem but also how they might learn adequate methods for resolving it that can be applied to similar situations in the future. If parents do not learn methods that can be applied throughout the child's growing years, they may win battles but lose wars. For instance, parents may have found that promising their child a treat when she is in the middle of a temper tantrum will stop the tantrum, but it will certainly not prevent other tantrums from occurring in the future (and in fact, may encourage them). Health visits are opportunities to provide guidance on healthy coping techniques for parents. In addition, a nurse's own communication skills with toddlers serve as a model for healthy communication behavior.

EVALUATION

Evaluation of care goals must be frequent during the toddler period as children learn so many new skills during this time that their abilities and associated parental concerns can change from day to day.

Examples of outcome criteria that might be established are:

- Parents state child maintains a consistent bedtime routine by 2 weeks.
- Parents state they have childproofed the home by putting a lock on household product's cupboard by next clinic visit.
- Grandmother states she has modified usual activities in order to conserve strength to care for toddler granddaughter by one week.

Nursing Assessment of Growth and Development of the Toddler

Physical Growth

While toddlers are making great strides developmentally, their physical growth actually begins to slow.

Weight, Height, and Head Circumference

Weight and height should be plotted on a standard growth chart at each health care visit (Appendix E) to determine if progress is normal for that individual child. A child gains only about 5 to 6 lb (2.5 kg) and 5 in (12 cm) a year during the toddler period. Subcutaneous tissue, or baby fat, begins to disappear toward the end of the third year as the child changes from a plump baby into a leaner, more muscular little girl or boy. The toddler's appetite decreases accordingly, yet adequate intake of all nutrients is essential to meeting the toddler's energy needs (see Chapter 34).

Head circumference equals chest circumference at 6 months to 1 year of age. At 2 years, chest circumference is greater than that of the head. Head circumference increases only about 2 cm during the second year compared to about 12 cm during the first year.

Body Contour

Toddlers tend to have a prominent abdomen—a pouchy belly—because, although they are walking, their abdominal muscles are not yet strong enough to support abdominal contents as well as they will later (Figure 30-1*A*). They also have a forward curve of the spine at the sacral area (**lordosis**). As they walk longer, this will correct itself naturally. The toddler walks with a wide stance, as a sailor does on a listing ship (Figure 30-1*B*). This stance seems to increase the lordotic curve, but it keeps the child on his or her feet.

Body Systems

Body systems continue to mature during this time: respirations slow slightly but continue to be mainly abdominal; the heart rate slows from 110 to 90 beats/min; blood pressure increases to about 99/64 mm Hg. In the nervous system, the brain develops to about 90% of its adult size. In the respiratory system, the lumens of vessels increase progressively so that the threat of lower respiratory infection is less. Stomach capacity increases to the point that the child can eat three meals a day. Stomach secretions become more acid; therefore, gastrointestinal infections also become less common. Urinary and anal sphincter control become possible with complete myelination of the spinal cord.

In the immune system, IgG and IgM antibody production becomes mature at 2 years of age. The passive

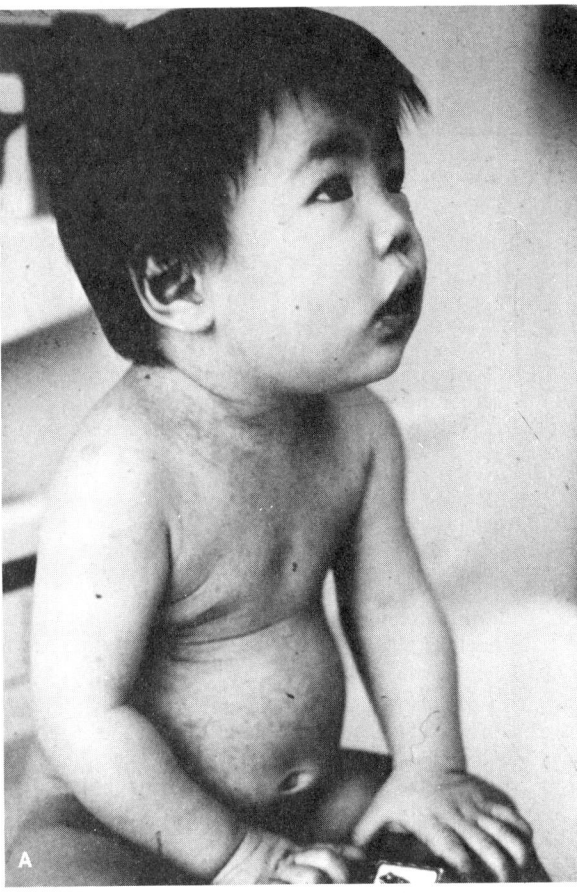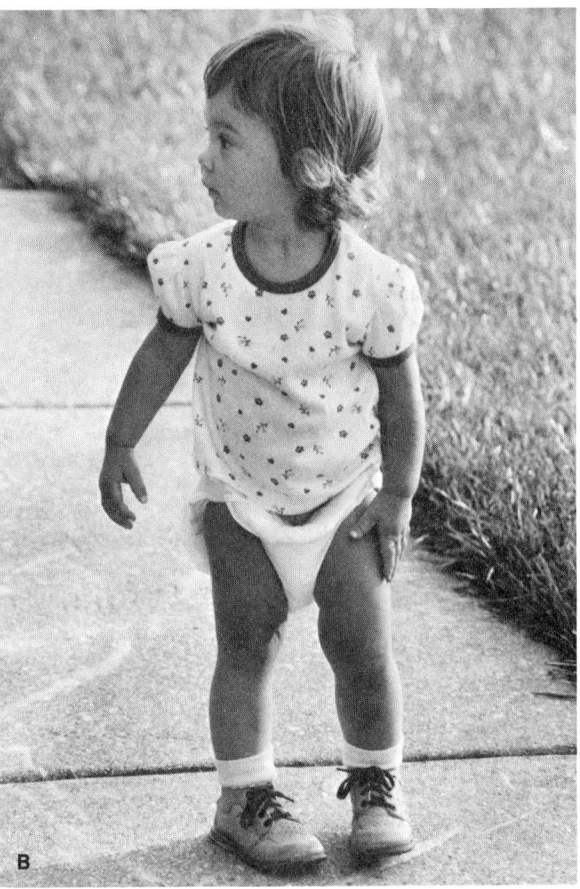

FIGURE 30-1
*Physical characteristics of toddlers. (**A**) Toddlers typically have a prominent abdomen. (Courtesy of the Centers for Disease Control, Atlanta, GA.) (**B**) Toddlers typically walk with an unsteady gait for better stability. (Courtesy of Brian Smistek.)*

immunity effects from intrauterine life are no longer operative.

Teeth

Eight new teeth (the canines and the first molars) erupt during the second year. All 20 deciduous teeth are generally present by 2½ to 3 years of age.

Developmental Milestones

The developmental milestones of the toddler years are less numerous but no less dramatic than those of the infant year, as this is a period of slow and steady, not sudden, growth. Toddler development is influenced to some extent by the amount of social contact and the number of opportunities the child has to explore and experience new degrees of independence. It is strongly influenced by individual readiness; when the child is developmentally ready for a new skill, he or she will acquire it. Table 30-2 highlights growth and development milestones of gross and fine motor, language, and play development of the toddler years.

Language Development

Toddlerhood is a critical time for language development (Prizant et al., 1993). To best master language, the child needs to practice talking. A child who is 2 years old and does not talk in 2-word noun-verb simple sentences should be examined to assess the cause. This is beyond a point of normal development.

A word that is used frequently by toddlers and that is a manifestation of developing autonomy is *no*. Toddlers may say no to mean they are refusing a task, or they do not understand it, or they may only be practicing a sound that they have noticed has potent effects on those around them.

To learn other words, children need exposure to conversation and they should be read to often. Language develops most quickly if the child grasps the use of language and if parents respect what the child has to say. Always answering the child's questions is a good way to do this. Answers for toddlers should be simple and brief so that the child can focus his or her short attention span on them (see Table 30-2).

Parents can do a great deal to encourage language

Table 30-2. *Milestones of Toddler Growth and Development*

Age (months)	Fine Motor	Gross Motor	Language	Play
15	Puts small pellets into small bottles. Scribbles voluntarily with a pencil or crayon. Holds a spoon well but may still turn it upside down on the way to mouth	Walks alone well; can seat self in chair; can creep upstairs.	4–6 words	Can stack 2 blocks; enjoys being read to; drops toys for adult to recover (exploring sense of permanence)
18	No longer rotates a spoon to bring it to mouth	Can run and jump in place. Can walk up and down stairs holding onto a person's hand or railing. Typically places both feet on one step before advancing.	7–20 words, uses jargoning; names 1 body part	Imitates household chores, dusting, etc.; begins parallel play (playing beside not with another child)
24	Can open doors by turning doorknobs, unscrew lids	Walks up stairs alone still using both feet on same step at same time.	50 words, 2-word sentences (noun-pronoun and verb), such as "Daddy go," "me come"	Parallel play evident
30	Makes simple lines or strokes for crosses with a pencil	Can jump down from chairs.	Verbal language increasing steadily. Knows full name; can name 1 color and holds up fingers to show age	Spends time playing house, imitating parents' actions

development by being certain to name objects as they play with the child (ball, block, music box, doll) or when they give him or her something ("Here is your drink of water," "Let's put on these pajamas," and so on). This helps the child grasp the concept that words are not meaningless sounds; they apply to people and objects, and they have uses.

Some children may not develop language because they are not called on to use it. When they point at an object, someone hands it to them; when they climb into their highchair, someone places a meal in front of them. To assess whether or not parents are encouraging language development, ask them what the child does when he or she wants something. Do they give the child opportunities to ask for things before they supply them? Children should not be made to name an object before they can have it (because their vocabulary is so limited, the objects they could have would be restricted to 10 or fewer), but parents can reinforce language by rewording a question, for example, "You want the ball?" Reading aloud strengthens vocabulary in the same way. Reading the exact words in a book is not as important to toddlers as pointing to the pictures that accompany them, however. For example, Dick threw the ball ("See Dick throwing the ball?") or the dog ran away with the ball ("Look, that dog took the ball!").

The child who is very active may use fewer words than the child who is less active. The first child is too

busy doing to describe what he or she is doing; he or she may be too busy obtaining objects to ask for many things. Such a child probably has a large unexpressed vocabulary; that is, the child understands more words (comprehensive vocabulary) than he or she can express (expressive vocabulary).

Because children learn language from imitating what they hear, they will speak like those around them. If they are spoken to in baby talk, their enunciation of words may be poor; if they hear examples of bad grammar, they will not use good grammar. Remind parents that pronouns are difficult for children to use correctly; many children are 3½ or 4 years of age before they can separate the different uses of *I, me, him,* and *her.*

Emotional Development

Developmental Task: Autonomy Versus Shame or Doubt

According to Erikson (1986), the developmental task of the toddler period is to learn a sense of **autonomy** or independence versus shame or doubt. Children who have learned to trust themselves and others during the infant year are better prepared to do this than those who cannot trust themselves or others.

To develop a sense of autonomy is to develop a sense of independence. Although toddlers enjoy the feeling of control that comes with being independent, they also feel some shame for wanting control and some doubt as to whether they can do all the things they want to try. Children who are constantly told not to try things because they will hurt themselves may be left with a stronger sense of doubt than confidence at the end of the toddler period. Children who are made to feel that it is wrong to be independent may leave the toddler period with a stronger sense of shame than autonomy. A healthy level of autonomy is achieved when parents are able to encourage independence while still maintaining consistently sound rules for safety.

Infants appear to have difficulty differentiating between their bodies and those of others; they think of their bodies as extensions of their parents or their primary caregivers. When infants approach toddlerhood, they begin to make the differentiation. As they recognize that they are separate individuals, they realize they do not always have to do what others want them to do. From this realization comes the reputation that toddlers have for being negativistic, obstinate, and difficult to manage.

This reputation is little deserved, however, and exists largely because parents misinterpret a child's cues. For example, a child's refusal to accept help putting on his shoes is seen by a parent as disobedience, whereas the child sees this as insisting on performing an act he can and does like to do himself. It is a positive expression of autonomy.

Socialization

Once he or she is walking well, a toddler becomes resistant to sitting in laps and being cuddled. This is not lack of a desire for socialization but a function of being independent. The 15-month-old is still very anxious to interact with people if they will follow him or her to where he or she wants to go.

By 18 months, toddlers imitate the things they see a parent doing, such as "study" or "sweep" so seeks out parents to observe and initiate interactions. By 2 or more years, children become aware of gender differences and may point to other children and identify them as "boy" or "girl."

Play Behavior

All during the toddler period, children play beside the children next to them, not with them. This side-by-side play (often called **parallel play**) is not unfriendly but a normal developmental sequence that occurs during the toddler period (Figure 30-2). Caution parents that if two toddlers are going to play side by side, they must provide duplicate toys or an argument over one toy will occur.

The toys toddlers enjoy most are those that they can play with by themselves and that require action. Trucks they can make go, squeaky frogs they can squeeze, waddling ducks they can pull, horses they can ride, pegs

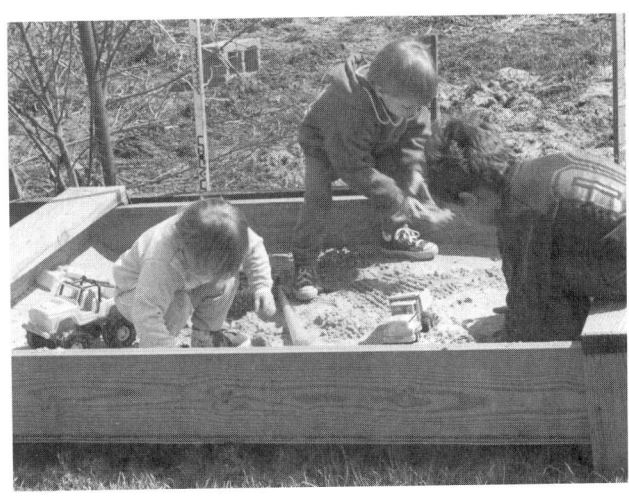

FIGURE 30-2
Toddlers play beside but not with other children (parallel play).

they can pound, blocks they can stack, and a toy telephone they can talk on are all favorites. These are all toys that children can control, giving them a sense of power in manipulation, an expression of autonomy (Figure 30-3).

Some parents are not prepared for this change of play habits in their child. They wonder why a child who used to play quietly in her crib is now more interested in banging trucks together. However, they need only watch a toddler tug a pull-toy, stop to see if it is following, walk again, and stop and look to see if it is still following to understand the feeling of accomplishment involved in manipulating toys.

A 15-month-old is still in a put-in, take-out stage, so he or she continues to enjoy stacks of boxes or balls that fit inside each other. He or she enjoys throwing toys out of a playpen or from a highchair tray as long as someone will pick them up and return them again.

The 18-month-old enjoys pull toys. Toys should be strong enough to take a great deal of abuse, as there are many things in the world toddlers do not recognize or know about. This causes them to use toys in other ways than those for which they were designed. (Whereas the infant sat and softly stroked a stuffed cat, the toddler picks it up by the tail and swings it, pounds it, or pulls at it.) Parents should not correct a child about the way a toddler is using a toy as long as it appears to give satisfaction. If a toddler finds a toy frustrating because he or she is holding or using it incorrectly, showing the child the right way will ease frustration.

By 2, toddlers begin to spend time imitating adult actions in their play, for example, wrapping a doll and putting it to bed; "setting the table"; or "driving the car." They use fewer toys than before; imitating actions they see parents doing has replaced them. Both boys and girls begin to like rough-housing and spend at least part of every day in this very active, stimulating type of play.

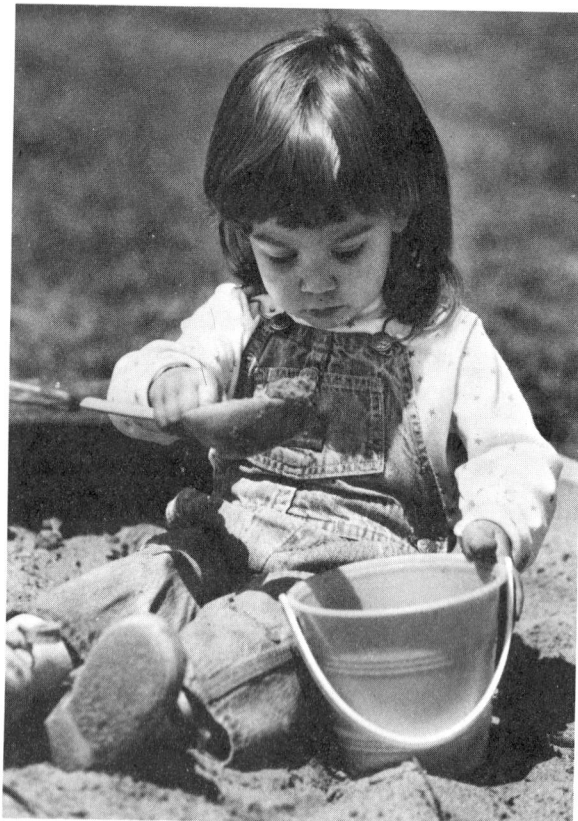

FIGURE 30-3
Toddlers enjoy toys that they can manipulate. (Courtesy of Brian Smistek.)

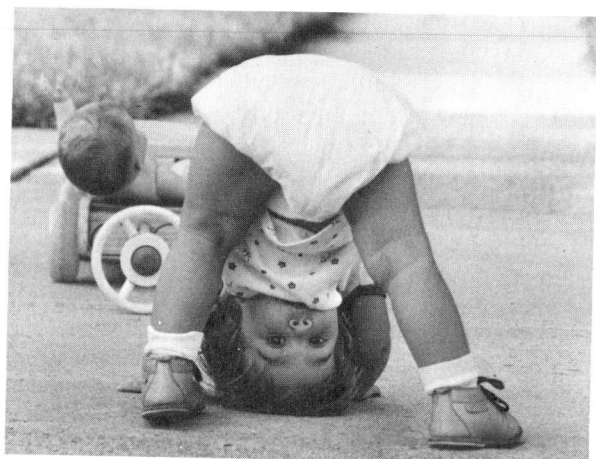

FIGURE 30-4
Toddlers usually enjoy rough and tumble play. (Courtesy of Brian Smistek.)

This type of play (Figure 30-4) is generally best scheduled for the outdoors where vases or other prized possessions cannot be broken. Because of this rough activity, most toddlers have at least one black-and-blue mark all the time from tripping over their feet while trying to run too fast or jumping or bumping into a chair or doorway. The child who feels a need for active play is unable to sit down and eat, fall asleep, or play quiet games. It is good to explore with the parents the amount of outside or roughtime activity the child has each day. A trip in a stroller is not the same kind of activity as walking and running. Stroller walks are good because they provide fresh air and sunshine, but the child must also have time to meet the need to engage in strenuous activity.

Cognitive Development

The toddler enters the fifth and sixth stages of sensorimotor thought (Table 30-3). Piaget referred to stage 5 as a **tertiary circular reaction stage**, describing the toddler in this stage as "a little scientist" because of the child's interest in trying to discover new ways to handle objects or new results different actions can achieve (Wadsworth, 1989). For instance, by trial and error, a toddler discovers that cats do not like baths and that cookies on the center of a table can be reached by crawling up onto the table or pulling on the table cloth. Obviously, this type of investigating can lead to errors or in-

jury. The toddler has also advanced beyond what he or she could do as an infant in terms of dropping objects and watching where they roll. As an infant, to retrieve an article that rolled under a chair, he or she would crawl under the chair along the same path the object took. Many children at 15 months are able to follow a different path (walk in back of the chair) to obtain the object. This results from increased awareness that the object is permanent and, even if it follows a different direction from the one the child must take, it will be there to retrieve.

Along this same line, the child is able to receive comfort from a parent's voice apart from his or her presence. This means that parents can call reassurance from their bedroom at night rather than having to go into the child's room. By stage 6, toddlers advance to being able to try out various actions mentally rather than having actually to per-

Table 30-3. *Cognitive and Emotional Development of the Toddler*

Age in Months	Stage	Task
Cognitive		
12–18	Sensorimotor 5	Child experiments by trial and error methods
18–24	Sensorimotor 6	Can pretend and use deferred imitation; object permanence is complete
24	Preoperational thought	Able to use assimilation or change situation to fit thoughts
Emotional		
24–36	Autonomy vs. shame or guilt	Learn independence and the beginning of problem solving

(From Piaget, J. [1961]. *The growth of logical thinking from childhood to adolescence.* New York: Basic Books; and Erikson, E. H. [1986]. *Childhood and society.* New York: W. W. Norton; with permission.)

form them—the beginning of problem solving or symbolic thought. Children at this stage are also able to remember an action and imitate it later (**deferred imitation**); they are able to do such things as pretend to drive a car or put a baby to sleep. Object permanence is complete.

At the end of the toddler period, children enter a second major period of cognitive development: **preoperational thought**. During this period, children deal much more constructively with symbols than they did while still in the sensorimotor period of cognition. They begin to use a process termed **assimilation**. They are not able to change their thoughts to fit a situation; therefore, they have to change the situation (or how they perceive it) to fit their thoughts. This ability is what causes toddlers to use toys in the "wrong" way. For example, if they are given a toy hammer, instead of pounding with it, they might shake it to see if it rattles, using the toy in a way that

they had previously played (the child has changed the toy's use to fit his or her thoughts, or used assimilation).

Planning and Implementation for Health Promotion of the Toddler and Family

The toddler tends to develop many upper respiratory and ear infections but otherwise comes to a health care facility most often for health maintenance visits (recommended at 15, 18, and 24 months) and the immunizations important during this time. These visits allow a nurse to focus on health promotion and provide an opportunity for early detection of any growth and development delays. Table 30-4 provides a schedule listing specific areas to assess during these visits.

Table 30-4. *Health Maintenance Schedule, Toddler Period*

Area of Focus	Methods	Frequency
Developmental milestones	History, observation	Every visit
	Formal Denver Developmental Screening Test (DDST II)	18th month visit
Growth milestones	Height, weight plotted on standard growth chart; physical examination	Every visit
Nutrition	History, observation; height/weight information	Every visit
Parent–child relationship	History, observation	Every visit
Behavior problems	History, observation	Every visit
Vision and hearing defects	History, observation	Every visit
Dental health	History, physical examination; first dental appointment	Every visit; first at 24 months
Anemia	Hematocrit	24th month visit
Lead screening	Erythrocyte protoporphyrin	18th month visit
Tuberculosis	Tine test	Depending on prevalence in community
Urinalysis	Clean catch urine	24th month visit
Immunizations		
Measles, mumps and rubella	Check history and past records; inform caregiver about any risks and side effects	15th month visit
Haemophilus influenzae type B (HiB)	Administer immunization in accordance with health care agency policies	15th month visit
Diphtheria, tetanus, and pertussis; trivalent oral poliomyelitis		18th month visit
Anticipatory Guidance		
Toddler care	Active listening and health teaching	Every visit
Expected growth and developmental milestones before next visit		Every visit
Poison and accident prevention	Provide syrup of ipecac to be used in case of poisoning; counseling	Every visit
Problem Solving		
Any problems expressed by caregiver during course of the visit	Active listening and health teaching regarding temper tantrums, toilet training	Every visit

Routine health maintenance visits also provide an opportunity to help parents through the normal crises of the toddler period. By listening carefully to their concerns, asking questions that will help to separate the objective circumstances surrounding a problem from the parents' possible emotional biases, and providing some guidelines for how to handle specific problems, the nurse encourages parents to promote the healthy development of independence in their toddler (Curry & Duby, 1994).

Promoting Toddler Safety

Accidents are the major cause of death in children, and toddlers are at greatest risk for accidental ingestions (Dershewitz, 1993). Poisoning often occurs from ingestion of cleaning products. It can also occur with ingestion of prescription drugs (Morelli, 1993) and poisonous plants. Childproofing the house by putting all poisonous products and drugs out of reach should have been completed by the time the infant is crawling (see Chapter 29). Aspiration or ingestion of small objects such as watch batteries, pencil erasers, or crayons is also a major danger for children of this age. Other accidents common to toddlers include motor vehicle accidents, burns, and playground injuries. These occur because a toddler's motor ability jumps ahead of his or her judgment, and toddlers can walk surely and swiftly enough so that if they are left outside to play, they can very quickly travel a block away. Because they have no judgment concerning moving cars, they must never be left outside alone unsupervised. To prevent serious injury, parents must be alert and know what their toddler is doing at all times (Dye et al., 1990). They should be certain their toddler uses a toddler-size car seat for safety in automobiles (Figure 30-5) and wears a helmet as soon as he or she begins riding a tricycle (Wilson & Testani-Dufour, 1993).

The Focus on Family Teaching box summarizes accident prevention measures to encourage parents to take with their toddler. Some 15-month-olds who are able to climb over the side rails of their cribs like to explore the house early in the morning before anyone else is awake. Parents might have to move the child to a regular bed with a side rail as early as 15 months to keep him or her from falling when he or she climbs out of the crib. A safety gate on the door of the room may keep the toddler contained and safe.

As the child reaches 2 years of age and begins to imitate housework or repairing the car, parents must be sure that he or she does not use real cleaning compounds or sharp tools.

Lead Screening

All children between the ages of 1 and 5 who live in communities with houses built before 1950 should be tested periodically for the presence of too much lead in

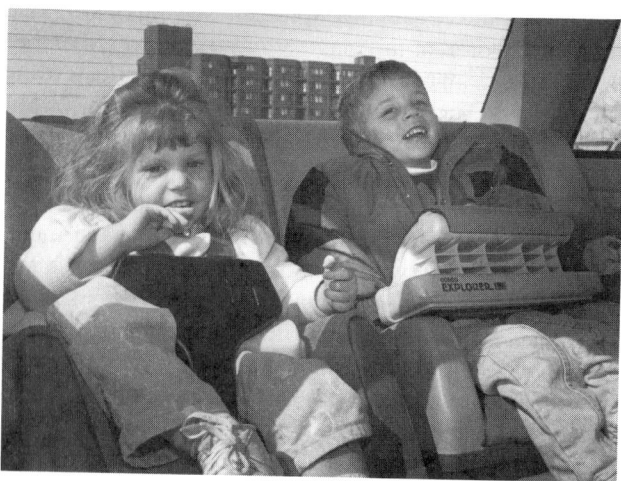

FIGURE 30-5
Toddlers and preschoolers should use a car seat for safety while riding in an automobile.

the body (lead poisoning). Lead poisoning is caused by eating, chewing, or sucking on objects such as windowsills, paint chips, or furniture that are covered by lead paint (Figure 30-6). Although federal law has prohibited the use of lead in the manufacture of interior and exterior paints since the mid-1970s, many older houses still contain lead paint. Soil around the exterior of the house can also contain high amounts of lead (thus possibly contaminating food grown there) as can dust or fumes created by home renovation. Other sources of lead poisoning include pottery made with lead glazes, colored print in newspapers, old water pipes, and lead-based gasoline. Children who live in high traffic areas are at high risk for contamination by lead fumes. Children may also be exposed when parents who work with lead products bring lead dust home on their clothes. A diet high in fat and low in calcium, magnesium, iron, zinc, and copper may increase the absorption of lead.

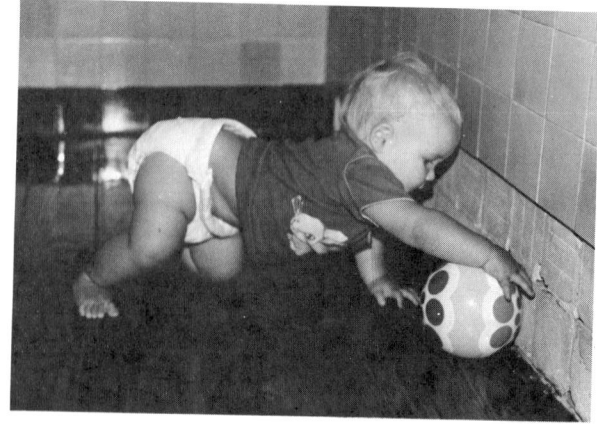

FIGURE 30-6
Chips of paint or plaster in a play area are a potential hazard because of the danger of lead poisoning.

FOCUS ON FAMILY TEACHING

Q. My child is 2 and "into everything." What actions should I take to help prevent poisoning or accidents?

A. The toddler period is high risk for harmful accidents because of the child's new independence. Actions you can take to prevent accidents are listed below.

Potential Accident	Prevention Measure
Motor vehicles	Maintain child in car seat; do not be distracted from safe driving by a child in a car.
	Do not allow child to play outside unsupervised. Do not allow child to operate electronic garage doors.
	Supervise toddler who is too young to be left alone on a tricycle. Teach safety with pedaling toys (look before crossing driveways; do not cross streets) but do not expect that toddler will obey these rules at all times (in other words, stay close by).
Falls	Keep house windows closed or keep secure screens in place.
	Place gates at top and bottom of stairs. Supervise at playgrounds.
	Do not allow child to walk with sharp object in hand or mouth.
	Raise crib rails and check to make sure they are locked before walking away from crib.
Aspiration	Examine toys for small parts that could be aspirated; remove toys that appear dangerous.
	Do not feed toddler popcorn, peanuts, etc.; urge children not to eat while running. Do not leave a toddler alone with a balloon.
Drowning	Do not leave toddler alone in a bathtub or near water (including buckets of cleaning water).
Animal bites	Do not allow the toddler to approach strange dogs.
	Supervise child's play with family pets.
Poisoning	Never present medication as candy. Buy medications with childproof caps; put away immediately after use.
	Never take medication in front of child.
	Place all medication and poisons in locked cabinets or overhead shelves where child cannot reach.
	Never leave medication in parents' purse or pocket, where child can reach.
	Always store food or substances in their original containers.
	Know the names of house plants and find out if they are on the list of poisonous plants. (Call regional poison control center for the information.)
	Hang plants or set them on high surfaces beyond toddler's grasp.
	Post telephone number of nearest poison control by the telephone.
	In all first-aid boxes, maintain supply of syrup of ipecac, an emetic, with proper instructions for administering if poisoning should occur. Never administer ipecac without medical authorization, since it is contraindicated in the treatment of some poisonous ingestions.
Burns	Buy flame-retardant clothing.
	Cook on the back burners of stove if possible and turn handles of pots towards back of stove to prevent toddler from reaching up and pulling them down.
	Use cool-mist vaporizer rather than steam vaporizer or remain in room when vaporizer is operating so that child is not tempted to play with it.
	Keep screen in front of fireplace or heater.
	Monitor toddlers carefully when they are near lit candles.
	Do not leave toddlers unsupervised near hot-water faucets.
	Check temperature setting for hot water heater and turn down thermostat if it is over 125°F.

(continued)

FOCUS ON FAMILY TEACHING (continued)

Potential Accident	Prevention Measure
General	Do not leave coffee/tea pots on a table where child can reach them.
	Never drink hot beverages when a child is sitting on your lap or playing within reach.
	Do not allow toddlers to blow out matches (teach that fire is not fun); store matches out of reach.
	Keep electric wires and cords out of toddler's reach; cover electrical outlets with safety plugs.
	Know whereabouts of toddlers at all times. Toddlers can climb onto chairs, stools, etc., that they could not manage before; can turn door knobs and go places they could not go before.
	Be aware that the frequency of accidents increases when the family is under stress and therefore less attentive to children. Special precautions must be taken at these times.
	Be aware some children are more active, curious, and impulsive and therefore more vulnerable to accidents than others.

Because lead is toxic to body tissue, lead poisoning can cause serious damage to the brain and nervous system, kidneys, and red blood cells. High levels may result in convulsions, mental retardation, coma, and even death. Levels as low as 10 to 15 μg/dL can cause learning and behavioral problems (Daniel et al., 1990).

Symptoms of lead poisoning include irritability, headaches, fatigue, and abdominal pain. Often, however, there are no symptoms, which is why periodic blood screening is so essential (Friedman & Weinberger, 1990). The CDC has recommended universal screening for all children between the ages of 6 months and 6 years (Dershewitz, 1993). A small amount of blood taken by a finger prick is analyzed. A positive result (over 10 μg/dL) must be confirmed by further testing.

Promoting Toddler Development in Daily Activities

The toddler's new independence and developing abilities in self-care, such as dressing, eating, and to a limited extent, hygiene, present special challenges for the parents. Learning how to promote autonomy yet maintain a safe, healthful environment is a major goal for the family caregivers. Toddler nutritional needs and changing patterns of feeding are discussed in Chapter 34. Other daily needs and activities are explored below.

Dressing

By the end of the toddler period, most toddlers are able to put on their own socks, underpants, and undershirt. Some may also be able to pull on slacks, pullover shirts (the sleeves of a shirt often confuse the toddler) or simple dresses. Parents may be guilty of being reluctant to encourage toddlers to dress themselves. It is often much easier and quicker to put their clothes on for them, and the toddler who is dressed by parents will (usually) be wearing clothes in the correct way. When toddlers dress themselves, they invariably put shoes on the wrong feet and shirt and pants on backwards. Encourage parents to give up perfection for the benefit of the child's developing sense of autonomy. If the child does end up with underpants or shirt on backwards, in most instances it does not make that much difference, and the toddler is not likely to feel independent and confident if his or her attempts at dressing are criticized. If the parents feel they must change the child's clothes, they should begin with a positive statement, such as "You did a good job," before making the switch.

During a health assessment, ask parents if their child can put on any of his or her own clothes. Those who allow this will name those the child can manage. Parents who do not allow self-dressing will probably describe the daily battle they have over dressing: "She puts up such a fuss, I don't think she will ever do it on her own." These parents may need help to understand the situation: the child may be resisting because she wants to dress herself. Don't judge how much independent exploration parents encourage by what they do in a physician's office or pediatric clinic. They may dress the child quickly after a physical examination to show the child that the examination is over, or they may simply be in a hurry to get home.

Shoes continue to be a controversial item all during childhood. As soon as children are up on their feet and walking, they need shoe soles that are firm enough to provide protection on rough surfaces. However, toddlers do not need extremely firm or ankle-high shoes. Because the toddler's arches are still developing, it is better for the arches to provide foot support rather than having it provided by shoes. Sneakers are an ideal toddler shoe because the soles are hard enough for rough surfaces and arch support is limited.

Sleep

The amount of sleep children need gradually decreases as they grow older. They may begin the toddler period napping twice a day and sleeping 12 hours each night, and end it with one nap a day and only 8 hours' sleep at night. Parents who are not aware that the need for sleep declines at this time may view a child's disinterest in sleeping as a problem. A parent's insistence that the child get more sleep may lead to sleeping problems or refusal to sleep at all. If the child is unable to fall asleep at night, maybe she is ready to omit or shorten her afternoon nap. If she is so short tempered at dinner time that she is impossible, perhaps she needs two naps a day.

Toddlers naturally fall asleep when they are tired. They may begin to resist naps, however, as well as nighttime sleep because they are aware for the first time that activities go on while they are asleep, and they do not want to miss anything. Parents must be sure that when they say, "We'll do this after naptime," that they wait until then to do it. Otherwise, the child will be reluctant to nap the next day for fear of missing another activity. Also, parents must be sure that older siblings do not point out to the toddler all the exciting things he or she missed while napping.

Some toddlers resist naptime as part of their developing negativism. Parents might minimize this by including a nap as part of lunchtime routine, not as a separate activity: the child always goes from the table directly to bed. The parent can state simply, "It's naptime now," and then give a secondary choice: "Do you want to sleep with your teddy bear or your rag doll?" Toward the end of the toddler period, many children are ready to omit their afternoon naps. They may be agreeable to a "shoes-off" or quiet-play period, however, until they begin to attend school full time.

As with any other activity of this period, the toddler loves a bedtime routine: bath, pajamas, a story, toothbrushing, being tucked into bed, having a drink of water, choosing a toy to sleep with, and turning out lights. Parents must be careful, however, that a child does not maneuver them into such a long procedure that sleep is considerably delayed past the time initially set. Although toddlers need to be independent, they also need a feeling of security. Just as adults like to know there are guard rails along steep mountain roads, toddlers must be sure that parents are firm, consistent people who can be counted on to be reliable.

Many toddlers are ready to be moved out of a crib into a youth bed or regular bed with protective side rails or a chair strategically placed beside it. Moving children to a more grown-up bed is usually preferable to forcing them to sleep in a crib if they no longer feel they should

be there. Either the child will not fall asleep in the crib or will scale the side rails and perhaps fall.

Children need to understand that sleeping in a regular bed does not give them the right to get in and out of bed as they choose because they cannot roam about the house at night unsupervised. Some toddlers do well if they are allowed to sleep in a regular bed and a folding gate is placed across the door to their room. This arrangement gives them a feeling of independence, but they are still safe from harm. When first moved to a bed without side rails, many children are found sleeping on the floor of the room in the morning. There is no harm in a child's sleeping on the floor unless it is cold or drafty. Dressing the child in warm pajamas or putting a blanket on the floor might be solutions to help parents accept this behavior.

Bathing

The time for a toddler's bath should depend on the parents' and the child's wishes and schedule. Some parents prefer to bathe a toddler before the evening meal because it has a quieting effect and prepares the child for eating; others prefer to give it at bedtime because it has a relaxing effect and helps the child sleep. The time, however, is not as important as the attempt to establish a sense of routine, a sense that life has order. The schedule should not be so rigid that the child feels lost and will not sleep without a bath, but learning to be independent is sometimes frightening; there is security in knowing that certain events are predictable.

Parents may have to be reminded that although toddlers can sit well in a bathtub, it is still not safe to leave them there unsupervised. They might slip and get their head under water or reach and turn on the hot water faucet and scald themselves. Toddlers usually enjoy bath time, and parents should make an effort to make it fun by providing a toy, such as a rubber duck, boat, or plastic fish. Bath time is usually so enjoyable for toddlers that parents can use it as a recreation activity or something to do on a rainy day when they can find nothing else to interest the child.

Care of Teeth

Between-meal snacks are important to a growing child. Parents should be encouraged, however, to offer fruit (bananas, pieces of apple, orange slices) or protein foods (cheese or pieces of chicken) rather than more traditional high-carbohydrate items. Such foods are not only nutritious but also reduce dental decay by limiting exposure of the child's teeth to carbohydrate. Calcium (found in large amounts in milk, cheese, and yogurt) is especially important to the development of strong teeth (see Chapter 34 for an in-depth discussion of the toddler's nutritional needs). In addition, children should continue to drink fluoridated water, if it is available, so that all new teeth form with cavity-resistant enamel.

Toddlers should have a toothbrush they recognize as their own. Toward the end of the toddler period, they can begin to do the brushing themselves under supervision (children need some supervision until about age 8). Remind parents that it is better for a child to brush thoroughly once a day, probably at bedtime, than to do it poorly many times a day. After brushing, parents should use dental floss to clean between the child's teeth and to remove plaque.

Urge parents to schedule a first visit to a dentist skilled in pediatric dental care by 2 years of age for assessment of dentition and a first fluoride application if needed (AAP, 1986). Parents can prepare their child for this first and subsequent visits by maintaining a positive attitude about the visit, avoiding the use of frightening words like *drill* or *shot,* and answering their child's questions about the dentist honestly without going into too much detail.

Promoting Healthy Family Functioning

Learning self-reliance is the primary goal of the child during the toddler period. Because of this fact, some parents who enjoyed caring for their child as an infant may find it difficult to have their authority challenged by a toddler. Help parents to understand that their responses to these attempts at independence are crucial to the healthy development of their child. Although the child still needs firm limits to feel secure, he or she must be given some room to make independent decisions in areas that the parents feel they do not necessarily need to control. An outside person, such as a nurse, can provide an important perspective on this issue.

If parents punish excessively at each move toward independence, a child will not fight them indefinitely. Instead, the child will begin to feel guilty that he or she wants to do things for himself or herself. Almost everyone knows an adult who feels this way about independent thought. This person may follow orders well, but when the job calls for a new program or function, the individual cannot reach into unknown areas without a great deal of consultation and help.

Some parents must be cautioned not to begin to function at the same level as their toddler. An easy reaction to a toddler's refusal to allow a parent to help is "You won't let me help you with this, I won't do anything for you." This is a defense mechanism that prevents people from feeling rejected. Teach parents that refusing to accept help is not refusing to accept love. Refusing to let mother put on a shoe is an instance of refusing to let mother put on a shoe, nothing more.

At bedtime or naptime or anytime they are tired, toddlers may become much more like their old selves, wanting to sit on a parent's lap and be rocked or picked up and carried. Parents may have to be reminded that this does not signal babyish behavior or regression in the toddler. It is a natural state between infant and preschool ages.

Parental Concerns Associated With the Toddler Period

Toilet Training

Toilet training is one of the biggest tasks the toddler must achieve. There are as many theories concerning toilet training as there are experts to write them, and understanding the procedure thus becomes one of the biggest tasks of this period for parents. Most first-time parents ask when to start toilet training, when the training should be completed, and how to go about it. The answer is that toilet training is an individualized task for each child. It should begin and be completed according to a child's ability to accomplish it, not according to a set schedule (Hauck, 1991). When it is started can be culturally determined (see the Focus on Cultural Awareness box).

Before children can begin to be toilet trained, they must have reached two important developmental levels, one physiologic and the other cognitive: (1) they must have control of rectal and urethral sphincters, and (2) they must have a cognitive understanding of what it means to hold urine and stools until they can release them at a certain place and time.

Because physiologic development is cephalocaudal, the rectal and urethral sphincter are not mature enough for control in most children until at least the end of the first year, when tracts of the spinal cord are myelinated to the anal level. A good way for a parent to know that a child's development has reached this point is to wait until the child is able to walk well independently.

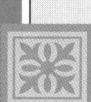

FOCUS ON CULTURAL AWARENESS

The toddler period is a time in the United States when toilet-training is usually introduced. Like so many other aspects of childrearing, the time when parents begin these activities is culturally determined. In other countries toilet training may be started as soon as the child can sit, at about 6 months. Although praise is used as a common means in the United States of encouraging toddlers to learn new tasks, other cultures believe praise will bring a child harm by releasing evil spirits. Strategies of shame or strict discipline are used instead (Geissler, 1994). Being aware that childrearing practices are not consistent across the world is a help in understanding why parents approach childrearing problems differently and why childrearing advice must be individualized.

Toilet training should not start this early, however, because cognitively, many children do not understand what is being asked of them until they are 2 or even 3 years old. The markers of readiness are subtle, but as a rule children are ready for toilet training when they can understand what their parents want them to do and when they begin to be uncomfortable in wet diapers. They may begin to pull or tug at diapers; they may bring a parent a clean diaper after they have soiled so that they can be changed (Figure 30-7).

When a toddler is 18 months to 2 year olds, parents can plan 1 or 2 weeks of "readiness" activities. They can be sure that the child sees them or older children in the family using the toilet. A mother could say, "Mommy is going to the bathroom. Soon you'll be big enough to do this, too, and not have wet pants any more." It is best not to suggest that urine and feces are dirty or distasteful, but simply to make it clear that bigger people customarily leave these materials in the toilet. Urine and feces, after all, come from the child; it is difficult for a toddler to see the difference between a parent's not liking him and not liking something that comes from him.

Training pants should be introduced during the

same week that the concept of using the bathroom is introduced. As a father is folding laundry he might say, "These are Daddy's underpants. He wears this kind because he goes potty in the bathroom." These types of readiness activities are important because they make completing the task of toilet training a step toward being grown up. If this preparation is not done, toilet training can seem to be something that only toddlers do, and the child may react to it with extreme negativism.

Teach parents not to underestimate what it is that they expect their child to achieve. Infants live by a pleasure principle: they want what they want when they want it. Before they can complete toilet training, children must be able to give up an immediate pleasure—relieving themselves whenever they have the urge—to gain other pleasure later on—improved physical comfort and another step in growing up.

It is easier for toddlers to comprehend the issue if parents attempt bowel training before bladder training. Stool is so much more evident than urine that the child grasps more easily what a parent is describing. As soon as the child is trained for bowel movements (about 1 week if the child is ready), the parents can then describe urine as a substance that also should be saved and expelled in the toilet or potty.

Some parents may have to be cautioned not to introduce morality into toilet training or to equate good with being dry and bad with being wet. Help them to think of it as analogous to walking. To say a child is "good" because he walks and "bad" because he has not yet learned to walk doesn't make sense. If the child begins to view excrement as a dirty substance, he may also begin to think that all physical functions are distasteful and that he must be careful in all aspects of life so that he does not get dirty and therefore displease a parent. Such an attitude may cause a child to become reluctant to participate in new activities; if the activity is not neat, it may be better not to try it. Finally, such a child may become an adult who lacks spontaneity or creativity.

Parents can purchase either a potty chair that sits on the floor or an infant seat that is placed on the regular toilet. The potty chair has the advantage of being low, and a child is less likely to be frightened by sitting on it. Because it must be emptied and cleaned after each use, however, some parents do not like to use one. If parents choose an infant seat, they should place a footstool in front of the toilet so that the child has some support for his or her feet. Be sure parents are careful not to flush the toilet while the child is sitting on it. Two-year-olds have poor space concepts, and they are unable to realize that they will not be flushed away. This experience is so frightening to some toddlers that they refuse to use an infant toilet seat, in which case the parents must respect that wish.

After parents have introduced the toddler to training pants and using the bathroom, they should put him or

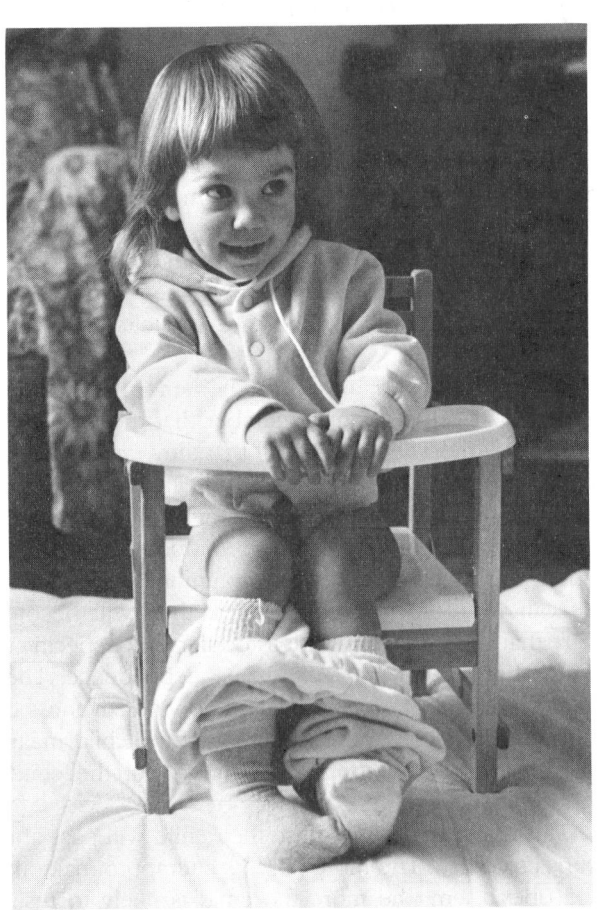

FIGURE 30-7
Toddlers are interested in toilet training as an expression of autonomy. (Courtesy of Brian Smistek.)

her on the potty chair or toilet at regular intervals, such as when the child wakes up in the morning, after breakfast, midmorning, before lunch, after lunch, and so forth. If the child does urinate or defecate, he or she should be praised. Remind parents that the child should not remain on the potty chair for much longer than 10 minutes and less than that if he or she is resistant. Also, the child should not sit on the chair to eat or use it as a play table because he or she will become confused as to its purpose.

If the child is ready for toilet training, within 1 to 2 weeks he or she will be using the bathroom independently, with help only in undressing and dressing and using toilet paper. Parents should check that training pants pull down readily and that slacks are free of complicated buttons or grippers; otherwise, the child will have accidents because he or she cannot undress quickly enough.

If, after a 2-week trial period, a child does not seem to be any drier than when training first began, parents would be wise to accept the fact that he or she is not yet ready for this skill and return to diapers with no feeling of having failed or of the child's being "bad." During the next month, they can continue to allow the child to see people using the bathroom for elimination and point out that adults do not have to wear diapers. They can reintroduce training pants and attempt toilet training again in another month.

Many children stay dry during the night at the same time they learn to be dry during the day. Others, perhaps those with physically smaller bladders, have difficulty remaining dry at night until they are 3 to 4 years old. Parents should not put pressure on a child to try and accomplish nighttime dryness but assume that the child is doing the best he or she can.

Parents can put the child into diapers for the night (keeping bedding drier and reducing sheet washing) by explaining (not punitively) that it is hard to keep dry during the night. Then, after the child has been dry during the daytime for about 1 month, they may begin to leave the child in training pants.

It is generally ineffective to wake children during the night and carry them to the bathroom to void. This system may keep them dry during the night, but it does not help them stay dry for long periods of time. It may even prolong nighttime wetness because it conditions children to void every 4 hours or so instead of retaining urine for 12 hours while they sleep.

Some toddlers smear or play with feces, often at about the same time that toilet training is started. This occurs because they become aware of body excretions but have no adult values toward them; stools are little different from the play dough that they play with. This activity can be minimized by providing toddlers with play substances of similar texture and by changing diapers immediately after defecation. Teach parents to ac-

cept this behavior for what it is: enjoyment of the body, of self, and the discovery of a new substance. After a child is fully toilet trained, this activity rarely persists.

Ritualistic Behavior

Although toddlers spend a great deal of time every day investigating new ways to do things and doing things they have never done before, they also enjoy ritualistic patterns. They will use only "their" spoon at meal time, only "their" washcloth at bathtime. They will not go outside unless mother or father locates their favorite cap.

The child who seems to need an excessive number of objects to cling to or an excessive number of routines, however, may be trying to say, "I need more guidelines, more rules. Don't let me be quite so independent."

Negativism

As part of establishing their identities as separate individuals, toddlers typically go through a period of extreme negativism. They do not want to do anything that a parent wants them to do. Their reply to every request is a very definite "No."

It is easy for parents to feel that their authority is being questioned when this happens and worry that the child is becoming so disrespectful that he or she will have difficulty getting along in the world. They can be baffled by the extreme change from a happy, cooperative infant who lived to please them to this irritating, uncooperative child. They may need some help to realize that this is not only a normal phenomenon of toddlerhood but a positive stage in development. It means that a toddler is seeing himself or herself as a separate individual with separate needs. It is important that toddlers do this if they are to grow up to be persons who are independent and able to take care of their own needs and desires.

Parents who went away from home for the first time to college or camp might remember that they have behaved similarly. They may recall that they rarely slept or ate sensibly; they tried, in effect, to break every rule that their parents used to enforce on them. Most regained their equilibrium in time to find a midpoint between irresponsible independence and common sense. If parents can recall such circumstances, they will become aware that this behavior in their toddler is not specific to the age but to the first feeling of independence. They can also remember that they meant no vindictiveness by their behavior, so they can realize that the child means none. This understanding can help to put the child's "No" in perspective.

This extreme negativism in their child will pass after it runs its course. The more parents attempt to make the child obey them, the more the child is likely to resist. Some long-term parent–child interaction problems begin during this period because parents insist on being obeyed totally.

A toddler's "No" can best be eliminated by limiting the number of questions asked of the child. A father does not really mean, for example, "Are you ready for dinner?" He means, "Come to the table. It's dinner time." A mother asks, "Will you come take a bath now?" She means, "It's time for your bath." Making the statement instead of asking the question can avoid a great many negative responses.

A toddler needs experience in making choices, however. To provide the opportunity to do this, a parent might give a *secondary* choice. "No" is not allowed for the major task, so the parent states, "It's bathtime now" but then says, "Do you want to take your duck or your toy boat into the tub with you?" Other examples would be "It's lunch time. Do you want to use a big or little plate?" or "It's time to go shopping. Do you want to wear your jacket or your sweater?" Although this solution is simple, it is one that parents may not arrive at themselves, because finding a solution is always more difficult for the person in the middle of a problem than for an objective observer. Once they are helped to practice this approach, however, parents usually find it definitely helpful in smoothing out the friction caused by the negativism of the toddler period (see the Focus on Nursing Research box).

Discipline

Some parents ask during the last part of the infant year or the early toddler period when they should start to discipline their child or when he or she will be old enough so that it is all right to punish him or her. Remind parents that **discipline** and **punishment** are not interchangeable terms. Discipline means setting rules or road signs so that the child knows what he or she is expected to do. Punishment is a consequence that results from a breakdown in discipline, from the child's disregarding the rules he or she has learned.

It is important that parents begin to instill some sense of discipline early in life because part of it involves setting safety limits and protecting others or property. The child must stay away from the fireplace or heater; she must not go in the street; she must not hit other children, for example. These actions, however, arise out of the day-to-day interaction with the child, out of the rhythm of child care, not out of a set procedure such as, "Today, I'm going to teach discipline." A general rule to follow is that rules are learned best if children's right behavior is praised rather than wrong behavior punished.

Separation Anxiety

As discussed in Chapter 29, fear of being separated from parents begins at about 6 months of age and persists throughout the preschool period. This universal fear of this age group is known as *separation anxiety*. For this reason, toddlers have difficulty accepting being sepa-

FOCUS ON NURSING RESEARCH

Which Toddlers Have the Most Difficult-to-Manage Temperament?

Toddlers have a reputation for being difficult for parents to manage ("terrible twos"). To see if being born preterm and cared for in a neonatal intensive care unit causes infants to have a more difficult-to-manage temperament than term infants, three nurse researchers performed a secondary analysis on three studies on temperament. All of the infants in these studies had been cared for in Level III (intensive care) nurseries in the United States.

Results of the secondary analysis revealed that as a group, preterm infants were significantly more difficult to care for than comparison groups of term infants but those infants who were the smallest, sickest, and exposed longest to the ICN environment were not necessarily the infants with the most difficult temperaments. Good interviewing to determine an infant's birth circumstances is important in understanding later behavior.

Gennaro, S., Medoff-Cooper, B., & Lotas, M. (1992). Perinatal factors and infant temperament: A collaborative approach. *Nursing Research, 41*, 375.

rated from their primary caregiver to spend a day at a day care center or if their mother is hospitalized to give birth to a new baby or they are hospitalized. Nursing responsibility for care of toddlers in the hospital as well as the reactions of toddlers to the separation caused by hospitalization and the methods used to minimize these reactions are discussed in Chapter 35.

Toddlers sometimes resist staying with baby sitters or at day care because of separation anxiety. Parents may ask a nurse what they can do about this problem. They feel they have a right to leave the child in a baby-sitter's or center's care, but how can they tolerate the crying at the door in order to do this? Most toddlers react best to separation if a regular baby-sitter is employed or the day care center is one with consistent caregivers. Many are more comfortable if they are cared for in their own home. It helps if they have fair warning that they will have a baby-sitter. For example, they might be told, "Mommy is fixing dinner early because Mommy and Daddy are going to visit some friends tonight. Marsha is going to come and baby-sit with you. She'll put you to bed. When you wake up in the morning, Mommy and Daddy will he here again."

No matter how well prepared a toddler is, he or she may cry when the baby-sitter actually appears or may greet her warmly only to cry when his or her parents reach for their coats. It helps if parents say goodbye firmly, repeat the explanation that they will be there when the child wakes in the morning, and then leave.

Prolonged goodbyes only lead to more crying. Sneaking out prevents crying and may ease the parent's guilt, but it may lead to the development of a grave fear of abandonment and should be discouraged. This applies to termination of hospital visits as well.

Nursing Diagnoses and Related Interventions

> ***Nursing Diagnosis:*** High risk for family coping, compromised, related to toddler behavior
>
> ***Goal:*** Family will learn better methods for coping with temper tantrums.
>
> ***Outcome Criteria:*** Family will state temper tantrums occur less than 2 times daily.

Temper Tantrums

Almost every toddler has a temper tantrum at one time or another. The child may kick, scream, stamp feet, and shout, "No, no, no," lie on the floor and flail arms and legs and bang the head against the floor. Children may even hold their breath until they become cyanotic and slump to the floor.

Temper tantrums are a natural consequence of toddlers' development. Toddlers are independent enough to know what they want, but they do not have the vocabulary or the wisdom to express their feelings in a more socially acceptable way. For example, temper tantrums occur most often when children are tired, just before naptime or bedtime or during a long shopping trip or visit. The tantrums are often a response to an unrealistic request by a parent: asking a child to comb his hair before he is coordinated enough to do so, asking her to pick up her toys before she has a feeling of family responsibility, or asking him to share before he is able to understand what is wanted. Also, they may occur if parents are saying no too frequently with regard to such things as touching the coffee table, getting dirty, using a spoon, or running and jumping; thus, the child feels constantly thwarted. A tantrum may be a response to difficulty making choices or decisions or to pressure from activities such as toilet training. Such a child needs to express feelings some way and does so with temper tantrums.

To help parents manage a toddler's temper tantrums, explore with them the reasons for the behavior. If tantrums always occur just before bedtime, the parents will probably realize what the answer is: schedule an earlier bedtime or an afternoon nap. If they occur every time the parent goes shopping, perhaps it would help to schedule two shorter trips each week rather than one long one. If they occur whenever the parent asks the child to do something, investigate whether or not the child is being asked to perform age-appropriate tasks. If tantrums occur in response to decision making, parents

may have to limit the number of choices they are giving the child.

After you know which circumstances generally lead to temper tantrums, ask parents to describe the behavior. Does it sound like a tantrum or something more? Is there a possibility a parent is mistaking seizure activity for temper tantrums? Could a parent be confusing neurologic breath holding with a temper tantrum?

Some children deliberately hold their breath to obtain something they want. This is manifested by a distended chest (a halt after inspiration), often air-filled cheeks, and increasing distress as the child's body registers oxygen want. This is harmless breath holding; ignoring it will make it ineffective and the child will give it up. True breath holding is a neurologic problem in which the child appears to "forget" to breathe. At the peak of anger, he or she breathes out and then does not breathe in again (a halt on expiration). This type of breath holding tends to be familial. Although it may have a neurologic basis, the child generally has normal electroencephalographic findings and is healthy in every other way (D'Mario et al., 1990).

The cessation of breathing in seizure activity occurs as part of generalized convulsive activity (see Chapter 49). Guidelines that are helpful in differentiating these activities are outlined in Table 30-5.

Assess next what the parents do when the child has a tantrum. It is rarely effective for parents to give either material or emotional bribes (e.g., "Come and get a cookie," or "Stop and I'll give you a kiss"). If they accede to the child's wishes, the child is generally encouraged to have more tantrums because they are so successful. Nor should a parent punish the child. Toddlers have a right to express opinions; they need to be guided to learn a more controlled and mature way of expressing them.

Parents should also make sure that they demonstrate adult behavior in managing a toddler's temper tantrums. If the child bites, the parent should not bite back; if the child shouts or kicks, the parent must not be triggered into saying, "I can shout as loud as you. I can kick as hard as you!" Instead of showing the child a better way to express feelings, this reinforces the way he or she is responding.

Probably the best approach is for parents to tell the child simply that they disapprove of the tantrum and then ignore it. They might say, "I'll be in the bedroom. When you're done kicking, you come into the bedroom, too." The child who is left alone in the kitchen will usually not continue a tantrum but will stop after 1 or 2 minutes and rejoin his or her parents. They should then accept the child warmly and proceed as if the tantrum had not occurred. This same approach works well for nurses caring for hospitalized toddlers.

Helping parents to correct problems early may limit the number of tantrums they must deal with; it will not

Table 30-5. *Differentiating Temper Tantrums, Breath Holding, and Seizures*

Assessment	Temper Tantrums	Breath Holding	Seizures
Provocation	Usually provoked—parent can state a reason for it (she asked toddler to come to dinner, but he wanted to finish an activity)	Usually provoked; child very angry	Not provoked
Appearance of cyanosis	Child holds breath, becomes cyanotic, then slumps to floor	Child breathes out, becomes cyanotic, then slumps to floor	Child slumps to floor first, then becomes cyanotic

totally prevent them, however, because parents cannot anticipate all the circumstances that will cause this reaction. In fact, parents should not feel they must prevent all of them; they are, after all, parents, not mind readers.

As the child matures and is capable of better responses to stress situations, tantrums begin to fade by themselves. These episodes are taxing for the parents; they are also energy consuming for the child (see the Nursing Care Plan).

Unique Concerns of the Family With a Disabled or Chronically Ill Toddler

It may be difficult for a child with a handicap to achieve a sense of autonomy or independence because of specific limitations. It is important for these children to develop a strong sense of autonomy so that they will see themselves as independent and become increasingly self-sufficient as they grow older (Figure 30-8). It takes courage for an adult to do such things as move a wheelchair through a busy airport or a concert crowd. Nursing actions designed to help the disabled or chronically ill child develop a sense of autonomy are outlined in Table 30-6. If a toddler has physical limitations, he or she may be unable to explore freely or may not have the physical ability to pound and manipulate toys as the average toddler does. If on a special diet, the child may not be allowed to eat finger foods; if he or she is tube fed, the child receives no experience with finger foods at all. For these toddlers, parents should try to provide other, comparable experiences in independence, such as letting them choose where they prefer to eat or what food they would like to eat first.

The toddler with a long-term illness or disability can be expected to exhibit normal toddler behaviors, such as temper tantrums, and to have normal outlooks, such as negativism. Parents whose child is uncoordinated or has neurologic disease may mistake temper tantrums for seizure activity. Investigate such activity carefully, and explain to parents the difference between the two. Parents may also mistake a disabled toddler's insistence on having his or her own way as a manifestation of illness. They can be reminded that the behavior is more often an indication of age and development than of illness and that they must respond with firmness.

Toilet training is difficult for a child who is hospitalized at periodic intervals. Success requires a consistent caregiver, and hospitalization can result in regressive behaviors. If a handicapped or chronically ill child also has

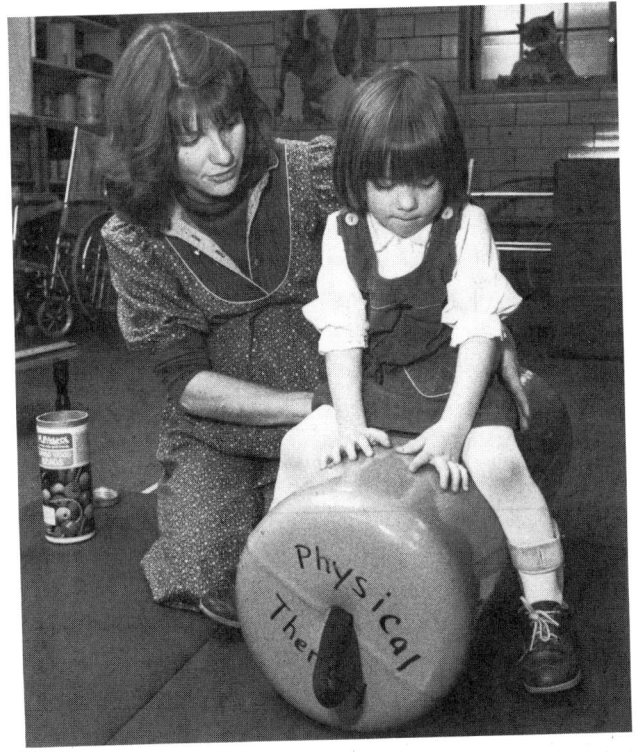

FIGURE 30-8
A toddler with leg braces practices leg-strengthening exercises. (Courtesy of the Department of Medical Photography, Children's Hospital, Buffalo, NY.)

Nursing Care Plan

A Health Maintenance Visit for a Toddler

Barita is a 2-year-old you see at a health maintenance clinic. The following is a nursing care plan designed for her.

Assessment: Mother states that Barita has temper tantrums at least 20 times a day during which she lies on the floor and pounds her head. They occur "over nothing" such as mother telling her that she cannot help her cook dinner. Mother states she doesn't know what to do to manage them. She picks Barita up immediately for fear she'll hurt her head or worse (she believes a neighbor's child became blind from falling and hitting her head on a sidewalk). Family consists of mother, Barita, and grandmother. Mother is primary caregiver.

Nursing Diagnosis: Health-seeking behaviors related to method for handling (and reducing the number of) child's temper tantrums

Defining Characteristic: Mother states she would like to know how to manage temper tantrums.

Goal: Mother will demonstrate increased ability to manage temper tantrums within 2 weeks.

Outcome Criteria: The number of temper tantrums Barita attempts decreases to less than three per day. Mother states she accepts that Barita will have some tantrums as a normal stage of her development, but that she can help reduce the number and severity of them.

Nursing Orders	Rationale
1. Ask mother to describe further when temper tantrums occur, what seems to trigger them, and what they consist of.	1. Understanding what factors contribute to the tantrums and how they are expressed will help both the nurse and the parent develop strategies for limiting them.
2. Assess for possible abnormal neurologic development and refer to physician if appropriate.	2. A parent may mistake seizure activity for a tantrum. Further assessment will help to rule out a neurologic problem.
3. Teach mother that children rarely hurt themselves during temper tantrums; they are the child's nonverbal way of expressing fatigue or frustration.	3. Understanding that the child is not likely to hurt herself during a tantrum will relieve some of the mother's anxiety during each episode, which will in turn help her to take a more objective view of her child's behavior.
4. Teach mother the technique of offering secondary choices to child.	4. This mother needs some methods for preventing tantrums, which are often related to the child's feelings of frustration and lack of control. Providing Barita with secondary choices will give the child a better sense of control and independence.
5. Suggest some actions that might be taken for the next week, such as ignoring tantrum if it occurs in the living room or bedroom (both have rugs on the floor) and picking up child only if she could actually hurt herself.	5. These interventions give the mother immediate and practical strategies for dealing with tantrums when they do occur.
6. Instruct mother to plan a time every day for reading or engaging in an enjoyable activity with child.	6. Planning a routine time for the mother and daughter to spend together reassures the child that she will have her mother's full attention during a time when she exhibits positive behavior (not when she is engaged in negative behavior, such as during a tantrum).
7. Mother to telephone in 1 week with record of child's behavior and effect on child of mother ignoring tantrums.	7. Encouraging a follow-up call lets the mother know that she still has someone to turn to for back-up and support on this issue.

Table 30-6. *Nursing Interventions to Help the Disabled or Chronically Ill Child Develop a Sense of Autonomy*

Area	Nursing Actions
Nutrition	A special diet may limit typical finger foods. Use imagination to offer other foods not usually eaten this way as finger foods. Allow child to help pour liquid diet for a tube feeding. Toddlers are frightened by vomiting because they have no control over it. Check for possibility of nausea; toddlers have no way to express this other than by not eating.
Dressing changes	The child can hold pieces of tape or put tape in place to maintain sense of control. The child can remove an old bandage if it is not contaminated. Allow the child to view his or her incision and watch dressing changes; explaining each step of a procedure as you perform it helps the child maintain control. Restrain only those body parts necessary during a procedure to allow the child a sense of control. Remove all supplies *after* a procedure, or the child may "redo" the dressing.
Medication	Allow children no choice as to whether a medicine will be taken. Do allow a child to choose a "chaser," such as milk or juice, after oral medicine. Do not ask a toddler to indicate a choice of site for an injection or intravenous insertion; this is too advanced a decision for a toddler to handle.
Rest	Locate or create a ritual for bedtime (put child into bed, tuck him in, say, "Goodnight, Bobby." Tuck in bear. Say, "Goodnight, Bear."). Allow a choice of toy or cover but not a choice of bedtime or naptime hour.
Hygiene	Allow the child a choice of bathtub toy or clothing. Allow the child to wash face and hands to gain control of the situation. Allow the child to put toothpaste on a brush, but you should brush or "touch up" teeth afterward to ensure that all plaque has been removed.
Pain	Encourage a child to express pain ("Say 'ouch' when I pull off the tape"). Help channel the child's self-expression to what is acceptable (e.g., the child may shout but may not kick).
Stimulation	Provide a toddler with a toy that can be manipulated, such as boxes that fit inside one another and can be taken out again, trucks that can be pushed, and pegs that can be pounded. In a health care setting, items can usually be found that fit together (boxes from central supply or plastic vials from the pharmacy). Another action toy: blow up a rubber glove and tie it to the crib side to be used as a punching bag; another one tied to the foot of the crib can serve as a leg exerciser.
Elimination	A child who is toilet trained needs to be encouraged to use a potty chair or toilet during an illness. Help children with ureter or bowel stomas to help with changing bags so they are as independent in bowel function as possible.

difficulty with ambulation, soiling accidents may occur beyond the usual age for them because the toddler's neurologic development is not sufficient or because of inability to reach the bathroom easily.

Some parents tend to protect and shelter an ill child, and you may have to remind them that even though chronically ill, a toddler will demand independence and has the right to explore. A child who uses a lower-extremity prosthesis, for example, might prefer to crawl somewhere rather than wait for help to put the prosthesis in place. Although this degree of independence is good, parents may have to limit how it is expressed so the child will learn how to use the prosthesis (for example, they could make a rule that the child must use the prosthesis to walk but can choose whether or not to use a spoon when eating.)

Key Points

- Toddlers make great strides forward in development but their physical growth slows.

- A critical milestone of toddler development is being able to form two-word sentences by 2 years of age.
- Erikson's developmental task for the toddler period is to form a sense of autonomy or independence vs. shame or doubt.
- Toddlers are capable of preoperational thought or are able to deal much more constructively with symbols than they could while still infants.
- Important aspects of care are promoting toddler safety, including screening for lead poisoning; promoting toddler development, such as promoting daily activities; and healthy family functioning.
- Common concerns of parents during the toddler period are toilet training, ritualistic behavior, negativism, temper tantrums, discipline, and separation anxiety.
- Promoting autonomy in the child who is disabled or chronically ill calls for creative planning, as there may be many tasks that must be done for the child to be certain they are done safely.

Critical Thinking Exercises

1. Bryan is a 2-year-old whose mother tells you has at least three temper tantrums a day. She asks you how to deal with these when they happen while shopping. What would you advise?

2. People with a sense of autonomy are capable of independent function. Describe the actions of someone who does not have a good sense of autonomy. Would you enjoy working with this person as a fellow nurse?

3. Many working mothers are concerned that toilet training will be especially difficult because their child has two or three caregivers every day. What suggestions could you offer to make toilet training easier under these circumstances?

References

American Academy of Pediatrics, Committee on Nutrition (1986). Fluoride supplementation. *Pediatrics, 77,* 758.

Curry, D. M., & Duby, J. C. (1994). Developmental surveillance by pediatric nurses. *Pediatric Nursing, 20,* 40.

Daniel, K., et al. (1990). Childhood lead poisoning, New York City, 1988. *Morbidity and Mortality Weekly Report, 39,* 1.

Department of Health and Human Services. (1991). *Healthy people 2000.* Washington, DC: Public Health Service.

Dershewitz, D. A. (1993). *Ambulatory pediatric care* (2nd ed.). Philadelphia: J.B. Lippincott.

D'Mario, F. J., et al. (1990). Pallid breath-holding spells. *Clinical Pediatrics, 29,* 17.

Dye, D. J., et al. (1990). Toddlers, teapots and kettles—beware of intraoral scalds. *British Medical Journal, 300,* 597.

Erikson, E. H. (1986). *Childhood and society.* New York: W. W. Norton.

Friedman, J. A., & Weinberger, H. L. (1990). Six children with lead poisoning. *American Journal of Diseases of Children, 144,* 1039.

Geissler, E. M. (1994). *Pocket guide to cultural assessment.* St. Louis: C. V. Mosby.

Gennaro, S., Medoff-Cooper, B., & Lotas, M. (1992). Perinatal factors and infant temperament: A collaborative approach. *Nursing Research, 41,* 375.

Hauck, M. R. (1991). Mothers' descriptions of the toilet training process. *Journal of Pediatric Nursing, 6,* 80.

Morelli, J. (1993). Pediatric poisonings: The ten most toxic prescription drugs. *American Journal of Nursing, 93,* 27.

Prizant, M., et al. (1993). Communication and language assessment for young children. *Infants and Young Children, 5,* 20.

Wadsworth, B. J. (1989). *Piaget's theory of cognitive and affective development.* New York: Longman.

Wilson, P. D., & Testani-Dufour, L. (1993). Bicycle safety programs: Targeting injury prevention through education. *Pediatric Nursing, 19,* 343.

Suggested Readings

Ahmann, E. (1994). Family-centered care: The time has come. *Pediatric Nursing, 20,* 52.

Canam, C. (1993). Common adaptive tasks facing parents of children with chronic conditions. *Journal of Advanced Nursing, 18,* 46.

Gillis, A. J. (1990). Nurses' knowledge of growth and development principles in meeting psychosocial needs of hospitalized children. *Journal of Pediatric Nursing, 5,* 78.

Heersema, D. J., & Vanhofvandium, J. (1990). Age norms for visual acuity in toddlers using the acuity card procedure. *Clinical Visual Science, 5,* 167.

Malfair, A. (1992). Supporting the child with special needs. *Canadian Nurse, 88,* 17.

Marino, B. L. (1991). Studying infant and toddler play. *Journal of Pediatric Nursing, 6,* 16.

McConachie, H. (1990). Early language development and severe visual impairment. *Child Care, Health and Development, 16,* 55.

Chapter 31

The Family With a Preschooler

Objectives

After mastering the contents of this chapter, you should be able to:

1. Describe normal growth and development and common parental concerns of the preschool period.

2. Assess a preschooler for normal growth and developmental milestones.

3. Formulate nursing diagnoses related to preschool growth and development and common parental concerns.

4. Plan nursing care to meet the preschooler's growth and development needs, such as planning age-appropriate play activities.

5. Implement nursing care related to normal growth and development of the preschooler, such as preparing a preschooler for an invasive procedure.

6. Evaluate outcome criteria established for care to be certain normal growth and development goals have been achieved.

7. Identify National Health Goals related to the preschool period that nurses can be instrumental in helping the nation to achieve.

8. Identify areas related to care of the preschool-age child that could benefit from additional nursing research.

9. Use critical thinking to analyze additional ways in which growth and developmental problems of the preschool child can be prevented and care can be family centered.

10. Synthesize knowledge of preschool growth and development with nursing process to achieve quality maternal and child health nursing care.

Adele Pillitteri: MATERNAL AND CHILD HEALTH NURSING, 2nd Edition. © 1995 Adele Pillitteri.

The preschool period is traditionally defined as including ages 3, 4, and 5 years. Although physical growth slows considerably during this period, personality and cognitive growth are substantial.

This is also an important period of growth for parents. They may be unsure about how much independence and responsibility for self-care they should give their preschooler. Most children of this age want to do things for themselves—choose their own clothing and dress by themselves, feed themselves completely, wash their own hair, and so forth. As a result, parents of a preschooler may find their child dressed in one red and one green sock, going to school with unwashed ears, or trying to eat soup with a fork. They need some reassurance that this behavior is typical and is helping the child develop more initiative and control of his life. They may also need some guidance in separating those tasks that the preschooler can accomplish independently from those that still require some adult supervision. Sensible limits must be set so that children do not harm themselves or others while participating in all the interesting experiences available to them. The Focus on National Health Goals box lists National Health Goals related to the period.

⊠ NURSING PROCESS OVERVIEW
for Healthy Development
of the Preschooler

ASSESSMENT

Regular assessment of the preschooler includes obtaining a health history and performing both a physical and developmental evaluation. Preschoolers speak very little during a health assessment; they may even revert to baby talk or babyish actions such as thumb-sucking if they find a health visit stressful. A history that details their usual performance level is therefore very important for accurate evaluation (see Focus on Cultural Awareness display).

Assess the child's weight and height according to standard growth charts (Appendix E). Keep in mind that these charts are based on average weights and heights of white American children, and that children from other ethnic or cultural backgrounds may not follow these norms. For instance, Asian children are often seen at the low end of the charts; children with exceptionally tall parents tend to fall at the higher ranges. Also assess the child for general appearance. Does the child appear to be alert? happy? active? healthy? (Colds are frequent in all children; the average preschooler may have from 10 to 12 a year.) Ask whether the child is able to attend a half-day session at a preschool or day care center without becoming exhausted. Are teeth cavity free? Is the child's gait symmetric?

NURSING DIAGNOSIS

A wellness-oriented nursing diagnosis used in health promotion of the preschooler is

- Health-seeking behaviors related to developmental expectations

Other nursing diagnoses that relate to the developmental stage of the preschooler include

- High risk for injury related to increased independence outside the home
- Altered growth and development related to frequent illness

- High risk for poisoning related to maturational age of child
- Parental anxiety related to lack of understanding of childhood development

PLANNING

Planning for care of the preschooler often begins with establishing a schedule for discussing normal preschool development with parents (which should be done at all health maintenance visits). For many parents, this is a difficult time, because the child is at an in-between stage: no longer an infant, though not yet ready for school. In addition, it is important to keep in mind that when asking parents to incorporate adventurous activities or messy material into a preschooler's play, you may be asking them to do something they don't personally enjoy. Most parents successfully initiate activities with a child if they believe they are important, but some are able to do this better than others. Allowing children choices may also be difficult for parents, because they may want to protect their children from making errors.

IMPLEMENTATION

Preschool children imitate moods as well as actions. An important nursing intervention, then, is role playing a

FOCUS ON
National Health Goals

A number of National Health Goals are designed to target the preschool population:

- Reduce infectious diarrhea by at least 25% among children in licensed child care centers.
- Reduce acute middle ear infections among children age 4 and younger, as measured by days of restricted activity or school absenteeism.
- Extend requirements of the use of effective head, face, eye, and mouth protection to all organizations, agencies, and institutions sponsoring sporting and recreation events that pose risks of injury (DHHS, 1991).

Nurses can be instrumental in helping the nation achieve these goals by serving as consultants at day care and preschool settings to be certain that protection from the spread of infectious diseases in these settings is provided and by advocating for parents to fit their children with helmets before beginning bicycle riding.

A number of questions could benefit from additional nursing research, such as, What practices seem most effective in reducing the spread of respiratory illnesses in day care settings? What are the barriers to parents buying helmets for this age child? What proportion of parents know the signs and symptoms of common illnesses their child might contract at a child care setting?

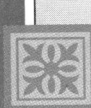

FOCUS ON CULTURAL AWARENESS

Whether preschool children remain home during this period or attend day care or preschool is, in part, culturally determined. Traditionally, a child this age remained at home. So, the more traditional the culture, the more a day care or preschool experience may be viewed as inappropriate for this age group. This can create differences in how social or comfortable children are in interacting with strangers in a health care setting.

Whether children are allowed to ask questions or not is also culturally determined. In a society in which children are expected to be seen and not heard, a child may not have the same expressive vocabulary as a child who has been encouraged to ask questions. Recognition that differences among cultures can affect levels of development alerts the nurse to individualized assessment, that is, assessment that is meaningful in terms of the cultural milieu.

mood or attitude you would like a child to learn. To project an attitude toward health assessment as an enjoyable activity, you might ask "Would you like to listen to your heart?" or "Can you hear my watch ticking?" as one type of positive role modeling.

EVALUATION

Evaluation of established goals should be continuous and frequent. Because growth during this period is more cognitive and emotional than physical, parents may report little growth. Evaluating specific areas helps them to see progress has occurred. Examples of outcome criteria might be:

- Child states importance of holding parent's hand while crossing street.
- Parent states realistic expectations of 3-year-old.
- Mother reports she has prepared 4-year-old for new baby by next visit.

Nursing Assessment of Growth and Development of the Preschooler

Physical Growth

There is a definite change in body contour during the preschool years. The wide-legged gait, prominent lordosis, and protuberant abdomen of the toddler change to slimmer, taller, and much more childlike proportions. Contour changes are so definite that future body type— **ectomorphic** (slim body build) or **endomorphic** (large body build)—becomes apparent. At least 90% of brain growth is achieved: handedness is beginning to be obvious. A major step forward is the child's ability to learn extended language, which is affected not only by motor but by cognitive development. Children of this age who are exposed to more than one language or who live in a bilingual family have a unique opportunity to master two languages with relative ease because of this increased cognitive ability.

Lymphatic tissue begins to grow, particularly tonsils, and levels of IgG and IgA antibodies increase. These changes tend to make preschool illnesses more localized (an upper respiratory infection remains localized to the nose without systemic fever).

Physiologic splitting of heart sounds may be present for the first time on auscultation; innocent heart murmurs may be heard. Murmurs occur due to the changing size of the heart in reference to the thorax. The anteroposterior and transverse diameters of the chest reach adult proportions. Pulse rate decreases to about 85 bpm; blood pressure holds at about 100/60 mm Hg.

The bladder remains palpable above the symphysis pubis; voiding is frequent enough (9 to 10 times a day)

that play is interrupted and accidents may occur if the child becomes absorbed in an activity.

The child who earlier in life had an indeterminant longitudinal arch in the foot generally demonstrates a well-formed arch now. Muscles are noticeably stronger and make activities such as gymnastics possible. Many children this age exhibit **genu valgus** (knock-knees), which disappears with skeletal growth.

Weight, Height, and Head Circumference

Weight gain is slight during the preschool years. The average child gains only about 4.5 lb (2 kg) a year. Appetite remains as it was during the toddler years, which is considerably less than some parents would like or expect. Parents may bring their preschooler to the health care facility because they fear their child is losing weight. When the child's weight is plotted on a growth chart, however, it becomes evident that he or she is indeed putting on some weight; what parents were noticing was the age-appropriate change in body shape from rounded to slim. Nutritional needs of the preschooler are discussed in Chapter 34.

Height gain is also minimal during this period; only 2 to 3.5 inches (6 to 8 cm) a year on average. Head circumference is not routinely measured at physical assessments on children over 2 years of age (see Appendix E for averages).

Teeth

Children generally have all 20 of their deciduous teeth by 3 years of age. Rarely do new teeth erupt during the preschool period.

Developmental Milestones

Each year during the preschool period marks a major step forward in gross motor, fine motor, and language development. Play activities also change focus as the preschooler learns new skills and understands more about his or her world (Figure 31-1). Table 31-1 summarizes the major milestones of the period.

Language Development

A 3-year-old has a vocabulary of between 300 and 900 words. They are used to ask questions constantly, mostly "how" and "why" questions, such as "Why is snow cold? Does the dog sleep at night? What does your tongue do?" A child needs simple answers so that curiosity, vocabulary building, and questioning are encouraged and also because the depth of the child's understanding is often deceptive. For example, if a parent tells a child that shoes should go on with the buckles on the outside, the child may seem to understand, but he or she may return in a few minutes to ask, "Why do I have to go outside to put on my shoes?" Words with double and triple meanings can be truly confounding to children of

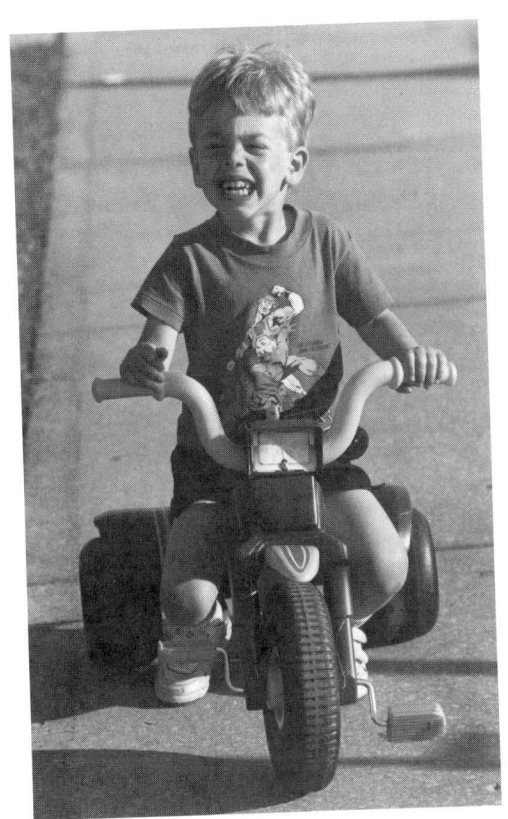

FIGURE 31-1
*Learning to ride a tricycle is a major milestone for the preschooler.
(Courtesy of Brian Smistek.)*

lives. They enjoy games that use imitation, such as playing house. If there are older siblings who can act as teachers, preschoolers play school very well even though they have not experienced it. They imitate what they see parents doing: eating meals, mowing the lawn, cleaning house, arguing, and so forth. Many preschoolers have imaginary friends (Lyytinen, 1991).

Four-year-olds divide their time between roughhousing and imitative play. Imaginary friends often exist until children begin school formally. Five-year-olds continue the rough-and-tumble play they participated in at age 4. Five-year-olds are also interested in group games that they have learned in a kindergarten or play group.

Emotional Development

Developmental Task: Initiative Versus Guilt

The developmental task for the preschool age child is to achieve a sense of initiative versus guilt (Erikson, 1986). The child with a well-developed sense of initiative has discovered that learning about new things is fun.

If children are criticized or punished for attempts at initiative, they develop a sense of guilt for wanting to try new activities or have new experiences. Those who leave the preschool period with guilt may carry it with them into new situations, such as starting school. They may even have difficulty later in life making decisions about everything from changing jobs to choosing an apartment, because they cannot envision that they are capable of solving associated problems.

Preschoolers need exposure to a wide variety of experiences and play materials so that they can learn as much about the world as possible. They are ready to reach outside their homes for new experiences, such as a trip to the zoo or playground (Figure 31-2), and are interested in seeing new places, for example, when they accompany the family on vacation. These types of experiences lead to increased vocabulary; preschoolers not only learn words, such as *giraffe, elephant,* and *bear,* but they learn to transfer them from abstract concepts to the objects to which they relate.

Preschoolers should have exposure to play materi-

this age. Four- and 5-year-olds continue to ask many questions. They enjoy participating in mealtime conversation and are able to describe something from their day in great detail.

Preschoolers are self-centered, so they define objects in relation to themselves (a key is not a metal object but "what I use to open a door," and a car is not a means of transportation but "what Mom uses to take me to school").

Play

Preschoolers do not need many toys. Their imaginations are keener than they will be at any other time in their

Table 31-1. *Summary of Preschool Growth and Development*

Age (yr)	Fine Motor	Gross Motor	Language	Play
3	Undresses self	Runs; climbs steps one at a time	Vocabulary of 300–900 words	Able to take turns; very imaginative
4	Draws a cross Can do simple buttons	Stands on one foot Constantly in motion; jumps; skips	Vocabulary of 1500 words	Pretending is major activity
5	Draws a 6-part man	Throws overhand	Vocabulary of 2100 words	Likes games with numbers or letters

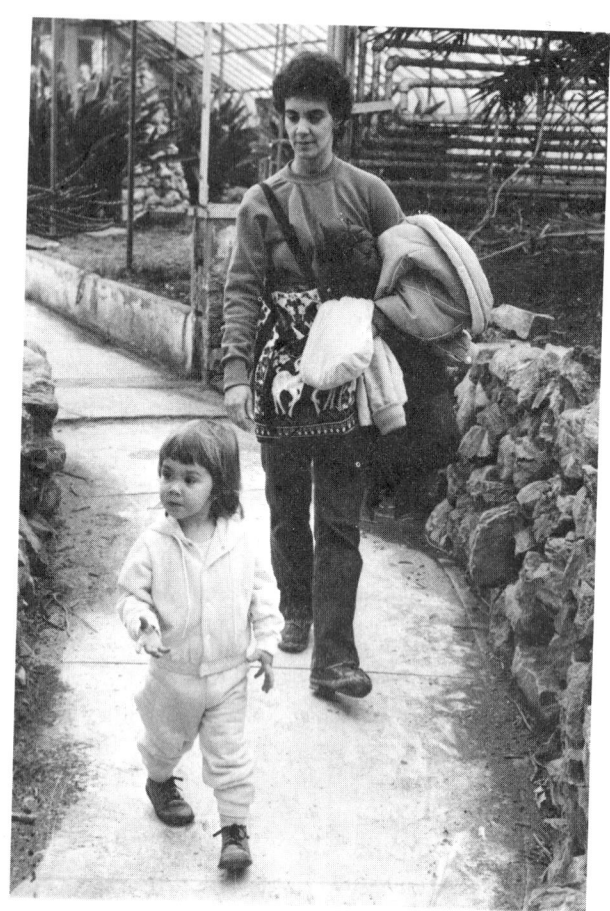

FIGURE 31-2
Preschoolers like exposure to new events and places. Here, a 3-year-old explores a park. (Courtesy of Brian Smistek.)

Imitation. Preschoolers need free rein to imitate the roles of the people around them. Again, role play should be fun and does not have to be accurate. If a child is a police officer and is busy putting out fires, or a firefighter and is stopping playmates from speeding, the fact that he is freely imitating a role is more important than the fact that he is absolutely certain of the adult role. If a parent is concerned that the child should separate these two roles accurately, it is usually best not to stop the play to do so. Rather, the next time they are driving past the fire station, the parent could explain that this is where firefighters work who put out fires or that the police station is where people work who make certain that other people drive safely.

Children generally imitate activities they see their parents performing at home. A young girl will set the table for breakfast, eat with her "husband," help clean off the table, and leave for work. A young boy might cook, pretend to feed a doll, and put the doll to bed as he has seen his father do with a younger sister. Many aspects of life in the 1990s prevent children from imitating adult roles. The pace of life is faster than ever before; parents find their weekend schedules so full with home projects that they overlook the need to take a preschooler to visit their work environment. Such visits are recommended, when possible, because they provide a visual context for the parent's job and let the child give form to such words as *photocopier, cash register,* and *file cabinet.* Another difficulty arises when a parent works in the city but lives in the suburbs or country an hour's train ride away. Taking the child to see the store or office then becomes a problem of scheduling and logistics.

Today, as many as 90% of mothers of childbearing age work outside the home at least part-time. Remind a mother to introduce her preschooler to her "other" self—as secretary, telephone repair person, or lawyer—in the same way that the child is exposed to the father's work side.

Fantasy. Preschoolers may become so intense about a fantasy role that they are afraid they have lost their own identity—that they have become "stuck" in their fantasies. Parents sometimes strengthen this feeling without realizing it: they (and you) must be careful in this regard. A preschooler, for example, may pretend that she is a white rabbit delivering Easter eggs. Her mother walks into the room, is aware of the game, and decides to participate. She says, "That's strange, I don't see Cindy anywhere. All I see is a white rabbit." Then she leaves the room. Cindy may be frightened that she has actually become a white rabbit. She worries that her mother will not fix dinner for her or will not want her to live in the house any more.

A better response for the mother would be to support the imitation—this is age-appropriate behavior and a good way of exploring roles—but help the child main-

als such as finger paints, soapy water to splash or blow into bubbles, mud to make pies, sand to build castles, and modeling clay or homemade dough to mold into figures and make into pretend cookies. These are messy activities, and many parents are not able to let a child indulge in them more than once a week, but any experience with free-form play is helpful.

Preschoolers have such active imaginations that they need little guidance in play. They smear both hands into clay or finger paint and create instinctively. Urge parents to support this kind of play and not try to take it over. If a parent draws a tree with finger paint, for example, and says, "Now you draw one," a child may decide it is no fun to finger paint. He knows that his tree will not look as good as his parent's. As he is not ready for competition, he will drop out of the activity rather than be shown up as inferior.

Preschoolers may make nothing recognizable out of clay or finger paint, preferring simply to handle the medium. As long as they enjoy the feel of the material, they do not need to make anything. Pressure to make things is not fun and can discourage their interest in learning.

tain a difference between pretend and real. She might say, "What a nice white rabbit you're pretending to be," thus supporting the fantasy and yet reassuring the child that she is still herself.

In a health care setting, it is particularly important that you let children know they are still recognizable. When examining the ears of a girl who thinks she is a rabbit, you can comment that her ears are all better again, rather than play to the make-believe with remarks about long, furry (rabbit) ears.

Oedipus and Electra Complexes

Although the development of Oedipus and Electra complexes may have been overstated by Freud because of gender biases, many children do appear to manifest such behavior (Robinson, 1993). **Oedipus complex** refers to the strong emotional attachment of a preschool boy to his mother; **Electra complex** is the attachment of a preschool girl to her father. Each child competes with the same-sex parent for the love and attention of the other parent. Parents who are not prepared for this behavior may feel hurt or rejected. For example, a daughter prefers to sit beside her father at the table or in the car; she asks her father to tuck her in at night. She is "Daddy's girl." The mother may feel left out of the family interaction when this happens. On the other hand, a boy will ask his mother for favors. He wants to sit beside her, to have her read to him, and to tuck him in for the night, and the father may feel left out.

Parents can be reassured that this phenomenon of competition and romance in preschoolers is normal. Parents may need help in handling feelings of jealousy and anger, particularly if the child is vocal in expressing feelings toward a parent. It is difficult for a mother to reply calmly to a 3-year-old daughter who is shouting at her, "I hate you! I only love Daddy!" Understanding this reaction is easier if the parent realizes that the child is providing a clue how to answer calmly—for example, "Well, I don't like to be shouted at, but I still love you."

Gender Roles

Preschoolers need exposure to an adult of the opposite gender so they can become familiar with opposite gender roles. Single parents should offer opportunities for their children to spend some time with adults other than themselves, perhaps an aunt or an uncle, for this exposure. A nursery school teacher may serve as this person. As most nursery school teachers are women, the mother may have to look elsewhere to find an adult male role model. If the child is hospitalized during the preschool period, a male nurse could help fill this role.

Children's gender-typical actions are strengthened by parents, strangers, nursery school teachers, other family members, and other children. Parents who do not want their child to grow up as they did, with a fixed role as a result of gender stereotyping, should be aware that they reinforce such attitudes by their actions as well as by their words. For example, a woman who won't balance a checkbook may be saying that math is not a woman's province; a man who will not do dishes no matter how many pile up in the kitchen is saying that managing a household is not a man's job.

Socialization

Because 3-year-olds are capable of sharing, they play with other children their age much more agreeably than do toddlers, which is a reason why the preschool period is a sensitive and critical time for socialization. Children who are exposed to other playmates have an easier time learning to relate to people than those, for instance, who are raised in a rural area where they never see other children of the same age (Figure 31-3).

Although 4-year-olds continue to enjoy play groups, they may become involved in arguments more, especially as they become more certain of their role in the group. This development, like so many others, may make parents worry a child is regressing. It is really forward movement, however, involving some testing and identification of their group role.

The 5-year-old begins to develop "best" friendships, perhaps on the basis of who he walks to school with or who lives closest to him. The elementary rule that an odd number of children don't play well together pertains to children at this age. Two or four will play; three or five will quarrel.

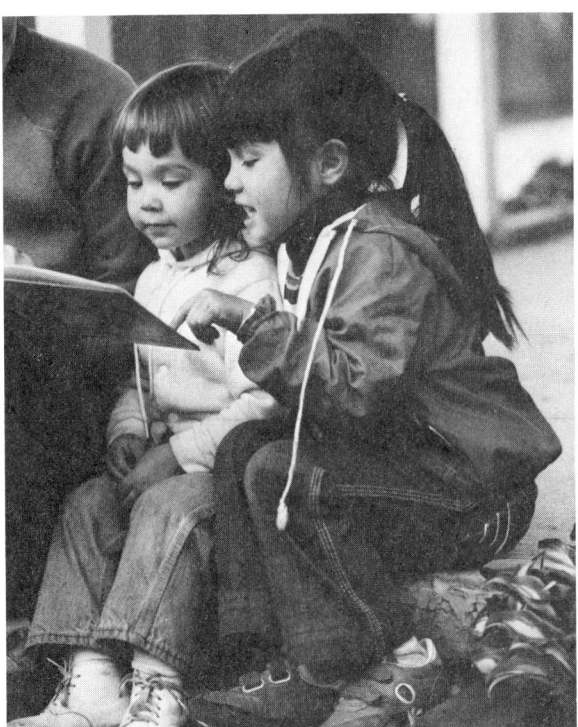

FIGURE 31-3
Preschoolers are interested in sharing activites with other children, such as listening to a story. (Courtesy of Brian Smistek.)

Cognitive Development

At age 3 years, cognitive development is still preoperational (Wadsworth, 1989). Although children at this period do enter a second phase called **intuitional thought,** they lack the insight to view themselves as others see them or put themselves in another's place. The preschooler is unable to make this kind of mental substitution; therefore he feels he is always right. He argues with the forcefulness that comes from knowing he is 100% correct. This is an important point for you to remember when explaining procedures to a preschooler. He cannot see your side of the situation; he cannot hurry because you must have something done by 10 o'clock; he cannot sit still just because you want him to.

Also, preschoolers are not yet aware of the property of **conservation.** This means that if they have two balls of clay of equal size, but one is squashed flatter and wider than the other, preschoolers will insist that the flatter one is bigger (because it is wider) or that the intact one is bigger (because it is taller). They are unable to see that only the form, not the amount, has changed. This inability to appreciate conservation has implications for working with preschoolers. Using the same theory, you will find that the preschooler cannot comprehend that a procedure done two separate ways is the same procedure. Thus, if the nurse before you told a child to turn on his right side and then his left side while his bed was made, you may have to allow him to turn these same ways, too.

Moral and Spiritual Development

Children of preschool age determine right from wrong based on their parents' rules. They have little understanding of the rationale for these rules or even whether the rules are consistent. If asked the question, "Why is it wrong for you to steal from your neighbor's house?" the average preschooler answers, "Because my mother says it's wrong." When pressed further, he justifies that conviction with, "It just is, that's all."

Because the preschooler depends on parents to supply rules for him, when faced with a new situation he has difficulty seeing that the rules he knows may also apply to a new situation ("Don't steal from stores" also applies to "Don't steal from a hospital").

Preschoolers begin to have an elemental concept of God if they have been provided some form of religious training. Belief in an outside force aids the development of conscience (Kohlberg, 1981); however, preschoolers tend to do good out of self-interest rather than because of strong spiritual motivation. Children this age enjoy the security of religious holidays, prayers, and grace said before meals, since these rituals can offer them the same reassurance that a familiar nursery rhyme read over and over does.

Planning and Implementation for Health Promotion of the Preschooler and Family

Promoting Preschooler Safety

As the preschooler broadens her horizons, safety issues also grow. By age 4, a child may project an attitude of independence and the ability to take care of her own needs. Part of this is pseudo-independence; she still needs supervision to be certain she does not injure herself or other children while roughhousing and to ensure that she does not stray too far from home. Her imitative interest in learning adult roles may lead her into exploring the blades of a lawn mover or an electric saw. She must be reminded repeatedly of automobile safety. Her thought "I want to play with Mary across the street" can be so quick and so intense that she will run into the middle of the street before she remembers "Watch out for cars" or "Don't cross the street."

Because he imitates adult roles so well, a child may imitate taking medicine if he sees family members doing so. A good rule for parents is never to take medicine in front of children. Safety points for the preschool period are summarized in the Focus on Family Teaching display.

Keeping Children Safe, Strong, and Free. The preschool years are not too early a time to educate children about the potential threat of harm from strangers or even how to address bullying behavior from people (children or adults) they know. This includes warning a child never to talk with or accept rides from strangers; how to call for help in an emergency (yelling or running to a designated neighbor's house if outside, or dialing 911 if near a phone); what police officers look like and that police officers are their friends, not their enemies; and that if children or adults ask them to keep secrets about anything that has made them uncomfortable, they should tell their parents or another trusted adult, even if they have promised to keep the secret.

It is often difficult for parents to impart this type of information to a preschooler, since parents can't imagine their children will ever be in such situations, nor do they want to terrify their children about the world around them. However, if discussed in a calm yet serious manner, children can begin to use the information to build safe habits that will help them later on when are old enough to walk home from school alone or play with their friends, unsupervised, at the playground.

Motor Vehicle and Bicycle Safety. With more and more cars being equipped with air bags and passive restraint systems, it has become easier for parents to make sure that their children are safely buckled up when rid-

Q. I have a 3-year-old who is very adventurous. What measures should I take to help prevent accidents?

A. Preschoolers are prone to accidents because they are so eager to explore. Here are some common safety measures to take:

Possible Accident	Prevention Measure
Motor vehicles	Maintain child in car seat; do not be distracted by child while driving.
	Do not allow preschooler to play outside unsupervised.
	Do not allow preschooler to operate electronic garage door.
	Teach safety with tricycle (look before crossing driveways; do not cross streets).
	Teach child to always hold hands with a grownup before crossing a street.
	Teach parking lot safety (hold hands with grownup; do not run behind cars that are backing up).
	Children should wear helmets when riding bicycles.
Falls	Supervise preschooler at playgrounds.
	Help child to judge safe distances for jumping or safe heights for climbing.
Drowning	Do not leave child alone in bathtub or near water.
	Teach beginning swimming.
Animal bites	Do not allow child to approach strange dogs.
	Supervise child's play with family pets.
Poisoning	Never present medication as a candy.
	Never take medication in front of a child.
	Never store food or substances in containers other than their own.
	Post telephone number of local poison control center by the telephone.
	Stock each first-aid box with syrup of ipecac, with proper instructions for administering.
	Teach child that medication is a serious substance and not for play.
Burns	Buy flame-retardant clothing.
	Turn handles of saucepans toward back of stove.
	Store matches in closed containers.
	Do not allow preschooler to help light birthday candles, fireplaces, etc. (fire is not fun or a "treat").
	Keep screen in front of a fireplace or heater.
Community safety	Teach preschooler that not all people are friends ("Do not talk to strangers or take candy from strangers").
	Define a stranger as someone child does not know, not someone odd looking.
	Teach child to say "no" to people whose touching he does not enjoy, including family members. (When a child is sexually abused, the offender is usually a family member or close family friend.)
General	Know whereabouts of preschooler at all times.
	Be aware that frequency of accidents is increased when parents are under stress. Special precautions must be taken at these times.
	Some children are more active, curious, and impulsive and therefore more vulnerable to accidents than others.

ing in the car. Many preschoolers outgrow their car seats during this period (when they reach 40 to 44 pounds), but they may still be too small for regular seat belts. The shoulder harness should not be worn if it goes across the child's face or throat. During this stage and until the child is large enough for the shoulder harness to fit properly, a booster seat is the safest method for restraining the child.

This is also the right age to promote bicycle safety (Wilson & Testani-Dufour, 1993). Head injuries are a major cause of death and injury to preschoolers, and bicycle accidents are among the major causes of such injuries. Some parents may have already purchased a helmet for the child when he was a toddler and riding in a bicycle seat. Once the child begins riding on his own, however, he will need a lighter safety helmet that has been approved for children his age and size. (ANSI and Snell Memorial Foundation are two organizations that have set safety standards for bicycle helmets.) Encourage parents who ride bicycles to demonstrate safe riding habits by wearing helmets as well. A parent who routinely wears her helmet may well prove to be the most compelling reason for the preschooler to wear his.

Promoting Development of the Preschooler in Daily Activities

The preschooler has often mastered the basic skills needed for most self-care activities, including self-feeding, dressing, washing (with supervision), and tooth-brushing (again, with supervision). Changes in nutritional needs, food preferences, and feeding habits are discussed in Chapter 34.

Dressing

Many 3-year-olds and most 4-year-olds are able to dress themselves except for difficult buttons, although there may be a conflict over what the child will wear. Preschoolers prefer bright colors or prints and may select items that do not match. As with other preschool activities, however, children need the experience of choosing their own clothes. One way for parents to solve the problem of mismatching is to fold together shirts and pants that go together so the child sees them as a set rather than individual pieces. If children insist on wearing mismatched clothes, parents should make no apologies for their appearance. A simple statement, such as "Mark chose his own clothes today," explains the situation. Anyone who understands preschoolers knows that the experience children gain in being able to select their own clothing is worth more than perfect appearance by adult standards.

Sleep

Many toddlers going through a negative phase resist naps no matter how tired they are. Preschoolers, on the other hand, are more aware of their needs; when they are tired, they often curl up on a couch or soft chair and fall asleep. Many preschoolers, particularly those who attend afternoon play groups or preschools, give up afternoon naps. Encourage parents to learn whether the school requires children to take a nap. If they rest there, the child may have some difficulty getting to sleep at the usual bedtime established at home.

Children in this age group continue to have problems with refusing to go to sleep and night waking. Preschoolers may have difficulty sleeping in a dark room and may need a night light when they did not need one before. This is a normal phenomenon because the preschooler's imagination is at a peak. A helpful suggestion for parents is to maintain enjoyable activities to reduce stress before bedtime.

Exercise

The preschool period is an active phase during which the child receives a great deal of exercise. Roughhousing is a good way of getting rid of tension and should be allowed as long as it does not become destructive or harmful. Also, preschoolers love games such as ring-around-the-rosy, London Bridge, or other more structured games that they were not ready for as toddlers.

Bathing

Although preschoolers certainly sit well in the bathtub, they should still not be left unsupervised at bathtime. They may decide to add more hot water and scald themselves or to practice swimming and slip and be unable to get their head out of the water. Most preschoolers enjoy soaking in the bathtub to get clean and enjoy having a bubble bath or playing with soap crayons. Some girls develop vulvar irritation (and perhaps bladder infection) from exposure to these products, however, so parents must use common sense in using them. Preschoolers do not clean their fingernails or ears well, so these areas often need "touching up" by a parent or older sibling.

Hair washing can be a problem. The preschooler is too heavy for a parent to hold over the sink to rinse hair. Children are also unable to close their eyes well enough or long enough (because they insist on opening them to see whether the parent is finished) to keep soap out while they have their hair rinsed in an upright position. Try washing hair in the tub and asking them to look at a toy hung from the ceiling. Use a shampoo that does not sting the eyes. If that doesn't help, parents may want to purchase a soap guard (plastic visor) to keep shampoo out of the eyes. Patience with this in-between age is the parent's greatest help, however.

Because preschoolers like to imitate adults, they begin to be interested in taking showers rather than baths as they see their parents doing. Although their children may not get too clean the few times they try showering, parents do not usually have to be concerned because most preschoolers shower only a few times, then return to tub soaking, which allows them to play with bath toys.

Preschoolers can wash and dry their hands perfectly adequately if the water faucet is regulated for them (again, so that they do not scald themselves with hot water). When possible, parents should turn down the temperature of the water heater to under 120°F. Children this age are not paragons of neatness, however, and may clean hands at the expense of a bathroom towel.

Care of Teeth

If independent toothbrushing was not started as a daily practice during the infant or toddler years, it should be during the preschool years. The child should continue to drink fluoridated water or receive a prescribed oral fluoride supplement if this is not provided in the water supply. Supplemental fluoride application treatments every 6 months are also beneficial in preventing decay.

One good toothbrushing period a day, with parents helping them use dental floss to clean between the teeth, is often more effective than more frequent half-hearted brushings. Although many preschoolers do well brushing their own teeth, parents must check that all tooth surfaces are cleaned. They should floss the teeth, because this is a skill beyond a preschooler's motor ability.

Toothbrushing is generally well accepted by preschoolers because it imitates adults. Electric or battery-operated toothbrushes are favorites because of the adult responsibility involved in handling them. Children must be supervised when using an electric toothbrush and must be taught not to use it or any other electrical appliance near a basin of water.

Encouraging children to eat apples, carrots, celery, chicken, or cheese for snack foods rather than candy or sweets is yet another way to attempt to prevent tooth decay. When a child is introduced to chewing gum, it should be the sugar-free variety.

Children should have made a first visit to a dentist by 2 years of age for evaluation of tooth formation. Because this age usually shows no caviues, this should have been a pain-free visit and implanted the idea that dentists like to help rather than hurt. If parents did not take the child for this previously, it should be done during the preschool period.

It is important that deciduous teeth be preserved to protect the dental arch. If teeth are pulled as a result of disease, the permanent teeth can drift out of position or the jaw may not grow enough to accommodate them.

Night Grinding. **Bruxism**, or grinding the teeth at night (usually during sleep) is a habit of many young children. Teeth grinding may be a way of "letting go," similar to body rocking, that children do for a short time each night to release tensions and allow themselves to

fall asleep. Children who grind their teeth extensively may have anxiety of a greater degree than the average child. Children with cerebral palsy may do it because of spasticity of jaw muscles. If the grinding is extensive, the crowns of the teeth can become abraded. It is possible for the condition to advance to such an extent that the tooth nerves are exposed. If the problem seems to stem from anxiety, identifying and relieving the source of the anxiety is essential for treatment. If some damage is evident, refer families to a pedodontist so the teeth can be evaluated, repaired (capped), and conserved.

Promoting Healthy Family Functioning

Some parents who enjoyed maintaining a rhythm of care for an infant and allowed for ritualistic behavior of a toddler may have difficulty being the parents of a preschooler, because more flexibility and creativity are required. Others come into their own as the parents of a preschooler. They delight in encouraging imaginative games and play.

A major parental role during this time is to encourage vocabulary development. One way to do this is to read aloud to the child; another is to answer questions so that the child sees language as an organized system of communication. Answering a preschooler's questions is often difficult because the questions are frequently philosophical, for example, "Why is grass green?" The child may listen to an explanation of chlorophyll but then repeat the question, regardless of the clarity of the explanation, because the parent underestimated the extent of the question. The child did not want to know what makes grass green, but why, philosophically, it is not red or blue or yellow. The obvious answer to that is "I don't know." Many parents, however, have trouble making such an admission to a child. Those who are confident can give this answer without feeling threatened. Parents who are less sure of themselves may feel extremely uncomfortable when they do not know the answers to a 4-year-old's questions.

Discipline

Preschoolers have definite opinions on things such as what they want to eat, where they want to go, and what they want to wear. This may bring them into opposition with their parent's opinions of what they should eat or wear, or where they should go. It is important for parents to guide a child through these struggles without discouraging the child's right to have an opinion. A technique commonly recommended is the use of "time out." The child has to sit by himself or herself without talking for a short designated time period, such as 1 minute per year of age or no more than 10 minutes. The technique of time out allows parents to discipline without using physical punishment. It allows the child to learn a new way of behavior without extreme stress.

Parental Concerns Associated With the Preschool Period

Common Health Problems of the Preschooler

The mortality of children during the preschool years is low and becoming increasingly lower every year as more infectious diseases are preventable. The major cause of death is automobile accidents, followed by poisoning and falls (DHHS, 1990).

The number of minor illnesses in preschoolers is exceptionally high, more than that of any other age. There is no appreciable difference in the distribution of illnesses between girls and boys; a high percentage of them involve the respiratory tract. Colds, ear infections, and flu abound. Children who live in homes in which parents smoke have a higher incidence of ear (otitis media) and respiratory infections than others (Kligman & Narce-Valente, 1990). Children who attend day care or preschool programs have an increased incidence of, most notably, diarrhea (Alexander et al., 1990).

This may be the parents' first experience with illness in a child; many find it easier to cope with major illnesses than with constant minor ones. Thus, stress may arise between parent and child, an almost monthly battle of "Stay indoors until your cold is better," conflict over day care, or frequent whining and clinging behavior because the child's stomach is upset. Such illnesses may cause parents to perceive a child as sickly or not able to cope with everyday life. Whereas parents encouraged independence before, they may now begin to overprotect, to shelter to too great a degree. They need reassurance that frequent minor illnesses are common in preschoolers. As they become more experienced in handling these conditions, their perception of whether or not an illness is a problem will change.

Table 31-2 shows the usual health maintenance schedule for preschoolers. Table 31-3 lists problems that parents may have in evaluating a preschooler's illness.

Common Fears of the Preschooler

Fear of the Dark. The tendency to fear the dark is heightened by the child's vivid imagination: a stuffed toy by daylight becomes a threatening monster in the dark. Children may awaken screaming if they are roused by a

---

Table 31-2. *Health Maintenance Schedule, Preschool Period*

Area of Focus	Methods	Frequency
Assessment		
Developmental milestones	History, observation	Every visit
	Formal Denver Developmental Screening Test (DDST II)	Prior to start of school
Growth milestones	Height, weight plotted on standard growth chart; physical examination	Every visit
Hypertension	Blood pressure	Every visit
Nutrition	History, observation; height/weight information	Every visit
Parent–child relationship	History, observation	Every visit
Behavior problems	History, observation	Every visit
Vision and hearing defects	History, observation	Every visit
	Formal Preschool E and audiometer testing	Prior to start of school
Dental health	History, physical examination	Every visit
Tuberculosis	Tine test	Prior to start of school
Immunizations		
Diphtheria, pertussis, and tetanus; trivalent oral poliomyelitis	Check history and past records; inform caregiver about any risks and side-effects; administer immunization in accordance with health care agency policies	Prior to start of school
Rubeola		Prior to start of school
Anticipatory Guidance		
Preschool care	Active listening and health teaching	Every visit
Expected growth and developmental milestones before next visit		Every visit
Accident prevention	Counseling about street and personal safety	Every visit
Problem-solving		
Any problems expressed by caregiver during course of the visit	Active listening and health teaching regarding temper tantrums, toilet training	Every visit

Table 31-3. *Parental Difficulties Evaluating Illness in the Preschool Child*

Difficulty	Helpful Suggestions for Parents
Evaluating seriousness of illness or condition	Preschoolers are eager to please and tend to answer all questions such as, "Does your stomach hurt?" with a yes. Observing the child for signs of illness—refusing to eat, holding an arm stiffly, having to go to the bathroom frequently—is often more productive as an evaluation technique.
Evaluating bowel and bladder problems	Preschoolers are independent in toilet habits for the first time, so parents do not have diaper contents to evaluate. Frequent trips to the bathroom, rubbing the abdomen, and holding genitals are the usual signs of bowel or bladder dysfunction.
Evaluating nutritional intake	Preschoolers begin to eat away from home at friends' houses or at day care, or to stay overnight with grandparents, so parents do not observe daily food intake as accurately as before. Observing whether the child is growing and active is better than monitoring any 1 day's food intake.
Evaluating bed-wetting	Many preschoolers continue to have occasional enuresis at night until school age. If other signs are present—pain, low-grade fever, listlessness—the child should have a urine culture, as persistent bed-wetting can indicate a low-grade urinary tract infection.
Evaluating activity vs hyper-activity	Many lay magazines have articles on hyperactivity in children. Parents often wonder whether their active child is truly hyperactive. As a rule of thumb, if a child can sit through a meal (when he is hungry), watch a half-hour television show (that is his favorite), or sit still while his favorite story is read to him, he is not hyperactive.
Age-specific diseases to be aware of	Preschool age is a time for vision and hearing assessment. For the first time the child is able to be tested by a standard chart or by audiometry.
	Urinary tract infections tend to occur with a high frequency in preschool-age girls.
	Language assessment should be done if the child is not able to make his wants known by complete, articulated sentences by age 3 (exceptions are transposing *w* for *r* and broken fluency: "I want-want-want to go").

nightmare. They may be reluctant to go to bed or to go to sleep by themselves unless a light is on.

If parents are prepared for this fear and understand that it is a phase of growth, they will be better able to cope with it. It is generally helpful if they monitor the stimuli their children are exposed to, especially around bedtime. This includes television, adult discussions, and frightening stories. Parents are sometimes reluctant to leave a child's light on at night because they do not want to cater to the fear. Burning a dim nightlight, however, may solve the problem and costs only pennies. Children who awake terrified and screaming need reassurance that they are safe, that whatever was chasing them was a dream and is not in their room. They may require an understanding adult to sit on their bed until they can fall back to sleep again. Most preschoolers do not remember in the morning that they had such a dream; they remember for a lifetime that they received comfort when they needed it (see the Nursing Care Plan).

If parents take sensible precautions against fear of the dark or nightmares and a child continues to have this kind of disturbance every night, it may be a reaction to undue stress. In these instances, the source of the stress should be investigated. Giving sleep medication to counteract the sleep disturbance does not help solve the basic problem, so is rarely recommended. Fear of the dark can become intensified in a hospital setting and requires careful planning to relieve.

Fear of Mutilation. Fear of mutilation is significant during the preschool age. That it exists is revealed by the intense reaction of the child to even a simple injury such as falling and scraping a knee (see the Focus on Nursing Research box). The child cries not only from the pain but also from the sight of the injury. Preschoolers often lift a bandage to peek at a surgical incision to see if healthy healing is taking place underneath it. They dislike invasive procedures, such as needlesticks, rectal temperature assessment, otoscopic examination, or having a nasogastric tube passed into their stomach (Kuttner, 1991).

Fear of Separation or Abandonment. Fear of separation continues to be a major concern for preschoolers. Their sense of time is still so distorted that they are not comforted by assurances such as "Mommy will pick you up from preschool at noon." Their sense of distance is also limited, making a statement such as "I'll be just next door" not reassuring. Their imagination is so keen that they feel they are being deserted when they are not.

Caution parents to be sensitive to such fears when they talk about missing children or if they have their preschooler's fingerprints taken for identification. A child whose chief fear is that he will be abandoned or kidnapped may not hear that fingerprints are being taken to keep him safe, only that he might be taken away from his parents.

Karen is a 3½-year-old girl. The following is a nursing care plan designed for her.

Assessment: Three-year-old girl whose father is concerned because she appears "rangy" and uncoordinated for her age. Father reports she can't tie her shoes as yet, although her older brother could at the same age. She prefers roughhousing with the boy next door rather than playing with dolls. Child is afraid father will not pick her up after day care; cries if he is not there immediately. Often wakes at night screaming because of a bad dream. Father admits feeling frustrated by own lack of sleep. Children live with father following divorce; father admits to having difficult time raising children alone, "especially a girl." Father works full-time; Karen spends day (7 to 3) at day care center; 7-year-old brother attends school. Weight: 14 kg (20th percentile); height: 95 cm (50th percentile). Hematocrit: 39%. Denver Developmental Screening Test (DDSTII) results are within normal limits.

Nursing Diagnosis: Parental anxiety related to lack of knowledge about variations in normal growth and development among children

Defining Characteristic: Father reports concerns about child's developmental progress.

Goal: Father will voice confidence about child's progress and abilities as expected for age by next visit.

Outcome Criteria: Father states that he understands that Karen's growth and development are within normal limits; is able to list skills she has mastered as well as those she is practicing.

Nursing Orders	**Rationale**
1. Review normal fine and gross motor range of accomplishments of preschoolers and emphasize that it is not expected for a 3-year-old to tie shoes.	1. Parent needs information about developmental milestones and range of normal.
2. Explain results of DDSTII to father.	2. Knowing that his daughter has tested within normal limits may help dispel his anxiety about her abilities.
3. Explore other areas that possibly distress parent; anticipate further guidance needed.	3. Parents, even those with other children, profit greatly from some discussion of what they can expect to happen next in their child's growth.

(continued)

A hospital admission or going to a new school often brings a child's fear of separation to the forefront. Preschoolers should be thoroughly prepared for these experiences so that they may survive them in sound mental health.

Behavior Problems

Telling Tall Tales. Stretching stories to make them more interesting is a problem frequently encountered in this age group. It arises from the child's overactive imagination. Following a trip to the zoo, for example, if you ask a child of this age a question such as "What happened today?," the child perceives that you want something exciting to have happened, so might answer "A bear jumped out of his cage and ate up the boy next to me." This is not lying, but merely supplying an expected answer. Caution parents not to encourage this kind of storytelling, and instead help the child separate fact from fiction by saying "That's a good story, but now tell me what really happened." This conveys the idea that the child has not told the truth, yet does not squash her imagination or initiative.

Imaginary Friends. Many preschoolers have an imaginary friend who plays with them. They tell a parent to "wait for Eric" or "set a place at the table for Lucy." Although imaginary friends are a normal, creative part of the preschool years and can be constructed by children who are surrounded by real playmates as well as by those who have few friends, parents may find them disconcerting. If so, ask parents to make sure that their child has exposure to real playmates. As long as the

Nursing Diagnosis: Fear of abandonment related to normal developmental trait of preschool period

Defining Characteristic: Child voices fear of abandonment.

Goal: Child will demonstrate reduced fear by next visit.

Outcome Criteria: Father reports that child does not appear as fearful after school, and waking at night has decreased to 1 time per week.

Nursing Orders	*Rationale*
1. Review with parent that fear of abandonment is a common preschool fear.	1. Reassures parent that his daughter is experiencing a normal preschool phenomenon, not something he might be responsible for.
2. Review with father specific measures to take to help reduce fear. a. Assure Karen that father will pick her up daily; will telephone center if there is any problem. b. Urge father to use nightlight; limit frightening stimuli close to bedtime. c. Urge father to spend time on weekends or in evening with daughter to build better and more secure parent–child relationship.	2. Ending the visit with specific measures to help reduce child's fear will give the father some confidence about his ability to address this problem and help his daughter.

imaginary playmates don't take center stage in a child's mind and prevent him from socializing with other children, they should not pose a problem and often leave as quickly as they come. In the meantime, they may provide an outlet for the child to express his innermost feelings or serve as a handy scapegoat for behavior about which the child has some conflict (Schuster & Ashburn, 1991).

Parents can help their preschooler to separate fact from fantasy by saying "I know Eric isn't real, but if you want to pretend, I'll set a place for him." This response helps the child to understand what is real and what is made up, yet does not restrict imagination or creativity.

Difficulty Sharing. Sharing is a concept that first comes to be understood around the age of 3 years. Prior to this, children engage in parallel play (two children need two toys and two spaces to play, because they cannot pass one toy back and forth or play together). Around 3 years of age, children begin to understand that some things are theirs, some belong to others, and some can belong to both. For the first time they are able to stand in line to wait for a drink, interact at a sandbox, and share a box of crayons. Sharing does not come easily, however; children who are ill or under stress have even greater difficulty with it.

In relation to this, preschoolers must have experience in learning property rights: "This is my private drawer and no one touches what is in it except me." "That is your dresser top and no one touches the things on it but you." "A shovel is ours and can be used by everyone playing in the sandpile." Defining limits and

FOCUS ON NURSING RESEARCH

What Is the Effect of Decorative Adhesive Bandages on Pain Intensity in Preschoolers?

As imagination is at its peak in the preschool child, it would seem that after a painful experience such as a fingerstick, a simple distraction technique such as applying a brightly colored decorative bandage should be able to soothe a child and decrease the amount of pain felt. To investigate if this is so, three nurse researchers asked 50 children ages 3 to 6 years who were having fingersticks for preoperative or diagnostic tests in an outpatient department to rate their pain immediately after a fingerstick for blood and then again after the application of an adhesive bandage.

Findings of the study indicated that the sight of blood increased the child's pain intensity rating; and the intervention of the attractive bandage was not sufficient to decrease the perceived pain intensity.

This is an important study in that it reveals the fright and pain children feel from even simple procedures and how such pain must be taken seriously by health care providers.

Johnston, C. C., Stevens, B., & Arbess, G. (1993). The effect of the sight of blood and use of decorative adhesive bandages on pain intensity ratings by preschool children. *Journal of Pediatric Nursing, 8,* 147.

exposing the child to these three categories (mine, yours, ours) can teach him or her to separate out which objects belong to which category.

Most parents become concerned if their child does not share readily. They can be reassured that this is a difficult concept to grasp and that, as with most skills, preschoolers need practice to understand it.

Regression. Some preschoolers, generally in relation to stress, revert to behavior they previously outgrew, such as thumb-sucking, negativism, loss of bladder control, or inability to separate from their parents. Although the stress that causes this may take many forms, it is usually the result of such things as a new baby in the family, a new school experience, marital difficulties between the parents, or separation caused by hospitalization.

If parents understand that regression in these circumstances can be normal, that the child's thumb-sucking is no different from the parent's reaction to stress (smoking many cigarettes, nail-biting, overeating), it is easier for them to accept and understand. Obviously, removing the stress is the best way to help the child discontinue this behavior. The stresses mentioned, however, are not easily removed. New babies cannot

be returned; irreparable marriages cannot be patched together; and hospitalizations do occur.

Techniques for minimizing stress of hospitalization for preschoolers are discussed in Chapter 35. Children's reactions to severe and prolonged stress are discussed in Chapter 54. The child undergoing less severe stress must be assured that although situations are changing, the important aspects of her life—that someone still loves her, someone will continue to take care of her—are not. Thumb-sucking or other manifestations of stress are best ignored; calling them to the child's attention merely causes more stress, because it makes the child aware that she is not pleasing her parents in addition to experiencing the primary stress.

Sibling Rivalry. Jealousy of a brother or sister may first become evident during the preschool period, partly because this is the first time that children have enough vocabulary to express how they feel (know a name to call) and partly because preschoolers are more aware of family roles and how responsibilities at home are divided. For many children this is also the time when a brother or sister is born.

A firstborn child is rarely allowed the privileges of a second child. The parents are untried, unsure of how far they should let the child venture or what level of responsibility the child can accept. The firstborn serves as the trial run for all the children who come after. This phenomenon can lead to sibling rivalry, because preschool children sense that a younger sibling is allowed behavior that is not tolerated in them. They are little appeased by the explanation that "Leslie is a baby."

To give them security and help promote their self-esteem, preschoolers should be given a private drawer or box for their things that parents or other children do not touch. This can help defend them against younger children who do not appreciate their property rights.

Preparing for a New Sibling

Preschoolers must be prepared for a new baby's coming just as for all new anticipated experiences. There is no fast rule for when this preparation should begin, but it should be prior to the time when the child begins to feel the difference the new baby will make. This is perhaps when the mother first begins to look pregnant. It is certainly before parents begin to make physical preparations for the new child. It is always less frightening for a child of any age to understand why things are happening, no matter how distasteful they may be, than to hear people whispering or having parents obviously evading the issue. The unknown is something to fear, whereas a definite event can be faced and conquered.

The meaning of a bed to a preschool child cannot be underestimated. It is security, consistency, and "home." If the preschooler has been sleeping in a crib that is to be used for the baby, it is usually best if he is moved to a bed about 3 months in advance of the birth, with the announcement that he is sleeping in a new bed because he is a big boy. The fact that he is growing up is a better reason for such a move than because a new brother or sister wants the old bed. The latter is surely the route to sibling rivalry and jealousy.

If the child is to start preschool or day care, she should do so either before the baby is born or 2 or 3 months afterward, if possible. That way, she can perceive starting school as a result of her maturity and not because she is being pushed out of the house by the new child.

If the mother will be hospitalized for the birth, she should be certain that the child is prepared for this separation in advance. This preparation must be done in advance, because the mother is likely to go to the hospital during the night, and the child deserves better than to wake in the morning, find mother gone, and be expected to be happy that she has a new brother. Some communities offer preparation-for-birth classes for preschoolers, the same as for parents, or include children in adult preparation courses (Spadt et al., 1990).

Mothers should try to maintain contact with their preschooler during the short time they are hospitalized for birth. Some preschoolers may react very coldly to their mothers, turning their head away and refusing to come to them after such a separation. This is a reaction not to the new baby but to the separation, the same phenomenon that may occur when a child returns home after being hospitalized (see Chapter 35).

When the baby is brought home from the hospital, it is helpful if someone other than the mother can bring the baby inside, so that she can devote her attention to greeting her older child. The new baby should be put to bed with as little fuss as possible, and time should be spent with the preschooler (and older children) renewing relationships. It is helpful when friends and family visit the new baby if they all spend some special time with the preschooler. It is considerate of those who bring gifts to bring a small one for the preschooler as well. It is not necessary or wise, however, for the preschooler to receive a gift every time the baby does. Parents who begin this practice during the preschool years will find themselves actually building sibling rivalry rather than preventing it, because thereafter children will expect equal gifts. It is better for the child to help open gifts and participate in giving than to receive presents herself. It can be explained to her that it is literally the baby's birthday and on the preschooler's birthday she will receive gifts, too.

An occasional preschooler is able to voice her attitude toward a new baby: "Can we take him back now?" Most are unable to do this, however, and pocket their emotions inside and manifest them as thumb-sucking, bed wetting, stammering, and night terrors. Don't ask preschoolers a question such as "Do you like your new brother?" It is better to express a feeling such as "New babies cry a lot. It's hard to get used to that, isn't it?" It is reassuring for a preschooler to realize that she is not unique, that what bothers her bothers others, too, and that what she is facing—this strange uncomfortable feeling of jealousy—others have faced as well.

Urge parents to be certain that they provide special time for the preschooler during each day, so that when they say "Mother and Daddy love you just the same," it seems real. This might be a quiet time for talking or reading. Because a great deal of jealousy occurs when the baby is being fed, the mother might be able to read to the preschooler while she nurses the baby or tell stories that are so well known she does not need to turn pages. Some children enjoy feeding a doll while a parent feeds the baby or giving a doll a bath while the baby has his. Ask pregnant women what kind of preparation they are making for their other children; ask the mother of a new baby how everything is working out. Most parents find that the problem of jealousy is bigger than they anticipated and welcome a few suggestions about how to provide more time for their preschooler during the day and which activities a preschooler would especially enjoy (Figure 31-4).

Sex Education

Children during the preschool age become acutely aware of the difference between boys and girls, possibly

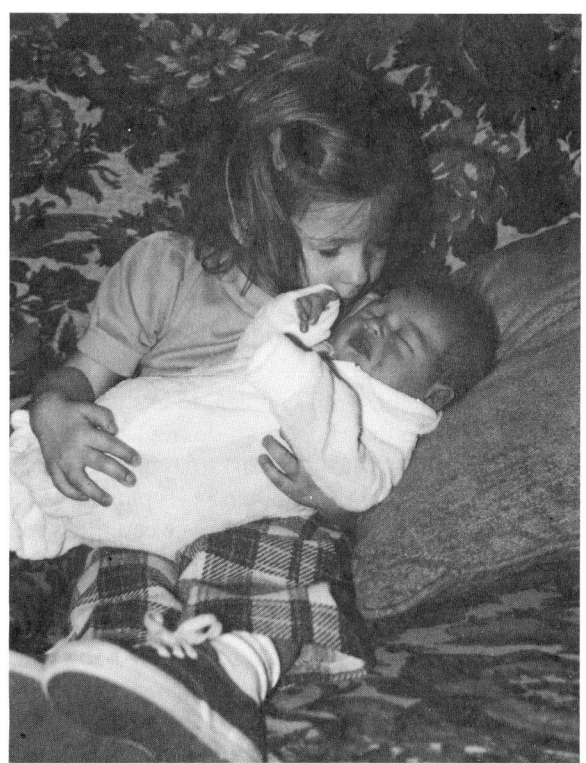

FIGURE 31-4
A preschooler greets a new baby sister. The situation may not always be this welcoming because of natural sibling rivalry.

because it is a normal progression in development, possibly because this may be the first time in their lives they are exposed to the genitalia of the opposite sex. They watch while a new brother or sister has diapers changed, they see other children using the bathroom at a preschool, or they see a parent nude.

Preschoolers' questions about genital organs are simple and fact finding, for example, "Why does Bobby look like that?" or "How does Judy pee?" Explanations should be just as simple: "Boys look different from girls. The different part is called a penis." It is important for parents to not convey that these body parts are never to be talked about, so that sexual questions are not suppressed. Occasionally, girls attempt to void standing up as they have seen boys doing; boys may try sitting down to void.

Preschoolers may engage in masturbation while watching TV or being read to or before they fall asleep at night. The frequency may increase under stress, as does thumb-sucking. If observing the child doing this bothers parents, suggest that they explain to the child that certain things are done in some places but not in others. Children can relate to this kind of direction without feeling inhibited, just as they can accept the fact that they use a bathroom in private or eat only at the table. Calling unnecessary attention to the act can increase anxiety and cause increased, not decreased, activity.

An important part of sex education for preschoolers is helping them learn rules to help them avoid sexual abuse. They are also taught that they do not have to allow anyone to touch their body unless they agree it is all right (see Box 32-1).

Because this may be the first time a new brother or sister comes into the family, it is also the most likely time for questions such as "Where do babies come from?" Because the child is asking a simple fact-finding question, a simple factual answer is best: "Babies grow in a special place in a mother's body called a uterus." It is better to use this term rather than "tummy" so that children do not envision babies and food all mixed together in their mother's stomach (Figure 31-5).

It is so natural for preschoolers to ask about where babies come from that those who do not ask are exceptions. Preschoolers who don't ask may be reticent because they sense from a preliminary exploratory question that the subject is closed. A parent could introduce the subject by visiting a new baby in the neighborhood with the child or pointing out a neighbor who is pregnant. The birth of kittens or puppies may also offer the chance to introduce the subject. If the new baby will be born at a birthing center or at home, many parents allow preschoolers to watch the birth of a new brother or sister. Encourage parents to prepare children well for this experience or else the sight of their mother in pain and the wonder of birth may be overwhelming for them.

Preschool children generally do not ask how babies

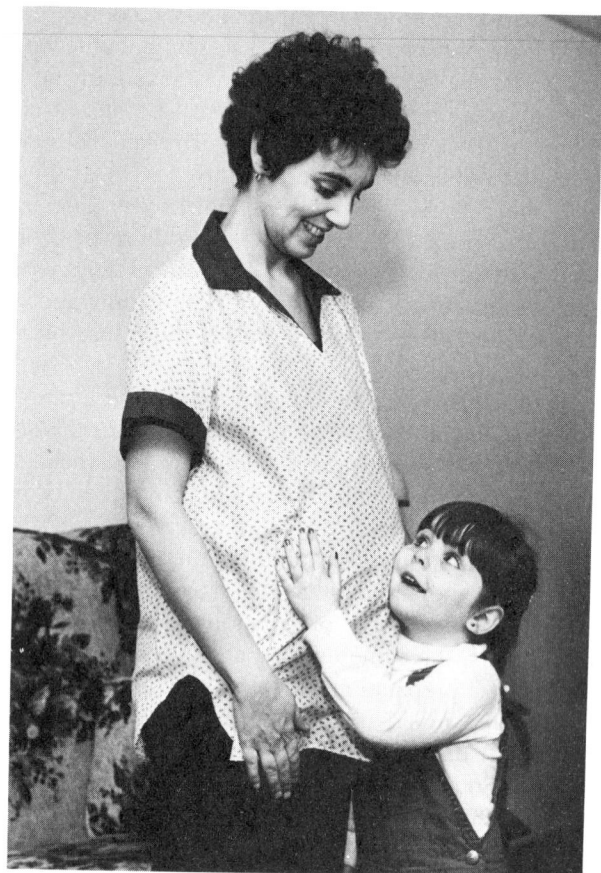

FIGURE 31-5
Preschool children are interested in learning where babies grow and have beginning sexual awareness. (Courtesy of Brian Smistek.)

get inside mothers to start growing or how babies get out at the end of the process. Should they ask, a suitable explanation might be, "When a woman and a man love each other and decide they want a baby, the man plants a seed inside the woman. The man's seed and the woman's seed grow together in the special place inside the mother into a new baby." Some parents prefer to say "God plants a seed." This answer may leave preschool boys feeling cheated that men have such a little role in this wondrous process. Perhaps a compromise statement would be "God helps the man plant a seed." If preschoolers ask how the baby gets out, an answer might be "The woman goes to the hospital and the doctor or nurse helps the baby get out from the vagina."

Many new books for children explain where babies come from, including descriptions of sexual relations and orgasm. These are helpful for parents to read to the child to increase understanding.

Choosing a Preschool or Day Care Center

The terms *day care center, preschool,* and *nursery school* are often used interchangeably—so often that parents cannot depend on the name of a school to define its structure. Traditionally, the day care center is a facility whose main purpose is to provide child care while parents work or are otherwise occupied. The preschool or nursery school is dedicated to stimulating children's sense of creativity and initiative and introducing them to new experiences and social contacts they would not ordinarily receive at home. Headstart programs and many modern day care centers can achieve both functions. Peer exposure appears to have a positive effect on preschoolers. Those who have learned to be comfortable in a group approach school comfortably and ready to learn; children who have played only infrequently in groups during the preschool age are forced into this new situation in kindergarten or first grade. They may be so busy adjusting to this gross concept that they are left behind in finer components. The effect of early interaction in groups can be demonstrated throughout life as well. Persons who are gregarious, interact comfortably with persons around them, and compete—and society is competitive—generally had early peer exposure.

If there are other 3- or 4-year-olds in the neighborhood with whom the child has almost daily contact and if some parent can supervise organized play and projects (providing peer interaction, in which working together is the key), a preschool program may not be necessary.

On the other hand, if all the neighborhood children are either older or younger or there is only one other child available to play with during the day, a preschool experience will probably be beneficial. Parents with large families point out that their child gets ample exposure to groups, that every meal is a "group session." This is not a peer group, however. Older siblings give in to the 3- or 4-year-old, and younger siblings are not capable of peer competition. This situation does not offer the same experience that preschool does.

Parents need to investigate preschools or day care centers carefully before they enroll their child in one. Guidelines to aid parents in their assessment of day care centers are shown in Table 31-4.

To continue to evaluate the experience for the child, urge parents to make a habit of asking children regularly what happened at school, what they learned, and the names of new friends. For the remainder of the growing years, schools will have important effects on the child's development. Parents must take an active role in providing input into education to influence what and how their child learns.

Day care centers are often blamed for the spread of infectious disease among the 5-and-under population and for sexual abuse (Kelley et al., 1993). Bringing together children from many different homes to one setting each day does increase the risk of spreading contagious disease. Most illnesses are spread through fecal–oral and respiratory transmission (Pauley & Gaines, 1993). For instance, some day care centers where infants as well as older children are enrolled have a high preva-lence of hepatitis A infection, which is caused in part by changing diapers on a table that is not washed after each use. The disease may be subclinical in the preschooler, but other members of the preschooler's family may develop overt symptoms as the illness spreads. Preschoolers may also develop frequent upper respiratory infections or gastrointestinal illnesses from a preschool or day care setting (Reves & Pickering, 1990). Outbreaks of cytomegalovirus and human parvovirus (fifth disease) make working in such centers a particular hazard to pregnant women (Gillespie et al., 1990).

Preparing the Child for School

At the end of the preschool period, children will begin a formal school experience. Parents may wonder whether their child is old enough for this, especially if the child's birthday is late in summer or early fall. Parents are well advised to discuss their concern with school officials to determine whether the child should be registered for kindergarten or delayed for a year. As school will involve a great deal of a child's time and influence his or her future greatly, parents should take time to prepare a preschooler for the experience.

Basic to this preparation is the parent's attitude. If school is always discussed as something to look forward to, as an adventure that will be satisfying and rewarding, a child will begin to perceive early on that it will be a positive experience. If school is presented as a punishment ("Wait until you get into first grade—your teacher will make you sit up and behave"), there can be little delight in anticipating it.

Some parents may have to change their child's daily routine a few months in advance of beginning school to accustom him or her to waking earlier and going to bed earlier, especially if they have encouraged the child to sleep late in the morning. School itself has so many new components that it is wise to try to eliminate as many distractions as possible.

If the child is to ride a bus to school, a parent might try to take the child on a municipal bus (if one exists in their community) as an introduction to this form of transportation. If the child is to walk, a trial walk is in order. In either instance, safety should be stressed: "Don't walk behind buses because the driver can't see you" and "Wait for the crossing guard to help you cross streets."

If the child will be required to take a lunch to school, the parent can introduce her to this new experience by preparing a school lunch at home some noon. Wrapping her usual sandwich in paper and serving soup in a Thermos will eliminate another strange experience. If the child is to purchase lunch at school, she can play "cafeteria" at home. A parent could serve a meal buffet-style and let her practice walking from one dish to another and selecting what she wants.

Some kindergartens suggest that the child know

Table 31-4. *Questions to Use in Evaluating Day Care Centers*

Question	Finding
Management	
How long has the center been in operation?	Length of operation does not necessarily indicate quality, but it allows you to locate other parents who have used the center to ask about their experience there.
Is the center licensed, registered, approved, or inspected by the appropriate agency?	Ask in your local community what agency has the responsibility for licensing day care centers. If not licensed, its quality is suspected.
What are the qualifications of staff members?	If staff members are teachers, more learning activities will be provided; staff should be qualified to perform cardiopulmonary resuscitation.
Is there a fast turnover rate of staff?	A fast turnover rate means little continuity of care will be provided (and probably suggests dissatisfaction with center administration).
What is the child–staff ratio?	A ratio of 3 or 4 children to 1 staff member provides time for quality interaction.
What is the center's policy on parental visits?	Parents should be able to drop in at any time. Be wary of facilities that restrict parental visiting in any way.
Physical Environment	
Is there adequate space in the center?	There should be opportunities for rough-and-tumble play and naptime as well as table activities.
Does the space appear safe?	Stairways should be fenced. No paint should be peeling.
Can children get in and out of the building easily?	A first-floor plan is safest. Fire exits should be well marked. An evacuation plan should be practiced.
Is there a safe play area for children outside?	Find out how often children are taken outside (once or twice a day) or only occasionally for "outings."
Is there a quiet place for naps?	Ask if a child can nap if tired or has to wait until a set naptime?
Can the bathroom be reached easily?	Both potty chairs and small toilet seats should be available.
Staff Philosophy	
Are the workers warm and affectionate towards the children?	Watch how they greet children. They should ask questions and listen to answers.
Do caretakers spend more of their time performing janitorial tasks (cleaning) and reprimanding children, or can they devote their time to the children?	It is best if cleaning staff is separate from care staff.
Is each child assigned to a particular caregiver on a continuing basis?	Ask staff to describe their care pattern; if this is not planned, little continuity of care results.
Are the children provided stimulating toys and equipment?	Imaginative items, such as a puppet theater, finger paint, and water play, should be included.
How do the staff discipline children? Do they yell or treat the children roughly?	The method should reflect the parents' philosophy. Staff should be able to talk to children calmly without raising their voices in anger.
Is there a planned curriculum?	There should be specific individualized goals the staff hopes to accomplish.
Can the child pursue an individual interest?	Play or learning activities should be individualized.
Health Care Protocols	
How does the center care for an ill child?	There should be access to a nurse. Staff should be able to evaluate for illness. They should know actions to take in an emergency.
What precautions does the staff take to prevent spread of infection?	Counter where diapers are changed should be wiped with a disinfectant; tissues and handwashing facilities should be present.
Does the center follow good sanitary practices?	Be sure the center requires waterproof disposable diapers to minimize contamination of the environment and other children, and separates diaper-changing area from other activities, especially anything related to food handling. Observe adult caregivers changing diapers. Do they wash hands after each change?
Under what conditions are children not allowed to attend the center?	A center should have a very specific policy on what illness symptoms require a child to be kept home—and they should enforce this policy strictly. For instance, a runny nose may be acceptable, but a fever is not; children with chickenpox should be kept at home until the scabs are healed over.
	Talk to parents whose children have been at the center long enough to have experienced some illnesses, and find out what the family did and how the center responded.
Children's Behavior	
Do the children appear happy and relaxed?	Observe for at least 1 morning.
Do they rush to greet any new visitors?	This could be a sign of boredom with their center's activities and a strong need for adult attention.

how to tie shoes, name basic colors, and print her name before she begins. Parents should familiarize themselves with any such suggestions from the school, but the wisdom of requiring these skills can be questioned. Identifying colors should be established by this age, but some children are not coordinated enough at 4½ to tie shoes or print. A better contribution for parents to make toward their child's achievement in school is to instill in her the concept that learning is fun, that she will not always be able to do all the things the other children around her can do, but that she should try to do her best. Trying to make a child complete fine motor tasks for which she is not developmentally prepared does not instill that concept.

For children to do well in a formal school setting, they must be able to follow instructions and sit at a table and chair for a short work period. Some parents are surprised to realize how few instructions they give their child to follow in a day. They put on his coat, pick up his toys, and lead him to the table for dinner. Similarly, they never encourage the child to spend any time in a chair, which is something he will do for at least short periods of time in school. Coloring at a table rather than on the floor will introduce this situation without any problem.

Finally, going to school is a form of separation if the child has not attended day care or preschool, so parents must make preparations for this. To do this, it might be good to arrange to have the child stay with another caregiver for part of a day. Staying at school can then be compared with that event.

These are minimum preparations parents can complete to ready their child for school. Both parents and children should understand, however, that not absolutely everything can be anticipated; school will bring some new happenings the parents cannot predict.

If the child has been led to believe that learning is fun and new experiences are enjoyable (creating a strong sense of initiative), these unpredictable instances can be accepted as fun. That concept will prepare the child not only for a first day at school but for thousands of profitable days and experiences afterward.

Broken Fluency

Developing language is such a complicated process that children from 2 to 6 years of age typically have some speech difficulty that parents may interpret as stuttering. The child may begin to repeat words or syllables, saying, "I-I-I want a n-n-new spoon-spoon-spoon." This is called **broken fluency** (repetition and prolongation of sounds, syllables, and words). It is often referred to as **secondary stuttering**, because the child begins to speak without this problem and then, during the preschool years, develops it. Unlike the adult who stutters, the child is unaware that he is not being fluent unless it is called to his attention. It is a part of normal

development and, if accepted as such, will pass. The parent who knows a chronic stutterer, however, or who was a chronic stutterer at one time, may react to this normal broken fluency of the preschooler in a more emotional way than the problem deserves. It is resolved most quickly if parents follow a few simple rules as shown in Box 31-1. If the child becomes conscious of a disrupted speech pattern, it is less likely that the problem will correct itself. Many preschoolers imitate their parents or older children in the family so well during this time that they incorporate swear words into their vocabularies. Parents may have to be reminded that the child does not understand what the words mean; he has simply heard them, just as he has heard hundreds of other words and decided to use them. Correction should be unemotional, for example, "That's not a word we like to hear you use. When you're angry, why don't you say 'fudge' (or whatever)." The correcting is no different from that involved when the child uses poor grammar. If parents become emotional, the child realizes the value of such words and may continue using them to get attention.

Box 31-1

Suggestions for Parents on How to Help Limit Stuttering in the Preschool Child

1. Do not discuss in the child's presence the difficulty he is having with speech. Do not label him a "stutterer." This makes him conscious of his speech patterns and compounds the problem. If you have to think about every word you say, it is difficult not to have difficulty speaking.
2. Listen with patience to what the child is saying. Do not interrrupt or fill in a word for him. Do not tell him to speak more slowly or to start over. These actions make the child conscious of his speech, and his broken fluency increases.
3. Talk to him in a calm, simple way. It is difficult for the child to keep up with adult speech. If adults talk slowly to him, he sees no need to rush and so speaks more clearly.
4. Protect space for him to talk if there are other children in the family. Rushing to say something before a second child interrupts is the same as rushing to conform to adult speech.
5. Do not force the child to speak if he does not want to. Do not ask him to recite or sing for strangers.
6. Do not reward him for fluent speech or punish him for nonfluent speech. Broken fluency is a developmental stage in language formation, not an indication of regression or a chronic speech pattern.

Unique Concerns of the Family With a Disabled or Chronically Ill Preschooler

Learning how to do things when you have physical limitations can be frustrating. Being unable to understand how to do things because of physical or mental limitations can be even more so. To learn problem-solving, however, is part of developing a sense of initiative. A preschooler with a disability such as cerebral palsy has a greater need for skill in problem-solving than the average child, because even simple procedures such as eating or getting dressed can be difficult if a physical handicap limits the options.

Experiences with eating help children reinforce their own sense of initiative. Chronically ill or disabled preschoolers who are limited in the foods they can eat (e.g., a diet of soft foods), or in the ability to help with food preparation, may miss this reinforcement. If their ap-

petite is diminished because of illness to the point where they take little or nothing orally, it is important that they continue to join the family at meals. In most households, this is a time for socialization, and preschoolers are ripe for the learning that goes with this type of day-by-day interaction with others.

Preschoolers with a handicap or chronic illness should attend a preschool program if at all possible. Many of the learning activities that preschoolers enjoy, such as playing with paint, clay, or soap bubbles, are messy. If the child must remain in bed, the parents may not offer these types of experiences. A large tray of dry oatmeal or other breakfast cereal with sand shovels or cars and trucks is a good substitute activity for such a child. Although not necessarily neat, these substances (which are available even in a hospital setting) can be swept away easily at the finish of play. Table 31-5 lists the nursing actions that aid a disabled or chronically ill child to solve problems and develop a sense of initiative.

Table 31-5. *Nursing Actions That Encourage a Sense of Initiative in the Disabled or Chronically Ill Preschooler*

Consideration	Nursing Actions
Nutrition	Serving toast or sandwiches cut into animal shapes with cookie cutters, cereal in the form of alphabet characters, or food arranged on a plate to make a face appeals to the imagination and may make a preschooler more interested in food.
	Respect child's food preferences.
Dressing change	Allow preschooler to measure and cut tape or draw a face on it.
	Allow him to see incision site. Explain steps of dressing change as you work to reduce unknowns and areas of fear.
	Provide extra bandages to put on a doll so child can see that bandages themselves are not to be feared.
Medicine	Allow child to choose a chaser such as juice or milk after oral medicine.
	Choosing sites for injection or intravenous line is too advanced for the preschooler; do not allow such choices.
Rest	Provide a light in the room or bring child's bed into hallway so fear of the dark is reduced and she can deal with only reality problems.
	Identify sounds the preschooler might hear in the hospital, such as an air conditioner turning on.
Hygiene	Allow child to choose bathtub toys, clothing.
	Allow child to wash own hands and face.
	Allow child to splash in water as a play activity as well as for cleanliness.
Pain	Encourage preschooler to express pain.
	Allow child to handle syringe or suction catheter, and give "shots" or suction to a doll to alleviate anger or fear.
	Encourage child to ask for analgesic if necessary.
Stimulation	Guessing games encourage a sense of initiative. Draw a dog or a house and ask child to close her eyes while you add one more detail to the drawing, such as an ear or a chimney; ask child to identify new item. Reverse the game and ask child what you erased from the drawing or allow child to do own drawing.
	Provide manipulative toys, such as finger paint, soapy water, play dough, or dry cereal to use as sand.
	Allow preschooler to accompany you to other departments as a way of teaching more about the hospital.
	Use Simon Says games not only for socialization but also to urge treatments, such as deep-breathing exercises.
	Encourage use of playroom for socialization.
	Encourage child to interact with family by drawing pictures for siblings or telephoning home.

Key Points

- Although preschoolers grow only slightly and gain just a little weight, they seem much taller than when they were toddlers because their contour changes to more childlike proportions.
- Erikson's developmental task for the preschool period is to gain a sense of initiative or learn how to do things. Play materials ideal for this age group are those that stimulate creativity such as modeling clay or colored markers.
- Promoting childhood safety is a major role, since preschoolers' active imaginations can lead them into dangerous situations.
- Common parental concerns during the preschool period are with "broken fluency," imaginary friends, difficulty sharing, and sibling rivalry.
- Preschool is often the time when a new sibling is born. Good preparation for this is necessary to prevent intense sibling rivalry.
- Preschoolers have a number of universal fears, including fear of the dark, mutilation, and abandonment. All care provided for this age group must include active measures to reduce these fears as much as possible.
- Preschoolers are still operating at a cognitive level that prevents them from understanding conservation (objects have not changed substance although they have changed appearance). This means they need an explanation, for example, of how they will be the same person postoperatively as they were preoperatively.
- Preschoolers are self-centered (egocentric). This makes it difficult for them to share and view someone else's side of a problem. They need good explanations of how a procedure will benefit them before they can agree to it.
- Many preschoolers begin preschool programs or day care. Late in the preschool period, they may be enrolled in kindergarten. Parents often appreciate guidance in how to orient their children to these new experiences.
- Preschoolers who are disabled or who have chronic illnesses may have difficulty achieving a sense of initiative, because they may be limited in their ability to participate in activities that stimulate initiative. They may need special play times set aside for stimulation and learning.

Critical Thinking Exercises

1. Marty is a 3-year-old who is going to start day care because his mother is returning to work. Specify the suggestions you could make to his mother about choosing a safe setting. How should she prepare Marty for the experience?
2. Kathy is a preschooler. Her parents tell you that Kathy keeps the entire family awake at night because she is so afraid of the dark. Formulate a plan of action to enable her family to help Kathy sleep.
3. Barry is a 4-year-old you see in a well child conference. His mother tells you she cannot stand messy activities. Explain the activities you could suggest to Barry's mother that would stimulate a sense of initiative but not be messy.

References

Alexander, C. S., et al. (1990). Acute gastrointestinal illness and child care arrangements. *American Journal of Epidemiology, 131,* 124.

Curry, D. M., & Duby, J. C. (1994). Developmental surveillance by pediatric nurses. *Pediatric Nursing, 20,* 40.

Department of Health and Human Services. (1990). Death rates by age and sex: United States. *Monthly Vital Statistics Report,* No. 39, 3.

Department of Health and Human Services. (1991). *Healthy people 2000.* Washington, DC: Public Health Service.

Erikson, E. H. (1986). *Childhood and society.* New York: W. W. Norton.

Gillespie, S. M., et al. (1990). Occupational risk of human parvovirus B19 infections for school and day-care personnel during an outbreak of erythema infectiosum. *Journal of the American Medical Association, 263,* 2061.

Kelley, S. J., et al. (1993). Sexual abuse of children in care centers. *Child Abuse and Neglect, 17,* 71.

Kligman, E. W., & Narce-Valente, S. (1990). Reducing the exposure of children to environmental tobacco smoke. *Journal of Family Practice, 30,* 263.

Kohlberg, L. (1981). *The philosophy of moral development: Moral stages and the idea of justice.* New York: Harper & Row.

Kuttner, L. (1991). Helpful strategies in working with preschool children in pediatric practice. *Pediatric Annals, 20,* 120.

Lyytinen, P. (1991). Development trends in children's pretend play. *Child Care, Health and Development, 17,* 9.

Pauley, J. G., & Gaines, S. K. (1993). Preventing day-care related illnesses. *Journal of Pediatric Health Care, 7,* 207.

Reves, R. R., & Pickering, L. K. (1990). Infections in child day care centers as they relate to internal medicine. *Annual Review of Medicine, 41,* 383.

Robinson, P. (1993). *Freud and his critics.* Berkeley: University of California Press.

Schuster, S., & Ashburn, A. (1991). *The process of human development: A holistic life span approach* (3rd ed.). Philadelphia: J.B. Lippincott.

Spadt, S. K., et al. (1990). Experiential classes for siblings to be. *MCN: American Journal of Maternal Child Nursing, 15,* 184.

Wilson, P. D., & Testani-Dufour, L. (1993). Bicycle safety programs: targeting injury prevention through education. *Pediatric Nursing, 19,* 343.

Wadsworth, B. J. (1989). *Piaget's theory of cognitive and affective development.* New York: Longman.

Suggested Readings

Canam, C. (1993). Common adaptive tasks facing parents of children with chronic conditions. *Journal of Advanced Nursing, 18,* 46.

Lee, E. J., et al. (1990). Survey of accidents in a university day-care center. *Journal of Pediatric Health Care, 4,* 18.

Malfair, A. (1992). Supporting the child with special needs. *Canadian Nurse, 88,* 17.

Nehring, W. M. (1994). The nurse whose specialty is developmental disabilities. *Pediatric Nursing, 20,* 78.

Prizant, B. M., et al. (1993). Communication and language assessment for young children. *Infants and Young Children, 5,* 20.

Sullivan, M., et al. (1990). Reducing child hazards in the home: A joint venture in injury control. *Journal of Burn Care and Rehabilitation, 11,* 175.

Terr, L. C. (1991). Childhood traumas: an outline and overview. *American Journal of Psychiatry, 148,* 10.

Yates, S. R. (1992). The school nurse's role: early intervention with preschool children. *Journal of School Nursing, 8,* 30.

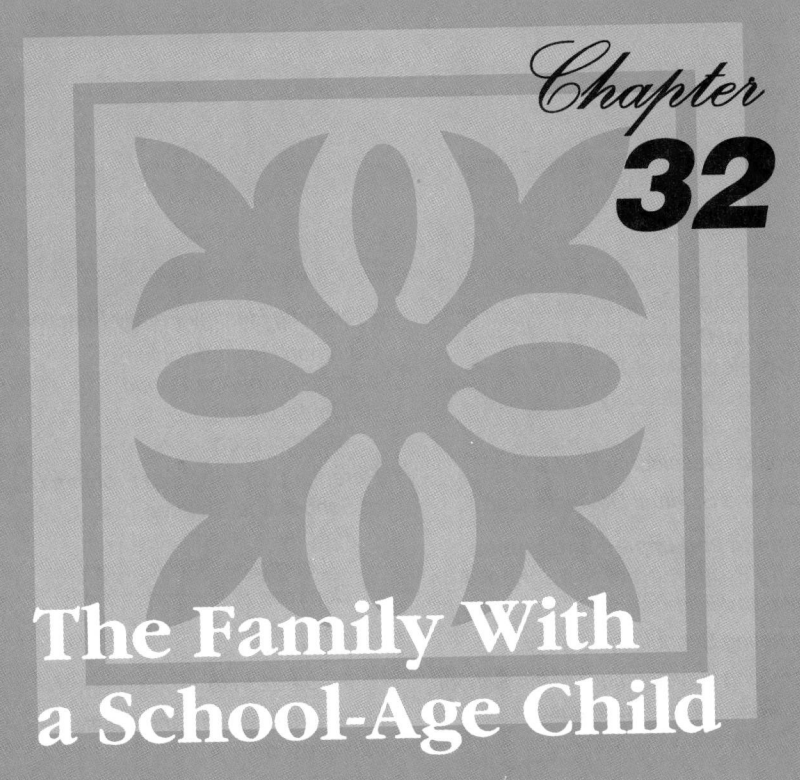

Chapter 32

The Family With a School-Age Child

Objectives

After mastering the contents of this chapter, you should be able to:

1. Describe the normal growth and development pattern and common parental concerns of the school-age period.

2. Assess a school-age child for normal growth and development milestones.

3. Formulate nursing diagnoses for the family of a school-age child.

4. Plan anticipatory guidance to prevent problems of growth and development in the school-age child (e.g., teaching about normal puberty).

5. Implement nursing care to help achieve normal growth and development of the school-age child, such as counseling parents about helping their child adjust to a new school.

6. Evaluate outcome criteria to be certain that goals of care have been achieved.

7. Identify National Health Goals related to the school-age child that nurses can be instrumental in helping the nation achieve.

8. Identify areas related to care of school-age children that could benefit from additional nursing research.

9. Use critical thinking to analyze ways in which the care of the school-age child can be more family centered.

10. Synthesize knowledge of school-age growth and development with the nursing process to achieve quality maternal and child health nursing care.

Adele Pillitteri: MATERNAL AND CHILD HEALTH NURSING, 2nd Edition. © 1995 Adele Pillitteri.

*I*n this chapter, the term *school age* refers to children between the ages of 6 and 12. Although the school-age years represent a time of slow physical growth, cognitive and developmental growth proceed at rapid rates. Because of this, it is important to keep in mind that there are many differences among children from one year to the next. Seven- and 10-year-olds have very different needs and outlooks, as do 11- and 12-year-olds. It is important to assess all children as individuals; to try to understand the particular developmental needs of each child based on his or her own developmental status, not based on where you think he or she should be.

The school-age period is usually the first time that children are making truly independent judgments. This may create some conflicts with parents if they are unable to keep up. Unlike the infant or toddler, whose progress is marked by new abilities and skills (e.g., ability to sit up or roll over; ability to speak a full sentence), the development of the school-age child is more subtle. Progress may, in fact, be marked by mood swings; what the child enjoys on one occasion may not be acceptable on another. This may precipitate crises in the family. For instance, a child may ask parents for a guitar and lessons, and then after the family has invested in these, the child quickly loses interest. The child of school age is also more influenced by the attitudes of his friends. He may choose not to do something he has previously

done well because none of his friends are interested in that activity. Parents who make too much of these likes and dislikes may find themselves engaged in unnecessary conflicts with their child. The Focus on National Health Goals box lists National Health Goals related to the school-age period.

⊠ **NURSING PROCESS OVERVIEW**
for Healthy Development
of the School-Age Child

ASSESSMENT

Growth and development of the school-age child should be assessed with both a history and physical examination. Be certain that the history includes an account of school activities and progress. School-age children are interested and able to contribute to their own health history; it is useful to interview children 10 years or older, at least in part, without their parents being present. During the physical examination, show your awareness of and respect for the fact that modesty is at an adult level by having children use a cover gown.

Yearly health visits for the school-age child and parents will often bring up behavioral issues or conflicts. Some parents feel they are losing contact with their children during these years and so may misinterpret a normal change in behavior, especially if they are not pre-pared for what to expect from their child.

When problems are discussed in the health care set-ting, it is important not only to take the history from the parent but also to allow the child to express the problem by him- or herself. Parents may consider a child who be-haves differently from siblings as "abnormal" when he is just expressing his own personality. It may be necessary to obtain the opinion of school personnel regarding the problem or even just determine whether they feel a problem exists. In rare instances, a law officer's opinion may be sought. If the problem is related to a medical condition, its effect on the family should also be as-sessed, because the illness of a child will certainly affect the functioning of the family unit.

NURSING DIAGNOSIS

Common nursing diagnoses regarding growth and de-velopment during the school-age period include:

- Health-seeking behaviors related to normal school-age growth and development
- Potential for enhanced parenting related to improved family living conditions
- Anxiety related to slow growth pattern of child
- High risk for injury related to parental knowledge deficit about safety precautions for a school-age child

PLANNING

In planning care, keep in mind the school-age child's tendency to enjoy small or short-term projects rather than long, involved ones. A child in her early school years with diabetes, for example, may gain a sense of achievement by learning to assess her own serum glu-cose level, but she may have difficulty continuing serum assessment on a long-term basis.

Behavior problems need to be well defined before interventions are planned for their solution. Often, it is enough for parents to accept the problem as one consis-tent with normal growth and development.

IMPLEMENTATION

School-age children are interested in adult roles. Be aware that they watch you to see your attitude as well as your actions in a given situation.

When giving care, keep in mind that children this age feel more comfortable knowing the how and why of an action. They may not cooperate at all with a proce-dure until they are satisfied with an explanation of why it must be done.

EVALUATION

Yearly health visits covering both physical and psy-chosocial development are important at this age. It may be useful for parents to look back at problems identified at the last visit and discuss if and how they were re-solved. Often, some problems and conflicts fade away without anyone really noticing. As some problems re-cede, however, others may emerge. At times, the same concerns of parents and the child may appear to be unresolved at each visit. It is important to make sure no underlying problem exists that prevents resolution. The following are examples of outcome criteria:

- Child sustains no injury from sports activities during summer.
- Child voices that he understands his growth is nor-mal, even though he is the shortest boy in his eighth grade class.

FOCUS ON
National Health Goals

A number of National Health Goals address the health of the school-age population, including these three:

- Increase to at least 30% the proportion of people age 6 and older who engage regularly, preferably daily, in light to moderate physical activity for at least 30 minutes per day.
- Reduce deaths caused by motor vehicle accidents to no more than 5.5 per 100,000 children age 14 years and younger.
- Reduce dental caries so that the proportion of children with one or more caries (in permanent or primary teeth) is no more than 35% among children ages 6 through 8 years (DHHS, 1991).

Nurses can be instrumental in helping the nation achieve these goals by such actions as urging children to begin and maintain a consistent exercise program, brush teeth and go for dental checkups regularly, and follow safety rules both in and around automobiles. Additional nursing research is needed to strengthen knowledge about the following: What is the ideal exercise program that is interesting enough to children that it will hold their attention for a long span of time? What are effective ways to teach street safety to children in the early school years? What strategies are most effective in helping school-age children to brush teeth daily?

Nursing Assessment of Growth and Development of the School-Age Child

Physical Growth

School-age children mature slowly but steadily. Their annual average weight gain is approximately 3 to 5 lb (1.3 to 2.2 kg); the increase in height is 1 to 2 inches (2.5 to 5 cm). Children who did not lose the lordosis and knock-kneed appearance of toddlers during the preschool period lose this now. Posture becomes more erect. Nutritional needs of the school-age child are discussed in Chapter 34.

By age 10 years, brain growth is complete. As a result, fine motor coordination becomes refined. As the eye globe reaches its final shape at this same time, the adult vision level is achieved. If the eruption of permanent teeth and the growth of the jaw do not correlate with final head growth, malocclusion with teeth malalignment may result.

The immunoglobulins IgG and IgA reach adult levels, and lymphatic tissue continues to grow in size up until about age 9. The resulting abundance of tonsillar and adenoid tissue in the early school years is often mistaken for disease during respiratory illness. It may also result in temporary conduction deafness from eustachian tube obstruction until this tissue recedes normally. The appendix is also lined with lymphatic tissue, and swelling of this tissue in the narrow tube can lead to trapped fecal material and inflammation (appendicitis) in the early school-age child. Frontal sinuses develop at about 6 years, and sinus-caused headache becomes a possibility. Before then, headache in children is rarely caused by sinus problems.

The left ventricle of the heart enlarges so as to be strong enough to pump blood to the growing body. Innocent heart murmurs may become apparent owing to the extra blood crossing heart valves. The pulse rate decreases to 70 to 80 bpm; blood pressure rises to about 112/60 mm Hg. Maturation of the respiratory system leads to increased oxygen–carbon dioxide exchange, which increases exertion ability and stamina.

Sexual Maturation

At a set point in brain maturity, the hypothalamus transmits an enzyme to the anterior pituitary gland to begin production of gonadotropic hormones, which activate changes in testes and ovaries. Timing of this maturity varies widely, between 10 and 14 years of age (Cunningham et al., 1993). Hormone changes that occur with puberty are discussed in Chapter 4. Table 32-1 describes the usual order for secondary sex characteristics.

Sexual Concerns

Changes in physical appearance lead to problems and worries for both children and their parents. This is a time for parents to discuss sexual responsibility with children and to reinforce previous teaching with children that their body is their own to be used only in the way they choose. Specific measures for children to help prevent sexual abuse are discussed later in the chapter.

Concerns of Girls. In both sexes, changes occur in the sebaceous glands. Under the influence of androgen, glands become more active, setting the stage for acne (DeWitt, 1990; see Chapter 33). Vasomotor instability commonly leads to blushing; perspiration increases.

Although these changes begin with preadolescence, they continue for a number of years. Puberty or sexual

Table 32-1. *Chronologic Development of Secondary Sex Characteristics*

Age (yr)	Boys	Girls
9–11	Prepubertal weight gain occurs.	Breasts: elevation of papilla with breast bud formation; areolar diameter enlarges.
11–12	Sparse growth of straight, downy, slightly pigmented hair at base of penis Scrotum becoming textured; growth of penis and testes begins. Sebaceous gland secretion increases. Perspiration increases.	Straight hair along the labia. Vaginal epithelium becomes cornified. *p*H of vaginal secretions acid; slight mucous vaginal discharge present. Sebaceous gland secretion increases. Perspiration increases. Dramatic growth spurt
12–13	Pubic hair present across pubis Penis lengthens. Dramatic linear growth spurt Breast enlargement occurs.	Pubic hair grows darker; spreads over entire pubis. Breasts enlarge; still no protrusion of nipples. Axillary hair present Menarche occurs.

maturation in girls occurs between 12 and 18 years, in boys between 14 and 20. Puberty is occurring increasingly earlier, however, and, in a class of 11-year-old sixth graders, it is not unusual to discover that more than one half of the girls are already menstruating. Even some 9-year-old girls are menstruating. In light of this fact, in order to be effective, sex education as a part of the school curriculum must be introduced not in high school or junior high but in grade school.

Prepubertal females are usually taller, by about 2 inches (5 cm) or more, than preadolescent males, because their typical growth spurt occurs earlier. In a culture in which boys are expected to be taller than girls, this can cause difficulties. Sometimes a girl notices the change in her pelvic contour when she tries on a skirt or dress from the year before and realizes her hips are now too broad to fit. She may misinterpret this finding as a gain in weight and attempt a crash diet. She can be reassured that broad bone structure of the hips is part of an adult female profile.

Females are usually conscious of breast development. A girl who is developing ahead of her peers may tend to slouch or wear loose clothing to hide the fact. Another girl studies herself in front of the mirror and wonders whether her breasts are going to develop enough. Breast development is not always symmetric, and it is not unusual for a girl to have breasts of slightly different sizes. She can be reassured, after the condition has been checked during a physical examination, that this development is normal—that one breast is not filled with a tumor to make it bigger or the other diseased in some way to make it smaller. Supernumerary (additional) nipples may darken or increase in size at puberty. It is important for girls to understand that a supernumerary nipple is affected by hormones in her body in the same way as other breast tissue. Otherwise, she may think of it as a growing mole and be afraid she has cancer.

As part of preparation for menstruation, girls should be told that vaginal secretions will appear. If this is not explained, a child may fear she has an infection and worry needlessly. Explain, too, that any secretions which are enough to cause vulvar irritation should be evaluated at a health care facility.

Concerns of Boys. Boys who are not prepared for physical changes worry about them in the same way as girls. Just as girls are keenly aware of breast development, boys are aware of increasing genital size. If they do not know that testicular development precedes penis growth, they can worry that their growth is inadequate. There is a tendency for men to measure their manliness by penis size, which can make a male who develops late feel inferior.

Hypertrophy of breast tissue (gynecomastia) occurs most often in stocky or heavy boys. A youth with this condition may be concerned that a breast tumor is present. He can be reassured that this is a transitory phenomenon and that, although it makes him self-conscious, will fade as soon as his male hormones become more mature and active.

Some boys are also concerned, because although they have pubic hair, they cannot yet grow a beard or do not have chest hair—the outward, easily recognized signs of maturity. It can be reassuring for them to learn that pubic hair normally appears first and that chest and facial hair may not grow until several years later.

As seminal fluid is produced, boys may begin to notice ejaculation during sleep—so-called **nocturnal emissions**. If they have not been prepared for these experiences, they may worry that they have contracted a disease. An old notion, often perpetuated by sports coaches, may lead preadolescents to believe that loss of seminal fluid is debilitating; also, boys may have heard the term *premature ejaculation* and worry that this is a forewarning of a problem in years to come. Both are fallacies.

Teeth

Deciduous teeth are lost and permanent teeth erupt during the school-age period (Figure 32-1). The average child gains 28 teeth between 6 and 12 years of age: the

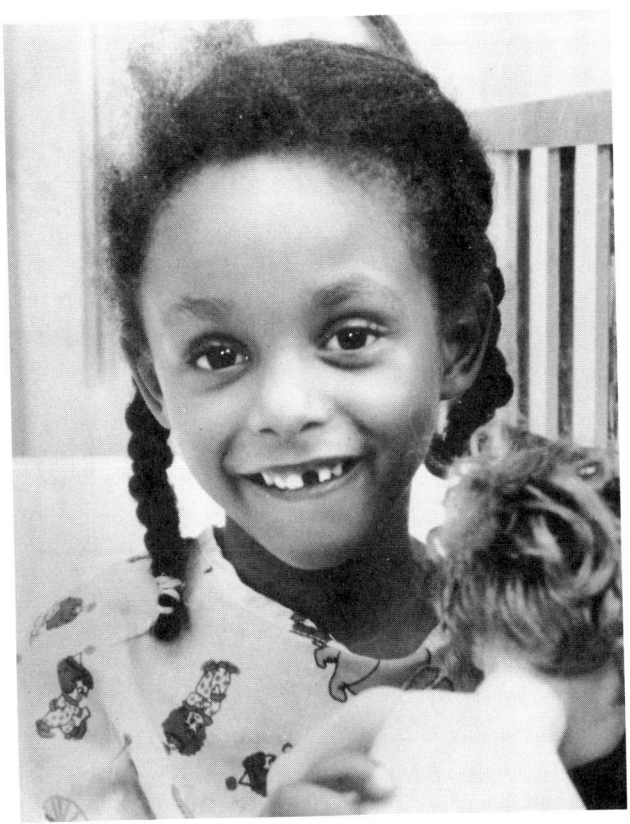

FIGURE 32-1
Early-school-age children typically have a missing upper incisor as deciduous teeth are replaced by permanent teeth. (Courtesy of the Department of Medical Photography, Children's Hospital, Buffalo, NY.)

central and lateral incisors; first, second and third cuspids; and first and second molars (Figure 32-2).

Developmental Milestones

Gross Motor Development

School-age development is summarized in Table 32-2. Six-year-olds endlessly jump, tumble, skip, and hop. They have enough coordination to walk a straight line. Many are able to ride a two-wheel bicycle. They can skip rope with practice. A 7-year-old appears quiet compared with a rough-and-tumble 6-year-old. Seven-year-olds usually have enough accuracy in jumping to play hopscotch and to skip rope well. Gender differences usually become manifest in play: there are "girl games," such as dressing dolls and jumping rope, and "boy games," such as pretending to be pirates.

The movements of 8-year-olds are more graceful than those of younger children, although as their arms and legs grow, they may stumble on furniture or spill milk and food. They ride a bicycle well and enjoy sports, such as gymnastics, soccer, and hockey.

Nine-year-olds are on the go constantly, as if they always have a deadline to meet. They have enough eye–hand coordination to enjoy baseball, basketball, and volleyball. By 10 years of age, girls become less tomboyish. Boys are more interested in perfecting sporting skills than previously (see Focus on Family Teaching display).

At 11, children are just as active as they were at age 10, although many are awkward because of their growth spurt and thus do less well at sports. This deficiency may bother the ones who see sports as the key to popularity. They may drop out of sports activities at this time rather than compete and look ungainly in their attempts. Energy is channeled into constant motion: drumming fingers and tapping pencils or feet.

Twelve-year-olds plunge into activities with inten-

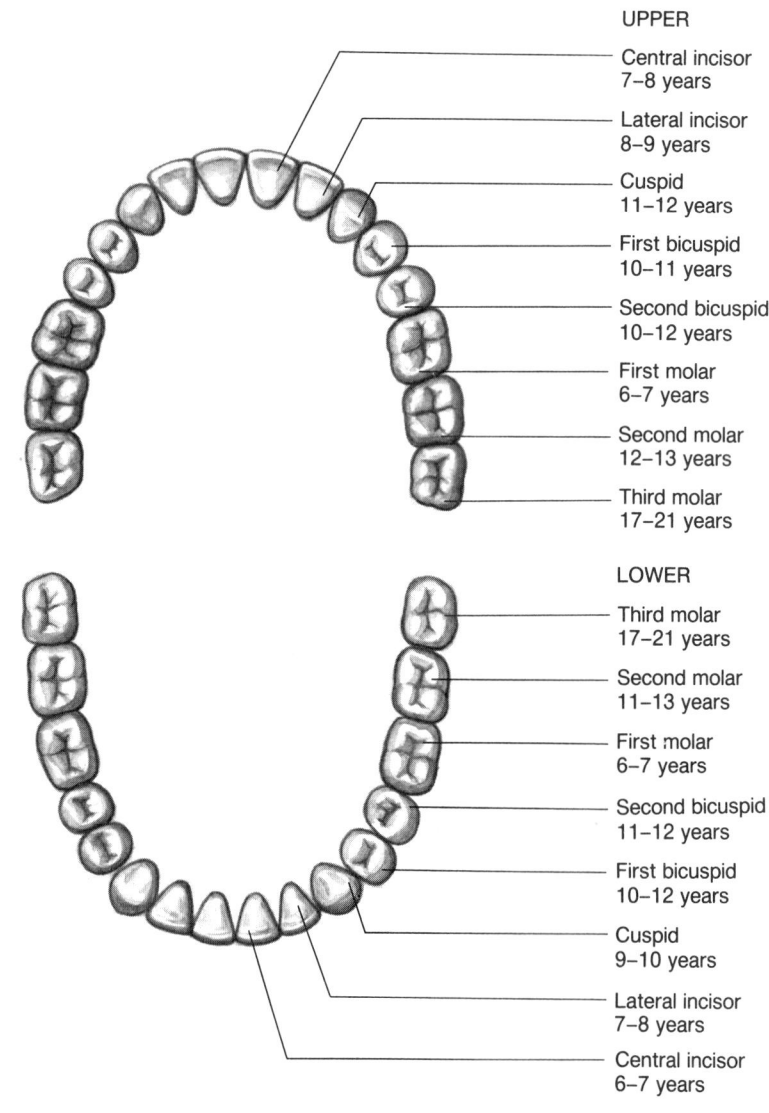

UPPER

Central incisor
7–8 years

Lateral incisor
8–9 years

Cuspid
11–12 years

First bicuspid
10–11 years

Second bicuspid
10–12 years

First molar
6–7 years

Second molar
12–13 years

Third molar
17–21 years

LOWER

Third molar
17–21 years

Second molar
11–13 years

First molar
6–7 years

Second bicuspid
11–12 years

First bicuspid
10–12 years

Cuspid
9–10 years

Lateral incisor
7–8 years

Central incisor
6–7 years

FIGURE 32-2
Eruption pattern of permanent teeth.

Table 32-2. *Summary of School-Age Development*

Age (yr)	Physical Development	Psychosocial Development
6	A year of constant motion; skipping is a new skill; first molars erupt.	First-grade teacher becomes authority figure; adjustment to all-day school may be difficult and lead to nervous manifestations of fingernail biting, etc. Defines words by their use: a key is to unlock a door, not a metal object.
7	Central incisors erupt; difference between sexes becomes apparent in play (video games vs. dolls); spends time in quiet play	A quiet year; striving for perfection leads to this year being called an *eraser* year. Conservation (water poured from tall container to a wide, flat one is the same amount of water) is learned; can tell time; can make simple change.
8	Coordination definitely improved; playing with gang becomes important; eyes become fully developed.	"Best friends" develop; whispering and giggling begin; can write as well as print; understands concepts of past, present, and future.
9	All activities done with gang	Gang age; a 9-year-old club is formed to spite someone, has secret codes, is all boy or all girl; gangs disband and reform quickly.
10	Coordination improves.	Ready for camp away from home; collecting age; likes rules; ready for competitive games.
11	Active, but awkward and ungainly	Insecure with members of opposite sex; repeats off-color jokes.
12	Coordination improves.	A sense of humor is present; is social and cooperative.

sity and concentration. They often enjoy participating in sports events for charities (e.g., walk-a-thons). They may be refreshingly cooperative around the house, able to handle a great deal of responsibility and complete given tasks.

Fine Motor Development

Six-year-olds can easily tie their shoelaces. They can cut and paste well and draw a person with good detail. They can print, although they may routinely reverse letters. Seven-year-olds concentrate on fine motor skills more than previously. This has been called the "eraser year," because children are never quite content with what they have done. They set too high a standard for themselves and then have difficulty accomplishing goals. By 7 years of age, children's eyes are developed enough so that they can read regular-size type. This makes reading a greater pleasure and school more enjoyable (Figure 32-3).

Eight-year-olds learn to write rather than to print. They enjoy showing off this new skill in cards, letters, or projects. By age 9, their writing begins to look mature and less awkward.

Older school-age children begin to evaluate their teachers' ability and can perform at varying levels, de-

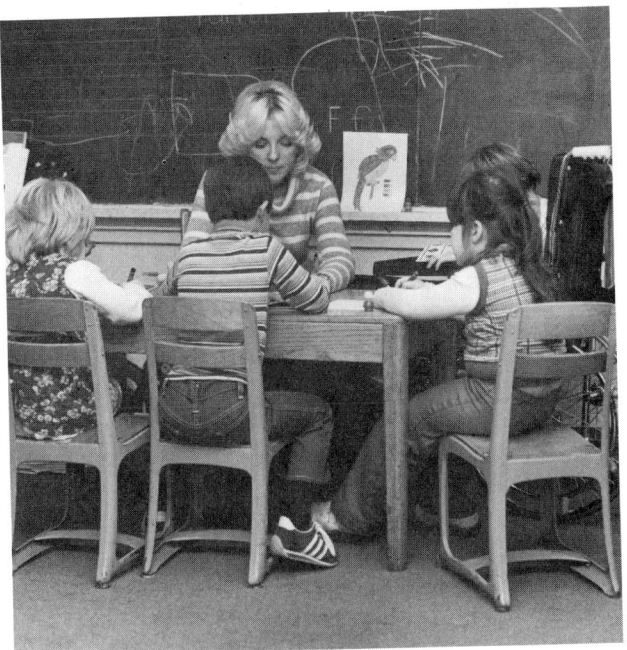

FIGURE 32-3
One of the biggest discoveries of childhood is that reading and writing are fun. Reading and writing are activities that can help a child pass the hours of hospitalization. (Courtesy of the Department of Medical Photography, Children's Hospital, Buffalo, NY.)

FOCUS ON FAMILY TEACHING

Q. My 10-year-old has become extremely independent. What safety measures do I need to stress with him to be certain he's safe?

A. Ten-year-olds can be so independent they neglect to be cautious of their own safety. Here are some common measures to teach school-age children:

Accident	Preventive Measure
Motor vehicle accidents	Encourage children to use seat belts in a car; role model their use.
	Teach street-crossing safety; stress that streets are no place for roughhousing, pushing, or shoving.
	Teach bicycle safety, including advice not to take "passengers" on a bicycle and to use a helmet.
	Teach parking lot and school bus safety (do not walk in back of parked cars, wait for crossing guard, etc.).
Community	Teach to avoid areas specifically unsafe, such as train yards, grain silos, back alleys. Teach not to go with strangers (parents can establish a code word with child; child does not leave school with anyone who does not know the word).
	Teach to say "no" to anyone who touches them whom they do not wish to do so, including family members (most sexual abuse is by a family member, not a stranger).
Burns	Teach safety with candles, matches, campfires—fire is not fun. Teach safety with beginning cooking skills (remember to include microwave oven safety, such as closing door firmly before turning on oven; not using metal containers).
	Teach not to climb electric poles.
Falls	Teach that roughhousing on fences, climbing on roofs, etc., is hazardous.
	Teach skateboard safety.
Sports injuries	Wearing appropriate equipment for sports (face masks for hockey, knee braces for football, batting helmets for baseball) is not babyish but smart.
	Teach not to play to a point of exhaustion or in a sport beyond physical capability (pitching baseball or toe ballet for a grade-school child).
	Teach to use trampolines only with adult supervision to avoid serious neck injury.
Drowning	Children should learn how to swim; dares and roughhousing when diving or swimming are not appropriate.
	Teach not to swim beyond limits of capabilities.
Drug	Teach to avoid all recreational drugs and to take prescription medicine only as directed.
Firearms	Teach safe firearm use. Parents should keep firearms in locked cabinets with bullets separate from gun.
General	Teach school-age children to keep adults informed as to where they are and what they are doing.
	Be aware that the frequency of accidents increases when parents are under stress and therefore less attentive. Special precautions must be taken at these times.
	Some children are more active, curious, and impulsive and therefore more vulnerable to accidents than others.

pending on each teacher's expectations. The junior or middle school level of curriculum involves more challenging science and mathematics courses than previously, and covers good literature. This may be a child's first exposure to reading as a fulfilling and worthwhile experience rather than just as an assignment.

Play

Play continues to be rough; however, when children discover reading as an enjoyable activity that opens doors to other worlds, they will begin to spend momentary quiet times with books. Many children spend hours playing increasingly challenging video games.

By 7 years of age, children require more props for play than when they were younger. To be a cowboy, a boy needs a hat and gun, when before he needed only a pointed finger. The girl needs real food for tea parties, when before she played with empty plates. This is the start of a decline in imaginative play, which will continue unless the child receives adequate stimulation and is encouraged to use the imagination.

Many girls prefer teenage dolls, and their coordination is good enough for them to button the miniature dresses and pull on the tiny boots. Keeping track of the dolls' wardrobes is difficult all throughout childhood.

The collecting age begins: baseball cards, straws, rocks, marbles. The type of item is not as important as the quantity.

School-age collections become structured as the child reaches 8 years of age. Time is spent sorting and cataloging. Most girls and boys of this age enjoy helping in the kitchen with jobs such as making cookies and salads and frosting cakes. They start to be more involved in simple science projects and experiments.

Eight-year-olds like table games but hate to lose, so tend to avoid competitive games. They may change the rules in the middle of the game to keep from losing.

Many children of this age enter a phase of reading comic books. These can be read quickly, so they complement a sense of industry, the developmental crisis of the school-age years. If parents forbid comic-book reading, the child may read the comics under the covers at night or at other children's houses. Parents would do better to set good reading examples and patiently wait out an acute interest in comic books. Their child *is* reading and will eventually seek out other types of books as well.

Nine-year-olds play hard. They wake in the morning, squeeze in some activity before school, and plan something the moment they arrive home. They have difficulty going to bed at night because they want to play just one more game. Play is rough, as children are not as interested in perfecting skills as they will be in another year. Nor are they as interested in skills as some parents or coaches would hope.

Many school programs begin music lessons for children at about 9 years of age. Children do well if others in their group are taking similar lessons. Talent for music or art becomes evident, and children respond with new interest in school or wherever they are exposed to these arts.

Many 10-year-olds spend most of their time playing television remote-control games. Boys' and girls' play remains separate at 10, although interest in the opposite sex is apparent. Boys show off as girls pass their group; girls talk loudly or giggle at the sight of a familiar boy. Girls spend time washing their hair, fussing with curlers, and choosing their clothing. They may feel old enough for nylons and lipstick for special occasions. Slumber parties for girls and camp-outs for boys are increasingly

popular. The children talk, giggle, and roughhouse into the middle of the night.

The tenth year is a year when children are very interested in rules and fairness. Before this time, they gave younger children breaks in games, allowing extra turns or hints. Now they strictly enforce rules (Figure 32-4). Club activities become structured, with president, secretary, and rules of order.

Eleven- and twelve-year-olds enjoy table games and are accommodating enough to be able to play with younger siblings who need rules modified to their advantage. Time with friends is often spent just talking. If the older school-age child uses his bedroom as a place to meet with friends, he becomes more interested in seeing that it is picked up (but do not look in the closet or under the bed). Girls may be interested in listening to popular music and learning how to dance to it. Both boys and girls seem to feel that they are on the verge of something great—their teens—and the year when they are age 12 is aimed toward preparing for that.

Language Development

Six-year-olds talk in full sentences, using language easily and with meaning. They no longer sound as though talking is an experiment but appear to have incorporated language permanently. They still define objects by their use: a key is to unlock a door; a fork is to eat with.

Most 7-year-olds can tell the time in hours, but they may have trouble with concepts such as *half past* and *quarter to*, especially with the prevalence of digital clocks and watches. They know the months of the year and can name the months in which holidays fall. They can add and subtract and make simple change (if they have had experience), so they can go to the store for simple purchases. Much of children's talk is concerned with these concepts as they practice them and show them off for family or friends.

As children discover "dirty" jokes at about age 9, they like to tell them to friends or try to understand

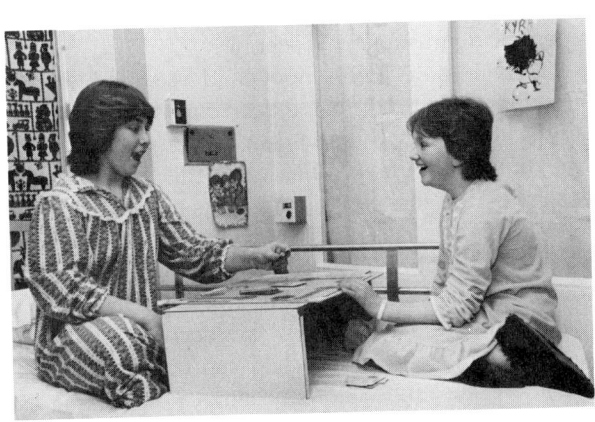

FIGURE 32-4
By 10 years of age, children are ready for competition. These two hospitalized children enjoy a board game. (Courtesy of the Department of Medical Photography, Children's Hospital, Buffalo, NY.)

those told by adults. They use swear words to express anger or just to show other children they are growing up. They may have a short period of intense fascination with "bathroom language," as they did during preschool years. As before, parents should make it clear that they find such language unacceptable and refrain from using it in their child's presence.

Twelve years of age is often described as the "lull before the storm," or a time of quiet readying for the teen years. A sense of humor is apparent and the child can carry on an adult conversation, although stories are limited because of their lack of experience.

Emotional Development

Ideally, children enter the school-age period with the ability to trust others and with a sense of respect for their own worth. They are able to accomplish small tasks independently, without feeling guilty, because they want to be independent (a sense of autonomy). They should have practiced or mimicked adult roles and had the opportunity to explore a preschool environment. At the same time, they should have learned to share and to have discovered that learning is fun and an adventure, and that doing things is more important and more rewarding than watching things being done.

Developmental Task: Industry Versus Inferiority

During the early school years, children attempt to master yet another developmental step: learning a sense of industry or accomplishment versus inferiority (Erikson, 1986). If gaining a sense of initiative can be defined as learning how to do things, then gaining a sense of industry is learning how to do things *well*.

If children are prevented from achieving a sense of industry or do not receive rewards for accomplishment, they develop a feeling of inferiority or become convinced that they cannot do things that they actually can do. These children can have difficulty tackling new situations later in life (new job, new school, new responsibility), because they cannot envision how they could be successful in handling them. This can result in children experiencing frustration in school.

The questions a preschool child asks are how, why, and what, questions that reflect curiosity. During the early school years children also demonstrate their concentration on the "how" of tasks: "Is this the right way to do this?" "Am I making this right?" "Is this good?"

Making decorated cookies with a preschooler is fun because the child revels in the feel of the dough, the excitement of watching shapes form, the color of the frosting, and the novelty of the decorations. Making cookies with a school-age child can become less pleasurable because the child concentrates on making each one perfect or right. "Do red sprinkles go with yellow frosting?" "How do I decorate a wreath?" "Do you like this one?" and the inevitable "I can't do anything right," because their cookies do not look perfect or fall short

of expectations. School-age children need reassurance that they are doing things correctly. This reassurance is best if it comes frequently rather than infrequently after long waits.

The best type of book for school-age children has many short chapters: children feel a sense of accomplishment when they finish each chapter, rather than having to wait until the end of the book. Small chores that can be completed quickly also give this type of reward. Children can survey their finished work and see that they have done a good job. A child may dislike vacuuming, for instance, because the rug may not look very different when he has finished. Picking up the scattered contents of a toy box, however, is a more obvious task that clearly makes a difference in the appearance of the room.

Hobbies and projects also are enjoyed best if they are small and can be finished within a short time. Most school-age children, for example, prefer putting together two or three fairly simple model-car kits to assembling one extremely complicated kit. The three kits offer three rewards; the involved one delays the reward so long that the child may become bored and never complete it. With adolescence will come more respect for quality. Children will realize that if they want the better model, they will have to spend the extra energy and attention—quality products involve work.

Home as a Setting to Learn Industry. Parents of a school-age child must take a step forward in development, along with the child. For the first time, the child does not accept them as complete authorities, but asks questions that parents may not be able to answer, because many school curriculums include new concepts and methods. Explaining to a 6- or 7-year-old that he does not understand what the child is doing can be demeaning for an unsure adult. Instead, an adult can say, "That looks interesting; can you explain it to me?" Most children love the chance to play "teacher."

Parents who enjoyed fostering individuality in a preschooler may feel frustrated when the school-age child begins to conform to rules and insists on the "right way to do things." They may feel they have failed to encourage the child's creativity, but conformity is vital to children at this age.

Eight- or 9-year-olds begin to spend more and more time with their peers and less time with their family. They forget to do household chores that they once enjoyed, such as setting the table or taking out the garbage, or they may do the work sloppily so as to have more time with their friends. Although this may seem like a regression in learning how to become responsible, it is actually a step of independence away from their parents and into the larger world, a developmental task that will help them become emotionally mature. This is an example of a new role the child is trying out, one of many he will try in the process of reaching adolescence and maturity when he will eventually find a role that is right for him.

School As a Setting to Learn Industry. Adjusting to school is one of the major tasks for this age group. Ideally, a child's teacher will think of learning as fun, and encourage him to plunge into new experiences. Unfortunately, parents have to monitor most teachers and school activities to make sure their children are being led this way, while not being pushed too hard.

Schools are increasingly assuming responsibility for education about sex, safety, avoidance of abusive substances, and preparation for family living. These discussions are generally superficial, however, and if the classes are large, may raise more questions than they can successfully answer. Such classes should not replace parental teaching in these areas. If given adequate encouragement and preparation by health care providers, most parents will be eager to maintain such responsibility. Others, however, do not believe their children should receive sex education at this age, and object to even the amount offered in the schools.

Structured Activities. Girl Scouts, Boy Scouts, Campfire Girls, and 4-H clubs are respected school-age activities, and if the local chapters are well run by leaders who understand children's needs, they can provide hours of constructive activity and strengthen a sense of autonomy. Merit badge systems are geared to the needs of school-age children, offering small but frequent rewards. As with school activities, parents should take responsibility to determine the worth of each organization for their individual child.

Competitive sports must be evaluated carefully. Before children can compete successfully, they must be able to lose a game without feeling devastated, to be able to say "I lost because I played badly," not "I lost because I am a bad person." Children do not usually develop sufficient ego strength to do this until they are about 10 years old.

Another problem to consider with organized contact sports is the possibility of athletic injuries. Encourage parents to consider their child's maturity and the risk of athletic injuries (see Chapter 51) before they decide whether team competition is advisable.

Problem-Solving. An important part of developing a sense of industry is learning how to solve problems. Parents and teachers can help children develop this skill by encouraging practice. When the child asks "Is this the right way to do this?" the parent can say "Let's talk about possible ways of doing it."

The world depends on machinery, so mishaps and breakdowns (and therefore sudden changes) do occur. The child who can create an indoor playhouse with a card table and blanket when it is too wet or cold to use her outdoor playhouse will be able as an adult to find

another solution to her data distribution problem when her computer malfunctions. Problem-solvers become adults who rarely say, "It can't be done." This attitude of optimism rather than pessimism improves the state of humankind. Just as important, it leaves these adults with confidence and a sense of pride, feeling good about themselves because they have control of their environment and abilities.

Learning to Live With Others. School-age children are sometimes so interested in tasks and in accomplishing physical projects that they forget they must work with people to achieve these goals. During the early school years, when children are first exposed to large groups of other youngsters, is a good time to urge them to learn compassion and thoughtfulness toward others by, for example, writing thank-you letters or shoveling an older neighbor's sidewalk.

Learning to give a present without receiving one in return or doing a favor without expecting a reward is also a part of this process, and can be taught by example. Children should see their parents doing such things with an attitude not of "What will I get?" but "What can I contribute?"

Children may show empathy towards others as early as 20 months, but cognitively are unable to relate others' experiences to their own until about 6 years of age. Therefore, it is usually ineffective to lecture a child with "That was cruel to call Mary names." The child may feel she had every right to do so. A better technique is to ask the child to put herself in Mary's place for a minute and imagine how she would feel if she were Mary. The school-age child will generally be able to do this and understand why name-calling hurts and makes children feel rejected. A simple "It doesn't feel good to be called names, does it?" may suffice.

Socialization

Six-year-old children play in groups, but when they are tired or under added stress, they prefer one-to-one contact. In a first-grade classroom, students compete actively for a few minutes of special time with the teacher. At the end of a day they enjoy time spent individually with parents. You may have to inform parents that this is not babyish behavior but that of a typical 6-year-old.

A 7-year-old is increasingly aware of family roles and responsibility. Promises must be kept, because 7-year-olds view them as definite, firm commitments. These children tattle, because they have a strong sense of justice. This tattling may dissolve play groups quickly.

The 8-year-old actively seeks the company of other children. Most 8-year-old girls have a close girlfriend; boys have a close boyfriend. Girls begin to whisper among themselves, annoying parents and teachers.

The 9-year-old takes the values of his peer group very seriously. He is much more interested in how other children dress than in what his parents say is proper.

This is typically the *gang age,* and children form clubs, usually "spite clubs." This means if there are four girls on the block, three form a club and exclude the fourth. The reason for exclusion is often unclear; it might be that the fourth child has a chronic disease, that she has more or less money than the others, that she was at the dentist's the day the club was formed, or simply that the club cannot exist unless there is someone to exclude. Such clubs typically have a secret password and secret meeting place. Membership is generally all girls or all boys. If an excluded child does not react badly to being shut out, the club will probably disband because its purpose is lost. The next day the excluded member may meet with two others and snub a different child. Parents have to be careful not to intervene with this type of play, because loyalties shift quickly. The child they defend today may be excluded tomorrow.

Nine-year-olds are ready for camp activities away from home. They can take care of their own needs and are mature enough to be separated from their parents for this length of time. Going to camp before this age usually results in homesickness and a negative introduction to a first experience away from home.

Although 10-year-olds enjoy groups, they also enjoy privacy. They like having their own bedroom or at least their own dresser, where they can put possessions and know they are free from parent's or siblings' eyes. One of the best gifts for a 10-year-old is a box that locks.

Girls become increasingly interested in boys and vice versa by 11 years. Parties tend to be mixed rather than single-sex ones. Children of this age are particularly insecure, however, and girls tend to dance with girls while boys talk together in corners. Better socialization patterns need not be rushed. Just as infants crawl before they walk, so 11-year-olds must attempt many awkward and uncomfortable social experiences before they become comfortable forming relationships with the opposite sex.

Twelve-year-olds are more social than they were the year before. This is because their easygoing manner makes others seek out their company. Boys experience erections on small provocation and may feel uncomfortable being pushed into boy–girl situations until they know how to control their bodies better. Girls are very aware of which friends have begun menstruating and which have not.

Cognitive Development

The period from 5 to 7 years of age is a transitional stage when children undergo a shift from the preoperational thought they used as preschoolers to concrete operational thought, or the ability to reason through any problem that they can actually visualize (Piaget & Infelder, 1969; Figure 32-5). Children are able to learn this because, unlike the preschooler, they can **decenter,** or focus on other views besides their own. This ability to

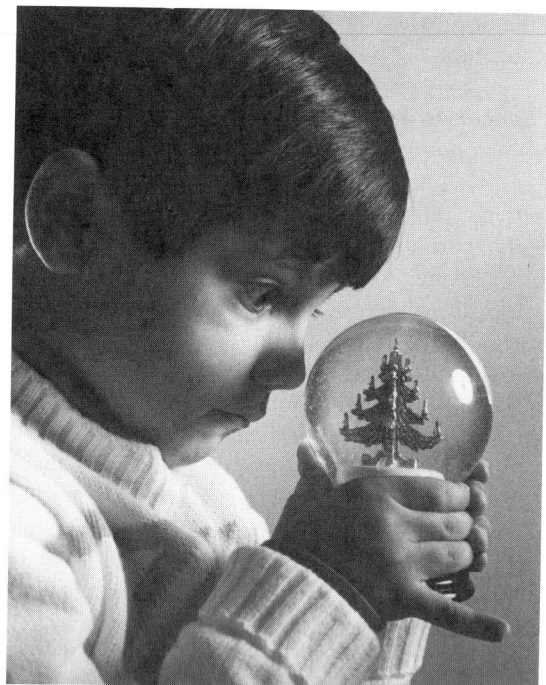

FIGURE 32-5

School-age children learn concrete operational thought or concentrate on phenomena they can actually see occurring. (Courtesy of the Department of Medical Photography, Children's Hospital, Buffalo, NY.)

project the self into other people's situations and see the world from their viewpoint is a refreshingly adult concept and makes the school-age child capable of a compassion that was not possible in younger years.

Accommodation, or the ability to adapt thought processes to fit what is perceived, is also learned during the school years. Prior to learning this, children are forced to change their impression of the situation to fit their thought processes—because Father always shaves before going to work, a child concludes that whenever she sees him shaving, he is getting ready for work. A boy who saw you making his hospital bed yesterday before giving him an injection might start to cry today when you make his bed, believing an injection will follow. However, the child who is able to accommodate is able to perceive that there can be more than one reason for other people's actions (Father shaves from habit or because company is coming, not only because it's a work day).

Learning **conservation** is yet another step in cognitive thought learned during this time. This is the ability to appreciate that a change in shape does not necessarily mean a change in size. If you pour 30 mL of cough medicine from a tall, thin glass to a short, wide one, a preschool child will say that the first glass held more (the cough medicine was higher in the glass). At about 7 years of age, children can realize that changing the shape of the substance this way does not change its quantity. This is an important concept, because the child is not fooled by perceptions as often as before. Sibling arguments over food (your piece of pie is bigger than mine, his glass of cola is bigger than mine) decrease during the school-age years as the child learns conservation.

School-age children also learn **class inclusion**, or the concept that objects can belong to more than one classification. A preschool child is able to categorize items in only one way—stones and shells found on the beach are objects gathered out of the sand. The school-age child is able to categorize them in many ways: stones are different from shells, they can be flat or round, colored or plain, smooth or rough. Shells come in different shapes and sizes as well as textures. This ability to classify objects leads to the collecting activities of the school-age period, and it is also necessary for learning mathematics and reading—systems that categorize numbers and words. Until children are able to grasp class inclusion, they confuse concepts from different categories, such as "If brothers and sisters are children, then grownups cannot be brothers or sisters."

Moral and Spiritual Development

School-age children begin to mature in terms of moral development as they enter a stage of **preconventional reasoning**, sometimes as early as 5 years of age (Kohlberg, 1981). During this stage, if asked "Why is it wrong to steal from your neighbor?" school-age children will answer "The police say it's wrong," or "Because if you do, you'll go to jail." They concentrate on "fairness" and cannot see yet that stealing hurts their neighbor, the highest level of moral reasoning.

School-age children begin to learn about the rituals and meaning behind their religious practice, so that the distinction between right and wrong becomes more important to them than it was when they were preschoolers. Parent role-modeling is also important (Walker & Taylor, 1991). Remember that school-age children are rule oriented; when they pray, they may expect their God to follow rules also (if you are good and pray for something, you should receive it). This makes children of this age confused if a prayer is not immediately answered. Because they are still limited in their ability to understand others' views, they may interpret something as being right because it is good for them, not because it is right for humanity as a whole.

Planning and Implementation for Health Promotion of the School-Age Child and Family

Promoting School-Age Safety

School-age children are allowed time on their own without direct adult supervision. This causes some accidents because the child doesn't always use common sense. As

with adults, accidents tend to occur when children are under stress (Grey, 1993). School programs to encourage safety are most effective if they address specific actions children should take in the course of their daily activities. The Focus on Family Teaching display lists common measures helpful in preventing accidents in this age group.

Sexual abuse is an unfortunate and all too common hazard in our society. Teaching points to help children avoid sexual abuse are summarized in Box 32-1. (See also Chapter 55.)

Promoting Development of the School-Age Child in Daily Activities

With life centered on school activities and friends, the school-age child still needs parental guidance for most activities of daily life. Habits and lifestyle patterns gained during this period can form the basis for healthy (or unhealthy) patterns of living later in life. Nutrition is still a major area of focus for health promotion. While parents may have less to say about what the school-age child eats, it is important that the increasing energy requirements which come with this age (often in spurts) are met with foods of high nutritional value. Chapter 34 discusses the nutritional needs, food preferences, and eating patterns for the school-age child.

Box 32-1
Teaching Points to Help Children Avoid Sexual Abuse

1. Your body is your property and you can decide who looks at it or touches it.
2. Secrets are fun things to keep. If a person asks you not to tell about something that was done to you that you didn't like, it's not a secret. It's all right to tell about it.
3. Don't go anywhere with a stranger (a stranger is someone you do not know, not someone "strange"). Don't be fooled by people asking you to show them directions or to go with them because your mother is sick or hurt.
4. Being touched by someone you like is a good feeling. You don't have to allow anyone to touch you in a way you don't like. Don't allow yourself to be left alone with a person you are uncomfortable with because he or she touches you in a way you don't like.
5. A "private part" is the part of you a bathing suit touches. If anyone asks you to show them a private part or touches a private part, tell them to stop, and tell someone else.
6. If the person you tell doesn't believe you, keep telling people until someone believes you.

Others areas of concern for the school-age child and family include sleep needs, dressing, exercise, hygiene, and dental care.

Dress

Although school-age children are capable of fully dressing themselves, they are not capable of taking care of their clothes until later in the school-age years—clothes taken off are dropped on the floor rather than placed in a hamper or a drawer. This is the right age (if not started already) to teach children the importance of caring for their own belongings. School-age children have definite opinions about style of clothing, often based on the likes of their friends rather than the preferences of their parents. Parents must be aware that the appropriate dress for school has changed since they were young. Where once school-age children wore uniforms or dresses and blazers, most schools now allow jeans and sweatshirts. Insisting that a child dress differently from classmates is unfair and even cruel. A child who wears different clothing may become the object of exclusion from a school club or group.

Sleep

Sleep needs vary among individual children. Younger school-age children generally require 12 hours of sleep each night, and older ones require about 10 hours. Most 6-year-olds are too old for naps but do require a quiet time after school to get them through the remainder of the day. Nighttime terrors may continue during the early school years and may actually increase during the first-grade year, as the child reacts to the stress of beginning school.

During the early school years, many children enjoy a quiet talk at bedtime. At about age 9, when friends become more important, children generally are ready to give up nighttime talks with parents. Some parents react strongly to this change and feel rejected. They may need some help to take at face value their child's statement, "I'm tired. I'd rather go to sleep."

Exercise

School-age children need daily exercise, and it is not true that because they go to school all day, they automatically receive this. School is basically a sit-down activity, and gym periods are not provided every day. Children who are bused to and from school may therefore return home without having spent much time in active exercise.

Exercise need not involve organized sports. It can come from neighborhood games or from bicycle riding. As children enter preadolescence, those with poor coordination may be reluctant to exercise. They should be stimulated to work off some calories in some daily exercise, or else obesity, which is a preteen problem, can result.

Hygiene

Children of 6 or 7 years of age still need help in regulating bath water temperature and in cleaning ears and fingernails. By age 8, children are generally capable of bathing themselves, but may not do it well because they are too busy to take the time or because they do not find bathing as important as their parents do.

Both boys and girls become interested in showering as they approach their teens. When girls begin to menstruate, they may be afraid to take baths or wash their hair during their period; they need information on the importance and safety of good hygiene during their menses.

Care of Teeth

With proper dental care, the average child today can expect to grow up cavity free. To ensure that this happens, school-age children should visit a dentist at least twice yearly for a checkup, cleaning, and possibly a fluoride treatment to strengthen and harden the tooth enamel (Figure 32-6). Some children develop a fear of dentists and, if the dentist hurts them, want to avoid going at all. The advantage of frequent visits is that if cavities are

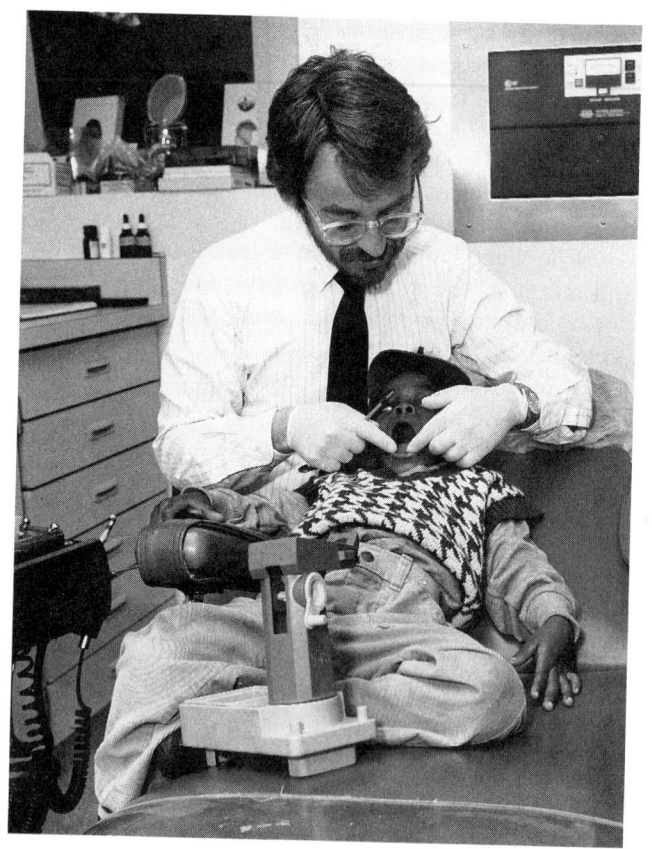

FIGURE 32-6

Dental caries are the number-one health problem in school-age children. Children need to be taught dental health measures and encouraged to visit a dentist twice a year. (Courtesy of the Department of Medical Photography, Children's Hospital, Buffalo, NY.)

filled when they are small, the drilling required is minimal and little pain is involved. If cavities are not treated promptly in this way but are allowed to grow large, the drilling hurts, causing these children to refuse to go back to the dentist. More large cavities then grow, and a vicious circle develops. Pedodontists specialize in caring for children's teeth and understand the developmental level of their patients. Children who tend to develop caries might be encouraged to visit a pedodontist if one is available and affordable.

School-age children have to be reminded to brush their teeth daily. If brushing becomes an area of conflict for the family, brushing well once a day may be more effective than brushing more often but doing an inadequate job. For effective brushing, the child should use a soft toothbrush, fluoride-based toothpaste, and dental floss to clean between teeth to help remove all plaque with each brushing.

Between-meal snacks are best limited to high-protein foods such as chicken and cheese, rather than snacks such as candy. If the child does eat candy, a type that is eaten quickly and dissolves quickly such as a plain chocolate bar is better than slowly dissolving or sticky candy, which stays in contact with the teeth longer. Fruit and vegetable snacks should be encouraged. Cereal, which is fortified with minerals and vitamins, can be a fun after-school snack for this age group (see also Chapter 34).

Promoting Healthy Family Functioning

At 6 years of age, most children have passed through a preschool phase of attraction for the parent of the opposite sex and identify with the parent of the same sex (Freud, 1962). Children from one-parent homes, or those with a parent who has difficulty being a good role model, may need help in finding a suitable adult to serve as this important person in their life.

To their parents' annoyance, many children often quote their teacher as the final authority on all subjects. This may be the first time the parents see someone surpassing them in their child's eyes, and accepting the situation can be painful. Children also cite their friends as guides for behavior: "Mary Jane doesn't have to go to bed until 10 o'clock," or "Billy's mother lets him go to the movies every Saturday." Parents may require help to realize that these remarks are a normal consequence of being exposed to other adults and children. A simple "There are all kinds of ways of doing things, but in our house, the rule is this" shows no criticism of Billy's or Mary Jane's or Miss Smith's way of life, yet conveys a special "our house" feeling and offers security to the child.

Parents often must be reminded that even the simplest tasks of everyday life require repeated practice before they can be accomplished well, and that good manners and grammar are not instinctive and must be learned in the same way as other tasks. The way parents correct a child as she learns simple tasks can influence her opinion of herself and her ability to continue learning new tasks. "Putting all the silverware in a pile is one way of putting them away; another way would be to divide spoons, forks, and knives separately" is always preferable to "What a silly way to put away silverware!" Comments such as "Can't you do anything right?" or "Why don't you ever do what I say?" should always be avoided, as children will rise only to the level expected of them. A child who is constantly told that he or she is stupid or thoughtless, bad or ill-behaved, may begin to act that way to conform to the parents' expectations.

If parents have difficulty telling what a child's completed project is supposed to be, the time-honored "Tell me about it" is preferable to "What is it?" It is good for parents to find a redeeming characteristic in a project, no matter how shakily put together it is: "I like the bright color you painted it" or "That must have been fun to make" does this. Actively displaying and using their gifts are part of having school-age children in a family. A finger painting hung on the refrigerator door will enhance, not detract from, the most elegant home. The best-dressed woman looks even more radiant wearing her child's necklace made of macaroni and paste. Both examples are gestures of love, a gesture that goes well with everything.

In talking to parents of school-age children, the following are good questions for you to ask to estimate the degree of interaction that occurs in the home and whether the parents are strengthening the child's sense of accomplishment: How do you correct John when he does something such as show poor manners at the table? ("It looks better to swallow food before you talk" or "Don't you ever do anything right? Swallow before you talk.") Do you hang up his drawings? Does he have chores that are his to accomplish?

Common Health Problems of the School-Age Period

Children in their early school years have one of the lowest rates of death and serious illness of any age group. The two leading causes of death that do occur are accidents and cancer. Illness is due largely to dental caries, gastrointestinal disturbances, and respiratory disorders, usually of an infectious origin. Chickenpox will continue to be a common infection in this age group until immunization is available and common.

Table 32-3 shows the usual health maintenance pattern for these children. Table 32-4 lists problems that parents may have in evaluating illness in the school-age child. Many communities are establishing school-based community health care clinics to improve the health care available for school-age children (Igoe, 1993).

Table 32-3. *Health Maintenance Schedule, School-Age Period*

Area of Focus	Methods	Frequency
Assessment		
Developmental milestones	History, observation	Every visit
Growth milestones	Height, weight plotted on standard growth chart; physical examination	Every visit
Hypertension	Blood pressure	Every visit
Nutrition	History, observation; height/weight information	Every visit
Parent–child relationship	History, observation	Every visit
Behavior or school problems	History, observation	Every visit
Vision and hearing disorders	History, observation	Every visit
	Formal Snellen or Titmus testing	At 7–8 yr and 10–12 yr
	Audiometer testing	At 6 yr and 10–12 yr
Dental health	History, physical examination	Every visit
Scoliosis	Physical examination	Yearly after age 8 yr
Thyroid	Physical examination, history	Every visit after age 10 yr
Tuberculosis	Tine test	Depending on prevalence of tuberculosis in community
Bacteriuria	Clean catch urine	At 6–7 and 10–12 yr
Anemia	Hematocrit	At 11–12 yr
Immunizations		
Rubeola, mumps, and rubella	Check history and past records; inform caregiver about any risks and side-effects; administer immunization in accordance with health care agency policies	At 12 yr
Anticipatory Guidance		
School-age care	Active listening and health teaching	Every visit
Expected growth and developmental milestones before next visit	Active listening and health teaching	Every visit
Accident prevention	Counseling about street and personal safety	Every visit
Problem-solving		
Any problems expressed by caregiver during course of the visit	Active listening and health teaching regarding cigarette smoking, drug abuse, school adjustment	Every visit

Dental Caries

Caries (cavities) are progressive, destructive lesions of the tooth calcium. As many as 80% of preschool children and 90% of school-age children have one cavity. The cause of dental decay is decalcification of the tooth enamel and dentine. When the *p*H of the tooth surface drops to 5.6 or below (which happens after children eat readily fermented carbohydrates, such as sucrose), acid microorganisms (acidogenic lactobacilli and aciduric streptococci) found in dental plaque attack the organic cementing medium of teeth and destroy it. Plaque tends to accumulate in deep grooves of the teeth and contact areas between teeth, making these areas most susceptible to dental decay. The enamel on primary teeth is thinner than on permanent teeth, making them more susceptible to destruction. The distance from the enamel to the pulp is shorter also, so destruction of the tooth nerve can occur quickly. Neglected caries also result in poor chewing and, therefore, poor digestion, abscess and pain, and, sometimes, osteomyelitis (bone infection).

As stated earlier, dental caries are largely preventable with proper brushing and fluoride application. When they do occur, it is important that they be treated quickly and that the child's dental hygiene practices are evaluated and improved, if that is deemed necessary. Most important, the child must feel that he has a stake in the health or disease of his teeth, so that he willingly undertakes the self-care measures necessary to ensure healthy teeth, with parental support rather than parental command.

Malocclusion

The upper jaw in children matures rapidly in early childhood along with skull growth; the lower jaw forms more slowly, which forces teeth to make a prolonged series of changes until they reach their final adult alignment and

Table 32-4. *Parental Difficulties Evaluating Illness in the School-Age Child*

Difficulty	Helpful Suggestions for Parents
Evaluating seriousness of illness	For the first time, a school-age child may view illness as a way to avoid unpleasant activities (school, a coach who asks too much, household chores). Evaluating whether the child has symptoms when he is asked to do something he likes to do often reveals the difference between exaggeration and an ill child (too sick to eat spinach, not too sick to eat ice cream; too sick to go to school, not too sick to go ice skating). If the child uses symptoms of illness as a means of avoiding situations, parents must evaluate what it is that the child wants so badly to avoid and see if some change should be made in expectations.
Evaluating nutritional intake	Many school-age children eat lunch at school; they may spend weekends away from home and weeks away at camp. As with all ages, noting whether they are growing and active is better than monitoring any 1 day's food intake.
Evaluating puberty changes	There is a wide variation in the time that secondary sex characteristics occur (9–17 yr for girls; 10–18 yr for boys). Children should be examined if and when they or their parents are concerned that pubertal changes are delayed.
Age-specific diseases to be aware of	School age is a time to evaluate vision; children normally develop vision changes as maturity of the eye globe increases. Squinting, rubbing eyes, or poor marks in school may be signs of poor vision.
	Streptococcal sore throats occur with a high frequency in early-school-age children. Those with sore throats should be examined by a health care provider to prevent complications, such as glomerulonephritis or rheumatic fever, from developing. Girls, in particular, must be evaluated for scoliosis (curvature of the spine). Mothers detect this by noticing that the girl's skirts hang unevenly or bra straps are uneven.
	Parents may need to be cautioned that vomiting or headache in the morning that passes fairly quickly (at about the same time the school bus leaves) may be a symptom of school phobia, but physical examination is in order because these are also symptoms of other conditions.
	Absence seizures, a neurologic condition that typically arises in school-age years, can be confused with behavior problems if observation is not thorough.

position. Good tooth occlusion, in which the upper teeth overlap the lower teeth by a small amount and teeth are evenly spaced and in good alignment, is necessary for optimum formation of teeth, health of the supporting tissue, optimum speech development, and a pleasant physical appearance for high self-esteem. **Malocclusion** (a deviation from the normal) may be congenital and related to conditions such as cleft palate, a small lower jaw, or familial traits tending toward malocclusion. The condition can result from constant mouth breathing or abnormal tongue position (tongue thrusting). Thumb-sucking appears to have little role in malocclusion as long as the thumb-sucking does not persist past the time of eruption of the permanent front teeth (6 to 7 years). The loss of teeth due to extraction or accident may lead to malocclusion if not properly treated to maintain alignment.

Malocclusion may be either crossbite (sideways) or anterior or posterior. Children with a malocclusion should be evaluated by an orthodontist to see if braces or other orthodontic work is necessary. Teeth braces are not only expensive, but they also cause pain for children when they are first applied and at periodic visits when they are tightened to maintain pressure for further straightening. Some children develop mild, shallow ulcerations (canker sores) of the buccal membrane

from friction of a metal wire. Rubbing the offending wire with dental wax dulls the surface and gives relief. Ora-Jel (an over-the-counter drug) rubbed on the ulceration also gives relief. Children who wear braces need to have their teeth assessed frequently to see that they are brushing properly around the braces (a Water Pik is often recommended for thorough cleaning) and that they are using dental floss to remove plaque from around wires.

Following the removal of braces, many children must wear retainers to help maintain the correction the braces achieved. Although braces are wired into place, retainers are not. Wearing a retainer can prove troublesome for the child, as it must be removed when eating (e.g., in the school cafeteria or in a restaurant). Show appropriate sympathy and help the child problem-solve if he or she is bothered by the appearance of braces or wearing a retainer. For instance, if removing the retainer in front of friends is truly embarrassing for the child, perhaps he or she could remove the retainer in the bathroom before going to the cafeteria each day. Braces and retainers have become a common feature of life for children of school age. Most children will find some comfort in not being the only one to suffer this indignity and, once used to their own appliances, will experience little reluctance in letting their classmates see them.

Parental Concerns of the School-Age Period

Problems Associated With Language Development

The common speech problem of the preschool years is broken fluency. The most common problem of the school-age child is articulation. The child has difficulty pronouncing *s, z, th, l, r,* and *w* or substitutes *w* for *r* ("west" instead of "rest") or *r* for *l* ("radies" instead of "ladies"). This is most noticeable during the first and second grades; it usually disappears by the third grade.

Common Fears and Anxieties of the School-Age Child

Anxiety Related to Beginning School. Adjusting to grade school is a big task for a 6-year-old. Even if he or she attended preschool, this is different. The rules are firmer and the elective feeling ("If he doesn't like it, we'll take him out of it") is gone. School is for keeps until age 16 or longer, a time span hard for the child to imagine. Whereas preschool learning was carried out through fun activities, part of every day in grade school involves obvious work (see the Focus on Cultural Awareness box).

Because school is an adjustment, a health assessment of all school-age children should include an inquiry about progress in school. You can obtain information by asking the parent, "How is Susan doing in school?" followed by a second question, "How does her teacher say she is doing?" If there is a discrepancy between the answers, the situation bears study. The answer to the first question reveals the parent's attitude toward the child's progress. The answer to the second may indicate that the child is having trouble adjusting to a structured school environment. Some parents have to alter their expectations to conform with their child's actual ability. This can be difficult.

FOCUS ON CULTURAL AWARENESS

The United States is a culture that supports education for all children, and thus it is usually assumed that all parents will be interested in seeing that their child attends school regularly. However, education is not viewed as important in all cultures and some parents do not value it highly or enforce school attendance strongly. It is important to be aware of this when planning care for a school-age child, since the child who sees attending and doing well in school as important will usually be more anxious to finish a rehabilitation program than the child who does not see hurrying back to school as a priority.

One of the biggest tasks of the first year of school is learning to read. It is best if parents have prepared their child for this by reading to him since infancy, pointing to the words and pictures as they went along. This helps children to realize that sentences flow from left to right and that the words, not the pictures, tell the story. Adults can set an example by being seen reading, so the child associates learning to read with adult activity. If adults spend most of their free time watching television, the child will think reading is mainly for children and assume that it is not important. Six-year-olds are very interested in imitating adults, and can be influenced toward or away from reading, depending on the behavior of adults around them.

If first graders have difficulty grasping the importance of reading because their school books tell uninteresting stories, a parent can make it more fun by encouraging the practical use of reading, such as asking the child to read recipes while the parent cooks or to read road signs during a car trip. A parent can also help by playing a game, such as treasure hunt in which the parent hides a small object, such as a favorite toy, then writes simple clues on slips of paper—"Look under a lamp," then, under the lamp, "Look in a book," and so on until the child has been led to the hidden object. Such games help the child see reading as an important means of obtaining information. He can develop writing skills by playing the same game for the parent to follow.

Many first-grade children are capable of mature action at school but appear less mature when they return home. Their pseudosophistication of the day is gone. They may bite their nails, suck their thumb, or talk baby talk. Some develop tics (irregular movements of isolated muscle groups), such as wrinkling the forehead, shrugging the shoulders, twisting the mouth, coughing, clearing the throat, or frequently blinking or rolling the eyes. Such movements may occasionally be confused with seizure activity. Tics, however, disappear during sleep and occur mainly when the child is subjected to stress or anxiety. Scolding, nagging, threatening, or punishing does not stop either tics or nail biting; it invariably makes these problems worse. Methods such as using bad-flavored clear nail polish and restraining the child's hands to prevent nail-biting are also ineffective.

To stop these behaviors, the underlying stress should be discovered and alleviated. Urge parents to spend some time with the child after school or in the evening, so that he or she continues to feel secure in the family and does not feel pushed out by being sent to school. If such behavior manifestations persist despite attempts to eliminate their cause, the child may need to be referred for counseling.

School Phobia. *School phobia* is fear of attending school (Castiglia, 1993). Children who resist attending school this way may develop physical signs of illness, such as vomiting, diarrhea, headache, or abdominal pain on school days. This lasts until after the school bus has left or the child is allowed to stay home for the day. The cause of resistance to school must be determined before it can be cured. In some instances it may be fear of separation from the parents. The child may be reluctant to leave home because she feels that younger brothers or sisters will usurp her parents' affection while she is at school. The child may also be reacting to a particular teacher or to a particular situation, such as a test or having to shower in gym class.

The anxiety of separation may be the child's or the parents'. The child may be overdependent, but the parent may be overprotective. One parent may overprotect the child to hide ambivalent feelings about her, while another parent may overprotect because the child has a physical problem, such as diabetes, recurrent convulsions, or a heart defect.

If a child is reacting to a particular teacher or a special situation such as gym showers, the parents should investigate the matter. The child's fear may be well grounded. Counseling may help the child accept the situation. If not, parents should attempt to have her transferred to another classroom or perhaps excused from a disliked situation such as showering. Because the problem of school phobia is usually only partly the child's, the entire family generally requires counseling to resolve the issue. As a rule, the child should continue to attend school once it has been established that he or she is free of any illness that would prevent this. Firmness on the part of parents should prevent the development of problems such as school failure, peer ridicule, or a pattern of avoiding difficulties. The child may benefit from a gradual program of school involvement, such as walking to school but not going in, then going to school but staying for only 1 hour, staying for half a day, and so on, until she can stay all day every day. Parents should treat the illness matter-of-factly (a great deal of reassurance that these symptoms are not major will be necessary) and take her firmly to the bus or to the classroom.

Handling school phobia requires coordination among the school, school nurse, and health care provider who diagnoses the problem. A nurse is the ideal person to coordinate such efforts and to help the parents allow the child some independence not only in going to school but in other activities. Counseling may be necessary to help parents realize that this is partly their problem and that they need to allow the child to develop some independence. A few children require psychiatric therapy to resolve their difficulties with school. See the Nursing Care Plan: Health Maintenance Visit for a School-Age Child.

Latchkey Children
Latchkey children are school children who are without adult supervision for a part of each weekday. The term

alludes to the fact that they generally carry a key so they can let themselves into their home after school (Doak & Hobbie, 1991).

Latchkey children have become a prominent concern because in as many as 90% of families today, both parents work at least part-time outside the home. Few of these parents have work hours so flexible that they can always be at home when the child leaves for or returns from school. Extended family members who once watched children after school are often working as well or may no longer be close at hand; many communities are no longer close-knit enough to have neighbors who can be depended on to help out with informal child care.

A major concern is that latchkey children feel lonely and have an increased tendency to have accidents, delinquent behavior, and decreased school performance from lack of homework supervision. For those children who feel safe in their community, however, a short period of independence every day may actually be beneficial, because it encourages problem-solving in self-care.

A number of helpful suggestions for parents whose children must spend time alone before or after school are shown in Box 32-2. Many communities offer special afterschool programs for such children. Nurses are in a position to educate parents about such services so that their children can feel both safe as well as stimulated creatively during this time. Both the Boy Scouts of America and the Council of Campfire Girls offer programs to help children adjust to being home alone. Many communities are organizing hot-line numbers that a child who is alone can call if a problem arises. At health visits, assess whether parents or the child appear to have a problem with, or are uncomfortable about, after-school arrangements. For the child who is extremely fearful or impulsive or who finds problem-solving difficult, time alone after school may not be appropriate. Determine the individual circumstances, and recommend changes when possible.

Preparation for Adolescence
For children to be prepared for their teens, it is important that they be educated about puberty changes and responsible sexual practices.

Menstruation. Most girls have some menstrual irregularity during the first year after menarche (the start of menstruation). This occurs primarily because menstruation is anovulatory at first. With maturity and the onset of ovulation, the cycle becomes more regular (Cunningham et al., 1993).

Early preparation for menstruation is important preparation for future childbearing and for the girl's concept of herself as a woman. A girl who is told that menstruation is a normal function that occurs every month in

Beth is a 7-year-old girl who is seen in an ambulatory care clinic for a yearly health maintenance visit. The following is a nursing care plan you might design for her.

Assessment: Seven-year-old who nods in response or answers only with short attempts to direct questions. Her mother is concerned because she "hates" school and has started refusing to ride school bus. Family consists of mother, three older siblings (ages 12, 15, and 17 years). Mother states Beth enjoyed school last year. States child prefers to practice baton twirling rather than read (has won two ribbons in state competition). Physical examination: within normal limits.

Nursing Diagnosis: Parental anxiety related to beginning school phobia in child

Defining Characteristic: Parent states she is concerned about child's reluctance to attend school.

Goal: Mother will report improved behavior in child by 6 months' time.

Outcome Criteria: Mother voices satisfaction with child's progress and attendance.

Nursing Orders	*Rationale*
1. Explore possible reasons for child's reluctance to attend school.	1. Identifying the reason for the problem can be the beginning of problem-solving (e.g., is another child bullying her on the bus to and from school?).
2. Assess Beth for vision and hearing; do physical exam.	2. Child's interest in large motor rather than fine motor activities can be indication of vision difficulty; a hearing deficit can interfere with understanding speech of those around her, causing child to feel embarrassed and withdrawn.
3. Stress importance of child attending school even though she resists (assuming physical exam reveals healthy child).	3. The longer a child stays out of school, the harder it is to return.
4. Suggest mother meet with child's teacher to discuss problem.	4. Encouraging school attendance should be a joint effort between family and school.
5. Suggest mother telephone with report of concern in 2 weeks; reschedule routine health assessment for 6 months.	5. School phobia can be an extensive problem that requires ongoing support.

all healthy women has a different attitude toward her body than the girl who wakes up one morning to find blood on her pajamas and is told bluntly, "You'd better get used to that. You're going to have to put up with it for the rest of your life." In the first instance, the girl can trust her body: it is doing what every woman's body does. In the second instance, she feels that her body is beyond her control. How can she accept and enjoy growing up if it involves something so unpredictable? In addition to an explanation of the reason for menstrual flow, a girl needs an explanation of good hygiene and reassurance that she can bathe, shower, and swim during her period. She can use either sanitary napkins or tampons, although if she uses tampons, she must take precautions to avoid toxic shock syndrome (see Chapter 47).

The significance of menstrual irregularity should not be dismissed lightly. A girl needs to know when her period will occur, so that she can grow used to this new phenomenon and learn to trust her body. An older girl in college can matter-of-factly explain that she prefers not to go to the beach today because she has her menstrual period and does not want to use tampons. For a preadolescent, this topic is too sophisticated and too emotionally charged to discuss openly. She wants to be able to plan activities to avoid making such explanations.

A girl may fear that irregular periods indicate a hor-

Box 32-2
Teaching Points for the Parents of Latchkey Children

Safety Teaching for the Child

Always to lock doors and never to show keys to others or indicate that he or she stays home alone.

To answer the telephone and say a parent is busy, not absent from home.

What to do in event he or she loses key (stay with a neighbor, etc.).

Not to go into the house if the door is open or a window is broken.

Fire safety (practice a fire drill from all rooms of the house).

To check in with parents by telephone when he or she first arrives home from school.

To identify a caller before opening the door. Agree on a secret code word; child should not open the door or go with a person unless the person knows the word.

How to change light bulbs safely if it will be dark before parents return home. If appropriate, teach child how to change fuses or reset circuit-breaker switches.

How to report a fire and telephone police (practice this with the child).

Safety Responsibilities of Parents

Prepare a safety kit and keep it filled; include a flashlight in case of a power failure so that the child does not need to light candles.

Plan after-school snacks that do not require cooking to prevent burns.

Keep firearms locked with the key in a place unknown to child. Instruct in firearm safety.

Keep a list of emergency telephone numbers (including parents' work numbers) by the telephone.

Arrange with a neighbor who is usually home during the late afternoon for the child to stay there in an emergency.

If an older child will be watching a younger one, be certain both children understand the rules laid down and the degree of responsibility expected.

Be certain the child understands that rules that apply during other times (never swim alone; do not play by the railroad tracks) also apply during independent time.

Parental Actions to Prevent Loneliness

Urge the child to telephone either parent every day to touch base (be sure the child has work telephone numbers).

Be certain to make additional time available at home after work so that the child is able to describe his or her day.

Each morning help the child plan an activity for that day so that he or she has something purposeful to look forward to during time alone.

Allow special privileges such as listening to music that other members of the family do not like as well; allow extra television hours during this time.

Consider a pet. Even a caged animal, such as a hamster or a bird, offers companionship in a quiet house.

Call the child if there will be a delay in arriving home; unexpected time alone is very frightening to a child.

Leave messages on the refrigerator or in the bathroom that just say hi.

Leave a tape or video recorded message for the child to play (make sure it is not full of tasks to do, but is a welcoming message).

Encourage the child to read; fictional characters serve as friends as well as help to pass time.

Urge the child to network with other latchkey children as to how they use time effectively; talking on the telephone to another child reduces loneliness for both.

Parental Actions to Increase Socialization

Help the child plan after-school activities such as joining a science club for 1 afternoon a week.

Explore sports programs at school or in the community, as these often are held after school.

Explore latchkey groups at the school the child attends, a public library, or a church.

Network with other parents (nurse can help) or ask for flex time so that child supervision can be alternated after school.

Be sure the child socializes with friends on weekends or on days when either parent is home.

Parental Actions to Increase Self-Esteem

Praise the child for the ability to take care of himself or herself for short time intervals (rather than scold that there are cracker crumbs on the carpet).

Walk with the child through the empty house and together identify sounds (the click of the furnace turning on, the refrigerator starting to defrost, etc.), so that he or she can problem-solve the cause of sounds when home alone.

Help the child to view quiet time as beneficial time in which he or she can do some things more efficiently than at noisy times (e.g., homework).

Do not allow child to use the latchkey role to provoke parental guilt. Allow the child to have some say in family spending and thus see how his or her time alone (which allows both parents to work) contributes to family unity and progress.

mone imbalance and worry about her future ability to conceive, or she may be ill-informed about how conception occurs and fear that irregularity of her periods means she is pregnant. Other causes of irregular periods are malnourishment and obesity. Emotions can also affect menstruation. If irregularity continues beyond the first year, a careful history of the girl's school, social, and home adjustment should be taken. (Dysmenorrhea, or painful menstruation, is discussed in Chapter 47.)

For a nominal charge, manufacturers of sanitary napkins will mail an introductory kit of their products, together with well-illustrated, factual booklets, to introduce girls to menstruation. Such kits are useful if they supplement a parent's or a nurse's discussion, but they should not take the place of individual discussion.

Sex Education. Preteenagers should have adults they can turn to for answers to questions about sex. Ideally, this should be their parents, but because sex is an emotionally charged topic, some parents may be extremely uncomfortable discussing it with their children. As a result, health care personnel often become resource persons for this (Braverman & Strasburger, 1994).

Teach children to understand not only the new functions of their bodies but the social and moral implications of sexual maturity. A sex education course that includes films and discussions is helpful but never answers all a preteen's questions. (Most youngsters would rather avoid asking a question than risk appearing ignorant in front of their peers.)

Handing children booklets or showing films with the words, "If you have any questions after you've read (or watched) this, come and ask me" is ineffective teaching. It implies that they should have no questions. Watch films or read booklets with children to show that you are truly available.

Teach reproductive organ function. Discuss secondary sexual characteristics so that children will know what is going on in their bodies. Describe the physiology of reproduction so that they understand what menstruation is and why it occurs. Explain male sexual functioning, including why the production of increased amounts of seminal fluid leads to nocturnal emissions. Assure preadolescent boys that these emissions are normal.

Both girls and boys should have an explanation of the physiology of pregnancy and the possibility that comes with sexual maturity for starting unplanned or unwanted pregnancies. The American Academy of Pediatrics recommends that sex education be incorporated into health education throughout the school years in a manner that is appropriate to age and development (AAP, 1990). For preadolescents, this may include guidance concerning birth control measures and the principles of safer sex, since some may already be sexually active (Swenson, 1992; see Chapter 4 and the Focus on Nursing Research display).

FOCUS ON NURSING RESEARCH

How Early Do Children Begin Sexual Relationships?

To answer this question, a nursing researcher studied the records of 183 adolescents, age 15 years or younger, who had attended a metropolitan teen family planning clinic. Of these children, 13% had yet to experience their first sexual experience. Twenty-eight percent had had their first experience before the age of 12; 41% between 12 and 13 years of age, and 18% between 14 and 15 years. Twenty-six percent had already experienced three or more sexually transmitted diseases.

This study documents the early age at which children are beginning to be sexually active. The researcher cautions that the population of this study was of a large metropolitan area and may not be representative of all communities.

Swenson, I. E. (1992). A profile of young adolescents attending a teen family planning clinic. *Adolescence, 27,* 647.

Nursing Diagnoses and Related Interventions

Nursing Diagnosis: Parental anxiety related to behavior of school-age child

Goal: Parent will voice he feels less anxious by next health supervision visit.

Outcome Criteria: Parent states that undesired behavior has decreased in frequency; parent feels less stress about child's health or future.

Stealing. During early school age, most children go through a period in which they steal loose change from their mother's purse or father's dresser. This usually happens at around 7 years of age, when they are learning how to make change and discovering the importance of money. Part of the reason for a 7-year-old's stealing is that, although the child is gaining an appreciation for money as she learns to make change and perhaps is sent to the store for minor purchases, this appreciation is not yet balanced by strong moral principles.

The reason for the stealing should be explored. Do other children on the block receive an allowance and thus have money for small items? Did the child make a bet he must pay off? Is he buying a bully's friendship by purchasing gum or candy for him? Does the child view money as security? The matter is best handled without a great deal of emotion. The child should be told that the money is missing. The importance of property rights should be reviewed: mother's and father's money is theirs; the child's money is the child's. They are not interchangeable. Youngsters who continue to steal much past 9 years of age may require counseling, because they should have progressed beyond this normal developmental step by this age.

Some shoplifting occurs at age 7, but the major problem with this arises during preadolescence. Some shoplifting occurs for the same reason that past generations tipped over outhouses or untied the preacher's horse and buggy: it is a public act of rebellion against authority, a "coming of age" ritual. It occurs due to peer pressure, when the child feels he *must* have a certain type of clothing to belong to the "in" crowd; it can be an initiation ritual to a gang. It is also hard for children to envision how a large store can be hurt by one missing article. The principle that keeps them from stealing from individuals is more difficult to apply here.

Children must be warned that shoplifting is a punishable crime, not a prank. Just as money missing from a purse should not be ignored, shoplifting should be confronted immediately to prevent the child who succeeds once from taking something even bigger the second time. She should be asked how she came to possess the article and should not be allowed to use it. The child should then be denied access to stores until she demonstrates more responsibility. A child who shoplifts more than once may need counseling; it reflects more than simple confusion about property rights.

As an overall principle, parents must set good examples if they expect their child to be honest. If one parent takes money from the other without permission, neither should be surprised to find their child attempting to do the same. If a parent changes price tags or unwraps items and eats them without paying for them in the supermarket, he or she cannot expect the child to do otherwise.

Recreational Drug Use. What was once considered a college or high school problem is now a problem of early school age. Illegal drugs are available to children as early as elementary school and certainly by the time they reach the seventh and eighth grades.

The use of hard drugs and alcohol and ways to encourage children to avoid that use are discussed in Chapter 33. Cocaine is becoming increasingly easy for children to obtain (Muramoto & Leshan, 1993). Two substances that are easily available to school-age children, and so uniquely abused by them, are rubber cement and airplane glue (toluene; Schulz, 1993). Children do not become physically addicted to glue but do become psychologically dependent on it. To achieve the desired effect, they drop quantities of the glue into a paper bag, then sniff the fumes and experience a feeling of exhilaration or giddiness. This may seem a harmless procedure, but in high concentrations the fumes can cause extensive liver damage or pulmonary edema that can be fatal.

Parents should suspect glue sniffing or some other form of recreational drug use if their child regularly appears irritable, inattentive, or drowsy. School health personnel should be aware of the increase in this practice among students and look for warning signs.

Abuse of steroids to improve muscle mass can be found in children as young as sixth grade. Children need to be counseled against this, since abuse of steroids leads to cardiovascular irregularities, uncontrollable aggressiveness, and possible cancer in later life.

Cigarette smoking can also begin in school-age children. With the sure knowledge that cigarette smoking plays a large part in the development of lung cancer and other serious respiratory illnesses, many parents assume that their children will not begin to smoke. Unfortunately, smoking is still considered by children to be an adult activity, so adopting the habit is thought to be a giant step on the road to adulthood. Because cigarette advertisers are increasingly targeting young people as consumers, it might be helpful to teach school-age children to recognize advertising manipulation aimed at them. Children also need to be cautioned against experimenting with smokeless tobacco, which leads to mouth and throat cancer. As many as 30% of boys try this after seeing baseball players using it (Hill et al., 1992).

Both nurses and parents should be role models of excellent health behaviors when caring for school-age children, in hopes that these adults of tomorrow will follow their example.

Unique Concerns of the Disabled or Chronically Ill School-Age Child

One of the biggest problems facing a school-age child with a long-term illness or disability is time lost from school. This not only threatens academic achievement but the child's relationships with peers. It may make him or her the "odd person out" with respect to making friends or joining gangs. Whether the child is confined to the home or hospitalized, helping him or her to keep in contact with friends by telephone or letter writing fosters the socialization that is important to continued development. A parent (or a school friend) can obtain schoolwork and help the child with homework so that the child is able to progress with learning and continue to build self-esteem.

Most disabled children attend regular schools and take classes with healthy children (termed **inclusion**) because federal law (PL 99-457) stipulates that all children must receive equal education in the least restrictive situation possible (Downey, 1990). Placement in classrooms is determined by a committee in each school system. You may need to advocate for a child with such a committee to demonstrate, for example, that although confined to a wheelchair or needing continuous oxygen, he or she can participate in a regular classroom setting;

or that a child would benefit from a period each day with a special resource teacher. It may be necessary to meet with a school nurse, teacher, or the child's classmates to increase their understanding and acceptance of the child's illness.

Children with a disability need to be assigned household chores as are other children and to participate in activities such as Girl or Boy Scouts, in which accomplishment is encouraged. It is important for the disabled or chronically ill school-age child to develop a sense of industry or accomplishment so that she can persevere in measures that will help her to be as independent as possible (Figure 32-7). For example, the child may practice muscle-strengthening exercises over and over again to prevent loss of muscle through atrophy.

When you are caring for a school-age child with a chronic illness or disability, choose short-term activities that can be completed independently. Conversely, be careful not to insult a child with tasks that are obviously not age-appropriate. Table 32-5 describes some nursing actions that can help to foster a sense of industry in disabled or chronically ill school-age children.

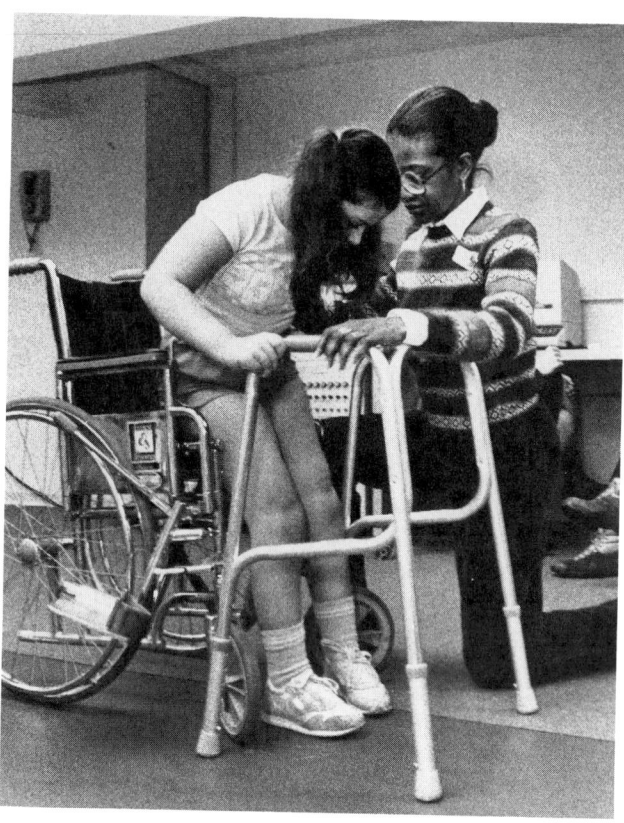

FIGURE 32-7
Helping school-age children who have physical disabilities to learn to ambulate goes far toward helping them gain a sense of industry. (Courtesy of the Department of Medical Photography, Children's Hospital, Buffalo, NY.)

Key Points

- School-age children mature slowly but steadily. Their annual average weight gain is 3 to 5 lb; their increase in height, 1 to 2 inches.
- At about age 10, children begin to develop secondary sex characteristics. Preparation for this helps them to accept these changes positively.
- Deciduous teeth are lost and permanent teeth erupt during the school-age period.
- Erikson's developmental task for the school-age period is to gain a sense of industry, or how to do things well.
- Common health problems during the school-age period include minor respiratory and gastrointestinal infections as well as dental caries and malocclusion.
- Common parental concerns about the school-age child are language development, fears and anxieties, and behavior problems such as stealing and using recreational drugs.
- As many as 90% of parents of school-age children are dual-earner families. This means many school-age children return home before their parents. Counseling families on ways to turn this into a positive experience is a nursing responsibility.
- Children in a concrete stage of operational thought are limited to understanding concepts they can actually see. When health teaching, use concrete examples (actually let them hold a syringe, don't just talk about it) to increase their understanding.
- School-age children thrive on set rules. It is confusing for them when rules are changed (medicine will now be taken four rather than three times a day) unless they have a clear explanation why the change is occurring.
- School-age children are looking for good adult role models; it is hard for them to feel confidence in an adult who isn't honest with them or who fails to live up to their expectations by not following through on promises.

Critical Thinking Exercises

1. Martha is a 6-year-old who tells you she "hates school." What areas would you want to explore with her to document the extent of the problem? What are suggestions you might make to her parents to make school more appealing?
2. Debbie is a 9-year-old you see at a health maintenance visit. Her father tells you she is a "behavior problem" in school. What special physical assessments would you want to make of Debbie? What questions would you want to ask to discover the extent of the problem?
3. Russell is a 12-year-old who is confined to a wheel-

Table 32-5. Nursing Actions That Encourage a Sense of Industry in the Disabled or Chronically Ill School-Age Child

Category	Actions
Nutrition	Allow choices of food and respect food preferences.
	Provide small food servings that child can finish, encouraging sense of accomplishment.
Dressing	Allow child to make out requisitions for supplies.
	Ask for suggestions as to how bulky the child wants dressing, where to apply tape.
Medicine	Teach child name and action of medicine.
	Encourage child to keep track of medication times by clock or record.
	Child may feel more in control of injections or intravenous insertions if allowed to choose the site from among options offered.
	Allow child to choose oral medicine form (capsules or liquid) if possible.
Rest	Establish clear rules for rest periods (reading or watching television is all right; playing a game is not, etc.).
Hygiene	Respect modesty of school-age child at an adult level.
	Allow as much choice as possible (e.g., own clothing, timing of self-care).
Pain	Encourage child to express pain.
	Encourage child to use distraction techniques, such as counting backward from 100 or imagery, during episodes of pain.
	Explain source and cause of pain to give child sense of mastery.
Stimulation	Encourage school work.
	Encourage activity that ends in a product (putting together a picture puzzle rather than listening to a record).
	Encourage paper-and-pencil games, such as connect the dots, tic tac toe.
	Card games provide social interaction and also encourage simple addition skills (make a deck from paper if one is not available).
	Do not suggest competition games for children less than age 10 yr.
	Encourage using playroom for socialization.
	Encourage child to keep in contact with school friends by telephoning or writing notes to them.

chair from muscular dystrophy. Why might developing a sense of industry be particularly difficult for him? What are specific suggestions you might make to encourage this?

References

American Academy of Pediatrics (AAP). (1990). Contraception and adolescents. *Pediatrics, 86,* 135.

Braverman. K., & Strasburger, V. C. (1994). Adolescent sexuality: the practitioner's role. *Clinical Pediatrics, 33,* 100.

Castiglia, P. T. (1993). School phobia/school avoidance. *Journal of Pediatric Health Care, 7,* 229.

Cunningham, F. G., et al. (1993). *Williams obstetrics* (19th ed.). Norwalk, CT: Appleton and Lange.

Curry, D. M., & Duby, J. C. (1994). Developmental surveillance by pediatric nurses. *Pediatric Nursing, 20,* 40.

Department of Health and Human Services. (1991). *Healthy people 2000.* Washington, DC: Public Health Service.

DeWitt, S. (1990). Nursing assessment of the skin and dermatologic lesions. *Nursing Clinics of North America, 25,* 235.

Doak, S., & Hobbie, C. (1991). Latchkey children. *Journal of Pediatric Health Care, 5,* 110.

Downey, W. S. (1990). Public Law 99-457 and the clinical pediatrician. *Clinical Pediatrics, 29,* 158.

Erikson, F. H. (1986). *Childhood and society.* New York: W. W. Norton.

Freud, S. (1962). *Three essays on the theory of sexuality.* New York: Hearst Corporation.

Grey, M. (1993). Stressors and children's health. *Journal of Pediatric Nursing, 8,* 85.

Hill, M. E., et al. (1992). Predictors of smokeless tobacco use by adolescents. *Research in Nursing and Health, 15,* 359.

Igoe, J. (1993). School-linked family health centers in health care reform. *Pediatric Nursing, 19,* 67.

Kohlberg, L. (1981). *The philosophy of moral development: Moral stages and the idea of justice.* New York: Harper & Row.

Muramoto, M. L., & Leshan, L. (1993). Adolescent substance abuse. *Primary Care, 20,* 141.

Piaget, J., & Infelder, B. (1969). *The psychology of the child.* New York: Basic Books.

Schulz, J. G. (1993). Illicit drugs of abuse. *Primary Care, 20,* 221.

Swenson, I. E. (1992). A profile of young adolescents attending a team family planning clinic. *Adolescence, 27,* 647.

Walker, L. J., & Taylor, J. H. (1991). Family interactions and the development of moral reasoning. *Child Development, 62,* 338.

Suggested Readings

Ahmann, E. (1994). Family-centered care; the time has come. *Pediatric Nursing, 20,* 52.

Gortmaker, S. L., et al. (1990). Chronic conditions, socio-economic risks, and behavioral problems in children and adolescents. *Pediatrics, 85,* 267.

Katz, P. A., & Walsh, P. V. (1991). Modification of children's gender-stereotyped behavior. *Child Development, 62,* 338.

Kornguth, M. L. (1990). School illnesses: Who's absent and why? *Pediatric Nursing, 16,* 95.

Loman, D. G. (1993). Child care problems of nurses. *Journal of Nursing Education, 23,* 5.

Malfair, A. (1992). Supporting the child with special needs. *Canadian Nurse, 88,* 17.

Malloy, C. (1992). Children and poverty: America's future at risk. *Pediatric Nursing, 18,* 553.

Wilson, P. D., & Testani-Dufour, L. (1993). Bicycle safety programs: targeting injury prevention through education. *Pediatric Nursing, 19,* 343.

Chapter 33

The Family With an Adolescent

Key Terms

- adolescence
- comedones
- formal operations
- identity
- puberty
- role confusion
- substance abuse

Objectives

After mastering the contents of this chapter, you should be able to:

1. Describe the normal growth and development pattern and common parental concerns of the adolescent period.

2. Assess adolescents for normal growth and development milestones.

3. Formulate nursing diagnoses for the family of an adolescent.

4. Plan nursing care related to growth and development concerns of the adolescent, such as planning health teaching necessary to accept puberty changes.

5. Implement nursing care related to growth and development or special needs of the adolescent, such as organizing a discussion group on ways to prevent drug abuse.

6. Evaluate outcome criteria to be certain that nursing goals were achieved.

7. Identify National Health Goals related to the adolescent that nurses could be instrumental in helping the nation to achieve.

8. Identify areas related to care of adolescents that could benefit from additional nursing research.

9. Use critical thinking to analyze ways in which care of the adolescent could be more family centered.

10. Synthesize knowledge of adolescent growth and development with nursing process to achieve quality maternal and child health nursing care.

Adele Pillitteri: MATERNAL AND CHILD HEALTH NURSING, 2nd Edition. © 1995 Adele Pillitteri.

Adolescence is the time period between 13 years and 18 to 20 years which serves as a transition period between childhood and adulthood. It can be divided into an early period (13 to 14 years), a middle period (15 to 16 years), and a late period (17 to 20 years). However, adolescence is defined not so much by chronologic age as by physiologic, psychological, and sociologic factors. The drastic change in physical appearance and the change in expectations of others (especially parents) may lead to both emotional and physical health problems.

Adolescents invariably feel a sense of pressure throughout this period. Parents expect them to think for themselves, yet set early evening curfews. The adolescent's sexual interests are awakening, but personal or parental prohibitions discourage him or her from becoming sexually active. These are examples of the major dilemma for adolescents—they are mature in some respects but still young in others—a dilemma that leads to the many growth and developmental concerns of the age.

There is such a strong adolescent subculture today that parents may feel that the minute their child enters the teenage years, all communication stops. Parents may expect difficulty controlling the child or understanding teenage values, as though entering this period locks the adolescent into a shell or pulls down a curtain between child and parents. This can become a self-fulfilling prophecy, whereby the parents actually cause the communication breakdown. At other times, of course, a communication problem can begin when a teenager refuses to respect parents' opinions and stops asking for them. Many of the problems adolescents bring to health care personnel arise from this communication impasse, no matter how it started. They often come to health care facilities with many misconceptions, seeking adult help and guidance. National Health Goals related to adolescence are shown in the Focus on National Health Goals display.

⊞ **NURSING PROCESS OVERVIEW**
*for Healthy Development
of the Adolescent*

ASSESSMENT

Parents rarely bring adolescents for health maintenance visits, and adolescents generally don't come to health care facilities on their own unless they are ill; as a result, these children are not seen for health assessments as often as they were when younger. When adolescents are accompanied by their parents at health visits, it is best to obtain their health history separately from parents to promote independence and responsibility for self-care. When performing physical examinations on adolescents, be aware that they may be very self-conscious. They also need health assurance and appreciate comments such as "Your hair has a nice, healthy feel," or "This is an accessory nipple. Have you ever wondered about it?" (see the Focus on Cultural Awareness display).

FOCUS ON
National Health Goals

Health teaching in the adolescent years is important, because healthy habits begun at this time can influence health over a life time. For this reason, a number of National Health Goals relate to adolescent health:

- Reduce the number of overweight adolescents to a prevalence of no more than 1.5% among adolescents ages 12 through 19 from a baseline of 15%.
- Reduce to no more than 15% the proportion of people age 6 and older who engage in no leisure-time physical activity from a baseline of 24%.
- Reduce smokeless tobacco use by males ages 12 through 24 to a prevalence of no more than 4% from a baseline of 8.9% in males; 6.6% in females.
- Reduce deaths caused by alcohol-related motor vehicle accidents to no more than 18% among people ages 15 to 24 from a baseline of 21.5%.
- Reduce suicide to no more than 8.2 per 100,000 youths ages 15 to 19 from a baseline of 10.3 per 100,000.
- Reduce homicides to no more than 1.4 per 100,000 individuals ages 15 to 34 from a baseline of 1.7 (DHHS, 1991).

Nurses can be instrumental in helping the nation achieve these goals by educating adolescents against cigarette, smokeless tobacco, alcohol, drug abuse, and violence and by acting as support people for adolescents during times of crisis to help prevent suicide. Areas in which additional knowledge is needed that could benefit from additional nursing research are identifying effective programs that reduce the use of smokeless tobacco or cigarette smoking, documenting the best actions for nurses to take in emergency rooms when adolescents are admitted following suicide attempts, and constructing rapid surveys to identify adolescents who are abusing drugs.

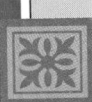

FOCUS ON CULTURAL AWARENESS

In the United States, as in most developed countries, adolescence covers a long time span. In developing countries, in contrast, adolescence tends to be much shorter because adolescents must take full-time jobs to help support their families. Socioeconomic factors definitely influence the length of adolescence across all cultures. Recognizing that adolescents may have differing responsibilities and life experiences based on cultural expectations can be useful to the nurse when making an assessment. In a family in which an adolescent is expected to begin working full-time or to marry at an early age, the nurse may need to make a broader health assessment that includes such factors as occupational hazards or the effects of job, family, and financial stress on the adolescent.

NURSING DIAGNOSIS

Frequent nursing diagnoses related to adolescents and their families are:

- Health-seeking behaviors related to normal growth and development
- Self-esteem disturbance related to facial acne
- Anxiety related to concerns about normal growth and development
- High risk for injury related to peer pressure to use alcohol and drugs
- Potential for enhanced parenting related to increased knowledge of teenage years

PLANNING

When planning with adolescents, respect the fact that they have a desire to exert independence and do things their own way. They are not likely to adhere to a plan of care that disrupts their lifestyle or makes them appear different from others their age. Including them in planning is essential so that the plan will be accepted. Establishing a contract (i.e., the adolescent agrees to take medication daily) may be the most effective means to reach a goal.

Adolescents are very present-oriented; a program that provides immediate results, such as focusing on short-term goals such as increased respiratory function, will be carried out well. Conversely, a regimen oriented toward the future, with long-term goals such as preventing hypertension, may not be as successful. This is not to say that it is not important to teach adolescents about the necessity for maintaining a healthy lifestyle—eating well, *not* smoking, and generally taking care of their bodies—but that information should be geared as much as possible to specific, short-term benefits to their health.

These organizations may be of use for possible referral:

American Association of Suicidology
2459 S. Ash Street
Denver, CO 80222

Partnership for a Drug-Free America
405 Lexington Avenue
New York, NY 10174

Children of Alcoholic Parents
23425 N. W. Highway
Southfield, MI 46075

Planned Parenthood Federation of America, Inc.
810 Seventh Avenue
New York, NY 10019

Sexual Information and Education Council
of the United States (SIECUS)
130 W. 42nd St., Suite 2500
New York, NY 10036

Tough Love
P.O. Box 1069
Doylestown, PA 18901

IMPLEMENTATION

Adolescents do poorly with tasks that someone else tells them they *must* do. If they help to plan tasks, however, they can carry them out successfully and implementation goes smoothly. Adolescents have little patience with adults who do not demonstrate the behavior they are being asked to achieve; a parent or nurse who smokes and asks an adolescent not to smoke may not get very far. Evaluate how an intervention appears from the adolescent's standpoint before initiating instructions.

EVALUATION

Evaluation of goals should include not only whether desired outcomes have been achieved but whether adolescents are pleased with their accomplishments. Individuals will have difficulty accomplishing desired goals as adults unless they have high self-esteem that includes feeling secure in body image.

The following are examples of outcome criteria that might be established:

- Client states he has not ingested alcohol for 2 weeks.
- Client states she is able to feel good about herself even though she is the shortest girl in her class.
- Parents voice they feel more confident about their ability to parent an adolescent.

Nursing Assessment of Growth and Development of the Adolescent

Physical Growth

The major milestones of development in the adolescent period are the onset of puberty and the cessation of body growth. Between these milestones, physiologic growth is rapid and the development of adult coordination is slow. At first, the gain in physical growth is mostly in weight, leading to the stocky, slightly obese appearance of prepubescence; later comes the thin, gangly appearance of late adolescence. Nutritional needs of the adolescent are discussed in Chapter 34.

Most girls are 1 to 2 inches (2.4 to 5 cm) taller than boys coming into adolescence and generally stop growing within 3 years from menarche. Thus, those girls who start menstruating at 10 years of age may reach their adult height by age 13.

Boys grow about 4 to 12 inches (10 to 30 cm) in height and gain 15 to 65 lb (7 to 30 kg) during adolescence. Girls grow 2 to 8 inches (5 to 20 cm) in height and gain 15 to 55 lb (7 to 25 kg). Growth stops with closure of the epiphyseal lines of long bones. This occurs at about 16 or 17 years in females and about 18 to 20 years in males.

The increase in body size does not occur in all organ systems at the same rate. For example, the skeletal system grows faster than the muscles, and muscle mass increases more rapidly than heart size. These differences in growth rates lead to lack of coordination and possibly to poor posture. It makes adolescents appear long-legged and awkward during a rapid growth spurt, because their extremities elongate first, followed by trunk growth. Because the heart and lungs increase in size more slowly than the rest of the body, blood flow and oxygen supply is reduced. Thus, adolescents may have insufficient energy and become fatigued trying to do the various activities that interest them.

Both sexes may lack coordination. The 13-year-old, for example, typically reaches to pick up a glass of milk at the dinner table and spills it, having reached beyond it because the arm is longer than the child realized.

Pulse rate and respiratory rate decrease slightly (to 70 bpm and 20 breaths/min, respectively), and blood pressure increases slightly (to 120/70 mm Hg), reaching adult levels by late adolescence. With adulthood, blood pressure becomes slightly higher in males than females because more force is necessary to distribute blood to the larger male body mass.

All during adolescence, androgen stimulates sebaceous glands to extreme activity, sometimes resulting in acne, a common adolescent skin problem. The formation of apocrine sweat glands (glands present in the axillae and genital area) occurs shortly after puberty. Apocrine sweat glands produce a strong odor in response to emotional stimulation. Therefore, adolescents begin to notice they must shower or bathe more frequently than they once did in order to be free of body odor.

Teeth

Adolescents gain their second molars at about 13 years of age and their third molars (wisdom teeth) between 18 and 21 years of age. Third molars may erupt as early as 14 to 15 years of age; however, the jaw reaches adult size only toward the end of adolescence. As a result, adolescents whose third molars erupt before the lengthening of the jaw is complete may experience pain and may need these molars extracted because they do not fit their jawline.

Puberty

Adolescence is the physiologic period between the beginning of puberty and the cessation of bodily growth. **Puberty** is the stage at which the individual first becomes capable of sexual reproduction. A girl has entered puberty when she begins to menstruate; a boy enters puberty when he begins to produce spermatozoa. These events usually occur between ages 11 and 14 years.

Secondary Sex Changes

Secondary sex characteristics, for example, body hair configuration and breast growth, distinguish the sexes from each other but play no direct part in reproduction. The secondary sex characteristics that begin in the late school-age period (see Chapter 32) continue to develop during adolescence. The typical stages of sexual maturation are shown in Table 33-1.

Sexual maturity in males and females is classified according to Tanner stages, named after the original researcher on sexual maturity (Tanner, 1955). Stages of female sexual development are shown in Figure 33-1; stages of male genital growth are shown in Figure 33-2.

Developmental Milestones

Thirteen-year-olds are beyond the age of spending time in any form of childhood play. Both sexes do spend a great deal of time playing sports. Team (or school) loyalty is intense, and following a coach's instructions becomes mandatory. This attitude is similar to the loyalty that 6-year-olds show toward their first-grade teacher.

Young adolescents who do not have the physical ability to compete successfully in sports may avoid these activities. Urge parents to encourage youngsters to play sports for their own health and well-being and the companionship involved, even though they do not excel. If not successful at sports, the young adolescent needs a sympathetic person to listen to frustrations and to be encouraging about trying other activities in which they may excel, such as science, music, or art. Overuse injuries from athletics occur in early adolescence until adolescents learn more about their limits and begin to respect the advice of adults on being well prepared and trained for sports participation.

Most adolescents spend a great deal of time just talking with peers. Some parents disapprove of the number of hours spent in this activity, afraid their children are wasting important time, or at least exchanging a great deal of trivial conversation. For the adolescent, however, talking is no more a waste of time than was pulling a toy back and forth across a rug as a toddler or

Table 33-1. Sexual Maturation in Adolescents

Age (yr)	Males	Females
13–15	Growth spurt continuing; pubic hair abundant and curly; testes, scrotum, and penis enlarging further; axillary hair present; facial hair fine and downy; voice changes happening with annoying frequency	Pubic hair thick and curly, triangular in distribution, breast areola and papilla form secondary mound; menstruation is ovulatory, making pregnancy possible
15–16	Genitalia adult; pubic hair abundant and curly; scrotum dark and heavily rugated; facial and body hair present; sperm production mature	Pubic hair curly and abundant (adult); may extend onto medial aspect of thighs; breast tissue adult and nipples protrude; areolas no longer project as separate ridges from breasts; may have some degree of facial acne.
16–17	Pubic hair curly and abundant (adult), may extend along medial aspect of thighs; testes, scrotum, and penis adult in size; may have some degree of facial acne; gynecomastia (enlarged breast tissue), if present, fades	End of skeletal growth
17–18	End of skeletal growth	

(From Tanner, J. M. [1955]. *Growth at adolescence*. Springfield, IL: Charles C Thomas; with permission.)

A

2

3

4

5

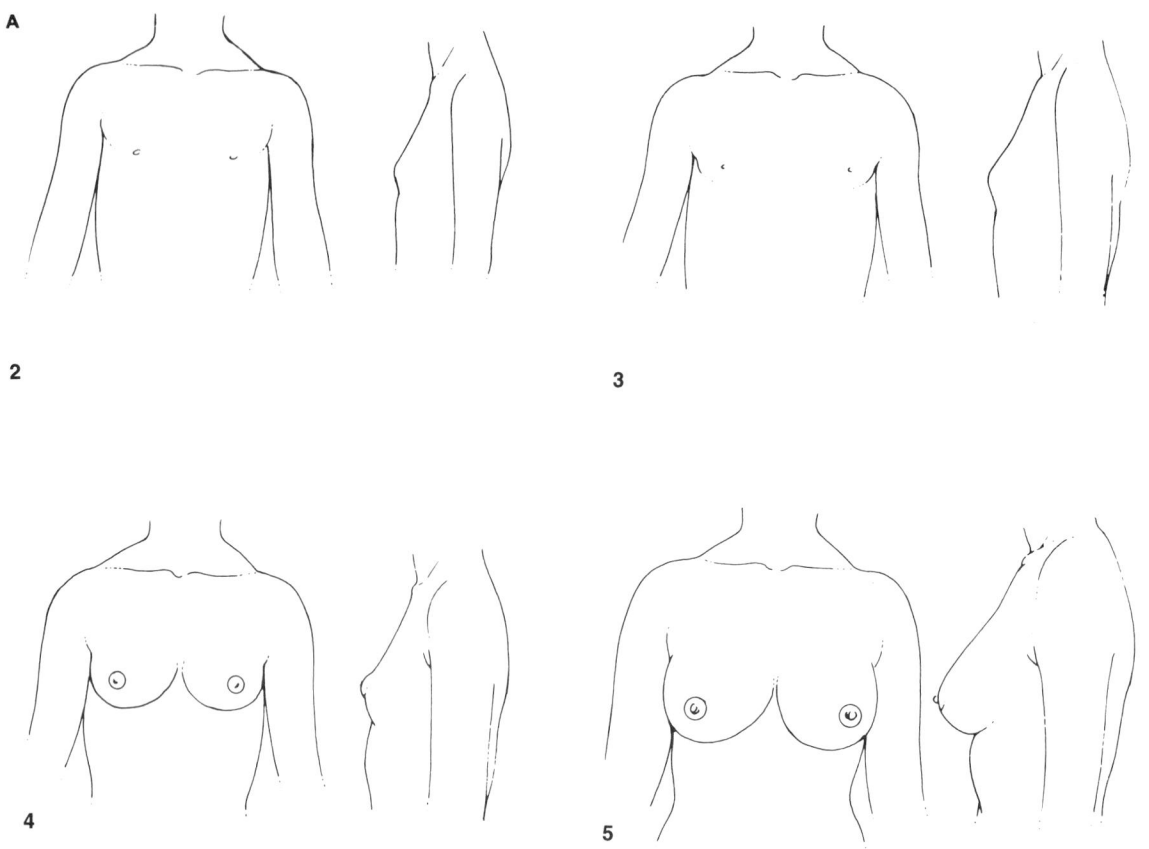

FIGURE 33-1

(**A**) *Female breast development. Sex maturity rating 1 (not shown): prepubertal; elevation of papilla only. Sex maturity rating 2: breast buds appear; areola is slightly widened and projects as small mound. Sex maturity rating 3: enlargement of the entire breast with no protrusion of the papilla or the nipple. Sex maturity rating 4: enlargement of the breast and projection of areola and papilla as a secondary mound. Sex maturity rating 5: adult configuration of the breast with protrusion of the nipple; areola no longer projects separately from remainder of breast.*

working with a model airplane or dressing a doll as a school-age child.

Fifteen-year-olds may spend a great deal of time in their room or, if they do not have a room of their own, in a quiet corner of the home away from traffic and conversation areas. If they cannot find privacy somewhere in the house, they tend to spend time elsewhere.

Beginning at age 16, most adolescents want part-time jobs to earn money. In addition, such jobs teach young persons how to work with others, accept responsibility, and spend money wisely.

When families were larger, each older child had responsibility for a younger sibling and baby care was a natural activity. With small nuclear families, many adolescents have never had the responsibility of caring for anyone younger than themselves. For their own sake and that of the children they care for, adolescents who plan to baby-sit should learn some basic rules of child care and safety. Many schools or Red Cross organizations offer courses in baby-sitting.

Many adolescents engage in charitable endeavors during middle to late adolescence. They learn that they are strong and capable enough not only to take care of themselves but also to help less fortunate people in their community. Adolescents do well organizing and supervising swimming or gym programs for disabled children, cooking and delivering food to older shut-ins, or raising money to purchase equipment for a hospital. High school clubs may be organized to send money to children overseas. These activities fulfill the adolescent's need for satisfying interaction with others and are indications of maturity and willingness to accept adult roles.

Emotional Development

Developmental Task: Identity Versus Role Confusion

According to Erikson (1986), the developmental task of youngsters in early and mid-adolescence is to form a sense of **identity** versus **role confusion**, that is, to decide who they are and what kind of person they will be. In late adolescence, the task is to form a sense of inti-

B

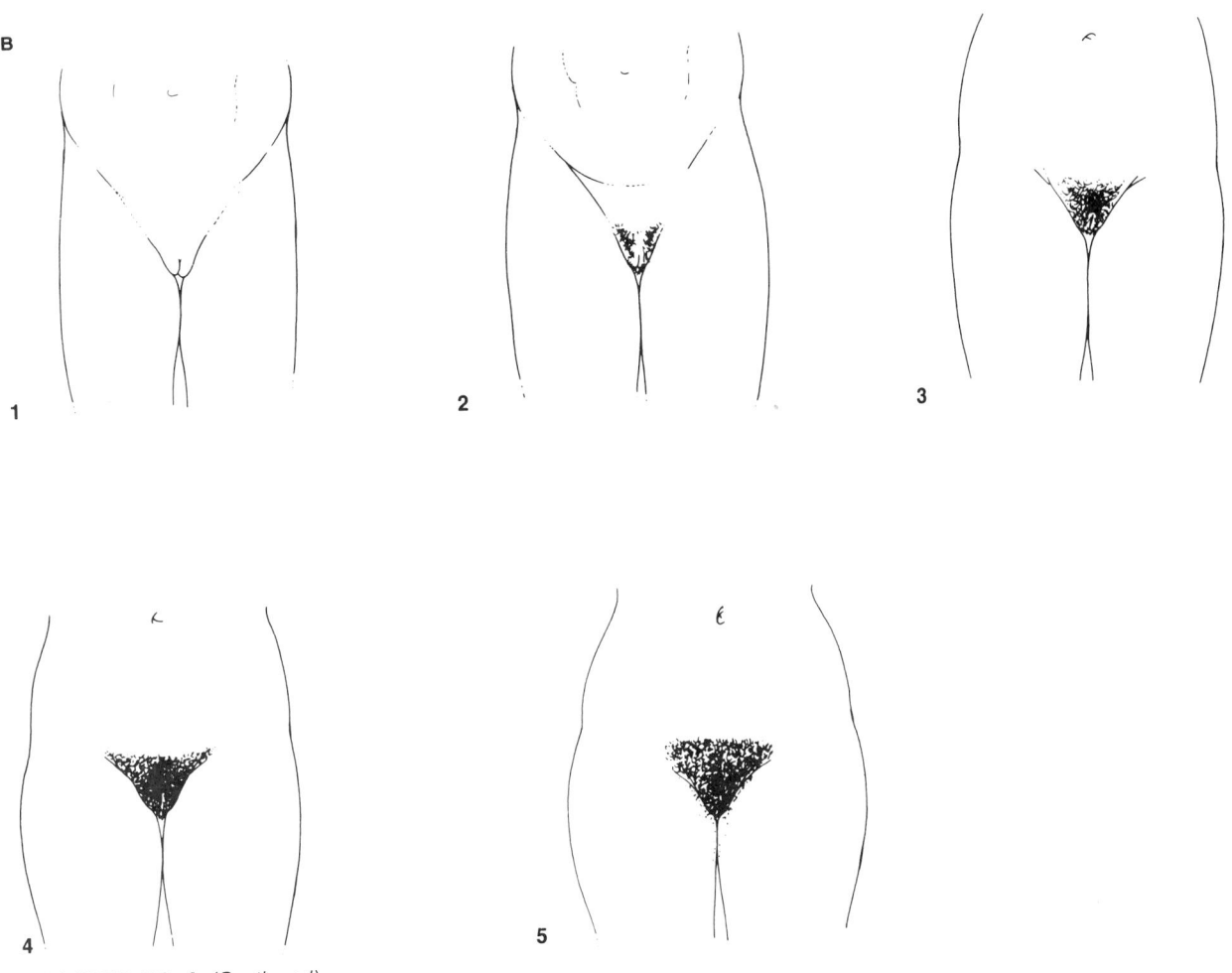

FIGURE 33-1 *(Continued)*
(B) *Female pubic hair development.* Sex maturity rating 1: *prepubertal; no pubic hair.* Sex maturity rating 2: *straight hair extending along the labia and, between rating 2 and 3, begins on the pubis.* Sex maturity rating 3: *Pubic hair increased in quantity, darker, and present in the typical female triangle but in smaller quantity.* Sex maturity rating 4: *pubic hair more dense, curled, and adult in distribution but less abundant.* Sex maturity rating 5: *abundant, adult-type pattern; hair may extend onto the medial part of the thighs. (From Fuller, E. [1979]. A physician's guide to sexual maturity.* Patient Care 13, *122; with permission. Copyright 1979, Patient Care Publications, Inc. Darien, CT. All rights reserved.)*

macy versus isolation or form close relationships with persons of the opposite as well as the same sex. It is the concentration on these two tasks which leads to typical adolescent behavior. The four main areas in which adolescents must make gains to achieve a sense of identity are (1) accepting their changed body image; (2) establishing a value system or what kind of person they want to be; (3) making a career decision; and (4) becoming emancipated from their parents.

If young persons do not achieve a sense of identity, they can have little idea what kind of person they are (Erikson, 1986). They have difficulty achieving effectively as adults, because they are unable, for example, to decide what stand to take on a particular issue or how to approach new challenges or situations. Some adolescents may become delinquent or exhibit acting-out (attention-getting) behavior, because they feel it is better to be socially unacceptable than to be nobody at all.

Body Image. Adolescents who have developed a strong sense of industry have learned to solve problems and are best equipped to adjust to their new body image. Nurses who care for adolescents can do much to educate them about their bodies and help them to accept the changes that mark maturity. Some adolescents, for example, are disappointed with their final height; they had hoped to be 6 ft in height and are only 5 ft, 6 inches tall. In other instances, they have seen themselves as ugly ducklings and dream they will emerge as beautiful swans. They are depressed to find, at the end of adolescence, that they have not turned into the image they fantasized. Adolescents are usually their own worst critics, never pleased with any aspect of their bodies. Children with low self-esteem may need parental support and help to understand that a person's worth is based on more than physical appearance, that the characteristics that make someone creative, compassionate,

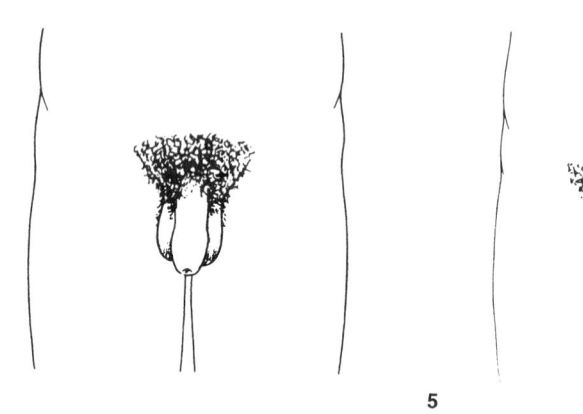

FIGURE 33-2

Male genital and pubic hair development. Ratings for pubic hair and for genital development can differ in a typical boy at any given time, since pubic hair and genitalia do not necessarily develop at the same rate. Sex maturity rating 1: prepubertal; no pubic hair; genitalia unchanged from early childhood. Sex maturity rating 2: light, downy hair develops laterally and later becomes dark; penis and testes may be slightly larger; scrotum becoming more textured. Sex maturity rating 3: pubic hair has extended across the pubis; testes and scrotum are further enlarged; penis is larger, especially in length. Sex maturity rating 4: more abundant pubic hair with curling; genitalia resemble those of an adult; glans has become larger and broader, scrotum is darker. Sex maturity rating 5: adult quantity and pattern of pubic hair, with hair present along inner borders of thighs; testes and scrotum are adult in size. (From Fuller, E. [1979]. A physician's guide to sexual maturity. Patient Care, 13, 122; with permission. Copyright 1979, Patient Care Publications, Inc. Darien, CT. All rights reserved.)

and fun to be with are the qualities on which lasting relationships are built.

Help parents understand how important it is to adolescents to make the high school basketball team, for example, or have a date for the senior prom. Parental comments, such as "When you're older, these things won't be so important," are not likely to erase the hurt that comes from being 16 years old and not being included in such major events. Compassionate understanding ("It's hard to be left out") is a better communication technique.

Self-Esteem. Like body image, self-esteem may undergo some major changes during the adolescent years. Self-esteem, however, can be challenged by *all* the

changes that occur during adolescence, including changes in one's body and physiologic functioning, changes in feelings and emotional focus, changes in social relationships (including relationships with both family and friends), and changes in family and school expectations of the adolescent. All of these factors will have an effect on the adolescent's feelings about himself or herself, sometimes resulting in crisis.

In recent years, a number of researchers have looked at the differences in the way boys and girls handle these emotional crises of adolescence. Several researchers have proposed that adolescence is a period of particular crisis to girls who are trying to find a place in a male-dominated society. The psychologist, Carol Gilligan, and her colleagues interviewed more than 500 girls between the ages of 7 and 16 over a 5-year period and found that many girls who, at age 11, were feisty, confident, and eager to speak their minds, became, by age 13, 14, or 15, hesitant and reluctant to voice their opinions aloud, having pushed their earlier resistance "underground" (Gilligan et al., 1990). Gilligan ties this change to a growing realization among girls during adolescence that their forthrightness may get them into trouble; they begin to self-censor to prevent this from happening. At the same time, girls are expected to grow up and to value independent and academic (or athletic) success over close relationships, a situation which conflicts with the girl's need to maintain personal connections. This scenario presents a double-edged sword for the developing adolescent whose concern with relationships is not valued by others and who can no longer necessarily rely on her former outspokenness to get across her concerns and opinions.

Although the turmoil of adolescence can be just as confusing to boys as it is to girls, Gilligan and other researchers have found that there may be less pressure on boys, who may have already learned to be competitive, independent, and separated from feelings (Bass, 1990). Gilligan describes the rearing of boys as including separation from emotions and feelings at an earlier age, whereas girls are encouraged to maintain their concern for people throughout their childhood. Girls are thus at risk for more conflicting feelings throughout adolescence (Bass, 1990).

Parents can help their adolescent girls deal with these conflicts by encouraging them to maintain their honesty and forthrightness. According to Gilligan, however, this option puts the adolescent at risk for criticism from other adults. The cost of going underground, by repressing one's views and feelings, may, however, be higher. Long-term psychological problems, notably eating disorders, which by some statistics are said to affect as many as one in five women in the United States, may be one unfortunate result of such repression.

Value System. Adolescents need to be able to talk to peers as they develop values. They also need an attentive adult ear, someone who will listen to their fears, hopes, dreams, and the pressure they feel to be somebody, the pressure of wanting to do something and yet not knowing what or how.

In early adolescence, girls tend to band together with girls and boys with boys. They dress identically with other members of the group: jeans and sweatshirts, special jackets, or whatever the fashion may be. On the surface, this makes adolescents appear to be losing their identities rather than finding them (Figure 33-3). Adolescents who are considered to be different for whatever reason (e.g., they are overweight or they come from a different socioeconomic, racial, or cultural background) often are excluded from groups in the same way that

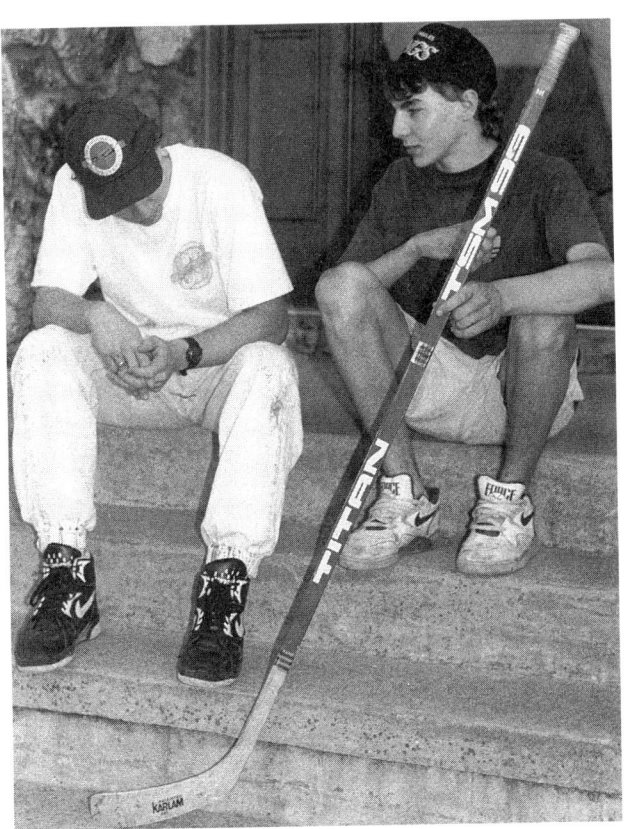

FIGURE 33-3
Adolescents have a need to interact with peers to learn more about themselves and others.

they were from clubs as 9-year-olds. This behavior may seem immature, but, like banding together, it is a necessary way for adolescents to establish a sense of identity. They know they are like the rest of the group because they dress, talk, and think the same way and go to the same places. They also know they are not like the excluded member. Knowing who they are *not* is one step in discovering who they are. Helping adolescents to appreciate it is not fair to exclude others on the basis of superficial characteristics helps them move more quickly through this stage.

Some parents may be concerned about an early adolescent's lack of interest in the opposite sex. Occasionally, they worry about an intensely close girl–girl or boy–boy relationship. Teach parents that adolescents must feel secure and pleased with their own sex before they can relate comfortably to the opposite sex.

Career Decisions. Part of the feeling of knowing what kind of person you are is knowing what kind of job you can do. Because of the varieties of opportunities available, making a career decision can be difficult.

Some guidance counselors suggest that adolescents wait until they have been in college for 2 years before making a career choice. This delay may be an advantage because of the wide range of available options. It delays settling on a concrete goal until about 20 years of age, however, and therefore puts off a choice that strengthens the adolescent's sense of identity. Some school-age children do poorly in school during preadolescence, but, as adolescents, show increased interest in learning as they select a job field at the high school level and come to see education as relevant to their future.

Emancipation From Parents. Emancipation from parents can become a major issue during the middle and late adolescent years for two reasons. Some parents may not yet be ready for their child to be totally independent, and some adolescents may not yet be sure that they want to be on their own. They may fight bitterly for a right—for example, to stay out until midnight or later on a weekend—then never use the privilege once they have gained it. Winning the battle is more important than exercising the newly won right.

In some instances, the closer the tie that adolescents feel with their parents, the more severe is their struggle. Because they love and feel loved, severing bonds is difficult. As long as parents are reasonable in their restrictions, the amount of noise being made is proof that the ties are strong and that separation or emancipation is not easy.

Encourage parents to give adolescents more freedom (e.g., allowing them to buy their own clothes, use their own judgment about allotting time for studying, choose their friends, join clubs, or choose after-school activities); at the same time, help parents continue to place some restrictions on adolescent behavior (e.g., "You must drive the car safely or you can't use it," or "You must continue to take responsibility for household chores"). These are not unreasonable rules and actually help adolescents to accept the responsibility that must come with independence.

Emancipation should be a gradual reeling-out process. Some parents err on one side or the other, either by neglecting to let out the line at all until adolescents, feeling trapped, have no other choice but to break free and swim away; or letting it all out at once, leaving adolescents to flounder because they cannot yet swim effectively on their own. The increasing number of adolescents who run away from home reflects how difficult a time adolescence is (Pennbridge et al., 1990).

In some instances, friction and misunderstandings may arise because the parents had such traumatic experiences as adolescents that they fear seeing their children reach this stage. Their own experiences may cause them to react so strongly that they are unable to discuss anything with their children. Adolescents then often feel they have offended the parents in some way. They do not understand that the parental attitudes are based not on anything they may have done, but on old, unresolved conflicts that are being brought to the surface. In

other instances, parents may feel threatened. Seeing their adolescent grow up may make them feel old, or if a marriage is not strong, fear that once their child becomes independent they no longer need to stay together. They may strive to keep their child immature (thus producing conflict) in an effort to keep these thoughts from entering the corners of their minds.

Both parents and adolescents may need help to understand that emancipation does not mean severance but a change in a relationship. Persons who are independent of one another may have even better relationships than those who are dependent on one another. This step is actually no different from the one children accomplished when they grew from infants to toddlers, when they changed from wanting to be held and rocked to wanting to run. If parents can think of it in this light, they will gain a better perspective and may begin to see that they will like their children as independent adults.

By the time children are 18 years of age, they have survived leaving high school. They are in college or have found a beginning job and have begun to manage their own lives, perhaps even their own apartment. They are like swimmers who have discovered that the water is not as cold as they thought it would be.

It is so much fun to be 18 years old that most of these young persons find it difficult to understand why adults they know have not achieved more in life. A little more maturity will help them to realize that initial success does not necessarily guarantee additional success, that beginning adult life may be far easier than the years ahead.

Sense of Intimacy. Once adolescents have achieved a sense of identity in early or mid-adolescence, they are ready to work on a second personality task, that of achieving a sense of intimacy (Erikson, 1986). The ability to form intimate relationships is strongly correlated with the sense of trust, which is the first developmental task in infancy. Infants who are unable to form a sense of trust may be unable to relate to others on a deep enough level to form lasting and close relationships as adults.

Some adolescents require help from parents or other adults to differentiate between sound relationships and those that are based only on sexual attraction. Never do adolescents need an adult to listen to them more than when they are struggling with the heart-rending feelings of young love or wondering whether a particular love relationship is temporary or lasting. Some parents may not be able simply to listen without interjecting their own opinions, because they worry that love between adolescents may involve a sexual relationship. Parents should feel an obligation to inform their children fully of their feelings about adolescent sexual relationships. They also should be realistically aware that some adolescents will not follow their advice. It is important for parents to keep the lines of communication open on the subject of sexuality. Rates of teenage pregnancy and sexually transmitted diseases, including human immunodeficiency virus (HIV), are high and still rising (Moore et al., 1993). If parents suspect that their adolescent is sexually active, they must at least make sure their child is knowledgeable about the prevention of sexually transmitted diseases and the use of birth control. If they are going to have sexual relationships, adolescents should establish a monogamous relationship and use condoms to try to prevent sexually transmitted diseases. (See Box 4-2 for guidelines regarding safer sex.)

Parents or health care personnel who counsel adolescents need to remember that first love hurts. The yearning sensation may make adolescents feel that it can be alleviated only by a sexual act. They can be reassured that they are pleasant people to be with because of the many fine qualities they possess and that sexual intercourse can be delayed until two persons have come to know these qualities in each other and have made a mutual commitment based on a deeper level than simply physical passion.

Intimacy involves developing a sense of compassion or concern for other persons. It means being able to discern when words will hurt, when a companion is unhappy and needs encouragement, when a friend is floundering and needs support.

In our busy modern society in which adolescents can engage in such a variety of activities, they may need help learning how to project themselves into another person's situation and to ask themselves how the world looks from that position. This ability, *empathy*, is feeling for another in its finest form.

Socialization

Early teenagers may be full of self-doubt. As teenagers, they feel they should look grown up but, instead, they still look like children. The voices of most boys have not yet dependably deepened; thus, they cannot trust their voices to carry the serious tone they wish to convey. Most girls' bodies have not yet fully developed; they may look at themselves in a mirror and compare their profiles with those of girls in popular magazines and feel inadequate.

Both male and female 13-year-olds tend to be loud and boisterous, particularly when peers of the opposite sex, whose attention they would like to attract, are nearby. They are impulsive and very much like 2-year-olds in that they want what they want immediately, not when it is convenient for others.

Many 13-year-olds fall "in love," a painful kind of love. At this age, however, they spend more time longing for someone of the opposite sex than they do instituting an in-depth and rewarding relationship. They have too little experience with life, too limited a frame of reference to know how to offer a deep commitment to another or accept one from that person.

Fourteen-year-olds are often quieter and more introspective than 13-year-olds. They are becoming used to their changing bodies, have more confidence in themselves, and feel more self-esteem.

Adolescents watch adults carefully, searching for good role models with whom they can identify. They usually have a hero—a film star, writer, scientist, doctor, or athlete—whom they want to grow up to be like. Fourteen-year-olds often form a friendship with an older adolescent of the same sex, trying to imitate that person in everything from thoughts to clothing. If the older adolescent has dropped out of school, the younger person may express a wish to drop out, too.

Idolization of famous people or older adolescents fades as adolescents become more interested in forming reciprocal friendships. Attachments to older adolescents are often severed abruptly and painfully as the older teenagers make it clear they are more interested in being with persons their own age. Rejection by an older member of a pair forces the younger member to turn to friends of his or her own age and ends the intense hero worship so typical of early adolescence.

Most 15-year-olds fall in love five or six times a year. Many are sexually attracted to the opposite sex, however, because of physical appearance, not because of inner qualities or characteristics that are necessarily compatible with their own. Such infatuation can lead to extremely intense but brief attachments that fade once the two young people discover that they really have little in common. However, falling in love this often does not mean their feelings are any less strong or that they feel any less pain when the relationship ends.

Sweet sixteen describes the general attitude of the 16-year-old. Boys are becoming sexually mature (although they continue to grow taller until 18 years of age). Both sexes are better able to trust their bodies than they were the year before. By age 17, they tend to be quieter and thoughtful about interactions. They have left behind the childish behaviors they used in early adolescence—shoving and punching—to get the attention of the opposite sex.

Cognitive Development

The final stage of cognitive development, the stage of **formal operations**, begins at age 12 or 13 years and grows in depth over the adolescent years (Wadsworth, 1989). It involves the ability to think in abstract terms and use the scientific method to arrive at conclusions. The problems that adolescents are asked to solve in school depend on this type of thought (e.g., a boy rowing upstream at 5 miles per hour against a current of 2 miles per hour will go how far in 1 hour?). Problem-solving in any situation depends on the ability to think abstractly and logically.

With the ability to use scientific thought, adolescents

can plan their future. They can create a hypothesis (What if I go to college? What if I don't go to college?) and think through the probable consequences. Thinking abstractly is what allows adolescents to project themselves into the minds of others and imagine how others view them or their actions.

Moral and Spiritual Development

Because adolescents enlarge their thought processes to include formal reasoning, they are able to respond to the question, "Why is it wrong to steal from your neighbor's house?" with "It would hurt my neighbor by requiring him to spend money to replace what I stole," rather than with the immature response of the school-age child, "The police will punish me." Some adolescents, however, may have difficulty envisioning a department store or a large corporation as capable of suffering economic loss from stealing, which may contribute to the frequent practice of petty shoplifting at this age.

Almost all adolescents question the existence of God and any religious practices they have been taught (Kohlberg, 1981). This questioning is a part of forming a sense of identity and establishing a value system at a time in life when they draw away from their families.

Planning and Implementation for Health Promotion of the Adolescent and Family

Promoting Adolescent Safety

Accidents, most commonly those involving motor vehicles, are the leading cause of death among adolescents. Although adolescents are at the peak of physical and sensorimotor functioning, their need to rebel against authority or to gain attention leads them to take foolish chances while driving, such as speeding or driving while intoxicated (see Focus on Family Teaching display).

In the interest of the adolescent's safety and that of others, parents should have the courage to insist on emotional maturity rather than age as the qualification for obtaining a driver's license. Encourage adolescents to take driver education courses to learn not only the techniques of driving but also a sense of responsibility

---

FOCUS ON FAMILY TEACHING

Q. My adolescent seems more reckless every day. What measures can I take to help prevent accidents in this age?

A. Adolescents run a high risk for accidental injury because of their impulsiveness. Some steps to take to help prevent accidental injury are listed below.

Accident	*Health Teaching Measure*
Motor vehicle	Use seat belts whether as driver or passenger.
	Do not drink alcohol while driving, and refuse to ride with anyone who has been drinking.
	Wear helmet and long trousers as driver or passenger on a motorcycle.
	Accepting dares has no place in safe driving.
	Take driver education courses to learn safe driving habits for both two-wheel and four-wheel vehicles.
Firearms	Always consider all guns loaded and potentially lethal.
	Learn safe gun handling before attempting to clean a gun or hunt.
Drowning	Adolescent should learn safe water rules, such as never swimming alone, no diving into shallow end of swimming pools, no hyperventilating before swimming under water, no swimming beyond own limit.
	Taking dares has no place in water safety.
	All adolescents should learn how to swim.
Sports	Use protective equipment, such as face masks for hockey, pads and knee braces for football.
	Do not attempt participation beyond physical limits.
	Careful preparation for sports through training is essential to safety.
	Recognize and set own limit for sports participation.

toward others. The use of seat belts should also be demanded. Adolescents tend to dismiss seat belts as childish, and they need convincing that it is only sensible to use every precaution available when in a motor vehicle.

Equally dangerous for adolescents are motorcycles, motorbikes, and motor scooters, which are appealing because of their low cost and convenience in parking. Both drivers and riders should wear safety helmets to prevent head injury and full body covering to prevent leg burns from exhaust pipes and arm and shoulder abrasions in case of an accident. Adolescents who choose this form of transportation should be as familiar with safety rules as automobile drivers. They should be prevented from driving motorcycles or scooters until they are emotionally mature enough to use sound driving judgment.

Drowning is one of the chief accidents of adolescence, even though it is largely preventable. Teaching all children to swim is not the only preventive measure, because some drownings occur when good swimmers go beyond their capabilities on dares or in hopes of impressing friends. Teaching water safety, such as not attempting to swim alone or swimming when tired, is as important as teaching the mechanics of swimming.

Gunshots are another source of injury or accidental death in adolescents. Accidental injuries increase in early adolescence, often for the same reason that drowning increases: youngsters want to impress friends. Some 13- to 15-year-olds even play Russian roulette. The second most common cause of death in adolescents is homicide. Both water and firearm safety must be taught creatively to adolescents by encouraging problem-solving rather than lecturing, because they tend to rebel against such lectures or claim that they have heard it all before.

Athletic injuries tend to occur during adolescence because of the vigorous level of competition that occurs. In early adolescence, overuse injuries result from poor conditioning. Athletic injuries are discussed in Chapter 51. Health teaching measures to prevent accidents and athletic injuries are summarized in the Focus on Family Teaching Box.

Promoting Development of the Adolescent in Daily Activities

Adolescents are in a stage of rapid physical growth (second only to the rate of growth during infancy). Maintaining adequate nutrition to support this growth is essential to continued healthy development, as discussed in Chapter 34. Maintaining adequate sleep, hygiene, and exercise is also important and should become the adolescent's responsibility rather than the parents'. Parents can, however, encourage adolescents to engage in healthy patterns of living—primarily through role-modeling.

Dress and Hygiene

Adolescents are capable of total self-care, and because of their body awareness, they may even be overly conscientious about personal hygiene and appearance. They often wash their hair every day, then grow dissatisfied because their hair has lost so much natural oil that it is dull and stringy. Both sexes try many types of shampoo, deodorant, breath fresheners, and toothpaste. They may take seriously (without admitting it) the content of ads showing toothpastes or deodorants helping to win an attractive person of the opposite sex or instant success. Remember this when caring for hospitalized adolescents. Providing time for self-care, such as shampooing hair, is important to include in an adolescent's nursing care plan.

Adolescents are acutely aware of what their peers are wearing. When adolescents cannot trust or are disappointed in their bodies, it is very reassuring to be dressed exactly like everyone else. When they first begin to work, many adolescents spend their first paychecks entirely on clothing. This seems inappropriate to many parents; they want their child to learn to spend money on more lasting items or to show an interest in saving. Adolescents may have to mature fully, however, before they make the same discovery as the emperor who wore his invisible suit: the real person shows through the clothing.

Remembering how important clothing is for adolescents also helps you plan care for them during a hospitalization. Most teenagers seem to improve markedly when allowed to wear their own clothing rather than a hospital gown.

Care of Teeth

Adolescents are generally very conscientious about toothbrushing because of a fear of developing bad breath. They should continue to use a fluoride paste rather than a brand advertised as providing white teeth. They tend to snack a great deal, so their teeth are always exposed to bacterial erosion. Some may develop cavities for the first time during this period. Those individuals with braces must be extremely conscientious in toothbrushing to prevent plaque buildup on tooth surfaces.

Sleep

Although it is widely believed that adults need 8 hours of sleep a night, some need more and others can adjust to considerably less. Protein synthesis occurs most readily during sleep. Because of this, adolescents need proportionately more sleep than school-age children to support the growth spurt during this time which demands the formation of so many new cells. In addition, because this is a stress period similar to first grade, adolescents may sleep restlessly as their mind reworks the day's tensions; sleep may not leave them feeling refreshed.

Many adolescents attempt to get by with too little

sleep, because they are constantly busy and because staying up late is a symbol of the adult status they long for. Frequent lack of sleep can lead to chronic fatigue. Adolescents admitted to a hospital for even a minor illness may sleep as if exhausted for the day to make up for what they have lost at home.

Exercise

Adolescents need exercise every day to maintain muscle tone and to provide an outlet for tension. Although they are constantly on the go, they often receive little real exercise. They ride a bus to school, sit for classes, sit at a mall after school and talk to friends, sit and watch a basketball game in the evening. They have put in a full day from 7:00 in the morning until 11:00 at night, yet they have had little exercise compared with the amount they used to get when they came home from school and played tag or hide-and-seek for several hours before dinner. Adolescents who have had an injury and must learn an activity such as crutch-walking should do muscle-strengthening exercises at first, just as adults must.

Adolescents who are involved in structured athletic activities do receive daily exercise. If they have not participated in competitive sports before, they may need advice on increasing exercise gradually so that they do not overdo and consequently develop muscle sprains or other injuries. Those who are used to daily exercise periods may feel trapped by hospitalization if some form of exercise is not available to them.

The Nursing Role in Health Promotion of the Adolescent and Family

Promoting Healthy Family Functioning

During early adolescence, children may have many disagreements with parents that stem partly from wanting more independence and partly from being disappointed in their bodies. It is frustrating for a child to be told by parents that she is too old to behave in a certain manner when she still doesn't feel or look older. At other times, just when she begins to accept her maturing appearance, parents tell her she is too young to do something. It may be helpful to counsel parents to appreciate that although it is not easy to live with a teenager, it is equally difficult to be the teenager.

At about age 15, parent–child friction tends to reach a peak. By 15, adolescents have discovered from careful observation that most adults are far from perfect. The teachers they previously thought of as all-knowing may be revealed to have very human shortcomings: they may not be able to answer every question; some may make it clear they do not have time for questions. Even a fa-

vorite coach may be discovered to be imperfect. School marks may slump as a reflection of this "fallen angel" syndrome.

Adolescents find even more fault in their parents and wonder how they can exist with their outdated ideas. They have trouble respecting parents who are so obviously imperfect. These adolescents may follow health advice poorly because they view health care personnel in the same light.

By the time they are 16 years old, adolescents generally become more willing to listen and to talk about problems. As a result, they may learn that adults are not as inadequate as they previously thought. Their parents, for example, may not be exactly the kind of persons these adolescents might wish they were, but generally, 16-year-olds can understand that adults are this way because they had to compromise their dreams somewhere along the way. This changed perception does not mean that the adolescent of 16 is calm and quiet, free of parent–child discord. Adolescents may comprehend how hard it was for parents to get where they are, but they may not understand, for example, why they themselves are not allowed to stay out beyond midnight on weekends.

Seventeen-year-olds who have stayed in school are usually seniors, and for most, this year is likely to be stormy. Looking ahead to leaving a school system with which they have been involved since they were very young may give some 17-year-olds a feeling of losing security. Even if going away to college or beginning a full-time job seems exciting, it may also be an unwelcome change from the persons and routines that they feel so comfortable with to new contacts and new regulations that appear strange and even hostile.

The ambivalence that such feelings create make 17-year-olds difficult to understand. They like to see parents perpetuating family traditions: a vacation in an old familiar place, the house decorated for a holiday in the same way, or the traditional birthday meal. Parents should appreciate that clinging to security this way is not the step backward it may seem to be. Instead, this behavior may be the preliminary working through of a time of separation that will be a major milestone in growing up.

To prove that they are old enough to leave high school and to enter into a more mature college or work world, adolescents may experiment with drugs or alcohol, sometimes interpreting their use as the mark of being an adult.

Common Health Problems of the Adolescent

A health maintenance schedule for the adolescent period and the assessments to be included at visits are shown in Table 33-2.

Table 33-2. *Health Maintenance Schedule, Adolescent Period*

Area of Focus	Methods	Frequency
Assessment		
Developmental milestones	History, observation	Every visit
Growth milestones	Height, weight plotted on standard growth chart; physical examination	Every visit
Hypertension	Blood pressure	Every visit
Nutrition	History, observation; height/weight information	Every visit
Hypercholesterolemia	Cholesterol level	During adolescence for children with family members with the disorder
Parent–child relationship	History, observation	Every visit
Behavior or school problems	History, observation	Every visit
Vision and hearing disorders	History, observation	Every visit
	Formal Snellen or Titmus testing	At 16 yr
	Audiometer testing	At 16 yr
Dental health	History, physical examination	Every visit
Scoliosis	Physical examination	Every visit to 16 yr
Thyroid	Physical examination, history	Every visit
Tuberculosis	Tine test	Depending on prevalence of tuberculosis in community
Bacteriuria	Clean-catch urine	At 16 yr
Anemia	Hematocrit	At 14–16 yr
Cervical or vaginal cancer	Pap test, pelvic examination	Every year for sexually active females or those whose mothers received diethylstilbestrol while in utero
Immunizations		
Tetanus & diphtheria (Td)	Check history and past records; inform caregiver about any risks and side-effects; administer vaccine in accordance with health care agency policies	At 14–16 yr or 10 yr since last booster
Anticipatory Guidance		
Adolescent care	Active listening and health teaching	Every visit
Expected growth and developmental milestones before next visit	Active listening and health teaching	Every visit
Accident prevention	Counseling about street and personal safety	Every visit
Problem-solving		
Any problems expressed by caregiver during course of the visit	Active listening and health teaching regarding cigarette smoking, drug abuse, school adjustment	Every visit

Hypertension

Hypertension is present if blood pressure is above the 95th percentile, or 127/81 mm Hg for 16-year-old girls; 131/81 for 16-year-old boys (see Appendix G). Adolescents who are obese, black, eat a diet high in salt, or have a family history of hypertension are most susceptible to developing the disease (see Chapter 41). All children over 3 years of age should have their blood pressure taken routinely at health assessments, although elevated levels often are not manifested until adolescence.

Poor Posture

Adolescents almost always demonstrate poor posture, a tendency to round shoulders and a shambling, slouchy walk. This is due in part to the imbalance of growth, the skeletal system growing a little more rapidly than the muscles attached to it. Poor posture particularly seems to develop in adolescents who reach adult height before their peers. They slouch to appear no taller than anyone around them. Girls, especially, may slouch so as not to appear taller than boys in the belief that males will only date females shorter than themselves. Girls may also slouch to diminish the appearance of their breast size if they are developing more rapidly than their friends.

Both sexes should be urged to use good posture during the rapid-growth years. Tall adolescents of both sexes are generally picked out by basketball or track coaches and thus may have the incentive, if properly guided, to maintain good posture. Assess posture at all adolescent health appraisals to detect the difference between normal posture and the beginning of scoliosis (lateral curvature of the spine; see Chapter 51).

Fatigue

So many adolescents complain of fatigue to some degree that it can be considered normal for the age group. Because fatigue may be a beginning symptom of disease, however, it is important that it be investigated as a legitimate concern and not underestimated. The adolescent's diet, sleep patterns, and activity schedules should be assessed, because all can contribute greatly to fatigue. Take a careful history, noting when the fatigue began. A short period of extreme tiredness is more likely to suggest disease than a long, ill-defined report of always feeling tired.

If an adolescent's sleep and diet appear to be adequate, the activity schedule is reasonable (in an attempt to be popular, some adolescents take on a schedule that would exhaust three people) and physical assessment suggests no illness, then the fatigue may be of emotional origin. It can be a means of avoiding school, avoiding conflict with parents (when children appear ill, parents are more sympathetic), or avoiding social situations. Those who are understimulated by school may develop fatigue as a sign of boredom.

Blood tests may be indicated to rule out anemia and the disease that is so common in adolescents, infectious mononucleosis (see Chapter 43). Some adolescents become so concerned about fatigue that they do not sleep well at night. They can be assured that they are healthy (after appropriate investigation has confirmed this) and then offered guidance to solve the problem with better diet, more sleep, fewer activities, and development of better problem-solving techniques to relieve tensions.

Menstrual Irregularities

Menstrual irregularities can be a major health concern of adolescent girls as they learn to adjust to their individual body cycles. Chapter 47 discusses these problems in detail.

Acne

Acne is a self-limiting inflammatory disease that involves the sebaceous glands that empty into hair shafts (the pilosebaceous unit) mainly of the face and shoulders (Lowe, 1993). It is the most common skin disorder of adolescence, occurring slightly more frequently in boys than girls. The peak age for the lesions to occur in girls

is 14 to 17 years; for boys, 16 to 19 years. Although not proven, genetic factors may influence the development of acne (Pochi, 1990). Cigarette smoking may increase the number of inflammatory lesions (Mills et al., 1993).

Prior to the rapid increase in androgen secretion with puberty, the sebaceous glands that enter into hair follicles are small and relatively inactive, so acne is nonexistent. As androgen levels rise in both sexes, sebaceous glands become active. Abnormal keratinization (cell growth) of the lining of the ducts occurs; this overgrowth obstructs the ducts. In addition, the output of sebum increases. Sebum is largely composed of lipids, mainly triglycerides. If all of the material formed cannot be eliminated to the skin surface due to the narrow gland ducts, the glands enlarge, and trapped sebum causes whiteheads, or closed **comedones**. As trapped sebum darkens from accumulation of melanin and oxidation of the fatty acid component on exposure to air, blackheads, or open comedones, form. Bacteria (generally, *Propionibacterium acnes*) lodge and thrive in the retained secretions, forming papules. Leakage of free fatty acid from triglycerides causes a dermal inflammatory reaction. If glands rupture, sebum is extruded into adjacent skin, which produces reddened inflammatory cysts. Acne is categorized as mild (comedones are present), moderate (papules and pustules are also present), or severe (cysts are present).

The most common locations of acne lesions are the face, neck, back, upper arms, and chest (Figure 33-4). Flare-ups are associated with emotional stress, menstrual periods, or the use of greasy hair creams or makeup that can further plug gland ducts. Lesions are less noticeable in summer months, probably because of increased exposure to the sun, which increases epidermic peeling, and the reduction of stress, possibly as a result of being out of school.

Assessment. Always ask adolescents at health assessments if they are troubled with acne and to what extent it interferes with their self-image. Inspect for facial, chest, and back lesions on physical examination.

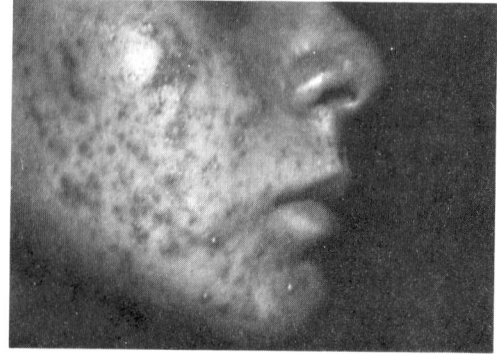

FIGURE 33-4
Facial acne in an adolescent. (From Arndt, K. Manual of dermatologic therapeutics. *Boston: Little, Brown.)*

Therapeutic Management. The goal of therapy is threefold: (1) to decrease sebum formation, (2) to prevent comedones, and (3) to control bacterial proliferation.

External Medication. Medications that are applied externally peel away the superficial skin layer to prevent sebum plugs from forming and are sufficient if only comedones are present. The most frequently prescribed medication is tretinoin (Retin-A cream). This reduces keratin formation and plugging of ducts. When using a vitamin A cream, adolescents should be cautioned to avoid prolonged sun exposure or to use a sunblock of SPF 15 or higher, since the preparation makes their skin more susceptible to ultraviolet rays. A second, frequently prescribed topical medication is benzoyl peroxide gel, an oxidizing agent. Caution adolescents that for the first week or two of therapy, peeling or oxidizing may make the complexion actually appear worse rather than better. Topical antibiotic creams such as erythromycin and clindamycin may be prescribed to reduce the bacterial level on skin, but usually only after oxidizing agents have not succeeded; these creams may sensitize adolescents unnecessarily to antibiotics.

Systemic Medication. In pustular and cystic acne, systemic (oral) antibiotics are helpful. Tetracycline (500 mg twice daily the first week, then tapered to 250 mg daily for maintenance) is effective against the anaerobic bacteria that breaks down sebum to form irritating acids. Improvement is not generally seen for 2 weeks, so adolescents must be supported to continue to take the medication during the waiting period. Without noticeable improvement, adolescents have a tendency to continue taking the higher dose or even increase the dose, hoping to initiate an effect. Tetracycline is not prescribed for children under age 12, because it can cause permanent staining of teeth. Since tetracycline may interfere with oral contraceptives, adolescent girls should use another method of birth control while on the antibiotic. Tetracycline should not be given to females who may be pregnant, because it causes faulty bone growth in a fetus.

Because food impairs the absorption of tetracycline, the drug should be taken on an empty stomach (2 hours before or after eating). Adolescents must be certain of the date of expiration of the drug; outdated tetracycline breaks down into an extremely toxic composition. Females taking systemic antibiotics for long periods of time become very susceptible to developing candidal vaginitis and must be instructed about the symptoms of this: a white, pruritic vaginal discharge. Alternative antibiotics prescribed are erythromycin, minocycline, or clindamycin (Pochi, 1990). Although these drugs avoid the complications of tetracycline, they may not produce the same results.

A new oral drug, isotretinoin (Accutane), a form of vitamin A, is an extremely effective drug for reducing sebum production and abnormal keratinization of gland ducts; it is prescribed for cystic acne. The drug must be prescribed with caution in adolescent girls because it is highly teratogenic (destructive to fetal growth) if taken during pregnancy; girls should have a pregnancy test before treatment. During therapy, serum levels of both triglycerides and cholesterol and liver function studies should be obtained, since both tryglycerides and cholesterol serum are raised by the drug.

Isotretinoin is extremely drying to skin; caution adolescents to discontinue all other acne medications during isotretinoin therapy to reduce this effect. Adolescents should continue to avoid sunlight or use a sunblock. If eyes become too dry, the use of contact lenses may need to be discontinued. An adverse effect of isotretinoin is neurologic damage. Adolescents with severe headache or visual disturbances should report these symptoms and the medication should be discontinued (Loeb, 1993).

Other Treatment Methods. If inflammatory reactions from acne are extreme, a corticosteroid such as prednisone or a nonsteroidal antiinflammatory drug may be prescribed. Steroids must be used with caution in growing adolescents, since they can lead to stunted growth. Cortisone may be injected directly into cystic lesions to reduce them rapidly. This type of injection may reduce keloid formation, which is why it is usually reserved for adolescents who are prone to this permanent form of scarring.

Estrogen, alone or in combination with progesterone, suppresses sebaceous gland activity and is therefore useful therapy in some girls. However, it is rarely prescribed today, because high estrogen levels tend to close epiphyseal centers of long bones causing bone growth to stop, and long-term therapy does have dangerous side-effects, including embolism and thrombophlebitis. Isotretinoin is prescribed instead.

Nursing Diagnoses and Related Interventions

Nursing Diagnosis: High risk for self-esteem disturbance related to development of acne during adolescence and lack of knowledge regarding treatment possibilities

Goal: Adolescent will express positive self-evaluation by next health maintenance visit.

Outcome Criteria: Adolescent verbalizes positive aspects of self; states that acne does not effect his or her positive self-image; or if client admits to feelings of negative self-esteem, is able to discuss feelings and concerns about condition with nurse; describes ways to prevent or reduce acne outbreaks and states realistic short- and long-term goals of treatment.

It is important to respect what acne means to the adolescent. The actual extent of the condition often is not as important as an adolescent's feelings about it. When one's face is constantly covered by red marks, it is

Jack is a 16-year-old who has come to an adolescent clinic for an annual health maintenance visit. The following is a nursing care plan you might design for him.

Assessment: Chief concern: "Acne for 6 months." States he has been washing face with Lava soap 6 times a day; is covering lesions with cocoa butter twice a day. Lesions seem to be growing worse instead of better. States he "dreads going to school" because of the way his face looks. Mother states, "I told him there wasn't anything to do for acne; just stay away from chocolate and wait it out." Physical assessment reveals scattered pustules and comedones on forehead, very prominent on nose and both cheeks. Two lesions of right cheek have large erythematous base; very tender to touch.

Nursing Diagnosis: Adolescent and parental knowledge deficit related to cause and current therapy for acne

Defining Characteristic: Parent and client both express misconceptions about condition.

Goal: Parent and Jack will voice more informed concepts concerning acne by close of visit.

Outcome Criteria: Parent and Jack voice agreement on treatment plan for acne on at least a trial basis.

Nursing Orders	Rationale
1. Discuss cause and treatment options for acne.	1. Both Jack and his mother need to understand what does and does not cause acne in order to appreciate the plan of treatment.
2. Teach client to use mild soap for face washing twice daily.	2. Irritation of lesions can worsen the condition.
3. Review prescription from physician for oral tetracycline and retinoic acid cream. Caution to watch expiration date on tetracycline and to take on empty stomach; avoid sun exposure while taking retinoic acid.	3. Understanding the drug therapy well is a crucial factor in compliance.
4. Explain that there is no diet restriction.	4. Neither chocolate nor any other food causes acne. Jack and parent must be educated about this; otherwise, they may place unnecessary blame on Jack for acne, which could damage his self-esteem.
5. Help to make out compliance chart for bedroom mirror.	5. Compliance is essential to successful treatment and may be very difficult for a busy adolescent to maintain.
6. Return to clinic in 2 weeks for re-evaluation.	6. A 2-week follow-up allows for additional education and review of compliance.

extremely difficult for an individual to feel good about oneself (see the Nursing Care Plan).

When carrying out interventions, remember that acne is a potentially destructive disease that, if left untreated, can cause irreparable physical and emotional scarring. Parents and adolescents should therefore be advised to seek medical treatment rather than self-medicate if the condition is severe. At the same time, overconcern may lead to undue self-consciousness that affects performance in school and establishment of social relationships. Health teaching measures for the prevention and treatment of acne are summarized in Box 33-1.

Concerns Regarding Sexuality and Sexual Activity

Because of increasing exposure to and acceptance of premarital sexual relations in society today, more adolescents than ever before engage in sexual intercourse. Because of this, as part of routine health assessment of

Box 33-1
Health Teaching Guidelines for the Prevention and Treatment of Acne

1. Diet does not influence the development of acne lesions. Eat a healthy, well-balanced diet for good general health.

2. Do not pick or squeeze acne lesions, which ruptures glands and spreads sebum into the skin, thus increasing symptoms. The times you are most likely to do this are during period of stress, such as when you are taking a test. When you find your hand on your face, distract yourself with some other motion, such as interlocking your fingers.

3. Makeup, greasy hair preparations, or tight sweatbands can plug ducts of glands and increase comedone formation. Avoid these, if possible. Using medicated makeup both covers and helps lesions heal.

4. Topical acne preparations work by unplugging glands. You must use them consistently to make them effective. Plan enough time in the morning before school and a time in the evening to apply these. Post a chart by your bathroom mirror to remind yourself.

5. Washing daily to remove irritating fatty acids is helpful. Excessive washing is not necessary to prevent lesion formation. Excessive washing can actually harm healing by rupturing glands.

6. Oral medications work by reducing sebum secretions or preventing bacterial invasion. These only work if you take them conscientiously. Make a chart to post in your bathroom or kitchen to remind yourself to take these, also. Remember that tetracycline must be taken on an empty stomach or it is not effective.

7. If you are taking oral vitamin A (Accutane), do not take another source of vitamin A in a tablet. Accutane is very harmful to fetal growth. Take measures to prevent pregnancy while taking the drug and for 1 month afterward. If you should become pregnant while taking the drug, stop taking it immediately and notify your physician.

8. Both topical and oral vitamin A make your skin very sensitive to sunlight. Avoid long exposures to sunlight, or you will sunburn readily.

9. No acne medication works immediately. While you are waiting for lesions to heal, keep yourself occupied with a new activity (join a school club, try dancing lessons). When your skin is clear once more, these experiences will help make you an interesting person as well as one with clear skin.

---

adolescents and preadolescents, you should ask about their sex lives.

Adolescents usually want to discuss this matter with a health care provider because they are concerned that they are exposing themselves to HIV infection or other sexually transmitted diseases and to pregnancy. Some adolescents may feel trapped into engaging in sex even though they are unwilling, because they perceive it as a way of having friends. Counseling can help them improve their perspective and learn how to say no. In contrast, some would like to be sexually active but are not, because they believe myths: early sexual relations will drain their strength and make them poor athletes; having sex too early in life will stretch the vagina and make sexual relations later on unenjoyable. Unless these falsehoods are explored through discussion, the adolescents who believe them may never be comfortable with sexual relationships.

Sometimes adolescents use a mild cold or a mild acne condition as a reason to come to a health care facility, where they hope that someone will stumble onto their real concern of sexual activity. After asking adolescents at health maintenance visits if they are sexually active, ask if they have any questions or problems

they want to discuss with you about this. Ask if they are interested in learning more about contraception. Be certain they are practicing safer sex measures (see Chapter 4 and Box 4-2). Overall guidelines on counseling the adolescent with respect to sexual activity are summarized in Box 33-2. Be certain to provide information on rape prevention as well, because a majority of rape victims are in the adolescent age group (Box 33-3; see also Chapter 55).

Substance Abuse

Substance abuse refers to the use of chemicals to improve the mental state or induce euphoria. As many as nearly 50% of high school seniors report having experimented with some form of drug (Muramoto & Leshan, 1993). Drug use occurs in adolescence from a desire to expand consciousness or to feel more confident and mature; it also can be a response to peer pressure or a form of adolescent rebellion. This type of rebellion is more emotionally charged than acts such as staying out late or wearing clothes other than those approved by parents, because it is not only harmful but also illegal. Stages of

Box 33-2
Health Teaching Guidelines for Adolescents Regarding Sexuality

1. It is your choice whether or not to participate in sexual relations. Do not be influenced by friends who may be exaggerating stories to impress you or who ask you for involvement you do not want. When you say no, be firm and clear about your wishes.
2. Pregnancy can occur with *any* sexual encounter unless you use some prevention to avoid it. Be direct with a sexual partner in discussing abstinence or birth control measures.
3. Sexual relations neither add to nor detract from your physical strength or general wellness.
4. The mark of an adult sexual relation is that the activity is pleasurable to both partners. If a sexual partner is not interested in your enjoyment as well as his or her own, you should reconsider the relationship.
5. There is no "normal" mode of sexual expression. Any activity that is pleasurable to both partners is normal.
6. Learn about safe sex techniques. Practice them (see Box 4-2).

substance abuse that have been identified are shown in Table 33-3.

Types of Abused Substances

Cigarettes. Although it is well documented that cigarette smoking leads to increased cardiovascular and respiratory illnesses by middle age, as many as 20% of adolescents smoke (Muramoto & Leshan, 1993). Although at one time proportionately more males than females smoked, adolescent girls now are the population most likely to begin smoking. Adolescents smoke because the habit conveys a stamp of maturity; it may be viewed as especially desirable by those who are having difficulty demonstrating maturity in other areas.

Most school systems have extensive programs as early as grade school, cautioning children against cigarette smoking. Unfortunately, the ultimate danger of illness or death in middle age is not a strong threat to young persons who are interested only in the present. One of the strongest determinants of whether adolescents will begin smoking is whether their friends smoke (Bertrand & Abernathy, 1993).

More effective, therefore, might be campaigns that point out that cigarette smoking causes foul-smelling hair, clothes, and breath and thus detracts from physical appearance and that smoking involves groups of adoles-

cents rather than single individuals. Emphasizing that being able not to smoke is a sign of true maturity may also be effective, as would helping adolescents to find other methods to demonstrate their maturity, such as allowing them opportunities for increased decision-making.

Remember that adolescents are very reluctant to follow instructions that are given from a "do as I say, not as I do" standpoint. Nurses who smoke themselves, therefore, will have extreme difficulty launching an effective campaign against the habit with adolescents.

Stopping smoking is especially difficult during periods of stress or inactivity. Trying to introduce such an action during exam week or the first week of summer vacation is not good planning. During an illness is also a bad time, unless not feeling well has reduced the urge to smoke. A return visit for follow-up and health maintenance care might be a better time to introduce the topic.

Adolescents should be urged to quit cigarette smoking through enrolling in a formal cigarette withdrawal program. Prescription of nicotine gum, clonidine, or a mild antidepressant are all possibilities to help with withdrawal (Glassman & Covey, 1990).

Another source of nicotine that school-age children and adolescents may abuse is "smokeless tobacco," or chewing tobacco. Many baseball players use this form of tobacco, and adolescents who admire them may be particularly drawn to this tobacco source. Although chewing tobacco does not have the potential dangers of smoking tobacco in relation to lung disease, it can lead to lip and mouth cancer. Smokeless tobacco can be just as habit-forming as cigarette tobacco.

Alcohol. As many as 90% of high school seniors report having used alcohol. Despite the fact that its use is correlated with motor vehicle accidents, homicide, and suicide in adolescents, alcohol does not carry the stigma of many other drugs (see Focus on Nursing Research display). Some parents are actually relieved when they realize that their child's strange behavior on returning home from a party is caused by drunkenness and not illegal drugs. Alcohol use cannot be taken lightly because it is linked to liver disease such as cirrhosis and cognitive impairment.

Heredity may play a role in alcohol addiction (Slap, 1990). Parents should be certain to set good examples for adolescents in the use of the drug and not drink indiscriminately.

Most adolescents will admit they use alcohol if asked two specific questions: (1) Have you had a drinking problem? and (2) When was your last drink? Adolescents who answer yes to the first and "within the last 24 hours" to the second need further assessment (Maly, 1993).

Once adolescents face the fact that they are alcohol dependent, organizations such as Alcoholics Anony-

Box 33-3
Measures to Teach Adolescents to Prevent Rape

Home

1. Do not advertise that you stay alone while a parent works or is on vacation.
2. Ask for identification from meter readers or repairmen before admitting them into the home.
3. Insist on adequate lighting for hallways in an apartment building or around your own home.
4. Have your house key in your hand when you approach your door, do not stand fumbling for it by the doorway.
5. Keep your doors and windows locked when you are alone at home.

Car

1. Avoid isolated parking places; park near a building or in a lot with a parking attendant.
2. Lock you car when waiting in it and after parking it.
3. Look in the back seat before unlocking and entering your car.
4. Have your car key ready when you approach your car; do not stand fumbling for it.

Work or School

1. Do not enter an elevator with a stranger.
2. Lock the outside door, and do not admit people you do not know when working alone at night.
3. Ask for security protection to walk out to your car.
4. When going to and from school or work after dark, walk in the street rather than next to shrubs or dark buildings.

Personal Actions

1. Do not wear chains around your neck that could be used to strangle you.
2. Learn self-defense; scratch the attacker to obtain skin and blood specimens under fingernails.
3. Be aware that an attacker could take any weapon away and use it on you; use caution carrying a weapon or Mace.
4. Fight or struggle cautiously to prevent harm to you beyond the rape itself. Actions such as kicking or gouging eyes may not be effective and may cause more violence.
5. If an attack occurs, observe the attacker's appearance as carefully as possible. Note identifying characteristics, such as a birthmark, scar, tattoo, words, or manner of speech, to be able to identify the individual later.
6. Press charges in court to make rape a crime of extreme magnitude and as an opportunity to fight back.
7. Work to provide rape prevention information and a united front against rape in your community.

mous are invaluable in helping them to stop drinking. The remainder of the family should be encouraged to join Al-Anon, the organization for families of alcoholics. Both children and families must restructure their lives to find satisfaction without the use of alcohol.

Many adolescents are not primary alcohol abusers but are the children of alcoholic parents. Efforts should be made to identify this group of children as well, not only to prevent them from becoming users of alcohol, but to help them build self-esteem and coping abilities for the difficulties they face living in a disorganized household (Scheitlin, 1990).

Anabolic Steroid Abuse. As many as 9% of high school athletes may abuse anabolic steroids (Du Rant et al., 1993). Such drugs are derivatives of the natural

Table 33-3. Stages of Substance Abuse

Stage	Name	Characteristics
0	Preabuse	Curious about drugs, need for peer acceptance; anger or boredom
1	Experimentation	Learning the high; little behavior change except lying; commonly used drugs: tobacco, alcohol, and marijuana; use is confined to social situations on weekends in the company of others, with others supplying the drugs.
2	Early regular use	Adolescent actively seeks the drug-induced mood swing; drugs are no longer just on social occasions but to relieve everyday stress. Use is frequent and may be solitary, regularly on weekends and occasionally on weekdays. Adolescent has his or her own supply. Drugs used include stimulants, sedatives, and inhalants. Behavior changes include change in dress, friends, deteriorating school performance, mood swings, lying, and stealing.
3	Late regular use	Dependent on substance of abuse; deteriorating behavior, fighting, lying, stealing, prostitution; often depressed, suicidal ideation, self-destructive or risk-taking behaviors
4	End stage	Substance use to avoid dysphoria; withdrawal; continued deterioration of behavior and mental state

(Muramoto, M. L., & Leshan L. [1993]. Adolescent substance abuse. *Primary Care, 20,* 141.)

hormone, testosterone (common names are stanozolol, an oral compound, and testosterone propionate, an injectable form). Students take steroids (obtained illegally) with the thought that they will enhance lean body mass and muscular development and so improve their athletic ability. Steroids also have the side-effects of euphoria and lessened fatigue, which make them doubly appealing.

To obtain maximum effects, teenagers may take up to 30 times the therapeutic dose. This leads to adverse effects, such as early closure of the epiphyseal line of long bones, acne, elevated triglycerides, hypertension, aggressiveness, and perhaps psychosis (Burnett & Kleiman, 1994). If taken orally, abnormal liver function and perhaps liver cancer may occur.

Students using steroids need to be identified so they can be cautioned that the use of such drugs is illegal in sports competition and is also detrimental to their health. There is also concern that the use of such drugs serves as a gateway to additional drug use, and if they are sharing needles, can contract hepatitis B and HIV infection (Du Rant et al., 1993).

Marijuana. Marijuana (widely known as *pot* or *grass*) is derived from the leaves and stems of the Indian hemp plant, *Cannabis sativa.* It is generally rolled into cigarettes ("joints" or "reefers") and smoked, although it can be mixed with food or sniffed. Scraping the resin from the flowering leaves produces a much stronger substance called *hashish. Sinsemilla* is a seedless form that

is even more potent. All forms of marijuana are euphoric, or consciousness-altering agents. They may temporarily impair coordination or motor activities, such as operating a motor vehicle (Schulz, 1993). Breakdown products of marijuana are not readily eliminated from the body but remain in the fatty cells of the brain. This residue results in synaptic gaps that delay electrical brain waves and memory storage. There may be loss of memory for recent events (up to 1 hour's time). Long-term pulmonary effects include sinusitis, bronchitis, emphysema, and, perhaps, lung cancer (Tashkin, 1990). These can develop after only 1 year of continual use compared with 20 years of use for cigarette smoking. Marijuana use may also lead to lack of sperm formation or infertility in males. Withdrawal symptoms include irritability, drowsiness, or cravings for high-carbohydrate snacks. Despite its known dangers, marijuana is the most commonly used illicit substance, next to alcohol, in adolescents. Help adolescents to realize that marijuana is a drug and not an amusing leisure-time activity and thus put its use into true perspective.

Amphetamines. The amphetamines are a group of drugs sometimes used in the treatment of hyperactivity and narcolepsy, among other central nervous system disorders. Their use without a prescription is illegal. Amphetamines are called *uppers* or *speed* because they give the user a false sense of well-being, alertness, or self-esteem. A newer, stronger form that produces intense symptoms is known as *ice.* Some of the side-effects that

FOCUS ON NURSING RESEARCH

Can Nurses Working in Emergency Rooms Identify Adolescents Who Are at High Risk for Alcohol Abuse?

As nurses in emergency rooms care for adolescents following automobile or other accidents, they are in an advantageous position to identify adolescents who might be at risk for abusing alcohol if it could be established there is an association between risky driving behavior and alcohol use. To investigate whether such a correlation exists, two nurse researchers asked 23 adolescent drivers, 16 to 18 years of age, to fill in questionnaires on their risk-taking behaviors, driving practices, and alcohol use. The results of the study indicate that risky driving practices are positively correlated with alcohol use. The researchers advise that when emergency room nurses identify adolescents who have engaged in risky driving practices, an index of suspicion about irresponsible alcohol use should be raised and appropriate counseling instigated.

Kidd, P. S., & Holton, C. (1993). Driving practices, risk-taking motivations and alcohol use among adolescent drivers: A pilot study. *Journal of Emergency Nursing, 19,* 292.

can occur are aggressive or demanding behavior, paranoia, and extreme restlessness. Because amphetamines suppress the appetite, adolescents may lose weight or eat only sporadically while taking them.

Cocaine. Cocaine is one of the most commonly used recreational drugs in the United States today (Schulz, 1993). It is difficult to document how many adolescents use cocaine, because the drug disrupts their lives so dramatically that they often drop out of school and become lost to statistical surveys. Estimates range from 3% to 9% (Muramoto & Leshan, 1993). Common street names for cocaine are *snow* and *white lady*, because it is supplied as a fine white powder that can be inhaled or injected. A stronger form, called "crack," is manufactured by heating cocaine powder with baking soda and water. This preparation process is dangerous in itself because it involves using volatile solvents that can ignite or explode. The resulting crack, often called "freebase" or "rock," is so strong it can cause immediate cardiac and respiratory arrhythmias (Povenmire, 1990).

Cocaine that is inhaled or smoked is absorbed through the mucous membrane into the bloodstream. After absorption, blood levels rise rapidly for the first 20 minutes, peak at 60 minutes, and then decline over the next 3 hours. Although a toxic dose of cocaine is usually considered to be 600 to 700 mg, toxicity has been reported with as low as 20 mg (a single line).

Cocaine produces both physical and psychological effects. The physical effects are increased pulse and respiration rates, increased temperature, and increased blood pressure. The psychological effects are euphoria and increased sociability; hallucinations may occur. Toxic symptoms include seizures, tachyarrhythmias, tachypnea, hypertension, increased deep tendon reflexes, and decreased response to stimuli.

Cocaine is rarely ingested orally, but occasionally adolescents swallow it when trying to hide a supply from parents or school personnel. Gastric acid destroys the action of cocaine so that it is potentially harmless when swallowed. Cocaine has been swallowed in plastic pouches with the idea of recovering it later in the stool; it can pass harmlessly through the gastrointestinal tract. However, if peristaltic action in the intestine causes the bag to break, the cocaine will be absorbed into the bloodstream at toxic levels. This can lead to sudden cardiac and respiratory arrest.

Teach adolescents that although cocaine sniffing may be fascinating and offer temporary pleasure, it causes psychological dependency and is potentially extremely dangerous because of its cardiac and respiratory effects. Chronic inhalation of cocaine can cause ulceration in the mucous membranes of the nose, and injection of the substance exposes the adolescent to the risk of AIDS, hepatitis, and other diseases contracted through contaminated equipment. Fluoxetine treatment may be helpful in successful withdrawal from cocaine (Pollack & Rosenbaum, 1991).

Hallucinogens. Examples of hallucinogenic drugs are lysergic acid dimethylamide (LSD), dimethyltryptamine (DMT), 2,5-dimethoxy-4-methylamphetamine (STP), and phencyclidine hydrochloride (PCP), and methaqualone (Quaalude). These drugs cause bizarre mind reactions such as distortions in vision, smell, or hearing. Adolescents report seeing colors more vivid than they have ever seen before, hearing sounds so clear they cause physical pain, and perceiving themselves as being impervious to harm.

The effect of such drugs can be extremely pleasurable (described as a "good trip") or extremely terrifying (a "bad trip"). Recurrences or flashbacks of drug-induced experiences may unfortunately recur at unpredictable times and in unexpected places. Such a flashback can be dangerous, especially if it occurs while driving a motor vehicle; it can be so frightening that it causes some users to believe they are becoming mentally deranged.

The use of LSD has increased substantially since the 1960s when it first became popular among young people, because it is a drug that can be manufactured by an informed adolescent in a "kitchen lab."

It is illegal to produce, sell, or possess hallucinogens in the United States. A hallucinogen related to mescaline, MDMA (known as *ecstasy*), has been added to Schedule I of the Controlled Substances Act because it was found to cause brain damage, and it is now illegal. It was previously used by some psychotherapists to make patients more receptive to therapy.

Opiates. Opiates are drugs such as heroin, meperidine, and morphine. Although they are not drugs typically used by adolescents, they can be extremely dangerous when used. Addiction can cause such a physiologic craving for opiates that a person will steal, defraud, turn to prostitution, and resort to any method available to secure enough money to buy a day's supply. Methadone or LAAM (levo-acetyl-alpha-methadol) programs may be prescribed to help adolescents wean themselves from opiates (Tobias et al., 1990). The users report to a center every day and receive an oral dose of methadone, which fulfills the same physiologic need as heroin. Methadone is a narcotic itself, but because adolescents do not have to pay for it, they no longer have to steal or prostitute themselves to obtain it. They receive help to return to school or to a job and become productive citizens. LAAM is gradually substituted for methadone. The advantage of LAAM over methadone is that its effect lasts longer—72 hours rather than 24 hours—so less frequent administration is necessary.

In addition to the direct danger of opiates, adolescents who use them risk the danger of contracting HIV and hepatitis B infection if they share contaminated needles.

Assessment of Substance Abuse

If adolescents trust health care personnel who are giving them care, they will generally admit that they have engaged in drug experimentation. Some common findings on the health history of a drug-abusing adolescent are failure to complete assignments in school, demonstration of poor reasoning ability, decreased school attendance, frequent mood swings, deteriorating physical appearance, recent change in peer group, and expressed negative perceptions of parents. These are not necessarily diagnostic findings, however, since they can also be part of an adolescent's search for identity. Substance abuse may be suspected, however, in an adolescent who is hospitalized for serum hepatitis or who is HIV positive and overly anxious to leave a facility, as well as one who appears to receive no benefit from the usual analgesic agents. General physical symptoms that indicate drug abuse are summarized in Table 33-4.

Nursing Diagnoses and Related Interventions

Nursing Diagnosis: High risk for injury related to peer pressure to use alcohol or illegal chemical substances

Goal: Adolescent will refrain from chemical experimentation by 1 month's time.

Outcome Criteria: Adolescent states that he or she is not experimenting with drugs; can demonstrate a way to respond to peers who encourage such use; shows no evidence of drug use (such as lethargy, confusion, positive urine drug screen, or parental suspicion).

In addition to any physical damage that chemicals may cause, one of the greatest dangers of early drug experimentation is that it affects the adolescent's ability to solve problems, with a consequent delay in maturity. The adolescent may cling to peers to shield drug use, stay away from adults who may detect it, and thus remove themselves from exposure to adult role models. It is important to help adolescents plan ways that they can feel satisfaction in life without substance use, such as how to feel secure enough to interact with others without propping themselves up with cocaine or marijuana, or how to accomplish activities to increase self-esteem so that alcohol is not needed.

Remember when setting goals with adolescents who are chemically dependent that it is difficult for them to appreciate how much they depend on a drug until they try to stop using it. A goal of not using a drug for 24 hours at a time may be the only one possible at first.

Adolescents should be cautioned against substance abuse in the same way as they are concerning the unwise use of motor vehicles or swimming beyond their personal limits. Scare stories (soft drugs automatically lead to hard drugs, marijuana rots your brain, drug addicts are sex perverts) cloud the issue and make adolescents dismiss all advice given them about drugs as worthless.

To maintain a realistic approach to the problem, health care personnel and parents must remember how very difficult it is for adolescents to say no to peer pressure. They need to be counseled (not lectured) that substance abuse is both illegal and harmful. Important teaching points to preventing substance abuse are summarized in Box 33-4.

Therapeutic communities or 24-hour facilities in which adolescents can live while they recover from chemical dependency may be necessary for some adolescents. The aim of all these programs is to increase adolescents' sense of self-esteem, improve problem-solving ability, realign them with society's values, and increase their self-awareness so that they can function normally without the aid of abusive substances. Unfortunately, campaigns against substance abuse for adolescents have not been very successful, and the problem continues. Adolescents who are no longer chemically dependent should be evaluated by a history and physical examination at all health care visits, because if the circumstances that initially caused them to become chemically dependent are repeated, they may return to a dependency pattern. A continuing relationship with

Table 33-4. *Symptoms to Help Identify Drug Abusers*

Drugs Used	Symptoms of Use	Dangers
Glue	Violence, drunken appearance, dreamy or blank expression Glue smears on clothing or fingers; tubes of glue, paper bags in possession	Lung, brain, or liver damage; death through suffocation or choking; anemia
Heroin, morphine, codeine	Stupor, drowsiness, needle marks on body, watery eyes, loss of appetite, bloodstains on shirt sleeve, runny nose Needle or hypodermic syringe, cotton, tourniquet string, burnt bottle caps or spoons, glassine envelopes in possession	Death from overdose; addiction; liver and other infections due to unsterile needles
Cough medicine containing codeine and opium	Drunken appearance, lack of coordination, confusion, excessive itching Empty bottle of cough medicine in possession	Addiction
Marijuana	Sleepiness, wandering mind, enlarged pupils, lack of coordination Strong odor of burnt leaves, small seeds in pocket lining, cigarette paper, discolored fingers	Psychological dependence
Hallucinogens (LSD, DMT, PCP)	Severe hallucinations, feelings of detachment, incoherent speech, cold hands and feet, laughing and crying, vomiting Possession of cube sugar with discoloration in center, strong body odor	Suicidal tendencies, unpredictable behavior; chronic exposure may have neurologic effects
Stimulants (amphetamine, cocaine)	Aggressive behavior, giggling, silliness, rapid speech, confused thinking, no appetite, extreme fatigue, dry mouth, shakiness, insomnia Pills or capsules of varying colors in possession; absence of nasal hair; possession of a glass pipe	Death from overdose; hallucinations; psychosis
Depressants (barbiturates, alcohol)	Drowsiness, stupor, dullness, slurred speech, drunken appearance, vomiting Pills or capsules of varying colors in possession; odor of alcohol on breath	Death or unconsciousness from overdose; addiction; convulsions from withdrawal

health care personnel not only allows time for this evaluation but also provides concrete role models of nonchemical, productive behavior.

Suicide

Suicide is deliberate self-injury with the intent to end one's life. Successful suicide occurs more frequently in males than in females, although more females apparently attempt suicide than males (about 8:1). Adolescent suicides are attempted most often in the spring or the fall, reflecting school stress at these times of year, and between 3 PM and midnight, reflecting depression that increases with the dark. Suicide is so common in adolescents that it ranks third as a cause of death in the 15- to 19-year-old group; as many as 6% of adolescents attempt suicide each year (Ackerman, 1993). The statistics may be underestimated because some well-meaning coroners or physicians tend to report these deaths as accidents to spare the family additional pain.

Incest, increased chemical dependency, marital in-

Box 33-4
Health Teaching Guidelines for the Prevention of Substance Abuse in Adolescents

1. All chemicals are harmful to the body, at least to some extent (alcohol, for example, causes liver disease).
2. Relying on drugs to give you courage to solve problems (or help to forget you have problems) prevents you from learning to handle life situations and maturing.
3. The bottom line of drug abuse is that you have the final say: you are the only one who can stop chemical dependency from happening.
4. Whether a drug is inhaled, swallowed, or injected, it still is absorbed and enters your body.
5. Despite its social acceptability, alcohol is a drug. A month of daily alcohol use can make you addicted.

stability in the family, and poor problem-solving ability are reasons that may lead the adolescent to the decision that death may be easier than coping with overwhelming problems. Most have difficulty communicating with parents (Magnussen, 1991). Drug and alcohol use may contribute to suicide by further impairing judgment (Muramoto & Leshan, 1993). Some accidents, such as those with motor vehicles, may be attempts at self-destruction; in addition, some homicides may be caused by deliberately provoking another person in the hope of being killed.

Adolescents who have been abused are at higher risk of suicide than others (Riggs et al., 1990). They tend to have reduced problem-solving ability (Orbach et al., 1990). Loss is the trigger that most often precipitates suicide. Some degree of depression is present in most adolescents, because they are not only losing their parents at this time as they grow apart from them, they are also losing their carefree childhood. If school failure or a loss of a friend or competition is superimposed on an existing depression, the pressure may be great enough to cause some adolescents to attempt suicide. Some other reasons for attempting suicide include anger with others, trying to get even, and manipulation (psychologic blackmail) as a way of having one's needs met. Loss of a parent through death or divorce; of a girlfriend or boyfriend; of a community because of moving away; or of self-esteem, for instance, through not making a coveted spot on a sports team are all significant losses. Because some adolescents may be unable to believe that a parent was at fault in the case of divorce or that the death of a parent could not have been prevented, they believe, instead, that they somehow caused the parent to leave or to die. The loss of a girlfriend or boyfriend is particularly significant because it involves two types of loss: friendship and self-esteem.

Assessment

A thorough physical examination should be performed at all health maintenance visits to assure adolescents they are in good physical health. Watch for signs of depression during health appraisals such as anorexia, insomnia, excessive fatigue, or weight loss. In younger adolescents, depression is most often manifested by behavior problems such as disobedience, temper tantrums, truancy, and running away from home. Self-destructive behavior or accident proneness may be noted. Difficulties in school may be a clue to depression. There may be acting out with chemicals, alcohol, or sexual promiscuity, or trouble with legal authorities. Occasionally depressed adolescents find it hard to be alone and may seek constant activity as a means of escape. Some may withdraw from contact with other persons and become isolated. Either behavior may be detected through assessment of activity and interaction levels.

Adolescents who attempt suicide often have a history of frequent school absence, uncompleted assignments, and failing grades. They tend to be loners or to have difficulty expressing their feelings to others and therefore do not receive emotional support from friends. Others are "perfect" students. The stress of trying to achieve continually at this level, however, is the trigger that provokes suicide.

Because suicide usually reflects a problem in family interaction, family assessment is necessary. A thorough history may reveal conflict with one or both parents. Many adolescents express a desire to get even with them. "They'll be sorry when I'm dead" is frequently expressed. Flag the medical charts of adolescents who express these thoughts even if no suicide attempt has been made so that you can further assess the depth of the emotion at a follow-up visit.

If another member of a family or a close friend has committed suicide, the chance that an adolescent will do so is greater. Adolescents see this method of coping and use it. The anniversary of a family member's suicide is an emotional time and may be especially difficult for an adolescent; wishing to join the dead family member appears attractive.

When one adolescent in a high school commits suicide, there is a good chance that another will take similar action soon afterward (Milin & Turgay, 1990). In some communities, adolescent suicide rates reach epidemic proportions after a popular student's suicide. School friends may often be aware that an adolescent is contemplating suicide before the parents. Caution parents not to discount reports of friends who tell them they are concerned about their child.

Close to the chosen time of suicide, some adolescents may demonstrate characteristic behaviors that show they are making preparations to end their life (Becker-Fritz et al., 1993). If a history reveals a personal loss, inquire further to see if any of these behaviors are present. Typical danger signs include the following:

Giving away prized possessions

Organ donation questions, such as "How do you leave your body to a medical school?"

Sudden, unexplained elevation of mood. Mood elevation may indicate that the individual has reached a decision about the suicide and feels relief.

Accident proneness, carelessness, and death wishes

A statement such as "This is the last time you will see me."

Decrease in verbal communication

Withdrawal from peer activities or previously enjoyed events

Previous attempt (80% of all completed suicides have been preceded by a failed attempt)

Preference for art, music, and literature with themes of death

Recent increase in interpersonal conflict with significant others

Running away from home

Inquiring about the hereafter

Asking for information (supposedly for a friend) about suicide prevention and intervention

Almost any sustained deviation from the normal pattern of behavior

After an actual suicide attempt, a health history should include asking enough questions so that you know whether or not the adolescent made a detailed plan to kill himself. A young person who took four aspirins and left the empty aspirin container conspicuously on the kitchen counter just before he knew his mother was due to arrive home from work is more likely to be only crying for help; the one who took 100 aspirins and hid the container under the bed just after her mother left for 8 hours of work is making a serious attempt. You may be the first person in a health care facility to realize that an adolescent talking about suicide is not "just talking" (it is a fallacy that people who talk about suicide do not attempt it) but has a definite, well-thought-out plan to accomplish it. The adolescent who has been admitted to a hospital unit after a serious aborted suicide attempt may formulate a new plan that will be successful the next time unless some action is taken and the adolescent's life is changed in some way.

Nursing Diagnoses and Related Interventions

Nursing Diagnosis: High risk for violence, self-directed, related to symptoms of depression or expressed desire to hurt oneself

Goal: Client will not harm self; will demonstrate other means of solving problems by 1 week's time.

Outcome Criteria: Client expresses feelings of depression to health care providers or other adults; states that she will contact support person should the desire to commit suicide become overwhelming.

Be aware that establishing goals with adolescents who are contemplating suicide or who have made an attempt will be difficult because they are often too depressed to come up with an alternative (their goal is to kill themselves, not problem-solve). Crisis intervention for adolescents who are contemplating suicide includes trying to alleviate their pain and depression and counseling them in an effort to help them change their perspective on the value of life.

Try to find out the things in life that are still important to adolescents; build a plan that will help them see that life is worth living enough to work through problems. Show them that no one can change everything, but everyone can make one or two changes that will make a difference. After these small changes are made, a domino effect can be created to change more and more of one's circumstances.

Because adolescents resort to suicide as a method of solving problems, helping them in this area is a prime intervention strategy. Ask them "what would happen if" questions. Suppose you did fail a course, what would happen? Are there ways you can reverse the finality of the problem? (Talk to a teacher about make-up assignments? Ask a friend for help in reviewing material? Buy a review book that will help in studying?) Be realistic in planning. Do not count on everyone being willing to help out. A high school teacher may feel that to be asked to do outside tutoring is an imposition, and for you to advise adolescents to seek this kind of help will only add to their depression if the teacher refuses. You may have to make these contacts yourself (with the adolescent's permission) because, generally, persons who are depressed have difficulty initiating this type of action and do not believe that anyone cares about them.

A general measure is to help them speak honestly about thoughts of suicide and the problems that have led them to thinking death is a solution. Most problems begin to seem manageable if they can be put into words in this way. It is important not to underestimate the adolescent's determination to end his or her life. In most instances, an adolescent needs referral to a consultant well versed in suicide prevention to provide additional therapy. Therapy will aim to improve self-image and offer alternative solutions to problems.

For the adolescent's safety, a period of observation in a hospital setting is desirable after a suicide attempt to prevent him from injuring himself and to allow him to be evaluated in a neutral setting, away from the stress that precipitated the attempt. This can take place in an adolescent service rather than a psychiatric service.

Antidepressant medicine alone, a therapy used with depressed adults, may be of little value in treating depressed children and adolescents. Continuing evaluation by both history-taking and physical examination is necessary for the adolescent who has attempted suicide, because the young person may attempt it again if support people and better problem-solving ability are not available at another time.

Runaways

A *runaway* is commonly an adolescent between the ages of 10 and 17 years who has been absent from home at least overnight without permission of parent or guardian. The frequency of running away may be as high as one in eight adolescents. Most do not go far or stay away long (under 1 week). Unfortunately, about 1 in 20 adolescent runaways stay away as long as 1 year; some never return home. Runaway adolescents are most likely from low- or high-income families. Unemployment, alcoholism, sexual abuse, and poverty are frequent characteristics of their families. They are slightly more likely to be male than female.

Assessment

Running away is usually preceded by an argument with parents that is often the last straw after a number of long-term disagreements. Other reasons may be personal concerns such as loneliness, pregnancy, and problems with friends, school, or the police. Incest can also be a precipitating cause, as can other parental abuse. A school history often reveals frequent truancy, failing grades, possible drug use, and runaway behavior by friends. It is a sad fact that some adolescents are "throwaways" or have been rejected by their families.

Common health reasons for which runaway adolescents are seen at health care facilities are sexually transmitted diseases, including HIV, rape, pregnancy, substance abuse, hepatitis, and vaginitis. They have a high incidence of suicide attempts (Rotherman-Borus, 1993). When caring for adolescents with these concerns, be certain to secure a thorough history, so that the fact they are no longer living at home will not be missed. To obtain an accurate history of an adolescent runaway, be nonjudgmental in questioning. Revealing that you are shocked by the report—that he or she has slept overnight on a park bench for 2 months, has been robbed, steals to obtain money, and spends most of it on alcohol—will prevent you from learning even greater concerns, such as having a sexually transmitted disease or being pregnant. Many adolescent runaways want to return home, but are afraid to do so or do not know how to take the first step back toward their parents.

Nursing Diagnoses and Related Interventions

Nursing Diagnosis: Ineffective individual coping related to stress of adolescent period and inadequate family resources

Goal: Adolescent will demonstrate adequate coping mechanisms by 1 month's time.

Outcome Criteria: Adolescent states that stress level at home is manageable; is able to describe how he can use family and community resources to help solve problems and aid in a crisis.

Adolescents may run away because they are unable to solve a problem in any other way; setting goals, therefore, may be difficult. A short-term goal to stay home through a holiday rather than a long-term one of finishing high school may be all that you can achieve.

Because adolescent runaways usually lack references for jobs and do not necessarily qualify for public assistance programs, they generally do not have a sound

source of income. Both males and females may resort to prostitution to support themselves, or they may resort to stealing to eat. Police consider them to be juvenile delinquents and therefore are required to return them to their homes if discovered. Following this, they may be sentenced to an institution for care; unfortunately, these facilities are often crowded and do not have the means to meet adolescent needs other than food and clothing (Podschum, 1993).

Educate runaway adolescents about the national Youth Crisis Hotline that they can telephone day or night: 1-800-448-4663 (1-800-HIT HOME). When planning health teaching, remember that many runaways have associated school failure and may be poor readers; discuss the information with them when giving them a pamphlet.

Try to put yourself in their circumstances to ascertain whether your instructions are sensible for their lifestyle. Giving them instructions to eat a high-protein diet or iron-rich foods, for example, may be ludicrous. They may not have a source of running water, and thus washing or changing a dressing may be difficult. They may have no way to pay for health care, making it impossible to obtain a prescription medication, so giving them a sample of a drug is often more practical. They may not have means of transportation so are unable to return to a health care facility for frequent follow-up visits. Meet as many of the runaway's needs as possible, therefore, at one visit.

Be certain adolescents know they can telephone the national runaway number at any time they want to return home. Remember also that they are runaways because, for some reason, their home was intolerable. Even though they agree to return home, they may not remain there unless circumstances change.

Nursing Diagnosis: Altered parenting related to inability of family to adjust to adolescent needs

Goal: Family will demonstrate increased ability to make necessary adjustments for family living within 1 month.

Outcome Criteria: Parents can list definite changes they have made in family life to better accommodate an adolescent, such as providing increased privacy or using "contracting" with adolescent.

In some instances it is impossible for a family to reestablish itself after a child has run away because the family is dysfunctional (incest or abuse has occurred). In other instances, family life can be modified to welcome the runaway adolescent back home.

So that parents and the adolescent can learn to communicate better, it is helpful to insist that they establish ground rules for communication (shouting or threats are not allowed; no subject is too difficult to be discussed calmly; no emotion or feeling is to be called "foolish"). Once ground rules are laid, parents and the adolescent should meet to discuss how difficult it is to be an adolescent and how equally difficult it is to be the parent of an adolescent; in the past, they became so engaged in arguing that they did not appreciate the other side of the controversy.

Helping parents and adolescents establish a contract for behavior can be effective (for the right to have her own private room, the adolescent can't do drugs; for the right to stay overnight at a friend's house on Friday, she must eat with the family all other nights, for example). Contracting is effective with adolescents, but it does carry the responsibility for parents of being certain that they are abiding with their half of the contract (not invading the private room) and of being prepared to enforce the contract.

Some families benefit by calling on a mediator (a relative, a close friend, a minister or rabbi) to listen to both sides of an issue and make a ruling. If, after a fair trial of trying to make adjustments, parents are still unable to maintain a functional home life, they will need help to make other arrangements for safe care of the adolescent (e.g., the adolescent could live with a relative or a friend's family).

Unique Concerns of the Family With a Disabled or Chronically Ill Adolescent

Achieving a sense of identity may be difficult for adolescents who have spent much of their life with an illness or disability. It is vital, however, for such individuals to look past their particular condition to their real selves. For example, a 16-year-old in a wheelchair must perceive herself as a teenager who is normal intellectually, is a good conversationalist, has a good sense of humor, enjoys watching football, and only incidentally is in a wheelchair.

Some of the biggest problems of chronically ill or disabled adolescents are likely to be difficulties in being as independent as they would like, achieving in school, and establishing intimate relationships. Those who cannot learn to drive when their friends are learning to do so, who are not invited to dances and parties, or are too hesitant to ask someone to go with them, may feel a loss of self-esteem. Moreover, the loss of many hours of school due to illness or frequent hospitalization may result in the inability to pursue a desired career, at least without a delay. Adolescence may be the first time these children realize that certain occupations or opportunities, such as a military career, may be closed to them. As they prepare to leave the security of a familiar school system, it may be the first time they examine just how they will be able to function on their own. Some may come to realize that they will never be able to do so completely independently.

Chronic hospitalization or a disabling condition can cause depression in adolescents, placing them at high risk for substance abuse or suicide. Helping these adolescents realize that many people must compromise in making life decisions for other reasons (e.g., lack of money, lack of ability or qualifications, extra personal responsibilities) can help them feel they are not so different from others. This type of guidance can be time consuming, but sometimes the fact that an adult is willing to make this level of commitment is enough to give these adolescents the self-esteem they need to alter aspirations and plans and find a future role that is consistent with their own capabilities. Nursing actions that encourage a sense of identity in the adolescent with a long-term illness are summarized in Table 33-5.

Key Points

- The major milestones of development in the adolescent period are the onset of puberty and the cessation of body growth. Between these milestones, physical growth is rapid and the development of adult coordination and thought processes is slow.
- The development of secondary sex characteristics is completed during adolescence. These are rated according to Tanner stages.
- The developmental task of the adolescent according to Erikson is to establish independence from parents through gaining a sense of identity versus role confusion. Adolescents, therefore, usually respond best to health care personnel who respect their attempts at independence and allow them as many choices as possible in care.
- Adolescents reach a point of cognitive development termed formal operational thought. At this stage, they are able to think in abstract terms and use the scientific method to arrive at conclusions.
- To appear older than they are, some adolescents present an assured, "I know that" attitude. To be effective, health teaching may have to be introduced with "I know you know this, so I'll just review it" approach that allows the adolescent to maintain a mature front, while gaining additional information.
- Being an adolescent is difficult in today's world. Be aware that to reduce stress, some adolescents begin to use abusive substances. Asking about an adolescent's drug experiences, if any, during a health assessment is not intruding on privacy; it is conducting safe health assessment.
- Promoting adolescent safety is an important nursing role. Motor vehicle accidents, homicide, and suicide are leading causes of death in this age group.
- Common health problems in the adolescent are sometimes minor and include poor posture, fatigue,

Table 33-5. *Nursing Actions That Encourage a Sense of Identity in the Disabled or Chronically Ill Adolescent*

Category	Actions
Nutrition	If adolescent is on special diet, discuss role of his or her food preferences with dietitian (hot dogs, pizza, etc.). Respect food preferences.
Dressing change	Allow adolescent to order supplies.
	Ask for suggestions as to final appearance of dressing.
	If soaks are included, have adolescent time the treatment.
	Allow adolescent to choose time for dressing change.
Medicine	Offering the adolescent a choice of site for injection or intravenous insertion encourages a sense of control.
	Teach name, action, and possible side-effects of medicine.
Rest	Contract with adolescent for time and length of rest periods.
Hygiene	Respect modesty of the adolescent as being at adult level.
	Contract with adolescent for extent of self-care (will give own bath and make bed, not medicate self).
Pain	Encourage adolescent to express pain; teach distraction technique for sharp pain, such as deep breathing, counting backward from 100.
	Encourage adolescent to ask for analgesics as needed.
Stimulation	Provide tapes of favorite music with earphones.
	Provide a radio for adolescent to listen to talk show to foster active involvement.
	Encourage school work, crossword puzzles (you may need to help adolescents divide up school assignments so that they do not become overly fatigued and frustrated).
	Provide cards for games to increase socialization (make or have the adolescent make a card deck from pieces of paper if one is not available).
	Encourage adolescents to network with one another.
	Encourage adolescents to keep in contact with school friends through telephoning or writing notes to them.

or acne; they can also be serious such as beginning hypertension, substance abuse, and suicide. Identifying these problems and referring the adolescent for help are important nursing actions.

Critical Thinking Exercises

1. Kenneth is a 16-year-old whom you meet in an ambulatory clinic. He tells you during history-taking that he does not smoke, but you smell cigarette smoke on his clothing. Although he says he doesn't use drugs, a number of blue and white capsules fall out of his shirt pocket when he unbuttons his shirt. Devise a plan of action to help you determine if Kenneth is smoking cigarettes or using drugs. Describe your next action if Kenneth does admit he is not only heavily into drugs but does not intend to stop using them.

2. Mary is a shy, quiet 14-year-old you care for in a hospital setting. She tells you she is concerned because she has not menstruated as yet. This is making her feel "left out" at school. How would you

counsel Mary? What if she were 16 and had the same concern?

3. Harry is a 15-year-old who enjoys rap music and has been collecting baseball cards since he was 8. He has recently started listening to classical music and he gave his collection of cards away to a neighbor boy because he "wouldn't need them where he's going." Why might you be concerned about Harry? What additional questions might you ask him? If you learned Harry is about to leave to be an exchange student in England, how would this affect your assessment of the situation?

References

Ackerman, G. L. (1993). A congressional view of youth suicide. *American Psychologist, 48*, 183.

Bass, A. (1990, Oct. 22). It's not easy being a girl. *The Boston Globe*, pp. 23, 26, 27.

Becker-Fritz, T., et al. (1993). What are the warning signs for suicidal adolescents? *Journal of Psychosocial Nursing and Mental Health Services, 31*, 37.

Bertrand, L. D., & Abernathy, T. J. (1993). Predicting cigarette smoking among adolescents using cross sectional and longitudinal approaches. *Journal of School Health, 63,* 98.

Department of Health and Human Services (1991). *Healthy people 2000.* Washington, D. C.: Public Health Service.

Du Rant, R. H., et al. (1993). Use of multiple drugs among adolescents who use anabolic steroids. *New England Journal of Medicine, 328,* 922.

Erikson, E. H. (1986). *Childhood and society.* New York: W. W. Norton.

Gilligan, C., et al. (1990). *Making connections: The relational worlds of adolescent girls at Emma Willard School.* Cambridge, MA: Harvard University Press.

Glassman, A. H., & Covey, L. S. (1990). Future trends in the pharmacological treatment of smoking cessation. *Drugs, 40,* 1.

Kohlberg, L. (1981). *The philosophy of moral development: Moral stages and the idea of justice.* New York: Harper & Row.

Loeb, S. (1993). *Nurse's handbook of drug therapy.* Springhouse, PA: Springhouse.

Lowe, J. G. (1993). The stigma of acne. *British Journal of Hospital Medicine, 49,* 809.

Maly, R. C. (1993). Early recognition of chemical dependence. *Primary Care, 20,* 33.

Magnussen, M. G. (1991). Characteristics of depressed and nondepressed children and their parents. *Child Psychiatry and Human Development, 21,* 185.

Milin, R., & Turgay, A. (1990). Adolescent couple suicide: Literature review. *Canadian Journal of Psychiatry, 35,* 183.

Mills, C. M., et al. (1993). Does smoking influence acne? *Clinical & Experimental Dermatology, 18,* 100.

Moore, J., et al. (1993). Selected behaviors that increase risk for HIV infection, other sexually transmitted diseases and unintended pregnancy among high school students. *Journal of School Health, 63,* 116.

Muramoto, M. L., & Leshan, L. (1993). Adolescent substance abuse. *Primary Care, 20,* 141.

Orbach, I., et al. (1990). Styles of problem solving in suicidal individuals. *Suicide and Life-Threatening Behavior, 20,* 56.

Pennbridge, J. N., et al. (1990). Runaway and homeless youth in Los Angeles County, California. *Journal of Adolescent Health Care, 11,* 159.

Pochi, P. E. (1990). The pathogenesis and treatment of acne. *Annual Review of Medicine, 41,* 187.

Podschum, G. D. (1993). Teen peer outreach-street work project: HIV prevention education for runaway & homeless youth. *Public Health Reports, 108,* 150.

Pollack, M. H., & Rosenbaum, J. F. (1991). Fluoxetine treatment of cocaine abuse in heroin addicts. *Journal of Clinical Psychiatry, 52,* 31.

Povenmire, K. I. (1990). Recognizing the cocaine addict. *Nursing, 20,* 46.

Riggs, S., et al. (1990). Health risk behaviors and attempted suicide in adolescents who report prior maltreatment. *Journal of Pediatrics, 116,* 815.

Rotherman-Borus, M. J. (1993). Suicidal behavior and risk factors among runaway youths. *American Journal of Psychiatry, 150,* 103.

Scheitlin, K. (1990). Identifying and helping children of alcoholics. *Nurse Practitioner, 15,* 34.

Schulz, J. G. (1993). Illicit drugs of abuse. *Primary Care, 20,* 221.

Slap, G. B. (1990). Substance abuse by adolescents. *Hospital Practice, 25,* 19.

Tanner, J. M. (1955). *Growth at adolescence.* Springfield, IL: Charles C Thomas.

Tashkin, D. P. (1990). Pulmonary complications of smoked substance abuse. *Western Journal of Medicine, 152,* 525.

Tobias, J. D., et al. (1990). Methadone as treatment for iatrogenic narcotic dependency in pediatric intensive care unit patients. *Critical Care Medicine, 18,* 1292.

Wadsworth, B. J. (1989). *Piaget's theory of cognitive and affective development.* New York: Longman.

Suggested Readings

Antwerp, C. V., & Spaniolo, A. M. (1991). Checking out children's lifestyle. *MCN: American Journal of Maternal Child Nursing, 16,* 144.

Bar J. H., & Tzuriel, D. (1990). Suicidal tendencies and ego identity in adolescence. *Adolescence, 25,* 215.

Braverman, P. K., & Strasburger, V. C. (1994). Adolescent sexuality: the practitioner's role. *Clinical Pediatrics, 33,* 100.

Cromwell, P. & LeMoine, A. (1992). Identifying substance abuse: an assessment tool for the school nurse. *Journal of School Nursing, 8,* 6.

Curtis, S. (1992). Promoting health through a developmental analysis of adolescent risk behavior. *Journal of Pediatric Health Care, 7,* 3.

Donovan, C. (1990). Adolescent sexuality. *British Medical Journal, 300,* 1026.

Henry, C. S., et al. (1993). Adolescent suicide and families: an ecological approach. *Adolescence, 28,* 291.

Hobbie, C. (1993). Teen pregnancy and teen parenting. *Journal of Pediatric Health Care, 7,* 96.

Remafedi, G., et al. (1992) Demography of sexual orientation in adolescents. *Pediatrics, 89,* 714.

Rickert, V. I., et al. (1993). A companion of methods for alcohol and marijuana anticipatory guidance with adolescents. *Journal of Adolescent Health, 14,* 225.

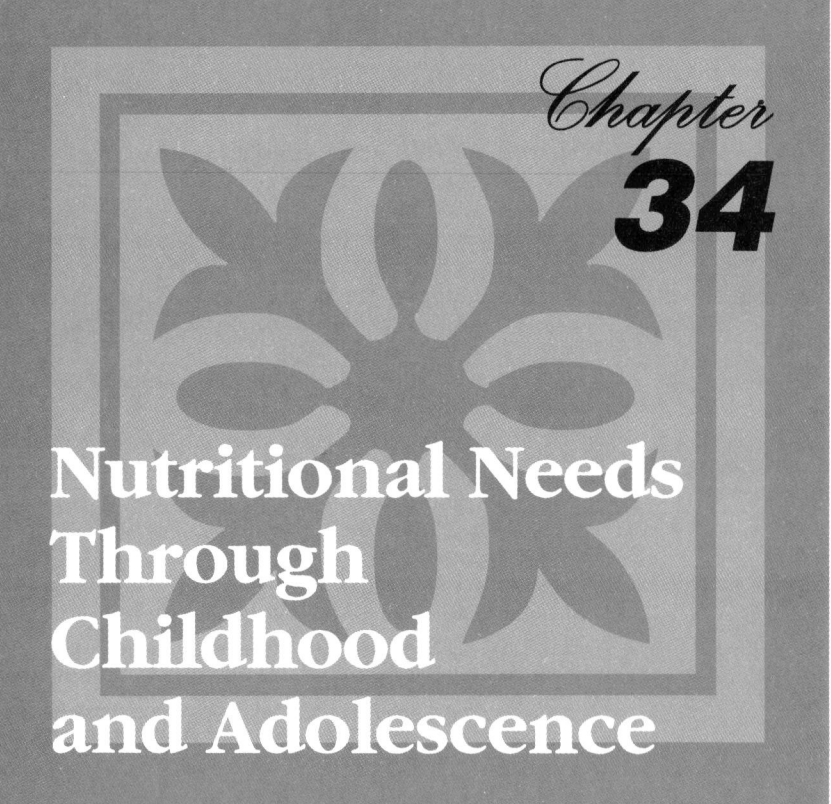

Chapter 34

Nutritional Needs Through Childhood and Adolescence

Key Terms

- adipocytes
- calorie counting
- gavage
- glycogen loading
- lacto-ovovegetarian
- lactose intolerance
- lactovegetarian
- macrobiotic diet
- macronutrient
- micronutrient
- ovovegetarian
- total parenteral nutrition
- vegan

Objectives

After mastering the contents of this chapter, you should be able to:

1. Describe the differences in nutritional needs of children during the infancy, toddler, preschool, school-age, and adolescent periods.

2. Assess a child's eating patterns and determine nutritional needs.

3. Formulate nursing diagnoses regarding nutritional needs of the well child.

4. Plan nursing care for the specific nutritional needs of a hospitalized or well child.

5. Implement nursing care to meet the specific nutritional needs of the child with special needs, such as administering total parenteral nutrition (TPN).

6. Evaluate outcomes established for care to ascertain whether goals have been achieved.

7. Identify National Health Goals related to nutrition and children that nurses could be instrumental in helping the nation to achieve.

8. Identify areas related to nutrition and children that could benefit from additional nursing research.

9. Use critical thinking to analyze methods that will help parents and children improve nutrition throughout the life span.

10. Synthesize the elements of knowledge about childhood nutrition with the nursing process to achieve quality maternal and child health nursing care.

Adele Pillitteri: MATERNAL AND CHILD HEALTH NURSING, 2nd Edition. © 1995 Adele Pillitteri.

Good nutrition is essential to the health of the fetus throughout intrauterine life, and nutrition continues to play a major role in the health of children, particularly in the first 2 years of life when bones, muscles, and body systems are still undergoing major growth, and in adolescence when another growth spurt pushes the child to adult height and weight. Although specific dietary needs of children vary according to growth needs, the value of a healthy, balanced diet at any age cannot be overestimated. Good nutrition not only helps in the prevention of illness during childhood, but may also help to prevent illness such as cardiovascular disease later in life. National Health Goals related to sound nutrition during childhood are shown in the Focus on National Health Goals display.

 NURSING PROCESS OVERVIEW
for Promoting Nutritional Health
During Childhood

ASSESSMENT

Assessment of a child's nutritional health provides important details relating to the child's overall health status, emphasizes to children and parents the importance of nutrition in health maintenance, and provides an important opportunity for education and counseling. For example, many toddlers eat little at specified mealtimes, but if parents are offering nutritious snacks (e.g., cut-up pieces of ham or cheese, orange sections, or pieces of hard-boiled egg), the child may be consuming an adequate daily diet. Inquiring about the child's intake of snacks reminds parents that snacks do not have to be empty calories but can be a way to ensure that their child's food intake is adequate. It may also allow them to relax and stop urging the child to eat.

NURSING DIAGNOSIS

Nursing diagnoses related to nutritional health of the child often focus on lack of knowledge about nutritional needs and healthy patterns of eating. The following are some examples:

- Health seeking behaviors related to nutritional needs of the infant
- Altered nutrition, less than body requirements, related to parental knowledge deficit regarding adolescent's need for high protein intake
- Knowledge deficit related to potential long-term effects of obesity in the school-age child
- Altered nutrition, more than body requirements,

related to child's desire to gain weight to qualify for sports team
- Altered nutrition, less than body requirements, related to inability to ingest food orally

PLANNING

Planning for improved nutrition must be a collaborative effort among the nurse, the child (when old enough), and the child's parents. The plan must address the family's cultural background, lifestyle, and economic ability as well as the child's particular likes and dislikes. Even toddlers are adept at revealing food dislikes or signaling when they have had enough (both a manifestation of autonomy and decreased caloric need). Teaching parents to observe for these cues will help them develop a nutritional plan that is likely to succeed.

Nursing planning for improving preschooler nutrition should involve teaching parents to design creative ways to present food so that meals are an exciting part of the day. Such preparation is important when a child is ill and finds food unappealing or if parents have a limited food budget.

IMPLEMENTATION

Nursing interventions for establishing nutritional health range from child and parental education to administering parenteral or enteral nutrition. When caring for children in a hospital setting when appetites may be lower than normal, always keep in mind that children learn through imitation and imagination. For example, if the parents of a preschooler dislike a basic food such as toast, their child may decide to dislike it as well. A piece of toast cut into the shape of a truck, however, may be more exciting. A dish of oatmeal might be boring; a raisin face on it might make it appealing.

EVALUATION

Whether nutritional intake is adequate or improved is evaluated by observing changes in weight and height. When nutrition is severely compromised, blood values can also be used (see Appendix F). Evaluating the success of education may be a long-term process. It is important to follow up with children and their families at each health care visit to be certain they are continuing to follow healthy nutritional habits between visits.

The following are examples of outcome criteria:

- Child reports she eats one vegetable a day even though it is not her favorite food.
- Parents state they are starting to phase out high-

FOCUS ON
National Health Goals

With good nutrition so important for the formation of growing bodies, investment in sound nutrition with children is essential to protect the future health of the country. National Health Goals related to nutrition and children include the following:

- Reduce growth retardation among low-income children age 5 and younger to less than 10%.
- Reduce dietary fat intake to an average of 30% of calories or less and average saturated fat intake to less than 10% of calories among children age 2 and older.
- Reduce overweight to a prevalence of no more than 15% among adolescents ages 12 through 19.
- Reduce iron deficiency to less than 3% among children ages 1 through 4.
- Increase calcium intake, so at least 50% of youth ages 12 through 24 consume three or more servings daily of foods rich in calcium (DHHS, 1991).

Nurses can be instrumental in helping the nation achieve these goals by improving nutrition education for parents and children. Additional nursing research could shed light on such questions as, What is the average length of time parents continue to feed infants iron-fortified cereal? Are school-based programs effective at weight control? What are effective methods to teach adolescents to reduce their saturated fat intake?

carbohydrate, non-nutritive snacks for their preschooler.
- Child states he is doing a half hour of aerobic exercises daily and following prescribed diet to reduce weight to 50th percentile on growth chart.

Importance of Nutrition to Health

In the past 20 years, nutrition has become a major focus of disease prevention in the United States. Many health care professionals, including the surgeon general, believe that diet is the cornerstone to health. Nutrition plays such a vital role in the body's susceptibility to disease that when suffering from an infectious disease, nutritional status can determine how well or how quickly the body fights off the illness; deficiencies can increase morbidity and mortality.

Diet also plays a major role in chronic illness. Of the eight leading causes of death in adult age groups, six have been linked to dietary excesses: heart disease, cancer, cerebrovascular disease, diabetes mellitus, cirrhosis, and arteriosclerosis. It is clear, too, that dietary habits have a cumulative effect; for example, although heart disease is not one of the top causes of death in the child, it is the number one cause of death in both men and women older than age 55 years. Increased consumption of food, alcohol, decreased levels of exercise, and smoking all lead to greater incidence of these diet-related diseases in adult life. Establishing healthy eating patterns early in life can contribute to better health in the adult years (Sparks, 1992).

Governmental Guidelines for a Healthy Diet

The importance of a healthy diet beginning at birth and continuing throughout a person's life cannot be over-emphasized (Splett & Story, 1991). Basic guidelines for

this healthy diet have been outlined by a variety of governmental groups, including the Surgeon General, the U.S. Department of Agriculture, and the U.S. Department of Health and Human Services. These guidelines are described with reference to children in the following paragraphs.

Eat a Variety of Foods
Choices from all food pyramid groups—dairy, meat and poultry, fruits, vegetables, cereals and grains—should be included in the diet every day (Figure 34-1). Table 34-1 lists recommended servings for children from the five pyramid food groups.

Maintain Ideal Weight
Although the tendency for obesity may be inherited, being overweight in infancy may also play a role. Although infants and toddlers need to receive all the nutrients they need for the substantial growth they are undergoing (including a high percentage of fat important for myelination of nerves), it is important that they not be overfed.

Avoid Too Much Fat, Saturated Fat, and Cholesterol
The American diet has changed substantially over the past 10 years to reflect this important goal. Many adults are consuming low-cholesterol diets, substituting nonfat milk for whole milk, decreasing their consumption of eggs and other high cholesterol sources, and reducing their consumption of meat. It is important that infants and toddlers receive 30% of their calories from fat, but it is not necessary for proper growth for these fats to be high in cholesterol.

Eat Foods With Adequate Starch and Fiber
Foods with starch and fiber are more beneficial for gastrointestinal function than more processed foods. Fiber,

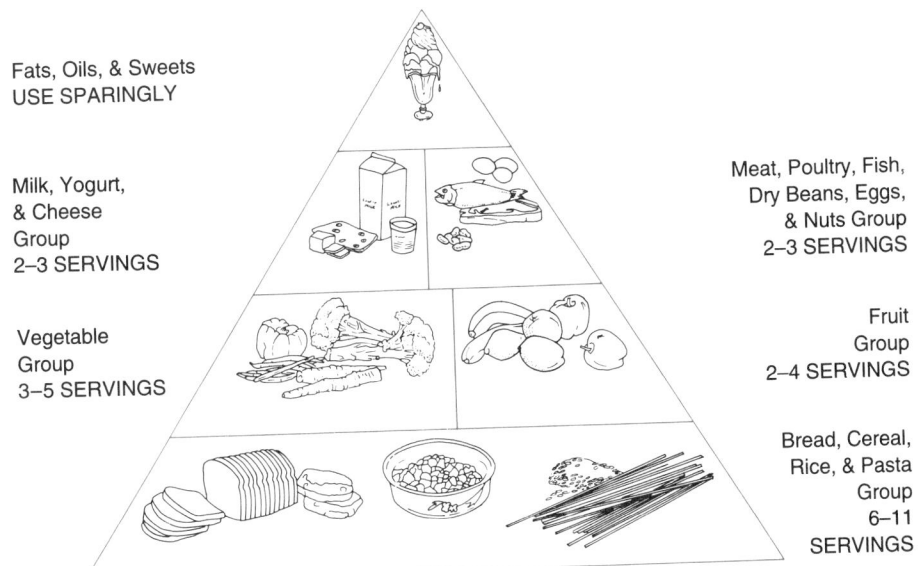

FIGURE 34-1
The food pyramid. (Dudek, S.G. [1993]. Nutrition handbook for nursing practice [2nd ed.]. Philadelphia: J.B. Lippincott.)

Table 34-1. *Servings of the Five Pyramid Food Groups*

Group	Foods	Recommended Daily Amounts				Major Nutrients Provided
		Toddler	Preschool	School-age	Adolescent	
Dairy	Whole milk and other milk products except butter	16 oz	2–4 cups	2–4 cups	4 cups or more	Calcium, phosphorus, complete protein, riboflavin, niacin, vitamin D (if vitamin D–fortified milk used)
Meat	Muscle meats (veal, beef, pork, lamb, mutton, venison); fish; poultry	1 serving	2 or more (2-oz serving)	2 or more (2–3 oz serving)	2 or more (2–3 oz serving)	Complete protein, iron, thiamin, riboflavin, niacin, vitamin B_{12}
Vegetables	Vegetables (yellow and green)	2–3 servings	2 servings	2 servings	2 servings	Vitamin A, iron, calcium (include vitamin A source at least every other day)
Fruits	Fruit	2 servings	2 servings	2 servings	2 servings	Vitamin C (include vitamin C daily)
Bread, cereals	Whole-grain and enriched	2 servings	4 or more servings	4 or more servings	4 or more servings	Thiamin, niacin, riboflavin (if enriched); iron (if enriched); incomplete protein

in particular, has been linked to the lowered incidence of a variety of illnesses such as intestinal polyps. Fiber can be introduced as early as during the infant year in the form of whole-grain cereals and raw fruits such as mashed bananas.

Avoid Too Much Sugar

Too high a consumption of sugar can contribute to dental caries and obesity. Refined sugar such as that used in soft drinks, prepared foods, candy, and chocolate represents "empty" calories, because it is high in calories yet provides no essential nutrients. Although children need adequate carbohydrate for energy, families can give their children a good start by preventing an excessive sugar intake.

Drink Alcohol in Moderation

Adolescents are at increased risk of establishing unhealthy patterns of alcohol use. Educating them on the importance of healthy nutrition for growth is as important as educating them about the long-term consequences of alcohol use (see Chapter 33).

Components of a Healthy Diet

Eating a variety of foods from all five pyramid food groups is a way of guaranteeing the intake of a balanced diet of proteins, carbohydrates, fats, vitamins, and minerals (Figure 34-2).

Protein

Protein is the major component of bones, skin, hair, and muscle, and is responsible for a wide variety of essential functions in the body. Protein is built from amino acids,

some of which are made in the body and some of which must be obtained from the daily diet.

Carbohydrate

Carbohydrates are the main and preferred fuel of the body, essential to the functioning of most body systems, the neurologic system in particular. This is why carbohydrates are so essential to infants and toddlers whose brain cells are actively growing.

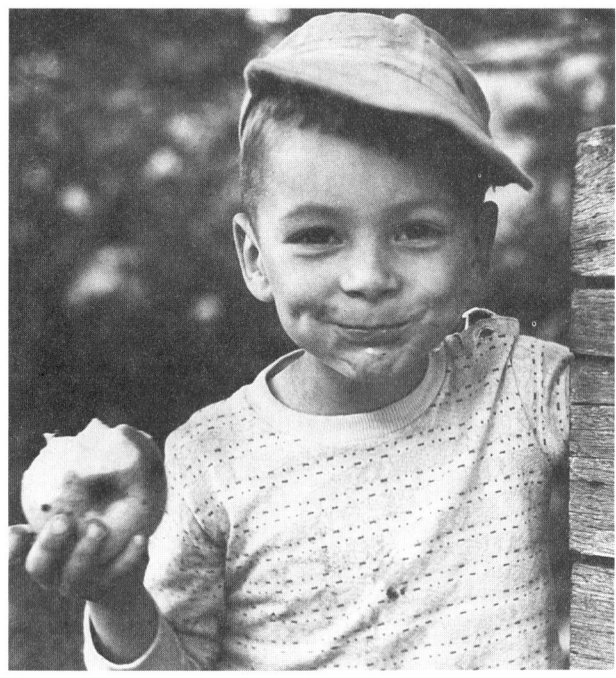

FIGURE 34-2
Good nutritional habits developed early in life provide a child with a health advantage. (Courtesy of USDA.)

Fat

Dietary fat is also a source of energy to the body. It can be an immediate energy source or stored if not used, then released when energy is required. Some fat deposits also serve as insulating material for subcutaneous tissues.

Vitamins

Vitamins are organic compounds that are essential for specific metabolic actions in cells. They do not produce energy but are essential in order for cells to be able to do so. The sources of fat-soluble vitamins (A, D, K, and E) are mainly plant oils and fish oils. Such vitamins are able to leave the gastrointestinal tract only by being absorbed with fat molecules. Once absorbed, they are used by the cells for growth or are stored in the liver and fat cells for later use. Because fat-soluble vitamins can be stored by the body, it is possible for an infant or child to ingest too many of them. Water-soluble vitamins (B complex and C) are not stored well in the body so must be taken daily to maintain effective levels in the blood.

Sources and functions of essential vitamins and results of their deficiency are summarized in Table 34-2.

Minerals

Minerals are necessary to build new cells and are therefore vital to the health of a growing infant or child. They are classified according to amounts needed daily. If more than 100 mg is needed daily, a mineral is a **macronutrient**, or major mineral. If the amount needed is less than 100 mg, it is a **micronutrient**, or minor mineral. Trace minerals refer to those needed in only extremely small amounts (Milner, 1990). Sources and functions of various minerals and results of their deficiency are listed in Table 34-3.

Recommended Daily Dietary Allowances Throughout Childhood

Because children's nutritional needs vary from infancy through adolescence, the recommended requirements of calories, protein, vitamins, and minerals also vary

Table 34-2. *Vitamins Essential for Health*

Vitamin	Selected Dietary Sources	Function in Body	Results of Deficiency
Fat-Soluble*			
A (retinol)	Liver, carrots, spinach	Important for night vision and corneal integrity and growth	Keratinization of the eye (xerophthalmia) and blindness
D	Egg yolk, margarine, salmon	Regulates absorption of calcium and phosphorus for bone growth	Rickets (bone deformity) in growing children
E	Margarine, corn oil, peanuts	An antioxidant that protects red blood cells from destruction by oxygen	In immature infants, severe anemia from destruction of red blood cells
K	Cabbage, spinach, pork	Aids blood clotting (synthesis of prothrombin)	Bleeding from lack of sufficient clotting action
Water-Soluble			
B complex: Thiamin	Wheat germ, yeast, pork	Important for use of glucose in cells	Beriberi, a disease that causes nerve paralysis
Riboflavin	Beef, chicken, liver, avocados, eggs, oats	Breaks down fatty acids and amino acids for energy	Red swollen tongue, inflamed eyes, fissures of lips
Niacin	Peanuts, rice bran, liver	Converts glucose to energy	Pellagra (diarrhea, mental confusion, dermatitis, death)
B$_6$ (pyridoxine)	Liver, herring, salmon	Metabolizes amino acids and glucose	Neuritis, depression, nausea, vomiting
B$_{12}$ (cobalamin)	Lamb, beef kidney, egg yolk	Blood formation	Pernicious anemia (large, nonfunctioning red blood cells)
Folic acid (folacin)	Liver, asparagus, bran	Red and white blood cell structure	Poor red cell formation
C (ascorbic acid)	Broccoli, collards, citrus fruit	Collagen structure	Scurvy (weakness, easy bleeding, joint pain)

*All fat-soluble vitamins can be absorbed only in the presence of lipids and can be transported only in the presence of protein.

Table 34-3. Minerals Essential for Health

Mineral	Selected Dietary Sources	Function in Body	Results of Deficiency or Excess
Macronutrients			
Calcium	Milk, hard cheese	Formation of bone and teeth; muscle contractility	Improper bone growth and maintenance shown by diseases such as rickets in children
Phosphorus	Milk, meats	Formation of bone and teeth; used in cell structure; aids use of glucose	Deficiency unlikely as long as calcium and protein needs are met
Sodium	Table salt	Regulates fluid volume and pH	Deficiency rare but excess leads to hypertension in genetically determined individuals
Chloride	Table salt	Formation of hydrochloric acid; regulates body fluid with sodium	Deficiency rare except with vomiting, which causes loss of hydrochloric acid
Potassium	Meats, dried fruits	Major cation of cells; essential for electrical conduction in muscle and therefore in heart action	Deficiency leading to muscle weakness and heart irritability occurs in people taking diuretics, because potassium is excreted with urine
Sulfur	Milk, meat, eggs	Essential for protein formation and cell growth	Deficiency rare as long as protein intake is adequate
Magnesium	Cocoa, nuts, green leafy vegetables	Relaxation of muscles after contraction	Deficiency leads to muscle contraction
Micronutrients			
Iodine	Seafood, dairy	Formation of thyroxine and regulation of metabolic rate	Reduced basal metabolic rate and goiter (enlarged thyroid gland)
Iron	Meats, fish, dried fruits, nuts	Formation of hemoglobin; transport of oxygen to body cells	Deficiency leads to microcytic (small) and hypochromic (pale) red blood cells (iron-deficiency anemia); excess leads to infiltration of tissue (hemosiderosis)
Copper	Nuts, raisins, legumes	Formation of collagen and nerve fiber	No deficiencies known
Fluoride	Water	Reduces dental caries and demineralization from bone	Dental caries
Zinc	Meat, eggs, seafood	Formation of eye, male reproductive organs, insulin, and taste sensation	Diabetes-like symptoms due to decreased insulin production; poor taste sensation leading to poor food intake
Manganese	Nuts, grains, legumes	Formation of enzymes	Deficiency unlikely
Molybdenum	Organ meats, grains	Mobilizes iron in body	Deficiency apparently unknown
Cobalt	Many sources	Formation of red blood cells in bone marrow	Deficiency rare as long as animal food sources are ingested
Selenium	Seafood, kidney, liver	Immunoglobin formation and prevention of oxidation of cells	Deficiency unknown
Chromium	Meat, cheese, grains	Glucose metabolism	Deficiency seen only in severe malnutrition
Silicon	Many sources	Aids growth of connective tissue and bone	Retarded growth and bone deformity
Nickel	Many sources	Duplication or growth of cells	Deficiency rare
Vanadium	Many sources	Lipid metabolism	Deficiency rare on a well-balanced diet
Tin	Many sources	Blood formation	Deficiency rare

with each period of development. Table 34-4 lists the recommended dietary requirements for children of different ages.

The Infant

The entire first year of life is one of rapid growth, requiring a high-protein, high-calorie intake. Calorie allowances can be reduced during the year from a level of 120 per kilogram of body weight at birth to approxi-mately 100 per kilogram of body weight at the end of the first year. It is important that the number of calories be gradually reduced during the first year; otherwise, babies tend to become overweight (Sherman & Alexander, 1990).

Although heredity plays a role, a baby who is overweight during the first year of life is more likely to become an obese adult than one whose weight is within normal limits. Overfeeding in early life produces large

Table 34-4. *Recommended Daily Dietary Allowances for Children, From Birth Through Adolescence*

	0–6 mo	*6–12 mo*	*1–3 yr*	*4–6 yr*	*7–10 yr*	*11–14 yr* Boys	Girls	*15–18 yr* Boys	Girls
Calories	650 kcal/d	850 kcal/d	1300 kcal/d	1800 kcal/d	2000 kcal/d	2500 kcal/d	2200 kcal/d	3000 kcal/d	2200 kcal/d
Protein	13 g	14 g	16 g	24 g	28 g	45 g	46 g	59 g	44 g
Fat-Soluble Vitamins									
A	375 μg RE*	375 μg RE*	400 μg RE*	500 μg RE*	700 μg RE*	1000 μg RE*	800 μg RE*	1000 μg RE*	800 μg RE*
D	7.5 μg†	10 μg†	10 μg†	10 μg†	10 μg†	10 μg†	10 μg†	10 μg†	10 μg†
E	3 mg α-TE‡	4 mg α-TE‡	6 mg α-TE‡	7 mg α-TE‡	7 mg α-TE‡	10 mg α-TE‡	8 mg α-TE‡	10 mg α-TE‡	8 mg α-TE‡
K	5 μg	10 μg	15 μg	20 μg	30 μg	45 μg	45 μg	65 μg	55 μg
Water-Soluble Vitamins									
Ascorbic acid (vitamin C)	30 mg	35 mg	40 mg	45 mg	45 mg	50 mg	50 mg	60 mg	60 mg
Folic acid	25 μg	35 μg	50 μg	75 μg	100 μg	150 μg	150 μg	200 μg	180 μg
Niacin	5 mg	6 mg	9 mg	12 mg	13 mg	17 mg	15 mg	20 mg	15 mg
Riboflavin	0.4 mg	0.5 mg	0.8 mg	1.1 mg	1.2 mg	1.5 mg	1.3 mg	1.8 mg	1.3 mg
Thiamine	0.3 mg	0.4 mg	0.7 mg	0.9 mg	1.0 mg	1.3 mg	1.1 mg	1.5 mg	1.1mg
Vitamin B_6	0.3 mg	0.6 mg	1.0 mg	1.1 mg	1.4 mg	1.7 mg	1.4 mg	2.0 mg	1.5 mg
Vitamin B_{12}	0.3 μg	0.5 μg	0.7 μg	1.0 μg	1.4 μg	2 μg	2 μg	2 μg	2 μg
Minerals									
Calcium	400 mg	600 mg	800 mg	800 mg	800 mg	1200 mg	1200 mg	1200 mg	1200 mg
Phosphorus	300 mg	500 mg	800 mg	800 mg	800 mg	1200 mg	1200 mg	1200 mg	1200 mg
Iodine	40 μg	50 μg	70 μg	90 μg	120 μg	150 μg	150 μg	150 μg	150 μg
Iron	6 mg	10 mg	10 mg	10 mg	10 mg	12 mg	15 mg	12 mg	15 mg
Magnesium	40 mg	60 mg	80 mg	120 mg	170 mg	270 mg	280 mg	400 mg	300 mg
Zinc	5 mg	5 mg	10 mg	10 mg	10 mg	15 mg	12 mg	15 mg	12 mg
Selenium	10 μg	15 μg	20 μg	20 μg	30 μg	40 μg	45 μg	50 μg	50 μg

*Retinol equivalents: 1 retinol equivalent = 1 μg retinol or 6 μg β carotene.
† As cholecalciferol: 10 μg cholecalciferol = 400 International Units of vitamin D.
‡ α-Tocopherol equivalents: 1 mg d-α-tocopherol = 1 α-TE.
(From National Academy of Sciences, Food and Nutrition Board. [1989]. *Recommended dietary allowances.*
[10th ed.] Washington, DC: National Academy Press, with permission.)

numbers of excess fat cells (**adipocytes**) used to store fat. Because these cells are permanent and remain filled with fat, once they are present, weight regulation can become difficult throughout life.

The Toddler

Because growth slows abruptly after the first year of life, the toddler's appetite is smaller than the infant's. A child who ate hungrily 2 months or 3 months earlier will now sit and play with food.

The actual amount of food eaten daily will vary from one child to another. Therefore, it is usually wisest if parents place a small amount of food on a plate and allow the child to eat it and ask for more rather than serve a large portion that he or she cannot finish. One tablespoonful of each food served is a good start. Also, cleaning a plate gives the child a feeling of independent

functioning, whereas leaving food uneaten may suggest to the child that parents expected something more.

Toddlers usually do not like food that is "mixed up" such as casseroles (except maybe spaghetti); they often prefer that different foods do not touch one another on their plate. Frequently they eat all of one item before going on to another. They enjoy finger foods because they can be eaten independently.

The Preschooler

Like the toddler period, the preschool years are not a time of fast growth, so the child is not likely to have a ravenous appetite. Offering small servings of food is still a good idea, so that the child is not overwhelmed and is allowed the successful feeling of cleaning a plate and asking for more. Parents should offer varied sources of calcium to ensure good bone growth (Chan, 1991).

Many parents ask whether their preschooler needs to take supplementary vitamins. As long as the child is eating foods from all five pyramid food groups and meets the criteria for a healthy child (i.e., alert and active, with height and weight within normal averages), additional vitamins are unnecessary.

If parents do give vitamins, they must remember that the child will undoubtedly view the vitamin as candy rather than medicine because of the attractive shapes and colors of preschool vitamins. Vitamins must be stored out of reach with other medicines. Caution parents not to give more than the recommended daily amount or else poisoning from high doses of fat-soluble vitamins and iron can result. Poisoning from excessive ingestion is an increasing problem among toddlers and preschoolers (CDC, 1993).

The School-Age Child

During the late school years, the recommended daily dietary allowances begin to be separated into categories for girls and boys (see Table 34-4), because boys require more calories and other nutrients at this time. Both girls and boys require more iron in prepuberty than they did between the ages of 7 years and 10 years. Adequate calcium and fluoride intake remain important to ensure good teeth.

The Adolescent

Because adolescence is a time of rapid growth, the adolescent's appetite increases so much that he or she may always seem hungry. As shown in Table 34-4, males continue to need more calories than females during this period. One of the most important things adolescents can learn about nutrition is that just filling their stomachs will not provide adequate nutrition. Foods that supply the necessary carbohydrates, vitamins, protein, and minerals are essential.

The nutrients that are most apt to be deficient in both male and female adolescent diets are iron, calcium, and zinc. Large amounts of iron are necessary in order to meet expanding blood volume requirements; increased calcium is necessary for rapid skeletal growth; zinc is necessary for sexual maturation and final body growth. Good sources of iron are meat and green vegetables; calcium is abundant in milk and milk products; meat and milk are also high in zinc. Females require a high iron intake not only because of increasing blood volume needs but also because iron begins to be lost with menstruation. Girls with a heavy menstrual flow (menorrhagia) may need to take an additional iron supplement to prevent iron-deficiency anemia (see Chapter 47).

Assessment of Nutritional Health

Begin nutritional assessment by taking a history and performing a physical examination. Take height and weight measurements and plot them on a standard growth curve to see if they are within normal limits (see Appendix E). Characteristics of a nutritionally healthy child that can be revealed by assessment are summarized in Table 34-5.

Measuring Food Intake

Taking a history of a child's food intake can help determine whether there are any foods missing in a typical meal plan or whether any quantities seem excessive. Be certain to assess not only the quantity of food taken but the quality as well (e.g., for the infant, cereal should be iron fortified; Treiber et al., 1990).

To do this, ask parents to describe a typical day (24-hour recall), listing what the child ate for each meal and in-between meals as well. With an older child, the 24-hour recall can be a joint parent–child venture. Providing this history can be difficult, however, when the child consumes some meals at home and others at day care or school. It may be necessary to ask for a weekend history to get a complete picture.

After taking the history, determine whether the child is receiving foods from the five pyramid groups. Remember that children do not have to eat food from all groups every meal, as long as they eat from them every week. If parents think in terms of weeks rather than days, they may exert less pressure on a child at each meal.

Assessment of the adolescent's diet includes evaluation of lifestyle and food preferences. Take a 24-hour recall nutritional history without a parent present, if possi-

Table 34-5. *Physical Signs of Adequate Nutrition*

Assessment	Finding
Overall impression	Alert, with good energy level; positive mood
Hair	Shiny, strong, with good body.
Eyes	Good eyesight, particularly at night; conjunctiva moist and pink
Mouth	No cavities in teeth; no swollen or inflamed gingivae; no cracks or fissures at corners of mouth; mucous membrane moist and pink; tongue smooth and nontender
Neck	Normal contour of thyroid gland
Skin	Smooth; normal color and turgor; no ecchymotic or petechial areas present
Extremities	Normal muscle mass and circumference; normal strength and mobility; no edema present; no tender joints; normal reflexes; legs not bowed
Gastrointestinal	No diarrhea or constipation is present
Finger and toenails	Smooth, pink; not cracked or broken
Height and weight	Within normal limits on growth chart
Blood pressure	Normal for age

ble. Adolescents may add extra foods to a food intake history in front of a parent or leave out foods they have eaten (e.g., milk shakes, potato chips, or pizza) to avoid a lecture later.

Do not appear critical of an adolescent's diet. If you convey dismay at erratic eating habits, they may begin to fabricate their food history to make it seem more acceptable, or leave out items because they may enjoy the obvious disapproval—a game that can appeal to them as part of their rebellion against adult authority.

When evaluating a completed food list, take into account the adolescent viewpoint. For example, although you might not view a hamburger with lettuce, onion, and tomatoes on a bun, french fries, and a chocolate milkshake as an ideal meal, it does include the five pyramid food groups (meat, bread, fruit, vegetable, milk).

Cultural and Social Considerations

It is important to consider the role of cultural variations when assessing food intake or developing a nutritional plan. The number of meals eaten at home versus outside the home, form and content of traditional meals cooked at home, and the pattern of meals should all be considered. Any religious dietary restrictions should also be determined (see the Focus on Cultural Awareness box).

Budgetary restrictions can also play a major role in dictating the dietary patterns of a family. If an essential nutritional component, such as protein, is consistently missing from the daily meals, and finances are determined to be responsible, simply recommending that protein be added will not help solve the problem. Brainstorming with the parent to determine foods high in protein that are not so costly and ways to prepare those foods will be much more helpful. A pleasant environment and adult supervision both influence how well children eat (Stanek et al., 1990; Klesges et al., 1991).

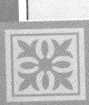

FOCUS ON CULTURAL AWARENESS

In addition to personal likes and dislikes, nutritional practices are culturally determined. Children whose religions prevent them from eating meat, for example, will be vegetarians. Some families prepare food with many spices, some blandly. Some families use corn as a dietary stable, some rice, and some potatoes or wheat. Lactose intolerance prohibits many Asian children from drinking milk. The main meal of the day is also culturally determined; for some families this is the noon meal; for others it is the evening meal (Geissler, 1994). Assessment is always necessary in order to understand the meaning of food to a particular family.

Pregnant and lactating women with infants and children up to 5 years of age, who meet income guidelines and who are at nutritional risk, qualify for the Supplemental Food Program for Women, Infants, and Children (WIC). If eligible, the family is given a voucher that is exchanged for milk, orange juice, eggs, iron-fortified cereal, iron-fortified formula, or cheese. An important part of WIC programs is periodic scheduled health care visits, which must be kept to continue to qualify. This further protects the health of this high-risk group (Batten et al., 1990).

Promoting Nutritional Health Throughout Childhood

The Infant

The best food for the infant during the first 6 months of life (and the only food necessary during this time) is breast milk (see Chapter 24). With breast-feeding, as long as the mother is ingesting an adequate diet, no additional supplements such as added iron or vitamins are necessary, except for fluoride if it is not included in the water supply (American Academy of Pediatrics [AAP], 1986). If the infant will not be receiving exposure to sunshine, vitamin D may also be prescribed. How long mothers continue to breast-feed is an individual choice. It is recommended through the entire first year; prolonged breast-feeding into the preschool period may impair child growth (Grummer-Strawn et al., 1993).

For infants whose mothers do not choose to breast-feed, a commercial iron-fortified formula may be used (see Appendix B). Supplementation is unnecessary with commercial formula unless the water supply does not contain fluoride (AAP, 1980). Infants who are changed to cow's milk before 1 year of age (a practice that is not recommended) should receive a supplementary form of vitamin C to make up for the deficiency of vitamin C in cow's milk. The introduction of cow's milk before 1 year may lead to such intestinal irritation that slight but continuous gastrointestinal bleeding can occur, possibly resulting in anemia (AAP, 1983).

Introducing Solid Food

Most parents are eager to begin feeding their infant solid food. Although it has not been shown to be successful, some parents believe that the introduction of food helps their child sleep through the night.

From a nutritional standpoint, a normal full-term infant can thrive on a commercial iron-fortified formula or breast milk without the addition of any solid food until age 6 months (AAP, 1980). Delaying solid food until this time helps to prevent obesity and the overwhelming of infant kidneys by a heavy solute load; it may also delay the development of food allergies in susceptible infants. Some parents do begin food before this time (without apparent ill effects), but much of it is probably not processed by the gastrointestinal tract (it passes through undigested due to immaturity of the digestive system and decreased amylase and lipase secretion).

Generally speaking, an infant is physiologically ready for solid food when he or she is taking more than 32 oz (960 mL) of formula a day and does not seem satisfied, or is nursing vigorously every 3 to 4 hours and does not seem satisfied. Teach parents that infants are not ready to digest complex starches until amylase is present in saliva at approximately 2 to 3 months. Before beginning to eat, however, an infant must also achieve a certain developmental maturity. Biting movements begin at approximately 3 months. Chewing movements do not begin until 7 to 9 months; thus, foods that require chewing should not be given until this age (see the Focus on Family Teaching display).

Loss of Extrusion Reflex

The extrusion reflex is a life-saving reflex that prevents an infant from swallowing or aspirating foreign objects that touch the mouth. When anything is placed on the anterior third of the newborn's tongue, it is automatically extruded or thrust out of the mouth by the tongue

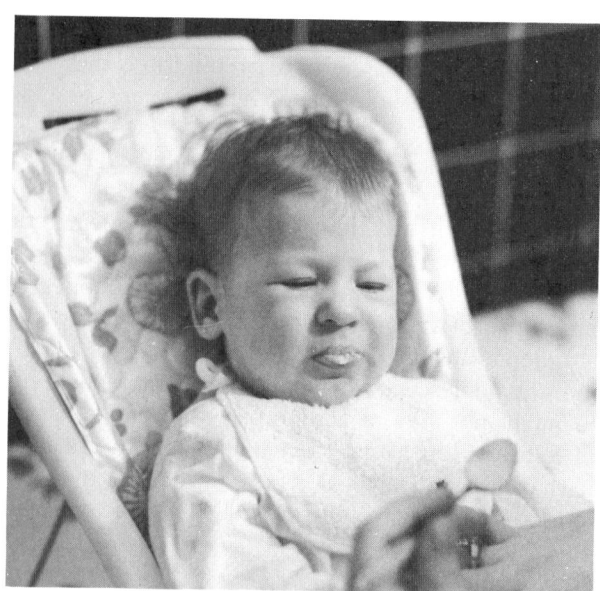

FIGURE 34-3
A 4-month-old baby demonstrates an extrusion reflex. Caution parents not to interpret this action as a food dislike but recognize it as the reflex action that it is.

(Figure 34-3). Thus, the infant automatically extrudes the food when a spoonful is placed on the tongue. The reflex fades at 3 to 4 months. Until this time, it may be difficult to get a child to eat solids.

Techniques for Feeding Solid Food

Table 34-6 shows the usual times and patterns for introducing solid food. Teach parents to offer new foods one at a time; allow the child to eat that item for 1 week before another one is given. This system helps parents to discern food allergies. For example, if they start egg yolk on Monday and by Tuesday evening the child is breathing noisily or has a rash, they might suspect that the child is allergic to eggs. If two new foods had been started on Monday, it would be hard to know which one was suspect. Introducing foods one at a time also helps to establish a sense of trust in infants, as it minimizes the number of new experiences in any 1 day.

It is best for the first solid food feeding if the infant is held in the parent's arms as if for bottle- or breast-feeding. This reduces the newness of the experience and minimizes the amount of stress associated with it. Some infants accept new experiences of this type readily, whereas other infants resist heartily. If an infant does not take readily to solid food, advise parents to wait a few days and then try again. Parents should not feel that they have to compete with friends to see whose child takes cereal, vegetables, or fruit first.

Even after the extrusion reflex has faded, an infant may appear to be spitting out food, because he or she has never experienced anything but liquid. Infants drink from a bottle or breast by pressing their tongue and the

FOCUS ON FAMILY TEACHING

Q. *My baby is 5 months old. What are guidelines to use to introduce solid foods?*

A. Infants are ready for solid food at 5 to 6 months of age. These tips can help with introducing your baby to his first solid foods.

- Introduce one food at a time, waiting 5 to 7 days between new items.
- Introduce the food before formula- or breast-feeding when the infant is hungry.
- Introduce small amounts of a new food (1 or 2 tsp) at a time.
- Respect infant food preferences; a child cannot be expected to like all new tastes equally well.
- Use a minimum of salt and sugar on solid foods to keep the number of additives to a minimum.
- Remember that the extrusion reflex is present for the first 4 to 6 months of life, which means that any food placed on an infant's tongue will be pushed forward.
- To prevent aspiration, do not place food in bottles with formula.
- Introduce foods with a positive, "You'll like this" attitude.

Table 34-6. *Suggested Schedule for Introduction of Solid Foods*

Age (mo)	Food to Introduce*	Rationale
5–6	Iron-fortified infant cereal mixed with breast milk, orange juice, or formula	Helps prevent iron-deficiency anemia; the least allergenic type of food; an easily digested food
7	Vegetables	Good source of vitamin A; adds new texture and flavors to diet
8	Fruit	Best source of vitamin C, good source of vitamin A; adds new texture and flavors to diet
9	Meat	Good source of protein, iron, and B vitamins
10	Egg yolk	Good source of iron

*Wheat, tomatoes, oranges, fish, and egg white should be omitted if there are allergies in the family, because these foods are most likely to cause allergies.

nipple against their hard palate. When an infant tries to manage solid food in this same way, it appears that the child is spitting it out. Babies have distinct taste preferences even at young ages and may spit out a food because they do not like the taste. A parent who knows an infant's cues will be able to distinguish taste preferences from inadequate management of solid food. The Focus on Family Teaching box lists pointers to help make the introduction of solid foods a positive experience.

Quantities and Types of Food

Children take different quantities of food according to their preferences and needs. A newborn stomach can hold approximately 2 tablespoons (30 mL); at 1 year, the stomach can hold approximately 1 cup (240 mL). For this reason, when they begin eating solid food, infants rarely take more than 2 tablespoons (30 mL) at a time.

Cereal. The first food generally given to infants is cereal fortified with B vitamins and iron. Infant cereals are precooked, fine dry powders to which orange juice, expressed breast milk, or infant formula is added. Orange juice is a good liquid to add because the iron in the cereal is absorbed best from an acid medium, which the orange juice supplies.

Cereal should be mixed in a small bowl with enough fluid to make the mixture fairly liquid. As the infant adjusts to eating food from a spoon, parents can thicken it gradually. It is unnecessary to add sugar to cereal; the infant eats it either way, and extra sugar in the diet can lead to diarrhea in young infants and beginning caries in older infants.

Fortified cereal costs no more than unfortified cereal, so remind parents to buy the fortified product. The first cereal introduced is usually rice cereal, because fewer children are allergic to rice products than to wheat and corn products. Cereal is usually offered twice a day,

morning and evening. Once the child has taken rice cereal for 1 week, another kind may be tried.

Some parents mix cereal with the infant's formula and give it to the child from a bottle. Caution parents that this is not a good practice because (1) it is necessary to cut a larger hole in the nipple for the cereal and milk mixture to flow freely, and there is a danger that the infant may aspirate if too big a hole is cut; (2) there is a real danger of aspiration if the parent then uses that nipple for formula without cereal added; and (3) it denies the child the opportunity of learning to eat from a spoon and appreciate different food tastes.

Infant cereal is so rich in iron that parents should be encouraged to continue feeding it at least through the first year; the American Academy of Pediatrics recommends feeding it through age 18 months (AAP, 1983). Ideally, children should eat infant cereal until age 3 or 4 years. Although children usually prefer the popularly advertised products by this time, few of these can match the nutrients of infant fortified cereal.

Vegetables and Fruit. Because their iron content is generally higher than that of fruits, vegetables are usually the second food added to the diet (at approximately age 7 months). Parents who have a blender, strainer, or grinder can prepare their own. They simply cook a vegetable and then blend or strain it so that it does not have to be chewed. Caution parents not to add butter or salt to the preparation, because infants have difficulty digesting fats until almost the end of the first year, and the intake of too much sodium may lead to hypertension later in life. Additional sugar is also unnecessary. By filling ice-cube trays with the blended vegetables, parents can make a 1-week supply and defrost a cube at a time. An ice cube is approximately 1 oz, or one fourth the size of a jar of baby food.

If parents use commercial food, they should feed it

from a dish rather than directly from the jar, because the spoon carries salivary enzymes from the infant's mouth to the food, which will liquefy what remains in the jar. Also, there is danger of transferring bacteria (principally streptococci) from the infant's mouth to the jar. Then, if the parent keeps the jar for another feeding in the next 24 hours, bacteria will multiply rapidly, because the contents serve as a culture medium. Infant food jars should be refrigerated once they are opened, and manufacturers recommend that they be used no later than 48 hours after they have been opened.

When vegetables are added to the diet, they are usually offered at the noon meal. Remind parents to offer both green and yellow vegetables. Help them to remember that their own dislike of a particular vegetable does not mean that their child will feel the same way about it. If they convey a distaste for the food, the child will pick up the feeling and the thing the parents feared will happen: the child will not like the vegetable.

Fruit is usually offered one month after vegetables (at approximately age 8 months). It can be given in addition to cereal for breakfast and dinner. Raw mashed banana is easy to prepare with just a fork; peaches are easily prepared in a blender. As with vegetables, parents should plan a selection so that the infant is exposed to different tastes and textures.

Meat and Eggs. Meat is usually introduced at 9 months and egg yolks at 10 months. Parents can grind a portion of the meat they have prepared for their own meal so it is tender, or use commercially prepared products. If they use commercial baby meat, urge them to use the plain meat products, not vegetable and meat dinners, since these contain mostly vegetables and, often, sodium. Chicken has less iron than beef or pork, so parents should not make chicken the most frequently offered meat (it has the advantage of being low in cholesterol, but this is not a priority with infants). When meat is added to the infant's diet, it is usually added as part of the evening meal in place of cereal.

Be certain parents understand the difference between the yolk and white of eggs. The egg yolk contains the bulk of the iron content of an egg; the white contains the bulk of protein. Egg yolk alone should be given at first, because the protein of the egg white can lead to allergy or be difficult for the infant to digest. Eggs may be prepared by hard-boiling (then adding a little formula to the mashed yolk to make it more liquid). Soft-boiling or poaching is not usually recommended, because salmonella, the chief offending microorganism in eggs, may not be fully killed by these methods. Egg yolk can also be purchased in commercial baby food jars. Eggs must always be well cooked, because raw eggs carry the danger of *Salmonella* infection. Also, cooking makes protein easier to digest.

If there is increased frequency of atherosclerosis in

the family, an infant probably should not be offered an egg daily, but only two or three times a week. An infant who is taking an iron-supplemented formula and eating vegetables and cereal—foods high in iron—does not need an egg every day.

Table Food. With the introduction of solid food, parents should arrange for their child to be eating three meals a day, if that is the family's pattern, and join the family at the table if he or she has not been introduced to this custom yet. It is generally better to encourage parents to use homemade foods rather than rely on commercially prepared junior foods, for economic as well as nutritional reasons: commercial dinners may contain little meat and, unlike infant foods, junior foods may have a high sodium content. Mashed potatoes or peas and cut-up meatloaf are examples of table foods that infants older than age 6 months like to eat. If hot dogs are offered, caution parents always to cut them into bite-size portions. Otherwise, being cylindrical and the diameter of the trachea, they can be especially dangerous if aspirated. As infants begin teething, they enjoy dried bread, teething biscuits, or zwieback.

Some infants are too distracted by the activity at a family table to eat well. Parents may find that these children eat more if they are fed first and then allowed to have a small amount to "feed themselves" or a cracker to chew on while just sitting at the table and being with the family.

Remind parents, as necessary, that high chairs are one of the most dangerous pieces of baby equipment they own. Urge them always to fasten the straps and never leave an infant unattended in a high chair, because even a 6-month-old can squirm out of the straps with little effort. This must also be kept in mind when feeding infants in a hospital setting.

Establishing Healthy Eating Patterns

Some parents may need reminders that there are no hard-and-fast rules for infant feeding. The rules are only guidelines based on what seems to work well with the majority of infants. Parents should individualize their approach according to the cues the child is giving them for readiness.

A child who adapts to change poorly can have difficulty accepting the first solid food and may have difficulty with each new food. The parents of such a child may need support to remember that the child is not conducting this struggle out of a desire for conflict but because this is a characteristic of temperament. Giving food to others is interpreted by many persons as giving love, so refusing food is equated with refusing love. Help parents to understand that this is not what is happening. Refusing a teaspoonful of carrots is refusing a teaspoonful of carrots, nothing more.

Most infants eat hungrily; thus, feeding problems generally are reported more frequently as a second-year or toddler problem than an infant concern. If an infant does refuse to eat, explore with the parents what foods they are offering. Have them list exactly the types and amounts of foods the child ate the day before (a 24-hour dietary recall history). When this is done, it may be apparent that enough is being eaten in a day's time; the parents' expectations are unrealistic for the child's age.

If intake is inadequate and the child is, indeed, a fussy eater, explore further to uncover the parents' methods of feeding. Ask if they are offering a bottle first and then infant food, for example. Infants generally accept the new experience of eating from a spoon when they are hungry, not when their stomach is full. Other babies, particularly those with an intense temperament, may be so hungry at mealtime that they cannot tolerate the frustration of spoon-feeding until some of their hunger is relieved. They may need to drink 2 or 3 oz of formula or nurse at the breast for a few minutes before they will eat a spoonful of food.

An infant who is fatigued or overstimulated may not eat well. Providing a quiet environment away from older brothers or sisters before mealtime may solve this problem.

Encourage parents not to force infants to eat. Healthy, happy infants will be hungry at mealtime and will eat. Those who refuse a meal may be tired, distracted, or perhaps ill. Forcing only leads to regurgitation or, if they are ill, vomiting. It also can result in feeding problems or a situation in which infants refuse to eat altogether. Infants who are eating and not thriving or not eating and therefore not thriving should be examined to determine the cause. Causes include metabolic disorders and failure to thrive (see Chapters 48 and 55).

Weaning

Infants are capable of approximating their lips to a cup effectively at about 6 months of age. The sucking reflex begins to diminish in intensity between ages 6 months and 9 months, which makes this the time to consider weaning. In actual practice, parents wean at varied times (Barness, 1990).

Infants usually need more fluid during hot weather than cold weather because of increased perspiration. Thus, it may be more difficult to introduce a new method of drinking during summer months. To wean from formula or breast, the mother chooses one feeding a day and then begins offering fluid by the new method at that feeding. She should choose a time of day that is not the infant's fussy period for best cooperation, but other than that the time is immaterial. After approximately 1 week, when the infant has become acclimated to the one change, the mother changes a second feeding. Should illness such as an upper respiratory infection occur or should the child have teething discomfort, there will be setbacks, so no set number of weeks should be prescribed to complete weaning.

Breast-fed infants are usually easier to wean than bottle-fed infants because, although it is comforting and enjoyable to breast-feed, the breast serves mainly as a food source, not as a toy or comforter the way a bottle may. Infants who have been given a pacifier appear easier to wean from a bottle than those who have not, but they may then be difficult to wean from a pacifier.

Self-Feeding

At approximately 6 months of age, infants become interested in handling a spoon and beginning to feed themselves; however, they are much more adept at feeding themselves with their fingers (Figure 34-4). Their coordination, unfortunately, has not developed enough for them to use a spoon without a great deal of spilling. One solution for parents concerned with neatness is to spread newspapers or a towel on the floor around the high chair to catch most of the dropped food, and then let the child practice. When an infant becomes fatigued or frustrated by attempts at self-feeding, a parent can then quietly help without making an issue of it. Parents who insist on continuing to spoon-feed can cause the infant to balk and eat nothing. Often, a compromise is helpful. If a parent gives an infant a spoon, the child can poke at a cereal dish with it while the parent continues to offer the child bites from a second spoon. In this way, the child is "in charge" of the feeding yet receptive to taking food from the parent.

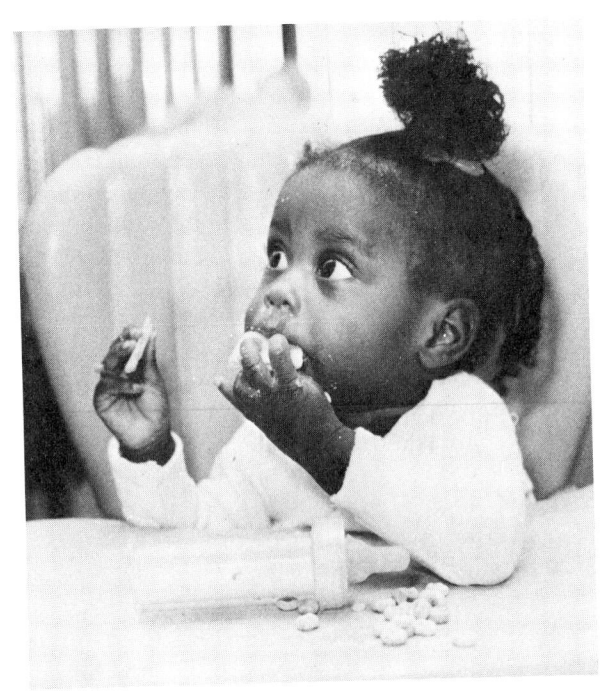

FIGURE 34-4
Self-feeding is not always a neat process for an infant. (Courtesy of the Department of Medical Photography, Children's Hospital, Buffalo, NY.)

When infants no longer attempt to feed themselves at a meal but merely begin to play with their food, by squeezing it through their fingers or dabbing it in their hair, it is time to end the meal. They are saying they have had enough.

The Toddler

Toddlers insist on feeding themselves and will resist eating if a parent insists on feeding them. They enjoy finger foods and eat best if some form of these is offered at every meal. Pieces of chicken are a good meat finger food; slices of banana are an example of a fruit; pieces of cheese are from the milk group; and crackers are a bread source. Milk should be whole milk until age 2 years, after which 2% milk can be introduced.

If feeding problems begin, it is often because parents are unaware that their toddler's appetite has decreased and food consumption is less. When they try to feed the child, he or she resists (toddler autonomy); the child may react to repeated attempts by refusing to eat at all. It is important to educate parents while the child is still an infant that this decline in food intake will occur so that they will not be concerned when it happens.

Self-feeding is a major way to strengthen independence in a toddler. Offering finger foods and allowing a choice between two types of fruit are ways to achieve this.

The Preschooler and School-Age Child

A child's appetite at any meal is influenced by the day's activity. If the child had a full day of activities, he or she may come to the dinner table ready to eat anything. If the day was full of frustration—the child received a poor mark in school, had an argument with a friend, or has a big game to think about—he or she may pick and poke at the food. This is no different from the way adults feel at times and should be respected (Figure 34-5).

Establishing Healthy Eating Patterns

School-age children need breakfast to provide enough energy to get them through active mornings at school. This means that parents must get up in the morning with their children to prepare breakfast and eat some themselves. Children react badly to the instruction, "Do as I say, not as I do." (See the Nursing Care Plan: Promoting Nutritional Health in a Preschooler.)

Many school children qualify for a free or reduced-price school lunch and breakfast. A government-regulated school lunch (type A) provides milk (8 oz); protein (2 oz); one starch serving; vegetable (¾ cup); and fruit (¾ cup), or supplies one third of a child's recommended allowances for a day. Check that children are actually eating school lunches, not trading items they do not want, so they receive the full benefit of the program.

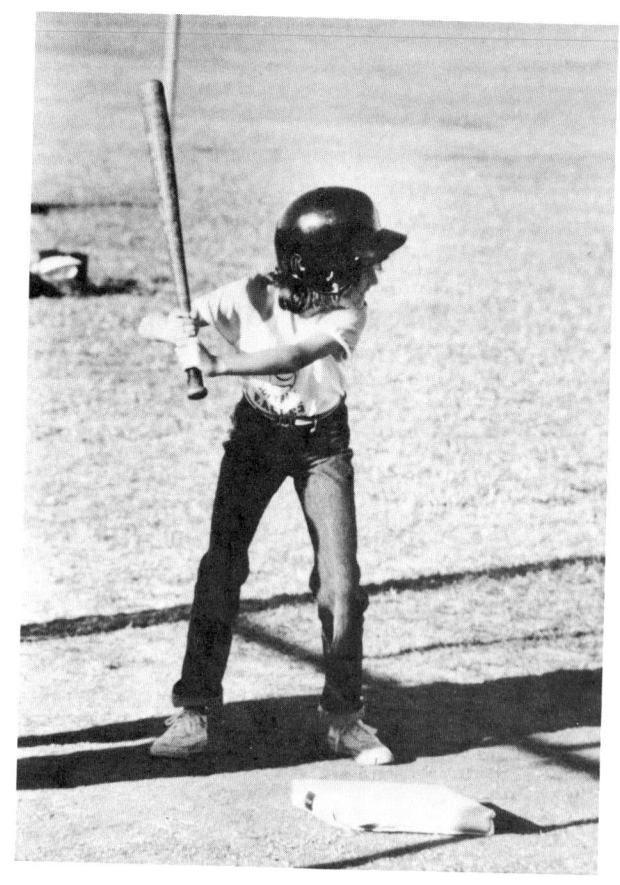

FIGURE 34-5
The school-age child's appetite varies, depending on the amount of activity he or she has in any day.

If children take a packed lunch to school, urge parents to allow them some say in what type of meal it is to be, since packed lunches become tedious for everyone after a while. Whether they take lunch or buy it at school, school-age children should know some elementary facts of nutrition so that they do not trade a sandwich for cake or choose only desserts from the cafeteria. Ideally, children should receive guidance from school personnel, but this often is impossible in a busy lunchroom. Health care personnel, therefore, should play an active role in nutrition education at health maintenance visits.

Most children are hungry after school and enjoy a snack when they arrive home. Because sugary foods may dull a child's appetite for dinner, urge parents to make the snack nutritious: fruit, cheese, juice, or milk, rather than cookies and a soft drink.

School-age children may develop strong prejudices about foods. As a 4-year-old, a child may have eaten spinach readily. As a 6-year-old, after the child has learned that children are not supposed to like spinach, he or she may refuse to touch it.

Teach parents to make every attempt to make mealtime a happy and enjoyable part of the day for every-

Lynn is a 3-year-old girl you see at a pediatrician's office. The following is a nursing care plan designed for her regarding nutrition.

Assessment: Female, age 3 years; weight: 14 kg (20th percentile); height: 95 cm (50th percentile). Father is concerned that child has cancer because she looks so thin. Child is active but takes two naps daily. Hematocrit: 39%. Father's 24-hour nutritional recall reveals that child ate no breakfast yesterday (no one in the family eats breakfast). Ate lunch at day care center. Parent is unaware of the usual day care center menu. Dinner was macaroni and cheese with ketchup, a "bite" of ice cream, and glass of fruit drink. Bedtime snack was a dish of ice cream.

Nursing Diagnosis: High risk for altered nutrition, less than body requirement, related to poor daily intake

Defining Characteristic: Father describes poor nutritional intake in child; length and height are not in same percentile.

Goal: Child to demonstrate improved nutrition within 1 month.

Outcome Criteria: Child has increased food intake to include breakfast and foods from all pyramid food groups daily.

Nursing Orders	Rationale
1. Complete health history and physical examination.	1. Performing a thorough health assessment is necessary to rule out illness.
2. Demonstrate 20th percentile weight on growth chart to parent.	2. Examining growth chart helps parent to realize child's inadequate weight.
3. Discuss with father the importance of the child eating a good breakfast (at least cereal or toast and fruit juice) and knowing the contents of the daily meal at the day care center.	3. Children need breakfast to have energy for their day. Knowing child's intake for lunch is important for nutritional planning.
4. Remind parent of importance of role modeling for a preschool child.	4. A child tends to imitate adult eating habits and likes and dislikes; eating a balanced diet is an important example for a parent to set.
5. Review with father the importance of including the five pyramid food groups daily in meal planning; review food groups with parent.	5. Educating father regarding good nutritional practices is necessary for planning.
6. Schedule a return appointment for 1 month to evaluate and reassess food intake and weight. Father to keep daily food record and to call in 2 weeks if child's intake has not improved.	6. As nutrition deficits take time to improve, follow-up care is necessary.

one. Some school-age children learn to eat as quickly as possible (and thus incompletely) to escape from the table before something unpleasant happens, such as an argument that they know is brewing.

Fostering Initiative and Industry

Initiative, or learning how to do things, can be strengthened by allowing a child to prepare simple foods, such as making a sandwich or spreading jelly on toast. As a part of fostering industry, school-age children usually enjoy helping to plan meals. They can prepare foods such as instant pudding, Jello, salads, scrambled eggs, and sandwiches. They may eat meals that they have planned or prepared more willingly than ones that are just set in front of them.

Most parents would like children to develop better table manners. Because they are in a hurry to finish eating, school-age children tend to gulp their food. Many meals are interrupted by spilled milk. As children become teenagers and are more aware of the impression they make on others, manners often improve dramatically. It is some comfort for parents to know that a child usually displays better table manners in other people's homes than in his or her own.

The Adolescent

Adolescents are undergoing so much growth that they may always feel hungry (Figure 34-6). If the adolescent's eating habits are unsupervised, however, he or she will tend to eat faddish or quick snack foods rather than more nutritionally sound ones. One form of rebellion is to refuse to eat foods parents believe are good for them ("I do not like your advice or have to listen to it"). Some adolescents may turn away from the five pyramid food groups to eat great quantities of sweets, soft drinks, or empty-calorie snacks, which leaves them poorly nourished despite the large intake. Parents who stock their kitchens with more nutritious foods, always keeping plenty of milk, juice, and healthy snacks such as fruit and vegetables on hand, and who are willing to meet their adolescents halfway in terms of food preferences (e.g., serving pizza once a week) will be more certain their child is eating nutritious foods during the day. Giving the adolescent some responsibility for food planning or meals (e.g., making dinner every Wednesday night) may teach some important lessons about nutrition without conflict.

Adolescents who are slightly obese because of prepuberty changes may begin low-calorie or starvation diets to lose excess weight. A weight-loss diet may be appropriate during adolescence, but it must be supervised to ensure that the adolescent consumes sufficient calories and nutrients for growth. For example, many adolescents omit breads and cereals entirely to lose weight rather than just reducing the amounts they consume. Diets such as these may be deficient in thiamine and riboflavin. Any weight-reduction diet should be

carefully evaluated before the adolescent follows it for any length of time.

Promoting Adequate Nutritional Intake in Varied Diets

Vegetarian Diets

Increasing numbers of adults of childrearing age are vegetarians; therefore, many children will eat such diets during their years of most rapid growth. Although a balanced vegetarian diet can be sufficient during childhood, careful assessment is necessary to ensure that it is adequate for growth.

There are four main types of vegetarian diets. A **lacto-ovovegetarian** diet includes dairy products (lacto), eggs (ovo), and vegetables. An **ovovegetarian** diet includes eggs but excludes dairy products. A **lactovegetarian** diet includes dairy products but excludes eggs. These three types are usually just described as vegetarian diets. A **vegan** diet excludes all animal products and thus consists of vegetables, fruits, and grains. A **macrobiotic** diet falls between vegetarian and vegan diets. Its main sources of protein are grains, seeds, and nuts, but small quantities of egg, fish, and wild game can be added. Macrobiotic diets have different levels of restrictions. In the 1960s, a popular Far Eastern version consisted only of cereal and restricted fluid; it was so restricted it caused death from starvation and nutrient inadequacy (and created a bad reputation for macrobiotic diets). This strict level is rarely seen currently; more lenient macrobiotic diets are adequate for children.

Families may select vegetarian diets for many reasons: economic (vegetables and grains are less expensive than animal food); ecologic (if everyone ate lower on the food chain, world hunger could be reduced); medical or health-related (avoiding animal foods stops the ingestion of hormones and chemicals used in meat production and probably lowers serum cholesterol, thereby reducing the frequency of atherosclerosis and obesity; avoiding red meat may reduce the likelihood of developing intestinal cancer); philosophic (belief that killing animals for food is unnecessary); or religious (many Hindus and Seventh-Day Adventists are vegetarians). Because of the association between red meat and bowel cancer and atherosclerosis, the number of families avoiding red meat will probably increase in the future.

Assessment

A typical vegetarian diet should contain daily one serving of seeds and nuts, two servings of vitamin B_{12}–fortified vegetable protein or soy milk, three servings of vegetables, four servings of fruits, and five servings of grains. Assess a 24-hour recall history to be certain that a

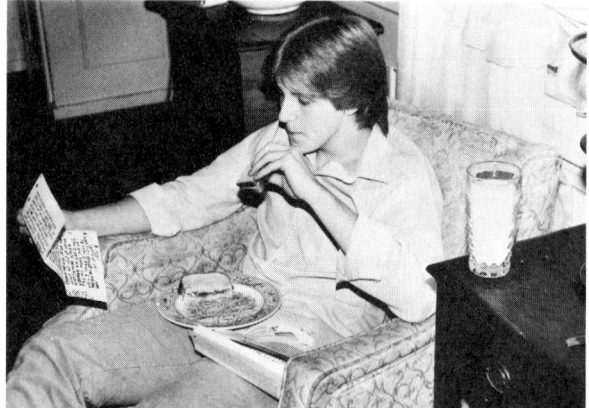

FIGURE 34-6
Adolescents experience rapid physical growth; typically, they are always hungry.

family has not just adopted a reduced-meat diet, thinking this is an adequate vegetarian diet.

Particular areas to assess are the sources of protein, calcium, iron, vitamin B$_{12}$, riboflavin, vitamin D, zinc, and iodine, as well as total calories.

Protein. Lacto-ovovegetarian, ovovegetarian, lacto-vegetarian, and liberal macrobiotic diets provide all of the essential amino acids for growth (both eggs and dairy products provide complete proteins). A vegan diet must include complementary proteins, that is, cereal and legume combinations such as peanut butter and wheat bread, corn and lima beans, pasta and beans, corn tortillas and beans, or chick peas and sesame seeds.

Calcium. Dairy products such as milk and cheese supply calcium. When these are not eaten, calcium must be obtained from other sources, such as green leafy vegetables (e.g., broccoli) or grain products such as tofu or soy flour.

Iron. Meats are good sources of iron. With meat omitted from a diet, iron must be included from foods such as legumes, whole grains, dark green leafy vegetables, or dried fruits. Vitamin C enhances the absorption of iron from the stomach, so eating fruits aids iron absorption.

Vitamins. Vitamin B$_{12}$ is unique among vitamins because it is present almost totally in animal products. This includes eggs and milk. Children who totally omit animal sources need to supplement this vitamin with a synthetic form daily.

Riboflavin is normally supplied by fortified milk. However, it may be supplied by soy milk, vegetables, or brewer's yeast, all of which contain all the B vitamins except B$_{12}$. Thus, it is usually present in a vegetarian diet daily without additional supplementation.

Vitamin D is necessary for calcium and phosphorus metabolism and is normally supplied in fortified milk. It is not present in plant foods, and therefore it must be supplemented in a vegan or ovovegetarian diet by vitamin D drops or tablets. Exposure to sunshine is an inadequate source (Wilson, 1994).

Minerals. Zinc is present primarily in animal foods but is also present in brewer's yeast, nuts, and wheat germ. Iodine is supplied normally by seafood or iodized table salt. In a vegan or vegetarian diet, it can be supplied by seaweeds and iodized table salt. Many families add a small amount of powdered kelp (a seaweed) to food two or three times a week to ensure an adequate iodine intake.

Total Calories. Plant foods have lower total calories than meats. As a rule, therefore, vegetable portions must be larger than meat portions to provide the same total calories necessary for childhood growth.

The Infant and Toddler

The infant eating a vegetarian diet should continue to be breast-fed or ingest an iron-fortified, balanced, commercial formula for the entire first year. If milk products are restricted, a soy-based formula can be used. When solid foods are added at 6 months, an assortment of foods should be provided, including vegetables such as avocados, potatoes, and broccoli; fruits such as apples, prunes (high in iron), and bananas; infant cereal; tofu; wheat germ; legumes; brewer's yeast; and synthetic vitamin D. Feeding a fortified cereal through the first year will ensure that iron stores are built. If the diet is to include dairy products, these can be added toward the end of the first year as usual.

Because vegetarian diets are high in fiber, they may cause infants to have more frequent and looser-than-normal bowel movements. Urge parents to change diapers frequently to avoid skin irritation. Using less fibrous, more concentrated forms of protein such as tofu and powdered nuts rather than cereal mixtures can minimize this problem.

A sound vegetarian diet can be easily designed for the child who prefers finger foods, because many vegetables, fruits, and grains (e.g., pieces of oranges, peaches, raisins, chick peas, tomatoes, and crackers) are all easily eaten this way. The use of fortified soy milk prevents both fluid and protein deficiencies.

The Preschooler and School-Age Child

A vegetarian diet is usually colorful and therefore appeals to the preschooler. Many vegetables, fruits, and grains are also good snack foods and so are convenient for the child who eats frequently during the day.

School-age children who are raised in vegetarian homes must be taught aspects of vegetarian nutrition if they are going to eat in a school cafeteria. Unfortunately, many school lunch programs offer mainly milk and meat or cheese foods, such as sloppy joe sandwiches, macaroni and cheese, or pizza. This forces children who are vegetarian to carry packed lunches to maintain their diet. These could consist of cucumber or tomato, or peanut butter sandwiches on whole-grain bread, hot soups, salads packed in small insulated containers, vegetable sticks, and fruit.

School-age children often eat at other children's houses and attend parties. Those who are vegetarians need to be educated to notify a host that they eat a special diet or to choose correctly from foods they are served.

A potential problem to assess with vegetarian school-age children is whether they are obtaining enough protein and calcium. Foods high in calcium are green leafy vegetables (e.g., spinach and turnip greens), prunes, nuts, enriched bread, and cereals. Soybeans, legumes, nuts, grains, and immature seeds (e.g., green beans, lima beans, and corn), are relatively high in protein.

The Adolescent

An adolescent needs an increased number of calories to maintain a rapid period of growth. Because vegetables generally contain fewer calories than meat, intake must therefore be ample with a vegetarian diet.

Textured vegetable protein is made from wheat or soy protein. When added to casseroles, it increases the amount of protein supplied and helps meet adolescent growth needs. Some adolescents may find it difficult to follow a vegetarian diet because it makes them different from their peers and limits foods they can eat at parties or at school, such as pizza, meat tortillas, or hot dogs. Whether to continue to follow this type of diet is a decision the adolescent must make as part of achieving a sense of identity.

Glycogen Loading

Athletes need more carbohydrate or energy than do people who do not engage in strenuous activity, and the source of carbohydrate that best sustains athletes comes from the breakdown of glycogen. **Glycogen loading** is a procedure used to ensure there is adequate glycogen to sustain energy through an athletic event. Several days before a sports event, athletes lower their carbohydrate intake and exercise heavily to deplete muscle glycogen stores and then switch to a diet high in carbohydrate. With the renewed carbohydrate intake, muscle glycogen is stored at approximately twice the usual level. The effects of frequent glycogen loading are unknown and it is not particularly recommended for adolescents, who need nutrients for growth. As a rule, the goals of nutrition that are best for everyone, such as eating a well-balanced diet, are also the best rules for athletes, rather than diets that interfere with carbohydrate, fluid, or fat intake (Wilson, 1994).

Common Childhood Nutritional Disorders

Lactose Intolerance

Lactose (the sugar in milk) is broken down in the intestine by the enzyme lactase. Few Caucasian infants have a deficiency of lactase and so can digest lactose easily. Significant numbers of African-American, Asian, and Mexican-American children do have lactase insufficiency and therefore have **lactose intolerance**.

Because this condition may be present in infancy, it must be considered in infants who fail to thrive on nor-

mally recommended infant formulas or breast milk. Usually, however, it develops with additional age. Approximately 50% of African-American and Mexican-American children are lactose intolerant at 4 to 5 years of age; as many as 70% to 80% are lactose intolerant by age 18 years.

The degree to which children notice symptoms varies (AAP, 1990). Symptoms are abdominal pain, flatulence, bloating, diarrhea, and, over time, failure to gain weight. After an episode of acute gastroenteritis, infants may temporarily develop lactose intolerance and show these symptoms. Such infants have to be weaned back to formula or breast milk gradually. Infants with true lactose intolerance must be given a lactose-free formula to receive adequate nutrition.

Preschool or school-age children with lactose intolerance generally show a dislike for milk or frequently leave it untouched. School lunch programs should be designed to furnish beverages other than milk for these children. Adequate calcium can be obtained by eating dark green vegetables and legumes.

Obesity

Obesity in Infants

Obesity in infants is defined as a weight greater than the 90th to 95th percentile on a standardized height/weight chart. Obesity occurs when there is an increase in the number of fat cells due to excessive calorie intake. It is important that obesity be prevented in infants, because the extra fat cells formed at this time are likely to remain through childhood and even into adulthood. If the child becomes obese because of overingesting milk, iron-deficiency anemia may also be present because of the low iron content of both breast and commercial milk. Once infant obesity begins, it is difficult to reverse; preventing it is the key.

Overfeeding in infancy often occurs because parents were taught to eat everything on their plate, and they continue to instill this concept in their children. This appears to be the case most often with formula-fed infants whose parents have urged them to empty their bottle or finish a cereal serving. It can occur any time parents automatically feed an infant when the child cries, rather than investigating what the cries might really mean. Infants should not be placed on low-fat diets, because they need fat for maturation of the nervous system and body growth (Finberg, 1990). An infant should not be taking more than 32 oz of formula daily, so that when solid food is introduced, a bottle of water can be substituted for formula at one feeding. All commercial infant formula contains 20 cal/mL. Advance, a formula fortified with iron for older infants and toddlers, contains 20% fewer calories than other formulas and therefore can be used to prevent extra weight gain. Skim milk should not be given, because it contains so little fat that essential fatty acid requirements may not be met well enough to ensure cell growth (Fomon et al., 1990).

Another way to help prevent obesity is to add a source of fiber such as whole-grain cereal and raw fruit to the infant's diet. These prolong stomach emptying time and can thus help reduce food intake. Caution parents about giving obese infants foods with high amounts of refined sugars such as pudding, cake, cookies, and candy. Encourage parents to learn more about balanced diets and to provide them for their entire family.

Obesity in School-Age Children

Many preteenagers, particularly boys, become overweight. Some have been overweight since infancy; their prepubertal natural weight gain makes them obese. Children with an endomorphic build (a natural tendency to accumulate body fat) are more likely to be obese at any time of life than those with a mesomorphic (normal) or ectomorphic (slender) build. Children of obese parents are also inclined to obesity and have difficulty losing extra weight. Perhaps genetic influences have some bearing. Certainly, if parents ingest a diet full of excessive calories, the child is encouraged to eat similarly; thus, environmental factors play a role. Many families currently rely on fast-food meals several times a week. Such foods tend to be high in calories and fat and can lead to obesity.

Obese children begin to develop many of the same health problems as obese adults, such as hypertension and elevated total cholesterol level with possible atherosclerosis. They also may be ridiculed for their size. This is strong evidence for the need for active measures to help preteenagers regulate their weight.

Those who become so obese that friends leave them out of activities or who are unable to compete in activities because they grow tired quickly may develop such a poor self-image that they have little motivation for self-improvement.

A weight-reduction program for school-age children should contain two aspects: (1) a diet of about 1200 calories designed to reduce weight and (2) an active exercise program. Total caloric intake cannot be too reduced, because children need calories to form new body tissue in order to continue to grow appropriately. If carbohydrate is restricted too greatly, protein is broken down for body energy and a negative nitrogen balance is produced. Caution children not to try faddish high-protein diets (as most adults should not), because those diets do not supply enough carbohydrates and may produce a heavy renal solute load (the breakdown product of proteins) for the kidneys.

Surgical techniques such as an intestinal bypass are obviously extreme measures and inappropriate for children. Obese children might request one, however, in an attempt to avoid the not insignificant difficulty of long-term dieting.

Nursing Diagnoses and Related Interventions

Nursing Diagnosis: Noncompliance with weight reduction plan related to lack of motivation to reduce weight

Goal: Child will demonstrate understanding and importance of weight loss and regular exercise to his or her own health by 1 month and state plan for losing weight.

Outcome Criteria: Child states reasonable weight loss and exercise goals; discusses feelings with nurse about being overweight and reactions from schoolmates; expresses positive feelings about self-worth.

Preteenagers often have little regard for what will happen to them in the future. They are not upset when told that obese people do not live as long as slimmer persons and have more heart attacks. They do, however, have a great respect for adults who are sympathetic to their problems. They are also aware that slim children are usually the most popular, and they wish they could look that way, too. They follow better dietary regimens, therefore, if they are asked to do so by a respected adult, such as a nurse, or if they fear being left out of social interactions. Because children follow adult examples, adults who are overweight have a responsibility to improve their own health before they attempt preadolescent counseling in this area.

Overweight school-age children often do well if a dieters' club is formed. They are not too young to participate in formal weight control organizations. Having tangible support from other group members helps them to follow a tedious and monotonous diet. There are also indications that behavior modification can be useful in teaching children how to eat healthier diets.

It helps if children aim to lose 5 lb over a short time rather than 50 lb over a year. This short-term goal coincides better with the task of developing industry. Because preadolescents do not prepare their own food, the person in the home who does (mother, father, or another) requires as much information on the planned weight loss as the child. The old concepts that used to hold ("A clean plate is good; How can you leave food when people in other countries are starving?") may have to be changed so children reduce their intake appropriately.

As a way of increasing daily activity, preadolescents do well with formal exercise classes, because they enjoy the support from other children. In addition, encourage them to exercise such as walking to and from school, if possible. Encourage coaches of childhood sports to accept obese children as part of a team, not because they will necessarily benefit the team, but because the exercise will benefit the children. Exercise burns up calories, and if children's daylight hours are filled with activities and friends, they have less time to spend eating.

Obesity in Adolescents

Most obese adolescents have obese parents, suggesting that inheritance plays a part to some extent; the majority of such adolescents continue to be obese as adults. It can be difficult for adolescents to learn to like themselves (achieve a sense of identity) if they do not like their reflection in a mirror. It is equally difficult if they are always excluded from groups because of their weight. Some adolescents may be unaware that their food intake is excessive, because they have been told that they need excess nutrients for healthy adolescent growth.

A reducing diet of fewer than 1400 to 1600 cal per day can rarely be tolerated by adolescents. This provides insufficient protein and may also be deficient in vitamins. If adolescents eat a low-protein diet for any length of time, they can develop an inadequate nitrogen balance and their growth will be impaired seriously. They generally will adhere to a diet of 1800 calories per day with less cheating.

Nursing Diagnoses and Related Interventions

> ***Nursing Diagnosis:*** Ineffective individual coping related to stresses of adolescent period that have led to obesity
>
> ***Goal:*** Adolescent will determine cause of stress and demonstrate healthy ways of dealing with it by 1 month.
>
> ***Outcome Criteria:*** Adolescent identifies stressful situations in his or her life that lead to overeating; describes ways he or she might avoid those situations or other methods for coping with them.

Adolescents who are overweight because of stress need support until their pleasure in eating diminishes and their satisfaction with themselves as a "new" person or their friends' satisfaction with them can sustain them. They may have to visit a health care facility once or twice a week for encouragement and praise for their efforts. Weight control organizations are good if other adolescents also attend the meetings. They are ineffective if all the other members are adults because adolescents generally cannot relate to adult problems.

In addition, encourage activities that use up calories, such as swimming and participation in gym classes and other school activities. Adolescents could perhaps walk to school rather than ride, or walk the dog for three blocks rather than one. These activities are generally preferable to formal exercises, such as sit-ups and push-ups, which can be viewed as punishment.

Adolescents who continually cope with stress by overeating rarely succeed in losing weight. They may require psychological counseling rather than diet counseling if they are to develop a more mature emotional response. Behavior modification is sometimes successful with adolescents as a means of helping them lose weight, but it is rarely recommended for obesity alone. If the obesity is causing serious body image problems, lowered self-esteem, and depression, behavior modification might be suggested (see Chapter 36).

Measures such as making a detailed log of the amount they eat, the time, and the circumstances (including how they felt while they were eating); always eating in one place (the kitchen table) instead of while walking home from school or watching television; slowing the process of eating by counting mouthfuls, putting the fork down beside the plate between bites; and being served food on small plates so that helpings look larger may help an adolescent. They may be of little use, however, unless they are combined with a suitable diet and adequate activities.

Despite all these interventions, weight reduction may not always be effective with adolescents. For some, a more realistic goal might be to prevent additional weight gain.

Disease Prevention

Hypertension

Although evidence exists that hypertension occurs mainly because of a genetic predisposition, a high intake of sodium such as that in table salt may increase the chances of developing the disorder in susceptible children by the time they reach late childhood (APA, 1981). If infants are never introduced to high-sodium foods, perhaps by the time they are selecting their own meals they will continue to eat a diet prudent in sodium amount and prevent the development of hypertension in later life.

Under public pressure, baby food manufacturers have stopped adding salt and monosodium glutamate to infant food. Commercial toddler foods may still be high in sodium, however.

The food group that constitutes the highest proportion of salt in the average daily intake is bread and grains. Salt is used in these products as a flavor enhancer and aids in controlling fermentation in yeast doughs. Puffed wheat and rice products are cereals low in salt, as are unleavened foods such as corn tortillas and matzos, zwieback (a cracker often used for teething), and graham crackers. Meats vary widely in sodium content per serving, mostly because of the amount used in processing. Any meat that is smoked, salted, dried, canned, or cured is higher in sodium than those that are not. Luncheon meat and hot dogs have high sodium content, as do canned soups, instant dehydrated potato products, and cheese. One serving of a soft cheese such as mozzarella has a lower sodium content (104 mg) than cheddar (197 mg) or Swiss (199 mg); cheese spreads contain the highest levels (200 to 300 mg).

Remind parents that children imitate parents' food habits. If parents salt food generously at the table, children will learn to do this also, which adds an extra burden of sodium to their diets. Many of the foods considered fun and "social," such as potato chips, pretzels, pepperoni, and salted french fries, are foods to avoid. Encourage children to plan social occasions with low-sodium substitutes, such as fruit and vegetable pieces.

Cardiovascular Disease

A diet high in saturated fat has been implicated in the development of cardiovascular disease in adults. How early in life children should be screened for hypercholesterolemia and when they need to begin restriction of total fat or cholesterol have not been determined (Nolan, 1994). It is particularly important that fat intake not be restricted in infants since they need the calories the fat provides for brain growth (Wilson, 1994).

School-age children should consume a diet with 30% to 40% of total calories as fats. In adolescents the amount should be 30%. The use of vegetable oils in place of saturated fat should begin when children start solid food. The AAP (1989) suggests that children from a high-risk family (some family members have had early myocardial infarctions) should be regularly screened for cholesterol level beginning at 2 years. Children with values above 176 mg/dL should be considered for dietary counseling in addition to a regular exercise program.

Promoting Nutritional Health in the Hospitalized Child

Nursing responsibilities related to nutrition for the hospitalized child include maintaining optimal nutritional status in the face of illness or treatment that interferes with adequate intake; correcting nutritional deficiencies or otherwise aiding children and families to follow the nutritional care plan devised by the health care team; and educating the child and family regarding specific nutritional needs as well as overall sound nutritional health.

Nursing Diagnoses and Related Interventions

Nursing Diagnosis: High risk for altered nutrition: potential for less than body requirements related to lack of appetite secondary to hospitalization

Goal: Child will continue to follow weight percentile or stay at same weight level while in hospital.

Outcome Criteria: Child maintains skin turgor and age- and size-determined weight pattern; ingests 80% of prescribed diet daily.

An acute illness in children, such as pneumonia, is often accompanied by a loss of appetite; gastrointestinal illnesses often cause nausea and vomiting. Because most acute illnesses only last a few days, there is no need for children to eat more than a small amount during this time as long as they can drink fluid. Trying to force them to eat will only increase nausea and vomiting, which increases the possibility of creating an electrolyte imbalance. When an illness lasts for more than a few days, however, providing adequate nutrition becomes increasingly important, because children need nutrients not only to repair ill or diseased tissue but to maintain normal childhood growth.

Important points to address when planning nutrition for ill children are summarized in Table 34-7. Children who are hospitalized often tolerate hospital-prepared food, which can be repetitious and bland, better than

Table 34-7. Areas to Consider When Planning Nutrition for Hospitalized Children

Area	Importance
Meaning of food	Early in life infants learn to associate eating with being held and loved; if they cannot eat for some reason (e.g., nothing by mouth for surgery), they may view the restriction as punishment or restriction of love.
Opportunity for socialization	Mealtime is often a time of the day when children socialize with other family members; they may feel lonely eating alone, and consequently may have a poor appetite.
Level of stress	Children under stress may either feel a loss of appetite or experience a need always to snack; planning is necessary to see that children maintain adequate intake if not hungry and that their snacks are nutritious.
Custom	Custom is important: for example, many children like foods served separately and resist them if mixed into a casserole.
Culture	Most children best eat those foods with which they are familiar; in many instances, parents can bring in favorite foods from home to provide culturally preferred items.
Environment	Hunger is associated with the sight and sounds of food; many children are normally in the kitchen while meals are being prepared; they may not be hungry when food is served to them without their having seen and smelled it being prepared.

adults do. Provided that it is the kind of food they like, such as hot dogs and hamburgers, it appeals to children more than the elaborate dishes with spices and sauces preferred by adults (Figure 34-7).

Measure Fluid Intake and Output. Fluid is an essential element of nutrition because of the water supplied and because it can also be a source of calories and vitamins. To document fluid balance, some children may have fluid intake and output measured and recorded. This is especially true for children with vomiting, diarrhea, burns, hemorrhage, dehydration, cardiac and kidney disease, draining wounds, gastrointestinal suction, edema, and diuretic or intravenous therapy.

Intake. Estimating the intake of infants who are formula-fed is simply a matter of estimating the kind and amount of fluids that were swallowed. Intake in breast-fed infants is merely recorded as "breast-fed." If it is necessary to estimate the amount more closely than this, the infant can be weighed before and after a feeding. The difference in weight in grams is the number of milliliters of breast milk ingested. This measurement is not very accurate, however, because if the child voided or had a bowel movement, weight would be affected by these losses.

With preschool children, be certain to record fluids ingested during snacks, because children this age usually have many during the day. At approximately 10 years of age, children can be depended on to record

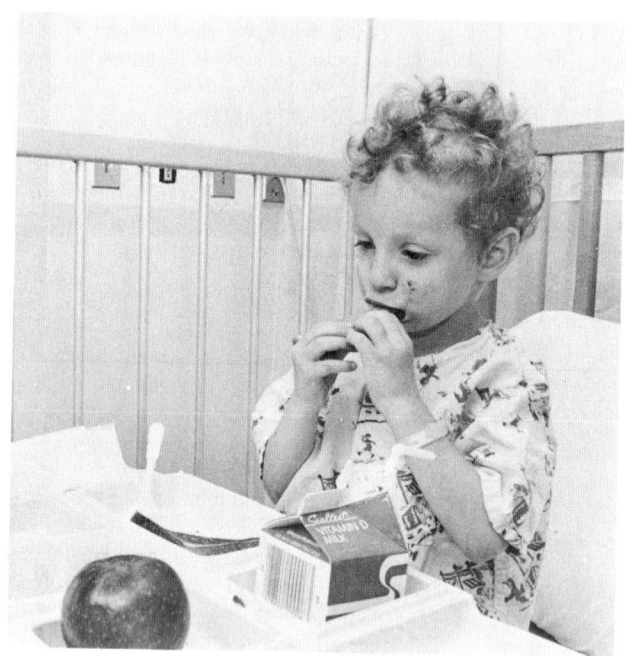

their own intake as long as they have a list of how many milliliters are contained in each glass or cup they use (an average cup is 150 mL; a glass, 180 mL). Be certain to check that they remember that soup, flavored frozen ice such as Popsicles, and sherbet are liquids and should be counted.

Output. Diapers can be readily used as a method of measuring urine output. Weigh the diaper before it is placed on the infant and record this weight conspicuously (mark it on the front of the plastic covering with a ballpoint pen). Reweigh the diaper after it is wet and subtract the difference to determine the amount of urine present. This difference will be in grams. Because 1 g = 1 mL, the amount can be recorded in milliliters. In infants who have liquid stools, it is difficult to separate stool from urine because these blend together in a diaper. Separate urine from stool by applying a urine collector; check it frequently for filling.

Girls often void along with bowel movements when they use a toilet, which means that a urine specimen is easily lost. To separate urine from bowel movements, teach older children to void first.

Encourage Fluid Intake. Increasing oral fluid intake has traditionally been termed "forcing fluid." It is better to avoid this term with children, because they can interpret the instruction to mean someone is physically about to force them to swallow fluid. A physician's order should state in detail the amount of fluid a child is to receive during 24 hours, because the amount differs so much for different ages. The following are some practical guidelines for encouraging fluid:

- Offer small, full glasses frequently rather than half-full larger glasses; children are mid-school age before they evaluate the amount of fluid in a container rather than the size of the container.
- Determine the child's favorite fluid, and then offer it.
- Try changes of temperature in fluid offered (hot cocoa, then cold juice, then hot soup) for variety.
- Broth can be a nice change of liquid (many commercial types are quick to prepare, but be aware of their high sodium content).
- Popsicles and Jello are fluids.
- Children can drink more of a clear fluid (ginger ale, water) than a thicker fluid (milk shakes or cream soups), because thicker fluids are absorbed from the stomach more slowly.
- Children with mouth lesions may be unable to drink fruit juices because the acid content stings their mouths; carbonated beverages may also cause discomfort. More soothing are ready-to-mix beverages such as Kool-Aid, Tang, or milk.
- Because ice melts to one half its volume, a glass of ice chips is only a half-full glass of fluid.

- Let children drink fluids with a straw; this is a novelty to many who do not use these at home and encourages intake.
- Introduce a game, such as "Simon Says" (Simon says, "Drink") or one in which a child takes turns and with each turn takes a drink.

Measure Food Intake. Calorie counting, as the name implies, involves counting the number of calories that children ingest in 1 day. When doing this, the nurse's usual responsibility is to list all the foods that a child eats during each 24-hour period, being certain to include snacks, candy, or gum. A dietitian then determines the caloric intake. Be certain to describe the types of food and their amount clearly (not "some toast," but "half slice of whole wheat toast"). Be sure that parents are aware that calories are being counted so that they also record the amount eaten by the child.

Nursing Diagnosis: Altered nutrition: less than body requirements related to inability to take in nutrients

Goal: Child will ingest adequate nutrients for needs by 3 days.

Outcome Criteria: Skin turgor is elastic with rapid recoil; no signs of dehydration. If newborn, no more than 10% weight loss in first 3 days of life; continued weight gain after this point. Urine output is maintained at 1 to 3 mL/kg/h; specific gravity of urine is maintained at 1.003 to 1.030.

Provide Enteral Feedings. Enteral feedings (nasogastric tube feedings) are a common means of supplying adequate nutrition to an infant who is unable to suck or tires too easily when sucking, or to an older child who cannot drink. In infants, such feedings are traditionally called **gavage feedings**. To prepare for an enteral feeding, the space from the bridge of the infant's nose to the earlobe to a point halfway between the xiphoid process and the umbilicus is measured against a no. 8 or no. 10 feeding tube (Figure 34-8). For children older than 1 year of age, measure from the bridge of the nose to the earlobe to the xiphoid process. The tube is marked at this point by a small Kelly clamp or piece of tape. It is important that the tube be measured in this way to ensure that it enters the stomach after it is passed. A tube passed too far will curl and end up in the esophagus; a tube not passed far enough will also be in the esophagus. Both situations could cause the feeding to be aspirated into the lungs. The tip of the catheter is next lubricated with water.

An infant may have to be loosely swaddled to be sure that the arms will be out of the way. An oil lubricant should never be used. Although the tube is going to be passed into the stomach, it is occasionally passed into

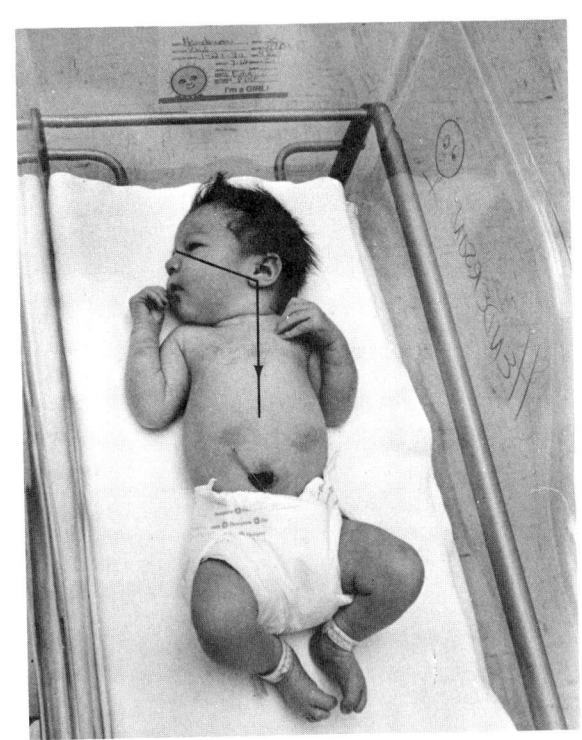

FIGURE 34-8
A nasogastric tube in an infant is measured from the bridge of the nose to the earlobe to a point halfway between the umbilicus and the xyphoid process.

the trachea accidentally; oil left in the trachea could lead to lipoid pneumonia, a complication that a child already burdened with a disease may be unable to tolerate.

Whether enteral catheters should be passed through the nares or the mouth is controversial. Because newborns are nose breathers, it seems reasonable that passing the catheter through the mouth will lead to less distress than passing it through the nose. This can also decrease the possibility of striking the vagal nerve and causing bradycardia. If the tube is to be left in place, however, it may be passed through a nostril. Insertion through a nostril is easier for the older child.

The catheter is passed with gentle pressure to the point of the clamp or tape. If the catheter is inadvertently passed into the trachea rather than the esophagus, the child usually has some dyspnea; the catheter should be withdrawn and replaced. The catheter must be checked for position (that it is not in the trachea) before any feeding is given. Checking may be done by either of the two ways described in Table 34-8. With some infants, it is important to evaluate whether the entire previous feeding has been absorbed. Testing for tube placement by aspiration allows you to both test placement and evaluate stomach contents in one step. If the amount aspirated is only a small amount (a few milliliters), it is merely replaced at the beginning of the feeding. If it is a large amount (large is determined by a

Table 34-8. *Methods to Determine Proper Gavage Tube Placement*

Method	Considerations
Attach syringe to the tube and aspirate stomach contents.	In most instances, stomach contents aspirated this way are returned to the stomach before the feeding; in small infants, the amount of stomach contents is subtracted from the prescribed amount of feeding; because stomach contents are highly acid, discarding them at each feeding can lead to alkalosis.
Inject 5 mL of air into the gavage tube and listen over the stomach with a stethoscope to the sound of injected air.	The injected air is heard as a whistling or growling sound; do not use an adult size stethoscope on small infants to listen for it; the diaphragm of the stethoscope will be partially over lung, and where one is hearing the air injection is unknown.

physician's order), it will be replaced through the tubing and the amount of the feeding then reduced by that amount. Replacing stomach secretions rather than discarding them is important to prevent electrolyte loss.

Once it is certain that the catheter is in the stomach, attach a syringe or special feeding funnel to the tube. Be certain the child's head and chest are slightly elevated to encourage fluid to flow downward into the stomach (Figure 34-9). Then add the specific kind and amount of feeding ordered to the syringe or funnel and allow it to

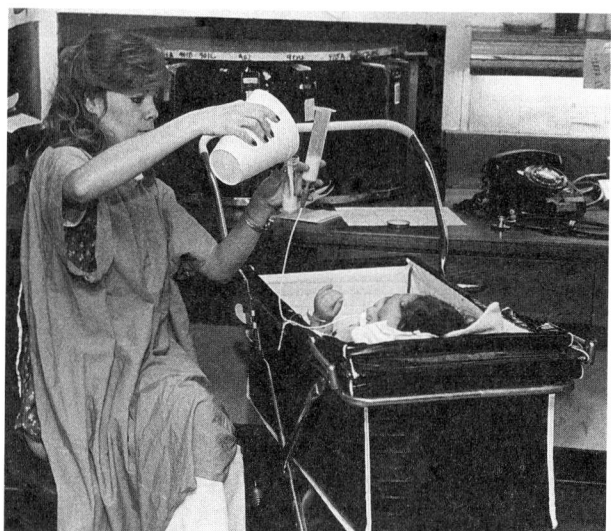

FIGURE 34-9
A gavage feeding. Formula enters the gavage tube by the force of gravity only. (Courtesy of the Department of Medical Photography, Children's Hospital, Buffalo, NY.)

flow by gravity drainage into the child's stomach. The fluid should be at room temperature to prevent chilling. The syringe end of the tube should not be elevated more than 12 inches above the child's abdomen so that the gravity flow is not too fast. Feedings should never be hurried by using the plunger of the syringe or a bulb attachment for more pressure. The result could be stomach overflow and aspiration.

Offering a pacifier (non-nutrient sucking) during the feeding may make the feeding experience more normal for the infant and supply the normal sucking time the infant would otherwise be missing by being gavage-fed. When the total feeding has passed through the tube, the tube is reclamped securely and then gently and rapidly withdrawn. Clamping the tube before it is withdrawn is important, because this prevents any milk remaining in the tube from flowing out as the tube is removed and, again, reduces the risk of aspiration. If the tube is to remain in place, it should be flushed with 1 to 5 mL of clear water and capped to seal out air. If it is to remain in place, tape it below the nose and to the cheek. Do not tape it to the forehead or pressure can be put on the anterior naris and cause ulceration there. Children with long-term neurologic disabilities may have enteral tubes left in place and continual feedings administered by a pump (Gruver, 1993).

A baby should be bubbled after an enteral feeding, just as after a bottle- or breast-feeding. This extra handling not only prevents regurgitation of formula along with bubbles after the infant is laid down but gives the close contact so essential to the baby's development. Both infants and older children should be unswaddled and placed on the right side with the head slightly elevated after a feeding or held and rocked in this position.

Older children fed by nasogastric tube require mouth care at least twice a day, or their mouths become dry and ulcers may form.

Provide Gastrostomy Tube Feedings. Children who may have gastrostomy tubes placed as a method of feeding include, for example, those who cannot swallow and those with esophageal atresia, severe gastro-esophageal reflux, or esophageal stricture. With the use of regional or general anesthesia, the tube is inserted through a puncture wound in the abdominal wall into the stomach (Figure 34-10). The tube used in children is usually a Foley catheter rather than a true gastrostomy tube. This is because a Foley catheter can be removed easily and changed if it should become plugged, and the balloon is small enough not to obscure and fill the small stomach space.

As with nasogastric feedings, gastrostomy feedings should be at room temperature to prevent chilling. Before a feeding, elevate the child's upper trunk 30 to 40 degrees so the food will remain in the stomach and not flow upward into the esophagus and possibly cause as-

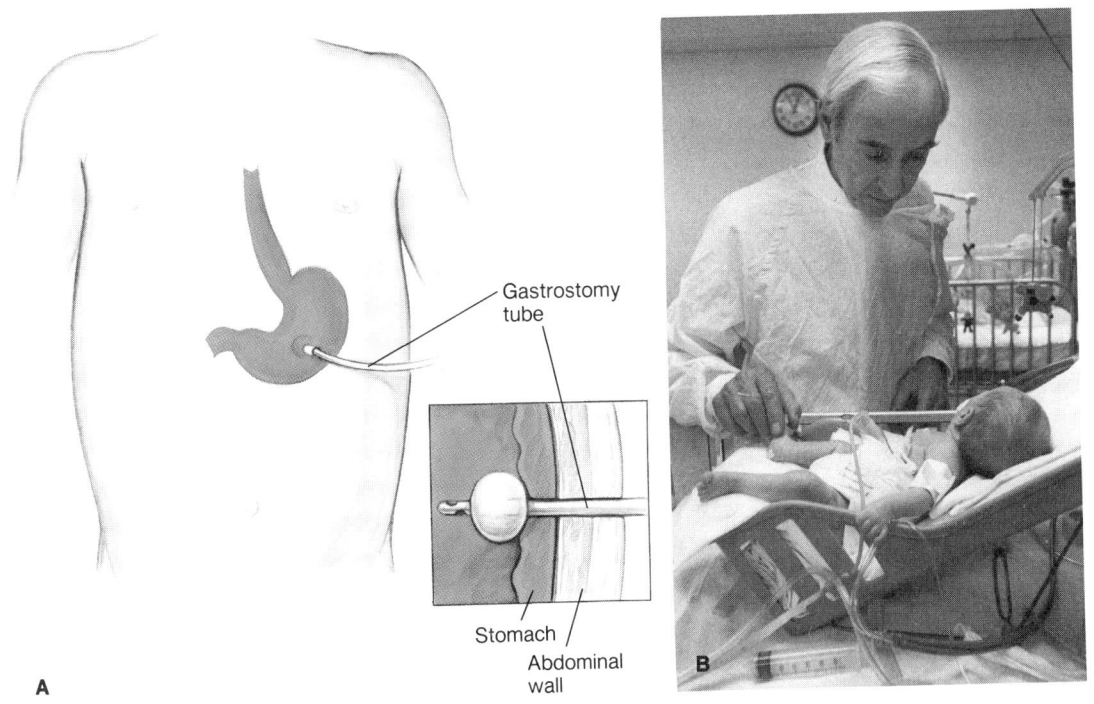

FIGURE 34-10
Children who are ill often need supplemental feeding by nasogastric or gastrostomy tube feedings.
*(**A**) Internal placement of a gastrostomy tube. (**B**) An infant with a gastrostomy tube in place. Used here*
for drainage, it also can be used for feeding. (Courtesy of the Department of Medical Photography,
Children's Hospital, Buffalo, NY.)

piration. Do this by holding an infant in the lap or placing him or her in an infant seat; for an older child, use pillows or elevate the head of the bed. Use a syringe to aspirate the tube for any stomach residual. After noting the amount, replace this fluid. To administer the feeding, attach a syringe to the tube; allow the specified amount to flow by gravity drainage only (again, to prevent reflux and possible aspiration). (See the Focus on Nursing Research display.)

After the feeding, flush the tube with a specified amount of clear water and either clamp or suspend the tube in an elevated position. Leaving the tube unclamped and elevated ensures that if the child should vomit, vomitus will be evacuated by the stomach from the tube rather than the esophagus. If a tube is left elevated and unclamped, cover it with a clean piece of porous gauze to prevent bacteria from settling into it. Leave the child in a head-elevated position for at least 1 hour after a feeding.

Infants who are fed by gastrostomy tube miss the pleasure of sucking. Offer a pacifier to suck on during the procedure. Talk or sing to the child as if the feeding were being given orally.

The biggest problem with gastrostomy tubes is that often they do not fit snugly, and formula or gastric secretions can leak around the tube onto the abdominal skin. These secretions are irritating because of their high hydrochloric acid content. Place stomadhesive around

the tube to protect skin. One method of helping to provide a snug fit for the tube is to place a soft nipple used with premature infants (enlarge the nipple opening slightly) over the catheter (nipple tip up) so the base of the nipple fits against the stomadhesive on the skin. Tape the tube to the nipple at the tip, which brings the balloon of the tube up against the stomach wall and prevents leakage. Tape the nipple to the skin and stomadhesives securely using nonadhesive tape. Clean the skin around the nipple daily with half-strength hydrogen peroxide; change the stomadhesive every 2 to 3 days. At the time of the change, expose the skin to air for approximately 1 hour.

The most important complication of a gastrostomy tube is that it can move into the duodenum through the pyloric sphincter and cause obstruction. Observe and report any vomiting, abdominal distention, or brown or green tube drainage (duodenal secretions that would suggest the tube has moved). Testing residual aspiration fluid to see that it is acid is a guarantee that the tube is in the stomach (stomach secretions are acid; duodenal secretions are alkaline). Putting a mark on the tube with a ballpoint pen just above the nipple lets you check that the tube has not migrated into the stomach but is remaining securely in place.

Tubes are replaced approximately every 6 weeks (Skale, 1992). To replace a tube, deflate the Foley balloon by withdrawing the water in it and gently pull the

FOCUS ON NURSING RESEARCH

Are There Differences in Skin-Level Gastrostomy Devices?

Frequently inserted devices for gastrostomy feedings are skin-level devices such as The Button (Bard Interventional Products) and MIC-KEY (Medical Innovations Corporation). In this study, these two devices were compared as to cost, size, appearance, feeding set adaptability, ease of removal, routine care needed, and whether an anti-reflux valve was included. The researchers concluded that although the MIC-KEY was more difficult to dry after a bath (the researchers suggest a hair dryer set on a low setting be used), it scored more favorably on the other measures. Nurses can be helpful in evaluating medical equipment this way, both in terms of whether it is best for nursing care and whether it is easiest for parents to use to give care at home.

Hass-Beckert, B., & Heyman, M. B. (1993). Comparison of two skin-level gastrostomy feeding tubes for infants and children. *Pediatric Nursing, 19,* 351.

tube free. Insert a clean Foley catheter into the stomach opening approximately 1 inch beyond the balloon; inflate the balloon with 2 to 4 mL of water. Attach a nipple and tape in place.

Most children who have gastrostomy feedings will have the tube in place for an extended time. Teach the parents how to feed their child this way, how to remove and to replace a tube, and the danger signs to watch for (e.g., vomiting, abdominal discomfort, or skin excoriation). Help parents to see this as an alternative way of feeding, not a totally different one. Be certain that they are comfortable with the procedure before the child is discharged from the hospital, so that they can feed the child by this method. Be certain they understand that it does not hurt the child to have the tube replaced or to have pressure put against the tube, so that they need not worry about holding the child snugly. Many children on long-term gastrostomy feedings have gastrostomy buttons implanted for easier stomach access (Haas-Beckert & Heyman, 1993; Figure 34-11). With this in place, only a small access device is visible, not a large bulky tube.

Nursing Diagnosis: Altered nutrition: less than body requirements related to malabsorption of nutrients

Goal: Child will receive adequate nutrients for physiologic needs during course of illness.

Outcome Criteria: Skin turgor is good; no signs of dehydration are present; child loses no weight during hospitalization.

Provide Total Parenteral Nutrition. Total parenteral nutrition (TPN) has become one of the most important therapies for children who have gastrointestinal illnesses that prevent proper absorption of basic caloric or fluid requirements (Cady & Yoshioka, 1991). Traditional intravenous therapy contains fluid, electrolytes, and sugars but not protein and fat, which are essential for the maintenance and growth of body tissues. With TPN (also called hyperalimentation), all of a child's nutritional needs can be met by intravenous therapy, because the solution consists of glucose, vitamins, electrolytes, trace minerals, and protein. An Intralipid solution (emulsified fat able to be administered intravenously) given once or twice a week supplies needed fatty acids. Children with chronic diarrhea or vomiting, bowel obstruction, anorexia, or extreme immaturity are examples of children who benefit greatly from TPN (Meguid & Muscaritoli, 1993; Figure 34-12).

Solutions may be administered into central intravenous or peripheral intravenous sites. If a central line is chosen, a catheter is inserted through the right external jugular vein into the superior vena cava or directly into the subclavian vein under strict aseptic conditions (see Figure 37-21). The catheter is secured at the site of insertion with sutures and covered with a sterile dressing to help reduce bacterial contamination. A major vein of this type is chosen to avoid inflammation reactions and resulting venous thrombosis from the high-caloric and high-osmotic fluid that will be infused.

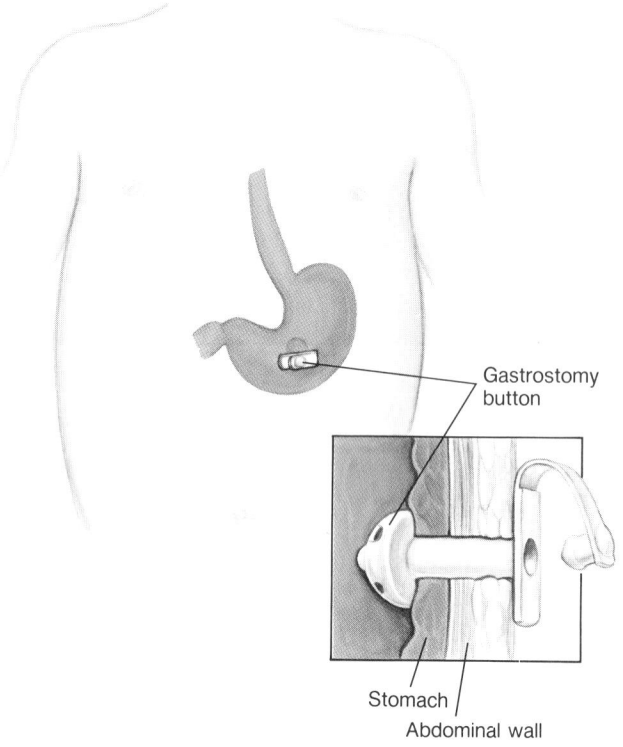

Gastrostomy button

Stomach

Abdominal wall

FIGURE 34-11
Placement of a gastrostomy button.

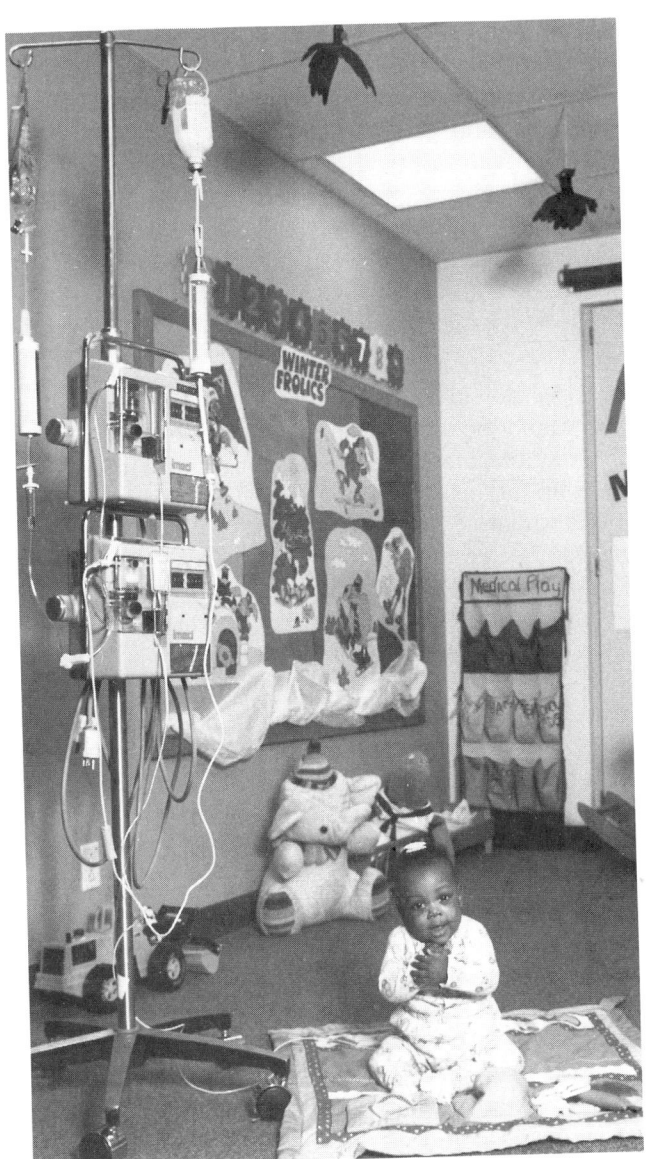

FIGURE 34-12
An infant receiving total parenteral nutrition. One pump controls the flow of a hyperalimentation solution, the other a lipid solution. (Courtesy of the Department of Medical Photography, Children's Hospital, Buffalo, NY.)

intravenous tubing are changed every 1 to 2 days to avoid infection; the tubing should not be used for drawing blood or for adding medications (unless a double-barreled tube is used), because either process may introduce infection. Sterile technique is required in changing bottles of solution so that the tubing is not contaminated. (Some health care facilities require nurses to wear both masks and gloves while doing this to avoid airborne and direct contamination.) The insertion site should be inspected at the time of the dressing change for indication of local infection: redness, tenderness, or discharge.

A second major problem that can occur with TPN is dehydration. A TPN solution contains approximately twice the amount of glucose normally administered in an intravenous solution to ensure that the amino acids in the solution will be used not for energy but for protein synthesis. Dehydration may occur as the body tries to reduce the amount of glucose recognized by the kidneys as excessive by excreting it (the same phenomenon that leads to high urine output in persons with diabetes mellitus). Urine should be tested for glucose and for specific gravity with each voiding. If two or more consecutive samples reveal a 3^+ or 4^+ glucose level, either the rate of the infusion or the amount of glucose in the solution should be decreased or insulin added to the solution to counteract the excess glucose. Generally, decreasing the concentration of glucose and then gradually increasing it again allows the child's body to adjust to the glucose overload.

After the first few days of TPN, a rebound effect (the child's body produces increased insulin) may cause hypoglycemia. A urine sample that suddenly is negative for glucose after a series that has been highly positive is therefore not necessarily an encouraging sign, but may be a warning that the child's glucose level is dangerously low. The TPN solution should not be discontinued abruptly but gradually tapered or a glucose rebound effect will occur. If a TPN catheter should be accidentally pulled by a child, the child must be immediately assessed for hemorrhage from the insertion site and closely observed in the next first few hours for signs of hypoglycemia (i.e., lethargy, incoordination, fidgetiness, or seizures).

Remember that to a child, eating is more than a means of receiving nourishment. It is a means of receiving love. Even though a child is able to voice the reason he or she must have TPN and appears to understand that he or she is receiving all the needed nutrients, the child still may miss eating food and the natural social interaction that comes with it. He or she may be upset by the smell of food from a kitchen or by the fact that his playmates have to leave him in order to eat a meal. Finding an activity for the child while other children eat (e.g., helping to check supplies on the emergency cart or stamping laboratory slips) may be helpful in supply-

The TPN solution is prepared in the hospital pharmacy under sterile conditions according to prescription. A millipore filter, which removes small particles present in the solution that might cause an embolus to form, is inserted into the tubing. The solution should be administered by means of a constant infusion pump so that the rate can be governed. If the rate should fall behind, do not increase it the next hour to make up the amount of fluid, because serious cardiovascular overload may result due to the concentrated fluid being administered. Infection is a major danger of TPN; the solution is a perfect medium for the growth of bacteria or *Candida* organisms. The dressing over the insertion site and the

ing the interaction the child misses. Ask the physician if the child can be allowed chewing gum or occasional hard candy for chewing and taste sensations. Tooth-brushing twice a day is necessary to keep the oral mucous membrane healthy because the child is not chewing. An infant needs sucking pleasure from a pacifier.

Many children on long-term total parenteral nutrition are discharged from a health care facility to home care (Bendorf et al., 1993). Careful coordination with the home care agency is necessary to ensure that parents are familiar with the system and are prescribed fluid before discharge so the child's care continues safely.

Nutrition and the Disabled Child

The Infant and Toddler

Nutrition is often a concern for the infant who is born with a disability or who is ill at birth. The infant who has an elevated temperature because of illness may have increased metabolic needs and require more calories than he would normally. To compound the problem, the child may become too fatigued to be able to take adequate feedings. If any degree of neurologic involvement is present, sucking and swallowing reflexes may not be coordinated; with gastrointestinal involvement, feeding may be impossible.

To ensure adequate calorie and protein intake, the infant may be maintained on TPN or nasogastric tube or gastrostomy feedings. These methods reduce the amount of opportunity for sucking, and because sucking provides pleasure as well as satisfies thirst, this is a major loss; the infant should be provided with non-nutritive sucking experiences if possible.

An infant who is ill for a long time may take poorly to solid foods once they are introduced, because he or she is not hungry enough to be interested in a new eating method. Children who have had esophageal tracheal surgery can reach 2 years of age without ever having tasted solid food. Help parents to experiment with different foods to find a taste that does appeal to the child or teach them to limit foods to only those the child appears to like most from all five pyramid food groups.

Toddlers need experience with feeding themselves if at all possible. Help parents accept the accidents that occur with self-feeding if the child has difficulty with coordination; suggest the use of finger foods if possible.

The Preschooler

Experiences with eating help to reinforce in preschoolers a sense of initiative. Chronically ill or disabled preschoolers who are limited in the foods they can eat (e.g., they have to maintain a diet of soft foods) or in their ability to help with food preparation may miss this reinforcement. If their appetite is diminished because of

illness to the point where they take little or nothing orally, it is still important that they continue to join the family at meals. In most households, this is a time for socialization, and preschoolers are ripe for the learning that goes with this type of daily interaction. Encourage parents to include the disabled or ill child in family meals and in other social occasions whenever possible.

The School-Age Child

Food preparation and dishwashing time are also times for socializing in most households. The school-age child who cannot be involved in these activities because of a disability or illness needs extra time during the day to make up for these lost socializing experiences, such as a specific hour set aside for talking or sharing a project that can be accomplished in one sitting.

When eating in cafeterias or at a friend's home, a child who must eat a special diet is usually tempted to select the same food as everyone else rather than limit what he chooses. The child may decline invitations rather than admit to a special diet or needing help with eating. Ask at health care visits if any of these problems are present. Help children with special diets to plan ways they could be comfortable in social food-based settings (e.g., brown-bagging a party snack that is easily eaten and appropriate for the child or politely declining particular foods). Help children who are hospitalized to select a diet that is enjoyable as well as nutritious.

The Adolescent

Adolescents whose disability involves lessened mobility must be aware of their total calorie intake, so that as growth needs decline at the end of adolescence they do not become obese. They should also be knowledgeable about good nutrition, so that they can participate in meal planning and feel a sense of control over this area of their life. Assess how often disabled adolescents have a chance to eat at fast-food restaurants; although this is not a source of excellent nutrition, eating there occasionally provides an important social experience and a chance to be like their peers.

Key Points

- Children need to follow basic guidelines for a healthy diet, such as eating a variety of foods; maintaining ideal weight; avoiding too much fat, saturated fat, and cholesterol; eating foods with adequate starch and fiber; avoiding too much sugar; and drinking alcohol in moderation, the same as adults.

- The best method for assessing nutritional intake is to take a 24-hour-recall history. Cultural and social considerations must be respected before assessing or planning nutrition for children.

- Solid food is generally introduced into the infant's diet at 5 to 6 months of age. Before infants can eat solid food effectively, they must lose their extrusion reflex.
- Infants are weaned from breast or bottle beginning at 6 to 9 months of age, depending on the parent's time preference. By 6 months, infants can begin to use a spoon to feed themselves.
- Toddlers are interested in finger foods as these can be eaten independently. The preschooler and school-age child enjoy helping prepare food and plan menus. Encouraging them to plan their school lunch helps them maintain a healthy diet during the school year.
- Adolescents are interested in eating what their friends eat. Nutrition planning must be creative to include basic food groups within this pattern.
- Vegetarian diets are adequate for children. Vitamin B_{12}, because it is found almost exclusively in animal sources, may need to be supplemented.
- Glycogen loading is inappropriate for children until the long-term consequences of carbohydrate deprivation are better studied.
- Children of African-American, Asian, and Mexican-American children may have lactase insufficiency and therefore lactose intolerance. They are unable to drink milk or eat milk products if this is present.
- Preventing obesity is an important concern in childhood nutrition. All children should be urged to engage in regular exercise and eat a sensible diet.
- Illnesses such as hypertension and hyperlipidemia occur during childhood. Measures such as reducing salt or saturated fat in the diet can be implemented to reduce symptoms. Children under 2 years of age should not have fat restricted to assure proper myelination of nerve cells.
- Actions that are necessary for promoting nutritional health in the hospitalized child include measuring fluid intake and output and providing enteral, gastrostomy, and total parenteral nutrition.

Critical Thinking Exercises

1. Renie is a 2-year-old whose mother tells you that she "eats nothing." What would be the best way to assess what she eats? What suggestions could you make to her mother to increase the amount of food she eats daily?
2. Sam is a 12-year-old whose mother wants him to take a meat sandwich for lunch at school daily. He refuses to take anything but a peanut butter and pickle sandwich. They argue about this daily. How could you help them resolve this conflict?
3. Karen is a preschooler. Her parents want her to follow a vegetarian diet but she doesn't seem to like any vegetables. What suggestions could you make to them to help Karen improve her nutrition?

References

American Academy of Pediatrics, Committee on Nutrition. (1980). On the feeding of supplemental foods to infants. *Pediatrics, 65,* 1178.

American Academy of Pediatrics, Committee on Nutrition. (1981). Sodium intake of infants in the United States. *Pediatrics, 68,* 444.

American Academy of Pediatrics, Committee on Nutrition. (1983). The use of whole cow's milk in infancy. *Pediatrics, 72,* 253.

American Academy of Pediatrics, Committee on Nutrition. (1986). Fluoride supplementation. *Pediatrics, 77,* 758.

American Academy of Pediatrics, Committee on Nutrition. (1989). Indications for cholesterol testing in children. *Pediatrics, 83,* 141.

American Academy of Pediatrics, Committee on Nutrition. (1990). Practical significance of lactose intolerance in children. *Pediatrics, 86,* 643.

Barness, L. A. (1990). Bases of weaning recommendations. *Journal of Pediatrics, 117,* S84.

Batten, S., et al. (1990). Impact of the Special Supplemental Food Program on infants. *Journal of Pediatrics, 117,* S101.

Bendorf, K., et al. (1993). Transition from the hospital to the home for the infant requiring total parenteral nutrition. *Journal of Perinatology and Neonatal Nursing, 6,* 80.

Cady, C., & Yoshioka, R. S. (1991). Using a learning contract to successfully discharge an infant on home total parenteral nutrition. *Pediatric Nursing, 17,* 67.

Centers for Disease Control. (1993). Toddler deaths resulting from ingestion of iron supplements. *Morbidity & Mortality Weekly Report, 42,* 111.

Chan, G. M. (1991). Dietary calcium and bone mineral status of children and adolescents. *American Journal of Diseases in Children, 145,* 631.

Department of Health & Human Services. (1991). *Healthy people 2000.* Washington, DC: Public Health Service.

Finberg, L. (1990). Modified fat diets: do they apply to infancy? *Journal of Pediatrics, 117,* S132.

Fomon, S. J., et al. (1990). Formulas for older infants. *Journal of Pediatrics, 116,* 690.

Geissler, E. M. (1994). *Pocket guide to cultural assessment.* St. Louis: C. V. Mosby.

Grummer-Strawn, L. M. (1993). Does prolonged breast-feeding impair child growth? A critical review. *Pediatrics, 91,* 766.

Gruver, J. (1993). Selecting an enteral feeding pump. *American Journal of Nursing, 93,* 66.

Haas-Beckert, B. & Heyman, M. B. (1993). Comparison of two skin-level gastrostomy feeding tubes. *Pediatric Nursing, 19,* 351.

Klesges, R. C., et al. (1991). Parental influences on food selection in young children and its relationship to childhood obesity. *American Journal of Clinical Nutrition, 53,* 859.

Meguid, M. M., & Muscaritoli, M. (1993). Current uses of total parenteral nutrition. *American Family Physician, 47,* 383.

Milner, J. A. (1990). Trace minerals in the nutrition of children. *Journal of Pediatrics, 117,* S147.

Nolan, R. (1994). Childhood hypercholesterolemia: implications for nurse practitioners. *Pediatric Nursing, 20,* 46.

Sherman, J. B., & Alexander, M. A. (1990). Obesity in children: a research update. *Journal of Pediatric Nursing, 5,* 161.

Skale, N. (1992). *Manual of pediatric nursing procedures.* Philadelphia: J. B. Lippincott.

Spark, A. (1992). Children's diet and health requirements: preschool age through adolescence. *Comprehensive Therapy, 18,* 9.

Splett, P. L., & Story, M. (1991). Child nutrition: objectives for the decade. *Journal of the American Dietetic Association, 91,* 665.

Stanek, K., et al. (1990). Diet quality and the eating environment of preschool children. *Journal of the American Dietetic Association, 90,* 1582.

Treiber, F. A., et al. (1990). Dietary assessment instruments for preschool children. *Journal of the American Dietetic Association, 90,* 814.

Wilson, M. H. (1994). Feeding the healthy child. In Oski, F. A., et al. *Principles and practice of pediatrics.* Philadelphia: J. B. Lippincott.

Suggested Readings

Arnold, W. C. (1990). Parenteral nutrition and fluid and electrolyte therapy. *Pediatric Clinics of North America, 37,* 449.

Beckholt, A. P. (1990). Breast milk for infants who cannot breast-feed. *Journal of Obstetrical, Gynecological and Neonatal Nursing, 19,* 216.

Dear, P. R. (1992). Total parenteral nutrition of the newborn. *Care of the Critically Ill, 8,* 252.

Estoup, M. (1994). Approaches and limitations of medication delivery in patients with enteral feeding tubes. *Critical Care Nurse, 14,* 68.

Hegsted, D. M. (1990). Trends in food consumption: implications for infant feeding. *Journal of Pediatrics, 117,* S80.

Hill, A. S., et al. (1993). The care and feeding of the low-birth-weight-infant. *Journal of Perinatal and Neonatal Nursing, 6,* 56.

Huddleston, K. C., et al. (1993). Nutritional support of a critically ill child. *Critical Care Nursing Clinics of North America, 5,* 65.

Lechky, O. (1990). If children are developing poorly, ask what they had for breakfast. *Canadian Medical Association Journal, 143,* 210.

Lucas, A., et al. (1990). Early diet in preterm babies and development status at 18 months. *Lancet, 335,* 1477.

Mills, A. F. (1990). Surveillance for anaemia: risk factors in patterns of milk intake. *Archives of Disease in Childhood, 65,* 428.

Pridham, K. F. (1990). Feeding behavior of 6 to 12 month old infants: assessment and source of parental information. *Journal of Pediatrics, 117,* S174.

Trowbridge, F. L., & Wong, F. L. (1990). Surveillance of severe pediatric undernutrition: conceptual and practical issues. *Journal of Nutrition, 120,* 943.

Ziegler, E. E. (1990). Milks and formulas for older infants. *Journal of Pediatrics, 117,* S76.

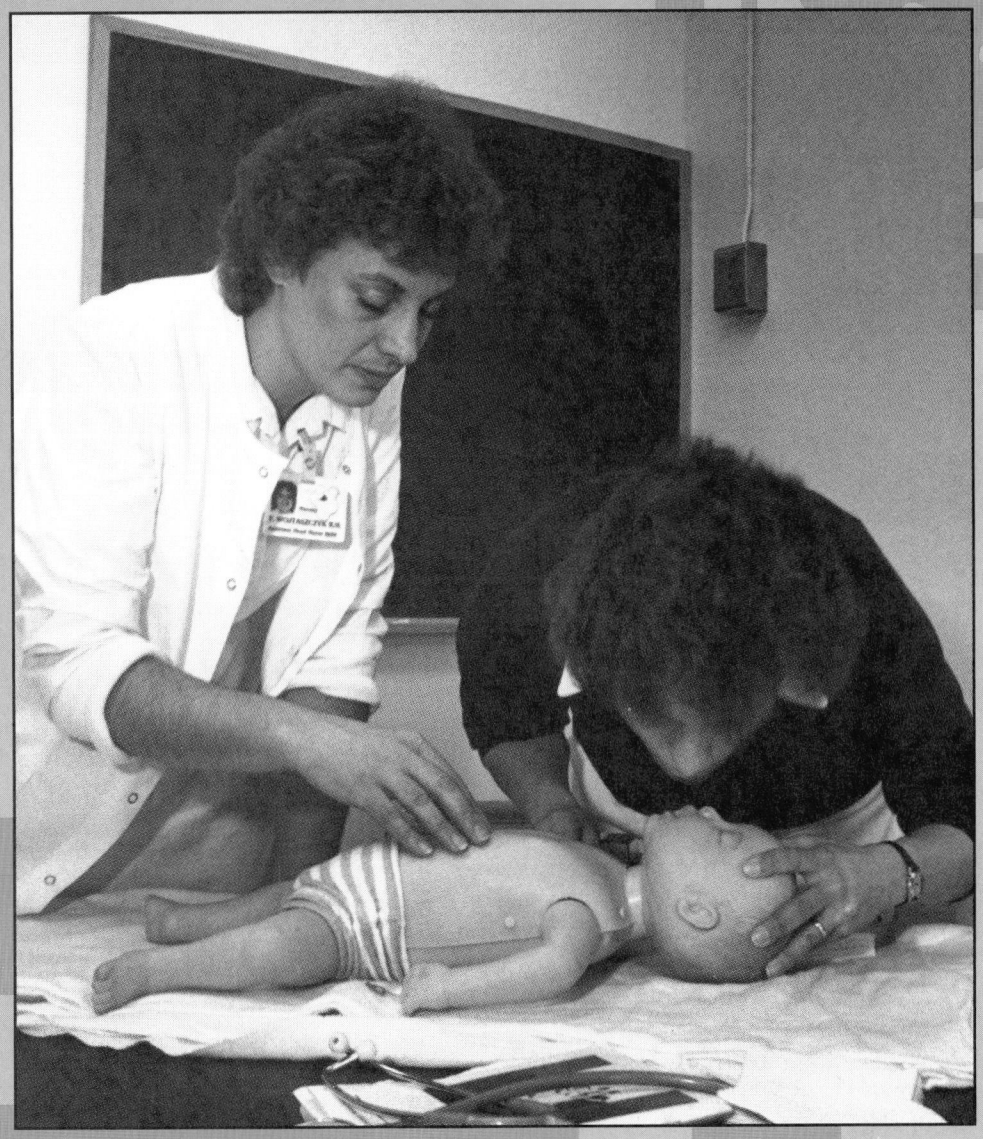

The Nursing Role in Supporting the Health of Ill Children and Their Families

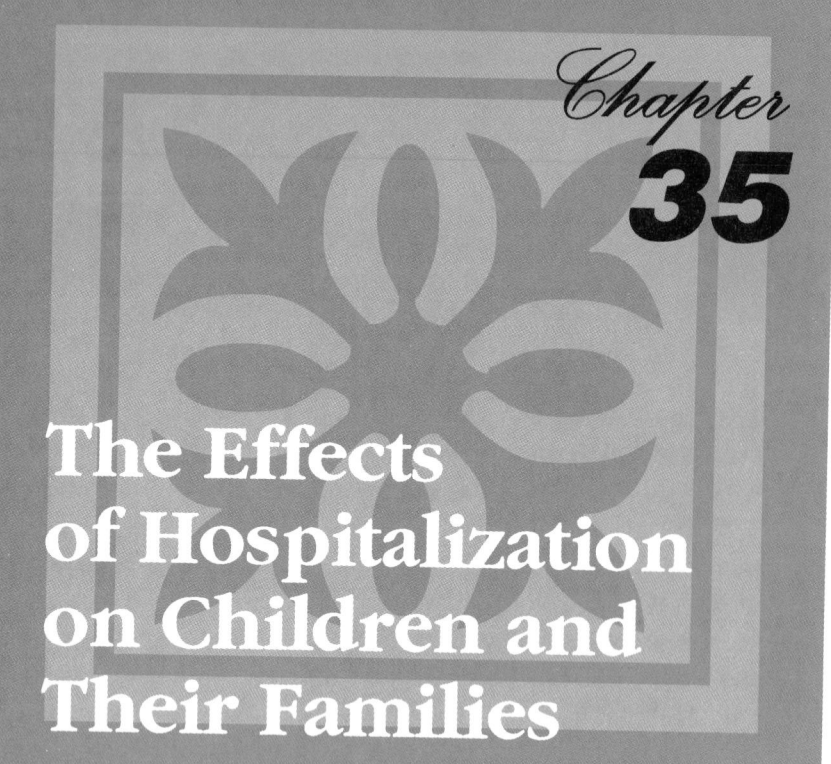

Chapter

35

The Effects of Hospitalization on Children and Their Families

Key Terms

- accommodation
- assimilation
- case management nursing
- play therapy
- primary nursing
- therapeutic play

Objectives

After mastering the contents of this chapter, you should be able to:

1. Describe the meaning of ambulatory and in-hospital experiences to children.

2. Assess the impact of a health care visit or hospital stay on a child.

3. Formulate nursing diagnoses related to the stress of a health care visit or hospital stay.

4. Plan nursing care to reduce the stress of a health care visit or hospital stay, such as helping parents plan for the experience.

5. Implement measures such as orientation, education, and therapeutic play to reduce the stress of health care visits.

6. Evaluate outcome criteria to be certain goals established for care were achieved.

7. Identify National Health Goals related to hospitalization or health care that nurses can be instrumental in helping the nation to achieve.

8. Identify areas related to hospitalization or health care of children that could benefit from additional nursing research.

9. Use critical thinking to analyze ways in which a hospital experience can be made more family centered and less traumatic for children.

10. Synthesize knowledge about the child's response to illness and hospitalization with the nursing process to achieve quality maternal and child health nursing care.

Adele Pillitteri: MATERNAL AND CHILD
HEALTH NURSING, 2nd Edition. © 1995
Adele Pillitteri.

---

*I*llnesses that require hospitalization are experiences outside the usual occurrences of childhood, so most children have little knowledge about them. Helping a child and family prepare for or adjust to such an experience is a fundamental nursing role. This role goes well beyond providing information on what to expect from a hospitalization. Nurses can work to provide orientation programs before admission and advocate for more open parental visiting and overnight stay policies whenever these are not already in effect. For individual families, nurses can carry out a number of interventions that promote comfort and security for the child and parents and also can make the difference between a successful and unsuccessful hospital experience. Play is one of the more powerful tools available to the nurse in working toward this objective. National Health Goals related to children and hospitalization are shown in the National Health Goals box.

■ NURSING PROCESS OVERVIEW
for Promotion of a Positive Health Care Experience

ASSESSMENT

A child's level of preparation for a hospitalization should be assessed at an ambulatory visit prior to an elective admission and again on admission to the facility. Carefully assess daily the child's continuing reaction. Be aware of not only what the child is orally describing but also what facial expressions or nervous manifestations reveal.

The way that children deal with hospitalization is based on the same factors that determine how they deal with any crisis: perception of the event, support people available, and effectiveness of past coping experiences or skills. After assessment, analyze if a child's coping ability will be enough to balance the hazards of hospitalization.

NURSING DIAGNOSIS

Nursing diagnoses often used with families of children seen in ambulatory settings who will be hospitalized shortly include the following:

- Health-seeking behaviors related to lack of knowledge regarding hospital routine
- Anxiety related to pending hospital admission
- High risk for social isolation related to hospitalization

PLANNING

Planning for hospitalization begins as soon as parents know that hospitalization will be necessary. Some parents may be so concerned about the reason for hospitalization that they are unable to begin this type of preparation until they are better prepared themselves. Reviewing with them any literature the hospital has sent them and answering their questions are important actions. An organization that offers additional information on hospitalization of children is:

Association for the Care of Children's Health
7910 Woodmont Avenue, Suite 300
Bethesda, MD 20814

IMPLEMENTATION

Five hazards that may occur with all hospitalizations regardless of the reason or length of stay are (1) harm or injury, such as physical discomfort, pain, mutilation, and death; (2) separation from routines, parents, peers, and respected adults; (3) facing the unknown (new and strange sights and sounds and happenings); (4) facing uncertain limits (unclear definition of acceptable and expected behavior while in the hospital); and (5) loss of control (loss of competence or loss of the ability to make decisions).

It is important for the nurse to be aware of these potential problems in order to guard against those that are preventable and to reduce the child's anxiety associated with those that cannot be prevented (such as facing new sights and sounds). Discussing these hazards with older children is important so that implementations to reduce their impact can be tailored to each individual child. Good preparation, reading to the child, role playing, and puppetry are all useful techniques for easing the younger child's hospital experience. Be certain that the techniques used are appropriate not only to the child's age but to his or her individual learning style as well.

FOCUS ON
National Health Goals

Hospitalization can be a major stress to children and thus a major threat to mental health. Two National Health Goals address the mental health of children:

* Reduce to less than 10% the prevalence of mental disorders among children and adolescents from a baseline of 12%.

* Increase to at least 75% the proportion of providers of primary care for children who include in their clinical practices assessment of cognitive, emotional, and parent–child functioning with appropriate counseling, referral, and follow-up (DHHS, 1991).

Helping with assessment of children's stress level and reducing the stress of hospitalization or health care are ways that nurses can help the nation achieve these goals. Areas where additional nursing research could aid understanding are: What measures do parents want taken to be able to feel most comfortable in a hospital setting; what are the deterrents to therapeutic play on hospital units and how could these be removed; and are there additional contributions nurses could make to shortening hospital stays for children?

EVALUATION

Outcome criteria for evaluation of hospitalization should include specific measures such as whether discomfort was kept to a minimum during the experience. Long-term criteria should include whether the child was able to return to his or her usual behavior after the experience.

The following are examples of outcome criteria regarding hospital preparation that might be devised:

* Parents state their level of anxiety regarding hospitalization of their infant is now at a tolerable level.
* Parents effectively change work schedules to be able to stay with child in hospital.
* Social isolation of toddler is reduced to a minimum through primary care nursing assignment.

Illness in Children

Meaning of Illness to Children

The response of children to illness depends on their cognitive development, past experiences, and level of knowledge. From early school age, children generally know quite a bit about the workings of their major body parts. As general guidelines, early grade school children are usually able to name the function of the heart, lungs, and stomach. They may not be able to do that for kidneys or bladder. This lack of information may reflect the difficulty some parents have in discussing elimination with their children.

Early grade school children may think the cause of illness is magical (no one knows where it comes from), or it occurs as a consequence of breaking a rule (e.g., walking in the rain or eating candy after school). With this perspective, they can think that getting well again is possible only if they follow another set of rules, such as staying in bed and taking medicine. By fourth grade, children are generally aware of the role of germs in illness but may be fooled by thinking that all illness is caused by germs. Because of this, they may see a passive role for themselves in getting well, because illness came from outside influences. At about eighth grade, children are able to voice an understanding that illness can occur from several causes, such as being susceptible to germs from walking in the rain, and that they can take an active role in getting better. These concepts parallel cognitive development (see Chapter 27).

Knowing how children view illness has implications for planning nursing care (Vessey et al., 1990). In a classic study of children's reactions to illness, Perrin and

Gerrity (1981) use the example "There's edema in your belly" being interpreted by a child as "There's a demon in your belly" to illustrate how confused children can be by technical explanations. Other examples are saying you are going to "stick" the child for blood work (interpreted as meaning you are actually going to put a stick in him or her), or saying the child will receive a dye for a test (interpreted as the child will "die" during the procedure). Children who think illness comes as punishment for breaking rules can interpret nursing procedures (e.g., taking a rectal temperature or giving an injection) as punishment. They can be confused about explanations of procedures because some words sound alike or have double meanings (e.g., "drawing" as in making a picture vs. drawing blood). Because of these distorted perceptions, explanations of procedures do not always successfully relieve children's stress level.

Differences in Responses of Children and Adults to Illness

Children are not just small adults. This is important to keep in mind when evaluating how children react to illness, perceive an illness, or react to health care (Figure 35-1). Their body images, as evidenced in their drawings, are different from those of adults. They can have difficulty telling which body parts are indispensable and which are not (why it is wise to talk to preschool and early school-age children about "fixing" body parts rather than "taking them out").

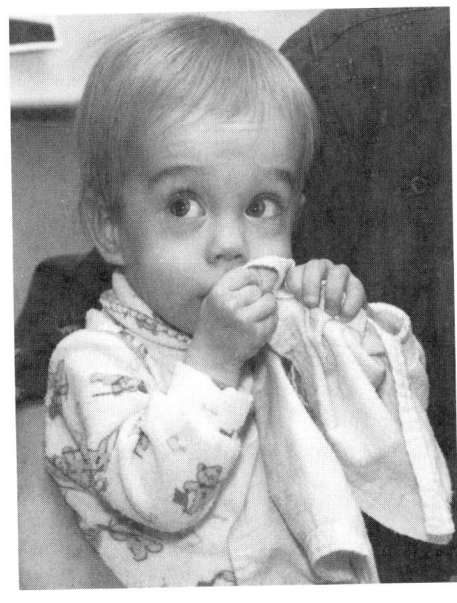

FIGURE 35-1

Hospitalization is potentially traumatic because of the unknown and pain and discomfort that may be involved. Children need extra attention and reassurance to calm their fears. (Courtesy of the Department of Medical Photography, Children's Hospital, Buffalo, NY.)

Inability to Communicate

Very young children do not have the vocabulary to describe symptoms. Headache is an example of a symptom that children younger than 5 years have a great deal of difficulty describing. Dizziness and nausea can be equally bewildering because children this age do not know the words to express these phenomena.

By the time they reach school age, most children can describe symptoms with accuracy. They may intensify their concerns, however, if they feel that someone expects symptoms to be more serious. They may minimize symptoms if they are afraid illness will interfere with an activity.

Determine a child's symptoms as much by observation as by the child's report. The crying, whining preschooler who is "just not herself" probably has a symptom she cannot describe. The school-age child who guards her abdomen (keeps abdominal muscles rigid) is in pain just as clearly as the child who verbalizes the source of discomfort. Considerable observational ability is necessary to ascertain the extent of a child's illness at any given time.

Inability to Monitor Own Care and Manage Fear

Adults who are hospitalized often ask about medication or procedures they are scheduled to undergo. For example, if a man knows he is to receive a diuretic three times a day and by 10:00 AM has not been given it, he usually reminds someone of the oversight. School-age and younger children are unable to monitor their own care this way because they may not know which medicine or procedures they are to receive. If they do know, they may be confused about the schedule for therapy. These children require conscientious nursing care.

In addition, children have fears that adults do not. The infant, for example, fears separation above all else; the toddler and preschooler fear such things as separation, the dark, the unknown, intrusive procedures, and mutilation of body parts. The school-age child and adolescent are concerned about the loss of body parts, loss of life, and loss of friends. Adults have fears also, but most have learned to cope with them. Children in a strange environment (such as a hospital) require more support and active intervention to cope with their stress and fears.

Nutritional Needs

In addition to psychological differences, there are major physiologic differences in the way illness affects children compared to adults. This is because children have different physiologic needs and respond to imbalances in different ways.

Children need more nutrients (calories, protein, minerals, and vitamins) per pound of body weight than adults, for example, because their basic metabolic rate is faster and they must take in not only enough to maintain body tissues but also enough to allow for growth. The infant requires 120 kcal per kilogram of body weight per day; the adult requires only 30 to 35 kcal/kg/day. An ill child who must limit food intake because of nausea or vomiting, therefore, may require hospitalization that would be unnecessary for an adult under the same circumstances.

Fluid and Electrolyte Balance

In the adult, extracellular water (in plasma and outside body cells) composes approximately 23% of total body water; in a newborn, extracellular water is closer to 40%. This means an infant does not have as much water stored in the cells as an adult and thus is more likely to lose a devastating amount of body water with diarrhea or vomiting. Because of this, there is no such thing as "only diarrhea" or "simple diarrhea" in a child younger than 1 year. The full implications of both vomiting and diarrhea are discussed in Chapter 45.

Systemic Response to Illness

Because their bodies are immature, children tend to respond to disease systemically rather than locally. The child with pneumonia, for example, may be brought to an emergency room not because of a cough (although the child has one) but because of accompanying systemic symptoms such as fever, vomiting, and diarrhea. Nausea and vomiting, in fact, occur so frequently in children with any type of illness that these symptoms do not have the diagnostic value they have in adults. Systemic reactions can delay diagnosis and therapy and cause increased fluid and nutrient loss, circumstances that compound an initial illness and can result in hospitalization.

Age-Specific Diseases

Because of their growth requirement and their immaturity, children are susceptible to some diseases that do not affect adults. For example, because infants are growing, a lack of vitamin D will cause rickets, but this same lack does not affect adults. Most adults have achieved immunity to diseases; children, however, are susceptible to childhood diseases such as measles, mumps, and chickenpox because of lack of immunity. Children younger than 5 years who have a high temperature may respond with generalized convulsions (febrile seizures), a phenomenon that rarely occurs after this age. Children younger than 1 year of age are subject to iron-deficiency anemia, because fetal red blood cells are destroyed after birth and are replaced by mature red blood cells very slowly.

Effects of Separation on Children

Problems of separation are especially important in children because they do not understand time. Statements such as "Mom will come tomorrow" or "Dad will be here

Thursday" are meaningless to children younger than 5 years of age because they do not know when tomorrow or Thursday is. Although many children attend day care and have had prior experiences with separation, others may have had only limited experiences. Being hospitalized may be the first time they are away from their parents. If this is so, many preschoolers may wonder whether they will ever live with their parents again.

It is difficult to explain the meaning that a primary caregiver has for a child, but the intensity of the relationship can be demonstrated. As early as 4 months of age, an infant will register disapproval if his or her primary caregiver walks away. As early as 5 months of age, the infant begins to register anxiety when strangers are present or when people other than the usual caregiver pick up the infant. The infant fixes his or her eyes on the stranger, becomes restless, perhaps thrashes arms or legs, and begins to cry. This activity reaches a peak at approximately 8 months of age and is commonly called *8-month anxiety*. It is a developmental milestone in that it reveals an infant is able to distinguish the primary caregiver from other persons. It also means that a child has reached a stage in emotional development at which he or she reacts poorly to separation or to the threat of it.

Today, hospitals welcome parents who room-in with children and thus keep separation to a minimum. In order to appreciate why preventing separation this way is so important, it is helpful to review the research that stimulated this method of care. Spitz (1945) was one of the first researchers to document the effects of separation on children. He observed children in a penal nursery as well as in a foundling home who were separated from their mothers for both short and long periods. Children older than 6 months began to show definite symptoms if separated from their mothers. Their first response was to cry—a loud, demanding sound—suggesting the children were reaching out for help or comfort. Spitz observed that this response lasted for the entire first month of separation. During the second month of separation, children tended to withdraw when approached. They sometimes reacted to a person approaching them by screaming, which was a different sound from the demanding cry they evidenced at first. They often lost weight and their level of development declined.

During the third month of separation, children characteristically assumed a position of lying flat on their abdomen. They seemed not to want contact with the world; if they were disturbed, they screamed incessantly. Children continued to lose weight and developed insomnia. They seemed prone to minor ailments and infections. Their intelligence quotients (IQs) typically tested 12 points lower than before separation.

Children who had shown these changes in a separation of less than 3 months and who were then returned to their mothers usually regained their normal relationships within a few days. If the separation was for a longer period, however, the changes were not so easily reversed and may have had a lasting effect.

During the fourth month of separation, facial expressions of the children became flat. They no longer screamed; their cries became wails—a pathetic, sad sound. Measured IQs continued to fall. Children lost previously acquired skills. If they had once been able to walk around their crib by holding on, they now stopped that activity; they sometimes even did not attempt to sit. During the fifth month of separation, the changes of the fourth month became progressively worse. These 2 months appeared to be a transition period: in some children, changes still were reversible; in others, they were not.

After more than 6 months of separation, irreversible changes occurred. The children became silent. Their faces became rigid and fixed. Among the 50 children in the foundling home Spitz studied, there was now a dramatic, overwhelming silence. These are startling responses, which occurred because the foundling home offered almost no motherly nurturing (primary caregiving). The infants were changed and kept clean, but the feeding bottles were propped. Staff people had no time to talk to the children, play games, or interact with them in other ways.

In another classic study, Bowlby (1966), an English psychoanalyst, observed children who were removed from London to the countryside during World War II to keep them safe from nightly bombing raids. It might seem that the psychological health of these children should have been better than that of children who stayed in London. The opposite appeared to be true. Although free of the threat of bombings, the children in the country suffered from maternal deprivation, which was reflected in affectionless, flat facial expressions.

Robertson (1958) is a researcher who has studied the effect of hospitalization on children and has supplied labels for the effects noted by Spitz. The first stage, in which the child cries loudly and demandingly, Robertson called *protest*. An ill child may pass through this phase in a few hours or in several days. The child rejects the attention of nurses or substitute primary caregivers during this time. The child wants only one person to come to him or her, and that is the primary caregiver.

The second stage, in which the child becomes less active and the cry changes to a monotonous one or a wail, is *despair*. The child is in a state of mourning. This is sometimes called "settling in" by people unaware of the psychological process at work. Be careful not to assume in a hospital that a quiet child is a contented child; he or she may be a child too overcome with grief to express true feelings.

The third stage of separation deprivation is called *denial*. In this phase, the child again seems to show interest in surroundings. This is done, however, by repressing feelings for the absent primary caregiver by

saying, for example, "I don't love her anymore. If I don't love her, I can't be hurt by her anymore." Denial can be a helpful defense mechanism to protect a child or adult from anxiety. When it is used to repress feelings of love, however, it is destructive, because children may use it to protect themselves against all close relationships. If this happens, they become the affectionless, traumatized person described by Bowlby. In later life, such children may have difficulty forming intimate relationships (they do not dare to offer love and risk being so overwhelmingly hurt again); they may have difficulty forming close parent–child relationships. Their children, who are not well loved, may not love well, either, and so cannot form lasting parent–child relationships. If there are lasting negative effects of a child's stay in any hospital, therefore, they could affect emotional health in future generations.

Separation is most damaging to a child between the ages of 5 months and a year. Stages of separation anxiety are summarized in Table 35-1.

In yet another classic study, Prugh and coworkers (1953) attempted to identify the amount of maternal deprivation during a hospital experience that would profoundly affect a child. Researchers studied 100 children admitted to an American hospital. On average, the children stayed 8 days.

A control group of 50 children were managed according to the hospital practice that was standard in the early 1950s. Parents could visit once weekly for a 2-hour period; they were not encouraged to participate in the care of their child. Of this group of children, 92% had significant difficulty in adapting to the hospital. On returning home, 92% of this group continued to show a significant disturbance in behavior that was not present before their hospitalization. Three months later, 58% of the group still showed disturbed behavior.

An experimental group of 50 children was managed by a new program that included daily visiting by and participation of parents in the care of their child. A spe-

Table 35-1. Stages of Separation Anxiety

Stage	Manifestations
Protest	The child cries loudly and demandingly; rejects any attempts to be comforted.
Despair	The child wails rather than cries; may turn away from parent's approach; often lies on abdomen, facial expression flat; may lose weight and develop insomnia; loses developmental skills; prone to minor ailments such as upper respiratory infections; IQ will measure lower than previous measurement.
Denial	The child is silent, face expressionless; deterioration in developmental milestones is apparent; may respond quickly but superficially to all caregivers; may have difficulty forming close relationships later in life.

cial play program, early ambulation, and psychological preparation for and support during procedures were carried out. Of these children, only 68% showed significant disturbances in the hospital; the same percentage remained significantly disturbed after discharge. After 3 months, 44% were still disturbed.

The study was one of the first done to show that specific measures carried out to minimize the effect of hospitalization can have worthwhile effects. It is interesting, however, that although the improvement in children's management greatly reduced the number, the percentage of disturbed children was still high. It is one of the reasons that increased changes such as encouraging parents to stay overnight are so important.

Nursing Diagnoses and Related Interventions for the Hospitalized Child and Family

Nursing Diagnosis: Parental health-seeking behaviors related to preparation for hospitalization

Goal: Parents and child will be prepared for hospital experience at a level appropriate to child's age and developmental stage by day of hospital admission.

Outcome Criteria: Parents and child both state they feel adequately prepared for hospitalization; child has brought some personal items important to herself. Preschooler or older child describes with accuracy and detail appropriate to age the reason for hospital stay; asks questions and expresses feelings (to some extent) about hospitalization with health care providers.

Many childhood illnesses such as febrile convulsions, appendicitis, poisonings, and asthma attacks strike suddenly, making advance preparation for hospital admission impossible. However, when hospitalization is planned ahead of time for orthopedic or cosmetic corrections, placement of tympanic tubes, or diagnostic work-ups, for example, preparation is possible. As a rule, parents eagerly seek guidance from nurses on what and how much to tell their children about an anticipated admission. The preparation a parent makes for a child obviously varies according to the child's age and individual experience. No matter what the child's age, however, parents should be encouraged to above all convey a positive attitude. Statements such as "They'll make you behave in the hospital" or "Wait until you have to stay in bed all day" should be avoided.

Children can worry unnecessarily if they are told about their approaching hospitalization too far in advance. On the other hand, few things are more frightening for children than to hear conversation halt as they enter a room or to hear adults spelling out unknown words. As a rule, therefore, children between 2 and 7 years should be told about a scheduled hospitalization as many days before the procedure as the child's age in years. For example, a 2-year-old should be informed 2 days before hospitalization; a 4-year-old, 4 days before, and so forth. Children older than 7 years should be told as soon as the parents are aware of it.

Preparing the Infant. Because an infant cannot understand explanations of surgery or treatments, preparation is minimal. Special items such as a favorite toy, blanket, or pacifier should be packed. These objects provide a special kind of security for which there is no substitute. Older infants, toddlers, and preschoolers cling to such objects as if they were symbols of the longed-for return home. Parents may need help in realizing the importance of packing favorite toys for hospitalization, no matter how worn they are. Some parents buy a new toy to replace the child's favorite one, because they feel ashamed of a teddy bear with one ear or one eye missing. A new bear may mean nothing to the child, however, and clinging to it may not comfort him or her.

Parents can be assured that hospital personnel appreciate the value of such items and think of them as well-loved objects. Some children prefer odd items such as pots or pans from the kitchen cupboard. If this is the child's preference, parents should not feel any more foolish packing this than a teddy bear.

When making hospital beds or straightening up a child's unit, be careful to watch for ragged blankets and threadbare stuffed animals that can cling to sheets and be easily discarded with linen. Throw nothing away without first asking the child or parent if it is all right. What looks like a useless alphabet block may be extremely important to the child.

When children are admitted in an emergency, they rarely have toys with them. In these instances, it helps if a parent gives the child a familiar object, such as the parent's wallet (money and papers removed) or a sweater. The child will hold these in the same way as a favorite toy. The child's outside shoes can serve this same purpose: encourage the parent to leave them.

Infants sense a parent's anxiety keenly. As part of preparation, the parent should ask questions about the hospitalization so they become as familiar as possible with what will happen. If they are well informed in this way, they will (at least theoretically) have as low an anxiety level as possible. If they arrive at a hospital unit with questions unanswered, fill in gaps immediately.

A primary caregiver should consider spending a great deal of time in the hospital with an infant. For rooming-in, he or she needs to make plans for older children or a spouse ahead of time.

Preparing the Toddler and Preschooler. Three chief fears of the toddler or preschooler are fear of the unknown, fear of abandonment, and fear of mutilation. These children, therefore, need preparation clearly aimed at alleviating these fears. Before parents can begin to prepare a child this way, they themselves must be instructed about what to expect.

Some parents are reluctant to take a physician's time to ask questions about hospitalization or surgery; most physicians, however, are eager to spend time explaining thoroughly to parents what a hospitalization entails. They know that frightened children do poorly under anesthesia, and frightened, misinformed parents radiate fear to children. Advise parents to ask about things such as how anesthesia will be given, length of hospital stay, and what kind of dressings or other equipment will be used. If practicing in a doctor's office or clinic where surgery or a hospital admission is first proposed, become familiar with these facts in order to serve as the parents' backup informant. Many parents ask a nurse for their main information or ask to have the physician's explanation clarified to be certain they have understood it correctly.

It is helpful if a hospital or doctor provides written instructions or reminders for special procedures. A child undergoing diagnostic tests, for example, must be oriented to the x-ray room or the need to swallow "special medicine."

Helpful books about hospitalization are available for parents. These can be obtained from local bookstores or libraries or by writing directly to the publishers (Box 35-1). A parent could read one of these books to a child, adapting the story to include information received from health care providers. Some books fail to orient children well to hospitalization because they are too sweet (as if they were preparing the child for a picnic rather than surgery) or because they omit pertinent facts, such as that surgery involves some pain (stress that the child can be given medicine so that the pain will go away) or that when bed rest is required, the child will have to use a bedpan. Using a bedpan is difficult for toddlers and preschoolers to accept, because they may have been toilet-trained only recently and have been told repeatedly that they must use only the bathroom.

Because the imagination of preschoolers is at a peak, "playing" is an effective means of preparing a child of this age for a new experience. The parent might pretend at home that they are walking into the hospital. The child changes into pajamas and gets into bed. The parent could act out a physical examination; a meal in bed; a bedpan (a round cake pan simulates this); or anesthesia administration (a strainer can be used for an induction mask). At the end of the session, the parent should stress that when the child's tummy or throat is better, he or she will change back to street clothes and come home. Remind parents that it is always better to use the word "fix" rather than "cut" when talking about surgery with young children, because "cut" automatically suggests pain and mutilation.

Preparing the School-Age Child and Adolescent. Both school-age children and adolescents need factual explanations of what will happen in the hospital. This also includes what will not happen: for example, surgery will require a small abdominal incision, but it will not create a scar that will show when wearing a bathing suit.

A hospital orientation program in which facts of hospitalization are discussed may be carried out in community settings with children's groups or school groups. There is a great deal of benefit in such a program in that it lays a foundation for all children about what to expect in a hospitalization; then, if they must be admitted on an emergency basis, they will not be so frightened. The program can be offered by nurses at the hospital or on visits to children's groups or schools (Figure 35-2). Box 35-2 provides guidelines for setting up hospital tours for early school-age children.

For parents to give factual explanations to school-age children, they must have good information themselves. If they do not know the answer to a question, caution them that the best response is simply "I don't know" rather than a guess. This prevents a child from feeling betrayed when the real answer is different. At approximately 9 years, when children first begin to understand the full meaning of death, take care again to explain that an anesthetic causes a "special" sleep. Knowing of another child who has undergone the same experience and come through it all right also helps to prepare school-age children and adolescents for hospitalization. Although parents cannot usually supply such a person in advance, on admission to the hospital, a visit to a recovering patient is often possible and is a constructive way to give reassurance.

Box 35-1
Books on Hospitalization for Children

Butler, D. (1991). *First look in the hospital.* Milwaukee, WI: Gareth Stevens, Inc. (Grades 1 and 2)

Ciliotta, C., & Livingston, C. (1992). *Why am I going to the hospital?* New York, NY: Caroll Publishing Group. (Grades K–7)

Howe, J. (1994). *The hospital book.* New York, NY: Morrow Junior Books. (Grades 1–8)

Krall, C. B., & Jim, J. M. (1987). *Fat Dog's first visit: A child's view of the hospital.* Atlanta, GA: Pritchett & Hull Associates. (Preschool)

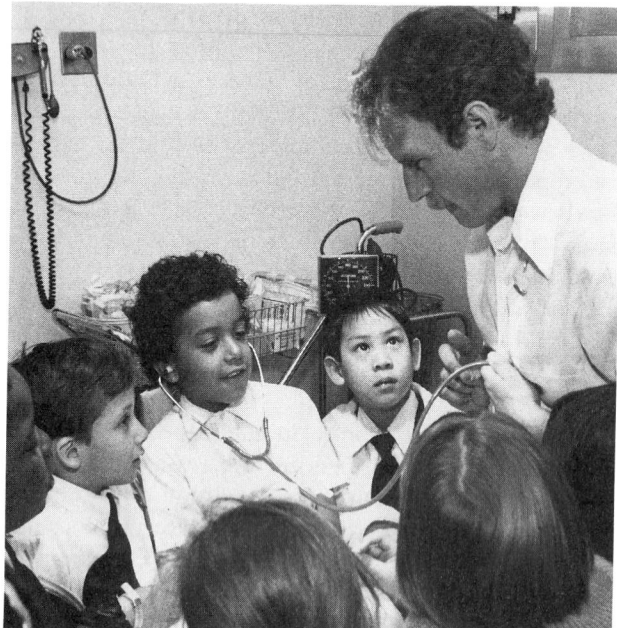

FIGURE 35-2
A nurse helps children learn what to expect from hospitalization during a prehospital program. (Courtesy of the Department of Medical Photography, Children's Hospital, Buffalo, NY.)

If hospitalization is to be more than 1 week long, a parent must think about continuing the child's schooling. Advise the parents to ask the physician at what point the child will be able to do homework. Many school systems provide tutors; children's hospitals often have their own teachers from the local school system to carry out this service.

Preparing the Child of a Different Cultural Background. Perhaps the most important consideration for a nurse who is preparing for admission of a child from a different cultural background is that it is the *nurse* who seems different to the child and family. The second most important consideration is that biased expectations about a family based on its cultural identity should not interfere with a thorough assessment, and, in fact, may do more damage to the nurse–patient relationship in the long run than not addressing cultural differences. Asking appropriate questions and practicing good listening technique can provide more information about the particular needs of a child and family than any textbook description of their cultural habits. When cultural differences do exist, a nurse is often the one to act as a liaison between the family and the health care team. If language is a problem, a translator may be brought in for this preparation phase. As with all families, conflict, confusion, and unnecessary fears can be avoided by providing the opportunity for parents to voice their fears and ask questions before the hospitalization or treatment begins. In the case of families who speak a different language or who are unfamiliar with hospital routine, more time and more opportunities should be given for this process to occur (see the Focus on Cultural Awareness display).

Preparing the Disabled or Chronically Ill Child. Disabled or chronically ill children come frequently to ambulatory health care settings for care, are often admitted to a hospital for care, and may remain in a hospital for extended visits. Think through ways in which a new hospitalization or visit will be like past ones and other ways in which it will be different to determine how to best prepare a child. Help children to maintain contact with their families and school friends during a long hospitalization by encouraging telephone calls and letters and open visiting.

Nursing Diagnosis: Parental knowledge deficit related to reason for child's hospitalization

Goal: Parents will demonstrate understanding of child's condition and treatment plan in one day.

Box 35-2
Guidelines for Conducting Hospital Tours With Early School-Age Children

1. Keep groups small (about 10 children per group) so individual reactions to the presentations can be assessed.
2. Allow or encourage parents to join the tour so their anxiety about the hospital can also be relieved.
3. Conduct the tour for only 20 to 30 minutes to meet the short attention span of children.
4. Use an indirect method to present various aspects of a hospital, such as puppets, films, or a slide show, to decrease anxiety.
5. Present the features of a hospital in a nonthreatening environment, such as the hospital playroom. Avoid the emergency room, ICUs, or operating rooms while touring, because these are anxiety-producing areas for children. Talk about these areas by using slides or photographs instead.
6. Present explanations about hospitalization in concrete terms and at the child's level of understanding. Include only what the child will see, hear, and feel.
7. Avoid dwelling on unpleasant and threatening events or intrusive procedures, such as blood drawing or anesthesia, that may create anxiety.
8. Allow children opportunities to ask questions.
9. Allow children opportunities to play with dolls and hospital equipment both to decrease anxiety and satisfy curiosity.

FOCUS ON CULTURAL AWARENESS

Although play is a universal activity of children, not all parents realize how important it is to children. Also, play activities vary greatly depending on cultural and socioeconomic circumstances. However, more and more parents are becoming aware of the value of reading to young children, and many bring favorite books to the hospital along with games and teddy bears. Encourage parents also to bring toys that a young child can manipulate independently in order to give parents a break from the child or the time to talk with the child's health care team about progress.

When a child does not understand English and that is the language of health care providers, games such as stacking blocks or building with tinker toys can be played despite communication difficulty. Playing tapes or records of well-loved children's songs can also be effective, because the child doesn't need to be able to understand the words to enjoy the music or clap with the rhythm.

Outcome Criteria: Parents state accurately the reason for child's hospital admission and therapy child will receive.

Providing Basic Information on Admission. On admission to the hospital, parents need basic information about their child's condition: Is he or she seriously ill, moderately ill, or minimally ill? If the diagnosis is uncertain, what steps are being taken to confirm a sure one? It helps if these steps are named specifically: for instance, blood work, radiographic studies, observation, recording of vital signs, or calling in a consultant. What is the tentative plan for the child? Complete bed rest or isolation until the results of blood work or cultures are back? Special diet? Special procedures? If the physician has written no orders yet, be honest: "The specific plan of care isn't written yet. I'll let you know as soon as I'm sure what it will be." Although this answer does not provide parents with information, it does tell them that health care providers appreciate how difficult and bewildering it is for parents to have their child admitted to a hospital (Hickey & Rykerson, 1992).

Reassuring parents this way is important because frightened, worried parents automatically transmit their emotions to their children, who are sensitive to the parents' tone of voice. Even though parents may say, "Don't worry, everything will be all right," a child will sense if parents really do not believe that everything will be all right, a situation that may hamper progress toward recovery (Ogilvie, 1990).

For an emergency admission, parents may have little understanding of the child's condition or the treatment plan. On the other hand, someone might have taken a great deal of time to explain what was happening while the child was being cared for in the emergency room. Do not stereotype or categorize people or situations. Ask parents if they have any questions about their child's condition or the course of treatment that they want to discuss with the health care team.

Orienting to Hospital Unit. A child coming to a hospital for an elective admission generally arrives at a reception area where significant factual information is obtained, such as name, age, address, and hospital insurance coverage. The child and parents are then brought to the hospital unit where the child is to stay. Remember that first impressions count. If parents are left standing at the desk while nurses chat, they may feel that no one appreciates their concern and that possibly their child will not receive good care. It is true that at certain times on a children's unit all nurses may be busy finishing the treatments for other children before they can take the time to admit a new child. Even so, one nurse should take the time to introduce himself or herself and find a comfortable place for the family to wait until someone is available.

When introducing yourself to children, stoop down so that your face is level with the child's face (Figure 35-3). Call the child by name or ask for a nickname. Call-

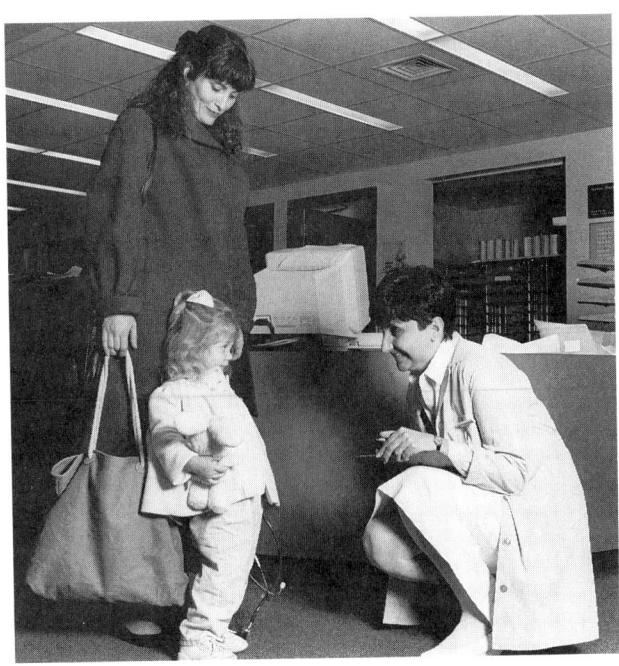

FIGURE 35-3
A child is admitted to a hospital unit. Notice how the nurse stoops to greet the child at the child's own level. (Courtesy of the Department of Medical Photography, Children's Hospital, Buffalo, NY.)

ing all children "Honey" or "Pumpkin" can worry children that they have been confused with another child.

Interview parents on hospital admission for a nursing history to obtain the information needed to plan nursing care (Chapter 28 describes a full child data base interview history). Many hospitals have checklists for parents to fill out while they wait. This way of obtaining information is highly efficient but not nearly as satisfying to worried parents as having a nurse take a few minutes to ask questions personally. Also, some parents may not understand the written items, and the information can be recorded wrongly if they are not asked personally. The information necessary to obtain about a child is shown in Table 35-2. It is included in the child's nursing care plan as a vital step of assessment. In addition, it assures parents that someone will be taking a personal interest in their child in the hospital. In some instances it may be advantageous to take a complete history in segments so the child or parents are not overwhelmed by so many questions.

Any medication or food allergies or reactions should be noted both on the child's nursing care plan and posted by the bed because, unlike an adult, a child cannot call these to the attention of health care personnel when food or medication is offered.

The child's temperature, pulse, and respirations should be taken and recorded. Height and weight should be measured to determine overall growth and to allow for determination of surface area, an important factor when computing medicine dosage. Whether blood pressure is taken or not depends on the age and condition of the child. A specimen for urinalysis should be taken. Explain all equipment used and allow the child to touch and handle it to help him or her reduce anxiety (Figure 35-4).

Inspect for gross motor ability when weighing the child and measuring height. Listen for language ability (although children in strange situations may say nothing). Perform a physical examination (see Chapter 28) to gain information needed for a nursing diagnosis and planning. Despite all the information needed, it is advisable that a child spend as little time as possible in a treatment room. The bravado of young children may be broken by being left too long in such a threatening setting.

If parents must leave rather than remain with a child, be certain to show them the child's room before they leave. This is important in convincing the child that the parents know where they can find him or her when they return. If there are other children in the room, introduce the new child to them. Let the child wear his or her own clothes if possible rather than change to a hospital gown.

Provide Opportunities for Parents to Participate in Child's Care. An important assessment to make all during hospitalization is the quality of parenting. This

Table 35-2. *Information Necessary for Nursing Care Plan on Admission*

Area of Information	Specific Knowledge
Chief concern	What is the parents' understanding of why the child is being admitted? (This view may differ widely from the physician's view regarding the reason the child is being admitted.) What has the child been told about the reason for hospitalization?
Family profile	Obtain child's name and birthday. Who lives at home (include pets)? Ask about parents' occupation and education levels. Who is the child's primary caregiver? Have there been any disruptive happenings lately in the child's life, such as a move or a divorce, that would make the child particularly insecure at this time? Will a parent be staying with the child? If parents are separated or divorced, what will arrangements be? Who has legal authority to sign medical permission?
Past experience with illness or separation	Ask about previous hospital experiences and how the child feels about them. Has there been a recent hospitalization for anyone in the family that resulted in a bad outcome? Has the child been away from the parents before? Overnight at a grandparent's? Summer camp? What is the child's past experience with taking medicine? Has the child swallowed pills before? Does the child have any known allergies to food or medications? (Document these by asking for exact symptoms and happenings.)
Daily routines	Ask about the child's regular bedtime and sleep times. Does the child nap? Does the child have a bedtime ritual? What type of bed does he or she sleep in? Does the child sleep with a favorite toy or blanket? What is his or her bathtime routine? Does the child brush his or her own teeth and hair or need help? What words does the child use for voiding and defecating? Is the child completely toilet-trained? If a preschooler, is the child accustomed to using a potty chair or toilet? Does the child have enuresis (bedwetting)? What is the child's usual meal plan? Are there foods the child does not eat? What is the child's favorite toy? Does he or she have it with him or her? What are the child's favorite games and hobbies or interests? Are there television programs the parents especially like the child to see or not see?
Developmental survey	Does child feed self? Use a spoon, cup, bottle? Dress self? If school age, what is grade in school?
Special information	Is there any special information about the child that would make him or her more comfortable in the hospital?

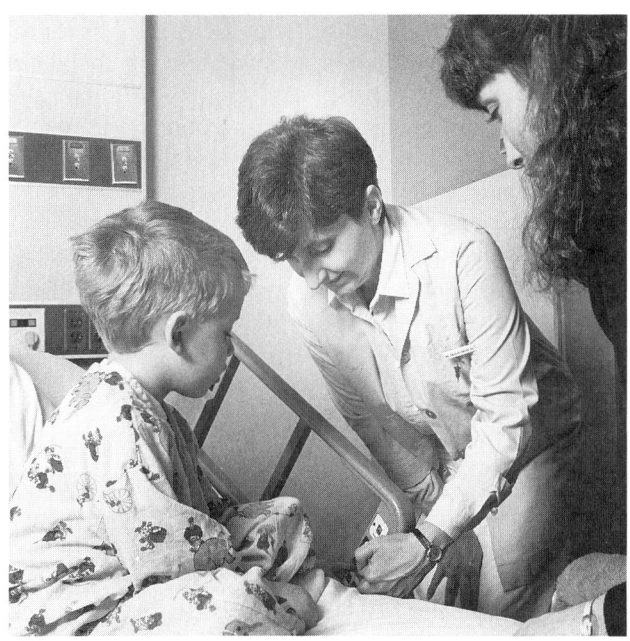

FIGURE 35-4
Orientation to a hospital room should include equipment that will be used, such as the push buttons of an electric bed. (Courtesy of the Department of Medical Photography, Children's Hospital, Buffalo, NY.)

can be assessed by observing parent–child interactions (the concerned parent asks questions of health care providers, plays with and comforts the child). To strengthen parent–child interaction, provide opportunities for parents to care for their child during a hospital stay to the extent that they are comfortable in doing so (Ahmann, 1994). This will depend on the child's condition and the parents' wishes. Most parents require instruction in some of the tasks they will be able to do. Mothers who change diapers or feed children should know if the number of diaper changes or the amount of food intake is being recorded; they can either report when they do these things or chart them on a flow sheet attached to the child's door or crib (Robbins, 1991).

Nursing Diagnosis: Anxiety of child related to separation during hospitalization

Goal: Child will demonstrate little evidence of separation anxiety during hospitalization.

Outcome Criteria: Child actively relates with nurses, physicians, and hospital routine in ways appropriate to particular child's age and stage of development.

Although some separation anxiety is unavoidable, reducing the ill effects of separation and hospitalization should be a high priority for health care providers. Nurses play a major role in reducing anxiety in children on both direct care and management levels.

Limiting Admissions. Only children who cannot successfully be managed on an ambulatory basis are now admitted to the hospital. This was not always true. For example, most children with head injuries automatically stayed overnight for observation. Currently, unless a child is unconscious or shows other signs of neurologic injury, he or she is sent home to be observed by parents for signs of increased intracranial pressure. This policy requires that time be spent in teaching parents skills such as how to take a pulse or evaluate consciousness. Teaching them requires patience because parents under stress can have difficulty comprehending instructions; however, because psychological trauma is prevented by allowing a child to return home, it is important teaching.

Limiting Hospital Stay. Hospitalization should be limited to the shortest time possible. At one time, all children having tonsillectomies and herniorrhaphies were admitted at least overnight. Currently, these types of surgery can be performed early in the morning, and after a short recovery period the child is able to return home. Again, parents must receive a great deal of education to make them aware of the danger signs to look for in the child, without becoming alarmed unnecessarily.

Be certain that diagnostic procedures are scheduled in such a way that no child's stay in a hospital is unnecessarily prolonged. Procedures should be scheduled for the child's, not the hospital's, convenience. Pressure from concerned nurses can make a big difference in a department's willingness to cooperate with scheduling.

Reducing or Eliminating Pain. Some pain and discomfort is unavoidable in association with health care. Limit this whenever possible by such measures as advocating the use of intermittent infusion devices such as heparin locks (see Chapter 37) to eliminate multiple punctures for intravenous medication or blood sampling, administering ample analgesia, including techniques such as imagery to distract the child from pain, providing traditional comforts such as a change of clothing or position, reading to the child, and planning a special project. Children do not always express discomfort as freely as adults; therefore, closer assessment may be necessary to reveal what they feel. Since anxiety increases pain, reducing a child's anxiety with good preparation and encouraging a sense of control can also help to eliminate discomfort.

Promoting Open Parent Visiting. When possible, children younger than 5 years should have their primary caregiver room in with them when they are in the hospital. Children younger than 10 to 12 years also enjoy the feeling of security that this provides. This policy is expensive for a hospital because a bed or cot must be provided for this person as well as for the child, and despite the presence of this person, no reduction in nurs-

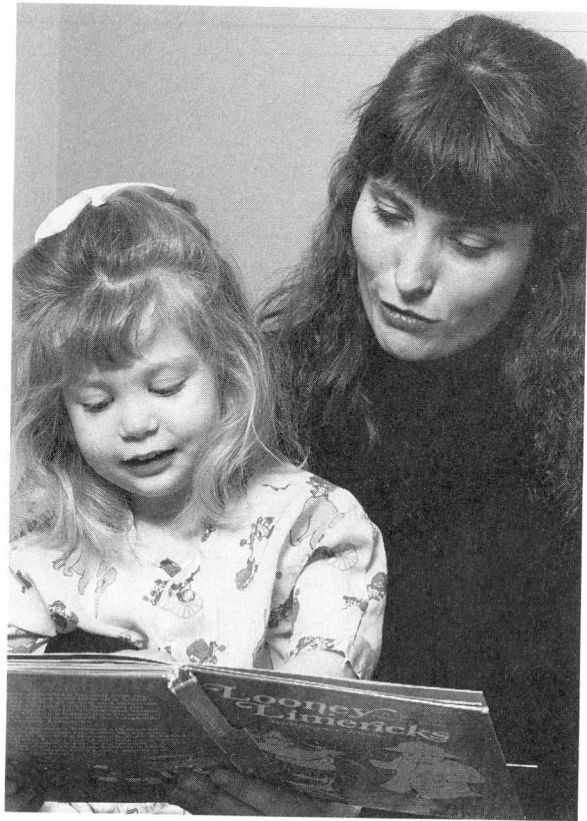

FIGURE 35-5
Parents should be encouraged to give as much care as possible. Here, a mother reads to her daughter to pass the time during intravenous medication therapy. (Courtesy of the Department of Medical Photography, Children's Hospital, Buffalo, NY.)

ing staff is possible. In many instances, because so much parental education is needed, requirements for health care personnel actually increase. Encourage parents to give as much care as possible during a hospitalization, such as bathing or feeding the child, giving oral medicine, or helping with procedures such as warm soaks. Do not be concerned with keeping parents busy. Their most important role is being parents. Sitting and rocking or reading to the child and just being there is their best role in minimizing the adverse effects of hospitalization, as well as reducing their own stress (Heuer, 1993) (Figure 35-5).

Supporting Sibling and Grandparent Visitations. Sibling visitation refers to the policy of allowing brothers and sisters of hospitalized children to visit. In the past, visitation by children younger than 12 to 14 years was restricted because of the danger that they would spread communicable diseases to the ill sibling or other patients. Currently, with effective immunization, a child runs no more risk of spreading a childhood disease other than chickenpox than do staff members or adult family members. With a vaccine for chickenpox on the horizon, soon even this will not be a problem.

Allowing siblings and grandparents to visit an ill child alleviates loneliness on both sides and helps prevent the children at home from imagining the ill child to be more sick than what they have been told. It helps the ill child continue to feel part of the family and allows grandparents to offer much-needed support. Sound policies governing sibling visitation need to be established: to assess siblings for immunization status; to help parents divide their time between the ill child and siblings during a visit (short, frequent visits may be better for young children than long, sustained ones); and to ensure that the ill child's room is safe for younger children's visits (e.g., no poisonous substances or electric wires within reach).

Providing a Substitute Parent. To expose children to as few substitute care people as possible, nursing assignments should be made so that one nurse gives as much care to the same child as possible (**primary** or **case management nursing;** Figure 35-6). These staffing patterns allow one nurse to admit the child, take the nursing history, establish nursing diagnoses, set goals for care in cooperation with the parents and the child, implement the bulk of care, and evaluate whether progress toward achieving goals is being made. This type of staffing pattern allows children, therefore, to have one main nurse to whom to relate. It allows parents to establish valuable contact with hospital staff and maintains continuity of care planning and implementation.

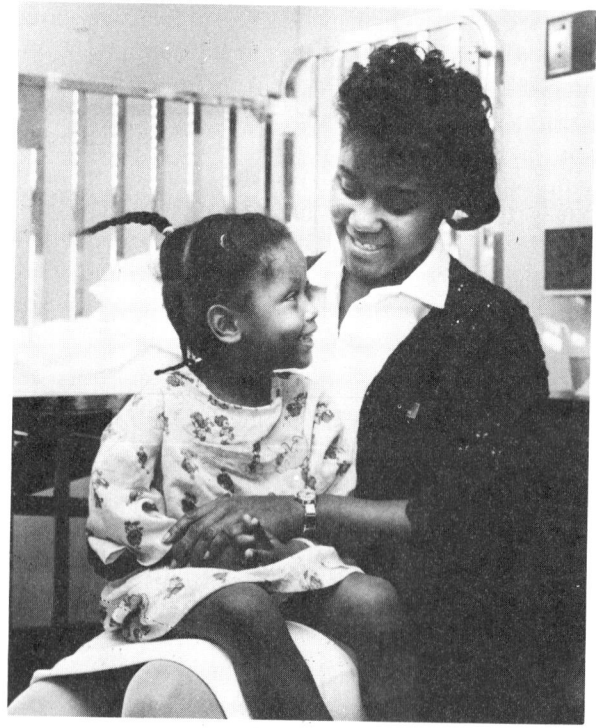

FIGURE 35-6
Each hospitalized child should have one nurse who is "his" or "hers" to minimize the effect of separation from parents (primary care nursing). (Courtesy of the Department of Medical Photography, Children's Hospital, Buffalo, NY.)

Dressing Positively and Having a Positive Attitude.
Children of all ages react more positively when the staff
is dressed in colorful clothing rather than white uniforms. School-age children and adolescents tend to see
nurses who are dressed this way as more friendly
and less authoritarian. Older children feel more comfortable about saying they are worried, asking questions
about what will happen to them when they go to
surgery, or discussing their fear that when they return to
school, no one will like them anymore. Concerns such
as these are much easier to voice to someone whose
everyday, non-uniform appearance suggests that he or
she is a regular person with feelings, rather than someone who is efficient and "in charge." For these reasons,
then, most pediatric nurses choose not to wear white
uniforms. In the final analysis, however, it is the nurse's
attitude of being a warm, caring person that will make
the most difference (see the Focus on Nursing Research
display).

Providing Adequate Play Facilities. Play is the
medium through which children learn. To continue to
develop during hospitalization, children need to be able
to play as normally as possible, no matter how long their
stay. They should have a playroom or play space in
which they can feel secure and in which they will not be
hurt. No medical procedures, not even painless ones,
should be carried out in this area (Figure 35-7). Children
who are in bed need toys or crafts with them there. In
addition, because hospitalization is a traumatic experience, children need the opportunity to express their
feelings through therapeutic play. The uses of play and

FOCUS ON NURSING RESEARCH

What Type of Uniform Do Children Prefer Nurses to Wear?

To answer this question, a nurse researcher asked 100 children 3, 4, and 5 years of age to look at photos of a nurse dressed in a traditional uniform with cap, a white pantsuit, street clothes, street clothes covered by a white lab coat, or white pants covered by a colorful smock top. Fifty of the children had been hospitalized prior to the study and 50 had not. After viewing the photos, children were asked, "Which nurse do you want to take care of you?" and "Is there a nurse you are afraid of?" Results of the study showed that the favorite choice of uniform for both the hospitalized and nonhospitalized children was the smock top. The traditionally uniformed nurse was the one chosen most often as a person to be afraid of. The researcher suggests that nurses caring for children should be aware that their attire can influence how children perceive them and modify their attire appropriately.

Meyer, D. (1992). Children's responses to nursing attire. *Pediatric Nursing, 18,* 157.

guidelines for providing therapeutic play are discussed
later in this chapter. (See the Nursing Care Plan: A
Preschooler Hospitalized With Pneumonia.)

Maintaining the Bed as a Safe Area. To assure children that their bed is an area that is safe, all painful pro-

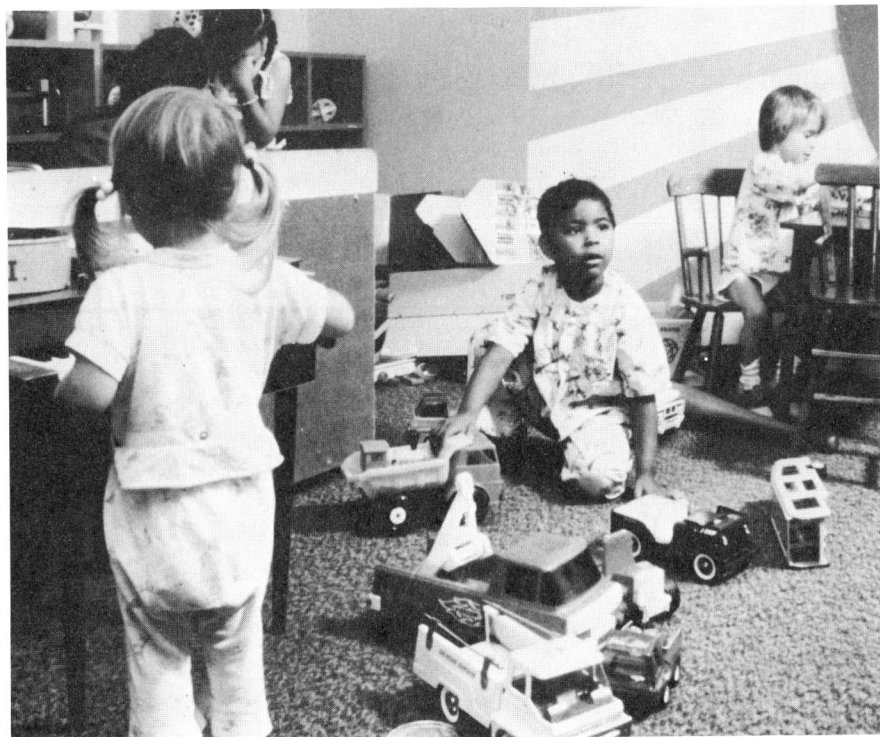

FIGURE 35-7
A hospital playroom. Children need such a free play area in the hospital where painful procedures are not performed. (Courtesy of the Department of Medical Photography, Children's Hospital, Buffalo, NY.)

Nursing Care Plan
A Preschooler Hospitalized With Pneumonia

Sally is a 3-year-old-girl admitted to the hospital for pneumonia. She will have continuous oxygen administration and intermittent antibiotic intravenous therapy. The following is a nursing care plan devised for her regarding hospital adjustment.

Assessment: Child has never been separated from parents longer than overnight; mother will room in. Mother has talked about and read Sally a book about hospitalization since admission. Favorite toy: Raggedy Ann doll. Words for voiding and stool: "pee-pee" and "poopy." Mother's concern: child is modest; will dislike procedures that expose her. Is afraid of the dark. Child appears fearful. Cried when nurse took her temperature by tympanic membrane. Refused to void. Presently lying on back with oxygen prongs in place soundlessly crying. No toys in bed with her. Stretching neck to see television set over her head (turned to adult game show). Shouted, "I want out! I'm going home!" when she saw the nurse.

Nursing Diagnosis: Anxiety related to new surroundings and medical procedures

Defining Characteristic: Child appears fearful; mother confirms she is apprehensive.

Goal: Child will experience minimal stress during hospitalization.

Outcome Criteria: Child voices reason for procedures being done for her; parents voice satisfaction with rooming-in as a means of support for the child.

Nursing Orders	Rationale
1. Admit to room 405B; identification band in place. Introduce to roommate.	1. Orients the child and mother to new room and other client.
2. Needs light on at night (door marked); cot for mother requested.	2. These measures help reduce fear to minimal level.
3. Keep favorite doll in bed for comfort.	3. A favorite toy is a strong support object.

(continued)

cedures should be done in a treatment room, away from the child's bed. Be sure that this rule is not broken "just once," since only one painful experience at the bedside can be enough to significantly increase a child's anxiety. This also increases the anxiety of another child in the room. This rule should include finger pricks for blood work that, although done quickly, cause pain and stress. In addition, dressing changes, although not necessarily painful, can cause stress and so should also be done in a treatment room, not at the child's bedside.

Helping Children To Maintain Control. Events are always more frightening if they appear to occur without a child's ability to control them. Explaining to children what will happen to them (i.e., what they will feel or what they will see) and helping them to make choices whenever possible limits the fear of hospitalization because it offers a sense of control. In almost any procedure that is carried out, there is some choice a child can

make (use a straw to drink or not, decide what size of tape to use on a bandage, or walk one way in the hall or the other). Letting a child participate in signing a consent form is part of helping the child to maintain control (Figure 35-8).

Nursing Diagnosis: High risk for altered growth and development related to effects of hospitalization

Goal: Child will demonstrate increased growth and development during hospitalization.

Outcome Criteria: Child, depending on age and stage of development, demonstrates only limited signs of regression to previous stage; is able to continue doing the thing he or she most recently accomplished.

Hospitalization represents a crisis event. In a crisis state, children, like adults, are susceptible to change and

1026

Nursing Orders	Rationale
4. Admission urinalysis is still needed. Mother to obtain, since child does not void for strangers.	4. Encourages mother to be an active support person.
5. Provide therapeutic puppet play to orient to procedures.	5. Playing with puppets may allow this child to express her fears openly, to which the nurse can then therapeutically respond.

Nursing Diagnosis: High risk for altered growth and development related to lack of play opportunity

Defining Characteristic: Child has no toy or game readily available.

Goal: Child will increase play time within 24 hours.

Outcome Criteria: Child actively engages in play at least 3 hours out of every 24 hours.

Nursing Orders	Rationale
1. Introduce initiative-producing materials, such as modeling clay or finger paint.	1. These materials are age appropriate.
2. Provide a 1-hour playtime morning and afternoon; 30 minutes after dinner.	2. Knowing playtime is scheduled may give Sally something to look forward to and will ensure that she gets the play time she needs.
3. Ask parents about favorite (or desired) television programs and position so television is visible.	3. Involves parents in decision-making.
4. Provide therapeutic play for 30 minutes in the morning and evening; introduce doll with oxygen and intravenous tubing in place (child receives an antibiotic intravenously 6 times daily).	4. Therapeutic play can be effective means of relieving fear in a preschooler.

growth with only the slightest intervention. Without intervention, they are likely to be overwhelmed.

Promoting Growth and Development of the Infant.
When an infant is admitted to a hospital, ask parents what type of bed the child sleeps in at home. A child who is used to sleeping in a bassinet may feel loose and insecure in a large crib. Such a child should be swaddled in a receiving blanket in a large crib to give him or her the close, bound feeling of a smaller sleeping area.

The infant's diet should be changed as little as possible. Unless the child is admitted for failure to thrive or because he or she is obviously underweight, hospitalization is not an ideal situation in which to introduce new foods or formula. Unless their physical condition warrants a change, infants who breast-feed should continue to do so for as many feedings as are possible for the mother. Expressed breast milk can be given by bottle for other feedings.

Children 6 months and older often protest strongly if they are separated from their parents. As they are taken from a parent's arm at the door of the treatment room, they may begin to cry loudly and without pausing until they are returned to the parent. The child is too angry and frightened in these surroundings to be comforted, particularly after having been hurt by a health care procedure. There is rarely any reason a parent cannot accompany an infant into the treatment room to undress the infant and help with measuring weight and height and with temperature taking. Most importantly, the mother or father can comfort the child in strange surroundings.

When a parent leaves a child to eat a meal or go home for the night (if the parent is not sleeping in), an infant may begin loud, intense crying. When this happens, a parent often needs help in saying goodbye. It may help to remind parents that they have been preparing their infant for separation from the time the child

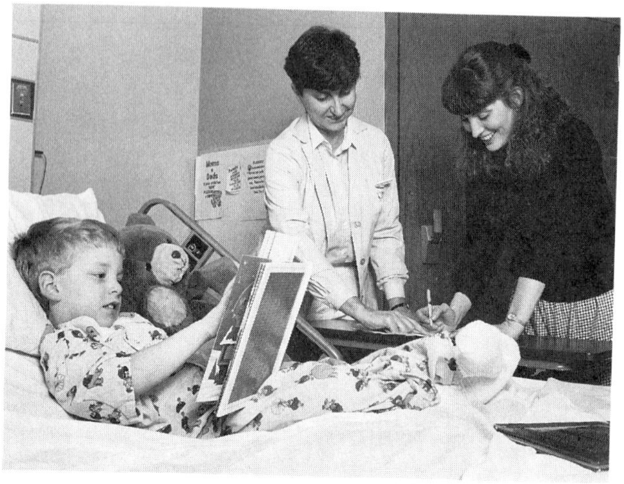

FIGURE 35-8
Children should be included in procedures whenever possible as a way of maintaining control. Here, a nurse helps a mother sign a consent form. The child gets acquainted with the hospital orientation book. (Courtesy of the Department of Medical Photography, Children's Hospital, Buffalo, NY.)

was 9 or 10 months old by playing games such as peek-a-boo. Be sure to assure parents while they are still in the hospital that although someone will not be in the infant's room every minute, he or she will be well cared for. Go into the room a few minutes before the parents leave and hold or play with the infant. Help a parent to say once, "I have to go now," and then go. Prolonged departures only delay the process and do not reduce the amount of crying that may occur. After a parent leaves, an infant may cry until he or she falls asleep from exhaustion. Hold and rock the child, letting him know that although his parents are not there, he will be safe.

Promoting Growth and Development of the Hospitalized Toddler and Preschooler. Toddlers and preschoolers can be as affected by separation as an infant. In some instances they express their feelings better and louder and longer than the infant. They cry for their parents and are unable to understand why they do not come. Such children startle at the slightest noise that could be interpreted as a parent's coming. They may suck their thumb, bang their head against the crib, clutch a blanket, or masturbate to try to achieve some comfort for their loss.

Other toddlers, after a short period of protest, move into a quiet, withdrawn attitude (despair). They lie quietly in their crib, come to nurses and other health care personnel readily, and sit at small tables to eat. They are literally "too good to be true." In reality, some of these children are in such distress that they cannot express their feelings. Quietness this way, therefore, is not necessarily being good or adjusting well; it may be the

numbness of grief. A toddler who is in despair may be crying just before a parent's arrival. When the toddler sees the parent, the first reaction is not to rush into his or her arms, however; often the opposite happens. The child sees the parents but does not move or acknowledge them, and may even look away. This is a defense mechanism: "I won't show them that I love them until they show me that they love me; that way I won't be hurt again."

Mothers and fathers may need help in recognizing this behavior in toddlers. Otherwise, their first reaction to being treated this way may be anger. If this makes parents go and play with a child in the next bed—a "well, be that way then" reaction—this behavior fulfills the toddler's worst fears: his parents do not love him anymore. Parents may also experience jealousy when their child goes toward the nursing staff instead of them. They may suspect the child actually likes the hospital better than home.

Fortunately, toddlers and preschoolers cannot maintain an emotionless front for more than a few minutes. If the parents speak to them for a few minutes, they generally reach out to be comforted. If the child turns toward the back of the crib, parents can usually interest him or her in a toy or a game. The child will watch the parents play with it for a moment, then ask to sit in the mother's or father's lap.

Fortunately, because the average parent stays overnight with a child, the problem of separation anxiety from limited visiting times is minimized. Those parents who cannot stay may grow dismayed because their child cries every time they visit. They ask whether it would be less traumatic if they stayed away. The answer is absolutely not. Children cry when they see their parents because it reminds them of how much they miss them. As disturbing as it is to be greeted with tears, the reaction shows that the child's emotions are still alive and that the child cares.

Parents of toddlers or preschoolers, like those of infants, should be asked on admission what type of bed a child sleeps in. Children who are not used to sleeping in cribs may resent being put in a crib unless the reason is explained to them ("All our beds here have side rails"). Toddlers must be watched closely to see that they do not climb over crib rails to get out of bed. A child who does try may be safer in a bed than a crib.

As with infants, hospitalization is a poor time to change the eating habits of toddlers and preschoolers. Because children of this age insist on self-feeding, they generally do poorly eating in bed. They often do better sitting at low tables. Many child-care units organize tables for toddlers and preschoolers to eat together. Some children do well at these tables. Others are too distracted by the activity and the noise and may need a separate low table by their bed.

Hospitalization is also a poor time to begin toilet-training, even if it is appropriate to the child's age. If the parents have begun toilet-training, it should be continued with a routine as close as possible to that at home.

If the parents of a toddler or preschooler have to leave, they should be urged first to give a warning that they will soon have to go: "I will have to leave in a minute to fix dinner for Jodie." When the time to go has come, the parent should say firmly that he or she must go and explain when he or she will return. Time for a preschooler should be measured in terms of events rather than clock hours. "I'll be back after you've eaten supper," "after you wake up tomorrow," or "after nap time" gives the child a concrete event by which to measure time.

Toddlers need someone with them when their parents leave; they like to be held or played with so that they know they are not alone.

Promoting Growth and Development of the Hospitalized School-Age Child. School-age children react better than younger children to the separation imposed by hospitalization because they have past experiences to draw on. They have been to school for whole days; perhaps they have stayed with a grandparent or a friend overnight. As long as they are given firm reassurance and definite times that parents will visit ("about 9:00 tomorrow morning," not "sometime tomorrow"), hospitalization may actually be a time for developing self-esteem and confidence in the ability to be independent.

Remember that children who are ill are not at their best and may not act as maturely as usual. In these circumstances, a 7-year-old whose parent describes her as very mature may not appear mature at all, but may seem to function at the level of a 5-year-old. Children of any age should not be held to chronologic age when they are ill. For the same reason, school-age children who do well with competition at home often do poorly with competition in a hospital. In planning games or entertainment, remember that they often enjoy experiences that at home they would dismiss as too young for them. School-age children enjoy sharing a room with another child close in age.

School-age children and adolescents should continue schooling if they are hospitalized for a long time, provided their condition will allow it. Children in the hospital do well with school activities or working with a tutor. This is such a normal, everyday activity for them that it provides security in an otherwise insecure environment and reassures them that they are expected to get better and to return to school when this is over. School-age children also find comfort in spiritual practices. Ways to assist with spiritual needs are shown in Box 35-3.

Promoting Growth and Development of the Adolescent. Hospitalization is difficult for adolescents because peer relationships are so important to them. They may miss being chosen for a school play, a sports team, or the cheerleader squad or competing for a scholarship. A girlfriend or boyfriend may fall in love with somebody else while the adolescent is away. They will miss out on the funny prank in history class or an "in" joke from chemistry, and feel excluded and hurt. For these reasons, they need visitors from their peer group as badly as infants need visits from parents.

Adolescents appreciate being hospitalized in a special adolescent unit or at least in rooms free of childish decor. Such units should be organized with the same considerations for visiting parents as other children's units; parents should be able to stay overnight if they and the adolescent wish. Remember that the anxiety and pain of separation are not limited to the under-13 set. Because parents often do not remain overnight with them, adolescents appreciate knowing that their parents are concerned about their welfare and continually checking that they are being cared for and that they are getting well. They also enjoy being separated from their parents (if everything is going all right).

Often adolescents convey a blasé attitude toward procedures: having radiographs taken is nothing, surgery is a cinch, or a cast change is a snap. Listen carefully to make certain that adolescents really feel this way. They may be trying to convince themselves that a procedure is harmless. Adolescents are extremely worried about their body parts. Make sure they know what is going to happen in surgery and in the radiology department. It is easy to assume from their attitude that they know more than they do.

Adolescence, like school age, covers a wide age range. A 13-year-old is a teenager, as is an 18-year-old, but they are little alike in terms of ability to handle new situations.

Nursing Diagnosis: Parental health-seeking behaviors related to care for child at home after hospital discharge

Goal: Parents will demonstrate ability to care for child at home before discharge.

Outcome Criteria: Parents state accurately the care their child will need at home; describe and demonstrate any procedures they will need to carry out with child.

Many children, particularly those having surgery, are hospitalized for only a number of hours and as soon as they are able to take and retain fluid and have voided once, they are discharged. Preparation for discharge must start even before they are admitted to the hospital.

Box 35-3
Nursing Interventions to Meet Children's Spiritual Needs

Action	Implementation
Prayers	Ask on hospital admission whether a child says grace with meals or a prayer at bedtime. Write it on the nursing care plan so that nurses can help with this. Remember that saying grace also applies to unconventional meals, such as a tube feeding. Bedtime prayers may be especially important by lending security in a strange environment.
Religious services	Many children of school age and older enjoy attending a religious service in a hospital chapel. Include time for this in a nursing care plan and be certain that transportation by wheelchair or cart is available.
Visits from clergy	Many school-age children and adolescents enjoy an active recreation or social program at a church facility when well. They enjoy a visit from clergy when they are ill, not so much for its religious importance as for support from a respected adult. Free the child's time as necessary for such visits.
Religious articles	A child's parent may wish to attach a religious article to the child's clothing or pillow or to post it over the bed. Be careful when changing linen that you do not throw away such articles. Mark their presence and importance on a care plan.

If a child has been admitted on an inpatient basis, preparation for discharge should begin on the day of admission. If some procedures must be done later at home, allow parents to perform them in the hospital so that they can become comfortable with the techniques and discover any problems while help is still available. Urge parents to think through problems they might have with the procedures at home. Suppose a parent will be doing warm sterile soaks to an open lesion at home. How does he or she sterilize water? Where can the parent buy dressings like those used in the hospital? Can the parent afford them? What can he or she use to keep the soaks warm for 20 minutes? What suggestions would be helpful to give the parent for keeping the child quiet and content for 20 minutes, so that the child does not move a great deal and knock off the dressing? These are real problems that must be worked out before a parent can carry out the procedure at home. Do not leave this kind of instruction until the last day, because then there will not be time left to solve such problems.

Discharge planners can be indispensable in helping ready parents for home care. In a general hospital setting, however, if the discharge planner is unfamiliar with specific procedures (or children), he or she may not be helpful on a practical level. Some parents require follow-up help in their homes that can be provided by a community or home health care nurse. Do not leave the full responsibility for teaching to these nurses, however. Teach the parents what they must do on the first day they are at home before further help arrives. Be certain they know who to contact if plans do not work out as anticipated and that they have a definite return appointment for follow-up care.

Many preschool children manifest behavior problems such as thumb-sucking, bed wetting, temper tantrums, and nightmares after returning home from a hospital stay; school-age children may manifest these behaviors to a lesser extent. Parents can be told that they are part of the child's normal response to hospitalization. These behaviors do not happen because the child has been "spoiled" by the hospital staff or by the parents during the illness but because the experience was too intense for the child to handle, even with all the precautions taken to prevent stress. As children realize that they are safely back home and the experience is over, these behavior reactions become less frequent and eventually disappear.

Value of Play to the Hospitalized Child

Play, which has often been described as the "work" of children, is an invaluable component of hospital care. Providing a space and opportunity for play can help a child feel more comfortable in the hospital environment and allow for an important release of energy for a child who is confined to a room or bed. Play may also be used to help assess a child's level of knowledge and feelings about his or her condition so that more individualized nursing care can be planned. Depending on the child's age, play can also be a useful tool in health teaching (see Chapter 36).

Defining play is not a simple task, because play activities vary greatly from child to child and among different age groups. A common definition is that play is any voluntary activity engaged in for the purpose of enjoyment. If a child views an activity as enjoyment, therefore, no matter what it is and whether it would be fun for an adult, it is play. According to Piaget (Wadsworth, 1989), children master tasks by **accommodation** (a child changes his or her perceptions to conform to reality) and **assimilation** (adapting stimuli to adjust to what the child already knows). Piaget has defined *play* as pure assimilation, or the repetition of a behavior or skill solely for the pleasure of performing the skill. An activity, therefore, can be work during the accommodation stage and become play as it is mastered and enjoyed.

Play is clearly the means by which children develop increasing cognitive, psychomotor, and social capabilities. Touching a soft rabbit, passing colored blocks from one hand to the other, pounding with a plastic hammer, feeding a doll, and playing board games are all ways in which children are exposed to and learn about different textures and different colors, experience the feeling of possessing and owning, and learn about competition, winning, and losing. A soft toy tells the child more clearly than can be described that this is what the word "soft" means. Colored blocks show him or her how parts can join to make a whole, how things stacked too high will fall (there are limits one cannot go beyond), and that practice makes perfect. As the child talks with playmates during play, he or she develops both language and social skills. The repetitive acts involved in most games encourage the development of musculoskeletal skills. Play is not something a child does when he or she has nothing else to do; it is something the child *has* to do. In a hospital setting, it provides a feeling of security because it is an activity that has continuity with home life (LeVieux-Anglin & Sawyer, 1993).

Types of Play

The manner in which children play differs as they mature. Types of play and the age groups in which these types are seen most frequently are shown in the Focus on Family Teaching display.

Assessing Child Health Through Play

Children who are acutely ill do not play or play very little. They have neither the strength, the attention span, nor the interest in activities that are required for play. Once children are over the acute phase of an illness,

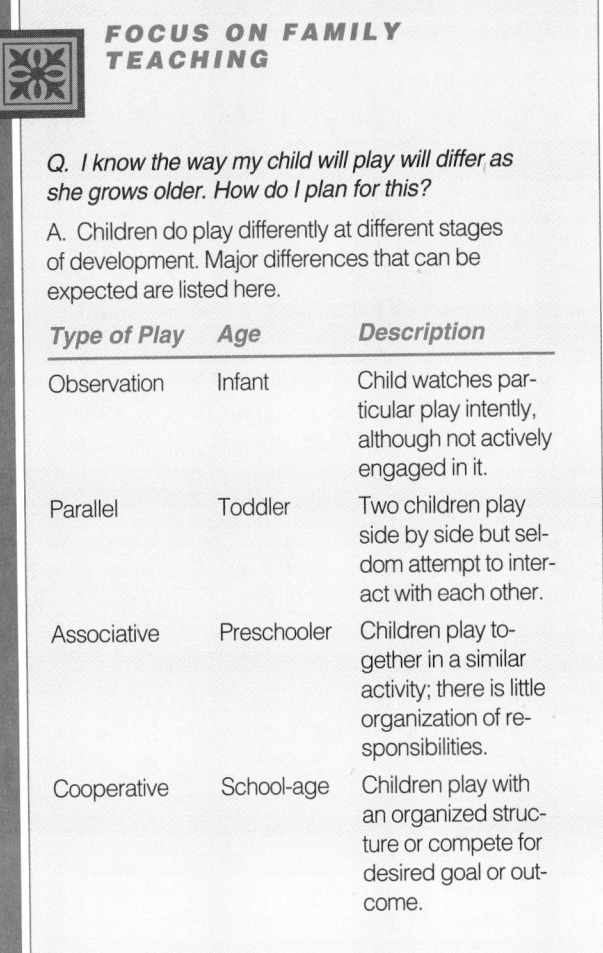

FOCUS ON FAMILY TEACHING

Q. I know the way my child will play will differ as she grows older. How do I plan for this?

A. Children do play differently at different stages of development. Major differences that can be expected are listed here.

Type of Play	Age	Description
Observation	Infant	Child watches particular play intently, although not actively engaged in it.
Parallel	Toddler	Two children play side by side but seldom attempt to interact with each other.
Associative	Preschooler	Children play together in a similar activity; there is little organization of responsibilities.
Cooperative	School-age	Children play with an organized structure or compete for desired goal or outcome.

however, interest in play usually returns. Whether a child is spontaneously playing or not, then, is a good index of health. The toys a child uses at play are a good indication of growth and development level and of emotional state.

Questions about the child's play patterns should be included in a health assessment interview. Ask such questions as "Has John been as active as usual? Has he been playing as usual?" A play history can also help document the duration of illness. When describing their child's illness, many parents say at first, "Susie has been ill since this morning." When asked about play, the parent will say, "Well, she hasn't been herself for the past 2 days." That is the prodromal period (the initial, sometimes symptomless period) of disease, and it indicates the time at which Susie actually became ill.

The average parent knows a child's play preferences and his or her current favorite game or toy. Asking for this information helps to assess the child's developmental level and whether it is age appropriate. It also helps to assess the quality of parenting (if parents view play as important or are familiar with the child's activities).

Providing Space, Time, and Equipment for Play

Play space and equipment for play should be provided in both ambulatory and inpatient settings wherever children are cared for.

Ambulatory Settings

Children in ambulatory departments are under a great deal of stress. They sit in a waiting room and glance fearfully at the door that leads to the examining room. They hear children crying beyond the door and wait in terror for what lies in store for them when it is their turn.

Most parents know that when their child is coming to a hospital to be admitted, they should pack the child's favorite toy. Often they do not think of an ambulatory visit as a sufficiently threatening circumstance to warrant bringing a favorite toy, however, so the child has nothing to play with. Having a parent sit beside them is so comforting that they may ignore or hesitate moving 4 feet away to get attractive toys furnished by the health care facility unless urged to do so.

Ambulatory departments should be stocked with toys that can be played with quickly and by single children. The departments should have low tables and chairs so that a parent can come to a table to play with a child. Examining rooms should have toys also—they may be needed to distract a child while a procedure such as an ear examination is performed, and because the wait in an examining room may be as long as the wait in a waiting room. Well siblings who accompany a parent and sick child to the facility should have toys to distract them as well so that the parent can concentrate on the ailing child. Some hospitals furnish computer games for older children for this reason. Specific examples of ways that play can be used in an ambulatory care setting are shown in Table 35-3.

Inpatient Settings

Children who are hospitalized on an inpatient basis need to have play periods built into their day. The length of time of play and the toys individual children can play with depend on age and physical and emotional states. Ways that play can be incorporated into inpatient care are shown in Table 35-4.

Infants need toys in their cribs, such as mobiles, blocks, soft toys, and rattles. They also need to be out of cribs, sitting on a parent's or a nurse's lap or sitting in strollers or swings. They need some time on the floor (with a sheet under them) to practice crawling or walking. At age 3 months, when an infant discovers the hands, those are his or her "toys." For a child learning to crawl or "cruise" or walk, that activity is his or her toy or interest for the month.

Toddlers need put-in and take-out types of toys such as blocks that can be repeatedly dropped into a

Table 35-3. *Ways to Incorporate Play Into Ambulatory Nursing Care*

Nursing Care	Play Activity
Aid with physical assessment	Distract child's attention with puppet during respiratory and cardiac assessment.
	Play "Simon Says" to encourage child to take deep breaths for respiratory assessment.
	Allow child to listen to own heart with stethoscope.
	Play "Follow the Leader" to assess gait.
	Draw a face on the tongue blade used to assess throat.
	Show child how to "blow out" the otoscope light.
	Draw child's outline on the table examining paper and give it to him or her to take home to color.
Health teaching	Use puppets as teacher.
	Create word scrambles or crossword puzzles.

bottle or that can be stacked to play with in bed; they enjoy listening to tapes of songs and nursery rhymes. Toddlers are in constant motion; they need to be out of bed as much as their physical condition allows, playing with take-apart, put-together, or pull-and-push toys. Preschoolers need creative materials such as modeling clay or sand.

School-age children need quiet games such as books or crayons or magic markers by their bedside. While in bed, they enjoy radios, compact disk players, or tapes. Most activities for hospitalized children must be short-term projects because children are called away for treatments or procedures, and because they are ill their attention span is shorter than usual. Short-term projects always appeal to the school-age child because they help this age child achieve a sense of industry.

Television watching is a nonparticipant activity and may not be the best activity for children. However, there is some value in watching nature programs or "after-school specials" that often depict school-age children in real-life situations coping with problems common to many of their peers. The nurse can watch a game show with a school-age child and help the child guess the solution to a puzzle or watch "Sesame Street" with a preschooler to make the activity a participatory one. Watching a soap opera with an adolescent and then discussing the people and their problems can also turn television watching into active participation. Table 35-5 lists possible games that require no equipment other than that readily available on a nursing unit for children who have brought nothing of their own to play with or who have grown bored with existing games.

Table 35-4. *Ways to Incorporate Play Into Inpatient Children's Nursing Care*

Care Measure	Play
Bathing	Allow child to play in bathtub with water toys.
	Play game such as "I Spy" while giving a bed bath.
Encouraging fluid	Hold a "tea party" for a preschooler and drink "tea" with important but imaginary guests.
	Play a board game with a school-age child in which each turn starts with taking a drink.
	Draw a circle and let child color in a section each time he or she drinks until the circle is full.
	Play "Simon Says," in which Simon says, "Drink."
Deep breathing exercises	Have child blow up a rubber glove.
	Have child blow soap bubbles in a glass of soapy water with a straw.
	Have child blow a cotton ball across the surface of a bed-side table.
	Play "Simon Says," in which Simon says, "Take a deep breath."
	Allow the child to score points for reaching a high number on an incentive spirometer.
Muscle strengthening exercises	Have child throw bean bags at a wastebasket.
	Play "Simon Says," in which Simon says, "Raise your arms," and so forth.
	Have child throw and catch a ball.
	Have child squeeze and mold modeling clay.
	Allow a tricycle for a preschooler.
	Encourage child to kick balloon suspended near foot of bed.
	Help a preschooler pretend he or she is a butterfly, airplane, and so forth.
Procedure such as blood transfusion	Save a favorite game or activity only for these times.
Health teaching	Use puppets as teacher.
	Make up board games, word scrambles, and crossword puzzles.

Space and Supervision

Ideally, all hospital units where children are cared for should have play space big enough for the majority of children on the unit. It should have enough space to accommodate children who are not fully ambulatory, such as those with casts or wheelchairs. Tables for board games and play materials such as crayons and paints should be available. Children can release a great deal of anger or tension by splashing water, squeezing or pouring sand, or smearing finger paint.

School-age children need to be provided with a game such as shuffleboard or sand bags to toss for tension relief and competition. Adolescents enjoy table tennis and pool tables. A great deal of older school-age and adolescent "play" centers around conversation with peers (Figure 35-9).

Children who are hospitalized for 1 week or more may enjoy putting on a puppet show or playing school, store, or house. A corner of a playroom should be de-voted to this kind of imaginative play: a structure that will serve as either a store front, puppet stage, house, or school; dolls, cribs, empty food boxes and cans, and puppets should also be provided. Large blocks, 6 inches by 12 inches, are available for playrooms so that such structures can be built and rebuilt each day. For ill children, the blocks must be made of cardboard, not wood, because ill children tire easily when lifting heavier wood blocks.

Providing play equipment and supervision for a recreational play program in most instances is economically feasible through donations and volunteers. Toys for a playroom can generally be secured through donations from men's or women's clubs in the community. For safety reasons, children need to be supervised while they play. Because they do not feel well in a hospital or are shy in the surroundings, they enjoy having a concerned adult to watch over them and suggest new activities. Such adults may be volunteers. Supervision is an

Table 35-5. *Games and Activities Using Materials Available on a Nursing Unit*

Age	Activity
Infant	Make a mobile from roller gauze and tongue blades to hang over a crib.
	Ask the pharmacy or central supply for different size boxes to use for put-in, take-out toys. (Do not use round vials from pharmacy; if accidentally aspirated, these can completely occlude the airway.)
	Blow up a glove as a balloon; draw a smiling face on it with a marker.
	Play "patty cake," "So Big," "Peek-a-boo."
Toddler	Ask central supply for boxes to use as blocks for stacking.
	Tie roller gauze to a glove box for a pull toy.
	Sing or recite familiar nursery rhymes such as "Peter, Peter, Pumpkin Eater."
Preschool	Play "Simon Says" or "Mother, May I?"
	Draw a picture of a dog; ask child to close eyes; add an additional feature to the dog; ask child to guess the added part, repeat until a full picture is drawn.
	Make a puppet from a lunch bag or draw a face on your hand with a marker.
	Cut out a picture from a newspaper or a magazine (or draw a picture); cut it into large puzzle pieces.
	Pour breakfast cereal into a basin; furnish boxes to pour and spoons to dig.
	Furnish chart paper and a magic marker for coloring.
	Make modeling clay from 1 cup salt, 1/2 cup flour, 1/2 cup water from diet kitchen.
	Play "Ring-Around-the-Rosey" or "London Bridge."
School-age	Play "I Spy" or charades.
	Make a deck of cards to play "Go Fish" or "Old Maid;" invent cards such as Nicholas Nurse, Doctor Dolittle, Irene Intern, Polly Patient.
	Play "Hangman."
	Furnish scale or table paper and a magic marker for a huge drawing or sign.
	Hide an object in the child's room and have the child look for it (have the child name places for you to look if the child cannot be out of bed).
Adolescent	Color squares on a chart form to make a checker board.
	Have adolescent make a deck of cards to use for "Hearts" or "Rummy."
	Compete to see how many words the adolescent can make from the letters in his or her name.
	Compete to guess whether the next person to enter the room will be a man or woman, next car to go by window will be red or black, and so forth.
	Compete to see who can name the most episodes of the television shows "Star Trek" or reruns of "The Brady Bunch."

excellent after-school activity for members of a future nurses' association. Ideally, child life or play specialists fill such roles (Dolan, 1993).

If play supervisors are unavailable through other sources, the nursing staff must free such personnel as necessary to lead play activities. This will demonstrate that nurses view play as being important, and that they believe that supervising finger painting is as important a duty for an aide as straightening beds, or that organizing a puppet show for long-term clients is as important a duty for a nurse as giving a bed bath. If play is considered a luxury or an activity that is provided only after all the other things are done, there will never be time for it. If it is included in nursing care plans, finger painting becomes as important for a child as going to physical therapy. That is reality; in terms of mental health, it is just as important. A clear sign that the nurses on a particular children's unit understand little about their young patients' needs is a locked playroom door and the explanation, "We have no one to staff it."

Safety With Play

Be certain to screen all toys for safety: no sharp edges and no small parts that could be swallowed or aspirated.

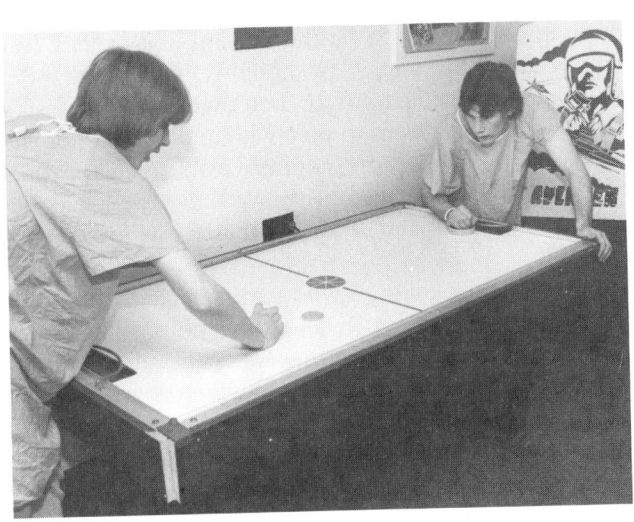

FIGURE 35-9
A lounge for adolescents is comfortable and set apart from the play area for smaller children. (Courtesy of the Department of Medical Photography, Children's Hospital, Buffalo, NY.)

A cylinder 1 inch in diameter, such as a rubber hot dog, is the most dangerous size for a toy because it totally occludes the trachea if it is aspirated. A toy smaller than this would only partially cause obstruction; something larger would not be inhaled into the trachea.

Be certain that a toy will not lead a child into danger. Tossing a ball generally is a safe activity for a toddler. One who has a large cast in place, however, might lean over to retrieve a dropped ball and fall out of bed.

If children become bored with a toy because it is not stimulating enough or they have had it for too long a time, they may begin to use the toy in an unsafe way. After a toddler grows tired of stacking blocks, for example, he or she may begin to throw them or, if the child is in an oxygen tent, drop them down the oxygen inlet pipe. Children who normally play safely with modeling clay but who are on a restricted diet may eat it because they are hungry. Knowing where children are and what activity they are engaged in at all times is the best prevention against unsafe play.

Child Life Programs

A child life department is currently an integral feature of a children's hospital. A child life specialist is one who can offer children the opportunity to reenact and thereby master the anxiety associated with hospitalization. Through therapeutic play, child life specialists provide programs that prepare children for hospitalization, and once hospitalized, prepare children for surgery or for procedures that could be painful. These specialists help children air their frustration about painful or intrusive procedures, prevent social isolation of children by means of an active recreation program, and ensure that the total environment of the hospital is conducive to children's well-being.

Such a program not only aids in promoting children's mental health but leads to more cooperative responses of children to treatments or procedures. It is complementary to play programs initiated by nurses.

Therapeutic Play

Any occurrence almost automatically becomes less threatening when a person can talk about it. Many children are unable to talk about what is happening to them during a hospital experience because of fear or because their vocabulary is so limited that they are unable to describe their feelings.

Because play is the language of children, children who have difficulty voicing their thoughts in words can often speak clearly through play. **Play therapy** is a psychoanalytic technique used by psychiatrists to help children understand their feelings and thoughts and motivations better. **Therapeutic play** is a *play technique* used by a play therapist or nurse to better understand children's feelings and thoughts. In play therapy, a therapist attempts to interpret both the child's verbal and nonverbal cues. Interpreting nonverbal cues and helping the child understand them requires the skill of a psychiatric nurse-clinician or others with specialized training. This level of expertise is not necessary to respond to *verbal* cues, however, so that is the purpose and the nursing role in therapeutic play. Therapeutic play can be divided into three types: (1) energy release, (2) dramatic play, and (3) creative play.

Energy Release

Any time people are anxious, action feels good. Children release anxiety by pounding, hitting, running, punching, or shouting. Furnishing children with materials helps them release anxiety in a hospital setting. Toddlers might pound pegs with a plastic hammer or pretend to cut wood with a toy saw. Other examples include modeling clay for a preschooler (an anxious child often pounds it flat; a relaxed child, however, will build it into shapes) and a balloon tied to an overbed trapeze for a school-age child or adolescent to punch.

Dramatic Play

Dramatic play is acting out an anxiety situation. It is most effective with preschool children because they are at the peak of imagination. In a hospital setting the situations about which children need to express feelings are hospital related, and therefore the equipment needed for therapeutic play is common hospital equipment: dolls, doll beds, play stethoscopes, intravenous equipment, syringes, masks, and gowns. Puppets of doctors, nurses, mothers, fathers, and children help young children express their feelings. Anatomically correct dolls are used to help children describe their feelings about sexual abuse.

It is good to have a play session with a child near the beginning of his or her hospitalization to see if the child communicates through play any fears concerning this experience. This initial session also serves as a way of preparing the child for events that will occur during the hospitalization (Figure 35-10). A play session should be repeated after any painful or traumatic procedure such as surgery so that the child can express new feelings. A list of procedures that fall into this category is shown in Table 35-6. If such play sessions reveal fears, a child should be scheduled for other play sessions, perhaps one daily during a hospital stay.

Furnish children with a wide range of hospital equipment and then let them choose those items with which they wish to play.

Children invariably choose a piece of equipment that has been used with them. They poke at a doll with a syringe or enjoy giving it a "shot." They wrap the doll in bandages or put tubes into its mouth or stomach, acting out things that were done to them or that they saw

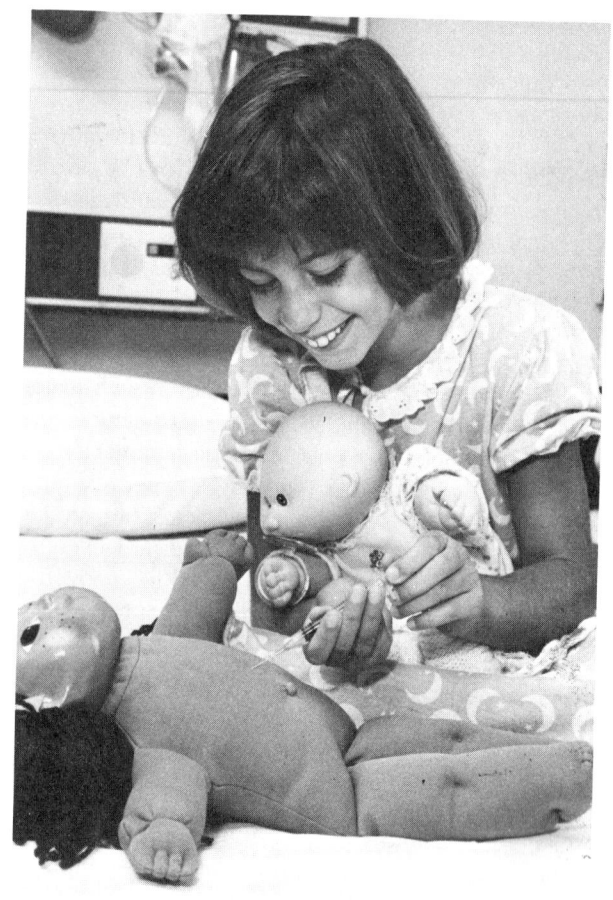

FIGURE 35-10
Therapeutic play allows children the opportunity to voice their fears of painful procedures. Notice the obvious delight a young girl takes in giving a doll a "shot." (Courtesy of the Department of Medical Photography, Children's Hospital, Buffalo, NY.)

done to other children on the nursing unit or they fear will be done to them. Play should be nondirective (let the child proceed at his or her own pace, choosing freely what equipment to play with and what he or she wants to do with the equipment). As a child works through an experience this way, the experience becomes less fearful and he or she masters increased control of it.

Observe for children who may be using equipment in an unusual way, such as hitting dolls with stethoscopes or poking them in the eye with a thermometer (suggesting they are confused about the purpose of such equipment). Such behavior alerts health care providers to the importance of explaining the purpose of equipment to children. Listen to what children say as they play. A comment such as "I'm giving shots to all the bad dolls" suggests the child thinks injections are punishment. It would be important to stress the next time the child needs an injection that medicine is to make the child feel well again. A comment such as "This doll is going to surgery so you won't have her anymore" could suggest the child thinks she will not return from surgery (she may have heard a family member describe someone who died following surgery and is asking for reassurance that such a thing is not going to happen to her). Do not be surprised about the force with which children insert nasogastric tubes into dolls. In part, this reflects how they perceive these procedures, but it also represents energy or anxiety release, in the way that pounding or hitting releases anger.

To better understand how the child feels, repeat what the child says verbally: "You're giving the bad dolls shots?" or ask the child to tell you more about what he or she said: "Do you think that's the only kind of children who get shots? Bad children?" Don't rush to reassure ("Don't worry—that isn't going to happen to you"). Quick reassurance rather than being reassuring tells the child that he or she should not ask any more questions or that the topic is not open for discussion.

Sometimes even children who seem well prepared may be taken by surprise during a procedure. For example, 7-year-old Becky, admitted for a diagnostic work-up following a urinary tract infection, showed little interest in dolls and syringes and tubing. She had been prepared by her mother for the experience and seemed to understand what would happen during various x-ray procedures. After returning from the x-ray room where she had a voiding cystourethrogram, however, she was obviously upset, although she denied that anything about the procedure had upset her. Her nurse brought her a rag doll, a doctor and a nurse figure, a play x-ray machine, and some tubing that could simulate a urinary catheter and encouraged Becky to play with them. Becky picked up the girl doll and put her under the x-ray machine. She imitated the doctor doll shouting, "Pee in front of everybody!" Becky's mother had not realized that she would have to void during a cysto-

Table 35-6. *Therapeutic Play Techniques for Children After Procedures*

Procedure	Play Activity
Radiograph	Provide a doll and table and box labeled "x-ray machine"; children sometimes worry that x-rays have injured them the same as laser rays in science fiction shows do.
Blood drawing .	Provide a doll and syringe, alcohol wipes, tourniquet, or finger lancets; remember that finger pricks are as frightening for children as are needles.
Clean-catch urine	Provide a doll (anatomically correct), alcohol wipes, and a collection cup; children are often more embarrassed by urine collection than adults realize.
Intravenous therapy	Provide a doll with intravenous tubing, as well as restraints and armboard; some children are as angry about being restrained as having the needle inserted.
Bronchograms, cystograms, and so forth	Provide a doll and catheters or a penlight to simulate a scope.
Scans	Scans usually require the intravenous injection of isotopes; provide a doll and intravenous fluid and tubing.
Bone marrow	Provide a doll, alcohol wipes, syringe.
Electroencephalogram, electrocardiogram	Provide a doll and electrode leads that attach to a box; children might be afraid of these procedures because of their fear of electricity.
Surgery	Provide a doll, an anesthesia mask, and a blunt kitchen knife; watch and listen for where the child cuts and how he or she describes the experience.
Dental examination	Provide a doll, a suction catheter, a penlight to simulate a drill, and a 4 × 4 piece of plastic; some children are angered by the use of plastic in their mouth.
Dressing changes	Provide a doll, gauze, and adhesive tape.
Cast application or removal	Provide plaster to soak and apply; simulate a cast cutter with an electric razor or hair dryer.
Nasogastric tube, enema, catheterization	Provide a doll and tubes.
Temperature taking	Provide a doll and thermometer.

urethrogram. Becky felt betrayed by not being really prepared for this embarrassing situation. Her play brought her emotion out in the open where it could be talked about and handled. When Becky was scheduled the next day for ureteral reflux surgery, her nurse was alerted to make the preparation absolutely thorough.

Children older than 9 and 10 years find playing with dolls too childish to be of benefit. They enjoy handling syringes, however, and being able to see and handle such equipment as nasogastric tubes in advance of their being placed. Active handling helps to eliminate fear because it identifies exactly what the child has to face.

Creative Play

Some children are too angry to be able to act out their feelings through dramatic play. However, they may be able to draw a picture that expresses their emotions or conveys the extent of their knowledge (Wilson et al., 1990). To encourage this, give a child a blank paper and crayons or markers. If a child seems reluctant to draw something spontaneously, suggest a topic: "Why don't you draw a picture of yourself?"

Some children are so concerned with particular parts of their bodies that when asked to draw pictures of themselves, they draw only the body parts about which they are worried. Such a child generally is saying that he or she needs to talk about that part of the body, to be given reassurance that it is going to be all right. Figure 35-11*A* shows a picture drawn by a 9-year-old who was admitted to the hospital for débridement of a campfire burn on her left foot. She stated on admission that she was being admitted to have the burn on her foot "cleaned out." This sounds like a child who understands what débridement involves. Note, however, that the

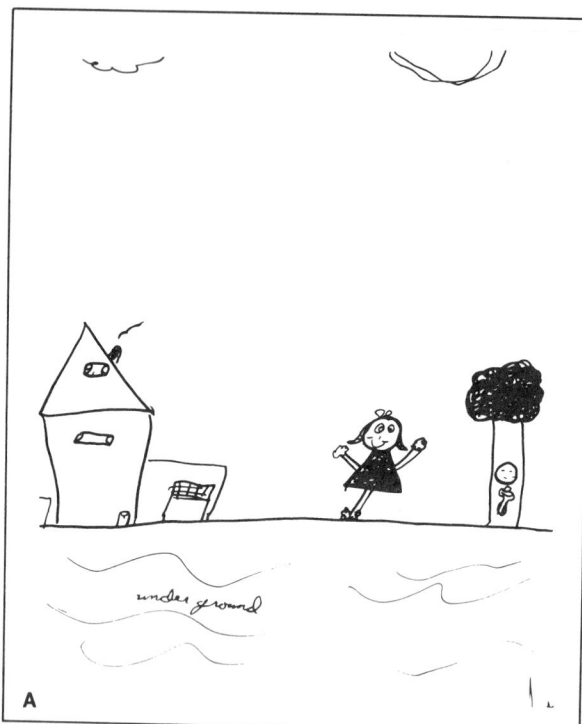
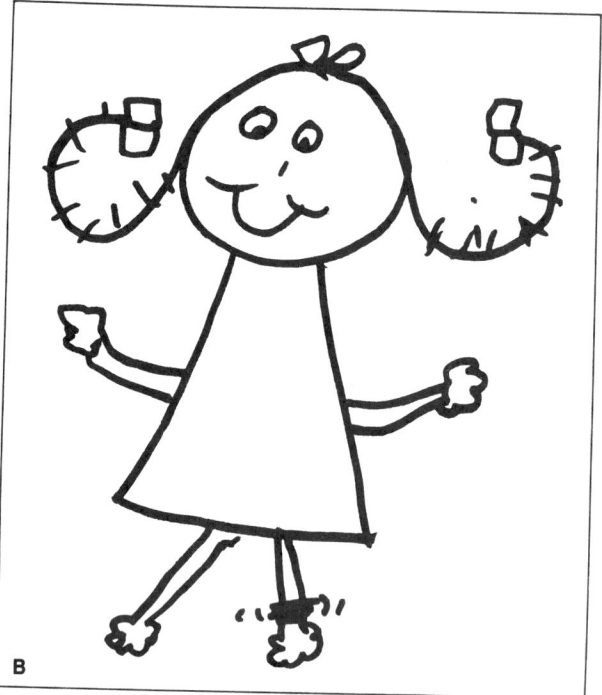

FIGURE 35-11

(**A**) *Children who are concerned about body parts may draw pictures with that part missing or exaggerated. Note the missing left leg here.* (**B**) *After reassurance that her leg will be all right, the girl who did the drawing in **A** now draws a girl with two legs.*

figure she drew has no left leg. One has to wonder whether she was concerned that she was going to surgery to have more than débridement. After the word *débridement* was explained to her, she drew the picture in Figure 35-11*B*. The child in the drawing now has a left and a right leg, the left leg covered by a bandage. Through a drawing, this child was able to say something she could not express without this help.

Many children in a hospital draw pictures that reflect punitive images: a boy or girl tied to a bed or shut behind bars, doctors and nurses frowning at them, obviously unhappy with them. Such children may need assurance that they are not hospitalized because they are being punished; they are in the hospital to be made well (Figure 35-12). Other children draw pictures that are symbolic of death: airplanes crashing, boats sinking, buildings on fire, children in graveyards. They need assurance that they will not die.

Preschoolers are usually filled with fear of abandonment and mutilation. They may draw a child in one corner of a picture and an adult in a far corner. They may comment that the parent cannot find the little child. They need to be reassured that their parents know where they are and will visit them after work.

Older school-age children and adolescents may not be interested in drawing but can be interested in making a list of procedures or experiences they like and dislike.

Examine the dislike list for hospital procedures such as "shots" or "chemo." Mark the nursing care plan for nurses to take special time to explain these procedures and to offer special support when they must be done.

Guidelines for Conducting Therapeutic Play

It is important to use common sense when conducting therapeutic play. Be certain not to interpret a child's

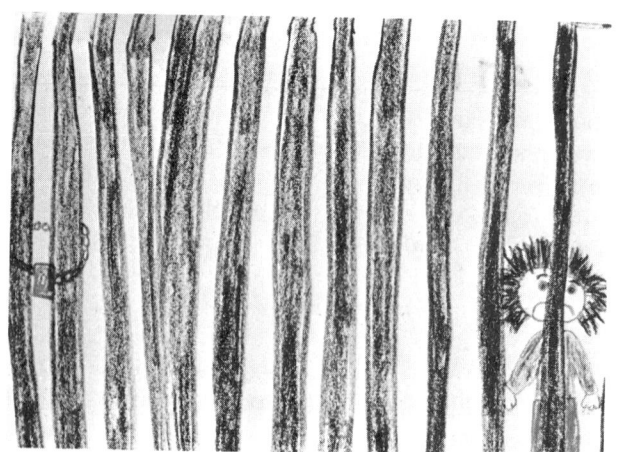

FIGURE 35-12

A picture drawn by a hospitalized child. Note the prison-like appearance of the crib. (Courtesy of Rita Crever.)

Box 35-4
Guidelines for Therapeutic Play

1. Allow a child to choose the articles with which he or she wants to play (something may be too frightening for a child to play with immediately; he or she needs time to work up to the activity).
2. Provide the materials specific to the child's experiences of which you, the nurse, are aware (e.g., nasogastric tube, syringe, or bandages), but do not supply only those things; a child may have misunderstandings and fears of situations you cannot know about.
3. Allow play to be unstructured or let the child use the materials however he or she wishes. If a child seems uninterested in materials, then begin to play with her (e.g., give a doll an injection) to see if this reduces her anxiety enough to be able to handle items.
4. If a child cannot manipulate materials himself (due to such things as a cast or traction), ask the child what he would like you to do with it.
5. Reflect only what the child expresses (verbal expression).
6. Do not criticize play; this inhibits further expression.
7. Use a therapeutic response, not "Don't worry, that won't happen," but "Are you worried that could happen?"
8. Ask children to describe paintings, not "That's a good picture of yourself," but "Tell me about your picture."
9. Do not be reluctant to use real equipment (e.g., real catheters and blood lancets). Handling real equipment best helps to reduce stress.
10. Supervise the therapeutic play, because some equipment could cause an accident (and therapeutically responding to the child's comments is necessary).

---

black and gloomy drawing as meaning the child is depressed when a black marker was the only one available. Many children 4 to 5 years of age draw a person lacking many body parts because that is the best human form they can draw. Many children younger than 6 years are unable to draw people with more than three body parts.

Remember, too, that all children occasionally treat dolls badly. A 2-year-old pounding and banging a rag doll may not be expressing anger toward the doll image at all, but may be intent on discovering the feel of a new texture and is unaware for the moment that the object is a doll.

A conference with health care team members, including the hospital psychologist or a psychiatric nurse specialist, may be called for if a child continues to express mutilating behavior after normal reassurance. Guidelines for conducting therapeutic play are summarized in Box 35-4.

Key Points

- Hospitalization may be more traumatic for children than for adults because of their inability to communicate and monitor their own care and because they have different nutritional, fluid, and electrolyte needs.
- Separation from parents can have permanent psychological effects on children. Methods to reduce this include keeping hospital stays as brief as possible, promoting open parent and sibling visiting, and providing primary or care management nursing.
- Preschoolers may have the most difficult time during a hospital experience because they have so many fears. Preparation and promotion of therapeutic play are essential to reduce trauma to a tolerable level.
- Currently, many medical procedures can be done on an ambulatory basis. Advocating for care to be done in such settings is a nursing responsibility.
- The presence of parents during health care can help reduce trauma to children. Making parents as welcome as possible makes it possible for them to room in. Include the parents in both the planning and implementation of care. Parents reinfect children with fear if their own fear is not reduced.
- Because hospitalizations currently are so brief, parents need good discharge instructions to continue to care for children safely at home. Providing clear instructions and danger signs for parents to watch for are nursing responsibilities.

Critical Thinking Exercises

1. Devon is a 3-year-old who had emergency surgery while on vacation with her single mother. Her mother has returned home because of work responsibilities, so Devon will have no family with her for a week. What measures could you take to help make hospitalization and separation less traumatic for her?

2. The administrator of a hospital has asked you to help plan a playroom on a hospital unit for toddlers and preschoolers. What toys would you suggest?

3. Many people suggest that children be allowed to play with syringes with actual needles attached. How do you feel about this? What would be some of the advantages and disadvantages?

References

Ahmann, E. (1994). Family-centered care: the time has come. *Pediatric Nursing, 20,* 52.

Bowlby, J., et al. (1966). *Maternal care and mental health.* New York: Schocken Books.

Department of Health & Human Services. (1991). *Healthy people 2000.* Washington, DC: Public Health Service.

Dolan, A. (1993). A day in the life of a hospital play specialist. *British Journal of Theatre Nursing, 3,* 31.

Heuer, L. (1993). Parental stressors in a pediatric intensive care unit. *Pediatric Nursing, 19,* 128.

Hickey, P. A., & Rykerson, S. (1992). Caring for parents of critically ill infants and children. *Critical Care Nursing Clinics of North America, 4,* 565.

LeVieux-Anglin, L., & Sawyer, E. H. (1993). Incorporating play interventions into nursing care. *Pediatric Nursing, 19,* 459.

Ogilvie, L. (1990). Hospitalization of children for surgery: The parent's view. *Children's Health Care, 19,* 49.

Perrin, E. C., & Gerrity, P. S. (1981). There's a demon in your belly: Children's understanding of illness. *Pediatrics, 67,* 841.

Prugh, D. G., et al. (1953). A study of the emotional responses of children and families to hospitalization and illness. *American Journal of Orthopsychiatry, 23,* 70.

Robbins, M. (1991). Sharing the care . . . family centered care in the paediatric ward. *Nursing Times, 87,* 36.

Robertson, J. (1958). *Young children in hospitals.* London: Tavistock.

Spitz, R. A. (1945). Hospitalism: An inquiry into the genesis of psychiatric conditions in early childhood. *Psychoanalytic Study of the Child, 1,* 53.

Vessey, J. A., et al. (1990). Teaching children about their internal bodies. *Pediatric Nursing, 16,* 29.

Wadsworth, B. J. (1989). *Piaget's theory of cognitive and affective development.* New York: Longman.

Wilson, D., et al. (1990). An introduction to using children's drawings as an assessment tool. *Nurse Practitioner, 15,* 23.

Suggested Readings

Adams, J., et al. (1991). Child health; reducing fear in hospital. *Nursing Times, 87,* 62.

Alcock, D., et al. (1990). Parents of long-stay children. *Canadian Nurse, 86,* 20.

Brown, J., et al. (1990). Nurses' perceptions of parent and nurse role in caring for hospitalized children. *Children's Health Care, 19,* 28.

Gillis, A. J. (1990). Hospitalized preparation: The children's story. *Children's Health Care, 19,* 19.

Graves, J. K., et al. (1990). Parents' and health professionals' perceptions concerning parental stress during a child's hospitalization. *Children's Health Care, 19,* 37.

LaMontagne, L. L., et al. (1992). Parental coping and activities during pediatric critical care. *American Journal of Critical Care, 1,* 76.

Nehring, W. M. (1994). The nurse whose specialty is developmental disabilities. *Pediatric Nursing, 20,* 78.

Palmer, S. J. (1993). Care of sick children by parents: a meaningful role. *Journal of Advanced Nursing, 18,* 185.

Sadler, C. (1990). Child's play: Play for children in hospital. *Nursing Times, 86,* 16.

Youngblut, J. M., et al. (1993). Child and family reactions during and after pediatric ICU hospitalization: a pilot study. *Heart Lung, 22,* 46.

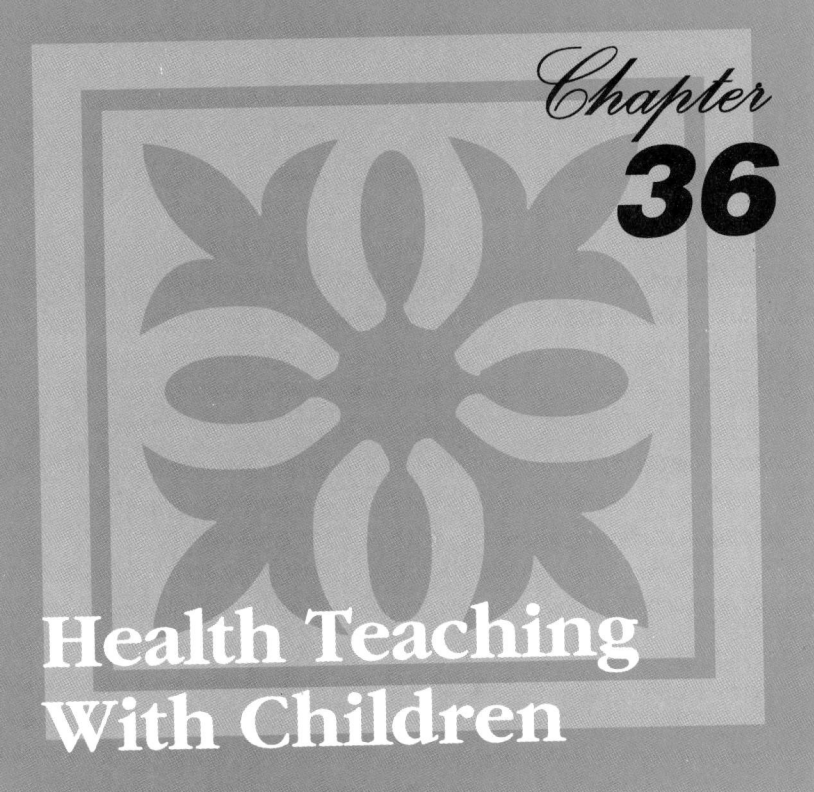

Chapter 36

Health Teaching With Children

Key Terms

- *affective learning*
- *behavior modification*
- *cognitive learning*
- *demonstration*
- *positive reinforcement*
- *psychomotor learning*
- *redemonstration*
- *teaching plan*

Objectives

After mastering the contents of this chapter, you should be able to:

1. *Describe principles of teaching and learning and their specific application to health teaching with children.*

2. *Assess children for their readiness to learn.*

3. *State nursing diagnoses related to health teaching and children.*

4. *Establish health teaching priorities for a specific child based on the child's age, developmental maturity, emotional needs, and learning style.*

5. *Implement health teaching (e.g., devising a puppet show) using principles of teaching-learning.*

6. *Evaluate outcome criteria to be certain that nursing goals established for care have been achieved.*

7. *Identify National Health Goals related to teaching and children that nurses could be instrumental in helping the nation achieve.*

8. *Identify areas of care related to health teaching of children that could benefit from additional nursing research.*

9. *Use critical thinking to analyze ways that health teaching can be further incorporated into the nursing care of children and families.*

10. *Synthesize knowledge of teaching-learning with the nursing process to achieve quality maternal and child health nursing care.*

Adele Pillitteri: MATERNAL AND CHILD HEALTH NURSING, 2nd Edition. © 1995 Adele Pillitteri.

H ealth teaching is an independent nursing action that accompanies all nursing care. It is probably the most frequently used intervention for nurses working with child-bearing and childrearing families for whom health promotion is such a priority. Health teaching is as important as any intervention for families experiencing some type of illness or injury; it is especially important when preparing a child for surgery or some other medical procedure. New areas that require teaching are constantly arising (Beier et al., 1993).

Health teaching may be offered to an individual or to a group of children with similar learning needs. It is offered both formally (e.g., teaching a group of pre-schoolers about hospitalization) and informally (e.g., when a nurse assures a parent that his or her child is getting enough nutrition, even though the child snacks rather than sits down to regular meals). The same principles of effective teaching and learning apply whether teaching is informal or formal, or offered to an individual or to a group. National Health Goals regarding health teaching and children are shown in the Focus on National Health Goals display.

☒ **NURSING PROCESS OVERVIEW**
for Health Teaching

ASSESSMENT

Although health teaching in itself is a nursing intervention, it cannot be effectively accomplished unless it is placed within the context of the nursing process. Learner needs and characteristics that will affect learning, such as learning style, must be assessed to formulate nursing diagnoses that clearly state the specific health needs that teaching will address.

NURSING DIAGNOSIS

The following are examples of common nursing diagnoses related to health teaching:

* Knowledge deficit related to importance of taking medicine daily
* Health-seeking behaviors related to ways to minimize stress
* Anxiety related to perceived amount of material needed to be learned for home care of child

PLANNING

After formulation of a nursing diagnosis, an individualized teaching plan is constructed. A plan should detail not only what is to be learned but also methods that will be used for teaching and evaluation.

IMPLEMENTATION

The step of implementation involves the actual teaching of the plan. Teaching children is not always easy and requires practice and knowledge of a child's particular developmental level.

EVALUATION

As a final step of teaching, what was learned is evaluated. A new plan may need to be developed to continue teaching if learning was less than optimal. These are examples of outcome criteria:

- Child demonstrates self-injection of insulin.
- Child lists foods to include in a high-protein diet.
- Parents demonstrate effective cardiopulmonary resuscitation technique at home visit.

The Art of Teaching

Teaching is more than presenting information; it is presenting information to increase someone's knowledge or insight. Before teaching can be considered effective, learning has to have occurred. Conversely, before learning occurs, teaching must have occurred in some form (Figure 36-1). Common principles of teaching are summarized in Table 36-1.

Types of Teaching

Formal Versus Informal Teaching
A successful health educator needs to be able to do both formal and informal teaching. Telling children who insist they are not hungry that their body needs more fluid,

FOCUS ON
National Health Goals

A number of National Health Goals address health teaching, because it is such an important mechanism of preventive health care. These include:

- Increase to at least 75% the proportion of the nation's elementary and secondary schools that provide planned and sequential quality school health education for kindergarten through 12th grade.

- Increase to at least 50% the proportion of counties that have established culturally and linguistically appropriate community health promotion programs for racial and ethnic minority populations.

- Increase to at least 90% the proportion of hospitals, health maintenance organizations, and large group practices that provide patient education programs, and to at least 90% the proportion of community hospitals that offer community health promotion programs addressing the priority health needs of their communities (DHHS, 1991).

Nurses can be instrumental in helping the nation achieve these goals by consulting with schools and health care organizations to develop health teaching programs and by teaching such programs. Areas that could benefit from nursing research include ways in which busy health care providers can better incorporate health teaching into care; what special techniques are needed to be certain that minority populations are addressed; and whether different teaching techniques are necessary for material with immediate application than for material for long-term care.

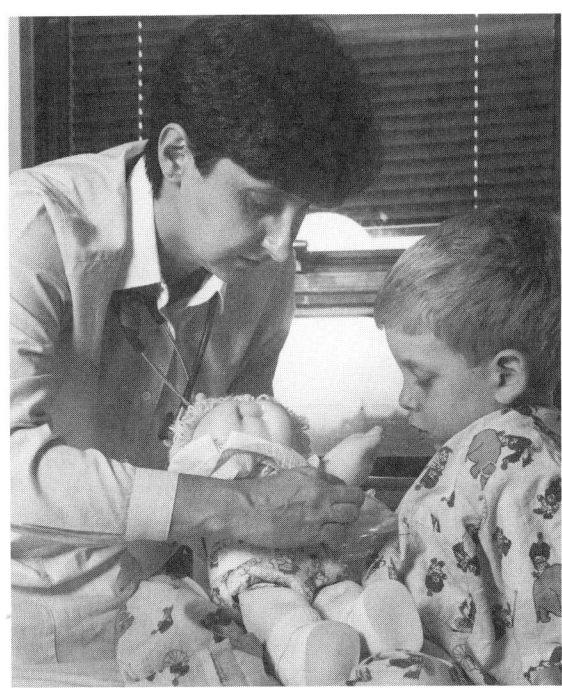

FIGURE 36-1
Health teaching is a major nursing intervention with children. Here a child learns how a colostomy appliance will look. (Courtesy of the Department of Medical Photography, Children's Hospital, Buffalo, NY.)

Table 36-1. *Principles of Teaching*	
Principle	**Rationale**
Know the subject.	To effectively teach children, you must be able not only to present material but also to answer questions about it. Children's questions can be as probing as an adult's and they can often be more frequent, because children are used to asking questions of a teacher or a parent.
Know the audience.	Children vary a great deal in cognitive development depending on their age group. To teach preschoolers about health, you might choose to teach how to brush teeth using puppets as a teaching aid. The same clever puppet and tooth brushing presentation likely would not be well received among adolescents, however.
Know yourself.	Analyze which teaching techniques (lecture, role playing, small group discussion, audiovisual aids) fit your teaching style. Using techniques that are comfortable allows teaching to be most effective.
Assess individual learning styles.	Most children respond well to visual images (seeing a demonstration or drawing) to complement learning. Assessing individual learning styles helps to meet each child's best way of learning.
Define teaching goals.	Teaching goals serve as guidelines to help you select from all you know about a subject that part which is most pertinent to an individual child. Instruction on how to walk using crutches for an early school-age child would include how to carry school books while using crutches; for an adolescent, instruction would include how to board a city bus so he or she could get to and from a part-time job.
Provide an environment conducive for learning.	Children are easily distracted from learning because of so many new experiences in their world. Divide material into segments to keep teaching sessions short; avoid competing factors such as television or mealtime.
Be consistent.	Nothing is more confusing to a person learning something for the first time than to be told two different ways to do it. Choose one method that should work best for a child and then consistently stress that method. After a child has learned the one method, then suggest alternative methods if the child is interested.
Be honest.	Abstract concepts such as "little white lies" cannot be understood by children younger than adolescents.
Recognize that actions teach as much as verbal statements.	Children watch facial expressions and nonverbal gestures as much as they listen. Be certain that a nonverbal statement is not contradicting a verbal one.
Teach from the simple to the complex.	Fundamentals must be grasped before extensive learning can proceed. Many children have little idea of body anatomy. Often you need to begin with the basics; when these are mastered, you can proceed to teach about a disease condition.
Teach principles.	Teaching a child the principle behind why he or she is doing something gives the child reason to do it. It expands learning in that it allows the child to modify and change to an alternative method as long as the principle is fulfilled.
Teach what the child should do, not what the child should not do.	Teaching from a positive standpoint makes learning more enjoyable. Because health care information should last a lifetime, thinking of it in a positive way makes it applicable to lifetime use.
Include evaluation as a final step.	The only way to determine the effectiveness of teaching is to test or evaluate if learning has occurred. Structure the time and method of evaluation when first establishing a teaching plan.

and that if they would at least try to drink something it would help them get better, is an example of informal teaching.

Be careful not to equate informal teaching with disorganized, or unnecessary, teaching. It is just as important as formal teaching; it is just communicated in a less structured way. Informal teaching requires that teaching and learning principles (i.e., know the subject, recognize

individual learning styles, provide an effective environment, limit time span, and so forth) are followed, just as with more formal teaching. Sometimes informal teaching occurs so spontaneously that it is easy to be unaware of it. It may occur, for example, in response to a question such as "How long will I have to take this medicine?" If a nurse answers, "For 2 weeks," he or she is just answering a question. If the nurse says, "For 2 weeks because . . ." he or she is teaching. Helping a postoperative child to do deep breathing is performing a psychomotor skill. Telling a child why it is important to do the deep breathing is teaching. Careful assessment is necessary to determine whether formal or informal teaching would be the best technique for a given situation (Good-Reis et al., 1990). Table 36-2 lists ways to incorporate informal teaching into care.

Group Teaching

Although most health teaching is done on an individual basis, teaching groups of children is common in some situations. Group teaching is more economical than individual instruction and can add depth to learning as children discuss information within the group. Childbirth preparation classes for adolescents are usually taught in groups, because it is as helpful to hear fellow adolescents share their experiences or concerns as it is to hear a nurse point out the stages of birth.

Consider the following four important guidelines when group teaching: (1) assess for common interests and goals in order for information to appeal to as many in the group as possible; (2) be certain all members of a group can see and hear all others; (3) encourage all members of the group to participate in discussions by calling on them if necessary; and (4) limit any one person from dominating the group by a statement such as "That's a good point, Reneé. Has anyone else had a similar experience?"

Behavior Modification

Typically, learning occurs best with **positive reinforcement** (a child tries to understand a new procedure, is praised for the effort, and tries even harder). **Behavior modification** is a term used for a system aimed at *erasing* some form of behavior that interferes with health functioning. It was originally designed to help mentally ill people erase socially unacceptable behavior; currently, it has many uses, including controlling disruptive classroom behavior. The basic premise of behavior modification is that the child is rewarded for healthful behavior, whereas unhealthful behavior is ignored or unrewarded. A mentally retarded child may have a socially unacceptable habit of constantly rocking back and forth.

Table 36-2. *Ways to Incorporate Teaching Into Care*

Activity	Type of Teaching
Medication administration	Children as young as early school age should know the type and action and any expected side-effects of all medication they are taking. Present medicine not by saying, "Here is your pill" but "Here is your [name of medication], medicine to help your temperature come back to normal. After you take this, you might feel yourself start to sweat."
Vital sign measurement	When taking vital signs such as blood pressure, temperature, and pulse, tell children what normal levels are: "Your blood pressure is 100/70. That's normal."
Any procedure	Always tell children the purpose and principle of procedures, not "You need to drink a lot of fluid," but "You need to drink a lot of fluid because . . ."
Dressing changes	Dressing changes provide an opportunity to teach the danger of introducing infection into an open wound. The parents or child may not change this dressing, but they will apply many adhesive bandages to small cuts and will benefit from teaching.
Mealtime	Provide information about nutrition: "I know you're not hungry enough to eat the entire sandwich, but could you try the meat? Meat is high in protein and that's important for healing."
Hygiene	Emphasize the necessity of good perineal hygiene to decrease the possibility of urinary tract infection.
Physical assessment	Explain aspects of self-breast or self-testicular examination and describe "normal" findings as both education and reassurance.
Positioning	Teach the hazards of immobility and how change of position and ambulation increase circulation and respiratory function.
Sleep	Teach that sleep is a healing therapy and should not be considered a waste of time.
Bowel elimination	Many adults are concerned about their intestinal elimination pattern, because they do not appreciate that their pattern is normal. Teach children that elimination patterns vary; there is a wide range of "normal."

The child is not scolded or criticized for rocking, but the action is ignored. On the other hand, preferred behavior (sitting for 15 minutes without rocking) is praised. As another example, a child might be ignored while biting her fingernails, then praised for not biting them for an hour. Children respond best to behavior modification if, in addition to praise, they receive a tangible reward such as a star on a chart or an extra privilege of some sort for good behavior.

A behavior modification program must be discussed with the child before it is begun, because no behavior can be modified, just as no new behavior can be learned, until the child truly wants a change to occur. It might be necessary to ask the child to sign a learning contract to be certain that both teacher and learner agree on the method to be used. Many older children are able to use self-rewards to reinforce a behavior modification program (e.g., rewarding themselves with a novel or movie for an afternoon of efficient studying or an hour of doing breathing exercises).

Behavior modification is a technique that must be used with common sense and concern so that children are not being manipulated more than they are being helped to achieve a more healthful lifestyle. It is a legitimate device to use in helping an overactive child sit still long enough to eat a meal or learn in school. It can be helpful in encouraging children to do as much self-care as possible.

Trying to modify beliefs or values by behavior modification is unethical and a reason that behavior modification is often criticized as a learning technique. It is a learning technique to be familiar with, however, because it does apply to health education in limited spheres.

Teaching in the Home

Client teaching is just as important in the home as it is in health care agency settings. Teaching in the home may focus on medication regimens, dressing changes, or measures to prevent complications of a particular illness. It may also involve helping a child and parents adapt a procedure to the home setting, such as accommodating a wheelchair at home. Be certain that parents have obtained the necessary supplies for the procedure they need to learn. Always include evaluation as a step of teaching so the child can feel confident that the procedure was successfully adapted to the home environment.

Teaching in the home offers the advantage of being able to assess the child's environment, interactions with other family members, and overall family functioning. This may yield data that will prove useful to further planning and implementation of care. It may also provide an opportunity to include other family members—siblings, grandparents, and so forth—in the teaching plan, which will strengthen the impact of teaching and ensure that all family members understand procedures in the same way.

The Art of Learning

Learning is a two-step process involving both the acquisition of knowledge and a change in behavior based on the new knowledge. Learning has not really occurred unless the change in behavior is measurable. For example, a parent teaching a child about the need to brush teeth daily must not only elicit the child's statement that daily brushing is important but also watch that the child is, in fact, brushing her teeth every day. If the topic is abstract, such as helping a child change a concept of chronic illness, change can still be measured (the child talks about the illness or begins to take action to prevent complications). Principles of learning are summarized in Table 36-3.

Types of Learning

There are many types of learning. Learning the mathematical formula necessary to determine the height of a triangle, for example, is different from learning how to skateboard. Learning to be kind to animals is yet another type. Before teaching can begin, it is important to analyze the type of learning desired. This will help in setting goals and designing teaching strategies.

Cognitive Learning

Cognitive learning involves a change in the individual's level of understanding or knowledge. Learning the principle behind why a particular medicine must be injected into a muscle, as opposed to subcutaneous tissue, is cognitive learning. Cognitive learning requires adequate development, intelligence, and attention span. It can be gained through exposure to any teaching technique but is usually learned through lecture, reading, and audiovisual aids. Techniques for teaching when cognitive learning is the goal must be based on the learner's cognitive ability. During the school-age years, learning capability is concrete (a child has difficulty picturing body parts functioning unless he or she actually sees them doing this); during the adolescent years, it becomes possible to learn abstract concepts (a child can accept that liver enzymes are released with liver damage even though he or she never sees this occur).

Psychomotor Learning

Psychomotor learning requires a change in an individual's ability to perform a skill. Learning to hold a syringe, draw up medicine, and inject it into muscle is an example of psychomotor learning. Acquiring psychomotor skills depends on muscle and neurologic coordination. It is mastered best through demonstration and redemonstration.

Affective Learning

Affective learning involves a change in a person's attitude. It is the most difficult area in which to bring about

Table 36-3. Principles of Learning

Principle	Rationale
Learning occurs best when a child is ready to learn.	Interferences with learning may be physical (e.g., pain or hunger) or psychologic (e.g., fear or anxiety). The first time a child is told that he or she must inject insulin daily, for example, the child may be too anxious to learn about it.
Learning occurs most quickly if the child can see how the new information will benefit him or her.	Sixteen-year-olds learn how to drive a car quickly because they grasp readily that being able to drive will immediately enlarge their world. A child is not ready to learn insulin injections until he or she can see an advantage of giving them. Make a habit of including the benefit of learning in the introduction of learning.
Learning occurs best if rewards, not penalties, are offered.	Notice the amount of shoulder patting and back slapping that high school coaches engage in (rewarding by praise). Giving positive reinforcement immediately like this makes it more effective than if such reinforcement is delayed. If you must criticize the way a task was done, first compliment the child on some aspect he or she did well and then explain the part that needs improvement. This increases self-esteem and allows the child to feel good enough about himself or herself so that the child can accept the criticism. Never be reluctant to praise in public; always criticize in private.
Children learn best by actively participating in learning.	Active participation requires involvement in learning. Ask questions to involve participation; allow children to touch and handle equipment to increase participation.
Learning occurs best in a nonstressful and accepting environment.	No one wants to take a chance redemonstrating a procedure or asking a question if he or she feels that actions or opinions will not be respected. People do learn from "top sergeants," but the learning experience has so many unpleasant memories attached to it that they do not retain the learning. Health teaching is too important to be presented in a way that will lead to its being quickly discarded.
Children learn best those things that hold a particular interest for them.	Everyone is more interested in something than others. A child with diabetes mellitus who enjoys dancing might be most interested in learning regulation of insulin for exercise; a child anxious to leave for college might be most interested in selecting a diabetic diet from a cafeteria.
Learning ability plateaus.	Children learn to the point of saturation; learning and interest in learning halts at that point and does not continue until the material learned is thoroughly digested and understood. Wait until information is processed and at that point the child will be interested once more.

change. To successfully teach a child the reason for and the skill of giving a self-injection, for example, may be easy; teaching the child to *like* giving a self-injection may never be possible. Affective learning is gained best though role modeling, role-playing, or shared-experience discussion.

Influence of Age and Stage on Ability to Learn

Infant

An infant learns by exploring the environment with his or her senses. The infant learns best from his or her primary caregiver because that is whom the infant most wants to please. Few health care points are taught at this age. Any that are taught must be presented not as a structured activity but as a game or an amusing or attractive activity for the child. An infant could be taught to exercise a leg by showing the child how to kick a balloon tied to a crib rail or rolling a ball and encouraging the child to move and creep after it, for example.

Toddler

Children during the toddler period are developing a sense of autonomy (i.e., learning to be independent). Trying to teach a 2-year-old a new activity such as eating a new food or brushing his or her teeth may be met with a sharp "No!" as the child exerts this new independence. The retort does not mean that the activity is not appealing to the child, but merely that the child is aware that he does not have to do everything he is told. Toddlers also sometimes resist a change in routine because they need rituals to feel secure. If an activity will allow the child to increase a level of independent functioning he or she will usually learn it rapidly. Teaching activities such as exercise or deep breathing by having a child imitate the action is an effective teaching method because it presents the activity as a game (so there is nothing to be resisted) and can be seen as a ritual.

Preschooler

Preschool children are interested in learning, because developing a sense of initiative is the main developmental task of the period. Provided that instructions are geared to their still small vocabularies, they "soak up" new methods of doing things. Because they are so imaginative and uninhibited, they have few reservations about the "right" way to do things. They will both watch eagerly and freely redemonstrate a skill.

Remember that in terms of cognitive development, preschool children "center," or are able to learn only one characteristic of an object. This may limit their ability to learn all aspects of care or more than one method of doing something on any one day.

Preschoolers are frightened of intrusive procedures (e.g., rectal temperature taking, bladder catheterization, or nasopharyngeal suction). They typically remove adhesive bandages minutes after application to check on the condition of the skin underneath (that it has not disappeared); they worry that any blood removed is the last they have. Teaching this type of procedure or explaining to the child why it is necessary calls for clear explanations. Use dolls to help the child visualize details whenever possible (Figure 36-2).

Preschool children ask many questions about equipment and procedures. Keep explanations short and words simple; a preschooler's attention span rarely exceeds 5 minutes.

School-Age Child

School-age children enjoy short projects that offer an immediate reward. They learn best if a procedure is broken down into different stages, therefore, and presented as separate short procedures rather than one long one. They enjoy games; playing "Simon Says" may be an effective way to have a child learn deep breathing.

School-age children are used to learning things and accept learning a new procedure or new information as just another experience in a busy day. The "staying power" of school-age children is notoriously short, however; the ability to continue to perform at the level taught tends to decrease sharply if learning is not reinforced. Be certain that a backup person in the home knows the health care information as well as the child, in order that the person can reinforce it or carry out a procedure of care if necessary.

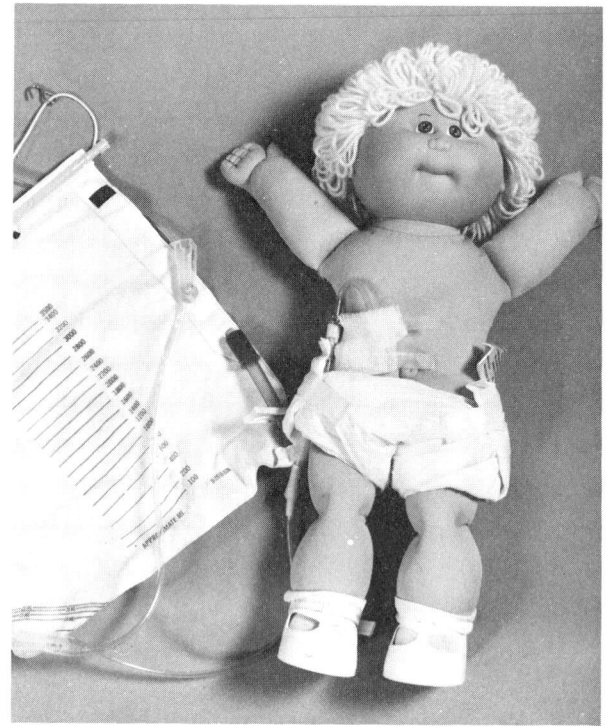

FIGURE 36-2
Teaching with dolls can help to make procedures seem less frightening. Here a doll is used to illustrate peritoneal dialysis. (Courtesy of the Department of Medical Photography, Children's Hospital, Buffalo, NY.)

Toward the end of the school-age period, children become interested in doing only those things that their friends are also doing. The child may interpret as unreasonable a request to do something after school (come home and take a medication) that is different from what all his or her friends are doing (e.g., stopping at the playground). Modify a teaching plan as necessary to help the child fit what he or she must learn into a school and social schedule, or else the teaching will be short-lived.

School-age children thrive on rules or the "right way" to do things. Be certain that if two or more people are going to be involved in teaching that they are consistent. It is frustrating for a school-age child to not have a "right way" to do something.

Adolescent

Adolescents, struggling for identity, like to learn things separately from their parents. Adolescents can be responsible for their own self-care as a rule; if they understand how the new actions they have been taught will directly benefit them, unlike school-age children, they will continue to carry those actions out conscientiously. Adolescents have a strong need to be exactly like their friends, however; they will not continue any action that makes them different or conspicuous in front of their friends. They focus best on things they can do rather than on things they cannot (Goldberg, et al., 1991).

Adolescents are present oriented; they learn procedures and new information best if they can see how it will immediately benefit them. They learn poorly if the only benefit of new information presented to them occurs at some future date. Rotating insulin injection sites, for example, prevents "pockmark" formations (*lipoatrophy*) in the skin when the person reaches approximately 30 years of age. Given this information, an adolescent tends not to rotate injection sites because the benefit is not relevant to him or her at the moment. An explanation such as "Rotating injection sites will ensure insulin absorption and dependability and allow you to play basketball this semester" (an equally true statement) is a better adolescent motivator.

Developing and Implementing a Teaching Plan

The first step in developing a **teaching plan** consists of assessing the child's current level of knowledge, ability to learn new knowledge, and your ability to teach the new knowledge.

Areas of Assessment

Child's Current Knowledge

Begin a teaching plan by assessing how much a child currently knows about the health area in question. Some children have had excellent anatomy and health classes as part of their school science curriculum. A child may have lived with another family member with an illness and may already know what home care problems occur with that particular illness; on the other hand, what the child knows about the illness may be accompanied by so many misconceptions that the child needs a great deal of teaching so that he or she is not hampered by half-truths or unnecessary restraints. A helpful method of assessment is asking the child to list what he or she knows about the health area on one side of a piece of paper and what he or she wants to know more about on the opposite side. A young child can be asked to draw a picture of himself, of someone with his illness, or of a good thing to do to keep well (Vessey et al., 1990).

Child's Physical Capabilities

If a procedure such as medicine injection that requires a certain level of psychomotor skill will be necessary for care, assess the child's physical ability to perform the procedure. If this is not present, the procedure will be frustrating for the child, who cannot perform above his capabilities. Assess vision and hearing ability and right- or left-hand dominance; these are important considerations for determining not only whether a child can accomplish the procedure but also how the material will be presented.

Child's Psychological or Emotional Capabilities

Children, like adults, may have difficulty learning about aspects of their care that they find distasteful. A child who uses food as comfort, for example, may have trouble learning about a restrictive diet because it conflicts with the way the child views food. A child with a urinary or bowel disorder may have difficulty learning about these body parts if he or she views them as "dirty" or distasteful. School-age and adolescent children may have difficulty discussing and asking questions about a reproductive tract illness not only because they lack knowledge of the subject but also because they sense sexual functioning is not an "open" topic.

Children with low self-esteem are less capable of learning self-care than others. For some children, it may be necessary to plan ways to increase self-esteem first before planning active teaching.

Child's Sociocultural Traits

Different cultures have different values about what good health means (Wenger, 1993). If a child from a family that values sports develops an illness that impairs her ability to run, for example, the family might consider the disability overwhelming. If the family believes that being able to write and read well are the cues to succeeding in life, the physical leg impairment might not be viewed as being that important. Studying each family individually is important in determining which aspect of health would be most important to emphasize when teaching (see the Focus on Cultural Awareness display).

Child's Attention Span

The attention span of a child and the capability to comprehend concepts and perform psychomotor skills differs a great deal depending on age. In general, the younger the child, the shorter the attention span and the more "attention-getting" teaching must be to hold attention.

Child's Cognitive Intellectual Capability

Intellectual capability, in many instances, can be inferred from educational level (i.e., the child is attending the age-appropriate class in school), but not necessarily. Be certain to assess mental age, not chronologic age, before beginning health teaching. With illness, most children regress at least slightly; what one would normally expect from a 10-year-old may be impossible for an *ill* 10-year-old.

Child's Lifestyle

Lifestyle refers to the common pattern of a child's life. A child who attends school daily, for example, has a fairly consistent lifestyle. An adolescent who has dropped out of school may have a varied pattern of activity every day.

Knowing family patterns helps to plan the timing of such activities as medication administration or exercise

FOCUS ON CULTURAL AWARENESS

Cultural differences between the teacher and the learner can sometimes complicate evaluation of the effectiveness of health teaching. Even when language is not a barrier, the way a child shows that she is listening or comprehending may vary from culture to culture. Looking directly at a speaker, for example, is considered disrespectful in many Asian countries. A traditional "OK" sign in Spain is interpreted as a vulgar one, not a positive one. In South Africa or some Middle Eastern countries, a "thumbs up" sign is insulting. In India, the way people shake their head to express yes and no are opposite those used in the United States (Geissler, 1994).

 Being aware of these cultural differences is important when planning health teaching for diverse cultural groups so that neither teaching nor reactions to teaching are misinterpreted.

or meal times. If both parents work during the day, for example, and do not return home until 6:00 PM, medication may have to be administered after this time; exercises may have to be supervised in the evening. A family that goes camping every weekend will need to plan ways to carry out a health routine at remote camp sites.

Child's Learning Style

Some children learn well from oral descriptions. Others have to see a statement in print before they can fully comprehend it. Still others are visually oriented: if they see a picture or a diagram, they grasp the explanation almost immediately. These different learning styles vary from child to child. Few children are aware of their own learning style, so they are unable to explain what it is. After caring for them for a time, it becomes easier to detect the way children learn best. Tailor a teaching plan to a learning style for the most effective learning situation.

Nurse's Own Strengths and Limitations

When formulating a teaching plan, be honest about your capabilities. If you feel uncomfortable teaching a child about surgery with clever puppets dressed in surgical scrub suits, it might be better to avoid this approach to teaching; in the wrong hands, such a method can sound so flat that the child is left feeling more frightened by the presentation than comforted. The use of humor is effective in teaching health care (White & Lewis, 1990). Assess whether this is a teaching strength for you. Attempting to use a teaching method that is uncomfortable may cause children to interpret apparent insecurity as evidence that there is something wrong with them, not with the method.

Some health teaching involves giving instructions in areas of care that may be personally embarrassing (instructing a member of the opposite sex how to obtain a clean-catch urine specimen, for example). Proceeding blindly may not result in effective teaching, because the child may be so embarrassed by the discomfort that he or she cannot concentrate on the instructions. In doing this type of teaching, nothing serves as well (as in any client contact) as honesty. Admit to the child or adolescent that you are not used to giving this type of instruction. This approach will probably evoke from the adolescent that he or she is not used to having anyone talk about it. Once the nurse and child have found common ground (this is not the most comfortable discussion for either party), there is a basis for effective health teaching. Honesty also allows a child to know that your discomfort is not from lack of knowledge on the subject (the child can trust what is being said) and not the child's fault (i.e., the subject, not the child, is the disturbing factor).

Formulating the Plan

Preparing Learning Goals

Preparing a teaching plan begins with preparing learning goals. Learning goals should reflect the type of learning desired: cognitive, psychomotor, or affective. They help to establish both content and time guidelines. They should be consistent with both the child's cognitive ability to learn and the time frame it will take to learn. It is unnecessary (and often overwhelming) for a child to learn everything about his or her illness in the first day or week following the diagnosis. Information on how to stay well does not need to be presented in one setting. In many instances, it is effective to teach only part of the information needed; another nurse in another setting such as a community health facility might teach the remainder. State teaching goals as behavioral objectives (outcome criteria) or as the activity the child is expected to demonstrate when the child has learned the new knowledge—not "Tim will understand the importance of deep breathing exercises daily" but "Tim will do deep breathing exercises daily."

Determining Teaching Strategies

Because children's attention spans tend to be short, strategies of teaching are most effective when they are intermixed and when they are selected in response to the individual situation and child to be taught. The more interactive the method, the better (Barber, 1994).

 Lecture. Lecture (or directly explaining information) is the most efficient and time-saving method of offering information to both individual children and to groups. A lecture, however, does not allow for participation and it is effective only in short, well-structured time spans. It is rarely effective for children who are not yet school age.

Demonstration. **Demonstration** is actually performing a procedure such as a dressing change or instillation of eye drops so that the child can see clearly how the procedure should be done. Never demonstrate a procedure unless all equipment necessary is present. If someone stops in the middle of a demonstration to say, "Be sure to use a sterile syringe, not what I'm doing," the poor technique demonstrated may be the lesson learned, not the good technique the child is expected to learn. The purpose of demonstration is to show how the procedure actually is done; having to imagine steps is little different from reading about it. School-age children, because of their stage of cognitive development (concrete operations), learn best by demonstration.

Redemonstration. To determine if a child has truly grasped a demonstration, ask the child to redemonstrate, or exactly imitate the procedure. **Redemonstration** is best if it immediately follows demonstration. Praise the effort to redemonstrate even if the redemonstration is not of the quality desired. No one likes to be put on the spot, and the child may be unwilling to expose himself or herself again by a second demonstration if criticized. Be aware that there are many different ways to do almost everything. The child may not have to follow the motions exactly, as long as the child's technique accomplishes the same goal. An effective way to correct a wrong action is to say, "That's one way of doing that; most children, however, find it easier to. . . ." This type of criticism is nonthreatening because it acknowledges the child's effort in a positive way before offering a correction.

Discussion. Discussion is a shared learning experience in which the child asks questions about particular concerns and these are answered based on the child's individual circumstances, or the child is asked questions about some problem, such as how the child anticipates managing some aspect of his or her care, and together the problem is solved. At the beginning of health education, children tend to ask few questions because they do not know enough about an illness or problem to anticipate concerns. As the child's knowledge increases, so does the ability to project and modify information to fit his or her own lifestyle. Remember that children tend to work in the present. A problem that will arise tomorrow is usually more important to a child than one that can be predicted to arise repeatedly in years to come. School-age and adolescent children enjoy discussion.

Role Modeling. Role modeling is demonstrating a certain attitude or behavior important for the child to learn. Be certain when health teaching to not only present facts but also radiate a positive attitude. Showing frustration at getting a bubble out of medicine in a syringe demonstrates, for example, that giving injections is frustrating; a bored attitude toward diet instructions im-

plies that nutrition information is boring. The child picks up the role modeling cues more readily than the spoken message. Role modeling is also an important technique used to teach new parents newborn care; as they watch a nurse hold, comfort, and talk to their newborn, they quickly learn to model these behaviors.

Visual Aids. "A picture is worth a thousand words" is not an idle quotation but a realistic one (Kuhn, 1990). Because small children know little about their bodies or where body organs are located, using visual aids such as drawings or photographs of anatomy can be helpful. Figure 36-3 shows internal abdominal contents as an example of such a drawing. Copyright laws prohibit anyone from copying this type of illustration for group distribution, but it can be done for use as an individual teaching aid. Use such an illustration to show a preschooler where he or she will be washed before surgery or where the child will have his or her stitches after the surgery.

Do not be afraid to draw a picture of a heart, a kidney, a bladder, or any other organ to make a point about anatomic structure. Children are more interested in understanding procedures or the reason for a health maintenance measure than criticizing your artwork (they likely do not know anatomy well enough to be able to tell if a drawing is distorted).

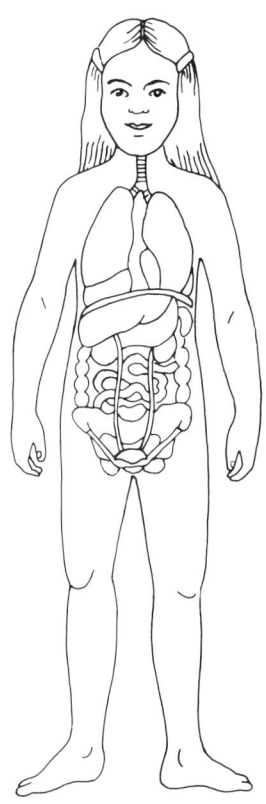

FIGURE 36-3
Anatomic drawings are helpful to illustrate what a procedure will entail.

Pamphlets. *Pamphlets* are helpful teaching aids with adolescents because they usually contain brief, easily understood information and are often cleverly illustrated with cartoon characters to make them enjoyable. Be certain to read any pamphlet before offering it to children to be certain that the information included in it is accurate. Medical advances are made so quickly that a 1-year-old pamphlet may contain a gross inaccuracy in the light of subsequent knowledge.

If a pamphlet has some statements in it that are inaccurate or that do not apply to the client, do not simply cross out the information that would be contradictory before offering it (most children deliberately read what they have been told not to); take the time to explain why it doesn't apply. Also, do not be misled into believing that because someone is given a clever pamphlet, they will necessarily read it and learn from it. Sit with a school-age child and read the pamphlet together; talk with an adolescent about the pamphlet's contents later to ensure compliance.

Learning Games. For memorizing certain kinds of information, such as what foods are high or low in potassium or sodium, the use of flash cards is a helpful learning action. Many children enjoy playing trivia-type board games. Instead of the usual categories of information, make up new cards with a question such as "Where is insulin produced in your body?" If the child can answer the question correctly, he or she is allowed to advance a designated number of spaces on the board. Children learn information quickly this way because the reward for learning is so immediate. Having parents play the game with their child educates the parents at the same time.

Word scrambles are easy games to develop. As an example, the crossword puzzle in Figure 25-6 might be altered to address the activities that are important for a child to do after surgery.

Videotapes, Slides, and Films. Many health care agencies have videotape playback equipment or slide or film projectors that can be used to show a short tape, film, or slide presentation as part of a health education program. As with pamphlets, view the material first before showing it; be certain to check that the vocabulary used is appropriate for an individual child.

Puppetry. Using puppets to teach health practices is helpful with preschool children, because a child this age can believe the puppet is actually talking to him or her. Teaching preschool children about what to expect from a hospital experience is often taught by using a series of puppets to represent different hospital personnel such as a surgeon, a nurse, and a nurse's assistant.

Mass Media. Television and radio are examples of effective mass media that reach many children on topics about self-help or self-care health. Consulting on the topics to present or helping develop material used in health messages can be an important role for nurses. Messages originated for these media must be attention-getting and brief to compete with the programs and commercial messages that precede or follow them.

Health Fairs. *Health fairs* are displays presenting health-related information to large numbers of people. They are effective with children if they encourage active participation such as playing computer games.

Preparing Supplies

To avoid having to reorganize equipment or instructions each time a procedure is taught, put together a basket or box of supplies that contains all the information and equipment needed to teach a particular task. This helps ensure that the teaching will be done and is economical in that everyone on a unit is not opening new equipment for demonstrations. It also helps to ensure that everyone is teaching the same information. Nothing is more confusing to anyone learning a new skill than to be taught two different principles for doing it or two different techniques.

Implementing the Plan

Health teaching can begin immediately and flow easily if goals have been developed well and strategies for teaching have been designed carefully.

Resource People

Many health care agencies have specific people who are available for health teaching about specific subjects (e.g., diabetes, colostomy care, or respiratory exercises). Using such people is helpful because they know all the "tricks of the trade" for teaching that particular subject.

Some children do not learn well from such designated teachers because they see them infrequently, whereas they see the primary nurse daily. Some parents react badly to the thought that it takes an expert to tell them about the care needed (if care is so complicated, how can they possibly learn it?). Health teaching is a part of nursing care, and it is unfair to parents to be told that their questions cannot be answered until the following day when the appropriate person is available to answer them.

Parent Education

With very young children, it is not the child but the parents who need teaching (Haskins et al., 1990). It is good practice with all children to be certain that at least one adult in the household has the necessary information or can perform the required skill as well as the child. Let the child, as a rule, choose this person. The individual who everyone assumes is a child's chief support person may not be the person the child perceives as the most reliable choice and therefore not the one he or she wants as a health care backup. This person, when identified, needs as much information as the child does about why the health measure is important. If diet modification is necessary, be certain to speak with the person who will prepare the food. See the Focus on Nursing Research display regarding the effectiveness of audiovisual teaching aids.

Evaluating the Effectiveness of Teaching

Evaluation, or assessing whether teaching has been effective, is the final step of teaching.

There is some advantage in asking children questions before and after teaching to prove that teaching was effective and the child has safely learned a new health care measure. Demonstration of a change of behavior or attitude, however, is the real proof that learning has occurred.

Health Teaching for the Surgical Experience

Teaching to prepare a child for surgery requires planning for several stages of learning. The child and the child's parents often feel anxious about the surgery and its results, so teaching must first address this anxiety. Do not downplay the family's fears but allow the child and family caregivers an opportunity to express their concerns as part of the teaching–learning process.

Assessing Current Level of Knowledge

On the child's admission, discuss with parents the preparation they have made for this experience and what specifically they have told the child. It is good to ask also whether the child's concerns about the experience seem more or less than parents had anticipated. Ask if there has been an unpleasant surgery or hospitalization in the family that the child might have heard discussed. Has the child seen anything recently on a medical show on television that might have upset him or her?

A good way to check the knowledge of a child younger than 7 years is through the use of a play telephone. Many children are shy about talking with nurses; this shyness, in addition to their concern about what will happen to them, may make it difficult for them to discuss or explain what they know about their intended surgery. They may be able to open up to an uncritical telephone, however.

Cindy, for example, is a 4-year-old admitted for repair of a birth anomaly (syndactyly, or webbed fingers). The nurse might call her on her play phone to begin the conversation.

FOCUS ON NURSING RESEARCH

Can Parents Effectively Learn CPR From an Audiovisual Tape?

It is becoming increasingly important that parents whose children are cared for in neonatal intensive care units learn cardiopulmonary resuscitation (CPR) before they can safely care for their infant at home. To see if they can learn this as well from an audiovisual tape as from a nurse lecture, a nurse researcher asked 30 parents (17 mothers and 13 fathers) who had an infant in a neonatal intensive care unit to attend either a lesson on CPR by lecture or by an audiovisual tape. At the end of each session, parents were asked to complete a 10-question cognitive test based on American Heart Association criteria. Their psychomotor resuscitation skills were assessed by a 20-point checklist and by having them return a demonstration of CPR on an infant mannequin.

Findings of the study revealed no significant differences between the traditional lecture and audiovisual tape groups on cognitive or psychomotor testing. The researcher concludes that using audiovisual tapes can be an effective method of teaching parents CPR skills; it could be a viable method of helping parents periodically update skills during home care or at follow-up visits.

Long, C. A. (1992). Teaching parents infant CPR—Lecture or audiovisual tape? *MCN: American Journal of Maternal Child Nursing, 17,* 30.

Nurse: Hello, nurse. I'm the doctor. Could you tell me what the little girl named Cindy is going to have done in surgery?
Cindy: Cindy's going to have her fingers fixed.
Nurse: How long do you think she'll be in the hospital?
Cindy: Three days.

Cindy has given evidence that she understands what is going to happen and the limit of her experience. Contrast her response to that of Bobby, admitted for the same treatment.

Bobby: He's going to have his hand cut off.
Nurse: Why is that going to happen?
Bobby: He's been really bad.

Such a child needs quick assurance and information about what is really going to happen.

Having children talk to puppets is equally effective with the preschool group. Their imagination is so great that puppets easily become real.

Formulating and Implementing the Plan

Be certain to prepare a preschooler for surgery or hospitalization in stages. A child this age cannot possibly absorb everything at once, and creating confusion only leaves him or her more frightened than before. A picture of a little girl or boy, such as that shown in Figure 36-4, is a good tool to use while naming body parts. Pointing to a figure drawing and saying, "This is the part of your tummy the doctor will fix," is less threatening than actually pointing to the child's abdomen. Clarifying body parts is important, because young children have no clear understanding of where a body part such as a hand ends and an arm begins.

When the child is ready for a second step in preparation, a helpful means of explaining postsurgery items, such as oxygen tents, monitors, bedpans, or intravenous feeding equipment, is to furnish a doll with such equipment as shown in Figure 36-5. It would be overwhelming to a preschooler to be taken to an intensive care unit and be shown actual monitors and respirators; doll-size toys, however, can be manipulated. The doll should be made of rubber or cloth so that the child can practice

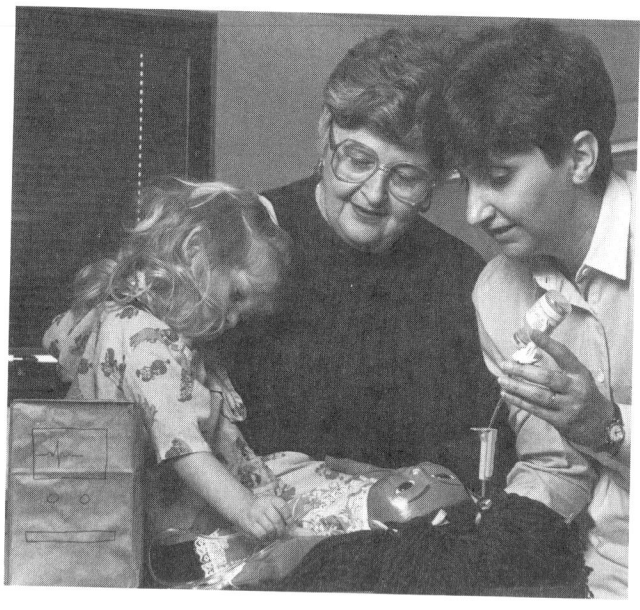

FIGURE 36-5

A nurse prepares a preschool child for heart surgery by explaining equipment that will be used postoperatively. Such play equipment can be handmade from boxes and medicine bottles. (Courtesy of the Department of Medical Photography, Children's Hospital, Buffalo, NY.)

giving it "shots" or submitting it to the procedures the child will experience (see Chapter 35 for a discussion of therapeutic play).

The doll could be prepared for surgery: its abdomen washed, an injection given to make it sleepy, and a hospital gown put on. It could be carried to a cart made from a cardboard box. After saying goodbye to its parents, the doll could be wheeled to surgery by a puppet nurse. It is important for preschoolers to be warned that nurses and doctors in surgery and perhaps the x-ray department dress differently from those they are used to seeing. Stress particularly that nurses and doctors in surgery wear surgical masks. The toddler and preschooler should be assured that the persons behind the masks are doctors and nurses, some of whom the child has probably already met. The puppet nurse could change clothes to convey the impression that nurses are nurses no matter how they dress.

The doll could next be given an anesthetic by mask and allowed to fall asleep. It is important to emphasize that anesthetized sleep is "special" sleep. Otherwise, toddlers or preschoolers may be reluctant to fall asleep after surgery and for a long time after discharge from the hospital for fear that people will come and do strange things to them. Do not say a child will be "put to sleep." Dogs and cats that are put to sleep are not seen again.

The surgery procedure itself should be minimized in play. "After you're sleeping, the doctor will fix your tummy. You won't feel anything the doctor is doing because of the special sleep. When you wake up, you'll be in a room called a recovery room where you'll stay until

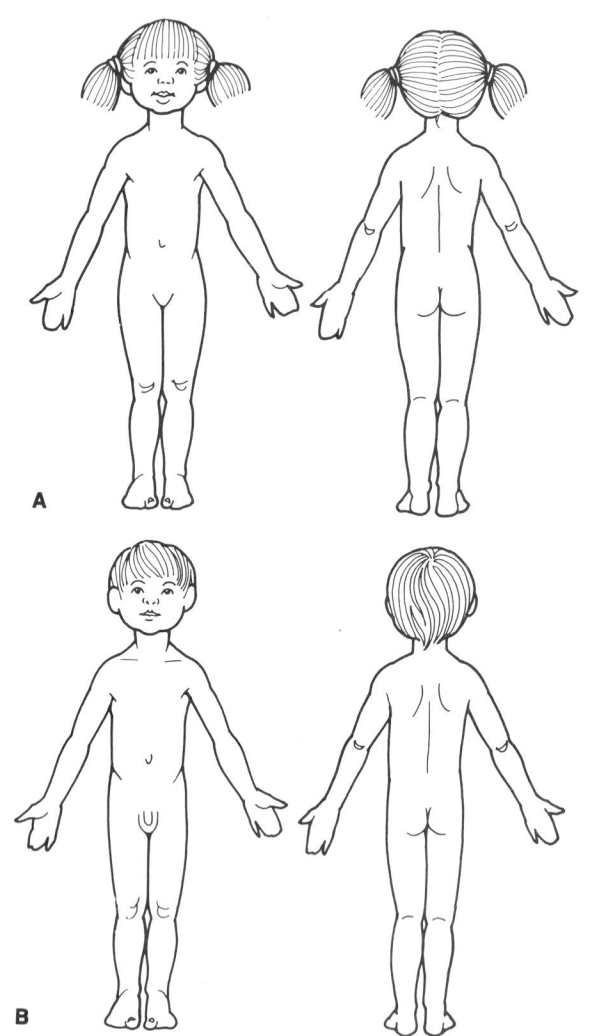

FIGURE 36-4

A simple line drawing such as this can be used to explain to a child exactly what part of his or her body will be "fixed" in surgery. For many children, having this pointed out on a drawing seems much less intrusive than having it pointed to on their own bodies.

Nursing Care Plan

A Preschooler Undergoing Surgery

Kim is a 3-year-old admitted to the hospital for revision of scar tissue on her right hand from a burn she accidentally received as an infant. She is unable to open her right hand completely or hold a crayon securely because of scar contraction. She is frightened of surgery despite preparation by her parents for the experience. When nervous or frightened, she has a habit of biting the scar tissue on her hand; she has done this constantly since admission. The following is a teaching plan to prepare her for surgery.

Teaching Points: Mother states child learns best from her rather than her father (father tends to be authoritarian). Ask mother to reinforce preparation (to help Kim go to the operation because it is a helping experience, not because Kim has to). Mother states Kim learns readily; "cocks head" when puzzled.

Nursing Diagnosis: Knowledge deficit related to surgery

Defining Characteristic: Child manifests behaviors that suggest she does not know what will happen in surgery.

Goal: Child will be prepared for surgery in 24 hours.

Outcome Criteria: Child voices happenings and outcomes of surgery. Demonstrates a minimum of nervous behaviors such as biting hand, can play "Simon Says" and describe how pain will be relieved by "special button" (patient-controlled analgesia).

Nursing Orders	Rationale
1. Assess Kim's and parents' knowledge of surgery.	1. It is important for the nurse to know how much information the child and parents already have, so that teaching can begin at *their* baseline.
2. Assess Kim's cognitive level.	2. An understanding of the child's ability to learn will help the nurse plan a teaching method that is most suitable for Kim's learning needs.
3. Using puppets, teach that hand must be washed for surgery and that Kim will be NPO, will ride in cart, will have intravenous line, patient-controlled analgesia after surgery, etc.	3. Puppets provide an excellent prop for teaching children Kim's age.
4. Introduce dressing and the way hand will be suspended postoperatively by letting Kim dress and suspend doll's hand.	4. Therapeutic play provides an excellent medium for teaching and learning with toddlers and preschoolers.
5. Introduce postoperative hand exercises she will need to do by playing "Simon Says."	5. Games are another appealing way to keep the preschooler interested and motivated.
6. Introduce the fact that Kim will have pain after surgery but that it can be relieved by a "special button" on her intravenous line.	6. Preparing the child for postoperative pain and teaching how this will be relieved before surgery (when the child still feels well) will reduce the amount of learning the child needs to accomplish after surgery, when she doesn't feel well.

you're wide awake." It is good to mention recovery rooms, because this may be an area that parents neglected to mention. In fact, parents may not be aware that they will not be allowed in the recovery room and may have promised the child, "When you wake up, I will be there." Clarify the parents' misconceptions about recovery rooms, and reiterate that the child will get to see the parents back in his or her own room once he or she is fully awake. This makes the parents' preparation correct and saves the child from feeling deceived. Be honest concerning pain: "Your tummy will feel sore afterward, but I'll give you something to make it feel better" is a fair statement.

The Nursing Care Plan: A Preschooler Undergoing Surgery illustrates the teaching process used for preparing a preschooler for surgery.

Key Points

- Children's cognitive development must be evaluated to ensure that material being presented can be easily comprehended. Preschoolers, for example, are egotistic and are only able to see situations from their standpoint, not others. They "center" and are able to grasp only one idea from a visual aid. School-age children are concrete thinkers. They learn best what they can see and touch and handle. Abstract concepts cannot be grasped until adolescence.

- The type of teaching used with children varies depending on the child's age. Various types to consider are: formal versus informal, single or group teaching, lecture, discussion, and role playing.

- Behavior modification is a special technique aimed at erasing some form of behavior that interferes with health functioning.

- There are three types of learning: cognitive, psychomotor, and affective. In order for something to be learned well, all of these areas must be involved.

- To individualize a teaching program for a child, assess the child's attention span, cognitive intellectual capability, lifestyle, learning style, and your own teaching strengths and limitations.

- In many instances there is a great deal of material that a child must learn about an illness. If taught all at once, however, this could be overwhelming. Divide material into lessons that must be taught immediately and lessons that can be taught at spaced return health visits.

- Remember that children are present-oriented. They learn information that they can see will immediately benefit them more easily than information that has future benefits.

- Children are learning many other things besides health information every day. This may make the retention of information not as great as you would like. Frequent reviews and updates may need to be scheduled to keep their information current.

Critical Thinking Exercises

1. Bobby is a 10-year-old with asthma who has to learn how to monitor his medication needs by using a peak flow meter at least once daily. How would you teach this skill? Suppose he states that he has no intention of learning how to read the meter because his mother can do it for him. Would your teaching plan be different?

2. Chuck is an adolescent who has familial hypercholesterolemia. His physician has prescribed a low cholesterol diet for him. What are teaching techniques that would be especially effective in introducing a new diet to Chuck? His mother has to learn this, too. Would you teach her any differently?

3. Mary is a preschooler who will be having surgery in a week for bilateral syndactyly. Her mother asks you how to prepare her for this. What suggestions would you make? Mary will be left with a noticeable scar and some lack of function following surgery, so she cannot be reassured that everything will be all right. Will this affect your teaching?

References

Barber, K. (1994). Expanding your teaching repertoire. *Journal of Nursing Staff Development, 10,* 12.

Beier, B., et al. (1993). AIDS/HIV teaching ideas. *Journal of Health Education, 24,* 47.

Department of Health & Human Services. (1991). *Healthy people 2000.* Washington, DC: Public Health Service.

Geissler, E. M. (1994). *Pocket guide to cultural assessment.* St. Louis: C. V. Mosby.

Goldberg, I., et al. (1991). Anabolic steroid education and adolescents: do scare tactics work? *Pediatrics, 87,* 283.

Good-Reis, D. V., et al. (1990). Structured vs unstructured teaching: A research study. *Association of Operating Room Nurses Journal, 51,* 1334.

Haskins, D. R., et al. (1990). Perioperative teaching of parents: A unit based study. *Association of Operating Room Nurses Journal, 51,* 1566.

Kuhn, M. E. (1990). Teaching materials: Ways to enhance visual aids in staff development programs. *Association of Operating Room Nurses Journal, 51,* 539.

Vessey, J. A., et al. (1990). Teaching children about their internal bodies. *Pediatric Nursing, 16,* 29.

Wenger, A. F. (1993). Teaching families from diverse cultural backgrounds. *Neonatal Network, 12,* 69.

White, L. A., & Lewis, D. J. (1990). Humor: A teaching strategy to promote learning. *Journal of Nursing Staff Development, 6,* 60.

Wright, S., et al. (1989). Retention of infant CPR instruction by parents. *Pediatric Nursing, 15,* 37.

Suggested Readings

Barnes, L. P. (1993). What kind of materials belong in a family resource library? *MCN: American Journal of Maternal Child Nursing, 18,* 181.

Discenza, D. J. (1993). A systematic approach to selecting and evaluating instructional materials. *Journal of Nursing Staff Development, 10,* 31.

Faris, M. A., & Steele, P. H. (1993). Airway support management: a teaching module. *Journal of Pediatric Nursing, 8,* 265.

Martin, R., & Coleman, S. (1994). Playing games with cardiopulmonary resuscitation. *Journal of Nursing Staff Development, 10,* 31.

Martinez, M., et al. (1993). Using a student constructed baby model to teach health subjects to learning disabled children. *Journal of School Health, 63,* 158.

Wojtowicz, C. G. (1993). An introductory activity for adolescent communication and intimacy. *Journal of Health Education, 24,* 50.

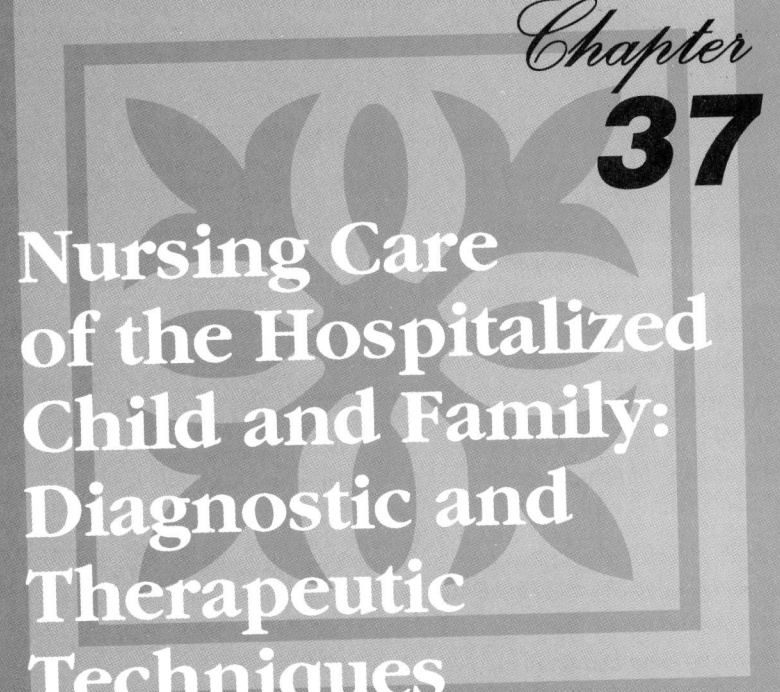

Chapter 37

Nursing Care of the Hospitalized Child and Family: Diagnostic and Therapeutic Techniques

Objectives

After mastering the contents of this chapter, you should be able to:

1. Describe common nursing interventions used in the health care of children to aid diagnosis and therapy.

2. Assess children as to developmental stage and knowledge level before beginning any diagnostic technique, therapeutic procedure, or other nursing intervention.

3. Formulate nursing diagnoses related to common diagnostic therapeutic techniques used with children.

4. Plan nursing interventions to aid in diagnosis or therapy for children, such as obtaining specimens or administering medicine.

5. Implement nursing procedures such as beginning intravenous therapy, while respecting the individuality and special needs of each child.

6. Evaluate outcome criteria to be certain that nursing goals related to diagnostic and therapeutic techniques were achieved.

7. Identify National Health Goals related to care of children that nurses could be instrumental in helping the nation achieve.

8. Identify areas related to nursing procedures with children that could benefit from additional nursing research.

9. Use critical thinking to analyze ways that procedures can be modified to meet the needs of children of all ages.

10. Synthesize knowledge of common procedures with nursing process to achieve quality maternal and child health nursing.

Key Terms

- aspiration studies
- barium contrast studies
- bronchoscopy
- central venous access devices
- clean-catch urine specimen
- computed tomography (CT)
- distraction
- electrical impulse studies
- endoscopy
- gating theory
- intermittent infusion devices
- magnetic resonance imaging (MRI)
- nocturnal enuresis
- non-rapid-eye movement (NREM) sleep
- positron emission tomograph (PET)
- radiopharmaceutical
- rapid-eye movement (REM) sleep
- sensory overload
- single photon emission computerized tomography (SPECT)
- sleep deprivation
- ultrasound
- venipuncture

Adele Pillitteri: MATERNAL AND CHILD HEALTH NURSING, 2nd Edition. © 1995 Adele Pillitteri.

The impetus for shortened hospital stays, although beneficial for the child and family in many respects, can make hospitalization more stressful, especially if it is necessary to crowd many diagnostic and therapeutic procedures into 1 or 2 days. When this happens, it leaves less time for teaching and preparation than once available, so good planning and follow-through are essential. Chapter 35 describes measures to make the hospital experience a positive one. Health teaching, discussed in Chapter 36, is a cornerstone in this process. However, everything that nurses do with and for children in the hospital will have a major influence on the child's progress toward health as well as on the child and family's perception of the hospital experience and ability to carry out healthful practices in the future. This includes therapeutic techniques aimed at promoting safety, comfort, and adequate sleep and nutrition, as well as administering medication and assisting with diagnostic procedures and specimen collection.

Many nursing actions offer an opportunity to accomplish several goals: providing the toddler with age-appropriate stimulation, for instance, not only promotes healthy development for the child while hospitalized but may also give the child's parents some ideas for stimulating activities that can be continued when the child goes home. Supporting the child and family during a diagnostic procedure can not only aid in efficient diagnosis but may also help establish a trusting relationship between the family and health care providers that will make all future interactions more successful. This chapter describes the most common diagnostic and therapeutic techniques used in the care of hospitalized children, including modifications needed to make these procedures safe and reduce associated stress, depending on the child's age and outlook. National Health Goals that address this area of child health practice are shown in the Focus on National Health Goals display.

NURSING PROCESS OVERVIEW
for Care of the Hospitalized Child and Family

ASSESSMENT

Before carrying out procedures such as assisting with a diagnostic test, collecting laboratory specimens, or teaching a child distraction techniques to counter pain, it is important to first carefully evaluate the child's age and developmental stage, as well as any special needs the child may have. Even the most common and painless procedures produce a certain amount of stress for the

child and parents. During complex diagnostic procedures, this stress level is almost certain to increase. Unfamiliar doctors and nurses, high-tech supplies and equipment, and strange surroundings all add up to a frightening experience for most adults; imagine how frightening they can seem to children.

Assess the child's level of anxiety associated with unfamiliar equipment and circumstances and strange surroundings as well as the child's knowledge concerning a technique before initiating a procedure or beginning health teaching. It may be possible to increase cooperation by acknowledging and respecting the child's past experience with the procedure.

FOCUS ON
National Health Goals

A basic part of carrying out procedures with children is keeping them safe during procedures. One National Health Goal concerns keeping patients safe from nosocomial infection:

- Reduce by at least 10% the incidence of surgical wound infections and nosocomial infections in intensive care patients.

A second concern for health care providers is to feel safe themselves from infection while carrying out procedures involving possible exposure to blood or body secretions. A National Health Goal also addresses this:

- Extend to all facilities where workers are at risk for occupational transmission of HIV, regulations to protect workers from exposure to bloodborne infections, including HIV infection (DHHS, 1991).

Nurses can be instrumental in helping to prevent nosocomial infection by enforcing measures such as frequent handwashing and being certain to use sterile technique for dressing changes. They can be instrumental in reducing the possibility of health care provider exposure to infection by being certain that they and their coworkers are following universal precautions, especially proper needle containment. Areas related to these goals that could benefit from additional nursing research are whether the type or thickness of surgical dressings or length of hospital stay effect the incidence of incision infections; whether allowing parents or children to change dressings affect the incidence, and under what circumstances breaks in universal precautions are most apt to occur and how this could be prevented.

NURSING DIAGNOSIS

Common nursing diagnoses related to diagnostic procedures or the hospital environment are as varied as the procedures and environment but include:

- Fear related to new and strange surroundings
- Pain related to lumbar puncture
- Knowledge deficit related to technique for 24-hour urine collection
- Diversionary activity deficit related to lack of appropriate toys in required setting
- Sleep pattern disturbance related to timing of medication administration
- Altered nutrition, less than body requirements related to lack of familiar foods
- High risk for infection related to presence of nosocomial infections within hospital environment

PLANNING

Hospitalization in itself creates anxiety in the child; unless the child is helped to feel comfortable and safe, every procedure can result in even more stress. To carry out interventions with the least degree of anxiety possible, plan specific ways to prepare children in advance. Planning should include the best way to explain the procedure to a particular child and also how to ensure that the child is not overwhelmed by the number of diagnostic or therapeutic procedures carried out in any one day. With small children, if financial circumstances allow, it may make more sense to stagger diagnostic tests over a number of days in order to preserve the child's coping ability. On the other hand, some older children (and parents) do better if they can complete all necessary tests in 1 day, so that they do not have to anticipate more testing over a long period. Use nursing judgment and data from periodic assessment to help primary care providers determine what sort of schedule is in the child's and family's best interest.

IMPLEMENTATION

Whether assisting with a procedure or carrying out a therapeutic intervention, it is necessary to function in several roles at the same time: performing (or assisting with) the procedure, providing active support to the child, and observing and then documenting the child's reactions. Providing support is a major role and there are many ways to do this, such as holding a child's hand or placing a hand on the child's shoulder. Playing a distracting game with an older child can also be helpful. Important observations to be made are signs of discomfort, changes in vital signs, or other signals of distress such as pallor or dizziness. Maintain a flowsheet of observations during a procedure. Following a procedure, the procedure and the child's reaction and specimens obtained can then be documented accurately and efficiently in the child's record.

As a final follow-through step, think of therapeutic play techniques to introduce that would be helpful in relieving stress caused by the procedure.

EVALUATION

Evaluating goals related to procedures not only helps in determining the effect of the procedure but also helps in planning, should other procedures be required. Recording that a particular child who did not appear nervous during a procedure later admitted to being "more scared than he'd ever been before," for example, can help another nurse provide reassurance to this child, even when the child is successfully masking his emotions the next time. Examples of outcome criteria might be:

- Child eats three meals brought in from home daily.
- Child is given scheduled time for 1 hour of active play daily.
- Child sleeps a minimum of 4 uninterrupted hours at night.

Diagnostic Techniques

Nursing Responsibilities

Responsibilities of the nurse in assisting with diagnostic procedures performed on children include the following: helping to obtain consent as needed; explaining the procedure to the child and his or her parents to prepare them psychologically; scheduling the procedure; preparing the child physically; obtaining equipment; accompanying the child to the treatment room or hospital department where the procedure will be performed; providing support during the procedure; assessing the child's response to the procedure; and providing care to the child and specimens obtained once the procedure is completed.

Obtaining Consent
Consent to perform a procedure must be obtained if the procedure carries any risk that would not be present if it were not performed. For a parent to sign a consent form, he or she must be informed about the content of the procedure and the risks of having or not having it performed. Although actually obtaining this is the physician's responsibility, seeing that it is obtained is a nursing one. Be certain that the rights of emancipated minors are respected and that in single-parent families the custodial parent has given the permission (Greve, 1990).

Explaining Procedures
In order to be able to explain procedures clearly and answer questions about them appropriately, it is important to see as many procedures performed as possible. Asking a child following any procedure what sensations he or she experienced not only helps the child work through a possibly frightening situation (often called

"debriefing") but also increases your knowledge of common procedures.

As a general guide, a child needs an explanation of why a procedure is performed (e.g., "The doctor needs to look at your blood to see why you're so sick") as well as a detailed description of the procedure ("I'll clean your finger. You will feel a small pinprick . . ."); where the procedure will be done (e.g., the x-ray department or a treatment room); any unusual sensations to be expected during the procedure (e.g., alcohol for cleaning skin will feel cold); a fair description of any pain involved (e.g., a needle will sting); any strange equipment used (e.g., a large x-ray machine); the approximate length of time the procedure will take; and any special care following the procedure ("You will need to lie quietly for 15 minutes afterward").

Be careful not to use words that might be confusing during an explanation, such as "transducer" or "electrode," without defining them. Try to associate the procedure with something with which the child is already familiar and comfortable (e.g., an x-ray machine is a "big camera").

If unfamiliar with what a procedure entails, do not guess: nothing is more confusing to a child than being told two different versions of something. Most technical personnel will take the time to describe important information over the telephone that a child should know about a study or procedure, as having a well-informed patient makes their job easier. Be certain that parents also receive an explanation of the procedure. A child has difficulty relaxing if parents are still anxious because he or she does not understand what is going to happen. Encourage parents to stay with the child during most procedures, because they can be extremely helpful in reducing a procedure's threatening aspects.

Try not to use the word "test" in explanations. School-age children associate the word "test" with a "pass/fail" situation. This can make them unduly worried following a procedure about whether they have "passed" it or not.

Scheduling

Procedures should be scheduled so that a child's stay in a health care facility is no longer than necessary; on the other hand, advocate so that a child is not overloaded with too many tests in 1 day. Try to arrange for the child to have time for meals and some free play time between procedures. If food or fluid must be restricted for procedures, monitor the child's degree of discomfort and physiologic needs related to this; advocate as necessary for a time lapse between examinations or improved coordination in scheduling to decrease the time spent without food or fluid.

Physical Preparation

Physical preparation varies depending on what procedure is to be performed. In many instances, preparing a

child for an examination (e.g., barium enema) involves another procedure (a saline enema), so physical preparation becomes education for the real examination. In all instances, be certain to explain both the preparative and actual procedures.

Accompanying the Child

It is difficult for children to come to a hospital for care. Once they have grown accustomed to the staff of a particular care unit, it is equally difficult for them to leave the unit to go to another department for procedures or care. Ideally, a primary care nurse should accompany a child to another department to minimize his or her reluctance and remain with the child for the procedure, or at least until the child has met a primary person who will be with him or her during the assessment. Older children do well without being accompanied as long as they have been introduced in advance to the new person who will give them care. A parent who can accompany a child is of invaluable help.

Before leaving the patient unit, have the child void for comfort unless this is a contraindication to the procedure. Check for any medication or a specific assessment procedure such as a blood pressure recording that should be given or done before leaving the unit for another department, in case the child is away from the primary unit for an extended time. Check also that the child's identification band is securely in place and readily visible despite any intravenous equipment. If there will be a considerable wait in another department, ask the child if he or she would like some activity during a wait, such as a game or book. Hallways can be cool. Provide adequate blankets for comfort, especially for infants. Always use cart straps and siderails for safety.

Providing Support

Children do well with diagnostic and evaluative procedures as long as they have adequate support from a concerned provider or parent. Provide this both verbally (explain what is going to happen; assure a child he or she is sitting still effectively) and nonverbally (a hand on the arm or a nearby presence).

Providing Care Following Procedures

After a procedure, assess how well a child reacted to it by both observation and history. Allowing the child to explain what happened helps the child retrace the procedure in his or her mind so he or she can conquer the fear of it. Fill in gaps in information as necessary to improve the child's perception of the procedure. Providing therapeutic play is another measure to reduce anxiety (see Chapter 35).

Be certain that tissue samples obtained following a procedure such as bone marrow aspiration are sent to the proper department for analysis as soon as possible. Guard against specimens being dropped or improperly labeled; children do not have extra body fluids such as blood to sacrifice for specimen collection.

Be careful not to leave supplies used for a procedure in a child's room. Cleaning agents such as alcohol or povidone-iodine are potential poisoning sources; syringes and needles can cause puncture injuries.

Modifying Procedures According to the Child's Age and Developmental Stage

A child's age and potential understanding of procedures must be considered when planning the number and order of tests as well as the way they are carried out.

The Infant

The number of painful or uncomfortable procedures done on infants should be kept to a minimum to avoid interfering with the infant's developing a sense of trust. Parents should be allowed to accompany their child to hospital departments and remain during procedures to offer support. Some parents may ask to hold their child during a procedure that causes pain, but don't ask parents to restrain the child during such a procedure. Their role should be a supportive and comforting, not pain-causing one.

Infants need to be picked up and comforted following procedures (a child of any age likes a hug or honest compliment for cooperation). Be aware that blood drawing (which can deplete blood stores) and x-rays (which are possibly harmful to bone marrow) should both be kept to a minimum in infants. Help parents understand why these procedures are being limited, so they do not feel that their infant's care is being compromised by few diagnostic procedures.

The Toddler and Preschooler

Toddlers and preschoolers resist any diagnostic testing that involves any degree of discomfort or pain. Children this age need short explanations of what to expect from procedures. Such explanations should be given close to the time of the procedure so that little time can be spent worrying over it.

The School-Age Child and Adolescent

School-age children are interested in the theory and reason for procedures; they often can be persuaded to cooperate for a procedure by being promised a look at their x-ray or laboratory report afterward. Be careful when promising children that they can see these results that this is actually possible. Otherwise, it can be difficult to obtain any further cooperation. Adolescents may project an air of maturity or sophistication beyond their years in order to remain in control of themselves in the face of frightening procedures. Do not be misled into thinking a child this age would not appreciate an explanation or a comforting hand on a shoulder during a procedure.

Common Diagnostic Procedures

Electrical Impulse Studies

Electrical impulse studies are those that include electrical conduction. Children need special preparation for studies such as electrocardiograms (ECGs) or electroencephalograms (EEGs) because they have been warned not to play with electric wires and may worry about being burned or electrocuted. They can be reassured that the electricity passes from their body to the machine, not the other way around; except for electromyelograms, children can be assured that these tests are painless. Electrodes are attached to the body by paste, which is easily removable. Give the child a portion of the test strip afterward as a souvenir (Figure 37-1).

Radiologic Studies

A variety of radiologic studies are used to inspect internal body tissues. These range from the simple x-ray to the more complicated CT scan or dye contrast study.

Flat-Plate X-Rays. Children accept radiographs well as a rule because an x-ray machine can be compared with a camera, an instrument with which they are familiar (Figure 37-2). Caution children that although you or a parent may be able to accompany them to the x-ray department, you will not be allowed to stay in the room while the picture is actually taken. If it is necessary for you to remain in the room to restrain a child, do not do this without lead apron and lead glove protection. Such protection is also necessary for portable x-rays taken by a child's or infant's bedside.

Dye Contrast Studies. To visualize a body cavity, some type of radiopaque dye may be swallowed or injected into the cavity and then examined on x-ray. **Barium contrast studies**, for example, are used to observe the outline of the gastrointestinal tract. Barium

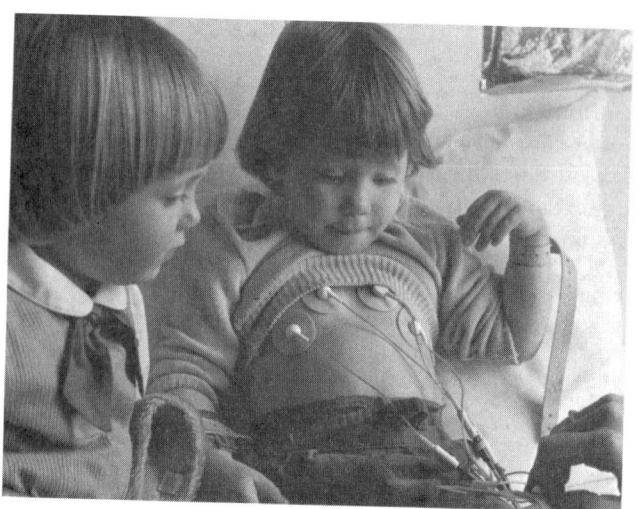

FIGURE 37-1
Administering an ECG. Children can be assured that this is a painless procedure. (Courtesy of Lori Bennett.)

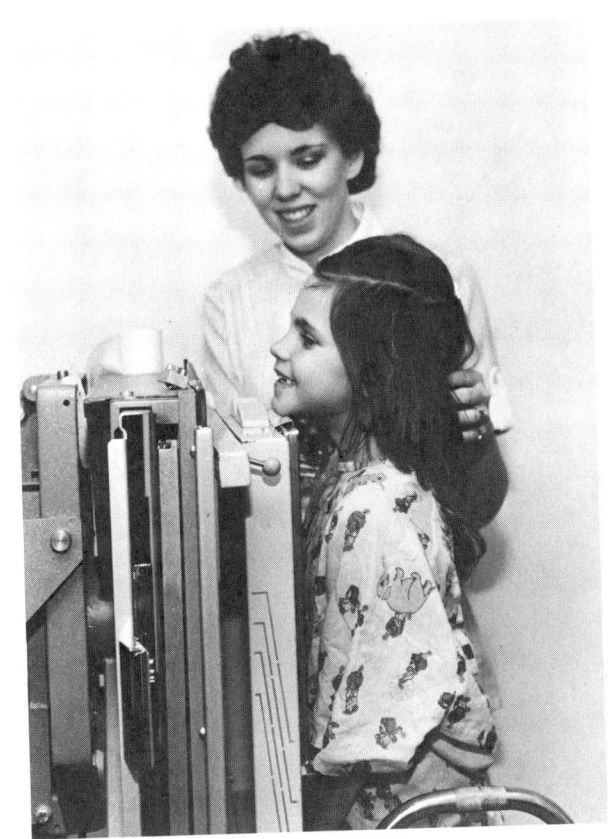

FIGURE 37-2
Positioning of a child for a chest film. (Courtesy of the Department of Medical Photography, Children's Hospital, Buffalo, NY.)

may be swallowed to outline the upper GI tract or instilled by enema to outline the lower. Caution the child that barium, even if flavored, does not taste terribly good. In studies such as an intravenous pyelogram (IVP), dye is injected intravenously; as it circulates to the kidneys, an x-ray is taken. Children must be thoroughly prepared for dye contrast procedures. Check if they are allergic to iodine as this is incorporated in the dye. At the time of an intravenous injection for such a study, the child may feel a hot flush, a sensation almost as frightening as the pain of the injection if the child is unprepared for it. Try not to use the word "dye" while describing the procedure to prevent a young child from worrying he or she will be dyed like a colored egg or "die." Use "medicine" instead.

Children easily grow bored with this type of procedure because of the time involved waiting for the dye to reach the specific organ to be studied. Take along an activity for the child to make the time pass faster. If a child should not eat for the duration of a long procedure, be certain he or she receives supervision or else, not realizing the importance of this, the child may decide to snack. Be certain that parents understand that the child will not be "radiating" x-rays or radioactivity following the procedure, so they will not be afraid to hold the child closely for comfort.

Computed Tomography. **Computed tomography**, or **CT** scan, is an x-ray procedure in which many views of an organ or body part are made to represent what the organ would look like if it were cut into thin slices. As with any x-ray, dense structures appear white and less dense structures appear gray to black on the films.

The procedure may require injection of an iodine-based contrast medium. If a radioisotope is added, the study is referred to as **positron emission tomography (PET)** or **single photon emission computerized tomography (SPECT)**.

Because a CT scan involves so many films, it is a lengthy procedure. The machinery is complex, large, and potentially frightening (Figure 37-3*A*). Children must lie still during the long procedure to avoid creating shadows on the film. In order to help them to lie still for an extended period, they may be administered a sedative such as chloral hydrate before the procedure (Slovis et al., 1993). Parents can be assured that although the radiation exposure occurs over a long period, such low doses are used that the actual exposure is less than during a regular x-ray.

Magnetic Resonance Imaging

Magnetic resonance imaging (MRI) combines a magnetic field, radio frequency, and computer technology to produce diagnostic images. The child lies on a moving pallet that is pushed into the core of the machine—the magnet. When the magnetic field surrounding the child is turned on, it causes tissue atoms to line up in a parallel fashion. As radio waves are turned on and off, the atoms change position. This change is sensed and converted into a visual display on a computer screen.

The procedure has an advantage over x-ray in that it has no apparent ill effects, it can reveal astonishingly clear structural defects in soft tissue, and if a contrast medium is required, it is not iodine-based, so the danger of a reaction is minimal (Plankey & Knauf, 1990). Because metal may deflect the magnetic waves, children with a metal prosthesis or metal dental braces may be poor candidates for the procedure. Hairpins and eye makeup (which often has a metallic base), watches, or other jewelry should be removed. Be certain the child's gown does not have a metal snap at the neckline (Figure 37-3*B*).

When the radio waves are turned on and off during the procedure, a booming noise occurs. Prepare the child for this sound (often compared with the sound of drums). Because the procedure may take up to 45 minutes, some children need a sedative prescribed beforehand so they can lie quietly for the duration.

Nuclear Medicine Studies

Radiopharmaceuticals are radioactive-combined substances that, when given orally or by injection, flow to designated body organs. When a scintillation machine (a form of Geiger counter) is passed over the organ

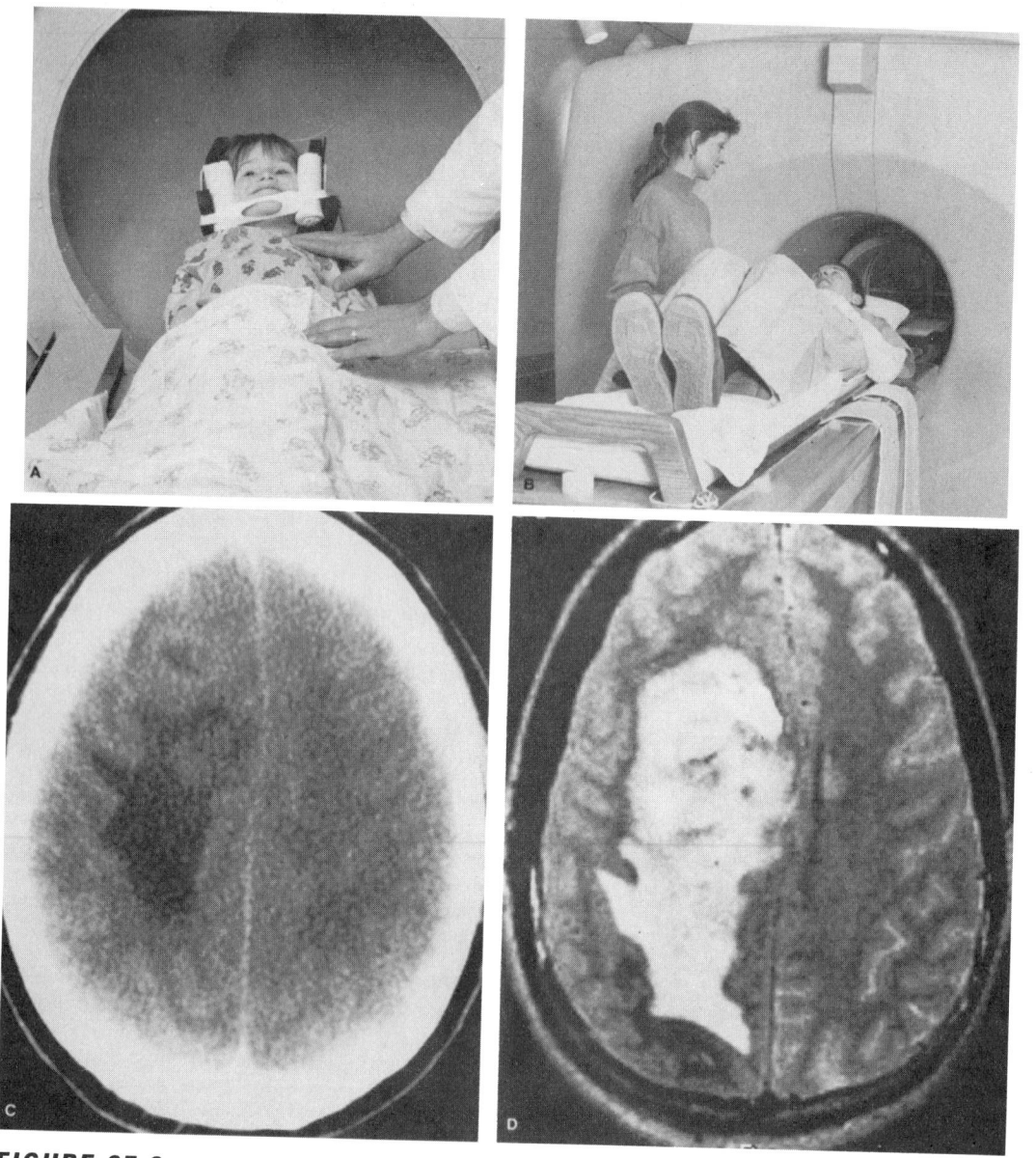

FIGURE 37-3
*Some procedures are potentially frightening because of the size of the machinery used. (**A**) A CT scanner. (**B**) An MRI scanner. (**C**) A CT scan of the ventricles. (**D**) An MRI of the ventricles. (Courtesy of the Department of Medical Photography, Children's Hospital, Buffalo, NY.)*

where the radiopharmaceutical has collected, the pattern of the collected material outlines the organ; the pattern can be produced as a screen image or a photograph.

Parents may worry that a child will be harmed by such exposure to a radioactive substance. They can be assured that the dose of radiation in these studies is no greater than that used for diagnostic x-ray, so this is not a danger. Tagged iodine (iodine 131) is frequently the medium used for such studies. Iodine will go immediately to the thyroid gland when injected intravenously, with the result being that enough concentrated radioactivity could accumulate to destroy the thyroid gland.

For this reason, a blocking agent such as potassium perchlorate that prevents thyroid gland accumulation may be given before the test. This prevents the radioactive substance from concentrating in the thyroid and protects the gland. Always check whether a blocking agent is required before transporting a child to the nuclear medicine department.

Ultrasound

Ultrasound is a painless procedure in which pictures of internal tissue and organs are produced by sound waves. Because it is noninvasive, children accept ultrasound easily and may even enjoy watching the oscilloscope screen during the procedure; the transducer that is passed along the body surface to pick up internal images can be compared with a television camera (Figure 37-4). Explain to parents that ultrasound is not an x-ray and appears to have no long-term effects. Tell the child that a clear gel will be applied to the skin over the body part to be studied to aid sound conduction, and it can feel cold and sticky.

Direct Visualization Procedures

Direct visualization procedures involve the observation of an internal body cavity by way of a thin tube inserted through a body surface opening. Types of direct visualization include **endoscopy**, in which an endoscope is passed through the mouth to examine the gastrointestinal tract; **bronchoscopy**, in which a bronchoscope is passed through the nose or mouth to observe the larynx, trachea, bronchi, and alveoli; and colonoscopy, in which a colonoscope is passed through the anus to examine the rectum or colon.

Endoscopy. Endoscopy has become a common method of diagnosis for gastrointestinal disorders in children. When first developed, endoscopes were straight, stiff, metal instruments, which limited their use. Currently, endoscopes are *fiberoptic* (a flexible, easily maneuvered, brightly lit tube), so these examinations are more common and not as uncomfortable as before.

The procedure is often frightening, however. A child can easily understand an explanation of the procedure

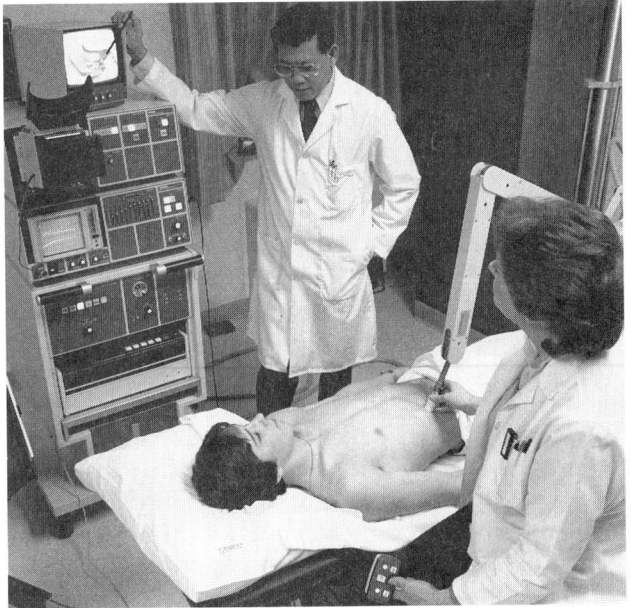

FIGURE 37-4
Sonography can be potentially frightening for children. Seeing the image on the television screen helps to relieve their fright. (Courtesy of the Department of Medical Photography, Children's Hospital, Buffalo, NY.)

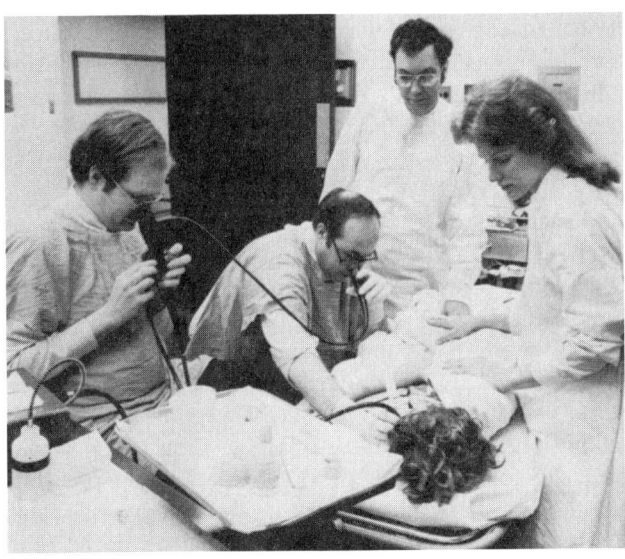

FIGURE 37-5
Examination with a flexible fiberoptic endoscope. (Courtesy of the Department of Medical Photography, Children's Hospital, Buffalo, NY.)

(the physician will extend the child's head and pass a tube down into the child's stomach for direct observation), but the child is uncomfortable at the thought of someone doing it. A child may need a sedative before the procedure so he or she can lie quietly for the time needed. Good support during the procedure is also important (Figure 37-5). Ask if the child can have a Polaroid photo taken during the procedure, to keep as a souvenir. Endoscopy is also used as an emergency measure to remove objects such as quarters or safety pins swallowed by children.

Following an endoscopy study, edema may occur from pressure of the scope on the esophagus and pharynx. After-care consists of close assessment to see that edema is not interfering with a vital function such as respiration or causing discomfort.

Bronchoscopy. Bronchoscopy is the direct visualization of the larynx, trachea, and bronchi through a lit, flexible, fiberoptic tube (a bronchofiberscope). The procedure is used with children who have aspirated a foreign object such as a peanut or to take culture and biopsy specimens. Before the procedure, the child may be administered atropine by injection to reduce bronchial secretions and encourage bronchial relaxation. A sedative or general anesthesia may also be administered because the procedure is so frightening it is difficult for the child to cooperate. As any manipulation of the airway has the potential to cause increased bronchial secretions and edema leading to narrowing of the airway, children need to be observed closely for respiratory function for 4 hours following the procedure. An ice bag applied to the neck often helps reduce the possibility of bronchial edema. Ice will also relieve throat discomfort. If children receive a local anesthetic, observe them carefully the first time they drink following the procedure to be certain their gag reflex has returned.

Aspiration Studies

Aspiration studies (removal of body fluids such as lumbar puncture or bone marrow aspiration) are always frightening procedures; not only are they painful, but looking at the size of the needle is frightening. A child may be worried that the needle will slip and puncture a vital organ. A child may need a sedative before the procedure so he or she can lie quietly. Support the child by talking and touching. Assess for bleeding at the puncture site following the procedure and apply pressure as needed. Remind children to lie quietly following lumbar puncture to help prevent spinal headache (see Chapter 49).

Vital Sign Assessment

Vital signs differ according to the size and age of children. Appendix G shows the average pulse rates, respiration rates, and blood pressures, respectively, for children of different ages.

Pulse Rate

As the child grows older, the heart rate slows and the range of normal values narrows.

If possible, both pulse and respirations should be measured with the child at rest. An apical pulse (listening at the heart apex through a stethoscope) is taken in children younger than 1 year because their radial (wrist) pulse is too faint to palpate accurately. In an infant, the point of maximum intensity, or the point on the chest wall where the heartbeat can be heard most distinctly, is just above and outside the left nipple (just lateral to the midclavicular line at the 3rd or 4th interspace). This point gradually becomes more medial and slightly lower until by 7 years of age it is at the 4th or 5th interspace at the midclavicular line. For greatest accuracy, pulse rate should be counted for 1 full minute.

Respiration Rate

Respirations should be measured before an infant is disturbed because respiration rate increases with crying. Take this while the child is sitting in the parent's lap or lying quietly in a crib before lowering the side rail. Infants tend to breathe with their abdominal muscles; therefore, it is as accurate to take respirations by counting movements of the abdomen as it is to count chest movements. Again, for greatest accuracy, respirations should be counted for 1 full minute.

Temperature

Temperature values in children are the same as in adults: axillary, 97.6°F (36.5°C); oral, 98.6°F (37.0°C); and rectal,

99.6°F (37.6°C). Electronic thermometers are ideal for assessing temperature in children because they register within 15 seconds or less and therefore cause less fear in the child because he or she does not have to be restrained for long. Thermometers that assess tympanic membrane temperature are also ideal because they register in 2 seconds by infrared emissions from the tympanic membrane (Figure 37-6A).

Newborns should always have their temperature taken in the axilla or by tympanic membrane because of the danger of damaging their rectal mucosa with a rectal thermometer (Figure 37-6B). Because preschoolers generally fear intrusive procedures, consider taking axillary temperatures in children until 4 years of age, although this may not be as reliable as a rectal one (Ogren, 1990). By 4 years, children are usually old enough to close their mouth sufficiently for oral temperature recording by electronic thermometer.

For an axillary recording, place the tip of an electronic thermometer in the axilla and hold the child's arm down to the side to keep the thermometer firmly in place. For the rare occasions when a rectal temperature must be taken, insert a thermometer only to the length of the bulb (½ inch) in infants and not over one inch in older children (Figure 37-6C).

All equipment used with children should be explained and demonstrated before use. Be certain that children understand that a thermometer is a painless measuring device and not an injectable needle (see the Focus on Nursing Research box).

Blood Pressure

Blood pressure should be included in the routine physical assessment of all children older than 3 years of age. Offer a good explanation of the procedure, especially to young children, because wrapping their arm and applying pressure can be frightening if they are not prepared for it.

Blood pressure is difficult to measure in infants because of mechanical problems. The cuff used should be no more than two thirds and not less than half the length of the upper arm; a wider cuff (larger bladder size) gives a lower reading; a narrower cuff gives a higher reading.

Systolic pressure in children is read as the manometer pressure is being lowered, at the moment that sound first appears. The point at which the sound becomes muffled, rather than the point at which it disappears, should be considered the diastolic pressure in children (Barness, 1994).

A thigh blood pressure can be recorded by wrapping the cuff over the thigh and palpating or auscultating the popliteal pulse (posterior knee). In infants younger than 1 year, the thigh and arm blood pressure should be equal. In children older than 1 year, the systolic pressure in the thigh tends to be 10 to 40 mm Hg

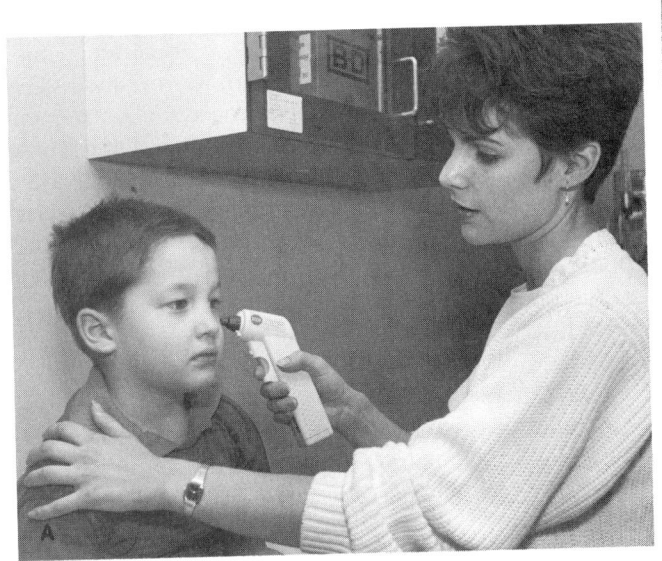
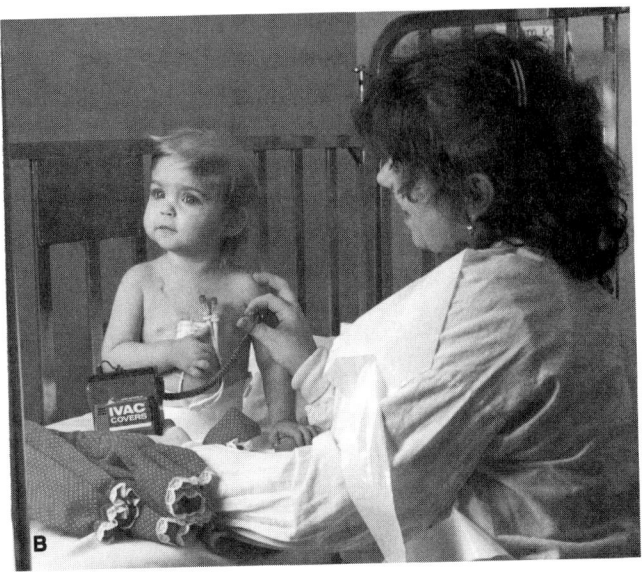
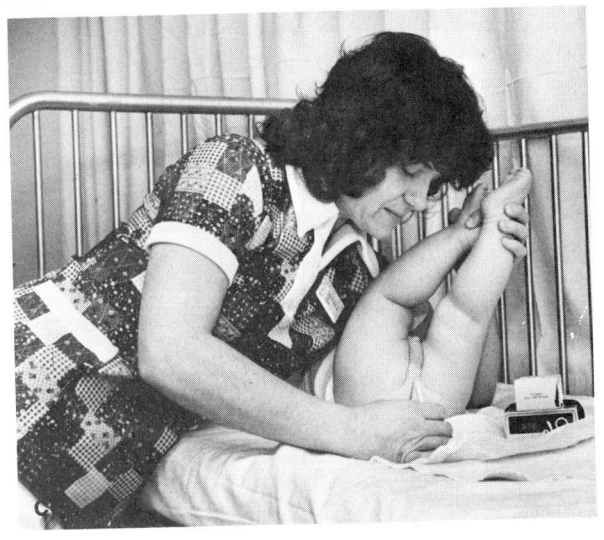

FIGURE 37-6
Temperature taking. (**A**) *Tympanic membrane temperature.* (**B**) *Axillary temperature.* (**C**) *Rectal temperature. (Courtesy of the Department of Medical Photography, Children's Hospital, Buffalo, NY.)*

higher; diastolic pressure remains the same. If pressure in the thighs of a child is lower than that in the arms, coarctation of the aorta or an interference with circulation to the lower extremities should be suspected.

When assessing blood pressure, be certain to pay attention to the pulse pressure—the difference between systolic and diastolic readings. Unusually wide (more than 50 mm Hg) or narrow (less than 10 mm Hg) ranges may both suggest congenital heart disease. An abnormally narrow pulse pressure, for instance, is a sign of aortic stenosis. An abnormally low diastolic pressure (causing a wide pulse pressure) occurs with patent ductus arteriosus.

A Doppler ultrasound blood pressure is especially effective with infants. This technique bounces high-frequency sound waves off body parts; the rate and pitch at which they return depends on the density of the body part that is struck. If a Doppler lead is placed over an artery, either the movement of the blood (pulse wave) or its tension (blood pressure) can be registered in a digital readout or monitor print. Dopplers can be adapted

to broadcast the sound of the pulse waves for auscultatory assessment.

Electronic blood pressure recording is most helpful when a continuous assessment is necessary, although it can be used for a single recording. It is helpful in infants whose blood pressure is difficult to obtain by usual methods. Watching the digital readout numbers is interesting for preschoolers. Direct measurement (intraarterial monitoring by an indwelling catheter into the radial or femoral artery) is used with children who are critically ill. This technique is reviewed in Chapter 41.

Specimen Collection

The collection of body fluids, secretions, and excretions is a collaborative nursing function essential to the complete assessment of a child. Elements of these fluids can be measured by a variety of means and compared with baseline standards of health. Findings may be used to help diagnose an illness, evaluate the progress of a particular disease, or evaluate a child's response to therapy.

FOCUS ON NURSING RESEARCH

How Reliable Are Different Types of Thermometers in Measuring Children's Temperatures?

To answer this question, nurse researchers compared the results of 960 temperature measurements taken on 89 febrile and 83 nonfebrile children 3 months to 6 years of age in a hospital emergency room. According to a set protocol, each child had his or her temperature taken by a standard glass-mercury thermometer and then three newer types of thermometers: an electronic one, a flexible plastic strip single-use thermometer, and a tympanic thermometer that was inserted in the child's ear. Children who were febrile and received Tylenol also had their temperature repeated at 1/2, 1 1/2 and 3 hours after the medication administration.

Findings of the study revealed that:

The plastic strip thermometer was the most accurate, followed by the tympanic membrane thermometer. Age, behavior, febrile status, or tympanic membrane bulge did not significantly affect the accuracy of any of the instruments. The most accurate sites for taking temperature were oral, axillary, ear, and rectal.

The precision of all instruments was highest for children without fevers. The researchers stress that decisions as to what equipment is used for procedures should be research based; nurses should be active in helping to conduct the research on which such decisions are made.

Pontious, S. L., Kennedy, A., Chung, K. L., Burroughs, T. E., Libby, L. J., and Vogel, D. W. (1993). Accuracy and reliability of temperature measurement in the emergency department by instrument and site in children. *Pediatric Nursing, 20,* 58.

Obtaining Blood Specimens

Never underestimate how frightening blood drawing is to children. For most children, any experience of losing blood has been from a nosebleed or a cut knee, which they remember as causing discomfort or pain. They have had injections for immunizations also, so they know that injections sting. Putting the two experiences together makes having blood taken an extremely frightening procedure. For this reason, blood specimens should always be drawn somewhere other than at the child's bedside, to keep the bed a safe area, and the child needs good preparation and support.

Venipuncture. Even for very small infants, the usual sites for **venipuncture** (entrance into a vein) are the same as for adults: the superficial veins of the dorsal surface of the hand or the antecubital fossa. In a few instances, the jugular or femoral vein is used. Give the child a simple explanation of what will be done. "I need to take some blood from your hand. You'll feel a pinprick, but that's all." Let the child know you understand how difficult it is to agree to the procedure. A statement such as "No one likes to have blood taken; I'm going to do this as quickly as possible to get it over", is always a better approach than "Be a big girl" or "Come on, show me how much of a big boy you can be," as the second approach shames a child who is unable to hold still. Try not to use the phrase "drawing blood." This sounds as if an activity with crayons is being proposed, not a procedure that will hurt.

Preschoolers may have to be restrained for blood sampling, because no matter how cooperative or brave they might be initially, the minute they see the needle, they are overwhelmed with fear.

Capillary Puncture. Capillary blood is often obtained for glucose and hematocrit determinations by a fingertip or a heel puncture. The technique for this is described in Nursing Procedure 37-1. For fingertip punctures, be certain to use the side of the finger, not the center, to reduce discomfort afterward; for heel punctures, use the lateral aspect of the heel to avoid striking the medial plantar artery or the periosteum of the bone (Figure 37-7).

Obtaining Urine Specimens

Depending on the type of test required, urine may be collected following a usual voiding, after the external

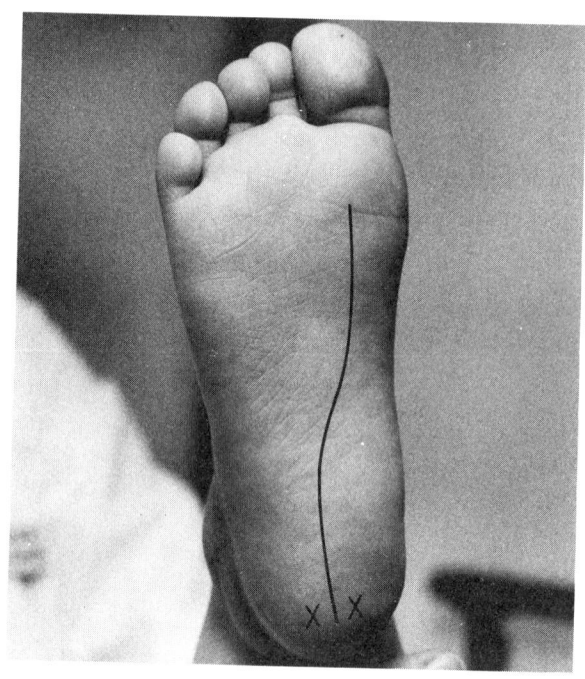

FIGURE 37-7
Sites for puncture on an infant's heel (outer aspect of heel). These sites avoid puncture of the medial artery or the calcaneus bone.

NURSING PROCEDURE 37-1
Technique for Fingertip or Heel Capillary Puncture

Purpose

To remove a sample of blood by sterile puncture from the capillary circulation, for laboratory analysis.

Plan	*Principle*
1. Wash your hands; identify child; explain procedure to child.	1. Prevents spread of microorganisms from you to child. Promotes safety and well-being.
2. Assess child's status.	2. Site must be warm and free of lesions.
3. Analyze appropriateness of procedure; adjust plan to individual circumstances.	3. Nursing care is always individualized based on professional judgment of client need.
4. Plan and give health teaching and preparation information as necessary.	4. Health teaching and preparation is an independent nursing action always included in care.
5. Implement care by assembling equipment: gloves, alcohol swab, lancet, collecting capillary blood tube, dry compress or cotton ball, adhesive bandage.	5. Conserve energy through organization and preparation.
6. Fingertips and heels must be warm so blood flows freely. Warm by holding finger or heel in your hand for a moment or two.	6. Warming heels or fingers by immersing them in warm water or covering with a warm compress is not advised, because these methods increase the flow of blood so much that values become comparable with arterial, not venous, values.
7. Select puncture site: sides of tip of finger; right or left of medial artery of heel (Fig. 37-7). Allow child to choose finger if appropriate.	7. Use child's nondominant hand to avoid child having to use tender finger on dominant hand afterward. Allowing choices adds to child's feelings of control and self-esteem.
8. Apply gloves. Swab site with alcohol; puncture with a quick thrusting movement; wipe away first drop of blood with dry cotton ball.	8. Wipe away first drop so alcohol does not contaminate or dilute specimen.
9. Hold heel or finger lower than proximal extremity; touch capillary tube to puncture site and tip to encourage flow. Do not squeeze tissue around site.	9. Capillary action will quickly fill the collecting tube; squeezing causes tissue injury.
10. After filling required number of blood tubes, apply dry compress to site; apply adhesive bandage.	10. Applying dry compress to site halts bleeding.
11. Label specimen appropriately and send to proper laboratory for analysis.	11. Ensures continuity of care.
12. Evaluate effectiveness, efficiency, cost, safety, and comfort aspects of procedure; record procedure and child's reaction.	12. Documents nursing care and client status.

meatus has been cleaned (a **clean-catch specimen**), by catheterization, or by suprapubic aspiration. The test may require a single specimen or collection of all voidings in a 24-hour period.

Routine Urinalysis. Routine urinalysis requires a single voiding specimen. The term "urinalysis" refers to assessment for appearance, glucose, specific gravity, and microscopic analysis of urine. Specimens for this must be collected in clean containers to prevent contamination by additives.

The Infant or Toddler. A child who has not been toilet

trained cannot be expected to urinate on command, so it is necessary to attach a collecting device to a girl's perineum or a boy's penis and scrotum, then wait for the infant to void. Be certain to wash and dry the site of attachment well so that no ointment or powder gets on the skin (Figure 37-8*A*) and to keep the sticky adhesive surface of the urine collector from adhering to the skin. If the infant attempts to loosen the collector, cover the device with a diaper to keep it out of reach. Otherwise, leave it visible so that it can be observed for voiding. Offer the child something to drink. Most infants void shortly after a feeding, so if the collector is put in place

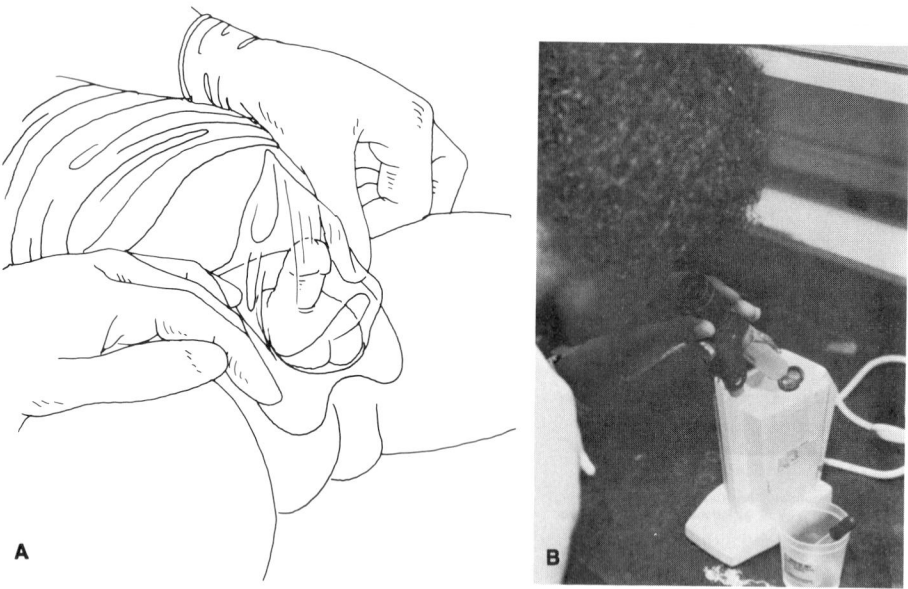

FIGURE 37-8

(**A**) *Urine collector for infants. The trick to making the collector adhere is to be certain that the child's skin is dry.* (**B**) *Testing specific gravity of urine with a refractometer. The advantage of this is that only one drop of urine is required. (Courtesy of the Department of Medical Photography, Children's Hospital, Buffalo, NY.)*

just before a regular feeding, voiding will probably result. Remove the collector as soon as the infant voids and transfer the specimen to a specimen cup by clipping a bottom corner of the bag.

Urine may be aspirated from diapers for tests such as specific gravity, dipstick protein, *p*H, or glucose (Figure 37-8*B*). This does not pull enough lint into the specimen to change its specific gravity (Lybrand et al., 1990). With disposable diapers, urine tends to be pulled into the diaper and is best available for testing if the diaper is torn apart. Placing cotton balls inside the diaper can be a help as they can be squeezed for additional urine.

The Preschooler or School-Age Child. It may be difficult to obtain routine urine specimens from preschoolers or toilet-trained toddlers because they can only void when they feel a definite urge to do so, not on command. Another problem is language. It is not unprofessional to use words such as "pee-pee" if this is what the child will understand. Provide a potty chair if one is available; if not, put a dutch cap collector on a toilet. Offer the child a glass of water or other fluid, and ask a parent to reinforce the request to void so that the child knows a parent approves. A generally successful approach with a child this age is to act as if voiding is not a difficult procedure. A school-age child is usually able to void when asked, although the child may find it more difficult than the adult. Do not encourage children to drink more than one glass of fluid to induce voiding, however, or else their urine production may be so diluted that the specific gravity, protein, and glucose levels will be inaccurate.

The Adolescent. Adolescents are usually knowledgeable and cooperative about providing urine specimens. As with adults, give them a clean specimen container and tell them what is needed. Unless they have voided recently, they are able to void "on command." Remember, however, that adolescents are concerned and self-conscious about body functions and therefore are often reluctant to carry a urine specimen through a crowded waiting room or desk area. They may be too self-conscious to void if they know someone is nearby—just outside a curtain, for example. Send them to a nearby bathroom with a closed door, or leave the area to give them privacy.

Some adolescents are suspicious that a urine specimen is being requested for drug testing; providing a good explanation of its actual purpose relieves this fear.

Adolescent girls may be embarrassed to mention that they are menstruating; ask them about this so that the presence of any red blood cells in a urine specimen can be explained.

To avoid having a urine specimen contaminated by menstrual blood (which changes the specific gravity, protein, and red blood cell analysis), ask the girl who is menstruating to wash her perineum well with soap and water and rinse and dry it to remove menstrual blood. Next, supply a sterile cotton ball for her to insert gently into her vagina just before voiding (and remove again following voiding). Mark the specimen "possibly contaminated by menstrual blood" even though it does not appear discolored, because red blood cells may be present microscopically.

Twenty-Four-Hour Urine Specimens. Although urinalysis of a single urine specimen will reveal the presence of such substances as protein or glucose, a *24-hour urine specimen* is necessary to determine the quantitative amount of many substances or how much of a substance is excreted during a day (quantitative analysis). To begin a 24-hour urine collection, ask the child to void (with an infant, attach a collecting bag and wait for the child to void). This specimen (the discard specimen) is then thrown away so that a specific time for the ensuing collection is known. If the urine collection was started early in the morning and this first specimen was counted as part of the collection, the urine collected during the next 24 hours would include urine that had been forming all night, resulting in an approximately 32-hour collection period that would distort the analysis.

Record the start of the collection period as the time of the discard urine. Save all urine voided for the next 24 hours and place it in one collection bottle. Have the child void (or watch for an infant to void) at the end of the 24-hour period and add the final specimen to the collection bottle. Record the time of the collection as being from the time of the discarded urine to the final specimen added to the collection.

Infant and Toddler. For an infant, use a 24-hour urine collector. A collector will adhere for this length of time only if the child's perineum is thoroughly dry at the time of application. Applying tincture of benzoin to toughen the perineal skin and make removal of the collector easier is helpful; tincture of benzoin also makes the perineum slightly sticky and aids in firm contact. Commercial sprays that encourage adhesiveness are also available. Place an infant in a semi-Fowler's position, if possible, to encourage urine to flow freely into the collector. Make certain that the tubing from the collector is pinned out of the infant's reach or the infant may pull the collector free. It may be necessary to place a diaper on the infant to keep the apparatus out of sight. Provide activities; make sure the parents understand that they can pick up the infant and hold him or her during this time, as long as they take care not to kink or pull the tubing.

To keep bacterial count to a minimum, 24-hour collections are generally kept refrigerated or on ice during the 24-hour period and until they are transported to the laboratory for analysis.

With active infants, fitting them with a colostomy bag applied to cover the urinary meatus may be more effective than using a collector with tubing (Figure 37-9). Puncture a small hole in the corner of the top of the bag. Insert a small feeding tube through this into the bottom of the bag. When the child voids, attach a syringe to the feeding tube and aspirate the urine. Transfer the specimen to the collection bottle. This type of urine collector has an advantage in that it allows the child to be ambu-

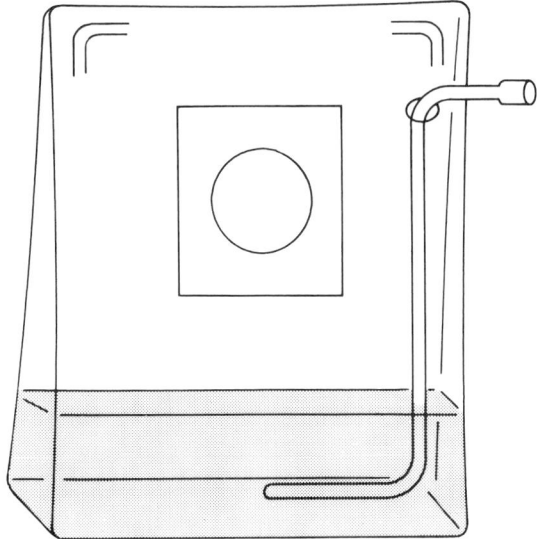

FIGURE 37-9
A 24-hour urine collector made from a colostomy bag. When the infant voids the bag fills with urine, which can be aspirated from the bag by the inserted feeding tube.

latory. For the active toddler, this collector may be the only type that is acceptable to the child.

Second-Voided (Double-Voided) Specimens. A *second-voided specimen* is sometimes used to better determine the amount of a product such as glucose or protein that kidneys are currently spilling rather than the amount they have been spilling during a number of hours. To obtain a second-voided specimen, ask the child to void and discard the specimen; then ask him or her to void again 20 to 30 minutes later. Test this specimen. Second-voided specimens are seldom used now because there is little difference between first- and second-voided specimens.

Children younger than 8 to 9 years of age have difficulty voiding when told to do so. Test the first specimen obtained as a backup in case the child is unable to void a second time. Mark it "not double-voided."

Clean-Catch Specimens. A clean-catch urine specimen is ordered when a urine culture for bacteria is desired. The objective of the specimen is to obtain urine that is uncontaminated by external organisms that increase the organism count of the urine, by cleaning the urinary meatus and the surrounding structures before voiding. Specimens used for protein or blood analysis may be ordered as clean-catch specimens because this careful cleaning also reduces the possibility of vaginal or foreskin secretions, which contain protein or blood, from being added to the specimen.

The technique for clean-catch urine collection is described in Nursing Procedure 37-2. Clean-catch urine specimens have a major advantage over catheterized

NURSING PROCEDURE 37-2
Obtaining a Clean-Catch Urine Specimen on a Young Child

Purpose
To obtain a urine specimen suitable for culture.

Plan	*Principle*
1. Wash your hands; identify the child; explain the procedure.	1. Prevents spread of microorganisms; promotes child's safety and well-being.
2. Assess child's status; analyze appropriateness of procedure; plan modification of procedure and health teaching as appropriate.	2. If child is old enough to be able to wash self thoroughly, give instructions for washing and allow child to carry out procedure by self. Health teaching is an independent nursing action always included as a part of care.
3. Implement care by assembling supplies: gloves, commercial clean-catch urine specimen kit, sterile emesis basin. Provide privacy.	3. Solution for cleaning differs in various health care agencies. Thorough cleansing appears to be more important than solution used.
4. Position female in dorsal recumbent position; male supine. Apply gloves. Moisten three cotton balls in antiseptic solution and clean urinary meatus by washing front to back, right side of meatus, left side of meatus, directly over meatus in female; three times in circular motion around and over meatus for males, using each cotton ball only once and then discarding it.	4. Cleansing front to back in females prevents bringing rectal contamination forward. Discarding cotton balls also prevents contamination.
5. Wipe away antiseptic solution using sterile water and same technique.	5. Wiping away antiseptic prevents it from entering specimen and, by germicidal action, decreasing bacterial growth and accurate analysis.
6. To obtain a urine specimen on a young child, ask the child to kneel over a sterile emesis basin on a bed while he or she begins to void and then dip a sterile container into the urine stream to obtain the specimen.	6. The flow of urine washes away bacteria from meatus. It is not always possible to obtain a midstream urine with young children because if they void only a small amount, there is not time to obtain it. This is the advantage of using a sterile emesis basin; the specimen is still salvageable; simply mark it "not midstream" for the laboratory.
7. After 10 to 20 mL is obtained in specimen cup, allow child to finish voiding in sterile basin.	7. If intake and output are being recorded, be certain to collect remainder of urine.
8. Cap specimen container; label with child's identification and list of antibiotics child is receiving. Mark "midstream" on label.	8. Prevents patient's results from being confused with someone else's.
9. Evaluate effectiveness, efficiency, cost, safety, and comfort of procedure.	9. Evaluation leads to improved nursing care.
10. Document that specimen was obtained, amount of urine obtained, and any abnormalities with voiding or urine.	10. Documents the child's status and the nursing care given.

Modification of Procedure for Infants

Wash the genitalia and apply a sterile urine collector. A specimen obtained this way is never a midstream; mark it as such for the laboratory. If an infant does not void within 2 hours, remove the collecting bag, recleanse the perineum or penis, and reapply a new sterile bag; some microorganisms will have collected after this amount of time.

specimens—they are not intrusive so they carry no risk of introducing a bladder infection. A clean-catch specimen with a bacterial colony count of more than 100,000 per mL is considered a positive specimen, or evidence that a urinary tract infection exists. If clean-catch specimens are obtained with care, they practically eliminate the need for catheterization specimens (an invasive procedure).

It is almost impossible for young girls to wash their perineum thoroughly because they cannot see it well, so they usually need assistance. Young boys must also be washed until they have enough coordination to do it themselves. Be aware that this is embarrassing for children. Ask a parent to confirm for the child that the procedure is all right as they have been told not to let adults touch this part of their body.

To be certain that school-agers and adolescents understand the procedure, have them repeat the instructions given to them; then send them to a nearby bathroom to carry out the procedure by themselves.

Suprapubic Aspiration. *Suprapubic aspiration* involves the insertion of a sterile needle into the bladder through the anterior wall of the abdomen and withdrawal of urine. It is used to obtain urine for culture in infants who cannot void on command. It is a procedure usually done by physicians, although nurses in specialty units may perform it. For the procedure, the anterior abdominal wall is cleaned with an antiseptic, and the urinary meatus is blocked by gloved finger pressure. A needle is inserted just above the pubis into the bladder; urine is aspirated through the needle into a sterile syringe. Although suprapubic aspiration for urine appears complicated, it is not. The bladder is the most anterior of abdominal organs and, when distended with urine, is easily accessible just under the abdominal wall (Figure 37-10). Parents may not have heard of this procedure, however, and may wonder why their child had urine drawn by needle and syringe instead of by catheter. The method is used because theoretically the risk of bladder infection from needle insertion is less than that from catheter insertion.

Catheterization. Bladder catheterization is accomplished most easily in females up to school age if a small (no. 5 or no. 8) feeding tube is used instead of a urinary catheter. This thin tube passes readily through the meatus of even an infant. Before beginning catheterization, be certain to observe the perineum of females to locate the urinary meatus. It is not as readily observable in infants and young children as it is in adult women. Cleanse the perineum well before inserting the tube to reduce the risk of infection.

Catheterization is an invasive procedure, so all children must be prepared in advance. Caution children that the catheter will sting for an instant as it is inserted and they will have to lie still until the urine specimen is ob-

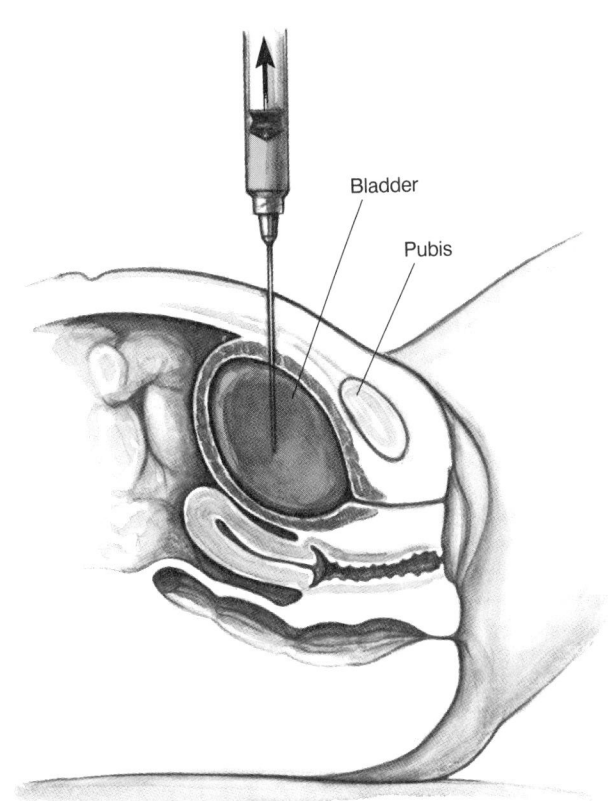

FIGURE 37-10
A suprapubic aspiration. The full bladder is easily accessible by an abdominal puncture.

tained. They need both support to submit to the procedure and praise afterwards for their cooperation.

Obtaining Stool Specimens

Obtain stool specimens from children who are toilet trained by asking them to use a potty seat or by placing a dutch cap on a toilet. For effective communication, be certain to know the word the child uses for stool. Transfer the specimen to a collection cup with tongue blades. To obtain a specimen from a child who is not toilet trained, scrape stool from a diaper using tongue blades and place it in a stool collection cup.

Be certain that stool specimens are sent to the laboratory promptly so that they do not have to be collected a second time, as they are difficult to obtain. If the stool specimen is for ova and parasites, see that it arrives in the laboratory in less than 1 hour. Do not refrigerate ova and parasite specimens because refrigeration destroys the organisms to be analyzed.

Medication Administration

Nursing Responsibilities

Safe medication administration is always a concern in child health nursing because "children" vary from 7-lb newborns to 150-lb 18-year-olds, and this weight range combined with the relative immaturity of body systems in children means that there is rarely a "standard" pediatric dosage of a particular drug. In order to administer drugs safely, it is important for a nurse to have a good understanding of *pharmacokinetics* (the way a drug is absorbed, distributed throughout the body, and inactivated). Each drug, each dose, and each child must be carefully and individually evaluated to ensure that the six rights of medicine administration—(1) right medicine, (2) right client, (3) right dose, (4) right route, (5) right time, and (6) right client instructions—have been fulfilled.

Pharmacokinetics in Children

Before a drug can be used by the body, it must be *absorbed* (transferred from its point of entry in the body into the bloodstream); *distributed* (moved through the bloodstream to the specific site of action); and then *biotransformed* (converted into an active form). A drug is then *inactivated* (and evacuated) through metabolism and *excretion* of raw drug or drug metabolites, a process that largely prevents drugs, when administered properly, from becoming toxic. The immaturity of body systems in infants and children (and especially in newborns) plays a major role in drug action in any of the aforementioned steps.

Absorption. Drug absorption is influenced by the route of administration as well as by the concentration and acidity of a drug. Some routes of administration in children are limited (e.g., children younger than school age do not hold tablets under their tongue for sublingual administration, and small muscle size limits sites for intramuscular injection). Moreover, gastrointestinal absorption may be immature at birth, so oral absorption in newborns may be reduced. Vomiting and diarrhea are frequent symptoms of childhood illnesses; these interfere with absorption because drugs do not remain in the gastrointestinal tract long enough for absorption when these symptoms are present.

Distribution. Many drugs are distributed by the bloodstream bound to serum albumin (manufactured by the liver). This binding action limits the amount of free drug in the circulation and therefore protects against toxic levels of the drug. As free drug is used, the bound drug is released to maintain the functioning level. Newborns have sluggish peripheral circulation, so distribution in infants this young may be affected. Any child with cardiovascular disease may also have limited distribution of drugs. Newborns with immature liver function may not have enough serum albumin to transport drugs readily. This is particularly true if elevated bilirubin is present, because bilirubin is also carried by serum albumin. Bound to serum albumin this way, bilirubin is harmless. In free form, however, it can leave the blood-

stream and enter other body tissues; if it enters the brain cells, it destroys their ability to function (*kernicterus*). If a newborn who has a high level of bilirubin from destruction of fetal hemoglobin receives a drug such as sulfonamide that competes for albumin binding sites, a large quantity of bilirubin may be left unbound and the infant may develop kernicterus.

Inactivation. Because a child's basic metabolic rate is faster than an adult's, certain drugs are metabolized (inactivated) faster in children. This means that the drug must be administered more frequently than in adults to maintain effective drug levels. Some drugs such as the salicylates and chloramphenicol are metabolized directly by liver enzymes. Because liver enzymes are not fully developed in newborns, these drugs cannot be metabolized, and will reach toxic levels rapidly. Older children with liver disease who have impaired liver enzymes also have decreased ability to inactivate drugs.

Excretion. The excretion of drugs such as penicillin by the kidneys is potentially limited until the age of 12 months, when kidney function becomes mature. If a child has kidney disease, excretion potential is limited at any age. A small number of drugs are excreted in bile (e.g., digitoxin). In the newborn with sluggish bile formation, excretion of these drugs is questionable. Monitoring intake and output is important in children receiving drugs to be certain that urine excretion is adequate.

Adverse Drug Reactions in Children

Children respond to drugs in much the same way as adults, but they may experience unique or exaggerated side effects due to physiologic factors during rapid growth and development. Drugs affecting the endocrine system are particularly likely to cause unique reactions in the child (Swonger & Matejski, 1991). The newborn may also suffer adverse effects from drugs administered to (or taken by) the mother prenatally or from drugs taken by the breastfeeding mother.

Determination of Correct Dosage

The dosage of most drugs is based on body surface area, using a nomogram such as the one shown in Figure 37-11. To calculate surface area using such a chart, find the child's height in the left-hand column (e.g., 40 cm); next, find the child's weight in the right-hand column (e.g., 20 kg). Hold a ruler or straight edge to connect the two points. The mark at which the ruler crosses the center column is the child's body surface area (0.38 m² in the example). Obtaining and recording height and weight measurements at health visits or on a hospital admission (or as frequently as daily during an admission) is important to supply this information for dose calculation.

Before administering any medication to a child, re-

Height		Surface Area	Weight	
Feet	Centimeters	Square meters	Pounds	Kilograms

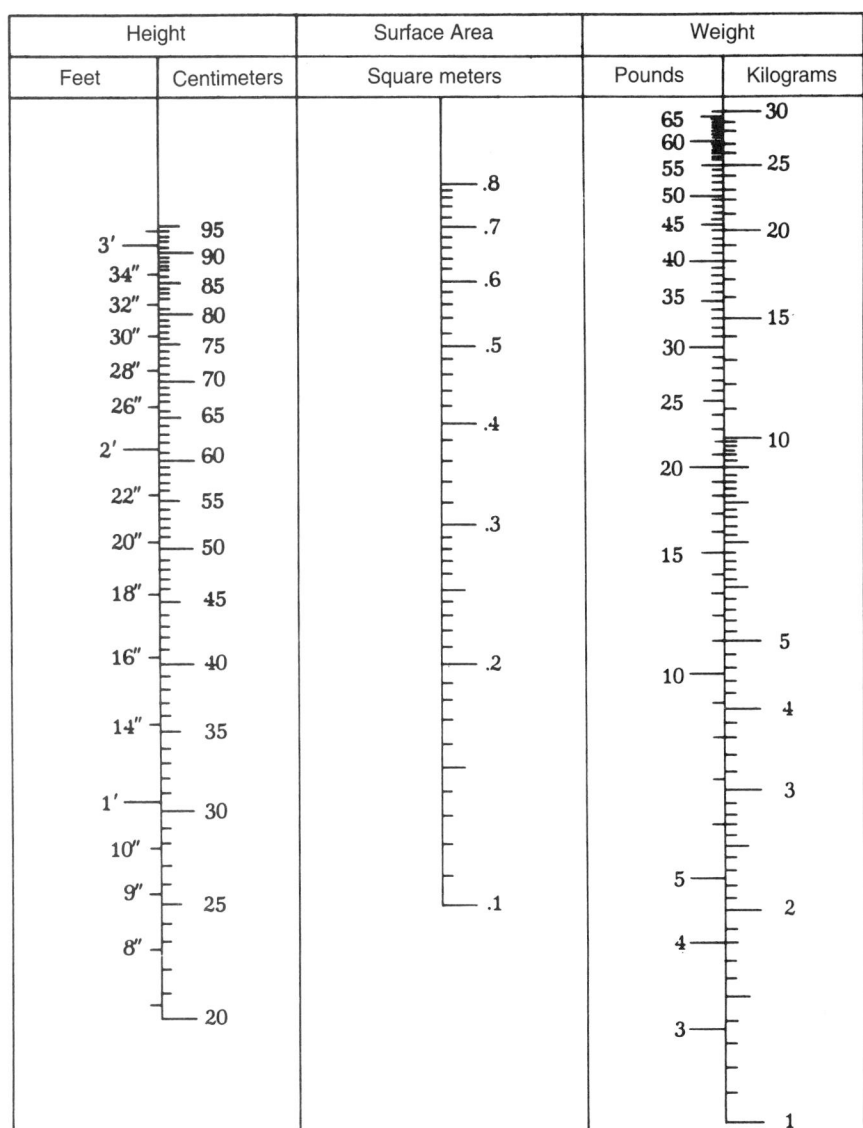

FIGURE 37-11

A nomogram to estimate body surface area. To use such a chart, draw a line from the child's height to the child's weight. The point at which it crosses the middle line is the child's surface area. (From Talbot, N. B., et al. [1980]. Functional endocrinology from birth to adolescence. *Cambridge, MA: Harvard University Press, with permission.)*

confirm that the dose ordered is correct for the child's weight or body surface. Every pediatric unit should have a drug reference, such as a *Physician's Desk Reference,* for this purpose. Remember that there are always exceptions to a rule: for example, a child with a gunshot wound may receive more than the usual dose of antibiotics because the risk of infection is so great; a 3-year-old weighing only as much as a 1-year-old would receive a dose of an antibiotic consistent with that given to a 1-year-old (not the child's actual age), because of small body size. Because of such exceptions, an ordered dose that does not conform to the standard dose may not be incorrect. The dose must be rechecked for accuracy with the prescribing physician or nurse practitioner, however, before it is administered.

Although most medication currently is supplied in unit doses (often supplied in oral feeding syringes), child health nurses may still need to calculate fractional dosages. Appendix I reviews the calculation of fractional dosages of drugs and intravenous flow rates. By verifying drug dosages, the nurse serves as a child's first line of defense against dosage error.

Identification of the Child

Children cannot be counted on to give their correct names before drugs are administered. Therefore, identification bands must be checked before medicine is offered. Anxious to please, a preschooler will answer the question, "Are you Johnny Jones?" with a "Yes." The child may also agree with any other name proposed. A school-age child who is anxious to avoid taking any medicine may deny that he or she is the person whose name is called. To prevent these types of errors, never ask children their names for identification. Instead, read their arm bands and compare them with the medication sheet that accompanies the medicine.

Administering Oral Medication

Children younger than 9 years old often have difficulty swallowing tablets. For children younger than age 3 years, this is virtually impossible. Most oral medication for young children, therefore, is furnished in liquid form.

In infants, oral medication can be given with a medicine dropper or a syringe (without a needle). Gently restrain the child's arms and head by holding the child against your body (Figure 37-12). Never give medicine with the child lying completely flat or the child may choke and aspirate. If the child is crying, he or she actively opens the mouth. If not, gently open the mouth by pressing on the child's chin. Press the bulb of the medicine dropper or use the plunger of the syringe to gently allow the fluid to flow slowly into the child's mouth. The end of the syringe or dropper should rest at the side of the infant's mouth to help prevent aspiration (some infants prefer to suck the contents of the syringe into their mouth). An infant may also be given fluid from a small glass or spoon. Allow the fluid to flow a little at a time so that the child has time to swallow between small sips.

Because firm pressure is used with the infant, he or she may be frightened afterward. Take time to sit and comfort the child or let a parent do this. The comfort is not a nicety—something to do only when there is extra time—but is as important as checking the correct dosage of the drug. Protecting a child's mental health is as important as protecting the child's physical health.

Preschoolers and early school-agers respond well to rewards such as stickers that they can paste into a book each time they take their medicine.

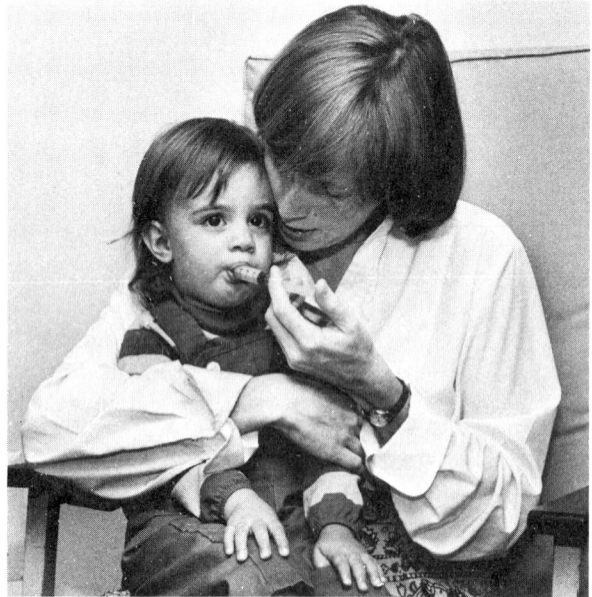

FIGURE 37-12
To administer oral medicine with a syringe, place the medicine at the side of the tongue. (Courtesy of the Department of Medical Photography, Children's Hospital, Buffalo, NY.)

For older children, hand them the glass of medicine as if they are expected to take it. Offer a "chaser" if necessary. If children have difficulty swallowing tablets, they can be crushed and added to a teaspoonful of applesauce or a flavored syrup. If pills are not to be chewed (capsules or enteric-coated tablets), the child must be instructed not to chew them. Some children are old enough to swallow tablets but have never done it before. To teach a child how to swallow them, it is often easier to use small bits of ice for practice; they melt rapidly and do not stick in the back of the child's throat or esophagus. Have the child put the ice on the back of the tongue, take a sip of water, and swallow the water. Once the child knows how to do this, he or she will not believe it was ever hard to do. Children who master this adult skill under a nurse's tutelage have a right to be proud of their accomplishment.

Techniques for Administering Oral Medicine

A number of techniques are helpful to remember when administering oral medication to children.

Do not say, "*Can* you drink this for me?" If an adult seems unsure whether a child can do it, the child may develop grave doubts himself or herself. Do not say, "*Will* you drink this for me?" This leaves the child the opportunity to say no and creates the awkward position of having to admit that the child really does not have a choice in the matter; the child *must* take the medicine. Instead, state firmly, "It's time for you to drink your medicine now." Give the child a secondary choice that allows him or her a sense of control: "It is time to drink your medicine now; do you want a drink of milk or water to swallow after it?" is a suitable choice, assuming both milk and water are compatible with the medication.

Children expect honesty from adults. Do not lie about the taste of medicine. If in doubt about the taste, taste it (with the obvious exception of drugs such as digitoxin). Most children's medicines are artificially flavored with raspberry, orange, or cherry syrup to improve their taste.

If a medicine tastes bitter, mix it with a spoonful of strained applesauce or a teaspoonful of flavored syrup. Do not mix medicine with a full jar of baby food because the child will then have to eat the entire jar of food to get all of the medicine. As a rule, encourage children to take medicine straight, then follow it with a pleasant-tasting drink to take away any bitter taste.

If a medicine is supplied in tablet form, it can be crushed or dissolved in water and mixed with syrup or applesauce for a better taste. Be certain before removing the particles from a capsule that the medicine will work properly when not in capsule form. Some are encapsulated to keep them from dissolving in the stomach and to bring them into the intestine where they have their therapeutic effect. The same precaution must be followed when handling enteric-coated tablets.

Never refer to medicine as candy. Children swallow medicine in fatal amounts when they think it is candy. (When everyone's back is turned, they help themselves to more "candy.")

Never leave medicine on a bedside stand for a child to take "in a minute" or "after your shower." Children may become involved with another activity "in a minute" and will not take it, or when he or she is not looking, a smaller child on the unit could find the medicine appealing and swallow it.

Do not bribe children to take medicine. Bribing may work for one dose, but when a second dose is due, the child will ask for a bigger bribe; for a third dose, an even bigger one. At some point (generally reached quickly), it is impossible to supply such large bribes and therefore it is impossible to enforce the rules.

Do not threaten. Statements such as "Take this quickly or I'll make it into a shot" cannot be followed through. The child calls the bluff (acetaminophen, for example, does not come in a form that can be injected intramuscularly), and once more the child is in control. A statement such as "Take this or I'll call your doctor" is unfair to a colleague (the physician has been made the villain) and ultimately undermines authority (it is obvious a person must not have much power or he or she would not need help).

Administering Nose Drops

It is uncomfortable to have someone drop medicine into the nose. Explain to the child that you understand this but that the medicine is important because it will help the child get better. Inform the child of the procedure: "I'm going to drop two drops of medicine into your nose. Then I want you to sniff for me [demonstrate]. Then I'll drop two drops into the other side of your nose and I want you to sniff again."

Place the child on his or her back. A school-age child could extend the head over the side of the bed so that it is lower than the trunk. Preschoolers generally are too frightened by this strange position and do better with a pillow under their shoulders so that their head extends over the pillow and rests downward. An infant generally must be restrained in a mummy restraint for nose drop administration (see the discussion of restraints later in the chapter).

Drop the appropriate number of drops into one nostril. Turn the child's head to the side—to the left after the left nostril, to the right after the right nostril—so that the medicine stays in the nose longer. If the child is a preschooler or older, ask him or her to further sniff the medicine. Have the child remain in the head-flat position for at least 1 full minute to let the medicine come in contact with the mucous membrane of the nose. If the child gets up immediately, the medicine will flow out and will be less effective.

Give the child high praise even if he or she did not cooperate at all. Praise tells the child you understand how hard it was to remain still.

Administering Eye Drops

Eye drops are uncomfortable and frightening to children who have been warned many times never to put anything into their eyes.

Infants and preschoolers generally must be restrained in a mummy restraint for eye drop administration. Place the child on the back. Open the eyes of infants and preschoolers. Do so by gently but firmly pressing on the lower lid with the thumb and on the upper lid with the index finger. A school-age child or adolescent will open his or her eyes cooperatively but may need to have a hand rested on the eyelid to keep an eye open long enough for the drug to be administered (Figure 37-13). Be sure that your fingernails are short to avoid inadvertently scratching the cornea.

Drop the correct number of drops of medication into the conjunctiva of the lower lid. Allow the eyelid to close. Try not to put drops directly on the cornea because that may be painful. To prevent the conjunctiva from drying, do not hold the eyelids apart any longer than is necessary. After the child has blinked two or three times, allow the child to get up. Praise the child for his or her cooperation even if cooperation was not evident.

Administering Ear Drops

Ear drops, like eye drops, are difficult for children to accept because they have been told not to put anything into their ears. Ear drops are generally administered for

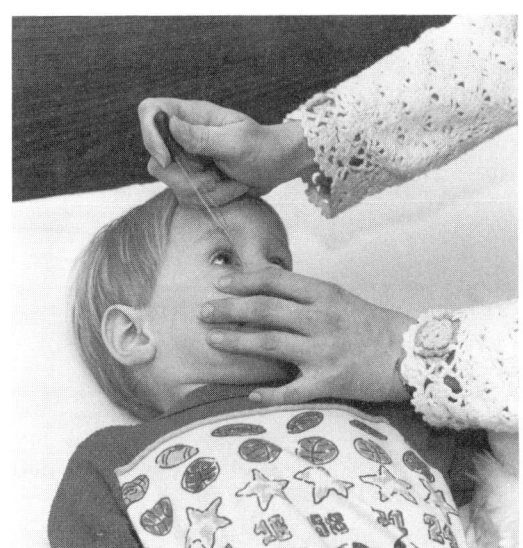

FIGURE 37-13
Administering eye drops. Resting the hand on the forehead prevents the dropper from striking the eye if the child should move the head. (Courtesy of the Department of Medical Photography, Children's Hospital, Buffalo, NY.)

earache, which is sharp, excruciating pain. A child may worry that having medicine put into the ear will make the pain worse. Also, he or she cannot watch what is happening. If health care providers have been honest with the child up to this point, the child can be reminded of this: "Remember how I told you that the injection would hurt a little? Well, if this would hurt, I'd tell you now too. But this doesn't hurt." Remind the child that ear drops can feel funny, as if someone were tickling the ear. The odd sensation of drops of fluid running into an ear may be frightening in itself.

Place the child on the back, in a mummy restraint if necessary. Turn the head to one side (Figure 37-14). The slant of the ear canal in children is shown in Chapter 50. If the child is younger than age 2 years, straighten the external ear canal by pulling the pinna down and back. If the child is older than age 2 years, pull the pinna of the ear up and back. Drop the specified number of drops into the ear canal. Hold the child's head in the sideways position for at least 1 full minute to ensure that the medication fills the entire ear canal. Ear drops must always be used at room temperature or warmed slightly. Cold fluid, such as medication taken from a refrigerator, causes pain and may cause severe vertigo as it touches the tympanic membrane. Praise the child for cooperation after the procedure.

Administering Rectal Medication

A good route for administering medication to children is by rectal insertion, because this allows the drug to be absorbed across the mucous membrane of the intestine.

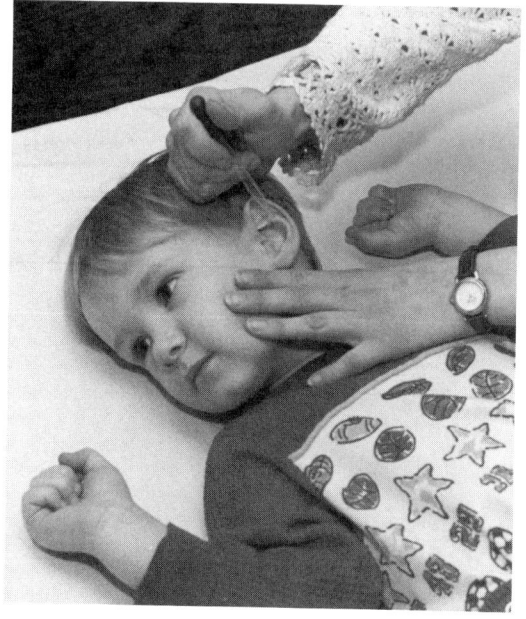

FIGURE 37-14
Administering ear drops. (Courtesy of the Department of Medical Photography, Children's Hospital, Buffalo, NY.)

Some medications are given by rectal suppository; a few are given by retention enema (Dieckmann, 1994).

Because the child cannot see what is happening, it is easy to be frightened by this procedure. Show the child the medication so that he or she can be certain it is not an injection. Having been honest with the child up to this point will be helpful again: "If it were anything else, I would tell you so."

Use a glove and insert a well-lubricated suppository gently but quickly beyond the rectal sphincters (as far as the first knuckle of the little finger for infants, and the first knuckle of the index finger for older children). Withdraw the finger and press the child's buttocks together firmly for approximately a count of 10 until the child's urge to evacuate the suppository passes. If a suppository is not prelubricated, dip the tip of it into a water-soluble lubricant such as K-Y jelly before insertion.

Invasive procedures are particularly threatening to the preschooler. Give lavish praise for cooperation.

If the medication is to be administered by enema to a child of this age, it must be given in as small an amount as possible so the child will retain it. Press the child's buttocks firmly together after administering the enema, using usual enema technique, for approximately 15 seconds or a child will expel the solution and the medicine will be lost. Using a distraction technique, such as asking the child to count backward or saying the alphabet backward, can help a defecation reflex to pass.

Administering Intramuscular and Subcutaneous Injections

Intramuscular injections are rarely prescribed for children as children do not have sufficient muscle masses for easy deposition of medication, and IM injections are painful. For intramuscular injections in infants, the mandatory site for administration is the quadriceps muscle of the anterior thigh (Figure 37-15*A*). Be certain to use the lateral aspect of the anterior thigh rather than the extremely tender medial portion, where an injection would cause more pain. Using the gluteal muscle in children younger than age 1 year is extremely hazardous. The muscle is not well developed until the child walks, so the sciatic nerve occupies a larger portion of the area than later on, and could become permanently damaged by gluteal injections. Figure 37-16 demonstrates an effective restraining technique for giving injections to infants. In older children, as in adults, the deltoid muscle (Figure 37-15*B*) or a ventrogluteal site (Figure 37-15*C*) may be used.

Do not give injections to sleeping children in the hope that they will not wake up and notice what is happening. They will wake terrified at being attacked. Instead, always give a short explanation: "I have some medicine for you, Lynn. I'm going to put it into your leg.

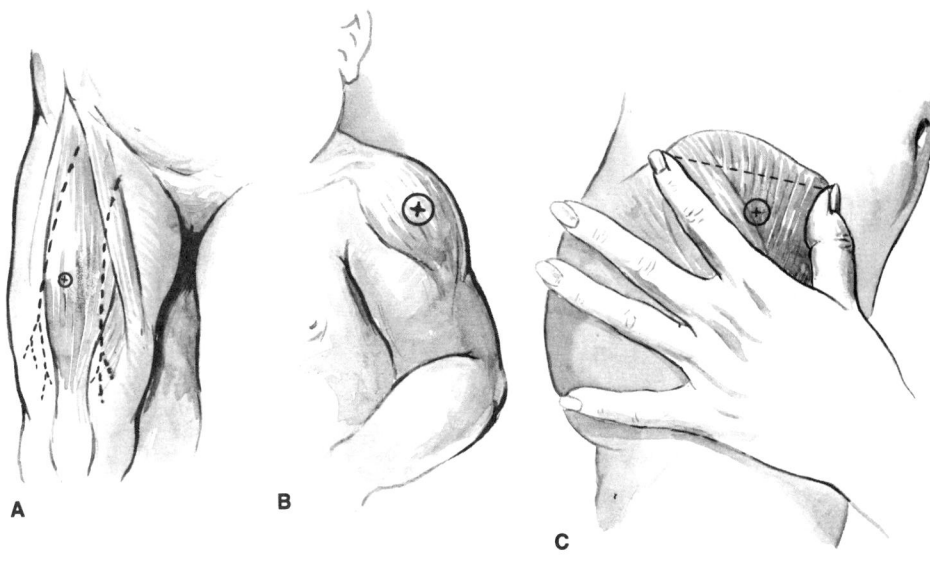

FIGURE 37-15
*Sites for intramuscular injections.
(**A**) For infants under walking age,
use the lateral aspect of the anterior
thigh. (**B**) In older children, the deltoid muscle is an acceptable site.
(**C**) A ventrogluteal site may also be
used in older children. Place a thumb
on the child's anterosuperior iliac
crest and spread the fingers. The
space between the index finger and
thumb is the correct site.*

It will sting for a second just like a pinprick. Then it will be over." Be honest about the pain involved; try to describe it accurately so that the child knows it has limits (a small amount of pain for a short time). Most children react well to injections if it is acknowledged that injections hurt. A statement such as "I know you don't

like medicine this way, but this is going to make you better" does not relieve the discomfort but it does let the child know that people are trying to appreciate his or her feelings.

Once the explanation is given, do not delay giving the injection further by trying to distract or convince the child it will not be bad. The suspense the child feels during this time is worse than the actual injection. Give the injection quickly but always use good technique. Do not hurry so much that aspirating the syringe is neglected. Quickness counts, but safety is your priority. Massage the area briefly after the injection to ensure absorption of the medication, but remember that the rubbing may be as painful as the actual injection.

Statements such as "Don't cry" are not therapeutic. If the child is hurt, he or she should be able to cry. Tell them they can say "ouch" when the needle is inserted. They will appreciate being given approval to vent their feelings this way.

If necessary, ask for help in restraining a child when giving an injection as having an extra pair of hands available may ensure safe administration. School-age children, however, may be proud that they are able to lie still. Being restrained would shame them. Be certain to hold and comfort the young child after all painful procedures, or let a parent do this. Record the site of an intramuscular injection as well as the medicine injected, so that sites can be rotated for better absorption.

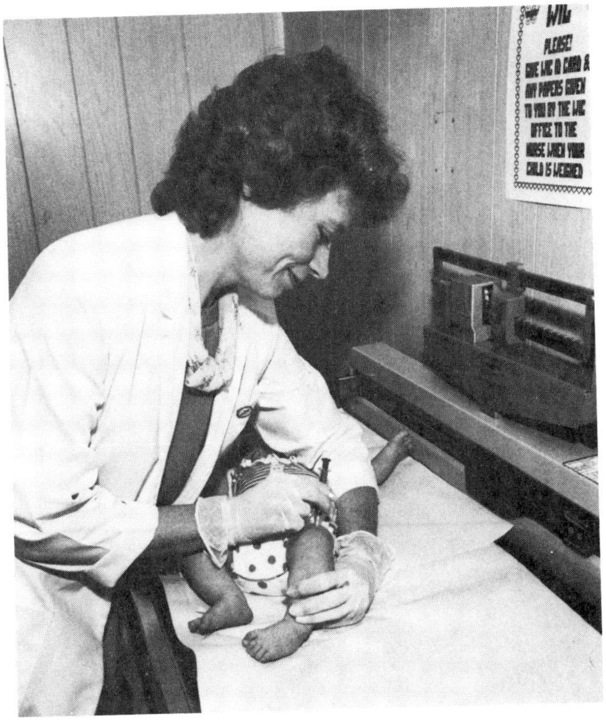

FIGURE 37-16
*Technique of administering an intramuscular injection to an infant.
Because the nurse needs to restrain only one leg, the rest of the
body is left free. This is a safe restraint and allows the nurse to give
injections in the lateral aspect of the anterior thigh without assistance. (Courtesy of the Department of Medical Photography,
Children's Hospital, Buffalo, NY.)*

Intravenous Therapy

Intravenous therapy is the quickest and most effective means of administering fluid or medicine to the ill infant and child and, as such, is a relatively common pediatric therapy. It has several major uses, including maintenance of fluid and electrolyte balance in the dehydrated child; as an avenue to bring drugs quickly up to therapeutic levels in the body; for nutritional support (by way of a peripheral or central line); and as a route for administration of chemotherapy drugs (Blatz & Paes, 1990). Intravenous fluid may be infused into a peripheral vein, a central access device, or a peripherally inserted central catheter (Goodwin & Carlson, 1993). The amount, type, and rate of intravenous fluids for children are prescribed carefully. It is important to understand the principles of intravenous therapy, including the fluid and caloric needs of the child (which differ significantly from those of the adult) in order to act as a second level of protection against overhydration or underhydration during intravenous fluid therapy.

Fluid and Caloric Needs of the Child

A formula that can be used to easily calculate water need in children is: for every 100 kcal expended in metabolism, the child must replace 115 mL water, 3 mEq sodium, and 2 mEq potassium.

Table 37-1 shows a method of calculating caloric expenditure. Fluids administered using this table should contain 25 mEq of sodium and 20 mEq of potassium per liter and 5% dextrose. Common intravenous solutions and oral electrolyte formulas used with infants (Pedialyte and Lytren) contain these proportions. According to Table 37-1, a child weighing 45 kg would have a caloric expenditure of 2000 cal; the child would need 2300 mL of a maintenance solution containing 5% dextrose, 25 mEq sodium, and 20 mEq potassium per liter. A flow rate would be calculated for this amount (2300 mL fluid in 24 hours = 95 mL/h).

Obtaining Venous Access

Sites frequently used for intravenous insertion in young children or infants are the veins on the dorsal surface of the hand or on the flexor surface of the wrist. Leg and foot veins may be used also.

Another site for intravenous infusion is a scalp vein over the temporal area (Figure 37-17). Seeing an infusion placed in a scalp vein can be frightening to parents; it seems a much more serious procedure than an infusion administered into an arm. Explain that this is an effective site for administering fluid or medicine in infants and ultimately causes the least discomfort for their child because needles there do not infiltrate readily.

An infant must be restrained adequately during a scalp vein insertion. Use a mummy restraint as it is physically exhausting to try to hold the infant's arms and legs still. Press the child's head to the side and hold it firmly in that position, one hand on the occiput, the other securing the front of the head. Be certain that the hand resting over the child's face does not obstruct the child's breathing.

The site over the temporal bone must be lathered with a soap solution and carefully shaved of hair. This reduces the possibility of infection and allows a clear view of the insertion site. Parents can be assured that the hair will grow in quickly after the procedure (ask parents if they want to save the clippings of hair if it is their child's first haircut). After the area is shaved, it is washed with an antiseptic solution. A rubber band is placed around the infant's head at the level of the forehead to serve as a tourniquet. A special small scalp vein needle or polytetrafluoroethylene (Teflon) catheter is then inserted. Scalp vein needles have protruding plastic "wings" (often referred to as butterflies) on the sides to allow easy manipulation. Continue to hold the infant firmly until the needle is securely taped in place, and until satisfied that the infusion is running well. Cover the

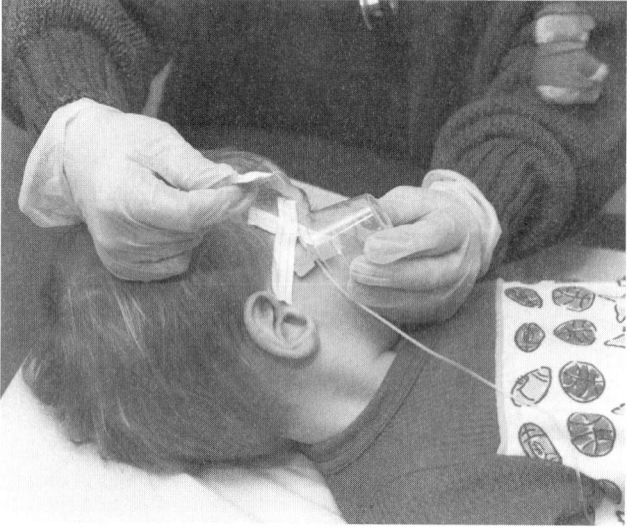

FIGURE 37-17

A scalp vein used for intravenous administration. The medicine cup protects the insertion site if the child turns over onto it. (Courtesy of the Department of Medical Photography, Children's Hospital, Buffalo, NY.)

Table 37-1. A Method to Calculate Caloric Expenditure	
Body Weight	*Caloric Expenditure per 24 h*
Up to 10 kg	100 kcal/kg
11–20 kg	1000 kcal + 50 kcal/kg for each kg more than 10 kg
More than 20 kg	1500 kcal + 20 kcal/kg for each kg more than 20 kg

(Siegel, N. J., Carpenter, T., & Gaudio, K. M. [1994]. The pathophysiology of body fluids. In F. A. Oski et al. *Principles and practice of pediatrics.* Philadelphia: J. B. Lippincott)

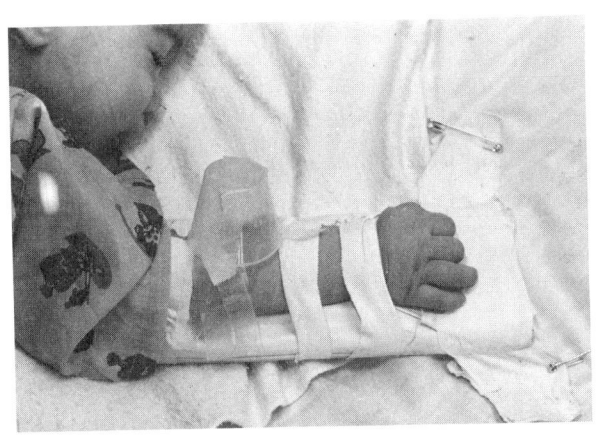

FIGURE 37-18
A peripheral site for intravenous infusion. A medicine cup protects the site; "wings" on the armboard are pinned to the bed. (Courtesy of the Department of Medical Photography, Children's Hospital, Buffalo, NY.)

infusion needle with a piece of gauze (a paper medicine cup taped onto the site provides additional protection) to keep the infant from brushing the needle out of place when he or she turns the head (Figure 37-18). Putting sandbags at both sides of the child's head can further help to keep the head straight.

Some infants with scalp vein infusions must have their arms restrained to keep them from brushing at the site. One way to do this is to pin their shirt sleeves to the sides of their diapers. An infant who is old enough to be able to turn over may need a trunk or jacket restraint to prevent turning.

The infant may be frightened by the pinprick of the needle insertion, as well as by having been held so firmly for a length of time. Spend some time comforting the child, talking and smiling at him or her, and lightly touching and stroking. Many infants enjoy sucking a pacifier after painful procedures; being held and rocked is the best comfort.

Preschoolers and older children often express some preference as to where they want an infusion inserted. Offer a choice, if possible, or suggest the nondominant hand. Remember that a doctor or intravenous therapy nurse who comes to insert an infusion may not know the child's preferences as well as a primary care nurse does. Act as the child's advocate and see that his or her wishes are respected.

Children who have intravenous infusions for long periods may require the placement of an *intracath* (a slim, pliable catheter threaded into a vein). The advantage of these is that the child can usually move about more freely because the intracath cannot be dislodged as easily as a normally inserted intravenous needle (Holder & Alexander, 1990). For all children (including adolescents), intravenous infusions must be secured in place with an armboard. Although children may say that

they will be careful not to move their arms, without an armboard it is easy to move unintentionally to turn off the television set or reach for something falling off their bed, and accidentally dislodge the needle. Tape a board to the arm of an older child with the words, "This is just to remind you to hold it still"—an explanation more acceptable than if the child thinks you doubt his or her ability to hold the hand still.

Determining Rate and Amount of Fluid Administration

Because children's hearts and circulatory systems are smaller than adults, intravenous fluid must flow more slowly into a child. If administered at an adult rate, it would quickly overload a child's system and cause cardiac overload. Automatic rate flow infusion pumps facilitate the infusion of potent medications (Ritter, 1990). They should be mandatory for small children because they regulate the flow accurately to a few drops per minute (Figure 37-19A). Overloading of intravenous fluid in infants and children can be further prevented by use of fluid chambers (Figure 37-19B), devices that allow only 50 to 100 mL of fluid into the drop chamber at a time. Even if the pump fails with these in place, only the amount in the drip chamber will be allowed to enter the child's circulation, not the entire contents of the bag suspended above the child's head.

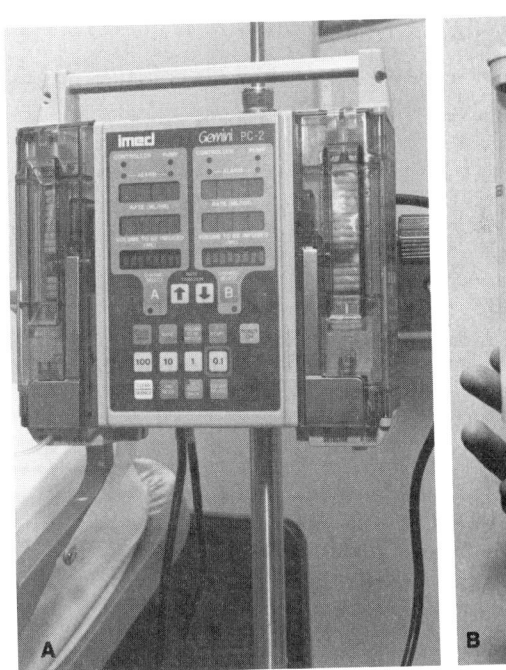

FIGURE 37-19
*Safety features used with children's intravenous lines. (**A**) An infusion pump. (**B**) A calibrated infusion chamber. A minidropper to reduce the size of drops protrudes into the drip chamber. (Courtesy of the Department of Medical Photography, Children's Hospital, Buffalo, NY.)*

A third fluid safety measure is a mini-dropper, a device that reduces the size of the drop in the control chamber to 60 drops per mL (usually there are 10 to 15 drops per mL) (Figure 37-19*B*). With a normal dropper in place, an infusion regulated to administer 30 mL/h drips at a rate of 7 to 8 drops per minute and is therefore difficult to regulate. With a mini-dropper in place, the drops are smaller; the same infusion (still providing the same amount of fluid per hour) drops at 30 drops per minute. This flow is easier to regulate and provides more accurate intravenous administration (calculating flow rates by mini-drops is reviewed in Appendix I).

It is important to keep a careful record of both rate and amount of intravenous fluid administered so that the child's circulatory system is not overloaded (Weinstein, 1990). At least once an hour, record the type and amount of fluid; the rate of flow (including the number of drops per minute); and, for a cross-check, the amount of fluid remaining in the bag. Signs of fluid overload are those of congestive heart failure: increased pulse rate and blood pressure. As the heart fails from excessive fluid, blood pressure falls and signs of edema develop. Be on guard for changes in vital signs such as these when children are receiving intravenous fluid. In addition, assess the specific gravity of urine at least every 4 hours to detect extremely dilute urine (specific gravity under 1.003) or whether the child is excreting a large quantity of fluid in an effort to reduce circulating volume.

It is difficult for children to lie still and wait for an infusion to finish. They need to be provided with activities and allowed out of bed as much as possible. Infants and preschoolers may have to have their other arm restrained to keep them from playing with the infusion needle. Infants who receive total fluids by intravenous infusion generally enjoy sucking on a pacifier during the day to fulfill their oral needs.

Intermittent Infusion Devices

Intermittent infusion devices, or *heparin locks*, are devices that maintain open venous access for medicine administration, yet allow children to be free of intravenous tubing so that they can be out of bed and more active (Figure 37-20). The vessels of the back of the hand are generally chosen as the intravenous site. Scalp vein tubing is used and capped at the end with a specially designed rubber stopper or a commercial trap. The tubing is filled with a dilute solution of heparin or normal saline through the rubber stopper and flushed again with solution every 2 to 8 hours (depending on hospital policy) to keep it patent. Intravenous medication can be added as needed. The tubing and stopper must be firmly secured to the wrist and an armboard taped in place to remind the child to protect the site from careless trauma.

Children who are hospitalized or on home care for a

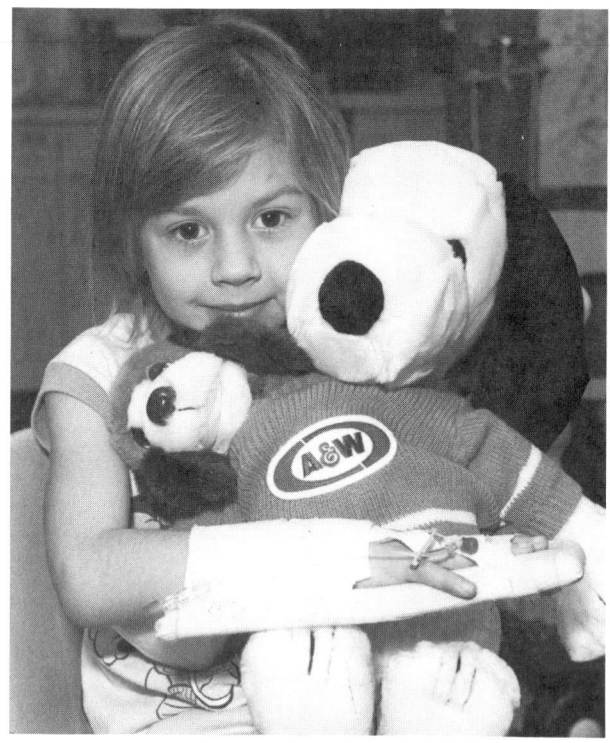

FIGURE 37-20
An intermittent infusion device (heparin lock) in place. Advocating for this type of apparatus minimizes pain. (Courtesy of the Department of Medical Photography, Children's Hospital, Buffalo, NY.)

long time and who need only intravenous medication, not additional fluid, are good candidates for such devices. Heparin locks can also be used with children when frequent venous blood samples are required. If blood is drawn from the already inserted tubing, the child is pricked only once (when the device is originally placed) no matter how many samples are drawn. Similar devices may be inserted into arteries when arterial blood is required—for example, for the child who is having blood gases monitored frequently.

Venous Access Catheters and Devices

Venous access for long-term intravenous therapy can be gained by insertion of a catheter into the vena cava just outside the right atrium; the catheter exits the chest just under the clavicle (Figure 37-21*A-D*). Typical catheters used in this way are Broviacs, Hickmans, or Groshongs. Such catheters have a wrinkle-resistant fabric (Dacron) cuff that adheres to subcutaneous tissue and helps to seal the catheter in place and keep infection out. Care of the catheters (depending on agency policy) consists of daily or weekly changes of dressings over the exit site and periodic irrigation with heparin or saline to ensure patency.

Such catheters have the advantage of not involving any further skin punctures, so they cause no further dis-

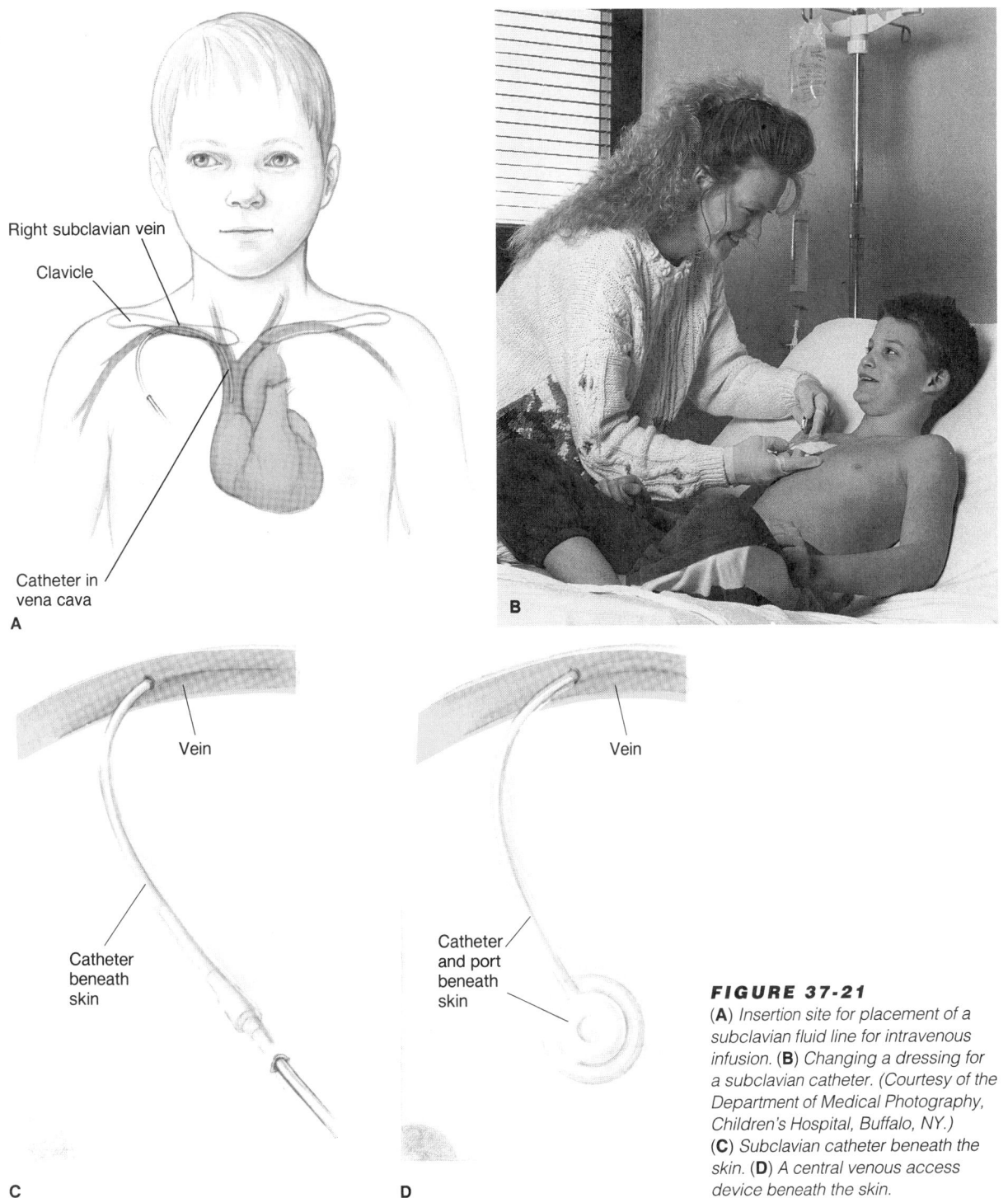

FIGURE 37-21

(**A**) *Insertion site for placement of a subclavian fluid line for intravenous infusion.* (**B**) *Changing a dressing for a subclavian catheter. (Courtesy of the Department of Medical Photography, Children's Hospital, Buffalo, NY.)* (**C**) *Subclavian catheter beneath the skin.* (**D**) *A central venous access device beneath the skin.*

comfort. One disadvantage is that the catheter could be snagged on something and accidentally pulled out. It is an emergency if this happens because the child could lose an appreciable amount of blood from the point of entrance into the vena cava. Children with a catheter in place are usually not allowed to swim or take showers, to avoid infection.

Central venous access devices (infusion ports that can be implanted) are small plastic devices that are implanted under the skin, usually on the anterior chest just under the clavicle (Albanese & Wiener, 1993) (Figure 37-21D). A small catheter threads from the port internally into a central vein. Common brands are Port-a-cath, Infus-A-port, and Groshong Venous Port. Blood samples can be removed or medication can be injected by a puncture through the chest skin into the port. Although this device requires a skin puncture (causes pain), it may be well accepted by children because it is not as visible as a central venous catheter, no dressing is required, and it allows a full range of activities such as showering and swimming. Be certain when accessing these ports to use only the needle supplied by the manufacturer. A regular needle has the tendency to "core" or remove a small circle of the membrane over the port and destroy the integrity of the device (Kandt, 1991).

Intraosseous Infusion

Intraosseous infusion (IO) is the infusion of fluid into the bone marrow cavity of a long bone, usually the distal or proximal tibia, the distal femur, or iliac crest (Skale, 1992). Because the bone marrow communicates directly with the circulatory system, the time at which fluid reaches the blood stream when administered this way is the same as if it were administered intravenously. All fluids that can be administered intravenously, including whole blood or medicine, can also be administered by this route.

Intraosseous infusion is used in an emergency when it is difficult to establish usual IV access or in a child with such extensive burns that the usual sites for intravenous infusion are not available (Guy et al., 1993).

Intraosseous infusion is a temporary measure until a usual route of administration can be opened because of the danger of osteomyelitis, a devastating infection with long-term effects to bone marrow. It must be initiated with sterile technique, and if continued for an extended time, the infusion point is rotated about every 2 to 3 days to try and minimize infection.

To begin the infusion, the skin over the chosen site is cleaned with betadine and anesthetized with a local anesthetic. A small incision is then made into the skin with a scalpel blade. A large hypodermic or bone marrow needle is inserted through the incision into the cavity of the bone. To ensure that the needle tip has reached the bone marrow cavity, a syringe is attached to the needle and aspirated for bone marrow. If bone marrow is obtained, the syringe is removed and intravenous tubing, including a filter and the fluid to be administered, is attached to the needle and opened to a gravity flow. A dressing with additional iodine is then applied over the needle site. Tubing must be changed about every 48 hours and the dressing over the site about every 24 hours—again, to try to reduce the possibility of infection.

A restraint is applied to the leg to help the child hold the leg still. Assess for a distal pulse and adequate temperature and color of the leg every hour during the length of the infusion to ensure that circulation to the leg is not becoming impaired. If the needle should become dislodged, symptoms of circulatory impairment or pain and taut skin over the site will occur.

Occasionally during the course of fluid administration, a bone chip or thick marrow will occlude an intraosseous needle and slow the infusion. If this occurs, a stilette passed through the needle clears it and allows for continued fluid administration.

Intraosseous infusion is painful as the needle first enters the bone marrow cavity or at the time of the bone marrow aspiration. Prepare the child for this and offer support.

Subcutaneous (Hypodermoclysis) Infusion

Before safe intravenous infusion was perfected with infants, fluid was given to them subcutaneously (perfusing fluid into subcutaneous skin layers by means of an intravenous infusion set). The technique may still be appropriate when an infant is extremely dehydrated and needs immediate replacement of fluid and it is impossible to locate a vein suitable for an intravenous infusion. Children with thalassemia anemia, a blood disorder, receive a medication to remove stored iron from their body by this route. Sites used for hypodermoclysis are generally the pectoral region, the back, or the anterolateral aspects of the thighs. The intravenous needle is inserted into the subcutaneous layer of the skin and the infusion apparatus opened. The rate is governed by the rate of absorption by the subcutaneous layer of skin, not a set rate.

Hot and Cold Therapy

Children who sustain muscle sprains or procedures such as bronchoscopy or tonsillectomy may have cold applications prescribed to prevent inflammation and edema (Figure 37-22). If inflammation or edema is already pres-

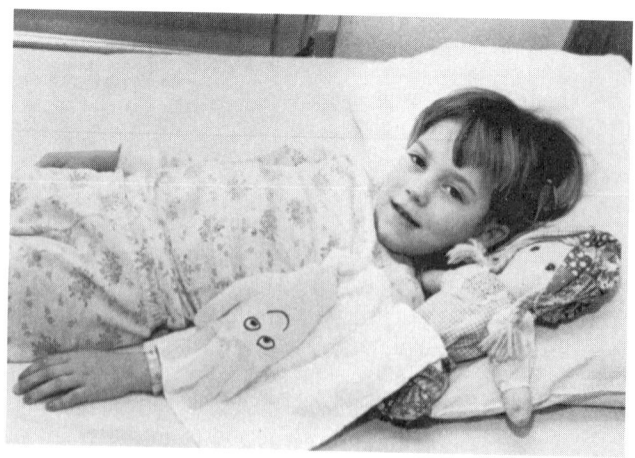

FIGURE 37-22
A rubber glove used as an ice pack. The face on it helps to make it seem friendlier. (Courtesy of the Department of Medical Photography, Children's Hospital, Buffalo, NY.)

ent, application of heat may be prescribed to help it re-solve. It is important to implement measures to prevent both burns and boredom in the child during treatments. Guidelines for hot and cold applications are shown in Box 37-1.

Aiding Elimination

Two aspects of intestinal elimination that require special care are administration of enemas and ostomy care.

Administering Enemas

Enemas are rarely used with children unless they are a part of preoperative preparation or are required for a radiologic study. If an enema is necessary, offer a careful explanation of what the child can expect to experience. The usual amounts of enema solutions used are as follows:

> Infant: Less than 250 mL (exact amount should be stipulated by physicians's order)
>
> Preschooler: 250–350 mL
>
> School-age child: 300–500 mL
>
> Adolescent: 500 mL

For an infant, use a small, soft catheter (no. 10 to 12 French) in place of an enema tip to prevent rectal trauma. Infants and children up to ages 3 or 4 years are unable to retain enema solutions, so they must rest on a bedpan during the procedure. Pad the edge of the pan so that it is not cold or sharp. Place a pillow under the infant's or young child's upper body for positioning and comfort. Lubricate the catheter generously with a water-soluble jelly and insert it only 2 to 3 inches (5 to 7 cm) in children and only 1 inch (2.5 cm) in infants. Be certain to hold the solution container no more than 1 foot above the level of the sigmoid colon (12 to 15 inches above the bed surface) so the solution flows at a con-trolled rate. If the child experiences intestinal cramping, clamp the tubing to halt the flow temporarily and wait until the cramping passes before instilling any more fluid. An older child can be asked to take a deep breath to help the cramping sensation pass. The amount of so-lution used in infants is so small that it is not usually a problem. If the enema solution is to be retained, such as an oil solution, hold the child's buttocks together after administration.

Until late school age, children cannot retain an enema as adults can (rarely more than 5 to 10 minutes). Be certain the bathroom the child will use is available before administering the enema.

Fleet enemas are not routinely administered to chil-dren younger than 2 years because of the harsh action of the sodium biphosphate and sodium phosphate they

---

1. Neither heat nor cold should be applied for longer than 20 minutes unless prescribed other-wise, because after this time, the vasoconstriction caused by cold and the vasodilatation caused by heat is reversed.
2. When using electrical sources of heat with tod-dlers and preschoolers, never make a game of plugging in and pulling out the apparatus that makes the light come on or a dial glow. Other-wise, the child may play with it after you leave.
3. Supply a special activity for a child to enjoy while a hot or cold application is in place (playing a board game or reading a story to the child) so that the procedure is not viewed as a chore but as a pleasant time to look forward to because of the accompanying enjoyable activity.
4. Put tape on the gauge of an electric appliance at the point where you want it so that a child can-not change the setting.
5. Always test the warmth of solutions or heat sources with your inner wrist before applying them to the child, to be certain they are not too hot.
6. Do not apply ice packs or ice directly to the skin. Cover the pack or ice with a towel or other cover to prevent frostbite and cell damage from cold.
7. Be cautious about heat or cold applications with a child who is receiving an analgesic because the child's perception of heat or cold may be reduced and he or she could easily be burned.

---

contain. Tap water is not used because it is not isotonic and causes rapid fluid shifts of water in body compart-ments, leading to possible water intoxication. Normal saline (0.9% sodium chloride) is the usual solution. It can be made by parents at home by adding 1 teaspoon-ful of salt to 1 pint (500 mL) of water.

After enema administration, praise the child for cooperating. Allow a preschooler an opportunity for therapeutic play, because this is a frightening procedure for a child of this age (Vessey & Mahon, 1990).

Providing Ostomy Care

An *ostomy* is an opening of the bowel on the surface of the abdomen. Ostomies in newborns are created to re-lieve bowel obstruction caused by conditions such as ileal atresia, necrotizing enterocolitis, and imperforate anus. In older children they are constructed for such conditions as inflammatory bowel syndrome. If an os-tomy is created in the ileum (an *ileostomy*), the stoma is located on the right side of the abdomen and drains liquid stool, which is extremely irritating to the skin because of the digestive enzymes it contains. If an ostomy is created in the sigmoid portion of the bowel (*colostomy*), the stoma is on the left lower abdomen and passes normally formed stool (Figure 37-23).

An ileostomy requires the use of a collecting ostomy appliance to contain acid stool and prevent excoriation of the abdominal skin; older children also may use an appliance with a colostomy. For an infant colostomy, parents may choose (with support and advice) whether to use an appliance or not.

There are two basic problems to using an ostomy appliance with an infant: it may be difficult to locate one small enough to contain liquid drainage without leaking, and the skin under the appliance may become extremely irritated. Clear plastic colostomy bags without a ring can be useful because they can be cut more easily to fit the size of the stoma and the contour and size of an infant's abdomen. A commercial skin sealant is helpful to harden the skin surrounding the stoma. Apply according to the brand directions and fan to dry. If a spray is used, protect the infant's face so that he or she does not inhale the solution. Apply the chosen stoma collection appliance. Tuck it inside the diaper.

Check the appliance or bag for collecting stool at least every 4 hours. To protect the underlying skin, do not remove a self-adhering bag if it is full, but drain collected stool from the bottom of the appliance into a basin or paper cup for disposal. To reduce odor, flush the appliance bag with a warm water and soap solution, using an asepto syringe, and rinse with clear water. Change the bag no more frequently than the point at which leakage occurs (perhaps as long as 1 week) to reduce skin irritation. To remove a bag that was placed with a sealant, be certain to use the designated solvent

to prevent pulling or harming underlying skin. The solvent must then be washed away with soap and water or it will become an irritant itself. Because most infants enjoy tub bathing, a long, soaking bath is also an excellent way to loosen an appliance.

If an appliance or bag is not used, stool will be discharged onto the abdomen three or four times a day (no different than a usual newborn or infant stool pattern). To care for a colostomy without using an appliance, wash and dry the stoma and surrounding skin area well; apply karaya powder, A&D ointment, or a stomadhesive to protect the skin. Apply ample absorbent gauze (fluffed) and an absorbent pad. Secure in place with nonadhesive tape or a binder. Check the dressing approximately every 4 hours. Remove and replace it when soiled, washing the skin well or ointment as necessary. Without an appliance in place, stool is kept from touching the skin only by the protection of the ointment and frequent changing of the dressing. Turning an infant from side to side after every feeding keeps stool from always flowing to one side and may be helpful. Leaving the abdominal skin exposed to air for at least 1 hour per day is helpful.

Stress that caring for an infant with an ostomy is little different than usual. All parents must change their infant's diapers frequently and clean the diaper area. Stress that the stoma has no nerves so that a parent can feel free to wash it without hurting the child and that compression against the stoma will not hurt so the parents feel comfortable laying the infant on his or her abdomen or holding the infant closely against their body for comfort.

Colostomies are rarely irrigated in children. On occasion, to prepare a child for second-stage abdominal surgery, irrigation of a colostomy may be ordered. If a *"blind-end"* bowel (bowel between the rectum and

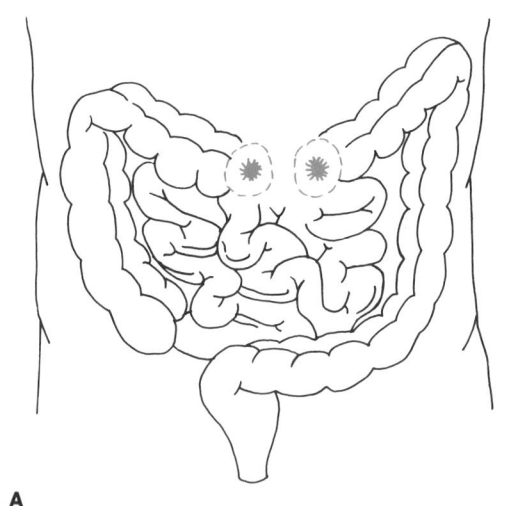
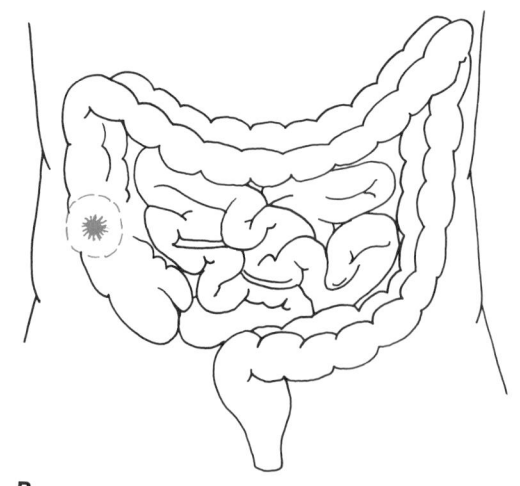

A   **B**

FIGURE 37-23
*Different sites for ostomies. (**A**) A double-barrel colostomy. (**B**) A single-barrel colostomy.*

colostomy) is present, that portion of bowel may be ordered irrigated daily to keep it lubricated and to maintain bowel tone. The exact amount of fluid to be used should be specified by the physician, but it is only a small amount (40 to 100 mL in infants). Tap water should never be used because it can lead to water intoxication as it is not isotonic. Normal saline (0.9% sodium chloride) is the usual preferred solution.

Children who have had a colostomy since infancy adapt well to it, because they have never known another method of defecation. In contrast, school-age children often have a great deal of difficulty adjusting to one. Encourage children to perform self-care as fully as possible. Preschool children usually benefit from therapeutic play that helps them work through their feelings (see Figure 36-11). Provide some time for older children to discuss concerns about being accepted by others and how to answer questions about a colostomy for other children. Adolescents with a colostomy may have questions regarding sexuality. They may appreciate open discussion of how they see this affecting their life.

Preparing a Child for Surgery

Preparing a child for surgery is a major responsibility for the child health nurse as surgery is a potentially very frightening procedure. Such preparation differs according to the type of surgery being performed, but certain activities apply to all surgery and all children. Psychological preparation is aimed at reducing the child's fears about the procedure and consists primarily of providing health teaching and opportunities for therapeutic play. Physical preparation includes providing for restrictions on food and fluid intake before surgery, preparing the incision site on the child's skin, and arranging for transportation of the child to surgery. Preparation must also include informing the parents about the details of the preparation techniques, the surgery, and the postoperative period.

Emotional Preparation

Preparing a child emotionally for surgery requires the prevention of fears common to all children (e.g., fear of separation, fear of mutilation, or fear of death). This can be accomplished by familiarizing the child with the procedure and describing the specific equipment and techniques that will be used, such as anesthesia, eye bandages, nasogastric tubes, sutures, or special aftercare. A teaching plan is essential for explaining all these features of surgery to the child (see Chapter 36). Preparation must be appropriate to age. Most children undergoing surgery will receive a general anesthetic, rather than a local or regional anesthetic as might be used with adults, because this minimizes their fears of intrusive or mutilat-

ing procedures, and because children who are not yet adolescents are not mature enough to cooperate adequately during surgery.

Physical Preparation

Most children will be on nothing by mouth (NPO) status for surgery. The length of the time the child will remain NPO depends on the child's age. Adolescents and school-age children may be restricted from food or fluid from midnight until the time of surgery the following morning; if infants younger than 6 months are held NPO for as long a time as this, they can be taken to surgery in dehydration. Because surgery means that the child will be NPO for a while afterward, this combined period on restricted fluids could cause the child to become extremely dehydrated. Therefore, infants younger than 6 months may be kept NPO for as little as 4 hours. At the end of the 4 hours, however, as the infant becomes hungry, he or she will begin to cry and fuss for fluid. Parents are not at their best at these times. They need an explanation that infants who vomit during surgery because of recent feedings may aspirate and therefore must be restricted from fluid. Infants who are used to pacifiers can be offered them, although a hungry child will usually not suck on one for long.

Preparing the Incision Area

Preparation of surgical sites varies. In most instances, shaving of the area and final cleansing are done in a holding room adjacent to the operating room after the child is anesthetized. A betadine wash may be ordered prior to transport to the operating room. Washing a particular body part this way can be interpreted as an intrusive procedure by a preschooler. He or she needs a great deal of assurance that the solution being used will not sting.

Transportation

The child should have his or her identification band checked to see that it is legible and secure. If not, it must be replaced or secured before surgery.

Immediately before transport, remove barrettes and bobby pins from the child's hair and check the mouth for loose teeth (particularly in children ages 6, 7, and 8 years who are losing their central and lateral incisors) or for dentures. It is rare to find a child with full dentures but not uncommon to find a "post" or screw-in tooth that may have to be removed before surgery or a "retainer" used to maintain an orthodontic correction following brace removal. Teeth braces do not need to be removed. Make certain the anesthesiologist knows about any loose teeth before an airway for surgery is inserted (a loose tooth could be knocked totally free and aspirated during the procedure).

Just before surgery, the child should be dressed in a hospital gown and underpants only. For some children, having to give up their own pajamas or their bedroom slippers or outside shoes is one of the most terrifying moments of hospitalization. Giving up underpants is a step that many preschool and early school-age children cannot tolerate, so children should be allowed to keep them on until they are under an anesthetic.

The cart that the child will ride to surgery should have been introduced during preparation. A child needs help in getting up onto a cart safely. The child should have a restraining strap fastened for safety (presented with "Here's your seat belt; it's just like going in a car"). Preschoolers may need a favorite toy or blanket to ride to surgery with them. Ideally, they should be allowed to keep this with them until they are under an anesthetic. Parents should be allowed to accompany their children to the operating suite. Some parents can accompany their child into an anesthesiologist's induction room; for others, this is asking more than they are capable of doing. A nurse whom the child knows should accompany the child to the operating room and remain there until the child is under the anesthetic. The bravest child can feel his or her courage fail at the moment the nurse who has cared for the child for the past 2 days says goodbye at the door of surgery and turns the child over to a green-dressed, firmly-capped stranger (even if the child has been well prepared for the exchange of personnel).

Although it may not be cost-effective to have a staff nurse wait with a child until he or she is under the anesthetic, the nurse's wait will probably not be long if the child has been called for surgery when the surgical suite is almost ready. The psychological benefit of a primary nurse's comforting presence is well worth it.

Preventing Injury in the Hospitalized Child

Nursing Diagnoses and Related Interventions

Nursing Diagnosis: High risk for injury related to maturational age of hospitalized child

Goal: The child will not sustain any injury during the hospital stay.

Outcome Criteria: Child does not fall from bed or sustain injury from hospital equipment.

Safety on a children's unit is the responsibility of everyone, from the administrator of the institution to part-time health care personnel. Because nurses are the ones most concerned with client care, the ultimate responsibility for safety rests most directly with them.

Fire Precautions

Ensure that there is a plan of action in case of a fire on a children's unit and that everyone on a unit knows it. Adults can usually take responsibility for removing themselves from a burning structure; children depend on care providers.

The average children's unit has respiratory and cardiac monitors, radiant heat warmers, special-care equipment, and even electrical thermometers, all of which must be plugged in. Do not use equipment with frayed cords or equipment that is not properly grounded. Plugs should be three-pronged for extra safety; do not overload circuits with additional plugs. Electrical outlets should have safety caps to cover them when they are not in use so that toddlers cannot poke objects into them and electrocute themselves.

Awareness of Children's Whereabouts and Actions

Always be sure of the location of all children. Ensure that doors or gates are provided near stairways and elevators. Windows should be covered by screens or guards so that children cannot climb up on sills and fall out.

Check that side rails are secured and in good repair. Bedside stands should be pushed away from cribs so that a child cannot climb over the railing and use the stand as a step down. Nothing should be within the child's reach that would be unsafe to eat (e.g., antiseptic, medication, or cleaning solution). If the child has a restraint in place, it should be assessed frequently as slipped restraints can occlude circulation; a jacket restraint can occlude the child's airway if it slips up to the neck.

Bathrooms

Ensure that electrical cords or appliances are not used in bathrooms where they will come in contact with water. Remind adolescents not to use a hair dryer or radio near a filled bathtub or sink. Never leave children under 5 years alone in a bathtub because they can turn on the hot water and scald themselves or slip under the water and drown.

Safety During Procedures

Children tend to fuss with equipment to see what will happen if they turn a knob or spin a dial. They need close monitoring while procedures are carried out to ensure that they do not increase the rate of infusions or in other ways accidentally harm themselves. After a procedure, be sure to remove all equipment from a room. Children pick up scissors or forceps left at bedsides and incur eye injuries; they drink antiseptics left at bedsides and poison themselves.

The Use of Restraints

No one likes to think about restraining children, because they may have difficulty distinguishing between restraint and punishment. Using restraints is a basic part of child safety, however (Masters et al., 1990).

Restraints should never be left in place longer than necessary. They should be checked every 15 minutes to see that they are not occluding circulation; they should be removed every hour so that the body part can be exercised (providing the exercise does not dislodge an infusion or interfere with a treatment). No other part of the child's body than what is necessary should be restrained. When a child has a scalp vein infusion in place, for example, the child's arms may need to be immobilized so that he or she does not touch the infusion, and the trunk may be immobilized so that the child does not turn. The child's lower extremities do not have to be restrained, however, so he or she can still actively kick and exercise them. Parents must be given careful explanations about why their child has a restraint in place (it is safer for their child). When the nurse or a parent are with the child, in most instances a restraint can be removed.

Types of Restraints

Bedside Rails. Some health care facilities require that all children have side rails raised at night. All children should have bedside rails raised after receiving preoperative or sedative medication.

Crib Rails. Crib sides should always be fully raised when a child is inside. Half-raised rails are more dangerous than completely lowered rails because the child climbs up to get over them and falls farther. A crib rail should be tested after it is raised to ensure that the lock has caught and it is firmly placed. Newly designed cribs have high added tops to them (climber cribs) to prevent children from climbing over rails (Figure 37-24).

High Chairs. An infant should not be left in a high chair (at home or in a hospital) without someone close enough to reach the child if he or she should fall from the chair. It is a good plan to use high-chair restraints with all infants in the hospital (or not to use high chairs). A restraint should tie around the back of the chair and also between the child's legs to keep the child from both climbing out and slipping out of the chair.

Wheelchairs and Carts. If a child needs to be transported in a wheelchair, he or she may need a restraint to

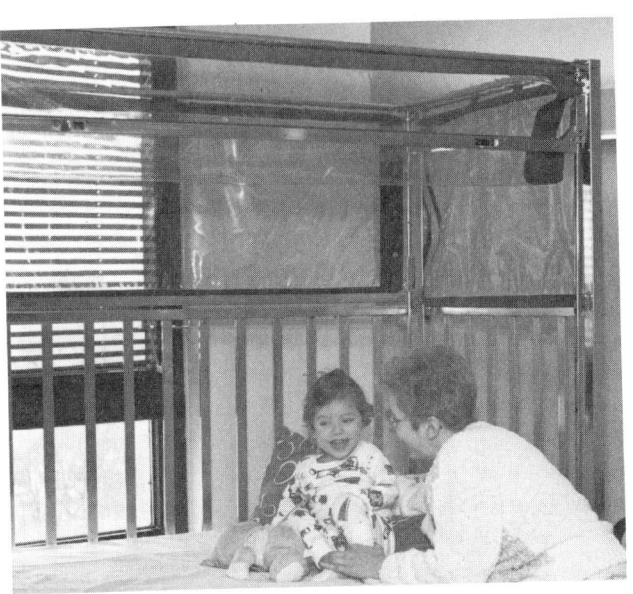

FIGURE 37-24
A climber crib with extended plastic sections at the top for safety. (Courtesy of the Department of Medical Photography, Children's Hospital, Buffalo, NY.)

be reminded to stay there. This is similar to a high-chair restraint. All children transported by a cart must have a restraint in place to prevent them from rolling off. It is generally just a restraining belt plus the side rails for the cart. Even with restraints in place, a child should not be left unattended in hallways outside departments in a wheelchair or on a cart. Not only is this unsafe because the child may attempt to get down from the cart or wheelchair, but the anxiety of waiting in a strange department for a procedure is too acute for him or her to handle.

Clove-Hitch Restraints. If a child is to have a procedure such as an intravenous infusion, the arm receiving the infusion must be kept still. Steps to keep the child's opposite arm out of the way so that the child does not fuss with the infusion may also be necessary.

To restrain arms and legs, use disposable wrist restraints or a clove-hitch restraint (Figure 37-25). Soft muslin is used for restraints because it "gives" a little if the child exerts pressure against it so it will not pull too tight and reduce circulation or cause pain.

If a child struggles against wrist restraints, fold several layers of soft gauze around the wrist or ankle under the restraint. Secure the restraint to the underpart of the bed. Never tie restraints to side rails: when a side rail is lowered, it will jerk the child's arm or leg and possibly cause an injury.

Release arm and leg restraints whenever someone can be with the child to keep the limb in the desired position.

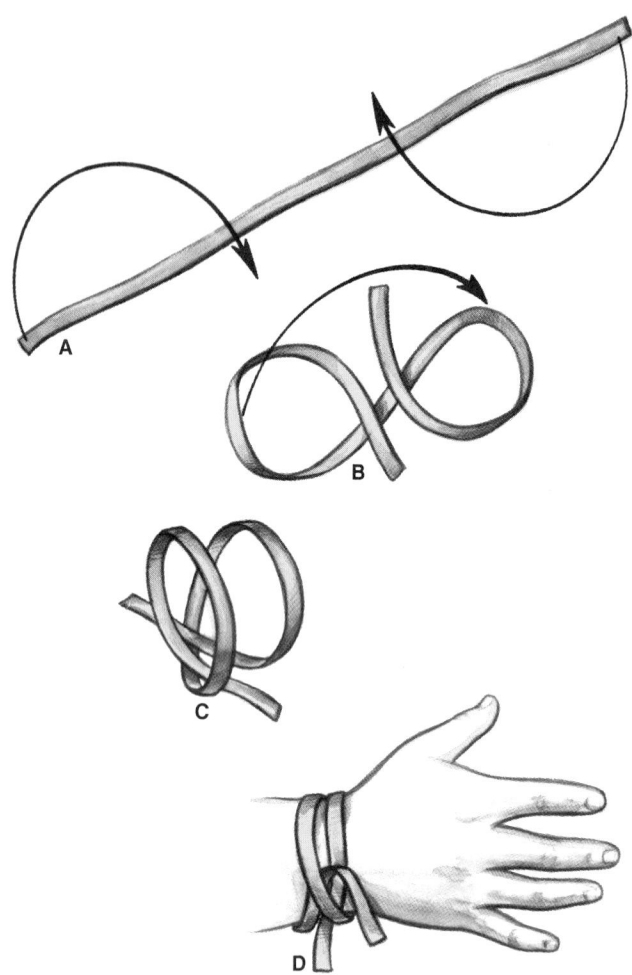

FIGURE 37-25
A clove-hitch restraint. A soft strip of cloth is formed into a figure 8, with both ends of cloth on top of the figure 8. Bring the loops together and pull the two ends to adjust the loop to the size of the child's wrist or ankle.

Jackets. A jacket restraint is a small jacket that ties at the child's back. Strips attached to the sides of the jacket are tied under the mattress to keep the child in one position. This is effective with children younger than 6 months. Older children are too active: they squirm and maneuver so much that there is a real danger of squirming out of the jacket or putting so much pressure on the trachea that they suffocate.

Elbow Restraints. The elbow restraint is used to prevent infants from touching scalp vein infusions and to keep infants with facial surgery, such as cleft lip or cleft palate repairs, from touching the suture line. Older children may have their arms immobilized to keep their hands from equipment or infusions.

There are a number of ways to restrain a child's elbows. Put an infant in a long-sleeved gown and pin the arms of the gown at the sides to the diaper. *No-No sleeves* are a commercial type of elbow restraint that slips

up over the infant's arms and is secured by Velcro strips (Figure 37-26). The baby should wear a long-sleeved infant shirt under the sleeves to prevent irritation. The child must be observed, as with all restraint devices, to be certain the sleeves are not too tight and interfere with circulation.

Mummy Restraints. A mummy restraint is used when young children must be temporarily immobilized—for example, during insertion of a nasogastric tube or drawing blood (Figure 37-27). Because this is a total body restraint, it is used only for the duration of the procedure, then removed. If the child is exceptionally strong, a few safety pins can be used to hold the restraint even more firmly. "Papoose Boards" are commercial restraints used in this same way as full or mummy restraints for newborns or infants. A mummy restraint can be folded so the chest is exposed for the infant who needs continuous observation for respiratory function.

Limits on Behavior

The average child is motivated to follow instructions and rules and demonstrate good behavior during a hospital stay because he or she wants to get well again and return home again as soon as possible. The occasional child who does misbehave in a hospital setting usually does so because he or she lacks a clear understanding of what is expected or is demonstrating that personal needs have not been appropriately recognized and met.

A child who needs frequent reminders to stop running in the hallway, for example, is probably bored with staying in a room. Providing more activities (playing a

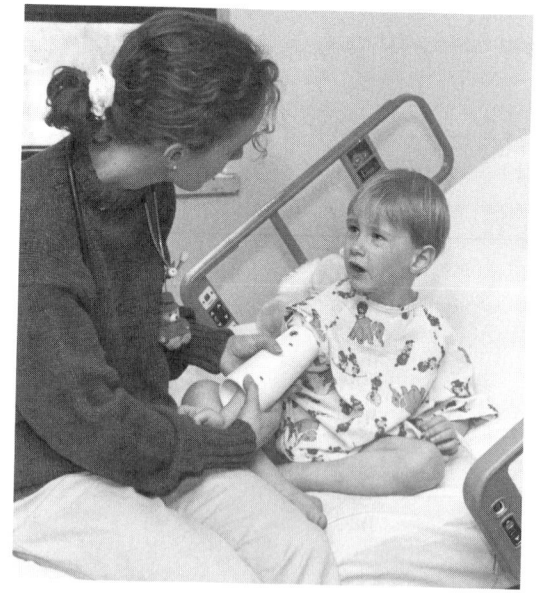

FIGURE 37-26
A No-No sleeve or commercial elbow restraint. (Courtesy of the Department of Medical Photography, Children's Hospital, Buffalo, NY.)

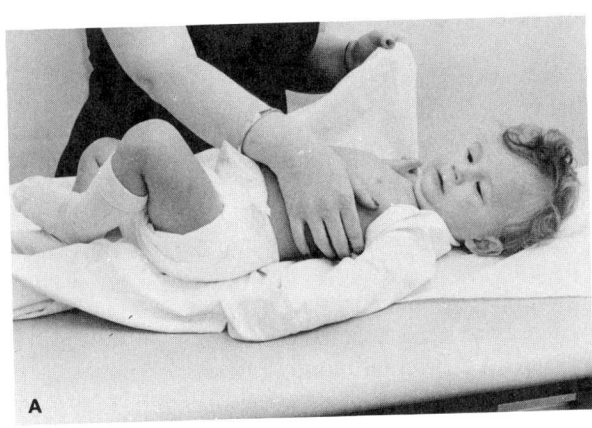
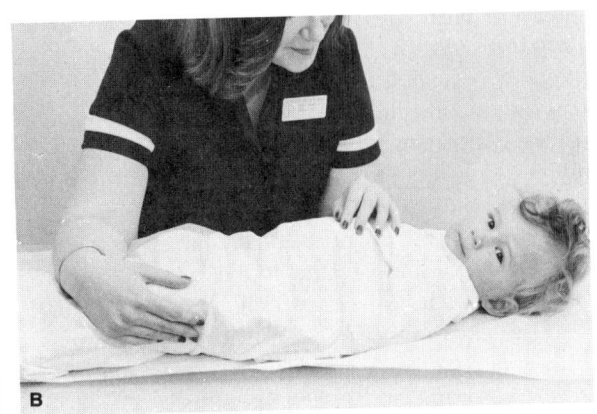

FIGURE 37-27
*A mummy restraint. (**A**) The child is placed on the back. The restraint (a draw sheet wide enough to circle the child twice or a towel for very young babies) is brought over one arm and anchored underneath the child by the weight of the child's own body. (**B**) The mummy restraint is completed by bringing the other side of the restraint over the top surface of the child and again anchoring it under the child by the weight of the body. (Courtesy of the Department of Medical Photography, Children's Hospital, Buffalo, NY.)*

game with the child) or allowing more structured exercise (letting the child accompany a nursing aide to take a blood specimen to a laboratory) prevents further unsafe activity.

Children who refuse to cooperate for procedures are generally acting out of fear of the unknown rather than deliberately misbehaving. For potentially painful procedures such as a bone marrow aspiration, lumbar puncture, blood sampling, or cast removal, any behavior short of hysterical screaming can be considered "good" behavior. The better prepared they are for such procedures, the better children are able to accept them (Mansson et al., 1993).

If limit setting is necessary, such as with a child who hits or bites other children, confer with parents about the need for limit setting and what measures they would suggest; gain their cooperation and approval. Using "time out" periods or removing the child to a nonstimulating area for a short time is an effective measure (Christophersen, 1992). Be certain the child understands the rules (if the child bites or hits, he or she will have to sit alone for a designated period). The next time the child misbehaves, give one warning that the behavior is against the rules; if the behavior does not improve, take the child to the "time out" designation. If the child is disruptive, begin timing the period from when the child quiets down. When the child has been quiet for the specified duration, he or she can leave the time out place and rejoin activities.

Assuring Client Identity

On admission to a health care facility, all children should have an armband attached giving their name, address, and hospital chart number. Because their hands are not much larger than their wrists and their feet are not much larger in diameter than their ankles, neonates (infants younger than 1 month of age) should have two bands in place as an extra safeguard. Never tape bands just to the crib or bedside stand; it is not adequate protection. If an infant is placed in the wrong crib by mistake, he or she may be given a medicine that is lethal before the mistake is realized.

If an armband must be removed because it interferes with an intravenous infusion site, cut it away but immediately anchor it to another extremity with adhesive tape. Ask the admissions department to provide a new armband as soon as possible. Do not leave the old one off while waiting for a replacement band. This leaves the child susceptible to the danger of mistaken identity during the waiting period.

Before giving any medication or food or before performing any procedure, look at the identification band. This check serves as a basic safety precaution.

Prevention of Nosocomial Infection

Children frequently have a dressing or bandage in place during a hospital stay, to cover a surgical incision or sutured laceration. Such dressings differ from adult dressings in terms of material, size, and methods used to secure them. Keeping a dressing dry in infants and toddlers who are not toilet trained can be a major problem (Braren, 1990). In many instances following surgery, collodion (a clear substance similar to nail polish) is applied to a suture line to serve as the dressing. This keeps the suture line from being contacted by urine or feces and, because it is clear, allows good visualization of the healing surface. Parents need to be assured that such a covering is adequate and actually preferable if the incision is in the groin from surgery such as a hernia repair.

If a gauze dressing is used, it can be covered with plastic, securely held in place with nonadhesive, waterproof tape. Be certain when cutting plastic to cover a dressing not to leave an extra piece behind in the crib; the child could pull it over his or her head and suffocate.

Infants and young children usually have skin that is too sensitive for adhesive tape to be used to secure dressings. Use nonadhesive tape (silk or paper) instead or secure a dressing with a nonadhering bandage (Kling) or roller gauze. Young children, as a rule, find bandages comforting and accept them as a "badge of courage," displaying them proudly. Apply adhesive bandages (Band-Aids) generously after venipuncture or finger punctures for this reason. Preschool children have little concept of how long it takes healing to occur. They are often surprised that their incision or wound has not yet healed the day after surgery. Preschoolers are often worried that a part of their body under a dressing is missing and find it reassuring to see that the body part is still there (they may pull a dressing away to do this). It is better to know what something is like than to worry about the unknown. Therefore, do not discourage children from looking at their incision during dressing changes. Even if the area looks raw and unhealed, it may look better than what the child has envisioned was under the dressing.

Promoting Adequate Sleep for the Hospitalized Child

Nursing Diagnoses and Related Interventions

Nursing Diagnosis: Sleep pattern disturbance related to timing of medication or hospital environment

Goal: Child will maintain regular sleep pattern during hospital stay.

Outcome Criteria: Child sleeps through the night without interruption (when therapeutic regimen allows); is alert and active during the day; is able to take nap during the day if that is part of usual sleep schedule.

Ill children need adequate rest and sleep so that their body tissues can effectively use nutrients for repair and normal growth can continue. Children may not sleep well in a hospital because it is a strange setting; they may have to undergo so many procedures that they do not even nap or rest as much as usual. For children to receive adequate rest and sleep, a nursing care plan must include measures to promote this.

Sleep Patterns

Sleep is influenced by anxiety level, state of health, habit, medication, and environment at the time of sleep. Figure 37-28A shows the pattern of normal sleep. During sleep, there is a decrease in the tone of the musculoskeletal system. Heart rate, respiratory rate, systolic blood pressure, and body temperature all decrease. Less urine forms during sleep owing to a falling basal metabolic rate. A child uses less oxygen during sleep than when awake; because of the recumbent position, there is increased cerebral blood flow.

During a night, sleep comprises repeated cycles of 60 to 120 minutes (average, 90 minutes) in length. These cycles are shortest in the newborn (45 to 60 minutes) and become longer (90 to 120 minutes) by adolescence. During an average night's sleep of 7 to 8 hours, four to six sleep cycles occur.

As a sleep cycle begins, a child first enters **non-rapid-eye movement (NREM) sleep**. This type of sleep occurs in up to 80% of total sleep time. As a child falls deeper and deeper asleep, he or she passes from stage I to stage II, III, and IV of NREM sleep over a period of 20 to 30 minutes. **Rapid-eye movement (REM)** sleep follows. A description of stages of sleep is shown in Table 37-2 with the importance to nursing care.

In infants, most of sleep time is REM sleep, whereas young adults have the least. If a child is awakened from sleep, he or she begins again with NREM sleep stage I as the child falls asleep again, not the pattern from which the child was awakened. The sleep pattern of a child who is awakened frequently during the night for procedures would resemble that shown in Figure 37-28B.

Children who are recovering from trauma such as injuries from a car accident or burns may be unable to sleep for fear the accident will happen again. They may suffer sleep deprivation in the same way as a child who is frequently awakened for procedures during the night. Encourage parents to stay with these children for support and comfort.

The purpose of NREM sleep is rest and restoration of the body; it keeps body cells functioning and healthy. During the periods of stage III and IV NREM sleep, the secretion of growth hormone (somatotropic hormone) from the pituitary is at its highest level. Growth hormone is necessary for protein synthesis and growth of new cells and for repair and maintenance of all cells. Corticosteroids and adrenaline from the adrenal gland, which are instrumental in the catabolism or breakdown of cells, are at their lowest levels. This balance of hormones is the ideal combination for protein synthesis and cell growth and repair.

The purpose of REM sleep is less clear. The rapid eye movements may serve to coordinate binocular vision; dreams that occur during this time apparently serve as a release of tension or help to integrate new knowl-

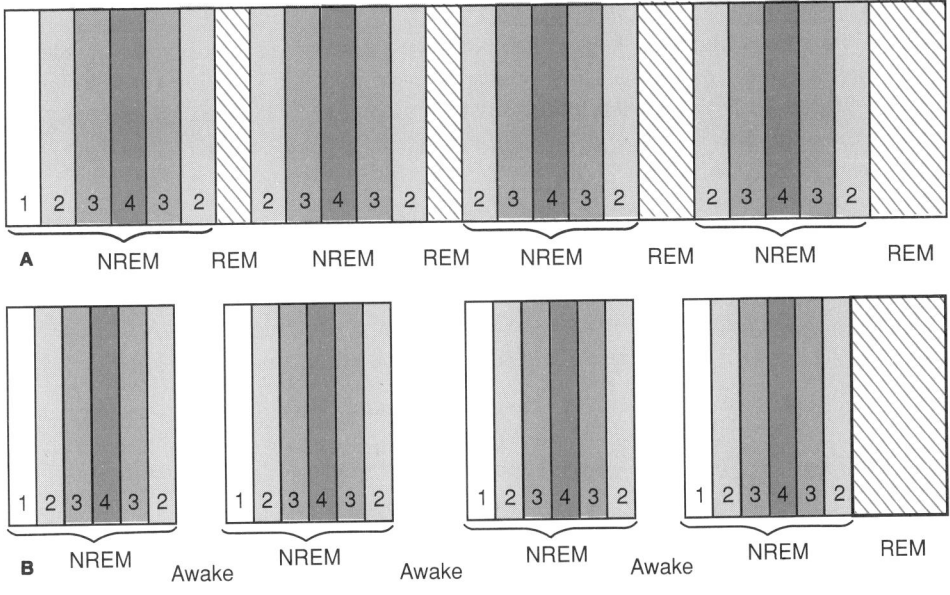

FIGURE 37-28
Sleep patterns. (A) Normal sleep pattern. Notice how the periods of REM sleep increase in length during the last half of the night. (B) The sleep pattern of a child who has been awakened frequently during the night. Notice how little REM sleep is present.

edge and experience with old in the brain's memory system. During REM sleep, vital signs rise to near-normal levels. These periods of REM sleep interspersed with NREM sleep may be a fail-safe measure to prevent vital signs from falling too low during sleep.

Sleep Problems

Sleep Deprivation

Like adults, children who do not receive enough sleep can suffer **sleep deprivation**. After approximately 4 days without sleep, they show difficulty in concentrating and experience episodes of disorientation and misperception; they are generally irritable and can manifest feelings of persecution and marked physical fatigue.

If the sleep loss is mainly REM deprivation, children mainly show symptoms of irritability and difficulty concentrating. Lack of stage IV NREM sleep tends to cause apathy and depression. This can happen in adolescents if they are studying for exams, or in younger children during a hospital stay if they are awakened frequently for treatments.

Table 37-2. *Stages of Sleep in Children*

Stage	Description	Nursing Implications
NREM		
I	A feeling of drifting or falling. Often described as twilight sleep. Temperature and heart rate decrease slightly; EEG waves show peaked, frequently occurring waves (alpha waves).	A child can be roused easily from this early sleep by the slightest noise or even the silent presence of another person in the room. Reduce noise level in room to promote sleep.
II	Sleep deepens. Temperature and heart rate decrease slightly more.	It is more difficult to wake a child from sleep when this point has been reached.
III	Sleep deepens still further. An EEG tracing reveals mixed spindle and delta (slow-moving) waves. Temperature and heart rate decrease further. This period lasts about 10 min.	It is very difficult to wake a child from stage III sleep. Use patience to wake a child fully to offer medicine.
IV	Approximately 20 min to 30 min after beginning to fall asleep, a child enters stage IV sleep. Respirations are slow and deep, temperature and heart rate slow even more, and blood pressure decreases; EEG shows delta (slow, steady) waves. A child remains at a stage IV sleep level for approximately 30 min, then progresses back through stages III and II until he or she then passes into a phase of REM sleep.	A child will be confused and unable to orient himself/herself readily if awakened from stage IV sleep. Use patience until a child is fully awake, particularly if asking a question.
REM	Eyes move in rapid, involuntary motions. Respirations are irregular; body turnings, movements, and penile erections may occur. Lasts 10 min to 30 min and then a new sleep cycle with NREM sleep begins.	Dreaming occurs during REM sleep. Although the child appears to be close to waking because of the active eye movements, he or she is really very soundly asleep. A child may wake afraid and crying, disturbed by a frightening dream.

Nocturnal Enuresis

Involuntary urination is *enuresis;* when it occurs at night it is **nocturnal enuresis** or bedwetting (Hamburger, 1993). Bedwetting occurs most frequently during the deep stage IV of NREM sleep or with the shift into an REM sleep pattern. Children who have difficulty with nocturnal enuresis at home can be expected to continue it in a hospital setting. Ask on a hospital admission if the child has this problem. Although bedwetting is frequently associated with small bladder capacity, it can also occur with a urinary tract infection. Interventions for bedwetting are discussed in Chapter 46.

Somnambulism

Sleepwalking (*somnambulism*) is a second sleep problem that occurs in childhood (Clore et al., 1993). Sleepwalking apparently occurs during NREM sleep, probably during the deepest stage, IV. It is frightening for a child to wake and realize that he or she has been sleepwalking; the child is confused because he or she is waking from such a deep stage of sleep. In a hospital setting, sleepwalking may be dangerous because, while getting out of bed, the child may dislodge intravenous tubing or fall. It is untrue that a sleepwalker should not be wakened; instead, the sleepwalker should be wakened gently, helped to get reoriented, and then returned to bed after being reassured that he or she is safe. Be certain that side rails are raised on the bed of a child who tends to sleepwalk. It may be necessary to move a child's bed out into the hallway near the nurse's desk at night if a parent will not be sleeping over, so the child can be observed for sleepwalking.

Sleeptalking

Sleeptalking seems to occur during REM sleep. Dreaming of some frightening or puzzling situation, a child calls out a name or instructions such as "Stop!" Because hospitalization is a stressful situation that increases anxiety, sleeptalking may occur at an increased rate during this time. It is unnecessary to wake a child who is sleeptalking unless the child is thrashing around and would dislodge equipment such as intravenous tubing. Because sleeptalking usually results from a frightening dream, waking the child gently is comforting. Parents may need to be assured that sleeptalking is harmless and will subside when their child returns to a more secure environment.

Night Terrors

A number of children are prone to night terrors, and wake screaming approximately 20 minutes after they fall asleep. Comforting them when they wake and calming other children who are frightened by the noise helps everyone return to sleep. In the morning, children rarely remember the incident.

Sleep Apnea

Sleep apnea is the cessation of respirations during sleep for 20 seconds or more and is a possible cause of sudden infant death syndrome (SIDS) (see Chapter 26).

Offering Stimulation in the Hospitalized Child

Nursing Diagnoses and Related Interventions

> **Nursing Diagnosis:** Diversionary activity deficit related to lack of appropriate toys and peers in hospital environment.
>
> **Goal:** Child will receive age-appropriate stimulation while in hospital.
>
> **Outcome Criteria:** Child remains alert and interested in self-care and hospital activities; if well and old enough, expresses interest in participating in hospital-sponsored activities or spending time in play-activity room.

Children are in constant interaction with both internal environment (body) and external environment (surroundings) by means of the five senses and the central nervous system. Thus, they can respond to changes in environment and by so doing meet basic needs. Both sensory deprivation and sensory overstimulation can occur because of hospitalization.

Sensory Deprivation

Sensory deprivation is the condition of being deprived of, or lacking, adequate sensory, social, physical, or cognitive stimulation. Children with this condition tend to lose the ability to make decisions and become easily confused and depressed. Some children are more prone to sensory deprivation than others.

Children at any age (most noticeably those younger than age 5 years) interact at a deeper level with their parents than with other people around them. As discussed in Chapter 35, when separated from parents, their level of cognitive interaction may fall markedly (maternal deprivation).

Children who have poor interaction with their parents generally receive less-than-normal cognitive stimulation. If this happens to a preschool child, he or she may show the same symptoms of failure to thrive due to maternal deprivation as the child whose parent is not actually present. Such children need a warm, reassuring relationship with health care personnel and cognitive stimulation to develop normally.

Adolescents who are having a particularly difficult time relating to their parents can manifest a hunger to relate with other adults to fulfill their need for interaction. They may discuss issues with nurses that they can no longer discuss with their own parents.

Children with hearing or visual deficits are prone to sensory deprivation. Children with forms of sensory nerve loss or who are having chemotherapy may lose their sense of touch, taste, or proprioception (sense of where they are in space). After losing these forms of perception, children may also draw back from interaction with other people because they are self-conscious about the loss, and thus be deprived of social and cognitive stimulation. The techniques for interacting with sensory deprived children are discussed in Chapter 50.

Some children receive medication to lessen awareness of the stimulating factors in their environment. To ensure that they do not suffer sensory deprivation, give them definite orientation measures, such as always mentioning the time of day and the day of the week in conversations with them. At the same time, they often must have overly stimulating factors reduced, such as the number of visitors, so that perceptions can be interpreted clearly.

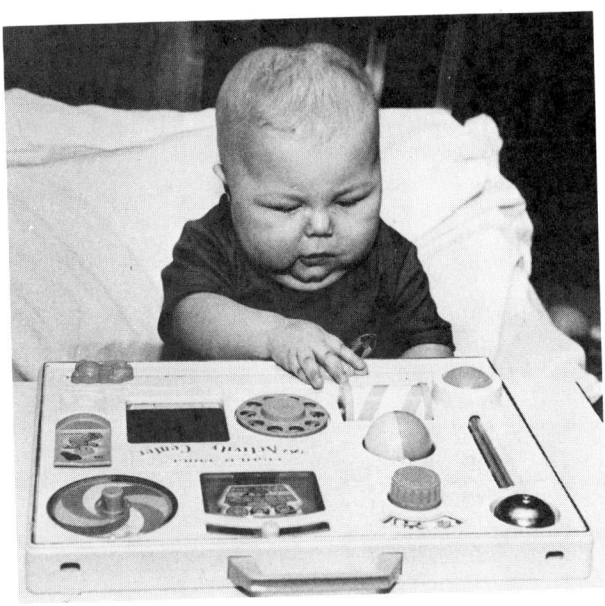

FIGURE 37-29
Children on bedrest need stimulation. Here, an infant enjoys a "busy board." (Courtesy of the Department of Medical Photography, Children's Hospital, Buffalo, NY.)

Stimulation for Children on Bedrest

Children on bedrest are unable to secure materials for cognitive stimulation by themselves or to participate in physical stimulation except to a limited degree. A room where walls and windows offer no visual appeal and therapeutic equipment provides the only sound offers them little sensory stimulation. If no one comes into the room, they may suffer from social deprivation. When possible, let the child sit in a wheelchair. This will provide some mobility and transportation to a place of interest, such as near a window or the nursing desk. Watching television, a common activity for children on bedrest, provides little cognitive stimulation after the first 24 hours when the novelty has worn off. For the average adolescent, many television programs are not stimulating enough.

Occasionally, a child must remain in bed to reduce stimulation (e.g., to rest the heart or to increase kidney function), but generally bedrest is prescribed mainly to inactivate one part of the body, such as a fractured bone. When possible, other stimulation, such as a favorite toy, games, books, or simply talking with someone, must be provided for the child to maintain physical bedrest; otherwise, he or she will become bored and irritable and will thrash and turn instead of lying still (Figure 37-29). Most parents are aware that a child will receive more rest on a living room couch where he or she can participate in the family's activities than in a distant bedroom where the child constantly calls out for attention or interaction. This principle applies to hospitalized children as well. A toddler may rest better in a parent's lap than in a bed.

Stimulation for Children in Isolation

Children who are isolated because of the possibility of contagious illness may experience severe sensory deprivation if everyone who enters the room must wear a gown and mask and if the number of visitors is kept to a minimum. If gloves are part of precautions, the child can experience a significant loss of skin-to-skin contact. Isolation techniques are discussed in Chapter 43. Careful planning must be done to ensure that a child in isolation is not psychologically isolated and that every possible measure is carried out to maintain sensory, social, physical, and cognitive stimulation. For example, try to visit with a child in addition to those times in which procedures are performed; place the bed so the child can see out; encourage him or her to telephone home; make posters for walls; bring toys such as electronic games from home and so forth. For ideas on providing stimulation to children in specific age groups, refer to Chapters 29 to 33.

The Child With Sensory Overload

Sensory overload, in contrast to deprivation, occurs when a child receives more stimulation than he or she can tolerate or process. This may occur in a room where the lights are too bright or the sound too loud. Children with sensory overload react similarly to those with sensory deprivation (i.e., they are confused, unable to make decisions, and severely fatigued). Sometimes it is difficult to determine the cause of these symptoms (whether they are caused by sensory deprivation or overload) unless assessed carefully.

The lights in intensive care units (ICUs), for example, are never turned out; although children may find this comforting, excessive stimulation may also result. In addition to constant light, there is excessive sound (e.g., whir of machines, buzzing of ventilators, ringing of alarms, or mix of voices in consultation). Most ICUs have no windows because the wall space is used for monitoring equipment; therefore night and day are not easily distinguished. It is easy for a child to become confused about time and place. An important nursing role is reducing sensory stimulation due to overload. Orient children to the time of day by making frequent references to it and by providing calendars and clocks. If necessary, provide eye covers or ear plugs to reduce stimulation.

Promoting Comfort in the Hospitalized Child

Nursing Diagnoses and Related Interventions

Nursing Diagnosis: Pain related to pathologic process or surgery

Goal: Child will experience nothing more than tolerable level of pain and discomfort during hospital stay.

Outcome Criteria: Child voices he or she is experiencing tolerable level of comfort and can describe ways to reduce pain when it returns; infant demonstrates little or no crying.

Many childhood illnesses and accidents are accompanied by pain. As in adults, pain in children occurs for one of four reasons: (1) reduced oxygen in tissues from impaired circulation, (2) pressure on tissue, (3) external injury, or (4) overstretching of body cavities with fluid or air. Pain is difficult to define, but McCaffery's (1980, p. 26) classic description is the most useful to use with children: "The sensation is whatever the person experiencing it says it is, and it exists whenever he or she says it does."

The purpose of acute pain is to warn that the body has been injured; this allows a person to group resources and get help. As soon as healing begins again, pain decreases. Unfortunately, some childhood illnesses, such as malignancy and juvenile arthritis, bring chronic pain as the child's body continues to sound a warning of danger for the entire length of the illness. Acute pain stimulates the sympathetic nervous system and increases heart rate, respiratory rate, and peripheral vasoconstriction. Chronic pain can lead to depression because it is

always present (Bullock & Rosendahl, 1992). Common myths about children and pain are shown in Table 37-3.

Assessing Type and Degree of Pain

Pain is often a confusing sensation to children. In addition, acute pain is frightening, and chronic pain is exhausting. With either, children may feel that their caregivers are letting them down because no one is able to give them relief from pain.

Determining when pain is present and its extent is difficult with children because they may be unable to describe it with their limited vocabularies (Johnston et al., 1990). Words such as "sharp," "nagging," or "aching" have no meaning in relation to pain until the child has experienced each type. Children who think concretely (preadolescents) can have difficulty envisioning that a word like "sharp" applies both to knives and to the feeling in their abdomen. Some children compound pain or suffer with it rather than report it, for fear of more unpleasant treatments such as injections. Some do not appear to be in pain because they distract themselves by such methods as concentrating on play. Some children may sleep, not from comfort but from the exhaustion caused by pain.

Adult scales such as the McGill Pain Questionnaire are available to rate pain in adolescents (Figure 37-30) (Melzack, 1975). With young children, use an easier concept such as asking them to evaluate their level of pain on a scale of 1 to 5, as a color, as a number of poker chips, or by looking at a row of frowning to smiling

Table 37-3. Myths and Facts About Pain in Children

Myth	Fact
Young children, particularly newborns, do not feel pain	Newborns and children do feel pain
A child who resumes usual activity cannot be in pain	Some children distract themselves with play while in pain
Because of the possible adverse effects, narcotic analgesics are too dangerous for young children	Narcotics can be used safely in children, including low-birth-weight infants
Unless a child tells you he or she is in pain, the child is not feeling pain	Children may assume you know they are in pain
If a child denies he or she is feeling pain, you should believe him or her	Children may deliberately deny pain to avoid an injection
Experiencing pain will not harm an infant or young child	Newborns with pain can become cyanotic and bradycardic; no one knows the psychological stress of pain at this age

(From McCaffery, M., & Beebe, A [1990]. Myths and facts about pain in children. *Nursing, 20,* 81, with permission.)

McGill-Melzack
PAIN QUESTIONNAIRE

Patient's name _____ Age_____

File No._____ Date_____

Clinical category (e.g., cardiac, neurological, etc): _____

Diagnosis: _____
_____
_____

Analgesic (if already administered):

1. Type_____
2. Dosage_____
3. Time given in relation to this test_____

Patient's intelligence: circle number that represents best estimate

1 (low)   2   3   4   5 (high)

****

This questionnaire has been designed to tell us more about your pain. Four major questions we ask are:

1. Where is your pain?
2. What does it feel like?
3. How does it change with time?
4. How strong is it?

It is important that you tell us how your pain feels now. Please follow the instructions at the beginning of each part.

Part 1.   Where Is Your Pain?

Please mark on the drawings below, the areas where you feel pain. Put E if external, or I if internal, near the areas which you mark. Put EI if both external and internal.

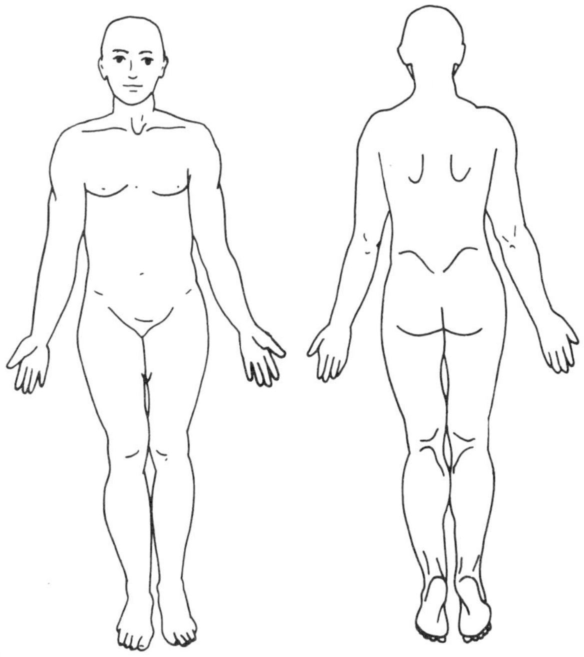

Part 2.   What Does Your Pain Feel Like?

Some of the words below describe your present pain. Circle ONLY those words that best describe it. Leave out any category that is not suitable. Use only a single word in each appropriate category—the one that applies best.

1	2	3	4
Flickering	Jumping	Pricking	Sharp
Quivering	Flashing	Boring	Cutting
Pulsing	Shooting	Drilling	Lacerating
Throbbing		Stabbing	
Beating		Lancinating	
Pounding			

5	6	7	8
Pinching	Tugging	Hot	Tingling
Pressing	Pulling	Burning	Itchy
Gnawing	Wrenching	Scalding	Smarting
Cramping		Searing	Stinging
Crushing			

9	10	11	12
Dull	Tender	Tiring	Sickening
Sore	Taut	Exhausting	Suffocating
Hurting	Rasping		
Aching	Splitting		
Heavy			

13	14	15	16
Fearful	Punishing	Wretched	Annoying
Frightful	Gruelling	Blinding	Troublesome
Terrifying	Cruel		Miserable
	Vicious		Intense
	Killing		Unbearable

17	18	19	20
Spreading	Tight	Cool	Nagging
Radiating	Numb	Cold	Nauseating
Penetrating	Drawing	Freezing	Agonizing
Piercing	Squeezing		Dreadful
	Tearing		Torturing

Part 3.   How Does Your Pain Change With Time?

1. Which word or words would you use to describe the pattern of your pain?

1	2	3
Continuous	Rhythmic	Brief
Steady	Periodic	Momentary
Constant	Intermittent	Transient

2. What kind of things relieve your pain?

3. What kind of things increase your pain?

Part 4.   How Strong Is Your Pain?

People agree that the following 5 words represent pain of increasing intensity. They are:

1   2   3   4   5
Mild Discomforting Distressing Horrible Excruciating

To answer each question below, write the number of the most appropriate word in the space beside the question.

1. Which word describes your pain right now? _____
2. Which word describes it at its worst? _____
3. Which word describes it when it is least? _____
4. Which word describes the worst toothache you ever had? _____
5. Which word describes the worst headache you ever had? _____
6. Which word describes the worst stomach-ache you ever had? _____

FIGURE 37-30

The McGill Pain Questionnaire. (From Melzack, R. [1975]. The McGill Pain Questionnaire. Major properties and scoring methods. Pain, 1, 277, with permission).

 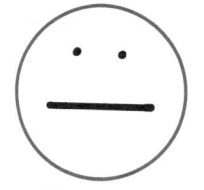  

Really bad pain   A lot of pain   Some pain   A little pain   No pain

FIGURE 37-31

A pain rating scale for children. The child indicates which face best represents his or her degree of pain.

faces and rating each face in comparison with how they feel (Price, 1990; Savedra, 1993) (Figure 37-31). Evaluating pain in infants is especially difficult as they are unable to voice or rate their pain by any method (Shapiro, 1993). Cultural differences also influence how pain is expressed (see the Focus on Cultural Awareness box).

The Infant

Infants respond to pain by diffuse body movements and intense crying. They are instinctively able to guard a body part with pain by holding an extremity still or tensing their abdomen. A mark of pain in infants is that when pain is present, they cannot be completely comforted.

The Toddler and Preschooler

Toddlers have enough understanding of the word "pain" to be able to point to what hurts. Pain is such a strange sensation to them, however, that aside from crying in re-

sponse to it, they may react aggressively (pounding and rocking) as if to fight it off.

Preschool children cry with acute pain; they continue to have difficulty describing the intensity. They are able to begin to use comforting mechanisms, such as gritting teeth, pressing a hand against a forehead, holding the throat, rubbing an arm, or grimacing, to control or express pain. A nursing problem with children this age is that they do not have a perception of time. Soothing statements such as "It's only for a minute" are discomforting to the preschooler who does not know how long that is.

The School-Age Child and Adolescent

School-age children use adult mechanisms for controlling pain, and some are more stoic in the face of pain than adults, trying to avoid the stereotypes of "cry-baby" or "chicken." Assess for pain in the child by body motions such as clenched hands, clenched teeth, rapid breathing, and guarding of body parts. Asking them to rate their pain by pointing to sketches of faces helps them tell the degree of pain they are experiencing. Children as young as early school age are able to describe pain in this way and localize it. They can understand that if pain will last only an instant, such as that of an injection, it can be controlled.

Use of Pain Management Techniques

Measures to alleviate pain are summarized in the Focus on Family Teaching box. These guidelines are based primarily on the gating theory (which is also described in detail in relation to childbirth in Chapter 13).

Gating Theory Techniques

The most effective specific method for pain relief, outside of the use of analgesics, is using a **gating theory** technique. This technique is based on the idea that gating mechanisms in the substantia gelatinosa of the spinal cord are capable of halting an impulse at the level of the spinal cord so that a pain impulse is not received at the brain level. Gating mechanisms can be stimulated by three techniques: (1) cutaneous stimulation, (2) distraction, and (3) reduction of anxiety.

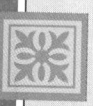

FOCUS ON CULTURAL AWARENESS

Procedures must always be adjusted to meet the individual needs or wishes of children and families. They must also be adjusted because of cultural influences. Pain, for example, is difficult to assess in children not only because they may not have the words to express how they feel but because how pain is expressed is culturally determined. In South American countries, pain may be expressed very freely. In Asian or northern European countries, children are expected to be more stoic about pain. In the Philippines, pain is thought to be the will of God. In Turkey, tolerating and not reporting pain is expected. In China, children may not accept something offered for pain relief until it has been offered twice (Geissler, 1994).

Because the expression of pain is culturally determined, two children having the same degree of pain may express it very differently. Assessment for pain must therefore be individualized for each child.

Q. *My 6-year-old has had almost continual pain since she became ill. Besides giving an analgesic, what can I do to make her more comfortable?*

A. Pain is a subjective symptom so only your daughter knows how much pain she has and what works best at relieving it. In addition to analgesic administration, some suggestions for helping reduce pain are:

- Administer pain medicine before pain becomes intense to help *prevent* pain rather than just relieve it.

- Use a positive approach: "This medicine will take away the pain," not "Let's see if this works or not."

- Never *just* give an analgesic; straighten sheets, offer a backrub, and so forth.

- Ask your daughter about measures she thinks will be helpful such as an additional pillow, the television turned on, her favorite toy next to her.

- Help your daughter to talk about and describe her pain. This can help to make it more concrete and not as psychologically frightening.

- Relieve anxiety if possible about other phases of life. Relaxation reduces muscle strain and tension that add to pain.

- Pain never seems as bad when a support person is present. Letting your daughter know that she is loved and you will be there for her can be one of the greatest helps.

Pain impulses are carried by small peripheral nerve fibers. If large peripheral nerves next to an injury site are stimulated, the ability of the small nerve fibers at the injury site to transmit pain impulses appears to decrease. Therefore, rubbing an injured part and applying heat or cold to the site are effective maneuvers to suppress pain. Rubbing an injection site afterward is another example. This technique is effective with children because the rubbing is not only comforting from a physical standpoint but also conveys psychological warmth.

If the cells of the brain stem that register an impulse as pain are preoccupied with other stimuli, a pain impulse will not register. Having a child focus on an action or a thought (**distraction**) accomplishes this. Telling a child to say "ouch" while an injection is administered is the simplest use of this technique.

Pain impulses are perceived more quickly if anxiety is also present, so anxiety should be reduced, if possible. Teaching a school-age child what to expect of a procedure is a means of achieving this. As well as knowing when something is going to happen, children should

know when nothing is going to happen. Being told that a morning will be free of painful procedures allows a child to relax and feel safe.

Substitution of Meaning

Substitution of meaning is helping the child to place another meaning (an unpainful one) on a painful procedure. Children are more adept at this than adults because their imagination is less inhibited. A venipuncture, for example, could be viewed as a silver rocket probing the moon to transport specimens back to earth or a submarine diving under the water to escape torpedoes just in time. Be certain a child thinks of a *specific* image. Help him or her elaborate on the image to make it more concrete and concentrate on it at the time of the procedure (Kachoyeanos & Friedhoff, 1993).

Incompatible Imagery

In *incompatible imagery*, the child recalls or images a pleasurable experience incompatible with pain. Ask the child to think of something that is pleasurable (e.g., waiting in suspense to learn he or she has won an art prize, walking up on stage while everyone applauds, or running a race and feeling the finish line tape snap as the child's chest strikes it). Have the child walk through the event with closed eyes so he or she remembers every detail. During a painful procedure, have the child "rerun" the event as many times as it takes to last throughout the procedure.

Thought Stopping

Thought stopping is a technique whereby children are taught to stop anxious thoughts by substituting positive or relaxing thoughts. Anticipatory anxiety is a negative force because it increases the pain experienced during a procedure and makes the time before it full of anxiety also. For this technique, help the child to think of a set of positive factors about the approaching feared procedure. For a bone marrow aspiration, for example, this might include, "It doesn't take long, the doctor and nurse who do it are nice, it's important to help me get better." Next, tell the child that when he or she starts to think about the impending procedure, to stop whatever he or she is doing and recite the list of positive thoughts (to himself or herself if others are present or out loud if the child is alone or important support people are present). The child can then return to the activity. Every time the anxious thoughts appear, however, the child should stop and recite the exercise.

Thought stopping is an effective technique because it allows a child to feel in control of his or her thoughts, which is different from merely saying "Don't think about it." This technique does not suppress thoughts; it changes them into positive ones. Some children can use thought stopping after only one teaching session; others take several sessions. The secret is for the child to use the technique *every* time the disturbing, anxious thought appears, even if at first such thoughts crowd in as frequently as every few minutes.

Administering Analgesia

Children need analgesic agents in addition to distraction techniques for pain relief. As children cannot voice a need for this, it is a nursing role to advocate for children to be certain they receive adequate amounts. *Patient-controlled analgesia* (PCA) is a form of analgesia that allows a child to self-administer intravenous narcotic doses with a medication pump (see also Chapter 19). Most children self-administer less medication by this method than what they would need in intramuscular doses. It has been shown to be a satisfactory method of pain relief for children (Weldon et al., 1993). To reduce the pain of procedures such as venipuncture and lumbar puncture, a new local anesthetic cream (EMLA) is available. This is applied to the skin and covered with a dressing 1 hour before an expected procedure (Nagengast, 1993). Single-dose epidural morphine injection has the potential for offering 12 to 24 hours of pain relief for children (Serlin, 1991).

Reducing Elevated Temperature in Children

Nursing Diagnoses and Related Interventions

Nursing Diagnosis: High risk for hyperthermia related to illness affecting temperature regulation, medications, or surgery

Goal: Child's temperature will return to normal with appropriate interventions within 2 hours.

Outcome Criteria: Child's temperature is at 98.6°F (37°C) orally.

Many illnesses cause elevated temperatures. Because children's temperature-regulating mechanism is immature, fever tends to be more marked in them than in adults and may even be out of proportion to the seriousness or extent of the disease. An increased temperature occurs because the child's temperature regulating point (*set point*) has been elevated. The temperature cannot be reduced until the set point returns (or is returned) to normal. An important nursing intervention with infants and young children is helping to reduce high temperatures, or giving a parent instructions on how to reduce the temperature at home. Any infant

younger than age 3 months with a fever should be seen by a physician or nurse practitioner as soon as possible because of the high incidence of febrile convulsions in infants.

Acetaminophen (Tylenol) is an excellent *antipyretic* (i.e., it acts to reduce temperature set point), and is the drug most often prescribed to reduce fever in children. Parents often do not give enough of an antipyretic such as acetaminophen to be effective because they are afraid the child will have a bad reaction to it. They must be encouraged to give the full dose every 4 hours up to five doses a day until their child's temperature is reduced. Acetaminophen is generally ordered for any child whose oral temperature is more than 101°F (38.4°C) or whose rectal temperature is more than 102°F (39.0°C) (Table 37-4).

Teach parents that fever is actually a body protection measure, and unless it is exceptionally high (more than 41.1°C, or 106°F) it does no specific harm. In fact, there is some evidence that fever may be of value in helping to combat infection, because it aids in destroying microorganisms (Reeves-Swift, 1990). In addition to acetaminophen administration, children with fever should be dressed in lightweight clothing, such as summer pajamas. All clothing but the diaper can be removed from an infant. Many parents dress febrile children warmly in flannel nightgowns to "keep them from getting a chill." This increases the child's temperature and does not prevent the shaking, trembling reaction that comes with high fever. Sponging children to lower the temperature is no longer recommended because it can lead to extreme chilling and shock to an immature nervous system (see the Nursing Care Plan).

Table 37-4. Calculating Acetaminophen (Tylenol) Doses

Age	Dosage	Frequency
0–3 mo	40 mg	every 4–6 h
4–12 mo	80 mg	every 4–6 h
12–24 mo	120 mg	every 4–6 h
2–4 y	160 mg	every 4–6 h
4–6 y	240 mg	every 4–6 h
6–9 y	320 mg	every 4–6 h
9–11 y	400 mg	every 4–6 h
11–12 y	480 mg	every 4–6 h
More than 12 y	325–1000 mg	every 4–6 h

Nursing considerations:
Dosage may be repeated 4–5 times daily.
Always assess degree and type of pain before administering any analgesic.
Profuse diaphoresis will follow administration if used with fever.
Not an effective antiinflammatory agent.
(From Deglin, J. H., & Vallerand, A. H. [1991]. *Nurses' med. deck* [2nd ed.]. Philadelphia: F. A. Davis, with permission.)

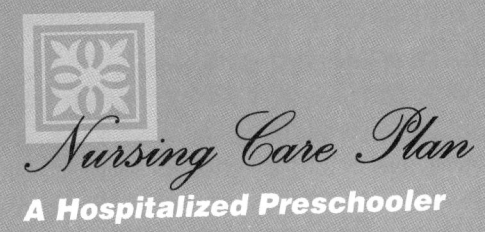

Nursing Care Plan

A Hospitalized Preschooler

Beth is a 4-year-old girl admitted to the hospital with a temperature of 104°F (orally). She is scheduled to have a number of painful diagnostic tests such as blood sampling (daily for 5 days), intravenous therapy, and bone marrow aspiration. The following is a nursing care plan you might design in relation to this.

Assessment: Client states, "I hate needles. Don't stick me with a needle!" Kicked and bit technician who approached her for finger puncture for blood sample. Covers ears with hands so she does not have to listen to explanations. Mother asks that Beth not be told anything in advance of procedures so she will not worry about them.

Nursing Diagnosis: Fear related to painful procedures

Defining Characteristic: Child states she is afraid of procedures.

Goal: Child will demonstrate acceptance of procedures necessary for diagnosis by 24 hours.

Outcome Criteria: Child limits protesting to verbal responses.

Nursing Orders	Rationale
1. Talk to parent about the advantage of being honest with Beth about procedures rather than surprising her with them.	1. Explanations can help the parent to establish better long-term relationship with child.
2. Take child to treatment room for painful procedures.	2. Avoiding doing painful procedures by the bedside can keep bed a safe area for girl.
3. Contract with child for suitable response: shouting is fine; kicking and biting are not.	3. Four-year-olds often need help expressing anger in acceptable ways.
4. Remain with child for entire length of procedures.	4. A support person can aid greatly in helping a child maintain control.
5. Encourage therapeutic play with syringes and teaching doll following procedures.	5. Therapeutic play is an effective technique to allow child to express anger at intrusive procedures.

Nursing Diagnosis: Hyperthermia related to undiagnosed disease process

Defining Characteristic: Child's temperature is 104°F (orally).

Goal: Child's temperature will return to a normal level by 1 hour.

Outcome Criteria: Child's temperature is reduced to less than 100°F orally.

Nursing Orders	Rationale
1. Administer acetaminophen 240 mg every 4 hours for fever of more than 102°F orally.	1. Acetaminophen is an effective hypopyrexia agent.
2. Keep child dressed in loose clothing (no flannel pajamas).	2. Loose clothing allows for evaporation and additional cooling.
3. Remake bed with only a top sheet (no blankets, heavy spread and so forth).	3. Light bedding allows for evaporation and additional cooling.
4. Encourage child to drink fluid (at least 330 mL a shift).	4. Additional fluid helps prevent dehydration from increased perspiration.

Key Points

- Preparing children for procedures reduces anxiety. Prepare a child by trying to relate a procedure to something he or she is already familiar with, such as comparing an x-ray machine to a camera.

- Include parents in both the planning and implementation of care. Parents reinfect children with fear if their own fear is uncontrolled. Give explanations on two levels: "I'm going to change the dressing on her suture line" for a parent; "I'm going to put a clean bandage on your tummy" for the child.

- Reduce painful procedures to the minimum possible (combine blood sampling procedures, if possible).

- Perform any procedures that will cause pain in a treatment room or away from the child's bedside so the bed remains a "safe place."

- Perform treatments without chilling or exposure. Be aware that even small children expect modesty to be respected.

- Allow the child to voice anger or fear of a procedure. Provide therapeutic play following a procedure to help reduce anger or fear.

- Identify a child well before a procedure; children do not monitor their own care as do adults.

- Children enjoy adults who are secure in their actions. Practice as necessary the steps of a procedure before you begin so you radiate confidence in your manner.

- Once you have announced that a procedure needs to be done, proceed to do it; waiting for something to happen is often as stressful as actually having it done.

- Respect time for play for children. This is not "free" time to be filled with procedures but a time for learning.

- Involve children in procedures because this gives them a sense of control. Allow a child to examine electrodes or apply lubricant for electrode contact. Give the child a portion of an ECG strip as a badge of courage following the procedure, or let the child apply his or her own adhesive bandage.

- Praise children for cooperation even if none was visibly obvious. For painful procedures, any behavior short of hysterical screaming counts as cooperation.

Critical Thinking Exercises

1. John is a 2-year-old who is very frightened of dark places. He is scheduled to have an MRI of his head done, which means he will be wheeled into a huge, dark, hollow tube. How could you prepare him for this?

2. Megan is a 6-year-old who has to have debridement for burns done daily, a very painful proce-

dure. She screams from fright when you bring in an analgesic injection to give her, however. Which would be better: to give the injection and risk frightening her, or not give it and allow her to experience more pain?

3. Jeff is an adolescent who is scheduled for a series of diagnostic tests for chronic abdominal pain. He always says, "I'm not a kid, you know," and refuses to listen when you start to explain any procedure. Later, he acts angry because he feels he has been "tricked" into having a procedure. How could you give explanations to Jeff without offending him? Why do you think he acts this way?

References

Albanese, C. T., & Wiener, E. S. (1993). Venous access in pediatric oncology patients. *Seminars in Surgical Oncology, 9,* 467.

Barness, L. A. (1994). The pediatric history and physical examination. In F.A. Oski et al. *Principles and practice of pediatrics* (pp. 29–44). Philadelphia: J.B. Lippincott.

Blatz, S., & Paes, B. A. (1990). Intravenous infusion by superficial vein in the neonate. *Journal of Intravenous Nursing, 13,* 122.

Braren, V. (1990). Care of hypospadias dressings. *Journal of Urology Nursing, 9,* 835.

Bullock, B. L., & Rosendahl, P. P. (1992). *Pathophysiology* (3rd ed.). Philadelphia: J.B. Lippincott.

Christophersen, E. R. (1992). Discipline. *Pediatric Clinics of North America, 39,* 395.

Clore, E. R., et al. (1993). The parasomnias. *Journal of Pediatric Health Care, 7,* 12.

Department of Health & Human Services. (1991). *Healthy people 2000.* Washington, DC: Public Health Service.

Dieckmann, R. A. (1994). Rectal diazepam for prehospital pediatric status epilepticus. *Annals of Emergency Medicine, 23,* 216.

Geissler, E. M. (1994). *Pocket guide to cultural assessment.* St. Louis: C. V. Mosby.

Goodwin, M. L., & Carlson, I. (1993). The peripherally inserted central catheter: A retrospective look at three years of insertions. *Journal of Intravenous Nursing, 16,* 92.

Greve, P. (1990). The smaller the patient, the greater the risk: How to handle the hazards of pediatric nursing without injury or liability. *RN, 53,* 77.

Guy, J., et al. (1993). Use of intraosseus infusion in the pediatric trauma patient. *Journal of Pediatric Surgery, 28,* 158.

Hamburger, B. (1993). Treating nocturnal enuresis. *Canadian Nurse, 89,* 26.

Holder, C., & Alexander, J. (1990). A new and improved guide to IV therapy. *American Journal of Nursing, 90,* 43.

Johnston, C. C., et al. (1990). Pain assessment in newborns. *Journal of Perinatology/Neonatology Nursing, 4,* 41.

Kachoyeanos, M. K., & Friedhoff, M. (1993). Cognitive and behavioral strategies to reduce children's pain. *MCN: American Journal of Maternal Child Nursing, 18,* 14.

Kandt, K. A. (1991). An implantable venous access device for children. *MCN: American Journal of Maternal Child Nursing, 16,* 88.

Lybrand, M., et al. (1990). Periodic comparisons of specific gravity using urine from a diaper and collecting bag. *MCN: American Journal of Maternal Child Nursing, 15,* 238.

Mansson, M. E., et al. (1993). The effect of preparation for lumbar puncture on children undergoing chemotherapy. *Oncology Nursing Forum, 20,* 39.

Masoorli, S., & Angeles, T. (1990). PICC lines: The latest home care challenge. *RN, 53,* 44.

Masters, R., et al. (1990). The use of restraints. *Rehabilitation Nursing, 15,* 22.

McCaffery, M. (1980). Understanding your patient's pain. *Nursing, 10,* 26.

Melzack, R. (1975). The McGill Pain Questionnaire: Major properties and scoring methods. *Pain, 1,* 277.

Nagengast, S. L. (1993). The use of EMLA cream to reduce and/or eliminate procedural pain in children. *Journal of Pediatric Nursing, 8,* 406.

Ogren, J. M. (1990). The inaccuracy of axillary temperatures measured with an electronic thermometer. *American Journal of Diseases of Children, 144,* 109.

Physician's desk reference (1994). Oradell, NJ: Medical Economics Co.

Plankey, E. D., & Knauf, J. (1990). What patients need to know about magnetic resonance imaging. *American Journal of Nursing, 90,* 27.

Price, S. (1990). Pain: Its experience, assessment and management in children. *Nursing Times, 86,* 42.

Reeves-Swift, R. (1990). Rational management of a child's acute fever. *MCN: American Journal of Maternal Child Nursing, 15,* 82.

Ritter, H. T. (1990). Evaluating and selecting general-purpose infusion pumps. *Journal of Intravenous Nursing, 13,* 156.

Savedra, M. C., et al. (1993). Assessment of postoperative pain in children and adolescents using the adolescent pediatric pain tool. *Nursing Research, 42,* 5.

Serlin, S. (1991). Single-dose caudal epidural morphine in children: Safe, effective and easy. *Journal of Clinical Anesthesia, 3,* 386.

Shapiro, C. R. (1993). Nurses' judgments of pain in term and preterm newborns. *Journal of Obstetric, Gynecological and Neonatal Nursing, 22,* 41.

Skale, N. (1992). *Manual of pediatric nursing procedures.* Philadelphia: J. B. Lippincott.

Slovis, T. L., et al. (1993). Pediatric sedation: Short term effects. *Pediatric Radiology, 23,* 345.

Swonger, A. K., & Matejski, M. P. (1991). *Nursing pharmacology: An integrated approach to drug therapy and nursing practice* (2nd ed.). Philadelphia: J.B. Lippincott.

Vessey, J. A., & Mahon, M. M. (1990). Therapeutic play and the hospitalized child. *Journal of Pediatric Nursing, 5,* 328.

Weinstein, S. M. (1990). Math calculations for intravenous nurses. *Journal of Intravenous Nursing, 13,* 221.

Weldon, B. C., et al. (1993). Pediatric PCA: The role of concurrent opioid infusions and nurse-controlled analgesia. *Clinical Journal of Pain, 9,* 26.

Suggested Readings

Beyer, J. E., et al. (1992). The creation, validation, and continuing development of the Oucher, a measure of pain intensity in children. *Journal of Pediatric Nursing, 7,* 335.

Broome, M. E., et al. (1990). Influences on nurses' management of pain in children. *MCN: American Journal of Maternal Child Nursing, 15,* 158.

Fletcher, K. R. (1990). Restraints should be a last resort. *RN, 53,* 52.

Harrison, M. B, et al. (1993). Children with central lines: Evidence-based practice. *Canadian Nurse, 89,* 18.

Kachoyeanos, M. K., et al. (1993). Cognitive and behavioral strategies to reduce children's pain. *MCN: American Journal of Maternal Child Nursing, 18,* 14.

Kennedy, W. C. (1990). Vital signs: Reading the essentials. *Journal of Emergency Medical Services, 15,* 26.

Krasner, D. (1990). What's wrong with this stoma? *American Journal of Nursing, 90,* 46.

McClowry, G. (1993). Pediatric nursing psychosocial care: A vision beyond hospitalization. *Pediatric Nursing, 19,* 146.

McConnell, E. A. (1990). How to tape a dressing. *Nursing, 20,* 23.

Palmer, S. J. (1993). Care of sick children by parents: A meaningful role. *Journal of Advanced Nursing, 18,* 185.

Pomfret, E. A., & Blackburn, G. L. (1994). Central venous access risk factors. *Critical Care Medicine, 22,* 196.

Strauch, C., et al. (1993). Implementation of a quiet hour: Effect on noise levels and infant sleep states. *Neonatal Network, 12,* 31.

Tourangeau, A., et al. (1993). Tap in on ear thermometry. *Canadian Nurse, 89* 24.

Weatherly, K. S., et al. (1991). Needle stick injury in pediatric hospitals. *Pediatric Nursing, 17,* 95.

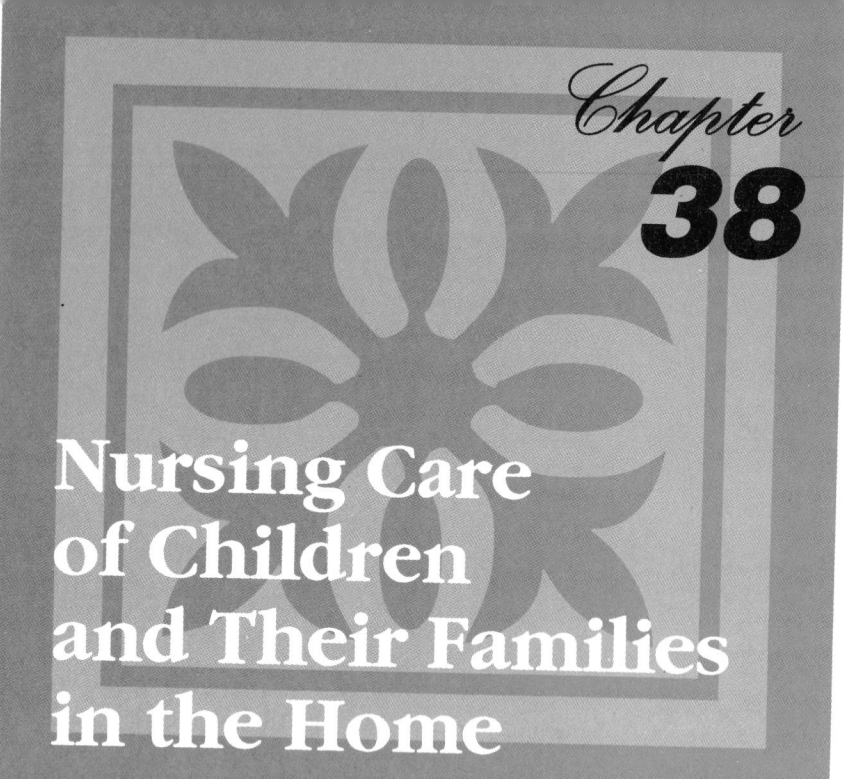

Chapter 38

Nursing Care of Children and Their Families in the Home

Objectives

After mastering the contents of this chapter, you should be able to:

1. Outline the advantages and disadvantages of home care.

2. Assess the appropriateness of home care for a particular child and family.

3. Formulate nursing diagnoses related to care of a child at home.

4. Plan modifications of nursing care such as administration of intravenous therapy for the home setting.

5. Implement care (e.g., supervising safe oxygen administration) for a child in the home.

6. Evaluate goal criteria to be certain that nursing goals were achieved.

7. Identify National Health Goals related to home care that nurses can be instrumental in helping the nation to achieve.

8. Identify areas related to home care that could benefit from additional nursing research.

9. Use critical thinking to analyze ways that nursing interventions can promote healthy family functioning when care is delivered in the home, as well as ways that the link between hospital and home care can be strengthened.

10. Synthesize principles of home care with nursing process to achieve quality maternal and child health care.

Adele Pillitteri: MATERNAL AND CHILD HEALTH NURSING, 2nd Edition. © 1995 Adele Pillitteri.

More and more emphasis is being placed on the home as an alternative setting for health care of children. The home has always been a traditional health care setting, especially in health promotion: new mothers receive postpartum care and early infant education in the home, families receive mental health counseling in the home, and elderly people receive assistance with medication schedules and support in activities of daily living (Spradley, 1990). In recent years, the need for home health care services has grown substantially. Acute care or postsurgical clients, including children, are released from the hospital so early they often require regular home nursing visits through a rehabilitation period. Children with chronic conditions such as bronchial pulmonary dysphasia, cystic fibrosis, and childhood cancer are being cared for at home rather than in hospital settings when at all possible. There are some clear benefits associated with caring for ill preterm infants in the home (Zahr et al., 1993). In addition, a number of children with terminal diseases are being cared for at home (**hospice care**).

Several factors have contributed to the success of the home as a health care setting. Technologic advances have made it possible for potentially complicated procedures, such as the administration of total parenteral nutrition and ventilation therapy, to be carried out safely at home. There is also a strong economic incentive to provide care in the home (it is less costly for health care plans). Moreover, consumer pressure to make the home a viable health setting has had a great effect in convincing once-reluctant physicians and nurses that care in the home can be successful. Perhaps the greatest benefit of home care for children is the opportunity it brings to include the entire family in health care planning and the ability to focus not only on a specific health problem but also on promoting healthy behaviors for the entire family. National Health Goals related to home care of children are shown in the Focus on National Health Goals display.

Chapter 13 discusses the home as a setting for childbirth, and Chapter 16 covers the home as a setting for care of the high-risk pregnant woman. This chapter discusses the advantages of the home for health care of children as well as ways in which nursing techniques developed for hospital care can be adapted to the home setting.

⌧ NURSING PROCESS OVERVIEW
for Care of the Child at Home

ASSESSMENT

Nursing assessment of the child at home is similar to assessment of the child in a hospital setting. Being in the home may actually allow data on the family and family functioning to be more easily obtained. Assessment in the home also requires continuous assessment of the suitability of the home environment for continued health care. Even though health care providers have initially established that the family is able to provide home care for the child, the situation may change—the child's condition may require more monitoring than originally believed, or the demands may be too great for the family to bear. For this reason, include an assessment of overall family functioning and coping ability in every visit.

If an in-depth history or physical examination is

necessary, be sure to provide the same level of privacy for the child that he or she would be provided in a clinic or hospital. It may be necessary to find a room or space that is quiet and free from the distractions of normal family activity.

NURSING DIAGNOSIS

Nursing diagnoses established in the home are the same as those that would be established with the same findings in a health care facility. Often, however, because of the participation of the family necessary for home care, nursing diagnoses are more family oriented. Home care can place a heavy burden on the family. The stress of being responsible for an ill child's daily health status can damage a parent's self-esteem or a couple's marital relationship, or it can prevent parents from spending time with their other children. Examples are:

- Family coping: Potential for growth related to increased time together because of home care
- Health-seeking behaviors related to skills needed to continue home care
- High risk for altered growth and development related to lack of usual childhood activities
- Parental role conflict related to need to provide constant care to home-bound child
- Altered family processes related to dependence of ill child
- Hopelessness related to prolonged care-giving responsibilities and perceived lack of health care alternatives
- Coping: Disabled, related to changes in family routine brought about by home care needs of ill child

PLANNING AND IMPLEMENTATION

Nursing interventions for home care often involve teaching family members how to give care. This may include encouraging members to voice the frustration they feel at being constantly confined at home or what they perceive to be a lack of progress in their child's condition. If the child has a terminal illness, parents need support to express their grief and not grow discouraged, because the work they are accomplishing is making the child comfortable before death.

EVALUATION

The goals of nursing care in the home need to be evaluated to determine if they are being met. Because a home setting is less structured than a health care facility setting, some goals will be more difficult to accomplish; for the same reason, because there is more room for inno-

vation at home, some goals will be more easily accomplished.

Examples of outcome criteria might be:

- Parents state they have been able to make adjustments to accommodate care of ill child at home.
- Child states he or she enjoys respite care in hospice setting 1 weekend a month.
- Parents state they feel they are supplying adequate growth experiences for siblings in light of home care of oldest child.

The Home as a Health Care Setting

Home care is care of children in their own home, provided by or supervised through a certified home health care or community health care agency. Home care agencies may be free standing or allied with a health care facility. Specialized services such as providing supplies for

FOCUS ON
National Health Goals

Specific National Health Goals are concerned with health promotion activities in the home or community. Examples of these are:

- Reduce to no more than 20% the proportion of children aged 6 and younger who are regularly exposed to tobacco smoke at home.
- Enact in 50 states comprehensive laws on clean indoor air that prohibit or strictly limit smoking in the workplace and enclosed public places.
- Eliminate or severely restrict all forms of tobacco product advertising and promotion to which youth younger than age 18 are likely to be exposed (DHHS, 1991).

Nurses can be instrumental in helping the nation achieve these goals by teaching the dangers of tobacco smoke in homes (increased otitis media and upper respiratory infection in children), and monitoring communities for adherence to cigarette advertising and public smoking laws. Additional nursing research that could be of benefit includes whether home care of a child serves as an impetus for a parent to stop smoking (or increase smoking because of the additional stress); effective programs that school nurses can initiate to encourage children never to begin tobacco use; and what methods of cigarette advertising appeal most to children (so should not be used)?

total parenteral nutrition, oxygen therapy, or laboratory analysis may be furnished by special service companies. Voluntary agencies often provide services such as transportation, with vans transporting children to and from health care agency assessments, or "respite" care so parents can have a break from continual care.

An adult caregiver must be strongly committed to home care and prepared to work in conjunction with health care providers for pediatric home care to be effective.

Advantages of Home Care

Although home care of children is not without drawbacks, it has two clear advantages.

Reduced Cost
The rising cost of health care is an undisputed problem. The introduction of diagnosis-related groups (DRGs) into hospital care has mandated that hospitals receive only a set fee for each client's care. The earlier the client can be discharged from the facility, the more cost-effective the care.

Although DRGs do not apply to the care of children, child care has been affected by them. Home care methods originally designed to help care for adults in homes have been adapted to care for children.

As with adults, in most instances it is less costly to care for a child at home than in a hospital setting; if the child does not need intensive nursing care, home care achieves cost containment. Cost containment must be weighed against safety and quality of care, however. Because not all home settings are safe for care and not all parents have the commitment necessary for home care, it is not an alternative for all families. In addition, although home care is cost-effective for health care agencies, it may not be cost-effective for the family. Costs that health insurance would have paid for had the child been hospitalized may no longer be covered once the child is transferred to home care (Harris, 1990).

Comfort and Support
Unlike a child who is isolated in a hospital facility, a child being taken care of at home has family and friends nearby. For children who are acutely but not terminally ill, this extra emotional support may not be as immediately important as physical care, but for those who are chronically ill or dying, being close to their family and friends may be the most important aspect of their care. For these children, home care is ideal.

Disadvantages of Home Care

There are some disadvantages to home care that make it a poor option for some families. Sometimes the physical care required (for example, suctioning or a complicated

medication regimen) can be overwhelming. The financial strain of at least one parent being at home full-time and not earning an income, the social isolation, and the disruption of normal family life are other major disadvantages that can outweigh the benefits of home care (McAnear, 1990).

Responsibilities of the Nurse in Home Care

The care that a child receives at home depends on his or her physical condition and stage of illness. Often, nursing responsibility begins with determining whether a child *should* be cared for at home.

Assessment to Determine Viability of Home Care

Assessment begins with investigation to determine whether the child's condition is compatible with home care as well as whether the family is capable of handling the stress of home care. A number of important aspects need to be included in an assessment.

Identification of Primary Care Provider
Assessment begins with identification of the child's primary caregiver. Although this is often the mother, if a father works more flexible hours, he may be the best candidate to give the bulk of care. In some homes, a grandparent or an older sibling will be the person primarily responsible for care. It is important to include this person in planning and problem solving because this person knows best what strategy of care will be most effective with the child as well as what strategy would be most appropriate in light of the physical layout of the home, the family's financial ability, and the family's lifestyle (Leonard et al., 1993).

Knowledge Level of Family
Before a child can be cared for at home, teaching will be required so that the family understands the child's illness. A teaching plan for the family should include those things to be learned immediately and additional care measures that can be taught after the child is home.

Available Resources
The term "resources" refers not only to material objects (e.g., hospital bed, portable oxygen, or glucometer but also whether family members are able to deal with the chronic stress of fatiguing, around-the-clock nursing care. Often, a parent has to quit work to become a home health care provider. This disrupts the family's current as well as future financial state because job seniority and promotions are lost. Assess physical surroundings: Is there adequate floor space for a hospital bed, oxygen

equipment, and so forth? Is a fire company nearby in case cardiopulmonary resuscitation (CPR) is needed? Is a power backup resource available if a blackout should occur? Does the family have a telephone? Does the family have available transport to a health care facility for follow-up care? Do parents understand the importance of the care they will give? Table 38-1 lists additional assessments to make depending on the age of the child.

Current Level of Family Functioning

The family that is supportive of all family members and provides an environment conducive to each member's continued growth and development is more likely to be able to manage home care than a family that has a history of ineffective or destructive coping strategies—that is, a family in which parents have unrealistic expectations of family members, one with a history of abusive relationships, or one that is coping ineffectively with other stressors in their lives. Even a family that appears to be functioning well, however, may be so adversely affected by the stress of home care that its members' ability to be successful with home care is limited. For example, the loss of employment income of the primary care provider or cramped living space could put the family at risk for ineffective coping; not only the family's current status but how it will be affected must be considered when determining the advisability of home care. It is important to remember that every family operates differently and handles stress in different ways. Events that to the nurse may seem overwhelming may actually be easy for the family to handle. On the other hand, problems that seem minor could be disruptive enough to affect the

family's ability to provide adequate care for their child at home (Dolan et al., 1990) (see the Focus on Cultural Awareness box).

Planning and Implementing Care

Nursing in the community requires a great deal of independent judgment because neither a nursing supervisor nor an attending physician is on the premises to offer advice. It also calls for creativity in adjusting procedures to the confines of a home and the lifestyle of the family. In addition, it requires nurses to be assertive enough to help a family secure adequate funding and resources for home care.

Care at home may include **direct care**, in which a nurse remains in continual attendance or visits frequently and actually administers care, or **indirect care**, in which a nurse plans and supervises care given by others such as home health care aides or the parents. Nursing care is considered **skilled home care** if it includes physician-prescribed procedures such as dressing changes, administration of drugs, health teaching, and observation of the client's progress or status through such measures as monitoring vital signs or measuring fluid intake and output. In many instances, classifying nursing care as skilled or not determines whether it will be paid for by third-party reimbursement.

The care a child needs at home depends on his or her physical condition and stage of illness. There are a number of common care priorities to be considered, however, when planning home care.

Table 38-1. Assessment Criteria for Home Care by Age Group

Age	Points to Assess
Infant	Is there a suitable sleeping place? Do side rails of a crib lock securely? Can the infant be heard from the parents' room at night? Is there a functioning refrigerator if formula will be used? Is there protection from mosquitoes? Is the home free of rodents that might attack a small infant?
	Are there adequate three-pronged plugs for the care equipment needed? If oxygen will be used, is there a sign to omit smoking in the room? Is the oxygen away from a fireplace, gas space heater, or stove? Does the family know not to light candles near oxygen in a power failure or for a birthday?
Toddler and preschooler	Is there a safe area for play free from stairs and poisoning possibilities? Are there screens or locks on windows to prevent child from crawling onto a ledge? Is there provision for stimulation and learning activities?
	Is there adequate space for supplies? If a special diet is necessary, does the person who will cook have adequate knowledge of food preparation? Do caregivers know the emergency call system procedure in their community? How to reorder supplies? Has the power company been notified if an electrical appliance is necessary for life support? What would be the caregiver's actions in a power failure? What emergency steps should the caregiver take if the child is suddenly worse?
School-age child and adolescent	What is the provision for schooling (possibly an intercom with a regular classroom or home tutor)? Is peer interaction possible? If adolescent is self-medicating, will reminder sheets or some other reminder system be necessary?

Providing a Therapeutic Environment

Children cared for at home often require a room similar to that provided in a health care agency. Hospital beds can be rented from medical supply companies. If a family cannot afford one, they can elevate a house bed on wooden or concrete blocks. Many home mattresses are not firm; a piece of plywood slid under the mattress improves firmness. A cardboard box or additional pillows can be placed under the mattress to elevate the head of a regular bed to a gatch position. Bed trays can be purchased at any department store or cut from a cardboard box.

If the bedroom is away from the main home activities, a child can become lonely. Encourage family members to include the ill child in as many family activities as possible—bring the television set into the child's bedroom so the entire family gathers there, or set up a card table in the room so everyone can eat there—or encourage the child to join the rest of the family for activities by resting on the couch in the living room or in a lounge chair in the back yard or sitting in the kitchen (Figure 38-1).

To be certain the home is safe, a smoke detector on each floor is a wise precaution. A downstairs bedroom is not only safest in case of a fire but allows the child more self-care ability. Fire departments supply free decals for the bedroom windows of children or those with a disability. Encourage parents to contact their local fire departments for this safety measure. The average wall telephone is too high for a child to reach from a wheelchair, particularly if a counter is in front of it. Installing a counter telephone enables the child to telephone for emergency help and also increases socialization.

Make sure that in a health emergency, the family would be able to transport their child to a health care fa-

cility or make arrangements for an ambulance to come to their home.

Providing for Adequate Nutrition

Children who are on home care need as much or more nursing supervision of their diet as those in health care agencies because they may not have a dietitian planning meals to assure adequate nutrition. Assess not only quantity but quality of food to ensure that intake is optimal.

Home Enteral Nutrition. Children who require enteral feedings may be cared for at home with nasogastric, nasoduodenal, or gastrostomy tubes or buttons (see Chapter 34). Medicine as well as feedings may be

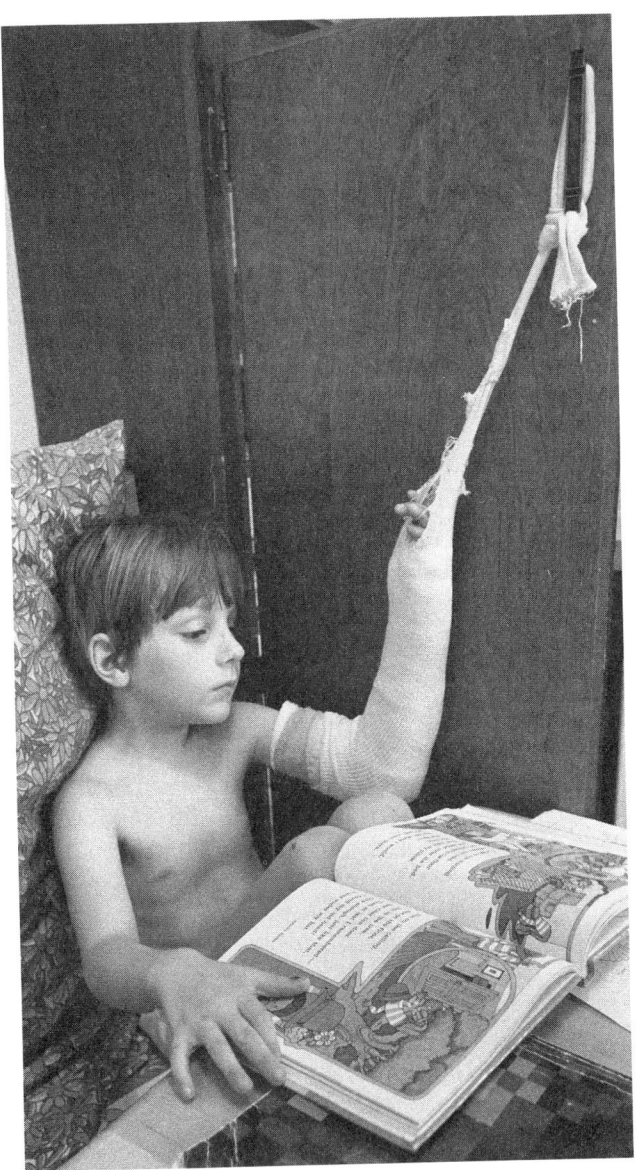

FIGURE 38-1
Procedures at home need to be modified to adjust to the setting. (Courtesy of Stock, Boston.)

administered by this route (Estoup, 1994). The supplies necessary for enteral feedings (feeding tubes and enteral pumps) are available for rent or purchase through pharmacies or medical supply houses. The type needed depends on the volume of feedings and whether they are continuous or intermittent (Gruver, 1993). Children and their family members can be taught to remove and reinsert feeding tubes as appropriate. Tubes are usually changed every 2 weeks to 4 weeks. The family may purchase a commercial formula for home feeding or prepare its own. Home-blended formulas may require large-bore feeding tubes; be certain that formula is prepared with clean utensils and kept well refrigerated until used.

It is just as important to check for proper tube placement before a feeding and to maintain an elevated head position during and after feedings at home as in a health care facility. Teach the child or family to add a designated amount of water at the end of each feeding to prevent formula from standing in the tube. To prevent clogging of feeding tubes, irrigation with half-strength cranberry juice is suggested once a day. The acidity of this solution also helps to reduce the bacterial level in tubes.

Parents need to assess the skin around a gastrostomy button or tube to be certain it is not excoriated (Hagelgans & Janusz, 1994). To assess that the child is receiving an adequate diet, he or she should be weighed daily; parents should keep a record of urine output and bowel movements as well. Laboratory analysis of electrolytes such as sodium and potassium will be ordered periodically.

Total Parenteral Nutrition. Children who are unable to absorb or metabolize food by their gastrointestinal system may be placed on total parenteral nutrition (TPN) at home (Bendorf et al., 1993). Parents need to be well informed of the special dangers of total parenteral nutrition (it flows into a central vessel such as the subclavian) and be knowledgeable about what to do in case the fluid line becomes dislodged (put pressure on the site with a sterile piece of gauze and telephone their home care nurse) (see Chapter 34 for a complete discussion of TPN therapy).

Total parenteral nutrition formula can be ordered through a private vendor who will deliver the formula, tubing, and clean dressings, or can be purchased or rented through a pharmacy or medical supply house.

Total parenteral nutrition solutions should be stored in the refrigerator until 1 hour to 2 hours before use. Removing them 1 hour before use allows them to warm to room temperature before being administered. Because it is important that total parenteral nutrition solutions are administered at a steady rate, the family is advised to rent an automatic pump for administration.

Some children receive total parenteral nutrition solutions during the night while they sleep and then have the central line catheter capped during the day so they are free of equipment for play. Be certain that parents use new tubing every night to ensure sterility. The dressing at the catheter site should be changed approximately every 48 hours or at any time it becomes soiled or moist. Catheter caps should be changed approximately every 3 days.

Be certain that the child who has a total parenteral nutrition catheter capped during the day does not engage in activities that might dislodge the cap, such as active roughhousing. Swimming or tub bathing with the water above the level of the catheter is contraindicated.

Administering the infusion during the night while the child sleeps is easiest for the child but not necessarily for parents. Help parents to determine a time that will be agreeable for them as well as the child, such as during a favorite television program, when the child is inactive yet parents are awake and able to monitor the infusion. A common side effect of total parenteral nutrition is hypoglycemia. Children's urine should be tested approximately twice daily to detect this. Assess that parents are aware of accompanying signs of hypoglycemia such as dizziness or nervousness. Assess that they are aware of steps they should take if hypoglycemia should occur (Feed some orange juice? Call their health care provider?).

Children on TPN will have periodic blood work done to assess, for instance, potassium and calcium levels. Be certain that parents understand the importance of these tests and have transportation available to take the child to a health care facility or have made arrangements for an ambulatory service to come to the home.

To be certain that the central line site is not becoming infected, the child's temperature should be taken approximately twice daily. When the dressing is changed, the site should be inspected for any erythema or drainage. Be certain that parents have an emergency telephone number to use if they have concerns during the night when fluid is infusing.

Providing Intravenous Therapy

Intravenous therapy may be implemented in the home as well as in a health care facility (Brown, 1990). Blood transfusions can also be administered. Intravenous therapy calls for strict aseptic technique on the part of parents or child. A major responsibility in discharge planning is to allow parents to become comfortable enough with the therapy that they feel confident in their ability to infuse fluid at home. The site for home therapy could be a peripheral vein using a short intracath or a central line using a double-lumen catheter such as a Broviac. The advantage of a central line is that it does not infiltrate as readily as a peripheral site. Unfortunately, it involves dressing changes and the risk of hemorrhage should it become dislodged. Be certain parents understand and are skilled at related procedures such as instillation of heparin or normal saline flushing (see Chapter 37).

It is helpful if a pump is used with home intravenous therapy so overhydration does not accidentally occur. This is particularly important if the intravenous solution contains electrolytes, such as sodium or potassium, or a medication. Infusion pumps can be rented from medical supply houses. Bags of intravenous fluid can be purchased through the same supply houses or pharmacies.

Children receiving intravenous therapy need to be evaluated periodically by a home care nurse. Frequent laboratory analysis is also necessary to see that electrolyte imbalances are not occurring. Be certain that parents understand the importance of this and how to schedule these assessments.

Teach parents to wash their hands well before touching an intravenous site or changing bags of fluid. Children can shower with both intermittent infusion devices (heparin locks) or continuous infusions in place. Covering the site with a plastic bag protects the tape from getting wet and loosening.

Be certain that parents have a "trouble-shooting" telephone number to call should they have a problem with an infusion. Most problems can be handled over the telephone. If parents feel that a peripheral site is infiltrating, they are usually advised to *slow* the infusion to a "barely dripping" rate and call their home care nurse rather than completely halt the infusion. Caution them not to administer any medication through the line until it has been checked by their nurse to avoid deposition of any medication in subcutaneous tissue.

For intravenous medication administration, the medication can be mixed in a "piggy-back" infusion bag by the home care nurse and then frozen in the home freezer for safe storage. Frozen bags should be defrosted approximately 12 hours before use so they are at room temperature to prevent chilling and to ensure a good mixture of the medication through the solution (Hammond et al., 1991). Parents may also add medication directly to an intravenous line through an infusion chamber or specially designed infusion system.

Another type of delivery service is the syringe pump, which is small and easily portable by belt or shoulder holster. Syringe pumps work as the pump compressor periodically decompresses the plunger of a medication-filled syringe, instilling a fixed rate of medication (McCoy & Feenan, 1990).

If the child's therapy will be intermittent rather than continuous, such as receiving an antibiotic three or four times a day, the use of an intermittent infusion device (heparin lock) or venous access device allows for mobility and freedom from tubing (Baranowski, 1993). Parents need to take the responsibility of flushing an inter-

mittent infusion device to maintain patency. This is safest if normal saline is used rather than heparin, to prevent accidental overdose of heparin.

Administering Medication
Most children on home care receive some type of medicine. The Focus on Family Teaching display summarizes guidelines for safe home administration of oral drugs.

Encouraging Self-Care
Children should be encouraged to carry out as much of their own personal care as possible in order to maintain a sense of control and wellness. It is helpful if the child's bedroom is located close to a bathroom so he or she can reach it easily. Help parents devise supplies for hygiene as necessary, such as providing a basin for bathing; a portable shower head with a flexible hose is helpful so that a child can sit on a chair in the tub or shower. To help an adolescent shave or put on makeup while sitting in a wheelchair, provide an angled mirror at eye level.

Caution parents that bathing can easily cause their child to become chilled, especially if their home is cold. If the family turns the heat down at night, bathing may have to be delayed until late morning or afternoon when the house has warmed up.

Urge parents to continue to stress teeth brushing while a child is ill. A toothache from a cavity is an easily preventable additional discomfort.

Providing for Adequate Mobility
If a child is confined to a wheelchair, parents must determine what adaptations of their home will be necessary. A local carpenter can build a ramp across the house steps to provide for wheelchair access. Unless the child will be using a motorized wheelchair, the ramp should have a railing for the child to grasp to pull himself or herself upward or to stop the wheelchair from moving down too fast; the child then can enter and leave the house independently. Wheelchair lifts or elevators can be purchased and mounted by house steps, but they are obviously more expensive.

It is difficult to move a wheelchair across a high pile carpet; covering the carpet with plastic is helpful. Throw rugs usually have to be removed as they become tangled in the wheels. Placing furniture along the walls allows for increased safe turning space for a wheelchair.

In the kitchen, it is impossible to reach high shelves from a wheelchair. To encourage the child to help with meal preparation, parents could move supplies the child will use often, such as boxes of cereal, to a lower cabinet. Purchasing a pair of tongs can help to reach supplies in upper cupboards. If the counter is too high to work to prepare foods, placing a board across the wheelchair arms provides a work space. A stove with controls at the back is difficult for a person in a wheelchair to use. Caution parents that if the child attempts

FOCUS ON FAMILY TEACHING

Q. My child needs to take five different kinds of medicine daily. What are safe guidelines for home administration of medicine?

A. Safe medicine administration requires both safe storage and administration techniques. Some suggestions are:

Oral Medication

- Store medicine in its original labeled container; the label is a safeguard against medicine error.
- Do not store unused and outdated portions of drugs because their composition may change over time. Do not discard them in the garbage because there is a possibility that children might find and ingest them. Discard them by flushing them down a toilet.
- Keep oral medication in a different storage area from medication to be used externally so external medicine will not be ingested accidentally.
- Keep all medicine up out of reach of young children so they do not help themselves to it; encourage self-medication, following prescribed instructions, for older children.
- Refrigerate all drugs that require refrigeration.
- Insist that the pharmacist put the name of the drug on the label of the medication. Having the name of the drug on the label helps prevent medicine errors and, in case of accidental poisoning or an untoward effect, it allows proper interventions to be started quickly.

- Do not prepare drugs in the dark because you will be unable to read and identify the label accurately.
- Make out a reminder chart so that doses are checked off as they are taken so doses are not forgotten or given twice.
- Set up all medication to be taken for the day in envelopes marked 10 AM, 2 PM, and so forth, first thing in the morning. This prevents missed doses or duplication of doses (if the envelope is empty at the end of the day, you know the medication was taken; if still full, a dose was missed).
- Do not use over-the-counter medicine with prescribed medication to prevent inadvertently causing a drug interaction.

Intravenous Medication

- Be sure to assess the site for infiltration before adding medication to avoid injuring subcutaneous tissue.
- Be certain medications are diluted properly or else they can injure veins.
- Be sure to maintain sterility; infection from an intravenous line is always serious.
- Dispose of needles and syringes in a covered container such as a coffee can so they can be disposed of properly by a health care provider.

---

to reach across a hot burner, he or she could be badly burned. A microwave oven placed on a low table allows a child to warm up meals and prepare snacks independently.

In the bathroom, installing a safety rail by the toilet helps the child to be able to transfer from wheelchair to toilet. A chair placed in the bathtub alongside safety rails allows the child to transfer to the bathtub.

Federal law mandates that all public buildings provide easy access for people in wheelchairs. In some small cities, buildings may not be equipped this way because no one has ever asked for the service before. Urge parents to contact their city council if the problem exists. Advocate for children if parents' approach is met with less than prompt action so that the child (and other people who use wheelchairs) will have access to facilities such as the public library, zoo, museums, and shopping malls.

Promoting Respiratory Function

Children with respiratory illnesses on home care are prescribed incentive spirometry as well as ventilator and oxygen support (Figure 38-2). They may have tracheotomies and need tracheotomy suction. They may need continuous apnea monitoring.

Children with respiratory illness should not be exposed to irritating substances such as cigarette smoke, dust, hair sprays, or room fresheners. Family members who do smoke should make an attempt to stop or smoke only outside, or at least in a room where the child does not spend an appreciable length of time. Damp dusting helps to remove dust from the air.

If suctioning is required, either a sterile or clean technique may be recommended depending on the length of time suctioning will be needed and the child's susceptibility to infection. *Sterile technique* requires the use of disposable catheters or reuse of catheters after they have been boiled or soaked in a bactericidal solution. *Clean technique* involves the reuse of catheters after they have been washed with soap and water. Because there are fewer pathologic bacteria in homes than in health care institutions, clean technique is adequate for most children. Parents should wash their hands well both before and after suctioning. Homemade saline so-

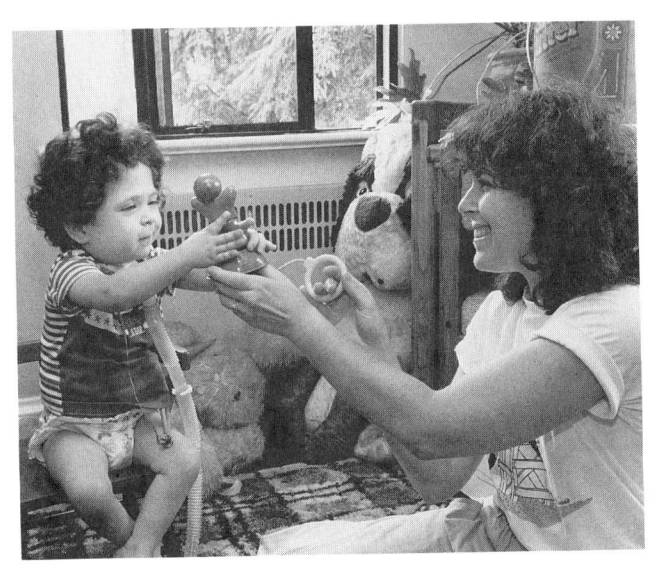

FIGURE 38-2
*Oxygen administration at home has become a common therapy.
(Courtesy of Michael Weisbrot and family and Stock, Boston.)*

lution for rinsing the catheter during suctioning can be prepared by mixing 1 teaspoon of salt with 1 pint of tap water. If sterile technique is being used, a 1-quart jar of saline can be placed in a pan with a few inches of water and boiled for 25 minutes (the same technique as terminal sterilization of baby formula). The unused solution can be stored in the refrigerator for 1 week and then replaced if not used by that time.

Oxygen for home use is supplied by medical supply houses or specialized oxygen supply firms. It comes in the same tanks as those used in health care facilities, or in liquid form. Either type must be stored away from heat, flames, or any flammable materials such as oil or grease; smoking should not be permitted in the same room where oxygen is being stored or used. Remind parents not to use candles in a room with oxygen supplies. A reminder during the winter holidays or on birthdays is appropriate.

Children who are ventilator dependent or who need suctioning must have their bed positioned near an electrical power outlet. If a ventilator is in use, the local electric company should be notified. This allows them to notify the family if for some reason they plan to disrupt service for repairs. Sufficient battery power to sustain the function of the ventilator in the event of a power shortage should be available for the family or a manual resuscitator such as an Ambu bag should be available. The local community emergency agency (i.e., police or fire department) should also be notified that a ventilator will be in use so they can respond quickly in an unexpected power failure.

Be certain that parents are aware of the signs and symptoms that suggest the need for emergency medical intervention to sustain respiratory function and what

steps to take should this occur. Possibilities are to call the hospital for an ambulance, or call the local fire department or 911.

When a child is ventilator dependent, parents need a home care nurse in constant attendance until they are absolutely comfortable with the ventilator, as it is frightening for parents to care for a child who is this ill at home (Anas, 1990). They often grow fatigued from lack of sleep and the daily stress of responsibility. It severely limits their ability to leave the house even for necessary trips such as grocery shopping (see the Focus on Nursing Research box).

The use of apnea monitors is discussed in Chapter 26. Be certain to evaluate whether parents can hear the monitor alarm from all parts of their house and whether the alarm can be heard over the sound of household ap-

 **FOCUS ON
NURSING RESEARCH**

What Is the Impact on Families Caring for Very Ill Children at Home?

More and more very ill children are being cared for at home. To investigate the impact of such care, three nursing researchers asked 57 families to complete a questionnaire designed to elicit psychological distress.

Children's ages ranged from 1 to 18 years with a mean of 4.6 years. Families were mainly middle-class; 91% of them were two-parent families; 58% of the mothers were employed. The majority of children had a central nervous system disorder and were technology dependent.

A score of over 63 on the psychological distress test indicated a need for psychiatric intervention. Seventy-five percent of families had a test score of 63 or greater or showed enough psychological distress to warrant psychological consultation. Father's psychological distress increased with a mother's employment outside the home, the presence of siblings in the family, high dependency in the child, and having a private third-party payer. Mother's increased distress was associated with increased homemaker hours, employment outside the home, and father's increasing care hours.

Although it has been suspected since the advent of extensive home care for children that this places a substantial strain on parents, this study is the first to document how extensive and deep the problem may be. The researchers stress that maternal outside employment is a factor that nurses must be prepared to address. Although this supplies additional, much-needed financial help to the family, mothers may feel guilty that such employment causes them to neglect their mothering role. They may need counseling to juggle both roles.

Leonard, B. J., Brust, J. D., & Nelson, R. P. (1993). Parental distress: Caring for medically fragile children at home. *Journal of Pediatric Nursing, 8*, 22.

pliances such as the vacuum cleaner or blender. If not, a parent will have to limit his or her activities when alone in the house so the alarm can be heard. Parents with children who have respiratory problems should learn CPR. Reviewing the steps of CPR with them monthly is important so that their skills remain current.

Promoting Elimination

If children are on bedrest at home, parents can purchase or rent a bedpan from a medical supply house or a local pharmacy. The addition of an overbed trapeze allows children to raise and lower themselves in bed and help with self-care. A portable commode to sit beside the bed may also be rented or purchased.

If the child can walk to the bathroom but has difficulty doing so, attaching a railing in the hallway that leads to the bathroom helps him or her accomplish this. Attaching a railing to the wall beside the toilet is also helpful.

Bladder catheterization to alleviate urinary retention is usually performed in the home by a nurse, but parents can be taught this procedure if it will be done frequently. Supplies such as catheters and tubing can be purchased at medical supply houses or many pharmacies. The odor of urine in leg bags or other collecting bags can be controlled by first cleaning the bag with warm, soapy water, then soaking it in a vinegar-and-water solution (1½ cups white vinegar in 2 quarts water) for approximately 2 hours. Many children are taught intermittent clean catheterization to eliminate the need for continuous catheterization (this is discussed in Chapter 46).

With a catheter in place, stress that periurethral care (i.e., washing the perineum with soap and water) should be performed twice daily; the rectal area should be cleansed with soap and water after each bowel movement, being careful always to wash away from the urethra in girls.

Caution parents that hot water bottles should be filled with water no hotter than they would like placed on the inside of their wrist. As a general rule, heating pads should not be set above a "medium" temperature. A washcloth should be placed between a chemical hot pack or a hot water bottle and the child's skin to help prevent burning and skin maceration. Parents should not use electric heating pads near sources of water (wet dressings) unless the heating pad is specifically marked as being designed for this. When using heating pads with very young children, parents should tape the heat dial to the safe temperature setting so the child will not play with the dial and increase the heat beyond a safe limit. catheter in place. With females, the presence of a catheter should not interfere with penile–vaginal intercourse because the catheter is pliable and compresses easily. Males can be taught to remove the catheter and replace it with a second sterile one after intercourse.

Children with inadequate renal function are often managed on continuous ambulatory peritoneal dialysis at home. The technique for this is discussed in Chapter 46.

Changing Wound Dressings

If children are discharged from health care facilities following surgery or need to have wound dressings for other reasons changed at home, parents need to be taught good aseptic technique. Dressings can be purchased at medical supply houses or pharmacies. Teach parents to wash their hands well before and after changing a dressing to reduce the possibility of introducing infection. In an effort to save money on dressings, parents may skip some dressing changes. To prevent infection from accumulating secretions at a wound site, however, it is better for them to use a thinner dressing and continue to change it frequently as a way of minimizing cost. If the dressing will be changed often, they should use Montgomery's straps or secure the dressing with roller gauze to help reduce skin irritation from removal of tape.

Providing Hot and Cold Applications

Hot and cold applications may be prescribed for children on home care to reduce inflammation. Supplies such as chemical hot packs or hot water bottles are available from pharmacies or medical supply houses. For a sustained period of warmth, teach parents to cover the hot pack with a piece of plastic. K-pads (pumps that circulate hot water to rubber pads) and electric heating pads can be rented from medical supply houses for a sustained source of heat.

Caution parents that hot water bottles should be filled with water no hotter than they would like placed on the inside of their wrist. As a general rule, heating pads should not be set above a "medium" temperature. A washcloth should be placed between a chemical hot pack or a hot water bottle and the child's skin to help prevent burning and skin maceration. Parents should not use electric heating pads near sources of water (wet dressings) unless the heating pad is specifically marked as being designed for this. When using heating pads with very young children, parents should tape the heat dial to the safe temperature setting so the child will not play with the dial and increase the heat beyond a safe

Heat treatments are ineffective after 20 minutes. Parents may need to be reminded of this limit or they will keep the heat continuously in place, thinking this increases the effectiveness.

Parents should always observe the site where the heat is to be applied before and after heat is used. Redness, blistering, or pain are signs of burning, and no further heat should be applied until their home care nurse has been notified and has inspected the site.

Cold applications are available as chemical cold packs, or ice can be placed in a hot water bottle or a plastic bag. Children need to have a washcloth placed between the cold pack and their skin the same as with heat treatments to protect their skin from frostbite and injury. Cold, like heat, should be limited to 20-minute applications.

Supporting Home Phototherapy for the Newborn

Well newborns who develop physiologic jaundice and need only a few days of phototherapy may be cared for safely at home rather than remaining in the hospital (Murphy et al., 1992). Bilirubin lights are rented from medical supply houses or a specialized phototherapy service.

Home phototherapy allows for uninterrupted contact between the parents and the newborn and therefore has the potential to aid bonding. Important considerations are that the lights are set so that they are a full 12 inches away from the infant to prevent burning and that the infant continuously wears eye patches and a diaper during phototherapy to protect the retinas of the eyes and the ovaries or testes.

The infant should have the eye patches removed when away from the lights for feeding for a period of visual stimulation and interaction. The point at which infants are most apt to dislodge eye patches is when they cry as they wake for a feeding. Urge parents not to allow an infant under bilirubin lights to cry for a sustained period to avoid having this happen.

The infant's progress can be measured daily by a transcutaneous bilirubinometer. This is a hand-held fiberoptic light that is placed against the infant's skin. The intensity of the yellow color of the skin is measured by the meter and a numerical level of bilirubin is calculated.

A newer innovation for hyperbilirubinemia management is the **phototherapy blanket**, a fiberoptic blanket that is wrapped around the baby (Rose, 1990). Light generated by the blanket has the same effect on bilirubin levels as banks of overhead lights. The advantages of a blanket are that the infant can be held for long periods without an interruption in the phototherapy, and eye patches are unnecessary.

Promoting Growth and Development

Children on home care may need a stimulation program designed for them so they do not spend all day watching television or napping. If their medical condition allows, home tutoring or contact with their school classroom by intercom should be arranged. During the times the child will not be attending school, working on projects such as needlecraft, helping plan family menus, writing for brochures about the place the family plans to vacation next year, or viewing videotapes on science or nature (rented for a minimum fee for a home videotape recorder) are suggestions that not only help pass the time but encourage learning.

Children should be encouraged to carry out self-care and to contribute to the household routines, such as helping with dishes and picking up after themselves, as much as they are able. This takes some burden off caregivers and makes the child feel an intrinsic part of the family.

Promoting Healthy Family Functioning

Although many families are good candidates for home care, they continue to need nursing care that helps them adapt constructively to the crisis of illness and home management, as a child's illness represents an automatic stressor to every family. Physical care requirements can disrupt the normal family routines and shift the focus of attention onto the ill child and away from other children in the family (Figure 38-3). The needs of the parents may also be neglected. Help these families by promoting communication and encouraging family members to identify and share their feelings about the new situation at home. Continued successful coping will require that the family acknowledge and take seriously the impact of home care on each family member and work together to solve identified problems. They may need to renegotiate roles and responsibilities within the family or seek outside help (see the Focus on Nursing Research display and the Nursing Care Plan: Home Care for a Ventilator-Dependent Infant).

When the family is not functioning well to begin with or has not adjusted to the child's illness, nursing measures to support family functioning are even more important. A family whose coping strategies are mal-

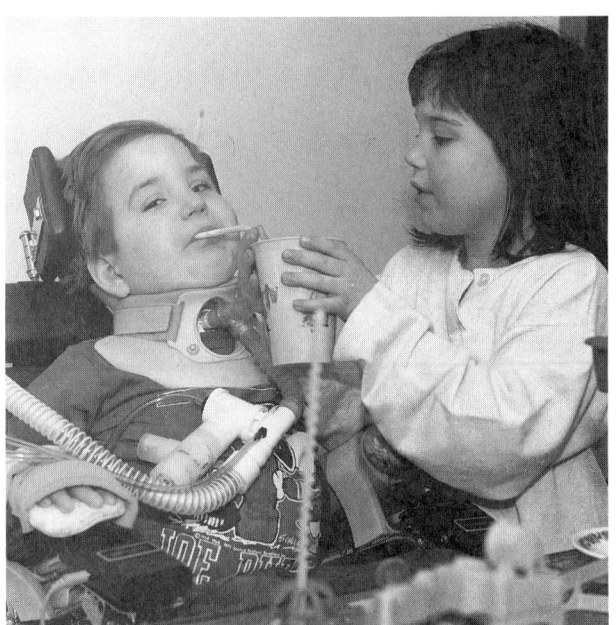

FIGURE 38-3
Home care of a child is family care. Here a sister helps a ventilator-dependent sibling with dinner. (Courtesy of the Department of Medical Photography, Children's Hospital, Buffalo, NY.)

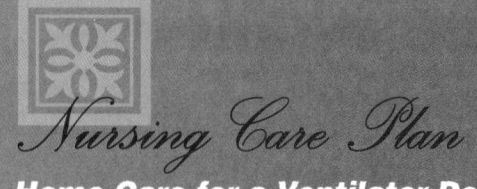

Nursing Care Plan

Home Care for a Ventilator-Dependent Infant

Kevin is a 3-month-old boy with bronchopulmonary dysplasia. He is ventilator dependent, receives feedings by a gastrostomy, and is on home care. The following is a nursing care plan designed for him.

Assessment: Child lives with two parents and a 4-year-old brother. Father is primary caregiver during the day while the mother works; mother is caregiver at night while the father works. Kevin needs continuous ventilator care; oxygen concentration at 40%. Has a gastrostomy button in place for feeding; present formula used is Enfamil with iron, 150 mL, six times a day.

Mother states that she and husband are managing adequately at present, but voices apprehension at continuing such close health surveillance for an extended time. States, "We have no life of our own any more. I feel like a slave to the ventilator." Also concerned because she never has time for 4-year-old son; states, "He might as well be an orphan."

Nursing Diagnosis: Powerlessness related to prolonged caretaking responsibilities for ventilator-dependent child

Defining Characteristic: Parent states that she feels "like slave" and "with no life of her own."

Goal: Parent will demonstrate positive expectations about the future by next clinic visit.

Outcome Criteria: Parents share their feelings with each other and with health care providers; state realistic goals for the future; identify ways they can spend time with each other and older child and maintain outside interests.

Nursing Orders	*Rationale*
1. Discuss possibility of parents employing a home health care provider at least 1 day a week.	1. Parents need to know they can count on being freed from their caregiving responsibilities on a regular basis.
2. Discuss necessity for parents to maintain contact with each other, not just spell each other in giving care.	2. Emphasizes to parents that their relationship is just as important as their family responsibilities.
3. Discuss ways and times that both parents could spend additional time with older sibling (a special time for reading while gastrostomy feeding infuses, for example). An alternative solution might be to enroll sibling in a preschool program to achieve additional stimulation and special activities for him.	3. A sibling's growth and development needs do not vanish with the arrival of new family responsibilities. Brainstorming ways to meet this child's needs as well can help the parents turn their focus away from their ill child in a positive way.

Nursing Diagnosis: High risk for altered nutrition related to gastrostomy feedings

Defining Characteristic: Child receives feeding by a gastrostomy button.

(continued)

adaptive and ineffective may not be able to care for a sick family member at home for long.

Key Points

- Home care is increasing as a way of providing care to chronically ill children. It has advantages of being cost effective and providing meaningful comfort and

ready support to the child. Disadvantages are that parents can become fatigued, the loss of a job for the primary caregiver can cause financial hardship, and social isolation and disruption of normal home life may occur.

- Not all homes are ideal for home care. Assess that a primary care provider is present; the family is knowledgeable about the care necessary; neces-

Goal: Child will receive adequate nutrition by gastrostomy feedings until able to ingest oral food satisfactorily.

Outcome Criteria: Child follows present curve on growth chart; appears satisfied following feedings (no excessive crying or sleeplessness).

Nursing Orders	Rationale
1. Review procedure with father (primary daytime caregiver), stressing necessity for handwashing before procedure.	1. Allows father to confirm/revise his technique and ask questions that may have come up since the baby was discharged from the hospital.
2. Review necessity for feeding with infant in upright position.	2. Keeping infant upright during feeding will help prevent esophageal reflux.
3. Review care of gastrostomy button (wash with soap and water); stress importance of reporting any erythema on skin or leaking of formula following feedings.	3. Proper care techniques and hygiene will help maintain skin integrity.

Nursing Diagnosis: High risk for impaired gas exchange related to child's inability to breathe independently

Defining Characteristic: Child is receiving oxygen by assisted ventilation.

Goal: Child will maintain adequate respiration by ventilator until he is able to manage needs independently.

Outcome Criteria: Child is not cyanotic, pulse is 100–120 beats/min; periodic blood gases obtained are PCO_2 under 40 mm Hg; PO_2 over 60 mm Hg.

Nursing Orders	Rationale
1. Review with parents necessity to assess temperature, pulse, and respirations and to suction endotracheal tube twice daily by clean technique.	1. These assessment measures and techniques will help prevent infection.
2. Review necessity to keep sources of heat or fire away from oxygen source.	2. Oxygen must be stored carefully to prevent accidents, as it supports combustion.
3. Assess that parents have contacted power company that they have a child on continuous ventilation.	3. It is important for the power company to know about the family's need for a continuous power source in the event of planned power outages.
4. Review technique of chest percussion to be done twice daily.	4. Chest percussion is important in the prevention of mucus build-up that could lead to respiratory obstruction or infection.
5. Review steps of cardiopulmonary resuscitation parent will take in case of respiratory emergency.	5. Parents need to be able to provide basic life support.

sary resources are available; and safety features such as a smoke detector, a safe area for oxygen storage, and a safe refrigerator for food or medicine are present.

• Important elements to consider when planning home care are ways to provide a therapeutic environment; provide for adequate nutrition and mobility; meet care requirements for respiratory function and elimination; administer medication; and encourage self-care.

• Be certain parents truly are comfortable and skilled at performing procedures by asking them to demonstrate how to perform a procedure such as a gastrostomy tube feeding. This is a rewarding time for them if they are comfortable and skilled; if they are not, it provides a time to review the skill.

- Home care can be exhausting for parents. Be certain they devise a schedule of care that allows them enough rest.
- To allow parents to sleep, advocate for medicine schedules that allow for administering medications during the day rather than a schedule that requires medication administration at night.
- Parents may need respite care to continue to be effective care providers, just as professionals need time off. Help parents to relieve each other so each has some free time during a week. Urge them to do something they truly enjoy during this time (read a good book, go to a movie, try a new recipe, jog, etc.). It is important for a couple to have some respite time together. Encourage families who are caring for an ill child at home to reach out to friends and family for help in managing the household from time to time so that the parents can go out alone together. Hiring a home health care provider once a week or once a month is another option.
- Home health care can continue for years. Help parents to discover ways to meet the child's growth and development needs during this time. Adult caregivers also have growth needs. If feasible, both child and parents might take a continuing education course, read library books, or learn a new hobby together to fulfill all their growth needs.

Critical Thinking Exercises

1. Terry is a 4-year-old on home care for chronic respiratory disease. His parents state that they are exhausted because of the necessity of round-the-clock care. What suggestions could you make to them to make care easier?
2. Celeste is a 14-year-old who will be cared for at home following orthopedic surgery. She is concerned that because her home stay will be lengthy, she will be cut off from her friends for a long time. What suggestions could you make to Celeste to help her maintain contact with friends?
3. Mario is a newborn who will be cared for at home because of hyperbilirubinemia. His parents tell you that they are inexperienced and are worried they are not up to providing care to an ill newborn. How would you support them until they grow more confident?

References

American Academy of Pediatrics, Ad Hoc Task Force on Home Care of Chronically Ill Infants and Children. (1984). Guidelines for home care of infants, children, and adolescents with chronic disease. *Pediatrics, 74,* 434.

Anas, N. (1990). Discharge planning and home management for the ventilator-assisted infant. *Journal of Home Health Care Practice, 2,* 53.

Baranowski, L. (1993). Central venous access devices: Current technologies, uses, and management strategies. *Journal of Intravenous Nursing, 16,* 167.

Bendorf, K., et al. (1993). Transition from the hospital to the home for the infant requiring total parenteral nutrition. *Journal of Perinatology and Neonatology Nursing, 6,* 80.

Brown, J. M. (1990). Home care models for infusion therapy. *Caring, 9,* 24.

Department of Health & Human Services. (1991). *Healthy people 2000.* Washington, DC: Public Health Service.

Dolan, M. G., et al. (1990). Evaluation of home visits using a nursing process approach. *Journal of Community Health Nursing, 7,* 69.

Estoup, M. (1994). Approaches and limitations of medication delivery in patients with enteral feeding tubes. *Critical Care Nurse, 14,* 68.

Geissler, E. M. (1994). *Pocket guide to cultural assessment.* St. Louis: C. V. Mosby.

Graver, J. (1993). Selecting an enteral feeding pump. *American Journal of Nursing, 93,* 66.

Hagelgans, N. A., & Janusz, H. B. (1994). Pediatric skin care issues for the home care nurse. *Pediatric Nursing, 20,* 8.

Hammond, L. J., et al. (1991). Cystic fibrosis, intravenous antibiotics, and home therapy. *Journal of Pediatric Health Care, 5,* 24.

Harris, M. D. (1990). Restructuring: Specifics for home health. *Nursing Economics, 8,* 257.

Leonard, B. J., Brust, J. D., & Nelson, R. P. (1993). Parental distress: Caring for medically fragile children at home. *Journal of Pediatric Nursing, 8,* 22.

McAnear, S. (1990). Parental reaction to a chronically ill child. *Home Healthcare Nurse, 8,* 35.

McCoy, P. A., & Feenan, L. M. (1990). Alterations in respiratory function. In P. A. McCoy & W. L. Votroubek, *Pediatric home care* (pp. 57–100). Rockville, MD: Aspen.

Murphy, B. N., et al. (1992). Home phototherapy for the jaundiced full-term newborn. *Journal of Home Health Care Practice, 5,* 26.

Rose, B. S. (1990). Phototherapy: All wrapped up? *Pediatric Nursing, 16,* 57.

Spradley, B. W. (1990). *Community health nursing.* Glenview, IL: Scott, Foresman.

Zahr, L. K., et al. (1993). The benefits of home care for sick premature infants. *Neonatal Network, 12,* 33.

Suggested Readings

Chu, N. L., & Schmele, J. A. (1990). Using the ANA standards as a basis for performance evaluation in the home health care setting. *Journal of Nursing Quality Assurance, 4,* 25.

Cohen, M. R., et al. (1994). Twelve ways to prevent medication errors. *Nursing 94, 24,* 34.

Everett, D. (1990). For a child with pneumonia, there's no place like home. *RN, 53,* 85.

Kenner, C., et al. (1993). Issues and controversies: The home visit. *Neonatal Network, 11,* 46.

Leonard, B. J., et al. (1993). Parental distress: Caring for medically fragile children at home. *Journal of Pediatric Nursing, 8,* 22.

Scannell, S., et al. (1993). Negotiating nurse-patient authority in pediatric home health care. *Journal of Pediatric Nursing, 8,* 70.

Wong, D. L. (1991). Transition from hospital to home for children with complex medical care. *Journal of Pediatric Oncology Nursing, 8,* 3.

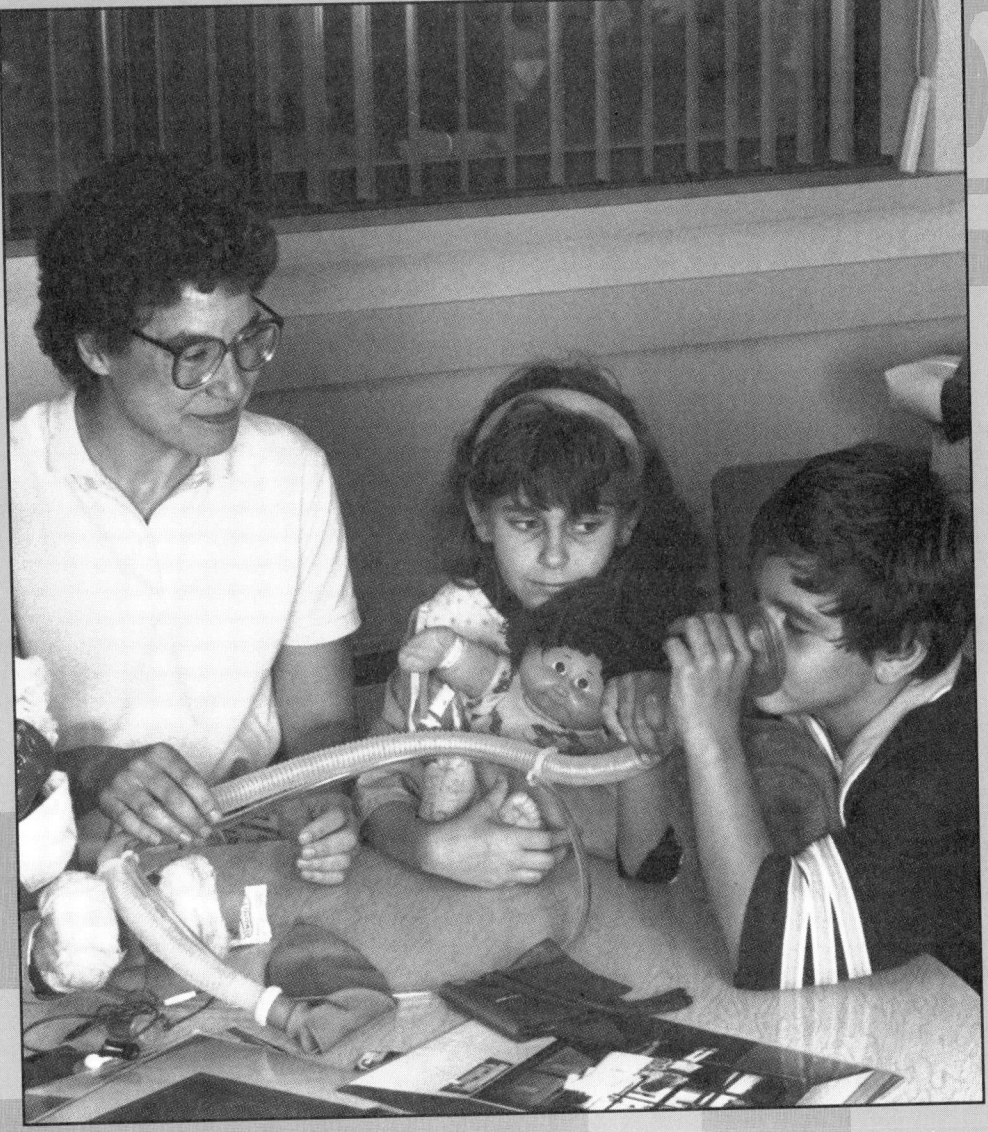

The Nursing Role in Restoring and Maintaining the Health of Children and Families With Physiologic Disorders

Unit

8

Chapter

39

Nursing Care of the Child Born With a Physical Developmental Disorder

Objectives

After mastering the contents of this chapter, you should be able to:

1. Describe common physical birth disorders.

2. Assess a newborn who is born with a physical developmental disorder.

3. Develop nursing diagnoses for the child born with a physical developmental disorder.

4. Plan nursing care related to meeting the established goals of care, such as planning ways to improve parent–child relationships.

5. Carry out nursing interventions in the care of children born with physical developmental disorders, such as preventing infection in the child with spina bifida.

6. Evaluate outcome criteria to be certain that established goals for care have been achieved.

7. Identify National Health Goals related to children born with physical disabilities that nurses could be instrumental in helping the nation achieve.

8. Identify areas related to infants with developmental disabilities that could benefit by additional nursing research.

9. Use critical thinking to analyze the impact on the family of a child born with a developmental anomaly and ways to make care more family-centered.

10. Synthesize knowledge of congenital physical anomalies with the nursing process to achieve quality maternal and child health nursing care.

Adele Pillitteri: MATERNAL AND CHILD HEALTH NURSING, 2nd Edition. © 1995 Adele Pillitteri.

F ew things, other than hemorrhage in the mother during delivery, can change the expectant, usually joyous tone of a birthing room faster than the birth of a baby with a developmental defect. Physicians or nurse-midwives who are used to saying "perfect boy" or "beautiful girl" and holding up the infant for the parents' first glance, are suddenly without words. The nurse is in the same predicament. Words of congratulations hang, unsaid, in the air.

When a child is born with an apparent physical developmental defect, the nursing role in support and education of the parents is especially important. Some disorders are easily repaired; others require surgery but the prognosis is good; some disorders, however, represent serious, even life-threatening problems for the infant and may result in long-term care needs. This chapter covers the physical congenital disorders that are appar-

ent at birth or soon after. Such disorders primarily involve the gastrointestinal, neurologic, and skeletal systems. Congenital disorders of the cardiovascular system, which also represent life-threatening problems for the infant, are addressed in Chapter 41. National Health Goals related to children with congenital anomalies are shown in the Focus on National Health Goals box.

⊠ **NURSING PROCESS OVERVIEW**
for Care of the Child Born With a Physical
Developmental Disorder

ASSESSMENT

Nursing assessment of the child born with a physical defect focuses on determining the immediate physiologic requirements of the child to sustain life and the immediate emotional needs of the parents to promote bonding between child and parents. The nurse should evaluate how the anomaly affects the infant's eight primary needs: establishment and maintenance of adequate respiration, establishment of extrauterine circulation and body temperature control, ability to take in adequate nourishment, establishment of waste elimination, prevention of infection, development of an infant–parent bond, and exposure to adequate stimulation. The parents' response to the diagnosis of a congenital defect must also be assessed. Anomalies that affect the child's appearance may have the most immediate effect on the parents' ability to establish a positive feeling about their child. It is important, however, not to jump to conclusions about parents' responses; assessment of the family's stated and nonverbal responses must be as thorough and objective as assessment of the infant's health status.

FOCUS ON
National Health Goals

Many congenital anomalies such as omphalocele and spinal cord defects can be detected during intrauterine life. The following National Health Goal addresses the importance of prenatal care and counseling:

- Increase to at least 90% the proportion of women enrolled in prenatal care who are offered screening and counseling on prenatal detection of fetal abnormalities.

Another National Health Goal emphasizes the importance of the coordination of services for complex disorders such as cleft lip and palate:

- Increase to at least 40 from a baseline of 25 states that have an effective system for recording infants with cleft lip and palate and referring them to craniofacial anomaly teams (DHHS, 1991).

Nurses can be instrumental in helping the nation achieve these goals by being certain that appointments for follow-up care or further diagnosis made at prenatal visits or in the newborn period are arranged at times convenient for parents so that such visits are kept.

Additional nursing research in this area is needed concerning what factors determine which women will continue their pregnancy after a congenital anomaly is discovered in their fetus; how far is reasonable to ask parents to travel for follow-up care for a newborn; and what measures do parents feel were most helpful to them at the time of a fetal or newborn anomaly diagnosis.

NURSING DIAGNOSIS

Many nursing diagnoses established for children born with congenital anomalies address their effect on body function or family interaction. The following diagnoses are examples:

- Altered nutrition, less than body requirements, related to inability to take in adequate nutrition secondary to physical defect
- Impaired physical mobility related to congenital anomaly
- High risk for altered parenting related to birth of child with anomaly
- Grieving (parental) related to loss of "perfect" child

PLANNING

When planning care, be certain to consider both the short- and long-term needs of the newborn and how these needs will affect the family. Consider, also, the family's resources—both emotional and practical—and devise a plan of care with these in mind. A parent or parents with supportive family members nearby may be able to accept the limits of the child's disorder and turn their attention to the planned treatment regimen or care priorities sooner than those who have no close friends or relatives to whom they can turn for comfort and support. For the latter, you may need to act not only as a source of information and support but also as a sounding board and advocate until the parents can begin to develop positive coping mechanisms that will help them come to terms with this unexpected turn of events. The following organizations may be helpful sources of support for parents:

National Easter Seal Society
70 East Lake Street
Chicago, IL 60601

Spina Bifida Association of America
4590 MacArthur Blvd., Suite 250
Washington, DC 20007

American Cleft Palate–Craniofacial Association
1218 Grandview Avenue
Pittsburgh, PA 15211

IMPLEMENTATION

Nursing interventions for the newborn with a physical anomaly include immediate life-sustaining measures such as providing for adequate intake of nutrients when a defect prevents the infant from sucking. Educating the parents regarding pre- and post-treatment procedures and encouraging them to hold, touch, and talk with their babies are interventions especially important to the future emotional well-being of the child and family.

Parents may have difficulty caring for a child with a congenital anomaly because they suffer a loss of self-esteem at the child's birth. They feel as if the baby is proof that something in the combination of their genes or the prenatal environment they provided was inadequate. They need to hear positive comments about themselves and be given support until they can realize that by caring for the child they are accomplishing more—not less—than other couples (see Focus on Cultural Awareness box).

Parents can be expected to move through the same stages of grief as those whose child died at birth. Chapter 56 describes those stages and helpful nursing interventions in more detail.

Parents are acutely aware of what people think of their children. They watch closely how the nurse handles the baby to see if he or she is giving as much attention to their baby as to other babies. It is important for the baby with an anomaly, and for the parents' acceptance of their child, that the nurse rock the baby after feeding and coo and talk to the baby as much as she talks to the other babies in the nursery; otherwise, parents may think that if a professional finds their child distasteful, how will they dare show the child to their family and friends? If a nurse is able to look past the anomaly to the whole child, however, they begin to do so, too. A nurse is setting the stage for healthy parent–child interaction every time he or she handles an infant born with a congenital anomaly.

EVALUATION

Evaluation should focus on goals established for the child's physical health and developmental needs, as well as the family's ability to cope with whatever special care and growth needs the child may have in the future. Be sure that parents have numbers to call for questions and follow-up care.

Outcome criteria may include these:

- Child is ambulatory with walker in 3 months.
- Parent voices positive features of child by 2 weeks.
- Parents voice they accept talipes anomaly as a correctable condition by 1 month.

Responsibilities of the Nurse at the Birth of an Infant With a Physical Anomaly

Most physicians and nurse-midwives believe that bearing the news of congenital physical anomalies to parents is their responsibility. However, because the physician or nurse-midwife must deliver the placenta and suture the perineum if an episiotomy was used for birth, if a neonal specialist is not immediately available, 10 minutes may pass before this person is ready to make a second inspection of the baby, assess the true extent of the anomaly from the physical symptoms present, and tell the parents about the defect and the baby's prognosis. This delay does one of two things to the parents: It leaves them believing for 10 minutes either that they delivered a perfect child among people who do not share their enthusiasm or that they have just given birth to a child so deformed that all the professionals in the room find it too horrible to even talk about. Because parents are aware of the atmosphere in a birthing room, the second response is by far more likely. In terms of parent–child interaction, this response is unhealthy. Parents begin anticipatory grieving for a deformed child. Even when they are told later that the defect is not extensive, is easily correctable, and that as soon as the correction is made the child will be perfect, the anticipatory grief reaction may be hard to stop. They may continue to cut themselves off emotionally from the child.

Nurses should be familiar enough with the most frequently encountered physical anomalies to be able to make truthful statements about them and so explain the problem to parents. This transfer does not represent "passing the buck" by physicians; rather, the responsibility then falls to the person who at that moment in the delivery process is free to assume it. If a physician does not feel comfortable in allowing a nurse to take on this role, the nurse must be ready to serve as a back-up in-

FOCUS ON CULTURAL AWARENESS

The cause of most congenital anomalies is unknown, although they probably arise from a combination of environmental and genetic factors. Still, many people persist in believing that infants with congenital anomalies are born to people less deserving than others or who have sinned or have been looked on by someone with envy during pregnancy. Eating raisins during pregnancy causes brown spots and strawberries cause hemangiomas are beliefs that still proliferate. New parents need a chance to talk about why they believe their child's disorder occurred, to relieve their guilt that they were the cause and allow them to regain sufficient self-esteem to be able to parent a child with a congenital disorder.

The way that parents carry infants may contribute to the formation of hip dysplasia. Infants who are carried straddled on their parents' hips may have less hip dysplasia than those carried with their legs brought together.

formant, to answer the questions the parents will have after being told that their child has been born less than perfect. It is probably best to explain to parents what the defect is and what the prognosis for the defect is before showing the baby to them. Parents may find it hard to look at an infant with a cleft lip or palate or exposed abdominal contents and also listen to what the nurse is saying. Their minds are so jammed with the visual image their eyes are sending them, so unlike the child of their imagination, that they cannot hear. Provide, for example, the following explanation:

> Your baby's upper lip isn't completely formed. That's called a cleft lip. Your doctor will call one of the plastic surgeons here at the hospital to look at your baby. This is a problem that can be repaired so well surgically that you'll barely be able to tell your baby was born this way. I'll bring the baby over so you can see her. Remember when you look at her that this can be repaired. She seems perfect in every other way.

These statements define and limit the problem for the parents and give them direction about where and how they should proceed in thinking about it and in beginning to seek help for their child.

Anomalies of the Gastrointestinal System

Many of the most common congenital anomalies involve the gastrointestinal system. The gastrointestinal tract forms first as a solid tube, then undergoes canalization. If this subsequent canalization does not occur, a blockage or obstruction will be present in the system. Other defects of the tract, such as cleft lip and cleft palate, are the results of midline closure failure extremely early in intrauterine life.

Ankyloglossia (Tongue-Tie)

Ankyloglossia is an abnormal restriction of the tongue caused by a tight **frenulum**, which is the membrane attached to the lower anterior tip of the tongue. Most children adapt well to this condition, but if it causes speech problems later on or if the condition places destructive pressure on gingival tissue, surgical release may be performed (Kula, 1994). Because parents may be concerned, even if surgery is not indicated, they need a good explanation of the normal appearances of newborns' tongues. Normally the frenulum is short and near the tip of the tongue, but as the anterior portion of the tongue grows, the frenulum becomes located farther back. Showing them other newborns or photographs of normal tongues is helpful in convincing them that a short frenulum is normal. Explore with them why they are concerned. Is there a child in the family with a speech defect or a cleft lip and palate? Do the parents

need assurance in any other way that their child is all right?

Thyroglossal Cyst

A *thyroglossal cyst* arises from an *embryogenic fault* (a persistent opening to the anterior surface of the neck that did not close normally); it may be a dominantly inherited trait. A cyst may form at the base of the tongue, may involve the *hyoid bone* (the bone at the anterior surface of the neck at the root of the tongue), or may contain aberrant thyroid gland tissue. As the cyst becomes filled with fluid, the obstruction can cause respiratory difficulty. If infected, the cyst becomes swollen, appears reddened, and drains mucus or pus from the anterior neck (Todd, 1993).

Treatment is surgical removal of the cyst to avoid future infection of the space or, if thyroid tissue is present, the possibility of carcinoma. Observe infants closely in the immediate postoperative period for respiratory distress, because the operative area will have some edema near it. Position such children on their abdomens so secretions drain freely from their mouths. They will be administered fluid intravenously for a period following surgery until the edema at the incision recedes somewhat and swallowing is safe once more (approximately 24 hours). If the mother is breast-feeding, encourage her to express her milk supply manually for the feedings that the child is not taking orally to preserve her milk supply. Observe infants closely the first few times they take fluid orally to be certain that they swallow safely and do not aspirate. Be certain parents feed them before they are discharged from the hospital so they can see that they are swallowing safely. This is important to their development of confidence in themselves as parents and their ability to feed the infant at home in a relaxed and comfortable way.

Cleft Lip and Palate

The fusion of the maxillary and median nasal processes normally occurs between weeks 5 and 8 of intrauterine life. In infants with **cleft lip**, the fusion fails in varying degrees, with the defect ranging from a small notch in the upper lip to a total separation of the lip and facial structure up into the floor of the nose. Upper teeth and gingiva may be absent. The nose is generally flattened, because the incomplete fusion of the upper lip has allowed it to expand in a horizontal dimension (Figure 39-1). The deviation may be unilateral or bilateral. Cleft lip is more prevalent among males than females. It occurs at a rate of approximately 1 in every 1000 live births. The incidence is approximately twice this in the Japanese population; it occurs rarely in African-Americans.

Cleft lip demonstrates a familial tendency or most

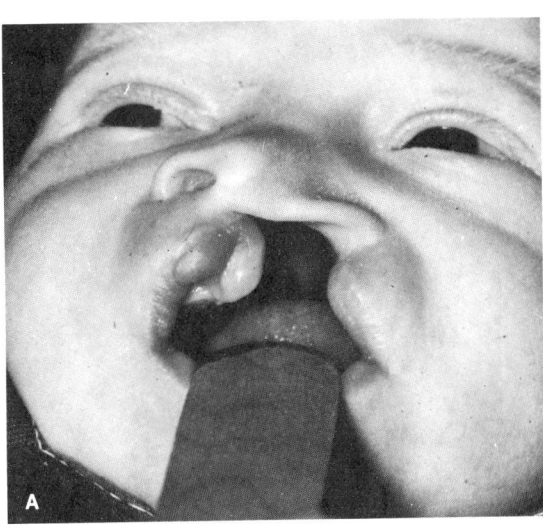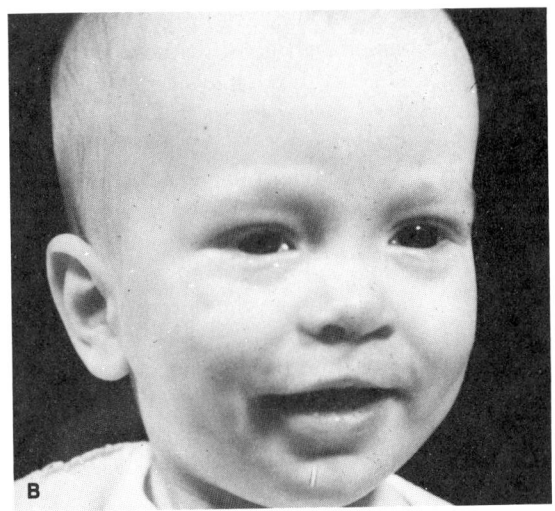

FIGURE 39-1
(**A**) *A 2-week-old infant with unilateral cleft lip.* (**B**) *Same child at age 14 months, showing surgical repair.*
(From Crowley, L. V. An introduction to clinical embryology. *Chicago: Year Book, with permission.)*

likely occurs from the transmission of multiple genes. Formation may be aided by teratogenic factors present during weeks 5 to 8 of intrauterine life such as avitaminosis or viral infection. Parents of a child with a cleft lip should be referred for genetic counseling to ensure that they understand that future children are at a greater risk than usual for this problem.

The palatal process closes at approximately weeks 9 to 12 of intrauterine life. A **cleft palate**, an opening of the palate, is usually on the midline and may involve just the anterior hard palate, or the posterior soft palate, or both (Figure 39-2). It may be a separate anomaly, but as a rule it occurs in conjunction with a cleft lip. As a single entity, it tends to occur more frequently in females than males; it appears, like cleft lip, to be the result of polygenic inheritance or environmental influences. In connection with cleft lip, the incidence is approximately 1 in every 1000 births; as a single entity, it occurs in approximately 1 in every 2500 births.

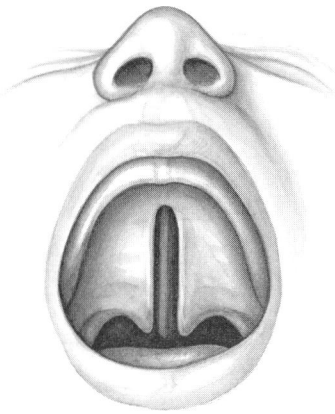

FIGURE 39-2
Cleft palate. Both the hard and soft palate are involved.

Assessment

Cleft lip may be detected by sonogram while the infant is in utero. The condition can be repaired by fetal surgery at this early time (Oberg et al., 1993). Both cleft lip and cleft palate are readily apparent on inspection at birth. A good light is necessary to reveal a cleft palate. Depressing the tongue with a tongue blade reveals the total palate and the extent of the defect. Because cleft palate is a component of many syndromes, a child with a cleft palate must be assessed for other congenital anomalies that would suggest it is only one of a combination of problems.

Therapeutic Management

A cleft lip is repaired surgically shortly after birth, sometimes at the time of the initial hospital stay and sometimes between 1 and 3 months. Because the deviation of the lip interferes with nutrition, infants may be a better surgical risk at birth than they are after a month or more of poor nourishment. Early repair also helps infants experience the pleasure of sucking as soon as possible. It is equally important from a psychological standpoint that these disorders be repaired early. Parents may find it extremely difficult to bond with an infant whose face is deformed in this way. This is not a sign of a "bad" parent. It is reality and a problem that should be dealt with as realistically as the actual oral construction.

The repair of cleft palate is usually postponed until the child is approximately age 4 to 6 months. If it is extensive, surgery may be postponed until the anatomic change in the palate contour that occurs during the first year of life has taken place. Repairs made before this change (the palate arch increases) may be ineffective and have to be rescheduled.

Currently, the results of surgical repair of cleft lip

and cleft palate are excellent. It is helpful to show parents photographs of babies with good repairs (see Figure 39-1) to assure them that their child's outcome can also be good. The older term for this condition, "harelip," should not be used when talking with parents about the problem. Before modern surgical techniques were available, children were left with large lip scars, gross speech impediments, and a poor appearance after surgery. Harelip tends to be associated with these negative outcomes rather than with the current positive outlook.

Some infants with a cleft lip have an accompanying deviated nasal septum, which may need to be repaired in later years for good air exchange. Some have a flattened, slightly distorted nose contour, which they may choose to have corrected for cosmetic appearance later in life.

Because palate repair narrows the upper dental arch or because the original cleft may have involved the dental arch, there may be less space in the upper jaw for the eruption of teeth, causing a defect in teeth alignment. These children need follow-up treatment by a pedodontist or a dentist skilled in children's dental problems, so that as the children grow, extractions or realignment of teeth can be done as indicated (Eliason, 1991).

Nursing Diagnoses and Related Interventions

Nursing Diagnosis: High risk for altered nutrition, less than body requirements, related to feeding problems caused by cleft lip or palate

Goal: Child will take in adequate nutrition until anomalies are fully repaired.

Outcome Criteria: Child will ingest a diet of 50 kcal/lb in 24 hours and will not lose more than 10% of birth weight.

Preoperative Period. Before a cleft lip is repaired, feeding the infant is a problem. The child must take in an adequate amount of food and also be prevented from aspirating (Danner, 1992).

Various modifications may be used for feeding. The best method for the child with cleft lip appears to be to support the baby in an upright position and feed the child gently by a commercial cleft lip nipple (Figure 39-3). Be careful when feeding these infants. A hurried nurse or a hurried parent can easily cause the infant to aspirate.

It may be possible for an infant with a cleft lip to breast-feed, because the bulk of the breast tends to form a seal against the injured upper lip. Although the baby needs the enjoyment of sucking, some surgeons do not want the baby to breast-feed or suck on a nipple before surgical correction of the defect to avoid any local bruising of tissue. If this is so, infants can then be fed with a Breck feeder, an apparatus similar to an aseptic syringe.

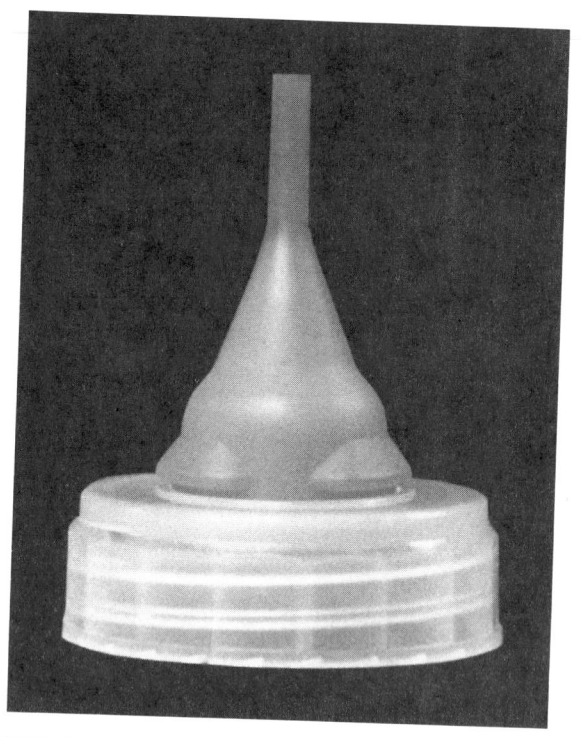

FIGURE 39-3
A commercial cleft lip nipple. (Used with permission of Ross Products Division, Abbott Laboratories, Columbus OH 43216. © Ross Products Division, Abbott Laboratories.)

Babies with extensive clefts are as unable to suck on a pacifier as they are on a nipple. If the surgical repair will be done immediately, the mother will be able to breast-feed as early as 7 to 10 days after surgery. Teach her how to pump or manually express breast milk to maintain a milk supply for this time. If surgery will be delayed for 1 month, she will need to decide whether or not she wants to continue to express milk for this period of time; if she chooses to do so, she may need continuing support and encouragement from the nursing staff.

The infant with a cleft lip needs to be held and bubbled well after feeding because of the tendency to swallow air caused by the inability to grasp a nipple or syringe edge securely with the mouth. If the cleft extends to the nares, the infant will breathe through the mouth; the mucous membrane becomes dry and the infant's lips may become dry, too. Small sips of fluid between feedings may help to keep the mucous membrane moist and prevent cracks and fissures that could lead to infection.

Infants with cleft palate cannot suck effectively, because pressing their tongue or a nipple against the roof of their mouth would force milk up into their pharynx and cause aspiration. The most successful method for feeding this infant, then, like the child with cleft lip, is to use a commercial cleft palate nipple with an extra flange of rubber to close the roof of the mouth. Breast-feeding may be possible if a breast shield with a cleft-lip nipple attached is used (Lawrence, 1994).

If surgery is delayed beyond age 6 months or the

time solid food is introduced, teach parents to be certain food offered is soft; particles of coarse food could invade the nasopharynx and cause aspiration. Infants whose surgery is delayed to this point can be fitted with plastic palate guards to form a synthetic palate and help prevent this.

Postoperative Period. Following surgery for both cleft lip and palate, the infant is kept on nothing-by-mouth (NPO) status for at least 4 hours. The infant is introduced to liquids (clear water or glucose water) at the end of this time; begin the process gradually to prevent vomiting.

No tension should be placed on a lip suture line to keep sutures from pulling apart and leaving a large scar. Both bottle- and breast-feeding is contraindicated during this immediate postoperative period. The infant is usually fed using a Breck feeder.

Following palate surgery, liquids are generally continued for the first 3 or 4 days, then a soft diet is given until healing is complete. Learn from parents what fluids the child prefers so that they can be ordered and will be available postoperatively.

When the child begins eating soft food, he or she should not use a spoon, because the child will invariably put it against the roof of the mouth. If being fed evokes an intense reaction, it is better to leave the child on a liquid diet, including milkshakes or concentrated formulas, until the sutures are ready to be removed. Be certain that milk is not included in the first fluids offered because milk curds tend to adhere to the suture line. Following a feeding, offer the child clear water to rinse the suture line and keep it as clean as possible (Wellman & Coughlin, 1991).

Nursing Diagnosis: High risk for ineffective airway clearance related to oral surgery

Goal: Child's airway will remain patent.

Outcome Criteria: Child's respiratory rate is between 20 and 30 respirations per minute without retractions or obvious distress.

Because of the local edema that occurs following cleft lip or palate surgery, observe children closely in the immediate postoperative period for respiratory distress (Litwack-Saleh, 1993). The infant with a cleft lip breathed through the mouth before surgery and now has to breathe through the nose; this may add to respiratory difficulty. This is not generally a problem, however, because newborns normally strictly breathe through the nose.

Infants may need suction to remove mucus, blood, and unswallowed saliva. Be gentle and do not touch the suture line with the catheter. Do not lie infants on their abdomen following cleft lip surgery to allow saliva to drain, because this would put pressure on the suture line and possibly tear it. Position them on their side or, as soon as awake, in an infant chair.

Nursing Diagnosis: Impaired tissue integrity at incision line related to cleft lip/cleft palate surgery

Goal: Child's incision will heal without incident.

Outcome Criteria: Incision line is free of erythema or drainage during postoperative period.

Tension on the suture line of a lip repair must be avoided or it will separate enough to cause a wide, obvious scar. The suture line is held in close approximation by a *Logan bar* (a wire bow taped to both cheeks) (Figure 39-4) or an adhesive bandage such as a Band-Aid simulating a bar. The Logan bar or Band-Aid–simulated bar must be checked after each feeding or cleaning of the suture line to be certain that it is secure and protecting the suture line. The infant should not be allowed to cry, because crying increases tension on the sutures. This means having to anticipate the infant's needs. Have formula ready and be ready to feed the infant on demand—do not wait until after the infant is awake and crying. The infant needs to be rocked, jiggled, carried, held, or whatever measure is necessary to make the child feel secure and comfortable. He or she also will need to be bubbled well after a feeding because of the tendency to swallow more air than the average infant, due to the nonsucking method of feeding used.

Nothing hard or sharp must come in contact with the cleft suture line. Observe infants after palate repair carefully to be certain that they do not put toys with sharp edges into their mouths. They should not use a straw to drink nor should they brush their own teeth—they will certainly brush the suture line accidentally. Keep elbow restraints in place when there is no adult present so that they do not put their fingers in their mouth and poke or pull at the sutures. Most children run

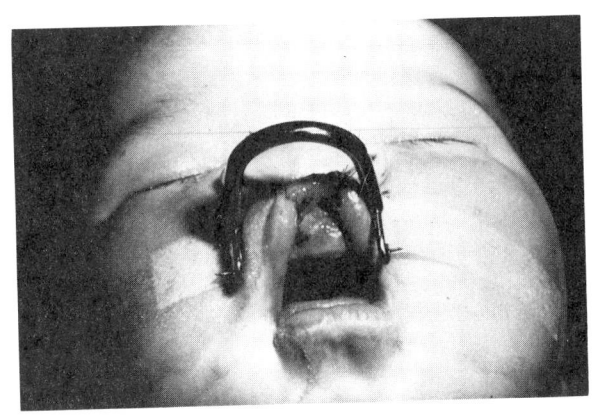

FIGURE 39-4
A Logan bar is placed to protect the surgical incision for a cleft lip repair. (From Fochtman, D., & Raffensberger, S. G. Principles of nursing care for the pediatric surgery patient. *Boston: Little, Brown, with permission.)*

their tongues over their sutures because of the odd feeling in the roofs of their mouths, and most children this age do not respond to a caution not to do this. Because children do this most when they have nothing to think about, reading, singing to them, and showing them things out the window are good ways to stop them from doing this.

Administration of acetaminophen (Tylenol) helps to keep children comfortable. Keeping infants contented after a cleft palate repair is much more difficult then keeping a newborn quiet following a cleft lip repair, because the older child is more aware of the strange hospital surroundings. They need a great deal of attention, holding, and active play. Encourage parents to stay in the hospital with them if at all possible.

Nursing Diagnosis: High risk for infection related to surgical incision

Goal: Infant will remain free of infection during postoperative period.

Outcome Criteria: Infant's temperature is below 37°C axillary; incision site is not erythematous or with drainage.

Infection may result if crusts are allowed to form on a cleft lip suture line. The line must be cleaned after every feeding and whenever serum forms. The procedure requires a sterile solution and sterile cotton-tipped applicators. The solution will depend on the individual surgeon's preference (e.g., sterile water, sterile saline, or 50% hydrogen peroxide in sterile water). It is applied by dabbing, not rubbing, the suture line with a cotton applicator. Rubbing loosens sutures, dabbing cleans them. If hydrogen peroxide is used, it will foam as it reacts with the protein particles at the suture line. Next, the suture line is rinsed with sterile water if a cleaning solution, such as half-strength hydrogen peroxide, was used. Again, dab, do not rub. The suture line is then dried by a dry cotton applicator. Remember that the infant has sutures on the inside of the lip that need the same meticulous care as those on the outside that show.

Nursing Diagnosis: High risk for altered parenting related to infant's congenital anomaly

Goal: Parents will demonstrate acceptance of infant by 48 hours postoperatively.

Outcome Criteria: Parents voice a belief in a positive outcome for child; they hold and help with infant care.

Parents need to interact with their child during the postoperative period. They should be cautioned that the incision does not look as good in the immediate postoperative period as it will eventually. As soon as the child's sutures have been removed, the infant may be fed by an ordinary bottle or breast-fed. The breast-feeding mother (who has been maintaining her milk supply through expression) needs assurance that the infant has never sucked before and will need time to learn, just as a newborn does. The infant may have an equally difficult time learning to suck from a bottle.

Notice whether the parents look at their baby's face while feeding the baby. Help them to understand that any negative feelings directed toward the child or themselves, such as sadness or anger that their baby was born this way, are normal. This does not instantly make them feel better about the child, but the knowledge that what they are experiencing is normal will help them to begin to deal with such emotions.

Nursing Diagnosis: High risk for self-esteem disturbance related to facial surgery

Goal: Child will demonstrate high self-esteem by age 3 years.

Outcome Criteria: Child participates in normal childhood activities that involve contact with other people; states activities he or she enjoys at healthcare visits.

If a scar remains after cleft lip surgery, the child may need to be introduced to the philosophy that what is inside people is more important than what shows on the surface, to strengthen self-esteem. As they reach adolescence, children need to have the inheritance pattern of cleft lip reviewed with them so they are informed of the risk of it occurring in their own children.

Nursing Diagnosis: High risk for ear infection related to altered slope of eustachian tube with cleft palate surgery

Goal: Child experiences no middle-ear infections during childhood.

Outcome Criteria: Parents state possible signs and symptoms of ear infection; state importance of early treatment; parents list signs of hearing loss.

Changing the contour of the palate also changes the slope of the eustachian tube to the middle ear. This can lead to a high incidence of middle ear infection (otitis media). Parents of children with a cleft palate must be alert to the signs of infection (e.g., fever, pain, pulling on the ear, or discharge from the ear). They need to report pharyngeal infection to the pediatrician so that it can be treated promptly before spread to the middle ear can occur. Because the eustachian tube may remain partially closed owing to its changed position, serous otitis media also tends to occur more frequently in these children than in others. The child needs routine screening for hearing loss during childhood, since this is a sign of serous otitis media. Parents should be cautioned to watch for signs of hearing loss (after being made aware that all children seem deaf when they are watching television or involved in play).

Nursing Diagnosis: High risk for altered pattern of communication related to cleft palate

Goal: Child will be able to communicate adequately enough to make needs known by 2 years.

Outcome Criteria: Family members voice satisfaction with child's speech; milestone of two-word sentences by age 2 years is met.

Infants with a cleft palate will begin to make speech sounds at the normal time (age 2 months); their speech may be guttural and harsh; at age 9 months, when other children begin to say meaningful words ("bye-bye," "mama," "dada"), assuming the cleft palate is still unrepaired, their sounds will be unclear. Some parents try to discourage their baby from talking, thinking that if he or she does not talk until after the cleft palate repair is made, a speech impediment will not develop. Speech occurs at a specified developmental time, however, and despite the unfused palate should be encouraged at these age-appropriate times. The child with a cleft palate can enunciate vowel sounds with the most clarity, so these are the sounds a parent should encourage the child to voice. Words such as "me," "they," "no," "mama," "home," "moon," "rain," "yell," and "row" are words consisting largely of vowel sounds and thus can be enunciated by the child before the cleft palate repair.

Almost all children with cleft palates continue to have accompanying speech problems following the repair. The soft palate must function for the child to pronounce *p* and *b* sounds. If cleft palate surgery is going to be delayed much past age 2 years (as might happen if the child has other congenital anomalies, such as heart disease), a plastic prosthesis to cover the palate defect may be prescribed. This allows children to articulate more normally. Such prostheses do not seem to stay in place and are not tolerated well by young toddlers; they may interfere with breathing (Minsley et al., 1991), so they are never a final solution to the problem.

If children learn to speak in a defective manner before the repair, they generally continue to speak this way following repair. Speech training by a speech therapist is usually necessary. Children may be asked to perform blowing games, such as blowing a feather or a table tennis ball (a blowing motion is what is required to pronounce *p* and *b*). Children do not spontaneously outgrow bad speech patterns. Without therapy, they continue to speak into adulthood as if the cleft were still present. Speech therapy is an important follow-up measure, therefore, not a luxury. No repair can be considered successful if children speak incoherently afterward.

Pierre Robin Syndrome

The Pierre Robin syndrome is a triad of *micrognathia* (small mandible); cleft palate; and *glossoptosis* (a tongue malpositioned downward; Kula, 1994). All infants with Pierre Robin syndrome need to be observed carefully to be certain that they are free of airway obstruction. They may need frequent nasopharyngeal suction to remove unswallowed saliva. Children with this syndrome are apt to have episodes beginning with birth in which they have difficulty breathing because, due to the small jaw, their tongue is too large for their mouth. This causes it to drop backward and obstruct the airway. This is most noticeable when they are lying in a supine position. No infant with this syndrome, therefore, should be placed in a supine position; they are in grave danger of anoxia if left in this position and should be positioned on the abdomen. Occasionally, infants have such an obstructed airway that attaching a suture to the anterior aspect of the tongue and pulling it forward is used to give relief. This position can be maintained if the suture is attached to the mucous membrane of the lower lip (creating an artificial tongue-tied condition).

Feed these infants with the same care and concern given all children with cleft palate. A gastrostomy tube may be inserted to relieve feeding difficulty (see Chapter 34). As the child grows older the jaw grows somewhat, although the mandible will always be small. Growth, coupled with a repair of the cleft palate, will decrease the respiratory embarrassment. Children with Pierre Robin syndrome may have associated disorders of congenital glaucoma, cataract, or cardiac disorders. They need thorough physical assessment to be certain that none of these associated disorders is present.

Parents of the child with Pierre Robin syndrome take on a great deal of responsibility when first assuming the infant's care. They need a health care provider to call when they have questions about care. Many of these parents grow exhausted during the first few weeks of the child's life, afraid they may fall soundly asleep at night and miss their child having respiratory difficulty. As their confidence grows in their ability to provide care, this problem lessens, but it may be months or even years before a high level of confidence is achieved.

Tracheoesophageal Atresia and Fistula

Between weeks 4 and 8 of intrauterine life, the laryngotracheal groove develops into the larynx, trachea, and beginning lung tissue, and the esophageal lumen is formed. A number of anomalies may be found in infants if the trachea and esophagus are affected by some teratogen that does not allow the esophagus and trachea to separate normally.

The five types of esophageal atresia (stricture) and **fistulas** (openings) are as follows:

1. The esophagus ends in a blind pouch; there is a tracheoesophageal fistula between the distal part of the esophagus and the trachea.
2. The esophagus ends in a blind pouch. There is no connection to the trachea.
3. A fistula is present between an otherwise normal esophagus and trachea.
4. The esophagus ends in a blind pouch. A fistula connects the blind pouch of the proximal esophagus to the trachea.
5. There is a blind end portion of the esophagus. Fistulas are present between both widely spaced segments of the esophagus and the trachea.

The three most common forms of esophageal atresia and tracheoesophageal fistula are illustrated in Figure 39-5. These are serious disorders because during a feeding, milk can fill the blind esophagus and overflow into the trachea or a fistula can allow milk to enter the trachea, resulting in aspiration. The incidence of tracheoesophageal fistula is approximately 1 in 3000 live births.

Assessment

Tracheoesophageal atresia must be ruled out in any infant born to a woman with hydramnios (excessive amniotic fluid). A normal fetus swallows amniotic fluid during intrauterine life. The infant with a tracheoesophageal atresia cannot swallow, so the amount of amniotic fluid

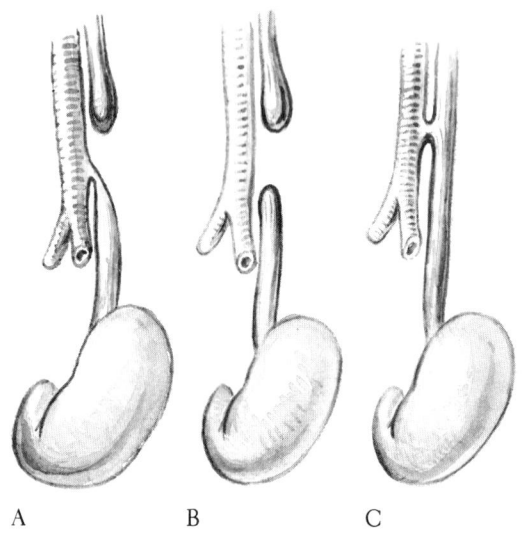

A   B   C

FIGURE 39-5
*Esophageal atresia and tracheoesophageal fistula. (**A**) In the most frequent type of esophageal atresia, the esophagus ends in a blind pouch. The trachea communicates by a fistula with the lower esophagus and stomach (approximately 90% of infants with the defect have this type). (**B**) Both upper and lower segments end in blind pouches (7% to 8% of infants with the defect have this type). (**C**) Both upper and lower segments communicate with the trachea (2% to 3% of infants with the defect have this type). (Courtesy of the Department of Medical Illustration, State University of New York at Buffalo.)*

may thus become abnormally large. Many infants are born preterm because of the accompanying hydramnios, which gives them the additional problem of immaturity. The infant needs to be examined carefully for other congenital anomalies that could have occurred from the teratogenic effect at the same week in gestation that caused the tracheoesophageal fistula, such as urologic, heart, or intestinal disorders (VATER syndrome).

Tracheoesophageal fistula can be diagnosed with certainty if a catheter cannot be passed through the infant's esophagus to the stomach and stomach contents are aspirated (be certain that catheters used this way are firm; a soft one will curl in a blind-end esophagus and appear to have passed). If a radiopaque catheter is used, it can be demonstrated coiled in the blind end of the esophagus on x-ray film. A flat plate film of the abdomen may reveal a stomach distended with the air, which is passing from the trachea into the esophagus and stomach. Either a barium swallow or a bronchial endoscopy examination will reveal the blind-end esophagus and fistula.

An infant who has so much mucus in the mouth that he or she appears to be blowing bubbles should be suspected of having tracheoesophageal fistula. The first time the infant is fed, he or she will cough, become cyanotic, and have obvious difficulty in breathing. This is the reason formula-fed infants are usually fed first with sterile water. A feeding of either glucose water or formula that is aspirated into the lungs is more dangerous to the infant because of the glucose or fat content. A breast-fed infant may be fed at the breast because colostrum is secreted in only small amounts at first, so that if a fistula is present no great amount of fluid can be aspirated.

Therapeutic Management

Emergency surgery for the infant with tracheoesophageal fistula is essential to prevent pneumonia from leakage of stomach secretions into the lungs, dehydration, or electrolyte imbalance from lack of oral intake. A gastrostomy may be performed (under local anesthesia) and the tube allowed to drain by gravity to keep the stomach empty of secretions and prevent reflux into the lungs. Upper right lobe pneumonia is one of the major complications of this disorder; thus, antibiotics also may be started to prevent this complication.

Surgery consists of closing the fistula and anastomosing the esophageal segments. It may be necessary to complete the surgery in different stages and to use a portion of the colon to complete the anastomosis if the esophageal segments are far apart from each other. Leaks occurring at anastomosis sites are a common complication, most frequently at postoperative days 7 to 10 when sutures dissolve. Fluid and air leak out into the chest cavity, and *pneumothorax* (collapse of the lung) occurs.

In most infants, some stenosis or stricture at the anastomosis site occurs and may necessitate esophageal dilatation at periodic intervals to keep the repaired esophagus fully patent. To do this, balloon endoscopy may be scheduled, or a string is passed from the mouth to the stomach through the esophagus and exits by the gastrostomy site in the stomach. For dilatation, a metal or plastic "bougie" or dilator is attached to the string and pulled through the esophagus. The string remains in place until the child has reached a point at which dilatation is no longer necessary.

Gastroesophageal reflux may also occur. This can lead to recurrent fistula formation.

The ultimate prognosis will depend on the extent of the repair necessary, the condition of the child at the time of surgery, and whether other congenital anomalies are present.

If surgery can be performed on the child before pneumonia develops and the defect is amenable to surgical correction, the prognosis is good. However, the mortality rate may be as high as 40%. This high mortality rate is associated with esophageal atresia or tracheoesophageal fistula in the presence of other congenital defects or low birth weight (Belknap & McEvoy, 1994).

Nursing Diagnoses and Related Interventions

Goals established for the child with tracheoesophageal fistula must be realistic in terms of the extent of the defect, the timing of anticipated surgery, and stage of grief or readiness for decision-making and planning that the parents have reached.

Nursing Diagnosis: High risk for altered nutrition, less than body requirements, related to incomplete esophagus

Goal: Child will ingest adequate nutrition during course of therapy.

Outcome Criteria: Child will not lose more than 10% of birth weight; will maintain weight in same percentile on growth curve.

Before surgery, an intravenous infusion supplies fluid and calories to the infant, because oral fluid cannot be given until the esophagus is repaired.

The infant is continued on intravenous fluid for a time after surgery until the possibility of vomiting from the anesthetic is decreased. The infant is then begun on feedings through the gastrostomy tube. The glucose water or formula ordered for a feeding should be introduced into the tube slowly and allowed to run by gravity, never by pressure, to prevent it from entering the esophagus and putting pressure on the suture line. After the feeding, the end of the tube should be elevated, covered by sterile gauze, and kept in that position, perhaps by suspending it from an intravenous pole. It should not be clamped. In this way, air introduced during the feeding will bubble from the tube and not enter the esophagus and pass the fresh suture line. This also helps to ensure that if the infant vomits the feeding, the vomitus will be projected into the gastrostomy tube and not contaminate the fresh sutures. Most newborns enjoy sucking a pacifier during gastrostomy feedings for sucking pleasure. If the mother wishes to breast-feed, she can manually express breast milk for the infant's feedings.

The infant may be given sips of clear fluid by mouth as early as the day after surgery, although some infants are kept on NPO status for 7 to 10 days until the suture line is healed. Early introduction of fluid may help to ensure patency of the esophagus, because it helps to decrease adhesions from the anastomosis and allows the infant the enjoyment and practice of sucking. The infant is introduced to a full oral fluid diet as soon as he or she begins to tolerate it and the suture line is healed. When the child is taking oral feedings satisfactorily, the gastrostomy tube is removed. If the child is to return home to await a second-stage operation, the gastrostomy tube will be left in place and the parents must be shown how to do gastrostomy feedings. If the gastrostomy tube is only a temporary measure for surgery, the parents do not need to learn the procedure. The parents' time with the child is better spent in holding him or her (in the Isolette, if necessary), gently stroking or talking to the child, and getting to know the child better.

Nursing Diagnosis: High risk for infection related to seepage of stomach secretions into lungs

Goal: Child will remain free of infection during course of therapy.

Outcome Criteria: Child's temperature remains below 37.0°C axillary; no chest rales on auscultation.

Preoperative Care. Before surgery, the infant should be kept in an upright position and on the right side to prevent gastric juice from entering the lungs from the fistula. Because the infant cannot swallow mucus, he or she needs frequent oropharyngeal suction to prevent aspiration of collected mucus. A catheter may be passed into the blind-end esophagus and attached to low suction (a sump pump) to keep this segment of the esophagus from filling with fluid and causing aspiration. Irrigation of the catheter may be necessary to keep it patent, because mucus tends to dry and plug it.

If surgery will be delayed, the infant may have a *cervical esophagostomy* (the distal end of the blind esophagus is brought to the surface just over the sternum so that mucus can drain). Use absorbent gauze around the opening to absorb moisture and prevent excoriation of the skin. Apply a protective ointment such as A & D Ointment or zinc oxide liberally to protect skin.

Keeping the infant in an Isolette with high humidity will both maintain body heat and liquefy bronchial secretions. The infant should be kept from crying to prevent air from entering the stomach from the trachea, distending the stomach, and thus causing vomiting into the lungs. A pacifier may help keep the baby calm.

Postoperative Care. After surgery, because the chest cavity was entered for the repair, the infant will have one or two chest tubes in place. The posterior tube drains collecting fluid; the anterior tube allows air to leave the chest space and the lung to expand again.

The infant must be observed closely for respiratory distress in the first few days following surgery. It will be necessary to continue to suction the child frequently because mucus tends to accumulate in the pharynx from surgery trauma. Suctioning must be done only shallowly, however, to prevent the suction catheter from touching the suture line in the esophagus. The child must also be turned frequently to discourage fluid from accumulating in the lungs. This turning and handling generally makes the child cry, and he or she *should* cry to help expand lung tissue (an older child or adult can be told to take deep breaths; the newborn cannot). An infant laryngoscope and endotracheal tube should be available at bedside in case extreme edema develops and the infant's airway is obstructed.

The newborn is generally cared for in an Isolette so that body warmth is maintained. The child may need oxygen and high humidity to keep respiratory secretions moist. It is best if the Pleurevac used for chest tube drainage is attached to the Isolette to allow it to move with the Isolette and not tip over or break (if it should break, room air will enter the chest, collapsing the lungs). Care of the child with chest tubes is discussed in Chapter 41.

Omphalocele

An **omphalocele** is a protrusion of abdominal contents through the abdominal wall at the point of the junction of the umbilical cord and abdomen. The herniated organs are usually the intestines, but they may include stomach and liver (Belknap & McEvoy, 1994). They are usually covered and contained by a thin transparent layer of peritoneum. The deviation is evident at birth and reflects an arrest of development of the abdominal cavity at weeks 7 to 10 of intrauterine life. At approximately weeks 6 to 8 of intrauterine life, the abdominal contents are extruded from the abdomen into the base of the umbilical cord. Omphalocele occurs when there is failure of the abdominal contents to return to the abdomen (Figure 39-6). The incidence of omphalocele is as rare as 1 in 5000 live births. The child may have accompanying defects that also were caused by the teratogen insult that prevented normal intestinal growth.

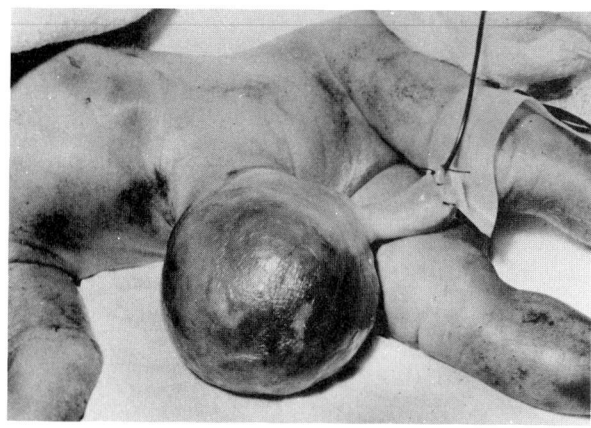

FIGURE 39-6
Omphalocele. This large example seen at birth contains intestine and liver. (Courtesy of the Department of Medical Photography, Children's Hospital, Buffalo, NY.)

Assessment

Omphalocele may be detected on sonogram during intrauterine life. Such infants are allowed to be born vaginally since there is no difference in the outcome for those delivered by cesarean birth (Tucci & Bard, 1990). The presence of omphalocele is obvious on inspection at birth. Record its general appearance and its size in centimeters.

Therapeutic Management

If the defect is small, infants will have immediate surgery to replace the bowel. If the defect is large, infants may be managed by topical application of silver sulphadiazine, which prevents infection of the sac, followed by delayed surgical closure (Adam et al., 1991). It is often difficult to replace the entire bowel immediately owing to the unusually small abdomen, which did not need to grow to accommodate the abdominal contents. If the total bowel were replaced, respiratory distress might result from the pressure of the visceral bulk. For this reason, the bowel may be contained by a Silastic pouch that is suspended over the infant's bed and gradually decreased in size as more bowel is gradually returned to the abdomen. During this time the infant can be fed by total parenteral nutrition.

Nursing Diagnoses and Related Interventions

Goals established must be realistic in terms of the extent of the defect, the timing of anticipated surgery, and stage of grief or readiness for decision-making and planning that the parents have reached. Omphalocele is a shock to parents, being an anomaly that is obviously severe and yet one that is generally unknown.

Nursing Diagnosis: High risk for infection related to exposed abdominal contents

Goal: Child remains free of infection until repair is complete.

Outcome Criteria: Child's temperature is below 37.0°C axillary; skin surrounding omphalocele is not erythematous; no foul drainage is present.

It is important that the lining of peritoneum covering the defect not be ruptured or allowed to dry out and crack; otherwise, infection and malrotation of the uncontained intestine will complicate the surgical repair. Exposure of intestine to air causes rapid loss of body heat; the baby should be placed immediately in a warmed incubator. Do not leave infants under a radiant heat source, because this will quickly dry the exposed bowel. A nasogastric tube will be inserted to prevent intestinal distention. To keep the sac moist, it is covered by either sterile saline-soaked gauze or a sterile plastic bowel bag until surgery. The saline used must be at body temperature: applying cold saline will lead to a decreased body temperature because so much intestinal surface is involved.

After the final surgical repair, the child with an omphalocele will be the perfect child his or her parents once envisioned, with the exception of a rather large abdominal scar. Even then, if the scar is a problem for the child in later life, plastic surgery can reduce the scar's appearance.

> ***Nursing Diagnosis:*** High risk for altered nutrition, less than body requirements, related to exposed abdominal contents
>
> ***Goal:*** Child's nutritional intake will be adequate for needs during course of treatment.
>
> ***Outcome Criteria:*** Child does not lose more than 10% of birth weight; skin turgor is good; specific gravity of urine is between 1.003 and 1.030.

The child must not be fed orally until the repair is complete; doing so would distend the exposed bowel and make the return to the abdomen more difficult. Some infants have an accompanying volvulus, which is another reason to omit oral feedings. After surgery, the infant is maintained on total parenteral nutrition; once the final stage of bowel repair is completed, a normal infant diet can be introduced gradually. Observe infants carefully for signs of obstruction when they begin eating (e.g., abdominal distention, constipation or diarrhea, or vomiting).

Infants with omphalocele will be hospitalized for a long time (a minimum of 1 or 2 months) waiting for a second-stage or even a third-stage operation. Parents need to be encouraged to visit frequently and hold them as much as possible. The infants should have a primary care nurse assigned to them so that they are exposed to a minimum number of caregivers. They need to be furnished toys for stimulation.

Many parents believe that surgeons can do anything and are distressed that their child's operation is being done in such small stages. They need support to accept that this treatment method is the only way to manage this type of intestinal disorder. Many children can be discharged from the hospital and cared for at home on total parenteral nutrition between surgery stages.

Gastroschisis

Gastroschisis is a condition similar to omphalocele, except that the abdominal wall defect is a distance from the umbilicus and abdominal organs are not contained by peritoneal membrane but rather spill from the abdomen freely. A greater amount of intestinal content tends to herniate, which increases the potential for volvulus and obstruction (Molenaar & Tibboel, 1993). Children with gastroschisis often have decreased bowel mobility and, even after surgical correction, they may have difficulty with absorption of nutrients and passage of stool.

Intestinal Obstruction

If canalization of intestine does not occur in utero at some point in the bowel, an **atresia** (complete closure) or **stenosis** (narrowing) of the bowel can occur. The most common site for this is the duodenal bowel portion.

Obstruction may occur because of a twisting (rotation) of the mesentery of the bowel as the bowel reenters the abdomen after being contained in the base of the umbilical cord early in intrauterine life, or because of severe twisting of the mesentery due to the looseness of the intestine in the abdomen of the neonate (this continues to be a problem for the first 6 months of life). Obstruction can also occur because of thicker than usual meconium formation.

Assessment

Intestinal obstruction may be anticipated if the mother had hydramnios during pregnancy (amniotic fluid could not be swallowed effectively) or if more than 30 mL of stomach contents can be aspirated from the stomach by catheter and syringe at birth. If the obstruction is not revealed by either of these findings, then symptoms of intestinal obstruction in the neonate are the same as at any other time in life: the infant passes no meconium or may pass one stool (meconium that formed below the obstruction) and then halt; the abdomen becomes distended. As the effect of the obstruction progresses, the infant will vomit. Obstructions are rare above Vater's ampulla or the junction of the bile duct with the duodenum, so vomitus will be bile-stained (greenish). Because meconium is black, vomitus may also be dark. Bowel sounds increase with obstruction owing to the increased peristaltic action as the intestine attempts to pass stool through the point of obstruction. Waves of peristalsis may be apparent across the abdomen. The infant may evidence pain by crying—hard, forceful, indignant crying—and by pulling the legs up against the abdomen. The child's respiratory rate will increase as the diaphragm is pushed up against the lungs and lung capacity decreases. On an abdominal flat plate x-ray study, there will be no air below the level of obstruction in the intestines. A barium swallow or barium enema x-ray film may be used to reveal the position of the obstruction.

Therapeutic Management

If bowel obstruction is established, an orogastric or nasogastric tube is inserted and then set to low suction or air to prevent further gastrointestinal distention from swallowed air (see Chapter 37). Always use low intermittent suction with decompression tubes with neonates. Pressure greater than this can break down the stomach lining.

The infant should be started on intravenous therapy to restore fluid and is scheduled for immediate surgery. A bowel obstruction is an emergency that must be treated before dehydration, electrolyte imbalance, or aspiration of vomitus occurs (Caty & Azizkhan, 1994).

Repair of the defect (with the exception of meconium plug syndrome) is done through an abdominal incision. The area of stenosis or atresia is removed and the bowel anastomosed. If the repair is anatomically difficult or the infant has other anomalies that interfere with his or her health, a temporary colostomy may be constructed and the infant discharged, with surgery rescheduled for age 3 to 6 months. Care of the child with a colostomy is discussed in Chapter 37. The final surgical procedure will restore the child to health.

Nursing Diagnoses and Related Interventions

> *Nursing Diagnosis:* High risk for fluid volume deficit related to vomiting
>
> *Goal:* Infant will maintain a normal circulating fluid volume during course of therapy.
>
> *Outcome Criteria:* Child's skin turgor is good; pulse rate is 100 to 120 bpm; no further vomiting occurs.

Once an obstruction is suspected, the child must be kept NPO to avoid compounding the problem and to prevent vomiting and aspiration. Vomiting in neonates is always serious not only because aspiration may occur but also because infants lose fluid rapidly, which results in dehydration. They also lose chloride from the hydrochloric acid of the stomach contents, and loss of chloride leads to alkalosis. The body attempts to compensate for the loss of chloride by excreting po-

tassium, which can cause infants to quickly become hypokalemic.

Remember that many neonates spit up feedings when burped. This rapid ejection of milk smells barely sour. True vomiting is usually sour smelling (stomach acid has acted on it) and occurs spontaneously without coughing or back patting.

Meconium Plug Syndrome

A **meconium plug** is an extremely hard portion of meconium that completely obstructs the intestinal lumen, causing bowel obstruction. Why this occurs is unknown but probably reflects normal variations of meconium consistency. If a meconium plug has formed, it is usually present in the lower end of the bowel; this is because this is the meconium that formed early in intrauterine life and has the best chance to become dry and inspissated.

Assessment

Because the obstruction is low in the intestinal tract, signs of obstruction such as abdominal distention and vomiting do not occur for at least 24 hours; the infant will be identified first as an infant who has had no meconium passage and is past age 24 hours. A gentle rectal examination may reveal the presence of hardened stool, although the plug may be too far removed to be palpated. An x-ray may reveal distended air-filled loops of bowel up to the point of obstruction. A barium enema study may not only reveal the level of obstruction but also be therapeutic in loosening the plug. The administration of saline enemas (never use tap water in newborns because it leads to water intoxication) may cause enough peristalsis to expel the plug. Instillation of acetylcysteine proteolytic enzyme (Mucomyst) rectally may dissolve the plug. Gastrografin is a highly osmotic radiographic substance that can be administered as an enema. The substance pulls fluid into the bowel because of its low osmotic pressure, allowing the stool to be softened and then passed.

Once the thickened portion of meconium has been passed, the infant should have no further difficulty and, over the next several hours, may pass a great amount of stool. The infant must be observed for further passage of meconium (should occur at least once daily) over the next 3 days, however, to be certain that additional plugs do not exist farther up in the bowel. If an infant is going to be discharged before this time, the parents need to be instructed on the importance of observing for meconium and the need to telephone the pediatrician should the child have no further defecation at home. The infant needs further assessment for aganglionic megacolon and cystic fibrosis (illnesses that present with constipation or meconium plugging) during health care visits during the first year of life.

Occasionally, a neonate passes a plug of hardened meconium—hard enough that it would have caused an obstruction except for the small size of the hardened particle—in the first 1 or 2 days of life. Be certain to record and report such a finding because the infant needs close observation for continued defecation, like the infant who actually had an obstruction, to rule out the presence of another larger and truly obstructing plug.

When a meconium plug is discovered, assess the family history for cystic fibrosis, a recessively inherited disorder (which may present as meconium ileus) or aganglionic megacolon, a polygenic inherited disorder (which also may present with absence of meconium). Hypothyroidism is another disorder that may present with constipation or hardened stool. Assess the infant for signs of hypothyroidism (i.e., large protruding tongue, lethargy, or subnormal body temperature). In most states, hypothyroid screening is done along with the phenylketonuria screen. Be certain that this blood test is obtained in any newborn with a meconium plug.

Meconium Ileus

Meconium ileus (obstruction of the intestinal lumen by hardened meconium) is a specific phenomenon that occurs most commonly in the infant with cystic fibrosis. With cystic fibrosis, the enzyme that moistens and makes all body fluids free flowing is absent. All body fluids are therefore thick and tenacious. Cystic fibrosis is most often thought of as a lung disorder, because the most severe manifestation of tenacious secretions is in the lung; tenacious lung fluid leads to stasis and infection and alveolar obstruction that reduces air exchange. Intestinal and pancreatic secretions are affected also, however, and this may be signaled at birth by hardened obstructive meconium at the ileus level from lack of trypsin secretion from the pancreas (meconium ileus). This will lead to the usual symptoms of bowel obstruction: no meconium passage, abdominal distention, and vomiting of bile-stained fluid. If the obstruction is too high for enemas to reduce it, the bowel must be incised and the hardened meconium surgically removed. The infant must be further assessed for cystic fibrosis in the following months. Cystic fibrosis is diagnosed by an abnormal concentration of chloride in sweat (a sweat test). Because a newborn does not sweat freely due to immaturity of his or her temperature regulating system, a sweat test may not be done until 4 to 6 weeks of age.

Diaphragmatic Hernia

A *diaphragmatic hernia* is a protrusion of an abdominal organ (usually the stomach or intestine) through a defect in the diaphragm into the chest cavity (Moreno et al., 1993). This usually occurs on the left side, and the heart is displaced to the right of the chest; the lung on the left side is collapsed. It occurs in approximately 1 in 3000 live births. There is no difference between male and female incidence.

Early in intrauterine life the chest and abdominal cavity are one; at approximately week 8 of growth, the diaphragm forms to divide them. If it does not form completely, the intestines will herniate through the diaphragm opening into the chest cavity (Figure 39-7).

Assessment

Diaphragmatic hernia may be detected in utero by sonogram. Surgery to remove the bowel from the chest may be attempted by fetoscopy while the fetus is still in utero (Harrison & Adzick, 1991).

Newborns with extensive diaphragmatic hernia will have respiratory difficulty from the time of birth, because at least one of their lungs is unable to expand satisfactorily (and may not have formed fully). They may also have cyanosis and intracostal or subcostal retractions. Their abdomen generally appears sunken because it is not as filled as in the normal newborn. Breath sounds will be absent on the affected side of the chest cavity by auscultation. These infants have a potential for developing persistent pulmonary hypertension because the blood is unable to perfuse readily through the unexpanded lung. This leads to right-to-left shunting through the foramen ovale in the heart or the ductus arteriosus outside the heart remaining patent. One condition, then, has led to another, and heart involvement complicates an already complicated lung picture. The mechanics of the right-to-left heart shunts are further discussed in Chapter 41.

Therapeutic Management

Unfortunately, the mortality rate of children with diaphragmatic hernia is 25% to 50%, with death often due to associated anomalies of the heart, lung, and intestine.

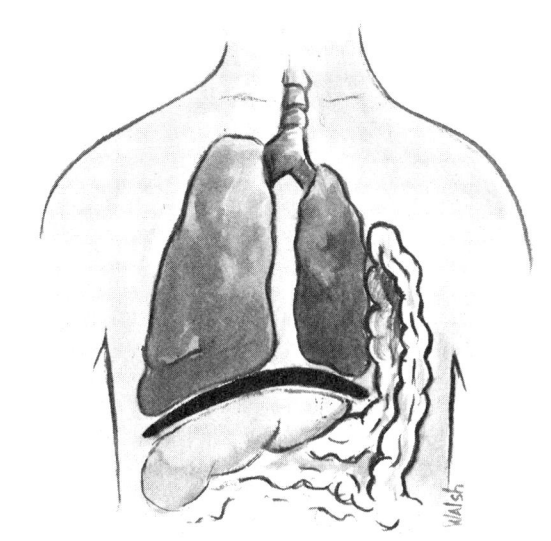

FIGURE 39-7
Diaphragmatic hernia. The bowel loop in the chest compresses the heart and lung on that side.

Treatment is immediate surgical repair of the diaphragm and replacement of the herniated intestine. Such a repair usually requires a thoracic incision and the placement of chest tubes. If the defect in the diaphragm is large, an insoluble polymer (Teflon) patch may be used in reconstruction. The repair is complicated if there is not enough room in the abdomen for the intestine to be returned. In these infants, the abdominal incision is not closed but left open to allow for the intestine to protrude abdominally. It is covered by silicone elastomer (Silastic) and left to be closed at a later date.

Over the next week, the compressed lung (if it is normal) will gradually expand and begin to function. If it is hypoplastic from the pressure of the intestine in utero, it will not expand and will be removed at the time of surgery.

Infants may be treated with nitric oxide or maintained on extracorporeal membrane oxygenation (ECMO) (a heart–lung machine) after surgery until lung tissue is able to function (Touloukian, 1994).

Nursing Diagnoses and Related Interventions

Nursing Diagnosis: High risk for ineffective airway clearance related to displaced bowel

Goal: Child will maintain adequate respiratory function through course of therapy.

Outcome Criteria: Child's respiration rate is 30 to 50 breaths per minute; PO_2 is 60 to 100 mm Hg; and PCO_2 is 30 to 35 mm Hg.

The infant with diaphragmatic hernia breathes better with the head elevated, which allows the herniated intestine to fall back as far as possible into the abdomen, providing a maximum of respiratory space. Turning the infant so that the compressed lung is down also allows the good lung to expand most completely and offers optimal aeration. A nasogastric tube or a gastrostomy tube is usually inserted to prevent distention of the herniated intestine, which would cause further respiratory difficulty. Be certain that the decompression strength is set to low to avoid injuring the lining of the stomach.

After surgery, the infant is kept in a semi-Fowler's position in an infant chair to keep pressure of the replaced intestine off the repaired diaphragm. The infant should stay in a warmed humidified environment to encourage lung fluid drainage and should be suctioned as necessary. Chest physical therapy helps to ensure that lung secretions do not pool and discourage pneumonia. Positive pressure ventilation may be ordered to increase lung expansion, although this pressure is kept to a minimum to prevent tearing the undeveloped or previously unopened lung tissue. Maintaining arterial oxygen (PO_2) at a high level of 100 mm Hg and the PCO_2 at the low level of 30 to 35 mm Hg helps prevent vasoconstriction of the arteries of the hypoplastic lung and increases lung function.

Nursing Diagnosis: High risk for altered nutrition, less than body requirements, related to NPO status

Goal: Child will receive adequate nutritional intake during course of therapy.

Outcome Criteria: Child's skin turgor is good; child does not lose more than 10% of birth weight; weight is maintained between a percentile curve on growth chart.

With diagnosis of diaphragmatic hernia, the infant is kept NPO, because filling of the intestine with food or active peristaltic motion will further impair lung function. If fed, the infant may vomit because of twisting and obstruction of the herniated bowel.

Postoperatively, to prevent pressure on the suture line in the diaphragm by a full bowel, intravenous or total parenteral nutrition may be maintained for 1 or 2 weeks. Be certain to bubble the infant well after feeding to reduce the amount of swallowed air and limit bowel expansion.

Umbilical Hernia

An *umbilical hernia* is a protrusion of a portion of the intestine through the umbilical ring, the muscle, and fascia surrounding the umbilical cord. The bulging protrusion under the skin at the umbilicus is rarely noticeable at birth while the cord is still present; it becomes noticeable at health care visits during the first year.

Umbilical hernias occur most frequently in African-American children and more often in girls than in boys. The structure is generally 1 to 2 cm (½ to 1 inch) in diameter but may be as big as an orange when children cry or strain. The size of the protruding mass is not as important as the size of the fascial ring through which the intestine protrudes. If this fascial ring is less than 2 cm, closure will usually occur spontaneously and no repair of the defect will be necessary. If the defect is more than 2 cm, surgery for repair will generally be indicated; this is done close to school age.

Old-fashioned remedies of taping an umbilical hernia in place or taping a penny against it to reduce it are ineffective and actually may be dangerous, because these practices may lead to strangulation of the bowel.

Surgery is generally accomplished on an ambulatory basis. The child returns from surgery with a pressure dressing that will remain in place for 7 days. Remind parents to sponge bathe the child until they return for a postoperative visit and the dressing is removed (Skinner & Grosfeld, 1993).

Imperforate Anus

Imperforate anus (Figure 39-8) is stricture of the anus. In week 7 of intrauterine life, the upper bowel elongates to pouch and combine with a pouch invaginating from the perineum. These two sections of bowel meet, the membranes between them are absorbed, and the bowel is then patent to the outside. If this motion toward each other does not occur or if the membrane between the two surfaces does not dissolve, imperforate anus occurs. The defect can be relatively minor, requiring just surgical incision of the persistent membrane, or much more severe, involving sections of the bowel that are many inches apart with no anus. There may be an accompanying fistula to the bladder in males and the vagina in females. The problem occurs in approximately 1 in 5000 live births, more commonly in males than females. Imperforate anus may occur as an additional complication of spinal cord defects, since both the external anal canal and the spinal cord arise from the same germ tissue layer (Belknap & McEvoy, 1994).

Assessment

Inspection of the perineum may reveal no anal formation or may be unhelpful because the anus is normal and the defect exists far enough inside to be missed on simple inspection. Occasionally, a membrane filled with black meconium can be seen protruding from the anus. It can be discovered in a newborn by the inability to insert a rectal thermometer or rubber catheter into the rectum. No stool will be passed, and abdominal distention will become evident. An x-ray or sonogram will reveal the defect if the infant is held in a head-down position to allow swallowed air to rise to the end of the blind pouch of the bowel. This method is also helpful in estimating the distance the intestine is separated from the perineum. If sensory nerve endings in the rectum are not intact, a "wink" reflex (touching the skin near the rectum should make it contract) will not be present.

Formerly, when all newborns stayed in the hospital 4 to 7 days after birth, imperforate anus was always discovered. When infants failed to pass stools after the first 24 hours, the reason was investigated. Currently newborns are discharged from health care facilities at age 1 day or even a few hours after birth, and possibly no one will notice that an infant has not passed a stool in that time. For an infant born in a birthing center or at home, follow-up must include assessment of whether the infant is defecating. The urine of all infants with imperforate anus should be collected and examined for the presence of meconium to determine whether the child has a fistula. Placing a urine collector bag over the vagina in females may reveal a meconium-stained discharge.

Therapeutic Management

The degree of difficulty in repairing an imperforate anus depends on the extent of the problem. If the rectum ends close to the perineum (below or at the level of the levator ani muscle) and the anal sphincter is formed, repair is not difficult. It becomes complicated if the end of the rectum is at a distance from the perineum (above the levator ani muscle) or the anal sphincter exists only in an underdeveloped form. All repairs are complicated if a fistula to the bladder or urethra is present. If the repair will be extensive, the surgeon may create a temporary colostomy, anticipating final repair when the infant is somewhat older (6 to 12 months). For successful repair, it is unnecessary for an internal rectal sphincter to be present as long as the subrectal muscle is judged to be intact.

Nursing Diagnoses and Related Interventions

> ***Nursing Diagnosis:*** Altered nutrition, less than body requirements, related to bowel obstruction
>
> ***Goal:*** Child will receive adequate nutritional intake during course of therapy.
>
> ***Outcome Criteria:*** Child does not lose more than 10% of birth weight; weight is maintained on a percentile curve on a growth chart; skin turgor is good.

Preoperatively, children must not be fed orally; an intravenous fluid line will be begun to maintain fluid and electrolyte balance. A nasogastric tube set to decompression will be inserted to relieve vomiting and prevent the intestine from putting pressure on other abdominal organs or the diaphragm.

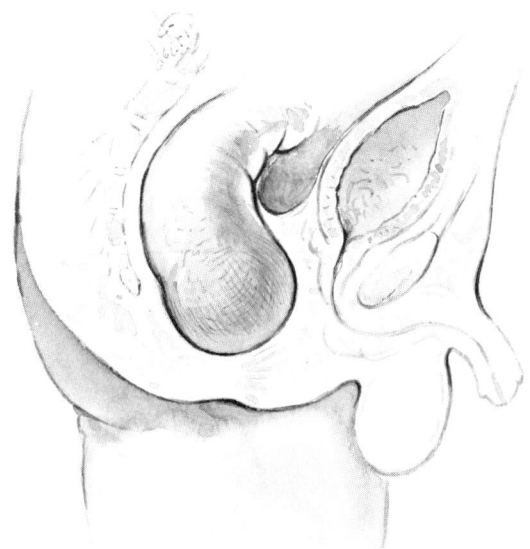

FIGURE 39-8
Imperforate anus. The lower bowel ends in a blind pouch.

Postoperative Care. The newborn will return from surgery with a nasogastric tube in place. When bowel sounds are present and the nasogastric tube is removed, small oral feedings, first of glucose water, then of half-strength formula, then of regular formula or breast-feedings, are begun.

Some infants, who are scheduled for repair in a second-stage operation and who have a temporary colostomy, are not permitted high-residue foods to lessen the bulk of stools. Although this is rarely a problem with infants because their diet naturally is a low-residue one, do not just assume that the parents know what low residue means; help them choose acceptable beginning foods (allow rice cereal, strained fruits and vegetables; avoid unrefined rice and grains or vegetables with fibers or fruits with peels).

> ***Nursing Diagnosis:*** Impaired tissue integrity at rectum related to surgical incision
>
> ***Goal:*** Surgical incision will heal without damage to sutures or new tissue by day 7.
>
> ***Outcome Criteria:*** Incision line is free of erythema or drainage by day 7 postoperation.

If a rectal repair was completed, remember that there is a fresh suture line at the rectum. Take axillary rather than rectal temperatures. Mark the crib well so that anyone taking temperatures cannot forget and take a rectal temperature by mistake. Infants should have no enemas or any other intrusive rectal procedures. They may be given a stool softener daily to keep the stool from becoming hard and tearing the healing suture line. The suture line must be cleaned well following bowel movements to keep infection to a minimum. Do this by irrigating the suture line with normal saline and an aseptic syringe. It is helpful to place a diaper under, not on, the infant so that bowel movements can be cleansed away as soon as they occur. Do not place the infant on the abdomen because in this position newborns tend to pull their knees under them, causing tension in the perineal area. A side-lying position is best.

The infant may need rectal dilatation done once or twice a day for a few months to ensure proper patency of the rectal sphincter. This technique (inserting a lubricated cot-covered finger into the rectum) must be demonstrated to the parents, and the parent must be able to perform it before the child is discharged. Be certain that the parents understand the importance of the procedure. The best surgical repair may end in failure if constriction occurs because the parent does not follow this procedure. If infants are to be discharged with a prescription for a daily stool softener, be certain that the parents understand why this is also important and have a plan for remembering the correct times and dosage.

> ***Nursing Diagnosis:*** High risk for altered parenting related to difficulty in bonding with infant who has been ill from birth
>
> ***Goal:*** Parents will demonstrate adequate bonding behavior during course of therapy.
>
> ***Outcome Criteria:*** Parents hold and comfort infant; voice positive characteristics of infant.

An imperforate anus may be a difficult anomaly for a parent to accept because it deals with a body area that they may not feel comfortable discussing. If it involves a temporary (or permanent) colostomy, learning to care for their infant may be difficult. Parents need a great deal of support. If a final surgical repair is successful, they can be assured their child will have normal bowel function thereafter. If a final repair could not be surgically achieved, they have the even harder task of caring for a child with a permanent ostomy. They can be assured that children who always have ostomies accept these well as they grow older, because they have never known any other method of defecation (see Chapter 37 for a discussion of care priorities for the child with an ostomy).

Physical Anomalies of the Nervous System

The most frequently seen defects of the nervous system include abnormal accumulation of cerebrospinal fluid (hydrocephalus), which has several causes, and abnormalities associated with a defect in neural tube closure.

Hydrocephalus

Hydrocephalus is an excess of cerebrospinal fluid (CSF) in the ventricles and subarachnoid spaces of the brain. In the infant whose cranial sutures are not firmly knitted, this excess fluid causes enlargement of the head. If there is passage of fluid between the ventricles and the spinal cord, the disorder is called *communicating hydrocephalus* or *extraventricular hydrocephalus*. If there is a block to such passage of fluid, the disorder is called *obstructive hydrocephalus* or *intraventricular hydrocephalus*. Hydrocephalus is also commonly classified as to whether it occurs at birth (congenital) or from an incident later in life (acquired).

An excess of cerebrospinal fluid may result from one of three main causes: (1) overproduction of fluid by the choroid plexus (rare), (2) obstruction of the passage of fluid somewhere between the point of origin and the point of absorption (the most frequent cause), or (3) interference with the absorption of the fluid from the subarachnoid space.

Overproduction is most frequently caused by a tumor in the choroid plexus. Obstruction generally occurs as a congenital atresia, usually along the narrow aqueduct of Sylvius. Other common sites are the foramina of Magendie and Luschka. Infections such as meningitis or encephalitis may leave adhesions that lead to obstruction. Hemorrhage or a growing tumor also may obstruct the passage of cerebrospinal fluid. An *Arnold-Chiari deformity* (elongation of the lower brain stem and displacement of the fourth ventricle into the upper cervical canal) may also lead to obstruction. Interference with absorption occurs following extensive subarachnoid hemorrhage when portions of the membrane absorption surface are obscured (Fishman, 1994).

Assessment

Hydrocephalus occurs at an incidence of approximately 3 to 4 per 1000 live births. When an obstruction is present, the excessive fluid accumulates and dilates the system above the point of obstruction. If the atresia is in the aqueduct of Sylvius, the first, second, and third ventricles will dilate. If it is at the exit from the fourth ventricle, all ventricles will dilate. Symptoms may develop rapidly or slowly, depending on the extent of the atresia.

Although hydrocephalus may be present prenatally and can sometimes be detected on sonogram (Tomda et al., 1990), it generally is not evident during pregnancy or even at birth but becomes evident in the first few weeks or months of life. The fontanelles widen and appear tense, the suture lines on the skull may separate, and the head diameter enlarges. As the fluid accumulation continues, the scalp becomes shiny and the scalp veins become prominent. The brow bulges in a typical appearance (*bossing*), and the eyes become "sunset eyes" (the sclera shows above the iris because of upper lid retraction rather than internal pressure on the orbit; Figure 39-9). Children show hyperactive reflexes, strabismus, and optic atrophy. Infants may become either irritable or lethargic, and they fail to thrive. They may have a typical shrill, high-pitched cry.

Hydrocephalus must be recognized early for treatment to be effective. Once intracranial pressure becomes so acute that brain tissue is damaged and motor or mental deterioration results, the best shunting procedure cannot replace and repair the damage already done. Detection of hydrocephalus can be an important role for the nurse in ambulatory child health settings. All children under age 2 years should have their head circumference recorded and plotted on an appropriate chart at health care visits, so a child whose head is growing abnormally can be detected early.

Measure the head circumference of all infants within an hour of birth and again before discharge from a health care facility. Children who have suffered head trauma severe enough to be seen in a medical facility

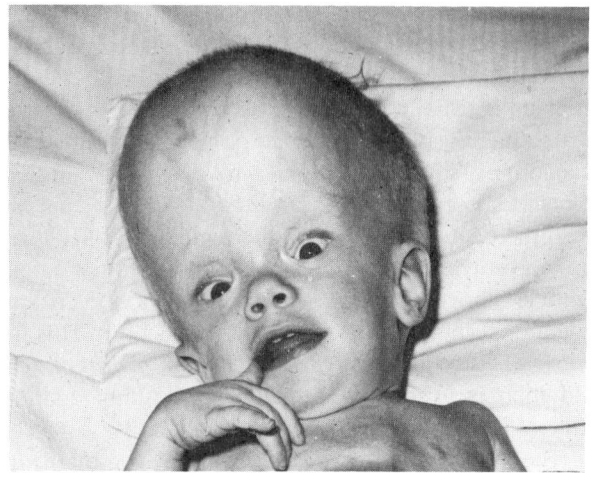

FIGURE 39-9
An infant with hydrocephalus. (From Marlow, D. Textbook of pediatric nursing. *Philadelphia: W.B. Saunders, with permission.)*

should have their head circumferences noted at the time of the accident; if other symptoms of increased intracranial pressure appear, head circumference can be added meaningfully to the store of information available concerning the child.

It is important to note in addition to the general enlargement of the head any asymmetry that is occurring, because this may suggest the point of obstruction. A skull that is enlarging anteriorly with a shallow posterior fossa, for example, suggests that the obstruction is in the aqueduct or third ventricle.

Motor function becomes impaired as the head enlarges, both because of neurologic impairment and atrophy caused by the inability to move, although as long as a child has more than 1 cm of cerebral tissue present, function is often not impaired. Even with an extremely enlarged head, children's intelligence may remain normal, although fine motor development may be affected.

Hydrocephalus is demonstrable by sonogram, computed tomography, and by magnetic resonance imaging. A skull x-ray film will reveal the separating sutures and thinning of the skull bones. **Transillumination** (holding a bright light such as a flashlight or a specialized light—a Chun gun—against the skull with the child in a darkened room) will reveal a skull filled with fluid rather than solid brain substance. If the hydrocephalus is a noncommunicating type, dye inserted into a ventricle through the anterior fontanelle will not appear in cerebrospinal fluid obtained from a lumbar puncture.

Therapeutic Management

The treatment of hydrocephalus depends on its cause and extent. If the hydrocephaly is caused by overproduction of fluid, destruction of a portion of the choroid plexus may be attempted. Acetazolamide is a drug that may be used to reduce the production of fluid. If a tumor in that area is responsible for the overproduction, removal of the tumor should provide a solution. Hydrocephalus is usually caused by obstruction, however, so the treatment usually involves bypassing the point of obstruction by shunting the fluid to normal or artificial points of absorption.

If the obstruction is along the aqueduct of Sylvius, a thin polyethylene tube might be passed from a lateral ventricle (above the point of obstruction) to the cisterna magna (a point below the point of obstruction). This is a *ventriculocisternostomy*, or *Torkildsen's operation*. The fluid then is absorbed normally by the subarachnoid space.

The fluid is most often shunted, however, by means of a polyethylene catheter from the ventricles to the peritoneum (Figure 39-10). It can be shunted to the right atrium or into a ureter, but these shunts are rarely used in favor of a peritoneal shunt, which allows the fluid to be absorbed across the peritoneal membrane and into the body circulation. This is the easiest shunt to place and tends to plug less readily. Unfortunately, the shunt has to be replaced as the child grows and it becomes too short. It may become enclosed in a fold of peritoneum and become obstructed. To encourage a free flow of

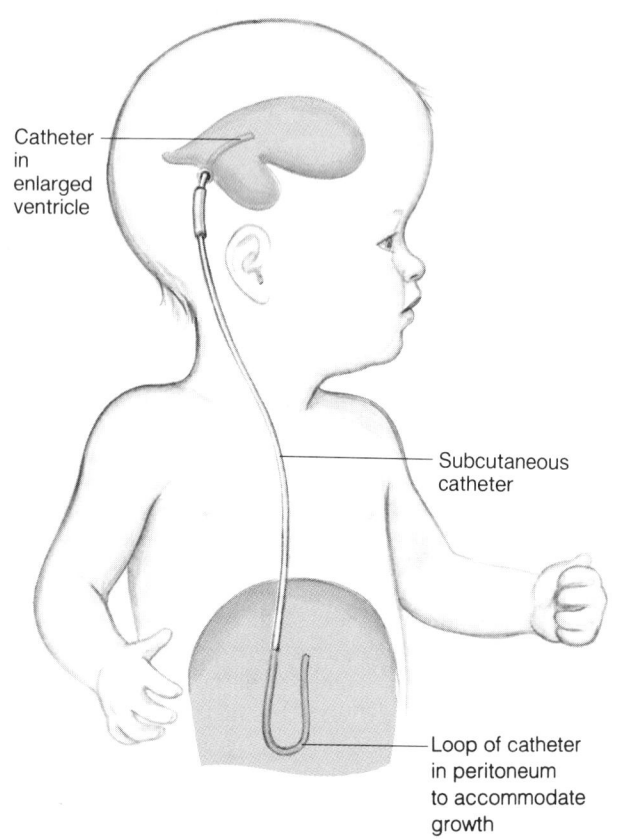

Catheter in enlarged ventricle

Subcutaneous catheter

Loop of catheter in peritoneum to accommodate growth

FIGURE 39-10

A ventriculoperitoneal shunt removes excessive cerebrospinal fluid from the ventricles and shunts it to the peritoneum. A one-way valve is present in the tubing behind the ear.

fluid, most shunts have a valve or pump incorporated into the catheter. This generally is placed just under the skin at the back of the child's ear. It must be "pumped" or pressed a number of times each day, depending on specific orders, to keep the tube patent and functioning.

Hydrocephalus is a potentially extremely serious defect; if left uncorrected, the intracranial pressure will eventually destroy brain tissue and leave the child severely mentally retarded and without motor nerve control. However, the prognosis for infants with hydrocephalus is improving every day as shunting procedures become more common and more effective. The ultimate prognosis for the child depends on whether brain damage occurred before shunting and whether the parents are able to recognize when the shunt needs replacing to reduce the possibility of increased intracranial pressure.

Nursing Diagnoses and Related Interventions

Nutrition and parent–child bonding are two major concerns in the infant with hydrocephalus. The Nursing Care Plan: The Child With Hydrocephalus illustrates these and other concerns, as do the following important nursing diagnoses:

Nursing Diagnosis: High risk for altered cerebral tissue perfusion related to increased intracranial pressure

Goal: Child will not demonstrate signs of increased intracranial pressure during childhood.

Outcome Criteria: Child shows no increased temperature and blood pressure, or decreased pulse rate, decreased respiratory rate, or decreased level of consciousness.

After a shunting procedure, the infant's bed is usually left flat or only slightly raised (approximately 30 degrees) so that the head remains level with the body. If the child's head is raised excessively, cerebrospinal fluid may flow too rapidly through the shunt, and decompression may occur too rapidly with possible tearing of cerebral arteries.

The valve is built to open when cerebrospinal fluid has increased in pressure owing to an accumulating bulk of fluid; it closes when enough fluid has drained to reduce the pressure. The surgeon who performed the shunting procedure will write specific orders about how often the infant is to be turned and to what side following surgery. Often infants are not turned to lie on the side with the shunt to prevent putting pressure on the valve, which might cause it to open and cause rapid decompression.

Orders may be written for the valve to be pressed a number of times a day to force fluid through the catheter in order to prevent any clot formation in the tubing. Be sure to follow the orders exactly: excessive pumping of the valve could decrease the pressure in the head too rapidly.

It is important to assess for signs of increased intracranial pressure following shunt insertion: tense fontanelles; increasing head circumference; irritability or lethargy; decreased level of consciousness; poor sucking; vomiting; an increase in blood pressure (difficult to measure accurately in infants unless Doppler instrumentation is used); increasing temperature; and a decrease in pulse and respiratory rates. Symptoms of infection (i.e., increased temperature, increased pulse rate, general malaise, and signs of meningitis such as a stiff neck and marked irritability) must also be assessed (see the Focus on Family Teaching box).

Nursing Diagnosis: High risk for altered nutrition, less than body requirements, related to increased intracranial pressure

Goal: Child will ingest an adequate nutritional intake following shunt placement.

Outcome Criteria: Child's weight remains within 5th to 95th percentile on height/weight chart; no vomiting occurs.

Because an abdominal incision is involved to thread the catheter into the peritoneum, most children have a nasogastric tube placed during surgery. They are kept NPO until bowel sounds return postoperatively and the tube can then be removed. Introduce fluid gradually in small quantities following removal of the tube. Vomiting that results from the introduction of fluid too soon after any surgery causes increased intracranial pressure.

If possible, infants with hydrocephalus should be held when fed. Be certain to support infants' heads well when moving them. Hold their head with the whole palm, not just the fingertips, because the skull is thinned to some degree and could actually puncture with a stiff, forceful touch. Use a rocking chair with an armrest to provide support for your arm. Otherwise, the infant's head will be so heavy that you may not want to spend as much time holding the infant after the feeding as you might spend with other infants the same age. There is no reason why mothers cannot breast-feed the infant with hydrocephalus. Encourage them as you would any other mother.

Note how the child sucks. Increased intracranial pressure may be noted first because of poor or ineffective sucking. Vomiting after feeding, without nausea (difficult to detect in a small infant), is also a sign of increased intracranial pressure.

Observe for constipation, because straining at passing stool causes increased intracranial pressure. This is not usually a problem of infants who are totally breast- or formula-fed. It can be a problem when children re-

turn for shunt replacement at an older age. Urge parents to maintain the child on a high fluid and roughage diet to prevent this.

Nursing Diagnosis: High risk for altered skin integrity related to immobility of head

Goal: Child's skin will remain intact during course of illness.

Outcome Criteria: Child's skin does not appear erythematous or ulcerated.

The head of the infant with hydrocephalus is so heavy it cannot be freely moved. The skin of the head is stretched thin, and skin decubitus ulcers tend to occur on the pressure points. Wash the child's head daily. Change position of the head approximately every 2 hours so that no portion of the head rests against the mattress for a long period. A foam rubber or synthetic sheepskin pad or an alternating air mattress may help to relieve pressure points. If a Kling or gauze bandage is used to hold the head dressing in place, place a piece of gauze or cotton behind the child's ear before the bandage is put in place to prevent skin surfaces from touching and becoming excoriated. Observe that the bandage does not become wet from oral secretions draining backward.

Nursing Diagnosis: Knowledge deficit related to home care needs of child with hydrocephalus

Goal: Parents will demonstrate understanding of shunt placement and voice confidence in their ability to care for child by hospital discharge.

Outcome Criteria: Parents state fears regarding ability to provide care well; state signs of increased cranial pressure for which to watch.

Caring for a child with a shunt in place is a continuing responsibility for parents. If parents do not seem to be asking many questions about the child's care after surgery, do not assume this is because they are taking the child's care in stride; it may be because they are too frightened or too bewildered to ask questions. A question such as "Most parents are a little frightened when they think about taking a child home with a shunt in place; do you feel that way?" gives them an opportunity to admit how they feel. For many people, being able to talk about a problem suddenly brings it down to manageable size. Talking about how frightened they feel about the responsibility will not immediately make them more comfortable with the child's care. It may make them more comfortable with their emotions, however. Assure them that the nurse and the other personnel caring for their child are interested in helping and supporting them.

(*text continues on page 1145*)

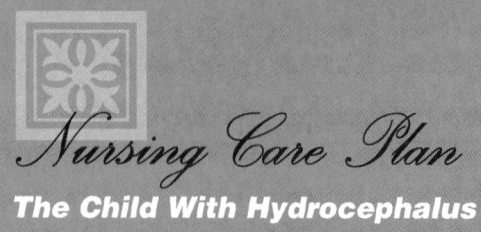

Nursing Care Plan

The Child With Hydrocephalus

Billy is a 3-month-old boy with hydrocephalus. The following is a nursing care plan designed for him.

Assessment: Child's head circumference was normal at birth (40th percentile). Measurement at 6-week check-up was 60th percentile; today, it is 80th percentile. Mother states that pregnancy was normal except for symptoms of hypertension of pregnancy late in pregnancy (blood pressure rose to 160/100 and mother was placed on complete bed rest). Delivery was vaginal; Apgar score 9/10. Child's forehead is bossed; sclera is evident above pupils of eyes (sunset eyes). Child had one episode of forceful vomiting yesterday. Blood pressure: 100/40; pulse rate: 120 bpm; respiration rate: 20 breaths/min; temperature: 37.0°C axillary.

Preoperative Care

Nursing Diagnosis: Altered cerebral tissue perfusion related to increased intracranial pressure from hydrocephalus

Defining Characteristic: Child has increased head circumference, forceful vomiting, and sunset eyes.

Goal: Infant will not develop any permanent effects of increased intracranial pressure during course of therapy.

Outcome Criteria: Child's temperature, respiratory and pulse rates, and blood pressure remain within normal limits for age group; head circumference follows normal growth curve; child meets developmental milestones.

Nursing Orders	Rationale
1. Measure and record head circumference daily.	1. Increasing head circumference occurs with increased collection of cerebrospinal fluid.
2. Assess temperature, pulse rate, respiratory rate, and blood pressure q4h.	2. Increased blood pressure and temperature and decreased respiratory and pulse rates are signs of increased intracranial pressure.
3. Assess anterior fontanelle for tenseness (in sitting position) and measure size q8h.	3. Increasing size of fontanelle is a sign of increasing intracranial pressure.
4. Assess for distended scalp veins, progression of sunset eye sign, and pupillary reaction q4h.	4. Document signs of increasing intracranial pressure.
5. Assess for level of consciousness (an infant "attunes" to your voice or a musical toy); assess for lethargy or irritability q4h.	5. Decreasing level of consciousness is a sign of increased intracranial pressure; lethargy or irritability may also be.
6. Provide oxygen and suction equipment for ready use.	6. The nurse should be prepared for respiratory emergency with this child.
7. Secure ventricular tap tray for emergency use.	7. A ventricular tap may be necessary to immediately remove excess cerebrospinal fluid if respiratory or heart function should be impaired.

Nursing Diagnosis: High risk for altered nutrition, less than body requirements, related to difficulty sucking and vomiting secondary to increased intracranial pressure

Defining Characteristic: Child has vomiting.

Goal: Child will ingest an adequate nutritional intake during course of illness.

Outcome Criteria: Specific gravity of urine is between 1.003 and 1.030; skin turgor is good; weight follows growth curve.

Nursing Orders	**Rationale**
1. Encourage breast-feeding if infant can suck effectively. Urge mother to support head when holding for feeding; use rocking chair for feeding.	1. Breast-feeding provides opportunity for mother–infant interaction in addition to nutritional benefits. Mother should be relaxed and comfortable so that the child's weight does not tire her and shorten the feeding.
2. Assess intake and output.	2. Fluid volume deficit is a concern when there is inadequate nutritional intake.
3. Place on side after feeding.	3. Side position is best for preventing aspiration from vomiting.
4. Refeed if vomiting occurs.	4. Maintains adequate fluid intake.

Nursing Diagnosis: High risk for ineffective family coping: compromised, related to child's chronic illness

Defining Characteristic: Adjusting to chronic illness in a child is a strain on family functioning.

Goal: Family will demonstrate adequate coping measures for present crisis within 1 week.

Outcome Criteria: Family members voice satisfaction in their ability to respond to present crisis; demonstrate ability to care for and meet child's needs.

Nursing Orders	**Rationale**
1. Review anatomy with parents. Allow them to voice concern or grief over child's condition.	1. Understanding the disorder can be the beginning of acceptance for the parents.
2. Encourage parents to care for child as much as possible. Help them to maintain contact if infant is transferred for care.	2. Promote parent-child bonding.
3. Attempt to increase parents' self-esteem by praising things they do well.	3. High self-esteem is an aid to coping.
4. Help with community health nurse referral as necessary; ascertain that parents have follow-up care for continued health care of the child and emotional support.	4. Child will need long-term follow-up for shunt care.

Postoperative Care

Nursing Diagnosis: High risk for infection related to surgical procedure

Defining Characteristic: Meningitis is a potential complication of shunt insertion.

Goal: Child will remain free of infection until surgical incision is healed.

Outcome Criteria: Child does not show symptoms of central nervous system infection (e.g., nuchal rigidity, elevated temperature or seizures); incision sites are free of erythema or drainage.

(continued)

Nursing Orders

1. Change incision dressings as prescribed; keep head incision dressing dry from oral secretions.
2. Observe incisions for drainage or redness.
3. Do not put infant in bathtub until abdominal incision site is healed.
4. Assess temperature q4h.

Rationale

1. Moisture can cause bacterial growth.

2. Drainage and redness are signs of infection.
3. Incision line needs to remain dry to prevent growth of bacteria.
4. Increased temperature is a sign of infection.

Nursing Diagnosis: High risk for altered cerebral tissue perfusion related to obstructed shunt

Defining Characteristic: Plugging of a shunt will lead to increased cerebral pressure.

Goal: Child's shunt will remain patent following insertion.

Outcome Criteria: Child's temperature, respiratory and pulse rates, and BP remain within normal limits for age group; head circumference follows normal growth curve; child meets developmental milestones.

Nursing Orders

1. Position infant as prescribed (shunt side down); keep head at level prescribed (flat or only slightly elevated).
2. Pump shunt 4 times as prescribed three times daily.

3. Assess for signs of increased intracranial pressure, increased temperature and blood pressure, decreased pulse and respiratory rate, loss of consciousness, decreased motor or sensory function, and decreased pupillary constriction every hour.

Rationale

1. Prescribed positioning allows for a constant level of drainage.

2. Regular pumping helps prevent plugging of cerebrospinal fluid.
3. Increased cerebral pressure can be the result of shunt obstruction, a serious occurrence requiring immediate attention.

Nursing Diagnosis: High risk for diversional activity deficit related to difficulty moving head

Defining Characteristic: Children with decreased mobility may suffer lack of stimulation.

Goal: Child will receive adequate stimulation for age following shunt insertion.

Outcome Criteria: Infant engages in at least one period of stimulation daily.

Nursing Orders

1. Provide a mobile for visual stimulation; vary visual stimuli.
2. Teach parents to maintain a continuing program of stimulation.

3. Encourage parents to participate in child's care, particularly by using comforting and stimulating measures (e.g., holding, cuddling, singing, and talking to the infant).

Rationale

1. Visual stimulation is a major way that infants relate to the world.
2. If a child's head is heavier than usual, he or she has difficulty turning it readily to seek stimulation; parents need to provide a variety of stimuli, since the infant cannot vary stimuli for himself.
3. Participation promotes parent–child bonding and initiation of a sense of trust by the infant in the parents.

Parents must be certain that their child understands that this strange object implanted behind an ear is not to be felt continually. A child nervously fidgeting with a pressure pump can inadvertently evacuate cerebrospinal fluid from the ventricles at a dangerously rapid rate.

Before an infant is discharged, be certain that the parents have ample opportunity to feed and care for the child, so that they can be comfortable and feel that they "know" him or her. Because irritability, lethargy, vomiting, and a change in the baby's cry are signs of increased intracranial pressure, the parents must report these symptoms immediately to their physician. Before parents can report a change in the infant's disposition in this way, they must know the infant well.

Nursing Diagnosis: High risk for altered growth and development related to potential neurologic impairment
Goal: Child will achieve developmental growth to the maximum of his or her potential.
Outcome Criteria: Child demonstrates regular observable growth and achieves developmental milestones.

Remember that the mental functioning of a child with hydrocephalus may remain intact despite extreme thinning of the brain cortex. Following a shunting procedure, the head may remain larger than normal but intelligence may be normal. Like all children, children with hydrocephalus need stimulation—to be talked to, smiled at, played with. If the child's head is enlarged, turning it and looking at things around him or her is difficult. It may be necessary to reposition mobiles or pictures so that the child receives adequate visual stimuli. Role-model talking and singing to the child to help parents more quickly include these actions in their care (see the Focus on Nursing Research box).

On the child's discharge from the hospital, be certain parents have a telephone number of the person they should call if they have a question or concern about the child's condition or care; they also need an appointment for the child's first checkup. This helps to assure them, again, that they are not being left alone just because they are leaving the hospital. Infection of the shunt is a possibility and a severe complication because it leads to meningitis. If this should occur, parents should look for signs of intracranial pressure as well as those of infection, such as increased temperature. The child will be admitted to the hospital and administered intravenous antibiotics. An extraventricular shunt to promote drainage will be inserted. This allows antibiotics to be administered directly to the cerebral fluid and ensures that infected cerebrospinal fluid is not draining to the peritoneal cavity where it could cause peritonitis (Scheinblum & Hammond, 1990).

As the child reaches preschool and school age, plans for school need to be made. Conferences with the school nurse may need to be arranged, to make him or her aware that the child has a shunt in place and that the child wears special head protection, if necessary, for sports activities (Failla et al., 1992).

Dandy-Walker Syndrome

Dandy-Walker syndrome is cystic dilatation of the fourth ventricle due to obstruction of the foramina of Luschka and Magendie (the outlets of the fourth ventricle). This results in so much pressure early in intrauterine life that the cerebrum of the brain develops only to a rudimentary form, resulting in severe mental and motor retardation. Children with this condition will have a shunt implanted to prevent their head from expanding any further, but this will not increase their prognosis for a normal life. It can be diagnosed during prenatal life by sonogram.

Neural Tube Disorders

Because the neural tube forms in utero first as a flat plate and then molds to form the brain and cord, it is susceptible to malformation. The term *spina bifida* (Latin for "divided spine") is most often used as a collective term for all spinal cord defects, but there are well-defined degrees of spina bifida involvement, and not all

neural defects involve the spinal cord. All these disorders, however, occur because of lack of fusion of the posterior surface of the embryo in early intrauterine life. They can be compared with cleft palate or cleft lip—these are also closure defects.

The incidence is approximately 1 to 3 per 1000 live births. No specific cause for many such disorders can be isolated, but poor nutrition, especially a diet deficient in vitamins, appears to be a contributing factor. Such disorders may occur as a polygenic inheritance pattern. The risk of bearing a second child with a neural defect once one child is born with such a defect increases to as much as 1 in 20. For this reason, women who have had one child born with a spinal cord defect are advised to have a maternal serum assay or amniocentesis to determine if such a defect is present in a second pregnancy.

Types of Defects

Anencephaly. *Anencephaly* is absence of the cerebral hemispheres. It occurs when the upper end of the neural tube fails to close in early intrauterine life. This is revealed by an elevated level of alpha-fetoprotein (AFP), a protein produced by the liver, in maternal serum or the amniotic fluid. Serum assessment is done at week 15 of pregnancy when AFP reaches its peak concentration and is a routine test in many prenatal settings. If the result is elevated, an amniocentesis will be done to assess the level of AFP in amniotic fluid. A sonogram is also helpful to determine that anencephaly is present in utero.

Infants with anencephaly may have difficulty in labor, because the malformed head does not engage the cervix well; many such infants present in a breech delivery position. On visual inspection at birth, the disorder is obvious (Figure 39-11). Children cannot survive with this disorder, because they have no cerebral function. Because the respiratory and cardiac centers are located in the intact medulla, however, they may survive for a number of days after birth.

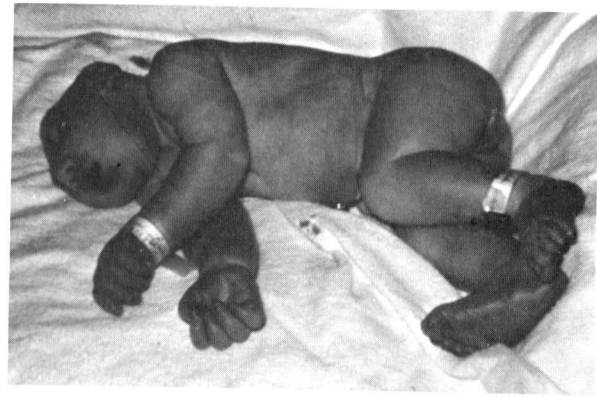

FIGURE 39-11
An infant with anencephaly. (Courtesy of the Department of Medical Photography, Children's Hospital, Buffalo, NY.)

When the condition is discovered prenatally, parents are offered the option of abortion. An ethical problem has arisen in a number of instances when parents, aware that the child cannot survive, elect to carry the infant to term so its organs can be used for transplant. Nurses need to think through their feelings about caring for such infants, since it can be difficult to give care to a child who has been born only to help others live (Van Cleve, 1993).

Microcephaly. *Microcephaly* is a disorder involving brain growth so slow that it falls more than three standard deviations below normal on growth charts. The cause might be a defect in brain development associated with maternal phenylketonuria or an intrauterine infection such as rubella, cytomegalovirus, or toxoplasmosis. It is apparent at birth in these instances. Microcephaly may also result from severe malnutrition or anoxia in early infancy.

Microcephaly generally results in mental retardation because of the lack of functioning brain tissue. True microcephaly must be differentiated from *craniosynostosis* (normal brain growth but premature fusion of the cranial sutures), which also causes decreased head circumference. Infants with craniosynostosis have abnormally closed fontanelles and often show bulging (bossing of the forehead and signs of increased intracranial pressure). Such children must be identified, because with surgery, craniosynostosis can be relieved and brain growth will be normal.

The prognosis for a normal life is guarded in children with microcephaly and depends on the extent of restriction of brain growth and on the cause (Fishman, 1994).

Dermal Sinus. A *dermal sinus* is a small pinpoint opening from the external surface of the back into the subarachnoid space of the spinal cord. The outer point of origin may be marked by a dimple in the skin or an abnormal tuft of hair. This opening is potentially dangerous because it can allow bacteria to enter the cerebrospinal fluid, leading to meningitis. Dermal sinuses generally occur in the lumbosacral area, although they may occur at any point along the spinal canal. Those appearing in the low sacral area are more frequently blind-end pouches (*pilonidal sinuses*) and thus do not carry the danger of cerebrospinal fluid contamination. If a dermal sinus does connect with the spinal cord, it must be surgically incised to prevent later infection.

Spina Bifida Occulta. *Spina bifida occulta* occurs when the posterior laminae of the vertebrae fail to fuse. This occurs most commonly at the fifth lumbar or first sacral level but may occur at any point along the spinal canal. The normal spinal cord is shown in Figure 39-12*A*. The defect may be noticeable as a dimpling at the point of poor fusion; abnormal tufts of hair may be present (Figure 39-12*B*). Simple spina bifida occulta is a benign defect; it occurs as frequently as in one of every four children.

The term *spina bifida* is often used wrongly to denote all spinal cord anomalies. Because of this wrong usage, parents, when told that their child has a spina bifida occulta, may interpret this as meaning that the child has an extremely serious defect. Health professionals should use the terms correctly to reduce confusion.

Meningocele. If the meninges covering the spinal cord herniate through unformed vertebrae, a *meningocele* occurs. The anomaly appears as a protruding mass, usually approximately the size of an orange, at the center of the back (Figure 39-12*C*). It generally occurs in the lumbar region, although it might be present anywhere along the spinal canal. The protrusion may be covered by a layer of skin or only the clear dura mater.

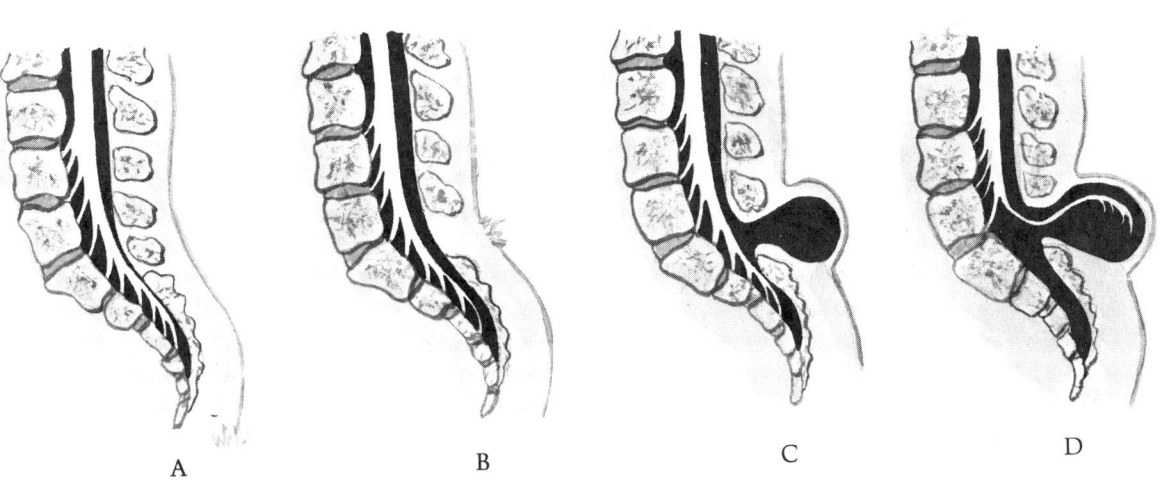

A B C D

FIGURE 39-12
Degrees of spinal cord anomalies. (**A**) *Normal spinal cord.* (**B**) *Spina bifida occulta.* (**C**) *Meningocele.*
(**D**) *Myelomeningocele.*

Myelomeningocele. In a *myelomeningocele*, the spinal cord and the meninges protrude through the vertebrae defect. The spinal cord often ends at the point of the defect, so motor and sensory function is absent beyond this point (Figure 39-12D). Because this results in lower motor neuron damage, the child will have flaccidity and lack of sensation of the lower extremities and loss of bowel and bladder control. The infant's legs are lax and he or she does not move them; urine and stools continually dribble because of lack of sphincter control. Children often have accompanying *talipes* (clubfoot) defects and subluxated hip (Ment & Fishman, 1994). Hydrocephalus may accompany myelomeningocele in as many as 80% of infants; the higher the myelomeningocele occurs on the cord, the more likely hydrocephalus will accompany it. It is generally difficult to tell from the gross appearance of the myelomeningocele whether it is the simpler meningocele (Figure 39-13).

Encephalocele. An *encephalocele* is a cranial meningocele or meningomyelocele. The defect occurs most often in the occipital area of the skull but may occur as a nasal or nasopharyngeal defect. Encephaloceles generally are covered fully by skin, but they may be open so that infection will occur. It is difficult to tell from the size of the encephalocele how much brain tissue is trapped in the defect. Transillumination of the sac will reveal solid substance or fluid in the sac. X-ray or sonography will reveal the size of the skull defect.

Assessment

All types of neural defects except spina bifida occulta are readily visible at birth. They may be discovered during intrauterine life by sonography, fetoscopy, amniocentesis (discovery of AFP in amniotic fluid), or analysis of AFP in maternal serum. When infants are detected as

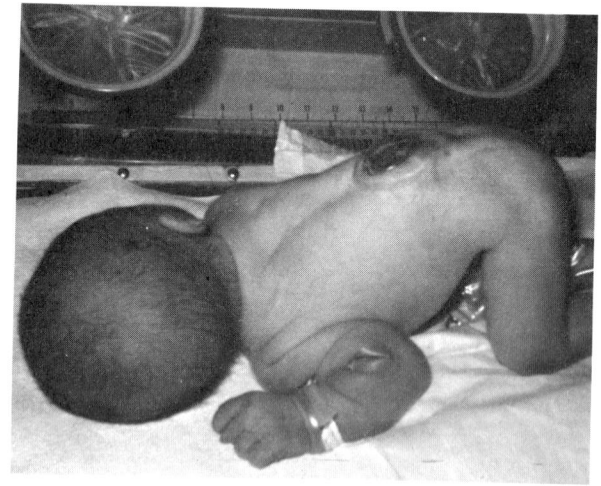

FIGURE 39-13
A myelomeningocele. (Courtesy of the Department of Medical Photography, Children's Hospital, Buffalo, NY.)

having meningocele or myelomeningocele, they are usually delivered by cesarean birth to avoid pressure and injury to the spinal cord (Luthy et al., 1991). Observe and record whether an infant born with a meningomyelocele has spontaneous movement of lower extremities and the nature and pattern of voiding and defecation. A normal infant appears to be "always wet" from voiding but actually voids in amounts of approximately 30 mL and then is dry for 2 or 3 hours before voiding again. An infant without sphincter control voids continually. This pattern is the same for defecating. Observing these features aids in differentiating between meningocele and myelomeningocele. Differentiation may be further established by sonography.

Therapeutic Management

Children with spina bifida occulta need no immediate surgical correction. The parents should be made aware of its existence, however, so that they are not surprised when someone points it out to them later on. Some children may eventually need surgery to prevent vertebral deterioration due to the unbalanced spinal column.

Treatment for a meningocele, myelomeningocele, or encephalocele is surgery to replace contents that are replaceable and to close the skin defect to prevent infection. The child with myelomeningocele will continue to have paralysis of lower extremities and loss of bowel and bladder function. Table 39-1 provides a classification of motor function disability. In the past, this surgery was done after the infant had survived the newborn period; currently, it is done as soon after birth as possible (usually within 24 hours) so that infection does not occur. Parents need to be cautioned that the surgery is not without risk and that brain defects accompanying an encephalocele may limit the child's potential.

The future prognosis will depend on the extent of the defect. The loss of meninges by surgery may limit the rate of absorption of cerebrospinal fluid; it may build up in amount, and hydrocephalus may develop following repair. Parents need a great deal of support to care for a child with a myelomeningocele because their child has a multiple disability. Some parents ask if it would not be better to allow a child born with myelomeningocele to die rather than undergo palliative surgery to close the defect. This poses an ethical problem: Whose rights should be honored, the parents' or the child's, and how will these rights be determined?

Nursing Diagnoses and Related Interventions: Immediate Concerns

It is difficult for parents to accept a diagnosis this severe. However, until they have accepted the diagnosis, it is difficult for them to make concrete plans. Some parents are advised against surgery by well-meaning friends. It may be necessary to advocate for surgery or counsel

Table 39-1. Motor Function Disability in Myelomeningocele	
Spinal Cord Lesion	**Dysfunction**
T6–12	Complete flaccid paralysis of the lower extremities; weakened abdominal and trunk musculature in higher lesions; kyphosis and scoliosis common; ambulation with maximal support
L1–2	Hip flexion present; paraplegia, ambulation with maximal support
L3–4	Hip flexion, adduction, and knee extension present; hip dislocation common; some control of hip and knee movement possible; ambulation with moderate support
L-5	Hip flexion, adduction, and varying degrees of abduction; knee extension and weak knee flexion; paralysis of the lower legs and feet; ambulation with moderate support
S1–2	As above, with preservation of some foot and ankle movement; ambulation with minimal support
S-3	Mild loss of intrinsic foot muscular function possible; ambulation without support

(From Kupka, J., et al. [1990]. Comprehensive management in the child with spina bifida. *Orthopedic Clinics of North America, 9,* 97, with permission.)

about the range of alternatives available before goal-setting can be realistic.

Even though they are told before surgery that the spinal deformity is a type that means motor and sensory function are absent in the child's lower extremities, parents do not necessarily hear this information. Only after surgery do they begin to comprehend the extent of their child's disability. When the child is discharged from the hospital, they need to be certain of the next step in follow-up care. This prevents them from feeling deserted when they most need support—the time when they begin to appreciate what this problem will mean to them in the coming years, and what it will mean to the child throughout life.

Nursing Diagnosis: High risk for infection related to rupture of neural tube sac

Goal: Child will not develop an infection before surgery.

Outcome Criteria: The neural tube sac remains unruptured; the child's temperature remains below 37.0°C.

If the sac should be allowed to dry, it might crack and allow cerebrospinal fluid to drain and microorganisms to enter. Pressure on the protruding mass might cause rupture of the sac, leading to quick decompression of the cerebrospinal fluid (which can led to herniation of the brain stem into the spinal cord and interference with respiratory and cardiac centers) and possibly to infection (meningitis). Such pressure may also force cerebrospinal fluid from the sac into the spinal column and, therefore, increase intracranial pressure.

Preoperative Positioning. Before surgery, infants should be positioned carefully so that pressure on the spinal defect does not occur. They can be placed in a prone position or supported on their side. When they are on their side, if a rolled blanket or diaper is placed behind their upper backs (above the defect) and a separate one behind their lower back (below the defect), no pressure will be exerted on the lesion, and the infant will be protected from rolling backward onto it. Placing infants on their abdomen has the added advantage of keeping the flow of feces and urine away from the defect as well as keeping the lesion free from pressure. This is important because in many instances the skin covering of the defect is incomplete. A folded towel under the abdomen helps to flex the hip, reduce pressure on the sac, and ensure good leg position. If an infant is on his or her side, putting a folded diaper between the legs prevents skin surfaces from touching and rubbing (and also helps to keep the hips from internally rotating). Notice the position of the infant's legs. If they are paralyzed because of lack of motor control, the infant cannot move and straighten them.

Placing a piece of plastic or sturdy plastic wrap below the meningocele on the child's back like an apron and taping it in place is another method of preventing feces from touching the open lesion. A sterile wet compress of saline, antiseptic, or antibiotic gauze over the lesion may be used to keep the sac moist. Rather than remove this to wet it again and risk rupturing the sac, merely add additional fluid.

Although no pressure should be exerted on the open lesion by a top sheet, make certain that the child is warm enough. He or she may need to be kept in an Isolette to maintain body heat if a large area of the back cannot be covered. Use caution when placing the infant under a radiant heat source for warmth. Radiant heat can dry the lesion and cause cracking. Any seepage of clear fluid from the defect should be reported promptly, because this is probably escaping cerebrospinal fluid.

Postoperative Care. Following surgery, a child is again placed on the abdomen until the skin incision has healed (7 to 14 days). The same careful precautions against allowing urine or feces to touch the incision area must be taken.

Nursing Diagnosis: High risk for altered nutrition, less than body requirements, related to difficulty assuming normal feeding position

Goal: Infant will take in adequate nutrition during period of healing.

Outcome Criteria: Infant has good skin turgor; loses no more than 10% of birth weight; specific gravity of urine remains between 1.030 and 1.003.

To maintain nutrition, the infant should be held in as normal a feeding position as possible. Make certain that the supporting arm does not press against the lesion. When bubbling the infant, remember not to pat the back over the defect. If the defect is large and the risk in picking up the infant is too great, the infant may be fed while lying on his or her side in bed or prone on a Bradford frame. Raise the infant's head slightly by slipping a folded diaper under it. Stroke the head, arms, or upper back while the infant sucks to give the child the same comfort and assurance at feeding time as a baby receives while being held. Talk to the infant and let him or her know that someone loves and cares for him or her. The infant may enjoy a pacifier after feeding, because the child does not experience the enjoyment of sucking while feeding that would be experienced if he or she could be held and cuddled. Every new mother has some difficulty getting comfortable with feeding an infant. The mother who must feed her child in this unusual position or with the infant on a support frame will have even more difficulty. She needs to observe a warm, comforting role model so that she can begin a positive mother–child interaction.

If a mother planned on breast-feeding and the infant can be held, urge her to do this. Caution her not to allow the incision line to press against her arm.

Children with increased intracranial pressure tend to suck poorly. If this complication develops following the surgery, nursing may be difficult. Parents need a realistic explanation of treatment planned for the child so that they can decide whether to continue to plan on breast-feeding. If it is necessary to forgo breast-feeding for this child, assure parents that the child will thrive on commercial formula.

Nursing Diagnosis: High risk for altered cerebral tissue perfusion related to increased intracranial pressure

Goal: Infant will not experience symptoms of compression from increased intracranial pressure or an increase in skull circumference during childhood.

Outcome Criteria: Infant's head circumference remains within present percentile on growth chart.

Preoperative Care. Increasing head size from poor absorption of cerebrospinal fluid (hydrocephalus) is a complication of neural tube disorders. To detect increased head size (development of hydrocephalus), measure head circumference once daily (or more frequently if ordered) in the preoperative period. Head circumference measurements are only accurate if the tape measure is placed on the same points of the child's head each time. Placing a ballpoint pen mark on the forehead just above the eyebrows and at the most prominent point of the occiput allows different people to measure the head during the day and yet be sure that they all measure at the same point.

Postoperative Care. Children may develop hydrocephalus following surgery, probably because of additional interference with subarachnoid absorption of cerebrospinal fluid. The child must be observed frequently for signs of increased intracranial pressure, such as changes in vital signs, neurologic signs such as pupillary changes, or an increase in head circumference or bulging fontanelles, as well as behavioral changes such as irritability or lethargy.

Nursing Diagnosis: High risk for altered skin integrity related to required prone positioning

Goal: Infant will not experience disruption in skin integrity during preoperative or postoperative period.

Outcome Criteria: Infant's skin remains intact without erythema or ulceration.

Preserving skin integrity is a major problem because of frequent dressing changes and because the constant prone position puts pressure on the infant's knees and elbows. Laying the infant on a synthetic sheepskin helps reduce friction; use nonadhesive tape for dressing changes or place Stomahesive on the skin under the area where the tape will touch. Change diapers frequently to prevent excessive contact of acid urine with skin. If hydrocephalus has developed, the head will be heavy and pressure areas at the temples can occur if the head is not turned every 2 hours.

Nursing Diagnoses and Related Interventions: Long-Term Concerns

Nursing Diagnosis: Impaired physical mobility related to neural tube disorder

Goal: Child will be mobile within the limits of nerve involvement following surgery.

Outcome Criteria: Child ambulates with the least amount of accessory equipment possible.

Parents need a great deal of support to care for a child with a myelomeningocele. They must provide normal stimulation and activities for the child because his or her mobility is limited. They need to be encouraged to take the infant to the places a child would normally accompany parents—relatives' homes, shopping, the zoo, and so forth. They need to encourage the child to be as independent as possible so that he or she can lead as normal a life as possible (Figure 39-14).

If a child has impaired lower-extremity motor control, parents will need to perform passive exercises to prevent muscle atrophy and formation of contractures. The child may need braces to help maintain good alignment and make walking with crutches possible in childhood. Parents are generally anxious to do something for their child and follow routines of passive exercises well if they are given sufficient support for their accomplishments at health care visits. As the child grows older, tendon transplants and osteotomy may be necessary to prevent contractures and poor bone alignment. Because these children have no sensation in their lower extremities, parents must make a routine of inspecting the child's lower extremities and buttocks daily for any area of irritation or possible infection. Teach children as they grow older to do this themselves; be certain to teach that as they sit in a wheelchair they must press with their arms on the armrests to raise their buttocks off the wheelchair seat, which will allow adequate circulation to lower extremities, at least once every hour.

Nursing Diagnosis: High risk for altered elimination related to neural tube disorder

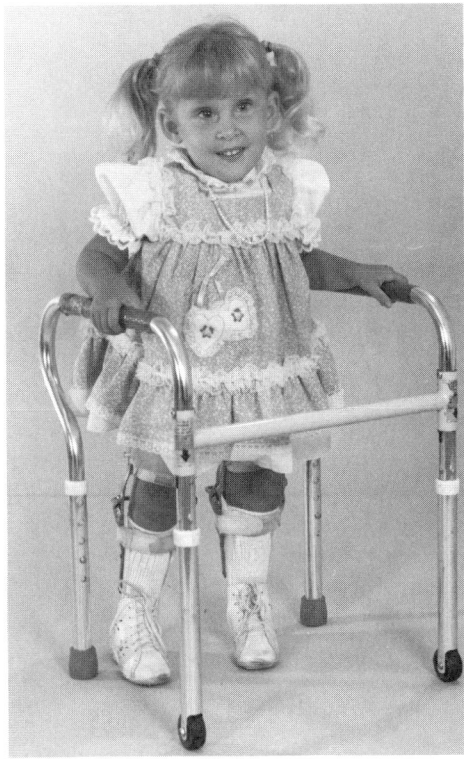

FIGURE 39-14
A child born with a neural tube impairment demonstrates her ability to walk using braces and a walker. (Courtesy of the Department of Medical Photography, Children's Hospital, Buffalo, NY.)

Goal: Child will achieve a satisfactory method of elimination by school age.

Outcome Criteria: Child demonstrates ability to independently manage bowel and bladder elimination.

To ensure bladder emptying, the Credé method of bladder evacuation is taught to parents when the infant is discharged from the hospital (a parent presses on the abdomen just under the umbilicus, sliding on down to press on the bladder and empty it every 2 to 3 hours). As the child grows older, toilet-training becomes a concern. In some children, a continent urinary reservoir or ureterosigmoidostomy (see Chapter 46) is constructed to bypass the nonfunctioning bladder. As the child reaches preschool age, the parent can learn to do catheterization. As the child reaches school age, he or she can be taught clean self-catheterization (inserting a clean catheter every 4 hours to drain urine from the bladder) (Box 39-1). It is possible for artificial bladder sphincters to be placed to help establish continence.

Arnold-Chiari Deformity (Chiari II Malformation)

The Arnold-Chiari deformity is caused by overgrowth of the neural tube in weeks 16 to 20 of fetal life. The specific anomaly is a projection of the cerebellum, medulla oblongata, and fourth ventricle into the cervical canal. This causes the upper cervical spinal cord to jackknife backward, obstructing cerebrospinal fluid flow and causing hydrocephalus. A lumbosacral myelomeningocele is also present in approximately 50% of children with this anomaly.

The prognosis for the child with an Arnold-Chiari malformation depends on the extent of the defect and the surgical procedure possible. Because of the upper motor neuron involvement, gagging and swallowing reflexes may be absent; this makes the child susceptible to tracheal aspiration.

Skeletal Anomalies

A number of physical developmental defects result in skeletal deformities in the newborn.

Absent or Malformed Extremities

Congenital bone defects may result from drug ingestion, virus invasion during pregnancy, or amniotic band formation in utero (Figure 39-15). If a child is born with a bone deformity, record a careful pregnancy history, although in most instances the cause of the anomaly cannot be established. Children born without an extremity

Box 39-1
Instructions for Self-Catheterization

1. The purpose of self-catheterization is to keep the bladder empty through using clean technique and frequent emptying so that microorganisms do not have time to grow in urine in the bladder. It is important that you always use clean equipment and that you self-catheterize at least every 4 hours to accomplish this.

2. Always carry your self-catheterization equipment with you (a plastic bag containing a clean catheter and water-soluble lubricant). This enables you to stay longer away from home if you wish. If you will be using a public lavatory, you might want to include a presoaped washcloth rather than have to use rough paper towels.

3. To begin self-catheterization, wash your hands in warm soapy water. This reduces the chance that you will introduce germs from your hands into the bladder.

4. Next wash your perineum or penis with a clean washcloth and warm soapy water. Rinse the washcloth and wash again with clear water. This reduces the chance that germs on your skin will be pushed into the bladder.

5. Coat a clean catheter with a water-soluble lubricant. This reduces friction and makes the catheter slide into the bladder easily.

6. Females use one hand to spread the lips of the perineum so the bladder entrance is exposed. Locate the urinary meatus and gently but quickly insert the catheter approximately 1 inch (males insert the catheter approximately 4 inches). Urine should begin to flow immediately through the catheter. Let this drain into the toilet.

7. When urine stops flowing, gently remove the catheter. Clean the catheter with soap and water, rinse with clear water, and replace in the plastic bag with the lubricant.

8. Examine your schedule at the beginning of each day and plan ways that you will be able to use a bathroom or school lavatory every 4 hours.

9. Be certain that on special days (e.g., school trips or vacation) that you do not forget the importance of self-catheterization.

10. Ask your parents to telephone your health care provider if urine is ever blood tinged, smells foul, or is cloudy rather than clear; if you have pain in your abdomen or lower back; or if you have an elevated temperature, because these may be symptoms of a urinary tract infection.

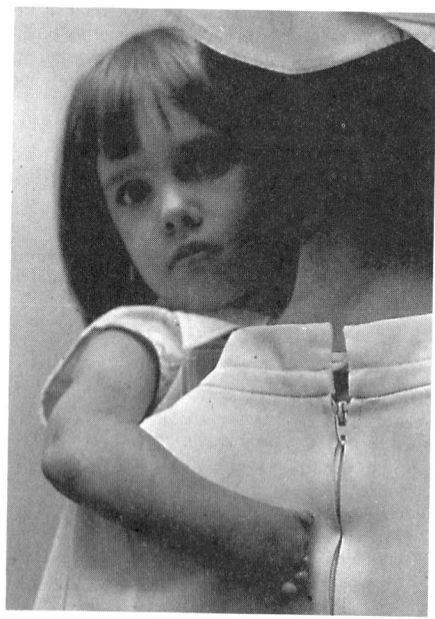

FIGURE 39-15
A child with absent fingers from an amniotic band in utero. (Courtesy of March of Dimes Birth Defects Foundation.)

or with a malformed extremity can be fitted with a prosthesis early in life. In most instances, children will have better function if the malformed portion of an extremity is amputated before a prosthesis is fitted. This is a difficult decision for parents to make and one that they cannot undo later on. They need assurance that arms that appear like seal flippers, for example, will not later grow to become normal. A well-fitted prosthesis that a child learns to use at an early age will provide more function and allow a more normal childhood and adult life than if the original deformity is left unchanged (Figure 39-16A). Lower-extremity prostheses are fitted as early as age 6 months (so that an infant will learn to stand at the normal time). Upper-extremity prostheses are fitted this early also, so that an infant will handle and explore objects readily.

Introducing a prosthesis early also prevents a child from adjusting to a missing extremity, such as writing with the feet or sliding across a floor rather than walking. Children can become so proficient at these adjustments that later in life they do not see the advantage of a prosthesis and refuse to use one. Although these self-

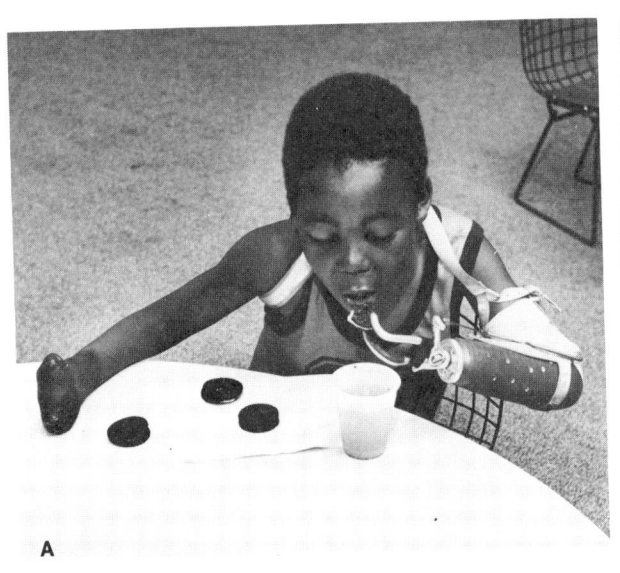
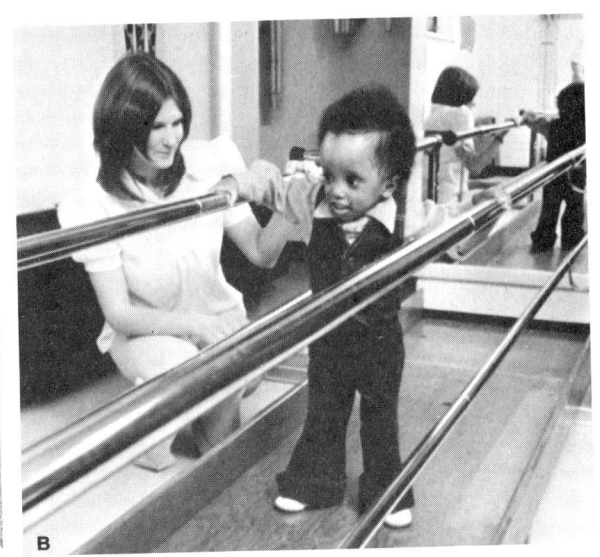

FIGURE 39-16
(**A**) *A child with a prosthesis learns to feed himself.* (**B**) *A child learns to ambulate with a leg prosthesis.*
(Courtesy of the Department of Medical Photography, Children's Hospital, Buffalo, NY.)

adjustments are cute in infants, in the long run they greatly limit their potential.

Learning to use a hand prosthesis takes weeks to months; help parents to think of interesting activities to introduce so a child uses a prosthesis to accomplish something rather than feeling he or she is only undergoing a ritual. Gait training for use of lower-extremity prostheses begins by use of parallel bars and proceeds to independent walking and mastery of steps (Figure 39-16B). Children who are born with an absent extremity need help not only in mastering the use of a prosthesis but also in mastering a positive body image of themselves as whole.

Parents often feel devastated at the child's birth and search to discover the cause of the defect. They should be introduced to a rehabilitation team in the newborn period if possible. Further steps then will be outlined

for them to help them move past the helplessness they feel to more positive action. Visiting with a child who uses a prosthesis well can be a great help in convincing them that their child can lead a normal life. Children with a congenital extremity loss do not grieve over the lost extremity as do adults or older children, which means they are often better prepared to quickly move on to rehabilitation.

Finger Conditions

Polydactyly is the presence of one or more additional fingers (Figure 39-17A). When this occurs, the supernumerary finger is usually amputated in infancy or early childhood. These extra fingers are often just cartilage or skin tags, and removal is simple and cosmetically sound. In **syndactyly** (two fingers are fused) the fusion is usu-

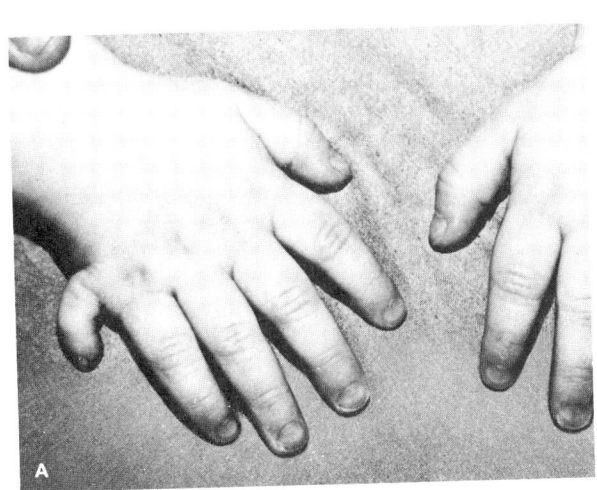
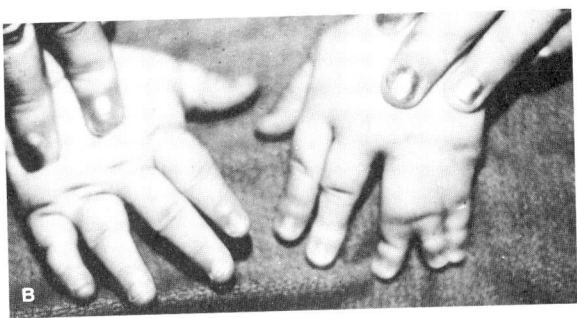

FIGURE 39-17
(**A**) *Polydactyly.* (**B**) *Syndactyly. (From Mead Johnson Company, Evansville, IN, with permission.)*

ally caused by a simple webbing (Figure 39-17*B*); separation of the fingers into two sound and cosmetically appealing ones is usually successful. In other instances, the bones of the fingers are also fused, and the cosmetic appearance and function of fingers will always be impaired.

These hand anomalies are always upsetting to parents (one of the first things that new parents do is count the fingers and toes of newborns). Parents need time to air their feelings and concerns. They need reassurance at health maintenance visits throughout the child's development that he or she is normal in other ways so that they can accept and love the child. Children need this same type of assurance so they can think of themselves as well people.

Sprengel's Deformity

Sprengel's deformity is a congenital deformity of the scapulae. One scapula is turned horizontally; it appears higher than the opposite bone. Children with this defect cannot raise the arm on the affected side above a right angle with the body. They may hold their head inclined toward the affected side. As they reach school age, scoliosis tends to develop.

Surgical correction will relieve Sprengel's deformity. The procedure is extreme, however, and may not be advised solely for cosmetic reasons.

Pectus Excavatum

Pectus excavatum is an indentation of the lower portion of the sternum (Figure 39-18). This usually occurs congenitally; it may also occur following chronic obstructive lung disease or rickets. The defect results in decreased lung volume and displacement of the heart to the left. Surgery can be done for cosmetic reasons or to expand lung volume.

Torticollis (Wry Neck)

Torticollis is a term derived from *tortus* (twisted) and *collum* (neck). Torticollis (wry neck) occurs as a congenital anomaly when the sternocleidomastoid muscle is injured during birth. This tends to occur in newborns with wide shoulders when pressure is exerted on the head to deliver the shoulder. The infant holds the head tilted to the side of the muscle involved; the head rotates to the opposite side. The injury may not be noticeable in the neck of the newborn and may become evident only as the original hemorrhage recedes and fibrous contraction occurs at age 1 to 2 months. A palpable mass will be present.

Treatment consists of passive stretching exercises and encouraging the infant to look in the direction of the affected muscle. A mother could encourage this by holding the child to feed in such a position that the child must look in the desired direction. When the parents are

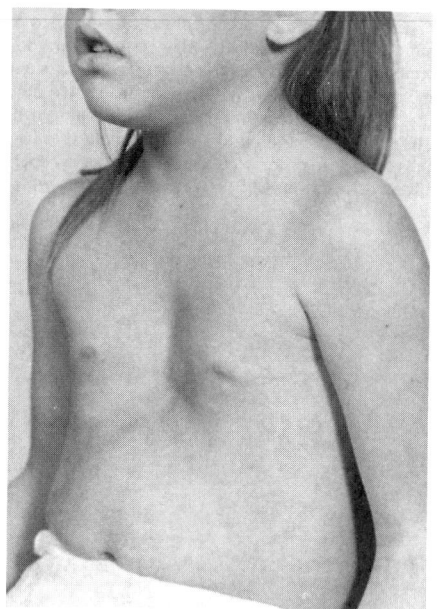

FIGURE 39-18
Pectus excavatum. (Courtesy of the Department of Medical Photography, Children's Hospital, Buffalo, NY.)

working in the kitchen they could place the infant in an infant seat and speak to the child from the affected side. A mobile on the child's crib should be placed to encourage the child to look toward the affected side. The parents should hand the child objects always from the affected side to make the child look that way.

If the parents do this consistently, further treatment usually is not necessary. It is important that parents understand that this is important therapy. It seems so simple that they otherwise may not take it seriously and may not carry it out. In the few instances in which simple exercises are not effective and the condition still exists at a year, surgical correction followed by a neck immobilizer will be necessary (Staheli, 1992). Torticollis can lead to the one shoulder continuing to be elevated. This has the potential to lead to scoliosis later in life.

Craniosynostosis

Craniosynostosis is premature closure of the sutures of the skull. This may occur in utero; it may occur early in infancy because of rickets, or irregularities of calcium or phosphate metabolism; and it also may occur without any known cause. It occurs more often in males than females.

It is important that craniosynostosis be detected early, because premature closure of the suture line will compromise brain growth. When the sagittal suture line closes prematurely, the child's head tends to grow anteriorly and posteriorly. If the coronal suture line fuses early, the child's face becomes deformed. The orbit of the eyes becomes misshapen, and the increased intracranial pressure may lead to exophthalmos, nystagmus, papilledema, strabismus, and atrophy of the optic nerve and consequent loss of vision. Premature closure of the coronal suture line is associated with syndactyly, so all infants with syndactyly should be observed closely for head circumference. Cardiac anomalies, choanal atresias, or defects of elbows and knee joints are also associated with craniosynostosis.

Head circumference should be measured on all children age 2 years or younger at all health maintenance visits and compared with normal head circumference charts. The posterior fontanelle closes normally at age 2 months, the anterior fontanelle at age 12 to 18 months. All children with premature closure of fontanelles must be observed closely for craniosynostosis.

Craniosynostosis can be established by x-ray film, which reveals the fused suture line. If the suture line is the sagittal one, treatment may involve only careful observation; if the coronal suture line is involved, it will need to be surgically opened (Persing et al., 1990).

Measuring head circumference at health maintenance visits is a nursing responsibility. Thoughtful comparison of an infant's head circumference with past measurements and with standard measurements can be important in detecting craniosynostosis and preventing brain compression.

Achondroplasia

Achondroplasia (chondrodystrophia) is a form of dwarfism inherited as a dominant trait. It involves a defect in cartilage production in utero. The epiphyseal plate of long bones cannot produce adequate cartilage for longitudinal bone growth, which results in both arms and legs being stunted.

Because the bones of the cranium are of membranous origin, they continue to grow normally; children's heads will therefore appear unusually large in contrast to extremities. The forehead is prominent and the bridge of the nose is flattened. Because it is a cartilage—not a brain—problem, intelligence generally is normal. Children's trunks are of near-normal size, but a *thoracic kyphosis* (outward curve) and *lumbar lordosis* (inward curve) of the spine may be present.

Achondroplasia dwarfism can be diagnosed in utero or at birth by comparing the length of extremities to the normal length (in the average child, the arms can be extended to the distance of the midthigh) or by x-ray film, which will reveal characteristic abnormal flaring epiphyseal lines. People with achondroplasia dwarfism rarely reach a height of more than 4½ ft (140 cm). Women with this condition will have difficulty with childbearing because of the deformed pelvis and generally have their children by cesarean birth. A course of growth hormone may be helpful to increase height (Yamate et al., 1993).

Children with achondroplasia become aware of their unusual appearance as early as during the preschool years. They are apt to become acutely aware of it

during school age, when they realize they do not "fit in" with the neighborhood children. Ideally such children have parents who have adjusted well to short stature in themselves and therefore have developed good self-esteem and are able to implant these qualities in a child. The child nearing reproductive age must be informed that, as with all dominantly inherited disorders, there is a high probability that any children will inherit the disorder. Adolescence may be a particularly difficult time for these children, and continued guidance or counseling can help them to emerge from this period feeling good about themselves as adults.

Talipes Deformities

Talipes is a Latin word formed from the words *talus* and *pes,* meaning "foot" and "ankle," respectively. The talipes deformities are ankle-foot deformities, popularly called *clubfoot.* The term "clubfoot" implies permanent crippling to many people and should not be used when discussing talipes deformities with parents. With good orthopedic correction techniques currently available, correction should leave the child with no permanent deformity of the foot.

Approximately 1 in every 1000 live-born children has a talipes deformity; it occurs more often in males than females. It probably is inherited as a polygenic pattern; it usually occurs only as a unilateral problem.

It is difficult for any new parents to learn that their newborn child has a congenital anomaly, but the stigma attached to a condition such as a talipes deformity often makes it particularly difficult to accept. Every parent knows of an older person in the community who had a correction for talipes years ago, before techniques for correction were perfected; this person still limps or wears awkward orthopedic shoes. It is easy for parents to equate this mental picture with their newborn.

Some newborns have a pseudo talipes deformity from their intrauterine position. In these infants the foot looks to be turned in but can be brought into a good position by manipulation: in a true defect, the foot cannot be properly aligned without further intervention. Be certain to demonstrate to parents that if a pseudodeformity is present, the foot can easily be brought into line or is not deformed. Otherwise, the first time parents fit booties or shoes on the infant, they will notice this and worry that the foot is misshapen.

A true talipes deformity can be one of four separate deformities: (1) *plantar flexion* (an equinus, or "horse-foot" position); (2) *dorsiflexion* (the heel is held lower than the foot or the anterior foot is flexed toward the anterior leg); (3) *varus deviation* (the foot turns in); or (4) *valgus deviation* (the foot turns out). Most children with talipes deformities have a combination of these conditions, or have an equinovarus (Figure 39-19) or a *calcaneovalgus* deformity (a child walks on the heel with the foot everted).

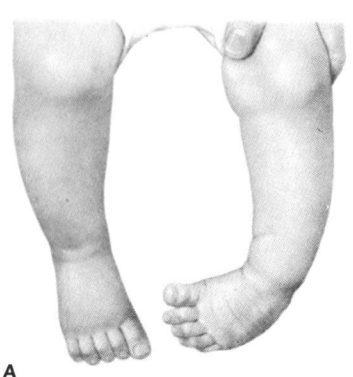
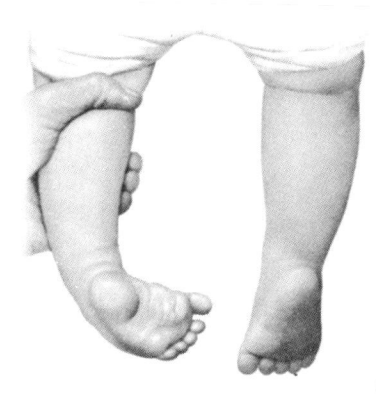
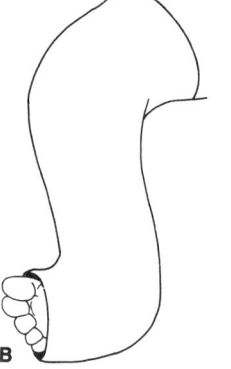
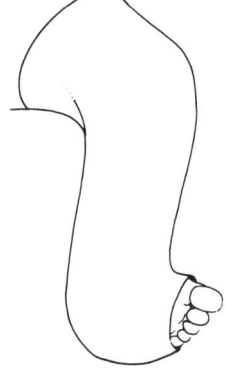

FIGURE 39-19

(**A**) *Talipes equinovarus. (Used with permission of Ross Products Division, Abbott Laboratories, Columbus OH 43216 from Clinical Education Aid No. 15. © 1965 Ross Products Division, Abbott Laboratories).*
(**B**) *Casts for bilateral equinovarus.*

Assessment

The earlier a true deformity is recognized, the better the correction. Make a habit of straightening all newborn feet to the midline as part of initial assessment to detect this defect.

Therapeutic Management

Correction is achieved best if it is begun in the newborn. This is usually accomplished by the foot being placed in a cast in an overcorrected position while the child is under a general anesthetic. Although the deformity involves the ankle, the cast extends above the infant's knee to ensure firm correction (Figure 39-19*B*). Caution parents that the cast will reach high on the leg (over the knee) but that the size of the cast does not mean that the child's problem is extensive.

Care of the child in a cast is discussed in Chapter 51. Talipes casts are high on the leg; diapers should be changed frequently to prevent a wet diaper from touching the cast and causing it to become soaked with urine or meconium. Review with parents how to check the infant's toes for coldness or blueness and how to blanch a toenail bed and watch it turn pink. Because a newborn is unable to report pain except by generalized crying, crying episodes in the infant must be evaluated carefully. Such crying may be due to colic, hunger, or wet diapers; it might also be due to the tingling feeling of circulatory compression (as when a foot is "asleep").

Because infants grow so rapidly in the neonatal period, casts for talipes deformities must be changed almost every week or every 2 weeks. If a mother has a complication of childbirth or is exhausted from childbirth (depression due to the child's having been born with a congenital defect may manifest itself as exhaustion), she may have to make arrangements for another family member to bring the infant to the hospital for cast changes.

After approximately 6 weeks (the time varies depending on the extent of the problem), the final cast is removed. After this, parents may need to perform passive foot exercises such as putting the infant's foot and ankle through a full range of motion several times a day for several months. These seem like simple maneuvers, so their importance must be impressed on the parents; otherwise, they will do them haphazardly or not at all. The infant may have to sleep in Denis Browne splints at night up to age 1 year (see Figure 51-12). Although a successful correction cannot be guaranteed, the prognosis with correction is good. For those children who do not achieve correction by casting, surgery can be performed to achieve a final correction.

Developmental Hip Dysplasia

Developmental **hip dysplasia** (often referred to as *congenital hip dysplasia*), is improper formation and function of the hip socket. It may be evident as subluxation or dislocation of the head of the femur (Figure 39-20).

A flattening of the acetabulum of the pelvis is present, which prevents the head of the femur from remaining in the acetabulum and rotating adequately. In **subluxated hip**, the femur "rides up" because of the flat acetabulum; in **dislocated hip**, the femur rides so far up that it actually leaves the acetabulum. Why the defect occurs is unknown, but it may be from a polygenic inheritance pattern; it may also occur from a uterine position that causes less than usual pressure of the femur head on the acetabulum.

Hip dysplasia is found in females six times more frequently than in males, possibly because the hips are normally more flaring in females and possibly because the hormone relaxin causes the pelvic ligaments to be more relaxed and so the femur does not press as effectively into the acetabulum during intrauterine life. It is usually, but not always, a unilateral involvement. It occurs most often in children of Mediterranean ancestry. Sociocultural methods of childrearing may promote or

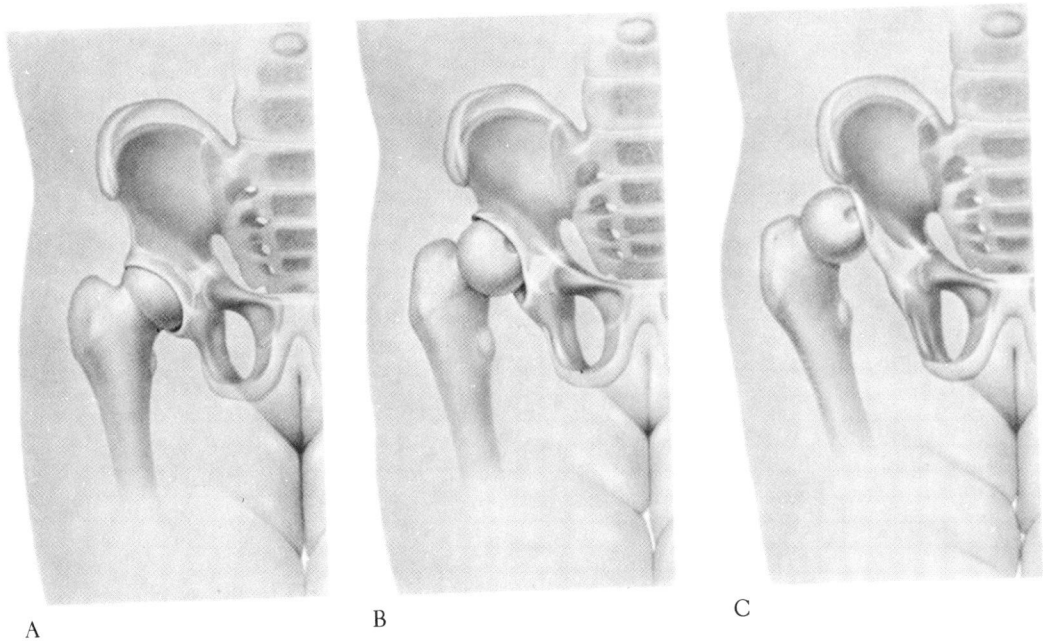

FIGURE 39-20
*Hip dysplasia. (**A**) A normal femur head and acetabulum. (**B**) A subluxated hip. The femur head is "riding high" in the shallow acetabulum. (**C**) A dislocated hip. The femur head is not engaged in the shallow acetabulum. (Used with permission of Ross Products Division, Abbott Laboratories, Columbus OH 43216 from Clinical Education Aid No. 15. © 1965 Ross Products Division, Abbott Laboratories).*

decrease the extent of the involvement (see the Focus on Cultural Awareness box).

Assessment

It is important that hip dysplasia be detected in the newborn because the longer it goes undetected, the more difficult it is to correct. Sometimes the affected leg may appear slightly shorter than the normal one because the femur head rides so high in the socket. This is most noticeable if the child is laid supine and the thighs are flexed to a 90-degree angle toward the abdomen. One knee will appear to be lower than the other (Figure 39-21*A*). An unequal number of skin folds may be present on the posterior thighs (Figure 39-21*B*). This finding is unreliable, however, because some infants with normal hips have an uneven number of posterior thigh skin folds (Way, 1991).

Subluxated or dislocated hip is best assessed by noting whether the hips abduct. To demonstrate this, lay the infant in a supine position and raise the knees, with the legs flexed to 90 degrees at the hips. Place your middle fingers over the greater trochanter of the femur

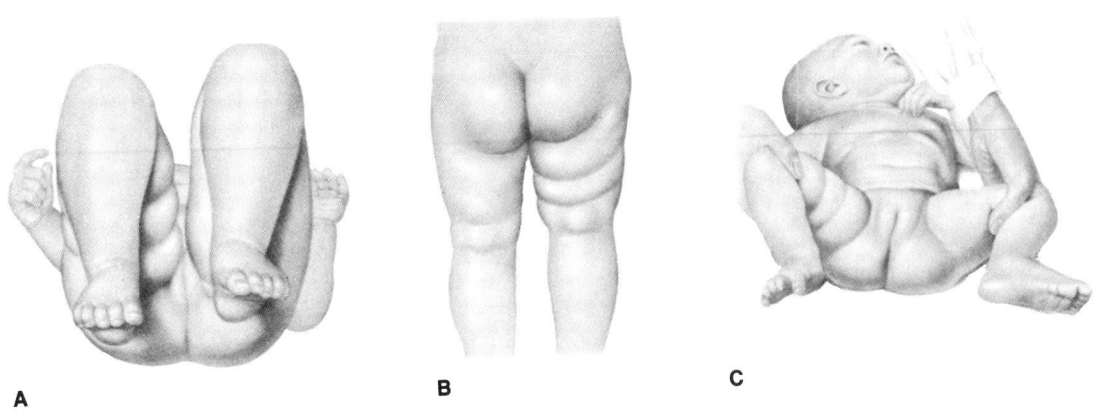

FIGURE 39-21
*Signs of subluxated hip. (**A**) With child in a supine position, the right knee on the side of the subluxation appears lower than the left because of malposition of the femur head. (**B**) Asymmetry of skin folds and prominence of the trochanter on the right side. (**C**) Limitation of the right hip. (Used with permission of Ross Products Division, Abbott Laboratories, Columbus OH 43216 from Clinical Education Aid No. 15. © 1965 Ross Products Division, Abbott Laboratories).*

and your thumb on the internal side of the thigh over the lesser trochanter. Abduct the hip. In the newborn normal infant, hips should abduct to approximately a full 180-degree angle, or so far that the knees touch the mattress at the side of the infant. With subluxated hip, the affected hip will not abduct fully because the femoral head cannot rotate fully (Figure 39-21*C*). An audible sound (a dull click or "clunk") may be heard as the femur slides to the top of the acetabulum (Ortolani's sign). By pressing down and laterally on the thigh it is possible to feel that the hip socket is unstable or the femur head actually slides out of the socket (Barlow's sign).

In some infants, the hip abducts properly at a newborn assessment, but at the time of the first health maintenance visit at approximately age 4 to 6 weeks, a secondary shortening of the adductor muscles will have occurred, and the defect will be evident. Tight adductor muscles occur in children with cerebral palsy, so this disorder must be ruled out. An x-ray film or sonogram will reveal the shallow acetabulum and a more lateral placement of the femur head than is ordinarily seen.

Hip dysplasia is difficult to detect at birth in an infant who delivered from a footling or frank breech presentation, because the knees are stiff and do not flex readily.

Therapeutic Management

Correction of subluxated and dislocated hip involves positioning the hip into a flexed, abducted (externally rotated) position to press the femur head against the acetabulum and deepen its contour by the pressure. Either splints, halters, or casts may be used. The small number of children who do not achieve a correction by these methods will have surgery and a pin inserted to stabilize the hip (Harris et al., 1992).

Nursing Diagnoses and Related Interventions

Nursing Diagnosis: Parental knowledge deficit related to splint, halter, or cast correction for hip subluxation

Goal: Parents will demonstrate increased knowledge of the care of the child in a splint, halter, or cast by discharge from the health care agency.

Outcome Criteria: Parents correctly demonstrate application and removal of splint or halter or cast.

Multiple Diapers. Often splint correction (to hold the legs in a frog-leg, or abducted, externally rotated position) is begun during the newborn's initial hospital stay by placing not one but two or three diapers on the infant. The extra bulk of cloth between the child's legs effectively separates and spreads them. Many brands of disposable diapers are cut narrow between the legs;

thus, they do not offer this much bulk and will not work as well as cloth diapers.

Parents should handle their infant enough before discharge from the hospital to become familiar with the equipment they will be using. If only bulky diapers are required, be certain that parents understand that, although this may not seem to be an important measure (as might a more complicated splint or cast), it is important that they continue to use the extra diapers. Parents are taught that swaddling babies tightly is comforting for the baby; be certain these parents understand that bringing the child's legs together with a tight swaddling blanket will not be good for him or her. Some Native American parents still use a swaddling board for their child. Be sure these parents know not to straighten the child's legs to swaddle him or her with a board.

Frejka Splint. A Frejka splint is made of plastic and buckles onto the child as a huge confining diaper (Figure 39-22*A*). Make certain that parents understand the importance of keeping the splint in place at all times, except when changing diapers or bathing the infant. This is a simple method of treatment, and the parents may not appreciate its importance unless it is made clear to them. Provide them with a telephone number to call for advice if they have any difficulty applying a splint. Although firm pressure may be needed to abduct the hip to place the splint correctly, forcible abduction might compromise the blood supply to the leg or the femur head and so should never be attempted.

Wearing the splint continually leads to the same problem that arises if an infant continually wears plastic pants: severe diaper rash. Teach parents to wash diapers in a mild soap and rinse them well if they use cloth diapers. If they use disposable diapers, they may have to try a number of different brands before they find one that does not cause a rash. The infant's diaper area should be washed with clear water after voiding or defecation. Applying an ointment such as A & D Ointment, Vaseline, or Desitin at each diaper change will protect the skin from urine irritation. Diapers should be changed as frequently as the infant voids or defecates.

Pavik Harness. A *Pavik harness* is an adjustable chest halter that extends the length of the legs and is the method of choice for long-term therapy (Figure 39-22*B*). Soft plastic stirrups (booties) with quick-fastening closures such as Velcro attach to the leg extension straps and hold the hips flexed, abducted, and externally rotated. At a health care setting the infant is laid supine, the thighs are grasped and abducted to place the femoral head into the acetabulum, and the harness is put in place. The harness is worn continually (infants must be sponge bathed). Diaper care is not a problem with the harness in place. Encourage parents to use

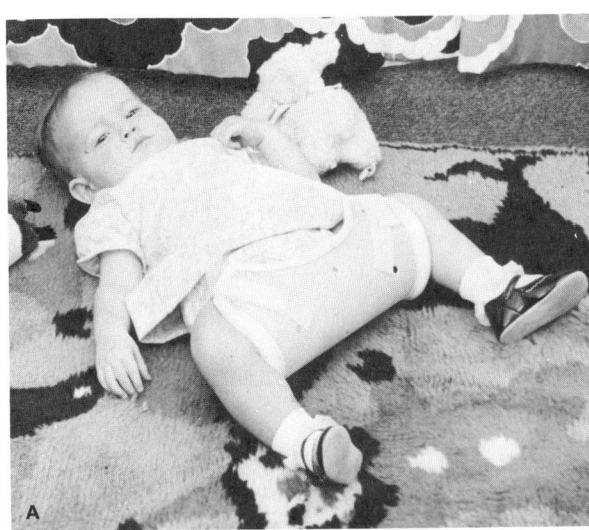

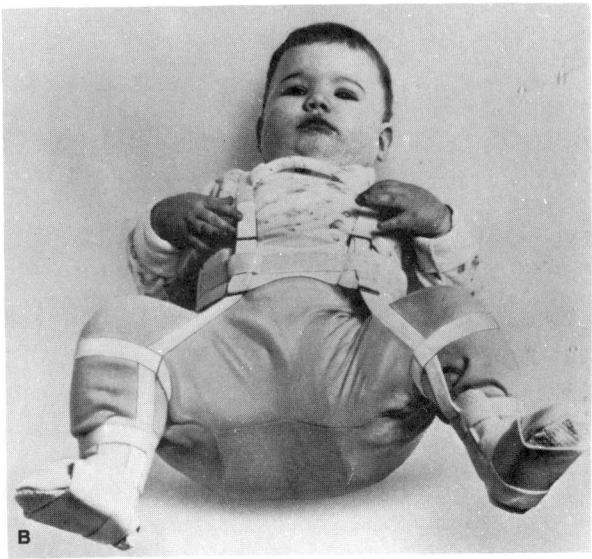

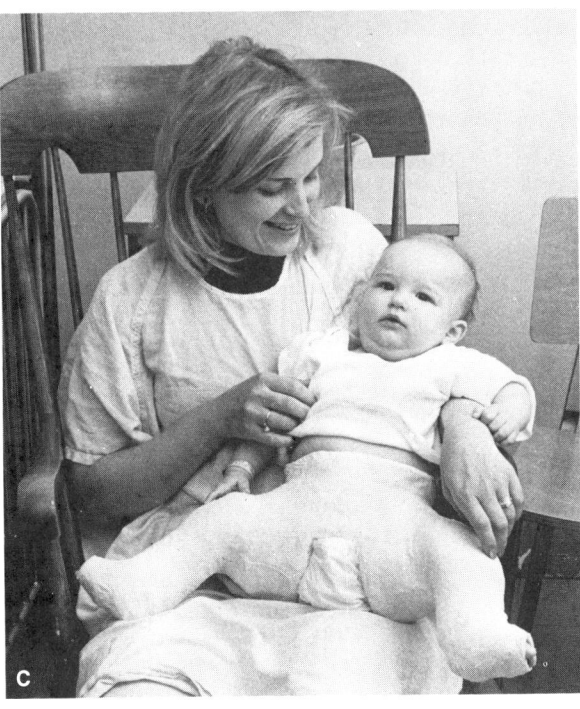

FIGURE 39-22

(**A**) *Hip abduction splint (Frejka splint) holds the hips in an abduction position, forcing the femur head into the acetabulum.* (**B**) *A Pavlik harness.* (**C**) *A hip abduction cast for correction of subluxation of the hip.* (**A** and **C** *courtesy of the Department of Medical Photography, Children's Hospital, Buffalo, NY;* **B** *from Mulley, D. A. Harnessing babies dysplastic hip.* American Journal of Nursing, 84, *1006. Courtesy of Durr-Fillauer Medical, Inc.)*

plastic pants that snap on the sides to keep the harness clean. Parents should assess the skin under the straps daily for irritation or redness. Because the harness does not show under a shirt and long trousers, many parents prefer a Pavik harness as a means of correction.

An advantage of a Pavik harness is that it promotes gentle reduction of the hip. A disadvantage may be that it is not firm enough if a hip is completely dislocated. It will be ineffective if parents remove it. With a few children whose hip is only mildly subluxated, parents may be taught to remove the harness for bathing and to reduce the hip again before it is replaced in the harness.

Spica Cast. If the hip is dislocated or the subluxation is severe, the infant may be placed immediately in a "frog-leg" cast or a spica cast to maintain the externally rotated hip position. The child may first be placed in Bryant's traction for a week to position the hip better. The hip is then placed in an abducted position (usually under general anesthesia) and a large hip spica cast or an A-line cast is applied (Figure 39-22*C*). These casts are heavy and are so wide that dressing infants or containing them in an infant car seat or bassinet is difficult. Newborns are unable to report that a cast is causing circulatory constriction, which necessitates assessing them hourly for the first 24 hours the cast is in place and daily thereafter (see Table 51-1). Teach parents how to do a neurocirculatory assessment before they take an infant home from the hospital to prevent circulatory compression from a rapidly growing limb outgrowing a cast. Parents must understand that casts need to be changed but maintained for 6 to 9 months.

General Care Guidelines. Teach parents from the beginning that the double-diapering may or may not work; the splint or harness may or may not work; surgery may be necessary even after the child has worn casts for a long period. Awareness of these possibilities prevents parents from thinking that their child's condition is so serious that usual methods of treatment have failed. It helps them from becoming discouraged or dissatisfied with health care. It helps them to accept from the beginning that this condition may require long-term correction. Some children are 2 years old before the final cast is removed.

The child and parents will be visiting their orthopedist frequently during these early years. Assess that the parents also schedule general health maintenance visits for routine immunizations and overall growth and development assessment. Spend time during health maintenance visits talking with the parents about infant stimulation. Teach parents to hold their child for feeding and to rock and cuddle the infant, even though the large casts or a harness may be bulky and awkward. Teach parents to bring experiences to the infant, because the child is unable to crawl and walk toward interesting objects in the environment. A child's wagon makes for convenient and fun transportation. The child may also be able to lie prone and move about on a large skate board. Many parents worry that the child who is still in a large cast at the normal age for walking (12 months) won't ever learn to walk. They can be assured that this is not a problem; when the cast is removed, the child will quickly catch up on this developmental step.

Congenital Dislocation of the Hip

In congenital dislocation of the hip (less common than hip subluxation) the femur head is completely dislocated from the acetabulum. The symptoms are the same as those of hip subluxation, but they are generally more extensive and more easily recognized. Abduction is limited; Ortolani's sign invariably is present; shortening of the leg may be evident; the inguinal crease may be deeper than normal.

If children with dislocated hip are not detected before they begin to walk, they walk with a peculiar rolling or "pull-toy" gait, because the femur head moves in and out of the acetabulum. Treatment of dislocation of the hip is by immobilization in a hip spica cast or open reduction followed by casting, as in hip subluxation.

Key Points

- The earlier parents learn about a child's health problem, the easier it is for them to adjust to it. Advocate for parents by helping them obtain as much information as they need.

- Cleft lip and palate result from the failure of the maxillary process to fuse in intrauterine life. The chief nursing diagnoses for these conditions are High risk for altered nutrition: less than body requirements, Ineffective airway clearance, Impaired tissue integrity, Infection, Altered parenting, Self-esteem disturbance, and Altered patterns of communication. Surgical repair is possible early in life with good prognosis for both these conditions.

- Tracheoesophageal atresia and fistula occur from failure of the trachea and esophagus to divide appropriately in intrauterine life. The nursing diagnoses most frequently identified for these conditions are High risk for altered nutrition: less than body requirements and Infection. Surgical intervention often needs to be completed in several procedures.

- Omphalocele is the protrusion of abdominal contents through the abdominal wall at birth, protected only by a peritoneal membrane. When the membrane is not present, this is gastroschisis. Nursing diagnoses most frequently identified are High risk for infection and Altered nutrition. Although several stages of repair are often necessary, surgical correction has a good outcome.

- Intestinal obstruction can result from atresia (complete closure) or stenosis (narrowing) of a part of the bowel. It is associated with hydramnios in pregnancy. The nursing diagnosis most frequently identified is High risk for fluid volume deficit related to vomiting.

- A meconium plug occurs when an extremely hard portion of meconium blocks the lumen of the intestine. Infants with meconium plug syndrome need to be observed for continued bowel function and may have a sweat test done for cystic fibrosis, since meconium plug is often a symptom of this.

- Diaphragmatic hernia occurs when the abdominal organs protrude through a defect in the diaphragm into the chest cavity. This prevents the lungs from fully expanding at birth. The nursing diagnoses for this condition include Ineffective airway clearance and Altered nutrition: less than body requirements related to the misplaced bowel. These infants are critically ill at birth and need extensive surgical correction.

- Imperforate anus is stricture of the anus resulting in inability to pass stool. Nursing diagnoses include Altered nutrition: less than body requirements, Impaired tissue integrity following surgery, and Altered parenting related to a lengthy hospitalization. The infant may have a temporary colostomy done before a final surgical correction.

- Physical anomalies of the nervous system include hydrocephalus (excess of cerebrospinal fluid in the ventricles) and spina bifida (incomplete closure of the spinal cord). Nursing diagnoses identified for the infant with hydrocephalus are High risk for altered nutrition: less than body requirements, Altered skin integrity, Altered cerebral tissue perfusion, Knowledge deficit, and Altered growth and development. Nursing diagnoses for the infant with spina bifida include High risk for infection, High risk for altered nutrition: less than body requirements, Altered cerebral tissue perfusion, Altered skin integrity, Impaired physical mobility, and Altered elimination. Infants with hydrocephalus have a shunt implanted from their ventricles to the peritoneal cavity to remove excess cerebrospinal fluid. Children with myelomeningocele, the most severe form of spinal cord defect, face a permanent loss of lower neuron function that requires continued habilitation.

- Absent or malformed extremities which may occur range from absence of a finger to absence of an entire limb. Children may need physical therapy and teaching on how to use a prosthesis to have full function.
- Hip dysplasia is the improper formation and function of the hip socket; talipes deformities are foot and ankle deformities. Children may need extensive bracing and casting to correct these disorders.
- Parent–infant bonding is often difficult to establish when the child is hospitalized at birth. Assess family relationships at health maintenance visits to see that bonding has occurred.

Critical Thinking Exercises

1. Joshua is a newborn who has been diagnosed with a tracheoesophageal fistula and is waiting transport to an intensive care nursery. What would be important assessments to make? How would you explain this disorder to his parents? They ask you how this could have happened. What would be your answer?

2. Children with subluxated hip may be in casts for a full year or more. What suggestions could you make to a parent to help her instill a strong sense of trust in her child? A sense of autonomy?

3. You notice that the 16-year-old mother of a child born with a cleft lip is obviously upset at the child's appearance. She doesn't want to feed the baby and voices the thought of placing her for adoption. The child's father, a 22-year-old, in contrast, handles the baby warmly and asks questions about surgery. No grandparents visit. What interventions would you want to begin with this family?

References

Adam, A. S., et al. (1991). Evaluation of conservative therapy for exomphalos. *Surgery, Gynecology and Obstetrics, 172,* 394.

Belknap, W. M., & McEvoy, C. (1994). Developmental disorders of gastrointestinal function. In Oski, F. A., et al. *Principles and practice of pediatrics*. Philadelphia: J. B. Lippincott.

Caty, M. G., & Azizkhan, R. G. (1994). Acute surgical conditions of the abdomen. *Pediatric Annals, 23,* 192.

Danner, S. C. (1992). Breastfeeding the infant with a cleft defect. *NAACOGS Clinical Issues in Perinatal and Women's Health Nursing, 3,* 634.

Department of Health & Human Services. (1991). *Healthy people 2000.* Washington, DC: Public Health Service.

Eliason, M. J. (1991). Cleft lip and palate: developmental effects. *Journal of Pediatric Nursing, 8,* 107.

Failla, S., et al. (1992). Planning for a child with hydrocephalus: a guide for the school nurse. *Journal of School Health, 62,* 107.

Fishman, M. A. (1994). Developmental defects. In Oski, F. A., et al. *Principles and practice of pediatrics.* Philadelphia: J. B. Lippincott.

Harris, I. E., et al. (1993). Use of the Pavlik harness for hip displacements. *Clinical Orthopaedics and Related Research, 281,* 29.

Harrison, M. R., & Adzick, N. S. (1991). The fetus as a patient: surgical considerations. *Annals of Surgery, 213,* 279.

Kula, K. (1994). Dental problems. In Oski, F. A., et al. *Principles and practice of pediatrics* (2nd ed.). Philadelphia: J. B. Lippincott.

Lawrence, R. A. (1994). *Breastfeeding: A guide for the medical profession* (4th ed.) St. Louis: C. V. Mosby.

Litwack-Saleh, K. (1993). Practical points in the care of the patient post cleft lip and palate repair. *Journal of Post Anesthesia Nursing, 8,* 35.

Luthy, D. A., et al. (1991). Cesarean section before the onset of labor and subsequent motor function in infants with meningomyelocele diagnosed antenatally. *New England Journal of Medicine, 324,* 882.

Ment, L. R., & Fishman, M. A. (1994). Neuroembryology. In Oski, F. A., et al. *Principles and practice of pediatrics* (2nd ed.). Philadelphia: J. B. Lippincott.

Minsley, G. E., et al. (1991). The effect of cleft palate speech aid prostheses on the nasopharyngeal airway and breathing. *Journal of Prosthetic Dentistry, 85,* 122.

Molenaar, J. C., & Tibboel, D. (1993). Gastroschisis and omphalocele. *World Journal of Surgery, 17,* 337.

Moreno, C. N., et al. (1993). Congenital diaphragmatic hernia. *Neonatal Network 12,* 19.

Oberg, K. C., et al. (1993). Perspectives in cleft lip and palate repair. *Clinics in Plastic Surgery, 20,* 815.

Scheinblum, S. T., & Hammond, M. (1990). The treatment of children with shunt infections: extraventricular drainage system care. *Pediatric Nursing, 18,* 139.

Skinner, M. A., & Grosfeld, J. L. (1993). Inguinal and umbilical hernia repair in infants and children. *Surgical Clinics of North America, 73,* 439.

Staheli, L. T. (1992). *Fundamentals of pediatric orthopedics.* New York: Raven Press.

Todd, N. W. (1993). Common congenital anomalies of the neck: embryology and surgical anatomy. *Surgical Clinics of North America, 73,* 599.

Tomda, P., et al. (1990). Hydrocephalus and porencephaly: prenatal diagnosis by ultrasonography and MR imaging. *Journal of Computer Assisted Tomography, 14,* 843.

Tonnis, D. (1990). Surgical treatment of congenital dislocation of the hip. *Clinical Orthopedics, 258,* 33.

Touloukian, R. J. (1994). Surgical considerations and postoperative care of the newborn. In Oski, F. A., et al. *Principles and practice of pediatrics.* Philadelphia: J. B. Lippincott.

Tucci, M., & Bard, H. (1990). The associated anomalies that determine prognosis in congenital omphalocele. *American Journal of Obstetrics and Gynecology, 163,* 1646.

Van Cleve, L. (1993). Nurses' experience caring for anencephalic infants who are potential organ donors. *Journal of Pediatric Nursing, 8,* 79.

Way, S. (1991). Midwifery: screening for congenital dislocation of the hip. *Nursing Times, 87,* 36.

Wellman, O. O., & Coughlin, S. M. (1991). Preoperative and postoperative nutritional management of the infant with cleft palate. *Journal of Pediatric Nursing, 8,* 154.

Yamate, T., et al. (1993). Growth hormone treatment in achondroplasia. *Journal of Pediatric Endocrinology, 6,* 45.

Suggested Readings

Birdsall, C., & Grief, L. (1990). How do you manage extra ventricular drainage? *American Journal of Nursing, 90,* 47.

Bordarier, C., & Aicardi, J. (1990). Dandy-Walker syndrome and agenesis of the cerebellar vermis: Diagnostic problems and genetic counseling. *Developmental Medicine and Child Neurology, 32,* 285.

Carroll, N. C., & Gross, R. H. (1990). Operative management of clubfoot. *Orthopedics, 13,*1285.

Fisher, J. C. (1991). Feeding children who have cleft lip or palate. *Western Journal of Medicine, 154,* 207.

Gleeson, R. M. (1990). Bowel continence for the child with a neurogenic bowel. *Rehabilitation Nursing, 15,* 319.

Hack, C. H., et al. (1990). Seizures in relation to shunt dysfunction in children with meningomyelocele. *Journal of Pediatrics, 118,* 57.

Johnson, R. V. (1990). Recent developments in care of the newborn. *American Family Physician, 41,* 1783.

Lewis, M. B. (1993). Unilateral cleft lip repair. *Clinics in Plastic Surgery, 20,* 647.

Moody, B. L. (1993). Continuing nursing needs of newborns with myelomeningocele and their families. *Home Healthcare Nurse, 11,* 29.

Moss, G. D., et al. (1991). Routine examination in the neonatal period. *BMJ (British Medical Journal), 302,* 878.

Rescorla, F. J., & Frosfeld, J. L. (1993). Contemporary management of meconium ileus. *World Journal of Surgery, 17,* 318.

Romanczuk, A. N. (1993). Urological issues with the spina bifida population. *Journal of Urology Nursing, 12,* 333.

Sauter, E. R., et al. (1991). Is primary repair of gastroschisis and omphalocele always the best operation? *American Surgery, 57,* 142.

Schaming, D., et al. (1990). When babies are born with orthopedic problems. *RN, 53,* 82.

Takahashi, H., et al. (1994). Eustachian tube compliance in cleft palate. *Laryngoscope, 104,* 83.

White, M. (1990). Continence: independence for the handicapped child. *Nursing Times, 88,* 89.

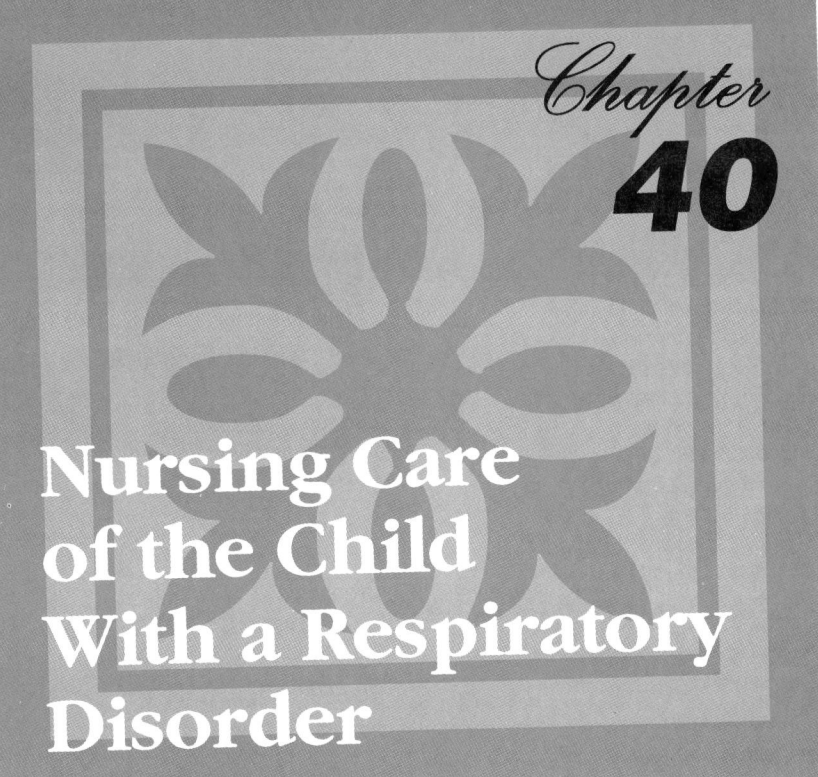

Chapter 40

Nursing Care of the Child With a Respiratory Disorder

Objectives

After mastering the contents of this chapter, you should be able to:

1. Describe common respiratory illnesses in children.

2. Assess the child with a respiratory illness.

3. Formulate a nursing diagnosis related to respiratory illness in children.

4. Plan the nursing care of the child with a respiratory illness, such as planning times for postural therapy.

5. Implement nursing care (e.g., providing oxygen therapy) for the child with a respiratory illness.

6. Evaluate outcome criteria to be certain that nursing goals established for care have been achieved.

7. Identify National Health Goals related to children with respiratory disorders that nurses could be instrumental in helping the nation achieve.

8. Identify areas related to care of children with respiratory disorders that could benefit from additional nursing research.

9. Use critical thinking to analyze ways that nursing care for a child with a respiratory illness could be more family centered.

10. Synthesize knowledge of respiratory illness in children with nursing process to achieve quality maternal and child health nursing care.

Key Terms

- adventitious sounds
- aspiration
- atelectasis
- bronchial breathing
- clubbing
- cupping
- cyanosis
- expiration
- hypoxemia
- hypoxia
- inspiration
- paroxysmal coughing
- percussion
- pneumothorax
- postural drainage
- rales
- retraction
- stridor
- tachypnea
- vesicular breathing
- wheezing

Adele Pillitteri: MATERNAL AND CHILD HEALTH NURSING, 2nd Edition. © 1995 Adele Pillitteri.

Respiratory diseases are among the most frequent causes of illness and hospitalization in children. Because the diseases range from minor illnesses such as a simple upper respiratory tract infection to life-threatening lower-respiratory tract diseases, such as pneumonia, and because they can change in acuteness quickly, respiratory diseases are often hard for parents to evaluate. Overall, respiratory dysfunction in children tends to be more serious than in adults because the lumens in the child's respiratory tract are smaller and therefore more likely to become obstructed in disease. Both the child and parents need a great deal of nursing support when disease interferes with the function of breathing. Early diagnosis and treatment are essential in preventing a minor problem from turning into a more serious disease.

Management of respiratory disease may require, among other treatments, the administration of oxygen, a potentially frightening procedure for children and parents. Care and support from skilled, confident health care personnel are essential; even very young children can panic when breathing becomes labored.

National Health Goals related to children with respiratory illnesses are shown in the Focus on National Health Goals box.

NURSING PROCESS OVERVIEW
for Care of the Child
With a Respiratory Disorder

ASSESSMENT

Respiratory illness can begin at birth when the newborn has difficulty breathing the first breath or establishing regular respirations (see Chapter 23). The Apgar score will help you and other health care personnel to quickly identify the infant who may be experiencing respiratory difficulty at this early stage.

Infants and children are prone to upper respiratory infections. As a nurse in a well-child clinic or health maintenance organization, you are often the first health care provider to talk to a parent about a child's respiratory illness; it is important to establish both onset and duration of the problem so that its seriousness can be determined. Infants who cannot finish a bottle feeding because of exhaustion or rapid breathing and children who cannot run with other children because they do not have enough breath, for examples, should be suspected of having respiratory disease. An episode of acute coughing is suggestive of an acute respiratory disorder.

The child admitted to the hospital with a respiratory illness is usually in an acute stage of the illness; the child's condition may worsen rapidly in the first few

hours until a prescribed antibiotic or bronchodilator begins to take effect. Your assessment that a child is developing tachypnea or retractions may be the first assessment of a child's worsening condition.

NURSING DIAGNOSIS

Nursing diagnoses established for the child with a respiratory illness focus both on the alteration in mechanisms of breathing and on the emotional distress such problems can create. "Ineffective airway clearance" is a common diagnostic category used in this area. The problem may be related to any one of a variety of factors, such as ineffective cough, fatigue, weakness, viscous secretions, pain, aspiration of foreign body, or lack of knowledge about importance of coughing.

The diagnostic categories "Impaired gas exchange"

FOCUS ON
National Health Goals

A number of National Health Goals focus on respiratory illness in children:

- Reduce the initiation of cigarette smoking by children and youth so that no more than 15% have become regular cigarette smokers by age 20 from a baseline of 30%.

- Reduce asthma morbidity as measured by a reduction in asthma hospitalizations to no more than 225 per 100,000 children under 14 years of age, from a baseline of 284 per 100,000.

- Reduce pneumonia-related days of restricted activity in children age 4 and younger to 24 days per 100 children, from a baseline of 27 days per 100 children.

- Reduce tuberculosis to an incidence of no more than 3.5 cases per 100,000 people from a baseline of 9.1 per 100,000 (DHHS, 1991).

Nurses can be instrumental in helping the nation achieve these goals by teaching children to avoid beginning cigarette smoking, teaching programs to help children with asthma learn ways of increasing activity and steps to take to reduce the severity of an attack, and reminding parents to come for child health maintenance visits so that children receive screening for tuberculosis.

Additional nursing research is needed on the accuracy of parents in reading and interpreting tine tests; what motivates children to keep participating in asthma exercise programs; and what new parents need to know to better manage respiratory illness in infants.

and "Ineffective breathing pattern" may also be used, although because the nurse does not generally prescribe definitive treatment for these problems (except when caused by hyperventilation), it may be more appropriate for a nursing diagnosis to focus on the effects of impaired gas exchange or ineffective breathing on daily activities and psychosocial health (Carpenito, 1992). Additional nursing diagnoses include the following:

- Activity intolerance related to insufficient oxygenation
- Fatigue related to impaired gas exchange
- Fear related to inability to breathe without effort
- Impaired social interaction related to difficulty in keeping up with physical activities of peers

PLANNING

If the child is experiencing an acute respiratory problem, the plan of care will focus on supporting the child and family through prescribed therapy and keeping parents informed about their child's health status and response to treatment. Often the treatment period for respiratory illness may be prolonged, and parents of children with chronic conditions need to learn how to continue therapy at home. Helping parents to plan programs of exercise, postural drainage, and continuing medication is an important nursing activity. Parents also need to understand that their approach to these programs must change as their children grow older. With an infant, they simply need to carry out the prescribed procedures. Toddlers may be ready to learn how to do some things for themselves and preschoolers should be ready. A game might be a good way to get across the necessary information ("Simon says cough. Simon says take 5 deep breaths"). Exercise programs for school-age children must be planned around the school day. If a home program is not well designed, an exercise or medication schedule may be so difficult for some parents to maintain that they may carry out the program only sporadically or not at all. Including other family members, such as older siblings (within reason) or grandparents, in this program may help to diffuse the burden of care and also to unite the family in working toward a common goal.

Some organizations to recommend as support to parents of the child with a respiratory disorder include the following:

American Lung Association
1740 Broadway
New York, NY 10019-4374

National Easter Seal Society
70 E. Lake Street
Chicago, IL 60601

IMPLEMENTATION

Collaborative nursing interventions in the care of the child with respiratory dysfunction include suctioning to remove respiratory secretions, administering oxygen, and providing humidification and expectorant therapy to help the child maintain a clear airway. Some of the most important nursing interventions in this area are independent nursing functions: placing the child in an upright position to help her cough more effectively; providing an interesting game to teach her the importance of strengthening chest muscles; supporting the child and family through the anxiety created when the child is not breathing normally; and teaching parents of the child with chronic respiratory dysfunction the basics of percussion techniques. All of these interventions require sound nursing judgment and skill.

EVALUATION

An acute respiratory illness such as pneumonia is extremely frightening for parents. After the child has recovered, talk with the parents to determine if they have come to terms with their fear and are able to treat the child as a well child again. Overprotection of children by their parents may result in well but dependent children. This pattern is one that nursing evaluation can help to prevent.

Evaluating goals for the child with chronic respiratory disease is an ongoing process that will change along with goals as the child grows and develops. No matter what the specific concerns are, however, evaluation should always include examination of how well the child individually and the family as a whole has adapted to manage the constraints of the illness while maintaining a lifestyle that fosters growth and development for all family members.

Expected outcomes may include the following:

- Infant maintains respiratory rate of at least 20 breaths/min.
- Child voices a reduced program of school activities he will maintain in order to reduce fatigue.
- Child's Pao_2 is maintained at 60 to 100 mm Hg in room air.
- Child lists steps he will take if breathing becomes impaired while at school.

Anatomy and Physiology of the Respiratory System

The respiratory system is usually separated into two divisions for discussion: the upper respiratory tract composed of the nose, paranasal sinuses, pharynx, larynx, and epiglottis; and the lower tract composed of the bronchi, bronchioles, and lungs. Through inspiration of air, the respiratory system delivers warmed and moistened air to the alveoli; transports oxygen across the alveolar membrane to hemoglobin-laden red blood cells; and allows carbon dioxide to transfuse from red blood cells back into the alveoli. Through exhalation, carbon dioxide–filled air is discharged to the outside. Levels of oxygen and carbon dioxide in the lungs, blood, and body cells are shown in Figure 40-1.

The respiratory center is located in the medulla of the brain. Changes in body acidity, percentages of carbon dioxide and oxygen, temperature, and blood pressure all stimulate the respiratory center to slow or increase respiratory activity. In the pons, an inhibitory center halts inspiratory impulses before the lungs become overextended. Depth of respiration is influenced by proprioceptors located in the lung periphery that register lung fullness and in the oxygen concentration and *p*H of arterial blood. Children who have chronic lung disease may become so acclimated to a chronically high P_{CO_2} level that reception sites in the blood vessels no longer register this as abnormal. In these instances, the main stimulus for respiration is a low oxygen level. In such children, administering high levels of oxygen may be dangerous, because it alleviates oxygen want and respiratory stimulus.

Respiratory Tract Differences in Children

Embryologic development of the respiratory tract is discussed in Chapter 9. The ethmoidal and maxillary sinuses are present at birth; the frontal sinuses (those sinuses most frequently involved in sinus infection) and the sphenoidal sinuses do not develop until 6 to 8 years of age. Tonsillar tissue is normally enlarged in early school-age children.

Respiratory mucus generally functions as a cleaning agent; newborns produce little respiratory mucus, which makes them more susceptible to respiratory infection than older children. Excessive production of mucus in children up to 2 years of age can readily lead to obstruction because the lumen is so narrow in a child of this age.

After 2 years of age, the right bronchus becomes shorter, wider, and more vertical than the left. For this reason, inhaled foreign bodies more often lodge in the right bronchus. Inhalation is possible in infants only by the use of the abdominal muscles. The change to thoracic breathing begins at 2 to 3 years of age and is

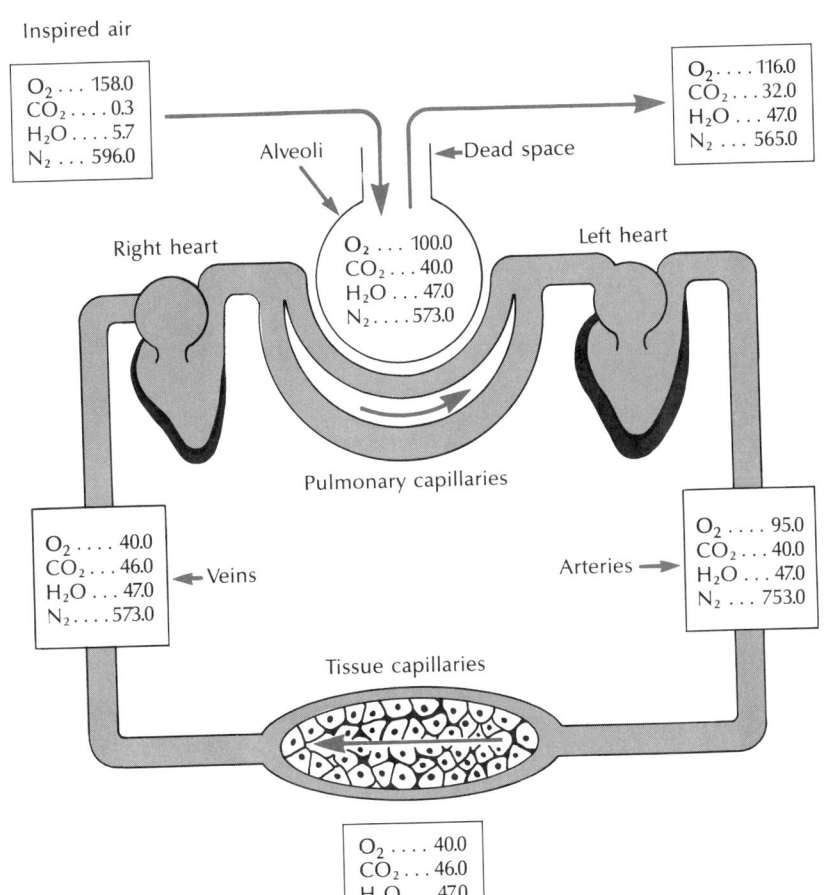

FIGURE 40-1

Partial pressure of gas (mm Hg) as measured in peripheral and systemic circulation. (From Seikurt, E. Basic physiology for the health sciences [2nd ed.]. Boston: Little, Brown, with permission.)

complete at 7 years. Because accessory muscles are used more in children than adults, weakness of these muscles from disease may result in respiratory failure.

In infants, the walls of the airways have less cartilage than in older children and adults and are more likely to collapse following expiration. A lessened amount of smooth muscle in the airway means that an infant does not develop bronchospasm as readily as an older child or adult. Wheezing, the sound of air being pushed through constricted bronchioles, therefore, may not be a prominent finding in infants even when the lumen of the airway is severely compromised.

Assessing Respiratory Illness in Children

Assessment of respiratory illness in children will include an interview, physical examination, and laboratory testing. If the child is in acute distress, the interview and health history may cover only the most important details: when the child first became ill and what symptoms are present. It is important, however, to get as accurate a picture as possible, because the problem could be the result of a variety of causes (Figure 40-2).

Common terms used to describe respiratory dysfunction are given in Table 40-1. It is important to take a thorough history because the symptoms of **hypoxemia** (deficient oxygenation of the blood) are often insidious (see the Focus on Cultural Awareness box). There is peripheral vasoconstriction (a mechanism to save the available oxygen for central life-sustaining body organs) that leads to a pale appearance. Tachypnea and tachycardia (efforts to oxygenate better), anxiety, and confusion (due to limited brain perfusion) may occur. A poor feeding pattern may be one of the first signs noted in the infant because an infant cannot suck and breathe rapidly at the same time. Cardiac arrhythmia may occur due to poor heart perfusion (James & Sharma, 1990).

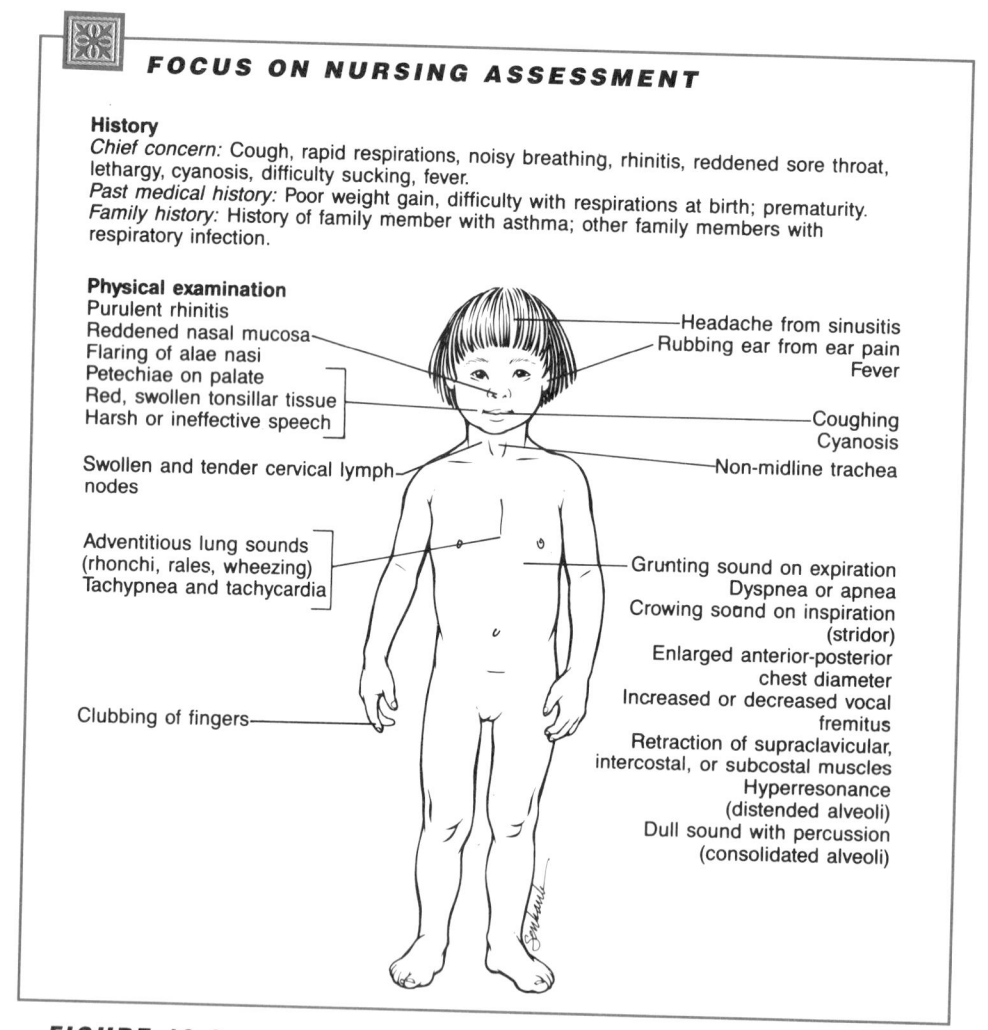

FOCUS ON NURSING ASSESSMENT

History
Chief concern: Cough, rapid respirations, noisy breathing, rhinitis, reddened sore throat, lethargy, cyanosis, difficulty sucking, fever.
Past medical history: Poor weight gain, difficulty with respirations at birth; prematurity.
Family history: History of family member with asthma; other family members with respiratory infection.

Physical examination
Purulent rhinitis
Reddened nasal mucosa
Flaring of alae nasi
Petechiae on palate
Red, swollen tonsillar tissue
Harsh or ineffective speech

Swollen and tender cervical lymph nodes

Adventitious lung sounds (rhonchi, rales, wheezing)
Tachypnea and tachycardia

Clubbing of fingers

Headache from sinusitis
Rubbing ear from ear pain
Fever

Coughing
Cyanosis

Non-midline trachea

Grunting sound on expiration
Dyspnea or apnea
Crowing sound on inspiration (stridor)
Enlarged anterior-posterior chest diameter
Increased or decreased vocal fremitus
Retraction of supraclavicular, intercostal, or subcostal muscles
Hyperresonance (distended alveoli)
Dull sound with percussion (consolidated alveoli)

FIGURE 40-2
Common signs and symptoms of respiratory dysfunction.

Term	Description
Apnea	Lack of respirations
Dyspnea	Difficulty in the force or rate of respiratory exchange
Tachypnea	Increased rate of respiration
Hypoxia	Low oxygen content in body tissues
Hypoxemia	Deficit oxygen content in the bloodstream
Anoxia	Reduction of oxygen in body tissues below physiologically adequate levels
Hyperventilation	Rapid, deep breathing
Hypoventilation	Shallow breathing

Table 40-1. *Commonly Used Respiratory Assessment Terms*

Physical Assessment

Physical assessment of the child with respiratory dysfunction includes observation of such presenting symptoms as cough, cyanosis, or pallor, as well as evaluation of respirations and lung sounds.

Cough

A cough reflex is initiated by stimulation of the nerves of the respiratory tract mucosa by the presence of dust, chemicals, mucus, or inflammation. The sound of coughing is caused by rapid expiration past the glottis. Coughing is a useful procedure to clear excess mucus or foreign bodies from the respiratory tract. It becomes harmful and needs suppression only when there is no mucus or debris to be expelled. This might occur with respiratory tract inflammation. A series of expiratory coughs following a deep inspiration is **paroxysmal coughing**; it occurs in children with pertussis (whooping cough). Coughing increases chest pressure and may decrease venous return to the heart. This lowers cardiac output and may lead to fainting (syncope). Paroxysmal coughing may increase the pressure in the central venous circulation to such an extent that there is bleeding into the central nervous system. Young children often vomit following a series of coughs and may be suspected first of having a gastric disturbance.

Rate and Depth of Respirations

Tachypnea is an increased respiratory rate. It is often the first indicator of airway obstruction in children. When assessing respiratory rate, particularly in infants, try to count the rate before waking an infant, since crying distorts respiratory rate. Assess also the depth and quality of respiration, which are also affected by anoxia.

Retractions

When children must inspire more forcefully than normally to inflate their lungs because of an airway obstruction or stiff, noncompliant lungs such as occur in newborns with pulmonary dysplasia, intrapleural pressure is decreased so much that the nonrigid parts of the chest (the intercostal spaces) draw inward, creating **retractions** (Figure 40-3). Retractions occur more often in the newborn and infant than in the older child, because the intercostal tissues are weak and underdeveloped in the young child. Retraction of upper chest muscles (supracostal or suprasternal) suggests upper airway obstruction; retraction of intercostal or subcostal muscles suggests lower airway obstruction.

Restlessness

When children or infants have difficulty securing adequate oxygen (**hypoxia**), they become anxious and restless. In infants, this restlessness along with tachypnea may be one of the first signs of airway obstruction. Be careful that you do not interpret the excessive movements of infants with respiratory distress as a sign that they are improving; anxious, restless stirring may be their only way of saying that their respiratory obstruction is becoming acute.

Cyanosis

Cyanosis, or a blue tinge to the skin, becomes apparent when Po_2 is under 40 mm Hg or the unoxygenated hemoglobin percentage increases over 3 g/100 mL, since incompletely oxygenated red blood cells in the circulation are what give blood a dark color. If children have a low red blood cell count, cyanosis may not be apparent because there are not enough red blood cells to give the arterial blood a blue (venous) color. This occurs at hemoglobin levels below 5 mg/100 mL. The degree of

FOCUS ON CULTURAL AWARENESS

Upper respiratory illnesses occur universally, making them a concern of parents the world over. Home remedies for such illnesses vary greatly, however. Hanging garlic around a child's neck is a frequent therapy in Mediterranean countries. Herbs may be used the same way by parents from the Far East or South America (Geissler, 1994). It is important to respect these remedies and not remove them when they are discovered. Although the therapeutic value of these remedies may not be proven, it is important to the nurse–patient and nurse–family relationships to respect family traditions.

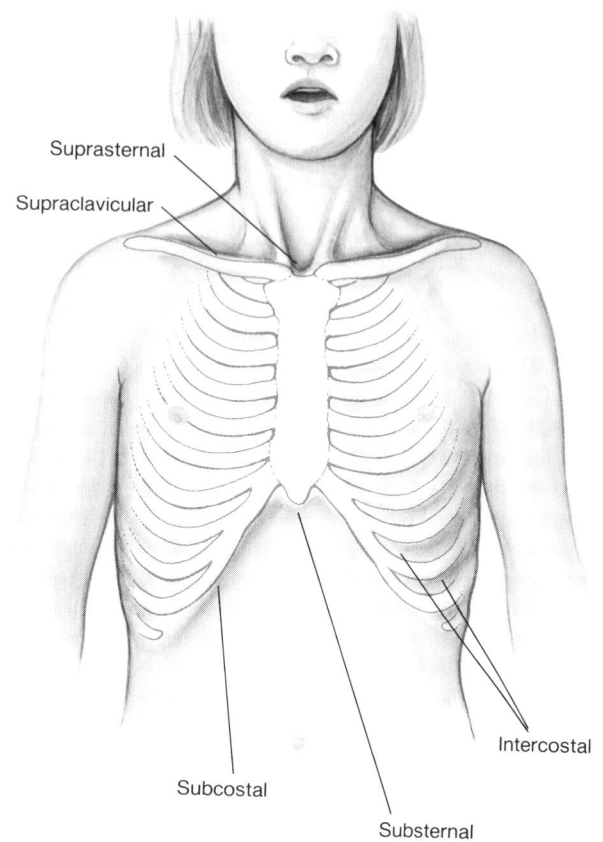

FIGURE 40-3
Sites of respiratory retraction.

cyanosis present, therefore, is not always an accurate indication of the degree of airway difficulty.

If children cannot inspire around an airway obstruction, they cannot provide sufficient oxygen to alveoli to saturate the arterial blood; cyanosis is the result. Children increase their respiratory efforts in an attempt to supply more oxygen. When they do this, the difference in pressure between the intralumen of the trachea and the surrounding tissue becomes so great that the trachea may collapse, compounding the obstruction problem. When children have accompanying peripheral vasoconstriction caused by shock, cyanosis of the extremities may not be apparent.

Clubbing of Fingers

Children with chronic respiratory illnesses develop **clubbing** of the fingers, a change in the angle of the nail to the fingertip because of increased capillary growth in the fingertips (Figure 40-4).

Adventitious Sounds

Adventitious sounds, or extra breathing sounds caused by pathology, heard on lung assessment in respiratory disease are shown in Table 40-2; their locations are shown in Figure 40-5. On auscultation, the inspiratory sound is normally softer and longer than the expiratory sound. This is referred to as **vesicular breathing**. Over the trachea, this pattern in terms of the length of **inspiration** (breathing in) and **expiration** (breathing out) is reversed. This is referred to as **bronchial** or **tubular breathing**. Bronchial breath sounds heard out in the periphery of the lungs, where normally you would expect to hear a vesicular pattern, indicate that gas exchange in peripheral alveoli is being compromised (such as happens in pneumonia) and you are listening to transmitted tracheal sounds.

Accessory sounds of respiration result from the vibrations produced as air is forced past obstructions such as mucus. If the obstruction is in the nose or pharynx, the noise produced is a snoring sound (rhonchi). If the obstruction is at the base of the tongue or in the larynx, a harsh, strident sound will be heard on inspiration. This is laryngeal **stridor**. It is often most marked when children are in a supine position, less marked when children sit upright. If the obstruction is in the lower trachea or bronchioles, it becomes most noticeable on expiration; the sound heard (**wheezing**) is an expiratory sound. If the alveoli become fluid filled, fine crackling sounds (**rales**) are heard. Respiratory sounds are heard best if children are not crying; therefore, infants should be soothed and held so they are quiet while their chests are being auscultated.

Chest Diameters

With chronic obstructive lung disease, children may be unable to expire, allowing air to be chronically trapped

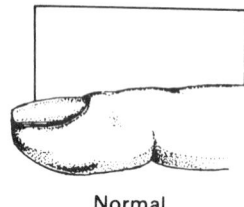
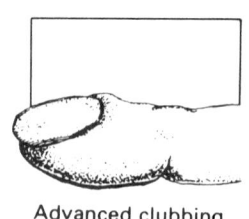

Normal   Early clubbing   Advanced clubbing

FIGURE 40-4
*Clubbing of the fingers. (**Left**) The angle between the nail and digit is about 20 degrees in a normal child. (**Center**) Flattened angle represents early stage of clubbing. (**Right**) In advanced clubbing, the nail is rounded over the end of the finger. Note also that the distal phalanx is bulbous and of greater depth than the proximal portion of the finger (interphalangeal depth). (From Buckingham, W. B. A primer of clinical diagnosis [2nd ed.]. Hagerstown, MD: Harper and Row.)*

Table 40-2. *Adventitious Findings Revealed by Auscultation and Palpation in Respiratory Disease*

Term	Definition	Finding
Rales	The sound of air passing through fluid in alveoli	Crackling sound, similar to the crinkling of tissue paper
Rhonchi	The sound of air passing through fluid in major airways	Loud, snoring sound
Wheezing	The sound of air being pushed through narrowed bronchi on expiration	Whistling sound
Stridor	The sound of air being pulled past a narrowed larynx on inspiration	Crowing-rooster sound
Resonance	The percussion sound heard over normal lung tissue	Loud, low tone
Hyperresonance	The percussion sound heard over hyperinflated lung tissue	Louder, lower sound than with resonance

in lung alveoli (hyperinflation). This produces an elongated anteroposterior diameter. There is an accompanying tympanic or hyperresonant (loud and hollow) sound heard on percussion over lung spaces.

Laboratory Tests

There are a number of laboratory tests that can be used to confirm or rule out the presence of a respiratory problem and to help identify the cause and severity of the problem. These include analysis of arterial blood gases, nasopharyngeal culture, sputum analysis, and sweat chloride analysis. The sweat chloride test, which is used in the diagnosis of cystic fibrosis, is discussed along with that disorder, later in this chapter. The other tests are described below.

Blood Gas Studies

Blood gas studies are important determinants of the effectiveness of ventilation and acid-base status. The normal values of blood gases are shown in Table 40-3.

Blood gas analysis provides important information about oxygenation of the blood. Values may indicate not only whether the PO_2 (peripheral oxygen) is adequate but also whether the hemoglobin saturation is adequate. The hemoglobin saturation level will fall if adequate oxygen cannot reach the bloodstream because of obstructive lung disease or if the hemoglobin is defective and cannot carry a full complement of oxygen (this occurs with sickle cell anemia or thalassemia major). If children have a severe anemia, the hemoglobin saturation may be adequate (97%), but body cells may not be receiving enough oxygen because of the limited number

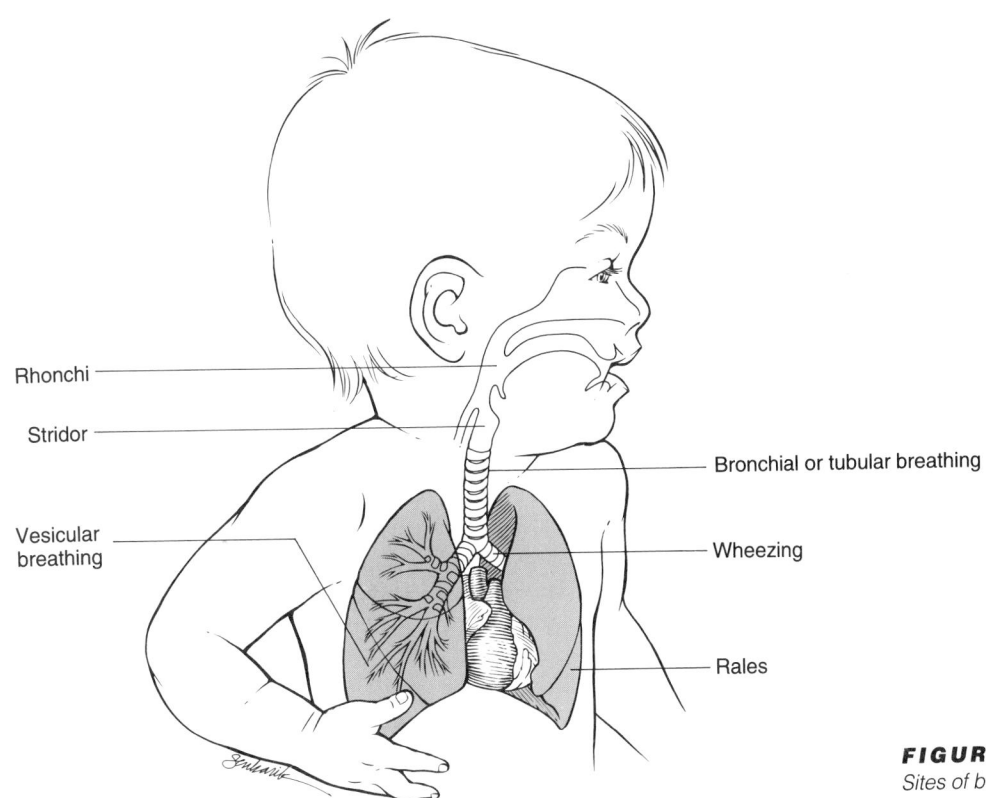

Rhonchi
Stridor
Vesicular breathing
Bronchial or tubular breathing
Wheezing
Rales

FIGURE 40-5
Sites of breathing patterns and lung sounds.

Table 40-3. *Blood Gas Values*

Measure	Definition	Normal Value	Clinical Significance
P_{O_2}	Partial pressure of oxygen in arterial blood	80–100 mm Hg	Will be decreased if child cannot inspire adequately
P_{CO_2}	Partial pressure of carbon dioxide in arterial blood	35–45 mm Hg	Will be increased if child cannot expire adequately
O_2 saturation	The percentage of hemoglobin carrying oxygen	96%–98%	Will be decreased if O_2 cannot reach red blood cells, if unoxygenated cells are being mixed with oxygenated ones, or if hemoglobin is defective
pH	The hydrogen ion concentration of blood	7.35–7.45	Value will be decreased if CO_2 is being retained as carbonic acid in blood
HCO_3	The bicarbonate concentration in blood	22–26 mEq/L	Will be decreased in compensated respiratory alkalosis; increased in respiratory alkalosis
Base excess	Bicarbonate available for buffering	−2.5 or +2.5 mEq/L	+ = alkaline excess − = alkaline deficit

of red blood cells present. With increased P_{CO_2} or decreased P_{O_2}, a low pH, or decreased temperature, the ability of hemoglobin to accept oxygen will diminish.

P_{CO_2} measures the efficiency of ventilation. Children who are hypoventilating will have an increased P_{CO_2}; children who are hyperventilating will have a decreased P_{CO_2}. When children cannot evacuate accumulated carbon dioxide because of an obstruction or hypoventilation, they show an increase in the partial pressure of carbon dioxide in the arterial blood, in the concentration of carbonic acid (formed when carbon dioxide dissolves in

plasma), and in the concentration of hydrogen ions. This can lead to acidosis (a decrease in serum pH or an increase in acidity; Anderson, 1990).

If an airway obstruction is partial, the body can compensate for a long time by increasing kidney tubular reabsorption of bicarbonate. When an airway obstruction is relieved (by removal of the obstruction or by assisted ventilation), the amount of bicarbonate present in the bloodstream may exceed the amount of acid factor produced and the child's condition may change to alkalosis. Alkalosis causes a decreased respiratory rate (to

Table 40-4. *Comparison of Respiratory Alkalosis and Respiratory Acidosis*

Acid-Base Condition	Cause	Findings

Respiratory alkalosis	Hyperventilation	Rapid, deep breathing
		Confusion, unconsciousness
		Elevated plasma pH (above 7.45)
		Elevated urine pH (above 7)
		Decreased P_{CO_2} (below 40 mm Hg)
		Plasma bicarbonate
		  Initially normal
		  Compensated: below 20 mEq/L
		Base excess: 0 or a negative reading such as −4

Respiratory acidosis	Hypoventilation trapping carbon dioxide in alveoli	Shallow breathing; inability to expire freely
		Confusion, disorientation
		Decreased plasma pH (below 7.35)
		Decreased urine pH (below 6)
		Elevated P_{CO_2} (over 40 mm Hg)
		Plasma bicarbonate
		  Initially normal
		  Compensated: above 25 mEq/L
		Base excess: 0 or a positive reading such as +4

conserve carbon dioxide), and periods of apnea may result. Children need to be observed carefully when this occurs. Blood gas and electrolyte determinations should be made so that the systemic changes can be reversed when they occur.

Respiratory alkalosis and respiratory acidosis are compared in Table 40-4. Box 40-1 shows steps for evaluating arterial blood gases.

To analyze blood gases, arterial blood rather than venous blood must be used (arterial blood will reflect how well the lungs are oxygenating the blood, whereas venous blood will only reflect the metabolism of the particular extremity from where the blood was drawn). In the young infant, the temporal artery may be used as a site; in newborns, an umbilical artery catheter can be positioned. In older children, the radial artery is the site of choice, because of the collateral circulation present at the wrist. (If clotting should occur in the radial artery, the hand would still be well nourished by collateral circulation; see the Allen Test in Box 40-2.) Blood is drawn by a heparinized syringe to prevent clotting in the sy-

ringe. After arterial puncture, the site must be compressed fully, or the pressure in the vessel punctured will cause seepage of blood into subcutaneous tissue. Large hematomas will form, obscuring the site for further assessment. A peripheral or subclavian arterial catheter may be inserted to allow frequent determinations to be made without additional punctures. Young children need to have a bandage over the point where the arterial catheter emerges so that they will not fuss with it. They may need a restraint, such as an elbow restraint, to keep them from dislodging this important assessment route.

In small infants, when it is impossible to obtain arterial blood directly, heel or finger pricks may be used. If the heel or finger is warmed for about 20 minutes in warm water before the procedure, local blood flow increases so much that the blood gas levels of the capillaries approach those of arteries.

Be certain to mark laboratory slips as to whether any oxygen was being used at the time and the percentage of liter flow as well as the site from which the spec-

---

Box 40-1
Interpreting ABGs

ABGs can be quite simple to understand if you follow a systematic format such as this one.

Step 1. Evaluate the *p*H: Normally, *p*H falls between 7.35 and 7.45. A *p*H below 7.35 reflects acidemia; one above 7.45 reflects alkalemia. If the patient has more than one acid-base imbalance at work, the *p*H identifies the process in control.

Step 2. Evaluate ventilation: The partial pressure of arterial CO_2 (PCO_2) normally lies between 35 and 45 mm Hg. A PCO_2 greater than 45 mm Hg indicates ventilatory failure and respiratory acidosis. A PCO_2 less than 35 mm Hg indicates alveolar hyperventilation and respiratory alkalosis.

Step 3. Evaluate metabolic process: A bicarbonate (HCO_3^-) less than 22 mEq/L and/or a base excess (BE) less than −2 mEq/L reflect metabolic acidosis. A bicarbonate level greater than 26 mEq/L and/or a BE greater than 2 mEq/L reflect metabolic alkalosis. Remember, if the two conflict, the BE is the better indicator of metabolic status.

Step 4. Determine primary and compensating disorder: Often, two acid-base imbalances coincide; one is primary, the other is the body's attempt to return the *p*H to normal. In most cases, when both the PCO_2 and the HCO_3^- are abnormal, one reflects the primary acid-base disorder and the other reflects the compensating disorder.

To decide which is which, check the *p*H. *Only a process of acidosis can make the pH acidic; only a process of alkalosis can make the pH alkaline.* For

example, if steps 2 and 3 indicate that the patient has respiratory acidosis and metabolic alkalosis and the *p*H is 7.25, the primary disorder must be respiratory acidosis. The remaining disorder is compensating for the primary problem.

When interpreting ABGs, keep in mind that three states of compensation are possible: *noncompensation,* reflected in an alteration of only PCO_2 or HCO_3^-; *partial compensation,* when both PCO_2 and HCO_3^- are abnormal and, because compensation is incomplete, the *p*H is also abnormal; and *complete compensation,* when both PCO_2 and HCO_3^- are abnormal but, because compensation is complete, the *p*H is normal. To identify the primary disorder when compensation is complete, consider a *p*H between 7.35 and 7.40 indicative of primary acidosis and a *p*H between 7.40 and 7.45 indicative of primary alkalosis.

Step 5. Evaluate oxygenation: Normally, PO_2 remains between 80 and 100 mm Hg. A PO_2 between 60 and 80 mm Hg reflects mild hypoxemia; between 40 and 60 mm Hg, moderate hypoxemia; and below 40 mm Hg, severe hypoxemia.

Step 6. Interpret: Your final analysis should include the degree of compensation, the primary disorder, and the oxygenation status, for example, "partially compensated respiratory acidosis with moderate hypoxemia."

Abbreviation: ABGs, arterial blood gases; BE, base excess.
(From Anderson, S. [1990]. ABGs: Six easy steps to interpreting blood gases. *American Journal of Nursing, 90,* 42.)

Before an arterial line is inserted into the radial artery, it is important to establish that the child has collateral circulation to the hand. Otherwise, the catheter will block the artery and effectively block blood flow to the hand.

To prove that there is collateral circulation, compress both the radial and ulnar arteries on the inner side of the wrist and elevate the hand until color disappears. Release the pressure over the ulnar artery and observe for a color change in the hand. If the hand does not pinken (proof the blood has flowed into the hand), the radial artery on that wrist should not be used for catheter insertion.

imen was obtained. Keep blood gas specimens on ice during transport to the laboratory to keep the sample accurate (carbon dioxide levels decline in room air).

Two *noninvasive methods* for measuring oxyhemoglobin saturation include transcutaneous oxygen monitoring and pulse oximetry, as described below.

Transcutaneous Oxygen Monitoring

Transcutaneous monitoring is a means of continuous, noninvasive measurement of blood gases. For the determination, electrodes heated to 44°C are attached to the infant's chest. The heat causes vasodilation underneath the skin and brings the peripheral arterial blood to the surface to be read for oxygen content. This is converted to millimeters of mercury for a monitor readout. The PO_2 read by this method correlates with intraarterial PO_2.

Pulse Oximetry

Pulse oximetry, like transcutaneous monitoring, is a continuous, noninvasive technique (Carroll, 1993). For the measurement, a sensor and photodetector are placed around a vascular bed, most often a finger. Infrared light is directed through the finger from the sensor to the photodetector. Because hemoglobin absorbs light waves differently when it is bound to oxygen than when it is not, the oximeter can detect the degree of oxygen saturation (SaO_2) in the hemoglobin.

Oxygen saturation is closely aligned with PO_2 (Figure 40-6). As can be seen in Figure 40-6, when PO_2 is within the normal range of 80 to 100 mm Hg, the oxygen saturation is 95%. When oxygen concentration has fallen to 60 mm Hg, the SaO_2 is 85% (Spyr & Preach, 1990).

Pulse oximetry works well with children because it is noninvasive. However, the sensor is small, and it must be checked frequently to see that it remains in place. Excess light in a room may distort the reading, so the sensor may need to be covered with a blanket in an intensive care unit or nursery.

Continuous monitoring allows you to modify your care appropriately. If an oxygen level begins to fall while you are handling an infant, for example, you would immediately stop care until the infant's PO_2 again returns to normal.

Nasopharyngeal Culture

When done efficiently, nasopharyngeal cultures cause little discomfort, but most children are terribly frightened by the taking of a nose and throat culture and resist accordingly. Firm, calm support during the procedure is essential. Nose and throat cultures can only reveal organisms present in the upper respiratory tract; they may not reveal organisms causing a lower respiratory tract infection. A throat culture will miss pathogenic organisms if the culture tip is not touched to the infected aspect of the pharynx.

Sputum Analysis

Children younger than school age cannot raise sputum with a cough, which makes sputum collection rarely feasible. Older children are able to cough and raise sputum and, with proper instruction as to what is needed (a specimen of what they are coughing up, not just clearing from the back of their throat), sputum samples for analysis can be obtained.

Diagnostic Procedures

There are also a number of diagnostic procedures commonly used to identify respiratory disease in children. Many of these procedures are also used with adults, but modified to take into account the physical and developmental differences of children. Bronchoscopy, which is

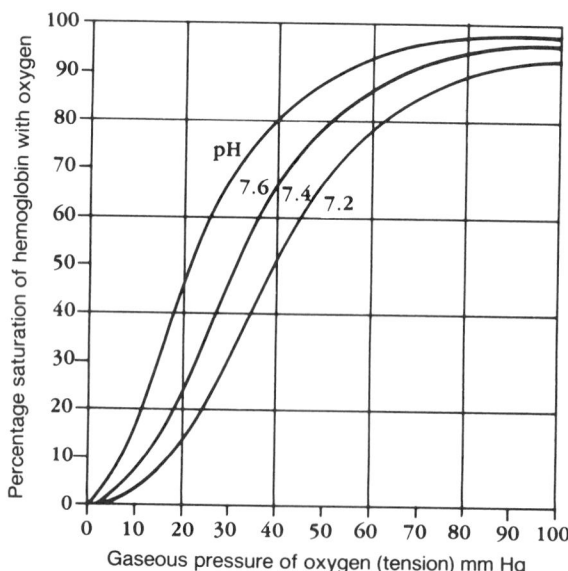

FIGURE 40-6

Oxyhemoglobin dissociation curve. (From Bullock, B. L., Rosendahl, P. P. [1992]. Pathophysiology: Adaptations and alterations in function *(3rd ed.) Philadelphia, J.B. Lippincott, p. 570.)*

visualization of the bronchi through a bronchoscope, is discussed in Chapter 37. Radiologic examination (chest x-ray and bronchography) and pulmonary function testing are discussed below.

Chest X-ray

Chest x-ray films will reveal areas of infiltration or consolidation in the lungs; if a foreign body is opaque, an x-ray study will reveal its location (Figure 40-7). Chest x-ray films are more difficult to take in infants than in older children, because infants cannot take a breath and hold it on instruction. It is therefore difficult to picture the lungs at their most expanded position. Computed tomography (CT) scans may be ordered for children with chronic lung disease (Lynch et al., 1990).

Bronchography

On a chest x-ray film, the air-filled larynx, trachea, and major bronchi are revealed. Any obstruction or distortion in the organs will be apparent. For further definition of structures, a radiopaque solution may be introduced into the respiratory tract by an ultrasonic nebulizer or by catheter before the x-ray study is made. Children may have an increase in mucus production after dye instillation from bronchial irritation by the dye. Observe children carefully after such a procedure for possible respiratory obstruction from accumulating mucus.

Pulmonary Function Studies

Alveoli of the lungs are never completely empty at the end of expiration because the bronchioles collapse, trapping air in the alveoli; they are never completely filled by inspiration because their potential for expansion exceeds that necessary for good respiratory function. Children with obstructive lung diseases such as asthma or cystic fibrosis have some difficulty moving air into the lungs; they have chronic difficulty moving air out of the lungs. Even if they can expire the same amount of air as the average child, they will expire it over a longer time period. Children with restrictive ventilatory disorders, such as neuromuscular disorders, will have equal difficulty with inspiration and expiration. (See Chapter 42 for further discussion of pulmonary function studies for children with asthma.)

A number of lung capacity studies can be done to determine the degree of obstruction or restricted ventilation ability. The child breathes into a *spirometer*, a device that records the air exchange, or a computerized vital capacity chamber (Figure 40-8). Common pulmonary function tests are outlined in Table 40-5.

Children under 4 years of age are usually unable to participate in pulmonary function tests because their cooperation is required. However, all children need good preparation and teaching because they must breathe forcefully through the mouth into a mouthpiece on cue. Some tests require that the nose be closed by a metal clamp or an assistant's hand while the child blows out. This is a frightening feeling for children with respiratory disease. They may need some trial runs to assure themselves that they can breathe with the metal clamp in place. Without good orientation to the equipment, they may become so anxious about their performance

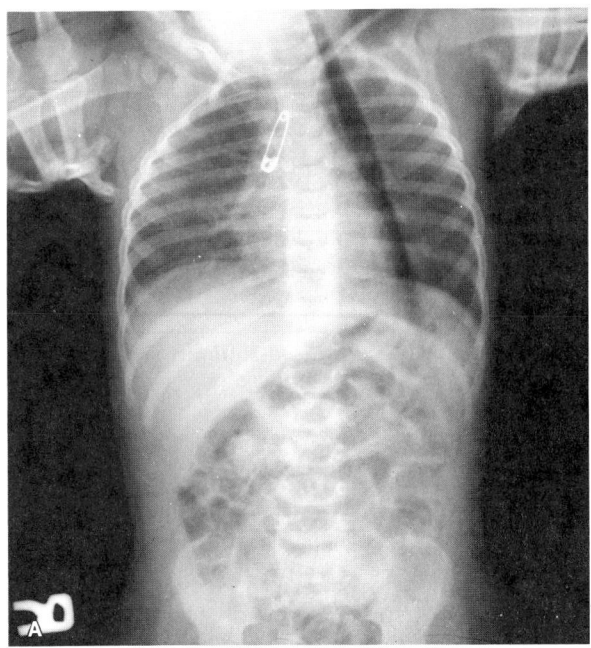
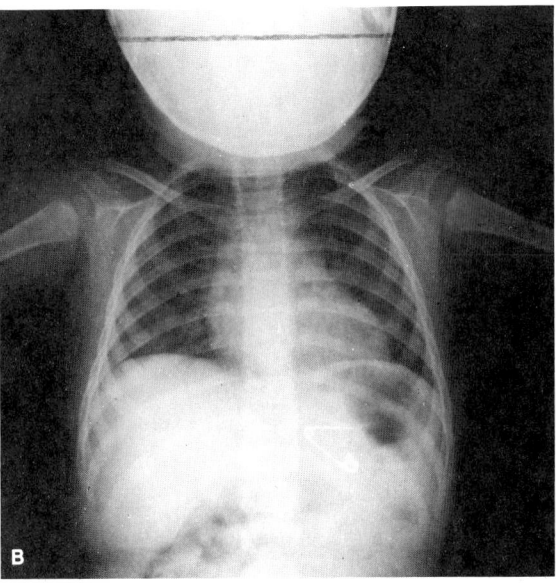

FIGURE 40-7
(**A**) *Chest x-ray film demonstrates a safety pin lodged in a bronchus.* (**B**) *A safety pin in the stomach.*
(Courtesy of J. P. Kuhn, M.D., Children's Hospital, Buffalo, NY.)

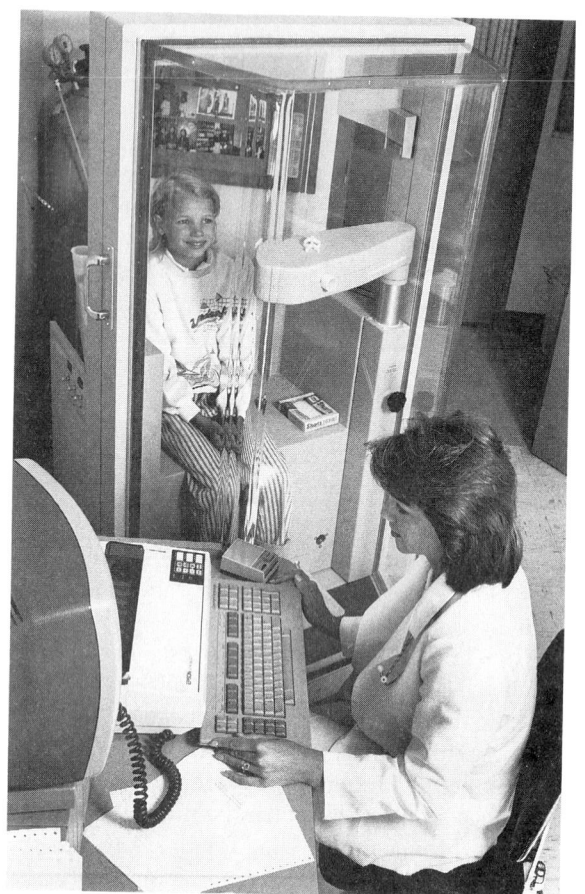

FIGURE 40-8
Assessing respiratory capacity by body plethysmography or use of a computerized vital capacity chamber. (Courtesy of the Department of Medical Photography, Children's Hospital, Buffalo, NY.)

that they have tachypnea and so do not inhale or exhale at their full capacity, thus skewing the test results.

The results of pulmonary function studies help determine the nature and extent of a child's respiratory problem and the best methods for achieving more effective ventilation.

Therapeutic Techniques Used in the Treatment of Respiratory Illness in Children

The primary goal of nursing interventions in the care of children with respiratory illness is to maintain or reestablish the airway to provide adequate oxygen to the blood. Often this will include interventions aimed at liquefying and removing mucus secretions so they do not clog the bronchial pathways; such clogging can prevent adequate oxygenation as well as contribute to the development of bronchial infections. Drugs commonly used in the treatment of respiratory disorders appear in Table 40-6.

Expectorant Therapy

Irritation of the respiratory tract causes the production of large amounts of mucus. The amount produced is often so great that the natural mechanisms for clearing it— coughing and upward cilia action—are not adequate. If children are breathing rapidly because of respiratory distress, the frequent passage of air over the mucus tends to dry it and make it more viscid. A number of measures may be employed to liquefy and raise mucus.

Oral Fluid

One of the best and most efficient means of lowering the viscosity of mucus is to keep the child well hydrated. Offering frequent sips of water or administering fluid intravenously will prevent dehydration. Keep careful intake and output records.

Liquefying Agents

Pharmacologic agents (expectorants) such as guaifenesin (Robitussin) can be administered to liquefy mucus. Instilling saline nose drops can be effective in liquefying dried mucus in the nose.

Table 40-5. Pulmonary Function Tests

Test	Measurement	Clinical Implications
Vital capacity (VC)	The maximum amount of air expelled after a maximum inspiration	Will be decreased if bronchial lumens are narrowed or obstructed
Tidal volume (TV)	The amount of air inhaled and exhaled in a normal respiratory movement	Will be decreased if bronchial lumens are constricted
Residual volume	The amount of air remaining in the lungs after a maximum expiration	Will be increased if there is air trapping in alveoli, as in obstructive lung disease
Functional residual capacity (FRC)	The volume of air remaining in the lungs after a normal expiration	Will be increased if ability to breathe out is impaired
Forced expiratory volume (FEV)	The amount of air expired in 1 sec	Will be decreased in obstructive disease that prevents free expiration

Table 40-6. *Drugs Commonly Used With Respiratory Disorders*

Classification	Example	Action	Nursing Responsibility
Antibiotics	Neomycin Polymyxin B sulfate	Decreases microorganisms by direct contact in respiratory tract	Ask if child has any known allergies to antibiotics.
Expectorants	Guaifenesin (Robitussin)	Helps to raise respiratory secretions	Monitor child for drowsiness.
Bronchodilators	Ephedrine Isoetharine (Bronkosol) Isoproterenol hydrochloride (Isuprel) Racemic epinephrine	Increases lumen of bronchial tubes	Monitor child for insomnia and anxiety.

Humidification

Humidification is the provision of a liquefying agent or moisture to the airway. Common methods of delivering moisture are by vaporizer, nebulizer, and mist tent.

Vaporizers. Vaporizers may provide either a cool or a warm mist. Most hospitals use only cool mist vaporizers, since warm mist moisturizers can cause a serious scald burn if children accidentally pull a vaporizer over on themselves. To avoid this type of accident when using any type of vaporizer, be certain it is never placed within reach of the child. Although cool mist can create a clammy atmosphere in a room, this can be an advantage if a child has a fever. Vaporizers should be returned to a central supply department for thorough cleaning following each use; any residual water can readily grow *Pseudomonas* organisms.

Nebulizers. Nebulizers are mechanical devices that provide a stream of moistened air into the respiratory tract. A nebulizer can be a simple hand-held apparatus (a metered-dose nebulizer) or can be attached to an electrical pump as a power source (Figure 40-9). Ultrasonic nebulization delivers such minuscule droplets into the respiratory tract that even the finest bronchioles can be moistened. Drugs such as detergents, antibiotics, or bronchodilators can be combined with the nebulized mist.

Many children find nebulizer treatments uncomfortable because they are frightened by the feel of the mist in their upper respiratory tract. Assure them that aerosol administration is the most effective route for medication to reach and cause an effect in the respiratory tract.

During aerosol medication administration, watch carefully for signs of both local tracheal or bronchial effect (spasm or edema) that might result from airway irritation or systemic symptoms that might result from absorption of a medication by the membrane.

Mist Tents. A mist tent is a plastic canopy that stretches over a child's bed; air enters the tent through a hose carrying nebulized water with it. Cool mist can be provided by an ice chamber or a refrigerator pump. Mist tents quickly become so filled with mist that it is impossible to see a child through the mist. Bedding becomes wet and cold easily. Be certain that children in mist tents have bedding changed frequently so they do not become chilled and arrange for an activity to occupy them. Parents (or you) can play a game with the child inside a tent to prevent the child from growing lonely.

Coughing

As a rule, coughing should be encouraged rather than suppressed in children because it is an effective method of raising mucus. A change in position, mild exercise, or deep breathing will initiate coughing. If a cough is causing irritation because mucus production is insufficient, dextromethorphan is an effective antitussive agent that suppresses cough but does not depress the respiratory rate as does codeine. If mucus in the back of the throat is causing a cough, a simple cough drop such as a glycerin and honey mixture is effective. It is important that parents not give adult cough syrups or cough drops to children. A number of adult cough syrups contain codeine in doses that are much too strong for children. If a cough is caused by mucus dripping from the nose because of nasal congestion, a decongestant such as pseudoephedrine (Sudafed) will best halt the draining mucus and therefore the cough.

Postural Drainage

Simple changing of a child's position helps mucus to move, initiate a cough reflex, and be expelled. When the child is positioned so the chest is lower than the abdomen, gravity aids the removal of mucus from the lower lobes and bronchi. When the child sits upright, gravity aids drainage from the upper lobes and bronchi. When lying supine, anterior bronchi drain; when prone, posterior bronchi drain. Frequent changes of position are important, therefore, to prevent pools of mucus from forming in a certain lung area. If the child has a localized mucus problem, lying predominantly in one position encourages drainage of that lung segment. When repositioned and the mucus drains into new bronchi, the child will often cough from irritation caused by this new drainage.

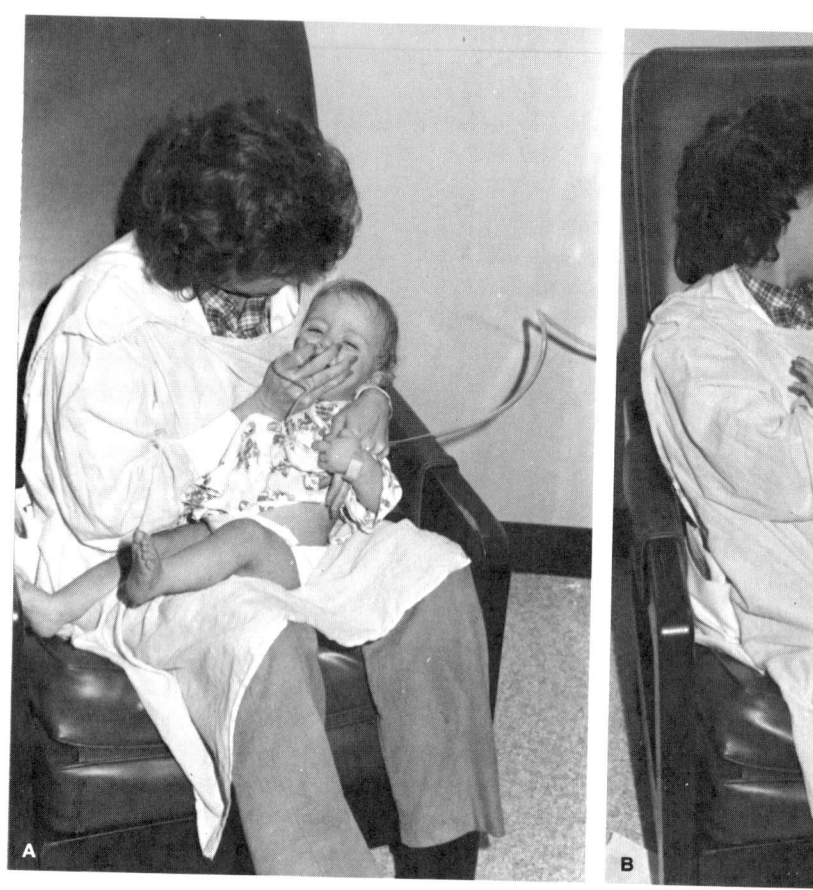

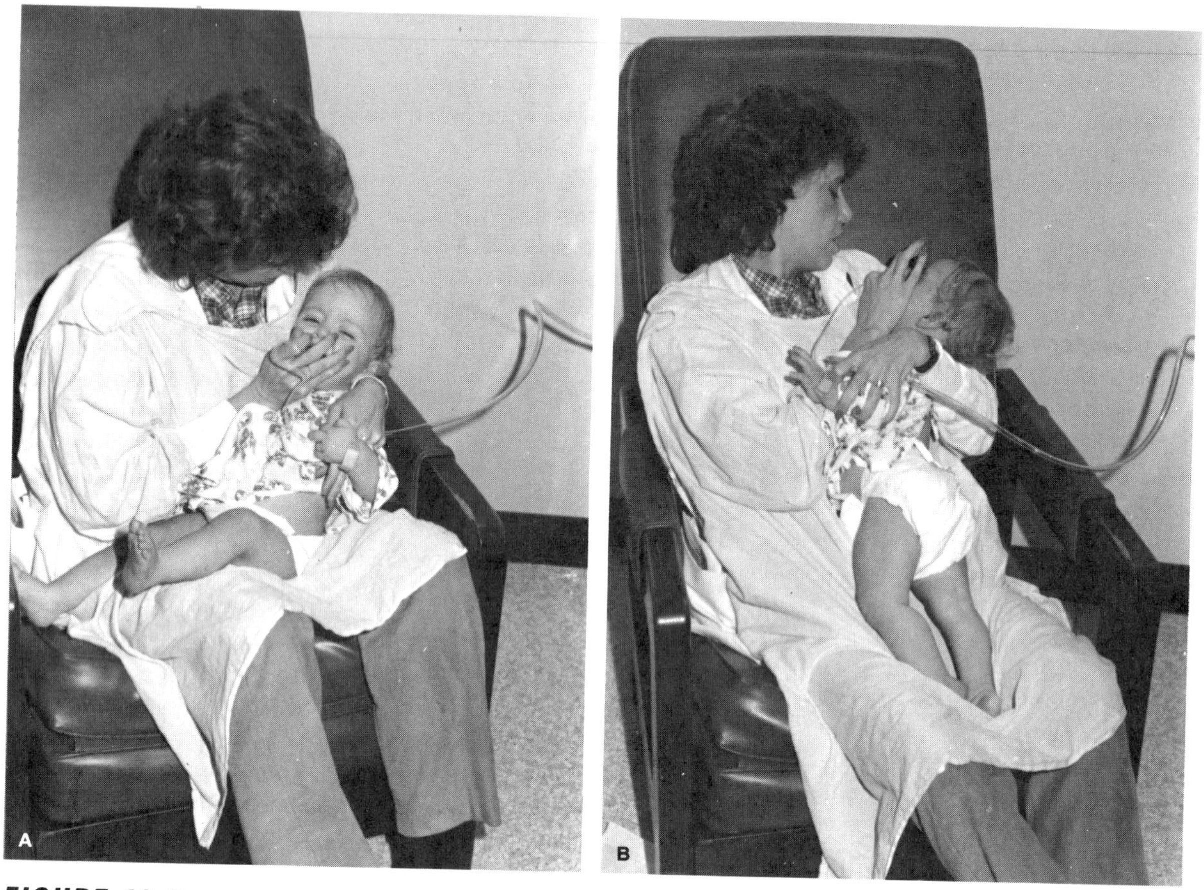

FIGURE 40-9

(**A**) *A respiratory therapist administers nebulizer therapy to a toddler.* (**B**) *Following the child to various positions offers the child a sense of control. (Courtesy of Bruce Hill.)*

Postural drainage, with cupping and vibration at set periods each day, may be prescribed to move mucus toward the main stem bronchus. Postural drainage should be done before meals or at least an hour after a meal, because the coughing this initiates may cause vomiting if the stomach is full. It should be limited to about 30 minutes, because the cupping and vibrating measures are tiring.

Technique. Common postural drainage positions for the infant are shown in Figure 40-10. An infant is positioned on your lap, whereas a slant board or other surface is needed for postural drainage with an older child. The technique is summarized in Nursing Procedure 40-1 and described below.

Cupping is percussion against the chest with a cupped or curved palm. This causes a loud, thumping noise that sounds as if it hurts. Parents need to be assured that it does not. *Vibration* is done by pressing a vibrating hand against a child's chest during exhalation. Like cupping, it mechanically loosens and helps move tenacious secretions. Vibration may also be accomplished by a mechanical vibrator or a vibrating vest. In infants, holding a nipple or small oxygen mask in your hand concentrates the motion and may increase the amount of mucus removed.

Following each position of postural drainage, the child is asked to cough. Children cough best if you demonstrate by taking a deep breath, blowing it out, taking a deep breath, blowing that out, taking a deep

FIGURE 40-10

Positions for bronchial drainage of major segments of all lobes in an infant positioned on a nurse's lap. Nurse's hand on chest indicates areas to be clapped or vibrated. (**A**) *Apical segment of left upper lobe.* (**B**) *Posterior segment of left upper lobe.* (**C**) *Anterior segment of left upper lobe.* (**D**) *Superior segment of right lower lobe.* (**E**) *Posterior basal segment of right lower lobe.* (**F**) *Lateral basal segment of right lower lobe.* (**G**) *Anterior basal segment of right lower lobe.* (**H**) *Medial and lateral segments of right middle lobe.* (**I**) *Lingular segments (superior and inferior) of left upper lobe. (From Skale, N. [1992]. Manual of pediatric procedures. Philadelphia J.B. Lippincott.)*

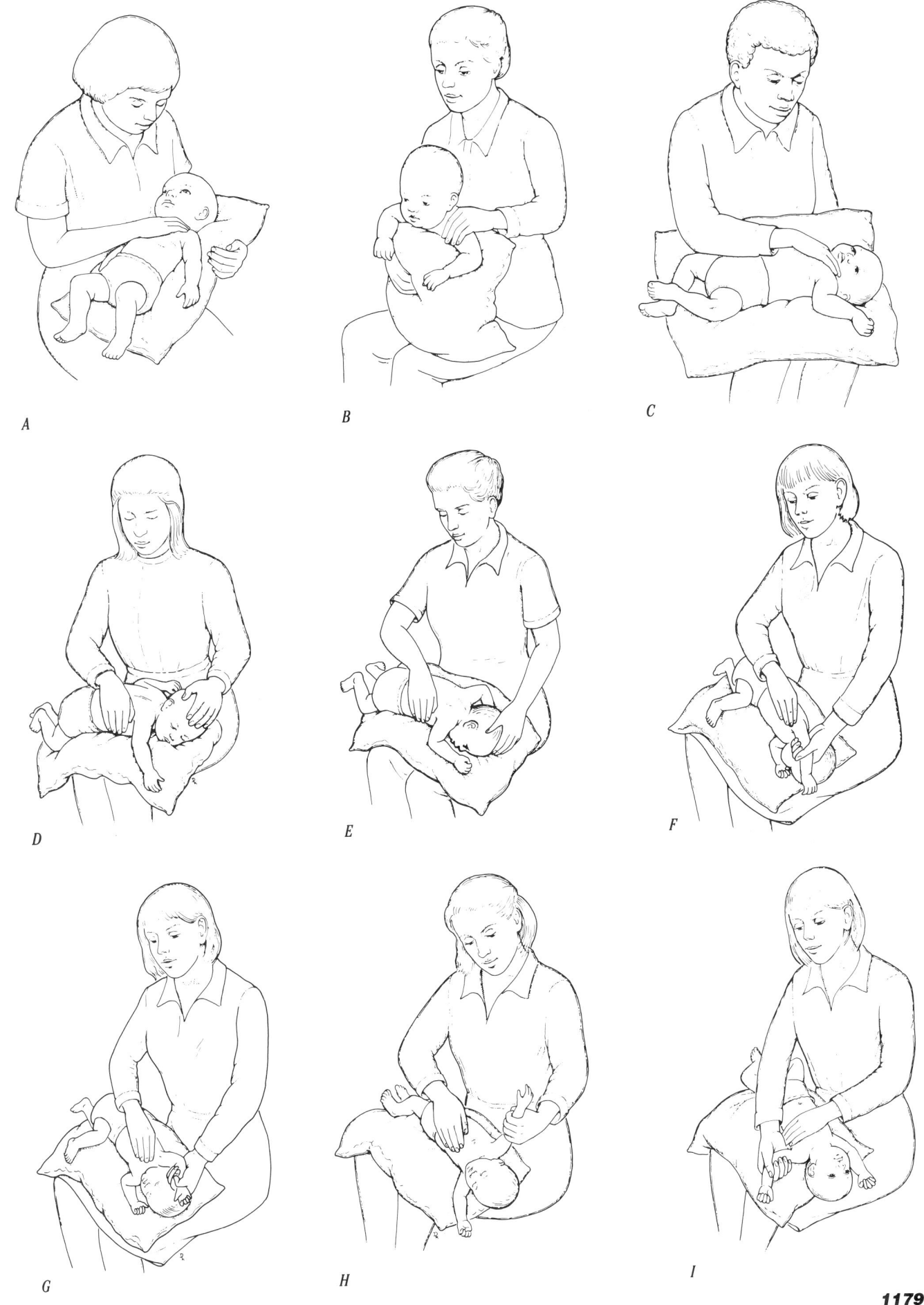

A

B

C

D

E

F

G

H

I

1179

NURSING PROCEDURE 40-1
Postural Drainage

Purpose
To encourage the loosening and raising of mucus from the respiratory tract through the use of gravity drainage and clapping and vibrating techniques.

Plan	Principle
1. Wash your hands; identify child; explain the procedure to the child.	1. Prevents spread of microorganisms; promotes child's understanding and compliance.
2. Assess child as to status; analyze appropriateness of procedure; modify plan as necessary.	2. Postural drainage is physically exhausting; can increase intracranial pressure when head is lowered in dependent position. Wait 1 h after meals to avoid inducing vomiting with coughing.
3. Implement procedure by assembling supplies: slant board, disposable tissues (sputum cup if specimen for culture is desired); nebulizer with correct fluid and medicine if prescribed.	3. Organizing care increases efficiency and helps prevent tiring child. Nebulization before postural drainage may be prescribed to dilate bronchials, dilute mucus, and aid mobility of secretions.
4. Select a drainage position (see Figure 40-12). Position child appropriately but comfortably. Auscultate and percuss lung area for baseline determinations.	4. Positions aid in the gravity drainage of secretions.
5. Use clapping technique for 1–2 min and vibrate during 4–5 exhalations the section of chest indicated for the position. Observe child closely for respiratory distress.	5. Clapping is forcefully striking the skin over a designated lung area with a cupped palm. Vibration is causing a quivering of tissue during exhalation. Both procedures loosen bronchial mucus and allow it to be coughed from the respiratory tract. As mucus moves, it may plug a bronchus; observe for cyanosis, tachypnea, dyspnea, and violent coughing as signs of this.
6. Ask child to deep breathe and cough to raise secretions. Auscultate lung section to ascertain clearing of secretions.	6. Coughing helps move secretions also.
7. Reposition and clap and vibrate the chest areas in additional drainage positions as prescribed. Continue to observe for signs of respiratory distress. Provide rest as necessary between positions.	7. Child may grow tired after repeated clapping/vibration.
8. At finish of prescribed positions return child to bed. Provide mouthwash if desired (and age appropriate); discard used tissues.	8. Coughed sputum may taste unpleasant.
9. Evaluate effectiveness, cost, comfort, and safety of procedure. Plan health teaching as necessary, such as benefit of procedure.	9. Health teaching is an independent nursing action always included in nursing care.
10. Record procedures, description of sputum raised, and child's reaction to procedure. If sputum specimen is obtained, route to laboratory for analysis.	10. Documents nursing care and child's status.

breath, and coughing. The irritation of mucus in the major airway by the third breath makes a cough happen almost spontaneously. Preschool children may respond best to a game such as "Simon says" when one of Simon's orders is "cough."

For postural drainage, position the child so that the lobe of the lung to be drained is in a superior position. Because clapping or vibrating is exhausting, the child may not have all lobes drained at each session. For example, before breakfast, the upper right and the left upper and lower lobes might be done; before lunch, the right lower lobe and right middle lobe might be done;

before supper or at bedtime, the upper and lower lobe on both sides might be done.

Postural drainage is usually done in a hospital setting by a respiratory therapist, but it is an important technique for nurses to know and be able to demonstrate to parents. One or both parents must learn the technique before their child is discharged so that it can be continued at home.

Therapy to Improve Oxygenation

Oxygen Administration

Oxygen administration elevates the arterial saturation level by supplying more available oxygen to the respiratory tract. Although using an oxygen tent is the most comfortable form of administration to use with children, the oxygen concentration in a tent rarely rises above 40%, a level inadequate to correct the oxygen need in many children. The moisture in oxygen tents may also harbor microorganisms and therefore be contraindicated.

Nursing care must be planned carefully when children are in tents. Opening of the tent should be minimized to keep the oxygen concentration as high as possible. A fussy, restless child causes the bottom of a tent to pull free. Because oxygen is heavier than air, a good deal of it can be lost through an improperly tucked tent.

Oxygen may be delivered to infants by flooding an Isolette or by using a plastic hood. This tight-fitting plastic enclosure can keep oxygen concentration at nearly 100% (Figure 40-11). A nasal catheter or nasal prongs, used with an oxygen flow of 4 L/min, provides a concentration of about 50%. Most children do not like nasal prongs because they are intrusive; assess the nostrils of

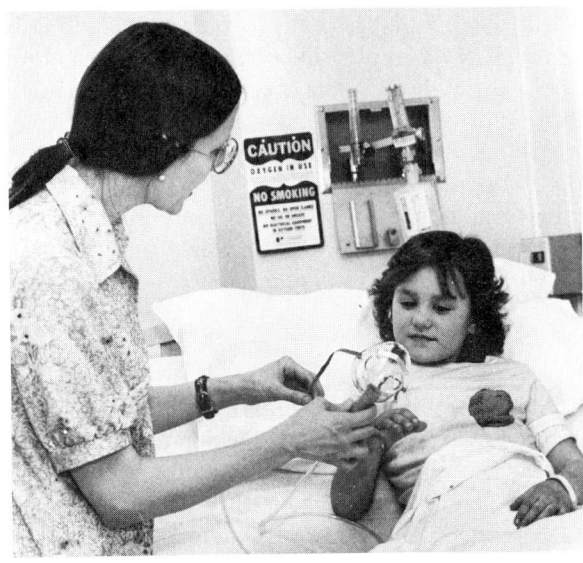

FIGURE 40-12
Orient children well to oxygen equipment such as oxygen masks. Here a school-age child manages a smile despite the new equipment. (Courtesy of the Department of Medical Photography, Children's Hospital, Buffalo, NY.)

infants carefully when using nasal prongs. The pressure of prongs can cause areas of necrosis, particularly on the nasal septum. A tight-fitting oxygen mask can supply nearly 100% oxygen. If necessary, let children hold a mask rather than strapping it in place to allow them more control (Figure 40-12).

Oxygen must be administered warmed and moistened, no matter what the route of delivery; dry oxygen will dry and thicken, not loosen, secretions (Bolgiano et al., 1990). Oxygen must be administered with the same careful observation and thoughtfulness as with any drug. If concentrations are too low, oxygen is not therapeutic; in concentrations greater than those desired, oxygen toxicity can develop (Kennedy & Warshaw, 1994). If newborns are subjected to a Po_2 of over 100 mm Hg for an extended time, retinopathy of prematurity can occur (see Chapter 26). In any child, administration of an oxygen concentration of 70% to 80% for an extended period may lead to a thickening of the lung alveoli and a loss of lung pliancy (oxygen toxicity or bronchopulmonary dysplasia). For these reasons, oxygen should not be given in high concentrations for long periods unless adequate facilities for blood gas analysis are available. Be certain, when caring for any child with any form of oxygen equipment, that you follow good safety rules. Blankets used in tents should be cotton, not wool or synthetic, so that sparks do not develop. A child's favorite blanket (if it is not cotton) can be placed outside a tent so that he or she can see it and feel it through the plastic covering. Because it contains a moisture source, oxygen equipment is also a source of microbial contaminants. Equipment should be changed at least once a

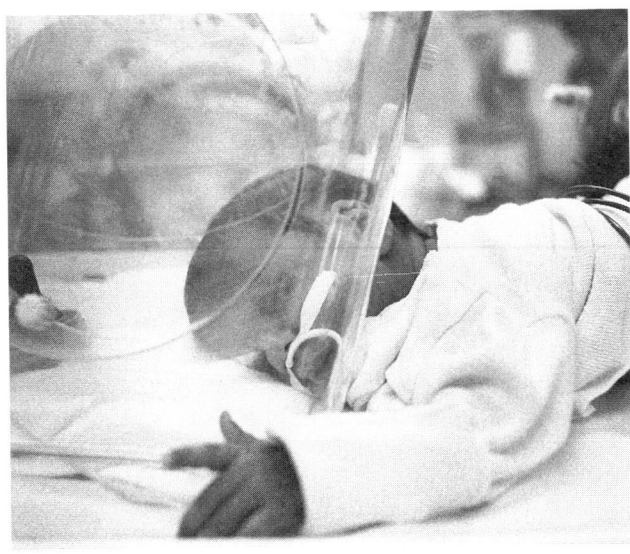

FIGURE 40-11
Infant with an oxygen hood in place. (Courtesy of the Department of Medical Photography, Children's Hospital, Buffalo, NY.)

week to keep bacterial counts within safe limits. Concentrations of oxygen should be measured and recorded and blood gas measurements obtained at any change in condition or oxygen flow.

Liquid Ventilation

Perfluorocarbons are substances used in industry to assess for leakage in pipes. When oxygen is bubbled through this, perfluorocarbons pick up and carry the oxygen with them. When perfluorocarbons are introduced into lungs that inflate poorly because they are deficient in surfactant, or in lungs damaged by trauma or disease, the weight of the fluid, which is heavy compared with air, helps to distend the lung. As the liquid moves into the lung, oxygen is carried along with it; as the liquid spreads over all lung surfaces, an exchange of gases occurs. The administration of liquid ventilation is being investigated in major research centers. It has promising applications for oxygen delivery in the future (Leach et al., 1993). An additional measure being researched is administration of nitric oxide. This causes pulmonary vasodilatation and can be very helpful when persistent pulmonary hypertension is present (Gross, 1994).

Extracorporeal Membrane Oxygenation (ECMO)

Extracorporeal membrane oxygenation was first developed as a means of oxygenating blood during cardiac surgery. Its current use is in the management of chronic severe hypoxemia in newborns with illnesses such as meconium aspiration, respiratory distress syndrome, pneumonia, and diaphragmatic hernia.

For the technique, blood is removed by gravity using a venous catheter advanced into the right atrium of the heart. The blood circulates from the catheter to the ECMO machine where it is oxygenated and rewarmed. It is then returned to the infant's aortic arch by a catheter advanced through the carotid artery. ECMO is typically used for 4 to 7 days (Haywood et al., 1993). ECMO has many potential complications, chief of which is intracranial hemorrhage possibly from the anticoagulation therapy that is necessary to prevent thromboembolism. Constant nursing care is required of the child receiving ECMO to be certain that the child's blood volume remains adequate, bleeding does not occur, and adequate oxygen is being supplied to the infant's body tissues.

Antihistamines

Swollen nasal mucosa can be constricted by the topical use of an antihistamine. Children are usually frightened by nasal spray medicine and will need support while it is administered. Most antihistamines cause a rebound action if used more than 3 days when they actually may begin to cause nasal obstruction and swelling. When giving instructions to parents, be certain to caution them

that continuing use of the medicine past 3 days will not increase but rather decrease their child's comfort.

Bronchodilators

The use of an effective bronchodilator increases the size of the airway lumen by about 25%. Common bronchodilators are listed in Table 40-6.

Incentive Spirometry

Incentive spirometers are manufactured in different configurations, but a common type consists of a hollow plastic tube containing a brightly colored ball that will rise in the tube when a child inhales on the attached mouthpiece and tubing. The deeper the inhalation, the higher the ball rises in the tube.

Children need instruction in how to use this type of device, since their first impression is that they should blow out against the mouthpiece rather than inhale. Such devices are helpful in encouraging children to inhale deeply and fully aerate their lungs (Figure 40-13A). Other methods for increasing aeration include asking the child to blow up a rubber glove or balloon, which requires the child to make a deep inhalation. Make this activity a game or contest rather than an exercise for best results (Figure 40-13B).

Tracheotomy

A tracheotomy is a temporary opening into the trachea to relieve respiratory obstruction that has occurred above that point. Tracheotomy also may be used when accumulating mucus causes lower airway obstruction, because the accumulated fluid can be suctioned through the tracheotomy. Tracheotomy interferes with the cleansing action of the mucous membrane lining the airway, and children with tracheotomies will need frequent suctioning to eliminate mucus. Tracheotomy also eliminates the warming and filtering action of the nose and pharynx, making children more susceptible to infection. For these reasons, tracheal intubation, not tracheotomy, has become the method of choice to relieve airway obstruction. The exception to this is obstruction in the pharynx, because it is impossible to pass an endotracheal tube beyond this point.

Emergency Intubation. Few medical emergencies are as frightening to a child or parents as an obstruction of a child's upper airway requiring a tracheotomy or intubation. The child suddenly becomes limp and breathless; color changes quickly from pink to pale; then systemic cyanosis develops. Tracheotomies are done more easily on a treatment room table than on a bed or crib, so it is generally best to carry the child immediately to the treatment room. If the child cannot be moved quickly, however, because of accessory equipment, no time should be lost in transport. For tracheotomy, the cricoid cartilage of the trachea is swabbed with an anti-

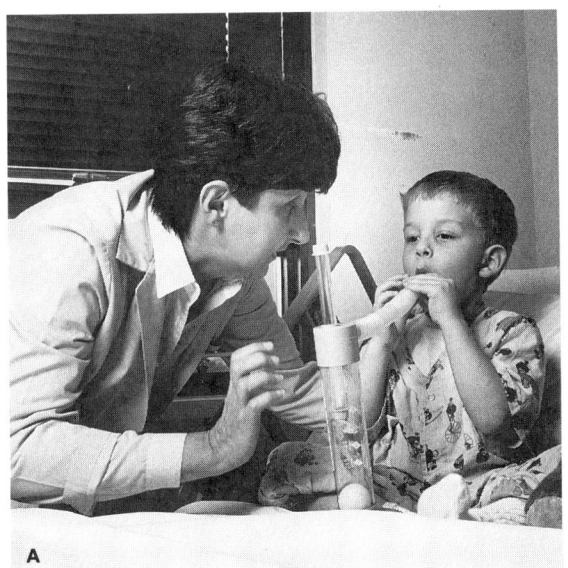
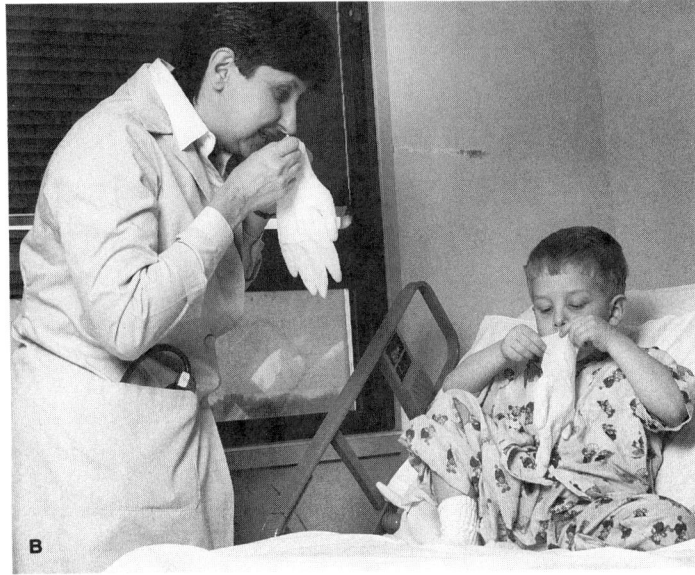

FIGURE 40-13
(**A**) *Incentive spirometry is an appealing method to encourage children to aerate their lungs.* (**B**) *Encouraging children to inflate rubber gloves or balloons is also an entertaining way to help children fully expand their lungs. (Courtesy of the Department of Medical Photography, Children's Hospital, Buffalo, NY.)*

septic; if readily available, a local anesthetic may be injected into the cartilage ring. (This is not necessary in the unconscious child.) An incision is made just under the ring of cartilage; a tracheotomy tube with its obturator in place is inserted into the opening. When the obturator is removed, the child is able to breath through the hollow tracheotomy tube. Suction equipment should be available for immediate use to clear any blood from the incision (this is minimal) and any obstructing mucus from the trachea.

The color change in children following tracheotomy is usually dramatic; they inhale deeply a number of times through the tube and color returns to normal. A few sutures may be necessary at the tube insertion site to halt bleeding or to reduce the size of the incision so the tube fits snugly (Hotaling et al., 1992).

As children begin to breathe normally and, if unconscious, regain consciousness, they often thrash and push at people around them. Part of this reaction stems from oxygen deficit, part from fright. Children try to cry for a parent but make no sound; their fright increases tenfold. Such a child needs to be assured that everything is all right. A school-age child can understand a simple explanation: she cannot speak at the moment because of the tube in her throat; if preschool age or younger, the comforting sound of someone saying that it is all right that they cannot speak will have a calming effect. As soon as the child's respirations are even and no longer distressed, the child can be shown that by placing a finger over the tracheotomy tube, air flowing past the larynx will allow the child to speak.

Explain to parents why the tube is in place. Assure

them that it is a temporary measure (providing this is true). Let them see the child as soon as possible after the procedure to assure themselves that their child is again all right. Explain well to parents why the tracheotomy was necessary. Children cannot relax and accept this strange new way of breathing until their parents can relax and accept it (Carabott et al., 1991).

Children with a tracheotomy need a great deal of support to accept this strange device (Figure 40-14*A*). Some children hyperventilate, not because of respiratory difficulty, but because of their fright of the tracheotomy.

Suctioning Technique. Most tracheotomy tubes used with children today are plastic, not silver, so they do not include an inner cannula that would require regular cleaning (Figure 40-14*B*). Most children, however, do require frequent suctioning (perhaps as often as every 15 minutes) to keep the airway free of mucus. Suction gently and yet thoroughly. Ineffective suction not only does not remove obstructive mucus but, because of irritation, causes more mucus to form. Be certain you know how deeply you should suction. Some children need only to be suctioned the length of the tracheotomy tube so that the catheter does not touch and irritate the tracheal mucosa. Others need to be deeply suctioned to reduce the possibility that mucus will become so copious or so thickened that it obstructs the trachea (Figure 40-15*A*).

Tracheotomy suctioning technique is shown in Nursing Procedure 40-2. Because suctioning removes air as well as secretions from the trachea, children may become very short of oxygen. "Bagging" them or adminis-

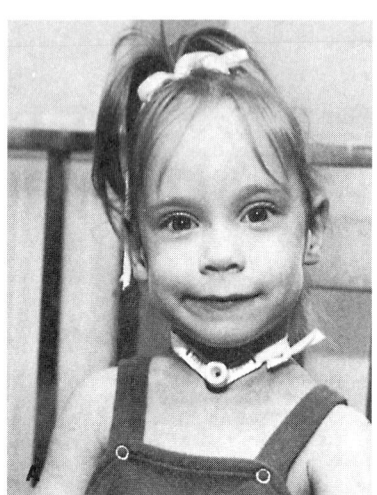
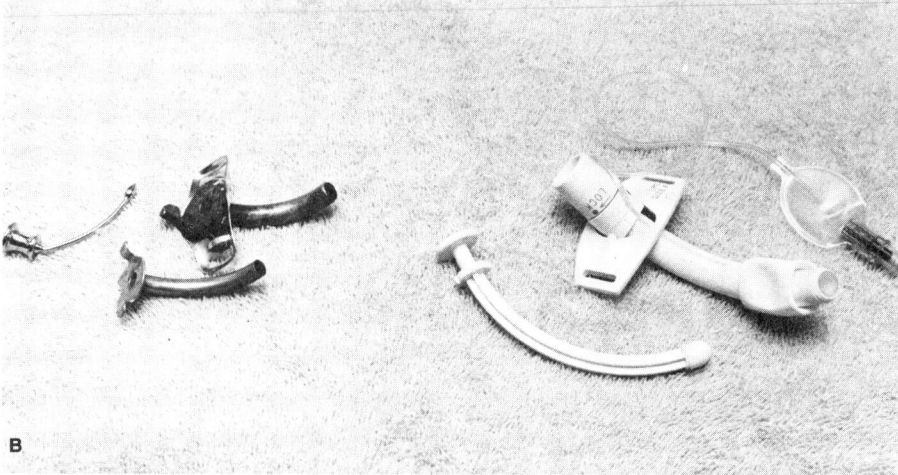

FIGURE 40-14
(**A**) *Child has a tracheotomy tube in place.* (**B**) *Tracheotomy tubes. (Left) A metal tube, inner cannula, and outer cannula; (right) a plastic, cuffed tube with obturator. (Courtesy of the Department of Medical Photography, Children's Hospital, Buffalo, NY.)*

tering oxygen for 5 minutes prior to the procedure helps reduce this problem (Figure 40-16*B*).

Dropping 1 or 2 mL of sterile saline into the tracheotomy tube prior to suctioning may be helpful in loosening secretions. This is a controversial procedure, however, because it induces violent coughing and may not actually aid the removal of secretions.

Young children may need to wear elbow restraints while they are suctioned, which helps to keep their hands away from the catheter. They may need to wear restraints at all times when they are alone to prevent them from fussing with the tracheotomy tube and accidentally removing it.

Although parents are capable of determining when their child needs tracheotomy suction and of doing the suctioning, there seems to be little merit in teaching parents how to do this procedure unless the tracheotomy tube is to be left in place after discharge from the hospital. It is never wise to ask a parent to hurt a child, and tracheotomy suction is a choking, hurting feeling. A better role for parents is to support children after the procedure. Make frequent checks on children with tracheotomies to make certain that they are not having respiratory difficulty. Make certain that you spend time playing with them or just sitting and rocking them so that they come to think of you in other ways than as the

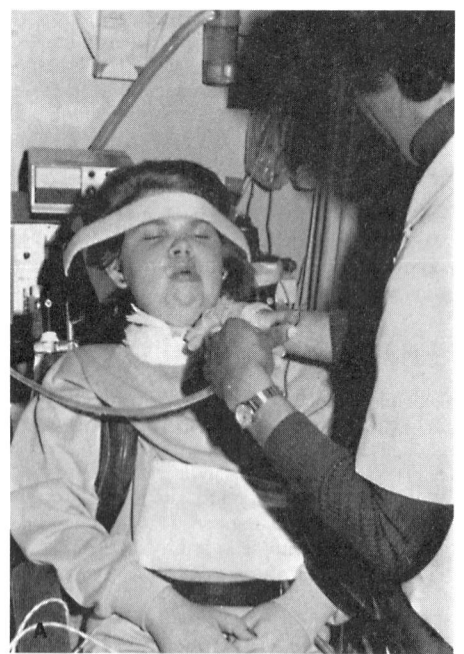
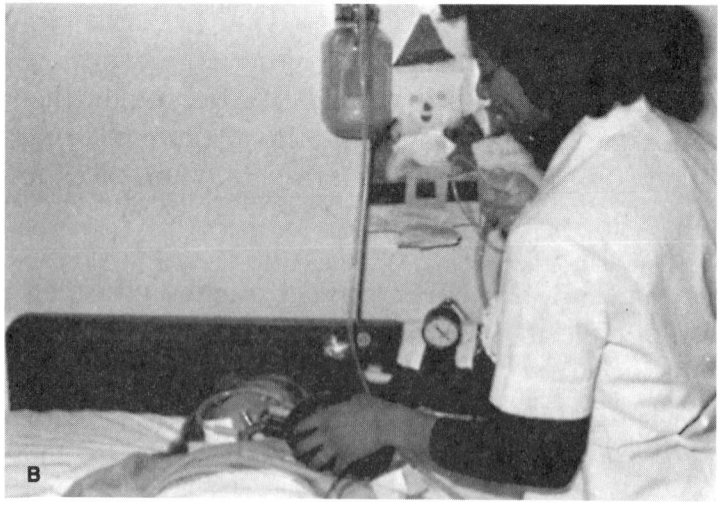

FIGURE 40-15
(**A**) *Suctioning a tracheotomy tube. This is not a pleasant sensation, as shown by the child's facial expression.* (**B**) *"Bagging" is done to increase oxygen concentration prior to tracheotomy suction. (Courtesy of Bruce Hill.)*

NURSING PROCEDURE 40-2
Tracheotomy Suction

Procedure	*Principle*
1. Wash hands, identify child, explain procedure to child.	1. Prevents spread of microorganisms; encourages cooperation.
2. Assess child; analyze appropriateness of procedure. Plan ways to modify care based on individual circumstances.	2. Nursing care is always individualized based on client need.
3. Implement care by assembling supplies: suction source, sterile suction catheter (#12 or 14F), sterile gloves, sterile bottle of normal saline, sterile medicine dropper or syringe, manual resuscitator. Plan method to keep child from touching sterile catheter (placing a restraint, distraction, or asking assistance from another nurse).	3. Organizing supplies will increase efficiency of procedure.
4. Open normal saline and suction catheter; put on sterile gloves.	4. Sterile technique is important to prevent introducing microorganisms.
5. Hold suction catheter with one gloved hand, suction tubing with other gloved hand, and attach tubing to sterile catheter; dip tip of catheter into normal saline and suction a small amount through catheter.	5. Note that once sterile glove touches suction tubing, it is no longer sterile. Suctioning normal saline ensures that the tubing and catheter are patent.
6. If necessary, instruct assistant to hyperoxygenate child with manual resuscitator.	6. Hyperoxygenation prevents child from developing anoxia during suctioning.
7. If necessary, drop prescribed amount of normal saline into tracheotomy tube with dropper or syringe, and observe child closely for respiratory distress.	7. Normal saline helps to keep secretions liquid enough to be suctioned readily.
8. Hold breath; introduce sterile catheter into tracheotomy tube to desired length. Apply suction and gently withdraw, rotating gently.	8. Holding breath helps you not to suction longer than is comfortable. Applying suction only on withdrawal allows catheter to pass freely without irritating the trachea.
9. Rinse catheter by dipping tip in normal saline and applying suction.	9. Rinsing catheter ensures that it remains patent.
10. Repeat procedure until airway sounds clear. Be careful not to suction longer than necessary.	10. Suctioning is fatiguing to child. Extended suctioning can lead to airway irritation and further mucus production.
11. Evaluate effectiveness and efficiency of procedure; plan teaching such as importance of procedure to parents; document procedure.	11. Teaching is an independent nursing care measure always included as part of care.
12. Comfort child; remain with child for support.	12. Suctioning is frightening; offer support and comfort after all such procedures.

person who comes to suction them. Make certain that parents are aware that you check on their child more frequently than necessary for suctioning alone, to assure them that if the child should have another episode of acute obstruction, someone will be nearby.

The tracheotomy tube is held in place by cloth ties that fasten at the back of the child's neck. Check these frequently to be certain they are secure; children tend to fuss with such things, whereas adults do not. For preschoolers or younger children, it is a good idea to cover the tracheotomy opening with a gauze square tied to the child's neck like a bib while they are eating. This prevents crumbs or spilled liquids from entering the tracheotomy. Do not give children small toys that could possibly fit into the lumen of the tube and cause obstruction (Carabott et al., 1991; see the Focus on Family Teaching box).

Tracheotomy tubes are generally sealed off partially for a day or two prior to removal then completely occluded (but not removed) for yet another day. In this

FOCUS ON FAMILY TEACHING

Q. My two-year-old daughter will be discharged from the hospital with a tracheotomy. What special measures do I need to do to prevent aspiration?

A. Caring for a child with a tracheotomy is a challenge until you have more experience. Here are some tips for preventing aspiration:

- Use a bib tied loosely over the tracheotomy when your daughter is eating to prevent food from entering the tube.
- Avoid buying toys with small parts that could be removed and dropped into the tube.
- Inspect stuffed toys to be certain they don't shed (fur could enter the tube).
- Supervise play with other children to be certain they don't place anything in the tube.
- Stay with your child in a bathtub to be certain water doesn't splash into the tube.
- Keep sprays such as perfume or room fresheners to a minimum, since they can be irritating to the trachea.
- Avoid cold air, since it can cause tracheal spasm (cover your daughter's throat with a loose scarf when out in cold weather).

way, suctioning is still possible if it is needed. Occasionally, children cough so forcefully that they dislodge a tracheotomy tube. You might be with a child when this occurs, or you might walk into the room and find the tube lying beside the child on the bedclothes. As long as a child is not in distress, this is not an emergency. The incision of a tracheotomy site usually does not close completely to occlude the tracheal opening when a tube is dislodged. Slide the obturator into the tube and gently replace it in the tracheal opening. If you do this quickly yet calmly, children are less likely to become alarmed and protest. If, however, they sense your excitement or if you indicate that something is terribly wrong, they may begin to cry and turn away; you will then have difficulty replacing the tube without another person's help.

If an inner cannula type is used, the inner cannula should be removed and cleaned as necessary, at least every 8 hours. Be certain that the school-age child who is old enough to understand this realizes that you are removing only the inner tube to clean it and this action will not interfere with breathing in any way. Wear sterile gloves and use sterile solutions to clean an inner cannula to prevent introducing bacteria to the trachea. If se-

cretions are moist and loose, a cotton-tipped applicator or tube brush dipped in sterile water may work well. If secretions are tenacious, they may soak away only in a solution such as half-strength hydrogen peroxide. Be certain that you dry an inner cannula well before you replace it in the outer tube, so that drops of water do not run from it into the trachea and add to the accumulating secretions.

Endotracheal Intubation

Endotracheal intubation (nasal or oral intubation) is another means of bypassing upper airway obstruction and allowing free entry of air to the trachea. Tracheotomy can be done with the child awake. Intubation, however, usually requires that the child (except the newborn) be lightly anesthetized. No anesthesia is necessary if the child is unconscious. Intubation tubes cause edema and local irritation and so are used only as emergency measures; they can rarely be left in place for longer than a week. Children cannot speak while intubated. Those old enough to write should be supplied with a pencil and paper for effective communication. Preschoolers may want to draw pictures to indicate what they need. It is helpful to have simple drawings that a child can point to (a drink, a straw, a blanket, the television turned on, a urinal) to make his needs known. Make sure that endotracheal tubes are carefully secured because a child can easily dislodge one, but avoid frequent changes of tape to protect the skin on the child's cheeks.

A capnometer is a device that measures the amount of CO_2 in inhaled or exhaled breaths. It uses infrared technology and is attached to the distal end of the endotracheal tube. By measuring the percentage of CO_2 in expired air, the arterial CO_2 can be estimated.

Assisted Ventilation

When it is not possible to improve oxygen saturation to sufficient levels by the methods described above, assisted ventilation may become necessary. Assisted ventilation can be based on positive or negative pressure.

Negative-Pressure Ventilators. A negative-pressure ventilator is a device that surrounds the chest area. When pressure in this "cage" is lowered to less than the pressure in the child's lungs, air flows out of the lungs (the child exhales). Automatic recoil of the lungs will then cause the lungs to fill again (the child inhales). Such ventilators were in use as early as the 1800s for respiratory illnesses. They fell into disuse in the 1950s because they are bulkier, allow only limited access to the client, and are not as effective as positive-pressure ventilators. They are coming back into use, however, because they have some advantages in home care (Dougherty, 1990).

The advantage of negative-pressure ventilators is

that a child does not need to be connected to the ventilator by intubation; suctioning can be done without interrupting ventilation. The most likely indications for their use are with children who have chronic respiratory disease, such as cystic fibrosis, or neuromuscular disease, such as muscular dystrophy.

Newer models are both compact and portable. Because they do not have an alarm, pulse oximetry is used to ensure adequate oxygen saturation.

Positive-Pressure Ventilators. Positive-pressure machines deliver moistened or nebulized air or oxygen to the lungs under enough pressure and with appropriate timing to produce artificial, periodical inflation of alveoli; they rely on the elastic recoil of the lungs to empty the alveoli.

Depending on the type of ventilator, the inspiration-expiration cycle is determined by a timed interval, a volume limit, or a pressure limit. Conventional mechanical ventilators supply high tidal volumes at a low frequency rate. High airway pressure is needed in this conventional system, which can, unfortunately, lead to bronchopulmonary disease. A newer method of ventilation depends on low tidal volumes delivered at high frequencies of 200 to 300 breaths/min. Hyperinflation of lungs can occur with high frequency ventilation, since there is not enough time for expiration to occur. For this reason, some high frequency ventilators are set so air is sucked out of the lungs rather than depending on the normal elastic recoil of the lungs. Ventilator rates can be set as high as 1800 breaths/min with these systems.

Pancuronium (Pavulon) may be administered intravenously to a point of abolishing spontaneous respiratory action in order to allow mechanical ventilation to be accomplished at lower pressures (there is no normal muscle resistance to overcome). Clearly, a child who has no spontaneous respiratory function needs critical observation and frequent arterial blood analysis, because he or she depends totally on the caregivers at that point. The effects of pancuronium decrease as the life of the drug expires; its effects can be interrupted by the administration of atropine or injectable neostigmine methylsulfate (Prostigmin Methylsulfate Injectable).

When pancuronium therapy is being used, the child's nursing care plan should be clearly marked to that effect, so that manual ventilatory assistance can be begun immediately in the event of a power failure.

Artificial ventilation for a prolonged period requires that children either have a tracheotomy performed or have an endotracheal tube passed. A cuffed tube must be used with a ventilator so the seal at the trachea is airtight. Infants need an nasogastric tube inserted to prevent stomach distension. Providing adequate nutrition may be difficult for the child on a ventilator. This can be provided by enteric (nasogastric) feedings or total parenteral nutrition. Providing a balance of rest and

stimulation for the child can be challenge for nursing personnel.

Children who need respiratory assistance are frightened; their parents are numb with fright. A nurse who is comfortable with ventilator care automatically conveys assurance that the child will be safe during ventilation. A great many children fight ventilators or refuse to lie quietly and let the ventilator breathe for them. Sometimes this anxiety may occur because the machine is set improperly (so it provides too much or too little oxygen). More often it results from children perceiving the nervousness of the people who are caring for them. Be certain that you are comfortable enough with the machinery being used that you can concentrate on providing total nursing care to the child (Figure 40-16 and Table 40-7).

Once children become accustomed to ventilator care, it is sometimes difficult to discontinue a device, even when there is no longer a clinical indication for it. This is most pronounced in adolescents who are aware of the role of oxygen and proper ventilation in life function. Children must have confidence in the people who care for them before they can be removed effectively from a ventilator. They may need a number of trial periods with someone remaining close by them, so that they can be certain that if they do have difficulty breathing, someone is standing by to help. For very anxious children, being supervised from across an intensive care unit may be interpreted as being "left alone." Anxiety in these instances will increase respirations; this may lead to hyperventilation and the distress they feared. Many children are too afraid to fall asleep on the first night off a ventilator unless someone is with them and has assured them that he or she will be there through the night.

Common problems experienced with assisted ventilation and associated nursing interventions are summarized in Table 40-8.

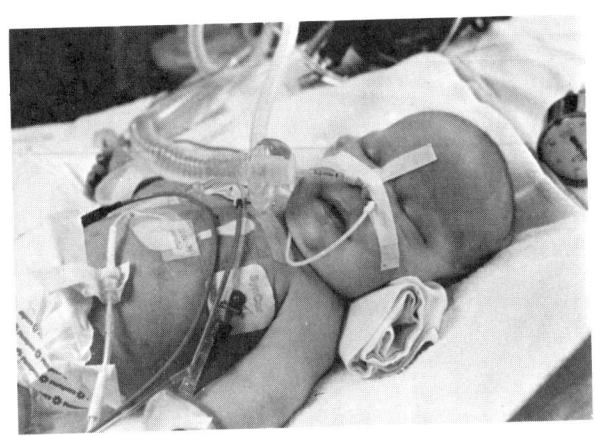

FIGURE 40-16
Infant is receiving assisted ventilation by endotracheal tube. The infant also has cardiac leads, a Broviac Catheter for a subclavian fluid line, and a nasogastric tube. (Courtesy of Mary Ormond.)

Table 40-7. *Terms Commonly Used With Ventilator Therapy*

Term	Definition	Clinical Application
IMV	Intermittent mandatory ventilation	Number of mandatory breaths the ventilator will deliver each hour. A child may breathe most of the time without assistance, but a set (mandatory) number of breaths per minute is delivered to ensure adequate lung expansion and oxygenation
PEEP	Positive end-expiratory pressure	Pressure delivered to lungs at the end of each expiration to keep alveoli from collapsing on expiration and ensuring adequate oxygenation
Sigh	A deep inhalation delivered by the ventilator	Used to fully inflate the lungs a number of times each minute
CPAP	Continuous positive airway pressure	A constant pressure exerted on the alveoli to keep them from collapsing on expiration
FIO_2	Concentration of oxygen the child is receiving (inspiring)	A child on oxygen therapy will have an FIO_2 from 22%–100%

Table 40-8. *Common Problems With Assisted Ventilation*

Assessment Finding	Probable Cause	Intervention
Sudden tachycardia, cyanosis, decreased PO_2, increased PCO_2	Tension pneumothorax	Notify physician. Prepare for emergency chest radiograph, thoracentesis, and insertion of needle or tube.
Cyanosis, breath sounds decreased bilaterally, inability to suction length of airway, decreased PO_2, increased PCO_2	Obstruction of airway	Notify physician. Instill 2–3 drops of normal saline into endotracheal or tracheotomy tube; attempt suction. Repeat if necessary, prepare for reintubation if no improvement. Support with 100% oxygen.
Decreased lung compliance, decreased PO_2, increased PCO_2, decreased breath sounds	Atelectasis	Notify physician. Initiate prescribed postural drainage technique (percussion and vibration) over affected area; change position frequently. Prepare to change ventilatory setting as prescribed (increased sighing function) or change position of endotracheal tube.
Decreased PO_2, increased PCO_2, cyanosis, change in marked point of endotracheal tube or tracheotomy tube, ability of child to vocalize, absent ventilator breath sounds bilaterally	Detubation	Notify physician. Remove displaced tube and administer oxygen at 100% by face mask; suction if necessary to clear airway. Prepare equipment for reintubation; evaluate why extubation occurred (possibly more restraint is needed).
Sudden cyanosis, alarm of ventilator rings	Electrical failure Ventilator disconnected accidentally	Manually resuscitate with bag and mask and 100% oxygen; evaluate why failure occurred. Assist with reinstitution of ventilation therapy.
Decreased PO_2, increased PCO_2, decreased lung compliance	Oxygen toxicity	Prepare for prescription of PEEP pressure to better oxygenate noncompliant lungs; prepare for chest radiograph.
Stool or aspiration from nasogastric tube tests positive for occult blood; pallor; anemia; restlessness from pain	Stress ulcer	Administer antacid or cimetidine as prescribed; monitor infusion of blood replacement therapy. Monitor vital signs as prescribed; assess stool and nasogastric tube aspirate for occult blood.
Decreased urine output, specific gravity above 1.030, decreased serum sodium, edema	Increased antidiuretic hormone secretion	Prepare blood-drawing equipment to measure serum osmolarity; reduce fluid intake as prescribed.
Rales on auscultation, fever, increased PCO_2, decreased PO_2, purulent or thick tracheal secretions	Infection	Prepare for blood sample for white blood cell evaluation; prepare for chest radiograph. Administer antibiotics as prescribed; change position frequently. Prepare to do postural drainage (percussion and vibration) over affected areas as prescribed.

Lung Transplant

Lung transplantation is a possibility for children with a chronic respiratory illness such as cystic fibrosis (Jenkinson & Levine, 1994). Because this procedure has been done only in limited numbers and the chance for tissue rejection is high, the mortality rate for the procedure is also high (about 33%). Lung transplantation may be done in conjunction with a heart transplant if chronic respiratory disease has caused ventricle hypertrophy.

Disorders of the Upper Respiratory Tract

The upper respiratory tract warms, humidifies, and filters the air that enters the body. As such, the structures of the upper respiratory tract constantly come into contact with a barrage of foreign organisms, including pathogens, which can sometimes lead to airway obstruction and illness. Congenital malformation of respiratory structures can also cause some upper respiratory tract disorders. Common childhood disorders of the upper respiratory tract are illustrated in Figure 40-17.

Choanal Atresia

Choanal atresia is the obstruction of the posterior nares, preventing a newborn from drawing air through the nose and down into the nasopharynx. The condition is congenital and is caused by an obstructing membrane or bony growth. It may be either unilateral or bilateral (Haywood et al., 1993).

Newborns up to about 3 months of age are naturally nose breathers. Infants with choanal atresia, therefore, develop signs of respiratory distress at birth or immediately after they quiet for the first time and attempt to breathe through the nose. Passing a soft No. 8 or 10 catheter through the posterior nares to the stomach is in many hospitals a part of delivery room procedure. If such a catheter will not pass bilaterally, the diagnosis of choanal atresia is confirmed.

To assess for choanal atresia, hold the newborn's mouth closed, then gently compress first one nostril, then the second. If atresia is present, infants will struggle as they experience air hunger when the mouth is closed. Their color improves when they open their mouth to cry. Atresia is also suggested if infants struggle and become cyanotic at feedings because they cannot suck and breathe through their mouth simultaneously.

Because infants with choanal atresia have such diffi-

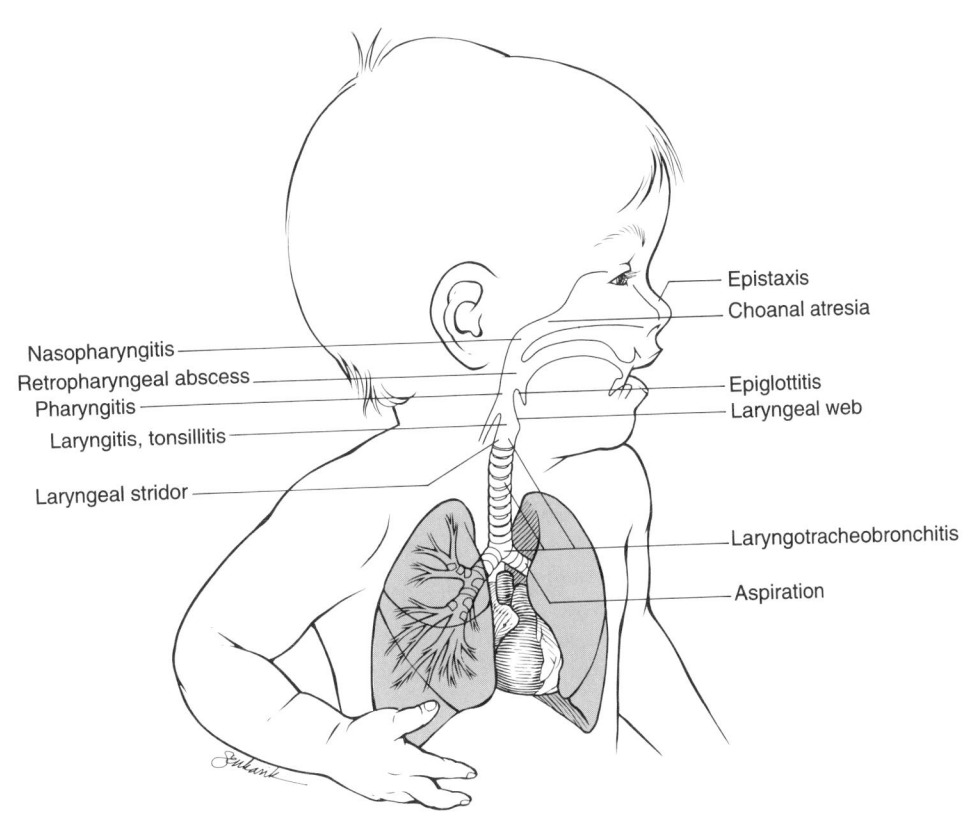

FIGURE 40-17
Sites of common upper respiratory diseases in children.

culty with feeding, they may receive intravenous fluid to maintain their glucose and fluid level until surgery can be performed. Some infants may need an oral airway inserted. The treatment for bilateral atresia is either local piercing of the obstructing membrane or surgical removal of the bony growth.

Acute Nasopharyngitis (Common Cold)

The common cold is the most frequent infectious disease in children. Toddlers have an average of 10 to 12 colds a year. School-age children and adolescents have as many as 4 to 5 yearly. The incubation period is about 2 days.

Acute nasopharyngitis (the common cold) is caused by one of several viruses, most predominantly by rhinovirus, coxsackievirus, respiratory syncytial virus, adenovirus, and parainfluenza and influenza viruses. Children are exposed to colds at school from other children. Those children who are in ill health from some other cause are more susceptible to the cold viruses than are well children. Stress factors also appear to play a role. Although it is difficult to document phenomena such as drafts, cold feet, or chilling as causative factors, they probably play a role in susceptibility.

Assessment

Symptoms begin with nasal congestion, a watery rhinitis, and low-grade fever. The mucous membrane of the nose becomes edematous and erythematous. Children experience difficulty in breathing because of this nasal edema and congestion. Posterior rhinitis, plus local irritation, leads to pharyngitis. Draining pharyngeal secretions may lead to a cough. Cervical lymph nodes may be swollen and palpable. In some children, a thick, purulent nasal discharge occurs because bacteria such as streptococci invade the irritated nasal mucous membrane and cause a secondary infection. The process lasts about a week and then symptoms fade.

Infants can be critically ill and not develop an increased temperature owing to their immature body systems, but when it comes to the common cold, they often develop a fever elevated out of proportion to the symptoms. Infants or toddlers may develop a fever of 102° to 104°F (38.8° to 40°C). Infants may also develop secondary symptoms such as vomiting and diarrhea. Because they cannot suck and breathe through their mouth at the same time, they refuse feedings. This can lead to dehydration. Older children will not develop as high a fever. Their temperature rarely exceeds 102°F (38.8°C). Because they can breathe through their mouth, the nasal congestion does not seem as acute.

Therapeutic Management

There is no specific treatment for a common cold. Antibiotics are not effective against a common cold unless a secondary bacterial invasion has occurred. If children have a fever, it should be controlled by an antipyretic such as acetaminophen (Tylenol). It is important for parents to understand that acetaminophen is to control the fever symptoms; Tylenol does not reduce congestion or "cure" the cold. It should not be given unless children have fever, generally defined as an oral temperature over 101°F (38.4°C).

If infants have difficulty nursing because of nasal congestion, saline nose drops may be prescribed to liquefy nasal secretions and help them drain. A bulb syringe, used before feedings to clear away nasal mucus, will allow infants to suck more efficiently. Caution parents that when they use a bulb syringe, they must compress the bulb first, then insert it into their child's nostril. If they insert the syringe first, then depress the bulb, they will actually push secretions further back into the nose, causing increased obstruction. Nose drops such as phenylephrine (Neo-Synephrine) cause constriction of the mucous membrane of the nose and, therefore, also free the airway.

There is little proof that oral decongestants relieve congestion with the common cold. Most parents feel that these products give relief, however, and feel better if one is prescribed for the child. It is not good policy to suppress the cough of a common cold, because a cough raises secretions, thus preventing pooling of secretions and consequent infection. Guaifenesin is an example of a drug that loosens secretions but does not suppress a cough. Parents may use a vaporizer to help loosen nasal secretions. The efficiency of home vaporizers is questionable, however, and safe use of a vaporizer, including proper cleaning, must be stressed. Be certain that parents place a warm mist vaporizer on a shelf where children cannot reach it. Children can be severely scalded from investigating a vaporizer to see where the steam is coming from.

Nursing Diagnoses and Related Interventions

Nursing Diagnosis: Parental health-seeking behaviors related to management of child's cold

Goal: Parents will demonstrate knowledge of what is and what is not helpful in the treatment of cold by end of health visit.

Outcome Criteria: Parents state intention to use cool mist vaporizer to loosen secretions, to encourage oral fluid, and to avoid cough medicine.

Parents generally ask if children should remain on bed rest. Children characteristically restrict their activity when ill. With acute cold symptoms, children naturally curl up on the couch and sleep. One of the best ways that parents can judge when children are improving is to note that they have begun to increase their activity or are "acting like themselves" again.

Children with a cold often show a loss of appetite. They may prefer simple liquids to solid food for the first few days of a cold.

Parents can be assured that a cold is only a cold and nothing more. Because the symptoms in infants are so out of proportion to the seriousness of the disorder, it is easy to be fooled into thinking that this is a more serious disorder than it is. A complication of a cold in children can be otitis media (middle ear infection). Symptoms of this are sudden elevated temperature and ear pain. If this occurs, a child needs antibiotic administration and further evaluation to protect against hearing impairment.

Pharyngitis

Pharyngitis is infection and inflammation of the throat. It may be either bacterial or viral in origin. It may occur as a result of a chronic allergy in which there is constant postnasal discharge and resulting secondary irritation. Some pharyngitis often accompanies a common cold. The peak incidence of pharyngitis occurs between 4 and 7 years of age. The nursing diagnosis most often used with pharyngitis is pain.

Viral Pharyngitis

If the causative agent of the pharyngitis is a virus, the symptoms are generally mild: a sore throat, fever, and general malaise. On physical assessment, regional lymph nodes may be noticeably enlarged. Erythema will be present in the back of the pharynx and the palatine arch. Laboratory studies will reveal an increased white blood cell count.

If the inflammation is mild, children rarely need more therapy than an analgesic such as acetaminophen. By school age, children are capable of gargling (before this, they tend to swallow the solution unless the procedure is well explained and demonstrated to them). Gargling with warm water may be soothing; warm heat may be applied to the external neck using a warm towel or heating pad.

Because children's throats are sore, they do not eat well. They often prefer liquid to solid food. Infants, especially, must be observed closely until the inflammation and tenderness diminish to be certain that they take in sufficient fluid to prevent dehydration.

Streptococcal Pharyngitis

Group A beta hemolytic streptococcus is the organism most frequently involved in bacterial pharyngitis in children 6 years old and older (Hammerschlag, 1994).

Assessment. Streptococcal infections are generally more severe than viral infections, although the fact that the symptoms are mild does not rule out streptococcal

infection. With a streptococcal pharyngitis, the palatine tonsils are usually markedly erythematous (bright red) and enlarged. There may be a white exudate in the tonsillar crypts. Petechiae may be present on the palate. The pharynx is erythematous; there may be high fever, extreme sore throat, and lethargy. The child appears ill and reports difficulty swallowing. The temperature is usually elevated to 104°F (40°C). The child may complain of headache, and swollen abdominal lymph nodes may cause abdominal pain. A throat culture confirms presence of the *Streptococcus* bacteria. An extremely virulent form of streptococci that actually necroses tissue, causing extensive tissue damage, has been identified.

Therapeutic Management. Treatment consists of a full 10-day course of an antibiotic such as clindamycin or amoxicillin. Parents should understand the importance of the full 10 days of therapy. The prolonged treatment is necessary to ensure that the streptococci are eradicated completely. If not, children may develop a hypersensitivity reaction to Group A streptococci that results in rheumatic fever (although the chance of rheumatic fever occurring is probably as low as 1%; Mayeux et al., 1990). To prevent this, help parents comply by making a reminder sheet to place on their refrigerator door.

Symptoms of acute glomerulonephritis (blood and protein in urine) may appear in 1 to 2 weeks after the pharyngitis (Tejani & Ingulli, 1990). There is no proof that antibiotic treatment prevents acute glomerulonephritis. If the strain of streptococci was a nephrogenic one, the chances are as high as 50% that kidney disease will develop.

Two weeks after treatment, children are asked to return to the health care facility with a urine specimen to be examined for protein so that developing acute glomerulonephritis can be detected. Because it is impossible for parents to discriminate between a pharyngitis caused by a virus (and needing no therapy other than comfort measures) and a streptococcal pharyngitis (needing definite therapy to prevent life-threatening illnesses), a child with pharyngitis always should be examined by health care personnel. "Simple" sore throats in children may not be simple at all.

Retropharyngeal Abscess

The lymph nodes that drain the nasopharynx are located behind the posterior pharynx wall. These nodes may become infected in an infant with an acute nasopharyngitis or pharyngitis. These nodes disappear by preschool age, so the problem is limited to young infants.

Assessment. Typically, children have an upper respiratory tract infection or sore throat for a few days. Suddenly, they refuse to eat. They may drool because they are unable to swallow saliva. They have a high fever.

They "snore" with respirations because of the occlusion of the pharynx. To allow themselves more breathing space, they may hyperextend their head, a very unusual position for infants.

On physical assessment, regional lymph nodes will be enlarged. The mass itself may not be visible in the posterior pharynx if it is below the point of vision. An x-ray study using a swallowed contrast medium will reveal the bulging tissue in the pharynx. Laboratory studies will reveal a leukocytosis.

Therapeutic Management. Because the most frequent cause of retropharyngeal abscess is group-A beta-hemolytic streptococcus, amoxicillin is the drug of choice for treatment. Infants' mouths may need to be suctioned to remove secretions, because they swallow poorly. Be careful not to touch the suction catheter to the posterior pharynx, because this might rupture the abscess. This, in turn, could lead to aspiration of the abscess contents (producing respiratory obstruction, or a pneumonia caused by the aspirated purulent material). Blood vessels invade some retropharyngeal abscesses, so that rupture of the structure can lead to profuse bleeding (dangerous to the child because of the loss of blood from major arteries such as the carotid artery and because the blood can be aspirated).

Infants need to be placed in a prone or side-lying position to allow difficult-to-swallow mouth secretions to drain forward. Food is generally restricted, and intake may be limited to fluids. Make certain that parents understand this so they do not offer a hard food such as a toast crust (a substance good for teething). The sharp edges could rupture the abscess.

If the mass in the pharynx is fluctuant, it may be incised by a surgeon. This is done in surgery with the child in a Trendelenburg position, so that drainage from the abscess can be suctioned away to prevent aspiration. After surgery, place the child in a Trendelenburg or a prone position to encourage further drainage and prevent aspiration. Observe infants carefully for vital signs. Increased respiratory rate suggests airway obstruction. Observe drainage from children's mouths to detect fresh bleeding. Frequent swallowing is also a sign of postpharyngeal bleeding.

In infants, oral fluid is introduced as soon as the swallowing and gag reflexes are intact after surgery. Although the throat is undoubtedly still sore, most infants suck eagerly and need supplemental intravenous fluid administration for only a short time.

Parents need to handle infants and care for them while in the hospital so that they can regain their confidence in themselves as parents. On admission they are thoroughly frightened by the extent of the child's symptoms (gurgling or snoring sound, high temperature, dyspnea). They need time and opportunity to work through their fright if they are to care for the child with confidence once again.

Tonsillitis

Tonsillitis is the term commonly used to refer to infection and inflammation of the palatine tonsils. *Adenitis* refers to infection and inflammation of the adenoid (pharyngeal) tonsils.

Tonsillar tissue is lymphoid tissue that acts to form antibodies and to filter pathogenic organisms from the head and neck area. The palatine tonsils are located on both sides of the pharynx; the adenoids are in the nasopharynx. Tubal tonsils are located at the entrance to the eustachian tubes. Lingual tonsils are located at the base of the tongue. All the tonsils may be referred to collectively as *Waldeyer's ring* (Figure 40-18).

Assessment

Infection of the palatine tonsils gives all the symptoms of a severe pharyngitis. Children drool because their throat is too sore for them to swallow saliva. They may describe swallowing saliva as swallowing bits of metal or glass because it feels so sharp. They have a high fever and are lethargic. On physical assessment, pus can be detected on or expelled from the crypts of the tonsils. Tonsillar tissue appears bright red and may be so enlarged that the two areas of palatine tonsillar tissue meet in the midline.

The symptoms of adenoidal tissue infection are a nasal quality of speech, mouth breathing, difficulty hearing, and perhaps halitosis, in addition to fever, lethargy, pharyngeal pain, and edema. The mouth breathing and change in speech come from the postpharyngeal obstruction by the enlarged tissue. The difficulty with hearing occurs because of eustachian tube obstruction. Eustachian tube blockage can contribute to both serous and acute otitis media (middle ear infection). Enlarged adenoidal tissue may be a cause of sleep apnea because of underaeration.

The organism causing tonsillitis is identified by a throat culture. The organism is generally a group-A beta-hemolytic streptococcus.

Therapeutic Management

As therapy for tonsillitis, children need an antipyretic for fever, an analgesic for pain, and a full 10-day course of an antibiotic such as clindamycin or amoxycillin. Caution parents that although the pain of the infection will subside a day or two after the antibiotic administration is begun, children need the full 10-day course of antibiotic to eradicate streptococci completely from the back of the throat. After a tonsillar infection, tonsillar tissue may remain hypertrophied or it may atrophy and appear smaller than normal.

Tonsillectomy. *Tonsillectomy* is removal of the palatine tonsils. *Adenoidectomy* is removal of the pharyngeal tonsils. In the past, tonsillectomy was a common therapy following tonsillitis. In current practice, however, tonsil-

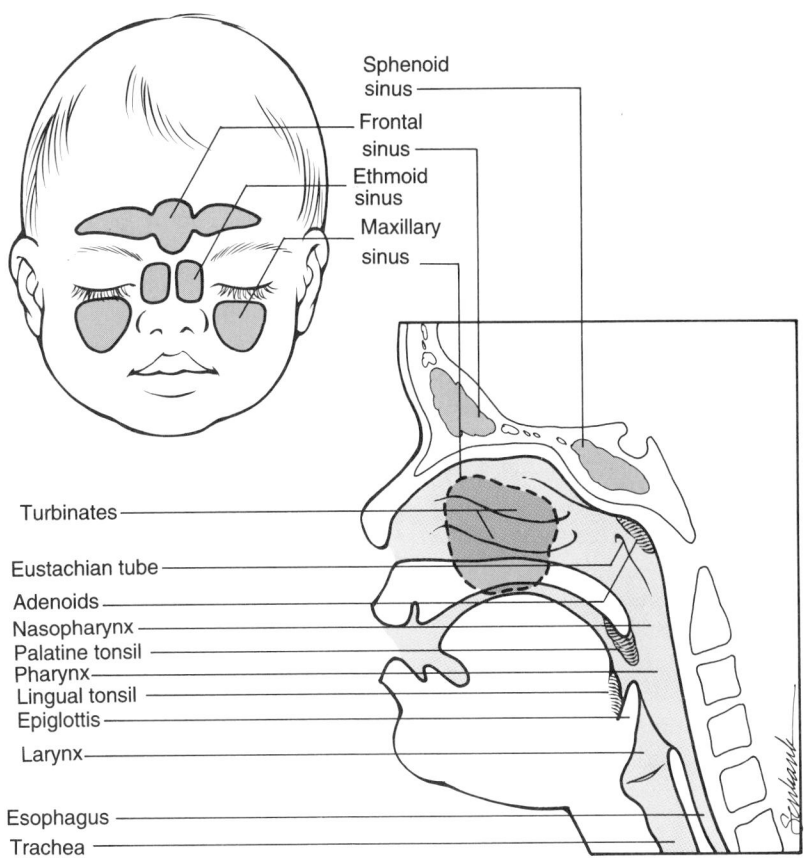

Sphenoid sinus
Frontal sinus
Ethmoid sinus
Maxillary sinus

Turbinates
Eustachian tube
Adenoids
Nasopharynx
Palatine tonsil
Pharynx
Lingual tonsil
Epiglottis
Larynx
Esophagus
Trachea

FIGURE 40-18
Anatomic features of upper respiratory tract.

lectomy is not recommended unless all other measures prove ineffective. Tonsillar tissue is removed by ligating the tonsil or by laser surgery (Stevens, 1990). Since sutures are not placed, the chance for hemorrhage after this type of surgery is higher than after surgery involving a closed incision. The danger of aspiration of blood at the time of surgery and the danger of a general anesthetic compound the risk.

Chronic tonsillitis is about the only reason for removal of palatine tonsils. Adenoids may be removed if they are so hypertrophied that they are causing obstruction. At one time, both adenoids and palatine tonsils were always removed together; today, depending on the symptoms and the extent of hypertrophy and infection, children may have a tonsillectomy, an adenoidectomy, or both.

Tonsillectomy or adenoidectomy is never done while the organs are infected, because an operation at such a time might spread pathogenic organisms into the bloodstream, causing septicemia. Parents often ask why an operation to remove tonsils must be delayed. They think that as long as the tonsils are sore, they should be immediately removed. They need an explanation of why this is not possible and why it is safer to schedule surgery for a later date.

Nursing Diagnoses and Related Interventions

Nursing Diagnosis: High risk for fluid volume deficit related to blood loss from surgery

Goal: Child will not experience significant fluid volume deficit during postoperative course.

Outcome Criteria: Child's pulse and blood pressure are normal for age group; no extensive bleeding is detected.

Prior to surgery for tonsillectomy, bleeding and clotting times should be recorded and a complete blood count and urinalysis should be made to verify general good health. These tests generally are done on an ambulatory basis, and children are admitted to the hospital only on the morning of surgery. Teach parents to use common sense in their child's care during the 2 weeks prior to hospital admission, so that the child does not have a cold or recurrent tonsillitis at the time planned for surgery. On the morning of surgery, the child receives a complete physical examination. An important aspect of assessment is for loose teeth that could be dislodged during surgery and aspirated. If loose teeth are present, mark this fact on the face of the child's chart and report it to the anesthesiologist.

After surgery, observe vital signs carefully to make certain that the child is not bleeding from the denuded surgical area. Place the child on the abdomen with a pillow under the chest so that the head is lower than the chest. This allows blood and unswallowed saliva to drain from the child's mouth rather than back to the pharynx, where it might be aspirated (Figure 40-19).

Because children will swallow any blood that is oozing from the surgical site, a child can be bleeding heavily and yet little blood is apparent. To detect bleeding, assess for subtle signs of hemorrhage: an increasing pulse or respiratory rate; frequent swallowing; throat clearing, and a feeling of anxiety. Hemorrhage following tonsillectomy can be acute and intense. A child's first line of defense is a nurse who recognizes these subtle signs of bleeding before the bleeding is so intense that symptoms of shock occur.

If bleeding does occur, elevating the child's head and turning him or her on the side reduces vascular pressure on the operative site yet continues to prevent obstruction. Physicians who examine the child need a good light source and a dentist's mirror so that they will have a good view of the posterior throat. Secure these items so the examination can be thorough and effective. If extreme hemorrhage of the surgical area occurs, the child may need to be returned to surgery for a suture or two to halt bleeding.

Occasionally, children have sufficient local bleeding and clot formation that a pharyngeal obstruction occurs. This event is accompanied by inspiratory stridor and an increased respiratory rate; the child may quickly become cyanotic and limp. If this occurs, notify the surgeon immediately. Extending a child's head and chest over the edge of the bed and striking the back sharply may dislodge the obstruction (AAP, 1991). If this is not effective, the child needs the back of the throat suctioned. Suctioning is potentially dangerous, because it may effectively remove the respiratory obstruction but initiate fresh bleeding.

The most dangerous periods following a tonsillectomy are the first 24 hours, when the clots covering the denuded surgical area are forming, and the fifth to seventh days, when the clots begin to lyse or dissolve. If new tissue is not yet present when the clots dissolve, hemorrhage from the denuded surface may result. If children have no complications from surgery, are able to swallow fluids, and have voided, they are generally discharged from the hospital later the same day of surgery or by the following morning. Parents need careful instruction concerning the danger signs to watch for in children during their first day home (frequent swallowing, clearing the throat, increasing restlessness). They are usually advised to restrict their child's activity until after the seventh day when firm healing should have taken place. The child needs a return appointment to a health care facility approximately 2 weeks after surgery for follow-up assessment that the surgical area has healed without complication.

Nursing Diagnosis: Pain related to surgical procedure

Goal: Child's level of discomfort will be limited to a tolerable level.

Outcome Criteria: Child states that level of pain is tolerable.

Tonsillectomy is an uncomfortable procedure for children. They need good preparation for the procedure and for sensations they will experience afterward. Although tonsils are removed, it is better to talk about tonsils being "fixed" rather than taken out; children may be extremely frightened to know that a body part will be removed, however small it is.

Most children are thirsty immediately after surgery. Swallowing fluid causes active pharyngeal movement, increasing the blood supply to the area and reducing edema and pain, so frequent sips of clear liquid or ice chips can be offered as soon as children have completely awakened from the anesthesia. Choose fluids carefully; dairy products tend to cling to the surgical site and make swallowing difficult; acid juices sting the denuded tissue, so are uncomfortable; and carbonated beverages irritate unless they are allowed to stand for a period of time to become "flat" (see the Focus on Nursing Research box).

Children are generally promised by well-meaning people that they can have all the ice cream they want

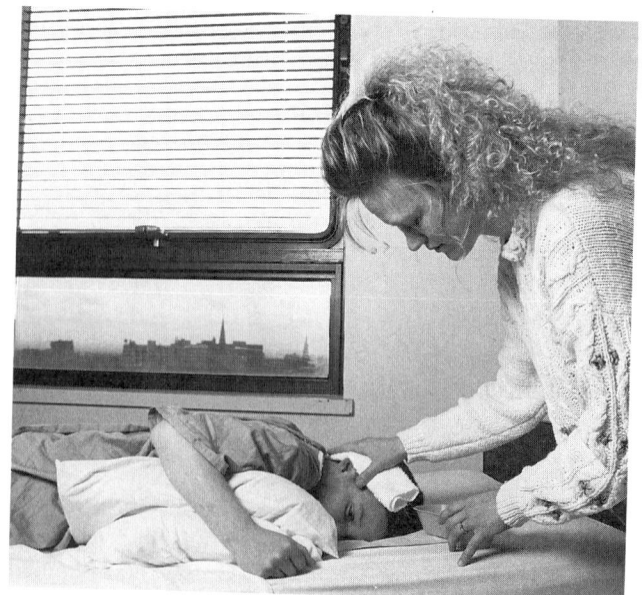

FIGURE 40-19

Positioning a child after tonsillectomy. The pillow under the chest helps secretions flow out of mouth. (Courtesy of the Department of Medical Photography, Children's Hospital, Buffalo, NY.)

FOCUS ON NURSING RESEARCH

Should Children Be Forced to Drink Fluid Following Tonsillectomy?

A child needs to drink enough fluid after surgery to remain well hydrated, and yet this can be very difficult because the child's throat is very sore. Prior to this study, post-tonsillectomy children under 20 kg were required to drink 700 mL of fluid before discharge; children over 20 kg were required to drink 1000 mL. If children did not drink readily, fluid was given into their mouths by syringe to ensure a high fluid intake. For this study, children admitted to the unit were divided into two groups: half were required to drink fluid according to the established routine; those in the second group were offered fluid but allowed to choose the rate at which they drank it.

Results of the study revealed that by 8 hours postoperatively, there was no significant difference in the amount of water taken by the two groups. This type of research is important for having questioned a nonscientific basis for a procedure and helping nurses determine their own rules for practice.

Carabott, J. A., Javaheri, Z., Keilty, K., & Manger, G. (1992). Oral fluid intake in children following tonsillectomy and adenoidectomy. *Pediatric Nursing, 18*, 124.

after a tonsillectomy, but because it forms tenacious secretions that are difficult to swallow, it is not a food of choice. A better treat is a Popsicle, which is a frozen clear liquid.

Children can be gradually put on a soft diet after 24 to 48 hours; they should continue to eat only soft foods for the first week. A selective diet can be given the second week (no toast crusts or other foods that could cause pharyngeal irritation if not chewed well). Be certain that parents know the telephone number they should call (clinic, hospital, or pediatrician) if they have a question or concern about a child's condition or care. Caution parents that some children develop a mild earache following tonsillectomy for the first week, probably caused by shifting pressure on the eustachian tube.

Epistaxis

Epistaxis (nosebleed) is extremely common in children. This usually occurs from trauma, such as picking at the nose, or from being hit on the nose by another child. In older homes that lack humidification, the hot dry environment makes children's mucous membranes dry, uncomfortable, and susceptible to cracking. In all children, epistaxis tends to occur during respiratory illnesses. It may occur after strenuous exercise. It is associated with a number of systemic diseases, such as rheumatic fever, scarlet fever, measles, or varicella infection (chicken-

pox). It can occur with nasal polyps, sinusitis, or allergic rhinitis. There apparently is a familial predisposition to epistaxis.

Nosebleeds are always frightening because of the visible bleeding and a choking sensation if blood should run down the back of the nasopharynx. The fear is generally out of proportion to the seriousness of the bleeding.

Keep children with nosebleeds in an upright position with their head tilted slightly forward to minimize the amount of blood pressure in nasal vessels and to keep blood moving forward, not back into the nasopharynx. Apply pressure to the sides of the nose with your fingers (Figure 40-20). Make every effort to quiet children and to help them stop crying, because crying increases pressure in the blood vessels of the head and prolongs bleeding. If these simple measures do not control the bleeding, epinephrine (1:1000) may be applied to the bleeding site to constrict blood vessels. A nasal pack may be necessary.

Every child has occasional nosebleeds. Chronic nasal bleeding, however, should be investigated to rule out a systemic disease or blood disorder. Parents who report that their child has "nosebleeds that just will not stop" are generally making the mistake of having the child lie down to treat the bleeding. Review with them the importance of keeping the child in an upright position and applying firm manual pressure.

Sinusitis

Sinusitis is rare in children under 6 years of age, because the frontal sinuses do not develop until age 6 (see Figure 40-20). This may occur as a secondary infection when streptococcal, staphylococcal, or *Hemo-*

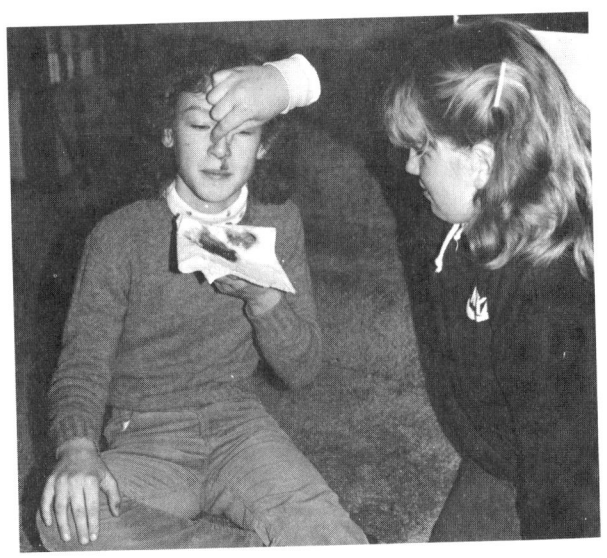

FIGURE 40-20
Emergency therapy for a nosebleed is to elevate the head and apply pressure to the sides of the nose.

philus influenzae organisms spread from the nasal cavity. Children will develop a fever, a purulent nasal discharge, headache, and tenderness over the affected sinus. Children should have a nose and throat culture taken to identify the infectious organism (Goldenhersh et al., 1990).

Treatment for acute sinusitis consists of an antipyretic for fever, an analgesic for pain, and an antibiotic for the specific organism involved. Nose drops such as phenylephrine or oxymetazoline hydrochloride (Afrin) to shrink the nasal congestion will allow drainage from the sinuses. Teach parents that the prolonged use of nasal drops or sprays can lead to nasal polyps. In order to avoid a rebound effect, they should be used for only 3 days at a time; otherwise, they actually cause more nasal congestion than originally. Warm compresses to the sinus area may both encourage drainage and relieve pain.

Sinusitis is considered by many adults to be a minor illness. It can have serious complications, however, if the infection spreads from the sinuses to invade the bone (osteomyelitis) or the middle ear (otitis media). Chronic sinusitis can interfere with school and social performance because of the constant pain.

Laryngitis

Laryngitis is inflammation of the larynx. It results in brassy, hoarse voice sounds or inability to make audible voice sounds. It may occur as a spread of pharyngitis or from excessive use of the voice, as in cheerleading. Laryngitis is as annoying for children as it is for adults. Sips of fluid (either warm or cold, whichever feels best) offer relief from the annoying tickling sensation often present. The most effective measure, however, is for children not to use their voice for at least 24 hours, until inflammation subsides. Be certain to meet infants' needs before they have to cry for things; older children simply need to be cautioned not to speak. Having children stay in bed is generally ineffective, because this requires them to shout to another room of the house to make their needs known; this merely adds to the irritation of the larynx.

Laryngeal Web

A web of tissue stretching between the vocal cords is an occasional congenital anomaly. Children will make a harsh crowing noise on inspiration (stridor). Under ordinary circumstances, the stridor may be absent; it will appear when children contract an upper respiratory tract infection and inflammation causes the web to swell and increase obstruction. If a web is large enough to cover the entire larynx, complete obstruction with cyanosis and death will result. Laryngeal webs are visualized by laryngoscopy. Treatment is surgical removal.

Congenital Laryngeal Stridor

Congenital laryngeal stridor (laryngomalacia) results when the child's laryngeal structure is weaker than normal and collapses more than usual on inspiration. The stridor is generally present from birth; it may be intensified when the child is in a supine position.

Assessment

The infant's sternum may become retracted on inspiration because of the increased effort to pull air into the trachea past the collapsed structure. The stridor may become most noticeable when infants suck. Most infants with this condition must stop sucking frequently during a feeding to maintain adequate ventilation. They may be exhausted easily and so interrupt their feeding to rest.

Therapeutic Management

Stridor is a frightening sound. Parents may worry that their child has aspirated something that should be removed surgically. When they wake at night and listen in a quiet house to the sound of stridor, it seems unbearably loud. They may need to be reassured at every health care visit that although the sound is raucous, it is safe for them to care for the infant at home. They need to see a weight chart that shows them that their child is growing and thriving despite this problem. Many parents sleep at night with a child's crib brought next to their bed or with one hand resting on the infant's chest so they can be assured during the night that the child is continuing to breathe. Assess at health care visits if parents are receiving enough sleep at night and are not becoming too exhausted to be able to continue work or give care.

Most children with congenital laryngeal stridor need no routine therapy other than to have parents feed them slowly, providing periods of rest as needed. The condition improves as children mature, because cartilage in the larynx becomes stronger at about 1 year of age.

Parents must be certain to bring the child for early care if signs of an upper respiratory tract infection develop. If not, laryngeal collapse will be even more intense during these times and complete obstruction of the trachea could occur. Any time stridor becomes more intense, infants should be seen by a physician, because generally this indicates beginning obstruction and probably the beginning of an upper respiratory tract infection. As parents become more used to the sound their infants make while breathing, they will become astute reporters of change in their infant's condition; listen to them carefully when they report a change so you do not miss this important information.

Croup (Laryngotracheobronchitis)

Croup (inflammation of the larynx, trachea, and major bronchi) is one of the most frightening diseases of early childhood. In children between 6 months and 3 years of age, the cause of croup is usually a viral infection such as parainfluenza virus; in children between 3 and 6 years, it may occur from *H. influenzae* (Skolnik, 1993).

Assessment

With croup, children typically have only a mild upper respiratory tract infection at bedtime; they have no fever or only a low-grade one. During the night they develop a barking cough (croupy cough), inspiratory stridor, and marked retractions. They wake in extreme respiratory distress. The larynx, trachea, and major bronchi are all inflamed. Cyanosis is rarely present, but the danger of glottal obstruction from the larynx inflammation is very real. The severe symptoms typically last a number of hours and then, except for a rattling cough, subside by morning. They may recur the following night. Pulse oximetry and transcutaneous CO_2 monitors are helpful measures to document if hypoxia is occurring.

Therapeutic Management

One emergency method of relieving croup symptoms is for a parent to run the shower or hot water tap in a bathroom until the room fills with steam, then keep the child in this warm, moist environment. If this does not relieve symptoms, the child should be transported to an emergency department for further evaluation and care. When a child is admitted to a hospital, cool moist air is supplied by means of a mist tent. Dextramethasone, a steroid, helps to reduce airway edema. Racemic epinephrine given by nebulizer causes effective bronchodilation and is prescribed to maintain a patent airway. Intravenous therapy may be begun to keep the child well hydrated.

Nursing Diagnoses and Related Interventions

Nursing Diagnosis: High risk for ineffective airway clearance related to edema and constriction of airway

Goal: Child will demonstrate adequate airway clearance by 1 hour.

Outcome Criteria: Respiratory rate is below 22 breaths/min; no cyanosis is present; Po_2 is 80 to 100 mm Hg.

Remain constantly with a child not only to observe closely but to reduce anxiety. Encourage a parent to remain constantly with the child for the same reason. It might be necessary for a parent to tuck his or her head into a mist tent with a child to keep the child content and not frightened by the plastic enclosure. Take vital signs as often as every 15 minutes, because extreme restlessness and thrashing, increased heart and respiratory rates, and cyanosis are symptoms of air hunger; tracheotomy or intubation may be necessary if these symptoms occur. (It is difficult to intubate children with croup

because of the severe respiratory tract edema.) Increasing stridor is also a good indication of increasing inflammation. Stridor may be deceptive, however, in the event that a child's air exchange begins to fall, because then insufficient air will pass through the respiratory tract to cause loud stridor. In some children, it is difficult to distinguish between fright from the newness of the experience (and their sense of their parent's fright) and the anxiousness that comes from oxygen want. Keep a continuous record of vital signs and activity as a way to easily demonstrate increasing respiratory rate and restlessness. A blood gas may be taken to assess for sufficient oxygenation if pulse oximetry is not being used.

Ensure that the child remains hydrated and secretions stay moist by offering frequent sips of oral fluid, unless the child has such rapid respirations that drinking is not possible. In this instance, the child will need intravenous therapy. Measure intake and output and urine specific gravity to evaluate hydration.

Laryngospasm with total occlusion of the airway is most apt to occur when a child's gag reflex is elicited or when the child is crying. Comfort to prevent crying; do not elicit a gag reflex of any child with a croupy, barking cough.

Croup is a frightening disease for parents, because the symptoms of distress appear so suddenly. If the severe symptoms disappear by morning, parents may feel foolish that they rushed to a hospital with the child in the middle of the night. Assure them that their judgment was correct. When they brought the child in at 2 AM, he or she was seriously ill. Parents may be reluctant to see children discharged in the morning; they may need to spend some time with them in the hospital the next morning before they are convinced that they are now well enough to go home (see the Nursing Care Plan: The Child With Croup).

Epiglottitis

Epiglottitis is inflammation of the epiglottis (the flap of tissue that covers the opening to the larynx to keep out food and fluid during swallowing; see Figure 40-19). Although occurring rarely, inflammation of the epiglottis creates an emergency situation because the swollen epiglottis is unable to rise and allow the airway to open. This occurs most frequently in children from 3 to about 6 years of age.

Epiglottitis can be either bacterial or viral in origin. *H. influenzae* type B is the most common bacterial cause of the disorder, but pneumococci, streptococci, or staphylococci may be responsible. Echovirus and respiratory syncytial virus also can cause the disorder (Bradford, 1993).

Assessment

Children's symptoms begin as those of a mild upper respiratory tract infection. After 1 or 2 days, as inflam-

Sylvester is a 12-month-old child admitted to your care unit with a diagnosis of croup. The following is a nursing care plan you might design for him.

Assessment: Father is out of town and unable to be contacted by telephone. Mother standing by desk area, crying. States, "Don't use an oxygen tent. My father smothered and died in a tent." States child had slight cold at bedtime. Woke an hour ago with difficulty breathing and bad cough. She tired to give him cough syrup, which he vomited with coughing. Respiratory rate; 50 breaths/min; loud stridor; sharp, barking cough; deep substernal retractions present; nasal flaring. Temperature: 39°C; apical pulse: 170 bpm; arterial blood gases: Po_2, 64 mm Hg; Pco_2, 48 mm Hg (room air).

Nursing Diagnosis: Ineffective airway clearance related to tracheal inflammation secondary to laryngotrachealitis

Defining Characteristic: Respiratory rate is 50 breaths/min; stridor and cough are present.

Goal: Child's respiratory distress will decrease with care measures by 1 h.

Outcome Criteria: Respiratory rate decreases to 20–24 breaths/min.

Nursing Orders	Rationale
1. Take and record respiratory rate q1/2h until below 40 breaths/min.	1. This data will help detect an increase in respiratory rate.
2. Tylenol, 1 gr, given for temperature over 39°C; repeat q4h PRN.	2. Tylenol will help reduce fever and make child more comfortable.
3. Child placed in mist tent; 30% oxygen prescribed. Keep chest exposed for easy viewing of respiratory rate.	3. Mist can be therapeutic in reducing airway inflammation.
4. Encourage fluid. Find out child's preferences and supply.	4. Good hydration can help prevent respiratory obstruction.
5. Assist respiratory therapist with racemic epinephrine therapy q1h. Hold child on lap for therapist.	5. Racemic epinephrine can enlarge airway lumen. Holding will help relieve child's anxiety and ensure effective administration.

Nursing Diagnosis: Parental fear related to obvious distress of child

Defining Characteristic: Mother voices fear at how ill her child has become and how father died in oxygen tent.

Goal: Mother will voice that she feels more comfortable about condition of child.

Outcome Criteria: Mother voices that croup is inflammation of major airway and use of cool mist will decrease inflammation, not harm son.

Nursing Orders	Rationale
1. Explain to parent procedures being used.	1. Knowledge of procedures can aid acceptance.
2. Encourage mother to participate in care.	2. Help mother gain sense of control and comfort child.
3. Encourage mother to stay in tent with child.	3. Mother can see for herself that tent is not suffocating. As the mother's fear subsides, so will her child's.

mation spreads to the epiglottis, they suddenly develop severe inspiratory stridor, a high fever, hoarseness, and a very sore throat. They may have difficulty swallowing, as evidenced by excessive drooling. They may protrude their tongues to increase free movement in the pharynx.

If the child's gag reflex were initiated with a tongue blade, the swollen and inflamed epiglottis would rise in the back of the throat as a cherry-red structure. It could be so edematous, however, that the gagging procedure would cause complete obstruction of the glottis and respiratory failure. Therefore, *children with symptoms of epiglottitis (dysphagia, inspiratory stridor, fever, and hoarseness) should never be gagged by a tongue blade unless a means of providing an artificial airway, such as tracheotomy or intubation, is readily available.* This is important for the nurse functioning in an expanded role, who performs physical assessments and routinely elicits gag reflexes.

Laboratory studies will reveal leukocytosis (20,000 to 30,000 mm^3) with the proportion of neutrophils increased. An arterial blood sample may be taken for analysis of blood gases and for a culture for septicemia. However, because excessive crying can precipitate entrapment of the epiglottis and obstruction, such tests may be delayed in preference to a lateral neck x-ray film or sonogram, which will reveal the enlarged epiglottis. Do not allow a child with possible epiglottitis to go to the x-ray department accompanied only by parents or a nursing aide, in case obstruction occurs while in the x-ray room.

Therapeutic Management

Children need moist air to reduce the epiglottal inflammation. If cyanosis is present, they need oxygen. An antibiotic, particularly cefuroxime or chloramphenicol (Chloromycetin) because either is effective against *H. influenzae,* may be prescribed until a throat culture indicates a specific antibiotic drug. Being unable to swallow, children need intravenous administration of fluid to maintain hydration. They may need a prophylactic tracheotomy or endotracheal intubation to prevent total obstruction. It is often difficult to intubate children with epiglottitis because the tube cannot be passed beyond the edematous epiglottis. After antibiotic therapy, the epiglottal inflammation recedes rapidly, and by 12 to 24 hours it has reduced in size enough that the airway may be removed. Antibiotic administration will continue for a full 7 to 10 days. Siblings of the ill child may be prescribed rifampin for prophylaxis.

The symptoms of epiglottitis are not unlike those of croup. Parents may not realize the extent of the occlusion in their child if the child has had croup on other occasions. They may question why a prophylactic tracheotomy was necessary this time when it was not used when the child had croup. Explain to them the difference between the two diseases (Table 40-9).

Some infants with epiglottitis die because obstruction occurs before a tracheotomy can be accomplished. If this should happen, parents need to be assured that they could not realize the seriousness of their child's symptoms. They may become overcautious, bringing other children to health care settings repeatedly for symptoms that are obviously not serious. It takes these parents time to regain confidence in themselves as parents and in their ability to judge a child's health again.

Aspiration

Aspiration is inhalation of a foreign object into the airway. Objects are most frequently aspirated by infants and toddlers. When a child aspirates a large foreign object, the immediate reaction is choking and hard, forceful coughing. Usually, this results in dislodging the object. However, if the cough becomes ineffective (no

---

Table 40-9. *Comparison of Laryngotracheobronchitis (Croup) and Epiglottitis*

Assessment	Laryngotracheobronchitis	Epiglottitis
Causative organism	Usually viral	Usually *Haemophilus influenzae*
Usual age of child	6 mo–3 yr	3–6 yr
Seasonal occurrence	Late fall and winter	No seasonal variation
Onset pattern	Preceded by upper respiratory infection; cough becomes worse at night	Preceded by upper respiratory infection; suddenly very ill
Presence of fever	Low grade	Elevated to about 103°F
Appearance	Retractions and stridor; prolonged inspiratory phase of respirations; not very ill appearing	Drooling; very ill appearing; neck is hyperextended to breathe. (Do not attempt to view enlarged epiglottis, or immediate airway obstruction can occur.)
Cough	Sharp, barking	Muffled cough
Radiographic findings	Lateral neck radiograph shows subglottal narrowing	Lateral neck radiograph shows enlarged epiglottis.
Possible complications	Asphyxia due to subglottic obstruction	Asphyxia due to supraglottic obstruction

sound with cough, or if there are signs of increased respiratory difficulty accompanied by stridor), some intervention is essential. A series of Heimlich subdiaphragmatic abdominal thrusts are recommended for children (but not for infants—see below; American Heart Association, 1992). Stand behind the child and place a fist just under the child's diaphragm (a point immediately below the anterior rib cage). Embrace the child, grip your fist with your other hand, and pull back and up with a rapid thrust. This action of pushing up on the diaphragm forces the aspirated material out of the trachea (Figure 40-21). If the child loses consciousness before the foreign body is expelled, the airway should be opened and rescue breathing attempted (American Heart Association, 1992).

If a child was lying on his or her back at the time of the aspiration, stand at the head of the bed or table, place your hands in the same position as just described for the Heimlich maneuver, and exert the same inward and upward thrust. A Heimlich maneuver may cause the child to vomit as well as expel an aspirated object. Turn the child's head to prevent aspiration of vomitus.

Heimlich thrusts are not recommended for infants because of the concern that they may cause laceration of the liver (American Heart Association, 1992). A combination of back blows and chest thrusts is considered the most effective method for relieving complete foreign

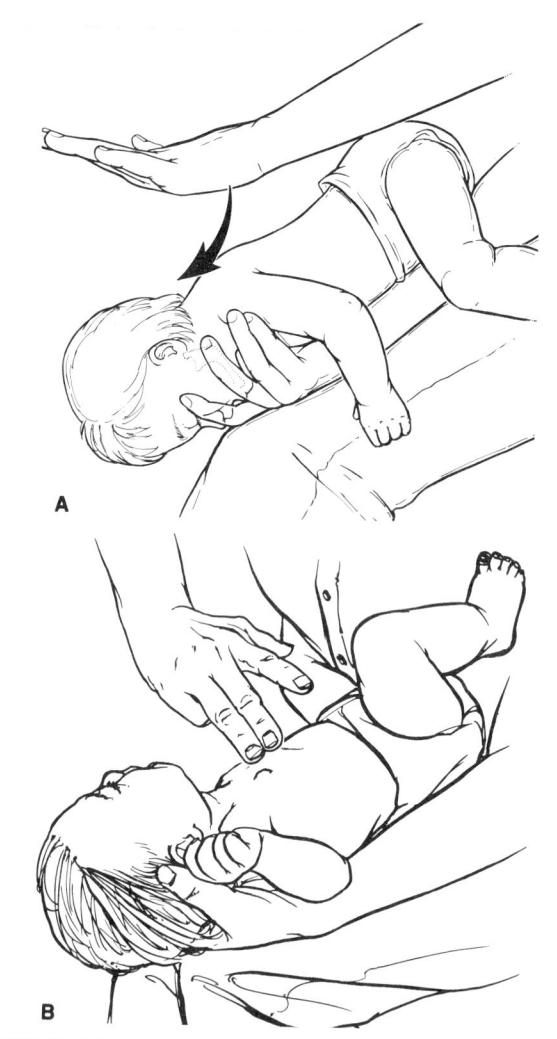

FIGURE 40-22

*Back blows (**A**) and chest compression (**B**) to relieve complete foreign body airway obstruction in an infant. (From American Heart Association. [1992] Pediatric basic life support. Journal of the American Medical Association, 268, 2251–2261, with permission.)*

body airway obstruction in infants. Turn the infant prone over your arm and administer up to five quick back blows forcefully between the infant's shoulder blades, using the heel of the hand (Figure 40-22A). If the object is not expelled, turn the infant while the head and neck are carefully supported and hold the infant in a supine position draped over your thigh. Provide up to five quick downward thrusts in the lower third of the sternum (Figure 40-22B; American Heart Association, 1992). This is generally enough to dislodge the foreign object. However, if this does not occur, rescue breathing may then be attempted. The infant will cough and expel the object.

Bronchial Obstruction

The right main bronchus is straighter and has a larger lumen than the left bronchus in children over 2 years of age. For this reason, an aspirated foreign object that is

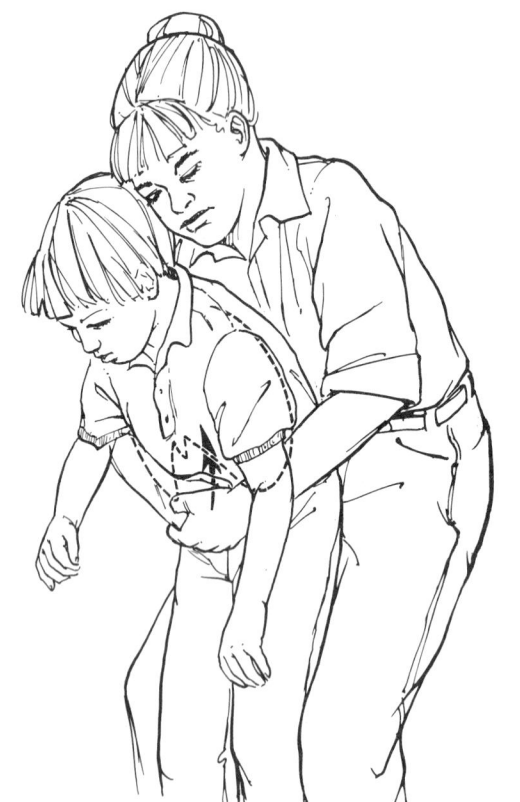

FIGURE 40-21

Heimlich maneuver on a school-age child. (From American Heart Association. [1992]. Pediatric basic life support. Journal of the American Medical Association, 268, 2251–2261, with permission.)

not large enough to obstruct the trachea may lodge in the right bronchus, obstructing a portion or all of the right lung. The alveoli distal to the obstruction will collapse as the air remaining in them becomes absorbed (atelectasis), or hyperinflation and pneumothorax may occur if the foreign body serves as a ball valve, allowing air to enter but not leave the alveoli (Figure 40-23).

Assessment

After aspirating a small foreign body, the child generally begins to cough violently and may become dyspneic. Hemoptysis, fever, purulent sputum, and leukocytosis will result if the object scratches the airway or infection develops. Localized wheezing (a high whistling sound on expiration made by air passing through the narrow lumen) may occur. Because it is localized, it is different from the generalized wheezing of a child with asthma.

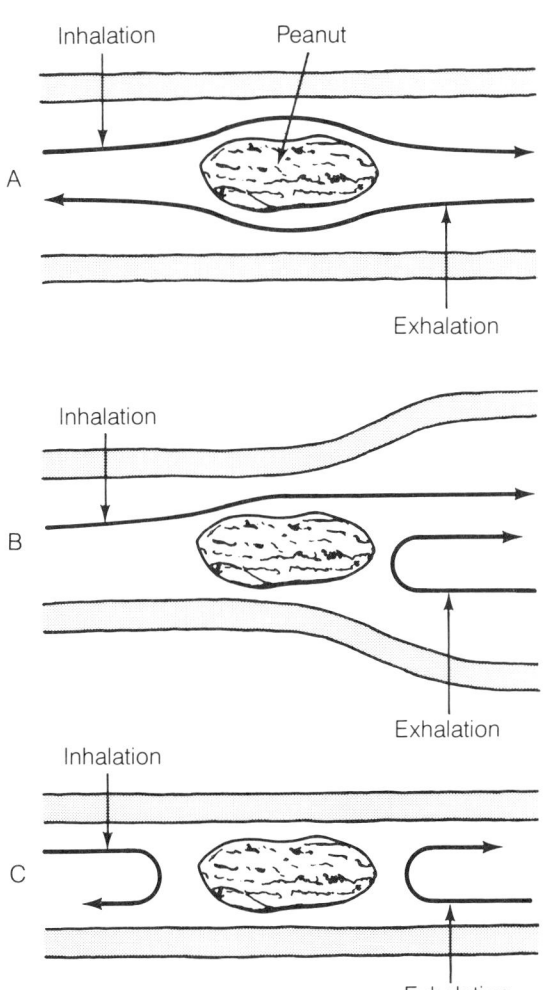

FIGURE 40-23
*Various effects of an aspirated foreign object in the airway. (**A**) The object is small enough that air can be both inhaled and exhaled around it. (**B**) The object is big enough to allow inhalation, but it obstructs exhalation. (**C**) The object has swollen, effectively halting both inhalation and exhalation.*

A chest x-ray film will reveal the presence of a radiopaque object. Objects most frequently aspirated are bones, nuts, coins, and safety pins (see Figure 40-6). As a rule, nuts or popcorn should not be given to children under school age, because these objects are so frequently aspirated. These objects are coated with oil, and as they swell with moisture in the respiratory tract, they cause not only obstruction but lipid pneumonia, a particularly difficult pneumonia to treat. Foreign bodies that are inhaled this deeply are rarely coughed up spontaneously, despite the severe coughing that ensues. Because objects such as bones and nuts cannot be visualized well on x-ray film, an x-ray study may be inconclusive. Most objects can be removed successfully by laryngoscopy or bronchoscopy.

Therapeutic Management

Children who are seen in emergency departments because of this type of aspirated foreign body are in distress from pain and are choking and coughing. Their parents are frightened by the degree of distress. They may have reason to feel badly about having offered a child (or allowing the child to reach) a food such as a peanut. Children need quick orientation to the treatment environment, because they may be taken immediately to the x-ray department, then to the operating room; they will be submitted very quickly to one new hospital environment after another. If possible, their parents should be allowed to go with them to x-ray and into surgery until the anesthetic is given.

Following bronchoscopy, the child must be observed closely and vital signs must be taken frequently to detect bronchial edema and airway obstruction. For details on the bronchoscopy procedure, see Chapter 37. The child is kept on NPO status for at least an hour; the first fluid must be given cautiously to be certain that the child does not aspirate it from difficulty swallowing. Cool fluid helps to reduce the soreness in the throat. Breathing cool, moist air or having an external ice collar applied may further reduce edema. Secretions that collect in the bronchus because of the irritation of manipulation can be kept moist and liquefied by placing the child in a mist tent.

Obviously, parents need to be cautioned about the danger of aspiration. Do not lecture, however. A parent whose child has just been through this experience recognizes the danger of aspiration and the need to be more careful in the future.

Disorders of the Lower Respiratory Tract

The structures of the lower respiratory tract are subject to infection by the same pathogens that can attack the upper respiratory tract structures. Inflammation and infection of the lungs, or pneumonia, is particularly troublesome and is seen in many different forms in children. Other illnesses that occur in the lower respiratory tract, such as cystic fibrosis, can lead to dangerous pneumonia infections.

Common disorders of the lower respiratory tract are illustrated in Figure 40-24. One of the most common childhood diseases, asthma, which is caused by a spasm of bronchial tubes, is discussed in Chapter 42 because of its connection to immune function. However, many of the same diagnostic and therapeutic tools and techniques, and certainly many of the nursing diagnoses and interventions for children with respiratory disorders described in this chapter, may also apply to the child with asthma.

Bronchitis

Bronchitis, or inflammation of the major bronchi and trachea, is one of the more common illnesses affecting preschool and school-age children (see Figure 40-24; Hanson & Shearer, 1994). It is characterized by fever and cough, usually in conjunction with nasal congestion. Causative agents include the influenza viruses, adenovirus, and *Mycoplasma pneumoniae*, among others.

Assessment

On auscultation, rhonchi and coarse rales can be heard. The child may have a mild upper respiratory tract infection for 1 or 2 days; the child then develops a fever and a dry, hacking cough that is hoarse and mildly productive in older children. The cough is serious enough to wake the child from sleep. These symptoms may last for a week, with full recovery sometimes taking as long as 2 weeks.

A chest x-ray film will reveal diffuse alveolar hyperinflation; there may be some markings at the hilus of the lung.

Therapeutic Management

Therapy is aimed at relieving the symptoms of illness, reducing fever and maintaining adequate hydration. An antibiotic will be prescribed if the infecting organism is a bacterium. If mucus is viscid, an expectorant may be helpful. It is important that children with bronchitis cough to raise accumulating sputum. Cough syrups to suppress the cough, therefore, are rarely indicated.

Bronchiolitis

Bronchiolitis is inflammation of the fine bronchioles and small bronchi. It occurs most often in children under the age of 2 years; the peak incidence is at 6 months of age. Incidence is highest in the winter and spring months. Many children who develop asthma later in life have numerous instances of bronchiolitis during their first year of life. Viruses, and the respiratory syncytial virus (RSV) in particular, appear to be the pathogens most responsi-

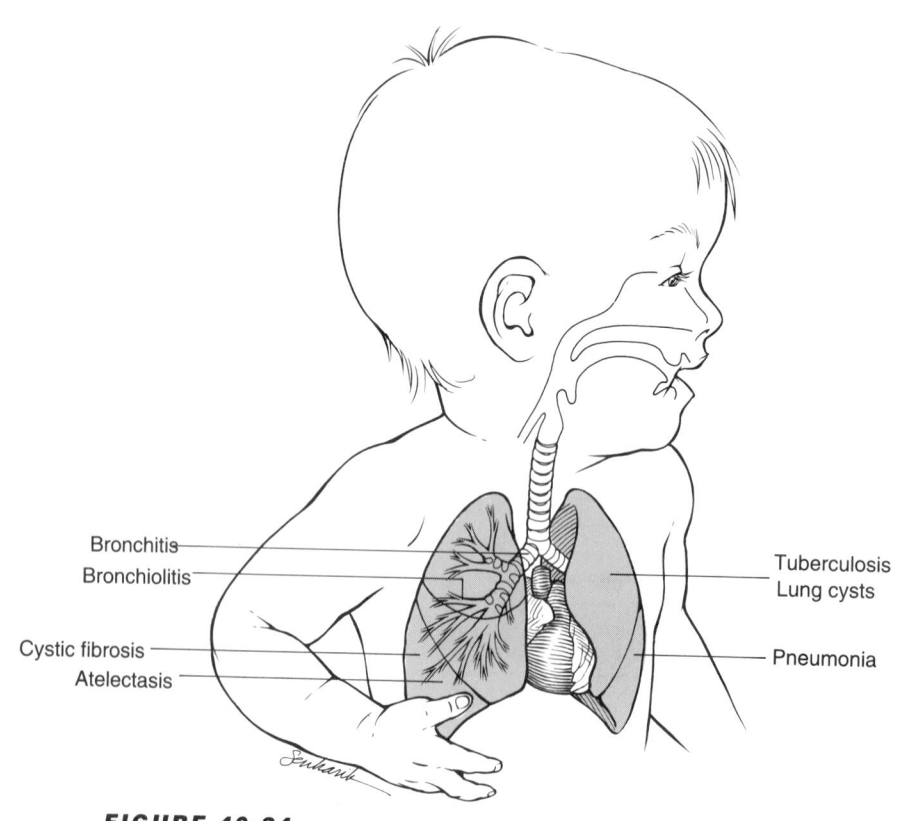

FIGURE 40-24
Sites of common lower respiratory tract disorders in children.

Bronchitis
Bronchiolitis

Cystic fibrosis
Atelectasis

Tuberculosis
Lung cysts

Pneumonia

ble for this illness. In fact, RSV is associated with most epidemic outbreaks of the illness (Hanson & Shearer, 1994).

Assessment

Typically, children have 1 or 2 days of an upper respiratory tract infection, then suddenly begin to have nasal flaring, intercostal and subcostal retractions on inspiration (Figure 40-25), and an increased respiratory rate. There is elongation of the expiratory phase of respiration; wheezing may be present. Mucus and inflammation block the small bronchioles, and air can no longer enter or leave alveoli freely. Most children develop hyperinflation of the alveoli because air enters more easily than it leaves inflamed, narrowed bronchioles. Following initial hyperinflation, areas of atelectasis may occur as alveoli are blocked and the air they contain is absorbed. Infants develop tachycardia and cyanosis from hypoxia. Soon they become exhausted from the rapid respirations. A chest x-ray film may show pulmonary infiltrates caused by a secondary infection or collapse of alveoli (atelectasis). Pulse oximetry reveals low hemoglobin saturation (Mulholland et al., 1990). They may have a mild fever, leukocytosis, and an increased erythrocyte sedimentation rate.

Therapeutic Management

Hospitalization is warranted for children in severe distress (e.g., if the child is tachypneic, has marked retractions, seems listless, or has a history of poor fluid intake; Hanson & Shearer, 1994). Oxygen, critical monitoring of vital signs and blood gas levels, and ventilatory support may be given. The use of bronchodilator therapy in infants with acute bronchiolitis is controversial, and studies have been published that both support and refute their positive effect. However, nebulized albuterol is sometimes used to help protect against progression to respiratory failure (Hanson & Shearer, 1994). For children with less severe symptoms, antipyretics, adequate

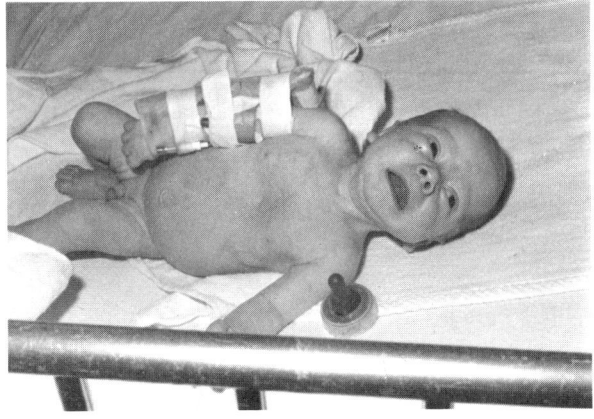

FIGURE 40-25
Infant displays prominent subcostal and mild intercostal retractions. (Courtesy of Bruce Hill.)

hydration, and maintaining a watchful eye on progression to more serious illness are recommended (Dorkin, 1993).

Antibiotics are not commonly used in the treatment of bronchiolitis, since bacteria is rarely a causative factor. Some severely ill children, infants under age 6 weeks, or children with congenital heart disease or immunodeficiency, may be treated with ribavirin by aerosol (given in a mask, hood, or tent) (Hanson & Shearer, 1994). Ribavirin is an antiviral agent effective against RSV and influenza viruses A and B.

Because ribavirin is given by aerosol, some of the drug escapes into the air. Nurses caring for children receiving the drug have reported headache and eye irritation. Ribavirin has the potential to be teratogenic to a growing fetus, although the incidence of this actually happening is difficult to document (Jury, 1993). In order to limit the amount of ribavirin in the air, a second oxygen canopy is suggested, to be used over the oxygen hood with the room door kept closed. It is also helpful if nurses discontinue nebulization for about 5 minutes before lifting the tent or oxygen hood. If the hood must be lifted frequently for care, health care providers and visitors can be fitted with respiratory masks. Wearing gowns and gloves can reduce the possibility of skin irritation.

In addition, all children need moist oxygen to counteract cyanosis and adequate hydration to keep respiratory membranes moist. A number of children may need assistance to achieve adequate ventilation. They all need to be carefully observed because respiratory syncytial virus may cause apnea. In some infants, extracorporeal membrane oxygenation (the same as that used for heart surgery) is necessary to maintain adequate oxygenation (Steinhorn & Green, 1990).

Infants are usually positioned in a semi-Fowler's position to facilitate breathing, although some appear to be more comfortable on their abdomen. The prone position allows the weight of the body to help empty the chest more completely on expiration. Feeding is often a problem; infants tire easily and, therefore, cannot finish a feeding. Intravenous fluids may be given for the first 1 or 2 days of illness to eliminate the need for oral feeding.

Health care providers who are pregnant or have asthma or chronic obstructive pulmonary disease should not routinely care for children with RSV infections. RSV is spread most easily by hand transmission. Health care providers should be certain to wash well after client care to avoid nosocomial infection.

Nursing Diagnoses and Related Interventions

Nursing Diagnosis: Parental anxiety related to respiratory distress in child

Goal: Parents will demonstrate reduced anxiety regarding child's illness by 24 hours.

Outcome Criteria: Parents state that anxiety level is tolerable as signs and symptoms of disease decrease.

Parents need a good explanation of the child's condition. Most parents are aware of bronchi but are unfamiliar with the word *bronchiole.* They may be unable to understand how a simple cold has become so severe. They wonder if they should have sought medical attention sooner. They need to be assured that bronchiolitis begins first as only a cold; they could not have known at that point that this cold would take a more serious turn.

Parents need to remain with the child and give as much care as possible. They can hold the child in the tent. As soon as possible, they need to begin offering feedings and to resume their care of the child. Most young parents lose confidence in themselves as parents when such a young infant becomes so severely ill. Before the child is discharged from the hospital, parents need support to gain confidence in their ability to evaluate the child's health and to care for him or her again.

The acute phase of bronchiolitis lasts 2 or 3 days. After this time, the child's condition improves rapidly. Although mortality from bronchiolitis is less than 1%, it is a serious disorder of infancy; without treatment, a larger number of infants certainly would die.

Bronchiectasis

Bronchiectasis is chronic dilatation of the bronchi. It may follow pneumonia, aspiration of a foreign body, pertussis, or asthma. It is often associated with cystic fibrosis.

Children develop a chronic cough that produces mucopurulent sputum. Young infants may have accompanying wheezing or stridor. If a large area of lung is obstructed, children may have cyanosis. As the disease becomes chronic, children may develop symptoms of chronic lung disease, such as clubbing of the fingers and easy fatigability. Their physical growth may become retarded. Their chest may become enlarged from overinflation of alveoli caused by the air trapped behind inflamed bronchi.

Postural drainage may be necessary to raise tenacious sputum. An antibiotic will be necessary if infection is present. The cause of the bronchiectasis must be identified and relieved before the chronic process can be relieved.

Pneumonia

Pneumonia is inflammation of the lung alveoli. Although far fewer children are hospitalized with pneumonia today than formerly, pneumonia is still an important cause of serious childhood illness. Pneumonia may be of bacterial origin (pneumococcal, streptococcal, staphylococcal, or chlamydial) or viral origin. Aspiration of lipid or hydrocarbon substances also causes pneumonia. Pneumonia is the most common pulmonary cause of death in infants under 48 hours of age. It occurs most often in late winter and early spring. Newborns who are born more than 24 hours after rupture of the amniotic membranes and those who aspirated amniotic fluid during delivery are particularly prone to developing pneumonia in their first few days of life (see Chapter 39). When it is known that the membranes have been ruptured for more than 24 hours before birth, prophylactic broad-spectrum antibiotics may be given to prevent pneumonia. Differences between bronchiolitis and pneumonia are summarized in Table 40-10. *Pneumocystis carinii* pneumonia, the type seen almost exclusively with human immunodeficiency syndrome, is discussed in Chapter 42.

Table 40-10. Comparison of Bronchiolitis and Pneumonia

Assessment	Bronchiolitis	Pneumonia
Cause	Usually respiratory syncytial virus	May be bacterial (pneumococcal, or *H. influenzae*), viral, or mycoplasmal; can occur from aspiration
Age of child	Under 2 yr	All through childhood
Onset pattern	Follows an upper respiratory infection	Follows an upper respiratory infection
Appearance	Fatigued, anxious, shallow respirations; increasing anteroposterior diameter of chest	Fatigued, anxious, shallow respirations
Cough	Paroxysmal, dry	Productive, harsh cough
Fever	Low grade	Elevated
Auscultatory sounds	Barely audible breath sounds; rales; expiratory wheezing	Decreased breath sounds; rales

Pneumococcal Pneumonia

The onset of pneumococcal pneumonia is generally abrupt and follows an upper respiratory tract infection. In infants, pneumonia tends to remain bronchopneumonia with poor consolidation (infiltration of exudate into the alveoli). In older children, pneumonia may localize in a single lobe, and consolidation may occur. With this, children may have blood-tinged sputum as exudative serum and red blood cells invade the alveoli. After 24 to 48 hours, the alveoli are no longer filled with red blood cells and serum but fibrin, leukocytes, and pneumococci; the child's cough no longer raises blood-tinged sputum but thick purulent material.

Assessment. Children develop a high fever, nasal flaring, retractions, chest pain, chills, and dyspnea. Some children report the pain as being abdominal (Modlin, 1994). The fever with pneumococcal pneumonia may rise so fast that a child has a febrile convulsion.

Children with pneumococcal pneumonia appear acutely ill. Physical assessment will reveal tachypnea and tachycardia; because lung space is filled with exudate, respiratory function is diminished. Breath sounds become bronchial (sound transmitted from the trachea) as air no longer or poorly enters fluid-filled alveoli. Rales will be present as a result of the fluid. Percussion will reveal dullness over a lobe in which consolidation has occurred. Chest x-ray films will reveal lung consolidation in older children and patchy diffusion in young children. Laboratory studies will reveal leukocytosis.

Therapeutic Management. Before antibiotic therapy was available for pneumonia, it was almost always a fatal disease, especially in infants, so parents may be more worried about a child's condition than is warranted. They need to be told of a child's favorable progress: "His temperature is down today; his breathing is slower than yesterday. These are good signs." They should begin to participate in caring for the child as the condition improves so that they can be assured that the child is getting better.

Therapy for pneumococcal pneumonia is antibiotics; penicillin G is the drug usually prescribed because it is extremely effective against pneumococci. Infants need rest to prevent exhaustion. Plan nursing care carefully to conserve a child's strength. Turn and reposition frequently to avoid pooling of secretions. Intravenous therapy may be necessary to supply fluid, especially in infants, because infants tire so readily with sucking that they cannot achieve a good oral intake. They may need an antipyretic such as acetaminophen to reduce fever.

Respirations will be less labored if the child breathes a cool, moist oxygen mixture. Postural drainage will encourage the movement of mucus and prevent obstruction. Older children may need to be encouraged to cough so that secretions do not pool and become further infected.

Following pneumonia, children usually have a period of at least a week when they tire easily and need frequent, small feedings. Parents need to be cautioned that this is an expected outcome and not a complication in itself. Children with chronic illness or who are immunocompromised receive a pneumococcal vaccine to prevent pneumonia.

Chlamydial Pneumonia

Chlamydia trachomatis pneumonia is most often seen in newborns up to 12 weeks of age. Symptoms usually begin gradually with nasal congestion and a sharp cough; children fail to gain weight. Symptoms continue to tachypnea with wheezing and rales audible on auscultation. Laboratory assessment will reveal an elevated level of IgG and IgM antibodies, peripheral eosinophilia, and a specific antibody to *C. trachomatis*. Such an infection is treated with erythromycin with good results.

Viral Pneumonia

Viral pneumonia is generally caused by the viruses of upper respiratory tract infection: the respiratory syncytial viruses, myxoviruses, or adenoviruses. The symptoms begin as an upper respiratory tract infection. After a day or two, symptoms (a low-grade fever, nonproductive cough, and tachypnea) begin. There may be diminished breath sounds and fine rales on chest auscultation, although few symptoms of lung disease may be noticed. Chest x-ray studies will reveal diffuse infiltrated areas. Respiratory syncytial virus may cause apnea.

Because this is a viral infection, antibiotic therapy is not effective. The child needs rest and, possibly, an antipyretic for the fever; intravenous fluid may be necessary if the child becomes exhausted from feeding. After recovery from the acute phase of illness, the child will have a week or two of lethargy or lack of energy, as occurs with bacterial pneumonia. Parents may be confused because their child is not receiving an antibiotic, despite the diagnosis being pneumonia. They need an explanation of the difference between viral and bacterial infections, so that they can better understand their child's therapy and plan of care.

Mycoplasmal Pneumonia

The *Mycoplasma* organisms are similar to, yet larger than, viruses. Mycoplasmal pneumonia occurs more frequently in older children (over 5 years) and more often during the winter months.

The symptoms of a mycoplasmal pneumonia make it difficult to differentiate from other pneumonias. The child has a fever and a cough and feels ill. Cervical lymph nodes will be enlarged; the child may have a persistent rhinitis.

Mycoplasmal organisms generally are sensitive to

erythromycin or tetracycline. Erythromycin is the preferred drug for children younger than 8 years of age, because tetracycline tends to stain teeth brown and possibly stunt long bone growth.

Lipid Pneumonia

Lipid pneumonia is caused by the aspiration of oily or lipid substances. It is much less common than it once was, because children are not given castor oil or cod liver oil as they were in the past. Lipid pneumonia may be caused by aspirated oily foreign bodies such as peanuts. A proliferative inflammatory response occurs when lung lipases act on the aspirated oil. This may be followed by diffuse fibrosis of the bronchi or alveoli. The area may become secondarily infected.

A child may have an initial coughing spell at the time of aspiration. A period follows during which the child is symptomless; then a chronic cough, dyspnea, and general respiratory distress will occur. A chest x-ray film will reveal densities at the affected site.

Antibiotic therapy is ineffective unless a secondary bacterial infection occurs. Surgical resection of a lung portion may be done to remove a lobe or segment if the pneumonitis does not heal by itself.

Hydrocarbon Pneumonia

A number of common household products such as furniture polish, cleaning fluids, turpentine, kerosene, gasoline, lighter fluid, and insect sprays have hydrocarbon bases. These products are a common cause of childhood poisonings and can result in hydrocarbon pneumonia.

Assessment. The child who has swallowed a hydrocarbon-based product will have gastrointestinal symptoms such as nausea and vomiting. The child may become drowsy due to inhalation of the vapors of the substance and may develop a cough as vapors from the stomach rise and are inhaled. As bronchial edema occurs from irritation and inflammation, the child's respirations become increased and dyspneic. Physical assessment will reveal an increased percussion sound caused by the presence of air trapped in the alveoli beyond the point of inflammation. There may be rales as air passes through collected mucus and diminished breath sounds because air does not reach and inflate the alveoli fully.

Therapeutic Management. Hydrocarbon aspiration may occur when children initially swallow the fluid. If they are given an emetic to induce vomiting, they may aspirate at the time of vomiting. This is why vomiting is never induced if a child has swallowed a hydrocarbon. Parents should telephone a poison control center to ask for advice before inducing vomiting if they do not know the substance ingested or are unsure whether it was a hydrocarbon. An oily substance such as olive oil or mineral oil may be administered by the parent to delay gastric absorption of the substance. Stomach lavage may be done by health care personnel with great care to remove the substance from the stomach.

The child is admitted to the hospital for observation. Vital signs and general appearance must be watched carefully for symptoms of increased respiratory tract obstruction. Careful observation for signs of increasing drowsiness or other symptoms of central nervous system involvement is also necessary. Cool, moist air with supplemental oxygen may decrease lung inflammation. If febrile, the child needs an antipyretic. Frequent changes of position will prevent pooling of secretions, which could lead to a secondary infection. Postural drainage will help to move secretions and reduce areas of stasis.

The initial inflammation reaction may lead to such occlusion that emphysema (pocketing of air in alveoli) occurs, causing rupture of the alveoli into the pleural space, with consequent pneumothorax and atelectasis.

Children who swallow a household cleaner or other substance are often aware that they should not have been handling substances kept under the sink. Such children cannot help but interpret the hospitalization, blood drawing, and other uncomfortable procedures as punishments for their action. They may benefit from therapeutic play with puppets or dolls that will help alleviate their guilt and anger at being "punished" so severely; you may see them treating the dolls roughly or poking them with needles.

After the illness, parents should be cautioned to put poisons in a safe place. They need a listening ear so they can explain that they did not mean this to happen and were unaware of the dangers of these everyday household products.

Atelectasis

Atelectasis is the collapse of lung alveoli. It may occur in children as a primary or secondary condition.

Primary Atelectasis

Primary atelectasis occurs in newborns who do not breathe with enough respiratory strength to inflate lung tissue or whose alveoli are so immature or so lacking in surfactant that they cannot expand. This is seen most commonly in immature infants or in infants with central nervous system damage. It may occur if infants have mucus or meconium plugs in the trachea (Figure 40-26).

When atelectasis occurs, the newborn's respirations become irregular, with nasal flaring and apnea. After a few minutes, a respiratory grunt and cyanosis may occur. The sound of a respiratory grunt is caused by the newborn's glottis closing on expiration. With this, pressure in the respiratory tract becomes increased, forcing more air into the alveoli in an attempt to inflate them. As cyanosis increases, the infant becomes hypotonic and

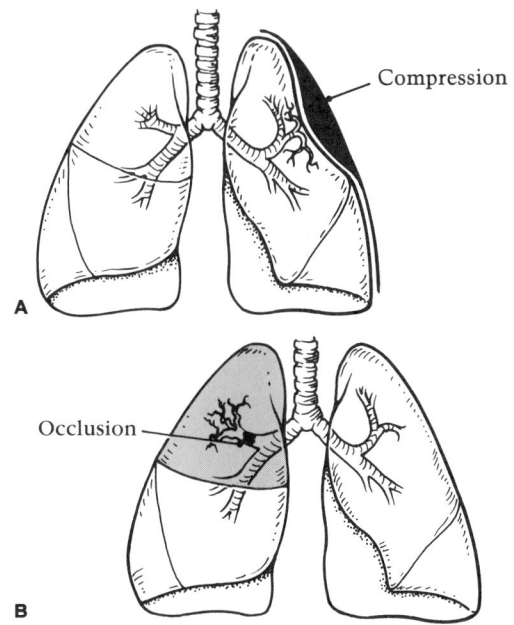

FIGURE 40-26
(**A**) *Atelectasis caused by compression of lung tissue.* (**B**) *Atelectasis caused by obstruction. (From Bullock, B. L., Rosendahl, P. P. [1992].* Pathophysiology: Adaptations and alterations in function *[3rd ed.]. Philadelphia: J.B. Lippincott, p. 582.)*

flaccid. The Apgar score (see Chapter 21) invariably will be low.

As infants cry, more alveoli become aerated and cyanosis may decrease. This distinguishes the condition from cyanotic heart disease, in which an affected infant may also be cyanotic at birth but tends to become *more* cyanotic with crying. The administration of oxygen may decrease cyanosis in both newborns with atelectasis and those with cyanotic congenital heart disease. The cause of the atelectasis must be established so that therapy directed to the specific cause can be initiated.

Secondary Atelectasis
Secondary atelectasis occurs in children when they have a respiratory tract obstruction that prevents air from entering a portion of the alveoli. As the residual air in the alveoli is absorbed, the alveoli will collapse. The causes of obstruction in children include mucus plugs that may occur with chronic respiratory disease and aspiration of foreign objects (see Figure 40-26*B*). In some children, atelectasis occurs because of pressure on lung tissue from outside forces, such as compression from a diaphragmatic hernia, scoliosis, or enlarged lymph nodes (see Figure 40-26*A*).

The signs of secondary atelectasis depend on the degree of collapse. Asymmetry of the chest may be noticed. Breath sounds on the affected side will be decreased. If the process is extensive, tachypnea and cyanosis will be present. A chest x-ray film will reveal the collapsed lung (a "white-out").

Children with atelectasis are prone to secondary infection because mucus continues to be secreted in the obstructed segment. Stasis of body fluid provides a good culture medium for bacteria.

Therapeutic Management
Atelectasis caused by inspiration of a foreign object will not be relieved until the object is removed by bronchoscopy. Atelectasis caused by a mucus plug will resolve itself with time. Children may need assisted ventilation to maintain adequate respiratory function during this time.

Make certain that the chest of a child with atelectasis is kept free from pressure so that lung expansion is as full as possible (to allow as much breathing space as possible). If restraints are being used to keep an infant positioned, make certain that body restraints are not crossing the chest area and interfering with chest expansion. Check clothing to be certain that it is loose and nonbinding. Make certain that children's arms are not positioned across the chest, where their weight will interfere with deep inspiration.

A semi-Fowler's position generally allows for the best lung expansion, because it depresses abdominal contents. The humidity of the child's environment should be increased to prevent further bronchial plugging; suction and postural drainage may be necessary to keep children's respiratory tracts clear and free of mucus. Children need close observation so that increased respirations or cyanosis can be detected. Atelectasis is a serious disorder in children of all ages. It must be considered as a possibility in all children with respiratory distress.

Pneumothorax

Pneumothorax is the presence of atmospheric air in the pleural space; its presence causes the alveoli of the lungs to collapse (Kharasch et al., 1990; Figure 40-27). Pneumothorax in children usually occurs when air seeps from ruptured alveoli and collects in the pleural cavity. It also can occur when puncture wounds allow air to enter the chest from the outside.

Pneumothorax occurs in about 1% of newborns, probably from the extreme intrathoracic pressure needed to initiate the first inspiration. The infant has tachypnea, grunting with respirations, flaring of the nares, and cyanosis. Auscultation will reveal absent or decreased breath sounds on the affected side. Percussion may not be revealing, despite the hollow air space; the sound may be hyperresonant. A more revealing sign may be the shift of the apical pulse away from the site of the pneumothorax and the resulting atelectasis. A chest film will reveal the darkened area of the air-filled pleural space.

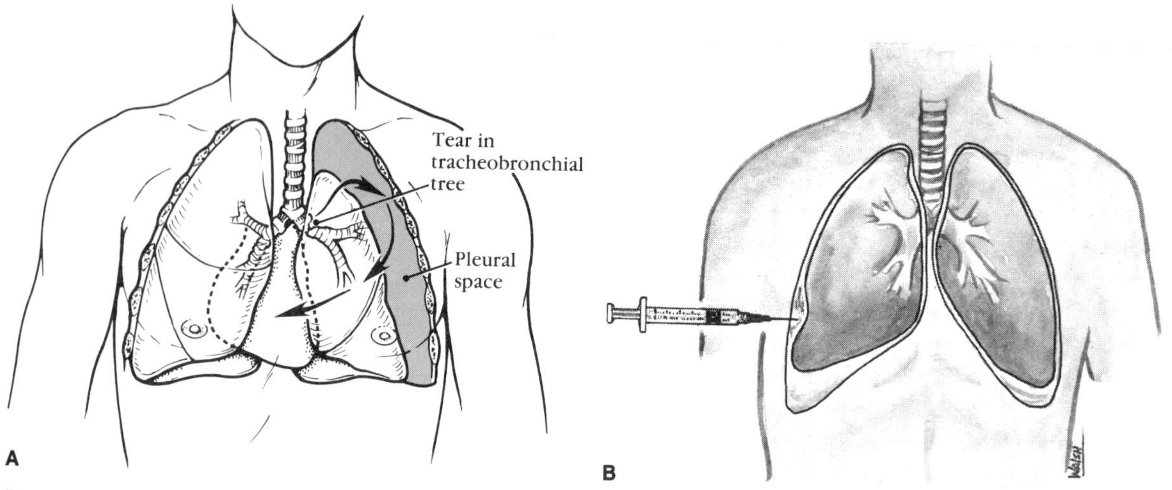

FIGURE 40-27

(**A**) *Pneumothorax. A tear in the tracheobronchial tree has caused air to move into the pleural space; the lung collapses and the mediastinum shifts to the unaffected side (From Bullock, B. L., Rosendahl, P. P. [1992].* Pathophysiology: Adaptations and alterations in function *[3rd ed.]. Philadelphia: J.B. Lippincott, p. 590). (**B**) Aspiration of air from the pleural space allows lung to reexpand after a pneumothorax.*

Children need oxygen therapy if they are in respiratory distress. A catheter or needle may be placed in the pleural space (thoracotomy), and low-pressure suction with water-seal drainage may be applied to remove accumulated air. In most children with pneumothorax, symptoms are relieved within 24 hours after suction is begun. The use of water-seal drainage with children is discussed in Chapter 41 (see Figure 41-12).

If the air in the pleural space is from a puncture wound, the chest wound must be covered immediately by an impervious material, such as petrolatum gauze, to prevent further air from entering. In an emergency, the impervious object can be your gloved hand.

Pneumothorax is always a serious respiratory problem. The extent of the symptoms and the outcome will depend on the cause of entry of air into the pleural space.

Lung Cysts

Lung cysts are fluid or air-filled spaces in the alveoli surrounded by definite walls. They may produce no symptoms. If they are large, they will produce signs of obstruction, such as coughing or wheezing. Children may have cyanosis if a cyst is occluding significant air space. Some cysts are congenital. Others form as a result of pneumonia or obstructive lesions of the airways. If the cyst is infected or causing obstruction, it is incised surgically. Small lesions that evidence no symptoms may be only observed.

The cause of lung cysts is often difficult to explain to parents, who may confuse cysts with tumors, which they associate with cancer. After surgery, parents need assurance that the growth was benign and that although the treatment included chest surgery, which is never undertaken lightly, the disorder is much less serious than they may have imagined.

Tuberculosis

Tuberculosis is a highly contagious pulmonary disease. The causative agent is *Mycobacterium tuberculosis* (tubercle bacillus). The mode of transmission is inhalation of infected droplets. The incubation period is from 2 to 10 weeks (AAP, 1991).

Children generally contract this disease from someone in the immediate family. When any member of a family contracts tuberculosis, all family members must have skin tests (tine or Mantoux) to screen for the disease. In some children, the contact is not known, and the disease is first detected when symptoms appear. Nonwhite children tend to be more susceptible than white children. Children with chronic illness or malnutrition are more susceptible than healthier children.

When *M. tuberculosis* invades the child's lung, there is primary inflammation. The child develops a slight cough. Leukocytes invade the area and are joined by a formation of new cells, effectively walling off the primary infection. The area calcifies and confines the organism permanently. This development of a primary focus is the most usual form of tuberculosis in children. If a child is in poor health or does not have adequate calcium intake for the body to confine the infection, tuberculosis may spread to other lung areas or to other parts of the body (miliary tuberculosis). As miliary tuberculosis develops, a child develops signs of anorexia, loss of weight, night sweats, and low-grade fever. Other body sites that may be affected are bones and joints, lymph nodes, kidneys, and the subarachnoid space (tuberculosis meningitis).

Assessment

The diagnosis of tuberculosis is suggested by the history of a recent contact. All children should have a tuberculin test as part of basic preventive health care at 9 to 12 months of age, and yearly thereafter if they live in an area in which there is a high risk of tuberculosis. The test should not be done following measles immunization or the test will read false-negative (a child with tuberculosis will be considered free of the disease). Also, the measles vaccine can cause a primary tuberculosis focus to become miliary; thus, it is important to have a negative tuberculin result before administration.

For a tine test, a small, four-pronged applicator, dipped in purified protein derivative (PPD) vaccine, is pressed against the inner aspect of the child's arm so that the prongs break the skin after the skin has been cleansed with acetone or alcohol. A parent inspects the area in 72 hours and notes the reaction. A positive reaction (the formation of one or more papules, 2 mm or larger in diameter) indicates that the child has been exposed to tuberculosis (has developed a sensitivity to the foreign products of the tuberculosis organism). Children with positive reactions need follow-up care, such as a chest x-ray film, to ascertain the importance of the reaction; that is, whether a current infection exists. Skin testing should not be done on children who are known to have had tuberculosis. Such a child will have such an intense reaction that the skin at the site of the test may slough off and necrose. A more definitive skin test is a Mantoux test, in which PPD vaccine is injected directly into the dermis layer of skin. The reaction is read by parents in the same way as a tine test.

As a second diagnostic procedure, sputum may be analyzed. Make certain that children understand that you want them to expectorate mucus raised from the lungs, not just from the back of the throat. Have the child demonstrate a deep cough to you, so that you can be sure you are both talking about the same thing. Infants and young children do not raise sputum but swallow it. In children under 9 or 10 years of age, therefore, sputum must be obtained by gastric lavage (because tuberculosis bacteria are acid-fast they are not destroyed by gastric secretions). Gastric lavage should be done early in the morning before the child eats. This prevents vomiting and should collect large numbers of organisms, because the child has been coughing sputum and swallowing it all night. A nasogastric tube is passed either nasally or orally. The stomach contents are aspirated and placed in a sterile container for laboratory processing. Gastric analysis is generally done for 3 consecutive days, because individual specimens may not contain organisms.

Having a large tube passed into the stomach is frightening. The feeling is uncomfortable—choking, gagging—and the concept itself is frightening. Children need support from people whom they know and trust. They need time to express their feelings about the procedure. They may enjoy playing with a plastic catheter and a doll, into which a tube can be inserted. It is revealing to see the force and the anger they use to insert the tube into the doll; this indicates how they envisioned the procedure being done to them.

In the early course of the disease, because the initial focus of the tuberculosis is so small, it may not be evident on a chest film. As local inflammation occurs, however, a cloudiness in the inflamed area will be noticeable on the film, as will calcification as it occurs.

Parents are concerned when their child is diagnosed as having tuberculosis. Before drug therapy became feasible, a diagnosis of tuberculosis meant a long-term hospital stay of about a year. Parents who believe that tuberculosis is still treated this way will need assurance that it is all right for their child to return home after only a short hospital stay and for him or her to attend regular school.

Therapeutic Management

The treatment of tuberculosis is based on the administration of a combination of specific antituberculin drugs (Jackson, 1993). Para-aminosalicylic acid (PAS) is bacteriostatic to *M. tuberculosis* and for a long time served as the mainstay of therapy. PAS administration may lead to such gastrointestinal disturbances in children that it is not used as much as in the past. If it is prescribed, it should be administered following meals and never on an empty stomach. Isoniazid (INH) is often now the drug of choice for therapy. INH may lead to peripheral neurologic symptoms if pyridoxine (vitamin B_6) is not administered concurrently. Rifampin is often used in combination with INH.

Ethambutol is used with older children. It is not used with infants because one side-effect is optic neuritis; inability to do adequate eye examinations in children under school age to discover this side-effect makes ethambutol unsafe for long-term use. Streptomycin is given only to children who have a severe or progressive infection, because it must be given intramuscularly, and long-term use may lead to eighth cranial nerve deafness. Parents need to be alerted to the symptoms of this possible ill effect: pulling at an ear; irritability; cocking the head; and vestibular dysfunction such as awkward or unsteady gait. In addition to drug therapy, children should receive a diet high in protein, calcium, and pyridoxine, especially if INH is used as therapy, in order to effectively wall off organisms in lung tissue (Richardson et al., 1991).

Children who have primary tuberculosis are not infectious, because they have a minimal pulmonary lesion and little or no cough. They need not be isolated. As soon as chemotherapy has been started and clinical symptoms have disappeared, children can return to regular activities, including school. Therapy may have to be continued, however, for up to 18 months.

Children should have a chest x-ray film at yearly intervals for the rest of their life to make certain that the disease does not become active later. A woman who had tuberculosis as a child must tell her obstetrician of this history when she becomes pregnant; lung changes that occur in pregnancy as a result of the pressure of the growing uterus against the lungs can break down calcifications and reactivate tuberculosis. Children who develop another chronic disease that interferes with appetite and, therefore, with calcium intake have a high risk of reactivation of calcium-contained tuberculosis.

Because children will be taking medicine for a long time, they need periodic health care facility visits to evaluate the extent of drug compliance. They must receive regular childhood immunizations so that they do not contract a second disease until they have fully recovered from tuberculosis. It is most important that pertussis (whooping cough) be prevented, because the paroxysmal cough caused by this illness could break and reactivate tuberculosis lesions.

The bacilli Calmette-Guerin (BCG) vaccine is available against tuberculosis, but it is not used routinely with children. It may be administered to children if there is active tuberculosis in the home. A skin test will be strongly positive after effective BCG vaccination. For this reason, most people advocate placing children on prophylactic INH when there is known tuberculosis in the home rather than vaccinating them against tuberculosis. As long as a repeat tine test remains negative, you know that they are disease free. After BCG vaccine, the value of skin testing is lost.

Cystic Fibrosis

Cystic fibrosis is a disease in which there is generalized dysfunction of the exocrine glands. Mucus secretions of the body, particularly in the pancreas and the lungs, have difficulty flowing through gland ducts. There is also a marked electrolyte change in the secretions of the sweat glands (chloride concentration of sweat is two to five times above normal). The cause of the disorder is the inability to transport small molecules across cell membranes; this leads to dehydration of epithelial cells in the airway and pancreas (Rosenstein, 1994).

The disorder is inherited as an autosomal recessive trait. The exact location of the specific gene at fault appears to be on chromosome 7. It occurs in about 1 in 2000 live births. It occurs most commonly in whites, rarely in blacks and Asians. Although the disease is fatal in early life, as many as 50% of children now live to be past 21 years of age. With the availability of lung transplants, life expectancy has increased (Frist et al., 1991).

Because the gene that causes the disorder can be isolated, chorionic villi sampling or amniocentesis can be done early in pregnancy to detect fetuses who have the disease.

Boys with cystic fibrosis may not be able to reproduce, as they have such tenacious plugging of the vas deferens from tenacious seminal fluid that blockage tends to occur. Girls may have such thick cervical secretions that sperm penetration is limited; artificial insemination can be accomplished if they desire to become pregnant (see Chapter 6).

Pancreas Involvement

The acinar cells of the pancreas normally produce lipase, trypsin, and amylase, enzymes that flow into the duodenum to digest fat, protein, and carbohydrate. With cystic fibrosis, these enzyme secretions become so tenacious that they plug the ducts; eventually, there is such back pressure on the acinar cells that they become atrophied and are then no longer capable of producing the enzymes. The islets of Langerhans and insulin production are little influenced by this process because they have endocrine activity (they are ductless cells) until late in the disease.

Without pancreatic enzymes in the duodenum, children are unable to digest fat, protein, and some sugars; the child's stools will be large, bulky, and greasy (steatorrhea). The flora of the intestine is increased in amount because of the undigested food and, combined with the fat in the stool, gives the stool an extremely foul odor often compared with that of a cat's stool. The bulk of feces in the intestine leads to a protuberant abdomen. Because children are benefiting from only about 50% of the food they ingest, they show signs of malnutrition—emaciated extremities and loose, flabby folds of skin on their buttocks. The fat-soluble vitamins, particularly A, D, and E, cannot be absorbed because fat is not absorbed, so children develop symptoms of low levels of these vitamins. These four symptoms—malnutrition, protuberant abdomen, steatorrhea, and fat-soluble vitamin deficiencies—are the same four symptoms that are part of celiac disease (malabsorption syndrome), so they are referred to as the *celiac syndrome* (see Chapter 45).

The meconium in a newborn is normally thick and tenacious. In about 10% of children with cystic fibrosis, it may be so thick, because pancreatic enzymes are lacking, that it obstructs the intestine (meconium ileus). The newborn will develop abdominal distention with no passage of stool. Meconium ileus should be suspected in any infant who does not pass a stool by 24 hours of life. This is discussed in Chapter 39.

Lung Involvement

Pockets of infection begin in pooled thick secretions of the bronchial tree, which obstruct the bronchioles. The organisms most frequently cultured from lung secretions in children with cystic fibrosis are *Staphylococcus aureus, Pseudomonas aeruginosa,* and *H. influenzae.* Secondary emphysema (overinflated alveoli) occurs because the air cannot be pushed past the thick mucus on expiration, when all bronchi are narrower than they are on inspiration. Bronchiectasis (bronchi dilated and filled with infected mucus) and pneumonia occur. Atelectasis (collapse of alveoli) occurs as a result of complete absorption of air from alveoli behind blocked bronchioles. Children's fingers become clubbed (square-tipped) because of the inadequate oxygenation of peripheral capillaries, which causes additional capillaries to form. Children's chests become distended in the anteroposterior diameter; they develop respiratory acidosis because obstruction renders them unable to exhale adequate amounts of carbon dioxide.

Sweat Gland Involvement
Although the sweat glands themselves do not appear to change in structure, the electrolyte composition of perspiration does change. In children with cystic fibrosis, the level of chloride to sodium is increased two to five times above normal. Some parents report that they knew their newborn had the disease before they had laboratory tests done, because when they kissed their child they could taste such strong salt in the perspiration.

Assessment
Cystic fibrosis is diagnosed by the history, the abnormal concentration of chloride in sweat, the absence of pancreatic enzymes in the duodenum, and pulmonary involvement.

The newborn with cystic fibrosis loses the normal amount of weight at birth (5% to 10% of birth weight), but then does not gain it back at the usual time of 7 to 10 days and perhaps not until 4 to 6 weeks of age. Failure to regain birth weight as a newborn is a significant sign, which nurses, who often weigh babies, may be the first to detect. As mentioned, at birth, meconium may be so tenacious that the baby has intestinal obstruction (meconium ileus) and so be unable to pass stool. All babies with meconium ileus should be tested for cystic fibrosis. This can be done by analysis of serum immunoreactive trypsin (IRT), which is elevated in newborns with the disease owing to obstruction in the pancreas as early as during fetal life.

Children may be seen in a health care setting at about 1 month of age because of a feeding problem. Using only about 50% of their intake because of their poor digestive function, they are always hungry. This causes them to eat so ravenously that they tend to swallow air. This is manifested as colic or abdominal distention and vomiting. Stools are large, bulky, and greasy; the stools may be loose and frequent. The appearance of the stools is an important finding as children with simple colic do not show changes in stool consistency.

Children may be seen by health care providers between 4 and 6 months of age because of frequent respiratory infections, a chronic cough, and failure to gain weight. On auscultation of the chest, wheezing and rhonchi may be heard.

By the time the child with cystic fibrosis is a preschooler, a cough is a prominent finding. On percussion, the chest will be hyperresonant, reflecting the emphysema present. Rales and rhonchi will be heard. Clubbing of the fingers may already be apparent. It is rare for a child to go undiagnosed beyond this time because the symptoms of the illness are becoming so persistent and evident.

Sweat Testing. A sweat test is a test for the chloride content of sweat. Infants may not be tested until 6 to 8 weeks of age because newborns do not sweat a great deal and interpretation of the test may not be accurate. With newer testing procedures, however, sweat testing may be done earlier than ever before.

For a sweat test, pilocarpine (a cholinergic drug that stimulates sweat gland activity) is dropped onto a gauze square. This is placed on the child's forearm, and copper electrodes are connected to it; a small electrical current is then applied to carry the pilocarpine into the skin. Because the electrical current is of such low intensity, it should be painless. Following the application of the electrical current, the area on the arm is washed with water and dried, and a filter paper is applied to collect the sweat that forms. The filter paper must be lifted by forceps rather than touched by your fingers, since the sweat from your skin could transfer to the paper and make the test analysis inaccurate.

A normal concentration of chloride in sweat is 20 mEq/L. A level of more than 60 mEq of chloride per liter in children is diagnostic of cystic fibrosis. Values between 50 and 60 mEq/L are suggestive of the disease and call for a repeat of the test in children.

Duodenal Analysis. Analysis of duodenal secretions for detection of pancreatic enzymes is done by passing a nasogastric tube nasally until it reaches the duodenum and then aspirating secretions for analysis. This test may take a considerable amount of time because the tube must pass through the pylorus and into the duodenum. You can tell a tube has passed from the stomach into the duodenum by aspirating secretions and testing them for *p*H. Stomach secretions are acid (less than 7.0); duodenal secretions are alkaline (more than 7.0). The initial insertion of the tube is frightening to children because they choke and gag as it passes the pharynx. Children, however, are generally surprised that once the initial insertion is done, the tube is not uncomfortable. They need a great deal of support during the procedure, however, because it is so unusual for them and initially so uncomfortable.

The secretions removed from the duodenum are sent to the laboratory for analysis of trypsin content, the easiest pancreatic enzyme to assay. The secretions must be kept cold and analyzed immediately for accurate results.

Pulmonary Testing. A chest x-ray film will generally confirm the pulmonary involvement of the disease. Pulmonary function tests may be done to determine the extent of the lung involvement.

Therapeutic Management

Therapy for children with cystic fibrosis consists of measures to reduce the involvement of the pancreas, lungs, and sweat glands as discussed below.

Nursing Diagnoses and Related Interventions

Nursing Diagnosis: Altered nutrition, less than body requirements, related to inability to digest fat

Goal: Child will absorb an adequate nutritional diet daily.

Outcome Criteria: Child's height and weight follow percentile growth curves.

Children with cystic fibrosis are placed on a high-calorie, high-protein, moderate-fat diet. Water-miscible forms of vitamins A, D, and E are supplemented. During the hot months of the year, extra salt may be added to food to replace that lost though perspiration. Medium-chain triglycerides are used with the diet because these are more readily digested than other oils.

Infants with cystic fibrosis are not generally breast-fed because there is not enough protein in breast milk for them (they need large amounts because they cannot make use of all the protein they ingest). Some of these children, unfortunately, are initially diagnosed as having a milk allergy and are treated by being placed on a soy-bean formula. This does not contain enough protein either, and their malnutrition will increase greatly while they are taking this formula. Probana, a high-protein formula, is generally the formula that should be recommended.

Cystic children have a ravenous appetite and eat well. Before each meal or snack they need to take a synthetic pancreatic enzyme, pancreatic lipase (Cotazym or Pancrease) to replace the enzyme they cannot produce. These synthetic enzymes are supplied in large capsules that must be opened for young children because they cannot swallow such a big capsule, and infants, in particular, may not have enough gastric acids to dissolve the capsule. The powder from the capsule is then added to a small amount (no more than a teaspoonful) of food. It should be added to warm, not hot, food or a large portion of enzyme activity will be destroyed. Also, it

must not be added to the infant's bottle of formula, because the infant may not drink the entire bottle and therefore will not receive the total benefit of the enzymes. When children are taking a synthetic source of pancreatic enzymes in this way, the size of stools and the accompanying foul odor decreases; children begin to gain weight. In adolescence, children may have a great deal of difficulty eating enough to maintain weight, since their growth spurt requires so many additional calories.

If the room of a child with cystic fibrosis becomes overheated, the child will begin to lose excessive sodium and chloride through perspiration and become dehydrated. Ensure that the room temperature is not above 72°F; offer water frequently.

Nursing Diagnosis: High risk for ineffective airway clearance related to inability to clear mucus from tract

Goal: Child's airway will maintain patency during course of illness.

Outcome Criteria: Child's temperature is below 38.0°C; Po_2 is 80 to 90 mm Hg; Pco_2 is 40 mm Hg.

Unfortunately, the pulmonary effects of cystic fibrosis progress despite supplementation with pancreatic enzymes; infection is always a possibility. It is therefore important to try to keep bronchial secretions as moist as possible so they can drain from the bronchial tree. This is done by frequent nebulization or aerosol therapy followed by postural drainage.

Provide Moistened Oxygen. Oxygen is supplied to children by mask, prongs, ventilators, or nebulizers and rarely by tent. Mist can be supplied by an ultrasonic compressor, which makes droplet size so small that the mist reaches the smallest bronchial spaces. A mucolytic, such as acetylcysteine (Mucomyst) can be added to the mist to aid in diluting and liquefying secretions. Children's coughs will become loose and productive after they have used aerosol therapy. Provide a box of tissues for them so they can cough up these loose secretions. Observe them to be certain they are able to cough and keep their airway clear. They must never be given cough syrups to suppress their cough, because getting secretions out is mandatory to air exchange. Likewise, they must never receive codeine as an analgesic, because codeine suppresses the cough reflex.

Provide Aerosol Therapy. Three or four times a day, children may be given aerosol therapy by means of a powered nebulizer. Antibiotics, bronchodilators, and decongestant drugs given by aerosol therapy this way reach tiny lung spaces. The most frequently prescribed antibiotic in aerosol therapy is polymyxin B sulfate, an antibiotic that is effective against *Pseudomonas*. Isoproterenol (Isuprel), a bronchodilator and expectorant, is another drug often given by nebulizer.

Hand nebulizers, such as those used by children with asthma, are not adequate for children with cystic fibrosis. They need nebulization by compressor to force the drug and nebulization mist into smaller bronchioles. Using this method, children place the tip of the nebulizer in their mouth and take deep breaths to assist the nebulizer (or to allow the nebulizer to assist them). It is frightening for children to use nebulizers with compression until they grow accustomed to them. They worry that they will suffocate from the mist. Holding children on your lap while they take this treatment will often help relieve this fear.

Provide Postural Drainage. Because the bronchial secretions with cystic fibrosis are so tenacious, even with liquefaction by mist or aerosol therapy, children are unable to raise them. To aid drainage of secretions, children need postural drainage about three times a day (see Figure 40-11).

Encourage Activity. Children with cystic fibrosis need frequent position changes in bed so that, at various times of the day, all lobes of their lungs will be encouraged to drain by being in a superior position. They should therefore alternately lie on either side, on their abdomen, and on their back. They should sit up part of the day to drain the upper lobes. This change in position also helps to prevent skin breakdown over bony prominences, and it helps to aerate their lungs by furnishing some activity for them.

Observe Child Frequently. Children require frequent observation during a hospital stay because their condition can change rapidly. If a portion of a lung becomes obstructed from a plug of mucus, they may quickly be in respiratory difficulty. Also, the right side of the heart enlarges in children with chronic respiratory disease because the congestion in the lungs increases pressure in the pulmonary artery. After a period of stress or exercise, children may begin to show signs of cardiac failure.

Provide Respiratory Hygiene. The sputum that children cough up may have a disagreeable taste or odor; they need frequent mouth care, tooth brushing, and a good-tasting mouthwash to make their mouth feel fresh.

Provide Adequate Rest and Comfort. Any child who has compromised lung function has a degree of dyspnea that leads to exhaustion. Children need to have nursing care planned so that they have long periods of rest during the day rather than being disturbed every few minutes. At the same time, they must not have too many procedures done all at once; many procedures done one right after another will exhaust them. They particularly

need a rest period before meals so that they are not too tired to eat. They may need a long stretch of rest before postural drainage so that it is not so tiring. Achieving a balance between allowing periods of rest and yet not doing all procedures at once is not an easy task.

Nursing Diagnosis: High risk for altered skin integrity related to acid stools
Goal: Child's skin will remain intact during course of illness.
Outcome Criteria: Child does not have areas of erythema or ulceration; rectal prolapse is not present.

Children who are not toilet-trained need to have their diapers changed immediately after they wet or stool so that they do not develop skin irritation and breakdown in the diaper area. Until children are regulated on pancreatic enzymes, the stool is particularly irritating because of its high fat content.

After a bowel movement, check the child's rectum for rectal prolapse. Because of weak musculature of the rectal area, this is a common complication. A prolapse of rectal mucosa appears as a bright red mass protruding from the anal sphincter. This mucosa must be replaced promptly before its blood supply is compromised. Place the child on the slant board used for physical therapy in a position with the head lower than the buttocks; then, with a lubricated, gloved hand, gently replace the prolapsed rectal mass. Afterward, tape the buttocks together to maintain gentle pressure on the anus. This is much less of a problem in children who are receiving pancreatic enzymes than in those who are not, since the incidence of rectal prolapse decreases with better nutrition.

Nursing Diagnosis: High risk for ineffective family coping, compromised, related to chronic illness in a child
Goal: Family members demonstrate an adequate level of coping ability during course of illness.
Outcome Criteria: Family members state they have adequate resources to cope with present circumstances.

The parents of these children are asked to assume a great deal of responsibility for care of their child. Discharge planning begins when a child is first admitted to a hospital in terms of what changes need to be made at home to accommodate the child's homecoming and to familiarize parents with the necessary care measures. For example, many children with this disorder sleep with oxygen by cannula at night when they are at home. Thus, parents will need to be taught the functions of oxygen and how to regulate the flow. The program is most effective if a little is taught every day (for example,

"Could you turn the oxygen on for me, Mrs. Smith? I'm ready to tuck Brian in to sleep" rather than a sit-down, let-me-tell-you-how-oxygen-works lecture given close to the day of discharge). Teach parents how to do postural drainage the same way.

The family will have to think through how the care of this child will affect their home life. They are going to be spending a great deal of time caring for the child. If both parents customarily work, one of them may have to give up a job now. If there are other young children in the family, parents may have to think about placing them in a day-care center or nursery school so that at least one parent will be free to spend time with the ill child.

Many parents become fatigued after the first week of having the child at home, because they are afraid to fall soundly asleep at night for fear of not hearing the child call if he or she should be in distress. As they grow more confident in their ability to evaluate the child's condition before bedtime, the apprehension will lessen, but real confidence may not come for months, even years. This may always be a problem for some parents.

Parents need the telephone number of the health care provider they should call when the pressure they are under is more than they can bear. Encourage parents to join a support group, so that there are other understanding people available to whom they can voice their concerns. At these times, one of the most important needs they have is to verbalize to someone what it feels like to be the parent of a child with cystic fibrosis.

Children need to attend regular school if that is at all possible. If not, a home tutor should be provided for them. They should participate to the extent that they can in physical fitness activities in school. Also, they must remember to take a pancreatic enzyme with them if they are going to be eating lunch in the school cafeteria. It is important that parents supervise what they are wearing to school so that they do not become chilled by neglecting a warm coat on a cold day or their boots on a rainy day. Their teacher needs to assume this responsibility for the trip home from school. Teach them to keep a sweater at school in case a fire drill is called on a windy or chilly day.

Children with cystic fibrosis need periodic health assessment the same as all children so that routine childhood immunizations can be given. It is not unusual for children with a chronic disease to fall behind in immunizations because they are hospitalized at the times they are routinely given. It is particularly important that these children be given pertussis and measles vaccine, because these two infections cause severe respiratory complications. Children also generally receive influenza, meningococcal, and pneumococcal vaccines to try to prevent them from contracting these illnesses.

If there are other children in the family with cystic fibrosis (not an uncommon occurrence), parents need

a great deal of support if the first child should die. Supporting parents after a child dies is discussed in Chapter 56.

Key Points

- Respiratory tract disorders tend to occur more frequently in children than adults, because the lumen of bronchi are narrow and obstruction can occur more easily.
- Acute nasopharyngitis (common cold) is the most frequently seen infectious disease in children. There is no specific therapy for a cold. The nursing diagnosis Health-seeking behaviors is usually most fitting because it describes the parents' response to illness in their child.
- Tonsillitis is infection and inflammation of the palatine tonsils. Adenitis is infection and inflammation of the adenoid tonsils. Two nursing diagnoses identified for this are usually High risk for fluid volume deficit and Pain because of the surgery required to remove the affected tonsils.
- Laryngotracheobronchitis (croup) is inflammation of the larynx, trachea, and major bronchi. Epiglottitis is inflammation of the epiglottis. Both of these conditions can cause severe impairment of the airway. The primary nursing diagnosis associated with these two disorders is High risk for ineffective airway clearance. Children with epiglottitis should never be gagged with a tongue blade or the elevated epiglottis can completely occlude the airway.
- Bronchitis is inflammation of the major bronchi and trachea. Bronchiolitis is inflammation of the fine bronchioles. Children are administered antibiotics and usually oxygen therapy.
- Respiratory syncytial virus infection is an infection that accounts for the majority of lower respiratory infection in young children. Infants with RSV infections must be observed closely because they are prone to apnea.
- Pneumonia may occur from a variety of organisms (viral, pneumococcal, chlamydial, mycoplasmal, lipid, and hydrocarbon). Children need specific antibiotics depending on the organism present.
- Tuberculosis is an illness growing in incidence. One strain is very resistant to the usual therapy and presents a risk to health care providers. Nurses are well advised to maintain a current PPD status so they can be aware if exposure occurs.
- Cystic fibrosis is a disease in which there is generalized dysfunction of the exocrine glands. Relevant nursing diagnoses include Altered nutrition, High risk for ineffective airway clearance, Altered skin integrity, and Ineffective family coping.
- Infants with respiratory illness need extremely close observation, because they cannot describe oxygen

hunger. Young children do not appreciate the fact that oxygen supports combustion. They need more observation than adults do to be certain that no flames, such as birthday candles, are brought within 10 ft of an oxygen source.

Critical Thinking Exercises

1. Mary is a 3-year-old who has a permanent tracheotomy tube in place. Her parents are going to enroll her in a preschool center. What precautions would you want to review with the parents to keep this experience safe for Mary?

2. Bryan is a 10-year-old who has just returned from tonsillectomy surgery. What observations would be important to make with Bryan? Why is the 7th day following tonsillectomy surgery a particularly important day?

3. Karen is a 16-year-old with cystic fibrosis. Her parents want to take her on an extended vacation in the Caribbean next summer. What anticipatory guidance would you give Karen and her parents?

References

Adams, D. A., & McFadden, E. A. (1990). Respiratory syncytial viral infection in infants: Nursing implications. *Critical Care Nurse, 10,* 74.

American Academy of Pediatrics (AAP), Committee on Infectious Diseases. (1991). *Report on the Committee of Infectious Diseases.* (16th ed.). Elk Grove, IL: AAP.

American Heart Association. (1992). Pediatric basic life support. *Journal of the American Medical Association, 268,* 2251–2261.

Anderson, S. (1990). ABGs: Six easy steps to interpreting blood gases. *American Journal of Nursing, 90,* 42.

Bolgiano, C. S., et al. (1990). Administering oxygen therapy: What you need to know. *Nursing, 20,* 47.

Bradford, B. J. (1993). Index of suspicion: Acute epiglottitis. *Pediatrics in Review, 14,* 281.

Carabott, J., et al. (1991). Teaching families tracheotomy care. *Canadian Nurse, 87,* 21.

Carpenito, L. (1992). *Nursing diagnosis: Application to clinical practice* (3rd ed.). Philadelphia: J. B. Lippincott.

Carroll, P. (1993). Clinical application of pulse oximetry. *Pediatric Nursing, 19,* 150.

Department of Health and Human Services. (1991). *Healthy people 2000.* Washington, DC: Public Health Service.

Dorkin, H.L. (1993). Bronchiolitis. In Dershewitz, R.A. (Ed.). *Ambulatory pediatric care* (2nd ed.). Philadelphia: J.B. Lippincott.

Dougherty, J. M. (1990). Negative pressure devices in pediatric practice. *Pediatric Nursing, 16,* 136.

Frist, W. H., et al. (1991). Cystic fibrosis treated with heart-lung transplantation: North American results. *Transplantation Process, 23,* 1203.

Geissler, E. M. (1994). *Pocket guide to cultural assessment.* St. Louis: C. V. Mosby.

Goldenhersh, M. J., et al. (1990). The microbiology of chronic sinus disease in children with respiratory allergy. *Journal of Allergy and Clinical Immunology, 85,* 1030.

Gross, I. (1994). Persistent pulmonary hypertension. In Oski, F. A., et al. (Eds.) *Principles and practice of pediatrics* (2nd ed.). Philadelphia: J. B. Lippincott.

Hammerschlag, M. R. (1994). Pharyngitis. In Oski, F. A., et al. (Eds.) *Principles and practice of pediatrics* (2nd ed.). Philadelphia: J. B. Lippincott.

Hanson, I.C., & Shearer, W.T. (1994). Lower respiratory tract infections. In Oski, F.A., et al. (Eds.). *Principles and practice of pediatrics* (2nd ed.). Philadelphia: J. B. Lippincott.

Haywood, J. L., et al. (1993). Assessment and management of respiratory dysfunction. In Kenner, C., et al. (Eds.). *Comprehensive neonatal nursing.* Philadelphia: W. B. Saunders.

Hotaling, A. J., et al. (1992). Pediatric tracheotomy: A review of technique. *American Journal of Otolaryngology, 13,* 115.

Jackson, M. M. (1993). Tuberculosis in infants, children and adolescents: New dilemmas with an old disease. *Pediatric Nursing, 19,* 437.

James, D. G., & Sharma, O. M. (1990). Respiratory diseases. *Postgraduate Medicine Journal, 66,* 1.

Jenkinson, S. G., & Levine, S. M. (1994). Lung transplantation. *Disease-a-Month, 40,* 1.

Jury, D. L. (1993). More on RSV and Ribavirin. (1993). *Pediatric Nursing, 19,* 89.

Kharasch, S. J., et al. (1990). Primary spontaneous bilateral pneumothorax in an adolescent: A case report. *Pediatric Emergency Care, 6,* 129.

Leach, C. L., et al. (1993). Perfluorocarbon-associated gas exchange. *Critical Care Medicine, 21,* 1270.

Lynch, D. A., et al. (1990). Pediatric pulmonary disease: Assessment with high-resolution ultrafast CT. *Radiology, 176,* 243.

Mayeux, A., et al. (1990). Rheumatic fever revisited. *Orthopedics, 13,* 477.

Modlin, J. F. (1994). Bacterial pneumonia. In Oski, F. A., et al. (Eds.) *Principles and practice of pediatrics* (2nd ed.). Philadelphia: J. B. Lippincott.

Mulholland, E. K., et al. (1990). Clinical findings and severity of acute bronchiolitis. *Lancet, 335,* 1259.

Richardson, V., et al. (1991). Tuberculosis screening and treatment in children. *Journal of Pediatric Health Care, 5,* 11.

Rosenstein, B. J. (1994). Cystic fibrosis. In Oski, F. A., et al. (Eds.) *Principles and practice of pediatrics* (2nd ed.). Philadelphia: J. B. Lippincott.

Skolnik, N. (1993). Croup. *Journal of Family Practice, 37,* 165.

Spencer, P. A. (1990). Pneumonia, diagnosed on the abdominal radiograph, as a cause for acute abdomen in children. *British Journal of Radiology, 63,* 306.

Spyr, J., & Preach, M. A. (1990). Pulse oximetry. *RN, 53,* 38.

Steinhorn, R. H., & Green, T. P. (1990). Use of extracorporeal membrane oxygenation in the treatment of respiratory syncytial virus bronchiolitis: The national experience. *Journal of Pediatrics, 116,* 338.

Stevens, M., II. (1990). Laser surgery of tonsils, adenoids, and pharynx. *Otolaryngology Clinics of North America, 23,* 43.

Tejani, A., & Ingulli, E. (1990). Poststreptococcal glomerulonephritis. *Nephron, 55,* 1.

Suggested Readings

Agrons, G. A., et al. (1993). Pulmonary tuberculosis in children. *Seminars in Roentgenology, 28,* 158.

Berkowitz, R. G., & Zalzal, G. H. (1990). Tonsillectomy in children under 3 years of age. *Archives of Otolaryngology Head and Neck Surgery, 116,* 685.

Brouillette, R. T., et al. (1990). Breathing control disorders in infants and children. *Hospital Practice, 25,* 82.

Davies, H., et al. (1990). Long term follow up after inhalation of foreign bodies. *Archives of Diseases of Childhood, 65,* 619.

Gill, S. (1993). Home administration of intravenous antibiotics to children with cystic fibrosis. *British Journal of Nursing, 2,* 767.

Greenspan, J. S. (1993). Liquid ventilation: A developing technology. *Neonatal Network, 12,* 23.

Hahn, K. (1990). Tips for giving oxygen therapy. *Nursing, 20,* 70.

Hess, D. L. (1993). Chlamydia in the neonate. *Neonatal Network, 12,* 9.

Lebenthal, E., et al. (1994). Enzyme therapy for pancreatic insufficiency. *Pancreas, 9,* 1.

Loch, W. E., et al. (1990). Sinusitis. *Primary Care, 17,* 323.

Miller, H. (1992). Respiratory syncytial virus and the use of ribavirin. *MCN: American Journal of Maternal Child Nursing, 17,* 238.

Reed, S. B. (1990). Potential for alterations in family process: When a family has a child with cystic fibrosis. *Issues in Comprehensive Pediatric Nursing, 13,* 15.

Roberts, A. (1991). The respiratory system. *Nursing Times, 87,* 53.

Rosenfeld, R. M., & Green, R. P. (1990). Tonsillectomy and adenoidectomy: Changing trends. *Annals of Otology, Rhinology and Laryngology, 99,* 187.

Swischuk, L. E. (1990). Cough and shortness of breath. *Pediatric Emergency Care, 6,* 145.

Tobin, M. J. (1990). Respiratory monitoring. *Journal of the American Medical Association, 264,* 244.

Whitney, J. D. (1990). The measurement of oxygen tension in tissue. *Nursing Research, 39,* 203.

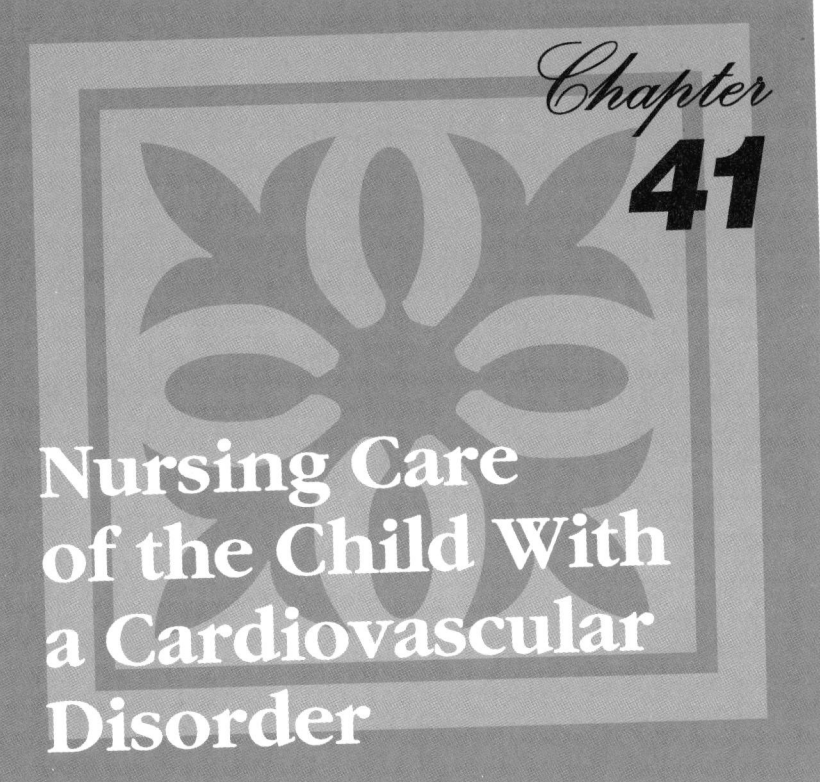

Chapter 41

Nursing Care of the Child With a Cardiovascular Disorder

Objectives

After mastering the contents of this chapter, you should be able to:

1. Describe the common cardiovascular disorders of childhood.

2. Assess a child with cardiovascular dysfunction.

3. Formulate nursing diagnoses for the child with a cardiovascular disorder such as congenital heart disease, rheumatic fever, and hypertension.

4. Plan nursing care for the child with a cardiovascular disorder, such as preparing a child for cardiac catheterization.

5. Implement nursing care, such as teaching parents how to administer a cardiac medication, for the child with a cardiovascular disorder.

6. Evaluate outcome criteria to be certain that nursing care goals were accomplished.

7. Identify National Health Goals related to cardiovascular disorders and children that nurses could be instrumental in helping the nation achieve.

8. Identify areas related to the care of children with cardiovascular problems that could benefit from additional nursing research.

9. Use critical thinking to analyze ways that nursing care of children with cardiovascular disorders could be more family centered.

10. Synthesize knowledge of cardiovascular disorders with nursing process to achieve quality maternal and child health nursing care.

Key Terms

- acyanotic heart disease
- afterload
- balloon stenotomy
- cardiac catheterization
- congestive heart failure
- contractility
- cyanosis
- cyanotic heart disease
- diastole
- echocardiography
- electrocardiogram
- extracorporeal membrane oxygenation
- fluoroscopy
- hypertension
- innocent heart murmur
- left-to-right shunt
- organic heart murmur
- phonocardiogram
- polycythemia
- postcardiac surgery syndrome
- postperfusion syndrome
- preload
- right-to-left shunt
- systole

Adele Pillitteri: MATERNAL AND CHILD HEALTH NURSING, 2nd Edition. © 1995 Adele Pillitteri.

The cardiovascular system is the body system on which all other systems depend. It consists of the heart, which acts as a reliable pump; the blood, which provides the fluid for transport; and the blood vessels. Through the regular pumping of the heart, oxygen and needed nutrients are delivered to cells and tissue waste products are removed from cells throughout the body. The cardiovascular system also transports regulatory materials such as hormones, enzymes, and antibodies to the body systems. It can adapt to changes in the body by adjusting the rate and force of heart pumping, changing the size of the blood vessels, and altering the volume and composition of the blood.

Most cardiovascular disorders in children occur as a result of a congenital anomaly; either the heart has developed inadequately in utero or the system is unable to adapt to extrauterine life. These disorders can lead to congestive heart failure or infection. Open heart surgery is often the only treatment that will correct the primary problem. Children also may experience acquired cardiovascular disorders, such as rheumatic fever or Kawasaki disease, which can severely compromise the functioning of the heart.

Cardiovascular disorders are frightening for children and adults alike. Even small children realize the importance of the heart in sustaining life, and they recognize the seriousness of any illness that undermines the heart's activity. For the families of children who are experiencing a cardiovascular disease, understanding the functioning of the heart and circulation is an important first step toward coping with the illness. National Health Goals related to cardiovascular illness and children are shown in the Focus on National Health Goals box.

NURSING PROCESS OVERVIEW
for Care of the Child
With a Cardiovascular Disorder

ASSESSMENT

Assessment of the child with a heart disorder includes both careful history-taking and physical examination, because many of the signs and symptoms of heart disease in children are subtle. A variety of diagnostic studies are used to confirm the diagnosis and prepare for surgery. Teaching and providing psychological support to children and their families are two major responsibilities of the nurse throughout the assessment process.

NURSING DIAGNOSIS

Examples of nursing diagnoses established for children with heart disease include the following:

- High risk for altered tissue perfusion related to inadequate cardiac output
- Fear related to lack of knowledge about child's disease
- Altered family processes related to stresses of diagnoses and care responsibilities
- Ineffective individual or family coping related to lack of adequate support
- Altered parenting related to inability to bond with critically ill newborn

If the concerns in the latter three diagnoses are not identified when the child is ill, they may continue long after the child is treated and returns home.

If the child will be undergoing surgery or cardiac catheterization, nursing diagnoses will focus on psychological needs of the child and family for preparation and postprocedure care as well as physical concerns after the procedure (e.g., Hypothermia related to cooling during surgery).

PLANNING

A great deal of nursing planning is necessary to help parents understand the necessity for diagnostic studies and to teach them to conscientiously administer cardiac drugs. An important nursing responsibility is to help parents set both short- and long-term goals (e.g., coping with their present fears and caring for the child at home). Parents may wish to contact the American Heart Association, 7272 Greenville Avenue, Dallas, TX 75231-4596, for educational materials and to look for family support groups in their area.

IMPLEMENTATION

Nursing interventions in the care of the child with a cardiovascular disorder include teaching, providing an opportunity for children and their families to express fears about the child's illness and treatment plan, psychologic support, and comfort measures for the child, such as helping the child find a position that is comfortable, administering oxygen, caring for the child in cardiac failure, and providing care after cardiac surgery. An equally important role is teaching prevention of heart disease. Measures such as promoting nonsmoking and exercise, maintaining an appropriate weight, and eating a low-fat diet are discussed in Chapter 32 with care of the school-age child.

 ### FOCUS ON
National Health Goals

Cardiovascular illness is a major health problem in adults, which makes it important to begin to take preventive measures early in childhood. A number of National Health Goals address ways children should modify nutrition or exercise to achieve cardiovascular health:

- Increase to at least 75% from a baseline of 65% the proportion of children and adolescents ages 5 through 17 who engage in vigorous physical activity that promotes the development and maintenance of cardiorespiratory fitness 3 or more days per week, for 20 or more minutes per occasion.

- Reduce dietary fat intake to an average of 30% of calories or less, and average saturated fat intake to less than 10% of calories, among people age 2 years and older (DHHS, 1991).

Nurses can be instrumental in helping the nation achieve these goals by educating parents and children about the importance of planned exercise and sound nutrition programs. It is equally important for nurses to caution parents not to begin reduced fat diets until their children are 2 years to allow for myelination of nerve cells.

Nursing research is needed as to what type of reduced fat foods make the best finger foods for preschoolers, what type of snacks could schools provide in snack machines that would have a reduced fat content and would also be eaten by children, and how to interest adolescents who do not participate in any type of organized sport in exercise programs.

EVALUATION

Evaluation should include long-term goals established for the family as well as short-term goals established for the child. Once treatment has ended, and even if long-term care is necessary, it is essential to evaluate whether the family is able to think of their child, not in terms of illness, but in terms of wellness. Providing the opportunity for parents to express their concerns about their child at follow-up visits may allow you to address any misconceptions about the child's future that may exist.

Expected outcomes may include the following:

- Child's heart rate remains between 80 and 100 bpm.
- Child states she feels able to cope with stress of cardiac surgery.
- Parent repeats guidelines for digoxin home administration.

The Cardiovascular System

Embryologic development of the heart is described in Chapter 9. Cardiac adaptations at birth are described in Chapter 23. After these adaptations, the heart can be thought of as consisting of two pumps: the right side pumps blood to the lungs, where it is oxygenated before returning to the left side of the heart; the left side pumps the oxygenated blood to the peripheral tissues through systemic arteries. After supplying these nutrients and collecting wastes, the blood returns through the veins to the right side of the heart where the cycle begins again. Contraction of the ventricles is termed **systole**, that of the atria as **diastole**.

Cardiac output (CO) is the volume of blood pumped by the ventricles per minute. It is calculated by multiplying stroke volume (the volume of blood a ventricle ejects during systole) by the heart rate (bpm). Cardiac output is affected by three main factors: preload, contractility, and afterload. **Preload** is the volume of blood in the ventricles at the end of diastole (the point just prior to contraction). **Afterload** refers to the resistance against which the ventricles must pump. **Contractility** is the ability of the ventricles to stretch and refers to the force of contraction generated by the myocardial muscle. The Frank-Starling law predicts that the stroke volume can be increased by increasing the stretch of the fibers. Excessive stretch, however, results in a decrease in cardiac output. Much of the therapy of heart disease is aimed at reducing preload and afterload and increasing contractility.

Most heart disease in children occurs because embryonic structures did not close at birth or the heart originally formed inappropriately. A septal defect between the right and left sides of the heart may remain open, and because contractility of the left side of the heart is greater than on the right side, the direction of the blood through the connective structure is invariably left to right, or from the area of stronger heart action to the area of weaker heart action. Normal heart anatomy is reviewed in Figure 41-1.

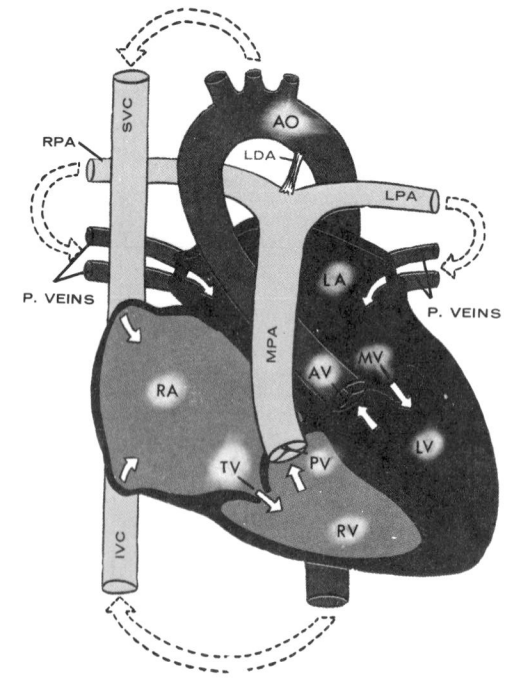

FIGURE 41-1

Circulation in the normal heart. (Used with permission of Ross Products Division, Abbott Laboratories, Columbus OH 43216 from Clinical Education Aid No. 7. © 1976 Ross Products Division, Abbott Laboratories.)

AO — Aorta

AV — Aortic valve

IVC — Inferior vena cava

LA — Left atrium

LPA — Left pulmonary artery

LV — Left ventricle

MPA — Main pulmonary artery

MV — Mitral valve

LDA — Ligamentum ductus arteriosus

PV — Pulmonary Valve

P. VEIN — Pulmonary vein

RA — Right atrium

RPA — Right pulmonary artery

RV — Right ventricle

SVC — Superior vena cava

TV — Tricuspid valve

Assessment of Heart Disorders in Children

The assessment of heart disease in children begins with a history and a physical assessment. More specific diagnostic studies, such as electrocardiography or echocardiography, are ordered as indicated. Since all children with heart disorders have an increased risk of poor blood perfusion, which may affect brain growth and development, developmental testing should be incorporated into assessment.

History

Heart disease is becoming increasingly recognized because of prenatal ultrasound, which shows poor heart action or a distended heart (Allan, 1993). Heart disease may not be detected in the newborn period because the newborn heart rate is so rapid that extra sounds of abnormal circulation cannot be heard. Because of relatively high pulmonary resistance, defects of the septum may not be readily apparent at birth. The infant may be brought to the physician's office by parents because the child is having difficulty feeding. Infants with heart disease generally have tachycardia and tachypnea. The infant who is breathing rapidly has to stop sucking on the bottle or breast frequently to breathe. The infant becomes easily fatigued because of ineffective heart action and has to stop sucking to rest before finishing a feeding.

The history should include a thorough pregnancy history to try to determine whether an intrauterine insult occurred. Some cardiac anomalies may occur as a result of an infection such as toxoplasmosis, cytomegalovirus, or rubella in intrauterine life. Ask if any medication was taken during pregnancy, if nutrition was adequate, or whether any radiation was used, since these may also contribute to congenital heart disorders.

Older children with heart disease also are easily fatigued. Ask in history-taking: How much activity does it take before the child becomes tired? An hour of strenuous play? A short walk? Be sure that parents are not confusing sedentary activities (the child who prefers to sit and read) with activities that are the result of fatigue (e.g., coming home from school and falling asleep day after day).

Ask about the child's usual position when resting: infants with cyanotic heart disease often prefer a knee-chest position; older children often voluntarily squat. These positions trap a blood supply in the lower extremities because of the sharp bend at the knee and hip and, therefore, allow the child to oxygenate the blood supply remaining in the upper body more fully and easily. Ask about frequency of infections, because children with heart disease have a higher incidence of lower respiratory tract infections than do other children. Children with left-to-right shunts tend to perspire excessively because of sympathetic nerve stimulation. Is there an indication of this? Edema is a late sign of congestive heart disease in children. If it does occur, periorbital edema generally occurs first. Urine is only produced when kidney perfusion is adequate. Ask if the infant is wetting diapers or if the older child is voiding normally.

Cyanosis (a blue tinge to the skin) will be reported as a sign in children with **cyanotic heart disease**. Such infants generally fail to thrive and are below normal height and weight on a standard growth chart. Children with coarctation of the aorta who have high blood pressure in the head and upper extremities have a history of nosebleeds and headaches. Because of corresponding low blood pressure in the lower extremities, such children may have pain in the legs on running (reported as "growing pains").

Some congenital heart disorders such as atrial septal defects may have a polygenic inheritance pattern. Ask if other family members have an incidence of heart disease. Cardiac anomalies often occur in conjunction with other disorders such as mental retardation and renal disease.

Physical Assessment

Physical assessment of the child with a suspected heart disorder begins with measurement of height and weight and comparison of these findings against standard growth charts. A thorough physical examination should then be done, with particular emphasis on certain body parts or systems (Figure 41-2).

General Appearance

Inspect the toes and fingers (particularly the thumbs) for clubbing (squaring of the end of phalanges; see Figure 40-4) and for color (if you press on a fingernail, it will blanch white and then quickly pinken in a child with good circulation and oxygenation; in a child with poor cell perfusion, the pink color returns slowly—over 5 seconds). Inspect mucous membranes of the mouth for color and evidence of cyanosis. Cyanosis is difficult to detect in black children; in them, the mucous membrane of the buccal membrane is often the best place to inspect.

Cyanosis can best be recognized in the tongue and mucous membrane of the newborn. Cyanosis persisting for over 20 minutes after birth (except for acrocyanosis) suggests serious cardiopulmonary dysfunction. If the cyanosis increases with crying, cardiac dysfunction is suggested (the child is unable to meet the increased circulatory demands); if the cyanosis decreases with crying, pulmonary dysfunction is suggested (crying deepens respirations and aerates more lung tissue). If the hemo-

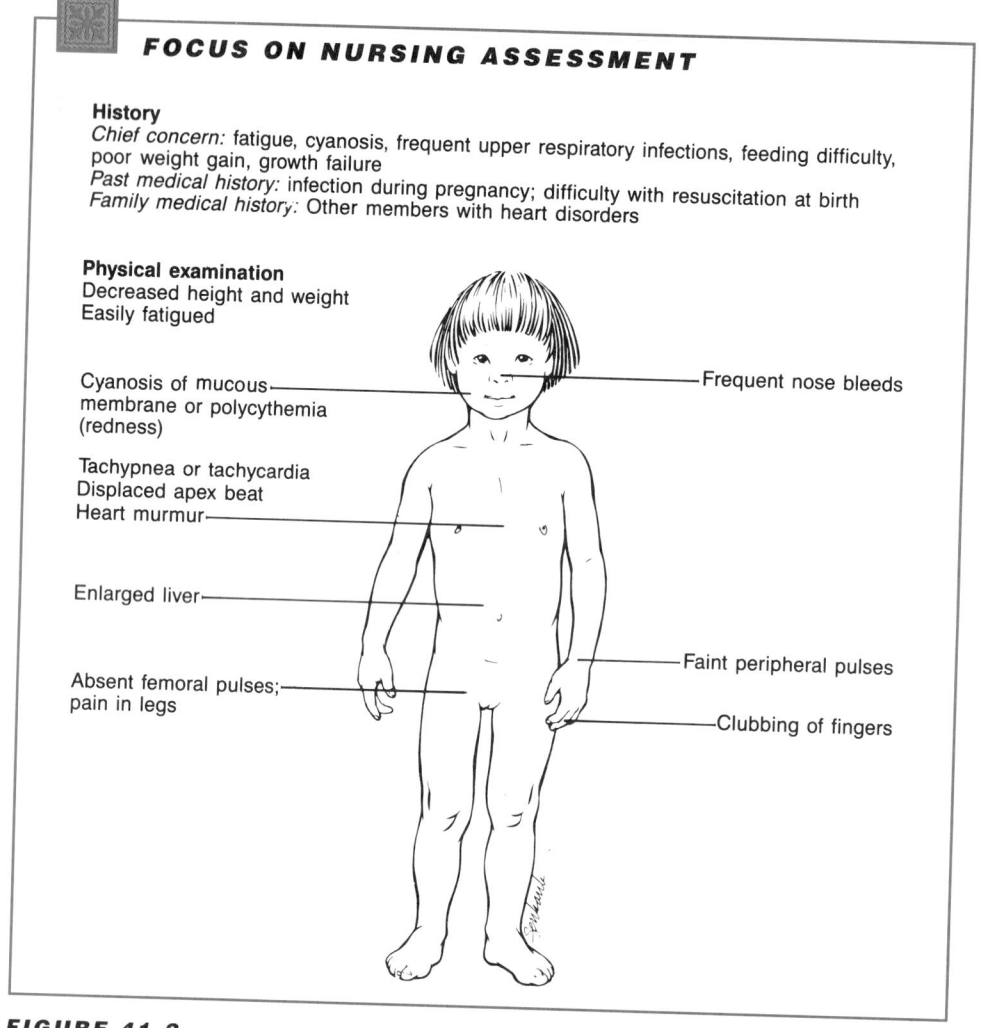

FOCUS ON NURSING ASSESSMENT

History
Chief concern: fatigue, cyanosis, frequent upper respiratory infections, feeding difficulty, poor weight gain, growth failure
Past medical history: infection during pregnancy; difficulty with resuscitation at birth
Family medical history: Other members with heart disorders

Physical examination
Decreased height and weight
Easily fatigued

Cyanosis of mucous membrane or polycythemia (redness)

Tachypnea or tachycardia
Displaced apex beat
Heart murmur

Enlarged liver

Absent femoral pulses; pain in legs

Frequent nose bleeds

Faint peripheral pulses

Clubbing of fingers

FIGURE 41-2
Common assessment findings in the child with a cardiovascular disorder.

globin is reduced below 4 to 6 g/100 mL, cyanosis is not present and severe anemia, therefore, must be ruled out.

A ruddy complexion may be present in some children with heart disease because the body overproduces red blood cells in an attempt to better oxygenate body cells. Observe children for lethargy, rapid respirations, or abnormal body posture, symptoms that the heart is an ineffective pump. Because a major part of the physical assessment will include inspection, palpation, and auscultation of the chest for heart function, children must be relaxed and not crying. Provide age-appropriate toys that will distract readily. Provide a bottle of glucose water in case an infant grows hungry. Play with children before the examination so that they know you.

Inspection of the chest may reveal a prominence of the left side and an obvious heart movement (apex beat, or point of maximum impulse). If a chest is extremely flat, loud innocent murmurs, accentuated heart sounds, and palpable cardiac activity may be very noticeable because of the proximity of the heart to the chest wall.

Pulse, Blood Pressure, and Respirations

The techniques for assessing pulse and blood pressure are described in Chapter 28. Normal findings for children of different ages are shown in Appendix G. *Tachycardia* is a pulse rate more than 160 bpm in an infant and more than 100 bpm at 3 years of age. An increase in pulse rate over this ratio needs further investigation. Tachycardia is particularly significant if it persists during sleep, when the possibility of excitement is removed. Abnormal pulse patterns that tend to occur in children with heart disorders are shown in Table 41-1.

Murmurs. Murmurs of no significance are termed *functional, insignificant,* or *innocent murmurs.* In discussing such murmurs with parents, the term **innocent murmur** is preferred, because it describes well the insignificance of the sound heard and strengthens the reassurance given parents that this is nothing to worry about. Innocent murmurs may become more pronounced during febrile illness, anxiety, or pregnancy;

Table 41-1. Abnormal Pulse Patterns

Pulse Pattern	Description
Water hammer	Very forceful and bounding pulse (Corrigan's pulse) and capillary pulsations may be apparent even in the fingernails; suggests cardiac insufficiency, as in patent ductus arteriosus
Pulsus alternans	A pulse of one strong beat and one weak beat; suggests myocardial weakness
Dicrotic	A double radial pulse for every apical beat; symptomatic of aortic stenosis
Thready	Weak and usually rapid pulse; suggests ineffective heart action

hence, they may become audible for the first time at a hospital admission. Such murmurs probably reflect a normal variation of vibration in the heart or pulmonary artery.

Parents should be told when children have innocent murmurs, because these sounds will undoubtedly be discovered again at a future health assessment. Teach parents that, although an innocent murmur is present, it is normal and is not a sign of any heart disease. Activities need not be restricted, and the child will require no more frequent health appraisals than other children. It is also important to teach parents that innocent murmurs do not turn into serious murmurs; otherwise, some parents see them as a prelude to future heart disease. At future health assessments, parents may need to be reassured again that the murmur is innocent.

If a murmur is the result of heart disease or a congenital defect, it is termed an **organic murmur.** A comparison of the usual characteristics of innocent and organic murmurs is shown in Table 41-2.

For assessment, any murmur heard should be described according to its position in the cardiac cycle (early systolic, midsystolic, late diastolic, etc.), duration, quality (blowing, rasping, rumbling), pitch, intensity, location where it is heard best (the point of maximum intensity), whether a thrill (a palpable purring sensation) is present, and the response of the murmur to exercise or

change of position. The intensity, or loudness, of the murmur is graded according to the standard criteria shown in Table 28-6.

Diagnostic Tests

The diagnostic studies performed on a child with suspected heart disease will vary with the specific lesion suspected.

Electrocardiogram

An **electrocardiogram** (ECG) provides information about heart rate, rhythm, state of the myocardium, presence or absence of hypertrophy (thickening of the heart walls), ischemia or necrosis, and abnormalities of conduction. It reflects the presence or effect of various drugs and electrolyte imbalance.

An ECG is a written record of the rising and falling voltages generated by the contracting heart. An upward tracing indicates a positive voltage, whereas a downward tracing indicates a negative voltage. The heart beat is initiated by the sinoatrial (SA) node in the right atrial wall near the entrance of the superior vena cava. From the SA node, the electrical impulse spreads over the atria while the atria are filling with blood; as the atria are filled, the electrical impulse reaches the valves; atria contract and empty. Electrical impulses reach the atrioventricular (AV) node, located in the lower right atrium and spread through the AV bundle (bundle of His) and the Purkinje fibers to the wall and septum of the ventricles while the ventricles are filling. At the point that the ventricles have filled, the electrical flow has reached a peak, causing the ventricles to contract.

A normal ECG consists of an atrial wave (the P wave), a brief inactive period, then the prominent ventricular peak (the QRS spike), a large slow wave caused by ventricular recovery (the T wave), and often an incompletely understood slow wave (the U wave; Figure 41-3). A long P wave suggests that the atria are hypertrophied and it is taking longer than usual for the electrical conduction to spread over the atria. A lengthened PR interval suggests that there is difficulty in coordination between the SA and AV nodes (first-degree heart

Table 41-2. Comparison of Innocent and Organic Murmurs

Characteristic	Innocent	Organic
Timing	Systolic	Systolic or diastolic
Duration	Short	Longer
Quality	Soft, musical	Harsh, blowing
Intensity	Soft	Loud
Position in which heard	Usually supine positions	Heard in all positions
Affected by exercise	Yes	Constant

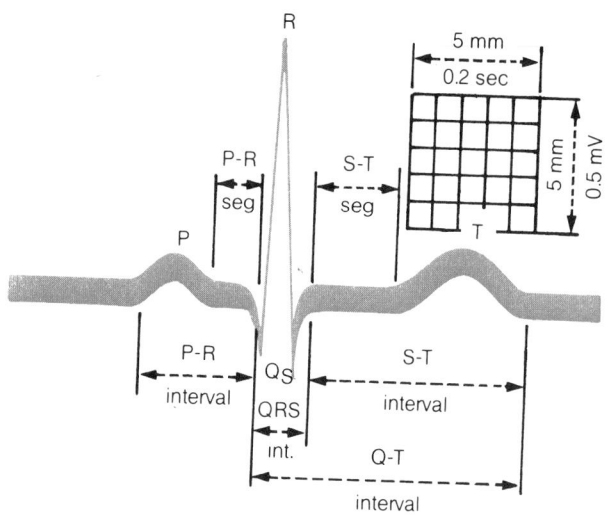

FIGURE 41-3

A normal ECG configuration. (From Suddarth DS. [1991]. The Lippincott manual of nursing practice [5th ed.]. Philadelphia: J.B. Lippincott, p. 365.)

block). A heightened R wave indicates that ventricular hypertrophy is present. An R wave that is decreased in height means that the ventricles cannot contract fully, as happens if they are surrounded by fluid (pericarditis). Elongation of the T wave occurs in hyperkalemia; depression of the T wave is associated with anoxia, and depression of the ST segment is associated with abnormal calcium levels. Figure 41-4 shows examples of these abnormal configurations.

Radiography

Radiography (x-ray) examination furnishes an accurate picture of the heart size and contour and size of heart chambers. It can reveal fluid collecting in the lungs from cardiac failure. It can be used to confirm the placement of pacemaker leads. In a posteroanterior view, if the cardiac width is more than half the chest width, the heart is usually enlarged. This measurement does not apply to infants, because the more horizontal position of the infant heart increases this ratio to more than half. Prominence of pulmonary blood flow may be evident.

Fluoroscopy, a form of radiograph, provides important information about the size and configuration of

the heart as well as of the great vessels, lungs, thoracic cage, and diaphragm. Because prolonged observation is necessary, however, special precautions must be taken to adjust accommodation of the eyes and to protect the child and health care personnel from radiation. Special techniques can be employed to reduce radiation to the child and also to provide a permanent motion picture record. The esophagus is so closely related to cardiac chambers that its visualization with barium also enhances cardiovascular structures. Interpretation of atrial or ventricular hypertrophy in infants and children by radiographic means is difficult. X-ray findings are, therefore, usually complemented by an ECG, a more sensitive and accurate measure of ventricular enlargement.

In *radioangiocardiography*, a radioactive substance such as technetium is injected intravenously into the bloodstream. As the substance circulates through the heart, it may be traced and recorded on videotape. The procedure involves a low dose of radiation and may be used to demonstrate, in particular, septal shunts.

Generalized *angiography*, or instillation of dye followed by radiographs, has little value in demonstrating pediatric heart defects. Selected *angiocardiography*, however, done as part of a cardiac catheterization, allows identification of specific abnormalities if followed by serial x-ray films. After a contrast medium has been introduced into a specific heart chamber, closed-circuit video equipment records the fluoroscopy pictures. Angiocardiography is not without hazard. Deaths have been reported from iodine sensitivity to the dye used, cardiac arrhythmias, and pulmonary edema.

Echocardiography

Echocardiography is ultrasound cardiography. High-frequency sound waves, directed toward the heart, are used to locate and study the movement and dimensions of cardiac structures, such as the size of chambers, thickness of walls, relationship of major vessels to chambers, and the thickness, motion, and pressure gradients of the valves. You may need to remind parents that echocardiography does not use x-rays. An advantage of the procedure is that it can be repeated at frequent intervals without exposing children to the possible risk of radiation. It may be done using a transesophageal probe to better reveal heart chambers (Stoumper et al., 1990).

FIGURE 41-4

*Abnormal ECG configurations. (**A**) Normal ECG. (**B**) Hypokalemia, showing a depressed ST segment, a prominent U wave, and a prolonged QT interval. (**C**) Hypercalcemia, demonstrating shortened ST segment and QT interval. (**D**) Hypocalcemia, demonstrating prolongation of the ST segment and QT interval.*

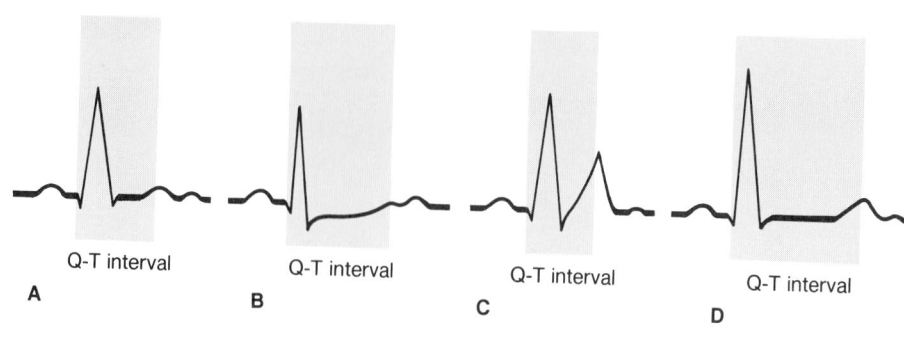

Fetal echocardiography can reveal heart anomalies as early as 18 weeks into a pregnancy. This can alert staff to be prepared with immediate resuscitation or other needed equipment at the baby's birth. *Magnetic resonance imaging* may also be used for studies to help reduce the amount of exposure to radiation (Kersting-Sommerhoff et al., 1990).

A **phonocardiogram** is a diagram of heart sounds translated into electrical energy by a microphone placed on the child's chest and then recorded as a diagrammatic representation of heart sounds. The technique can measure the timing of heart sounds that occur too quickly or at too high or too low a sound frequency for the human ear to detect by direct auscultation.

Exercise Testing

Exercise tests to demonstrate that the pulmonary circulation can increase to meet the increased respiratory demands of exercise may be performed with children following cardiac surgery. With heart defects that obstruct the flow of blood to the lungs (such as pulmonary stenosis), such accommodation is not possible, and the child will evidence exertional dyspnea. Such tests are difficult to perform with children because they require the child's cooperation. In infants, one of the earliest symptoms of exertional dyspnea is evident during feeding: the child tires before he or she can complete a feeding.

Laboratory Tests

Children with heart disease usually have a number of blood tests done to support the diagnosis of heart disease or to rule out anemia or clotting defects. Hematocrit or hemoglobin studies are performed with children who have cyanotic heart disease to assess the rate of erythrocyte production, which in these children is increased in the body's attempt to produce more oxygen-carrying red blood cells. If the increase in the number of red blood cells is extreme (this is termed **polycythemia**), there will be a corresponding increase in blood volume; there may be a decrease in blood viscosity. Newborns are normally slightly polycythemic. In a newborn, polycythemia may be defined as a hemoglobin over 25 g/100 mL or a hematocrit over 70%. In an older child, polycythemia may be defined as a hemoglobin over 16 g/100 mL or a hematocrit over 55%. An elevated erythrocyte sedimentation rate (ESR) denotes inflammation and is useful in documenting that an inflammatory process such as occurs with rheumatic fever, Kawasaki disease, or myocarditis is present.

Blood gas levels are also determined. To test for cyanotic heart disease, the child can be administered 100% oxygen for 15 minutes. If the infant still has a PO_2 less than 150 mm Hg after this time, cyanotic heart disease is suspected. Oxygen saturation levels are assessed; children with a cyanotic heart disease have a lower-than-normal oxygen saturation level in arterial blood. Normally, arterial blood oxygen saturation is 96% to 98%; oxygen saturation under 92% is indicative of cyanotic heart disease.

Prior to cardiac catheterization or surgery, blood clotting must be assessed. Prothrombin, partial thromboplastin, and platelet count studies can therefore be expected to be completed before the procedure. Some children with polycythemia from cyanotic heart disease have an associated reduced platelet count (thrombocytopenia). Because platelet formation is necessary for blood coagulation, the state of the platelet count must be corrected prior to cardiac surgery.

Serum sodium is assessed in children with congestive heart failure to be certain that an increased sodium level is not adding to edema formation. All children who are placed on diuretics to help their body evacuate edematous fluid must have serum potassium levels determined, since diuretics tend to deplete the body of potassium. Low serum potassium potentiates the effect of digitoxin and digoxin; thus, serum potassium levels must also be obtained in children receiving these medications.

Nursing Care of the Child With a Heart Disorder

Taking home an infant born with a heart defect is difficult for most parents. They have many questions that need to be answered fully before they feel confident enough to do this. Encourage parents to handle and feed their infant in the hospital so that they can feel secure in caring for him or her at home. It is important for parents to understand as much as possible about their child's disorder. The more they know the less they will assume that all children with congenital heart disease have the same disease. If this is not made clear to parents, they may unnecessarily limit a child's activity, assuming that because a neighbor's child was told not to do some activity, their child should not do it either.

Nursing Diagnoses and Related Interventions

Nursing Diagnosis: Parental health-seeking behaviors related to lack of knowledge about child's disorder

Goal: Parents will demonstrate a full understanding of child's illness and treatment plan before discharge.

Outcome Criteria: Parents state accurately the nature of the illness and unique needs of their baby; are able to name primary care providers who will be following child's progress and can be telephoned for emergencies.

Provide Information About Care

Parents generally ask, "Can we let the baby cry?" If infants have tetralogy of Fallot or another heart disorder in which cyanotic spells tend to develop, or if they have a severe aortic stenosis, they should not be allowed to cry for long periods of time (no baby should). Crying for a few minutes while a parent warms formula or fully awakens at night will, as a rule, not harm them.

"What do we feed him?" Babies with heart disorders are generally able to tolerate a normal diet. Only rarely is salt restricted during this period. Infants are generally given an iron supplement, either in formula or separately, to prevent iron deficiency anemia during the first year. This is especially important in children with heart disease, because anemia places a strain on an already overtaxed heart. They should receive supplemental vitamins with formula when breast-feeding is stopped, as should all infants. Because some infants with congenital heart disease tire readily, parents may need to give them frequent, small feedings during the day rather than the usual every-4-hour pattern of normal newborns. If children are extremely poor eaters, they may be placed on a high-calorie formula or fed by enteral or gastrostomy technique (Schwarz et al., 1990).

"How much activity can we allow the baby?" The answer to this question depends on the heart disorder and the extent of the defect. As a rule, infants or young children naturally limit their own activity. Parents need guidance, however, in setting limits of activity. Roughhousing with infants, such as tossing them up in the air and watching them squeal and laugh, is not advised. Playing games such as chasing a ball or placing them for long periods of time in infant walkers may be contraindicated. Encourage parents to spend time in the hospital with their infant to learn to recognize the first signs of respiratory distress and the point at which their child's activity is beginning to exceed his or her tolerance. Caution parents to observe the child carefully and thoughtfully as new activities are introduced and new interests are gained, so that the child's activity is limited to what the heart can accommodate. Children can travel in cars as long as the trip is a sensible length. Those with cyanotic disease may need oxygen supplementation during air travel.

"What do we do if he becomes ill?" Although children with congenital heart disorders are usually seen by a cardiologist for health supervision, it is important that they are also seen by health care personnel who can ensure that they are receiving normal childhood immunizations and health guidance. As a rule, infants with heart disorders need prompt treatment for minor illnesses. The fever that accompanies a cold, for instance, can increase the metabolic rate of a child who has a severe congenital heart defect to beyond the point at which the child's heart can compensate. Dehydration must be avoided in children with cyanotic heart disease;

the polycythemia they have will become so extreme that thrombophlebitis may result. It is important that infections be treated vigorously so that infectious endocarditis does not develop.

Such children need prophylactic antibiotic therapy before they have oral surgery (tooth extractions or tonsils removed), because streptococcal organisms generally present in the mouth are often involved in infectious endocarditis. It is a good rule for children to be placed on prophylactic antibiotic therapy before they visit a dentist at all, because parents cannot always anticipate what dentists will do at any one visit. Penicillin is the preferred prophylactic antibiotic; erythromycin is used when a child is sensitive to penicillin. Many parents need frequent reassurance that a child will not become immune to penicillin if it is taken over long periods of time. Children with congenital heart disease should receive routine immunizations and be considered for pneumonia and influenza vaccines.

Review Steps for Follow-Up Care and Emergencies

Before parents leave the hospital with their newborn, be certain they know whom they should call if they have a question regarding the infant's health (their own pediatrician or a clinic telephone number and an emergency telephone number as a back-up.) Review with them the steps to take if their child becomes cyanotic, such as placing him or her in a knee-chest position. Be certain they have an appointment for a first health assessment, so they can be reassured that the responsibility of caring for this child is not being placed solely on their shoulders but will be shared by concerned health care personnel through all the child's growing years. They need to be told that if they are unsure whether their child is in distress or ill, it is better to err on the side of caution by bringing the child to a physician. Everyone who cares for infants with heart disease appreciates the responsibility the parents feel and the difficulty they have in making health judgments about their child; in many instances they not only are the parents of this particular child but they also are new parents.

The parents may appreciate being referred to a community health nurse with whom they can discuss the sometimes frightening responsibility they feel and from whom they can obtain a second opinion of their child's health. They need to learn cardiopulmonary resuscitation (CPR). Parents of children with heart disease are highly motivated to learn CPR, knowing how necessary this skill could be.

The Child Undergoing Cardiac Catheterization

Cardiac catheterization is a procedure used to help diagnose specific heart defects in anticipation of surgery. A small radiopaque catheter is passed through a vein in the arm, leg, or neck into the heart to secure blood samples or inject dye. This allows the physician to evaluate the pressure of blood flow in any heart chamber as well as total cardiac output. Blood can be removed from the catheter for determination of oxygen saturation levels, or a contrast dye can be injected for angiography.

Children are generally kept NPO for 4 to 6 hours prior to a cardiac catheterization procedure to reduce the danger of vomiting and aspiration during the procedure. Children must have had a recent chest x-ray and ECG recorded and have blood typed and cross-matched ready for use. Because it is vitally important that the vessel site chosen for catheterization not be infected at the time of catheterization (or obscured by a hematoma), blood should not be drawn from the projected catheterization entry site. *Protecting this site is a nursing responsibility, especially on nursing units in which auxiliary personnel routinely draw blood.*

In the cardiac catheterization room, ECG leads are attached. The site for catheterization is locally anesthetized, and the vessel is opened by cutdown or entered through a large-bore needle. The vessel used will differ according to the individual technique being planned. In neonates an umbilical artery can be catheterized. Right-side heart catheterization is done by a venous approach. A right femoral vein or a vein in the antecubital fossa is used. Left-side heart catheterization can be performed by either a venous or an arterial approach. If done by the arterial route, a catheter is inserted into either the femoral or brachial artery. If a venous route is used, the catheter is inserted into the right femoral vein and advanced to the right atrium. The catheter then punctures the intraatrial septum and enters the left atrium (Figure 41-5).

Cardiac catheterization has a mortality rate of about 0.5%, so it is not without risk. Most fatalities with the procedure occur in infants under 7 months of age, usually because of cardiac perforation and arrhythmia.

Transient arrhythmias may occur during passage of the catheter through the heart chambers or during injection of a contrast medium. Such arrhythmias generally stop abruptly with withdrawal of the catheter. Perforation of the heart may occur during passage of the catheter. Other complications include bleeding from the insertion site, because of heparin introduced into the catheter to reduce the possibility of clot formation, and thrombophlebitis from irritation by the catheter (a foreign body). Because cardiac catheterization is necessary for the heart surgeon to visualize and plan a cardiac repair, however, the benefit of the procedure outweighs the risks.

Nursing Diagnosis and Related Interventions: Preprocedure Phase

Nursing Diagnosis: Anxiety related to lack of knowledge about cardiac catheterization procedure

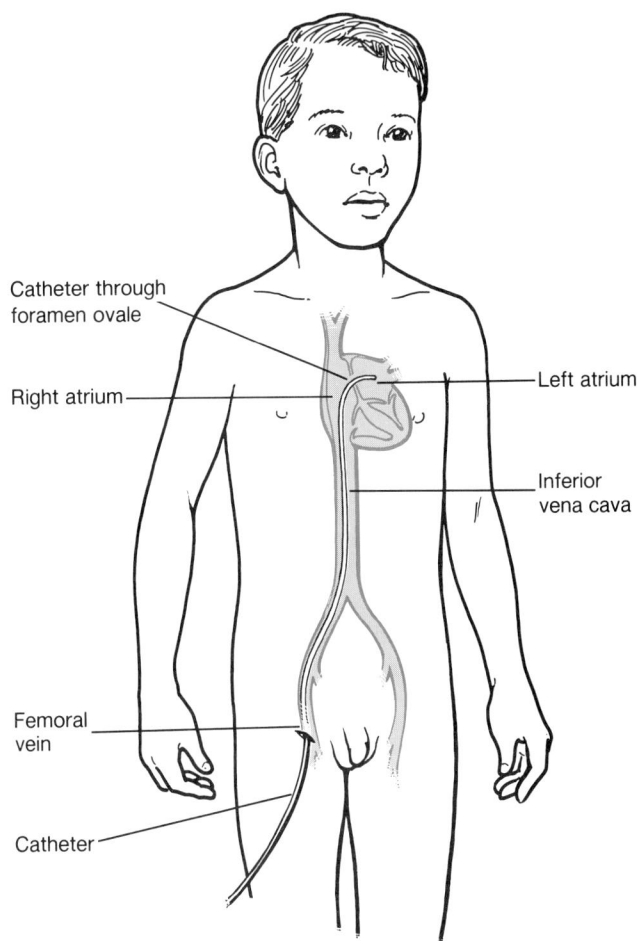

FIGURE 41-5
Cardiac catheterization. The catheter takes the path shown during cardiac catheterization to analyze pressure in the left heart.

Goal: Parents and child will demonstrate increased knowledge prior to procedure; will express confidence about need for and outcome of procedure.

Outcome Criteria: Parents and child (when possible) state goal of procedure and reasons for preparation and aftercare measures; state that anxiety is less after teaching.

Because most cardiac catheterizations are done with children awake but sedated with a combination of drugs such as chloral hydrate and meperidine, they may need more information about what is going to happen during the procedure than they would normally need for cardiac surgery. It is best to provide explanations for the children with parents present. Parents will then be able to help reinforce the information. Following this explanation, parents often prefer a more detailed explanation of the procedure for themselves and time to ask their own questions.

Be aware that consenting to a cardiac catheterization experience arouses the realization that cardiac surgery may be necessary. Parents may be so concerned with what the procedure may reveal that they are unable to listen well to explanations. Allow them to accompany their children to the catheterization room and remain there for support during the procedure if they so choose.

Prepare children for what they will see in the catheterization room (Figure 41-6). Because they may be overwhelmed by the sight of all the equipment, it may help if you build a facsimile room out of small cardboard boxes (representing the x-ray machine, the fluoroscopy screen, the ECG machine, etc.). A puppet or small doll might serve as the patient in the miniature room. Dress the puppets in "sterile surgery suits" and "masks" like those worn by cardiac catheterization personnel.

If children have never seen ECG leads or restraints before, let them touch and feel the equipment. Tell them that the procedure will be as long as 3 hours and that they will need to lie very still during this time.

Do not underestimate what children know about their heart's purpose and function; even preschoolers recognize that the heart is vital to the body. Reassure them that the doctors are only taking a look at their heart, not cutting it or removing any part of it.

Teach children that when the catheter is inserted, it will not hurt, but their heart may momentarily speed up, a feeling that is uncomfortable. When dye is inserted, they may feel a stinging sensation (but do not use the word "dye," which may frighten young children who may think that dying is exactly what this procedure is all about; say "medicine"). Caution them that lights will be turned off after the medicine is injected so that the doctor can watch the medicine on a television screen (fluoroscopy) as it passes through the heart. After the procedure, a pressure dressing will be placed over the catheter insertion site to reduce the risk of bleeding.

Parents often need to have a review of heart anatomy at their conference. Even though the cardiologist may have already done this, many parents appreciate being shown again the pathway the tubing must take during the procedure.

Nursing Diagnoses and Related Interventions: Postprocedure Phase

Nursing Diagnosis: High risk for altered tissue perfusion related to cardiac catheterization

Goal: Child will maintain adequate tissue perfusion during the recovery period.

Outcome Criteria: Child's vital signs are within normal limits; no dysrhythmia is present; no bleeding from catheterization site is present; pedal pulse is present distal to catheterization site.

When children return from the procedure, move them gently to their bed. Assess the dressing over the catheterization site to see that it is snug and intact and that there is no bleeding present. This is particularly important when an artery was used for catheterization; a loose dressing on an artery will cause a large blood loss in a very short time as well as allow bacteria to enter. A pulse distal to the bandage should be palpated to assure yourself that the blood flow in the extremity is not obstructed (dorsalis pedis pulse on the foot; Figure 41-7). For the same reason, assess the extremity distal to the entry site for color, temperature, and circulation (blanch the toe or fingernail and watch to see that it pinkens again readily). If there is bleeding at the entry site, firm, continuous pressure is generally the best method to control bleeding until the physician can check the site.

To reduce anxiety, children need an opportunity to describe their experience to an interested person. Saying out loud how frightened they were—by the x-ray machine being pushed in over them, by the thought of a tube going all the way into their heart, by a comment made by one of the personnel in the room—makes their fear much less and their acceptance of the procedure easier. They need to be praised for their cooperation.

Keep the child flat in bed for 3 to 4 hours. This is to prevent oozing at the insertion site and to prevent postural hypotension, which may occur when rising suddenly after lying flat for a long period of time. Assess pulse, blood pressure, and respirations at frequent inter-

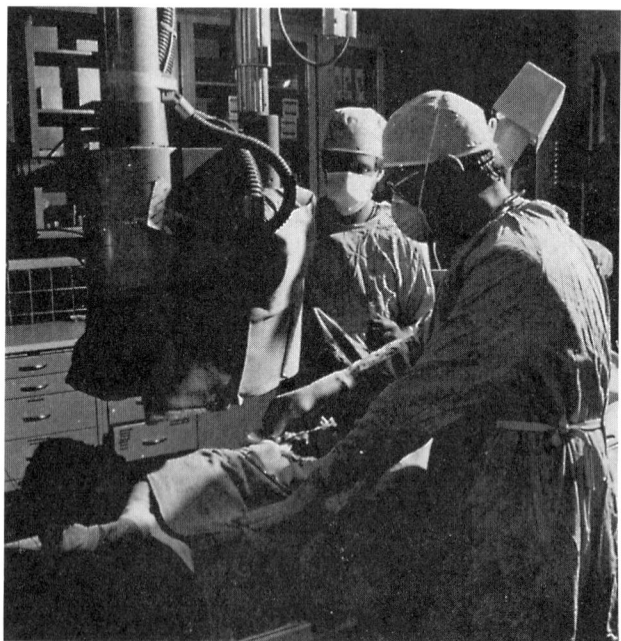

FIGURE 41-6

Children should be well prepared for the amount of equipment and the subdued lights in the cardiac catheterization laboratory. (Courtesy of the Department of Medical Photography, Children's Hospital, Buffalo, NY.)

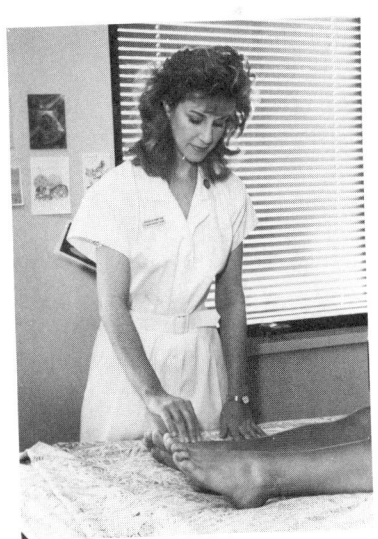

FIGURE 41-7
Assess a dorsalis pedis pulse following cardiac catheterization to ensure that circulation is intact distal to the catheter insertion site. (Courtesy of the Department of Medical Photography, Children's Hospital, Buffalo, NY.)

vals (about every 15 minutes) for the first several hours. In the immediate postcatheterization period, the blood pressure may be 10% to 15% lower than the child's precatheterization level because of the hypotensive effect of the radiopaque dye injected.

Cardiac arrhythmia and bradycardia may result from the mechanical action of the catheter having touched the conduction nodes of the heart. If the pulse is taken for a full minute, such arrhythmias will be more easily recognized than if the pulse is taken for a shorter time. Small children are unable to describe the feelings that accompany an arrhythmia; an older child might describe it as "heart fluttering" or "skipping beats." Therefore, increasing anxiety in the child after a catheterization is an important observation to report; it may be the child's way of saying these things.

Infants need fluid replacement to counteract the transient dehydration that results from being NPO for a period of time. If the infant has a cyanotic heart disease and is polycythemic, the increased fluid intake helps to avoid vessel thrombi. Infants may require intravenous (IV) fluid during the procedure and for a number of hours afterward to prevent dehydration. Regulate this carefully to prevent congestive heart failure from a fluid overload.

Adverse effects of cardiac catheterization may also be manifested by spells of apnea, sternal retractions, or dyspnea. If the infant received oxygen during the catheterization procedure, it may be continued for a period of time following the procedure to reduce the stress of respirations. Although arrhythmias, dyspnea, bradycardia, and blood pressure anomalies may be transient,

children with these signs need to be examined by a physician so that they can be evaluated further.

Nursing Diagnosis: High risk for infection related to presence of cardiac catheterization incision site

Goal: The child will not develop an infection following the procedure.

Outcome Procedure: The child's temperature is not above 38.0°C axillary; the catheter insertion site is not erythematous or with foul drainage.

If the dressing is over the femoral artery or vein, it is important to keep it clean of stool and urine. Waterproofing the dressing with plastic may be necessary. Temperature should be assessed immediately and then hourly for several hours after cardiac catheterization. Some children will have a transient elevated temperature due to physiologic dehydration from having been on NPO status for such a long period of time. Some children react to the injection of the dye by a rise in temperature. An elevated temperature caused by infection from the introduction of pathogens at the time of the procedure must be distinguished from a rise due to other causes.

Nursing Diagnosis: High risk for hypothermia related to cooling during procedure

Goal: Child's temperature will return to normal soon after the procedure.

Outcome Criteria: Child's temperature is above 36.0°C axillary 1 hour after the procedure.

Infants may have hypothermia afterward from being uncovered during the procedure. Respiratory and heart action are quickly compromised because, to raise body temperature, the infant's metabolic rate increases. This requires rapid breathing and increased heart action and can lead to exhaustion. Infants may need to be placed in warmed incubators or on radiant heat warmers so they can regain and maintain normal body temperature.

The Child Undergoing Cardiac Surgery

Open heart surgery is made possible by the use of pulmonary bypass techniques. The venous return to the heart is diverted from the right atrium or inferior and superior vena cava to a heart–lung machine, where it is artificially oxygenated. It is returned to the body's arterial system by way of the aorta bypassing the heart. This procedure is often referred to as **extracorporeal membrane oxygenation** (ECMO). The heart, practically bloodless, can be opened and operated on. Blood returns to the coronary and pulmonary arteries from the aorta so that, even though the heart is not pumping, it still receives an adequate blood supply for self-mainte-nance during the bypass procedure. Hypothermia (re-ducing the child's body temperature to 20° to 26°C) is used during surgery to reduce the child's metabolic needs. If extreme hypothermia is used (15° to 20°C), the body temperature drops so low that the heart stops beat-ing and the surgeon can work in a quiet as well as bloodless field. Very ill infants may be maintained on ECMO following surgery (Suddaby & O'Brien, 1993).

Preoperative Care

Prior to surgery, children will have vital signs (blood pressure, pulse, and respirations) taken several times a day. Some children may have pulse determinations done at several pulse points or blood pressures of both upper and lower extremities taken. It is important that these measurements be done accurately, because they will serve as a baseline for comparison of postoperative measurements. Have children rest for about 15 minutes prior to blood pressure recording; do the actual record-ing with children lying down. Count pulse and respira-tion rates for a full minute for accuracy. Height and weight need to be recorded, because these parameters are necessary for the estimation of blood volume for the heart–lung machine and for medication dosages. Weigh-ing will also be helpful in estimating blood loss or edema after surgery. Children who are receiving digitalis usually have their dose withheld 24 hours before surgery, because cardiac surgery may cause arrhythmias in the presence of digitalis.

The immediate surgical preparation of children varies from one institution to another but usually in-cludes an enema (to keep children from straining to pass stool in the immediate postoperative period and thus adding strain on the heart).

Nursing Diagnoses and Related Interventions: Preoperative Phase

Nursing Diagnosis: Fear related to outcome of cardiac surgery

Goal: Parents and child will demonstrate increased knowledge prior to procedure and confidence in their health care team.

Outcome Criteria: Parents and child accurately state the reason for surgery and expected outcome.

Bringing a child to the hospital for cardiac surgery is a large responsibility for parents. They want their child to be made well, yet they are aware that there is a defi-nite risk from this surgery. They may have been protect-ing and guarding their child for months or years. They feel no less protective this morning than usual. Parents of children being readied for cardiac surgery may watch preoperative procedures carefully, wanting nothing to go wrong that will interfere with surgery. They are usu-

ally anxious to help with preoperative measures them-selves to be sure that nothing is being done incorrectly. You need to review with them what they already know about the surgery to correct any misconceptions. Be cer-tain to prepare them for the amount of equipment that will surround their child after surgery; cardiac monitors, oxygen equipment, IV equipment, chest tubes, and a ventilator. Parents usually appreciate visiting the inten-sive care unit (ICU) where their child will go following surgery. Be certain that they have an opportunity to meet the ICU staff, especially if these nurses are not the same ones who are caring for the child preoperatively. Parents need to have confidence in the personnel who will be caring for their child so they can continue to offer support to the child (Hardingham, 1993; see Focus on Nursing Research box).

Explain Procedures to Parents and Child. Children undergoing cardiac surgery and their parents all need careful preparation. Do not underestimate how much

FOCUS ON NURSING RESEARCH

What Are the Most Intense Stressors That Parents Experience When Their Children Are Cared for in Intensive Care Units?

Many children with cardiovascular disorders are hospital-ized in intensive care units because they have had car-diac surgery. To investigate what particular stressors hospitalization in an ICU causes parents, a nursing re-searcher asked 32 parents (10 fathers and 22 mothers) whose child was hospitalized in such a unit to rate on a 6-point Likert scale the types of stresses they were feeling about such areas as their child's appearance, sights and sounds, procedures, professional staff, behaviors/emo-tions, their parental role, and social support. Parents' ages ranged from 20 to 53 years. Their children's ages ranged from 6 weeks to 15 years. Children's length of stay was 2 to 10 days with an average of 4 days. In this study, fathers rated their overall intensive care experience as more stressful than did mothers. Both mothers and father rated "tubes in my child" as the most stressful item on the list of procedures. Other concerns rated as major were being separated from their child and receiving different medical opinions from doctors.

The researcher suggests that the most important roles of a nurse in an intensive care unit should be to orient par-ents to the unit and procedures and to serve as a consis-tent health care professional in the midst of rotating staff personnel.

Heuer, L. (1993). Parental stressors in a pediatric intensive care unit. *Pediatric Nursing, 19*, 128.

children know about the importance of their heart or the seriousness of this surgery (Figure 41-8).

Some parents believe that their children will be frightened by explanations about the surgery and do not want them to be told anything about it; this stems from the extreme protectiveness the parents have harbored for so long. If you give these parents a clear, calm explanation of what is going to happen to their child, they usually find this step-by-step explanation a relief, and realize that so, probably, will their child. Remember when caring for these children preoperatively (or any time) not to make careless remarks, such as "These syringes never work right" (when all you mean is that you prefer another brand) or "Amy (an ICU nurse) is a real clown" (when you mean she is not only a competent nurse but has a good sense of humor besides). Anxious parents may interpret such statements to mean their child is in less than competent hands.

Encourage Child and Parents to Express Fears. Children are generally admitted one day before surgery is planned. This is so that blood oxygen saturation levels, chest films, ECG, or other additional diagnostic procedures can be completed prior to surgery. Blood to be used for pulmonary bypass must be typed and crossmatched. The early admission also helps to prevent children from contracting an upper respiratory infection just prior to surgery. This extra day in the hospital before

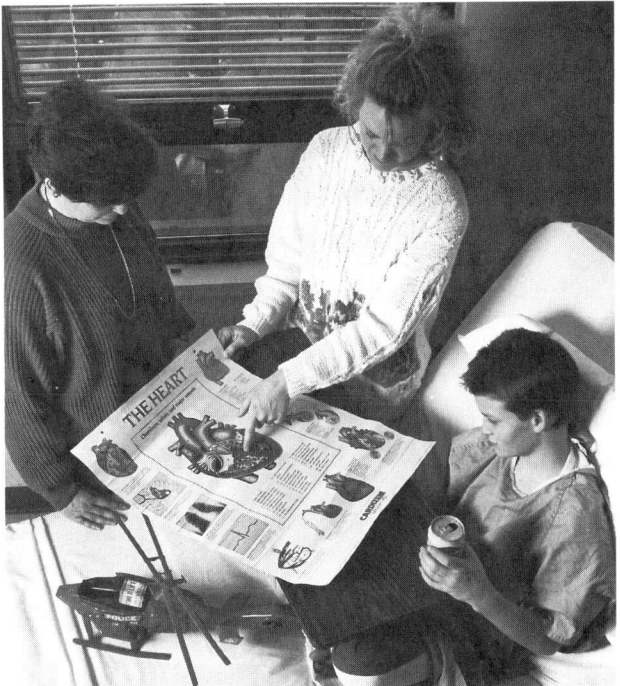

FIGURE 41-8
Orientation for cardiac surgery includes time for talking and learning more about the heart. (Courtesy of the Department of Medical Photography, Children's Hospital, Buffalo, NY.)

surgery provides an opportune time to prepare children psychologically for surgery. Because many children having cardiac surgery have had previous cardiac catheterizations, they need time to talk about their previous hospitalization experiences. Talking will reveal those things that they are most afraid of this time. Any misconceptions that they have about past experiences can be discussed and cleared away.

Prepare Child for Surgery and Postoperative Care. It is best if children are prepared for surgery with their parents present. This allows parents the opportunity to reinforce your teaching and shows children that their parents approve and feel secure with these surgery plans. Parents will then need additional time to discuss the surgical procedure with you and ask questions they might not have wished to ask in the presence of their child.

Both parents and the child may have questions about the difference between cardiac catheterization and cardiac surgery. One important difference is that children are sedated but awake for the former, but anesthetized for the latter. For some children, being awake is more reassuring; for others, it is more frightening. With the catheterization, they were aware the entire time that they were all right; asleep, how can they know? They need to express these feelings and receive reassurance that anesthetized sleep is a special sleep from which they will have no difficulty waking. Meeting the anesthesiologist and receiving reassurance directly from him or her that they will be watched over while they are asleep is often helpful.

As with cardiac catheterization, it may help to make models of the equipment that will surround the child postoperatively. Adolescents should be taken to the ICU where they will return after surgery and be shown the actual equipment. School-age or younger children may be too overwhelmed by seeing the actual room, so models (made from cereal boxes) or photographs will help familiarize them with the equipment without being too frightening. Puppets or small dolls can be used to explain how the equipment will be used.

After surgery, the child will need to cough and deep-breathe to help the lungs expand. It is good to introduce these exercises preoperatively to let the child know what is expected. Having children blow up a balloon is a helpful means of encouraging those who do not deep-breathe to do this well. In addition, introduce children to the form of oxygen therapy they will receive following surgery (tent, mask, cannula, or ventilator). Orienting children to oxygen equipment is discussed in Chapter 40.

Familiarize children with chest tubes and an underwater seal apparatus. Caution both children and parents that chest tubes must stay in place until it is time for them to be removed; if they want to turn over with tubes in place, they should ask for help to prevent the

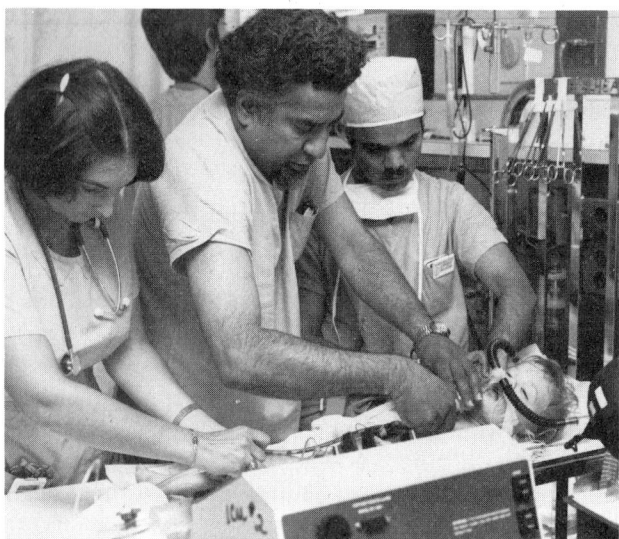

FIGURE 41-9
A child returning from cardiac surgery with an ET tube, chest tubes, nasogastric tube, urinary catheter, and CVP catheter in place. Children should be prepared carefully for all of these experiences. (Courtesy of the Department of Medical Photography, Children's Hospital, Buffalo, NY.)

tubes from being pulled out. Caution parents that a chest-tube drainage reservoir must remain below the level of the child's chest and must not be raised for any reason. If children are not familiar with ECG leads, introduce these to them as part of the preoperative preparation (Figure 41-9). Comparing these tubes or leads to being "hooked up" like an astronaut is often appealing to children.

Postoperative Care

Following surgery and before leaving the operating room, an x-ray film is taken and the child is weighed. Future estimates of lung expansion and weight will be checked against these two measurements.

Nursing Diagnoses and Related Interventions: Postoperative Phase

> ***Nursing Diagnosis:*** High risk for altered cardiopulmonary tissue perfusion related to cardiac surgery
>
> ***Goal:*** Child will maintain adequate tissue perfusion during the recovery period.
>
> ***Outcome Criteria:*** Vital signs are within normal limits; central venous pressure (CVP) or pulmonary artery wedge pressure are normal.

Taking accurate vital signs (as often as every 15 minutes) is a prime nursing responsibility in the immediate postoperative period. The child will have a continuous ECG recorded or cardiac monitor leads attached to

record heart rate and rhythm. Assisted ventilation with intubation is usually necessary. Blood pressure will probably be electronically monitored by means of an intraarterial catheter as well as by normal blood pressure recording (Figure 41-10). Hemodynamic monitoring by right and left heart catheters reveals information on chamber pressures and oxygen saturation.

That a child is voiding adequately after surgery means that the kidneys are receiving adequate circulation. A Foley catheter is usually inserted at the time of surgery so that urine output can be carefully recorded postoperatively (it should be 1 mL/kg/h). Individual samples are tested for specific gravity and pH. A specific gravity below 1.010 implies that the kidneys are not concentrating urine well, perhaps because of surgical shock. The pH should remain slightly acid; extreme acidity may indicate that metabolic acidosis is occurring. Be certain to mark the amount of urine drainage present when children first return from surgery so that lack of urinary drainage (kidney failure) will not be missed or misinterpreted.

All IV fluid given to children after heart surgery must be given with careful thought and control as to amount and rate of infusion. A heart newly operated on cannot stand the assault of overload from IV fluid given too rapidly. It is better if such fluid is administered by means of a mechanical pump in order to prevent accidental overloading.

For assessment of cardiac and respiratory function, children will have blood gases (Po_2 and Pco_2) determined along with hemoglobin, hematocrit, clotting time, and electrolytes (particularly sodium and potassium) during the postoperative course. Po_2 may be assessed by means of an arterial catheter or continuous transcutaneous tension or pulse oximetry. Sensors may be placed on the chest, abdomen, finger, or toe. A drug such as dopamine may be administered to improve cardiac output. Isoproterenol helps increase heart rate.

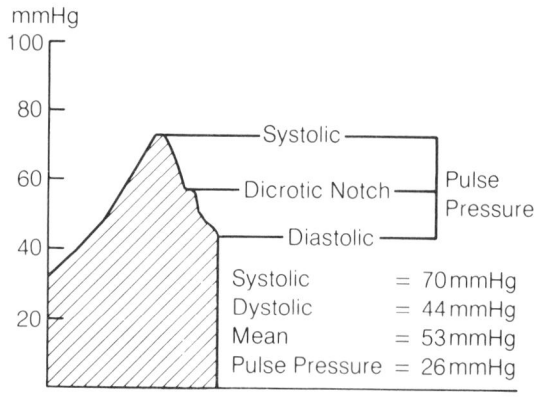

FIGURE 41-10
Systolic and diastolic points are indicated on an arterial pressure wave form. (From Nugent, J. [1983]. Intraarterial blood pressure monitoring in the neonate. Journal of Obstetric, Gynecologic, and Neonatal Nursing, 11, 281, with permission.)

Central Venous Pressure Monitoring. CVP may be recorded by inserting a catheter into a brachial vein and then into the left atrium (Figure 41-11). The exiting catheter is attached to a continuous infusion of IV fluid. A stopcock inserted in the tubing allows the fluid to be diverted from the IV fluid bottle into the tubing, catheter, or manometer where the pressure can be read. The manometer is taped to an IV pole beside the bed. With the child in a supine position, the zero reading on the manometer should be at the level of the right atrium (midaxillary line at the fourth intercostal space). CVP is an excellent guide to whether children's hearts are able to accommodate the blood arriving at them from the venous system. The pressure rises in congestive heart failure when a heart is not able to handle the blood arriving.

Directions for taking a CVP reading are as follows:

1. Turn the stopcock so that fluid from the IV bottle flows into the manometer until the fluid column measures about 25 cm H_2O; turn the stopcock to end the flow from the IV fluid to the manometer.
2. The fluid in the manometer will gradually fall as it infuses into the child until its pressure equals the child's CVP. Read the level at which it stops falling. The fluid level will fluctuate by 1 to 2 cm H_2O as the child breathes.
3. After a reading, reverse the stopcock and reopen the fluid flow between the IV fluid and the catheter. If this is not done, blood will clot at the tip of the catheter and may cause an embolus. Regulate the flow rate to that prescribed.

A normal CVP reading is 6 to 12 cm of fluid. If the reading is 0 to 6 cm, the child probably has hypovolemia; if the range is as high as 15 to 20 cm, he or she is in danger of cardiac failure. If you obtain a high reading, check to see that the tubing was not kinked, because this can cause false high readings. Be certain to include in your measurement of fluid that used to keep the CVP line open and that used to read the CVP; otherwise, total fluid input can be underestimated or fluid overload can occur.

Pulmonary Artery Pressure. In order to assess the pressure in the left side of the heart parallel to CVP measurement, a Swan-Ganz catheter is threaded through the venous circulation, through the right side of the heart, and into the pulmonary artery. The pressure, registered there as a waveform on a cardiac monitor, reflects both the resistance of the lungs to the passage of blood (pulmonary artery resistance) and the ability of the left side of the heart to handle the circulating fluid volume. Such catheters must be kept from clotting with frequent irrigation or with a constant infusion system. When withdrawing blood for sampling, it is important that no air be allowed to enter, since this would immediately flow into the left side of the heart and possibly to a cerebral artery as an embolus.

Combined Hemodynamic Monitoring. Many children have catheters inserted at the time of surgery into the right and left atria and the pulmonary artery. These exit through stab wounds in the anterior chest and are attached to a continuous IV infusion to keep them patent. Such catheters are used to monitor pressure and oxygen saturation in these locations. When such catheters are no

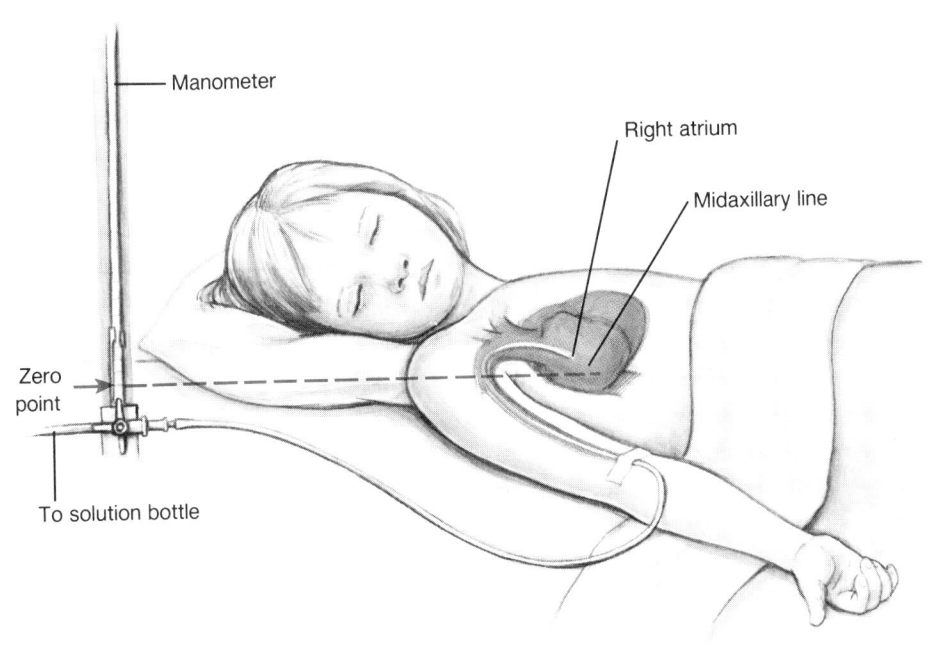

FIGURE 41-11

A CVP catheter may be inserted after cardiac surgery to monitor fluid volume. The zero point on the scale is at the level of the right atrium.

longer required, they are pulled gently through the skin incision. This is a dangerous point in the postoperative course, because bleeding into the pericardial sac (tamponade) from the heart incision area could occur. Close observation for signs of tachycardia, hypotension, and elevated intracardial pressures is critical.

Nursing Diagnosis: High risk for ineffective airway clearance related to unexpanded lung space and collection of lung excretions

Goal: Child will demonstrate adequate respiratory status during the recovery period.

Outcome Criteria: Child's respiratory rate will be normal for age group; no rales present; chest tube functions normally.

Measures to Prevent the Pooling of Secretions in the Lungs. As soon as the endotracheal tube is removed, encourage children to deep-breathe or use a spirometer at hourly intervals to prevent secretions from pooling in the respiratory system. Even though children practiced such procedures preoperatively, they have a great deal of difficulty carrying them out now because their chest is extremely painful when they cough or deep-breathe. It is helpful if a child's analgesia is given first; as soon as this takes effect (10 to 15 minutes), attempt to have the child deep-breathe. You generally have to demonstrate this again and sometimes deep-breathe with them. Be certain that parents understand that games such as blowing cotton balls or blowing up a balloon are not really "games" but important exercises in achieving lung expansion; otherwise, they may interpret these exercises as too tiring for their child and discourage them.

Most children and infants need suction to remove secretions. Postural drainage and percussion are prescribed to keep lung secretions mobile. Keep children placed in a semi-Fowler's position. Chest tubes drain better with children in this position and often there is less dyspnea as well, because abdominal contents do not press on the lungs (Hultgren, 1991).

Most children will have two chest tubes inserted. The upper tube will drain air, the lower one will drain fluid. These are connected to a water-seal drainage apparatus (a Pleur-Evac; Figure 41-12). If tubes should become clogged, air and fluid cannot drain from the chest and the lungs cannot expand. If the tube connections should become loose or the Pleur-Evac cracked or broken, air will enter the chest cavity through a tube and collapse the lungs (pneumothorax). To prevent fluid in the tube from re-entering the chest, the Pleur-Evac must never be raised above the level of the child's chest. Connections in the tubes should be sealed with extra adhesive tape and checked frequently to see that the connections remain airtight. It is important that Pleur-Evacs be marked "Do not empty" so that a person, not realizing

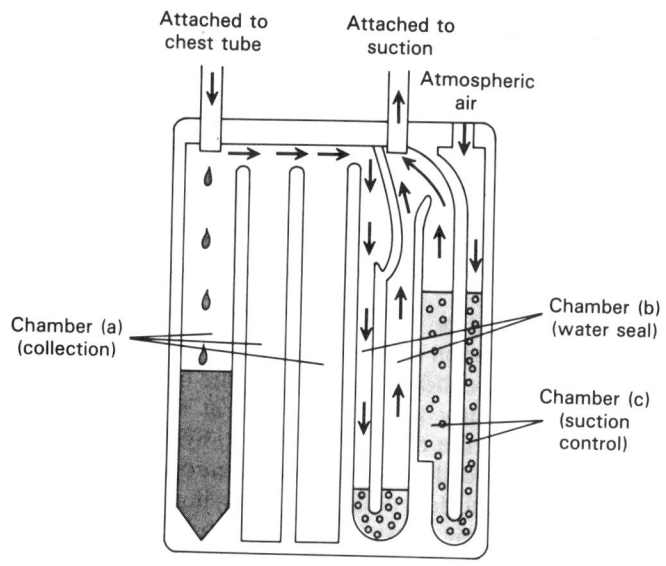

FIGURE 41-12

Pleur-Evac system for chest tube drainage. (From Earnest, V. [1993]. Clinical skills in nursing practice [2nd ed.]. Philadelphia: J.B. Lippincott Company, p. 760.)

the danger of this, does not attempt it and allow air to enter the tubes.

The purpose of chest tubes is to restore negative pressure to the pleural space so lungs can reexpand. Inspect tubes and collecting spaces closely. A Pleur-Evac consists of three chambers, one to collect drainage, one to furnish a water seal, and one that is attached to suction. The chest tube connects to the drainage compartment. Because of the water seal, atmospheric air cannot enter the chest tube and flow back to the pleural space. Note how much drainage is occurring and if the level of fluid fluctuates. On the third or fourth postoperative day, the fluctuation will cease, indicating that the lungs are fully expanded; then it is time for the tubes to be removed.

Clots can be removed from the tubes by "milking" them gently. If this is done hourly, it prevents clot formation. Be certain when you are milking chest tubes that you do not inadvertently pull on a tube and dislodge it. Place one hand on the tube to stabilize it, then milk with the other hand. Every time the child turns, make sure the chest tubes have not become caught under the child's body and become obstructed.

Record the amount of drainage from chest tubes hourly. It should not be more than 5 mL/kg/h. The water level in the collecting chamber should be marked in the operating room when the system is first established or immediately in the postoperative room. If a piece of adhesive tape is placed on the side of the Pleur-Evac, the level of fluid can be marked every hour and the hourly amount of drainage can be determined. The color and the presence of any clots in the drainage should be noted as well. Drainage fluid is blood-tinged but should not contain dark blood; if it does, this may be an indication that the heart incision is hemorrhaging.

Occasionally, despite being cautioned not to, children turn so suddenly following surgery that a chest tube is accidentally pulled out. This is an emergency situation, which may lead to pneumothorax with sudden dyspnea, tachycardia, cyanosis, and perhaps sharp chest pain. If a tube is only loosened or air is leaking through a connection, the symptoms may be less dramatic: restlessness and apprehension accompany gradually increasing dyspnea. If the air entering the chest is the result of air leaking into the tubing, the tube should be clamped close to the child's chest with a large clamp, such as a Rochester, to prevent further leakage. If the tube has been pulled out, the puncture wound to the chest must be closed immediately. This is best done by covering it with petrolatum gauze, which is impervious to air. If such gauze is not immediately available, placing your hand over the puncture wound and holding it snugly in place until help arrives is the best emergency procedure. Children may need emergency oxygen administration to counteract the decreased amount of air exchange space they have as a result of partial lung collapse.

When the chest tubes appear ready to be removed, a chest x-ray film will be made to confirm full lung expansion. The tubes are then removed by the physician while an impervious dressing is simultaneously applied to the puncture wound. Provide emotional support during chest-tube removal. Children know these tubes are important for their well-being; aside from worrying about the momentary pain of removal, they think something bad will happen once the tubes are removed. Don't change dressings over former chest-tube sites (lifting them to change them would allow air to enter). Leave them snugly in place until the incision has healed, so that air does not enter the chest cavity.

Nursing Diagnosis: High risk for infection related to surgical incision and tube sites

Goal: Child will not develop postoperative infection.

Outcome Criteria: Child's temperature will remain at or below 38.0°C axillary; incision site will not be erythematous or with foul drainage.

Some children begin a prophylactic course of a broad-spectrum antibiotic prior to surgery; this is continued postoperatively. Children may have the skin over the surgical incision area scrubbed with a povidone-iodine (Betadine) solution before surgery to ensure as clean a surgical field as possible. Most children and parents are startled to learn that cardiac surgery is generally performed through the sternal bone, not over the left side of the chest, and may question the area being prepared for the incision.

Postoperatively, assess the dressing of the surgical incision and the points of insertion of the chest tubes (thoracotomy tubes) frequently for drainage and erythema.

Nursing Diagnosis: High risk for hypothermia related to cooling during surgery

Goal: Child's temperature will return to normal by 4 hours after surgery.

Outcome Criteria: Child's temperature is above 36.0°C axillary.

If hypothermia was induced for surgery, the child's temperature will be low postoperatively and the child may need to be warmed by a hyperthermia blanket, covered by warm blankets, or administered radiant heat. Assess temperature accurately, because the child's temperature may elevate after recovery from hypothermia because of an inflammatory response; body temperature will gradually return to normal in a few days.

Nursing Diagnosis: High risk for fluid volume excess or deficit related to fluid shift accompanying cardiac surgery

Goal: Child will not experience fluid volume excess or deficit during the recovery period.

Outcome Criteria: Child maintains weight; skin turgor is good; central venous pressure or pulmonary artery pressure are within normal limits.

Children tend to develop hypervolemia following cardiac surgery because of increased production of aldosterone by the adrenal glands and an increase in antidiuretic hormone secretion by the pituitary gland; both are the body's responses to the shock of such extreme surgery. Also, if a heart–lung machine was used, some fluid may have been shifted from the intravascular system to the interstitial system during surgery; after surgery, this fluid returns by osmosis to the vessels, causing hypervolemia. On the other hand, the child may bleed excessively because of the heparin used during surgery and develop hypovolemia.

Intravenous fluid administration must be monitored carefully to prevent fluid overload. Oral fluid intake is withheld for at least the first 24 hours after surgery. After bowel sounds are present, oral fluids are introduced gradually.

Nursing Diagnosis: Parental anxiety related to lack of knowledge of postoperative routine and exercises

Goal: Family members demonstrate adaptive coping behaviors during the recovery period.

Outcome Criteria: Family members accurately state plans for child's postoperative recovery; relate less anxiety after teaching and support.

It is always surprising how quickly children recover from heart surgery. Passive range-of-motion exercises are prescribed the day after surgery. By the time the chest tubes are removed, children are up to sitting in a chair beside the bed. Encourage parents to do whatever they want to for their child's care during the postoperative period. It is difficult for them to accept the fact that the surgery is over and their child is now a well child (or will be at the end of the recovery period).

Offering the child sips of water or helping him or her take a bath (under supervision) helps parents to see that their child is returning to normal activities and doing well. It is important that children receive adequate rest in the first postoperative days. This requires you to monitor and regulate visits by staff and outside visitors to make sure the child is undisturbed for sustained rest periods. Parents might wish to read to children or play records for them as a way of providing quiet rest periods. Caution parents not to pick up an infant under the arms, as this pulls on the chest incision. Lift an infant by placing hands under the shoulders and buttocks instead.

Once children have passed the immediate postoperative period, they will be moved from the ICU of the hospital to a routine patient unit. This is often a difficult move for both children and their parents, because they have developed confidence in the ICU staff and are reluctant to entrust themselves to new personnel (even if the patient unit is the one to which the child was initially admitted before surgery). If the regular nursing staff has continued to visit the child daily in the ICU, the family will feel more comfortable making this transition back to the original patient unit. Parents frequently worry that no one will be watching their child closely on the regular patient unit. It is generally helpful to place children returning from the ICU in a room near the nursing station. Place the bed in the room so it can be easily seen from the hallway. Although you are not providing the constant attendance that the children received in the ICU, you can demonstrate that you are very observant and aware of their needs. Just stopping to look in every time you pass the room reassures the family that you are always close by. Parents need an opportunity to voice their concern over the change in personnel and surroundings. Accepting this change prepares them for the day of discharge when they will be observing and caring for their child on their own.

At discharge, parents need clear explanations of what activities their child will and will not be able to engage in. They need an appointment for a checkup for the child and the telephone number they should call if they have any questions regarding the care of their child. The protectiveness they felt for the child before surgery does not diminish instantly, even though surgery has been accomplished. They may find themselves saying, "Don't run" for months after the child has been allowed full activity. They may appreciate being referred to a community health nurse so they have a listening ear for their concerns, which may include feeling they are not as important to their child as they were when the child was ill. Such parents need reassurance that looking after a well child is just as important as nurturing a sick one and ultimately just as rewarding.

Complications

A number of complications may occur with cardiac surgery because of the use of pulmonary bypass and the extent of the surgery. The first of these is hemorrhage, because heparin is used to prevent blood coagulation during the pulmonary bypass. Although protamine (the antidote for heparin) is administered immediately postoperatively, some heparin is still present in the child's system. Hemorrhage may occur, especially in children with cyanotic heart disease, because of the prolonged coagulation time that is inherent with these defects. This is why the careful taking and recording of vital signs and observation of thoracotomy tube drainage are such important postoperative procedures.

Shock, which is manifested by hypotension, oliguria, acidosis, and cyanosis, may also occur. It may result from hypovolemia, cardiac tamponade (bleeding into the heart muscle or pericardium causing heart constriction), or from the effect of prolonged extracorporeal perfusion. It is treated according to individual needs, including artificial ventilation if that is necessary, until the child can begin breathing on his or her own again. Heart block or arrhythmias may occur as the result of edema or trauma compromising the effectiveness of the bundle of His. An artificial pacemaker may be needed to correct these problems.

Congestive heart failure may persist for a week or more after surgery if it was present before surgery. If it occurs as a new entity, it suggests that the surgery has caused a stricture to circulation at some point. Measures for treating postoperative congestive heart failure are those initiated in children who have this syndrome from any cause.

After the child returns home, a **postcardiac surgery syndrome** may develop at the end of the first postoperative week. This is a febrile illness with pericarditis and pleurisy that appears to be a response to the surgical procedure. The child needs salicylate therapy and bed rest; the course is generally benign. These symptoms may recur months after surgery.

Postperfusion syndrome may occur 3 to 12 weeks after surgery. The child develops a fever, splenomegaly, general malaise, and a maculopapular rash. Hepatomegaly may be present. The white blood count reveals a leukocytosis, in which lymphocytes are the predominant type of cell. Such a reaction is usually caused by a cytomegalovirus infection contracted from donor blood used in the heart–lung machine. The illness runs a short course with no permanent effect.

The Child With an Artificial Valve Replacement

A number of congenital heart anomalies such as aortic stenosis as well as diseases such as rheumatic fever or Kawasaki syndrome can require artificial heart valve replacement in children. This procedure is technically more complicated in children than adults because of the child's small heart size. As children have a longer life expectancy than adults, valve durability is a prime consideration. The advantage of long-term anticoagulation therapy must be weighed against the problem of bleeding from normal childhood accidents.

Artificial valves can be porcine (pig) or bovine (cow), prosthetic (synthetic material), or homograft (human donor). The majority of valves implanted today are made of synthetic materials because these appear to give the best long-term placement. Following placement of an artificial valve, the child must be placed on either anticoagulation or antiplatelet therapy to prevent thromboembolisms from forming at the valve implantation site. The drug prescribed most commonly for anticoagulation therapy is sodium warfarin. The dosage for this must be periodically monitored by blood analysis, which requires that children maintain follow-up visits. Antiplatelet therapy is most often aspirin and dipyridamole. Aspirin decreases platelet aggregation; dipyridamole decreases platelet adhesiveness.

In addition, children are placed on prophylactic antibiotic therapy against endocarditis. If bacteria are introduced into the child, they tend to cluster and colonize in the eddying blood at the valve site. Additional therapy is needed if the child is scheduled for dental or any other invasive procedure.

Adolescent girls need counseling about avoiding unplanned pregnancies, because the artificial valve may not be able to accommodate the increased blood volume that occurs with pregnancy. In addition, because sodium warfarin is teratogenic, any girl contemplating pregnancy needs to be changed to a heparin regime prior to conception. It is not recommended that girls with artificial valves in place use an estrogen-based birth control pill, because this can increase blood coagulation. They are also advised not to use an intrauterine device, which has been shown to cause an increased rate of pelvic inflammatory disease (Tong, 1992).

Hemolytic anemia is a complication of artificial valve replacement. This reaction is thought to be the result of the extreme turbulence of blood through the prosthetic valve, resulting in breakage of red blood cells. Blood replacement may be necessary if the hemolytic process persists.

The Child Undergoing Cardiac Transplant

Children who have a hypoplastic left ventricle or extensive cardiomyopathy from any cause are candidates for heart transplant (Boucek et al., 1993).

Transplant hearts are chilled immediately after removal from the donors. They can be maintained this way for 2 to 3 hours before being transplanted by pulmonary bypass technique. The aorta of the recipient is cross-clamped and his or her original heart removed except for the upper portion of the right atrium, which contains the SA node. Once the new heart has been transplanted, intrathoracic hemodynamic monitoring lines (right and left atria and pulmonary artery) as well as ventricle pacing wires are also implanted before closure.

The transplanted heart is able to respond normally except for autonomic nervous system control. This means it varies its rate in response to the amount of blood arriving rather than by nervous system control. An ECG will show two P waves (one from the residual original heart and one from the donor heart) because both sinoatrial nodes are intact.

Postoperative care is similar to that of any cardiac surgery patient. The child has the same potential problems: altered cardiac output, impaired gas exchange, high risk for infection, altered nutrition, and family coping. Children are prone to arrhythmias because of the possibility of injury to the SA node during transport or transplant. Cyclosporine A, prednisone, and azathioprine are drugs commonly used for immunosuppression (Lyons, 1993).

Rejection of the transplant is the number one cause of death in cardiac transplant patients. This can occur as hyperacute, acute, or chronic forms. *Hyperacute rejection* occurs immediately and is manifested by coronary thrombosis. *Acute rejection* occurs in about 7 days and is manifested by low-grade fever, tachycardia, and ECG changes. Cardiac catheterization is performed a week after transplant to biopsy the heart muscle for signs of acute rejection (tissue necrosis will have started to occur). Long-term or *chronic rejection* may begin at about a year's time. At any point that rejection is beginning, monoclonal antibodies may be infused to help stop the process.

Once past the rejection period, most children adjust well to cardiac transplant. They are able to participate in normal growth and development activities after the procedure. They return to the transplant center once yearly for a repeat cardiac catheterization and evaluation of their progress.

The Child With a Pacemaker

A child whose heart has ineffective SA node function or has difficulty in transmitting impulses from the SA node to the ventricles may have an artificial pacemaker inserted. Pacemakers control the heartbeat by stimulating the ventricles electronically (Figure 41-13). A pacing system consists of two components: a pulse generator containing the battery and programmed instructions, and the leads that connect to the heart. Most leads placed in children are an epicardial type and are attached to the epicardium by suture. This requires a median sternotomy incision to be made under general anesthesia. The generator will be placed in the subxyphoid or mid- or lower abdomen (Daberkow, 1992).

The types of pacemakers and functions are denoted by either a 3- or 5-letter code. With the 3-letter system, the first letter identifies the chamber paced, the second the chamber sensed, and the third the pacemaker's response to the intrinsic activity of the heart. For example, a pacemaker that is set to pace the *v*entricle, sense the *v*entricle, and be *i*nhibited (does not respond as long as the heart initiates a normal beat) is a VVI pacemaker. If a fourth letter is used, it denotes whether rate modulation is possible; a fifth letter denotes whether antitachyarrhythmia function such as the ability to produce a shock to defibrillate is possible.

Whether children have heart defects that will need pacing can be detected during intrauterine life by fetal monitoring. In these children, pacemakers can be implanted as soon as they are born.

Parents of the child with a pacemaker must be taught how to take the child's pulse accurately. They will need to do this daily at home and report any alterations in the pulse rate to their physician. They also are asked to telephone the health care center periodically and transmit a recording of their child's heart action to the center by way of a special telephone attachment.

Some parents stay awake at night worrying that their child's pacemaker batteries will suddenly stop operating; because of this, they may also be afraid to take vacations. Pacemakers usually contain lithium batteries, which have greater battery life than regular batteries. How long any individual pacemaker battery lasts is dependent on the percent of time pacing is needed (continuous or intermittent), battery energy output in amplitude (the amount of battery voltage needed to create each pacing impulse), and the pulse width (the length of time the impulse is being delivered). With an intermittent pattern, low amplitude, and narrow pulse width, a battery can last up to 15 years. Parents can be reassured that pacemaker batteries lose power slowly, not abruptly. They will have ample time to recognize weakening batteries through such signs in their child as dizziness, fatigue, fainting, or slow pulse rate and arrange to have the pacemaker replaced before the child's heart would fail.

Occasionally, pacemaker leads in the right ventricle of infants may lie in such close proximity to the diaphragm that they stimulate the diaphragm to contract with each ventricular contraction. This causes constant hiccupping. Another problem is that if prolonged hiccupping occurs, the infant should be seen by the physician. The leads may need a position adjustment. Another problem is that if the generator is not implanted deeply, it can trigger airport security systems.

Help parents learn to evaluate safe toys for children with pacemakers. Magnets should be avoided. Toys that emit an electrical current may interfere with a pacemaker's operation; parents should ask about this possibility before purchasing them. Most microwave ovens are safe to use with pacemakers in place. In the hospital, question the use of magnetic resonance imaging or electrocautery with these children.

Congenital Heart Disease

Five to ten percent of term newborns are born with a congenital cardiovascular abnormality; this rate is even higher in preterm infants. These defects affect equal numbers of male and female infants, but specific defects show a tendency toward sex differences. Patent ductus arteriosus and atrial septal defect, for example, are found more commonly in females. Conditions such as valvular aortic stenosis, coarctation of the aorta, tetralogy of Fallot, and transposition of the great vessels occur more often in males.

The usual cause of congenital heart disease is failure of a heart structure to progress beyond an early stage of embryonic development. Maternal rubella is associated with defects such as patent ductus arteriosus, pulmonary

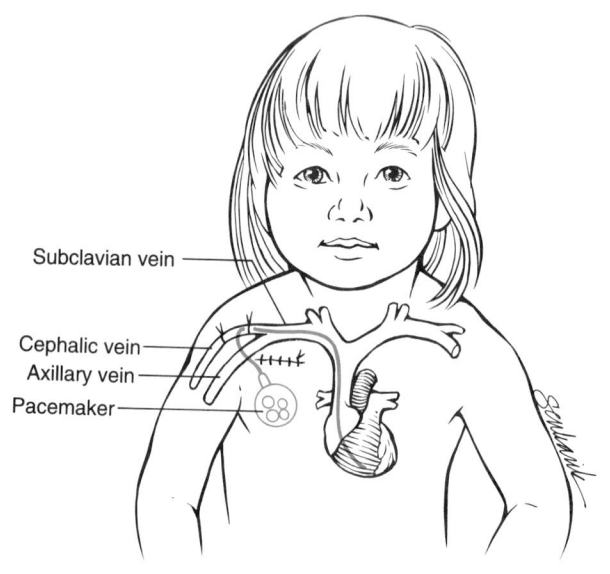

FIGURE 41-13
Children with abnormal conduction activity need pacemakers to regulate heart action. A conduction lead is shown threaded into the right ventricle, and the pacemaker is permanently implanted under the skin.

Subclavian vein

Cephalic vein
Axillary vein
Pacemaker

or aortic stenosis, atrial septal defects, ventricular septal defects, or pulmonary stenosis. Atrial septal and ventricular septal defects tend to be familial.

Acyanotic Heart Defects With Increased Pulmonary blood Flow

Acyanotic heart defects are heart or circulatory anomalies that involve either a stricture to the flow of blood or a shunt that moves blood from the arterial to the venous system (oxygenated to unoxygenated blood, or **left-to-right shunts**). These disorders cause the heart to function as an ineffective pump and make children prone to congestive heart failure. Previous to and following some repairs, depending on the extent of the repair, prophylactic administration of antibiotics to prevent infectious endocarditis must be conscientiously carried out.

Ventricular Septal Defect

Ventricular septal defects are the most common of all congenital cardiac defects. They account for about 25% of all congenital heart disease or about 2 in every 1000 live births. With this defect, an opening is present in the septum between the two ventricles. Because pressure in the left ventricle is greater than that in the right ventricle, blood will shunt from left to right across the septum. This impairs the effort of the heart, because blood that should go into the aorta and out to the body is shunted back into the pulmonary circulation. Right ventricular hypertrophy occurs from the shunted blood (Figure 41-14).

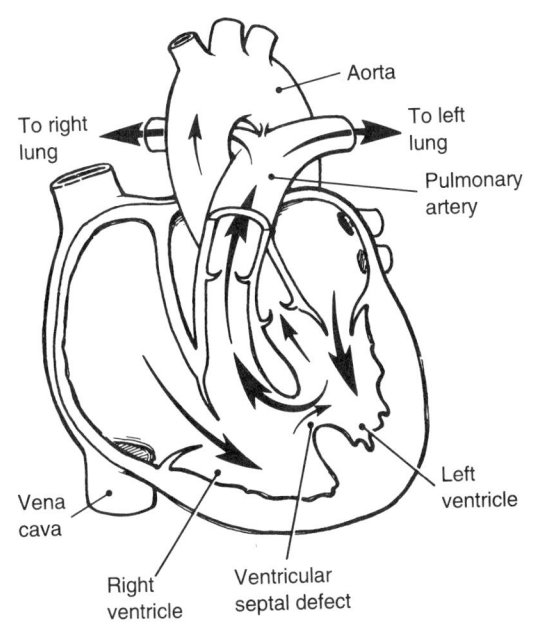

FIGURE 41-14
A ventricular septal defect.

Assessment. A ventricular septal defect may not be evident at birth. With incomplete opening of the alveoli, there is still high pulmonary artery resistance, causing little blood to be shunted through the defect. At about 4 to 8 weeks of age, a loud, harsh systolic murmur becomes evident along the left sternal border at the third or fourth interspace. This typical murmur is generally widely transmitted; a thrill may be palpable. The diagnosis of ventricular septal defect is based on examination by x-ray film, magnetic resonance imaging, or ultrasound, which will reveal right ventricular hypertrophy and possibly pulmonary artery dilatation from the increased blood flow. On cardiac catheterization, the oxygen saturation level of the right ventricle is higher than normal, because oxygenated blood is entering the ventricle through the defect. If the catheter is passed into the pulmonary artery and the pressure is measured there, it is generally increased above normal because of the increased flow in the vessel. On ECG, the right ventricular hypertrophy will be evident also.

Therapeutic Management. About 60% of small ventricular septal defects close spontaneously; the remainder require open heart surgery. In surgery, after cardiopulmonary bypass, the edges of the opening are approximated and sutured. If the defect is large, a Silastic patch is sutured into place to occlude the space. With time, septal tissue will grow across the gap and completely knit the patch in place.

Surgery requires use of extracorporeal circulation and a quiet heart. An important postoperative complication to assess is dysrhythmia, since edema in the septum may interfere with conduction (Moynihan & King, 1989). If there are no complications, the prognosis is good. Without surgery, infectious endocarditis and cardiac failure are risks.

If symptoms of ventricular septal defect develop in the first few months of life, pulmonary artery banding may be attempted to try to increase the resistance to blood flow. This will force a buildup of right ventricular pressure and prevent excess shunting. In most infants, the defect can be permanently corrected surgically during the first year of life (Gumbiner, 1994).

Atrial Septal Defect

An atrial septal defect is an abnormal communication between the two atria. It occurs more frequently in girls than boys. Blood flow is from left to right (oxygenated to unoxygenated) because of the stronger contraction of the left side of the heart. This increases the volume in the right side of the heart and generally results in ventricular hypertrophy (Figure 41-15).

Assessment. A harsh systolic murmur is heard over the second or third interspace (the pulmonic area) because of the extra amount of blood crossing the pul-

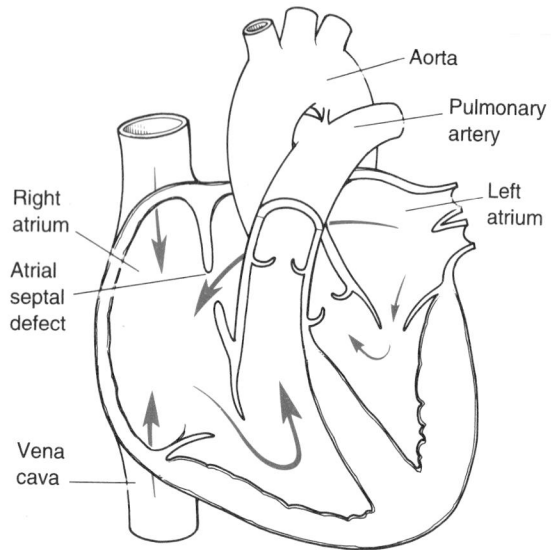

FIGURE 41-15
Atrial septal defect.

monic valve. As the volume of blood causes the pulmonic valve to close consistently later than the aortic valve, the second heart sound will be split (*fixed splitting*). Such a sound is almost always diagnostic of atrial septal defect.

Echocardiography will generally reveal the enlarged right side of the heart and the increased pulmonary circulation. Cardiac catheterization will reveal the separation in the atrial septum and the increased oxygen saturation in the right atrium.

Therapeutic Management. Management is by open heart surgery. After a cardiopulmonary bypass, the edges of the opening are approximated and sutured. If the defect is large, a Silastic patch may be sutured in place to occlude the space. Surgery requires use of extracorporeal circulation and a quiet heart. The child needs to be observed postoperatively for arrhythmias that may arise when edema of the atria interferes with the SA node function. With uncomplicated surgery, the prognosis is good. Without surgery, infectious endocarditis and eventual heart failure are risks. It is particularly important that atrial septal defects be repaired in girls, because they can cause emboli during pregnancy (Vick & Titus, 1994).

Endocardial Cushion Defects

An endocardial cushion defect (AV canal) occurs in the septum of the heart at the junction of the atria and the ventricles (Figure 41-16). It may involve the mitral and tricuspid valves as well. About one in nine children with trisomy 21 (Down syndrome) have this type of congenital cardiac defect (Marino et al., 1990). Cardiac catheterization and x-ray films will confirm the diagnosis. The management is surgical. Because the procedure may in-

volve a valve repair as well as a septal repair, mitral and tricuspid insufficiency may occur at a later date. Children need to be closely observed postoperatively for jaundice resulting from red blood cell destruction from the newly constructed valves; they may be placed on anticoagulation and antibiotic prophylactic therapy.

Patent Ductus Arteriosus

The ductus arteriosus is an accessory fetal vessel that connects the pulmonary artery to the aorta. If it fails to close at birth (closure should begin with the first breath but may not be completed until 3 months of age in some normal children) it will shunt blood from the aorta (oxygenated blood), because of increased aortic pressure, to the pulmonary artery (unoxygenated blood). The shunted blood returns to the left atrium of the heart, passes to the left ventricle, out to the aorta, and again to the pulmonary artery (Figure 41-17). This ineffective flow of blood puts a strain on the left ventricle and generally causes hypertrophy. There may be increased pressure in the pulmonary circulation from the extra shunted blood.

Assessment. On physical examination, the child usually has a wide pulse pressure (the difference between systolic and diastolic blood pressures). The diastolic pressure is low because of the shunt or runoff of blood, which reduces peripheral resistance. A typical continuous (systolic and diastolic) "machinery" murmur will be heard at the upper left sternal border or under the left clavicle in older children. In newborns, the murmur may not be quite so characteristic, perhaps a short grade II or III harsh systolic sound. The ECG is generally

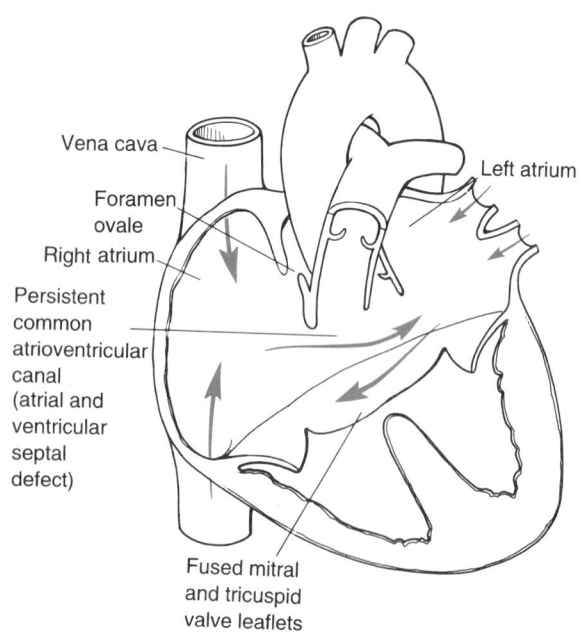

FIGURE 41-16
An endocardial cushion defect.

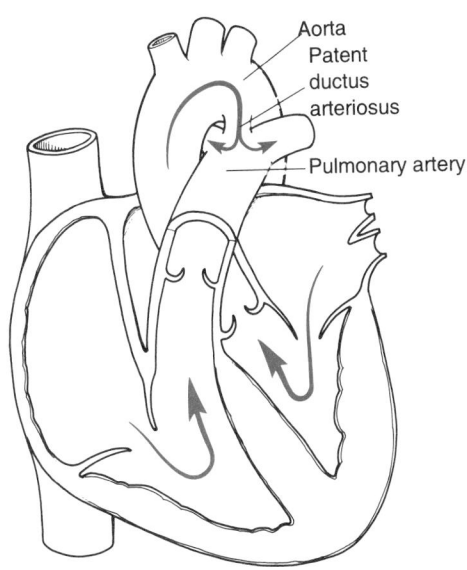

FIGURE 41-17
Patent ductus arteriosus.

normal, although it may demonstrate left ventricle en-largement if the shunt is large. A cardiac catheterization is generally not necessary for diagnosis but may be per-formed to rule out associated defects.

Therapeutic Management. One reason that the duc-tus arteriosus remains open in fetal life is stimulation by prostaglandins, particularly PGE$_1$, from the placenta and the low oxygen (Po$_2$) level of fetal blood. Following birth, when the PGE$_1$ level falls and oxygen level in-creases, the ductus arteriosus is stimulated to close. Medical management for the child may consist of the ad-ministration of oral or IV indomethacin, a prostaglandin inhibitor. This can be repeated as many as three times 12 to 24 hours apart. Side effects of indomethacin ther-apy are reduced glomerular filtration, impaired platelet aggregation, and diminished gastrointestinal and cere-bral blood flow.

If medical management fails to bring about closure of the ductus arteriosus, the defect can be ligated surgi-cally. Although the surgical procedure is a major opera-tion that involves opening the chest (thoracotomy) and manipulating the great vessels, it is not open-heart surgery and does not involve the use of extracorporeal circulation. If surgery is not done, the risks include con-gestive heart failure caused by the increased amount of blood pouring back into the pulmonary artery and infec-tious endocarditis developing from the recirculating blood and its potential stasis in the pulmonary artery.

In other countries, the ductus may be closed using a Rashkind umbrella technique during cardiac catheteriza-tion. A collapsed umbrella-like device is inserted into the femoral vein and advanced through the inferior vena cava, downward to the pulmonary artery, and, finally, to the ductus. Once it is in position, the "umbrella" is

opened and blocks the flow of blood through the vessel. This procedure can be done on a same-day surgery basis but is not yet approved in the United States (Mullins, 1994).

Acyanotic Heart Defects With Decreased Pulmonary Blood Flow

A number of congenital anomalies cause the blood flow to the pulmonary artery to be decreased. These are problematic defects in that they prohibit enough blood from reaching the lungs for adequate oxygenation.

Pulmonary Stenosis
Pulmonary stenosis is a stenosis, or narrowing, of the pulmonary valve or the pulmonary artery just distal to the valve (Figure 41-18). It accounts for 25% to 35% of congenital heart anomalies. Inability of the right ventri-cle to evacuate blood by way of the pulmonary artery with ease may lead to right ventricular hypertrophy.

Assessment. A typical systolic ejection murmur, grade IV or V crescendo-decrescendo in quality, will be heard, which is loudest at the upper left sternal border but may radiate to the suprasternal notch. A thrill may be present in the upper left sternal area or at the suprasternal notch. The second heart sound may be widely split because of the late closure of the pulmonary valve. The ECG will reveal right ventricular hypertrophy; x-ray studies may indicate this also. Cardiac catheteriza-tion will demonstrate the degree of the stenosis.

Therapeutic Management. The management of the defect depends on the severity of the stenosis and the

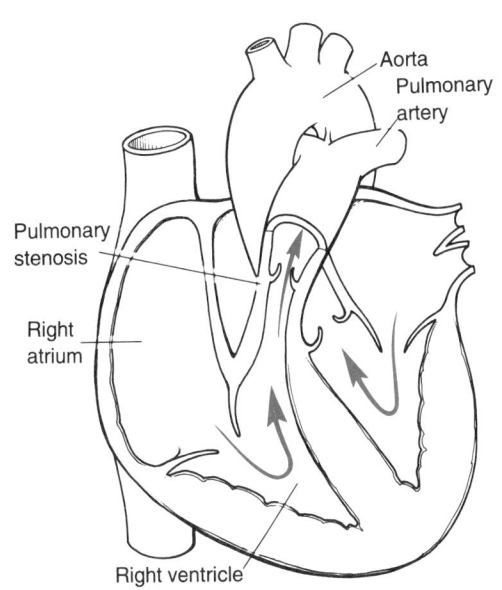

FIGURE 41-18
Pulmonary stenosis.

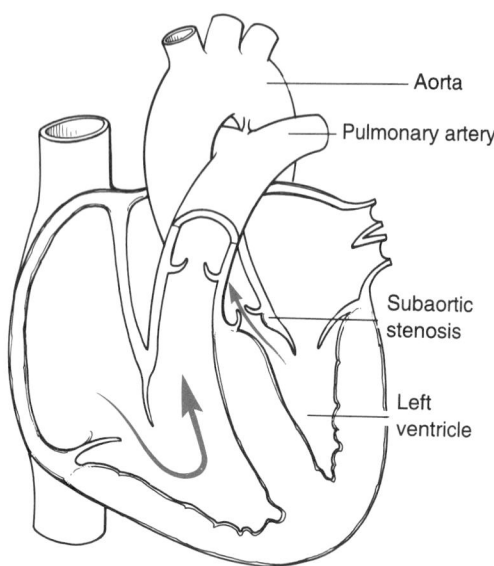

FIGURE 41-19
Subaortic stenosis.

child's age. When it is severe, the increased pressure in the right side of the heart may reopen the foramen ovale, and blood flowing from right to left chambers of the heart may produce mild cyanosis. A continuous infusion of PGE_1 helps to prevent closure of the ductus arteriosus, which will help supply more blood to the lungs to be oxygenated. **Balloon stenotomy** may be attempted. This consists of inserting a catheter with an uninflated balloon on the end of it by cardiac catheterization technique through the heart and into the stenosed valve. As the balloon is inflated, it breaks valve adhesions and may relieve the stenosis. Infants with a severe stenosis will have the defect repaired in early infancy; others, with lesser degrees of stenosis, can wait until they are 4 to 5 years of age when there is less surgical risk.

Aortic Stenosis

Stenosis, or stricture, of the aortic valve prevents blood from passing freely from the left ventricle of the heart into the aorta. It causes increased pressure in the heart as it attempts to force blood through the strictured valve and, therefore, leads to hypertrophy of the left ventricle (Figure 41-19). Aortic stenosis accounts for about 5% of congenital cardiac abnormalities.

Assessment. The child may be free of symptoms with aortic stenosis, but physical assessment will generally reveal a typical murmur, a rough systolic sound heard loudest in the second right interspace (the aortic space). The murmur transmits to the right shoulder, clavicle, and up the vessels of the neck; it may also transmit to the apex. A thrill may be present, particularly at the suprasternal notch. When the child is active, he or she may develop chest pain similar to angina. Sudden death

can occur when the amount of oxygen needed by the heart muscle on exertion far exceeds what is available because of the aortic stenosis.

The x-ray film and ECG will reveal left ventricular hypertrophy. Cardiac catheterization will reveal the degree of the stenosis.

Therapeutic Management. The management of aortic stenosis is balloon stenotomy or surgical repair, dividing the stenotic valve, or dilating an accompanying constrictive aortic ring (Landzberg & Lock, 1993). Such a repair may lead to aortic valve insufficiency in later life, at which time the operation may have to be repeated. Some children will need artificial valve replacement. If a prosthetic valve is used, children must continue anticoagulation or antiplatelet therapy and antibiotic prophylaxis against endocarditis for life.

Duplication of the Aortic Arch

Duplication of the aortic arch occurs because of the persistence of embryonic vascular precursors of the aorta and stem branches of the aorta (Figure 41-20). It produces symptoms of compression of the trachea or esophagus or both. Beginning in the first year of life, children with this defect have respiratory difficulty. They tend to extend their neck to obtain relief. They may have dysphagia (which is much more apparent with table food than with strained baby food). The diagnosis is made by the history and a barium esophageal x-ray study. The x-ray study will reveal constriction or devia-

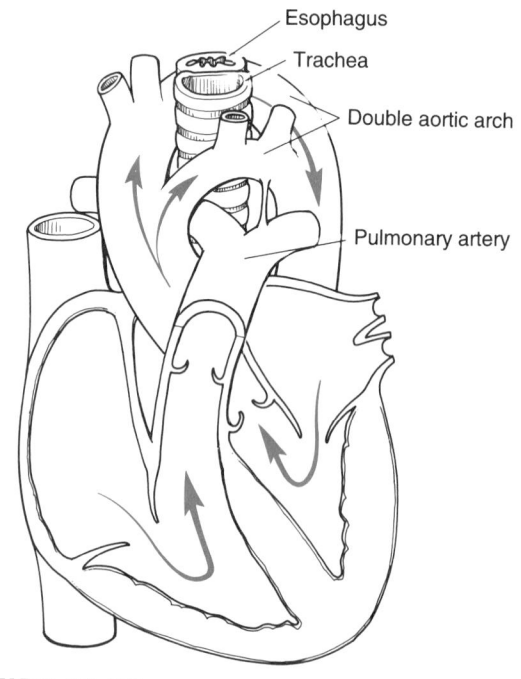

FIGURE 41-20
A duplicate aortic arch. This malformation puts pressure on the esophagus and trachea.

tion of the esophagus or the trachea or both. The management is surgical, involving the removal of the duplicated tissue. With uncomplicated surgery, the outcome and prognosis are excellent.

Coarctation of the Aorta

Coarctation of the aorta is a narrowing of the lumen of the aorta due to a constricting band (Figure 41-21). There are two locations in which this commonly occurs. The first is termed the *infantile,* or *preductal,* type; the constriction exists between the subclavian artery and the ductus arteriosus. The second is the *postductal* type; the constriction is distal to the ductus arteriosus.

Because it is difficult for blood to pass through the narrowed lumen of the aorta, pressure is high proximal to the coarctation and low distal to it. This results in increased blood pressure in the upper portions of the body because of increased pressure in the subclavian artery and decreased blood pressure in the lower extremities. High blood pressure of the upper body produces headache and vertigo. A child under 3 years of age cannot describe these sensations, but exceptional irritability may be a clue that these symptoms exist. Epistaxis (nosebleed) may occur. Cerebrovascular accident, an event not generally associated with pediatric conditions, can occur from this dangerously high blood pressure.

Assessment. If the coarctation is slight, absence of the femoral pulses may be the only symptom. Children who have an obstruction proximal to the left subclavian artery may have absent brachial pulses as well. Checking for femoral pulses should be included in any initial newborn assessment and admission inspection in the newborn nursery. As children with coarctation of the aorta grow older, they may experience leg pain on exertion; this is because of the diminished blood supply to the lower extremities. Because collateral circulation is necessary to allow blood to flow around the constriction, collateral arteries enlarge and may be seen on the ribs as obvious nodules as the child grows older.

The diagnosis of coarctation of the aorta may be made on history and physical assessment. On examination, the blood pressure in the arms will be at least 20 mm Hg higher than in the legs, a reversal of the normal pattern. In the normal child, lower extremity pressure is 10 to 40 mm Hg higher because of peripheral resistance. Radiographic examination of older children may reveal left-sided heart enlargement resulting from back pressure due to aortic constriction and also notching of the ribs from the enlarged collateral vessels. An ECG may also reveal left ventricular hypertrophy. Occasionally, a murmur may be present that is variable in position, intensity, and character. The most frequent type is a soft or moderately loud systolic murmur, especially prominent at the base of the heart and transmitted to the left interscapular area. The absence of a murmur, however, does not rule out coarctation of the aorta.

Therapeutic Management. Management of coarctation of the aorta is surgical. The narrowed portion of the aorta is removed, and the new ends of the aorta are anastomosed. A graft of transplanted subclavian artery may be necessary if the narrowing is so extensive that an anastomosis cannot be accomplished readily.

Planning a time for correction of the condition is important. It would be ideal if children could achieve the greater part of their adult height before surgical correction to prevent a strain on the incision line. At the same time, in terms of self-image, correction is best done before children begin to think of themselves as chronically ill or before they develop a complication, such as chronic hypertension. Girls must have the defect repaired before childbearing age or else the extra blood volume during pregnancy can cause congestive heart failure. Therefore, surgical repair is usually scheduled between 2 and 4 years of age. If the surgery is successful, without complications, the child can live a normal life. After surgery, abdominal vessels receive more blood than they did previously. This may result in abdominal pain or generalized abdominal discomfort, but it is a short-term problem.

Cyanotic Heart Defects With Increased Pulmonary Blood Flow

Cyanotic heart disease occurs when blood is shunted from the venous to the arterial system as a result of abnormal communication between the two (unoxygenated blood to oxygenated blood; **right-to-left shunt**).

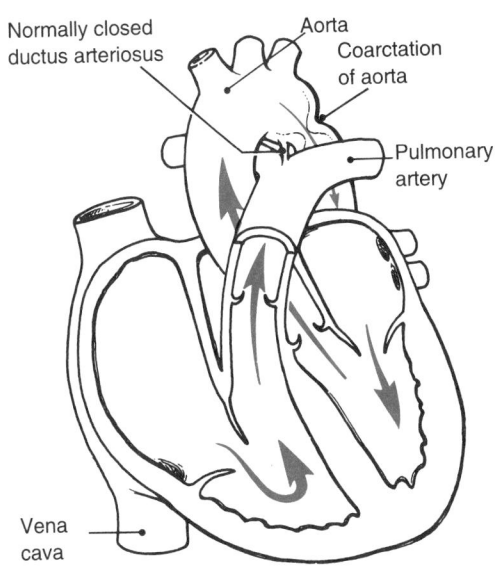

FIGURE 41-21
Coarctation of the aorta.

Until the heart is repaired, children with cyanotic heart disease are prone to congestive heart failure and anoxic episodes. Before and after some repairs, depending on the extent of the repair, prophylactic administration of antibiotics to prevent infectious endocarditis must continue. Those who have prosthetic valve replacements must continue with anticoagulant or antiplatelet therapy.

Transposition of the Great Arteries

In transposition of the great arteries, the aorta arises from the right ventricle instead of the left, and the pulmonary artery arises from the left ventricle instead of the right. Blood enters the heart from the vena cava to the right atrium, then to the right ventricle, and goes out into the aorta to the body completely unoxygenated; it enters the heart from the pulmonary veins, goes to the left atrium, left ventricle, and out the pulmonary artery to the lungs to be oxygenated, and returns to the left atrium, a second closed circulatory system (Figure 41-22). This severe defect is generally incompatible with life. In most instances, atrial and ventricular septal defects occur in connection with this transposition, making the entire heart one mixed circulatory system. It accounts for about 5% of congenital heart anomalies.

Assessment. Infants with this defect are usually cyanotic from birth. There may be no murmur, or there may be various murmurs, depending on the shunting of blood through atrial or ventricular defects or through the ductus arteriosus, which usually remains open.

An x-ray film will generally reveal an enlarged heart. An ECG may or may not reveal heart changes. Cardiac catheterization will reveal the low oxygen saturation resulting from the mixing of blood in the heart chambers.

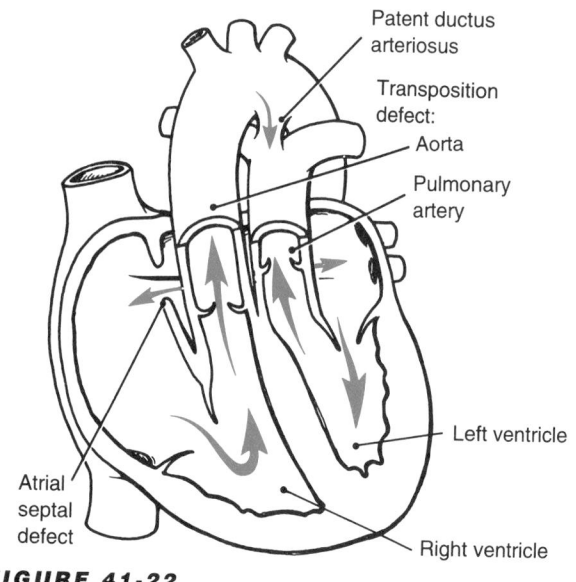

Patent ductus arteriosus

Transposition defect:
— Aorta

Pulmonary artery

Left ventricle

Atrial septal defect

Right ventricle

FIGURE 41-22
Transposition of the great vessels.

Therapeutic Management. If no septal defect exists or if the defect is too small to allow enough mixing of blood to sustain life, a pull-through operation may be done in the infant's first few days. At cardiac catheterization, a deflated balloon catheter is passed from the right atrium through the foramen ovale into the left atrium. The balloon is then inflated and the catheter is drawn back into the right atrium. This enlarges the opening of the foramen ovale and creates an artificial atrial septal defect. PGE$_1$ will be administered to keep the ductus arteriosus patent.

Complete correction of transposition of the great vessels is now available. A *Mustard procedure* involves restructuring of the heart to baffle blood entering the heart from the pulmonary veins into the right ventricle and thus into the aorta and the systemic circulation. Blood returning to the heart from the vena cava is baffled into the left ventricle and thus into the pulmonary artery and the lung circulation. In an *arterial switch procedure*, the major vessels are actually reversed in position. These procedures are done when the child cannot survive without further correction and only at major medical centers. The child will be transported to such a center for care as soon as the defect is diagnosed.

Total Anomalous Pulmonary Venous Return

In this disorder, the pulmonary veins return to the right atrium or the superior vena cava instead of to the left atrium as they normally would. For blood to reach the left side of the heart, it must be shunted across a patent foreman ovale or a patent ductus arteriosus (Figure 41-23). These infants are mildly cyanotic and tire easily. An absent spleen is often associated with this disorder.

Surgical therapy involves reimplanting the pulmonary veins into the left atrium. Until this can be carried out, the child will be maintained on a continuous IV infusion containing PGE$_1$ to help keep the ductus arteriosus open.

Truncus Arteriosus

In truncus arteriosus, one major artery or "trunk" arises from the left and right ventricles in place of a separate aorta and pulmonary artery (Figure 41-24). There is usually an accompanying ventricle septal defect. Repair involves restructuring of the common trunk to create separate vessels.

Hypoplastic Left Heart Syndrome

In hypoplastic left heart syndrome, the left ventricle of the heart is nonfunctional; there may be mitral or aortic valve atresia (Barber, 1994). The nonfunctioning left ventricle is unable to effectively pump blood into the systemic circulation; the right ventricle hypertrophies as it tries to maintain the entire heart action. Cyanosis becomes mild to moderate as unoxygenated blood is

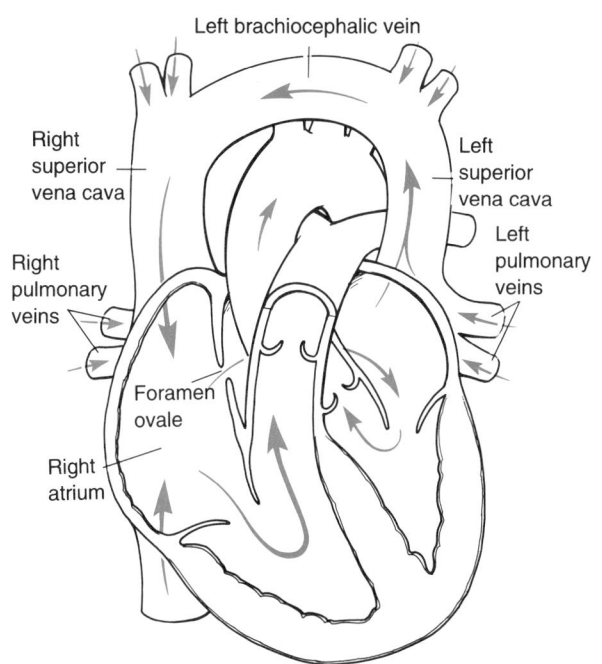

FIGURE 41-23
Total anomalous pulmonary venous return.

shunted across the foramen ovale. Prostaglandin therapy to maintain a patent ductus will be started. Attempts at surgery are of limited success with this syndrome, although a great deal of research is currently being done in this area and a Norwood procedure (restructuring of the heart) is possible. Children need to be screened for additional congenital anomalies, such as abnormal brain formation (Glauser et al., 1990). Heart transplant is a possible answer for prolonging the child's life, but the number of donor hearts available for newborns is limited. Without these measures, infants rarely live longer than 1 month.

Cyanotic Heart Defects With Decreased Pulmonary Blood Flow

Tricuspid Atresia

Tricuspid atresia is an extremely serious disorder because, as the name implies, the tricuspid valve is completely closed, allowing no blood to flow from the right atrium to the right ventricle. Instead, blood crosses through the patent foramen ovale into the left atrium, bypassing the lungs and the step of oxygenation. It reaches the lungs by being shunted back through a patent ductus arteriosus (Figure 41-25).

As long as these fetal shunts remain open, the child will obtain adequate oxygenation of blood. Prior to surgery, the child is maintained on an IV infusion of PGE$_1$. Surgery consists of the construction of a subclavian-to-pulmonary artery shunt, which deflects more blood to the lungs, or a Fontan procedure, which restructures the right side of the heart (Fontan et al., 1990).

Tetralogy of Fallot

Tetralogy of Fallot is the most common type of cyanotic congenital heart disease, representing about 10% of children with congenital cardiac disease. It is called a tetralogy because four anomalies are present: pulmonary artery stenosis, intraventricular septal defect, dextroposition (overriding) of the aorta, and hypertrophy of the right ventricle. Because of the pulmonary artery stenosis, pressure builds up in the right side of the heart; blood is

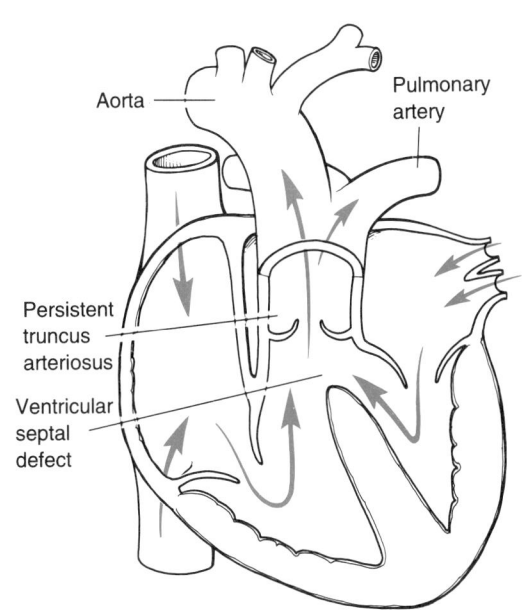

FIGURE 41-24
Truncus arteriosus.

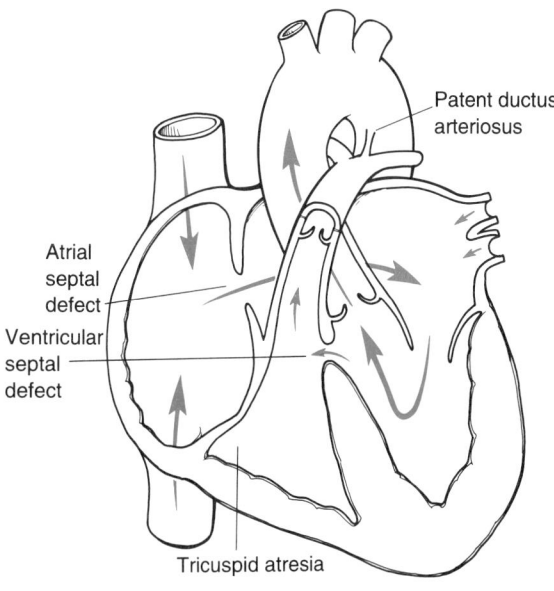

FIGURE 41-25
Tricuspid atresia.

then shunted from this increased pressure area into the left ventricle and the overriding aorta. The extra effort involved to force blood through the stenosed pulmonary artery causes the fourth deformity, hypertrophy of the right ventricle (Figure 41-26).

Assessment. Although this is an extremely serious form of heart disease, newborns may not exhibit a high degree of cyanosis immediately after birth. As they become more active, however, they will begin to appear cyanotic, their skin acquiring a bluish tint. A polycythemia (increase in the number of red blood cells) will occur as the body attempts to provide enough red blood cells to supply oxygen to all body parts. This is a potential danger to children because the increased concentration causes the blood to become too thick, and clots in blood vessels may occur, with consequent complications of thrombophlebitis, embolism, or cerebrovascular accident.

Children generally develop severe dyspnea and growth retardation. They tend to assume a squatting or a knee-chest position when resting, which normal children rarely do. Squatting gives physiologic relief to the overstressed heart. Unfortunately, this position leaves an insufficient amount of total circulating blood for the body to oxygenate and deliver to major body organs.

Children may develop syncope (fainting) and hypoxic episodes (sometimes called *tet spells*) caused by decreased blood supply to the brain; these usually follow prolonged crying or exertion. Mental retardation

may develop for the same reason. Clubbing of the fingers and toes (distended and flat tips) occurs because of an increase in the number of capillaries formed in the tips of extremities as the body attempts to send blood to all body parts.

Tetralogy of Fallot is diagnosed on the history and physical symptoms, x-ray film, and ECG. A loud, harsh, widely transmitted murmur or a soft, scratchy, localized systolic murmur in the left second, third, or fourth parasternal interspace may be present. It is a widely transmitted murmur, often heard as well in the left clavicular area. Posteriorly, it is heard in the interscapular space. The pulmonary second sound may be normal but is usually diminished in intensity or absent. Splitting of the second heart sound rarely occurs with tetralogy of Fallot (blood is forced through the shunt; the pulmonic valve does not, therefore, close later than the aortic valve).

An x-ray film shows the enlarged chamber of the right side of the heart, the decrease in the size of the pulmonary artery, and the reduced blood flow through the lungs. The heart as seen on x-ray film has been termed *boot-shaped*. Right ventricular hypertrophy is also revealed by ECG. Cardiac catheterization and angiography will permit a definitive evaluation of the extent of the defect, particularly the pulmonary stenosis and the ventricular septal defect (Link et al., 1993). Laboratory findings reveal polycythemia and reduced oxygen saturation of the blood.

Therapeutic Management. Management of tetralogy of Fallot is surgical, but because reconstructive measures are complicated, surgery may be postponed until 2 or 3 years of age if the child's condition warrants it.

If infants overexert themselves during the waiting period, they will lack enough oxygen for body cells and will develop anoxic episodes. If a baby begins to have a hypoxic episode, placing him or her in a knee–chest position and administering morphine sulfate is generally effective. If not, propranolol (Inderal, a beta blocker) may be prescribed to reduce heart spasm. A temporary or palliative surgical repair, called the *Blalock-Taussig procedure,* can create a shunt between the aorta and the pulmonary artery (a ductus arteriosus). This will allow blood to leave the aorta and enter the pulmonary artery, oxygenate in the lungs, and return to the left side of the heart, the aorta, and the body. Because the subclavian artery is used in a Blalock-Taussig procedure, the child will not have a palpable pulse in the right arm afterward (Tamisier et al., 1990).

A full repair that relieves the pulmonary stenosis, ventricular septal defect, and overriding aorta may be accomplished at a later date (a *Brock procedure*). In large medical centers, full repair is usually done as early in life as possible before the danger of hypoxic episodes occurs.

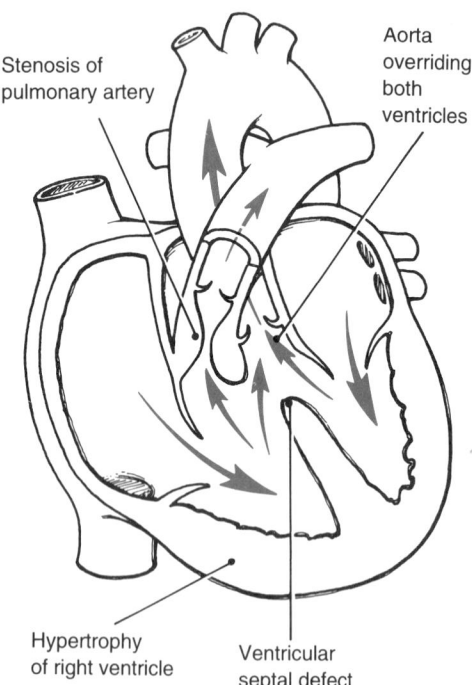

FIGURE 41-26
Tetralogy of Fallot.

Stenosis of pulmonary artery

Aorta overriding both ventricles

Hypertrophy of right ventricle

Ventricular septal defect

Acquired Heart Disease

The most commonly acquired heart disease in children is congestive heart failure, which usually occurs as a result of a congenital heart disorder or a disease such as rheumatic fever, Kawasaki disease, or infectious endocarditis.

Congestive Heart Failure

Congestive heart failure results when the myocardium of the heart cannot circulate and pump enough blood to supply oxygen and nutrients to body cells. Blood pools in the heart (excessive preload) or in the pulmonary or venous systems. This may be the result of a congenital defect that lessens the effectiveness of the heart's pumping action, or it may occur after cardiac surgery or rheumatic fever, which weakens the myocardium. Severe anemia, hypocalcemia, and myocarditis may contribute to the heart's inability to function effectively. Congestive heart failure occurs most often in children under 1 year of age (Gessner, 1993).

A heart can compensate in several ways to move blood forward. The muscle fibers can lengthen, causing the ventricles to enlarge and handle more blood with each heart stroke (ventricular hypertrophy). The rate of the strokes can also increase. As long as there is adequate cardiac output, the signs of heart failure are not immediately apparent. However, the heart's capacity for compensation is limited, particularly in infants. Eventually, the heart can dilate no further, and blood pools behind the section where dilation has stopped, unable to be pushed forward effectively.

As the renal blood flow decreases, glomerular filtration rate slows. Both fluid and sodium are then retained. When the body senses that its cells are not receiving adequate oxygen, aldosterone secretion by the adrenal glands further promotes sodium retention in an attempt to increase blood flow to the kidneys. Antidiuretic hormone secretion by the pituitary is also increased to help retain fluid. Sympathetic nervous system stimulation causes excessive sweating and pallor.

Assessment

One of the first signs of congestive heart failure is tachycardia as the heart attempts to beat faster to function more effectively; this is quickly followed by tachypnea. When children have primary right heart failure, there is increased venous pressure and hepatomegaly (enlarged liver) from back pressure in the portal circulation. Children may be irritable and restless from abdominal pain caused by the liver distention. Edema, usually a primary sign in adults, is often a late sign of congestive heart failure in children (Figure 41-27).

With left heart failure, blood accumulates in the pulmonary system. Dyspnea is usually the dominant symp-

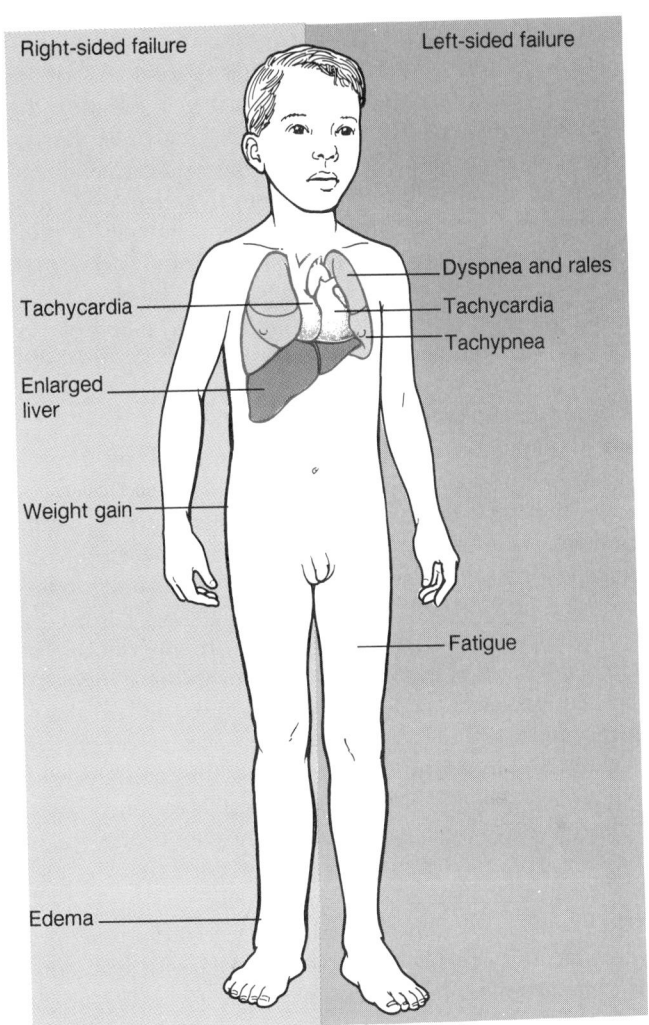

FIGURE 41-27
Signs of congestive heart failure.

tom, especially when children lie in a supine position (due to increased pulmonary congestion). Children may have rales and bloody sputum on coughing (from lung capillaries broken under increased pulmonary blood pressure). They may have cyanosis from interference with gas exchange in the alveoli, which begin to fill with fluid.

In an infant, congestive heart failure presents with very subtle signs. Infants are breathless from rapid respirations, tire easily, and have difficulty feeding because of the exhaustion and dyspnea present. If edema is present, it is generalized rather than dependent and often is first noticed as periorbital edema. An abrupt gain in weight may be the most obvious indication. On examination, infants will have an enlarged liver (a liver palpable more than 2 cm below the right costal margin).

Congestive heart failure may be confirmed by chest x-ray film or echocardiography, which reveals the enlarged size of the heart. Fluoroscopy may also reveal this enlargement. On physical examination, the apical heart beat will be displaced laterally and downward. As a rule of thumb, if the width of the heart is more than half the width of the chest (in a child over 1 year of age), the heart is enlarged. The presence of ventricular hypertrophy is confirmed by ECG. Physical assessment may reveal, in addition to the hepatomegaly, a gallop rhythm of the heart or the presence of an accentuated third heart sound. This sound occurs significantly later than that of a split second sound and is caused by the sudden distention of the ventricle during the rapid filling phase. Tachycardia and tachypnea are present.

Therapeutic Management

The therapeutic management of congestive heart disease consists of reducing the workload of the heart by measures such as evacuating the accumulated fluid (reduces preload), strengthening cardiac function (increases contractility) by administering an inotropic (heart-strengthening) drug, and reducing afterload by vasodilators.

Medications to reduce preload are prescribed for circulatory congestion resulting from either congenital or acquired heart disease. Common drugs used are furosemide, a diuretic which decreases reabsorption of sodium and therefore evacuates fluid, and nitroglycerin, which is a direct-acting venous vasodilator. Drugs used to increase contractility are dopamine, dobutamine, isoproterenol, and digoxin. Drugs that decrease afterload are arteriolar dilators such as hydralazine, a diuretic; nifedipine, a calcium channel blocker; nitroprusside, a direct-acting vasodilator; Captopril, an angiotensin-converting enzyme inhibitor; and prazosin, a blocking agent that also produces vasodilation (Baker & Alyn, 1992).

Nursing Diagnoses and Related Interventions

Be certain that goals established for care of the child with congestive heart disease are realistic. Your interventions will be aimed at supporting heart function and helping parents deal with this crisis until the child regains resources to help with strong heart action. The Nursing Care Plan: The Infant With Congestive Heart Failure and Cardiac Surgery summarizes care priorities for the infant with congestive heart failure.

Nursing Diagnosis: Altered cardiopulmonary tissue perfusion related to inadequate heart function

Goal: Child will maintain adequate tissue perfusion during the course of illness.

Outcome Criteria: Child's pulse, blood pressure, and rate of respirations are normal for age group; third heart sound is not audible.

Provide for Rest Periods. Rest is a major factor in helping the heart to handle blood adequately, since it reduces metabolic rate and the need for blood pumping.

Most children with congestive heart failure are more comfortable in a semi-Fowler's position than in a supine position, because the semi-Fowler's position lowers abdominal contents and allows for easier, more comfortable lung expansion. Babies are most comfortable in an infant seat, which supports them in a semi-Fowler's position (Figure 41-28). Sedation may be necessary to encourage bed rest in some children (e.g., morphine or barbiturates). Many children with congestive heart disease, however, automatically limit their activity, so sedation must be considered on an individual basis.

It is important that you organize nursing procedures to allow periods of sustained rest. At the same time, you cannot do too many procedures at once or you will exhaust the child. Use common sense and individualize your care for each child. Be certain that both you and the child's parents understand how much rest the child is to have each day. The term *complete bed rest* is often loosely used and has different connotations to different people. Does it mean that the child may eat by herself or must be fed? Does it mean bathroom privileges or not? Play time or not? Unless they are exceptionally exhausted, children need to be entertained or played with to remain on bed rest. Activities such as watching television, being read to, or listening to records can quiet a child and promote better rest than if they are expected to rest quietly without any diversion.

(*text continues on page 1254*)

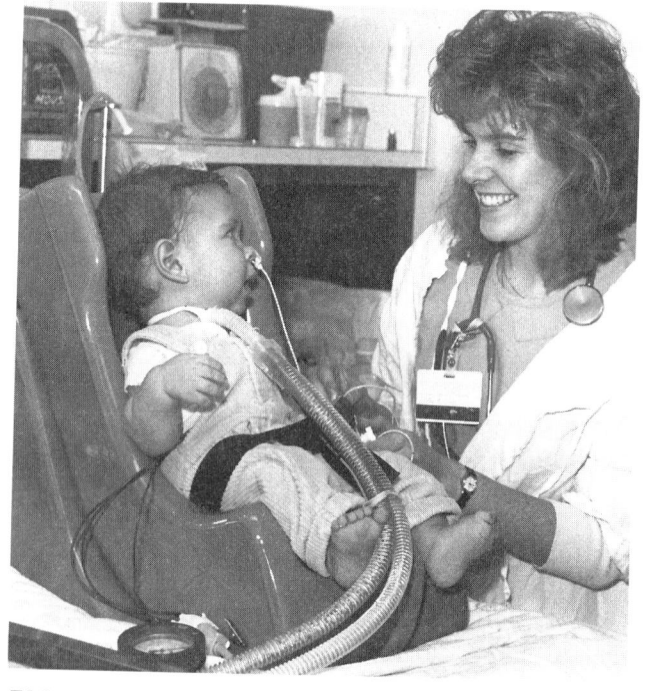

FIGURE 41-28

An infant seat provides a semi-Fowler's position for child with congestive heart disease. A tracheotomy tube with oxygen therapy and a nasogastric tube are in place. (Courtesy of the Department of Medical Photography, Children's Hospital, Buffalo, NY.)

Nursing Care Plan

The Infant With Congestive Heart Failure and Cardiac Surgery

> Brian is a 6-month-old boy who is admitted to your hospital unit for surgical repair of a ventricular septal defect. The following is a nursing care plan devised for him.

Assessment: Thin-appearing white male infant with periorbital edema admitted in mother's arms. Temperature: 97.6°F axillary; pulse: 150 bpm apically; respirations: 38 (crying). Pulse oximetry: Sao_2 = 40 mm Hg. Grade II systolic murmur heard on heart auscultation. Harsh rhonchi present on lung auscultation. Weight: 7.2 kg (20th percentile); height: 68 cm (50th percentile). Mother states infant is breast-fed; has just introduced rice cereal. Growth and development: Child turns both ways; says "ba-ba" (for brother); bears weight when held in standing position. Mother says he grows "exhausted" if playing games like "so big." "His chest heaves when he gets tired." Had cardiac catheterization at 4 months; admitted now in congestive heart failure for surgical repair. Both parents express concern over safety of surgery; father states, "If I thought he could make it through life without this, I'd never let it be done."

Nursing Diagnosis: Altered peripheral tissue perfusion, related to congestive heart failure

Defining Characteristic: Apical pulse = 150 bpm; child tires easily.

Goal: Child will experience adequate peripheral tissue perfusion during course of illness.

Outcome Criteria: Child's apical pulse is 100–120 bpm; Sao_2 is above 60 mm Hg.

Nursing Orders	Rationale
1. Obtain additional history to determine effect of illness on activities such as feeding and stimulation.	1. This information will help in planning Brian's care.
2. Elevate to semi-Fowler's position.	2. This position aids heart function.
3. Limit procedures to only those necessary; space them for periods of rest.	3. It is important that Brian's heart not be overly stressed with fatigue.
4. Anticipate child's needs so he does not cry.	4. Crying also contributes to fatigue, which should be avoided at all cost.
5. Caution caregivers not to play games that would tire child (so big, patty-cake, etc.).	5. Caregivers need specific reminders about the importance of not tiring the child unnecessarily.
6. Administer digoxin and diuretics as prescribed.	6. Digoxin slows the heart rate; diuretics aid fluid evacuation.
7. Monitor heart function by means of cardiac monitor q1h. Always use apical pulse rate for single assessments.	7. Using the same assessment site provides for consistency, leading to the most accurate results.
8. Assist with ECG assessment as necessary.	8. A familiar face may help to prevent Brian from crying when exposed to unfamiliar personnel.
9. Keep infant warm (be certain child is not exposed during procedures, physical examinations, blood drawing, etc.).	9. Maintaining an even temperature will help avoid an increase in Brian's metabolic rate, which could put further stress on his heart.

Nursing Diagnosis: Altered cardiopulmonary tissue perfusion, related to congestive heart failure

Defining Characteristic: Sao_2 is only 40 mm Hg.

Goal: Child will experience adequate cardiopulmonary tissue perfusion during course of illness.

Outcome Criteria: Child's respiration rate is between 20 and 25 breaths/min. Sao_2 is above 60 mm Hg.

(continued)

Nursing Orders	**Rationale**
1. Administer oxygen and humidity as prescribed (nasal prongs at 40%).	1. Oxygen and humidity are prescribed to improve heart function.
2. Remove constricting clothing from chest.	2. Removing tight clothing allows full lung expansion.
3. Perform pulmonary drainage as prescribed (percussion, clapping, and vibrating); divide therapy into lung segments to reduce the possibility of exhausting infant.	3. Postural therapy helps remove lung secretions without tiring infant.
4. If a cyanotic episode should occur, place child in knee-chest position.	4. Knee-chest is the best position to restore optimal cardiac function.

Nursing Diagnosis: Altered nutrition, less than body requirements, related to fatigue caused by congestive heart failure

Defining Characteristic: Weight of infant is at 20th percentile; height at 50th percentile.

Goal: Child will ingest adequate nutrition during course of illness.

Outcome Criteria: Child maintains present weight; follows percentile curve following surgery.

Nursing Orders	**Rationale**
1. Provide small, frequent feedings. If breast-feeding is exhausting, encourage mother to pump breast milk and feed with soft preemie nipple. Observe carefully that child's intake is 150 kcal/kg/24 h.	1. Infant may be exhausted from congestive heart failure.
2. Provide gavage feedings if infant cannot suck effectively.	2. Gavage feedings may be necessary if child is too exhausted to eat.
3. Assess chart for serum potassium levels.	3. Potassium may be depleted with diuretic administration.
4. Administer iron supplement as prescribed.	4. Iron supplementation will help prevent anemia because it increases heart action.
5. Assess intake and output.	5. Intake and output data are essential to a complete analysis of the infant's postsurgical status.
6. Weigh daily.	6. Weight data will help with fluid retention assessment.
7. Provide salt-poor formula if prescribed.	7. Salt-poor formula can aid fluid evacuation.

Nursing Diagnosis: Parental health-seeking behaviors related to need for cardiac surgery

Defining Characteristic: Parents voice they are not certain surgery is best therapy.

Goal: Parents will demonstrate increased knowledge of surgery within 24 hours.

Outcome Criteria: Parents state they understand importance of surgery and sign surgery consent.

(continued)

Nursing Orders	**Rationale**
1. Review anatomy of heart with parents.	1. Understanding heart anatomy may give parents better insight into their child's problem and the necessity of surgery.
2. Explain all procedures such as blood gases, chest preparation, etc.	2. Advance explanations of procedures will help prepare parents so that they can comfort their child.
3. Take parent to ICU and introduce to staff.	3. Knowing who will be caring for their child post operation and what the ICU looks like will give parents a better sense of trust and familiarity with the hospital setting.
4. Explain that postoperative care will include a ventilator, intravenous therapy, postural drainage, chest tubes, nasogastric tube.	4. These explanations will familiarize parents with expected procedures so there are no surprises later on.
5. Allow time for parents to express their concerns.	5. Expressing concerns and talking together with health care staff will help reduce stress about the procedure.
6. Advise surgeon of parent's concerns.	6. Keeps all health care team members informed and sensitive to parents' needs.

Following surgery for Brian, additional diagnoses were added:

Nursing Diagnosis: High risk for ineffective airway clearance related to anesthesia for surgery

Defining Characteristics: Potential for airway obstruction exists with any general anesthesia procedure.

Goal: Brian's airway will remain patent during recovery period.

Outcome Criteria: Respirations are within normal limits (20–22/min); no cyanosis is present.

Nursing Orders	**Rationale**
1. Keep oxygen hood with 40% oxygen in place for first 8 h per physician order.	1. Oxygen helps decrease heart function.
2. Assess for respiratory rate, dyspnea, tachypnea, retractions, and decreased breath sounds q15min × 4; then 1 h × 8.	2. Assessing vital signs allows for continuing data on Brian's progress.
3. Maintain chest tubes to underwater seal. Milk tubes q30min; mark drainage q1h; report drainage over 10 mL/h. Assess drainage for active bleeding. Keep 2 hemostats and extra endotracheal tube at head of bed for emergency use.	3. Underwater seal drainage is necessary to reinflate lungs. Strict adherence to procedure is essential.
4. Change infant's position q2h. Perform postural drainage for 10 min q4h.	4. Postural changes aid in evacuation of respiratory secretions.
5. Suction endotracheal tube q2h and PRN.	5. Suctioning keeps airway patent.

(continued)

Nursing Diagnosis: Hypothermia related to cardiac surgery

Defining Characteristic: Infant's temperature is decreased because of body cooling for surgery.

Goal: Child's temperature will return to normal by 24 h.

Outcome Criteria: Child's temperature is at 37.0°C axillary.

Nursing Orders	Rationale
1. Place infant on warming pad until temperature reaches 35.5°C.	1. Infant needs to be warmed to recover from hypothermia used for surgery.
2. Keep infant covered with 2 blankets (include head).	2. The head is an area that loses heat very quickly.
3. Assess temperature q1h axillary by 24 h postop.	3. It is important to be sure that the infant is warming as scheduled.

Nursing Diagnosis: High risk for fluid volume deficit related to cardiac surgery

Defining Characteristic: Blood loss occurs with cardiac surgery.

Goal: Fluid volume will remain adequate during recovery period.

Outcome Criteria: Pulse and respiration rates remain within normal limits; (100–120 bpm and 20–35 breaths/min); child does not lose more than 10% of presurgery weight.

Nursing Orders	Rationale
1. Maintain arterial line for blood gases and pressure readings. Assess q1h.	1. Arterial line allows for monitoring of blood pressure and blood gases continuously.
2. Assess dressing for drainage q30min; reinforce as necessary; report bright bleeding or excessive drainage.	2. Bleeding is a possible complication after cardiac surgery.
3. Foley catheter to gravity drainage. Measure q1h and test for specific gravity and hemoglobinuria. Notify physician if urinary output is under 1 mL/kg/h.	3. A falling urinary output suggests poor circulation in kidneys.
4. Weigh daily.	4. Increased weight can suggest fluid accumulation.
5. Maintain NPO for 24h; then begin sips of water if bowel sounds are present and child is extubated.	5. Bowel sounds are a sign that peristalsis has returned.
6. CBC with differential, electrolytes 1 h postoperatively.	6. Electrolyte concentration can suggest fluid volume.
7. Continue heart rate and pulse oximetry monitors; notify physician if under 100 or over 120 bpm or Sao_2 under 60 mm Hg.	7. Maintains continuous monitoring for continuing heart function.
8. Assess for liver size q1h to detect increased size.	8. An increase in liver size can be a sign of poor venous return.

(continued)

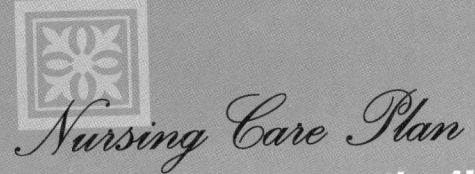

Nursing Diagnosis: Pain related to cardiac surgery

Defining Characteristic: Surgical incisions produce pain.

Goal: Child's pain will be at a tolerable level during recovery period.

Outcome Criteria: Child appears comfortable (sleeps and does not cry excessively).

Nursing Orders	***Rationale***
1. Administer morphine sulfate as prescribed. Assess if expiratory rate is under 16 breaths/min before administration.	1. Morphine is an analgesic. Slowed respiratory rate is a toxic reaction to this drug.
2. Move gently to avoid tension on suture line or thoracotomy tube insertion sites. Do not pick up child under arms.	2. Protect incision line from stress.
3. Encourage parents to hold and care for child.	3. A feeling of security for both child and parents can reduce overall stress.

Nursing Diagnosis: High risk for ineffective family coping, compromised, related to stress of major surgery in child

Defining Characteristic: Parents voice this undertaking has been very difficult to cope with.

Goal: Parents will demonstrate adequate coping behavior during recovery period.

Outcome Criteria: Parents state ways they are coping with current stress level.

Nursing Orders	***Rationale***
1. Keep parents informed of therapy so they understand reasons for procedures and care.	1. Understanding can be the beginning of acceptance.
2. Allow time for parents to voice concerns about their child's illness and begin to view child as a well child.	2. Changing concepts of wellness and illness requires time and thought.
3. Prepare parents for discharge (any restriction of activities, diet).	3. Discharge planning is important for follow-up care.
4. Teach prophylaxis for infectious endocarditis. Help parents to make a medicine reminder sheet to ensure compliance.	4. Endocarditis is a potential complication of cardiac surgery.
5. Be certain child has an appointment for a follow-up visit.	5. Maintains continuity of care.
6. Be certain parents have an emergency call number.	6. A name and emergency number provides a source of ready emergency help.
7. Contact support people such as hospital chaplain or social work personnel as indicated by parents.	7. Provide support network as necessary.

Provide Oxygen as Necessary. If children have dyspnea or cyanosis, they may need to be placed in an oxygen tent or receive oxygen by mask, cannula, or oxygen prongs. Assess the nostrils of the child with nasal prongs in place every 4 hours to make sure the prongs are not causing a pressure sore on the nostrils (this is a major problem in newborns). It is a strain for a child with congestive heart failure to be submitted to strange, frightening equipment. Talk about oxygen equipment before it is brought to the bedside. Help children to grow accustomed to a tent by placing your own head in the tent. Children generally experience such relief from dyspnea when they are receiving oxygen that their apprehension over its use is quickly dispelled.

Administer Drugs as Ordered to Strengthen Heart Action. Many children are discharged from the hospital on long-term administration of digoxin (Lanoxin). Digoxin is a cardiac glycoside made from digitalis, which acts directly on the heart to increase the contractility of the myocardium (and the force of contraction); it also slows the ventricular response in atrial dysrhythmias. Digoxin is a potent drug; parents must prepare doses with extreme accuracy. For safest administration, digoxin preparation should be prescribed with the dose designated in both milligrams and milliliters. When this is done, the milligram dose can be checked against the milliliter dose to be certain that the decimal point of the milligram dose has not been inadvertently misplaced, that is, 0.03 mg, not 0.3 mg. Digoxin may also be ordered in micrograms (μg)—for example, 0.02 mg equals 20 μg.

Digoxin preparations are administered parenterally first in a large dose (the digitalizing dose). Six to 8 hours later, one fourth of the initial dose is given; another one-fourth dose is given again in 6 to 8 hours. An ECG is generally obtained before the second or third dose of digoxin is administered. Maintenance doses are given once daily, or this could be divided into two doses given at 12-hour intervals. When effective, digoxin reduces heart rate, venous pressure, and liver size. Diuresis begins and relieves any edema present. Changes in ECG (a lengthening of the PR interval and a depression of the ST segment) confirm that digitalization has taken place. The "window" between effective digitalization and digitalis toxicity is very narrow. Symptoms of toxicity are anorexia, nausea and vomiting, dizziness, diarrhea, headache, and arrhythmia (Deglin et al., 1991). Before a dose of a digitalis preparation is administered, the child's apical pulse should be taken. As a rule, the pulse rate should be above 100 bpm in infants and above 70 bpm in older children. If the child vomits, do not repeat digitalis doses until a physician confirms that it is safe to do so; vomiting may be an early sign of digoxin toxicity.

If parents will be administering the digoxin after their child's discharge from the hospital, be certain that they understand the drug's importance and the need to space the daily doses carefully. Help them choose a specific time for administration to which they can adhere faithfully. Make out a reminder sheet to aid compliance. Instructions for home administration of digoxin are given in the Focus on Family Teaching display.

Diuretics such as furosemide (Lasix) may be administered to remove edema that is causing pulmonary failure (thus reducing postload), which is better than restricting salt and fluid in young children. Daily weights

---

FOCUS ON FAMILY TEACHING

Q. I'm going to be giving my 2-month-old son digoxin at home. What do I need to do to be sure I am giving such a potent medicine safely?

A. Administering digoxin safely calls for increased responsibility on your part. Follow these safety rules:

• Always assess an apical pulse before administration; do not administer the drug if your child's heart beat is below 100 bpm (or as specifically instructed as he grows older).

• Always use the same measuring device (spoon or dropper) each time so the dose given remains consistent.

• Do not change the amount or timing of the dose without specific instructions from your primary care provider.

• If a single dose should be omitted, give the next dose on time as prescribed.

• If more than one dose should be omitted, telephone your primary care provider for further instructions.

• Give digoxin 1 h before or 2 h after feedings to avoid a dose being lost with spitting up.

• If a dose is vomited within 15 min after administration, repeat the dose. If more than 15 min has passed since administration, do not repeat.

• Notify your primary care provider if the child vomits more than once each day, since vomiting is a sign of digoxin overdose (toxicity).

• Notify your primary care provider if administration of the medicine or timing of the dose is difficult for your lifestyle.

are a good way to gauge the diuretic's effectiveness. Be certain that children are weighed in the same clothing (or nude) every day so that any weight loss can be noted easily. Mercurial diuretics act by increasing the secretion of sodium. As large quantities of fluid are lost, potassium levels may be lowered as well. To monitor the potassium level, electrolyte levels must be assessed by blood drawing and analysis. Hydrochlorothiazide is a typical diuretic used for long-term therapy. With this, some children need to ingest a diet high in potassium and perhaps take oral potassium to maintain potassium levels. Liquid potassium is irritating to the gastrointestinal tract and must be given mixed with fruit juice. Be certain that children on diuretics are voiding. The infant's normal output is 1 to 2 mL/kg/h; normal output for the child is 30 mL/kg/h.

Nursing Diagnosis: High risk for altered nutrition, less than body requirements, related to fatigue

Goal: Child will ingest adequate nutritional intake during the course of illness.

Outcome Criteria: Child maintains percentile curve on growth chart; skin turgor is good.

Maintaining proper nutrition may be a problem for children with congestive heart failure. Eating six to eight small meals daily is often less tiring than eating three large meals. Smaller meals also prevent the child's stomach from pressing on the diaphragm and compromising an enlarged heart. If the infant is breast-fed, the mother may need to consult a lactation consultant. Sucking is hard work, and the infant may need to drink smaller amounts frequently to maintain an adequate fluid intake; using soft "preemie" nipples may be helpful. Low-salt formulas are available for the infant.

Nursing Diagnosis: Fear related to child's ill appearance and disease outcome

Goal: Parents and child will demonstrate accurate understanding of child's condition, treatment options, and prognosis during illness.

Outcome Criteria: Parents and child accurately describe disease and express confidence in treatment plan and health care team.

Children with congestive heart failure are often extremely knowledgeable about the seriousness of their condition. They have learned this from the frequent procedures and visits by cardiologists and from their exhaustion when their heart is not working well. They may lie stiffly in bed, afraid to move, afraid to burden their already overtaxed heart with simple activities such as turning pages in a book. Offer reassurance that although their heart is getting a little behind in its action, the oxygen and medication they are receiving will make it

stronger. Reassure them that people are checking on them frequently, observing them closely in between as well as during procedures.

Parents of a child with congestive heart failure need the same reassurance (provided, of course, the statements are true). They are as frightened by what a physician has told them as by their child's obvious ill appearance. It is often helpful to point out subtle signs of improvement in their child that they may not notice on their own, such as a slower heart rate or slower, less distressed respirations.

Review cardiopulmonary resuscitation techniques to be certain the parents know what to do in an emergency. Be certain that parents have a follow-up appointment scheduled and a telephone number they can call if they have any concerns on hospital discharge.

Rheumatic Fever

Rheumatic fever is an autoimmune disease that occurs as a reaction to a group-A beta-hemolytic streptococcus infection. The name is derived from the involvement of joints, as in rheumatic arthritis. The disease often follows an attack of pharyngitis, tonsillitis, scarlet fever, "strep throat," or impetigo, since the organism common to these infections is a group-A beta-hemolytic streptococcus. Although the incidence of rheumatic fever has declined greatly in recent years, it has not been eradicated. It occurs most often in children 6 to 15 years of age, with a peak incidence at 8 years. Because streptococcal infections recur, rheumatic fever can also recur. It is seen most often in low-socioeconomic urban areas (Ayoub, 1993).

In 95% of children with acute rheumatic fever, there is an elevation of one or more antistreptococcal antibodies, which is an indication of a recent streptococcal infection. The symptoms of the original infection subside in a few days with or without antimicrobial therapy. Children appear well again. After 1 to 3 weeks, however, if a child was not treated with an appropriate antibiotic for the original infection, the onset of rheumatic fever symptoms can occur. Currently, the average child is treated for the initial infection by appropriate antibiotic therapy, so that incidence of the disease has declined dramatically. Since nurses are the primary people who advise parents when to seek health care and how to comply with medicine administration, nurses have contributed greatly to the decline of this disorder.

Assessment

The signs and symptoms of rheumatic fever are divided into major and minor symptoms according to the Jones criteria (Figure 41-29). Of these manifestations, the heart involvement is the most serious. The child usually has a systolic murmur and prolonged PR and QT intervals on ECG due to inflammation. Chorea (sudden involuntary

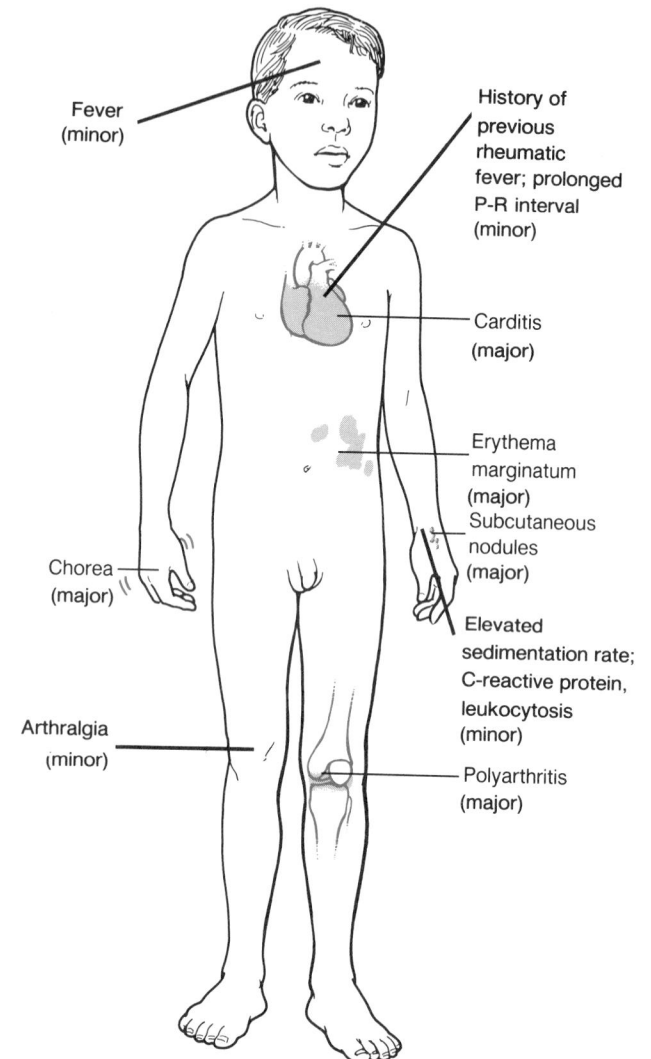

Fever (minor)

History of previous rheumatic fever; prolonged P-R interval (minor)

Carditis (major)

Erythema marginatum (major)

Subcutaneous nodules (major)

Chorea (major)

Elevated sedimentation rate; C-reactive protein, leukocytosis (minor)

Arthralgia (minor)

Polyarthritis (major)

FIGURE 41-29
Major and minor manifestations of rheumatic fever. The disease is diagnosed if two major or one major and two minor symptoms are present, plus a history of a streptococcal infection (Jones' criteria).

movement of the limbs) is the most striking symptom. This loss of voluntary muscle control occurs most often in children between 7 and 14 years of age (very rarely after age 20); it occurs more frequently in girls than boys. Dysfunctional speech from chorea may be demonstrated by asking the child to count rapidly. Children with chorea begin with clear speech, but then suddenly the sounds are garbled or they are unable to speak for several seconds. Hand grasp may be weak or may consist of spasmodic contractions and relaxation. If asked to protrude the tongue, children are unable to keep from making undulating, jerky movements. If asked to extend their arms in front of them, they soon hyperextend their wrists and fingers. If asked to smile, their facial expression may change rapidly from a "Cheshire cat grin" to a flat, expressionless affect or grimace. Subcutaneous nod-

ules are painless lumps on tendon sheaths by the joints. A sign of polyarthritis is that large joints become swollen and tender and the effect moves from one to another. Erythema margination is a macular rash found predominantly on the trunk. Important laboratory findings are increased erythrocyte sedimentation and C-reactive protein levels.

Therapeutic Management

The course of rheumatic fever is 6 to 8 weeks. Children are maintained on bed rest during the acute phase of illness until the erythrocyte sedimentation rate shows a decrease, and the C-reactive protein level and pulse rate return to normal. Bed rest guidelines are based on the degree of carditis present and ranges from 2 weeks to as long as heart failure is present. Because pulse rate is a valuable sign of improvement, taking vital signs is a prime nursing responsibility during the acute phase. This is best done by using an apical pulse: count it for a full minute. Apical pulse is often ordered to be taken when the child is asleep as well as when the child is awake in order to measure the effect of activity.

A course of penicillin is used to eliminate group-A beta-hemolytic streptococci completely from children's bodies. This can be given as a single intramuscular injection of a benzathine penicillin. Erythromycin is used for children who are sensitive to penicillin. Salicylates are helpful in reducing the inflammation and pain of accompanying symptoms; these are given orally. It is important to observe for symptoms of aspirin toxicity that may result from the high dosage; these include tinnitus, nausea, vomiting, headache, and blurred vision. If the aspirin dosage interferes with prothrombin synthesis, purpura may result. Corticosteroids are prescribed for children who are not responding to salicylate therapy by itself. Side-effects of corticosteroid therapy are hirsutism and a round moon face (Cushingoid syndrome).

Phenobarbital is effective in reducing the purposeless movements of chorea. If congestive heart failure is present, measures to reduce congestive heart failure will be prescribed.

The prognosis for the child with rheumatic fever depends on the extent of myocardial involvement. Valve destruction from formation of Aschoff's bodies (fibrin deposits) may leave permanent valve dysfunction, especially of the mitral valve. There are no aftereffects of joint or chorea involvement. If the cardiac muscle is not greatly affected, it can compensate for a long time. With severe myocarditis, the heart dilates and cannot maintain this compensation, eventually failing to function. Children may be left with mitral valve insufficiency, which is especially hazardous for girls, since it may lead to heart failure during pregnancy later on. Some children need mitral valve replacement to restore heart function (El-said 1994).

Nursing Diagnoses and Related Interventions

Nursing Diagnosis: High risk for noncompliance with drug therapy related to knowledge deficit about importance of long-term therapy

Goal: Child will maintain prophylaxis against reinfection for prescribed interval.

Outcome Criteria: Child takes oral penicillin daily; has no symptoms of throat infection.

Prevent Initial Attacks. The incidence of rheumatic fever can be greatly reduced by eliminating streptococci from the upper respiratory tract. After mild cases of streptococcal pharyngitis, rheumatic fever occurs in about 0.3% of children. After severe streptococcal infections, the attack rate may be as high as 1% to 3%. Amoxicillin or penicillin are used to eliminate streptococci from the upper respiratory tract. To be effective, a drug level must be maintained for 10 to 14 days. Erythromycin is used in children sensitive to penicillin; it, too, must be continued for at least 10 days. One intramuscular injection of a long-acting penicillin, such as Bicillin, should be used with children when there is doubt that the parent will give, or the child will take, the full course of oral penicillin. It is important that nurses repeat prescription orders for parents in ambulatory settings so that they understand how often and how much of a drug is to be given and that it is important for the drug to be given for the full 10 to 14 days. The child's symptoms will fade before then, and if the parents are not cautioned about the importance of this, they may give the drug only for 2 or 3 days and then discontinue it.

Prevent Recurrent Attacks. Children who have had rheumatic fever must be prevented from contracting the disease again. To do this, they must be maintained on prophylactic antibiotic therapy for at least 5 years after the initial attack, or until they are 18 years of age. Many physicians advocate maintaining the child on penicillin indefinitely. Penicillin may be prescribed as monthly injections of benzathine penicillin G or daily oral doses of aqueous penicillin.

Extra prophylactic measures should be instituted when dental or tonsillar surgery is planned, because most children have streptococci in their throats. With an open incision in the mouth, the risk of streptococcal invasion of the bloodstream increases.

Nursing Diagnosis: Self-esteem disturbance related to choreal movements secondary to rheumatic fever

Goal: Child will express confidence in self and tran-

sitory nature of the chorea; will continue with major part of self-care during the course of illness.

Outcome Criteria: Child expresses frustration with inability to control movements; continues to feed and dress self with help as needed.

Children may have difficulty feeding themselves because of chorea. They may also be emotionally unstable, cry easily, and resist being fed. Emphasize the transitory nature of the chorea, that it is frustrating to have to be fed and to be unable to use your hands meaningfully, but that this lack of coordination will pass without permanent effects. If chorea is present, provide toys and games for children that do not require fine coordination, because it may be frustrating to try to do something such as move checkers or chessmen on a board (an activity normally suited to bed rest). Children with chorea may need to have the bedrails padded so that they do not injure themselves from thrashing movements.

Kawasaki Disease

Kawasaki disease (mucocutaneous lymph node syndrome) is a febrile, multisystem disorder that occurs almost exclusively in children before the age of puberty. Peak incidence is in boys under 4 years of age; Asian Pacific children are at highest risk (Feigin et al., 1994). There is a higher incidence in late winter and spring. The disease occurs most frequently in middle and upper socioeconomic levels (Rowley & Shulman, 1993). Vasculitis is the principal (and life-threatening) finding, leading to formation of aneurysm and myocardial infarction.

The cause of Kawasaki disease is unknown but apparently develops in genetically predisposed individuals after exposure to an as yet unidentified infectious agent. Following the infection (perhaps an upper respiratory infection), altered immune function occurs. An increase in antibody production may create circulating immune (antibody-antigen) complexes that bind to the vascular endothelium and cause inflammation. The inflammation (vasculitis) of blood vessels leads to platelet accumulation and the formation of thrombi or obstruction in the heart and blood vessels.

Assessment

Kawasaki disease begins with an acute phase (stage I) of high fever (38.9° to 41.4°C) that does not respond to antipyretics (Figure 41-30). The child acts lethargic or irritable and may have reddened and swollen hands and feet. Soon, the bulbar mucous membrane of the eyes become inflamed (conjunctivitis) and the child develops a "strawberry" tongue and red, cracked lips (Roberts, 1991). A variety of rashes occur, often confined to the diaper area. Cervical lymph nodes become enlarged. As

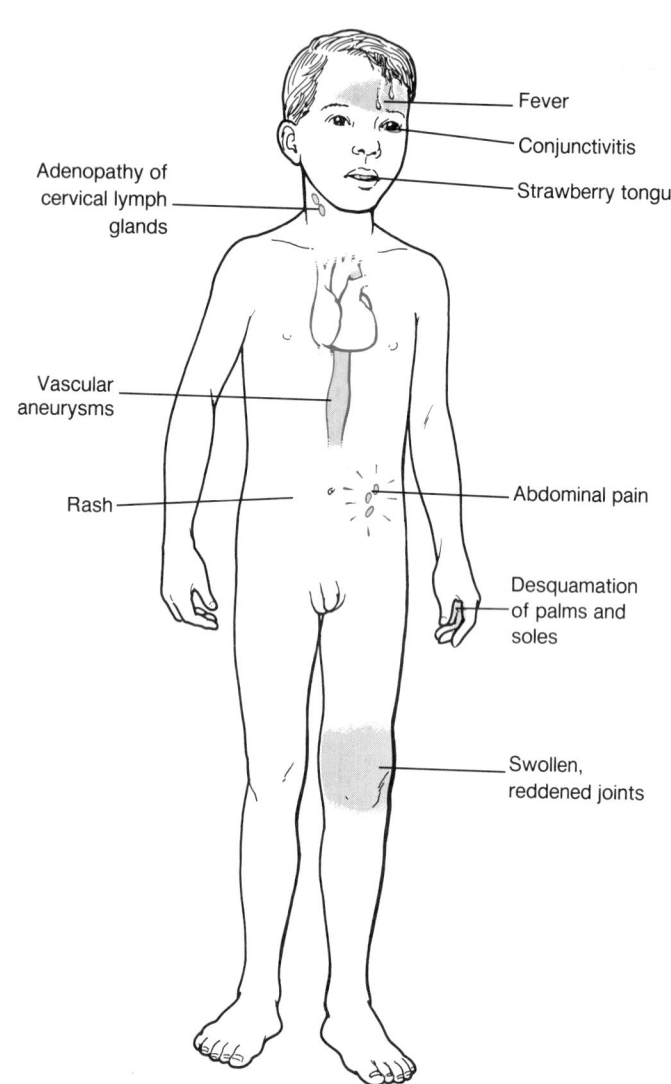

FIGURE 41-30
Common signs and symptoms of Kawasaki disease.

Labels (from diagram): Adenopathy of cervical lymph glands; Vascular aneurysms; Rash; Fever; Conjunctivitis; Strawberry tongue; Abdominal pain; Desquamation of palms and soles; Swollen, reddened joints

internal lymph nodes swell, children may develop abdominal pain, anorexia, and diarrhea. Joints may swell and redden as well, simulating an arthritic process. White blood cell count and erythrocyte sedimentation rate (ESR) are both elevated. Vasculitis is present in small arteries. At about 10 days after onset, a subacute phase begins. The skin desquamates, particularly on the palms and soles of the feet. The platelet count rises. This causes clotting and eventual necrosis, particularly in the finger tips. Aneurysms may form in coronary arteries. Vascular aneurysms may lead to sudden death from accumulating thrombi or rupture of the aneurysm, making this the most dangerous phase for the child. The convalescent phase (stage II) begins at about the 25th day and lasts until 40 days. Stage III lasts from 40 days until the ESR returns to normal. To be diagnosed with Kawasaki disease, a child must manifest fever and four of the typical symptoms shown in Table 41-3 and echogram confirmation of artery disease (Feigin et al., 1994). Children

Table 41-3. Criteria for Diagnosis of Kawasaki Disease

1. Fever of 5 or more days
2. Bilateral congestion of ocular conjunctivae
3. Changes of the mucous membrane of the upper respiratory tract, such as reddened pharynx; red, dry, fissured lips; or protuberance of tongue papillae (strawberry tongue)
4. Changes of the peripheral extremities, such as peripheral edema, peripheral erythema, desquamation of palms and soles
5. Rash, primarily trunkal and polymorphous
6. Cervical lymph node swelling

are followed by sequential echocardiograms to monitor if aneurysms are developing.

Therapeutic Management

The administration of salicylic acid (aspirin) should decrease inflammation and block platelet agglutination. This requires higher than normal dosages of aspirin (about 100 mg/kg/day). The serum level should be between 20 to 25 mg/dL to be therapeutic; during the subacute phase, this can be reduced to 10 mg/dL. Dipyridamole to increase coronary vasodilatation and decrease platelet accumulation may be given concurrently. Steroids, which may increase aneurysm formation, are contraindicated. IV gamma globulin is administered currently with aspirin to reduce the antigen-antibody reaction and the possibility of coronary artery disease. In children with particularly severe coronary findings, Coumadin or heparin, or fibrinolytic therapy such as streptokinase, urokinase or tissue plasminogen activator may be prescribed (Rowley & Shulman, 1993). If the child is left with coronary artery disease from stenosis of coronary arteries, coronary artery bypass surgery may be necessary in the future (Fukushige, 1994).

Nursing Diagnoses and Related Interventions

Nursing Diagnosis: High risk for altered peripheral tissue perfusion related to inflammation of blood vessels

Goal: Child will maintain adequate tissue perfusion during the course of illness.

Outcome Criteria: Child's pulse, blood pressure, and respiratory rate are normal for age group; capillary filling time in fingernails is less than 5 seconds.

Observe the child for signs of congestive heart failure such as tachycardia, dyspnea, rales, and edema. Monitor that thrombi are not forming and impairing circulation in the peripheral vessels by palpating for warmth and capillary filling in toes and fingers. If the child is developing myocarditis, chest pain, arrhythmias, and ECG changes will occur.

> ***Nursing Diagnosis:*** Pain related to swelling of lymph nodes and inflammation of joints
>
> ***Goal:*** Child will experience a tolerable level of pain during the course of illness.
>
> ***Outcome Criteria:*** Child voices that level of pain is tolerable.

A child with Kawasaki disease is uncomfortable from the joint involvement, the edema, the pruritic rash, abdominal discomfort, and the frequent blood sampling necessary to monitor the platelet count. Fortunately, the aspirin administered for its anti-inflammatory action helps reduce the pain and itchiness as well. Provide additional comfort measures such as rocking, holding, and reassurance that the child will get better. Protect edematous areas from pressure; make certain clothing is not constricting and irritating areas of rash.

Because the fever remains high, offer extra fluid to help maintain hydration and reduce mouth tenderness; keep the child free of heavy blankets or clothing and prevent overexertion.

Children with Kawasaki disease lose their appetite and generally eat poorly because of the systemic illness and mouth soreness from cracks and fissures. Monitor and carefully record the child's intake and output. Observe for possible signs of gastrointestinal obstruction, such as vomiting. Apply a soothing ointment such as petrolatum to the lips. Encourage the child to continue brushing teeth (use a soft toothbrush or a padded tongue blade), even though the oral mucous membrane is tender. Soft, nonirritating food may be better tolerated than food that requires chewing or orange juice that might sting.

Endocarditis

Endocarditis is inflammation and infection of the endocardium or valves of the heart. It may occur in the child without heart disease but more commonly occurs as a complication of congenital heart disease such as tetralogy of Fallot, ventricular septal defect, or coarctation of the aorta. The infection is generally caused by streptococci of the viridans type, although staphylococcal or fungal organisms may be at fault. The streptococcal infection tends to invade the body at a time of oral surgery, such as with dental extractions; it can enter from a urinary infection or a skin infection, such as impetigo. As the disease progresses, vegetation composed of bacteria, fibrin, and blood appears on the endocardium of the valves and heart chambers. This tends to occur more commonly on the left side of the heart, although if a heart defect is present, the erosion begins at the site of the defect. Over a period of time, the invading process destroys the endocardial lining of the heart. Underlying muscle and valves may also be affected.

Assessment

The onset of the illness is insidious. Children look pale; they may have anorexia and weight loss. Arthralgia, malaise, chills, or periods of sweating, especially at night, may occur. As the vegetative process begins to erode the heart's valves, significant murmurs will be audible. Signs of congestive heart failure will appear. Petechiae of the conjunctiva or oral mucosa or hemorrhages of the fingernails or toenails (that simulate a splinter inserted under the nail) may be present. The child may first complain of left upper quadrant pain from infarction of the spleen; on physical assessment, the spleen may be found to be enlarged. Laboratory studies may reveal proteinuria or hematuria; a normochromic, normocytic anemia may be present. There may be leukocytosis and an increased erythrocyte sedimentation rate. The diagnosis may be confirmed by a blood culture that reveals the presence of the invading organism. An echocardiogram shows vegetative growths on heart valves.

Therapeutic Management

The prognosis in children treated with intensive antibiotics is good. Therapy is directed toward the underlying infection and also includes support measures to reduce congestive heart failure. Because the invading organism is generally a *Streptococcus,* penicillin is prescribed. The penicillin may be given intravenously by means of a central catheter. Giving the drug into this large vessel allows quick dilution and distribution; therefore, large doses can be given without causing pain or risking infiltration. Children need long-term follow-up care to be certain that the invading organism is completely eliminated and the disease process has halted.

All children with congenital heart disease and who have had rheumatic fever should have prophylactic administration of penicillin before ear, nose, throat, tonsil, or mouth surgery (and before childbirth) to prevent infectious endocarditis (Dajani, 1993).

Hypertension

Although primary **hypertension** may occur in children, it usually occurs as a secondary manifestation of another disease such as a kidney disorder. It has a higher incidence among black children than in other ethnic groups and occurs in about 1% to 2% of school children and in about 11% of adolescents (see the Focus on Cultural Awareness box).

It is difficult to define hypertension in children because normal blood pressure varies with the age of the child. A systolic pressure reading of more than 2 stan-

---

FOCUS ON CULTURAL AWARENESS

Hypertension, hypercholesterolemia, and congenital heart disorders begin to occur at higher incidences in some adolescents than others because there is a tendency for these disorders to be familial. Hypertension, for example, occurs at a higher incidence in African-Americans than in other groups. Nurses have a responsibility to educate adolescents about the importance of maintaining a sensible sodium intake and reducing saturated fat and cholesterol intake. Knowledge of some cultural preferences in foods would be very useful to nurses in their role as health educators.

---

dard deviations above the mean (the 95th percentile) for a given age may be used as a practical criterion (Strong et al., 1993).

Assessment

Beginning at 3 years of age, blood pressure should be included in the routine assessment of children. Normal blood pressure and the technique of blood pressure recording in children is discussed in Chapter 28. Blood pressure should be taken with the child relaxed and after at least 1 or 2 minutes of rest. When children are discovered at routine physical assessments to have hypertension, the reading should be repeated at a successive visit to confirm that the abnormal reading is not a reaction to the stress of the examination or some other emotional event of that day. Levels of blood pressure that denote hypertension for different age groups are show in Appendix G.

When a child has hypertension, a number of additional studies are ordered to discover underlying disease conditions. The most common diseases associated with hypertension in children are renal and cardiac disease (coarctation of the aorta), Cushing's syndrome, primary hyperaldosteronism, adrenogenital syndrome, pheochromocytoma (a tumor of the adrenal gland), and brain tumor. Children should have blood pressure recorded in their lower extremities as well as upper extremities to rule out coarctation of the aorta (which results in low pressure in the lower extremities). A urine specimen should be obtained for analysis. The presence of red blood cells in urine suggests glomerulonephritis. White blood cells suggest pyelonephritis. Proteinuria suggests renal (nephron) disease. The abdomen should be auscultated with a stethoscope for an abdominal bruit, a murmur suggestive of renal vascular disease. Children should have a funduscopic examination to determine the presence of papilledema, spasm, or hemorrhage

from the constantly elevated blood pressure. If papilledema is present, children need immediate care to prevent optic nerve damage. Further studies to rule out adrenal or renal disease may be ordered if these preliminary assessment procedures do not reveal a cause for the hypertension.

Therapeutic Management

Therapy for hypertension will depend on the underlying primary disease. Although the underlying disease conditions that lead to hypertension are serious disorders, they are also ones that can respond to therapy, so hypertension must not be dismissed lightly.

If *idiopathic hypertension* is present (elevated blood pressure for no identifiable reason) and a child is obese, he or she is placed on a reducing diet and urged to increase the level of exercise. Salt intake is limited if it has been excessive; girls are advised not to use oral contraceptives, which elevate blood pressure. Unfortunately, because mild hypertension gives children few symptoms, they do not follow a diet well. For these children, a diuretic, a renin-angiotensin agent, or a calcium channel blocker such as verapamil may be prescribed. Again, because few symptoms are present, many children do not adhere well to taking a vasopressor and need continued counseling at health care visits.

Children with hypertension need to be educated about its long-term effects (increased risk of heart and blood vessel disease). Even if they can tell you why they must take measures to reduce their high blood pressure, they may not follow your advice because they are unable to see the long-term benefits of doing so.

Hyperlipidemia

Hyperlipidemia is increased fatty acid level in blood. All children of parents with premature coronary artery disease (disease before the age of 55) or a family history of hypercholesterolemia (parents with blood cholesterol level higher than 240 mg/dL) should be screened for total serum cholesterol, since there is an association between total cholesterol and low density lipoprotein (LDL) and the incidence of coronary artery disease (Glassman et al., 1990). This is particularly important if the child smokes, is obese, or has a sedentary lifestyle. Total cholesterol can be measured without the child fasting; LDL, in contrast, requires a 12-hour fasting period for accuracy.

Acceptable levels of total cholesterol and LDL cholesterol are less than 170 mg/dL and less than 110 mg/dL, respectively; levels are said to be borderline if they are between 170 and 199 mg/dL and 110 to 129 mg/dL. They are high if over 200 mg/dL and 130 mg/dL (Stone, 1993).

If the total fatty acid level, cholesterol, or LDL is found to be elevated, the child's diet should be regulated in an attempt to lower total cholesterol levels; exercise should be increased. Children should not be placed on total low-fat diets, because they need calories for growth. Infants under 2 years of age are rarely placed on a low-fat diet, since it may interfere with myelinization of the nerves and neurologic development. Low-cholesterol diets for children are discussed in Chapter 34. If the child is over 10 years of age and diet has not been effective in reducing the cholesterol level, a drug such as cholestyramine may be prescribed. It reduces the cholesterol level by binding bile acids and decreasing their absorption. Side-effects include large bulky stools and gastrointestinal discomfort. As cholesterolemia has no symptoms, it is difficult to motivate children to continue a special diet and take medication. They need continued counseling at health care visits or they will not remain in compliance.

Cardiopulmonary Arrest

Children with heart disease are at high risk for cardiopulmonary arrest, which is why nurses must know what steps to take in such an emergency. Because it may occur for other reasons as well—airway obstruction, accident trauma, anaphylactic allergic reactions, central nervous system depression, drowning, and electrocutions—all nurses should know resuscitation techniques. Management may vary according to the cause of the arrest and the age of the patient, but the basic considerations are the same.

Respiratory Failure

Respiratory failure is the most frequent cause of cardiac arrest (Hazinski, 1992). If the child was attached to a respiratory monitor before the arrest, the monitor will show no activity. If a monitor is not currently in place, do not waste time attaching one.

Cardiac arrest occurs as soon as the heart muscle is affected by anoxia. No audible heart sounds or pulses are obtainable. No blood pressure can be recorded (don't waste time trying to obtain one). If a cardiac monitor was attached prior to the arrest, it will show no ECG complex. This is a helpful assessment if available, but again, do not waste time attaching monitor leads if they are not already in place. It is better to err on the side of unnecessary resuscitation. The outcome for the child will depend to a great extent on the speed with which resuscitation is begun. The steps for resuscitation can be remembered as "ABC" (*A*irway, *B*reathing, and *C*irculation).

Airway

The first step in resuscitation is to shake the child and call the child's name. If the child does not respond to

this action, call for help. Turn the child onto his or her back and open the mouth. Tip the child's head backward slightly or place a rolled towel or other fairly firm object under the neck to hyperextend the head slightly (a "sniffing" position). Do not overextend the neck, however, or you will occlude, not clear, the airway.

Breathing

Emergency equipment such as breathing bags should be readily available in all hospital units, so that mouth-to-mouth resuscitation will not be necessary. Place the breathing bag over the child's face and administer two breaths, allowing time for exhalation in between breaths. If no breathing bag is available, use a protective one-way mask for mouth-to-mouth resuscitation to protect yourself from body secretions.

For small infants, place your mouth over the infant's mouth and nose, creating a seal; for large infants and children, make a mouth-to-mouth seal, pinching the child's nose tightly with the thumb and forefingers (Figure 41-31). Provide two slow breaths (1 to 1½ sec per breath), pausing after the first to take a breath to increase oxygen content and decrease CO_2 concentration in the delivered breaths. It may be necessary to adjust the head-tilt chin position to obtain optional airway patency (although this should not be done if neck or spine trauma is suspected; American Heart Association, 1992).

If oxygen is available, insert an oxygen catheter running at a rate of about 4 L/min into the child's mouth or attach it to the breathing bag. Do not wait for a catheter if one is not available. Room air contains an oxygen content of about 21%, so additional oxygen is helpful but not necessary for resuscitation.

Observe the child's chest with each of the breaths you administer to see if the child's chest rises. If it does not, the child's airway is obstructed and air cannot reach the lungs. Continued breaths should be at the rate of 20/min. When respiratory arrest has occurred and mechanical ventilation is anticipated, children need to be intubated to provide a free airway, as discussed in Chapter 40.

Circulation

After the two ventilations, feel for a carotid pulse (in an infant, the brachial pulse; Figure 41-32). It is better to use the carotid rather than a peripheral pulse as an indicator of cardiac function in older children, because with shock, the peripheral pulses may be absent while the heart is still beating. The carotid pulse is also the easiest to assess from your position near the child's head. In an infant, however, the neck may be too chubby for you to palpate the carotid pulses.

If you feel no pulse, begin cardiac massage by chest compression. In a newborn, enough pressure will be generated by two fingers or your thumb pressed on the midsternum about a fingerbreadth below the nipple line

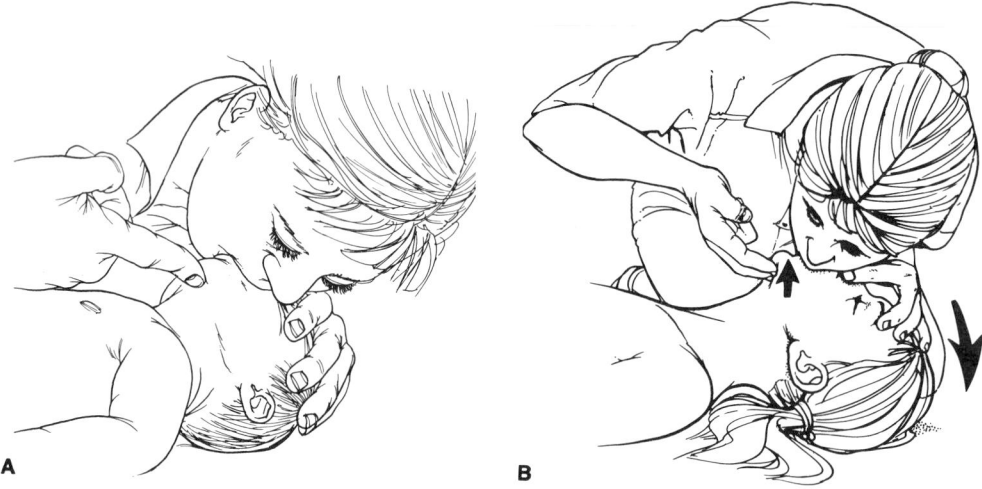

FIGURE 41-31
(**A**) *Rescue breathing in an infant. The rescuer's mouth covers the infant's nose and mouth, creating a seal. One hand performs head tilt while the other hand lifts the infant's jaw. Avoid head tilt if the infant has sustained head or neck trauma.* (**B**) *Rescue breathing in a child. The rescuer's mouth covers the mouth of the child, creating a mouth-to-mouth seal. One hand maintains the head tilt; the thumb and forefinger of the same hand are used to pinch the child's nose. (From American Heart Association [1992]. Pediatric basic life support.* Journal of the American Medical Association, 268, *2255; with permission.)*

(Figure 41-33). Midsternal compression is used with newborns and infants to prevent excessive pressure on the ribs and the possibility of breaking either a rib or the xiphoid process (which then might puncture the heart or liver). In the older child, you need to apply the heel of your palm over the sternum (measure one or two fingerbreadths up from the sternal-costal notch and place palm there; Figure 41-34). Massage the chest at a rate of 100 bpm in an infant, 80 to 100 bpm in an older child (Hazinski, 1992).

Breathing and cardiac compression must be carried out concurrently but not exactly at the same time. If there are two people available for resuscitation, one can breathe into the child while the other compresses the chest. If you are by yourself, you must do both. Breathe once, then compress the chest five times; breathe again, then compress the chest five more times, and so forth. This 1:5 ratio will effectively ventilate and circulate

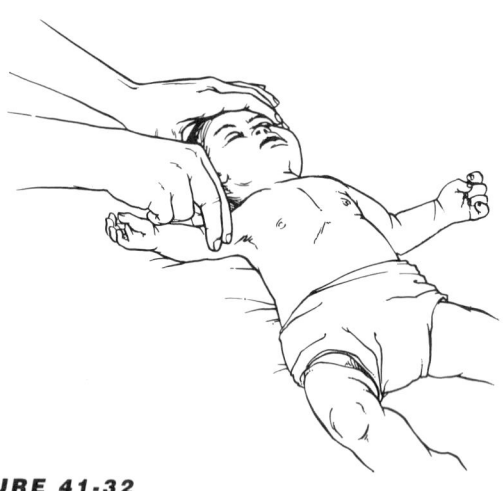

FIGURE 41-32
Assessing a brachial pulse in an infant. (From American Heart Association. [1992]. Pediatric basic life support. Journal of the American Medical Association, 268, *2256; with permission.)*

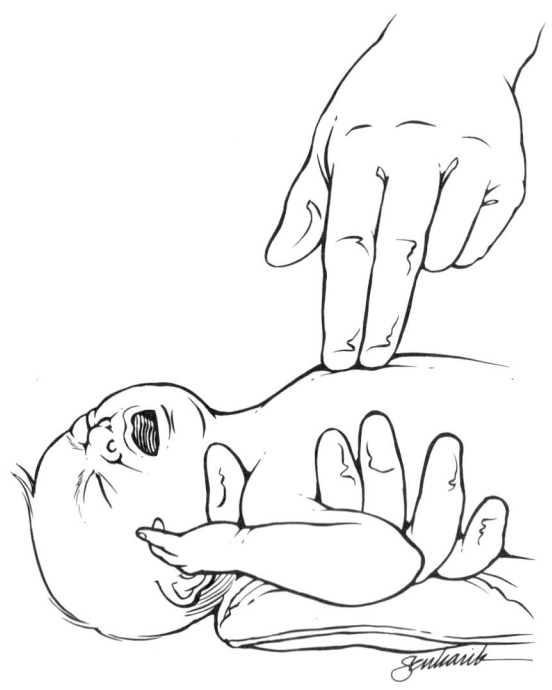

FIGURE 41-33
With cardiac resuscitation in a newborn or infant, chest compression is best done by pressing a thumb or two fingers on the midsternum. Notice the slight extension of the infant's head to maintain a patent airway.

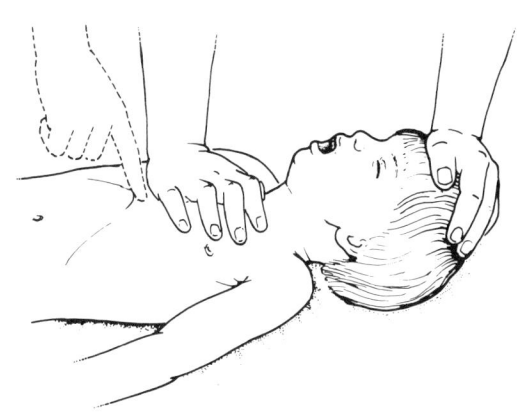

FIGURE 41-34
*Locating hand position for cardiac compression in an older child.
(From Skale, N. [1992]. Manual of pediatric nursing procedures.
Philadelphia: J.B. Lippincott.)*

blood. Do not attempt to inflate lungs and compress the chest at the same time; both efforts will be ineffective. Be certain that your hand comes completely away from the chest between compressions. This allows the heart to fill more readily. If the attempt is successful, the child's color will improve (especially the oral mucous membrane, which is readily visible) and the carotid pulse will become palpable. If two rescuers are working, continue to use a 1:5 ratio in the infant or a 2:15 ratio in the older child.

These three techniques (clearing the airway, ventilating the lungs, and circulating blood by cardiac compression) will provide adequate oxygenation to major body organs for several minutes until additional personnel arrive who can initiate further measures of resuscitation. The outcome of these secondary measures depends on how well and promptly the initial measures were performed.

Secondary Measures

Intravenous access must be accomplished for drug administration. If this is not possible in about a minute's time span, an intraosseous catheter should be inserted. Drugs administered through an intraosseous route reach the circulation as rapidly as IV administration because of the rich blood supply in bone. An endotracheal dose is calculated by multiplying the intravenous dose by 2 or 3. The drug is then diluted with normal saline, administered by a catheter inserted deeply into the tube, and followed by an additional 1 or 2 mL of normal saline and several positive-pressure breaths. A number of drugs are helpful in resuscitation procedures and should be available on an emergency resuscitation cart. Commercial tape measures are available to quickly estimate weight and height and drug dosages (Broselow tapes) (Schuman, 1991). When the child is stretched out beside the tape, accurate endotracheal tube size may be determined as well as emergency drug doses.

Epinephrine (Adrenaline)

Children who have had an anaphylactic reaction need epinephrine injected to counteract the effect of the allergic reaction. Because epinephrine strengthens or initiates cardiac contractions, and increases heart rate and blood pressure, it may be used in any resuscitation attempt. It can be given intravenously, intraosseously, through the endotracheal tube, or intracardially (directly into the heart). The third person arriving at the emergency scene can draw up a syringe, with the dose determined by the child's weight.

Atropine

Atropine reduces bronchial secretions, keeping the airway clear during resuscitation attempts. It also reduces vagus nerve effects, relieving bradycardia.

Calcium Chloride

Calcium increases heart contractility, so it may be administered in place of epinephrine. It causes less irritability than epinephrine, so it produces less ventricular fibrillation also. Doses of calcium chloride may be given concurrently with epinephrine to reduce the amount of epinephrine needed. A contraindication to its use is the presence of digitalis toxicity. Other common drugs that may be needed in a resuscitation attempt are glucose, isoproterenol (Isuprel), and lidocaine.

Psychological Support

A cardiopulmonary arrest is an acute emergency, and everyone who arrives at the scene should know what course of action to take (Ellstrum & Belle, 1990). Even after heart action has been initiated, the heart may be in ventricular fibrillation and will need to be defibrillated. As soon as children begin to respond to resuscitation, be aware that they begin to hear. They are obviously frightened by the number of people surrounding them and by cardiac monitor leads and IV tubing attached to them. They may have vivid memories of frightening body sensations just before going into cardiac arrest. They may regain consciousness struggling and fighting. They need to be assured that everyone is there to help them. They need to help by lying still. Someone on the cardiac arrest team should take the role of comforting the child and providing reassurance that everything is all right. Yet another person should assist, inform, and comfort the child's parents if they are present. It is extremely frightening for parents to see their child suddenly cease breathing. Although it is comforting to see emergency personnel arrive promptly and efficiently, parents are frightened to realize their child is ill enough to need such skilled personnel.

Parents can be allowed to observe a resuscitation attempt, or they can be given definite information on their child's condition as soon as it is available. They need to see the child as soon as possible after the resuscitation attempt is complete to assure themselves that their child is breathing and has heart function. They should be reassured that follow-up procedures such as ECG monitoring or blood-gas measurements are being undertaken to prevent another emergency.

Key Points

- Cardiovascular disorders in children may be either structural, such as congenital heart disease, or acquired, such as Kawasaki disease and rheumatic fever.

- Cardiac anomalies are the most frequently occurring type of congenital anomaly. Observing for cyanosis in newborns to help detect this is a major nursing responsibility. Assessing the femoral pulses in newborns helps rule out coarctation of the aorta.

- Assessment of children with heart disease includes history and physical examination. Cardiac catheterization is a procedure used frequently for diagnosis. Nursing diagnoses associated with this procedure include Anxiety, High risk for altered tissue perfusion, and Infection.

- Preoperative care is an important component of cardiovascular surgery. Nursing diagnoses commonly identified in connection with cardiac surgery are Fear, High risk for altered cardiopulmonary tissue perfusion, Ineffective airway clearance, Hypothermia, and Parental anxiety.

- Postcardiac surgery syndrome and postperfusion syndrome are two complications that may occur following cardiac surgery, which are related to the extracorporal circulation used during the procedure.

- There are a number of treatment possibilities for children with cardiac disease. For example, children such as those born with hypoplastic left heart syndrome may undergo cardiac transplant. Children born with ineffective SA node function may have pacemakers implanted to improve heart function.

- Common types of acyanotic heart defects include ventricular or atrial septal defect, coarctation of the aorta, patent ductus arteriosus, pulmonary or aortic stenosis, duplication of the aortic arch, and an endocardial cushion defect.

- Cyanotic heart defects commonly seen are tetralogy of Fallot and transportation of the great arteries, total anomalous pulmonary venous return, truncus arteriosus, tricuspid atresia, and hypoplastic left heart syndrome. Children with cyanotic heart disease are prone to "tet" or cyanotic episodes. The emergency intervention when this occurs is to place the child in a knee-chest position.

- The families of children undergoing cardiac surgery need a great deal of support so they can cope well enough with this major event to be a support for the child.

- Common signs of congestive heart failure seen in children are tachycardia, tachypnea, enlarged liver, dyspnea, and cyanosis. Signs tend to be subtle in infants and may be manifested chiefly by difficulty in feeding from exhaustion and dyspnea. Nursing diagnoses identified for congestive heart failure include High risk for altered nutrition, Altered cardiopulmonary tissue perfusion, and Fear.

- Rheumatic fever is an autoimmune disease that occurs following a group-A beta-hemolytic streptococcus infection. Common signs and symptoms are fever, chorea, arthralgia, polyarthritis, erythema marginatum, subcutaneous nodules, and an elevated sedimentation rate. Helping parents (and the child) remember to administer prophylactic penicillin following the illness until age 18 helps prevent further recurrence and cardiac involvement. Children with congenital heart disease may also need to maintain this same protective routine.

- Kawasaki disease results from altered immune function. An inflammation of blood vessels leads to platelet accumulation and the formation of thrombi.

- Infectious endocarditis is infection of the endocardium of the valves of the heart. It may be a complication of congenital heart disease.

- Children with cardiac disease may fall behind in developmental progress, because they do not have the energy to play the usual childhood games. Help parents to think of games that are intellectually or developmentally stimulating without being physically exhausting.

- Hypertension in children usually occurs as a secondary manifestation, not a primary one. Cardiac disease in adulthood can be reduced if children eat a moderate cholesterol diet, exercise regularly, and maintain a weight proportional to height. Counseling children to follow these "heart healthy" guidelines calls for tact and persistence.

- Children with heart disease are at high risk for cardiopulmonary arrest. Cardiac resuscitation in a newborn is done by a light touch: pressing a thumb or two fingers on the midsternum. Drugs commonly used in resuscitation procedures are epinephrine, atropine, and calcium chloride.

Critical Thinking Exercises

1. Joey is a newborn who has been diagnosed as having congenital heart disease. He will be living at home with his parents for a month before he returns for surgery. His doctor told his parents to "watch him carefully" during this time. They ask

you what this means. How would you answer them?

2. Heather, 10 years old, is a child who is recovering from rheumatic fever. She lives during the week with her mother and visits her father on the weekends. She will need to continue to take penicillin daily for the next 8 years. What steps would you take to ensure compliance over this long a period of time?

3. You have been asked to prepare a class for a group of parents on cardiopulmonary resuscitation for newborns. How would you teach this?

References

Allan, L. D. (1993). Fetal diagnosis of fatal congenital disease. *Journal of Heart and Lung Transplantation, 12,* S159.

American Heart Association (1992). Pediatric basic life support. *Journal of the American Medical Association, 268,* 2251–2263.

Ayoub, E. M. (1993). Rheumatic fever. In Gessner, I. H., & Victorica, B. E. *Pediatric cardiology.* Philadelphia: W. B. Saunders.

Baker, L. K., & Alyn, I. B. (1992). Pharmacologic manipulation of preload, afterload, and contractility in the young. *Journal of Cardiovascular Nursing, 6,* 12.

Barker, G. (1994). Hypoplastic left heart syndrome. In Oski, F. A., et al. (Eds.). *Principles and practice of pediatrics* (2nd ed.). Philadelphia: J. B. Lippincott.

Boucek, M. M., et al. (1993). Indications and contraindications for heart transplantation in infancy. *Journal of Heart and Lung Transplantation, 12,* S154.

Daberkow, E. (1992). Permanent pacemaker in children. *Journal of Cardiovascular Nursing 6,* 56.

Dajani, A. S. (1993). Endocarditis. In Gessner, I. H., & Victorica, B. E. *Pediatric cardiology.* Philadelphia: W. B. Saunders.

Deglin, J. H., et al. (1991). *Davis's drug guide for nurses* (2nd ed.). Philadelphia: F. A. Davis.

Department of Health & Human Services. (1991). *Healthy people 2000.* Washington, DC: Public Health Service.

El-said, G. M. (1994). Rheumatic heart disease. In Oski, F. A., et al. (Eds.) *Principles and practice of pediatrics* (2nd ed.). Philadelphia: J. B. Lippincott.

Ellstrom, K., & Belle, L. D. (1990). Understanding your role during a code. *Nursing, 20,* 36.

Feigin, R. D., et al. (1994). Kawasaki disease. In Oski, F. A., et al. (Eds.) *Principles and practice of pediatrics* (2nd ed.). Philadelphia: J. B. Lippincott.

Fontan, F., et al. (1990). Outcome after a "perfect" Fontan operation. *Circulation, 81,* 1520.

Fukushige, J. (1994). Cardiovascular aspects of Kawasaki disease. In Oski, F. A., et al. (Eds.) *Principles and practice of pediatrics* (2nd ed.). Philadelphia: J. B. Lippincott.

Gessner, I. H. (1993). Congestive heart failure. In Gessner, I. H., & Victorica, B. E. *Pediatric cardiology.* Philadelphia: W. B. Saunders.

Glassman, M., et al. (1990). Treatment of type IIe hyperlipidemia in childhood by a simplified American Heart Association diet and fiber supplementation. *American Journal of Diseases of Children, 144,* 973.

Glauser, T. A., et al. (1990). Congenital brain anomalies associated with the hypoplastic left heart syndrome. *Pediatrics, 85,* 984.

Gumbiner, C. H. (1994). Ventricular septal defect. In Oski, F. A., et al. (Eds.) *Principles and practice of pediatrics* (2nd ed.). Philadelphia: J. B. Lippincott.

Hardingham, K., et al. (1993). Nursing grand rounds; the pediatric cardiovascular surgery patient: a case study. *Journal of Cardiovascular Nursing, 7,* 80.

Hazinski, M. F. (1992). Advances and controversies in cardiopulmonary resuscitation in the young. *Journal of Cardiovascular Nursing, 6,* 74.

Hultgren, M. S. (1991). Pulmonary management of children after cardiac surgery. *Critical Care Nurse, 11,* 55.

Kersting-Sommerhoff, B. A., et al. (1990). Evaluation of complex congenital ventricular anomalies with magnetic resonance imaging. *American Heart Journal, 120,* 133.

Landzberg, M. J., & Lock, J. E. (1993). Interventional catheter procedures used in congenital heart disease. *Cardiology Clinics, 11,* 569.

Link, K. M., et al. (1993). Congenital heart disease. *Coronary Artery Disease, 4,* 340.

Lyons, M. (1993). Immunosuppressive therapy after cardiac transplantation: teaching pediatric patients and their families. *Critical Care Nurse 12,* 42.

Marino, B., et al. (1990). Atrioventricular canal in Down syndrome. *American Journal of Diseases of Children, 144,* 1120.

Mullins, C. E. (1994). Patent ductus arteriosus. In Oski, F. A., et al. (Eds.) *Principles and practice of pediatrics* (2nd ed.). Philadelphia: J. B. Lippincott.

Roberts, K. B. (1991). Kawasaki syndrome: in the eye of the beholder. *Contemporary Pediatrics, 8,* 126.

Rowley, A. H., & Shulman, S. T. (1993). Kawasaki syndrome. In Gessner, I. H., & Victorica, B. E. *Pediatric cardiology.* Philadelphia: W. B. Saunders.

Schuman, A. J. (1991). The Broselow tape: taking the guesswork out of resuscitation meds. *Contemporary Pediatrics, 8,* 101.

Schwarz, S. M., et al. (1990). Enteral nutrition in infants with congenital heart disease and growth failure. *Pediatrics, 86,* 368.

Stone, N. J. (1993). Diet, blood cholesterol levels and coronary heart disease. *Coronary Artery Disease, 4,* 871.

Stoumper, O. F., et al. (1990). Transesophageal echocardiography in children with congenital heart disease. *Journal of the American College of Cardiologists, 16,* 433.

Strong, W. B., et al. (1993). integrated cardiovascular health promotion in childhood. In Gessner, I. H., & Victorica, B. E. *Pediatric cardiology.* Philadelphia: W. B. Saunders.

Suddaby, E. C., & O'Brien, A. M. (1993). ECMO for cardiac support in children. *Heart and Lung, 22,* 401.

Tamisier, D., et al. (1990). Modified Blalock-Taussig shunts: Results in infants less than 3 months of age. *Annals of Thoracic Surgery, 49,* 797.

Tong, E. (1992). An overview of artificial heart valve replacement in infants and children. *Journal of Cardiovascular Nursing, 6,* 30.

Vick, G. W., & Titus, J. L. (1994). Defects of the atrial septum including the atrioventricular canal. In Oski, F. A., et al. (Eds.) *Principles and practice of pediatrics* (2nd ed.). Philadelphia: J. B. Lippincott.

Suggested Readings

Addonizio, L. J. (1990). Cardiac transplantation in the pediatric patient. *Progress in Cardiovascular Disease, 33,* 19.

Allen, H. D., & Franklin, W. H. (1993). Life style issues. In Gessner, I. H., & Victorica, B. E. *Pediatric cardiology.* Philadelphia: W. B. Saunders.

Alyn, I. B., & Baker, L. K. (1992). Cardiovascular anatomy and physiology of the fetus, neonate, infant, child and adolescent. *Journal of Cardiovascular Nursing, 6,* 1.

Mahoney, L. T. (1993). Acyanotic congenital heart disease. *Cardiology Clinics, 11,* 603.

Monroe, D. (1991). Patient teaching for x-ray and other diagnostics. *RN, 54,* 44.

Popp, R. L. (1990). Echocardiography. *New England Journal of Medicine, 323,* 165.

Rossiter, J. P., & Callan, N. A. (1993). Prenatal diagnosis of congenital heart disease. *Obstetrics and Gynecology Clinics of North America, 20,* 485.

Sciscione, A. C., & Callan, N. A. (1993). Congenital heart disease in adolescents and adults. *Cardiology Clinics, 11,* 701.

Stone, N. J. (1994). Secondary causes of hyperlipidemia. *Medical Clinics of North America, 78,* 117.

Sundel, R. P., & Newburger, J. W. (1993). Kawasaki disease and its cardiac sequelae. *Hospital Practice, 28,* 51.

West, D. W. (1990). Iron deficiency in children with cyanotic congenital heart disease. *Journal of Pediatrics, 117,* 266.

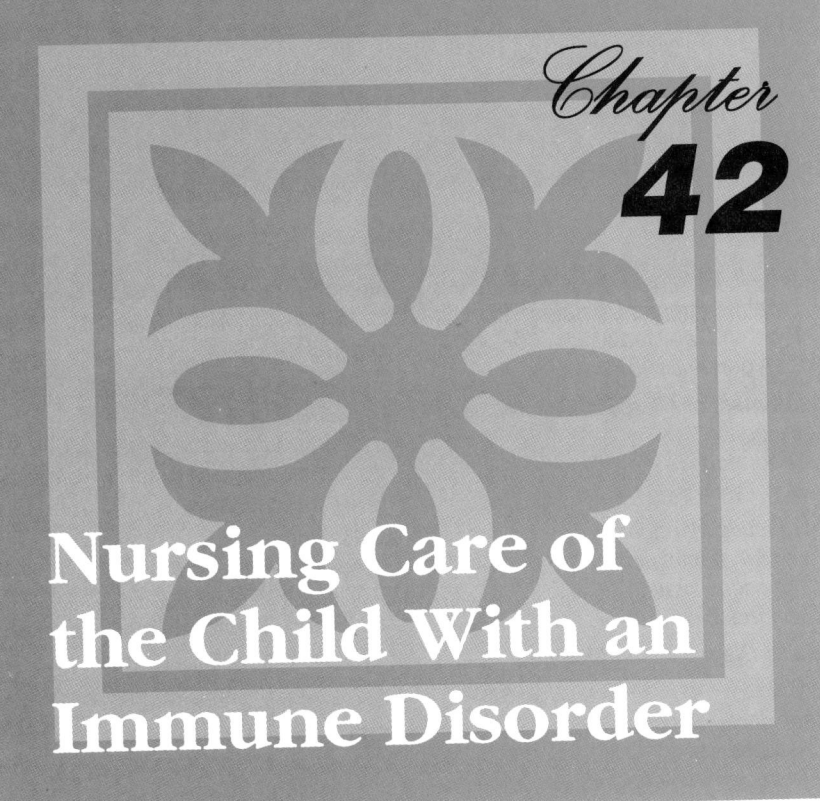

Chapter 42

Nursing Care of the Child With an Immune Disorder

Objectives

After mastering the contents of this chapter, you should be able to:

1. Describe the immune process as it relates to childhood illness.
2. Assess the child with a disorder of the immune system.
3. Formulate nursing diagnoses for the child with a disorder of the immune system.
4. Plan nursing care pertinent to the child with an immune system disorder such as teaching a parent ways to make a house environmentally safe for the child.
5. Implement nursing care for the child with an immune disorder, for example, teaching breathing exercises to a child with asthma.
6. Evaluate outcome criteria to be certain that goals established for care of the child with an immune disorder have been achieved.
7. Identify National Health Goals related to immune disorders and children that nurses could be instrumental in helping the nation achieve.
8. Identify areas related to care of the child with an immune disorder that could benefit from additional nursing research.
9. Use critical thinking to analyze ways that nursing care for the child with an immune disorder can be more family centered.
10. Synthesize knowledge of immune disorders and nursing process to achieve quality maternal and child health nursing care.

Key Terms

- allergen
- anaphylaxis
- angioedema
- antigen
- atopy
- autoimmunity
- B lymphocyte
- cell-mediated immunity
- chemotaxis
- complement
- contact dermatitis
- cytotoxic response
- delayed hypersensitivity
- environmental control
- hapten formation
- helper T cell
- humoral immunity
- hypersensitivity response
- hyposensitization
- immune response
- immunity
- immunocompetent
- immunogen
- killer T cell
- lymphokines
- lysis
- macrophage
- memory cell
- phagocytosis
- plasma cell
- specificity
- suppressor T cell
- T lymphocyte
- tolerance
- urticaria
- vaccine

Adele Pillitteri: MATERNAL AND CHILD HEALTH NURSING, 2nd Edition. © 1995 Adele Pillitteri

The immune system consists of a complex network of cells interacting to protect the body against invasion by foreign substances. The study of the immune system has grown immensely during the past decade, and almost every day brings a new finding. More diseases are being attributed at least in part to a malfunctioning of the immune system, all of which makes an understanding of how the immune system works in health and disease essential for safe nursing care. Disorders of the immune system include deficiencies of immune substances and function that affect the ability of the body to ward off infection (immunodeficiency disorders); abnormal and excessive immune response to foreign substances (hypersensitivity disorders, or allergies); and abnormal and excessive immune response to self (autoimmune disorders). Immunodeficiencies and allergic disorders are

described in this chapter. Autoimmune disorders, which include a wide range of illnesses affecting many body systems, are addressed in those chapters that discuss the affected system (e.g., rheumatoid arthritis, which affects the joints, is discussed in Chapter 51). National Health Goals related to immune disorders and children are shown in the Focus on National Health Goals box.

⊠ **NURSING PROCESS OVERVIEW**
for the Child With an Immune Disorder
ASSESSMENT

The immune system provides protection for the body from invading organisms (antigens). A deficiency of **im-munocompetent** cells (cells capable of resisting foreign invaders) or alteration in their function may limit protection. Assessment focuses on analysis of blood components, particularly the white blood cells, to determine exactly what components are missing or are not functioning properly. When the immune system operates excessively or inappropriately to the invasion of certain antigens, a thorough history and analysis of presenting symptoms is usually the best way to identify the problem and develop appropriate interventions.

NURSING DIAGNOSIS

High risk for infection related to altered immune response is the most relevant diagnosis when the immune system is unable to protect the body from infection. Nursing diagnoses for children experiencing allergic responses focus on their particular allergic symptoms, for example:

- Altered comfort (pruritus) related to infantile eczema
- Ineffective breathing patterns related to status asthmaticus
- Anxiety related to ongoing attack of asthma
- Powerlessness related to difficulty determining cause of allergy
- High risk for altered growth and development related to longevity of illness

PLANNING

Planning for the child with an immune disorder must address both short- and long-term goals. Relief of immediate symptoms or danger is the first priority. Planning for long-term care and prevention of future problems is the next and ongoing priority. Organizations useful to recommend to parents for information or support include the following:

American Lung Association
1740 Broadway
New York, NY 10019-4374

Asthma and Allergy Foundation of America
1125 15th Street NW. Suite 502
Washington, DC 20005

National Allergy and Asthma Network
3554 Chain Bridge Road, Suite 200
Fairfax, VA 22030-2709

Pediatric AIDS Foundation
2210 Wilshire Boulevard
Santa Monica, CA 90403-5784

Ryan White National Teen Education Program
for AIDS

c/o Athletes and Entertainment for Kids
P.O. Box 191, Building B
Gardena, CA 90248-0191

IMPLEMENTATION

A major nursing intervention in the care of children with immune disorders is client and family teaching. The family of the child with an immunodeficiency may need help in identifying ways to keep a child from contracting life-threatening infections while at the same time providing enough stimulation and social contact to promote normal growth and development. A similar teaching goal must be established for the child with a chronic al-

FOCUS ON
National Health Goals

Of the immunologic disorders, human immunodeficiency virus (HIV) is the most serious, not only because it is still ultimately fatal but also because its spread has been so difficult to stop. A number of National Health Goals address this problem:

- Increase to at least 60% from a baseline of 26% the proportion of sexually active, unmarried young women aged 15 to 19 whose partner used a condom at last sexual intercourse.

- Increase to at least 75% from a baseline of 57% the proportion of sexually active young men aged 15–19 who used a condom at last sexual intercourse.

- Increase to at least 50% from a baseline of 11% the estimated proportion of intravenous drug abusers who are in drug abuse treatment programs.

- Increase to at least 95% from a baseline of 5% the proportion of schools that have age-appropriate HIV education curricula for students in 4th through 12th grade (DHHS, 1991).

Nurses can be instrumental in helping the nation achieve these goals by educating children about the way the disease is spread (sexual relations and unclean intravenous needles) and protective measures they can take to avoid contracting the disease (using safer sex practices and not using intravenous drugs).

Nursing research that could add helpful information to the area includes research that attempts to answer the following questions: how can parents of schoolage children best be convinced that safer sex practices should be part of usual schoolage health awareness curricula? What methods used to educate adolescents about the danger of unprotected sex work best?

lergic disorder such as asthma. Parents need to learn ways to help their child avoid situations that may bring on an asthma attack, yet they must not keep the child so isolated or fearful that the child misses out on important experiences.

EVALUATION

Despite the long-term nature of many of these illnesses, it is important that short-term goals also be developed so evaluation can be ongoing. Examples of outcome criteria that might be established are:

- Child's respiratory rate is reduced to 20/min with minimal wheezing.
- Child and parent state they are able to cope with their present level of anxiety.
- Child lists three actions he or she takes daily to help feel in control in face of HIV-positive diagnosis.

Because the field of immunology is evolving so rapidly, theories about immune diseases and associated treatment may change from visit to visit. Be certain that parents are kept abreast of new developments in the field, especially those that will affect their ability to provide an environment that is safest for their child.

Immune System

The body (host) is protected from invasion by foreign substances at several levels. First, body surfaces such as the skin, cilia, and mucous membranes act as a physical protective barrier. When an invading pathogen gets through this barrier, the process of **phagocytosis** (destruction of invaders) begins. **Macrophages** (a type of white blood cell) engulf, ingest, and neutralize the pathogen. At the same time, the inflammatory response creates vascular and cellular changes that help to rid the body of dead tissue and inactivated antigens. The immune system maintains cells ready to attack whenever necessary, sometimes directing the efforts of macrophages and supplementing the inflammatory response as well. The immune system, however, is the only element of this defense quartet that is capable of **specificity**, directly interacting with invading antigens. As such, the immune system provides the basis of the body's immune protection.

Immune Response

The **immune response** is the body's ability to combat outside invading organisms or substances by leukocyte activity. An **antigen** is any foreign substance (molecule) capable of stimulating an immune response. Most antigens are proteins, but other large molecules such as polysaccharides may also function as antigens. Penicillin, although not antigenic by itself, may become anti-

genic when it combines with a higher weight molecule, usually a protein (a process called **hapten formation**). If an antigen is one that can be readily destroyed by an immune response, and **immunity** (the ability to destroy like antigens) results, the antigen may be referred to as a simple **immunogen**; if in the course of the immune response mediating substances are released that cause tissue injury, the antigen is termed an **allergen** and allergic symptoms result. Allergens may enter the body through a variety of routes: they may be ingested (e.g., foods such as eggs or wheat), inhaled (e.g., pollen, dust, or mold spores), injected (e.g., drugs), or absorbed across the skin or mucous membranes (e.g., poison ivy).

Immune System Organs and Cells

The organs of the immune system consist of the lymph nodes, thymus, spleen, and tonsils. Bone marrow produces lymphocytes, which are divided into **B lymphocytes** and **T lymphocytes**. These are primarily located in the lymph nodes and spleen, but travel throughout the lymphoid system. It is the T and B lymphocytes that recognize invading organisms and provide for attack of specific antigens (Figure 42-1).

B Lymphocytes

Originating in the bone marrow, the B lymphocytes divide into **plasma cells** and **memory cells** when exposed to antigens. Plasma cells secrete large quantities of immunoglobulins or antibodies, which are capable of binding to and destroying specific antigens. This process is termed *immunoglobulin-mediated* or **cell-mediated immunity**. When an antibody is formed in response to a particular antigen, it is specific to that antigen. An antibody against the pertussis antigen, for instance, will not have any effect on the tetanus antigen. Memory cells are responsible for retaining the formula or ability to produce specific immunoglobulins. Immunoglobulins involved in immunity are IgG, IgA, and IgM. IgM reaches adult levels at approximately age 1 year, IgG at age 4 years, and IgA at adolescence. IgE is the immunoglobulin primarily responsible for allergic or hypersensitivity responses. The functions of the immunoglobulins are described in Table 42-1.

T Lymphocytes

T lymphocytes account for 70% to 80% of blood lymphocytes. Responsible for long-term immunity, T lymphocytes are produced by the bone marrow but mature under the influence of the thymus gland (hence the term "T cells"). Distinctive receptors on their surfaces mark them as different from the structure of B cells. When mature, T cells leave the thymus to enter specific body regions (thymus-dependent zones) mostly in the lymph nodes and spleen. They can enter the blood circulation or extravascular spaces to contact antigens. When a T cell meets an antigen, it divides until there are enough

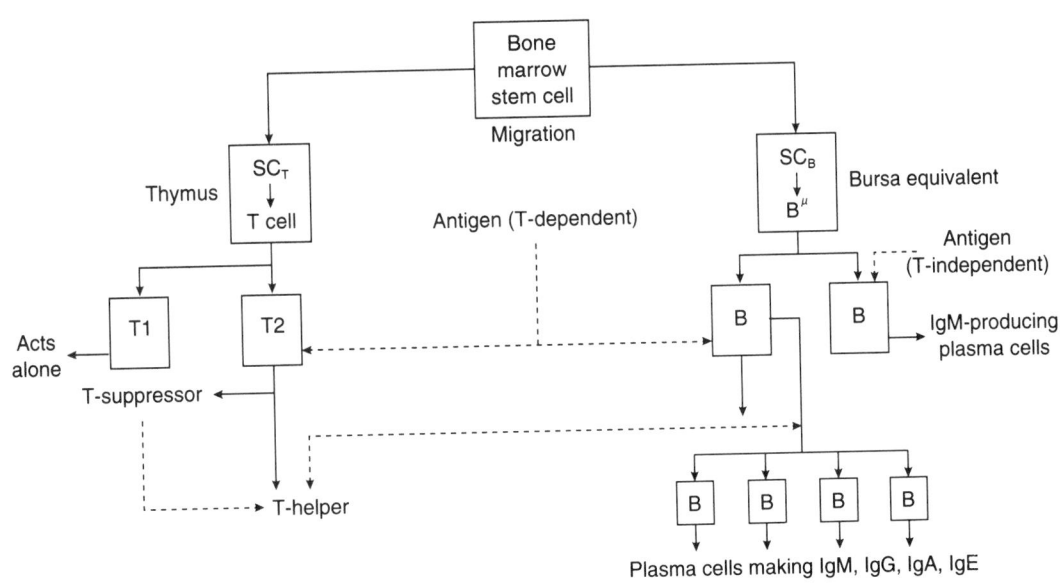

FIGURE 42-1
Origins of the immune response. Both T and B lymphocytes arise from the bone marrow stem cell (SC) and migrate to the thymus gland (T cell) or to unknown bursa equivalent areas (B cell) where they mature to immunocompetent cells. (From Bullock, B., & Rosendahl, P. [1992]. Pathophysiology. *Philadelphia: J.B. Lippincott.)*

Table 42-1. *Location and Function of Immunoglobulins*

Immunoglobulin	*Description*
IgM	Effective in agglutinating antigen as well as lysing cell walls; discovered early in the course of an infection in the bloodstream
IgG	Most frequently occurring antibody in plasma; during secondary response, it is the major immunoglobulin to be synthesized; it freely diffuses into extravascular spaces to contact antigens; in prenatal life, it diffuses across the placenta to supply passive immune protection to the fetus and until the infant can effectively produce immunoglobulins; it has the major responsibility for neutralizing bacterial toxins and in activating phagocytosis (destruction of bacteria)
IgA	Found in external body secretions such as saliva, sweat, tears, mucus, bile, and colostrum; provides defense against pathogens on exposed surfaces, especially those of the gastrointestinal tract and respiratory tract apparently by preventing adherence of pathogens to mucosal cells
IgD	Found in plasma; may be the receptor that binds antigens to lymphocyte surfaces
IgE	Involved in immediate hypersensitivity reactions; exists bound to mast cells on tissue surfaces; when contacted by an antigen, cellular granules are released; associated with allergy and parasitic infections

cells to destroy the antigen. T cells can be differentiated into three subtypes.

The first type, **killer T cells**, are T lymphocytes that have the specific feature of binding to the surface of antigens and directly destroying the cell membrane and therefore the cell. Killer cells secrete **lymphokines**, which help to prevent migration of antigens. Interferon is an example of a lymphokine important in preventing viral spread and helping to call leukocytes into the area (the property of chemotaxis).

The second type, **helper T cells**, stimulate B lymphocytes to divide and mature into plasma cells and begin secretion of immunoglobulins. IgA antibody response depends on helper T cells.

The third type, **suppressor T cells**, are T cells that reduce the production of immunoglobulins against a specific antigen. This prevents overproduction of immunoglobulins.

Types of Immunity

The action of B lymphocytes and T lymphocytes leads to two different types of immunity.

Humoral Immunity
Humoral immunity refers to immunity created by antibody production. Helper T cells recognize the antigen and cause activation of B lymphocytes (possibly by an intermediary macrophage). The specific B cells differentiate into plasma cells and begin secretion of specific immunoglobulins to mark the antigen for destruction (Figure 42-2*A*). A few antigens (e.g., *Escherichia coli*) are

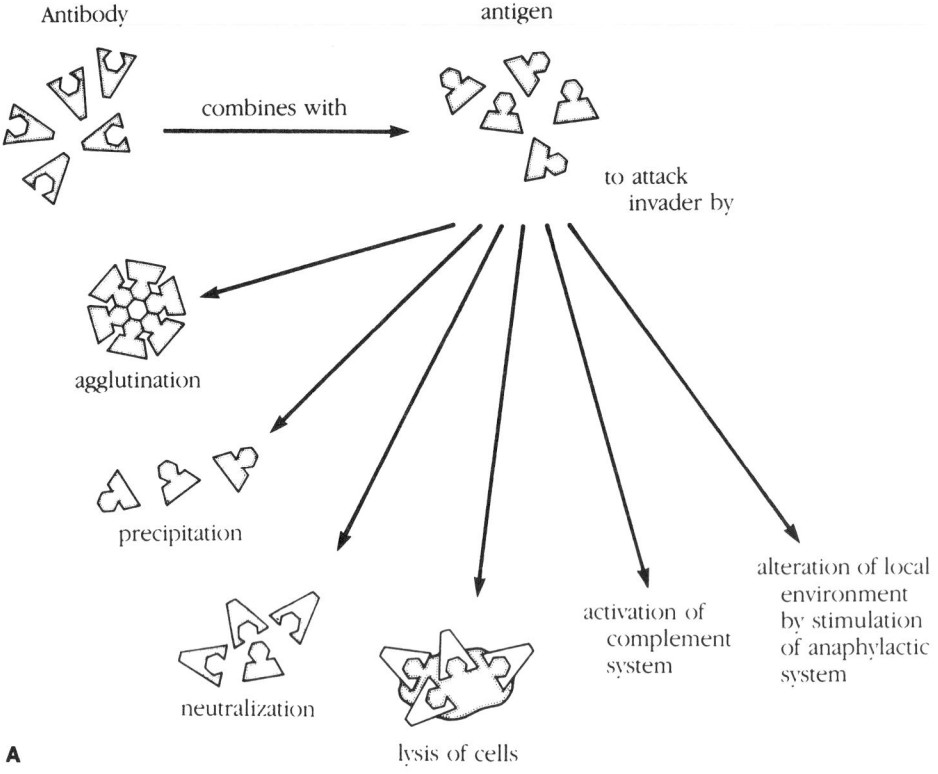

A

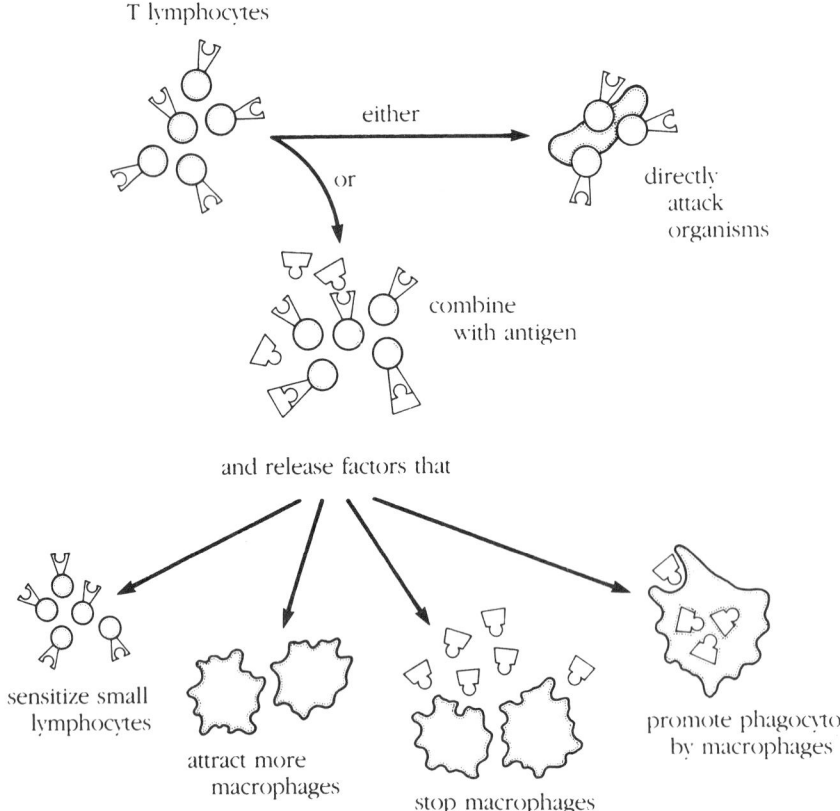

B

FIGURE 42-2
Mechanism of immunity response. (A) Humoral immunity. (B) Cell-mediated immunity. (From Beyers, M., & Dudas, S. The clinical practice of medical surgical nursing (2nd ed.). Boston: Little, Brown.)

capable of activating B-cell response without recognition by T cells.

Primary Response. The first time a specific antigen enters the body, B-cell differentiation and growth begins. Within 6 days, IgM antibodies specific to the antigen can be measured in the bloodstream. The production of IgM antibodies peaks at 14 days and then growth declines until, within a few weeks, there are few present. At approximately day 10, IgG production begins. IgG production remains high for several weeks (Figure 42-3).

Secondary Response. When a specific antigen enters the body a second or additional time, antibody production begins immediately because of memory cells. The type of immunoglobulin mainly produced in a secondary response is IgG (see Figure 42-3).

Complement Activation. **Complement** comprises 20 different proteins that are normally nonfunctional molecules; however, when activated by an antigen-antibody contact, these molecules begin a cascade response essential to promote an inflammatory reaction. Inflammation occurs because of increased vascular permeability; smooth muscle contraction; **chemotaxis** ("calling" leukocytes into the area); phagocytosis; and **lysis** (killing) of the foreign antigen. Although an inflammatory reaction causes some local harm to tissue around the antigen, it is helpful overall because it produces an environment harmful to the antigen. Complement reac-

tions that persist beyond the usual inhibition may be responsible for many of the autoimmune disorders.

Cell-Mediated Immunity

Cell-mediated immunity is the type of immune response due to T-lymphocyte activity. Killer T cells attack and destroy invading antigens through either the release of chemical compounds on the antigen membrane, injection of a toxin directly into the antigen, or secretion of lymphokines. A weal and flare response occurs due to accumulation of lymphocytes around small blood vessels, resulting in minor destruction to blood vessels (see Figure 42-2*B*). This response is termed **delayed hypersensitivity** if the T cell activity occurs solely without an accompanying humoral response. It is this response that causes transplant rejection.

Autoimmunity

Autoimmunity results from an inability to distinguish self from nonself, causing the immune system to carry out immune responses against normal host cells and tissue. Autoimmune responses may be organ specific, that is, limited to one organ, as in Hashimoto's disease (see Chapter 48) or generalized and systemic (non-organ specific), as in rheumatoid arthritis and systemic lupus erythematosus (see Chapter 51). There is currently much research oriented toward the study of autoimmune responses and their possible implication in a wide variety of disorders, including multiple sclerosis and hepatitis. Females are more likely than males to suffer from auto-

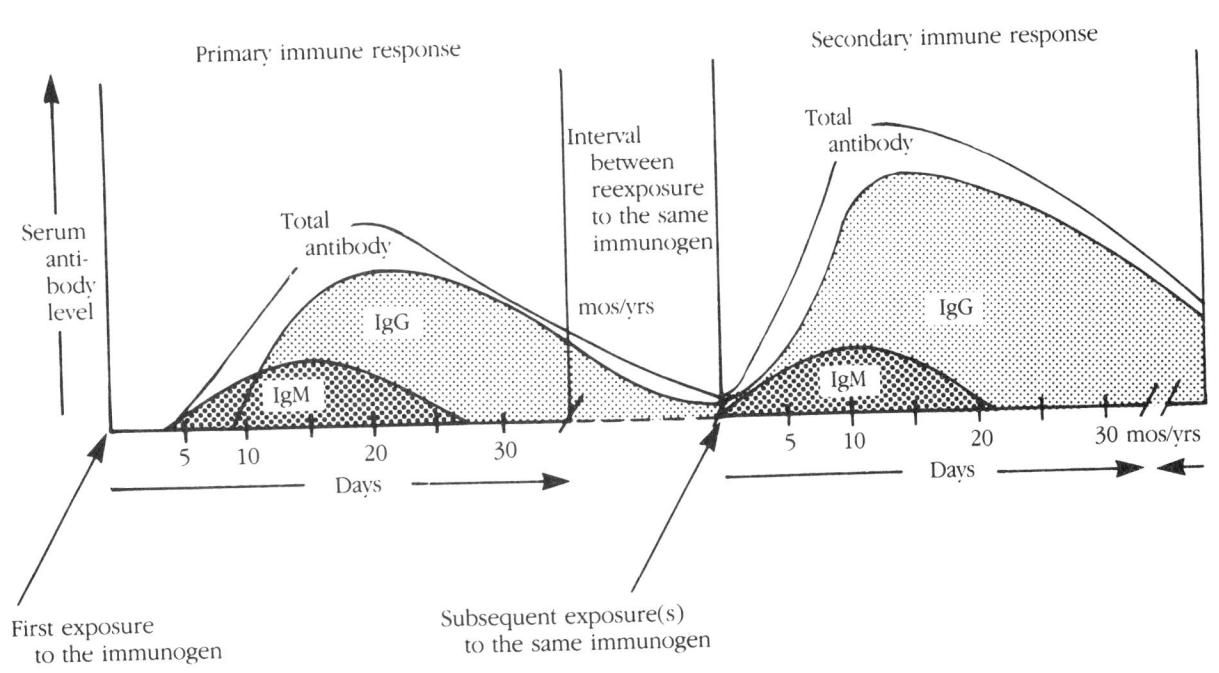

FIGURE 42-3
*Primary and secondary humoral responses. IgM is the first immunoglobulin to appear in the serum.
(From Beyers, M., & Dudas, S. The clinical practice of medical surgical nursing [2nd ed.]. Boston:
Little, Brown.)*

immune disorders, which may indicate a relationship between sex hormones and the immune response.

Immunodeficiency Disorders

The immune system is a complex, interlocking network of cells with specific functions. When any one portion is not functioning adequately, an immunodeficiency results, and the entire system may fail in its goal to protect the body from invading organisms. The immunodeficiency disorders may be primary (congenital) or acquired (secondary to viral invasion or exposure to a toxic substance).

Primary Immunodeficiency

Children with primary congenital immunodeficiencies are born without an essential immune substance or function or with inadequate amounts of immune substances. Usually these deficiencies become apparent relatively early in life, although it may take a few months for B-cell deficiencies to show up because a newborn is born with enough maternal IgG (which crosses the placenta during pregnancy) to supply protection for approximately the first 6 months of life (Zwetchkenbaum, 1990).

B-Cell Deficiencies
B-cell deficiencies involve abnormally low levels of immunoglobulins either selectively (as in an IgA deficiency) or in total, which is referred to as *hypogammaglobulinemia.*

Hypogammaglobulinemia. X-linked hypogammaglobulinemia is an inherited defect in the maturation of B lymphocytes, which results in abnormally low levels of all immunoglobulins. At approximately age 6 months, at the point passively transferred maternal antibodies fade, male infants begin to show susceptibility to bacterial infections and develop frequent respiratory, digestive, and throat infections. Autoimmune diseases such as rheumatoid arthritis and systemic lupus erythematosus occur in later life. Cellular or T-lymphocyte response remains adequate. This allows the child the ability to resist viral, fungal, and parasitic infections. Treatment is with monthly gamma globulin injections; bone marrow transplantation may be successful in restoring immune competency.

Selective Immunoglobulin Deficiencies. The most common disorder in this group is an inherited deficiency of IgA in surface secretions. There is a normal level of B lymphocytes but IgA production is reduced or absent, perhaps due to an increase of IgA suppressor cells or a defect in helper cells important for IgA synthesis. Without IgA, infection of surfaces exposed to the external en-

vironment and normally protected by mucus become common. Sinusitis, upper respiratory tract illness, ulcerative colitis, and malabsorption are apt to occur. There are associated atopic diseases (allergies); autoimmune diseases; and malignancy of the respiratory, gastrointestinal, and lymphoid systems. Systemic lupus erythematosus and rheumatoid arthritis occur at an increased rate. These effects occur because, without IgA on the surface mucosa, many more antigens than usual enter the body. This allows more antigens to interact with IgE and produce allergic symptoms. There is an increased risk that an antibody will cross-react with a self-antigen to cause autoimmune illness. Chronic irritation due to large numbers of antigens could predispose exposed tissue to malignant transformation. IgA deficiency can occur as a secondary type due to treatment with phenytoin and penicillamine. Gamma globulin contains little IgA so therapy with this does not greatly reduce symptoms.

T-Cell Deficiencies
T-cell immunodeficiencies involve inadequate numbers or inadequate functioning of the T cells, which affects cell-mediated immunity and which can also affect humoral immunity. DiGeorge syndrome and chronic mucocutaneous candidiasis are two disorders caused by T cell deficiency or malfunction.

Combined T- and B-Cell Deficiency
Severe combined immunodeficiency syndrome (SCIDS) is the most frequently seen disorder characterized by an absence or reduction of both humoral and cell-mediated immunity. SCIDS is inherited as an X-linked or autosomal recessive disorder and is caused by a developmental abnormality (sometimes but not always related to an absence of a particular enzyme), which prevents the formation of T lymphocytes (a stem cell abnormality). This in turn prevents the maturation of both T and B lymphocytes. Children are unable to respond to antigen invasion and no antibodies are produced. Bone marrow transplantation has proven to be the only effective treatment for this disorder.

Secondary Immune Deficiency

Secondary immune deficiency or loss of immune system response can occur from factors such as severe systemic infection, cancer, renal disease, radiation therapy, stress, malnutrition, immunosuppressive therapy, and aging. There can be complete or partial loss of both B- and T-lymphocyte response.

Stress appears to alter the immune response by interruption of a hypothalamus response; this decreases function of the thymus gland. Stress also increases production of corticosteroids; these suppress the inflammatory response by suppressing macrophage action. Immunosuppressive drugs and radiation are effective in that they limit or destroy rapidly growing cells. Because both T and B cell lymphocytes are rapidly growing and dividing cells, they are killed by these drugs or radiation. Extreme infection can result in a decreased immune response in that it exhausts the body's ability to continue to combat infection.

Malnutrition causes changes because rapidly growing cells need protein for synthesis; renal disease with protein loss will deplete the amount of protein available for new lymphocyte production. Lymphocytotic leukemia results in nonfunctional lymphocytes.

Acquired Immunodeficiency Syndrome

Acquired immunodeficiency syndrome (AIDS) is an acquired immunodeficiency spread by contact with the retrovirus HIV through blood and body secretions. The virus attacks the lymphoreticular system, in particular CD_4-bearing T lymphocytes. The virus replicates in lymphocytes, destroying CD_4 sites. This results in loss of ability to initiate a B-lymphocyte response. The immune response and screening and removing malignant cells from the body are lost. Because B cells or humoral immune function, which initiates the production of antibodies, is affected, antibody formation will be decreased (hypogammaglobulinemia). When monocytes and macrophages become affected as well, the person with HIV infection is unable to resist normal infection and is susceptible to malignant growths (Scott & Parks, 1994).

Transmission. In adults, HIV infection is spread primarily through sexual contact (especially anal intercourse) and through parenteral exposure to blood and blood products. Those at greatest risk include homosexual and bisexual men, intravenous drug users and their sexual partners, recipients of multiple transfusions such as children with hemophilia who received contaminated blood products, female and male sexual partners of HIV-infected individuals, and heterosexuals with multiple sexual partners. Transmission of HIV from mother to child by placental spread is the most common reason for childhood HIV. Transmission of the virus can occur during pregnancy, at delivery, and possibly during breastfeeding. Cesarean birth is not a protection (Caldwell & Rogers, 1991). When contacted during intrauterine life, up to 35% of children of infected women will develop the disease. A small number of children have acquired the infection through sexual abuse (Gutman, 1991). HIV is not transmitted through casual contact, such as in households, day care, or school. Administration of AZT to HIV-positive women during pregnancy may greatly reduce the rate of placental transmission.

The increasing rate of sexual activity and rapidly rising rate of sexually transmitted disease among adolescents makes this group vulnerable to growing rates of HIV. AIDS has become the ninth leading cause of death in children 1 to 4 years of age, and in some areas the number one cause of death in adolescents. The incidence is higher among African-American and Hispanic children than others (Borkowsky & Wilfert, 1992).

Risk to Health Care Providers. Because most carriers of HIV are asymptomatic, it is not always possible to know when a child has AIDS. To protect health care providers from contracting the disease, the Centers for Disease Control (CDC) recommends the use of universal precautions when providing care for all individuals. With universal precautions, all blood and body fluids from all clients are considered potentially infectious. These precautions include washing hands before and after patient care and wearing gloves to handle blood and other body fluids containing visible blood, semen, and vaginal secretions. Universal precautions also apply to tissues and to a number of body fluids: cerebrospinal fluid, synovial fluid, pleural fluid, peritoneal fluid, pericardial fluid, and amniotic fluid. Universal precautions do not apply to feces, nasal secretions, sputum, sweat, tears, urine, and vomitus unless they contain visible blood. However, because some of these fluids and excretions are potential sources of other pathogens, it is recommended that appropriate care be taken when handling them. Specimens should be labeled well and sent in an impervious container to protect transport and laboratory personnel. Any spills of body blood or secretions should be cleaned with sodium hypochlorite (bleach). If a child is coughing, respiratory isolation must be maintained.

The risk to nurses of exposure to HIV is low but real. Most blood exposures result from needle-prick accidents, so extreme care should be taken when handling any needle or sharp instrument (do not recap needles). Pregnant nurses and physicians should use strict precautions when caring for clients known to be infected with HIV, because the possibility of a secondary herpes, toxoplasmosis, or cytomegalic infection also being present is great.

Assessment. HIV has a long incubation period of years in adults; this may be reduced to months in children. During this time, children are HIV positive and may transmit the virus through blood or other body fluids to others. Antibody development significant enough to be detected generally takes about 4 to 12 weeks after exposure, with most developing antibody by 6 months. During this time, the child may have poor resistance to infection such as fever, swollen lymph nodes, and respiratory tract infections. The diagnosis of AIDS itself indicates a condition of immune suppression serious enough to cause life-threatening infections such as pneumonitis carinii and malignancies such as Kaposi's sarcoma. The CDC classification of HIV is shown in Table 42-2.

Because infants can retain maternal antibodies for

Table 42-2. CDC Classification System for HIV in Children	
Class P-0	Indeterminate infection
	Infants less than 15 months born to infected mothers but without definitive evidence of HIV infection or AIDS
Class P-1	Asymptomatic infection
Subclass A	Normal immune function
Subclass B	Abnormal immune function
Subclass C	Immune function not tested
Class P-2	Symptomatic infection
Subclass A	Nonspecific findings such as fever, failure to thrive, or recurrent diarrhea
Subclass B	Progressive neurologic disease
Subclass C	Lymphoid interstitial pneumonitis
Subclass D	Secondary infectious diseases
Category D-1	Bacterial, fungal, parasitic, viral opportunistic infections
Category D-2	Unexplained, recurrent, serious bacterial infections
Category D-3	Other infectious diseases
Subclass E	Secondary cancers
Subclass F	Other conditions possibly due to HIV infection such as hepatitis, cardiopathy, nephropathy, hematologic disorders, or dermatologic diseases

(Centers for Disease Control. [1987]. Classification for human immunodeficiency virus (HIV) infection in children under 13 years of age. *Morbidity and Mortality Weekly Report, 36,* 225.)

HIV infection for as long as 15 months, diagnosis of HIV infection in an at-risk infant (one whose mother is infected) is extremely difficult. After the child is 15 months old, positive antibody test results are considered to be reliable, as is a positive HIV culture (Karthas, 1989). A lower than usual birth weight is noted. More definite signs and symptoms of illness can occur at any time, but usually begin in the first 2 years of life. Failure to thrive (HIV wasting syndrome) is often the first indication of disease. Rather than losing weight, which is common in adults with HIV infection, infected infants fail to gain weight. They may have recurrent bacterial infections, chronic diarrhea, hepatomegaly, and splenomegaly. Infections include mycobacterium pneumonia, *Candida albicans* esophagitis and thrush, disseminated cytomegalovirus, herpes simplex virus infection, *Toxoplasmosis* infection, *Salmonella* bacteremia, and tuberculosis. *Pneumocystis carinii* pneumonia develops rapidly and severely and is often the cause of death in children with AIDS (as it is with adults) (Sanders-Laufer et al., 1991). However, children rarely develop the neoplasm Kaposi's sarcoma commonly seen in adults with AIDS. Diagnosis is confirmed by an ELISA or Western Blot technique of antibody testing (Krasinski & Borkowsky, 1991). A faster technique, PCR (or polymerase chain re-

action), is currently being developed (Borkowsky & Wilfert, 1992). The child's progress and response to therapy is followed by CD$_4$ levels.

Therapeutic Management. Many perinatally infected infants, whose life expectancy was thought at one time to be much shorter, now survive to school age. To prevent loss of weight, protein and caloric supplements may need to be given. These children and their families must maintain strict personal hygiene (e.g., frequent handwashing) and avoid close contact with those who have respiratory infections to prevent them from contracting dangerous opportunistic infections. When infections do occur, antibiotic and antifungal treatment should be prompt and aggressive. Prophylactic use of the antiviral drug zidovudine (AZT) increases growth and prolongs life. Other drugs that may contribute to prolonging life are dideoxyinosine (DDI), dideoxycytidine (DDC), and interferon, which interferes with the entry of viruses into cells. Trimethoprim-sulfamethoxazole (TMP-SMZ) or pentamidine are specific agents used to treat pneumocystis carinii pneumonia. Some children are being prescribed these drugs prophylactically as well as prophylactic immune globulin with good results.

Nursing Diagnoses and Related Interventions

Relevant nursing diagnoses include:

- High risk for infection related to immune system deficiency
- Altered nutrition; less than body requirements related to persistent oral candidiasis or decreased appetite
- Ineffective breathing patterns related to upper respiratory infection
- Altered growth and development related to neurological damage secondary to HIV infection
- Self-esteem disturbance related to exclusion from activities by peers and community

The most persistent problem for the family is related to the combined acute and chronic nature of the disease and to the child's prognosis. Even when one infection or crisis is averted, the family knows to expect additional infections or crises.

Children with HIV often have difficulty establishing normal lives because friends and neighbors, who are afraid that they also will develop AIDS, are unwilling to socialize with these children. School systems may attempt to deny children entry to school. AIDS victims and their families need counseling to maintain self-esteem in the light of this major disaster in their lives.

Nursing Diagnosis: High risk for ineffective family coping: compromised, related to diagnosis of AIDS in child

Goal: Family will demonstrate ability to care for child and maintain family functioning within 1 month.

Outcome Criteria: Parents state ability to continue providing child's physical care; identify outside resources for help with care and decision making.

The diagnosis of HIV in an infant or child can prove devastating for a family. When the disease is transmitted maternally, this diagnosis may be the first indication of the existence of HIV in the mother, and as such, signals tragedy for the whole family. If the child contracted HIV from a contaminated blood transfusion or organ donation (an occurrence less likely now with current protocols for donor screening), the family will feel betrayed and angry. Parents may be unwilling to cooperate with health care providers who, in their minds, are responsible for their child's illness. In any case, the family's coping skills, even if previously healthy, are sure to be seriously compromised. Siblings may be lost in the shuffle of hospital appointments and left alone with their fears of contracting the disease themselves. One of the first nursing priorities in the care of such a family should be to help the family reestablish their previous level of functioning so that they can turn their attention to their child's emotional and physical care needs and to their own needs as well (Clark, 1993).

Physical care requirements for the child with AIDS may be extensive, depending on the child's symptoms and disease progression; no matter what the child's physical needs, however, love and emotional support are essential to his or her well-being and psychologic health. Children should receive all immunizations with the exception of live polio vaccine. Encourage parents to seek medical care for their child at the first sign of illness or infection to prevent unnecessary hospitalization and pain. Parents or caregivers will need extensive support, education, and anticipatory guidance from nurses and other members of the health care team (Meyers & Weitzman, 1991). A number of infants who are HIV positive are abandoned in newborn nurseries by their mothers and left to be raised as "boarder infants" by the nursing staff. In these instances, nurses become their "family." The same difficulty of being unable to cope with the eventual prognosis occurs.

Allergy

Allergic diseases occur as a result of an abnormal antigen-antibody response. Approximately 1 in every 5 children suffer from some form of allergy. Allergy symptoms can be chronic and minor, such as those that occur with seasonal rhinitis, or acute and severe as in an anaphylactic reaction. Allergic disorders in childhood can disrupt a child's life and development and the life of the family. When the cause of an allergic response is difficult to pinpoint, the child and parents become frustrated. Even when the child has a known allergy, symptoms can vary from minor to acute without warning and ultimately disrupt family functioning.

Hypersensitivity

The underlying cause of all allergic disorders appears to be an excessive antigen-antibody response when the invading organism is an allergen rather than a simple immunogen. This is termed a type I response or a **hypersensitivity response** when it happens immediately. It can also occur as a type II, III, or IV response (Table 42-3). Types I, II, and III are mediated by antibodies (humoral response), whereas type IV is mediated by the T cells (cell-mediated response).

Table 42-3. *Classification of Hypersensitivity Reactions*

Type	Involved Cell	Mechanism	Effect
I Anaphylaxis	IgE	IgE attached to surface of mast cell triggers release of intracellular granules from mast cells on contact with antigens	Allergies, asthma, atopic dermatitis, anaphylaxis
II Cytotoxic	IgG or IgM	Antigen-antibody reaction leading to antigen destruction; complement is activated	Hemolytic anemia, transfusion reaction, erythroblastosis fetalis
III Immune complex disease	IgG or IgE	Antigen-antibody complexes precipitate; complement is activated leading to inflammatory response	Rheumatoid arthritis, systemic lupus erythematosus
IV Delayed	T lymphocyte	T cells combine with antigen to induce inflammatory reactions by direct cell involvement or release of lymphokines	Contact dermatitis, transplant graft reaction

Type I: Anaphylaxis or Atopy

Anaphylaxis is an acute reaction characterized by extreme vasodilation that leads to circulatory shock. **Atopy** is a hypersensitivity state that is inherited and results in a range of typical illnesses. In atopic disorders, the immune response is activated when IgE antibodies attached to the surface of mast cells bind to an antigen. Mast cells are specialized cells found in connective tissue, the mucous membranes, and skin. The IgE molecule triggers the release of intracellular granules. These contain histamine; slow-reacting substance of anaphylaxis (SRS-A); and chemotactic substances (substances to draw leukocytes into the area). Histamine leads to peripheral vasodilation and permeability of blood vessels. Vascular congestion and edema result. Smooth muscle constriction in the bronchioles occurs.

SRS-A causes extreme bronchial constriction and reduced vasodilation and permeability.

Type II: Cytotoxic Response

In a **cytotoxic (cell-destroying) response**, cells are detected as foreign and immunoglobulins directly attack and destroy the cells without harming surrounding tissue. Tumor cells may be destroyed by this process. Why this immune response fails when malignant cells begin to proliferate is not understood. Current research is attempting to devise ways to activate the natural immune response as a method of destroying malignant cells. Care of the child with a malignancy (neoplasm) is discussed in Chapter 53.

Type III: Immune Complex

A type III response is an IgG- or IgE-mediated antigen-antibody complex reaction that involves complement and initiates the inflammatory response. Complement reactions that persist beyond the usual inhibition may serve as the basis for many of the autoimmune illnesses such as glomerulonephritis and lupus erythematosus (see Chapter 46). Serum sickness also occurs as a result of a type III response.

Type IV: Cell-Mediated Hypersensitivity

In a delayed hypersensitivity response, T cells react with antigens and release lymphokines to call macrophages into the area. An inflammatory response occurs that helps to destroy the foreign tissue. A tuberculin test is an example of this. Redness and induration of the site does not begin initially but only after approximately 12 hours from the injection. The reaction peaks in 24 hours to 72 hours (a delayed response).

Contact dermatitis is another example of a delayed hypersensitivity response. Certain substances such as cosmetics, household products, or cured leather alter the protein of skin cells so that they become an antigen, or the foreign substance combines with the protein (hapten formation) to become an antigenic protein. Lympho-cytes and macrophages infiltrate the area and attempt to destroy the offending protein. Redness and vesicles may occur. Pruritus may be intense.

Assessment of Allergy in Children

History

Taking a health history of an allergic child is time consuming because many factors must be considered. A family history is important because there are familial tendencies with allergic diseases. Also, the exact symptoms of the allergy are important in helping to identify the allergen—rhinitis is probably due to an airborne antigen; **urticaria** (swelling and itching) is often caused by ingested antigens; and contact dermatitis (often a rash) must be from something that contacts the skin in that area. The time of the year that the allergy occurs may give a clue to its cause. If the child's allergy exists all year, the antigen must be one that is present all year (house dust, pet dander, or a common food). If it occurs in the spring, it is probably a tree pollen; in summer, a grass pollen; if it occurs just in August, ragweed is a prime suspect as the offending antigen.

Many symptoms of allergy are vague, described as "colds all winter," "itching," or "runny nose." Listen carefully to recognize that although no one symptom is acute, together such symptoms can interfere with a child's comfort, school experience, and long-term health. Helping parents and the child to keep a chart of when symptoms are worse and better is often an aid to identification of a specific allergen. Children with allergic rhinitis (hay fever), for example, have more symptoms on a day when the wind is blowing than when it is not, and fewer symptoms after a rainstorm than before (the rain washes pollen out of the air). A record that details when symptoms start—for example, on arising, or only after the child reaches school—may help to identify an allergen. Children are often poor reporters because they cannot remember clearly whether they had the same rhinitis and watery eye symptoms last summer as they do this summer.

Laboratory Testing

Few laboratory tests are helpful in establishing a diagnosis of allergy. A determination of IgE blood antibodies can be made. Most children with an allergy will have an increased eosinophil count; 5% or more of eosinophils on a differential count, or an eosinophil count of 250 or more cells per cubic millimeter, is considered to be significant. Another main cause of an increased eosinophil count is invasion by ova or parasite. Thus, a stool specimen for ova and parasites is generally collected to rule out these problems as the cause of the increased eosinophil count. A radioallergosorbent test (RAST) may be ordered. This is an indirect radioimmunoassay in which the child's serum IgE is allowed to react with specific allergens impregnated in laboratory disks. Only a few allergens are available for this type of indirect testing, so the use of a RAST assessment is limited.

Skin Testing

Skin testing is done to detect the presence of IgE in the skin, or to isolate an antigen (allergen) to which a child is sensitive. When an allergen is introduced into the child's skin, and the child is sensitive to that allergen, a weal or flare response appears at the site of the test. This is due to the release of histamine, which leads to local vasodilation. Because this reaction appears quickly, the test should be read in 20 minutes. Systemic or aerosol administration of an antihistamine or a theophylline derivative will inhibit the flare response, so the child should not receive these drugs for 8 hours before skin testing. Corticosteroid therapy does not affect immediate skin reactivity and so may be continued during skin testing.

Skin testing may be done by either a scratch or an intracutaneous injection technique. Scratch testing is done by placing a drop of allergen solution on the skin after the area has been washed with alcohol. The skin is then scratched with a sterile needle through the drop of liquid. A relatively concentrated extract of allergen must be used for scratch testing because little allergen enters the child's skin. This is the safest form of skin testing and is used with children who are thought to be highly sensitive to the solution being tested.

Intracutaneous injections are done by injecting a small amount of an aqueous solution of allergen below the epidermis of the child's skin. This is usually done on the child's forearm, so that if a sensitivity reaction does occur, a tourniquet can be applied proximal to the test site to prevent further absorption of the antigen. If the categories tested are extensive, the back can be used (Figure 42-4). Solutions used for intracutaneous injections are more dilute than those used for scratch testing (1:500 dilution compared with 1:5 for scratch testing). This means that the allergen extracts are not interchangeable from a group prepared for scratch testing to a group prepared for intracutaneous injections (or vice versa).

Because intracutaneous injections are given just below the epidermal layer of skin, they are painless. This is the same phenomenon as passing a needle or pin under the top layer of skin of a fingertip, a trick every school-age child does at least once to the horror of friends. The child needs a great deal of support for skin testing, however, because it looks as if it will be painful.

For both scratch and intracutaneous testing, the allergic reaction will be a weal and erythema (redness). The size of the reaction is measured and graded as 1+ to 4+ or as slight, moderate, or marked. The allergens chosen for skin testing will depend on the child's individual symptoms; few children need more than 30

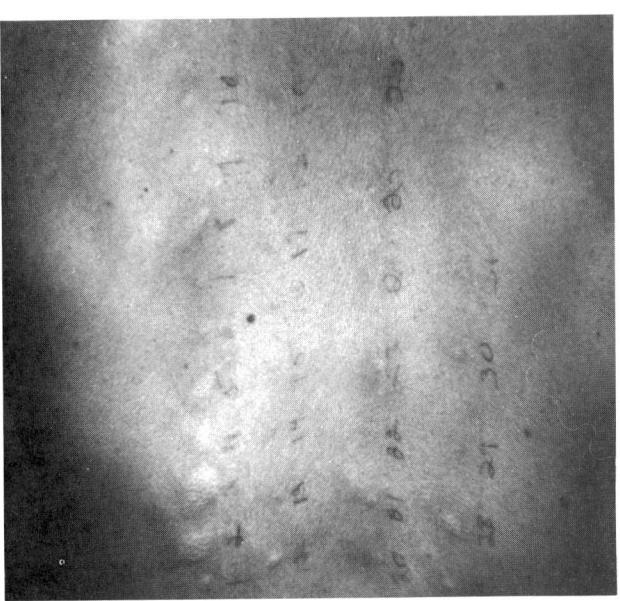

FIGURE 42-4
The back of a child following allergy testing. Each site is numbered. Note the large reactions by sites 2 and 3.

test media tried. This is because most allergies are worse at certain times of the year, and only those allergens prevalent at that time of year need to be tried.

Have a syringe filled with 1 mL of epinephrine (Adrenalin) 1:1000 on hand to counteract an unexpected, but entirely possible, anaphylactic reaction from skin testing. Epinephrine is given subcutaneously in doses of 0.01 mg/kg, up to 0.5 mg. Be sure the epinephrine is drawn up, not waiting beside the vial to be drawn up. The pennies that are wasted each time skin testing is done because of the epinephrine that is not used will be justified the day a reaction does result, and the medication is needed instantaneously to relieve bronchial constriction. Be certain all children stay in the health care setting for 30 minutes following skin testing so they are there during the time a reaction to the injected allergen is apt to occur.

Skin testing may be done by a passive transfer technique. For this, serum from the allergic child is injected intracutaneously into a number of sites on the back of a nonallergic person such as a parent. After 24 hours to 48 hours, the sites are challenged with suspected allergens. If the child's serum contained high levels of IgE, the injection sites will show a weal and erythema the same as in direct testing.

Skin testing with food extracts is ineffective. Food allergies are best identified by eliminating a suspected food from the diet and observing the child to see if there is an improvement in symptoms. After a time of improvement, the food is reintroduced. If it is one to which the child is allergic, symptoms, absent while it was omitted, will return with its reintroduction (often called "rechallenging").

Bronchial challenge testing may be used if skin testing reveals multiple positive reactions, and it is difficult to tell which allergens are clinically significant. For this, the child is asked to inhale powders of various allergenic extracts, and objective and subjective symptoms are recorded. In a child with asthma, pulmonary function tests may be done after the inhalation to demonstrate a change in bronchial capability.

Therapeutic Management

No matter what the symptoms of a child's allergy, there are three goals for therapy: (1) reduce the child's exposure to the allergen, (2) hyposensitize the child to produce a state of increased clinical **tolerance** (a state of not responding) to the allergen, and (3) modify the child's response to the allergen with a pharmacologic agent.

Reducing the child's exposure to the allergen is possible when the offending allergen is a drug, a food, or an irritant, such as a watchband. However, reducing exposure is much more difficult when children are found to be allergic to allergens such as molds, dust, feathers, or other substances found almost everywhere. Reducing children's exposure to allergens of this kind is termed **environmental control**. For some children who are allergic to substances such as mold, dust, or animal hair, environmental control is all that is necessary to control their symptoms and their disease.

Environmental Control

Environmental control means that as many allergens as possible are removed from children's environment. This begins in children's bedrooms, because they spend 8 to 10 hours a day there. Common measures of environmental control are shown in Table 42-4 and the Focus on Family Teaching box. Some parents carry out instructions to reduce potential allergens in their house without difficulty. For others, the process seems too involved to undertake. For example, the parent who envi-

sions his or her child sleeping in a ruffled canopy bed in a room surrounded by stuffed animals may have the most difficult time. Parents need to understand that environmental control may make a great deal of difference in their child's symptoms. If just environmental control is effective with their child, this will be preferable to hyposensitization, which will involve many doctor's visits and many injections.

Hyposensitization

Hyposensitization, or immunotherapy, is done when the child's allergy symptoms cannot be controlled adequately by avoidance of the allergen or by conventional drug therapy. It is expensive to undertake and may not be successful, so is usually considered only after environmental control has been tried.

Hyposensitization works by increasing the plasma concentration of IgG antibodies. IgG acts to prevent or block IgE antibodies from coming in contact with the allergen. After specific allergens have been recognized with skin testings, small amounts of the allergy extract (dilute enough to be clinically subreactive) are injected subcutaneously at 3- to 5-day intervals. The dose of antigen is increased in strength each time until a peak concentration is reached. The peak dose corresponds to the greatest strength that does not give clinical symptoms after injection. After hyposensitization has been achieved, the child will then need periodic injections every 3 weeks to 4 weeks to maintain hyposensitization to this allergen. If a child is going to have an anaphylactic reaction to the injected allergen, it generally occurs within 30 minutes after the injection. Therefore, the child should always wait in the health care setting for 30 minutes after the injection before going home.

Immunotherapy is generally continued for 2 years to 3 years. The longer it is used, the longer the period of relief from symptoms following the cessation of therapy. Be certain that parents know at the beginning of therapy that this therapy will not "cure" their child. It will make the child symptom-free or will decrease symptoms for a

FOCUS ON FAMILY TEACHING

Q. I know that helping my child avoid secondary smoke can help reduce allergies, but how do I do this?

A. You're right that avoiding secondary smoke can be important. Some suggestions for doing this are:

• Declare your home a smoke-free zone.

• If a family member smokes, ask them to use only one room in the house or the porch to confine secondary smoke.

• If at a restaurant, ask to sit in a no-smoking area.

• If staying at a hotel, ask for a nonsmoking room.

• Don't be reluctant to ask people around your child at a social gathering to stop smoking.

• Encourage your friends or a family member who smokes to take quit-smoking courses (for their own benefit as well as yours).

Area of Concern	Implementations
Child's bed	Encase the mattress and pillow in sturdy plastic to keep the child away from the dust that collects in pillows and mattresses. The presence of a minute mite can be demonstrated in house dust, and it may be this mite from which the child actually needs protection. A strip of adhesive tape that covers the zipper of the plastic pillow and mattress case will further keep the dust confined. Use only blankets made of smooth, synthetic material, not wool. Even though wool is not an item to which the child may be particularly sensitive, it is a good dust-collector and so should be removed. If a quilt is used, it must be stuffed with a synthetic material, not wool. Take down a canopy to prevent dust collection.
Flooring	Remove all carpets and use small, easily washable, synthetic throw rugs instead to avoid containers for dust (shag carpets, in particular, trap a great deal of dust). Some new houses do not have finished floors in the bedrooms because the builder anticipated that carpeting would be used. In these instances, the parents may not be able to remove the carpet. Caution them to check that it has a foam rubber, not an animal hair, pad under it. Stuffed chairs collect dust. Replace these with simple wooden ones. Venetian blinds also act as dust trappers and so should be removed. Curtains should be made of a synthetic, easy-to-launder material. All stuffed toys must be ones stuffed with synthetic material. Some very expensive stuffed toys are made from real animal fur. Suggest parents give these to a neighbor whose child does not need environmental control or donate them to a charity. Aquariums and plants both tend to harbor molds and so should be removed. The bedroom closet should be cleaned out so that it contains only currently used items, not clothing that is stored, waiting for the child to grow into it, nor out-of-season clothes. Parents should check the child's wardrobe to be certain that it contains only synthetic materials or cotton, not real fur or wool.

If the family owns a pet, it should not be allowed in the child's room. A new pet should not be purchased. The child should not use hair spray, perfume, or such things as scented stationery. If the bathroom is shared by the whole family, family members should not apply hair spray, deodorant, or cosmetics in the bathroom but, rather, in their own bedrooms.

The bedroom needs to be dusted daily. This is best done by using a wet dustcloth or dust mop rather than a dry one, so that dust is picked up, not just pushed around. Vacuuming removes even more dust. The child should not be assigned tasks of household dusting, mowing the lawn, or washing the dog. Some children have to be out of the house at the time of the cleaning because this is when dust is stirred about most. Dusting is an important aspect of control in all rooms. |
| Living room | Do not allow the child to sit on stuffed furniture (a potential source of dust); a wooden rocker that is the child's own chair solves the problem for some children. Other children insist on lying on the carpet in front of the television set. The child must not lie on the carpet, because even if vacuumed daily, it still contains a great deal of dust. Have parents place a large piece of linoleum or plastic laminate on the carpet in front of the television for a "special space." If the child is allergic to mold, a dehumidifier may be necessary to reduce the dampness of the house. Compounds to kill mold can be added to paint, and sprays or compounds to decrease mold spores can be used directly or added to cleaning compounds. Air-filtration devices are often helpful in reducing the amount of dust present. Such units are expensive, however, so parents can be advised to rent one for a month or two before purchasing one to be certain it is going to make a difference in their child's symptoms. Air conditioners filter outside air and so also may be helpful in decreasing the pollen and dust count in the house or a single room. In some children, however, cold air aggravates their symptoms. These children can have the air conditioner turned on to filter but not to cool. Also, the filter on the furnace must be changed frequently (once a month), and the ducts from the furnace to the rooms in the house may have to be cleaned to eliminate dust in these spaces. |
| School room | Suggest the child not sit near the blackboard (chalk dust) or caged animals or fishtanks. Caution the child to keep school locker free of collectibles. |

length of time, however, and it may prevent a disease such as hay fever (allergic rhinitis) from turning into asthma.

Pharmacologic Approach

A number of pharmacologic preparations can be used to reduce the symptoms of childhood allergies. Like hyposensitization procedures, none of these drugs changes the sensitivity to allergens; the drugs only relieve the symptoms. Common drugs are summarized in the Focus on Nursing Care box.

Corticosteroids stabilize mast cells and thus reduce

an inflammatory reaction. Antihistamines act to block the release of histamine. Drugs such as epinephrine and theophylline act to reverse the effects of histamine release.

Nursing Diagnoses and Related Interventions

Allergies may result in symptoms ranging from minor itching to life-threatening bronchospasm. Nursing diagnoses and related interventions address both short-term goals (to relieve immediate symptoms and discomfort)

FOCUS ON NURSING CARE

Nursing Actions for Drugs Used to Treat Allergy

Diphenhydramine Hydrochloride (Benadryl)

Action

Antihistamine. Does not stop the release of histamine, but reverses the effects of released histamine.

Nursing Actions

1. Antihistamines may cause drowsiness. If this is enough to interfere with school performance, the physician should be consulted for a change of medication or doses.

2. Should not be used with children with glucose-6-phosphate dehydrogenase deficiency because hemolysis may result.

3. Antihistamines have anticholinergic (drying) effects on mucous membrane so should not be used with lower respiratory illness when secretions must be kept moist to be raised.

Epinephrine

Action

An antagonist of histamine that acts on both alpha and beta receptor sites of sympathetic effector cells to cause the effects of increased blood pressure and heart rate, and constriction of arterioles. It relaxes smooth muscle of the bronchi and increases blood glucose.

Nursing Actions

1. Check dosage carefully because solution is available in different strengths.

2. Epinephrine deteriorates on exposure to air. Do not use if brown or contains a precipitate.

3. Obtain blood pressure, pulse rate, and respiration rate, and auscultate for breath sounds before and immediately following administration.

Albuterol Sulfate; Terbutaline Sulfate

Action

Beta$_2$-adrenergic stimulation resulting in bronchial dilatation.

Nursing Actions

1. Drug of choice for rapid relief of asthma symptoms.

2. May be administered by face mask nebulizer for children too young to use an inhaler effectively.

Disodium Cromoglycate (Comolyn Sodium)

Action

Reduces bronchoconstriction effects of histamine and serotonin released by antigen-antibody reactions by locally inhibiting secretion of histamine in the lungs. Used to prevent attacks of bronchospasm; because at the time of the attack, histamine has already been released, it is ineffective once an attack has started. It is not a stimulant, so it may legally be used before sports events to prevent exercise-induced bronchospasm. Because it must be administered by inhaler, it is not recommended for children younger than age 5 years.

Nursing Actions

1. Teach that capsules are used in inhaler only; they must not be swallowed. Capsules should not be handled too much because they soften with body heat. Demonstrate use of inhaler and observe child using it correctly before giving permission for the child to self-medicate.

2. If bronchospasm, severe coughing, or respiratory distress occur during administration, child should discontinue therapy and notify physician.

Oxymetazoline Hydrochloride (Afrin)

Action

A decongestant. A sympathomimetic amine that stimulates alpha receptors of vascular and smooth muscle to shrink mucous membrane to provide relief from nasal congestion in conditions such as sinusitis and allergic rhinitis.

Nursing Actions

1. Caution parents and children that rebound congestion may occur if nasal sprays or drops are used more than 3 days in succession.

2. Teach parents to remember that this is medicine, so cannot be treated lightly just because it is administered by nose, not mouth.

3. Teach correct method of administering nose drops or sprays (see Chapter 37).

4. Nasal application of medicine is usually frightening to children (they worry they will drown). Offer support until the child realizes he or she has nothing to fear.

Deglin, J. H. et al. (1991). *Davis's drug guide for nurses* (2nd ed.). Philadelphia: F. A. Davis.

and long-term goals (to help the child avoid allergens in the future). Education is paramount.

Nursing Diagnosis: Health-seeking behaviors related to dietary/exercise restrictions to prevent/relieve allergy symptoms

Goal: Family and child will demonstrate knowledge of symptom relief measures.

Outcome Criteria: Parents (and child) list foods to avoid; state plans for avoiding suspected inhaled allergens.

Educate Regarding Known Allergens

Children with allergies and their parents must understand how allergic reactions lead to symptoms and how important it is for children to play a role in their own therapy. If parents are going to prepare an allergy-free diet, they need to consider the child's likes and dislikes and to think through the child's weekly intake to assure that in one week the child receives all essential nutrients. If a child eats at school or has a meal prepared every day by a day care center, parents must be certain that the day care center, baby-sitter, or school dietitian are aware of the child's allergies. If a child is allergic to wheat products and cannot eat bread, preparing a bag lunch for school may be a difficult daily problem that only good planning can eliminate.

If a child's allergies involve pollen sensitivities, planning activities such as vacations at a time when the pollen count is low may make the vacation the most pleasant for the family. If desensitization against a pollen will be necessary, it is important to plan to start it so it will be effective by the time the pollen count of the offending allergen rises.

Educate Regarding Ways to Prevent Allergies

Although it is probably impossible to keep children with atopic allergies free of reactions and manifestations of allergies, parents who know of familial allergy patterns can take some preventive steps in this direction.

In families where there are allergies, infants should be breastfed if at all possible. Parents should introduce foods singly so that food allergies can be detected and offending foods eliminated from the child's diet. They should omit eggs and chocolate from the child's diet for the first year. They should begin environmental control when they first choose furniture for the child's room by eliminating wool blankets, choosing toys carefully, and keeping them free of dust. Teach parents to use a minimum of washing compounds to expose children to as few chemical products as possible and not to introduce pets into the house. Avoiding spray products such as air fresheners and discontinuing cigarette smoking also help.

These are sensible rules for parents to follow rather than waiting for a child to develop allergic rhinitis, asthma, or atopic dermatitis and then having to put more extreme measures into effect.

Anaphylactic Shock

Anaphylactic shock is an immediate hypersensitivity reaction. Within minutes of antigen invasion (being stung by an insect or receiving an injection of a drug to which a child has been sensitized), the symptoms of anaphylactic shock begin (O'Neill, 1990).

Assessment

A child may first become nauseated, with vomiting and diarrhea, because of the sudden increase in gastrointestinal secretions produced by the stimulation of histamine. This is followed by bronchospasm that is so severe the child becomes cyanotic and dyspneic. As blood vessels dilate, the blood pressure and pulse rate may fall. Convulsions and death may follow as soon as 10 minutes after the allergen was introduced into the child's body.

It is sometimes difficult to tell anaphylactic shock from fainting (syncope). Children as a rule do not faint at the sight of an injection or a bee stinging them. Syncope rarely occurs if a person is lying prone, so if the reaction occurred while the child was lying on the treatment table, it is most likely that the reaction is anaphylactic. With syncope, although the child falls and is momentarily unconscious, the pulse and blood pressure remain normal. The child appears pale and may have intense perspiration. However, he or she rouses readily after breathing amyl nitrite (smelling salts). The child with an anaphylactic reaction cannot be roused this way.

Therapeutic Management

Preventing anaphylaxis is as important as knowing how to respond to anaphylaxis when it occurs. Before giving drugs that are known to have a high incidence of anaphylactic reactions (e.g., penicillin, aspirin, or antitoxin serums), be certain to ask parents if the child has ever had a reaction to the drug before. If in doubt, withhold the drug until its safety can be confirmed. Check the child's chart to be certain that no prior reactions are noted. People, including children, who have hypersensitive reactions to any injectable substance should wear a bracelet or necklace identifying those drugs to which they are allergic to protect them from receiving the untoward solution. Some children object to these safety measures because they do not want to look conspicuous. They need health teaching to be assured that this is important. Those children who have hypersensitive reactions to insect stings should be given hyposensitization therapy.

Emergency interventions for anaphylactic shock are summarized in Box 42-1. If the anaphylaxis follows an injection or insect sting, give the epinephrine in the opposite arm. Place a tourniquet on the extremity of the allergenic injection or sting proximal to the injection site to prevent further absorption of the allergen. If a sensitized child receives an injection or is stung by an insect while at home, parents must be aware of the proper procedure to follow so that they can give their child immediate help. In place of a tourniquet they can apply ice to the injection or sting site to slow absorption. If the child is on an epinephrine medication or using an epinephrine inhaler, they should give this as prescribed. Then they should notify an emergency squad that their child is having a severe reaction. Caution them not to attempt to give an oral medication if the child is comatose. Parents may purchase an emergency kit (e.g., Ana-Kit), an insect sting treatment kit that contains two measured doses of epinephrine and an antihistamine.

Anaphylaxis is an emergency condition and fast action is necessary. This may be treated by the administration of aqueous epinephrine (Adrenalin) 1:1000 subcutaneously at a dosage of 0.01 mg per kilogram of body weight up to 0.5 mg. This relieves laryngeal edema and severe bronchospasm.

Aminophylline may be administered intravenously or a bronchodilator such as isoetharine (bronkosol) may be given by nebulizer to halt wheezing. Position the child with head even with the body to counteract hypotension.

Oxygen by mask or prong may be necessary if cyanosis is present; the cardiac arrest team should be notified because both respiratory and cardiac arrest may occur. Benadryl may be injected intramuscularly as a secondary medication, particularly if urticaria (itching and swelling) is present. If the child is convulsing, phenobarbital or diazepam may be required.

Keep the child and family members calm; anxiety adds to bronchospasm and decreases breathing ability.

Evaluation of the child following anaphylactic reaction involves not only physical evaluation but evaluation to help the child avoid such a serious reaction from occurring again. This involves health teaching about the substance that caused the reaction and related substances that could conceivably have the same effect.

Serum Sickness

Serum sickness is a type III hypersensitive response of the body to a foreign serum antigen or drug. Examples of foreign sera given to children are tetanus antitoxin, diphtheria antitoxin, and rabies antiserum. These are obtained from horse serum. Children may rarely have a serum sickness reaction to a drug, for example, penicillin.

Assessment

Symptoms of serum sickness begin 7 days to 12 days after the serum injection. If the child has received the same type of foreign serum previously, some symptoms may occur as early as 1 to 5 days. Children notice itching, edema, and erythema at the injection site. There is generalized urticaria (hives) with or without angioedema (generalized edema). Erythematous maculopapular rashes; *erythema multiforme* (a generalized macular eruption with dark red papules); or *purpura* (hemorrhage into the skin) may result.

Urticaria with pruritus is usually present. There may be fever, and *arthralgia* (joint pain) is present. Lymphadenopathy may be present, especially of the regional nodes near the site of the injection. The child may have weight gain, nausea, vomiting, and abdominal pain. In more extreme instances, the child's nervous system may be involved. There may be optic neuritis, stupor, and coma. If edema is severe, laryngeal edema will become the paramount symptom that needs treatment.

Therapeutic Management

Serum sickness lasts a matter of days or weeks. In its usual form (i.e., urticaria, edema, arthralgia, or pruritus) the treatment is only symptomatic because the condition will improve by itself with time. However, antihistamines or epinephrine may be helpful in relieving symptoms. Salicylates may be necessary to relieve the fever and joint pain.

Both anaphylactic reactions and serum sickness reactions are frightening to the child and parents. Parents need an explanation of why the reaction occurred (their child has a low threshold of sensitization to this particular substance), that it was not anyone's fault, and that it did not occur from administration of the wrong compound (assuming that proper precautions to ascertain sensitivity to the solution were taken before the incident). Because serum sickness mimics so many other diseases, parents need reassurance that it is not arthritis (the arthralgia may make them think it is) and that their child will not have long-term effects from it.

The child should not receive again the foreign serum or drug that was responsible for this primary occurrence of serum sickness; the next time the manifestation of the reaction may be anaphylaxis. The child should wear a bracelet or necklace stating the solutions to which he or she is hypersensitive. Children should have their immunizations (and records) kept current so that there is never a need to give sera such as tetanus or diphtheria antitoxins (Belcher, 1993).

Urticaria and Angioedema

Urticaria, or *hives*, refers to flat weals surrounded by erythema arising from the chorion layer of skin; they are intensely pruritic (often described as a burning sensation). This is an immediate hypersensitivity reaction created by the release of histamine from an antibody-antigen reaction (Ghosh et al., 1993). In chronic urticaria, no causative allergen may be found. There is dilatation of capillaries and venules with increased permeability. Hives may occur so close together they tend to coalesce (blend together).

Angioedema is edema of the skin and subcutaneous tissue. This occurs most frequently on the eyelids, hands, feet, genitalia, and lips—areas where skin is loosely bound by subcutaneous tissue. Angioedema can be distinguished from other edemas because it is not dependent, it is generally asymmetrically distributed, and it usually occurs with urticaria. In severe angioedema, the larynx may be involved, which is a serious consequence, because laryngeal edema may cause asphyxiation and death.

The allergens that most frequently cause urticaria and angioedema are drugs, foods, and insect stings. Exposure to hot or cold can also cause these reactions. The cause of the reaction should be identified so that it can be avoided in the future. Although hot and cold exposure is a rare cause of histamine release, children with this form must be identified because if they swim in cold water, the sudden release of histamine could cause such dizziness that they could drown. Therapy for urticaria or angioedema is subcutaneous epinephrine or an oral antihistamine.

Atopic Disorders

The atopic diseases include hay fever (allergic rhinitis); eczema (atopic dermatitis); and asthma. Although these diseases show a familial tendency, different diseases may be manifested in different family members. In one family, for example, the father may have allergic rhinitis, one child may have asthma, and another may have eczema.

The gene responsible for an immune response is located chromosomally near the human leukocyte antigen that is responsible for graft rejection. In certain children, a tendency to sensitivity to antigens or abnormality of this gene is apparently inherited. In these children, there is a higher than normal production of IgE antibody that makes them more responsive to allergens than other people. However, there is also a strong environmental component to this disease. Children whose parents smoke have twice the incidence of atopic disorders compared with children of nonsmoking parents (Sampson & Eggleston, 1991).

Allergic Rhinitis

Allergic rhinitis is caused by an immediate hypersensitivity immune response.

Assessment

Allergic rhinitis is manifested by sneezing, nasal engorgement, and a profuse watery nasal discharge. The conjunctivas of the eyes may be pruritic; the eyes may water. The conjunctiva often has a distinctive pebbly appearance (Figure 42-5). Children may constantly rub their noses, a motion termed an *allergic salute*. Over a long period, rubbing the nose this way leads to a horizontal crease across the tip of the nose, which is called an *allergic crease*. Because of congestion in the nose, there tends to be back pressure to the blood circulation around the eye orbit, which leads to blackened areas under the eyes, termed *allergic shiners* (Figure

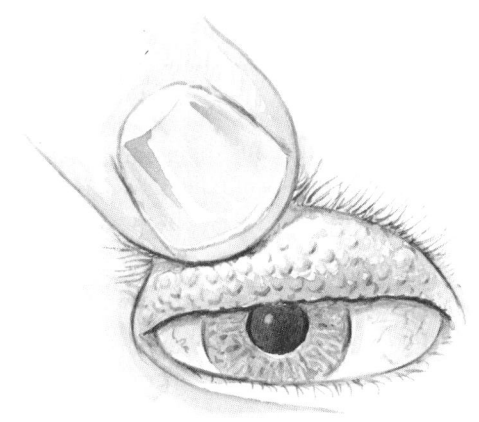

FIGURE 42-5
In children with allergic rhinitis (hay fever), the conjunctiva often shows a distinctive, pebble-like appearance. (Courtesy of the Department of Medical Illustration, State University of New York at Buffalo, Buffalo, NY.)

42-6). The mucous membrane of the nose is generally paler than normal. It may be edematous, adding to nasal congestion.

Children older than age 6 years (when frontal sinuses develop) may report a full frontal headache; this becomes more marked with adolescence. Some children are exhausted and lethargic and are unable to function well in school. As many as 50% of children with seasonal allergic rhinitis have a family history of eczema or asthma. Recurrent otitis media may occur due to the swollen pharyngeal tissue (eustachian tubes are blocked to the middle ear). A smear of the nasal discharge present will reveal an increased eosinophil count (more than 10% of the white cell count).

The allergens that cause allergic rhinitis are gen-

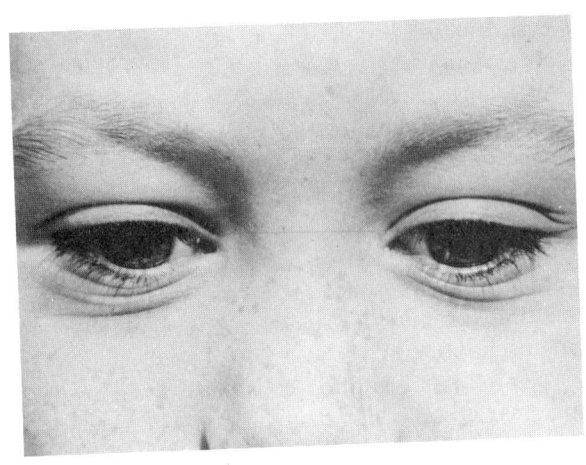

FIGURE 42-6
Back pressure to the blood circulation around the eye orbit from allergic rhinitis may lead to dark areas under the eyes (allergic shiners) or a peculiar horizontal crease (Dennie's line). (Courtesy of the Department of Medical Photography, Children's Hospital, Buffalo, NY.)

erally pollens or molds rather than food or drugs. Many of these children are brought to a health care setting during peak pollen months because parents think they have a "summer cold." However, with an upper respiratory infection, the mucous membrane of the nose is more apt to be reddened than pale; the secretions draining from the nose are apt to be thick white or yellow rather than the thin watery secretions of allergic rhinitis. Children with an upper respiratory infection often have a temperature; children with allergic rhinitis do not. With an upper respiratory infection, a sore throat and cervical adenopathy may be present; with allergic rhinitis, that is rare.

Therapeutic Management

Parents want to know when children should just be treated with antihistamines and when they should see an allergist about skin testing and definite treatment (which is an expensive, time-consuming, and potentially painful procedure). Individual circumstances must dictate the direction of treatment. As a rule, a child whose symptoms are increasing in intensity, who has associated lower respiratory tract involvement, or whose condition interferes with activities in which he or she wants to participate needs definitive testing and treatment.

Antihistamines are a group of drugs that reverse the action of histamine. If a child's symptoms are not severe, he or she may be treated with an antihistamine without initial skin testing. If symptoms are so severe that they interfere with the child's ability to function in school, skin testing to locate individual allergens may be done. Once identified, hyposensitization therapy against the responsible allergens is carried out. Antihistamines tend to cause sleepiness. Assess if this is interfering with schoolwork (Vuurman et al., 1993). Be certain that parents understand that if nasal antihistamine sprays are given for more than 3 days, a rebound effect may occur (the nasal mucosa becomes more edematous rather than less edematous).

Avoidance of allergens is rather ineffective with allergic rhinitis. If children always show symptoms at one particular time of the year, parents may be able to carry out environmental control for that period of the year. Some children with allergic rhinitis are more comfortable in air-conditioned buildings; others have strong symptoms in the presence of air conditioning (probably accounting for the high incidence of headaches that occur at school).

Allergic rhinitis is often considered a minor illness by parents, as something that children will grow out of. However, for children who have the condition, it may not be a minor illness and may keep them from interacting with other children during spring and summer months because they dread going outside and initiating symptoms.

Perennial Allergic Rhinitis

Allergic rhinitis is perennial (year round) when the allergen is one that is capable of affecting the child year round, such as house dust or pet hair. Although the child's symptoms may not result in the obvious distress associated with seasonal allergic rhinitis, they need treatment just as much because they occur constantly. Serous otitis media may be a serious consequence of perennial allergic rhinitis (see Chapter 50).

Because the agent that causes perennial allergic rhinitis is often house dust, environmental control plays a big role in the control of the disorder.

Atopic Dermatitis (Infantile Eczema)

Infantile eczema is primarily a disease of infants. Its signs begin as early as the second month of life and may last until age 2 to 3 years. It is apparently caused mainly by a food allergy because it tends to occur more often in formula-fed than in breastfed infants. Sweat, heat, tight clothing, and contact irritants such as soap increase the pruritus. Symptoms may be more annoying in the winter months when additional irritating clothing is present, with marked improvement in the summer months (Tunnessen, 1994).

Assessment

With infantile atopic dermatitis, there is capillary permeability with loss of serous fluid out into the tissues. Children have papular and vesicular skin eruptions with surrounding erythema. The vesicles rupture and exude yellow sticky secretions that form crusts on the skin as they dry. Because the lesions are extremely pruritic, the child scratches and further irritates the lesions, causing linear excoriations. Secondary infections of open lesions may then occur. As the infected lesions heal, the skin become depigmented and lichenified (shiny), and dry flaky scales form. If secondary infection occurs, local lymph nodes will be swollen. The child may have a low-grade fever. An increased eosinophil count will be present in blood serum.

The common sites for lesions are the scalp and forehead, the cheeks, neck, behind the ears, and the extensor surfaces of the extremities. The palms of the hands and the soles of the feet are uninvolved. Because the lesions are uncomfortable, children with infantile atopic dermatitis are fussy and irritable. They may not eat well due to this discomfort.

Although infantile atopic dermatitis is generally diagnosed while taking the family history (considering other allergic individuals in the family) and noticing the characteristic lesions and their patterns, it is sometimes difficult to distinguish it from seborrheic dermatitis (cradle cap) (see Chapter 23).

A comparison of the findings in seborrheic dermatitis and infantile atopic dermatitis is presented in Table 42-5. Seborrheic dermatitis is a fairly benign condition of infants, requiring little treatment other than frequently shampooing the hair and soaking the lesions in mineral oil and combing them away. A child with infantile atopic dermatitis, on the other hand, will not respond to these measures but must be referred to a pediatrician for treatment. Also, children with infantile atopic dermatitis should have a repeat test for phenylketonuria (PKU) done because children with PKU often have atopic dermatitis.

Although the allergen causing infantile atopic dermatitis is often a food allergen, it may also be caused by pollens, dust, or mold spores. For this reason, skin testing to isolate a causative allergen may be attempted. (Skin testing for food allergies is generally ineffective.) Direct testing is always preferable to passive transfer if there are areas of the skin that are lesion free. In most instances, the upper inner arm is clear and can be used for this purpose.

Therapeutic Management

The medical treatment of atopic dermatitis is aimed at reducing the amount of allergen exposure if such allergens can be identified. The most likely foods to which infants are allergic are milk, eggs, wheat, citrus juices, and tomatoes. The use of elimination diets to identify food allergens is discussed later in this chapter. A second major consideration in treatment is aimed toward reducing pruritus so that children do not irritate lesions and cause secondary infections by scratching. Hydrating the skin by applying wet dressings (wet with tap water or Burow's solution) is helpful. Be careful not to allow infants to become chilled if a large portion of the body is to be covered. Wet dressings can be held in place with gauze dressings. A stockinette dressing with holes cut out for the eyes, nose, and mouth pulled over the head will hold wet dressings in place on the face and neck. To prevent corneal irritation, be careful that such dressings do not come in contact with the eyes.

Topical steroids such as 1% hydrocortisone cream do a great deal to relieve the appearance and discomfort of lesions. If the lesions are dry, a corticosteroid ointment is most effective; if moist, a lotion may be most effective. Applying the cream or lotion and then covering the area with an occlusive dressing such as plastic wrap overnight may speed the healing process. If the lesions are secondarily infected, hydrocortisone mixed with an antibiotic (generally neomycin) and a suitable base is prescribed. Caution parents not to discontinue application of cortisone cream abruptly. Although absorption with topical application is limited, some does occur. This reduces adrenal gland functioning. If the cream is discontinued abruptly, the infant's adrenal response (ability to produce epinephrine) in an emergency might be limited.

Nursing Diagnoses and Related Interventions

Nursing Diagnosis: High risk for altered parenting related to feelings of inadequacy secondary to infant's chronic atopic dermatitis

Goal: Parents will demonstrate sound attachment behaviors throughout course of illness.

Outcome Criteria: Parents express confidence in their ability to follow recommended therapy; express positive aspects of infant and hold infant close and smile and talk to infant.

Parents of children with infantile atopic dermatitis need a great deal of support through the course of the disease. They may worry that they are not "good" par-

---

Table 42-5. *Comparison of Seborrheic Dermatitis and Infantile Eczema*

Finding	Seborrheic dermatitis	Infantile eczema
Age at onset	0–6 mo	2–6 mo
Length of disease	Rarely 1 y	2–3 y
Mood of child	Happy; parents happy	Irritable; parents tired
Location of lesions	Scalp, behind ears, near umbilicus	Cheeks, extensor surfaces, some flexor surfaces
Types of lesions	Salmon erythematous lesions with greasy scales	Papulovesicular erythematous lesions with weeping and crusting
Itching	No	Severe
Depigmentation	No	Yes
Lichenification	No	Yes
White dermographism	No	Yes
Eosinophilia	No nasal mucus or blood eosinophilia	Nasal mucus or blood eosinophilia
IgE serum levels	Low	High

ents because their child's skin looks dirty and crusty. They may worry that health care personnel think they did not keep the infant clean. If children are hospitalized at the first exacerbation of the disease, and, in the hospital, with the use of hydrocortisone ointment, the lesions clear, parents begin to think of the condition as cured. However, 1 week after their baby returns home, the lesions may reappear. They may feel inadequate because this happened. It is not easy for new parents to prepare an allergen-free diet. If a mother wanted to breastfeed and cannot because the child is allergic to milk, she feels doubly inadequate as a mother. How can her child be allergic to her milk? Children with infantile atopic dermatitis are irritable and fussy because of the constant pruritus. No matter how hard parents try, they cannot seem to make them happy. Where is all the fun, the happiness they thought being a parent would bring them? Parents need a "listening ear" so they can vent these concerns and maintain their self-esteem as parents.

> *Nursing Diagnosis:* Altered comfort (pruritus) related to infantile atopic dermatitis
>
> *Goal:* Infant will demonstrate decreased discomfort within 2 hours.
>
> *Outcome Criteria:* Infant does not scratch lesions; parents state infant is less irritable and easier to care for.

When lesions begin to heal, a skin emollient and moisturizer, such as Eucerin, or baths with a substance to lubricate the skin, such as Alpha-Keri, are prescribed. This helps to avoid excessive dryness of the skin. The infant should soak for approximately 15 minutes, then be patted, not rubbed, dry so that the lesions are not aggravated. Because soap is drying, it should not be used on the skin. A skin cleanser for soap-intolerant people, such as Cetaphil Cream, may be prescribed.

Trim infants' fingernails short to prevent effective scratching. Covering the hands with cotton socks prevents them from scratching effectively. An oral antihistamine, such as hydroxyzine hydrochloride (Atarax) may be helpful in relieving pruritus and relieving scratching and discomfort.

In most infants, the lesions of infantile atopic dermatitis clear by the time the child is age 3 years. Unless secondary infection with scarring resulted, the skin surface will not be marked. Approximately 50% of these children go on to develop other allergies, however, as they grow older. In the preschool years, children's parents may report that their children have "one cold after another" (allergic rhinitis). By early school years, the children may show signs of asthma. Exposure to herpes can cause a generalized reaction. Health care personnel with herpes simplex must not care for infants with active atopic dermatitis.

Atopic Dermatitis in the Older Child

Atopic dermatitis may occur at any age, but frequently it occurs at puberty, or ages 16 to 18 years. Atopic dermatitis that occurs at these later ages is prominent on the flexor surface of the extremities and on the dorsal surfaces of the wrists and ankles (Figure 42-7). It often occurs in the eyebrows and, if they scratch lesions, children may have scant eyebrows. Depigmentation or hyperpigmentation is usually present, and lichenification is marked. The fingernails of children often have a glossy sheen from the buffing action of rubbing and scratching. In some children, an itch-scratch cycle may lead to an exacerbation of symptoms. For example, a child begins to feel pressured in school or upset because he or she is left out of the neighborhood group of children. The child rubs his or her skin, a nervous, comforting mannerism with stress, and the rubbing or scratching leads to the formation of lesions. Then the lesions itch, and the child scratches vigorously because of discomfort. The more the child scratches the worse the lesions become; the more lesions there are, the more the child scratches, and so on.

Therapeutic Management

Atopic dermatitis is a difficult disease for older children. Because they can see that the scratching leads to depigmentation or lichenification, they can see that they should stop scratching to keep the disorder under control. The itching is so intense, however, that they wake at night scratching and cannot stop. Adolescents are acutely aware of their appearance, so this is an especially difficult illness for them. Suggestions to decrease discomfort are to encourage the child to shower rather than take tub-baths because water dries skin. Suggest not using soap or only a prescription soap for the same reason. Swimming in chlorinated pools may dry the skin. Encourage other summer sports if possible. Fol-

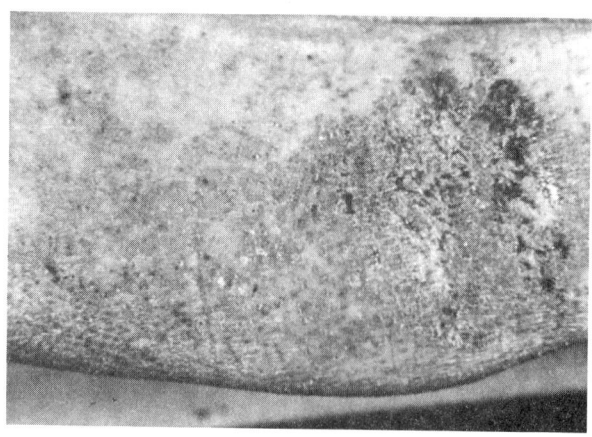

FIGURE 42-7
Atopic dermatitis. (Courtesy of the Centers for Disease Control, Atlanta, GA.)

lowing required swim periods in school, encourage children to shower well to remove chlorine from the skin and apply a skin emollient and moisturizer such as Eucerin. Following a period of activity in which sweating occurred, have the child take a shower to remove sweat, which is irritating to skin. Avoiding tight clothing at the flexor portions of the extremities may also help. Caution children not to use medication intended for acne cover-up on atopic dermatitis lesions as these medications are designed to dry skin.

Medical treatment is basically the same as for the infant with atopic dermatitis. Identifying allergens and any psychologic problems that are initiating an itch-scratch cycle is important.

Evaluation for the older child with atopic dermatitis should include not only evaluation of whether lesions are controlled but the adjustment of the child to school and family. A child who enters adulthood with poor self-esteem because of a chronic allergic disorder during childhood will not have high-level wellness.

Asthma

Asthma is an immediate hypersensitivity (type I) response. It accounts for many days of absenteeism from school and many hospital admissions each year. It tends to occur initially before age 5 years, although in these early years it may be diagnosed as frequent occurrences of bronchiolitis rather than asthma.

Asthma results in diffuse obstructive disease of the airway. Severe bronchoconstriction can be induced by cold air and irritating odors, such as turpentine or smog, as well as inhalation of a known allergen. Air pollutants such as cigarette smoke may lower the threshold for hypersensitivity reactions. Most children with asthma can be shown to have sensitization to inhalant antigens such as pollens, molds, or house dust; food may be involved. Although there may be a seasonal factor responsible for the child's symptoms, most of these children have multiple sensitivities and so are affected all year long. Some children with asthma, strangely, appear to have no immunologic cause for their clinical symptoms. This form is referred to as intrinsic asthma.

Mechanism of Disease

Asthma primarily affects the small airways and involves three separate processes: (1) bronchospasm, (2) edema of bronchial mucosa, and (3) increased bronchial secretions (mucus). All three processes act to reduce the size of the lumen of the airway, leading to distress. Bronchial constriction occurs because of stimulation of the parasympathetic nervous system (cholinergic mediated system), which initiates smooth muscle constriction. Bronchial dilatation occurs because of stimulation of the beta-2 receptors of the sympathetic nervous system (adrenergic-mediated system). Dilatation is always influ-

enced by epinephrine because epinephrine acts to convert precursors into cyclic adenosine monophosphate (cyclic AMP) necessary for cell metabolism and is capable of mediating beta-adrenergic influences. Acetylcholine acts on cyclic guanosine monophosphate (cyclic GMP) to mediate the effects of the cholinergic system.

Drugs prescribed for asthma act to increase the effect of either acetylcholine or epinephrine to change the balance of cyclic AMP or cyclic GMP. Epinephrine, for example, increases the production of cyclic AMP; theophylline inactivates the enzyme that destroys cyclic AMP, also resulting in an increased level of cyclic AMP.

Assessment

The word "asthma" is derived from the Greek word for "panting." The child notices chest tightness, dyspnea, wheezing, and a paroxysmal cough that produces thick, mucoid sputum. Because bronchioles are normally larger in lumen on inspiration than expiration even with bronchospasm, children may inhale normally. They are unable to exhale, however, without difficulty because they cannot force air through the narrowed lumen of the bronchioles filled with mucus. This causes the dyspnea and the wheezing (the sound caused by air being pushed forcibly through obstructed bronchioles). The child coughs up mucus, which is generally copious. The sputum produced after a severe attack may contain white casts bearing the shape of the bronchi from which they were dislodged. It is important to remember that wheezing is a sound of expiration. If a sound similar to wheezing is heard on inspiration, it is probably *stridor,* a sound prominent not in asthma as a rule, but in laryngospasm, an equally serious but different disorder.

History. Assessment should include a thorough history of the development of the child's symptoms and any factor that would have been involved in initiating the present attack. When an acute attack has passed, ask the parent or child to describe the home environment including any pets, the child's bedroom, outdoor play space, classroom environment, and type of heating in the house to see if inhalants in the environment could be eliminated.

Physical Assessment. A physical assessment includes general assessment of growth and development as well as specific symptoms of asthma. On auscultation, wheezing will be present. Bronchospasm will lead to CO_2 trapping and retention. Arterial O_2 may be decreased because of the inability to draw in full breaths.

As constriction becomes acute, the sound of wheezing may decrease because so little air is able to leave the alveoli; cyanosis will become severe. When blood gases show an increased CO_2 level, respiratory failure is imminent.

In many children, the wheezing is so loud that it can

be heard across a room. In others, it will be evident only by auscultation. Asthma affects all lobes of the lungs; thus, although the wheezing may be more prominent in one lobe than in another, it is generally audible in all lung fields. If wheezing is audible in only one lobe, it suggests that only one bronchus is plugged, which may indicate that a foreign body such as a peanut is responsible, rather than asthma. This possibility should be investigated (see the section on bronchial obstruction in Chapter 40).

During attacks, children with asthma are generally more comfortable in a sitting or standing position rather than lying down. If seated in a chair, they lean forward and raise their shoulders, to give themselves more breathing space. Do not urge children to "lie down and relax." This causes severe anxiety and increased difficulty in breathing. Children who do agree to lie down are either at the end of an attack and so beginning to feel less threatened by the dyspnea or are so exhausted by the paroxysms of coughing that they no longer have the strength to sit upright.

The lungs will be hyperresonant to percussion (i.e., they will make louder, hollower noise on percussion than usual) because of pockets of emphysema (trapped air) behind clogged bronchi. The length of expiration will be increased beyond normal limits. In normal respirations, the inspiration phase of breathing is longer than the expiration phase. During an attack of asthma, children must work so hard to exhale that the expiration phase becomes longer than the inspiration phase. Time the two phases to demonstrate this. To achieve full breaths, children use intercostal accessory muscles, producing retractions.

Over time, as the child has many bouts of asthma, the child's chest assumes a shieldlike or barrel shape from constant overinflation of air in alveoli. Clubbing of the fingers from lack of complete oxygenation in distal parts may be noticeable. If the child has been treated for a long period with steroids, growth may be stunted. On laboratory examination, the eosinophil count will be elevated and pulmonary function studies will be reduced.

Pulmonary Function Studies.
Good pulmonary function depends on good ventilation (drawing adequate air into the lungs and expelling it again); adequate transfer of gases across the alveolar capillary membranes; and the volume and distribution of pulmonary capillary blood flow.

The process of ventilation, or the work of breathing, involves three main forces: (1) an inertial force that must be overcome to change the speed and direction of air when the lungs change from exhalation to inhalation, or vice versa; (2) an elastic force to help the lungs expand with inhalation and "snap back" with exhalation; and (3) the flow resistance force or resistance to the movement of air through the bronchial tree that must be over-

come. Flow resistance must be at a minimum for best ventilation. It is increased when the bronchioles are narrowed or plugged with mucus. The forces of inertia, elasticity, and flow resistance are measured in pulmonary function tests.

Vital capacity is the total volume of air that can be expired following a normal inspiration. Vital capacity will be low in children who have bronchial asthma if there is atelectasis (collapsed alveoli) from air absorption behind bronchial plugging.

Forced vital capacity is measured by having the child expire rapidly. Both timed and forced vital capacities are compared with standard charts to see if the value is normal for a child of that age. The forced vital capacity should be 80% of that predicted for that age group for it to be considered normal. A child begins to have exertional dyspnea when the forced vital capacity falls below 60% of the normal level.

The procedure for pulmonary function testing is described in Chapter 40. In children with asthma, the vital capacity may be low or the capacity may be normal but, due to narrowed bronchioles as a result of bronchospasm, the expiratory rate may be abnormally long (more than 10 seconds rather than the normal 2 or 3 seconds). When a vital capacity test is abnormal, the child may have it repeated following an inhalation treatment or a subcutaneous injection of epinephrine. The epinephrine will cause dilatation of bronchioles and easier expiration. This gives an indication of whether the child's condition is reversible. A gross measure of vital capacity is to ask a child to blow out a match. A child with an average vital capacity should be able to do this when the match is held at 6 in. Some doctors may ask a child to use a home peak flow meter daily to measure gross changes in peak expiratory flow over time. This can help in the planning of an appropriate therapeutic regimen (Figure 42-8).

Therapeutic Management
Therapy for children with asthma involves planning for the three goals of all allergy disorders: (1) avoidance of the allergen by environmental control, (2) skin-testing and hyposensitization to identified allergens, and (3) relief of symptoms by the use of pharmacologic agents.

In the past, children with asthma were maintained on an oral preparation of a methylxanthine such as theophylline and administered epinephrine to relieve acute attacks. Today, adrenergic agonists such as albuterol, terbutaline, and metaproterenol are the drugs of choice for both maintenance and acute attacks (Eggleston, 1994). These drugs are available in oral, metered dose inhaler, or nebulizer form. Cromolyn sodium is yet another choice. This can be administered by metered dose inhaler to prevent attacks. It is important that if children are to receive medication by nebulizer or inhaler, that they learn to use these wisely. It is easy to take this type

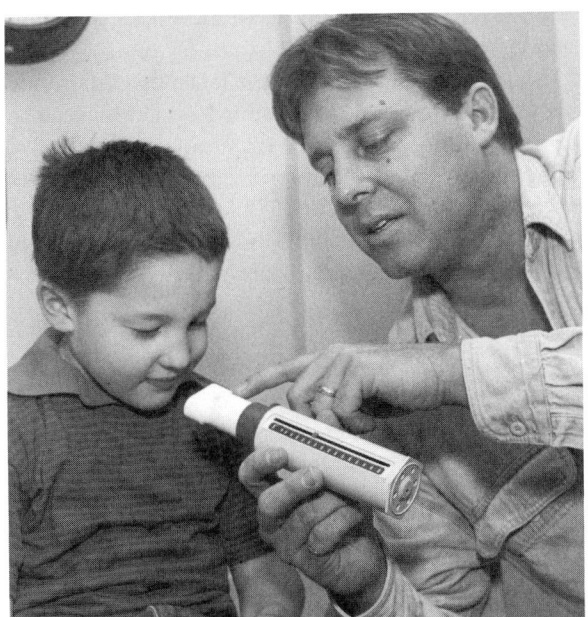

FIGURE 42-8
Children with any chronic illness require periodic evaluation and sometimes home monitoring. Children with asthma may use a home peak flow meter and track their peak expiratory flow readings on a daily or weekly basis. (Courtesy of the Department of Medical Photography, Children's Hospital, Buffalo, NY.)

of medication lightly (because it is "not really medicine"), and so overdose from constant use of nebulizers can occur. Metered dose inhalers require that the child trigger the inhaler at the same time he or she breathes in. As it is difficult for children under about 12 years to do this, placing a "spacer" tube between the inhaler and the mouthpiece eliminates this problem (Figure 42-9). Pulse oximetry is helpful to monitor oxygen saturation during an attack (Schweich, 1994).

Dehydration occurs rapidly in children during an asthma attack from decreased oral intake (children stop drinking because they are coughing or coughing makes them vomit and parents stop offering fluid) and increased insensible loss from tachypnea. If theophylline is administered, its diuretic effect contributes to fluid loss. Dehydration leads to increased mucus plugging and further airway obstruction. Encourage children to continue to drink oral fluid (ask what are favorite beverages and offer small sips of them). Avoid milk or milk products because they cause thick mucus and difficulty swallowing. In an emergency setting, an intravenous line will be established to supply continuous fluid therapy.

Following the initial therapy, aminophylline (the intravenous form of theophylline) or a corticosteroid such as methyl prednisolone may be also prescribed. The biggest problem children who are kept on corticosteroid therapy for long periods face is that their growth may be stunted. Prednisone given every other day seems to affect growth less than prednisone given every day. Those

children who have a large amount of secretions may need postural drainage daily (see Figure 40-11).

Nursing Diagnoses and Related Interventions

> ***Nursing Diagnosis:*** Fear related to sudden onset of asthma attack
>
> ***Goal:*** Parents and child will demonstrate ability to manage sudden attacks within 1 month.
>
> ***Outcome Criteria:*** Parents and child express confidence in their ability to prevent attacks and handle any that occur.

Asthma is a frightening disease. Parents may be afraid to allow children to attend school for fear that they will have an attack while in school and that they will not receive proper treatment there. Parents may be afraid to leave them alone with baby sitters or even relatives so that they may have evenings to themselves or enjoy a vacation. Help parents to allow a child enough freedom for growth and development while still being certain that he or she is safe ("Helping Your Child," 1991).

> ***Nursing Diagnosis:*** Health-seeking behaviors related to prevention of and treatment for asthma attacks
>
> ***Goal:*** Parents and child within 1 month will demonstrate understanding of ways to prevent attacks and measures to manage attacks when they occur.

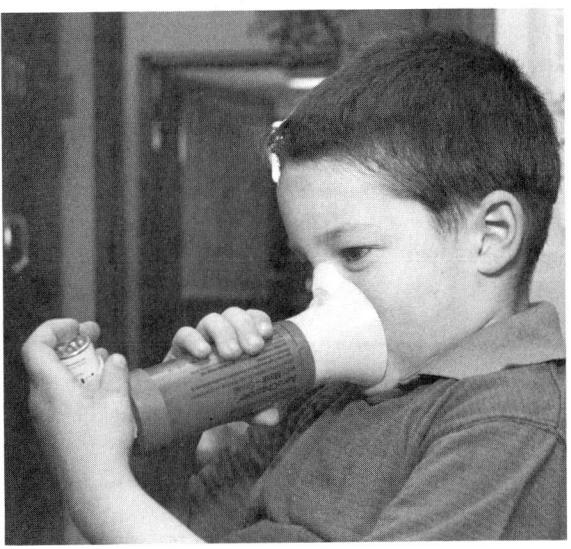

FIGURE 42-9
Many children with asthma use a metered dose inhaler to administer a bronchodilator to themselves. Be certain children respect such medicine as medicine and thus use sensible precautions. Younger children need a "spacer" with inhalers so they do not need to correlate administration with inhalation. (Courtesy of the Department of Medical Photography, Children's Hospital, Buffalo, NY.)

Outcome Criteria: Parents and child accurately state dietary restrictions; child correctly demonstrates breathing exercises and use of inhaler.

Children need to learn to be responsible for their own diets if there are foods they must avoid. Children as young as age 6 years can learn the foods they cannot eat. They may not understand why they cannot eat them, but they must take the responsibility to tell a friend's parent or a schoolteacher that they must not eat certain foods. They must learn to use a metered dose inhaler if that is prescribed for them. At the same time, they must not become inhaler dependent or carry the inhaler with them constantly, afraid to go anywhere without it. This will invariably result in their using the inhaler much more often than is necessary.

To prevent children with asthma from losing chest mobility and to decrease their tendency to develop a "barrel chest," they frequently are taught a number of breathing or mobility exercises to do daily at home. Mobility exercises consist of such activities as bending side to side, bending forward and touching the left foot with the right hand and swinging the arms rhythmically in front of the body like a windmill. These keep chest muscles supple.

Breathing exercises are aimed at increasing expiratory function (diaphragmatic or side-expansion breathing). These exercises can be incorporated into a bedtime or after-school routine. Parents (and nurses) who do the mobility exercises with the children find that the exercises help to reduce abdominal size, because they tighten abdominal muscles as well.

If a child will be receiving epinephrine to relieve acute attacks, parents of the child as well as the child as soon as he or she is old enough (age 9 to 10 years) must be taught how to administer this injection. Parents and the child both need enough practice so that they can do this comfortably in an emergency when their coordination and their thinking processes are not at their best. This is an excellent thing to review with parents at health maintenance visits. When the nurse teaches the parents of a child with diabetes mellitus to give an insulin injection, these parents then go home and do it every day and quickly become as competent as the nurse at giving injections. The parents of a child with asthma may only use this injection skill once in 3 months, many only once a year or once every 3 years. Thus, they need to review and practice the skill (e.g., injecting into an orange) at periodic visits.

The prognosis in children who develop asthma is good. The majority of them will be symptom-free as adults, probably because the lumen of major airways enlarges with adulthood; a small number will continue to have symptoms that they can control without loss of work time or activities; an even smaller proportion will continue to have asthma symptoms severe enough to incapacitate them (see the Focus on Nursing Research box).

In informing parents of these facts, be certain not to convey the impression that asthma is a disease that is outgrown. Although asthma may not always last into adulthood, the need for careful environmental control, conscientious administration of medication, and hyposensitization during childhood should not be diminished (see the Nursing Care Plan, p. 1294).

Status Asthmaticus

Under ordinary circumstances, an asthma attack responds readily to the aerosol administration of a bronchodilator such as albuterol. When children fail to respond and an attack continues, they are in status asthmaticus. This is an extreme emergency because if the attack cannot be relieved, the child will die from heart failure due to exhaustion, atelectasis, or respiratory acidosis from bronchial plugging.

Assessment

Status asthmaticus is often caused by pulmonary infection, which acts as the triggering mechanism for the prolonged attack. Cultures should be obtained from coughed sputum, and a broad-spectrum antibiotic will be ordered until the cultures are returned. Be sure the sputum obtained for culture is coughed from deep in the respiratory tract and not just from the back of the throat.

FOCUS ON NURSING RESEARCH

What Are the Needs of Chronically Ill Adolescents?

To answer this question, 24 adolescents cared for at a university health care center who had long-term conditions such as asthma were asked to identify what they viewed as their primary health care needs or concerns. The mean age of the sample group was 15.4 years; 14 members of the group were female and 10 members were male.

Those concerns identified by over 50% of the sample group were: "bored a lot," "wonder how my illness will affect me when I get older," "not able to do the things my friends do," "worried about my health," and "a lot of headaches."

The researcher stresses that these concerns may lead to depression (or result from depression already present). Helping adolescents with chronic illnesses define their fears and concerns might be a way to help them deal with or avoid depression about having a chronic illness.

Dragone, M. A. (1990). Perspectives of chronically ill adolescents and parents on health care needs. *Pediatric Nursing, 16,* 45.

Therapeutic Management

The child in status asthmaticus needs oxygen to reduce cyanosis and dyspnea. This is best given by face mask or nasal prongs in an emergency situation because these methods supply good oxygen concentrations and yet leave the child unobscured. To prevent drying of pulmonary secretions, oxygen must be given with humidification. Oxygen is best administered at a concentration of 30% to 40%, not 100%. Some children in severe status asthmaticus have such a carbon dioxide buildup (because they cannot exhale properly) that they develop carbon dioxide narcosis with no stimulation for inhalation. The child's respiratory stimulus, therefore, is hypoxia, or lack of oxygen. If 100% oxygen were administered, the oxygen lack would disappear and respirations would cease. The idea "if a little is good, a lot is better" does not apply here. After it has been ascertained that the child is not in acidosis (from blood gas and *p*H studies), oxygen levels may be increased, but, for initial therapy, keep the level at 30% to 40%.

By definition, the child in status asthmaticus has failed to respond to first-line therapy. Therefore, other drugs must be given in an attempt to cause bronchodilation. Epinephrine may be injected subcutaneously. Aminophylline, 4 to 6 mg/kg per body weight, given intravenously over 10 to 20 minutes, is also generally effective. Observe the child's respiratory rate and appearance (e.g., retractions, effort, nasal flaring, or inspiratory/expiratory ratio); auscultate for wheezing; and take blood pressure and pulse rate. Assist with blood gases as necessary. The chief danger with aminophylline is overadministration. Before any is given in an emergency room, be sure to ask the parents if they administered theophylline at home. If the child is becoming acidotic, sodium bicarbonate may be given intravenously. As soon as the acidosis is corrected, the child may respond to epinephrine again. Corticosteroids may give prompt relief in status asthmaticus. This is mostly true in children who are on continuous steroid therapy or who have been on it in the past.

Following an acute stage of status asthmaticus, children need increased fluid to keep airway secretions moist. Drinking tends to aggravate coughing, so they are unlikely to drink and they are often dehydrated on admission to the hospital. An intravenous infusion of 5% glucose in 0.45 saline is started to supply fluid. If the child is able to drink, do not offer cold fluids because these tend to aggravate bronchospasm. Also, the child should not be given any cough suppressants. As long as they continue to cough up mucus, they are not in serious danger. When they stop coughing up mucus, it forms thick mucus plugs that lead to pneumonia, atelectasis, and acidosis. Monitor intake and output; measure the specific gravity of urine. Under stress, antidiuretic hormone is released so fluid retention and overhydration may occur.

The Po_2 level is maintained at more than 60 mm Hg; an increasing Pco_2 level is a danger sign because it indicates the degree of hypoventilation. In severe attacks, ventilation with a respirator may be necessary to maintain effective respirations.

Nursing Diagnoses and Related Interventions

Nursing Diagnosis: Anxiety related to unrelenting respiratory distress and associated fatigue

Goal: Child will experience reduction of fatigue and anxiety by 1 hour.

Outcome Criteria: Child states ability to rest comfortably; states confidence in health care providers to stop attack.

Children need as much rest as possible to eliminate fatigue. This must be provided by allowing them to rest in an upright position. If they are admitted to a hospital unit, elevate the head of the bed. If they are in an emergency room, and the head of the examining table does not elevate, position the table against the wall so that they can rest against the wall for support, or have them sit upright supported by a parent or an aide.

Sedation may be ordered for the child who is hysterical from anxiety, but as a rule psychological assurance is preferable to sedation. Excessive sedation will make it difficult for the child to raise mucus. Thus, children need to have reassuring people around them, people who exude confidence that they are all right despite the respiratory distress.

Children having an asthma attack are so anxious and desperate that it is easy for them to communicate their anxiety to the people around them. Parents often need as much support in an emergency as the children. Be certain not to allow a child's anxiety and fright to interfere with the ability to act as a support person. Appreciate and respect children's fear, but do not spread it further.

Drug and Food Allergies

Drug Allergies

One of the hazards of giving any medication is the danger that a child may experience a reaction to it or exhibit allergic symptoms. Because reactions to drugs differ, it is important to be familiar with whether a child is showing symptoms of an allergic reaction, a toxic reaction, or a known side effect to a drug.

A *toxic reaction* is one that occurs when a child has received too much of a drug. *Side effects* of drugs are those effects that are known to occur in addition to a

(text continues on page 1296)

Nursing Care Plan
The Child With Asthma

Mandy is a 9-year-old admitted with asthma. The following is a nursing care plan devised for her.

Assessment: Mother states child had mild cold symptoms yesterday and today. At 3 PM, child came home from school with audible wheezing (had stopped on way home to play with a cat, although she is allergic to them). Mother administered usual medication (Quibron) with no relief. Child was breathing too rapidly to drink. Vomited small amount of medicine-stained, clear fluid. Seen in emergency room here; was administered terbutaline by nebulizer with minimal relief. Child disappointed because she was to be in a school play tomorrow. Mother concerned but also angry that child was so irresponsible with cat. Respiratory rate: 60 breaths/min. Wheezing present in all lobes by auscultation. Appears exhausted from breathing effort; blood gases drawn but not available yet. Intravenous line in place in left hand. D5½ NS infusing well at 50 mL/h.

Nursing Diagnosis: Ineffective airway clearance related to bronchospasm

Defining Characteristic: Child has wheezing and respiratory rate of 60 breaths/min.

Goal: Child will demonstrate relief from major symptoms within 1 hour.

Outcome Criteria: Respiratory rate is reduced to 20 breaths/min with minimal wheezing.

Nursing Orders

1. Maintain D5½ NS solution until child voids, then change to T5#2 at 30 mL/h as per physician's order. Keep nothing by mouth status.
2. Assess for cyanosis, pulse rate, and respiratory rate every 15 min. Assess blood pressure every 30 min. Assess temperature and auscultate chest every 1 h including lung sounds, depth of respirations, presence of retractions, nasal flaring, and inspiratory/expiratory ratio. Assist with blood gases as necessary. Prepare child for pulmonary function tests and assist as necessary.
3. Administer oxygen at 4 L by face mask (very resistant to nasal prongs).
4. Administer Solu-Medrol 30 mg IV and aminophylline 140 mg IV every 6 hours per MD order.
5. Maintain upright position by pillows and gatch bed.
6. Terbutaline therapy to be provided by inhalation therapist every 4 h. Assist with administration as necessary.
7. Give assurance that respiratory ability will soon improve and she will breathe more easily.
8. Perform (or teach parents to perform) postural drainage.

Rationale

1. Dehydration is likely to occur due to insensible loss from tachypnea as well as vomiting episode unless steps are taken to rehydrate the child.
2. It is essential to monitor for improving (or declining) respiratory function.

3. The face mask is an acceptable source of oxygen for this child.
4. Anti-inflammatory and bronchodilator agents can enlarge lumen of airway.
5. An upright position can ease breathing.
6. Bronchodilatation will continue to enlarge lumen of airway.
7. Relieving anxiety can help to slow respiratory rate.
8. Postural drainage will help to remove excess secretions from the bronchial passages to clear airway.

Nursing Diagnosis: Knowledge deficit related to cause of asthma

Defining Characteristic: Child played with a cat without concern of potential allergenic effects.

Goal: Child will demonstrate increased level of knowledge of asthma's cause and ways to prevent attacks by time of hospital discharge.

Outcome Criteria: Child voices that asthma symptoms occur from exposure to allergens.

(continued)

Nursing Orders

1. Obtain history.

2. Assist with sensitization testing as necessary.
3. Discuss effect of cat hair allergy on airway with Mandy when she has improved.

4. Discuss with mother that cats are attractive animals to children and so such incidents do occur.

Rationale

1. Identifies known allergens and family history of allergies.
2. Sensitization can help identify allergens.
3. Understanding how the cat hair can trigger an allergic reaction may help Mandy remember that cats are to be avoided the next time she sees one.
4. Promotes parental understanding of child's growth and development.

Nursing Diagnosis: High risk for anxiety related to severity of symptoms

Defining Characteristic: Shortness of breath is an anxiety-producing sensation.

Goal: Child's and parent's level of anxiety will be within controllable level within 24 hours.

Outcome Criteria: Child and parents voice that they are able to cope with present level of anxiety.

Nursing Orders

1. Provide explanation of procedures; teach cause and effect of disease.
2. Remain with child while she is having respiratory distress.
3. Encourage parents to provide care.

4. Encourage parents and child to discuss the effects of a long term and potentially frightening illness on their family life.
5. Refer parents to organizations devoted to sharing experiences and learning more about allergies.

Rationale

1. Increased knowledge of disease can reduce anxiety.

2. Assures child that she will not be left alone when ill.
3. Parents can serve as important support for hospitalized children; their presence is reassuring.
4. Better understanding of stress can help relieve anxiety.

5. Support groups can serve as important sources of support in times of stress.

Nursing Diagnosis: High risk for fluid volume deficit related to inability to take oral fluid

Defining Characteristic: Rapid breathing increases fluid loss and makes ingesting fluids difficult.

Goal: Child will maintain an adequate fluid intake during asthma attack.

Outcome Criteria: Child's skin turgor is good; is able to cough and expectorate secretions.

Nursing Orders

1. Encourage fluids when able to take orally.

2. Maintain and monitor IV infusion carefully.

3. Measure intake and output and specific gravity of urine.
4. When able, encourage child to eat a balanced, nutritious diet.

Rationale

1. Adequate fluid helps to keep airway secretions moist.
2. Protects against infiltration and assures administration of adequate fluid.
3. Documents that fluid intake is adequate.

4. Restores nutrients lost while NPO.

therapeutic effect. When an *allergic effect* occurs, unpredictable symptoms occur. The drug itself may not be an allergen, but when the drug combines with body protein, it becomes an allergen. This is why allergic responses occur not with the initial administration of a drug but only after the protein interaction (hapten formation or sensitivity) has occurred. When drugs are applied to skin or mucous membrane, the chance of drug allergy is most often encountered. It occurs most rarely in orally administered drugs. Children with atopic diseases appear to be most prone to having drug allergic reactions, although any person can show such a reaction.

Reactions to drugs differ, but skin manifestations seen frequently are urticaria, angioedema, allergic contact dermatitis, pruritus, and purpura. Respiratory symptoms may be asthma or rhinitis. There may be thrombocytopenia and hemolytic anemia. Anaphylactic shock and serum sickness may occur. Children with a known drug allergy should wear a medical identification bracelet indicating the drug to which they are sensitive. Some children feel these make them look conspicuous and need counseling on the importance of their safety.

A number of drugs used with children that are frequently involved in allergic reactions are discussed in the following sections. In most instances, just discontinuing the drug is the only therapy needed. In instances when urticaria or serum sickness has resulted, an antihistamine (such as diphenhydramine hydrochloride [Benadryl]) is needed to relieve the symptoms. If anaphylaxis resulted, the treatment would be the same as for any anaphylaxis.

Penicillin

Penicillin reactions occur almost entirely from parenteral injections, not oral administration. Urticaria and serum sickness are the symptoms that become evident. Anaphylactic shock from penicillin sensitivity is so severe it is often fatal before help can reach the child. Children who are allergic to one form of penicillin are generally allergic to all forms. Ampicillin is a synthetic penicillin and so may generally be given to children who are allergic to regular penicillin. It is advisable to check with a physician before administering it to children allergic to penicillin, however.

Be certain before administering penicillin to ask a child or parents, or both (depending on the child's age), if there is any reason to think the child is allergic to penicillin. If the child has exhibited symptoms in the past after receiving penicillin, do not give any until a physician can decide if those symptoms seem to indicate an allergic response. Many parents worry that children with penicillin allergies will be without antibiotic protection because of the allergy. Assure them that other drugs such as erythromycin, a broad-spectrum antibiotic, will protect children equally well in most instances.

Aspirin (Acetylsalicylic Acid)

Aspirin allergy is generally manifested as urticaria and asthma symptoms. This form of asthma is intractable, so children must not be given aspirin again once they demonstrate an allergy. An analgesic medication they can take, however, is acetaminophen (Tylenol) or propoxyphene (Darvon). Darvon must be plain, not Darvon compound, because the compound contains aspirin.

Vaccines

When a vaccine grown in egg media is injected into extremely egg-sensitive individuals, urticaria or anaphylactic shock may result. The vaccines in current use that are prepared from egg yolks are types of rubella and mumps vaccines.

If children are allergic to horse serum, they cannot receive the antitoxins prepared from a horse-serum base. These antitoxins are diphtheria and tetanus antitoxins. The use of these two compounds will never be required in children if their immunizations for diphtheria and tetanus are kept current. It is important for parents to understand that it is the antitoxin that their child cannot receive. Otherwise, they will not allow children to have normal immunizations. (Immunizations and specific vaccines are discussed in Chapter 43.)

Food Allergies

Food allergies manifest themselves differently from one child to another, but urticaria, angioedema, pruritus, stomach pain, respiratory symptoms, and atopic dermatitis are common symptoms.

A symptom such as urticaria begins to manifest itself only minutes after an offending food is eaten. Other symptoms may be delayed, making the offending food difficult to recognize. Whole protein is probably the cause of immediate reactions, whereas delayed reactions are a sensitivity to some protein breakdown product.

Skin testing is unreliable with food allergies because it is done with whole protein extracts; delayed reactions, therefore, will not be detected this way. The most common foods that cause immediate allergy symptoms are egg white, fish and other seafood, berries, and nuts. Delayed food reactions are caused by cereals (wheat and corn); milk; chocolate; pork; legumes; white potatoes; beef; food additives and colorings; and oranges. If children are allergic to milk, they are probably allergic to milk products as well. Children who are allergic to eggs often cannot eat any foods that contain egg, such as pudding or baked goods.

Assessment

Children with food allergies are often reported as being "fussy eaters." Young children are unable to describe why they do not enjoy eating because they do not have the word for "headache," "stomachache," or "itchiness," but they tend to avoid those foods that so affect them. However, this is not diagnostic of food allergies because children may refuse to eat foods as a form of toddler rebellion or may be reported as fussy eaters because parents are expecting them to eat more than their small size requires.

Therapeutic Management

Although not well documented, there is increasing evidence that some children with food allergies become hyperactive (unable to sit through a whole meal or the time it takes to listen to a favorite story) following ingestion of a food to which they are allergic. Some children may become aggressive or manifest behavioral problems in school after eating such a food. The foods that tend to cause these behavior changes most frequently are sugar, milk, wheat, and food colorings.

A food diary, which is a record of everything the child eats each day, kept by the child or a parent, may be the best way to spot offending foods. Each day is rated as either symptom free or a day when symptoms were strongly evident. A food that is found on lists when symptoms were few, but not on days when the child is in distress, is not an offending food. A food that appears only on "bad days," however, is strongly suspect as an allergen.

An elimination diet is another method used to detect food allergens. For this, parents are given a list of a few foods that are rarely causes of allergy, such as rice, lamb, carrots, peas, and sweet potatoes. One by one, at 2-day to 3-day intervals, foods that are suspected of causing allergy are added to the child's diet. When a food is introduced this way, the child must be encouraged to eat a lot of it that day. If symptoms occur, the food will be eliminated from the child's diet on a permanent basis. If no symptoms occur, the child can continue to eat the food.

The treatment of food allergy is to eliminate offending foods from the child's diet. This is relatively easy to do if there are only a small number of offending foods. It becomes exceedingly difficult when the foods are great in number or, like milk, wheat, or eggs, are found in a great many products. The parents of children with food allergies must learn to be careful shoppers, reading labels carefully to be certain that the foods they are buying do not contain products to which their child is sensitive.

Milk Allergy

The true incidence of milk allergy is probably not as high as the number of diagnoses made. Milk allergy is typified by failure to gain weight, diarrhea, perhaps vomiting, and abdominal pain. These symptoms may also occur in a gastroenteritis infection. Some infants with colic (characterized by abdominal pain, no change in stools, and no failure to gain weight) or those with lactase deficiency (they cannot ingest the lactose in milk) may also be incorrectly diagnosed as having a milk allergy. If milk allergy is suspected, children are placed on a casein hydrolysate formula. When this is done, symptoms are relieved dramatically. To establish whether the cause of the problem was truly a milk allergy, milk should be reintroduced again at a later date. If the problem was a true milk allergy, signs will recur at this reintroduction to milk.

Stinging Insect Allergy

Children may have severe hypersensitivity reactions to stings from bees, wasps, hornets, or yellow jackets. Although a serum sickness reaction may occur, the usual reaction to these stings is an immediate hypersensitivity reaction (anaphylaxis). The peak season for insect stings is August, and more boys than girls have allergic reactions to insect stings.

Assessment

The first time a child is stung, the total reaction is probably only local edema at the site. The second time, there may be generalized urticaria, pruritus, and edema. The third time, symptoms may progress to wheezing and dyspnea. The next time, the reaction could be so severe there is instant shock and death. The progression of symptoms may be slower than this (involving 10 to 12 stings); if the stings are received close together (1 day or 2 days apart, or even 3 weeks apart) the progression to fatal symptoms may be present as early as the second or third exposure.

The time interval between the fatal sting and death is extremely short, approximately 10 minutes. These children must be identified and given medication to combat shock immediately (there is not time to transport them for emergency care).

Therapeutic Management

The best way to protect children with allergies to stinging insects is to administer hyposensitization against insect stings following the first reaction (Reisman, 1992). An extract of wasp, yellow jacket, hornet, and honey bee is effective.

The child who has not been hyposensitized must be treated immediately following the sting. Pressurized aerosol inhalers containing epinephrine are effective; they give rapid relief and are easily administered while the child is transported to a health care facility for care.

Some children have such an intense reaction that subcutaneous administration of epinephrine is necessary to combat symptoms. If children are going on a hiking or camping expedition away from parents, they will need to be able to administer this to themselves. Someone at school should be given the responsibility of administering this if the child is stung during a recess or outside gym period. If a school nurse is in attendance, this certainly is his or her job. In schools where there is no full-time nurse, another person must be designated and taught how to give the injection. If children have antihistamine medication, this should be given also. Ice applied to the site minimizes the amount of venom absorbed; a tourniquet applied proximal to the sting may also retard absorption. The child should then be transported to the nearest hospital in case additional epinephrine is needed (the effectiveness of the initial injection will last only approximately 20 minutes).

Teach children who are allergic to stinging insects not to wear scented preparations such as hair spray or perfume because these attract bees and wasps. They should not go outside barefoot because bees are often found in ground clover. They should not be assigned such household chores as mowing the lawn or weeding flowers, which might stir up bees. Because insects tend to cluster around garbage containers, taking out the trash or garbage is also an inappropriate chore for these children. They should have a fast-acting insecticide handy when out of doors to use on flying insects that approach them.

Contact Dermatitis

Contact dermatitis is an example of a delayed or type IV hypersensitivity response; it is a reaction to skin contact with an allergen (a substance irritating only to the child with prior sensitization). The first reaction is generally erythema. Papules develop next, then vesicles. Pruritus is intense. The allergen is often suggested by the part of the child's body that is affected. Allergy to cosmetics, for example, appears on the face of the child at puberty when the child begins to use these compounds; oozing at the site of pierced ears suggests an allergy to the nickel used in earring posts; dermatitis from a diaper-washing compound appears in the diaper area; poison ivy appears on the hands and arms where the child brushed against the plant (Figure 42-10). A number of health care providers are developing reactions to latex gloves (Barton, 1993).

Assessment

Patch testing may be used to identify contact dermatitis allergens. For this, the skin of the upper arm is washed with alcohol and dried. A drop or two of the suspected

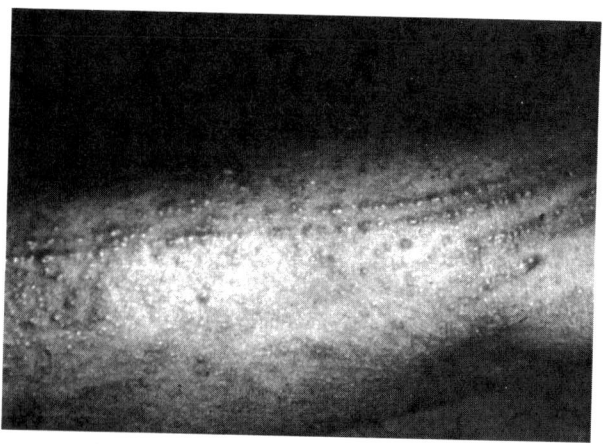

FIGURE 42-10
The lesions of poison ivy. Note the linear distribution. (Courtesy of the Centers for Disease Control, Atlanta, GA.)

allergen is placed on the skin; the site is covered by a gauze square, which is left in place for 48 hours. A child should not take adrenocorticotropic hormone or a corticosteroid at the time of patch testing because these drugs reduce delayed hypersensitivity reactions. However, a child may take antihistamines or sympatheticomimetic drugs because these do not interfere with delayed reactions. After 48 hours, the patches are removed and the reactions are graded 1+ to 4+, the same as in regular skin testing.

Therapeutic Management

Treatment for contact dermatitis consists of removing the identified allergen from the child's environment. In children, this is generally not difficult to do. In adults, because allergens are often job related, this is much more difficult.

For the reaction when it is present, dressings wet with water, saline, or Burow's solution relieve itching. Calamine lotion is a standby that is also generally effective. Corticosteroid lotions or creams reduce itching and also promote healing. Baths with baking soda or oatmeal in the water may be helpful if a large area of the child's body is involved. Some children need a sedative ordered to relieve their discomfort during the period of intense pruritus.

Key Points

- An antigen is a foreign substance capable of stimulating an immune response. The immune system protects the body from invasion by foreign substances by leukocyte activity.
- Humoral immunity refers to immunity created by antibody production. B cells are involved in this type of reaction.

- Autoimmunity results from an inability to distinguish self from nonself, causing the immune system to carry out immune responses against normal cells.
- Immunodeficiency disorders can be primary such as B-cell and T-cell deficiencies or secondary such as acquired immunodeficiency syndrome (AIDS). AIDS is spread by the retrovirus HIV through blood and body secretions. By following universal precautions, health care personnel can prevent the spread of this illness in the hospital setting.
- Allergic disorders occur as a result of an abnormal antigen-antibody response. About 1 in every 5 children suffer from some form of allergy.
- Immune disorders, as a category, are long-term disorders, and children must participate in their own care in order to remain well (avoiding allergens or a child at school with an infection, for example). Involving children from the start helps them achieve an active role in their own care.
- Anaphylactic shock is an acute reaction characterized by extreme vasodilation and circulatory shock. Know the procedure for care at your care site so you can act quickly to alleviate symptoms if this happens.
- Environmental control refers to ways to reduce the number of allergens to which children are exposed. Hyposensitization is increasing the plasma concentration of IgG antibodies to prevent or block IgE antibody formation and allergic symptoms.
- Atopic disorders include hay fever (allergic rhinitis), atopic dermatitis, and asthma.
- Asthma is a diffuse obstructive disease of the airway. Parents of children with asthma need to be well informed about emergency measures to take during an acute attack. Review these measures with them at health assessments, particularly if they will be administering an injection, so they remain well prepared to act in an emergency. Nursing diagnoses commonly identified for children with asthma include Fear, Health-seeking behaviors, and High risk for ineffective airway clearance.
- Promoting breastfeeding may be a prime intervention to help prevent allergies in allergy-prone families.

Critical Thinking Exercises

1. Jose is a 4-year-old who has a primary B-cell immune deficiency. His teacher calls you; she is afraid to have him in her classroom because he will spread the HIV virus to classmates. What would you want to explain to Jose's teacher about immune deficiency disorders?
2. Ellen is a 10-year-old who has allergic rhinitis (hay fever). She notices symptoms most strongly in the late spring while in school. What environmental control measures would you suggest to her parents to improve her symptoms?
3. Samuel is a 12-year-old with asthma you care for in the emergency room. His mother states the first thing she did when Samuel became ill was to bring him to the hospital even though she had been taught to inject epinephrine possibly to prevent a hospital admission. Why do you think the mother reacted this way? What steps could you take to help the mother follow a specified emergency protocol next time?

References

Barton, E. C. (1993). Latex allergy: Recognition and management of a modern problem. *Nurse Practitioner, 18,* 54.

Belcher, E. A. (1993). Prevention of childhood diseases through vaccination. *Neonatal Network, 12,* 35.

Borkowsky, W., & Wilfert, C. M. (1992). Acquired immune syndrome. In S. Krugman et al. *Infectious diseases in children.* St. Louis: Mosby.

Caldwell, M. B., & Rogers, M. F. (1991). Epidemiology of pediatric HIV infection. *Pediatric Clinics of North America, 38,* 1.

Clark, P. J., et al. (1993). Clinical issues in long-term pediatric HIV disease. *MCN: American Journal of Maternal Child Nursing, 18,* 164.

Department of Health & Human Services. (1991). *Healthy people 2000.* Washington, DC: Public Health Service.

Eggleston, P. A. (1994). Asthma. In F. A. Oski et al. *Principles and practice of pediatrics.* Philadelphia: J.B. Lippincott.

Ghosh, S., et al. (1993). Urticaria in children. *Pediatric Dermatology, 10,* 107.

Gutman, L. T. (1991). Human immune virus transmission by sexual abuse. *American Journal of Diseases of Children, 145,* 137.

Helping your child live with asthma. (1991). *Patient Care, 25,* 151.

Krasinski, K., & Borkowsky, W. (1991). Laboratory diagnosis of HIV infection. *Pediatric Clinics of North America, 38,* 17.

Meyers, A., & Weitzman, M. (1991). Pediatric HIV disease: The newest chronic illness of childhood. *Pediatric Clinics of North America, 38:* 169.

O'Neill, S. P. (1990). Anaphylactic shock. *American Journal of Nursing, 90,* 40.

Reisman, R. E. (1992). Stinging insect allergy. *Medical Clinics of North America, 76,* 883.

Sampson, H. A., & Eggleston, P. A. (1994). Allergy. In F. A. Oski et al. *Principles and practice of pediatrics.* Philadelphia: J.B. Lippincott.

Sanders-Laufer, D., et al. (1991). *Pneumocystis carinii* infections in HIV-infected children. *Pediatric Clinics of North America, 38,* 39.

Schweich, P. J. (1994). Emergency medicine except poisoning. In F. A. Oski et al. *Principles and practice of pediatrics.* Philadelphia: J.B. Lippincott.

Scott, G. B., & Parks, W. P. (1994). Pediatric AIDS. In F. A. Oski et al. *Principles and practice of pediatrics.* Philadelphia: J.B. Lippincott.

Tunnessen, W. W. (1994). Pediatric dermatology. In F. A. Oski et al. *Principles and practice of pediatrics.* Philadelphia: J.B. Lippincott.

Vuurman, E. F., et al. (1993). Seasonal allergic rhinitis and antihistamine effects on children's learning. *Annals of Allergy, 71,* 121.

Zwetchkenbaum, J. F. (1990). Hypogammaglobulinemia. *Annals of Allergy, 65,* 361.

Suggested Readings

Bobo, J. K., et al. (1993). Risk factors for delayed immunization in a random sample of 1163 children from Oregon and Washington. *Pediatrics, 91,* 308.

Boland, M. G., et al. (1991). Starting life with HIV. *RN, 54,* 54.

Bradford, B. J. (1991). Immunization: A 1991 update. *Journal of School Nursing, 7,* 18.

Burroughs, M. H., & Edelson, P. J. (1991). Medical care of the HIV-infected child. *Pediatric Clinics of North America, 38,* 45.

Businco, L., et al. (1993). Is prevention of food allergy worth-while? *Journal of Investigative Allergology and Clinical Immunology, 3,* 231.

Cox, K., et al. (1993). A creative approach to adolescent HIV. *AIDS Patient Care, 7,* 16.

Newacheck, P. W., & Stoddard, J. J. (1994). Prevalence and impact of multiple childhood chronic illnesses. *Journal of Pediatrics, 124,* 40.

Strudley, M., et al. (1990). Asthma in the classroom. *Nursing Standard, 5,* 49.

Tully, M. R. (1990). Banked human milk in the treatment of IgA deficiency and allergy symptoms. *Journal of Human Lactation, 6,* 75.

Vickers, P. (1990). Severe combined immunodeficiency syndrome. *Nursing, 4,* 32.

Chapter 43

Nursing Care of the Child With an Infectious Disorder

Key Terms

- anaerobic
- antitoxin
- chain of infection
- communicability
- complement
- convalescent period
- enanthem
- exanthem
- fomites
- gamma globulin
- immune serum
- incubation period
- interferon
- Koplik's spots
- means of transmission
- pathogen
- portal of entry
- portal of exit
- prodromal period
- reservoir
- septicemia
- susceptible host
- toxoid

Objectives

After mastering the contents of this chapter, you should be able to:

1. Describe the causes and course of common infectious disorders of childhood.

2. Assess the child with infection such as the common exanthems.

3. Formulate nursing diagnoses related to infection in children.

4. Plan nursing care, such as how to relieve the discomfort of a rash, for the child with an infection.

5. Implement nursing care specific to the child with an infection (e.g., administer an antibiotic intravenously).

6. Evaluate outcome criteria to be certain that nursing goals for care of the child with an infection have been achieved.

7. Identify National Health Goals related to infectious disorders and children that nurses could be instrumental in helping the nation achieve.

8. Identify areas of nursing care related to children with infectious disease that could benefit from additional nursing research.

9. Use critical thinking to analyze ways that care of the child with an infection can be more family centered.

10. Synthesize knowledge of infectious diseases and nursing process to achieve quality maternal and child health nursing care.

Adele Pillitteri: MATERNAL AND CHILD HEALTH NURSING, 2nd Edition. © 1995 Adele Pillitteri.

*I*nfectious disease is a leading cause of mortality in children and accounts for approximately 50% of all visits to child health settings. Nurses must be able to identify the symptoms of common infectious diseases of childhood because they occur so frequently and because nurses are often the first to see evidence of infection. For example, a school nurse is asked to be an expert on screening and isolating children who have potentially contagious infections such as chickenpox or measles. In health care settings, a nurse often performs triage, identifying children who must be seen immediately, those

who can wait to be seen, and those who should not stay in a waiting room because they may have an infectious disease. Occasionally, children admitted to an in-service unit for emergency care or surgery will break out in a rash soon after admission. If, for example, the rash begins as macular, then quickly becomes papular, and then vesicular and crusting, it is vital that the nurse quickly recognize the pattern of this exanthem as varicella (chickenpox) so that the child can be isolated and other children in the hospital protected. The varicella virus can be fatal, particularly to children who are receiving corticosteroids. National Health Goals related to infectious disorders and children are shown in the Focus on National Health Goals box.

NURSING PROCESS OVERVIEW
for the Child With an Infectious Disorder

ASSESSMENT

Many infectious diseases begin subtly. Parents report symptoms such as "he doesn't act like himself" or "she's so listless." These changes in behavior may be the first indication of an infectious process at work (Figure 43-1).

A large number of childhood infectious diseases involve an exanthem (a rash). Rashes can be difficult to identify, so it is important to obtain as full a description and history of the rash as possible.

NURSING DIAGNOSIS

Nursing diagnoses for children with infectious disease include:

- Pain (pruritus) related to viral rash
- High risk for infection transmission related to presence of contagious disease
- High risk for infection related to presence of contagious disease in sibling

Additional diagnoses when children must be isolated to prevent infection transmission include:

- Social isolation related to isolation precautions
- High risk for diversional activity deficit related to protective isolation

PLANNING

When planning goals for care, include those goals that help parents prevent another infection as well as help deal with a current infection; for example, teach about necessary vaccinations. Parents will ask about communicability to their other children as well as to the infected child's playmates or schoolmates. Planning care for a child who is in isolation requires thoughtful consideration to prevent boredom. An organization helpful for referral is:

National Foundation for Infectious Diseases
4733 Bethesda Avenue, Suite 750
Bethesda, MD 20814

IMPLEMENTATION

Nursing responsibilities for care of the child with an infection will depend on the setting in which the child is seen. Often, a child will not be brought into a clinic if the disease can be easily identified over the phone; counseling parents about techniques to relieve the irritation of rashes and other symptoms of infectious illness is paramount. Although it is good practice always to follow aseptic technique to prevent the spread of infection, preventing transmission of an infectious illness takes on new importance when a child is known to have a particular disease. Administering antibiotics and being alert for potential adverse effects is another major responsibility of the nurse.

EVALUATION

Evaluation of the child with an infectious disease should include not only whether the child is returning to wellness but whether the child and family have learned more about ways to prevent infectious diseases. If one member of the family is on steroid therapy or has a malfunctioning immune system, disease prevention is extremely important.

FOCUS ON
National Health Goals

Several National Health Goals address the prevention of infectious diseases:

- Increase basic immunization series among children under age 2 and 4 to at least 90% from a baseline of 70% to 80%.

- Increase basic immunization series among children in licensed child care facilities and kindergarten through post-secondary education institutions to at least 95% from baselines of 94% to 97%.

- Reduce postexposure rabies treatments to no more than 9000/year from a baseline of 18,000/year (DHHS, 1991).

Nurses can be instrumental in helping the nation achieve these goals by educating parents about the importance of immunization and actually administering immunizations to infants and children.

Nursing research that could increase understanding in this area includes studies aimed at answering questions such as: How soon in pregnancy are parents interested in learning about the immunizations their child will need? What precautions can summer camps or camp sites take to discourage children from petting wild animals that could be carrying rabies? Should parents be given more responsibility for knowing what and when immunizations are required?

FOCUS ON NURSING ASSESSMENT

History
Chief concern: Does child have a fever, general malaise, vomiting, or diarrhea? Was child recently exposed to someone with an infection?
Past medical history: Are child's immunizations current?

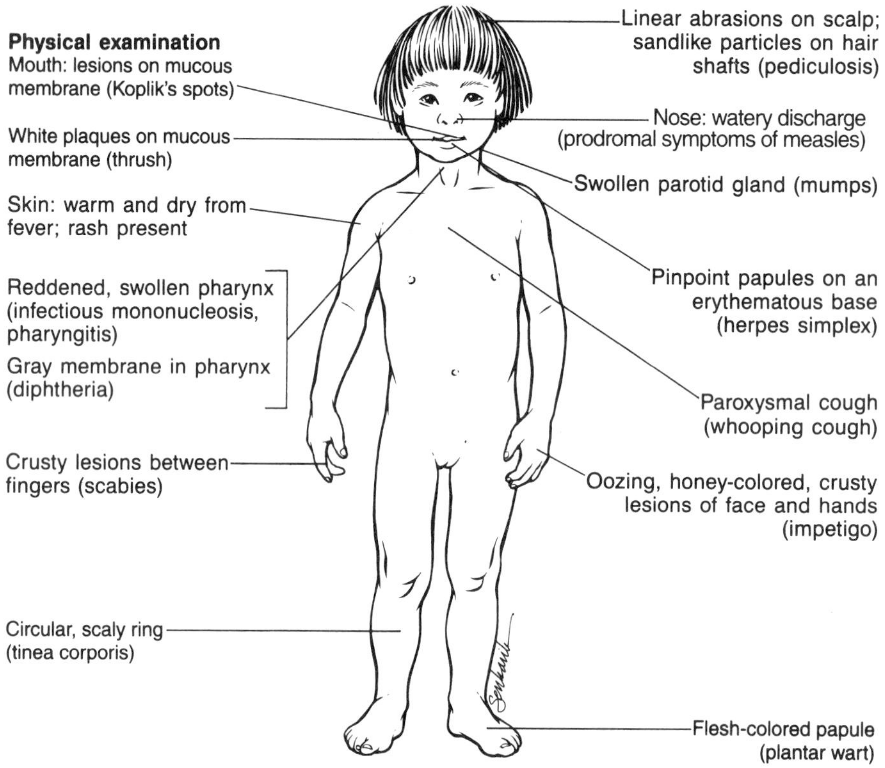

Physical examination
Mouth: lesions on mucous membrane (Koplik's spots)
White plaques on mucous membrane (thrush)
Skin: warm and dry from fever; rash present
Reddened, swollen pharynx (infectious mononucleosis, pharyngitis)
Gray membrane in pharynx (diphtheria)
Crusty lesions between fingers (scabies)
Circular, scaly ring (tinea corporis)
Linear abrasions on scalp; sandlike particles on hair shafts (pediculosis)
Nose: watery discharge (prodromal symptoms of measles)
Swollen parotid gland (mumps)
Pinpoint papules on an erythematous base (herpes simplex)
Paroxysmal cough (whooping cough)
Oozing, honey-colored, crusty lesions of face and hands (impetigo)
Flesh-colored papule (plantar wart)

FIGURE 43-1
Common signs and symptoms of infectious disease in children.

Examples of outcome criteria are:

- Child states pruritus from rash is at tolerable level.
- Sibling does not contract pertussis from sibling.
- Parent names activities he or she has planned to provide diversional activities.

Infectious Process

Organisms that cause disease in children are called **pathogens**. Pathogens can be classified into five types of microorganisms: (1) viruses, (2) bacteria, (3) rickettsiae, (4) helminths, and (5) fungi. The properties of these organisms are discussed in conjunction with the common diseases they cause.

Stages of Infectious Disease

Infectious diseases follow certain stages during which **communicability** (ability to be spread to others) or severity of the illness can be predicted (Figure 43-2). The **incubation period** is the time between the invasion of an organism and the onset of symptoms of infection. During this time, microorganisms grow and multiply. The length of the incubation period varies depending on the pathogen. A common interval is 7 to 10 days, but it can be longer; the incubation period for tetanus, for example, is from 2 to 21 days.

Invasion of organism
Return to wellness
Incubation period
Prodromal period
Clinical signs and symptoms
Convalescent period
Period of communicability

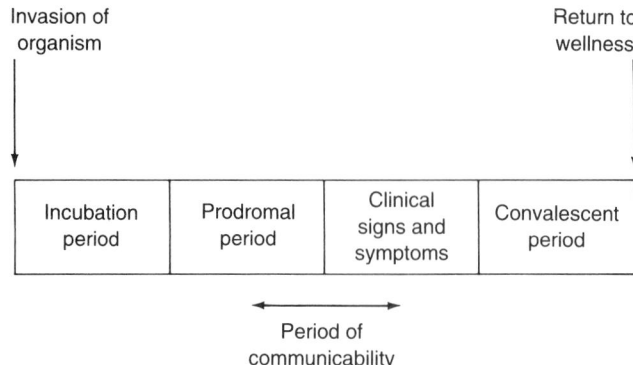

FIGURE 43-2
Time frame for infectious diseases. Period of communicability is the time during which the disease can be transmitted to other people.

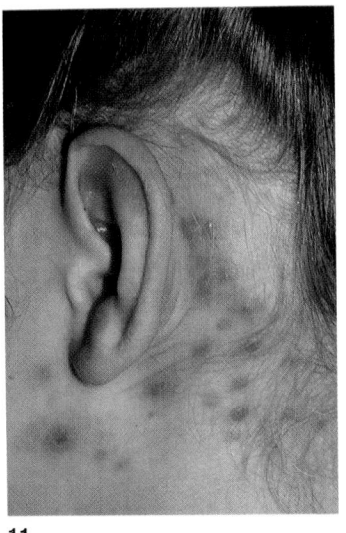

11

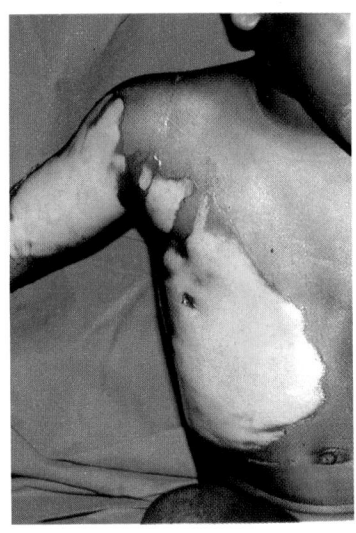

12

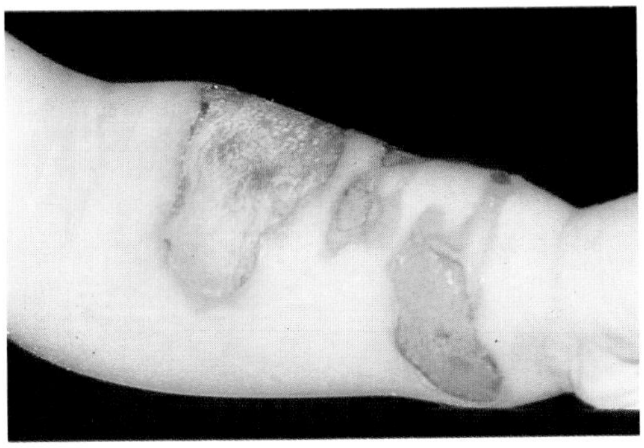

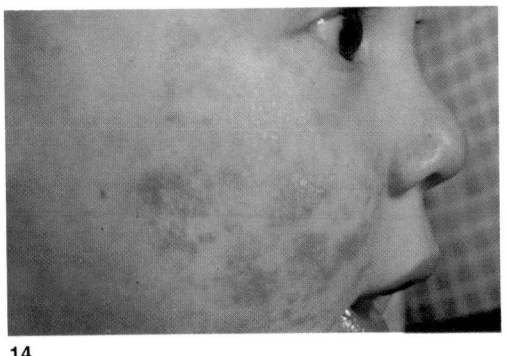

13

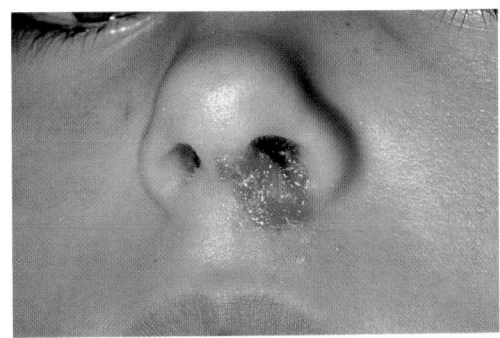

14

15

COLOR PLATE 11. *Child with chicken pox behind the ear.*
COLOR PLATE 12. *Tea scald on upper body of young child.*
COLOR PLATE 13. *Heat burn on infant's arm.*
COLOR PLATE 14. *Baby with eczema on cheek.*
COLOR PLATE 15. *Child with impetigo on nostril.*

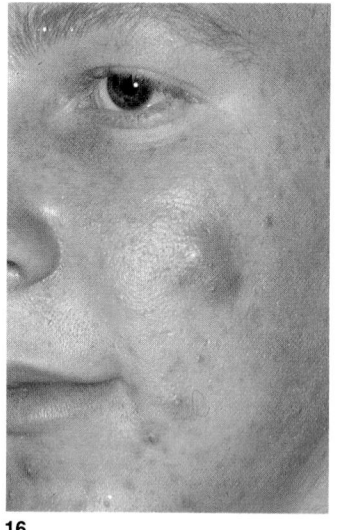
16

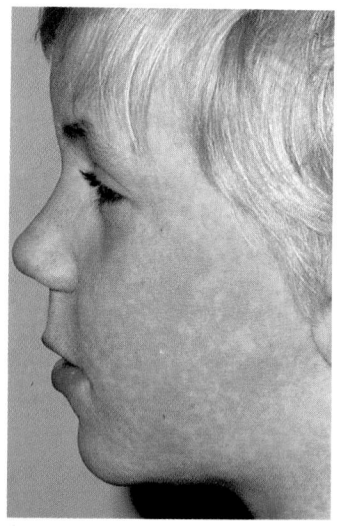
17

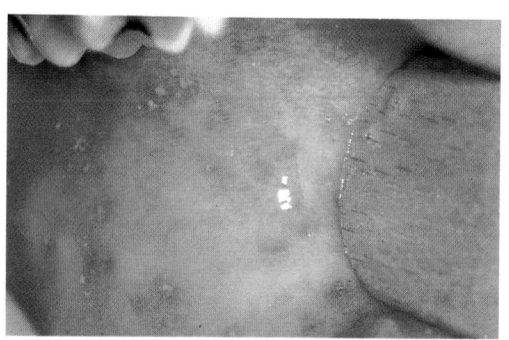
18

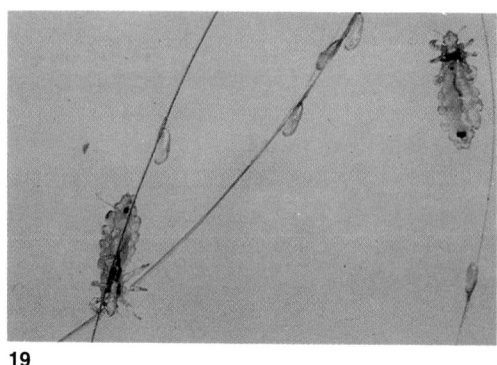
19

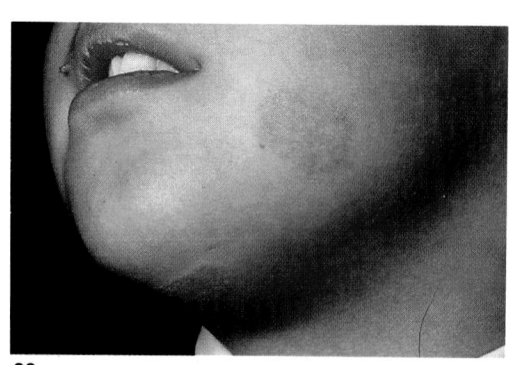
20

COLOR PLATE 16. *Adolescent with acne vulgaris.*
COLOR PLATE 17. *Child with measles on cheek.*
COLOR PLATE 18. *Child's mouth showing Koplik's spots.*
COLOR PLATE 19. *Head lice and nits.*
COLOR PLATE 20. *Ringworm on child's face.*

Systemic infections usually have a **prodromal period**, or a time between the beginning of nonspecific symptoms and specific symptoms. Nonspecific symptoms include lethargy, low-grade fever, fatigue, and malaise. During a prodromal period, infectious diseases spread readily through communities to any children not immunized. Children are infectious (capable of spreading the microorganisms to others) during this time, but because their symptoms are so vague, they do not generally take any precautions against spreading disease. Prodromal stages are generally short, ranging from hours to a few days.

Illness is the stage during which specific symptoms are evident. Most illnesses have local symptoms related to the body organ affected, and also systemic symptoms that affect the entire body, such as fever, increased white blood cell count, or headache. Many childhood infections have an accompanying rash on the skin (**exanthem**) or mucous membrane (**enanthem**).

The **convalescent period** is the interval between the period when symptoms begin to fade and the return to full wellness. Because fatigue is often an accompanying symptom of infection, the convalescent period, or the time until full energy is restored, is often longer than anticipated.

Chain of Infection

Chain of infection refers to the method by which organisms are spread and enter a new individual to cause disease (Bullock & Rosendahl, 1992). An important method of preventing infection is to break a chain of infection. Nurses are instrumental in teaching parents how to prevent the spread of infection in homes and how to carry out safe practices so infection does not spread in health care facilities.

Reservoir

The **reservoir** is the container or place in which organisms grow and reproduce. The source of a human pathogen could be another human with the disease, a human carrying the disease, or an animal. The more children are immunized, the less likely it is that organisms can use children as reservoirs for growth.

Portal of Exit

The **portal of exit** is the method by which organisms leave a child's body. This could be by upper respiratory excretions, feces, vomitus, saliva, urine, vaginal secretions, blood, or lesion secretions (Table 43-1). To break a chain of infection at this point, follow good aseptic technique and prescribed isolation procedures (e.g., wear gown, gloves, or mask as appropriate). Teach parents good handwashing technique following the use of a bathroom or after handling diapers. Supply an adequate number of disposable tissues so children can limit respiratory or airborne spread.

Means of Transmission

The **means of transmission** for the spread of pathogens can be by direct or indirect contact; by **fomites**, that is, inanimate objects such as soil, food, water, bedding, towels, combs, or drinking glasses; or by insects (*vectors*). Direct contact implies body-to-body touching. Sexually transmitted diseases (STDs) and skin disorders are spread this way. The most common means of indirect contact is the spreading of mouth and nose secretions (*droplet infection*) through talking, sneezing, coughing, breathing, and kissing. Some droplets containing pathogenic organisms are spread immediately to another individual in this way. Some droplets fall to the ground, where the organisms dry and then are spread by dust. If small, the organisms become suspended in

Table 43-1. Methods by Which Infections Spread

Exit from Body	Method of Spread	Portal of Entry	Prevention Measures
Blood	Arthropod vectors Blood sampling Transfusion	Injection into bloodstream	Decreasing vector incidence Careful handling of blood sampling equipment Screening of transfused blood for organisms such as human immunodeficiency virus (HIV) or hepatitis B
Respiratory secretions	Airborne droplets Fomites	Respiratory tract	Wearing mask Isolation Hand washing
Feces	Water, food Fomites Vectors such as flies	Gastrointestinal tract	Hand washing before eating, after using bathroom or handling diapers
Exudate from lesions	Direct contact Contact with soiled dressings	Skin, mucous membrane	Isolation from direct contact Self-screening for sexual contacts

the air and can infect people from a distance. The major childhood exanthems (e.g., chickenpox, measles, and rubella) are spread by indirect contact.

Head lice (tinia capitis) can be spread by a fomite such as a comb and passed from one child to another. Soil constantly contains some **anaerobic** organisms (those that grow without oxygen), such as tetanus bacilli. When a child receives a puncture wound, such as a puncture from a rusty nail, some dirt may be left in the closed wound and tetanus bacilli contained in the soil can begin to multiply in the closed area. Staphylococcal gastrointestinal disorders can be caused by improperly refrigerated food. Insects carry and spread rickettsial diseases. To break a chain of infection at this point, use isolation precautions as appropriate and wash hands between giving client care. Teach parents and children good hand washing technique.

Portal of Entry

The **portal of entry** through which a pathogen can enter a child's body can be by inhalation, ingestion, or breaks in the skin such as bites, abrasions, and burns. To break a chain of infection at this point, teach children to wash their hands before eating and after using a bathroom. Teach girls to wipe their perineum from front to back after defecation or voiding to prevent organisms spreading from the rectum to the urethra.

Susceptible Host

For infection to occur, a child must be **susceptible** to the infection (not have immunization against it). Certain characteristics make some individuals more prone to infection than others.

Age. Infectious processes occur most readily in the very young and the very old. Newborns have antibodies to those diseases for which the mother had sufficient levels of antibodies that crossed the placenta (IgG type). This usually includes measles, poliomyelitis, rubella, diphtheria, pertussis, and tetanus. Because the infant's immune response is not fully developed, however, he or she is more susceptible than others to common infections such as upper respiratory infection.

The immune system or ability to produce antibodies is immature for at least the first 2 months of life. This is why immunization is not begun until after this point. As infants begin to explore their environment, they tend to place any object they can into their mouths, thus introducing organisms.

Infants who are breastfed have fewer gastrointestinal infections than formula-fed infants because breast milk contains antibodies that protect against such infections. Because the eustachian tube in infants is short and more horizontal than in adults, an upper respiratory infection spreads easily to become an otitis media (middle ear infection). Toddlers and preschoolers are ex-

posed to more infections than infants because they contact more people, especially at day care or nursery school settings. They also have frequent mosquito bites or scratches that can easily become infected if scratched into open lesions.

Young school children contract a series of upper respiratory infections as they are exposed to new and different friends in school. Streptococcal infections may cause serious throat infection ("strep throat" or tonsillitis). Fungal infection of the outer ear canal is a frequent summer infection of school-age children. Childhood diseases (e.g., mumps, measles, and rubella) are becoming infrequent as greater numbers of children are immunized against these diseases. The incidence can increase in teenagers if this age group did not receive adequate immunization in childhood.

STDs are increasing in incidence and are at epidemic proportions in populations with a high number of adolescents or young adults.

Gender. Some infections occur more frequently in one sex than the other. Girls, for example, are more prone to urinary tract infections than boys.

Virulence of Invading Organisms. Virulence refers to the ability of organisms to cause disease. For an organism to be pathogenic, it must resist or overcome body defenses, effectively enter the body, multiply in significant quantities, and damage body tissues.

Body Defenses Present. Body defense mechanisms can be divided into physical, chemical, and immune types. The body's mucous membranes are protected by mucus that causes microorganisms to be extruded from the body. Because of its high sodium content, it kills many microorganisms. *Staphylococcus aureus,* however, is an organism usually found in large quantities on children's skin. It invades hair follicles to form boils or pustules, and it enters scratched mosquito bites or wounds to cause impetigo.

Chemical barriers include hydrochloric acid in the stomach and the acid pH of urine. Tears contain lysozyme, which dissolves many organisms attempting to invade the conjunctiva. Saliva is faintly bactericidal. The intestines are filled with microorganisms (normal bacterial flora) that destroy pathogenic organisms. Children who are on long-term antibiotic therapy may develop candidiasis or yeast infections of the intestinal tract due to the disturbance of this normal bacteria flora.

Immune Response to Organisms

When a foreign organism (antigen) is identified, it can be destroyed by the phagocytic (cell-engulfing) action of white blood cells or by activation of the body's immune system. Phagocytes are white blood cells that are capable of cell destruction. The cells chiefly responsible for this function are neutrophils. Monocytes serve as back-up cells in the action of phagocytosis. The action of white blood cells is summarized in Table 43-2.

The action of phagocytes on organisms produces pus (remnants of the organisms, phagocytes, and destroyed tissue). Children and parents alike may need a review of the purpose of pus because they think its presence indicates that an infection is becoming worse; it more likely indicates that phagocytosis is occurring and the infection is resolving.

If bacteria escape the action of the phagocytes, they enter the blood and lymph systems and are transmitted to other body locations, activating the immune system. Pathogenic organisms in the bloodstream create **septicemia**, always a serious development because it means that the organism is being spread systemically.

With activation of the immune system, B-cell (humoral immunity) and T-cell (cellular immunity) lymphocytes are produced. B-cell lymphocytes form antibodies specific to offending antigens that either actively destroy cells or produce **complement**, a special body protein that is capable of lysing cells.

T-cell lymphocytes (thymus dependent) can destroy antigens by direct contact and release of lymphokines. An example of a lymphokine is **interferon**, a substance that prevents cells from being host to more than one virus at a time so that two virus infections cannot be present in the body at the same time. This is why it is rare to see a child with two viral diseases (such as measles and chickenpox) at the same time, although it is not impossible to see a child with both a virus and a bacterial disease (e.g., scarlet fever and a common cold) at the same time. This is also the reason why two virus vaccines are not given to a child at the same time except under special circumstances. The exception to this rule is the combination measles-mumps-rubella vaccine,

which was so designed that interferon would not affect it. (See Chapter 42 for a more detailed discussion of the immune response.)

Immunization

Study of the immune response has led to the development of one of the most important elements of health promotion and disease prevention, namely, immunization. Based on what is known about the ability of the immune system to identify and respond to specific foreign substances, vaccines can provide artificial immunity to a number of dangerous infections, including measles, mumps, rubella, diphtheria, tetanus, pertussis, and poliomyelitis, among others. New influenza vaccines are developed regularly to help high-risk clients (e.g., infants, elderly people, and immunosuppressed individuals) ward off the influenza viruses. Research continues on the development of vaccines to combat other diseases, including varicella (chickenpox), pneumonia, and human immunodeficiency virus (HIV) (see the Focus on Cultural Awareness box).

Active Versus Passive Immunity

Immunity, the ability to destroy a particular antigen, may be either active or passive.

Active Immunity

When a child produce antibodies following the natural invasion of a pathogen (the child has the disease), the child is said to have naturally acquired active immunity. Active antibodies (or the child's ability to produce antibiotics rapidly when the specific antigen invades) last a lifetime. When pathogens are artificially injected into the child by immunization, the child receives artificially ac-

Table 43-2. *Types and Functions of White Blood Cells (Leukocytes)*

Type	Percentage of Total Count	Origin	Function
Granular Forms			
Neutrophils	60 at birth 33 at 2 y 60 thereafter	Bone marrow	Active in acute bacterial infections
Eosinophils	1–4	Bone marrow	Increased in parasitic infection
Basophils	0.0–0.5	Bone marrow	Increased with inflammation
Nongranular Forms			
Lymphocytes	30 at birth 50 at 2 y 30 thereafter	Bone marrow Divides into B cells and T cells	T cells (centered in thymus gland) react with antigens directly; B cells produce antibodies against antigens
Monocytes	5-10	Bone marrow	Act as backup for neutrophils in acute infection

FOCUS ON CULTURAL AWARENESS

Some cultures are much more aware of the role of communicable disease in childhood illnesses than others, so advocate for all children to be immunized against these disorders. Even if awareness about the danger of disease spread exists, however, it doesn't mean that all people in a community are conscientious about having their children immunized; other factors such as cost and convenience and ethical beliefs are also important.

Some religious groups, such as the Amish, discourage immunizations; in these communities, the prevalence of illnesses such as measles can rise to high numbers. Being aware that immunization rates are not consistent from place to place aids in understanding the importance of planning health education and health surveillance based on individual community needs.

quired active immunity: antibodies are produced against the pathogen that are just as lasting as those produced in naturally acquired active immunity.

Passive Immunity

IgG antibodies that a woman possesses either through immunization or through having had a disease are transferred across the placenta to a fetus in utero. Because the fetus does not make these antibodies but merely receives them, this is considered naturally acquired passive immunity. Passive immunity lasts only a matter of months. Some antibodies transferred across the placenta may have slightly longer lifetimes than this; measles antibodies, for example, have been isolated up to age 1 year, and that is why measles immunization must be delayed until age 15 months.

When children are exposed to a disease against which they have no antibodies, antibodies made synthetically or obtained from animal serum may be injected into the child to give them immunity (artificially acquired passive immunity). Like naturally acquired passive antibodies, these last only approximately 6 weeks.

Types of Immunizations

Vaccines are the solutions used to immunize children to provide artificially acquired active or passive immunity. They are prepared in a number of forms.

Attenuated vaccines are made from live organisms that have been reduced in virulence to a point where they will not cause active disease but will ensure a good antibody response. Because they are strong and effec-

tive solutions, a single dose usually gives a good degree of immunity.

Because some bacteria, such as diphtheria, cause disease by producing a toxin, the vaccine against such a disease, a **toxoid**, is actually an extract of the toxin reduced in virulence. The antibodies for toxin-producing bacteria are **antitoxins**. A solution given for passive immunity against diphtheria is an antitoxin.

Gamma globulin is serum obtained from the pooled blood of many people. Because it comes from many people, it contains the antibodies of many people and probably has antibody protection against measles, rubella, poliomyelitis, and infectious hepatitis among many other infectious diseases. It offers passive immunity.

Immune serum is serum removed from horses that have been given a disease. The usual preparations used are those against diphtheria, tetanus, the pit viper snake, and the black widow spider. Because these antibodies are prepared from horse serum, be certain before giving the serum to skin-test a child to ensure he or she is not allergic to horse serum. Equine serums are being replaced by synthetic preparations.

Administration of Vaccines

The schedule of immunizations for children recommended by the American Academy of Pediatrics (AAP) is shown in Table 43-3.

Diphtheria, Tetanus, Pertussis (DTP) Vaccines

Diphtheria, tetanus, and pertussis (whooping cough) vaccines are supplied in a single vial as DTP and given in one intramuscular injection. It is recommended that children receive a primary series of four immunizations with DTP between 6 weeks and 4 years of age. A booster is then given between ages 4 and 6 years, or before entry into school (Rennels, 1993).

There has been a great deal of controversy about the safety of the DTP vaccine, most of it directed at the pertussis component. Side effects include drowsiness, fretfulness, low-grade fever, and redness and pain at the injection site. More severe reactions, such as high fever, persistent crying, and, rarely, seizures, have been reported. However, these symptoms have not been associated with any long-term damage (Rennels, 1993), and the general medical consensus is that the risk of complications from contracting the disease is greater than the risk of a reaction to the vaccine. To avoid reactions to pertussis vaccine, an acellular or reduced strength product is now available and it is recommended that this strength (DTaP) be used for the 4th and 5th vaccinations at 15 to 18 months and 3 to 4 years.

Parents have the right to refuse immunizations for their children. However, children who are not immunized against pertussis (unless there is a medical con-

Table 43-3. *Schedule for the Routine Immunization of Healthy Infants and Children (Based on the Recommendations of the American Academy of Pediatrics and the CDCP)*

Recommended Age[1]	Immunization[2]	Comments
At birth	HBV[3]	Alternate schedule for HBV vaccination: 1–2 mo, 4 mo, and 6–18 mo.
1–2 mo	HBV	
2 mo	DTP,[4] HbCV,[5] OPV[6]	DTP and OPV can be given as early as 4 wk after birth in areas of high endemicity or during outbreaks.
4 mo	DTP, HbCV, OPV	A 2-mo interval (minimum of 6 wk) is desirable for OPV to avoid interference from the previous dose.
6 mo	DTP, HbCV	
6–18 mo	HBV	
15 mo	MMR[7] HbCV	MMR may be given at 12 mo of age in areas of recurrent measles transmission; if given at less than 12 mo, it should be given again at 15 mo.
15–18 mo	DTaP[8] or DTP, OPV	These vaccines may be given simultaneously with MMR at 15 mo.
4–6 yr	DTaP or DTP, OPV	At or before school entry.
11–12 yr	MMR	At entry to middle school or junior high school unless the second dose was previously given.
14–16 yr	Td[9]	Repeat every 10 yr throughout life.

[1] Recommended ages should not be construed as absolute.
[2] For all products used, consult manufacturer's package enclosure for instructions for storage, handling, and administration. Immunobiologics prepared by different manufacturers may vary, and those of the same manufacturer may change periodically.
[3] HBV = hepatitis B vaccine.
[4] DTP = diphtheria and tetanus toxoids and pertussis vaccine absorbed.
[5] HbCV = *Haemophilus influenzae* type b conjugate vaccine.
[6] OPV = poliovirus vaccine live oral; contains poliovirus strains types 1, 2, and 3.
[7] MMR = measles, mumps, rubella vaccine, live.
[8] DTaP = diphtheria, tetanus and acellular (reduced strength) pertussis vaccine.
[9] Td = tetanus and diphtheria toxoids adsorbed (adult type). Contains the same dose of tetanus toxoid as DTP or DT (diphtheria and tetanus) and a reduced dose of diphtheria toxoid.

traindication) may be refused admittance to preschool or beginning school programs. Parents should be so informed of this when they refuse to sign consent for immunization.

Pertussis vaccination is contraindicated in children who have a progressive or unstable neurologic disorder or who have had a severe allergic reaction to pertussis in a previous DTP vaccination. If pertussis immunization is contraindicated, the DT, or Diphtheria/Tetanus vaccine is substituted.

Pertussis is not generally given after age 6 because the side effects of the vaccine may be more common in older children (Rennels, 1993). The diphtheria toxoid is still given to children older than age 6 years, but the adult or more diluted form (d) is used after this age. After the fifth dose of DTP, the tetanus and diluted form of diphtheria (Td) are recommended to be given every 10 years.

Polio Vaccines

Oral polio vaccine (OPV) and inactivated polio vaccine (IPV) contain all three strains of poliovirus and are both available for use in the United States. The oral form of polio vaccine (Sabin's vaccine or OPV) is preferred, not for its convenience as most parents believe, but because it produces longer-acting immunity than the killed injectable type (Salk vaccine). However, OPV, which consists of live attenuated poliovirus, should never be administered to any child who is immunosuppressed; this could cause a rare form of paralytic poliomyelitis. Because OPV is shed in the stools, it should also never be administered to any child who may come in close contact with an immunosuppressed person, as these contacts would have a very small risk of developing the same OPV-paralytic disease (Rennels, 1993).

OPV or IPV is administered in a primary series of three doses and given along with DTP at 2, 4, and 18 months of age. A fourth booster dose is given between the ages of 4 and 6 years, before school entry.

Measles, Mumps, Rubella (MMR) Vaccines

Measles-mumps-rubella vaccine is furnished in one vial and routinely administered as a single injection. A first dose is given around the time of the 15 month check-up. A second dose of MMR is generally given between the ages of 11 and 12 years. It is usually recommended that the measles vaccine not be administered to children younger than age 15 months because children receive a great deal of passive immunity to this disease from their mother across the placenta. Until this passive immunity is destroyed by the child's body, the injected vaccine will be neutralized by passive antibodies and no immunity will result. For the same reason, children who have recently received immune globulin or other blood products that contain antibodies should defer the MMR for 3 months following such infusion, as the passively acquired antibodies could interfere with the child's immune response to the vaccine (Rennels, 1993).

Side effects of the measles vaccine include transient rashes and a fever which may begin 5 to 12 days after vaccination and last several days. Adverse reactions include low-grade fever, rash, and lymphadenopathy 5 to 12 days after vaccination. There have also been some reports of joint pain (Rennels, 1993).

Children should be skin-tested for tuberculosis before measles vaccine administration because measles virus can cause tuberculosis to become systemic. Tuberculosis skin tests may show false-negative reactions if given shortly after measles immunization (a child who has active tuberculosis will be wrongly identified as not having it).

Hepatitis Vaccine

The vaccine for hepatitis B (HBV) has recently been recommended for all infants in the United States. The AAP also recommends that adolescents receive universal immunization when resources permit (Rennels, 1993). In addition, HBV immunization is recommended for those population groups who are at increased risk for contracting hepatitis B infection, including (but not limited to) health care workers with significant exposure to blood, hemodialysis patients, hemophiliacs and other patients who receive clotting factor concentrates, illicit injectable drug users, sexually active homosexual and bisexual males, and heterosexual persons with multiple sexual partners.

There are currently two hepatitis B vaccines licensed for use in the United States. The dose varies depending on the formulation being used and the age and immune status of the recipient. Immunization is routinely first given to infants either at birth or at 1 to 2 months of age; it is essential that infants of women who are HBsAg (Hepatitis B surface antigen) positive be immunized as soon after birth as possible.

Haemophilus Influenzae Type B Vaccines

H influenzae type b conjugate vaccines (HbcVs) protect against *haemophilus influenzae* bacteria, and are one of the newest immunizations available for public use. There are several formulations of this vaccine available, and three of them are currently licensed for use in infancy. Depending on the individual vaccine, they are administered in a three-dose regimen at 2, 4, and 15 months or in a four-dose regimen, ordinarily at 2, 4, 6, and 12 to 15 months. Local reactions include tenderness

at the injection site; some systemic reactions such as crying and fever have been reported. Because of the ongoing research and licensing of these vaccines, it is important to read carefully the package insert and published data and to follow your health care facility's guidelines.

Assessment

Children who are seriously ill should not receive immunizations. A slight upper respiratory tract infection, however (a stuffy nose with no fever), is not a contraindication to immunization. So many infants and preschoolers have common cold symptoms (the average toddler has 10 to 12 colds a year) that if children are not immunized at health maintenance visits when they have slight cold symptoms, they will never receive basic immunizations. An exception to this may be measles-mumps-rubella vaccine. This appears less effective when children have upper respiratory infections (Krober et al., 1991). Box 43-1 describes other commonly held misconceptions about immunization administration.

Assess the immunization status of ill children at clinic or hospital admission to identify those who need their immunizations updated. Because children with chronic illness may be hospitalized when an injection is due, such children often fall behind schedule. Children who miss the scheduled time for an immunization do not have the series started over but are simply continued where they left off.

Physicians may choose to alter the sequence of immunization schedules if specific infections are prevalent at the time. For example, measles vaccine might be given on a first health maintenance visit (providing a child is older than age 14 months) if an epidemic was currently underway in the community.

Be sure to assess each child's health status before administering any vaccine. Children who are immunosuppressed, who are receiving corticosteroids, or who are on chemotherapy or radiation treatment cannot receive live virus vaccines. The live attenuated viruses (i.e., measles, rubella, oral polio, and mumps) also must not be given to girls who are pregnant because these vaccines could cross the placenta and cause the actual disease in the fetus.

Preparation and Storage

Be careful to follow manufacturer's recommendations for storage and handling of vaccines (e.g., whether to expose to light or whether to refrigerate). Failure to follow these precautions may significantly reduce the potency and effectiveness of vaccines.

Although measles, mumps, and rubella vaccines are prepared from chick embryo cultures, egg sensitivities are not likely to occur because egg albumin and yolk components of the egg are absent from the culture. Children with egg allergy should have their allergist's per-

Box 43-1
Misconceptions Concerning Contraindications to Vaccination

- A reaction to a previous dose of DTP vaccine with only soreness, redness or swelling in the immediate vicinity of the vaccination site or a temperature of less than 40.5°C (105°F)
- Mild acute illness with low-grade fever or mild diarrheal illness in an otherwise well child
- Current antimicrobial therapy or the convalescent phase of illnesses
- Prematurity (the appropriate age for initiating immunization in premature infants is the usual chronologic age; vaccine doses should not be reduced for preterm infants)
- Pregnancy in the mother or another household contact
- Recent exposure to an infectious disease
- Breast-feeding (the only vaccine virus that has been isolated from breast milk is rubella vaccine virus; no evidence indicates that the breast milk of women immunized against rubella is harmful to infants)
- A history of nonspecific allergies or relatives with allergies
- Allergy to penicillin or any other antibiotic agent, except anaphylactic reaction to neomycin (e.g., MMR-containing vaccines) or streptomycin (e.g., OPV). (None of the vaccines licensed in the United States contain penicillin.)
- Allergies to duck meat or duck feathers (no vaccine available in the United States is produced in substrates containing duck antigen)
- A family history of convulsions in children who require vaccination against pertussis or measles
- A family history of sudden infant death syndrome in children who require DTP vaccination
- A family history of an adverse event, unrelated to immunosuppression, after vaccination

American Academy of Pediatrics. (1991). *The red book.* Elk Grove Village, IL: AAP.

mission for immunization, however, to rule out the possibility of a hypersensitivity reaction.

Parent Education

A major reason that parents bring children for routine immunizations is that they do not know what is required (Salsberry et al., 1993). Fully inform parents of children (and children as soon as they are old enough) about what immunizations they are being given and what side effects may be expected (Belcher, 1993). Children may develop a low-grade fever following immunization. Parents may be counseled to give acetaminophen (Tylenol) for a fever of more than 101°F (38.4°C).

Parents should report any untoward symptoms of immunization. Unfavorable reactions are most likely to occur within a few hours or days of administration. With live attenuated virus vaccines, viruses can multiply, so reactions may occur up to 30 days later. With rubella vaccine, a reaction (serum sickness) may occur up to 60 days later.

The date, type of vaccine, vaccine manufacturer, lot number, and name and address of the provider must be recorded so that if a vaccine reaction should occur, the instance can be investigated. Make a copy and urge parents to keep such records at home as well. They will need this information to admit their child to school and in the event of an epidemic of a particular disease. They will need to know their child's record of tetanus immunization if their child should receive a puncture wound so the correct therapy can be given.

Preventing the Spread of Infections in the Hospital

Nosocomial infections represent a major threat to hospitalized children, a threat that nurses can play a major role in combatting. Nurses and other health care providers must also take precautions to protect themselves from acquiring communicable diseases, including HIV and hepatitis. Universal precautions to take in all clinical settings recommended by the Centers for Disease Control (CDC) are summarized in Table 43-4.

Table 43-4. *Universal Precautions to Prevent Infection*

Object	Procedure
Hands	Hands should always be washed before and after contact with clients, even when gloves have been worn; if hands come in contact with blood, body fluid, or human tissue, they should be washed immediately with soap and water
Gloves	Gloves should be worn when contact with blood, body fluid, tissues, or contaminated surfaces is anticipated
Gowns	Gowns or plastic aprons are indicated if blood spattering is likely
Masks and goggles	These should be worn if aerosolization or splattering is likely to occur, such as in certain dental and surgical procedures, wound irrigations, postmortem examinations, and bronchoscopy
Sharp objects	Sharp objects should be handled in such a manner to prevent accidental cuts or punctures; used needles should not be bent, broken, reinserted into their original sheath, or unnecessarily handled; they should be discarded intact immediately after use into an impervious needle-disposal box, which should be readily accessible; all needle-stick accidents, mucosal splashes, and contamination of open wounds with blood or body fluids should be reported immediately to the department supervisor and an accident report should be filed with employee health
Blood spills	Blood spills should be cleaned up promptly with an agency designated disinfectant solution such as 5.25% sodium hypochlorite diluted 1:10 with water
Blood specimens	Blood specimens should be considered biohazardous and be so labeled
Resuscitation	To minimize the need for emergency mouth-to-mouth resuscitation, mouth pieces, resuscitation bags, and other ventilatory devices should be located strategically and available for use in areas where the need for resuscitation is predictable

(From Centers for Disease Control. [1987]. *Morbidity and Mortality Weekly Report, 35,* 5, with permission.)

Nursing Diagnoses and Related Interventions

Nursing Diagnosis: High risk for infection related to incidence of nosocomial infections

Goal: Child will not contract infectious disease while hospitalized.

Outcome Criteria: Oral temperature is 98.6°F (37.0°C); no gastrointestinal symptoms such as vomiting or diarrhea are present; no erythema is present at incision site.

The overall rate of nosocomial, or hospital acquired, infection in children is between 0.2% and 7% (Allen & Ford-Jones, 1990). Children younger than age 2 years, children with a nutritional deficit, those who are immunosuppressed, those who have indwelling vascular lines or catheters, those on multiple antibiotic therapy, or those who remain in the hospital for longer than 72 hours are at highest risk for contracting a nosocomial infection. Nurses provide a second line of defense by always adhering to strict aseptic techniques, such as frequent and thorough hand washing, and by following protective isolation techniques when indicated (see the Focus on Nursing Research box).

Maintain Indicated Isolation Precautions

Requirements of isolation vary according to the route by which the pathogen concerned can be spread. Measles and pulmonary tuberculosis, for example, are diseases requiring only respiratory isolation.

Enteric isolation (used for diseases spread by urine or feces) is required for parasitic infestations. Strict isolation is required for diphtheria because of its extreme virulence.

Good isolation technique requires a well-marked room door so everyone is aware of the type of isolation being practiced, clearly written instructions of the necessary precautions, and availability of ample supplies so there is no delay in being able to put on the proper apparel for protection. Proper technique must be used when removing supplies from an isolation room.

Respiratory Isolation. Respiratory isolation is used to contain the spread of airborne microorganisms. Children must be in a private room; the door to the room must be kept closed. Anyone entering the room must wear a mask over the nose and mouth. Respiratory secretions should be handled only while wearing gloves, and be removed from the room by a double-bag technique. If caring for an infant who might drool, wear a gown to keep saliva off your uniform. If a child in respiratory isolation must be removed from the room, he or she should have a mask over the nose and mouth.

Enteric Isolation. Enteric isolation describes precautions used to limit the spread of microorganisms by urine or feces. Children are best cared for in a private room with a private bathroom (if their hygiene habits are poor, they *must* be in a private room). When giving direct care (touching client or bed), wear a gown if soiling is likely. Wear gloves to handle a bedpan. Specimens

FOCUS ON NURSING RESEARCH

What Would Be the Best Way to Influence Nursing Staff to Follow a New Infection Control Measure?

Social power is defined as the potential ability of a person to change the thoughts, attitudes, or behavior of another. It can be manifested as coercive power (influence by the ability to punish); reward power (influence by the ability to reward); legitimate power (influence because one holds a superior position to another); expert power (influence through superior knowledge); referent power (one person is used as a frame of reference for another); or informational power (ability to influence by persuasion).

To investigate which type of social power nurses respond to best in the area of infection control, researchers interviewed 142 nurses and 140 housekeeping staff in a major Hong Kong teaching hospital and asked them what source of power would be the most important to influence them to adhere to a change in infection control policy. Of the nurses, 55% (n = 78) stated they would be most influenced by informational power; 28% (n = 40) stated expert power. In contrast, 30% (n = 42) of housekeeping members stated they would be most influenced by legitimate power; 23% (n = 32) by informational power.

Although this study must be evaluated in light of the Hong Kong setting, the results indicate that a major need of staff nurses is adequate information before they will follow a new procedure; more important for many housekeeping persons would be assurance that their superior approved of the change.

Seto, W. H., Ching, T. Y., Chu, Y. B., & Seto, W. L. (1991). Social power and motivation for the compliance of nurse and housekeeping staff with infection control policies. *American Journal of Infection Control, 19,* 42.

of feces that are removed from the room to be analyzed in a laboratory must be double-bagged to protect laboratory personnel.

Drainage Secretion Precautions. Drainage secretion precautions, as the name implies, are designed to prevent transmission of microbes from drainage such as from an infected wound. Health care providers can walk into the room without precautions other than usual hand washing, but to give direct care, a gown must be worn if soiling is likely. Gloves are indicated for touching infectious material. Any object that has come in direct contact with the infected area must be double-bagged to be removed from the room.

Blood and Body Fluid Precautions. When children have a disease that is carried by the bloodstream or by body fluid (e.g., HIV or hepatitis B), special precautions are taken with blood and other fluids and with objects such as needles that have entered the bloodstream and syringes that have been contaminated with body fluids. Wear gloves if touching any body fluid. Wear a gown if soiling with fluid or blood is likely; wear eye covering such as goggles if the possibility of splattering is likely, such as while suctioning a tracheotomy. Be exceptionally careful not to prick a finger when handling contaminated needles. Do not recap injection needles after use; discard immediately into a designated container instead. The CDC recommends that these precautions be followed with all clients (universal precautions).

Contact Isolation. Contact isolation is required to contain diseases that are spread by close body contact, such as herpes simplex virus and impetigo. Masks are indicated for those who come close to the client; gowns are worn if soiling is likely. Gloves should be worn when touching infectious material. Contaminated articles should be discarded or bagged and labeled before being sent for decontamination and reprocessing. Hands must be washed after touching the client and potentially contaminated articles, and before taking care of another client.

Acid-Fast Bacterial Isolation. This type of isolation is for children with active pulmonary tuberculosis who have a positive sputum culture, or a chest radiograph that strongly suggests current, active disease. The child should be in a private room. Masks are indicated if the child is coughing and does not reliably cover his or her mouth; gowns are necessary to prevent gross contamination of clothing. Gloves are not required. Articles used in the room should be discarded and cleaned before being sent for decontamination and reprocessing. Hands must be washed after touching the child or potentially contaminated articles and before taking care of another client.

Strict Isolation. A few microorganisms are so virulent or so contagious by air or by contact (e.g., diphtheria and varicella) that maximum precautions are necessary to limit their spread. With strict isolation, a mask, gown, and gloves must be worn to give care. The child must be in a private room with the door kept closed. All articles removed from the room must be double-bagged.

Caring for the Child With an Infectious Disease

Nursing Diagnoses and Related Interventions

Nursing Diagnosis: Social isolation related to required isolation precautions

Goal: Child will not feel left out or lonely while in isolation.

Outcome Criteria: Child states reasons for being in isolation. Expresses interest in activities proposed by nurses or parents.

Infection control may lead to other client concerns. For instance, the child under strict isolation precautions will begin to feel lonely and depressed unless the child's stimulation and social needs are also met.

Children in isolation rooms are aware that they are shut inside a room and that other children are not allowed to enter. It is easy for children to associate isolation with being punished, and it is easy for them to become lonely in a room by themselves. Make as few trips as possible in and out of the room to limit pathogen spread, but do not run quickly in and out. If there is a procedure scheduled at 9:00 AM and another at 9:30 AM, stay in the room rather than leave and return again, if possible. Use the time to read a story to a child or play a card game or talk about how strange and lonely it feels to be isolated from other people.

Encourage parents to visit children who are in isolation. Many parents feel so self-conscious about having to gown and wash that they tend to stay away rather than visit. Remember that when children are admitted to a hospital, parents hear only half of what is said to them because of their anxiety over the admission. If gowning technique is explained on admission, therefore, do not expect parents to remember the next day what was said. Explain technique as many times as necessary.

Parents may be reluctant to give children in isolation their favorite toy, thinking that the hospital will insist on destroying it after the child is removed from isolation. There are few pathogens that are not destroyed by exposure to sunlight, and there are few articles that cannot be gas sterilized to ensure that pathogens have been removed from them. Check children's isolation rooms for favorite toys the same as in all rooms. Never leave children in an isolation room before checking that they have a toy to play with or an activity that will keep them busy for the length of time the child will be alone. "Diversional activity deficit related to monotony of confinement" is another nursing diagnosis associated with isolation. See Chapter 37 for a discussion of interventions that can be used to promote adequate stimulation for the child in isolation.

Nursing Diagnosis: Pain (pruritus) related to rash from infection.

Goal: Child's discomfort will be tolerable during course of illness.

Outcome Criteria: Child states that he or she is not too uncomfortable; child not scratching rash; no signs of excessive scratching or bleeding are present.

Providing comfort for rash is a major category of responsibility for many childhood infections. No matter what agent is causing the disease, a rash tends to be extremely itchy and uncomfortable. A number of remedies are available for reducing the discomforts of rashes. Because pruritus is a minimal form of pain, an analgesic, such as acetaminophen (Tylenol), is helpful in reducing itching. An antihistamine, such as diphenhydramine hydrochloride (Benadryl), is extremely helpful in reducing the discomfort of rash. A physician should be consulted for the appropriate dose. Colloidal baths—baking soda or oatmeal, approximately 1 cup to 3 inches of bath water—are soothing for some children (take precautions not to clog drains with oatmeal if it is used). The water should be only lukewarm, not hot, because heat usually increases itching. Bathing may not be as soothing for children as it is distracting; either way, the child, especially a preschooler, may splash for 15 minutes to 20 minutes in a bathtub without noticing the discomfort of a rash.

Many parents bundle up children with rashes, believing that the extra clothing brings out the rash, and that if a rash does not come out, it will go in and affect a child's heart or brain. In reality, bundling up only serves to make a rash more uncomfortable and probably increases any accompanying fever. Instead, dress the child in light summer clothing. Remove wool blankets from the bed. Cut the child's fingernails short so that scratching will not open up lesions, causing secondary infection. It may help to put cotton gloves on the child, especially at night. Calamine lotion is a nonprescription lotion that is cooling and soothing and often helps to relieve itching. Comfort measures for relieving the discomfort of rashes are summarized in the Focus on Family Teaching display.

None of these measures is foolproof; some measures may provide great relief to some children and little or no relief to others. Regardless of whether they offer direct relief, they do give a parent a constructive and comforting activity. When children are crying and uncomfortable with a rash, parents need to provide some care in an effort to soothe their children and themselves. This is, in part, how a sense of trust develops.

Most infectious diseases also involve fever. Measures to combat fever in children are discussed in Chapter 37.

Viral Infections

Viruses are the smallest infectious agents known, so small they cannot be seen through an ordinary microscope. A virus is not a true cell because it contains either ribonucleic acid (RNA) or deoxyribonucleic acid (DNA), but not both. Viruses increase in number not by independent fission but by replication inside bacteria, plant, animal, or human cell using the biochemical products of living cells to function. A cell may not be outwardly al-

tered by a virus invasion or may die because of lysis or rupture. Symptoms usually do not become apparent until many cells have been interrupted in function. Some viruses are capable of invading only specific cells. The Epstein-Barr virus, for example invades only B-lymphocytes; tracheal cells have receptor sites specific for influenzae viruses.

Viral Exanthems

The majority of childhood exanthems (rashes) are caused by viruses. Each of these diseases has specific symptoms and a specific distribution or pattern to the rash that allows it to be identified (Figures 43-3 and 43-4).

Exanthem Subitum (Roseola Infantum)
- Causative agent: Herpesvirus 6 (HHV-6)
- Incubation period: Approximately 10 days
- Period of communicability: During febrile period
- Mode of transmission: Unknown
- Immunity: Contracting the disease offers lasting natural immunity; no artificial immunity is available

Assessment. Roseola is a disease whose symptoms are out of proportion to its severity (i.e., it appears more severe than it is). It generally occurs in children ages 6 months to 3 years, mainly in the spring and fall, although it can occur any time of the year. The first symptom is a high fever (104°F to 105°F [40.0°C to 40.6°C]). Infants may be irritable and anorexic but rarely are as ill-appearing as this high fever suggests; they usually remain playful and alert. The pharynx may be slightly inflamed. There may be enlargement of the occipital,

cervical, and postauricular lymph nodes. The white blood count is usually decreased with the proportion of lymphocytes present increased (75% to 85%) (McMillan & Grose, 1994).

After 3 days or 4 days, the fever falls abruptly and a distinctive rash appears (Figure 43-4). The lesions are discrete, rose pink macules approximately 2 mm to 3 mm in size. They fade on pressure and occur most prominently on the trunk. The rash resembles that of rubella or measles, but it is darker in color, and children have no accompanying coryza (cold symptoms), conjunctivitis, or cough. Because it occurs mainly on the child's trunk, parents may report it as a heat rash. The rash lasts 1 to 2 days. The diagnosis of roseola is based on the physical signs and symptoms. The hallmark of roseola is the appearance of a rash immediately after the sharp decline in fever.

Therapeutic Management. Treatment is symptomatic relief of rash discomfort and fever. Isolation is unnecessary. The most frequent complication of roseola is a febrile convulsion with the onset of the disease. Management of this type of convulsion is discussed in Chapter 49. The fever will respond to acetaminophen (Tylenol), but after 4 hours it will again rise to the high level.

Rubella (German Measles)
- Causative agent: Rubella virus
- Incubation period: 14 to 21 days
- Period of communicability: 7 days before to approximately 5 days after the rash appears
- Mode of transmission: Direct and indirect contact with droplets
- Immunity: Contracting the disease offers lasting natural immunity

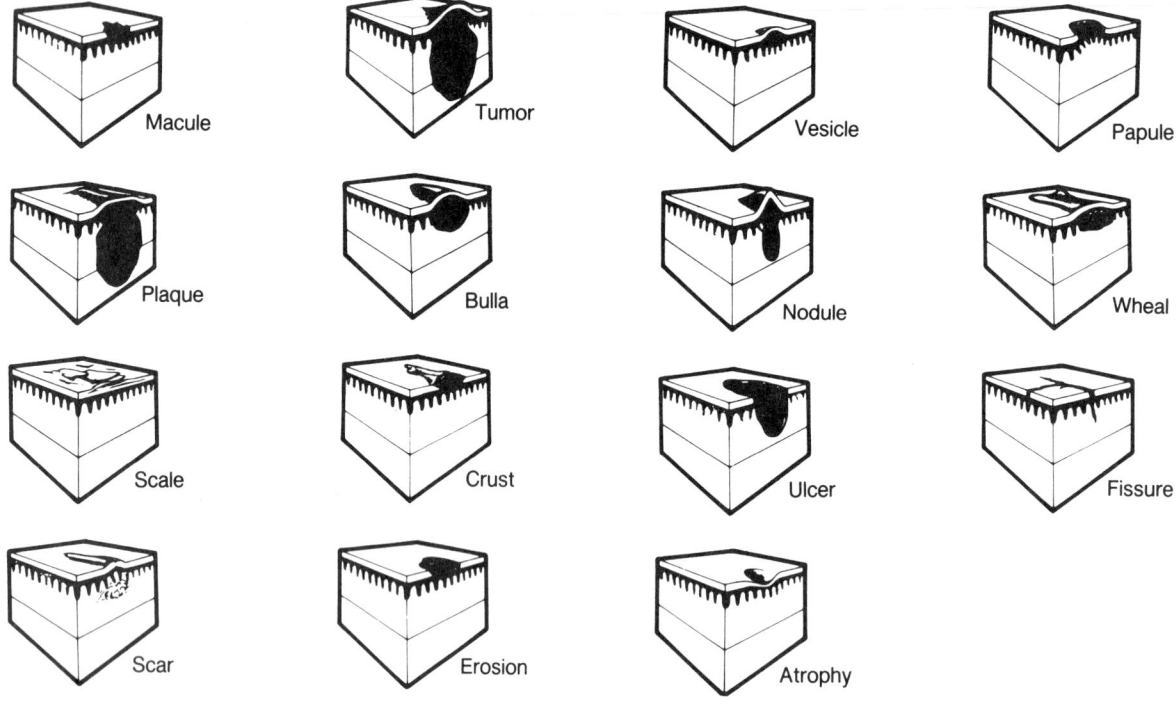

FIGURE 43-3
Primary and secondary skin lesions and their characteristics. (From Sana, J. M., & Judge, R. D. Physical assessment skills for nursing practice. *Boston: Little, Brown, with permission.)*

- Active artificial immunity: Attenuated live virus vaccine
- Passive artificial immunity: Immune serum globulin is considered for pregnant women

Assessment. Rubella is a disease of older school-age and adolescent children; it occurs most commonly during the spring. The symptoms of rubella begin with a 1- to 5-day prodromal period, during which children have a low-grade fever, headache, malaise, anorexia, mild conjunctivitis, possibly a sore throat, a mild cough, and lymphadenopathy. The nodes most noticeably affected are the suboccipital, postauricular, and cervical.

Following the 1 to 5 days of prodromal signs, a rash appears (Figures 43-4 and 43-5A). Many children have such slight prodromal symptoms that the rash is the first sign parents notice. The rash of rubella consists of discrete pink-red maculopapules. It begins first on the face, then spreads downward to the trunk and extremities. On the second day, the rash begins to fade from the face. It is still prominent on the trunk, however, and may even be intensified or coalesce (fuse together) on the trunk. On the third day, the rash disappears. There is generally no desquamation (peeling); if there is, it is only fine flakes.

Fever with rubella is not marked. Arthritis (joint pain) with effusion into the joints may occur in some children on the second or third day of the rash; these symptoms may last as long as 5 to 10 days. Rubella is di-

agnosed on clinical signs and symptoms. A high rubella antibody titer will reveal that children have recently had rubella.

Therapeutic Management. Children need comfort measures for the rash, and an antipyretic such as acetaminophen if a marked fever occurs. If arthritis occurs, acetaminophen will control this discomfort as well. If weight-bearing joints are affected, bedrest is generally advised until the discomfort subsides (2 to 3 days).

If rubella occurs during pregnancy, it is capable of causing extensive congenital malformation (see Chapter 26). Because of this, it can never be considered a simple disease. Girls especially should be immunized against it (Bakshi & Cooper, 1990).

Measles (Rubeola)
- Causative agent: Measles virus
- Incubation period: 10 to 12 days
- Period of communicability: Fifth day of incubation period through the first few days of rash
- Mode of transmission: Direct or indirect contact with droplets
- Immunity: Contracting the disease offers lasting natural immunity
  - Active artificial immunity: Attenuated live measles vaccine
  - Passive artificial immunity: Immune serum globulin

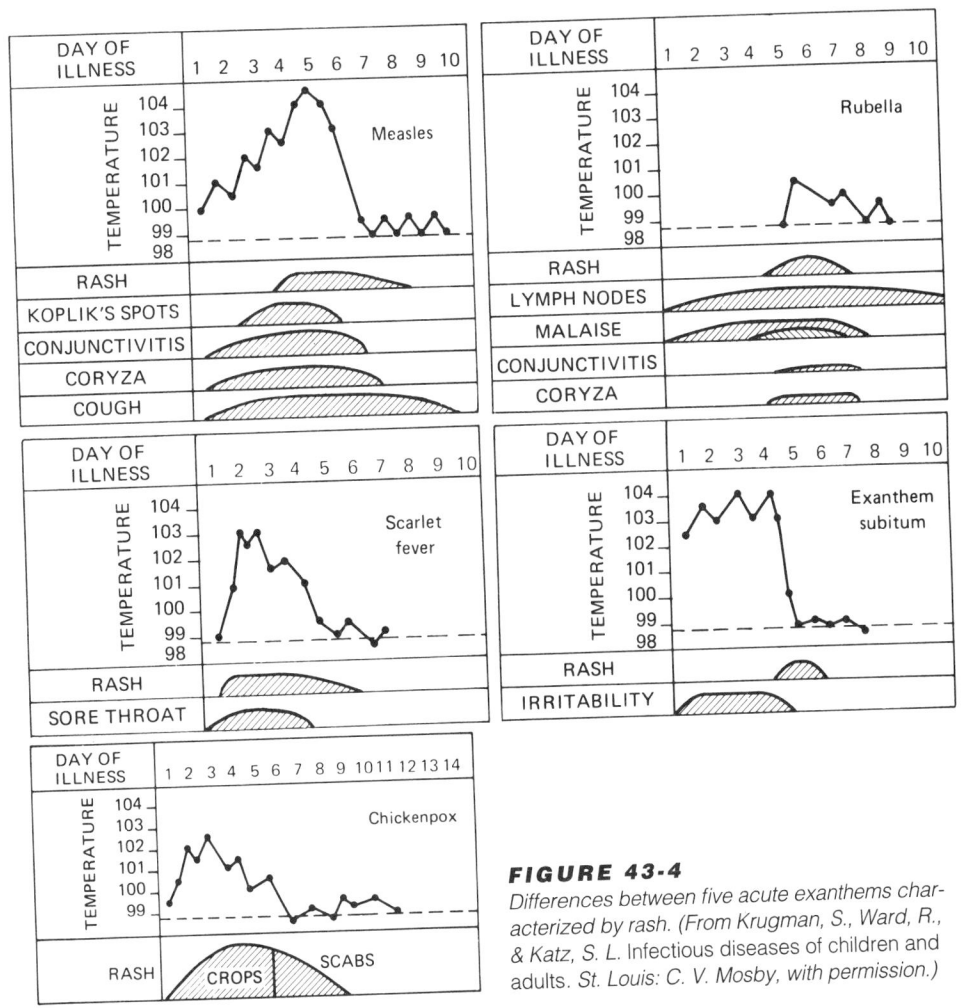

FIGURE 43-4

Differences between five acute exanthems characterized by rash. (From Krugman, S., Ward, R., & Katz, S. L. Infectious diseases of children and adults. St. Louis: C. V. Mosby, with permission.)

Assessment. Measles is sometimes called brown or black, regular, or 7-day measles to differentiate it from rubella (German, or 3-day, measles). It formerly occurred most frequently in children ages 5 to 10 years. Because most children of preschool and school age have now been immunized against measles, outbreaks currently most often occur in the college-age population. Incidence of the disease is highest in the winter and spring months.

Measles has a 10- to 11-day prodromal period. During this time, lymphoid tissue, particularly postauricular, cervical, and occipital lymph nodes, becomes enlarged. Children have a high fever (103°F to 104°F [39.5°C to 40.0°C]); they have malaise and appear ill. By the second day of the prodromal period, there is coryza (rhinitis and a sore throat); conjunctivitis with photophobia (sensitivity to light); and a cough. **Koplik's spots,** small, irregular, bright red spots with a blue-white center point, are present on the buccal membrane. The coryza of measles is indistinguishable from that of a common cold. Children have nasal congestion and a mucopurulent discharge. Their eyes water with the conjunctivitis; they blink at bright lights. Their cough is a deep, brassy,

bronchial cough caused by an inflammation reaction extending into the respiratory tract. Many children with measles are diagnosed as having a simple upper respiratory infection at this point.

Koplik's spots appear first on the buccal membrane opposite the molars, and then extend to cover the entire buccal surface (Figure 43-6). The raised base of the spots may coalesce so that the blue-white centers stand out as grains of salt on the erythematous membrane. Koplik's spots are diagnostic of measles. None of the other exanthems has this finding.

On the fourth day of fever, the rash appears (Figures 43-4 and 43-5*B*). On the fifth day, the fever drops and the Koplik's spots fade (Figure 43-7). The rash of measles is a deep-red maculopapular eruption. It begins first at the hairline of the forehead, behind the ears, and at the back of the neck. It then spreads to include the face, the neck, upper extremities, trunk, and, finally, the lower extremities. The rash on the upper part of the body, particularly the face, may be so intense that it coalesces; rash on the lower extremities generally remains discrete. After several days, the rash turns from a red to a brown color. While the rash is red, it fades on

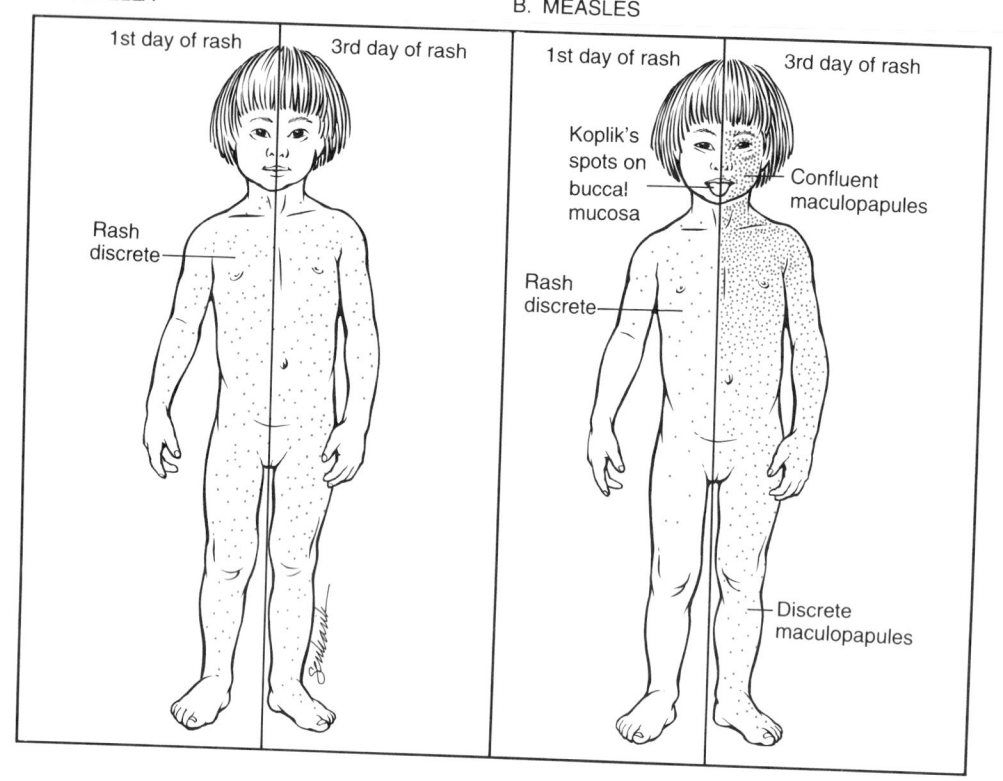

A. RUBELLA

1st day of rash   3rd day of rash

Rash discrete—

B. MEASLES

1st day of rash   3rd day of rash

Koplik's spots on buccal mucosa

Confluent maculopapules

Rash discrete—

Discrete maculopapules

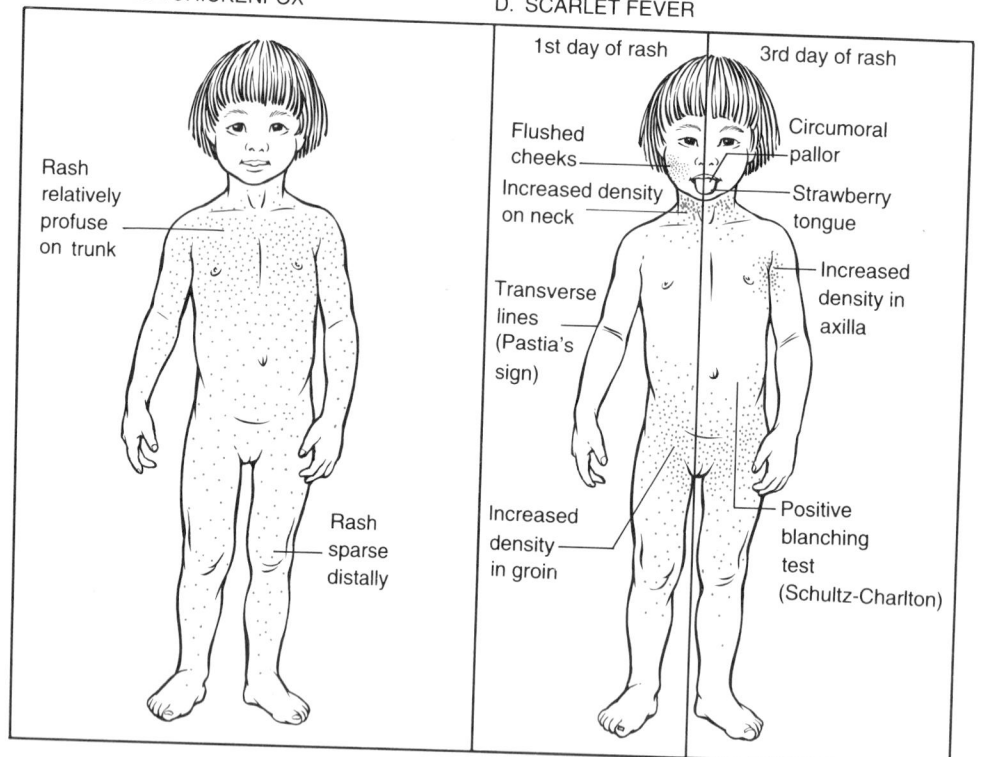

C. VARICELLA CHICKENPOX

Rash relatively profuse on trunk

Rash sparse distally

D. SCARLET FEVER

1st day of rash   3rd day of rash

Flushed cheeks

Circumoral pallor

Increased density on neck

Strawberry tongue

Transverse lines (Pastia's sign)

Increased density in axilla

Increased density in groin

Positive blanching test (Schultz-Charlton)

FIGURE 43-5

Differences in appearance, distribution, and progression of the rashes of rubella, measles, varicella, and scarlet fever.

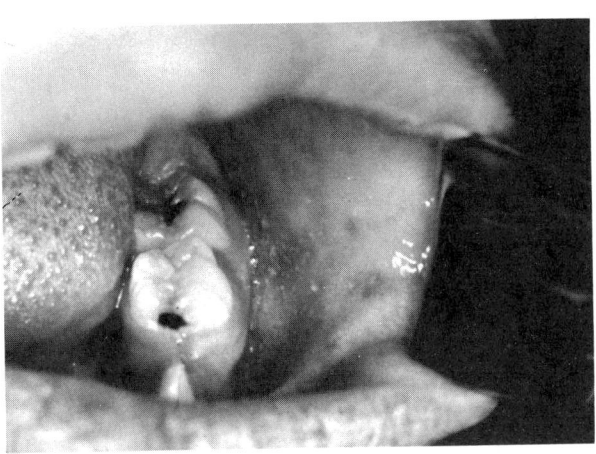

FIGURE 43·6
Koplik's spots on the oral mucous membrane. (Courtesy of the Centers for Disease Control, Atlanta, GA.)

pressure; when it is brown, it does not fade. This differentiates it from the rash of scarlet fever, which always fades on pressure. The rash lasts 5 to 6 days, then fades. There is a fine desquamation following this. Interestingly, the skin of the hands and feet does not desquamate, another feature that differentiates this rash from that of scarlet fever.

Children with measles appear very ill approximately the second day of the rash. Their cough is loud and frequent, the coryza is acute, the fever is high, and the rash is pruritic. On the third day or fourth day of rash, when

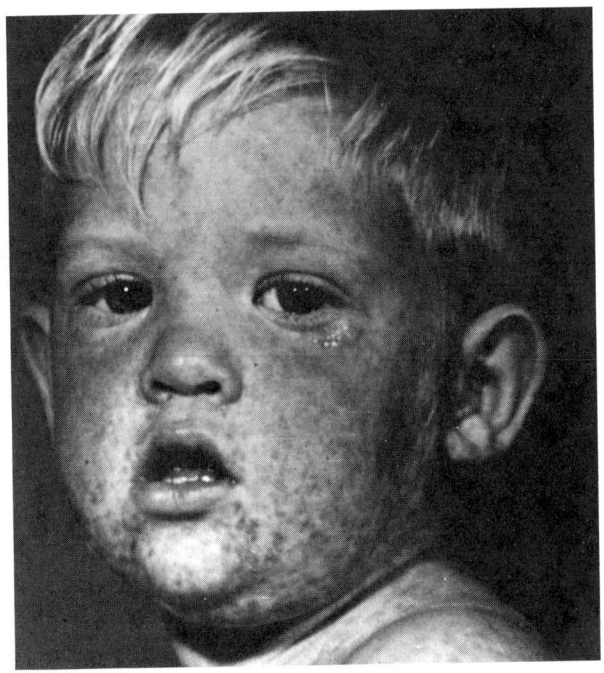

FIGURE 43·7
Typical rash of rubeola. (Courtesy of the Centers for Disease Control, Atlanta, GA.)

the temperature falls, the other symptoms clear quickly and children begin to feel better. Fever that lasts beyond the third or fourth day of rash generally suggests that a complication of measles has occurred (Brunell, 1990).

Therapeutic Management. Children with measles need comfort measures for rash, and they may need an antipyretic for the fever. The coryza does not respond to decongestants, but fortunately lasts only for a few days. The child's skin below the nose may become excoriated from the constant nasal drainage. Applying a lubricating jelly or an emollient (A and D ointment) to the area will prevent excoriation. The child may need a cough suppressant to control the cough; otherwise, the child's throat can become painful from frequent irritation. Because children with measles have photophobia, it is painful for them to look at bright lights; it may be painful for them to watch television. There is an old belief that children with measles must be kept in a dark room because exposure to bright light will lead to blindness. There is no truth to this. However, children are often more comfortable with the shades or curtains drawn or wearing dark glasses, so these measures should be instituted.

Complications. The complications of measles include otitis media (middle ear infection); pneumonia; airway obstruction; and acute encephalitis. Symptoms of otitis media are ear pain in the older child, and irritability and ear-pulling in the infant. Pneumonia is revealed by a chest x-ray and by dullness to percussion, rales, bronchial breathing, and suppression of breath sounds on auscultation. Some degree of hoarseness and a cough are inevitable symptoms of measles. If the inflammation process of the respiratory tract becomes acute and there is airway obstruction, children will have increased hoarseness, a barklike cough, inspiratory stridor, dyspnea, and tachycardia. Children with airway obstruction may need to be intubated to provide a patent airway. Administration of vitamin A appears to reduce the severity of complications such as pneumonia (Hussey & Klein, 1990).

Approximately 1 in 1000 children with rubeola develops measles encephalitis. Symptoms of acute encephalitis are increased fever, headache, vomiting, drowsiness, convulsions, and coma. Children may have a stiff neck or a positive Kernig's sign (pain on extending the leg after it has been flexed on the abdomen), which are signs of meningeal irritation. A lumbar puncture will reveal increased protein in the cerebrospinal fluid. The encephalitis of measles tends to be a severe fulminating type. Approximately 15% of children with this complication die; another 25% will be left with permanent brain damage, such as mental retardation, nerve deafness, hemiplegia, or paraplegia.

Chickenpox (Varicella)

- Causative agent: Varicella-zoster virus
- Incubation period: 10 to 21 days
- Period of communicability: 1 day before the rash to 5 to 6 days after its appearance, when all the vesicles have crusted
- Mode of transmission: Highly contagious; spread by direct or indirect contact of saliva or vesicles
- Immunity: Contracting the disease offers lasting natural immunity to chickenpox; because the same virus causes herpes zoster, it may be reactivated at a later time as herpes zoster.
  - Active artificial immunity: An experimental vaccine is available but has limited use due to side effects.
  - Passive artificial immunity: There is little passive placental immunity to chickenpox. Children with leukemia or who are being treated with corticosteroids are given varicella-zoster immune globulin (VZIG). This may prevent or modify chickenpox if given within 72 hours of exposure.

Assessment. Chickenpox occurs most often in the preschool or early school-age child (ages 2 to 8 years). Children first develop a low-grade fever, malaise, and, in 24 hours, the appearance of a rash (see Figures 43-4 and 43-5C). A chickenpox lesion begins as a macula, then progresses rapidly in a period of 6 to 8 hours to a papule, then a vesicle that first becomes umbilicated and then forms a crust. Each lesion is approximately 2 mm to 3 mm in diameter and is surrounded by an erythematous area. When the first crop of lesions appears, children's temperature may rise markedly to 104°F or 105°F (40.0°C or 40.6°C).

The greatest concentration of chickenpox lesions are on the trunk, although the face, scalp, palate, and neck are also involved. Lesions on the extremities are generally scant in number. Lesions appear in approximately three separate "crops" and move through progressive stages (Figure 43-8). At one time, all four stages of lesions—(1) macule, (2) papule, (3) vesicle, and (4) crust—will be present.

Therapeutic Management. If the scab from crusting is allowed to fall off naturally and lesions do not become secondarily infected, no scarring will result. Scabs removed prematurely may leave a white, round, slightly indented scar at the site. The rash of chickenpox is extremely pruritic, and because it is important that children not scratch and remove scabs, preventing scratching becomes a difficult problem for parents. A prescribed antihistamine will usually reduce the itchiness to a bearable level, and an antipyretic will counteract the high fever. Acyclovir may be prescribed to reduce the number of lesions and shorten the course of the illness (Grose, 1994).

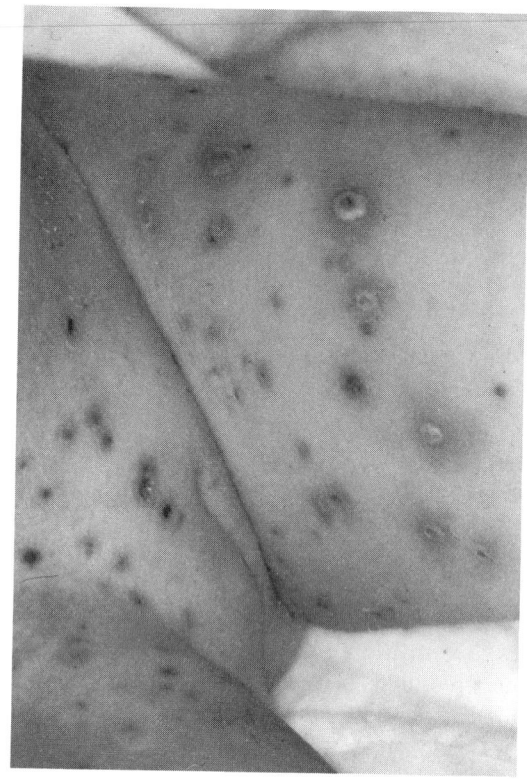

FIGURE 43-8
The lesions of chickenpox—maculas, pustules, vesicles, and crusts—are all present at the same time. (Courtesy of Brian Smistek.)

Complications of chickenpox are secondary infections of the lesions, pneumonia, and encephalitis. The encephalitis of chickenpox generally has a lower mortality associated with it than does measles encephalitis. The development of Reye's syndrome has been associated with aspirin use during varicella and influenza virus illness (see Chapter 49; Novak et al., 1994). Caution parents with all childhood exanthems to avoid aspirin and use acetaminophen (Tylenol) to control fever instead.

Although chickenpox is not as serious a disease as measles, it often seems to be a more severe disease because of the extreme itchiness accompanying it. Reviewing comfort measures for rashes is important for these parents (see also the Nursing Care Plan, p. 1322). Children may return to school as soon as all lesions are crusted; the crusts are not infectious. Chickenpox is extremely serious if it occurs in immunosuppressed children such as those with leukemia. A future vaccine will decrease the incidence of the disease (Hardy & Gershon, 1990).

Herpes Zoster

Herpes zoster is caused by the varicella-zoster virus, the virus of chickenpox. Apparently, the first time children are invaded by the virus, they have symptoms of chickenpox. Thereafter, herpes zoster symptoms may appear, due to reactivation of a latent virus or possibly due to a second or third exposure. Chickenpox tends to be a disease of preschoolers or of younger school-age children. Herpes zoster tends to occur in older children, although it can occur even in infants (Krause & Straus, 1990).

In adults, the first manifestations of herpes zoster are peripheral neuritis and cutaneous vesicular lesions on erythematous bases that follow the distributions of the lumbar and thoracic nerves (spread across the chest and upper face) (Figure 43-9). There is accompanying root pain and motor weakness. The only discomfort children appear to suffer is pruritus; in adults, herpes zoster may cause sharp constant pain at the site of the lesions (Cuzzell, 1990).

Therapeutic Management. Treatment for herpes zoster is basically symptomatic, consisting of an analgesic for pain. Acyclovir, which inhibits viral DNA synthesis, may be effective in limiting the disease. Varicella-zoster immune globulin (VZIG) may minimize symptoms.

Erythema Infectiosum ("Fifth Disease")
- Causative agent: Parvovirus B19
- Incubation period: 6 to 14 days
- Period of communicability: Uncertain
- Mode of transmission: Droplet
- Immunity: None

Assessment. Erythema infectiosum (the fifth important childhood exanthem) occurs most often in children ages 2 to 12 years. The first symptom is the rash, which erupts in three stages. It is intensely red and appears first

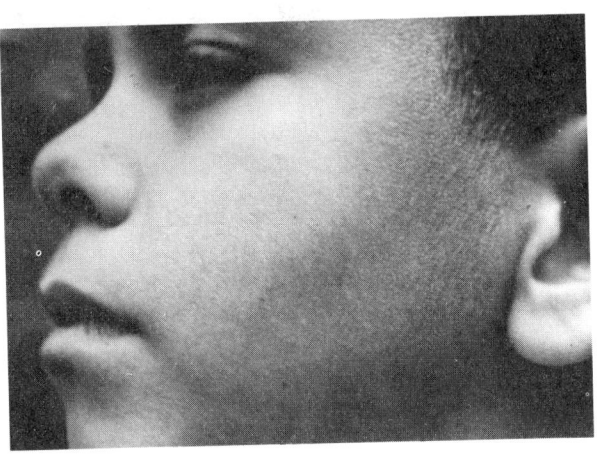

FIGURE 43-10
The typical facial patterns of a child with erythema infectiosum (fifth disease). (Courtesy of the Centers for Disease Control, Atlanta, GA.)

on the face. The lesions are maculopapular and coalesce on the cheeks to form a "slapped face" appearance (Figure 43-10). The circumoral area appears pale next to the reddened area. The facial lesions fade in 1 to 40 days.

A day after the facial lesions appear, a rash appears on the extensor surfaces of the extremities. One day later, it invades the flexor surfaces and the trunk. These lesions last for 1 week or more. When they fade, they fade from the center outward, giving the lesions a lace-like appearance. After the rash has faded, it may reappear if precipitated by skin irritation, such as trauma, sunlight, hot, or cold.

Therapeutic Management. Children may need comfort measures for the rash (see the Focus on Family Teaching box). There are no known complications of fifth disease for the child; it is teratogenic for a fetus.

Pityriasis Rosea
- Causative agent: Probably a virus
- Incubation period: Unknown
- Period of communicability: No evidence to suggest it is contagious
- Mode of transmission: No evidence to suggest it is contagious
- Immunity: Apparently none

Assessment. Pityriasis rosea occurs in school-age and older children. Children may have a short, mild prodromal period of fever and sore throat. A herald patch, an erythematous round lesion with a scaly border, usually appearing on the trunk, is the first obvious lesion (Figure 43-11). Approximately 1 week after the appearance of the herald patch, a generalized rash of papules, vesicles, or urticaria appears. This is generally also confined to the trunk. It follows skin lines, giving it the unique configuration of a Christmas tree.

(text continues on page 1324)

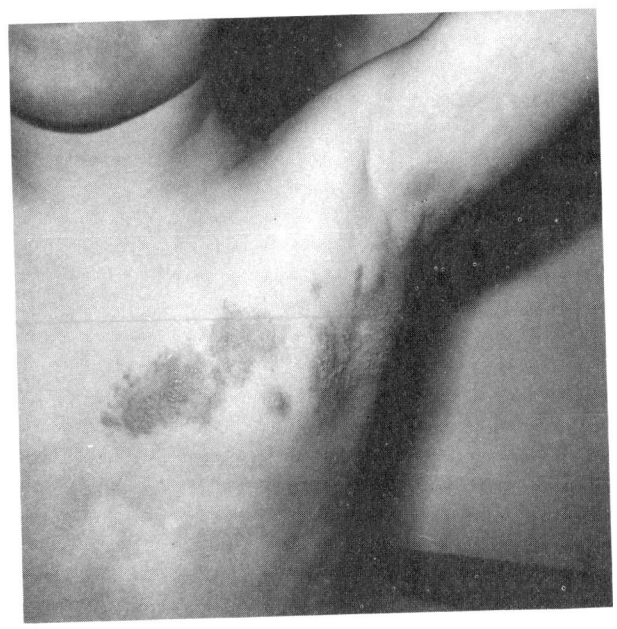

FIGURE 43-9
An adolescent with herpes zoster. Notice the typical distribution. (Courtesy of the Centers for Disease Control, Atlanta, GA.)

Melanie is a 4-year-old admitted to your hospital unit for an appendectomy. The day following surgery, she is diagnosed as having chickenpox (varicella). The following is a nursing care plan you might design for this phase of her care.

Assessment: Four hours after she returned from surgery, Melanie began to develop red macules on her chest and abdomen. By evening, lesions on her back were present and some were papules. By the next morning, lesions had changed to become pruritic, indurated vesicles. Child scratches lesions constantly. Temperature 101.2°F axillary. Mother is a single parent. She is unable to room in because of new 2-month-old at home. Parent's major concern is that the baby will also get chickenpox. Melanie observed soundlessly crying; listless. Stated, "I wish mommy could stay here. I have nothing to do. I'll never be able to go home again so Bobby doesn't get poxed." Wound and respiratory isolation begun.

Nursing Diagnosis: Social isolation related to infection precautions

Defining Characteristic: Child expresses loneliness and boredom.

Goal: Child will demonstrate understanding of the purpose and duration of isolation.

Outcome Criteria: Child states her understanding that her isolation is to prevent other children in the hospital from getting sick. States that chickenpox will go away soon; also states that she will go home when she is recovered from surgery and that by that time, she will no longer be contagious to other children or the new baby.

Nursing Orders	Rationale
1. Maintain respiratory and wound isolation precautions (e.g., closed door, mask, gown if holding child).	1. Prevents spread of infection to other children.
2. Encourage parent to visit. Stress to Melanie that she will be returning home when "tummy is better from surgery."	2. Decreases loneliness in isolation.
3. Allow to apply calamine lotion to lesions by self.	3. Provides a way for Melanie to gain a sense of control.
4. Identify contacts who may need prophylactic immune globulin.	4. Administration of varicella antibodies may help protect susceptible children.
5. Be aware that any children on unit who are immunosuppressed are susceptible to infection.	5. Children on corticotropins or with impaired immune systems following radiation or chemotherapy may easily contract viral infections.

(continued)

Nursing Diagnosis: High risk for altered growth and development related to isolation

Defining Characteristic: Isolation limits interaction with others.

Goal: Child will demonstrate normal growth and development during period of isolation.

Outcome Criteria: Child states she is able to adjust to isolation; relates to personnel and mother at visits.

1. Allow child to see your face before putting on mask to enter isolation room.
2. Provide therapeutic play with dolls, masks, and gowns.
3. Visit child at least hourly while in isolation; devise games that require few materials such as "I spy" or "What happens next" stories.
4. Encourage child to contact mother by telephone during isolation.

1. Helps child to identify personnel even when masked.
2. Therapeutic play helps child deal with fear of hospitalization.
3. Helps prevent loneliness.

4. Knowing that she can reach her mother by phone will help child feel safer and less lonely.

Nursing Diagnosis: Pain (pruritus) related to varicella rash

Defining Characteristic: Child states she is uncomfortable.

Goal: Child will not experience an intolerable level of discomfort.

Outcome Criteria: Child states level of discomfort is tolerable.

Nursing Orders

1. Assess temperature and administer antipyretic as prescribed for temperature of more than 101°F.
2. Administer acetaminophen (Tylenol) as prescribed.

3. Dress child in light clothing so that overheating does not occur. Change bed linen daily for comfort.
4. Offer adequate fluid.
5. Keep child's fingernails cut short.

6. Ask physician for antihistamine prescription; teach child to press on area or use cold cloths as necessary to relieve itching.

Rationale

1. Elevated temperature can be a source of discomfort.
2. Provides measure to reduce itching. To prevent Reye's syndrome, aspirin is never used as a routine analgesic if child has fever.
3. These measures will also help to alleviate discomfort.
4. Maintains hydration.
5. Prevents child from injuring herself when scratching.
6. An antihistamine or cold application can relieve itching.

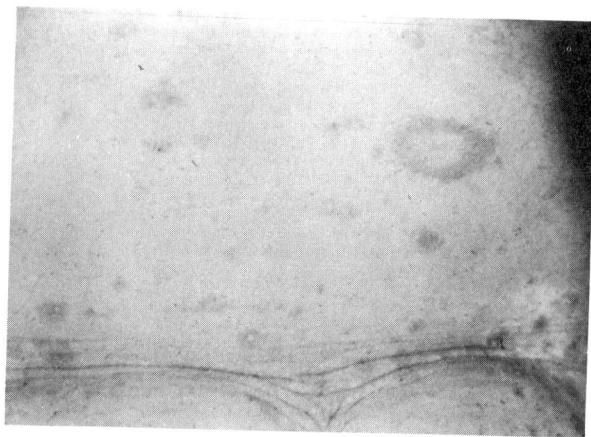

FIGURE 43-11
A herald patch that precedes pityriasis rosea. (Courtesy of the Centers for Disease Control, Atlanta, GA.)

The rash lasts for 6 to 8 weeks. It is pruritic and, because it lasts so long, is particularly worrisome to children and parents. Because the lesions, particularly the herald patch, are scaly at the edges, they are often confused with tinea corporis (ringworm). Treatment is limited to oral antihistamines and other comfort measures for rash.

Pityriasis rosea appears to have no sequelae or complications; in fact, it is difficult to demonstrate in what manner it is infectious. It is mentioned because it is sometimes a baffling rash of childhood and should be differentiated from serious (severe) exanthems (AAP, 1991).

Enteroviruses

The enteroviruses comprise three main types: echoviruses (33 subdivisions); coxsackievirus A (24 subdivisions) and coxsackievirus B (6 types); and polioviruses (3 subdivisions).

Echovirus Infections
The echoviruses are responsible for a number of childhood diseases, including aseptic meningitis, diarrhea, acute respiratory illness, and maculopapular rashes. Such infections are usually benign and self-limiting. Treatment is aimed toward supportive measures.

Coxsackievirus Infections
The coxsackievirus groups are responsible, like the echovirus groups, for a variety of diseases. One of the most frequently found diseases of children caused by coxsackievirus A is herpangina. With herpangina, children have an abrupt elevation of temperature, up to 104°F or 105°F (40.0°C or 40.6°C). This lasts for 1 to 4 days. Anorexia, difficulty swallowing, sore throat, and vomiting may be present. Children may have headaches and abdominal pain. Small lesions, generally discrete

grayish vesicles, pinpoint in size, appear on the fauces, soft palate, and uvula. They may be present elsewhere in the mouth or throat as well. The lesions gradually change to shallow ulcers surrounded by a red areola. The lesions disappear within a few days after the temperature returns to normal. There are generally no complications.

Children need to be maintained on soft or liquid foods while their mouth and throat are sore. They may need an antipyretic for the fever. A local anesthetic (Xylocaine Viscous) may be applied to ulcers by a cotton-tipped applicator to relieve local pain. Children must not swallow the anesthetic liquid; if they do, their throat will become anesthetized and they may then aspirate with swallowing.

Poliovirus Infections: Poliomyelitis (Infantile Paralysis)
- Causative agent: Poliovirus
- Incubation period: 7 to 14 days
- Period of communicability: Greatest shortly before and after onset of symptoms when virus is present in the throat and feces (1 week to 6 weeks)
- Mode of transmission: Direct and indirect contact
- Immunity: Contracting the disease causes active immunity against the one strain of virus causing the illness.
  - Active artificial immunity: Live attenuated virus vaccine
  - Passive artificial immunity: None

Poliomyelitis may be caused by any of the three strains of poliovirus, which is why children must be immunized with trivalent (three-strain) vaccine. Fortunately, because of effective immunization programs against the disease, it currently is rare. The World Health Organization has set a goal to make it extinct by the year 2000 (Robertson et al., 1990).

Assessment. The poliovirus enters children's gastrointestinal tract, where it multiplies. Children may develop the following symptoms: fever, headache, nausea, vomiting, or abdominal pain. Slight erythema of the throat may be seen during a physical assessment. Children have pain and stiffness of the neck, back, and legs. The cerebrospinal fluid (CSF) will generally show increased protein and lymphocytes.

These initial symptoms are followed by intense pain and tremors of extremities, and then paralysis, occurring either immediately or over a period of 1 to 7 days as the virus invades the central nervous system. Kernig's sign will be positive. Children show a tripod sign—when sitting on the floor or on an examining table, they are unable to sit without placing both their arms and hands behind them to brace themselves. Their deep tendon reflexes are hyperactive at first and then diminish.

Paralysis is generally asymmetric. Children's legs seem to be more susceptible than the arms. Respiratory problems occur when there is damage to the cells of the cervical and thoracic segments of the spinal cord. Bulbar paralysis involves the cranial nerves. With bulbar poliomyelitis, children may have difficulty swallowing or talking, and there will be laryngeal paralysis. Respiration halts as the respiratory center of the brain is involved.

Therapeutic Management. Treatment for poliomyelitis is bedrest. For the pain, moist hot packs are helpful. Passive movements and muscle therapy as soon as the pain and spasm are gone will offer best results. For long-term care, children need bracing to strengthen atrophied muscles. They may need muscle transplant operations to achieve better muscle function. Poliomyelitis, in its severest form, is such a crippling disease that it is mandatory that children receive immunization against it. If respiratory muscles were involved, long-term ventilation is necessary. Survivors tend to develop progressive muscle atrophy (postpoliomyelitis muscular atrophy syndrome) in late adulthood, further compounding their ability to be self-sufficient (Ravits et al., 1990).

Viral Infections of the Integumentary System

Viral infections of the skin include the herpes infections and warts (verrucae).

Herpesvirus Infections

Herpesviruses are responsible for a number of infections in children.

- Causative agent: Herpes simplex or herpes type 1 or type 2 virus
- Incubation period: 2 to 12 days
- Period of communicability: Greatest early in the course of the infection
- Mode of transmission: Direct contact
- Immunity: Immunity to a primary herpes response is gained after one incident. There is no immunity to recurrent herpes infections because the virus lies dormant in the body until it is activated by stress, sun exposure, fever, other illness, or menstruation.

Assessment. When children are first invaded by a herpesvirus, they have no antibodies against the virus, so a primary form of disease occurs. The virus remains latent in the neurons of local sensory ganglia or children become permanent carriers of herpes simplex.

Acute Herpetic Gingivostomatitis. Acute herpetic gingivostomatitis is the most common form of herpes simplex invasion in children; it is an example of the primary, not the recurrent, response. It occurs in children ages 1 to 4 years. Children have a high fever (104°F to 105°F [40.0°C to 40.6°C]), are restless, and have anorexia and a sore mouth. Their gumline is swollen and reddened and bleeds easily. White plaques or shallow ulcers with red areolae appear on the buccal mucosa, tongue, palate, and perhaps on the tonsillar fauces. The anterior cervical lymph nodes are enlarged and tender. The disease runs its course in 5 to 7 days.

Therapeutic Management. Children need an antipyretic to reduce fever. A local anesthetic (Xylocaine Viscous) may be applied to lesions by a cotton-tipped applicator to relieve pain. It is important that children not swallow this anesthetic. Children need soft, acid-free foods that they can eat with minimum irritation or abrasion.

Children with gingivostomatitis are often very ill; it is easy to think that this is, after all, just a reaction to herpes simplex and cannot be too serious. However, it can become very serious if children's mouths are so sore that they cannot swallow readily and they become dehydrated.

Herpes Simplex (Herpes Labialis). Herpes simplex infection is popularly known as a cold sore or fever blister. It represents the recurrent form of a type 1 herpesvirus invasion that has remained dormant in ganglia of the trigeminal or 5th cranial nerve. Herpes simplex typically appears as clusters of painful, grouped vesicles found on the lips or skin surrounding the mouth. After 2 or 3 days, vesicles crust, then gradually dry. Keeping lesions dry helps them to fade sooner, but keeping them lubricated with an ointment reduces pain. Application of topical acyclovir reduces pain and increases healing (Spruance et al., 1990). Children feel conspicuous about the appearance of herpes simplex lesions. They may need counseling to assure them that the lesions are not as obvious to others as they imagine.

Acute Herpetic Vulvovaginitis (Genital Herpes). Genital herpes is caused by the herpesvirus type 2, which remains dormant in the ganglia of the sacral nerves. Because this form is spread primarily by sexual contact, it is discussed in Chapter 47 with other STDs.

Eczema Herpeticum. Children with atopic dermatitis (infantile eczema) may have a generalized reaction if they contract a herpes infection. Children develop a fever as high as 104°F to 105°F (40.0°C to 40.6°C), irritability, and crops of vesicles that erupt at the sites of eczematous skin lesions. Lesions may occur at different times during the disease course of 7 to 9 days. Generally by day 10, all lesions are crusted.

In children with severe eczema, the number of lesions that appear may be extreme. Enough body fluid can be lost through the oozing of the vesicles to cause serious fluid loss; pain can be intense. The extent of the involvement can make children gravely ill.

Warts (Verrucae)

Warts are one of the most common dermatological diseases in children. They are caused by the papillomavirus that has an incubation period of between 1 month and 6 months. The mode of transmission is unknown, but it is probably by direct contact.

Warts are flesh-colored, dirty-appearing papules. They generally occur on the dorsal surface of the hands, although they may occur anywhere. Plantar warts appear on the soles of the feet and are painful when children walk. They may be differentiated from calluses in that they obliterate skin lines as they grow, whereas calluses do not.

Warts on the hands or the face are generally removed if they are cosmetically unattractive to children. Plantar warts may have to be removed because of the discomfort they cause. Application of 10% salicylic acid is relatively painless and usually effectively causes warts to atrophy. Parents can use over-the-counter wart remover preparations (e.g., Compound W) to apply to warts and dissolve them. Carbon dioxide snow, liquid nitrogen, electrodesiccation, and curettage are also effective for removal, but these methods are painful.

Children need some reassurance that people do not catch warts from frogs or toads. Also, many children are excluded from gym programs or swimming because they have plantar warts. There is no justification for such exclusion because warts are not that contagious (it may be necessary to advocate for a child to be allowed to join a swimming or gym class). If left without any treatment, warts eventually fade by themselves (AAP, 1991).

Viruses Causing Central Nervous System Diseases

Both encephalitis and meningitis may be caused by a number of viruses of the arbovirus group or by certain bacteria. These are discussed in Chapter 49.

Rabies

- Causative agent: Rabies virus
- Incubation period: 2 to 6 weeks and possibly as long as 12 months
- Period of communicability: 3 to 5 days before the onset of symptoms through the course of the disease
- Mode of transmission: The bite of rabid animals; rarely through saliva from infected animals being transferred to open lesions on a child's skin
- Immunity: Contracting the disease apparently offers active immunity (few people have ever survived the illness to verify this)

- Active artificial immunity: Human diploid cell rabies vaccine
- Passive artificial immunity: Human rabies immune globulin (HRIG)

Any warm-blooded animal can contract rabies. Wild animals, such as skunks, squirrels, and bats, constitute the most important sources of infection from rabies in the United States. However, children receive more bites and, therefore, more treatments for rabies from bites of dogs or cats. Bites of rodents are seldom found to be rabid; bites from other children are not rabid (although therapy is required because such bites usually contain streptococci). In the animal infected with rabies, the virus can be cultured from the central nervous system, saliva, urine, lymph, and blood. When a child is bitten by an infected animal, the virus migrates from the bite area to the central nervous system. Cranial nerve and spinal cord nuclei become acutely damaged. Negri bodies (cytoplasmic inclusion bodies) can be isolated from nerve cells.

Assessment. The diagnosis of rabies is established largely from the history of an animal bite and the clinical symptoms. Following the long incubation period of the virus, children begin to show prodromal signs of malaise, fever, anorexia, nausea, sore throat, drowsiness, irritability, and restlessness. They may notice numbness or hyperesthesia at the area of the bite and along the course of the involved nerves. The white blood cell count (WBC) will show slight leukocytosis. CSF is usually surprisingly normal, with perhaps only a slight elevation in protein and cells. As the symptoms increase, there is high fever, anxiety, and hyperexcitability. Involuntary twitching movements and generalized convulsions may occur. When children try to drink, there are violent contractions of the muscles of the mouth. They may drool saliva rather than swallow it because swallowing is extremely painful. These two phenomena give the disease its popular name hydrophobia ("water-fear").

As symptoms progress, children become comatose; they may have total body paralysis. Peripheral vascular collapse and death follow quickly in only 5 days or 6 days. Postmortem examination will reveal the diagnostic Negri bodies in brain cells.

Therapeutic Management. Once the disease process begins, rabies is invariably fatal; hope lies in preventing the active process. All children who receive an animal bite should be seen by a physician who can evaluate the circumstances surrounding the bite and decide whether to begin rabies prevention measures. The decision to treat must be made immediately if treatment is to be effective.

Taking a history of the incident to determine the type of animal is of primary importance. Most children are sure they know the type of animal if it was a dog; they may be unsure if it was a wild animal. Do not lead children into naming an animal just to please. If asked, "Was it a skunk? A raccoon? A squirrel?" children may choose an animal name because they think that is the answer expected. Instead, ask the child to describe the animal, and then, from that description, establish the kind of animal that bit them. It helps in rural health facilities if there is a picture book of animals handy so preschoolers, especially, can identify the animal in the book that looks like the one that bit them. A rabid animal usually does not act normally. It runs blindly, often staggering; it may dribble saliva rather than swallow it. It is easy to assess whether a household pet is acting this way. It is sometimes difficult to assess the actions of a wild animal because the fear it experiences at being trapped or cornered may make it run about frantically.

An unprovoked attack is more likely to mean the animal is rabid than if the bite happens during a provoked attack. Let children know that they are not going to be punished if they were provoking an animal so they feel free to say so. "I was only hugging him or feeding him" may sound innocent but may have constituted a provoked attack to the animal.

The kind of wound that children receive also is instrumental in deciding whether to begin treatment. A bite mark is much more serious than a scratch from an animal's claws. The immunization status of the animal should be checked if this is available. An animal that has been properly immunized against rabies will rarely transmit the virus. Whether rabies exists in the community at the time of the attack will also influence the decision. If there have been no other reported instances in domestic animals, the chance that this dog bite is serious in terms of rabies is smaller than if other dogs in the area with rabies have been reported.

When children are seen at health care facilities for bites, the wound must be inspected carefully to see whether it was caused by teeth marks or scratch marks. Wash the wound well with soap and water and a suitable antiseptic such as alcohol. If there are puncture wounds, the wound must not be sutured and closed, because tetanus may result. Tetanus organisms are anaerobic and grow in deep closed wounds where oxygen does not reach. The animal that caused the bite must be located if at all possible; it is then confined for 5 to 10 days. If it develops any signs of rabies during this period, it will be destroyed and the brain examined for evidence of rabies. It is important that people understand that domestic animals are not destroyed unless the animal shows signs of rabies. Not knowing this, they may resist surrendering an animal for observation.

If the animal is found to be rabid, children receive both rabies vaccine and antirabies serum. This applies also if the animal escapes and its condition is unknown (it is assumed to be rabid). Routine active immunization

procedure involves 5 days of injections given into the deltoid muscle on days 1, 3, 7, 14, and 28. HRIG is used in addition to the active immunization procedure. A portion of the dose is injected into the wound site; the remainder is given intramuscularly (CDC, 1990).

It may seem contradictory to give an active immunization serum (administering antigen to children) when they have received an animal bite (which administers antigen to them). This is done because rabies virus has a long incubation period before antibody production is stimulated; serum that is administered causes children to begin to form antibodies against the rabies virus immediately. By the time the rabies virus from the bite begins to have an effect (2 to 6 weeks after the bite), children have developed sufficient antibodies to combat it and prevent the illness.

Other Viral Infections
Mumps (Epidemic Parotitis)
- Causative agent: Mumps virus
- Incubation period: 14 to 21 days
- Period of communicability: Shortly before and after onset of parotitis
- Mode of transmission: Direct or indirect contact
- Immunity: Contracting the disease gives lasting natural immunity
  - Active artificial immunity: Attenuated live mumps vaccine
  - Passive artificial immunity: Mumps immune globulin

Assessment. Mumps is now a rare disease due to successful immunization programs. Mumps generally begins with fever, headache, anorexia, and malaise. Within a 24-hour period, children begin to complain of an "earache." When they point to the site of the pain, however, they point not to their ear, but to the jaw line just in front of the ear lobe. Chewing movements aggravate the pain. By the next day, the parotid gland (located just in front of the ear lobe) is swollen and tender. As the parotid gland swells, it displaces the ear upward and backward. The swelling will last for 1 to 6 days.

It is often difficult to differentiate mumps from submaxillary adenitis (swelling of lymph nodes). The best method of differentiation is to place a hand along the child's jaw line. If the major amount of swelling is above the hand, it is probably mumps. If the largest amount of swelling is below the hand line, it is probably adenitis (Figure 43-12) (Isaacs & Menser, 1990).

Therapeutic Management. Children may need to be kept on soft or liquid foods until the major portion of the swelling recedes, because chewing movements are so painful. It is also more difficult for them to swallow

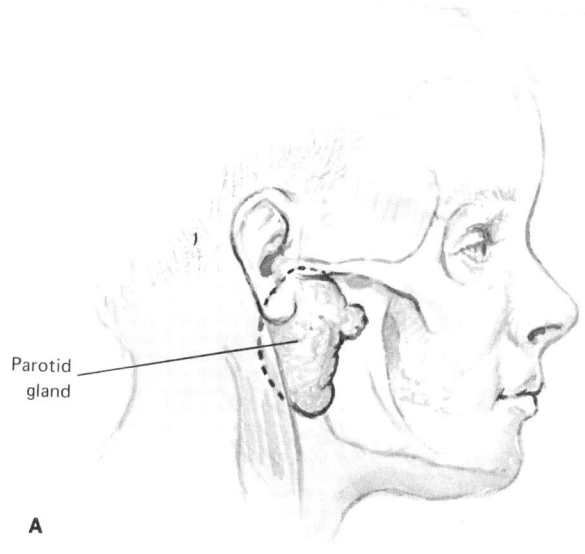

Parotid gland

A

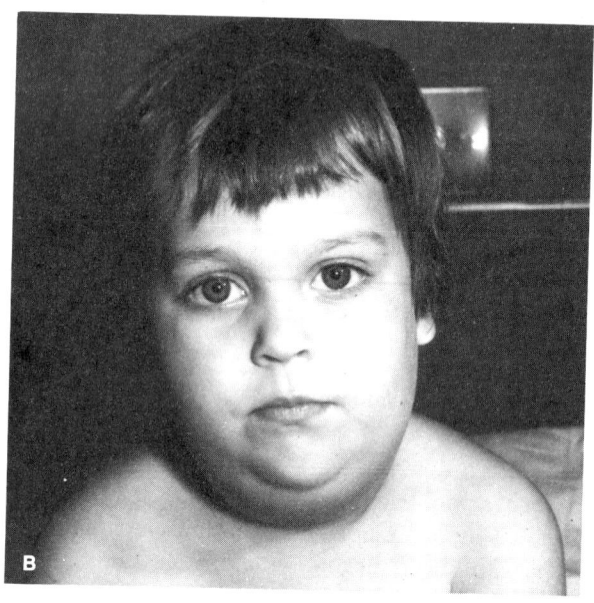

B

FIGURE 43-12

*Infectious parotitis. (**A**) The parotid gland is located just in front of the ear. (Courtesy of the Department of Medical Illustration, State University of New York at Buffalo, Buffalo, NY.) (**B**) The swelling in mumps is invariably above the jawline, which differentiates it from cervical adenitis.*

sour foods than sweet ones. They may need an analgesic for pain and an antipyretic for fever.

It is important to remember that one attack of mumps gives lasting immunity. Some parents report that children had mumps only on one side 1 year ago so they are afraid the child will develop mumps on the opposite side. Children who appear to have had mumps twice are children whose diagnosis was probably confused with cervical adenitis one of the two times.

Complications. A number of serious complications can arise from mumps. Between 20% and 30% of males

older than the age of puberty who develop mumps will develop the complication of orchitis (inflammation of the testes). Fortunately, mumps orchitis is generally unilateral. A single testis swells rapidly and is painful and tender. When the fever of the disease falls, the size of the testis will decrease also, but the tenderness may exist for weeks. Atrophy of the testis may result. The chance that mumps orchitis will lead to complete sterility is exaggerated, however, because the condition is usually unilateral. It is enough reason, however, to be certain that all males receive active immunization against epidemic parotitis before they reach puberty (Manson, 1990).

Meningoencephalitis may occur in a small number of children. The symptoms are increased fever, headache, vomiting, neck rigidity, and a positive Kernig's sign. Unlike the encephalitis of measles or chickenpox, this sequela rarely leaves lasting damage. Severe hearing impairment is a rare complication of mumps. This occurs because of neuritis of the auditory nerve, and it is permanent.

Infectious Mononucleosis

- Causative agent: Epstein-Barr virus
- Incubation period: Unknown; probably 2 to 8 weeks
- Period of communicability: Unknown; probably only during acute illness
- Mode of transmission: Direct and indirect contact
- Immunity: One episode apparently gives lasting immunity. No vaccination is available.

Infectious mononucleosis is also known as glandular fever or, because it was first discovered as a disease that is transferred readily from one person to another by kissing, the kissing disease. It occurs most commonly in adolescents, although it may occur in any age child (Sumaya, 1994).

Assessment. The beginning symptoms are chills, fever, headache, anorexia, and malaise. Children develop lymphadenopathy and a severe sore throat. The fever is generally high (103°F [39.5°C]), although young children may have a low-grade fever or no fever. The fever lasts approximately 6 days.

The cervical lymph nodes are those most markedly affected. They are firm and tender to the touch. The tonsils are not only painful but enlarged and erythematous. There may be a thick white membrane covering the tonsils (Figure 43-13). There are often petechiae on the palate. When mesenteric lymph nodes are enlarged, children may have abdominal pain so sharp it simulates appendicitis. The spleen is enlarged and a danger is that it may spontaneously rupture (Safran & Bloom, 1990). Hepatitis, skin manifestations (such as a maculopapular eruption similar to the rash of rubella), pneumonitis, and

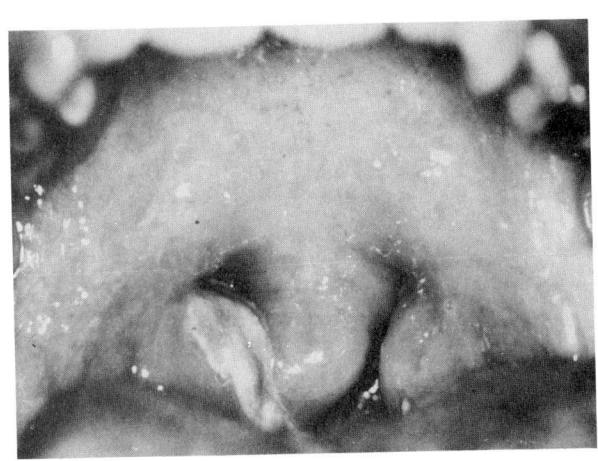

FIGURE 43-13
The pharynx of a child with infectious mononucleosis. Notice the thick, tenacious membrane suggestive of diphtheria. (Courtesy of the Department of Medical Photography, Children's Hospital, Buffalo, NY.)

central nervous system involvement (e.g., encephalitis, meningitis, or polyneuritis) may occur.

With infectious mononucleosis, there is such lymphocytosis that lymphocytes compose more than 50% of the total WBC. Of these lymphocytes, a significant number (more than 20%) are atypical; they are larger-than-normal, mature lymphocytes, and their nuclei are somewhat less dense. A serologic test, known as the heterophil antibody test, has its basis on the fact that the antibody produced in infectious mononucleosis will agglutinate sheep red blood cells. A technique known as the monospot test has also been developed, using horse red blood cells. This test can be performed in a matter of minutes and, if positive, along with the increased number of atypical lymphocytes apparent on a blood slide, confirms a diagnosis of infectious mononucleosis. Epstein-Barr virus antibodies can be recovered for a final diagnosis.

Therapeutic Management. Children with infectious mononucleosis are kept on bedrest during the acute stage of the illness (7 to 10 days), because with the splenomegaly, there is a danger of spleen rupture with any trauma to that area. Children who are extremely ill may be hospitalized. Be careful in helping children with this disease turn in bed so that no pressure is placed over the splenic area. If palpating the spleen as an assessment procedure, use extremely gentle technique to avoid possible rupture.

Administration of corticosteroids may reduce the extent and time span of the sore throat and prolonged fever. Teach children and parents the importance of maintaining a good fluid intake despite the sore throat; cool and nonacidic fluids can be tolerated best.

Children may notice weakness and general fatigue for up to 6 weeks following the illness. Caution them to avoid contact sports as long as the spleen is enlarged. Because infectious mononucleosis occurs primarily in young adults, it may interrupt school or career plans, especially if hospitalization is necessary. Help these young adults to voice their frustration with this illness; offer support to help them through this unexpected interruption in their life.

Cat Scratch Disease

- Causative agent: Cat scratch disease virus
- Incubation period: 3 to 10 days
- Period of communicability: Unknown
- Mode of transmission: Bite or scratch from a cat or kitten
- Immunity: One episode of disease gives lasting immunity; no passive artificial immunity

Cat scratch disease occurs most commonly in preschool children because children at that age play roughly with cats or pick them up against their will and thus receive scratches. Children with HIV are very susceptible to the virus. The organism of cat scratch disease is apparently similar to that of herpes simplex. The cat does not appear to be ill at the time the child contracts the disease. The first symptom is a single skin papule or pustule. This lasts 1 to 3 weeks. Approximately 2 weeks after the scratch, severe local lymphadenopathy develops. The nodes most markedly involved are those of the head, neck, and axilla. The node enlargement generally lasts 2 to 3 months. In some children, there is node suppuration (a node breaks open to the skin and drains sterile pus).

Some children have a low-grade fever and malaise. Occasionally, central nervous system involvement, such as encephalitis or meningitis, occurs. Children will have a positive reaction to a skin test of cat scratch disease antigen. This, with the history of a cat scratch and the aspiration of sterile pus from enlarged lymph nodes, is diagnostic. The treatment is relief of symptoms, although an antibiotic may be prescribed to help shorten the course of the disease. Children may need an analgesic for painful adenopathy; they may need to have the nodes aspirated to relieve pain.

Parents may ask if the cat should be destroyed. Because an attack of cat scratch disease gives lifetime immunity and fewer than 10% of children scratched by the same cat contract cat scratch disease, there is no need to destroy the cat (Boyer, 1994).

Hantavirus Infection

The hantavirus is a member of the arbovirus group. The virus infects small rodents and perhaps cats who have eaten mice. In the Far East, the virus produces an illness marked by extreme purpura from thrombocytopenia and severe gastrointestinal symptoms. In 1993, an outbreak of severe illness from a previously undiscovered hantavirus occurred in the United States; major symptoms were fever, muscle aches, thrombocytopenia, gastrointestinal symptoms, and hypotension. Death occurred from rapid progressive pulmonary edema (Duchin et al., 1994).

Although the mortality from this particular hantavirus infection has been high (about 75%), treatment with the antiviral agent ribavirin may be effective.

Bacterial Infections

Bacteria are usually single-celled organisms. They reproduce by fission, in which one cell enlarges and duplicates itself, then divides into two equal parts. Bacteria have three main shapes: (1) spheres (cocci), (2) rods (bacilli), and (3) corkscrews (spirochetes). Bacteria are independent, living organisms. They have a nucleus, cytoplasm, and a cell wall, and they contain both DNA and RNA.

Bacteria are most commonly observed under a microscope after being fixed to a slide by heating and then being stained. Those bacteria that stain violet are gram-positive organisms; those that stain red are gram-negative organisms. Those that cannot be decolorized with acid after being stained are acid-fast. As some bacteria grow, they produce exotoxin, or poison. Disease symptoms arise not from the bacteria themselves but from the effect of these toxins on the body. Tetanus, botulism, and diphtheria are diseases caused by the systemic spread of toxins produced by bacteria.

Some bacteria are capable of producing enzymes as they grow. Hemolytic streptococci, for example, produce streptokinase, which allows the bacteria to pass through blood clots. Penicillinase, an enzyme produced by certain bacteria, can destroy penicillin. Penicillin will be ineffective, therefore, against such organisms.

Streptococcal Diseases

Streptococci are gram-positive organisms. They are found normally in the respiratory, alimentary, and female genital tracts. The majority of severe diseases in children result from infection with *S. pyogenes* (beta-hemolytic streptococci, group A). Streptococcal pharyngeal infection is discussed in Chapter 40.

Scarlet Fever

- Causative agent: Beta-hemolytic streptococci, group A
- Incubation period: 2 to 5 days
- Period of communicability: Greatest during acute phase of respiratory illness
- Mode of transmission: Direct contact and large droplets
- Immunity: One episode of disease gives lasting immunity to scarlet fever toxin

Assessment. Scarlet fever occurs most commonly in the 6- to 12-year-old age group, although it may be seen in the preschooler. The incidence is highest in temperate climates, and it occurs usually in late winter or early spring months.

The symptoms of scarlet fever begin abruptly and are those of a streptococcal pharyngitis: fever, sore throat, perhaps headache, chills, and malaise. As the beta-hemolytic, group A streptococcus grows in children's bodies, it produces a number of toxins: erythrogenic toxin is the one that is responsible for the rash of scarlet fever. The rash appears 12 to 48 hours after the onset of the pharyngeal symptoms (see Figure 43-3). The fever is high (103°F to 104°F [39.5°C to 40.0°C]) on the first day of throat symptoms and again on the day the rash appears; it then falls gradually to normal (see Figure 43-6). The child's pulse rate may be increased out of proportion to the fever.

The rash of scarlet fever is both enanthematous and exanthematous (on both mucous membrane and skin; see Figures 43-4 and 43-5D). The tonsils are inflamed and enlarged and usually covered with white exudate. The uvula and pharynx are beefy red. The palate is usually covered with erythematous punctiform (pinpoint) lesions and perhaps scattered petechiae. The tongue, during the first 2 days of the illness, is white and furry-appearing. By day 3, papillae enlarge and protrude through the white coat, giving the tongue a white strawberry appearance. By day 4 or 5, the white coat disappears and the prominent papillae of the tongue give it a red strawberry appearance. A "strawberry tongue" is distinctive for scarlet fever and helps to differentiate the disease from other rashes.

The skin rash comprises red pinpoint lesions that blanch on pressure. Lesions are most dense on the trunk and in skin folds. They are few on the face. The area around the mouth tends to be abnormally pale (circumoral pallor). There are areas of hyperpigmentation in the folds of the joints (Pastia's sign). The rash persists for approximately 1 week; it desquamates with large areas of skin peeling off in fine flakes. A throat culture reveals streptococcus.

A particularly virulent form of group A streptococcus has been identified. Caution parents not to "self-treat" children with scarlet fever in case the streptococcus involved is this virulent strain.

Therapeutic Management. Children with scarlet fever are usually ill-appearing. They need a soft or liquid diet for a few days until their throat soreness has diminished. They may need an analgesic such as acetaminophen (Tylenol) for pain and an antipyretic for fever. The rash of scarlet fever tends to be pruritic, so children need comfort measures for rash. Because the underlying cause of the illness is a streptococcus infection, they will be prescribed a 10-day course of penicillin. Parents need to be cautioned to give the full amount prescribed for the full course to prevent the complications of beta-hemolytic, group A streptococcal infections (acute glomerulonephritis or rheumatic fever).

Children who are administered penicillin do not have the typical extreme rash, and obviously do not have as severe a systemic illness as those who do not receive penicillin. As a result, scarlet fever is currently popularly termed "scarlatina" (a small scarlet rash). Caution parents that no matter what name is applied to the disorder, the consequences of it can be grave and penicillin therapy is necessary.

The incidence of rheumatic fever and acute glomerulonephritis occur as sequelae to scarlet fever in only approximately 2% to 3% of children. This occurs 1 week to 3 weeks following the rash. The occurrence seems to be related not to the severity of the scarlet fever but to the body reaction to the toxins produced at the time of the illness.

Impetigo

- Causative agent: Usually beta-hemolytic streptococcus, group A; possibly staphylococcus
- Incubation period: 2 to 5 days
- Period of communicability: From outbreak of lesions until lesions are healed
- Mode of transmission: Direct contact with lesions
- Immunity: none

Impetigo is a superficial infection of the skin. It begins as a single papulovesicular lesion surrounded by localized erythema. More vesicles appear, and they become purulent, ooze, and form honey-colored crusts (Figure 43-14). They are found most commonly on the face and extremities. They are often seen as secondary infections of insect bites or in children who have pierced ears. If there are a number of lesions, children may have local adenopathy.

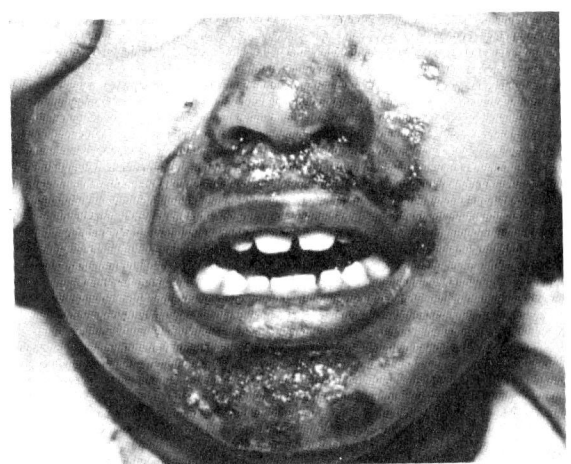

FIGURE 43-14
Typical lesions of impetigo. (From Hoekelman, R., et al. Principles of pediatrics: Health care of the young. New York: McGraw-Hill, with permission.)

Impetigo is only mildly infectious because it seems to be transmitted only by direct contact. It is not uncommon to see several children in a family with identical lesions, however. Parents may be upset at being told their child has impetigo, because at one time the lesions (dirty and crusty appearing) were associated with poor hygiene. Parents' first statement at being told the diagnosis may be, "But our children take baths every day." They can be assured that streptococcal organisms are so numerous that the cleanest child can contract this disease. The presence of the infection reflects on the number of organisms available, not on their child care.

Caution parents to seek health supervision for any lesion that appears reddened or filled with pus (infected), since the causative agent may be a particularly virulent form of streptococcus.

Therapeutic Management. Treatment is oral administration of penicillin or erythromycin or the application of mupirocin (Bactroban) ointment (McLinn, 1990) for a full 10-day period. The application of local antibiotic ointment is not as effective because it does not reduce the number of organisms as effectively and, therefore, reduce the toxin level. The lesions heal most quickly if a parent or the child washes the crusts daily with soap and water.

Impetigo may also occur as a staphylococcal infection, but it should be considered first as a streptococcal infection for treatment. Complications of rheumatic fever or acute glomerulonephritis may occur following impetigo as they may after other streptococcal infections, although this is rare.

Staphylococcal Infections

The staphylococcal organisms are gram-positive. Colonies of staphylococci are normally found on the skin, so they are generally the organisms involved in skin infections (pyoderma). Because the organisms grow rapidly in cream foods that are not well refrigerated, such as potato salad or cream pies, they are the organisms involved in food poisoning episodes during the summer months. Food poisoning leads to gastrointestinal symptoms; this is discussed in Chapter 45.

Furunculosis (Boils)

A furuncle is an infection of the hair follicle; a yellow pustule forms at the site. There is localized redness, pain, and edema of the surrounding skin. Children must be urged not to rupture these lesions but to allow them to run their self-limiting course so that the infection is not spread to surrounding tissue and does not become a cellulitis.

Cellulitis

Cellulitis is an inflammation of the deeper layers of skin. It occurs generally on the extremities or face, or surrounding wounds. The skin feels warm to the touch and is edematous and reddened. Cellulitis is treated with a systemic antibiotic. Warm soaks relieve pain and inflammation.

Scalded Skin Disease

Scalded skin disease (Ritter's disease) is a staphylococcal infection seen primarily in newborns. Children develop rough textured skin and general erythema. Large bullae (vesicles), filled with clear fluid, form. The epidermis separates from children in large sheets, leaving a red, glistening, scalded-looking surface. Children need intensive therapy with a penicillinase-resistant antibiotic such as methicillin and flucloxacillin to survive this extreme infection.

Other Bacterial Infections

Diphtheria

- Causative agent: *C. diphtheriae* (Klebs-Löffler bacillus)
- Incubation period: 2 to 6 days
- Period of communicability: Rarely more than 2 weeks to 4 weeks in untreated persons; 1 to 2 days in patients treated with antibiotics
- Mode of transmission: Direct or indirect contact
- Immunity: Contracting the disease gives lasting natural immunity
  - Active artificial immunity: Diphtheria toxin given as part of DTP vaccine
  - Passive artificial immunity: Diphtheria antitoxin

Assessment. When diphtheria bacilli become infected by a virus, they not only invade and grow in the nasopharynx of children, they produce an exotoxin (a potent protein poison) that causes massive cell necrosis and inflammation. The necrosing material lends itself well to the growth of the bacilli, so the bacilli reproduce rapidly. The inflammation and necrosing cells form a characteristic gray membrane on the nasopharynx. It may extend up into the nose and down into the major bronchi, causing a purulent nasal discharge and a brassy cough. The toxin is absorbed from the membrane surface and spread systemically by the bloodstream to affect the heart (it causes myocarditis with congestive heart failure and conduction disturbances) on approximately day 10 to 14 of the illness and the nervous system (severe neuritis with paralysis of the diaphragm and pharyngeal and laryngeal muscles) on day 3 to week 7 of the illness. Airway obstruction from the inflammation and the membrane is a possibility from the time it first forms. The diagnosis of diphtheria is made on clinical appearance and on a throat culture, which reveals the presence of the bacilli.

Therapeutic Management. Children are treated by intravenous administration of antitoxin in large doses. The antitoxin of diphtheria is grown from a horse-serum

base. Before it is administered, therefore, children must be given a skin or conjunctiva test to rule out a reaction to horse serum. For a conjunctiva test, a drop of the diphtheria antitoxin well diluted with saline is instilled inside the lower lid of one eye. A drop of saline is placed in the other eye as a control. In 20 minutes, both eyes are examined. If lacrimation or conjunctivitis is present in the eye that received the serum, it suggests the child is hypersensitive to horse serum. The antitoxin cannot be administered until the child is desensitized. For a skin test, a small amount of diluted diphtheria antitoxin is administered intracutaneously. After 20 minutes, a wheal 1 cm or more in diameter reveals sensitivity to horse serum. Again, the antitoxin cannot be given until the child is desensitized. Have a syringe of epinephrine prepared before horse-serum antitoxin testing or administration is begun in case a sudden anaphylactic reaction occurs with the serum administration.

In addition to the antitoxin, children are given penicillin or erythromycin for treatment. They need to be maintained on bedrest for the acute stage of the illness. They need careful observation to prevent airway obstruction. If this does occur, intubation may be necessary.

Because diphtheria vaccine is included in routine immunizations for infants, it is almost an extinct disease in the United States. Isolated instances do occur, however, and when they do, prompt recognition and treatment of the disorder is necessary.

Whooping Cough (Pertussis)

- Causative agent: *B. pertussis*
- Incubation period: 5 to 21 days
- Mode of transmission: Direct or indirect contact
- Period of communicability: Greatest in catarrhal stage
- Immunity: Contracting the disease offers lasting natural immunity
  - Active artificial immunity: Pertussis vaccine given as part of DPT vaccine
  - Passive artificial immunity: Pertussis immune serum globulin

Pertussis is a serious disease of childhood, particularly in the infant period. It occurs most often in children up to age 9 years. African-American and Native American children seem to be most susceptible. In older children, more girls than boys contract the infection. It occurs with no seasonal variation.

Assessment. Pertussis manifests itself in three stages: (1) catarrhal, (2) paroxysmal, and (3) convalescent. The catarrhal stage begins with upper respiratory symptoms such as coryza, sneezing, lacrimation, cough, and a low-grade fever. Children are irritable and listless. In some children, a mild cough is the only symptom during this stage. It lasts 1 to 2 weeks.

The paroxysmal stage lasts 4 to 6 weeks. During this time, the cough changes from a mild one to a paroxysmal one, involving five to 10 short, rapid coughs, followed by a rapid inspiration, which causes the "whoop," or high-pitched crowing sound, of whooping cough. Children are in obvious distress while coughing. They may become cyanotic or red faced, and their nose may drain thick, tenacious mucus. They often vomit following a paroxysm of coughing, and they are exhausted afterward from the effort. Attacks of coughing tend to be more severe at night than during the daytime.

During the convalescent stage, there is a gradual cessation of the coughing and vomiting. The cough may be present for some time, but as single, not paroxysmal coughs. During the next year, if children develop an upper respiratory infection, they may again have a return of the paroxysmal coughing with vomiting.

Pertussis is diagnosed by its striking symptoms, although in children younger than age 6 months the "whoop" of the cough may be absent, making it more difficult to diagnose. The *B. pertussis* bacillus may be cultured from nasopharyngeal secretions during the catarrhal and paroxysmal stages. WBC rises with whooping cough, particularly the lymphocyte count. WBC may be as high as 20,000 to 30,000 mm^3 at the end of the catarrhal stage (normal is 5,000 to 10,000 mm^3).

Therapeutic Management. Children with pertussis must be maintained on bedrest until the paroxysms of coughing subside. They need to be secluded from external factors such as cigarette smoke, dust, and strenuous activity that initiate coughing episodes. Nutrition may be a problem if the child is constantly coughing and vomiting. There is no nausea with this form of vomiting, so children can be fed again immediately after vomiting. As a rule, frequent small meals are vomited less than larger meals. Infants with pertussis may be admitted to a health care facility for observation because they may have such tenacious secretions with coughing episodes that they need airway suction. Some infants do well in a mist tent, which tends to loosen secretions. Placing an intercom in the infant's room allows personnel to listen for paroxysms of coughing even when not immediately near the child.

A full 10-day course of erythromycin or penicillin is prescribed. These drugs shorten the period of communicability and may shorten the duration of symptoms.

Complications of pertussis are pneumonia, atelectasis, or emphysema from plugged bronchioles. Convulsions from asphyxia as a result of severe paroxysms of coughing may occur. Subarachnoid bleeding from the forcefulness of coughing may occur. If sufficient fluid intake cannot be maintained, alkalosis and dehydration from the persistent vomiting can occur.

Prevention. Little passive immunity is transferred to the newborn, so children in their early months are par-

ticularly susceptible to this disease. Infants who are exposed may be administered pertussis immune serum globulin to protect them from contracting the disease. Currently, some parents ask not to have their children immunized against pertussis because of reports that the vaccine causes central nervous system damage. This has created a group of children who are susceptible to the illness (Brahams, 1990). As a rule, the risk of a complication from the vaccine is less then the risk of a complication from the illness and administration of a new acellular vaccine further reduces the risk. AAP (1991) recommends that all children receive immunization against pertussis.

Tetanus (Lockjaw)

- Causative agent: *C. tetani*
- Incubation period: 3 days to 3 weeks
- Period of communicability: None
- Mode of transmission: Direct or indirect contamination of a closed wound
- Immunity: Development of the disease gives lasting natural immunity
  - Active artificial immunity: Tetanus toxoid contained in DPT vaccine
  - Passive artificial immunity: Tetanus immune globulin

Tetanus is a highly fatal disease (the mortality rate is as high as 35%), caused by an anaerobic, spore-forming bacillus. The bacillus is found in soil and in the excretions of animals, and it enters the body through a wound. If the wound is deep, such as a puncture wound, where the distal end of the wound is shut off from an oxygen source, the tetanus bacilli begins to reproduce. The organism may also enter through a burn site, which crusts, creating an anaerobic environment. As the bacilli grow, they produce exotoxins that cause the disease symptoms by affecting the motor nuclei of the central nervous system.

The site of entrance of the bacillus does not appear infected (no pus or reddened area is present unless a secondary infection also exists). After the incubation period, the exotoxins have developed to such an extent, however, that they are capable of disrupting the nervous system.

Assessment. The first symptoms that are noticeable are stiffness of the neck and jaw (lockjaw). Within 24 to 48 hours, muscular rigidity of the trunk and extremities develops. Children's backs become arched (opisthotonos); their abdominal muscles are stiff and boardlike; and their faces assume an unusual appearance with wrinkling of the forehead and distortion of the corners of the mouth (a "sardonic grin" sign). Any stimulation such as a sudden noise, a bright light, or someone touching them causes children to have painful, paroxysmal spasms. Children's sensoriums are clear throughout the course of the disease, so they are aware of the pain associated with muscle spasms. As these spasms begin to include laryngospasm, respiratory obstruction, and a collection of secretions in the respiratory tract, they will lead ultimately to death by asphyxiation.

Fever is an ominous sign accompanying tetanus; those children who survive the disease rarely have more than a low-grade fever.

Therapeutic Management. Children need to be cared for in a quiet, stimulation-free room. If the wound has necrotic tissue, it may be debrided to ensure that no secondary infections arise. Tube feeding or total parenteral nutrition may be begun to prevent aspiration from laryngeal spasm. Children are administered tetanus immune globulin (human). This supplies passive antitoxins to combat the extent of the disease involvement.

Parenteral penicillin G or a form of tetracycline is administered to reduce the number of growing forms of the bacillus. Children must be given a form of sedation and a muscle relaxant to reduce the severity and pain of the muscle spasms. This may be done by administering d-tubocurarine, which produces systemic paralysis. Children need to be intubated and artificial ventilation begun to maintain respiratory function after administration.

Prevention. Tetanus is a serious disease, but is also a preventable one through active immunization and suitable booster immunization. Children routinely receive tetanus immunization as part of routine DPT immunization and a booster dose at school age; thereafter they should receive a booster dose every 10 years. At the time of a wound, the wound site should be cleaned well with soap and water and a suitable antiseptic. If the wound is deep, such as a knife stab, a nail puncture, or a dog bite, it should not be sutured but, rather, left open to heal by secondary intention. This reduces the possibility of an anaerobic pocket forming in the wound. If children received their basic immunization against tetanus (five doses) and it has been fewer than 10 years since the last injection, children need no booster or antitoxin management at the time of the wound.

If a child's immunization record cannot be obtained, or if it has been more than 10 years since the child received a booster injection, or an initial injection for tetanus, the child will probably be treated with a booster injection and tetanus immune globulin. A booster injection provides tetanus antigen to the child. If children received their initial immunization for this disease, the booster will cause their bodies to "remember" how to make tetanus antibodies, and their body will begin to produce them rapidly. By the time the invading tetanus organisms from the wound have passed their long incubation period (3 days to 3 weeks), children have antibodies in their system prepared to eradicate the organisms. If their initial immunizations were incomplete or are unknown, in addition to tetanus antigen they will also receive the passive antibodies included in tetanus immune globulin.

Other Infectious Pathogens

Rickettsial Diseases

Rickettsiae are organisms that resemble viruses both in size and in their inability to reproduce except inside the cells of a host organism. They reproduce by fission, however, as bacteria do; like bacteria, they are complete organisms in that they have both RNA and DNA in their makeup. They multiply inside ticks, lice, mites, or fleas (arthropods) without causing disease. They are transmitted to humans by the bite or feces of the infected arthropod. An exception is Q fever, which is spread by droplet infection. All rickettsial diseases include fever and almost all include a rash caused by rickettsial multiplication in the endothelial cells of small blood vessels. Rickettsiae invasion triggers an immune response.

Rocky Mountain Spotted Fever

- Causative agent: *R. rickettsii*
- Incubation period: 3 to 12 days
- Period of communicability: Not communicable from one person to another
- Mode of transmission: Wood, dog, or rabbit tick
- Active artificial immunity: Rocky Mountain spotted fever vaccine

This is the most common rickettsial disease seen in the United States. It is transmitted by a tick, so it is seen most often during the spring and early summer when ticks are most commonly seen. Children have a fever, severe headache, and a measleslike rash. The rash begins on the ankles and wrists, then spreads to the palms, soles, back, arms, thighs, and chest. The rash comprises bright red macules at first; as it spreads, it becomes hemorrhagic (Figure 43-15).

If untreated, Rocky Mountain spotted fever is fatal. The disease responds well to tetracycline, however.

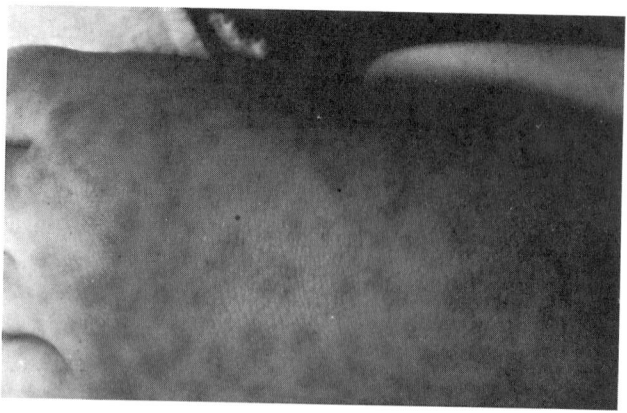

FIGURE 43-15
Typical rash of Rocky Mountain spotted fever. (Courtesy of the Centers for Disease Control, Atlanta, GA.)

Children can be actively immunized against the disease, but the efficiency of the vaccine is questionable and it is generally only administered to workers exposed to high occupational risk such as telephone line personnel (Fischer, 1990).

Rickettsialpox

Rickettsialpox is a disease of crowded urban areas because it is carried by a mouse mite. There is a local lesion at the site of the bite and a generalized rash over the entire body with the exception of the palms and soles. The illness responds to tetracycline.

Lyme Disease

Lyme disease is caused by a spirochete *Borrelia burgdorferi* that is transmitted by a tick often carried on deer. The disease is the most frequently reported vector-borne infection in the United States. It occurs most often in the summer and early fall. Almost immediately following the tick bite, an erythematous papule is noticeable at the site. This spreads over the next 3 to 30 days (the incubation period) to become a large round ring with a raised swollen border (erythema chronicum migrans). This is followed by systemic involvement that leads to cardiac, musculoskeletal, and neurologic symptoms. Cardiac involvement may be so severe that it includes heart block from atrioventricular conduction abnormalities. Neurologic symptoms are commonly stiff neck, headache, and cranial nerve palsy. Musculoskeletal symptoms occur in 50% of children and include painful swollen arthritic joints, particularly the knee (Stechenberg, 1990).

Oral penicillin is administered at the time of the bite to young children; tetracycline to those older than age 8 years. Anti-inflammatory agents and daily prednisone may be necessary to reduce the cardiac and arthritic effects.

Parents should be cautioned to inspect the skin of children who have been playing in wooded areas for possible tick bites when they return from play so this illness can be better identified before debilitating symptoms occur. Suggestions for avoiding Lyme disease are shown in Box 43-2 (Bresingham, 1990).

Murine Typhus

Murine typhus is seen almost exclusively in the southern United States. It is transmitted by mites and fleas that live on rats. It is almost identical in symptoms to Rocky Mountain spotted fever. It responds to tetracycline or a third generation antibiotic such as ciprofloxacin (Strand & Stroomberg, 1990).

Chlamydial Infections

Chlamydiae are gram-negative nonmotile organisms similar to rickettsiae. Chlamydiae vaginitis or pneumonia may occur (see Chapters 40 and 47). Psittacosis is a chlamydial infection commonly found in children.

> **Box 43-2**
> *Tips for Avoiding Exposure to Lyme Disease*
>
> - Wear protective clothing when hiking in wooded areas: long sleeves, high necklines, long slacks, Tuck bottom of slacks into socks or boots.
> - Wear light colored clothing so any tick present on clothing can be readily observed.
> - Inspect skin following hiking in woody areas for ticks. Remove any present with tweezers.
> - Report any area of inflammation that might be a tick bite to a health care provider for early diagnosis.

Psittacosis

Psittacosis is caused by *Chlamydia psittace*. It is a disease transmitted to children by birds, such as parakeets, lovebirds, parrots, chickens, turkeys, and pigeons. The bird has no apparent symptoms of illness. Children develop symptoms of an upper respiratory infection. They may have a low-grade fever, a dry cough, weakness, and anorexia out of proportion to the fever. An enlarged spleen may also be present. Children may develop patchy bronchopneumonia. The course of the disease is as long as 3 to 4 weeks. Treatment is with tetracycline.

Parasitic Infections

Parasites are organisms that live and obtain their food supply from other organisms.

Pediculosis Capitis

Head lice are commonly found among school-age children. The lice themselves are rarely visible, but the eggs are usually seen as small, white flecks on hair shafts (Figure 43-16). The lice cause intense pruritus, and scratching often leads to breaks in the skin that become secondarily infected. The use of lindane (Kwell shampoo) or pyrethrin effectively kills head lice. Following the shampooing, the eggs (nits) can be combed from the hair with a fine-tooth comb. Kwell should not be left on the scalp longer than the manufacturer recommends or else neurotoxicity can occur.

In addition to shampooing, children's bed sheets and all clothing worn recently should be laundered before being worn again. Lice are spread easily in classrooms because children exchange combs and towels after gym classes or touch heads while whispering secrets or tumbling on mats in gym class. Parents are often embarrassed when they learn their child has lice, afraid that health care personnel will think their home is dirty or they do not practice adequate hygiene. They can be assured that lice infestation can happen to any child.

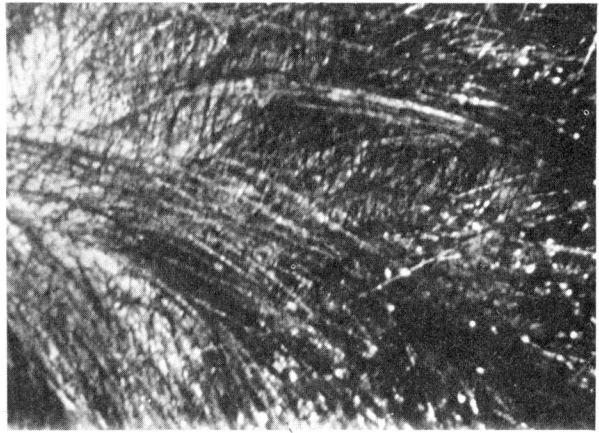

FIGURE 43-16
Nits (eggs) of pediculosis capitis (lice) on hair shafts. (Courtesy of the Centers for Disease Control, Atlanta, GA.)

Pediculosis Pubis

Pubic lice infect the pubic hair of children. Commonly called "crabs," they occur mostly in adolescents; they are spread most often by physical intimacy. Treatment is the same as with head lice.

Scabies

Scabies is a skin disorder caused by a female mite, *Acarus scabiei.* The mite burrows into the skin in areas that are thin and moist, particularly the areas between fingers and toes, the palms, in the axilla, and in the groin, although in the young child the sites may be much more scattered in location than this (O'Donnell et al., 1990). The female mite burrows into the skin to deposit eggs. Black-colored burrows, contaminated by mite feces, approximately ½ inch in length, are generally visible. Severe itching is present, and secondary infection due to scratching and breaks in the skin may occur. Washing the areas with lindane (Kwell lotion) or permethrin will destroy the mites.

Helminthic Infections

Helminth means worm and refers to pathogenic or parasitic ones. They may be roundworms (nematodes), flukes (trematodes), or tapeworms (cestodes). Most helminths begin life when the eggs or larvae are eliminated in feces or urine of humans. They are then transmitted to the oral cavity by unclean foods or hands. Because children tend to be careless about washing hands before eating or suck their thumbs, they are prone to these infections.

Roundworms (Ascariasis)

The roundworm parasite lives in the intestinal tract; eggs are excreted in the feces. If children eat food that is improperly washed or with hands that are improperly washed, eggs may be ingested by them along with soil.

Larvae, which hatch from the ingested eggs, penetrate the intestinal wall and enter the circulation. From there, they may migrate to any body tissue. Children have a loss of appetite and perhaps nausea and vomiting. Intestinal obstruction may occur from a mass of roundworms in the intestinal tract. Ascariasis can be prevented by the sanitary disposal of feces so this does not contaminate soil. A single dose of an anthelmintic such as pyrantel pamoate (Antiminth) controls the infection.

Hookworm

Hookworm eggs, like roundworm eggs, are found in human feces. They enter children's bodies through the skin and then migrate to the intestinal tract, where they attach themselves onto the intestinal villi. They suck blood from children's intestinal wall to sustain themselves. If a great number of hookworms are present, severe anemia may result. Treatment is with anthelmintics to destroy the worms. Children may also need therapy for the anemia.

Pinworms

Pinworms are small, white, threadlike worms that live in the cecum. At night, the female pinworm migrates down the intestinal tract and out the anus to deposit eggs in the anal and perianal region. The anal area itches and the child wakes at night crying and scratching. Some of the eggs are then carried from their fingernails to their mouths; they hatch in children's intestinal tract, and the cycle is repeated.

The worms are large enough that they can be seen if children's buttocks are separated when they are sleeping. Pressing a piece of cellophane tape against the anus and then looking at it under a microscope will generally reveal pinworm eggs.

Treatment is with a single dose of mebendazole (Vermox) or pyrantel pamoate (Antiminth); both drugs destroy pinworms effectively. All family members are treated for pinworm infestation because such worms are easily transmitted from person to person. Underclothing, bedding, towels, and nightclothing should be washed before reuse. Teach children to avoid nailbiting and to wash hands before food preparation or eating to avoid transfer of pinworm eggs to the GI tract.

Protozoan Infections

Protozoa are unicellular organisms. They absorb fluid through the cell membrane and are able to move from place to place by pseudopod, flagella, or cilia action. They are most pathogenic in the gastrointestinal, genitourinary, and circulatory systems. Some protozoa reproduce by simple binary fission; other forms have complex life cycles. Protozoa have the ability to form cysts or surround themselves with a resistant membrane. This makes them resistant to destruction.

Giardia Lamblia

Giardia lamblia is a protozoan infection that is responsible for epidemic outbreaks of diarrhea, particularly in travelers to Europe and in United States day care centers.

Transmission occurs when the child ingests the cysts of the organism on unclean hands. In the intestine, the cysts develop into the mature form of the organism causing symptoms such as diarrhea, weight loss, abdominal cramps, and nausea.

Diagnosis is made by history and recognition of the mature form of the organism in the stool or on duodenal aspiration. Therapy is with quinacrine hydrochloride (Atabrine) for 5 to 7 days or metronidazole (Flagyl) for 5 days. Be certain that parents of children know that Flagyl is contraindicated during pregnancy so a pregnant mother does not self-medicate.

Fungal Infections

Fungi are larger than bacteria; some are unicellular (yeasts), but generally they are multicellular (molds). Fungal infections are most often divided into groups according to the body tissue they infect. Deep mycoses invade internal organs. Transmission is by the inhalation of spores. Subcutaneous mycoses invade skin, subcutaneous tissue, and bone. Infections usually occur from introduction of the fungi into a wound. Superficial mycoses invade only the hair, skin, or nails.

Superficial Fungal Infections

Four superficial fungal infections are seen frequently in children.

Tinea Cruris. *Tinea cruris* (jock itch) occurs on the inner aspects of the thighs and scrotum. It is pruritic. Local application of tolnaftate liquid or powder is effective in destroying the infection.

Tinea Pedis. *Tinea pedis* (athlete's foot) produces lesions on skin between toes and on the plantar surface of the foot. Pruritic, pinpoint-size vesicles and fissuring, especially between the toes, may occur. It is treated with liquid preparations of tolnaftate (Pariser, 1990).

Tinea Capitis. *Tinea capitis* (ringworm) is a fungal infection that begins as an infection of a single hair follicle but spreads rapidly in a circular pattern to produce a lesion usually approximately 1 inch or so in diameter. The hairs involved in the lesion generally break off. The circle becomes filled with dirty-appearing scales. Some strains of tinea capitis may be detected because they glow green under a Wood's light. Newer strains of the organism do not do this, so the test is losing its accuracy. Treatment is with griseofulvin given orally. Teach adolescents not to use alcohol while taking this drug; this may cause tachycardia. Safety during pregnancy is not

established. Children should avoid strong sunlight during therapy, because photosensitivity may occur. Tinea capitis is not as contagious as was once assumed. Children should not be kept home from school, although they should be cautioned not to exchange towels or combs or other potential fomites. The course of the disease may be long; it may be 3 months before all lesions have faded (Figure 43-17).

Tinea Corporis. *Tinea corporis* is fungal infection of the epidermal layer of the skin. It presents as a scaly ring of inflammation with a clear area in the center. Treatment is with a topical antifungal agent such as clotrimazole (Tunnessen, 1994).

Candidiasis

Candida albicans is the fungus that is responsible for candidal (monilial infections). *Candida* organisms grow in the vagina of many adult women (candidal vaginitis). Newborns delivered vaginally may develop an infection of the mucous membrane of the mouth (thrush or oral *Candida* infection). Thrush is characterized by white plaques on an erythematous base on the buccal membrane and the surface of the tongue. It resembles milk curd left from a recent milk feeding. Thrush plaques do not scrape away, however, whereas milk curds do. The child's mouth is painful, and he or she does not eat well due to the inflammation and local pain. Adolescent girls may develop candidal vaginitis.

C. albicans also causes a severe, bright red, sharply circumscribed diaper-area rash (Figure 43-18). Stellite lesions also may appear. The rash is marked by its intense color, and it does not improve with the usual diaper-rash measures, such as application of talcum or a diaper rash remedy such as Desitin, frequent changing of diapers, or exposure to air.

Nystatin is an antifungal drug that is effective against

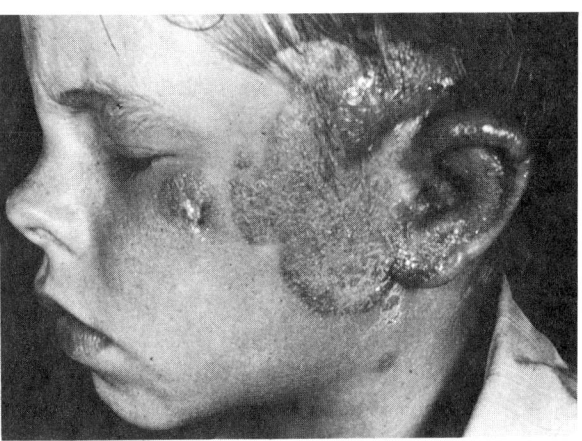

FIGURE 43-17
Tinea capitis (ringworm) of the scalp and face. (Courtesy of the Centers for Disease Control, Atlanta, GA.)

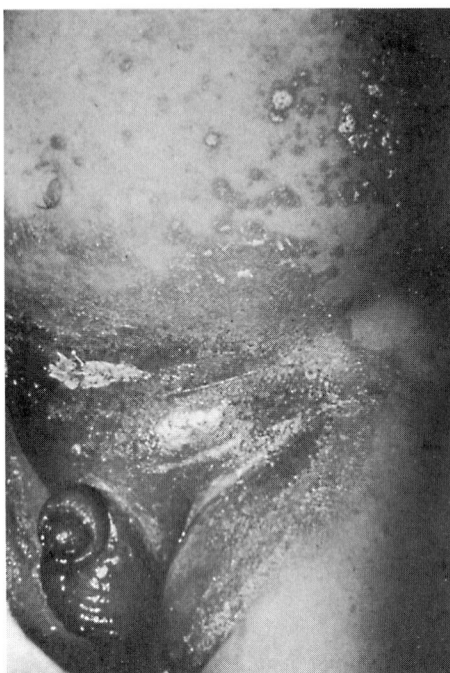

FIGURE 43-18
Monilial diaper area rash. (Courtesy of the Centers for Disease Control, Atlanta, GA.)

all three forms of this disease. For thrush, it is generally administered orally approximately 4 times a day. It should be dropped into infant's mouths following feedings so it will remain in contact with lesions for a time rather than being washed away immediately by a feeding. For diaper rash, a nystatin ointment is prescribed. For candidal vaginitis in the adolescent, vaginal suppositories of nystatin may be prescribed. Teach adolescents to continue use through the menstrual period. A sexual partner should use a condom to avoid reinfection. Itraconazole may be prescribed if the infection is persistent (Blatchford, 1990).

Candidiasis can become a generalized infection, especially in a newborn. There is a tendency to think of thrush as a common—almost something to be expected—disease of infants. It needs treatment, however, to prevent it from becoming more serious or systemic.

Key Points

- The incubation period of infectious disease is the time between the invasion of an organism and the onset of symptoms. A prodromal period is the time between the beginning of nonspecific symptoms and specific symptoms. Children are infectious during the prodromal period. Illness is the stage during which specific symptoms are evident. The convalescent period is the interval between the time symptoms begin to fade and the child returns to full wellness.

- The chain of infection depends on the presence of a reservoir, a portal of exit, a means of transmission, a portal of entry, and a susceptible host.

- Immunization depends on the activation of the immune system. Both B-cell (humoral immunity) and T-cell (cellular immunity) lymphocytes are involved. Immunity may be active (the child has developed the disease or had antigens of the disease administered), or passive (antibodies against the disease are administered to the child by vaccines or placental transfer).

- Common viral infections of childhood are exanthem subitum (roseola), rubella (German measles), measles (rubeola), chickenpox (varicella), herpes zoster, erythema infectiosum (fifth disease), pityriasis rosea, mumps (epidemic parotitis), infectious mononucleosis, and cat scratch disease. Other important viral infections are poliomyelitis (now almost extinct), herpesvirus infections, and verrucae (warts). Rabies continues to be a problem because of children's love of animals.

- Streptococcal diseases seen are scarlet fever and impetigo. Staphylococcal infections seen are furunculosis (boils), cellulitis, and scalded skin disease. Outbreaks of diphtheria, whooping cough (pertussis), and tetanus (lockjaw) still occur.

- Important rickettsial diseases seen are Rocky Mountain spotted fever and Lyme disease. Parasitic infections are pediculosis capitis (head lice), pediculosis pubis, and scabies. Helminthic infections are roundworm, hookworm, and pinworm. Fungal infections are tinea capitis and tinea corporis (ringworm).

- Teach parents and children that keeping immunizations up to date is the best protection against childhood communicable diseases.

- Teach children that careful handwashing and limiting the number of items shared in school can limit the spread of many childhood infections.

- Before a horse-based serum is administered, sensitivity testing must be done to rule out the possibility of anaphylactic shock.

Critical Thinking Exercises

1. Norman is a 2-year-old who is found to have pediculosis on a routine health exam. His mother tells you she can't believe the diagnosis because she thought only poor children developed head lice. She is also very concerned that her son will have his head shaved to cure him. How would you advise her?

2. Mrs. Torrance tells you that she does not intend to

have her newborn immunized because she feels the risk of developing a complication from vaccine administration is higher than letting her child contract simple childhood diseases. How would you counsel her?

3. Mrs. Bernicki's daughter developed chickenpox after attending a birthday party. She asks you why parents don't have enough common sense to keep an ill child at home so infectious diseases aren't spread this way. Is controlling infectious disease this simple? Can Mrs. Bernicki be certain her daughter didn't spread the disease to others before her disease became obvious?

References

Allen, U., & Ford-Jones, E. L. (1990). Nosocomial infections in the pediatric patient: An update. *American Journal of Infection Control, 18,* 176.

American Academy of Pediatrics, Committee on Infectious Diseases. (1991). *The red book.* Elk Grove Village, IL: Author.

Bakshi, S. S., & Cooper, L. Z. (1990). Rubella and mumps vaccines. *Pediatric Clinics of North America, 37,* 651.

Belcher, E. A. (1993). Prevention of childhood diseases through vaccination. *Neonatal Network, 12,* 35.

Blatchford, N. R. (1990). Treatment of oral candidiasis with itraconazole: A review. *Journal of the American Academy of Dermatology, 23,* 565.

Boyer, K. M. (1994). Cat-scratch disease. In F. A. Oski et al. (Eds.) *Principles and practice of pediatrics* (2nd ed.). Philadelphia: J.B. Lippincott.

Brahams, D. (1990). Pertussis vaccine litigation. *Lancet, 335,* 909.

Bresingham, I. (1990). Pediatric management problems: Lyme disease. *Pediatric Nursing, 16,* 280.

Brunell, P. A. (1990). Measles one more time. *Pediatrics, 86,* 474.

Bullock, B. L. & Rosendahl, P. P. (1992). *Pathophysiology: Adaptations and alterations in function* (3rd ed.). Philadelphia: J.B. Lippincott.

Centers for Disease Control. (1990). Compendium of animal rabies control. *Morbidity and Mortality Weekly Report, 39,* 7.

Cuzzell, J. A. (1990). Clues: Pain, burning and itching. *American Journal of Nursing, 90,* 15.

Department of Health & Human Services. (1991). *Healthy people 2000.* Washington, DC: Public Health Service.

Duchin, J. S., et al. (1994). Hantavirus pulmonary syndrome. *New England Journal of Medicine, 330,* 949.

Fischer, J. J. (1990). Rocky Mountain spotted fever. *Postgraduate Medicine, 87,* 109.

Grose, C. (1994). Varicella-zoster virus infections. In F. A. Oski et al. (Eds.) *Principles and practice of pediatrics* (2nd ed.). Philadelphia: J.B. Lippincott.

Hardy, I. R., & Gershon, A. A. (1990). Prospects for use of a varicella vaccine in adults. *Infectious Disease Clinics of North America, 4,* 159.

Hussey, G. D., & Klein, M. (1990). A randomized, controlled trial of vitamin A in children with severe measles. *New England Journal of Medicine, 323,* 160.

Isaacs, D., & Menser, M. (1990). Measles, mumps, rubella and varicella. *Lancet, 335,* 1384.

Krause, P. R., & Straus, S. E. (1990). Zoster and its complications. *Hospital Practice, 25,* 61.

Krober, M. S., et al. (1991). Decreased measles antibody response after measles-mumps-rubella vaccine in infants with colds. *Journal of the American Medical Association, 265,* 2095.

Manson, A. L. (1990). Mumps orchitis. *Urology, 36,* 355.

McLinn, S. (1990). A bacteriologically controlled randomized study comparing the efficiency of 2% mupirocin ointment (Bactroban) with oral erythromycin in the treatment of patients with impetigo. *Journal of the American Academy of Dermatology, 22,* 883.

McMillan, J., & Grose, C. (1994). Roseola and human herpesvirus type 6. In F. A. Oski et al. (Eds.) *Principles and practice of pediatrics* (2nd ed.). Philadelphia: J.B. Lippincott.

Novak, D. A., et al. (1994). Disorders of the liver and biliary system relevant to clinical practice. In F. A. Oski et al. (Eds.) *Principles and practice of pediatrics* (2nd ed.). Philadelphia: J.B. Lippincott.

O'Donnell, B. F., et al. (1990). Management of crusted scabies. *International Journal of Dermatology, 29,* 258.

Pariser, D. M. (1990). Superficial fungal infections. *Postgraduate Medicine, 87,* 205.

Ravits, J., et al. (1990). Clinical and electromyographic studies of postpoliomyelitis muscular atrophy. *Muscle Nerve, 13,* 667.

Rennels, M. B. (1993). Childhood immunizations. In R. A. Derstewitz. *Ambulatory pediatric care.* Philadelphia: J.B. Lippincott.

Robertson, S. E., et al. (1990). Worldwide status of poliomyelitis in 1986, 1987 and 1988 and plans for its global eradication by the year 2000. *World Health Statistics Quarterly, 43,* 80.

Safran, E., & Bloom, G. P. (1990). Spontaneous splenic rupture following infectious mononucleosis. *American Surgery, 56,* 601.

Salsberry, P. J., et al. (1993). Why aren't preschoolers immunized? *Journal of Community Health Nursing, 10,* 213.

Smith, D. G., Jr., et al. (1992). A protocol for foscarnet administration. *Journal of Intravenous Nursing, 15,* 274.

Spruance, S. L., et al. (1990). Treatment of recurrent herpes simplex labialis with oral acyclovir. *Journal of Infectious Diseases, 16,* 185.

Stechenberg, B.W. (1994). Lyme disease. In F. A. Oski et al. (Eds.). *Principles and practice of pediatrics* (2nd ed.). Philadelphia: J.B. Lippincott.

Steinberg, D. G., & Stollerman, G. H. (1989). Dangerous pyogenic skin infections. *Hospital Practice, 24,* 101.

Strand, O., & Stroomberg, A. (1990). Ciprofloxacin treatment of murine typhus. *Scandinavian Journal of Infectious Disease, 22,* 503.

Sumaya, C. V. (1994). Infectious mononucleosis. In F. A. Oski et al. (Eds.) *Principles and practice of pediatrics* (2nd ed.). Philadelphia: J.B. Lippincott.

Tunnessen, W. W. (1994). Pediatric dermatology. In F. A. Oski et al. (Eds.). *Principles and practice of pediatrics* (2nd ed.). Philadelphia: J.B. Lippincott.

Suggested Readings

Bennett, P., et al. (1992). Parents attitudinal and social influences on childhood vaccination. *Health Education and Research, 7,* 341.

Bobo, J. K., et al. (1993). Risk factors for delayed immunization in a random sample of 1163 children from Oregon and Washington. *Pediatrics, 91,* 308.

Gershon, A. A. (1990). Immunization practices in children. *Hospital Practice, 25,* 91.

Gurevich, I. (1990). Counseling the patient with herpes. *RN, 53,* 22.

Hall, A. J., et al. (1990). Modern vaccines: Practice in developing countries. *Lancet, 335,* 774.

Hammarsten, J. E., & Hammarsten, J. F. (1990). Histoplasmosis: Recognition and treatment. *Hospital Practice, 25,* 95.

Hayden, G. F., & Henderon, R. H. (1990). Worldwide control of disease through immunization. *Infectious Disease Clinics of North America, 4,* 245.

Holtan, N. R. (1990). Measles, forgotten but not gone. *Postgraduate Medicine, 88,* 95.

Jiminez, G. (1994). Index of suspicion: Infectious mononucleosis. *Pediatrics in Review, 15,* 39.

Katz, S. L. (1993). Prospects for childhood immunization in the next decade. *Pediatric Annals, 22,* 733.

Lynch, L., et al. (1993). Perinatal infections. *Current Opinions in Obstetrics and Gynecology, 5,* 24.

Malloy, M. B., & Perez-Wood, R. C. (1991). Neonatal skin care: Prevention of skin breakdown. *Pediatric Nursing, 17,* 41.

Nicholson, K. G. (1990). Modern vaccines: Rabies. *Lancet, 335,* 1201.

Poon, C. Y. (1992). Childhood immunization. *Journal of Pediatric Health Care, 6,* 370.

Wharton, M., et al. (1990). Measles, mumps and rubella vaccines. *Infectious Disease Clinics of North America, 4,* 47.

Zwolski, K. (1990). Lyme disease. *Orthopedic Nursing, 9,* 10.

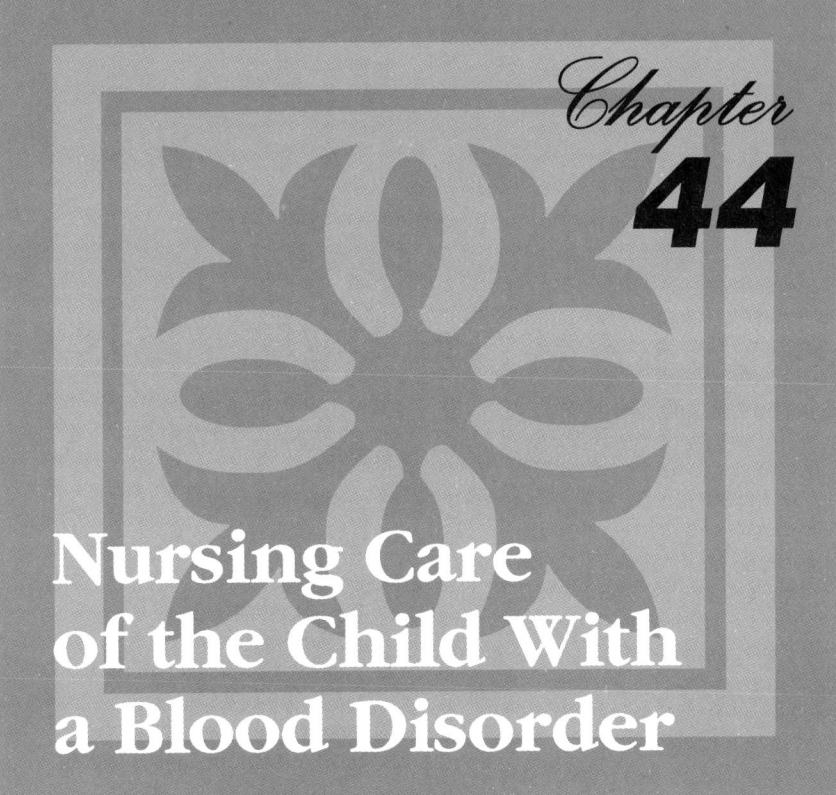

Chapter 44

Nursing Care of the Child With a Blood Disorder

Objectives

After mastering the contents of this chapter, you should be able to:

1. Describe the major blood disorders of childhood such as sickle cell anemia, iron-deficiency anemia, hemophilia, and thalassemia.

2. Assess the child with a blood disorder.

3. Formulate nursing diagnoses for the child with a blood disorder such as sickle cell anemia.

4. Plan nursing care for the child with a blood disorder, for example, helping parents plan an iron-rich diet.

5. Implement nursing care related to the child with a blood disorder (e.g., relieve pain in the child with sickle cell anemia).

6. Evaluate outcome criteria to be certain that nursing care goals have been achieved.

7. Identify National Health Goals related to children with blood disorders that nurses could be instrumental in helping the nation achieve.

8. Identify areas related to care of children with blood disorders that could benefit from additional nursing research.

9. Use critical thinking to analyze ways that nursing care for a child with a blood disorder could be more family centered.

10. Synthesize knowledge of blood disorders in children with nursing process to achieve quality maternal and child health nursing care.

Key Terms

- agranulocytes
- allogeneic transplantation
- aplastic anemias
- autologous transplantation
- bilirubin
- blood dyscrasias
- blood plasma
- erythroblasts
- erythrocytes
- granulocytes
- hemochromatosis
- hemoglobin
- hemolysis
- hemosiderosis
- leukocytes
- leukopenia
- megakaryocytes
- normoblasts
- pancytopenia
- petechiae
- polycythemia
- purpura
- reticulocytes
- sickle cell crisis
- sickle cell trait
- synergeneic transplantation
- thrombocytes
- thrombocytopenia

Adele Pillitteri: MATERNAL AND CHILD HEALTH NURSING, 2nd Edition. © 1995 Adele Pillitteri.

*T*he blood and blood-forming tissues that make up the hematologic system play a vital role in body metabolism—transporting oxygen and nutrients to body cells, removing carbon dioxide from cells, and initiating blood coagulation when vessels are injured. As a result, any alteration in the substance or function of blood and its components can have immediate and life-threatening effects on the functioning of all body systems. For instance, an alteration in the process of coagulation can result in death from acute and uncontrollable blood loss. Inadequate red cell formation results in decreased oxygenation in tissues.

Blood disorders, often called **blood dyscrasias**, occur when components of the blood either increase or decrease in amount beyond normal ranges or are formed incorrectly. Most blood dyscrasias originate in the bone marrow where blood cells are formed. National Health Goals related to hematologic disorders and

children are shown in the Focus on National Health Goals box.

⊠ **NURSING PROCESS OVERVIEW**
for the Child with a Blood Disorder

ASSESSMENT

Many of the symptoms of blood disorders begin insidiously, with pallor, lethargy, and bruising (Figure 44-1). These seem to be such minor symptoms that parents may not bring their child to a health care facility for some time. They are surprised to learn that subtle symptoms such as these can signify the presence of a serious disease.

Many blood dyscrasias are inherited. The diagnosis of the disease may cause guilt in parents or a period of blaming themselves or their partner for the child's disease. It is difficult for parents to support a child during an illness when they themselves need intensive support. Be certain children receive the support and comfort they need during painful diagnostic tests.

Asking at routine checkups about a child's dietary intake often reveals iron deficiency anemia. Many babies with this problem have been drinking too much milk and not enough iron-containing foods. This makes them iron deficient, but aside from paleness and irritability, they appear plump and "healthy." Their parents have not suspected that their baby's appearance masks a nutritional deficiency.

NURSING DIAGNOSIS

Nursing diagnoses that might be used with children who have blood diseases include:

- Knowledge deficit related to cause of illness
- Altered nutrition: less than body requirements related to parental lack of knowledge of need for iron rich diet
- Anxiety related to frequent blood sampling procedures
- Pain related to tissue ischemia
- Family coping, compromised, related to long-term care needs of child with chronic blood disorder

PLANNING

Be certain in helping parents plan goals that they are realistic. The number of blood sampling procedures, for example, cannot be reduced but the child can be helped to deal with the pain and anxiety the procedures cause through individual distraction techniques.

Children with blood disorders often are placed on long-term medication such as a corticosteroid. When a child is very ill, parents give such medicine well and conscientiously. When a child has a disorder with few symptoms, however, it is easy for parents to forget to give medication. Planning includes helping the parents devise ways to remember to give medicine over a long period.

Diet planning is another area that needs consideration. Parents of children with iron-deficiency anemia, for example, may need to modify meal plans not only for an anemic child but for the entire family as well. Remember that iron-rich foods tend to be the most expensive foods. A parent planning on a limited budget has a difficult time providing meals rich in iron content. If children are "fussy eaters," parents may need a great deal of support to insist on foods containing iron rather than giving children what they want. If children will be isolated for long periods because their immune system is compromised as a part of their illness, planning must include ways to keep the child interested in activities to promote development.

Three organizations helpful for referral are as follows:

Aplastic Anemia Foundation of America
P.O. Box 22689
Baltimore, MD 21203

National Association for Sickle Cell Disease, Inc.
3345 Wilshire Boulevard, Suite 1106
Los Angeles, CA 90010-1880

National Hemophilia Foundation
110 Greene Street, Suite 303
New York, NY 10012

IMPLEMENTATION

Nursing interventions for children with blood disorders include helping with blood sampling and assisting in blood or bone marrow transfusions. Remember that a finger prick for blood is often as painful as a venipuncture (and more painful afterward because the fingertip is irritated every time the child attempts to use it). Suggesting that blood be drawn by means of a heparin lock may help to reduce the number of times a child is subjected to venipuncture. Children may need some therapeutic play time with a syringe and a doll to express angry feelings about constant invasion by needles.

FOCUS ON
National Health Goals

A National Health Goal that addresses iron deficiency anemia, the most common blood disorder in children, is:

- Reduce iron deficiency in low-income children aged 1 to 2 years to less than 10% and among women of childbearing age to less than 3% from baselines of 21% and 5% (DHHS, 1991).

Nurses can be instrumental in helping the nation achieve this goal by educating parents about the importance of adding iron-rich cereal to infants' diets and women taking an iron supplement during pregnancy. Nursing research questions that could add important information for prevention include: what are ways of increasing compliance in pregnant women that would help insure that all women take an iron supplement during pregnancy; and do infants maintain higher iron levels when cereal is eaten with milk or orange juice?

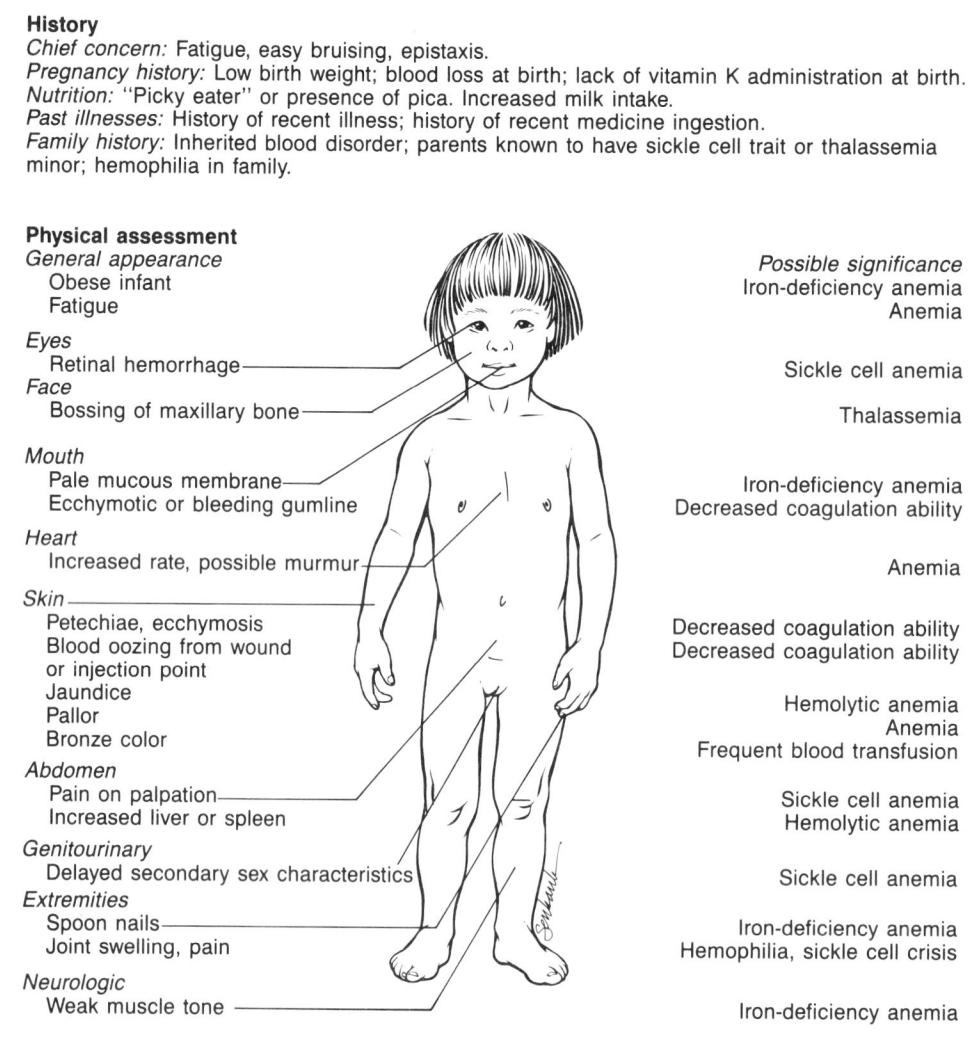

FIGURE 44-1
Possible symptoms of blood disorders in children.

EVALUATION

Evaluation will focus on the achievement of short-term goals (such as the moderation of pain or elimination of anxiety in the child undergoing testing or treatment) and progress toward the achievement of long-term goals (such as improving the ability of the family to manage the stress of raising a child with a chronic illness or deal with frequently occurring health crises—for example, the family with a child who has sickle cell anemia).

Examples of outcome criteria might be:

• Parents state increased knowledge of cause of iron deficiency anemia.
• Child states he or she feels better able to cope with blood sampling procedures through the use of imagery.

• Parents describes realistic plans they will take to ensure compliance of long-term medication administration.

Structure and Function of Blood

Blood Formation and Components

The formation of blood cells begins as early as week 2 of intrauterine life. The yolk sac is responsible for this early blood formation. By month 2 of intrauterine life, the liver and spleen begin forming blood components. At approximately month 4, the bone marrow becomes and remains the active center for the origination of blood cells. As in extrauterine life, the spleen then serves as the organ for the destruction of blood cells once their normal lifetime has passed.

The total volume of blood in the body is roughly proportional to body weight: 85 mL/kg at birth, 75 mL/kg at age 6 months, and 70 mL/kg after the first year. The **blood plasma** (liquid portion containing proteins, hormones, enzymes, and electrolytes) is in equilibrium with the fluid of the interstitial tissue spaces, and although important in diseases causing vomiting and diarrhea (when it may become depleted, leading to dehydration), plasma is not a major site of blood disease. The formed elements, the **erythrocytes** (red blood cells); **leukocytes** (white blood cells); and **thrombocytes** (platelets), are the portions most affected by blood diseases in children.

Erythrocytes (Red Blood Cells)

The chief function of erythrocytes is to transport oxygen to and carry carbon dioxide from body cells. Red blood cells are formed under the stimulation of erythropoietin, a hormone produced by the kidneys. An increase in erythropoietin is stimulated whenever a child has tissue hypoxia. Children with cyanotic heart disease have such systemic hypoxia that **polycythemia**, or an overproduction of red blood cells, is chronically present. Children with kidney disease often have a low number of red blood cells because erythropoietin secretion is inadequate in diseased kidneys.

Red blood cells form first as **erythroblasts** (large, nucleated cells), then mature through **normoblast** and **reticulocyte** stages to mature, nonnucleated erythrocytes; approximately 1% of red blood cells are in the reticulocyte stage at all times. An elevated reticulocyte count in children indicates rapid production of red blood cells; this is seen in children with iron-deficiency anemia once iron therapy is begun and the body is again able to produce red blood cells. The absence of a nucleus in the mature cell allows for increased space for oxygen transport; it also, unfortunately, limits the life of cells because metabolic processes are limited. At the end of their life span, erythrocytes are destroyed through phagocytosis by reticuloendothelial cells, found in the highest proportion in the spleen.

In infants, the long bones of the body are filled with red marrow and actively produce disc-shaped red blood cells. In early childhood, yellow marrow begins to replace this in long bones so blood element production is then carried out mainly in ribs, scapulas, vertebrae, and skull bones. The yellow marrow remaining in the extremities can be activated if necessary to produce additional blood products.

At birth, an infant has approximately 5 million red blood cells per cubic millimeter of blood. This concentration diminishes rapidly in the first months, reaching a low of approximately 4.1 million per cubic millimeter at age 3 to 4 months. The number then slowly increases until adolescence, when adult values of approximately 4.9 million per cubic millimeter are reached. These normal values, together with those of other formed blood elements, are listed in Appendix F.

Hemoglobin. The component of red blood cells that allows them to carry out the transport of oxygen is **hemoglobin**, a complex protein. Hemoglobin comprises globin, a protein dependent (like all protein) on nitrogen metabolism for its formation, and heme, an iron-containing pigment. Deficiency of either iron stores or nitrogen will interfere with the synthesis of hemoglobin. It is the heme portion that combines with oxygen and carbon dioxide for transport.

The hemoglobin in erythrocytes during fetal life is different from that formed after birth. Fetal hemoglobin serves the fetus well because it can absorb oxygen at the low oxygen tension that exists in utero. It comprises two alpha and two gamma polypeptide chains. At birth, between 40% and 70% of the child's hemoglobin is fetal hemoglobin (hemoglobin F), identified in the laboratory by its resistance to denaturation by alkali. Fetal hemoglobin is gradually replaced by adult hemoglobin (hemoglobin A) during the first 6 months of life. Hemoglobin A comprises two alpha and two beta chains. This is the reason that diseases such as sickle cell anemia or the thalassemias, which are defects of the beta chains, do not become apparent clinically until this hemoglobin change has occurred (at approximately age 6 months). They can be diagnosed even prenatally, however, because from early intrauterine life, some hemoglobin A is present.

The hemoglobin level of blood varies according to the number of red blood cells present and the average amount of hemoglobin each cell contains. Hemoglobin levels are highest at birth (between 13.7 and 20.1 g/100 mL); reach a low at approximately age 3 months (between 9.5 and 14.5 g/100 mL); and gradually rise again until adult values are reached at puberty (between 11 and 16 g/100 mL).

Bilirubin. Red blood cells have a life span of approximately 120 days. After this time, they disintegrate and their components are preserved by specialized cells in the liver and spleen (reticuloendothelial cells) for further use. Iron is released for reuse by the bone marrow to construct new red blood cells. As the heme portion is degraded, it is converted into protoporphyrin. Protoporphyrin is then further broken down into indirect bilirubin. Indirect bilirubin is fat soluble and cannot be excreted by the kidneys in this state. It is therefore converted by the liver enzyme glucuronyl transferase into direct **bilirubin**, which is water soluble and is combined and excreted in bile.

In the newborn infant, liver function is generally so immature that the conversion to direct bilirubin cannot be made. Therefore, bilirubin remains in the indirect form. When the level of indirect bilirubin in the blood rises to more than 7 mg/100 mL, it permeates outside the circulatory system, and the infant shows signs of yellowing from physiologic jaundice. If excessive **hemolysis** (destruction) of red blood cells occurs, as in disorders such as erythroblastosis or the thalassemias, the child will also show signs of jaundice.

Leukocytes (White Blood Cells)

Leukocytes are nucleated cells, few in number when compared with red blood cells (there is only approximately 1 white blood cell to every 500 red blood cells). Their primary function is defense against antigen invasion. There are two main forms of white blood cells: (1) **granulocytes** (those with granules in the cell cytoplasm) and (2) **agranulocytes** (those without granules in the cell cytoplasm). Granulocytes (often referred to as polymorphonuclear forms) are further differentiated as neutrophils, basophils, and eosinophils. The agranulocytic leukocytes are further differentiated as lymphocytes and monocytes (see Table 41-3).

The total white blood cell count in newborns is approximately 20,000 per cubic millimeter, a high level caused by the trauma of birth. In the newborn, granulocytes are the most common white blood cells. By 14 days to 30 days of life, the total white blood cell count falls to approximately 12,000 per cubic millimeter, and lymphocytes become the dominant type. By age 4 years, the white blood cell count reaches the adult level, and granulocytes are again the dominant type. Leukocytes are produced in response to need. The life span of leukocytes varies from approximately 6 hours to unknown intervals.

Thrombocytes (Platelets)

When blood is centrifuged in a test tube, plasma rises to the top as a clear yellow fluid; red cells sink to the bottom as a dark red paste. Between these two layers forms a thin white strip (often termed a buffy coat) that comprises the white blood cells and platelets. Platelets are round, nonnucleated bodies formed by bone marrow. Their function is capillary hemostasis and primary coagulation. The normal range is 150,000 to 300,000 per cubic millimeter after the first year. Immature thrombocytes are termed **megakaryocytes**. If large numbers of these are present in serum, it indicates rapid production of platelets is occurring.

Blood Coagulation

Effective blood coagulation depends on a complex series of events (Figure 44-2), including a combination of blood and tissue factors released from the plasma (the intrinsic system) and from injured tissue (the extrinsic system). The factors released from the plasma are factors

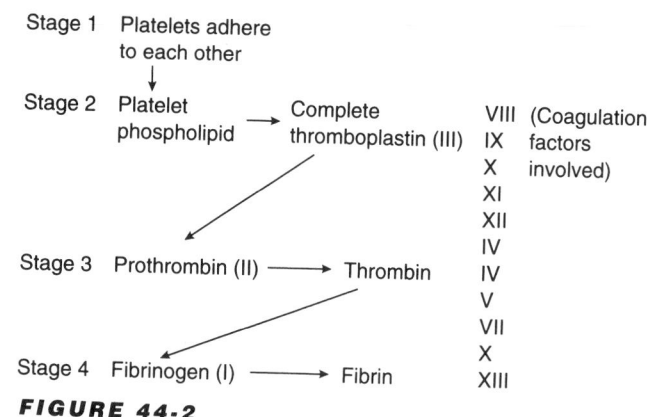

FIGURE 44-2
Steps in blood coagulation.

V, VIII, and IX through XII. Factors released from injured tissues are a tissue factor (an incomplete thromboplastin), plus factors V, VII, and X. The names for coagulation factors are given in Box 44-1. Factors are numbered not by the order in which they are used but for the order in which they were discovered. When a vessel is injured, one of the first responses is vasoconstriction in the area proximal to the injury. This narrows the lumen of the vessel and reduces the amount of blood that approaches the injured area. Platelets begin to adhere to the damaged vessel site and to one another, forming a platelet plug. This is the first stage, or phase, of clotting (see Figure 44-2).

In a second stage, factors from either the intrinsic or the extrinsic system combine with platelet phospholipid to form complete thromboplastin.

In a third stage, thromboplastin converts prothrom-

Box 44-1
Blood Coagulation Factors*

   I: Fibrinogen
  II: Prothrombin
 III: Thromboplastin
 IV: Calcium
  V: Labile factor (platelet phospholipids)
 VII: Stable factor
VIII: Antihemophilic factor
 IX: Christmas factor; antihemophilic factor B; plasma thromboplastin component
  X: Stuart factor
 XI: Plasma thromboplastin antecedent (antihemophilic factor C)
 XII: Hageman factor
XIII: Fibrin stabilizing factor

*Numbers refer to the order in which factors were discovered, not to the order of action in coagulation.

Table 44-1. Tests for Blood Coagulation

Test	Definition	Normal Value
Prothrombin time (PT)	Measures action of prothrombin after complete thromboplastin is added to the child's blood in a test tube; reveals deficiencies in prothrombin, factors V, VII, and X	12–15 sec
Partial thromboplastin time (PTT)	Measures activity of thromboplastin after incomplete thromboplastin is added to child's blood in test tube; reveals deficiencies in thromboplastin, factors VIII–XII	39–53 sec
Bleeding time	Time required for bleeding at site of earlobe incision to cease; reveals deficiencies in platelet formation and vasoconstrictive ability	3–6 min
Clot retraction	Interval from placement of blood in a tube to the point clot shrinks and expels serum; measures platelet function	Retraction at side of test tube in 1 h; complete in 24 h
Tourniquet	Response of tissue to application of tourniquet to forearm for 5–10 min; measures capillary fragility and platelet function	Under 10 petechiae per 2-cm area
Prothrombin-consumption time	Child's blood is allowed to clot and PT is then done on the serum; if clot formation used a great deal of prothrombin (as it should), serum prothrombin time will be low; increase denotes defects in thromboplastin function	Approximately 20 sec
Thromboplastin-generation time	Tests basic ability to form thromboplastin; difficult test to do; ordered rarely to distinguish factor VIII from factor IX defects	12 sec or less
Plasma fibrinogen	Level of fibrinogen in blood; measures stage 4 clotting process	200–320 mg/100 mL plasma
Venous clotting time (Lee-White)	Time it takes venous blood to clot in a test tube; measures factor defects in stages 2 and 4	9–12 min

bin (factor II) to thrombin if ionized calcium is present. The production of prothrombin and factors VII, IX, and X depends on the presence of vitamin K. This stage will be incomplete if any of factors VIII through XII or calcium is deficient.

In a fourth stage, thrombin converts fibrinogen (factor I) to fibrin. Fibrin strands form a mesh, incorporating red blood cells, white blood cells, and platelets to form a permanent protective seal at the site of injury. Factor XIII (fibrin stabilizing factor) acts to make the fibrin clot insoluble and permanent.

To prevent too much coagulation, plasminogen may be converted to plasmin (a fibrinolysin) near the injury. Blood coagulation problems will result if any step or factor in the process is inadequate. Common tests for blood coagulation are described in Table 44-1.

Assessment and Therapeutic Techniques Involving Blood and Blood Products

Bone Marrow Aspiration

Bone marrow aspiration provides samples of bone marrow for determination of type and quantity of cells present. The sites for aspiration in children are the iliac crests, or spines, rather than the sternum, as may be used in adults (Figure 44-3). These sites have larger marrow compartments during childhood, and the test performed there is less frightening for children. Because the procedure is threatening and involves pain, it should be done if possible in a treatment room, not at the child's bedside. In neonates, the anterial tibia can be used.

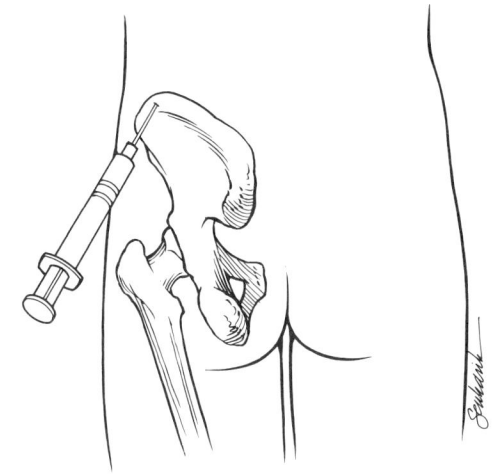

FIGURE 44-3
A common site used for bone marrow aspiration in children is the iliac crest. In neonates, the anterior tibia may be used.

The child lies prone on a treatment table. Use of a hard table is advantageous because pressure is needed to insert the needle through the surface of the bone into the marrow compartment.

The area of the aspiration is cleaned with an antiseptic solution such as povidone-iodine (Betadine); a sterile drape is positioned around the site. The overlying skin is infiltrated with a local anesthetic. After a few minutes, a large-bore needle with stylus is introduced through the overlying tissue into the bone. This involves considerable pressure. When the marrow cavity is reached, the stylus is removed; a syringe is attached to the needle; and bone marrow is aspirated (appears as thick blood in the syringe). The syringe is then removed and marrow is expelled onto a slide and allowed to dry. After being sprayed with a preservative, it is taken to the laboratory for analysis. The aspiration needle is removed and pressure applied to the puncture site to prevent bleeding. After another few minutes, a pressure dressing is applied.

The child feels the pain of the local anesthetic injection and the hard pressure while the needle is inserted; some report a sharp pain when the marrow is actually aspirated. Observe the dressing every 15 minutes for the first hour following the procedure to be certain that no bleeding is occurring; keep the child fairly quiet for the first hour by playing a quiet game or other activity. Assess the child's temperature at 12 hours and 24 hours to detect the possibility that infection has occurred. Allow young children an opportunity for therapeutic play with a doll and syringe to help them express the anger they feel at such a painful, invasive procedure.

Blood Transfusion

Transfusions of blood or its products are used in the treatment of many disorders, including the anemias and primary immunodeficiency disorders (see Chapter 42) and are given in a variety of forms: whole blood; packed red cells; washed red blood cells (as much "foreign" matter is removed as possible to reduce the possibility of blood reaction); plasma; plasma factors such as cryoprecipitate or proplex; platelets; white blood cell transfusion; and albumin. No matter what the blood product, it is important to be certain that it has been carefully matched with the child's own blood type. Blood must not be infused in the same tubing with an intravenous glucose or electrolyte solution but with a solution as nearly isotonic as possible (normal saline). If blood is given with a hypertonic solution, fluid will be drawn out of the red blood cells, causing them to shrink; if infused with a hypotonic solution, fluid will be drawn into the cells, and they will burst; in both instances, they will be worthless.

Blood must be infused through a blood filter, so that no impurities are infused. Packed red cells is the most common form of transfusion to prevent fluid overload. The usual amount of blood transfused to children is 15 mL/kg of body weight. The commonly accepted rate for transfusions in a child is 10 mL/kg/h unless the child has hypovolemic shock and volume equilibrium needs to be established. An infusion of packed red cells at a proportion of 15 mL/kg can be expected to raise the hematocrit level 5 points. Platelets last only approximately 10 days, so transfusion of these must be repeated every 10 days. A transfusion of platelets will elevate a platelet count by approximately 10,000.

Even if given slowly, blood transfusion is always a strain on a child's circulation beyond that of regular intravenous infusion, because the circulatory system must accommodate a thick, difficult-to-mobilize fluid. Other dangers include contracting hepatitis B (HBV) and hepatitis C (HCV), which can lead to liver disease later in life. HIV is also a potential risk, though with current screening standards, the risk is much lower than it was before screening was in place. According to one estimate, 1 in 250,000 units of donated blood will contain HIV and 1 in 200,000 units will contain the virus causing hepatitis B (Saltus, 1994).

Before any transfusion, vital signs are taken to establish a baseline, then every 15 minutes during the first hour and approximately every half hour for the remainder of the transfusion. Provide an enjoyable activity for the child during a transfusion. Without this, the child can become bored and attempt to increase the infusion rate. Common symptoms of blood transfusion reactions to observe for are shown in Table 44-2. Be certain that permission for blood transfusion is obtained to respect sociocultural or religious beliefs (Quintero, 1993).

Bone Marrow Transplantation

Bone marrow transplantation is the intravenous infusion of bone marrow to reestablish marrow function in a child with defective or nonfunctioning bone marrow. **Allogeneic transplantation** involves the transfer of bone marrow from an immune compatible (histocompatible) donor (through aspiration) and its intravenous infusion to the recipient (Gaiewski et al., 1990). The term **synergeneic transplant** is used when the donor and recipient are genetically identical (i.e., identical twins)(Geller, 1993). In **autologous transplantation,** the child's own marrow is used. The marrow is aspirated, treated to remove abnormal cells, and then reinfused (Robertson, 1993).

Bone marrow transplantation has become a relatively common procedure for children with blood disorders such as acquired aplastic anemia and leukemia and some forms of immune dysfunction. Bone marrow transplants are most successful when the recipients have not already received multiple blood transfusions that have sensitized them to blood products. Success also depends

Table 44-2. *Common Blood Transfusion Reaction Symptoms*

Symptoms	Cause	Time of Occurrence	Nursing Intervention
Headache, chills, back pain, dyspnea, hypotension, hemoglobinuria (blood in urine)	Anaphylactic reaction to incompatible blood; agglutination of red blood cells occurs; kidney tubules may become blocked, resulting in kidney failure	Immediately after start of transfusion	Discontinue transfusion; maintain normal saline infusion for accessible intravenous line; administer oxygen as necessary; physician may order diuretic to increase renal tubule flow and reduce tubule plugging; heparin to reduce intravascular coagulation
Pruritus, urticaria (hives), wheezing	Allergy to protein components of transfusion	Within first hour after start of transfusion	Discontinue transfusion temporarily; give oxygen as needed; physician may order antihistamine to reduce symptoms
Increased temperature	Possible contaminant in transfused blood	Approximately 1 hour after start of transfusion	Discontinue transfusion; blood culture may be obtained to rule out bacterial invasion
Increased pulse, dyspnea	Circulatory overload	During course of transfusion	Discontinue transfusion; give oxygen as needed; supportive care for pulmonary edema and congestive heart failure; physician may order diuretic to increase excretion of fluid
Muscle cramping, twitching of extremities, convulsion	Acid-citrate-dextrose anticoagulant in transfusion is combining with serum calcium and causing hypocalcemia	During course of transfusion	Discontinue transfusion; physician may order calcium gluconate administered intravenously to restore calcium level
Fever, jaundice, lethargy, tenderness over liver	Hepatitis from contaminated transfusion	Weeks or months after transfusion	Obtain transfusion history of any child with hepatitis symptoms; refer for care of hepatitis
Bronze-colored skin	Hemosiderosis or deposition of iron from transfusion in skin	After repeated transfusions	Support self-esteem with altered body image; iron-chelating agent (deferoxamine) may be ordered to help reduce level of accumulating iron

on the compatibility of donated marrow to a child's blood. An identical twin is the ideal donor; a parent or sibling may be next best, though compatibility is not guaranteed; donors registered with regional or national bone marrow "banks" have provided closer matches in some instances.

All potential donors are typed for human leukocyte antigen (HLA) compatibility. Parents who are found to be incompatible often feel guilty and frustrated that they could not do more for their child. If the most compatible person is a young sibling, health care personnel and parents alike may have some reservations about submitting a child to bone marrow aspiration (done under general anesthesia). There is no guarantee that the graft will be accepted by the diseased child, or that improvement

will occur, although with good tissue compatibility in the absence of infection, this can be effective in 80% of children.

Children who are scheduled for a bone marrow transplant are admitted to the hospital several days before the procedure. To prevent rejection of the newly transplanted marrow by the T lymphocytes, cyclophosphamide (Cytoxan) is administered intravenously to suppress marrow and T lymphocyte production. This may cause nausea and vomiting. Total body irradiation to destroy the child's marrow may be done as well; it is a difficult time for the child because total body irradiation causes extreme nausea, vomiting, and diarrhea.

On the day of the procedure, the donor is administered a general anesthetic and samples of bone marrow are obtained by multiple aspirations. The marrow is then treated and strained to remove fat and bone particles and any other unwanted cells; an anticoagulant is added to prevent clotting. It is infused intravenously into the recipient child's bloodstream. Because the infused solution is fairly thick, this infusion takes 60 to 90 minutes. The infusion set should not include the filter that is normally used for infusion of blood products because this would filter out marrow tissue. A cardiac monitor should be in place during the infusion to detect circulatory overload or pulmonary emboli from unfiltered particles.

Fever and chills are common reactions to bone marrow transplant infusion. Administration of acetaminophen (Tylenol); diazepam (Valium); and diphenhydramine hydrochloride (Benadryl) may be prescribed to reduce this reaction.

After the infusion, the child's temperature should be taken every 4 hours to detect infection that could occur because of nonfunctioning white blood cells from radiation. Strict handwashing should be reinforced. Diet is limited to cooked foods to reduce the presence of bacteria. White blood cell count must be measured daily; bone marrow aspirations or venous sampling are scheduled for regular intervals to assess the growth of the new marrow.

Almost immediately after the infusion, marrow cells begin to migrate from the child's bloodstream into the marrow. If engraftment occurs (the transplant is accepted), red blood cells can be detected in peripheral blood in approximately 3 weeks. White blood cells and platelet cells may not return to normal for up to 1 year posttransplant.

Nursing Diagnoses and Related Interventions

Nursing Diagnosis: Anxiety related to lack of knowledge about procedure for and expected outcome of transplant

Goal: Parents and child will demonstrate an understanding of transplant procedure and uncertainty of outcome during therapy by 24 hours.

Outcome Criteria: Parents state that they know transplant may not work, depending on immunologic factors that are not totally known to science, but are agreeable to procedure.

Bone marrow transplantation is an emotional experience not only for the child but for the parents and for the marrow donor as well. Be certain that the child who receives the transplant and the donor understand that they are not responsible for the outcome of the transplant. Its success does not depend on their behavior or what kind of person they are but on immunologic factors over which they have no control. If a sibling was the donor, he or she may become jealous of the recipient

child who is once again the center of attention. Be certain that donors know that although bone marrow donation is not painful because the aspiration is done under general anesthesia, donor sites will feel tender afterward. General anesthesia will make them feel exhausted for several days. Donors generally remain in the hospital for 24 hours to 48 hours until it is determined that aspiration sites are not infected (no local swelling, redness or intense pain, or elevated temperature is present).

Nursing Diagnosis: High risk for altered growth and development related to extended isolation in hospital and long-term isolation at home

Goal: Child will demonstrate age-appropriate growth in motor skills and social, cognitive, and emotional behaviors during course of therapy.

Outcome Criteria: Parents express satisfaction with child's ongoing development. Objective tests of developmental stage show child within age-appropriate ranges.

Be certain that children in protective isolation are not socially isolated as well. Visit the room frequently; provide gas-sterilized play materials. Most children grow tired of a restricted diet and may crave fresh fruits and vegetables that are usually not their favorite food. Thick-skinned fruits such as bananas and oranges can be given soon after the procedure. Be certain that children are well prepared for all procedures. Allow them to make as many choices as they can about their care to help them preserve a sense of control over their life. Children who receive a transplant need periods of therapeutic play incorporated into care so they can begin to express their anger and frustration at the number of intravenous therapies or follow-up bone marrow aspirations they require. Measures to help children cope with pain, such as imagery (see Chapter 35), can help a child to accept one more painful procedure. Encourage parents to spend time with their child during the long period of isolation as well as with other children at home.

Provisions for completing schoolwork need to be made as soon as the child has a return of red blood cells in peripheral blood (approximately 3 weeks). School books and papers can be gas sterilized for use in reverse isolation rooms. If children are prepared adequately for these painful procedures and supported throughout, they should have no long-term consequences. Not all transplants are successful, however, and some children will die of the original disease that required the transplant. Some children develop an infection despite all precautions and die in the weeks immediately following the transplant.

On the day of hospital discharge, parents may be surprised that the child's blood replacement is not totally complete and that they will need to continue isolating the child at home. Help them locate a support group in the community if possible. Be certain that they feel free to call the transplant center after discharge if they have any problems. Once isolation can be discontinued, parents may still be reluctant to allow their child outside, fearing that the child may still be susceptible to infection. Frequent follow-up for the next year is necessary to assure that the child is free of infection until white blood cells have risen to normal levels. Follow-up should also address the parents' commitment to allowing their child to pursue age-appropriate activities and avoiding overprotecting him or her.

Graft-Versus-Host Disease

Graft-versus-host disease (GVHD) is an immunologic response of donor T cells against the tissue of the recipient and can be a lethal complication of bone marrow transplantation. The symptoms range from mild to severe and include a rash and general malaise beginning 7 to 14 days posttransplant. Latent virus infections may become active. Severe symptoms include high fever and diarrhea, and liver and spleen enlargement.

Because there is no known cure for GVHD, prevention is essential. Careful tissue typing; intravenous administration of methotrexate or cyclosporine; and irradiation of blood products (which helps to inactivate mature T cells) before bone marrow infusion can all contribute to the reduction of this complication. Drugs such as methotrexate and cyclosporine kill all rapidly growing cells, including white blood cells and T lymphocytes, so administration of these drugs after transplantation cannot be continued because they would also slow the growth of the host's bone marrow. Depletion of mature T cells from donor bone marrow before infusion into the child seems to have the best results.

Disorders of the Red Blood Cells

Most red blood cell disorders fall into the category of the anemias, or a reduction in the number or function of erythrocytes. Polycythemia, or an increase in the number of red blood cells, can also occur, and may be as dangerous to the child as a reduction in red blood cell production (see the Focus on Cultural Awareness box).

Anemia occurs when the rate of red blood cell production falls below that of cell destruction, or when there is a loss of red blood cells, causing their number, or the hemoglobin level, to fall below the normal value for a child's age. Anemias are classified either according to the changes seen in red blood cell numbers or configuration, or according to the source of the problem. Although any reduction in the amount of circulating hemoglobin lessens the oxygen-carrying capacity, clinical symptoms of this are not apparent until hemoglobin

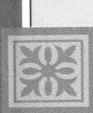

FOCUS ON CULTURAL AWARENESS

Blood dyscrasias do not occur at equal rates in all countries because many of them are inherited. Sickle-cell anemia occurs mainly in African-Americans; thalassemia occurs in children from Mediterranean countries. Iron deficiency anemia, an example of a noninherited disorder, tends to occur in children from lower socioeconomic areas of many countries because iron-rich foods are the most expensive foods for families to buy. Being aware of the differences in the incidence of blood dyscrasias can be helpful in planning care and health care services for an individual community.

reaches 7 to 8 g/100 mL. Average values for hemoglobin and red cell number are shown in Appendix F.

Normochromic, Normocytic Anemias

Normochromic, normocytic anemias are marked by impaired production of erythrocytes by the bone marrow, or by abnormal or uncompensated loss of circulating red blood cells as in acute hemorrhage. The remaining red blood cells are normal in both color and size; they are simply too few in number.

Acute Blood-Loss Anemia

Blood loss sufficient to cause anemia might occur from trauma such as an automobile accident with internal bleeding; acute nephritis in which blood is being lost in the urine; or, in the newborn, from disorders such as placenta previa, premature separation of the placenta, maternal-fetal or twin-to-twin transfusion, or trauma to the cord or placenta as might occur with cesarean birth.

Children are in shock from acute blood loss, and appear pale. As the heart attempts to push the reduced amount of blood through the body more rapidly, tachycardia will occur. Loss of red blood cells needed for oxygen transport causes body cells to register an oxygen deficit, and children experience tachypnea. Newborns may have gasping respirations, sternal retractions, and cyanosis. They will not respond to oxygen therapy because they lack red blood cells to transport and use the oxygen. Such infants will be listless and inactive.

This type of acute blood-loss anemia generally is transitory because sudden reduction in available oxygen stimulates a regeneration response in the bone marrow. The reticulocyte count becomes elevated, evidence that the bone marrow is trying to increase production of erythrocytes to meet the sudden shortage.

Treatment involves control of bleeding by addressing its underlying cause. The child or infant should be placed in a supine position to provide as much circulation as possible to brain cells. Keep the child warm with blankets; place an infant in an incubator. Blood transfusion may be necessary for an immediate increase in the number of erythrocytes. Until blood is available for transfusion, a blood expander such as plasma, or intravenous fluid such as saline or Ringer's lactate, may be given to expand blood volume and improve blood pressure.

Anemia of Acute Infection

Acute infection or inflammation, especially in infants, may lead to increased destruction of erythrocytes and therefore to decreased erythrocyte levels. Impaired production of erythrocytes due to the infection may also contribute to the anemia. Management involves treatment of the underlying infection. When this is reversed, the blood picture will return to normal. Common infections with which this occurs are osteomyelitis, ulcerative colitis, and advanced renal disease.

Anemia of Neoplastic Disease

Malignant growths such as leukemia or lymphosarcoma (common neoplasms of childhood) result in normochromic, normocytic anemias because invasion of bone marrow by proliferating neoplastic cells impairs red blood cell production. There may be accompanying blood loss if platelet formation also has decreased. The treatment of such an anemia involves measures designed to achieve remission of the neoplastic process and transfusion to increase the erythrocyte count.

Aplastic Anemias

Aplastic anemias result from depression of hematopoietic activity in bone marrow. The formation and development of white blood cells, platelets, and red blood cells are all affected.

Congenital aplastic anemia (Fanconi's syndrome) is inherited as an autosomal recessive trait. The child is born with a number of congenital anomalies, such as skeletal and renal abnormalities, hypogenitalism, and dwarfism. Between 4 to 12 years of age, children begin to manifest symptoms of **pancytopenia** (reduction of all blood cell components).

Acquired Aplastic Anemia. Acquired aplastic anemia is a decrease in bone marrow production that can occur if children have excessive exposure to radiation, drugs, or chemicals known to cause bone marrow damage. Chloramphenicol is the major drug involved in such an anemia. Other drugs are sulfonamides, arsenic (contained in rat poison, sometimes eaten by children), hydantoin, benzene, and quinine. Exposure to insecticides also may cause such bone marrow dysfunction.

Chemotherapeutic drugs temporarily reduce bone marrow production. A serious infection might cause autoimmunologic suppression of bone marrow.

Assessment. As symptoms begin, children appear pale; they fatigue easily and have anorexia. These symptoms reflect the lower red blood cell count (anemia) and tissue hypoxia. Because of reduced platelet formation (thrombocytopenia), children bruise easily or have **petechiae** (pinpoint macular, purplish red spots caused by intradermal or submucous hemorrhage); they may have excessive nose bleeds or gastrointestinal bleeding. As a result of a decrease in white blood cells, termed **leukopenia**, children may contract an increased number of infections; they will respond poorly to antibiotic therapy. Observe closely for signs of heart decompensation (e.g., tachycardia, tachypnea, shortness of breath, or cyanosis) from the long-term increased workload on the heart (see Figure 44-1). Ask about exposure to drugs, chemicals or recent infection.

Bone marrow samples will show a reduced number of hematopoietic forms; blood-forming spaces are infiltrated by fatty tissue.

Therapeutic Management. The goal of treatment for aplastic anemia is to suppress abnormal bone marrow with antithymocyte globulin (ATG) or antilymphocyte globulin (ALG) and to supplement blood elements being formed in abnormally low numbers (Loughran & Storb, 1990). Both ATG and ALG are given intravenously and must be administered cautiously, as an anaphylactic reaction to the products can occur. Packed red cell and platelet transfusions are generally necessary to maintain adequate hemoglobin. Any drug or chemical suspected of causing the bone marrow dysfunction must be discontinued at once. A red cell-stimulating factor (erythropoietin) that increases cell growth has been developed through recombinant DNA analysis (Kojima et al., 1991). Bone marrow transplantation is the treatment of choice (Gaiewski et al., 1990).

Some children with congenital aplastic anemia show improvement on an oral course of a corticosteroid (prednisone) and testosterone (oxymetholone). The testosterone acts to increase erythrocyte production in the bone marrow. Prednisone acts to decrease erythrocyte destruction and prolong closure of the epiphyseal lines of the long bones, reversing the early closure that would normally occur with administration of testosterone. Such therapy must be given for an extended period, usually approximately 1 year.

If children survive the first 6 months of aplastic anemia, their chances for complete recovery are good. A decreased platelet count may persist for years after other blood elements have returned to normal; hence, bleeding, especially petechiae or purpura, may be a long-term problem. If the disease was caused by exposure to a drug or chemical, children must never be exposed to that substance again.

Be certain, when discussing with parents the outcome of this disease, to be conservatively optimistic. For some children, the outcome will be fatal. It may be easier for parents to deal with this problem if they face only 1 day or one blood test at a time, rather than trying to predict the outcomes of all the blood tests to come. They need to feel that they can discuss with health care personnel their frustration and bitterness about continual abnormal results. Establishing good communication patterns with these parents does much to reestablish their trust in everyone caring for their child.

Nursing Diagnoses and Related Interventions

Children with aplastic anemia are apt to be irritable because of their fatigue and recurring symptoms. Their parents may feel that they caused the illness if it originated from exposure to a chemical such as an insecticide. Many parents will have less confidence in health care personnel if the illness followed treatment with a drug such as chloramphenicol. They feel that if one drug caused this illness, how can they trust another to cure it? How can they trust that their child will not be harmed further?

Nursing Diagnosis: High risk for infection related to dramatic decrease in number of white blood cells

Goal: Child will remain free of infection during treatment period.

Outcome Criteria: Child's temperature is below 38.0°C axillary; no symptoms such as cough, vomiting, or diarrhea are present.

Exposure to other children must be limited as long as white cell production is inadequate to prevent infection. Although the use of strict handwashing is replacing reverse isolation or care in rooms with a laminar air flow, these may be prescribed following bone marrow transplantation. Such children will be isolated for long periods; be innovative in supplying them with projects to keep them busy and occupied during this time (school books and reading material can easily be gas sterilized and brought into the room).

Devise games that can be played easily with children in isolation rooms and that do not require any materials (e.g., "I Spy," "Tic Tac Toe," or "charades").

On hospital discharge, teach parents to protect their child from exposure to infectious disease as much as possible, and to come for treatment promptly if the child shows symptoms of an infection. In the absence of granulocytes, however, antibiotic therapy may be ineffective, and severe septicemia can result. White blood cells (granulocytes) may be transfused for a severe infection.

Nursing Diagnosis: High risk for altered self-esteem related to changed body appearance that occurs as medication side effect

Goal: Child will demonstrate adequate self-esteem during therapy interval.

Outcome Criteria: Child voices that he or she thinks of himself or herself as a worthwhile person and is not excessively shy or reluctant to interact with peers.

Children who receive prednisone for a long period almost certainly will experience some of the side effects of corticosteroid therapy, such as a cushingoid appearance, hirsutism, hypertension, and marked weight gain. Masculinizing effects, such as growth of facial and body hair, the development of acne, and deepening of the voice, may occur as the result of long-term therapy with testosterone. Both child and parents need to be prepared that these effects may occur, that they are related to the medication being taken, and that they will fade when the medication is withdrawn.

Children need a chance to express their feelings about being made fun of because of their changed physical appearance. They can be assured that their appearance will not change who they are inside, and that true friends will like them anyway.

Nursing Diagnosis: High risk for fluid volume deficit related to ineffective blood clotting mechanisms secondary to inadequate platelet formation

Goal: Child will not experience excessive bleeding episodes while condition is resolving.

Outcome Criteria: Child is free of ecchymotic skin areas or epistaxis; stool tests negative for occult blood.

Techniques for reducing bleeding due to inadequate platelet formation are shown in the Focus on Nursing Care box; these measures require conscientious nursing care.

Hypoplastic Anemias

Hypoplastic anemias also result from depression of hematopoietic activity in bone marrow; they can be either congenital or acquired. Unlike aplastic anemias, in which white and red blood cells and platelets are affected, in hypoplastic anemias, only the red blood cells are affected.

Congenital hypoplastic anemia (Blackfan-Diamond Syndrome) is a rare disorder revealed in the first 6 to 8 months of life. It affects both sexes and is apparently caused by an inherent defect in red blood cell formation. There are no changes in the leukocytes or platelets. An acquired form is caused by infection with parvovirus,

Methods to Reduce Bleeding With a Diminished Platelet Count

1. Limit the number of blood drawing procedures necessary by combining samples whenever possible; use a blood pressure cuff rather than a tourniquet to reduce the number of petechiae.
2. Apply pressure to a puncture site for a full 5 minutes before applying an adhesive bandage.
3. Use a minimum of adhesive tape on the skin (pulling it to remove it may cause petechiae).
4. Pad siderails or crib rails to keep child from hitting against steel sides and bruising arms or legs.
5. Guard intravenous infusion sites carefully so they will not have to be removed and new puncture sites opened.
6. Investigate if medicine can be given orally or by continuous intravenous line rather than by injection to reduce the number of puncture sites.
7. Assess the diet of the child to be certain he or she can chew it without any mechanical irritation (e.g., no toast crusts).
8. Urge the child to use a soft tooth brush to prevent gingiva trauma.
9. Check toys for sharp corners that could cause a scratch. Urge the child to be careful with paper. A paper cut can bleed out of proportion to its size.
10. Assess whether routine blood pressure assessments are necessary (tightening a cuff could cause petechiae).
11. Distract from "roughhousing" play by suggesting stimulating but quiet play to prevent bruising.
12. Keep a record of blood drawn; do not draw extra amounts "just in case."

the infectious agent of fifth disease (Martin & Pearson, 1994).

The onset of hypoplastic anemia is insidious, and must be differentiated from iron-deficiency anemia. The blood cells will appear hypochromic and microcytic in iron-deficiency anemia; in hypoplastic anemia, they are normochromic and normocytic.

With acquired hypoplastic anemia, the reduction of red blood cells is transient, so no therapy is necessary. Children with the congenital form will show increased erythropoiesis with corticosteroid therapy. Long-term transfusions of packed red cells are needed to raise erythrocyte levels. So many transfusions will result in hemosiderosis (deposition of iron in body tissue) so an iron chelation program such as subcutaneous infusion (hypodermoclysis) of deferoxamine is begun concur-

rently with transfusions. Deferoxamine binds with iron and aids its excretion from the body in urine; it is given 5 or 6 days a week over an 8-hour period. Therapy can be administered by parents at home after careful instruction. The parent must assess that voiding is present and specific gravity is normal (1.003 to 1.030) before administration. For a subcutaneous infusion, an area beside the scapula or on the thigh is cleaned with alcohol; a short no. 25 needle is inserted at a low angle into only the subcutaneous tissue. The infusion is allowed to drip slowly for 6 to 8 hours (usually at night while the child sleeps). Infusion should be slow enough not to cause pain yet complete the infusion within the designated time frame. Periodic slit-lamp eye examinations should be scheduled to determine possible cataract formation, as this can occur as a drug side-effect.

Congenital hypoplastic anemia is a chronic condition, but approximately one fourth of affected children will undergo spontaneous permanent remission before age 13 years. Both the child and the parents need support from health care personnel to help them accept the many procedures and tests required in the care of a child with a potentially fatal, long-term disease.

Hypersplenism

Under normal conditions, blood is filtered rapidly through the spleen. If the spleen is enlarged and functioning abnormally, blood cells pass through more slowly and more are destroyed in the process. The increased destruction of red blood cells causes anemia and may lead to pancytopenia (deficiency of all cell elements of blood). Virtually any underlying splenic condition can cause this syndrome. Therapeutic management consists of treating the underlying splenic disorder, including possible splenectomy. Although the spleen's role in the body's defense mechanisms against infection is not well documented, the organ appears to be relatively important in early infancy. Its function decreases as the child grows older and may serve no function at all in adulthood. If the spleen is removed, there is no decrease in general immunity or in gamma globulin or antibody formation. With the removal of the spleen's filtering function, however, there seems to be an increased susceptibility to meningitis due to pneumococci. For this reason, a splenectomy may be delayed until after age 2 years, when the risk of meningitis decreases. Such children should receive immunization against pneumococci, as well as prophylactic penicillin for 2 years after the splenectomy.

Hypochromic Anemias

When hemoglobin synthesis is inadequate, the erythrocytes appear pale (hypochromia). Hypochromia is generally accompanied by a reduction in the diameter of cells (red blood cells are also microcytic).

Iron-Deficiency Anemia

Iron-deficiency anemia is the most common anemia of infancy and childhood, occurring when the intake of dietary iron is inadequate. This lack prevents proper hemoglobin formation (Martin & Pearson, 1994). Most iron in the body is incorporated in hemoglobin, but an additional amount is stored in the bone marrow to be available for hemoglobin production. With iron-deficiency anemia, red blood cells are both small in size (hypocytic) and pale (hypochromic) due to the stunted hemoglobin.

Children are at high risk for iron-deficiency anemia because they need more daily iron than adults in proportion to their body weight to maintain an adequate iron level. A daily intake of 6 to 15 mg iron is necessary. Iron-deficiency anemia occurs most often between ages 6 months and 2 years; its frequency rises again in adolescence when iron requirements increase for girls who are menstruating. As many as 25% of adolescent girls and 40% of infants are anemic.

Prevention. Iron-deficiency anemia can be prevented in infants by giving them iron-fortified formula or, if breastfed, iron-fortified cereal when solid foods are introduced in the first year. Fortunately, these cost no more than the plain foods. Occasionally, an infant will become constipated on iron-rich formula, but this is the exception rather than the rule.

Causes in Infants. When an infant's diet lacks sufficient iron, he or she usually has enough in reserve to last for the first 6 months; after that, if the infant continues to be iron deficient, he or she will have difficulty forming the red cells needed. Infants of low birth weight have fewer iron stores than those born at term because the iron stores develop near the end of gestation. As low-birth-weight infants grow rapidly and their need for red blood cells expands accordingly, they will develop an iron-deficiency anemia before 5 to 6 months. They are given an iron supplement at the time of hospital discharge or at the age they would have reached term to prevent this from happening.

Women with iron deficiency during pregnancy tend to give birth to iron-deficient babies, because they do not have iron stores to pass through the placenta. Low hemoglobin levels from iron-deficiency anemia lead to diffusion of plasma proteins such as albumin and gamma globulin out of the bloodstream by osmosis. The loss of transferrin, a plasma protein responsible for binding iron to protein to facilitate its transportation to bone marrow after absorption from the gastrointestinal tract, further depletes this system of iron transport.

Infants born with structural defects of the gastrointestinal system, such as chalasia (immature valve between esophagus and stomach resulting in regurgitation) or pyloric stenosis (narrowed valve between stomach and duodenum resulting in vomiting) are particularly prone to iron-deficiency anemia. Although their diet is adequate, they are unable to make use of the iron because it is never adequately digested. Infants with chronic diarrhea are also prone to this form of anemia, due to inadequate absorption.

Causes in Toddlers and Older Children. In children older than age 2 years, chronic blood loss is the most frequent cause of iron-deficiency anemia. This results from gastrointestinal tract lesions such as polyps, ulcerative colitis, Crohn's disease, protein-induced enteropathies, parasitic infestation, or frequent epistaxis.

Many adolescent girls are iron deficient because their frequent attempts to diet combined with over-consumption of snack foods results in low iron intake. Without sufficient iron, their body cannot compensate for the iron lost with menstrual flow.

Assessment. Common symptoms of iron-deficiency anemia are shown in Figure 44-4. Children with iron-deficiency anemia appear pale. Because the pallor develops slowly, however, parents may not realize how extensive it is. They may describe their child as "fair

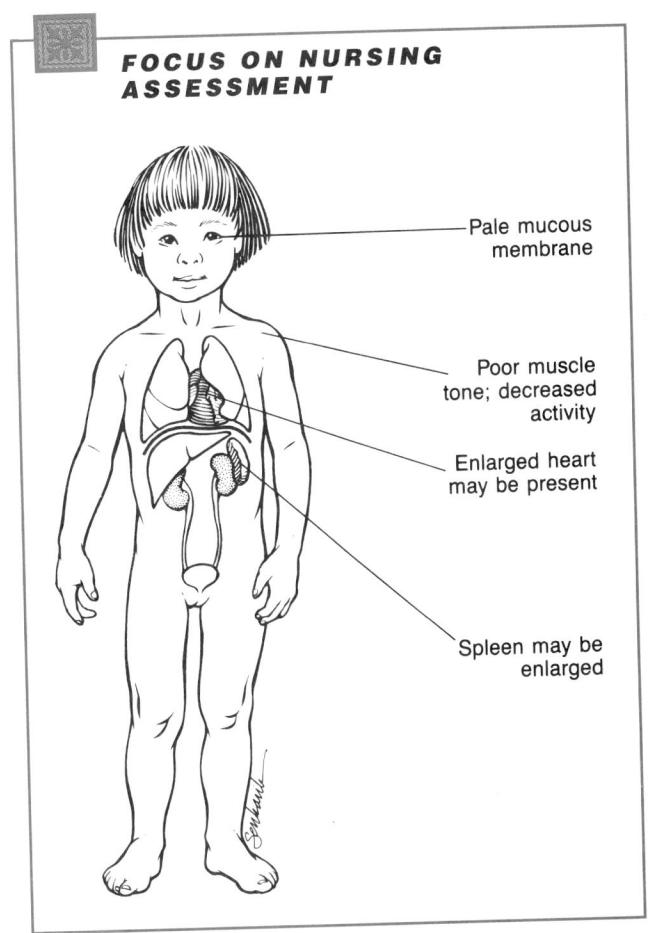

FOCUS ON NURSING ASSESSMENT

Pale mucous membrane

Poor muscle tone; decreased activity

Enlarged heart may be present

Spleen may be enlarged

FIGURE 44-4
Common symptoms of iron-deficiency anemia.

skinned" even though the child's pallor is so extreme that his or her skin is transparent. In dark-skinned infants, pallor of mucous membranes may be the most significant finding.

Infants may show poor muscle tone and reduced activity; they are generally irritable from fatigue. The heart may be enlarged, and there may be a soft systolic precordial murmur as the heart increases its action, attempting to supply blood cells better. The spleen may be slightly enlarged. Fingernails become typically "spoon-shaped" or depressed in contour.

A dietary history generally reveals an abnormally high milk intake. As a rule, infants should not ingest more than 32 oz of milk a day. Infants with iron-deficiency anemia may be drinking up to 50 oz a day. One quart of milk provides only approximately 0.5 mg of iron; in contrast, 1 tbs of iron-fortified baby cereal supplies 2.5 to 5.0 mg of iron.

With iron-deficiency anemia, laboratory studies reveal decreased hemoglobin (defined as a hemoglobin level less than 11 g per 100 mL of blood) and hematocrit levels (a level below 33%). Because the red blood cells are microcytic and hypochromic and possibly poikilocytic, the MCV will be low also. The MCH may be reduced. There is a low serum iron (normal is 70 µg/100 mL; with iron-deficiency anemia, the level is often as low as 30 µg/100 mL) with an increased iron-binding capacity (more than 350 µg/100 mL). The level of serum ferritin reflects the extent of iron stores (will be less than 10 µg/100 mL; normal is 35 µg/mL). Monoamine oxidase (MAO) is an enzyme important for central nervous system maturation. Iron is incorporated into MAO structure, so without iron, this necessary enzyme is absent. Without iron, heme precursors cannot be used, so free erythrocyte protoporphyrins increase to more than 10 µg/g from a normal of 1.9 µg/g. Iron-deficiency anemia is associated with infants who are more fearful, less active, less persistent, and less happy. When tested by a Bayley scale, iron-deficient infants demonstrate poor performance, restricted perception, and decreased attentiveness. School-age children with iron-deficiency anemia score less well on tests than their healthy counterparts and tend to be more inattentive and disruptive in class (Filer, 1990). Iron-deficiency anemia is also associated with pica (the eating of inedible substances such as dirt and paper). Eating ice cubes is common in adolescents. Until the anemia is corrected, parents need to supervise the child's environment to keep inedible materials out of the child's reach.

Therapeutic Management. Medical treatment of iron-deficiency anemia is treatment of the underlying cause. Sources of gastrointestinal bleeding must be ruled out. The diet must be rich in iron and should contain extra vitamin C that will enhance iron absorption. Infants should be given iron-fortified formula for a full year (Belkengren & Sapala, 1993). Ferrous sulfate is the drug of choice to improve red cell formation and replace iron stores.

Nursing Diagnoses and Related Interventions

Nursing Diagnosis: Altered nutrition; less than body requirements related to inadequate ingestion of iron

Goal: Child will increase his or her oral intake of iron by 24 hours.

Outcome Criteria: Infant ingests an iron-fortified formula plus two servings of iron-fortified cereal daily, and ferrous sulfate as prescribed; adolescent ingests a diet with iron-rich foods plus ferrous sulfate as prescribed.

When planning care for the infant with iron-deficiency anemia, minimize the child's activities to prevent fatigue, particularly at mealtime; it is vitally important that the infant eat well.

Parents need to be counseled on measures to improve their child's diet, such as adding iron-rich foods while decreasing milk intake to maintain the iron levels and prevent recurring anemia. If the child is not fond of meat, parents can substitute cheese, eggs, green vegetables, or fortified cereal. Though iron-rich foods are often expensive, parents must be reminded that these items are important, and that they should not substitute less expensive, high-carbohydrate foods.

Before iron therapy is started, alert parents to any possible side effects. If oral iron is not tolerated or if there is a doubt that the child will take it, an iron-dextran injection (Imferon) can be given intramuscularly. Imferon stains skin and is extremely irritating unless it is given by deep z-track intramuscular injection.

Of all age groups, adolescents do the least well with medicine compliance. Help them plan a daily time for taking their iron supplement with a medicine reminder chart. At first they may reject this as "childish," but you can tell them that everyone needs these charts, not just adolescents. Review with them the iron-rich foods they will need to eat daily; an iron supplement is effective only if taken with iron-rich foods.

After 7 days of iron therapy, the child usually returns on an ambulatory basis for a reticulocyte determination. If elevated, this means that the child is receiving adequate iron and that the rapid proliferation of new erythrocytes is correcting the anemia. Iron medication must be taken for at least 4 to 6 weeks after the red cell count is normal to rebuild iron levels in the blood. In some children, maintenance therapy may continue for as long as 1 year.

Chronic-Infection Anemia

Acute infection interferes with red blood cell production, producing a normochromic, normocytic anemia.

When infections are chronic, anemia of a hypochromic, microcytic type occurs. This is probably caused by impaired iron metabolism as well as impaired red blood cell production.

The degree of anemia is rarely as severe as that occurring with iron deficiency. Administration of iron has little effect until the infection is controlled.

Macrocytic (Megaloblastic) Anemias

A macrocytic anemia is one in which red blood cells are abnormally large. These cells are actually immature erythrocytes or megaloblasts (nucleated immature red cells). For this reason, these anemias are often referred to as megaloblastic anemias. They are uncommon in the United States.

Anemia of Folic Acid Deficiency

A deficiency of folic acid combined with vitamin C deficiency produces an anemia in which erythrocytes are abnormally large; there is accompanying neutropenia and thrombocytopenia. There will be an increased MCV and MCH and a normal MCHC. Bone marrow will contain megaloblasts, indicating inhibition of the production of erythrocytes at an early stage. Megaloblastic arrest may occur in the first year of life from the continued use of infant food containing too little folic acid. Goat's milk tends to be deficient in folic acid, so infants who are fed this are prone to megaloblastic anemia. Treatment is daily oral administration of folic acid. Response to treatment is dramatic.

Pernicious Anemia (Vitamin B$_{12}$ Deficiency)

Pernicious anemia is caused by deficiency or inability to use vitamin B$_{12}$. Vitamin B$_{12}$ is found primarily in food of animal origin, including both cow's milk and breast milk, so as a rule is readily available to infants. An adolescent may be deficient in vitamin B$_{12}$ if he or she is on a long-term, poorly formulated vegetarian diet.

For absorption of vitamin B$_{12}$ from the intestine, an intrinsic factor must be present in the gastric mucosa. Lack of the intrinsic factor is the most frequent cause of the disorder. Symptoms of intrinsic factor deficiency generally occur in the first 2 years of life (once the intrauterine stores of vitamin B$_{12}$ have been exhausted). The child appears pale, anorexic, and irritable, with chronic diarrhea. The tongue appears smooth and beefred in color due to papillary atrophy. In adults, neuropathologic findings such ataxia, hyporeflexia, paresthesia, and a positive Babinski reflex are common; in children, however, they are less noticeable.

Laboratory findings will reveal low serum levels of vitamin B$_{12}$. The rate and efficiency of absorption of vitamin B$_{12}$ can be tested by the ingestion of the radioactively tagged vitamin. The dose absorbed in the presence and absence of a dose of intrinsic factor can be measured (a Schilling test).

Pernicious anemia is treated with lifelong monthly intramuscular injections of vitamin B$_{12}$. Parents and the child need to understand clearly that lifelong therapy is necessary. Many people think anemia is always a minor illness. Help parents to understand that neurologic impairment can occur if vitamin B$_{12}$ is not administered conscientiously.

Hemolytic Anemias

Hemolytic anemias are those in which the number of erythrocytes decreases because of increased destruction of erythrocytes. This may be caused by fundamental abnormalities of erythrocyte structure or by extracellular destruction forces.

Congenital Spherocytosis

Congenital spherocytosis is a hemolytic anemia that is inherited as an autosomal dominant trait; it occurs most frequently in the white population. The life span of erythrocytes is diminished; the cells are small and defective, apparently due to abnormalities of the protein of the cell membrane that make them unusually permeable to sodium.

The disease may be noticed shortly after birth, although symptoms may appear at any age. The hemolysis of red blood cells appears to occur in the spleen, apparently from excessive absorption of sodium into the cell. The abnormal cell swells and ruptures and so is destroyed. Chronic jaundice and splenomegaly are present. The MCHC will be increased because the cells are small. Gallstones may be present in the older school-age child and adolescent because of the continuous hemolysis, bilirubin release, and incorporation of bilirubin into gallstones.

Infections may precipitate a "crisis" involving bone marrow failure. During such a period, the anemia increases rapidly as the hemolysis continues. Blood transfusion will be necessary to maintain a sufficient number of circulating erythrocytes.

The diagnosis of the disease is based on family history, the obvious hemolysis, and the presence of the abnormal spherocytes. The medical treatment is generally splenectomy at approximately 5 to 6 years. This measure will increase the number of red blood cells present but will not alter their abnormal structure. Children are susceptible to infection following splenectomy, particularly pneumococcal infections; be certain parents know to seek early treatment for beginning infections. Children may be placed on a prophylactic antibiotic such as penicillin or given pneumococcal vaccine to attempt to prevent infection.

Glucose-6-Phosphate Dehydrogenase (G6PD) Deficiency

The enzyme G6PD is necessary for maintenance of red blood cell life. Lack of the enzyme results in premature destruction of red blood cells if the cells are exposed to an oxidant. Deficiency of the enzyme occurs most frequently in children of black, Asian, Sephardic Jewish, and Mediterranean descent. The disease is transmitted as a sex-linked recessive trait or on the genes of the X chromosome. Approximately 13% of African American males and 2% of African-American females have the disorder (Martin & Pearson, 1994).

G6PD occurs in three identifiable forms. Children with congenital nonspherocytic hemolytic anemia have hemolysis, jaundice, and splenomegaly, and may have aplastic crises. Other children have a drug-induced form in which the blood patterns are normal until the child is exposed to fava beans or drugs such as antipyretics; sulfonamides; antimalarials; and naphthaquinolones (the most common drug in these groups is acetylsalicylic acid [aspirin]). Approximately 2 days after ingestion of such an oxidant drug, the child begins to show evidence of hemolysis.

A blood smear will show Heinz bodies (oddly shaped particles in red blood cells). The degree of red blood cell destruction depends on the drug and the extent of exposure to it. The child may have accompanying fever and back pain. Occasionally a newborn is seen with marked hemolysis because the mother ingested an initiating drug during pregnancy.

Drug-induced hemolysis usually is self-limiting, and blood transfusions are rarely necessary. G6PD deficiency may be diagnosed by a rapid enzyme screening test or electrophoretic analysis of red blood cells. Both parents and children must be told of the defect in the child's metabolism so that they can avoid common drugs such as acetylsalicylic acid.

Because the disease is sex linked, males of high-risk groups should be screened in infancy.

Sickle Cell Anemia

Sickle cell anemia is the presence of abnormally shaped (elongated) red blood cells. It is an autosomal recessive inherited defect of the beta chain of hemoglobin; the amino acid valine takes the place of the normally appearing glutamic acid. The erythrocytes become characteristically elongated and crescent shaped (sickled) when they are submitted to low oxygen tension (less than 60% to 70%), a low blood pH (acidosis), or increased blood viscosity such as occurs with dehydration or hypoxia. When red blood cells sickle, they do not move freely through vessels; blood stasis and further sickling occurs (a sickle cell disease crisis). Blood flow halts due to blocked vessels and tissue distal to the blockage becomes ischemic, resulting in acute pain and cell destruction.

Because fetal hemoglobin contains a gamma, not a beta, chain, the disease will not result in clinical symptoms until the child's hemoglobin changes from the fetal to the adult form at approximately 4 to 6 months.

The disease can be diagnosed prenatally by chorionic villi sampling or from cord blood during amniocentesis. The abnormal form of hemoglobin in this disorder is designated hemoglobin S. A child with sickle cell disease is said to have hemoglobin SS (homozygous involvement).

Sickle cell disease occurs almost exclusively among blacks. Both parents of the child with the disease will be carriers (heterozygous) of the **sickle cell trait**. A person who has the trait (heterozygous) is said to have hemoglobin SA. In people with the trait, approximately 25% to 50% of hemoglobin produced is abnormal; they produce enough normal hemoglobin to compensate for the defect and therefore show no symptoms. Sickle cell trait occurs in approximately 8% to 10% of African Americans. A child with the disease (homozygous) produces no normal hemoglobin and so shows characteristic symptoms of sickle cell anemia. Approximately 1 in 400 African Americans have hemoglobin SS disease.

Assessment. Screening for sickle cell anemia is a simple procedure. A test is available in which blood placed in a test tube with a test reagent is allowed to stand for 5 minutes and then is observed (a sickling test).

Unfortunately, all hemoglobin S cells sickle in a sickling test, so the test yields a positive result both for people with sickle cell disease and those with sickle cell trait. Further differentiation involves hemoglobin electrophoresis; in many states, all newborns are routinely screened for the disorder.

At approximately 4 to 6 months of age, children with SS disease will begin to show initial signs of fever and anemia. Stasis of blood and infarction may occur in any body part, leading to local disease. Some infants have swelling of the hands and feet (a hand-foot syndrome). This is probably caused by aseptic infarction of the bones of the hands and feet. Children with sickle cell anemia tend to have a slight build and characteristically long arms and legs; they may have a protruding abdomen because of an enlarged spleen and liver. In adolescence, the spleen size may be decreased from repeated infarction and atrophy. An atropic spleen leaves a child more susceptible to infection than normal because the spleen can no longer filter bacteria; pneumococcal meningitis and *Salmonella*-induced osteomyelitis are frequent illnesses. To prevent infection, many children are placed on prophylactic penicillin from about 6 months to 6 years of age. The liver may become enlarged from stasis of blood flow; eventually, cirrhosis (fibrotic degeneration) will occur from infarcts and tissue scarring. The kidneys may have subsequent scarring also, and kidney function will be decreased (Allon, 1990). The sclerae are generally icteric (yellowed) from chronic destruction of the sickled cells; small retinal occlusions may lead to decreased vision. Regular eye exams are necessary in children with sickle cell disease to detect this. Cell clusters in the blood vessel of the penis may cause priapism, or persistent, painful erection.

Sickle Cell Crisis. **Sickle cell crisis** is the term used to denote a sudden, severe onset of sickling. Symptoms of crisis occur from pooling of the many new sickled cells in vessels and consequent tissue hypoxia (a vaso-occlusive crisis). A sickle cell crisis can occur when a child has an illness causing dehydration or a respiratory infection that results in lowered oxygen exchange and lowered arterial oxygen level, or following extremely strenuous exercise (enough to lead to tissue hypoxia). Sometimes no obvious cause of a crisis can be found. Symptoms are sudden, severe, and painful. The child has fever and acute abdominal, back, and extremity pain; hands may be painful and swollen (Platt et al., 1991). There may be vomiting and abdominal tenderness due to visceral infarcts, as if the child had undergone surgery (Bonadio, 1990). The joints may be warm and swollen, simulating a rheumatic process. Aseptic necrosis of the head of the femur or humerus with increased joint pain may occur. Laboratory reports reveal a hemoglobin of only 6 to 8 g/100 mL. A peripheral blood smear will demonstrate sickled cells. White blood count is often elevated to 12,000 to 20,000/mm³. Bilirubin and reticulocyte levels will be increased.

If a cardiovascular accident occurs from a blocked artery, the central nervous system will be affected and the child may have coma, convulsions, or even death. If there is renal involvement, hematuria or flank pain may result. Common symptoms of the child in sickle cell crisis are shown in Figure 44-5. Less frequent forms of crisis may occur when there is splenic sequestration of red blood cells or severe anemia due to pooling and increased destruction of sickled cells in the liver and spleen. This leads to shock from hypovolemia; the spleen is enlarged and tender. An aplastic crisis is manifested by severe anemia due to a sudden decrease in production of red blood cells. This form usually occurs with infection. A megaloblastic crisis may occur if the child has folic acid or vitamin B₁₂ deficiency (new red blood cells cannot be fully formed due to lack of these ingredients).

Therapeutic Management. The child in sickle cell crisis has two primary needs: (1) pain relief and (2) adequate hydration and oxygenation to prevent further sickling and halt the crisis.

Acetaminophen (Tylenol) or narcotics are usually prescribed to control pain; administer as often as allowed. Once the child is pain free, his or her agitation will decrease, reducing the metabolic need for oxygen and ending the sickling. Hydration is generally accom-

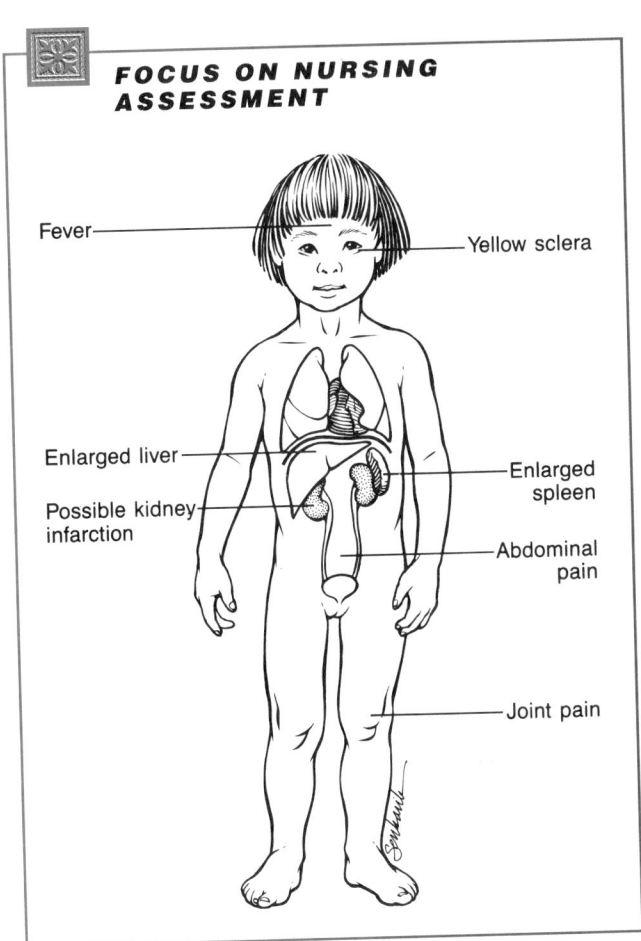

FOCUS ON NURSING ASSESSMENT

Fever — Yellow sclera

Enlarged liver — Enlarged spleen

Possible kidney infarction — Abdominal pain

Joint pain

FIGURE 44-5
Common symptoms of the child in sickle cell crisis.

plished by intensive intravenous therapy. Tissue hypoxia leads to acidosis; the acidosis must be corrected by electrolyte replacement. Some kidney infarction may have occurred. Do not administer potassium by intravenous line until the child has voided; otherwise, excessive potassium levels will lead to cardiac arrhythmias. Infection may cause a sickling crisis. If this occurs, blood and urine cultures, a chest x-ray, and a complete blood count will be taken and the infection treated by antibiotics.

Blood transfusion (usually packed red cells) may be necessary to maintain the hemoglobin above 12 g/dL (termed hypertransfusion). Although the blood supply is much safer due to improved screening and testing, there is still a small chance of acquiring HIV and hepatitis through blood transfusion.

If none of the above measures appears to be effective, children may be given an exchange transfusion to remove most of the sickled cells and replace them with normal cells. Exchange transfusion (see Chapter 26) must be done with small amounts of blood at each exchange; otherwise, the pressure changes can cause such irregularities in blood volume that heart failure results.

Nursing Diagnoses and Related Interventions

Nursing Diagnosis: High risk for ineffective tissue perfusion related to infarcts due to sickling

Goal: Child will not experience detrimental effects of sickle cell crisis during course of crisis.

Outcome Criteria: Child's respiratory rate is 16/min to 20/min; cyanosis is not present; $Pco_2 = 40$ mm Hg; $Po_2 = 80$ mm Hg to 90 mm Hg; urine output is greater than 1 mL/kg/h.

Oxygen may be administered by mask if blood gases reveal a low Po_2 level. Oxygen may not reach every distal body part effectively if blood flowing to the part is obstructed by the sickled cells. When hemoglobin S is below 40%, blood flow can be predicted to be adequate to body cells. High concentrations of oxygen are not used because hypoxia is a stimulant to erythrocyte production—production badly needed to replace damaged cells. Monitor the flow rate and extent of use carefully. Bedrest is necessary both to relieve the pain and reduce oxygen expenditure.

It is important to maintain accurate intake and output records, test urine specific gravity, and dipstick for hematuria to detect the extent or presence of kidney damage from infarcts.

Nursing Diagnosis: Altered health maintenance related to lack of knowledge regarding long-term needs of child with sickle cell anemia

Goal: Family will demonstrate ability to carry out necessary measures to maintain child's health in the future.

Outcome Criteria: Mother or father accurately describes disease process and special precautions they will take to prevent child from going into sickle cell crisis.

In many children, episodes of sickling grow less severe as the child reaches adolescence. These children may live a normal life span but still experience the stresses of chronic illness. Other children experience such devastating episodes in early childhood that the disease is fatal at an early age. Parents need support to supervise children carefully day by day when they are aware that, due to children's intense episodes, the children may die despite the parents' precautions.

Between crisis periods, care focuses on preventing recurring crisis. Although the hemoglobin level of children may remain as low as 6 to 9 g/100 mL, children adjust well to this chronic state. Children who are having frequent blood transfusions should not be given supplementary iron or iron-fortified formula or vitamins or they may receive too much iron; high levels of excess iron are deposited in body tissues (**hemosiderosis**) to a point of destroying them (**hemochromatosis**). Children are regularly prescribed oral folic acid to help them rebuild hemolyzed red blood cells.

Children with sickle cell anemia need to be followed at regular health care visits. They must receive childhood immunizations so that they are not vulnerable to common childhood infections such as measles or pertussis. They are also candidates for meningococcal and pneumococcal vaccines to attempt to prevent infection from these sources. Puberty may be delayed; both parents and children may need counseling to accept this. Once puberty changes do occur, they are adequate, just later than normal. Some boys who suffer severe priapism, however, may become impotent (Mykulak & Glassberg, 1990).

Caution parents to bring their child to a health care facility at the first indication of infection. Some parents are reluctant to do this, afraid that they will be labeled "overprotective." Assure them that health care personnel are knowledgeable about sickle cell anemia, and they know that a child with even a minor infection could become very ill. Respiratory illness will lead to sickling for two reasons: (1) the accompanying dehydration and (2) the lowered oxygen tension from altered oxygen–carbon dioxide exchange.

Parents must make decisions regarding children's activity levels. Children should attend regular school if at all possible and be allowed to participate in all school activities except contact sports (such as football) that could result in rupture of an enlarged spleen. Long-distance running is also inadvisable because it can lead to dehydration. Caution parents to give the child fluids on long hikes and at the beach. They should be cautioned against taking the child on board an unpressurized aircraft in which the oxygen concentration may fall during flight. During the summer months, parents need to be certain that they offer the child frequent drinks to prevent dehydration. The average child usually drinks adequate fluid without urging if fluids are available (see the Focus on Family Teaching box).

Some children who have had kidney infarcts and lessened ability to concentrate urine will have chronic nocturnal enuresis (bedwetting). One often recommended solution for alleviating bedwetting is to restrict fluids after dinner. This should be followed with caution in a child with sickle cell anemia. The fluid restriction combined with the kidney's inability to concentrate urine may lead to severe dehydration (Readett et al., 1990).

Children with sickle cell disease are under particular threat if they need surgery. The hours of being on nothing-by-mouth status, as well as being unable to eat afterward, may lead to dehydration; anesthesia may cause a transient hypoxia leading to sickling. Parents must be cautioned that even for such a simple operation as tooth extraction, they must alert health care personnel of their child's condition.

Q. My 4-year-old son has been diagnosed as having sickle-cell anemia. What special precautions do I have to take to keep him safe when he starts school next year?

A. Starting school is a major point in a child's life because he will be independent for such a long period during the day. Some suggestions for safety precautions are:

- Children with sickle-cell anemia need to maintain a high fluid intake to prevent blood from becoming thick. Be certain your child either takes fluid with him or buys adequate fluid for lunch.

- Provide additional fluid in the summer when dehydration is more apt to happen. Anticipate ways to provide fluid during long hikes or school trips; time spent on a hot beach may need to be limited.

- Learn about sources high in folic acid such as vegetables and fruit and be certain these are included in your son's diet every day.

- Encourage the child to get adequate sleep at night as a general measure to prevent illness.

- With the exception of contact sports (to avoid damage to an enlarged spleen) and long-distance running (to prevent dehydration), encourage your child to participate in normal school activities.

- Nocturnal enuresis may occur as part of the illness. Encourage your son to take baths in the morning if this occurs so his clothes don't smell of urine.

- Maintain routine health care such as immunizations to prevent common childhood illnesses such as measles and mumps.

- Call your primary health care provider at the first sign of illness such as an upper respiratory infection so therapy can be begun immediately.

Thalassemias

The thalassemias are anemias associated with abnormalities of the beta chain of adult hemoglobin (HgbA). Although these anemias occur most frequently in the Mediterranean population, they also occur in children of African and Asian heritage.

Thalassemia Minor (Heterozygous β-Thalassemia)

Children with thalassemia minor, a minor form of this anemia, produce both defective beta hemoglobin and normal hemoglobin. Because there is some normal production, the red blood cell count will be normal but the hemoglobin concentration will be decreased 2 to 3 g/100 mL below normal levels. The blood cells are moderately hypochromic and microcytic because of the poor hemoglobin formation.

Children may have no symptoms other than pallor. They require no treatment, and life expectancy is normal. They should not receive a routine iron supplement because their inability to incorporate it well into hemoglobin may cause them to accumulate too much iron. The condition represents the heterozygous form of the disorder or can be compared with children having the sickle cell trait.

Thalassemia Major (Homozygous β-Thalassemia)

Thalassemia major is also called Cooley's anemia or Mediterranean anemia. Because thalassemia is a beta-chain hemoglobin defect, symptoms do not become apparent until children's fetal hemoglobin has largely been replaced by adult hemoglobin during the second half of the first year. Effects of thalassemia on body systems are summarized in Table 44-3. Unable to produce normal beta hemoglobin, children show symptoms of anemia: pallor, irritability, and anorexia.

Red blood cells will be hypochromic (pale) and microcytic (small); fragmented poikilocytes and basophilic stippling (unevenness of hemoglobin concentration) will be present. The hemoglobin level will be less than 5 g/100 mL. The serum iron level will be high because iron is not being incorporated into hemoglobin; iron saturation will be 100%.

Assessment. To maintain a functional level of hemoglobin, the bone marrow hypertrophies in an attempt to produce more red blood cells. This may cause bone pain; the ineffective attempt often leads to the formation

Table 44-3. *Effects of Thalassemia*

Body Organ or System	Effect of Abnormal Cell Production
Bone marrow	Overstimulation of bone marrow leads to increased facial-mandibular growth
Skin	Bronze colored from hemosiderosis and jaundice
Spleen	Splenomegaly
Liver and gallbladder	Cirrhosis and cholelithiasis
Pancreas	Destruction of islet cells and diabetes mellitus
Heart	Failure from circulatory overload

of target cells or large macrocytes that are short lived and nonfunctional. As bone marrow becomes hyperactive, this results in characteristic change in the shape of the skull (parietal and frontal bossing) and protrusion of the upper teeth, with marked malocclusion. The base of the nose may be broad and flattened; the eyes may be slanted with an epicanthal fold as in Down syndrome (Figure 44-6). An x-ray of bone will show marked osteoporotic (lessened density) tissue; this may result in fractures (Johanson, 1990). The child may have hepatosplenomegaly due to excessive iron deposits and fibrotic scarring in the liver, and the spleen's increased attempts to destroy defective red blood cells. Abdominal pressure from the enlarged spleen may cause anorexia and vomiting. Epistaxis is common, as is diabetes mellitus due to pancreatic siderosis and cardiac dilatation with an accompanying murmur. Arrhythmias and heart failure are a frequent cause of death.

Therapeutic Management. Digitalis, diuretics, and a low sodium diet may be prescribed to prevent congestive heart failure, which could result from the decompensation that accompanies anemia, and from myocardial fibrosis caused by invasion of iron (hemochromatosis). Transfusion of packed red cells every 2 to 4 weeks (hypertransfusion therapy) will maintain hemoglobin between 10 and 12 g/100 mL. Within this level of hemoglobin, erythropoiesis is suppressed and cosmetic facial alterations, osteoporosis, and cardiac dilatation are kept to a minimum. Hypertransfusion therapy also reduces the possibility that splenectomy will be necessary. Frequent blood transfusions unfortunately increase the risk of hepatitis B and C, HIV, and deposition of iron in body tissues (hemosiderosis).

Splenectomy may become necessary to reduce discomfort from the markedly enlarged spleen; this will also reduce the rate of red cell hemolysis and the number of necessary transfusions. After a splenectomy, children become more susceptible to infection. They may be placed on a prophylactic antibiotic such as penicillin to reduce the possibility of infection or immunized with pneumococcal vaccine. Splenectomy is a major surgical procedure with a high level of postoperative pain, especially with coughing as the diaphragm presses on the suture line. Children may be afraid to cough deeply and risk developing pneumonia.

The overall prognosis of thalassemia is improving but still grave. Most children with the disease will die from cardiac failure during adolescence or as young adults.

Nursing Diagnoses and Related Interventions

Nursing Diagnosis: High risk for self-esteem disturbance related to changed physical appearance.

Goal: Child will demonstrate an adequate level of self-esteem during course of illness.

Outcome Criteria: Child states he or she can accept altered appearance, and interacts with peers.

Children with thalassemia major may have delayed growth and sexual maturation. They usually develop a marked change in facial appearance because of the overgrowth of marrow-producing centers. This can be demoralizing because these changes will be permanent. In addition, the child who receives frequent blood transfusions may develop such hemosiderosis that his or her skin appears bronze.

Children should be allowed as much activity as possible and should attend regular school if possible to maintain a nearly normal childhood. Discussions about other children's reactions to their changing facial appearance can be helpful.

Autoimmune Acquired Hemolytic Anemia

Occasionally, autoimmune antibodies (abnormal antibodies of the IgG class directed against the child's red cells) attach themselves to red blood cells and cause hemolysis. This may occur at any age, and its origin is generally idiopathic, although the disorder may be associated with malignancy, viral infections, or collagen diseases such as rheumatoid arthritis or systemic lupus erythematosus. A child may recently have had an upper respiratory infection, measles, or varicella virus infection (chickenpox). Such hemolysis may occur after the administration of drugs such as quinine, phenacetin, sulfonamides, or penicillin.

Why children form antibodies against their own cells is unknown but may involve a change in the red blood cells themselves, making them antigenic, or a change in antibody production, making antibodies destructive to other substances.

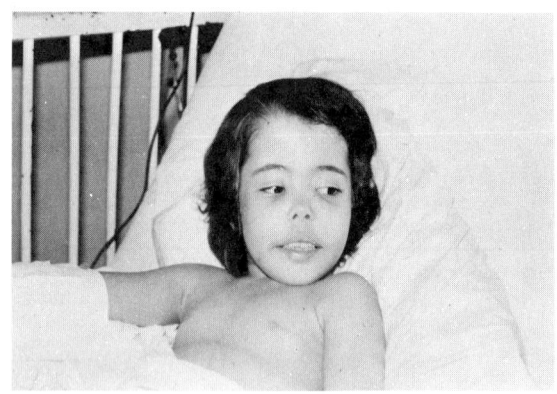

FIGURE 44-6
A child with the characteristic facies of thalassemia major. The maxilla becomes prominent, causing malocclusion. (From Mauer, A. M. [1969]. Pediatric hematology. *New York: McGraw-Hill, with permission.)*

Assessment. The onset of hemolytic anemia is insidious. Children have a low-grade fever, anorexia, lethargy, pallor, and icterus from release of indirect bilirubin from the hemolyzed cells. Both urine and stools appear dark because the excess bilirubin is being excreted. In some children, the illness begins abruptly with high fever, hemoglobinuria, marked jaundice, and pallor. There may be an enlarged liver and spleen.

Laboratory findings will reveal that the red cells are extremely small and round (spherocytosis), resembling hereditary spherocytosis. The reticulocyte count will be increased as the body attempts to form replacement red cells. A direct Coombs' test result will be positive, indicating the presence of antibodies attached to red cells. Hemoglobin levels will fall as low as 6 g/100 mL.

Therapeutic Management. In some children, the disease process runs a limited course and no treatment is necessary. In others, a single blood transfusion may correct the disturbance. It is difficult to cross match blood for transfusion for these children because the red cell antibody tends to clump or agglutinate all blood tested. If cross matching is impossible, the child may be given type O Rh− blood. Observe the child carefully during any transfusion for signs of blood reaction.

If the anemia is persistent, corticosteroid therapy (oral prednisone) is generally effective. If such therapy is effective, there will be an increase in the red blood cell count and increased hemoglobin concentration in a short period. If treatment with corticosteroids is ineffective, splenectomy may be necessary. For some children, immunosuppressive agents (such as cyclophosphamide [Cytoxan] or azathioprine [Imuran]) are effective in reducing antibody formation.

This is a distressing illness to parents because it is so difficult for them to understand the process. How could a child's body turn on itself? What caused this? How long will it last? What will stop it from happening again? There are no answers to these questions. The parents and child all need support as they wait for this unexplainable process to run its course and for the child to be well again.

Polycythemia

Polycythemia is an increase in the number of red blood cells that results as a compensatory response to insufficient oxygenation of the blood. With this disorder, erythropoiesis is increased to attempt to supply enough red blood cells to supply oxygen to cells. Chronic pulmonary disease and cyanotic congenital heart disease are the usual causes of polycythemia in childhood. It may occur from twin transfusion at birth (one twin receives excess blood while a second twin is anemic). Plethora (marked reddened appearance of the skin) occurs because of the increase in total red cell volume.

The erythrocytes are usually macrocytic (large); the hemoglobin content is high. This means that the MCH will be elevated; the MCHC, however, will be normal, indicating that although many in number, each erythrocyte is normally saturated with hemoglobin. The red blood cell count may be as high as 7.0 million/mm^3; hemoglobin levels may be as high as 23 g/100 mL.

Treatment of polycythemia involves treatment of the underlying cause. Because of the high blood viscosity, there is danger of cerebrovascular accident occurring or of emboli developing. The child is particularly in danger from these disorders if he or she becomes dehydrated, as occurs with fever or during surgery. Exchange transfusion to reduce the red blood cell count may be necessary.

Disorders of the White Blood Cells

Disorders Related to the Number or Proportion of White Blood Cells

Most disorders characterized by a decrease or increase in the number of white blood cells or specific white blood cell components occur in response to other disease (often infection or an allergic reaction) in the body. Laboratory values of white blood cells therefore provide one of the first objective indicators of disease, often aiding in specific diagnosis.

Neutropenia

Neutropenia refers to a reduced number of white blood cells. It may occur as a transient phenomenon with nonpyrogenic infections such as viral disease. It will occur predictably as a response to therapy with some drugs, such as 6-mercaptopurine or nitrogen mustard. It may also occur as a side effect from drugs such as phenytoin sodium (Dilantin); chloramphenicol, or chlorpromazine. A white cell count of less than 1500/mm^3 is always serious because absence of neutrophils lessens the child's protection against overwhelming infection (opportunistic infection), protection normally provided by phagocytosis. White blood cell transfusion may be used to restore a functioning cell level; prophylactic antibiotics may be prescribed.

Neutrophilia

Neutrophilia refers to an increased number of circulating white blood cells, primarily neutrophils. This occurs in the presence of infection or inflammation. Not only does the total number of cells increase but the proportion of mature neutrophils changes, with an increase in immature cells. The presence of many banded or immature forms is sometimes referred to as a "shift to the left." Infections that may cause neutrophilia in children are discussed in Chapter 43.

Leukemia

Leukemia, the uncontrolled proliferation of white blood cells, is discussed in Chapter 53.

Eosinophilia

Eosinophilia, an increase in eosinophils, is associated with many allergic disorders such as atopic dermatitis and with parasitic invasion. These disorders are discussed in Chapters 42 and 43, respectively.

Lymphocytosis

Lymphocytosis occurs normally in the preschool period when there is a marked predominance of lymphocytes in relation to neutrophils. Lymphocytes are abnormally elevated in childhood illnesses such as pertussis, infectious mononucleosis, and lymphoblastic leukemia.

Disorders of Blood Coagulation

A normal platelet level is 150,000/mm³. **Thrombocytopenia** (decreased platelet count) may be defined as a platelet count of less than 40,000/mm³. Because platelets are necessary for blood coagulation, platelet disorders limit the effectiveness of blood coagulation. In one disorder children are born with thrombocytopenia and also are missing the radius bone in the forearm (TAR [thrombocytopenia–absent radius] syndrome). Thrombocytopenia leads to purpura (Casella, 1994).

Purpuras

Purpura is a hemorrhagic rash or small hemorrhages occurring in the superficial layer of skin. Two main types of purpura occur in children.

Idiopathic Thrombocytopenic Purpura

Idiopathic thrombocytopenic purpura (ITP) is the result of a decrease in the number of circulating platelets, although adequate megakaryocytes (precursors to platelets) are present. The cause is unknown but it probably results from an increased rate of destruction of platelets due to an antiplatelet antibody that destroys platelets (making this an autoimmune illness).

In most instances, ITP occurs approximately 2 weeks following a viral infection such as rubella, rubeola, or an upper respiratory tract infection (Ruggenenti & Remuzzi, 1990). Congenital ITP may occur in the newborn of a woman who has had ITP during pregnancy. An antiplatelet factor apparently crosses the placenta and causes platelet destruction in the newborn. If it occurs in infants whose mother did not have ITP, the disease appears to develop in the same way as Rh incompatibility or hemolytic disease of the newborn: however, in ITP, the platelets, not the red blood cells, are sensitized (see Chapter 26).

Assessment. The hemorrhage manifestations begin abruptly. This may first be evidenced as miniature petechiae or as large areas of asymmetrical ecchymosis most prominent over the legs. Epistaxis may be present.

Laboratory studies reveal marked thrombocytopenia. The platelet count may be as low as 20,000/mm³. Bone marrow examination will show a normal number of megakaryocytes. A tourniquet test may be performed. For this, take the child's blood pressure, then reinflate the cuff on the child's arm to a point halfway between systolic and diastolic pressure; leave it inflated for 5 minutes. In a child with normal coagulation ability, this extended pressure should result in fewer than 10 petechiae marks on an area of skin on the forearm 2 cm square. The child with decreased platelets will have a greater number of petechiae. Table 44-1 lists other commonly used tests of coagulation ability.

Therapeutic Management. Medical treatment for the disease is the administration of oral prednisone. Platelet transfusion will temporarily increase the platelet count, but because the lifespan of platelets is relatively short, a platelet transfusion will have limited effect. Children with central nervous system bleeding are treated more vigorously, with initial splenectomy and then transfusion.

Salicylates should not be given to relieve joint pain from bleeding because salicylates interfere with blood clotting by preventing the aggregation of platelets at wound sites.

In most children, ITP runs a limited, 1- to 3-month course. A few children develop chronic ITP. A course of immunosuppressive drugs may be attempted if the chronic state persists; intravenous gamma globulin may be used to improve the platelet count. Plasmapheresis (transfusion of plasma) may be effective in some children (Welborn et al., 1990).

All children need to be vaccinated against the viral diseases of childhood so that diseases such as rubella and rubeola are eradicated and no longer lead to this defective coagulation process.

Nursing Diagnoses and Related Interventions

Nursing Diagnosis: Health-seeking behaviors related to injury prevention measures

Goal: Parents will demonstrate knowledge of ways to prevent injury that would result in bleeding during child's illness.

Outcome Criteria: Parents state precautions they will take to reduce possibility of bleeding injury; child's skin is free of ecchymotic areas.

The Focus on Nursing Care box earlier in the chapter summarizes measures that can be used to reduce the possibility of bleeding (e.g., padding the surfaces where the child plays). Parents cannot completely eliminate the possibility of a serious bleeding injury, however, until the platelet count returns to normal. The chief danger to the child from ITP, aside from the psychological stress of a perplexing illness, is intracranial hemorrhage. Fortunately, this rarely occurs. Signs of this would be persistent headache, nuchal rigidity, and lethargy.

Nursing Diagnosis: High risk for family coping, compromised, related to diagnosis of child's illness

Goal: Parents demonstrate ability to cope with life-threatening circumstances during course of illness.

Outcome Criteria: Parents state that they understand the nature of their child's illness and have identified ways to carry out daily activities despite the illness.

Because the symptoms (e.g., easy bruising) of ITP mimic the beginning ones of leukemia, parents may be extremely frightened. They can be assured that this bruising is not leukemia. If the ITP follows a long course (2 or 3 months), they need to be reassured that this process will not later become leukemia. A child may have so many bruises that the parents are initially suspected of child abuse. They may become very defensive and angry at health care personnel. They need time to express their anger and regain confidence in the health care team.

It is also bewildering for parents to be told that no one knows exactly what is causing their child's disease. To be convinced that health care personnel can manage their child's care without knowing the exact cause, they need careful explanations of all procedures.

Henoch-Schönlein Syndrome

Henoch-Schönlein purpura (also called anaphylactoid purpura) is caused by increased vessel permeability. Although no definite allergic correlation can be identified, Henoch-Schönlein purpura is generally considered to be a hypersensitivity reaction to an invading allergen. It occurs most frequently in children between 2 and 8 years of age, and more frequently in boys than girls. There is generally a history of mild infection before the outbreak of symptoms. The syndrome presents (because of the purpura) as a possible platelet disorder until a differential diagnosis is made.

Assessment. The purpural rash occurs typically on the buttocks, posterior thighs, and extensor surface of the arms and legs (Figure 44-7). The tips of the ears may be involved. The rash begins as a crop of urticarial lesions that change to pink maculopapules. These become hemorrhagic (bright red), then fade, leaving brown macular spots that remain for several weeks. The child's

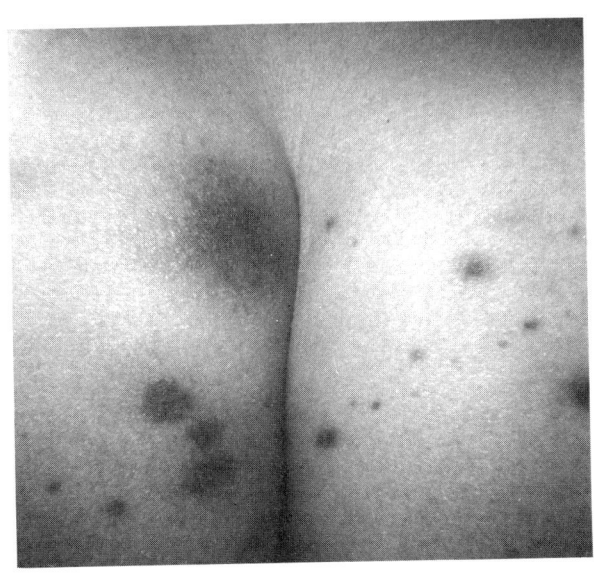

FIGURE 44-7
The typical pattern of ecchymotic spots of Henoch-Schönlein purpura.

joints are tender and swollen. The child may have gastrointestinal symptoms such as abdominal pain, vomiting, or blood in stools. Gross or microscopic hematuria may be present from kidney involvement. A biopsy shows granulocytes in the walls of small arterioles (Amitai et al., 1993).

Laboratory studies will show a normal platelet count; sedimentation rate, white blood count, and eosinophil count will be elevated.

Therapeutic Management. Treatment involves steroid therapy (oral prednisone) for a short period. Nose and throat cultures rule out continuing bacterial involvement. Urine should be assessed for protein and glucose to detect kidney involvement. The disease runs a typical course of 4 to 6 weeks. A few children will develop chronic nephritis as a complication.

Disseminated Intravascular Coagulation

Disseminated intravascular coagulation is an acquired disorder of blood clotting that results from excessive trauma or some similar underlying stimulus.

Normal blood clotting is a balance between the hemostatic (clotting) system and the fibrinolytic (dissolving) system of the bloodstream. Following a blood vessel injury, local vasoconstriction rapidly prevents additional blood loss at the site. With the tear in the vessel wall, the underlying collagen is exposed. This causes changes in platelets (they swell, become adherent, and irregular in shape). They release adenosine diphosphate, which attracts additional platelets and binds them together (platelet aggregation). This phenomenon results in a platelet plug to seal the vessel. The plug is strengthened by fibrin threads forming as a result of an intrinsic and extrinsic coagulation process into a firm, fixed structure. To prevent too much clotting from occurring, plasmin or fibrinolysin, a proteolytic enzyme, is formed from plasminogen; it digests fibrin threads and causes lysis of the clot along with consumption of blood clotting factors. As plasmin, fibrinogen, and fibrin are lysed, fibrin degradation products are formed. These products prevent the laying down of further fibrin and platelet aggregation.

With DIC, an imbalance occurs between clotting activity and fibrinolysis. Extreme clotting due to endothelial damage begins at one point in the circulatory system, depleting the availability of clotting factors such as platelets and fibrin from the general circulation; a secondary initiation of fibrinolysis begins as well. A paradox exists: the person has both increased coagulation and a bleeding defect at the same time. Many of the complications of pregnancy (abruptio placenta or death of a fetus) initiate DIC, so this is a common complication seen accompanying bleeding during pregnancy (see Chapter 15).

Assessment. A child begins to have uncontrolled bleeding from puncture sites from injections or intravenous therapy; ecchymosis and petechiae form on the skin. The child's toes and fingers may be cyanotic or mottled and cold because small blood vessels are so filled with coagulated blood that circulation to extremities is impaired. If coagulation is acute, neurologic or renal symptoms may occur from occlusion of vessels supplying the brain and kidneys. Observe all children with a serious illness carefully for signs of increased bleeding such as skin petechiae or oozing from blood-drawing sites.

Common blood coagulation values are shown in Appendix F. With DIC, laboratory tests usually show that the platelet count is depressed. The level depends on the rate at which bone marrow is able to replace the platelets. On a blood smear, many of the platelets appear large, evidence of their recent production, and they may appear fragmented from passing through meshes of collecting fibrin. As a rule, both PT and PTT are prolonged. Fibrinogen, the final factor necessary to make the clot, will have a markedly low level in serum (less than 100 mg/100 mL). Fibrin split (degradation) products are elevated.

Therapeutic Management. To stop the process of disseminated intravascular coagulation, the underlying insult that began the phenomenon must be halted. The marked coagulation can be ended by the intravenous administration of heparin. Although blood transfusion may be necessary to correct blood loss, it may be delayed until after heparin has been administered so that the new blood factors are not also consumed by the coagulation process. Fresh frozen plasma, fibrinogen, or

cryoprecipitate (which contains fibrinogen) may be administered. Cryoprecipitate is the blood product administered to a child with hemophilia and therefore may not be available in hospitals that do not routinely treat a large number of these children. Thus, if neither fibrinogen nor cryoprecipitate is available, fresh frozen plasma or platelets will aid in restoring clotting function.

With adequate therapy, blood coagulation studies will return to normal. If renal or brain cells were damaged from occluded capillaries, permanent injury to body cells could result.

Nursing Diagnoses and Related Interventions

Nursing Diagnosis: Knowledge deficit about blood clotting disorder related to its paradoxical nature

Goal: Client (or parents) will demonstrate increased knowledge of the illness by 1 hour.

Outcome Criteria: Client (or parents) accurately state nature of illness and proposed therapy.

Parents may be bewildered when a physician tells them one minute that their chief concern is the child's bleeding, and the next minute heparin has been ordered because coagulation is the problem. If they understand the action of heparin—to discourage blood coagulation—their child's need and the medication seem directly contradictory. Be certain that both children and parents are given a full explanation: The child has an increased risk of hemorrhaging because part of the coagulation system has begun coagulation; heparin is acting to stop coagulation. This effort will help maintain parents' confidence in caregivers.

Hemophilias

Hemophilia is an inherited interference with blood coagulation. There are numerous hemophilia types, each involving deficiency of a different blood coagulation factor.

Hemophilia A (Factor VIII Deficiency)

The classic form of hemophilia is caused by deficiency of the coagulation component factor VIII, the antihemophilic factor, which is transmitted as a sex-linked recessive trait. In the United States, the incidence is approximately 1 in 10,000 white males. The female carrier may have slightly lowered but sufficient levels of the factor VIII component so that she does not manifest a bleeding disorder. Males with the disease also have varying levels of factor VIII, and their bleeding tendency varies accordingly, from mild to severe.

Factor VIII is an intrinsic factor of coagulation, so the intrinsic system for manufacturing thromboplastin is incomplete. The child is not wholly without coagulation ability, however, because the extrinsic or tissue system remains intact. Thus, the child's blood will eventually coagulate after an injury.

Assessment. Hemophilia often is recognized first in the infant who bleeds excessively after circumcision. If the disease has not shown itself for several generations in a family, the parents may not know it existed. For this reason, all infants need careful and thoughtful observation following circumcision.

Because infants do not receive many injuries, the child's bleeding tendency may not become apparent until the child begins to walk. Suddenly the lower extremities (where the child bumps things) become heavily bruised. There is soft tissue bleeding and painful hemorrhage into the joints. The child holds the injured joint stiffly; it becomes swollen and warm. Repeated bleeding into a joint causes damage to the synovial membrane (hemarthrosis), and can result in severe loss of joint mobility.

Severe bleeding may also occur into the gastrointestinal tract, peritoneal cavity, or central nervous system. Interestingly, nosebleeds are common, but are not as severe as with the platelet deficiency syndromes. The child must be identified as having hemophilia before surgery is performed for any reason; otherwise, fatal bleeding could occur (Morgan et al., 1993).

With hemophilia, the platelet count and prothrombin time are normal. The whole blood clotting time is markedly prolonged or normal, depending on the level of factor VIII present. A thromboplastin generation test is abnormal. PTT is the test that best reveals the low levels of factor VIII.

Therapeutic Management. With even minor abrasions, bleeding must be controlled by the administration of factor VIII. This may be supplied by fresh whole blood or by fresh or frozen plasma, but it is best supplied by a concentrate of factor VIII or cryoprecipitate (the product is a precipitate of plasma and is then frozen). If plasma is to be given, it must be administered over a period of not more than 30 minutes because factor VIII loses its potency at room temperature. The child often needs large amounts of factor VIII to halt bleeding; the child would need so much whole blood or plasma to supply factor VIII that the circulatory system would become overloaded. Administering a concentrate of factor VIII alleviates this problem. One bag of concentrate per 5 kg of body weight is usually sufficient. This provides protection for approximately 12 hours; another transfusion may be necessary at that time. Newer powdered forms of factor VIII that can be stored at home and reconstructed as needed are available.

In a small number of children, antibodies (termed inhibitors) to factor VIII develop, rendering the factor ineffective. Epsilon-aminocaproic acid, a fibrinolytic enzyme that helps to stabilize clot formation and promote wound healing, can be self-administered every 6 hours if needed. Children with inhibitors to factor VIII can also be administered a factor IX concentrate (Proplex or Konyne). This concentrate enters the coagulation cascade after factor VIII and halts bleeding. Administration of any blood product, including factor replacement, exposes the child to a slight possibility of hepatitis B and C, and HIV. Before blood was screened for viral contaminants as is done currently, as many as 80% of hemophiliacs received contaminated blood through transfusions (Kleinert et al., 1990).

Nursing Diagnoses and Related Interventions

Nursing Diagnosis: Parental health-seeking behaviors related to strategies for protecting the child from injury

Goal: Parents will develop plan for preventing injury to the child and child will not experience major bleeding episodes during childhood.

Outcome Criteria: Child's skin is free of ecchymotic areas; frequent epistaxis is not present; blood pressure is normal for age group; no swelling or warmth at joints is present.

Prevention of injury is the most important intervention with these children. Help parents to set appropriate limits. An active infant may need his or her crib sides padded; all toys need to be inspected for sharp edges or parts.

Parents (and the child as soon as he or she is approximately 10 years old) can be taught to administer a replacement factor intravenously to prevent bleeding immediately after an injury (Figure 44-8). This action, combined with immobilization of the injured extremity and an ice pack applied locally, will almost always eliminate the need for hospital admissions. Pressure should be applied to a laceration to halt bleeding directly. Suturing of lacerations is avoided whenever possible, because the sutures make additional puncture sites that may bleed.

Nursing Diagnosis: Pain related to joint infiltration by blood

Goal: Child will experience a tolerable level of pain following injury.

Outcome Criteria: Child voices that pain is at a tolerable level.

The child with hemophiliac bleeding experiences discomfort because of the bleeding into joints and may be frightened because the parents are so frightened.

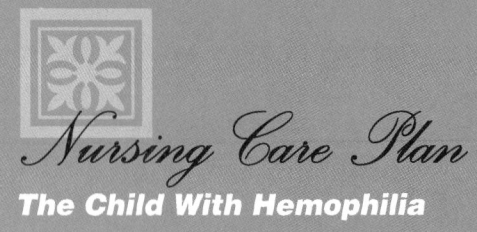

Nursing Care Plan
The Child With Hemophilia

Larry is a 7-year-old boy with hemophilia. The following is a nursing care plan designed for him.

Assessment: Child brought to emergency room by father and stepmother following a fall from his bicycle. Parents were divorced 1 year ago and father recently remarried; child has lived with father and stepmother since their marriage. Larry's stepmother admits that his disease "scares her" and states that although she has factor replacement at home, she did not feel confident enough to administer it and brought child to emergency room instead. Larry has changed school during last month because of move following remarriage; he is shy with strangers so has had difficulty adjusting. He has no siblings; Larry's stepmother states her husband has been hesitant to have another child for fear the disease will occur again.

Immunization record unknown. On physical exam, child's left knee is swollen and feels tender and warm to touch.

Nursing Diagnosis: Parental knowledge deficit related to inheritability of hemophilia

Defining Characteristic: Stepmother states that Larry's father is afraid to have other children.

Goal: Parent will demonstrate increased knowledge of illness by end of health care visit.

Outcome Criteria: Parent states she recognizes inheritance of disease was from Larry's mother, not father.

Nursing Orders	Rationale
1. Teach Larry's stepmother that this is a sex-linked condition so child's mother carried the recessive gene and not his father.	1. It is important to start with basics when educating families about an illness.
2. Refer for genetic counseling so parents and Larry are more familiar with disorder.	2. Genetic counseling can supply information parents need to make an informed reproductive choice.

Nursing Diagnosis: High risk for self-esteem disturbance related to chronic illness and recent family changes

Defining Characteristic: Mother states that child is shy with peers; has recently moved.

Goal: Child will demonstrate positive attitude about himself during childhood.

Outcome Criteria: Child expresses feelings about his illness and states that although he feels a little different from others because of it, he knows it does not affect his ability to interact with peers and do many of the same things his friends do; interacts well with peers and family.

(continued)

Immobilization of the affected joint not only decreases bleeding but also provides relief. Be certain that immobilized joints are in good alignment. Passive range of motion to maintain function will be ordered as soon as the acute bleeding has halted (approximately 48 hours). Neither aspirin nor ibuprofen (Advil) are ordered as analgesics because they may prolong bleeding. As soon as effective levels of factor VIII have been provided, the pain in the bleeding joint is generally relieved, despite the continued heat or swelling.

Nursing Diagnosis: High risk for altered family processes related to fears regarding child's prognosis and long-term nature of illness

Goal: Family members will demonstrate adequate coping behaviors by 1 month.

Outcome Criteria: Family members voice their feelings of fear regarding illness; state that they are able to cope despite stress level.

Parents of children with hemophilia are frightened

Nursing Orders	*Rationale*
1. Help child to select a lifestyle in which he can excel (join a computer club rather than play football).	1. Encourages development of hobbies and interests that can lead to high self-esteem.
2. Suggest summer camps for hemophiliac children.	2. A camp where Larry doesn't feel different from everyone else may improve his ability to form peer relationships.

Nursing Diagnosis: Parental knowledge deficit related to measures to prevent long-term injury secondary to ineffective blood coagulation

Defining Characteristic: Altered blood coagulation is hallmark of hemophilia. Parents need review of basic information about long-term effects of disease.

Goal: Both parents will demonstrate knowledge about measures to prevent and manage bleeding episodes. Child will not have permanent detrimental effects from current or future bleeding episodes.

Outcome Criteria: Parents state importance of prevention of bleeding; accurately state measures to manage any bleeding episode. Child maintains full range of motion in joints.

Nursing Orders	*Rationale*
1. Teach parents or child to apply pressure and cold compress to bleeding area; immobilize an extremity.	1. These measures reduce bleeding.
2. Teach parents or child to administer factor replacement at home.	2. It is important for parents to be comfortable in their ability to administer factor replacement in an emergency.
3. If school is far from home, allow him to keep factor replacement at school for rapid use.	3. Provides for rapid replacement of absent factor to reduce effects of poor coagulation.
4. Teach parents or child to follow emergency care with a medical checkup.	4. Long-term follow-up is necessary to prevent permanent joint injury.
5. Urge parents to allow child to have usual immunizations (apply pressure to site for 10 minutes following to help prevent bleeding).	5. Usual immunizations can be administered to children with hemophilia.
6. Urge careful tooth care (good brushing, preventive checkups, fluoride application, no high carbohydrate snacks between meals) to reduce possibility of dental surgery.	6. Oral surgery can cause extensive bleeding.

during a time of acute bleeding, not just because of what is currently happening, but also because they may have seen other family members or even a previous child die of the disease. Be certain to give them a chance to talk about how the bleeding began (e.g., "I should have noticed that toy had a sharp edge," "He fell from his bike. I should have watched him more closely"). Parents need assurance that it is extremely important that they allow their child to lead a normal life, with toys and bicycle riding, and that they cannot totally prevent an in-

jury. As the child reaches school age, the child must learn to monitor his or her own activities (see the Focus on Nursing Research display and the Nursing Care Plan).

Von Willebrand's Disease

Von Willebrand's disease is often referred to as angiohemophilia because there is not only a factor VIII defect but also an inability of the platelets to aggregate; nor can blood vessels constrict and aid in coagulation. It is inherited as an autosomal dominant disorder, affecting

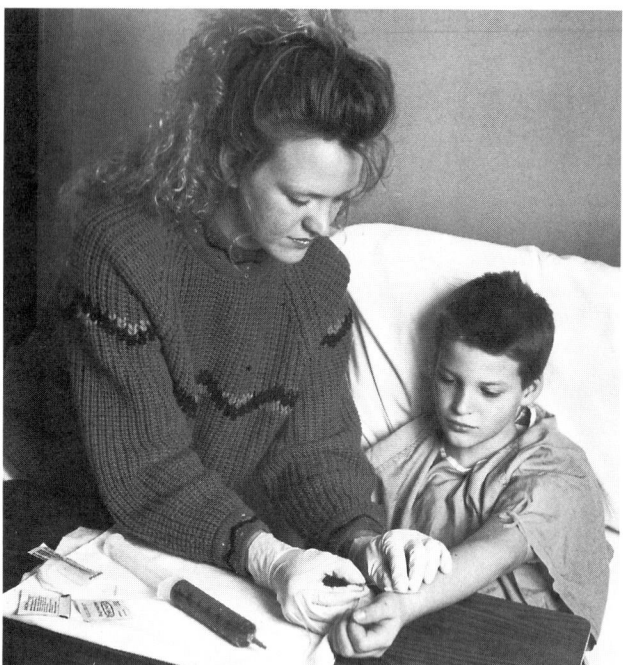

FIGURE 44-8

A nurse demonstrates self-administration of factor replacement for home care. (Courtesy of the Department of Medical Photography, Children's Hospital, Buffalo, NY.)

both sexes. There will be a prolonged bleeding time; most hemorrhages tend to occur from mucous membrane sites.

Epistaxis is a major problem, because children tend to rub or pick at their noses as a nervous mechanism. In girls, menstrual flow will be unusually heavy and cause embarrassment from stained clothing. Childbirth is obviously a risk for women with von Willebrand's disease. Bleeding is controlled with factor VIII replenishment as with hemophilia, or by administration of arginine desmopressin (DDAVP), a vasoconstricting agent (Miller, 1990).

Christmas Disease
(Hemophilia B, Factor IV Deficiency)

Christmas disease, caused by factor IX deficiency, is transmitted as a sex-linked recessive trait. Only approximately 15% of people with hemophilia have this form. Treatment is with a concentrate of factor IX, available for home administration.

Hemophilia C (Factor XI deficiency)

Plasma thromboplastin antecedent deficiency, caused by factor XI deficiency, is transmitted as an autosomal recessive trait and therefore occurs in both sexes. It tends to occur in Jewish children. The symptoms are generally mild compared with those in children with factor VIII or

factor IX deficiencies. Bleeding episodes are treated with the transfusion of fresh blood or plasma (Casella, 1994).

Key Points

- Bone marrow transplantation is the main therapy for a number of blood dyscrasias. Transplantation can be allogeneic (from a histocompatible donor) or autologous (using the child's own marrow).
- Disorders of the red blood cells which commonly occur in children are acute blood-loss anemia and anemia of acute infection. Aplastic and hypoplastic anemias occur from depression of hematopoietic activity in bone marrow. These anemias can be congenital or acquired.
- A major hypochromic anemia that develops in children is iron-deficiency anemia. The major nursing diagnosis associated with this illness is Altered nutrition: less than body requirements.
- Macrocytic anemias occur from folic acid deficiency and pernicious anemia (vitamin B_{12} deficiency).
- Hemolytic anemias are congenital spherocytosis, glucose-6-dehydrogenase deficiency, sickle-cell anemia, thalassemia, and autoimmune acquired hemolytic anemia. Sickle-cell anemia occurs most often in black children. Nursing diagnoses related

FOCUS ON NURSING RESEARCH

Are Children With Hemophilia Knowledgeable About Their Illness?

Hemophilia is a disorder that has no cure, but whose symptoms can be reduced in severity if children monitor the amount of trauma bones and joints receive and therapy is begun immediately if trauma should occur. It is generally assumed that the earlier children with the disorder learn the nature of the illness and understand why treatment is needed, the better they will be able to comply with treatment. To assess how well children with hemophilia understand their illness, a nurse researcher interviewed 20 children with hemophilia ages 6 to 12 years using 5 pictures of children as stimulants to discussion. Findings revealed that children knew less about their disease and the methods of therapy than would have been expected. One factor contributing to this lack of knowledge may be the difficulty school-age children typically experience in learning abstract concepts. These findings should alert health care providers to the amount of health instruction and review required by children of school age.

Spitzer, A. (1992). Children's knowledge of illness and treatment experiences in hemophilia. *Journal of Pediatric Nursing, 7,* 43.

to this disease are High risk for ineffective tissue perfusion and Altered health maintenance.

- Disorders of white blood cells that occur are neutropenia (reduced number of white blood cells) and neutrophilia (increased number). Neutropenia makes children susceptible to infection. Reverse isolation may be instituted to guard against this. Health care personnel and family members with infections should be restricted.

- Disorders of blood coagulation seen are the purpuras (idiopathic thrombocytopenic purpura, Henoch-Schönlein syndrome, and disseminated intravascular coagulation) and the hemophilias. Nursing diagnoses often developed for the hemophilias are Pain related to joint infiltration and Altered family processes related to the long-term nature of the illness.

- Children with blood coagulation disorders must be guarded carefully against injury. This includes monitoring types of toys and activities. It may include padding a crib or siderails.

- Children with anemia invariably fatigue easily because they are unable to oxygenate body cells well. Their care must include measures to keep them from tiring; oxygen administration may be necessary.

- Disorders of the blood tend to be long-term illnesses. Education of the parents and of the child is important so they can learn to adapt to the condition; long-term administration of medication needs planning so that it is consistently maintained.

Critical Thinking Exercises

1. Maria is a 12-year-old with sickle-cell anemia. You have noticed that every summer for the past five years while Maria has been home from school on summer vacation, she has had an acute episode of her illness. What assessments would you want to make of Maria's family before this summer? What precautions would you want to discuss with them?

2. Hillary is a 6-year-old who has developed neutropenia from chemotherapy. What precautions to prevent infection would you want to encourage her family to take while Hillary attends a family reunion?

3. Kevin is a 5-year-old with hemophilia. He wants to join a preschool soccer program. How would you counsel his family regarding this?

References

Allon, M. (1990). Renal abnormalities in sickle cell disease. *Archives of Internal Medicine, 150,* 501.

Amitai, Y., et al. (1993). Henoch-Schönlein purpura in infants. *Pediatrics, 92,* 865.

Belkengren, R. P., & Sapala, S. (1993). Pediatric management problems: Iron deficiency anemia. *Pediatric Nursing, 19,* 378.

Bonadio, W. A. (1990). Clinical features of abdominal painful crisis in sickle cell anemia. *Journal of Pediatric Surgery, 25,* 301.

Casella, J. F. (1994). Disorders of coagulation. In F. A. Oski et al. (Eds.). *Principles and practice of pediatrics* (2nd ed.). Philadelphia: J.B. Lippincott.

Department of Health & Human Services. (1991). *Healthy people 2000.* Washington, DC: Public Health Service.

Filer, L. J. (1990). Iron needs during rapid growth and mental development. *Journal of Pediatrics, 117,* S143.

Geller, R. B. (1993). Role of autologous bone marrow transplantation for patients with acute and chronic leukemia purged with cyclophosphamide. *Hematology/Oncology Clinics of North America, 7,* 422.

Johanson, N. A. (1990). Musculoskeletal problems in hemoglobinopathy. *Orthopedic Clinics of North America, 21,* 191.

Kojima, S., et al. (1991). Treatment of aplastic anemia in children with recombinant human granulocyte colony-stimulating factor. *Blood, 77,* 937.

Loughran, T. P., & Storb, R. (1990). Treatment of aplastic anemia. *Hematology/Oncology Clinics of North America, 4,* 559.

Martin, P. L., & Pearson, H. A. (1994). The hemolytic anemias. In F. A. Oski et al. (Eds.). *Principles and practice of pediatrics* (2nd ed.). Philadelphia: J.B. Lippincott.

Martin, P. L., & Pearson, H. A. (1994). The nutritional anemias. In F. A. Oski et al. (Eds.). *Principles and practice of pediatrics* (2nd ed.). Philadelphia: J.B. Lippincott.

Miller, J. L. (1990). Von Willebrand disease. *Hematology/Oncology Clinics of North America, 4,* 107.

Mortan, L. M., et al. (1993). Experience with the hemophilic child in a pediatric emergency department. *Journal of Emergency Medicine, 11,* 518.

Mykulak, O. J., & Glassberg, K. I. (1990). Impotence following childhood priapism. *Journal of Urology, 144,* 134.

Platt, O. S., et al. (1991). Pain in sickle cell disease: Rates and risk factors. *New England Journal of Medicine, 325,* 11.

Quintero, C. (1993). Blood administration in pediatric Jehovah's Witnesses. *Pediatric Nursing, 19,* 46.

Readett, D. R., et al. (1990). Nocturnal enuresis in sickle cell haemoglobinopathies. *Archives of Disease of Childhood, 65,* 290.

Robertson, K. A. (1993). Pediatric bone marrow transplantation. *Current Opinion in Pediatrics, 5,* 103.

Ruggenenti, P., & Remuzzi, G. (1990). Thrombotic thrombocytopenic purpura and related disorders. *Hematology/Oncology Clinics of North America, 4,* 219.

Saltus, R. (1994, March 21). Search is on for risk-free blood supply. *Boston Globe,* pp. 25, 27.

Welborn, J. L., et al. (1990). Rapid improvement of thrombotic thrombocytopenic purpura with vincristine and plasmapheresis. *American Journal of Hematology, 35,* 18.

Suggested Readings

Baynes, R. D., & Bothwell, T. H. (1990). Iron deficiency. *Annual Review of Nutrition, 10,* 133.

Bray, G. L., et al. (1994). Assessing clinical severity in children with sickle-cell disease. *American Journal of Pediatric Hematology-Oncology, 16,* 50.

Crocker, K. S., & Coker, M. H. (1990). Initiation of a home hemotherapy program using a primary nursing model. *Journal of Intravenous Nursing, 13,* 13.

Folkes, M. E. (1990). Transfusion therapy in critical care nursing. *Critical Care Nursing Quarterly, 13,* 15.

Furie, B., & Furie, B. C. (1990). Molecular basis of hemophilia. *Seminars in Hematology, 27,* 270.

Guinan, E. C., et al. (1990). A phase I/II trial of recombinant granulocyte-macrophage colony-stimulating factor for children with aplastic anemia. *Blood, 76,* 1077.

Harrington, W. J., et al. (1990). Is splenectomy an outmoded procedure? *Advances in Internal Medicine, 35,* 415.

Kasper, C. K. (1990). Hemophilia care in the near future. *Progress in Clinical Biology Research, 324,* 291.

Marder, E., et al. (1990). Discovering anaemia at child health clinics. *Archives of Disease of Childhood, 65,* 892.

Nordenberg, D., et al. (1990). The effect of cigarette smoking on hemoglobin levels and anemia screening. *Journal of the American Medical Association, 264,* 1556.

Pizarro, F., et al. (1991). Iron status with different infant feeding regimens: Relevance to screening and prevention of iron deficiency. *Journal of Pediatrics, 118,* 687.

Powers, D. R., & Brown, M. (1990). Sickle cell disease: Summer camp experiences of a 22-year community supported program. *Clinical Pediatrics, 29,* 81.

Rivers, R., & Williamson, N. (1990). Sickle cell anemia: Complex disease, nursing challenge. *RN, 53,* 24.

Slichter, S. J. (1990). Platelet transfusion therapy. *Hematology/Oncology Clinics of North America, 4,* 291.

Taft, E. G. (1990). Advances in the treatment of TTP. *Progress in Clinical Biology Research, 337,* 151.

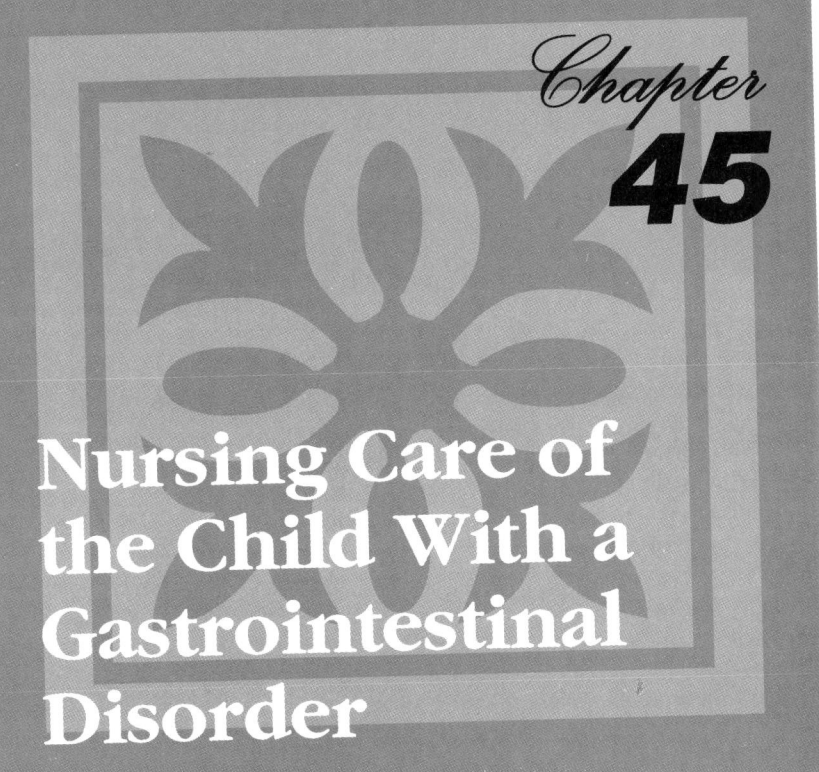

Chapter 45

Nursing Care of the Child With a Gastrointestinal Disorder

Objectives

After mastering the contents of this chapter, you should be able to:

1. Describe common gastrointestinal disorders in children, such as appendicitis, vomiting, and diarrhea.
2. Assess the child with a gastrointestinal disorder.
3. Formulate nursing diagnoses for the child with a gastrointestinal disorder.
4. Plan nursing care with specific goals for the child with a gastrointestinal disorder (e.g., a plan that teaches parents about a special diet).
5. Implement nursing care for the child with a gastrointestinal disorder, such as administering a gastrostomy feeding.
6. Evaluate outcome criteria to ensure that goals of nursing care were achieved.
7. Identify National Health Goals related to gastrointestinal disorders and children that nurses could be instrumental in helping the nation achieve.
8. Identify areas of care related to gastrointestinal disorders and children that could benefit from additional nursing research.
9. Analyze ways that nursing care of the child with a gastrointestinal disorder can be more family centered.
10. Synthesize knowledge of gastrointestinal disorders with nursing process to achieve quality maternal and child health nursing care.

Key Terms

- aganglionic megacolon
- appendicitis
- beriberi
- celiac disease
- chalasia
- dehydration
- hepatitis
- hiatal hernia
- hypertonic dehydration
- hypotonic dehydration
- inguinal hernia
- intussusception
- irritable bowel syndrome
- isotonic dehydration
- keratomalacia
- kwashiorkor
- liver transplantation
- Meckel's diverticulum
- metabolic acidosis
- metabolic alkalosis
- necrotizing enterocolitis
- nutritional marasmus
- overhydration
- pellagra
- peptic ulcer
- pyloric stenosis
- rickets
- steatorrhea
- ulcerative colitis
- volvulus
- xerophthalmia

Adele Pillitteri: MATERNAL AND CHILD HEALTH NURSING, 2nd Edition. © 1995 Adele Pillitteri.

The gastrointestinal tract is such a long body system that a multitude of possible disorders can occur in it, including both congenital defects and acquired illnesses. (Developmental physical defects that are discovered at birth are discussed in Chapter 39.) Because the gastrointestinal system is responsible for taking in and processing nutrients for all parts of the body, any problem can quickly affect other systems of the body and, if not adequately treated, can affect overall health, growth, and development.

Gastrointestinal illnesses, as a category, require a high level of health education. Many parents do not appreciate the seriousness of gastrointestinal illness; they are surprised to find that what they thought was a simple "stomach flu" has put their child in serious electrolyte imbalance and a life-threatening state. Some illnesses require both parents and child to learn about a new diet. When the child is young, the parents need education concerning the diet and other care measures. As the child grows older, counseling to help the child maintain self-esteem and learn diet requirements becomes important. National Health Goals related to gastrointestinal disorders and children are shown in the Focus on National Health Goals box.

FOCUS ON
National Health Goals

In the past, diarrhea was a major cause of death in infants. National Health Goals address this as well as hepatitis B. These goals are:

- Reduce viral hepatitis B in infants to 350/100,000 new carriers from a baseline of 500/100,000.

- Reduce infectious diarrhea by at least 25% among children in licensed child care centers and children in programs that provide an individualized education program (DHHS, 1991).

Nurses can be instrumental in helping the nation achieve these goals by serving as consultants to day care providers to reduce the spread of diarrhea in these settings and actively administering hepatitis B vaccine to infants to eradicate this illness in another generation. Nursing research on a number of areas could be helpful: Do the brand names of diapers used by children in day care influence the spread of infectious diarrhea; how many infants are not being brought for follow-up care and thus do not receive all three immunizations against hepatitis B; and do the majority of parents appreciate the devastating outcome that can result from diarrhea in infants?

NURSING PROCESS OVERVIEW
for the Child With Altered Gastrointestinal Function

ASSESSMENT

Children with gastrointestinal disorders quickly become dehydrated, especially if vomiting or diarrhea is one of the symptoms. They need to be assessed for signs of dehydration (e.g., poor skin turgor, dry mucous membranes, or lack of tearing) (Figure 45-1). When talking to parents about a child's symptoms, it is important to ask exactly what they mean when they say "spitting up" or "a little vomiting." For another measure of hydration, ask how many times a child has voided in the past 24 hours and if this is less than usual. Compare current weight with past weight measurements. Unless the child is an adolescent who has been actively dieting, there is never a normal reason for weight loss in children.

Ask parents to describe what they mean by diarrhea. Some parents mistakenly confuse normal newborn stools with diarrhea. As a rule, all children with diarrhea, especially small children, need to be seen by a health care provider because fluid and electrolyte changes occur rapidly in children.

For many children, a gastrointestinal tract disorder is diagnosed largely by presenting symptoms. In other instances, x-ray studies with a contrast medium (barium) are used to outline the bowel and confirm the presence of an anomaly. Ultrasound or magnetic resonance may be helpful. Another important assessment area is laboratory testing for electrolyte balance through serum analysis, or fluid concentration through urinalysis.

NURSING DIAGNOSIS

Nursing diagnoses relevant to children with gastrointestinal illness invariably center on altered nutrition, because most gastrointestinal diseases in some way alter the kind and amount of nutrients ingested or absorbed into the body. However, gastrointestinal illness also takes an emotional toll on the ill child and family. Feeding is one of the primary ways mothers establish a good bond with their newborn, and bonding can be seriously threatened when the infant suffers from a gastrointestinal disorder, especially when hospitalization is required. Eating and diet are also integral components of family life and culture, so any disruption caused by illness can place a strain on the entire family. Examples of nursing diagnoses are:

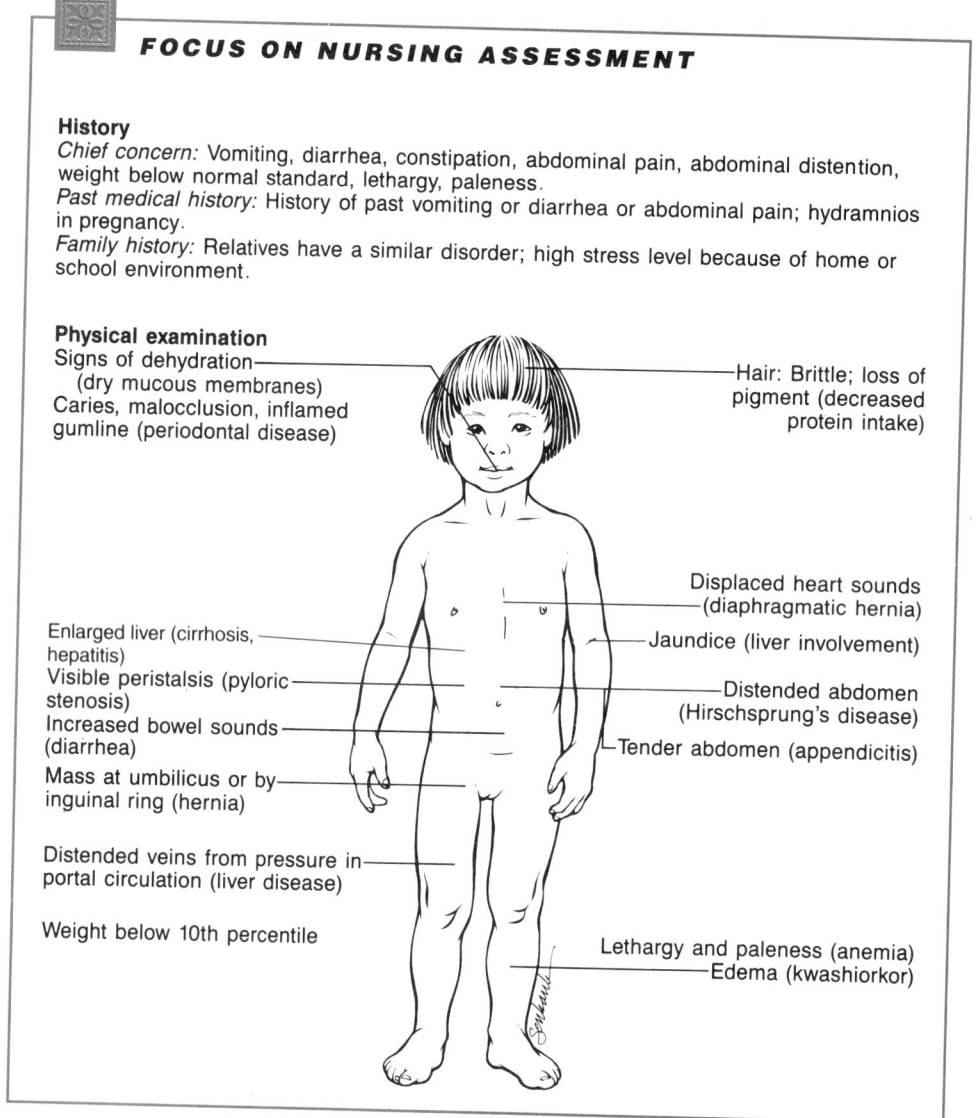

FOCUS ON NURSING ASSESSMENT

History
Chief concern: Vomiting, diarrhea, constipation, abdominal pain, abdominal distention, weight below normal standard, lethargy, paleness.
Past medical history: History of past vomiting or diarrhea or abdominal pain; hydramnios in pregnancy.
Family history: Relatives have a similar disorder; high stress level because of home or school environment.

Physical examination
Signs of dehydration (dry mucous membranes)
Caries, malocclusion, inflamed gumline (periodontal disease)

Hair: Brittle; loss of pigment (decreased protein intake)

Displaced heart sounds (diaphragmatic hernia)

Enlarged liver (cirrhosis, hepatitis)
Visible peristalsis (pyloric stenosis)
Increased bowel sounds (diarrhea)
Mass at umbilicus or by inguinal ring (hernia)
Distended veins from pressure in portal circulation (liver disease)
Weight below 10th percentile

Jaundice (liver involvement)
Distended abdomen (Hirschsprung's disease)
Tender abdomen (appendicitis)

Lethargy and paleness (anemia)
Edema (kwashiorkor)

FIGURE 45-1
Signs and symptoms of altered gastrointestinal function.

- Altered parenting related to difficulty in establishing parent–infant bond
- Altered family processes related to chronic illness in child
- Altered parenting related to difficulty in preparing child's special diet
- High risk for fluid volume deficit related to chronic diarrhea
- Altered nutrition, less than body requirements, related to malabsorption of necessary nutrients

PLANNING

Planning care for the child with a gastrointestinal disorder often includes diet planning with the child and parents. Be certain when helping to plan a diet that the person who actually prepares or supervises the child's diet is included in planning. In many instances, part of the diet is prepared by a baby sitter, day care center staff, the child's other parent, or a grandparent. Many children eat breakfast and lunch at school cafeterias. It may be necessary to contact school staff to ask them to make meal exceptions for the child or to supervise a choice of foods (or to see that a child eats only the packaged lunch he or she brought to school, not extra items the child traded for with friends).

Some parents are unfamiliar with the basic food groups and the importance of providing food from each group in children's diets. They may have little understanding of which foods have high or low fiber content, or which foods are "bland" or "clear." Many parents have difficulty keeping children "nothing by mouth" (NPO) for tests or to rest the gastrointestinal tract. They have been told that dehydration happens quickly in infants; they need support to follow the necessary restrictions when those restrictions are so opposed to basic parenting, which involves giving food.

If feedings will be given by nasogastric or gastrostomy tube, parents need enough practice time in the hospital to be comfortable with the equipment and the technique before they are given the responsibility of doing it alone at home. If a child is going to gag or become distressed when a new tube is passed, parents need to have this happen where there are calm support people nearby, not when they are by themselves at home. Agencies that might be helpful for referral are:

American Celiac Society
58 Musano Court
West Orange, NJ 07052

Crohn's and Colitis Foundation of America
444 Park Avenue South, 11th Floor
New York, NY 10016–7374

IMPLEMENTATION

Do not underestimate how difficult it is for family members to adapt to alternative nutrition methods such as total parenteral nutrition, enteric tubes for feeding, or care for a child with a colostomy. Parents need a great deal of support to adapt their busy life to these alternative methods of care. Help them plan the necessary adaptations to their lifestyle (e.g., Will day care center personnel do gastrostomy feedings? Will a nursery school accept a child with a colostomy?). Even on their busiest days, all families should be encouraged to eat at least one meal together so they can have time to share experiences and "touch base" with each other. For the family with a child who has a special feeding problem such as a gastrostomy feeding or total parenteral nutrition, this can be difficult. Urge such families to bring the child to the table for a social time even if the child cannot eat with the family. If watching family members eat while the child cannot is too difficult, urge the family to be certain to provide a "together" time in some other way so they do not miss out on this valuable family activity daily.

Insertion of a nasogastric tube and administration of an enema are discussed in Chapter 37. Administration of gastrostomy and enteral feedings is discussed in Chapter 34. Be certain to give excellent explanations and praise afterward for these procedures. Children can easily interpret enemas as punishment because of the extreme intrusiveness. Provide therapeutic play after these procedures to reduce children's anxiety.

EVALUATION

A major method of evaluation to see that nutritional goals have been met is evaluation of children's height and weight. Even if a diet is limited in a special way, if it

is adequate, children should gain weight and maintain growth.

Because children will ultimately be responsible for their own diet, evaluation often includes making certain that children are gradually learning more about their diet so they can become increasingly responsible for their own intake. Only when they are at this stage can their parents feel secure enough to let them stay overnight with a friend, visit a relative in a distant city, go to summer camp—activities that become important to children as they reach school age.

The saying "people are what they eat" has some relevance. Children who are on special diets need to be evaluated for self-esteem at periodic health visits. Does the child think of himself or herself as inferior to or different from others because of food restrictions? What kind of positive experiences can be offered to such a child, or what can parents do to provide the child with experiences that would improve the child's self-esteem?

Some examples of outcome criteria are:

- Child lists examples of bland foods that she could select from school cafeteria for lunch.
- Parent states steps she will take to seek medical care if child has a second episode of severe diarrhea.
- Family members state they have adjusted to care of a child with celiac disease.

Anatomy and Physiology of the Gastrointestinal System

Embryonic development of the gastrointestinal tract is discussed in Chapter 8. Digestion begins in the mouth where food is broken down into small-sized particles and mixed with saliva from the sublingual, submandibular, and parotid glands. Both gagging and swallowing reflexes are present even in newborns to prevent against aspiration with swallowing.

The esophagus serves as a passageway to the stomach; it pierces the diaphragm to do this (Figure 45-2). Occasionally, an infant is born with a portion of the bowel or stomach protruding through the diaphragm's esophageal opening (hiatal hernia). At the junction of the esophagus and the stomach is the cardiac sphincter. In some newborns, the cardiac sphincter is so lax that it allows regurgitation of fluid into the esophagus (chalasia). At the distal end of the stomach is the pyloric sphincter. In some infants, this valve is stenosed and does not allow food to flow out of the stomach freely (pyloric stenosis).

The small intestine comprises three divisions: (1) duodenum, (2) jejunum, and (3) ileum. The divisions of the large intestine are the cecum, ascending colon, transverse colon, descending colon, sigmoid colon, and rec-

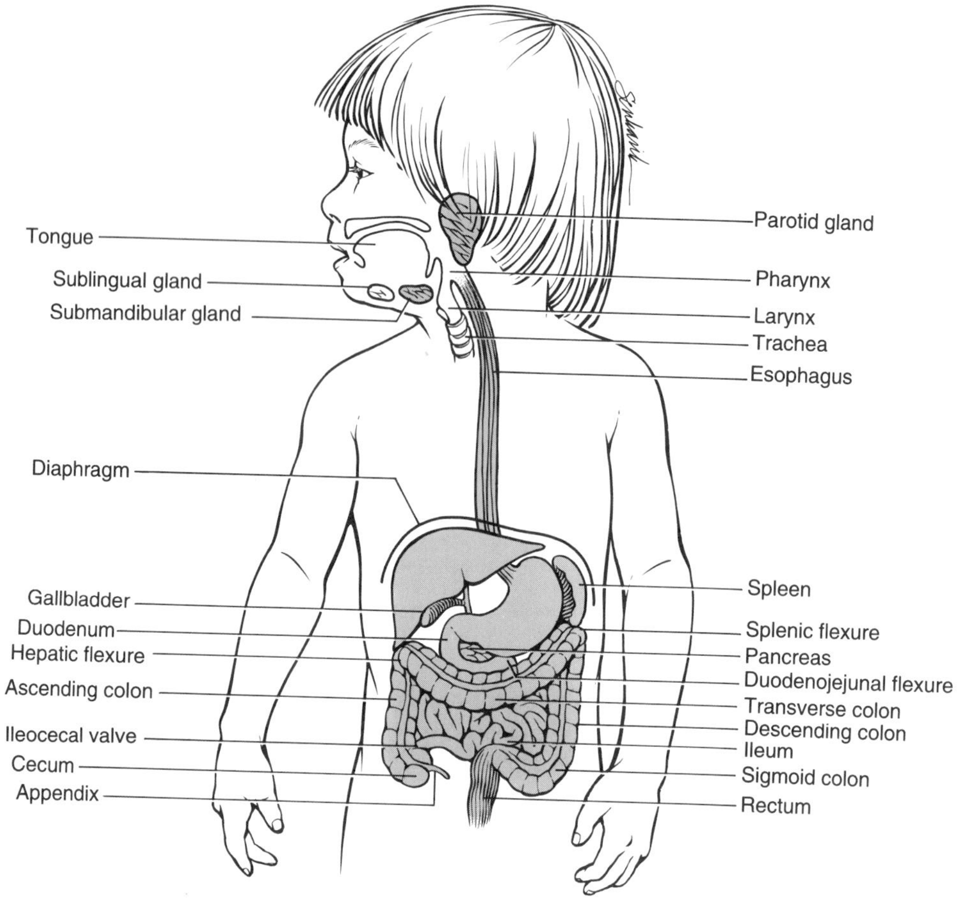

FIGURE 45-2
The gastrointestinal tract.

tum. The appendix, which frequently becomes diseased in children. is attached to the cecum.

Fluid and Electrolyte Balance

Fluid Balance

Fluid is of greater importance in the body chemistry of infants than adults because it comprises a greater fraction of the infant's total weight. In adults, body water accounts for approximately 60% of total weight; in infants it accounts for 70% to 75% of total weight.

Fluid is distributed in three body compartments: (1) intracellular (within cells), 35% to 40% of body weight; (2) interstitial (surrounding cells and bloodstream), 20% of body weight; and (3) intravascular (blood plasma), 5% of body weight. The interstitial and the intravascular fluid together are often referred to as the extracellular fluid (total 25% of body weight). In infants, the extracellular portion is much greater, up to 45% of total body weight (Figure 45-3).

Fluid is normally taken into the body by oral ingestion of fluid and by the water formed in the metabolic breakdown of food. The major amount of water is lost from the body in urine and feces. Minor losses (insensi-

ble losses) occur from evaporation from skin and lungs and from saliva (of little importance except in tracheotomized children or those with nasopharyngeal suction). Infants do not concentrate urine as well as adults; infants have a proportionally greater loss of water in their urine. In infants, the relatively greater surface area to body mass causes a greater insensible loss as well. Illness interferes with the ingestion of fluid in that a child may be nauseated and unable to take in fluid or may be vomiting and losing fluid ingested. When feces becomes diarrheal, or when a child becomes diaphoretic due to fever, the output of fluid can be markedly increased (Siegel et al., 1994). **Dehydration** occurs when there is an excessive loss of body water.

In an adult weighing 70 kg, the extracellular fluid volume is approximately 14,000 mL. Each day, the well adult ingests approximately 2000 mL of fluid and excretes approximately 2000 mL as urine. This means approximately 14% of his or her total extracellular fluid (2000 mL of 14,000 mL) is exchanged each day. In contrast to this, 7-kg infants have an extracellular fluid volume of only 1750 mL. They ingest approximately 700 mL daily and excrete approximately 700 mL daily. Therefore, they exchange approximately 40% of their volume daily.

With this higher exchange rate, the fluid exchange

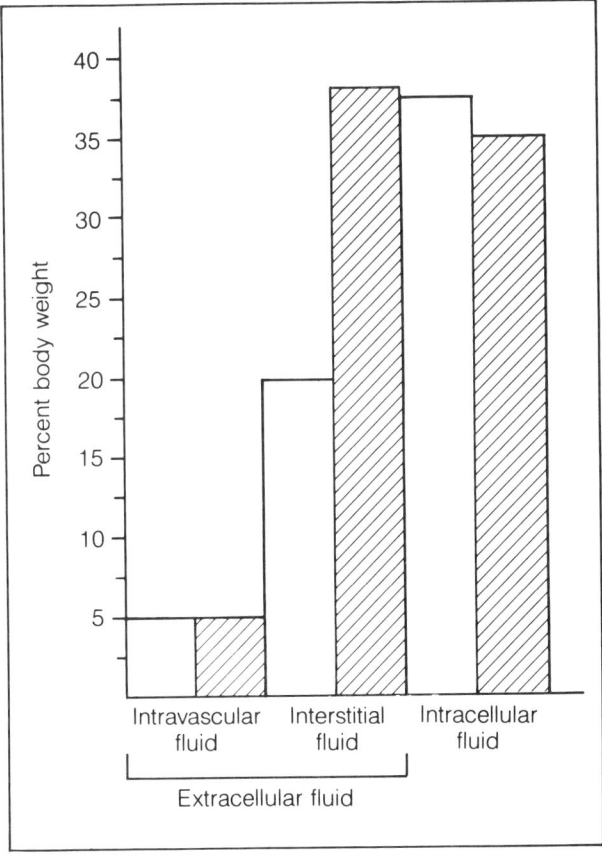

☐	= Adult
▨	= Infant

FIGURE 45-3
Distribution of fluid in body compartments.

balance of infants may be more critically affected when they are ill. Adults, when they do not eat for a day due to gastrointestinal upset, and whose kidneys continue to excrete at the normal rate, will have 14% less fluid in the extracellular space by the end of the day. Infants who do not eat for a day (providing kidney function remains constant) will be 40% short of extracellular fluid by the

end of the day. This is obviously a more critical loss of fluid than the same loss would be in an adult; thus, dehydration is always a more serious problem in infants than in older children and adults. Maintenance requirements of fluid for infants and children are shown in Table 45-1.

Isotonic Dehydration

When the body loses more water than it absorbs (due to diarrhea) or absorbs less fluid than it excretes (as in nausea and vomiting), the first result will be a decrease in the volume of blood plasma. The body compensates for this fairly rapidly by a shift of interstitial fluid into the blood vessels. The composition of fluid in these two spaces is similar, so the replacement by this fluid does not change plasma composition. However, this replacement phenomenon will only proceed until the interstitial fluid reserve is depleted—a danger point for the child because it is difficult for the body to replace interstitial fluid from the intracellular fluid (the fluids in these two compartments have different electrolyte contents). If an infant continues to lose fluid after this point, the volume of the plasma will continue to fall rapidly, resulting in cardiovascular collapse. The child will have weight loss; skin will be dry; skin turgor will be poor (when a ridge of skin is lifted instead of returning to place afterward, it remains raised); and eyeballs may be sunken from decreased intraocular pressure. The anterior fontanelle, if still patent, will be depressed. The child appears gray or ashen due to inadequate peripheral circulation. Pulse is rapid and weak; blood pressure is low. The child will have oliguria as kidneys attempt to retain body fluid. These signs of dehydration are summarized in Table 45-2.

Under most circumstances, water and salt are lost in proportion to each other (**isotonic dehydration**). Occasionally, water is lost out of proportion to salt (i.e., water depletion or **hypertonic dehydration**). Occasionally, electrolytes are lost out of proportion to water (**hypotonic dehydration**). Each of these abnormal states produces specific symptoms.

Table 45-1. *Maintenance Requirements of Fluid Based on Caloric Expenditure*

Body Wt (kg)	Caloric Expenditure	Fluid Requirement
3–10	100 cal/kg/d	100 mL/kg/d
10–20	1000 cal + 50 cal/kg for each kg of body wt more than 10 kg	1000 mL + 50 mL/kg for each kg of body wt more than 10 kg
More than 20	1500 cal + 20 cal/kg for each kg of body wt more than 20 kg	1500 mL + 20 mL/kg for each kg of body wt more than 20 kg

(From Siegel, N. J., et al. [1994]. The pathophysiology of body fluids. In Oski, F. A., et al. *Principles and practice of pediatrics* [2nd ed.]. Philadelphia: J. B. Lippincott.)

Table 45-2. Signs of Dehydration in Children

Assessment Area	Findings
Respirations	Rapid
Pulse	Rapid and thready
Skin	Pale; cold to touch; poor turgor
Mucous membranes	Dry; no tearing with crying
Fontanelles	Sunken
Eyes	Sunken-appearing; dark circles underneath
Weight	Wt loss less than 5% of normal wt = *mild* dehydration
	Wt loss between 5% and 10% = *moderate* dehydration
	Wt loss more than 10% = *severe* dehydration
Behavior	Irritable or lethargic; confused

Hypertonic Dehydration

Water is apt to be lost in a greater proportion than electrolytes when there is decreased fluid intake and increased fluid loss, such as might occur in a child with nausea (preventing fluid intake) and fever (increased fluid loss through perspiration); profuse diarrhea, where there is a greater loss of fluid than salt; or renal disease associated with polyuria (i.e., diabetes insipidus or nephrosis with diuresis).

When there is such an increased loss of fluid, electrolytes concentrate in the blood. Fluid is shifted from the interstitial and intracellular spaces to the bloodstream (from areas of less osmotic pressure to areas of greater pressure). Dehydration in the interstitial and intracellular compartments occurs. Children will be extremely thirsty and will have fever. Their skin will be dry and flushed; saliva and tears will be scant. The red blood cell count and hematocrit will be elevated because the blood is more concentrated than normally. Electrolytes (i.e., sodium, chloride, and bicarbonate) will also likely be increased. Because the shift in fluid has maintained adequate blood plasma volume, the child's blood pressure will be normal or only moderately low. Urine will be scanty and concentrated (an elevated specific gravity) because the child's body is attempting to conserve fluid and reverse the process of fluid loss. There will be increased chloride in the urine because the kidneys try to remove electrolytes to bring the child's electrolyte-fluid balance into line. Neurologic signs, such as stupor and irritability, may be present from loss of fluid from brain cells.

Hypotonic Dehydration

With hypotonic dehydration, there has been a disproportionately high loss of electrolytes relative to fluid lost. The plasma concentration of sodium and chloride will

be low. This could result from excessive gastrointestinal loss by vomiting or from low intake of salt associated with extreme losses through therapeutic diuresis. It also occurs when there is extreme loss of electrolytes in diseases such as adrenocortical insufficiency or diabetic acidosis. When low levels of electrolytes occur, the osmotic pressure in extracellular spaces decreases. The kidneys begin to excrete more fluid to decrease extracellular fluid volume and bring the proportion of electrolytes and fluid back into line. This may lead to a secondary extracellular dehydration.

Blood pressure may fall as the circulating blood volume decreases; cardiovascular collapse may occur. Renal blood flow will then be reduced, glomerular filtration will be affected, and oliguria or anuria may result. Because the kidneys stop excreting chloride as soon as the plasma level of chloride falls below normal, urinary chloride will be low or absent. Children's skin turgor will be poor; they will feel cold and clammy.

Overhydration

Overhydration is as serious as dehydration. It generally occurs in children who are receiving intravenous fluid. The excess fluid in these instances is usually extracellular. The condition is serious because the overload of extracellular fluid may result in cardiovascular overload and cardiac failure.

When large quantities of salt-poor fluid (hypotonic solutions) such as tap water are ingested or are given by enema, the body transfers water from the extracellular space into the intracellular space to restore normal osmotic relationships. This transfer results in intracellular edema. The symptoms of intracellular edema are headache, nausea, vomiting, dimness and blurring of vision, cramps, muscle twitching, and convulsions. A situation in which intracellular edema may occur is when tap water enemas are given in the presence of aganglionic disease of the intestine.

Acid-Base Balance

When acids, bases, and salts are dissolved in water they dissociate into positively charged particles (cations) and negatively charged particles (anions). Because these particles have positive or negative electric charges, they are termed *electrolytes*. The common cations found in blood are sodium (Na^+); potassium (K^+); magnesium (Mg^{++}); and calcium (Ca^{++}). The common anions found in blood are bicarbonate (HCO_3^-); phosphate (PO_4^{---}); sulfate (SO_4^{--}); and chloride (Cl^-).

Most ions have a single positive or negative charge. Others such as calcium (Ca^{++}) and sulfate (SO_4^{--}) have a double charge; these can be thought of as being twice as strong. In an electrolyte solution, the number of positive charges is matched with the number of negative charges. In a healthy person, the above-mentioned cations and anions of the blood will adjust themselves so that the number of positive charges present equals the number of negative charges present. Table 45-3 shows the maintenance requirements of sodium, chloride, and potassium.

pH

The abbreviation "*p*H" refers to two French words that mean the "power of hydrogen." Water (H_2O) can be dissociated into H^+ and OH^-. A solution is acid (*p*H below 7.0) if it contains more H^+ ions than OH^- ions. It is alkaline (*p*H above 7.0) if the number of OH^- ions exceeds that of H^+ ions. The *p*H of blood is normally 7.4, or slightly alkaline, and OH^- ions and H^+ ions are at a 20:1 proportion. If the number of anions (e.g., Cl^-) should decrease by 10 (as would occur in vomiting, when hydrochloric acid is lost), the number of H^+ ions must be decreased by 10 to keep the number of positive and negative charges in proportion (these are only hypothetical amounts). Because this makes the OH^- concentration in blood proportionately greater than the H^+ concentration, the plasma is more alkaline than normal, the typical picture in vomiting. Conversely, if the number of H^+ ions should increase by 10, the blood will become acidotic because there are then more H^+ ions present proportionately than OH^- ions. Hemoglobin is unable to carry as much oxygen in an acidic as in a normal *p*H state. A low *p*H also leads to vascular constriction, particularly of the pulmonary vessels. The *p*H levels, then, affect overall circulatory and oxygenation function.

There are three buffer systems in the body that work to try to keep the number of H^+ and OH^- ions at a 1:20 ratio so the *p*H remains at the usual point of near neutrality (normal serum *p*H is 7.35 to 7.45). A *p*H less than 7.0 or more than 7.8 is incompatible with life.

Buffer Salts

Buffer salts are basic or acidic substances that convert strong acids or bases into weaker ones. After being buffered, an acid that normally would yield many H^+ ions is changed into one that now ionizes only slightly to yield only a few H^+ ions. A strong base is converted to a substance that now yields only a few OH^- ions. By this mechanism, dramatic changes in blood *p*H are avoided because fewer H^+ ions or OH^- ions are added to the blood at one time.

Respiratory Excretion

The lungs are capable of removing excess H^+ ions from the blood. Hydrogen ions (H^+) combine with bicarbonate ions (HCO_3^-) to form carbonic acid (H_2CO_3). In the lungs, carbonic acid is converted to CO_2 and H_2O. The CO_2 is excreted from the lungs; the H^- ion is tied up in the production of H_2O and no longer affects the acidity of the blood ($H^+ + HCO_3^- = H_2CO_3 = CO_2 + H_2O$). Conversely, with a rising *p*H level, the lungs will retain CO_2, and the reverse equation results: CO_2 and H_2O combine to form carbonic acid, which then is converted into H^+ and HCO_3^- ($H_2O + CO_2 = H_2CO_3 = H^+ + HCO_3^-$).

Kidney Excretion

H^+ by itself or as NH_4^+ (ammonia) can be excreted in the urine in exchange for sodium and potassium. Conversely, when the serum HCO_3^- and serum *p*H rise, H^+ ion secretion stops and potassium excretion may be excessive.

Blood CO_2 as an Indicator of Blood *p*H

Disturbances in acid-base balance lead to acidosis or alkalosis (low or high *p*H, respectively). How much either of these is present is reflected in the measured blood CO_2 level.

The blood CO_2 represents all the CO_2 present in the plasma. Most of the CO_2 content of plasma is in the form of bicarbonate, with a small amount held at the intermediary stage as carbonic acid, which is actually dissolved CO_2. The CO_2 concentration is expressed as milliequivalents per liter. The normal value is 22 mEq/L to 28 mEq/L.

When excessive Na^+ ion is lost through diarrhea, the body conserves H^+ ions to keep the positive and negative charges equal in number. The child begins to become acidotic as the number of H^+ ions in the blood increases over the number of OH^- ions present. To correct the blood *p*H, the body can excrete H^+ ions by way of the kidney; the most rapid way is by combining H^+ ions with HCO_3^- ions in the blood to form carbonic acid and then CO_2 and H_2O to be eliminated by the lungs. As this continues for a time, the CO_2 level will fall lower and lower as the body uses up its store of bicarbonate. *In metabolic acidosis, therefore, the blood CO_2 value is invariably low.* The lower the blood CO_2 value, presumably the larger the number of Na^+ ions that have been lost.

When Cl^- ions are lost in vomiting, the body decreases the number of H^+ ions present so the number of positive and negative charges remains the same. The child is now nearing alkalosis; the number of H^+ ions is smaller than the number of OH^- ions present. To com-

Mineral	Requirement
Sodium	2.5 mEq/100 cal
Chloride	5.0 mEq/100 cal
Potassium	2.5 mEq/100 cal

Table 45-3. *Maintenance Requirements of Sodium, Chloride, and Potassium for Intravenous Therapy in Children*

pensate for this, the kidney can conserve H^+ ions; a more immediate solution is for the lungs to conserve CO_2. The child's respirations slow and become shallow (*hypopnea*). The excessive CO_2 accumulated is dissolved in the blood as carbonic acid and then is converted into H^+ and HCO_3^-. The total blood CO_2 content (HCO_3^- and carbonic acid) will rise. *In metabolic alkalosis, therefore, the blood CO_2 level will invariably be high.* The higher the number, presumably the larger the number of Cl^- ions that have been lost.

Fluid and Electrolyte Distribution in Body Compartments

Not only is the fluid in the body divided into different compartments, but electrolytes are compartmentalized as well. The major cation of the plasma and interstitial fluid (extracellular fluid) is Na^+; the anions in these compartments are mainly Cl^- and HCO_3^- (bicarbonate). In cell fluid, K^+ is the main cation and PO_4^{---} (phosphate) is the main anion.

Metabolic Acidosis

Metabolic acidosis occurs when there is rapid loss of base (cations) through intestinal secretions, as in diarrhea, or from an accumulation of acids, as when ketone bodies (acids or anions) accumulate in diabetes mellitus. The child will develop hyperpnea (the body attempts to "blow off" CO, to prevent it from combining with H_2O and releasing H^+ ions as H^+ and HCO_3^-). There is increased Cl^- (chloride ion) and ammonia formation in the urine as the kidney attempts to remove excess H^+.

The blood CO_2 level will be low, reflecting the large number of cations that have been lost.

Metabolic Alkalosis

Metabolic alkalosis can occur when there is excessive loss of Cl^- (chloride ion), such as occurs with persistent vomiting; or it can occur when there is potassium deficiency due to inadequate intake or excessive loss in stools or urine. To increase the number of H^+ ions in the blood, H^+ ions are released from cells in exchange for Na^+ or K^+. The kidneys excrete K^+ into urine to reduce the intracellular load. As a result of this loss of K^+ in urine, low K^+ levels invariably accompany alkalosis.

The child will evidence hypopnea (slowed respirations) as the body attempts to retain CO_2 in the lungs to further increase H^+ ions. The blood CO_2 will be above 40 mEq/L. Tetany may also occur with alkalosis because the increased carbonate ions (HCO_3^-) may combine with calcium ions (Ca^{++}). Metabolic acidosis and alkalosis are compared in Table 45-4.

Common Gastrointestinal Symptoms of Illness in Children

Vomiting and diarrhea are common symptoms in children because they occur as symptoms of disease of the gastrointestinal tract as well as symptoms of disease in other body systems. Pneumonia or otitis media, for example, may present first with vomiting or diarrhea. The danger of both is that they will lead to a disturbance in hydration or electrolyte balance. In many infants, these

Table 45-4. *Comparison of Metabolic Alkalosis and Metabolic Acidosis*

Acid-base Condition	Cause	Findings
Metabolic alkalosis	Vomiting with chloride loss	Slowed respirations
		Twitching or tremor of muscles
		Confusion
		Elevated plasma pH (more than 7.45)
		Elevated urine pH (more than 7)
		Elevated plasma bicarbonate (more than 25 mEq/L)
		Normal or elevated plasma CO_2 (more than 40 mEq/L)
		Base excess (a positive number, as +8)
		Decreased potassium in plasma (less than 3.6 mEq/L)
Metabolic acidosis	Diarrhea in which sodium is lost	Rapid, deep respirations (Kussmaul's respirations)
		Weakness, lethargy
		Confusion, coma
		Decreased plasma pH (less than 7.35)
		Decreased urine pH (less than 6)
		Decreased plasma CO_2 (less than 40 mEq/L)
		Decreased plasma bicarbonate (less than 20 mEq/L)
		Base deficit (a negative number, as −8)
		Potassium excess may be present (more than 5.5 mEq/L)

Table 45-5. *Differentiation Between Regurgitation and Vomiting*

Characteristic	Regurgitation	Vomiting
Timing	Occurs with feeding	Timing unrelated to feeding
Forcefulness	Runs out of mouth with *little force*	Forceful; often projected 1 ft away from the infant; *projectile vomiting* is projected as much as 4 feet; this is most often related to increased intracranial pressure in newborns; in infants age 4–6 wk, may be caused by pyloric stenosis
Description	Smells barely sour; only slightly curdled	Smells very sour, appears curdled, yellow, green, or clear water, or black; perhaps fresh blood or old blood staining from swallowed maternal blood in newborns
Distress	Nonpainful; child does not appear to be in distress and may even smile as if sensation is enjoyable	Child may cry just before vomiting as if abdominal pain is present, and after vomiting as if the force of action is frightening
Duration	Occurs once per feeding	Continues until stomach is empty and then dry retching occurs
Amount	1–2 tsp	Full stomach contents

secondary disturbances constitute a worse threat to the child than the primary disease.

Vomiting

Vomiting is one of the most common and most frightening symptoms of illness in children. Many children with vomiting are suffering from a mild gastroenteritis (infection) caused by a viral or bacterial organism. The condition is always potentially serious because a metabolic alkalosis may result.

Assessment

In describing symptoms of vomiting, be certain to differentiate between the various terms that are used (Table 45-5). It is important that vomiting be described correctly because different conditions are marked by different forms of vomiting and a correct description of the child's actions can aid greatly in diagnosis (see the Focus on Nursing Research display).

Therapeutic Management

The treatment for vomiting is to withhold food from the stomach for a period; if there is nothing in the stomach, vomiting cannot occur. Most parents treat vomiting in the opposite way: every time the child vomits, they attempt to feed the child again; the child vomits again; they feed again, and so on. This prolongs the vomiting and intensifies the potential for electrolyte imbalance.

Nursing Diagnoses and Related Interventions

Nursing Diagnosis: High risk for fluid volume deficit, related to vomiting

Goal: Child will maintain an adequate fluid volume until vomiting ceases.

Outcome Criteria: Skin turgor is good; specific gravity of urine is 1.003 to 1.030; urine output is more than 1 mL/kg/h.

To decrease vomiting, withhold food and fluid for a time, depending on the age of the child—3 hours to 6 hours are average times. In the older child, following this period of fasting, offer a few ice chips, then water in small amounts—approximately 1 tbs every 15 minutes, 4 times; then 2 tbs every 1/2 hour, 4 times. Popsicles can be substituted for water. If that is retained, children can be given small sips of clear liquids, such as tea or ginger ale. Children may become hungry and want whole glasses, but keeping the quantity to small sips prevents vomiting. On the second day, children can be offered portions of broth, clear soup, and skimmed milk in ad-

FOCUS ON NURSING RESEARCH

Can Nurses Accurately Measure the Volume of Infant Emesis?

Infant emesis, because it variably spills onto sheets or blankets and then spreads out or soaks into the cloth surface, is almost impossible to measure in actual milliliters.

When 109 student and practicing pediatric and nursery nurses were shown amounts of infant formula ranging in quantity from 1 mL to 50 mL poured onto receiving blankets, subjects were able to predict the correct amount of fluid in only 2.63 of 20 times (13%).

The researchers recommend that the practice of charting infant emesis in milliliters should be discouraged unless nurses indicate that the value was an estimation, not a true measurement.

Moss, J. R., & Craft, M. J. (1990). Accurate assessment of infant emesis volume. *Pediatric Nursing, 16,* 455.

dition to clear liquids. Dry crackers or toast will help hunger. By the third day, children can take a soft diet; by the fourth day, they should be back to their regular diet.

Introduce fluid to the infant after a fasting period of approximately 3 hours in the same slow manner: 1 tbs every 15 minutes for 2 hours, then 1 oz every 2 hours for the next 12 to 18 hours. Glucose water or a commercial electrolyte solution such as Pedialyte may be given as fluid during this time to help the infant maintain electrolyte balance. Infants progress, as do older children, gradually the next day to clear liquids or breast milk, then a soft diet, then a regular diet.

Teach parents the importance of following these slow routines of increasing fluid at intervals. Assure them that if children receive a small amount of fluid and do not vomit it they will ultimately receive more fluid than if they take a large amount but, because of a gastroenteritis, vomit that amount. Parents are capable of understanding that stomach secretions are lost along with vomitus each time, and the preservation of these stomach secretions is important to keep their child well. Antiemetics are rarely necessary for children (see the Focus on Cultural Awareness box.) Parents should not give over-the-counter preparations for vomiting to children; instead, they should control vomiting by dietary management to protect the child's electrolyte balance. Prochlorperazine (Compazine), used with adults to control vomiting, may result in bizarre behavior symptoms (toxicity) in children; thus, it is rarely prescribed for children who have not reached adolescence.

Diarrhea

Diarrhea is the major cause of infant mortality in developing countries. Although diarrhea in infants may result from other causes, its primary cause is viral or bacterial invasion of the gastrointestinal tract. The most common viral pathogens are rotaviruses and adenoviruses. The most common bacterial pathogens are *Campylobacter jejuni* and *Salmonella*. Diarrhea in infants is always serious because infants have such a small extracellular fluid reserve that sudden losses of water exhaust the supply quickly, rapidly leading to dehydration (Househam et al., 1990). Na^+ and K^+ ions are lost in stools as well as fluid. The loss of extracellular sodium leads to a decrease in plasma volume (additional water is excreted) and circulatory collapse. Renal failure results, with irreversible acidosis and death. Breastfeeding may actively prevent diarrhea, especially that caused by *Campylobacter* (Ruiz-Palacios et al., 1990).

Assessment of Mild Diarrhea

Normal and diarrheal stool characteristics are compared in the Focus on Family Teaching display. In mild diarrhea, fever of 101°F to 102°F (38.4°C to 39.0°C) may be present; children are anorectic and irritable and appear

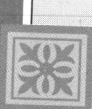

FOCUS ON CULTURAL AWARENESS

Gastrointestinal illnesses do not occur at the same incidence in all communities. Vomiting and diarrhea, for example, tend to occur in communities where refrigeration is less than optimal. Celiac disease occurs most frequently in children with north European ancestry. Because vomiting and diarrhea are so common, there are home remedies for these in every culture. To be certain that a child seen in a health care facility doesn't receive two forms of the same drug (one prescribed and one given in an herb form by a parent), always ask what home remedies have been given and document these on the child's nursing plan.

unwell. The diarrhea consists of 2 to 10 loose, watery bowel movements per day.

The mucous membrane of the infant's mouth with mild diarrhea will be dry. Pulse will be rapid and out of proportion to the low-grade fever. Skin feels warm; skin turgor is not yet decreased. Urine output is normal.

Therapeutic Management of Mild Diarrhea

At this stage, diarrhea is not yet serious, and children can be cared for at home. As with vomiting, treatment for diarrhea must involve resting the gastrointestinal tract, but this is only necessary for a short time. At the end of approximately 1 hour, parents can begin to offer water or an oral rehydration solution such as Pedialyte in small amounts on a regimen similar to that for vomiting (Laney & Cohen, 1993). If infants are breastfed, breastfeeding should continue. Again, it may be difficult for parents to restrict fluid for a short time if they think they should overfeed children to make up for the fluid loss. Children also need measures taken to reduce the elevated temperature. Caution parents not to use over-the-counter drugs such as diphenoxylate (Lomotil) or kaolin and pectin (Kaopectate) to halt diarrhea. As a rule, these are too strong for young children. Caution them also to wash their hands after changing diapers to prevent the spread of infection.

Infants may develop a lactase deficiency following diarrhea. This leads to lactose intolerance. With lactose intolerance, the child is unable to take formula or breast milk or new diarrhea will begin. Such an infant will need to be introduced to a lactose-free formula initially before being returned to the usual kind or to breast milk.

Assessment of Severe Diarrhea

Severe diarrhea may result from progressive mild diarrhea, or it may begin in a severe form. Infants with se-

FOCUS ON FAMILY TEACHING

Q. I know that diarrhea is serious in infants. How can I differentiate between diarrheal stool and normal infant stool that is also loose?

A. It can be difficult to differentiate between normal and diarrheal stool. Some contrasting characteristics are:

Characteristic	Normal Infant Stool	Diarrheal Stool
Frequency	1–3 daily	Unlimited number
Color	Yellow	Green
Effort of expulsion	Some pushing effort	Effortless; may be explosive
pH	More than 7.0 (alkaline)	Less than 7.0 (acidic)
Odor	Odorless	Sweet or foul-smelling
Occult blood	Negative	Positive, blood may be overt
Reducing substances	Negative	Positive

vere diarrhea are obviously ill. Rectal temperature is often as high as 103°F to 104°F (39.5°C to 40.0°C). Both pulse and respirations will be weak and rapid. The skin is cool to the touch; the infants appear pale. Infants may appear apprehensive, or they may be listless and lethargic. They have obvious signs of dehydration: a depressed fontanelle, sunken eyes, and poor skin turgor. The diarrhea will consist of a bowel movement every few minutes. The stool is liquid green, perhaps mixed with mucus and blood, and may be passed with explosive force. Urine output will be scanty and concentrated. Laboratory findings will show an elevated hematocrit, hemoglobin, and serum protein levels due to the dehydration. Electrolyte determinations will reveal a metabolic acidosis.

It is difficult to measure the amount of fluid the child has lost, but estimation of the amount can be derived from the loss in body weight if that is known. For example, if a child weighed 10.4 kg yesterday at a health maintenance visit and today weighs 8.9 kg, he or she has lost more than 10% of body weight. Mild dehydration occurs with a loss of 2.5% to 5% of body weight; severe diarrhea quickly causes a 5% to 15% loss. Any infant who has lost 10% or more of body weight is in serious difficulty and needs hospital admission and immediate treatment.

Therapeutic Management of Severe Diarrhea

Treatment consists of attempting to regulate the electrolyte and fluid balance, initiating rest for the gastrointestinal tract, and discovering the organism responsible.

All children with diarrhea will have a stool culture taken on admission to the hospital so that definite antibiotic therapy can be prescribed. Stool cultures may be taken from the rectum or from stool in the diaper or a bedpan. On admission, infants will have blood drawn for a hemoglobin level (an estimation of hydration as well as anemia); white blood cell and differential counts (to attempt to establish if infection is present); and determinations of CO_2, Cl^-, Na^+, K^+, and pH (to establish electrolyte needs). Before these results are obtained, they will have an intravenous solution such as normal saline or 5% glucose in normal saline begun. The solution will provide fluid in addition to sodium and calories for replacement. Although infants usually have a potassium depletion, potassium cannot be given until it is established that they are not in renal failure. Giving potassium intravenously when the body has no outlet for excessive potassium could lead to excessively high potassium levels and heart block. *Before this initial fluid is changed to a potassium solution, therefore, be certain that the infant or child has voided–proof that the kidneys are functioning.*

Fluid must be given to replace the deficit that has occurred for maintenance therapy and to replace the continuing loss until the diarrhea improves (Figure 45-4). If infants have lost less than 5% of total body weight, their fluid deficit is approximately 50 mL/kg of body weight. If infants have lost 10% of body weight, they need approximately 100 mL/kg of body weight to replace their fluid deficit. If the weight loss suggests a 12% to 15% loss of body fluid, they require 125 mL/kg of body weight to replace the fluid lost. This fluid will be given rapidly in the first 3 to 6 hours, then it will be slowed to a maintenance rate. Once infants void, a sodium lactate solution or a potassium additive may be begun to make up for potassium deficit.

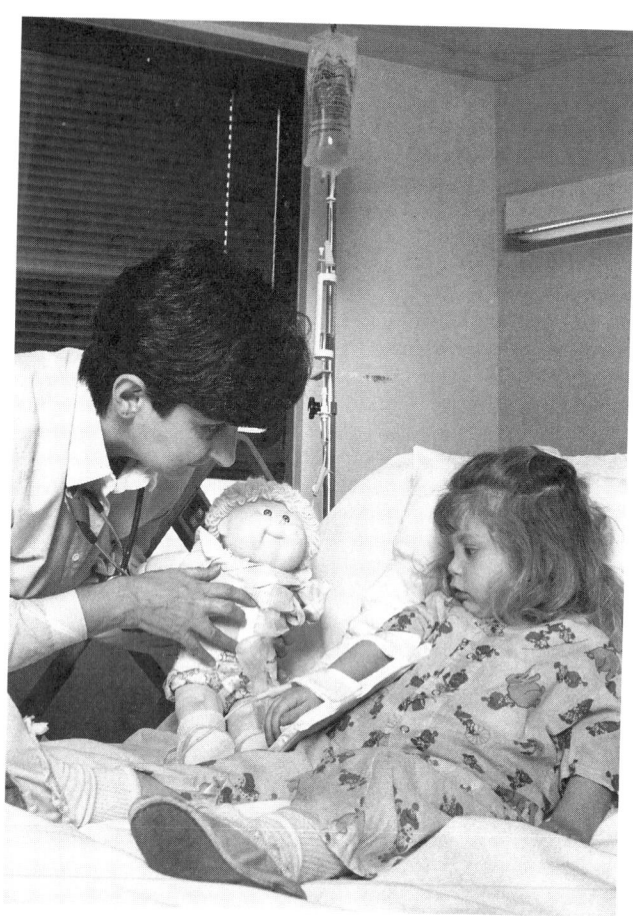

FIGURE 45-4
Restoring fluid loss is important in children with diarrhea. Therapeutic play helps ease fear of the therapy. (Courtesy of the Department of Medical Photography, Children's Hospital, Buffalo, NY.)

Nursing Diagnoses and Related Interventions

Nursing Diagnosis: Fluid volume deficit, related to loss of fluid through diarrhea

Goal: Child will maintain an adequate fluid balance until normal elimination pattern is restored.

Outcome Criteria: Skin turgor is good; specific gravity of urine is 1.003 to 1.030; urine output is more than 1 mL/kg/h, bowel movements are formed and fewer than four per day. Stool tests negative for reducing substances and blood. *p*H = more than 7.

Promote Hydration and Comfort. Although infants' mouths appear dry, be sure they are offered nothing by mouth. Vomiting at this point will compound the problem by adding to the dehydration. Wet the infant's lips with a moisturizing jelly (Vaseline) if they appear to be dry and cracking. Give them a pacifier to suck if this seems to comfort them. (They want to suck because

they are very thirsty, and if they have intestinal cramping with the diarrhea, they interpret this as hunger.)

After several hours, infants may be allowed small sips of clear fluid, an oral rehydration solution, or breast milk. Gradually, the infant's oral intake is increased, changing to a soft diet (sometimes called a BRAT diet because it comprises bananas, rice cereal, applesauce, and toast). If the child with severe diarrhea also has a fever, measures to reduce the fever will be necessary (see Chapter 37). A rectal thermometer should not be used to assess fever, because this could initiate more diarrhea.

Record Fluid Intake and Output. Much of the nursing care of children with diarrhea hinges on careful recording of fluid intake and output. Keep careful records of the kind, rate, and total amount of intravenous fluid given. Because children are admitted in dehydration, their intravenous therapy tubing serves as their lifeline. It is extremely important that it not become dislodged and thereby infiltrated, and that the tubing is not allowed to run dry so that clotting and plugging result. It may be necessary to restrain not only the infant's arm in which the intravenous line is inserted, but also the other arm and probably the trunk as well so that the infant does not turn or poke at the tubing. Because this tubing may remain in place for 2 or 3 days (until it is clear that taking oral fluids does not initiate the diarrhea again), children should have restraints released every hour and their arms passively exercised. Give parents an explanation of why the intravenous infusion is important so that they will understand the necessity of the restraint.

In children who are not toilet trained, put a plastic urine collector in place to enable separation of urine from feces. This makes it obvious that the child is voiding (to determine when potassium can be safely added to the intravenous infusion) and to confirm continuous kidney function. When urine is separated from stools, the appearance of stools or their water content can also be better judged. For each stool that children have, record its color, consistency, odor, size, and the presence of any blood or mucus. Weigh soiled diapers to reveal the number of grams of stool in the diaper. Testing the stool with litmus paper or a dipstick Reagent Strip to determine its acidity and with a Clinitest tablet for reducing substances (sugars) reveals how quickly the stool is passing through the irritated tract. A stool positive for sugar shows what little absorption has occurred as sugar is absorbed rapidly from ingested food. (Dilute stool with a few drops of tap water to make it liquid enough to drop for a Clinitest test). Acid stool (*p*H less than 7.0) shows the presence of unabsorbed sugar also (a process occurs similar to the process that causes acid to invade tooth enamel in the presence of glucose on teeth). Diarrhea stools are green from lack of time for bile to be modified in the intestine. As diarrhea improves and stool remains in the intestine for a longer period, the stool deepens in color, and the acid and sugar content fade. Testing stools for occult blood reveals the extent of bowel irritation that is occurring from the acid stool. Occult blood is also not found as the diarrhea improves and the irritation to the bowel lessens.

Nursing Diagnosis: High risk for altered skin integrity related to presence of diarrheal stool on skin

Goal: Child's skin will remain intact during period of diarrhea.

Outcome Criteria: Skin in diaper area is not erythematous or with ulcerations.

Change diapers immediately after infants stool (caution older children to wipe away stool thoroughly) because diarrheal stool is extremely irritating to skin. Wash the skin of the diaper area well after each stool and cover it with an ointment such as Vaseline or A and D to protect it from further irritation.

If infants already have skin excoriation on admission from the number of stools they have had at home, an ointment such as Desitin may be helpful in soothing the irritated skin. Lying infants on their abdomen and exposing their buttocks to air is generally helpful in healing irritation.

Nursing Diagnosis: High risk for anxiety related to hospitalization experience

Goal: Child will not suffer long-term effects of hospitalization.

Outcome Criteria: Child interacts with parents in age-appropriate way; is able to be comforted following painful procedures.

All children with diarrhea are assumed to have an infectious form of gastroenteritis and, therefore, are isolated until this is ruled out. They are uncomfortable from the diarrhea, exhausted, and confused with these new body sensations. They need the security of someone to stay with them in an isolation room. When an infant with severe diarrhea is admitted to the hospital, many emergency procedures must be performed: the intravenous route must be established, the urine collection must be started, and temperature reduction measures initiated. During all these procedures, try to remember how all of this must seem to the child in the bed. Be sure to take time during initial procedures to touch and soothe children and talk to them; once the initial admission procedures are done, sit by the bed and gently stroke the child's head or hold the child. Teach parents isolation room technique so that they feel welcome in an isolation room. Encourage them to give any care possible. Children need this support to counteract the strange world into which they have suddenly been plunged. Further care of the child in isolation is discussed in Chapter 43.

Bacterial Infectious Diseases That Cause Diarrhea and Vomiting

Salmonella

- Causative agent: One of the *Salmonella* bacteria
- Incubation period: 6 to 72 hours for intraluminal type; 7 to 14 days for extraluminal type
- Period of communicability: As long as organisms are being excreted (may be as long as 3 months)
- Mode of transmission: Ingestion of contaminated food

Salmonella is the most common type of food poisoning in the United States. Children with a *Salmonella* infection have symptoms of diarrhea, abdominal pain, vomiting, high temperature, and headache. They are listless and drowsy. The diarrhea is severe and may contain blood and mucus. *Salmonella* infection may remain as an intraluminal disease. When it does, it is treated, like severe diarrhea, with fluid and electrolyte replacement. It may also become systemic (extraluminal disease) and, in that instance, it is treated with an antibiotic such as amoxicillin. The diagnosis of the infection can be made from stool culture (AAP, 1991).

Salmonella infections are serious in childhood. Complications such as meningitis, bronchitis, and osteomyelitis may result. Although the source of *Salmonella* generally is infected food (contaminated chicken and eggs are common sources), it may be transmitted to children by infected turtles. To prevent this, teach children to wash their hands well after handling pet turtles or changing the turtles' water.

Shigellosis (Dysentery)

- Causative agent: Organisms of the genus *Shigella*
- Incubation period: 1 to 7 days
- Period of communicability: Approximately 1 to 4 weeks
- Mode of transmission: Contaminated food or milk products

Shigella organisms, like the *Salmonella* group, cause extremely severe diarrhea. In addition to the severe diarrhea, the stool may contain blood and mucus. Ampicillin or trimethoprim sulfamethoxazole are the preferred drugs for therapy (AAP, 1991). The child needs intense fluid and electrolyte replacement.

Staphylococcal Food Poisoning

- Causative agent: Staphylococcal enterotoxin produced by some strains of *Staphylococcus aureus*
- Incubation period: 1 to 7 hours
- Period of communicability: Carriers may contaminate food as long as they harbor the organism
- Mode of transmission: Ingestion of contaminated food

With staphylococcal food poisoning, the child has severe vomiting and diarrhea, abdominal cramping, excessive salivation, and nausea. It is often difficult to culture the causative organism from the contaminated food because, although the staphylococcus may have been destroyed by inadequate cooking, the enterotoxin that actually causes the disorder will not have been destroyed. The child needs intensive supportive therapy in the form of fluid and electrolyte replacement.

Disorders of the Stomach and Duodenum

Chalasia (Gastroesophageal Reflux)

Chalasia is a neuromuscular disturbance in which the cardiac sphincter and the lower portion of the esophagus are lax and, therefore, allow easy regurgitation of gastric contents into the esophagus (Sterling et al., 1993). It starts within 1 week after birth, as a rule. It may be associated with a hiatal hernia. The regurgitation occurs almost immediately after feeding or when the infant is laid down after a feeding. The process may result in aspiration pneumonia or esophageal stricture from the constant reflux of hydrochloric acid into the esophagus. If the reflux is a large amount, the infant does not retain sufficient calories and will fail to thrive.

Assessment

The diagnosis of chalasia is suggested by the history. This vomiting is effortless and nonprojectile and begins much earlier than pyloric stenosis vomiting. If a probe or catheter is inserted into the esophagus through the nose to the distal esophagus, and pH is determined from secretions, it can reveal whether gastric secretions are entering the esophagus (if pH is less than 7.0, then acid is present). An esophagography (barium swallow) will reveal the lax cardiac sphincter and the reflux of stomach contents into the esophagus, especially if the infant's head is tilted down. An esophagoscopy will directly reveal the reflux.

Therapeutic Management

The treatment of chalasia is to feed such infants a formula thickened with rice cereal while holding them in an upright position and to keep them in an elevated prone position for 1 hour after feeding. Elevating the baby's head and trunk after a feeding is important. An antacid or cimetidine may be prescribed three or four times daily to reduce the possibility of the stomach acid contents irritating the esophagus. Bethanechol or metoclopramide (Reglan) may be prescribed to hurry gastric emptying.

Chalasia is usually a self-limiting condition. As the esophageal sphincter matures and the child begins to eat solid food and is maintained in a more upright position, the problem disappears. It is a problem that needs

treatment, however, or serious consequences can result from dehydration, alkalosis, or damage to the esophagus. If medical therapy is ineffective, a surgical procedure (a Nissen fundoplication) may be scheduled to correct the cardiac sphincter. Following this, the child will return from surgery with a nasogastric tube inserted; it is usually irrigated with normal saline every 2 hours to ensure its patency. Assess nasogastric tube drainage for coffee-colored drainage (although this is normal for the first 24 hours) that would reveal bleeding from the incision. Following surgery, infants may display symptoms of abdominal discomfort and stomach distention because food can no longer enter the esophagus. This distention may be so extreme that it leads to bradycardia and dyspnea.

Nursing Diagnoses and Related Interventions

Nursing Diagnosis: High risk for altered nutrition, less than body requirements related to regurgitation of food with esophageal reflux

Goal: Infant will receive adequate nutrition during course of therapy.

Outcome Criteria: Skin turgor is good; specific gravity of urine is 1.003 to 1.030; intake is 50 cal/lb/24 h.

After a feeding, the infant should sit in an infant seat or lie prone on a slanted board (Figure 45-5). The average baby will fall asleep in either of these positions as easily as lying down. Use a sheepskin-like covering on a slant board to prevent knee and face irritation. Be certain parents understand how much cereal to mix with formula. Mothers who are breastfeeding may manually express breast milk and mix it with rice cereal for feedings.

Help parents to understand that this feeding difficulty was in no way their fault (they are not poor nurturers; the infant had an internal problem). Encourage

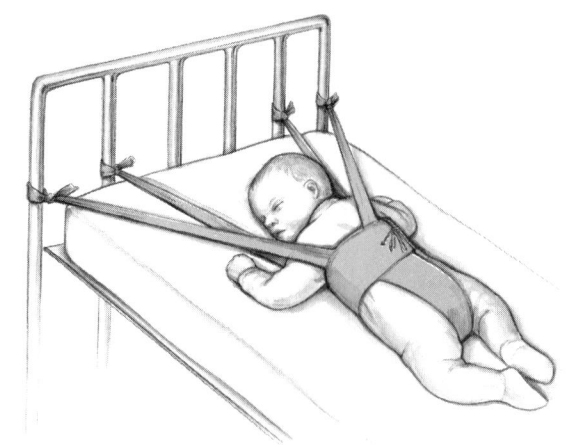

FIGURE 45-5
Positional treatment for gastroesophageal reflux.

them to feed the infant in the hospital and give care to regain confidence in themselves as parents.

Pyloric Stenosis

The *pylorus* is the valve between the stomach and the beginning portion of the intestine, the duodenum. If hypertrophy or hyperplasia of the muscle surrounding the valve occurs, it is difficult for the stomach to empty, a condition called **pyloric stenosis** (Figure 45-6). With this condition, at 4 to 6 weeks of age, children begin to vomit almost immediately following each feeding. The vomiting grows increasingly forceful until it is projectile; the vomitus may be projected as much as 3 to 4 feet. Pyloric stenosis tends to occur most frequently in first-born white male infants. The incidence is high, approximately 1:150 in males, 1:750 in females. The cause is unknown, but multifactorial inheritance is the likely cause (Belknap & McEvoy, 1994). Pyloric stenosis occurs less frequently in breastfed infants than in formula-fed infants. Infants fed on formula begin having symptoms at approximately 4 weeks of age; the breastfed infant begins developing symptoms at approximately 6 weeks because the curd of breast milk is smaller than that of cow's milk, and it passes through a hypertrophied muscle more easily.

Vomitus is marked by the force with which it occurs. It usually smells sour because it has reached the stomach and has been in contact with stomach enzymes. There is never bile in the vomiting of pyloric stenosis because the feeding does not reach the duodenum to become mixed with bile. The infant is usually hungry immediately after vomiting because he or she is not nauseated. It is difficult to assess whether nausea is present in infants, but some of its symptoms may be a disinterest in eating, excessive drooling, or chewing on the tongue.

Assessment

The diagnosis of pyloric stenosis is made primarily from the history. Whenever parents say that their baby is vomiting or spitting up, be certain to get a full descrip-

tion. What is the duration? What is the intensity? What is the frequency? What is the description of the vomitus? Is the infant ill in any other way? Many infants have signs of dehydration from the vomiting at the time they are first seen. Lack of tears (many infants younger than age 6 weeks do not tear); dry mucous membrane of the mouth; sunken fontanelles; fever; decreased urine output; poor skin turgor (when lifting a ridge of skin, instead of returning to place afterward, it remains raised); and loss of weight are common signs of dehydration. Alkalosis may be present because of the excessive loss of Cl^- ions from stomach fluid. The child will also have accompanying hypochloremia, hypokalemia, and starvation. The child will have hypopnea (slowed respirations) as the body attempts to retain CO_2 to increase the H^+ ion concentration and decrease the alkalosis. This will cause the CO_2 content of plasma generally to be above 30 mEq/L (normal is 22 mEq/L to 28 mEq/L). Tetany may occur with alkalosis because the increased HCO_3^- ions may combine with Ca^{++} ions, trying to effect homeostasis and thereby lowering the level of ionized calcium.

A definitive diagnosis is made by watching the infant drink. Before the child drinks, by palpating the right upper quadrant of the abdomen, it may be possible to palpate the pyloric mass. It feels round and firm, approximately the size of an olive. As the infant drinks, gastric peristaltic waves passing from left to right across the abdomen may be seen. The olive-size lump becomes more prominent; the infant vomits with projectile emesis. If the diagnosis is still in doubt, the child may have a sonogram or barium swallow x-ray ordered. The hypertrophied valve is obvious on sonogram; the obstruction at the pylorus will be revealed on x-ray—a diagnostic "shoestring" sign. Endoscopy may also be used for diagnosis.

Therapeutic Management

Treatment is surgical correction before electrolyte imbalance from the vomiting or hypoglycemia from the lack of food intake occurs. Before surgery, the electrolyte imbalance, dehydration, and starvation must be corrected by administration of intravenous fluid. No oral feedings are given so that vomiting will not further deplete electrolytes. An infant who is receiving only intravenous fluid generally needs a pacifier to fulfill the child's oral needs and be comfortable. The intravenous fluid offered is isotonic saline or 5% glucose in saline because this contains an excess of Cl^- ions. If tetany is present, calcium must be administered also. The infant needs additional potassium also, as a rule, but this must not be administered until it is ascertained that the child's kidneys are working (i.e., the child is voiding); otherwise, the potassium buildup will cause heart arrhythmia.

The surgical procedure for pyloric stenosis is pyloromyotomy (a *Fredet-Ramstedt operation*). The muscle of the pylorus is split, allowing for a larger lumen. Although the procedure sounds simple, it is technically

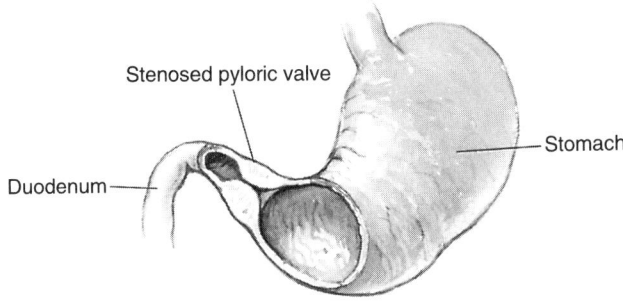

FIGURE 45-6
Pyloric stenosis. Fluid is unable to pass easily through the stenosed and hypertrophied pyloric valve. (Courtesy of the Department of Medical Illustration, State University of New York at Buffalo, Buffalo, NY.)

difficult to perform and there is high risk for infection afterward because the incision is near the diaper area.

The prognosis for infants with pyloric stenosis is excellent if the condition was discovered before the electrolyte imbalance occurred.

Nursing Diagnoses and Related Interventions

Nursing Diagnosis: High risk for fluid volume deficit related to inability to retain food

Goal: Infant will remain well hydrated until condition is corrected.

Outcome Criteria: Skin turgor is good; specific gravity of urine is 1.003 to 1.030; no further vomiting has occurred.

Preoperative Care. A baseline weight is essential for establishing the extent of dehydration. Note carefully the frequency of urination, the specific gravity of the urine, and the number of stools to help assess dehydration and starvation. Parents may be impatient with preoperative management. They need an explanation that infants cannot go to surgery with an electrolyte imbalance; these hours before surgery are as important to the welfare of their child as the operation itself.

Postoperative Care. Infants may return from surgery with an intravenous line in place. The feeding regimen postoperatively differs from one surgeon to another, but usually is based on a regimen requiring frequent feedings of small amounts of fluid, referred to as *Down's regimen.* Approximately 4 to 6 hours after surgery, children are given approximately 1 tsp of 5% glucose in saline hourly by bottle for four feedings; if no vomiting occurs, the amount is increased to 2 tsp hourly for four more feedings. Next, half-strength formula is begun every 4 hours. Finally, by 24 hours to 48 hours, infants are taking their full formula diet or being breastfed. They are usually discharged at the end of 48 hours.

It is important that infants be given no more than the amount ordered at a time so the newly operated-on pylorus is not overwhelmed. It is important that infants take these small amounts because a small quantity of fluid passing through the valve in the immediate postoperative days helps to keep adhesions of the incision from forming. As the amount taken orally increases, the intravenous fluid will be decreased and then discontinued. Infants should be bubbled well after a feeding so there is no pressure from air in the stomach; they should be laid on their side after feeding so if vomiting does occur, there is little chance of aspiration. Laying them on their right side possibly aids the flow of fluid through the pyloric valve by gravity. Daily weights are continued during this time to confirm that children are receiving adequate intake. Usually no vomiting occurs postoperatively. If vomiting does occur, it should be reported. The regimen of feeding will be slowed accordingly and the infant may be kept in the hospital longer. Some infants have a short-term diarrhea following surgery due to rapid functioning of the pyloric valve. A number of them may be colicky and fretful.

Nursing Diagnosis: High risk for infection at site of surgical incision related to proximity of incision to diaper area

Goal: Infant's surgical incision will remain free of infection until it is healed.

Outcome Criteria: Infant's temperature is below 37.0°C axillary; incision does not appear erythematous or with drainage.

The surgical incision for pyloric stenosis may be covered with collodion in surgery to help keep urine and feces from touching it. Keep diapers folded low to prevent the incision from being contaminated and change diapers frequently. If the incision should be exposed to feces, wash the collodion well with soap and water.

Nursing Diagnosis: High risk for altered parenting related to infant's feeding difficulty and illness

Goal: Parents will demonstrate adequate bonding behavior with the infant both pre- and postoperatively.

Outcome Criteria: Parents hold and feed infant; express positive characteristics about infant.

Encourage the parents of a baby this young who is hospitalized to room in during the hospitalization so that they can grow comfortable and confident in caring for their child again. When the child first began vomiting so forcefully, parents were frightened and may have felt they were doing something wrong. They began to lose confidence in themselves as parents. They will need an explanation that the vomiting was caused by a physical problem and was not their fault.

Hospitalization often occurs near the infant's second month, when the child would normally receive diphtheria-tetanus-pertussis, oral poliomyelitis, and *Haemophilus influenzae* immunization. Ask if this could be administered before discharge so the child's immunization status remains current. This might also serve to remind parents that getting back to normal means regular health care visits for vaccines and checkups.

Peptic Ulcer

A **peptic ulcer** is a shallow excavation formed in the mucosal wall of the stomach, the pylorus, or the duodenum. In children, ulcers are usually duodenal. Such ulcers occur because of oversecretion of gastric juices or failure of the mucosa to neutralize gastric secretions, so the acid is irritating to mucosa. They may be associated with infection by *C. jejuni*. A small ulceration of the gastric or duodenal lining will lead to symptoms of pain, blood in the stools, and vomiting (with blood). If left uncorrected, peptic ulcers can lead to bowel or stomach perforation with acute hemorrhage or pyloric obstruction. A chronic ulcer condition will lead to anemia from the constant slight blood loss.

Although peptic ulcers are most commonly seen in adults, they do occur in children as well; 2% to 18% of people with chronic duodenal ulcers date the onset of their symptoms to childhood. Peptic ulcers occur more frequently in males than in females, in whites more than in other races, and in urban rather than in rural populations.

Gastric ulcers may develop during the administration of adrenocorticotropic hormone or corticosteroids. Salicylates, similarly, may be instrumental in causing gastric ulceration. Ulcers in the neonatal period are associated with stress, perhaps prolonged or protracted labor, sepsis, or the trauma of intubation. Infants with these histories should be suspected of having peptic ulcer. Secondary ulcers may occur in children with stressful illnesses such as burns. In older children, genetic factors may be involved; some children with peptic ulcer have a positive family history for the disorder.

Assessment

An ulcer occurring in a neonate usually presents with hematemesis (blood in vomitus) or melena (blood in the stool). Such ulcers are usually superficial and heal rapidly, although they can lead to rupture with symptoms of respiratory distress, abdominal distention, vomiting, and, if extensive, cardiovascular collapse. If the ulcer occurs in the toddler, the first symptoms are usually feeding problems or vomiting. Bleeding follows in several weeks. If the ulcer begins when children are of preschool or early school age, pain may be the presenting symptom. Children experience pain on arising in the morning, and it is not necessarily relieved by the ingestion of food, milk, or an alkaline substance, as are adult peptic ulcers. Children may report pain as mild, severe, colicky, or continuous. It is often poorly localized, although it may be in the epigastric area as in adult clients. It may occur in the right lower quadrant and be confused with appendicitis.

In older school-age children and adolescents, the symptoms are generally those of the adult: a gnawing or aching pain in the epigastric area before meals that is relieved by eating. Vomiting (due to spasm and edema of the pylorus) occurs in a small number of children as well. On abdominal palpation, there is tenderness in the epigastric region.

A definitive diagnosis can only be made by x-ray study or endoscopy. Because childhood ulcers are shallow, however, they do not show well on x-ray, and so, even when present, they may not be diagnosed by this method. In many children, little increase in gastric activity is demonstrable by gastric analysis.

Peptic ulcer is increasing in frequency in children as a reflection of the stress that modern society puts on even its youngest members. Children with this condition must have blood tests done periodically to be monitored for hypochromic, microcytic anemia (blood loss anemia).

Therapeutic Management

Children with a peptic ulcer are treated with medications to suppress gastric acidity and perhaps antibiotics if infection is suspected. When a peptic ulcer is uncomplicated, it heals rapidly with therapy. The long-term prognosis may not be satisfactory, however; many of these children (up to 50%) develop an ulcer again in adult life.

The dangers of a peptic ulcer are perforation and intestinal obstruction. Perforation is rare but is most likely to occur in infancy. Perforation should be suspected if the child suddenly complains of back pain or if the abdominal pain, which previously was intermittent, becomes continuous. It may be possible to elicit tenderness over the sixth or tenth thoracic vertebrae if the perforation is posterior. Children will have epigastric tenderness and abdominal guarding if the perforation is anterior. In infants, extreme fussiness or crying from the increased pain, pallor, diaphoresis, or signs of shock from blood loss may be the signs noted. Repair of the perforation must be accomplished by immediate surgery.

Obstruction of the gastrointestinal tract may occur when edema and spasm of the duodenum and pylorus develops suddenly or gradually. The symptoms are those of intestinal obstruction: a feeling of fullness, nausea, and vomiting. The vomitus becomes projectile as the obstruction becomes complete. In these instances, children will need electrolyte replacement; a nasogastric tube will relieve stomach distention. Unless obstruction is complete, small frequent feedings are begun as soon as possible to supply nutrition.

Nursing Diagnoses and Related Interventions

Having a peptic ulcer, whether it is surgically treated (removing a part of the stomach, cutting a nerve) or medically treated (taking cimetidine four times a day) is difficult for children to accept. Loss of a body part is traumatic, even it is a part that never shows, such as the stomach. Remembering to take medicine daily is difficult for children.

Be certain that goals of care are realistic. It may not be possible to relieve symptoms of peptic ulcer immediately, for example. Children can be helped immediately to understand why the pain occurs and what they can do to help relieve it.

> **Nursing Diagnosis:** Pain related to ulceration in intestinal tract
>
> **Goal:** Child's pain will be kept at an acceptable level during course of illness.
>
> **Outcome Criteria:** Child states that pain is at a tolerable level; the infant appears comfortable without excessive crying.

Infants may receive frequent, small feedings or a slow, continuous nasogastric drip of combined formula and an antacid to provide pain relief and healing. The older child should be able to eat a normal diet, avoiding heavily spiced food such as pizza or sausage if such food causes discomfort. To decrease gastric acidity, the child is prescribed cimetidine (Tagamet) with meals and at bedtime, or antacids at these same times. Compounds that contain magnesium sulfate (e.g., Maalox) are less constipating antacids than aluminum hydroxide products (Amphojel, Gelusil, or Mylanta). For children in school, antacid tablets are less attention-getting and, although not as effective, may be taken more easily.

In addition to administering medications, explore with such children the terms on which they are asked to live at home and at school. For some, a hospital experience is a welcome relief because it temporarily removes them from stress. For others, it may increase the stress. If school pressure is a stress factor, for example, children may perceive a hospital stay as an escape from the pressure. Other children may perceive the days of missed classes in terms of all the material that must be made up, which heightens their stress. In either circumstance, children probably need help in learning coping mechanisms that will serve them better.

Hepatic Disorders

Hepatic disorders include both congenital disorders such as obstruction of the biliary duct and acquired disorders such as hepatitis or cirrhosis.

Liver Function

The liver lies immediately under the diaphragm of the child's right side. In infants, 1 or 2 cm of liver is readily and normally palpable. The organ is essential for the normal metabolism of all three types of foods. It plays a role in the maintenance of normal blood sugar level by changing glucose to glycogen and storing it as such until needed by body cells. It then reverses the process and changes glycogen back to glucose and releases it into the blood when cells require it.

The liver assists in the catabolism of fatty acids and protein and serves as a temporary storage space for both fat and protein. The liver, by the means of the enzyme glucuronyl transferase, converts indirect (or unconjugated) bilirubin into direct (or conjugated) bilirubin so that it can be excreted in bile and eliminated from the body. This is an important function in the newborn, and jaundice can result if the enzyme glucuronyl transferase is low in amount due to immaturity.

The liver manufactures bile, a secretion necessary for the digestion of fat; fibrinogen and prothrombin, substances essential for blood clotting; heparin, a substance necessary to keep blood from clotting in intact vessels; and blood proteins. It produces large amounts of body heat. It destroys red blood cells and detoxifies many harmful absorbed substances, such as drugs. Because the liver, a life-sustaining organ, performs all of these functions, liver disease is always serious. There are a number of common liver function tests used to diagnose the nature of liver pathology. These are summarized in Table 45-6.

Hepatitis

Hepatitis (inflammation and infection of the liver) is caused by the invasion of hepatitis A; hepatitis B; a non-A, non-B virus (hepatitis C); hepatitis D; or hepatitis E (West, 1990).

Hepatitis A
- Causative agent: Hepatitis A virus
- Incubation period: 25 days on average
- Period of communicability: Highest during 2 weeks preceding onset of jaundice
- Mode of transmission: Ingestion of fecally contaminated water or shellfish from such water; sexual transmission from anal intercourse; day care center spread from contaminated changing tables
- Immunity: Natural; one episode induces immunity for the specific type of virus
  - Passive artificial immunity: Immune globulin

Hepatitis B
- Causative agent: Hepatitis B virus
- Incubation period: 120 days on average
- Period of communicability: Later part of incubation period and during the acute stage
- Mode of transmission: Transfusion of contaminated blood and plasma or semen; accidental inoculation by a syringe or needle; may be spread to fetus if mother has infection in third trimester of pregnancy
- Immunity: Natural; one episode induces immunity for the specific type of virus
  - Active artificial immunity: Vaccine for the B virus
  - Passive artificial immunity: Specific hepatitis B immune serum globulin

Table 45-6. Liver Function Tests

Test	Description
Serum bilirubin	Indirect bilirubin found in large quantities in bloodstream indicates that the child is not converting it to direct bilirubin, hence liver cell function is impaired; the normal value of total bilirubin in serum is 1.5 mg per 100 mL; if large amounts of direct bilirubin are found in serum, it implies obstruction of the bile duct, preventing the excretion of the converted substance.
Stool and urine	If bile pigments can be obtained from stool (excreted as urobilinogen in stool and urine), it is evidence that bile is being manufactured and excreted from the liver; stool appears light in color (clay colored) without the presence of bile pigment.
Alkaline phosphatase	Alkaline phosphatase is an enzyme produced by the liver and bone that is excreted in the bile; when there is bile duct obstruction, there will be increased levels of alkaline phosphatase in the blood.
Leucine amino peptidase (LAP)	LAP is an enzyme produced exclusively by the liver; the level of LAP is elevated in the bloodstream, as is that of alkaline phosphatase, with bile duct obstruction.
Prothrombin time	In chronic liver disease, the level of prothrombin produced by the liver may fall so severely that the prothrombin time is increased; there is little change in prothrombin time in mild or short-term liver disease.
Serum glutamic oxaloacetic transaminase (SGOT)	SGOT is an enzyme found in the heart and liver; when there is acute cellular destruction to either organ, the enzyme is released into the bloodstream from the damaged cells; the blood levels are increased by 8 hours after injury; the level reaches a peak in 24 or 36 h and then falls to normal in 4 to 6 d.
Serum glutamic pyruvic transaminase (SGPT)	SGPT is an enzyme found mostly in the liver; it rises for the same reasons as SGOT but is not as sensitive an indicator of liver damage.
Lactic dehydrogenase (LDH)	LDH is another enzyme found in the heart and liver; it is a relatively insensitive indicator of liver destruction, however; infectious mononucleosis is the one disease in which increased levels of LDH seem to be seen frequently.
Serum proteins	Because albumin is chiefly synthesized in the liver, most acute or chronic liver disease will show decreased serum albumin.

Assessment

Hepatitis is a generalized body infection with specific intense liver effects (Mitchell, 1990).

Type A infectious hepatitis occurs in children of all ages. Hepatitis B tends to occur in adolescents following intimate contact or the use of contaminated syringes for drug injection. It has an unusually high incidence in the Asian population and in immunosuppressed children (AAP, 1991).

Clinically, it is impossible to differentiate from the signs the type of virus involved. All hepatitis viruses cause liver cell destruction leading to increased serum glutamic-oxaloacetic transaminase (SGOT) and alkaline phosphatase levels. There is decreased albumin synthesis and impaired bile formation and excretion. The type of virus causing the disease can be determined by the recognition of a specific hemagglutination reaction for hepatitis B virus (an HBsAg titer).

The onset of symptoms is usually abrupt. Children notice headache, vomiting, generalized aching, and right upper quadrant pain. They may have a low-grade fever and a sore throat or nasal discharge. They feel ill; they are irritable and fretful from pruritus. After 3 to 7 days of such symptoms, the color of the urine becomes darker (brown) due to the excretion of bilirubin. In another 2 days, children's eye scleras become jaundiced; soon

they have generalized jaundice. With the generalized jaundice, there is little excretion of bilirubin into the stool, so the stool color becomes white or gray. This icteric (jaundiced) phase lasts for a few days to 2 weeks. Some children have an anicteric form of infection, in which they develop the beginning symptoms but then never develop the jaundice. They are as infectious, however, as children with overt jaundice.

Laboratory studies will demonstrate elevations of SGOT and serum glutamate pyruvate transaminase (SGPT). Measurement of bilirubin in the urine shows increased levels. Bile pigments in the stool are decreased. Serum bilirubin levels will be increased.

Therapeutic Management

The treatment for infectious hepatitis is increased rest and maintenance of a good caloric intake. A low-fat diet, once recommended, is not required and in any event is difficult to enforce. Children are generally hungrier at breakfast than later in the day, so a good intake should be encouraged for breakfast. Children can be cared for at home. They should not return to school until the jaundice has completely disappeared and liver enzymes are no more than twice normal.

A complication of hepatitis is hepatic coma. Hepatic coma is ammonia intoxication caused by the inability of the liver to detoxify the ammonia being constantly produced by the intestine in the process of digestion. (It is normally detoxified to urea.) With hepatic coma, children show signs of mental aberrations, such as confusion, drowsiness, or disorientation. Untreated, it is fatal. Treatment is to reduce protein intake and administer lactulose to prevent absorption of ammonia in the colon or to administer nonabsorbable antibiotics, such as neomycin, to decrease the production of ammonia by the intestinal bacteria.

Children with type A involvement generally recover with no long-term effects. Of those with type B, 90% will also recover completely, but 10% will develop chronic hepatitis and become hepatitis carriers. Infants who contracted the disease at birth have an increased risk for liver carcinoma later in life.

Nursing Diagnoses and Related Interventions

Nursing Diagnosis: High risk for infection transmission to close contacts related to infectious nature of disease

Goal: Caregivers will take precautions to decrease spread during course of illness.

Outcome Criteria: Caregivers wash hands following changing of diapers; use precautions with blood samples and syringes.

Strict hand washing and isolation technique are mandatory when caring for children with infectious hepatitis. Feces must be disposed of carefully because the type A virus may be cultured from feces. Syringes and needles must be disposed of with caution because the type B virus can be transmitted by blood. Contacts should receive immune globulin (hepatitis A) or hepatitis B immune globulin (HBIG) as appropriate. All health care providers should receive prophylaxis against hepatitis by the hepatitis vaccine (AAP, 1991). All women should be screened during pregnancy for hepatitis B (HBsAg). Infants born of hepatitis positive mothers receive both HBIG and active immunization at birth to prevent their contracting the disease.

Nursing Diagnosis: Altered comfort (pruritus) related to effects of jaundice

Goal: Child will not experience extreme discomfort during course of illness.

Outcome Criteria: Child states level of itching is tolerable; no scratch marks on skin are present.

Jaundice commonly causes pruritus, and for some children this can result in extreme discomfort. Being certain that the child is not overheated and not perspiring reduces the itching. A cool bath is often comforting. Skin moisturizers such as Eucerin or an antihistamine may be prescribed. Teach the child distractive techniques such as putting pressure on a pruritic area or trying imagery to lessen the urge to scratch.

Obstruction of the Bile Ducts

Obstruction of the bile ducts in children generally occurs from congenital atresia, stenosis, or absence of the duct. It can occur from a plugging of biliary secretions, but this is rare. When the bile duct is obstructed, bile cannot enter the intestinal tract. It accumulates in the liver. Bile pigments (direct bilirubin) enter the bloodstream. Infants begin to appear jaundiced; the jaundice increases in intensity daily.

Assessment

Although bile duct obstruction is a congenital disorder, the chief sign of it or jaundice takes approximately 2 weeks to develop. This delay in signs differentiates it clinically from physiologic jaundice that occurs in almost all newborns on the third day of life or the jaundice of blood incompatibility, which typically occurs during the first 24 hours of life, respectively. Laboratory findings will also distinguish this type of jaundice. Physiologic jaundice and blood incompatibility jaundice occur from a rise in indirect bilirubin, whereas the jaundice of bile duct obstruction is direct bilirubin jaundice. Alkaline phosphatase levels will be elevated. SGOT will be normal in the early phase, then later will become abnormal, when prolonged obstruction and back pressure cause liver cell damage. In addition, because bile salts (necessary for fat absorption) are not reaching the intestine, absorption of fat and fat-soluble vitamins (i.e., vitamins A, D, E, and K) is poor. Absorption of calcium, which depends on vitamin D absorption, will be poor. Infant's stools will be white from lack of bile pigments. The pressure on the liver from the obstruction becomes so acute with time that cell destruction or cirrhosis occurs in the liver. Ultimately, without liver transplantation, death from liver failure will result.

Therapeutic Management

Before treatment is begun, the condition must be differentiated from jaundice due to infectious hepatitis; exploratory surgery under a general anesthetic is hazardous if the child does have infectious hepatitis. Appropriate blood work and a punch biopsy under a local anesthetic may be done to rule out infectious hepatitis. If a mucus plug in the duct is suspected, children may be given a course of magnesium sulfate (installed into the duodenum to relax the bile duct) or given dehydrocholic acid (Decholin) intravenously to stimulate the flow of bile. If atresia of the bile duct appears to be the problem, surgical correction is the treatment (a Kasai procedure) (Wood et al., 1990). With this surgery, a loop of bowel is sutured next to the liver to create a fistula for bile flow between the liver and intestine. A double-barreled colostomy is then created (enterostomy). Bile flows out of the proximal loop into a collecting bag. It is periodically returned to the distal loop of intestine by injection. After 6 to 12 weeks, the colostomy is closed when a normal bile flow has been established. Unfortunately, surgical correction is impossible in all infants with atresia because the atresia tends to occur too far back in the liver to be in an operable area. Liver transplant is needed for those children with extensive involvement (Coleman et al., 1991).

Nursing Diagnoses and Related Interventions

Nursing Diagnosis: High risk for altered nutrition; less than body requirements related to inability to digest fat

Goal: Child will ingest adequate nutritional requirements until surgical correction is complete.

Outcome Criteria: Infant's weight remains in same percentile on standardized growth curve; no signs of vitamin deficiency (e.g., cracked lips or altered bone growth) are present.

Preoperative Care. Infants who are admitted for surgery for bile duct obstruction are placed on a low-fat, high-protein preoperative diet. They are given water-miscible vitamins A, D, and K to improve vitamin levels. If their vitamin K level is too low, their coagulation ability will be low, and they will be a hazardous surgical risk. Vitamin K may be administered parenterally until the prothrombin level of the blood rises to normal limits. Infants will also be well hydrated with parenteral fluids.

Postoperative Care. Following surgery, infants are returned with a nasogastric tube in place. They must be observed carefully for abdominal distention because paralytic ileus is a frequent complication of this type of surgery. The nasogastric tube will be left in place until bowel peristalsis has returned. Children will then be gradually introduced to oral fluid and gradually will return to a normal diet. If the repair is successful, the stools of children change to a yellow and then brown (normal stool) color following surgery. Description of stools is therefore an important postoperative observation.

If bile flow is inadequate following surgery, a formula such as Portagen, which has medium chain fatty acids, may be started. Water-miscible vitamins may be necessary.

Cirrhosis

Cirrhosis is fibrotic scarring of the liver. Cirrhosis means "yellow" or the typical color of hepatic scar tissue. It occurs rarely in children, although it may be seen as a result of congenital biliary atresia or as a complication of

chronic illnesses such as protracted hepatitis, sickle cell anemia, or cystic fibrosis (Cochan, 1994).

When fibrotic infiltrates replace normal liver cells, liver function is impaired. There is decreased ability to detoxify toxic substances, decreased protein synthesis, inability to produce prothrombin, decreased ability to produce bile, and, possibly, hypoglycemia. Children will have large, fatty stools as a result of the decrease in bile production; avitaminosis of fat-soluble vitamins; symptoms of hemorrhage from decreased clotting ability; and anemia.

Fibrotic infiltration interferes not only with the function of liver cells but also with the hepatic blood flow. This leads to portal hypertension from the back pressure of blood that cannot flow readily through the scarred organ (Figure 45-7). Children will have compromised heart action; *ascites* (an exudate of fluid into the abdomen); possibly esophageal varices (back pressure causing them to dilate); and hypersplenism.

Once fibrotic infiltration begins, there is no way to reverse the changes. Nursing implementations are directed toward allowing children to be as comfortable as possible, providing adequate nutrition by a high-protein, high-carbohydrate, and medium-chain-triglyceride diet, and preventing further involvement until liver transplantation can be scheduled. Cholestyramine (Questran) may be prescribed to stimulate bile flow and reduce reabsorption of bile into the circulation (this will minimize jaundice).

Esophageal Varices

Esophageal varices can be a frequent complication of liver disorders such as cirrhosis. Varices are distended

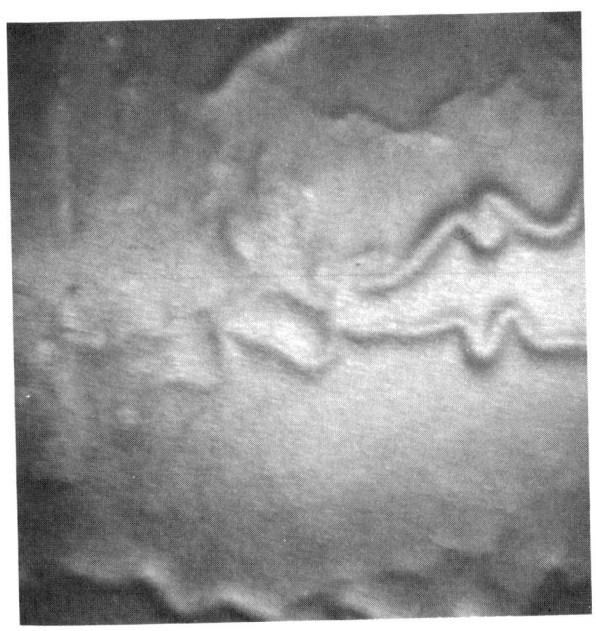

FIGURE 45-7
Tortuous veins on the abdomen from distortion of portal circulation with cirrhosis of the liver.

veins. Esophageal varices generally form at the distal end of the esophagus close to the stomach when there is back pressure on the veins from increased blood pressure in the portal circulation. Bleeding of varices may occur if children cough vigorously or strain to pass stool. Gastric reflux into the distal esophagus may irritate and erode the fine covering of the distended vessels and cause rupture.

Rupture of esophageal varices is an emergency situation; children can lose a large quantity of blood quickly from the ruptured, engorged vessels. Vasopressin or nitroglycerin may be given intravenously to lessen hypertension and reduce the hemorrhage (Teraes et al., 1990). Injection into veins to induce sclerosing may be attempted. Cold saline irrigation by nasogastric tube may be instituted to promote vasoconstriction. A Sengstaken-Blakemore tube or Linton-Nachlas catheter may be passed into the stomach. After it is inserted, balloons on the sides of the catheter are inflated and institute pressure against the bleeding vessels. As with an external tourniquet, the compression in such a catheter must be reduced for a 5- to 10-minute period every 6 hours to 8 hours, or tissue necrosis can result.

Children must be monitored for future bleeding episodes. Frequent vital sign measurements and testing of stool and any vomitus for the presence of blood will reveal new gastrointestinal system bleeding.

Liver Transplantation

Liver transplantation is the surgical replacement of a malfunctioning liver by a donor liver. Donor livers are not readily available and finding an acceptable child-sized liver may be a problem, although livers can be reduced in size for transplantation (Kocoshis et al., 1993). Often a child is extremely ill with ascites, gastrointestinal bleeding, extreme pruritus, hepatic encephalopathy, or renal dysfunction before the surgery can be accomplished. Nursing care after liver transplantation in a child is compounded because it involves taking care not only of a child who has had major surgery, but one who normally would be categorized as too ill to undergo surgery. Despite the severity of illness and the length of surgery, children tend to recover quickly after liver transplantation. Both children and parents must have thorough preoperative preparation so that they understand the seriousness of the surgery and the possibility that the graft will be rejected. It helps to introduce the parents to others whose children have successfully undergone the procedure so they have support people available.

Surgical Procedure

Liver transplantation requires a wide subcostal incision. The vena cava is temporarily clamped during the removal of the natural liver to prevent bleeding, which means that all intravenous lines must be placed in the upper extremities. Clamping the vena cava this way can result in renal failure due to the temporary halt of blood flow to the kidneys and dramatic shifts of fluid during surgery. The total operation takes 10 to 14 hours to complete.

Nursing Diagnoses and Related Interventions

Nursing care after liver transplantation surgery focuses on preventing complications that may arise from the surgery and postoperative medical management. Children require assisted ventilation for approximately 24 hours. Pulmonary complications such as atelectasis and pneumonia are likely to occur because the large abdominal incision makes deep breathing difficult. Ascites places pressure against the diaphragm, and pulmonary fluid may be present from presurgery edema. After extubation and discontinuation of ventilation, postural drainage may be begun to increase the mobility of lung secretions.

Assess blood pressure, capillary refilling, peripheral pulses, and skin color frequently in the postoperative period to be certain that cardiovascular function is adequate; this is important for good tissue perfusion of the transplanted liver. The child may have a central venous pressure line or Swan-Gantz catheter inserted to assess fluid and pressure adequacy further. Assess neurologic status hourly using a Glasgow coma scale (see Chapter 49).

The child is positioned flat for the first 24 hours to prevent cerebral air emboli from any air remaining in the transplanted liver. Children have a nasogastric tube inserted during surgery; it is attached to low suction postoperatively. Assess the gastric *p*H by aspirating stomach contents every 4 hours and, based on this assessment, administer antacids or cimetidine as prescribed to help prevent stress ulcer. If preoperative esophageal varices are present, nasogastric drainage must be assessed carefully for symptoms of bleeding (test the aspirated stomach contents with a Hemastix strip for occult blood). A T-tube for drainage allows the amount of bile being produced by the new liver to be evaluated. Liquids and then solid foods are introduced gradually after bowel sounds are present. If vomiting occurs persistently, total parenteral nutrition may be used for 3 or 4 days to rest the intestinal tract before fluid is reintroduced.

Hypoglycemia is a danger postoperatively because glucose levels are regulated by the liver and the transplanted organ may not function efficiently at first. Assess serum glucose levels hourly by finger puncture with a chemical test strip. A strong (10%) solution of dextrose may be necessary to prevent hypoglycemia.

Sodium, potassium, chloride, and calcium levels are evaluated approximately every 6 to 8 hours to be certain that an electrolyte balance is maintained. Even if a low potassium level is detected, potassium is rarely added to intravenous solutions because of the risk of renal failure due to the stress of surgery; if the graft begins to necrose, the breakdown of cells releases potassium, elevating the level. Children usually are monitored by electrocardiograph to detect hyperkalemia (hyperkalemia causes elevation of T waves or ventricular fibrillation; hypokalemia causes small T waves and the presence of a U wave).

The majority of children develop hypertension within 72 hours after surgery. This is due to alterations in the renin-angiotensin system of the transplanted liver, a side effect of cyclosporine and steroid therapy. Intravenous therapy with hypotensive agents such as hydralazine (Apresoline) and nitroprusside is usually necessary. Hypotension will occur if the transplanted liver becomes dysfunctional or there is bleeding due to poor blood coagulation. The child is high risk for bleeding because of the number of anastomosis sites included in the procedure. Observe and record abdominal girth, the incision line, and drainage from incision catheters to help detect bleeding (Gruppi et al., 1990).

Nursing Diagnosis: High risk for altered skin integrity related to possible presence of rectal hemorrhoids

Goal: Child will not experience any skin breakdown in rectal area.

Outcome Criteria: Skin remains intact.

Take axillary, not rectal, temperatures, because many children with liver damage have rectal hemorrhoids that could rupture from the trauma of a thermometer touching them. Maintain normal body temperature by preventing the child from being unnecessarily exposed during procedures. A warming blanket may be required postoperatively to maintain normal body temperature after the long exposure of surgery.

Nursing Diagnosis: High risk for infection related to administration of immunosuppressive medication

Goal: Child will not contract any infection while in hospital.

Outcome Criteria: Temperature remains within normal range; no presence of exudate or inflammation around abdominal incision.

Successful liver transplantation is possible because of the administration of cyclosporine A, which effectively suppresses T lymphocytes, the lymphocytes responsible for rejecting transplanted organs. Cyclosporine (Sandimmune) and steroids (Solu-Medrol) are administered intravenously immediately postoperatively to prevent rejection of the graft. Because children are prone to

infection while receiving immunosuppressive therapy, prevent their contracting an infection by using reverse isolation and careful hand washing. Clean the skin around any abdominal drains (usually a Jackson-Pratt) every 4 hours to prevent skin breakdown that opens a site for microorganisms to enter (Oleinik, 1990).

Children usually do not show signs of liver rejection until 5 to 7 days after surgery. Serum transaminases (SGOT and SGPT); alkaline phosphatase; serum bilirubin; and ammonia level are assessed daily to detect rejection. In addition to changes in these laboratory values, with liver rejection the child develops fever; abdominal width increases (from ascites); and the urine turns orange from increased urobilinogen excretion. If rejection appears to be occurring, doses of cyclosporine and steroids are increased to maximum levels.

Nursing Diagnosis: Altered family processes related to stress of surgery and unknown outcome of transplant

Goal: Child and family will demonstrate adequate coping techniques postoperatively.

Outcome Criteria: Child and family state that, although waiting is difficult, they are able to do so; identify ways they have changed their family life at home to accommodate child's illness and surgery.

Children and parents must have continued support during the postsurgery period while they wait to see if the graft will be rejected.

After successful liver transplantation, a child should be able to function normally, attending school and enjoying age-appropriate activities. Be certain by hospital discharge that parents have a return appointment for evaluation and are aware of the symptoms of graft rejection, such as jaundice, lethargy, and fever.

Intestinal Disorders

Intussusception

Intussusception is the invagination of one portion of the intestine into another (Figure 45-8). This generally occurs in the second half of the first year.

In infants younger than age 1 year, intussusception generally occurs for idiopathic reasons. In infants older than age 1 year, a "lead point" on the intestine likely cues the invagination. Such a point might be a Meckel's diverticulum; a polyp; hypertrophy of *Peyer's patches* (lymphatic tissue of the bowel that increases in size with viral diseases); or bowel tumors. The point of the invagination is generally the juncture of the distal ileum and proximal colon.

This condition is a surgical emergency: reduction of the intussusception must be done promptly by barium

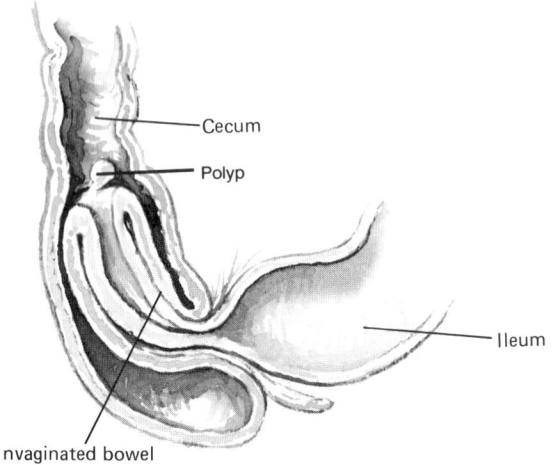

FIGURE 45-8
Intussusception. The distal ileal segment of bowel has invaginated into the cecum. A polyp serves as a lead point. (Courtesy of the Department of Medical Illustration, State University of New York at Buffalo, Buffalo, NY.)

enema or surgery before necrosis of the invaginated portion of the bowel results.

Assessment

Children with this disorder suddenly draw up their legs and cry as if they are in severe pain. They may vomit. Following the peristaltic wave that caused the discomfort, they are symptom free. They play happily. In approximately 15 minutes, the same phenomenon of intense abdominal pain strikes again. Vomitus will begin to contain bile because the obstruction is invariably below *Vater's ampulla,* the point in the intestine where bile empties into the duodenum. After approximately 12 hours, children develop blood in stool. This is described as having a "currant jelly" appearance. Their abdomen becomes distended as the bowel above the intussusception distends.

If necrosis has occurred, children generally have an increased temperature; peritoneal irritation (their abdomen will feel tender; they may "guard" it by tightening their abdominal muscles); an increased white blood cell count (WBC); and often a rapid pulse.

Diagnosis is suggested by the history. Any time a parent is describing a child who is crying, be certain to ask enough questions so that it is possible to recognize a history of intussusception. What is the duration of the pain? (It lasts a short time with intervals of no crying in between.) What is the intensity? (Severe.) What is the frequency? (Approximately every 15 to 20 minutes.) What is the description? (The child pulls up his or her legs with crying.) Is the child ill in any other way? (Yes. Vomits; refuses food; complains of his or her stomach feeling "full.")

Therapeutic Management

Therapy of intussusception is surgery to remove the invaginated portion, or reduction of the intussusception by a water-soluble solution or barium enema. A newer technique is to use air (pneumatic insufflation) (Zheng et al., 1994). If there is no lead point, just the pressure of a barium enema may successfully reduce the intussusception. Following a barium enema reduction, children are observed for 24 hours because a number of children will have a recurrence of the intussusception within 24 hours.

Nursing Diagnoses and Related Interventions

Nursing Diagnosis: High risk for pain related to abnormal abdominal peristalsis

Goal: Child's pain will be at a tolerable level throughout illness.

Outcome Criteria: Child is able to be comforted between spasms of pain.

Infants with intussusception have episodes of acute pain. They are bewildered by this type of pain because it is so different from any they have experienced before. Ordinarily, if they pinch a finger on a toy and it hurts, a parent picks them up, kisses their fingers, and the pain goes away. A parent picks them up now and the pain goes away; but it returns repeatedly. Infants need to be held and rocked and comforted in an attempt to relieve their frustration at this strange happening.

Nursing Diagnosis: High risk for fluid volume deficit related to bowel obstruction

Goal: Infant to maintain adequate fluid volume until bowel obstruction is relieved.

Outcome Criteria: Infant's skin turgor is good; pulse is 90 beats/min to 100 beats/min. Amount of diarrhea and blood loss in stool is minimal.

Preoperative Care. Infants are kept on NPO status before surgery. Because they have abdominal pain, they may find comfort in sucking a pacifier. Because they have been vomiting before admission to the hospital, they need to have an intravenous infusion begun promptly to reestablish their electrolyte balance and to supply adequate fluid to hydrate them.

Postoperative Care. Infants will return from surgery with a nasogastric tube in place and an intravenous infusion running. The nasogastric tube will remain in place until the suture line is healing and peristaltic function has returned. Infants will be introduced to oral feedings on a gradual schedule.

Nursing Diagnosis: High risk for altered parenting related to infant's illness

Goal: Parents will demonstrate adequate bonding behavior with the infant before and after surgery.

Outcome Criteria: Parents hold and talk to infant; express positive characteristics about infant.

Parents need to feed and hold infants postoperatively so that they have an opportunity to regain confidence in themselves as parents again. They need to be assured that this did not occur because of anything they did. Whenever a child's disorder begins with vomiting, many parents worry that the vomiting is somehow related to the child's method of feeding. They need to hold and be with the child as recovery occurs to reassure themselves that the child is now all right again.

Volvulus

A **volvulus** is a twisting of the intestine (Figure 45-9). The twist leads to obstruction of the passage of feces and compromise of the blood supply to the loop of intestine involved. This occurs most often because, in fetal

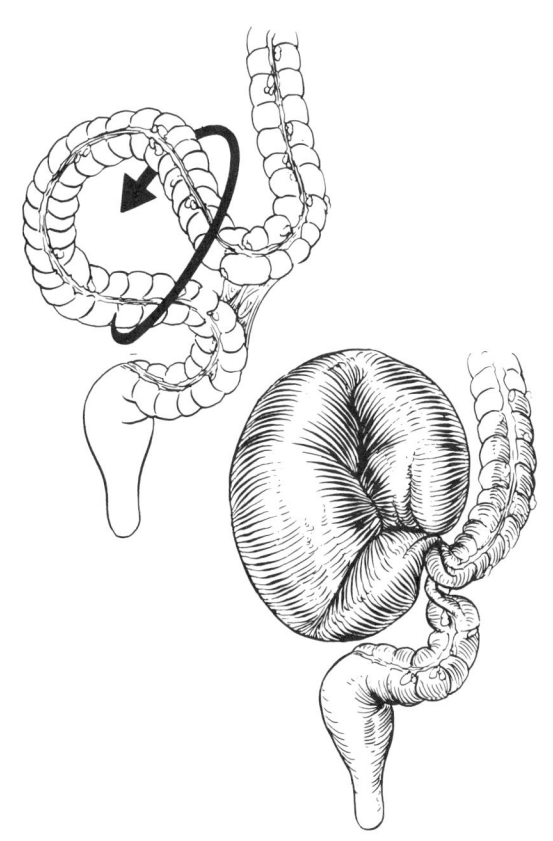

FIGURE 45-9
Volvulus of the sigmoid colon. (From Way, L. W. [Ed.]. [1985]. Current surgical diagnosis and treatment [7th ed.]. Los Altos, CA: Lange Medical Publications, with permission.)

life, a portion of the intestine first protrudes into the base of the umbilical cord at approximately age 6 weeks. At approximately age 10 weeks, it returns to the abdominal cavity. As the intestine returns to the abdominal cavity, it rotates to its permanent position. After the rotation, the mesentery becomes fixed in this position. In an instance of volvulus, the action is incomplete, so that the mesentery does not attach to a normal position. The bowel is left free to move and twist.

The symptoms are those of intestinal obstruction and usually occur during the first 6 months of life: intense crying and pain, pulling up the legs, abdominal distention, and vomiting. Diagnosis is made on the history and on abdominal examination, which reveals the abdominal mass. A barium x-ray also will demonstrate the obstruction. Treatment is surgery to relieve the volvulus and reattach the bowel so that it is no longer so free moving. This must be done promptly before necrosis of the intestine occurs from a lack of blood supply to the involved loop of bowel. Preoperative and postoperative care will be the same as for infants with intussusception.

Necrotizing Enterocolitis

Necrotizing enterocolitis (NEC) is a condition that develops in approximately 5% of all infants in intensive care nurseries. The bowel develops necrotic patches, interfering with digestion and possibly leading to a paralytic ileus. Perforation and peritonitis may follow.

The necrosis appears to result from ischemic or poor perfusion of blood vessels in sections of bowel. The ischemic process may occur when, owing to shock or hypoxia, there is vasoconstriction of blood vessels to nonessential organs such as the bowel. The entire bowel may be involved, or it may be a localized phenomenon. The incidence of NEC is highest in immature infants and those who have suffered anoxia or shock. Infants with infections may develop it as a further complication of their already stressed state.

Assessment

Signs that the condition is beginning usually appear in the first week of life. The abdomen becomes distended and tense. The infant does not empty the stomach by the next feeding time because of poor intestinal action, so if stomach contents are aspirated before a gavage feeding, a return of undigested milk of more than 2 mL will be obtained. Stool may be positive for occult blood. Periods of apnea may begin, or increase in number if they were already present. Signs of blood loss due to intestinal bleeding such as lowered blood pressure and inability to stabilize temperature may be present.

Abdominal x-ray films reveal a characteristic picture of air invading the intestinal wall; if perforation has occurred, there will be air in the abdominal cavity. That the abdomen is increasing in size can be ascertained by measuring the abdominal circumference every 4 to 8 hours. The measurement is made just above the umbilicus.

Therapeutic Management

The infant may need a temporary colostomy performed to relieve obstruction. If the area of necrosis appears to be localized, surgery to remove that portion of the bowel may be successful. If a large portion of the bowel is removed, the infant may be prone to "short-bowel" syndrome or have a problem with digestion of nutrients in the future.

NEC is a grave insult to an infant already stressed by immaturity. The prognosis is guarded until it can be demonstrated that the infant can again take oral feedings without bowel complication.

There is a lower incidence of the condition in infants who are fed breast milk than in those who are formula fed. Intestinal organisms grow more profusely with cow's milk than breast milk because cow's milk lacks antibodies. A response to the foreign protein in cow's milk may be a mechanism that starts the necrotic process. Encouraging breastfeeding, therefore, may prevent the disorder from developing.

Gavage or bottle feedings must be discontinued as soon as the condition is recognized, and the infant maintained on intravenous or total parenteral nutrition solutions to rest the gastrointestinal tract. A course of an antibiotic may be given to limit secondary infection. The abdomen must be handled gently to lessen the possibility of bowel perforation. Testing stool for occult blood helps determine whether the bowel is healing.

Appendicitis

Appendicitis is inflammation of the appendix. This is the most common cause of abdominal surgery in children. It is seen most frequently in school-age children, although it can occur even in newborns. The *appendix*, a blind-end pouch attached to the cecum, may become inflamed following an upper respiratory or other body infection, but the cause of appendicitis is generally obscure. In most instances, fecal material apparently enters the appendix, and hardens and obstructs the appendix lumen. Inflammation and edema develop, leading to compression of blood vessels, shutting off nutrition to appendix cells. Necrosis and pain result. If the condition is not discovered early enough, the necrotic area will rupture, and fecal material will burst out of the appendix, causing peritonitis—a potentially fatal condition.

Assessment

Most people assume that appendicitis begins with sharp pain, so they may dismiss their children's early symp-

toms for some time as a simple gastroenteritis. Actually, pain is a late symptom in appendicitis. The history typically begins with anorexia for 12 to 24 hours. Children do not eat and "just do not act like themselves." They may then report nausea and vomiting. The abdominal pain, when it does start, is at first diffuse. Gradually, it becomes localized to the right lower quadrant. The point of sharpest pain is often one-third of the way between the anterior superior iliac crest and the umbilicus (*McBurney's point*). If the child's appendix is displaced from the usual position, the pain will not be at this typical point, so pain at any other point does not rule out appendicitis. Fever is a late symptom. On laboratory findings, children usually have leukocytosis (WBC between 10,000 to 18,000 per cubic millimeter), which is actually low for the extent of the infection that may be present. Acetone in the urine is inordinately elevated as a symptom of starvation from poor intestinal absorption. It is important in history taking to document the progress of the disease. How was Joan on Monday? (Not herself. She was not eating.) How was she Monday night? (Had generalized abdominal pain.) Tuesday morning? (Had sharp localized pain.) Now? (Has localized pain, vomiting, and fever.) Until the pain becomes localized, appendicitis is difficult to distinguish from acute gastroenteritis. On abdominal examination, right lower quadrant tenderness may be elicited. It is difficult to palpate children's abdomens because they guard their abdomen and make it stiff and hard by tensing their abdominal muscles. Although this interferes with abdominal examination, it is in itself an important sign that children have abdominal pain. To assist in a diagnosis of a painful abdomen, always begin palpating a tender abdomen first at the portion where it is not tender. Approach the tender area gradually.

Rebound tenderness is a phenomenon in which the child feels relatively mild pain when the area over his or her appendix is palpated, but once the examiner's hand is withdrawn, the child experiences acute pain caused by the shifting of the abdominal contents. This is diagnostic for appendicitis, but should be done with children only when absolutely necessary because it does cause acute pain. Caution children that the maneuver may cause pain so that they do not lose confidence in health care personnel. On auscultation, bowel sounds will be reduced. Only one or two are heard in the same length of time 30 are normally heard. If there are no bowel sounds on auscultation, this suggests peritonitis, or an appendix that has already ruptured.

A rectal examination is done in addition to abdominal examination to establish the diagnosis of appendicitis. For this, a gloved finger is inserted gently into the rectum and then moved to the child's right. As it touches the area of the appendix, the tenderness will be acute. Pain in the right lower quadrant may occur as a manifestation of right lower lobe pneumonia. Therefore children may have a chest x-ray taken to rule out this source of pain. An abdominal sonogram may be taken to rule out a possible obstruction or possibly reveal a hardened fecal impaction and inflammation of the appendix.

Therapeutic Management

Therapy for appendicitis is surgical removal of the appendix before it ruptures. Achieving surgery before rupture occurs is easier in older children, who are more capable of relating the progression of symptoms. It is more difficult in young children, whose history is not as accurate, who do not have the words to describe their symptoms, or who will not relax their abdominal muscles enough to allow for manual examination. Also, the wall of the appendix is thinner and perforates more readily in young children. Appendicitis may be diagnosed and the inflamed appendix removed by laparoscopy (Miller, 1993). This shortens the hospital course and the amount of postoperative pain.

Nursing Diagnoses and Related Interventions

Goals for nursing care must be established quickly because this is an emergency situation and the child must be prepared immediately for surgery (see the Nursing Care Plan: A Toddler With Appendicitis, p. 1403).

Nursing Diagnosis: Pain related to inflamed appendix

Goal: Child will not experience pain above a tolerable level throughout course of therapy.

Outcome Criteria: Child voices that level of pain is tolerable.

In the period before surgery, analgesics must not be given because they obscure diagnostic signs such as tenderness and localizing pain. Cathartics and heat to the abdomen are also contraindicated because they may lead to rupture of the appendix. In adolescents, the abdomen and perineum must be shaved and washed with an antiseptic solution (unless this will be done in surgery). Be gentle with such a procedure. The abdomen is tender to touch and compression could cause an appendix to rupture. Use lukewarm, not hot water, because heat can increase the possibility of appendix rupture by increasing edema in the appendix.

Nursing Diagnosis: Parent and child fear related to emergency hospital procedure and potential outcome

Goal: Both parents and child will demonstrate confidence in health care providers during hospital stay.

Outcome Criteria: Parents and child voice they

understand what interventions are necessary and cooperate as necessary.

Admission for appendicitis occurs rapidly. A parent telephones the physician, who recommends hospitalization; the child is seen in the emergency room and scheduled for surgery. A mere 30 minutes may have passed from the time of the first phone call until a child is wheeled to surgery. The parent and child both need to be told exactly what is happening ("I'm going to take some blood; I'm putting your name tag on your arm"); they need to be told exactly who the people are who are caring for them ("This is Dr. Brown, the anesthesiologist. I'm Ms. Henry, a registered nurse.") Parents do not think clearly in this type of emergency, and their reactions to situations are not their usual reactions. Before antibiotics were available, a ruptured appendix meant certain death for children because of the resultant peritonitis. Parents are aware of many old tales ("His appendix ruptured 2 minutes before they got him to surgery and he died . . ."). They often leave food cooking on the stove or in the oven; some scoop up ill children so quickly to bring them to the hospital that they leave other children unattended at home; some of them park their cars in the center of the street in front of the hospital. They need some help to take a few minutes to think whether they have done any of these things. Explain that the procedures being done for their child (e.g., blood studies or a short wait while a surgery room is prepared) are necessary for safe surgery and that the danger of the appendix rupturing is not as acute a danger as they may have believed.

Remember that these children have had no preparation for hospitalization. The axiom "What they don't know won't hurt them" is not true of hospitalization. The fear of strange people and the strange situation hurts. Appendicitis is such a harrowing experience for both parents and children that, during the postoperative period, they may need some time to talk about how worried or frightened they were to learn of the diagnosis and a chance to work through these few days in their life so that they can put them in better perspective. Some parents are embarrassed by how rude they were to personnel on admission when they were so frightened that they misunderstood or misinterpreted a direction or explanation. They can be assured that no one is at their best in an emergency situation and can be praised for those things they did do well (recognized their child was ill and brought the child immediately for care).

Nursing Diagnosis: High risk for fluid volume deficit related to NPO status

Goal: Child will remain well hydrated during treatment period.

Outcome Criteria: Child's skin turgor is good;

pulse and blood pressure are within normal age limits; no weight loss occurs.

Obtain a urine sample for urinalysis and blood for a complete blood count preoperatively. An intravenous infusion to hydrate the child and maintain electrolyte balance needs to be begun. If children have been vomiting a great deal, they may need several hours of intravenous therapy before a balance of electrolytes is achieved and they are good candidates for surgery.

Following surgery, children will return with a nasogastric tube in place; they will be maintained on intravenous fluids until they can take adequate oral feedings (approximately 24 hours). With unruptured appendicitis, the postoperative course is uneventful; children are up a few hours after surgery and are discharged within a number of days. They generally return to school in another week.

Ruptured Appendix

If a child's appendix has already ruptured when admitted to the hospital or ruptures before emergency preparation for surgery can be made, the potential for peritonitis is great. When rupture occurs, children generally appear prostrate; WBC rises to more than 20,000 per cubic millimeter. Position them in a semi-Fowler's position so that infected drainage from the cecum drains downward into the pelvis rather than upward to the lungs to better contain it. They need a fluid line inserted for hydration; antibiotics will be begun preoperatively or at the point the ruptured appendix is confirmed.

Following surgery, children will have drains placed beside the surgery incision so any infectious material in the abdomen can continue to drain. Warm soaks to these dressings may be ordered three or four times a day to encourage drainage. Examine the wound carefully at each dressing change. Be certain not to dislodge drains while removing soiled dressings; report immediately any drain that is expelled; the surgeon may want to replace it to ensure a patent drainage route. Often drains are shortened with each dressing change to encourage initially deep areas, then areas closer to the skin to drain. Intravenous fluid and antibiotic therapy will be continued for as long as 7 to 10 days because it will be this long before full bowel function is restored (Putnam et al., 1990).

Signs of peritonitis include a boardlike (rigid) abdomen; generally shallow respirations (because breathing deeply puts pressure on the abdomen and causes pain); and increased temperature; these signs should be watched for closely during the postoperative period. Although the postoperative course is slower (approximately 3 weeks) following a ruptured appendix, the prognosis is still good. A local abscess or intestinal adhesions may result. A long-term effect could be that adhesion formation could interfere with fertility in females or cause bowel obstruction in both sexes later in life.

Meckel's Diverticulum

In embryonic life, the intestine is attached to the umbilicus by the omphalomesenteric (vitelline) duct. This duct becomes a vestigial ligament as infants reach term. In 2% or 3% of all infants, a small pouch off the ileum, approximately 18 inches from the ileum-colon junction, remains: a **Meckel's diverticulum**. In this structure, there may be some misplaced gastric mucosa, which secretes gastric acids that flow into the intestine and are irritating to the bowel wall. Ulceration and bleeding may result. Infants will have painless, tar-like (black) stools or grossly bloody stools. On occasion, the diverticulum may serve as a lead point and cause an intussusception. In some instances, a fibrous band extending from the diverticulum pouch to the umbilicus acts as a constricting band, causing bowel obstruction. The history of the child suggests the diagnosis. Because the pouch is small, it does not fill and, therefore, may not be evident on x-ray. Treatment is surgical exploration and removal of the vestigial structure.

Celiac Disease (Malabsorption Syndrome; Gluten-Induced Enteropathy)

Although gluten-induced enteropathy is a relatively rare condition, early recognition is essential to therapy and to provide early support and nutritional guidance for the parents. The illness occurs most frequently in children of a northern European background. It is apparently a dominantly inherited illness; incomplete penetrance results in children having different degrees of involvement. It is associated with Down syndrome and diabetes mellitus. The basic problem in **celiac disease** is a sensitivity or immunologic response to protein, particularly the gluten factor of protein found in grains—wheat, rye, oats, and barley. When such children ingest gluten, changes occur in the intestinal mucosa or villi that prevent the absorption of foods across the intestinal villi into the bloodstream. Children develop most noticeably an inability to absorb fat. Due to this, they develop **steatorrhea** (bulky, foul-smelling, fatty stools); deficiency of fat-soluble vitamins A, D, K, and E (the vitamins are not absorbed because the fat is not absorbed); malnutrition; and a distended abdomen from the fat, bulky stools (Figure 45-10). Because vitamin D is one of the fat-soluble vitamins, rickets may occur. Hypoprothrombinemia may occur from loss of vitamin K. In addition, children may have hypochromic anemia (iron deficiency anemia) and hypoalbuminemia from poor protein absorption.

Assessment

Children tend to be anorectic and irritable. They gradually fall behind other children their age in height and weight. They appear skinny with spindly extremities and wasted buttocks. Their face, however, in contrast to chil-

Nursing Care Plan
A Toddler With Appendicitis

Etta is a 2-year-old girl who was diagnosed as having a ruptured appendix; the following is a nursing care plan designed for her.

Assessment: Black, obviously distressed, well-proportioned female. Mother states Etta woke this morning looking listless and "not well." Refused all but orange juice and toast for breakfast. At 10 AM, Etta vomited small amount undigested food. Since 11 AM, has been crying that her "tummy hurts"; sits on mother's lap with legs pulled up against abdomen. Temperature 101.8°F axillary; rebound tenderness in lower right quadrant present; no bowel sounds present.

Nursing Diagnosis: Altered family processes related to emergency illness in child

Defining Characteristic: Mother states that she is concerned.

Goal: Parents will demonstrate adequate coping behavior during course of illness.

Outcome Criteria: Child and parents state they are able to cope with level of stress at this time.

Nursing Orders (Preoperative)	Rationale
1. Project a calm, controlled manner; explain cause of appendicitis and planned interventions.	1. Education can help with reducing anxiety and acceptance of surgery.
2. See that informed consent for surgery is obtained.	2. Even with emergency procedures, consent must be obtained.
3. Allow time for parents to discuss and work through anxiety over sudden surgery.	3. Discussion can help reduce level of anxiety.
4. Review use of nasogastric tube and intravenous fluid so parents understand therapy.	4. Education can help with acceptance of procedures.
5. Praise parents' recognition of child's symptoms and their coping ability in emergency.	5. Increasing self-esteem can aid with adjustment to emergency situation.

Nursing Diagnosis: High risk for infection related to ruptured appendix

Defining Characteristic: Ruptured appendix invariably leads to peritonitis.

Goal: Child will not develop infection in postoperative period although appendix is ruptured.

Outcome Criteria: No signs of peritonitis (e.g., pain, high temperature) are present. Abdomen soft; temperature below 99°F axillary.

Nursing Orders	Rationale
1. Document gradual progression of symptoms, time since child last ate (if recently, anesthesia is a risk); and if parent administered an analgesic for pain (could be masking amount of pain present).	1. Documentation of signs and symptoms assists in diagnosis of appendicitis.
2. Avoid palpating abdomen except as necessary to assist with diagnosis.	2. Palpating could lead to ruptured appendix.
3. Obtain a urine specimen for urinalysis and blood sample for complete blood count.	3. Establishes baseline values preoperatively.
4. Assess temperature, pulse, and respiration.	4. Establishes baseline values.
5. Do not apply heat to abdomen.	5. Heat could lead to rupture of appendix.
6. Do not administer an enema, laxative, or analgesia.	6. An enema or laxative could lead to rupture; analgesic could mask extent of pain.
7. Maintain position of comfort (often with legs drawn up onto abdomen).	7. Provides comfort measure for pain.

(continued)

Nursing Orders (Postoperative)	Rationale
1. Assess abdomen for softness.	1. Abdominal hardness is a sign of peritonitis.
2. Position in semi-Fowler's position.	2. Helps to contain any possible infectious material in lower abdomen.
3. Administer antibiotics as prescribed.	3. Helps prevent infection.
4. Apply Montgomery straps to sides of abdomen.	4. Protects skin integrity from frequent dressing changes.
5. Observe incision for inflammation and drainage.	5. Detects beginning signs of infection.
6. Initiate wound isolation precautions if drainage is present.	6. Protects spread of infection to personnel or other children.
7. Change dressing as ordered; protect drains (if present) when removing dressing; advance drains as prescribed.	7. Reduces level of contaminated drainage against suture line.
8. Child wears diapers; keep diaper folded below dressing.	8. Prevents infection of suture line.
9. Assess vital signs every 4 hours.	9. Detects signs of infection.

Nursing Diagnosis: High risk for altered nutrition: less than body requirements, related to bowel surgery

Defining Characteristic: Child has been ordered NPO.

Goal: Child will receive adequate nutrition.

Outcome Criteria: Child's weight is maintained in same percentile on growth curve; skin turgor is good.

Nursing Orders	Rationale
1. Maintain NPO as prescribed.	1. Reducing fluid intake can reduce vomiting with surgery anesthesia.
2. Assist with intravenous therapy; keep restraints in place to prevent child from dislodging needle.	2. Intravenous therapy can help restore fluid volume deficit.
3. Nasogastric tube will be present postoperatively; assess drainage of nasogastric tube q 1 h.	3. Monitoring for obstruction is important.
4. Assess for bowel sounds q 2 h postoperatively.	4. Bowel sounds indicate that bowel tone is returning.
5. Introduce oral fluids gradually when prescribed.	5. Prevents vomiting with reintroduction of fluid.
6. Maintain record of intake and output.	6. Documents fluid balance.

(continued)

dren with true starvation, may be plump and well-appearing.

Symptoms become noticeable between 6 and 18 months of age. Diagnosis is based on history; clinical symptoms; serum analysis of IgA antigliadin antibodies; and a biopsy of intestinal mucosa (done by endoscopy), which establishes the typical changes in intestinal villi (Valletta et al., 1990). Children may have a serum D-xylose absorption test to demonstrate that the intestine does not absorb nutrients. Stool may be collected for fat content.

In addition, response to gluten is observed by placing children on a gluten-free diet. In most instances, the response to this diet is dramatic. Children begin to gain weight, there is improvement in the steatorrhea, and the irritability fades (Kelly et al., 1990).

Therapeutic Management

Treatment is to continue children on a gluten-free diet for life because there is some suggestion that they are more prone to gastrointestinal carcinoma later in life if they do not continue the diet into adulthood. In addition

Nursing Diagnosis: High risk for ineffective airway clearance related to pooling of secretions from inactivity

Defining Characteristic: Stasis of any body fluid leads to infection.

Goal: Child's airway will remain patent during course of illness.

Outcome Criteria: Child's respiration rate is between 16/min and 20/min; no rales are heard on chest auscultation.

Nursing Orders	Rationale
1. Encourage deep breathing and turning every 2 hours (abdomen is painful so this is difficult).	1. Encourages air exchange.
2. Incorporate games as necessary to ensure cooperation.	2. Child is 2 years old and does not understand necessity for airway clearance.
3. Perform spirometry, percussion, and vibration as prescribed.	3. Provides methods of increasing air exchange.
4. Ambulate as early as prescribed.	4. Ambulation aids in effective air exchange.

Nursing Diagnosis: Pain related to surgical incision

Defining Characteristic: Surgical incisions always cause pain

Goal: Child will experience a tolerable level of pain.

Outcome Criteria: Child will state that level of pain is tolerable.

Nursing Orders	Rationale
1. Administer analgesia as prescribed and necessary.	1. Provides a means to reduce pain.
2. Support abdomen when turning.	2. Support can help reduce pain.

to this, children need to have water-miscible forms of vitamins A and D administered. Both iron and folate may also be necessary to correct any anemia present.

Nursing Diagnoses and Related Interventions

Be certain that goals established are realistic for the disease process. Villi changes cannot be made to heal instantly; parents can learn about a gluten-free diet immediately.

Nursing Diagnosis: Altered nutrition; less than body requirements related to malabsorption of food

Goal: Child will receive adequate nutritional intake on gluten-free diet.

Outcome Criteria: Child's weight is maintained on a percentile curve on a growth chart; skin turgor is good; steatorrhea is minimal.

Parents need a great deal of nutritional counseling when children are first placed on a gluten-free diet so

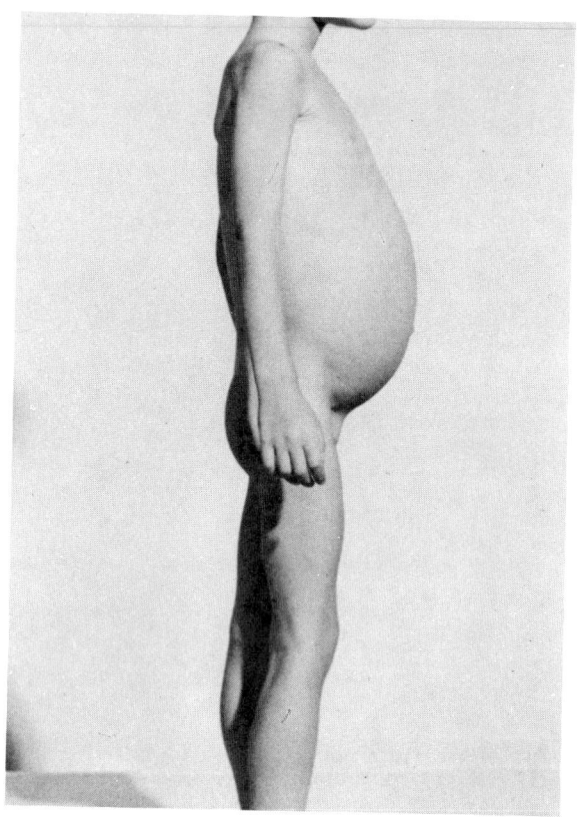

FIGURE 45-10
A child with celiac disease. Notice the extremely enlarged abdomen and the wasted extremities. (Courtesy of the Department of Medical Photography, Children's Hospital, Buffalo, NY.)

that they can recognize foods that contain gluten (i.e., wheat, rye, oats, and barley products). Guidelines for a gluten-free diet are shown in Table 45-7. Because gluten is a part of wheat flour, gravy, soups, sauces, and packaged and frozen foods usually contain gluten as fillers. Teach parents to be careful shoppers and read food labels carefully. Because children are anorectic when they are first introduced to the diet, getting them to eat it may be a problem. Remember that small servings are often eaten better by toddlers than large servings. If hospitalized, they need to eat where they are most comfortable: at a table with other toddlers or alone in their room with their parents or a nurse. Inviting dolls to "tea" or eating a picnic outside in nice weather might be incentives to eat. Accept anger at no longer being able to eat favorite foods such as hot dogs.

Chart carefully the consistency, appearance, size and number of stools children pass because the disappearance of steatorrhea is a good indicator that children's ability to absorb nutrients is improving. As children reach school age, preparing a diet grows more and more difficult, because favorite foods (e.g., spaghetti, pizza, hot dogs, cake, and cookies) are not allowed. Selecting a diet in a school cafeteria may be impossible. Holidays pose special problems—birthday cake, turkey stuffing, and holiday cookies are prohibited. Children

need to learn to recognize sources of gluten by early school age. Until they are able to recognize which foods they can or cannot eat, their parents cannot feel safe in letting them stay at friend's houses or go to summer camp—activities important to children's learning independence. Following approximately 12 months of a gluten-free diet, children may be challenged with gluten to assess the need to continue the diet.

> ***Nursing Diagnosis:*** Altered family processes related to chronic disease in the child
>
> ***Goal:*** Parents will demonstrate continuing adequate coping behaviors.
>
> ***Outcome Criteria:*** Parents express feelings about their child's disease to nurses; voice realistic plans for how they intend to care for child at home.

Encourage parents to spend time with children. Because they have been fussy, irritable children, parents may tend to hold and rock them a great deal, not allowing them time to explore and learn on their own as much as they would like. Some parents may have become so impatient with their children because nothing they did for them made them happy that they do not hold and comfort them as much as they should. Spending time with children as their children's dispositions improves helps parents find a middle ground of satisfying care. As children's dispositions improve, they find it more enjoyable to be with them.

Celiac Crisis

When children with celiac disease develop any type of infection, a crisis of extreme symptoms may occur. Both vomiting and diarrhea will become acute. Children can quickly move into electrolyte and fluid imbalance and need intensive therapy to replace electrolytes and fluids (see nursing care for children with vomiting and diarrhea earlier in chapter). Gradually, following such an episode, they are placed back on a high-protein, low-fat, gluten-free diet.

Disorders of the Lower Bowel

Constipation

Constipation, or difficulty passing hardened stools, may occur in children of any age. Constipation is distressing to a child because passing hardened stool is painful and may cause anal fissures. The child then represses the next urge to defecate because of pain. The rectum gradually becomes distended and adjusts to the ever-present bulk of stool. The urge to defecate becomes less frequent. When the child does pass stool, it is larger and firmer than before and causes even more anal pain. This vicious cycle continues until the child becomes severely constipated. Children may have episodes of diarrhea or *encopresis* (involuntary release of stool) when their rec-

Table 45-7. *Gluten-Restricted Diet*

Food Group	Foods Allowed	Foods to Avoid
Note: Because many processed foods contain wheat, rye, oats, barley, or flours from these grains, *labels should be read carefully*.		
Beverages	Milk, carbonated beverages, fruit-flavored beverages	Cereal beverages; malted milk
Breads	Breads made from cornmeal; corn, potato, rice, soybean, tapioca, and arrowroot flours	All bread and crackers containing wheat, rye, oats, or barley
Cereals	Cornmeal, rice, precooked rice cereal, dry cereals containing only rice or corn	All cooked and prepared cereals containing wheat, rye, oats, barley, malt, bran, or wheat germ
Desserts	Custard; gelatin desserts; fruit ice; puddings, cakes, cookies, and other desserts made with allowed flours or starches	Cakes, cookies, pastries, or commercial pudding mixes containing restricted flours; ice cream cones; fruit sauces thickened with wheat flour; commercial ice cream or sherbet containing a wheat stabilizer
Eggs	Baked, poached, soft or hard cooked, scrambled, fried	Creamed eggs, soufflé, or fondue unless made with allowed flours
Fats	Butter, margarine, cream, vegetable oils and shortenings, lard, bacon, salad dressings thickened with allowed flours or starches	Salad dressings or gravies containing wheat, rye, oats, or barley
Fruits, fruit juices	All fresh, frozen, canned, and dried	None
Meat, fish, poultry, cheese	Baked, broiled, roasted, or steamed beef, lamb, liver, pork, veal, poultry, fish; cottage cheese, cream cheese, nonprocessed cheeses	Meat, fish, poultry, or cheese products containing restricted cereals (the following foods frequently contain these cereals: meatloaf, meat patties; breaded meat, fish, or poultry; canned meat products; cold cuts unless guaranteed all meat; cheese spreads)
Potatoes or substitutes	White and sweet potatoes, rice, hominy, potato chips	Creamed or scalloped potatoes unless made with allowed flours, macaroni, noodles, spaghetti
Soups	Broth-based and cream soups made from allowed foods	Soups containing wheat, rye, oats, barley, or products made from these grains; soups thickened with flour
Sugar, sweets	Sugar, syrup, honey, jelly, molasses, candy, chocolate, chewing gum	Commercial candies containing wheat, rye, oats, barley, or malt
Vegetables, vegetable juices	All fresh, frozen, and canned	None
Miscellaneous	Salt, flavorings, spices, cider vinegar, peanut butter, coconut, popcorn, olives, pickles, catsup, mustard, chocolate, cocoa powder, gravy or cream sauce if thickened with allowed flours or starches	Pretzels, distilled white vinegar, gravy thickened with flours or starches other than allowed

Sample Menu for Gluten-Restricted Diet

Breakfast	Lunch	Dinner
1/2 cup orange juice	2 oz sliced chicken	3 oz roast beef
1/2 cup cream of rice cereal	1/2 cup rice	1/2 cup cubed white potato
1 egg, soft cooked	1/2 cup green beans	1/2 cup cooked carrots
Cornmeal muffin	1/2 sliced tomato on lettuce	3/4 cup tossed lettuce salad
1 tsp butter or margarine	Rice muffin	1 tbsp french dressing
1 cup 2% milk	1 tsp butter or margarine	Rice muffin
2 tsp sugar	Puffed rice bar	1 cup 2% milk
Coffee or tea	1 cup 2% milk	Coffee or tea
	Coffee or tea	

(From Dietary Department, University of Iowa. [1989]. *Recent advances in therapeutic diets* [4th ed.]. Ames, IA: Iowa State University Press.)

tum can hold no more. They may have abdominal pain from forceful intestinal contractions.

Some children begin holding stool for emotional reasons. Once the process begins, however, the hardened stool, the anal fissures, and the pain on defecation soon occur, and what began for an emotional reason becomes a physical ailment. This is important to understand, because with these children, the therapy is never just counseling to correct the initial problem but treatment of the physical symptoms as well.

Assessment

When taking a history of the condition, be certain to have parents describe what they mean by constipation. Some children have normal defecation habits of passing stool only every other day or even every 3 days. As long as the stool is not hard and there is no discomfort associated with passing stool, this is not constipation.

Children with constipation should be examined carefully to see if they have anal fissures. Constipation must be differentiated from aganglionic disease of the intestine. In constipation, on rectal examination, hard stool will be found in the rectum; in aganglionic disease of the intestine, no stool will normally be present.

Therapeutic Management

Treatment of chronic constipation is aimed at softening stool, so that it will pass painlessly, and helping children to form bowel habits so that they evacuate their bowels frequently enough that stool does not tend to become large and hardened before evacuation.

Nursing Diagnoses and Related Interventions

> **Nursing Diagnosis:** Constipation related to pain from anal fissure
>
> **Goal:** Child will achieve a normal elimination pattern by 2 weeks.
>
> **Outcome Criteria:** Child has a soft bowel movement without pain every other day.

For initial therapy, children may need an enema administered to loosen hard stool. Following this, a stool softener such as docusate sodium (Colace) is prescribed. Children need to ingest a high fiber, high fluid diet and be urged to evacuate their bowels at the same time every day to form a habit.

Hiatal Hernia

Hiatal hernia is the intermittent protrusion of the stomach through the esophageal opening in the diaphragm (Ellis, 1990). When this occurs, the volume of the stomach is suddenly restricted, leading to periodic vomiting very similar to that of gastroesophageal reflux. A difference is that with a hiatal hernia, pain usually accompanies the vomiting. Shortness of breath may occur from compression of the lung space by the stomach.

Hiatal hernia is diagnosed by history and a sonogram or barium swallow. A baby can be kept in an upright position to help prevent the condition; if it has not corrected itself by the time the infant is six months old and has been maintained in an upright position most of the day, surgery may be performed to reduce the size of the esophageal opening in the diaphragm.

Inguinal Hernia

Inguinal hernia is a protrusion of a section of the bowel into the inguinal ring. It occurs usually in males because as the testes descend from the abdominal cavity into the scrotum late in fetal life, a fold of parietal peritoneum also descends, forming a tube from the abdomen to the scrotum. In most infants, this tube closes completely. If it fails to close, descent of the intestine into it (hernia) may occur at any time when there is an increase in intra-abdominal pressure. In girls, the round ligament extends from the uterus into the inguinal canal to its attachment on the abdominal wall; an inguinal hernia may occur in girls due to a weakness of the muscle surrounding the round ligament.

Assessment

The hernia appears as a lump in the groin; about 60 percent of the time, this occurs on the right side. In some instances, the hernia is apparent only on crying (when abdominal pressure increases), and not when children are less active. Inguinal hernias are painless. Pain at the site implies that the bowel has become incarcerated in the sac, an emergency situation in which action must be taken to prevent bowel obstruction or compromise to the blood supply of the trapped bowel.

The diagnosis is established on history and physical appearance. When taking a history of a well child, be certain to ask parents if they have ever noticed any lumps in the child's groin area. The hernia may not be noticeable at the time of the visit, so unless asked specifically, parents may not mention it. If present, the herniated intestine may be palpated in the inguinal ring on physical examination.

Therapeutic Management

Treatment of inguinal hernia is surgery. The bowel is returned to the abdominal cavity and retained there by sealing the inguinal ring. Pneumoperitoneum (instillation of carbon dioxide into the perineal cavity) during surgery may be performed to reveal the presence of an enlarged inguinal ring on the opposite side. If this is the case, both sides may be repaired and the child will return from surgery with dressings in both groins.

Formerly, surgery for inguinal hernia was delayed until children were 3 or 4 years of age. Today, to prevent the complication of bowel strangulation—a surgical emergency—the newborn with inguinal hernia may be operated on before hospital discharge or at 1 to 2 months of age. If surgery is projected for children as a prophylactic measure, goal-setting may be difficult for parents as they weigh the value of surgical repair against the risk of anesthesia and surgery.

Following surgery, keep the suture line dry and free of urine or feces to prevent infection. Most incisions in this area are covered with collodion (which looks like clear nail polish) instead of a dressing. Collodion is waterproof and seals the incision from urine and feces. Even so, the infant will need frequent diaper changes and good diaper-area care. Assess circulation in the leg on the side of the surgical repair to be certain that edema of the groin is not compressing blood vessels and obstructing blood flow to the leg.

Hirschsprung's Disease (Aganglionic Megacolon)

Aganglionic megacolon is absence of ganglionic innervation to the muscle of a section of the bowel. In most instances, this is the lower portion of the sigmoid colon just above the anus. The absence of nerve cells means there are no peristaltic waves at this section to further the passage of fecal material through that segment of intestine. This results in chronic constipation or ribbon-like stools (stools passing through such a small, narrow segment look like ribbons). The portion of the bowel proximal to the obstruction dilates, distending the abdomen (Figure 45-11).

There is a familial incidence of aganglionic disease (it occurs at a greater incidence in siblings of a child with the disorder than in other children) and it occurs more often in males than in females. It is caused by an abnormal gene on chromosome 10 (Lyonnet et al., 1993). The incidence is approximately 1 in 5000 live births.

Assessment

Because newborn stools are normally soft, symptoms of aganglionic megacolon generally do not become apparent in the neonatal period, but only after 6 to 12 months of age. Occasionally, infants are born with such an extensive section of bowel involved that even meconium cannot pass. The defect is suggested if infants fail to pass meconium by age 24 hours and have increasing abdominal distention.

Infants with aganglionic disease of the intestine generally have a history of chronic constipation or intermittent constipation and diarrhea. A careful history helps to document the symptoms. What is the duration of the constipation? (With this disease it may be a problem from birth.) What do parents mean by constipation? (With this disease, children do not have a bowel movement more than once a week.) What is the consistency of the stool? (Ribbonlike or watery.) Is the child ill in any other way? (Children with aganglionic disease of the intestine tend to be thin and undernourished, sometimes deceptively so because their abdomen is large and distended.)

If a finger covered with a glove is inserted into the rectum of a child with true constipation, the examining finger will touch hard, caked stool. With aganglionic colon disease, the rectum is empty because fecal material cannot pass into the rectum through the obstructed portion. A barium enema is generally ordered to substantiate the diagnosis. The barium will outline on x-ray film the narrow, nerveless portion and the proximal distended portion of the bowel. Barium enema must be

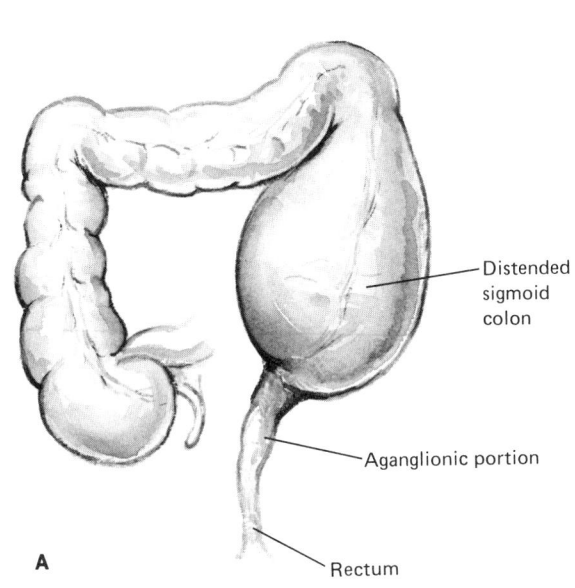

Distended sigmoid colon

Aganglionic portion

A

Rectum

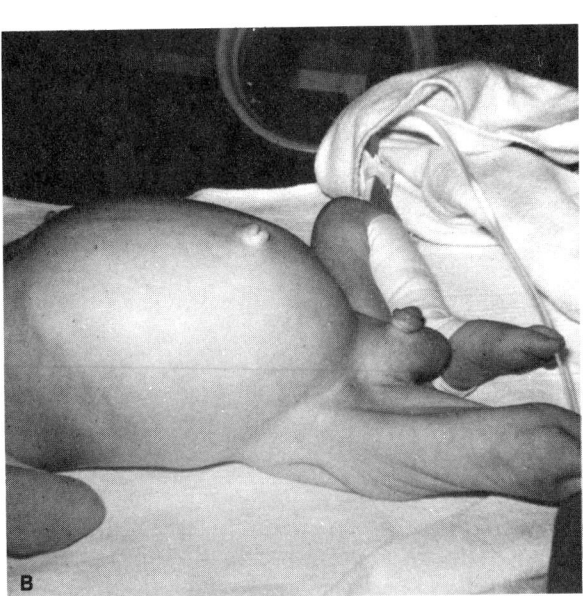

B

FIGURE 45-11

(**A**) *Aganglionic megacolon (Hirschsprung's disease). The distal portion of the bowel lacks nerve inner-vation. Because there is no peristalsis in this narrowed segment, the bowel distends markedly proximal to it.* (**B**) *Distended abdomen from Hirschsprung's disease. (Courtesy of the Department of Medical Photography, Children's Hospital, Buffalo, NY.)*

used cautiously because children cannot expel this afterward any more effectively than they can stool. The definitive diagnosis is by a biopsy of the affected segment to show the lack of innervation. *Anorectal manometry* is a technique to test the strength or innervation of the internal rectal sphincter by inserting a balloon catheter into the rectum and measuring the pressure exerted against it. Although this may be some help in diagnosis, it also has a high degree of false negative results.

Therapeutic Management

Repair of aganglionic megacolon involves dissection and removal of the affected section with anastomosis of the intestine. Because this is a technically difficult surgery to perform in a small abdomen, the condition is generally treated in the newborn by establishing a temporary colostomy, and the bowel is repaired at 12 to 18 months of age.

Following the final surgery, children should have a functioning, normal bowel. In those few instances in which the anus is deprived of nerve endings, a permanent colostomy may be established (Foster et al., 1990).

Nursing Diagnoses and Related Interventions

> *Nursing Diagnosis:* Altered bowel elimination related to reduced bowel function
>
> *Goal:* Child will accomplish adequate bowel elimination with some adaptation until normal bowel function can be established.
>
> *Outcome Criteria:* Child has a daily bowel movement through either a colostomy movement or by enema.

Before surgery, the child may be prescribed daily enemas to achieve bowel movements. It is important in infants that fluid used for enemas be normal saline (0.9% NaCl) and not tap water. Tap water is hypotonic; if it is instilled into the bowel, it moves rapidly across the intestine into interstitial and intravascular fluid compartments to equalize osmotic pressure (by the laws of osmosis, fluid moves from an area of less to greater concentration). This has led to death of infants from cardiac congestion or cerebral edema (water intoxication). Parents can buy a ready-made saline preparation at a pharmacy or they can prepare their own by mixing 2 tsp of noniodized salt to 1 quart of water. Adding salt to water does not seem important, so be certain that the parents understand why they must do this and that the proportion of salt to water is important.

Caring for a child with a colostomy is discussed in Chapter 37. Children may have an antibiotic solution or saline prescribed to be infused into the distal bowel to reduce the possibility of infection in the now unused segment and help maintain bowel tone.

> *Nursing Diagnosis:* Altered nutrition, less than body requirements, related to reduced bowel function
>
> *Goal:* Child will receive adequate nutrition during course of illness.
>
> *Outcome Criteria:* Child ingests a low-residue diet; weight follows a percentile curve on a growth chart.

Preoperative Care. Older children may be in poor physical health from poor food intake over a long period at the time the condition is diagnosed. If this is so, they may be hospitalized or returned home on a low-residue diet, stool softeners, vitamin supplements, and perhaps daily enemas until their condition improves. Total parenteral nutrition is helpful to offer a source of nutrition. If a child is to be cared for at home, help the parents learn about a minimal-residue diet (i.e., one that is low in undigestible fiber, connective fiber, and residue.) Milk, fried foods, and highly seasoned foods are omitted to eliminate chemical irritants from the intestinal tract. A list of minimal-residue foods is shown in Table 45-8. Help parents to make out a reminder sheet for the stool softener so it is given daily. During a time of a special diet is not a good time for parents to introduce new feeding methods, such as a cup or spoon, unless children are at that developmental point where they will quickly adapt to the new procedure and are, in fact, so anxious to feed themselves that they will actually eat better this way.

Postoperative Care. Following anastomosis of the colon to remove the aganglionic portion, infants will return with a nasogastric tube in place, an intravenous infusion, and probably a Foley catheter as well. Observe the infant for abdominal distention. Assess bowel sounds and observe also for passage of flatus and stools. As soon as peristalsis has returned (approximately 24 hours postsurgery), the nasogastric tube may be removed and children offered small, frequent feedings of fluids, such as water or gelatin. They are then introduced gradually to full fluids, a soft diet, then a minimal-residue diet, and finally, a normal diet for age. Children will usually have a barium enema performed before discharge from the hospital to be certain that the bowel empties well and that the anastomosis site is not leaking.

> *Nursing Diagnosis:* High risk for ineffective family coping, compromised, related to chronic illness in child
>
> *Goal:* Parents will demonstrate adequate coping behavior during course of child's illness.
>
> *Outcome Criteria:* Parents state they are able to cope with the level of stress present from their child's condition.

Table 45-8. *Minimum-Residue Diet*

Description: The purpose of the minimum-residue diet is to supply food that will provide more complete nourishment than a clear liquid diet, while producing a minimum of fecal residue in the lower bowel. To reduce indigestible carbohydrate to a minimum, all fruits and vegetables are omitted except strained fruit juice and tomato juice. Eggs, tender meat, or meat made tender in the cooking process are used. Milk as a beverage is not allowed.

Adequacy: This diet does not meet the Recommended Dietary Allowances for calcium, iron, vitamin A, riboflavin, or vitamin D.

Food Group	Foods Allowed	Foods to Avoid
Beverages	Cereal beverages, carbonated beverages, nondairy creamer, 1 oz cream/d	Milk, milk drinks
Breads	Saltine crackers, melba toast, rusk, zwieback; refined, enriched white bread	Bread or crackers containing whole grain flour or bran
Cereals	Cooked refined wheat, corn, or rice cereal; strained oatmeal; prepared cereals made from refined corn or rice	Whole grain cereals, barley
Desserts	Arrowroot and plain sugar cookies, angel food and sponge cakes, plain gelatin desserts, puddings made with strained fruit juice or water, popsicles, fruit ices and frappés made without milk; sugar and vanilla wafers	All products containing seeds, nuts, coconut, fruit, fruit pulp, and other foods to avoid
Eggs	Any except fried	Fried eggs
Fats	Butter, margarine, crisp bacon, bland salad dressings	None
Fruits, fruit juices	Strained fruit juices	All others
Meat, fish, poultry, cheese	Tender beef, chicken, lamb, liver, turkey, pork, veal, fish; cottage cheese; cream cheese; American cheese used only in cooking)	Fried meat, fish, poultry; cheese other than that allowed
Potatoes or substitutes	Macaroni, noodles, refined rice, spaghetti	Potatoes, hominy, whole grain or wild rice
Soups	Bouillon, broth, consommé	All others
Sugar, sweets	Plain candy, honey, jelly, marshmallows, sugar, syrup (all used in moderation)	Jam, marmalade, candy containing fruits or nuts
Vegetables, vegetable juices	Tomato juice	All others
Miscellaneous	Salt, mild spices in moderation, dilute vinegar, gravy in moderation	Catsup, chili sauce, peanut butter, coconut, garlic, horseradish, nuts, olives, pickles, relish, popcorn, herbs

Sample Menu for Minimum-Residue Diet

Breakfast	Lunch	Dinner
1/2 cup strained orange juice	1/2 cup tomato juice	3 oz roast beef
1/2 cup farina	1 oz sliced chicken	1/2 cup noodles
1 egg, soft cooked	1 cup rice	1/2 cup beef broth
2 slices refined white bread, enriched	2 slices refined white bread, enriched	2 slices refined white bread, enriched
2 tsp butter or margarine	2 tsp butter or margarine	2 tsp butter or margarine
1 tbsp grape jelly	1 tbs honey	1 tbs apple jelly
2 tsp sugar	1 slice angel food cake	1/2 cup orange gelatin
1/4 cup nondairy creamer	1 tsp sugar	3 vanilla wafers
3 arrowroot cookies	Coffee or tea	1/2 cup lemon pudding
1/2 cup grape juice	1 popsicle	1 tsp sugar
		Coffee or tea
		1/2 cup apple juice

(From Dietary Department, University of Iowa. [1989]. *Recent advances in therapeutic diets* [4th ed.]. Ames, IA: Iowa State University Press.)

Most parents feel tremendous relief after surgery that the surgery is over for their child and that a chronic illness is at last over. Caution parents that children may still remain "fussy" eaters for a few months because feeding problems that begin for physical reasons continue for emotional or psychologic reasons. Help parents to diminish the importance of meals gradually, to schedule periods of time during the day when they give their full attention to the child such as reading a story or putting a puzzle together, and to offer praise for pleasant, not difficult behavior. These measures will cause meal time problems to fade.

Inflammatory Bowel Disease: Ulcerative Colitis and Crohn's Disease

Two conditions are categorized as inflammatory bowel disease: ulcerative colitis and Crohn's disease. They both involve the development of ulceration of the mucosa or submucosa layers of the colon and rectum. They both occur most frequently in young adults and adolescents, although more and more frequently symptoms first appear during school age. Both diseases occur most frequently in Jewish children and in families with a tendency toward allergy, and they have a higher incidence in the white than in the nonwhite population.

The etiologies of these disorders is obscure, although they tend to be familial. They probably represent an alteration in immune system response or are autoimmune processes. There is an increased number of immunoglobulins IgA and IgG present on intestinal mucosa. IgE immunoglobulins and the eosinophil count may also possibly be elevated. Psychologic factors, if they are not instrumental in triggering inflammatory bowel disease, appear to cause exacerbation of the conditions; a gastroenteritis will do the same thing. Smoking is directly correlated with the occurrence of Crohn's disease.

Crohn's disease is an inflammation of segments of the intestine. Involved segments are separated by normal bowel tissue. The wall of the colon becomes thickened and the surface is inflamed, leading to a "cobblestone" appearance of mucosa. Usually, the areas of the bowel affected are higher in the intestine than is the involvement seen with ulcerative colitis. In **ulcerative colitis**, the entire lower bowel is involved.

As inflammation becomes acute, children develop abdominal pain from contractions of the irritated portions. These areas do not absorb nutrients or fluid well, so malnutrition develops. To reduce abdominal pain (which is most acute after eating when the bowel becomes active), children begin to omit meals. They may be malnourished and have a vitamin or iron deficiency at the time the condition is diagnosed.

A number of complications may occur during the course of the disease. Hemorrhage from bowel perfora-

tion during the active disease is a possibility. A relapse is apt to occur 6 to 12 months after therapy. With ulcerative colitis, there is an association between bowel carcinoma and the disease; approximately 10% of children can be predicted to develop bowel carcinoma 10 years after having the illness; as many as 25% will develop this after 20 years.

Assessment

Children develop diarrhea and steatorrhea from the irritation and the unabsorbed fluid. Inflamed portions may ulcerate, leading to blood in the stool. Perforation can occur, leading to peritonitis or the formation of fistulas between bowel loops. Rectal fistula is present in as many as 20% of children. Weight loss occurs; growth failure occurs in prepubertal children. A recurring fever may be present.

Diagnosis is established by sigmoidoscopy and barium enema. On sigmoidoscopy, the shallow ulcerations along the bowel can be seen; the mucosa is friable (easily irritated) and bleeds easily from inflammation. A biopsy may be made for definite diagnosis. Observe children carefully following a bowel biopsy to detect rectal bleeding from an internal bleeding point (take blood pressure and pulse and assess stool for occult blood).

Therapeutic Management

The child's bowel heals best if it is allowed to rest for a time. Total parenteral nutrition is usually provided for nutrition during the resting period. The child can return home during this period as long as parents have good orientation to the necessary home care (see Chapter 38).

When food is reintroduced after the resting period, a high protein, high carbohydrate, high vitamin diet is prescribed to replace nutrients. Children may eat cautiously at first to avoid reintroducing diarrhea; assess intake and output to be certain it is adequate. An anti-inflammatory drug, such as prednisone or *sulfasalazine* (*Azulfidine*)—a sulfonamide and salicylic acid—or mesalamine generally brings about a great improvement in symptoms. If medical therapy is ineffective, bowel resection may be necessary. In some children, a large portion of the bowel may be removed and a colostomy, or a continent ileostomy, constructed (an internal reservoir is created by a section of bowel and emptied by insertion of a catheter; Figure 45-12). This is a harsh step for a child, but because it removes the possibility of the child's developing intestinal cancer, is a needed one in children whose disease is running a long-term, debilitating, course that does not improve.

Nursing Diagnoses and Related Interventions

Nursing Diagnosis: High risk for ineffective individual coping related to chronic illness

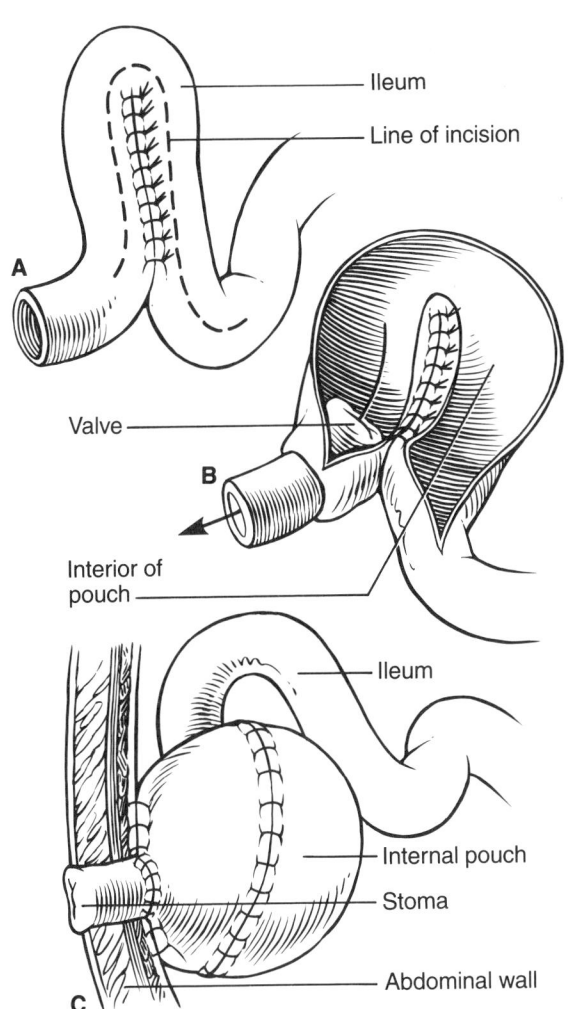

FIGURE 45-12
*A continent ileostomy. (**A**) Segment of bowel is anastomosed. (**B**) Pouch for stool collection is formed. (**C**) Liquid stool is contained in pouch until drained by catheter.*

Goal: Child will demonstrate adequate coping behavior during course of illness.

Outcome Criteria: Child expresses feelings; voices that he or she understands the disease and therapy, and suggests ways to minimize stress.

Caution children that side effects such as excessive weight gain and a round facial appearance may occur on prednisone therapy so they are not surprised by this. Assess blood pressure, intake and output, weight, and sleep patterns on any child taking prednisone. Caution children that sulfasalazine (Azulfidine) turns urine an orange-yellow so they do not mistake this color change as bleeding.

Provide time to listen so children have someone outside their family to talk to about their symptoms and family or stress problems. Some children with ulcerative colitis are described as having a certain personality pattern: passive, dependent, and rigid—children who have

difficulty expressing their aggression, anger, or fears; their parents may have the same personality traits. If this is so, the family may need to be referred to a family service agency or a psychologist for family counseling.

Irritable Bowel Syndrome

Irritable bowel syndrome is the presence of either intermittent episodes of loose stools or recurrent abdominal pain. It appears slightly more often in girls than in boys. It has an increased incidence at ages 5 to 6 years and again at ages 10 to 11 years. As many as 1 in 10 school-age children suffer from this phenomenon. The cause is unknown but it is associated with low fat intake (without fat slowing absorption, stool passes rapidly through the bowel) or excessive fluid intake.

Assessment

The symptoms are usually vague. The episodes of diarrhea or pain may occur several times a week or as infrequently as once a month. There is seemingly no relationship to meals. Children are rarely awakened from sleep by pain. The episodes of pain may last only 1 minute or may last for hours. The pain is generally mild or "annoying," rather than colicky or severe. It is generally poorly localized, although the area surrounding the umbilicus is a common site. The pain may radiate to bizarre sites. Nausea, pallor, dizziness, headache, and faintness may precede or accompany the episodes of pain.

Although irritable bowel syndrome may occur for purely physical reasons, a history of the pain generally reveals problems in the family such as marital discord, physical illness in parents or siblings, psychologic illness in parents, or an unsatisfactory parent-child relationship. Children may have difficulty handling aggression, anger, or sexual feelings. Other symptoms of stress, such as sleep disturbances, fears, or eating problems, may be present. Recurrent abdominal pain may be associated with school phobia or reluctance to attend school. School phobia tends to occur in firstborn children. It is often noticed that both parents and children may be reluctant to separate. Irritable bowel syndrome may be associated with food intolerance (Paganelli et al., 1990).

Be certain when history taking that, in the light of such family problems, a physical basis for the pain is not overlooked. Children whose parents have marital discord or psychologic illness also develop peptic ulcers, colitis, intestinal polyps, appendicitis, and other physical reasons for recurrent abdominal pain.

If the pain is psychogenic in origin, a physical assessment will produce no significant findings. There is no abdominal tenderness, distention, guarded abdomen, or muscle spasm. The physician may order a number of diagnostic procedures to rule out organic disease, such as a complete blood count to rule out infection and anemia; a urinalysis (urinary tract infection often presents with recurrent abdominal pain); a study of stool for ova, parasites, and occult blood; and a perineal evaluation for pinworms. Whether a barium swallow or enema, a flat plate of the abdomen, or other studies are ordered depends on specific symptoms and history.

Therapeutic Management

For some children, just having the opportunity to talk to an understanding person about the problem is all that is necessary to stop the attacks of pain. Other families need counseling regarding the underlying problem, such as allowing children to express their anger, reducing excessive demands on them, or giving them more attention. They may need to be referred to a family service agency or a psychiatrist to secure more extensive counseling. Calcium channel blockers may be helpful in treating irritable bowel syndrome (Sun et al., 1990).

Diseases Caused by Food, Vitamin, and Mineral Deficiencies

There are many underfed and malnourished children in every part of the world. Although extreme diseases of food or vitamin deprivation are rare in the United States, they do exist. Such children need early identification so that they can receive better nutrition before permanent damage occurs.

The average child does not develop a deficient intake of essential nutrients, because even if the child is occasionally a fussy eater, over 1 week, he or she does ingest foods from all food groups. Always assess carefully any child who has an interference in nutrition such as a gastrointestinal illness or the child placed on enteric feedings or total parenteral nutrition to see that nutrient deficiencies do not exist. Assess abused or neglected children well for nutrition deficiencies because they may not have been given adequate food.

Kwashiorkor

Kwashiorkor is a disease caused by protein deficiency. It occurs most frequently in children ages 1 to 3 years because this is an age group requiring a high protein intake. It is a disease found almost exclusively in developing countries such as Africa, Asia, and Latin America, although it does occur in the United States (Fischer, 1993). It tends to occur after weaning, when children change from breast milk to a diet consisting mainly of carbohydrate. Growth failure is a major symptom. Because edema is also a symptom, however, children may not appear light in weight until the edema is relieved. There is a severe wasting of muscles, but, again, this is masked by the edema.

Edema occurs because the hypoproteinemia causes

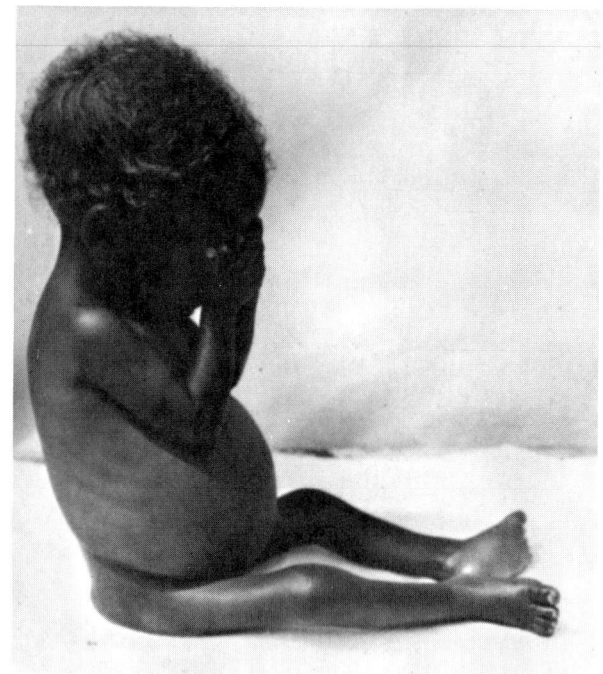

FIGURE 45-13
An infant with kwashiorkor. Notice the distended abdomen and emaciated lower extremities. (Courtesy of UNICEF.)

a shift of body fluid from the intravascular compartments to the interstitial space causing ascites (Figure 45-13). This is the same phenomenon that causes extensive edema in children with nephrosis. The edema tends to be dependent, so it is first noted in children's lower extremities. Children are generally irritable and uninterested in their surroundings. In addition, they may be behind other children of the same age in motor development.

If children had a period of good protein intake, then poor protein intake, then good intake again, soon individual hair shafts will have a striped appearance of brown, then white, and so on—a zebra sign. Children also have diarrhea, iron deficiency anemia, and hepatomegaly.

Kwashiorkor without treatment is fatal. For therapy, children need to be begun on a diet rich in protein. Even so, there is evidence to suggest that protein malnutrition early in life, even if corrected later, may result in failure of children to reach their full potential of intellectual and psychologic development.

Nutritional Marasmus

Nutritional marasmus is a disease caused by deficiency of all food groups. It is basically a form of starvation and, although it is seen most commonly in developing countries where food supplies are short, it is seen in grossly neglected children in the United States. These children are most commonly younger than age 1 year.

Children have many of the same symptoms as children with kwashiorkor: growth failure, wasting of muscles, irritability, iron deficiency anemia, and diarrhea. Whereas children with kwashiorkor are anorectic, children with nutritional marasmus are invariably hungry (starving) and will suck at any object offered them, such as a finger or their clothing. Treatment is to supply the children with a diet rich in nutrients. This condition generally results from poor maternal-child bonding in the United States. Care of children with failure to thrive from poor parent–child bonding is discussed in Chapter 54.

Vitamin A Deficiency

The earliest sign of vitamin A deficiency is night blindness, or the inability to see well in dim light. If the deficiency becomes severe, **xerophthalmia**, a condition in which the conjunctivae of the eye become dry and lusterless, occurs. **Keratomalacia** is the final result of severe vitamin A deficiency. With this stage, there is a necrosis of the cornea with perforation, loss of ocular fluid, and blindness. Children must have severe vitamin A deficiency for a prolonged period for these changes to occur. For this reason, keratomalacia is rarely seen in the United States. Treatment is administration of supplementary vitamin A (parenterally or orally) plus a diet rich in the vitamin. The effects of keratomalacia can be arrested at the point at which therapy begins, but existing damage is irreversible.

Thiamine Deficiency

Deficiency of thiamine (vitamin B₁) in children leads to **beriberi**, a disease primarily of people who eat polished rice as their dietary stable. It occurs because the B vitamin is contained in the hull of rice. When rice is polished or refined, the source of vitamin B₁ is removed.

Early signs of beriberi are tingling or numbness of the extremities, occasional heart palpitation, and exhaustion. Infants who are being breastfed by a mother whose diet is deficient in thiamine usually develop symptoms between 2 to 6 months of age. Infants may be thin and wasted; they may have diarrhea and vomiting. They may develop acute symptoms of dyspnea, cyanosis, and cardiac failure. Anesthesia of the feet and a peculiar ataxic gait may occur. Children have *aphonia*—they cry without making a sound. Edema and convulsions may occur in the terminal stage. Many older children have a symptom of edema first, occurring mainly in the legs, scrotum, face, and trunk.

Beriberi may be confused with cardiac or renal disease because of the presence of the edema. Treatment of beriberi is administration of thiamine (parenterally and orally). Children must then be maintained on a thiamine-rich diet.

Niacin Deficiency

Pellagra is a disease seen in people who eat corn as their main dietary staple because corn is not a good source of niacin. The disease is said to be characterized by four *D*s: (1) dermatitis, (2) diarrhea, (3) dementia, and (4) death.

The dermatitis in white children resembles the erythema of sunburn; in black children, it is marked by hyperpigmentation. After this first stage, the lesions become scaly, dry, and cracked. Children's tongues are often sore and raw-looking. The dementia is marked by loss of memory and irritability. Treatment is the administration of niacin (parenterally or orally). Children need to be maintained on a diet high in niacin thereafter.

Vitamin C Deficiency

Scurvy is rare today but results from vitamin C deficiency. In scurvy, the walls of the capillaries become fragile, and hemorrhage of vessels results. There is often muscle tenderness, petechial hemorrhage of the skin, nosebleeds, and swollen gums that bleed easily. Infantile scurvy occurs in infants 2 to 12 months of age, who are fed only milk. Infants with scurvy cry when they are moved due to muscle pain and tenderness. They often lie on their back with their legs held in a froglike position. Children may have hemorrhagic areas on the extremities that resemble bruises from trauma. Treatment is administration of supplementary vitamin C (parenterally or orally). Children need to be maintained on a diet rich in fresh fruits and vegetables to provide vitamin C.

Vitamin D Deficiency

Vitamin D is necessary for calcium to be absorbed by bones. Deficiency of vitamin D in children, therefore, leads to poor bone formation, or **rickets**.

Infants with rickets are often plump in appearance. However, their muscle tone is poor, and their motor development may be behind other children their age. Tooth eruption will be delayed. Children may have gastrointestinal upsets and excessive perspiration of the head. There is a swelling of the epiphysis of the long bones. The radius at the wrist may be the first sign of this. The costochondral junctions of the ribs swell and give the chest a beadlike appearance (rachitic rosary sign). *Craniotabes* (softening of the skull) may be a sign in young children. Failure of the anterior fontanelle to close and *bossing* (a protrusion) of the skull may also be present. When children begin to walk, bowlegs and knock-knee deformities result. Spinal deformities, such as kyphosis, may develop. In girls, severe pelvic contraction, a deformity that may interfere with future childbearing, may result. Calcium absorption from the intestine is regulated by vitamin D. Tetany, resulting from the decreased level of serum calcium, may be a symptom.

The diagnosis is confirmed by x-ray examination. On x-ray, the characteristic changes of the epiphysis of long bones will be apparent. Treatment of rickets is the administration of vitamin D along with sufficient quantities of calcium. Children need to be maintained on a diet high in vitamin D and exposed to sunlight, which also serves as a precursor to vitamin D formation. The disease will not progress further after therapy, but bone deformities discovered at the time of correction are irreversible.

Iodine Deficiency

A diet deficient in iodine may lead to hyperplasia of the thyroid gland (*goiter*). In the United States, areas where goiter is endemic are mainly the states bordering Canada, especially the Great Lakes area and those states between the Rocky Mountains and the Appalachians. When the thyroid gland does not have adequate iodine to make thyroxine, its chief hormone, the gland is overstimulated by the pituitary gland; the overstimulation leads to the hyperplasia. Goiter tends to occur most commonly in females at puberty and during pregnancy. An enlarged thyroid gland may lead to difficulty in breathing; some people with simple goiter from iodine deficiency develop symptoms of hypothyroidism. For treatment, they need supplemental iodine or synthetic thyroxine. Children must also be maintained on a diet adequate in iodine.

Key Points

- Remember that children lose proportionately more fluid with vomiting and diarrhea than adults. For this reason, they need rapid assessment and interventions to avoid dehydration.
- Both fluid and electrolyte imbalances tend to occur rapidly with vomiting and diarrhea. Vomiting leads to alkalosis. Diarrhea leads to acidosis. Nursing diagnoses associated with diarrhea are High risk for fluid volume deficit, Altered skin integrity, and Anxiety.
- Gastrointestinal disorders almost always interfere with nutrition at least to some degree. This is a greater problem in children than adults as children need to take in enough nutrients and fluid daily for growth as well as body maintenance.
- Chalasia (gastroesophageal reflux) is a neuromuscular disturbance in which the cardiac sphincter is lax, allowing for easy regurgitation of gastric contents into the esophagus. It is treated by feeding a thickened formula and positioning the infant prone with head elevated.
- Pyloric stenosis is hypertrophy of the valve between the stomach and duodenum. It impedes the passage

of feedings leading to vomiting. Nursing diagnoses associated with this are High risk for fluid volume deficit and Infection.

- Peptic ulcer may occur even in young children. This is a shallow excavation formed in the mucosal wall of the stomach. It is treated, like adult ulcers, with medications to suppress gastric acidity.
- Hepatic disorders seen in children are hepatitis A (caused usually by eating contaminated shellfish) and hepatitis B (caused by contaminated blood or placental spread). Nursing diagnoses associated with these disorders are High risk for infection transmission and Altered comfort.
- Congenital obstruction of the bile ducts occurs from failure of the bile duct to recanalize in utero. Cirrhosis is fibrotic scarring of the liver that occurs as a result of congenital biliary atresia. Most of these children need a liver transplant to restore liver function.
- Intussusception is the invagination of one portion of the intestine into another. Nursing diagnoses identified for this are High risk for pain, Fluid volume deficit, and Altered parenting.
- Necrotizing enterocolitis is the development of necrotic patches on the intestine. It occurs almost exclusively in immature infants.
- Appendicitis is inflammation of the appendix. It is always an emergency situation and is the most common cause of abdominal surgery in children. Therapy is surgery to removed the appendix before it ruptures. Nursing diagnoses identified for this are Pain, Fear, and High risk for fluid volume deficit.
- Celiac disease (gluten-induced enteropathy) is a change in the ability of the intestinal villi to absorb. It is apparently a dominantly inherited illness. Nursing diagnoses identified are Altered family processes and Altered nutrition.
- A number of hernias can occur in children such as inguinal and hiatal hernia. These are surgically corrected when recognized.
- Hirschsprung's disease (aganglionic megacolon) is absence of ganglionic innervation in a section of the lower bowel. The therapy is possibly a temporary colostomy followed by surgery. Nursing diagnoses identified for this are Altered bowel elimination, Altered nutrition, and High risk for ineffective family coping.
- Inflammatory bowel disease can occur as either ulcerative colitis or Crohn's disease. Children may have portions of their bowel removed to relieve these conditions.
- Kwashiorkor (protein deficiency), nutritional marasmus (starvation), vitamin A, D (rickets), B1 (beriberi), and C (scurvy) deficiencies occur in children when they are not provided or cannot absorb adequate nutrients. Although associated with developing countries, they can occur in a child in any community.

- Encourage children with nutrient disorders to join the family for mealtime if possible. Even if they cannot eat the same foods as other family members, they benefit from the social interaction.
- Some gastrointestinal disorders lead to long-term therapies such as colostomy or gastrostomy feedings. Because these disorders interfere with common body functions such as eating and elimination, they are difficult for children to accept without the support of concerned health care providers.

Critical Thinking Exercises

1. Anne is an 8-month-old girl admitted to the hospital with severe diarrhea. What emergency interventions does Anne need to prevent an electrolyte or fluid imbalance? What measures could you take to reduce her fear of the strange hospital environment?

2. John is a 12-year-old with Crohn's disease. He is being cared for at home with total parenteral nutrition. How can you help John keep pace with his friends at school? How can you help him maintain a sense of high self-esteem in light of many hospitalizations and home care?

3. Pamela is a 4-year-old who is being transferred to a distant city to have a liver transplant because of congenital biliary atresia. Her parents ask you what they can expect at the distant hospital. How would you prepare them for this?

References

American Academy of Pediatrics. (1991). *Report of the committee on infectious diseases*. Elkgrove Village, IL: American Academy of Pediatrics.

Belknap, W. M., & McEvoy, C. (1994). Developmental disorders of gastrointestinal function. In F. A. Oski et al. *Principles and practice of pediatrics* (2nd ed.). Philadelphia: J.B. Lippincott.

Cochan, W. J. (1994). Cirrhosis. In F. A Oski et al. *Principles and practice of pediatrics* (2nd ed.). Philadelphia: J.B. Lippincott.

Coleman, J., et al. (1991). Liver diseases that lead to transplantation. *Critical Care Nursing Quarterly, 13*, 41.

Department of Health & Human Services. (1991). *Healthy people 2000*. Washington, DC: Public Health Service.

Ellis, T. H. (1990). Diaphragmatic hiatal hernias. *Postgraduate Medicine, 88*, 113.

Fischer, P. R. (1993). Tropical pediatrics. *Pediatrics in Review, 14*, 95.

Foster, P., et al. (1990). Twenty-five years' experience with Hirschsprung's disease. *Journal of Pediatric Surgery, 25*, 531.

Gruppi, L. A., et al. (1990). Liver transplantation: Key nursing diagnoses. *Dimensions of Critical Care Nursing, 9*, 272.

Househam, K. C., et al. (1990). Factors influencing the duration of acute diarrheal disease in infancy. *Journal of Pediatric Gastroenterology and Nutrition, 10*, 37.

Kelly, C. P., et al. (1990). Diagnosis and treatment of gluten-sensitive enteropathy. *Advances in Internal Medicine, 35*, 341.

Kocoshis, S. A., et al. (1993). Pediatric liver transplantation. *Clinical Pediatrics, 32*, 386.

Laney, D. W., & Cohen, M. B. (1993). Approach to the pediatric patient with diarrhea. *Gastroenterology Clinics of North America, 22*, 499.

Lyonnet, S., et al. (1993). A gene for Hirschsprung disease maps to the proximal long arm of chromosome 10. *Nature Genetics, 4*, 346.

Miller, J. P. (1993). Laparoscopic appendectomy. *Pediatric Annals, 22*, 663.

Mitchell, G. W. (1990). Hepatitis A. *Emergency Medical Services, 9*, 36.

Oleinik, S. S. (1990). Care of the critically ill child after liver transplantation. *Focus on Critical Care, 17*, 300.

Paganelli, R., et al. (1990). Intestinal permeability in irritable bowel syndrome. *Annuals of Allergy, 64*, 377.

Putnam, T. C., et al. (1990). Appendicitis in children. *Surgery, Gynecology, and Obstetrics, 170*, 527.

Ruiz-Palacios, G. M., et al. (1990). Protection of breast-fed infants against campylobacter diarrhea by antibodies in human milk. *Journal of Pediatrics, 116*, 707.

Siegel, N. J., et al. (1994). The pathophysiology of body fluids. In F. A. Oski et al. *Principles and practice of pediatrics* (2nd ed.). Philadelphia: J.B. Lippincott.

Sterling, C. E., et al. (1993). Home management related to medical treatment of childhood gastrointestinal reflux. *Pediatric Nursing, 19*, 167.

Sun, W. M., et al. (1990). Effect of oral nicardipine on anorectal function in normal human volunteers and patients with irritable bowel syndrome. *Digestive Diseases and Science, 35*, 885.

Teraes, J., et al. (1990). Vasopressin/nitroglycerin infusion vs. esophageal tamponade in the treatment of acute variceal bleeding: A randomized controlled trial. *Hepatology, 11*, 964.

Valletta, E. A., et al. (1990). IgA anti-gliadin antibodies in the monitoring of gluten challenge in celiac disease. *Journal of Pediatric Gastroenterology and Nutrition, 10*, 169.

West, K. H. (1990). Non-A, non-B, and delta hepatitis: Hepatitis C and D. *Emergency Medical Services, 19*, 37.

Wood, R. P., et al. (1990). Optimal therapy for patients with biliary atresia: Portoenterostomy (Kasai procedure) versus primary transplantation. *Journal of Pediatric Surgery, 25*, 153.

Zheng, J. Y., et al. (1994). Review of pneumatic reduction of intussusception. *Journal of Pediatric Surgery, 28*, 93.

Suggested Readings

Blanchard, H., et al. (1990). Pediatric liver transplantation: The Montreal experience. *Journal of Pediatric Surgery, 24*, 1000.

Ford, J., et al. (1990). The incidence of viral associated diarrhea after admission to a pediatric hospital. *American Journal of Epidemiology, 131*, 711.

Kallen, R. J. (1990). The management of diarrheal dehydration in infants using parenteral fluids. *Pediatric Clinics of North America, 37*, 265.

Khoshoo, V., et al. (1990). Salmonella typhimurium-associated severe protracted diarrhea in infants and young children. *Journal of Pediatric Gastroenterology and Nutrition, 10*, 33.

Margolis, P. A., et al. (1990). Effects of unrestricted diet on mild infantile diarrhea. *American Journal of Diseases of Children, 144*, 102.

Reynolds, S. L., & Jaffe, D. M. (1990). Children with abdominal pain: Evaluation in the pediatric emergency department. *Pediatric Emergency Care, 6*, 8.

Stringer, M. D., & Drake, D. P. (1991). Hirschsprung's disease presenting as neonatal gastrointestinal perforation. *British Journal of Surgery, 78*, 188.

Zenn, M. R., & Redo, S. F. (1993). Hypertrophic pyloric stenosis in the newborn. *Journal of Pediatric Surgery, 28*, 1577.

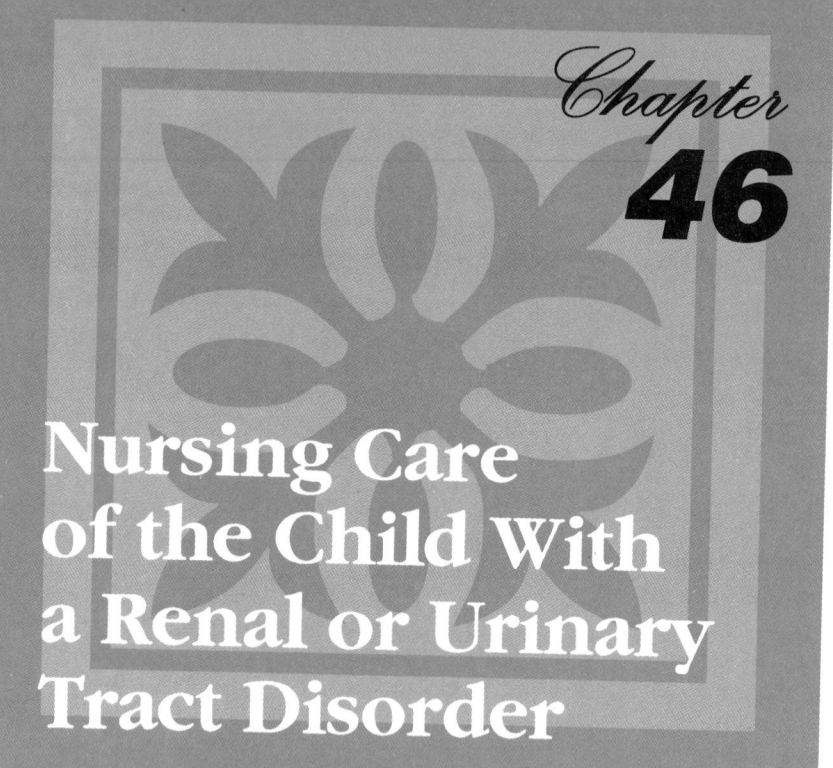

Chapter 46

Nursing Care of the Child With a Renal or Urinary Tract Disorder

Objectives

After mastering the contents of this chapter, you should be able to:

1. Describe common renal and urinary disorders that occur in children, such as urinary tract infection (UTI), nephrosis, and glomerulonephritis.

2. Assess a child for a renal or urinary tract disorder.

3. Formulate nursing diagnoses related to renal or urinary disorders.

4. Plan nursing care related to urinary or renal disorders, such as teaching about the importance of perineal hygiene to prevent infection.

5. Implement nursing care for the child with a renal or urinary disorder, such as assisting a child to plan a low protein diet.

6. Evaluate outcome criteria to ensure that nursing goals have been achieved.

7. Identify National Health Goals related to renal or urinary tract disorders and children that nurses can be instrumental in helping the nation achieve.

8. Identify areas related to care of the child with a renal or urinary disorder that would benefit from additional nursing research.

9. Use critical thinking to analyze methods for making nursing care of the child with a renal or urinary disorder more family centered.

10. Synthesize knowledge of renal and urinary tract disorders with the nursing process to achieve quality maternal and child health nursing care.

Adele Pillitteri: MATERNAL AND CHILD HEALTH NURSING, 2nd Edition. © 1995 Adele Pillitteri.

I n health, the urinary system maintains the proper balance of fluid (water) and electrolytes in the blood. In disease, with structural abnormalities or renal (kidney) malfunction, a child may be left with excessive amounts of fluid in the body or with an imbalance of minerals essential to the body's functioning. Disorders of the urinary system tend to be long term. They are always potentially life-threatening, because any urinary tract disorder can ultimately (if not originally) affect the kidneys, and kidney dysfunction can have potentially fatal consequences.

Unfortunately, children with urinary disorders may not be brought into a health care facility at the first sign of illness, because symptoms may be vague, or because the child or parents do not realize the seriousness of urinary disease or are embarrassed to discuss illness in this particular body system. Health education to increase awareness of the symptoms of kidney disease is an important area of family health teaching. National Health Goals related to renal or urinary tract disorders and children are shown in the Focus on National Health Goals box.

NURSING PROCESS OVERVIEW
for Care of the Child With a Renal or Urinary Tract Disorder

ASSESSMENT

Because the symptoms of many urinary tract disorders (e.g., mild abdominal pain, slowly growing edema, or low-grade fever) are subtle, parents may not bring their child to a health care facility as early in the disease as they might if symptoms were more definite. School nurses are in a prime position to recognize that a combination of minor symptoms can be serious and to see that children receive a proper referral for care.

Common findings from a health history and physical examination of the child with urinary system dysfunction are shown in Figure 46-1. If children have a urinary tract infection or have had bladder surgery, they may have pain on urination or pain from bladder spasms. The degree of pain must be assessed before an analgesic or antispasmodic can be administered. Techniques for obtaining urine samples (i.e., clean-catch, catheterization, 24-hour collections, suprapubic aspiration, and urinalysis) are described in Chapter 37.

NURSING DIAGNOSIS

Examples of nursing diagnoses for children with urinary tract disease include the following:

- Fluid volume excess related to decreased kidney function
- Fear related to outcome of kidney transplant
- Social isolation related to immunosuppressant therapy

Because the entire family becomes involved in chronic renal failure, other diagnoses may be appropriate:

- Altered family processes related to chronic illness in child
- Ineffective family coping: compromised, related to child's chronic illness

PLANNING

Be certain that goals established for care are relevant to the child's age and condition. Because renal disease may become chronic, goals should be modified frequently to meet changing needs.

Planning for the child with a urinary tract disorder often involves helping parents plan how to remember to give medicine. The child with nephrotic syndrome, for example, may be taking three or four different types of medicine every day at home. Inform parents about the types of medicine they are being asked to administer and the expected action of each. School-age children must have a schedule that allows them to take medicine before they leave home in the morning or after they return in the afternoon.

If a child has severe renal impairment, parents are asked to make decisions regarding kidney removal and transplant, and they need a great deal of time for discussion. If a kidney donor is sought among relatives, the parents must help decide whether the person whose tissue matches the child's really wants to donate a kidney or is being pressured to do so. Helping parents to schedule hospital visits or times for hemodialysis or peritoneal dialysis, to supervise continuous ambulatory peritoneal dialysis (CAPD), to care for their other children, and to provide a life apart from their child's requires nursing planning.

Two organizations that offer help in planning care are:

National Kidney Foundation
30 E 33rd Street, Suite 1100
New York, NY 10016

American Kidney Foundation
6110 Executive Boulevard, Suite 1010
Rockville, MD 20852

FOCUS ON
National Health Goals

Renal disease can lead to long-term illness. The following National Health Goal addresses prevention of long-term illness:

- Reduce to no more than 8% the proportion of people who experience a limitation in major activity due to chronic conditions from a baseline of 9.4% (DHHS, 1991).

Nurses can be instrumental in helping the nation achieve this goal by educating parents that children need a follow-up assessment for protein in urine after streptococcal infections. They also need to provide optimal care to children with renal disease.

Nursing research would be helpful on whether parents or children accurately self-assess for proteinuria after streptococcal infections, on the specific needs of children on ambulatory peritoneal dialysis, and on ways to make low-potassium diets more appealing to children with end-stage renal disease.

FOCUS ON NURSING ASSESSMENT

History
Chief concern: Child reports burning or cries on urination; blood or "dark" urine, frequency of urination; abdominal pain, flank pain, enuresis. Parents report increase in size of abdomen, periorbital edema, poor appetite, frequent thirst, weight gain, strong odor to urine; diaper rash in infants. A school-age child may be described as a behavior problem because he or she frequently asks to use the bathroom.
Family history: History of renal disease, such as polycystic kidney, enuresis; hypertension.
Pregnancy history: Exposure to nephrotoxic drugs (antibiotics) during pregnancy. Oligohydramnios at birth.
Past illness history: Child recently had a throat or skin infection.

Physical assessment

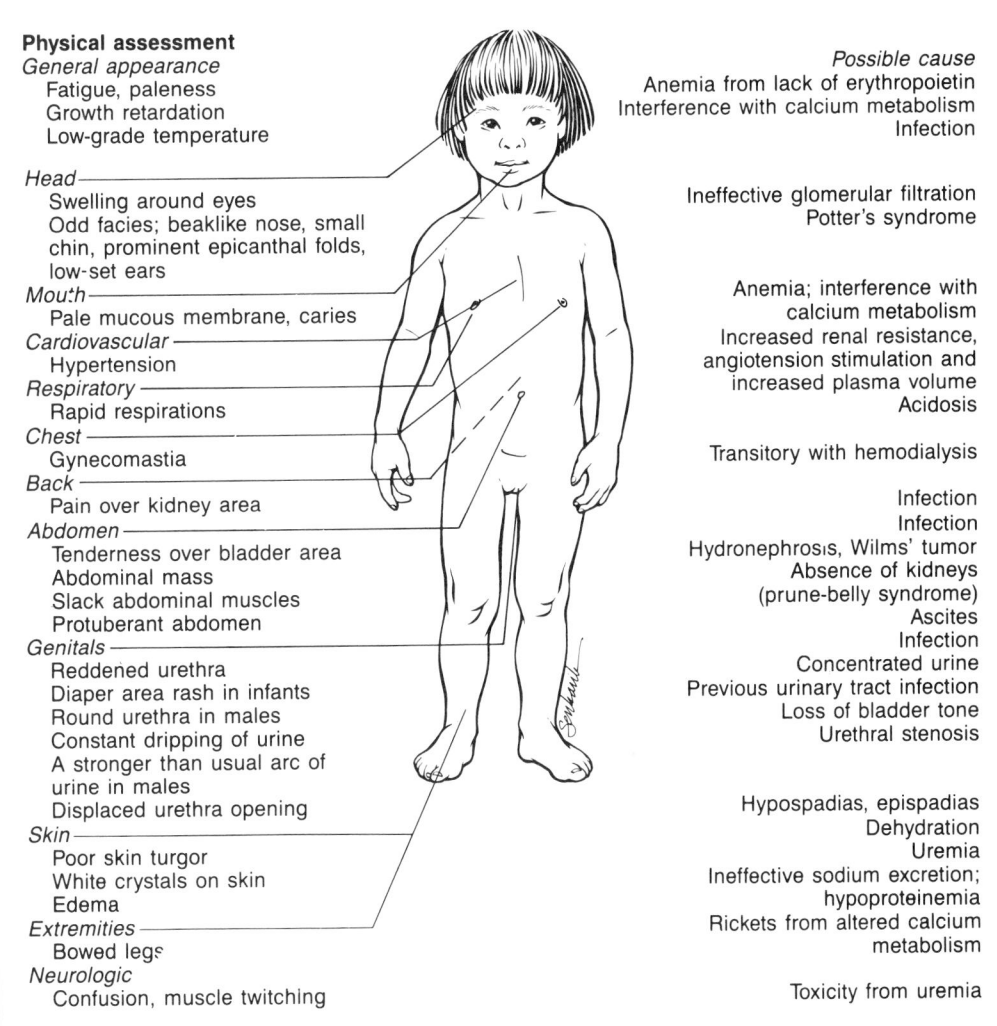

General appearance
  Fatigue, paleness
  Growth retardation
  Low-grade temperature

Head
  Swelling around eyes
  Odd facies; beaklike nose, small chin, prominent epicanthal folds, low-set ears
Mouth
  Pale mucous membrane, caries
Cardiovascular
  Hypertension
Respiratory
  Rapid respirations
Chest
  Gynecomastia
Back
  Pain over kidney area
Abdomen
  Tenderness over bladder area
  Abdominal mass
  Slack abdominal muscles
  Protuberant abdomen
Genitals
  Reddened urethra
  Diaper area rash in infants
  Round urethra in males
  Constant dripping of urine
  A stronger than usual arc of urine in males
  Displaced urethra opening
Skin
  Poor skin turgor
  White crystals on skin
  Edema
Extremities
  Bowed legs
Neurologic
  Confusion, muscle twitching

Possible cause
Anemia from lack of erythropoietin
Interference with calcium metabolism
Infection

Ineffective glomerular filtration
Potter's syndrome

Anemia; interference with calcium metabolism
Increased renal resistance, angiotension stimulation and increased plasma volume
Acidosis

Transitory with hemodialysis

Infection
Infection
Hydronephrosis, Wilms' tumor
Absence of kidneys (prune-belly syndrome)
Ascites
Infection
Concentrated urine
Previous urinary tract infection
Loss of bladder tone
Urethral stenosis

Hypospadias, epispadias
Dehydration
Uremia
Ineffective sodium excretion; hypoproteinemia
Rickets from altered calcium metabolism

Toxicity from uremia

FIGURE 46-1
Signs and symptoms of urinary tract dysfunction.

IMPLEMENTATION

Some parents are not knowledgeable about the function of the urinary system; for example, they confuse the words ureter and urethra. The nurse is in an excellent position to serve as a resource person to explain tests or procedures and the reason that they are being done.

Many children with kidney disease take steroids and develop a typical cushingoid appearance. They may have edema or ascites, which makes them appear obese. Classmates can be cruel to the child with a "different" appearance. Implementations may include contacting the school nurse or making the reason for the child's appearance known to the child's teacher. It may include talking to the child's siblings and helping them to understand the reason for so many tests and hospitalizations and why this one child in the family is receiving so much attention.

If kidney damage is extensive and the child's kidneys fail or a transplant is rejected, a family who has worked so hard trying to keep the child alive must now contemplate the death of the child. Nursing interventions can begin to prepare both the child and the parents for death (see Chapter 56).

EVALUATION

Children with urinary or renal disease need follow-up care after their acute illness. They also need comprehensive health maintenance care. Because they are followed by a specialty group or clinic, parents may assume that such care is being given when it is not. Check to see that children have received their routine childhood immunizations (remember that children on steroid or other immunosuppressive therapy should not receive live virus immunizations) and that the mother has had her questions about day-to-day child-rearing concerns answered.

Children returning to the hospital for reevaluation x-ray films or urine tests need as much preparation for procedures as those having them for the first time. Memory blurs events and sometimes confuses children. For example, they may recall that a particular test involved an injection when it did not. Parents wait anxiously for the results of reevaluation studies. They need to be given the results as soon as a comprehensive opinion of the child's progress is available. It may be necessary to point out to busy medical personnel how anxious a particular parent is to hear about the results of the reevaluation.

Examples of outcome criteria established for care might be the following:

- Family states they are able to cope with long-term illness in child.
- Child states the value of a low sodium diet and lists the ingredients of a low-sodium meal.
- Child states she can accept the necessity of a kidney transplant.

Anatomy and Physiology of the Kidneys

Embryonic development of the urinary tract is discussed in Chapter 9. Figure 46-2 identifies the structures of the tract.

Kidneys are more susceptible to trauma in children than in adults, because they are located slightly lower than in adults and are less protected by the ribs. They also do not have as much perinephritic fat to pad them.

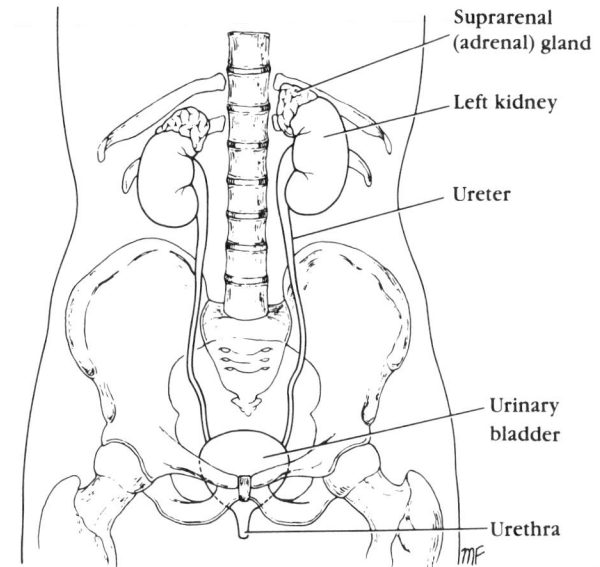

FIGURE 46-2
The urinary system. (From Snell, R. Clinical histology for medical students. Boston: Little, Brown, with permission.)

Nephron

A *nephron* comprises a glomerulus (a filtrating unit) and a complex set of tubules with accompanying blood supply (Figure 46-3). The *glomerulus* is a capillary tuft supplied by a large afferent (ingoing) and a small efferent (outgoing) glomerular artery. It is invaginated within a tubule with a proximal and distal portion. In the glomerulus, water and solutes are filtered from the blood. Passage of water and solutes from the blood into the kidney glomeruli in this way will be effective only as long as the blood pressure in glomerular arteries exceeds that in the tubule. The smaller efferent artery causes back-pressure in the glomerulus, increasing the existing pressure and usually filtration occurs readily. If blood pressure in the glomerulus should fall below the tubular pressure or the tubular pressure should rise so that it is above that of the artery, little or no filtration can occur. This is why renal function must be assessed carefully in children who are hemorrhaging or are in shock with lowered blood pressure for any reason.

This filtered solution passes through the proximal tubule, Henle's loop, and the distal tubule. There, water and electrolytes diffuse back into blood capillaries to such an extent that the volume of the filtrate is reduced by approximately 90%.

The glomerular filtrate enters the proximal tubule at a rate of approximately 120 mL/min. So much of it is reabsorbed that the final end product (urine) is excreted at a rate of only approximately 1 mL/min. The proximal tubules reabsorb most of the water, glucose, sodium chloride, phosphate (PO_4^-), sulfate (SO_4^-), and some bicarbonate (HCO_3^-) ions. This is a passive process, not particularly affected by body needs. The distal tubules have a selective function that responds to body needs. If

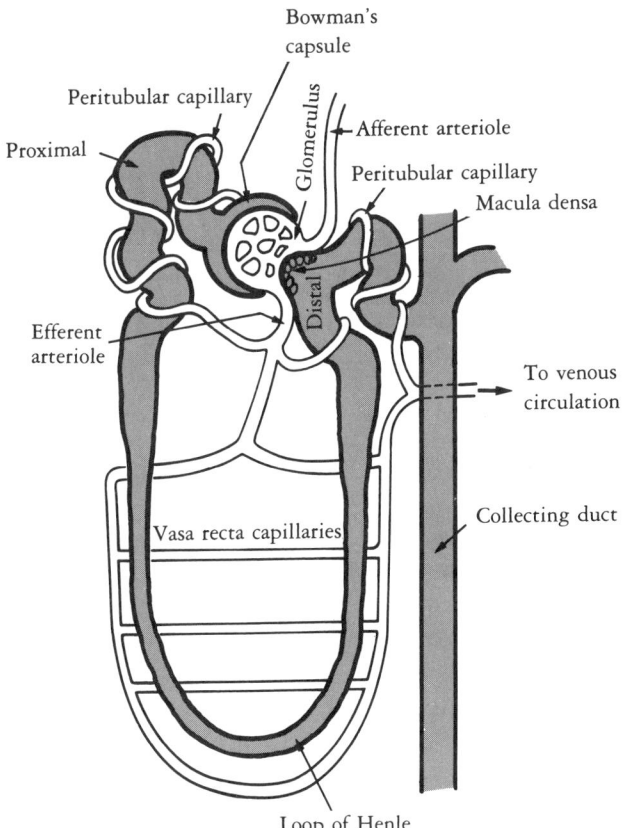

FIGURE 46-3
Basic structure of a nephron with its accompanying blood vessels. (From Richard, C. Comprehensive nephrology nursing. *Boston: Little, Brown, p. 14, with permission.)*

necessary, Na⁺ and HCO_3^- ions and additional water are reabsorbed. If tubular pressure increases (owing to back pressure in the ureters or pelvis) to become greater than glomerular pressure, little absorption can occur. The functions of the various kidney structures are summarized in Table 46-1.

Urine

The amount of urine excreted in a 24-hour period depends on fluid intake, state of kidney health, and age. Approximate urine output from different age groups is shown in Table 46-2. A significant decrease in urine production is termed *oliguria;* absence of urine production is termed *anuria.*

When renal disease occurs, and glomerular or tubular function becomes impaired, nonprotein nitrogenous substances such as creatinine, urea, ammonia, and purine bodies are not excreted but are retained in the blood. Urea is formed from the breakdown of amino acids by the liver; therefore, measuring the amount of urea in urine indirectly measures liver function.

Creatinine is released during cell metabolism. The concentration in urine remains constant, irrespective of the amount of protein in the diet. Its presence and

amount, therefore, can be used in comparing urine specimens. When kidney function is impaired, constituents that normally are retained will be allowed to enter the urine. These include albumin, glucose, blood, bile pigments, and casts. Bile pigments appear in the urine when the child has elevated levels of indirect or direct bilirubin in the blood plasma (hemolysis of red blood cells and obstructed jaundice will cause this). Bile pigments stain urine a greenish yellow-brown color. Casts are formed when there is an abnormal condition that causes the kidney tubule to become lined with a substance that hardens and forms a mold inside the tube. After urine washes the casts out, they can be detected by microscopic examination of urine. They may comprise red and white blood cells, epithelial cells, or fatty cells. Normal constituents of urine are shown in Table 46-3.

Table 46-1. *Kidney Functions*

Site	Activity
Glomerulus	Secretion of water and all solutes but protein from blood
Proximal convoluted tubule	Reabsorption of 80% of glomerular filtrated water, all of glucose, most of sodium, chloride, and ascorbic acid; secretion of creatinine occurs here
Descending and ascending Henle's loop	Reabsorption of additional water; fluid becomes neutral in reaction; specific gravity 1.010; additional sodium and chloride reabsorbed.
Distal convoluted tubule	Reabsorption of water, sodium, chloride, phosphate, and sulfate as needed; secretion of potassium, H⁺ ions, and ammonia (secretion of NH_4^+ and H⁺ ions conserves base because H⁺ ions are substituted for sodium ions; sodium is reabsorbed as sodium bicarbonate)

Table 46-2. *Average Urine Output in a 24-Hour Period in Children*

Age	Amount of Urine (mL)
6 mo–2 yr	540–600
2–5 yr	500–780
5–8 yr	600–1200
8–14 yr	1000–1500
Over 14 yr	1500

(From Behrman, R. E., et al. [1992]. *Nelson's textbook of pediatrics* [14th ed]. Philadelphia: W. B. Saunders, with permission.)

Table 46-3. Normal Urine Analysis Findings

Assessment	Normal Finding	Description
Color	Pale yellow	Color is influenced by urine concentration and ingredients; concentrated urine is more yellow than dilute urine; if fresh blood is present, urine may be red; if old blood is present, it may be brown or black.
Appearance	Clear	Bacteria, excessive crystals, or cells causes urine to be cloudy; if protein content is high, it foams like beer when it is poured from a collecting container to the laboratory collector.
pH	4.6–8.0	Urine becomes alkaline (pH more than 7) when urinary tract infection or severe alkalosis is present; urine left at room temperature becomes alkaline; thus, keep urine refrigerated.
Specific gravity	1.003–1.030	Specific gravity is elevated in dehydration as kidneys try to conserve fluid, and decreased in overhydration as they try to rid the body of fluid; it is important in analysis of protein content (concentrated urine specimen gives a higher protein concentration than a dilute specimen—a fixed amount of protein has been excreted; it is more concentrated in a smaller fluid volume).
Protein	0	In kidney disease (probably due to inflammation), protein molecules are allowed to pass into urine; in adolescent girls, protein in urine may occur as a result of pregnancy; some children (for poorly understood reasons) have *orthostatic proteinuria*, slight to mild proteinuria occurring only when they are standing; this can be detected by comparing an early morning urine specimen, taken just after the child rises, with one taken late in the day.
Ketones	0	Ketones are released following breakdown of body protein, generally because of starvation; diabetes mellitus, if not properly regulated, will also cause ketonuria.
Glucose	0	Glucose in urine can occur as a result of kidney disease; it occurs most frequently in children as a symptom of diabetes mellitus; in adolescent girls, glucosuria may occur with pregnancy.
Red blood cells	Less than 1 per high-power field Negative on dipstick	Blood may be present in urine from such diseases as glomerulonephritis, urinary tract infection, or trauma; renal calculi rarely cause blood in the urine of children; blood may also suggest systemic diseases such as leukemia or blood dyscrasias.

(continued)

Assessment of Urinary Tract Dysfunction

Laboratory/Diagnostic Tests

A variety of diagnostic tests may be performed, either in an ambulatory department or on an inpatient basis, to document urinary tract disease (see the Focus on Cultural Awareness box).

Urinalysis

One of the most revealing tests of kidney function is also one of the simplest: urinalysis. Urine collected for analysis should be fresh; urine that stands at room temperature for any length of time changes composition. Urine collectors for obtaining specimens in infants are described in Chapter 37; urine from diapers may also be analyzed (Gammage et al., 1993). The presence of glucose, protein, and occult blood can be detected and pH can be measured using a dipstick method. Specific grav-

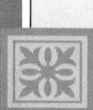

FOCUS ON CULTURAL AWARENESS

The ease with which parents and children are able to discuss illnesses of the kidneys or urinary tract is culturally influenced. As a general rule, this is not a body system that persons discuss as comfortably as they do illnesses of other body systems, because elimination functions are typically regarded as private. The more that modesty is stressed in a culture, the more difficult it may be for people to ask questions about kidney or urinary tract disorders and the later parents may bring a child for care. By being aware that this is a difficult area for parents to discuss health care personnel can observe whether added health education is needed when caring for a child with one of these disorders.

Table 46-3. *(Continued)*

Assessment	Normal Finding	Description
White blood cells	Less than 5 per high-power field	White blood cells are round, small configurations on a microscopic slide; they are present with bacteriuria.
Casts	0	Casts are protein configurations that outline the shape of the distal collecting tubules in which they formed; they are found most often in concentrated urine specimens; when there is cast formation, there is invariably proteinuria; casts comprise red blood cells, white blood cells, or desquamated renal epithelium; as an epithelial cast moves along the nephron, the cells begin to disintegrate, leaving a coarse granular cast; some coarse casts disintegrate still further to become fine granular casts. The last stage of the process is a configuration in the shape of the tubule, termed a waxy cast; waxy casts are translucent and may be shiny and reflect light. The stage of the cast is important in indicating the flow of urine through the kidney; a cast that has reached the waxy stage by the time it has reached the bladder means that there is fairly severe stasis of urine in the urine tubules. Hyaline casts are formations of protein; they appear dull and reflect light poorly; fatty casts are casts caused by the degeneration of tubular epithelial cells and are found in children with nephrosis. The significance of cast formation varies; red blood cells, white blood cells, and fatty casts are evidence of disease; other casts suggest urine stasis and probably proteinuria; the presence of these casts may become significant in the presence of other symptoms or may suggest that other findings should be investigated.
Crystals		Crystal formation may be an indication of urine *p*H; uric acid, cystine, and calcium oxalate crystals are examples of crystals found in acid urine; phosphate crystals tend to be present in alkaline urine. This is an important finding because infection (particularly *Proteus* infection) is the most usual cause of alkaline urine. Sulfur crystals may be present if the child is receiving a sulfa drug (Gantrisin).

ity is best determined by use of a refractometer, because this requires only a single drop (see Chapter 37). A small portion of urine is placed in a centrifuge for 5 minutes, and a portion of the sediment is placed on a microscope slide, where it can be examined for red and white blood cells, casts, or bacteria.

Glomerular Filtration Rate

Glomerular filtration rate is the rate at which substances are filtered from the blood in the kidneys. It is measured by the amount of creatinine (the breakdown product of creatine from muscle contraction) excreted in a 24-hour period. This is known as a creatinine clearance test. A venous blood sample is taken during the 24-hour period to use to compare with the urine findings. A normal creatinine clearance rate is 100 mL/min.

The administration of radioisotopes (a technetium scan) may also be used to assess glomeruli filtration ability. Radioactively tagged substances are given intravenously; the rate at which these substances can be observed flowing through the kidney is then scanned. Parents and the child can be assured that the level of radioisotopes used in these studies is small, and the substance is removed from the body immediately afterward.

Thus, parents do not need to feel that children remain radioactive; they should not be afraid to stay near them or, with infants, hold them after such a study (Kass & Fink-Bennett, 1990).

Urine Culture

The presence of UTI is established by urine culture. Because bladder catheterization can introduce bacteria into the bladder and is painful and intrusive, most urine specimens in children are obtained by a clean-catch procedure. This is an assessment used frequently in children, as discussed in Chapter 37.

The presence of bacteria in urine can be determined by microscopic examination of a specimen. A number of commercial kits for culturing urine are available for use in ambulatory settings. The procedure involved is simple: a specified amount of the urine specimen is added to a commercial vial of culture medium and then observed for a color change at a specified time interval.

Blood Studies

A blood urea nitrogen (BUN) test measures the level of urea in blood and, therefore, is a test of glomerular function. This level may not increase with kidney failure until approximately 50% of glomeruli are destroyed, because the remaining glomeruli are able to increase in size and function to accommodate urine production. A normal value is 5 to 20 mg per 100 mL.

Serum creatinine is equally useful as a measure of glomeruli function. A normal value is 0.7 to 1.5 mg per 100 mL. Creatinine, like urea, is excreted entirely by the kidneys and its level is directly proportional to renal excretory function.

Sonography and Magnetic Resonance Imaging

A *sonogram* (ultrasonic sound waves) or *magnetic resonance imaging* will detect differing sizes of kidneys or ureters and will differentiate between solid or cystic kidney masses (Jones et al., 1990). Parents can be assured that these techniques do not use x-rays, and so may be repeated at frequent intervals for follow-up without danger of radiation exposure to the child.

X-ray Studies

A plain flat-plate abdominal x-ray film will provide information about the size and contour of the kidneys. A small kidney revealed this way is generally a hypoplastic or underdeveloped organ. A large kidney may indicate hydronephrosis or a polycystic kidney. Such an x-ray may be referred to as a *KUB: k*idney, *u*reters, and *b*ladder.

Intravenous Pyelogram. An *intravenous pyelogram* (*IVP*) is an x-ray study of the upper urinary tract. A radiopaque dye is injected into a peripheral vein, circulates through the bloodstream, and is almost immediately identified as a foreign substance by the kidney and filtered out into the urine by the glomeruli. X-ray films taken at frequent intervals reveal the outline of collecting systems in the kidney and of the ureters (Figure 46-4; Monroe, 1990).

In preparing children for an IVP, tell them honestly that they will receive an injection. Say "medicine," not "dye" (or compare coloring kidneys to coloring Easter eggs); some children mistake "dye" for "die." Be sure they know that after this injection they must lie still in whatever position they are placed until all films are taken. This is not easy for children because x-ray tables are hard and cold and the x-ray camera overhead can be frightening. Compare x-ray machines to cameras to reduce this fright. Children may experience flushing of the face, warmth, and a salty taste in their mouth after the injection of dye. The dye used is iodine-based; ask if the child has a known allergy to iodine. This is rarely known in children, since they have had no previous studies of this kind.

Voiding Cystourethrogram. A *voiding cystourethrogram* (*VCUG*) is a study of the lower urinary tract. The urethra and bladder and the presence of reflux into the

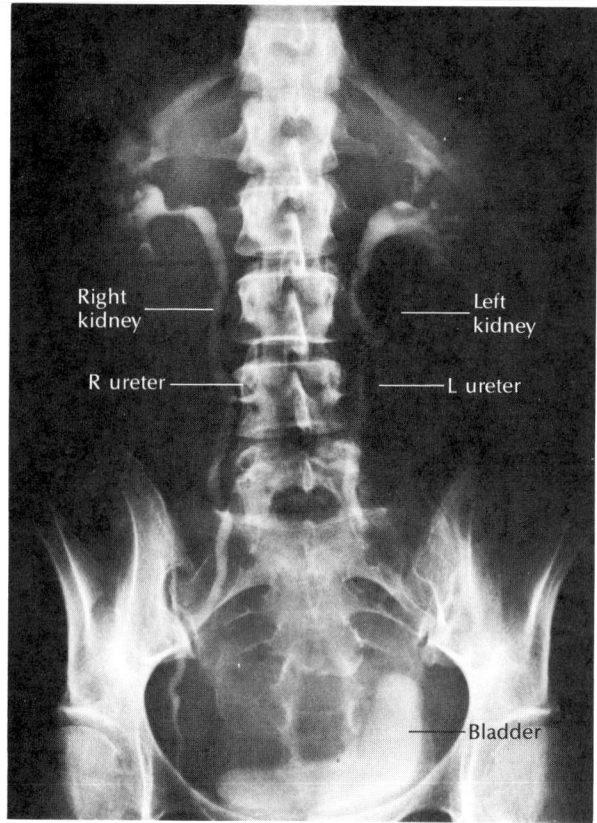

FIGURE 46-4
X-ray film of an intravenous pyelogram. Note how the left kidney fills more fully than the right (a hydronephrosis is present). (Courtesy of the Department of Medical Photography, Children's Hospital, Buffalo, NY.)

ureters are revealed. On the x-ray table, the child's bladder is catheterized, then radiopaque dye is injected into the bladder. The child is then asked to void while serial x-ray films are taken. Although the catheterization is unpleasant, being asked to void while they are observed on the x-ray table is the most stressful part of the procedure for most children. Voiding, after all, is considered a private act for most people. Children need to be told in advance that they will be asked to do this, that it is a necessary part of the study. Being certain that children are aware their parents approve of voiding on a table is helpful to some children (they have just been taught that the only proper place for voiding is a bathroom). Caution children that a first voiding after catheterization may be painful. A few children have difficulty voiding a second time after they return to their hospital room, because they worry that the second voiding will also sting. Sitting in a bathtub of warm water and voiding into the water may help relieve pain. Most children, once they void this second time and realize that it is not painful, have no further difficulty.

A VCUG should not be done if the child has an active UTI; there is danger that the radiopaque material injected into the bladder will spread, along with bacteria from the infection, into the ureters and kidneys. Any symptoms of UTI (i.e., frequency, pain on voiding, or low back pain) should be reported to the physician on admission. A clean-catch urine test may be ordered before the VCUG to rule out infection.

Computed Tomography. *Computed tomography* (*CT*) scans of the kidneys are used to reveal the size and density of kidney structures and adequacy of urine flow. Children may be given a sedative before a CT scan because they must lie still for an extended time during the procedure. The size of a CT scanner and the fact that it surrounds the child is frightening to small children, so they need to be well prepared for this. A dye may be injected before the procedure to better outline urine flow. Call the x-ray department to ask if this will be done to ensure that preparation will be adequate. X-ray studies always carry an extra threat to children, because a support person is not allowed to remain in the room during the procedure. Be certain that the preparation is so thorough that children can comfortably handle the procedure by themselves.

Cystoscopy

Cystoscopy, examination of the bladder and ureter openings with direct examination by a cystoscope introduced through the urethra, is done with children with possible vesicoureteral reflux or urethral stenosis. Because it is painful and requires the child to lie still for the procedure, it is usually done under general anesthesia. Children must have nothing by mouth for at least 4 hours before the procedure so that the general anesthesia can be administered safely. After the procedure, the first voiding may be painful. Urge the child to drink afterward so he or she urinates frequently to flush out any possible pathogens introduced at the time of the procedure.

Radiopaque dye may be introduced into the bladder at the time of cystoscopy so the bladder can be visualized on x-ray (cystography). Small catheters can also be threaded into the ureters and dye introduced into ureters to outline them (retrograde pyelography).

Renal Biopsy

Renal biopsy, which involves passing a thin biopsy needle into the kidney through the skin over the kidney, is used to diagnose the extent of renal disease and thereby predict disease outcome or progress or beginning rejection of a transplanted kidney. Renal biopsy may be done in the older child under only a local anesthetic; general anesthesia will be necessary for the younger child who cannot cooperate easily. The kidney is located first by sonogram to accurately locate the place of the biopsy. The child lies prone with a sandbag under the abdomen for firmness. If the procedure is done under a local anesthetic, prepare children for the feel of a pinprick as the

local anesthetic is injected; after this, they will not feel any further pain. They will feel pressure as the biopsy needle is inserted. Caution children that they need to lie still while the biopsy specimen is taken (if the child moved suddenly, the needle might puncture a renal artery or vein or tear vital glomeruli). It helps if a child's primary nurse can always accompany her for this procedure so that she has someone to hold her hand or touch her during the time she feels the pressure of the needle.

After the biopsy, a sterile gauze square is pressed against the site for approximately 15 minutes to halt bleeding, followed by a pressure dressing. Caution parents that a large dressing will be used and that the size of this dressing does not reflect the size of the specimen taken (the amount of tissue removed is no more than the lumen of the needle used or approximately the size of a pencil lead).

Urine voided after renal biopsy is invariably blood-tinged. Children are kept on complete bed rest for 24 hours or until no more hematuria is present. Keeping serial urine samples helps to detect whether hematuria is becoming more or less marked. Pour each voided urine into a separate container (or replace the collector at timed intervals if a catheter is in place); measure each specimen for volume, mark each specimen with the time of collection, and refrigerate each specimen. Compare each specimen with the previous one. When urine no longer appears bloody, test it with a dipstick for occult blood.

Vital signs should be measured and the biopsy site observed frequently (every 15 minutes for the first hour). Do not lift the dressing to assess bleeding because this destroys the protective function of the pressure dressing. Encourage children to drink a considerable amount of fluid during the first 24 hours to keep urine flowing freely and prevent blood clotting during this time. Play games with a child if necessary to encourage a high fluid intake (the child must take a drink each time before his or her turn at a game; play "Simon Says" and have Simon frequently say, "Drink").

A hematocrit is usually ordered 24 hours after the procedure to provide another assessment that bleeding is not occurring.

Structural Abnormalities of the Urinary Tract

Patent Urachus

When a bladder first forms in utero, it is joined to the umbilicus by a narrow tube, the *urachus.* When this fails to close properly during embryologic development, a fistula is left between the bladder and umbilicus (**patent urachus**). This occurs more commonly in males than females. The urachus remnant can be revealed on sonogram (Hawkins 1994). On close inspection, a clean, odorless fluid will be seen draining from the base of the cord. If the fluid is tested with Nitrazine Paper for *p*H, its acid content will identify it as urine.

A few patent urachus abnormalities heal spontaneously. The majority require surgical correction to prevent pathogens from entering the fistula site and causing persistent bladder infection. This can be done in the immediate neonatal period using only a small subumbilical incision.

Exstrophy of the Bladder

Exstrophy of the bladder is a midline closure defect that occurs during the embryonic period of gestation (first 8 weeks). It results in the bladder lying open and exposed on the abdomen. It occurs more frequently in males than females.

Assessment

Exstrophy can be revealed by fetal sonogram (Jaffe et al., 1990). With the condition, there is no anterior wall of the bladder and no anterior skin covering on the lower anterior abdomen (Figure 46-5). The bladder ap-

pears bright red and is unable to contain urine; thus, urine continually drains from it. In males, the penis is often unformed or malformed. Pelvic bone defects, particularly nonclosure of the pubic arch, and urethral defects such as *epispadias*—opening of the urinary meatus on the dorsal or superior surface of the penis—may also be present. The skin around the bladder quickly becomes excoriated owing to constant exposure to acid urine. Children with this disorder need to be observed as they begin to walk for a "waddling" gait that denotes the effect of the nonfused pubic arch.

Therapeutic Management

The surgical treatment of bladder exstrophy is surgical closure of the bladder and anterior abdominal wall if that is possible. In a second-stage operation, a urethra is created. Surgical repair may be unsuccessful because limited bladder tissue may be present. For this reason, in some instances, the bladder is surgically removed and a *continent urinary reservoir* (an artificial bladder) is constructed (Figure 46-6).

Formerly, children had ilioconduits constructed. This involved segmenting a section of the bowel, attaching the ureters, and then creating a stoma to the abdominal surface. Ilioconduits constantly drain urine and thus

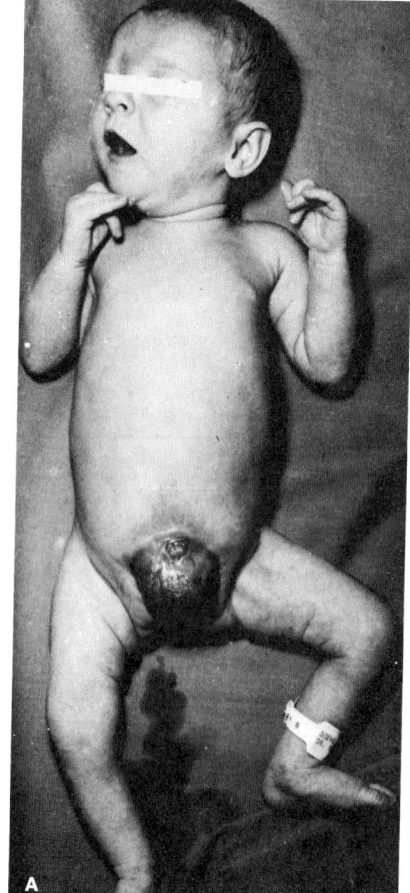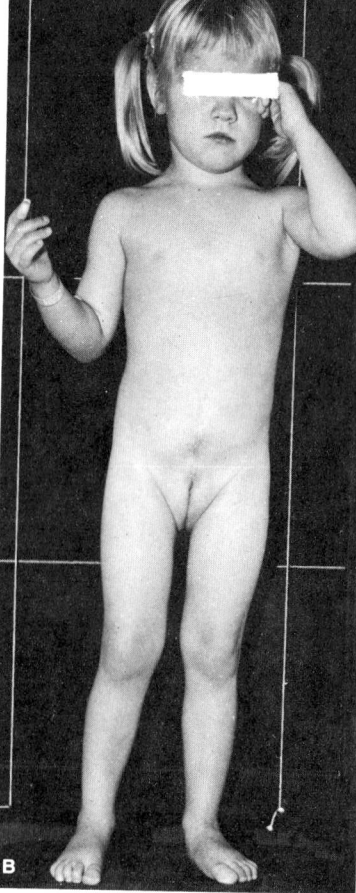

FIGURE 46-5

*Bladder exstrophy. (**A**) Characteristic appearance of exstrophy in a 6-month-old infant. (**B**) Same child at age 2 years, following surgical reconstruction. (From Crowley, L. V. An introduction to clinical embryology. Chicago: Year Book Medical Publishers, with permission.)*

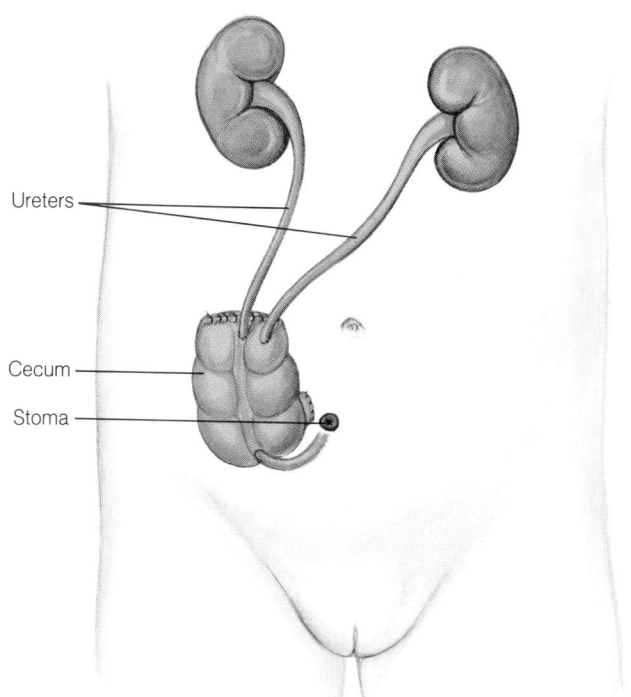

FIGURE 46-6
A continent urine reservoir. A portion of intestine is isolated; the attached ureters drain to it. The appendix creates an abdominal stoma for catheterization.

need to be covered by an ostomy bag to collect urine. For a continent urinary reservoir, a small segment of the intestine, usually the cecum, is separated from the intestinal tract. The intestinal tract is then anastomosed so that a normal gastrointestinal tract is maintained. The separated segment is attached to the internal abdominal wall using the appendix to create an artificial urethra. The ureters are anastomosed to this segment (Figure 46-6; Atta, 1991).

Urine drains from the kidneys into the ureters, and then into the collecting bowel segment. The child self-catheterizes the abdominal urethra three or four times daily to empty urine. Although the procedure is theoretically simple, it is technically difficult to accomplish. Parents need a good review of anatomy so that they understand well the procedure to be done. As the child reaches school age and begins school activities that expose the condition to others, such as showering, adjusting to a continent urinary reservoir may be difficult. The child needs follow-up care during the school years and in adolescence, to assess not only the function of the reservoir but also adjustment to it.

An older system of transplanting ureters directly into the intestine (a *ureterosigmoidostomy*) is little used currently because there is a possibility that ureterosigmoidostomy leads to the growth of adenocarcinoma in the bowel, caused by irritation from the urine (Husmann & Spence, 1990).

Nursing Diagnoses and Related Interventions

Preoperative Interventions. To minimize the possibility of infection, the exposed bladder is usually covered by sterile petrolatum gauze or a moist sheet of silicone elastomer (Silastic) membrane. This also prevents the bladder surface from adhering to bedclothes or diapers and the mucosal surface from being injured. Because the skin of the abdomen becomes excoriated from the constant irritation of urine, it must be protected by a substance such as A & D Ointment, Karaya Gum, or Maalox. To reduce pressure and prevent further separation of the symphysis, the infant's legs may be flexed and brought together and wrapped in Ace bandages to hold them in that position. Do not separate the infant's legs to place diapers. Diapers are usually just placed under the child rather than fastened in place. Be certain to change the diaper promptly after the infant defecates so that he or she does not move and bring feces forward to the open bladder. Position the infant on his or her side so that urine drains freely. The child is generally not placed in a tub for a bath but is sponge-bathed, so that bath water will not enter the ureters and become a source of infection.

Help parents to learn to care for the child. They need support to view their child as normal in all other ways but the unusual bladder formation. In some instances, the bladder repair will not be made immediately, so parents will need instructions on how to care for the child at home while waiting for surgery to be scheduled.

Postoperative Interventions. Surgery is often completed in a two-step procedure. In the first step, the bladder tissue is constructed; in the second a urethra is created. After bladder construction, the surgical incision over the bladder area must be kept free of infection. Position the infant on one side or the other or in an infant chair to prevent feces from coming forward and contaminating the incision line. A suprapubic tube for urine drainage will be in place to rest the newly constructed bladder. Urine draining from the tube may be blood-stained immediately after surgery but should clear after the first few hours. Children may notice sharp painful bladder contractions for the few few days following surgery. Analgesics and antispasmotics may be needed to keep the child comfortable. In order to prevent the nonfused pubic bone from separating and putting stress on the suture line, the child may be fitted with an external fixation device after the osteotomy to hold the pubic bones in approximation until they fuse (Gearhart, 1991).

After the second-stage urethra repair, children can be expected to experience some stress incontinence (loss of urine on physical exertion) from the constructed urethra.

Hypospadias

Hypospadias is a urethral defect in which the urethral opening is not at the end of the penis but on the ventral (lower) aspect of the penis (Figure 46-7*A*) (Coran & Polley, 1994). The meatus may be near the glans, midway back, or at the base of the penis. This anomaly is fairly common, occurring in approximately 1 in 300 male newborns. It tends to be familial and may occur from a multifactorial genetic focus. Epispadias is a similar defect occurring on the dorsal surface of the penis (Figure 46-7*B*).

Assessment

All male newborns should be inspected at birth for hypospadias. The degree of hypospadias may be minimal (on the glans but inferior in site) or maximal (at the mid-shaft or at the penal-scrotal junction). Many newborns with hypospadias have an accompanying short *chorda*—a fibrous band that causes the penis to curve downward (often called a cobra-head appearance; Figure 46-7*C*). Inspect boys with hypospadias carefully for *cryptorchidism* (undescended testes), often found in conjunction with hypospadias.

If the penis defect is so extensive that sex determination is unclear, a Barr body analysis from a buccal cell smear or full sex cell karyotyping (see Chapter 7) may be done. Hypospadias is a difficult medical diagnosis for most parents to accept. They may view it as a threat to the child's masculinity. They may have difficulty discussing this defect with relatives or health care personnel. Help them work through these feelings by allowing them to talk about the disorder and by answering their questions directly.

Therapeutic Management

In the newborn, a *meatotomy*—a surgical procedure in which the urethra is extended to a normal position—may initially be performed to establish better urinary function. When the child is older (age 12 to 18 months), adherent chordae may be released; if the plastic repair will be extensive, all surgery may be delayed until the child is age 3 to 4 years. In order to encourage penis growth and make the procedure easier, the child may have testosterone cream applied or an injection of testosterone given daily. Much or all of the surgery can be done in an ambulatory setting. It is important that hypospadias be corrected before school age so that the child appears normal to his school classmates. Later in life, a meatal opening at an inferior penile site will interfere with fertility, because it does not allow sperm to be deposited close to the female cervix as in normal coitus. Repair must be made before this time to prevent infertility.

Children with hypospadias should not be circumcised, because at the time of plastic repair, the surgeon may wish to use a portion of the foreskin for the repair (Snow et al., 1990).

After surgery for repair, a urinary drainage catheter (suprapubic or perineal) will be inserted to allow output of urine without tension against the urethral sutures. Parents need to be familiarized with this type of urinary catheter or they may worry that the correction differs from what they were told. The purpose of the correction is to make a normal urethra. A catheter that does not exit through the meatus suggests that the urethra is still not normal. The child may notice painful bladder spasms as long as the catheter is in place (1 week to 10 days). An antispasmodic medication such as propantheline bromide (Pro-Banthine) may be prescribed.

After a hypospadias repair, children can be expected to be normal both in urinary and reproductive function unless accompanying anomalies of the penis are present.

Infections of the Urinary System and Related Disorders

Urinary Tract Infection

UTIs occur most often in females. Of girls ages 5 to 15 years, 5% have at least one UTI during their school-age years. The incidence of infection is so high in preschool

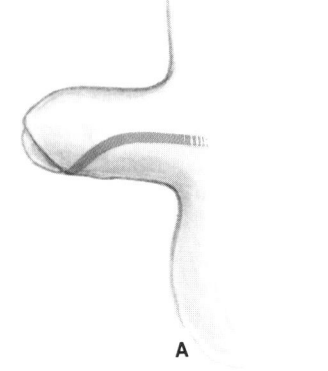
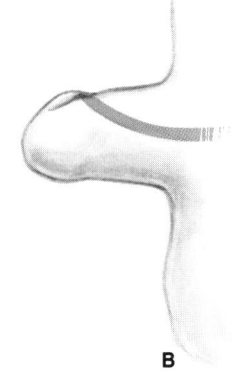
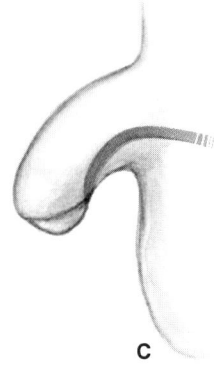

FIGURE 46-7
*Urethral defects. (**A**) Hypospadias. (**B**) Epispadias. (**C**) Hypospadias with chordee.*

A   B   C

girls that a routine clean-catch urine specimen is suggested at routine preschool health assessments.

UTIs need vigorous treatment in childhood so that they do not spread to involve the kidneys (pyelonephritis). Children with recurrent UTIs will be scheduled for a full diagnostic work-up to determine whether they may have a congenital anomaly such as urethral stenosis or bladder-ureter reflux that causes recurrent urine stasis. This is apt to be true in boys with UTIs.

Pathogens appear to enter the urinary tract most often as an ascending infection. Most urinary pathogens are gram-negative rods; *Escherichia coli* is a frequent offender. Antibody formation may occur if the infection involves the pelvis of the kidney; it is less likely if the infection is limited to the lower tract (Belkengren & Sapala, 1993).

Prevention

UTI occurs from ascending spread from the urethra to the bladder (Schlager & Lohr, 1993). They tend to occur more often in girls than boys probably because the urethra is shorter in girls and because it is located closer to the anus, from which *E. coli* spread. Girls should be taught early (when they are toilet-trained) to wipe themselves from front to back after voiding and defecating to avoid contamination of the urethra. There is a suggested correlation between the use of products such as bubble bath and UTI in girls. Infection also often occurs after first sexual intercourse. Use of these products as well as feminine hygiene sprays should be kept to a minimum. Measures to prevent UTI are summarized in the Focus on Family Teaching.

Assessment

The symptoms of UTI in children generally are not clear cut. The symptoms that occur in older children or in adults—pain on urination, frequency, burning, and hematuria—may not be present in young children. If the infection is confined to the bladder (cystitis), the child may have a low-grade fever, abdominal pain, and enuresis (bedwetting). Children under 2 years of age may demonstrate failure to thrive. If the infection is a pyelonephritis, the symptoms generally are more acute, with high fever, abdominal or flank pain, vomiting, and malaise. Some children are admitted to emergency rooms because of the high fever. Although it may be possible to locate a UTI precisely as urethritis, cystitis, ureteritis, or pyelonephritis, more often the exact location or extent of the infection is unknown, and so it is referred to simply as a UTI.

Urine for culture should be collected by a clean-catch technique, suprapubic aspiration, or catheterization, so that bacteria from the vulva or foreskin are not contained in the sample. Suprapubic aspiration is generally limited to newborns, because it is so frightening to older children. Catheterization may actually introduce infection as well as be frightening, so its use is limited in children of all ages.

Urine obtained from suprapubic aspiration is generally sterile, so any growth from this source is significant. A clean-catch urine specimen is said to be positive for bacteriuria if the bacterial colony count is more than 100,000 per milliliter. A count of less than 10,000 per milliliter is considered a negative culture. Counts between 10,000 and 100,000 per milliliter are repeated.

FOCUS ON FAMILY TEACHING

Q. My adolescent daughter has had two urinary tract infections in the past year. How can she better prevent these in the future?

A. Urinary tract infections usually occur because bacteria enter the urethra. Here are some common measures she can take to prevent this from happening:

- Drink periodically during the day, especially in warm weather or during exercise, to keep urine flowing freely and prevent stasis of urine in ureters.

- Void at least every 4 hours to prevent stasis of urine in bladder.

- Do not use bubble bath and feminine hygiene sprays; they cause vulvar and urethral irritation.

- Wipe front to back after defecation or urination to prevent moving rectal contamination forward to urethra.

- Void immediately after coitus to remove any bacteria forced into the urethra by pressure.

- Wear cotton, not synthetic, underwear to decrease perineal irritation.

- Wash vulva daily to lower the bacterial count on the perineum.

- When menstruating, change sanitary pads at least every 4 hours to reduce the possible growth of bacteria near the urethra.

- If symptoms of a urinary tract infection should occur (pain on urination, frequency, blood in urine), call your primary health care provider. If an antibiotic is prescribed it must be taken for the full prescribed course so all bacteria is completely eradicated. Otherwise, after a short time, bacteria will proliferate, and the infection will recur.

Usually the urine also is positive for proteinuria (due to the presence of bacteria). Microscopic examination may reveal the presence of red blood cells (hematuria) because of mucosal irritation. The presence of red or white blood cells and bacteria tends to make urine more alkaline; the *p*H will therefore be elevated (more than 7).

Therapeutic Management

The medical treatment for UTI is the oral administration of an antibiotic such as ampicillin or amoxicillin or parenteral therapy of cefotaxime or gentamicin.

In addition to the antibiotic, the child needs to drink a large quantity of fluid to "flush" the infection out of the urinary tract. Cranberry juice is often recommended as being highly effective in acidifying urine and making it more resistant to bacterial growth. In actual practice, there is little proof of its effectiveness, so offer any fluid the child drinks readily. If the child has such pain on urination that he or she refuses to void, sitting in a bathtub of warm water and voiding into the water may be helpful. A mild analgesic may help reduce pain enough to allow voiding.

The length of time that a child must remain on antibiotic therapy is fairly controversial. Treatment with antibiotics must be continued for a minimum of 10 days; some physicians prefer to continue use for 2 to 6 months so that all bacteria are completely eradicated. Parents need to be reminded that although the child's symptoms will fade in 1 or 2 days, the full course of treatment must be given. Create a reminder sheet to be posted on the refrigerator door to help ensure compliance. A repeat clean-catch urine is usually obtained at 72 hours to assess the effectiveness of the antibiotic treatment.

After antibiotic therapy is stopped, at least three sterile urine specimens must be obtained to prove that bacteria are not still present. At periodic health checkups for the next few years, a child should void a clean-catch specimen for culture or microscopic analysis.

If more than one infection occurs, in addition to removal of the bacteria causing the infection, an investigation as to the cause of infection will be scheduled, whether a congenital stricture or ureteral reflux. Studies such as an IVP and a VCUG are routinely done. A radioactive scan to show bladder filling may be done. Vesicoureteral reflux will be corrected surgically if this is the cause. Meatal or bladder neck obstruction is difficult to relieve in girls, although if the stenosis is extensive, surgery is necessary to relieve back pressure on the kidney as well as urine stasis.

"Honeymoon" Cystitis

Honeymoon cystitis refers to lower UTIs seen in young women shortly after they initiate a first sexual relationship. Such infections occur in connection with the local irritation and inflammation caused by initial sexual coitus. Cystitis of this nature is occurring more and more

frequently in young adolescent girls as more girls of this age group begin to engage in sexual relations. Such UTIs respond quickly to antibiotic therapy. Voiding as soon as possible following coitus may help to flush pathogenic organisms from the urethra and prevent such infections from occurring. When cystitis is seen in adolescent girls, it should alert health care providers to the possibility that a girl may be sexually active and, in addition to needing counseling about personal hygiene measures to prevent UTIs, may need information on sexually transmitted diseases, reproductive planning, and her responsibility for her maturing body.

Vesicoureteral Reflux

Normally, urine flows from the ureters into the bladder with almost no flow reentering the ureters from the bladder. **Vesicoureteral reflux** refers to retrograde flow of urine from the bladder into the ureters. This occurs because the valve that guards the entrance from the bladder to the ureter is defective either from birth or because of scarring from repeated UTIs, bladder pressure that is stronger than usual, or ureters that are implanted at abnormal sites or angles. This back flow of urine happens at micturition (voiding) when the bladder contracts (Figure 46-8; Hawkins, 1994).

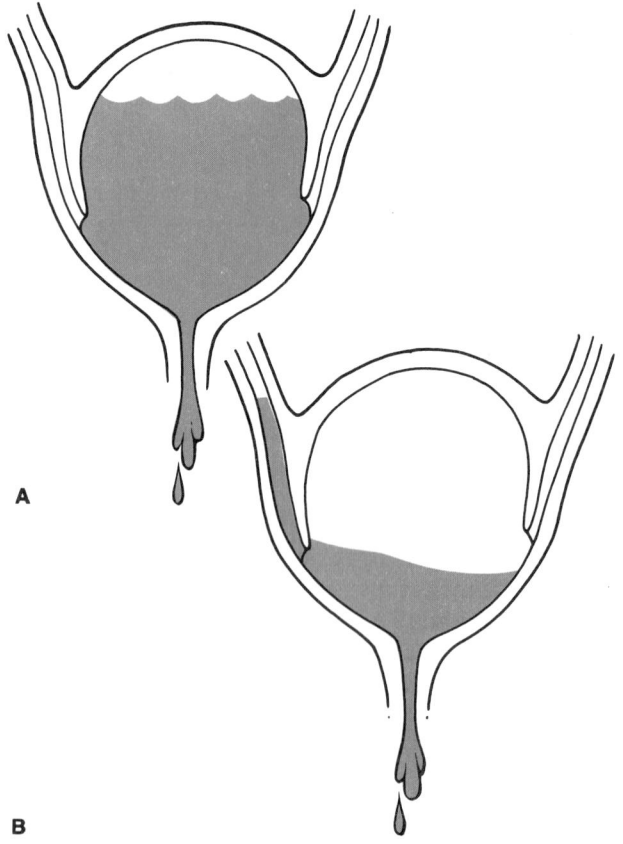

FIGURE 46-8
*Bladder reflux. (**A**) Normal voiding pattern. (**B**) Reflux into ureters with voiding.*

Reflux leads to bladder infection because with reflux, urine is retained in ureters after voiding. Stasis of this urine leads to infection. It also appears that the capacity for normal bladder tissue to lyse bacteria becomes reduced with reflux because of the large residual urine volume that is always present. In addition, reflux is a potentially serious condition because it can lead to back pressure on the kidneys, which destroys nephrons because of the high pressure; it can lead to hydronephrosis or dilatation of the renal pelvis. The condition is inherited as a polygenic disorder (Skoog & Belman, 1991).

Assessment

A child with reflux is usually first seen by health care personnel because of a history of repeated UTIs. A VCUG, isotope scan, cystoscopy, or cystography with contrast material will reveal the ureteral reflux.

Reflux is graded by degree as follows:

Grade 1: Reflux is only into the ureters. No dilatation of ureters is present.

Grade 2: Reflux reaches the renal pelvis. No dilatation of ureters is present.

Grade 3: Dilatation of ureters is present.

Grade 4: Both ureteral and renal pelvic dilatation is present.

Grade 5: Progressive ureteral and renal pelvic dilatation.

Therapeutic Management

UTIs must be rigorously treated to decrease the possibility of glomeruli scarring. Teaching double voiding (having the child void, then in a few minutes attempt to void again) may help to empty the bladder and prevent recurrent infection from stasis of urine. It may be necessary to maintain a child on prophylactic antibiotics to prevent bladder infection. The long-term maintenance with antibiotics is apparently as effective in reducing renal scarring as is surgical intervention (Walker, 1994).

If the reflux is minimal when first discovered, it can be corrected by endoscopy. Under a general anesthesia, a cytoscope is passed and polytetrafluoroethylene (Teflon) paste is injected to stabilize the ureter valves (O'Donnell, 1990). Surgery to correct the placement of ureters may be scheduled; this can be done by laparoscopy. The reason reflux does not normally occur is that ureters enter the bladder obliquely and a bladder skin flap or "valve" obscures the end of the ureter. Surgery reinserts ureters at a more oblique angle, creating this normal valve effect.

The child returns from reflux surgery with a suprapubic catheter in place to keep the bladder empty and prevent pressure against the surgical area. Two ureteral catheters (stents), threaded into the ureters to drain urine directly from the kidney pelvis also exit at the suprapubic tube site. In preparing children for this type of surgery, be certain to prepare them for the number of tubes that will be inserted. Explain that even with the tubes in place, the child will be allowed to walk and move about soon after the operation (and should do this). Both the child and parents must understand that it will be important to keep the urine collecting bags below the level of the child's bladder so they do not raise them when helping the child out of bed. Use a three-dimensional anatomic model to show the location of ureters and bladder. Many children are unaware of the purpose or location of these organs so cannot understand an explanation related to them unless they are shown models. Parents need a good explanation of the necessity for this type of surgery and of the potential seriousness of bladder reflux. Otherwise, they find this surgery so frightening that they may question whether it is necessary. Provide opportunities for therapeutic play (e.g., catheters, simulated x-ray machines, or soft dolls) to help children work through all the new experiences they have had to accept.

Both the ureter catheters and the suprapubic catheter must be observed closely for drainage; the color and the amount of urine must be carefully measured and recorded. This will be bloody initially, but will clear in 1 or 2 days. Assess drainage for clots (should not be over pinpoint in size). Check every hour for the first 24 hours and then every 4 hours that all three tubes are draining urine. The stents should drain an equal amount, to ensure that kidney production is equal on both sides; urine will drain primarily from the stents the first 3 days postsurgery; thereafter, drainage will flow around the stents and be mainly from the suprapubic tube.

The ends of both the suprapubic tube and splint tubes drain to closed collecting bags. It is extremely important that the ends of the catheters not become infected, because infection can then spread to the surgical area or the kidneys. An antibiotic solution such as povidone-iodine (Betadine) may be ordered placed in the drainage bags to limit the growth of bacteria in the collecting urine. Be certain any amount added is subtracted from the output amount. As soon as urine drainage from the splint catheters has decreased and blood has cleared, the splint catheters will be removed. To show that urine is clearing of blood, it is helpful to save a portion of urine each time that collecting bags are emptied; label with the time of removal. Comparing the color of these samples (serial urines) will show that urine is clearing of blood. School-age children can help with labeling such bottles and can achieve a real sense of accomplishment by showing this progress to parents. Many children become frightened when they learn the splint catheters will be removed. They can be assured that this does not hurt and can be done in a treatment room without anesthetic.

Children may have painful bladder spasms for the first 3 days postsurgery as well as incision line pain.

Antispasmodics may be prescribed to reduce bladder spasm; not touching or not moving the suprapubic tube also reduces spasms. The suprapubic tube is removed approximately on day 7 postsurgery (again, a nearly painless procedure). There will be slight urine leakage from the puncture site of the tube for 1 or 2 days after removal of the tube. Keep a sterile dressing in place to absorb the leaking urine. The child should not take tub baths until healing at the suprapubic tube site is complete.

A small number of children continue to have bladder reflux after ureter reimplantation. All children need follow-up care (i.e., repeated urine cultures or perhaps an IVP or VCUG at a later date) to establish that surgery was effective in halting the reflux.

Hydronephrosis

Hydronephrosis is enlargement of the pelvis of the kidney with urine as a result of back pressure in the ureter (Arent, 1994). The back pressure is generally caused by obstruction, either of the ureter or of the point where the ureter joins the bladder such as happens with vesicoureteral reflux. Although this may occur at any age, it occurs most often in the first 6 months of life. It may be revealed by fetal sonography (King & Hatcher, 1990).

Children with hydronephrosis are usually free of symptoms; they may have repeated UTIs from urine stasis (difficult to detect in a child this age except as general irritability or crying on voiding). Elevated blood pressure caused by increasing tubular pressure (which activates an angiotensin response) may be detected on a routine health assessment, although blood pressure is not taken routinely in a child of this age. With severe involvement, the infant experiences flank or abdominal pain. Abdominal palpation will often reveal an abdominal mass (the dilated kidney pelvis). An IVP will reveal the enlarged pelvis and the point of obstruction.

Hydronephrosis is a serious disorder, because if the pressure in the pelvis becomes too acute, back pressure on the kidney will interfere with tubular function or cause destruction of nephrons. The treatment is surgical correction of the obstruction before glomerular or tubular destruction occurs.

Disorders Affecting Normal Urinary Elimination

Enuresis

Enuresis is involuntary passage of urine past the age when a child should be expected to have attained bladder control. As this is expected at age 2 to 3 years for daytime, age 4 years for nighttime, enuresis is said to occur at about 5 to 7 years. Enuresis may be nocturnal, diurnal, or both. It is primary if bladder training was never achieved; acquired or secondary if control was established but was lost (Kurtz et al., 1993).

Functional nocturnal enuresis (that with no known cause) occurs in approximately 8% to 12% of children age 8 years or younger. It is found more frequently in boys than girls; it tends to be familial (if it is present in a child, one of the parents probably experienced it, too).

Assessment

Children who are older than age 5 years need an evaluation to determine if there is an organic cause for the disorder. Ask at history-taking how parents have tried to correct the problem; identify whether it is primarily a problem for the child or the parents (treatment will be most effective if the child wants the situation corrected). Assess the level of stress in the family. Stress factors may be parents who expect more mature behavior of a child than he or she can handle, a new brother or sister, an uncomfortable school situation such as being assigned to a "shouting" teacher, or marital discord between the parents.

If a child wets only on nights when he or she is exceptionally tired or troubled, a functional rather than an organic cause is suggested. If the child has symptoms other than bedwetting, such as abdominal pain, burning, or frequency, UTI is suggested (Williams et al., 1994). Some children who have allergies seem to have an increased incidence of bedwetting at times when their allergic symptoms are evident. If a child wets only when he or she is engrossed in an interesting activity, he or she may simply need more frequent reminding to empty the bladder. It is a common practice for many parents to get children out of bed every night when the parents go to bed to take them to the bathroom; at any point parents stop this practice, children may begin bedwetting because they have been conditioned to empty their bladder at this time of night.

Some children with enuresis have abnormal electroencephalographic patterns. Other children with the same abnormal patterns do not have enuresis, however, so this by itself is not a sufficiently specific finding to be helpful. In others, bedwetting seems to occur as children pass from a period of rapid eye movement sleep pattern to a type IV level, or it is primarily a sleep disorder. It may be associated with small bladder capacity (which would account for why the condition is familial).

To aid diagnosis, an IVP, VCUG, or sonogram may be done to rule out organic disease. A clean-catch urine should be collected to rule out bacteriuria. Specific gravity is assessed to rule out a defect in urine concentration; protein and glucose to determine basic kidney disease.

Therapeutic Management

The treatment of enuresis may be complex because the cause is generally unknown. If stress factors have been identified, an attempt should be made to correct these. Some stress factors such as birth of a new sibling cannot be changed, but frank discussion with children of what causes the stress and attempts to help children cope better with their daytime activities may improve enuresis. If allergy appears to be the cause, a restricted diet may be necessary.

It may help to limit fluids after dinner. Parents need to exercise common sense, however. A thirsty child is thirsty, and he or she may not be able to go every night without a drink from dinner until breakfast. Caution parents of children with sickle-cell anemia not to restrict fluid this way, because if such children become dehydrated, increased sickling of cells occurs.

Synthetic ADH (desmopressin) administered intranasally may be prescribed to reduce urinary output. Imipramine (Tofranil) is an anticholinergic drug that inhibits urination; given an hour before bedtime, it is often effective (see the Focus on Nursing Care box). Alarm bells that ring when children wet at night may be effective but are not widely encouraged. This type of system does not actually stop bedwetting; the alarm wakes the child, he or she stops voiding, and then the child gets up and uses the bathroom. Over time, this type of conditioning is effective. Once the urine alarm is removed, however, children may relapse to enuresis. If enuresis was a manifestation of stress in the child, parents may discover that although this method stops the bedwetting, the child develops another habit, such as stuttering or thumb-sucking. Bladder-stretching exercises—drinking a large quantity of water and then refraining from voiding as long as possible—to increase the functional size of the bladder may be helpful in some children. A bladder that can hold 300 to 350 mL of fluid will generally be large enough to contain urine during a night's sleep. As a general measure, children who wet their beds need to

---

FOCUS ON NURSING CARE

Medications Frequently Prescribed With Urinary or Renal Disorders

Ethacrynic Acid (Edecrin)

Action: Diuretic; inhibits reabsorption of sodium in loop of Henle, promoting increased production of urine
   Dose: 1–2 mg/kg/day given early in day
   Side-effects: Nausea and vomiting; anorexia, hypokalemia, hearing loss

Nursing Actions
1. Administer early in day so child does not have diuresis during the night.
2. Assess for hypokalemia (signs of muscle weakness, cardiac arrhythmia).
3. Assess for gastrointestinal effects (nausea and vomiting).

Imipramine Hydrochloride (Tofranil)

Action: A tricyclic antidepressant with anticholinergic effects, one of which is urine retention. Taken orally, it is absorbed from the gastrointestinal tract and carried to responsive organs highly bound to plasma protein. It can effectively reduce enuresis.
Caution: The product contains tartrazine (yellow dye no. 5) and should not be used with children allergic to this compound. Use with caution in children with a history of seizures, as it may activate these.
   Side-effects: Nervousness, sleep disorders, fatigue, mild gastrointestinal disturbance, constipation, photophobia.
   Dose: 2.5 mg/kg/day taken 1 hour before bedtime.

Nursing Actions
1. Monitor the child for constipation and adequate sleep.
2. Help the child remember to take the medicine daily by a reminder sheet.

Furosemide (Lasix)

Action: Diuretic; inhibits reabsorption of sodium in loop of Henle, promoting increased production of urine.
   Dose: 2–5 mg/kg per dose.

Nursing Actions
1. Monitor for excessive fluid and electrolyte loss.
2. Encourage consumption of a potassium-rich diet to maintain serum potassium level.
3. Store oral solution in the refrigerator to ensure stability and potency.

take baths in the morning rather than at bedtime so that the odor of urine does not cling to them during the day.

Nursing Diagnoses and Related Interventions

A nursing diagnosis specific for enuresis might be Self-esteem disturbance related to enuresis. If the situation is causing a family disruption, High risk for altered family processes related to child's bed wetting might be appropriate. Be certain that goals established are realistic. Some children will respond to therapy more quickly than others.

Enuresis is not a minor problem for either parents or for a child. Parents find it difficult to include the child on vacation trips; they may resent the daily linen washing. Children find they must exclude themselves from activities such as slumber parties or camping trips with friends, which might be embarrassing.

Enuresis may occur in hospitalized children because of the stress of their new surroundings; it occurs in preschool children because they are uncomfortable using strange bathrooms or do not understand which bathroom is theirs to use. They need good orientation on admission to the hospital to reduce these misunderstandings and anxieties. Once it has been established that there is no organic basis for the condition, placing as little stress or importance on the enuresis as possible during an illness is the best course.

Postural (Orthostatic) Proteinuria

Some children will spill albumin into the urine when they stand upright for an extended period. The amount of spilling decreases when they rest in a supine position. This condition, called **postural proteinuria** (postural albuminuria), may occur in 2% to 5% of children.

Many children with this condition have no apparent disease; the phenomenon is apparently due to the effect of gravity on glomerulus function. However, because a certain percentage (perhaps as many as one third) of these children develop some form of kidney disorder later in life, they should be investigated for primary kidney disease and should be followed for later reanalysis of urine.

To determine postural proteinuria, urine is collected after the child has been recumbent during the night (a first-voided specimen) and again after the child has been up and active for a number of hours. Make certain when you are collecting urine that you record the child's activity accurately. If the child stood by the crib rail crying for a parent or was held in a nurse's lap for most of the night, the urine may show protein in the morning specimen because it is not truly a "resting specimen." Likewise, for the specimen to be collected after the child has been active, make certain that he or she is up and active,

not lying in a supine position reading a book for most of the time. Play a game if necessary, such as follow the leader, so the child is active.

Disorders of Altered Kidney Function

Renal disorders occur because of faulty kidney formation or illness that causes glomeruli changes.

Kidney Agenesis

Agenesis means lack of growth (literally, lack of a beginning) or that no organ has formed in utero. Absence of kidneys in a newborn is suggested when the volume of amniotic fluid on sonogram or at birth is less than normal (oligohydramnios), because urine normally adds to the volume of amniotic fluid in utero. The infant with kidney agenesis often has Potter's syndrome or accompanying misshapen, low-set ears and hypoplastic (stiff, inflexible) lungs. He or she will void no urine. Bilateral absence of kidneys is obviously incompatible with life unless a renal transplant can be accomplished. The associated condition of inoperative lungs makes a successful transplant highly unlikely.

Polycystic Kidney

Polycystic kidney means that large, fluid filled cysts have formed in place of normal kidney tissue (Hawkins, 1994). The most frequent type of polycystic kidney seen in children is inherited as an autosomal recessive trait. With this, there is abnormal development of the collecting tubules. The kidneys are large and feel soft and spongy to palpation. If the disorder is bilateral, an infant will not pass urine. The mother will have had oligohydramnios during pregnancy. Children often have a typical appearance (i.e., *hypertelorism*—wide-spaced eyes, epicanthal folds, flattened nose; or *micrognathia*—small jaw), a "Potter facies." *Transillumination* (holding a bright light against the kidney area, which makes the fluid in the cysts glow) can demonstrate that the kidneys comprise fluid-filled cysts, or the cysts are revealed by sonogram. In many children, the liver is filled with identical cysts. This is most evident later in life when increased portal circulation occurs (blood cannot perfuse the cystic liver structures, either). Because this kidney disease is inherited, parents and children at adolescence need genetic counseling to fully inform them that future children may also have this problem.

If the condition is unilateral, rather than anuretic, urine production will be decreased (oliguria). Because kidneys are difficult to locate in newborns, a unilateral polycystic kidney may be missed until later in life, when, with increased kidney growth, an abdominal mass can be palpated. The cystic growth offers such resistance to blood circulation that systemic hypertension will result by school age.

The treatment for polycystic formation is surgical removal of a kidney if only one is cystic. If both kidneys are cystic, treatment is renal transplant (difficult in the young child, because few infant kidneys are available for transplant and because of the technical challenge of such small blood vessels).

Both the absence of kidneys and polycystic kidneys are congenital conditions. An important nursing responsibility is observing newborns for voiding (the average newborn voids within 24 hours of birth) to help to establish a diagnosis and prognosis for such infants.

Renal Hypoplasia

Hypoplasia means reduced growth. Hypoplastic kidneys contain fewer lobes than normal kidneys and are small and underdeveloped. The child with hypoplastic kidneys, in addition to having poor kidney function, may develop hypertension from stenosis of the renal arteries. If hypoplasia is bilateral, the child may need a kidney transplant performed in later life to maintain kidney function.

Prune Belly Syndrome

Prune belly syndrome is severe urethral obstruction in utero from abnormal urethral valves. Occurring mainly in males, it causes severe back pressure and destruction of kidneys (Hawkins, 1994). The infant is born with oligohydramnios and pulmonary dysplasia because of the tight pressure in utero. There is massive dilatation of the ureters and possibly a patent urachus.

Accompanying disorders such as undescended testes, cardiac abnormalities, malrotation of the bowel, and abnormal limbs are common. The infant's abdomen is wrinkled (like a prune) because of poorly developed abdominal muscles (Figure 46-9). Without therapy the prognosis is poor, because end-stage renal disease tends to develop. With surgery to correct obstruction in the ureters the prognosis is good. Parents need to be advised to protect children's abdomens from trauma that could be caused by lap belts or baby walkers, because their child lacks abdominal support.

Acute Poststreptococcal Glomerulonephritis

Glomerulonephritis is inflammation of the glomeruli of the kidney. It occurs as an immune complex disease after infection with nephritogenic streptococcus (most commonly subtypes of group-A beta-hemolytic bacteria). Tissue damage occurs from a complement fixation reaction in the glomeruli (*complement* is a protein that is activated by antigen-antibody reactions and actually

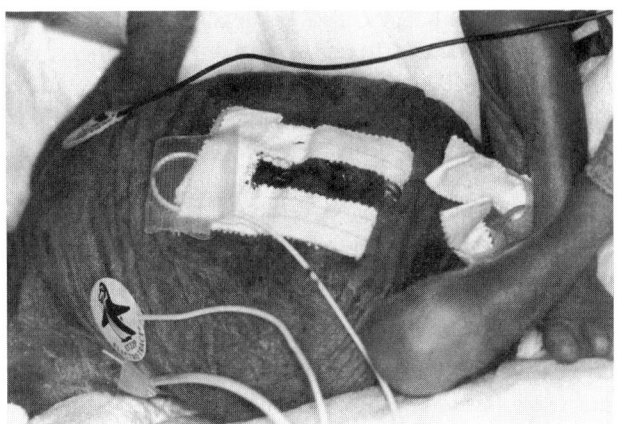

FIGURE 46-9
Prune belly syndrome. Notice the absence of abdominal tone. (Courtesy of the Department of Medical Photography, Children's Hospital, Buffalo, NY.)

plugs or obstructs glomeruli). IgG antibodies against *Streptococcus* may be detected in the bloodstream of children with acute glomerulonephritis, proof that the illness follows a streptococcal infection (Berry & Brewer, 1994).

Intravascular coagulation in minute renal vessels occurs. Ischemic damage leads to scar formation and decreased glomeruli formation. The result is a reduction in the glomerular filtration rate, leading to an accumulation of sodium and water in the bloodstream. Inflammation of the glomeruli will result in increased permeability, allowing protein molecules to escape into the filtrate.

Assessment

Acute glomerulonephritis is most common in the age group most susceptible to streptococcal infections: 5 to 10 years. Boys appear to develop the disease more often than girls; it occurs more often during the winter and spring months, as do pharyngeal streptococcal infections. The child typically has a history of a recent respiratory infection (within 7 to 14 days) or impetigo (within 3 weeks). All children who have had a "strep" throat, tonsillitis, otitis media caused by streptococcal infection, or impetigo caused by *Streptococcus* should have a urinalysis 2 weeks after the infection. Without frightening them unduly, tell parents that this is an extremely important test that they must not take lightly or forget.

Acute glomerulonephritis is characterized by a sudden onset of hematuria and proteinuria. The protein content both of individual urine specimens and of total 24-hour urine volume is measured. A dipstick test of a single specimen will show 1^+ to 4^+ protein; a 24-hour urine specimen may contain as much as 1 g of protein. Normal urine contains none.

The hematuria with acute glomerulonephritis is usually so gross that the child's urine appears reddish-brown or smokey. Urinary sediment will contain white blood cells; epithelial cells; and hyaline, granular, and red blood cell casts. After these initial urine changes, the child develops oliguria. Specific gravity of urine will be elevated. Hypertension from hypervolemia occurs. The child may have abdominal pain, a low-grade fever, edema, anorexia, vomiting, or headache. There may be cardiac involvement related to the difficulty in managing the excessive plasma fluid. Such children show signs of orthopnea, cardiac enlargement, enlarged liver, pulmonary edema, and a galloping heart rhythm. Heart failure may occur from an extreme circulatory overload. If the heart is involved, electrocardiographic changes such as T wave inversion and prolongation of the PR interval may be evident.

If blood pressure reaches 160/100 mm Hg as part of the acute process, encephalopathy may occur, with symptoms of headache, irritability, convulsions, vomiting, coma or lethargy, and perhaps transitory paralysis. The reason for the blood pressure increase is probably the expanded circulatory volume. The cerebral symptoms are caused by *cerebral ischemia* (vasoconstriction of cerebral vessels to reduce cranial pressure).

Blood analysis may reveal a lowered blood protein level (hypoalbuminemia) due to the massive proteinuria. Low serum complement will be present and, as the blood volume expands, a mild anemia. As in all inflammatory diseases, the erythrocyte sedimentation rate will increase. Because the glomeruli of the kidney cannot filter properly, concentrations of urea and nonprotein nitrogen (BUN) and creatinine in blood plasma will increase. The antistreptolysin O (anti-DNase B) titer or antibody formation against *Streptococcus* is generally elevated, indicating that a recent hemolytic streptococcal infection has occurred.

Therapeutic Management

The course of acute glomerulonephritis is 1 to 2 weeks. During this time, there is little therapy specific for the disorder. Antibiotics usually are ineffective because the disease is caused not by an active infection but by an antigen-antibody inflammatory response to a past infection. Diuretics are of little value because plugged glomeruli bases cannot be made to function; a course of ethacrynic acid may be tried. If congestive heart failure seems to be occurring, specific measures such as a semi-Fowler's position, digitalization, and oxygen administration may be necessary. If diastolic blood pressure rises to more than 90 mm Hg, antihypertensive therapy with a fast-acting vasodilator is necessary. Diazoxide or hydralazine are agents commonly used (Berry & Brewer, 1994).

Bed rest is unnecessary. Children should be encouraged to participate in quiet play activities. They are permitted to attend school and to engage in normal activities after 1 or 2 weeks, but competitive activity is limited until kidney function has returned to normal.

Diet is controversial. Although limiting protein intake reduces the amount of protein lost in urine, many children who are losing large quantities of protein need high-protein diets to supplement this loss. Salt restriction may be successful in reducing severe edema. Most children do well on a normal diet for their age, however, with normal salt and protein content. Weighing the child every day and calculating intake and output are important assessments in following the course of the disease. In most children, acute glomerulonephritis runs a limited, benign course. After most symptoms fade, proteinuria and impaired clearance of urea and creatinine may remain for as long as 2 months. Parents must be cautioned that the results of a test for protein in the urine will remain abnormal for several weeks, so that if their child has this test as a routine screening procedure at a health checkup, they should not worry that this finding means reinfection or the beginning of further disease. Approximately 2% of children will not completely recover from acute glomerulonephritis but will develop chronic nephritis. These children appear to suffer destruction from the initial inflammation that resulted in chronic renal insufficiency.

Nursing Diagnoses and Related Interventions

> ***Nursing Diagnosis:*** Situational low self-esteem, related to feelings of responsibility for onset of serious illness
>
> ***Goal:*** Child (Parent) will verbalize positive aspects about self and interact appropriately with others in 1 month.
>
> ***Outcome criteria:*** Child (Parent) states feelings about becoming ill; discusses future plans and ways to maintain health; participates in care.

Glomerulonephritis is a frightening disease for both child and parents. Children may be frightened by the initial hematuria; they may be upset at the appearance of periorbital edema, which makes their reflection in the mirror so strange to them. Children as young as early school age are aware that kidneys are necessary for life; they recognize the significance of kidney disease for life.

If children were prescribed penicillin for a pharyngitis 2 weeks before the development of the nephritis and refused to take it, they have reason to feel that they caused this disease. The parents feel guilty because they did not force the child to take the medicine. They worry that their child will develop chronic glomerulonephritis or die during the acute phase of this attack because of heart failure. These parents and children need to talk about their feelings. They need frequent reports of subtle positive changes in a child's condition (e.g., "His blood pressure is staying down by itself now; he does not need medicine for that anymore." "He weighs 2 pounds less today than when he was admitted; that generally means his kidneys are beginning to function more efficiently again").

If the child is discharged on limited activity, parents may appreciate suggestions about activities that kept him or her most interested for long periods while in the hospital. Before discharge, they need to know the date and place of a return visit for follow-up care. Be sure they have a telephone number to call if they have questions about their child's care or condition while the child is at home.

Acute glomerulonephritis can be avoided by the prevention or effective early treatment of group-A beta-hemolytic streptococcal infections. Acute glomerulonephritis tends not to recur with subsequent streptococcal infections, so prophylactic penicillin to prevent further streptococcal infections is unnecessary.

Chronic Glomerulonephritis

Although chronic glomerulonephritis (chronic renal failure) occasionally may follow acute glomerulonephritis or nephrotic syndrome, it also occurs as a primary disease (or following acute glomerulonephritis that was clinically so mild it was undiagnosed). The child is found to have proteinuria at a routine checkup. Further investigation may reveal hypertension and the presence of red cell or white cell casts and occult blood in urine. The specific gravity of the child's urine is below normal (below 1.003). Blood studies may reveal an increased BUN or creatinine level. A renal biopsy will establish permanent destruction of glomeruli membranes.

Chronic glomerulonephritis may be diffuse or local. In both instances, there is some nephron damage. The remaining functioning nephrons increase their glomerular filtration rate to compensate for those that are damaged. At some point in this chronic disease destruction process, however, compensatory mechanisms fail, and renal insufficiency or failure will result. **Alport's syndrome** is a progressive chronic nephritis inherited as an autosomal dominant disorder.

During the chronic course of glomerulonephritis, if the child has acute symptoms of edema, hematuria, hypertension, or oliguria, hospitalization with bed rest is necessary. If children have only a chronic manifestation such as proteinuria, and if they feel well, they can maintain normal activity, including attending school. Children should not engage in competitive activities such as contact sports, however, because of the danger of kidney injury.

Medical therapy is nonspecific, directed toward symptoms rather than the disease process itself, because the cause of chronic kidney destruction is unknown. Therapy with hypotensive drugs such as hydralazine (Apresoline) or with diuretics such as the thiazides may

be necessary. Corticosteroid therapy may reduce or halt the progress of the disorder by reducing inflammation. Children have difficulty accepting long-term corticosteroid therapy because of the side-effects, in particular, a typical moon face and extra body hair (Cushing's syndrome). Children need someone to talk to about these body changes and to be assured that these changes will be reversed when the drug is discontinued.

Children on corticosteroids are extremely prone to infection because their immunologic system is suppressed. They need protection from other children and health care personnel with infection. Parents need to learn to take their child's temperature and must recognize and report the earliest signs of infection.

Generally the prognosis in children with chronic glomerulonephritis is poor. Although the illness may run a long-term course, eventually it tends to lead to renal insufficiency or renal failure. Children may be maintained for long periods by peritoneal dialysis or hemodialysis. Kidney transplantation is a possibility.

Because children as young as early school age are aware of the importance of kidney function to life, most children with chronic renal disease are aware of the likely outcome of their disease. Most children are adolescents or young adults before the disease runs its ultimate course. They indicate that they appreciate having health care personnel face this outcome with them honestly if a kidney transplant cannot be obtained to prolong their life.

Nephrotic Syndrome (Nephrosis)

Nephrosis is altered glomeruli permeability due to fusion of the glomeruli membrane surfaces; it causes abnormal loss of protein in urine.

Immunologic mechanisms are involved in instigating the process; the cause may be hypersensitivity to an antigen-antibody reaction or an autoimmune process; a T-cell dysfunction may be responsible. Nephrotic syndrome in children occurs in three forms: (1) congenital; (2) secondary, as a progression of glomerulonephritis or in connection with systemic diseases such as sickle cell anemia or systemic lupus erythematosus (SLE); or (3) idiopathic (primary). In children, the idiopathic form is seen most commonly. Nephrosis can be further classified according to the amount of membrane destruction present. Minimal change nephrotic syndrome (MCNS) is the type most often seen in children; with this, as the name implies, little scarring of glomeruli occurs. Children with this degree of scarring respond well to therapy. Other types are focal glomerulosclerosis (FGS) and membranoproliferative glomerulonephritis (MBGN). Both types involve scarring of glomeruli. These children will have a poor response to therapy. Fortunately, the majority of children (80%) develop only MCNS.

The age of peak incidence of the idiopathic

nephrotic syndrome is 2 to 3 years; the syndrome occurs more often in males than females.

The four characteristic symptoms of nephrotic syndrome are (1) proteinuria, (2) edema, (3) low serum albumin (hypoalbuminemia), and (4) hyperlipidemia (increased blood lipid level). Proteinuria occurs because protein is lost owing to the increased glomeruli permeability. The result is hypoalbuminemia. With a low level of protein in the bloodstream, osmotic pressure causes fluid to shift away from the bloodstream into interstitial tissue, causing edema. As the blood volume decreases, the kidneys begin to conserve sodium and water, adding to the potential for edema. The hyperlipidemia occurs because the liver increases production of lipoproteins to try and compensate for protein loss. Lipids are too large to be lost in urine and thus rise to high levels in the blood serum (Thabet et al., 1993). Some children have such high cholesterol levels that when blood is drawn and placed into a test tube, a circle of white fat forms on the top of it. Figure 46-10 illustrates the process that leads to the common symptoms.

Assessment

Symptoms usually begin insidiously. Children develop edema around the eyes (periorbital edema), most noticeable when they wake in the morning from a head-dependent position. Parents may notice that clothing no longer fits a child around the waist, because edematous fluid is beginning to collect in the abdominal cavity (ascites). It is easy to dismiss these first symptoms as those of an upper respiratory tract infection and the normal "paunchy" belly of a toddler or preschooler. As edema progresses, the child's skin becomes pale and stretched taut. In boys, scrotal edema becomes extremely marked. Ascites becomes extensive enough that pressure on the stomach leads to anorexia or vomiting. Children may have diarrhea due to intestinal edema and poor absorption from the edematous membrane. Because of poor nutrition, growth may stop. The child may become malnourished but yet appear deceptively obese, because of

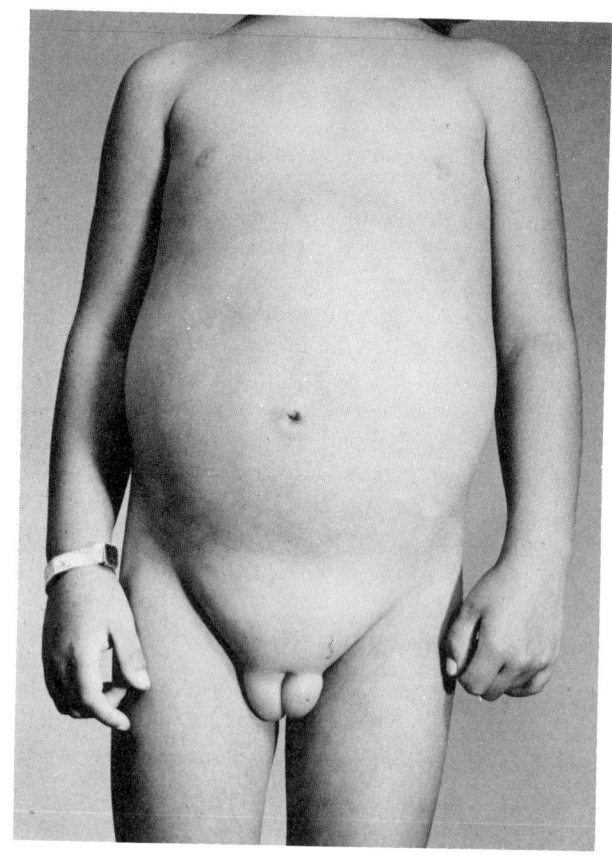

FIGURE 46-11

A child with nephrotic syndrome. Notice the distended abdomen caused by ascites and the edematous labia. (Courtesy of the Department of Medical Photography, Children's Hospital, Buffalo, NY.)

the extensive edema (Figure 46-11). When the ascites becomes even more extensive, children may have difficulty with respiration as the abdominal fluid presses against the diaphragm. Parents report that children are irritable and fussy, probably from the feeling of abdominal fullness and generalized edema. An increased clotting tendency can occur from the decreased intravascular fluid volume.

Laboratory studies will reveal marked proteinuria. A single dipstick test will reveal a 1^+ to 4^+ protein; a 24-hour total urine test will reveal up to 15 g of protein. The protein loss with nephrosis syndrome is almost entirely albumin, differentiating it from the proteinuria of glomerulonephritis, in which protein loss tends to be nonspecific. Some children with nephrotic syndrome have hematuria at the onset, but it is minimal in contrast to that seen with acute glomerulonephritis. The erythrocyte sedimentation rate (demonstrating the inflammation of the glomeruli membrane) is elevated. Features of acute glomerulonephritis and nephrotic syndrome are compared in Table 46-4.

A renal biopsy may be done to determine whether there is scarring of the glomeruli membrane.

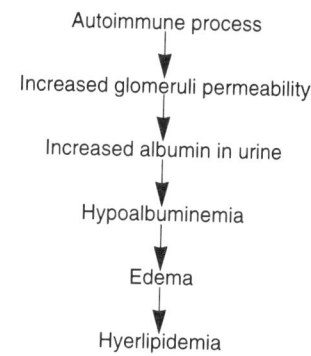

Autoimmune process

Increased glomeruli permeability

Increased albumin in urine

Hypoalbuminemia

Edema

Hyerlipidemia

FIGURE 46-10

The process that results in the signs and symptoms of nephrotic syndrome.

Table 46-4. *Comparison of Features of Acute Glomerulonephritis and the Nephrotic Syndrome*

Assessment Factor	Acute Glomerulonephritis	Nephrotic Syndrome
Cause	Immune reaction to group-A beta-hemolytic strepto-coccal infection	Idiopathic; possibly a hypersensitivity reaction
Onset	Abrupt	Insidious
Hematuria	Profuse	Rare
Edema	Mild	Extreme
Hypertension	Marked	Mild
Hyperlipidemia	Rare or mild	Marked
Peak age frequency	5–10 yr	2–3 yr
Interventions	Limited activity; antihypertensives as needed; symptomatic therapy for congestive heart failure	Corticosteroid administration; cyclophosphamide administration; possibly a diuretic and potassium supplement
Diet	Normal for age	High-protein, low-sodium
Prevention	Prevention or thorough treatment of group-A beta-hemolytic streptococcal infections	None known

Therapeutic Management

Medical treatment for the child with nephrotic syndrome is directed toward reducing the edema with a course of steroid therapy and keeping the child free of infection while the immune system is suppressed owing to the steroid therapy. Adrenocortical steroid therapy (oral prednisone) rapidly reduces proteinuria and consequently edema in most children. An initial dose of prednisone is given until diuresis without protein loss is accomplished; dosage is then reduced for maintenance.

This will continue for 1 to 2 months. Parents must test the first urine specimen of the day for protein with a dipstick method and keep an accurate chart showing the pattern of protein loss. Approximately once a week, they are usually asked to collect a 24-hour urine specimen so that total protein loss can be measured.

Prednisone is generally given every other day after the initial 4 weeks rather than every day. Prednisone has the potential to halt growth and to suppress adrenal gland secretion. However, growth is apparently not delayed when the drug is given on alternate days, and this method also prevents alteration of adrenal steroid production. Parents may need to be assured that therapy every other day is best to keep them from changing the schedule to every day or giving twice the calculated dose by adding extra tablets on alternate days. To help parents remember to give medication on alternate days, have them choose either even or odd calendar days as the day of administration. Help them design a reminder chart for the refrigerator or bathroom door. Prednisone tastes bitter; parents may welcome suggestions as to how to disguise the taste, such as by mixing it with applesauce.

Be certain both the parents and the child are aware that prednisone causes a cushingoid appearance (i.e., moon face, extra fat at the base of the neck, and increased body hair). Caution parents to plan ahead when getting refills of prescriptions, so that the prednisone therapy is not stopped abruptly because they ran out of medication. This abrupt stop can lead to adrenal insufficiency.

Diuretics are not commonly used to reduce the edema, because they tend to decrease blood volume, which is already decreased. This could lead to acute renal failure. Children who respond poorly to administration of prednisone alone may need diuretic therapy with furosemide (Lasix). When children are taking furosemide for extended periods, there is always a danger that too much potassium will be removed from their bodies with urine, causing hypokalemia. Children on long-term diuretic therapy need frequent blood studies to determine that the potassium level is adequate. They may need supplemental potassium and should have strong potassium sources included in their diet. Children may be administered intravenous albumin to temporarily correct hypoalbuminemia. As the serum albumin level rises, fluid shifts from subcutaneous spaces into the bloodstream. Children are then administered a rapidly acting diuretic to remove the extra fluid. It is important that the diuretic be administered after the albumin infusion or the child could develop a fluid overload and congestive heart failure.

A course of cyclophosphamide (Cytoxan), because of its immunosuppressant action, may be effective in reducing symptoms or preventing further relapses of the disease in children who do not respond to corticosteroid therapy. It is important to ensure adequate fluid intake with cyclophosphamide to prevent bladder irritation and bleeding. Cyclophosphamide is also used in chemotherapy for malignancy. (Table 53-2 in Chapter 53 describes this and other chemotherapeutic drugs.) Be certain that parents are not misled into believing that their child has cancer because he or she is receiving a chemotherapeutic drug. Cyclosporine (Sandimmune) is another immunosuppressant that may be used.

The prognosis in children with nephrotic syndrome varies. Almost all children with MCNS respond initially to steroid therapy and, although they may have a relapse, they will then remain free of the disease. Those with FGS and MBGN types will have relapses at frequent or infrequent intervals over the next several years. Children who have frequent relapses have a relatively poor chance of ever being free of the disorder. Many later develop renal failure. A kidney transplant is a possibility to sustain life.

Nursing Diagnoses and Related Interventions

Nursing Diagnosis: Altered nutrition, less than body requirements, related to poor appetite and restricted diet

Goal: Child will take in adequate nutrients for growth needs throughout course of illness.

Outcome Criteria: Child follows normal growth curve on standard assessment scale.

Because children with nephrosis have poor appetites, maintaining them on restricted diets is difficult. They need a good protein intake to offset protein loss. In some children, mild salt restriction during periods of acute edema is helpful. They need a good potassium intake (e.g., through consumption of fruits and fruit juices, particularly bananas) to maintain sufficient potassium concentrations. During acute phases of the disease, fluid may be temporarily restricted. If this is so, most children are happiest with many small glasses of fluid during the day, rather than several large drinks. It helps to make a chart showing the amount of fluid the child is allowed each day. As fluid is given, color in a portion of the chart corresponding to the amount given. The child can tell from the uncolored portion how much more he or she is allowed that day. This is easier for toddler and preschoolers (the age group usually affected by this disease) to understand than talking in terms of milliliters or even glassfuls.

Nursing Diagnosis: High risk for altered skin integrity related to edema

Goal: Child's skin will remain intact through course of illness.

Outcome Criteria: Child's skin is not broken or erythematous.

The edematous skin of children with nephrotic syndrome tends to break down easily, so they need frequent position changes while in bed. Check clothing to make certain that the elastic band at the waist of pajamas or other constricting parts is not tight. Check boys' scrotums. Soft gauze placed between skin surfaces tends to prevent skin irritation and breakdown. Edematous tissue does not heal well, so breaks in the skin easily become secondarily infected. The child who is not toilet-trained needs frequent diaper changes and thorough cleaning at each change to prevent skin breakdown in the diaper area.

Children are generally more comfortable if they sleep with their head elevated in a semi-Fowler's position. This reduces periorbital edema; if children sleep in a head-flat position, edema can be so severe by morning that children's eyes are swollen completely shut; their tongue is also swollen, so they cannot speak. Parents at home can provide a semi-Fowler's position by placing extra pillows on children's beds or slipping a cardboard box under the head of the mattress to raise the end of the mattress.

Because medications are poorly absorbed from edematous skin areas, intramuscular injections should be kept to a minimum; if one is necessary, it should not be given in the thigh or buttocks of children with edema. Use a deltoid site, which tends to be less edematous. Medication should be administered orally if possible. Weigh children daily to detect fluid accumulation (use the same scale with the child in the same clothing at the same time of day); measure intake and output accurately. Taking pulse rate and blood pressure every 4 hours will detect hypovolemia from excessive fluid shifts to interstitial tissue.

Nursing Diagnosis: Knowledge deficit related to chronic illness

Goal: Parents will demonstrate increased knowledge concerning nephrotic syndrome in 1 week.

Outcome Criteria: Parents describe course and nature of nephrosis and their role in care of child at home.

Parents often need support to manage children at home after the acute phase of the disease subsides. They need clear instructions about their at-home responsibilities: keeping the child free of infection, perhaps by limiting exposure to friends, and giving prednisone or oral diuretics and a potassium supplement. It is easy for parents to confuse these medications and give the wrong tablet on the wrong day or the incorrect dose. Review medication instructions with parents before discharge from the hospital; have the parents repeat the instructions. Make certain they understand when they are to return for a follow-up visit. Make certain they have a telephone number to call if they have a question or concern about their child's care or health.

Congenital Nephrotic Syndrome

Occasionally, nephrotic syndrome occurs in newborns or in infants younger than age 3 months. Such children are particularly resistant to steroid therapy and so have an extremely poor prognosis for recovery. This form of nephrosis occurs most often in Finnish people or those of Finnish descent; it is apparently inherited as an autosomal recessive trait (Figure 46-12). It can be detected during intrauterine life by an elevated alpha-fetoprotein level in maternal serum or by amniocentesis (Albright et al., 1990). The elevated value probably reflects an overproduction of protein to compensate for loss of protein in the urine.

The onset of the disorder is probably during intrauterine life; the child is born with poorly joined cranial sutures as though ossification processes have halted because of calcium metabolism difficulty. The placenta may be much larger than normal, suggesting a perfusion or fluid problem. Almost immediately, proteinuria is present. Renal biopsy will demonstrate some nephron changes. Immunologic studies suggest that the nephron changes may result from a sensitization between the mother and fetus.

The symptoms of congenital nephrotic syndrome are the same as for the syndrome in older children, but they are exaggerated in seriousness. As soon as this disease is diagnosed, a renal transplant is scheduled. These children tend to be steroid resistant, and they will die within months if no transplant is attempted.

Henoch-Schönlein Syndrome Nephritis

Henoch-Schönlein purpura is discussed in Chapter 44. Approximately one quarter of the children who develop this type of purpura develop renal disease as a secondary complication. The renal involvement becomes apparent within a few days after the manifestations of purpuric symptoms. Children may show only urinary abnormalities such as proteinuria or may have a rapidly progressing glomerulonephritis. Most children recover completely; only a few develop chronic symptoms. In those who do, long-term kidney disease develops.

Systemic Lupus Erythematosus

SLE is an autoimmune disease in which autoantibodies and antigens cause deposits of complement on the kidney glomerulus (see Chapter 14). Approximately two thirds of children with SLE develop symptoms of acute or chronic glomerulonephritis. This renal disease is the ultimate cause of death in many adults with SLE. Therapy with corticosteroids or cytotoxic agents may be effective in children with SLE renal disease (Berry & Brewer, 1994).

Hemolytic-Uremic Syndrome

With hemolytic-uremic syndrome, the lining of glomerular arterioles become inflamed, swollen, and occluded with particles of platelets and fibrin. Red blood cells and platelets are damaged as they flow through the partially occluded blood vessels. As the damaged cells reach the spleen, they are destroyed by the spleen and removed from circulation. This leads to hemolytic anemia (Louis, 1994). Hemolytic-uremic syndrome occurs most often in white children generally between the ages of 6 months and 3 years. In most children, no causative factor is known. However, the syndrome often follows a viral or rickettsial, gastrointestinal, or upper respiratory infection, which suggests that it is the result of an antigen-antibody reaction.

Assessment

The major symptom of hemolytic-uremic syndrome is oliguria with proteinuria, hematuria, and urinary casts in urine. The oliguria will lead to increased serum creatinine and BUN. Children will develop symptoms of lethargy and anorexia. They appear pale from the anemia; easy bruising may be present from *thrombocytopenia* (reduced platelet level). Laboratory studies will reveal fibrin-split products in the serum as the fibrin deposits in glomerular vessels are degraded. Thrombocytopenia is present because platelets are damaged by the irregular blood vessels. An increased reticulocyte count reveals that red blood cells are rapidly being replaced.

Therapeutic Management

The extreme oliguria can be treated with peritoneal dialysis; anemia can be corrected by careful transfusion of packed red cells. Peritoneal dialysis is not only frightening to parents because it involves penetration of their child's abdomen, but to many parents it seems to be unscientific (only a homemade therapy). Parents need support during the procedure. Be certain they understand

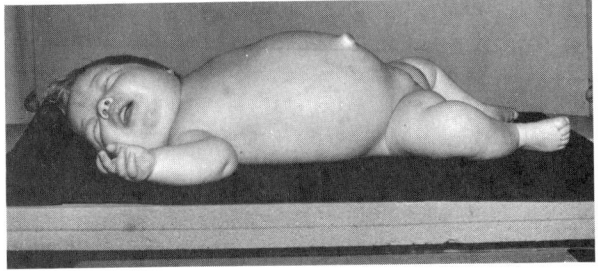

FIGURE 46-12
An infant with congenital nephrotic syndrome. Notice that she has extensive periorbital edema from sleeping with her head at a level with her body. It is a frightening feeling for the child to wake up in the morning unable to see because of such extensive edema. (Courtesy of the Department of Medical Photography, Children's Hospital, Buffalo, NY.)

that they can hold the child during the equilibrium period of dialysis and it does not cause pain. When kidney function begins to return, report the results, such as the improvement in serum creatinine levels. Help parents provide stimulating activities such as a play board, a ball to throw, or rings to stack for the infant on peritoneal dialysis (parents may envision the infant as so ill that lying still without an activity would be the best thing for him or her and so the child misses normal development milestones).

Before discharge from the health care facility, be certain that parents have an appointment for follow-up care. Help them begin to view the infant as well again so they do not continue to shelter him or her unnecessarily but allow for normal growth and development. Despite the extent of the illness, most infants (95%) with hemolytic-uremic syndrome recover completely. A number of children will unfortunately continue to have chronic renal involvement.

Alport's Syndrome (Familial Glomerulopathy)

Alport's syndrome is an autosomal dominant (possible X-linked) inherited disorder that involves ocular disorders, deafness, and chronic renal failure. The initial symptoms that begin in infancy are those associated with glomerulonephritis, such as hematuria, proteinuria, and mild edema. The process slowly increases in intensity until by adolescence the child is in chronic renal failure.

Parents and children should be offered genetic counseling so they are aware of the method by which the illness is inherited. Children can be supported by continuous peritoneal or hemodialysis followed by kidney transplantation.

Renal Insufficiency: Acute Form

Renal insufficiency (kidney failure) occurs in either an acute or chronic form. The acute form most often occurs owing to a sudden body insult; the chronic form from extensive kidney disease.

Children who undergo prolonged anesthesia, hemorrhage, shock, severe diarrhea leading to dehydration, or sudden traumatic injury may develop acute kidney failure. Acute failure also can occur in a child who is placed on a pump oxygenator while undergoing heart surgery or who receives common antibiotics (aminoglycosides, penicillin, cephalosporins, and sulfonamides). Children who swallow poisons such as arsenic (found in rat poison) or are exposed to industrial wastes such as mercury may develop renal insufficiency. The active course of acute glomerulonephritis may also cause kidney failure. All of these conditions appear to lead to renal ischemia, which ultimately leads to acute renal failure.

Assessment

One of the first symptoms noted with acute renal failure is *oliguria,* defined as a urine output of less than 1 mL per kilogram of the child's body weight per hour. To rule out the possibility that the problem is urinary retention in the bladder rather than kidney dysfunction that is causing the oliguria, a Foley catheter may be inserted to drainage.

Azotemia (accumulation of nitrogen waste in the bloodstream) will occur because of the oliguria. *Uremia* (extra accumulation of nitrogen wastes in the blood with additional toxic symptoms such as cerebral irritation) may occur. The BUN level rises progressively as renal insufficiency continues. A level of more than 80 to 100 mg per 100 mL is a toxic level that needs correction, usually by dialysis. Urine creatinine level is another measure that can be used as an indicator of function, because it is normally excreted at a uniform rate. A rate of less than 10 mg per 100 mL indicates severe renal failure. *Hyperkalemia* (elevated potassium level) will occur because potassium not only cannot be excreted but also is released into the bloodstream as cells are catabolized at a rapid rate to maintain plasma protein levels (Feld et al., 1990). Hyperkalemia is revealed by a weak, irregular pulse, abdominal cramps, lowered blood pressure, and muscle weakness. Acidosis will follow shortly from inability of H^+ ions to be excreted. As it becomes difficult to excrete phosphorus, this level will rise in the bloodstream. A high serum phosphorus leads to a low calcium serum level (these always exist in reverse proportion to each other). Severe hypocalcemia can lead to muscle twitching and convulsions (*tetany*); chronic hypocalcemia can lead to withdrawal of calcium from bones (*osteodystrophy*). As the kidneys become unable to dilute or concentrate urine, the specific gravity of urine often becomes "fixed" at 1.010.

An IVP or radioactive uptake scan may be ordered to substantiate the lack of kidney function. Parents and children need support for this type of study, because the results are disappointing and so different from what they hoped they would be. Some children with acute renal insufficiency will die before a kidney transplant can be performed.

Therapeutic Management

Because acute renal insufficiency is a reaction to body stress caused by acute disease or insult, attempts to correct sudden renal failure are aimed at supporting the child's body systems while correcting the underlying condition. If the child is dehydrated (as with diarrhea or hemorrhage), intravenous fluid will be given to replace plasma volume. Such fluid must be given slowly enough to avoid congestive heart failure (extra fluid cannot be removed by the kidneys because the kidneys are not functioning). The fluid should not contain potassium until it is established that kidney function is adequate;

buildup of potassium may otherwise cause heart block. Levels of blood potassium of more than 6 mEq/L are scheduled to be corrected either by the intravenous administration of calcium gluconate (as the glucose moves into cells, it carries potassium with it) or the oral administration of a cation exchange resin such as Kayexalate or by dialysis. Administering sodium bicarbonate may cause a shift of potassium from the bloodstream into cells, temporarily reducing the circulating potassium level. Administration of a combination of intravenous glucose and insulin may be effective (insulin helps glucose move into cells).

A diuretic such as furosemide or mannitol may be ordered in an attempt to increase urine production. Diet should be low in protein, potassium, and sodium and high in carbohydrate to supply enough calories for metabolism yet limit urea production, serum potassium, and fluid retention. Table 46-5 lists foods high in potassium. Fluid intake may be limited to prevent congestive heart failure from accumulating fluid that cannot be excreted. Weigh children daily (same scale, same clothing, same time of day) and maintain accurate intake and output recordings so fluid accumulation can be detected. If children are so ill that they cannot eat, total parenteral nutrition may be used. Regulate amounts carefully to prevent fluid overload (see Chapter 34 for total parental nutrition administration techniques).

When recovery from acute renal insufficiency begins, children generally have a degree of diuresis as the extra fluid accumulated by the body is cleared. The increase in urine must be noted, because children may need additional fluid intake to prevent hypovolemia, which could lead once more to renal insufficiency. Parents usually remain anxious for an extended period after acute renal insufficiency (they are afraid that the restoration of kidney function is only temporary). Give reassurance that urine output is remaining at a normal level; they can begin again to relax and interact effectively with their child.

Renal Insufficiency: Chronic Form

Chronic renal insufficiency results when acute failure becomes long-term or when chronic kidney disease has caused extensive nephron destruction. The nephrons that are not destroyed by long-term disease appear to function normally; they simply are inadequate in number to sustain kidney function. Glomeruli are capable of adjusting and, until 50% of nephrons are destroyed, they enable kidney function to continue normally. After this point, kidney function diminishes by degree until the child develops end-stage kidney disease.

Assessment

With loss of nephron function, kidneys are unable to concentrate the urine. The first sign is polyuria, which

Table 46-5. *Foods High in Potassium*

Food Group	Examples
Fruits	Bananas, peaches, prunes, raisins, oranges, and orange juice
Vegetables	Carrots, celery, lima beans, potatoes, collards, dandelion greens, spinach
Meat	Nuts, peanuts, red meat
Dairy products	Milk, whole or skim; low-sodium milk
Miscellaneous	Salt substitutes, chocolate and cocoa, bran

may be manifested as enuresis. The few functioning nephrons present are unable to reabsorb enough sodium to maintain a functioning level of body fluid so that dehydration occurs. As additional nephrons are lost, oliguria and anuria occur. Inability to excrete H^+ ions leads to acidosis. Part of the excess hydrogen is buffered by bone salts and the result is chronic *osteodystrophy* (calcium leaves bones). Hypocalcemia and hyperphosphatemia occur from inability to excrete phosphate. To compensate for the increased serum calcium level, the parathyroid glands become hyperactive, which leads to further osteodystrophy as calcium is withdrawn from bones to compensate. Kidneys are responsible for synthesizing vitamin D to its active form. With poor kidney function, vitamin D cannot be used; without this, calcium cannot be absorbed from the gastrointestinal tract and deposited in bones. Bones become so drained of calcium that growth halts and they lose strength (renal rickets).

Erythropoietin, formed by the kidneys, stimulates red cell production. When there is decreased erythropoietin production anemia develops. Pruritus may be present from skin irritation from excretion of nitrogenous wastes in sweat from high levels of BUN and serum creatinine. These changes are summarized in Figure 46-13.

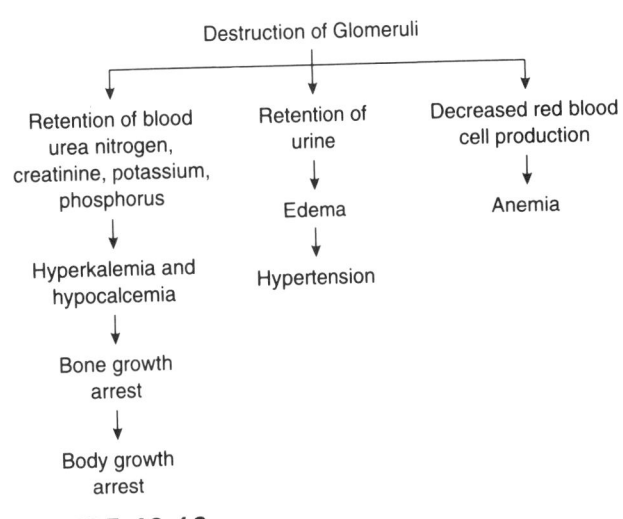

FIGURE 46-13
Pathology of end-stage renal disease.

Therapeutic Management

Children with chronic renal insufficiency are generally placed on a low-protein, low-phosphorus diet to prevent rapid urea and phosphate buildup. Children may take aluminum hydroxide gel with meals to bind phosphorus in the intestines and prevent absorption. Milk usually is not given because it is high in sodium, potassium, and phosphate—electrolytes children may have difficulty clearing. Vegetables such as beans are high in protein and should be eliminated from the diet. This is hard for parents and children to understand because they are taught that meats are high in protein but vegetables are not. Letting the child have some choice about foods they eat each day will help them to tolerate this diet longer. If children will be returning home on a low-protein diet, whoever prepares meals at home will need good instruction on selecting low-protein foods. Low-electrolyte, low-protein formulas such as Similac PM 60/40 and SMA Formula (S-26) are commercially available formulas for infants with renal insufficiency.

Daily fluid intake may need to be restricted, although restriction should be as slight as possible or it will present an area of tremendous conflict between the child and parents. Many children need sodium intake restricted; others require a normal sodium intake (but no excessively salty foods such as luncheon meats, potato chips, or pretzels); other children may actually need additional salt because, due to poor tubular reabsorption, they dump salt in urine. Low-sodium formulas such as Lonalac are recommended for children with congestive heart failure who require a low-sodium intake. They must be used cautiously with children with renal insufficiency, because their high potassium content can lead to toxic blood potassium levels. Diuretics may be ordered to help children regulate sodium and fluid levels and prevent edema.

As renal insufficiency becomes prolonged, the child may need supplemental calcium to prevent muscle cramping, rickets, tetany, or convulsions. As hypertension becomes more and more acute, a daily hypotensive drug may be ordered. A blood transfusion may be needed to correct anemia, but it must be given cautiously so that volume overload does not occur (extra fluid cannot be excreted). Recombinant human erythropoietin may be prescribed to stimulate red blood cell formation (Brown, 1992). Effective excretion of urea can be accomplished by dialysis or by replacing the nonfunctioning kidneys with a kidney transplant.

Nursing Diagnoses and Related Interventions

Nursing Diagnosis: High risk for altered family processes related to chronically ill family member

Goal: Family members will maintain functional system of mutual support for each other during course of child's illness.

Outcome Criteria: Family members express feelings about illness to each other and to nurses; participate in care of ill member.

Children with renal insufficiency grow poorly because of the alteration in calcium metabolism. Their height begins to fall below normal. It is easy for them to become depressed because of chronic fatigue and an unappetizing diet. If children are on corticosteroids or other immunosuppressive drugs, they may be angry or disheartened about their change in appearance.

Caring for a child with chronic renal disease is not only time-consuming but financially and socially devastating for parents. Parents caring for such children at home need opportunities at periodic health assessments to voice their frustrations about trying to keep a child happy (Frauman & Gilman, 1990). They need time to do those things important to them as individuals, whether take a weekend trip or attend an evening show or program. Ask parents at clinic or follow-up visits, "Do you ever get out of the house or have the opportunity to do anything for yourself?" "What can we do for *you?*" Help of this kind ultimately improves children's care, because it improves the lives and mental attitudes of those around them. Nursing care of the child with end-stage renal disease is summarized in the Nursing Care Plan, p. 1448.

Therapeutic Measures for the Management of Renal Disease

Peritoneal Dialysis

Dialysis is the separation and removal of solutes from body fluid by diffusion through a semipermeable membrane. *Peritoneal dialysis* uses the membrane of the peritoneal cavity to do this. It has the advantages of not requiring elaborate equipment or expense; it has the disadvantage of requiring more time than hemodialysis.

Peritoneal dialysis may be used as a temporary measure for children who experience sudden kidney failure due to trauma or shock. It is used for fairly long periods with children with chronic renal disease to allow them to live until a kidney transplant can be arranged (Alexander & Honda, 1993). It is usually begun when the serum creatinine level reaches 10 mg per 100 mL. Other indications are congestive heart failure; BUN of more than 100 mg per 100 mL; hyperkalemia (potassium of more than 6 mEq/L); and uremic encephalopathy (confusion or coma).

Steps of Procedure

Before peritoneal dialysis, weigh a child and take vital signs to provide baseline information. Ask the child to void to reduce bladder size so that the bladder occupies as little anterior space as possible. If a child cannot void, bladder catheterization can be done. The abdomen of the child is cleaned just below the umbilicus with an antiseptic solution and covered with a sterile drape. A local anesthetic is injected into the abdominal wall. A large-bore needle is inserted into the peritoneal cavity. If ascites fluid is present, a quantity of it is drained. A warmed hypertonic glucose solution (approximately 50 to 100 mL per kilogram of body weight) or a commercial dialysis solution is infused by gravity flow into the peritoneal cavity. This distends the abdominal wall and allows insertion of a peritoneal catheter, which will be sutured in place and covered with a sterile dressing (Figure 46-14). This catheter will remain in place for the period of dialysis.

A prescribed amount of dialysis solution is then infused into the peritoneal cavity by gravity drainage. This takes approximately 10 minutes and is recorded as inflow time. The infusion fluid needs to be warmed to room temperature to prevent the child from becoming chilled; moreover, warming the solution to near body temperature appears to improve diffusion efficiency. It can be warmed in a basin of warm water at the child's bedside. Heparin is generally added at least to the first infusion to keep any blood from the abdominal puncture from plugging the tube.

Infused fluid is allowed to remain in the child's peritoneal cavity for 15 to 60 minutes (called the *equilibrium time*). Because the infused solution is hypertonic, fluid from extracellular spaces will diffuse across the semipermeable peritoneal membrane to dilute the hypertonic solution. Urea and electrolytes will diffuse with this fluid. After this diffusion time, the fluid is drained from the peritoneal catheter into a collecting bottle (this takes approximately 10 minutes); this is recorded as outflow time. More fluid generally drains from the peritoneal cavity than is infused, because excessive fluid diffuses across the peritoneum, reducing edema. After a cycle of inflow, equilibrium, and outflow time, a new cycle is begun. Peritoneal dialysis may be continued for periods of 12 to 72 hours depending on the effectiveness of the procedure in restoring the serum creatinine and BUN levels to normal. A careful record of the amount of fluid

infused and recovered must be kept. Meaningful analysis of the figures (i.e., whether the amount of the fluid infused is recovered each time) is a nursing responsibility.

Monitor vital signs at least every hour while children are having peritoneal dialysis. Observe carefully during each new infusion period and during the time the solution is in the abdomen (the equilization period) for shortness of breath from upward pressure on the diaphragm. Elevating the head of the bed helps to increase breathing space and make respirations easier. Tachycardia or lowered blood pressure may indicate hypovolemia. An increasing temperature may indicate that infection of the peritoneum has occurred, a serious complication of peritoneal dialysis. Frequent blood studies are necessary during periods of peritoneal dialysis to determine electrolyte concentrations and if electrolyte imbalances occur, electrolytes may be added to the infusion solution or administered intravenously.

The longer the peritoneal catheter remains in place, the greater becomes the risk of peritoneal infection from the catheter insertion site. Assess the skin insertion site daily for signs of infection (i.e., redness or drainage). Wash the end of the catheter with an antiseptic solution such as povidone-iodine (Betadine) before attaching it to infusion tubing; at the finish of the procedure, if it will not be removed, reclean it and cover it with a secure sterile dressing or commercial cover. Children with peritoneal dialysis tubes in place should have their temperature taken every 4 hours. Ask them to report any abdominal pain or diarrhea. Assess for abdominal guarding or tenderness once daily by palpating their abdomen.

Nursing Diagnoses and Related Interventions

Nursing Diagnosis: Anxiety related to lack of knowledge regarding peritoneal dialysis procedure

Goal: Child will demonstrate comfort with procedure by 24 hours.

Outcome Criteria: Child (if age permits) states he or she understands procedure and ways to keep occupied and entertained during procedure.

As for any procedure, children need to be prepared for peritoneal dialysis. If the procedure is presented in a matter-of-fact way, it is accepted by children with no more apprehension than they have about intravenous therapy. Both procedures, after all, involve a needle penetration. Children can be assured that they will feel the initial prick of the needle that administers the local anesthetic; they will feel pressure after that as the peritoneal needle or catheter is inserted, but this is not pain. It is intrusive, however, and frightening (children have seen characters in movies stabbed or shot in the abdomen and die and cannot help but be worried they will

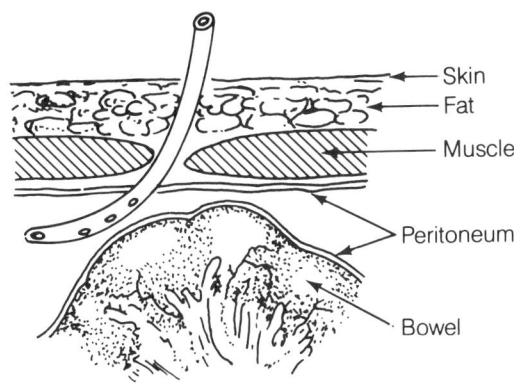

FIGURE 46-14
Insertion site for peritoneal dialysis catheter.

Skin
Fat
Muscle
Peritoneum
Bowel

(text continues on page 1450)

Nursing Care Plan

A Child With End-Stage Renal Disease

Jeanine is a 6-year-old girl with end-stage renal disease. She is cared for at home by her parents. Family consists of one older brother and a younger sister. Child has a home tutor and is visited weekly by a home care nurse. Mother completes peritoneal dialysis four times a week. Parents state their biggest concerns are that Jeanine is losing weight (only at 20th percentile on growth chart), that they lack time for themselves and other children and adequate finances. Mother had to quit her job to care for child.

Nursing Diagnosis: Altered nutrition, less than body requirements, related to end-stage renal disease

Defining Characteristic: Child's weight has been steadily decreasing on growth chart; now at 20th percentile.

Outcome Criteria: Child's weight is maintained at 20th percentile on a growth curve.

Nursing Orders	Rationale
1. Provide high-carbohydrate, low-protein, low-potassium, low-phosphate, low-sodium diet, and possibly decreased fluid.	1. Provides a diet easily digested that leaves little residue for kidneys to evacuate.
2. Supplement with vitamins D and C, folic acid, and pyridoxine as prescribed.	2. Additional vitamins may be needed because of limited intake.
3. Administer oral sodium polystyrene sulfate (Kayesalate) as prescribed for serum potassium over 6 mEq/L.	3. Kayexalate acts to reduce serum potassium.
4. Administer aluminum hydroxide gel as prescribed.	4. Reduces phosphorus absorption from gastrointestinal tract and osteoporosis.
5. Administer supplemental calcium as prescribed.	5. Additional calcium may be necessary to prevent withdrawal from bones.

Nursing Diagnosis: Knowledge deficit related to care of the child with end stage kidney disease

Defining Characteristic: Parents voice that they need increased knowledge of expected problems.

Goal: Parent will demonstrate increased knowledge of care of child.

Outcome Criteria: Parents demonstrate ability to care for child at home.

Nursing Orders	Rationale
1. Educate family about role of kidneys in body function.	1. Understanding can be the beginning of acceptance.
2. Prepare family for transplant when appropriate.	2. Adequate preparation can help family cope with new developments.

Nursing Diagnosis: Altered cardiovascular tissue perfusion related to increased blood pressure

Defining Characteristic: Child's blood pressure is 160/90 mm Hg.

Goal: Child's blood pressure will not increase in amount during illness.

Outcome Criteria: Child's blood pressure is maintained at 130/80 mm Hg.

(continued)

Nursing Orders	Rationale
1. Administer diuretics and antihypertensives as prescribed.	1. Helps reduce blood pressure
2. Assess fluid intake and output.	2. Monitoring intake and output provides early warning about fluid accumulation.

Nursing Diagnosis: High risk for altered growth and development related to chronic illness.

Defining Characteristic: Child is not exposed to normal experiences due to bed rest and frequent hospital admissions.

Goal: Child will meet developmental milestones during childhood.

Outcome Criteria: Child continues progress in school; relates well with family and peers.

Nursing Orders	Rationale
1. Encourage age-appropriate activities such as schoolwork or collecting.	1. Encourages normal growth and development.
2. Encourage interactions with peers through letters and telephone calls.	2. Provides opportunities for age-appropriate growth and development.
3. Avoid unnecessary dietary and activity restrictions.	3. Allows child to have as many choices as possible.
4. Allow child to help plan menus, to add I & O and peritoneal exchange totals, and so forth.	4. Encourages a sense of control.
5. Provide opportunities for therapeutic play (e.g., provide soft doll, peritoneal catheter, syringes, needles, or doll's bed).	5. Therapeutic play can be instrumental in reducing anxiety.

Nursing Diagnosis: Ineffective family coping: compromised, related to care of child with chronic illness

Defining Characteristic: Mother states that chronic illness of child is a stress to family.

Goal: Parents will demonstrate adequate coping behaviors during child's illness.

Outcome Criteria: Parents voice that they are able to cope with present level of stress; use community resources appropriately.

Nursing Orders	Rationale
1. Encourage parents and child to discuss feelings about renal disease.	1. Discussion can lead to better understanding of problems.
2. Help parents contact parent support group (or help form one).	2. Support from a parent's group could aid coping.
3. Plan an activity program based on the extent of the child's condition, a program in which all family members could participate.	3. Planning family activities can build a sense of family strength.
4. Help parents maintain a life and time that is their own through respite care or viewing themselves as important enough to arrange for other caregivers for the child.	4. A strong sense of self-esteem can aid ability to cope.

die with this procedure). Provide opportunities for therapeutic play (e.g., use a cloth doll, a dialysis tube, intravenous tubing, a doll's bed, or syringes and needles).

Once cycles of dialysis begin, children grow bored lying in bed waiting for this procedure to be finished. They need planned entertainment for these times—perhaps a toy or game that is allowed only during the procedure, so that it remains special. Children generally do not feel hungry while having peritoneal dialysis, because the bulk of peritoneal fluid causes pressure on the stomach and makes them feel uncomfortably full. They do well on a liquid diet during this time. So that children can have a sense of control over what is happening to them, let them help with the procedure by doing such things as recording the amount of solution infused and drained; allow them to select liquids they like for meals.

Peritoneal dialysis is such a simple concept that parents may not appreciate its effectiveness in relieving their child's edema or removing urea from the bloodstream. Help them to appreciate the importance so they can radiate a positive attitude toward it; the parents' acceptance of the procedure helps the child to accept it positively also.

Continuous Ambulatory Peritoneal Dialysis

Continuous ambulatory peritoneal dialysis (CAPD) allows a child to return home and go to school (Miller, 1990). A permanent dialysis tube is inserted and sutured into place on the abdomen. The child or parent attaches a bag of dialysis fluid and tubing to this and infuses a prescribed dialysis solution by gravity drainage; the bag and tubing are then rolled into a compact square and carried with the child. The infused solution remains in the child for 4 to 6 hours during the day (8 hours at night); the dialysate bag is then lowered and the solution drains from the peritoneal cavity into it; the bag and fluid are then discarded and a new bag of dialysate solution is attached and raised and new solution infused.

CAPD requires careful monitoring and attention on the part of the child's family. The parent or child must keep accurate records of infusions. Children can participate in gym programs but not contact sports; no swimming is allowed. Teach parents to think ahead for holidays or family trips so they have adequate supplies on hand.

Because CAPD is continuous, it maintains more constant levels of electrolytes in the bloodstream than periodic dialysis; it allows greater freedom because the child can return home and go back to school. Its cost is low because hospitalization is not required. However, there are disadvantages: infection can occur because of the long-term placement of the catheter and, because the tube constantly remains in place, the child is frequently reminded of the illness and may have difficulty accepting this change in body image. In addition, the peritoneal solution constantly distends the abdomen, making the child appear obese and clothing difficult to fit; dehydration may occur due to excessive fluid removal. Possible complications are listed in Table 46-6.

Hemodialysis

Hemodialysis removes body wastes by using an external membrane as the diffusion surface. For hemodialysis, a catheter is inserted into an artery and blood is removed

Table 46-6. *Possible Complications of CAPD*

Assessment	Problem	Implementations
Redness or pain or swelling at tubing insertion	Infection	Take culture at site; administer antibiotics as prescribed; continue site care (1/2-strength H_2O_2 two times daily); notify physician.
Abdominal pain, increased temperature, nausea and vomiting, cloudy return in drainage solution	Peritonitis	Notify physician; administer antibiotics as prescribed; auscultate for bowel sounds.
Cramps as fluid is infused	Irritation of peritoneal cavity	Infuse solutions more slowly; warm temperature of solution to body temperature.
Difficulty with infusion or drainage of fluid	Kinked or clotted tubing; malpositioned catheter	Assess tubing for kinking; change position of child; ask child to cough to increase abdominal pressure; add prescribed amount of heparin to dialysate bag (prevents clotting).
Weight increase; moist cough, shortness of breath	Fluid overload	Decrease sodium and fluid oral intake; assess blood pressure and weight; use 4.25% exchange solution until weight is again decreased.
Weight loss, hypotension, poor skin turgor, tachycardia	Fluid loss	Increase fluid and sodium intake; assess blood pressure and weight; do not use 4.25% solution.
Blood-tinged dialysis return	Ruptured blood vessel	Assess pulse and blood pressure; observe for further bleeding in drainage; flush catheter with prescribed amount of heparin to keep clots from forming.

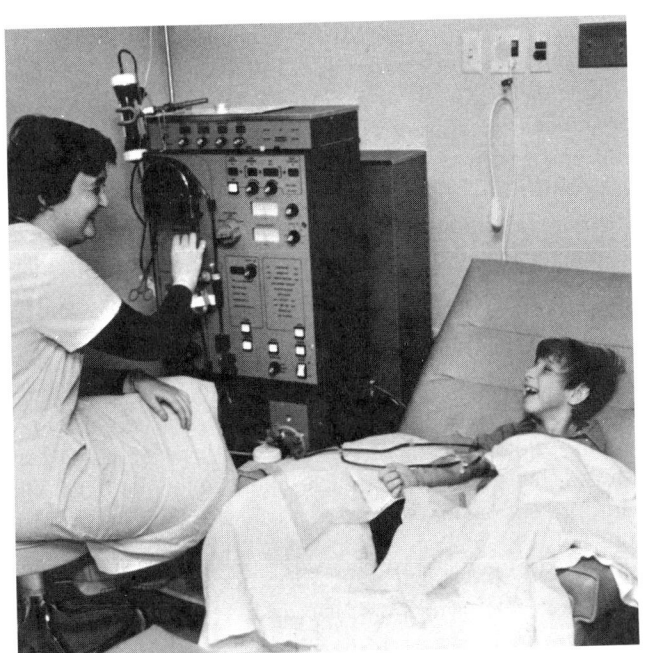

FIGURE 46-15
Hemodialysis. The artificial kidney is the barbell-shaped apparatus above the nurse's head. (Courtesy of the Department of Medical Photography, Children's Hospital, Buffalo, NY.)

from the child and circulated through a dialysis coil. Urea and electrolytes in the blood diffuse into the surrounding fluid bath as the blood passes through the coil. After diffusion is complete, the blood is returned to the child's venous circulation (Figure 46-15).

Hemodialysis is so effective that 3 hours of hemodialysis accomplishes as much as 12 hours of peritoneal dialysis. Children who have renal failure or whose kidneys have been removed can be maintained almost indefinitely in good electrolyte and fluid balance by hemodialysis two or three times a week. To establish

a site for blood removal, children may have polytetrafluoroethylene (Teflon) or silicone elastomer (Silastic) tubing inserted into a forearm vein and artery (Figure 46-16A); this is an external arteriovenous shunt. A sterile dressing is kept in place over the shunt site; the child must keep the arm out of water (swimming is prohibited, and the child must cover the dressing with a plastic bag before showering or washing hair). Serum collected at the shunt site should be washed away daily with a solution such as half-strength hydrogen peroxide and an antibiotic ointment applied. The site should be assessed daily for redness or warmth that suggests infection. At the time of dialysis, the tubing is cleaned with povidone-iodine (Betadine) and punctured to make the connection to the hemodialysis machine. External hemodialysis shunts established this way are only a temporary measure, because, over a long period, infection is apt to occur and the child has to be extremely careful that the external tubing does not dislodge and lead to hemorrhage from the exposed artery. It has one advantage and that is it prevents the child having to have a venipuncture at the time of dialysis. As a rule, take blood pressures in the arm opposite a hemodialysis shunt.

A permanent technique is subcutaneous anastomosis of a vein and artery (usually the brachial artery and brachiocephalic vein; Figure 46-16B). The possibility of infection is reduced with this method, although, unfortunately, two venipunctures, one from a low point in the shunt to remove blood and one high in the shunt to return it, are necessary for dialysis (use lidocaine first to reduce pain). Ability to feel a thrill (vibration) over the shunt is proof that the shunt is open and not plugged.

The risks of hemodialysis are infection introduced with venipuncture (severe because the infection automatically is septicemia) and blood clotting in the shunt, which can lead to emboli (Kohaut, 1994). During hemodialysis, children may begin to show signs of confu-

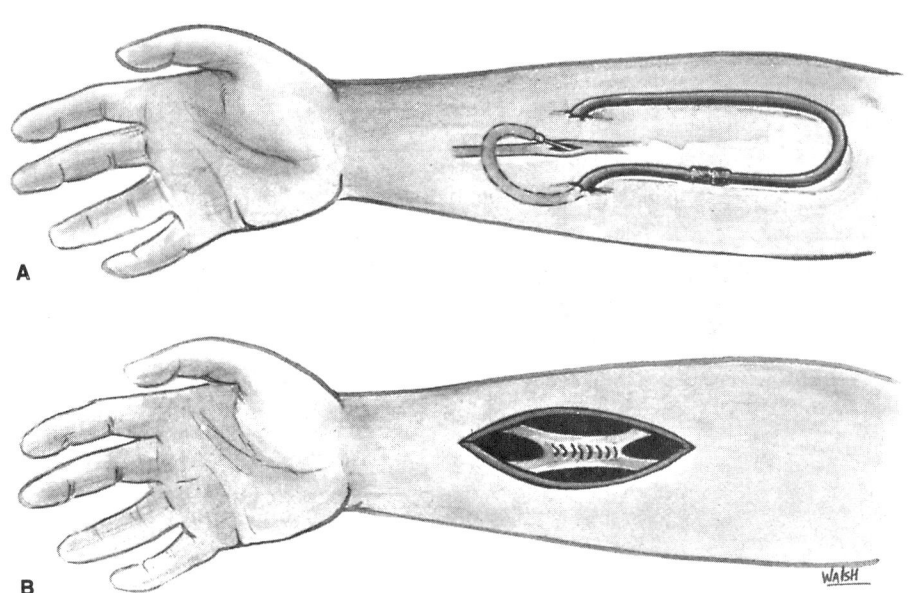

FIGURE 46-16
(A) *An external arteriovenous shunt.*
(B) *An internal arteriovenous fistula.*

sion, vomiting, visual blurring, or hallucinations from a *dialysis disequilibrium syndrome.* This occurs because the hemodialysis is removing urea from the blood at a rapid rate—faster than urea can be shifted from the brain to the blood. This causes fluid to shift into the brain, resulting in cerebral edema. The procedure must be temporarily halted to allow equalization to return. Muscle cramping may occur from sodium depletion. A "first use" syndrome (i.e., dizziness or muscle cramping) may occur from a reaction to the fibers in the artificial kidney.

Children grow bored during hemodialysis as they do during peritoneal dialysis. They need entertainment provided for them so the procedure remains acceptable. When children's kidneys are removed and they must remain on a continuous program of hemodialysis, they may come to resent a machine as "owning" or "controlling" them (see the Focus on Nursing Research box). They become aware that they cannot exist apart from it. Planning special activities to do during hemodialysis time helps to give them a feeling of control.

Kidney Transplantation

The ultimate possibility for prolonging the life of children with renal failure is kidney transplantation (Farrington & Sweny, 1990). With complete kidney failure, chil-

FOCUS ON NURSING RESEARCH

Is Behavior Modification an Effective Technique With Adolescents for Encouraging Compliance With Hemodialysis?

For this study, two male preadolescents and two male adolescents, ages 10 to 16 and all with end-stage renal disease secondary to congenital obstructions, were offered tokens for cooperating with hemodialysis. Subjects came for dialysis three to five times weekly. Tokens were awarded for displaying an absence of physical or verbal abuse toward staff and for maintaining a potassium level under 5.0 mg/dL. Tokens could be exchanged in the hospital gift shop for any desired item.

During the course of the study, subjects earned 76.6% of the tokens that were available. The cost to the dialysis unit was $549, or an average of $2.29 per patient per week. Although the sample was exceedingly small, the researchers concluded that this strategy could be an effective method for encouraging adolescents to better accept hemodialysis.

Wysocki, T., et al. (1990). Behavior modification in pediatric hemodialysis. *American Nephrology Nurses' Association Journal, 17,* 250.

dren who have extensive hypertension will have their kidneys removed and will be placed on periodic hemodialysis or CAPD to await a transplant kidney. Kidney removal is an important step for parents and the child; although they realize that the child's kidneys are no longer functioning, this step removes all hope that a miracle might happen and make them function once more. It may be viewed by some parents as a form of mutilation. They may ask whether it is possible to leave one kidney, since only one kidney will be transplanted (this is impossible, because the hypertension would continue). Parents need a thorough explanation of why hypertension is destructive (i.e., it will lead to cerebral vascular accident). They must understand that renal biopsy shows that, short of a miracle, their child's kidneys will not function again, so that removal of them is not a loss but only recognition of a loss.

Kidney transplants are most effective (the kidney is less likely to be rejected) if the kidney is taken from a twin or sibling. Rejection occurs at a higher incidence if a kidney comes from a cadaver or recently deceased child. If a relative's tissue-compatible kidney is used, the success rate is as high as 90%; it is approximately 80% with cadaver kidneys (Kohaut, 1994). Most people consider that children should be of legal age to give consent to supply a kidney for transplantation, so few children have a sibling who is eligible to donate such a kidney. Tissue studies done to determine the best donor (matched for human leukocyte antigens) may reveal that the person in a family most willing to donate a kidney is not the best person in terms of tissue compatibility. This may cause bitterness and hopelessness in the family, compounding an already stressed family life. Many children anticipate that the characteristics of the donor will be transmitted to them by the kidney, and thus they are reluctant to accept the kidney of a family member with a character trait they do not like (perhaps a bad temper). They need to be assured that transplanted organs do not carry this type of problem with them. Adult-sized kidneys may be transplanted into children, although if the child weighs under 10 kg, this large a kidney may lead to hypertension, excessive diuresis, and abdominal complications due to the lack of space this leaves in the abdomen (transplanted kidneys are placed in the abdomen, not the usual kidney space).

Tests that kidney donors can expect to have preoperatively are an HLA (human leukocyte antigen) typing, electrolyte blood analysis, complete blood count, bleeding time, urinalysis and urine culture, 24-hour urine for protein, renal arteriogram, and intravenous pyelography. People who are unable to donate a kidney are those with multiple bilateral small renal arteries, bilateral renal disease, renal infection, advanced medical illness, severe obesity, or hypertension. Donors must understand that removal of a kidney involves major surgery, and they can expect to feel exhausted afterward for approximately 2 weeks. Donors will have urine samples collected after surgery to assess that their remaining kidney is capable of maintaining full function and they are still in good health.

Before surgery, children who are to receive a transplant are dialyzed to clear their body of excessive potassium and fluid. If the donated kidney will be from a relative, there is adequate time for thorough preoperative preparation. If the donor kidney is from a cadaver, the announcement of surgery may be sudden and time for preoperative instruction limited.

Children who receive pretransplant blood transfusions have an improved chance of transplant success. Most children receive at least five blood transfusions while awaiting surgery. The mechanisms by which this operates are unclear, but transfusion-induced production of antibodies or immune complexes mediates graft survival.

HLA Typing

The presence of antigens on erythrocytes has been documented for years,since antigens serve as the basis for blood transfusion typing and reactions. HLA (human leukocyte antigens) is a group of antigens found on the surfaces of all cells with a nucleus, including blood components such as leukocytes and platelets. The name is derived from the fact that they were first identified on white blood cells. Such antigens are inherited from both parents and are specific for each individual. They denote tissue type or determine which tissue the immune system identifies as foreign tissue. They are carried on the short arm of chromosome 6 in each cell.

Such antigens also serve as the basis for paternity typing; they may cause reactions to blood product transfusions, bone marrow, and organ transplants. When two people have like HLA antigens, they are said to be *histocompatible.* Identical twins have complete histocompatibility, family members have partial compatibility; any two people can have histocompatibility at least on one antigen site.

For tissue typing, lymphocytes from both a donor and recipient are grown together in a culture medium for approximately 5 days and then examined for like characteristics. Whether certain HLA subgroups are present or not apparently influences what diseases people can contract. The presence of HLA-15, for example, is associated with the development of cervical cancer; in the person with Hodgkin's lymphoma, if Aw19 and B5 are present, the person has a poorer chance of responding to therapy than normally. The development of acute lymphoblastic leukemia may be associated with HLA antigens in this same way. Possibly the malignant antigen resembles the HLA antigen so closely that the body detects the antigen not as foreign but as "self." Children who are awaiting a kidney transplant are tissue typed, and this information is circulated to major medical

centers. When a kidney is available for transplant, the child's tissue type is compared with the donor kidney.

Postoperative Care

After surgery, children are cared for in an environment as near sterile as possible. In some institutions, children are cared for in a "life-island" or a plastic-enclosed sterile bubble or room. In others, children are cared for in reverse isolation. Parents will need to wear gowns and masks to stay with the child.

Children are placed on immunosuppressive therapy (administration of cyclosporine, azathioprine (Imuran), and methylprednisolone (Solu-Medrol) to reduce the possibility of kidney rejection. Antilymphocyte globulin and antithymocyte globulin may be administered to aid immunosuppression. This therapy makes children extremely susceptible to infection, particularly fungal and viral infections (Yadin et al., 1991).

Although some kidney transplants begin to function immediately, hemodialysis may continue until the implanted kidney can fully function after the insult of transplantation. Because surgery is retroperitoneal, recovery is rapid. In the weeks that follow surgery, both the parents and the child hope for transplant acceptance.

Transplant Rejection

Acute transplant rejection usually occurs within the first 3 months after transplant. Children begin to develop fever, proteinuria, oliguria, weight gain, hypertension, and tenderness over the kidney. Serum creatinine and BUN levels will increase. Increasing the dose of prednisone may be effective in relieving this type of rejection.

Rejection may also be *chronic*, in which the transplanted kidney gradually loses function (after 6 months). Hypertension and anemia result. A biopsy will reveal vascular changes such as narrowing of arterial lumens and interstitial changes such as fibrosis and tubular atrophy. This type of rejection is difficult to halt, although it may be such a slow steady process that it is 2 or 3 years before the kidney fails. If a kidney is rejected, it is removed, and a child is returned to a program of hemodialysis. Because one kidney was rejected does not mean that a second transplant will be rejected also. Unfortunately, however, the number of kidneys available for transplantation is limited, so kidney rejection becomes an ominous sign for the child's long-term survival.

The incidence of malignant disease is six times more frequent in transplant recipients than in the normal population, probably owing to the long-term immunosuppression. The original disease for which the child had the transplant may recur in the transplanted kidney. This is most apt to occur in glomerulonephritis. During adolescence, an age of poor medicine compliance, kidney recipients need to be followed closely to be certain they are taking their immunosuppressive therapy.

Parents cannot help but overprotect the child; they worry that a rough-housing session with a sibling or playing a game such as baseball may jiggle and injure the transplanted kidney. The child may be afraid to engage in any activity for the same reason.

It is important that children understand that acceptance or rejection of a kidney depends on a multitude of factors—the condition of renal veins and arteries, the transplanted kidney, or antigen–antibody formation—but none of these factors is related to whether the child is good or bad or deserves or does not deserve to have the transplant work. Children with transplanted kidneys who believe they will only be saved if they are good will never be whole people, because this belief limits what they can do and think and be.

Children with end-stage renal disease usually fail to grow despite treatment. Although the rate of growth is improved after a kidney transplant, they will probably never reach full height. Part of this growth retardation is related to corticosteroid maintenance.

Key Points

- Many urinary tract disorders such as cystic kidneys, urethral obstruction, and bladder exstrophy are evident on fetal sonogram. Early identification allows therapy to begin immediately at birth.

- Many urinary tract disorders such as infection or chronic renal insufficiency are long-term conditions requiring years of therapy. Be certain that parents are well informed about the child's condition so they can continue to participate in planning the child's care.

- Diminished kidney function leads to both fluid and electrolyte imbalances. Creative techniques are necessary to encourage children to continue to ingest a high protein diet to counteract protein losses in urine.

- Congenital structural abnormalities of the urinary tract are patent urachus, exstrophy of the bladder, hypospadias, and epispadias. Surgical correction is required for all of these.

- Urinary tact infections tend to occur more often in girls than boys. "Honeymoon cystitis" refers to a UTI occurring with first-time sexual relations.

- Vesicoureteral reflex is the backflow of urine into ureters with voiding. It occurs because the valve that guards the entrance to the ureters is defective. Surgical correction may be necessary to prevent repeated urinary tract infection.

- Renal dysfunction can occur for structural reasons such as kidney agenesis, polycystic kidney, and renal hypoplasia. Acute poststreptococcal glomerulo-nephritis is inflammation of the glomeruli after a streptococcal infection. It is characterized by an acute episode of hematuria and proteinuria.

- Nephrotic syndrome is an immunologic process that results in altered glomeruli permeability. Nursing diagnoses associated with this are Altered nutrition, High risk for altered skin integrity, and Knowledge deficit.

- Renal insufficiency can occur in an acute or chronic form. Peritoneal dialysis or hemodialysis may be used to remove body waste until kidney function can be restored.

- Kidney transplantation may be a therapy option for some children with kidney disorders. This is extensive surgery and requires the child to remain on immunosuppressive therapy to counteract transplant rejection.

Critical Thinking Exercises

1. Mary is a 12-year-old who is admitted to your hospital unit with her third urinary tract infection this year. Her mother asks you if there is anything she should be doing to help prevent these. How would you answer her?

2. Charlie is a child with end-stage renal disease awaiting a kidney transplant. He tells you he hopes he has been good enough to deserve being chosen for the next kidney available. What would you want to teach Charlie about the transplant selection process?

3. Beth is 6-year-old who has continuous ambulatory peritoneal dialysis. She wants to go to her church camp this summer. Her parents ask you if this would be a good experience for Beth. What factors would you want to know about the camp? About Beth? About her procedure?

References

Albright, S. G., et al. (1990). Congenital nephrosis as a cause of elevated alpha-fetoprotein. *Obstetrics and Gynecology, 76*, 969.

Alexander, G. R., & Honda, M. (1993). Continuous peritoneal dialysis for children: A decade of worldwide growth and development. *Kidney International, 40*, 665.

Arant, B. S. (1994). Renal and genitourinary diseases. In F. A. Oski, et al. *Principles and practice of pediatrics* (2nd ed.). Philadelphia: J. B Lippincott.

Atta, M. A. (1991). A new technique for continent urinary reservoir reconstruction. *Journal of Urology, 145*, 960.

Belkengren, R., & Sapala, G. (1993). Pediatric management problems: Urinary tract infection. *Pediatric Nursing, 19*, 184.

Berry, P. L., & Brewer, E. D (1990). Glomerulonephritis and nephrotic syndrome. In F. A. Oski, et al. (Eds.). *Principles and practice of pediatrics*. Philadelphia: J. B. Lippincott.

Brown, S. M. (1992). Recombinant human erythropoietin and renal failure. *Care of the Critically Ill, 8*, 12.

Casale, A. J. (1990). Early ureteral surgery for posterior urethral valves. *Urology Clinics of North America, 17*, 361.

Coran, A. G., & Polley, T. Z. (1991). Surgical management of ambiguous genitalia in the infant and child. *Journal of Pediatric Surgery, 26,* 812.

Department of Health and Human Services. (1991). *Healthy people 2000.* Washington, DC: Public Health Service.

Farrington, K., & Sweny, P. (1990). Nephrology, dialysis and transplantation. *Postgraduate Medical Journal, 66,* 502.

Feld, L. G., et al. (1990). Fluid needs in acute renal failure. *Pediatric Clinics of North America, 37,* 337.

Frauman, A. C., & Gilman, C. M. (1990). Care of the family of the child with end stage renal disease. *American Nephrology Nurses' Association Journal, 17,* 383.

Gammage, D., et al. (1993). The effects of diaper brands, urine volume and time on specific gravity measurement. *Journal of Pediatric Nursing, 8,* 10.

Gearhart, J. P. (1991). Failed bladder exstrophy repair. *Urology Clinics of North America, 18,* 687.

Hawkins, E. P. (1994). Renal malformations. In F. A. Oski, et al. (Eds.). *Principles and practice of pediatrics* (2nd ed.). Philadelphia: J. B. Lippincott.

Husmann, D. A., & Spence, H. M. (1990). Current status of tumor of the bowel following ureterosigmoidostomy: A review. *Journal of Urology, 144,* 607.

Jaffe, R., et al. (1990). Sonographic findings in the prenatal diagnosis of bladder exstrophy. *American Journal of Obstetrics and Gynecology, 162,* 675.

Jones, B. E., et al. (1990). Pitfalls in pediatric urinary sonography. *Urology, 35,* 38.

Kass, E. J., & Fink-Bennett, D. (1990). Contemporary techniques for the radioisotopic evaluation of the dilated urinary tract. *Urology Clinics of North America, 17,* 273.

King, L. R., & Hatcher, P. A. (1990). The natural history of fetal and neonatal hydronephrosis. *Urology, 35,* 433.

Kohaut, E. C. (1994). End-stage renal disease. In F. A. Oski, et al. (Eds.). *Principles and practice of pediatrics* (2nd ed.). Philadelphia: J. B. Lippincott.

Kurtz, M., et al. (1993). Daytime incontinence. *Journal of Pediatric Health Care, 7,* 92.

Louis, P. T. (1994). Hemolytic-uremic syndrome. In F. A. Oski, et al. *Principles and practice of pediatrics* (2nd ed.). Philadelphia: J. B. Lippincott.

Mandell, J., et al. (1990). Current concepts in the perinatal diagnosis and management of hydronephrosis. *Urology Clinics of North America, 17,* 247.

Miller, L. A. (1990). At-home help for the CAPD patient. *RN, 53,* 77.

Monroe, D. (1990). Patient teaching for x-ray and other diagnostics: Intravenous pyelogram. *RN, 53,* 43.

O'Donnell, B. (1990). Management of urinary tract infection and vesicoureteric reflux in children: The case for surgery. *BMJ, 300,* 1393.

Schlager, T. A., & Lohr, J. A. (1992). Urinary tract infection in outpatient febrile infants and children younger than 5 years of age. *Pediatric Annals, 22,* 505.

Skoog, S. J., & Belman, A. B. (1991). Primary vesicoureteral reflux in the black child. *Pediatrics, 87,* 538.

Snow, B. W., et al. (1990). Techniques for outpatient hypospadias surgery. *Urology, 35,* 327.

Thabet, M. A., et al. (1993). Hyperlipidemia in childhood nephrotic syndrome. *Pediatric Nephrology, 7,* 559.

Walker, R. D. (1994). Vesicoureteral reflux update: Effect of prospective studies on current management. *Urology, 43,* 270.

Williams, M. A., et al. (1994). The importance of urinary tract infection in the evaluation of the incontinent child. *Journal of Urology, 15,* 188.

Yadin, O., et al. (1991). Renal transplantation in children. *Pediatric Annals, 20,* 657.

Suggested Readings

Castillo, O. A., et al. (1991). Multilocular cysts of the kidney. *Urology, 37,* 156.

Covalesky, R. (1990). Myths & facts about peritoneal dialysis. *Nursing, 20,* 91.

Duckett, J. W. (1990). Advances in hypospadias repair. *Postgraduate Medical Journal, 66* (Suppl. 1), S62.

Dunn, S. A. (1993). How to care for the dialysis patient. *American Journal of Nursing, 93,* 26.

Gearhart, J. P., et al. (1991). Childhood urolithiasis: experiences and advances. *Pediatrics, 87,* 445.

Leonard, M. P., et al. (1990). Continent urinary reservoirs in pediatric urological practice. *Journal of Urology, 144,* 330.

Maizels, M., et al. (1990). Role of in-office ultrasonography in screening infants and children for urinary obstruction. *Urology Clinics of North America, 17,* 429.

O'Donnell, B. (1990). Progress in the management of vesicoureteric reflux. *Postgraduate Medical Journal, 66* (Suppl. 1), 544.

Pollack, C. V., et al. (1994). Suprapubic bladder aspiration versus urethral catheterization in ill infants: Success, efficiency and complication rates. *Annals of Emergency Medicine, 23,* 226.

Randles, J. (1992). An alternative to urinary conduit. *Nursing Standard, 6,* 33.

Rosenthal, J. T., et al. (1990). Technical factors contributing to successful kidney transplantation in small children. *Journal of Urology, 144,* 116.

Shannon, K. M. (1990). Recombinant erythropoietin in pediatrics: A clinical perspective. *Pediatric Annals, 19,* 197.

White, R. H. (1990). Management of urinary tract infection and vesicoureteric reflux in children: Operative treatment has no advantage over medical management. *BMJ, 300,* 1391.

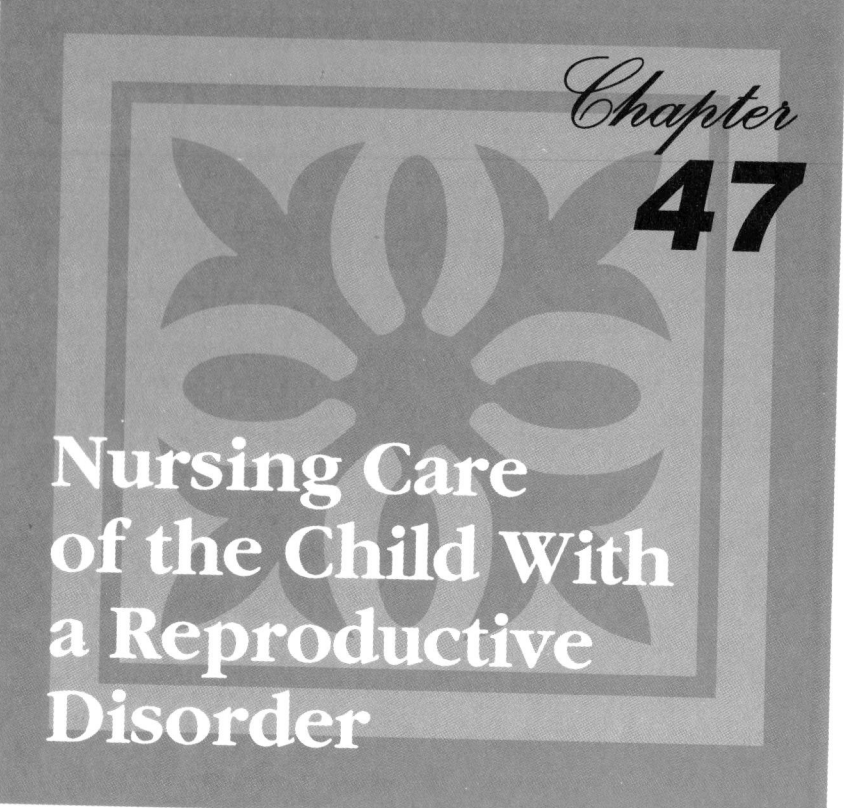

Chapter

47

Nursing Care of the Child With a Reproductive Disorder

Objectives

After mastering the contents of this chapter, you should be able to:

1. Describe common reproductive disorders in children.
2. Assess the child with a reproductive disorder.
3. Formulate nursing diagnoses related to a child's reproductive illness.
4. Plan nursing care related to preventing reproductive disorders in children, such as teaching ways to avoid vaginal infections.
5. Implement nursing care for the child with a reproductive disorder, such as caring for the child with undescended testes.
6. Evaluate outcome criteria to be certain that nursing goals have been accomplished.
7. Identify National Health Goals related to reproductive disorders and children that nurses can be instrumental in helping the nation to achieve.
8. Identify areas related to care of children with reproductive disorders that could benefit from additional nursing research.
9. Use critical thinking to analyze ways that nursing care for the child with a reproductive disorder can be more family centered.
10. Synthesize knowledge of reproductive disorders in children with the nursing process to achieve quality maternal and child health nursing care.

Key Terms

- adenocarcinoma
- adenosis
- amenorrhea
- anovulatory
- colposcopy
- cryptorchidism
- dysmenorrhea
- endometriosis
- fibrocystic breast disease
- gynecomastia
- hermaphrodite
- hydrocele
- menorrhagia
- metrorrhagia
- mittelschmerz
- orchiectomy
- orchiopexy
- pelvic inflammatory disease
- premenstrual syndrome (PMS)
- pseudohermaphrodite
- sexually transmitted disease (STD)
- toxic shock syndrome
- varicocele
- vulvovaginitis

Adele Pillitteri: MATERNAL AND CHILD
HEALTH NURSING, 2nd Edition. © 1995
Adele Pillitteri.

Reproductive disorders in children range from mild infections to serious anatomic malformations that can interfere with fertility. All of these disorders, however, require prompt and careful treatment so that the child will reach adulthood in reproductive health and with a positive sense of his or her sexual self.

Parents are not always as comfortable asking questions about disorders of the reproductive tract as they are inquiring about other disorders. Unless they have clear, thorough explanations of the disease process and prescribed therapy, their reluctance to pursue the subject may leave them confused or misinformed. Even young children can sense that illness affecting genitalia or reproductive ability is viewed by some adults as different from other diseases. As they reach puberty, they need honest explanations about any effect such a condition will have on interpersonal relationships, sexual

functioning, or childbearing. National Health Goals related to reproductive disorders and children are shown in the Focus on National Health Goals display.

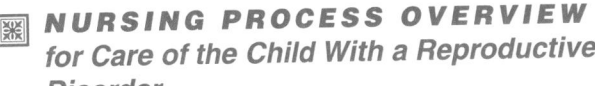

NURSING PROCESS OVERVIEW
for Care of the Child With a Reproductive Disorder

ASSESSMENT

Assessment of reproductive health begins with the first physical examination at birth and continues at health assessments during childhood (Figure 47-1). As with other parts of the health interview, questions regarding reproductive health and illness are generally addressed to the parents until the child is able to begin answering history questions reliably on his or her own. Once the girl has reached adolescence, a gynecologic history should be included in the health assessment (Box 47-1). Adolescents of both genders may prefer not to be accompanied by a parent to preserve privacy.

Adolescents may visit health care facilities on their own because they are worried that they have contracted a **sexually transmitted disease** (**STD**; a disease spread by sexual relations), have become pregnant, or wish to receive some form of contraception. Before they are able to admit their chief concern to health care providers, however, they may "test" the compassion of the health care staff by eliciting a reaction to a minor problem. Be aware that an adolescent who presents at a health care agency with a minor concern may only be misinterpreting symptoms and is truly worried that a minor symptom is serious; on the other hand, the adolescent may actually be seeking help for a bigger problem. Asking the adolescent, "Is there anything else that worries you? Any other way we can help you today?" may help you elicit the adolescent's primary concern.

A pelvic examination is unnecessary for girls who have not yet reached adolescence, but if vaginal walls need to be inspected (because of an inflammation or infection), an otoscope and ear tip can be used. Cotton-tipped applicators moistened with sterile normal saline can be used to take cultures without causing discomfort. For the adolescent girl the pelvic examination becomes an important part of the health assessment. The first pelvic examination can be frightening. Spend time with her before the procedure to teach her about what is being assessed. A three-dimensional model of internal organs may be more useful than a verbal description of anatomy. Let her look at and handle a speculum. A small speculum (a Graves, Hoffman, or Pederson) should be used for examining young girls. For their comfort, warm the speculum first.

Allow the adolescent to choose whether she wants a parent to remain in the room with her. Remaining beside her as a support person helps to make the examination less embarrassing. To protect her self-esteem, be sure the girl meets the person who will examine her before she is placed in a lithotomy position (see the Focus on Cultural Awareness display). A young adolescent may be uncomfortable in a lithotomy position and can be examined in a dorsal recumbent one instead (see Chapter 10 for technique for assisting with a pelvic examination).

NURSING DIAGNOSIS

Nursing diagnoses used for children with reproductive system problems include the following:

- Pain related to vaginal infection
- High risk for self-esteem disturbance related to early development of secondary sex characteristics
- Body-image disturbance related to fibrocystic disease
- Anxiety related to absence or irregularity of menstrual periods in adolescent
- Fear related to surgery on genital organs

PLANNING

Planning often begins with assessment of the child's knowledge about the reproductive tract and ways that illness can affect reproductive and sexual functioning. Educating the child about reproductive health may be

---

FOCUS ON
National Health Goals

Because sexually transmitted diseases not only cause short-term distress because of painful lesions but can also have long-term implications for fertility and future childbearing, a number of National Health Goals address them. These are:

- Reduce gonorrhea to an incidence of no more than 225 cases/100,000 people from a baseline of 300/100,000.

- Reduce primary and secondary syphilis to an incidence of no more than 10 cases/100,000 people from a baseline of 18 per 100,000.

- Reduce genital herpes from 385,000 to 142,000 first-time consultations per year.

- Reduce the incidence of pelvic inflammatory disease as measured by a reduction in hospitalizations for the condition from 311/100,000 to no more than 250/100,000 women aged 15 through 44 (DHHS, 1991).

Nurses can be instrumental in helping the nation achieve these goals by educating adolescents about effective ways to prevent STDs and recognize the signs and symptoms of these illnesses. Areas that could benefit from additional nursing research in this area include: what are the most effective ways to teach adolescents about safer sex practices; what are the reasons adolescents continue to believe that infectious diseases cannot occur to them; and what are strategies that would make it easier for parents to discuss this topic with adolescents?

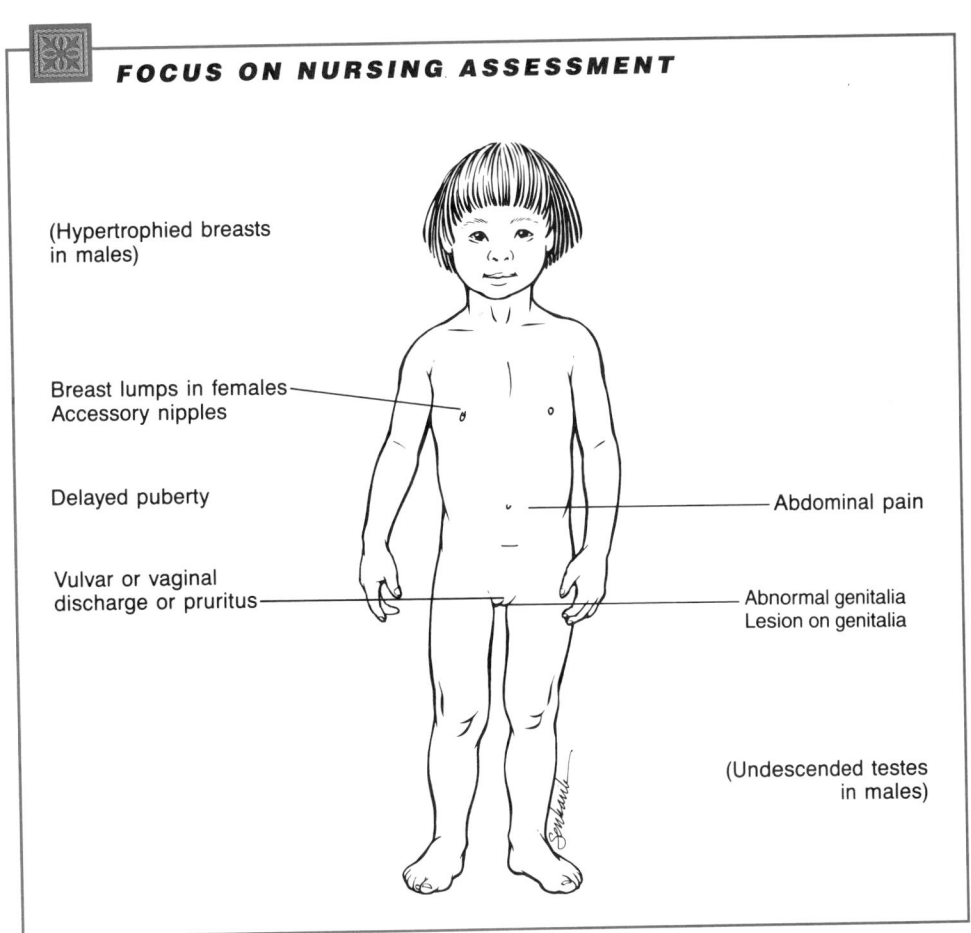

FOCUS ON NURSING ASSESSMENT

(Hypertrophied breasts in males)

Breast lumps in females
Accessory nipples

Delayed puberty

Vulvar or vaginal discharge or pruritus

Abdominal pain

Abnormal genitalia
Lesion on genitalia

(Undescended testes in males)

FIGURE 47-1
Signs and symptoms of reproductive disorders in children.

one of the next areas to plan. Remember when establishing goals with adolescents that it will be difficult to meet goals requiring a wholesale change in lifestyle. It may be more effective to plan for change one step at a time. An organization helpful for referral is:

National Women's Health Network
1325 G Street, NW
Washington, DC 20005

IMPLEMENTATION

Interventions for children with reproductive disorders should always include education about reproductive functioning and measures for maintaining reproductive and sexual health and preventing illness. Health education regarding the importance of testicular self-examination for adolescent males and breast self-examination for adolescent females should be stressed at all health care visits (see Chapter 28). (Guidelines for teaching about menstrual health and safer sex are covered in Chapter 4, Table 4-3, and Box 4-2, respectively.)

Essential nursing interventions also include support of parents and children through difficult decisions and frightening procedures and close observation and sympathetic counseling after surgery. Surgery for undescended testes is an example of a procedure that may be taken lightly by health care providers but one that can be traumatic for the child, especially if performed during a developmental stage in which he views such surgery as castrating. Being certain that the child receives good preparation for surgery and reassurance that he will not be mutilated is an essential nursing intervention.

EVALUATION

The responses of children to reproductive dysfunction vary both with the severity of the illness and the specific age and fears of the child. It is safe to assume, however, that children who have suffered from such an illness are at risk for a loss of self-esteem or confusion about their body image. Evaluation of goals must include long-term evaluation of the child's coping abilities and self-image. If the child suffers from an STD, evaluation should also address his or her knowledge about avoiding STDs in

---

Box 47-1
Gynecologic History Questions

Menstrual history	What was the girl's age at menarche?
	What is the frequency and duration of menstrual periods?
	What is the amount of menstrual flow? (Document by amount of pads or tampons used.)
	Does she experience discomfort? (Document if first day, all days, and so forth, and action taken to relieve it.)
	Does any female sibling or her mother have dysmenorrhea also (endometriosis is familial)?
	Does she experience premenstrual syndrome (e.g., irritability, moodiness, headache, or diarrhea) 1 or 2 days before menses?
	What were the dates of last two menstrual periods and the duration and type of flow?
Reproductive tract history	Has the girl had any vaginal discharge? (Document amount and whether pad is necessary or not—include duration, frequency, description, associated symptoms, actions taken.)
	Is there vaginal pruritus?
	Is there any vaginal odor?
	Has she had reproductive tract surgery?
Sexual history	Has she ever had an STD (include herpes, gonorrhea, and syphilis)?
	Is she currently sexually active? Heterosexually? Homosexually? Bisexually?
	Is there discomfort (dyspareunia) or postcoital spotting?
	Does she have any concerns (worried about frequency, position, partner's satisfaction with coitus)? Is orgasm experienced?
Contraception history:	What contraceptive currently is being used? (Document length of time used, satisfaction, any problems.)
	What types were used in the past?
Breast health	Has she ever noticed any abnormality (lump, discharge, pain)?
	Has she ever had breast surgery?
	Has she breast-fed a child?

---

the future and willingness to seek help should an infection be contracted once again. An STD infection in a young child should be investigated as possible sexual abuse.

These are examples of outcome criteria:

- Child states discomfort from vaginal infection is tolerable after beginning medication.
- Child states she is able to view self as competent in spite of fibrocystic disease.
- Child states she is able to wait 6 months without worrying about not yet having a menstrual period.

Disorders Caused by Altered Reproductive Development

Genetic sex or *biologic gender* (sex chromosome XX or XY) is determined at conception. However, development of the reproductive system, including external genitalia, occurs over two distinct periods: reproductive organs and genitalia begin to differentiate in utero by the 8th week, with growth and refinement occurring over the next several months. This period constitutes the first phase of reproductive development. The second phase

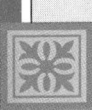

FOCUS ON CULTURAL AWARENESS

Different cultures have different attitudes toward reproductive disorders. Adolescents in Middle Eastern countries, for example, are extremely modest, and so are extremely uncomfortable having pelvic examinations done for reproductive disorders. Adolescents from these countries may be more comfortable if the examiner is a woman. The practice of always having a female health provider in an examining room when a woman is examined by a male physician has not been carried out for years in the United States. However, such a practice might be followed in order to make these adolescents more comfortable.

occurs with specific endocrine changes that are triggered during puberty; this is a period of maturation of primary and secondary sexual characteristics.

Two disorders related to reproductive development are discussed: ambiguous genitalia, a rare condition with different causes, which occurs during fetal development; and delayed and precocious onset of puberty.

Ambiguous Genitalia

In order to understand how ambiguous genitalia can occur, it is important to understand how reproductive organs develop in utero. Although external sexual characteristics generally follow from the XX or XY chromosome, it is possible under certain circumstances for structures generally considered "male" or "female" to develop in either chromosomal gender. Usually, a diagnosis of ambiguous genitalia means that external sexual organs in the child did not follow the normal course of development, so that at birth the external sexual organs are so incompletely or abnormally formed that it is impossible to clearly determine the child's sex by simple observation. For instance, a male infant with *hypospadias* (urethra opening on the underside of the penis) or *cryptorchidism* (undescended testes) may appear more female than male on first inspection. (See Chapter 46 for a discussion of hypospadias; cryptorchidism is described later in this chapter.) Alternatively, a chromosomal female (XX) fetus may become "masculinized" with exposure to androgen in utero (the clitoris is so enlarged that it appears more as a penis than a clitoris; labia may be partially fused so it is difficult to tell them from a male peritoneum; the urethra may be displaced so far forward that it is located on the clitoris); the newborn will appear to be a boy on initial inspection. Likewise, under certain conditions, a chromosomal male (XY) may become "feminized," with a lack of fusion of the labioscrotal

folds and an incompletely formed penis (Catlin & Crawford, 1994).

The most common cause of in vitro virilization of females is *congenital adrenocortical hyperplasia syndrome,* which is related to deficient activity of the 21-hydroxylase enzyme. The adrenal gland produces androgen instead of adequate cortisone, causing the clitoris to become the size of a typical newborn male's penis (see Chapter 48).

If testosterone was produced in utero but the müllerian duct development was not suppressed, a child may have both ovaries and testes (**hermaphrodite**) and, consequently, malformed external genitalia. Children with ambiguous genitalia are often termed **pseudohermaphrodites** because, although only either ovaries or testes are present (or neither is present), infants have some external features of both sexes.

Assessment

If there is any question about the child's gender, a simple sex chromatin (Barr body determination) test will help to establish whether the child is genetically male or female (see Chapter 7).

A more thorough chromosome examination, or *karyotype,* may also be performed. This involves drawing a specimen of blood, allowing the white blood cells to reach a division stage, then examining them (see Chapter 7). *Laparoscopy* (introduction of a narrow laparoscope into the abdominal cavity through a ½-inch incision) may determine if ovaries' or undescended testes are present. *Intravenous pyelography* is used to establish whether a male has a full urinary tract. *Laparotomy* (a full surgical exploration) may be necessary to establish whether gonads are present.

Therapeutic Management

Once the child's true gender is determined, the extent of necessary reconstructive surgery is determined in consultation with the parents. This may involve correction of a hypospadias or cryptorchidism, removal of labial adhesions, or surgical removal of an enlarged clitoris. When removal of an enlarged clitoris is involved, the parents must consider what the absence of this organ will mean to the girl in terms of later sexual enjoyment. Parents may be well advised to delay this type of surgery until the girl is able to decide for herself whether she wants it done. Nonfunctioning ovaries or testes are generally removed to prevent malignancy later in life. If an infant is chromosomally male but does not have an adequate penis, a decision to raise the child as a female might be made. The child will need estrogen administration at puberty for secondary sex characteristics to develop. She will, however, remain incapable of childbearing. An artificial vagina can be constructed for fuller sexual function.

Nursing Diagnoses and Related Interventions

When establishing goals, be aware that parents under stress may have difficulty making long-range plans. The birth of a child with a perplexing defect produces a particularly high level of stress, hampering parents' ability to think clearly and calmly about their situation.

> *Nursing Diagnosis:* Anxiety related to ambiguous sex of child at birth
>
> *Goal:* Parents will demonstrate confidence in health care team and increased knowledge about child's condition and necessary care.
>
> *Outcome Criteria:* Parents voice willingness to support treatment plan, including additional necessary tests, and state they are prepared to make decisions with guidance from health care team.

If the sex of the child is unclear, parents should be told this immediately. If told first that their child is a boy, only to be told 24 hours later that "he" is really a girl, parents will have difficulty accepting this drastic change. They may feel awkward having to tell friends and relatives that the child's sex is unclear. They may lack confidence in health care personnel. They may worry that there is something else wrong with the child. During this period when the baby's sex has not yet been determined, avoid calling the baby "it"; say "the baby" or "your child." Explain how sexual organs form in utero and that every child has the potential to be externally female or male. To promote bonding, help parents understand that their child is otherwise perfect.

Parents need frequent assurance at health care visits that a child with ambiguous genitalia is normal except in this one area (assuming that is true) so they can help their child achieve his or her potential. As the child grows, he or she may need additional counseling to adjust to an abnormal appearance or function.

Precocious Puberty

The development of breast or pubic hair before age 8 years or menses before age 9 years is considered to be precocious sexual development (Plotnick, 1994). Often, such development is expressed as isolated breast or pubic hair growth but can proceed to complete spermatogenesis and menstrual function. It occurs more often in girls than in boys.

Precocious puberty is caused by the early production of gonadotropins by the pituitary gland; gonadotropins stimulate the ovaries or testes to produce sex hormones. Such stimulation can occur because of a pituitary tumor, cyst, or traumatic injury to the third ventricle next to the pituitary gland. It also can occur because of estrogen-secreting cysts or tumors of the ovary or testosterone-secreting cysts of the testes. In rare instances, it occurs because of an estrogen- or testosterone-secreting adrenal tumor. In girls, ingestion of their mother's oral contraceptives can initiate menarche-like changes. The presence of a tumor must be ruled out. When no physical innervation such as a tumor is present, the phenomenon appears to occur only because the gonadostat of the hypothalamus was triggered several years too early.

Assessment

Children have increased breast development and accelerated skeletal maturation. Girls have vaginal bleeding with little pubic or axillary hair because of still low androgen secretion (Figure 47-2). The diagnosis of early puberty is confirmed by the analysis of serum for estrogen or androgen. These will be at adult levels in the child with precocious puberty.

Therapeutic Management

A synthetic analogue to luteinizing hormone-releasing hormone (LHRH) is currently available as Factrel. Ad-

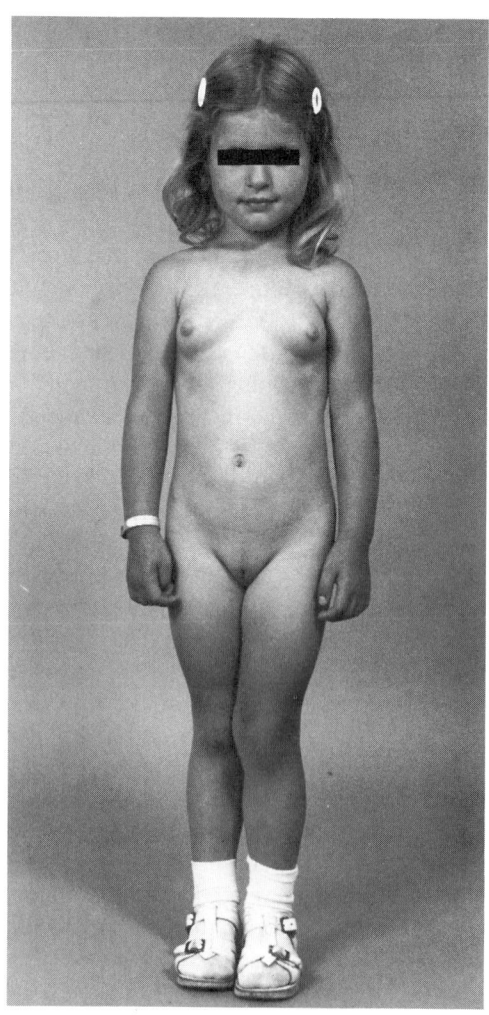

FIGURE 47-2
An 8-year-old with precocious puberty. (Courtesy of Brian Smistek.)

ministration of this analogue desensitizes the pituitary to the child's own prematurely elevated hypothalamic LHRH. It is administered subcutaneously daily. When discontinued at age 12 or 13 years, puberty progresses normally (Breyer et al., 1993).

Nursing Diagnoses and Related Interventions

Nursing Diagnosis: High risk for body image disturbance related to precocious puberty

Goal: Child will demonstrate adequate level of confidence in self and body in 3 months.

Outcome Criteria: Child voices she understands what is happening to her and does not evidence excessive shyness or reluctance to interact with peers.

Girls who develop precociously may have difficulty interacting with peers because they appear so different from other members of their group (Jackson & Ott, 1990). Their parents worry about the children becoming sexually active and possibly pregnant.

Parents may need reassurance that once the child reaches normal puberty age, he or she will again be the same as other children; the fact that the child's sexual growth started early does not mean the genitals will be out of proportion to the rest of the body.

Parents must also understand that the child is fully fertile and able to conceive when early puberty occurs. Oral contraceptives are not advisable for girls this young because the increased load of estrogen will hasten the closing of epiphyseal lines of long bones too early and stunt their growth permanently.

Parents may need to be reminded that, although their child appears to be much older, the changes are only in sexual characteristics. Household tasks, responsibility, and expectations must be geared to the child's chronologic age, not to outward appearance.

Delayed Puberty

A family history in many children reveals a family tendency for late maturation. If so, the child needs a thorough physical examination that will reveal whether some secondary sex characteristics are present or if endocrine stimulation is beginning.

If girls have not begun to menstruate by age 17 years and pathology has been ruled out, menstrual cycles can be started by the administration of estrogen. Many girls worry considerably about delayed menstruation, but once assured that development is merely delayed, they are usually willing to wait for menarche to occur on its own (Rosenfield, 1990). Boys who are distressed by their lack of development may be given testosterone supplements to stimulate hair and genital growth (Plotnick, 1994).

Reproductive Disorders in Males

Common reproductive disorders in males include structural alterations in the penis or testes such as phimosis and cryptorchidism, inflammation such as balanoposthitis, and, in adolescents, testicular cancer.

Balanoposthitis

Balanoposthitis is inflammation of the glans and prepuce of the penis. It is generally caused by poor hygiene, and may accompany a urethritis or a regional dermatitis.

Assessment

The prepuce and glans become red and swollen; a purulent discharge may be present (Vohra & Bedlani, 1992). The boy may have difficulty voiding because of crusting at the meatal opening and because acidic urine touching the denuded surface of the glans causes pain.

Therapeutic Management

Medical treatment is local application of heat; this can be carried out with warm wet soaks or sitz baths. A local antibiotic ointment may be prescribed. If *phimosis* (a tight foreskin) appears to be contributing to the condition, circumcision may be advocated after the inflammation has subsided to prevent the condition from occurring again.

Although balanoposthitis is painful, a boy may tolerate the discomfort for several days because he is too embarrassed to discuss problems in this part of his body. He may think it was caused by masturbation (which can contribute to the irritation) or sexual activity, and is reluctant to seek help for fear of being criticized. He can be assured that the problem is local and will have no long-range effect. Any discharge should be cultured to rule out gonorrhea.

Phimosis

In the normal infant, the foreskin is tight at birth and even held by adhesions, and generally cannot be retracted. After a few months of age, the adhesions should dissolve and the foreskin will become retractable. If not, the infant may have phimosis. With this, the foreskin remains so tight that it interferes with voiding, and balanoposthitis may develop because the foreskin cannot be retracted for cleaning. True phimosis is rare but can be corrected by circumcision (Wiswell et al., 1993). The technique of circumcision is discussed in Chapter 23.

Cryptorchidism

Cryptorchidism is failure of one or both testes to descend from the abdominal cavity to the scrotum. The testes descend into the scrotal sac during months 7 to 9

of intrauterine life. They may descend anytime up to 6 weeks after birth; rarely do they descend after that point.

The cause of undescended testes is unclear. Fibrous bands at the inguinal ring or inadequate length of spermatic vessels may prevent descent. Testes apparently descend because of stimulation by testosterone; hence, it is possible that a lower than normal level of testosterone production prevents descent. Many premature infants are born with undescended testes.

Assessment

Early detection of undescended testes is important, because the warmth of the abdominal cavity may inhibit development of the testes and affect spermatogenesis. After puberty, sperm production deteriorates rapidly in undescended testes, and the testes may undergo a malignant change. Anchoring the testes in the scrotal sac may not prevent malignancy but will allow the boy to perform preventive measures such as testicular self-examination (Hawkins, 1994).

It is more common for the right testis to remain undescended than the left one. In approximately 20% of all cases, both testes remain undescended. Some children may be diagnosed with undescended testes when, in fact, poor examining technique caused the testes to retract. If the child is supine or the examining room is chilly, the scrotal sac may appear to be empty. Excessive palpation or stroking the inner thigh may also stimulate the cremasteric reflex and cause retraction. Testes descend when the child is standing or after a warm bath.

An undescended testis may be at the inguinal ring (true undescended testis) or ectopic (still in the abdomen). Laparoscopy is effective in identifying undescended testes. Because testes arise from the same germ tissue as the kidneys, children with ectopic testes are usually evaluated for kidney function. A buccal smear may be done to determine true sex.

Therapeutic Management

Sometimes the testes descend spontaneously during the first year of life, so treatment is delayed until after this age (Kogan et al., 1990). Preschool children may be given chorionic gonadotropin hormone to stimulate testes descent, but this therapy is only approximately 20% successful. If necessary, surgery (**orchiopexy**) during infant or toddler years will correct the condition.

Nursing Diagnoses and Related Interventions

If an orchiopexy is scheduled, nursing goals focus on parent and child teaching, preoperative preparation, and postoperative care.

> **Nursing Diagnosis:** Parental and child knowledge deficit related to surgical procedure and postoperative treatment plan

> **Goal:** Parents and child (if old enough) will demonstrate increased level of knowledge about surgical procedure by time of admission.

> **Outcome Criteria:** Parents (and child) state what will be done during surgery.

Boys who are old enough to understand need good preparation for this type of surgery. Use an anatomically correct picture to point out exactly the location where surgery will be performed. Assure the boy that his penis itself will not be cut. The child may not voice a fear of mutilation, but you can assume that it exists, especially in preschool children.

During surgery, an internal suture may be inserted to hold the testis in place, or a suture may be inserted through the scrotum into the newly brought down testis and then connected to a rubber band taped to the child's thigh. If this is done, both the child and his parents need to be prepared for this apparatus. Although this device effectively keeps the testis within the scrotal sac and away from the inguinal ring, which has been sutured closed, it looks makeshift—as though the hospital ran out of the usual materials and someone substituted this instead. Parents need to be assured that this is the usual arrangement.

Although the child may be discharged from the hospital the same day, his activity will be limited until approximately the second day after surgery, when the tension suture is released.

> **Nursing Diagnosis:** High risk for altered self-esteem related to change in physical appearance

> **Goal:** Child will evidence an adequate level of self-esteem during surgical experience.

> **Outcome Criteria:** Child (if verbal) states he views self as whole person and interacts with peers without excessive shyness or hesitancy.

Postoperative evaluation should ascertain that the suture line is healing well and that both testes can be palpated in the scrotum. It should also address the boy's feelings about the surgery and the changes in his body. He may need an opportunity to express his fears about mutilation or castration by playing with puppets or dolls after surgery. When he reaches puberty, he can be taught testicular self-examination to assess any early symptoms of malignancy, such as nodules or growths (Clore, 1993) (see Chapter 28).

Hydrocele

When a testis descends into the scrotum in utero, it is preceded by a fold of tissue, the *processus vaginalis.* Fluid may collect in this space (**hydrocele**) and be present at birth. This causes the scrotum of the newborn to appear enlarged. On *transillumination* (the shining of a light through the scrotal sac), the area is illuminated by the water and shines or glows (Politoff et al., 1990). If the hydrocele is uncomplicated, the fluid will gradually be reabsorbed into the body and no treatment is necessary.

The child's parents can be assured that the hydrocele is only excess fluid and that the scrotal enlargement is not due to an abnormal testis, tumor, or hernia.

A hydrocele may form later in life due to *inguinal hernia* (abdominal contents extruding into the scrotum through the inguinal ring, with accompanying fluid). If this is the case, the hernia must be repaired in order for the hydrocele to be reabsorbed (see Chapter 45). Injection of a drug to decrease fluid production (*sclerotherapy*) may also be effective (Rencken et al., 1990).

Varicocele

A **varicocele** is abnormal dilation of the veins of the spermatic cord. It tends to occur most often on the left side. Identifying the presence of varicocele is important in adolescents because, although asymptomatic, the increased heat and congestion in the testicles can lead to infertility. No treatment is necessary for a varicocele unless fertility becomes a concern, at which time it can be surgically removed. There may be some local tenderness for a few days after surgery. Edema can be kept to a minimum by applying ice for the first few hours postoperatively.

Testicular Torsion

Testicular torsion (twisting of the spermatic cord) is a surgical emergency (Cilento et al., 1993). It occurs most frequently in early adolescence; it can be present in newborns. The boy apparently has less than normal testicular support, which allows the spermatic cord to twist. He notices severe scrotal pain and perhaps nausea and vomiting; the testis feels tender to palpation and edema begins to develop. If the condition is not recognized promptly (within 4 hours), irreversible change in the testes may occur from lack of circulation to the organ. Boys need to be educated about the phenomenon so that they report symptoms promptly.

Testicular Cancer

Testicular cancer is rare (only 1% of all malignancies). It usually occurs between ages 15 and 35 years and often in association with cryptorchidism (Brock et al., 1993). If discovered early, testicular cancer is one of the most curable cancers.

Symptoms include painless testicular enlargement and a feeling of heaviness in the scrotum. The disease metastasizes rapidly, leading to abdominal and back pain due to retroperitoneal node extension, weight loss,

and general weakness. **Gynecomastia** (enlargement of the breasts) may arise from human chorionic gonadotropins (HCG) produced by the tumor. HCG and alphafetoprotein can be detected in blood serum, serving as tumor markers.

Therapy for testicular malignancy is **orchiectomy** (removal of the testis) followed by radiation or chemotherapy. A gel-filled prosthesis may be inserted for a symmetric appearance. Infertility in the opposite testis results after radiation therapy. "Sperm banking," or preserving frozen sperm before the procedure, may be an appealing option.

Teaching testicular self-examination in boys for early detection is as important as teaching breast selfexamination for females (Goldenring, 1992) (see Chapter 28).

Reproductive Disorders in Females

The most frequent reproductive disorders in females involve vaginal or menstrual irregularities. Other disorders are caused by structural alterations of the reproductive organs, such as imperforate hymen, **pelvic inflammatory disease** (PID), or infections caused by STDs.

Menstrual Disorders

Because menstruation is an ongoing process throughout half of a woman's life, it affects her self-image significantly. An irregularity such as a painful cycle can exert a major influence on daily activities and should never be taken lightly; it is a health concern requiring as much time and attention as that given to other concerns.

Menstrual disorders generally fall into two categories: (1) menstruation that is painful or uncomfortable and (2) infrequent or too-frequent cycles.

Mittelschmerz
Some women may experience abdominal pain during ovulation and the release of accompanying prostaglandins. Some even notice irritation when a drop or two of follicular fluid or blood spills into the abdominal cavity. This pain, called **mittelschmerz**, may range from a few sharp cramps to several hours of discomfort. It is typically felt on either side of the abdomen (near an ovary) and may be accompanied by scant vaginal spotting.

The nurse can reassure women that mittelschmerz pain is benign, and one advantage is that it clearly marks ovulation. If pain is felt in the right lower quadrant, it can be differentiated from appendicitis by the lack of associated symptoms (i.e., nausea, vomiting, fever, abdominal guarding, and rebound tenderness) as well as by its occurrence in the menstrual cycle. Usually mittelschmerz is of limited duration and intensity.

Dysmenorrhea

Dysmenorrhea is painful menstruation. For generations, it was thought to be mainly psychological, needing no other treatment than reassurance that it was a normal phenomenon and something women should endure. Currently, it is recognized that the pain is due to the release of prostaglandins (primarily PF$_2$) in response to tissue destruction during the ischemic phase of the menstrual cycle. PF$_2$ causes smooth muscle contraction in the uterus.

Dysmenorrhea can also be a symptom of an underlying illness such as PID, *uterine myomas* (tumors), or *endometriosis* (abnormal formation of endometrial tissue; Wilson, 1994).

Assessment. As many as 80% of adolescents have discomfort with menstruation; approximately 10% have discomfort that seriously interferes with daily living. Dysmenorrhea is *primary* if it occurs in the absence of organic disease; it is *secondary* if it occurs as a result of organic disease. There may be a "bloating" feeling and light cramping 24 hours before menstrual flow. Pain is mainly noticed, however, when the flow begins. Colicky (sharp) pain and cyclic pain is superimposed on a dull, nagging pain across the lower abdomen. Accompanying this is an "aching, pulling" sensation of the vulva and inner thighs. Some women have mild diarrhea with the abdominal cramping. Mild breast tenderness, abdominal distention, nausea and vomiting, headache, and facial flushing may be present.

Therapeutic Management. These painful symptoms can generally be controlled by a common analgesic such as acetylsalicylic acid (aspirin). Acetylsalicylic acid works well as an analgesic for dysmenorrhea because it is a mild prostaglandin inhibitor. Although adolescents are generally advised not to take aspirin because of recent research linking it to Reye's syndrome, girls may take it safely at the beginning of a menstrual period as long as they do not have additional flu symptoms. A major breakthrough in the relief of menstrual discomfort is the discovery of ibuprofen (Motrin), a stronger prostaglandin inhibitor. Ibuprofen is currently available over the counter. Low-dose oral contraceptives to prevent ovulation may also be effective if pregnancy is not desired. One disadvantage of this is the possibly negative side-effects of long-term estrogen administration.

During the first year or two of menstruation dysmenorrhea rarely occurs, because early menstrual cycles are usually **anovulatory**. As ovulation begins, typical menstrual discomfort begins.

Nursing Diagnoses and Related Interventions

Nursing Diagnosis: Pain related to dysmenorrhea

Goal: Client will not experience pain above a tolerable level.

Outcome Criteria: Client states that she has some control over pain through nonpharmacologic or pharmacologic methods.

A number of nonpharmacologic solutions may help decrease the pain of dysmenorrhea. Decreasing sodium intake a few days before an expected menstrual flow by omitting salty foods such as potato chips, pretzels, ham and other luncheon meats, and by not adding salt to foods may help reduce "bloated" feelings. Abdominal breathing (breathing in and out slowly, allowing the abdominal wall to rise with each inhalation) may also be helpful. Applying heat to the abdomen with a heating pad or taking a hot shower or tub bath may relax muscle tension and relieve pain. Caution young girls not to apply heat to their abdomen for abdominal pain unless they are actually menstruating; if the pain is due to an inflamed appendix, heat can cause rupture of the appendix and life-threatening peritonitis. Resting may help to relieve vulvar pain; abdominal massage (effleurage or light massage) may feel soothing. Women who remain sexually active during their menses may discover that orgasm is helpful in relieving pelvic engorgement and therefore may relieve cramping.

Menorrhagia

Menorrhagia is an abnormally heavy menstrual flow. It may occur in girls close to puberty and in woman nearing menopause because of anovulatory cycles. Without ovulation and subsequent progesterone secretion, estrogen secretion continues and causes extreme proliferation of endometrium.

Assessment. It is difficult to determine when a flow is abnormally heavy, but one method is to ask the girl how long it takes her to saturate a sanitary napkin or tampon. A sanitary napkin or tampon holds approximately 25 mL of fluid. Saturating a pad or tampon in less than 1 hour means the flow is heavier than usual. There is often an unusual amount of flow in girls using intrauterine devices (IUDs). With oral contraceptives the flow is often light, but may seem alarmingly heavy once the pills are discontinued. Usually, however, this is just a return of the adolescent's normal flow.

A heavy flow can indicate endometriosis (see below), a systemic disease (anemia), blood dyscrasia such as a clotting defect, or a uterine abnormality such as a myoma (fibroid) tumor. It can be a symptom of infection such as PID or an indication of early pregnancy loss that is coincidentally occurring at the time of an expected menstrual flow.

It is important to determine the cause of menorrhagia because it can lead to anemia from excessive iron loss, thus requiring iron supplements to achieve sufficient hemoglobin formation. The adolescent who is losing excessive blood because of anovulatory cycles may be administered progesterone during the luteal phase to prevent proliferative growth during this phase of the cycle; if the ability to conceive is unimportant, adolescents may be placed on a low-dose oral contraceptive, which decreases the flow.

Metrorrhagia

Metrorrhagia is bleeding between menstrual periods. This is normal in some adolescents who have spotting at the time of ovulation ("mittelstaining"). This may also occur in women on oral contraceptives (breakthrough bleeding) for the first 3 or 4 months. Vaginal irritation from infection might lead to midcycle spotting. Spotting may also represent a temporarily low level of progesterone production and endometrial sloughing (dysfunctional uterine bleeding or a luteal phase defect), a condition that tends to occur near the end of the reproductive years.

If metrorrhagia occurs for more than one menstrual cycle and the client is not on oral contraceptives, she should be referred to a physician for examination, because vaginal bleeding is also an early sign of uterine carcinoma or ovarian cysts.

Endometriosis

Endometriosis is the abnormal growth of extrauterine endometrial cells, often in the cul-de-sac of the peritoneal cavity, the uterine ligaments, and the ovaries (Davis et al., 1993; see Figure 6-1). This abnormal tissue results from excessive endometrial production and a reflux of blood and tissue through the fallopian tubes during menstrual flow. As many as 25% of women in the United States have endometriosis. It tends to occur most often in white nulliparous women, but there is also a familial tendency. Daughters of women with endometriosis may develop symptoms of dysmenorrhea early in life and may be encouraged to have children before overgrowth of the endometrium becomes so extensive that it interferes with conception.

Etiology. The excessive production of endometrial tissue may be related to a deficient immunologic response. In many women, it appears to be related to excess estrogen production or a failed luteal menstrual phase. Many women with endometriosis do not ovulate or ovulate irregularly. Estrogen secretion continues through the cycle rather than becoming secondary to progesterone late in the cycle, as happens with normal ovulation. This proliferation of tissue then forces the blood back into the fallopian tubes.

Endometriosis causes dysmenorrhea when the abnormal tissue responds to estrogen and progesterone stimulation by swelling and then sloughing its layers in the same manner as the uterine lining. This causes inflammation of surrounding tissue in the abdominal cavity and an even greater release of prostaglandins. Abnormal tissue in the pelvic cul-de-sac may cause *dyspareunia* (painful coitus) because it puts pressure on

the posterior vagina. Infertility may result when the fallopian tubes become immobilized and blocked by tissue implants or adhesions, preventing peristaltic motion and ova transport (see Chapter 6).

Assessment. Pelvic examination may show that the uterus is displaced by tender, fixed, palpable nodules. Nodules in the cul-de-sac or on an ovary may be palpable as well. If the endometriosis is minimal, the woman will not experience any related symptoms. If the condition is moderate or extensive, she may experience dysmenorrhea or dyspareunia.

Therapeutic Management. Medical treatment for endometriosis can be medical or surgical, depending on the extent of the disease. Estrogen/progesterone-based oral contraceptives may stimulate implant regression as the tissue sloughs under the influence of the progesterone. Danazol, a synthetic androgen, also helps shrink the abnormal tissue. Laparotomy and excision by laser surgery is the most effective measure, but because it is a highly invasive procedure, a course of conservative medical treatment may be tried first.

Amenorrhea

Amenorrhea, or absence of a menstrual flow, strongly suggests pregnancy but is by no means definitively diagnostic. It may result from tension, anxiety, fatigue, chronic illness, extreme dieting, or strenuous exercise. Competitive swimmers, long distance runners (50 to 75 mi/week), and ballet dancers notice that intensive training causes their periods to become scant and irregular (Loucks, 1990). This appears to be associated with their low ratio of body fat to body muscle, which leads to excessive secretion of prolactin. An elevation in prolactin causes a decrease in LHRH from the hypothalamus, followed by a decline in follicle-stimulating hormone, follicular development, and estrogen secretion. Menstrual cycles generally return to normal, however, within 3 months of discontinuing strenuous training and conditioning (see the Focus on Nursing Research display).

Women who wish to maintain a normal cycle while training for a sports event may take bromocriptine (Parlodel), which can reduce high prolactin levels by acting on the hypothalamus and initiating menstruation each month; many women, however, view the absence of menstrual periods as a benefit during sports training. If a menstrual flow is delayed and pregnancy is suspected, bromocriptine should be discontinued, because it is potentially teratogenic. Side-effects of bromocriptine include nausea, headache, and dizziness. Nausea can be alleviated by taking the drug with meals.

Amenorrhea also occurs when women diet excessively, partially as a natural defense mechanism to limit ovulation and the chance of a poor pregnancy outcome, and as a means of conserving body fluid. Women with *anorexia nervosa* or *bulimia* (eating disorders described

FOCUS ON NURSING RESEARCH

When Women Run, Does It Influence the Length and Frequency of Periods?

Adolescents who engage in strenuous athletic exercises can develop erratic menstrual periods (athletic menstrual irregularity syndrome). To investigate the effect of running on women, 146 women who participated in various levels of running were asked to record exercise practices and menstrual cycle data as well as test for their day of ovulation using a rapid urine test for three consecutive months. Mean age of the women was 29.6 years; their range of weight was 93 to 218 pounds. Their activity levels ranged from nonrunning to over 30 miles weekly. Results of the study showed that runners had significantly more ovulatory disturbances than nonrunners. Researchers suggest nurses in fertility clinics be aware of the association between running and ovulatory disturbances so they are certain to assess patients' athletic level.

Estok, P. J., Rudy, E. B., Kerr, M. E., & Menzel, L. (1993). Menstrual response to running. Nursing Implications. *Nursing Research, 42,* 158.

in Chapter 54) often develop amenorrhea after approximately 3 months of excessive dieting or binging and dieting; as in athletes, this is due to an increase in prolactin.

Amenorrhea is primary if a woman has never menstruated and secondary if it occurs after normal menstrual periods. Amenorrhea as a sign of pregnancy is discussed in Chapter 8.

Premenstrual Syndrome

Premenstrual syndrome (PMS) is a condition occurring in the luteal phase of the menstrual cycle that has both behavioral and physiologic symptoms. Because of the variety of possible symptoms, the incidence of PMS can be considered quite high: it has been estimated that as many as 30% of women experience some degree of PMS, a cluster of symptoms that includes anxiety, fatigue, abdominal bloating, headache, appetite disturbance, irritability, and depression (Raja et al., 1992). For some women, these symptoms can be incapacitating.

The cause of PMS is unknown, but it may be due to the drop in progesterone just before menses. A syndrome similar to PMS may occur in women after tubal ligation. A decrease in the blood supply to the ovary apparently results in decreased luteal function and low progesterone levels. A vitamin B–complex deficiency may lead to estrogen excess, causing an abnormal ratio of estrogen to progesterone; other related causes may be poor renal clearance leading to water retention, an endometrial toxin from the presence of ischemic tissue,

hypoglycemia that leads to a surge of adrenaline, and low calcium levels.

Symptoms of PMS vary from cycle to cycle and throughout life. Therapy is aimed at correcting specific symptoms (Mortola et al., 1991).

Women who think they may have PMS should keep a diary of when symptoms occur. If they are aware of recurring patterns that indicate PMS, they will better be able to recognize the cause of their increased tension or heightened emotional reactions to everyday stresses. Some women benefit from vaginal progesterone suppositories to increase their progesterone level. They should be certain their diet is high in vitamins and calcium and low in salt. If they suspect they are pregnant, they should not use progesterone suppositories, since progesterone has the potential to harm the fetus. This syndrome needs to be studied in greater depth so that better diagnostic techniques and treatment can be developed.

Other Reproductive Disorders in Females

Imperforate Hymen

The *hymen* is a membranous ring of tissue partly obstructing the vaginal opening. An *imperforate hymen* totally occludes the vagina, preventing the escape of vaginal secretions and menstrual blood.

Before menarche, the child with an imperforate hymen generally has no symptoms. With onset, the menstrual flow is obstructed. It builds up in the vagina, causing increased pressure in the vagina and uterus and eventual abdominal pain. Palpation of the abdomen will reveal a lower abdominal mass. On vaginal examination, an intact, bulging hymen is evident.

The treatment is surgical incision or removal of the hymenal tissue. The girl may have local pain following the incision that can be relieved by a mild analgesic and warm sitz baths.

Careful explanation of this condition will help the girl understand that it will not interfere with sexual relations or future childbearing. Because most girls of early menstrual age have scant knowledge of anatomy, pictures of the reproductive tract will make it clear that this is a local and therefore inconsequential problem.

Adenosis

From 1940 to 1970, women experiencing bleeding in early pregnancy were often given diethylstilbestrol (DES), a nonsteroidal estrogen, to prevent spontaneous abortion. As many as 2 million women received the drug, which was later found to be ineffective and led to **adenosis** (the formation of vaginal cysts) in female offspring (Sharp & Cole, 1990).

In the normal female fetus, the upper vagina, exterior cervix, and endocervix are covered with columnar epithelium in early stages. During late fetal development, these areas gradually change to squamous epithelium, except in the endocervix, where the original columnar formation remains. When estrogen is taken by the mother, however, the change in tissue is inhibited and the fetus is left with only columnar epithelium. Only at puberty does the squamous epithelium begin to develop, growing so rapidly that it may lead to adenosis and possibly vaginal carcinoma (**adenocarcinoma**).

Males born of pregnancies in which DES was administered have a possibility of developing hypoplastic testes, epididymal cysts, and alteration in sperm production as they reach maturity.

Assessment. The girl with adenosis may notice no symptoms or have slight abnormal vaginal bleeding, a mucoid vaginal discharge, a sensation of warmth or heat in the vagina, dyspareunia, or discomfort on tampon insertion.

At a pelvic examination, miniature submucosal vaginal cysts (called "sand granules") may be palpable on the vaginal wall. On **colposcopy** (examination of the magnified vaginal tissue), it can be demonstrated that columnar epithelium rather than squamous epithelium is present on the cervix or vaginal walls. This columnar epithelium can also be identified because it will not stain with Lugol's (iodine) solution (a Schiller's test); such tissue is biopsied. Although by itself adenosis is a benign process, DES daughters may tend to have early pregnancy loss (Hricak et al., 1990). Because clear cell adenocarcinoma can occur, all females born of a DES pregnancy should have a screening pelvic examination at menarche, or at age 14 years if not menstruating, and thereafter be closely followed by yearly vaginal examinations. A Papanicolaou's (Pap) test may be normal in connection with adenosis, so a vaginal examination with Lugol's solution is also necessary. If adenosis is present, the girl should have an examination two or three times a year.

Therapeutic Management. If adenocarcinoma is discovered, local destruction of atypical cells can be achieved by excision, *cautery* (heat), or *cryosurgery* (freezing). If the adenocarcinoma is advanced, a hysterectomy, vaginectomy, pelvic lymph node resection, and vaginal replacement with a skin graft will be necessary. Fortunately, even when adenosis is present, the rate of malignant change is rare (only 0.1%). The girl should be cautioned not to use estrogen contraceptives or morning-after pills that might influence the malignant change. She needs some time to discuss feelings about possibly being a "time bomb" in whom vaginal epithelium changes may one day occur.

Toxic Shock Syndrome

Toxic shock syndrome (TSS) is an infection by toxin-producing strains of *Staphylococcus aureus* organisms. Organisms typically enter the body through vaginal

walls damaged by the insertion of tampons at the time of a menstrual period. As many as 70% of women in the United States used tampons in 1980, the year that TSS reached its peak incidence. The incidence of disease has fallen because women have become more cautious about heavy tampon usage (Patrick, 1994).

Assessment. The symptoms of TSS are shown in Box 47-2. Any female who develops fever with diarrhea and vomiting during a menstrual period should be suspected of having TSS. Remember that a number of adolescents have mild diarrhea as a normal accompaniment to dysmenorrhea.

Therapeutic Management. Women or adolescents with suspected TSS need a careful vaginal examination and removal of any tampon particles, as well as cervical and vaginal cultures for *S. aureus*. Iodine douches may reduce the number of organisms present vaginally. *S. aureus* is generally resistant to penicillin but not to penicillinase-resistant antibiotics (i.e., cephalosporins, oxacillins, or clindamycins). Intravenous fluid therapy to restore circulating fluid volume and increase blood pressure or vasopressors such as dopamine (Intropin) may be necessary to increase the blood pressure. Diuretic therapy to shift fluid back to the intravascular circulation and support of renal and cardiac failure may be neces-

---

> ### Box 47-2
> ### *Symptoms of TSS**
>
> - Temperature more than 38.9°C (102°F)
> - Vomiting and diarrhea
> - A macular (sunburn-like) rash that desquamates on palms and soles 1 to 2 weeks after illness
> - Severe hypotension (systolic pressure less than 90 mm Hg)
> - Shock, leading to poor organ perfusion
> - Impaired renal function with elevated blood urea nitrogen or creatinine at least twice the upper limit of normal
> - Severe muscle pain or creatine phosphokinase at least twice the upper limit of normal
> - Hyperemia of mucous membrane
> - Impaired liver function with increased total bilirubin and increased serum glutamic-oxaloacetic transaminase at twice the upper limit of normal
> - Decreased platelet count
> - Central nervous system symptoms of disorientation, confusion, severe headache
>
> *Three symptoms must be present for diagnosis.
> (From Centers for Disease Control. [1982]. Toxic shock syndrome: U.S. 1970–1982. *Morbidity and Mortality Weekly Report, 31,* 201.)

sary. Recovery occurs in 7 to 10 days; fatigue and weakness may be present for months afterward.

The rate of TSS recurrence is 28% to 64%, generally within 2 months of the first attack. Recurrence probably happens because the organism is not completely eliminated from the body (Broscious, 1991).

Nursing Diagnoses and Related Interventions

Nursing Diagnosis: Knowledge deficit related to safe tampon use

Goal: The client will demonstrate increased knowledge of tampon use by end of health care visit.

Outcome Criteria: The client states common rules such as not handling the portion of the tampon that will be inserted vaginally.

The risk of developing TSS is high in young women (ages 20 to 30 years). *Staphylococcus* is probably introduced by fingers or on insertion of the tampon (tampons are clean, but not sterile). The blood-saturated tampon then provides an ideal growth medium for bacteria. Vaginal mucosa may become abraded and inflamed due to a mild allergic or irritant reaction to the synthetic material in tampons (cellulose and polyester), or to ingredients included to reduce odor. "Superabsorbent" tampons containing cellulose may contribute to the problem because bacteria can break down cellulose

into glycogen, providing an ideal nutrient for growth. Tampon manufacturers are required to label tampons as superabsorbent (Nightingale, 1990). Teaching points to help women avoid TSS are shown in the Focus on Family Teaching display.

Vulvovaginitis

Vulvovaginitis is inflammation of the vulva or vagina (Vandeven & Emans, 1993). It is accompanied by pain, odor, pruritus, and a vaginal discharge. It may occur in a girl of any age but tends to be more frequent as the girl reaches puberty, and a change to adult *p*H and the presence of vaginal secretions make the vagina more receptive to infections. Common causes of vulvovaginitis and medical therapy are summarized in Table 47-1 and discussed later in this chapter. Table 47-2 lists common measures to relieve discomfort. See also the Nursing Care Plan: An Adolescent With Vulvovaginitis.

Preschool and School-Age Children. Vaginal discharge may occur before menarche, but bleeding is rarely seen. If bleeding is present, its cause must be determined. A cystitis can cause urethral bleeding; scratching from rectal pruritus will lead to rectal bleeding. The cause of true vaginal bleeding in this early age group is generally either irritation of an inserted foreign object in the vagina, infestation of pinworms, or *vaginitis* (inflammation or infection). Sexual abuse must also be investigated as a cause of any bleeding, tenderness, or infec-

---

FOCUS ON FAMILY TEACHING

Q. What are some tips on preventing toxic shock syndrome?

A. Toxic shock syndrome is caused by invasion of bacteria through an abrasion in the vagina. Prevention actions are aimed at avoiding injury to the vagina where germs could enter.

- Do not use tampons.
- Use only tampons made of natural materials such as cotton, not synthetics such as cellulose or polyester; do not use high-absorbency tampons.
- Change tampons at least every 4 hours during use.
- Alternate the use of tampons with sanitary pads (use tampons during the day, sanitary pads at night).
- Avoid handling the portion of the tampon that will be inserted vaginally.
- Do not use tampons near the end of a menstrual flow when they can cause excessive vaginal dryness from scant flow.

- Do not insert more than one tampon at a time to avoid abrasions and to keep the vaginal walls from becoming too dry.
- Avoid deodorant tampons, sanitary pads, and feminine hygiene sprays; these products can irritate the vulvar–vaginal lining.
- If fever, vomiting, or diarrhea occur during a menstrual period, discontinue tampon use and immediately consult a health care provider because these are symptoms of TSS.
- Anyone who has had one episode of TSS is well advised not to use tampons again or at least not until two vaginal cultures for *Staphylococcus aureus*, the usual bacteria responsible for TSS, are negative.

Table 47-1. *Common Vulvovaginitis Infections*

Causative Agent	Symptoms	Common Therapy
Candida	Vulvar pruritus; thick, white vaginal discharge	Nystatin or miconazole (Monistat) suppositories; bathing with dilute sodium bicarbonate solution may relieve pruritus.
Trichomonas	Thin, irritating frothy discharge; strong, putrid odor	Metronidazole (Flagyl) orally; douching with weak vinegar solution may reduce pruritus.
Herpesvirus type II	Painful pinpoint vesicles on an erythematous base with a watery vaginal discharge possible; voiding may be irritating and painful.	Bathing with dilute sodium bicarbonate solution, applying lubricating jelly to lesions or an oral analgesic such as aspirin may be necessary for pain relief; topically applied acyclovir (Zovirax) helps heal lesions.
Gardnerella	Edema and reddening of vulva	Metronidazole (Flagyl)
Chlamydia trachomatis	Watery vaginal discharge	Erythromycin or doxycycline
Neisseria gonorrhoeae	May be symptomless; may have profuse yellow-green vaginal discharge	Ceftriaxone and doxycycline
Enterobius vermicularis (pinworm)	Rectal pruritus, especially on rising in the morning	Oral administration of an anthelmintic
Treponema pallidum (syphilis)	Painless ulcer on vulva or vagina	Benzathine penicillin, administered intramuscularly
Foreign body	Vaginal discharge; odor	Removal of foreign body by pelvic examination

tion (see Chapter 55). Precocious puberty must also be ruled out.

Pinworms invade the vagina from the rectum. Treatment for this is discussed in Chapter 43. If there is a foreign body in the vagina, it should be removed. Vaginal examination is necessary first to locate the object and then to confirm that it has been fully removed. This may be difficult for girls to accept, and vaginal manipulation and stretching can be painful. A small speculum helps reduce the pain. A local antibiotic ointment or warm bath may be ordered to reduce accompanying infection and inflammation.

Sometimes daily bubble baths can cause vulvar irritation. This can be quickly remedied by discontinuing the bubble baths, because irritation from such a compound can lead not only to local discomfort but to urinary tract infection as well.

A few preschool or school-age children develop a vaginitis from *Escherichia coli* introduced from the anus by improper perineal care after voiding or bowel move-

Table 47-2. *Comfort Measures for Vulvitis*

Measure	Rationale
Wash vulva twice a day with mild, nonperfumed soap and water; pat dry front to back.	Removing secretions decreases irritation; washing front to back prevents spread of rectal contamination forward.
Apply cornstarch for comfort.	Talc should be used sparingly because it may be associated with ovarian cancer.
Take sitz baths or use warm moist compresses three times a day for comfort.	Warm moist heat is soothing in removing edema and keeping the area free of irritating discharge.
Follow instructions concerning a vaginal infection.	Only when the vaginal discharge is eliminated will the vulvitis clear.
Avoid bubble bath or feminine hygiene sprays.	Products may cause local irritation; bubble bath may contribute to urinary tract infections.
Take acetaminophen (Tylenol) every 4 h for comfort.	Itching is a minimal pain sensation, so analgesics reduce itching as well as pain.
Do not scratch the area; apply a cold compress to decrease the sensation of pruritus.	Scratching leaves abrasions that may be secondarily infected.
Use an anesthetic spray or hydrocortisone cream only as prescribed.	Some absorption occurs with topical application, so toxic systemic symptoms can occur.
Wear cotton underwear; sleep without underwear.	Nylon or silk underwear does not allow evaporation and keeps perineum moist.

Jennifer is a 15-year-old girl seen in an ambulatory clinic. Her chief concern is vaginal pruritus. The following is a nursing care plan designed for her.

Assessment: Client states that she has had pruritus and a thick white vaginal discharge for 10 days. Her perineum appears excoriated. White discharge is present at vaginal opening. The clinic physician has made a diagnosis of candidiasis.

Nursing Diagnosis: Pain related to vulvovaginitis

Defining Characteristic: Client states she has pain.

Goal: Client will experience reduced pain in 24 hours.

Outcome Criteria: Client will voice pain is at tolerable level through use of common comfort measures.

Nursing Orders	Rationale
1. Teach Jennifer how to insert a miconazole (Monistat) suppository for 7 days and to continue even if menses begins.	1. Correct use of medication is essential to complete eradication of the candidal organisms.
2. Teach Jennifer additional comfort and prevention measures:	2. A vaginal infection can be quite uncomfortable. These measures will reduce irritation and may also help to prevent recurrent infections.
Take acetaminophen (Tylenol) every 4 h.	
Wash vulva twice daily with mild nonperfumed soap and water. Apply cornstarch afterward.	
Take sitz baths or apply warm moist compresses three times a day.	
Avoid bubble bath, feminine hygiene sprays or contraceptive creams and jellies.	
Do not scratch the area. Apply a cold compress to decrease the sensation of pruritus.	
Wear cotton underwear. Sleep without underwear.	
Refrain from coitus or urge sexual partner to wear a condom.	

ments. A tight hymen then traps the microorganisms in the vagina and leads to infection. The girl needs to be reminded to wipe from front to back following voiding or bowel movements.

Adolescents. As a girl enters puberty, she may notice a slight vaginal discharge due to increased vaginal secretions. She can be reassured that this is normal. To keep from developing vulvar irritation, girls should wear cotton underpants rather than nylon (so moisture is absorbed better) and dry the vulva thoroughly after bathing or swimming.

Some girls may develop vulvar irritation from personal hygiene sprays that supposedly keep the body smelling fresh. These products are unnecessary. Good hygiene can be achieved by daily washing and frequent changing of tampons or pads during menstruation. This will prevent chafing or stasis of menstrual blood and help avoid irritation and excessive odor.

Pelvic Inflammatory Disease

Pelvic inflammatory disease (PID) is infection of the pelvic organs: the uterus, fallopian tubes, ovaries, and their supporting structures. The infection can extend to cause pelvic peritonitis. Gonorrheal infections are the most frequent cause (Dodson, 1990). Although sexual transmission accounts for approximately 75% of all PIDs (gonorrhea and chlamydia are frequently the organisms responsible), infections from other causes such as *E. coli* and *Streptococcus* are beginning to occur more frequently and may be as severe. There is a higher incidence of PID in women using IUDs, a compelling reason for not recommending IUDs for adolescents (Siner et al., 1990).

PID begins with a cervical infection that spreads by surface invasion along the uterine endometrium and then out to the fallopian tubes and ovaries. It is most apt to occur at the end of a menstrual period, because menstrual blood provides an excellent growth medium for bacteria and there is loss of the normal cervical mucus barrier.

Assessment. As peritoneal tissue becomes inflamed and edematous, a purulent exudate forms. If the process is untreated, it enters a chronic phase and fibrotic scarring with stricture of the fallopian tubes will result. With acute PID, the adolescent notices severe pain in the lower abdomen. She may have an accompanying heavy purulent discharge. As the infection progresses, she will develop a fever. Leukocytosis and an elevated sedimentation rate will be present on laboratory testing. On a pelvic examination, any manipulation of the cervix causes severe pain. It may be difficult to palpate the ovaries because of tenderness and abdominal guarding. If the PID enters a chronic phase, the abdominal pain lessens but dyspareunia and dysmenorrhea may be extreme. If the ovaries are affected, intermenstrual spotting may occur. Diagnosis can be aided by sonogram and laparoscopy.

Therapeutic Management. Therapy involves administration of analgesia for comfort plus specific antibiotics such as cefoxitin, doxycycline, or clindamycin and analgesics. Limiting activity helps relieve the pain. In some women, a pelvic abscess forms, which must be drained through the cul-de-sac before healing will occur.

Women who have had one episode of PID have an increased chance of a second occurrence, because the immune protection of the tubes and ovaries may be damaged. They should not have coitus with an infected partner, and they should avoid coitus during menstruation, when their protective mechanisms are lowest. Early childbearing may be recommended if they plan to have children, because extensive tubal scarring could impair fertility. It is important for adolescents to recognize the symptoms of PID and to seek early help for the best outcome (Spence et al., 1990).

Breast Disorders

Males have few breast disorders. Breast tissue may enlarge temporarily in preadolescent boys in response to rising estrogen. Particularly noticeable in obese males,

this reaction fades with a normal increase in testosterone production. Breast disorders that concern adolescent females include additional nipples, benign lesions such as cysts, infections, and injury.

Accessory Nipples

As the name implies, *accessory nipples* are additional breast nipples. They occur along the mammary lines (Figure 47-3) and are generally not as protuberant as true nipples and lack areolar pigmentation. Many girls are unaware that they have an accessory nipple, and think it is a large mole. Accessory nipples are present at birth, and parents should be told what they are so they can inform their daughters later. Some growth in accessory nipples often occurs at puberty or during pregnancy in response to estrogen stimulation.

In a few instances, actual breast tissue is present beneath the accessory nipple. If so, it is subject to the same diseases as other breast tissue. If the accessory nipple or accessory breast tissue is cosmetically distressing to the

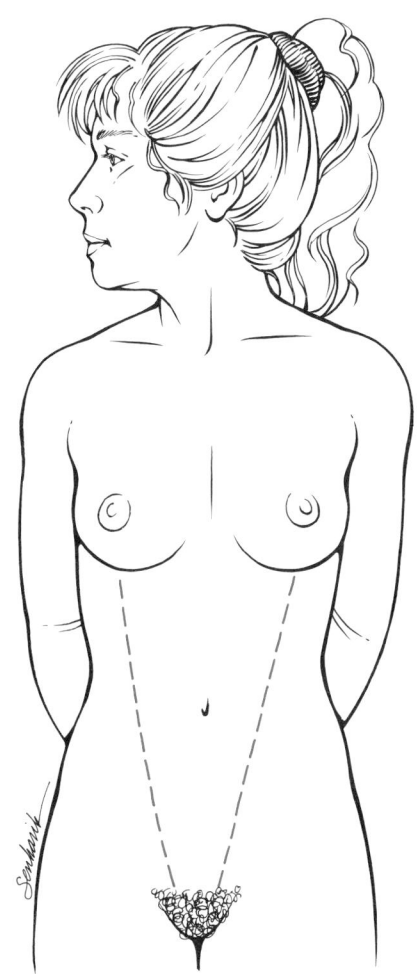

FIGURE 47-3
Nipple lines along which supernumerary nipples occur.

adolescent, it can be removed by simple surgical excision.

Breast Hypertrophy

Breast hypertrophy is abnormal enlargement of breast tissue. In the average girl, breast development halts soon after puberty as soon as progesterone levels rise to mature strength. Progesterone levels remain low until menstruation cycles are fully established. If this process is a lengthy one, breast growth may last for several years.

Breast hypertrophy leads to both physical and emotional stress. The girl may feel pain and fatigue in the back or shoulders from attempting to maintain good posture with heavy breast tissue in front. She may feel self-conscious and try to minimize her breast size by slouching and developing poor posture or rounded shoulders.

Adolescent girls with large breasts may find it difficult to adapt to such a new appearance. They may be treated as provocative sex objects, and feel they should live up to this image. This can make it difficult for them to find their own identity. They may hear comments such as "I wish I had your problem" rather than receiving support and understanding from parents, peers, and health care providers.

If breast hypertrophy is interfering with the girl's physical and emotional well-being, she can have surgical breast reduction. Adolescents need to seriously consider the consequences of this procedure before undertaking it. If a large amount of glandular tissue is removed, breast-feeding may no longer be possible. The adolescent needs to be told realistically that changing her physical appearance will reduce physical discomfort, but changing her self-concept must come from within. An adolescent with large breasts must conscientiously perform breast self-examination, because it is easier for a cancerous lesion to escape detection in large amounts of breast tissue than in a smaller breast. Pregnancy and lactation may be a particularly difficult time because breasts that are already large become even heavier with milk.

Breast Hypoplasia

Breast hypoplasia is stunted growth of fatty tissue, resulting in less-than-average breast size. In most instances, this does not represent a decreased amount of glandular or functional breast tissue, and as a rule, will not interfere with breast-feeding. If an adolescent feels that having small breasts interferes with self-esteem, she can have surgical augmentation to increase breast size, although currently this is not advised until the final results of the safety of breast implants are in. For augmentation, an incision is made under the breast and a silicon implant is inserted under the breast tissue next to the musculus pectoralis major. It is important for the adolescent to realize that her breast tissue is not being replaced by the implant; she still needs to do monthly breast self-examination. Because the original breast tissue is in front of the implant, she will be able to perform self-examination, as well as breast-feeding without difficulty.

Breasts with implants in place may feel firmer than normal on palpation due to the formation of a fibrotic band or capsule around the implant. The girl may notice decreased nipple sensation for approximately 1 year after the procedure. As with breast reduction, adolescents need to be cautioned that although surgery will alter their breast size, a change in self-concept must come from within.

Some women elect not to breast-feed with implants in place because a breast infection would necessitate removal of the implant. A traumatic blow to the breast such as from an automobile accident requires examination by the augmentation surgeon to be certain that the implant did not rupture and cause silicon to leak from the implant. Free-floating silicon could escape into the bloodstream and cause an embolus. In addition, women with implants should have yearly examinations to guard against the gradual absorption of silicon into the breast tissue.

Breast Tenderness or Fullness

Many women notice a day or two of premenstrual breast fullness and tenderness each month. Some may find palpable granular or fine nodular lumps in their breasts during this time. This is a benign occurrence and part of the monthly change in hormone stimulation. For accurate assessment, breast self-examination should be done after, not before, a menstrual period. If a lump or tenderness persists, the woman should consult a health care provider for additional assessment and care, because it might suggest a more extensive change than simple menstruation cycle fluctuation.

Fat Necrosis

If struck during a fall or an automobile accident, breast tissue will show tenderness, pain, local erythema, and perhaps ecchymotic bruising. A few days later, necrosis or disintegration may occur in the fatty layer. As the area heals, fibrotic scar tissue forms. This may leave a firm, palpable lump in the breast. It is not freely movable; it may cause skin or nipple retraction or dimpling on the skin surface. Unlike malignant breast growths, post-traumatic breast lumps tend to be well delineated.

It is generally recommended that such fibrotic areas be biopsied and then excised. The surgical procedure usually leaves little scarring and the woman no longer needs to worry about the lump in her breast. Although at one time breast trauma was thought to be a precipitating factor of breast carcinoma, no direct correlation between the two has been established. The association may exist because a woman who examines her breasts after an injury may find an already existing carcinoma.

Fibrocystic Breast Disease

Fibrocystic breast disease is the most common benign breast disease in women of all ages (Hockenberger, 1993). It can occur as early as puberty when estrogen rises to adult levels, but is found most commonly in women between the ages of 20 and 45 years. Round, fluid-filled cysts form in the connective breast tissue (Figure 47-4). The woman is able to palpate freely movable, well-delineated breast lumps. Lumps may also be visible on the surface of the breasts, and they often occur in the upper outer quadrant. The consistency of these lesions varies with the menstrual cycle, changing from firm and hard to soft and flexible, depending on the amount of serous fluid present. Oral contraceptives help reduce the incidence and size of cysts. The lesions tend to shrink or even disappear during pregnancy and lactation, and they totally disappear with menopause.

Fibrocystic breast disease can be painful; the breasts may feel tender and "stretched," interfering with active sports. This discomfort can be relieved with a simple analgesia such as acetaminophen (Tylenol) or warm compresses. Decreasing sodium intake as well as short-term use of a mild diuretic can reduce the fluid retention just before menses.

The formation of fibrocystic lesions appears to be associated with the use of methylxanthines found in caffeine, theophylline, and theobromine (Bullough et al., 1990). Inform women with fibrocystic lesions that they should avoid the caffeine in coffee, cola drinks, tea, chocolate, and some toffee candy, and medications such as aspirin compound or Excedrin. Discontinuing smoking can also decrease the occurrence of fibrocystic lesions. A supplement of vitamin E may be helpful.

If these measures do not decrease the fibrocystic

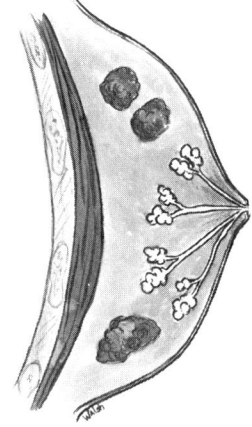

FIGURE 47-4
Round, fluid-filled cysts form in breast tissue in fibrocystic breast disease.

symptoms, cysts may be aspirated under a local anesthetic by injection of a thin sterile needle attached to a small syringe. This procedure not only reduces the size of the cyst but also provides fluid for biopsy.

Danazol (Danocrine) is a synthetic androgen that helps reduce the symptoms of fibrocystic breast disease by suppressing estrogen formation in the ovaries. Danazol is contraindicated in pregnancy; its side-effects are virilization, fluid retention, and estrogen withdrawal symptoms such as sweating or hot flashes. Danazol should not be taken in conjunction with an ovulation suppressant form of birth control, because the androgen stimulation might render the contraceptive ineffective.

In addition to being physically distressing, fibrocystic breast disease can cause women to worry that each lump may turn out to be malignant. They can be reassured that the disease itself does not lead to breast carcinoma, as was previously thought. Breast carcinoma can occur in a woman with fibrocystic disease, however, and may even metastasize before she seeks health consultation, having assumed that all her breast lesions are benign. As a result, she needs more consultation than the average woman. In addition to a yearly breast examination, she needs to perform monthly breast self-examinations, and have an annual mammogram (breast x-ray study). An alternative method of early diagnosis is the breast sonogram, which involves no x-ray exposure and can efficiently locate fluid-filled cysts.

Fibroadenoma

Fibroadenomas are tumors consisting of both fibrotic and glandular components that occur in response to estrogen stimulation. They tend to occur in young black women and are rarely seen after menopause. The tumors may increase in size during adolescence and during pregnancy and lactation, or when a woman takes an estrogen source such as an oral contraceptive.

Unlike fibrocystic lesions, fibroadenomas are round and well delineated, feeling firmer and more rubbery than fluid-filled cysts. Occasionally they calcify and feel extremely hard. They are typically painless, freely movable, and tend not to cause skin retraction. As with fibrocystic lesions, they do not become malignant.

Such tumors can be surgically excised so that the woman no longer has to worry about them. Because the incision is small, it leaves little scarring at the site.

Sexually Transmitted Diseases

STDs are those diseases spread through sexual contact. They range in severity from easily treated infection (such as trichomoniasis) to life-threatening disease (such as human immunodeficiency virus [HIV]; Rosenberg, 1993).

A condom provides the best protection against STDs and should always be used in addition to washing the genitals well with soap and water, voiding immediately after coitus, and choosing sexual partners who are at low risk for infection (avoiding intravenous drug users and prostitutes). None of these practices guarantees protection, however. Educate adolescents that little immunity develops from STDs, which means such diseases can be contracted repeatedly. Being treated once for an STD does not ensure that a person will not contract that disease again. The effects of STDs on pregnancy and the fetus are discussed in Chapter 14.

Candidiasis

The candidal organism is a fungus that thrives on glycogen. As many as 40% of adult females have asymptomatic candidal vaginal infections; this rate rises even higher during pregnancy when high estrogen levels lead to glycogen levels that produce a favorable environment for fungal growth. Because oral contraceptives produce a pseudopregnancy state, pill users also have frequent vaginal candidal infections. When a woman is being treated with an antibiotic (which destroys normal vaginal flora and lets fungal organisms grow more readily), she is particularly susceptible to this infection. Incidence is also strongly associated with diabetes mellitus.

Assessment

Due to the scant mucus production in the premenses period, symptoms may be most acute at this time. The adolescent notices vulvar reddening, burning and itching, and even bleeding from hairline fissures. The vagina sometimes shows white "patches" on the walls that are adherent and cannot be scraped away without bleeding. A thick, cream cheese–like discharge can usually be observed at the vaginal introitus. The adolescent may notice pain on coitus or tampon insertion. Candidal infections may also be present at other body sites, such as the oral cavity or a wet moist area such as the umbilicus.

Candidal infections are diagnosed by removing a sample of discharge from the vaginal wall and placing it on a glass slide; three or four drops of a 20% potassium hydroxide (KOH) solution are then added and the mixture is protected by a coverslip. Under a microscope, typical fungal hyphae indicate the presence of *Candida* organisms (Figure 47-5*A*).

Therapeutic Management

Therapy for candidal infections includes vaginal suppositories or cream applications of antifungal preparations such as miconazole (Monistat), nystatin, and clotrimazole, usually once a day for 7 days. These are generally administered at bedtime so the drug does not drain from the vagina immediately afterward. During the day, the girl might want to wear a sanitary napkin to avoid staining from vaginal discharge. Although sexual contact is not the usual means of contracting the initial candidal infection, a reinfection cycle may occur through sexual activity. If the adolescent is sexually active, treatment of the male partner may be necessary to break the cycle, although abstinence or condom use would be wiser to prevent the risk of contracting other STDs. Treatment should not be interrupted until it is complete, even during a menstrual period.

If a girl has frequent candidal infections, her urine should be tested for glucose to rule out diabetes mellitus. She should be assessed to see if she is high risk for HIV. If she is using an oral contraceptive, she might be counseled to use another contraceptive method.

Trichomoniasis

Trichomonas vaginalis is a single-cell protozoan that is spread by coitus. Up to 25% of adult men and women have asymptomatic *Trichomonas*. The incubation period is 4 to 20 days.

With a trichomonal infection, the girl will notice vaginal irritation and a frothy white or grayish-green vaginal discharge. The frothiness of the discharge is an important typical finding. The upper vagina is reddened and may have pinpoint petechiae. Extreme vulvar itch-

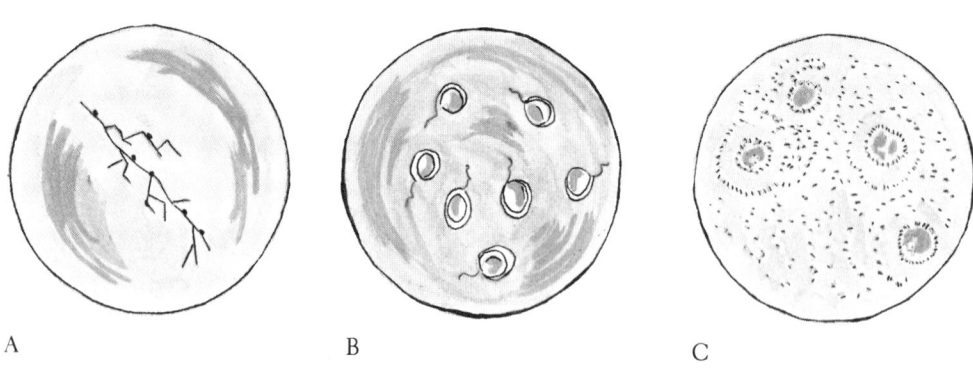

FIGURE 47-5
Microscopic appearance of common organisms causing vaginitis. (**A**) Candida. (**B**) Trichomonas.
(**C**) Gardnerella.

ing is present. By contrast, males with the same infection rarely show any symptoms.

Assessment

The infection is diagnosed by microscopic examination of vaginal discharge combined with Ringer's lactate solution or normal saline. Trichomonads typically appear as rounded, mobile structures (see Figure 47-5B).

Therapeutic Management

Oral metronidazole (Flagyl) eradicates trichomonal infections. Because Flagyl causes acute nausea and vomiting with alcohol, the adolescent should not drink during the course of treatment. A pregnancy test should be prescribed before Flagyl is prescribed, because this drug may be teratogenic. Treatment with Flagyl and use of condoms by her sexual partner will help prevent recurrence of *Trichomonas* in both parties. Be aware that *Trichomonas* infections cause such inflammatory changes in the cervix or vagina that a Pap test taken during this time may be misinterpreted as showing abnormal tissue. If the woman is pregnant, an alternative treatment is douching with a povidone-iodine (Betadine) or vinegar solution.

Bacterial Vaginosis

Bacterial vaginosis is the invasion of *Gardnerella* or *Haemophilus*. These organisms thrive in the vagina, a body area with a reduced oxygen level. The associated discharge is milk-white to gray and has a fishlike odor. Pruritus may be intense. Microscopic examination of the discharge in normal saline shows gram-negative rods adhering to vaginal epithelial cells, which are termed "clue cells" (see Figure 47-5C).

The treatment is oral metronidazole or clindamycin for 7 days; the woman's sexual partner should also be treated to prevent recurrence of the infection.

Chlamydia Trachomatis Infection

Chlamydia trachomatis infections are becoming increasingly common. Symptoms include a heavy grayish-white discharge and vulvar itching. The incubation period is 1 to 5 weeks. Diagnosis is made by culture of the organism. Therapy is oral doxycycline or tetracycline for 7 days. *Chlamydia* infection in a mother may cause eye infection or pneumonia in her newborn (see Chapter 40). During pregnancy, the infection is treated with erythromycin, since tetracycline is teratogenic.

Genital Warts

Genital warts are lesions caused by the human papilloma virus. They are rapid-growing structures on the vulva, vagina, or cervix. Large growths may be excised by cautery or cryotherapy, since they can lead to carcinoma (Lilley & Schaffer, 1990). Small growths may be removed by application of podophyllin (see Chapter 14).

Herpes Genitalis

Genital herpes is caused by the herpesvirus *hominis* type 2 (HSV-2). This is one of four similar herpes viruses: cytomegalovirus, Epstein-Barr, varicella-zoster, and herpes type 1 and type 2. Genital herpes occurs in epidemic proportions in the United States, and its incidence appears to be growing yearly (more than 500,000 new cases reported annually). Unlike most other STDs, there is no known cure. The disease involves a lifelong process and is associated with cervical cancer. The virus is spread by skin-to-skin contact, entering a break in skin or mucous membrane. For the newborn, it can be systemic and even fatal (see Chapter 26).

Assessment

Herpes is diagnosed by a culture of the lesion secretion from its location on the vulva, vagina, cervix, or penis or by isolation of HSV antibodies in serum. The incubation period is 3 to 14 days. On first contact, extensive primary lesions originate as a group of pinpoint vesicles on an erythematous base. Within a few days, the vesicles ulcerate and become moist, draining, open lesions. The client may have accompanying flulike symptoms with an increased temperature; vaginal lesions may cause profuse discharge. Pain is intense on contact with clothing or acid urine. After the primary stage that lasts approximately 1 week, the virus generally lingers in a latent form, affecting the sensory nerve ganglia. It will flare up and become an active infection during illness, PMS, fever, overexposure to sunlight, or stress. A secondary response usually produces local rather than systemic symptoms. Herpes may be transmitted to a newborn at birth through active lesions. To avoid this, a cesarean birth can be scheduled.

Women with a herpes type 2 infection have an increased chance (eight times higher than normal) of developing cervical cancer.

Therapeutic Management

Acyclovir (Zovirax) destroys the virus by interfering with deoxyribonucleic acid reproduction and decreasing symptoms, and is available as a topical ointment. When applying this, protect yourself with a finger cot so that you do not contract the virus or absorb the drug. Soothing sitz baths three times a day, keeping the lesions clean and dry, and applying a soothing substance such as cornstarch to reduce discomfort, may be helpful. An emollient (A & D Ointment) also reduces discomfort, but its moisture tends to prolong the active period of the lesions. Ointments should be used sparingly to keep the area dry and promote healing.

Because of the association with cervical cancer, any female with genital herpes should have a yearly Pap test for the rest of her life. Annual Pap tests are recommended for all women, so this is a standard precaution to follow. Condoms will help prevent the spread of herpes among sexual partners.

People with herpes may have difficulty establishing sexual relationships for fear of infecting a partner. Because herpes is communicated only by direct contact, infected individuals need to inform their partner when they have any active lesions and take extra precautions to decrease the danger of spreading the virus.

Hepatitis B

Hepatitis B can be spread by semen and is considered an STD. It is discussed in Chapter 45 with other forms of hepatitis.

Gonorrhea

Gonorrhea is transmitted by *Neisseria gonorrhoeae,* a gram-positive diplococcus that thrives on columnar transitional epithelium of the mucous membrane. Symptoms begin after a 2- to 7-day incubation period, and, in males, include *urethritis* (pain on urination and frequency of urination) and a urethral discharge. Without treatment, the infection may spread to the testes, causing scarring of the tubules that results in permanent sterility. Untreated, the infection is easily spread among sexual partners.

Although symptoms of gonorrhea in females are not as visible, there may be a slight yellowish vaginal discharge. Bartholin's glands may become inflamed and painful. If left untreated, the infection may spread to pelvic organs, most notably the fallopian tubes (PID). Tubal scarring can result in permanent sterility. In both males and females, untreated gonorrhea can lead to arthritis or heart disease from systemic involvement (May & Clasen, 1990).

An infant may contract gonorrhea from its mother in the birth canal. This leads frequently to gonorrheal ophthalmia (discussed in Chapter 26).

Assessment

A culture for gonococcal bacillus should be done on all children with vulvovaginitis or urethral discharge. In males, a first voiding may reveal gonococci if a midstream specimen is inconclusive.

Therapeutic Management

The treatment for gonorrhea is one intramuscular injection of ceftriaxone or oral amoxicillin plus oral doxycycline for 7 days. Sexual partners should receive the same treatment.

Approximately 24 hours after treatment, the gonor-

rhea is no longer infectious. Approximately 7 days after treatment, a client should return for a follow-up culture to verify that the disease has been completely eradicated (few people take this precaution). A sexually active client should be given a serologic test for syphilis along with the gonorrheal culture. If the dose of ceftriaxone and doxycycline has effectively eliminated the gonorrhea, no additional treatment for syphilis will be necessary. Most states require that gonorrhea be reported to the health department; adolescents are asked to name sexual contacts.

Nursing Diagnoses and Related Interventions

Nursing Diagnosis: Anxiety related to having contracted a reportable STD

Goal: Client will demonstrate reduced anxiety by end of health care visit.

Outcome Criteria: Client voices confidence in ability to cope with this problem; demonstrates understanding of both illness and treatment regimen.

People who seek treatment for STDs need to feel they can trust health care personnel and reveal information without fear of criticism. Assure the client of absolute confidentiality in naming his or her sexual contacts. Without being told who put them at risk, these people can then be notified by a health department investigator that they have been exposed to a particular STD. This vital information will help prevent further spread of the disease.

Some people are reluctant to seek treatment for gonorrhea because they have heard stories that therapy involves 10 to 15 days of intramuscular injections. Because they have no symptoms, some girls may avoid going for what they think will be extremely painful treatment. Alert them that this is an insidious disease, and even though no symptoms are apparent, it can have disastrous long-term effects if left untreated.

Syphilis

Syphilis is a systemic disease caused by the spirochete *Treponema pallidum.* It is transmitted by sexual contact with a person who has an active spirochete-containing lesion; it is also reportable.

Following an incubation period of 10 to 90 days, a typical lesion appears, generally on the genitalia (penis or labia) or on the mouth, lips, or rectal area from oral-genital or genital-anal contact. The lesion (termed a *chancre*) is a deep ulcer and generally painless despite its size. Lymphadenopathy may be present but is unlikely to be noticed by the affected individual. A lesion in the vagina may not be immediately evident. Without treatment, a chancre lasts approximately 6 weeks and then fades.

Approximately 2 to 4 weeks after the chancre disappears, a generalized macular copper-colored rash becomes evident. Unlike many other rashes, it affects the soles and the palms. A serologic test for syphilis yields a positive result at this time. There may be secondary symptoms of generalized illness such as low-grade fever and adenopathy. With or without treatment, this stage of syphilis will also fade.

The next stage is a latency period that may last from only a few years to several decades. The only indication of the disease is the serologic test, which continues to yield a positive result.

The final stage of syphilis is a destructive neurologic disease that involves major body organs such as the heart and the nervous system. Typical symptoms are blindness, paralysis, severe crippling neurologic deformities, mental confusion, slurred speech, and lack of coordination. This third stage should be identified before it becomes fatal.

Assessment

Syphilis is diagnosed by the recognition of the various symptoms of the three stages and by serologic serum tests, usually VDRL (Venereal Disease Research Laboratory), ART (automated reagin test), RPR (rapid plasma reagin test), or FTA-ABS (fluorescent treponemal antibody absorption test).

Therapeutic Management

The therapy effectively arrests the disease at whatever stage it has reached. Benzathine penicillin G given intramuscularly in two sites is effective therapy. For the adolescent sensitive to penicillin, either oral erythromycin or tetracycline can be given for 10 to 15 days. As with gonorrhea, contacts are treated in the same way as the person with the active infection.

Because syphilis can be treated so easily, one would think it would be easy to eradicate. In reality, however, because the primary chancre is painless, many individuals are either unaware of it or choose to ignore it, thereby transmitting the disease to unsuspecting partners. Adolescents, in particular, need accurate information about STDs to become aware of the symptoms. They should be able to feel they can report the disease to health care personnel and that they can name sexual contacts without fear of being criticized.

Human Immunodeficiency Virus

HIV is carried by semen as well as other body fluids, and is considered an STD. Invasion of the virus is discussed with other immune disorders in Chapter 42, and in relation to pregnancy in Chapter 14.

Key Points

- The cause of ambiguous genitalia is unknown but may be related to the level of testosterone produced in utero. The true sex of children is established by a sex chromatin test (Barr body determination) or a karyotype of chromosomes.
- Precocious puberty is the development of breast or pubic hair before age 8 years. Girls may be treated with a synthetic analogue to luteinizing hormone releasing hormone to reduce development. Such children are high risk for body image disturbance without effective support.
- Delayed puberty is the failure to develop secondary sex characteristics by age 17 years. Girls may be administered estrogen to promote development; boys may be administered testosterone.
- Balanoposthitis (inflammation of the glans and prepuce) and phimosis (constricted foreskin) are conditions seen in boys. Phimosis can be treated with circumcision.
- Cryptorchidism is failure of one or both testes to descend during intrauterine life. The condition is surgically corrected to prevent malignancy development later in life.
- Testicular cancer is a rare malignancy but tends to occur in young adults. Boys need to be taught testicular self-examination for early detection.
- Dysmenorrhea is a menstrual disorder that occurs frequently in adolescent girls. Therapy for this is a prostaglandin inhibitor such as ibuprofen.
- Endometriosis (the abnormal growth of extrauterine endometrial tissue) can lead to infertility later in life if not treated. Therapy is administration of Danazol, a synthetic androgen, or surgery to reduce the size of the abnormal tissue.
- Children whose mothers took diethylstilbestrol (DES) while the child was in utero may be susceptible to adenosis or vaginal cancer if girls; cystic testes if boys. They need regular follow-up examinations for early detection of these disorders.
- Vulvovaginitis (inflammation of the vulva) or pelvic inflammatory disease are infections that can occur in adolescents. Therapy to prevent scarring of fallopian tubes and infertility later in life is essential.
- Breast disorders such as fibrocystic breast disease can occur in adolescents. Adolescent girls need to learn breast self-examination to detect abnormalities that could mean breast cancer.
- Sexually transmitted diseases such as candidiasis, trichomoniasis, *Chlamydia trachomatis,* genital warts, herpes genitalis, gonorrhea, and syphilis are increasing in incidence in the adolescent population. An important health teaching area with children is the need to follow safer sex practices. Girls

need to be taught, in addition, ways to avoid toxic shock syndrome.

- It is important when teaching about STDs to stress that STDs do not confer immunity and thus can be contracted more than once.
- Children who are born with a reproductive tract disorder frequently adjust well when young. They may need counseling at puberty or when they become aware of the impact of their disorder on their sexual functioning or their ability to reproduce.

Critical Thinking Exercises

1. Ralph is a 16-year-old who tells you he is sexually active but is not practicing safe sex practices because he does not believe he will contact a disease with only sporadic sexual relations. What are the measures you would want to discuss with Ralph?
2. Chris is a 15-year-old girl who has no breast development and also has not menstruated as yet. She asks you if it is time to worry. How would you counsel her?
3. Timothy is a 12-year-old who was born with undescended testes. He had surgery for this at age 2 years. He is concerned now that he is at high risk for testicular cancer. How would you counsel him?

References

Breyer, et al. (1993). Gonadotropin-releasing hormone agoinsts in the treatment of girls with central precocious puberty. *Clinical Obstetrics and Gynecology, 36,* 764.

Brock, D., et al. (1993). Testicular cancer. *Seminars in Oncology Nursing, 9,* 224.

Broscious, S. K. (1991). Toxic shock syndrome and its potential complications. *Critical Care Nurse, 11,* 28.

Bullough, B., et al. (1990). Methylxanthines and fibrocystic breast disease: A study of correlations. *Nurse Practitioner, 15,* 36.

Catlin, E. A., & Crawford, J. D. (1994). Neonatal endocrinology. In Oski, F. A., et al. *Principles and practice of pediatrics* (2nd ed.). Philadelphia: J. B. Lippincott.

Cilento, B. G., et al. (1993). Cryptorchidism and testicular torsion. *Pediatric Clinics of North America, 40,* 1133.

Clore, E. R. (1993). A guide for the testicular self-examination. *Journal of Pediatric Health Care, 7,* 264.

Davis, G. D., et al. (1993). Clinical characteristics of adolescent endometriosis. *Journal of Adolescent Health, 14,* 362.

Department of Health and Human Services. (1991). *Healthy people 2000.* Washington, DC: Public Health Service.

Dodson, M. G. (1990). Optimum therapy for acute pelvic inflammatory disease. *Drugs, 39,* 511.

Goldenring, J. M. (1992). Testicular self-exam: A lifesaver. *Patient Care, 26,* 62.

Hawkins, E. P. (1994). The genitourinary system. In Oski, F. A., et al. *Principles and practice of pediatrics* (2nd ed.). Philadelphia: J. B. Lippincott.

Hockenberger, S. J. (1993). Fibrocystic breast disease: Every woman is at risk. *Plastic Surgery Nursing, 13,* 37.

Hricak, H., et al. (1990). Cervical incompetence: Preliminary evaluation with MR imaging. *Radiology, 174,* 821.

Jackson, P. L., & Ott, M. J. (1990). Perceived self-esteem among children diagnosed with precocious puberty. *Journal of Pediatric Nursing, 5,* 190.

Kogan, S. J., et al. (1990). Efficacy of orchiopexy by patient age 1 year for cryptorchidism. *Journal of Urology, 144,* 508.

Lilley, L. L., & Schaffer, S. (1990). Human papillomavirus: A sexually transmitted disease with carcinogenic potential. *Cancer Nursing, 13,* 366.

Loucks, A. B. (1990). Effects of exercise training on the menstrual cycle. *Medical Science of Sports and Exercise, 22,* 275.

May, J. G., & Clasen, M. E. (1990). The patient with gonococcal infection. *Primary Care, 17,* 59.

Mortola, J. F., et al. (1991). Successful treatment of severe premenstrual syndrome by combined use of gonadotropin-releasing hormone agonist and estrogen/progestin. *Journal of Clinical Endocrinology and Metabolism, 72,* 252A.

Nightingale, S. L. (1990). New requirements for tampon labeling. *American Family Physician, 41,* 999.

Patrick, C. C. (1994). Staphylococcal infections. In Oski, F. A., et al. *Principles and practice of pediatrics* (2nd ed.). Philadelphia: J. B. Lippincott.

Plotnick, L. P. (1994). Puberty and gonadal disorders. In Oski, F. A., et al. *Principles and practice of pediatrics* (2nd ed.). Philadelphia: J. B. Lippincott.

Politoff, L., et al. (1990). Does hydrocele affect later fertility? *Fertility and Sterility, 53,* 700.

Raja, S. N., et al. (1992). Prevalence and correlates of the premenstrual syndrome in adolescence. *Journal of the American Academy of Child and Adolescent Psychiatry, 31,* 783.

Rencken, R. K., et al. (1990). Sclerotherapy for hydroceles. *Journal of Urology, 143,* 940.

Rosenberg, J. (1993). Sexually transmitted diseases: What women should know for the 90s. *National Women's Health Report, 15,* 1.

Rosenfield, R. L. (1990). Diagnosis and management of delayed puberty. *Journal of Clinical Endocrinology and Metabolism, 70,* 559.

Sharp, G. G., & Cole, P. (1990). Vaginal bleeding and diethylstilbestrol exposure during pregnancy: Relationship to genital tract clear cell adenocarcinoma and vaginal adenosis in daughters. *American Journal of Obstetrics and Gynecology, 162,* 994.

Siner, S. K., et al. (1990). Preventing IUD-related pelvic infection: The efficacy of prophylactic doxycycline at insertion. *British Journal of Obstetrics and Gynaecology, 97,* 412.

Spence, M. R., et al. (1990). Pelvic inflammatory disease in the adolescent. *Journal of Adolescent Health Care, 11,* 304.

Vandeven, A. M., & Emans, S. J. (1993). Vulvovaginitis in the child and adolescent. *Pediatrics in Review, 14,* 141.

Vohra, S. & Bedlani, G. (1992). Balanitis and balanoposthitis. *Urology Clinics of North America, 19,* 143.

Wilson, M. D. (1994). Menstrual disorders. In Oski, F. A., et al. *Principles and practice of pediatrics* (2nd ed.). Philadelphia: J. B. Lippincott.

Wiswell, T. E., et al. (1993). Circumcision in children beyond the neonatal period. *Pediatrics, 92,* 791.

Suggested Readings

Cokkinades, V. E., et al. (1990). Menstrual dysfunction among habitual runners. *Women and Health, 18,* 59.

Cook, R. R., et al. (1994). The breast implant controversy. *Arthritis and Rheumatism, 37,* 153.

Eschenbach, O. A., et al. (1992). Managing problem vaginitis. *Patient Care, 26,* 187.

Felten, B. S. (1990). The lingering tragedy of DES. *RN, 53,* 35.

Levine, G. I. (1991). Sexually transmitted parasitic diseases. *Primary Care, 18,* 101.

McCann, J., et al. (1990). Genital findings in prepubertal girls selected for nonabuse: A descriptive study. *Pediatrics, 86,* 428.

Nolan, J. R., et al. (1990). Acute management of the zipper-entrapped penis. *Journal of Emergency Medicine, 8,* 305.

Olsen, C. G., & Gordon, R. E. (1990). Breast disorders in nursing mothers. *American Family Physician, 41,* 1509.

Quinn, R. M., et al. (1990). Secondary changes in the scrotal testis in experimental unilateral cryptorchidism. *Journal of Pediatric Surgery, 25,* 402.

Rosenfield, R. L., & Barnes, R. B. (1993). Menstrual disorders in adolescence. *Endocrinology and Metabolism Clinics of North America, 22,* 491.

Swanson, J. M., & Chenitz, W. C. (1990). Psychosocial aspects of genital herpes: A review of the literature. *Public Health Nursing, 7,* 96.

Turek, P. J., et al. (1994). The absent cryptorchid testis: Surgical findings and their implications for diagnosis and etiology. *Journal of Urology, 151,* 718.

Yarber, W. L. et al. (1992). Adolescents and sexually transmitted diseases. *Journal of School Health, 62,* 331.

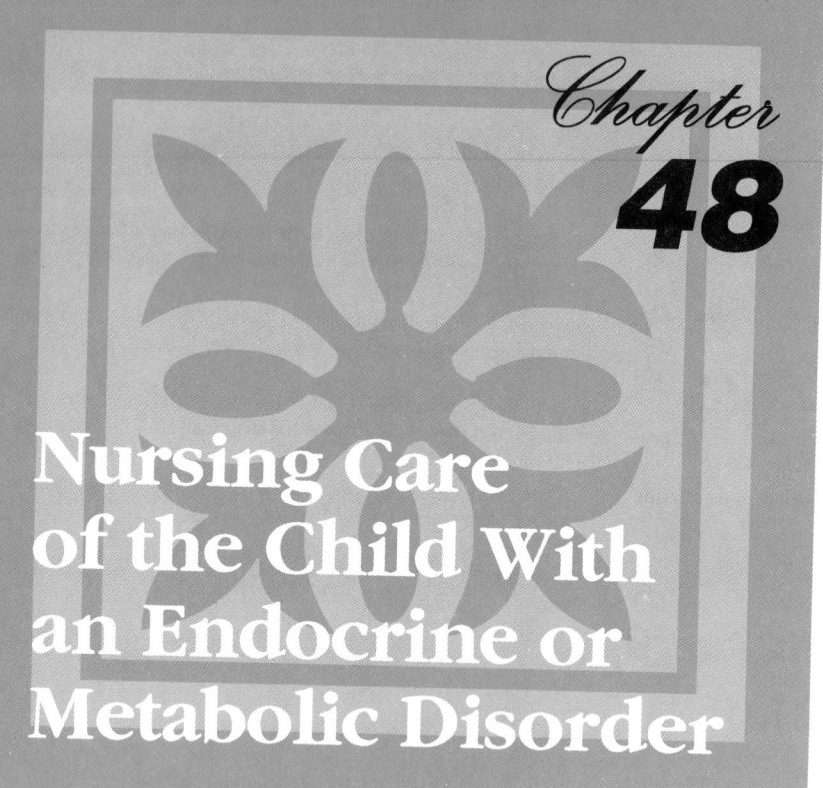

Chapter 48

Nursing Care of the Child With an Endocrine or Metabolic Disorder

Key Terms

- carpal spasm
- exophthalmos
- glycosuria
- hormones
- hyperfunction
- hypofunction
- hypoglycemia
- hypothalamus
- ketoacidosis
- latent tetany
- manifest tetany
- pedal spasm
- polydipsia
- polyuria
- sella turcica
- Somogyi phenomenon

Objectives

After mastering the contents of this chapter, you should be able to:

1. Describe the different endocrine glands and their functions.

2. Assess a child with a disorder of endocrine function.

3. Formulate nursing diagnoses for the child with altered endocrine function.

4. Plan nursing care for the child with altered endocrine function, such as planning health teaching for the child with hypopituitary dysfunction.

5. Implement nursing care for the child with endocrine dysfunction, such as teaching insulin administration to the child with diabetes mellitus.

6. Evaluate outcome criteria established to be certain that goals of nursing care were achieved.

7. Identify National Health Goals related to endocrine disorders and children that nurses could be instrumental in helping the nation achieve.

8. Identify areas related to care of children with endocrine disorders that could benefit from additional nursing research.

9. Use critical thinking to analyze ways that care of the child with altered endocrine function can be family centered.

10. Synthesize knowledge of endocrine dysfunction and the nursing process to ensure quality maternal and child health nursing care.

Adele Pillitteri: MATERNAL AND CHILD HEALTH NURSING, 2nd Edition. © 1995 Adele Pillitteri..

The endocrine system is composed of a small group of glands that work together with the neurologic system to regulate and coordinate all body systems (Figure 48-1). The glands produce chemicals called **hormones**, which are expelled into surrounding tissue and picked up by the bloodstream where they act individually and in concert to affect various organ systems. (The word *hormone* is from the Greek *hormaein*, which means "to set in motion.") Each gland of the endocrine system has specific functions that are necessary for regulation of body processes; each hormone secreted acts on a specific target or designated organ.

Dysfunction of the glands or action of the hormones results in a variety of disorders, most of which have long-term implications. Parents—and children themselves as soon as they are old enough—need to understand these diseases to the best of their ability and to participate in the long-term plan of care. National Health Goals related to endocrine disorders and children are shown in the Focus on National Health Goals box.

NURSING PROCESS OVERVIEW
for Care of the Child
With an Endocrine Disorder

ASSESSMENT

Endocrine disorders as a group often cause changes in normal growth or activity patterns. This is often detected when height and weight are assessed and compared with standards for the child's age at all health visits. Obese children may have thyroid deficiencies. Short children may have pituitary difficulties. An acute loss in weight is often the first symptom of diabetes mellitus in children.

Taking a day history (asking the parent or child to describe all the child's actions on a typical day) will help you distinguish between a normal "quiet" child and one with decreased endocrine function that is making the child chronically fatigued and inactive. (The quiet child lies down after school and reads; the ill child lies down and sleeps.) Taking a day history also differentiates between a child who is merely active and one who is overly active because of hyperthyroidism. (The healthy child appears to "go constantly" but is able to sit through a favorite television program or a meal; the child with increased thyroid production may not be able to sit quietly at all.)

Assess dietary and elimination habits. Extreme thirst or appetite may occur with endocrine malfunction. Frequent voiding in children most often reflects a urinary tract infection but may be evidence of excessive urinary excretion (polyuria), as occurs with pituitary dysfunction or diabetes mellitus.

On physical examination, the child's general appearance should be inspected for excessive tiredness, scaling or dry skin, drooping eyelids or protrusion of eyes (**exophthalmos**), or poor muscle tone (Figure 48-2).

NURSING DIAGNOSIS

Nursing diagnoses relevant to children with endocrine disorders include these:

- Fluid volume deficit related to constant excessive loss of fluid through urination
- High risk for altered nutrition, less than body requirements, related to inability to use glucose
- Altered self-concept related to abnormal height
- Health-seeking behaviors related to self-administration of insulin

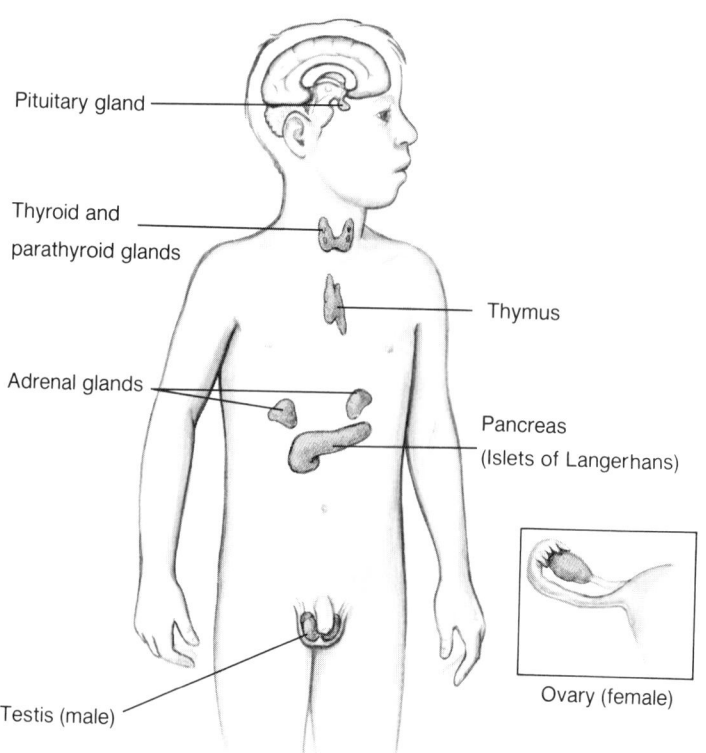

FIGURE 48-1

Location of the endocrine glands.

- Knowledge deficit related to treatment needs
- Fear related to illness outcome
- Grieving related to acceptance of long-term illness
- Altered family processes related to child's chronic illness

PLANNING

Although most endocrine disorders have long-term implications, parents and children may find it easier to work with short-term goals at first; they are still reacting too strongly to the diagnosis to be able to accept the long-term nature of the disorder. Because symptoms are often not acute, it is easy for children and parents to forget medications. Helping parents make out reminder charts is an effective measure to increase compliance.

The school situation must be carefully evaluated for any child with chronic illness. Teachers may have to be alerted to the child's health problem so they do not make excessive or inappropriate demands (e.g., insisting that the child with hyperthyroidism submit neat handwriting assignments when she cannot do so).

Organizations for referral include the following:

American Diabetes Association
P.O. Box 25757
1160 Duke Street
Alexandria, VA 22314

Little People of America
7238 Piedmont Drive
Dallas, TX 75227-9324

National Tay-Sachs and Allied Disease Association
2001 Beacon Street
Brookline, MA 02146

IMPLEMENTATION

Interventions for children with endocrine disorders must always be carried out with the long-term aspects of care in mind. Bribing children to take a medicine, for example, is never good practice. It has no place with children who must continue to take a medication for the rest of their lives (it quickly becomes ineffective). As children grow older and are better able to understand their disorder, explanations of why they must continue to take medication should become more detailed.

EVALUATION

Children with disorders of endocrine function need to be evaluated periodically all during childhood; growth and activity will necessitate changes in medication dosages or schedules. These checkups provide good opportunities for health teaching to equip children to meet new situations that arise as they gain more maturity. Body appearance becomes increasingly important as children enter adolescence, for example. Being like, not unlike, their peers, grows even more important. Seemingly well-adjusted school-age children may now have extreme difficulty accepting their illness. Compliance with a medication program may be erratic during adolescent years. Only by periodic reevaluation can these problems be identified so that health care plans can be modified and adapted to the child's needs, enabling the child and family to once more cope with a long-term illness.

The following are examples of outcome criteria:

- Child states reasons for complying with medication regimen.
- Child's blood pressure and pulse are within normal limits for age; specific gravity of urine is between 1.003 and 1.030; skin turgor is good; child states thirst is not excessive.
- Parents demonstrate correct insulin injection technique and state they are comfortable injecting their child.

FOCUS ON
National Health Goals

Diabetes mellitus is a disorder with serious consequences in both children and pregnant women. A number of National Health Goals address reducing the incidence of this disease:

- Reduce diabetes-related deaths to no more than 34/100,000 people from a baseline of 38/100,000.
- Reduce the most severe complications of diabetes such as perinatal mortality to 2% from a baseline of 5%, and major congenital malformations from the illness from 8% to 4%.
- Reduce diabetes to a prevalence of no more than 25 per 1000 people from a baseline of 28/1000 (DHHS, 1991).

Nurses can be instrumental in helping the nation achieve these goals by educating women about the possible effects the illness can have on pregnancy and educating children about ways to prevent the long-term effects of the illness. Nursing research could shed additional light on these goals by asking questions such as, how should women be taught that fetal anomalies from hyperglycemia occur very early in pregnancy so they must be certain to enter pregnancy in good glucose control? Long-term effects of diabetes are not noticeable in childhood, but how can children be educated to plan a healthy lifestyle to prevent these effects in adult life? How soon in life can children be expected to be responsible for glucose monitoring and insulin injection? What methods are best for encouraging children to be in charge of their own diet?

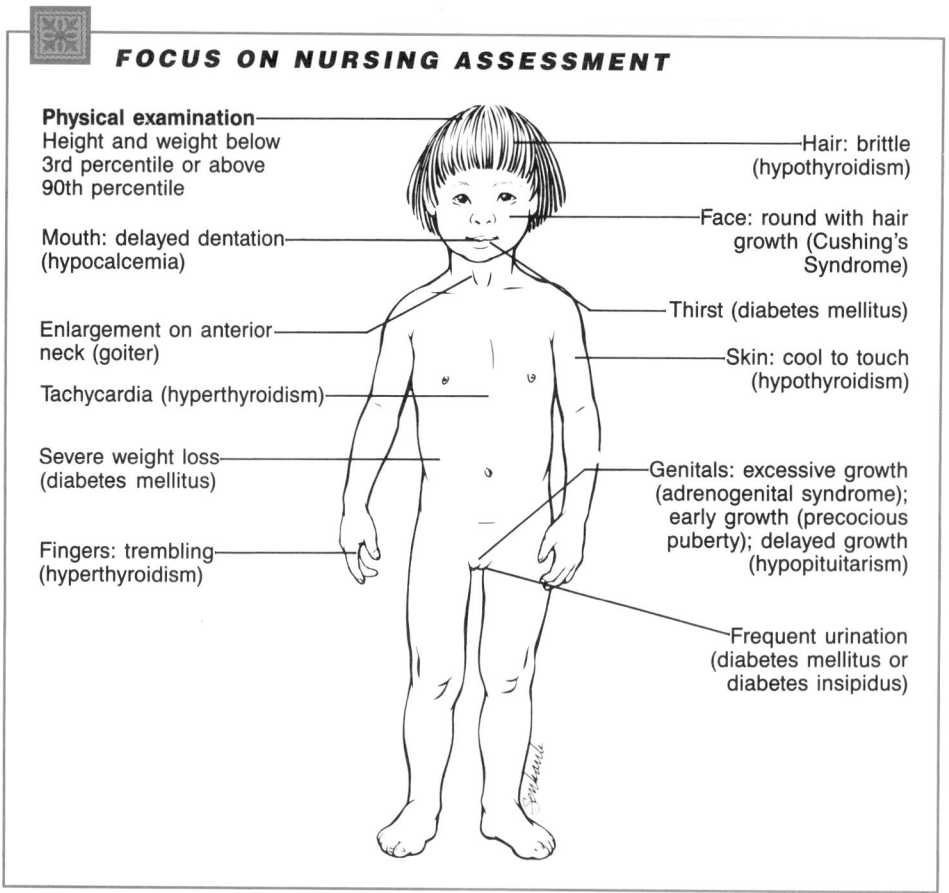

FOCUS ON NURSING ASSESSMENT

Physical examination
Height and weight below
3rd percentile or above
90th percentile

Mouth: delayed dentation
(hypocalcemia)

Enlargement on anterior
neck (goiter)

Tachycardia (hyperthyroidism)

Severe weight loss
(diabetes mellitus)

Fingers: trembling
(hyperthyroidism)

Hair: brittle
(hypothyroidism)

Face: round with hair
growth (Cushing's
Syndrome)

Thirst (diabetes mellitus)

Skin: cool to touch
(hypothyroidism)

Genitals: excessive growth
(adrenogenital syndrome);
early growth (precocious
puberty); delayed growth
(hypopituitarism)

Frequent urination
(diabetes mellitus or
diabetes insipidus)

FIGURE 48-2
Assessment of the child with an endocrine disorder.

The Pituitary Gland

The work of the pituitary gland is directed by the **hypothalamus**, an organ that is located in the brain and serves as the regulator of the autonomic nervous system. About 1 cm long, 1.0 to 1.5 cm wide, and 0.5 cm thick, the pituitary rests in the **sella turcica**, a depression of the sphenoid bone. It is covered by a tough membrane, which also joins the gland to the hypothalamus.

There are several distinct regions of the pituitary: the anterior lobe, or *adenohypophysis*; the posterior lobe, or *neurohypophysis*; and the intermediate lobe (*pars intermedia*), which lies between the anterior and posterior lobes. Each of these regions appears to have its own function and secretes specific hormones.

Pituitary Hormones

The regions of the pituitary gland store and release eight hormones; four of these are prominently involved in childhood illnesses.

Antidiuretic Hormone

Antidiuretic hormone, or ADH, is secreted by the neurohypophysis. The kidneys are the target organs for ADH.

In the presence of ADH, the distal tubules and collecting ducts of the kidney nephrons decrease urine output by increasing water reabsorption. This leads to an increased amount of extracellular fluid, which causes a vasopressor effect (increased blood pressure). When the concentration of the plasma is increased or there is decreased overall circulating vascular volume, additional ADH will be released. If blood is pooling in the body periphery, decreasing core body volume, ADH will be released. A change from a supine to a standing position, exposure to high temperature (blood is shifted to the periphery to begin cooling), and positive-pressure respiration (there is decreased blood volume in the vena cava) all stimulate ADH release. Other factors that increase release are trauma, pain, and anxiety. With a lowered amount of ADH, little or no water is reabsorbed, which increases urinary output. The consumption of alcohol causes inhibited secretion of ADH, and as a result urine output increases.

Thyrotropin

Secreted by the adenohypophysis, thyrotropin (also called TSH) stimulates the thyroid gland to produce thyroid hormones (thyroxine and tri-iodothyronine). A deficiency of TSH will lead to atrophy and inactivity of the thyroid gland; an excess of TSH will cause hypertrophy (increase in size) and hyperplasia (increase in the number of cells) of the gland. A feedback message of increased thyroid secretion will lower production of TSH; decreased thyroid production will increase thyrotropin production.

Corticotropin

Corticotropin, or ACTH, which is also secreted by the adenohypophysis, stimulates the adrenal gland to produce glucocorticoid and mineralocorticoid hormones. Increased production of adrenal gland secretions decreases production of ACTH and vice versa. If a child is given synthetic ACTH or a corticosteroid, the production of natural ACTH is temporarily depressed. If these synthetic substances are given for a long time, then stopped abruptly, the lessened amount of natural ACTH may not be enough to stimulate adrenal gland activity; the child will then show symptoms of adrenal insufficiency. This is an important concept for nurses, who administer medicine. Administration of ACTH and high doses of corticosteroids must always be tapered; to protect adrenal function, the medication should never be stopped abruptly.

Somatotropin

Somatotropin (also known as growth hormone [GH]) has no specific target organ but acts on all body cells. It is released from the adenohypophysis based on a release factor from both the hypothalamus and the liver. The amount of secretion is influenced by exercise, sleep, nutrition, and thyroid and adrenal function. GH acts to increase growth in bone and cartilage and increases gastrointestinal absorption of calcium. It causes decreased catabolism of protein in cells by freeing fatty acids for energy; this frees glucose for glycogen storage (it is both protein and glucose sparing). Production is increased with **hypoglycemia** (an abnormally low concentration of glucose in the blood) and during sleep. If decreased in amount, dwarfism will occur. If increased in amount, gigantism or overgrowth will occur.

Disorders Caused by Pituitary Gland Dysfunction

Illnesses caused by pituitary malfunction result from tumor growth of the pituitary or hypothalamus, interference with circulation to the gland, trauma, inflammation, structural abnormalities, erratic or nonfunctional feedback mechanisms, and, possibly, autoimmune responses.

Growth Hormone Deficiency

When production of human GH (somatotropin) is deficient, children remain short of stature (Plotnick, 1994a). Such children are well proportioned but simply minia-

ture in size. This may be caused by a nonmalignant cystic tumor of embryonic origin that causes pressure on the pituitary gland or from increased intracranial pressure from another cause. In most children with hypopituitarism, the cause of the defect is unknown.

It is difficult to predict exactly what height will be reached in the untreated child because this varies with each individual. Without treatment, however, the child will not reach a height over 3 or 4 feet.

Assessment

The child with deficient production of GH is generally normal in size and weight at birth. Within the first few years of life, however, the child begins to fall below the third percentile of height and weight on growth charts. The face appears infantile because the mandible is recessed and immature; the nose is usually small. The child's teeth may be crowded in a small jaw (and may erupt late). The child's voice may be high-pitched, and there is a delayed onset of pubic, facial, and axillary hair and genital growth.

History, physical findings, and a decreased level of circulating GH contribute to the diagnosis. Evaluate the family history for traits of short stature or to detect if the main problem is constitutional delay (innocent late development). If at all possible, obtain estimates of the parents' height and siblings' height and weight during their periods of growth. Assess thoroughly the child's prenatal and birth history for suggestion of intrauterine growth retardation or severe head trauma at birth, which could have injured the pituitary gland. Assess the past health history for signals of chronic illness, such as heart, kidney, or intestinal disorders, that could contribute to the decreased level of growth. Take a 24-hour nutrition history and ask carefully about urinary and bowel function. Parents often report that their child is a "picky eater," yet the 24-hour history does not reveal a poor appetite to be extensive enough to halt growth.

The presence of a pituitary tumor as the cause of the decreased production of GH must be ruled out. If a child has suddenly halted growth, a tumor is suggested; gradual failure suggests an idiopathic involvement. A history of loss of vision, headache, increase in head circumference, nausea, and vomiting is suggestive of a pituitary tumor. The history of a child with hypopituitary dwarfism typically reveals a well child except for the abnormal lack of growth.

A physical assessment, including a funduscopic examination and neurologic testing, should be done to detect the presence of a lesion or tumor. Blood studies for hypothyroidism, hypoadrenalism, and hypoaldosteronism are done, because these conditions also influence growth. The wrist is examined by x-ray film to determine bone age. Epiphyseal closure of long bone is delayed with growth hormone deficiency but is proportional to the height delay. A skull series, computed tomography (CT) scan, magnetic resonance imaging, or ultrasound scan will be performed to detect possible enlargement of the sella turcica, which would suggest a pituitary tumor.

Normally, GH level rises after a period of sound sleep or a period of activity. If the level is low during these test periods, the hormone's response to artificial stimulation can be tested. If normal children are given a test dose of insulin, for example, they will become hypoglycemic. Hypoglycemia stimulates the release of circulating GH. Intravenous infusion of arginine or oral administration of clonidine or propranolol will have the same effect. In children with GH deficiency, an increase in the level of GH does not occur in these instances.

These studies obviously call for careful nursing attention so that children do not become extremely hypoglycemic or refuse to cooperate with the number of blood samples and the intravenous line necessary for the studies. If the child is not concerned about being short, these studies may not seem important; it may be difficult to tolerate the pain associated with the procedures. Encourage the use of a heparin lock so that blood sampling will involve as few venipunctures as possible; provide enjoyable activities during the testing period.

Therapeutic Management

Growth hormone deficiency is treated by the administration of intramuscular human GH injection two or three times a week. Fortunately, because these children have delayed epiphyseal closure, they will still be able to grow to normal height. When human GH was in short supply, available only from cadavers, few children were able to receive treatment for their condition; today, however, advances in recombinant DNA synthesis have made adequate amounts of synthetic GH available to all who need it. Some children, unfortunately, develop antibodies to GH, and its effect is therefore decreased. Other treatment will depend on accompanying pituitary dysfunctions. Some children may need supplements of gonadotropin or other pituitary hormones as well.

Nursing Diagnoses and Related Interventions

Nurses routinely assess height and weight of children, and in so doing, they become instrumental in first recognizing disturbances of growth. It is important that these assessment tasks be done responsibly and that the results are interpreted meaningfully in order to identify early those children with growth hormone deficiency and other growth disorders. Obtain a history that details not only the child's growth rate but also the child's reaction to being so short. Some children display an aggressive personality (making up for being small by being "tough"). The child's response to the problem must be included in the plan of care.

Nursing Diagnosis: Altered self-esteem related to short stature

Goal: Child will demonstrate adequate self-esteem by the end of the treatment period.

Outcome Criteria: Child speaks positively about self; identifies friends and activities with peers.

If a girl has been consistently behind in growth since early life, parents may simply assume she is petite and become concerned only when she reaches puberty and fails to develop secondary sex characteristics. When investigation reveals the child's true problem, parents may feel guilty that they did not become alarmed earlier. They feel resentment toward health care personnel who did not alert them to the problem. Parents should be encouraged to discuss these feelings and will need support accepting their child in this new light (see the Focus on Cultural Awareness box).

Children may need some help in accepting themselves at the ultimate height they achieve, especially if this is only in the fifth percentile, not the fiftieth. You may need to remind parents to assign duties and responsibilities to children that match their chronologic age, not physical size, to promote their feelings of maturity and self-esteem.

Pituitary Gigantism

An overproduction of GH before the epiphyseal lines of the long bones have closed may cause excessive growth. Weight is excessive also, but it is proportional to

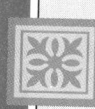

FOCUS ON CULTURAL AWARENESS

How people view endocrine disorders can be culturally influenced. Since many of these disorders are inherited, they lead to cluster in various populations so that people either have a high incidence of the conditions in family or friends or else know nothing about the conditions. In the past, because many endocrine disorders lead to changes in body appearance, particularly overgrowth or undergrowth, and because the reason for these changes was poorly understood, children with these disorders were poorly accepted by many people. Before insulin was available for treatment of diabetes, children with the disorder didn't live to adulthood. Being aware of the way that these diseases used to be viewed aids the nurse in understanding a parent's anxiety at diagnosis of these disorders and helps with nursing care planning to include reassurance and modern concepts of therapy in education.

height. Such excessive growth generally becomes evident at puberty. *Acromegaly* (enlargement of the bones of the head and soft parts of the hands and feet) may accompany the excessive growth in stature. Acromegaly becomes more pronounced after the epiphyseal lines of the long bones close and linear growth is no longer possible. The skull generally has a circumference that is greater than normal, and the fontanelles may close late or not close at all. The tongue may be so enlarged and thickened that it protrudes from the mouth, giving the child a dull, apathetic appearance. X-ray films or ultrasound scans of the skull will reveal enlargement of the sella turcica. Untreated, a child may reach a height of over 8 feet. Overproduction of GH is generally caused by a tumor of the anterior pituitary (an adenoma).

If the cause of the increased hormone production is a tumor, surgery to remove the tumor or cryosurgery (freezing of tissue) is the primary treatment. If no tumor is present, irradiation or radioactive implants of the pituitary may be successful in reducing the GH production. To halt GH secretion, other hormones may also be affected. It may be necessary in later life to supplement thyroid extract, cortisol, and gonadotropin hormones.

It is difficult for a child always to be bigger and taller than playmates, and the problem continues to be very real and embarrassing in adulthood. These children need to be identified during regular health screening so that the cause of such excessive growth can be determined and some form of treatment offered.

Diabetes Insipidus

Diabetes insipidus is a disease in which there is decreased release of ADH by the posterior pituitary gland (Yarber et al., 1992). This causes less reabsorption of fluid in the distal kidney tubules. Urine becomes extremely dilute, and a great deal of fluid is lost from the body. Diabetes insipidus may be an autosomal dominant trait or it may be transmitted by a sex-linked recessive gene; it may result from a lesion, tumor, or injury to the posterior pituitary; it may have an unknown cause. A very rare type of diabetes insipidus results from adequate pituitary function, but the kidney nephrons are not sensitive to ADH.

Assessment

The child with diabetes insipidus evidences excessive thirst (**polydipsia**), relieved only by drinking water, not breast milk or formula, and excessive urination (**polyuria**). The specific gravity of the urine will be low (1.001 to 1.005); the normal values are more often 1.010 to 1.030. Urine output may reach 4 to 10 L in a 24-hour period (the normal is 1 to 2 L), depending on age.

Diabetes insipidus usually presents gradually. The polyuria may be noticed first as bedwetting in the toilet-trained child. Weight loss from the large loss of fluid oc-

curs. Untreated, the child will lose such a quantity of water that dehydration and death may result.

Diabetes insipidus is diagnosed by a urine concentration test. In the average child, when fluid is severely restricted for a period of hours, urine will become concentrated. Such concentration does not occur in this child. Such a test is very difficult for children, because they quickly grow thirsty and uncomfortable. X-ray film, CT scan, or ultrasound study of the skull will reveal whether a lesion or tumor is present.

A further test is the administration of vasopressin (Pitressin). Pitressin initiates its effect by decreasing the blood pressure, alerting the kidney to retain more fluid to maintain vascular pressure. If the fault is with the pituitary, not the kidney, vasopressin should decrease urine output.

Therapeutic Management

If a tumor is present, it is removed by surgery. If the cause is idiopathic, the condition can be controlled by the intramuscular or intranasal administration of desmopressin (DDAVP), an arginine vasopressin. When this is given as an intranasal spray, it can be placed on a cotton ball and held against the mucous membrane of the nose for 3 to 5 min one or two times a day. Nasal irritation may result from intranasal administration; it will not be effective if the child has an upper respiratory infection and swollen mucous membranes. The child will notice an increasing urine output just before the next dose is due. In an emergency, vasopressin can be given intravenously (Ralston & Butt, 1990).

Vasopressin is not effective if the kidney tubules are resistant to ADH. Excessive thirst can be relieved by lowering the child's intake of sodium and protein and by administering a diuretic that reduces reabsorption of sodium ions.

Nursing Diagnoses and Related Interventions

> **Nursing Diagnosis:** High risk for fluid volume deficit, related to constant, excessive loss of fluid through urination
>
> **Goal:** Child will maintain adequate fluid volume during the illness.
>
> **Outcome Criteria:** Child's blood pressure and pulse are within normal limits for age; specific gravity of urine is between 1.003 and 1.030; skin turgor is good; child states thirst is not excessive.

Teach parents about long-term therapy; at least one parent must learn injection technique if intramuscular medication is required. Explain the difference between diabetes insipidus and diabetes mellitus, the disorder most people think of when they hear the word *diabetes*. Caution parents that they should always notify health care providers that the child has diabetes insipidus when seeking any type of health care. Surgery poses particular dangers because of the fluid restrictions that accompany most procedures. Encourage children to wear a Medic-Alert tag identifying them as having diabetes insipidus. With the child's and parent's permission, inform school personnel that the child will need to use the bathroom frequently; help the child make plans to include frequent bathroom stops and adequate fluid intake on long trips.

The Thyroid Gland

The thyroid gland is responsible for controlling the rate of metabolism in the body through production of thyroxine (T_4) and tri-iodothyronine (T_3) by the follicular cells of the thyroid.

Another thyroid hormone, thyrocalcitonin, is produced by the interstitial cells of the gland. Thyrocalcitonin is released if a high serum calcium level occurs; the hormone inhibits bone resorption, thereby slowing the rate of release of calcium from bone to plasma and a resulting lowered serum calcium level. It reflects the reverse action of parathyroid hormone, which elevates serum calcium levels.

Assessment of Thyroid Function

Radioimmunoassay of T_4 and T_3 is a specific blood study to determine how much protein-bound iodine (PBI) is present. If a child has recently taken large amounts of cough medicine containing iodide or had a contrast-media study, such as urography or bronchography, the PBI level may be abnormally elevated. The small amount of iodine ingested from iodized salt does not affect PBI levels.

Children who have low circulating albumin levels will have abnormally low PBI levels, because iodine is carried bound to protein. Phenytoin (Dilantin), a common medication given to children with recurrent convulsions, may displace thyroxine from binding globulin and further contribute to these low PBI levels.

Another test of thyroid function is a radioactive iodine uptake test. Children are given an oral dose of a solution containing radioactive iodine (^{123}I). The thyroid gland "traps" this iodine, and 24 hours later, after the maximum amount has been trapped, the amount of radioactive iodine present can be determined. It is important in this type of test that the child swallow all the solution. In infants, this is generally given as a gavage feeding so that accuracy of the dose can be ensured.

An uptake of less than 10% of the test dose is suggestive of hypothyroidism. If children vomit after ingesting the substance, this event should be recorded and called to the attention of the physician; it will obviously result in a lower uptake value, because only a part of the actual dose was available for uptake. Be certain the child does not receive iodine or thyroid extract in any other form during the test time; it will compete with the uptake of the radioactive iodine and, again, the value will be falsely low.

Disorders of the Thyroid Gland

Congenital Hypothyroidism (Thyroid Dysgenesis)

Thyroid hypofunction causes reduced production of both T_4 and T_3. Congenital hypothyroidism occurs as a result of an absent or nonfunctioning thyroid gland. The condition may not be noticeable initially, because the mother's thyroid hormones maintain adequate levels in the fetus during pregnancy. The symptoms of congenital hypothyroidism become apparent, however, during the first 3 months of life in a formula-fed infant and at about 6 months in a breast-fed infant (Rovet, 1990).

Assessment

Parents may begin to notice that their child sleeps excessively. The tongue becomes enlarged, causing respiratory difficulty, noisy respirations, or obstruction (Figure 48-3). The child may develop trouble feeding because of sluggishness or choking. The skin of the extremities is usually cold, and the overall body temperature may be subnormal because of slowed metabolism. A slow metabolic rate is also revealed by a slow pulse and respiratory rate. Prolonged jaundice, due to the immature liver's inability to conjugate bilirubin, may be present. Anemia may increase the child's lethargy and fatigue.

This disorder occurs in 1 in 4000 live births and about twice as often in girls as in boys (Donohoue, 1994a). If the condition is not recognized from these early symptoms, retardation of both mental and physical development will occur. The neck becomes short and thick; the facial expression is dull and open-mouthed because of mental retardation and the child's attempts to breathe around the enlarged tongue. The extremities are short and fat, with hypotonic muscles, giving the infant a floppy, rag-doll appearance. Deep tendon reflexes are slower than normal. Generalized obesity usually occurs. Hair is brittle and dry. Dentition is delayed, or teeth may be defective when they do erupt.

The hypotonia affects the intestinal tract as well, so that the child has chronic constipation; the abdomen enlarges because of poor muscle tone. Many infants have an umbilical hernia. Overall, the skin is dry and perhaps scaly, and the child does not perspire. Infants will have low radioactive iodine uptake levels, low serum T_4 and T_3 levels, and elevated thyroid-stimulating factor. Blood

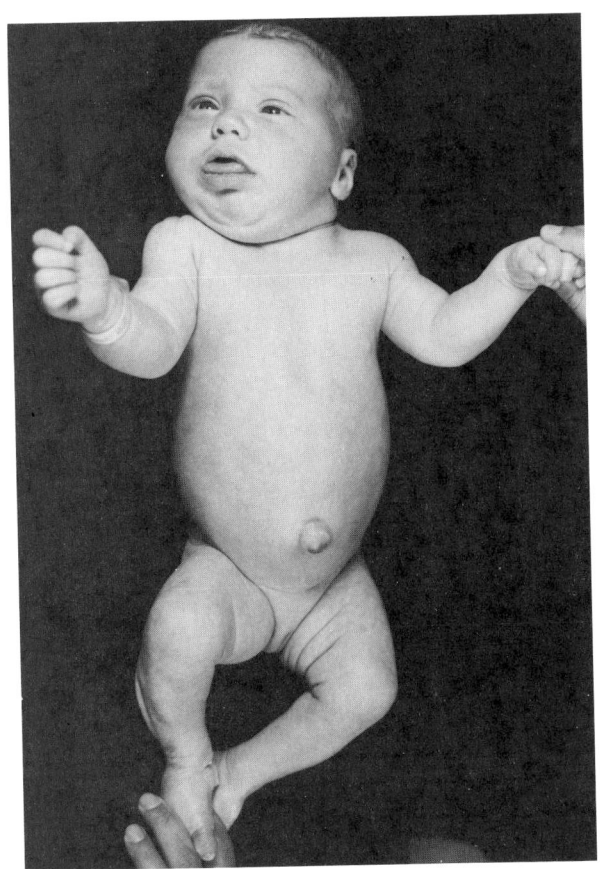

FIGURE 48-3
An infant with congenital hypothyroidism. Notice the prominent tongue and the dull expression. (Courtesy of John Crigler, Jr., MD.)

lipids will be increased; x-ray films may reveal no femoral epiphyseal line or delayed bone growth.

In most states, a screening test for hypothyroidism is mandatory at birth (using the same few drops of blood obtained for a Guthrie or phenylketonuria test).

Therapeutic Management

The treatment for hypothyroidism is oral administration of synthetic thyroid hormone, sodium levothyroxine (Gruters, 1992). A small dose is given at first, and then the dose is gradually increased to therapeutic levels. The child will need to continue on medication indefinitely. Supplemental vitamin D may also be given to prevent the development of rickets when, with the administration of thyroid hormone, rapid bone growth begins.

Further mental retardation can be prevented as soon as therapy is started, but any retardation already present cannot be reversed. Congenital hypothyroidism, therefore, is a serious disorder because it results in permanent mental retardation if not recognized early.

Helping parents administer medication is a major nursing role. Be certain that parents know the rules for long-term medication administration with children, as shown in Box 48-1. Periodic monitoring of T_4 and T_3 will

help to ensure an appropriate medication dosage. If the dose of thyroid hormone is not adequate, the T_4 level will remain low, and there will be few signs of clinical improvement. If the dose is too high, the T_4 level will be increased, and the child will show signs of hyperthyroidism: irritability, fever, rapid pulse, and perhaps vomiting, diarrhea, and weight loss.

Thyroiditis (Hashimoto's Disease)

Thyroiditis is the most common form of acquired hypothyroidism in childhood (Donohoue, 1994a); the age of onset is often 10 to 11 years, and there may be a family history of thyroid disease. It occurs more often in girls than in boys. The decrease in thyroid secretion is caused by the development of an autoimmune phenomenon that interferes with thyroid production. TSH stimulation from the pituitary increases when thyroid hormone production decreases in an attempt to cause the thyroid to be more effective.

Assessment

In response to TSH, there is hypertrophy of the thyroid (goiter). Growth is impaired by lack of thyroxine; children tend to become obese and lethargic and sexual development is delayed.

Box 48-1
Teaching Points for Long-Term Medicine Administration

1. Educate parents and children about the type and purpose of medicine they will be taking. Knowing the purpose of something maintains interest and compliance.
2. Always be certain to anticipate obtaining prescriptions so a ready supply is on hand before vacations, summer camp, holidays.
3. Don't use bribes to achieve compliance. After a period of time, the size of a bribe becomes too big to be maintained.
4. The earlier that children can be involved in their own administration, the sooner they can achieve an independent lifestyle.
5. Be aware of the life span of the medicine being administered so outdated medication is not used.
6. Don't become careless with storage of medicine. Consider all medicine a potential poison and keep it out of the reach of small children.
7. Use a reminder system such as a chart on the refrigerator, bathroom door, or school locker.
8. Plan times for medication administration that allow for a normal lifestyle (no getting up at 2 AM, having to interrupt a school class for an injection, etc.).

Antithyroid antibodies are present in serum. The enlarged thyroid may become nodular in response to the oversecretion of TSH. Although in childhood a nodular thyroid is usually benign, an investigation into the possibility of thyroid malignancy must be considered. For diagnosis, children are administered radioactive iodine. If the nodes are benign, there is generally a rapid uptake of radioactive iodine ("hot nodes"). If there is no uptake ("cold nodes"), carcinoma is a much more likely diagnosis (extremely rare at this age).

Therapeutic Management

Treatment for thyroiditis is the administration of synthetic thyroid hormone (sodium levothyroxine), the same as for congenital hypothyroidism (Lafranchi, 1992). With adequate dosage, the obesity will fade and growth will begin again. It is important that the disease be recognized as early as possible, so that there is time to stimulate growth before the epiphyseal lines close at puberty.

Hyperthyroidism (Thyrotoxicosis or Graves' Disease)

Hyperthyroidism is oversecretion of thyroid hormones by the thyroid gland. Thyrotoxicosis is the body's response to excessive production of thyroid hormones. Thyrotoxicosis in children usually occurs at the time of puberty or during adolescence and is more common in girls than in boys. Overactivity of the thyroid gland can occur from the gland being overstimulated by the thyrotropic hormone of the pituitary (TSH) due to a pituitary tumor. More frequently, hyperthyroidism and thyrotoxicosis in children is caused by an autoimmune reaction that results in production of IgG class immunoglobulins that stimulate the thyroid gland (Foley, 1992). An exophthalmos-producing pituitary substance causes the prominent-appearing eyes that accompany hyperthyroidism in some children.

Assessment

Graves' disease often follows a viral illness or a period of stress. Some children may have a genetic predisposition to development of the disorder. With overproduction of T_3 and T_4, children gradually develop nervousness, loss of muscle strength, and easy fatigue. Their basal metabolic rate is high; blood pressure and pulse are increased. They perspire freely. They are always hungry and, although they eat constantly, they do not gain weight and may even lose weight owing to the increased basal metabolic rate. Bone age, on x-ray examination, will be seen to be advanced beyond the chronologic age of the child. This means the child will not be able to reach normal adult height, because epiphyseal lines of long bones will close before normal height is attained.

The thyroid gland is usually prominent on the anterior neck (goiter) and can be confirmed by ultrasound. When the child protrudes the tongue or extends the hands, fine tremors are noticeable. In a few children, the eye globes will be prominent (exophthalmos), giving the child a wide-eyed, staring appearance. Laboratory tests will show elevated T_4 and T_3 levels and an increased radioactive iodine uptake level. TSH level will be low or absent because the thyroid is being stimulated by antibodies, not by the pituitary gland.

Therapeutic Management

Therapy consists first of a course of a beta-adrenergic blocking agent such as propranolol to decrease the antibody response. After this, the child is placed on an antithyroid drug such as propylthiouracil or methimazole (Tapazole) to suppress the formation of thyroxine. While taking the drug, the child must be monitored to prevent a depressed white blood cell level (leukopenia) from occurring as a side-effect. If serious leukopenia should result, the drug should be discontinued and the child isolated until the white blood cell count returns to normal, so that he or she does not contract an infection.

Because the thyroid stores considerable thyroid hormone that must be used up first, it will take about 2 weeks for these drugs to have an effect. The child will generally have to take the drug for a period of years before the condition "burns itself out." The exophthalmos may not recede but will not become worse from the time therapy is instituted.

If the child has a toxic reaction to medical management (lowered white blood cell count) or is noncompliant about taking the medicine, radioiodine ablative with I^{131} to reduce the size of the thyroid gland can be accomplished. Surgical removal of part or almost all of the thyroid gland may be necessary in a young adult. After both radioiodine ablative therapy and thyroidectomy, supplemental thyroid hormone therapy will be needed indefinitely.

Nursing Diagnoses and Related Interventions

> ***Nursing Diagnosis:*** Altered self-esteem related to lack of coordination and presence of prominent goiter
>
> ***Goal:*** Child will demonstrate adequate self-esteem by the end of the treatment period.
>
> ***Outcome Criteria:*** Child states positive traits about self and identifies friends and activities enjoyed.

Hyperthyroidism begins gradually and may become fairly involved before it is detected. Children at puberty should be suspected of having hyperthyroidism if they are losing weight or having behavior problems in school because of new hand tremors and tongue tremors that make it hard for them to write or speak. Behavior problems may also arise because of the nervousness and inability to sit still during class.

The parents need support in giving the medication or making sure that the child takes the medicine every day. Caution them not to stop medicine abruptly or a thyroxine crisis (sudden onset of symptoms) can occur (Lammon & Hart, 1993). Some parents ask if their child can have surgery as a cure so that long-term administration of medicine will not be required. Help them understand that surgery will not relieve them of the responsibility of giving medicine to the child, it will simply be of another type. If a large portion of the thyroid gland is removed, it may be necessary to give medicine indefinitely to make up for the missing gland. In any event, it is preferable to try a course of medical management before resorting to surgery.

Because the onset of hyperthyroidism is gradual, children themselves may be aware of their difficulties in school before their parents realize what is happening. Increasing exophthalmos may lead to an appearance that the other children make fun of. After therapy, these children need to be encouraged to go back to activities that require fine coordination or social interaction and to think of themselves as well again.

The Adrenal Gland

The two adrenal glands are located retroperitoneally just above each kidney. (Because of their location, they are also referred to as suprarenal glands.) The adrenal glands are made up of two distinct parts, which differ not only in tissue origin but also in function. The *adrenal medulla* is a small core surrounded by the *adrenal cortex.* Although each of these parts has different functions and releases different hormones, together they protect the body against acute and chronic forms of stress.

Adrenal Hormones

The adrenal cortex produces cortisol (a glucocorticoid), androgen, and aldosterone (a mineralocorticoid)—three hormones important in childhood illness. Norepinephrine and epinephrine, hormones important for maintaining blood pressure, are produced by the adrenal medulla.

Cortisol
Cortisol is released by the adrenal cortex in response to ACTH stimulation from the pituitary gland. ACTH is strongly influenced by biorhythm or circadian rhythms. In the hours just prior to and after waking, ACTH

reaches its highest peak. The level decreases again gradually throughout the day and night. The level of ACTH secretion also increases during a period of emotional stress, leading to increased production of cortisol. Severe trauma, major surgery, hypotension, extreme cold, and acute or chronic illness also increase production of cortisol.

Glucocorticoids are named for their ability to regulate serum glucose and protein levels. This regulation is accomplished primarily by increasing the amount of glucose formed by the liver (gluconeogenesis) and decreasing utilization of glucose by tissue. Free fatty acids are released from tissue stores into the plasma, making them available for energy. Protein synthesis in cells is halted, which frees up amino acids for liver production of protein. Cortisol is necessary during a time of stress to allow the body to have glucose and protein available for emergency processes.

Cortisol is also important in decreasing an inflammatory response. In the bloodstream, it causes a reduced number of eosinophil and lymphocyte numbers while red blood cell and platelet production is increased. A drawback of this response is that the decreased number of lymphocytes may allow infection to occur.

Aldosterone
Aldosterone is secreted in response to renin-angiotensin, serum potassium, and sodium levels.

Renin is released from kidney nephrons in response to a lowered blood pressure; shortly thereafter, it is converted to angiotensin II. In the presence of angiotensin II, aldosterone is released from the adrenal cortex. At the point that angiotensin is decreased, the production of aldosterone stops. When serum potassium levels are elevated, aldosterone secretion is increased. Lowered levels of potassium decrease aldosterone secretion. Sodium influences aldosterone by a reverse process (when sodium levels are low, aldosterone secretion is increased; and an increased sodium concentration inhibits aldosterone secretion).

The action of aldosterone is to cause salt to be retained by the body; as sodium is retained, fluid is also retained. Aldosterone plays a direct role in the stabilization of blood volume and pressure because of its role in maintaining sodium balance. Infants born with an inability to produce aldosterone will very quickly become dehydrated, and their life will be in immediate danger.

Disorders of the Adrenal Gland

Disorders of the adrenal gland include those related to hypofunction, which can lead to acute or chronic insufficiency, and those related to **hyperfunction**, which most often leads to overproduction of androgen.

Acute Adrenal Cortical Insufficiency

Insufficiency (**hypofunction**) of the adrenal gland may be either acute or chronic. In many adrenal syndromes only one hormone is involved, and the symptoms are directly related only to that hormone. In acute adrenal cortical insufficiency, the entire cortical adrenal gland function suddenly becomes insufficient. This occurs generally in association with severe overwhelming infections in which there is hemorrhagic destruction of the adrenal glands. It is seen most commonly in meningococcemia. It can occur when corticosteroid therapy, which has been maintained at high levels for long periods of time, is abruptly stopped.

Assessment

The symptoms of acute adrenal cortical insufficiency are acute and sudden. The blood pressure drops to extremely low levels; the child appears ashen gray and may be pulseless. Temperature is elevated; dehydration and hypoglycemia are marked. Sodium and chloride blood levels will be very low, but serum potassium will be elevated, because there is usually an inverse relationship between sodium and potassium values. The child is prostrate, and convulsions may occur. Without treatment, death may come abruptly.

Therapeutic Management

Treatment involves the immediate replacement of cortisol (intravenous Solu-Cortef) as well as deoxycorticosterone acetate (DOCA), the synthetic equivalent of aldosterone, and intravenous 5% glucose in normal saline to restore blood pressure, sodium, and blood glucose levels. A vasopressor may be necessary to elevate the blood pressure. Potassium replacement may be necessary to replace potassium lost with diuresis to prevent cardiac arrhythmias.

Acute adrenal cortical insufficiency is a medical emergency. Although seen less often than in the past because of antibiotics that quickly halt the course of infectious disease, it is not an obsolete entity. Now that more conditions are being treated with corticosteroids, the chances that acute adrenal cortical insufficiency will occur from sudden withdrawal of steroids is actually increasing.

Adrenogenital Syndrome (Congenital Adrenal Hyperplasia)

Adrenogenital syndrome is inherited as an autosomal recessive trait. The primary defect is an inability to synthesize cortisol from its precursors. This fault ordinarily occurs at the 21-hydroxylase level. When the adrenal gland is unable to produce cortisol, the amount of pituitary adrenotropic hormone increases, stimulating the adrenal glands to improve function. The adrenals become hyperplastic (enlarged) but, still unable to produce hydrocortisone, overproduce androgen.

Assessment

The excessive androgen production masculinizes the female child or increases the size of genital organs in male infants (Figure 48-4). This process begins during fetal life, so that the female is born with a clitoris so enlarged it appears more like a penis. As her labia are often fused as well, the girl resembles a boy with undescended testes and hypospadias. Internal female organs are generally normal, although a sinus between the urethra and vagina may be present (see discussion of ambiguous genitalia in Chapter 47). If the condition is not recognized at birth and the child is not treated, pubic and axillary hair and acne will appear precociously and a deep masculine voice will develop. At puberty there will be no breast development or menstruation.

The male child may appear normal at birth, but by 6 months of age signs of sexual precocity appear. By 3 or 4 years of age boys will have enlargement of the penis, scrotum, and prostate and the presence of pubic hair. They may have acne and a deep, mature voice. The testes do not enlarge, however, and although they are normal in size, appear small in relation to the size of the penis. Spermatogenesis does not occur, so the child is not fertile (New et al., 1990).

Children with adrenogenital syndrome will have increased levels of testosterone in the plasma, an important point for diagnosis. By determining the amount of other adrenal enzymes, the exact level of the metabolic defect in the production of cortisol can be measured. The bone age is usually advanced, and the epiphyseal line of the long bones therefore closes early. This closure will prevent the child from reaching adult height unless treatment is undertaken.

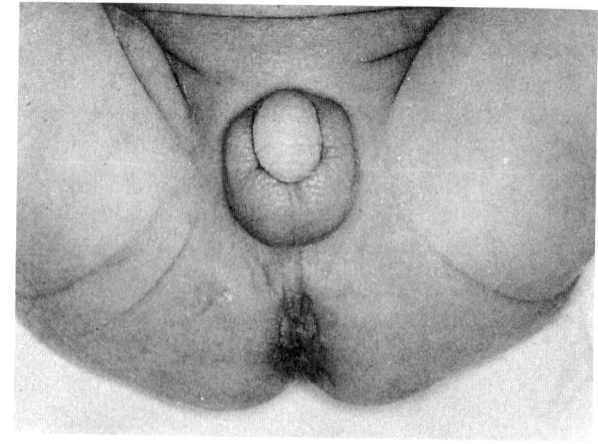

FIGURE 48-4

An infant with adrenogenital syndrome. Note the abnormally enlarged clitoris. (Courtesy of the Department of Medical Photography, Children's Hospital, Buffalo, NY.)

Therapeutic Management

Both male and female infants are placed on oral hydrocortisone to replace what they cannot produce naturally (Young & Hughes, 1990). When corticosteroids are given to the child in this way, the production of androgen will return to normal limits and no further masculinization will occur. Corticosteroid therapy needs to continue indefinitely. The child will need periodic analysis of serum and growth measurements to estimate the effectiveness of the therapy.

It is possible to identify the fetus with congenital adrenal hyperplasia as early as at 6 to 8 weeks of pregnancy by means of chorionic villi sampling (see Chapter 7). Treating the mother with dexamethasone (a corticosteroid), which will cross the placenta to the fetus, can prevent masculinization in the female fetus for the remainder of pregnancy (Speiser et al., 1990).

Nursing Diagnoses and Related Interventions

Nursing Diagnosis: Altered self-esteem related to genital formation at variance with true gender

Goal: Child will demonstrate adequate self-esteem throughout life.

Outcome Criteria: Child identifies positive traits about self and describes activities enjoyed with peers; expresses satisfaction with gender identity.

When children with adrenogenital syndrome are not closely scrutinized at birth, they can be wrongly identified as males when they are actually chromosomally female. It is sometimes recommended that a girl's enlarged clitoris be reduced by plastic surgery early in life. This treatment has been controversial, however, because clitoral reduction can also result in reduced clitoral sensation. Fortunately, with new surgical techniques, this problem is now minimal (Gonzalez & Fernandes, 1990).

Parents of females with adrenogenital syndrome need a great deal of support during the first few days of their child's life as they may feel that their child is imperfect in an embarrassing, hard-to-explain way. When they are told the results of a Barr body test (the child has an extra Barr body present, indicating the presence of two X chromosomes; see Chapter 7), parents may react with grief for the loss of the son they thought was born to them. They may be embarrassed to call friends and tell them the sex of the child is different from what they first reported. Neighbors may view the child suspiciously as if there is something perverted or provocative about the child. Parents need support from health care personnel who recognize that the child is simply lacking a completely formed hormone.

Nursing Diagnosis: Health-seeking behaviors related to lack of knowledge about long-term treatment needed to sustain adequate growth and development

Goal: Parents will understand the importance of giving prescribed medication through the child's growing years.

Outcome Criteria: Parents state plans for ways they will incorporate medication administration into daily routine as well as other occasions (e.g., trips away from home).

Parents, and the children themselves as they grow older, need to understand the importance of continuing to take the oral medication prescribed. When the condition is first diagnosed, it is easy for parents to remember to give the drug. As the years pass, however, it becomes difficult to keep the child on the regimen, especially when plans are made for summer camp or vacation away from home; special arrangements for regular medicine administration must be made. Cortisol is necessary for glucose and fat metabolism, and the body needs adequate levels to allow it to react to both physical and emotional stress. Thus, children may need to have a routine dose increased when they are undergoing periods of stress, such as surgery or infection.

Salt-Losing Form of Adrenogenital Syndrome

When there is a complete blockage of cortisol formation, aldosterone production will also be deficient. Without adequate aldosterone, salt is not retained by the body, and fluid is lost as well. Within the first month of life, infants begin to have vomiting, diarrhea, anorexia, loss of weight, and extreme dehydration. If these symptoms are untreated, the extreme loss of salt and fluid will lead to collapse and death as early as 48 to 72 hours after birth.

About one third of children with adrenogenital syndrome are affected by this complete deficiency. Because boys with this syndrome appear normal at birth, it may be incorrectly diagnosed as pyloric stenosis, intestinal obstruction, or failure to thrive. In females, because of the ambiguous genitalia, the correct diagnosis can be made more easily.

Assessment

Even though this form of adrenogenital syndrome is rare, it must be detected in infants before they reach an irreversible point of salt depletion. Thus, it is necessary to weigh newborn infants daily for the first few days of life and to weigh each infant accurately at each health checkup. In males, the inability to gain back their birth weight may be the first sign of the syndrome. With this disease, weighing is not merely routine work but a lifesaving assessment tool.

Therapeutic Management

Children with the salt-losing form of adrenogenital syndrome need to take not only supplements of hydrocortisone but also a high amount of salt and DOCA, a synthetic aldosterone, to maintain a balance of fluid and electrolytes. A long-acting form of DOCA can be given once a month intramuscularly. Capsules of DOCA can be implanted subcutaneously as another form of long-acting therapy. As the child grows older, fluorohydrocortisone (Florinef) may be given orally to aid salt retention.

Nursing Diagnoses and Related Interventions

Nursing Diagnosis: High risk for fluid volume deficit, related to loss of body fluid

Goal: Child will remain well hydrated throughout childhood.

Outcome Criteria: Child's skin turgor remains good; specific gravity of urine is between 1.003 and 1.030.

Parents need to be taught about the body's critical need to balance aldosterone, salt, and water, so that they understand the drastic consequences if their child skips his or her medication. They need to understand that although salt seems to be an "extra" in their own diet, it is as vital to their child's metabolism as digitalis is to heart disease or insulin is to diabetes.

Cushing's Syndrome

Cushing's syndrome is caused by the overproduction of the adrenal hormone, cortisol, which may result from benign increased ACTH production but generally is associated with a malignant tumor of the adrenal cortex (Donohoue, 1994b). Overproduction of cortisol results in increased glucose production. The child becomes obese and hypertensive. Fat tends to accumulate on the cheeks and chin, caus-ing a moon-faced look, but there is little fat on the extremities. Protein loss occurs, leading to muscle wasting. Osteoporosis occurs in bones. Humoral immunity is decreased, leaving children susceptible to infection. Hyperpigmentation occurs from melanin-stimulation properties of ACTH. The child's face is unusually red, especially the cheeks. Signs of abnormal masculinization or feminization may occur from overproduction of androgen or estrogen. Purple striae resulting from collagen deficit appear on the child's hips, abdomen, and thighs, similar to those seen in pregnancy (Figure 48-5).

Polyuria develops from increased glucose levels in serum. Growth ceases and, if the condition is not reversed before epiphyseal lines close, short stature will result.

Children who receive high doses of synthetic corti-

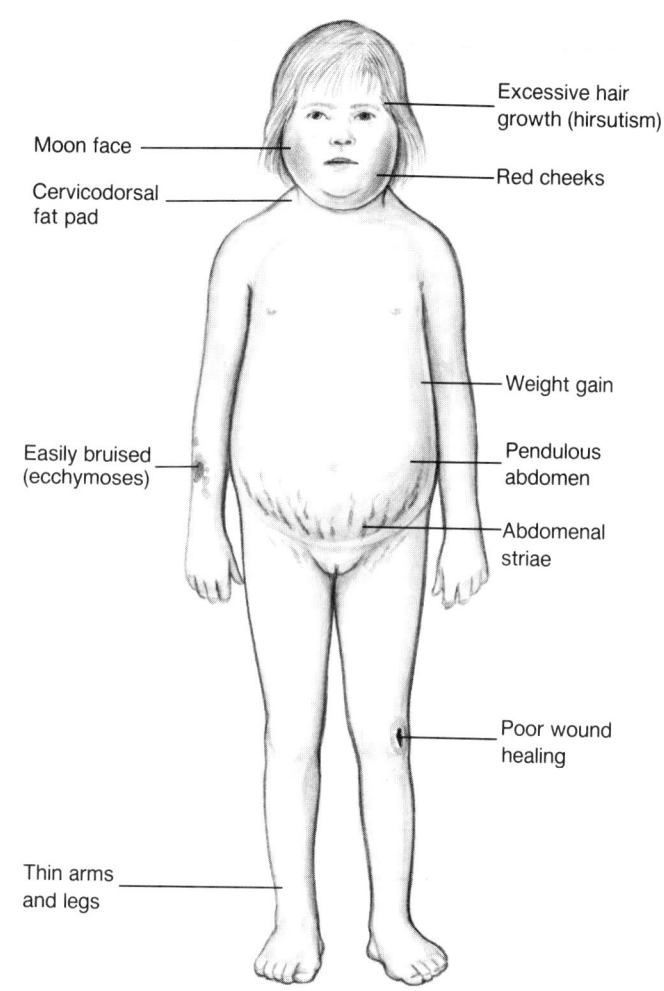

FIGURE 48-5
Signs and symptoms of Cushing's syndrome.

costeroids such as prednisone for a long period of time may develop the same symptoms as in Cushing's syndrome. Such children are said to have a *cushingoid appearance*. Cushing's syndrome is often suspected as the cause of obesity in children; some obese children do have elevated levels of plasma corticosteroids, a fact that complicates the diagnosis. These elevated levels of corticosteroids, however, are secondary to the obesity, not the cause. Children with natural obesity are generally tall; those with Cushing's syndrome are short.

Assessment

Children with Cushing's syndrome have elevated plasma cortisol and increased urinary free-cortisol levels. A dexamethasone suppression test confirms the diagnosis. If a normal child is given a test dose of dexamethasone (a glucocorticoid), the plasma level of adrenal cortisol will fall. It will not fall in children with adrenal cortical tumors because the tumor continues to stimulate the adrenal glands to oversecretion. If Cortrosyn (synthetic ACTH) is administered, plasma cortisol levels will normally rise; with an adrenal tumor, the gland is already functioning at full capacity so no cortisol elevation occurs. A CT scan or ultrasound will reveal the enlarged adrenal gland. Thus, these tests can be used to confirm the diagnosis.

Therapeutic Management

Treatment of Cushing's syndrome is surgical removal of the causative tumor. The prognosis will depend on whether the tumor is benign or malignant; carcinoma of this type tends to metastasize rapidly. If a major part of the adrenal gland is surgically removed, the child will need replacement cortisol therapy indefinitely.

The Pancreas

The pancreas is a unique organ in that it has both endocrine (ductless) and exocrine (with duct) types of tissue. The *islets of Langerhans* form the endocrine portion; these cells are scattered throughout the exocrine cells like small islets, hence their name. The islet cells compose only about 1% of the total weight of the pancreas. Alpha islet cells secrete glucagon; beta cells secrete insulin.

Insulin is essential for carbohydrate metabolism and important to the metabolism of fats and protein. It is formed by two amino acid chains from a precursor, *proinsulin,* at a rate of 35 to 50 U/day in adults. The amount of insulin produced is regulated by serum glucose levels. When serum glucose that passes through the pancreas exceeds 100 mg/100 mL, beta cells immediately increase insulin production. When blood serum levels are lowered, production decreases. Both the ability to secrete additional insulin and the action to decrease production are immediate responses.

Also important in the secretion of insulin is the presence of gastrointestinal hormones such as gastrin that rise when the stomach is full, since these stimulate the pancreas to produce the necessary insulin. Other hormones that stimulate insulin production are glucagon, cortisol, growth hormone, progesterone, and estrogen. In contrast, increasing levels of epinephrine or norepinephrine inhibit the secretion of insulin.

The principal childhood disorders associated with pancreatic dysfunction are diabetes mellitus and cystic fibrosis. Because the nursing care for children with cystic fibrosis includes many respiratory care procedures, it is discussed in Chapter 40.

Diabetes Mellitus (Insulin Dependent)

Diabetes mellitus is caused by a deficiency in the production of insulin. It occurs in as many as 1 out of 500 children, and its incidence is increasing (Sperling, 1990). This is because susceptibility to the disease is apparently inherited, and as therapy becomes more advanced, more children with diabetes are living long enough to mature and pass on the tendency to their children.

There are two main types of diabetes, as shown in Table 48-1. Type I diabetes, formerly referred to as *juvenile diabetes,* most commonly occurs in childhood. Children with this type are insulin dependent, or must take insulin to replace what their pancreas can no longer produce (Hirsch & Farkas-Hirsch, 1993). This is a separate disease from type II diabetes, in which pancreatic function diminishes with aging and insulin secretion slows. Many people with type II diabetes do not need daily insulin, since their disease can be managed with diet and oral hypoglycemic agents. When type II diabetes occurs in young adults, it may be referred to as *maturity-onset diabetes of the young.*

Etiology

The exact cause of insulin-dependent diabetes mellitus (IDDM) is not known but appears to result from autoimmune destruction of islet cells in predisposed persons. Children with IDDM have a high frequency of specific human leukocyte antigens (HLA). If HLA-DR3 and HLA-DR4 are present, children have a seven to ten times greater chance of developing diabetes mellitus (Sperling, 1990).

Specific HLA antigens predispose a child to developing diabetes but do not always result in the actual disease. An environmental factor, such as a viral infection, may act to trigger active pancreatic dysfunction through an autoimmune process. Symptoms of the disease generally do not manifest until preschool or school age but can occur as early as 6 months of age. The peak age of incidence in children is either 5 to 7 years of age or at puberty.

If one child in a family has diabetes, the chance of a sibling also developing the illness is higher than normal, because siblings also tend to have one of the specific HLA antigens that lead to the development of the disease. Because no prevention measures are currently available to stop diabetes from developing, children are not routinely tissue typed for the disorder, although this may be done experimentally. Administration of immune suppressors to stop destruction of insulin-secreting cells may be possible in the future.

Progress of Disease

Insulin can be thought of as a compound that opens the doors to body cells, allowing them to admit the glucose they need. Without insulin, the cell's doors are closed; when glucose is unable to enter body cells, it builds up in the bloodstream (hyperglycemia). Insulin does not increase glucose transport into the brain, erythrocytes, leukocytes, intestinal mucosa, or epithelium of the kidney. These cells can survive insulin deficiency but not glucose deficiency.

Table 48-1. *Comparison of Type I and Type II Diabetes*

Assessment	Type I (Insulin Dependent)	Type II (Non-Insulin Dependent)
Age of onset	5–7 yr or at puberty	40–65 yr
Type of onset	Abrupt	Gradual
Weight changes	Marked weight loss is often initial sign	Associated with obesity
Other symptoms	Polydipsia	Polydipsia
	Polyuria (often begins as bedwetting)	Polyuria
	Fatigue (marks fall in school)	Fatigue
	Blurred vision (marks fall in school)	Blurred vision
	Glycosuria	Glycosuria
	Polyphagia	
	Pruritus	Pruritus
	Mood changes (may cause behavior problems in school)	Mood changes
Therapy	Hypoglycemia agents never effective; insulin must be administered	Managed by insulin injection or diet alone; oral hypoglycemic agents a possibility
	Diet only moderately restricted; no dietary foods used	Diet tends to be strict
	Common-sense foot care for growing children	Good skin and foot care necessary
Period of remission	Period of remission for 1–12 months generally follows initial diagnosis	Not demonstrable

When the kidneys detect the increased level of glucose in the bloodstream (above the renal threshold of about 160 mg/100 mL), they attempt to lower it to normal levels by excreting the excess into the urine, which results in **glycosuria**. In attempting to excrete this excess glucose, the body excretes a large amount of fluid as well (polyuria). Potassium and phosphate pass from body cells into the bloodstream. As they are evacuated, the body moves toward electrolyte depletion.

Because the body cells are unable to use glucose but still need a source of energy, they begin to break down protein and fat for cell utilization. When large amounts of fat are metabolized this way, ketone bodies, the acid end-product of fat breakdown (a simple example is acetone), begin to accumulate in the bloodstream and spill into the urine. Because the blood bicarbonate cannot effectively continue to buffer the high acid levels, the *p*H of the blood becomes acidic, resulting in severe acidosis. The breakdown of fat metabolism also leads to increased serum cholesterol levels.

Untreated diabetic children are acidotic because of the buildup of ketone bodies in their blood, dehydrated because of the loss of water, and experiencing an electrolyte imbalance because of the loss of electrolytes in urine. Because large amounts of protein and fat are being used for energy instead of glucose, these children will remain short in stature and underweight since they lack the necessary components for growth.

Assessment

Although children may be prediabetic for some time, the onset of symptoms in childhood is generally abrupt

(Betschart, 1993). The first symptoms likely to be reported are increased thirst (polydipsia) and increased urination (polyuria). Increased urination may begin as bedwetting (enuresis) in the previously toilet-trained child. Although adults are often overweight at the time of the onset of diabetes, children are more likely to be underweight. They may have constipation because of the dehydration.

Laboratory Studies. In some children, diabetes is detected only at a routine health screening. For others, the disease has such an abrupt onset that they will be in coma from acidosis and hyperglycemia by the time it is detected. Laboratory studies usually show an elevated blood glucose level (above 200 mg/100 mL; normal is 70 to 130 mg/100 mL fasting and 100 to 180 mg/10 mL not fasting) and glycosuria (Table 48-2).

A glucose tolerance test confirms the abnormality in glucose metabolism. An intravenous glucose tolerance

Table 48-2. *Acceptable Target Blood Glucose Levels for Young Children*

Timing	Value
Preprandial	70–130 mg/dL
1 hour postprandial	100–180 mg/dL
2 hours postprandial	80–150 mg/dL
2 and 4 AM	70–120 mg/dL

(Hirsch, I. B., Farkas-Hirsch, R., & Skyler, J. S. [1990]. Intensive insulin therapy for treatment of type I diabetes. *Diabetes Care, 13,* 1265.)

test is preferred to an oral test, because it avoids the possibility of children vomiting after drinking a heavily concentrated glucose preparation (Glucola). A dose of glucose is administered intravenously into a fasting child over several minutes. Blood samples are then taken at 30, 60, 90, 120, and 180 minutes.

A fasting tolerance test is difficult for children to undergo, because it requires the child to fast as well as submit to painful, intrusive procedures. Water in small amounts is allowed during the procedure and will help the child tolerate the fasting time.

If children are preschool or early school age, they will need to have their arms restrained for the intravenous infusion so that the dose can be given accurately and will not be lost through infiltration. Even though the procedure takes only a few minutes, an armboard will help the child keep the arm still and will be easier for the child to accept than an adult's overpowering grip.

In a normal child, the blood glucose level will rise rapidly after the intravenous injection. The sugar will be metabolized equally rapidly, and the glucose level will then fall back to normal. In the child with diabetes, the level of glucose will rise and stay elevated because there is not enough insulin to aid its distribution to the body's cells.

The blood samples can be obtained by finger puncture rather than by venipuncture (see Chapter 37 for finger puncture technique). Do not underestimate the amount of pain involved in a finger puncture. This can hurt as much as having blood drawn intravenously. Children need a great deal of encouragement to come back to the treatment room five times during this procedure. Approach them positively and assume that they will be able to cooperate; praise them generously even if they do not fully comply. Do not bribe children into cooperating, because this will not sustain them in the long run. Instead, you can reward them by having their breakfast tray waiting for them immediately after the test, perhaps including their favorite breakfast food.

Blood for frequent glucose testing may also be obtained by means of a *heparin lock* (see Chapter 37), which eliminates many painful procedures for children and makes the initial adjustment to diabetes much easier. Suggesting that locks be used to eliminate discomfort is a nursing responsibility. You cannot take blood for glucose analysis from a functioning intravenous tubing, because the glucose in the intravenous solution will cause the serum reading to be abnormally high.

Other Diagnostic Tests.
In addition to the glucose level test, the diagnostic work-up includes blood samples for serum acetone, *p*H, Pco$_2$, sodium, potassium, a white blood cell count, and glycosylated hemoglobin. Normally, red blood cells carry only a trace of glucose incorporated into the hemoglobin. If the serum glucose is excessive, however, it attaches itself to hemoglobin

molecules, causing glycosylated hemoglobin. The higher the serum glucose level, the higher the hemoglobin A$_{1c}$ becomes. In nondiabetic children, the usual hemoglobin A$_{1c}$ value is 1.8 to 4.0. A value above 8.0 reflects an excessive level of serum glucose. Measuring glycosylated hemoglobin provides information about what the child's glucose levels have been during the preceding 2-month period, since red blood cells have a life span of less than 120 days.

If the potassium level of the blood is low, children may have an electrocardiogram to observe for T-wave abnormalities. The white blood cell count of a child with diabetes may be elevated even though no infection is present, apparently as a response to the ketoacidosis. The presence of infection must always be suspected, however, because it is often a precipitant to a diabetic crisis. For this reason, nose and throat cultures may be taken as well.

Therapeutic Management
Children with newly suspected diabetes mellitus are usually admitted to the hospital for diagnosis, regulation of insulin dosage, and education. Intensive management (frequent insulin injections and conscientious dietary control with regulation of exercise) can reduce the incidence of complications such as retinal and cardiovascular disease. Therapy includes teaching children and parents about the disease and the care, administration of insulin, and urine and blood testing. Electrolyte and fluid replacement, depending on the severity of the condition when the disease is first detected, may be necessary. Be certain that goals established for care are realistic. It will take time for parents and children to adjust to an illness that requires as much constant vigilance as diabetes mellitus does.

Initial Regulation of Insulin.
When children are first diagnosed with diabetes, they are generally hyperglycemic and perhaps ketoacidotic. To correct metabolism imbalance, they are given insulin. This is usually administered intravenously at a dose between 1 and 2 U/kg of body weight, depending on the severity of the symptoms. This initial administration of insulin is followed by further doses at 1 to 2 hours, again at 6 to 8 hours, and again at 12 to 18 hours. The amount of these doses will depend on the change in the acidosis and the degree of glycosemia and ketonuria. Ideally, by 12 hours' time, the acidosis is considerably less than when the child was admitted to the hospital, and the serum glucose is close to the normal range. The insulin given for emergency replacement is always regular (short-acting) insulin, because regular insulin takes effect more quickly.

It may seem that in the diabetic child in a state of acidosis, the administration of glucose would not be warranted. Because children are being administered insulin, however, body cells are now ready to use glucose. If it is not provided, cells will continue to break down fats and protein, and the acidosis will increase, not decrease. Therefore, an intravenous infusion of lactated Ringer's (half-strength) solution with a small amount of glucose (2.5%) is usually begun on admission. This intravenous infusion also serves to open a lifeline for the administration of intravenous insulin and fluid to arrest dehydration. As soon as the blood glucose falls below 200 mg/100 mL, the amount of glucose in the infusion is generally increased to 5%.

A large amount of intravenous fluid is administered to combat dehydration. After 24 hours, as the child begins to improve, oral feedings may replace the intravenous route. Further management of the child in the days following this first crucial 24-hour period will be based on the urine and blood determinations. Children will remain on regular insulin alone (given three or four times a day, depending on blood and urine findings) for the first 1 or 2 days and then will be changed to a short-acting and intermediate-acting combination, so that only two injections of insulin (one before breakfast and one before dinner daily) are needed.

Insulin Administration. Before insulin was discovered in 1920, few children with diabetes lived to adulthood. Even after its discovery, not all children responded well to its administration, because early insulin was manufactured from a pork or beef base that caused them to develop antibodies, making the treatments less effective than predicted. Today, insulin is manufactured by a recombinant DNA technique to simulate human insulin (Humulin), largely eliminating the problem of antibody reaction. Types of insulin vary as to their time of onset, their peak action, and their duration of action depending on the type of insulin and whether the preparation is an animal or recombinant DNA source. These differences are shown in Table 48-3.

Regular insulin is usually referred to as a short-acting insulin; NPH and lente are examples of intermediate-acting insulins; ultralente is long-acting. Children are regulated on a variety of insulin programs, but most receive a dose of 0.7 to 1.0 U/kg daily in two divided intervals (one before breakfast and one before dinner); adolescents may need as much as 1.2 U/kg daily. The most common mixture of insulin used with children is a combination of an intermediate insulin and a regular insulin; this is usually mixed at a ratio of ⅔ unit of the intermediate insulin to ⅓ unit regular insulin and given in the same syringe, although this prescription may vary for individual children. The morning dose is ⅔ the total daily dose; the evening dose is the remaining ⅓. The peak effects of the short-acting insulins are at 3 to 4 hours (see Table 48-3). This means that the child who takes insulin before breakfast will notice a peak effect between 10 AM and 12 PM; that is the time of day when hypoglycemia (a reaction to an excessive insulin level) is most apt to occur. The peak effect period of the intermediate insulins is 8 to 14 hours, or late afternoon, just before dinner. This is another prime time for hypoglycemia.

Some children require a program of insulin that includes three injections daily (a short-acting and intermediate-acting insulin before breakfast, a short-acting insulin before supper, and a bedtime injection of an intermediate-acting insulin). Still others may receive an injection of regular insulin before each meal followed by a bedtime injection of intermediate insulin (a total of four injections daily). Although a regimen with the fewest injections daily at first seems advantageous, multiple injections allow for greater variation in activity and meal consumption.

In the past, children were prescribed fixed doses of insulin and parents were advised not to vary the dose. Today, parents are educated to be able to vary the dose based on an insulin algorithm or protocol.

Table 48-3. *Common Types of Insulin*

Preparation	Effect Begins (Hours)	Peak Effect (Hours)	Duration of Effect (Hours)
Animal Insulin			
Regular	0.5–2.0	3–4	6–8
NPH	4–6	8–14	20–24
Lente	4–6	8–14	20–24
Ultralente	8–14	Minimal	24–36
Human Insulin			
Regular	0.5–1.0	3–3	4–6
NPH	2–4	4–10	14–16
Lente	3–4	4–12	16–20
Ultralente	6–10	12–16	20–30

(Hirsch, I. B., & Farkas-Hirsch, R. [1993]. Type I diabetes and insulin therapy. *Nursing Clinics of North America, 28*, 11.

How much insulin is needed is determined by the child's level of activity, the size of meals consumed, and the time of the injection. The time between the insulin injection and a meal is known as "lag time." If a child's premeal blood glucose is found to be above a target range, parents learn that increasing the lag time will help prevent hyperglycemia. If the blood glucose is low at a premeal test, decreasing the lag time could help prevent hypoglycemia. If it is anticipated that the child will eat an unusually large meal (a birthday dinner, for example), parents can increase the size of the premeal regular insulin injection. If the child will participate in an extra-strenuous sport in the afternoon, the regular insulin injection can be decreased.

Injection Technique. When insulins are mixed in one syringe, the regular or short-acting insulin should be drawn into the syringe first. Then, if mixing accidentally occurs in the bottle, the time of effectiveness of the short-acting insulin (which needs to be kept short-acting for emergency treatment) will not be lengthened by the addition of the intermediate-acting insulin.

Insulin is always injected subcutaneously except in emergencies, when half the required dose may be given intravenously. Children are usually urged to rotate sites in a pattern based on their planned activity. Absorption is increased if the muscle is exercised after the injection, so it is best to choose muscles that will not be exercised soon after the injection. Injection sites generally chosen are the two deltoid muscles and the outer aspects of the thighs (Figure 48-6). Adults often use the abdominal muscles as injection sites. Many children, however, do not have suitable musculature for abdominal injections. If a child will be jogging after an injection he or she probably should not use a thigh for injection (a muscle that will be exercised). If the child will be playing tennis, he or she should not use the dominant arm.

The nursing staff on a hospital unit must work out a plan of rotation for each child so that every nurse on the unit knows what injection site should be used next. The injection site should be recorded in the child's chart or nursing care plan so that you can check it before an injection and not repeat an injection site. If sites are not rotated, a great deal of subcutaneous atrophy (lipodystrophy) will occur at the injection site, causing deep, obvious pockmarks, although this is less of a problem now that synthetic human insulin is available.

Children learn quickly that if they continuously give injections in one site, scar tissue (lipohypertrophy) will form there and no pain will be felt on injection. This is a dangerous practice, however, because insulin no longer absorbs well from this site; the child will have to increase the dose beyond what he or she actually needs for glucose metabolism, because a portion of each dose is "locked" in the tissue. Should the child then inject this larger dose of insulin into a new site, there is a potential for overdose (which would cause hypoglycemia).

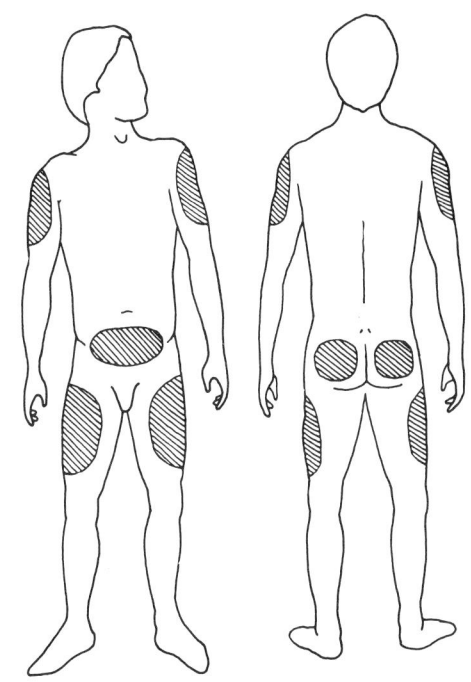

FIGURE 48-6
Commonly used injection sites for insulin. (From Beyers, M., & Dudas, S. The clinical practice of medical-surgical nursing. *Boston: Little, Brown, with permission.)*

Insulin should be given at room temperature, not refrigerated. This diminishes subcutaneous atrophy and ensures its peak effectiveness. Parents may keep additional bottles in the refrigerator to increase the insulin's shelf life.

When a low-dose insulin syringe is used, the needle is so short (about 0.5 in) that children can administer insulin by bunching skin at the site and giving the injection to themselves at a 90-degree angle, a technique more closely resembling that of intramuscular than subcutaneous injection. With this technique, because the needle is so short, the insulin is deposited in the subcutaneous tissue. This technique is easier for children to learn because it takes less coordination to administer an injection at a 90-degree angle than at a 45-degree subcutaneous angle (Figure 48-7). Automatic injection devices are easy for children to use and allow early independence (Figure 48-8).

Insulin Pumps. An insulin pump is an automatic device approximately the size of a transistor radio. A syringe of regular insulin is placed in the pump chamber; a thin polyethylene tubing leads to the child's abdomen where it is implanted into the subcutaneous tissue by a small-gauge needle (see Figure 14-8). Throughout the day, the pump edges the syringe barrel forward, infusing insulin at a continuous rate into the subcutaneous tissue. Before a snack or meal, the parent or child presses a button on the pump and forces a bolus of insulin forward to increase the insulin injection for managing these

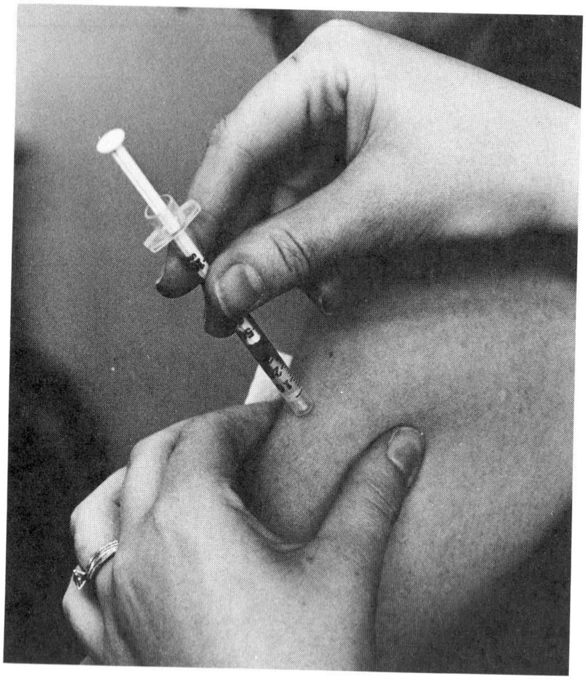

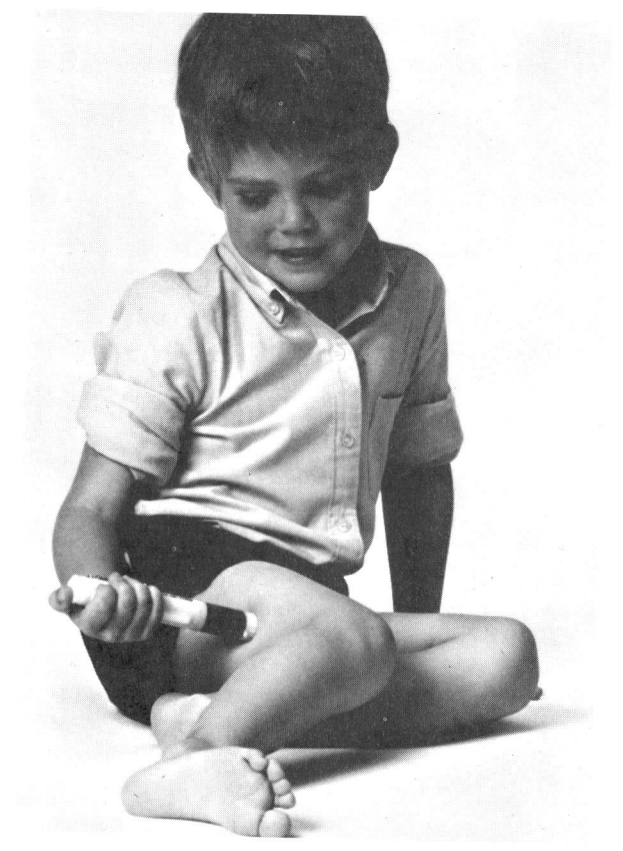

FIGURE 48-7

Insulin is usually injected at a 90-degree angle. Using a short needle, this angle places the insulin in the subcutaneous space.

times of high carbohydrate intake. The site of the pump insertion is cleaned daily and covered with sterile gauze; the site is changed every 24 to 48 hours to ensure that absorption is still optimum.

Restrictions with pump therapy include keeping it dry; a child must remove the pump (not the syringe and tubing) while showering. The needle and syringe must be removed to bathe or swim (caution children not to leave it disconnected for over an hour or they will become hyperglycemic). A disadvantage of pump therapy is that the pump is always present. Children usually prefer to wear clothing that hides the pump's outline (it can be held against the abdomen by an over-the-shoulder sling or hung from a belt around the waist). To assess the pump's delivery of insulin, the child must do blood glucose determinations throughout the day. When pump therapy first begins, a parent must wake at night and test a 2 AM blood glucose, since this is such a vulnerable time for hypoglycemia (the pump is delivering insulin, but the child has not eaten since bedtime).

Nutrition. Children with IDDM need to consume a diet appropriate for their age with a proportion of 50% carbohydrate, 20% protein, and 30% fat. The meal pattern should be three spaced meals with a snack in the midafternoon and evening.

Urine Testing. Urine testing has the disadvantage of not being as accurate as blood serum testing, and is now used only to test for ketonuria when the child is ill or to detect nocturnal hypoglycemia. An Acetest tablet or dip-

stick technique may be used. Warn parents and children that Acetest tablets are poisonous. They must be kept out of the reach of smaller siblings.

If acetone appears in the urine, it is a sign that fat is being utilized for energy; it occurs with infection or when not enough food has been ingested.

Serum Monitoring. Children as young as early school age can learn the technique of finger puncture and reading a computerized monitor. Using a spring-loaded puncture device helps minimize pain, and an automatic readout monitor such as a Glucometer simplifies the procedure and gives a more accurate reading than matching the shade of blood on a test strip to the colors on the test strip container (Figure 48-9). When blood is analyzed by these test strips, a whole blood value is being measured, not the serum glucose level. This means that the result will be about 15% higher than a serum determination, that is, a blood determination of 115 mg/100 mL equals 100 mg/100 mL of serum.

The "Honeymoon" Period. After the child's diagnosis has been confirmed and he or she has been initially regulated on insulin, there invariably follows a honeymoon period when only a minimal amount of insulin, or none

FIGURE 48-8

Injection of insulin by an automatic dispenser. (Courtesy of Ulster Scientific, Inc., Highland, NY.)

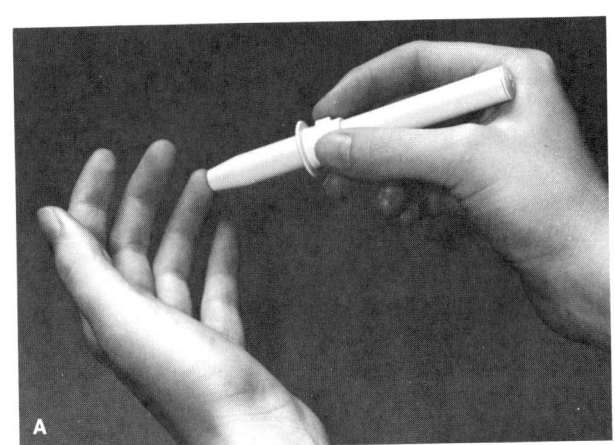

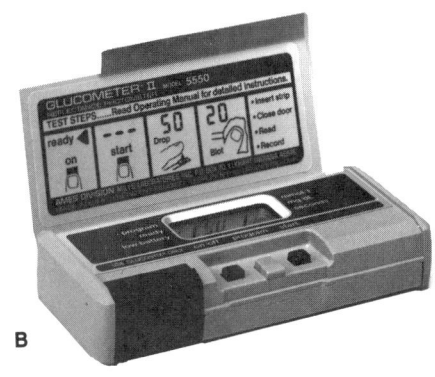

FIGURE 48-9
(**A**) *An automatic lancet for blood sampling. (Courtesy of Palco Laboratories, Santa Cruz, CA.)* (**B**) *A Glucometer for evaluating blood glucose values. (Courtesy of Ames Laboratories, Elkhart, IN.)*

at all, is needed for glucose regulation. Apparently, the presence of exogenous insulin stimulates the islet cells to produce natural insulin, as if they are being reminded of their true function. Unfortunately, after a month or even up to a year, the islet cells begin to fail once again, and diabetic symptoms recur. This is upsetting to parents who have begun to believe that the child was wrongly diagnosed and that diabetes is really not present or that a cure has taken place. The parents and child need to be warned that symptoms will inevitably recur. Sometimes the child is maintained on a minimum amount of insulin during this period to keep everyone from having unrealistic expectations of the child's being cured.

Complications of Diabetes Mellitus

Whenever children with diabetes undergo a stressful situation, either emotionally or physically, they may need increased insulin to maintain glucose homeostasis. When seen at health care facilities for periodic checkups, they should be asked not only whether they are having any difficulty with blood testing or insulin injection but how things are at home and at school. Interview children separately from their parents so that they can feel free to talk about anything that may be happening

or going wrong. There must be cooperation between primary health care personnel and school health care personnel so that conflicts over the children's regimen do not cause problems or tensions. You may have to meet with schoolteachers to prevent them from treating diabetic children as invalids. Sometimes children are embarrassed to have to do serum testing in school, especially in the public lavatory. It may be easier for them if they can go to the nurse's office for privacy when testing. Diabetic children may want to play a team sport very badly, but the school coach may not believe they should play sports. If parents have taken the stand that the school knows best, children may need an advocate to listen to their problem and intervene on their behalf.

When a child with diabetes contracts an infection, the temperature increases, the metabolic rate increases, and the body needs more sugar and insulin to make the sugar usable. Teach parents to notify their physician when their child appears to be ill (particularly if the child is vomiting or has nausea) for careful observation and a change in insulin dosage if necessary. If a child with diabetes is scheduled for surgery, careful regulation on the day of surgery and in the immediate postoperative period is essential, especially while oral fluids are restricted.

A number of long-term body changes are secondary to diabetes but may not be a part of childhood management because their onset does not begin until late adolescence or adulthood. Among these changes are arteriosclerosis (hardening of artery walls), thickening of retinal capillaries, and cataract formation from irritation of hyperglycemia that ultimately may lead to blindness. Some children may notice blurriness of vision when their disease is not in control, but this should not be confused with the final retinopathy that may result with older age. It is a temporary change in infraction ability related to hyperglycemia.

Because girls with diabetes eventually develop some degree of arteriosclerosis in adulthood, they are encouraged to have children relatively early if they plan to do so. This does not mean they should conceive their first child at age 16, but somewhere in their early 20s is best. Because the estrogen in birth control pills tends to interfere with blood glucose regulation, young women with diabetes mellitus are usually counseled to use alternative measures of birth control such as the diaphragm or vaginal foam along with condoms for their sexual partners. Care of the woman with diabetes mellitus during pregnancy is discussed in Chapter 14.

Pancreas Transplant

For children with severe kidney disease or retinopathy, a pancreas transplant may be considered. Unlike other organ transplants, the original pancreas is not removed entirely. The half that supplies digestive enzymes is still functioning and is left in place. During surgery, the new pancreas is grafted to the iliac artery and vein to allow insulin from the new organ to enter the systemic circulation. For this reason, pancreatic replacement is more accurately called *grafting*.

The digestive enzymes of the new pancreas can be diverted into the intestine or bladder, or the pancreatic ducts can be sclerosed so the digestive enzymes do not leave the transplanted organ. Grafts may be taken from cadavers or from live donors, who can lose up to 45% of their pancreas and still maintain a functioning organ for themselves.

To reduce their immune response and protect against graft rejection, children are administered drugs such as antilymphocyte globulin, cyclosporine, prednisone, or azathioprine (Imuran) after surgery. If rejection does start to occur, they are then given monoclonal T-cell antibodies (OKT3).

Pancreatic transplant is a last-resort solution for children, because the outcome is guarded (about 50% of transplanted organs will be rejected) and the outcome—continuous immune-suppressive medication for life—is not a big improvement on the original illness, for which they would take continuous daily insulin for life.

Nursing Diagnoses and Related Interventions

Nursing Diagnosis: Health-seeking behaviors related to self-administration of insulin, exercise, and hygiene

Goal: Child will demonstrate ability to self-administer insulin and identify an exercise and hygiene program by 3 days' time.

Outcome Criteria: Child demonstrates insulin injection technique to nurse; describes steps correctly as well as exercise and hygiene program.

Self-Administration of Insulin. From about 9 years of age, children can be taught to administer their own insulin (Figure 48-10). Many children younger than this age do not have the dexterity to handle a syringe or an understanding of the importance of sterile technique and proper dosage. Do not underestimate how difficult it is for children to learn to give injections to themselves. After you have been giving injections for some time, it seems as if it is a two-step process: (1) draw up the medication, and (2) give it. In actuality, there are over 25 steps involved.

When children have to mix insulins, the number of steps increases. Besides lacking dexterity and adult-level fine motor skills, children have to face *injecting themselves*. There is no such thing as getting used to injections. Children grow used to the *idea* of self-injection, not the injections themselves.

There is little advantage in teaching children younger than 9 years of age to give their own insulin in-

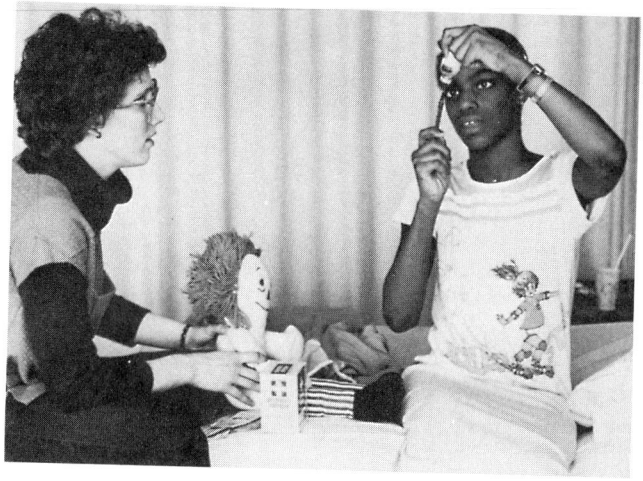

FIGURE 48-10

A school-age child is taught insulin administration using a teaching doll for practice. (Courtesy of the Department of Medical Photography, Children's Hospital, Buffalo, NY.)

jections. Although younger children may learn to master the process, they are not able to understand the principles behind it and are not responsible enough to determine the dosage of insulin. Although they might project an image of knowing all about their disease, its process, and its consequences, they are in reality doing little more than a mechanical procedure of transferring medicine from a vial into a syringe and then into their body.

Even if children are taught to give their own insulin from the beginning, at least one adult in the family should be taught to give it as well. There will be days when children refuse to administer their own insulin or are not feeling well and need to have or appreciate having someone else do it. Parents may have a hard time giving their child a painful injection; teaching them to view it as a helping action will alleviate their distress.

Exercise. Exercise is an important component of care, since it uses carbohydrates and so helps reduce hyperglycemia. No type of exercise need be restricted for children with diabetes.

A problem that arises with vigorous exercise, however, is the development of hypoglycemia because of the increased absorption of insulin from the injection site. One way of minimizing this effect is to choose an injection site least likely to be exercised. Another method is to take an additional carbohydrate exchange or decrease the regular insulin injection according to an established protocol (algorithm) prior to exercise.

The child should design a daily exercise program that is constantly maintained. Caution children that once they establish a daily program (running the length of the school track every day after school or 10 minutes of aerobics before school) they have to continue this type of exercise every day (on weekends, too), or they will be hyperglycemic on those days.

Hygiene. Skin care and, particularly, foot care is extremely important to adults with diabetes, because arteriosclerosis causes loss of circulation to the feet; and decreased circulation leads to poor healing ability. This is not as important a concern with IDDM, but children should be taught to cut their toenails straight across to prevent ingrown toenails (as should all children). Cuts and scrapes should be tended to promptly so that healing can begin right away. Properly fitting shoes are essential. Girls may need to be reminded of good perineal care to prevent vaginal infection.

Nursing Diagnosis: Parental anxiety related to newly diagnosed diabetes mellitus in a child

Goal: Parents will demonstrate a full understanding of disease process and their role in child's care and state ability to deal with new responsibilities by 1 month's time.

Outcome Criteria: Parents accurately describe child's illness and treatment and ways the disease will affect their lifestyle; state specific plan for daily routine measures for child's care; identify potential problems in schedule and ways these can be handled.

It is a big responsibility for parents to take home a child with diabetes after the initial diagnosis. Parents need the telephone number of the health care facility, liaison, or home care person to call for the first few days of home management. During the first few days at home, most parents appreciate having someone to check with before they give insulin, for reassurance that they are giving the correct dose.

Allow Parents to Express Fears About Disease. Preparation for discharge begins on the day of admission. Although parents may be aware of the disease occurring in other family members, they may be surprised to see it in their child. Both parents and the child need time to describe their perceptions of diabetes. If there are other family members with the illness, they may have heard many false stories about the disorder; these misconceptions need to be corrected before parents can begin to accept the diagnosis and view their child as basically well except for the illness.

Teach Parents About Disease and Principles of Care. Review general principles of care, including the fact that insulin injections, limited intake of food, and exercise will decrease blood glucose, and increased intake of food will raise it. Infection and emotional upset also increase the requirement for insulin. If this process is not explained, parents will attempt to keep the child relatively quiet, not appreciating the fact that exercise is actually good for him or her. They may limit candy in hopes that the child will then not need to have blood continually tested. Teach them that all foods are capable of raising blood glucose to some extent, so they must be monitored regularly.

Teach that hypoglycemia is an extremely serious condition and must be prevented. Otherwise, parents may view continuous low blood glucose as a positive sign rather than as a potentially threatening condition.

Hypoglycemia is potentially dangerous because it deprives body cells of glucose; if early signs are not recognized and treated, they will lead to coma and convulsions. Severe glucose depletion will lead to permanent brain damage with mental and motor impairment, because brain cells need glucose for metabolism.

Parents need an opportunity to practice insulin injection and serum testing while their child is hospitalized so they become familiar with the procedure and any accompanying problems before the child is discharged. A fair appraisal of what their child will be able to undertake for himself or herself must be made. It is often better to limit the child's share of care to one serum test and one self-administered insulin injection per day. This will help parents not to expect too much from their child and not to grow frustrated when the child does not meet their expectations; successfully managing their child's diabetes should be a rewarding experience rather than a chore.

Teach parents what type of insulin they will be using with their child, but do not give too much confusing detail about all the different types. If the insulin is changed at a later date, the new form can be described in greater depth at that time. Also, the parents or the child should begin keeping a log of serum test results in a permanent notebook so that these numbers can be evaluated for any unusual patterns at periodic checkups.

Establish Mechanism for Long-Term Supervision and Support. Children with diabetes need frequent health supervision visits. Those who appear to accept their diagnosis initially may have difficulty later on when their true feelings about their disorder surface. Adolescents who are rebelling against a multitude of things may choose to rebel against serum testing and insulin administration. Children with diabetes need good friends as well as good teaching from health care personnel. It is not easy to be a child with diabetes. Sometimes what is needed most from health care personnel is understanding and appreciation of this fact.

Serving as an active support person to parents is an important nursing role. Often, at the first hospital admission, parents are so concerned with learning the techniques of insulin administration and serum testing that they are not aware of other problems of everyday living with friends and neighbors that will arise later on. Make sure at hospital discharge that the parents can identify support people and whom to contact if they have problems or questions (see the Focus on Nursing Research box).

Nursing Diagnosis: High risk for altered nutrition, less than body requirements, related to decreased insulin level

Goal: Child will demonstrate ability to plan nutrition to achieve normal serum glucose values within 1 month.

Outcome Criteria: Child's growth follows percentile curve on standard growth chart; serum glucose is between 70 and 130 mg/100 mL fasting; child states that nutrition and exercise program are being followed.

Plan Nutrition Program With Child and Family. At one time, children with diabetes were placed on rigidly specified diets in which each food item had to be weighed. Then followed a period when children were allowed free diets and any resulting glycosuria was managed by increasing insulin doses. Today, it is generally accepted that conscientious diet modification is necessary, since chronic hyperglycemia can lead to vascular disease (Brenchley, 1993). American Dietary Association food exchange lists should be used. General guidelines for good nutrition are shown in the Focus on Family Teaching box.

 FOCUS ON NURSING RESEARCH

What Is the Effect on a Family When an Adolescent Daughter Has Diabetes?

For this study, 12 couples from two diabetes clinics whose daughters had juvenile-onset insulin-dependent diabetes of at least 1 year's duration were interviewed about the impact of the disease on their daughter, the family as a whole, and themselves as a marital unit. The age of the daughters in the study ranged from 11 to 15 years of age. Results of the study showed that most parents believed their daughter's diabetes had drawn the family closer together because everyone had to pitch in to help with monitoring the illness. In contrast, spouse relationships were sacrificed and strained.

The researcher suggests that, although diabetes in adolescents can improve family integrity, it can distance parents from each other and perhaps interfere with the adolescent developing a sense of identity, as the natural progression of families during the adolescent period is to pull apart, not draw closer together.

Dashiff, C. J. (1993). Parents' perceptions of diabetes in adolescent daughters and its impact on the family. *Journal of Pediatric Nursing, 8,* 361.

Teach Parents Signs of Hypoglycemia. Symptoms of hypoglycemia occur when the blood glucose level falls to about 60 mg/100 mL. At this point, there will be no glycosuria. Parents, and children as soon as they are old enough to understand, must be very aware of the reasons for hypoglycemia and what measures they must take to counteract it if it occurs.

Hypoglycemia can result from the administration of too much insulin, excessive exercise (because exercise uses up glucose), or failure to eat enough food, as might occur with illness. Typically, beginning symptoms are nervousness, weakness, dizziness, sweating, or tremors. In many children, the first signs of hypoglycemia are behavior problems: temper tantrums, stubbornness, silliness, irritability, or simply "not acting like himself." A few children become insensitive to the symptoms of hypoglycemia (termed *hypoglycemia unawareness*) and are then unable to recognize that it is occurring. Such children need more blood glucose determinations built into their routine than others.

When the signs of hypoglycemia are recognized, the child needs an immediate source of sugar. This can best be furnished in the form of about five sugar cubes or half a glass of orange juice with added sugar. It is easy for children always to carry single lumps of sugar with them and have them available for these times. If, after 15 minutes following sugar administration, there is no improvement in symptoms, more sugar or orange juice should be given. Parents should telephone the health care agency to let them know about the incident.

If children are in coma when they are first discovered or are too upset or uncooperative to take oral sugar, parents can be taught to inject a specified dose of glucagon hydrochloride. This converts glycogen that is stored in the liver to glucose. Generally, enough glycogen is converted after the drug injection to bring the child out of coma so that an oral form of glucose can then be given. The drug is not effective if the child has a depleted supply of glycogen.

If parents are unable to give their child an injection and oral sugar cannot be given, a solution of Karo syrup given as an enema is a good source of glucose. The enema is prepared by emptying a Fleet enema container and refilling it with 1 oz of dark Karo syrup and about 2 oz of water. The sugar in the syrup is readily absorbed across the intestinal mucosa upon administration. Particularly with a very young diabetic child, it is helpful to have this source of sugar on hand. Parents can prepare the enema container, fill it with just the syrup beforehand, and keep it refrigerated. They then add 2 oz of warm tap water just before administration to dilute and warm the syrup. As soon as children are out of coma or are again cooperative, they must take a source of oral sugar to further discourage hypoglycemia. The physician needs to be notified of the incident, so that the cause of

FOCUS ON FAMILY TEACHING

Q. My 8-year-old daughter has just been diagnosed with diabetes mellitus. What nutrition guidelines do I need to use when cooking for her?

A. Nutrition for the child with diabetes mellitus is based on a few simple rules. These are as follows:

- Diet should be well balanced and appealing; the calories should be appropriate for the age group.
- Three meals should be provided spaced throughout the day plus snacks. Total daily caloric intake is divided to provide 20% as breakfast, 20% as lunch, 30% as dinner, and 10% as afternoon and evening snacks. Distribution of calories should be 50% carbohydrate, 30% fat, and 20% protein.
- Don't use dietetic food. This is more expensive and not necessary.
- Urge your daughter not to omit meals. This calls for creative dietary planning so she likes the foods served and eats readily.
- Stress the foods your daughter is allowed to eat, not those she cannot, to maintain a positive mood.
- Your child's diet should not include concentrated carbohydrate sources such as candy bars; adequate fiber should be included, since this helps prevent hyperglycemia.
- The amount of aspartame (NutraSweet) included in the diet should be limited until the safety of this product is firmly established.
- Complex carbohydrates may need to be eaten before exercise such as swimming or a softball game to provide sustained carbohydrate.
- Children should learn dietary allowances so they can manage their own diet in a school cafeteria or at friends' homes in order to increase independence.

it can be determined and steps can be taken to prevent it from occurring again.

Parents need to anticipate occasions when hypoglycemia is likely to occur and take preventive measures against this themselves. Hypoglycemia is most likely to occur at the peak effective time of the insulins being given, that is, just before lunch or just before dinner. Many children who are attending school need to be scheduled for the first lunch period, not the second, or need a sugar cube snack before lunch. They should eat dinner at a regular time or have a snack to tide them over until dinnertime. If children are going to engage in an active sport, such as swimming, tennis, or basketball, they should take a source of sugar prior to participation. This precaution is extremely important before swimming, because a child who suddenly becomes weak in the middle of a pool cannot reach the side of the pool and safety. Although eating before swimming is something that children are taught not to do, the child with diabetes must be taught to break this rule (sensibly, of course; before swimming, the child

eats a complex carbohydrate such as crackers, not a full-course meal).

Occasionally, insulin overuse and persistent hypoglycemia cause a rebound hyperglycemic response referred to as the **Somogyi phenomenon**. Children who show hypoglycemia during the night and a high hyperglycemia early in the morning should be suspected of having this. They actually need less insulin, not more, to correct their problem.

Teach Parents Signs of Ketoacidosis. It is often difficult to distinguish between *hypoglycemia* (occurring from too much insulin) and *hyperglycemia* (occurring from too little insulin for the level of glucose present in the bloodstream). Hyperglycemia leads to **ketoacidosis** with symptoms of vomiting and abdominal pain and the same kind of behavior changes exhibited with hypoglycemia. The differentiation can be made readily if children void and the urine is tested for glucose. In hypoglycemia, the glucose level will be zero; in ketoacidosis, occurring from too little insulin, glycosuria will be extreme. When children cannot void, however, there may be a real question as to what is happening. In this instance, when a parent does not know the cause of the upset, children should be offered sugar as if the problem were hypoglycemia. The added carbohydrate will do no harm if the problem is already hyperglycemia, but giving insulin would do harm if the cause were hypoglycemia. The fact that children cannot void helps to establish the fact that the problem is hypoglycemia. With hyperglycemia, urine output is copious—one of the primary signs of diabetes. Assessing a serum glucose level by a finger prick solves the problem of whether symptoms relate to hypoglycemia or hyperglycemia.

When ketoacidosis is severe, children's respirations become deep and rapid (Kussmaul breathing) in an attempt to "blow off" carbon dioxide and lessen the acid state. Breath smells sweet because of the presence of ketone bodies, and the pulse may be rapid. Children may have signs of dehydration: dry mucous membranes and skin, sunken eyeballs, and no tears. This is the picture when children with diabetes are first diagnosed. It is often seen in children with diabetes who develop a gastroenteritis and hence eat poorly for a number of meals. Because the child is not eating well, parents may omit giving insulin. In actuality, because of an increased metabolic rate due to fever, children may need more insulin and glucose than usual during these times.

A comparison of hypoglycemia and hyperglycemia reactions is shown in Table 48-4. See also the Nursing Care Plan: A Child With Insulin-Dependent Diabetes Mellitus.

The Parathyroid Glands

The parathyroid glands (four of them) are located posterior and adjacent to the thyroid gland. The function of the parathyroid glands is to regulate serum levels of calcium in the body and control the rate of bone metabolism by the secretion of parathyroid hormone. This hormone is not under the control of the pituitary gland but is related to negative feedback of the circulatory serum levels of calcium. If calcium levels fall, parathyroid hormone secretion is increased; if calcium levels increase, hormone production is decreased (Mimouni & Tsang, 1990).

Vitamin D is necessary for calcium absorption from the gastrointestinal tract into the bloodstream, and it also influences parathyroid hormone secretion. Calcitonin (thyrocalcitonin) secreted by the thyroid gland opposes the action of parathyroid hormone and therefore decreases blood calcium levels.

Hypocalcemia

Hypocalcemia is a lowered blood calcium level. Phosphorus and calcium levels are maintained in indirect proportion to each other in the bloodstream. That is, if phosphorus levels rise, calcium levels decrease; if calcium levels rise, phosphorus levels decrease. Hypocal-

Table 48-4. Comparison of Hypoglycemia and Hyperglycemia Symptoms

Comparison Factor	Hypoglycemia	Hyperglycemia
Cause	Excessive insulin injection Excessive exercise Limited food intake	Inadequate insulin injection Excessive food intake Stress from infection, surgery, etc.
Symptoms	Hunger Lethargy Sensorium changes Convulsions Coma	Glycosuria and ketonuria Polyuria, polydipsia Kussmaul respirations Sweet (acetone) breath Decreased CO_2 combining power Dehydration Lowered sodium, potassium, bicarbonate, chloride, and phosphate levels Vomiting, abdominal pain Coma
Danger	Brain cells need glucose for function and survival	Fatty acids are utilized and acidosis develops
Major nursing interventions	Administration of source of glucose by oral, rectal, or intravenous route Education to prevent occurrences	Re-establishment of electrolyte balance and hydration Education to prevent occurrences

Noreen is a 9-year-old girl newly diagnosed as having insulin-dependent diabetes mellitus (IDDM) who is admitted to your hospital unit. The following is a nursing care plan designed for her.

Assessment: Pale-appearing, well-proportioned 9-year-old admitted by ambulance after being found unconscious by mother. Mother states that Noreen had been playing basketball in driveway when she suddenly acted dizzy and slumped unconscious to the pavement. No past illnesses but chickenpox at age 3, although mother states she "hasn't seemed well" for 2 weeks; has lost weight over past month. Grandmother had diabetes (died 1 yr ago). Mother states Noreen only knew her grandmother as "always sick and for the last 3 years almost blind." Mother admits to knowing nothing about management of disease. Serum glucose on admission: 620 mg/dL. Child regained consciousness following administration of regular insulin IV in emergency department.

Blood glucose levels: 7:00 AM = 220; 11:00 AM = 160. Urines consistently 4+ (2%) and moderate for acetone. Continuous intravenous infusion with 2.5 U regular insulin in 500 D5W begun at 8:00 AM.

Child states, "I'm never going to like giving myself shots." Cries readily at being asked to help with urine testing. Refuses to try insulin injection or even watch injection by nurse.

Nursing Diagnosis: Knowledge deficit related to importance of balancing insulin and diet

Defining Characteristic: Child is newly diagnosed as having diabetes mellitus; parent states she knows almost nothing about the disease.

Goal: Parent and child will demonstrate increased knowledge about disease process within 1 month.

Outcome Criteria: Parents and child state they have a beginning understanding of disease process; child and parent will demonstrate insulin injection technique.

Nursing Orders	Rationale
1. Teach parents function and importance of insulin.	1. Understanding role of insulin is important for administration compliance.
2. Demonstrate insulin injection technique using 5/8-inch needle and 90-degree injection technique; stress importance of rotating sites.	2. Learning is best achieved by watching and then practicing the technique.
3. Teach parents and child the technique of blood glucose monitoring.	3. Documentation and analysis of serum glucose levels is part of daily insulin and administration routine.
4. Teach technique of urine monitoring.	4. Urine monitoring can detect ketosis.
5. Help parents establish a blood monitoring and insulin administration record that is easy yet accurate to maintain. Stress that the most important component of the record is what really occurred, not a correct-looking record. Design a column to add signs of illness, level of exercise, unusual eating patterns, and other comments.	5. A monitoring record will help parents and child keep track on a daily and long-term basis.

(continued)

cemia, therefore, may be caused by changes in either calcium or phosphorus metabolism.

Assessment

Hypocalcemia tends to occur in infants who had birth anoxia (phosphorus is released with anoxia), immature infants (the parathyroid gland is immature), and infants of diabetic mothers (it tends to accompany hypoglycemia). It may be caused by the imbalance between phosphorus and calcium in milk (such an imbalance does not exist in breast milk and is modified in commercial formulas).

Nursing Diagnosis: High risk for injury related to hypoglycemia, infection, or poisoning

Defining Characteristic: Glucose is necessary for cell function; healing is delayed by altered glucose metabolism; Acetest tablets are poison.

Goal: Child will experience no injury related to hypoglycemia, infection, or poisoning.

Outcome Criteria: Child voices steps to take to prevent injury.

Nursing Orders	Rationale
1. Stress that urine-testing materials are poison and must be kept safe from young children.	1. It is important to know which substances are poisonous in order to keep them away from young children.
2. Teach importance of hygiene to prevent vaginitis or urinary tract infection.	2. Because of increased glucose in urine, girls are susceptible to urinary tract infection and vulvovaginitis.
3. Teach importance of regular dental care and maintaining general good health through childhood immunizations and periodic health care assessment; advise health care personnel at the first sign of illness.	3. An increased metabolic rate that comes with illness could lead to hypoglycemia.
4. Teach the symptoms of hypoglycemia (hunger, dizziness, sleepiness) and to obtain a blood glucose sample to document the hypoglycemia occurrence.	4. If the child knows the early symptoms of hypoglycemia, she can take readily absorbed sugar to prevent more serious symptoms.
5. Administer a readily absorbed sugar such as orange juice if hypoglycemia is apparent.	5. Carbohydrate will increase serum glucose.
6. Help child plan what source of emergency carbohydrate will be easiest to take to school.	6. Encourage the child to think about daily routine and ways to prevent hypoglycemia.
7. Help child obtain a Medic-Alert tag for safety.	7. A bracelet will alert health care personnel of the child's illness.
8. Teach the importance of reporting any eye changes.	8. Constriction of retinal arteries is a long-term effect of diabetes mellitus.

Nursing Diagnosis: Altered nutrition, less than body requirements, related to decreased insulin production

Defining Characteristic: Weight loss over last month; lack of energy; elevated glucose level.

Goal: Child will obtain adequate nutrition following prescribed diet.

Outcome Criteria: Fasting serum glucose remains between 60 and 100 mg/dL; weight loss halts.

(continued)

Latent Tetany. The chief sign of hypocalcemia is neuromuscular irritability, often referred to as **latent tetany**. This is accompanied by a serum calcium level less than 7.5 mg/100 mL of blood. Newborns with latent tetany are jittery when they are handled, or they cry for extended periods.

There are four ways to produce the clinical manifestations of tetany for diagnosis of hypocalcemia; these are shown in Table 48-5. These are all useful tests to determine or suggest whether newborn jitteriness is from hypocalcemia, a central nervous system problem, or some other cause.

If tetany is caused by cow's milk, it occurs at about the seventh day of life. A community health nurse making a follow-up visit after a home birth might be the one to recognize the problem initially.

Manifest Tetany. If the serum calcium level falls well below 7 mg/100 mL of blood, **manifest tetany** may result. Muscular twitching and carpopedal spasms

Nursing Orders

1. Assist with glucose tolerance test as necessary.
2. Obtain blood glucose samples as prescribed.

3. Assess intake and output.

4. Plan blood sampling and insulin administration to correlate with times meals are served.

Rationale

1. Glucose tolerance test helps with diagnosis.
2. Blood glucose samples provide for continuous health monitoring.
3. I & O data provide a way to monitor fluid balance.
4. Timing must be well coordinated.

Nursing Diagnosis: High risk for ineffective family coping, compromised, related to care of child with long-term illness

Defining Characteristic: Parents have to make long-term adjustments in lifestyle.

Goal: Family will demonstrate adequate coping behavior by 1 week.

Outcome Criteria: Family members state they are able to cope with present stress level.

Nursing Orders

1. Provide time for voicing concerns about having a chronically ill child at health care visits.
2. Help parents contact a formal support group, such as parents of diabetic children or the American Diabetic Association.
3. Help parents devise ways to incorporate child with a chronic illness into their lifestyle.

4. Help parents anticipate changes that will occur as child matures, such as coping with rebellion against insulin administration during adolescence.

Rationale

1. Discussion of a problem can be the beginning of problem-solving.
2. Parent groups can be a strong source of support.

3. Chronic illness can place a huge burden on a family by requiring constant alterations in plans. If the family learns creative ways to manage the child's care concerns and still maintain their usual activities, they will be well on the way to coping with the stress of chronic illness.
4. Anticipating change makes planning easier.

---

are the usual signs of this kind of tetany. A **carpal** (hand) **spasm** involves abduction of the hand and flexion of the wrist with the thumb positioned across the palm. In **pedal** (foot) **spasm**, the foot is extended, the toes flex, and the sole of the foot cups. Generalized seizures may occur. There may be spasm of the larynx. Because of this spasm, the infant emits a high-pitched, crowing sound on inspiration because of the constricted airway. If the spasm is prolonged, respirations may cease.

Therapeutic Management

Treatment is aimed at increasing the serum calcium level in the blood to the point above the level that leads to latent tetany. Calcium may be administered orally as 10% calcium chloride if the infant can and will suck. It can be given intravenously as a 10% solution of calcium gluconate if the tetany has progressed to a point at which the child does not have enough muscular coordination to take oral fluid safely. Calcium gluconate should not be given intramuscularly or subcutaneously, because

1511

Table 48-5. Assessment for Hypocalcemia

Sign	Description
Chvostek's	When skin anterior to external ear (just over sixth cranial nerve) is tapped, facial muscles surrounding eye, nose, and mouth contract unilaterally.
Trousseau's	When upper arm is constricted by tourniquet for 2–3 min and area becomes blanched, carpal spasm is elicited (hand abducts, wrist flexes, thumb is positioned across cupped palm).
Peroneal	When fibular side of leg over peroneal nerve is tapped, foot abducts and dorsiflexes.
Erb's	This test is a dramatic one to see demonstrated, although it requires a mild galvanic current so is not used routinely. A person with tetany has greater muscular irritability than a person with a normal calcium level; therefore, when a mild current is applied over the perineal nerve just below the head of the fibula, the foot on that side will abduct and dorsiflex.

necrosis may occur at the injection site. Newborns who are having generalized seizures may require sodium phenobarbital in addition to the calcium gluconate to halt the seizures. Emergency equipment for intubation to relieve laryngospasm should be available.

Following immediate therapy to increase the low serum blood levels, infants will be placed on oral calcium therapy until their calcium level has been shown to be regulated. Because vitamin D is necessary for the absorption of calcium and phosphorus from the gastrointestinal tract, the infant also may be given a vitamin D supplement.

Metabolic Disorders

So far in this chapter we have seen how overproduction or underproduction of certain hormones can seriously hinder body metabolism, creating such problems as hypothyroidism, adrenogenital syndrome, and diabetes mellitus. We have seen, too, that there are many causes for hormonal deficiency or excess, most of which are related to the endocrine glands and a highly complex system of feedback and communication between these glands and the hypothalamus. The neuroendocrine regulation of hormonal balance is so sensitive that it is affected by both the body's internal and external environments, that is, injury, stress, and emotional changes.

We now move to a group of hereditary biochemical disorders that also affect metabolism, but which are caused largely by some specific defect in the body biochemistry that disrupts one step of the metabolic process. The term *inborn errors of metabolism* is used to refer to these disorders. Most of them are caused by a

lack of or deficiency in a particular enzyme, which seriously impairs the ability of the body to properly metabolize the components of food for energy.

Inborn errors of metabolism affect amino acid and protein, carbohydrate, and lipid metabolism. Many of these disorders are evident at or soon after birth and can cause severe symptoms quite rapidly. Early detection and treatment are essential to the prevention of irreversible mental retardation and early death.

Phenylketonuria (PKU)

Phenylketonuria (PKU) is a disease of metabolism inherited as an autosomal recessive trait. Absence of the liver enzyme phenylalanine hydroxylase prevents conversion of phenylalanine, an essential amino acid, into tyrosine (a precursor of epinephrine, thyroxine, and melanin). As a result, excessive phenylalanine builds up in the bloodstream and tissues, causing permanent damage to brain tissue and severe mental retardation.

The metabolite phenylpyruvic acid (a breakdown product of phenylalanine) spills into the urine to give the disorder its name. This causes urine to have a typical musty or "mousy" odor. This is a very strong odor that often pervades not only the urine but the entire child.

Tyrosine is necessary for building body pigment and thyroxine. Without it, body pigment fades and the child becomes very fair skinned, blonde, and blue eyed. The child fails to meet average growth standards owing to the lack of thyroxine production. Many children develop an accompanying seizure disorder. The skin is prone to eczema (atopic dermatitis). There is such a strong association between these two disorders that all infants with atopic dermatitis need to be rescreened for PKU.

Phenylketonuria is found in 1 in 10,000 births in the United States. It occurs rarely in people of black or Jewish ancestry. Untreated, the child with PKU will have an IQ that is generally below 20. In addition, about one third of affected children have recurrent convulsions, and about half have muscular hypertonicity and spasticity. PKU cannot be detected by amniocentesis or percutaneous umbilical cord blood analysis as a routine screening measure, because the phenylalanine level does not rise in utero while the infant is still under the control of the mother's enzyme system. Recombinant DNA techniques can be used for carrier detection and prenatal diagnosis (Wappner & Brandt, 1994).

Assessment

Early identification of the disorder is essential to the prevention of mental retardation. Infants should be screened close to birth. After two full days of feedings (at least 120 mL of formula at a concentration of 20 calories per ounce, or the equivalent amount obtained by breast-feeding), the infant's heel is pricked with a blood lancet, and a few drops of blood are allowed to fall onto a specially prepared filter paper. The filter paper is then analyzed by a bacterial inhibition process for the amount of phenylalanine contained in the infant's blood (the Guthrie test). If an infant is born at home or discharged from a hospital or birthing center before the second day of life, the parents will need to bring the child to the health care facility for the test on the second or third day after birth. If the infant is being breast-fed and there is a question as to whether or not he has received only colostrum, he should be screened by the second week of life by a repeat Guthrie test at a health care visit.

Therapeutic Management

Infants in whom this disease is detected in the first few days of life can be placed on an extremely low phenylalanine formula (e.g., Lofenalac). If the diet is begun this early, mental retardation can be prevented. A dietitian may recommend a small amount of milk in the infant's diet every day so that the child does receive some phenylalanine (this essential amino acid is necessary for growth and repair of body cells). As a result, a mother who wants to breast-feed may be able to do this on a limited basis.

Parents of children with phenylketonuria need a realistic prognosis of their child's potential. If the disorder was detected in the first few days of life and the child's diet is well controlled so that he or she never has abnormally high levels of phenylalanine, the child's IQ will not be adversely affected. On the other hand, if the disorder was not detected until some brain damage or other symptoms were noticeable, such symptoms cannot be reversed.

Preparing a diet for a child with PKU is a difficult task. There is no natural protein with both a low phenylalanine concentration and a normal concentration of other essential amino acids. A diet of just protein restriction, therefore, would result in restriction of all essential amino acids—a diet that is incompatible with life. Lofenalac is a synthetic compound that fills the needs of phenylketonuric children. It has a low phenylalanine concentration but contains enough other essential nutrients that, with the exception of some additional milk, it is the only food required in early infancy. Lofenalac has a rather disagreeable taste. When infants are placed on this in the first few days of life, however, they do not seem to react to the taste and will drink it readily into adulthood. The infant on Lofenalac may have stools that are looser than the average child's. As children grow older, they will have solid foods added to their diet. These foods must be low in phenylalanine, so that the phenylalanine level of the blood stays below 9 mg per 100 mL.

Foods highest in phenylalanine are protein-rich foods: meats, eggs, and milk. Low phenylalanine foods include orange juice, bananas, potatoes, lettuce, spinach,

and peas. Lofenalac can be used to make treat foods, such as ice cream, milk shakes, birthday cakes, and puddings (foods that would otherwise be forbidden).

Children need blood and urine monitored frequently for phenylalanine levels. Hemoglobin levels should also be closely monitored to be certain the child is not becoming anemic.

Parents need an opportunity to express their feelings about the difficulty of maintaining a young child on such a restricted diet. It is not easy to refuse a piece of turkey for Thanksgiving dinner, a slice of ham for Easter dinner, or a piece of a brother's birthday cake.

How long the child should remain on the diet is controversial. It is generally agreed that the child should remain on a restricted phenylalanine diet to keep the phenylalanine serum level below 9 mg/dL until past 5 years of age, at which time 90% of brain growth is complete. Perhaps the diet can be modified at this time to include more foods so the serum phenylalanine level rises to 15 mg/dL. Because of reports of progressive neurologic deterioration in children no longer following a restricted diet, however, current advise is now generally for children to follow the diet indefinitely (Wappner & Brandt, 1994). A woman who has PKU must anticipate when she wants to have children as an adult and return to a low phenylalanine diet for about 3 months before conception and remain on the diet during pregnancy. If not, the fetus will be exposed to high levels of phenylalanine during pregnancy and be born mentally retarded (see Chapter 14).

Maple Syrup Urine Disease

Maple syrup urine disease is a rare disorder, inherited as an autosomal recessive trait, in which there is a defect in amino acid metabolism leading to cerebral degeneration similar to that of phenylketonuria. The infant appears well at birth but quickly begins to show signs of feeding difficulty, loss of the Moro reflex, and irregular respirations. The symptoms progress rapidly to *opisthotonos*, generalized muscular rigidity, and convulsions. Untreated, the child may die of the disease as early as 2 to 4 weeks of age.

Although the disorder is rare, it is mentioned here because it is relatively easy to detect: by the first or second day of life the urine of the child develops the characteristic odor of maple syrup, hence the name of the disease. The odor is due to the presence of ketoacids, the same phenomenon that makes the breath of diabetic children in severe acidosis smell sweet. Since nurses are the people most likely to detect the characteristic urine odor in the first few days of life, it is a disorder that any nurse who cares for newborns should be aware of so she or he does not discount the pleasant urine odor as an innocent finding.

Prenatal detection is possible. If maple syrup urine

disease is diagnosed in the first day or two of life and the child is placed on a well-controlled diet high in thiamine and low in the amino acids leucine, isoleucine, and valine, the cerebral degeneration can be prevented, just as it can be prevented in phenylketonuria. Such a diet is extremely difficult to maintain, however, because of its low protein content, and parents will need intensive diet counseling. Hemodialysis can be used to temporarily reduce abnormal serum levels at birth or during a childhood infection when catabolism of cells releases increased amino acid into the bloodstream (Wappner & Brandt, 1994).

Galactosemia

Galactosemia is a disorder of carbohydrate metabolism characterized by abnormal amounts of galactose in the blood (*galactosemia*) and in the urine (*galactosuria*). It most often occurs as an inborn error of metabolism, transmitted as an autosomal recessive trait, in which the child is deficient in the liver enzyme galactose 1-phosphate uridyl transferase (Goodman & Greene, 1991).

Lactose (the sugar found in milk) is broken down into galactose and glucose; galactose is then further broken down into additional glucose. Without the galactose 1-phosphate uridyl transferase enzyme, this second step, the conversion of galactose into glucose, cannot take place, and galactose builds up in the bloodstream and spills into the urine.

Assessment

Galactosemia occurs in about 1 in 62,000 births. Symptoms appear when the child begins formula- or breast-feeding: lethargy, hypotonia, and perhaps diarrhea and vomiting. Next, the liver enlarges and cirrhosis develops. Jaundice is often present and persistent; bilateral cataracts develop. The symptoms begin abruptly and worsen rapidly. Untreated, the child may die by 3 days of age. Untreated children who do survive beyond this time may have mental retardation and bilateral cataracts.

Diagnosis is made by measuring the level of the affected enzyme in the red blood cells. A screening test (the Beutler test) can be used to analyze cord blood when the child is known to be at risk for the disorder.

Therapeutic Management

The treatment of galactosemia consists of placing the infant on a diet that is free of galactose or on a formula made with milk substitutes like casein hydrolysates (e.g., Nutramigen). Once the child is regulated on this diet, symptoms of the disease do not progress; however, any neurologic or cataract damage already present will persist. The duration of the restricted diet is controversial, but it should be followed at least past 8 years of age.

Glycogen Storage Disease

Glycogen storage disease is actually a group of genetically transmitted disorders involving altered production and use of glycogen in the body. All but one of the 13 types described are inherited as autosomal recessive traits; one is a sex-linked disorder.

Glycogen is normally stored in the liver as a reserve supply of glucose. When the body needs glucose for energy, this glycogen is transformed back to glucose. In children with glycogen storage disease, glycogen is deposited normally, but an enzyme deficiency prevents retransformation of the glycogen back to glucose. Children with this disorder are susceptible to periods of hypoglycemia because their only source of ready glucose is oral intake. The liver becomes enlarged because it must store such a large supply of glycogen; consequently the abdomen becomes protuberant. Over a long period of time, the child's growth is stunted because there is not enough glucose for any function but immediate energy. If hypoglycemic episodes have been severe, brain damage may result. Many children have a tendency toward epistaxis or hemorrhage and are at risk when having surgery performed because of impaired clotting ability.

Therapeutic Management

Children with glycogen storage disease need to be maintained on a high-carbohydrate diet with snacks between meals in order to prevent hypoglycemia. In addition, a continuous glucose nasogastric or gastrostomy feeding during the night may be necessary in order to prevent hypoglycemia while sleeping. Uncooked cornstarch in a water suspension may be used with older children every 6 hours to maintain serum glucose levels (Wappner & Brandt, 1994). Liver transplantation may be a future answer for improving glucose regulation (Kirschner et al., 1991).

In one form of this disorder (type II or Pompe's disease), children deposit large stores of glycogen not only in the liver but in the muscle and heart as well. The muscles begin to feel hard to palpation from the deposits of glycogen. The heart will be enlarged and many children have an arrhythmia. They will usually die of heart failure before they reach adulthood.

Tay-Sachs Disease

Tay-Sachs disease is an autosomal recessive inherited disease in which the infant lacks *hexosaminidase A,* an enzyme necessary for lipid metabolism. Without this enzyme, lipid deposits accumulate on nerve cells, leading to mental retardation when deposits are on brain cells, and blindness when deposits are on optic nerve cells.

Assessment

Tay-Sachs disease is found primarily in the Ashkenazic Jewish population (Eastern European Jewish ancestry). Children generally appear normal in the first few months of life except for an extreme Moro reflex and mild hypotonia. At about 6 months of age, they begin to lose head control and are unable to sit up or roll over without support. On ophthalmoscopic examination, a cherry-red macula is noticeable (caused by lipid deposits).

By 1 year of age, children have developed symptoms of spasticity and are unable to perform even simple motor tasks. By 2 years of age, generalized convulsions and blindness have occurred. Most children die of cachexia (malnutrition) and pneumonia by 3 to 5 years of age.

Unfortunately, there is no cure for Tay-Sachs disease. The disorder may be detected in utero by amniocentesis. Carriers for the disease trait may be identified by hexosaminidase A assay (Kaback et al., 1993).

Key Points

- Growth hormone deficiency results in children who are short in stature. Therapy for children is the injection of human growth hormone. Children can experience altered self-esteem if they do not receive adequate emotional support from significant others.
- Other pituitary disorders are pituitary gigantism and diabetes insipidus. With gigantism there is overproduction of growth hormone. With diabetes insipidus there is decreased release of antidiuretic hormone. Urine becomes dilute and large amounts are excreted. Therapy is administration of desmopressin (DDAVP), an arginine vasopressin. Children with this are at high risk for fluid volume deficit.
- Congenital hypothyroidism occurs as a result of an absent or nonfunctioning thyroid gland. The condition is discovered by a blood test at birth. The therapy is oral administration of synthetic thyroid hormone.
- Thyroiditis (Hashimoto's disease) is an autoimmune phenomenon that interferes with thyroid gland function. Therapy is administration of synthetic thyroid hormone.
- Acute adrenal cortical insufficiency can occur in children from causes such as an overwhelming infection in which there is hemorrhagic destruction of the adrenal gland. A more common disease in children is congenital adrenal hyperplasia. Girls are born masculinized; either sex may be unable to retain sodium, which results in rapid fluid loss. Therapy is administration of corticosteroids. Without therapy, children are prone to altered self-esteem and high risk for fluid volume deficit.

- Cushing's syndrome is overproduction of cortisol by the adrenal gland. This usually results from a tumor in the gland. Children appear abnormally obese. Therapy is surgical removal of the tumor.
- The most frequently seen pancreatic disorder is type I diabetes mellitus. This may be an autoimmune process in which there has been destruction of insulin-producing islet cells. Therapy is a combination of diet, exercise, and administration of insulin.
- Hypocalcemia, a parathyroid gland disorder, results in lowered blood calcium. Children develop tetany. Therapy is the administration of calcium.
- Various disorders of metabolism that interfere with carbohydrate, amino acid, or fat metabolism occur in children. Representative of these are phenylketonuria, galactosemia, and Tay-Sachs disease.
- Endocrine disorders are almost all long-term disorders. helping parents and children remember to take medicine on a long-term basis is an important nursing responsibility.
- Children with endocrine disorders often develop height or weight discrepancies. Help children continue to feel high self-esteem by concentrating on those things they are able to do despite growth lag.
- Children with endocrine disorders are often identified first through routine height and weight measurements. Weighing babies at birth may detect the salt-losing form of adrenal genital syndrome. That makes this measurement one of the most important ones that nurses make. Weight loss is often an early sign of diabetes mellitus in children and may be identified first by a nurse at a pediatric clinic or office. School nurses may be the first to discover hypopituitary growth problems through yearly school assessments.

Critical Thinking Exercises

1. Lea is a 12-year-old girl with growth hormone deficiency. She is only 3 feet tall at present and probably will achieve a final growth of not over 4 feet, 6 inches. Her parents tell you they find her "cute" so do not want her to receive growth hormone. How would you approach this family? How much should Lea be able to contribute to this decision?
2. Caroline is a newborn diagnosed as having salt-losing adrenogenital syndrome. What would be the most important measure to teach her parents before Caroline is discharged from the hospital? How will having a child with this disorder change their lives?
3. Shawn is a 16-year-old who has been diagnosed as having diabetes mellitus since he was 7. You have been following him in an ambulatory clinic. You notice that although he was in good control for

years, over the last 6 months he has "forgotten" to take his insulin at least once a week. Since he obtained his driver's license, he has been eating many meals away from home and indulges in rich desserts. What health teaching does Shawn need? Why is this happening at this time of life?

References

Betschart, J. (1993). Children and adolescents with diabetes. *Nursing Clinics of North America, 28,* 35.

Brenchley, S. (1993). Children with diabetes: current dietary advice. *Professional Care of Mother and Child, 3,* 32.

Department of Health and Human Services. (1991). *Healthy people 2000.* Washington, DC: Public Health Service.

Donohoue, P. A. (1994a). The thyroid gland. In Oski, F. A., et al. (Eds.) *Principles and practice of pediatrics* (2nd ed.). Philadelphia: J. B. Lippincott.

Donohoue, P. A. (1994b). The adrenal cortex. In Oski, F. A., et al. (Eds.) *Principles and practice of pediatrics* (2nd ed.). Philadelphia: J. B. Lippincott.

Foley, T. P. (1992). Thyrotoxicosis in childhood. *Pediatric Annals, 21,* 43.

Gonzalez, R., & Fernandes, E. T. (1990). Single-stage feminization genitoplasty. *Journal of Urology, 143,* 776.

Goodman, S. I., & Greene, C. L. (1991). Inborn errors as causes of acute disease in infancy. *Seminars in Perinatology, 14,* 431.

Gruters, A. (1992). Congenital hypothyroidism. *Pediatric Annals, 21,* 15.

Hirsch, I. B., & Farkas-Hirsch, R. (1993). Type I diabetes and insulin therapy. *Nursing Clinics of North America, 28,* 9.

Kaback, M., et al. (1993). Tay-Sachs disease–carrier screening, prenatal diagnosis and the molecular era. *Journal of the American Medical Association, 270,* 2307.

Kirschner, B. S., et al. (1991). Growth in adulthood after liver transplantation for glycogen storage disease type I. *Gastroenterology, 10,* 238.

Lafranchi, S. (1992). Thyroiditis and acquired hypothyroidism. *Pediatric Annals, 21,* 43.

Lammon, C. A., & Hart, G. (1993). Action STAT! Recognizing thyroid crisis. *Nursing, 23,* 33.

Mimouni, F., & Tsang, R. C. (1990). Parathyroid and vitamin D-related disorders. In Kaplan, S. A. (Ed.). *Clinical pediatric endocrinology.* Philadelphia: W. B. Saunders.

New, M. I., et al. (1990). The adrenal cortex. In Kaplan, S. A. (Ed.). *Clinical pediatric endocrinology.* Philadelphia: W. B. Saunders.

Plotnick, L. P. (1994a). Growth, growth hormone and pituitary disorders. In Oski, F. A., et al. (Eds.) *Principles and practice of pediatrics* (2nd ed.). Philadelphia: J. B. Lippincott.

Plotnick, L. P. (1994b). Insulin-dependent diabetes mellitus. In Oski, F. A., et al. (Eds.) *Principles and practice of pediatrics* (2nd ed.). Philadelphia: J. B. Lippincott.

Ralston, C., & Butt, W. (1990). Continuous vasopressin replacement in diabetes insipidus. *Archives of Diseases of Childhood, 65,* 896.

Rovet, J. F. (1900) Does breast-feeding protect the hypothyroid infant whose condition is diagnosed by newborn screening? *American Journal of Diseases of Children, 144,* 319.

Speiser, P. W., et al. (1990). First trimester prenatal treatment and molecular genetic diagnosis of congenital adrenal hyperplasia. *Journal of Clinical Endocrinology and Metabolism, 70,* 838.

Sperling, M. A. (1990). Diabetes mellitus. In Kaplan, S. A. (Ed.). *Clinical pediatric endocrinology.* Philadelphia: W. B. Saunders.

Wappner, R. S., & Brandt, I. K. (1994). Disorders of amino acid metabolism. In Oski, F. A., et al. (Eds.) *Principles and practice of pediatrics* (2nd ed.). Philadelphia: J. B. Lippincott.

Yarber, B., et al. (1992). Early diagnosis and treatment of diabetes insipidus in a newborn infant: a case study. *Neonatal Network, 11,* 17.

Young, M. C., & Hughes, I. A. (1990). Response to treatment of congenital adrenal hyperplasia in infancy. *Archives of Diseases of Childhood, 65,* 441.

Suggested Readings

Aronson, R., et al. (1990). Growth in children with congenital hypothyroidism detected by neonatal screening. *Journal of Pediatrics, 116,* 33.

Brenchley, S. (1993). Children with diabetes: current dietary advice. *Professional Care of Mother and Children, 3,* 32.

Drass, J., et al. (1990). Caring for the diabetic patient who takes insulin. *Nursing, 20,* 98.

Foley, T. P. (1992). Thyrotoxicosis in childhood. *Pediatric Annals, 21,* 43.

Germak, J. A., & Foley, T. P. (1990). Longitudinal assessment of L-thyroxine therapy for congenital hypothyroidism. *Journal of Pediatrics, 117,* 211.

Haas, L. B. (1993). Chronic complications of diabetes mellitus. *Nursing Clinics of North America, 28,* 71.

Hahn, K. (1990). Teaching patients to administer insulin. *Nursing, 20,* 70.

Kestel, F. (1993). Using blood glucose meters: what you and your patient need to know. *Nursing, 23,* 34.

Martin, R., et al. (1994). The infant with diabetes mellitus: a case study. *Pediatric Nursing, 20,* 27.

Mercer, M. E. (1990). Myths and facts about diabetes insipidus. *Nursing, 20,* 20.

Robertson, C. (1990). The new challenges of insulin therapy. *RN, 52,* 34.

Rosenbloom, A. L., et al. (1990). Growth hormone by daily injection in patients previously treated for growth hormone deficiency. *Southern Medical Journal, 83,* 653.

Savinetti-Rose, B. (1994). Developmental issues in managing children with diabetes. *Pediatric Nursing, 20,* 11.

Tomky, D. (1989). Diabetes now: Tapping the full power of insulin pumps. *RN, 52,* 46.

Westphal, S. A., & Goetz, F. C. (1990). Current approaches to continuous insulin replacement for insulin-dependent diabetes: Pancreas transplantation and pumps. *Advances in Internal Medicine, 35,* 107.

Young, M. C., & Hughes, I. A. (1990). Dexamethasone treatment for congenital adrenal hyperplasia. *Archives of Diseases of Childhood, 65,* 312.

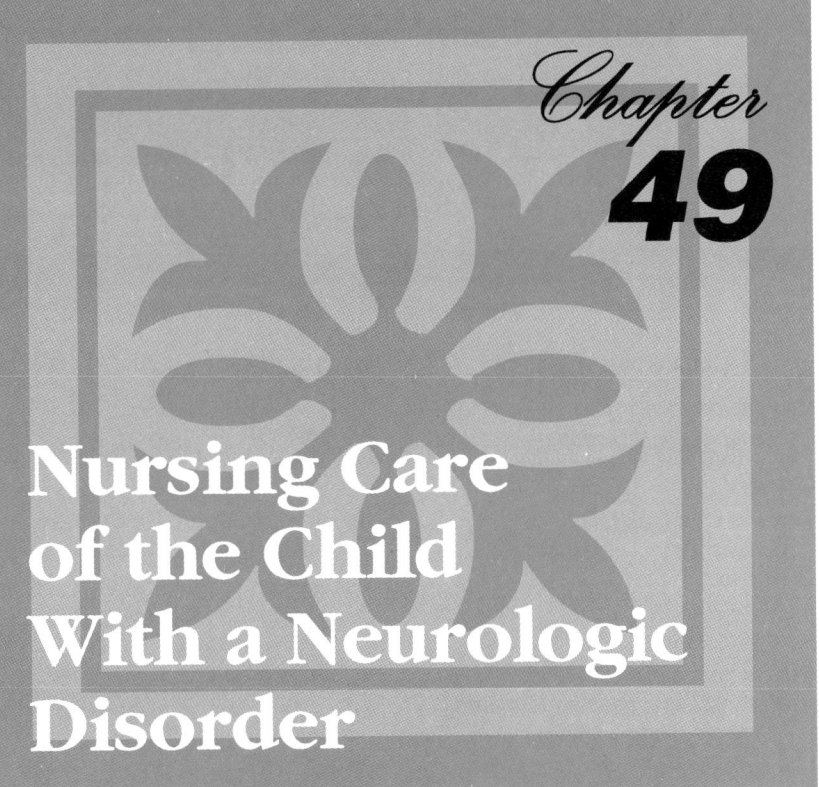

Chapter 49

Nursing Care of the Child With a Neurologic Disorder

Objectives

After mastering the contents of this chapter, you should be able to:

1. *Describe common neurologic disorders in children.*

2. *Assess a child with a neurologic disorder.*

3. *Formulate nursing diagnoses for the child with a neurologic disorder.*

4. *Plan nursing care for the child with a neurologic disorder, such as teaching a child about the importance of taking anticonvulsant medication consistently.*

5. *Implement nursing care (e.g., perform a neurologic assessment) for the child with a neurologic disorder.*

6. *Evaluate outcome criteria to be certain that nursing goals were achieved.*

7. *Identify National Health Goals related to neurologic disorders and children that nurses could be instrumental in helping the nation achieve.*

8. *Identify areas related to care of children with neurologic disorders that could benefit from additional nursing research.*

9. *Use critical thinking to analyze ways that care of the child with a neurologic disorder can be optimally family centered.*

10. *Synthesize knowledge of neurologic disorders and the nursing process to achieve quality maternal and child health nursing care.*

Adele Pillitteri: MATERNAL AND CHILD HEALTH NURSING, 2nd Edition. © 1995 Adele Pillitteri.

Neurologic disorders encompass a wide array of problems resulting from congenital defects, acquired dysfunction, infection, or trauma. Many of these disorders can cause severe illness, and even the minor problems carry life-threatening complications. In addition, because neural tissue does not have the regenerative power of other body tissue, any nervous system degeneration is permanent. Whenever possible, prevention must be the highest priority for keeping the nervous system healthy. When degeneration has already occurred, nursing care often focuses on helping the child and family develop strategies for dealing with the associated loss in mental or physical functioning, in making the child comfortable, and in providing an environment conducive to the child's growth and self-esteem. National Health Goals related to neurologic disorders and children are shown in the Focus on National Health Goals box.

 NURSING PROCESS OVERVIEW
*for Care of the Child With a Neurologic
System Disorder*

ASSESSMENT

Neurologic disorders often present with vague symptoms of something being wrong. Parents may indicate that their child "seems to be walking strangely" or is "just not herself." A thorough history and neurologic examination together provide the best source of information regarding the cause of the child's problem. Figure 49-1 illustrates possible findings. The neurologic examination covers six areas of neurologic functioning and includes mental or cognitive processes as well as motor and sensory functioning. When more information is needed, a battery of diagnostic laboratory tests may be ordered. The parents and child will need considerable support throughout the assessment process. Although the neurologic examination may be made "fun" for a child, other procedures such as the computed tomography (CT) scan and lumbar puncture can be frightening. The anxiety of not knowing what is wrong and fearing the worst can make this waiting period especially difficult for the child's parents.

NURSING DIAGNOSIS

Nursing diagnoses for children with neurologic disorders vary according to the child's needs. Initially, the child may need emergency care and constant observation, and the parents may need to discuss their fears about their child's illness. If the child undergoes surgery, nursing diagnoses should address preoperative and postoperative care, as well as long-term goals such as home care, taking into account the child's specific limitations and health care needs. Two nursing diagnoses should be kept in mind throughout these treatment phases:

- High risk for disuse syndrome related to neurologic deficit affecting one area of functioning
- Altered family processes related to child with neurologic dysfunction

Other nursing diagnoses are described along with specific disorders in this chapter.

PLANNING

Be realistic when establishing goals. Children who have permanent limitations will not be able to achieve in some areas. When neurologic disorders are first diagnosed, parents are ready to look at only short-term goals: the child will survive meningitis; the child has stopped convulsing. Later, they may need help to look at long-term goals: Will they need assistance to care for the child at home? What type of education can be obtained? What type of exercise program will be required?

Before a diagnosis is confirmed, parents may attribute their child's functional deficits to immaturity (she is not walking yet because she is simply too young). They insist that with age, her ability to function will improve. They are unable to make plans because they have not accepted their child's neurologic deficits. Until they face the truth, they will not be ready for specific planning. When parents begin to adjust to the new reality, they will need support and help in solving problems.

Organizations concerned with children with neurologic disorders include the following:

Epilepsy Foundation of America
4351 Garden City Drive
Landover, MD 20785

National Information Center for Children and Youth with Disabilities
Box 1492
Washington, DC 20013

FOCUS ON
National Health Goals

Bacterial meningitis and head injuries are major causes of neurologic damage in children. Three National Health Goals have to do with reducing the incidence of neurologic disorders from these sources:

- Reduce bacterial meningitis to no more than 4.7 cases/100,000 people from a baseline of 6.3/100,000.

- Reduce the incidence of secondary disabilities associated with injuries of the head and spinal cord to no more than 16/100,000 and 2.6/100,000 people from baselines of 20/100,000 for serious head injuries and 3.2/100,000 for spinal cord injuries.

- Increase use of helmets to at least 80% of motorcyclists and at least 50% of bicyclists from a baseline of 60% of motorcyclists and 8% of bicyclists (DHHS, 1991).

Nurses can be instrumental in helping the nation achieve these goals by educating children and parents about the use of helmets for bicycle and motorcycle safety, by administering and teaching paramedical personnel to administer safe care at accident scenes so that children's heads and necks are protected, and by decreasing the possible spread of bacterial meningitis by using good handwashing or isolation techniques in hospitals.

Topics of nursing research that might help in the prevention of neurologic injury or disease include: What kind of programs can school nurses initiate that would effectively teach bicycle safety? Could serious outcomes of bacterial meningitis be reduced if parents were educated about the symptoms of meningitis and thus were able to bring children with such symptoms to health care facilities earlier?

National Spinal Cord Injury Association
600 W. Cummings Park, Suite 2000
Woburn, MA 01801

Spina Bifida Association of America
4590 MacArthur Blvd., NW, Suite 250
Washington, DC 20007

United Cerebral Palsy Association
1522 K Street NW, Suite 1112
Washington, DC 20005

IMPLEMENTATION

Nursing interventions for the child with a neurologic problem must address both short- and long-term needs. For instance, while feeding an infant with increased intracranial pressure, you can demonstrate a caring attitude by showing her parents how to handle her gently.

For parents of a child with seizures, you can explain that turning him gently to his side will prevent him from choking; this will help them feel less anxious about future seizures. The child, too, will feel more in control of her illness if she believes both she and her parents will be able to handle any acute symptoms. Providing nursing care that meets everyone's needs takes a great deal of sensitivity and planning.

EVALUATION

Evaluation of the child with a neurologic disorder should address not only the child's progress in regaining physical function but also his or her level of self-esteem. Further planning to increase the child's self-esteem will be necessary for a long-term neurologic disorder.

These are examples of outcome criteria:

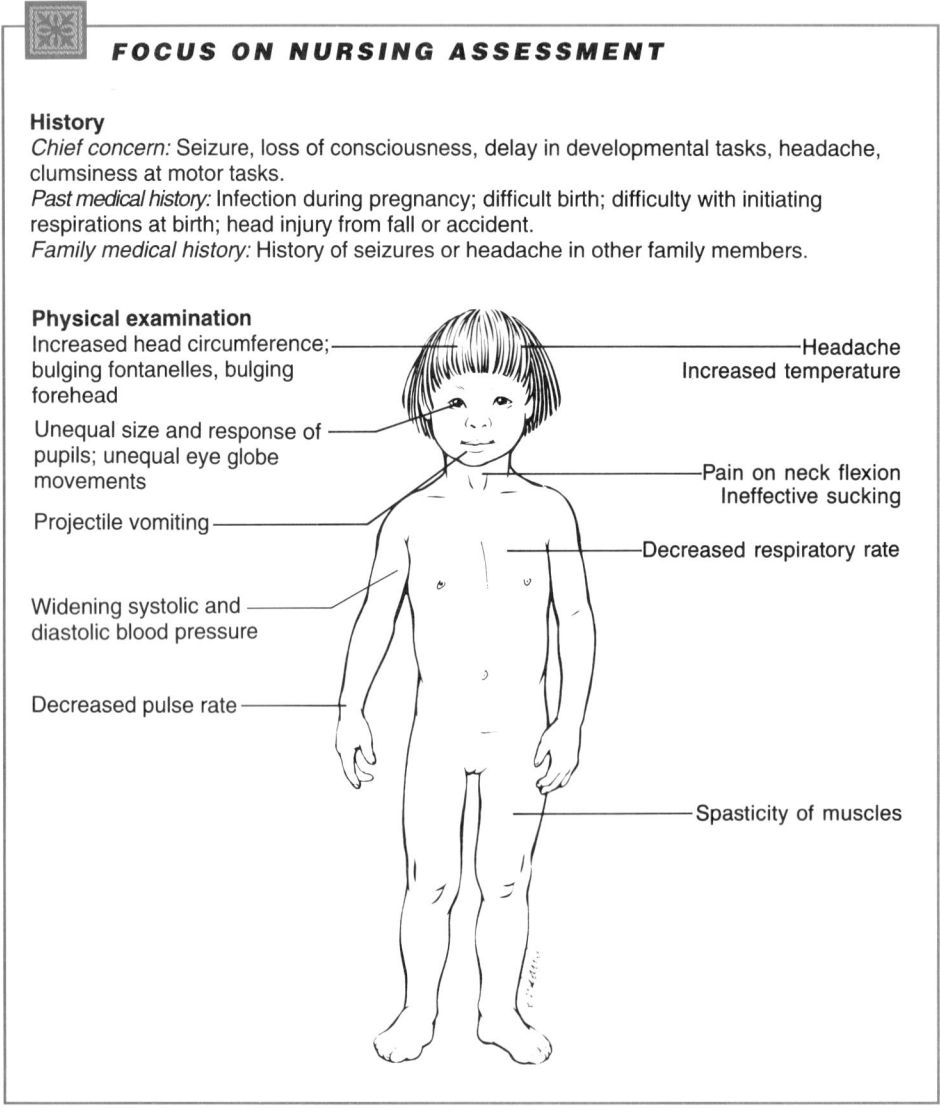

FOCUS ON NURSING ASSESSMENT

History
Chief concern: Seizure, loss of consciousness, delay in developmental tasks, headache, clumsiness at motor tasks.
Past medical history: Infection during pregnancy; difficult birth; difficulty with initiating respirations at birth; head injury from fall or accident.
Family medical history: History of seizures or headache in other family members.

Physical examination
Increased head circumference; bulging fontanelles, bulging forehead

Unequal size and response of pupils; unequal eye globe movements

Projectile vomiting

Widening systolic and diastolic blood pressure

Decreased pulse rate

Headache
Increased temperature

Pain on neck flexion
Ineffective sucking

Decreased respiratory rate

Spasticity of muscles

FIGURE 49-1
Common signs and symptoms of the child with a neurologic disorder.

- Child is aware of potential for injury related to recurrent convulsions.
- Family members state they are able to maintain family cohesiveness yet maintain contact with hospitalized child.
- Child practices exercises daily to reduce possibility of contracture from disuse syndrome.

Anatomy and Physiology of the Nervous System

Nerve cells (**neurons**) are unique among body cells in that instead of being compact, they consist of a cell nucleus and two long "arms." The *dendrite* transmits impulses to the cell nucleus; the *axon* transmits impulses from the cell nucleus to body organs. These cells range from a few inches to several feet long, reaching from distant body sites such as the feet, through the spinal cord, and to the brain. Although their great length is vital to motor and sensory function, nerve cells are more susceptible to injury than other body cells.

The nervous system continues to mature through the first 12 years of life. It actually consists of two separate systems: the **central nervous system (CNS)** and the **peripheral nervous system (PNS)**. The PNS consists of the cranial nerves, the spinal nerves, and the autonomic system.

The central nervous system consists of the brain, the spinal cord, and the surrounding membranes or meninges that protect the delicate tissues from normal trauma; these are also protected by the skull, the vertebral column, and the **cerebrospinal fluid (CSF)**, the fluid in the subarachnoid space, which serves as a cushion (Roberts, 1993).

The brain is covered by three membranes: the *dura mater* (a fibrous, connective tissue structure containing many blood vessels), the *arachnoid membrane* (a delicate serous membrane), and the *pia mater* (a vascular membrane; Figure 49-2).

Four fluid-filled cavities, or ventricles, lie within the brain (Figure 49-3). CSF forms in the two lateral ventricles in the *choroid plexus* of the pia mater and flows through the foramina of Monro into the third ventricle,

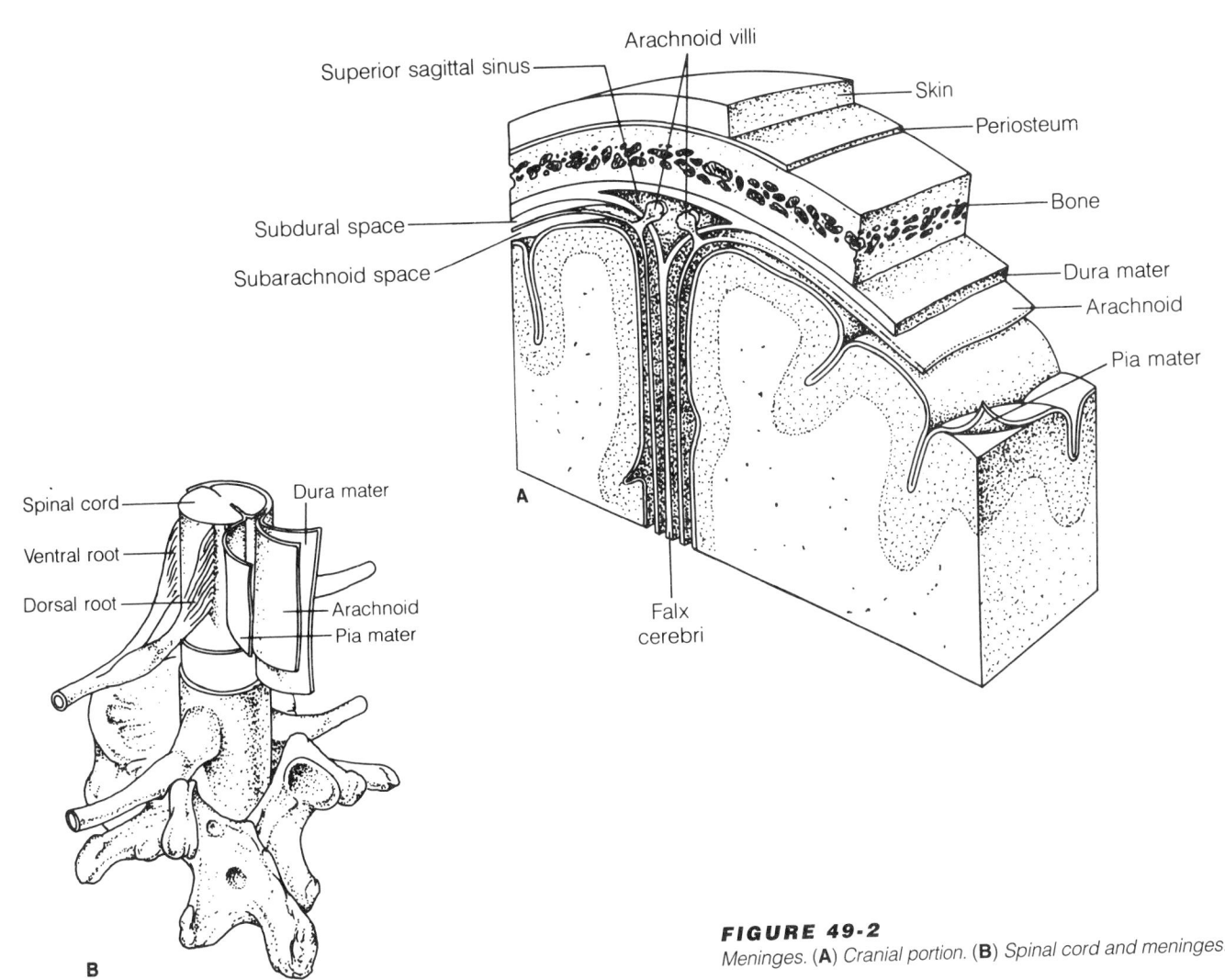

FIGURE 49-2
Meninges. (**A**) *Cranial portion.* (**B**) *Spinal cord and meninges.*

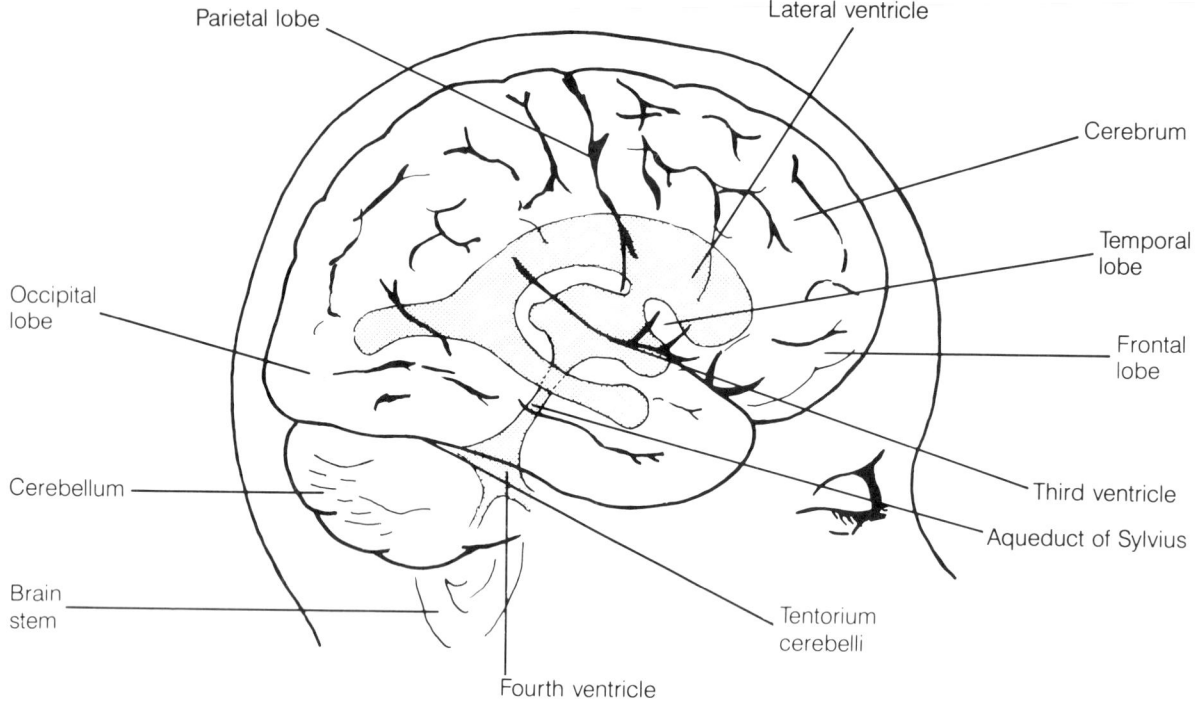

FIGURE 49-3
Ventricles and portions of the brain. Cerebrospinal fluid flows from the lateral ventricles into the third ventricle, then through the narrow aqueduct of Sylvius to the fourth ventricle. (From Snell, R. Clinical neurology for medical students. Boston: Little, Brown; with permission.)

then through a narrow canal (the aqueduct of Sylvius) to the fourth ventricle. It leaves the fourth ventricle by the foramen of Magendie and the two foramina of Lushka and into the cisterna magna, a collection pool at the base of the skull. From the cisterna magna, the fluid circulates to the subarachnoid space of the spinal cord, bathing both the brain and spinal cord. The fluid is then absorbed by the arachnoid membrane; the time span for replacement is about 6 hours.

The properties of cerebrospinal fluid are shown in Table 49-1. It is basically a colorless, alkaline fluid with a specific gravity of about 1.004 to 1.008, containing traces of protein, glucose, lymphocytes, and body salts. The fluid circulates downward to the second sacral vertebral level (S2). In infants, the spinal cord ends at the third lumbar vertebra (L3); in adolescents and adults, at L1 or L2. Thus, a space near the cord base contains CSF that can be tapped safely (lumbar puncture) without fear of causing damage.

Assessing the Child With a Neurologic Disorder

Neurologic symptoms are often insidious (headache; a tendency to walk with an unsteady gait; lethargy). Parents need support during diagnostic procedures. They may need help in understanding test results and becoming familiar with the terminology of brain anatomy.

Health History

The child's history may be the first clue in assessing a neurologic disorder. Many neurologic problems result from injury to the fetus; the mother's pregnancy history, therefore, is important to obtain.

At primary care visits, parents should be asked about their child's developmental milestones and ability to perform age-appropriate tasks successfully. The Denver Developmental Screening Test can reveal whether a parent's concern about a preschool child is well founded. Ability to perform well in school is important documentation for the older child.

Neurologic Examination

A complete neurologic examination takes at least 20 minutes. It requires patience and skill to keep the child's attention while observing all the features that indicate neurologic disease. Six areas should be assessed: cerebral, cranial nerve, cerebellar, motor, sensory, and reflex function.

Cerebral Function

Both general and specific cerebral functions are evaluated. General cerebral function is indicated by level of

Table 49-1. *Normal Findings of Cerebrospinal Fluid*

Assessment	Finding	Possible Significance
Opening Pressure	60–160 cmH₂O	Lowered pressure generally indicates that there is subarachnoid obstruction in the spinal column above the puncture site.
		Elevated pressure suggests intracranial compression, hemorrhage, or infection.
		Pressure will increase if a child coughs or pressure is applied to the external jugular vein (Valsalva maneuver).
Appearance	Clear and colorless	If cloudy, possible infection and an increased number of white blood cells
		If reddened, probably red blood cells
Cell count	0–8/mm³	Granulocytes are suggestive of CSF infection.
		Lymphocytes suggest meningeal irritation and inflammation.
		A few of both red and white blood cells are present in the newborn from the trauma of birth.
Protein	15–45 mg/100 mL	Elevated count (over 45/100 mL) occurs if red blood cells are present.
		If both protein content and red blood cell count are elevated, meningitis or subarachnoid hemorrhage is suggested. If protein content alone is elevated it is more suggestive of a degenerative process such as multiple sclerosis.
Glucose	60%–80% of serum glucose level	Decreased glucose level suggests that a glycolytic process is occurring.
		Bacterial meningitis causes a marked decrease in CSF glucose; invasion of fungi, yeast, tuberculosis, or protozoans into the CSF will result in some decrease in glucose level.
		Viral infections do not cause a decrease in CSF glucose level and may occasionally cause a slight increase.
A/G	8:1	Increase suggests infection or A/G ratio neurologic disorder.

A/G = albumin/globulin.
(Behrman, R. C., & Vaughan, R. C. [1992]. *Nelson's textbook of pediatrics* [14th ed.]. Philadelphia: W. B. Saunders.)

consciousness, orientation, intelligence, performance, mood, and general behavior (Sullivan, 1990).

Evaluate the child's level of consciousness through conversation. Note any drowsiness or lethargy and whether the child is oriented to his surroundings. Allow the child to answer questions without prompting, and listen carefully to what he says; this is more than "just conversation."

Orientation refers to whether a child is aware of who he is, as well as where he is and what day it is. Be careful to take into account the child's age and development, however; children less than 4 years of age may not know both their first and last names. They may be of school age before they know their address. Children younger than 7 or 8 are confused about days of the week and confuse "yesterday" with "today" or "tomorrow." Generally, you will be able to sense whether they are in touch with their surroundings and have a clear sense of self.

Intellectual performance can be determined by the child's score on a standard intelligence test. Estimates of intellectual function can be made by asking the child questions on several topics. *Immediate recall* is the ability to retain a concept for a short time. Ask the child to repeat numbers after you. The child who is 4 years old can usually repeat three digits; the child of over 6 can repeat five digits. *Recent memory* covers a slightly longer period. Show the preschool child an object such as a key and ask him to remember it, because later you will ask him to tell you what it was. After about 5 minutes, ask him if he remembers what object you showed him. Ask the older child what he ate for breakfast.

Remote memory is long-term recall. Ask preschoolers what they ate for breakfast that morning (to them, it was a long time ago); ask older children the name of their first-grade teacher. Most people will remember this for their entire life.

Specific cerebral function can be measured by assessing language, sensory interpretation, and motor integration. Listen to the child's ability to articulate. Remember that many preschoolers substitute "w" for "r," saying "west time" instead of "rest time."

Stereognosis means the ability to recognize an object by touch. Ask the child to close her eyes; place a familiar object, such as a key, a penny, or a bottle cap, in her hand and ask her to identify it.

Graphesthesia is the ability to recognize a shape that has been traced on the skin. Ask a preschooler to close his eyes, then trace first a circle, then a square, on the back of his hand; ask him if the shapes are the same or different. (First show him two keys and a bottle cap to see if he understands the concept "different.") For the older child, trace a number (8, 3, 0, and 1 work well) and ask the child to identify each one.

Kinesthesia is the ability to distinguish movement. Have the child close her eyes and extend her hands in front of her. Raise one of her fingers and ask her if it is up or down. Hold the finger by its sides so that your other fingers do not brush against the child's palm or the back of her hand, as this will reveal the finger position. Repeat the same movement with a toe on each foot. (For preschoolers, first determine whether the child understands the concept of up and down.)

Measure motor integration by asking the child to do a complex motor skill, such as folding a piece of paper and putting it into an envelope. A child of 4 years and older should be able to do this neatly.

Children do best when these tests are presented as a game. Be certain to convey that there are no right or wrong answers. A child who feels that he has failed these tests may not respond well to further testing.

Cranial Nerve Function

Testing for cranial nerve function consists of assessing each pair of cranial nerves separately (Table 49-2).

The first cranial nerve (olfactory) is responsible for the sense of smell. Assess its function by asking the child to identify a familiar odor, such as peanut butter, chocolate, and oranges. Occlude one of the child's nostrils at a time, and ask her to name one of the smells. Make a note if the child has a cold or any allergies that may interfere with the sense of smell.

The second cranial nerve (optic) is responsible for vision. Test visual acuity and function by asking the child to read a vision chart, such as a Snellen chart or preschool E chart (for children 3 years and older; see Chapter 28).

Measure visual fields (Figure 49-4) by asking the child to sit directly opposite you. Tell him to close his right eye and look directly at your nose. Close your left eye; hold your fingers just beyond the edge of your peripheral vision; wiggle one finger and bring it into your upper right vision quadrant. Ask the child to tell you when he first sees it. Assess his visual fields against your own; when you see the finger, he should

---

Table 49-2. *Cranial Nerve Function*

Nerve	Function	Assessment
I (olfactory)	Sense of smell	Assess child's ability to recognize common odors (e.g., peanut butter or an orange) while eyes are closed.
II (optic)	Vision	Assess vision fields and visual acuity, and examine retinas.
III (oculomotor)	Motor control and sensation for eye muscles and upper eyelid elevation	Assess ability to move eyes to follow an object in all directions. Note nystagmus (jerking motion). Assess size, equalness, and reaction to light of pupils.
IV (trochlear)	Movement of major eye globe muscles	As above
V (trigeminal)	Mastication muscles and some facial sensations	Assess ability to discern light touch to test sensory component; assess symmetry and strength of bite to test motor component.
VI (abducens)	Movement and muscle sense of eye globe	As with nerves III and IV
VII (facial)	Impulses for hyoid and facial muscles, salivation, and taste	Assess motor strength by asking child to close eyes while you attempt to open them. Note symmetry of facial expression and movement. Assess taste by asking child to identify salt or sugar.
VIII (acoustic)	Equilibration and hearing	Assess hearing by the response to a whispered word. Equilibrium is not tested routinely.
IX (glossopharyngeal)	Motor impulses to heart and other organs; sensation from pharynx, thorax, and abdominal organs	Assess gag reflex by pressing on rear of tongue with tongue blade. Note midline uvula.
X (vagus)	Swallowing and gag reflexes	Assess ability to swallow; elicit gag reflex by pressing a tongue blade on posterior tongue.
XI (accessory)	Impulses to striated muscles of pharynx and shoulders	Ask child to turn head to the side; try to turn it to center. Ask the child to elevate shoulders while you press down on them.
XII (hypoglossal)	Motor impulses to tongue and skeletal muscles; sensation from skin and viscera	Ask child to protrude tongue. Assess for tremors. Ask child to press on side of cheek with tongue; assess tongue strength.

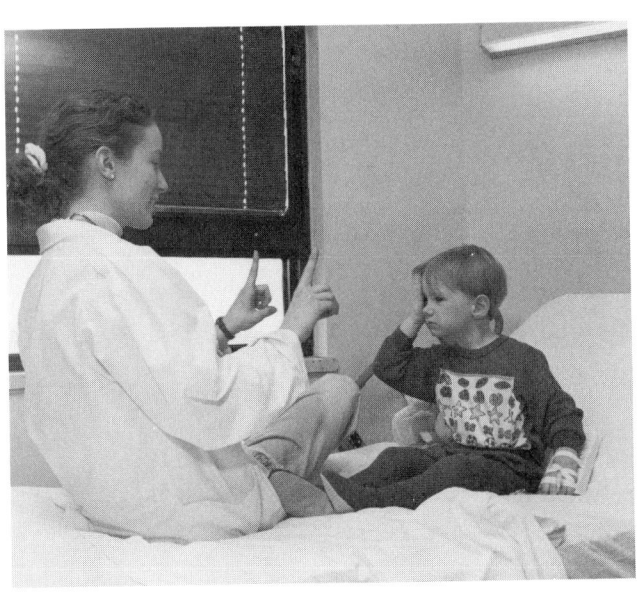

FIGURE 49-4
Testing visual fields. Nurse assesses second cranial nerve function. (Courtesy of the Department of Medical Photography, Children's Hospital, Buffalo, NY.)

see it too. Do this in all four quadrants; repeat it with the other eye.

The third, fourth, and sixth cranial nerves (oculomotor, trochlear, and abducens) are responsible for ocular movements. They are tested together. The oculomotor nerve innervates the superior, inferior, and medial rectus; inferior oblique; and levator palpabrae muscles. The trochlear innervates the superior oblique; the abducens innervates the lateral rectus muscles.

To test oculomotor nerve function, hold the child's chin steady; ask her to follow your finger as it moves through the six cardinal positions of gaze: superior, inferior, medial, lateral, and superior and inferior oblique. Some children show slight nystagmus as they look directly sideways; sustained nystagmus or inability to look at any point of vision is pathologic.

The fifth nerve (trigeminal) is responsible for motor and sensory innervation of the face and the muscles of mastication. This nerve must be tested for both sensory and motor components. The motor component is tested by asking the child to bite on a tongue blade. Palpate the jaw to see that it closes evenly; try to withdraw the tongue blade to test the strength of the bite.

The sensory component is tested by touching the child's forehead, cheek, and jaw with a light touch or a wisp of cotton (while the child's eyes are closed); ask him to tell you when and where he feels the touch.

Touch the child's cornea with a wisp of cotton to test the corneal reflex. The child will blink, because the cornea is sensitive to the pain of touch. It is often best to leave this part of the examination until last, because it does cause momentary pain, and the child may not be willing to close her eyes for any more testing. She may be afraid that you will hurt her again if she does not watch you. In any event, give fair warning: tell her that you know this will cause momentary discomfort.

The seventh cranial nerve (facial) also has a sensory and motor component. The sensory component is responsible for taste sensation for the anterior two thirds of the tongue; the motor component is responsible for facial expression. Test the sensory component by asking the child to stick out his tongue; place a substance such as sugar or salt on it and ask the child to identify the taste. Be certain the child protrudes his tongue so the substance touches only the forward two thirds. The preschooler cannot necessarily name these substances, but he can tell you whether the taste is good or bad. Test the motor component by asking a child to smile (look for symmetry). Ask him to wrinkle his forehead. Ask him to close his eyes and hold them closed while you attempt to open them.

The eighth cranial nerve (acoustic) is responsible for hearing (cochlear branch) and balance (vestibular branch). The cochlear branch is tested by an audiometer on another occasion. Gross hearing can be assessed by the child's response to the whispered or spoken word.

A Weber test or a Rinne test (see Chapter 28) may differentiate between conductive and nerve hearing loss. The vestibular branch of the eighth nerve is not routinely tested in children.

The ninth (glossopharyngeal) and tenth (vagus) cranial nerves innervate the oropharyngeal muscles, so they are tested together. Observe the pharynx for a midline uvula and difficulty in swallowing.

The 11th nerve (accessory) innervates the sternocleidomastoid and trapezius muscles. To test the strength of the sternocleidomastoid muscle, gently push the child's head to one side and, while pressing on his jaw, ask him to push back against your hand; repeat on the other side. To test the trapezius muscle, push down on the child's shoulders; ask him to raise his shoulders or push up against your force. Assess symmetry and strength.

The 12th nerve (hypoglossal) controls motor function of the tongue. Test it by asking the child to extrude her tongue. Inspect it for tremors. Next place a finger against the child's cheek; ask the child to press against your finger with her tongue. Compare the sides for strength of the tongue force.

Cerebellar Function

Tests for cerebellar function are tests for normal balance and coordination. Observe the child walking. Does he do so naturally and freely? (Most children walk self-consciously when being observed.) Ask the child to stand on one foot. A child as young as 4 years should be able to do this for as long as 5 seconds. Ask him to attempt a tandem walk (walk a straight line, one foot directly in front of the other, heel touching toe) (Figure 49-5*A*). A

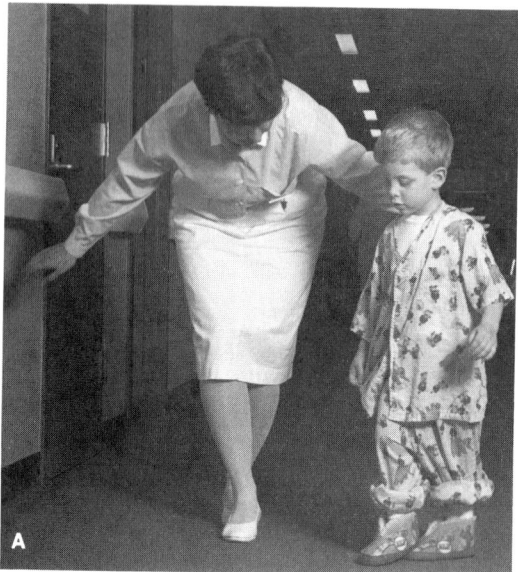
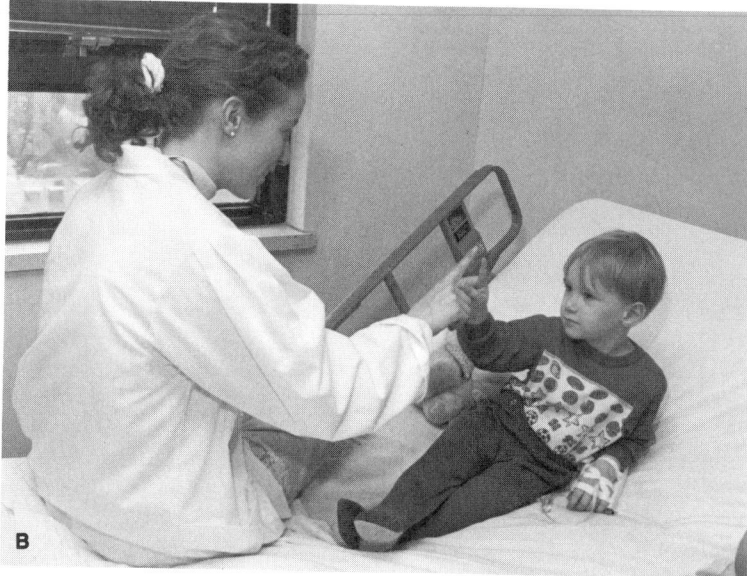

FIGURE 49-5

(**A**) *Observing a child attempt a tandem walk.* (**B**) *Nose-to-finger test is an assessment of cerebellar function. (Courtesy of the Department of Medical Photography, Children's Hospital, Buffalo, NY.)*

child over 4 years should be able to do this for about four consecutive steps. Ask the child to touch his nose with his finger, then touch your finger (held about 1½ feet in front of him; Figure 49-5*B*). Tell him to repeat this action; move your finger to a new position each time. The average child rarely reaches past your finger.

Ask the child to pat one knee with the palm of her hand, then quickly turn the hand over and pat the knee with the back of her hand; repeat over and over. She should be able to do this rapid, coordinated motion without much difficulty. Ask her to do this one hand at a time. Preschoolers will mirror the movement of the actively moving hand by moving the inactive hand as well. Older children should not demonstrate this (or should show only a small amount of movement).

Ask the child to touch each finger on one hand with the thumb of that hand in rapid succession. Ask him to run the heel of one foot down the front of his other leg while he is lying supine (he should be able to do this without "running off" the leg). While he is still lying on the examining table, ask him to close his eyes and to draw a circle or figure 8 in the air with his foot.

Tests of cerebellar function are all fun for a child to do, as long as he knows that there are no passes or failures. Show approval for his effort even if he is having difficulty with the task, so that he has confidence to try another one.

Motor Function

Muscle size, strength, and tone are part of motor system assessment. Compare the size of the extremities on each side. If in doubt, measure the circumference of the calves or thighs or upper and lower arms for comparison. Feel muscles for tone. Move the extremities through passive range of motion; evaluate for symmetry, spasticity, and flaccidity. Ask the child to extend her arms in front of her and resist your action as you push down or up on her hands, or push them out to the side. Do the same with the lower extremities.

Sensory Function

If a child's sensory system is intact, he should be able to distinguish light touch, pain, and vibration, hot and cold. Have the child close his eyes and point to the spot where you touch him with an object. Light touch is tested by a wisp of cotton, deep pressure by pressure of your finger, pain by a safety pin, temperature by test tubes filled with hot or cold water. Vibration is tested by touching the child's bony prominences (iliac crest, elbows, knees) with a vibrating tuning fork. Warn the child that on pin testing, he will feel a momentary prick. Otherwise, he may be unwilling to close his eyes again for further testing.

Reflex Testing

Deep tendon reflex testing, which is part of a primary physical assessment (see Chapter 28), is also a basic part of a neurologic assessment. In newborns, reflex testing is especially important, because the infant cannot perform tasks on command to demonstrate the range of his neurologic function (see Chapter 23).

Diagnostic Testing

A variety of diagnostic tests may be ordered to provide more information should any abnormalities be detected in the health history, physical examination, or neurologic examination. Many of these tests are invasive, and it is best to try to schedule the least invasive procedures first, before the painful or more frightening procedures are done. Preparing the child and the child's family for these procedures is an important nursing responsibility. When explaining tests, the nurse must take into account not only the child's chronologic age but also the child's level of cognitive functioning, or else explanations may not be well understood. Be sure also to provide an explanation that includes a description of all the sensory experiences the child might undergo, that is, not only what will be done but also how the child might feel, or what he or she might see or hear or even smell or taste (if appropriate).

Lumbar Puncture

Lumbar puncture is the introduction of a needle into the subarachnoid space (under the arachnoid membrane) at the level of L4 or L5 to withdraw cerebrospinal fluid for analysis. The procedure is used most frequently to diagnose hemorrhage or infection in the central nervous system or to diagnose an obstruction of CSF flow. Lumbar puncture is contraindicated if the needle insertion site is infected (to avoid introducing pathogens into the CSF) or if there is a suspected elevation of CSF pressure. In this case, the increased pressure in the subarachnoid space may cause the brain stem to be drawn down into the spinal cord space, compressing the medulla and compromising the action of the cardiac and respiratory centers.

For the procedure, the newborn is seated upright with her head bent forward. The older infant or child is placed on his side on the examining table. His head is flexed forward, his knees are flexed on his abdomen, and his back is arched as much as possible. This position opens the space between the lumbar vertebrae, facilitating needle insertion (Figure 49-6). The child's back should be aligned with the edge of the table. Children under school age need to be held in this position, because they may be frightened by someone working on their back unseen; they may try to turn over or turn their head to see what is happening. It helps a school-age child or adolescent if you stand by the table facing him and gently rest your hand on the back of his head, keeping it bent forward. This does not convey the impression that you are restraining him, but it does keep him in good position.

Children need good preparation for a lumbar puncture, because they cannot see what is happening. They need to be cautioned that the physician will wash their back (that feels cold) and inject a local anesthetic (that stings like a mosquito bite). They will feel pressure but not pain as the lumbar puncture needle is inserted. They need to be reminded to remain absolutely still throughout the procedure. You might describe the position as "rolling into a ball" or "folding up like an astronaut in a small spaceship."

Occasionally during a lumbar puncture, the needle

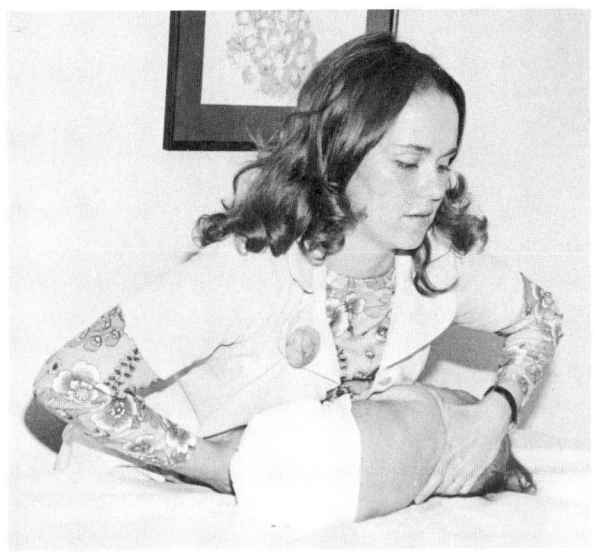

FIGURE 49-6
Restraining an infant for a lumbar puncture. (Courtesy of the Department of Medical Photography, Children's Hospital, Buffalo, NY.)

will press against a dorsal nerve root and the child will experience a shooting pain down one leg. He needs quick assurance that this feeling passes quickly and does not indicate an injury. When the insertion stylet is removed and CSF drips from the end of the needle, the procedure has been successful. An initial pressure reading is made, typically three tubes of 2 to 3 mL of CSF are collected, a closing pressure reading is taken, and the needle is withdrawn. Samples are usually sent for culture, sensitivity, glucose, and red blood cells. A *colloidal gold test* determines whether there is an alteration in the albumin-globulin ratio of CSF. An increased level of gamma globulin is suggestive of multiple sclerosis or meningitis. The first sample obtained may contain blood or skin pathogens from the puncture, so it should not be sent for determination of blood cell content or culturing.

Lumbar puncture involves at least momentary pain, so children need to be comforted afterward. The child should lie flat for at least 1 hour after the procedure. Drinking fluids will reduce spinal headaches that may come on as a result of the reduction in CSF volume or invasion of a small air pocket during the puncture. Lying flat helps prevent cerebral irritation caused by air rising in the subarachnoid space, and a quick intake of fluids will increase the amount of CSF in the body. Some children may have a headache despite these precautions; they will need an analgesic for pain relief.

The opening pressure of CSF varies with the child's age. To confirm that the subarachnoid space in the cord is patent with that in the skull, the examiner may ask a child who is older than 3 years to cough, or ask you to press on the child's external jugular during the procedure (a Valsalva maneuver). Either of these measures will cause an increase of CSF pressure if fluid can flow freely through the subarachnoid space.

Sterile technique must be strictly observed for lumbar punctures to ensure that a clean sample of fluid is sent for culture.

If a child had minimally increased CSF pressure at the time of the puncture, she must be observed closely afterward to prevent respiratory and cardiac difficulty from medulla pressure. Take vital signs every 15 minutes for several hours. An increase in blood pressure or a decrease in pulse and respiration is an important sign of increased intracranial compression. Other important signs are a change in consciousness, pupillary changes, or decrease in motor ability.

Ventricular Tap
In infants, CSF may be obtained by a subdural tap into the ventricle through the coronal suture or anterior fontanelle. The scalp over the insertion site must be shaved or the hair clipped and the area prepared with an antiseptic. The infant's head must be held firmly while in a supine position so that he does not move during the procedure, which could cause the needle to strike and lacerate meningeal tissue.

Fluid must be removed from this site slowly rather than suddenly, to prevent a sudden shift in pressure that could cause intracranial hemorrhage. After the procedure, a pressure dressing is applied to the site, and the infant is placed in a half-sitting position in an infant seat to prevent prolonged drainage from the puncture site. After the procedure, comfort the infant to both reduce the stress of a painful procedure and prevent him from crying excessively, an action which could increase intracranial pressure.

X-ray Film Techniques
A flat-plate skull x-ray film may be used to obtain information about increased intracranial pressure or skull defects such as fracture or craniosynostosis (premature knitting of cranial sutures). Increased intracranial pressure is suggested when skull sutures are separated. When the process is chronic, other subtle changes such as a flattening of the sella turcica or an increase in the convolutions of the inner table of the skull may be present.

Cerebral Angiography. Cerebral angiography is an x-ray study of cerebral blood vessels by the injection of a contrast material into an extracranial artery. X-ray films are taken in series as the dye flows through the blood vessels of the cerebrum. The injection site chosen is often a femoral artery, although a carotid artery may be used. The study will reveal any space-occupying lesions that are occluding blood vessels or defects in vessels themselves.

Myelography. Myelography is an x-ray study of the spinal cord by the introduction of a contrast material

into the CSF by lumbar puncture. It is used to reveal the presence of space-occupying lesions of the spinal cord. Keep the head of the child's bed elevated after the procedure to prevent contrast medium from reaching the brain.

Computed Tomography. CT is a brain scan that reveals densities at different levels or layers of brain tissue. It is helpful in confirming the presence of a brain tumor or other encroaching lesions. The study is discussed in further detail in Chapter 37. Single photon-emission computed tomography (SPECT) is a similar procedure used mainly for blood flow evaluation (Caplan, 1991).

Positron Emission Tomography. The diagnostic technique of positron emission tomography (PET) is similar to CT or MRI, involving imaging after injection of positron-emitting radiopharmaceuticals into the brain. It is extremely accurate in identifying seizure foci ("Assessment: Positron Emission Tomography," 1991).

Brain Scan
For a brain scan, a radioactive material is injected intravenously, and after a fixed time during which the injected material is deposited in cerebral tissue, radioactivity levels over the skull are measured. If the blood–brain barrier is not functioning, the radioactive material will accumulate in specific areas, suggesting possible tumor, subdural hematoma, abscess, or encephalitis.

Echoencephalography
Echoencephalography is the projection of ultrasound (high-frequency sound waves above the audible range) toward the child's head (a sonogram). Sonography may be used to outline the ventricles. Because this technique of scanning is noninvasive, produces no discomfort, and has no known complications, it may be repeated frequently to follow change in the size of ventricles.

Magnetic Resonance Imaging
Magnetic resonance imaging (MRI) is the use of magnetic fields to demonstrate differences in tissue composition (Barnes, 1990). It reveals normal versus abnormal brain tissue very effectively. This is discussed in greater detail in Chapter 37.

Electroencephalography
The electroencephalogram (EEG) reflects the electrical patterns of the brain. It summarizes the physical and chemical interaction within the brain at the time of the test. Normally, a tracing reveals four types of waves: delta (1 to 3 waves/sec), theta (4 to 7 waves/sec), alpha (8 to 12 waves/sec), and beta (13 to 20 waves/sec) (Figure 49-7).

To reduce extraneous movements of the eyes, head, or muscles that will affect the tracing, children must be

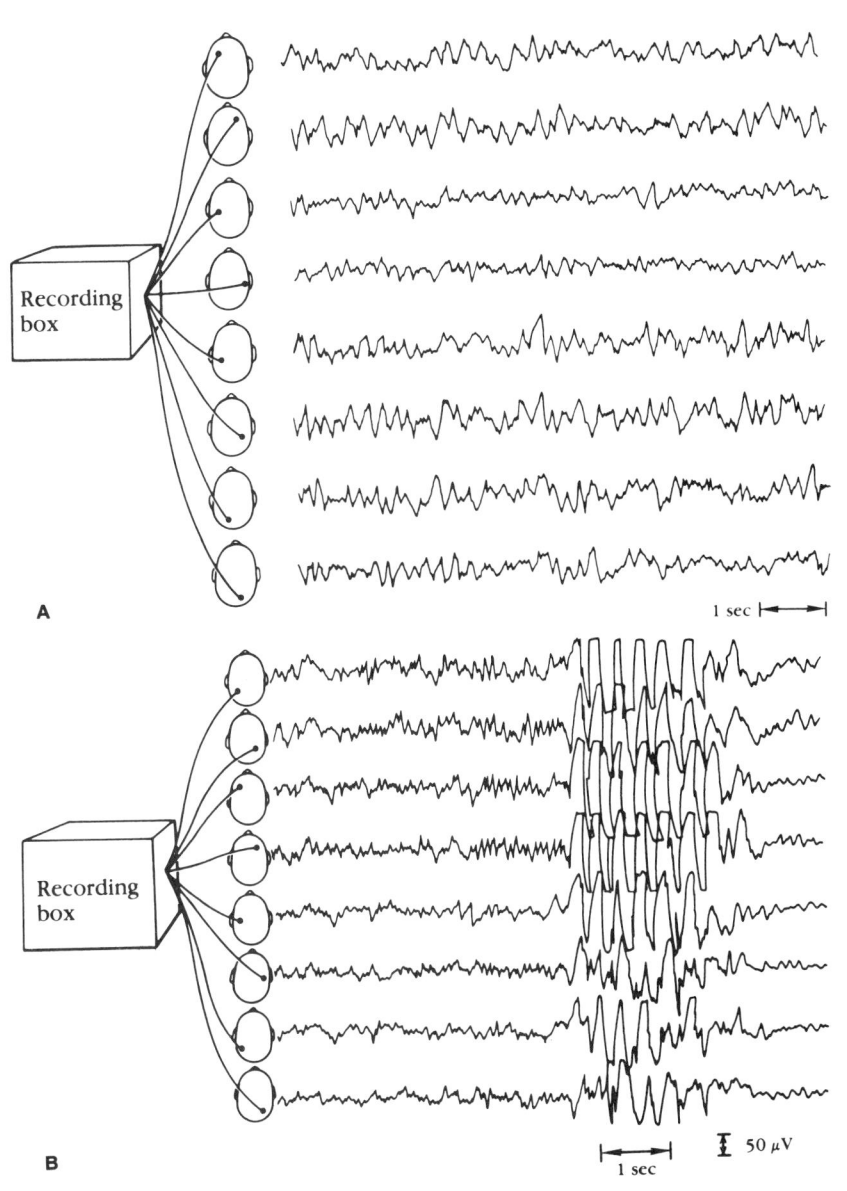

FIGURE 49-7
(**A**) *A normal EEG tracing in a child.* (**B**) *EEG during a tonic-clonic seizure. (From Bullock, B., & Rosendahl, P. P. [1992].* Pathophysiology. *Philadelphia: J. B. Lippincott.)*

cooperative and quiet. And for that they will need good preparation and encouragement. Caution them that the room will probably be darkened to help them rest; the electrode wires attached to their scalp with adhesive paste can be compared to those attached to astronauts in space and are not painful. Be careful not to use the word *electrical*; children as young as 3 years know that electrical wires are ordinarily dangerous and can hurt them. They cannot relax if they are worried that they may be shocked or even electrocuted.

If children are unable to lie still and cooperate even after careful explanation, they may need sedation. The sedation alters the electrical pattern of the cortex, so it is avoided if possible. Chloral hydrate, for example, may increase the fast activity of brain waves; chlorpromazine (Thorazine) may increase slow activity. Because phenobarbital and phenytoin sodium (diphenylhydantoin; Dilantin) also cause an increase in fast activity, it is im-

portant that the person interpreting the recording knows what medication the child currently is receiving. Check to see if anticonvulsant medication should be withheld on the morning of an EEG to reduce the effect of medications on tracings.

Although EEGs can reveal important information about brain activity, they are not necessarily helpful. For example, approximately 15% of children who are absolutely normal clinically will demonstrate some abnormality on an EEG. Most brain tumors in pediatric patients are in the posterior fossa. The activity of this region does not show up well on an EEG. An EEG may appear normal even when there is a brain tumor, unless the tumor is pressing on more distal brain portions. On inspecting the symmetry of hemispheres, local lesions may be suggested. Where there is a lesion, there will be slower waves, a higher voltage pattern, and an overall more irregular pattern. A subdural lesion (perhaps from a hematoma) can interfere with the transmission of the electrical impulses, and the voltage pattern will be lower.

An EEG is the most beneficial in diagnosing absence seizures. The typical pattern with this disorder is discussed under Recurrent Convulsions.

Visual stimulation, such as having children look at a whirling disk, may be used in connection with EEG, because various types of electrical discharges increase with rapid eye movements. In a child who is sensitive to this type of stimulation, the testing may produce a seizure. The child may be very disturbed and disoriented after the procedure, so you can describe what has happened and help him relax.

Following an EEG, children will be sleepy if they have been sedated. They should be allowed to sleep as long as needed.

Increased Intracranial Pressure

Increased intracranial pressure (IIP) is not a single disorder but a syndrome arising with many neurologic disorders. When caring for a child with a potential neurologic disorder, it is important to observe him or her closely for signs of this syndrome.

Increased intracranial pressure may occur when there is an increase in the CSF volume, when blood enters the CSF, when cerebral edema is present, or when there are space-occupying lesions such as tumors. Examples that lead to IIP in the newborn are birth trauma or hydrocephalus; in the infant or preschooler, head trauma or infection; in the school-age child or adolescent, brain tumor or Guillain-Barré syndrome. The rate at which symptoms develop depends on the cause and on whether the child's skull can expand to accommodate the increased pressure. Children with open fontanelles can withstand more pressure without brain damage than older children whose suture lines and fontanelles are already closed.

Assessment

Assessment for neurologic function may involve only a few rapid procedures: vital signs, pupil response, level of consciousness, and motor and sensory function, or more elaborate electronic monitoring. Signs and symptoms of intracranial pressure are shown in Table 49-3. With increased intracranial pressure, symptoms are often subtle at first and include irritability or restlessness. The child may have a headache but may not report it. Infants with a headache become increasingly fussy. Changes in vital signs may be strongly indicative of intracranial pressure. Growing pressure on the brain stem, which controls respiration and cardiac activity, causes pulse and respirations to slow down. Compression of cranial vessels leads to a compensatory increase in blood pressure (or pulse pressure, the widening gap between systolic and diastolic). Pressure on the hypothalamus, the temperature-regulating center of the body, causes an increase in temperature. These changes may occur gradually, so a single measurement may not reveal the extent of the change. Always compare the new recording against all recordings taken in the last 24 hours or since the child's hospital admission.

Children with increased intracranial pressure typically may assume a knee–chest position (Straussberg et al., 1993). Changes in the eye may indicate increased pressure posterior to the eye globe. One obvious abnormality may be a dilated pupil that suggests third cranial nerve compression. Test pupil reactivity by shining a light into each eye; the pupil should constrict. The room need not be completely dark, but there should not be an

---

Table 49-3. *Signs and Symptoms of Increased Intracranial Pressure*

Sign	Symptom
Increased head circumference	An increase greater than 2 cm/mon in first 3 months of life, >1 cm/mon in the second 3 months, and >0.5 cm/mon for the next 6 months
Fontanelle changes	Anterior fontanelle is tense and bulging; will close late.
Vomiting	Occurs in the absence of nausea, on awakening in morning or after nap. Will become projectile
Vision changes	Diplopia (double vision) occurs from pressure on abducens nerves; white of sclera evident over pupil (setting sun sign); limited visual fields, papilledema
Vital sign changes	Elevated temperature and blood pressure; decreased pulse and respiration rates
Pain	Headache, often present on awakening and standing. Increases with straining at stool or holding breath (a Valsalva maneuver)
Mentation	Irritability, altered consciousness

overhead light shining directly into the child's eyes. In a newborn nursery, dim the lights before testing an infant's pupillary response. To elicit the most dramatic and sudden response, bring your light to the child's eye from the side or down from the forehead, to make it appear suddenly rather than gradually. Repeat this with the other eye.

Consensual constriction should also be noted: as you shine the light on the right pupil, the left pupil should constrict as well, and vice versa. Note not only whether the pupils both constrict but also whether they constrict equally.

If the child is alert and able to cooperate, have him follow your light through positions of gaze: up, down, obliquely, and laterally; to test convergence, have him follow it to his nose. Note any tendency toward strabismus, nystagmus, "sunset eyes" (white sclera showing over the top of the cornea), or inability to follow the light into any quadrant. Chart and report carefully the exact abnormality you note. "Inability to follow light" is not nearly as informative as "inability to follow light into left superior oblique field; vertical nystagmus noted as child follows light into other fields."

While lying supine, a normal child will turn his eyes to the left if you turn his head rapidly to the right, and vice versa. If the child has increased intracranial pressure, this phenomenon (a doll's eye reflex) will be absent. (This is useful in assessing a comatose child who is unable to cooperate by following a light.) An older child may be able to report symptoms such as diplopia. On funduscopic examination, papilledema may be detected.

Assess the child's level of consciousness. Signs of confusion, in which the child is alert but unable to comprehend surroundings, time, or place, may be the first indication of increased intracranial pressure, followed by a pseudoawake state, in which the child is awake but unable to follow light or noise. Finally, the child may be comatose, unable to be roused by any stimuli. Levels of coma are rated by a Glasgow coma scale. This is discussed in Chapter 52 in connection with assessment for head injury.

Children, like adults, generally become disoriented about time first, then place, then self. It is useful, therefore, to assess that the child is alert enough to answer these questions. Explain that you will be asking these seemingly simple questions periodically to make sure the child can answer them accurately each time. Otherwise, the child will quickly become annoyed with your questions and may refuse to answer them or make up silly answers instead. She may pretend to be asleep to avoid being asked. If she does not understand why you are asking her name and what time it is over and over, she may think you are not smart enough to take good care of her.

Be certain that you ask questions appropriate to a child's age. A preschooler does not usually know the day of the week or concepts such as *morning* or *night*. They do not necessarily know their whole name. With children of this age, it is often more helpful to identify an area of knowledge they are familiar with (colors, for instance). Every half hour or hour, show them a colored block and ask them its color. Even if they give the wrong answer, your main concern is that they understand your request and respond to it appropriately.

Remind parents that you are asking these questions to assess their child's level of consciousness, not to quiz him for right answers or to be intrusive. Remind them not to answer for the child.

A good way to test an infant's level of consciousness is to see if he or she will respond to a music box or voices or will reach for an attractive object. Be aware that many children, even when healthy, are groggy when they first wake up, and until fully awake may not be able to say who or where they are. This happens especially when the child is awakened from a dream. Make sure the child is fully awake before attempting to determine his or her level of consciousness.

Evaluate motor ability by asking a child to perform some simple motor task such as squeezing your hands; evaluate whether she can do this symmetrically. Have her push against your hand with both feet. Can she do this with equal strength? Have her perform rapid, alternating hand movements, such as turning her hand over and back several times. Is she able to do this as well as last time? Evaluate cranial nerves grossly by having her make a face, close her eyes tightly, and show you her teeth. Can she do this symmetrically?

Test deep tendon reflexes, which decrease in intensity with decreased level of consciousness. Carefully observe the child's resting posture. When motor control grows weaker owing to loss of cell function, characteristic posturing (primitive reflexes) occurs. Cerebral loss is shown mainly by **decorticate posturing**; a child's arms are adducted and flexed on the chest with wrists flexed, hands fisted; lower extremities are extended and adducted (Figure 49-8*A*). **Decerebrate posturing**, which occurs when the midbrain is not functional, is characterized by rigid extension and pronation of the arms and legs (Figure 49-8*B*).

Observe the child carefully for any seizure activity, as this is a late sign of increased intracranial pressure.

Intracranial Pressure Monitoring

Intracranial pressure can be measured by several methods: an intraventricular catheter inserted through the anterior fontanelle, a burr hole in the skull, a fiberoptic sensor implanted into the epidural space, or a hollow subarachnoid screw (Figure 49-9*A,B*). The most accurate of these is the intraventricular catheter (Figure 49-9*C*). It is threaded into the lateral ventricle, filled with normal saline, and then connected to an external pressure mon-

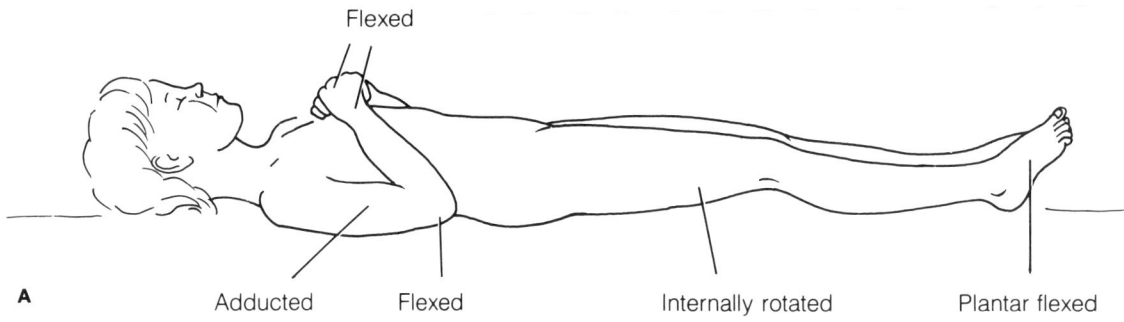

Flexed

A   Adducted   Flexed   Internally rotated   Plantar flexed

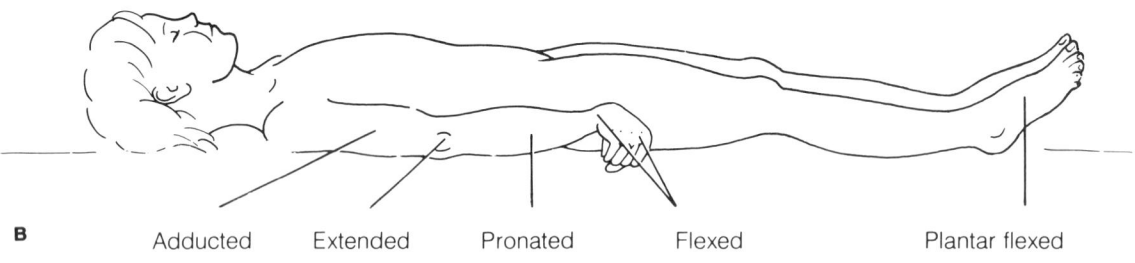

B   Adducted   Extended   Pronated   Flexed   Plantar flexed

FIGURE 49-8
(**A**) *Decorticate rigidity.* (**B**) *Decerebrate rigidity.*

itor. As pressure in the ventricle changes, it is registered through the filled catheter on an oscilloscope screen and a written printout. An additional advantage of this method is that medication can be administered through the catheter.

A normal intracranial pressure reading is 1 to 10 mm

Hg. A level of over 15 mm Hg is considered abnormal. As blood pressure rises and falls with the influx of blood through vessels, so does intracranial pressure. On a monitor it appears as A waves (plateau waves) or transient paroxysmal elevations that last for 5 to 20 minutes; their amplitude is 50 to 100 mm Hg. If brain ischemia is

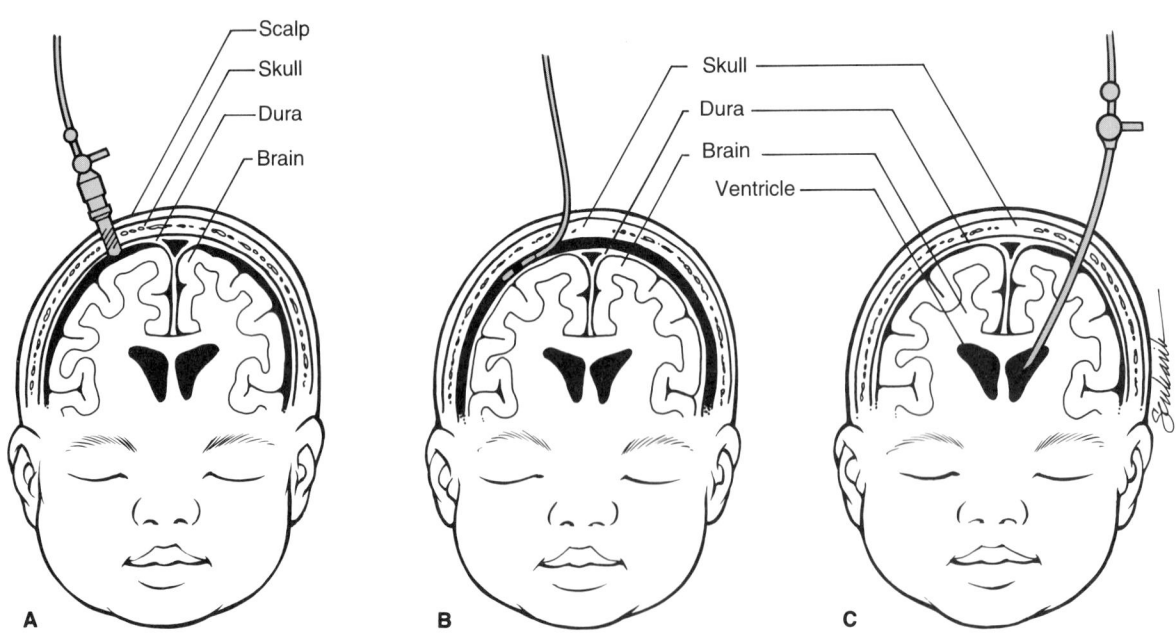

Scalp
Skull
Dura
Brain

Skull
Dura
Brain
Ventricle

A   **B**   **C**

FIGURE 49-9
Devices used to monitor intracranial pressure. (**A**) *Subdural screw.* (**B**) *Epidural sensor.* (**C**) *Intraventricular catheter. (Modified from* Massachusetts General Hospital Department of Nursing manual of nursing procedures. *Boston: Little, Brown; with permission.)*

present, these waves increase before other signs, such as a change in blood pressure or pulse rate, become apparent. B waves are short-duration waves (½ to 2 minutes) with low amplitude (up to 50 mm Hg). C waves are small, rhythmic waves at a frequency of about 6 waves/min. They are related to deviations in the arterial blood pressure. Because A waves appear to reflect brain ischemia, they can be used to signal when the child needs more oxygen (Figure 49-10).

Intracranial pressure monitoring can also be used to estimate cerebral perfusion pressure or cerebral blood flow. This is calculated by subtracting the mean intracranial pressure from the mean arterial pressure. Mean arterial pressure is determined by subtracting the diastolic reading from the systolic reading, dividing this by 3, then adding that sum to 80. The mean arterial pressure of a blood pressure of 100 over 70 is 90 mm Hg (100 − 70 = 30 ÷ 3 = 10 + 80 = 90). If a child had a blood pressure of 100/70 and an intracranial pressure of 10, his cerebral perfusion pressure would be 80 mm Hg (90 − 10). Normal cerebral perfusion pressure is at least 50 mm Hg. Cerebral circulation ceases if intracranial pressure ever exceeds arterial pressure, because blood vessels become obstructed (Rosman, 1994).

Parents have difficulty accepting procedures such as the insertion of intraventricular catheters or screws. Explaining the brain's anatomy will help them see that the catheter or screw does not puncture or tear brain tissue and is a helpful assessment tool, not an injurious one.

Therapeutic Management

In children the source of increased intracranial pressure must be identified and removed as quickly as possible; severe elevation of pressure will compress the brain stem and lead to cardiac and respiratory failure. Actions such as coughing, vomiting, and sneezing will increase the intracranial pressure; these should be kept to a minimum if possible. When bubbling infants with increased intracranial pressure, do not put pressure on the jugular veins, because this will increase the intracranial pressure.

Hyperventilation may be induced to lower intracranial pressure. The rate of intravenous fluid administration in such children must be monitored carefully, because overhydration will increase intracranial pressure. The child may be placed in a semi-Fowler's position (use an infant seat for babies) to reduce cerebral pressure. A steroid such as dexamethasone (Decadron) may effectively reduce cerebral edema and pressure. An osmotic diuretic, such as mannitol, may be given intravenously to reduce pressure from cerebral edema. Mannitol causes a shift of fluid from extravascular compartments into the vascular stream, where it can be eliminated by the kidneys. Children generally have a urinary catheter inserted before starting this therapy, so that bladder distention does not result from rapid diuresis. If excessive fluid accumulates in the brain's ventricles, a ventricular tap may be necessary for immediate reduction of pressure. High doses of barbiturates may also be therapeutic.

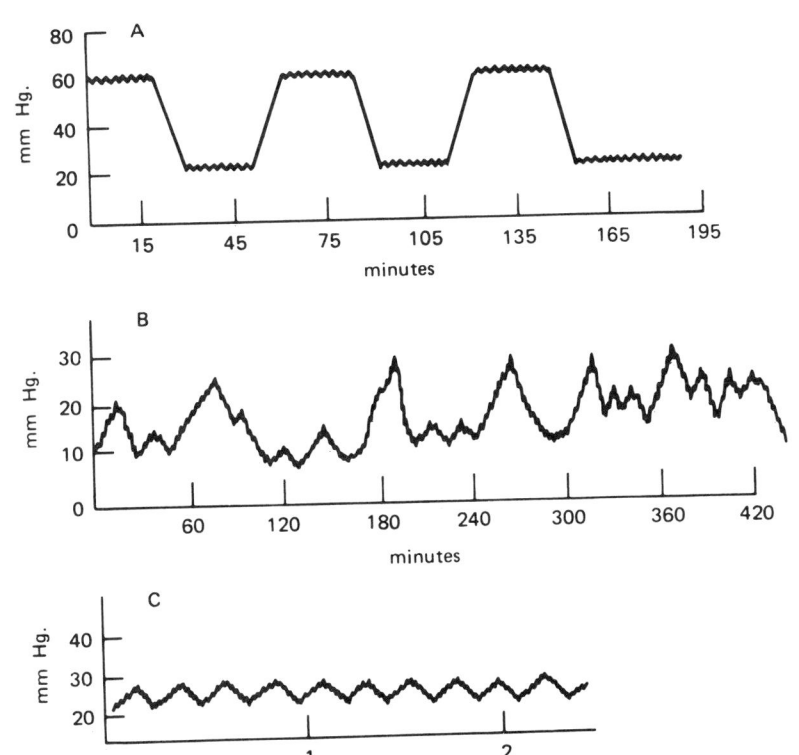

FIGURE 49-10
Generalized shapes of the three types of intracranial pressure waves: A waves or plateau waves (top), *B waves* (middle), *and C waves* (bottom). *(From Hamilton, A. Critical care nursing skills. New York: Appleton-Century-Crofts, with permission.)*

Neural Tube Disorders

The neural tube is the embryotic structure that matures to form the central nervous system. Because this forms in utero first as a flat plate, then molds to form the brain and cord, it is susceptible to malformation. Neural tube disorders, including spina bifida, are discussed in Chapter 39.

Neurocutaneous Syndromes

Neurocutaneous syndromes are characterized by the involvement of skin or pigment disorders with central nervous system dysfunction.

Sturge-Weber Syndrome

Sturge-Weber syndrome involves a congenital port-wine stain on the skin of the face that extends to the meninges and choroid. The skin manifestation follows the distribution of the fifth cranial nerve (trigeminal nerve). Because the defect is generally unilateral, the port-wine stain ends abruptly at the midline. In many children, only the ophthalmic branch of the nerve is involved, so the lesion is confined to the upper aspect of the face.

Due to involvement of the meningeal blood vessels, blood flow is sluggish, and anoxia may develop in some portions of the cerebral cortex. The child may have symptoms of hemiparesis from destruction of motor neurons on the side opposite the lesion. Intractable convulsions and mental deficiency, as well as blindness from glaucoma, may result. A CT scan or MRI of the skull will generally reveal calcification in the involved cerebral cortex. Such calcification follows a diagnostic "railroad track" or double-groove pattern.

Sturge-Weber syndrome is a bewildering disease for parents. They may find it hard to believe that the defect is more extensive than the skin lesion. They may ask to have the lesion surgically removed in the belief that this will correct their child's condition completely.

Children need careful follow-up as they grow so that they can be treated for symptoms such as convulsions. Surgery to relieve seizures may be possible in some children (Holmes, 1993).

Neurofibromatosis (Von Recklinghausen's Disease)

Neurofibromatosis is the unexplained development of subcutaneous tumors. The disorder is inherited as an autosomal dominant trait carried on the long arm of chromosome 17; it occurs in approximately 1 in 4000 live births. The famous "Elephant Man" is thought to have had an extreme case of multiple neurofibromatosis involving skeletal changes as well. As an infant, the child with neurofibromatosis has excessive skin pigmentation; later in childhood, pigmented nevi or "café-au-lait" (coffee with cream) spots appear. These café-au-lait spots tend to follow the paths of cutaneous nerves. The presence of more than five spots larger than 1 cm in diameter is suggestive of neurofibromatosis (Roach, 1992). A newborn often has extreme bowing of the tibia and disfigurement of the sphenoid wing. By puberty, multiple soft cutaneous tumors begin to form in the child's skin along nerve pathways. Subcutaneous tumors occur by young adulthood. The eighth cranial nerve, the acoustic nerve, is frequently involved, leading to hearing loss. Involvement of the optic nerve causes vision loss. About 15% of children will develop neurologic complications such as seizures. About 10% will develop mental retardation from cerebral deterioration. Symptoms and growth of tumors increase at puberty and during pregnancy.

If lesions are causing acoustic or optic degeneration, surgical removal may be attempted. The mast cell blocker ketotifen may slow the growth rate of the tumors. No other therapy is effective; the parents and child will need emotional support through the disease's invariably fatal course. Prenatal diagnosis is available.

Cerebral Palsy

Cerebral palsy is a group of nonprogressive disorders of upper motor neuron impairment that result in motor dysfunction. A child may also have speech or ocular difficulty, seizures, and mental retardation or hyperactivity.

Cerebral palsy may be caused before, during, or shortly after birth. It is most frequently caused by brain anoxia that leads to cell destruction. If intrauterine anoxia occurs for some reason (such as faulty placental implantation, placenta previa, or abruptio placentae), brain cell dysfunction may result. Nutritional deficiencies, drugs, or maternal infections (such as cytomegalovirus or toxoplasmosis) may also cause intrauterine damage.

Cerebral palsy occurs in approximately 1 in 1000 births. It occurs most frequently in very-low-birth-weight infants or those who are small for gestational age. Twenty percent to 25% of infants with cerebral palsy weigh less than 2500 g (5½ lb) at birth. Cerebral palsy occurs more frequently in infants born from occipitoposterior rather than anterior birth positions. In these instances, anoxia and resulting brain damage may occur with delivery. In all instances, however, the damage may already have occurred. This may be why the infant is born abnormally early or presents in an unusual position. It is increasing in incidence because of the number of very-low-birth-weight infants who survive today (Bhushan et al., 1993).

During the neonatal period, kernicterus from neonatal hyperbilirubinemia can cause cerebral palsy. This usually produces the athetoid type of cerebral palsy (slow writhing, involuntary movements). Children may have associated defects such as deafness, mental retardation, and significant difficulty with upward gaze. Infections such as meningitis or encephalitis in the newborn also may result in cerebral palsy. Severe dehydration in the newborn, with resulting venous thrombosis, may also lead to these symptoms.

Types of Cerebral Palsy

Cerebral palsy traditionally is divided into two main categories based on the type of neuromuscular involvement: pyramidal or spastic (about 50% of affected children) and extrapyramidal. Extrapyramidal is further subdivided into ataxic (about 5%), athetoid (about 20%), and mixed (25%) (Shapiro & Capute, 1994). A newer classification rates children according to their degree of motor involvement, regardless of the specific type of involvement present.

Spastic Type

Spasticity is excessive tone in the voluntary muscles (loss of upper motor neurons). The child with spastic cerebral palsy has hypertonic muscles, abnormal clonus, exaggeration of deep tendon reflexes, abnormal reflexes such as a positive Babinski reflex, and continuation of neonatal reflexes, such as the tonic neck reflex, past the age at which these usually disappear. When infants with cerebral palsy are held in a ventral suspension position, they arch their backs and extend their arms and legs abnormally. They fail to demonstrate a parachute reflex if lowered suddenly, failing to hold out their arms as if to break their fall. Children tend to assume a "scissors gait." Tight adductor thigh muscles cause their legs to cross when they are held upright. This adductor thigh involvement may be so severe that it leads to a subluxated hip. Tightening of the heel cord usually is so severe that children walk on their toes, unable to stretch their heel to touch the ground (Figure 49-11).

Spastic involvement may affect both extremities on one side (**hemiplegia**), all four extremities (**quadriplegia**), or primarily the lower extremities (**diplegia** or **paraplegia**). When a child has hemiplegia, the arm is usually more involved than the leg. This may be demonstrated by asking the child to extend his arms and pronate them. When asked to supinate the arm, the child's elbow flexes on the involved side. The involved arm may be shorter than the other and may have a smaller muscle circumference. Most children with hemiplegia have difficulty identifying objects placed in their involved hand when their eyes are closed (**astereognosis**).

In older children, leg involvement may be detected most easily by examining the child's shoes. One heel

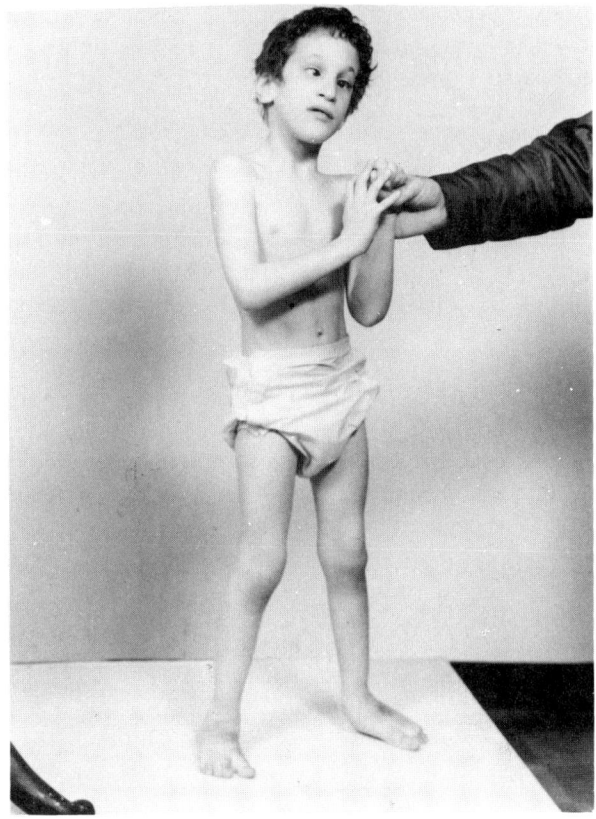

FIGURE 49-11
A child with spastic form of cerebral palsy. Notice the rigidly held arms and strabismus. (Courtesy of the Department of Medical Photography, Children's Hospital, Buffalo, NY.)

will be much more worn than the other because the child does not put the heel all the way down on the involved side. On physical examination, it may be difficult to adduct the involved hip fully, extend the knee, or dorsiflex the foot.

A child with quadriplegia invariably has impaired speech (pseudobulbar palsy). Swallowing saliva may be so difficult that the child drools continually and has difficulty swallowing food as well. Mental retardation may accompany quadriplegia as well. Diplegia tends to occur most commonly in children who have a low birth weight. The upper extremity involvement may be limited to an abnormal, awkward hand movement. If there is no involvement of the arms at all, this is a true spastic paraplegia, and a spinal cord anomaly rather than cerebral anomaly is suggested.

Athetoid Type

This type of cerebral palsy involves abnormal involuntary movement. *Athetoid* means "wormlike." Early in life, the child is limp and flaccid; later, in place of voluntary movement, he or she makes slow, writhing motions. This may involve all four extremities as well as the face and neck. The movements increase under stress or anxiety. Because of poor tongue and swallowing movements, the child drools and speech is difficult to understand.

Ataxic Type

Children with ataxic involvement have an awkward, wide-based gait. On neurologic examination, they are unable to perform the finger-to-nose test or perform rapid, repetitive movements (tests of cerebellar function); this is apparently a cerebellar rather than cerebral disorder.

Mixed Type

Some children show symptoms of both spasticity and athetoid movements. Ataxia and athetoid movements also may be present together. This combination results in a severe degree of impairment.

Assessment of Cerebral Palsy

The diagnosis of cerebral palsy is based on history and physical assessment. On history, an episode of possible anoxia during prenatal life or at birth should be docu-

mented. Determining the extent of involvement in an infant can be difficult. The full extent of the disorder may be recognizable only when children are older and attempt more complex motor skills such as walking. All infants need careful neurologic assessment during the first year of life, however, so that the accumulation of small signs of impairment can be tracked and also so that the child can be followed closely for further testing and assessment. Important physical findings that suggest cerebral palsy are shown in Table 49-4.

Children with cerebral palsy may have sensory disturbances such as strabismus, refractive disorders, visual perception problems, and visual field defects, as well as speech disorders such as abnormal rhythm or articulation. They may show an attention deficit disorder as well. Deafness caused by kernicterus occurs in connection with athetoid cerebral palsy.

Twenty-five percent to 75% of children with symptoms of cerebral palsy have mental retardation, which occurs most frequently in spastic or mixed types. As many as 20% to 25% of children with cerebral palsy have recurrent convulsions.

A cranial x-ray film or sonogram may reveal cerebral

Table 49-4. *Physical Findings That Suggest Cerebral Palsy*

Finding	Description
Delayed motor development	Children with this disorder generally do not meet motor developmental milestones such as sitting, walking, saying sentences, or changing objects from hand to hand when they should, especially if there is associated mental retardation.
Abnormal head circumference	The child's head circumference may be smaller than normal for age, because the head grows as the brain grows. If the brain cortex is severely involved, it grows more slowly than normal.
Abnormal postures	When infants lie on their back, they usually flex their legs; infants with cerebral palsy straighten or "scissor" them; they often hold feet plantar flexed (toes down). Scissoring is also evident when the infant is held upright and you try to make him or her bear weight. In a prone position, an infant tends to raise the head higher than normal because of arching of the back. The child may flex arms and legs abnormally under trunk.
Abnormal reflexes	Newborn reflexes tend to be persistent or last long past the point they should fade: tonic neck reflex or grasp reflex beyond 5 months, Moro beyond 6 months. Hyperreflexia (extreme reflexes) is also present. Ankle clonus (persistent movement of the ankle after you have repeatedly flexed it) often occurs.
Abnormal motor performance	These infants often show abnormal use of muscle groups. They often tend to move about not by crawling on their abdomen but by scooting on their back. When they begin walking, they walk by placing their toes down first. Tight adductus muscles at the hip (which also causes scissoring) tend to pull the femoral head out of the acetabulum so that subluxation of the hip occurs not because of faulty bone formation but because of muscle spasticity.

asymmetry, but generally the skull shape is normal. A CT scan will be negative. The EEG usually is abnormal. The abnormality may be asymmetry or a spike seizure discharge, but the EEG pattern is highly variable with cerebral palsy. An abnormality is noteworthy but not diagnostic in itself.

Nursing Diagnoses and Related Interventions

Be certain that goals established for care are realistic. Parents who are reacting to the revelation that their child has multiple physical disabilities find it difficult to make long-range plans. They are functioning well if they are even able to focus effectively on short-term goals.

Nursing Diagnosis: Knowledge deficit related to understanding of complex disease condition

Goal: Parents will demonstrate increased knowledge of cause and prognosis of cerebral palsy by next visit.

Outcome Criteria: Parents state they understand that cause of disease is unknown and that disease is not progressive.

It is important for parents to understand that cerebral palsy is a nonprogressive disease. The brain damage that occurred during pregnancy or at birth will not recur. The child's condition may seem to grow more apparent with age, however. Motor deficits of the upper extremities, for example, may not be strikingly evident until the child attempts fine motor tasks in school; without follow-up care, contractures from spasticity may result, further reducing existing motor function.

Caution parents also that cerebral palsy is a single name for a wide variety and extent of diseases. Although the child next door may have such severe cerebral palsy that he has no useful function in his extremities, their own child may not be affected to the same extent. Conversely, although they know someone with cerebral palsy who is able to hold a full-time job, their child may not necessarily be able to do as well some day. Each child's potential must be evaluated individually.

Nursing Diagnosis: High risk for disuse syndrome related to spasticity of muscle groups

Goal: Child will achieve maximum mobility possible during childhood.

Outcome Criteria: Child walks with a minimum of support or equipment; skin and tissue remains intact.

Important goals in caring for the child with cerebral palsy are to promote any function that is not already impaired and to prevent any further loss of function. Major

areas to be addressed are self-care, communication, ambulation, education, safety, nutrition, support of the parents, and establishment of self-esteem in the child.

Learning to be ambulatory is an important part of self-care. This is difficult to achieve because of lack of muscle group coordination. Surgery to lengthen heel tendons may be needed even after the continuous use of leg braces (Figure 49-12; Brucker, 1990). Medication to reduce spasticity has little effect, although baclofen (Lioresal) may be prescribed for some children to improve motor function. Cerebellar pacemakers may reduce spasticity in some children.

Preventing contractures is important. Formerly children were fitted with extensive braces. The weight of these braces, however, often impeded muscle movement and prevented children from learning to walk. This added to their disability. Partial leg braces, however, are used to encourage children to bring their heels down and keep the heel cords from tightening. If leg braces are prescribed, parents may need some encouragement and support to insist that their children wear them. If

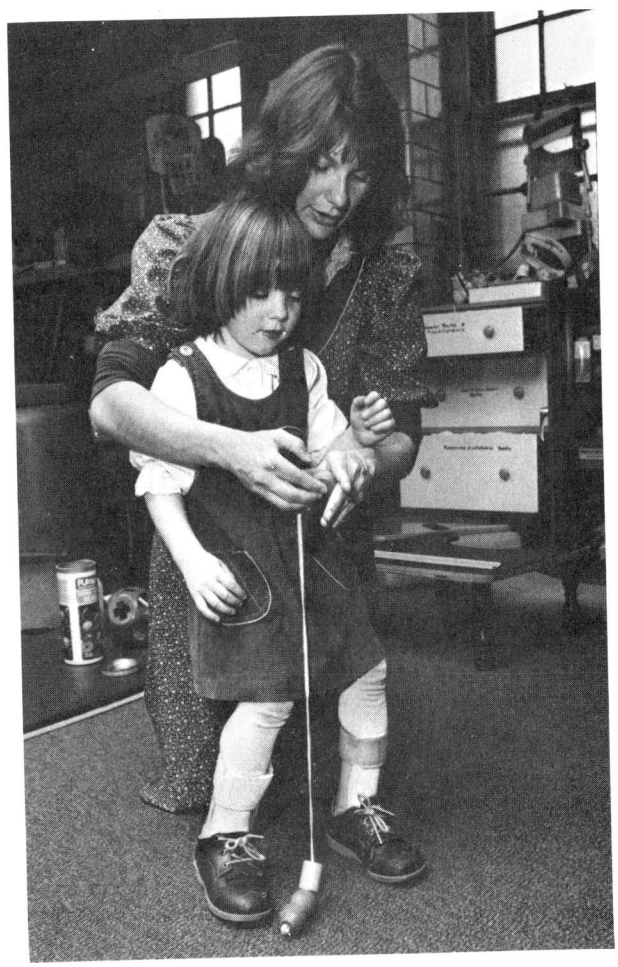

FIGURE 49-12
Leg braces give a child added stability for walking and keep heel cords from shortening. (Courtesy of the Department of Medical Photography, Children's Hospital, Buffalo, NY.)

braces are presented with a casual attitude early in life ("This is all part of your shoe"), children generally do not have difficulty accepting them. Remind parents that partial leg braces for stretching the heel cords should be worn for long periods during the day to be effective; just putting them on when the child is going outside is not enough.

Passive and active muscle exercises also are important in preventing contractures. Parents can be taught to do passive exercises and to play games with the child that encourage active exercise. At health care visits, remind parents that these exercises are an important part of their child's therapy and are not just for fun; they must be done consistently each day.

Nursing Diagnosis: High risk for self-care deficit related to impaired mobility

Goal: Child will achieve independent self-care by puberty.

Outcome Criteria: Child feeds and dresses self and manages elimination independently.

Children need to learn self-care measures such as dressing, toothbrushing, bathing, and toileting so they can gain self-esteem from accomplishing these tasks. They may need modifications such as straps attached to their toothbrush so they can hold it more securely. During a bath, they should always be supervised because their lack of coordination could cause them to slip underwater and drown. You can, however, encourage them to scrub themselves and wash their hair. Toileting is often difficult because they do not have the muscle group coordination to achieve successful bowel evacuation. A high-roughage diet will prevent constipation and aid bowel evacuation. Voiding may be equally difficult because the child lacks sufficient voluntary muscle control.

Nursing Diagnosis: High risk for altered growth and development related to activity restriction secondary to cerebral palsy

Goal: Child will receive age-appropriate stimulation throughout childhood.

Outcome Criteria: Child's environment is stimulating; child expresses interest in people and activities around him; child attends school setting as free of restrictions as possible.

Children with cerebral palsy may be unable to pursue stimulating activities and surroundings. Therefore, these things must be brought to them. Some children may need more stimulating activities than others because they have difficulty concentrating on one activity for any length of time. An activity should be neither too difficult nor too easy for the child. Choose toys and activities appropriate to the child's intellectual, developmental, and motor levels.

A preschool program is essential for providing exposure to the outside world. If at all possible, school-age children with cerebral palsy should be mainstreamed so that they can be among able-bodied children. Under federal law, children with disabilities must be provided an education in the least restrictive setting possible. If they are mentally retarded, their combined mental and motor deficits may severely limit their abilities, making school placement difficult. You may need to advocate that a child be placed in a school setting that is consistent with his or her intellectual abilities.

Nursing Diagnosis: High risk for altered nutrition, less than body requirements, related to difficulty sucking in infancy and in feeding self as older child

Goal: Child will ingest an adequate nutritional intake throughout childhood.

Outcome Criteria: Child's weight will remain within 5th to 95th percentile on height-weight chart; skin turgor remains good; specific gravity of urine is 1.003 to 1.030.

Providing adequate nutrition to children with cerebral palsy is often difficult. As infants, they often suck poorly because of uncoordinated movements of the tongue, lips, and jaw; tongue thrust causes them to push food out of their mouth (a retained primitive reflex), their lip and tongue control is poor, and they have weak or uncoordinated jaw muscles. Older children have difficulty holding and controlling a spoon to bring food to their mouth. Spasticity causes children to hyperextend the head when leaning forward to take a bite, so they never feel comfortable while eating. Parents need guidance in finding a feeding pattern that works for their child. If children cannot chew or swallow well, they should have a diet of liquid or soft food. Other children can handle solids and finger foods but may take longer to eat than the average child. Because it is hard for them to stay neat while eating, they will need better protection for their clothing and the floor. It may take longer for them to eat than the rest of the family, so people will need to wait patiently for them to finish.

A hyperactive gag reflex may cause children to vomit after feeding. Be certain that infants are positioned on their side or upright after feeding to prevent vomitus aspiration.

Nursing Diagnosis: Impaired verbal communication related to neurologic impairment

Goal: Child will achieve satisfactory communication with caregivers and significant others by school age.

Outcome Criteria: Child can verbally make needs known to strangers and family members.

Most children with cerebral palsy benefit from speech therapy; this helps them learn to speak slowly and coordinate their lips and tongue to form speech sounds. Be patient with children, and allow them to form words deliberately; if they try to hurry to please you, their speech will be much less clear and communication will be impaired. For the child who cannot speak clearly, provide an alternative form of communication, such as flash cards or a picture board. Touch-screen computer programs are often used in school settings to aid communication.

Discharge Planning for Home Care

Because cerebral palsy is not always diagnosed early in infancy, parents may not learn that their child has a chronic disease until nearly 2 to 4 years later. They will need a great deal of support to help them cope with their grief and disappointment.

Help parents encourage children with cerebral palsy to reach their fullest potential within the limits of their disorder. Evaluations at health care visits should note not only whether the child is achieving this goal but also whether he and his family members find satisfaction and acceptance in his achievements. Listen to parents during health care visits and encourage them to discuss the difficulties of daily living, such as feeding problems. They may grieve because their child is not able to accomplish all the major things they had wished for during pregnancy, and they may feel defeated by the day-to-day strain of caring for the child's multiple special needs. Care of the child with a chronic illness is discussed further in Chapter 56.

Infection

Nervous system tissue is as susceptible to infection as all other body tissue. The five major infections covered here are meningitis, encephalitis, Guillain-Barré, Reye's syndrome, and botulism.

Bacterial Meningitis

Meningitis is an infection of the cerebral meninges. In the United States (except in newborns), it is caused most frequently by *Haemophilus influenzae* type B. *Neisseria meningitidis* (meningococcal meningitis) or *Diplococcus pneumoniae* (pneumococcal meningitis) are less frequently occurring types. In newborns, group B *Streptococcus* is becoming the most common cause of meningitis. In children with myelomeningocele who develop meningitis, *Pseudomonas* infection is common. Children who have had a splenectomy are particularly susceptible to meningococcal meningitis.

Meningitis occurs most often between the ages of 1 month and 5 years; half of these cases occur in children less than 1 year old. Although the disease may occur in any month, its peak incidence is in the winter (Feigin, 1990).

Pathologic organisms generally are spread to the meninges from upper respiratory tract infections, by lymphatic drainage possibly through the mastoid or sinuses, or by direct introduction by a lumbar puncture or skull fracture. Once organisms enter the meningeal space, they multiply rapidly and spread throughout the CSF. Organisms invade brain tissue through meningeal folds that extend down into the brain itself. An inflammatory response may lead to a thick, fibrinous exudate that blocks CSF flow. Brain abscess or invasion of the infection into cranial nerves may result in blindness, deafness, or facial paralysis. Pus that accumulates in the narrow aqueduct of Sylvius may cause obstruction that will lead to hydrocephalus. Brain tissue edema puts pressure on the hypopituitary gland, causing increased production of antidiuretic hormone. This causes increased edema because the body cannot excrete adequate urine. The current routine immunization of children with *H. influenzae* vaccine has limited the number of those who contract meningitis (Feigin, 1994). Meningococcal vaccine is recommended for children over 5 years of age who have been exposed to someone with this form of meningitis or for children who have had their spleen removed.

Assessment

The symptoms of meningitis may occur insidiously or suddenly. Children generally have 2 or 3 days of upper respiratory tract infection. They become increasingly irritable and complain of headaches. They may have convulsions. In some children, convulsions or shock are the first noticeable signs of illness. As the disease progresses, signs of meningeal irritability occur. Children resist neck flexion (Figure 49-13); their back may become arched and their neck hyperextended (opisthotonos). There may be cranial nerve paralysis (most typically of the third and sixth nerves, so that children will not able to follow a light through full visual fields). If the fontanelles are open, they will feel bulging and tense; if they are closed, children may develop papilledema. If the meningitis is caused by *H. influenzae*, children may develop septic arthritis. If it is caused by *N. meningitidis*, a papular or purple petechial skin rash may develop.

In the newborn, the symptoms are often vague: poor sucking, weak cry, and lethargy. After this generalized beginning, sudden cardiovascular shock, convulsions, or apnea may occur. Because the infant has open fontanelles, nuchal rigidity appears late and is not as useful a sign for diagnosis as in the older child.

Meningitis is diagnosed by history and by analysis of CSF obtained by lumbar puncture. A child with a febrile convulsion should be assumed to have meningitis until

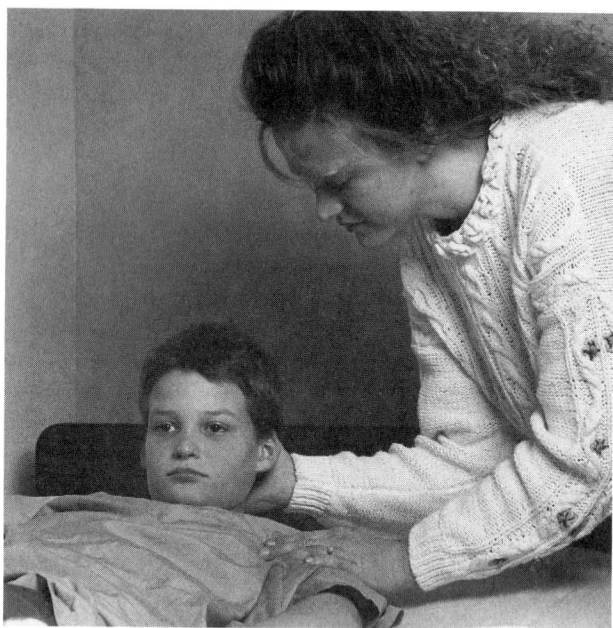

FIGURE 49-13
Testing a child for pain on flexion of the neck. (Courtesy of the Department of Medical Photography, Children's Hospital, Buffalo, NY.)

normal CSF findings prove otherwise. CSF results that indicate meningitis include an increase in white blood cell and protein level and a lowered glucose level (bacteria have fed on the glucose). In a healthy child, the glucose level in the CSF is equal to the serum glucose level. Because meningitis often spreads and causes septicemia, a blood culture is done as well. A fulminating meningitis often leads to leukopenia. If children have had close association with someone with tuberculosis, a tuberculin skin test to rule out tuberculosis meningitis will be done. A CT scan, MRI, or ultrasound may be ordered to examine for abscesses. Intracranial pressure will be measured (often over 300 mm H_2O).

Therapeutic Management

Treatment is an antibiotic as indicated by sensitivity studies; this is given intravenously for rapid effect. Intrathecal injections (directly into the CSF) may be necessary to reduce the infection, because the blood–brain barrier may prevent an antibiotic from passing freely into the CSF. If the organism identified is *H. influenzae*, ampicillin generally is the drug of choice; in other instances, cefotaxime, ceftriaxone, or chloramphenicol may be used. Therapy will be continued for a minimum of 8 to 10 days; in some children, it will take a month before the CSF cell count is back to normal. A corticosteroid such as dexamethasone or the osmotic diuretic, mannitol, may be administered to reduce intracranial pressure and help prevent hearing loss.

Children with meningitis are placed on respiratory isolation for at least 24 hours of antibiotic therapy to prevent spread of the infection.

The siblings of the ill child may be prescribed an antibiotic, such as rifampin, prophylactically. One side-effect is that this drug stains urine, tears, and sweat a deep orange color, so that contact lenses cannot be worn or they will become stained. Rifampin is also unsafe to use during pregnancy.

Meningitis is always a serious disorder. It can run a rapid, fulminating, often fatal course, although if symptoms are recognized early enough, and if treatment is effective, the child will recover with no sequelae. For a good outcome, children must receive rapid diagnosis and treatment. Neurologic sequelae, such as learning problems, convulsions, hearing impairment, mental retardation, and inability to concentrate urine must be assessed after the infection.

Nursing Diagnoses and Related Interventions

When a child has meningitis, the parents may feel responsible for the illness. They knew the child had a cold, and they wonder if they could have prevented meningitis if only they had taken him to a physician as soon as the cold symptoms started. Assure them that the symptoms of meningitis occur insidiously and that no one could have predicted the full extent of the disease from the first signs.

Encourage parents to care for the child during the illness, both to help make the child more comfortable and to help them manage their own anxiety. Teach them good isolation technique so they can perform these tasks safely.

> **Nursing Diagnosis:** Pain related to meningeal irritation
>
> **Goal:** Child will experience a tolerable degree of pain during the course of illness.
>
> **Outcome Criteria:** Child states that pain is tolerable; shows no facial grimacing or other signs of discomfort.

The hospital course for a child with meningitis is not easy. The child has a lumbar puncture on admission, so his initial impression of the hospital is of people who restrain him for a painful procedure. Continuous intravenous infusions contribute to that impression. Remember that the child feels pain when his head is flexed forward and will usually be more comfortable without a pillow. Be careful not to flex the child's neck when turning or positioning him.

On admission, a child may be extremely irritable; and although he would benefit from puppet play or drawing that would help him express how he feels about so many intrusive procedures, he is too uncomfortable to play; nothing seems to appease him. This is the result of the disease process, and he cannot help feeling this way. It is important that all health care personnel are aware of this so that they do not interpret the child's withdrawal as unfriendliness and feel hurt when their advances are rebuffed. Parents also need to understand that this is because of the disease. The child needs a good explanation of everything that is happening. He needs extra attention from health care personnel and not just when they perform painful procedures. As the child recovers, he will become less irritable and will show more interest in communicating his feelings. Promote rest for the child by keeping stimulation in his room to a minimum.

> *Nursing Diagnosis:* High risk for altered tissue perfusion (cerebral), related to increased intracranial pressure
> *Goal:* Child will not demonstrate symptoms of altered tissue perfusion during course of illness.
> *Outcome Criteria:* Child's vital signs return to normal; motor, cognitive, and sensory function are not impaired; specific gravity of urine is 1.003 to 1.030.

Observe the child carefully for signs of increased intracranial pressure. The rate of all intravenous infusions must be monitored carefully to prevent overhydration. Urine should be measured for specific gravity to detect oversecretion or undersecretion of antidiuretic hormone from pituitary pressure. Measure the child's head circumference and weigh him daily.

Monitor hearing acuity (reduced if there is compression of the eighth cranial nerve) by asking the child a question or observing if the infant listens to a music box or your voice.

Group B, Beta-hemolytic Streptococcal Meningitis

The major cause of meningitis in newborns today is the group B, beta-hemolytic streptococcal organism. Between 50 and 300 infants in every 1000 live births display a positive culture for this organism. The organism is contracted either in utero or from secretions in the birth canal at delivery. It can spread to other newborns if good handwashing technique is not used.

Group-B, beta-hemolytic streptococci colonization may result in early-onset or late-onset illness. With the early-onset form, symptoms of pneumonia become apparent in the first few hours of life. The infant will have tachypnea, apnea, and signs of shock, such as decreased urine output, extreme paleness, or hypotonia. He may develop an expiratory grunt that is made by air being forced past contracted vocal cords. This is a compensatory mechanism in newborns to maintain pressure in their alveoli on expiration and prevent alveolar collapse. Pneumonia may develop so rapidly that as many as 40% of infants who contract the infection die within 24 hours of birth.

The late-onset type often leads to meningitis instead of pneumonia. At about the age of 2 weeks, the infant may gradually become lethargic, developing a fever and upper respiratory symptoms. The fontanelles will bulge from increased intracranial pressure. Mortality from the late-onset type is lower (15% compared to 40% in early-onset type), but neurologic consequences such as hydrocephalus may occur. Gentamicin, ampicillin, and penicillin G are all effective against group-B, beta-hemolytic streptococcal infections.

It can be difficult for parents to understand how their infant suddenly became so ill. They may need considerable support in caring for the infant who is left neurologically disabled.

Encephalitis

Encephalitis is an inflammation of brain tissue and, possibly, the meninges as well. It can arise from protozoan, bacterial, fungal, or viral invasion. Enteroviruses are the most frequent cause, followed by arboviruses. A number of encephalitis viruses, such as St. Louis encephalitis and eastern equine encephalitis, are borne by mosquitoes, and in endemic areas mosquito repellents are strongly suggested; these forms of encephalitis are seen most during the summer months. Encephalitis can also result from direct invasion of the CSF during lumbar puncture. It may occur as a complication of common childhood diseases, such as measles, mumps, or chickenpox; it is crucial, therefore, that children receive immunization against these childhood diseases.

Assessment
Symptoms of encephalitis may begin gradually or suddenly. These include headache, high temperature, and signs of meningeal irritation, such as nuchal rigidity and Kernig's sign (pain on extending the knee when the thigh is bent on the abdomen; Figure 49-14). There may be symptoms of ataxia, muscle weakness or paralysis, diplopia, confusion, or irritability. The child becomes increasingly lethargic and eventually comatose.

The diagnosis is made by the history and physical assessment. Laboratory studies of CSF generally reveal an elevated leukocyte count and elevated protein and glucose levels. An EEG shows widespread cerebral involvement.

Therapeutic Management
An antipyretic is given to control fever. Take and record vital signs frequently, because brain stem involvement may affect cardiac or respiratory rates. Mechanical ventilation may be required to maintain the child's respirations during the acute phase. If the cause is viral, antibiotics will not be effective. Anticonvulsants may be prescribed for seizures; some commonly used drugs are listed in Table 49-5. A steroid such as dexamethasone

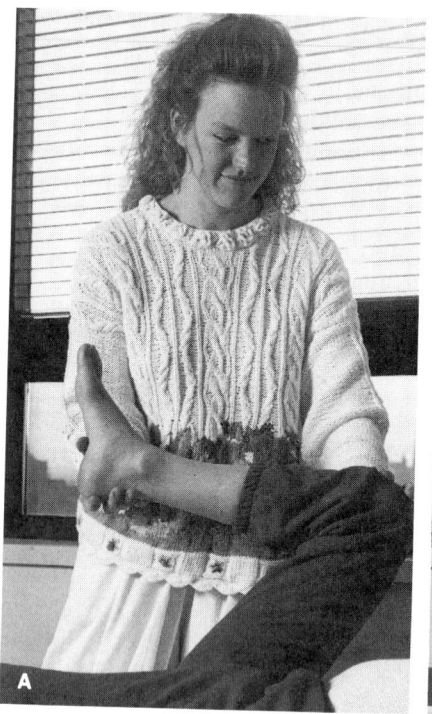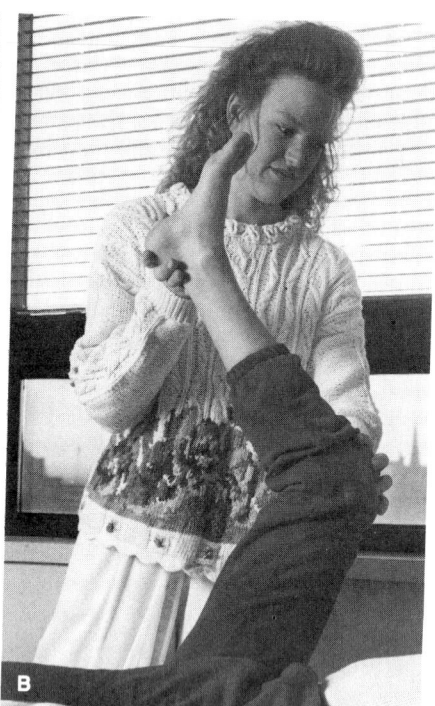

FIGURE 49-14
Testing for Kernig's sign. (A) Flex leg on abdomen. (B) Straighten leg. If child has pain, meningeal irritation is suggested. (Courtesy of the Department of Medical Photography, Children's Hospital, Buffalo, NY.)

may be prescribed to decrease brain edema and intracranial pressure.

Encephalitis is always a serious diagnosis because, even though the child may recover from the initial attack, there may be residual neurologic damage, such as seizures or mental retardation. Parents may find it hard to believe that their child is seriously ill (she only seemed tired and had a slight headache). They will find it even harder to accept a diagnosis of permanent impairment such as mental retardation. They will need follow-up care after the hospitalization to help them deal with their grief, shock, and anger. Although complete recovery is possible, many parents will find themselves with a child whose health and abilities have been changed forever.

Reye's Syndrome

Reye's syndrome is acute encephalitis with accompanying fatty infiltration of the liver, heart, lungs, pancreas, and skeletal muscle. It occurs in children from 1 to 18 years of age. There is no difference in sex distribution; a sibling has an increased risk of developing the disease, perhaps because of a genetic susceptibility.

The cause of Reye's syndrome is unknown, but it generally occurs after a viral infection such as varicella (chickenpox) or an upper respiratory infection, so it may be caused by viral invasion of the tissues or specific toxic reactions to a virus. Research has confirmed the association of acetylsalicylic acid (aspirin) intake during the viral infection with the onset of Reye's afterward

Table 49-5. *Anticonvulsants*

Drug	Action	Side-Effects
Carbamazepine (Tegretol)	Control partial, generalized, and mixed seizures	Leukopenia, thrombocytopenia, drowsiness, abdominal distress
Ethosuzimide (Zarontin)	Depresses motor cortex to prevent absence seizures	Rare blood dyscrasias, drowsiness, nausea
Phenobarbital	Controls generalized tonic-clonic seizures, cortical focal seizures, and status epilepticus	Rare blood dyscrasias, hyperkinesis, drowsiness
Phenytoin (Dilantin)	Inhibits motor cortex to inhibit tonic-clonic and psychomotor seizures and status epilepticus	Rare blood dyscrasias, gingival hyperplasia, hirsutism, ataxia, fetal hydantoin syndrome
Primidone (Mysoline)	Mechanism of action is unknown, but it controls tonic-clonic, psychomotor, and focal seizures	Severe megaloblastic anemia possible
Valproic acid (Depakene)	Controls absence seizures	Leukopenia, thrombocytopenia, drowsiness, abdominal distress

(Porter et al., 1990). It is a perplexing disease, and its seriousness is difficult for parents to grasp when it follows such common infections.

Assessment

After seeming to recover from an initial viral illness, children may become ill again 1 to 3 weeks later, with lethargy, vomiting, agitation, anorexia, confusion, and combativeness. The vomiting may be so severe it leads to dehydration. Symptoms in adolescents may mimic those of drug intoxication (inappropriate language, visual hallucinations, pupillary dilation, slurred speech, and staggering gait). Liver infiltration involves mitochondrial fatty droplet infiltration, enzyme abnormalities, particularly serum glutamic-oxaloacetic transaminase (SGOT) and serum glutamic-pyruvic transaminase (SGPT), and hypothrombinemia. Hypoglycemia will be present, and blood ammonia levels will be elevated because of poor liver function. Although CSF findings remain normal, cerebral symptoms progress from confusion to stupor to deep coma, with seizures and respiratory arrest resulting from pressure on the brain stem.

If left untreated, Reye's syndrome is rapidly fatal. Without acute respiratory support, as many as two thirds of children with the disease die within 2 or 3 days of onset. Fortunately, those who recover do so quickly and generally without residual neurologic effects. In addition, because health care providers are aware of the link between acetylsalicylic acid and Reye's syndrome, they can advise parents to give their children acetaminophen (Tylenol) for fever instead. School-age children should know this as well, and the rule applies to persons up through 21 years. Because Reye's syndrome can be so easily prevented, it is now relatively rare.

Laboratory diagnosis of Reye's syndrome is confirmed by an elevated SGPT and SGOT liver function test, elevated serum ammonia, normal direct bilirubin, delayed prothrombin time and partial thromboplastin time, decreased blood glucose, elevated blood urea nitrogen, elevated serum amylase, elevated short-chain fatty acids, and an elevated white blood count. A lumbar puncture to rule out other infection is done. CSF findings are normal, except for slightly elevated opening pressure. A skull CT scan or sonogram will be normal at first; later this will show cerebral edema and decreased ventricle size. An EEG may be ordered. A liver biopsy will reveal fatty infiltration, but this is optional because of the risk of hemorrhage from the delayed prothrombin time (Louis, 1994).

Therapeutic Management

The child is not infectious at the onset of Reye's syndrome. Therapy is directed toward supporting respiratory function, controlling hypoglycemia, and reducing brain edema. He or she will be started on a 10% or 15% dextrose solution to reduce cerebral edema and to correct hypoglycemia. Mannitol or a corticosteroid may also be ordered.

Reye's syndrome is categorized by stages of involvement from 1 to 5, depending on the amount of the child's lethargy or presence of coma. Frequent neurologic evaluations need to be performed to evaluate that a child is not entering a more serious stage of involvement. Blood sugar, electrolytes, and prothrombin level are monitored carefully. Sedating children who are combative (struggling against procedures, thrashing wildly) is controversial because it renders the neurologic evaluation invalid, but phenobarbital is given occasionally.

If children progress to stage III involvement, fluid intake must be carefully regulated to prevent overload and increased cerebral edema. A central venous pressure line or Swan-Ganz catheter may be inserted to monitor venous pressure and cardiac capability, and intracranial pressure needs to be monitored as well. A Foley catheter may be inserted. A nasogastric tube may be inserted to prevent vomiting and aspiration. If the child seems in danger of respiratory arrest, an endotracheal tube and artificial ventilation may be tried to maintain Pco_2 between 20 and 25 mm Hg. A low Pco_2 causes cerebral vessel constriction and lowered intracranial pressure. It may be necessary to administer pancuronium bromide to paralyze respiratory muscles, which will allow maximum ventilation. If the child wakes from coma in an intensive care unit, she will need to be oriented to her surroundings, since her last clear memory may be the day before she became ill.

Guillain-Barré Syndrome

Guillain-Barré (inflammatory polyradiculoneuropathy) is a perplexing syndrome involving both motor and sensory portions of peripheral nerves. It affects both sexes and occurs most often in school-age children and adolescents.

The cause of the condition is unknown, but it is suspected that the reaction is immune mediated, following upper respiratory and gastrointestinal illnesses and immunization. Inflammation of the nerve fibers apparently causes temporary demyelinization of the nerve sheaths. (Murray, 1993).

Assessment

Children experience peripheral neuritis several days after the primary infection. Tendon reflexes are decreased or absent. Muscle paralysis and paresthesia (loss of sensation) begins first in the legs and then spreads to involve the arms and trunk and head. Cranial nerve involvement leads to facial weakness and difficulty in swallowing. As the respiratory muscles become involved, spontaneous respirations are no longer possible. Ten percent to 20% of those who develop the syndrome will have respiratory involvement severe enough to warrant mechanical ventilation.

A significant laboratory finding is an elevated CSF protein level. An EEG may show denervation and decreased nerve conduction velocity.

Therapeutic Management

The therapy for Guillain-Barré syndrome is supportive care until the process runs its course (paralysis peaks at 3 weeks, followed by gradual recovery). A course of prednisone to halt the autoimmune response may be tried, but its use is controversial. Plasmapheresis or transfusion of immune serum globulin may shorten the course of the illness (Epstein & Sladky, 1990; Shahar et al., 1990). Care of the totally paralyzed child includes preventing all the effects of extreme immobility while guarding respiratory function. The child's cardiac and respiratory function must be closely monitored. A Foley catheter is usually inserted to monitor urine output. The child may be fed by total parenteral nutrition or by enteral stomach tube to prevent tracheal aspiration. If the child has discomfort from neuritis, adequate analgesia can be administered.

To prevent muscle contracture, the child should have passive range of motion exercises every 4 hours. Turning and repositioning the child every 2 hours is important to protect skin integrity. Providing adequate stimulation for the long weeks when the child is unable to perform any care for himself or herself is also important. Ninety-five percent of children recover completely, without any residual effects of the syndrome. This can be credited to conscientious nursing care that wards off complications during the course of the illness.

Botulism

Botulism occurs when spores of *Clostridium botulinum* colonize and produce toxins in the immature intestine. The source of the spores is generally unknown, but honey and corn syrup are frequent contaminants. The disease is not infectious and generally occurs in infants under 6 months of age.

With infant botulism, symptoms occur within a few hours of ingestion of contaminated food. Almost immediately there is generalized weakness, hypotonia, listlessness, a weak cry, and a diminished gag reflex. This is followed by a flaccid paralysis of the bulbar muscles that leads to diminished respiratory function. The organism can be cultured from stools or serum. Electromyography may be helpful to support the diagnosis.

Treatment is supportive care. The antitoxin for botulism is rarely given to infants because it is made from a horse serum base and can cause a hypersensitivity reaction; it is generally not necessary for full recovery. Infant botulism may account for some fatalities from sudden infant death syndrome (Carroll & Loughlin, 1994).

Paroxysmal Disorders

A paroxysmal disorder is one that occurs suddenly and recurrently. Convulsions, headaches, and breath-holding spells are the most frequent types seen in childhood.

Recurrent Convulsions

A *convulsion* is an involuntary contraction of muscle caused by abnormal electrical brain discharges. About 2% to 4% of children will have at least one convulsion by the time they reach adulthood (Hauser, 1994). These episodes are always frightening to parents and other children. Although convulsions may be idiopathic (without cause), they can also be attributed to infection, trauma, or tumor growth. Familiar or polygenic inheritance may be responsible. Fifty percent of seizures are unexplainable. They are not so much a disease as symptoms of an underlying disorder and should be investigated carefully (see the Focus on Cultural Awareness box).

The term *epilepsy* comes from a Greek word meaning "to take hold of" and refers to a person with chronic convulsions. The preferred terms now are *seizures* or *convulsions,* since epilepsy carries the stigma of mental retardation, behavioral disorders, institutionalization, or just unexplainable strangeness. This is unfair for children who have episodic seizures.

The types and causes of seizures vary according to the child's age. They have been categorized by the International League Against Epilepsy as partial seizures and generalized seizures (Box 49-1). With partial seizures, only one hemisphere of the brain is involved; with generalized seizures, the disturbance involves the entire brain. Loss of consciousness will occur. It is important that seizures be differentiated by their degree of

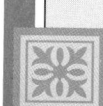

FOCUS ON CULTURAL AWARENESS

The degree of understanding about the cause of disorders such as recurrent seizures varies in different cultures. Because the cause of recurrent seizures is often unknown (idiopathic), it has in the past been attributed to an invasion by evil spirits. Many people today still fear that recurrent seizures will lead to mental retardation. Adults with recurrent seizures may be refused jobs because they are viewed as undependable. Being aware of these common misconceptions helps the nurse understand parents' anxiety about the diagnosis of recurrent seizures. It can accentuate the need for careful planning to maintain self-esteem in the child.

Box 49-1
Classifications of Seizures

I. Partial Seizures
  A. Elementary symptomatology
    1. With motor symptoms
    2. With sensory symptoms
  B. Complex symptomatology
    1. With impairment of consciousness only
    2. With cognitive symptoms
    3. With affective symptoms
    4. With psychosensory symptoms
    5. Compound forms
  C. Partial seizures secondarily generalized
II. Generalized Seizures
  A. Absence seizures
  B. Myoclonic
  C. Atonic
  D. Clonic
  E. Tonic-clonic

(International League Against Epilepsy. [1981]. Proposal for revised clinical and electroencephalographic classification of epileptic seizures. *Epilepsia, 22,* 489.)

severity so that dosages of seizure medication can be adjusted accordingly. See Box 49-2 for a summary of anticonvulsant medications.

Causes of Seizures in the Newborn Period

Seizure activity in the newborn period may be difficult to recognize because it may consist only of twitching of the head, arms, or eyes; slight cyanosis; and perhaps respiratory difficulty or apnea. Afterward, the infant may appear limp and flaccid. Whereas older children often have seizures of unknown etiology, 75% of seizures in neonates have a known cause. These include perinatal injury, effects of anoxia, or a metabolic disorder.

EEGs in the newborn may be normal, despite extensive disease, owing to the nervous system's immaturity. A noticeably abnormal EEG, therefore, generally means a poor prognosis, indicating that the involvement this early in life must be severe. Lumbar puncture in newborns is also not too revealing, because nearly 20% of all newborns have abnormal CSF as measured by adult standards. Protein is increased, and there may be a few red blood cells from rupture of subarachnoid capillaries under the pressure of birth.

A high dosage of anticonvulsant medicine may be needed to control convulsions in newborns because they metabolize drugs more rapidly than older infants. In adults, for example, phenobarbital may be administered in the range of 1.5 mg per kilogram of body weight per day. In newborns, the dose might be as high as 3 to 10 mg/kg/day.

Trauma. The birth process normally involves head trauma of some degree. An unusually tight maternal cervix, poor use of forceps, or placenta previa that results in anoxia may lead to seizure disorders. Subdural hematomas resulting from birth pressure do not usually cause convulsions, because the skull suture lines are so expandable at this age that pressure on the brain is not severe.

Metabolic Disorders. Although newborns have a greater resistance to hypoglycemia-induced seizures than older children, they are susceptible in some instances. If glucose levels fall below 30 mg/100 mL in full-term infants (20 mg/100 mL in infants born prematurely), the infant is at risk for seizures. Babies of diabetic mothers are particularly prone to hypoglycemia and should be observed carefully (see Chapter 26). Hypocalcemia and lack of pyridoxine (vitamin B_6) can also cause seizures. In all these situations, therapy will be aimed toward replacing the metabolic deficit with sufficient amounts of glucose, calcium, or vitamin B_6. If the deficiencies causing hypocalcemia and pyridoxine deficiency are corrected promptly, the prognosis is good. With hypoglycemia, the prognosis is more guarded, however, because lack of glucose in the brain cells may have caused permanent brain damage. Hypocalcemia and hypoglycemia are discussed further in Chapters 26 and 48.

Neonatal Infection. Occasionally, neonates will have infections of the central nervous system that are evi-

Box 49-2
Safe Administration of Anticonvulsants

- Many anticonvulsants cause drowsiness. Caution children to be careful around motor vehicles.
- Many cause thrombocytopenia. Observe for easy bruising.
- Caution adolescents not to drink alcohol while taking anticonvulsant agents as the effect can by synergistic (accentuated).
- Safety during pregnancy has not been established for most anticonvulsants. Phenytoin is a known teratogen.
- If gastrointestinal upset occurs, administer with food.
- Many anticonvulsants are metabolized by the liver. Use caution administering such drugs to children with liver disease.
- Caution parents and children not to discontinue anticonvulsant therapy abruptly, since this can lead to status epilepticus.

denced by convulsions. Convulsions that occur after the third day of life are much more likely to be caused by infection than by trauma. Newborns whose membranes were ruptured for more than 24 hours prior to delivery are more prone to infection than those whose membranes were ruptured at or close to delivery.

Kernicterus. *Kernicterus* is the buildup of indirect bilirubin in brain tissue. It occurs most commonly in infants born with a blood incompatibility, such as an Rh or ABO incompatibility. When brain cells are invaded by indirect bilirubin, seizures may occur. In this instance, the accompanying jaundice is a warning sign of buildup. Blood incompatibility is discussed in Chapter 15.

Causes of Seizures in the Infant and Toddler Periods

Infantile Spasms. Infantile spasms are classified as generalized seizures—"salaam" and "jackknife"—or infantile myoclonic seizures, characterized by very rapid movements of the trunk; the infant suddenly slumps forward from a sitting position or falls from a standing position. These episodes may occur as frequently as 100 times a day.

The cause is unknown, but the spasms apparently result from a failure of normal organized electrical activity in the brain. Sometimes, the seizures accompany a pre-existing form of neurologic damage. About 95% of these infants are mentally retarded. In about 50% of affected infants, there is an identifiable cause such as trauma or a metabolic disease such as phenylketonuria. In the other 50%, there may be no identifiable cause. They may follow invasion by viruses such as herpes or cytomegalovirus (Riikonen, 1993).

In infants whose development was previously normal, intellectual development appears to halt and even regress after seizures start. Children with infantile spasms demonstrate a high-voltage chaotic discharge called *hypsarrhythmia* on an EEG tracing.

Seizures can be reduced somewhat with drug therapy such as valproate, phenytoin, phenobarbital, ACTH, and steroids such as prednisone. The infantile seizure phenomenon seems to "burn itself out" by 2 years of age. The associated mental retardation or developmental lag remains, however, so children need follow-up planning and care (Kongelbeck, 1990).

Febrile Convulsions. Convulsions associated with high fever (102° to 104°F; 38.9° to 40.0°C) are the most common in preschool children, or between 5 months and 5 years of age, although seizures may occur as early as 3 months and as late as 7 years. There generally are no more than five to seven such episodes in the child's life. The seizure shows an active tonic-clonic pattern, which lasts 15 to 20 seconds. The EEG tracing is normal. There usually is a history of other family members having had similar convulsions (Rylance, 1990).

It is unclear whether seizures are initiated by a consistently high fever or a sudden spike of temperature, which brings about a generalized tonic-clonic seizure (Berg, 1993). The seizure subsides quickly once the fever is lowered.

Prevention of Febrile Convulsions. Because these convulsions arise with sudden high fever, they are largely preventable. If acetaminophen is given to keep fever below 101°F (38.4°C), convulsions rarely occur. They happen most often when children develop a fever at night, when the parent is not aware of it, until the temperature is already high, or when a parent is reluctant to give acetaminophen in large enough doses to be therapeutic. See Table 37-4 for recommended dosages of Tylenol. Although this type of seizure can be prevented by phenobarbital, it is useless to give the drug preventively during an upper respiratory infection. Phenobarbital takes 2 or 3 days to reach blood levels high enough to be effective. By this time, convulsions would already have occurred. In addition, phenobarbital may reduce cognitive function in children (Farwell et al., 1990).

The child who has one febrile convulsion usually is not given further treatment, but parents should be counseled not to let the child develop a second high fever. A child who has had two or more febrile seizures may be placed on a maintenance dose of phenobarbital, although whether this prevents further seizures is unproved and may make the child so sleepy he or she is unable to achieve well in school. For this reason the practice is controversial. Teach parents that every child who has a febrile seizure must be seen by a physician. A good rule is to assume that the child in this situation has meningitis until it is ruled out by a complete neurologic workup.

Therapeutic Management. Teach parents that after the seizure subsides, they should sponge the child with tepid water to reduce the fever quickly. They should not put the child in the bathtub, however, since it would be easy for the child to slip underwater during a second seizure. A parent might not be able to hold the convulsing child's head above water. Alcohol or cold water is also not advisable; extreme cooling causes shock to an immature nervous system, and alcohol can be absorbed by the skin or the fumes inhaled in toxic amounts, compounding the child's problems. Parents should not attempt to give oral medications such as acetaminophen, because the child will be in a drowsy, or *postictal,* state following the seizure and might aspirate the medicine. If attempts to reduce the child's temperature by sponging are unsuccessful, advise parents to put a cold washcloth on the child's forehead and transport the child, lightly clothed, to a health care facility for immediate evaluation.

Additional treatment will depend on the underlying cause of the fever. A lumbar puncture will be performed to rule out meningitis. Antipyretic drugs to keep the fever below seizure levels will be administered. Appropriate antibiotic therapy will be started, depending on the type of infection.

Many parents need to be assured that febrile convulsions do not lead to brain damage and that their child is almost always completely well afterward.

Poisoning or Drugs. The possibility of poisoning must be considered in all children who have a first seizure. Although poisoning is most likely in the age group between 6 months and 3 years, it must be considered again in adolescence when drugs may be intentionally self-administered. Seizures can also be a late symptom of encephalopathy caused by lead poisoning.

Types of Seizures in Children Over 3 Years of Age

Over half of children who have recurrent seizures before puberty have an idiopathic type—the cause of the seizures cannot be discovered. Fortunately, even without a clearly understood cause, medication controls these idiopathic seizures in almost all affected children. Other seizures in this age group occur because of organic causes. They generally result from focal or diffuse brain injury that has left residual damage. The injury may have been the result of laceration of brain tissue in a car accident or fall, hemorrhage due to blood dyscrasia, infection (meningitis or encephalitis), anoxia, or toxic conditions such as lead poisoning. The possibility that a growing brain tumor is causing brain irritation must be considered.

Psychomotor Seizures. Psychomotor seizures vary greatly in extent and symptoms and tend to be the most difficult to control. They are classified as partial seizures and occur apparently because of dysfunction in the temporal lobe. A CT scan may show scar tissue. The child may have a slight aura, but it is rarely as definite as that seen with tonic-clonic seizures.

As an example, the seizure may begin with a sudden change in posture, such as an arm dropping suddenly to the side. The child slumps to the ground, unconscious. He may have circumoral pallor. He regains consciousness in less than 5 minutes. He may be slightly drowsy afterward but does not have an actual postictal stage as in tonic-clonic seizures. The child with psychomotor seizures generally has a normal EEG.

Common drugs used are phenytoin, carbamazepine, and primidone. If these are not effective, surgery to remove the epileptogenic focus may be attempted (Wheless, 1991).

Focal Seizures. Focal seizures originate from a specific brain area. A typical focal seizure begins in the fingers and spreads to the wrist, arm, and face in a clonic contraction. If the movement remains localized, there will be no loss of consciousness. When the spread is extensive, the seizure becomes generalized; it is then impossible to differentiate this type of seizure from a tonic-clonic convulsion. Thus, it is important to observe children carefully as a convulsion begins. Focal seizures may be due to something as specific as a rapidly growing brain tumor. Documenting the spread (a Jacksonian march) can help localize the spot where the seizure first began.

Absence Seizures. Absence seizures, formerly known as *petit mal,* are classified as generalized. They usually consist of a staring spell that lasts for a few seconds. A child might be reciting in class when he pauses and stares for 1 to 5 seconds before continuing the recitation; he is unaware that time has passed. Rhythmic blinking and twitching of the mouth or an extremity may accompany the staring. Absence seizures can occur up to 100 times per day. An EEG usually demonstrates a typical 3 wave/sec spike and slow-wave discharge. Such seizures tend to occur more frequently in girls than boys. The usual age of occurrence is 6 to 7 years (Porter, 1993).

Children with absence episodes may be accused of daydreaming in school and may be referred to the school nurse for behavior problems. These children generally have normal intelligence, although if they have frequent episodes, they may be doing poorly in school because they are missing so much instructional content.

Absence seizures can usually be demonstrated in children by asking them to hyperventilate and count out loud. If they are susceptible to such seizures, they will breathe in and out deeply, possibly 10 times, stop and stare for 3 seconds, then continue to hyperventilate and count, unaware that they paused.

No first aid measures are necessary for absence seizures. Downplaying the importance of these episodes will help children maintain a positive self-image.

Absence seizures can be controlled by ethosuximide (Zarontin) or by valproate. If seizures are fully controlled by medication, children can participate in normal school activities and ride a bicycle. They should not swim alone, but no child should swim alone in any case. If seizures cannot be controlled fully, parents need to anticipate potentially hazardous situations during the child's day, such as crossing a busy street on the way to school or learning to drive. This is crucial for adolescents who are eager to get a driver's license; their tendency to seizures should be evaluated carefully, for their own safety as well as others'.

About one third to one half of all children with absence seizures "outgrow them" by adulthood. This does not mean that treatment is not necessary during childhood. Absence seizures usually occur independently of tonic-clonic seizures, although it is possible for children to manifest both types. Some children's seizure pattern changes from absence involvement to tonic-clonic involvement as they approach adulthood.

Tonic-Clonic Seizures. Typical tonic-clonic seizures (formerly termed *grand mal seizures*) are generalized, consisting of four stages. There may be a *prodromal* period of hours or days, an *aura,* or warning, immediately before the seizure, the tonic-clonic convulsion, and finally, a postictal state. Not all four stages occur with every seizure.

The prodromal period may consist of drowsiness, dizziness, malaise, lack of coordination, or tension. Parents may observe simply that the child is "not himself." As the child reaches school age, he may be able to predict from these vague preliminary feelings when he is going to have a seizure.

The aura, or second phase, may reflect the portion of the brain in which the seizure originates. Smelling unpleasant odors (often reported as feces) denotes activity in the medial portion of the temporal lobe. Seeing flashing lights suggests the occipital area; repeated hallucinations arise from the temporal lobe; numbness of an extremity relates to the opposite parietal lobe; and a "Cheshire cat grin" is from the frontal lobe. Young children, unable to describe or understand an aura, may scream in fright or run to their parent with its onset. Note exactly what symptoms the child experiences during this time, because this may help to localize the involved brain portion.

The third phase is the tonic stage. All muscles of the body contract, and the child falls to the ground. Extremities stiffen; the face distorts. This phase lasts only about 20 seconds, but because the respiratory muscles are contracted, the child may experience hypoxia and turn cyanotic. Contraction of the throat prevents swallowing, so saliva collects in the mouth. The child may bite his tongue when his jaws contract.. As the chest muscles contract initially, air is pushed through the glottis, producing a guttural cry.

The convulsion then enters a clonic stage, in which muscles of the body rapidly contract and relax, producing quick, jerky motions. The child may blow bubbles or foamy saliva and, if he bit his tongue when his jaw spasmed shut, he may have blood in his mouth. He may be incontinent of stool and urine. This phase also lasts about 20 seconds.

Following the tonic-clonic period, the child falls into a sound sleep (coma), called the *postictal period.* He will sleep soundly for 1 to 4 hours and will rouse only to painful stimuli during this time. When he awakens, he often experiences a severe headache. He has no memory of the seizure.

Convulsions may occur only at night. The child wakes in the morning with a bitten tongue, blood on the pillow, or a bed wet with urine. In the child with persistent bedwetting, the possibility of nocturnal seizures must be considered.

Children with this type of convulsion generally have an abnormal EEG pattern, although this is not always the case. Other family members may have similarly abnormal EEG patterns without any symptoms.

Therapy usually includes the daily administration of oral phenobarbital, which has the advantage of being inexpensive. If the dosage is too heavy, the child may be drowsy and too sleepy to do well in school. Phenobarbital dosages should be tapered, never stopped suddenly, since the body becomes dependent on it. Rapid withdrawal will bring on a convulsion.

Children with tonic-clonic convulsions also may be given phenytoin sodium (Dilantin) to control seizures. One nontoxic side-effect of phenytoin is painless hypertrophy of the gums. This necessitates good oral hygiene and can be a problem when a child is having an orthodontic appliance fitted. Unless the gum hypertrophy is extensive, however, it is not sufficient reason to discontinue Dilantin. Other commonly prescribed drugs are valproate (Depakane) and carbamazepine (Tegretol; Glaze, 1994). Medications are usually continued until the child has been seizure free for 2 to 3 years.

Some children may be placed on a ketogenic diet (Gasch, 1990). This diet is high in fat and low in protein and carbohydrate. It causes the child to have a high level of ketones, which decreases myoclonic or tonic-clonic seizure activity. Because a ketogenic diet is monotonous for children and difficult for parents to prepare, however, it is hard to maintain for very long.

Status Epilepticus. Status epilepticus convulsions occur in rapid succession without pause. This is potentially serious because the child does not have a chance to aerate his lungs well. Intravenous diazepam (Valium) followed by intravenous phenytoin halts seizures dramatically. Diazepam must be administered with extreme caution, however, because any accidental infiltration into subcutaneous tissue causes extensive tissue sloughing. Status epilepticus convulsions may also be relieved by intravenous phenobarbital sodium. Lorazepam, a long-acting benzodiazepine, may also be used. Oxygen administration helps to relieve cyanosis. Parents may administer diazepam by enema at home (Dieckmann, 1994).

Assessment of the Child With Seizures

A thorough pregnancy history is obtained on children with seizures. Events immediately prior to the seizure as well as an accurate description of the seizure itself should also be recorded. Overall behavior in the last few weeks should be documented. Is the child an A student who has been getting Ds lately? Has the parent noticed bedwetting? These might be signs of small seizures occurring in school or at night. The child should have a complete physical and neurologic examination as well as blood studies to rule out metabolic or infectious processes. A lumbar puncture will be done to rule out meningitis or bleeding in the CSF. A CT scan, skull x-ray film, or EEG will be done if indicated. During the EEG, the child may be given stimulation such as rhythm patterns and flashing lights or may be asked to hyperventilate to see if a seizure can be provoked.

Nursing Diagnoses and Related Interventions

Nursing Diagnosis: High risk for injury related to tonic-clonic seizure

Goal: Child will not be injured during seizure.

Outcome Criteria: Child experiences no aspiration or traumatic injury.

The child must be protected from hurting himself during a tonic-clonic convulsion (see the Focus on Family Teaching box). Restraining the child's thrashing extremities is not advisable, since it is difficult for the adult and could result in injury to either person because of the amount of force needed to keep the child still. It is particularly important that a tongue blade not be used in early school-age children, who tend to have loose anterior teeth that are on the verge of falling out.

Remaining calm is also important; be aware that people are frightened by the sight of a child convulsing, because the action is so forceful and violent. It is reassuring for them to see someone calm and in control of the situation and that there is no reason to be afraid. If the child passes rapidly from one convulsion into another (status epilepticus), he will need supplemental oxygen and therapy to counteract this.

Nursing Diagnosis: Altered family processes related to diagnosis of long-term illness in child

Goal: Family will maintain functional system of support for each member throughout the course of the illness.

Outcome Criteria: Child, parents, and other family members express fears and questions about disease to health care team; parents discuss ways to accommodate illness in their daily life (e.g., medication schedules, school, sports activities, ‚plans for vacation, and discipline).

As soon as the diagnosis of a convulsive disorder is made, parents and children need to be told it is likely to signify a long-term disease. Although the seizures can be controlled with medication, the disease is not cured. If the child neglects her medication, seizures are apt to recur. Most children are given tablets rather than liquid medication, because the latter tends to settle at the bottom of the bottle, resulting in overdiluted or overconcentrated doses that might allow seizures to break through. Parents must plan to have enough medication

FOCUS ON FAMILY TEACHING

Q. My 10-year-old son has begun having tonic-clonic convulsions. What steps do I need to take to keep him safe during a seizure?

A. The main way a child could hurt himself during a seizure is injuring an extremity by striking it against a nearby object or aspirating mouth secretions. The following are recommended preventive measures.

• Remain calm.

• Move away furniture or any sharp object.

• Turn your son gently on his side or abdomen with his head turned to the side to prevent aspiration of unswallowed mouth secretions.

• Don't restrain him other than to keep his head turned to the side so that mouth secretions continue to drain. Restraining the child could result in injury because of the amount of force necessary.

• Do not attempt to place a stick or padded tongue blade between the child's teeth. Trying to force a tongue blade into the mouth this way could break the tongue blade or loosen teeth.

• A convulsing child is an abnormal sight and always attracts a crowd. Ask people who are only interested spectators to move away.

• A child having this type of convulsion may have some slight cyanosis during the tonic and clonic stages, but these stages are so short that administering oxygen is not needed.

• Following any convulsion, telephone your primary care provider and notify him or her of the convulsion so arrangements for any necessary follow-up care can be made.

• If your child should pass rapidly from one convulsion into another (status epilepticus), he may need supplemental oxygen and you may need to administer diazepam. If this happens, telephone your emergency medical service number.

for a trip away from home or for summer camp. Abrupt discontinuation of seizure medications (particularly phenobarbital) may result in severe seizures.

The child will need to be monitored frequently during childhood to be certain that a medication dosage is adequate. He or she will need periodic blood sampling to ascertain whether therapeutic blood levels of the medication are being maintained.

Parents should be given as much information as possible about the cause of their child's seizures. This will help them feel that they are dealing with a known disease, not an unexplainable and unpredictable illness. If the cause of the seizures is unknown, parents can be reassured that the treatment is known. Their child can be expected to respond to anticonvulsant medication as well as the child whose seizures have a known cause such as recent trauma.

Parents need to make a strong effort to treat children with seizures as a normal member of the family. They need to know that scolding the child, asking her to do household chores, or insisting that she do her homework will not cause seizures. A few children with absence seizures can initiate them by hyperventilating and may try to manipulate those around them to gain sympathy. Like the 2-year-old who throws temper tantrums to try to get his way, the child who deliberately has an absence seizure should be ignored and his demands should not be met. The few children who use this extreme form of manipulation are disturbed emotionally and should be referred for counseling.

Parents need to be assured that occasional seizures in children are not harmful. Unless status epilepticus occurs and the child becomes anoxic, the chance that their child will be injured during a seizure is remote. They need not worry about the child becoming mentally retarded nor heed other popular misconceptions about seizures. Although some children who have seizures are also mentally retarded, the retardation and the seizures were caused by the same event; the seizures did not cause the retardation. At every health care visit, parents need time to ask questions about their child's care and to express any concerns they have. There are so many "scare stories" about convulsions that every parent is likely to believe some of these stories unless counseled otherwise.

As a rule, children with convulsions should attend regular school and participate in active sports. Many teachers are frightened of the responsibility of having a child with convulsions assigned to their classes. They need to become well informed about seizure control. Children with seizures should participate in gym classes. Being physically active tends to reduce the frequency of seizures and is healthier than being sedentary (see the Nursing Care Plan, p. 1552).

In many children, seizures increase at puberty. This may be the result of glandular changes or of sudden growth and the need for an increased medicine dosage. It may result in part from adolescent rebellion against prescribed routines of medicine-taking. An adolescent who rebels in this way needs help to channel his feelings (which must be respected—he cannot become an independent adult until he frees himself of dependence) toward less harmful means of expression.

All anticonvulsant medications are potentially teratogenic. Adolescent girls must be made aware of this. They may choose to delay childbearing until later in life when their medication can be reduced or even discontinued.

Breath-Holding

Breath-holding is a phenomenon that occurs in young children when they are stressed or angry. The child breathes in and, because he is upset, does not breathe out again or else breathes out and then does not inhale again. As brain cells become anoxic, the child becomes cyanotic and slumps to the floor, momentarily unconscious. With loss of consciousness, the child begins breathing again. Color returns to normal and he is revived. The child needs no therapy except reassurance that he is all right. Breath-holding is frightening but represents the immaturity of the child's neurologic control. This differs from a temper tantrum in which a child deliberately attempts to hold his breath and pass out (see Chapter 30).

Headache

Headache in children under school age is extremely rare, although children may complain of "headache" in imitation of their parents. Preschoolers may have headache with a fever, however, because of increased cerebral blood flow and intracranial pressure. As the child reaches school age, headaches may occur as a result of conditions as minor as eyestrain and sinusitis or as serious as a brain tumor. Headache pain results from meningeal or vascular irritation. The brain itself is insensitive to pain, so a cerebral tumor may be present for a long time before meningeal irritation occurs and pain symptoms are apparent. With a brain tumor, pain becomes evident on changing body position, so a young child who reports headache after getting up should be carefully evaluated. Pain from a brain tumor is also generally occipital, so asking the child to indicate where it hurts will help determine whether there is a tumor.

Migraine Headache

Migraine headache refers to a specific type of headache that begins with an aura of visual disturbance such as diplopia or a zigzag pattern across the visual field. The pain that follows is generally unilateral and extremely intense. It is usually accompanied by nausea and vomiting (Singer & Rowe, 1992).

The cause of migraine headache in any age group is not well understood. It probably results from abnormal constriction of intracranial arteries; this leads to a temporarily reduced blood supply to cerebral tissue, followed by overdistention of cranial blood vessels. The aura accompanying such headaches is the result of the temporary ischemia, and the headache is the result of the overdistention. Some children who have migraine headaches have an abnormal EEG.

Most children with migraine headache have a positive family history. This syndrome may be inherited as a dominant trait.

Assessment. Obtain a thorough history of when the headache generally occurs; the events preceding it (to detect an aura); its duration, frequency, intensity, description, and associated symptoms; and the actions taken to treat the headache. The child needs a thorough physical examination, including funduscopic examination, to rule out papilledema. Blood pressure must be measured to rule out hypertension. If an aura is documented, an EEG will be ordered.

Therapeutic Management. The specific drug therapy for migraine headache in children is ergotamine tartrate (Cafergot), which constricts cerebral arteries. Sumatriptan, a serotonin agonist approved for adults, will be available to children in the future. Sleep or lying down may be necessary to relieve the pain and vomiting. Frequent headaches interfere with a child's ability to achieve in school. Children need to be reassured that migraine headaches are benign, although painful and incapacitating, and not signs of a developing brain tumor. They may need a number of follow-up visits to confirm that there is no progressive disease.

If other family members have migraine headaches, they need to be counseled that how they react to their headaches influences their child's reaction to his or her own headaches. If the mother goes to bed for the day when she has a migraine headache, she cannot expect her child to go to school when he has one. Prophylactic use of propranolol may prevent further headaches (Prensky, 1994).

Tension Headache

When children are studying intently or taking a test, contraction of their neck muscles from tension may cause temporary ischemia. This is experienced as a dull, steady pain in the head. Children with these symptoms should have their vision tested, because poor eyesight may be causing them to hunch over their books. Tension is relieved by simple analgesics, such as acetaminophen, or by sleep (Prensky, 1990).

Sinus Headache

Sinus headache in children under 6 to 8 years of age is rare, because the frontal sinuses are not fully developed before this. Sinusitis is discussed in Chapter 40.

Ataxic Disorders

Ataxia is the failure of muscular coordination, or irregularity of muscle action. Ataxic disorders are often manifested by an awkward gait or lack of coordination. Causes of ataxias differ, but degeneration of cerebellar or vestibular function is always involved.

Ataxia-Telangiectasia

Ataxia-telangiectasia is a primary immunodeficiency disorder that results in progressive cerebellar degeneration; it is transmitted as an autosomal recessive trait due to a defect of the 11th chromosome (Sanai et al., 1990). This is a multisystem disease with neurologic and immunologic aspects. In addition, endocrine abnormalities may occur, and there is an increased risk of cancer, particularly brain tumor. Telangiectasia (red vascular markings) appear on the conjunctiva and skin at the flexor creases (Hong, 1994).

Both immunologic and neurologic symptoms of this disorder vary in severity and onset. Serum IgA and IgE levels may be low, and there is often evidence of reduced T-cell function. Children generally develop frequent infections (primarily sinopulmonary) because of the immunologic deficits. Tonsillar tissue in the pharynx is scant.

Neurologic symptoms from the degeneration process can usually be detected in early infancy when developmental milestones are not met. Children develop an awkward gait when they begin to walk. Choreoathetosis (rapid, purposeless movements), nystagmus, an intention tremor, or scoliosis may develop. They may be unable to move their eyes on demand or follow through visual fields. Eye changes (conjunctival telangiectasia) develop by 5 years of age. Children with this disorder often die in late adolescence from infection, respiratory failure, or a malignant brain tumor.

Friedreich's Ataxia

Friedreich's ataxia is a variety of degenerative symptoms, carried on the short arm of the ninth chromosome as an autosomal recessive trait (Hanauer et al., 1990). Symptoms occur in late adolescence. There is progressive cerebellar and spinal cord dysfunction. The children develop a progressive gait disturbance or a lack of coordinated arm movements. They tend to have a high-arched foot (pes cavus), hammer toes, and scoliosis. The combined symptoms of a positive Babinski reflex, absence of deep tendon reflexes in the ankle, and ataxia are strongly diagnostic. Neurologic examination reveals difficulty in recognizing foot position (whether the foot is moved up or down). Death occurs in young adulthood from myocardial failure due to cardiac muscle fiber degeneration.

Spinal Cord Injury

Because of the resilience of their vertebrae, children have fewer spinal cord injuries than adults. Because more adolescents are having motorcycle accidents that

(text continues on page 1554)

Nursing Care Plan

A Child With Recurrent Convulsions

John is a 12-year-old boy who is admitted to the hospital following a tonic-clonic convulsion. The following is a nursing care plan you might design for him.

Assessment: Well-proportioned white male sleeping soundly on left side. Respiratory rate, 20. Mother reports child was diagnosed as having tonic-clonic seizures 3 years ago. Takes phenobarbital ¼ gr and Dilantin 50 mg 4 times daily. Six months ago, parents were divorced. John (man of the family now) took responsibility for his own medication administration. Was sitting watching television this morning when he said, "The light hurts my eyes. Everything is turning orange." Child then fell to floor and "began shaking." Mouth slack and drooling blood-flecked saliva; incontinent of urine. Has been sleeping soundly since episode (about 20 min ago). Brought to hospital by ambulance. Phenobarbital blood serum level drawn in emergency department.

No history of seizures for 2 years, although mother states she has noticed blood flecks on child's pillow two times in last week and now wonders if child had a seizure during night. Questions whether child has been taking medication regularly (leaves for school when she does at 7 AM; returns home on last school bus at 6 PM after baseball practice).

Child attends 7th grade; is a B student. Plays on school baseball team; good with 7-year-old sister except for occasional arguments. Physical examination: Lumbar puncture done by physician with normal opening and closing pressures; samples sent for cell and glucose and culture. DTRs depressed; level of consciousness; reacts to painful stimuli only.

Nursing Diagnosis: High risk for injury related to reduced level of consciousness during seizures

Defining Characteristic: Child's seizures are marked by a loss of consciousness.

Goal: Child will remain free of injury during future seizures.

Outcome Criteria: Child and parent state safety measures to prevent injury; the child does not experience aspiration or any traumatic injury.

Nursing Orders

1. If an aura can be identified, help the child to the floor during this time.
2. Provide for privacy.
3. Turn the head to the side.
4. Stay with child and observe for respiratory distress; provide oxygen if cyanosis should occur.
5. Perform neurologic assessment q15min until full consciousness returns.
6. Provide a resting environment following the seizure.
7. After a seizure, orient the child to what occurred to decrease confusion.

Rationale

1. Provides for safety against falling.
2. Helps the child avoid embarrassment.
3. Prevents aspiration of saliva.
4. Monitoring for respiratory sufficiency is crucial after a seizure.
5. Periodic neurologic assessment helps provide information on extent of involvement.
6. Tonic-clonic seizures are followed by a period of deep sleep.
7. With no memory for event, child can awake confused.

Nursing Diagnosis: Noncompliance related to age, lack of knowledge, and lack of supervision

Defining Characteristic: Mother questions whether child has been taking medicine.

Goal: Child will take responsibility for self-medication at hospital discharge.

Outcome Criteria: Child's serum levels of anticonvulsants are maintained at therapeutic levels.

(continued)

Nursing Orders

1. Administer medication as prescribed during hospitalization.
2. Review seizure medications with child and parent so they understand action and importance of routine administration.
3. Caution child and parent to measure dosage accurately and to be certain to administer medication on time.
4. Educate child and parent about avoiding alcohol, fatigue, excess stress, poorly adjusted television, audiovisual games, and strobe lights.
5. Discuss a medication schedule that will fit child's long school day.
6. Help John make out a reminder chart for medicine administration.
7. Review with mother the necessity for supervision of 12-year-old's medicine administration.

Rationale

1. Provides for therapeutic serum levels while in hospital.
2. Understanding should result in better compliance.
3. Both child and parent need to understand importance of maintaining therapeutic serum levels while at home.
4. Educate about stimuli that can provoke convulsions.
5. Medication schedule needs to be spaced before 7 AM and after 6 PM to suit child's daily routine.
6. A reminder sheet could help with compliance.
7. Age 12 appears too young for John to assume total responsibility.

Nursing Diagnosis: Knowledge deficit related to recurrent convulsions

Defining Characteristic: Parent states she didn't recognize possible seizures child was having.

Goal: Child and parent will demonstrate increased knowledge of condition by hospital discharge.

Outcome Criteria: Child and parent accurately state etiology, current therapy, and prognosis of recurrent convulsions.

Nursing Orders

1. Review what is known about seizures with child and parent so they do not view this as an uncontrollable, perplexing disorder.
2. Child and parent should be aware that seizure activity can increase with adolescence.
3. Inform child and parent that all states allow children with seizures to obtain a driving license after they are seizure-free 1 to 3 years; help them learn laws of their own state.
4. Counsel parent and child that vocational counseling should stress occupations that will be safe in light of seizures (no multistory construction work, etc.).
5. Encourage child and parent to obtain a Med-Alert bracelet or tag that identifies child as one who has seizures for health care personnel.

Rationale

1. Increasing knowledge can increase compliance with medicine regimen.
2. Helps family plan for future growth and development needs.
3. Obtaining a license is something many children highly value; this information may provide John with some extra motivation to follow medication regimen.
4. John and his mother need this information for planning in the future.
5. A Med-Alert bracelet will help to ensure John's safety when he is away from home.

leave them paralyzed, however, spinal cord injuries in this age group are becoming more common. Another major cause of spinal cord injury is diving into too-shallow water. Any patient with multiple traumatic injuries should be assessed for spinal cord damage. Spinal cord injury without radiographic abnormality (SCIWRA syndrome) may occur. Stabilizing the neck is the best protection against further injury when this happens (Lang & Bernards, 1993).

Recovery Phases

Spinal injuries result when the cord becomes compressed or severed by the vertebrae; further cord damage can be caused by hemorrhage, edema, or inflammation at the injury site as the blood supply becomes impeded. Table 49-6 summarizes functional ability after spinal cord injury. The first questions asked by the parents or the child following the injury are, How much damage is there? Will our child be able to walk again? Predictions of useful body function cannot be made at the time of the accident, however. First, two phases of recovery must take place (Richmond, 1990).

First Recovery Phase

Immediately after the injury, the child experiences spinal shock syndrome or loss of **autonomic nervous system** function (anterior nerve fibers traveling through the anterior horn of the spinal canal). This leads to loss of motor function, sensation, reflex activity, and flaccid paralysis in body areas below the level of the injury. If a cervical injury is present, this will mean loss of respiratory function due to flaccidity of the diaphragm. In high thoracic lesions, use of accessory muscles of the chest is lost, so the child has difficulty maintaining effective respirations. The child has no ability to sweat or shiver to change body temperature below the level of the lesion because of loss of autonomic nerve control; hypothermia or hyperthermia becomes a threat. Blood vessels below the level of the injury are no longer able to constrict, so blood tends to pool in the lower body, leading to hypotension, especially if the upper body is elevated.

Table 49-6. *Functional Ability After Spinal Cord Injury*

Injury Site	Highest Key Functions Still Present	Abilities on Which to Set Nursing Goals
C1–3	Head and neck muscles intact	Respiratory paralysis from loss of phrenic nerve innervation; will need ventilatory assistance
		No voluntary motion below chin
		Can learn to use mouth to control pen for writing and mouthstick to reach objects
C4	Diaphragm intact	Loss of motor function of upper and lower extremities and trunk
		Can learn to use abdominal muscles to breathe independently
C5	Shoulder control; biceps, deltoid function	Can feed self and operate wheelchair if fitted with self-care aids
C6	Forearm pronation; wrist extension	Use of upper extremities for self-care. Can transfer to wheelchair and so have increased independence
C7	Triceps function	Able to transfer to wheelchair readily; increasing independence
C8	Thumb and finger function	Ability to do fine motor tasks increases self-care ability
T1–7	Intercostal muscle (able to breathe with chest, not abdominal, muscles)	Has full use of upper extremities but is still dependent on wheelchair
		May drive car with hand controls
		May have high leg braces fitted for standing
T10–L2	Abdominal muscles	Ambulatory with long leg braces and four-point crutch
L2–4	Hip flexion Leg extension	Ambulatory with long or short leg braces
L5–S1	Gluteus maximus	Walks without aids
S4	Bladder and anal sphincter control	Control of bladder and bowel function
		Penile erection and ejaculation

Areflexia, or loss of bladder control, will occur (when flaccid, the bladder overdistends and continually empties). The bowel becomes equally distended, and bowel sounds are absent. This phase of spinal cord injury lasts from 1 to 6 weeks. As a rule, the shorter the phase of spinal shock, the better the final outcome.

Second Recovery Phase

During the second phase of recovery, the flaccid paralysis of the shock phase is replaced by spastic paralysis. Normally, motor impulses begin in the brain cortex, are transmitted to the medulla, where they cross to the opposite side of the cord, and then travel down the descending motor tracts of the spinal cord. They synapse in the anterior horn of the spinal cord and travel by way of the spinal and peripheral nerves to the designated muscle group, which they set in motion. The nerve

pathways of the brain and the descending tracts are termed *upper motor neurons*. Those in the anterior horn cells and the spinal and peripheral nerves are termed *lower motor neurons*. Whether a motor neuron has upper or lower function, therefore, does not depend as much on its height in the spinal tract as on its position in relation to an anterior horn (between the brain and the anterior horn, it is an upper motor neuron; between the anterior horn and the point of innervation, it is a lower motor neuron; Figure 49-15).

Spasticity in the second phase is due to the loss of upper level control or transmission of meaningful innervation to the lower muscles. Lacking upper motor neuron function because of a severed cord, lower motor neurons or reflex arcs cause the muscles to contract and remain that way. Parents and children are quick to interpret the sudden spastic movement of a lower extremity

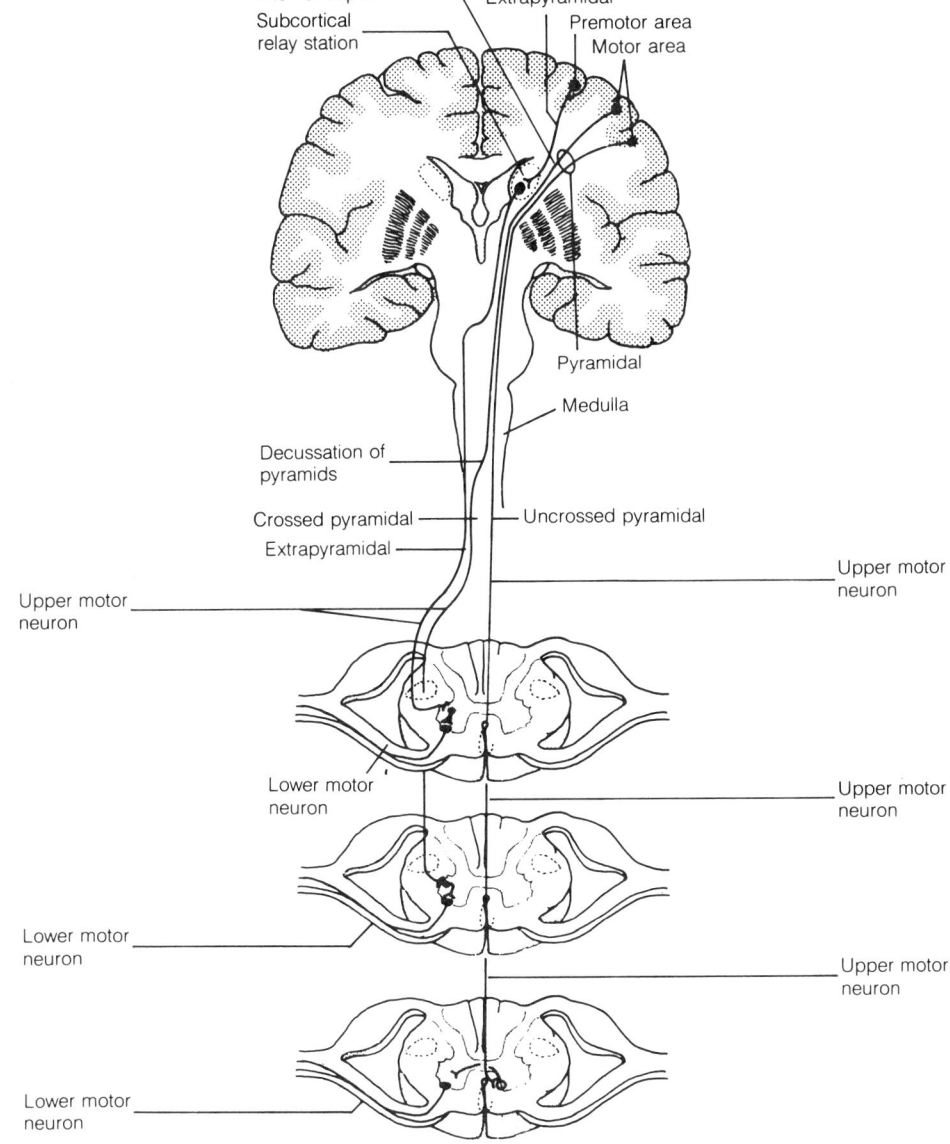

Internal capsule
Subcortical relay station
Extrapyramidal
Premotor area
Motor area

Pyramidal

Medulla

Decussation of pyramids

Crossed pyramidal
Uncrossed pyramidal
Extrapyramidal

Upper motor neuron

Upper motor neuron

Lower motor neuron

Lower motor neuron

Upper motor neuron

Lower motor neuron

Upper motor neuron

FIGURE 49-15

Diagram of motor pathways between the cerebral cortex, one of the subcortical relay stations, and lower motor neurons in the spinal cord. Decussation (crossing of fibers) means that each side of the brain controls skeletal muscles on the opposite side of the body.

as meaningful activity. This is particularly easy to believe with an infant, who cannot tell you that he has no control over his leg movement. Differences between upper and lower neuron damage are listed in Table 49-7. If the injury is very low in the spinal tract, affecting mostly lower motor neurons, muscles will remain flaccid, since lower motor neurons cannot send impulses for contraction.

During this phase, if the child's bladder is allowed to fill, the resultant sensory stimulation relayed to the damaged cord will initiate a powerful sympathetic reflex reaction (autonomic dysreflexia), and the child will show signs of hypertension, tachycardia, flushed face, and severe occipital headache. This is an emergency situation, and if the severe hypertension is not relieved, cerebral vascular accident can result.

Third Recovery Phase
The third phase of recovery from spinal cord injury is the final outcome, or permanent limitation of motor and sensory function. If the compression of the spinal cord is due to edema that is then relieved, no permanent motor and sensory disability will occur.

Assessment of Spinal Cord Injury

Spinal cord injury should be suspected whenever a child has sustained a forceful trauma of any kind. The signs of spinal cord injury vary according to the level of the injury. The cervical and thoracolumbar areas of the spine are the ones most likely to sustain injury.

It is important that a child with suspected spinal cord injury not be moved until the back and head can be supported in a straight line to prevent further injury to the spinal column from twisting or bending. In the emergency department, do not attempt to move the child from the admission stretcher to an examining table until spinal x-ray films are done. This will reduce any unnecessary movement. When moving the child onto the x-ray table, log-roll him gently so that additional injury does not result. If resuscitation is necessary, main-

tain the head in a neutral position; do not hyperextend it. To keep the neck immobilized, do not remove a child's football helmet or neck brace.

The child will need a thorough neurologic assessment to determine the level of injury. Help maintain spinal immobilization during procedures.

Nursing Diagnoses and Related Interventions

During the first phase of recovery, the child's major problems are those resulting from almost complete immobility: pressure sores on bony prominences; loss of appetite (thus poor nutrition) from depression or being in the supine position; urinary calculi from excessive calcium loss; atrophy of flaccid muscle groups; and urinary retention and bladder infection. These effects of immobility are shown in Figure 49-16.

> ***Nursing Diagnosis:*** Altered mobility related to spinal cord injury
>
> ***Goal:*** Child will achieve optimal mobility possible following injury.
>
> ***Outcome Criteria:*** Child is ambulatory with a minimum of artificial support and equipment.

Children may be placed in cervical traction with Crutchfield tongs and a traction belt (Figure 49-17) or by halo traction (see Chapter 51). Having tongs inserted into the skull is a very frightening procedure for children. They are afraid that the tongs will burrow into their skull and strike their brain. Children need someone they know and trust to help them lie still during the procedure. To relieve edema at the injury site and prevent further injury, corticosteroids may be administered.

To promote circulation and prevent loss of calcium that results from inactivity, full range-of-motion exercises must be done approximately three times per day. These are time consuming but important in maintaining joint function.

T a b l e 49-7. *Characteristics of Upper and Lower Motor Nerve Lesions After Spinal Shock Phase*

Finding	Upper Motor Lesion	Lower Motor Lesion
Spasticity	Present	Absent (flaccidity present)
Clonus	Present, increased	Absent
Tendon reflexes	Increased	Absent
Babinski reflex	Present	Absent
Reflexes below level of lesion	Present	Absent
Reflex at level of lesion	Absent	Absent
Atrophy of muscles	Absent or present only to slight degree	Present (muscle fasciculations may be present)

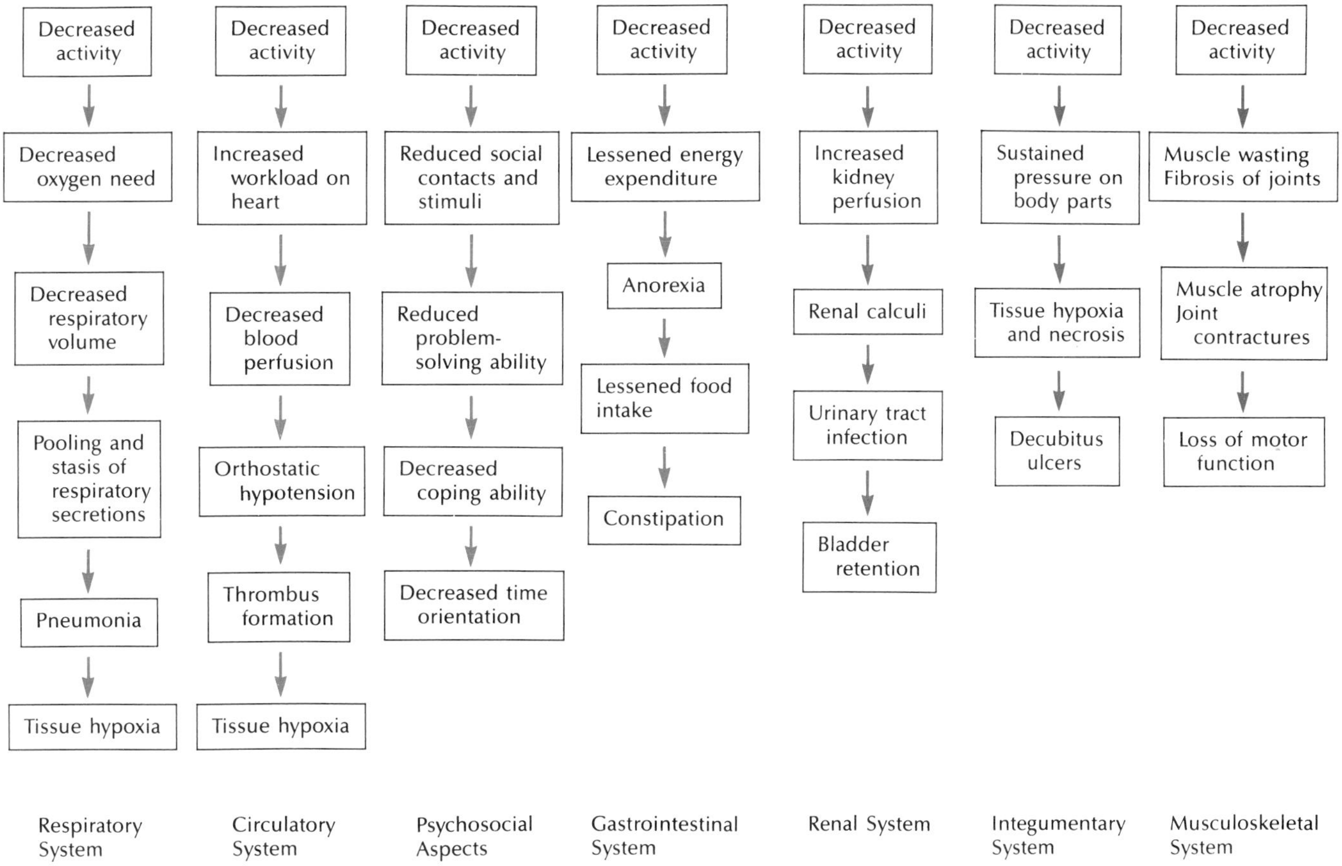

Decreased activity	Decreased activity	Decreased activity	Decreased activity	Decreased activity	Decreased activity	Decreased activity
↓	↓	↓	↓	↓	↓	↓
Decreased oxygen need	Increased workload on heart	Reduced social contacts and stimuli	Lessened energy expenditure	Increased kidney perfusion	Sustained pressure on body parts	Muscle wasting Fibrosis of joints
↓	↓	↓	↓	↓	↓	↓
Decreased respiratory volume	Decreased blood perfusion	Reduced problem-solving ability	Anorexia	Renal calculi	Tissue hypoxia and necrosis	Muscle atrophy Joint contractures
↓	↓	↓	↓	↓	↓	↓
Pooling and stasis of respiratory secretions	Orthostatic hypotension	Decreased coping ability	Lessened food intake	Urinary tract infection	Decubitus ulcers	Loss of motor function
↓	↓	↓	↓	↓		
Pneumonia	Thrombus formation	Decreased time orientation	Constipation	Bladder retention		
↓	↓					
Tissue hypoxia	Tissue hypoxia					

Respiratory System	Circulatory System	Psychosocial Aspects	Gastrointestinal System	Renal System	Integumentary System	Musculoskeletal System

FIGURE 49-16
Effects of immobilization.

During the second phase of recovery, when spasticity of muscle groups occurs, preventing contractures becomes an important nursing responsibility (Figure 49-18). A muscle relaxant, such as diazepam, may be ordered to prevent painful muscle spasm. Holding legs and arms at the joints helps reduce the spasms. If children have upper extremity mobility but will be left with lower extremity paralysis, exercises to strengthen the upper extremity muscle groups will be started. Strengthening the arms will help children be able to lift them-

selves from bed to wheelchair or raise themselves with a trapeze over the bed when changing positions.

One major problem of ambulation following spinal cord injury is helping a child's body readjust to a vertical position after being maintained in the supine position for so long. When the child is raised, blood tends to pool in dilated blood vessels below the level of the lesion. This pooling of blood results in a pseudohypovolemia and hypotension, and the child may faint. Gradually increasing the angle of the bed will help the child become acclimated to the upright position without experiencing vascular pooling.

Nursing Diagnosis: Self-care deficit related to spinal cord injury

Goal: Child will be able to perform as many activities of daily living as possible.

Outcome Criteria: Child states intention of taking over self-care; practices using equipment for eating, bathing, and toileting.

As soon as possible, children should be introduced to self-help methods for activities of daily living. Most parents need to be encouraged to allow the child to be-

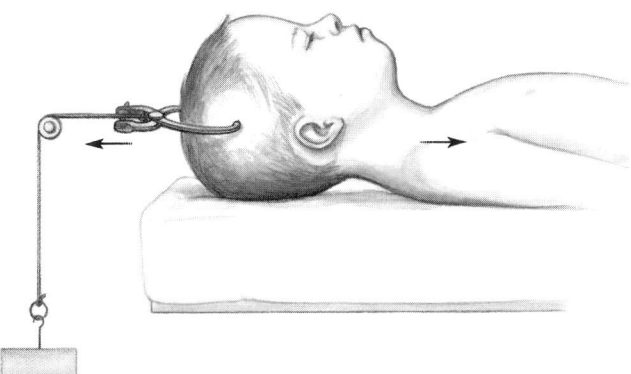

FIGURE 49-17
Crutchfield tongs used to create spinal traction.

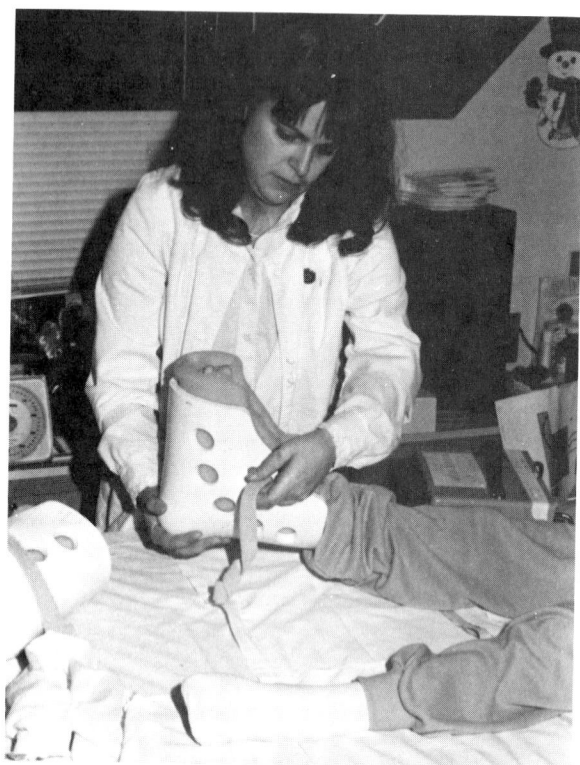

FIGURE 49-18
A plastic boot is applied to prevent foot drop contracture in a child with a spinal cord injury. (Courtesy of Bruce Hill.)

come as self-sufficient as possible and not to take over her complete care. The child may well outlive them and will some day need to be able to function as independently as possible.

With autonomic nervous system dysfunction, the child will be unable to sweat and will become hyperthermic if covered too warmly; if not covered warmly enough, the capillaries will dilate and he will lose considerable heat into the environment. If the room temperature cools at night, be careful to dress the child appropriately for sleeping.

For some children and parents, the first day of using a wheelchair is exciting (proof they can be partially ambulatory). For others, it is the day they must face the reality that they cannot undo the results of the accident and that this is a lifelong disability. For some parents who have nearly overcome their grief and almost accepted their child's disability, the day they are introduced to a symbol of disability such as a wheelchair or long-leg braces may bring new grieving and a sense of loss (see the Focus on Nursing Research box).

When the child reaches sexual maturity, limitations in this area may become apparent. If a male has had an upper motor neuron injury, he will not be able to achieve spontaneous erection or ejaculation. With manual stimulation of the penis, however (stimulation of lower motor neuron function), he can achieve an erection and engage in coitus. Ejaculation and fertility remain limited. At the time of injury, lack of lower ex-

tremity motor control may seem the greatest loss. In adolescence, loss of normal sexual function may become even more disturbing. With most spinal cord injuries, a female is not able to experience orgasm but is nonetheless able to conceive and bear children.

The limitations caused by a spinal cord injury will become especially evident to the child (and the parents) when choosing a vocation and selecting an appropriate school program (children cannot be denied normal schooling by federal law in the United States, even with a severe physical disability).

Nursing Diagnosis: High risk for altered respiratory function related to spinal cord injury

Goal: Child will achieve optimum respiratory function possible.

Outcome Criteria: Child breathes independently following third recovery phase.

If the cervical level of the cord is involved, the child will need ventilatory assistance. He may be intubated at first, but orotracheal or nasotracheal intubation can only be left in place 4 or 5 days. It must then be replaced by a tracheotomy tube to prevent sloughing of pharyngeal tissue from the pressure of the intubation tube. A phrenic nerve pacemaker may be used to stimulate the diaphragm to contract and initiate respirations (Figure 49-19). If

---

**FOCUS ON
NURSING RESEARCH**

Do Adolescents With Spinal Cord Dysfunction Demonstrate the Same Degree of Autonomy as Healthy Adolescents?

It is important for children with disabilities to develop a strong sense of autonomy as well as the ability to cope with new situations; they need to do self-care in order to be independent. To see if adolescents with spina bifida demonstrate the same degree of autonomy as adolescents without disabilities, two groups of 22 adolescents (12 female and 10 male), one with spinal cord impairment and one without, were asked to complete questionnaires that examined autonomy, coping, and self-care.

Results of the study showed that the adolescents with limited mobility scored significantly lower on measures of autonomy than healthy adolescents; there were no differences on coping or self-care ability. The findings of this study are not unexpected, since during the time when autonomy should have been developing, these children were undoubtedly very dependent. Deepening their sense of autonomy to help them be more independent should be an important facet of nursing care.

Monsen, R. B. (1992). Autonomy, coping, and self-care agency in healthy adolescents and in adolescents with spina bifida. *Journal of Pediatric Nursing, 7,* 9.

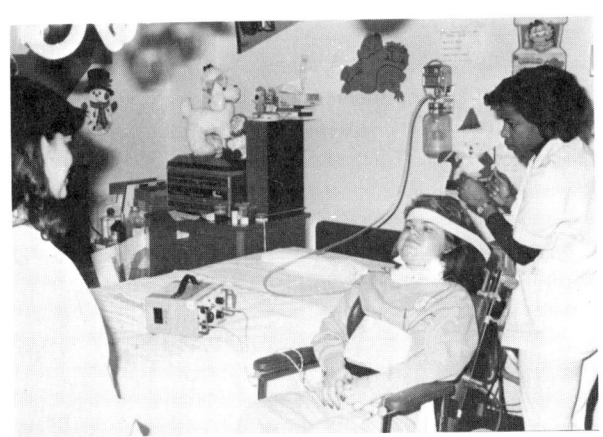

FIGURE 49-19
A 9-year-old girl with a C2–3 spinal injury. The box on the bed is a phrenic pacemaker to initiate contraction of the diaphragm. (Courtesy of Bruce Hill.)

the child has a thoracic level injury (this is rare, since the rib cage gives extra strength to thoracic vertebrae), the child will be able to breathe on her own but will have reduced vital capacity. Periodic intermittent positive pressure breathing treatments may be necessary to encourage increased lung filling. Be careful when positioning the child that you are not compromising any chest movement with sandbags or other restricting objects.

Nursing Diagnosis: High risk for altered skin integrity related to immobility

Goal: Child's skin will remain intact.

Outcome Criteria: Child's skin develops no erythema or ulcerations.

To prevent skin breakdown, the child should be turned about every 2 hours (always be sure to log-roll or maintain immobilization with a striker frame or Circo-Electric bed). The use of an alternating-pressure mattress or sheepskin is helpful. With loss of sensation in body parts, the child is unable to report skin irritation from a wrinkled sheet or wet clothing. If he or she is incontinent, the bedding must be changed immediately to prevent skin breakdown. Once they begin to be ambulatory, their legs and buttocks should be checked regularly to prevent pressure sores from sitting in a wheelchair or using leg braces.

Nursing Diagnosis: High risk for altered urinary and bowel elimination related to spinal cord injury

Goal: Child will achieve adequate elimination.

Outcome Criteria: Child manages bowel and bladder elimination independently.

To prevent urinary retention during the first phase of recovery, a Foley catheter will be inserted, or the bladder can be emptied by periodic suprapubic aspira-

tion, catheterization, or Credé maneuver (pressing on the bladder to evacuate it). Second-stage spasticity causes periodic reflex emptying. This rarely empties the bladder completely, however, so the same problems of stasis and infection continue. Encouraging a child to drink cranberry juice will help acidify the urine and limit bacterial growth. Ascorbic acid tablets can be substituted for cranberry juice. To live independently, the child will need to learn self-catheterization or the Credé maneuver to empty the bladder (see Chapter 39).

Bowel movements may be regulated by inserting a bisacodyl (Dulcolax) suppository once a day at the same time to establish a defecation pattern. If the stool tends to be hard, a stool softener such as ducosate (Colace) will aid in complete stool evacuation.

Nursing Diagnosis: Grieving related to loss of function secondary to spinal cord injury

Goal: Child and parents will express their grief regarding spinal cord injury during recovery period.

Outcome Criteria: Child and parents openly discuss their feelings about injury and its effect on their lives.

The second recovery phase is the time for parents and children to begin thinking about what this degree of disability will mean to them and to face its full extent. Children and parents typically react to the initial diagnosis with grief. They may still be in denial or shock when the second phase begins. With no sudden miracle cure in sight, they may begin to move through stages of anger, bargaining, depression, and then acceptance (the accident happened; we must go on from this point) (Figure 49-20). Both the parents and the child may need counseling to reach this point.

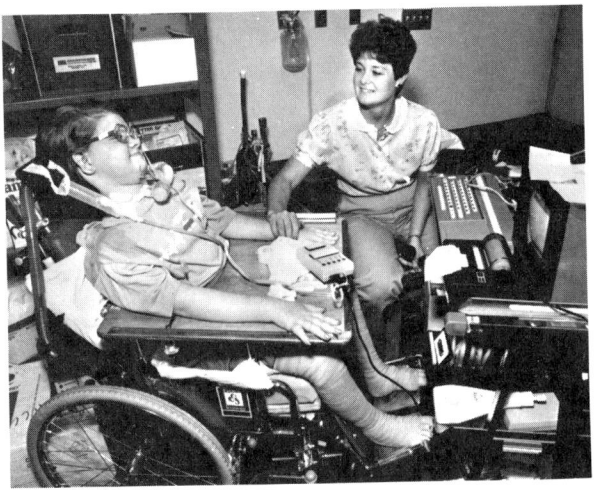

FIGURE 49-20
A child with a cervical spinal injury. Note the tracheostomy for ventilatory assistance, gastrostomy tube for feedings, and Ace bandages on her legs to reduce vasodilation. Learning to work a computer offers her an opportunity to communicate and learn. (Courtesy of Bruce Hill.)

Key Points

- Increased intracranial pressure arises from an increase in the CSF volume or from blood accumulation, cerebral edema, or space-occupying lesions. Neurologic changes such as increased temperature and blood pressure and decreased pulse and respirations that occur with this are subtle. Always compare assessments to previous levels to detect that a consistent, although minor, change is occurring.

- Cerebral palsy is a nonprogressive disorder of upper motor neurons. The exact cause is generally unknown, but the condition is associated with anoxia before, during, or shortly after birth. Four major types are identified: spastic (there is excessive tone in the voluntary muscles), athetoid (abnormal involuntary movement), atonic (decreased muscle tone), and mixed (symptoms of both spasticity and athetoid movements are present).

- Meningitis is infection of the cerebral meninges. It is caused most frequently by bacterial invasion. Nursing diagnoses commonly identified for this illness are Pain and High risk for altered tissue perfusion. Children need follow-up afterward to monitor for hearing acuity and undersecretion of antidiuretic hormone.

- Encephalitis is inflammation of brain tissue. This is always a serious diagnosis, because the child may be left with residual neurologic damage such as seizures or mental retardation.

- Reye's syndrome is acute encephalitis with accompanying fatty infiltration of the liver, heart, and lungs. Once common, the disease is now rarely seen, since it tends to follow the administration of acetylsalicylic acid (aspirin) to a child who has a viral infection. Cautioning parents not to administer aspirin has caused the decline in incidence.

- Guillain-Barré syndrome is inflammation of motor and sensory nerves. The reaction may be immune mediated, after an upper respiratory illness. Temporary demyelinization of the nerve sheaths occurs with loss of function.

- Botulism occurs when spores of *Clostridium botulinum* produce toxins in the intestine. Because honey and corn syrup may be sources of the organism, they should not be given to infants.

- Recurrent convulsions are involuntary contractions of muscle caused by abnormal electrical brain discharges. Common types seen in children are infantile spasms, focal, absence, and tonic-clonic. Seizures may occur from fever in children under 7 years of age. Therapy is administration of anticonvulsant drugs. Nursing diagnoses associated with recurrent convulsions are High risk for injury and Altered family processes.

- Spinal cord injury is occurring at increased rates in children from sports and motor vehicle accidents. Children pass through a first, second, and third recovery phase following the injury. Nursing diagnoses associated with spinal cord injury are High risk for altered mobility, Self-care deficit, Altered respiratory function, Altered skin integrity, Altered urinary and bowel elimination, and Grieving.

- Many neurologic disorders cause problems with balance. Be certain that children are capable of ambulating safely before allowing them out of bed without assistance. Some children need to wear a helmet to protect their head from trauma if they should fall.

- Nerve cells are unique in that they do not regenerate if damaged. This makes neurologic disease a long-term type of illness. Parents and children alike need support from health care providers to cope with problems that continue to occur over a long period of time.

Critical Thinking Exercises

1. Beverly is a 2-year-old diagnosed with bacterial meningitis. She has severe neck pain when she is moved. Her mother asks you not to worry so much about intake and output so her daughter can rest. How would you answer her mother? Suppose you call Beverly and she doesn't answer you? Why is this a particular cause of concern with a child with meningitis?

2. Bill is a high school senior and your neighbor. He tells you that he thinks he has the flu and that he took some aspirin for it. When you tell him it isn't wise for children to take aspirin for flulike symptoms, he tells you that advice is "just for babies." Would you pursue the matter with Bill?

3. A spinal cord injury can cause severe disability in adolescents. If you were designing a program to teach measures to prevent spinal cord injury, what topics would you include in your presentation?

References

Assessment: Positron emission tomography. (1991). *Neurology, 41,* 163.

Barnes, P. D. (1990). Magnetic resonance in pediatric and adolescent neuroimaging. *Nursing Clinics of North America, 8,* 741.

Berg, A. T. (1993). Are febrile seizures provoked by a rapid rise in temperature? *American Journal of Diseases of Children, 147,* 1101.

Bhushan, V., et al. (1993). Impact of improved survival of very low birth weight infants on recent secular trends in the prevalence of cerebral palsy. *Pediatrics, 91,* 1094.

Brucker, J. M. (1990). Selective dorsal rhizotomy: Neurosurgical treatment of cerebral palsy. *Journal of Pediatric Nursing, 5,* 105.

Caplan, L. R. (1991). Question-driven technology assessment: SPECT as an example. *Neurology, 41,* 187.

Carroll, J. I., & Loughlin, G. M. (1990). Sudden unexplained death and apparent life-threatening events. In Oski, F. A., et al. (Eds.).

Principles and practice of pediatrics (2nd ed.). Philadelphia: J. B. Lippincott.

Department of Health & Human Services. (1991). *Healthy people 2000.* Washington, DC: Public Health Service.

Dieckmann, R. A. (1994). Rectal diazepam for prehospital pediatric status epilepticus. *Annals of Emergency Medicine, 23,* 216.

Farwell, J. R., et al. (1990). Phenobarbital for febrile seizures: Effects on intelligence and on seizure recurrence. *New England Journal of Medicine, 322,* 364.

Feigin, R. D. (1994). Bacterial meningitis beyond the newborn period. In F. A. Oski, et al. (Eds.). *Principles and practice of pediatrics* (2nd. ed.). Philadelphia: J. B. Lippincott.

Gasch, A. T. (1990). Use of the traditional ketogenic diet for treatment of intractable epilepsy. *Journal of the American Dietetic Association, 90,* 1433.

Glaze, D. G. (1994). Epilepsy. In Oski, F. A., et al. (Eds.) *Principles and practice of pediatrics* (2nd ed.). Philadelphia: J. B. Lippincott.

Hanauer, A., et al. (1990). The Friedreich ataxia gene is assigned to chromosome 9q13-q21 by mapping of tightly linked markers and shows linkage disequilibrium with 09S15. *American Journal of Human Genetics, 46,* 133.

Hauser, W. A. (1994). The prevalence and incidence of convulsive disorders in children. *Epilepsia, 35,* 51.

Holmes, G. L. (1993). Surgery for intractable seizures in infancy and early childhood. *Neurology, 43,* S28.

Hong, R. (1994). Combined immunodeficiency diseases. In F. A. Oski, et al. (Eds.). *Principles and practice of pediatrics* (2nd ed.). Philadelphia: J. B. Lippincott.

Kongelbeck, S. R. (1990). Discharge planning for the child with infantile spasms. *Journal of Neurology Nursing, 22,* 238.

Lang, S. M., & Bernards, L. M. (1993). SCIWORA syndrome: Nursing assessment. *Dimensions of Critical Care Nursing, 12,* 247.

Lockman, L. A. (1990). Treatment of status epilepticus in children. *Neurology, 40,* 43.

Louis, P. T. (1994). Reye's syndrome. In Oski, F. A., et al. (Eds.) *Principles and practice of pediatrics* (2nd ed.). Philadelphia: J. B. Lippincott.

Murray, D. P. (1993). Impaired mobility: Guillain-Barré syndrome. *Journal of Neuroscience Nursing, 25,* 100.

Niijima, S., & Wallace, S. J. (1989). Effects of puberty on seizure frequency. *Developmental Medicine and Child Neurology, 31,* 174.

Parke, J. T. (1994). Peripheral neuropathy. In Oski, F. A., et al. (Eds.) *Principles and practice of pediatrics* (2nd ed.). Philadelphia: J. B. Lippincott.

Porter, J. D., et al. (1990). Trends in the incidence of Reye's syndrome and the use of aspirin. *Archives of Disease of Childhood, 65,* 826.

Porter, R. J. (1993). The absence epilepsies. *Epilepsia, 34,* S42.

Prensky, A. L. (1994). Headaches. In F. A. Oski, et al. (Eds.). *Principles and practice of pediatrics* (2nd ed.). Philadelphia: J. B. Lippincott.

Richmond, T. S. (1990). Spinal cord injury. *Nursing Clinics of North America, 25,* 57.

Riikonen, R. (1993). Infantile spasms: Infectious disorders. *Neuropediatrics, 24,* 274.

Roach, E. S. (1992). Neurocutaneous syndromes. *Pediatric Clinics of North America, 39,* 591.

Roberts, A. (1993). The nervous system. *Nursing Times, 89,* 57.

Rosman, N. P. (1994). Intracranial pressure measurements. In Oski, F. A., et al. (Eds.) *Principles and practice of pediatrics* (2nd ed.). Philadelphia: J. B. Lippincott.

Rylance, G. W. (1990). Treatment of epilepsy and febrile convulsions in children. *Lancet, 336,* 488.

Sanai, O., et al. (1990). Further mapping of an ataxia telangiectasia locus to the chromosome 11q23 region. *American Journal of Human Genetics, 47,* 860.

Singer, H. S. & Rowe, S. (1992). Chronic recurrent headaches in children. *Pediatric Annals, 21,* 369.

Shapiro, B. K., & Capute, A. J. (1994). Cerebral palsy. In Oski, F. A., et al. (Eds.) *Principles and practice of pediatrics* (2nd ed.). Philadelphia: J. B. Lippincott.

Straussberg, R., et al. (1993). Knee-chest position as a sign of increased intracranial pressure. *Journal of Pediatrics, 122,* 99.

Sullivan, J. (1990). Neurologic assessment. *Nursing Clinics of North America, 25,* 795.

Wheless, J. (1991). Evaluation of children for epilepsy surgery. *Pediatric Annals, 20,* 41.

Suggested Readings

Bell, W. E. (1992). Bacterial meningitis in children: selected aspects. *Pediatric Clinics of North America, 39,* 651.

Boyle, C. A., et al. (1994). Prevalence and health impact of developmental disabilities in U.S. children. *Pediatrics, 93,* 399.

Clevenger, V. (1990). Nursing management of lumbar drains. *Journal of Neuroscience Nursing, 22,* 227.

Crumrine, P. K. (1993). A trio of pediatric neurological emergencies. *Emergency Medicine, 25,* 103.

Davis, B. D., & Steele, S. (1991). Case management for young children with special health care needs. *Pediatric Nursing, 17,* 15.

Engel, N. S. (1990). Phenobarbital for pediatric febrile seizures: Risk-benefit update. *MCN: American Journal of Maternal Child Nursing, 15,* 257.

Listernick, R., & Charrow, J. (1990). Neurofibromatosis type 1 in childhood. *Journal of Pediatrics, 116,* 845.

Martin, J. (1990). Pediatric management problems: Epilepsy. *Pediatric Nursing, 16,* 394.

McKhann, G. M. (1990). Guillain-Barré syndrome: Clinical and therapeutic observations. *Annals of Neurology, 27,* 513.

Oehler, J. M., et al. (1993). How to target infants at highest risk for developmental delay. *MCN: American Journal of Maternal Child Nursing, 18,* 20.

Pueschel, S. M., et al. (1991). Seizure disorders in Down syndrome. *Archives of Neurology, 48,* 318.

Scheller, J. M., & Nelson, K. B. (1994). Does cesarean delivery prevent cerebral palsy or other neurologic problems of childhood? *Obstetrics and Gynecology, 83,* 624.

Selekman, J. (1991). Pediatric rehabilitation: From concepts to practice. *Pediatric Nursing, 17,* 11.

Symposium: Cerebral palsy. (1990). *Clinical Orthopaedics, 251,* 1.

White, M. (1990). Continence: Independence for the handicapped child. *Nursing Times, 86,* 69.

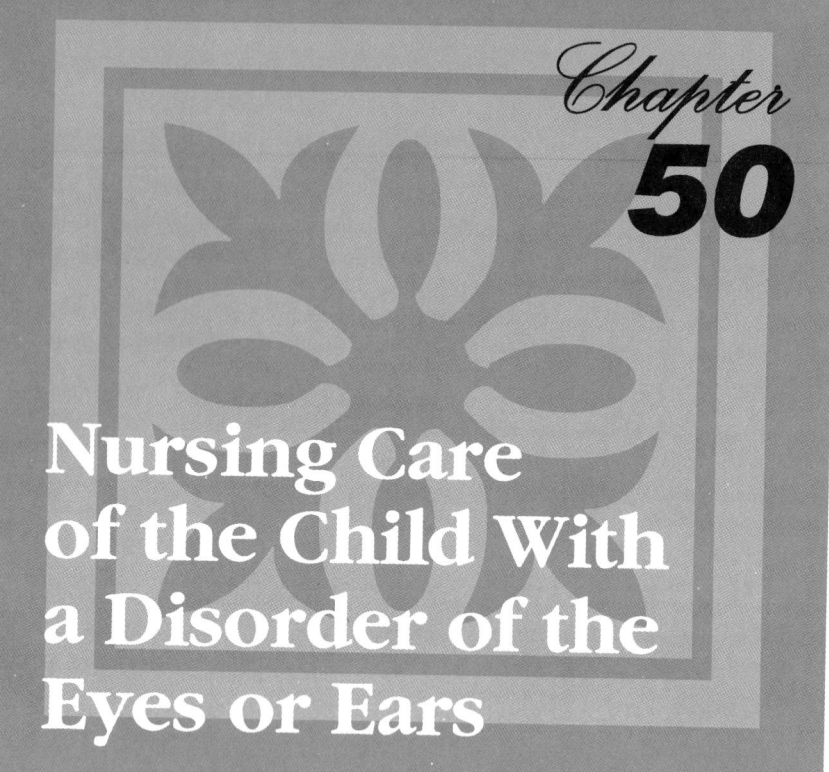

Chapter 50

Nursing Care of the Child With a Disorder of the Eyes or Ears

Key Terms

- accommodation
- amblyopia
- astigmatism
- chalazion
- cones
- convergence
- diplopia
- fovea centralis
- globe
- goniotomy
- hyperopia
- light refraction
- myopia
- myringotomy
- nystagmus
- orthoptics
- photophobia
- ptosis
- rods
- stereopsis
- strabismus
- stye
- tympanocentesis

Objectives

After mastering the contents of this chapter, you should be able to:

1. Describe the structure and function of the eyes and ears and disorders of these organs that affect children.

2. Assess the child who has a disorder of vision or hearing.

3. Formulate nursing diagnoses related to the child with a disorder of vision or hearing.

4. Plan nursing interventions for the child with a disorder of vision or hearing, such as teaching parents about eye patching.

5. Implement nursing care to meet the specific needs of the child who has a disorder of the eyes or ears, such as preparing the child for eye surgery.

6. Evaluate outcome criteria to be certain that goals of nursing care have been achieved.

7. Identify National Health Goals related to vision and hearing disorders and children that nurses could be instrumental in helping the nation achieve.

8. Identify areas related to care of children with vision or hearing disorders that could benefit from additional nursing research.

9. Use critical thinking to analyze ways that nursing care of children with dysfunction of vision or hearing could be more family centered.

10. Synthesize knowledge of childhood disorders of the eyes or ears with the nursing process to achieve quality maternal and child health nursing care.

Adele Pillitteri: MATERNAL AND CHILD HEALTH NURSING, 2nd Edition. © 1995 Adele Pillitteri.

NURSING PROCESS OVERVIEW
for Health Promotion of Vision and Hearing
ASSESSMENT
NURSING DIAGNOSIS
PLANNING
IMPLEMENTATION
EVALUATION

Vision

Stereopsis

Accommodation

Disorders That Interfere With Vision

Refractive Errors

Astigmatism

Nystagmus

Amblyopia
  Assessment
  Therapeutic Management
  Nursing Diagnoses and Related
    Interventions
Color Vision Deficit (Color Blindness)

Structural Problems of the Eye

Coloboma

Hypertelorism

Ptosis

Strabismus
  Assessment
  Therapeutic Management

Infection or Inflammation of the Eye

Stye (Hordeolum)

Chalazion

Blepharitis Marginalis

Conjunctivitis
  Inclusion Blennorrhea
  Acute Catarrhal Conjunctivitis
  Herpetic Conjunctivitis
  Allergic Conjunctivitis

Keratitis

Periorbital Cellulitis

Dacryostenosis

Dacryocystitis

Traumatic Injury to the Eye

Assessment
  Nursing Diagnoses and Related
    Interventions
Foreign Bodies

Contusion Injuries

Eyelid Injuries

Inner Eye Conditions

Congenital Glaucoma
  Assessment
  Therapeutic Management
  Discharge Planning and Follow-Up
Cataract
  Assessment
  Therapeutic Management

The Child Undergoing Eye Surgery
  Nursing Diagnoses and Related
    Interventions
The Child With Vision Impairment in the Hospital
  Nursing Diagnoses and Related
    Interventions

Structure and Function of the Ears

Physiology of Hearing Loss

Hearing Impairment
  Hearing Aids
  Speech Therapy

Disorders of the Ear

External Otitis
  Assessment
  Therapeutic Management
  Nursing Diagnoses and Related
    Interventions
Impacted Cerumen

Acute Otitis Media
  Assessment
  Therapeutic Management

Serous Otitis Media
  Assessment
  Therapeutic Management

Cholesteatoma

The Hearing-Impaired Child in the Hospital

Impairment of the eyes or ears always poses a threat to normal growth and development, because so much of how a child learns about the world is achieved through these sensory organs. Infants first learn how to interact with others by watching their parents' faces; they learn to speak by listening to words spoken to them. They continue to depend on sensory input for stimulation throughout life.

Eye and ear disorders may be transitory (e.g., a stye or external otitis infection), but they always have the potential for becoming long-term illnesses if they permanently affect vision and hearing. This is an area in which health promotion (e.g., teaching eye safety), illness prevention (e.g., detecting early hearing problems), and health rehabilitation (e.g., helping parents of a child with a vision or hearing impairment gain the expertise they need to care for their child) are all important phases of nursing care. National Health Goals related to vision and hearing disorders and children are shown in the Focus on National Health Goals box.

NURSING PROCESS OVERVIEW
for Health Promotion of Vision and Hearing

ASSESSMENT

All newborns should be assessed for their ability to focus on or see an examiner's face and to follow an object from the periphery of vision to the midline. Be sure to observe the infant so you are certain that the newborn's interest is evoked by sight, not sound. Newborn vision can be further tested by optokinetic nystagmus testing (the infant is shown alternating black and white stripes), visual-evoked potential testing (similar but checkerboard-appearing pictures are shown) and forced-choice preferential looking testing (the infant is shown a pattern and a plain picture; the seeing child focuses on the pattern; Traboulsi & Maumenee, 1994). Assessing newborn infants for hearing loss is an equally important part of newborn care. Newborns should quiet to the sound of a soothing voice. (For this you need to stay out of sight so you are certain the infant is not quieting to your face.) Newborns should startle or attune to a loud noise made near them. Instruments for testing newborn hearing are currently being developed which will provide for better documentation of the newborn's ability to respond to a noise.

Children should be assessed for vision problems and hearing loss by history throughout childhood. (Is a parent or teacher concerned about vision? Does a parent worry that a child may not be hearing well? Is a child having any difficulty in school?) Vision should also be assessed by inspection: Do the child's eyes follow a moving light into all six fields of vision? Is a red reflex present? Do the child's eyes appear to be in straight alignment? Both vision and hearing acuity should be checked periodically (Figure 50-1). Children should also be assessed for their ability to speak clearly and age appropriately, since language is influenced by hearing. Detailed vision and hearing assessment is discussed in Chapter 28 with other aspects of physical assessment. Magnetic resonance imaging is helpful after eye injury to locate internal globe bleeding or the presence of a foreign body. Brain stem auditory evoked response is a technique used for children who are unconscious or are unable to respond to hearing assessment for some other reason (Pagana & Pagana, 1993).

NURSING DIAGNOSIS

Health promotion in regard to safety measures for eye and ear health is a major responsibility of the nurse. Related nursing diagnoses include the following:

- Health-seeking behaviors related to prevention of trauma to eyes or ears
- Knowledge deficit related to importance of early diagnosis and treatment of ear infection

Nursing diagnoses for the child with vision or hearing impairment should focus on the child and parents' responses to loss of sight or hearing, not on the deficit itself (Carpenito, 1993). Such nursing diagnoses might include these:

- Self-care disturbance related to impaired visual acuity
- High risk for injury related to hearing loss
- High risk for altered self-esteem related to long-term vision deficit
- Impaired verbal communication related to congenital hearing deficit
- Social isolation related to hearing loss
- Dysfunctional grieving related to child's loss of sight
- Family coping, potential for growth, related to child's traumatic injury and subsequent loss of vision in one eye

PLANNING

Be certain that goals established are realistic and address areas in which you can have some impact. You may not

FOCUS ON
National Health Goals

Adequate vision and hearing ability are necessary to normal growth and development; three National Health Goals address improvements in these areas:

- Reduce acute middle ear infections among children aged 4 and younger, as measured by days of restricted activity or school absenteeism, to no more than 105 days per 100 children from a baseline of 131 days per 100 children.

- Reduce significant hearing impairment to a prevalence of no more than 82/1000 people from a baseline of 88.9/1000.

- Reduce significant visual impairment to a prevalence of no more than 30/1000 people from a baseline of 34.5/1000 (DHHS, 1991).

Nurses can be instrumental in helping the nation achieve these goals by screening for vision and hearing at all well child assessments, paying particular attention to those children who have been cared for in neonatal intensive care units. Nursing research questions that might yield helpful information include: Can infants who are prone to hearing and vision disorders be better identified before discharge from a neonatal intensive unit? What are effective techniques for teaching adolescents to avoid excessive sound levels, such as those associated with loud music? What are effective ways to teach school-age children to avoid eye injury?

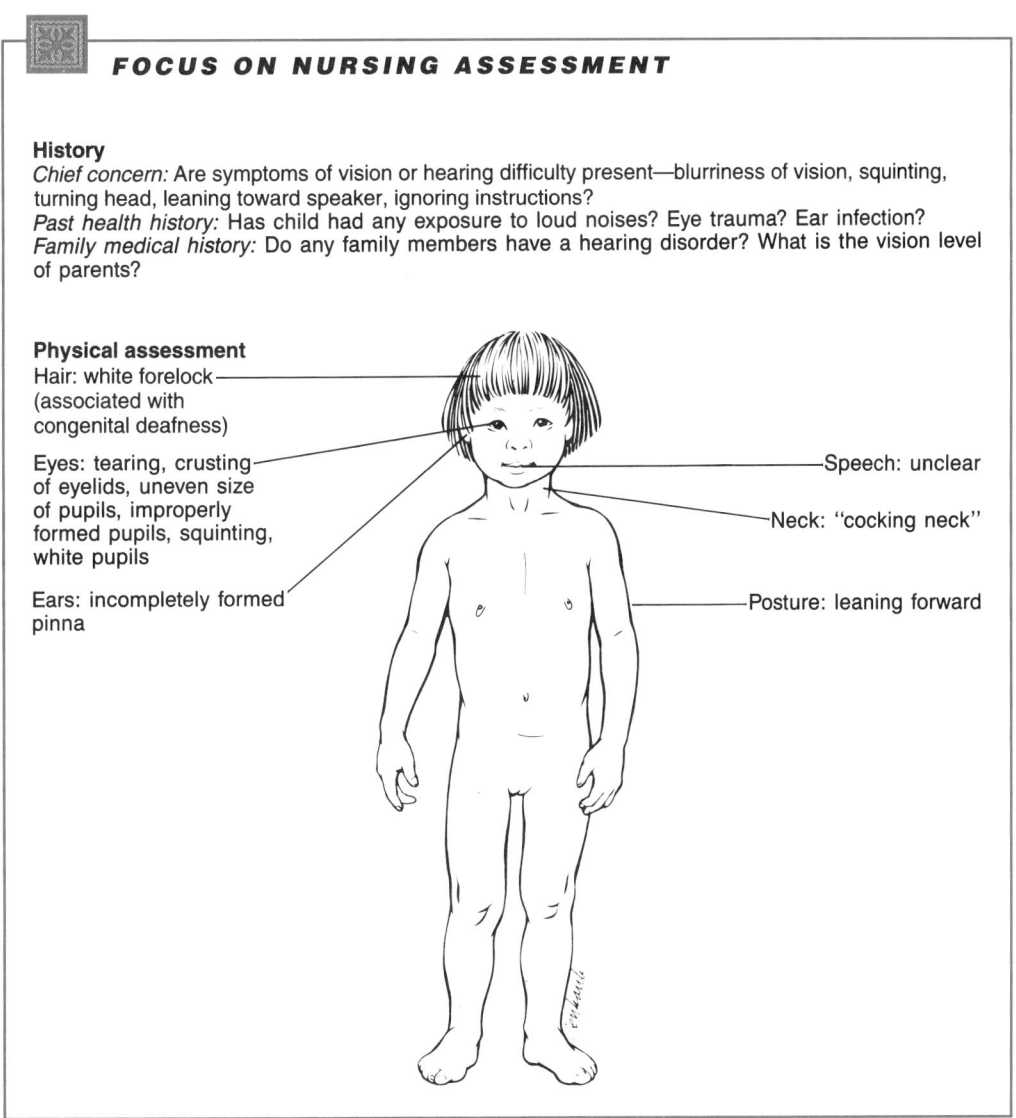

FOCUS ON NURSING ASSESSMENT

History
Chief concern: Are symptoms of vision or hearing difficulty present—blurriness of vision, squinting, turning head, leaning toward speaker, ignoring instructions?
Past health history: Has child had any exposure to loud noises? Eye trauma? Ear infection?
Family medical history: Do any family members have a hearing disorder? What is the vision level of parents?

Physical assessment
Hair: white forelock (associated with congenital deafness)

Eyes: tearing, crusting of eyelids, uneven size of pupils, improperly formed pupils, squinting, white pupils

Ears: incompletely formed pinna

Speech: unclear

Neck: "cocking neck"

Posture: leaning forward

FIGURE 50-1
Signs and symptoms of vision or hearing disorders in children.

be able to increase an infant's vision or hearing, but you can help to increase the child's ability to function effectively by listening attentively to parents' concerns and providing useful anticipatory guidance. Many eye and ear disorders cause pain. Helping parents reduce pain is a major nursing responsibility. Goals should always address preventive aspects of care in all areas of daily living.

When parents learn that a child has a vision or hearing impairment, they generally need help in planning schooling for the child and such activities as toilet-training and self-care. You need to discuss with these parents the importance of talking to and touching their infant; of teaching her how to communicate and learn about the world around her through touch as well as through her other functioning senses.

Children with sensory impairment generally need

very early preschool education programs so that they are exposed to interesting and stimulating tasks when their sense of initiative is strongest and so they can accomplish learning tasks despite their disability. It may be difficult for parents to relinquish their children to such programs during the day, especially at such an early age. It takes careful planning to enable parents to accept this separation.

Parents of children with hearing impairments may need to be encouraged to talk to their children, even in infancy. Although the infant may not be able to hear what the parents are saying, observing facial expressions and spontaneous body movements that accompany verbal speech will help him or her learn important aspects of communication. The older child may not be able to hear her mother say, "I'm so proud of you," but she can see the happiness on her mother's face.

IMPLEMENTATION

Nursing interventions for the child with a disorder of the eye or ear range from providing anticipatory guidance and teaching children and parents measures to promote eye and ear health to preparing a child for surgery. The Focus on Family Teaching box summarizes safety measures for preventing eye injuries and hearing loss in children. Nursing interventions also include helping a child and parents adjust to aids that will improve hearing, speech, or sight. Referrals to organizations that can provide information and support to parents of children with vision or hearing impairment can be particularly useful, especially when the impairment will be long term. Some of the organizations concerned with sensory impairment are the following:

Alexander Graham Bell Association for the Deaf
3417 Volta Place NW
Washington, DC 20007

American Foundation for the Blind
15 West 16th Street
New York, NY 10011

American Speech-Language-Hearing Association
10801 Rockville Pike
Rockville, MD 20852

National Association for the Visually Handicapped
22 West 21st Street
New York, NY 10010

National Federation of the Blind
1800 Johnson Street
Baltimore, MD 21230

Recording for the Blind
20 Roszel Road
Princeton, NJ 08540

EVALUATION

As stated before, a disorder of the eyes or ears can turn from an acute, one-time illness into a chronic and developmentally debilitating condition if steps are not taken to treat the initial problem quickly and completely. Even the most rigorous preventive care and attention, however, cannot avert the occurrence of some serious disorders affecting vision and hearing. Nursing care must

---

FOCUS ON FAMILY TEACHING

Q. We have such an active family, I'm concerned that someone's eye or hearing may be accidentally injured. What are some safety measures I should take to avoid this?

A. Protecting children's vision and hearing is important. Some common measures to take to avoid eye injury are the following:

- Infants and small children should use a car seat (older children, a seat belt) in a car to prevent hitting the dashboard or front seat in an accident.

- Don't allow infants to hold sharp objects. If an infant is holding such an object in his hand, there is the danger that the object could strike his eye as he brings his fist to his mouth to suck his thumb.

- Don't allow toddlers to carry sharp objects such as lollipop sticks in their hands while walking. They fall readily because of their unsteady gait.

- Don't allow older children to run with sharp objects in their hands, since they can fall while running and puncture an eye.

- Caution older children to use eye-protection measures, such as goggles, when working with projects such as soldering metal in school.

- Encourage the use of face masks for hockey players.

- Teach children not to place any medication in their eyes not prescribed by a health care provider; don't use outdated eye medication, since it may become contaminated with bacteria or change in composition with time.

- Caution children that chemicals can cause burns to the eye; alert them to the emergency shower installations in science rooms to use to wash away any spilled chemical from their eye. Chemical burns may be worse in children with contact lenses in place, because chemicals may flow under the lens and remain longer in contact with the cornea.

- Teach children not to wear contact lenses for longer intervals than recommended by the manufacturer to prevent drying and lack of oxygen to the cornea.

To prevent hearing loss:

- Teach children to avoid chronic exposure to loud noises, such as can occur with radios and using earphones.

- Secure prompt treatment for symptoms of otitis media (fever and ear pain) and administer any antibiotic prescribed for the full prescribed course to prevent damage to the middle ear from infection.

- Be certain children's immunizations are up to date, since illnesses such as parotitis (mumps) or bacterial meningitis can lead to hearing loss.

then focus on helping the child and parents adjust to this condition and making sure that the child receives the stimulation needed to grow and develop on a normal continuum.

Continuous follow-up is essential, too, to be sure that other long-term goals are being met. Self-esteem is an important factor to be evaluated. Does the child see herself as well or ill; as a person able to do things or as helpless? Plans to promote self-esteem may have to be devised. Some parents may require help with their own feelings of worth. (Feeling inferior to other parents is common in parents of children with disabilities.) They may need help in letting go as children begin school. The growth of parents in allowing their child to be independent is just as important to evaluate as the child's own progress toward independence.

The following are examples of outcome criteria:

- Parent voices importance of giving full 10-day supply of antibiotic to child for otitis media therapy.
- Parents state concrete plans for enrolling child in preschool program.
- Child wears corrective lenses for major portion of each day.

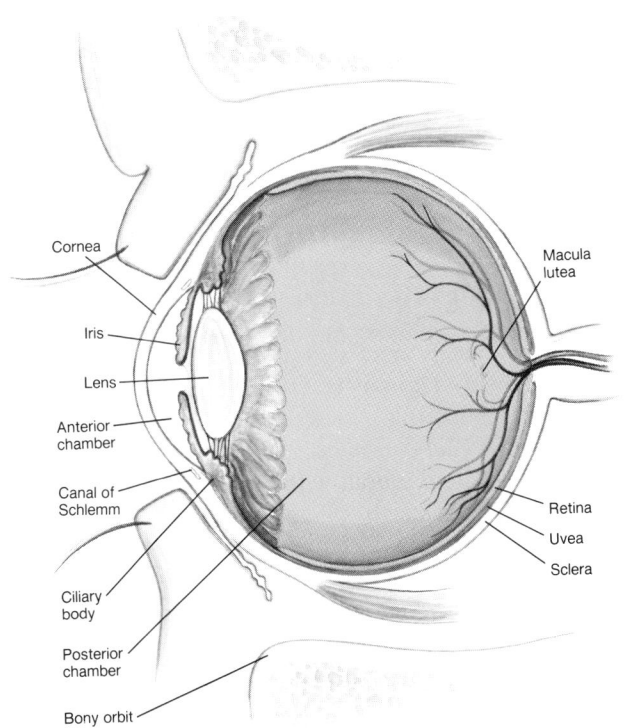

FIGURE 50-2
Anatomy of the eye.

Vision

Vision occurs because light rays reflect from an object through the corneas, aqueous humors, lenses, and vitreous humors to the retinas (Figure 50-2). If any of these structures have defects, light rays may not be able to reach the retinas or focus correctly there, resulting in a vision disturbance. The retinas are studded with **rods**, which are instrumental for night vision and movement in the visual field, and **cones**, which register daylight and color vision. Rods and cones join in a major network to register at the optic nerve. The **fovea centralis** (the center of the macula) is an area of closely packed cones on the retinas where color is best perceived.

It is not enough that each globe develops good central and peripheral vision. *Fusion* must occur; that is, both eyes must interpret a visual image as one image, fusing a visual perception into a single image. This is called *single binocular vision*. Infants with poor eye alignment cannot establish single binocular vision but have **diplopia**, or double vision.

Stereopsis

Stereopsis is depth perception, or the ability to locate an object in space relative to other objects. The right eye sees more of the right side of an object, the left sees more of the left side. This makes the object appear to be three-dimensional. Children with vision loss in one eye do not develop stereopsis and consequently reach far-

ther than or closer to an object to grasp it; they have difficulty learning to ride a bicycle and have great difficulty driving a car safely. Children without stereopsis do not realize that their sight is different from that of other people. The fact that one eye is not functioning is revealed on a routine screening test. A simple test for depth perception is available, the *Stereo-Fly* test. This is a specially constructed picture of a large fly. When asked to touch the fly's wings, a child with good depth perception touches them accurately. A child with poor depth perception touches a spot 2 or 3 inches above the fly's wings.

Accommodation

To focus the image of a close object, eyes must make an active contribution to focusing. This is done by contraction of the ciliary body that changes the curvature of the lens, or **accommodation**. Not only do eyes accommodate (by the action of the ciliary body) for near vision, but eyes also converge (look medially) and the pupil constricts. This action is tested by having children follow a penlight as it moves in toward their nose. Children should be able to follow a light toward their nose by 6 months of age and older. It is **convergence** that you see being actively demonstrated with this test, but convergence does not occur without accommodation. Children who are not able to accommodate will have double vision (diplopia) or be unable to focus on objects near their eyes.

Disorders That Interfere With Vision

Eye disease in children is always potentially serious; if permanent vision impairment occurs, a child's functioning at many everyday tasks may be severely compromised.

Refractive Errors

The largest category of vision defects in children is refractive errors. **Light refraction** refers to the manner that light is bent as it passes through the lens. Normally, this bending causes a ray of light to fall directly on the retina. Because the depth of the eye globe in infants and children increases with age, the light rays do not always focus onto the retina accurately, but at a point behind the retina (Figure 50-3). This results in **hyperopia** (farsightedness) in which vision is blurry at a close range and clear at a far range. The normal hyperopia of a preschooler needs no correction. It is important that you keep this in mind when performing vision screening with children this age. At about 5 years of age, as a result of developmental changes, hyperopia begins to diminish. In some children, however, eyesight does not change in the early school years, and so they remain hyperopic. Focusing on close objects requires such strong accommodation that these children often have headaches or dizziness after completing schoolwork. A finding of hyperopia in a school-age child is cause for referral so that the child may get a prescription for reading glasses.

About 10% of school-age children have eye changes that result in **myopia** (nearsightedness), meaning that the light rays focus at a point in front of the retina. These children are able to read a book immediately in front of them but are unable to read the blackboard clearly in a classroom; they have difficulty reading signs across the street or playing baseball. Once myopia begins, it often progresses into the teen years, when it levels off. Children with myopia need corrective lenses to enable them to see at a distance.

Myopia tends to be familial; If both parents are myopic, children should be screened yearly during the early school years. Any child who complains of difficulty seeing or who shows mannerisms suggestive of refraction errors—rubbing eyes, tearing, red-rimmed eyes, blinking, squinting, or pressing on their eyes—should be screened for visual difficulty. These children try to focus on objects by squinting and rubbing their eyes, which changes the shape of their eye globe.

Teach both children and parents that there is no cure for simple refractive errors of vision, only correction by properly fitted glasses or contact lenses (Figure 50-3*B,C*). Occasionally, a parent will ask if eye exercises or surgery will help; as a rule exercises do not. Eye exercises strengthen eye muscles but do not change the depth of the eye globe.

Parents should be advised to choose glasses fitted with plastic or safety glass (shatterproof) lenses. Contact

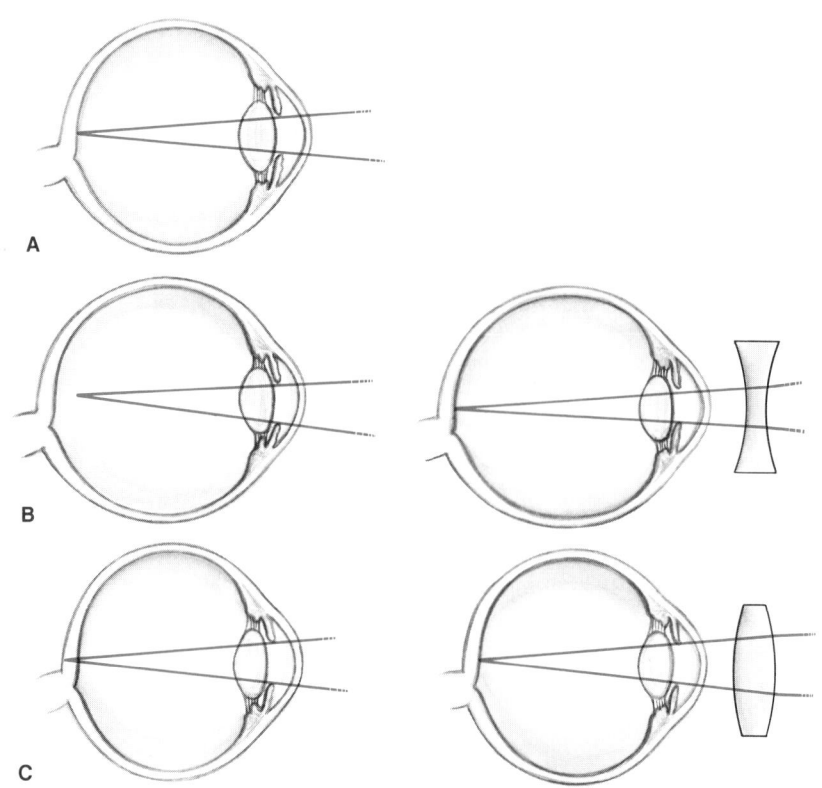

FIGURE 50-3

*Corrective lenses for refractive errors of vision. (**A**) Normal vision. (**B**) Concave lens for myopia (nearsightedness). (**C**) Convex lens for hyperopia (farsightedness).*

lenses can be fitted for infants, and children as young as 5 years of age are capable of putting in and taking out contact lenses if taught properly. Children this age tend to lose the lenses, however, during vigorous physical playing. Contact lenses are a big responsibility requiring conscientious cleaning to prevent eye irritation or infections. Until children are about 12 years of age or older, they generally cannot be relied on to take care of contact lenses independently.

Although wearing glasses is more acceptable today, children still may face being called "geek" or "four-eyes." You may have to encourage them to give glasses a fair try. In most instances, glasses improve vision so much that after trying them, children will continue to wear them. Surgery to improve myopia is improving but is not recommended for children until the technique is further refined.

Astigmatism

Astigmatism is congenital or acquired unevenness of the curvature of the cornea so that not all light rays coming to the retina are refracted in the same way, resulting in an uneven quality of vision. When children with astigmatism look at the letter T, for example, they see the crossbar but not the letter stem. If they focus on the stem, they cannot see the crossbar. On any given page of print, therefore, they may see only half the letters. Because of this, they will have difficulty reading or following written instruction. They report headache and vertigo after doing close work. Their vision may appear deceptively normal by vision screening, because by tilting their head, they may be able to see all numbers on a chart enough to pass a vision screening test. They need to be referred to an ophthalmologist, however, on the basis of their other difficulties: vertigo, headaches, and difficulty with reading. Corrective lenses for close work relieve the symptoms and restore functional vision. Contact lenses may be even more helpful because they actually smooth out the curvature of the cornea.

Nystagmus

Nystagmus is rapid, irregular eye movement. It is not a disease in itself but rather a symptom of an underlying disease condition. Ocular nystagmus is seen in children with vision-impairing lesions, such as congenital cataracts. It also occurs in a neurologic form when there is a lesion of the cerebellum or brain stem. Children with nystagmus must be referred to a physician so that the underlying cause of the symptom can be determined.

Amblyopia

Amblyopia is "lazy eye," or subnormal vision in one eye. Children use only one eye for vision while "resting" the other eye. If this process continues for too long a pe-

riod of time, children fail to develop central vision (or the central vision that had developed fades) and they become functionally blind in one eye. This occurs if children have a refractive error in one eye that is significantly different from that of the other eye. Because one eye focuses more readily than the other, children come to depend on only the easily focused eye.

Amblyopia can also develop from **strabismus** (crossed eyes). With strabismus, one eye looks straight ahead; the other "wanders." Children whose one eye wanders will constantly be looking at two separate images rather than one fused image. To make sense out of what they see, they suppress one visual image. This leads to suppression of central vision in that eye, or amblyopia. The same phenomenon occurs if the vision in one eye is obscured due to a lid that does not open fully (**ptosis**).

Assessment

All preschool children should be screened for amblyopia by vision testing with a preschool E chart (see Chapter 28). The child with amblyopia will have 20/50 vision (normal for preschool age) in one eye. The other eye will show lessened vision (perhaps 20/100). The Worth 4-Dot Test is one designed specifically to test for amblyopia. For the test, children wear specially colored glasses. When they look at a series of dots, they see four dots if both eyes are functioning; they see three if their right eye is not functional and two if their left eye is not functioning (Figure 50-4).

Therapeutic Management

Amblyopia is correctable if treated during the preschool period. After 6 years of age, the prognosis for correction

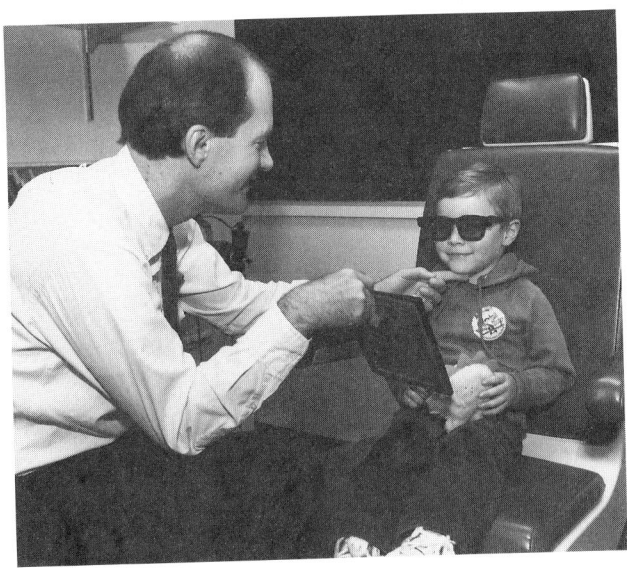

FIGURE 50-4
Screening for amblyopia using a Worth 4-Dot Test. Children should be well prepared for eye examinations so that they do not perceive them as "tests." (Courtesy of the Department of Medical Photography, Children's Hospital, Buffalo, NY.)

is considerably diminished; after 8 years, little improvement in vision can be achieved. For treatment, the good eye is covered by a patch held firmly in place with Elastoplast. This forces a child to use her poor eye to develop vision in that eye. She generally has some difficulty initially adjusting to the patch. She cannot see well from the unpatched eye and may develop headaches and dizziness. Only constant attempts to see with the poor eye, however, can improve binocular vision. A newer treatment is administration of levodopa/carbidopa in addition to occlusion therapy; this may offer longer effects (Leguire et al., 1993).

Nursing Diagnoses and Related Interventions

Nursing Diagnosis: Knowledge deficit related to need for consistent wearing of patch

Goal: By 1 week, parents and child will demonstrate understanding of the importance of early and constant wearing of patch to achieve correction of amblyopia.

Outcome Criteria: Parents state that the reason for child to wear a patch over the good eye is to improve vision in the poorly functioning eye.

Parents need support to be firm with their child about keeping the patch on. The child may beg to remove the patch for special occasions, such as a birthday party or a family wedding, or just for an hour, because she finds the patch embarrassing and uncomfortable. Soon, however, the "special occasions" become so frequent that she ends up wearing the patch only half the time. Remind parents that this correction is not like dental braces. If a child does not wear his retainer half the time, this means he will eventually need to wear the retainer about 50% longer but will still achieve a good correction. Children with amblyopia do not have this luxury. If their amblyopic eyes are not corrected by 6 years of age, the time for correction runs out. Teach them to keep patches in place constantly. If amblyopia occurs secondary to another defect (strabismus, ptosis, or refraction error), this primary problem will need to be corrected also; otherwise, the amblyopia will recur after the patching is completed.

Color Vision Deficit (Color Blindness)

Color blindness is the inability to perceive color correctly. It occurs because one of the sets of cones of the retina that perceive red, green, or blue is absent. It is inherited as a sex-linked disorder and occurs in about 8% of males. There is a high incidence of color vision deficit in children with hemophilia, congenital nystagmus, and glucose-6-phosphate dehydrogenase deficiency.

The vision problem may involve the inability to see red and green or blue and yellow; a small proportion of children have inability to see all colors. Ishihara color plates may be used to detect color deficit in children as young as preschool age. Children with normal vision see numbers on these plates; children with a color vision deficit see only a jumble of dots.

There is no therapy for color blindness, but the condition should be detected early so that children are not asked to complete color identification assignments in school and so they can be educated about traffic signals and other color-dependent signs.

Some children associate color blindness with total "blindness" and fear that they will eventually lose their eyesight. They need to be reassured early on that although color blindness is not a normal condition, it will not destroy their vision.

Structural Problems of the Eye

Coloboma

A *coloboma* is a congenital incomplete closure of the facial cleft. The incomplete closure may involve only the lower eyelid (there is a notch in the lid); it may involve the iris, which will appear as a keyhole, not a circle (Figure 50-5). It may involve the ciliary body, the lens, the choroid, the retina, and the optic nerve. Children with any degree of coloboma should be referred to an ophthalmologist for further investigation so that the extent of the condition can be accurately determined. Children with retina and optic nerve coloboma will have a degree of vision impairment in the affected eye.

Hypertelorism

Hypertelorism is congenital, abnormally wide-spaced eyes. Children with wide epicanthal folds by the inner canthus may appear to have wide-spaced eyes, but

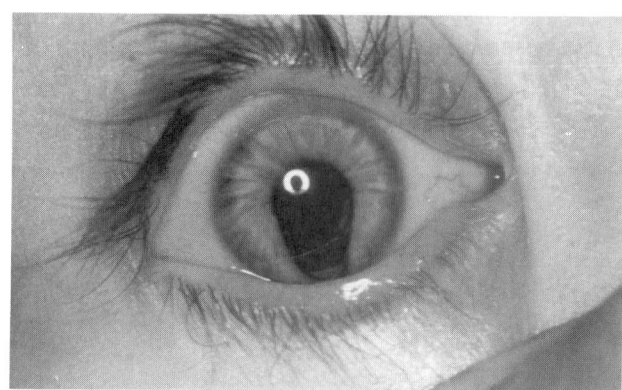

FIGURE 50-5
Coloboma. In this photograph, the inferior portion of the iris is incompletely formed, leaving a "keyhole" pupil. (Courtesy of Brian Smistek.)

when the distance between the pupils is measured and compared with standards for that age, the true condition is revealed. It is important that true hypertelorism in children be detected because it is associated with chromosomal abnormalities, most notably Waardenburg's syndrome, which involves congenital hearing impairment as well. These children also have a white forelock of hair (not always noticeable in newborns who have little hair), different-colored irises (not always noticeable in newborns whose irises are always blue), and eyebrows that tend to grow together in the center line (again, not always present in the newborn). The wide-spaced eyes, because of a broad-bridged nose, then, is the chief clue in the newborn that the child can hear no sound.

Ptosis

Ptosis is the inability to raise the upper eyelid normally so that it always remains slightly closed (Figure 50-6). The condition may be congenital or acquired. The congenital type is frequently hereditary and tends to be bilateral. Acquired ptosis is generally unilateral. It may have a neurogenic origin (injury to the third cranial nerve) or be caused by injury to the lid or levator muscle. When the cause is neurogenic, there is generally paralysis of one or more of the other muscles supplied by the third cranial nerve (children have a dilated pupil; are unable to rotate the eye globe upward, medially, or downward; and have weakness of accommodation [looking at near objects]). Myasthenia gravis, which produces generalized muscle weakness, must always be ruled out as the cause of bilateral ptosis.

Children with ptosis tend to wrinkle their forehead and raise their eyebrows more than usual in an attempt to lift the eyelid further. Also, they may cock their heads back to see under the lowered lid.

Correction for ptosis is usually by surgery after careful investigation of the cause has been completed. The correction is usually important to the child from a cosmetic standpoint, but more important, if the lid obstructs vision, early surgery is necessary to prevent the development of amblyopia (from lack of use of the eye). It is important that parents understand this; otherwise, they may insist on delaying a corrective procedure "until the child is older." When the child is older, the ptosis can be corrected but the amblyopia cannot.

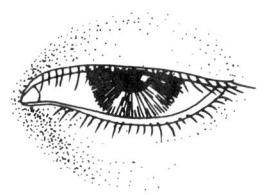

FIGURE 50-6
Ptosis, or drooping of the upper eyelid.

Strabismus

Strabismus is unequally aligned eyes (cross-eyes). About 1% to 2% of children have some degree of strabismus; the condition occurs without regard for sex, social status, or geographic area. About 50% of children with strabismus have a history of someone else in the family having a similar strabismus. When there is a family history of strabismus, children need to be observed and examined yearly for this problem.

The movement of each eye globe is controlled by extraocular muscles. These can be compared in movement to the handling of reins of a horse. The superior rectus muscle turns the eye up and medially. The inferior rectus muscle turns the eye down and medially. The medial rectus muscle turns the eye inward. All three muscles receive their nerve innervation from the oculomotor (third cranial) nerve. The lateral rectus muscle turns the eye out; nerve innervation of this muscle is the abducens (or sixth cranial) nerve. The superior oblique muscle turns the eye down and laterally. This muscle receives its nerve innervation from the trochlear (or fourth cranial) nerve. The inferior oblique muscle turns the eye up and laterally. Innervation is from the oculomotor (or third cranial) nerve (Figure 50-7).

Normally, with good eye alignment, the resting position of the eyes is straight. This is largely the result of muscle or nerve influences that the child cannot control. In strabismus, the resting position of one eye may be *divergent* (turned out) or *convergent* (turned in). One pupil may be higher than the other (vertical strabismus). The strabismus may be monocular, in which the same eye deviates constantly; or it may be an alternating strabismus, in which first one eye deviates, then the other.

Both the resting position of eyes and the amount of turning necessary to read small print depend on the eyes' ability to fuse and see only one image. The ability to do this is slight in infancy; it becomes stronger with practice and, in adulthood, it is automatic. If children do not learn to fuse vision effectively early in life, they are never able to achieve it later on or to maintain good eye position.

It takes muscular effort to look medially (turn an eye in toward the nose). When children read small print, they turn both eyes medially, or *converge,* to focus at the short distance. If they are farsighted in one eye, they have to turn the affected eye in more than the other, causing strabismus. If they have one eye that is nearsighted, they will not need to turn that eye in as far as the other one; this results in divergence of that eye. Although these children have good eye alignment at rest, they "cross their eyes" when attempting to focus at a reading distance.

Assessment

Infants' eyes may cross occasionally until 6 weeks of age. If infants demonstrate strabismus past this age, they

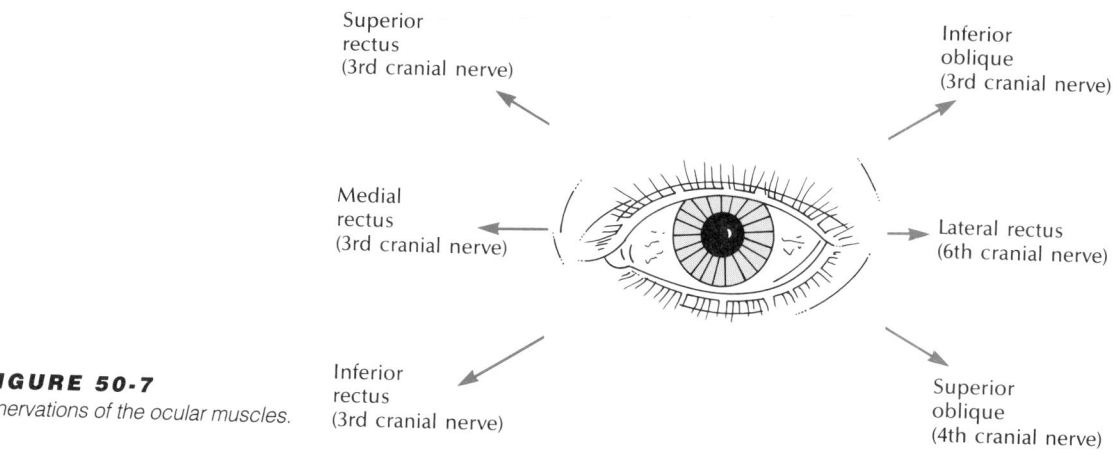

FIGURE 50-7
Innervations of the ocular muscles.

should be referred for diagnosis and treatment. Infants who demonstrate a constant strabismus before 6 weeks of age need referral right away.

Definite deviations will be obvious (Figure 50-8). These can be *exotropia* (eye turning out), *esotropia* (eye turning in), or *hypertropia* (eye turning up). If the deviation is not so obvious but only occurs when the child is fatigued or ill, and therefore less able to maintain fixation, the terms used are *exophoria, esophoria,* and *hyperphoria.* If the parents report that the deviation only occurs when the child is tired or sick, ask them to come for assessment when the child will most likely be tired and the deviation will be most striking.

Children who have flat, broad-bridged noses, a narrow interpupillary distance, and an epicanthal fold or

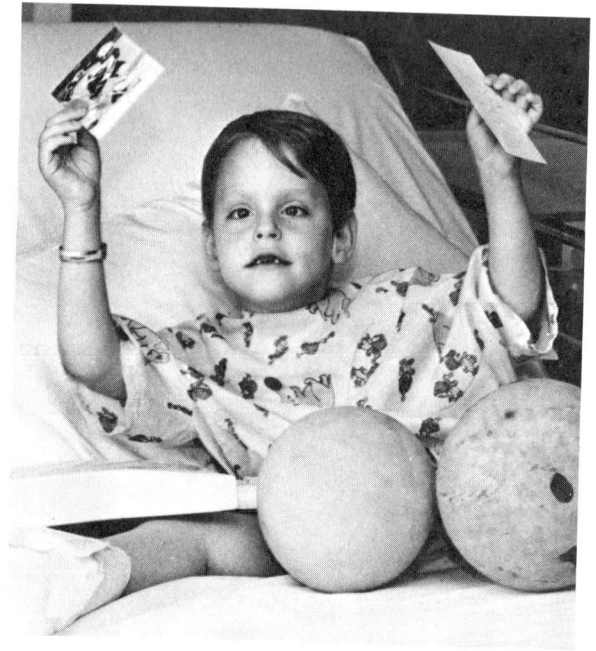

FIGURE 50-8
A child with strabismus. The child has an esotropia of the right eye. (Courtesy of the Department of Medical Photography, Children's Hospital, Buffalo, NY.)

oval-shaped palpebral fissures may appear to have strabismus when they truly do not (pseudostrabismus). When you observe these children, you see less white sclera in the inner margin of the eye than normally, and so the eye appears to be turned in (*pseudoesotropia*).

Some children have a latent strabismus, but because they are able to maintain fusion, the strabismus is not overt. They maintain this fusion at the expense of eyestrain, however. They experience headaches; tired, irritated eyes; and perhaps even nausea and vomiting.

A cover test will reveal the latent deviation. For this test, ask a child to look at an object about 5 feet in front of him. Cover the suspected eye with a 3 × 5 card. While it is covered, the eye will move to its deviated position. After 5 seconds of covering, remove the card. The deviated eye will move back to a good alignment as the child refixes on the object (Figure 50-9). This movement of an eye after a cover test is evidence of a latent strabismus. In pseudostrabismus, the covered eye will not move—it is straight. It only appears turned medially because of the obscured sclera at the inner canthus.

Another method of detecting strabismus is to shine an otoscopic light into both the child's eyes (Hirshberg's test; Figure 50-10). If the eyes are in alignment, the reflection of the light will be at the same point on each pupil. If the light reflects on the edge of the pupil on one eye and on the sclera of the other eye, the eyes are not in alignment. Once a strabismus is detected, it is important to attempt to discern whether it is concomitant (measures the same in all directions of gaze) or nonconcomitant (greater in one direction than another, often called *paralytic strabismus*).

Paralytic strabismus is caused by paralysis of a muscle or nerve, perhaps from an injury or invading lesion; it can occur from a birth injury. The eyes appear straight except when they are moved in the direction of the paralyzed muscle; then double vision occurs, and the crossed eye is evident. Such children often close one eye or tilt their head to see better to decrease the double vision. They may tilt their head so much they appear to

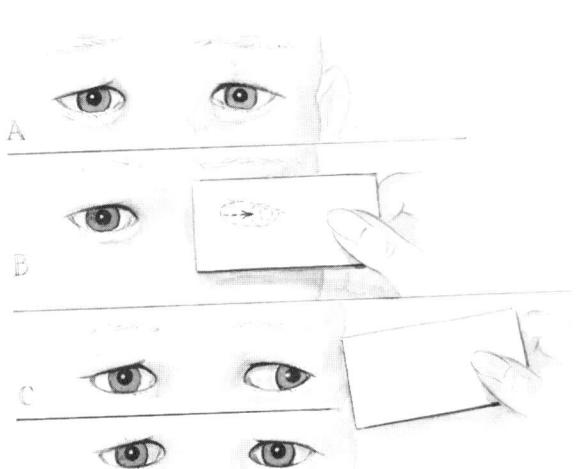

FIGURE 50-9
*Cover test. (**A**) The child's eyes appear to be in good alignment. (**B**) The left eye is covered for 5 sec. (**C**) When the card is removed, the left eye is seen to move perceptibly back to good alignment. This movement indicates that the eye drifted into a deviant position while covered.*

have a torticollis, or "wry neck"—an orthopedic rather than an eye problem. They are often fussy or clumsy because of the diplopia. They cannot see well and may be too young to describe what is happening to them through any other means than fussiness.

Concomitant (nonparalytic) strabismus is the most usual type found in children. All the muscles of the eye are capable of function, but they are not functioning together. This deviation is equally apparent in all directions of gaze.

Therapeutic Management

The therapy for strabismus depends on the cause of the problem. If the fusion mechanism is weak, eye exercises (**orthoptics**) may be necessary to correct the problem. If eyes are diverging with convergence because of far-sightedness or nearsightedness, the child needs glasses to correct the basic visual defect. If the misalignment is caused by unequal muscle strength, eye-muscle surgery is generally necessary to correct it. Nursing care for the child having eye surgery is discussed in the section The Child Undergoing Eye Surgery. No eye patches are required for strabismus surgery. Parents will need to apply antibiotic ointment to the eye for 2 to 3 days. Muscle surgery may give the child some pain on eye movement for the first day postoperatively.

Children need a follow-up visit after surgery to see that their surgical repair was successful. Retest them periodically at health maintenance visits to be certain that their vision remains equal and eye alignment remains straight.

Because strabismus causes the eyes to be viewing two different fields of vision, diplopia, or double vision, occurs. To prevent this, the child suppresses the vision in one eye or only looks with one eye (amblyopia). Even if diplopia is not present, the lack of fusion leads to the same consequence. For this reason, eye correction for strabismus must be done early in life, before 6 years of age. It is true that some children whose eyes are crossing because of an accommodation problem caused by hyperopia in one eye will outgrow the condition as the normal hyperopia of the preschooler lessens; but this cannot be counted on. Even if the child's eyes appear to be straighter later, an amblyopia may be present that could have been prevented by earlier treatment.

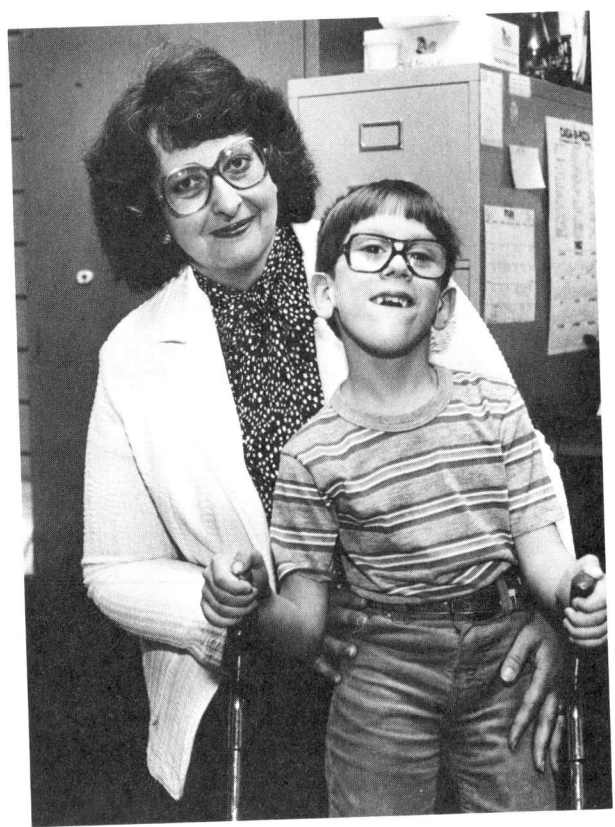

FIGURE 50-10
Testing for good eye alignment by Hirshberg's test. Notice how the light reflects at the same point on both of the nurse's pupils and at different points on the child's pupils, indicating that the child's are misaligned. (Courtesy of the Department of Medical Photography, Children's Hospital, Buffalo, NY.)

Infection or Inflammation of the Eye

Stye (Hordeolum)

A **stye** is an infection of a ciliary gland (a modified sweat gland) that enters into the hair follicle at the lid margin (Figure 50-11*A*). The organism responsible for such an infection is generally *Staphylococcus*. Children note pain and redness at a localized point on the lid

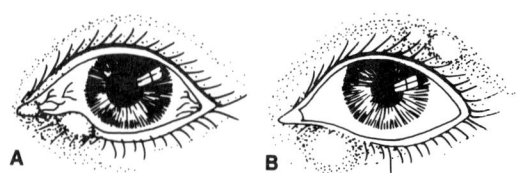

FIGURE 50-11
(**A**) *A stye, or infection of a ciliary gland.* (**B**) *A chalazion, or inflammation of a meibomian gland.*

margin. The lid may become edematous out of proportion to the severity of the disease. The regional lymph node (preauricular) may become swollen and tender.

Hot, wet compresses, applied for 15 to 20 minutes four times a day, help to relieve the pain of the inflammation and hasten the self-limiting process. An antibiotic ointment may be prescribed to be applied after the compresses. When the stye points (develops a head), it is ready to be incised and drained. This is a frightening procedure for children, because they worry that the physician's hand will slip and cut their eye. Also, their eyes are so painful from the infection that they are very reluctant to let anyone touch them.

Children who have repeated styes should have a general health assessment, as styes tend to occur in the setting of debilitating disease such as diabetes mellitus or anemia. The nose and throat should be cultured for *Staphylococcus* as well. Although styes are not associated with refraction error, they occur when children rub their eyes excessively because of this, so vision acuity should be assessed.

Chalazion

A **chalazion** is a low-grade granulation tissue tumor of the *meibomian,* or tarsal, gland on the eyelid (Figure 50-11*B*). The cause is unknown, but it may occur as a result of a low-grade infection produced by retained secretion in the gland. A small, slow-growing, hard-but-painless nodule appears on the lid. The skin is freely movable over it. It is not inflamed nor is edema present. A chalazion may resolve itself spontaneously and evacuate itself onto the conjunctival surface of the lid. Incision and curettage of the lesion may be necessary if spontaneous remission does not occur. Antibiotic ointment may be prescribed to prevent a secondary infection of the gland after incision and drainage. This is applied in a strip along the rim of the lower eyelid; when the child closes his eye, ointment is swept over the eye globe to the chalazion opening on the lid.

Although a chalazion is painless, its presence is frightening to parents. An abnormal growth on the body is one of the seven danger signs of cancer. Both parents and child may need to be reassured that the growth is only a swollen gland and that the lesion is confined to the lid, not involving the eye.

If a chalazion is large enough to cause a ptosis or presses on the cornea to cause an astigmatism, it may lead to amblyopia. In young children (under 8 years), therefore, a chalazion is removed surgically early instead of waiting for it to resolve spontaneously.

Blepharitis Marginalis

Blepharitis marginalis is inflammation of the eyelid margin. The margin appears reddened and may be covered by hard, dirty-yellow crusts that stick tenaciously to the lid margin and lashes. The cause is a local infection generally caused by *Staphylococcus* organisms (Weiss, 1993). It may be an extension of seborrheic dermatitis (cradle cap). Treatment generally consists of the application of an antibiotic ointment six to eight times a day to the lower conjunctival rim. The crusts may be removed with a moistened cotton applicator after the lid margins have been covered by wet compresses for 10 to 15 minutes.

Styes may be present secondary to the presence of *Staphylococcus*. If the condition persists, the child may be prescribed a systemic antibiotic to reduce the presence of *Staphylococcus* on the skin surface. Although blepharitis marginalis is a small local problem, it is a big problem for the child because it is so unsightly; it can spread and become conjunctivitis.

Conjunctivitis

Conjunctivitis is inflammation of the conjunctiva, the mucous membrane that covers the anterior surface of the eye globe and the inner surface of the eyelid. With this, the eye waters, the conjunctiva becomes reddened, and the eye may be sensitive to light; the eyelid may become stuck shut with a pustular drainage. There are a number of common causative agents of conjunctivitis in children. The most serious of these, ophthalmia neonatorum, is caused by exposure to the gonococcus bacillus (Hammerschlag, 1993). This is discussed in Chapter 26, as it tends to occur only in newborns.

Inclusion Blennorrhea
Inclusion blennorrhea usually occurs on the fifth to the fourteenth day after birth from contact with chlamydial organisms. The inflammation is acute; the conjunctiva is reddened, and tearing occurs. The diagnosis is made by the staining of cytoplasmic basophilic inclusion bodies from the eye discharge. The treatment consists of a systemic antibiotic such as erythromycin. Older children may contract this as "swimming pool conjunctivitis."

Acute Catarrhal Conjunctivitis
Catarrhal conjunctivitis is caused most frequently by two common organisms: *Hemophilus influenzae* and *Streptococcus pneumoniae* (Lohr, 1993). Commonly called "pinkeye," this type of conjunctivitis may also be caused

by a virus or irritation from a foreign body. The conjunctiva turns fiery red, is painful, and tears readily. Treatment consists of the administration of antibiotic drops or ointment three or four times a day for 7 days. Parents need to be reminded to give the antibiotic for the full 7 days. Because the redness disappears by 48 hours, parents may not realize that it is important to continue giving the medication. As with any antibiotic, if treatment is discontinued too early, the infection may not be completely eradicated and may recur in another week. Be certain infection is not spread from the first eye to the second one when the child rubs his or her eyes on application of ointment or drops. Don't use an occlusive dressing on the eye, because the dark will increase the growth potential of organisms.

Herpetic Conjunctivitis

Conjunctivitis from the herpes simplex virus may occur along with development of a facial herpes lesion (Persaud et al., 1993). A series of pinpoint vesicles appear on the conjunctiva. If the conjunctiva is touched with a strip of paper impregnated with fluorescein stain, the vesicles stain bright green and are readily evident. Because this is a viral infection, antibiotic drops are ineffective as treatment. The child should be referred to an ophthalmologist for care, however, because herpetic conjunctivitis can spread easily and become a corneal infection with resultant opacity and permanent scarring. Steroids should never be used with herpetic conjunctivitis because they may spread the infection to the cornea. Idoxuridine or trifluorothymidine, drugs specific for herpes virus, may be effective in limiting corneal involvement.

Allergic Conjunctivitis

When children become hypersensitive to a specific allergen, conjunctival changes may occur as part of a hypersensitivity reaction. With this reaction, there is generally edema of the eyelids and conjunctiva, profuse tearing, and severe itching. This will occur seasonally as a rule, because the allergen is most often a pollen. The itching is far more intense than in infectious conjunctivitis. Care of children with allergies is discussed in Chapter 42.

Keratitis

Keratitis is inflammation and infection of the superficial layers of the cornea. It may accompany or be a complication of conjunctivitis. It may result when a foreign body strikes the cornea. The invading organism may be fungal, bacterial, or viral in origin. When the cornea becomes infected, symptoms of pain, tearing, **photophobia** (intolerance to light), and redness become acute. Children with keratitis must be referred to an ophthalmologist for therapy because the infection could lead to scarring of the cornea, resulting in vision impairment

when light rays are no longer able to enter the eye normally.

Periorbital Cellulitis

Cellulitis (infection of subcutaneous tissue) most often occurs in children as an extension of a superficial infection after an open break in the skin. If a child has a mosquito bite or scratch by the eye, cellulitis may develop and spread around the eye. Because the eye globe fits snugly into the orbit in children, periorbital cellulitis is always serious. The infection must be brought under control before the eye globe or the optic nerve at its point of insertion is compressed by swelling and permanently damaged.

The extent of the inflammation can be detected by sonogram. Children with periorbital cellulitis are usually hospitalized and begun on intravenous antibiotic therapy. A cellulitis may not look serious enough to parents to warrant this extensive therapy. Give them a good explanation of why therapy is so important, so they can help their child with compliance.

Dacryostenosis

In many newborns a membrane obscures the distal end of the nasolacrimal duct, or the duct that drains eye secretions into the nasopharynx is plugged by epithelial debris. When this happens, the normal secretions of the lacrimal gland have nowhere to empty, so the eye tears (Lavich & Nelson, 1993). The condition is called *dacryostenosis* (Figure 50-12). You may be able to palpate a painless lump in the inner canthus of the infant's eye—this is the filled lacrimal duct. To help clear debris from the duct, teach a parent to apply gentle pressure to the inner aspect of the eye at each feeding, gently "milking" secretions down into the nasolacrimal duct, in hopes of clearing epithelial debris that is lodged there. If a child reaches 6 months of age and there is no spontaneous correction of the problem, it is usually necessary for an ophthalmologist to probe the gland duct with a thin metal stylet after inserting anesthetic eye drops to clear the tract. Probing before this time is not usually recommended because it is difficult to do. The lumen of the duct is very small, and irritation may lead to scar formation at the site, which will cause further blockage.

Dacryostenosis is not a serious condition, but it is a cause for concern. Parents may not be sure of how

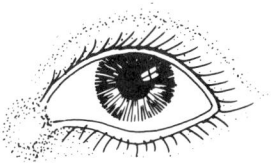

FIGURE 50-12
Dacryostenosis, or blockage of the lacrimal duct.

much pressure they can safely apply to the duct. They need to have the procedure demonstrated so they can learn how to do it safely at home.

Dacryocystitis

Dacryocystitis is an inflammation of the nasolacrimal duct. This may occur secondary to dacryostenosis because of the stasis of fluid. It may occur in school-age and adolescent children with sinusitis when nasal mucosa is swollen and infected mucus is forced back into the nasolacrimal duct. Pressure on the sac may result in the extrusion of pus into the inner canthus of the eye. Children will develop acute pain in the inner canthus from the presence of the infected sac. They usually describe pain as not being in the inner canthus but in the back of the eye and sometimes in the eye itself. Both children and parents need assurance that this is an infection of an organ surrounding the eye and does not affect vision. Therapy includes local and systemic antibiotics. The duct may need to be probed to be freed of obstructing debris and to allow for free drainage.

To prevent further occurrences, a child with chronic allergies or sinusitis may be placed on an antihistamine to keep nasal mucosa from becoming edematous and pressing on the distal end of the duct.

Traumatic Injury to the Eye

The primary cause of vision impairment in children today is from ocular trauma, such as dirt or sand, baseballs, pieces of broken plastic toys, or flying glass in car accidents that strike and even enter the eye globe. Fights with other children, cigarette burns, and fingernail scratches are also causes.

Assessment

Children who have eye injuries are generally in acute pain immediately after the accident. Their eyes tear and are sensitive to light and they blink rapidly. Vision may be blurred or lost in the affected eye. Because of the pain and the fright of not being able to see clearly, most children are very reluctant to let anyone touch their injured eye for examination. They may need a few drops of a topical anesthetic placed in the eye to relieve the pain and to help them allow their eye to be opened for examination. Even after the anesthetic is applied, they need a great deal of explanation of what is happening and that an examiner is "just looking" (providing this is the case). Even after anesthetic application, children may not be able to open their eye readily for inspection, because the acute pain of the injury can cause the eyelid to close by reflex spasm. Edema may form quickly in the eyelid as well, preventing the eye from opening. Do not

confuse these physical problems with a child's unwillingness to open an eye.

To visualize the inner surface of the lower lid and bottom half of the eye globe, press firmly on the lower lid with your finger tip until it turns out. The inner surface of the upper lid and the upper portion of the eye globe can best be visualized if the upper eyelid is everted. Ask the child to look downward. Grasp the eyelash and gently stretch the upper eyelid downward; place the stick of a cotton-tipped applicator horizontally against the center of the upper lid; still grasping the eyelash, pull the eyelid upward and over the stick until it is everted (Figure 50-13). Everting an eyelid is a task that often is done best by a health care provider with small hands; a female member of the emergency team may be able to do this best. Gently press the everted eyelid against the eyebrow to maintain the everted position. Be careful not to exert pressure on the eye globe during the procedure in case a penetrating injury from a foreign body is present. Pressure would further embed the object in the eye globe. Be certain your fingernails are cut short before the procedure so you do not cause corneal abrasions by a scratch during the procedure.

A foreign body, such as a speck of dirt or a fragment of glass, often clings to the inside of the upper lid and can be readily removed by being touched with a moistened, cotton-tipped applicator with the lid everted in this way. Keep an eyelid everted no longer than is necessary for diagnosis and treatment because the eye globe tends to become dry when it is exposed.

Nursing Diagnoses and Related Interventions

Nursing Diagnosis: Parental role conflict related to feelings of guilt about accident affecting child's vision

Goal: Parents will demonstrate confidence in their ability to care for child and verbalize feelings of guilt about the accident by 1 hour.

Outcome Criteria: Parents accurately state child's treatment plan and expected outcome; child and parents talk openly about accident and ways to

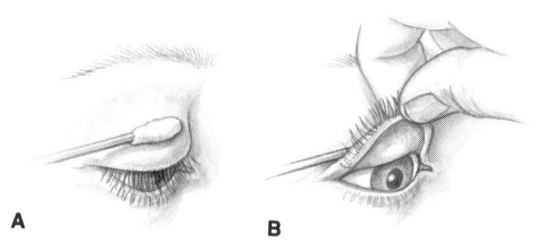

A   B

FIGURE 50-13
*Technique for everting the upper eyelid for examination and foreign body removal. (**A**) Place a cotton applicator across the upper eyelid. (**B**) Pull the eyelid outward and upward over the applicator.*

prevent future ones; parents participate actively in child's care while in hospital and in decision-making with health care providers regarding long-term care.

Eye injuries are almost always serious in children because of the pain and the potential threat to vision. Both parents and children are apt to feel guilty about the accident (aware they should have been more careful). Children remember that they have been told many times to be careful of their eyes. Parents may have difficulty handling this emergency because they feel angry at their children and even more angry at themselves for not supervising them or teaching better eye safety. Children may need help in understanding that although this accident might have been prevented, accidents do happen. This helps them to maintain a sense of self-esteem. Parents may need counseling to understand that accidents can happen even under the most watchful care; this will help them reestablish their feelings of worth as parents.

Following eye trauma, the degree of vision in the child's affected eye, as well as the status of the parent–child relationship, needs to be evaluated. As long as either parent or child feels guilt over the accident, it is difficult for them to have a smooth relationship. After an eye injury, most children do not need future warnings about protecting their eyes.

Foreign Bodies

Foreign bodies such as sand or dirt that are loose on the conjunctiva can be removed by irrigation with a sterile normal saline solution or by gentle wiping with a well-moistened, cotton-tipped applicator after the eyelid is everted, as in Figure 50-13. After the removal, if the conjunctiva is touched with a strip of filter paper impregnated with fluorescein stain, any corneal ulceration or abrasion from the foreign body will stain green and be readily apparent. If the foreign body is easily removed and no corneal ulceration or injury is present, no further treatment is necessary. Children will blink a few times after their upper lid is returned to place, but in a matter of minutes, they will report feeling "fine" again. If the fluorescein stain reveals any corneal ulceration, refer the child to an ophthalmologist for follow-up care.

If a foreign body adheres to the cornea, it needs to be removed by an ophthalmologist. This may be done with an electronic magnet. If the foreign body is metallic, and it has been in contact with the cornea for a period of hours, a rust ring forms around the particle. This rust ring must be removed as well as the original particle or it will continue to act as a foreign body. After corneal injury, corneal tissue will regenerate. To allow for this, the eye is washed with an antibiotic solution and then closed and patched. The patch must be secure enough to keep the eyelid closed yet not put undue pressure on the eye. Caution children that it must be left in place to

prevent the delicate regenerating corneal epithelium from being rubbed off until it is well healed and secure once more.

If a foreign object is a large one such as a BB bullet, a lollipop stick, or a piece of broken glass, the fact that it has punctured the eye globe is usually apparent on first inspection. In these instances, children also need to be examined by an ophthalmologist. Surgery may be necessary to explore the depth of the puncture and save the child's sight in that eye.

If the ciliary body was involved in a penetrating injury, an extremely serious complication called *sympathetic iritis,* or inflammation of the opposite eye, may result, and blindness in the noninjured eye may occur (Kraus-Mackiw, 1990). This complication can be prevented by removal (enucleation) of the injured eye. If the vision in the injured eye appears to be destroyed, a decision for removal is not difficult for parents to make. If the vision is not totally destroyed, however, deciding to remove the injured eye is extremely difficult for parents. Fortunately, immediate treatment with corticosteroids and antibiotics has significantly reduced the incidence of this complication today.

Contusion Injuries

Many eye injuries happen not from a sharp object striking the eye but from blunt trauma: a baseball, a fist, or an automobile dashboard striking the eye. With this type of injury, the eyelid and the surrounding tissue, including the intraorbital tissue, may hemorrhage and become edematous.

The simplest form of contusion injury is a "black eye." After this occurs, the eye globe should be inspected (including a funduscopic examination). Assess vision in the eye. If a vision chart is not available, vision can be assessed by having children tell you how many fingers they can count at a distance of about 6 feet (assuming they are old enough to count accurately) or by having them read a printed page at reading distance (assuming they are old enough to read). Ask children if they have difficulty seeing. Check the range of motion of the eye globe to determine whether or not the extraocular muscles are functioning adequately. Children should be able to look up and down, left and right, upward obliquely, and downward obliquely—the six cardinal positions of gaze.

In children who have no apparent eye injury, good ocular movement, and normal vision (for them), an ice pack applied to the eye to minimize swelling is the only treatment necessary (20 minutes on, 20 minutes off, and repeat). Reabsorption of hemorrhage in the tissue surrounding the eye will take place over the next 1 to 3 weeks. Often, tissue hemorrhage extends across the nose and surrounds the other eye the day after the injury. You can assure both parents and child that this is not a worsening of the condition but mainly evidence of the severity of the initial blow.

If children have limited eye movement or report diplopia (double vision), evidence is strong that a "blow out" fracture of the floor of the orbit (the maxillary bone) has occurred. This fracture line is trapping intra-orbital tissue and preventing the eye globe from moving freely. Children with this sign need to be referred to an ophthalmologist. They need surgery to free the entrapped tissue, prevent interference with vascular flow, and restore normal eye movement.

After a blunt contusion to the eye globe, a number of serious findings besides limited motion may be present. These are disturbances of the pupil, such as a dilated, fixed, or cloudy pupil; cloudy lens or cornea; loss of vision in the eye; and visible blood in the anterior chamber (hyphema), all of which may indicate dislocation of the lens or retina detachment. Children with these signs must also be referred to an ophthalmologist for care.

Eyelid Injuries

Eyelid injuries may accompany eye globe injuries or may be the only finding present after a foreign body has struck the eye. Although such injuries appear to be trivial, don't dismiss them lightly but refer the child to an ophthalmologist for care. A deep laceration of the eyelid can cause a permanent ptosis; a laceration to the inner canthal area may disrupt the lacrimal drainage system (dacryostenosis).

Inner Eye Conditions

Congenital Glaucoma

Glaucoma is increased intraocular pressure in the eye globe because of inadequate or blocked drainage of aqueous humor. Aqueous humor is produced by the ciliary body; it flows from the posterior chamber through the pupil to the anterior chamber and is excreted through the canal of Schlemm at the lateral angle into the venous circulation (Figure 50-14). When glaucoma is congenital, a developmental anomaly in the angle of the anterior chamber prevents proper drainage at the canal. Later in life, glaucoma occurs when the canal becomes blocked. The increased fluid content causes the globe of the eye to increase in size. After the eye globe has increased in size to the extent that it can, the pressure in the eye globe continues to rise, and the optic nerve is compressed and destroyed. Glaucoma (meaning "gray") gets its name from the color of the retina or red reflex (gray to green) in the eye after the sight has been lost. The condition occurs as often as 1 in 30,000 live births.

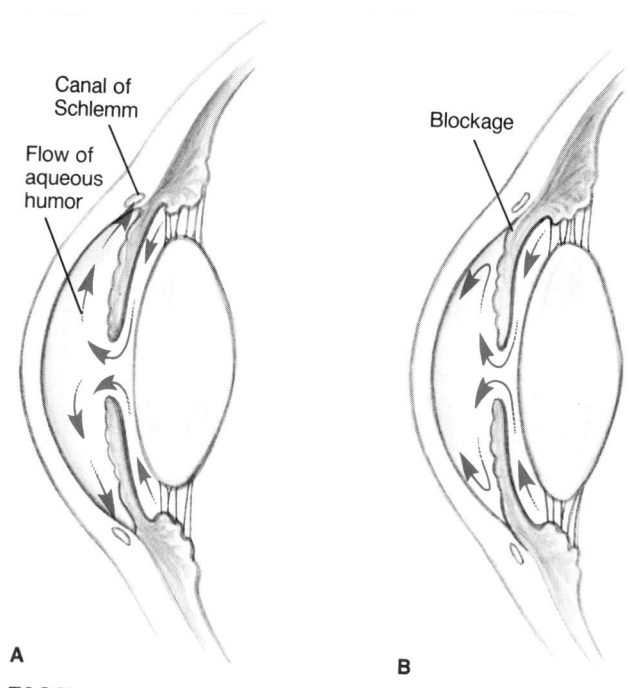

FIGURE 50-14
(**A**) *Circulation of aqueous humor.* (**B**) *Blockage of canal of Schlemm in glaucoma.*

Assessment

Congenital glaucoma is a rare disease but one that must be assessed for in infants; it accounts for vision impairment in 5% to 13% of children in schools for the visually impaired. It is caused by a recessive gene inheritance pattern (Traboulsi & Maumenee, 1994). In most infants, the condition is usually bilateral. In about 50% of children with this condition, symptoms are noticeable shortly after birth; in 80% to 90%, glaucoma is apparent at 1 year of age. The cornea appears enlarged; it may be edematous and hazy. Most newborn corneas measure 10 mm or less; at 1 year, they measure 12 mm. A newborn with a cornea measurement of over 11 mm and a child at 1 year with a cornea measurement over 12 mm should be investigated for glaucoma. In addition to the enlarged cornea, the newborn may have tearing, pain, and photophobia, which are all difficult to identify in a newborn. The eye globe may feel tense to finger palpation.

Eye pressure is measured by means of a *tonometer*, a pressure-sensitive device that is placed against the anterior eye globe, usually under anesthesia in infants. Normal tension is 12 to 20 mm Hg. Tension above this is suggestive of glaucoma. A new tonometry apparatus allows a pressure recording to be made (similar to an electrocardiogram strip) that can be included in the chart as a permanent record. If tonometry is done under local anesthesia, caution children not to rub their eyes after the procedure. Restrain an infant's arms to prevent eye rubbing for about 4 hours after an examination under a local anesthesia, or else corneal abrasions may occur because of the cornea's lack of sensitivity.

Therapeutic Management

Immediate surgery—a **goniotomy**, in which a new opening to the canal of Schlemm is constructed—is scheduled for the infant. A drug such as acetazolamide (Diamox), a carbonic anhydrase inhibitor that suppresses the formation of aqueous humor, or a miotic agent to increase aqueous humor drainage may be used as a temporary measure to attempt to reduce eye pressure before the surgery can be scheduled, but it is never a long-range solution in children. Newer surgery techniques include laser therapy.

It is important that the infant does not receive a drug that dilates the pupil prior to surgery (this will further occlude the canal of Schlemm). Question an order such as atropine sulfate for preoperative medication. After surgery, the child is usually placed on bed rest with an eye patch in place. Contact sports or "roughhousing" in younger children is restricted for 2 weeks.

Some infants may need three or four operations before the new opening for drainage of fluid is adequate to keep tension of the eye globe at a normal level. Parents need to be told of this possibility when surgery is first proposed, so that they will not think that additional surgery is being scheduled because the first operation was inadequate or was done incorrectly.

Discharge Planning and Follow-Up

Eye examination in infants and children at regular intervals is important so that congenital glaucoma can be recognized before damage to the optic nerve occurs. Glaucoma may occur following eye trauma if there is scarring at the canal of Schlemm. Children who have eye injuries are usually asked to return for a follow-up appointment in a month for the pressure in their eye to be assessed. Stress the importance of this visit without alarming parents or child about the possible complication.

Cataract

A *cataract* is a marked opacity of the lens. This may be present at birth or may become apparent in early childhood. It can occur as a result of trauma to the eye if the lens is injured. When the opacity is on the anterior surface of the lens, the cause is thought to be birth injury or possibly contact between the lens and the cornea during intrauterine life. When the opacity is located at the edge of the lens, it may be the result of nutritional deficiency during intrauterine life, such as rickets or hypocalcemia. Infants who contract rubella prenatally may develop central cataracts. Some central cataracts are familial.

Assessment

When you inspect the pupil of a child with a cataract, the pupil opening appears to be white, not black (leukocoria). The red reflex elicited by shining a light into the pupil appears white, not red. Older children report blurred vision from cataract formation; in the infant, this can be detected by a lack of response to a smile or inability to reach and grasp a nearby object. The infant will also demonstrate nystagmus, being unable to focus the eye on objects. A few other conditions simulate this appearance: retinoblastoma, retinopathy of prematurity, or an abscess of the posterior chamber. In congenital glaucoma, the lens may be opaque from edema. This can be differentiated from simple cataract by the accompanying enlargement of the eye and pupil opening.

Therapeutic Management

Treatment of childhood cataract is surgical removal of the lens. If the total lens is involved, this may be done as early as 3 months of age. If this is not done before 6 months of age, amblyopia may result.

During the immediate postoperative period, the infant's eyes may be covered with patches, although with newer surgical techniques the incision is so small that this may not be necessary. Infants may be given a sedative to keep them still for 24 hours. Introduce fluids cautiously after eye surgery so that nausea and vomiting do not occur; vomiting increases intraocular pressure, which could injure the suture line. Encourage parents to stay with the infant and help with care so the infant does not cry following surgery, because this also increases eye pressure. Infants can be expected to have some discomfort but generally should not have acute eye pain after surgery. If they are unusually restless, fussy, or crying and seem to be in pain, notify the physician immediately. Although this could be caused by an unrelated reason, this may be a sign of increased intraocular pressure from hemorrhage or from occlusion of the canal of Schlemm, causing a developing glaucoma.

As a rule, children will be given a mydriatic (to dilate the pupil) and steroids to prevent adhesions of the pupil from developing postoperatively. They will be fitted with contact lenses to give them accommodative power shortly after surgery. If the eye that had the cataract is now amblyopic, patching of the normal eye may be necessary in addition to the use of eyeglasses to restore vision.

Parents of children with congenital cataracts need support to carry out the procedures necessary and to give the long-term medication and corrective measures needed. Evaluation should include not only the child's current vision status but also whether the child views himself or herself as well despite this early life problem.

The Child Undergoing Eye Surgery

Cataract or glaucoma operations in childhood are generally performed on infants; thus, preparation for this surgery primarily consists of helping the baby to adjust to the strange environment of a hospital and encouraging parents or a primary care person to spend as much time with the baby as possible. This is particularly important if eyes will be patched after surgery. Strabismus operations are often done during the preschool period. Such surgery is generally done on an ambulatory basis so the child does not have to stay overnight in the hospital. The operation can be explained to the preschooler through the use of puppets or dolls. As with all surgical procedures, talk about the child's affected parts, in this case, the eyes, being "fixed" or "made better," never "cut." Even a very young child knows how important his or her eyes are and will agree to having them made better, but not cut (see the Focus on Nursing Research box).

Nursing Diagnoses and Related Interventions

Nursing Diagnosis: Anxiety related to lack of knowledge about eye surgery and postoperative experience

Goal: Child will demonstrate confidence in and cooperate with health care providers postoperatively.

Outcome Criteria: Child asks questions and expresses fears about surgery; child states plans for postoperative period and practices putting on eye patches, if appropriate.

If the child's eyes are going to be patched after surgery, you can accustom him to the feeling of the patches beforehand. Even when only one eye is going to be operated on, it is not unusual for both eyes to be patched after strabismus repairs because eyes move conjugately. When your right eye looks to the right, so does your left eye. The repaired eye, therefore, will only stay immobile under a bandage if both eyes are patched.

Show the child a doll with eye patches, and let the child try wearing them. Compare this sensation to something familiar. Most preschoolers have played games such as "pin the tail on the donkey" or "blindman's bluff"; if not, describe the rules of these games and play them with the child, to help her associate the feeling of covered eyes with fun. Another helpful game is to have the child pull out familiar objects from a paper bag—a key, an orange, a spoon, and a penny—and with her eyes covered, try to guess what they are.

Be certain that you speak with the child preoperatively so that she can recognize your voice afterward. Practice having the child identify your voice by covering her eyes and then alternate talking with a parent, so the child can guess which of you said what.

Some young children will have not only patches in place after surgery but also arm restraints, to prevent them from pressing on their eyes or removing the patches. If that is the plan, introduce these preopera-

FOCUS ON NURSING RESEARCH

How Can the Anxiety of Mothers Following A Child's Unplanned Hospitalization Be Reduced?

An unplanned hospitalization such as can occur from an eye injury can be a frightening experience for both a child and parent. To investigate whether parent anxiety can be reduced in this situation by providing more information to parents, a nurse researcher asked 108 mothers whose children had been admitted for unplanned hospitalization to participate in a research study. Mothers' ages ranged from 21 to 44 years. Eighty-three percent of mothers had high school educations. Nearly all of them chose to room-in with their hospitalized child. The age range of the children was 24 to 71 months. Over 90% of them had been admitted to the hospital through the emergency room.

For the study, mothers were divided into four groups: one which received no additional information other than that routinely given to parents, a second group which listened to a 7-minute audiotape on typical ways that children react to hospitalization, a third group which listened to a 7-minute audiotape on the active role that parents can play in their child's care, and a fourth groups which listened to both audiotapes (14 minutes).

Mothers filled in questionnaires rating their level of anxiety and the level at which they participated in their child's care. Nurses in the unit rated how active mothers were in supporting their child during an intrusive procedure. Results of the study showed that mothers who heard either audiotape had less anxiety, participated more in their child's care, and were able to support more effectively during an intrusive procedure than those who heard no tape. Mothers who received the combined information were the most effective at supporting children. After hospitalization, mothers who had received the child behavioral tape or the combined tapes had the least anxiety about the hospital experience and their child had the least negative behavior changes from hospitalization of all the groups.

This is an important study because it documents that a few minutes spent in active preparation of mothers at an unplanned hospital admission can be effective in making hospitalization a more positive experience for both child and parent.

Melnyk, B. M. (1993). Coping with unplanned childhood hospitalization: Effects of informational interventions on mothers and children. *Nursing Research, 43,* 50.

tively as well. Children who wake from an anesthetic and find their arms tied down will be extremely frightened and may feel they are being punished.

Postoperatively, be sure the young child's favorite toy is within easy reach if his or her eyes are patched. It is difficult for any young child to be in a hospital, but to be continually in the dark without a parent nearby is frightening. Encourage parents to stay with their child overnight and as much as possible during the day.

The Child With Vision Impairment in the Hospital

Like other children, those with vision impairment experience disorders such as lacerations, appendicitis, and pneumonia, which may require being hospitalized. Children with severe vision impairment or those who are blind can have increased difficulty adjusting to a hospital environment. Children are said to have poor vision when they test 20/60 to 20/200 in the better eye on a standard eye examination. They are legally blind if their vision is less than 20/200 or their peripheral vision is less than 20 degrees.

Nursing Diagnoses and Related Interventions

Nursing Diagnosis: Powerlessness related to difficulty adjusting to strange environment, secondary to vision impairment

Goal: Child will feel secure and confident during hospitalization.

Outcome Criteria: Child identifies specific fears and concerns; is able to make age-appropriate decisions regarding self-care.

Vision impairment can range from very mild to total blindness. Assess children carefully for the degree of their vision impairment so you can gauge your care to their abilities, neither helping them too much or not enough. Children who are blind need to feel secure in a strange hospital environment so they need extremely thorough orientation to the experience. Remember that they may think that a parent has left them when the parent has only moved a few feet away. Assure visually impaired children as much as necessary that parents are nearby.

Before you approach a child who is blind, be certain to speak to avoid startling her. She is very aware of another person's presence in the room and may be frightened if you slip in quietly to straighten another child's bed or pick up some equipment without speaking to her. A quick, "Hi, Mary Ann. I'm Miss Collins. I'm going to take your dinner tray back to the kitchen," lets the child know who you are and what you are doing.

Remember that the sounds of a hospital are strange sounds to any child. The whirring noise of a floor-polishing machine or another child's oxygen tent, the hissing of a ventilator, or the clanking of waste baskets being emptied can be frightening sounds if you do not know what they are. Stand by the child's bed and explain the sounds you both hear. Sound is a major way in which visually impaired children experience their environment.

Children who are blind need to learn self-care like other children; they can be taught to bathe themselves, brush their teeth, brush their hair, and put on their clothes like other children their age. Toilet-training may come later, since they cannot see the excretions that parents are asking them to dispose of in a special place. They must be able to understand cognitively what is expected of them.

Blind children often want to be told what is on their food tray when it is first presented to them. Name the foods so that they can identify tastes with names. Do not hesitate to use food colors: "Those are green beans; this is an orange; those are red beets." These words are names as well as colors. Visually impaired preschoolers enjoy the same finger foods as sighted children; they can easily feed themselves. If a food must be eaten by a spoon, it is easier for the blind child to use a small bowl rather than a plate (that is true for sighted toddlers as well). Children with severe vision impairments have difficulty getting food from spoons or forks to their mouths neatly. They should not be fed just because it is neater and faster, however; eating is important self-care for the blind child to learn to be independent as an adult.

When children over 7 years of age are hospitalized for eye surgery and have temporary eye patches in place, you can help them locate food on their plate by comparing it to a clock face. They have usually learned to tell time by now and enjoy being told that their meat is at 9 o'clock, peas are at 6 o'clock, mashed potatoes are at 3 o'clock, and so forth. Although learning to tell time is difficult for children who are permanently visually impaired, this technique will still work well if they have learned to identify the numbers on a Braille clock face.

Blind children need to be given frequent descriptions of what is being offered them or done for them. They cannot see their surgery bandage, but they can feel it; they cannot see the intravenous infusion, but they can feel the tubing and the armboard that is holding their arm in place.

Parents of a severely visually impaired child generally plan to room in with their child during a hospitalization experience. Demonstrate to them that you are competent to care for their child by using good techniques with the child in their presence and by relating to him or her warmly. This will help parents feel they are able to leave to eat lunch or dinner or just spend some time away from the hospital. Ask the parents about the child's routines at mealtime and bedtime, his or her favorite toy, what word is used for voiding, and so on, and pass the information on to the entire nursing staff. Only when parents have confidence in you and the other staff members will they be able to leave their child in your care.

Structure and Function of the Ears

Ear anatomy is shown in Figure 50-15. Most ear disease in children involves the external and middle portions.

Physiology of Hearing Loss

Hearing loss is termed a *conduction loss* if there is interference with sound reaching the inner ear (difficulty with the external canal, the tympanic membrane, or the ossicles). It is termed *nerve* or *sensorineural loss* if the inner ear or the nerve is affected. Conduction loss can occur if the external canal is obstructed with cerumen (wax) or a foreign object, the tympanic membrane is damaged or immobile, or the middle ear is filled with fluid, as occurs in *serous otitis media*. Sensorineural loss occurs from disease that affects the transmission of sound sensation to the cerebral cortex or pathology of the cochlea. In children, this condition is usually congenital, although it can occur from drug therapy or infection from an illness such as meningitis. It can occur from exposure to loud sound.

Hearing Impairment

Hearing impairment occurs in many different degrees and can be rated by levels of severity. Usual classifications are shown in Table 50-1. About 1 in 1000 children in the United States are profoundly hearing impaired: 25 of 1000 children have a moderate to severe hearing impairment. As much as 50% of severe hearing impairment is inherited; prenatal rubella infection accounts for another large percentage. Treacher Collins syndrome, otosclerosis, osteogenesis imperfecta, and Waardenburg's syndrome, all diseases transmitted by autosomal dominant inheritance, are examples of diseases causing congenital deafness. Causes of slight hearing impairment are serous otitis media, trauma, or untreated acute otitis media with rupture of the tympanic membrane.

Children with congenital hearing impairment should be enrolled in special programs for hearing-impaired children as soon as the hearing loss is discovered. They need this early exposure to a speech and hearing therapist to learn effective speech (Figure 50-16). For children who have conductive losses (interference with sound waves reaching the inner ear), an improvement in hearing can generally be achieved by use of a hearing aid (which intensifies the level of sound waves). Children who have inner ear or nerve deafness cannot expect this kind of improvement. Parents of children with neural deafness need an explanation of the difference so that they do not continue to search for a "cure" for their child or spend a great deal of money for hearing aids, hoping a different brand or model will help their child. Acupuncture, often recommended to parents by friends as therapy for nerve deafness, has no

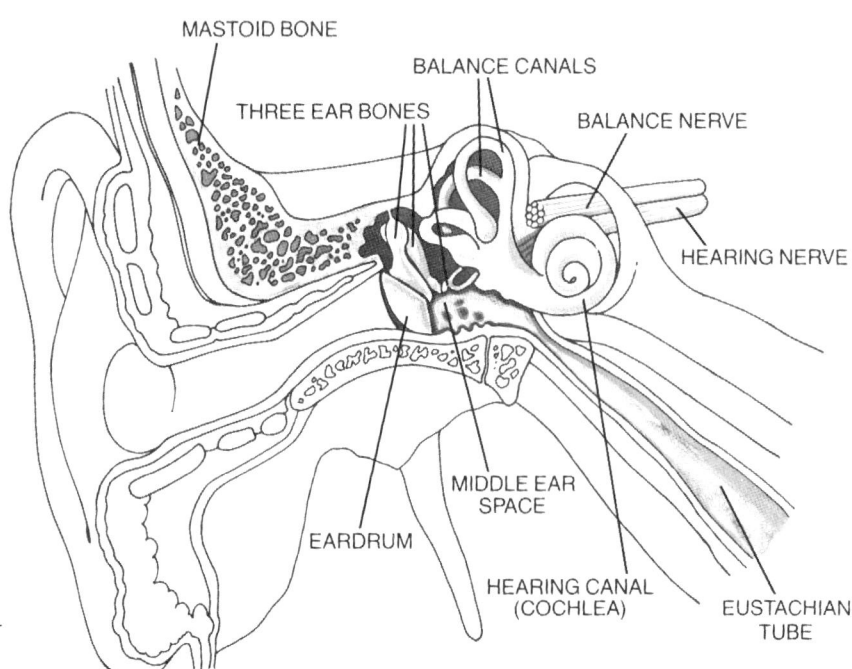

FIGURE 50-15
Structure of the middle ear. (From Ear Anatomy Chart, *copyright Ross Laboratories. Reprinted with permission of Ross Laboratories, Columbus, OH.)*

Table 50-1. *Levels of Hearing Impairment*

dB level	Hearing Level Present
Slight (<30)	Unable to hear whispered words or faint speech
	No speech impairment present
	May not be aware of hearing difficulty
	Achieves well in school and home by compensating by leaning forward, speaking loudly
Mild (30–50)	Beginning speech impairment may be present
	Difficulty hearing if not facing speaker; some difficulty with normal conversation
Moderate (55–70)	Speech impairment present; may require speech therapy
	Difficulty with normal conversation
Severe (70–90)	Difficulty with any but nearby loud voice
	Hears vowels easier than consonants
	Requires speech therapy for clear speech
	May still hear loud sounds, such as jets or train whistles
Profound (> 90)	Hears almost no sound

documented effect. Cochlear transplants are now available to replace a nonfunctioning inner ear. After a transplant, hearing is often reported as "muffled" but adequate. Hearing-impaired adults may be reluctant to consent to a cochlear transplant in their child, feeling that to move from hearing-impaired to non-hearing-impaired status would remove the child from their culture. Children who spoke with an impediment prior to a transplant usually need speech therapy afterward to restore their speech pattern.

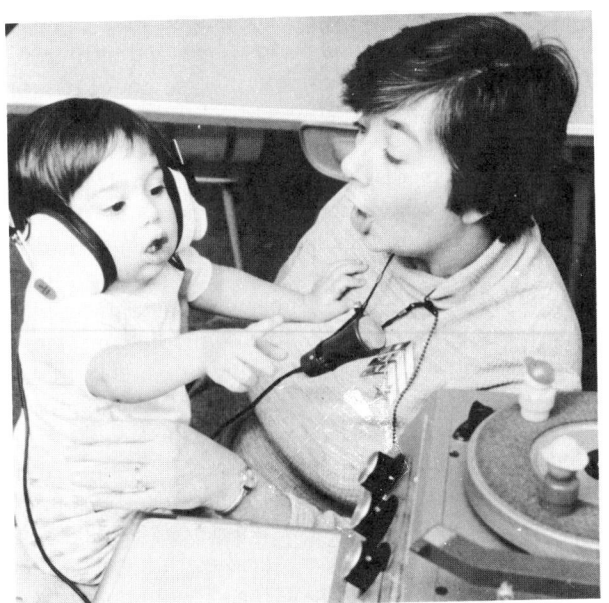

FIGURE 50-16
Hearing-impaired infants should have speech therapy early in life so that they can learn to appreciate as many sounds as possible. (Courtesy of the Department of Medical Photography, Children's Hospital, Buffalo, NY.)

Because the diseases that lead to inherited hearing impairment are all autosomal dominant, there is a strong chance that they will occur in future siblings of the hearing-impaired child. Parents need to be made aware of this through genetic counseling.

Hearing Aids

Hearing aids pick up sound through a microphone, convert sound waves into electrical impulses, and amplify them across the tympanic membrane. They are powered by batteries that must be changed periodically (Weinstock, 1990).

Hearing aids are designed to be as inconspicuous as possible so that children will not feel self-conscious wearing them. The receiver of the hearing aid may be incorporated into eyeglasses, molded into a plastic form that fits behind or in the ear, or housed in a small box resembling a small transistor radio that children wear on a cord around their neck or carry in a blouse or shirt pocket (Figure 50-17). Teach children to remove hearing aids before washing their hair or showering so that hearing aids do not get wet. Hearing aids should be turned off when removed to preserve the life of the batteries.

Children with a hearing impairment may grow self-conscious about wearing a hearing aid during school years. For girls, encouraging them to wear their hair long so that it covers the device behind their ear may be helpful. A long-range goal, however, should be to encourage such children to view themselves as whole persons despite their need for such devices, rather than as someone with something to hide.

Speech Therapy

If children with a hearing impairment are to interact as fully as possible with the world around them, they need

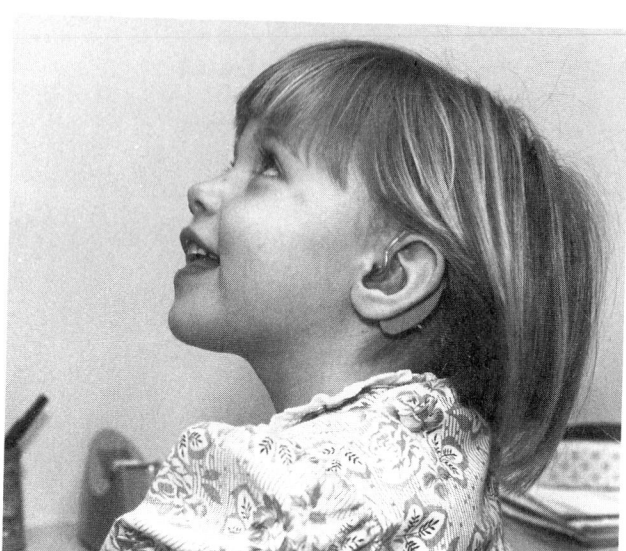

FIGURE 50-17
Children may need encouragement to accept hearing aids until they realize their value for communication. The type shown here is barely visible. (Courtesy of the Department of Medical Photography, Children's Hospital, Buffalo, NY.)

an intensive program of speech therapy. Some therapists feel that learning sign language early is helpful in that it allows children to express their needs early. Others feel that by learning sign language, children decrease their need to learn to articulate speech sounds or to lip read and, for this reason, learning sign language should not be encouraged. It is true that for real independence and to perform in regular school classes, children need to communicate by means other than sign language. For children with a profound impairment, however, learning speech sounds may be such a long-term process that sign language is necessary for contact with the world around them until they learn to speak.

Disorders of the Ear

Ear disease is always serious in children because hearing is such an important function for the growing child. Some parents need to be cautioned that there is no such thing as "only an earache." "Only an earache" today may mean "only a hearing impairment" when the child reaches maturity. Assessment of hearing is discussed in Chapter 28.

External Otitis

External otitis is inflammation of the external ear canal. Although external ear inflammation rarely threatens hearing or causes permanent damage, it does cause discomfort in the form of itching and sometimes extreme pain.

Assessment
The history of children with external otitis generally reveals that they have recently been swimming, which is why this condition is popularly called *swimmer's ear*. It can occur if a young child pushes a foreign object, such as a peanut, into the ear canal. Unlike middle ear infection (otitis media), there is no history of a recent respiratory infection. Children first notice itching of the canal, then pain. When you touch the external ear, the pain becomes acute. The moisture in the canal left from swimming has caused inflammation; a secondary infection may occur in the closed space. *Pseudomonas* and *Candida* are frequent agents involved in infection. If you look into the external canal through an otoscope, only a sharply localized, tender swelling of a furuncle may be present; the entire canal may be swollen shut and tender to the touch. This could be from multiple furuncles or a generalized cellulitis of the skin lining the canal. If a fungal infection is present, the entire canal may appear brown or black. If the inflammation is from a foreign body such as a peanut or the tip of a cotton applicator being present, white or gray debris may surround the object; the skin under the object is moist, red, and eroded.

It is extremely important in external otitis that the tympanic membrane be visualized, so that it can be ascertained that there is no extension of the external otitis into the middle ear. In some instances, the eardrum is so inflamed from the external infectious process that it is difficult to tell whether or not the middle ear is free of disease. Before the tympanic membrane can be visualized, it is often necessary to remove superficial debris from the canal. A Weber test (discussed in Chapter 28) should show that, once all debris is cleaned from the external canal, a tuning fork held in the center of the forehead will be heard equally well in both ears. A tuning fork vibration that sounds louder in the affected ear suggests that otitis media (middle ear infection) is present.

Removal of debris from an infected external canal requires patience and skill. Foreign material should not be irrigated until it is shown that the tympanic membrane is intact; otherwise, infected material could be washed through a rupture into the middle ear. Material should be removed by an ear curette using extremely gentle pressure. Children must be well restrained for the procedure to avoid sudden turning of the head, causing the curette to puncture their tympanic membrane. If the debris is hard and difficult to remove, it can be softened and loosened by touching it with a peroxide-soaked soft cotton applicator, or 2% acetic acid can be instilled into the canal and allowed to stand for a few minutes.

Therapeutic Management
The treatment of an external otitis differs according to the organism causing the infection. If the canal is so swollen shut that ear drops will not be able to flow back

into the canal, a cotton wick moistened with Burow's solution may be threaded into the canal. The cotton extending out into the auricle is kept moistened by rewetting it for 24 hours with Burow's solution. This generally reduces the swelling of the canal to such a point that further treatment can be initiated.

The parents of children are then instructed to use ear drops containing a hydrocortisone and an antibiotic or an antifungal mixture. Hydrocortisone reduces inflammation; the antibiotic or antifungal preparation will reduce the infection. Some ear drops have an additional alcohol base, which serves to dry the external canal further. Drops are administered about two times a day for 7 to 10 days. If ear pain is present, an analgesic such as acetaminophen may be necessary to control discomfort. Children must keep the ear canal dry, omitting swimming or hair washing during this time. If children shower, they should first insert cotton into the external meatus.

Nursing Diagnoses and Related Interventions

Nursing Diagnosis: Knowledge deficit related to technique for ear drop instillation and preventive care measures

Goal: Parents will demonstrate effective ear drop administration technique by 1 hour.

Outcome Criteria: Parents properly demonstrate instilling ear drops and state the importance of continuing prescribed treatment to completion.

Putting in ear drops is not easy. Show parents how this is done (see Chapter 37) before they leave the health care facility. Encourage them to give the medication for the full time period prescribed; otherwise, because ear drops are difficult to give, they may give them only until the pain subsides (24 to 48 hours); a week later, the infection, never really cured, will recur. Caution parents not to put anything but the ear drops into their child's ear. Some parents, in an effort to "get the ear really dry," will put in cotton with bobby pins or crochet hooks, and, by accident, rupture the tympanic membrane.

Follow-Up

Evaluation after an ear infection should include not only whether the inflammation and pain has decreased but also whether children are aware of how to prevent the condition in the future. This includes knowing not to put any object into the ear canal. Instillation of a dilute alcohol or acetic acid solution by dropper following swimming is a prophylactic measure that helps keep the ear canal dry. This is often recommended for children who participate on a swimming team and spend a great deal of time in water.

Impacted Cerumen

Cerumen (ear wax) serves the important function of cleansing the external ear canal as it gradually moves outward, bringing with it shed epithelial cells and any foreign objects. Parents are often concerned that ear wax will lead to loss of hearing (or view it as dirty) and will ask to have it removed. Wax accumulation rarely is enough to interfere with hearing, and it does serve a protective function, so it should not be removed. Caution parents not to clean ears with cotton-tipped applicators as a regular practice because they may scratch the ear canal, causing an invasion site for a secondary infection. This practice may also push accumulated cerumen farther into the ear canal, causing a true plugging of wax.

If cerumen accumulates to such an extent that hearing is affected, the wax can be softened by the instillation by dropper of mineral oil or a commercial softening compound. Some physicians advise a dilute solution of hydrogen peroxide to dissolve cerumen. This may be done once in a while, but again, should not be done regularly because this will keep the ear canal constantly moist, an environment that leads to external otitis. For most children, the basic rule of thumb—never put anything smaller or more liquid than an elbow in a child's ear—is the best rule.

Acute Otitis Media

Inflammation of the middle ear (otitis media) is the most prevalent disease of childhood after respiratory tract infections. It occurs most often in the child 6 to 36 months of age and again at 4 to 6 years. It occurs most frequently in males, Alaskan and American Indians, and children with cleft palate. There is a higher incidence of otitis media in formula-fed infants than those who are breast-fed because of the more slanted position that formula-fed infants are held in while feeding. This allows milk to enter the eustachian tube. The incidence of otitis media is highest in the winter and spring. It is higher in homes in which a parent smokes cigarettes (Charlton, 1994).

Otitis media is an extremely serious disease of childhood because, if it is not treated and cured, permanent damage can occur to middle ear structures, leading to hearing impairment.

Assessment

Acute otitis media generally follows a respiratory infection. Children have a "cold," rhinitis, and perhaps a low-grade fever for a number of days. Suddenly, they have a fever of about 102°F (38°C) and a sharp, constant pain in one or both ears. Older children voice pain; the infant becomes extremely irritable and frequently pulls or tugs at the affected ear in an attempt to gain relief from pain.

The external canal is generally free of wax because the warmth of the inflammation and fever melts the wax and moves it more readily out of the canal. In contrast to an external ear canal infection, the discomfort does not increase on manipulation of the auricle; the mastoid process behind the ear should not be tender to touch; if it is, the infection probably has spread out of the middle ear into the mastoid cells, a very serious complication (Myer, 1991).

The appearance of a normal eardrum shows the outline of the malleus (see Chapter 28). With infection, on otoscopic examination, the tympanic membrane appears inflamed. It may be seen bulging into the external canal. The light reflex of the otoscope will not be as definite as usual because of the convex shape of the eardrum. The landmarks of the tympanic membrane, the malleus and incus, will not be present or can only be poorly visualized. There will be decreased mobility on a pneumatic examination.

A **tympanocentesis** (withdrawal of fluid from the middle ear through the tympanic membrane) may be performed by a physician to obtain fluid for culture at the time of assessment, although this is usually not necessary unless the infection is resistant to usual antibiotics (Hoekelman, 1991). For this procedure, the tympanic membrane is cleaned with alcohol, a spinal needle attached to a syringe is introduced, and any fluid in the middle ear is aspirated.

Therapeutic Management

Most middle ear infections are caused by *Pneumococcus, H. influenzae* (especially in children under 5 years), or hemolytic streptococci. For this reason, most children with otitis media are treated with ampicillin and gentamicin or amoxicillin (antibiotics that eliminate *H. influenzae* organisms). With more and more organisms becoming ampicillin-resistant, erythromycin and a sulfonamide may be added to the therapy. Chronic otitis media may be caused by *Staphylococcus,* which would require treatment with an antibiotic that is effective against *Staphylococcus,* such as cephalothin (Keflin) (Kline, 1994).

Caution parents to give the prescribed antibiotic for the full length of treatment (10 days); otherwise, parents may give it only until the pain is gone (24 to 48 hours), and the child will return in about 2 weeks with recurrent otitis media. It is actually still the first infection, which was not properly eradicated. Also, because the cause of the infection may be *Streptococcus,* children are susceptible to the complications of streptococcal infection (rheumatic fever or glomerulonephritis) unless properly treated (see the Focus on Cultural Awareness box).

During the course of otitis media, most children have a conductive hearing loss. Many children will have some conductive hearing impairment for up to 6 months after an acute infection. Caution parents about this so that they will not think the infection is growing worse if

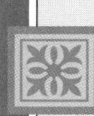

FOCUS ON CULTURAL AWARENESS

Vision and hearing are both senses that are respected worldwide, and eye or ear injuries are universally considered as major threats to children's health. Not all parents are aware of the importance of antibiotics in curing infections, however, so despite their desire to see an eye or ear illness resolve quickly, they may not administer an antibiotic conscientiously. Being aware of this helps you understand the parents' level of anxiety when either vision or hearing is threatened.

they first notice the impairment after they arrive home from the health care facility. They also need to know about the hearing loss so that if children are routinely screened for hearing in school during the next 6 months, they can account for the loss. If children still have a conductive hearing loss after 6 months (or have other symptoms), they should be examined again to see if a new infection or serous otitis media is present.

Children need an analgesic such as acetaminophen (Tylenol) ordered for the relief of pain. Some physicians prescribe decongestant nose drops to open the eustachian tubes and allow air to be admitted to the middle ear; although not proven, this may be helpful in preventing the infection from becoming a serous or long-term otitis media. Nasal decongestant drops are only given for 3 days or they may have a rebound effect with an increase in mucous membrane size caused by edema (see the Nursing Care Plan).

Myringotomy. **Myringotomy** is a surgical incision of the tympanic membrane. It is done when the middle ear is so full of purulent effusion from an infection that the eardrum bulges forward and looks as if it is about to rupture. Incising the eardrum to relieve the pressure against it will cause a small, neat opening; if the eardrum should rupture by itself, the tear might be larger, and the tympanic membrane might not adhere again afterward, causing a permanent hearing loss (Cotton, 1991).

Because it is a painful procedure, myringotomy is best done under a general anesthetic in small children. To avoid the risks of general anesthesia, however, it may be done as an office procedure with the use of a local anesthetic. To avoid damage to the membrane during the procedure, however, children must remain or be held absolutely still. The incision is made on the lower posterior quadrant of the tympanic membrane, a portion of the eardrum that is not important in conduction of sound, so a small scar there does not affect hearing. This is a good fact to include in health teaching for parents so they do not worry that the procedure is leaving their

Nursing Care Plan

A Child With Otitis Media

Jason is a 6-month-old boy who is seen at an ambulatory clinic with a history of two previous ear infections in the last 8 months. The following is a nursing care plan designed for him.

Assessment: Jason is bottle-fed. He has had an upper respiratory infection for 3 days. Today, his temperature is 38.2°C. He sits in his mother's lap crying from apparent discomfort; he tugs at his left ear. Mother states frustration with chronic ear infections. Assessment reveals a reddened and bulging left tympanic membrane. He is diagnosed as having a left otitis media. His physician has prescribed amoxicillin orally q6h for 10 days and acetaminophen 5 mg prn q4h for pain.

Nursing Diagnosis: Pain related to ear infection

Defining Characteristic: Child is crying and pulling at ear.

Goal: Child's pain will be reduced to a tolerable level within 20 min.

Outcome Criteria: Child has stopped crying and tugging at earlobe.

Nursing Orders	Rationale
1. Administer analgesic as prescribed. *Caution*: if sudden relief of pain occurs, rupture of the tympanic membrane may have occurred.	1. Analgesic will provide pain relief, but sudden relief may indicate rupture.
2. Instruct mother about preventing pressure on affected ear (position on other side). If the tympanic membrane has ruptured, child should be positioned with affected ear down.	2. Pressure on the infected ear will lead to increased pain. However, if the tympanic membrane has ruptured, pressure will be quickly relieved and the child can rest on affected ear without pain. This will allow fluid to drain from the middle ear.
3. Instruct mother to offer only liquids or soft food if chewing is painful because of movement of eustachian tube.	3. Decreasing movement of eustachian tube will reduce pain.

child with damage to the eardrum. After a myringotomy, the contents of the middle ear—pus or blood—will drain from the ear.

With the prompt administration of therapy for otitis media, a myringotomy is now rarely required. Educate parents to recognize the symptoms of otitis media and to regard it as a serious disorder so that they come for early care. That way infection can be arrested before myringotomy is necessary.

Serous Otitis Media

Serous otitis media is a result of chronic otitis media. Normally, the middle ear is an air-filled cavity, air being supplied to it by the eustachian tube. The tube opens with swallowing, yawning, or chewing. If the source of air to the middle ear is shut off, the epithelial cells of the middle ear tend to change in function to become secretory cells. The middle ear fills with these secretions. Over time, the fluid becomes so thick and tenacious that it is described as "gluelike." Some children notice a feel-

ing of fullness or the sound of popping or ringing in their ears. There may be a drop in hearing of 20 to 40 dB because of the fluid content. Because the loss is gradual, parents and children may not be aware of it until it is noticed on a routine hearing screening. Involvement is generally bilateral. It occurs most frequently in children 3 to 10 years of age.

Assessment

Examination of the ears may show a level of fluid behind the tympanic membrane. This is visible, however, only if there is also a quantity of air in the middle ear as well, to contrast with the fluid line. As the collected fluid becomes thick, it tends to retract the eardrum. This makes the malleus more prominent and perhaps displaced to a horizontal angle as the membrane is retracted around it; the light reflex from the otoscope light becomes distorted. If a pneumatic otoscope is used, when air is gently introduced against the eardrum, there is no movement of the tympanic membrane (as there would be normally).

Air can be blocked from reaching the middle ear if the eustachian tube is closed by inflammation from allergy (the child generally, but not necessarily, has an accompanying allergic rhinitis). Blockage may also be due to enlarged adenoidal tissue or, possibly, to insufficient treatment of an episode of acute otitis media (Sadae & Luntz, 1991).

Therapeutic Management

Therapy for serous otitis media may involve a long-term process (Pulec, 1993). If the condition appears to be caused by inflammation from an allergy, measures to control the allergy must be instituted: avoidance of the allergen, hyposensitization, or pharmacologic alteration of the allergic response. Treatment of children with allergies is discussed in Chapter 42.

Definitive medical treatment is aimed at supplying air to the middle ear. For mild involvement, the daily administration of an antihistamine or a nasal decongestant to shrink the mucous membrane of the eustachian tube may be enough to achieve this. In a few children, the eustachian tube is blocked by enlarged adenoids, and their removal is indicated. This is not often needed, however. Fluid from the middle ear can be removed by tympanocentesis (withdrawal) of fluid by injection of a needle attached to a syringe through the tympanic membrane. Fluid usually returns, however, unless some intervention to introduce air to the middle ear (tubal myringotomy) is undertaken.

Tubal Myringotomy. A source of air can be supplied to the middle ear by the insertion of small plastic (Teflon) tubes through the tympanic membrane (a tympanostomy). The insertion of such tubes is done after a myringotomy at a point in the tympanic membrane that is not instrumental for hearing, in order not to interfere with hearing (Figure 50-18). Placing myringotomy tubes can be done as an ambulatory procedure following the local injection of lidocaine (Xylocaine), although many surgeons prefer to insert them under a general anesthetic. Tubes tend to be extruded after 6 to 12 months. For many children, this period of time is enough to halt the secretory process of the middle ear. In others, tubes must be reinserted to continue the aeration.

With myringotomy tubes in place, children cannot allow water to enter their ears. This means neither diving underwater nor playing water-splashing games is allowed. Most physicians prefer children to bathe rather than shower, but using ear plugs in their ears while showering may be allowed. Hair washing should be done with ear plugs in place.

Serous otitis media runs a long-term course in many children. Teach parents to continue giving medications as prescribed. They often need a great deal of support to accept the insertion of myringotomy tubes. They are afraid that cutting the eardrum will do more harm than if they just leave the situation alone. Because the course

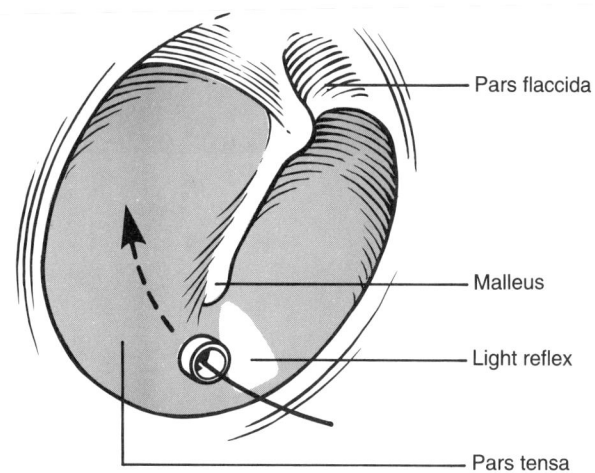

FIGURE 50-18
A myringotomy tube provides air to the middle ear to prevent serous otitis media.

of the process is long, the hearing impairment associated with it may also be long term. Have the parents notify the school nurse of the problem. Children may need to be changed to a front seat in a classroom so that they do not miss important class content or discussion. They need support through a puzzling and annoying condition.

Cholesteatoma

Cholesteatoma is a lesion of the pars flaccida or upper portion of the tympanic membrane (Powell, 1990). A retraction cyst forms, and there is necrosis of the pars flaccida with foul-smelling drainage from the ear. If the retraction cyst is not discovered and treated (surgically removed) at this point, it grows gradually deeper and deeper until it eventually invades the mastoid cells. It can progress to mastoiditis, meningitis, and possibly facial nerve paralysis.

This is obviously a serious ear problem. Any child with foul-smelling drainage from the ear should be referred to a physician for further investigation of the problem to be certain it is not this condition. If you are inspecting children's tympanic membranes during health maintenance visits, be certain to inspect the pars flaccida area (see Figure 28-18) as well as the pars tensa to detect cholesteatoma.

The Hearing-Impaired Child in the Hospital

Children who have a hearing loss greater than 50 dB have a hearing impairment great enough to interfere with hearing normal conversation and developing language (Kravitz, 1992). Like visually impaired children, children are rarely admitted to a hospital or seen in an ambulatory setting just for hearing impairment. They are seen for other health problems, however.

It is difficult to prepare children who cannot hear for hospitalization. Words such as *surgery, tonsils, hurts, operating room,* and *recovery room* are new to them. Show a child a book with good pictures demonstrating what is going to happen and allow them time to play with dolls or puppets to help them understand hospital routine. Because children with hearing impairment may not be as well prepared for hospitalization as hearing children, extra effort must be made on admission to a health care facility to see that they receive such instruction (Harrison, 1990).

Be certain that hearing-impaired children see you before you touch them. They will not find this nearly as intrusive as being touched without warning. If children are sleeping when you approach them, wake them gently with a light touch. Some children turn off their hearing aid while they sleep. You may need to turn it on before you call them to wake them. Children as young as 2 years of age are effective lip readers as long as you are facing them. Position yourself at eye level to the child so he can view your face. In a group, help a child follow conversation by directing him to who is speaking. Assign a primary nurse to decrease the number of persons with whom a child must attempt to communicate. Have a staff person accompany him and stay with him in all departments to help with communication. Do not underestimate the intelligence level of hearing-impaired children. Because they do not speak clearly and may not be given information that the average hearing child receives, such as explanations of how things work, they often appear to be slightly mentally retarded. This is deceptive. On a hospital unit, hearing-impaired children, locked in a silent world, are unable to express how they feel about procedures. They need help from health care personnel who understand this and take more than the usual amount of time to offer them explanations and support.

Ask parents of children with hearing impairments to draw pictures or demonstrate the sign language symbols children use for important words such as *pain, drink,* and *bathroom.* Encourage children to draw pictures of what they want if they are still too young to write words and you cannot understand what they are saying.

Key Points

- Refractive errors of vision such as myopia and hyperopia are the most common eye disorders in children. Amblyopia (lazy eye) is subnormal vision in one eye. Children with these disorders need correction at the time the disorder is recognized to prevent further vision distortion.
- Coloboma is congenital incomplete closure of the pupil or lower eyelid. Ptosis is the inability to open the upper eyelid normally. Ptosis needs correction to avoid development of amblyopia.

- Strabismus is unequally aligned eyes. Like ptosis, it may lead to amblyopia if not corrected.
- Infections of the lids such as styes or chalazions can occur in children. Conjunctivitis (inflammation of the conjunctiva) often presents with acute symptoms. An antibiotic is necessary for therapy.
- Children need to be taught to avoid eye injuries by using proper eye protection during sports or work. Eye injuries such as penetration by a foreign body need follow-up after treatment to be certain that vision remains adequate.
- Children with either vision or hearing impairment need special preparation and orientation for a hospital or ambulatory health visit so they can fully understand what is going to happen during the visit.
- Help children with vision impairment work through new experiences by letting them feel equipment as much as possible. Guide their hands through the steps of a new procedure you are teaching them.
- Otitis media (middle ear infection) is a common childhood illness. Children need therapy with antibiotics to correct this. With serous otitis media, some children have myringotomy tubes placed to relieve pressure and supply air access to the middle ear.
- Use photos, drawings, or demonstration with hearing-impaired children to help them learn new skills. Contact a signing interpreter as appropriate to be certain the children understand instructions.
- Teaching preventive measures to avoid eye and hearing injuries (wearing goggles or ear protection as appropriate) and screening children for sensory impairments are important nursing roles.

Critical Thinking Exercises

1. Jody is a 4-year-old who is going to have eye surgery. What special steps in preparation for surgery would you want to make for her? Is Jody old enough to appreciate the importance of seeing?
2. Fred is a 14-year-old who is deaf from developing meningitis as a preschooler. He uses sign language to communicate. How could you communicate effectively with Fred while he's hospitalized? What are Fred's rights as a patient in regard to having an interpreter provided for him?
3. You are going to teach a first-grade class on ways to prevent eye and hearing injuries. What would you include in your class? Would this be different if the class was for 16-year-olds?

References

Carpenito, L. J. (1993). *Nursing diagnosis: Application to clinical practice* (5th ed.). Philadelphia: J. B. Lippincott.

Charlton, A. (1994). Children and passive smoking: A review. *Journal of Family Practice, 38,* 267.

Cotton, R. T. (1991). The surgical management of chronic otitis media with effusion. *Pediatric Annals, 20,* 628.

Department of Health and Human Services. (1991). *Healthy people 2000.* Washington, DC: Public Health Service.

Hammerschlag, M. R. (1993). Neonatal conjunctivitis. *Pediatric Annals, 22,* 346.

Harrison, L. L. (1990). Minimizing barriers when teaching hearing-impaired clients. *MCN: American Journal of Maternal Child Nursing, 15,* 113.

Hoekelman, R. A. (1991) A pediatrician's view: Do you do tympanocenteses? *Pediatric Annals, 20,* 585.

Kline, M. W. (1994). Otitis media. In Oski, F. A., et al. (Eds.) *Principles and practice of pediatrics* (2nd ed.). Philadelphia: J. B. Lippincott.

Kraus-Mackiw, E. (1990). Sympathetic ophthalmia: A genuine autoimmune disease. *Current Eye Research, 9,* 1.

Kravitz, L., et al. (1992). Understanding hearing loss in children. *Pediatric Nursing, 18,* 591.

Laguire, L. E., et al. (1993). Longitudinal study of levodopa/carbidopa for childhood amblyopia. *Journal of Pediatric Ophthalmology and Strabismus, 30,* 354.

Lavrich, J. B., & Nelson, L. B. (1993). Disorders of the lacrimal system apparatus. *Pediatric Clinics of North America, 40,* 767.

Lohr, J. A. (1993). Treatment of conjunctivitis in infants and children. *Pediatric Annals, 22,* 359.

Myer, C. M. (1991). The diagnosis and management of mastoiditis in children. *Pediatric Annals, 20,* 622.

Pagano, K. D., & Pagano, T. J. (1990). *Diagnostic testing and nursing implications.* St. Louis: C. V. Mosby.

Persaud, D., et al (1993). Serious eye infections in children. *Pediatric Annals, 22,* 379.

Powell, M. A. (1990). Cholesteatoma. *Journal of the American Academy of Nurse Practitioners, 2,* 83.

Pulec, J. L. (1993). Serous otitis media. *Ear, Nose and Throat Journal, 72,* 193.

Traboulsi, E I., & Maumenee, I. H. (1994). Eye problems. In Oski, F. A. (Ed.). *Principles and practice of pediatrics* (2nd ed.). Philadelphia: J. B. Lippincott.

Weinstock, C. P. (1990). Hearing aids: A link to the world. *FDA Consumer, 24,* 18.

Weiss, A. H. (1993). Chronic conjunctivitis in infants and children. *Pediatric Annals, 22,* 368.

Suggested Readings

Baker, R. C. (1991). Pitfalls in diagnosing acute otitis media. *Pediatric Annals, 20,* 591.

Bocking, H., et al. (1990). Making sense of artificial eyes. *Nursing Times, 86,* 40.

Donnenfeld, E. D., et al. (1993). Conjunctivitis: Update on diagnosis and treatment. *Patient Care, 27,* 22.

Faye, E. E., et al. (1994). Help people with disabilities help themselves. *Patient Care, 28,* 65.

Garber, N. (1990). Health promotion and disease prevention in ophthalmology. *Journal of Ophthalmic Nursing and Technology, 9,* 186.

Gigliotti, F. (1993). Acute conjunctivitis of childhood. *Pediatric Annals, 22,* 353.

Kaye, B. (1990). The cure for lazy eye. *Journal of Ophthalmic Nursing and Technology, 9,* 90.

Scherbanske, J. M., et al. (1990). Cutaneous and ocular manifestations of Down syndrome. *Journal of American Academy of Dermatology, 22,* 933.

Silverstein, H., et al. (1992). Diagnosis and management of hearing loss. *Clinical Symposia, 44,* 2.

Tuft, S. J., et al. (1991). Clinical features of atopic keratoconjunctivitis. *Ophthalmology, 98,* 150.

Wuest, J., et al. (1992). Adolescent hearing behavior: A school health promotion program. *Journal of School Health, 62,* 436.

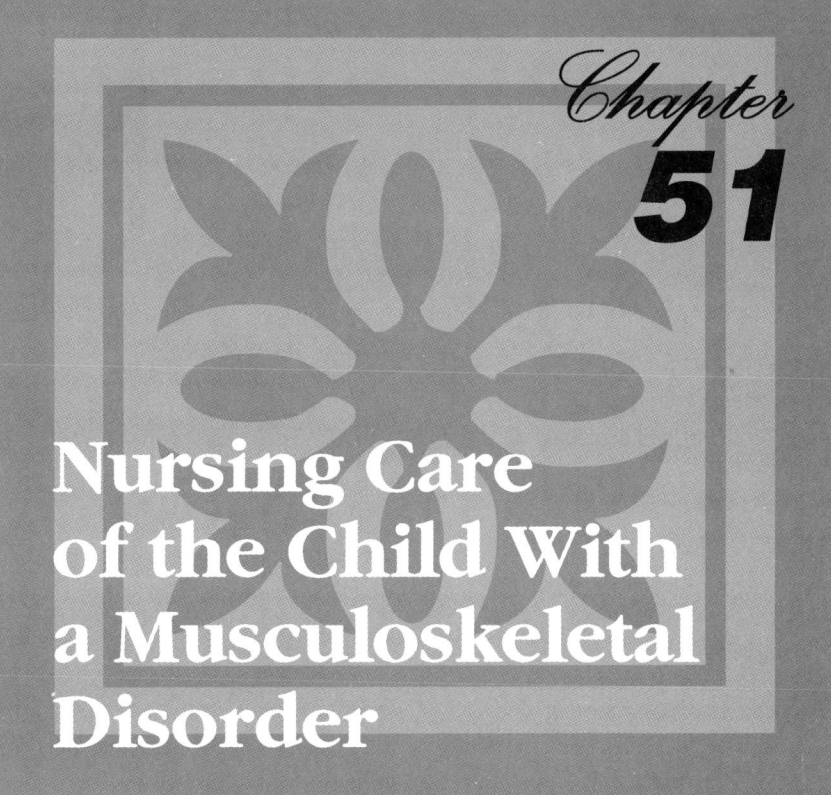

Chapter 51

Nursing Care of the Child With a Musculoskeletal Disorder

Objectives

After mastering the contents of this chapter, you should be able to:

1. Describe common musculoskeletal disorders in children.
2. Assess the child with a musculoskeletal disorder.
3. Formulate nursing diagnoses related to the child with a musculoskeletal disorder.
4. Plan nursing care such as age-appropriate diversional activities for the child with a musculoskeletal disorder.
5. Implement nursing care for the child with a musculoskeletal disorder (e.g., explain cast care to a school-ager and parents).
6. Evaluate outcome criteria to be certain that goals established for care were achieved.
7. Identify National Health Goals related to musculoskeletal disorders and children that nurses can be instrumental in helping the nation to achieve.
8. Identify areas related to care of the child with a musculoskeletal disorder that could benefit from additional nursing research.
9. Use critical thinking to analyze ways that care of the child immobilized by a cast or traction can be more family centered.
10. Synthesize knowledge of musculoskeletal disorders with nursing process to achieve quality maternal and child health nursing care.

Adele Pillitteri: MATERNAL AND CHILD HEALTH NURSING, 2nd Edition. © 1995 Adele Pillitteri.

The skeletal system, composed of more than 200 bones connected by the joints and tendons, provides a structural casing or protective armor for the internal organs of the body. Skeletal muscles, attached to the bones by connective tissue, tendons, and ligaments, allow for voluntary movement—including gross motor activity such as running and fine motor activity such as writing. Together, the skeletal and muscular systems support the body and make coordinated movement possible.

Because their bones and muscles are still growing, children suffer from disorders of the musculoskeletal system more frequently than adults. With fractures, the fact that bones are still growing works on the child's behalf—healing occurs much more quickly for the child than for the adult. If a growth plate is injured, however, an injury that would be simple in an adult becomes serious in a child. Because many musculoskeletal system disorders lead to problems with locomotion, they can threaten a child's ability to develop' optimally in other ways. Some problems of locomotion are slight and self-limiting; others are extensive and incapacitating. In either instance, because children gain much of their knowledge by interacting with people and exploring the environment around them, a problem of locomotion can be a serious impairment during childhood. When caring for such children, it is important for nurses to try to bring some of the world to the child so that the same sorts of stimuli are received that might be experienced if the child were able to move around independently. National Health Goals related to musculoskeletal disorders and children are shown in the Focus on National Health Goals display.

 NURSING PROCESS OVERVIEW
*for Care of the Child With
a Musculoskeletal Disorder*

ASSESSMENT

Unlike many other diseases in children, disorders of the skeletal system usually present with specific, localized symptoms, and parents bring children to health care facilities early in the course of such illnesses. On the other hand, disorders of the muscles or joints (such as juvenile rheumatoid arthritis) may present insidiously, and when the disorder is diagnosed, parents may feel guilty for not having sought health care earlier.

One condition whose seriousness parents may underestimate greatly is a childhood limp. A limp is never normal and may be the first manifestation of a serious hip or knee problem. When weighing or measuring a child, you have ample opportunity to assess gait (whether the child walks naturally or stiffly, tiptoes or walks on the whole foot; whether the feet are in good alignment; whether the back is held straight). By such assessment, you may be the first person to detect that a child who has been brought to a health care center because of an upper respiratory condition, for example, has another, perhaps more important, musculoskeletal problem that should be brought to the attention of the child's primary care provider.

School nurses have direct responsibility for instituting scoliosis screening programs in their schools, as this is a common spinal deformity of children that needs to be detected at its earliest appearance.

NURSING DIAGNOSIS

The nursing diagnostic categories most frequently applied to children with musculoskeletal disorders include those that deal with pain, lack of mobility, long periods of bedrest because of a cast, and a need for diversional activities. Children, especially adolescents, requiring braces or other equipment to aid in skeletal support or locomotion may encounter problems with self-concept. Some common nursing diagnoses include

- Pain related to chronic inflammation of joints
- Impaired mobility related to cast on leg
- Diversional activity deficit related to need to restrict activity for 4 weeks
- Self-esteem disturbance related to need to continuously wear body brace

PLANNING

Be certain that goals established are realistic. Despite current therapies, some disorders will leave the child with a permanent disability. Many orthopedic problems

---

FOCUS ON
National Health Goals

In order to maintain a healthy musculoskeletal system, proper exercise is necessary. Several National Health Goals address this issue:

- Increase to at least 30% the proportion of people aged 6 and older who engage regularly, preferably daily, in light to moderate physical activity for at least 30 minutes per day.

- Increase to at least 50% from a baseline of 36% the proportion of children and adolescents in 1st through 12th grades who participate in daily school physical education.

- Increase to at least 50% from a baseline of 30% the proportion of primary care providers who routinely assess and counsel their patients regarding the frequency, duration, type and intensity of each patient's physical activity practices (DHHS, 1991).

Nurses can be instrumental in helping the nation achieve these goals by educating children about the importance of physical activity, serving as consultants for school systems in designing physical education programs and being certain to ask children about their usual activity level at health maintenance visits. Nursing research that would be helpful in adding to nursing knowledge in this area includes whether children sustain interest longer in group or single person exercise programs; whether adolescents are accurate in reporting the time and intensity of exercise in which they engage; and whether designing exercise programs for children with chronic illness can be a nursing role.

in children require long-term care. Before children are discharged from an ambulatory or inpatient setting, help parents plan how they will care for the child at home. At first, a cast on an arm seems exciting to a school-ager—a cast to show off; an injury to describe; a place for autographs; an excuse not to write in school. After a few days, the cast becomes more frustrating than enjoyable, however, if you do not take the time to review what wearing it will mean to the child in everyday situations. (The cast will not fit through blouses with tight cuffs—will dressing for school be a problem? She cannot swim with it on—can she help manage the swim team rather than be a swimming member of it this year? Her home chore is to do dishes—will she have to trade chores with a sibling for the next 4 weeks?) Planning transportation for the child with a large cast (it will not fit in the front seat of a compact car) may be a problem. If the child will have to stay home from school, plans for tutoring need to be made. If both parents work, child care will have to be arranged.

You do not have the answers to all these problems because the answers differ, depending on the child's individual and family's collective circumstances; however, taking time to sit down with the parents and asking them whether or not these things will be problems helps parents begin to plan and prepare solutions. Doing this with a concerned nurse is not as difficult as doing this all by themselves at home. Organizations that can be used for referral are:

Muscular Dystrophy Association of America, Inc.
3300 E. Sunrise Drive
Tucson, AZ 85718

National Scoliosis Foundation, Inc.
72 Mt. Auburn Street
Watertown, MA 02172

Osteogenesis Imperfecta Foundation, Inc.
5005 W. Laurel Avenue, Suite 210
Tampa, FL 33607-3836

American Juvenile Arthritis Organization
1314 Spring Street, NW
Atlanta, GA 30309

IMPLEMENTATION

Many nursing interventions for children with musculoskeletal disorders involve care of a child in a cast or in traction or teaching about common concerns such as posture or children's shoes. Parents and children who are kept well informed in these matters are much more likely to be able to cope with changing circumstances.

EVALUATION

Children with musculoskeletal disorders invariably need follow-up care after discharge from an ambulatory visit or inpatient care, because bone healing is a slow process. Parents may ask to have x-rays taken frequently so that they can be assured that healing is occurring. They may need to be reminded that x-rays are never taken on children unless there is a documented need for them (excessive radiation is possibly associated with the development of leukemia in children).

Both parents and children may need support at reevaluation visits to continue exercises or on learning that a cast or brace must stay on a while longer. Praise for how well they have managed thus far is an effective intervention for helping parents realize that they can cope with the situation in the future.

Part of the time in reevaluation visits should be spent assessing a child's body image and self-esteem. Does a child view himself or herself as a well person with (by the way) a right leg shorter than the left leg, or as a deformed person, inferior to others? Bone healing is incomplete if a child's concept of self is not as whole as the bone.

Some examples of outcome criteria include:

- Child states he or she feels no pain or numbness in extremity.
- Parents accurately state child's care needs to be met both in and outside of the hospital.
- Child states positive aspects of self; participates in activities; establishes friendships with peers.

The Musculoskeletal System

Bones and Bone Growth

Bones are generally classified as long, short, flat, or irregular. **Long bones** are the bones of the extremities, and they are the bones in which most childhood bone disorders are found. The short bones are the bones found in the wrist; flat bones are found in the skull and ribs; and irregular bones are found in the vertebrae.

Long bones are composed of a long central shaft (the **diaphysis**), a rounded end portion (the **epiphysis**), and a thin area between them (the **metaphysis**) (Figure 51-1). Increase in the length of long bones occurs at the cartilage segment (the **epiphyseal plate**) between the metaphysis and epiphysis. As **cartilage** (connective tissue) cells grow away from the shaft, they are replaced by bone, thereby increasing bone length. Injury to this area in a growing child is always potentially serious, because it may halt growth, stimulate abnormal growth, or cause irregular or erratic growth. The central shafts of long bones are covered by an outer sensitive layer of **periosteum**. Bone width increases by growth at the inner surface of the periosteum. Injury to the periosteum, such as may occur with osteomyelitis, can also threaten bone growth.

Although it is easy to think of bones as rigid, solid structures, they are, in fact, living tissue, for which nutri-

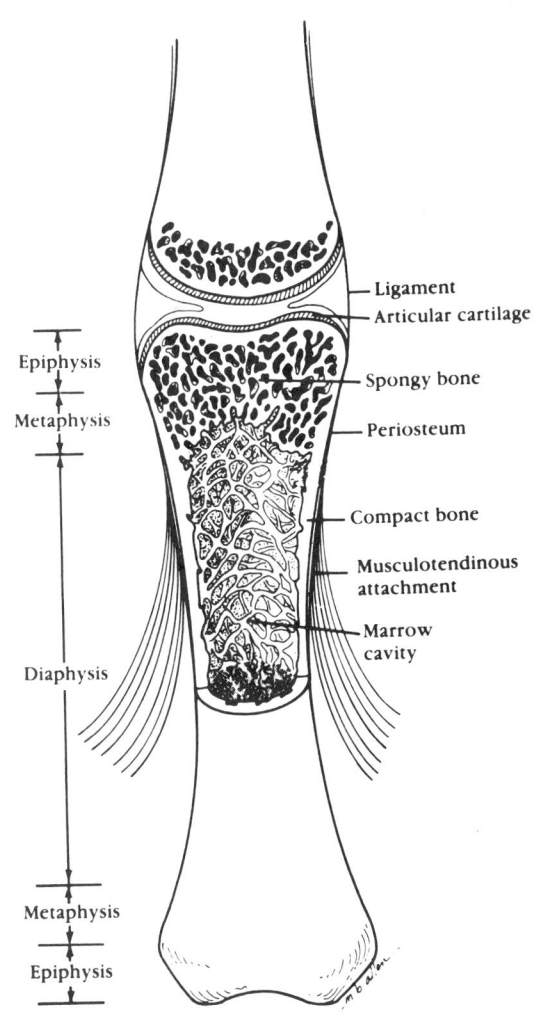

FIGURE 51-1
Structure of a bone. (From Borysenko, M., et al. Functional histology. Boston: Little, Brown, with permission.)

ents for growth must be supplied. Calcium, one of the main components of bone, is constantly reabsorbed and then laid down. The rate of this process is governed by parathyroid hormone. "Bone age" can be determined by an x-ray of the wrists that shows the ossification level of bones. The inner core of long bones is filled with marrow, which is responsible for red blood cell production. The blood supply to bones is abundant so that the marrow can actively supply enough red blood cells for the body. As with other tissues, if the blood supply is cut off, bone cells die.

The bones of children tend to be more resilient than the bones of adults. This means that accidents that might result in severe breaks to adult bones are apt to result in lesser breaks or only torsional twists in children. Bones tend to heal more quickly in children than in adults, so children are incapacitated for a shorter time following an injury. As an example, a broken femur in a 2-year-old child will heal in about 4 weeks; in an adult, a similar fracture would require up to 20 weeks to heal.

Muscle

The skeletal muscular system is composed of one type of muscle, called **striated muscle**, which is the predominant muscle in the body (and differentiated from **smooth muscle**, which is responsible for, among other things, gastrointestinal peristalsis). Activation of skeletal muscle occurs with innervation from a motor nerve. **Myopathy**, or disease in the muscular system, can be inherited (as in muscular dystrophy) or acquired (as in myasthenia gravis).

Assessment of Musculoskeletal Function

Diagnostic tests frequently ordered for children with musculoskeletal dysfunction include x-rays and bone scans, bone and muscle biopsy, and electromyography. Ultrasound and magnetic resonance studies may be used to reveal soft tissue disease.

X-ray or Bone Scan

Because bones are opaque, they outline well on x-ray. A bone scan is a study of the uptake of intravenously injected radioactive substances by rapidly healing portions of bones. If a child is in pain, lying still on an x-ray or examining table in an uncomfortable position for such studies may be very difficult. Before a bone scan, you may be asked to administer potassium percholate to prevent the radioactive substance from concentrating in the child's thyroid. Be certain always to check for such an order before any scanning procedure.

Electromyography

Electromyography studies the electrical activity of muscle motor units. For the test, needle electrodes are inserted into muscle masses; the electrical activity of the muscle at rest and in motion is detected by audioamplification and recorded on an oscilloscope. Normally, resting muscle is quiet; if defects in muscle, such as fasciculations, are present, abnormal noises or oscilloscope spikes will be observed.

Although the needle electrodes are small, the test is frightening for children because they are pricked by needles, so they need support from someone they know during the procedure. Following the examination, they may need an opportunity to play with a rag doll and a needle to express their anxiety at the procedure.

Muscle Biopsy

Muscle biopsy is generally done under a local anesthetic, but if children cannot cooperate, it may be done under a general anesthetic. Caution children that they will feel the initial prick of an anesthetizing needle; then, as the actual biopsy needle enters the muscle mass, they will feel an additional momentary pain. They can be assured that the amount of tissue taken from them is no larger than the inner bore of the biopsy needle or the lead in a pencil.

Therapeutic Management of Musculoskeletal Disorders in Children

Casting

Casts may be used in the treatment of a variety of musculoskeletal system disorders—from simple fractures in the extremities to correction of congenital structural bone disorders (see Chapter 39 for a discussion of the latter).

Casting Procedure

Casts are created from either plastic or fiberglass. Fiberglass is an attractive material to use for childrens' casts as it is light, comes in color, and is water resistant. Unfortunately, it is more expensive, so it may not be practical for casts that need frequent changing.

Children need an explanation of what they can expect in the process of casting. To maintain alignment of body parts, a physician gently exerts a pull on the body part being casted during cast application. If a large body cast is being applied, children may be positioned on a special cast table with traction apparatus at the chin and pelvis. These tables are stark, steel tables; they may resemble torture racks children have seen in horror movies. It helps if they have a nurse accompany them to a cast room, so they know they have a friend to stand by them and perhaps hold their hand while the chin straps or pelvic traction is applied. Most children (and adults)

are unaware that traditional casts are formed from strips of gauze impregnated with plaster of paris (Figure 51-2). The normal curiosity of children as they watch a cast grow and mold to their body part makes casting a pleasant procedure. Some children look forward to having a cast put in place (it may be a badge of courage, a conversation piece, an "autograph book").

Caution children that when wet strips of plaster of Paris are first applied, they feel cool. Almost immediately, the strips begin to generate heat as evaporation begins, and children's body parts feel warm. If the cast is a full-body cast, children may be uncomfortably warm and sweat may run from their forehead. Assure them that this warmth is never enough to burn and is a transient phenomenon.

After a cast has been applied, children will be transferred to a stretcher and then to bed if they are to stay in the hospital. When moving a child in a wet cast, always use open palms to move the cast. Fingers indent the cast and may cause pressure points that will result in pressure sores under the cast. Support the cast on soft pillows so that you do not dent the undersurface (Figure 51-3). A cast should be left uncovered by clothing or bedclothes so that it dries as rapidly as possible. Turn children about every 2 hours to allow the underside of the cast to dry. The use of heaters or fans to dry the cast is not advised because they can cause uneven drying and because heat can cause a burn under the cast (McConnell, 1993).

Nursing Diagnoses and Related Interventions

Nursing Diagnosis: High risk for altered peripheral tissue perfusion related to pressure from cast

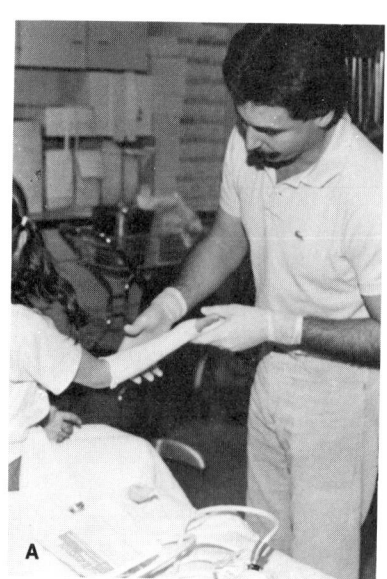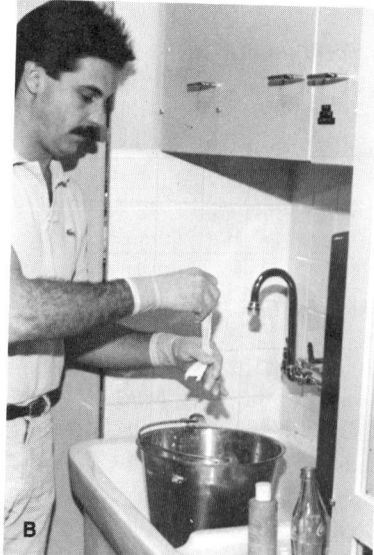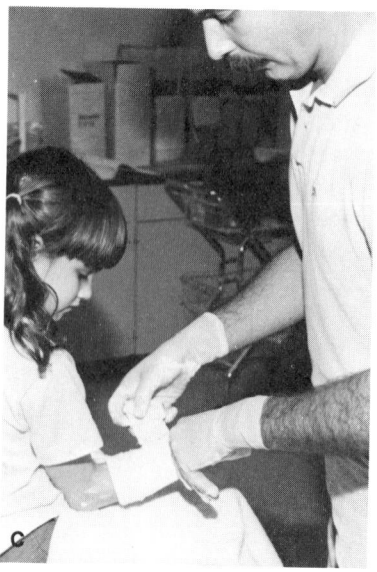

FIGURE 51-2

*Application of a cast. (**A**) Applying stockinet. (**B**) Soaking plaster of paris strips. (**C**) Molding plaster of paris for the cast. (Courtesy of Bruce Hill.)*

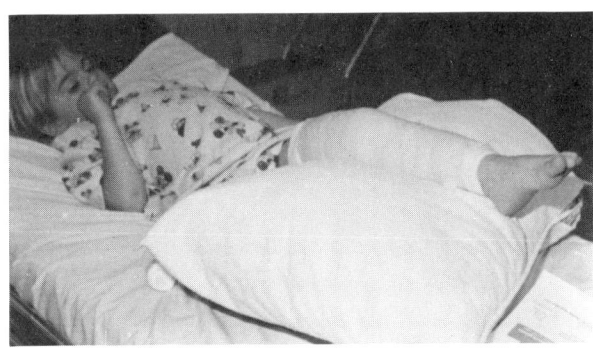

FIGURE 51-3
Elevating a newly casted leg on a pillow helps to prevent edema. (Courtesy of Bruce Hill.)

Goal: Child will not experience impaired circulatory function during the time the cast is in place.

Outcome Criteria: Child states he or she feels no pain or numbness in extremity; distal nail bed blanches and refills in less than 5 seconds.

If an extremity has been casted, keep it elevated to prevent edema in the part. Check circulation frequently (every 15 minutes during the first hour; hourly for the first 24 hours; every 4 hours thereafter) (see Figure 41-7). Signs of impaired neurologic or circulatory function are blueness or coldness of a distal part, lack of a peripheral pulse, edema that does not improve with elevation, pain in the casted part, or numbness or tingling in the part as if it were "asleep." (Children under 6 or 7 years of age have difficulty describing this feeling; they may whine or cry with the discomfort of the sensation, however.) Any of these symptoms requires immediate attention, because circulatory impairment will lead to nerve ischemia and destruction, which could cause permanent paralysis of an extremity (Table 51-1).

Nursing Diagnosis: High risk for impaired tissue integrity related to pressure from cast

Goal: Child's skin will remain intact during time cast is in place.

Table 51-1. *Neurocirculatory Assessment for the Child in a Cast*

Temperature	Distal body part should feel warm to the touch
Color	Distal body part should have normal skin color
Pulse	Distal pulse should be palpable
Pain	Child should not experience pain or tingling in distal body part
Blanching	If blanched white, a distal finger or toenail should pinken again in less than 5 sec

Outcome Criteria: Child reports no pain under cast; cast remains dry and free of stains; skin is intact and not erythematous following cast removal.

When a cast is dry, edges that are not smooth or covered by a fold of stockinet must be smoothed by applying adhesive tape strips to prevent skin irritation. This is termed **petaling** (Figure 51-4).

If a cast surrounds the genital area, cover the cast with plastic to prevent urine from impregnating it. Placing an infant on a Bradford frame while the cast is in place may help urine and feces to drain away from the cast. Pin diapers so that they do not cover areas of the cast not protected by the plastic covering; otherwise, a soaked diaper will wet the cast. Instead, fold the diaper so that it fits a smaller area. In some children, a sanitary pad absorbs urine well and keeps the cast dry. Plastic pants should not be used over a cast because they tend to hold the moisture and urine, preventing drying. Using a urine collector is not a good plan, because the tape required to keep it in place for a long period of time will cause skin irritation.

Keeping children in a semi-Fowler's position by using pillows or a raised bed helps to direct urine and feces downward and prevents soaking of the back of a body cast. Because a cast is heavy, an infant tends to slip down a great deal and so needs frequent repositioning to keep in the raised position.

Once urine has penetrated a cast, there is no way to remove it, so prevention is of the utmost importance. A urine-soaked cast becomes very odorous; not only is the odor unappealing, but it may mask the odor of a pressure sore under the cast. Heavy soaking tends to weaken the cast, causing loss of support.

Make certain that when children are being fed or are feeding themselves, they have a bib or a cover over the top edge of a cast so that crumbs and fluid are not spilled inside. Toys should be chosen carefully for the same reason. A piece of food inside a cast will mold and macerate the skin; a small part of a toy dropped inside a cast can cause irritation and a pressure ulcer.

If a child spills food on a cast, or if the cast becomes soiled, it can be cleaned with a damp cloth. Scouring powder without a chlorine base (such as Bon Ami) may be used. Using chlorine-based scouring powder causes the plaster to deteriorate and weaken.

Nursing Diagnosis: Parental health-seeking behaviors related to home care of child with cast

Goal: Parents will demonstrate confidence about their ability to care for child following cast application.

Outcome Criteria: Parents state plans for adapting home environment and lifestyle to accommodate child with cast.

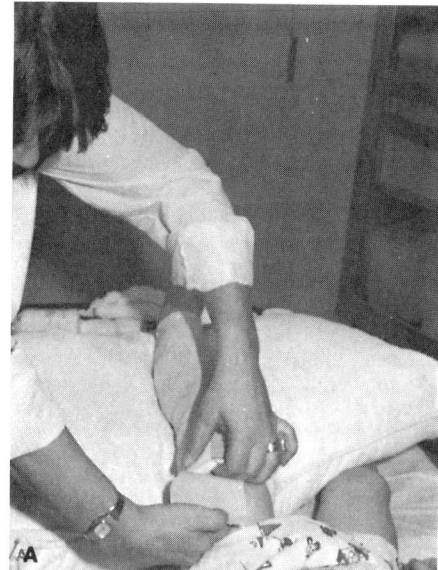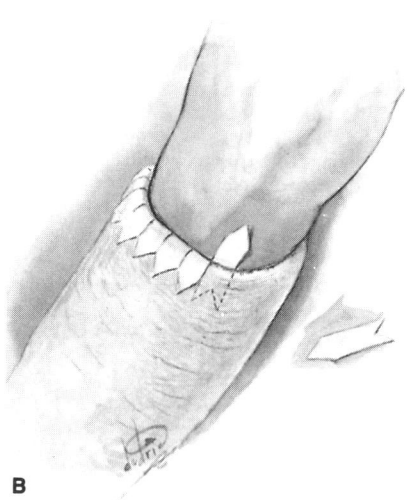

FIGURE 51-4
(**A**) *Technique for petaling a cast with adhesive tape. This smooths the rough edges and prevents irritation of the child's skin.* (**B**) *A petal in place. (Courtesy of Bruce Hill.)*

Handling a child in a large cast is a major task for parents. For many, it may seem so overwhelming that they do not see how they will be able to care for the child at home. Assure them that the child is quite comfortable in the cast, despite its awkward, constricting appearance. Allow them to observe you moving the child and positioning him or her before they are ready to attempt these maneuvers themselves. Be sure to caution them that if an abduction bar is used with a cast, it must never be used as a handle for lifting a cast. Such use can break the bar from the cast or weaken its support.

A body cast is heavy, so parents may need to be cautioned to use good body mechanics (lift with the thighs, not the back) when turning or positioning the child (and they should see you role modeling this type of lifting). Be certain that parents have had adequate handling and positioning practice before a child is discharged from a health care facility, so that they can care for a child confidently. If a cast is bulky, parents may appreciate suggestions on ways to help move the child from room to room, such as using a toy wagon with a flat board on top or using a skateboard for the child to propels himself or herself. It is important to point out that all children thrive on being touched. Children in a large body cast need their head and arms stroked (or any areas of the body that are not covered by a cast). Demonstrate how even a child in a large hip spica cast can be held, cuddled, and supported for feeding. Otherwise, parents may tend to neglect this aspect of total care.

Many children complain of itching inside a cast at about the end of the first week the cast has been in place. If the area is immediately under the edge of the cast, the itching is probably the result of dry skin caused by the drying effect of the plaster. Reaching a hand

under the edge of the cast and massaging the area generally relieves the itching. Applying hand lotion may relieve the dryness. If the area is unreachable, blowing cool air through the cast with a fan, a hair dryer set on cool air, or a vacuum cleaner attachment may relieve the uncomfortable feeling. Caution the child and parents not to use implements such as a coat hanger or knitting needle to scratch the area. These can injure the skin, causing infection under a cast.

Transporting the child in the car, particularly fitting a bulky cast into an infant car seat, can be a major problem (Stout et al., 1992). Before a child is discharged, give parents a telephone number to call if they have any questions about their child's care or condition. Do not underestimate how difficult it is for parents to provide care at home for a child in a large, bulky cast.

Cast Removal

Most casts remain in place for 4 to 8 weeks and are then removed, using an electric cast cutter with a rapidly vibrating, circular disk (Figure 51-5). The disk makes a very loud noise as it cuts through plaster. To the child, the disk appears capable of cutting through not only the plaster but an arm or leg as well. The physician who removes the cast generally demonstrates that the disk does not cut skin by touching a thumb to the edge of it (if not, you can demonstrate this). Not all children are totally convinced by the demonstration, however, and may require your support while the disk moves from one end of a cast to the other, such as saying, "It's all right to cry; I know this looks scary" or by holding your hands over the child's ears to lessen the noise.

The skin of the child's extremity looks macerated and dirty after the cast is removed; a good bath usually washes away most of this. If the arm has been casted in

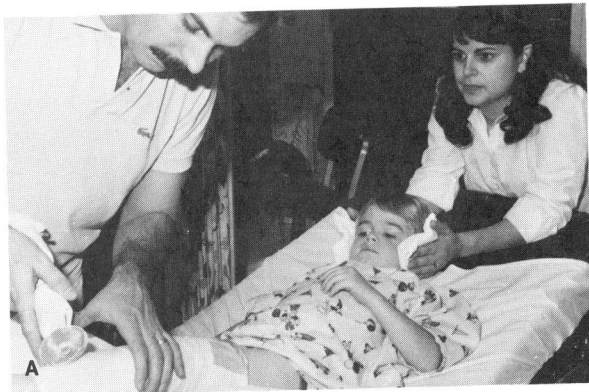

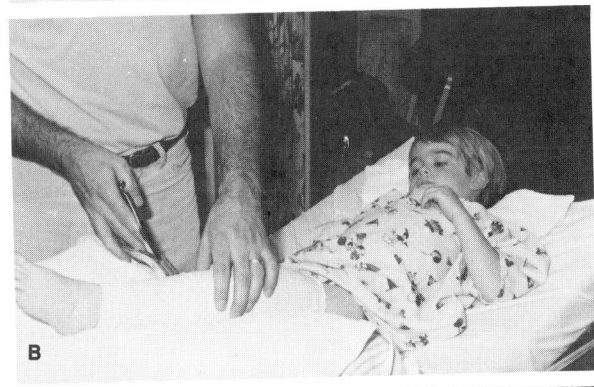

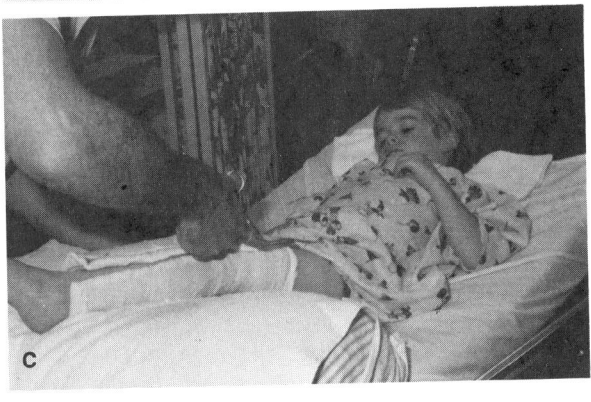

FIGURE 51-5
*Cast removal. (**A**) A cast cutter. (**B**) Pliers break the sections apart. (**C**) Scissors cut the stockinet. Notice how the nurse is holding wash-cloths over the child's ears to make the noise of a cast cutter less frightening. (Courtesy of Bruce Hill.)*

flexion, the elbow feels stiff and even sore as the child is asked to extend it for the first time. Children use extremities with caution after a cast has been removed; therefore, advise parents to allow the child to begin using the extremity again at his or her own pace. Neither passive exercises to loosen up an arm or leg nor the old method of carrying heavy weights to pull out an arm is recommended. As children naturally play and reach for objects, they gradually forget to favor the arm or leg; full function then returns. Once healing has taken place, the extremity is as strong as it was before the fracture. The child does not need to continue to favor the extremity to protect it from a second fracture.

Crutches

Crutches are prescribed for children for one of three reasons: to keep weight off one or both legs, to support weakened legs, or to maintain balance. Usually, a physical therapist measures crutch length and gives beginning instruction in crutch walking. You need to be familiar with the measurement of crutches and the supervision of crutch walking to offer emotional support to children as they learn and to assess progress at ambulatory return appointments or during a visit in the home.

Fit and Adjustment

If crutches are properly fitted, there should be a space of 1 to 1½ in between the axilla crutch pad and the child's axilla. When the child stands upright and places his hands on the handrests of the crutches, the elbows should flex about 20 degrees. This degree of flexion assures you that when the child bears weight on the crutch, the body weight will be borne by the arm, not axilla. Pressure of a crutch against the axilla could lead to compression and damage of the brachial plexus nerves as they cross the axilla, resulting in permanent nerve palsy. Teach children not to rest with the crutch pad pressing on the axilla but always to support their weight at the hand grip.

Always assess the tips of crutches to see that the rubber tip is intact and not worn through. The tip prevents the crutch from slipping when it is in place. Be certain that the child is walking with the crutches placed about 6 in to the side of foot. This distance furnishes a wide, balanced base for support.

Explore with children any problems crutches will cause in their day. If they carry books to school, for example, they may prefer to wear a backpack until they are free of crutches so they can leave their hands free for the handrests. Caution parents to clear articles such as throw rugs and small footstools out of the paths at home. If there are small children at home, the parents will need to keep the traffic areas free of toys to prevent an accident.

Crutch Walking

Two main crutch-walking patterns are used (Figure 51-6). A two-point gait is a crutch-walking pattern used when a child needs support for weakened muscles or balance but may bear weight on both lower extremities. The child places the right crutch and left foot forward, then left crutch and right foot forward, and so on. Using the crutch opposite a foot provides a wider base of support than using the crutch next to the foot. Caution children to take small steps until they feel confident.

A three-point swing-through gait is used when no weight bearing is allowed on one foot. For this, the crutches are both brought forward. The weight of the body is shifted forward as both legs are swung through the crutches. The child bears weight on the good leg

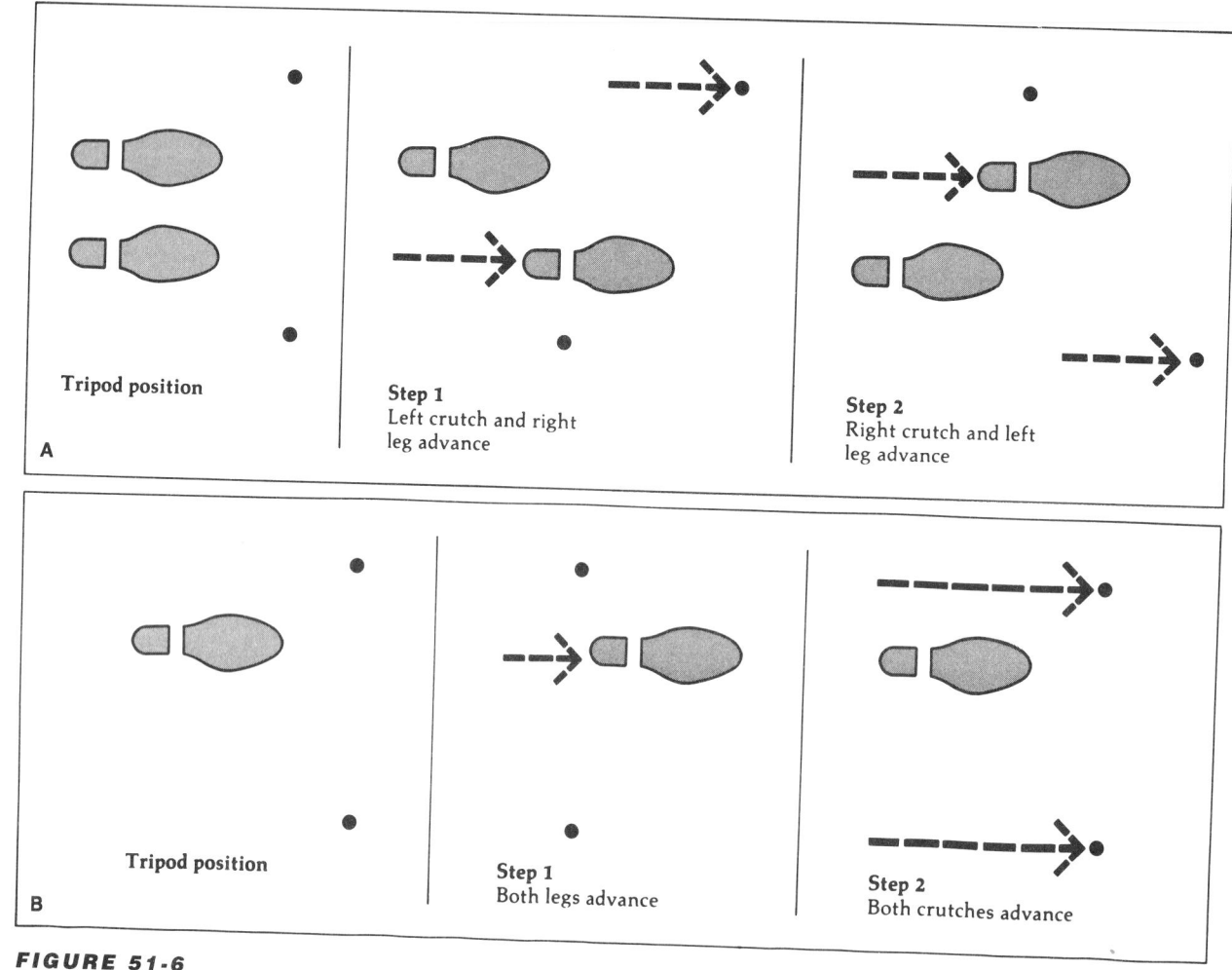

FIGURE 51-6
Crutch-walking patterns. (**A**) *Two-point gait.* (**B**) *Swing-through gait. (From Belland, K. H., & Wells, M. A.*
Clinical nursing procedures. *Boston: Jones and Bartlett Publishers, with permission.)*

and moves the crutches forward again. It takes strong arm support to bear full weight on crutches this way. Be certain the child is bearing weight on the hands and not the axillae when swinging through. Some children use a swing-through gait rather recklessly and need to be advised to slow their pace to a safer one.

To walk downstairs using a swing-through gait, children place the crutches on the lower step, then swing the good foot forward and down to that step. To go upstairs, they place their good foot on the elevated step, then raise the crutches onto the step and lift themselves up. To help children remember this pattern, a saying—"angels" (the good foot) go up; "devils" (the bad foot with the crutches) go down—is traditionally used.

Traction

Traction is used to reduce dislocation and immobilize fractures. Although it is still necessary for some conditions, its use is declining. It involves pulling on a body part in one direction against a counterpull exerted in the opposite direction. In straight traction, a child's body

weight serves as the counterpull. In suspended or balanced traction, the body part is suspended by a sling, and the counterpull, as well as the primary pull, is accomplished by pulleys and weights. Skin traction (in which skin provides the counterpull) or skeletal traction (in which bone provides the counterpull) may be used. Skin traction is used when only minimal traction is necessary; the child's skin must be in good condition for this procedure. Skeletal traction is used when a longer period of traction or greater strength of traction is needed. Types of traction are illustrated in Figure 51-7. Home traction, which allows the child to interact with family members, should be encouraged.

Skin Traction

Bryant's traction, used for fractured femurs in younger children (under 2 years of age), is an example of skin traction (Figure 51-8). It is also used as preparation for surgical repair of congenital developmental defects, such as developmental dysplasia of the hip (see Chapter 39). Buck's extension is an example of skin traction used for immobilizing fractures in older children (Figure 51-9).

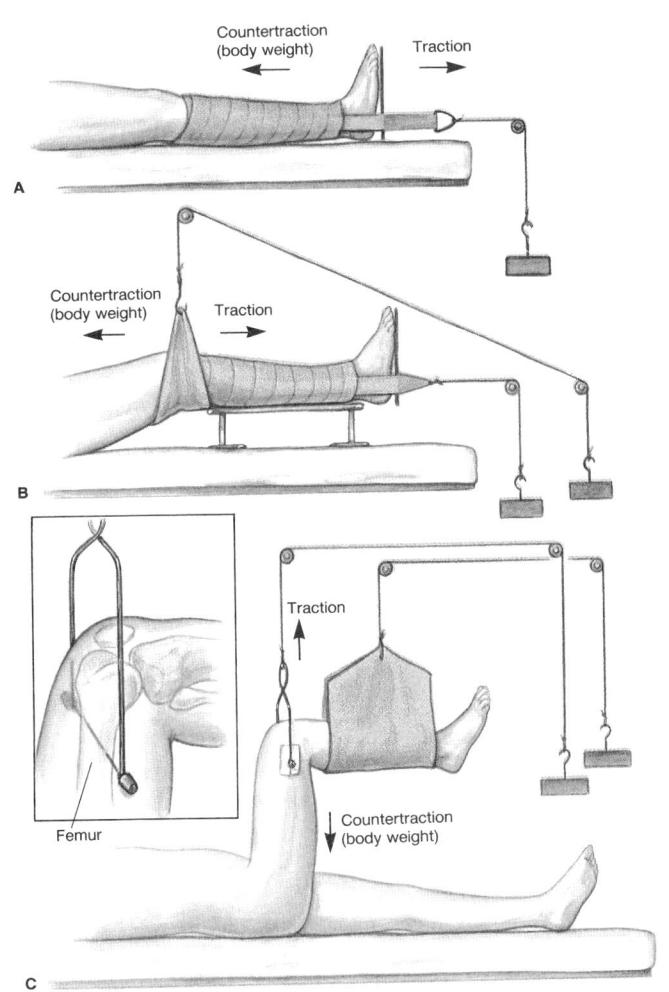

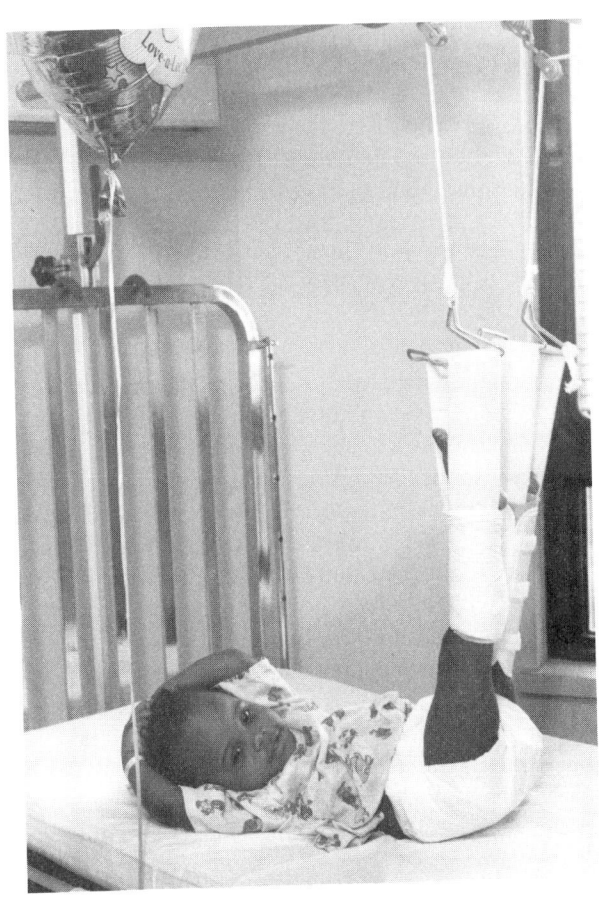

FIGURE 51-7
*Types of traction. (**A**) Buck's extension, a form of skin traction. (**B**) Russell traction, a type of skin traction. Two lines of traction (one horizontal and one vertical) allow for good bone alignment for healing. (**C**) 90 degree–90 degree (skeletal) traction. A wire pin is inserted into the distal femur.*

FIGURE 51-8
An infant in Bryant's traction. Notice that the infant's buttocks are far enough off the bed for a hand to slide underneath them. This ensures that traction is exerted on the legs and hips. (Courtesy of the Department of Medical Photography, Children's Hospital, Buffalo, NY.)

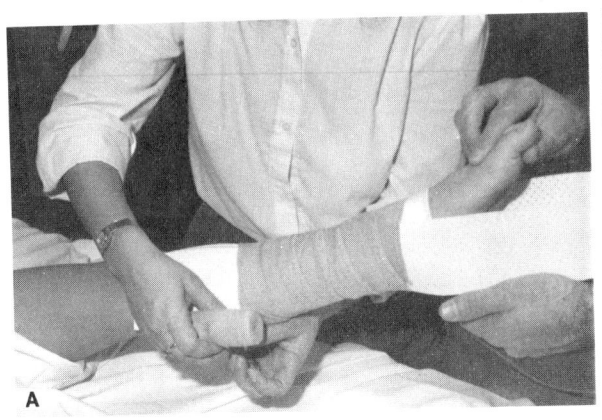

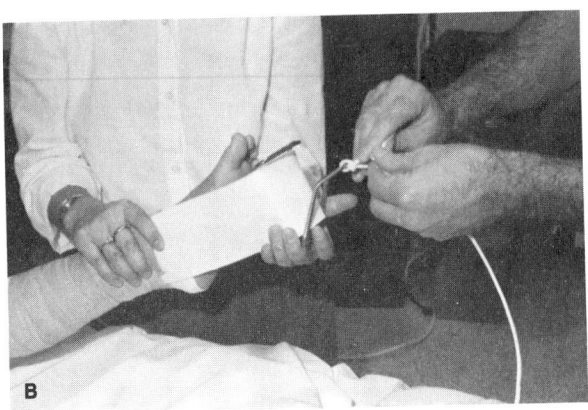

FIGURE 51-9
*Applying Buck's extension traction. (**A**) Wrapping an Ace bandage over gauze and traction supports. (**B**) Attaching the rope and end plate. (Courtesy of Bruce Hill.)*

The child's skin usually is prepared for skin traction by being coated with tincture of benzoin, which toughens the skin and becomes tacky or sticky as it dries. Moleskin or adhesive-backed strips, which are soft and nonirritating and adhere to the tacky skin, are then molded to the extremity. The moleskin and a metal or wooden foot plate are held in place by an elastic bandage wrap. Ropes are attached to the wood or metal plate at the distal end of the extremity. These ropes pass over pulleys attached to an orthopedic frame over the bed, and weights attached to the end of the ropes exert traction or pull on the extremity.

Skeletal Traction

Skeletal traction involves the use of a Steinmann pin or a Kirschner wire passed through the skin into the end of a long bone. The area of insertion is shaved and prepared with an antiseptic. The pin can be inserted in an emergency department under local anesthesia if the child can hold absolutely still, but usually it is done under general anesthesia in the operating room. Children return to their room with cotton gauze squares placed around the ends of the pin. Observe the site daily for drainage. Odorous or excessive drainage or erythema may be a sign of infection at the pin site. With skeletal traction, ropes strung over pulleys and attached to weights exert a pull on the extremity at the pin site (Figure 51-10).

Children in traction need to be assessed carefully for circulatory or neurologic impairment, as do children in casts. The extremity in traction should be checked every 15 minutes during the first hour, hourly for 24 hours, and every 4 hours thereafter for signs of blueness, coldness, tingling, lack of peripheral pulse, edema, or pain (see Table 51-1). Traction can lead to hypertension because the head typically is positioned lower than the lower extremities. Assess once a day for this.

Be careful when changing the child's bed or carrying out other nursing functions that you do not move the weights or in any other way interfere with the traction. Provide good skin care on the child's back, elbows, and heels, which tend to become irritated. A trapeze suspended over the bed provides a great deal of mobility and assists children in using a bedpan and positioning themselves in bed.

Being in traction is not as dramatic for children as being placed in a cast. There is nothing for people to autograph. There is an unspoken feeling from other children that "if what you have is really serious, you'd have a cast on." Children need an explanation so that they understand why this type of treatment is best for them. Keep them informed of x-ray reports: "Callus formation is beginning," "The fracture is being held in just the right position," and so on. Although they cannot see progress, they can be assured that it is happening.

Children need to maintain contact with their school friends through cards, letters, or tape-recorded messages. If hospitalized, their bed should be located so that they can see unit activities. Whether at home or in the hospital, they should be allowed to have visitors their own age, so that they do not lose their place among their friends during this long period of hospitalization or home care.

Children in traction are generally not "ill" children. They feel well except for the leg or arm being held in correct position. Therefore, they have the energy and need the stimulation of well children. Keeping them occupied and exposed to activities appropriate to their age group is a major part of nursing planning for such children.

Disorders of Bone Development

Flat Feet (Pes Planus)

The term *flat feet* refers to relaxation of the longitudinal arch of the foot. Many parents worry that their children have this problem; only rarely, however, does this occur. Parents become concerned because, normally, a newborn's foot is flatter and proportionately wider than an adult's. A transverse arch rarely is visible; a longitudinal arch may not be present until a child has been walking for months. Parents notice that when their child walks in the sand or makes wet tracks on the bathroom floor, he or she makes an impression of a "flat foot."

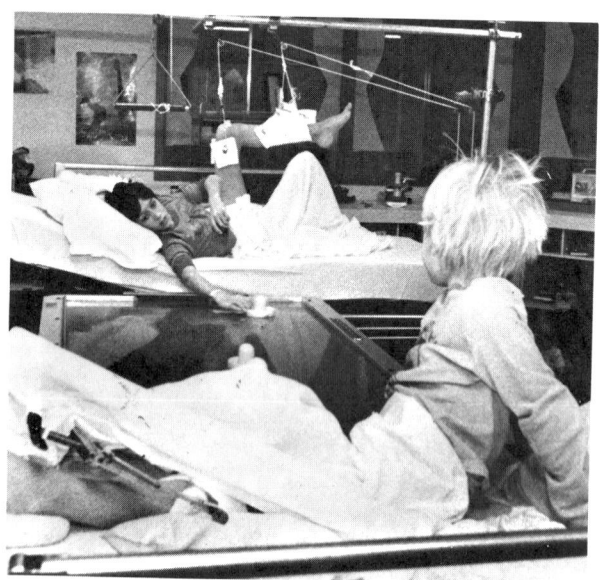

FIGURE 51-10
The boy in the rear bed has skeletal traction with a Steinmann's pin through the distal portion of the femur (90 degree–90 degree traction). The gauze dressing at the pin's insertion is stained with povidone-iodine. He is playing ski ball with a boy in skeletal traction in the near bed. Notice the overhead trapeze to facilitate movement. (Courtesy of the Department of Medical Photography, Children's Hospital, Buffalo, NY.)

Evaluate children's feet for this by having them stand on tiptoe. In this position, a longitudinal arch should be visible. If they can stand on their heels with the soles of the feet off the ground, the feet probably are normal. Examine the ankle joint to be certain a full range of motion is present to demonstrate that the Achilles tendon is not shortened. Tarsal and metatarsal joints should normally show a full range of motion.

Some children complain of foot pain at the end of the day. This probably occurs not from lack of a longitudinal arch but from poor arch development. The arch can be strengthened and the pain usually can be eliminated if the child walks on tiptoe for 5 to 10 minutes daily or practices picking up marbles with the toes. For an older child, standing pigeon-toed (toes pointed in) and throwing the weight forward onto the lateral aspect of the feet tends to strengthen arches.

Teach parents that children do not need a hightop or rigid shoe for foot development. Shoes with strong foot support may actually prevent the arch from forming adequately and so should be avoided (Staheli, 1992).

Genu Varum (Bowlegs)

Genu varum is usually said to be present if, when the malleoli of the ankles are touching, the medial surface of the knees are over 1 in apart (Figure 51-11*A*). A number of children develop this condition as they grow as part of normal development. It is seen most commonly in 2-year-olds. Record the extent of the bowing at health

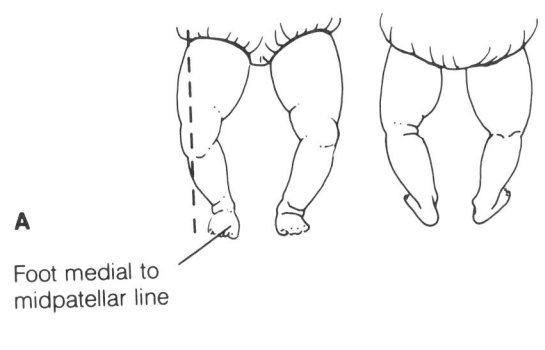

A

Foot medial to midpatellar line

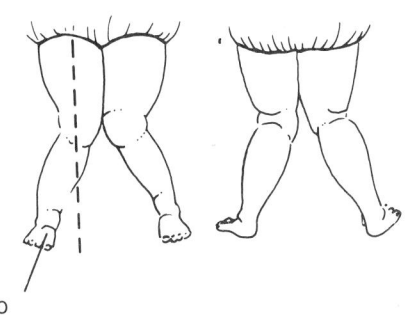

B

Foot lateral to midpatellar line

FIGURE 51-11
(**A**) *Genu varum.* (**B**) *Genu valgum.*

maintenance visits by approximating the medial malleoli of the ankles and measuring the distance between the patellas (knees) to see if it is increasing or not.

Genu varum gradually corrects itself by about 2 years of age and at the latest by school-age. If the problem is becoming rapidly worse or persists beyond this time, children need referral to an orthopedist for further evaluation (Heath & Staheli, 1993).

Blount's Disease (Tibia Vara)

Blount's disease is retardation of growth of the epiphyseal line on the medial side of the proximal tibia (inside of the knee). This results in bowed legs. Blount's disease, unlike the normal developmental aspect of genu varum, however, is a serious disturbance in bone growth and requires treatment.

Because it is not possible to rule out Blount's disease by appearance alone, almost all children with bowed legs have an initial x-ray to determine whether the problem is Blount's disease. With Blount's disease, the medial aspect of the proximal tibia will show a sharp, beaklike appearance on x-ray.

Bracing or osteotomy may be necessary to correct this deformity or prevent it from becoming more severe. Parents need an explanation of why their child requires treatment or surgery when another child on the block with a similar appearance (developmental genu varum) is expected to outgrow his or her problem.

Genu Valgum (Knock Knees)

Genu valgum is said to be present if, when the medial surfaces of the knees touch, the medial surfaces of the ankle malleoli are separated by more than 1 in (Figure 51-11*B*). The severity of the deformity should be measured at regular health maintenance visits by approximating the medial aspects of the knees and measuring the distance between the medial malleoli of the ankles.

This is seen most commonly in children aged 3 to 4 years. No treatment is necessary for genu valgum. The problem tends to correct itself as the child grows. By school age, few children continue to have the problem. Those children who do, or those in whom the abnormality is becoming more pronounced, need a referral to an orthopedist for further evaluation.

Toeing-In

Toeing-in (pigeon toe) in children may occur as a result of foot, tibial, femoral, or hip displacement. Assess for this when a parent describes a child as "always falling over her feet" or "awkward."

Metatarsus adductus is turning in of the forefoot. The heel is in good alignment; only the forefoot is turned in. This may develop or become more pronounced in infants who sleep prone with feet adducted or older children who watch television by kneeling, resting on their feet, and turning their feet in. If the child stands on a copying machine and a print is made, the turning in of the foot is well demonstrated.

Most instances of metatarsus adductus resolve without therapy. Those that persist beyond one year can be corrected by passive stretching exercises. Wearing shoes on the opposite feet may help some infants. Wearing a Denis Browne splint at night may be necessary. A Denis Browne splint consists of a pair of shoes connected by a metal or plastic rod. The shoes are positioned to keep the foot in the correct alignment and are then held firmly to the rod by metal or plastic plates (Figure 51-12). Most infants wear these only at night because walking with them in place is impossible. Parents must be cautioned not to unscrew and reposition a shoe. The toes of the shoes are cut away so that children have ample room for growing without the shoes needing to be replaced.

A few infants with extremely rigid, incorrect foot posture may require casts rather than splints for correction. Treatment for metatarsus adductus is most effective if it is begun before an infant walks, so early detection is important. When treatment begins early, the prognosis is excellent.

Inward tibial torsion also may be evidenced as toeing-in. This condition is diagnosed when a line drawn from the anterior superior iliac crest through the center of the patella intersects the fourth or fifth toe (or a position even more lateral) (Figure 51-13). Ordinarily such a line should intersect the second toe.

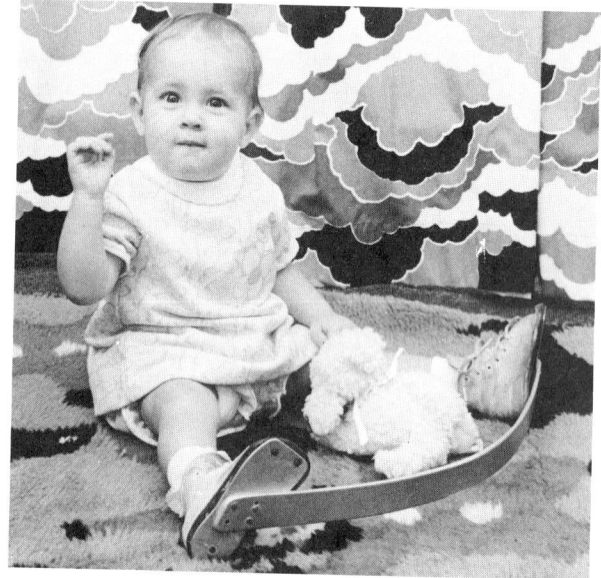

FIGURE 51-12

A Denis Browne splint. Although at first glance this looks cumbersome, children adjust to these splints readily and accept them well. (Courtesy of the Department of Medical Photography, Children's Hospital, Buffalo, NY.)

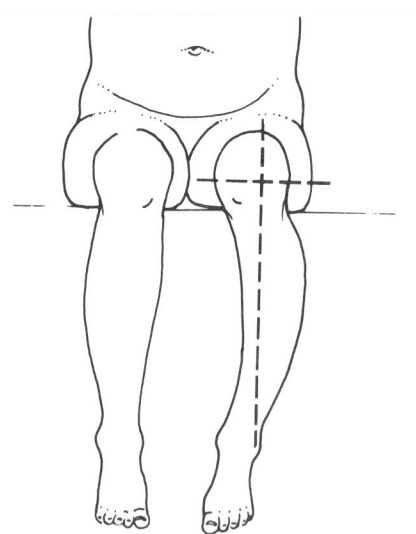

FIGURE 51-13

Toeing-in caused by inward tibial torsion. In good alignment, a line drawn from the anterosuperior iliac crest through the patella should intersect the second toe.

Tibial torsion is a normal developmental finding. It will improve as the tibia grows and so needs no treatment. Parents will need a good explanation of why no treatment is necessary. They may need reassurance at periodic health maintenance visits that patience and time will correct tibial torsion.

Inward femoral torsion can be detected if you have a child lie supine and attempt to rotate his or her leg internally and then externally at the hip. Normally, internal rotation is about 30 degrees and outward rotation is about 90 degrees. With inward femoral torsion, the legs rotate so far inward that the degree of internal rotation is closer to 90 degrees. In some children, the femur rotates so far that the patellar bones face each other. As with tibial torsion, no treatment for this is necessary. Inward femoral rotation will not correct itself, but a compensating tibial torsion will develop and make feet appear straight.

A fourth cause of toeing-in may be improper hip placement or hip dysplasia, a problem that is very serious and needs early therapy for correction (see Chapter 39).

Limps

All children should be observed walking as a part of health assessment at health maintenance visits. Gait is a variable characteristic. You probably know at least one friend you can recognize from a distance simply by a characteristic walk. Limping is never normal, however, and although it may reflect a simple problem (a recently stubbed toe), it may also reflect serious bone or muscle involvement, such as occurs in osteomyelitis or cerebral palsy.

History is important in determining the cause of the limp. When children have pain in lower extremities, they protect their extremities by limping—stepping gingerly and quickly on an affected leg. Although children may seem to be favoring an ankle or a knee, ask them specifically what hurts. They may be favoring a hip; because a hip hurts, they may be walking gingerly on the leg and causing pain in a knee.

The lower extremities need careful, thoughtful examination, including inspection, measurement of leg length, range of motion, palpation, and a neurologic examination. X-ray or bone scan may be necessary to rule out a pathologic process (Staheli, 1992).

Growing Pains

Listen to parents carefully when they state that their child has "growing pains"; what they are reporting may be symptoms indicative of rheumatic fever or juvenile rheumatoid arthritis rather than of a simple, transient phenomenon. Growing pains occur most frequently in the muscle of the calf. They never occur in a joint. Children wake at night because of the pain. Such cramping generally is associated with a day of vigorous activity or wearing of new shoes with a heel of a different height than before. Children with genu varum (bowlegs) tend to have more of such pain than other children. Growing pains should never be taken lightly but should be evaluated seriously at health maintenance visits to detect possible symptoms of disease.

Osteogenesis Imperfecta

Osteogenesis imperfecta is characterized by the formation of brittle bones (Weaver, 1994). It occurs in two main forms: a severe form that is recognized at birth (osteogenesis imperfecta congenita) and a form that occurs later in life (osteogenesis imperfecta tarda).

Children with the congenital form are born with countless fractures. They develop many more fractures during childhood. This condition appears to be inherited as a recessive trait. Children with the late-occurring form may have associated deafness, dental deformities, and an unusual blueness of the sclera because of poor connective tissue formation. This disorder is inherited as a dominant trait. X-ray reveals a particular ribbonlike or mosaic pattern in bones, which aids in diagnosis.

In both instances, the major clinical manifestation is a tendency to fracture easily due to poor collagen formation. In some children, their bones are so fragile, fracture results not only from trauma, such as occurs in a fall, but from simple walking. It can occur from the force of birth.

As such children grow older, the multiple breaks tend to cause limb and spinal column deformities, which

interfere with alignment or growth. Growth hormone may be administered to stimulate growth. There is no additional therapy except to protect children from trauma, to treat and align fractures, and to educate children to develop a lifestyle that is productive yet results in little trauma. Lightweight leg braces or intermedullary rods may be effective in strengthening bones.

Always be careful when caring for such children to raise side rails on cribs or beds. Keep floors dry; remove objects that could cause falls from the pathway to avoid injury. Always lift children gently; do not lift them by a single arm or leg.

Legg-Calvé-Perthes Disease (Coxa Plana)

Legg-Calvé-Perthes disease is avascular necrosis of the proximal femoral epiphysis. This occurs more often in males than females; the peak age of incidence is between 4 and 8 years of age (Sponseller, 1994).

The affected child notices pain in the hip joint. There is much spasm and limitation of motion. X-ray studies are used to distinguish between Legg-Calvé-Perthes disease and a simple synovitis (inflammation of the hip joint), which begins with the same symptoms. X-ray changes may not be apparent when a child is first seen; they appear after about 3 weeks. For this reason, most children seen for a synovitis of the hip joint are asked to return in 3 weeks for a repeat x-ray.

Legg-Calvé-Perthes disease passes through four stages. First is the synovitis stage, or period of painful inflammation. Following this is a necrotic stage during which bone in the femur head becomes smaller and shows increased density on x-ray. This stage lasts 6 to 12 months. A third stage is a fragmentation stage. Resorption of dead bone occurs over a 1- to 2-year period. The fourth stage, a reconstruction stage, marks final healing with deposition of new bone occurring.

Treatment for Legg-Calvé-Perthes disease in the past required a child to avoid bearing weight. Preventing an active 4- to 10-year-old child from bearing weight for up to 18 months was obviously a demanding task for parents. It was difficult for children not to "cheat" and walk "just a little bit." Today, children are treated with "containment" braces. These braces contain the femur head in the acetabulum socket by abducting the leg (Staheli, 1992). In this position, the acetabulum maintains the correct shape of the femur head as it remolds. Parents need to be certain that the child is wearing the brace. Without the apparatus, the femur head tends to remold in a mushroom shape. This makes the hip unstable thereafter. Because the shape does not conform well to the acetabulum, degenerative changes may occur later in life, leading to chronic pain and reduced mobility of the hip joint.

A reconstructive surgery technique (an osteotomy to center the femur head in the acetabulum followed by cast application) is available that limits the time of containment to 3 to 4 months (Coates et al., 1990).

Following surgery, children are placed in a large, full-leg-abduction spica cast. Although it is difficult to do, children can ambulate with crutches with this bulky cast in place and so can return to school. Depending on the reliability of parents and children, they eventually can be graduated to crutches without the cast.

It is difficult for children to accept the extended treatment period involved with this disorder, so be certain that both parents and children know the long-term consequences. With restriction of weight bearing now, children will develop no sequelae from the condition. If children do not meet these requirements, however, they can develop degenerative changes in a hip joint and permanent disability.

Osgood-Schlatter Disease

Osgood-Schlatter disease is thickening and enlargement of the tibial tuberosity resulting from microtrauma (Dunn, 1990) (Figure 51-14). Children notice pain and swelling over the tibia tubercle; pain is aggravated by running and squatting. This tends to occur in early adolescence or preadolescence in children who are athletic, probably because of rapid growth at these times.

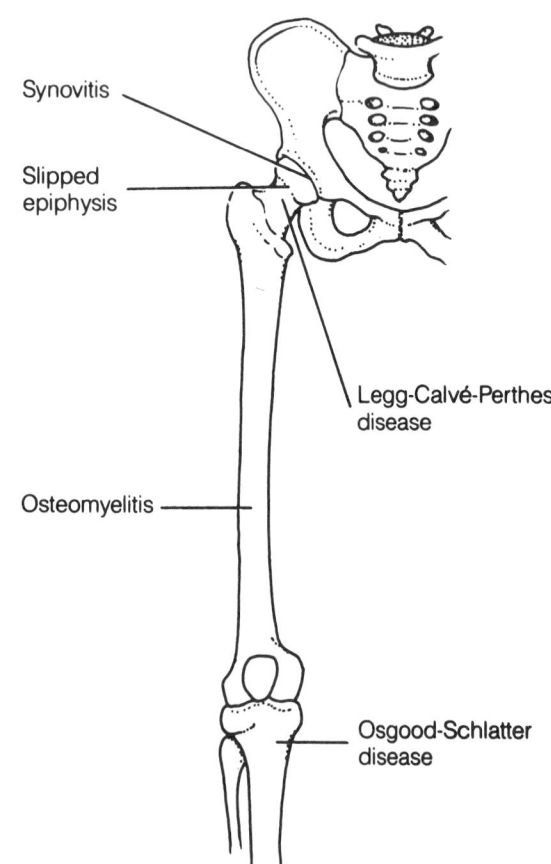

Synovitis

Slipped epiphysis

Legg-Calvé-Perthes disease

Osteomyelitis

Osgood-Schlatter disease

FIGURE 51-14
Common sites of bone disease in children.

Depending on the extent of the bone changes, therapy may require no more than limitation of strenuous physical exercise or could require immobilization of a leg in a walking cast or immobilizer for about 6 weeks.

Slipped Capital Femoral Epiphysis

Slipped epiphysis is, as the name implies, a slipping of the femur head in relation to the neck of the femur at the epiphyseal line (Morrissy & Selman, 1991) (see Figure 51-14). The cartilage covering the femur head may be destroyed by necrosis; this will result in permanent loss of motion of the femur head. An avascular necrosis similar to Legg-Calvé-Perthes disease may occur. With both complications, surgical reconstruction of the hip joint will be necessary. It occurs most frequently in preadolescence; it is twice as frequent in blacks as other races and twice as frequent in boys as in girls. It is seen more commonly in obese or rapidly growing children than others. This suggests it occurs due to the influence of growth hormone in the preadolescent.

The onset of symptoms is gradual. On inspection, you often notice children holding their leg externally rotated to relieve stress and pain in the hip joint; they may complain first of pain in their knee, because the way they are favoring their hip joint puts abnormal stress on the knee. On physical examination, internal rotation of the hip is difficult and painful. X-ray will reveal the slipped epiphysis at the femur head.

Correction is easiest if it is attempted before the condition has progressed to epiphyseal destruction, so early detection is important. Treatment is by surgical internal fixation to stabilize the femur head. Adolescence is a difficult time of life to be confined to bed following surgery. Adolescents need to be kept in touch with school friends. They need to understand that this is a potentially serious condition so that, although they may not like being confined in this way, they can accept it as necessary to maintain good healing and function of the hip joint.

Although this condition usually is unilateral, about 30% of affected children later develop the same condition in the opposite hip. All children with a slipped epiphysis, therefore, need follow-up care, with careful attention to the condition of the opposite hip (Sponseller, 1994).

Infectious and Inflammatory Disorders of the Bones and Joints

Osteomyelitis

Osteomyelitis is infection of the bone. It is most often caused by *Staphylococcus aureus* in older children and *Hemophilus influenzae* in younger children and is carried to the bone site by septicemia (blood infection). It may follow extensive impetigo, burns, or something as simple as a furuncle (skin abscess). Children with sickle cell anemia have a special susceptibility to *Salmonella* invasion in long bones (Sponseller, 1994). If strict aseptic technique is not used, it can be caused by heel punctures for blood sampling (Borris, 1992).

Osteomyelitis begins typically as a metaphysis infection because the blood supply is sluggish in that portion of the bone (see Figure 51-14). An abscess forms and spreads along the shaft of the bone under the periosteum. It may extend and penetrate to the bone marrow. Sinuses may form between the marrow and the periosteum or between the infected bone and the skin above. If the epiphyseal plate is infected, altered bone growth may result.

Assessment

Osteomyelitis generally begins with acute symptoms. Children show systemic malaise, fever, and irritability. They may have sharp pain at the bone metaphysis. By the second day, the area of skin over the infected bone will feel warm to the touch; edema will be present. Edema reduces the blood supply to vast expanses of bone, causing death of bone tissue. This dead bone tissue appears dense on x-ray; it is referred to as **sequestrum**.

Blood studies will reveal an increased white blood cell count and sedimentation rate, and the blood culture generally is positive. X-ray may not reveal bone changes (formation of sequestrum) until 5 to 10 days after the beginning of the infection. Some children with osteomyelitis are not seen at health care facilities as soon as they might be, because parents account for the pain as "growing pain." Children with systemic symptoms, such as fever, malaise, and joint pain, must be evaluated carefully so that developing osteomyelitis, if present, can be detected early.

Therapeutic Management

Medical treatment is limitation of weight bearing on the affected part and administration of an antibiotic as indicated by the blood culture. The antibiotic generally is administered intravenously for 3 to 6 weeks and orally for 2 weeks thereafter.

Nursing Diagnoses and Related Interventions

Nursing Diagnosis: Parental health-seeking behaviors related to care of the child with osteomyelitis

Goal: Parents demonstrate understanding of child's care needs by 24 hours.

Outcome Criteria: Parents accurately state child's care needs to be met both in and outside of the hospital.

When planning nursing goals for the child with osteomyelitis, be certain that the long-term immobilization necessary for care will be considered. Parents may need to make major changes in their lifestyle to remain in a hospital with a child or give care at home for such an extended length of time.

Parents have many questions when osteomyelitis is diagnosed because, at first, the defect does not show on x-ray. They are startled to hear their physician talking about 6 weeks of home care. They ask to see an x-ray to prove to themselves that a pathologic process is present. They may be suspicious of the physician's or the hospital's actions (or yours) when they are told that the x-ray does not yet show the defect, afraid that hospitalization and administration of intravenous fluid are really unnecessary.

At the point that the x-ray reveals the process, they will become more supportive and appreciative of the care that has been given their child.

Handle the extremity gently when giving care because the child has pain. Offer a diet high in calcium and protein for bone healing. If there is pus formation under the periosteum, this will be aspirated, using a technique with a needle and syringe similar to bone marrow aspiration; following this, a drainage tube to suction may be inserted to evacuate the subperiosteum area. Because such a drain evacuates infected material, institute wound precautions while it is in place.

If the child is discharged with instructions for follow-up oral antibiotic care at home, be certain that parents understand the importance of giving medication even though the child's symptoms have completely disappeared. If osteomyelitis is not entirely eradicated with the initial treatment, it will return and result in a chronic infectious process with open, draining sinuses and bone deformity in years to come. Growth plates can be destroyed, leading to shortening of an extremity.

Synovitis

Synovitis, an acute, nonpurulent inflammation of the synovial membrane of a joint, occurs most commonly in the hip joint in children (see Figure 51-14). The peak age of incidence of this condition is between 2 and 10 years. Children notice pain in their groin, the lower portion of the thigh or knee, or the buttocks. Pain is intense and most noticeable in the morning when they first awaken. Children may wake at night or in the morning, crying from the pain of turning over. Pain again becomes worse later in the day when children become tired.

Aside from the localized pain, children feel well except they generally hold the joint flexed in a position of comfort. On physical examination, range-of-motion exercises will cause pain. An x-ray may reveal capsular swelling at the involved joint.

The treatment of synovitis is bedrest until muscle spasm from pain has passed. Some children have such flexion contractures that countertraction as well as bedrest may be necessary.

In most children, 3 days of bedrest will reduce the synovitis; some children may need 10 to 14 days. Synovitis must be differentiated from septic arthritis restricted to one joint. With septic arthritis, the child tends to be systemically ill, and blood studies will reveal an increased white blood cell count.

It is important that children and parents understand that synovitis is a simple inflammation process and will heal without sequelae. Bedrest is important for this recovery, however, and so must be enforced.

Apophysitis

Adolescents who are growing rapidly are prone to apophysitis, or inflammation of the epiphysis of a heel bone. The heel feels tender, and pain on walking may be acute.

Pain generally can be relieved by adding a lift to the heel of the adolescent's shoe; this puts reduced tension on the heel cord. When pain has subsided, adolescents need to practice exercises to stretch the heel cord. This can be accomplished by having an adolescent stand on a slanting board, which elevates the foot and toes above the level of the heel, for 20 minutes about three times a day.

Apophysitis is an annoying condition, particularly for adolescents who feel a need to excel in sports to win peer approval. They need assurance that although this annoying pain may persist for months, it is not a serious disorder. It helps to put the slant board by the telephone or somewhere where they will be reminded of it daily; many adolescents are so busy they do not feel they have time for such an exercise three times a day unless they can combine it with another activity, such as talking on the telephone or watching television.

Disorders of Skeletal Structure

Scoliosis: Functional (Postural)

Scoliosis is a lateral (sideways) curvature of the spine. It may involve all or only a portion of the spinal column. It may be functional (a curve caused by a secondary problem) or structural (a primary deformity).

Functional scoliosis occurs as a compensatory mechanism in children who have unequal leg lengths and sometimes in those children with ocular refractive errors that cause them constantly to tilt their head sideways. The pelvic tilt caused by unequal leg length or the neck tilt results in a spinal deviation in order for the child to stand upright. The curve that occurs in functional scoliosis tends to be a C-shaped curve, in contrast to that in structural scoliosis, which tends to be S-shaped (composed of two separate curves). There is little change in the shape of vertebrae on x-ray with functional curves.

To rectify functional scoliosis, the difficulty causing the spinal curvature must be corrected. A lift inserted in one shoe will correct unequal leg length (leg length is measured from the anterior iliac spine to the bottom of the medial malleolus). Correcting ocular refractive errors will improve problems caused by head tilt. In addition, children must be reminded to maintain good posture during everyday activities. Walking with a book on the head for 10 minutes, three times a day, or hanging by the hands from a door frame (chinning themselves) stretches the back and is often helpful. Sit-ups and push-ups are good exercises. Swimming also is good exercise, because the reaching involved stretches the spine.

Both parents and children need to be assured that functional scoliosis is a disorder that can be corrected. Children need to be certain of this so they maintain a good body image. Caution parents about nagging children of this age to do exercises or maintain good posture. Puberty is an age of rebellion, and parents do not want children to choose this area of life as an area of rebellion. It helps with some children to be frank and spell out rules. Tell them you understand that children of their age feel they do not have to do everything their parents want them to do. Help them to find another area, such as cleaning up their rooms, in which to rebel.

Scoliosis: Structural

Structural scoliosis is idiopathic, permanent curvature of the spine; damaging vertebral changes occur (Renshaw, 1993). The spine assumes a primary lateral curvature, and to allow children to hold their head level, a compensatory second curve develops. This gives the spine an S-shaped appearance. The primary curve is often a right thoracic convexity. As the original curve becomes severe, rotation and angulation of vertebrae occur. The thoracic rib cage will rotate to become very protuberant on the convex curve. Vertebral growth may halt because of extreme pressure changes.

A family history of curvature of the spine is found in up to 70% of children with scoliosis, although no specific inheritance pattern has been documented. It is five times more common in females than males. The age of peak incidence is 8 to 15 years.

As long as children are growing, the spinal curves will become more severe. This is why the symptoms become most marked at prepuberty, a time of rapid growth.

Assessment

All children over 10 years of age should be assessed for scoliosis at all health assessment visits.

The condition develops insidiously and may be very prominent before it is noticed, because during pre-puberty and adolescence, girls usually are modest and rarely undress in front of family members. A parent might notice when doing laundry that the daughter's bra straps are adjusted to unequal lengths. The parents might notice that the girl finds it difficult to buy jeans that fit correctly because of her uneven iliac crests. They might notice that the girl's skirts or dresses hang un-evenly.

The diagnosis of structural scoliosis is made on physical examination. Spinal deformities are more obvi-ous in thin children than obese children. Thin children also are more likely than obese children to participate in sports programs where coaches or gym teachers observe them. Obese children, therefore, need careful considera-tion and inspection at health assessment.

To assess for scoliosis, observe children from a pos-terior view when they are undressed except for under-pants. Ask children to hold their arms at their sides. In-spect for unequal shoulder or hip level, prominence of one scapula, or a curved spinal column (Figure 51-15A). Compare the level of the elbows in relation to the iliac crests. In normal children, the elbow falls above the iliac crest; in children with scoliosis, it will be at the level of the crest or closer to the crest on the one side.

Ask children to bend over and touch their toes while you continue to observe their back. As they bend, the rotation of the spine accompanying scoliosis be-comes more prominent. The scapula on one side (the convex side of the curve) becomes prominent; the other side becomes hollow (Figure 51-15B). Steps in screening for scoliosis are summarized in Box 51-1.

X-rays and photographs must be taken to estimate the extent of the deformity and to serve as a baseline de-scription. Children's bone age is established by x-ray of

---

Box 51-1
Screening Procedure for Scoliosis

With the child standing straight, look at the back. Ask yourself the following:

Is one shoulder higher than the other? (The shoul-der on the convex side of a scoliotic curve will be elevated.)

Is one shoulder blade more prominent than the other? (The scapula may be high on the convex side of the curve.)

When the arms are hanging down at the sides, is the distance between one arm and body greater than on the other? Are elbows uneven?

Does one hip seem higher or more prominent than the other?

Does the child seem to lean to one side?

Does the spinal column appear curved?

With the child bending forward, look at the back. Ask yourself the following:

Is there a hump in the back in the rib area? (A hump will appear on the convex side of a scoliotic curve.)

Does the spinal column appear curved?

If the answer to any of these questions is yes, the child should be referred to a physician for further examination.

---

the wrists. If children have a vertebral rotation causing rib imbalance, lung function studies and a chest x-ray may be done to provide further baseline information. If bone growth is complete or nearly complete, little more deformity will result, and so no correction may be nec-essary. On the other hand, if children have a year or two

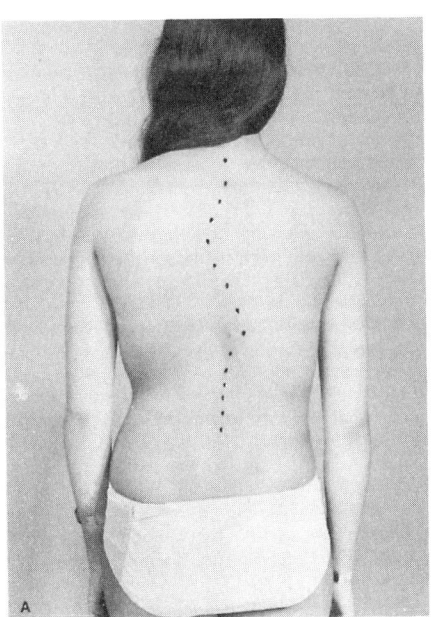
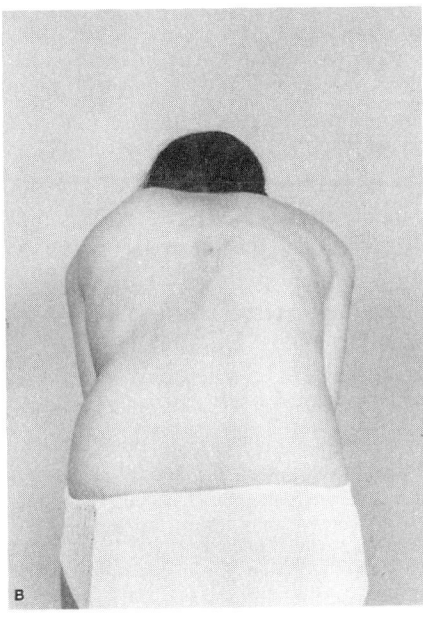

FIGURE 51-15
*Scoliosis. (**A**) Standing. (**B**) When the child with a structural scoliosis bends forward, the severe rotation of the spine is more clearly apparent. (Courtesy of the Department of Medical Photography, Children's Hospital, Buffalo, NY.)*

of bone growth still to go, some correction will surely be undertaken.

Therapeutic Management

If the spinal curve is less than 20 degrees, no therapy is usually required except for close observation until the child reaches about 18 years of age.

If the curve is greater than 20 degrees, treatment may be by a conservative, nonsurgical approach using bracing or traction, or surgery, or a combination of both. No matter what type of treatment is chosen, the child must be prepared for it to be long term. The goal of both surgery and mechanical bracing is to maintain spinal stability and prevent further progression of the deformity until bone growth is complete.

During prepuberty and adolescence, children are very concerned about body image and are very impatient with scoliosis correction. They want their problem corrected immediately. They need a great deal of support at health care visits to endure the years the correction is expected to take.

Transcutaneous electrical nerve stimulation (TENS) is a form of treatment being used experimentally. Leads are applied with a lubricant along the convexity of the spinal curve. Low pulsating current from a battery is applied for 6 to 8 hours a night while the child sleeps. This reduces muscle tension and creates less pull on the vertebrae. The effects of TENS are probably equal to bracing but need further study. Its advantage is that bracing, with its resultant problems of body image, is not necessary.

Bracing. If the curve is greater than 20 degrees but less than 40 degrees and the child is still skeletally immature, bracing may be the proposed therapy. The Milwaukee brace is the brace used most frequently to improve spine alignment (it does not correct spinal curves but does prevent them from growing greater). A Milwaukee brace is a torso brace consisting of an anterior rod, two posterior rods, leather pads, and a plastic torso piece. A ring with a padded throat mold encircles the neck (Figure 51-16). Milwaukee braces are made individually for each child according to his or her specific dimensions. Before a brace is designed, children may be hospitalized or placed on home care in supine head and pelvic traction for about 2 weeks. This brings the spine into good alignment and makes the brace more effective. To have a brace designed, children have a body cast applied from the chin to the hips. When this cast dries, it is cut and broken open to serve as the mold into which a form is poured. The brace is designed against this form in a procedure similar to the way a dressmaker's dummy is used for fitting clothes.

Children and parents need good instructions on how to apply the brace. It helps if the proper strap holes are marked with a ballpoint pen at first so that the child

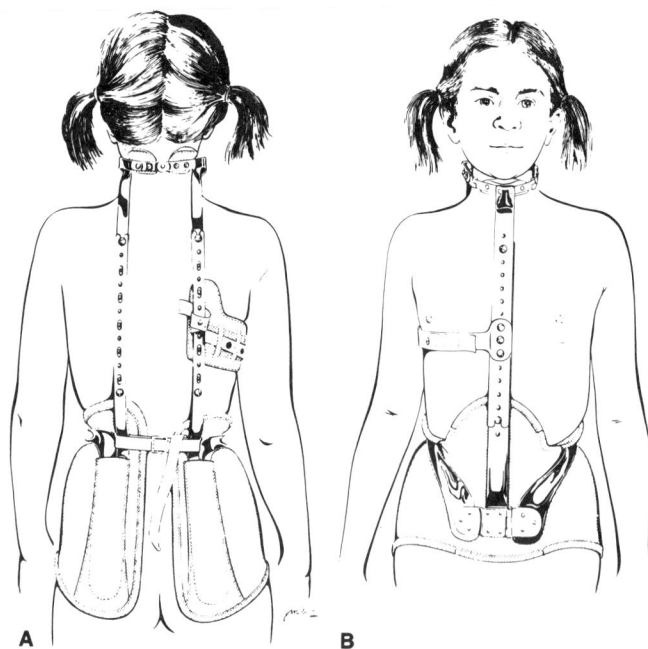

FIGURE 51-16
*A Milwaukee brace. (**A**) Posterior view. (**B**) Anterior view. (Courtesy of W. P. Blount, M.D.)*

always uses the correct holes. Children must make frequent health care visits following application of the brace to check that it fits snugly without rubbing on body prominences such as the iliac crests. Caution children that if rubbing does occur, they must be seen by the orthopedist; they should not just loosen straps to decrease the discomfort. This makes the brace fit loosely, and it will not exert adequate compression and traction this way.

During the first 2 weeks they wear the brace, children may notice slight muscle aches resulting from the new alignment. If neck and pelvic traction were applied beforehand, this aching is minimized. A mild analgesic will decrease the discomfort in most children. Rest also provides considerable relief. Children need to be cautioned not to remove the brace during this time; removing it will compound the problem of discomfort by prolonging the period of adjustment.

A Milwaukee brace must be worn constantly (23 hours a day, 7 days a week) for maximum correction. It is worn over a tee shirt to prevent the leather and plastic pads from touching skin surfaces. Leather tends to deteriorate when exposed to sweat, and skin excoriation may occur with long exposure to leather or plastic. Children can remove the brace once a day to bathe or shower. In addition, children may be able to remove it for an hour every day while they swim because this strengthens muscles. If the hour is for swimming, children must be certain to spend the hour actively swimming, not suntanning on the beach or poolside.

In addition to wearing the brace, children are taught

a series of exercises to do several times a day. To increase pelvic tilt, children should stand against a wall and push the small of their back (lumbar area) toward the wall. This swings the superior portion of the pelvis backward and the inferior portion of the pelvis forward. Children can tell they are doing this effectively if this movement brings the abdomen away from the anterior portion of the brace. They should do this exercise about three times a day and should attempt to walk in this manner at all times. For lateral strengthening, children stand straight and move their body away from the major pad of the brace. To correct thoracic lordosis, children stand as tall as they can and push back against the posterior bars of the brace with their posterior chest. This places the prominent side of the thorax against the pads, the spine rotates, and the lordotic side touches the pad also. These exercises may be taught to children before the brace is applied, but they should always be done with the brace in place after it is fitted. The brace checks the compensatory curve of the spine; without the brace in place, such exercises actually may increase the spinal deformity by increasing the extent of the minor curve.

Nursing Diagnoses and Related Interventions

> **Nursing Diagnosis:** Self-esteem disturbance related to bracing for scoliosis
>
> **Goal:** Child will demonstrate positive self-concept by 1 week.
>
> **Outcome Criteria:** Child states positive aspects of self; participates in activities; establishes friendships with peers.

It is easier for children to accept Milwaukee braces today than it once was because the braces are made more compact, and because teenage clothing tends to be more casual and looser than ever before. Even though choosing clothes is easier than it once was, it may still be a major problem for some children. They need time at health care visits to voice concerns about their appearance. Sweat shirts are loose and come with colorful pictures and slogans to wear over braces. Encourage children to voice what it feels like to have to wear a brace of this size constantly. Help them to concentrate not on those things they cannot do because of the brace (play basketball, make the track team) but on those that they can do (have friends over for a party, join the drama club—why can't Juliet wear a loose-fitting gown this season?—or be a cheerleader who doesn't help build pyramids).

Encourage children in Milwaukee braces to be as active as possible. They may comment at first that they feel awkward or "so much taller" that they are afraid that they will fall. The only way to get comfortable with this feeling is to walk and get used to the new sensation of

actually being a little taller. Braces may be awkward at school if chairs are attached to desks; advocate for the child with the school nurse for seating arrangements that are comfortable.

Friends are going to ask questions about what has happened to a child. The sooner children expose themselves wearing a brace to friends and family, the sooner these beginning questions will be out of the way. The brace is adjusted about every 3 months to accomplish more alignment. Children may need more frequent visits than this, however, to be able to express the problems they are having with social and school adjustment. Again and again, children may need to be reminded that people who really care about other people can see through such things as Milwaukee braces and look at the person inside. On the other hand, do not underestimate an adolescent's ability to adjust to new situations. Children can see by looking in a mirror that their spine is curved. They want this corrected. They will endure a great deal of discomfort if they have hope that they will emerge at the end of the correction period without an obvious physical deformity (see the Focus on Cultural Awareness box).

Parents must be firm about insisting that the child wear the brace continuously. When parents begin allowing the child to take it off once a week for a special occasion, there soon may be two or three and then six or eight such occasions weekly and the benefits from wearing the brace will be reduced. If bracing does not work, children must have spinal alignment and fusion surgery. Be certain that children do not think spinal surgery is a simple, quick procedure, similar to an appendectomy, and therefore preferable to bracing. If children think this, they may avoid wearing the brace, hoping that surgery will then be prescribed. (On the other hand, do

FOCUS ON CULTURAL AWARENESS

The way that parents or a child react to the diagnosis of a musculoskeletal disorder can be culturally influenced. In a culture in which athletic prowess is paramount, for example, a disorder such as muscular dystrophy might be viewed as more severe than it would be in a culture in which mental prowess is more respected. In a culture in which beauty and looking similar to others are important values, being asked to wear a Milwaukee or halo brace would be very hard to accept. Because an adolescent culture is often one that respects athletics, beauty, and conformity, adolescence may be a very difficult time for a child to maintain body image and self-esteem when a musculoskeletal disorder is present.

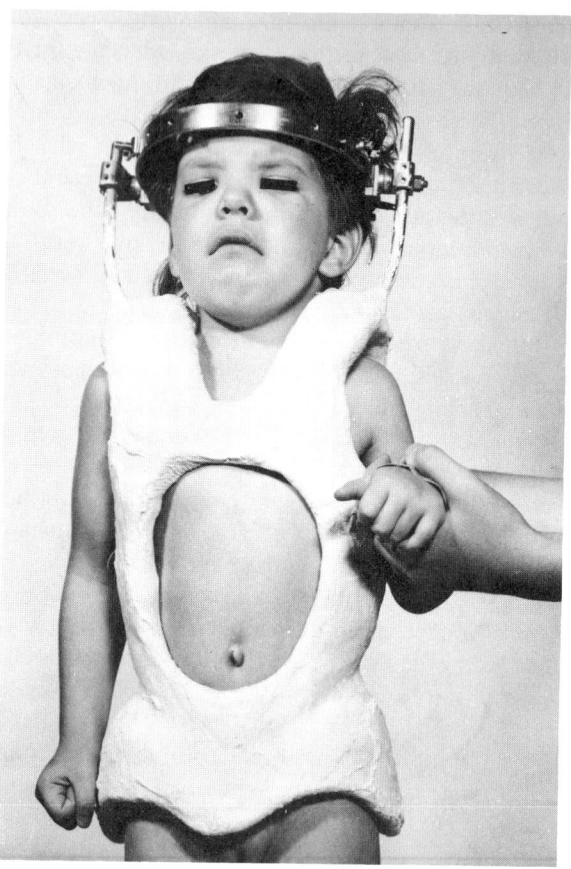

FIGURE 51-17
Halo traction applied to a body cast. Although this appears top-heavy, the child can ambulate with the traction in place. (Courtesy of J. H. Moe, M.D.)

looks frightening. Children have some real fear that when the pins are inserted into their skull (done under general anesthesia), the pins will slip and penetrate their brain. They may worry that the apparatus will be so heavy that it will strain or break their neck.

Halo traction is generally used when children have respiratory involvement, cervical instability, a high thoracic deformity, or decreased vital capacity from severe spinal curvature and rotation. Children need to see photographs of the apparatus or talk to children who have the apparatus in place before having it applied. They need time to express their feelings about being placed in such a cumbersome device. Children may react to the apparatus with nausea, diarrhea, or chronic sadness until they see that they can adjust to it. Orientation must be as thorough for the parents as it is for the child. Parents may show symptoms of nausea like the child's for the first few days after the application of such traction. They are generally too unsure of themselves to care for a child during the first week, so they need support to parent during this time.

When caring for the child, careful explanations about what you will do before you begin care help reduce anxiety. Stressing positive aspects, such as what the child can do, not what he or she cannot do, and that the traction will help the spinal curvature may encourage children to begin to accept such extreme traction (see the Focus on Nursing Research display).

not oversell the horrible aspects of surgery; in some children, the scoliosis continues to worsen despite good bracing, and surgery will be necessary.)

A Milwaukee brace that is effective will be worn until the child's spinal growth stops (about 14½ years in girls, 16½ years in boys). This point can be demonstrated by spinal x-ray. Bracing is not discontinued abruptly, but when this point is reached, children are weaned from it gradually. They may wear the brace at night for a prolonged period (1 to 2 years). Children are weaned gradually from the brace because some demineralization of vertebrae may have occurred during the long period of bracing. Gradual resumption of activity allows remineralization and continued spinal support.

Halo Traction. Traction is the use of opposing forces to straighten and reduce spinal curves. Halo traction is achieved using a ring of metal (a halo) held in place by about four stainless steel pins inserted into the skull bones. Counteraction is applied by pins inserted into the distal femurs or iliac crests (Figure 51-17).

A halo traction apparatus is a bulky apparatus that

**FOCUS ON
NURSING RESEARCH**

*How Do Children in Halo Braces
Maintain Their Self-Concept?*

For this study, 38 young adults (17 females and 21 males) who had worn a halo brace at some time during the previous 8 years answered a questionnaire as to their feelings on body image and self-concept. Seventy-nine percent of subjects reported that the halo brace affected how they felt about themselves. Common words used to describe their feelings were fear, anger, guilt, embarrassment, and depression.

The researchers suggest that nurses can be most helpful to patients in halo braces by actions such as inspiring hope and trust, promoting self-care and enhancing knowledge, displaying nonverbal reassurance, encouraging healthy support systems, providing encouragement and positive feedback, and promoting laughter and humor.

Olson, B., Ustanko, L., & Warner, S. (1991). The patient in a halo brace: Striving for normalcy in body image and self-concept. *Orthopaedic Nursing, 10,* 44.

For application of the apparatus, the area of the skull where pins will be placed is shaved and prepared with an antiseptic. The actual application takes only about 30 minutes. For the first 24 hours afterward, children generally experience pain at the pin insertion sites; generalized headache may occur, requiring analgesia. Accepting halo traction is difficult enough, even without this pain. Offer adequate analgesia for comfort.

Children in halo traction need frequent shampoos to keep the pin sites clean. Crusting around the pin sites can be reduced by washing around the pins daily with half-strength hydrogen peroxide or other appropriate solution. Children should be encouraged to be as self-sufficient as possible (Olson & Ustanko, 1990). Be certain that parents or children have a telephone number they can call for help or questions as to what activity will be safe after the child returns home.

When optimal spinal correction has been achieved, halo traction equipment is removed easily. The pin sites in the skull heal within a week without obvious scarring.

Surgical Intervention: Spinal Instrumentation.

Surgical correction is generally necessary when the degree of curvature is greater than 40 degrees. Stainless steel rods are placed next to the spinal column to provide firm reduction of the curvature; the spine is then fused in the corrected position. Bone from the iliac crests may be used to strengthen the fusion procedure.

Preoperative Nursing Care. To place such rods, a posterior surgical approach is used. Extensive x-rays will be taken to plan the exact location of the rods. Introduce children to deep-breathing exercises, incentive spirometry, or intermittent positive-pressure breathing treatments before surgery if these will be used to increase lung function postoperatively. Deep-breathing exercises are particularly important in children whose scoliosis has caused chronically reduced lung capacity.

Children need a good explanation of what they can expect after surgery. This surgery involves bone destruction, so they can expect to have pain. It is a major operation, so they can expect to feel tired and "not themselves" for a number of days. Teaching children of this age about these events helps them to accept them in the postoperative period. They appreciate being treated like adults. Be aware, however, that an early adolescent is not an adult, and although they seem eager to breathe deeply and cooperate with routines before surgery, these requests may be pretty overwhelming for them postoperatively, and their behavior may not be nearly as adult as they anticipate. Allowing children to use a patient-controlled analgesia system offers both pain relief and a feeling of control.

The type of rods used depends on the degree of spinal curvature and the age of the child. Harrington rods were the first such rods manufactured, so the surgery is frequently referred to as Harrington rod place-

ment even though newer types of rods are now more commonly used. Luque rods and Wisconsin segmental spinal instrumentation are types that use a segmental approach. Cotrel-Dubousset rods are the type most often used today (Drummond, 1991; Dubousset & Cotrel, 1991). These are attached to the vertebrae using hooks or screws (Figure 51-18).

Postoperative Care. Following surgery, the child's bed must not be gatched, because once rods are in place and the spinal fusion has been done, the back must not be bent. Tape the gatch of the bed in place or unplug electric controls so that the bed cannot be raised by accident by a parent or by uninformed auxiliary personnel. In some instances, a child may be cared for postoperatively on a Stryker frame. If this will be so, introduce a frame preoperatively. A nasogastric tube generally is inserted prior to surgery to prevent abdominal distention; major surgery may cause paralytic ileus and lack of bowel tone.

When the child returns from surgery, he or she must lie flat and must be log-rolled (always by two people) to a side-lying position every 2 hours to enhance respiratory status unless segmented rods were used (Figure 51-18B). Appropriate checks of lower-extremity neurologic function must be made every hour for the first 24 hours. Feel the lower extremities for warmth. Ask the child if he or she can feel you touch a foot. Ask the child to wiggle his or her toes. Neurologic dysfunction may result from bleeding or compression caused by a bone particle dislodged during the spinal fusion. Vital signs must be recorded carefully; there is extensive blood loss during spinal fusion surgery. A Hemovac drainage system is usually inserted next to the incision to evacuate any accumulating drainage (Figure 51-18C). The procedure itself or the blood loss may cause shock. Circulatory pressure changes resulting from realignment of the chest cage and reduced rotation of the spine may result in circulatory impairment.

The child is kept NPO until bowel sounds indicate that paralytic ileus is not present. A Foley catheter is generally in place because voiding may be difficult due to the horizontal position that must be maintained and the edema at the lower spinal cord innervation points.

Even though the parents have been prepared for the fact that spinal fusion is major surgery, they may be shocked by the child's appearance after surgery. They are afraid to touch the child to comfort her. They may not be aware that although their child may be 14 or 15 years old, she would probably enjoy being touched now because she feels so ill and frightened by the thought of the stainless steel rods in her back.

Gradually, pain is reduced; the child can take fluids, then solids. Because of the need to maintain a dependent position following surgery, there may be a rapid release of calcium from bones. Calcium intake should, therefore, be moderate at first rather than extensive to prevent renal calculi.

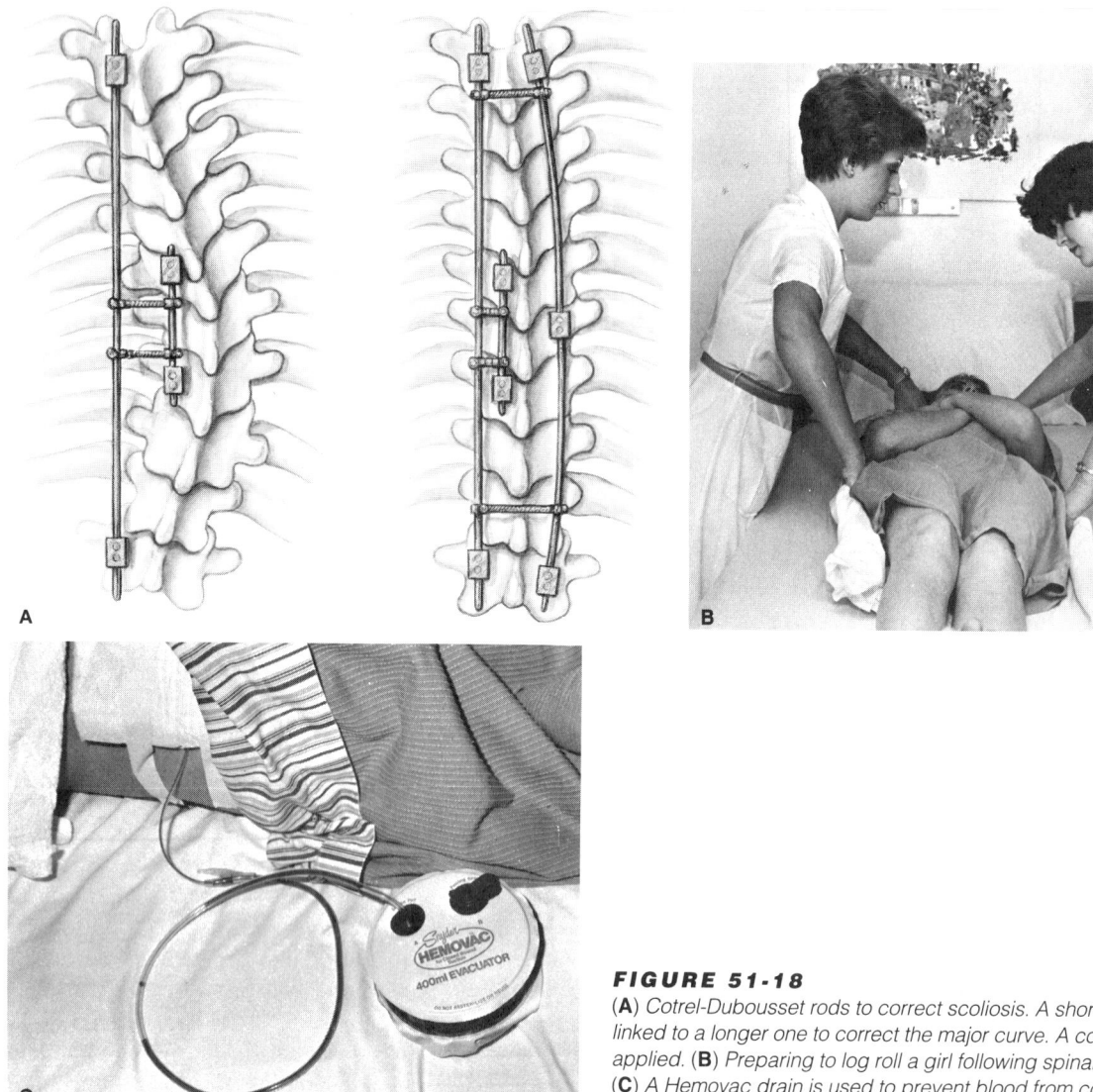

FIGURE 51-18
(**A**) *Cotrel-Dubousset rods to correct scoliosis. A short distraction rod is linked to a longer one to correct the major curve. A convex rod is then applied.* (**B**) *Preparing to log roll a girl following spinal rod insertion.* (**C**) *A Hemovac drain is used to prevent blood from collecting at the incision site.*

After 2 or 4 days, the child is allowed out of bed to sit up. He or she may feel very dizzy at first and must get used to sitting by attempting it for short periods at a time. Some children will have a body cast applied before hospital discharge to help ensure spinal fusion. Activity will be allowed gradually.

Instrumentation rods are left in place permanently unless they cause irritation later. Removing the rods is as extensive a procedure as inserting them. The average child will never be aware that they are in place. They must always be conscious of good posture, however (slumping in chairs is not allowed; they must stoop, not bend, to pick up objects from the floor). Extremely active gymnastics or trampoline work are contraindicated. The rods do not interfere with other sports or childbearing in girls.

Children may be afraid to move or behave normally following spinal fusion, because they have been in some type of restraining device for such a long time. They need time to readjust to the freedom of normal body movement. They may need to be assured again and again that, with the spinal fusion, their problem finally is corrected. No further curvature can occur after this point, so it is safe for them to be without support.

Correction of scoliosis may have taken years. Following surgery, children need an opportunity to talk at health care assessments about how they feel to be free of this problem. If the correction was not as complete as the child wished (children with severe scoliosis cannot expect 100% correction), they need time to talk about their disappointment and to adjust to their new appearance. They may feel that they have missed adolescence or "the best time of their lives." They may need assurance that true friends are more interested in what type of person they are inside than they are in their physical appearance and that many positive experiences in life are yet to come.

Disorders of the Joints and Tendons: Collagen-Vascular Disease

Collagen is protein composed of bundles of fibers forming the connective tissue of the tendons, ligaments, and bones. Because this tissue is found throughout the body, collagen diseases are systemic; they also tend to be long term.

Juvenile Rheumatoid Arthritis (JRA)

JRA primarily involves the joints of the body, although it also affects blood vessels and other connective tissue. To be classified as JRA, symptoms must begin before 16 years of age and last longer than 3 months. The peak incidence occurs at two times in childhood: 1 to 3 years and 8 to 12 years. The cause of JRA is unknown, although it is probably an autoimmune process or the child has developed circulating antibodies (immunoglobulins) against his or her own body cells. This is revealed by an antinuclear antibody level. T lymphocytes may also be involved in the process or change to attack and destroy body cells, or ineffective lymphocytic-inhibition cells are unable to halt lymphocyte production. A genetic predisposition may make it apt to happen in some people more than others. JRA can occur in children as young as 6 months of age. It is slightly more common in girls than boys. Acute changes rarely continue past 19 years.

Three separate types of JRA exist. Major distinctions of these types are outlined in Table 51-2. Types differ mainly by the type of joint affected and the severity of systemic effects.

Polyarticular Juvenile Rheumatoid Arthritis

Polyarticular JRA may develop at any age. It affects multiple joints, including small joints such as fingers and toes. The beginning symptoms are stiffness and minimal swelling in joints leading to limitation of motion caused by synovial thickening of joints (Figure 51-19). Few systemic effects are present, although fatigue, malaise, anorexia, and poor weight gain may be noticed.

Polyarticular JRA can be differentiated from other types in that a rheumatoid factor (actually IgM antibodies) is present in as many as 20% of children. This tends to be a more reliable finding in female adolescents; it may be negative in males between 5 and 10 years of age. The prognosis for the disease is worse in those with the factor. Antinuclear antibodies (antibody formation against cell nuclei) may be present. Total white blood cell count, complement, and sedimentation rate may be elevated.

Monarticular or Pauciarticular Juvenile Rheumatoid Arthritis

Monarticular (one joint) or pauciarticular (few joints) JRA is the most common form of JRA. This form involves one to four major joints such as knees, ankles, and elbows; small joints are rarely involved. Joints swell painlessly; there is little redness present, although joints may feel warm. Few systemic symptoms, such as increased temperature and anemia, are present, although a child may be irritable, fatigue easily, and have a diminished appetite. A child typically wakes in the morning with stiffness in a knee and refuses to bear weight on the leg.

Table 51-2. *Characteristics of Different Types of Juvenile Rheumatoid Arthritis*

Characteristic	Polyarthritis	Pauciarticular	Systemic
Frequency of occurrence	40–50%	40–50%	10–20%
Number of joints involved	5 or more	4 or less	Variable
Sex ratio (F:M)	3:1	5:1	1:1
Systemic involvement	Moderate	Not present	Prominent
Uveitis	5%	20%	Rare
Seropositivity			
Rheumatoid factors	10%	Rare	Rare
Antinuclear antibodies	40–50%	75–85%	10%
Course	Systemic disease is generally mild; articular involvement may be unremitting	Systemic disease is absent; major cause of morbidity is uveitis	Systemic disease is often self-limited; arthritis is chronic and destructive in 50%
Prognosis	Guarded to moderately good	Excellent except for eyesight	Moderate to poor

(From Cassidy, J. T. [1994]. Connective tissue diseases and amyloidosis. In Oski, F. A. et al. [Eds.]. *Principles and practice of pediatrics* [2nd ed.]. Philadelphia, J. B. Lippincott; with permission.)

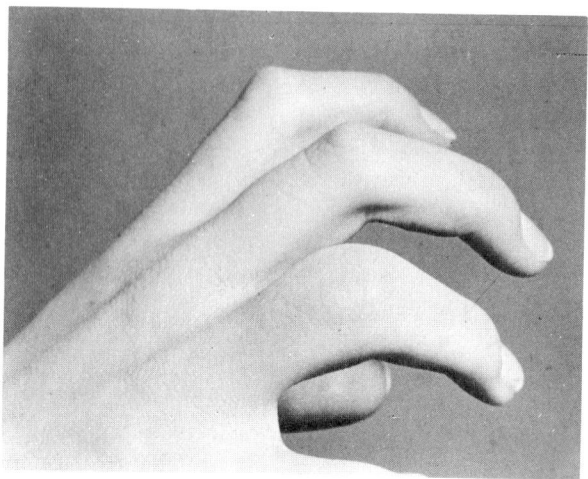

FIGURE 51-19

Fingers of a child with juvenile rheumatoid arthritis. Note the peculiar spindle shape. (Courtesy of the Department of Medical Photography, Children's Hospital, Buffalo, NY.)

As the day progresses, the knee appears to have less joint discomfort. About 30% of females under 3 years of age who have a positive antinuclear antibody titer develop uveitis (inflammation of the iris). This can be extensive before signs such as redness or eye pain are present. To detect this, a slit-lamp examination should be routine in children with pauciarticular JRA every 3 months until 19 years of age.

Boys with pauciarticular JRA appear to have a greater incidence of a human leukocyte antigen (HLA-B27) than would normally occur. These children have a high incidence of developing involvement of the sacroiliac joint. This leads in later life to ankylosing spondylosis (immobility of the joint). Those who are prepubertal with a negative rheumatoid factor and negative antinuclear antibody titer may develop swelling only in the joints of the lower extremities.

If children have only one joint affected, they may have the joint aspirated and any fluid in the joint cultured to rule out septic (infectious) arthritis. A white blood cell count and differential are obtained as these also offer information as to whether an infectious process is present (white blood cell count would be elevated with septic arthritis and normal with monoarticular JRA).

Systemic Juvenile Rheumatoid Arthritis

One third of all children with JRA develop a systemic form. It occurs equally in boys and girls. The rheumatoid factor or antinuclear antibody is rarely present. All children develop a high fever (spiking fevers to 103°F twice daily) for at least 3 to 4 weeks at the beginning of the disease. There is multiple joint swelling; in addition, children may have a pale, red, macular rash on the trunk and extremities, enlarged lymph nodes, an elevated white blood cell count, enlarged liver or spleen, and

fluid-filled joints. Children are irritable during the periods of high fever and may have accompanying malaise, increased fatigability, pleuritis, enlarged spleen and liver, pericarditis, and profound anemia. Any of the systemic symptoms may be present for as long as 3 months before joint involvement occurs. Uveitis does not occur. The joint involvement may fade after 2 or 3 years or may continue to become destructive synovitis with limitation of motion requiring total joint replacement in later years (Cassidy, 1994).

Assessment

Children with systemic JRA are often admitted to a hospital unit for diagnosis of their persistent fever and rash as these may be present before joint involvement is present. When arthritis is diagnosed, parents may be surprised, believing that arthritis is a disease of only older adults. Assess children not only for signs and symptoms of the disease but for the effect their disease is having on self-care (do they need help eating? dressing? ambulating? toileting?). Assess also the child and parents' understanding of the illness and planned therapy. Children do not remain for long periods in health care facilities. Children and parents will have to be responsible for carrying out therapy at home.

Therapeutic Management

JRA is a long-term illness. Therapy includes a balanced program of exercise, rest, and medication administration.

Exercise. With synovitis, children develop limitation of motion and muscle atrophy near joints. To preserve muscle and joint function, a set program of physical activities to strengthen muscles and put joints through a full range of motion should be instituted. To reduce joint destruction, however, activities that place excessive strain on joints should be avoided. Running, jumping, prolonged walking, and kicking should be avoided if active lower extremity synovitis is present. School-age children can cooperate to avoid these activities. Parents of preschool children will need to create alternative activities that are so interesting the child avoids these motions.

Extremes of immobilization should also be avoided. To prevent this, children need to perform full range-of-motion exercises twice every day. It is best if these exercises can be incorporated into a dance routine or a game such as "Simon says" with a parent. This will make the exercise a family participation time to be anticipated rather than a dull routine that must be done. Swimming and tricycle or bicycle riding are excellent activities to encourage as these provide smooth joint action.

Encourage children to do as much self-care as they are capable of because the natural motions of dressing, brushing teeth, and so forth exercise joints.

Children should attend school if possible. Active children tend to show fewer contractures and less decalcification of bones than do inactive children. Children with JRA fatigue easily, however, so they may need to have a school day shortened to reduce fatigue. If a school day is to be shortened, it is often better if the starting time is moved to midmorning. This allows the child time for a warm bath in the morning before school, which reduces the pain and increases movement of involved joints. An activity such as sitting on a toilet may be uncomfortable if hip and knee joints are painful (elevating the seat may be helpful in that it reduces bending); children may be unable to dress themselves independently as they cannot manage buttons or zippers with painful finger joints. Modifying these activities not only helps children feel good about themselves but increases their overall level of activity.

Acutely inflamed joints should be rested both passively and actively during the period of acute inflammation. To maintain muscle strength during this time, children may do isometric exercises (exercises that do not change the length of muscles), but not active exercises. Support inflamed joints in good body alignment. This may be achieved with large joints by positioning pillows for support. To further prevent contractures, encourage children to sleep prone rather than curled into a ball.

Heat Application. Heat acts to reduce pain and inflammation in joints and therefore increases comfort and motion. Heat can be applied by the use of warm water soaks for 20 to 30 minutes. Scheduling a hot bath on arising can help to eliminate stiff joints and make a child feel well enough to begin to function for the morning. Paraffin soaks can be useful for wrist and finger inflammation.

Splinting. Splinting is used to immobilize a joint in good body alignment (Figure 51-20). These are worn continuously during periods of active inflammation, even during sleep. If splints are removed, joints tend to assume a flexed, more comfortable position, and contracture may occur in this position. Splints should not be worn past a period of inflammation because the splint can actually cause a contracture and deformity with extended use.

Nutrition. Children with JRA, as with almost all chronic diseases, eat poorly because of anorexia, joint

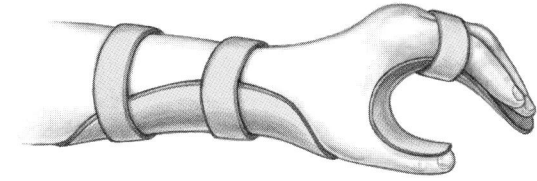

FIGURE 51-20
A full-hand resting splint used for juvenile rheumatoid arthritis.

pain, and fatigue. Help parents plan mealtimes for "best times" of the day to try and overcome these problems.

Medication. The drug of choice for children with JRA is aspirin because it is both analgesic and antiinflammatory. This is given in a usual dose of 80 mg/kg/day in four divided doses. Educate parents that aspirin should not be given on an empty stomach because it tends to cause gastrointestinal bleeding (have the child drink a glass of milk first). Most parents think of aspirin as a drug to give children only when they have pain. Teach that they should continue to give it even if the child has no noticeable pain at the time of administration as its antiinflammatory action is important in preventing pain. There is currently a great deal of discussion on the safety of giving aspirin to children because this has been associated with the development of Reye's syndrome. Teach that although normally children should receive acetaminophen (Tylenol) for fevers, the child with JRA needs aspirin because of the antiinflammatory effect. Aspirin administration is usually continued for 6 months beyond any signs of inflammation.

Nonsteroidal antiinflammatory drugs (NSAIDS) may be used as well with children. Those approved for use in children include tolmetin sodium, naproxen, and indomethacin. NSAIDs reduce joint swelling, joint discomfort, and morning stiffness. They may contribute to improvement in malaise and irritability.

Steroids may be added to the drug therapy, although they are avoided if at all possible. Prednisone is not continued for a long time because it can lead to gastrointestinal bleeding and devascularization with aseptic necrosis of joints and growth retardation. Children who do not have improvement on aspirin and a NSAID are candidates for gold therapy. Intramuscular gold injections may shorten the duration of the disease and reduce joint involvement but not the systemic symptoms. This is used with children who are becoming prednisone dependent or who cannot take aspirin. Therapy with an immunosuppressant such as methotrexate may be instituted (Fife, 1993).

Nursing Diagnoses and Related Interventions

Nursing Diagnosis: Knowledge deficit related to care necessary to control disease symptoms

Goal: Parents and child will demonstrate increased knowledge of care regimen by 1 week.

Outcome Criteria: Parents and child follow instructions regarding exercise and medication.

Both parents and children need to know about the necessity for them to take an active role in therapy. Help them schedule exercise and medication programs around school and other activities; help them make out reminder sheets as necessary so therapy periods are not forgotten.

Be certain that goals established are realistic. Children with JRA are irritable and fatigue easily. They may not be able to achieve the goals that you would like to establish for them because of this.

Children with JRA need ongoing evaluation to be certain that they continue to view themselves as well again following such a long period of pain and illness. Children who are left with joint contractures may have soft-tissue surgery, such as contracture release, tendon reconstruction, and synovectomy, or orthopedic surgery, such as equalization of leg length and orthoplasty, done at a later date. Surgery may be delayed until growth is complete so further growth will not influence the outcome.

About half of children with JRA will recover without joint deformity. One third will continue to have the disease into adulthood. About one sixth will be left after several years with severe, crippling deformities. Children need a great deal of support to perform exercises, wear splints, and take daily medication as prescribed. They need time set aside at health care visits to talk about how it feels to discover that the joints of the hands are gradually becoming more and more useless. Provide hope for recovery; children may not be able to follow a regimen of therapy if they see nothing ahead except complete disability.

Disorders of the Skeletal Muscles

Myasthenia Gravis

For nerve conduction to cause muscles to contract effectively, a neurotransmitter, acetylcholine, must be released at synaptic junctions. Myasthenia gravis is an interference in this process, leading to symptoms of progressive muscle weakness. The fault may be the impaired synthesis or storage of acetylcholine, insufficient acetylcholine release, blockage of acetylcholine factor present at motor end plates, or opposition of acetylcholine by an antiacetylcholine factor. The defect is probably a motor end plate insufficiency (a decreased number of acetylcholine receptors present). This probably occurs from an autoimmune process (autoantibodies may block receptor sites for acetylcholine) (Parke, 1994). There is some evidence that a tendency for the condition may be inherited; the thymus gland is usually enlarged in persons with the condition, suggesting that thymopoietin may be overproduced, leading to neuromuscular block.

Assessment

If a mother has myasthenia gravis, an infant may evidence transient disease symptoms at birth from transfer of antibodies (Tzartos et al., 1990). The newborn is "floppy," sucks poorly, and has weak respiratory effort. Ptosis (drooping eyelids) may be present. The symptoms disappear within 2 to 4 weeks, but if not recognized when they occur, they may prove fatal because of respiratory difficulty.

If myasthenia gravis does not occur in the newborn period, the onset generally is delayed until the child is about 10 years old. The condition occurs more frequently in girls than boys (about 5:1). The child begins to notice symptoms of blurred or double vision (diplopia). Ptosis is present because of weakness of the extraocular muscles. Symptoms grow more intense as facial, neck, jaw, swallowing, and intercostal muscles become affected. There is extreme fatigue, becoming more noticeable as the day progresses. Symptoms are increased with emotional stress, fatigue, menstruation, respiratory infections, and alcoholic intake. In the most severe form, all muscles, including those of respiration, become paralyzed.

Obtaining an accurate history is important in diagnosis. On physical examination, children are asked to perform repetitive movements. If you ask a child to look upward and hold that position, he or she will gradually demonstrate ptosis. Most children will have myography performed to document the poor muscle function. Chest x-ray and a computed tomography scan are done to demonstrate an enlarged thymus gland. Administration of Tensilon (edrophonium), which prolongs the action of acetylcholine and therefore increases muscle strength, causes renewal of exhausted muscles in a few minutes. If this occurs, the diagnosis is positive for myasthenia gravis.

Therapeutic Management

Myasthenia gravis is treated by the administration of anticholinesterase drugs such as neostigmine (Prostigmin), which prolong acetylcholine action. The dose of these agents must be individually determined. Assess for side effects such as bradycardia, increased peristalsis, abdominal cramping, sweating, and miotic pupils (parasympathetic nerve action) with these drugs. If a toxic effect of these drugs occurs, it is similar to the symptoms of the original disease. Atropine is the antidote for an overdose of anticholinesterase drugs and should be available when dosage is first being determined. In some children, prednisone may be added to their medication regimen to decrease the amount of anticholinesterase medication required. In some children, plasmapheresis to remove immune complexes from the bloodstream is effective in reducing symptoms. Excision of the thymus gland is rarely performed under 12 years of age because there is an increased risk of children developing neoplastic growths without a thymus gland.

Teach both parents and children that symptoms become worse under stress. Parents will need to prepare children well for new experiences (menstruation, high school, a parental divorce, surgery) to keep this to a minimum. Help children plan their day to include rest periods (you may have to advocate for a special school schedule that allows for this). If chewing and swallowing are difficult, a rest period should proceed meals. Children may need to eat a soft diet and to learn to eat slowly and cautiously to avoid choking and aspiration. Scheduling medication administration for about an hour before mealtime is often helpful. If symptoms of muscle weakness suddenly become very severe, children should be seen at a health care facility, because paralysis of intercostal muscles may lead to respiratory arrest.

Dermatomyositis

Dermatomyositis involves degeneration of skeletal muscle fibers. The cause of the disorder is unknown. Symptoms generally begin insidiously with muscle weakness. Children are unable to perform tasks that they could manage previously, such as competing in gym classes, lifting objects, or climbing onto a high stool. Skin symptoms are present (swollen upper eyelids, a confluent rash on the cheeks that increases to become telangiectatic and scaling). Subcutaneous calcifications may appear, making the skin feel unusually firm. Muscle breakdown causes creatinine to appear in the urine. A muscle biopsy will reveal lack of electrical activity in muscle fibers.

Corticosteroids improve muscle strength; immune globulins may also be helpful. Children who survive beyond the first year after diagnosis have a good prognosis for prolonged remissions. Unfortunately, many adults with dermatomyositis develop neoplastic complications.

Muscular Dystrophy

Muscular dystrophy is progressive degeneration of skeletal muscles from an as yet unknown biochemical defect within the muscle. It is not a single disorder but a group of disorders that leads to gradual degeneration of muscle fibers. All the disorders are inherited (Griggs et al., 1990).

Congenital Muscular Dystrophy

Congenital muscular dystrophy is inherited as an autosomal recessive trait. The disease process begins in utero. The infant may be born with severe myotonia; muscle degeneration may make respiratory muscle movement difficult. Diagnosis is by serum enzyme analysis and muscle biopsy. Most of these infants die before they are 1 year old because they cannot sustain respiratory function.

Facioscapulohumeral Muscular Dystrophy

Facioscapulohumeral muscular dystrophy is inherited as a dominant trait, carried on the number 4 chromosome (Wijmenga et al., 1990). Symptoms begin after the age of 10. The predominant symptom is facial weakness. The child is unable to wrinkle his or her forehead and cannot whistle. Serum enzyme analysis and muscle biopsy are used in diagnosis. The symptoms generally progress so slowly that a normal life span is possible.

Pseudohypertrophic Muscular Dystrophy (Duchenne's Disease)

Duchenne's disease, the most common form of muscular dystrophy, is inherited as a sex-linked recessive trait; it occurs, therefore, only in boys.

Assessment. Children generally have a history of meeting motor milestones, such as sitting, walking, and standing, later than the average infant. At about 3 years of age symptoms become acute and obvious. It is difficult to lift the young child with this condition by placing your hands under the axillae. The child seems to slip through your hands because of the lax shoulder muscles. In contrast, calf muscles are hypertrophied (measure larger than normal) because the muscles become so degenerated they are replaced by fat and connective tissue.

Children have a waddling gait and have difficulty climbing stairs. They can rise from the floor only by rolling onto their stomachs, then pushing themselves to their knees. To stand, they press their hands against their ankles, knees, and thighs (they "walk up their front"); this is Gower's sign. They may walk on their toes and therefore develop a short heel cord. Speech and swallowing become difficult. Many boys with this type of muscular dystrophy show delays in meeting developmental milestones (Smith et al., 1990).

As the disease progresses, the muscle weakness becomes more and more pronounced. Scoliosis of the spine and fractures of long bones may occur from abnormal muscle tension and lack of muscle support. By junior high school age, most boys are confined to a wheelchair, unable to walk independently. Tachycardia occurs as heart muscle weakens and enlarges. Pneumonia develops easily as the child's cough reflex becomes weak and ineffective. Death from congestive heart failure occurs at about age 20.

The diagnosis is based on the history and physical findings, on muscle biopsy showing fibrous degeneration and fatty deposits, and on an elevated level of serum creatine phosphokinase.

Therapeutic Management. Boys with muscular dystrophy should be encouraged to remain ambulatory as long as possible. Help the child plan a program of both active and passive range of motion exercises to do daily; help make reminder sheets so exercises are done daily. Splinting and bracing may be necessary to maintain lower extremity stability and avoid contractures. If children become overweight, remaining ambulatory becomes more difficult for them. Encourage a low-calorie, high-protein diet to avoid this. To prevent constipation, encourage a high-fiber and high-fluid diet; advocate for a stool softener prescription if necessary.

Be certain when establishing goals that they are realistic. The disease is progressive, so any goal that aims at total wellness again cannot be achieved. Help children and parents locate a parent support group. The Muscular Dystrophy Association can be helpful in supplying information on the disease and support through the long period of illness.

Injuries of the Extremities

Finger Injuries

Few children make it through childhood without one finger injury from a slammed car door. This injury causes a crushing blow to the tip of the finger and is excruciatingly painful. The fingernail may be lacerated and detached. Blood accumulates under an attached fingernail and continues to be very painful. Pain is relieved by an incision under the distal end of the nail or a stab wound through the attached nail. Fingernails often are lost following these injuries, but they grow back readily with little scarring. Parents should understand that although fingernails may be lost, the cosmetic effect will invariably not be a problem.

Parents are embarrassed and feel guilty when they bring in a child for this type of injury. The accident is usually their fault, because they closed a door without looking for the child's finger. They appreciate how much this hurts and are angry with themselves for being so careless. Parents can be assured that this is a common childhood injury; there is hardly a parent who has not done this once.

The fingertip will be x-rayed to make certain that the tip of the distal phalanx is not broken. The rule "If the child can bend it, it's not broken," does not apply to this injury, because the fracture is often distal to the last phalangeal joint. Any open wound should be cleaned well. A splint should be applied to the finger if the distal phalanx is fractured. The child needs a follow-up visit to make certain that healing has taken place.

Bicycle-Spoke Injuries

Children who ride in infant seats or over the back wheel of a bicycle can catch a foot or ankle between the spoke and the frame of the bicycle. This causes a crushing, lacerating injury that quickly becomes edematous. Other children injure their fingers in bicycle spokes. Children need an x-ray to rule out a fracture.

The wound usually is contaminated with spoke grease. Clean it with an appropriate antiseptic. It may be necessary to soak the area first with a solution of lidocaine, a local anesthetic, because of the amount of pain present. Sutures may be necessary. The area may need a splint, and, if a foot, the child may need to limit weight bearing by using crutches.

Soft-tissue injuries are painful. Edema and ecchymosis will be extensive. Raising the body part (propping it on pillows) tends to reduce the pain because it tends to reduce the edema. Such a major tissue injury may take up to 6 weeks to heal; parents should be advised of this at the time of the injury. Otherwise, they may worry that the child's injury is not healing.

Fractures

A **fracture** is a break in the continuity or structure of bone (Monk, 1993). Because children have a lot of falls during their years of growing up, fractures of long bones are common childhood injuries. Many fractures in early childhood are the greenstick variety (one side of a bone is broken, the other is only bent) because of the high resilience of immature bone. These fractures cause minimal pain, swelling, or deformity, the usual hallmarks of fracture. The various types of fractures are described in Table 51-3 and illustrated in Figure 51-21. Fractures in children tend to be different than in adults because bone in childhood is fairly porous (allowing bone to bend rather than break); the periosteum is thick (causes greenstick fractures); epiphyseal lines may cushion a blow so bone does not break; and healing is rapid as a result of overall increased bone growth (Barrett & Bryant, 1990).

Many fractures in children occur at the epiphyseal line. These are always serious fractures because bone growth occurs at this point. Damage to the area may lead to complications of bone growth (undergrowth, overgrowth, or uneven growth resulting in angulation). If a child is involved in an accident that causes severe trauma, such as an automobile accident, compound (open) fractures may result. These are always serious injuries because the severed bone may lacerate nerves or blood vessels. The open wound may become infected, and correction will involve a surgical procedure with the risk involved in anesthesia.

If a fall is from a high distance or caused by a violent force, such as a speeding automobile, breaks may be complex or the formation may be compounded (the bone pierces the skin) or comminuted (the parts of the bone are fragmented).

Fractures heal relatively slowly compared with other body injuries. Immediately following a fracture, a hematoma forms at the site of the break; over the next several days this is infiltrated by capillaries to lay down granulation tissue. Over the next several weeks, osteoblasts invade the new tissue and calcium is deposited (termed *callus*) to form new bone. When callus forma-

Table 51-3. *Types of Fractures*

Type	Description	Implications for the Child
Comminuted	Bone is broken into fragments	Open reduction surgery will probably be necessary to set the bone
Compound	The bone is broken and piercing the skin	The child is open to developing osteomyelitis from outside contamination
Compressed	One bone is forced or pressed against another	A term used to describe vertebral injuries
Displaced	The ends of the broken bone are not in good alignment for healing	Such a break may require a pin or tracuon to approximate the break if healing is to take place
Greenstick	An incomplete fracture—the periosteum is divided only on one side	A fracture that heals quickly
Pathological	A fracture that occurs because of a bone defect such as at the site of a bone neoplasm	Mending the fracture is only a small part of repairing the basic problem or illness
Simple	The fracture is straight and in good alignment	Healing time will be fairly short
Spiral	A fracture that results from a twisting motion	May be difficult to bring the bone segments into good alignment for healing

tion is extensive (enough for movement at the fracture site to be impossible), clinical healing or clinical union has occurred. Complete healing does not occur until all the temporary callus formation has been replaced by mature bone cells and the bone has once more regained its normal shape and contour.

A number of complications may occur following traumatic fractures. One is fat embolus or the release of fat from the broken bone into the blood stream (Fleischer, 1993). This can travel to the brain and cause symptoms of confusion or hallucinations; it could become a pulmonary embolus producing dyspnea, tachycardia, and cyanosis. A second problem is compartment syndrome. This occurs when excessive swelling around the injury site causes increased pressure. The child notices severe pain which is aggravated by passive stretching. Color and warmth of the extremity may remain normal. The child needs a constricting device such as a cast removed to reduce the pressure in the compartment. A long-term complication of fracture may be interference with growth if the growth plate of the bone was involved. Some children need bone lengthening or shortening procedures later in life.

Open Reduction

Open reduction is a surgical technique used to align and repair bone. If there is a spinal fracture, or if both bones of a forearm or lower leg are fractured, open reduction

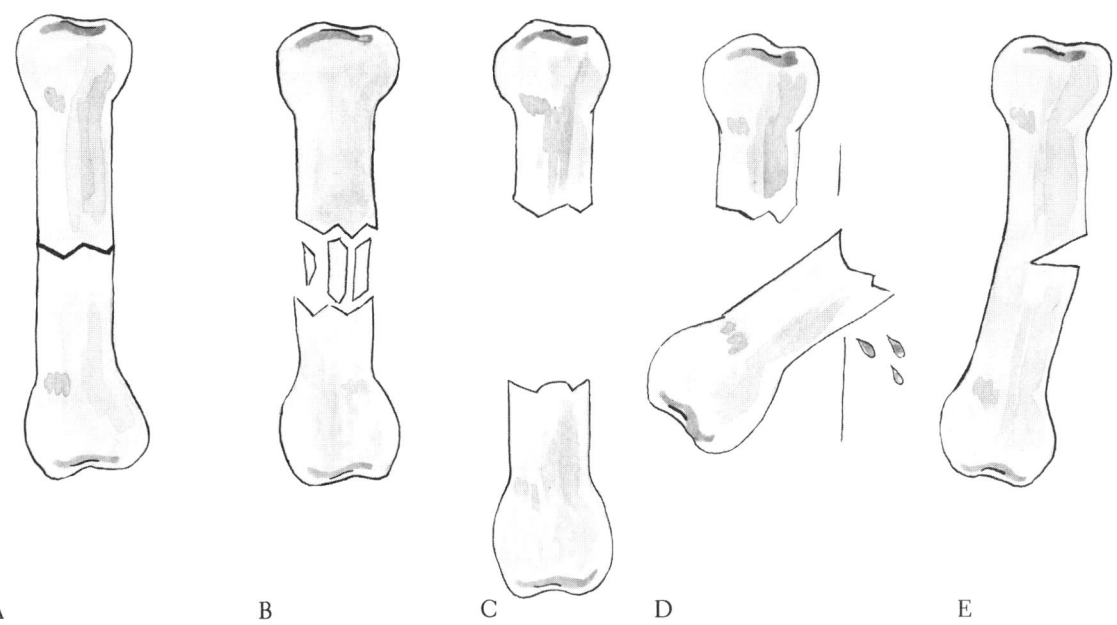

FIGURE 51-21
Types of fractures. (**A**) *Simple.* (**B**) *Comminuted.* (**C**) *Displaced.* (**D**) *Compound.* (**E**) *Greenstick.*

may be necessary to stabilize the bones. Internal fixation, ie, the use of rods or screws, is employed rarely with children.

Once an open reduction is completed, the area is generally casted to provide support. Invariably, serosanguineous fluid oozes from an open-reduction site. Any stain on the cast that suggests oozing from a surgical incision should be outlined with a ballpoint pen so that an increase in the size of the mark can be noted. Do not use a magic marker for this, because the fluid tends to penetrate through the cast. Noting the time you make the pen mark on the cast allows you to tell how rapidly the spot is increasing in size. Children with an open-reduction incision are prone to incision infection as is any child after a surgical incision. Be aware of systemic symptoms of infection (increased pulse, increased temperature, lethargy) as well as local signs (edema, pain, tingling, blueness or coolness of the distal extremity).

Assessment

When children are seen in an emergency department for multiple trauma, the extremities should be observed closely for signs of fracture (deformity, edema, pain). If a fracture is suspected, splint the extremity to avoid further trauma to the fracture site. Splinting also serves to reduce pain, because it prevents further movement of the bone. If the extremity is so seriously deformed by the break that it will not conform to the contour of a splint, do not attempt to move it into a splint position. Place sandbags on the sides of the arm or leg to immobilize it, and leave it in that position. Splints are applied so that they reach a joint above and a joint below the suspected fracture site (for a fracture of the forearm, the splint should reach above the elbow and below the wrist, for example). Immobilizing the joint below and above the injury prevents movement and muscle tension and thus further dislocation of the fracture. Take a thorough history of the accident. Some fractures in childhood occur from child abuse; this must be ruled out with all accidents.

Therapeutic Management

All children with a suspected fracture will need an x-ray to determine whether a fracture actually is present and to determine the alignment and apposition of the fractured segments of bone. Apposition (the amount of end-to-end contact of the bone fragments) is not as important in children as in adults. Bayonet or side-to-side apposition may be established or left in children up to 10 to 12 years old, because as the child grows and remodeling occurs, the bone will develop with normal contour and length. Side-to-side apposition results in a rapid, strong union and actually is the preferred position in some fractures.

If skin has been broken, children may need antitetanus vaccine. A hematocrit determination to estimate blood loss and crossmatching for replacement therapy may be necessary. An intravenous line is generally established to provide a route for fluid or blood replacement or for administration of an intravenous antibiotic to reduce the possibility of infection through the open wound.

All children with fractures are in some pain. They generally are thoroughly frightened not only from the pain and the appearance of the fracture and from their inability to use the extremity but also from the frightening situation that led to the fracture (a fall, an automobile accident). Time in the emergency department is well spent comforting and helping children to realize that they are now safe, that they will not be injured further. If they can relax enough to lie still and not move the fractured extremity, they will feel less pain. When children have a compound fracture, they are as frightened at the sight of blood as they are of the deformity and pain. However, children and parents can both be assured that unless the bone has been crushed, the bone fragments can be brought back into line. After this, the bone will heal with the same strength as before.

Forearm Fractures

Because a child often falls on an outstretched arm, fractures of the forearm are common. In children, most fractures of the forearm involve the distal third; a smaller number of such accidents occur in the middle or proximal third. The injury may involve a fracture of the radius, a fracture of both the radius and ulna, or a displacement of the epiphyseal plate of the radius. In young children, the injury generally is a greenstick fracture. Sometimes greenstick fractures are broken completely before casting to prevent the bone's resuming its "bent" position within the cast. Refer to this as "straightening" the bone, rather than "breaking" the bone—how much confidence can a child or parent have in a physician who, instead of helping a bone heal, breaks it further?

If a greenstick fracture is slight, so that the degree of angulation is not great, it may not be reduced or brought into a straight line. As callus is formed and the bone remodels itself, it will naturally straighten into good alignment.

If the fracture is complete and overriding is excessive, traction to the fingers may be employed as a part of the cast. This "banjo" traction is cumbersome and limits the use the child has of that hand. With almost all casts, the hand is covered up to the first phalangeal knuckle to prevent the child from moving the hand excessively and damaging the edge of the cast, which will loosen it and put the arm into poor alignment (see the Focus on Family Teaching box).

Volkmann's Ischemic Contracture

When an arm is flexed and put into a cast, the radial artery and nerve may be compressed at the elbow, caus-

Q. My 6-year-old just had a cast applied to her arm in the emergency room. How do I take care of her until this is removed?

A. The most important care necessary for a child with a cast is to protect the cast and arm from further injury. Some important steps to take are:

- Keep the arm elevated on a pillow for the first day to decrease swelling in the arm.

- Avoid touching the cast with other than your palm (no sharp fingers) until it is dry to avoid denting it.

- Observe the fingers for swelling or blueness and ask your child to move her fingers about every 4 hours for the first 24 hours; if she is unable to move her fingers or swelling, blueness, or pain is present, telephone your health care provider (this could mean the cast is pressing on a nerve or constricting a blood vessel).

- Monitor strenuous activities such as roughhousing while the cast is in place; urge usual activities so your child remains active.

- Ask your child to think through how wearing a cast will change her day, such as making it difficult to eat in a cafeteria at school or carry books to classes, and brainstorm how to solve these problems.

- Be certain your child knows not to put anything inside the cast. If itching occurs inside the cast, blowing some cool air into it from a hair dryer can be comforting.

- Be certain your child keeps the cast dry (cover with a plastic bag to shower); no swimming is allowed.

- Be certain to keep your return appointment for follow-up care. Because children grow so rapidly, they can outgrow a cast rapidly. This could put pressure on nerves and lead to permanent disability.

ing nerve injury or severe impairment of circulation. If the fracture is in the proximal third of the radius, the child generally is admitted to the hospital for 24 hours so that signs of circulatory or nerve impairment can be observed for carefully.

If symptoms of compression are present but are not detected within 6 hours, permanent damage to the arm will result. The arm is left permanently flexed at the elbow; the wrist is hyperextended, and the fingers assume a flexed, clawlike, useless position, a Volkmann's contracture. If a child is going to be discharged following application of a cast, parents must be made aware of the symptoms of compression so that its development

can be detected. If a child is admitted to the hospital for 24 hours, the radial pulse (if palpable at the edge of the cast) should be taken hourly along with checks for coldness, blanching, and color for the first 8 hours. In some instances, the cast will be applied incompletely for 24 hours, the elbow portion just being splinted and wrapped with elastic bandages. After 24 hours, when edema has subsided and the chance of compression is less, the plaster is applied to the rest of the arm.

Elbow Fractures

If a child falls and stops the fall with a hand, the elbow may hyperextend, transmitting the force of the blow to the distal humerus and causing supracondylar fracture of the humerus. The fracture of the humerus is reduced and stabilized with an arm cast, a splint, or traction, depending on the position of the fracture. Although the fracture may be minor, the child is usually admitted to the hospital for overnight observation; a close watch is kept for circulatory stasis so that Volkmann's contracture does not occur. Elevate the cast on pillows or suspend the hand by a strip of gauze or traction apparatus to reduce edema.

Explain to parents why the child needs to be hospitalized, so that they can keep the accident in perspective. The child is not being admitted because this is a serious fracture that will take an unusually long time to heal but because of the possibility of an immediate complication. If there is no indication of a complication within 24 to 48 hours and the arm can be casted, the child will be discharged.

Epiphyseal Separations of the Radius

When children break a fall with an outstretched arm, they may cause a separation of the epiphysis of the distal radius. When this occurs, the wrist must be casted to restabilize the epiphysis. Although epiphyseal injuries are always serious, because injury to an epiphysis may cause growth disturbances, distal radial injury rarely causes serious sequelae in children. Advise parents that it is important to keep appointments for follow-up visits, however, so growth disturbances can be detected early and correction started. Stapling the epiphysis may be done to arrest abnormal growth if it occurs; stimulation of the epiphyseal line may increase growth if growth retardation occurs.

Clavicle Fractures

When young children fall and catch themselves with an outstretched arm, the force of the blow may be transmitted to the clavicle, causing fracture of the clavicle rather than of the arm. Clavicles also may be fractured during birth, particularly in infants with broad shoulders.

Swelling is often present at the site of the break. The child refuses to use the arm, and it hangs at the side. In the newborn, a Moro reflex is demonstrated only on the unaffected side. Newborns are treated by having the arm on that side immobilized against the chest. Following x-ray diagnosis, an older child is placed in a figure-eight splint of stockinet wound over the shoulders and under the armpits that keeps the arm adducted and flexed across the chest (Figure 51-22). This is left in place for about 3 weeks. The child should keep it dry—no swimming or showering during this time. The parent often needs to tighten it every morning to keep it firmly in place. These stockinet wraps tend to get extremely dirty in 3 weeks. Parents are usually apologetic about the appearance of the stockinet when they return for a repeat x-ray after 3 weeks, worried that the soiled appearance of the splint reflects the quality of their housekeeping or child care. Assure them that the soiled splint proves that they followed instructions well and left the splint in place for 3 weeks, that the soiled appearance is proof of their concern and the high quality of their care.

Parents may need reassurance that this splint is adequate therapy. The bone is broken, after all—why is the child not being placed in a cast? Acknowledging their concern with a statement such as "Most people think that when there is a broken bone, a cast is needed—this is an exception" allows parents to voice their concern and receive further assurance.

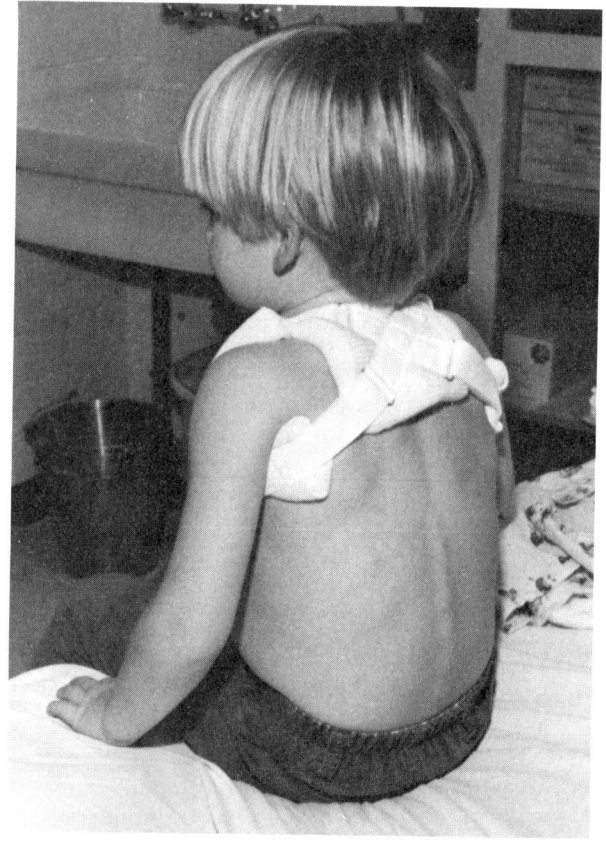

FIGURE 51-22
A splint for a broken clavicle. (Courtesy of Bruce Hill.)

Fracture of the Femur

Children who are involved in automobile accidents or who fall from considerable heights and land on their feet may suffer a fractured femur. Child abuse should be considered in an infant who sustains a fractured femur as there are few normal instances when this could occur in an infant.

Even if these fractures are closed so the skin is not broken, blood loss may be extensive because of the size of the bone broken. As the child lies on the examining table in the emergency department, the child holds the leg externally rotated; the thigh may appear abnormally short or deformed. The child is in a great deal of pain. He or she may be in shock from pain and blood loss. Children are always frightened from the force of the accident that caused such a severe injury.

Fractured femurs usually cannot be casted at first, because strong tendon spasm causes poor alignment and overriding of the femur segments. Therefore, alignment must be initiated first by traction.

For a child less than 2 years old, Bryant's traction is used (see Figure 51-8). For the older child with a fractured femur, skeletal traction with a pin through the distal femur is used. When muscle spasm has been reduced enough to allow close approximation of the bone edges, and when callus formation is good (7 to 14 days), the child is removed from traction and placed in a hip spica cast. A young child will remain in a cast for an additional 3 to 4 weeks. In older children, healing of a fractured femur requires an extended time. In a child who is 12 years old, firm union of the bone fragments will take about 12 weeks. Help the child and family identify ways for the child to continue school work and contact with friends if he or she is unable to attend school because of the large cast during this time.

Dislocation of the Radial Head

If a small child is lifted by one hand, as happens when a parent pulls on one arm to lift the child over a curb or up a step, the head of the radius may escape the ligament surrounding it and become dislocated (nursemaid's elbow). The child holds the arm flexed at the elbow; the forearm is held pronated. The child winces with pain when the radial head is palpated (Jackson, 1994).

A simple dislocation of the radial head can be reduced by a physician, using gentle pressure on the radial head while the arm is flexed and supinated. Relief of pain is immediate, and the child begins to use the arm again.

Assure parents that this is a common injury in small children. Parents feel guilty because they caused this dislocation. They rarely need to be cautioned that lifting a child in this manner is not wise; the proof of it is standing in front of them. Be aware, however, that a dislocation of the radial head can occur from extremely rough handling as is seen in child abuse.

Athletic Injuries

Knee Injuries

Participation in sports such as football, skiing, or track can cause knee injuries in children. As football becomes a more popular sport for young children, more and more knee injuries are occurring. These injuries generally involve the ligaments surrounding the knee. The ligaments may be the medial, lateral, posterior, or cruciate ligaments (figure-eight ligaments that stabilize the knee). Following the injury, the child has severe pain in the knee. There will be localized edema. An x-ray will be taken to rule out fracture (Landry, 1994).

If the injury is mild (only a few torn fibers), bedrest with ice applied to the knee is often the only therapy needed. Local infiltration of an anesthetic may be necessary to minimize pain. After 24 hours, heat is applied to the leg to hasten healing.

If the injury is more severe, the knee joint may fill with fluid. The child will need bedrest. The abnormal synovial fluid will be aspirated, and a compression dressing will be applied to discourage accumulation of further fluid. Ice will be applied to the joint. After 24 hours, heat treatments will be started to hasten healing.

If the injury is severe, a cast may be applied for complete immobilization. It takes as long for a severe ligament injury to heal as it does for a bone fracture, so the cast will remain in place for about 8 weeks. Arthroscopy is the observation of knee ligaments by means of a narrow scope. Surgery done through an arthroscope makes repair of ligaments or cartilage a minor procedure and limits the necessity for immobilization and a cast.

A severe twisting motion to the knee may cause a dislocation of the kneecap (it moves to the posterior surface of the knee). The knee appears deformed, and the child is in acute pain. Immediate treatment for a dislocated kneecap is to slide it again to the front of the knee. Following this, the child will usually have to use a leg immobilizer for 1 week. If the problem is chronic or occurs frequently, surgery to strengthen the ligaments may be necessary.

Throwing Injuries

Throwing places repeated stress on the upper extremity, particularly the elbow joint. The injury tends to occur during the forward motion of the arm or the follow-through. Children are unable to extend their elbow completely because of minute tears and fibrous contractures in the muscle. They notice pain and tenderness and loss of complete elbow extension for 24 to 48 hours after the injury. Resting the arm and applying ice packs for 15 to 20 minutes three times a day relieves the pain. Phenylbutazone (Butazolidin) given systemically may be helpful. A limited number of cortisone injections into the elbow musculature may be helpful. Exercises to strengthen flexor muscles help to prevent this type of injury.

"Little Leaguer's elbow" is epiphysitis of the medial epicondylar epiphysis. Stress in this area is increased by throwing curves and breaking pitches because of the forceful flexion and pronation required. An x-ray of the elbow may reveal increased growth, separation, and fragmentation of the medial epicondylar epiphysis. This injury may occur in as many as 95% of Little League pitchers between the ages of 9 and 14.

Children generally need extra protection against injury until the epiphyseal growth centers at the elbow have fused at 14 to 17 years of age. Children who participate in Little League sports need coaches who understand that this is just a game; children should have proper warm-up times; they should throw no curves or breaking pitches and should be limited to pitching about six innings per week. They should have a 3-day rest between games. Treatment for Little Leaguer's elbow is rest and immobilization until pain, tenderness, and limitation of movement have passed. If the injury is not treated adequately, permanent damage to the epiphyseal line and elbow deformity can occur.

Strains and Sprains

A strain is a muscle-tendon injury. A sprain is a ligament injury. Strained or sprained ankles are common but difficult childhood injuries. The joint is painful and swollen. When the x-ray reveals no fracture, the child may feel as though someone has said that the injury is not serious, but "just a sprain." He or she finds the extension of the swelling and pain baffling. Some children may be accused by parents of "putting on" pain, because the injury is "only a sprain."

Help the child and parents to understand that strains and sprains are truly painful. Because a cast is not used and an ankle is not immobilized completely, strains and sprains are often more painful than fractures, which are casted.

If the injury is recent, an ice pack should be applied for approximately 20 minutes to attempt to reduce edema at the site. An elastic bandage may be applied to give firm support. The child may be given crutches to limit weight bearing for the next 3 or 4 days. Make certain that the parents of the child understand how the elastic bandage has been applied, so that it can be rewrapped if it loosens, and that the child is using the crutches properly before being discharged from the emergency department.

Key Points

- Many children have casts applied to allow broken bones to heal. Nursing diagnoses identified in connection to cast care are High risk for altered peripheral tissue perfusion, Impaired tissue integrity, and Parental health-seeking behaviors.
- Volkmann's ischemic contracture is a complication that occurs when an arm is casted in a bent position and a radial artery and nerve are compressed at the elbow. Frequent assessments that finger color and warmth are remaining adequate are safeguards that this is not occurring.
- If broken bones are not easily aligned, children are placed in traction. Nursing diagnoses commonly associated with this are High risk for altered nutrition, Impaired physical mobility, Altered skin integrity, High risk for infection, and Altered growth and development.
- Developmental disorders that occur in children are flat feet (pronation), genu varum (bowlegs), and genu valgum (knock knees). The majority of these disorders are corrected naturally by normal growth.
- Slipped epiphysis is slipping of the femur head in relation to the neck of the femur at the epiphyseal line. It occurs most frequently in obese or rapidly growing boys.
- Osteomyelitis is infection of the bone. It can result in extensive destruction of the bone. Antibiotic therapy is necessary to combat the infection.
- Scoliosis is a lateral curvature of the spine. It is treated by bracing or surgery. Nursing diagnoses commonly identified for this are Knowledge deficit, High risk for altered skin integrity, and Altered self-concept.
- Juvenile rheumatoid arthritis (JRA) occurs in a number of different forms: polyarthritis, pauciarticular, and systemic. Therapy is exercise, heat application, splinting, and administration of nonsteroidal anti-inflammatory drugs, methotrexate, or aspirin.
- Myasthenia gravis can occur in a transient form at birth from transfer of antibodies from a mother with the illness or as a primary form later in childhood. Therapy is administration of anticholinesterase drugs such as neostigmine (Prostigmin) that prolong acetylcholine action.
- Muscular dystrophy is the inherited progressive degeneration of skeletal muscles. Different types that can occur are congenital, facioscapulohumeral, and pseudohypertrophic. Children and parents alike need long-term support through the course of this long-term illness. Fortunately, due to new progress in gene replacement therapy, research is close to revealing a cure for this disease.
- A fracture or bruise of soft tissue could have resulted from child abuse. Be certain to secure a detailed history of an injury to be certain that the history is consistent with the degree of injury.
- Bone and muscle disorders tend to be long-term disorders. Help children and their families to think through how the disorder will affect tasks of daily living to help the child better adjust to a cast or brace. Help children plan self-diversional activities as necessary so they continue to grow developmentally while confined to a cast or traction.
- As a rule, if a bone is broken, children need additional calcium in their diet to aid bone healing. If they are on strict bedrest, however, this should only be a moderate addition to their diet to prevent renal calculi from forming.

Critical Thinking Exercises

1. Judy is a 14-year-old who wears a Milwaukee brace 23 hours a day for scoliosis. During the last month, she turned down an invitation to the high school prom and has dropped out of the high school band and the one after-school club she belonged to. She tells you she is dropping activities to have more "time to study." Would you be concerned about Judy?
2. Dominic is a 3-year-old with juvenile rheumatoid arthritis. You notice when he returns for a follow-up visit to the arthritis clinic that the inflammation in his joints is worse than at his last visit. He has a great deal of pain. His mother tells you she has been giving him acetaminophen instead of aspirin for therapy because her primary doctor said not to give aspirin to children under 18. How would you explain these contradictory instructions? Why do children with JRA receive aspirin?
3. Mrs. Howard has three athletically inclined boys in grade school. She is concerned with guiding them into sports that will be safe for them during their growing years. What advice would you give her?

References

Barrett, J. B., & Bryant, B. H. (1993). Fractures: Types, treatment perioperative implications. *Association of Operating Room Nurses Journal, 52,* 755.

Borris, L. C. (1992). Complications of heel pad punctures for blood sampling in the newborn. *Neonatal Intensive Care, 5,* 63.

Cassidy, J. T. (1994). Connective tissue diseases and amyloidosis. In Oski, F. A., et al. (Eds.) *Principles and practice of pediatrics* (2nd ed.). Philadelphia: J. B. Lippincott.

Coates, C. J., et al. (1990). Femoral osteotomy in Perthes' disease. *Journal of Bone and Joint Surgery, 72,* 581.

Davis, P. (1989). The principles of traction. *Nursing, 3,* 5.

Department of Health and Human Services. (1991). *Healthy people 2000.* Washington, DC: Public Health Service.

Drummond, D. S. (1991). A perspective on recent trends for scoliosis correction. *Clinical Orthopaedics and Related Research, 232,* 90.

Dubousset, J., & Cotrel, Y. (1991). Application technique of Cotrel-Dubousset instrumentation for scoliosis deformities. *Clinical Orthopaedics and Related Research, 232,* 103.

Dunn, J. F. (1990). Osgood-Schlatter disease. *American Family Physician, 41,* 173.

Fife, R. S. (1993). Methotrexate use in juvenile rheumatoid arthritis. *Orthopedic Nursing, 12,* 32.

Fleischer, E., et al. (1993). Fat embolism syndrome. *Nurse Anesthesia, 4,* 18.

Gerber, L. H., et al. (1990). Rehabilitation of children and infants with osteogenesis imperfecta. *Clinical Orthopaedics and Related Research, 251,* 254.

Griggs, R. C., et al. (1990). Mechanism of muscle wasting in myotonic dystrophy. *Annals of Neurology, 27,* 505.

Heath, C. H., & Staheli, L. T. (1993). Normal limits of knee angle in white children: Genu varum and genu valgum. *Journal of Pediatric Orthopaedics, 13,* 259.

Jackson, K. V. (1994). Acute pediatric orthopedic conditions. *Pediatric Annals, 23,* 240.

Landry, G. L. (1994). Sports medicine. In Oski, F. A., et al. (Eds.). *Principles and practice of pediatrics* (2nd ed.). Philadelphia: J. B. Lippincott.

McConnell, E. A. (1993). Providing cast care. *Nursing, 23,* 19.

Monk, H. L. (1993). Fractures are never simple. *RN, 56,* 30.

Morrissy, R. T., & Selman, S. (1991). Slipped capital femoral epiphysis. *Orthopedic Nursing, 10,* 11.

Olsen B., et al. (1991). The patient in a halo brace: Striving for normalcy in body image and self-concept. *Orthopaedic Nursing, 10,* 44.

Olson, B., & Ustanko, L. (1990). Self-care needs of patients in the halo brace. *Orthopedic Nursing, 9,* 27.

Parke, J. H. (1994). Diseases of the neuromuscular junction. In Oski, F. A., et al. (Eds.). *Principles and practice of pediatrics* (2nd ed.). Philadelphia: J. B. Lippincott.

Renshaw, T. S. (1993). Idiopathic scoliosis in children. *Current Opinion in Pediatrics, 5,* 407.

Smith, R. A., et al. (1990). Early development of boys with Duchenne muscular dystrophy. *Developmental Medicine and Child Neurology, 32,* 519.

Sponseller, P. D. (1994). Bone, joint and muscle problems. In Oski, F. A., et al. (Eds.). *Principles and practice of pediatrics* (2nd ed.). Philadelphia: J. B. Lippincott.

Staheli, L. T. (1992). *Fundamentals of pediatric orthopedics.* New York: Raven Press.

Stout, J. D., et al. (1992). Transportation resources for pediatric orthopaedic clients. *Orthopaedic Nursing, 11,* 26.

Tzartos, S. J., et al. (1990). Neonatal myasthenia gravis: Antigenic specificities of antibodies in sera from mothers and their infants. *Clinical Experiments in Immunology, 80,* 376.

Weaver, D. D. (1994). Skeletal dysplasias. In Oski, F. A., et al. (Eds.) *Principles and practice of pediatrics* (2nd ed.). Philadelphia: J. B. Lippincott.

Wijmenga, C., et al. (1990). Location of facioscapulohumeral muscular dystrophy gene on chromosome 4. *Lancet, 336,* 651.

Suggested Readings

Barnes, L. P. (1990). Teaching self-care to children. *MCN: American Journal of Maternal Child Nursing, 16,* 101.

Betz, R. R., et al. (1990). Treatment of slipped capital femoral epiphysis: Spica-cast immobilization. *Journal of Bone and Joint Surgery, 72,* 587.

Campbell, L. S., & Campbell, J. D. (1991). Musculoskeletal trauma in children. *Critical Care Nursing Clinics of North America, 3,* 445.

Davis, B. D., & Steele, S. (1991). Case management for young children with special health care needs. *Pediatric Nursing, 17,* 15.

Dickson, J. H., et al. (1990). Harrington instrumentation and arthrodesis for idiopathic scoliosis. *Journal of Bone and Joint Surgery, 72,* 678.

Heckman, J. D. (1991). Fractures: Emergency care and complications. *Clinical Symposia, 43,* 2.

Herron, D. G., & Nance, J. (1990). Emergency department nursing management of patients with orthopedic fractures resulting from motor vehicle accidents. *Nursing Clinics of North America, 25,* 71.

Jones-Walton, P. (1991). Clinical standards in skeletal traction pin site care. *Orthopedic Nursing, 10,* 12.

Kostuik, J. P. (1990). Operative treatment of idiopathic scoliosis. *Journal of Bone and Joint Surgery, 72,* 1108.

Mason, K. J. (1991). Congenital orthopedic anomalies and their impact on the family. *Nursing Clinics of North America, 26,* 1.

Pons, V. G. (1991). Osteomyelitis: The case for aggressive diagnoses and treatment. *Consultant, 31,* 23.

Richardson, A. (1992). Rheumatoid arthritis in pregnancy. *Nursing Standards, 6,* 25.

Selekman, J. (1991). Pediatric rehabilitation: From concepts to practice. *Pediatric Nursing, 17,* 11.

Volpon, J. B. (1994). Footprint analysis during the growth period. *Journal of Pediatric Orthopaedics, 14,* 83.

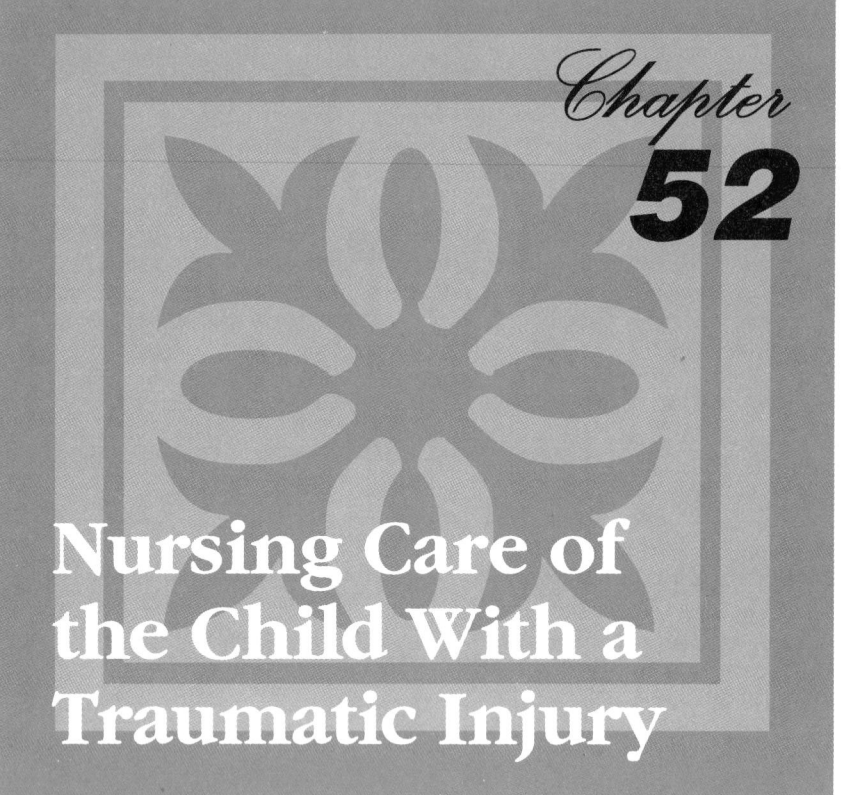

Chapter 52

Nursing Care of the Child With a Traumatic Injury

Key Terms

- allografting
- autografting
- bougie
- contrecoup injury
- debridement
- drowning
- escharotomy
- heterografting
- homografting
- near drowning
- stupor

Objectives

After mastering the contents of this chapter, you should be able to:

1. Describe the causes and consequences of common accidents and injuries in childhood as well as measures to prevent them.

2. Assess a child injured from an accident such as poisoning or burning.

3. Formulate nursing diagnoses related to the injured child.

4. Plan nursing care related to the injured child such as teaching poisoning prevention.

5. Implement nursing care for the child with an injury such as assessing circulation following casting.

6. Evaluate goal outcomes to be certain that nursing goals were achieved.

7. Identify National Health Goals related to children and trauma that nurses can be instrumental in helping the nation to achieve.

8. Identify areas related to care of children with traumatic injuries that could benefit from additional nursing research.

9. Use critical thinking to analyze ways that accidents and injuries can be prevented in childhood.

10. Synthesize knowledge of injuries in childhood with nursing process to achieve quality maternal and child health care.

Adele Pillitteri: MATERNAL AND CHILD HEALTH NURSING, 2nd Edition. © 1995 Adele Pillitteri.

Accidents cause more deaths in the 1- to 4-year age group than the next six most prevalent diseases combined; in the 15- to 24-year age group, they cause more deaths than all other combined causes. If accidents could be prevented, a major cause of childhood morbidity and mortality would be eliminated. Accident reduction is certainly a realistic goal to strive for; total elimination, however, may not be possible, as many children believe that accidents will not happen to them and so do not take sensible precautions against them. Some parents lead children into accidents by overestimating their development and giving them responsibility beyond their capabilities (for example, allowing a child to light a fire in the fireplace before he or she appreciates the danger of fire). Family stress plays a large role in childhood poisoning accidents. In a classic study, Sobel

(1970) compared the home environments of children who had poisoned themselves with those of matched children with no poisoning history. This study looked at the availability of poisons and the presence of stress in the house. The results showed that both types of houses had poisons available. The families in which poisonings occurred, however, had more stress factors such as illness in the mother, marital discord, or illness in another family member. Eliminating accidents in children, therefore, is not a simple procedure, because it involves reducing family stress as well. National Health Goals re-

FOCUS ON
National Health Goals

A number of National Health Goals are concerned with trauma and children. These are:

- Reduce homicides to no more than 3.1/100,000 in children aged 3 and younger and 1.4/100,000 in persons aged 15–34 from baselines of 3.9 and 1.7/100,000, respectively.

- Reduce assault injuries among people aged 12 and older to no more than 10/1000 people from a baseline of 11.1/1000.

- Reduce by 20% the incidence of weapons-carrying by adolescents aged 14 through 17.

- Reduce residential fire deaths to no more than 3.3 per 100,000 children aged 4 and younger from a baseline of 4.4/100,000.

- Reduce drowning deaths to no more than 2.3/100,000 children aged 4 and younger from a baseline of 4.2/100,000.

- Increase to at least 50% the proportion of primary care providers who routinely provide age-appropriate counseling on safety precautions to prevent unintentional injury (DHHS, 1991).

Nurses can be instrumental in helping the nation achieve these goals by being primary care providers who provide counseling on safety precautions to parents and children. Additional nursing research would be helpful in areas such as the following: what are effective ways to communicate safety information to parents at well child visits when time is at a premium; what ways should safety teaching given after an accident to prevent a further accident be different from that given as primary prevention; and is there an association between children setting fires and their exposure to fire experiences with fireplaces or candles?

Table 52-1. *Most Frequent Accidents in Children by Age Group*

Age (yr)	Type of Accident
0–1	Falls, inhalation of foreign objects, poisoning, burns, drowning
1–4	Falls, drowning, motor vehicles, poisoning, burns
5–9	Motor vehicles, bicycle accidents, drowning, burns, firearms
10–14	Motor vehicles, drowning, burns, firearms, falls, bicycle accidents
15–18	Motor vehicles, drowning, falls, firearms

lated to children and trauma are shown in the Focus on National Health Goals box.

The frequency of different types of accidents varies according to age group (Table 52-1). Because the anatomy and physiology of children is different from that of adults, they are affected by accidents differently than adults.

NURSING PROCESS OVERVIEW
for Care of the Child With a Traumatic Injury

ASSESSMENT

When children are seen at health care facilities because of accidents, neither they nor their parents may be at their best because of the stress of the situation. They may be apprehensive and frightened not only about what *has* happened but also about what could have happened if, for instance, the knife had slipped a fraction of an inch further or the child had swallowed a different substance. Children often feel guilty and are afraid that they will be scolded or punished. After all, they had been told many times not to play with knives (or climb on kitchen counters, or touch the bottles under the sink). Their parents feel guilty. If they were really "good" parents, they would have been watching more closely or put the knife or the poison up out of the way. They may feel defensive because they are worried that they will be criticized. Remember that people under stress do not hear well and may not perceive correctly the information given to them; information they receive in the emergency department may be grossly misinterpreted or not heard at all.

Children are likely to be in pain. They are frightened not just from the pain of the injury but also from the circumstance of the injury. Children count on their parents to keep them safe, and yet they have been hurt. The trust is broken momentarily. How can they be safe here if their parents no longer are protecting them?

Assess children's conditions quickly when they are first seen. They may be seriously hurt and yet not cry because they are in shock; they may be hemorrhaging, but if they are bleeding internally, blood may not be evident. Because the emergency department nurse is often the first person who sees a child after an injury, be ready to make a preliminary assessment of the extent of the child's injury before a physician arrives. Accidents become fatal when lung, heart, or brain function becomes inadequate. These three body systems, therefore, must be evaluated first. Table 52-2 lists signs and symptoms to assess to determine the respiratory, cardiovascular, and neurologic status of an injured child.

While you conduct a preliminary assessment of a child's major body systems, take a brief history of the accident. What happened? How long ago did it happen? What have the parents done? If the child fell, how far did he or she fall? (A fall from the top of a ladder is more likely to be serious than a fall from a lower rung.) What body part did the child land on? (A head injury is more likely to be serious than an ankle injury, although a child may be in more pain and have more obvious symptoms with the lesser injury.) Ask parents what they think are a

child's major injuries. Children may complain about one body part at first, but then a small cut elsewhere begins to bleed, and they focus on the minor bleeding as their major injury. If parents say, "At first, he acted as if his stomach hurt," this may be the first suggestion that he has a splenic rupture.

It is often difficult to evaluate children in an emergency department, because they are so frightened that they cannot stop crying to report which body parts are painful or to indicate which parts should be assessed first. A few minutes spent attempting to calm children and get them past this initial fright is time well spent unless symptoms of major body system disturbances require that you direct your immediate efforts elsewhere. Parents need frequent explanations of care given or planned, because as long as they are worried and tense, children cannot be calmed easily.

A proportion of traumatic injuries in children result from child abuse (Pike, 1993). Ask yourself if this could be a possibility (see Chapter 55).

NURSING DIAGNOSIS

The nursing diagnostic category used most frequently with injured children is Pain. Depending on the particular injury, a number of other nursing diagnoses are relevant, as well as those that relate to the suffering that parents experience when their child is injured:

- Ineffective airway clearance related to burned esophageal tissue
- Impaired mobility related to severe burn injury
- Body image disturbance related to change in physical appearance with thermal burns
- Parental fear related to outcome after head injury in child
- Altered family processes related to child's accident

PLANNING

Parents in an emergency department are rarely ready for long-term planning; they have great difficulty in coming up with answers even to the most straightforward questions. Establishing goals is often difficult with injured children because both they and their parents are too frightened to plan. Long-term goals may have to be delayed until the immediate concern of the injury has passed.

On discharge from the emergency department, parents need printed instructions as to the child's care at home (change the dressing or not; take the child's temperature or not) and whom to call if they have questions about care or progress; they also need an appointment (or the number to call for a return appointment) for follow-up care. If the child is admitted to the hospital from the emergency department, it is helpful if the nurse who cared for the child in the emergency department can ac-

Table 52-2. *Important Assessments on Initial Examination of an Injured Child*

Body System	Assessment
Respiratory system	Quality of respirations (labored or even?)
	Rate of respirations
	Sound of obstruction (wheezing, stridor, retractions, coughing?)
	Color (cyanotic?)
	Oxygen hunger (restlessness, inability to lie flat?)
Cardiovascular system	Color (pallor from hemorrhage or cardiovascular collapse?)
	Gross bleeding
	Pulse rate (increases with hemorrhage)
	Blood pressure (decreases with hemorrhage)
	Feeling of apprehension from altered vascular pressure
Nervous system	Level of consciousness (child answers questions coherently?; infant attunes to parent's voice?)
	Pupils (equal and reacting to light?)
	Bumps or bruises on head or spinal column
	Loss of motion or sensory function in a body part

company him or her to the hospital unit. The first people who care for a child after an injury become very important to the child and parents. Parents have difficulty letting them go and accepting new caregivers. A transition period, a "passing on of care," helps a parent to accept the child's new caregivers as just as dependable and trustworthy as the emergency department staff.

IMPLEMENTATION

The extent of a child's injury depends on the injuring agent, the part of the body injured, and often the immediate care, including both physical and psychological management at the time of the injury and at the health care facility where the child was seen.

The diameter of the airway in children is smaller than in adults, so an injury to this body area almost always will result in a greater danger of airway closure than in adults. This could happen from the child inhaling a substance such as water that directly obstructs the airway or from inhaling toxic fumes that cause inflammation along the lining of the airway and resulting obstruction. A blow to the neck can result in such edema of surrounding tissues that the airway is pushed closed.

Most injuries involve some blood loss. Fortunately, a child's circulatory system is capable of rapid compensation for blood loss by vasoconstriction. Because the total volume of blood in a child is reduced, however, blood loss in children is always potentially serious.

Often, large portions of the child's body must be exposed to view so that care can be easily given. This means that rapid cooling can occur. Because of the large surface area of children in relation to weight, always be conscious of body temperature and take active measures to decrease cooling by keeping the child covered as much as possible during examination times.

Parental consent must be obtained for treatment procedures even in an emergency, except for life-saving actions such as cardiopulmonary resuscitation procedures. In these instances, action can and should be taken to save the child's life with or without parental permission (it is assumed that parents would consent to life-saving procedures). Delaying emergency procedures until parents can be located may result in permanent disability or death. Remember to use universal precautions in emergency situations, the same as at any other time.

A part of nursing intervention in an emergency department should be helping parents to understand why an injury happened (a 3-year-old child is too young to understand that matches are dangerous; the parent must keep matches out of the child's reach) and helping the parents plan ways to make their house or community safe for children. If seat belt use could be reinforced, for example, it is estimated that infant deaths in motor vehicle accidents could be reduced by 91% and infant injury by 78%.

EVALUATION

After an injury, children need follow-up care to be certain that the immediate interventions were adequate and that healing is taking place. Evaluation visits are also the time to determine if the child's environment has been changed and is safer now than at the time of the accident (if applicable). At that time, parents may have been too anxious to hear health supervision information. Now, with the accident behind them, they are ready for such information and prepared to make changes.

When an injury happens that could not be anticipated (a child was ice skating and fell and broke his or her arm), parents appreciate hearing one more time that such an accident could not have been avoided, that they are good parents. This helps them maintain adequate self-esteem to continue to function well as parents.

Examples of outcome criteria are:

- Child is able to swallow fluids without distress following esophageal burns.
- Child states pain is at tolerable level by half hour.
- Child has full range of motion in hand following thermal injury.

Head Trauma

Children receive head injuries when they are involved in multiple trauma accidents, such as automobile accidents. Falls from swing sets, porches, and bunk beds also cause many head injuries. Sometimes children are struck on the head by an object such as a baseball, rock, or hockey puck, or fall from a bicycle (see the Focus on Nursing Research box).

Head injuries are serious not only because they cause an immediate life threat to the child but also because a number of complications may follow head injury (Romig, 1993). If there was a depressed skull fracture, the incidence of recurrent seizures after the injury is as high as 30% to 60%. Recurrent seizures occur primarily in children who were unconscious for longer than 24 hours or who had convulsions during the acute phase of illness (Rosman, 1994). Many of these children show focal abnormalities on an electroencephalogram (EEG). A number of children with seizure involvement will have a normal EEG, however, so by itself EEG is of limited value in predicting posttraumatic seizures.

Some children experience memory deficits or minor personality changes after head injury. Symptoms such as headache, irritability, and postural vertigo (posttrauma syndrome) also may occur. Behavior manifestations may include aggressiveness or poor school performance. It often is difficult to determine whether these symptoms are organic or result from being treated differently than usual by anxious parents.

FOCUS ON NURSING RESEARCH

Are Bicycle Injuries a Major Cause of Injury in Childhood?

Bicycling is becoming an increasingly popular sport for both adults and children; unfortunately, when they are injured in bicycle accidents, children's injuries can be severe.

To investigate the extent of the problem in one community, hospital records were reviewed to document how many children had been seen for bicycle injuries in the past year. Thirty-seven children were identified who had had a bicycle injury. The majority of these children were less than 10 years of age; 70% were male, 30% female. Twenty-five children (67%) had been admitted because of head injury. Other injuries included lacerations, contusions, and abrasions, plus fractures of the femur, humerus, patella, mandible, ribs, tibia, fibula, radius, and ulna. Fourteen children had injuries severe enough that they were admitted to the intensive care unit. None of the children were wearing helmets at the time of the accident.

The researchers stress that 67% of these injuries probably could have been prevented if children had been wearing helmets. They urge nurses to be active in teaching bicycle safety, especially the use of safety helmets, to grade-school children to help reduce the number of serious bicycle injuries.

Wilson, P. D., & Testani-Dufour, L. (1993). Bicycle safety programs: Targeting injury prevention through education. *Pediatric Nursing, 19,* 343.

Immediate Assessment

All children with head trauma need an assessment of neurologic function as soon as they are seen and at continuing frequent intervals to detect increased intracranial pressure. Increasing pressure will put pressure on the respiratory, cardiac, and temperature centers and cause dysfunction in these areas. With increased pressure, the pupils become unable to react immediately, both level of consciousness and motor ability decrease, pulse rate decreases, respiratory rate decreases, temperature level increases, and pulse pressure (the distance between systolic and diastolic blood pressure) increases.

Determine vital signs to detect changes in these, and observe children's pupils to be certain that they are equal and react to light. Assess children's level of consciousness (ask children a question they must answer) and motor function (ask children to grasp your fingers and to push against your hands with their feet). Stabilize the neck with a brace until cervical trauma has been ruled out (Rosman, 1990).

Immediate Management

After a head injury, brain edema is likely to occur because fluid rushes into the inflamed and bruised area. A central venous line and arterial line will be established. Intracranial monitoring may be begun (see Chapter 49). A CT scan will be ordered to determine areas of edema or bleeding. An attempt may be made to decrease brain edema by the administration of a hypertonic solution such as mannitol intravenously; this will increase intravascular pressure and cause a shift of edema fluid back into the blood vessels. Steroids such as dexamethasone may be added to decrease inflammation and edema. Intubation and hyperventilation (keeping the PCO_2 below 25 mm HG) is also effective in reducing intracranial pressure.

Nursing Diagnoses and Related Interventions

Nursing Diagnosis: High risk for fluid volume excess related to administration of hypertonic solution

Goal: Increased fluid load will not overtax the child's system during the course of treatment.

Outcome Criteria: The child's respiratory rate remains between 16 to 24 per minute; specific gravity of urine between 1.003 and 1.030; pulse remains between 60 to 100 beats per minute; blood pressure will remain consistent for age group.

When hypertonic solutions are being infused into children, it is important to asses vital signs frequently to be certain that the fluid load being called into the intravascular system does not overtax it. This fluid must be excreted by the kidneys to keep the vascular system from being overloaded. Keep accurate intake and output records, and test the specific gravity of urine to detect the development of pituitary compression and resultant overproduction or underproduction of antidiuretic hormone from the posterior pituitary. Positioning children with their head slightly elevated also helps to decrease cerebral edema (Glaze, 1994).

Nursing Diagnosis: High risk for altered growth and development related to late sequelae of head injury

Goal: Child will maintain normal function following head trauma.

Outcome Criteria: Child shows no evidence of any alteration in thought processes, seizure activity, or memory at follow-up visits; cognitive and physical development are appropriate to age.

Helping care for the child with a head injury may be difficult for parents because they are so worried. Offer information on the child's progress as it is available to you. Urge parents to help care for the child, if possible, to increase their sense of control.

It is important during the acute phase of illness that parents be informed about the dangers of trauma. If they ask about the possibility that personality changes or seizures will develop later in life, their questions should be answered truthfully. At the same time, don't give unnecessary warnings about observing the child carefully in the months to come. Head injuries by themselves are worrisome enough to parents and children without adding to their burden.

Skull Fracture

A skull fracture is a crack in the bone of the skull. It is important that skull fractures be recognized in children, because associated cerebral injury often occurs under the fracture. Many skull fractures are simple linear types, most often involving the parietal bones. In some children, the skull does not fracture, but the suture lines separate. This occurs more commonly in the lambdoid suture line; a coronal suture separation is much more rare and, if present, indicates severe trauma.

Assessment

If the base of the skull is fractured, children generally have orbital or postauricular ecchymosis. They may have rhinorrhea or otorrhea (clear fluid draining from the nose or ear). This is escaping cerebrospinal fluid—a serious finding, because it means the child's central nervous system is open to infection. Nasal discharge may be tested with a glucose reagent strip if there is doubt about the source of the drainage. Cerebrospinal fluid will be positive for glucose, whereas the clear, watery drainage of a beginning upper respiratory tract infection will not.

Skull fractures are confirmed by skull x-ray. Take a careful history of the accident so that the strength of the blow to the head can be judged. Shock rarely occurs with an isolated head injury. If children are in shock, bleeding points other than the head injury should be investigated.

If a skull fracture is linear, with no underlying pathology, no treatment except for observation and prescription of an analgesic is necessary. In about 3 weeks, children need a repeat x-ray to confirm that healing has taken place. Parents can be assured that a second x-ray this soon is not harmful but necessary.

If a fracture is depressed (a bone fragment is pressing inward) or compounded (bone is broken into pieces), surgery will be necessary. Cranial surgery is discussed in Chapter 49.

Therapeutic Management

If there is drainage of cerebrospinal fluid from the nose, children will be hospitalized. Keep them in a semi-Fowler's position so fluid drains out, not inward, to reduce the possibility of introducing infection. Make certain that they do not attempt to hold their nose or pack their nostrils with something to halt the drainage. Coughing and sneezing may allow air to enter the meningeal space, so coughing may be suppressed by medication. If the drainage is excoriating to the upper lip, coat the space with petrolatum. Children may be placed on a prophylactic antibiotic to reduce the danger of meningitis. If the drainage does not stop within a few days, surgery will be necessary to repair the fracture and reduce the danger of meningitis. Air that enters intracranial spaces generally is absorbed rapidly. If x-rays at 72 hours still show air in the cerebral spaces, it implies that a skull defect remains; surgery may be indicated to close the defect.

Potential Complications

A long-term complication of even a linear fracture may be a *leptomeningeal cyst.* This results from projection of the arachnoid membrane into the fracture site. With the interfering tissue, bone cannot heal and actually erodes, so that the fracture site becomes progressively larger, not smaller. This will be evident on a follow-up x-ray. It may be suspected if a child develops focal seizures or symptoms of increased intracranial pressure. The defect may be palpated on the skull as an underlying indentation. Surgical resection will be necessary to remove the cyst.

Subdural Hematoma

Subdural hematoma is venous bleeding into the space between the dura and arachnoid membrane (Figure 52-1*A*). It occurs when head trauma lacerates minute veins in this area. The collection of blood generally is bilateral.

Subdural hematomas tend to occur in infants more than older children. Symptoms may occur within 3 days of trauma or as late as 20 days. Infants generally have symptoms of increased intracranial pressure. Seizures, vomiting, hyperirritability, and enlargement of the head may occur. Anemia from the substantial blood loss is a prominent sign. Angiocardiography or sonogram will reveal the extent of the hematoma.

In infants, accumulated subdural blood may be removed by a subdural puncture through the lateral aspect of a patent anterior fontanelle. The procedure is similar to a lumbar puncture. Infant's heads are shaved over the anterior fontanelle. The site is prepared with an antiseptic solution and draped. A long, thin needle is then inserted through the fontanelle into the subdural space and the collected blood is allowed to drain (Rowe, 1994). Infants must be held extremely still during the procedure so that they do not move and cause the aspiration needle to be inserted incorrectly. Half of the success of subdural puncture depends on the competence of the person holding the child.

Subdural punctures may have to be repeated daily

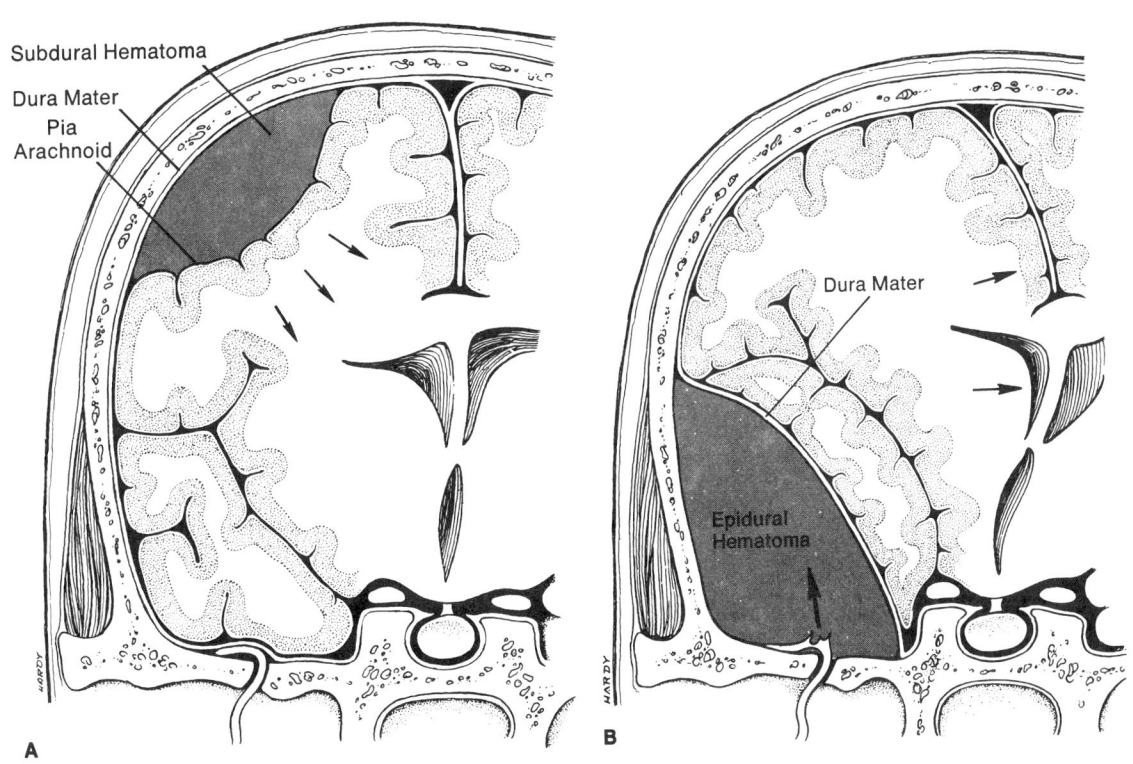

FIGURE 52-1
(**A**) *Subdural hemotoma. The dark area in the upper left area of the drawing is the hematoma. Note the shift of structures.* (**B**) *Epidural hematoma. The dark area in the lower left area of the drawing is the hematoma. Note the broken blood vessel and the shift of midline structures. (From Cosgriff, J. H., & Anderson, D. L. [1975].* The practice of emergency nursing. *Philadelphia: J.B. Lippincott, with permission.)*

to empty the subdural space. When the space is empty, it will be occluded by expanding brain tissue. If the space has not been occluded after 2 weeks of daily punctures, active bleeding is still present, and surgery generally is necessary to reduce the space and halt bleeding.

In older children, surgery generally is necessary because the anterior fontanelle is closed, and the space cannot be reached by puncture.

Epidural Hematoma

Epidural hematoma is bleeding into the space between the dura and the skull (Figure 52-1*B*). It happens when head trauma is severe. Subdural hemorrhage is generally venous bleeding, but epidural hemorrhage is usually a result of rupture of the middle meningeal artery and is arterial bleeding. It is intense and causes rapid brain compression.

At the time of the injury, children are usually momentarily unconscious. They then regain consciousness and, to the untrained eye, appear to be well for minutes or hours. Then signs of cortical compression—vomiting, loss of consciousness, headache, convulsions, or hemiparesis (paralysis on one side)—are observed. On physical examination, unequal dilatation or constriction of

the pupils may be present. Decorticate posturing (spasticity of an arm with the hand fisted and the thumb tucked under the fingers) (see Figure 49-8) may be seen, indicating that there is extreme pressure on upper cortical centers. If the pressure is allowed to continue unchecked, cortical compression may be so great that brain stem, respiratory, or cardiovascular function is impaired.

As a rule, the closer to the time of the injury that symptoms of compression occur, the more extreme is the amount of blood loss. The treatment is surgical removal of the accumulated blood and cauterization or ligation of the torn artery. The earlier the process is recognized and treated, the less is the chance of residual damage from extreme pressure or anoxia to a brain portion.

Concussion

Concussion is defined as a head injury from a hard, jarring shock. Concussion may occur on the side of the skull that was struck (a *coup injury*) or on the opposite side of the brain (a **contrecoup injury**; Figure 52-2). As the brain recoils from the force of the blow and strikes the posterior surface of the skull, this second injury occurs. Children have at least a transient loss of conscious-

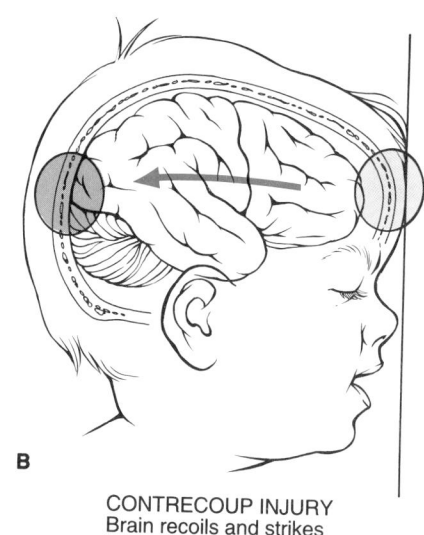

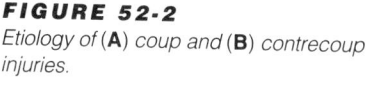

FIGURE 52-2
Etiology of (A) coup and (B) contrecoup injuries.

COUP INJURY
Anterior of brain strikes skull and is injured

CONTRECOUP INJURY
Brain recoils and strikes posterior skull, so is injured twice

ness at the time of the injury. They may vomit and may show irritability after regaining consciousness. They may have a convulsion within minutes of the trauma. They typically have no memory (amnesia) of the events leading up to the injury or at the time of injury. For some children, being asked questions about the accident is extremely upsetting because they do not remember anything that happened and feel a frightening loss of control. The child requires a skull radiograph to rule out skull fracture and observation for 24 hours to rule out severe brain trauma, edema, or laceration. The child usually can be observed at home by the parents, who are instructed to rouse him or her every 1 to 2 hours to check the level of consciousness.

To be certain that children are alert, they should be asked to name a familiar object, such as a favorite toy, or to name the color of some object shown to them. Telling parents their name or where they live is equally revealing. Occasionally, parents are instructed not to keep waking children because multiple wakings are disorienting and can be confused with unconsciousness. Parents should wake the child at least once during the night, however, and assess that the pulse rate is more than 60 beats per minute.

Give parents the telephone number to call if they have any questions about their child's care. Advise them to call if their child's behavior changes in any way that makes them suspicious. Many parents will need to set an alarm clock to wake themselves every 2 hours during the night to assess their child's status. There is an old belief that if children fall asleep following a head injury, they will die in their sleep; thus, some parents may keep shaking children awake or make them walk continuously. Be certain they understand that it is all right for children to sleep, but they must wake them at least once

to assess their status. It is not sleeping that kills children following a head injury but the unnoticed neurologic symptoms that develop while they sleep.

Contusion

A brain contusion occurs when there is tearing or laceration of brain tissue (Figure 52-3). The symptoms are the same as for concussion except they are more severe. In addition, there are specific symptoms related to the lacerated brain area (focal seizure, eye deviation, loss of speech). Surgery may be necessary to halt bleeding. The child's prognosis depends on the extent of the injury and effectiveness of therapy.

Coma

Coma (unconsciousness from which children cannot be roused) or **stupor** (grogginess from which children can be roused) may be present in children following severe head trauma. Coma and stupor are both symptoms of underlying disorders; a history of injury must be obtained so that treatment can be directed specifically toward the cause.

Obtain a history to determine the circumstances immediately prior to the time the child became comatose. Assess children in coma carefully and completely so that the cause of the decreased consciousness can quickly be determined.

Assessment

Although head injury is most likely to be the underlying cause of coma, seizure, metabolic disturbances such as diabetes mellitus, dehydration, severe hemorrhage, or drug ingestion also must be considered as possible

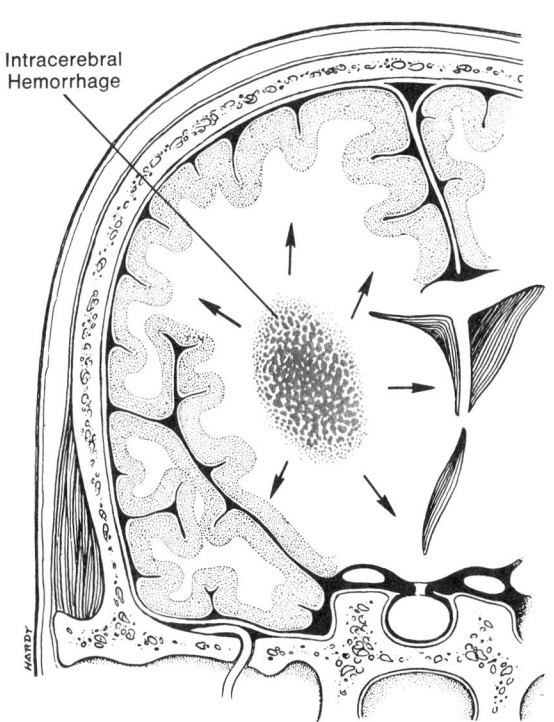

Intracerebral
Hemorrhage

FIGURE 52-3
Intracerebral hemorrhage. The central large dark area represents the hemorrhage. Note the midline shift. (From Cosgriff, J. H., & Anderson, D. L. [1975]. The practice of emergency nursing. Philadelphia: J.B. Lippincott, with permission.)

causes. Vital signs often provide good clues. A child with increased intracranial pressure will show a decreased pulse rate, decreased respiratory rate, and increased blood pressure. Diabetes leads to increased respirations. Hemorrhage leads to an increased pulse rate and a decreased blood pressure. Drug ingestion may lead to increased or decreased measurements, depending on the drug ingested.

Undress children completely so that all body parts can be inspected. Irregular breathing such as hyperventilation may occur from medullary pressure from brain injury. If bulbar (brain stem) compression is present, children cannot swallow effectively or safely. Turn them on the side to keep from aspirating saliva. Count respirations and pulse and measure blood pressure to establish baseline values. Observe for eye signs of increased intracranial pressure. If both pupils are dilated, irreversible brain stem damage is suggested, although such a finding may be present with poisoning from an atropine-like drug. Pinpoint pupils suggest barbiturate or opiate intoxication. One pupil dilated more than the other suggests third cranial nerve damage. The eye may be deviated downward and laterally as well. This may be caused by a tentorial tear (the membrane between the cerebellum and cerebrum) and herniation of the temporal lobe into the torn membrane. This situation requires immediate surgery to correct temporal compression.

The retina of the eye should be examined for papilledema. If increased pressure is long-standing (more than 24 to 48 hours), papilledema will be present; if the increased pressure is of a shorter duration, papilledema may not be present. Lack of a doll's eye reflex (when the child's head is suddenly moved one way, the eyes move in the opposite direction) suggests that compression of the oculomotor nerves (third, fourth, or sixth) or the brain stem is involved. Observe for posturing, such as a decerebrate sign (see Figure 49-8), that suggests cerebral compression and dysfunction.

Coma is usually graded according to a standard scale so changes can be evaluated accurately. Figure 52-4 shows a Glasgow scale, a commonly used evaluation system. As this system was devised to be an adult assessment scale, it must be modified for use with children; such a modification is shown in Box 52-1.

A score of 3–8 suggests severe trauma (under 5 carries a very severe prognosis); a score of 9–12, moderate trauma; and 13–15, slight trauma. A number of laboratory studies are helpful in determining the cause of coma. Blood glucose, blood electrolytes, blood urea nitrogen (BUN), liver function tests, blood gas studies, lumbar puncture, and toxicology tests may be ordered to rule out bacterial meningitis or hemorrhage.

Therapeutic Management

If children are unconscious for more than a transient period, they generally are admitted to the hospital for observation. Place children who are comatose on their side so that saliva drains from their mouths and tracheal aspiration does not occur. They may need oral suction to remove mucous from their mouths and pharynx. If children have acute signs of respiration difficulty, they may be intubated or have a tracheotomy done to ensure respiratory function.

An intravenous route is established so that when specific measures are determined (blood replacement, electrolyte replacement, fluid replacement), a route for immediate administration will be available. Blood will be drawn for a complete blood count, electrolyte determination, toxicology tests, and crossmatching. If the cause of the coma is unknown, a lumbar puncture and EEG may be done. Skull x-rays or a computed tomography scan may be taken.

Lumbar puncture has little value at first in predicting the severity of a head injury, because any degree of cerebral contusion generally leads to an increased cerebrospinal fluid pressure, and lumbar punctures cannot be done with increased intracranial pressure or brain stem compression can result. Children's vital signs and also their neurologic signs, such as state of consciousness and the ability of pupils to react to light, should be taken every 15 to 20 minutes. These must be taken accurately and recorded carefully so that a picture of gradual change will become apparent.

Glasgow Coma Scale			A.M.	P.M.						A.M.					
Assessment	Reaction	Score	8	10	12	2	4	6	8	10	12	2	4	6	8
Eye Opening Response	Spontaneously	4	X							X	X	X	X	X	
	To speech	3		X				X							
	To pain	2			X	X	X								
	No response	1													
Motor Response	Obeys verbal command	6	X							X	X	X	X	X	
	Localizes pain	5		X	X										
	Flexion withdrawal	4				X		X							
	Flexion	3					X								
	Extension	2													
	No response	1													
Verbal Response	Oriented ×3	5	X							X	X	X	X	X	
	Conversation confused	4		X				X							
	Inappropriate speech	3			X										
	Incomprehensible sounds	2				X	X								
	No response	1													

FIGURE 52-4

Glasgow Coma Scale scoring for a child. A score of 3 to 8 denotes severe trauma; 9 to 12, moderate trauma; 13 to 15, slight trauma. Notice the gradual improvement from coma in this example.

A child's prognosis following coma depends on the initial cause of the coma. If the increased intracranial pressure can be relieved before any permanent brain damage results, the effects of the coma will be transient. Prognosis is always guarded, however, because coma in itself reflects a major health problem to children.

Nursing Diagnoses and Related Interventions

Care of the child in coma is directed toward maintaining body function in an optimum state until the child reawakens.

Nursing Diagnosis: High risk for ineffective airway clearance related to brain stem pressure

Goal: Child's airway will remain unobstructed during course of illness.

Outcome Criteria: Child's respiratory rate is between 16 and 20 breaths per minute; no retraction or sound of obstruction is present.

Some children who are comatose will have an endotracheal tube or tracheotomy placed to ensure an open airway. Some will be placed on ventilator care. Maintaining the PCO_2 level below 30 mm Hg may help reduce cerebral edema. Oxygen may be prescribed if blood gases do not reveal good oxygenation of body cells (PO_2 below 55 mm Hg). Endotracheal tubes are replaced with a tracheotomy after 3 or 4 days to prevent necrosis of the pharynx from pressure of the tube.

Nursing Diagnosis: High risk for impaired skin integrity related to lack of mobility

Goal: Skin will remain intact during the period of coma.

Outcome Criteria: No areas of broken or irritated skin are present.

Bathe children who are comatose daily to stimulate skin circulation. Include the hair as part of the bath about every 3 days. Position for a comatose child should always be on the side or abdomen, to prevent aspiration from pooling unswallowed mouth secretions. Some children need oral suction to remove this danger. Change position at least every 2 hours, so that pressure points to skin do not develop and hydrostatic pneumonia from pooled secretions does not occur. When turning, assess skin for reddened points and massage the areas to increase circulation to the part. Keep linen dry and free from wrinkles. Passive range-of-motion exercises help to maintain muscle tone and prevent contractures, if done about three times a day. Be certain that exercises are thorough, not merely including a few motions. Without thoroughness, this type of exercise does not prevent

Box 52-1
Scoring for Glasgow Coma Scale

Eye Opening

4. Child opens his or her eyes spontaneously when you approach.
3. Child opens his or her eyes in response to speech (spoken or shouted).
2. Child opens his or her eyes only in response to painful stimuli such as pressure on a nail bed.
1. Child does not open his or her eyes in response to painful stimuli.

Motor Response

6. Child can obey a simple command such as "hand me a toy" (infant smiles or attunes).
5. Child moves an extremity to locate a painful stimuli applied to the head or trunk and attempts to remove the source.
4. Child attempts to withdraw from the source of pain.
3. Child flexes his or her arms at the elbows and wrists in response to painful stimuli to the nail beds (decorticate rigidity).
2. Child extends his or her arms (straightens the elbows) in response to painful stimuli (cerebrate rigidity).
1. Child has no motor response to pain on any extremity.

Verbal Response

5. Child is oriented to time, place, and person (child over age 4 years knows name, date, and where he or she is; infant appears to recognize parent).
4. Child is able to converse, although not oriented to time, place, or person (does not know who or where he or she is; infant says words but does not appear to differentiate parents from others).
3. Child speaks only in words or phrases that make little or no sense ("I want frazzle no"; infant's vocabulary is less than it is normally).
2. Child responds with incomprehensible sounds, such as groans.
1. Child does not respond verbally at all.

Source: Modified from Teasdale, G., & Bennett, B. (1974). Assessment of coma and impaired consciousness: A practical scale. *Lancet, 2,* 81.

contractures and wastes nursing time. Using sheepskin, an egg carton, or an alternating pressure mattress also can be important in decreasing pressure points.

Nursing Diagnosis: High risk for altered nutrition, less than body requirements, related to inability to take oral food or fluid

Goal: Child will remain well nourished during period of coma.

Outcome Criteria: Child's skin turgor is normal; there is no loss of weight; urine output remains over 2 to 3 mL/kg/h.

Children who are unconscious cannot be fed orally or they might aspirate. Nutrition, therefore, must be maintained by nasogastric feedings, gastrostomy tube, intravenous fluid, or total parenteral nutrition. Intravenous fluid is only a short-term answer as adequate protein and fat cannot be supplied solely by this route. Nasogastric feedings or gastrostomy is effective. Always aspirate the tube for stomach contents before giving a feeding to assess that the child is digesting the prescribed amount of feedings and to check placement of the tube. Always return any amount of stomach residue aspirated because if this is discarded each time, the child will lose a large amount of stomach acid, possibly leading to alkalosis. Check whether the amount of the feeding should be reduced by the amount of fluid remaining in the stomach before feeding the full amount of prescribed formula.

Give mouth care at least twice daily with clear water and a padded tongue blade. Coat lips with petrolatum to prevent drying and cracking. If the child's eyes tend to dry, close them to prevent corneal ulceration. Artificial tears (methylcellulose) may be prescribed to keep eyes from drying. Gauze patches over eyes will keep them closed and moist.

Abdominal Trauma

When children are brought to a health care facility after suffering multiple trauma, several medical specialists may be called to see them: a neurosurgeon for consultation about a head injury; an orthopedic physician for consultation about a fractured extremity; a thoracic surgeon to intubate or investigate lung trauma. The nurse may serve the important function as the person who is best able to observe a total child and recognize subtle signs of abdominal trauma.

Assessment

Abdominal trauma can result from an object such as a knife or metal fence post penetrating the abdomen (Plaisier et al., 1993). In young children, abdominal trauma is generally nonpenetrating and occurs from a direct blow to the abdomen from an object such as a baseball bat or an automobile dashboard. All children who have multiple trauma such as happens in automobile accidents need observation for abdominal injury (Grant, 1992). Monitor vital signs frequently until they are stable.

Hypotension (under 80 mm Hg systolic pressure in older children; under 60 mm Hg in infants) generally suggests hemorrhage, which may well be hidden abdominal bleeding. In addition, children may have increasing pallor and rapid respirations. Blood pressure will show little improvement when intravenous fluid is administered if internal bleeding is present.

When abdominal trauma is suspected, a nasogastric tube is passed and a syringeful of stomach contents aspirated to be checked visually for blood as well as tested for occult blood. Attach the tube to low suction if the presence of blood is established. A Foley catheter is next passed so urine can be examined for blood. This may indicate accompanying kidney or bladder trauma. If the urine contains blood, an emergency intravenous pyelogram may be ordered. Be aware that having nasogastric tubes or catheters passed is always frightening for children (unsure of their anatomy, they have no clear idea where the tubes are going); following an accident, when they are already frightened, they need a great deal of support to accept this.

An abdominal x-ray may be ordered to rule out a fractured pelvis, a condition that could contribute to blood loss. Air under the diaphragm on the x-ray suggests gastric or intestinal rupture and escape of air from these organs into the peritoneal cavity. Free fluid in the abdomen, shown on x-ray when children are turned on their side, suggests leakage of bowel fluid or splenic rupture and pooling of blood. If the x-ray does not suggest the source of the fluid, an abdominal paracentesis may be done. This procedure is very frightening to children not only because it is intrusive but also because children's abdomens are likely to be tender. Parents may be so frightened by the sight of the procedure that they are unable to remain with a child while this is done. A nurse, therefore, needs to be present to offer this main support.

For a paracentesis, children are placed in a sitting or side-lying position; their abdomen is cleaned with an antiseptic and covered with a sterile drape. Caution children that they will feel a pinprick as a local anesthetic is inserted into their abdominal wall. They will feel pressure as the paracentesis needle is inserted (Figure 52-5) but no more pain or pressure after that. Appreciate children's concern. It is almost impossible for them to lie still while the procedure is being done. Comments such as, "Don't cry. Be a good boy," are not therapeutic. "It's all right to cry; I know this is scary," is much more comforting and achieves better results, because it lets children know that you understand what you are asking of them.

It is often difficult for parents to appreciate the seriousness of abdominal trauma, because the signs are not as dramatic or obvious as those of fractured extremities or lacerations. They may ask why an x-ray is necessary. When children are asked to turn on the x-ray table so that an abdominal fluid level can be revealed, they may

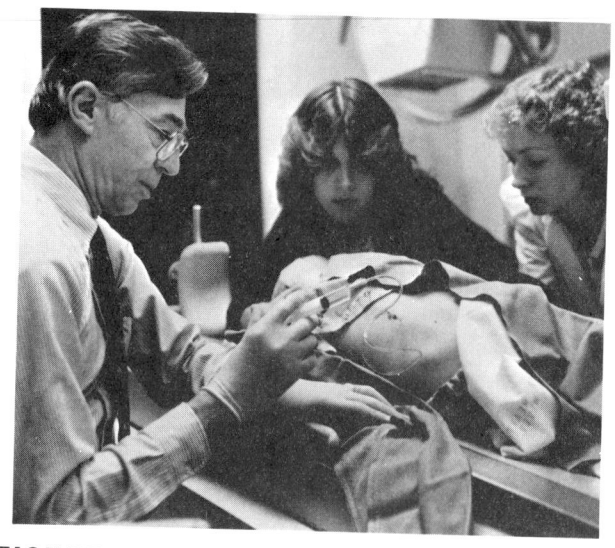

FIGURE 52-5
Abdominal paracentesis. Children require support and comfort during this procedure. (Courtesy of the Department of Medical Photography, Children's Hospital, Buffalo, NY.)

perceive this as unnecessary manipulation of an injured child. Some parents may not bring a child to an emergency department immediately following abdominal trauma, because they are unaware that serious injury can result to this part of the body. Without frightening them, explain that an injury need not be obvious at first glance to be serious and to need care.

Nursing Diagnoses and Related Interventions

Nursing Diagnosis: Pain related to abdominal injury

Goal: Child will experience a tolerable level of pain during period of recovery.

Outcome Criteria: Child states that level of pain is tolerable; does not grimace when thinks he or she is not being observed.

Most children with abdominal trauma have pain because they are not routinely administered an analgesic following abdominal trauma so the location of the pain can help to identify which organs may be injured. If parents did not recognize that the child was injured, guilt and fear compound the problem. Goal setting is usually concerned with the immediate diagnostic procedures or surgery that is anticipated. Interventions differ according to the specific injury present.

Splenic Rupture

The spleen is the organ most frequently injured in abdominal trauma because in children this is usually palpable under the lower rib. Children with splenic injury will have tenderness in the left upper quadrant. They notice this especially on deep inspiration, when the diaphragm moves down and touches the spleen. They may hold their left shoulder elevated to keep the diaphragm raised on the left side to keep this from happening. Occasionally, children will notice radiated left shoulder pain when they lie in a supine position (Kehr's sign). An abdominal x-ray will show little about the spleen itself but perhaps will reveal a broken rib over the spleen, suggesting the extent of the trauma to that area. Fluid in the abdomen will suggest bleeding from some source. Obtaining blood on abdominal paracentesis strongly suggests splenic rupture.

An intravenous line is immediately placed to begin fluid replacement and an intravenous pyelogram will be done to rule out damage to the left kidney, which, because of its location in that area, probably also suffered trauma. A complete blood count is done to estimate the extent of the blood loss. Blood is typed and crossmatched so blood for replacement can then be readied if necessary. Children will be admitted to a hospital unit for observation if the blood loss from rupture appears mild; they will be scheduled for immediate surgery if the blood loss is severe. Partial or total splenectomy may be necessary to halt bleeding and save their life.

If a spleen is removed, children are very susceptible to infection, particularly pneumococci infections, afterward. Following splenectomy, therefore, most children are immunized with pneumococci vaccine to prevent this possibility.

Liver Rupture

Children with liver rupture or laceration usually have severe abdominal pain, most marked on inspiration when the diaphragm descends and touches the liver. They show symptoms of blood loss: tachycardia, hypotension, anxiety, and pallor. Their hematocrit value will be low or falling. Such children need to be prepared for immediate surgery, because the liver is a highly vascular organ and blood loss from it is acute and damaging.

Occasionally, a communication between an artery and a bile duct occurs at the time of trauma. With this, symptoms are not immediate, but gastrointestinal (GI) bleeding, such as hematemesis, or melena may occur in a few days. The child may have colicky upper abdominal pain that may be relieved by emesis. Liver studies, such as a liver arteriogram, will be necessary to reveal the extent of the problem.

Following both liver and spleen surgery, children need careful observation for return of bowel function, assessment for the possibility that peritonitis may develop, and careful reintroduction of oral nutrition.

Dental Trauma

Injuries to teeth occur most often from falls in which children strike their upper front incisors and from blows to the face by objects such as baseball bats or hockey sticks. They are always potentially serious as they can lead to aspiration or malalignment of future teeth (Krasner, 1992).

When a tooth is knocked out, parents should rinse the tooth in water and replace it in the child's mouth or drop the tooth in a salt solution or milk and bring it to the emergency department with them. If permanent teeth that have been knocked out recently are washed with saline in the emergency department and replaced, there is a good chance that they will reimplant successfully. Some dentists advocate immersing the tooth in an antiseptic and then an antibiotic solution before replacing it. If a tooth is replaced, it generally is wired into place to hold it in good alignment. Children receive a 10-day course of oral penicillin to prevent infection. They must eat only soft food until the tooth has firmly adhered.

If a blow to a child's teeth was extensive, an x-ray may be taken to rule out a mandibular or maxillary fracture. If a portion of a tooth cannot be located, the possibility of aspiration must be considered and confirmed or ruled out by a chest x-ray. In young children, often a tooth is not knocked out but is pushed back up into the gum. These teeth gradually regrow, and although they may darken in color, they usually are healthy. If the affected tooth is a deciduous tooth, the permanent tooth is rarely injured even though it is already formed in the gum. At the appropriate time, the permanent tooth will erupt normally.

Near Drowning

Drowning is defined as death due to suffocation from submersion in liquid. Inhaled water fills and therefore blocks the exchange of oxygen in the alveoli. More than 3500 children die from drowning annually. The term **near drowning** is used to describe the person with a submersion injury who requires emergency treatment and who survives the first 24 hours postinjury (Norris, 1993).

Drowning accidents occur most frequently in the summer months, when more children are swimming and boating. Toddlers and preschool-age children who cannot swim are the most frequent victims of drowning and near-drowning accidents, although children (and adults) of all ages and swimming abilities are at risk. Small children may fall into neighborhood swimming pools or adolescents may take dares to swim farther than their ability or swim under the influence of alcohol, which impairs their decision-making ability as well as their physical coordination.

Pathophysiology of Drowning

If children hyperventilate prior to swimming underwater, excess carbon dioxide is blown off; during an extended period of underwater swimming, carbon dioxide levels rise, but not adequately to cause children to experience distress. This results in decreased oxygen levels with drowsiness and listlessness (children drown without struggling or realizing their danger).

When children first inhale water, they cough violently from the irritation of the water in their nose and throat. If children cannot get their head out of water at that point, water will enter the larynx. The larynx will go into spasm, preventing any air from entering the trachea, and asphyxia will result. If children are ventilated at this point, treatment generally is very effective because there is little water in the lungs; the condition more closely simulates the asphyxia that occurs with croup or when a foreign body, such as a nut, lodges in the larynx and stops air flow.

If treatment is not given at this point (if children are not discovered and taken out of the water immediately), the larynx relaxes from the asphyxia, and water enters the lungs. Children can no longer exchange oxygen, because the alveoli fill with water. Hypoxia deepens, and cardiac arrest occurs.

Additional changes that occur when water enters the lungs depend on whether the water is fresh or salt. The osmotic pressure of the hypertonic salt solution in salt water causes fluid to diffuse from the bloodstream and enter the alveoli, increasing the amount of fluid in the lung tissue. Tachycardia and decreased blood pressure from hypovolemia will result; blood viscosity will be increased (increased hematocrit level); the presence of pulmonary edema will cause increased hypoxia. In fresh water, which is hypotonic, fluid in the lungs is absorbed into the bloodstream (Figure 52-6). This may lead to hemolysis of red blood cells, a dilution of plasma, and

possible hypervolemia with tachycardia and increased blood pressure. If the release of potassium from destroyed red blood cells is great enough with fresh-water drowning, cardiac arrhythmias may occur. In both instances, loss of surfactant from the lung alveoli, caused by introduction of water, will cause alveolar collapse.

Very young children display a mammalian diving reflex when they plunge under cold water: immediately, a life-saving bradycardia and shunting of blood away from the periphery of their body to their brain and heart occurs. This is triggered when water is 70°F (21°C) or less and their face is submerged first. If the water is very cold (0°C to 15°C; 32°F to 60°F), children have fully recovered after being submerged up to 40 minutes.

Emergency Management

When children are pulled from the water following drowning, mouth-to-mouth resuscitation should be started at once. If cardiac arrest has occurred with the hypoxia, simultaneous measures to initiate cardiac action must be taken. The techniques of cardiopulmonary resuscitation for infants and children are discussed in Chapter 41.

Assuming that cardiopulmonary resuscitation is effective, children next need follow-up care at a health care facility, because they are certain to be acidotic from accumulated PCO_2 and hypoxic from lack of oxygen because of the water in the alveoli.

Follow-up care aims to increase children's oxygen and carbon dioxide exchange capacity, using the lung areas that are not filled with water. Children are intubated with a cuffed intratracheal tube; mechanical ventilation with positive end-expiratory pressure may be necessary to force air into the alveoli. Because children swallow as well as aspirate water, vomiting usually occurs as the child is revived. The cuff of the intratracheal tube prevents vomitus from being aspirated. Children are given 100% oxygen so that as much space as possible in the available lung alveoli can be used. Generally, either isoproterenol, albuterol, or racemic epinephrine is administered by aerosol to prevent bronchospasm and, again, to allow children to make maximum use of the oxygen administered. Intravenous aminophylline may also be used to discourage inflammation. If a child aspirated salt water, plasma may be administered to replace protein loss into the lungs and prevent hypovolemia.

If the child's body temperature is very low, gradual warming (not using a warming blanket) is advised so metabolism need does not rise sharply before alveolar space is ready to accommodate this. Extracorporeal membrane oxygenation may be used (Kallas & O'Rourke, 1993).

Unfortunately, neurologic damage occurs in as many as 21% of near-drowning incidents. If the child is

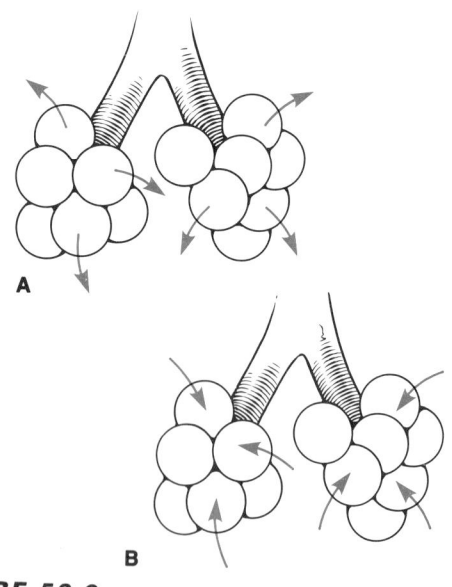

FIGURE 52-6
*The differing fluid shifts in lung alveoli after drowning: (**A**) fresh water; (**B**) salt water.*

awake or only lethargic at the scene of the accident and immediately afterward in the hospital, the prognosis is greatly improved over that of the child who is comatose.

Nursing Diagnoses and Related Interventions

Nursing Diagnosis: High risk for infection related to foreign substance in respiratory tract

Goal: No symptoms of infection will develop following near drowning.

Outcome Criteria: Child's temperature remains below 37.0°C orally; no rales are present on lung auscultation.

Children may be placed on a prophylactic antibiotic to prevent pneumonia and additional airway interference. Assess vital signs and auscultate lung sounds for adventitious sounds, such as rales or fine rhonchi. Turning the child every 2 hours if on bedrest and encouraging deep breathing every hour helps to aerate the lungs fully and prevent the accumulation of fluid, which invites infection.

Nursing Diagnosis: Fear related to near-drowning experience

Goal: Child will demonstrate that he or she can manage this degree of fear.

Outcome Criteria: Child discusses fears; states that he or she understands that, although frightening, the experience is over and he or she is now safe.

Children must be admitted to the hospital for observation and for monitoring of blood gases until water from the alveoli is absorbed and they once again can ventilate effectively on their own. Children may wake at night while in the hospital from a nightmare that they are drowning. They need frequent reassurance that they are now all right and definitely out of the water. Near-drowning is a thoroughly frightening experience. Children need to verbalize this fright. They will need support from parents before they will go swimming again after such a frightening experience.

Poisoning

Poisoning occurs most commonly between the ages of 2 and 3 years and in children in all socioeconomic groups. Common agents in childhood poisoning are soaps, detergents or cleaners, and plants. It can occur from over-the-counter drugs such as vitamins, iron compounds, aspirin or acetaminophen, or prescription drugs such as antidepressants (Morelli, 1993). Poisoning is entirely preventable. Parents must be educated regarding the high

risk for poisoning and strategies for maintaining a home environment that is safe for children of all ages.

Nursing Diagnoses and Related Interventions

Nursing Diagnosis: High risk for poisoning related to maturational age of child

Goal: Child will not ingest a poison during childhood; if so, help is sought immediately.

Outcome Criteria: Parents identify poisonous/ toxic items in the home and describe how they are stored safely; they know local poison control center number.

Emergency Management of Poisoning at Home. Teach parents that if they discover that a child has swallowed a poison, they should immediately call the emergency number in their community used by the poison control center. Information they need to provide is the child's name, telephone number, address, weight, and age. How long before did the poisoning occur? What was the route of poisoning (oral, inhaled, sprayed on skin)? How much of the poison has the child taken? This is often difficult for parents to judge as they don't know how much was in the bottle. If they just answer, "a whole bottle," ask them to read from the bottle how much that is. If the poison was in pill form, are there pills scattered under a chair, or are they all missing and presumed swallowed? What was swallowed? If the name of a medicine is not known, ask what it was prescribed for and a description of it (color, size, shape of pills). Determine the child's present condition (sleepy? hyperactive? comatose?). If one child has swallowed a poison, parents must investigate whether other children have also poisoned themselves. A preschooler often gives a younger sibling some of the "candy" he or she has been eating. Ask if parents have transportation to the health care facility or if they need an ambulance.

Parents should keep a bottle of syrup of ipecac (an emetic) with their emergency first aid supplies (see Focus on Nursing Care box). Before they administer this emetic, however, they should call a poison control center to make certain that vomiting is desirable. Unless the poison was a caustic, corrosive, or a hydrocarbon, vomiting is the most effective way to remove the poison from the body—more effective even than lavage. The recommended dosages of syrup of ipecac parents should administer are 15 mL to an adolescent, school-age child, or preschooler; and 10 mL to an infant (15 mL = 1 tbsp; 5 mL = 1 tsp). This should be followed by about 200 mL (or about 1 cup) of fluid. It is important to give the fluid so that the child has something to vomit effectively. The type of fluid is unimportant; the parents should offer whatever fluid they think the child will drink most readily. In 90% of children, vomiting will

FOCUS ON NURSING CARE

Drugs Used to Counteract Poisoning

Ipecac Syrup

Action: An oral emetic to cause vomiting after drug overdose or poisoning.

If poisoning occurs, telephone the nearest poison control center for instructions before administering drug, because not all poisons should be vomited. Dosage: Children < 1 year: 5–10 mL followed by 1 glass of water. Repeat dosage one time if vomiting does not occur in 20 min.

Nursing Implications:

1. Ipecac syrup will not be effective if the swallowed substance is an antiemetic. This will cause absorption of the ipecac syrup and possible cardiac arrhythmia.

2. Do not administer if swallowed substance would be harmful when vomited, such as a caustic lye.

3. Administer before activated charcoal is given because the charcoal will inactivate ipecac syrup.

4. Caution adolescents that ipecac syrup should not be used to induce vomiting as a weight-reduction measure. It has extreme cardiotoxic properties when used frequently that can lead to arrhythmia and death.

EDTA (edetate calcium disodium)

Action: A chelating agent to reduce level of blood serum and deposited stores of lead through excretion in urine. Dosage: 50 to 75 mg/kg/day in 2–4 divided dosages. Add 1% procaine 0.5 mL to injection to minimize pain at injection site.

Nursing Implications:

1. Because drug is excreted in urine, assess that specific gravity of urine is within normal range (1.003–1.030) before administering.

2. Give deep IM in large muscle group to help reduce pain of injection.

3. Check drug label carefully. Edeteate disodium is also a calcium chelating agent with almost same name.

---

occur within 20 minutes. If vomiting does not occur in 30 minutes, another dose of ipecac can be given. Parents should, however, begin transport to a health care facility for follow-up treatment as soon as the first dose of ipecac is given.

If parents do not have ipecac in the house, making children vomit by placing a finger in the back of the throat (gagging them) is effective. Administering a substance such as mustard is rarely effective, because children will not swallow enough of it to serve as an emetic. Administering a "universal antidote" of burned toast,

milk of magnesia, and charcoal is not nearly as effective as induced vomiting, so it should not be tried. Ask parents to bring any vomited material to the health care facility with them so it can be analyzed for content.

Emergency Management of Poisoning at the Health Care Facility. At the health care facility, further removal of the poison may be carried out by gastric lavage. For this, a large-bore nasogastric tube is passed through the nares into the stomach. Approximately 50 to 100 mL of saline is flushed into the tube and then aspirated; this procedure is continued until the return is clear. When lavaging, always place the first specimen returned in a separate specimen container or emesis basin to save for a toxicology analysis. Later specimens are often too dilute for an analysis of them to be effective (Nursing Procedure 52-1).

After lavage, activated charcoal may be administered, either through the lavage tube or orally. Activated charcoal is supplied as a fine black powder that is mixed with water for administration. It combines with the poison and inactivates it. As the charcoal is excreted through the bowel over the next 3 days, stools will appear black. Never administer activated charcoal before ipecac as it will inactivate the ipecac. Never administer it if acetylcysteine (Mucomyst; the specific antidote for acetaminophen poisoning) will be used, as charcoal inactivates acetylcysteine.

Yet another way to speed removal of a poison from the body is to administer a saline cathartic. Saline cathartics are harsh laxatives, however, so are used with caution in young children as severe dehydration and electrolyte imbalance could occur.

Always follow emergency measures with an education program to prevent poisoning from happening again. Specific measures for each age group are shown in earlier chapters with problems and concerns of the age group.

Salicylate Poisoning

About 25% of childhood poisonings are salicylate (aspirin) poisonings, although this percentage is decreasing because of safety packaging and less use of aspirin for childhood fever (to prevent Reye's syndrome).

Assessment

An overdose of salicylate causes a myriad of metabolic consequences: increased metabolic rate, interference with the utilization of carbohydrate, decreased prothrombin production, and stimulation of the respiratory center of the brain, causing hyperventilation (hyperpnea and tachypnea). Hyperventilation will lead to respiratory alkalosis as excessive amounts of carbon dioxide are "blown off." Because of the increased metabolic rate and an inability to utilize carbohydrates, the body begins to

---

NURSING PROCEDURE 52-1
Gastric Lavage

Purpose
To dilute and remove toxic contents from the stomach

Procedure	*Principle*
1. Wash your hands; identify the child; explain the procedure.	1. Prevents spread of microorganisms; encourages client compliance and cooperation.
2. Assess child for current status; analyze appropriateness of procedure.	2. If child is vomiting, stomach lavage may be unnecessary. Lavage should not be begun if the ingested substance was a flammable liquid or caustic until an antidote is administered.
3. Implement procedure by organizing supplies: nasogastric (NG) tube, normal saline, basin, tape, asepto or barrel syringe with catheter tip.	3. Organization speeds emergency care.
4. Restrain child as necessary. Pass NG tube into stomach using usual technique, then position child on side with head slightly elevated. Aspirate all stomach contents possible.	4. Aspirating before diluting stomach allows you to secure a sample of the contents for laboratory analysis. Positioning on side reduces possibility of aspiration if child vomits.
5. Remove plunger from syringe; attach barrel to NG tube, and elevate about 12 in over the child's stomach level.	5. Proper technique allows procedure to be carried out efficiently.
6. Pour a designated amount of irrigating solution into syringe; allow it to flow into the stomach by gravity.	6. Don't force irrigating solution into the stomach as this might force the poison into the small intestine or cause vomiting with aspiration.
7. Remove the syringe and lower the end of the NG tube. Allow the stomach contents to drain by gravity into the basin. If necessary, attach syringe and apply gentle suction.	7. Aspiration can injure the stomach lining if the catheter rests against the stomach wall. Notify the child's physician if the return fluid is bloody as it suggests a caustic poison.
8. Repeat the procedure until the stomach contents return clear (about 10 times).	8. It is important to remove as much of the toxic contents as possible.
9. Remove the NG tube. Position the child comfortably.	9. Keeping the child on the side helps prevent aspiration if further vomiting occurs.
10. Evaluate procedure in terms of effectiveness, cost, and efficiency. Record the type and amount of irrigating solution used and the child's reaction to the procedure.	10. Evaluation allows the nurse to determine whether procedure has been successful. Documentation allows further follow-up based on previous results.
11. Plan health teaching such as safe rules for household poisons.	11. Health teaching is an independent nursing action always included in care and will help prevent future accidents.

---

use protein and fat sources for energy; this causes the initial alkalosis to be quickly replaced by metabolic acidosis. The increased metabolism will also lead to a high fever and dehydration. Within 2 hours of ingestion, children have marked tachycardia, tachypnea, and perhaps hypoglycemia. They may have fever, vomiting, and diarrhea. They may have central nervous system signs such as restlessness, stupor, convulsions, or coma. Because salicylate also interferes with the formation of prothrombin, areas of purpura may appear on the child's skin. Irritation to the gastric lining may lead to stomach ulcer.

Tinnitus (ringing in the ears), a specific toxic effect of salicylate overdose, may occur.

Symptoms increase in severity, depending on the amount of aspirin ingested (Table 52-3). Symptoms begin when children ingest 150 to 200 mg of salicylate per kilogram of body weight. The peak blood level is reached within 2 to 3 hours of ingestion.

A simple test for detecting salicylate poisoning is to test a urine specimen with a strip of Phenistix. If there is salicylate secretion in the urine, the strip will turn brownish purple. Phenistix may also be used as a quick

Table 52-3. *Levels of Salicylate Poisoning*

Dose Ingested (mg/kg)	Symptoms
<150	None
150–300	Mild to moderate hyperpnea, lethargy and excitability, metabolic acidosis that can be compensated
300–500	Severe tachypnea and hyperventilation; possible convulsions; uncompensated metabolic acidosis; pyrexia
>500	Coma, uncompensated metabolic acidosis; convulsions, severe pyrexia

test of blood serum. If the strip turns tan when a blood sample is placed on it, the serum salicylate level is less than 70 mg/100 mL; if purple, the serum level is more than 70 mg/100 mL.

Therapeutic Management

With salicylate poisoning, parents should administer syrup of ipecac to induce vomiting. If a child has not vomited by the time he or she is seen at a health care facility, a repeat dose of ipecac or gastric lavage will be initiated.

Next, implementations are begun to support metabolic and respiratory function and encourage salicylate elimination. If the serum salicylate level is more than 50 mg/100 mL, children usually are admitted to a health care facility for observation. Offer fluid orally to dilute the poison and prevent dehydration. If children will not drink, intravenous fluid will be administered. Administering sodium bicarbonate to create an alkaline urine (*p*H over 8) aids salicylate excretion. With some children, hemodialysis may be necessary to remove the salicylate load and maintain normal potassium levels (potassium is exchanged for H^+ in urine so it reaches high levels).

Continue to monitor vital signs every 4 hours. Test urine for *p*H. Even though the child's temperature is elevated, a method of decreasing temperature (administering aspirin) is obviously contraindicated following aspirin intoxication. Dress children lightly; sponging with tepid water or using a cooling blanket may be prescribed. Test stool for occult blood to see if gastric irritation from aspirin is occurring. Observe especially for signs of hypoglycemia (coma, profuse sweating, disorientation) or metabolic acidosis (rapid, deep breathing; disorientation). Blood serum for glucose may be ordered at periodic intervals based on clinical signs of hypoglycemia.

The prognosis of the child with salicylate poisoning depends on the amount of salicylate ingested and the speed with which treatment was begun. Some parents

do not call for aid immediately after aspirin poisoning, because they do not think of aspirin as a harmful drug. They may think that the dose was too small to cause a problem. In addition, they may be guilt-filled because they realize they were careless about putting the bottle of medicine away after use.

Nursing Diagnoses and Related Interventions

Nursing Diagnosis: High risk for altered self-esteem related to child's poisoning

Goal: Parents demonstrate confidence in their ability to provide safe care for the child (and other family members) by 24 hours.

Outcome Criteria: Parents state guidelines for continued assessment of child at home. State ways they can improve "childproofing."

After the child is stabilized, take some time to talk to parents about how they feel about this event. Remember that poisoning tends to happen in homes where there is stress. If stress was already present, how has this poisoning added to it? Some parents are so distraught when they discover their child has swallowed something that they scoop up that child and bring him or her to a health care facility, leaving other children unattended at home. Be sure to ask them where their other children are.

Outcome criteria that would assure you that the child is excreting the salicylate would be a positive Phenistix test; a urine *p*H above 8; respiratory, cardiac rates, and temperature level returning to normal; no progression of ecchymotic or petechial areas; and return of a normal serum glucose level.

Before children are discharged from a health care facility, be certain parents are comfortable with any further assessment measures they will need to continue at home (temperature taking, urging a high fluid intake). Talk to the parents about childproofing their home. Do not nag or scold. These parents usually are acutely aware that they have not been as careful as they should have been with poisons. Make them aware of their error and yet leave them enough self-esteem to be good parents in the future.

Acetaminophen Poisoning

Parents are now using acetaminophen (Tylenol) as a substitute for aspirin for childhood fevers, so it is now more available than aspirin in many homes. Told that acetaminophen is safer than aspirin, parents may not be as careful about putting this substance away as they were with aspirin; if their child swallows acetaminophen, they may delay bringing him or her for help, thinking it is a harmless drug. They may feel guilty because they may have even referred to such pills as "candy" and realize they led the child into taking a lethal dose.

Acetaminophen in large doses is not an innocent drug, as it can cause extreme liver destruction. Immediately after ingestion, the child will experience anorexia, nausea, and vomiting. Soon, serum glutamic-oxaloacetic transaminase (SGOT) and serum glutamic-pyruvic transaminase (SGPT) liver enzymes become elevated. The liver may be tender. Liver toxicity occurs at an acetaminophen load greater than 200 μg/mL by 4 hours and 50 μg/mL by 12 hours.

Syrup of ipecac is administered to induce vomiting. This can be followed by acetylcysteine every 4 hours for 72 hours orally. This prevents hepatotoxicity by binding with the breakdown product of acetaminophen so it will not bind to liver cells (Mariscalco, 1994). Acetylcysteine, unfortunately, has an offensive odor and taste. Administer it in a carbonated beverage to help the child swallow it. In small children, it is administered directly into the nasogastric tube following lavage to avoid this difficulty. If the child is admitted to the hospital for observation, continue to observe for jaundice and tenderness over the liver; assess SGOT and SGPT reports.

Caustic Poisoning

Ingestion of a strong alkali, such as lye (which is contained in toilet bowl cleaners or hair care products), causes burns and tissue necrosis in the mouth, esophagus, and stomach (Stenson & Gruber, 1993).

Assessment

After a caustic ingestion, the child has immediate pain in the mouth and throat and drools saliva from an inability to swallow. The mouth turns white immediately from the burn; later, the mouth turns brown as edema and ulceration occur. There may be such marked edema of the lips and mouth that it is difficult to examine them. The child may immediately vomit blood, mucus, and necrotic tissue. The loss of blood from the denuded, burned surface may lead to systemic signs of tachycardia, tachypnea, pallor, and hypotension.

A chest x-ray is ordered to determine if pulmonary involvement has occurred from any aspirated poison or an esophageal perforation has allowed poison to seep into the mediastinum. An esophagoscopy under anesthesia may be done to assess the esophagus. This may be omitted as there is a possibility an esophagoscope might perforate the burned esophagus. After 2 weeks, a barium swallow may be done to reveal the final extent of the esophageal burns.

Therapeutic Management

Parents should always call a poison control center to ask for advice on how to proceed. *With caustic poisoning, vomiting should not be induced, because the corrosive substance will burn as it comes up just as it did going down.* Diluting the poison with milk or water is a good emergency measure. Parents should not waste time trying to get children to swallow anything, however. They should immediately take them to a health care facility for treatment.

There is a high possibility that pharyngeal edema will be severe enough to obstruct children's airway by even 20 minutes after the burn. Intubation may be necessary to provide a clear airway.

To detect respiratory interference, assess vital signs conscientiously, especially respiratory rate. In infants, increasing restlessness is an important accompanying sign of this. Assess children for the degree of pain involved. A strong analgesic may need to be ordered and administered to achieve pain relief.

Nursing Diagnoses and Related Interventions

Nursing Diagnosis: High risk for ineffective airway clearance related to burns of esophagus and mouth

Goal: Child will maintain adequate respiratory function. (This is an emergency concern, so care goals must be established quickly to meet the child's needs immediately.)

Outcome Criteria: Child's respiration rate will remain within 16 to 20 breaths per minute.

Starting therapy immediately with a steroid such as dexamethasone (Decadron) and continuing it for about 4 weeks will reduce the chance of permanent esophageal scarring to as low as about 5%. Children may be placed on a prophylactic antibiotic to reduce the possibility of infection and additional inflammation in the denuded mouth and esophageal area.

Those children who respond well to steroid therapy will recover with no important sequelae. Those children who do not receive steroid therapy for some reason may have such scarring of the esophagus that it becomes completely obstructed. To correct complete obstruction, repeated surgical procedures are necessary; sometimes transplantation of intestinal tissue or a synthetic graft is required to replace stenosed esophageal tissue. If partial obstruction is present, a string is passed through the nose and esophagus and exited through a gastrostomy opening to form a continuous loop. **Bougies** (flexible, cylindrical, metal instruments) are tied to the string and pulled through the esophagus to dilate it and increase the lumen size. This may be done as often as once or twice a week up to 1 year following the burn.

Nursing Diagnosis: High risk for altered nutrition, less than body requirements, related to esophageal stricture from burn scarring

Goal: Child will ingest an adequate intake for age following ingestion.

Outcome Criteria: Child's diet meets recommended-daily-allowance requirements for age.

Oral intake will be a problem for the first week because of the soreness of the child's mouth. Observe children carefully the first time they drink to observe for signs that an esophageal perforation has occurred (coughing, choking, cyanosis). Intravenous fluid may need to be given as a supplement. If a child is totally unable to swallow, total parenteral nutrition may be necessary; a gastrostomy may be performed for feeding. When children are able to take food, they should begin by taking a liquid diet. Liquid passing through the burned and scarring esophagus tends to maintain esophageal patency and so is therapeutic for the burn as well as nutritious for the child.

Hydrocarbon Ingestion

Hydrocarbons are substances contained in products such as kerosene and furniture polish. Because these substances are volatile, fumes rise from them, and their major effect is respiratory irritation (see Chapter 40).

Iron Poisoning

Iron is frequently swallowed by small children as it is an ingredient in vitamin preparations, particularly pregnancy vitamins. When it is ingested, it is corrosive to the gastric mucosa, and the symptoms of iron ingestion reflect this irritation. The immediate effects of iron toxicity are nausea and vomiting, diarrhea, and abdominal pain. After 6 hours, these symptoms fade and the child's condition appears to improve. By this time, however, hemorrhagic necrosis of the lining of the GI tract has occurred. By 12 hours, melena (blood in stool) and hematemesis (blood in emesis) will be present as well as lethargy and coma, cyanosis, and vasomotor collapse. Coagulation defects may occur; hepatic injury also can result. Shock from an increase in peripheral vascular resistance and decreased cardiac output can occur. Long-term effects can be gastric scarring from fibrotic tissue formation.

Assessment

Generally, it is difficult to estimate the amount of iron a child has swallowed, because parents can only guess at the number of pills in the bottle and the amount of elemental iron in compounds varies. Serum iron and iron binding concentration should be measured. A level of more than 500 μg/100 mL serum iron is a significant level. A toxic dose is 20 to 30 mg per kilogram of body weight; 60 to 180 mg/kg is a potentially lethal amount.

Therapeutic Management

Having children vomit by taking syrup of ipecac helps to remove any iron not yet absorbed. This may be followed by stomach lavage with a bicarbonate solution to convert the remaining ferrous iron to a less absorbable carbonate compound. A cathartic may be given to help a child pass enteric-coated iron pills. Activated charcoal has no effect.

A child who has ingested a potentially toxic dose (40 to 60 mg per kilogram of body weight of elemental iron) is admitted to the hospital for therapy with a chelating agent such as intravenous or intramuscular deferoxamine. Chelating agents combine with metal and allow metal to be excreted from the body. Deferoxamine causes urine to turn orange as iron is excreted. An exchange transfusion (see Chapter 26) is yet another way that excess iron can be removed from the body. An upper GI series and liver studies will be done a week after ingestion to screen for long-term effects. The hope is that the iron load was removed from the stomach in time so that not all of it was absorbed.

Assisting with emergency measures, such as stomach lavage, and administering chelating agents are important nursing measures. Test any stool passed for the next 3 days for occult blood to assess for stomach irritation. Be certain that parents understand the importance of follow-up studies if any of these are prescribed.

Nursing Diagnoses and Related Interventions

Nursing Diagnosis: Parental knowledge deficit related to the danger of iron as a poison

Goal: Parents will acknowledge iron is a dangerous substance to children in toxic dosages following the ingestion.

Outcome Criteria: Parents state ways they have safeguarded their child from iron exposure.

Iron poisoning occurs frequently because parents do not think of iron pills as real medicine. As mentioned, poisoning tends to happen when a family is under stress. Pregnancy in the mother is a form of stress, and almost all pregnant women take iron compounds. The 9 months of pregnancy are therefore a likely time for iron poisoning to occur in an older sibling. When you instruct parents to use an iron supplement for themselves or their children, stress that overdoses can be fatal to small children. Teach them to think of iron as they would any other medicine and keep it out of the reach of small children.

Lead Poisoning

The effect of lead in the body is to interfere with red blood cell function by blocking the incorporation of iron into the protoporphyrin compound that makes up the heme portion of hemoglobin in red blood cells. This leads to a hypochromic, microcytic anemia. Kidney destruction may occur, causing excess excretion of amino acids, glucose, and phosphates in the urine. The ultimate result will be lead encephalitis or inflammation of brain cells from the toxic lead content. Lead poisoning (plumbism), like all forms of poisoning in children, tends to occur most often in the toddler and preschool child. It occurs most frequently during the summer (Schwartz & Levin, 1991). It is a largely preventable disease (DeRienzo-DeVivio, 1992). Sources of lead poisoning are described in Chapter 30, along with guidelines for its prevention.

Assessment

The usual source of ingested lead is ingested paint chips or paint dust. Paint tastes sweet, and a child will pick chips up off the floor or off the walls over and over again. If a crib rail is painted with lead paint, a child will ingest it as he or she teethes on the rail. Chewing on window sills is also common. Poisoning may occur from environmental contamination such as gasoline or industry (Levallois et al., 1991). Restoring an older home saturates the air with lead dust. In such homes, lead plumbing may contaminate the drinking water with lead.

All children who live in old housing (built before 1940) should be screened for plumbism yearly. The most widely used method of screening for lead levels is the blood lead determination. Unfortunately, this test requires using atomic absorption spectrophotometry, which is a costly procedure that is not available in all communities. Free erythrocyte protoporphyrin (FEP) tests are a simple screening procedure, involving only a finger prick. Cleansing the skin before taking a blood sample is extremely important in lead-level analysis, because there may be enough lead in the dust on a child's finger to contaminate the sample. Because protoporphyrin is blocked from entering heme by lead, it will be elevated in lead poisoning.

Many children with fairly high blood lead levels are asymptomatic; others show insidious symptoms of anorexia and abdominal pain from the presence of lead in the stomach. One of the major effects of excessive lead levels is encephalopathy. The child usually has beginning symptoms of lethargy, impulsiveness, and learning difficulties. As the child's blood level of lead increases, severe encephalopathy with seizures and permanent mental retardation will result.

Basophilic stippling (an odd striation of basophils) may be apparent on a blood smear. An x-ray of the abdomen may reveal paint chips in the intestinal tract (Figure 52-7A). "Lead lines" (areas of increased density) may be present near the epiphyseal line of long bones (Figure 52-7B). The thickness of the line shows the length of time lead ingestion has been occurring. Damage to the kidney nephrons from the presence of lead leads to proteinuria, ketonuria, and glycosuria. Cerebrospinal fluid may have an increased protein level.

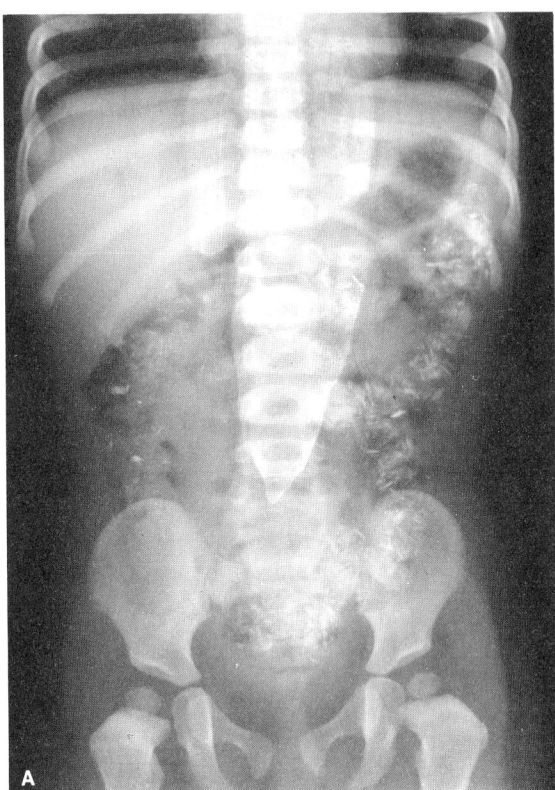
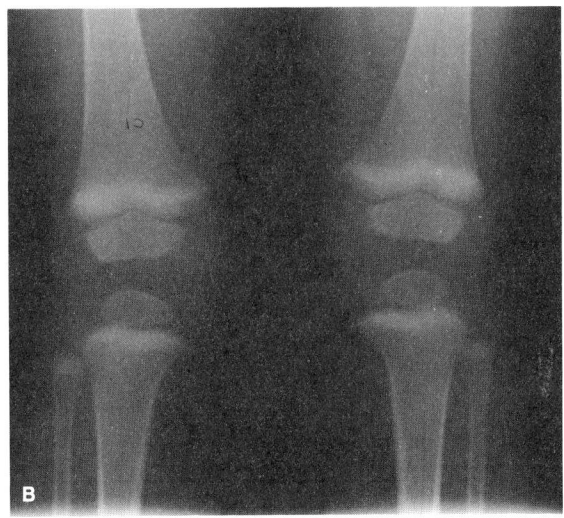

FIGURE 52-7
(**A**) *Ingested paint chips (white crescents) in the intestinal tract.* (**B**) *A radiograph of the long bones of a child with chronic lead ingestion showing the characteristic "lead line" or white marking at the epiphyseal line. (Courtesy of Dr. Jerald P. Kuhn, Children's Hospital, Buffalo, NY.)*

Lead poisoning is usually said to be present when the child has two successive blood lead levels greater than 10 μg/dL. A classification of levels of lead poisoning is shown in Table 52-4.

Therapeutic Management

A child with a blood lead level between 10 and 14 μg/dL needs to be rescreened to confirm the level. If the

Table 52-4. Classification of Lead Poisoning Risk

Class	Blood Level Concentration (μg/dL)
Class I (low risk)	Lead under 9
Class IIa (rescreen)	Lead 10–14
Class IIb (moderate risk)	Lead 15–19
Class III (high risk)	Lead 20–44
Class IV (urgent risk)	Lead 45–69
Class V (urgent risk)	Lead greater than 70

(Centers for Disease Control. [1991]. *Preventing lead poisoning in young children.* Washington, DC: U.S. Department of Health and Human Services, Public Health Service.)

lead level is 15 or above, the child needs active interventions to prevent further lead exposure. All children with lead levels over 25 μg/100 mL require treatment. A major part of treatment is removing the child from the environment containing the lead source or removing the source of lead from the child's environment. Removing the lead source may be difficult; if the family lives in a rented apartment, however, the landlord may be legally obligated to remove the lead. Simple repainting or wallpapering does not remove a source of peeling paint adequately. After some months, the new paint will begin to peel because of the defective paint underneath. The walls must be covered by paneling or masonite. Plastic-covered contact paper can be used temporarily and is less expensive than paneling.

Until such repairs are made, children may be removed from the home for hospital care or foster home placement. Children with blood lead levels of greater than 30 μg/100 mL may be admitted to the hospital for chelating therapy with agents such as dimercaprol (BAL) or edetate calcium disodium (CaEDTA), one of the most commonly used chelating agents (see the Focus on Nursing Care box earlier in this chapter).

Chelating agents act to remove the lead from soft tissue and bone (although not from red blood cells) and eliminate it in the urine. EDTA is administered for 5 days, then not for 2 days (to allow time for renal excretion), then restarted as necessary for another 5 days. Injections of EDTA, which must be given intramuscularly into a large muscle mass, are so painful that it is generally combined with 0.5 mL of procaine. (Pull the procaine into the syringe last so it enters the child first.) EDTA also removes calcium from the body; therefore, serum calcium must be measured periodically to determine whether it is at a safe level. Intake and output must be measured for assurance that kidney function is adequate to handle the lead being excreted. BUN, serum creatinine, and protein in urine may also be assessed. If kidney function is not adequate, EDTA may lead to nephrotoxicity or kidney damage.

BAL has the advantage of removing lead from red blood cells, but because of severe toxicity is only used with children who have severe forms of lead intoxication. Penicillamine is an experimental drug for lead poisoning. It is given orally following BAL or EDTA. Weekly complete blood count and renal and liver function tests are done accompanying the administration of penicillamine. It may be given for as long as 3 to 6 months.

Nursing Diagnoses and Related Interventions

Goal planning can be difficult when parents are angry at a landlord or with themselves for exposing their child to a source of lead. They may experience a loss of self-esteem and sense of powerlessness when realizing that their financial circumstances or lifestyle has hurt their child.

> **Nursing Diagnosis:** Knowledge deficit related to the dangers of lead ingestion
> **Goal:** Parents will acknowledge the danger of lead ingestion to their child and potential sources of lead in their environment.
> **Outcome Criteria:** Parents state ways they have safeguarded their child against further lead ingestion.

Teach parents about the risk of lead poisoning. Teach them to keep toddlers away from windowsills and other common sources of lead paint. Placing the television or an overstuffed chair against the windowsill may be effective as a temporary measure. As a rule, children's cribs should be placed about 3 ft away from walls in older homes so that there is no tendency for children to pick at loose wallpaper when they first wake in the morning or before they fall asleep at night (plaster, which contains lead, clings to the wallpaper).

All children with elevated lead levels need careful follow-up care to determine the seriousness of their condition and to ensure that they are kept from a lead source (parents may move from one poorly maintained apartment to another, and exposure to lead continues). Because children who recover from symptomatic lead poisoning have a high incidence of permanent neurologic damage, all children with elevated blood lead levels need appropriate follow-up care to evaluate development and intelligence, so that proper school placement and a realistic plan for the child's future can be determined.

Insecticide Poisoning

Children can be poisoned by insecticides (1) by accidental ingestion or (2) through skin or respiratory tract contact when playing in an area that has recently been sprayed with one. Long-term exposure may result from exposure to a parent's clothing if he or she comes home covered with insecticide spray. Once thought to be only a rural problem, the increase in the use of lawn sprays by commercial companies now makes this a suburban problem as well.

Many insecticides have an organophosphate base that leads to an accumulation of acetylcholine at neuromuscular junctions. Within a few minutes to 2 hours of exposure, children develop nausea and vomiting, diarrhea, excessive salivation, weakness of respiratory muscles, confusion, depressed reflexes, and possibly seizures.

Vomiting should be induced by syrup of ipecac or gastric lavage. Activated charcoal may be helpful in neutralizing any poison remaining. If clothing is contaminated, it should be removed and the child's skin and hair washed. To prevent contacting the insecticide yourself, wear gloves while giving such a bath.

Intravenous atropine is an effective antidote to reverse symptoms. Pralidoxime also may be effective.

Plant Poisoning

Plant poisoning (ingestion of a growing plant) occurs because parents do not think of plants as being poisonous. Common plants to which children may be exposed and the effect when they are ingested are shown in the Focus on Family Teaching box. In addition to teaching parents about such plants, teach them to childproof their home against these. Teach children not to eat any substances such as attractive berries on a bush unless a parent or trusted adult has deemed them acceptable for eating (McIntire et al., 1991).

Recreational Drug Poisoning

Adolescents (and, more and more frequently, grade-school children) are brought to health care facilities by parents or friends because of a drug overdose or a "bad trip" caused by an unusual reaction or the effect of an unfortunate combination of drugs.

Children are often extremely disoriented following this form of ingestion. They may be having hallucinations of people attacking them, objects hurting them, or bugs crawling over them. Obtaining a history may be difficult because children may have no idea what they took except that it was a red or a yellow capsule. They may know but be reluctant to name a drug if it was obtained illegally. They may have been "slipped a mickey" (a drug in a drink) by a joke-playing friend and may have no idea what they have taken. The feeling of not being in control of their body is extremely frightening to anyone. Children have certainly heard many scare stories about drug abuse and may be very worried (often rightly) that this drug reaction will be fatal.

FOCUS ON FAMILY TEACHING

Q. I've heard that some house plants can be poisonous to children. What are some examples of ones that are?

A. Before purchasing a new plant for either inside or as shrubbery for outside the house, it is good to ask if poisoning would be a problem. A number of common plants that can lead to poisoning in children, and the symptoms they produce, are:

English Ivy	Nausea, vomiting, excess salivation, diarrhea, abdominal pain
Holly (berries)	Vomiting, diarrhea, abdominal pain
Hydrangea	Nausea, vomiting, muscular weakness, convulsions, dyspnea
Lily of the valley	Vomiting, abdominal pain, diarrhea, cardiac disturbances
Mistletoe	Vomiting, diarrhea, bradycardia
Morning glory (seeds)	Nausea, diarrhea, hallucinations
Philodendron	Swelling of the tongue, lips, irritation of mouth
Poinsettia	Nausea, vomiting
Rhubarb (leaves)	Irritant action on gastrointestinal tract
Rhododendron	Nausea, vomiting, abdominal pain, convulsions, limb paralysis

Assessment

Even though the child may not appear to hear well or may not seem coherent, try to elicit a history from him or her. Avoid shouting or aggravating, however: children who are having a paranoid reaction will be unable to cope rationally with this approach. If friends accompany an ill child, point out that your role is not that of a law enforcer. Your role is to help the child, and you cannot do that effectively unless the drug is identified. Approaching a child's friends this way is more likely than a threat to result in their naming the drug. If a child is brought in by parents who have no idea what drug could possibly have been taken, ask them to have someone at home check the child's bedroom for drugs (provided the child became ill while at home).

Try to determine whether the ingestion was an accident (a child was unaware that two drugs would react this way or took a wrong dose) or whether a child was actually attempting suicide. In the first instance, children will need better counseling about drug use or about which drugs do not mix. If the incident was an attempted suicide, children will need observation and counseling toward more effective coping mechanisms in self-care. All poisonings or drug ingestions in children older than 7 years of age should be considered potential suicides until established otherwise.

Blood should be drawn so that blood electrolytes can be measured and a toxicology scan completed. If a child is vomiting, save vomitus for analysis also.

Therapeutic Management

Children need supportive measures for their specific symptoms: oxygen administration; electrolyte replacement (particularly if there is accompanying nausea and vomiting); and perhaps intravenous fluid administration in an attempt to dilute the drug.

Children who have swallowed a recreational drug need immediate treatment followed by sympathetic investigation into the events leading to the poisoning. This potentially lethal ingestion may act as a turning point in the child's life, as it alerts the child and family to the fact of a drug problem and the need for help. Outcome criteria to ensure that goals have been reached would include factors such as reduction of fear and anxiety and increased coping mechanisms, and knowledge of the effects of drug use and sources of referral for a drug problem.

Foreign Body Obstruction

Foreign bodies can become lodged in the throat or other body openings, causing stasis of secretions and infection. Direct obstruction or laceration of the mucous membrane may also result, with serious consequences.

Whether a foreign substance is inhaled or embedded elsewhere, nursing interventions will focus first on comforting the child and aiding in the substance's removal, and then on teaching the child and parents ways to avoid such occurrences in the future.

Foreign Bodies in the Ear

Any child with a history of draining exudate from the ear canal needs an otoscopic examination to establish the reason for the drainage. In toddlers and preschoolers, the drainage often is the result of a foreign body in the ear canal. The object might be a small piece of a toy, a piece of paper, a transistor battery, or food, such as a peanut.

Removing foreign bodies from the ear is difficult because children are afraid that the instrument used will hurt them and so have difficulty lying still for the procedure. If there is reason to think that the tympanic membrane is intact, a physician may attempt to irrigate the object from the ear canal with a syringe and normal saline. This should not be done if the object is a substance such as a peanut that will swell when wet. If it is possible that the tympanic membrane is ruptured, the ear canal must not be irrigated or fluid will be forced into the middle ear, possibly introducing infection (otitis media).

Often, it is better to wait for an otolaryngologist to care for the child, because trauma to the ear canal in an attempt to remove a foreign body will increase the edema and make removal even more difficult.

Teach children the importance of never placing anything in their ear canal to avoid this type of problem.

Foreign Bodies in the Nose

Foreign objects stuffed into the nose eventually cause inflammation and purulent discharge from the nares. The odor accompanying such impaction is often the first sign noticed by a parent. Objects pushed into the nose generally can be removed with forceps. A local antibiotic might be necessary after removal if ulceration resulted from the local irritation.

Teach children not to put anything in their noses to avoid this problem.

Foreign Bodies in the Esophagus

Children tend not to chew food well and to swallow portions that are too big to pass safely through the esophagus. Candy Lifesavers are common objects caught in the esophagus. Intense pain at the site where the object is lodged will result. If it is an object that will dissolve, such as a Lifesaver or a piece of digestible meat, offer the child fluid to drink to help flush the object into the stomach. Even after the object dissolves or passes into the stomach, children will feel transient pain at the original site of the obstruction.

An object that is a part of a toy or a chicken bone (other objects frequently swallowed) that will not dissolve and should not be passed is removed by esophagoscopy under a general anesthetic (or a sedative, with adolescents). Quarters (often swallowed by adolescents playing a drinking game with quarters in beer) do not pass readily and usually must be removed by esophagoscopy. Other coins, such as pennies and dimes, generally pass by themselves without difficulty.

Parents (or children themselves if adolescents) should observe stools over the next several days to determine when the coin passes through the GI tract (this takes about 48 hours). Without frightening them, caution parents to observe for signs of bowel perforation or obstruction—vomiting or abdominal pain—until an object has passed. If there is any doubt, an x-ray taken 3 days to a week after ingestion will establish whether the object has been evacuated from the body.

Subcutaneous Objects

Children receive many wood splinters in hands and feet. These usually are removed easily by a probing needle and tweezers following cleaning with an antiseptic solution. If the penetrating object is metal, such as a sewing needle or nail, its presence can be detected by x-ray. If the object is one that would have been in contact with soil, such as a rusty nail, the child needs tetanus prophylaxis following extraction of the object (Inaba, 1993).

Trauma Related to Environmental Exposure

Frostbite

Frostbite is tissue injury caused by freezing cold. Cells at the site actually die. Cold exposure leads to peripheral vasoconstriction, so oxygen supply is cut off to surrounding cells. In children, the body parts involved are usually the fingers or toes.

Assessment
The affected part appears white or erythematous with edema and feels numb. Degrees of frostbite are summarized in Table 52-5. Explore the cause of frostbite by careful history taking. It occurs most frequently in children who are skiing or snowmobiling for long periods whose parents failed to provide adequate clothing because they underestimated the degree of cold outside. The possibility of neglect or child abuse must be ruled out as a cause.

Therapeutic Management
Always warm frostbitten areas gradually. (Sudden warming will increase the metabolism rate of cells; without adequate blood flow to the area because of still-present

Table 52-5. *Degrees of Frostbite*

Degree	Description
First	Mild freezing of epidermis; appears erythematous with edema
Second	Partial- or full-thickness injury; appears erythematous with blisters and pain occurring after rewarming
Third	Full thickness (epidermis, dermis, and subcutaneous tissue); appears white
Fourth	Complete necrosis with gangrene and possible ultimate loss of body part

vasoconstriction, additional damage will be done to cells.)

Occasionally in the summer months, toddlers eating popsicles suffer frostbite on the buccal membrane because they hold a popsicle against the side of the mouth and cheek. The area appears red and swollen. Because this is invariably mild frostbite, no treatment is necessary except to offer soft food for a day or two. There are no permanent effects.

Nursing Diagnoses and Related Interventions

Nursing Diagnosis: Pain related to frostbite damage to cells

Goal: Child will experience a minimum amount of pain following injury.

Outcome Criteria: Child states that pain is controlled at a tolerable level.

As soon as warming begins, the area becomes painful from cells that are injured, but not destroyed, registering their anoxic state. Children may need an analgesic at this point for pain. The pain is usually extreme; do not underestimate its extent.

During the next few days after severe frostbite, necrosis of destroyed tissue will occur and affected tissue will slough away. Apply a dressing as necessary to avoid secondary bacterial contamination of a necrotic injury site. Assess body temperature conscientiously to detect early symptoms of infection.

Bites

Mammalian Bites

Dog bites account for approximately 90% of all bites inflicted on humans, and children and adolescents are involved in one third to one half of reported incidents. Cat bites, wild animal bites, and human bites also constitute a threat, although less common to children. All of these bites can cause abrasions, puncture wounds, and lacerations, as well as crushing injuries related to the size of the animal and location of the bite. The biggest concerns associated with animal bites are the possibility of long-term scarring and disfigurement and the possibility of infection, especially rabies, from the presence of microorganisms in the mouth of the animal. This latter subject is discussed in Chapter 43.

Snakebite

Most fatal snakebites in the United States are copperhead (found in Eastern and Southern states) and rattlesnake bites (found in almost every state). A few bites occur from cottonmouth moccasins (found in Southeastern states) or coral snakes (also found in Southeastern states). The effect of rattlesnake, copperhead, and cottonmouth bites is to cause a failure of the blood coagulation system; children die of intracranial hemorrhage. Coral snakes are known for the small coral, yellow, and black rings encircling their body; fortunately, they are shy and seldom bite. The effect of venom injected through the bite of these snakes is to cause neuromuscular paralysis.

Assessment

Snakebites tend to occur during the warm months of the year, from April to October. Reaction to a poisonous snakebite is almost immediate: a white wheal forms at the site, showing the puncture marks, and there is excruciating pain at the site; purplish erythema and edema begin to extend rapidly from the site.

By the time children are seen at a health care facility, sanguineous fluid may ooze from the bite. Systemic symptoms, such as dizziness, vomiting, perspiration, and weakness, may be present. As snake venom interferes with blood coagulation, children may have bloody vomiting or bleeding from the nose, intestines, or bladder from subcutaneous or internal hemorrhage. The pupils may be dilated, showing the potent effect on cerebral centers. If children are not treated, convulsions, coma, and death may result.

Emergency Management at the Scene

At the scene of a snakebite, apply a cold compress to the bite in the hope of slowing the spread of the venom and to reduce the formation of edema (Snyder & Knowles, 1991). Urge the child to lie quietly to slow circulation; keep the bitten extremity dependent, again to slow venous circulation. Commercial snakebite kits have rubber suction cups in them to use to suction out venom. These should be used. Excising the bite with a knife and sucking out the venom orally (often shown in old western movies) is of questionable value and contradicts rules of universal precautions. If the person administering the treatment has open mouth lesions such as carious teeth, the procedure may be dangerous to

that person (venom is not dangerous when swallowed, only when absorbed through open lesions). Excising the bite may lead to secondary infection, and if done too vigorously may injure tendon or muscle. No time should be wasted before children are taken to a health care facility for treatment.

Emergency Management at the Health Facility

In the emergency facility, ask the child or a person who was with him or her to describe the snake. In areas where snakebites are frequent, keep available photographs of the venomous snakes in the area. Even a preschooler may be able to identify the snake by pointing to a photograph. Specific antivenin will be administered. Because rattlesnakes, copperheads, and cottonmouth moccasins are all one type of snake (pit vipers), one form of antivenin acts against all these bites. Specific antivenin is prepared for coral snake or cobra bites and is kept at most zoos. If the child receives antivenin promptly after a bite, the prognosis for full recovery is good. Tetanus prophylaxis is instituted if the child's immunization status is unknown or if it has been more than 10 years since a tetanus immunization was given.

Antivenin contains a horse-serum base. Therefore, before the serum is injected intramuscularly or intravenously, a skin test is first performed to prevent the child from having an anaphylactic reaction to the serum. If the serum is given intramuscularly, it should not be injected into an edematous body part because medication is absorbed poorly from edematous areas. Giving antivenin in the limb opposite the bitten limb will be just as effective as administering it into the bitten limb.

Nursing Diagnoses and Related Interventions

> ***Nursing Diagnosis:*** Fear related to seriousness of child's condition
>
> ***Goal:*** Parents and child will demonstrate ability to keep fear within manageable limits.
>
> ***Outcome Criteria:*** Parents and child voice that they are able to cope with the degree of fear present.

Children with snakebites are extremely frightened. Their parents who have seen old cowboy movies showing the agony of snakebite also are thoroughly frightened. Children need a great deal of support from health care personnel because parents may be too frightened (or guilty—they should have protected the child better; or angry—they never should have gone camping) to offer the support they would like to offer at this time.

As a final care measure, teach children safety rules for avoiding snakebites, such as look for snakes before stepping into underbrush; don't lift up rocks without looking at what could be under them; listen for the telltale sound of a rattlesnake; be aware that snakes sun on rocks; and be knowledgeable of the markings of poisonous snakes.

Burn Trauma

A burn is injury to body tissue caused by excessive heat. They commonly occur in children of all ages after infancy. They are the second cause of accidental injury in children 1 to 4 years of age and the third cause in children 5 to 14 years. Toddlers are often burned by turning pans of scalding water over on themselves or by biting into electrical cords. Older children are more apt to suffer burns from flames when they move too close to a campfire, heater, or fireplace or if they play with matches. Some burns are symptoms of child abuse. As many as 50% of burns could be prevented with improved parent and child education, as most burns occur because children are temporarily unsupervised.

With a thermal burn, tissue damage occurs when heat is greater than 40°C. Any thermal burn tends to be more serious in children than in adults because the same size burn covers a larger surface of a child's body.

Assessment

When children are brought to a health care facility with a thermal injury, the first questions must be, "What is the extent of the burn? What is the depth of the burn? Where is the burn?" Burns are classified according to criteria of the American Burn Association as major, moderate, or minor burns. These classifications are shown in Table 52-6. It is important that not only the size and depth but also the location of the burn are assessed. Face and throat burns are particularly hazardous because the child probably inhaled hot flames or air and so has burns in the respiratory tract; resulting edema will lead to respiratory tract obstruction. Hand burns are also hazardous, because if the fingers and thumb are not positioned properly during healing, adhesions will inhibit full range

of motion in the future. Burns of the feet and genitalia often become secondarily infected if the child is sent home after only initial treatment. Genital burns are also hazardous because edema of the urinary meatus may prevent a child from voiding: a Foley catheter might be necessary to maintain urinary function in such situations.

With adults, a "rule of nine" is a quick method of estimating the extent of a burn: each upper extremity represents 9% of body surface; each lower extremity represents two 9s, or 18%; the head and neck represent 9%. Because the body proportions of children are different from those of adults, this rule does not always apply and is misleading in the very young child. Data for determining the extent of burns in children are shown in Figure 52-8.

Depth of Burn

Assessing the depth of burns is not always easy. Descriptions of tissue at different burn depths appear in Table 52-7 and are illustrated in Figure 52-9. *Partial thickness* burns are first- and second-degree burns. A first-degree burn involves only the superficial epidermis. The area appears erythematous. It is painful to touch and blanches on pressure (Figure 52-10). Scalds and sunburn are examples of first-degree burns. Such burns heal by simple regeneration and take only 1 to 10 days to heal.

A second-degree burn involves the entire epidermis; sweat glands and hair follicles are left intact. The area appears very erythematous, blistered, and moist from exudate. It is extremely painful. Scalds can cause second-degree burns (see Figure 52-10). Such burns heal by regeneration of tissue but take 2 to 6 weeks to heal.

A third-degree burn is a full-thickness burn involving both skin layers, epidermis and dermis. It may also involve adipose tissue, fascia, muscle, and bone. The burn appears either white or black (Figure 52-11). Because the nerves as well as sweat glands and hair follicles have been burned, third-degree burns are not painful. Flames lead to third-degree burns. Such burns cannot heal by regeneration because even underlying layers of skin are destroyed. Skin grafting is usually necessary; healing will take months. Scar tissue will remain at the healed site.

In estimating the depth of a burn, use the appearance of the burn and the sensitivity of the area to pain as criteria. Many burns are compound, involving first-, second-, and third-degree burns. There may be a central white area that is insensitive to pain (third degree) surrounded by an area of erythematous blisters (second degree) surrounded by yet another area that is erythematous only (first degree).

Undress children with burns completely so that the entire body can be inspected for burns. A first-degree burn is painful, whereas a third-degree burn is not; therefore, a child may be crying from a superficial burn

Table 52-6. *Classification of Burns*

Classification	Description
Minor	First-degree burn or second degree < 10% of body surface or third degree < 2% of body surface; no area of the face, feet, hands, or genitalia is burned.
Moderate	Second-degree burn between 10–20% or on the face, hands, feet, or genitalia or third-degree burn < 10% body surface or if smoke inhalation has occurred
Severe	Second-degree burn > 20% body surface or third-degree burn > 10% body surface.

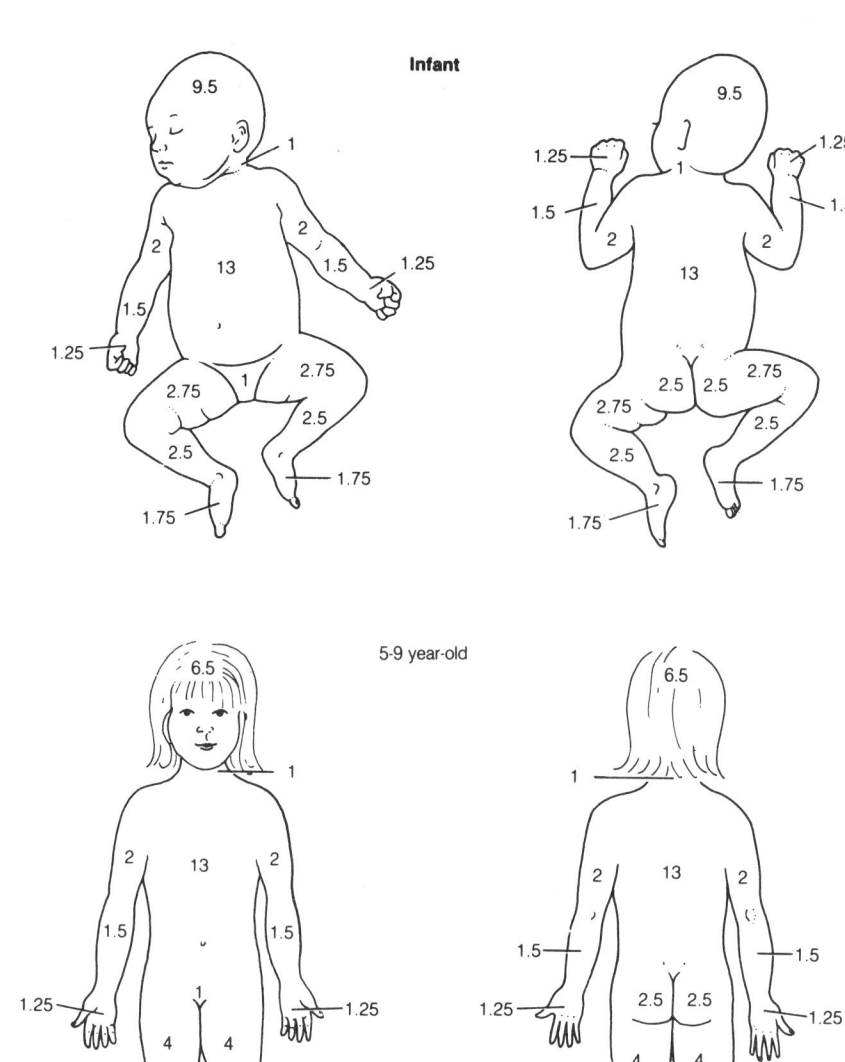

FIGURE 52-8
Determination of extent of burns in children.

Table 52-7. Characteristics of Burns

Severity	Depth of Tissue Involved	Appearance	Example
First degree (partial thickness)	Epidermis	Erythematous, dry, painful	Sunburn
Second degree (partial thickness)	Epidermis Portion of dermis	Blistered, erythematous to white	Scalds
Third degree (full thickness)	Entire skin, including nerves and blood vessels in skin	Leathery; black or white; not sensitive to pain (nerve endings destroyed)	Flame

Depths of burns   Skin grafts

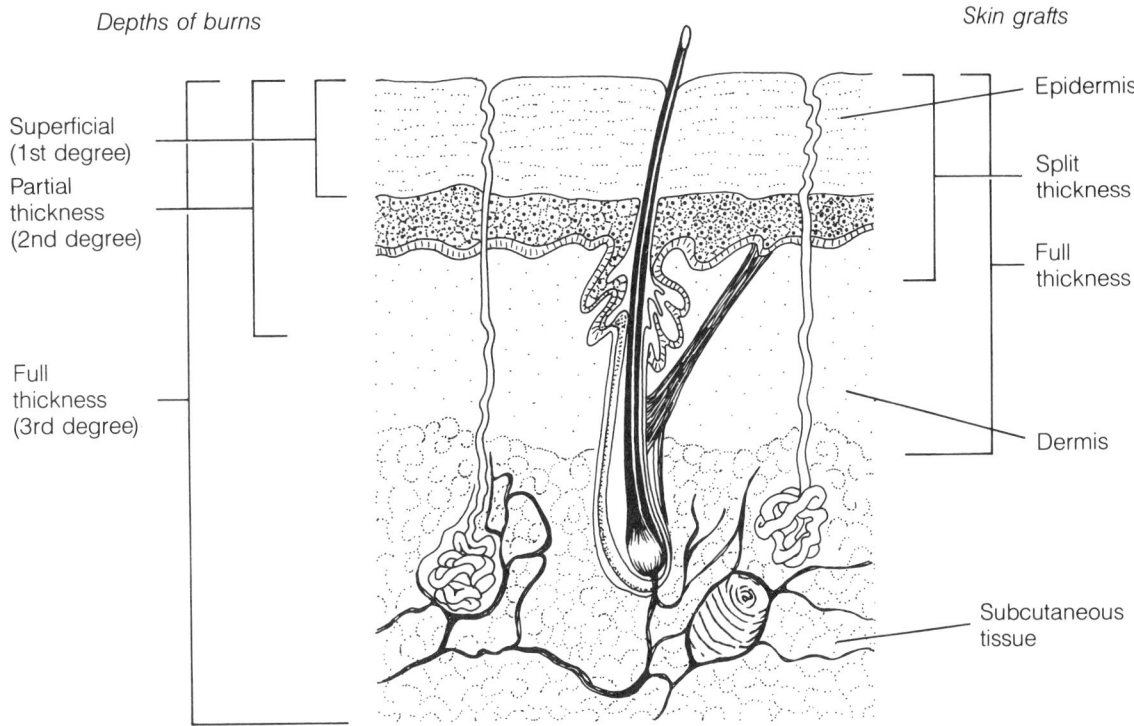

FIGURE 52-9
Depths of burns.

that is obvious on the arm, although the condition needing the most immediate attention is a third-degree burn on the chest, which is covered by a jacket.

Ask what caused the burn, because different materials cause different degrees of burn. Hot water, for example, causes scalding, a generally lesser degree of burn than is caused by flaming clothing. Ask where the fire happened. Fires in closed spaces are apt to cause more respiratory involvement than fires in open areas (Ruddy, 1993).

Ask if the child has any secondary health problem. In the anxiety over the present burn, parents forget to report such important facts as, for example, that the child has diabetes or is allergic to a common drug. Following a fire, parents often pick up the burned child and bring him or her to a health care facility, leaving other children unprotected at home. Ask about other children and where they are. Parents may have burned hands from putting out the fire in the child's clothes and need equal care, but in their anxiety over the child's condition

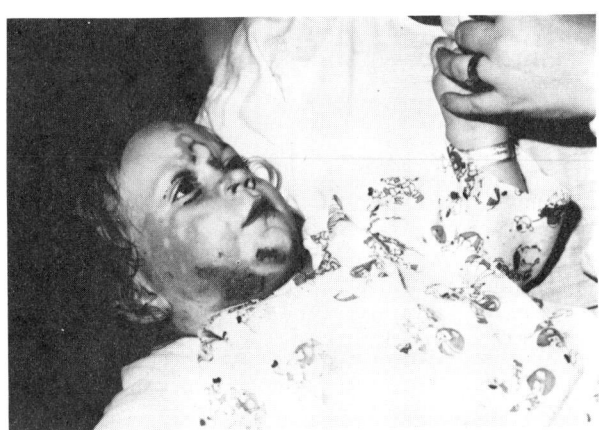

FIGURE 52-10
First- and second-degree burns of the face. (Courtesy of Bruce Hill.)

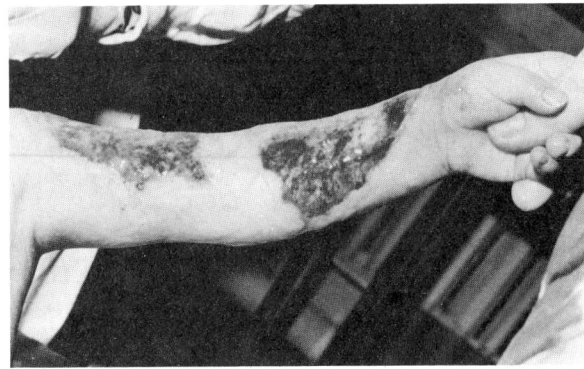

FIGURE 52-11
Second- and third-degree burns of the arm caused by hot grease. (Courtesy of the Department of Medical Photography, Children's Hospital, Buffalo, NY.)

will not mention this. Ask who put out the fire. Were any other family members or close friends hurt? Does anyone else need care?

Emergency Management

Mild (First-Degree) Burns

Although first-degree partial-thickness burns are the simplest type of burn, they involve pain and death of skin cells and so must be treated seriously. Cleanse the area with an antiseptic. Apply an analgesic and antibiotic ointment and a gauze bandage to prevent infection. Don't break any blisters that are present because this invites infection. Broken blisters may be debrided (cut away) to remove possible necrotic tissue. The child should return in 2 days to have the area inspected for a secondary infection and to have the dressing changed. Caution parents to keep the dressing dry (no washing or getting the area wet while bathing for 1 week). A first-degree burn heals in about that time.

Moderate and Severe Burns

The child with a moderate or severe burn is severely injured and needs swift, sure care to survive the injury without a disability caused by scarring, infection, or contracture (see the Nursing Care Plan: A Toddler With a Second-Degree Burn, p. 1660).

Nursing Diagnoses and Related Interventions

Because severe burns affect every body system, the nursing diagnoses and interventions that follow are divided by body system.

Neurologic System. Children who have smoke inhalation may be unconscious from brain anoxia immediately following a burn. Most children, however, are awake and very aware of the pain and treatments involved, so need immediate care to relieve this. After the first week following a major burn, some children develop symptoms of delirium, seizures, and coma that result from toxic breakdown of damaged cells as well as sensory deprivation, isolation, and lack of sleep. Nursing care aimed at reducing unnecessary stimuli helps to prevent these late symptoms from occurring.

Nursing Diagnosis: Pain related to trauma to body cells

Goal: Child will experience the minimum amount of pain possible (be certain that goal established is realistic; you cannot eliminate *all* pain).

Outcome Criteria: Child states that pain is at a tolerable level.

A child needs an analgesic to relieve pain and to help prevent shock. Morphine sulfate or meperidine (Demerol) are drugs commonly given. These can be given intramuscularly, but because circulation is impaired in children with shock, intravenous administration is most effective. Daily debridement that follows emergency care is a painful procedure. Whirlpool treatment, which precedes the debridement, may at first be painful but quickly becomes a pleasant part of the day, because the swirling water is soothing to burned areas. It is difficult for a child really to enjoy it, however, because as soon as it is over, the painful debridement will begin.

For most of every day, children may be required to remain in awkward positions to keep joints overextended. If their anterior throat is burned, for example, their head will be hyperextended to keep scar tissue that forms on the anterior neck from pulling their chin down against their chest in a contracture. It is difficult for children to watch television in this position or even to view activities on the unit. If they have burns at extremity joints, they may have splints applied over burn dressings to maintain joints in extension. Again, this makes activities very difficult for them.

Circulatory System. Immediately following a severe burn, the child's circulatory system becomes hypovolemic, because a great deal of plasma is lost through the burn site and a great deal of fluid is sequestered in edematous tissue at the site. The outpouring of plasma, caused by increased permeability of capillaries (or damage to capillaries), is most marked during the first 6 hours after a burn; it continues to some extent for the first 24 hours. To replace this, the child may have intravenous albumen ordered (12.5 g/L of intravenous fluid).

Accompanying the hypovolemia that is occurring will be a marked reduction in cardiac output. Part of this decrease apparently results from a primary response of the myocardium to the shock of thermal injury. Even with relatively minor burns, vital signs must be followed closely, so that this reaction can be detected. The child may be severely anemic because of injury to red blood cells by heat and loss at the wound site, and he or she may have severe electrolyte abnormalities as a result of fluid shifts (Table 52-8). The large amount of sodium lost with the edematous burn fluid and the release of potassium from damaged cells lead to an immediate hyponatremia and hyperkalemia.

Nursing Diagnosis: Fluid volume deficit related to fluid shifts with severe thermal burn

Goal: Child will maintain normal balance of fluid and electrolytes during period of therapy.

Outcome Criteria: Skin turgor is good; urine output is greater than 1 mL/kg/hr, with specific gravity between 1.003 and 1.030.

Table 52-8. *Fluid Shifts After Thermal Injury*

Fluid Shifts in First 24 Hours	Remobilization of Fluid After 48 Hours
Burn ↓	Edematous tissue surrounding burn area ↓
Increased capillary permeability ↓	Intravascular compartment ↓
Hypoproteinemia	
Hyponatremia	Hypervolemia
Hyperkalemia	Hypernatremia
Hypovolemia	Hypokalemia

Lactated Ringer's solution is the commercially available solution most compatible with extracellular fluid and so is one of the first fluids usually begun for fluid replacement, although normal saline may be used. The child may also need plasma replacement and additional fluid such as 5% dextrose in water. Potassium must not be administered immediately after a burn because kidney function must first be tested. Intravenous fluid is generally administered by the most convenient vein that can be entered so that morphine sulfate can be administered to relieve pain. A more stable fluid line may then be inserted by means of an intracath or a cutdown. The amount of fluid necessary is calculated carefully, based on predicted insensible fluid loss and loss due to the burn. A common formula used to calculate fluid needed is:

$$2000 \text{ mL/m}^2 \text{ of body surface/24 h}$$
$$+ 5000 \text{ mL/m}^2 \text{ of body surface } burned/24 \text{ h}$$

This fluid is administered rapidly for the first 8 hours (half of the 24-hour load), then more slowly for the next 16 hours (the second half). It is important that it be continued beyond the time of increased capillary permeability (at least the first 24 hours). The administration site, therefore, must be safeguarded carefully so that it does not become infiltrated or infected. A central venous pressure catheter helps to determine whether adequate fluid is being given.

About 48 hours after the burn, the extracellular fluid at the burn site begins to be reabsorbed into the bloodstream. The edema begins to subside; the child will have diuresis and lose weight. The heart rate will increase because of temporary hypervolemia. The hematocrit level will be low because red blood cells will be diluted. The child will need frequent blood electrolyte determinations to establish the effectiveness of fluid balance during this period. Potassium supplements may be necessary to maintain normal heart function, because although potassium is released into serum from destroyed

cells, it is rapidly excreted by the kidneys. If the child needs continued electrolyte replacement at this time, the rate of flow of fluid must be monitored carefully so that the blood volume does not exceed the child's tolerance. The child may need packed red blood cells to maintain an adequate hemoglobin level.

> ***Nursing Diagnosis:*** High risk for altered tissue perfusion related to cardiovascular adjustments following thermal injury
>
> ***Goal:*** Child's cardiovascular system will satisfactorily adjust to fluid shifts during therapy.
>
> ***Outcome Criteria:*** Child's vital signs stay within normal limits; urine output remains greater than 1 mL/kg/h.

Take height, weight, and vital signs on admission; continue to take vital signs every 15 minutes until they are stable. The pulse, blood pressure, and central venous pressure should be recorded hourly until the child passes the immediate danger of shock. At 48 hours when fluid is returning to the bloodstream is another important period. Make certain you evaluate vital signs and urine output carefully. Gradual changes may be as informative as sudden changes.

A complete blood count, blood typing and cross-matching, electrolyte and BUN determinations, and blood gas studies to ascertain blood levels of oxygen and carbon dioxide are also important.

Respiratory System. If the child breathed in smoke from a fire, the injury from the smoke inhalation can be more serious than the skin surface burns. Smoke coming from a fire is at the temperature of the fire; breathing this in is therefore the same as exposing the upper respiratory tract to open fire. In addition, toxic substances and soot given off from fire may be extremely irritating to the respiratory tract (Sockrider & Seilheimer, 1994). Carbon monoxide is absorbed from smoke; this enters red blood cells in place of oxygen, shutting off oxygen supply to body cells. Smoke inhalation leads to loss of consciousness because of the lack of oxygen to brain cells. Edema fluid will pass into the injured bronchioles and trachea, causing pulmonary edema or obstruction. This leads to dyspnea and stridor. The edema may be so extensive that it reduces lung function substantially. About a week after the smoke inhalation, the possible development of pneumonia because of denuded tracheal and bronchial tract areas becomes a major problem. That inhalation of smoke or flame from a fire can be more serious than the skin burns the child suffers is rarely appreciated by parents. They are relieved if they learn that the child has suffered only smoke inhalation. They need an

(text continues on page 1664)

Jeanette is a 2-year-old girl admitted to your hospital unit with burns. The following is a nursing care plan designed for her.

Assessment: Child admitted through emergency department. Mother states she put out new candles on the dining room table, then went downstairs to change clothes in washing machine in basement while child was watching television. She heard child scream. Child ran to her from kitchen with her hair and upper clothes on fire (had been lighting candles as a "surprise" for mother). Mother rolled child in cotton sheet to put out flames, poured cold water from laundry tub on top to put out smoldering clothing. Called emergency number. Child admitted to emergency department within 20 min of burn.

Pulse: 110 beats/min; respirations: 26; blood pressure: 80/40 mm Hg. Child lying on examining table soundlessly crying. Mother states child's voice sounded "hoarse" in ambulance.

Burns estimated as 20% of body, second and third degree. Lower face, chin and neck, chest, back of head, and left arm are burned. Mother became hysterical in emergency department. Screamed that God was punishing her for recent divorce. Presently sitting by child's bedside, sobbing. Seems unable to support child because of her own unmet needs.

Nursing Diagnosis: Pain related to thermal injury

Defining Characteristic: Child is crying and appears uncomfortable.

Goal: Pain will be reduced to tolerable level in 10 min.

Outcome Criteria: Child is able to be comforted and stops crying.

Nursing Orders	Rationale
1. Intravenous (IV) line begun in dorsal surface of right foot. Morphine sulfate, 2mg, administered by IV push.	1. Provides relief from pain.
2. Assess respiratory function q 15 min for first hour because of morphine administration.	2. Morphine administration can reduce respiratory rate.
3. Encourage mother to redirect attention to child to reassure child that she is now safe.	3. Mother's concern for child's needs will help both mother and child to calm down; child receives psychologic support.
4. Administer analgesic to child (morphine 2 mg) daily before hydrotherapy and debridement therapy. Accompany child to physical therapy department for support.	4. Debridement is painful. Analgesic prior to therapy decreases pain.

Nursing Diagnosis: Self-esteem disturbance related to feelings of guilt about child's accident.

Defining Characteristic: Parent stated she felt accident was her fault.

Goal: Mother will view herself as worthwhile adult during recovery period.

Outcome Criteria: Mother identifies positive steps she took in emergency situation; participates in child's care (comforting, etc.).

(continued)

Nursing Orders	Rationale
1. Assure mother that she took normal precautions against an accident (saw child was occupied before leaving momentarily) and was able to respond with correct actions in an emergency (rolled child in sheet, called emergency squad).	1. Helps mother maintain high self-esteem.
2. Help mother locate a support person to give her enough support to be able to comfort child.	2. Mother needs support during a crisis period.
3. Provide time for mother to talk about the accident and voice that, while one must always try, it is not always possible to prevent all accidents.	3. Helps mother maintain high self-esteem through venting feelings.

Nursing Diagnosis: High risk for ineffective airway clearance related to inflammation caused by smoke inhalation

Defining Characteristic: Child's voice was hoarse in ambulance; silent crying in emergency room.

Goal: Child's airway will remain unobstructed.

Outcome Criteria: Respiratory rate is under 20/min; no stridor present; no temperature elevation to suggest pneumonia.

Nursing Orders	Rationale
1. Assess respiratory rate and quality of respirations q 15 min × 1, then q 1/2 h × 4.	1. Assessment helps determine degree of irritation from smoke inhalation.
2. Assess lungs for adventitious sounds with each vital sign assessment.	2. Abnormal sounds may indicate beginning of fluid accumulation in lungs.
3. Have emergency endotracheal tube tray at bedside and be prepared to assist with procedure.	3. Emergency interventions may be necessary.
4. Assist with blood gasses as necessary.	4. Hypoxemia can be detected by measuring blood gasses.
5. Begin postural drainage (percussion and vibrating) for 5 min q 1 h, modified because of location of burns on chest.	5. Postural drainage can help raise fluid formed as a result of smoke irritation.
6. Schedule chest x-ray as ordered.	6. Assists with detection of inflammation from smoke inhalation.
7. Oxygen by nasal cannula at 6 L to be administered until blood gas reports are returned.	7. Prevents hypoxemia.
8. Prevent hypothermia by keeping child warm.	8. Hypothermia can lead to respiratory distress.

Nursing Diagnosis: High risk for fluid volume deficit related to second-degree burn

Defining Characteristic: Second-degree burns cause fluid shifts because of increased permeability of blood vessels and inflammation process.

Goal: Child will maintain fluid and electrolyte balance during course of illness.

Outcome Criteria: Child's skin turgor is adequate; serum potassium from 3.5–5 mEq/L; serum sodium remains between 136 and 145 mEq/L; urine output remains greater than 1 mL/kg/h with specific gravity between 1.003 and 1.030.

(continued)

Nursing Orders

1. Assist with placement of IV therapy; maintain Ringer's lactate at 50 mL/h.
2. Weight for baseline weight q 12 h.
3. Assist with electrolyte and hematocrit determinations as necessary.
4. Test all urine specimens for amount and specific gravity.
5. Assess blood pressure and pulse q 15 min × 4 then q 1/2 hour × 4 h.
6. Assess peripheral pulses and capillary filling distal to burns on left arm q 1/2 h.
7. Assist with insertion of central venous pressure line; notify physician if reading is below 7.

Rationale

1. Provides increased fluid to prevent hypovolemia.
2. Weight loss may suggest hypovolemia.
3. An increasing hematocrit may suggest hypovolemia.
4. Urine output becomes inadequate in face of hypovolemia.
5. Decreased blood pressure and increased pulse suggests hypovolemia.
6. Alerts nurse to development of constricting eschar from burn.
7. A reduced central venous pressure level suggests hypovolemia.

Nursing Diagnosis: High risk for altered pattern of urinary elimination related to thermal injury

Defining Characteristic: Kidney failure is a possibility with any sudden body trauma.

Goal: Child will maintain a normal urinary output during therapy.

Outcome Criteria: Child's urine output remains greater than 1 mL/kg/h; tests negative for glucose, acetone, and protein.

Nursing Orders

1. Insert foley catheter.
2. Measure amount, specific gravity, protein, and acetone of urine every hour.

Rationale

1. Provide means to measure urine output.
2. Adequate urine output and normal specific gravity and protein and acetone levels indicate normal renal function.

Nursing Diagnosis: High risk for altered nutrition, less than body requirements, related to thermal injury

Defining Characteristic: Healing of burns requires more than normal intake of calories and protein.

Goal: Child will ingest an adequate diet for both maintenance and healing during course of illness.

Outcome Criteria: Child will ingest a high-protein, high-calorie diet.

Nursing Orders

1. Keep child NPO for first 24 h.
2. Insert nasogastric tube as prescribed.

Rationale

1. Delay food until bowel obstruction is ruled out.
2. Prevents vomiting and aspiration.

(continued)

Nursing Orders

3. Assess bowel sounds q 1 h.

4. Administer Maalox 10 mL q 1/2 h; assess any emesis for occult blood; assess stool daily for occult blood.
5. If bowel sounds are present at 24 h, begin liquid, high-protein, high-calorie diet.
6. Encourage parent to visit at mealtime to make it a social occasion.
7. Discourage child from refusing food as a way of maintaining independence (contracting with child may be helpful).
8. Schedule mealtime before, not immediately following, hydrotherapy.
9. Encourage child to feed herself as much as possible despite dressings.
10. Record intake and output.

Rationale

3. Indicates whether normal bowel sounds are present.
4. Helps prevent stress ulcer, monitors for development of stress ulcer.

5. High-protein, high-calorie diet is necessary for healing of burned tissue.
6. Encourages child to eat better.

7. Adequate caloric intake is an important part of the healing process.

8. Exhaustion following hydrotherapy can dull the child's appetite.
9. Allows the child to maintain some control over the environment.
10. Monitors kidney function.

Nursing Diagnosis: High risk for infection related to thermal injury

Defining Characteristic: Alteration in skin integrity leaves an open portal for invasion of microorganisms.

Goal: Child will not develop an infection of burned area during healing period.

Outcome Criteria: Child's temperature remains below 37.0°C rectally; skin surface surrounding burn is not erythematous or warm.

Nursing Orders

1. Establish and maintain isolation as necessary.
2. Wear sterile gloves and mask (strict aseptic technique) when burned area is exposed during dressing change.
3. Apply silver sulfadiazine cream 15% to all burned areas daily following hydrotherapy. Cover with sterile Kling gauze.
4. Use extreme care when changing dressings.
5. Protect burned area or graft site from trauma (hitting a burned area against a siderail, sleeping on burned arm, etc.)
6. Encourage activity to tolerance.

7. Obtain wound cultures as prescribed or if obvious drainage or erythema is present.

8. Administer mouth care 3 times daily to reduce oral microorganisms.
9. Administer antibiotics (gentamicin by IV q 6 h) as prescribed.

Rationale

1. Reduces level of microorganisms near burned areas.
2. Reduces level of microorganisms near burned areas.

3. Protects against microorganism invasion.

4. Protects against injuring new tissue.
5. Protects against injuring new tissue.

6. Promotes circulation and supplies nutrients to burned areas.
7. Provides early warning of infection; allows identification of appropriate antibiotic for the organism that is cultured.
8. The mouth normally harbors a high level of microorganisms.
9. Provides prophylaxis against infection.

(continued)

1663

Nursing Diagnosis: Impaired physical mobility related to thermal injury

Defining Characteristic: Treatment of thermal injury requires bedrest and positioning.

Goal: Child will experience no permanent interference with mobility during rehabilitation.

Outcome Criteria: Child demonstrates a full range of motion in left arm and neck.

Nursing Orders	**Rationale**
1. Determine which areas are most apt to develop contractures (burns over a body joint, for example).	1. This complication is preventable.
2. Encourage the child to be active and give self-care.	2. Active motion could help prevent contractures.
3. Establish a program of active or passive exercises 4 × daily; use a reminder sheet to aid compliance.	3. Range of motion exercises can help prevent contractures.
4. Include games such as "Simon Says" in exercise program.	4. Age appropriate motivation technique will increase compliance.
5. Maintain overextended body alignment in neck and left elbow.	5. Prevents joint contractures.
6. Apply and maintain a splint over dressing on left elbow continuously.	6. Prevents joint contractures.

Nursing Diagnosis: High risk for body image disturbance related to thermal injury

Defining Characteristic: Child verbalizes negative feelings about how scar tissue will look.

Goal: Child will demonstrate positive perception of self at end of burn therapy.

Outcome Criteria: Child states that she sees herself as well again; participates in activities; is able to look at injured skin and does not keep burned areas always covered by clothing.

(continued)

explanation of the physiologic consequences that can result from pulmonary injury.

> **Nursing Diagnosis:** High risk for altered breathing patterns related to edema from thermal injury

> **Goal:** Child will maintain respiratory function during course of illness.

> **Outcome Criteria:** Child's respiratory rate stays within 16 to 20 breaths per minute; lung auscultation reveals no rales.

Obtain a history to assess if the fire occurred in a closed space, such as a garage. Assess for burns of the face, neck, or chest, which meant fire was near the nose and respiratory tract. Assess the quality of the child's voice (will be hoarse if the throat is irritated from smoke). The respiratory rate of all burned children should be monitored carefully, because the respiratory rate increases with respiratory obstruction. The child may become restless and thrash because of oxygen lack. Measurement of blood gases will demonstrate the degree of hypoxia present from carbon monoxide intoxication. Administering 100% oxygen is the best therapy for displacing carbon monoxide and providing adequate oxygenation to body cells once more. The child may need intubation or tracheotomy with assisted ventilation. Intubation is best because this child is even more prone to pneumonia than the average child with a tracheotomy. Symptoms of smoke inhalation may not occur immediately but only after 8 to 24 hours. A chest x-ray

Nursing Orders	**Rationale**
1. Allow time to discuss why the burn occurred.	1. Child may feel an accident is her fault.
2. Encourage child to talk about appearance if scar tissue will be present; teach that how people are inside is more important than physical appearance.	2. Child will maintain positive body image.
3. Encourage activities the child can do, not those she cannot.	3. Helps increase positive feelings in the child.
4. Help family to be supportive of their child's feelings.	4. Family support will encourage child to maintain positive body image.
5. Allow the optimum amount of decision making possible.	5. Provides the child with a sense of autonomy.
6. Encourage child to express resentment of painful procedures.	6. Helps child maintain control by expressing feelings.
7. Accept regressive behavior as a normal reaction to stress.	7. Helps child to deal with stress of body image change.
8. Facilitate adjustment to compression dressing by stressing its importance.	8. Understanding the value of the dressing in reducing deformity may increase compliance.

Nursing Diagnosis: Parental knowledge deficit related to what is safe home environment for toddler

Defining Characteristic: Mother left candles and matches within easy reach.

Goal: Parent will demonstrate increased knowledge of safe home environment.

Outcome Criteria: Parent identifies steps she has taken to make home a safer environment for toddler.

Nursing Orders	**Rationale**
1. Discuss fire safety in relation to toddler age group.	1. Increases mother's awareness of fire hazards in the home.
2. Discuss normal growth and development of toddler and the potential dangers that children of this age group are prone to (poisoning, falls).	2. Mother will be knowledgeable about how to child-proof her home.

taken at this time will reveal collecting edematous fluid and decreased aeration ability. Continue to assess the child's temperature every 4 hours for the first week after the injury to detect lung infection. The cause of fever may relate to infection in the burn area; if the burn occurred in a closed area so that the child inhaled smoke, pneumonia must also be considered as a possible reason for increasing temperature. Bronchodilators to increase respiratory tract lumens and antibiotics to decrease the possibility of pneumonia will be prescribed. High-frequency ventilation may be helpful to keep alveoli functioning.

Urinary System. Because the child's blood volume decreases immediately following a burn, renal function is threatened by kidney ischemia just when renal function is needed to rid the body of breakdown products from burned cells. If the child is burned over 10% of his or her body surface, urinary output may decrease immediately. Blood volume must be maintained by intravenous fluid administration to establish good urinary output once more. Urine output should be 1 mL per kilogram of body weight per hour. The specific gravity of urine also should be monitored to determine whether the kidneys can concentrate urine to conserve body fluid (failing kidneys lose this ability rapidly). In the days following the burn, as products of necrotic tissue and toxic substances must be evacuated by the kidney, kidney function may fail again. There are also increases in antidiuretic hormone and aldosterone. Diuresis occurs at 48 hours.

Nursing Diagnosis: High risk for altered urinary elimination related to thermal trauma

Goal: Child will not experience decreased urine output during course of illness.

Outcome Criteria: Child's urine output will be greater than 1 mL per kilogram of body weight per hour.

A Foley catheter should be inserted and an immediate urine specimen obtained for analysis. A specific gravity determination performed immediately in the emergency department is helpful. Observing urinary output will be a major nursing responsibility in the days to come.

Urine output less than 1 mL/kg/hour suggests renal insufficiency. Free hemoglobin from destroyed red blood cells can plug kidney tubules and lead to kidney failure (acute tubular necrosis). When this is occurring, urine will be red to black from the hemoglobin present. A diuretic such as mannitol may be administered to flush this from the kidneys. If effective, urine returns to its usual straw color.

Gastrointestinal System. The metabolic rate increases in children following burns as their body begins to pool its resources to adjust to the insult. If the child does not receive enough calories in intravenous fluid, he or she will begin to utilize protein. This is particularly dangerous since the child needs protein now for burn healing, and he or she will become acidotic.

Nursing Diagnosis: High risk for altered nutrition, less than body requirements, related to thermal trauma

Goal: Child will ingest adequate nutrients for increased metabolic needs during therapy.

Outcome Criteria: Child's weight remains within normal growth percentiles; skin turgor remains normal; urine specific gravity remains between 1.003 and 1.030.

A nasogastric tube may be inserted and regulated to low suction as prophylactic therapy to prevent aspiration of vomitus. The tube must remain in place until bowel sounds are detected. This usually occurs within 24 hours but may take as long as 72 hours in severely burned children. The suction from a nasogastric tube may be tinged with blood (coffee-ground fluid) due to bleeding caused by stomach vessel congestion. This drainage must be observed closely for a change to fresh bleeding, which can be caused by a stomach ulcer (Curling's ulcer). This type of ulcer results from stress. It is prevented by administering cimetidine (Tagamet) in an attempt to reduce gastric acidity and ulcer formation.

If a bleeding ulcer occurs, gastric lavage with iced saline may be necessary. A blood transfusion should be prepared, because the blood loss from a GI ulcer can be rapid and severe.

When children have burns over more than 30% of the body surface, paralytic ileus may occur. If this happens, within hours of the burn, symptoms of intestinal obstruction (vomiting, abdominal distention, colicky pain) will appear.

Children with severe burns are usually kept NPO for 24 hours because of the danger of paralytic ileus. After this, most burned children are able to eat, and oral feedings are begun as soon as possible. To supply adequate calories for increased metabolic needs and spare protein for repairing cells, the diet is high in calories and protein (1800 cal/m^2/24 h plus 22 cal per square meter of burned areas per 24 hours); children may also need vitamin (particularly B and C) and iron supplements. High-protein drinks may be necessary in between meals to ensure an adequate protein intake.

Because adequate nutrition is important, it may be necessary to supplement the child's diet with intravenous or hyperalimentation solutions or nasogastric tube feeding. Don't ever use these methods of supplying nutrition as threats (caution parents not to do this either); present them if they are needed as just another way of being fed. As additional methods of stimulating interest in eating, you can encourage school-age children to help add intake and output columns; help the dietitian add a calorie-count list; or keep track of their own daily weight (taken at the same time each day with the same clothing on). It may be helpful to make contracts with older children for a good nutritional intake.

Immune System. There appears to be some defect in the ability of neutrophils to phagocytize bacteria following thermal injury, and formation of IgG antibodies apparently fails. For these reasons, the child has reduced protection against infection. *Staphylococcus aureus* and streptococci are the gram-positive organisms and *Pseudomonas aeruginosa* is the gram-negative organism most likely to invade burn tissue. Children are usually prescribed parenteral penicillin to prevent β-hemolytic streptococcal infection and tetanus toxoid to prevent tetanus.

Bacteria penetrate the burn eschar readily, so this offers no protection from infection, although it does offer protection from fluid loss. Fortunately, granulation tissue, which forms under the eschar 3 to 4 weeks after the burn, is resistant to bacterial invasion.

Nursing Diagnosis: High risk for infection related to denuded skin surfaces and lowered resistance to infection with thermal injury

Goal: Child will not develop an infection during time of denuded tissue.

Outcome Criteria: Child's temperature remains below 37°C; skin areas surrounding burned areas show no signs of erythema or warmth.

Because the child has lost the integumentary defense against infection, prophylactic treatment is important to prevent infection. Antibiotics are not very effective in controlling burn-wound infection, probably because the burned and constricted capillaries around the burn site cannot carry the antibiotic to the area. Equipment used with the child must therefore be sterile. Personnel caring for the severely burned child should wear caps, masks, gowns, and gloves, even for emergency care. Children are placed on a sterile sheet on the examining table. Nose, throat, and wound cultures may be done.

Even though their burns may be covered by gauze dressings, children generally are kept isolated until adequate granulation tissue has formed to serve as a barrier against massive infection. Cultures of the burned area are taken about every third day so that invading organisms can be identified and specific therapy planned. Helping children maintain their self-esteem and keeping them from withdrawing from social contacts is one of the most difficult nursing roles in caring for a burned child during the isolation period.

Endocrine System. In response to injury, the adrenal gland releases epinephrine and norepinephrine. This may lead to compensatory hypertension. Both aldosterone and antidiuretic hormone levels rise in an attempt to conserve fluid.

Integumentary and Musculoskeletal Systems. Because third-degree burns heal with fibrous scarring, contracture of the joint may occur if the burn was over a movable body part. Joints are positioned carefully, often overextended, so that if some contracture occurs, the joint will eventually remain in good position. Extremities are elevated to decrease edema and tissue pressure. The overextension positions are difficult to maintain because they become uncomfortable for the child, who needs support to accept these measures. You must be certain that you understand the need for these positions, so that you can reinforce their importance (Figure 52-12).

Therapy for Severe Burns

Once the child has been given immediate care and is thoroughly assessed to determine the effects of the injury on all body systems, planning for burn treatment can begin.

Second- and third-degree burns may be cared for by open treatment, leaving the burned area exposed to the air, or by a closed method, covering the burned area with an antibacterial cream and many layers of gauze. These two methods are compared in Table 52-9. As a rule, burn dressings are applied loosely in the first 24 hours to prevent circulation from being interfered with as edema forms. Be certain not to allow two burned body surfaces such as the sides of fingers or the back of the ears and the scalp to touch, because as healing takes place, a webbing forms between these surfaces. Don't use adhesive tape as it is painful to remove and can leave excoriated areas, additional areas for infection.

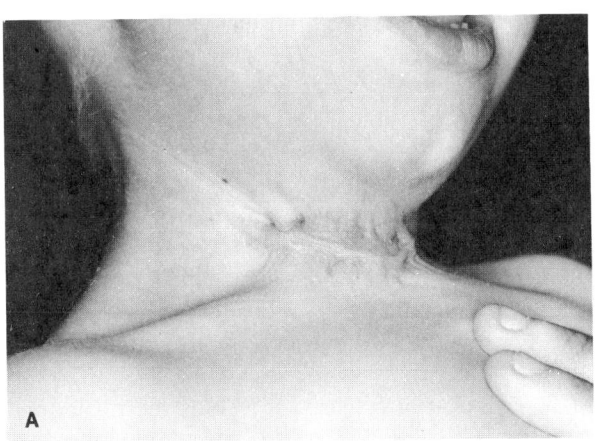

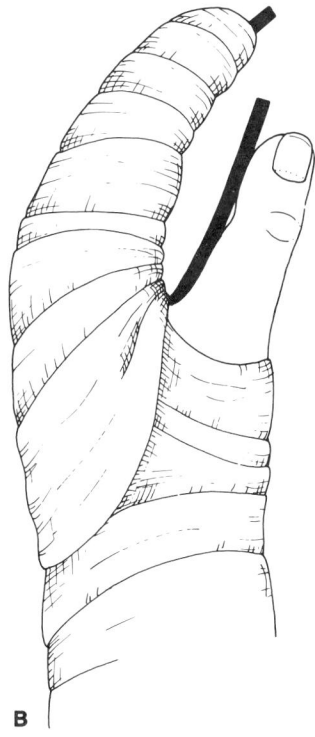

FIGURE 52-12
(**A**) A contracture caused by a third-degree burn of the neck. The child has limited ability to hyperextend his head. (Courtesy of the Department of Medical Photography, Children's Hospital, Buffalo, NY.) (**B**) A hand splint to maintain normal position held in place by Kerlex over a burn dressing.

Table 52-9. *Comparison of Open and Closed Burn Therapy*

Method	Description	Advantages	Disadvantages
Open	Burn is exposed to air; used for superficial burns or body parts that are prone to infection, such as perineum	Allows frequent inspection of site; allows child to follow healing process	Requires strict isolation to prevent infection; area may scrape and bleed easily and impede healing
Closed	Burn is covered with nonadherent gauze; used for moderate and severe burns	Better protection from injury; easier to turn and position child; allows child more freedom to play	Dressing changes are painful; possibility of infection may increase because of dark, moist environment

Netting is useful to use to hold dressings in place as it expands easily and needs no additional tape.

Topical Therapy

Silver sulfadiazine (Silvadene) is the drug of choice for burn therapy to limit infection at the burn site. It is applied as a paste to the burn, and the area is covered with a few layers of mesh gauze (Figure 52-13). Silver sulfadiazine is an effective agent against gram-negative and gram-positive organisms as well as secondary infectious agents such as *Candida*. It is soothing when applied and tends to keep the burn eschar soft, making debridement easier. It does not penetrate the eschar well, which is its one drawback.

Povidone-iodine (Betadine) may be used to inhibit bacterial and fungal growth. Unfortunately, iodine stings as it is applied and stains skin and clothing brown. Dressings must be kept continually wet to keep them from clinging to and disrupting the healing tissue. An occlusive dressing with topical antibiotic therapy may be used.

Pseudomonas is a pathogen commonly found in burn wounds. If it is detected in cultures, gentamicin (Garamycin) cream may be applied. If a topical cream is not effective against invading organisms in the deeper tissue under the eschar, daily injections of specific antibiotics to the deeper layers of the burned area may be necessary. Staphylococcus or proteus are other common contaminates.

If a burned area cannot be readily dressed, such as the female genitalia, it can be left exposed. The danger of this method is the potential invasion of pathogens.

Escharotomy

An eschar is the tough, leathery scab that forms over moderately or severely burned areas. Fluid accumulates rapidly under eschars, putting pressure on underlying blood vessels and nerves. If an extremity or the trunk has been burned so both anterior and posterior surfaces have eschar formation, this may form a tight band around the extremity or trunk, shutting off circulation to the distal body portions. Distal parts feel cool to the touch and appear pale; the child notices tingling or numbness. Pulses are difficult to palpate and capillary refill is slow (more than 5 seconds). To alleviate this problem, an **escharotomy** (cut into the eschar) is performed. Some bleeding following escharotomy will occur. Packing the wound and applying pressure usually relieves this.

Debridement

Debridement is the removal of necrotic tissue from a burned area. Debridement reduces the possibility of infection because it reduces the tissue present for microorganisms to live on. Children usually have 20 minutes of hydrotherapy before debridement to soften and loosen eschar (Figure 52-14), which can then be gently snipped away with forceps and scissors. Debridement is painful, and some bleeding occurs with it. Help children use a distraction technique (discussed in Chapter 37) during the procedure to reduce the level of pain. Transcutaneous electrical nerve stimulation therapy may be helpful to reduce the pain of debridement. Praise any degree of cooperation. Plan an enjoyable activity afterward.

There are very few times when being a nurse is not rewarding or enjoyable. Unfortunately, helping with burn debridement is one of them. Children need to have a "helping" person with them, to hold their hand, to stroke their head, and to offer some verbal comfort: "It's all right to cry; we know that hurts. We don't like to do this, but it's one of the things that makes burns heal." Nursing personnel need a great deal of talk time to voice their feelings about assisting with or doing debridement procedures. Be careful in serving as the "helping" person that you do not project yourself as the healer and the comforter and a fellow nurse as the hurter, the "bad guy." It helps if people alternate this chore so that on alternate days each serves as the protector and the comforter. Kavanagh (1990) has found that when children are given some control over the process of debridement (e.g., piercing blisters), they are much better able to cope with the procedure and much less likely to suffer from depression later.

If eschar tissue is debrided in this manner day after day, granulation tissue forms underneath. When a full

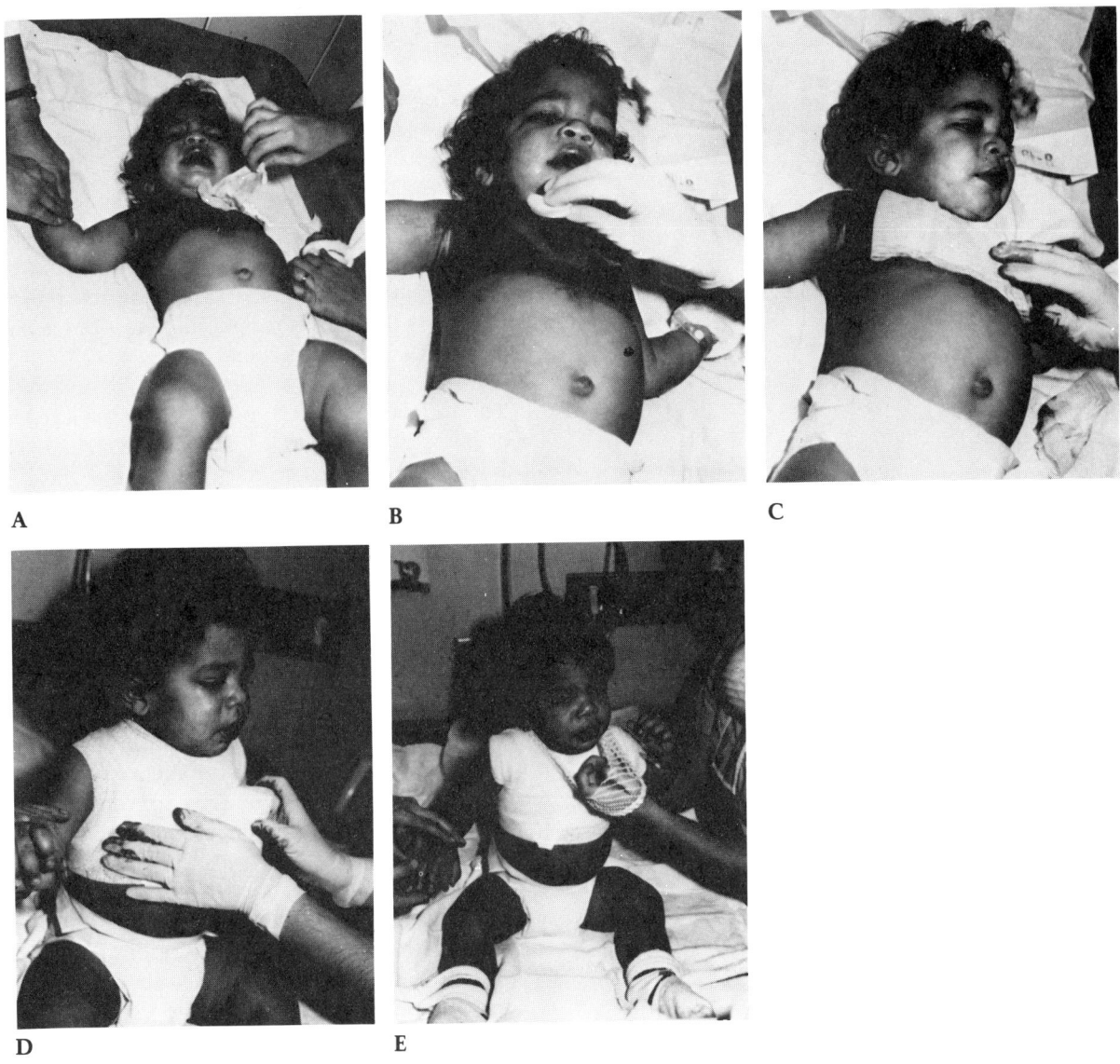

A B C

D E

FIGURE 52-13
*Changing a burn dressing: (**A**) removing the old dressing; (**B**) cleaning the burned area; (**C**) iodine gauze placed under the chin to prevent skin surfaces from touching; (**D**) Kerlex; (**E**) net tubing. (Courtesy of Bruce Hill.)*

bed of granulation tissue is present (about 2 weeks after the injury) the area is ready for skin grafting. In some burn centers, this waiting period is avoided by immediate surgical excision of eschar and placement of skin grafts. A newer trend in debridement is the use of Travase, an enzyme that can dissolve tissue.

Grafting
Homografting (also called **allografting**) is the placing of skin (sterilized and frozen) from cadavers or a donor on the cleaned burn site. These grafts do not grow but provide a protective covering for the area. In small children, **heterografts** (also called *xenografts*) from other sources such as porcine (pig) skin may be used. **Autografting** is a process in which a layer of skin of both

epidermis and a part of the dermis (called a *split-thickness graft*) is removed from a distal, unburned portion of the child's body and placed at the prepared burn site, where it will grow and replace the burned skin. Postage stamp–sized grafts of split-thickness skin are often used. Larger areas require mesh grafts (a strip of partial thickness skin that is slit at intervals so that it can be stretched to cover a larger area) (Figure 52-15). The advantage of grafting is that it reduces fluid and electrolyte loss, pain, and the chance of infection.

Following the grafting procedure, the area is covered by a bulky dressing. So that the growth of the newly adhering cells will not be disrupted, this should not be removed or changed. The donor site on the child's body (often the anterior thigh or buttocks) is also

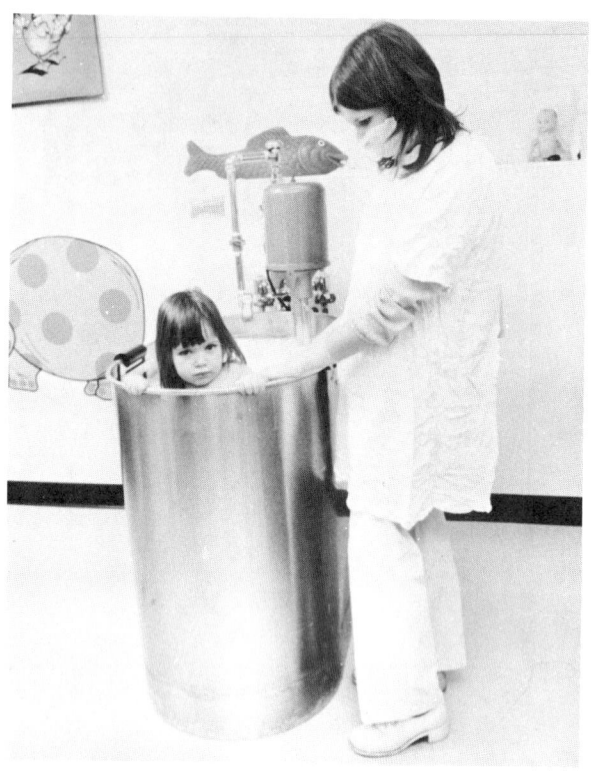

FIGURE 52-14

A child with burns receiving a whirlpool treatment. Notice the apprehension on her face because of this strange bathtub. (Courtesy of the Department of Medical Photography, Children's Hospital, Buffalo, NY.)

covered by a gauze dressing. Both donor and graft dressings should be observed for fluid drainage and odor. Observe the child to see if he or she has pain at either site, which might indicate infection. The child's temperature should be taken every 4 hours; a rise in systemic temperature may be the first indication that there is infection at the graft or donor site. Autograft sites can be reused every 7 to 10 days, so any one site can provide a great deal of skin for grafting.

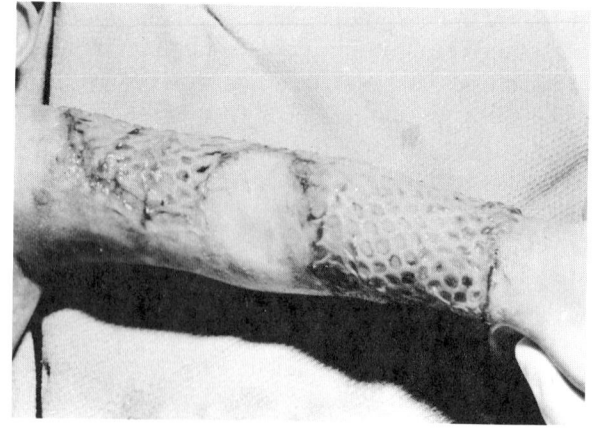

FIGURE 52-15

Skin grafting: a mesh graft in place. (Courtesy of the Department of Medical Photography, Children's Hospital, Buffalo, NY.)

Nursing Diagnoses and Related Interventions

Nursing Diagnosis: Social isolation related to reverse isolation necessary to control spread of microorganisms

Goal: Child will demonstrate that he or she is able to cope with degree of isolation necessary during course of illness.

Outcome Criteria: Child states that he or she understands the reason for isolation and can accept it as a necessary part of therapy.

The isolation involved in the care of children with major burns is more than just isolation in a single room; all the people who come into the room wear gowns, masks, caps, and sterile gloves. The child, therefore, is doubly isolated: by distance and by strangers who never touch him or her directly.

It is easy for children with burns (who were told not to play with matches or go too close to the fireplace) to interpret this isolation as punishment. Make every effort to make their environment as warm and comforting as possible, despite the isolation procedures. Place children's beds so that they can see as much unit activity as possible. Decorate walls in front of them with cards they receive or with a changing gallery of pictures (gas sterilized) drawn by staff members of things in which the children appear interested.

Children need to be able to discuss their feelings about being kept in a room by themselves. A question such as, "It's hard to understand a lot of things about a hospital; do you understand why your bed is in this special room?" gives children a chance to express their feelings. The answer from young children is invariably, "Because I was bad." You should explain that although they might have been bad (playing with matches), they are being kept in this special room now to make their burns heal so that they can go home as quickly as possible. It is important that burned children do not view their hospitalization as one long punishment for being burned. If children were so "bad" that they must be punished as much as this, how can they ever think of themselves as "good" again? How can they ever achieve anything in life after this experience?

Encourage parents to put on their gowns and masks and come into the room to give as much care as possible. Parents often do not ask to do these things spontaneously when their children are severely burned. They are in a state of grief. They do not react in a normal manner. They may believe the bulky dressings make it impossible for them to hold the child. Actually, the closed bulky dressings on the wound make it *possible* for the child to be held. If it is not possible for children to be held, help parents to see that stroking a child's face or touching a hand (even with rubber gloves in place) gives the child a feeling of still being loved.

Nursing Diagnosis: Altered family processes related to severe burns in family member

Goal: The family will remain intact and functional during the period of rehabilitation.

Outcome Criteria: Family voices that they are able to cope effectively with the degree of stress they are subjected to.

Children with severe burns always have a difficult hospitalization because it involves pain, isolation, and (at some point) awareness of the disfigurement that accompanies major burns.

Some parents grieve so deeply over the child's condition or are so concerned with other upsetting factors in their lives (many burns happen because of situational crisis in the family) that their interaction with the child seems to falter or proves very difficult for them. They may avoid visiting because the sound of the child's crying when they leave is more than they can endure at the same time they have lost their home and possessions to fire. They may need help in establishing priorities. It may be important that they wait at home one morning for an insurance inspector to make an estimate on damage caused by the fire to their house or furniture. Other tasks, however, such as shopping or housecleaning, could possibly be done by relatives or neighbors, leaving them time to visit the child.

Nursing Diagnosis: Diversional activity deficit related to restricted mobility following severe burn

Goal: Child remains interested in age-appropriate activities during rehabilitation.

Outcome Criteria: Child expresses interest in obtaining school homework; communicates with friends and relatives via telephone or letters.

Remember that although children's chest, abdomen, and hands are burned, they do not stop thinking. If they lie for hours, days, or months with nothing to do, however, it is as though their mind were as burned and functionless as their body. They need stimulation in their isolated environment. A television set is good for passing time but should not be the child's main communication with the outside world. Listening to favorite records, having stories read to him or her, talking about what is going on at home or what the child normally does at school, and doing schoolwork are important, too.

Most toys or play material can be sterilized by gas autoclave and brought into isolation units. They should be cultured periodically and sterilized frequently to prevent their becoming a source of infection. When a child is in pain, as severely burned children are, the presence of a favorite toy in the room becomes extremely important.

Make certain to visit the child just to talk to him or her, or come to play a game at times other than proce-

dures or treatment times. The child may be hospitalized for a long time. He or she needs to view the nursing staff as friends as well as caregivers. Frequent visits, even though they are short, convey to a child that he or she is not alone, that people are aware of the child and his or her needs. This usually prevents the child from developing a whining, demanding manner, the consequence of feeling that if he or she does not demand attention, no one will come.

Nursing Diagnosis Body image disturbance related to changes in physical appearance with thermal injury

Goal: Child will maintain self-esteem during rehabilitation period.

Outcome Criteria: Child expresses fears about physical appearance; demonstrates desire to resume age-appropriate activities.

Children with burns are often forced to become extremely dependent on the nursing staff because of the position in which they must lie and because of bulky dressings that cover their arms or hands and prevent them from feeding themselves. They respond to this forced dependence at first with gratitude. They are hurt, and someone is taking care of them. After a period, however, the response may become less healthy. The young school-age child or preschooler may revert to bedwetting or baby talk. Older children respond by becoming openly aggressive to counteract their feelings of helplessness. They attempt to reestablish independence in the ways that they can, often by refusing to eat or to lie in a position that is best for them. Although good nutrition is vitally important for rapid healing, it may suffer because of children's need to assert their independence. Make certain when caring for burned children (and all children) that you allow independent decision making whenever possible. Children must take their 10 o'clock medicine, but they can choose the fluid they want to swallow after it. They must be fed meals because of the bulky dressings over their hands, but they can decide which food they will be fed first. They must have their dressings changed, but they can choose the story you will read them afterward.

Be careful that you do not give choices when there really are none to give. "Can I change your dressing now?" "Do you want dinner now?" "Will you swallow this pill?" are inappropriate questions; you do not really mean to give children a choice about these things.

Immediately after a severe burn, children (if they are old enough to understand), parents, and probably the hospital staff are most concerned with whether or not they will live. When body systems have stabilized and it seems appropriate to assure parents that the child will live, thoughts turn to the child's cosmetic appearance. At first it is easy for children and parents to ignore this problem because the burned areas are covered by dressings. Even when the dressings are removed for debridement or whirlpool, it is easy for children to assume that the appearance of the burned area is only temporary and the area will eventually heal and have a good appearance. They have probably never seen anyone with a scar from a second- or third-degree burn and so have no reason to worry about it (Figure 52-16).

When children see others on the unit with burn scars, they begin to realize what healing will look like. Depending on the extent and the site of the burn, parents and children will have varying degrees of difficulty accepting this. They may lose confidence in the health care personnel (it seems that with all the advances in medicine, a burn should heal with a better appearance).

Parents and children need time to talk about their feelings. A girl may be extremely concerned if her chest is burned because she is worried that breast tissue will not develop (a very real concern, depending on the extent of the burn). Her parents may be most concerned because they can see that although a blouse can cover her chest, her right hand will not have full function. Do not assume, therefore, that what you are most concerned about is what the child and parents are most concerned about. A father who dreamed his son would be a great track star may be most concerned about a leg scar; the child may be most concerned about a facial burn.

Children watch you as you care for them to see if you find them unattractive. As dressings are removed, children may expose parts of their body seemingly inappropriately, to see if you are shocked or revolted by them. It is easy to think that you will not react this way, but for everyone the first sight of a severe burn is a shock and it is difficult not to react accordingly. Imagining how the child feels, realizing that this mutilated skin

is his or hers, helps health care providers maintain a professional attitude.

Returning to school is difficult for children who have been hospitalized or on home care for a long time. Their old friends have new friends, so they may feel cut out of school activities. They look different if they have burn scars. The appearance of scar formation can be improved by the application of pressure dressings that the child wears 24 hours a day. If the child has facial burns, facing friends with a compression bandage in place may be difficult. They need a great deal of support from health care personnel at health care visits to be able to endure this. Some children may need referral for formal counseling. Some parents may need formal counseling as well to help them accept the child's changed appearance.

Electrical Burns of the Mouth

If children put the prongs of a plugged-in extension cord into their mouth, their mouth will be burned severely. Electrical current from the plug is conducted for a distance through the skin and underlying tissue so a tissue area much larger than where the prongs actually touched is involved (Linebaugh & Koka, 1993).

Tissue will be destroyed at the entry site, leaving an angry-looking ulcer. If blood vessels were burned, active bleeding will be present. The immediate treatment for electrical burns is to unplug the electric cord and control bleeding. Pressure applied to the site with gauze will usually control this. Most children are admitted to a hospital for at least 24 hours of observation following electrical burns of the mouth because edema in the mouth may lead to airway obstruction.

Clean the wound about four times a day with an antiseptic solution, such as half-strength hydrogen peroxide, to reduce the possibility of infection (a real danger in this area because bacteria are always present in the mouth).

Eating will be a problem for children because their mouth is so sore. They may be able to drink fluids from a cup best. Bland fluids, such as artificial fruit drinks, flat ginger ale, or milk products, are best.

Electrical burns of the mouth turn black as local tissue necrosis begins. They will heal with white, fibrous scar tissue, possibly causing a deformity of the lip and cheeks with healing (Figure 52-17). This can be minimized by the use of a mouth appliance, which helps maintain lip contour (Kula, 1994). Some children may have difficulty with speech sounds because of resulting lip scarring. They need follow-up care by a plastic surgeon to restore their lip contour and function again. Obviously, you need to review with parents the importance of not leaving "live" electrical cords where young children can reach them.

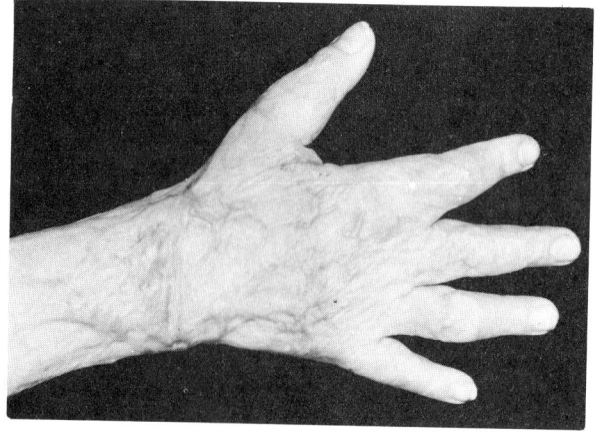

FIGURE 52-16

Scars remaining from a third-degree burn on the back of the hand. Notice the good finger alignment and function despite the extent of this burn. (Courtesy of the Department of Medical Photography, Children's Hospital, Buffalo, NY.)

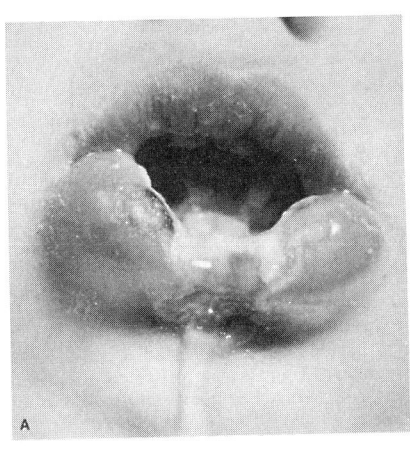 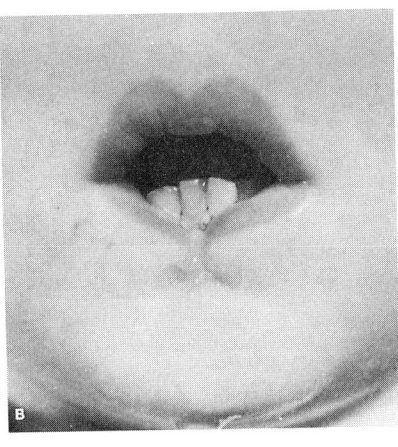

FIGURE 52-17
*An electrical burn of the mouth from a plugged-in electrical cord. (**A**) Two weeks after the accident, a portion of the lower lip is missing because of tissue necrosis. (**B**) The lower lip after 6 months. Plastic surgery will be necessary to achieve full function. (Courtesy of the Department of Medical Photography, Children's Hospital, Buffalo, NY.)*

Nursing Role in the Prevention of Accidents

Nurses in every care setting have the unique opportunity among health care professionals of providing patient/family teaching concerning the prevention of accidents. Even in the acute care setting when an accident has already occurred, nurses can provide invaluable instruction to families on safeguarding their children against future accidents. In the community setting, nurses have a greater opportunity for assessment of the unique threats present in particular environments, for example, lead-based paint in older homes, the presence of kerosene heaters in a home, the risk of drowning in a home that has a swimming pool, and so on. Nurses therefore need to be knowledgeable about both interventions utilized when accidents occur and preventive measures. Instructing families in prevention requires a broad awareness of age-old as well as modern threats in the environment.

Key Points

- Children need total body assessment following a traumatic injury, as they may be unable to describe other injuries besides a primary one they may have suffered. Be certain that aseptic technique is maintained when caring for trauma victims so the child doesn't develop an additional unnecessary infection.
- Head injuries are always potentially serious in children. Skull fractures, subdural hematoma, epidural hematomas, concussion, and contusions can occur. Nursing diagnoses identified in association with this are High risk for fluid volume excess and Altered growth and development.
- Coma (unconsciousness from which children cannot be roused) may be present in children following severe head trauma. Nursing diagnoses related to this are High risk for ineffective airway clearance, Altered skin integrity, and Altered nutrition.

- Abdominal trauma resulting in splenic or liver rupture may occur in connection with multiple trauma.
- Near drowning can occur from salt or fresh water. Nursing diagnoses identified with this are High risk for infection and Fear. The physiologic basis for complications following drowning differs as to whether the water was fresh or salt water.
- Common substances children swallow which result in poisoning are acetaminophen (Tylenol) and salicylic acid (aspirin). Teach parents to keep the number of the local poison control center next to their telephone and always to call first before administering an antidote for poisoning.
- Lead poisoning most frequently occurs from the ingestion of lead chips from older housing. Preventing this is a major nursing responsibility.
- Burns are divided into three types—first degree, second degree, and third degree—depending on the depth of the burn. Burns produce systemic body reactions. Nursing diagnoses identified with this are High risk for altered tissue perfusion, Altered breathing patterns, Altered urinary elimination, Altered nutrition, Infection, Social isolation, Altered family processes, Diversional activity deficit, and Body image disturbance.
- Be aware that some trauma in children occurs from child abuse. Screen for this by history and physical examination.

Critical Thinking Exercises

1. Jeremy is a 6-year-old who is admitted to the hospital in coma. What special precautions would you want to take to insure that he maintains a patent airway? That he maintains skin integrity?
2. Susan is a 3-year-old seen in the emergency room for acetaminophen poisoning. Her father tells you they normally lock all medicine away carefully. His wife left acetaminophen on the counter because she was hurrying to take some and lie down be-

cause she had a migraine headache. Would you want to discuss the necessity of poisoning prevention with these parents or should they have learned from this experience that their actions were not safe?

3. Chris is a 10-year-old who has third-degree burns on her legs from lighting a fire to burn leaves. She will probably have a lengthy hospitalization and may need skin grafts to improve healing. What precautions does Chris need to prevent infection until healing is complete?

References

Department of Health & Human Services. (1991). *Healthy people 2000.* Washington, DC: Public Health Service.

DeRienzo-DeVivio, S. (1992). Childhood lead poisoning: Shifting to primary prevention. *Pediatric Nursing, 18,* 565.

Glaze, D. G. (1994). The comatose child. In F.A. Oski et al. (Eds.) *Principles and practice of pediatrics* (2nd ed.). Philadelphia: J.B. Lippincott.

Grant, T. A. (1992). Pediatric abdominal trauma. *Emergency, 24,* 36.

Inaba, A. S. (1993). The rusty nail—and other puncture wounds of the foot. *Contemporary Pediatrics, 10,* 138.

Kallas, H. J., & O'Rourke, P. P. (1993). Drowning and immersion injuries in children. *Current Opinion in Pediatrics, 5,* 295.

Kavanagh, C. (1990). Psychiatric mental health nursing with the patient in intensive care. In F. Gary & C. Kavanagh (Eds.), *Psychiatric mental health nursing.* Glenview, IL: Scott, Foresman.

Krasner, P. (1992). Management of dental injuries. *Journal of School Nursing, 8,* 20.

Kula, K. (1994). Electrical burns. In F. A. Oski et al. (Eds.) *Principles and practice of pediatrics (2nd ed.).* Philadelphia: J. B. Lippincott.

Levallois, P., et al. (1991). Blood lead levels in children and pregnant women living near a lead reclamation plant. *Canadian Medical Association Journal, 144,* 877.

Linebaugh, M. L., & Koka, S. (1993). Oral electrical burns. *Journal of Prosthodontics, 2,* 136.

Mariscalco, M. M. (1994). Acetaminophen overdose. In F. A. Oski et al. (Eds.) *Principles and practice of pediatrics* (2nd ed.). Philadelphia: J.B. Lippincott.

McIntire, M. S., et al. (1991). Philodendron—an infant death. *Journal of Toxicology and Clinical Toxicology, 28,* 177.

Morelli, J. (1993). Pediatric poisonings: The ten most toxic prescription drugs. *American Journal of Nursing, 93,* 27.

Norris, M. K. (1993). Pediatric near-drowning. *Nursing, 23,* 33.

Pike, K. M. (1993). When a child cries. *Emergency, 25,* 39.

Plaisier, B. R., et al. (1993). Management of penetrating abdominal trauma. *Topics in Emergency Medicine, 15,* 51.

Romig, L. E. (1993). Assessment of the traumatized child. *Emergency, 25,* 35.

Rosman, N. P. (1994). Acute head trauma. In F. A. Oski et al. (Eds.) *Principles and practice of pediatrics* (2nd ed.). Philadelphia: J.B. Lippincott.

Rowe, P. C. (1994). Pediatric procedures. In F. A. Oski et al. (Eds.) *Principles and practice of pediatrics* (2nd ed.). Philadelphia: J.B. Lippincott.

Ruddy, R. M. (1993). Smoke inhalation injury. *Pediatric Clinics of North America, 41,* 317.

Schwartz, J., & Levin, R. (1991). The risk of lead toxicity in homes with lead paint hazard. *Environmental Research, 54,* 1.

Snyder, C. C., & Knowles, R. P. (1991). Snake bites: Guidelines for practical management. *Postgraduate Medicine, 83,* 52.

Sobel, R. (1970). The psychiatric implications of accidental poisonings in childhood. *Pediatric Clinics of North America, 17,* 653.

Sockrider, M. M., & Seilheimer, D. K. (1994). Respiratory burns. In F. A. Oski et al. (Eds.) *Principles and practice of pediatrics* (2nd ed.). Philadelphia: J. B. Lippincott.

Stenson, K., & Gruber, B. (1993). Ingestion of caustic cosmetic products. *Otolaryngology, 109,* 821.

Suggested Readings

Barker, P. O., & Lewis, D. A. (1990). The management of lead exposure in pediatric populations. *Nurse Practitioner, 15,* 8.

Bubulka, G. M., & Cipolla, F. (1991). Preparing for pediatric emergencies. *Journal of Emergency Nursing, 17,* 236.

Cox, D. M. (1993). Keeping score: Triage for organized patient care and evaluation. *Emergency, 25,* 42.

Fleischer, E., et al. (1993). Fat embolism syndrome. *Nurse Anesthetist, 4,* 18.

Henry, P. C., et al. (1992). Factors associated with closed head injury in a pediatric population. *Journal of Neuroscience Nursing, 24,* 311.

Johnson, C. A. (1991). The management of snakebite. *American Family Physician, 44,* 174.

Jones, N. E. (1992). Prevention of childhood injuries: Recreational injuries. *Pediatric Nursing, 18,* 619.

Manoguerra, A. S. (1992). Pediatric poisoning. *Emergency, 24,* 19.

Monk, H. L. (1993). Fractures are never simple. *RN, 56,* 30.

Reynolds, E. A. (1992). Controversies in caring for the child with a head injury. *MCN: American Journal of Maternal Child Nursing, 17,* 246.

Schoenfeld, P. S., et al. (1993). Management of cardio-pulmonary and trauma resuscitation in the pediatric emergency department. *Pediatrics, 91,* 726.

Weiss, B. D. (1994). Bicycle-related head injuries. *Clinics in Sports Medicine, 13,* 99.

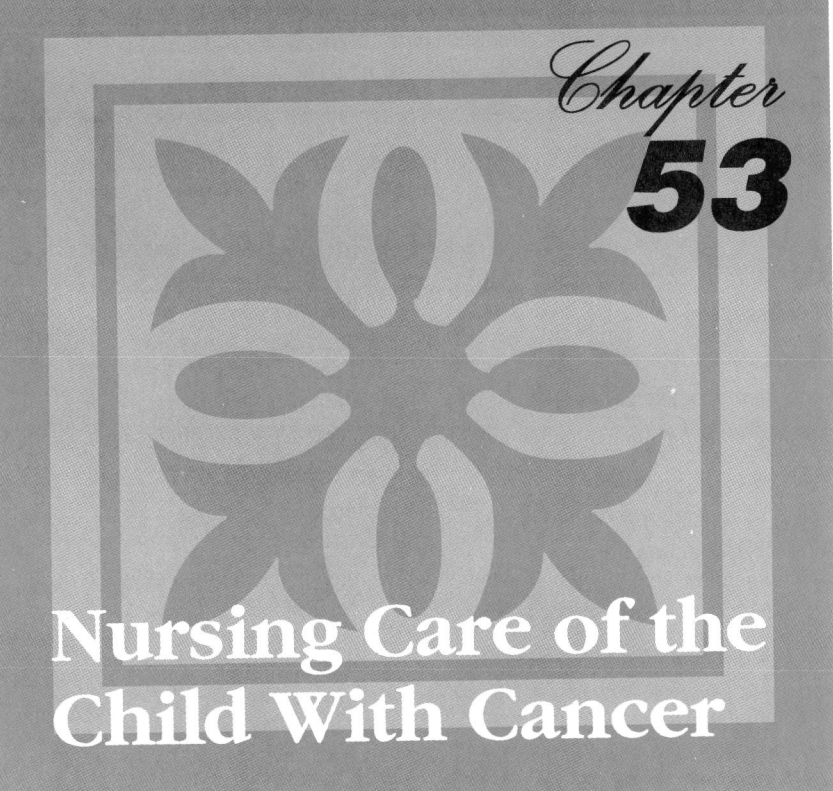

Chapter 53

Nursing Care of the Child With Cancer

Key Terms

- benign neoplasm
- biopsy
- chemotherapeutic agent
- Ewing's sarcoma
- leukemia
- lymphoma
- malignant neoplasm
- metastasis
- neoplasm
- neuroblastoma
- oncogenic virus
- osteogenic sarcoma
- rhabdomyosarcoma
- sarcoma
- tumor staging

Objectives

After mastering the contents of this chapter, you should be able to:

1. Define terms related to tumor growth such as neoplasm, benign, malignant, sarcoma, and carcinoma and describe normal cell growth and theories that explain how cells are altered to become neoplastic in children.

2. Assess the child with a neoplastic process such as a rhabdomyosarcoma, neuroblastoma, Wilms' tumor, and leukemia.

3. Formulate nursing diagnoses related to the child with a malignancy.

4. Plan nursing care specific to the child with a neoplasm such as measures to prevent nausea and vomiting from chemotherapy.

5. Implement nursing care for the child undergoing cancer therapy such as providing mouth care for the child with stomatitis.

6. Evaluate outcome criteria to be certain that nursing care goals were achieved.

7. Identify National Health Goals related to the care of the child with cancer that nurses can be instrumental in helping the nation to achieve.

8. Identify areas related to care of children with cancer that could benefit from additional nursing research.

9. Use critical thinking to analyze ways that nursing care for the child with a neoplasm can be more family-centered.

10. Synthesize knowledge of abnormal cell growth in children with nursing process to achieve quality maternal and child health nursing care.

Adele Pillitteri: MATERNAL AND CHILD
HEALTH NURSING, 2nd Edition. © 1995
Adele Pillitteri.

The terms *malignant* and *cancerous* refer to cells growing and spreading in a disorderly, chaotic fashion. In adults, cancer usually presents in the form of a solid tumor (abnormal growth); in children, the most frequent type of malignancy is that of a blood cell overgrowth, or leukemia.

Many parents assume that the diagnosis of cancer means that the child's life will be very limited. Because of the giant strides in cancer research and treatment over the last 20 years, however, the prognosis for children with cancer has been improving daily. To help parents and children adjust to this illness, nursing support is necessary at the time of diagnosis and throughout the long-term therapy required. National Health Goals re-

lated to cancer and children are shown in the National Health Goals box.

⊠ **NURSING PROCESS OVERVIEW**
for Care of the Child With Cancer

ASSESSMENT

The symptoms of cancer in children are often insidious and hard to define. Weight loss, headaches, or pain at a particular body site can often be explained away by other factors. Weight loss, however, is a common symptom of malignancy. A child's height and weight should be plotted and analyzed at every health care visit. Although pain and swelling could be attributed to injury, be sure to refer children with swelling of major joints to a physician for further assessment so that bone malignancies will not go undetected. Figure 53-1 illustrates common signs and symptoms of malignancy in children.

NURSING DIAGNOSIS

Nursing diagnoses established for the child with a malignancy address specific symptoms caused by the cancer, side effects of the cancer treatment process, or coping abilities of the child and family.

- Pain related to neoplastic process in bone
- Altered nutrition: less than body requirements, related to malignancy
- High risk for infection related to immunosuppressive effects of chemotherapy
- Body image disturbance related to loss of hair following radiation treatment
- Family coping, compromised, related to long term chemotherapy program

FOCUS ON
National Health Goals

A number of National Health Goals concern cancer prevention and children. These are:

- Reduce rise in cancer deaths to achieve a rate of no more than 130/100,000 people.
- Increase to at least 60% the proportion of people of all ages who limit sun exposure, use sunscreens and protective clothing when exposed to sunlight and avoid artificial sources of ultraviolet light (e.g., sun lamps, tanning booths) (DHHS, 1991).

Nurses can be instrumental in helping the nation achieve these goals by careful history taking at health assessments to reveal the symptoms of cancer, as these are often subtle in children, and active teaching to stimulate children to begin self-examination measures such as breast and testicular examination and measures to avoid excessive sun exposure.

Areas that could benefit from additional nursing research are effective ways to teach adolescents about the dangers of tanning booths or excessive sun exposure, reasons adolescents give for avoiding self-examination, and reasons parents give for avoiding bringing a child for health assessment after they have discovered an abnormal growth or recognize easy bruising or loss of weight.

PLANNING

When a neoplasm is first diagnosed in a child, parents may be able to deal with only short-term goals and plans. They may concentrate on learning about the effect or toxic responses of a particular chemotherapeutic drug given their child; they may ask how long the child's surgical incision will be. Dealing with such specifics helps them to control their anxiety. It prevents them from dealing with the overall picture or prognosis: that their child has a potentially lethal condition. When planning, sit down with parents and discuss the treatment protocol and measures they will need to take to make their child more comfortable during therapy (not forcing food if the child is nauseated, playing games or reading stories while intravenous fluid is administered).

Parents are eager for results of diagnostic tests. They may need support while waiting until all the reports have been assembled for an accurate assessment of staging and prognosis. Establishing a primary relationship with both the child and parents is important, so no matter how many hospitalizations are necessary, they know a support person is waiting to help them through this long-term illness. Multidimensional therapy is expensive, so planning should include consideration of the family's financial capabilities to help them make any necessary financial arrangements for care. The siblings of the child with cancer should be included in the planning of the care for a child who has cancer not only because of the seriousness of the illness but also because the treatment may last for an extended period of time, adding additional stress on the family.

Parents will hear of many questionable cancer cures from newspapers or friends during the course of the illness. Help them to voice their hope for these cures as they hear them. Open discussion helps parents keep such cures in perspective and not put more faith in them than they warrant. If these so-called cures can't be discussed with health care personnel, they appear to grow in importance and parents may turn to them in preference to established therapy.

Parents can be expected to undergo grief responses when the prognosis is poor for their child. They move slowly through stages of denial, anger, bargaining, depression, and acceptance. Planning with parents must take into account the stage of grief they are in (see Chapter 56).

Organizations that may be helpful in supplying information to parents include the following:

American Cancer Society
1599 Clifton Road NE
Atlanta, GA 30329

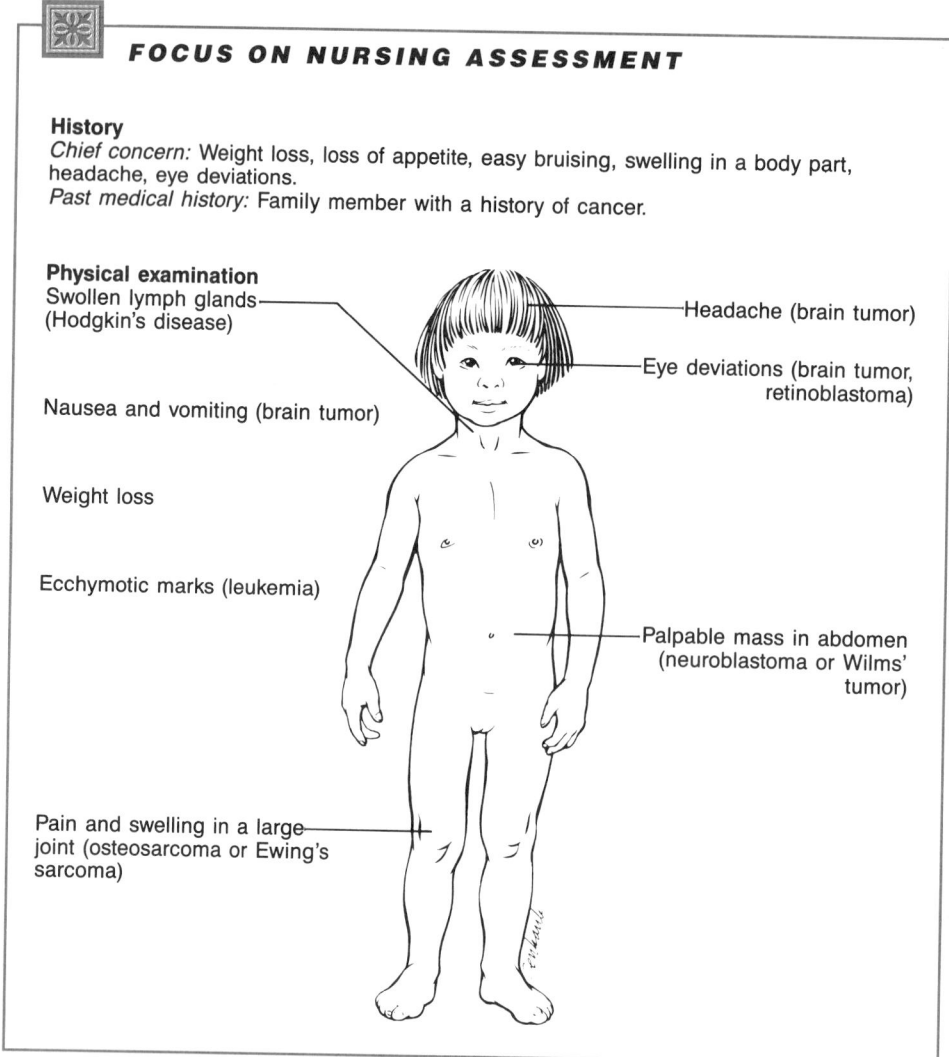

FOCUS ON NURSING ASSESSMENT

History
Chief concern: Weight loss, loss of appetite, easy bruising, swelling in a body part, headache, eye deviations.
Past medical history: Family member with a history of cancer.

Physical examination
Swollen lymph glands (Hodgkin's disease)

Nausea and vomiting (brain tumor)

Weight loss

Ecchymotic marks (leukemia)

Pain and swelling in a large joint (osteosarcoma or Ewing's sarcoma)

Headache (brain tumor)

Eye deviations (brain tumor, retinoblastoma)

Palpable mass in abdomen (neuroblastoma or Wilms' tumor)

FIGURE 53-1
Common signs of malignancy in the child.

Cancer Information Service/National Institutes of Health
Building 31
9000 Rockville Pike
Bethesda, MD 20892

Candlelighters Childhood Cancer Foundation
7910 Woodmont Avenue, Suite 460
Bethesda, MD 20814

Leukemia Society of America, Inc.
600 3rd Avenue
New York, NY 10016

IMPLEMENTATION

Nursing interventions for the child with a neoplasm include supporting the child and parents from the time of the diagnosis of the disorder through procedures such as surgery, radiation therapy, and chemotherapy and con-

tinued health supervision. This is a long-term process because chemotherapy may be continued for 2 to 3 years following diagnosis. Increasingly, cancer treatment is offered on an ambulatory basis to keep hospitalization to a minimum. Keep in mind that the stress of long-term treatment may put the child and family at risk for developmental or family coping problems. The nurse can be a positive force in encouraging healthy adaptation to the demands of the child's illness. Reassess to be certain the child is receiving appropriate stimulation for developmental growth during therapy. Providing comfort and alleviation of pain is often a primary concern in oncology nursing. Measures for pain relief are discussed in Chapter 37.

EVALUATION

Because cancer therapy includes long-term care, children must be evaluated periodically to be certain that nursing goals are being met and are still current. When evaluating nursing care, be certain you are using specific outcome criteria such as the following:

- Child keeps all appointments for chemotherapy treatments.
- Child maintains passing grades in school in spite of interruptions for therapy.
- Parents voice that they are able to keep anxiety level at an acceptable level between clinic appointments.

Children with cancer need the same well-child maintenance care that all children do, with the exception that while they are on chemotherapy, they should not receive live-virus vaccines.

Returning for health care visits for follow-up care causes anxiety. The child seems well, but parents are apprehensive while the physician palpates the child's abdomen and while blood is drawn. Some parents may find the strain of returning for follow-up visits too great and so may miss appointments (not to know seems better than to be told bad news). Such parents need help in understanding that second remissions can be achieved and that maintenance therapy must be continued. Children who receive chemotherapy or radiation are more prone to develop a second malignancy later in life than others. Follow-up is essential to detect the occurrence of these second malignancies.

Parents of the child with cancer may bring their other children for health maintenance care or evaluation of minor illness more often than other parents would. This is because they are worried that what seems just a minor symptom is actually a sign of cancer in that child also. They need more assurance than the average parent that their other children are well.

Some parents of a child with a fatal illness want to take the child home to care for themselves rather than to keep the child in a hospital. These parents need good preparation for home care (see Chapter 38). They need to maintain close contact with health care personnel so that they do not feel abandoned. When the child dies, they may feel a need to return to their primary caregiver for support. This allows for their adjustment to the child's death to be evaluated and help given if needed. Being with a child who dies at home appears to make death a more understandable phenomenon for siblings and, in many instances, can be advocated. Hospice care is another option for the child in whom a remission cannot be achieved (see Chapter 56).

Neoplasia

All body tissue undergoes growth specific to that type of tissue. Normally, the body is able to maintain that proliferation necessary to replace old cells that die and sustain physical growth needs. Malignant or cancerous tissue, however, is unable to maintain this balance and begins to proliferate in disorderly, chaotic ways.

The word **neoplasm** means "new growth"; it is most often used to refer to a new *abnormal* growth that does not respond to normal growth-control mechanisms. Whether this process is one that will form a solid tumor or one that involves blood-forming elements, growth begins insidiously. The process may have been ongoing for some time before parents or a child realize that it is present. Even after parents or children themselves are aware that a change exists, it may be some time before they realize that the changes are serious enough to require health care, because changes are not well defined.

Although cancer in children is rare, it still remains the leading cause of death due to disease in children between the ages of 3 and 14 years. The American Cancer Society estimates that 6000 new cases of cancer occur in children under 15 years of age in the United States each year (Fernbach, 1994); approximately 1600 deaths occur annually from this cause. Fortunately, the overall survival rate for children with cancer today is greater than 50%. Knowing the processes involved in cell growth—both normal and abnormal—is essential to help parents understand what is happening to their child and why specific treatment measures planned for their child are necessary.

Cell Growth

A normal cell growth cycle has two main divisions: an interphase (resting phase) and a mitosis, or dividing, phase. The interphase is divided into four periods: G0, G1, S, and G2. Activity during these periods is summarized in Table 53-1. The time span for a life cycle differs from a short one of 10 hours for a bone cell to a person's lifetime for nerve cells. The rate of cycles is slowed by outside stimuli such as hypoxia, genetic and immunologic factors, and physical and chemical agents. Normally, both resting and active cells are always present.

How body cell growth is determined (how many new liver cells, skin cells, and so on are needed) is poorly understood, but apparently the space that cells have to grow in and the point at which they touch other cells aids in limiting cell growth.

Cells have the ability to recognize their own type, possibly by recognizing surface enzymes or glucose particles on cell membranes. Normally, cells of like types do not migrate away from each other because they recognize and adhere to each other to form a solid mass. In neoplastic cells, the ability to keep together is defective. This may be related to decreased calcium in the cell membrane or an increased negative charge that repels other cells rather than bonds them together.

Like cells appear to be able to recognize when they

Phase	Activity
G (interphase)	*G* refers to gap, or the phase between mitosis and synthesis.
G0	*G0* refers to the cell at rest. Cells remain in this state until some stimulant, such as death of surrounding cells, triggers the cell to enter an active phase; it is difficult to destroy cells in this resting state.
G1	Period until DNA stabilization is complete; it remains difficult to destroy cells in this phase.
S (synthesis)	Period (6–8 h) during which DNA and chromosomes are duplicated or a cell readies itself for division of the cell into 2 daughter cells.
G2	Cell doubles in size preparatory to dividing into 2 daughter cells; if protein synthesis can be stopped at this point so that the cell cannot reach a "critical mass," mitosis, or cell division, cannot take place.
M (mitosis)	Period of cell division into 2 like daughter cells.

Table 53-1. Phases of the Cell Cycle

are being crowded for the space they must occupy and apparently communicate with one another to halt growth. Neoplastic cells do not respond to this communication or cannot receive it, so despite how crowded they are, they continue to grow. By the time a tumor mass is detected by palpation, it has probably doubled from its original aberrant cell about 30 times. In many instances, for the entire mass to be destroyed, it may be necessary to kill as many as a billion cells.

Neoplastic Growth

Neoplasms can be either **benign** (growth is limited) or **malignant** (cancerous). Even when a tumor is benign, however, it may not be completely harmless. It can cause damage by pressing on adjacent tissue (for example, brain tumors in children are often benign but can cause extensive respiratory center depression).

Causes of Neoplastic Growth

The exact origin of neoplastic growth is unknown, and any growth may actually involve more than one cause. In adults, tumors may grow because cell growth has been altered due to environmental irritation, such as chronic exposure to chemical irritants or cigarette smoke. Tumors of the skin, bladder, lung, and intestines all involve organs exposed to such outside influences and irritation. In children, tumors most frequently occur in organs unexposed to the environment: leukemia of the blood stream, Wilms' tumor of the kidney, brain tumors, and neuroblastoma in the abdomen. Because many tumors occur in children under 5 years, exposure to environmental carcinogens is limited (unless exposure occurred in utero), so this cause of tumors is probably not a great influence in childhood cancer. One substance to which children may be exposed is asbestos, which leads to lung cancer. Children are exposed to asbestos if their school building is insulated with it or if a parent works at an asbestos plant.

A child who has survived one malignancy appears to be at higher than normal risk for a second malignancy (possibly as much as a 12% chance). Radiation exposure used to treat the first malignancy may be responsible for this. There may be a predisposition to cancer in some families.

Another common theory of why neoplasms grow is the cell mutation theory. This suggests that carcinogenic agents and hereditary susceptibility combine to alter the nature of cells, leading to abnormal growth. A first stage of *initiation* may take place that marks the cells for abnormal growth. A second stage of *promotion* actually begins abnormal growth. Carcinogens can be living (viral), physical (radiation), or chemical (diethylstilbestrol [DES]). Radiation during intrauterine life has been established as a documented cause of leukemia. Radiation of the thyroid in infancy may cause thyroid cancer later in life. Intrauterine exposure to DES may lead to clear cell adenocarcinoma of the vagina in girls. There may be an association between barbiturate administration and brain tumors as well as fetal hydantoin syndrome and neuroblastoma. Treatment of aplastic anemia with androgenic steroids may lead to hepatocellular cancer.

This theory explains why the growth of neoplastic cells is irreversible (the cells cannot return to a normal state because they are intrinsically changed) and why neoplasms occur in some people but not in others (both an intrinsic and extrinsic factor or an inherited tendency and an environmental insult must be present). It is difficult to document this process because two separate steps are probably necessary for a cell to become cancerous. If there is a lengthy time span between these steps, the cause-and-effect relationship is difficult to trace.

Yet another theory is that oncogenic (cancer-causing) viruses are responsible for tumor growth. According to the viral theory, **oncogenic viruses** have the ability to change the structure of DNA or RNA in cells to a neoplastic type. C-type RNA viruses may be implicated in development of leukemia. Epstein-Barr virus, a DNA virus, may be associated with Burkitt's lymphoma. This theory is supported by the fact that an immunodeficient state increases the risks of developing a neoplastic growth. With this state, both viral surveillance and removal of abnormal cells are lost; therefore, virus invasion and abnormal cell growth begin. Still another theory is that tumor suppressor cells exist in some individuals and not in others (Helman & Thiele, 1991).) Retinoblastoma may occur when such cells are not present.

Assessing Children With Malignancies

The distribution of various types of pediatric cancers is shown in Figure 53-2. The beginning signs of malignancy in children (as in adults) are subtle. Children need routine health assessment during their growing years that includes screening for signs or symptoms of neoplastic growth.

History

A thorough history is helpful in identifying growths that are not yet clinically present. Symptoms of obstruction (such as constipation) or pressure (such as headache) may be revealed first by this method. As malignant tumors grow, they tend to cause systemic effects in the child. Cachexia (loss of weight, anorexia) may be present if the tumor is growing so rapidly that it is taking nu-

---

Box 53-1

The Seven Danger Signs of Cancer

1. A change in bowel or bladder habits
2. A nonhealing sore
3. Unusual bleeding or discharge
4. A thickening or lump in the breast or other body part
5. Indigestion or difficulty swallowing
6. An obvious change in a wart or mole
7. A nagging cough or persistent hoarseness

Source: The American Cancer Society, 1599 Clifton Road NE, Atlanta GA, 30329.

---

trients from normal cells. Excessive hormone production (overproduction of antidiuretic hormone or adrenocorticotropic hormone) may occur because of tumor growth. Although the seven danger signs of cancer listed by the American Cancer Society (Box 53-1) apply primarily to cancer in adults, they should be kept in mind when assessing children, too (see the Focus on Cultural Awareness box).

Physical and Laboratory Examination

Any suspicion of a malignancy requires a thorough physical examination. Assessing height and weight of children is important, because weight loss is a common

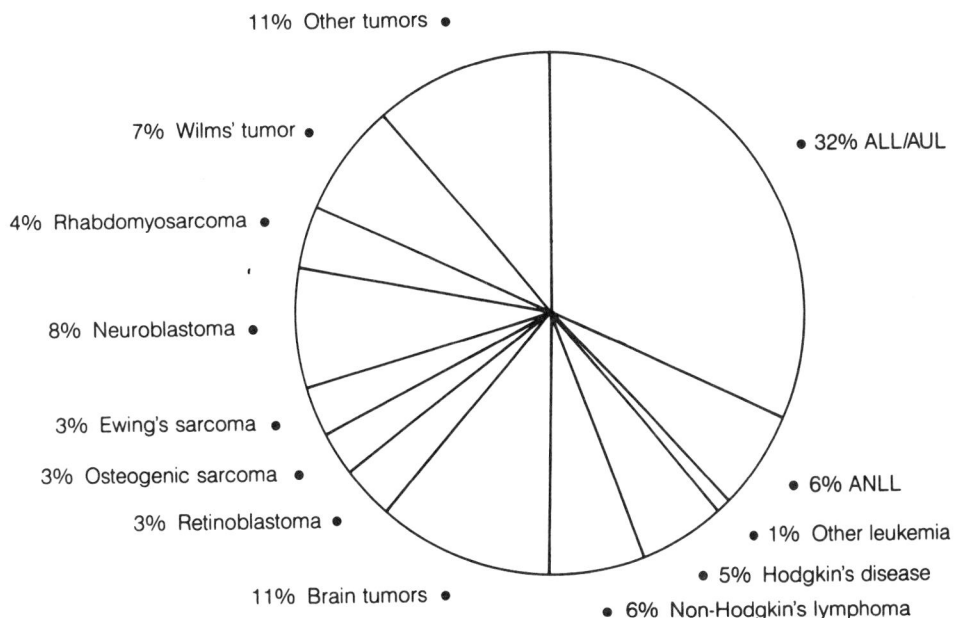

FIGURE 53-2
Approximate percent distribution of common pediatric malignancies.

symptom of malignancy in both children and adults (see Figure 53-1). To confirm a diagnosis, a number of diagnostic procedures may be used including x-ray, sonogram, magnetic resonance screening, blood analysis, and biopsy.

Biopsy

A **biopsy** is the surgical removal of tissue cells for laboratory analysis. Most children with a possible diagnosis of cancer will have a biopsy done on admission to the hospital. Although biopsies are classified as only minor surgery, don't treat them lightly. They carry a definite surgical risk because of the general anesthesia used and because they are an anxiety-producing procedure for the parents and the child. Up to this point, parents can convince themselves that the child has something innocent; a biopsy breaks this hope because the word *biopsy* implies that cancer is at least a possibility. For this reason, parents and children need thorough preparation for the biopsy procedure and the care the child will need following the procedure. Anxious parents do not "hear" well and may need to have postoperative instructions repeated thoroughly at a later time. Bone marrow aspiration is a frequent type of biopsy used with children. Although this is done with local anesthesia, it is equally frightening (see Chapter 44).

Staging of Malignancy

Tumor staging is designating the extent of a solid tumor malignant process. This is necessary to design an effective treatment program and to establish an accurate prognosis. In staging systems, stage I refers to a tumor that can be completely resected surgically. Stage II refers to a tumor that cannot be completely resected. Stages III and IV designate tumors that have extended beyond the original site or have spread systemically (**metastasis**). A second method for staging tumors is a TNM system. A TNM system is one that denotes a tumor's (T) size, lymph node (N) involvement, and presence of metastasis (M) (cancerous spread). A TNM system is most applicable to carcinoma. Because most childhood tumors are sarcomas, the system is not as applicable to childhood tumors as a simple staging system.

Overview of Cancer Treatment Measures Used With Children

The treatment of a child with a malignancy centers on devising ways to kill the growth of the abnormal cells while protecting normal surrounding cells. This can be done by radiation or chemotherapy.

Radiation Therapy

Radiation therapy acts to change the DNA component of a cell nucleus to a point where the cell cannot replicate DNA material and so cannot divide and grow further. Radiation is not effective on cells that have a low oxygen content (a proportion of cells in every tumor mass); it is not effective at the time of cell division (mitosis). Radiation schedules therefore are designed to take place over 1 to 6 weeks so that cells that are not in a susceptible stage on one day will be in a susceptible stage on another. Tumors that require such a massive dose of radiation that normal tissue through which the radiation must pass to penetrate the tumor would be destroyed in the process are said to be radioresistant.

Immediate Side Effects

Radiation has both systemic and localized effects. Radiation sickness (anorexia, nausea, vomiting) is the most frequently encountered systemic effect. This occurs if the gastrointestinal tract is radiated. It also can occur to a lesser degree from the release of toxic substances from destroyed tumor cells. The child may need an antiemetic ordered to be given before each procedure to tolerate the discomfort. Extreme fatigue is also very common.

Long-Term Side Effects

The long-term side effects of radiation are becoming more apparent as increasing numbers of children who have had intense radiation survive (Gootenberg & Pizzo, 1991). Because radiation damages all cells in its path to some extent, any body tissue could be affected. Asymmetric growth of bones, easy fracturing, scoliosis, kyphosis, or spinal shortening can occur. Bones are most vulnerable during times of rapid growth, such as the first year of life or during a prepubertal growth spurt. Scoliosis and kyphosis can be avoided if the entire vertebra is radiated rather than one side or the other; this means that a larger area of bone may be radiated than formerly so that both sides of the vertebra are in the radiation path.

Radiation to the head can result in long-term thyroid, hypothalamic, and pituitary gland dysfunction. This may result in growth hormone deficiency or hypothalamic-pituitary stimulation to the thyroid gland. Children's growth and thyroid function should be evaluated every 6 months for the next 3 years to detect these changes. Both hypothyroidism and hypopituitary growth failure can be treated with hormone replacement in coming years. Radiation to ovaries or testes can result in infertility. Girls may develop lack of estrogen production, preventing secondary sexual changes from developing; lack of testosterone production occurs only rarely in boys. Pretreatment sperm banking may be advocated for a boy past puberty before undergoing radiation to the testes.

Long-term effects of radiation to the nervous system are demyelination and necrosis of the white matter of the brain. This can result in symptoms of lethargy, sleepiness, and seizures. Effects on the gray matter can result in learning disabilities. There may be abnormal electroencephalograph (EEG) tracings; the child may have low-intensity headaches, cataracts, salivary gland damage, and a chronic change in or loss of taste. Radiation to the lungs may result in a chronic pneumonitis and pulmonary fibrosis or thickening. Heart effects may be pericardial thickening and reduced heart expandability. Radiation to the gastrointestinal system can result in chronic malabsorption from changes in intestinal villi. Hepatic fibrosis can result in reduced liver function. Radiation to the kidney and bladder can result in nephritis and chronic cystitis.

Children who have intense radiation treatments may develop a secondary malignancy later in life, apparently from oncogenic changes in cells.

The possibility of these long-term effects of radiation should be explained to parents when radiation is initially discussed as a part of obtaining informed consent. At the early stage of diagnosis, however, parents rarely are concerned with these long-term effects. Their thoughts are understandably filled with such short-term goals as the achievement of a remission or destruction of the tumor.

Nursing Diagnoses and Related Interventions

Nursing Diagnosis: Parental and child anxiety related to radiation procedure

Goal: Parents demonstrate reduced anxiety about radiation by time of therapy.

Outcome Criteria: Parents voice that they understand necessity of therapy and can help support child during therapy.

The points where radiotherapy will be directed are marked on the child's skin in ink. Be careful not to wash these marks away during bathing until the course of therapy is over. As a rule, no cream or lotion should be applied to radiation areas until a radiation series is complete. Creams may distort or interfere with the entrance of radiation.

Most children have had prior x-rays taken at the point that radiation therapy is begun and so are not frightened by the procedure. Because, however, the procedure requires them to lie still for about 20 minutes on an uncomfortable table, in a room away from personnel or their parents, they do not particularly like the procedure. Assure parents and the child that during the treatment, just as there is no feeling from x-ray exposure, the child will experience no sensation from radiation exposure. Infants are usually prescribed a sedative before therapy to insure that they will lie still during the procedure. To make this approach effective, keep the child fairly active early in the day and introduce calming activities after the sedative is administered so the child is sleepy and actually falls asleep during radiation. It is helpful for an older child if you help him or her plan an activity to think about during radiation, such as which 10 friends would be picked to take on a camping trip (and why); if 10 places could be visited next year, what would they be, etc.

If the head area is involved in therapy, a child may develop alopecia (hair loss). Radiation may reduce salivary gland function, leading to a constantly dry mouth. If a child needs dental work done during the time of radiation, parents should be certain to tell the dentist of the radiation therapy as healing may be slowed. Tooth growth may be halted due to root atrophy. Radiation to bone marrow may cause depression of white blood cell and platelet production. Children undergoing radiation therapy need their leukocyte and platelet counts monitored to be certain that these remain adequate during the course of therapy. Nursing care priorities to maintain skin integrity are summarized in the Focus on Nursing Care display.

Chemotherapy

A **chemotherapeutic agent** is one that is capable of destroying malignant cells. In many instances, not one but a combination of chemotherapeutic agents is used to cause multiple damage to cells and thereby increase the chances that cells will no longer be able to reproduce. Like radiation, chemotherapy is scheduled over a period of time so that all cells can eventually be destroyed (cells undergoing meiosis and therefore not susceptible to the chemotherapeutic agent on one day will be susceptible on the next).

Types of Chemotherapeutic Agents

There are several categories of chemotherapeutic agents available. When preparing such agents, wear gloves and

FOCUS ON NURSING CARE

Guidelines for Care of the Child Receiving Radiation

Promote Skin Integrity

1. Keep radiation area exposed to the air as much as possible. Avoid exposing the area to direct heat or sun exposure or dramatic temperature changes. Prevent clothing such as a tight waist band from rubbing the area.

2. Avoid soaking the skin area in water for long intervals such as soaking baths or swimming. The chlorine in swimming pools may irritate the skin area so use of pools should be discontinued.

3. Do not wash off the red or purple marks that designate the radiation area. If marks are accidentally removed, do not attempt to redraw them.

4. If the head is being radiated, use only a mild shampoo to wash hair. Do not use a hair dryer as the skin area can burn readily. Do not rub hair to dry it; pat it gently.

5. Supply soft toothbrush for child to prevent excoriation of gumline. Teach parent to schedule a dental referral following radiation therapy to assess condition of teeth (intense radiation may lead to root atrophy and loosening of teeth).

6. Salivary gland secretions may decrease with cranial radiation. Provide frequent sips of water and a mouthwash to rinse mouth 3–4 times daily. If ulcers are present in mouth (stomatitis), supply bland and nonacid food to prevent pain.

7. If a radiated area appears dry, do not apply creams or lotions unless specifically prescribed by the radiation department. The products could interfere with radiation penetration through the skin.

8. Don't refer to any reddened area as a burn, but merely as a "radiation area."

Maintain Nutrition

1. Administer antiemetic as prescribed.

2. Encourage adequate calories for breakfast and before treatment, when child is apt to be less nauseated.

3. Ask child to identify and try to supply favorite foods and drinks.

4. Allow the child to have as much choice about food as possible; allow parents to bring favorite foods or beverages from home.

5. Praise the child for eating; avoid urging to eat more to keep mealtime a positive experience.

Prevent Fluid Loss

1. If the intestinal tract is radiated, diarrhea may occur. Provide good skin care at diaper changes to prevent skin irritation.

2. Reduce fresh fruit and vegetables concentrated in cellulose.

3. Eliminate apple juice from diet.

4. Administer antidiarrheal medication as prescribed.

5. Administer and monitor intravenous fluid replacement as prescribed.

Prevent Infection

1. Use precautions for child with neutropenia (see page 1695).

Prevent Fatigue

1. Provide adequate rest periods; protect child from being awakened frequently at night.

2. Provide activities that provide stimulation yet do not physically tire child.

3. Radiation to long bones may weaken the bone. Caution children not to bear weight or lift weights with high-risk extremity.

4. Radiation may lead to long-term effects of linear growth retardation, enzymatic growth disturbances, pulmonary abnormalities, sterility, and, possibly, chromosomal damage. Assess children at health maintenance visits for possible abnormalities.

Promote Self-Esteem

1. Prepare child and parents for effects of radiation therapy. If a child's head is being radiated, hair will probably fall out. A scarf or "dust cap" may be acceptable for children. Stress that what a person is like inside is more important than what shows outside.

2. Introduce a bald Cabbage Patch doll for a new friend.

3. Prepare for radiation procedure by a tour of the radiation department or play with miniature x-ray machines and tables.

4. Provide opportunities for therapeutic play with a doll, a radiation machine, and a table.

5. Some children may need a sedative administered before radiation so they can lie quietly during the procedure. Provide active games before sedative, quiet games afterward.

6. Help child devise a "mind activity" to use during procedure such as listing 10 friends he or she would take on a camping trip, 10 friends he or she would not, etc.

wash your hands well afterward to prevent skin exposure and absorption of the drug.

Alkylating Agents. Alkylating agents interfere with DNA synthesis. They are cycle specific, that is, they are most effective against cells in the G1 and S phases of growth. Alkylating agents commonly used with children are cyclophosphamide (Cytoxan) and chlorambucil (Leukeran).

Antimetabolites. Antimetabolites are drugs that so closely resemble natural products that a cell incorporates them into its structure. They are not the natural product, however, so the cell cannot function with them in its structure and will die. They act only in the S (synthesis) phase of the cell cycle. Methotrexate, a folic acid antagonist, is an example.

Plant Alkaloids. Plant alkaloids interfere with cell mitosis (M phase). Two commonly used plant alkaloids are vincristine (Oncovin) and vinblastine (Velban).

Antibiotics. A number of antibiotics are effective in destroying malignant cells by impairing DNA synthesis. These are not cell cycle specific, which means the agents can be effective at any cell phase (resting or dividing). Dactinomycin and doxorubicin (Adriamycin) are examples.

Nitrosourea Compounds. The action of nitrosoureas is similar to that of antibiotics in that these agents interfere with DNA synthesis. Nitrosoureas are not used extensively in chemotherapy with children.

Enzymes. Body cells need a ready supply of L-asparagine (an essential amino acid) to grow. L-asparaginase, a chemotherapeutic agent, is an enzyme that converts L-asparagine into L-aspartic acid, thereby making L-asparagine unavailable for leukemia cell growth.

Steroids. The addition of a corticosteroid (most frequently prednisone) binds to DNA to inhibit mitosis in cells and probably RNA synthesis, preventing the formation of new cells.

Immunotherapy. Immunotherapy is the stimulation of the body's immune system to attempt destruction of foreign or malignant cells. The administration of bacillus Calmette-Guerin vaccine (the vaccine for tuberculosis) is an example of this type of therapy. The presence of the tuberculin antigen stimulates the immune system to identify and destroy an antigen; it is hoped that the system "recognizes" that foreign tumor cells are also present and acts against these as well. Interferon is an antiviral agent that, when present, prevents growth of viruses; stimulation of interferon or interferon therapy may be used to attempt to halt malignant cell growth.

Active immunotherapy can be attempted by the injection of tumor cells taken from the child (or a child with a similar tumor type). Passive immunotherapy using serum from children with a like type of cancer is a possibility.

Unfortunately, although the theory of immunotherapy is sound, results have been disappointing. The immune system may be so altered by the malignant process that it is not able to respond when stimulated. It is also possible that the immune response to malignant cells is so different from the response to invading microorganisms that immunotherapy is unable to stimulate it.

Side Effects and Toxic Responses of Chemotherapy

All chemotherapeutic agents have both side effects and toxic responses. Table 53-2 lists commonly used chemotherapeutic agents and the specific side effects and potential toxic responses for each agent. Malnutrition, nausea and vomiting, hair loss, stomatitis, constipation, diarrhea, cushingoid appearance, and susceptibility to infection are side effects common to almost all these agents. One particularly harmful toxic response is tissue necrosis. Nursing diagnoses and related interventions associated with these side effects are described below.

If an intravenous infusion of a chemotherapeutic agent infiltrates into the subcutaneous tissue, there is apt to be extensive tissue sloughing. Intravenous infusions of chemotherapeutic agents must be watched very carefully to prevent this from happening. The infusion should be discontinued if infiltration occurs; an ice pack applied to the site will induce vasoconstriction and prevent further spread of the toxic solution. Hyaluronidase injected into the site may speed absorption. Following this, warm compresses will hasten absorption and clearance of the solution from subcutaneous tissue.

Nursing Diagnoses and Related Interventions

Nursing Diagnosis: Altered nutrition: less than body requirements, related to nausea, vomiting, or anorexia resulting from chemotherapy

Goal: Child will take in adequate nutrients for needs during therapy period.

Outcome Criteria: Child is able to eat frequent, small meals; calorie intake is adequate for age.

It is easy for the child with cancer to become malnourished. The fast-growing malignant cells take more than their share of nutrients from normal cells. Nausea and vomiting from chemotherapy make it difficult for the child to maintain an adequate oral intake. If stomatitis occurs as a result of chemotherapy, eating becomes

Table 53-2. *Commonly Used Chemotherapeutic Agents*

Drug	Classification	Method of Administration	Side Effects and Toxic Responses	Special Considerations
Asparaginase (Elspar)	Enzyme; deprives leukemic cells of asparagine, leading to cell death	IV	Anorexia, weight loss, nausea, vomiting, hepatotoxicity, central nervous system toxicity, anaphylactic reaction	Stay with child for first hour of infusion; take vital signs q15 min for first hour to detect anaphylactic reaction
Azacytidine	Interferes with nucleic acid metabolism (antimetabolite)	IV	Nausea, vomiting, diarrhea, bone marrow depression, hepatotoxicity	Sensitivity to sunlight occurs
Carmustine (BCNU) (BiCNU)	Nitrosourea compound; crosses blood-brain barrier	IV	Nausea, vomiting, bone marrow depression (after 3–4 weeks), hepatotoxicity	Child may notice burning sensation along vein during administration due to alcohol diluent
Chlorambucil (Leukeran)	Nitrogen mustard derivative	Oral	Bone marrow depression	Monitoring of white blood cell count is necessary
Cisplatin (Platinol)	Reacts with and injures cell nucleus	IV	Bone marrow depression, nephrotoxicity (renal dysfunction), nausea, vomiting, loss of taste, tinnitus, high-frequency hearing loss	Infusion bottle must be covered with aluminum foil to keep out light, or decomposition will result
Cyclophosphamide (Cytoxan)	Alkylating agent (nitrogen mustard derivative)	IV, oral	Bone marrow depression, anorexia, nausea, vomiting, stomatitis, alopecia, cystitis, (hemorrhagic) hepatotoxicity	Encourage fluids; maintain intravenous line to limit bladder irritation; test urine for blood and specific gravity
Cytosine arabinoside (Ara-C)	Antimetabolite (pyrimidine analog)	IV, SC, intrathecal	Nausea, vomiting, bone marrow depression, stomatitis, alopecia, photosensitivity	
Dactinomycin (Cosmegen)	Antibiotic; inhibits DNA synthesis	IV	Nausea, vomiting, bone marrow depression, stomatitis	Causes tissue inflammation if it infiltrates into tissue
Dacarbazine (DTIC)	Alkylating agent	IV	Bone marrow depression	Infiltration causes severe tissue damage
Daunorubicin (Cerubidine)	Antibiotic	IV	Alopecia, bone marrow depression	Infiltration causes severe tissue damage
Doxorubicin (Adriamycin)	Antibiotic; inhibits DNA synthesis	IV	Nausea, vomiting, bone marrow depression, alopecia, stomatitis, possible heart toxicity	Urine may turn red; take pulse for full minute to detect arrhythmia; tissue necrosis if infiltrated.
Lomustine (CCNU) (CeeNu)	Alkylating agent (nitrosourea compound)	Oral	Nausea, vomiting in 6 h, bone marrow depression (after 3–4 weeks)	Should be taken on an empty stomach for best absorption

(continued)

difficult due to mouth pain. Not only is the oral cavity affected but the stomach and intestines also have like ulcers, interfering with absorption. Changes in fatty acid metabolism may alter the responsiveness of body cells to insulin metabolism; unable to use glucose effectively, cells cannot function at an optimum level. This may account for the frequently reported sense of fatigue children with cancer report. Anorexia may occur from a factor produced by the tumor that acts directly on the center for hunger in the hypothalamus, reducing sensations of hunger and altering taste perception. Cyclophosphamide is associated with taste changes. For many children, foods taste very bitter; foods are not described as sweet until they are very sweet. Because of these taste changes, foods the child used to enjoy no longer taste good; unwilling to try new foods, the child decreases his or her oral intake. To counteract these taste changes, you may need to suggest different foods or methods of

Table 53-2. *Continued*

Drug	Classification	Method of Administration	Side Effects and Toxic Responses	Special Considerations
Mercaptopurine (Purinethol)	Antimetabolite (purine analog)	Oral	Bone marrow depression, nausea, vomiting, stomatitis, hepatotoxicity	Allopurinol delays the degradation of mercaptopurine and thus increases toxicity; question order if both are to be administered
Methotrexate (Methotrexate)	Antimetabolite	Oral, IV, intrathecal	Stomatitis, bone marrow depression, nausea, vomiting, alopecia, hepatotoxicity, nephrotoxicity at high dosage	Decreased effect if administered with salicylates; often followed by leucovorin to decrease toxicity to normal cells
Prednisone (Prednisone)	Corticosteroid; suppresses lymphocyte production	Oral	Weight gain, cushingoid facies, depressed systemic response to infection	
Procarbazine (Matulane)	Interferes with DNA and RNA synthesis	Oral	Nausea, vomiting, bone marrow depression	May cause blurriness of vision; avoid foods with high tyramine content
Thioguanine	Antimetabolite	Oral	Bone marrow suppression	Monitoring of hepatic function tests is necessary
Vinblastine (Velban)	Plant alkaloid	IV	Alopecia, anorexia, bone marrow depression, nausea, vomiting, constipation	Tissue necrosis if infiltrated
Vincristine (Oncovin)	Plant alkaloid	IV	Constipation, alopecia, joint and muscle pain, muscle weakness	Paresthesis of fingers and toes, footdrop may occur; may need stool softener; tissue necrosis if infiltrated
Additional Agents				
Allopurinol (Allopurinol, Lopurin, Zyloprim)	Prevents formation of uric acid from destroyed cells	IV, oral	Nausea, vomiting	
Bacillus Calmette-Guerin (BCG) vaccine*	Stimulates immune system	Intradermal	Local inflammation	
Leucovorin (Citrovorum)	Folinic acid given to neutralize the toxicity of methotrexate	IV, IM, oral		
Interferon	Antiviral agent	IV, intrathecal	Fever	
Filgrastin	Granulocyte-colony-stimulating factor	IV	Nausea, vomiting	Increases leukocyte count

IV = intravenous; IM = intramuscular; SC = subcutaneous.
*Otherwise used to vaccinate against tuberculosis.

food preparation. Chicken, for example, often tastes less bitter than beef or pork. Adding brown sugar on cereal gives a different sweet taste than plain sugar. Many children believe that sugar is bad for them so are reluctant to use a lot of it to make foods taste good. Assure them that eating is the most important thing to think about now and careful brushing of teeth after eating will preserve teeth even if they eat a great deal of sugar. Don't recommend honey as a sweetener. Botulism organisms may grow in honey, and the immunosuppressed child has little resistance to these.

Make mealtime a pleasant time; serve food that is appetizing in taste, color, and temperature. Allow the child to make choices of food whenever possible. Assess what are favorite foods and urge the nutritionist (in the hospital) or parents (if at home) to supply these; parents may be able to bring in foods to the hospital from home (Figure 53-3).

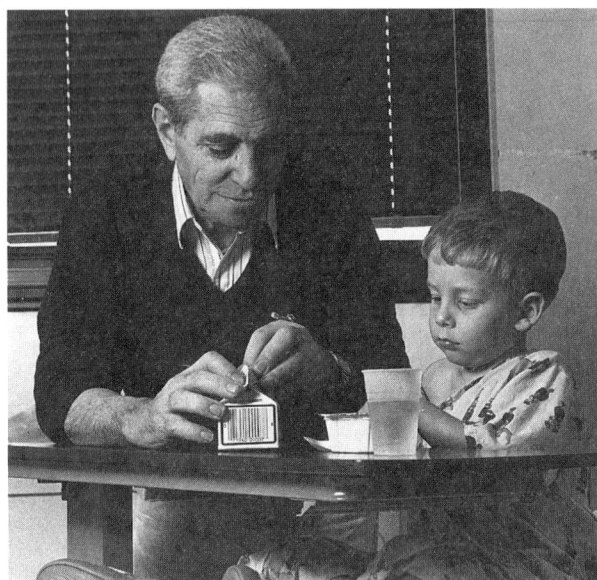

FIGURE 53-3
Children receiving radiation or chemotherapy often have reduced appetites. Here a grandfather helps with lunch to try and stimulate his grandson's appetite. (Courtesy of the Department of Medical Photography, Children's Hospital, Buffalo, NY.)

A small meal that can be finished is more satisfying than a large meal half finished. Urge parents to make snack foods nutritious (a malted milkshake rather than a cola beverage). Additional good advice is to plan larger meals for early in the day before chemotherapy is begun, when the child is apt to be less nauseated.

> *Nursing Diagnosis:* High risk for fluid-volume deficit related to nausea and vomiting resulting from chemotherapy
>
> *Goal:* Child will not become dehydrated during therapy period.
>
> *Outcome Criteria:* Skin turgor is good; mucous membranes are moist; vomiting does not occur more than once a day.

Nausea and vomiting are common side effects of chemotherapy because the cells lining the stomach are fast growing and so are irritated by drugs. Nausea and vomiting can often be prevented by the administration of hydroxyzine (Atarax) or phenobarbital prior to chemotherapy and at 4-hour intervals during the course of therapy. These drugs will effectively reduce the occurrence of nausea and vomiting in children but will not necessarily relieve it once it is present. It is necessary, therefore, to give these medications prophylactically. Parents are usually aware that chemotherapy agents cause extreme nausea. They may believe that chemotherapy will not be effective unless nausea occurs. Offer an explanation that antiemetic drugs do not halt the

chemotherapy action, only the systemic reaction from the injured stomach-lining cells.

Do not encourage children to eat if they are nauseated. Encourage them to take clear fluids, however, as this helps prevent uric acid buildup in the kidneys from the malignant cells being destroyed. If children are vomiting or cannot take even clear fluid, intravenous therapy for hydration may be started. With a drug such as cyclophosphamide, known to cause cystitis when fluid intake is reduced, an intravenous line for adequate fluid intake must be started.

Antiemetic suppositories such as trimethobenzamide (Tigan) are of limited help and not normally used with children. Many children have intense reactions to prochlorperazine (Compazine), so it is not often administered to them. Techniques for increasing nutrition during chemotherapy are discussed in the Nursing Care Plan: A School-Age Child With Leukemia (p. 1690).

> *Nursing Diagnosis:* High risk for self-esteem disturbance related to changes in physical appearance caused by chemotherapy
>
> *Goal:* Child will accept side effects affecting appearance as *temporary,* inevitable components of treatment that do not affect how people feel about him or her by 1 week.
>
> *Outcome Criteria:* Child discusses feelings about appearance changes with nurse and parents; states that although he or she doesn't like them, they don't alter him or her in any other way.

Alopecia. *Alopecia,* or hair loss, is a side effect that occurs with almost all chemotherapeutic drugs because hairs are fast-growing cells that are easily killed. Even when warned that such a consequence is likely, most children and parents are surprised at the suddenness of the hair loss (entire curls may fall out at a time; the child can be totally bald in 2 to 3 days). Hair loss is often a greater problem for the parents than the child. A boy may view his hair loss as a very modern, macho condition. Although girls are less apt to view alopecia as a positive occurrence, they may still react to it with less apprehension than their parents. Wearing a wig or scarf may be a solution. Buying them a doll like the Cabbage Patch doll that has no hair helps them to feel not so alone. Being reminded that people are liked for what is inside them helps most (Figure 53-4). It may be possible to reduce the amount of alopecia by placing ice packs on the scalp during chemotherapy. This prevents a large uptake of drug by hair follicles. Do not use this technique with children who have leukemia, as it may prevent destruction of leukemic cells near hair follicles.

Cushingoid Appearance. Children on long-term corticosteroid (prednisone) therapy will develop typical

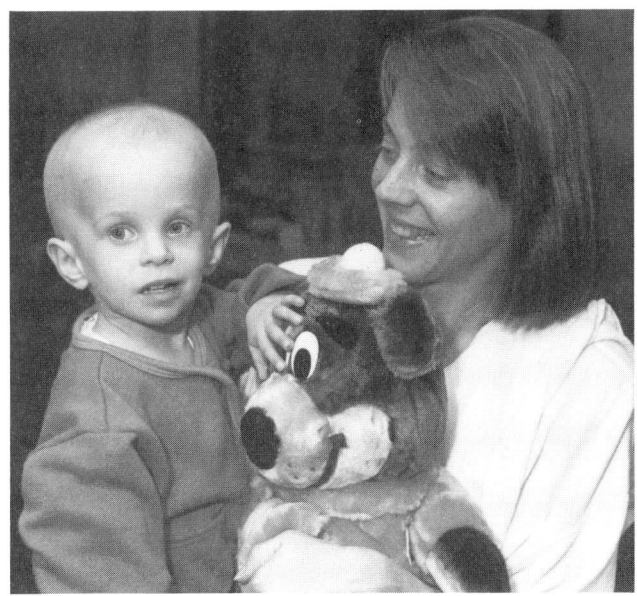

FIGURE 53-4
A child with alopecia poses with a staff nurse. It helps the child to know that hair loss does not prevent warm interactions with people. (Courtesy of Children's Medical Center, Dayton, OH.)

"moon face," red checks, and increased body hair. Like the loss of body hair, a cushingoid appearance may be devastating to children, the final insult in light of all the other things happening to them. Assurance that appearance will revert to normal when they are no longer on therapy may help, as will telling them that people care more about the kind of person they are rather than how they look.

Nursing Diagnosis: Altered oral mucous membrane related to effects of chemotherapy

Goal: Child will not experience severe discomfort from stomatitis during course of chemotherapy.

Outcome Criteria: Child states that mouth discomfort is at tolerable level; no signs of ulceration are present.

Stomatitis, or ulcers of the gumline and mucous membranes of the mouth, often occurs with antimetabolic drugs. The child may need a soft or light diet for comfort. Brushing the teeth with a soft swab rather than a brush or having the child just rinse the mouth with half-strength hydrogen peroxide and water is helpful. Viscous lidocaine (Xylocaine) may be prescribed to be swabbed on individual lesions for comfort. Lidocaine can cause paralysis of the gag reflex if it is swallowed, so it must be swabbed on individual lesions, *not* used for rinsing out the mouth as it is in adults. (Children under 8 years of age are apt to rinse and swallow.) Measures to reduce stomatitis are summarized in the Focus on Family Teaching box.

Because mucous membrane ulcers may occur throughout the gastrointestinal tract, children on antimetabolic therapy should not have rectal temperatures taken to avoid aggravation or perforation of rectal ulcers.

Nursing Diagnosis: High risk for altered patterns of bowel elimination related to effects of chemotherapeutic agents

Goal: Child will not experience constipation or diarrhea during course of treatment.

Outcome Criteria: Child maintains usual pattern of bowel elimination; reports (and nurse confirms) no existence of hard or watery stools.

Constipation. Some chemotherapeutic agents, particularly vincristine, cause constipation. Children are placed on a stool softener such as docusate sodium (Colace) to prevent exacerbation of rectal ulceration by hard stools. The frequency of bowel movements should be recorded so that constipation is recognized early in its course.

Diarrhea. Diarrhea may occur from effects on the absorption surfaces of the intestine. Keep careful

FOCUS ON FAMILY TEACHING

Q. My son has had a constant sore mouth since he's been on chemotherapy. What actions can I take to make him more comfortable?

A. Stomatitis is an unfortunate accompaniment to many chemotherapeutic agents. Some tips for improving comfort when this happens are:

• Encourage good oral hygiene using a soft toothbrush to keep the number of germs in his mouth to a minimum and hopefully prevent infection.

• Suggest soft foods rather than hard ones such as toast crusts or crunchy cereal to avoid further abrasions to tender gumlines.

• Encourage your child to rinse his mouth with lukewarm water 3 times a day (half strength H_2O_2 may be prescribed) both for comfort and to encourage healing.

• Encourage your child not to eat acidic foods, such as fruit juice, as they can sting if abrasions are present.

• Encourage your child to maintain a good fluid intake as this helps to keep lips from cracking.

• Keep his lips well lubricated with vaseline or a commercial product as this also prevents cracking.

Beth is a 6-year-old girl admitted to the hospital with a diagnosis of acute lymphoblastic leukemia to be started on chemotherapy. The following is a nursing care plan you might devise for her.

Assessment: Pale-appearing 6-year-old screaming at sight of needle for blood sampling. One 2 × 3 inch ecchymotic area on right ankle; scattered petechiae on both arms. Cervical lymph glands enlarged bilaterally. Linear abrasion on right thumb is reddened with a pustular discharge. Systemic temperature is 101°F. Child lives with father and two brothers (12 and 14) following a divorce of her parents 6 months ago. Father states that Beth has been chronically fatigued since divorce; not interested in softball competition she previously enjoyed very much. He encourages this as it is a family activity. Brought to health center because a note from her teacher last week stated that Beth's school work has not been done well lately and she wondered if Beth was depressed. Father observed sitting crying by daughter's bedside. States he is concerned that the stress of the recent divorce caused the leukemia; embarrassed that teacher was more aware his daughter was ill than he was. Bone marrow completed: 80% blast cells obtained.

Nursing Diagnosis: Knowledge deficit related to origin of disease

Defining Characteristic: Father states he wonders if depression has caused disease.

Goal: Father demonstrates improved knowledge about cause of leukemia by 1 week's time.

Outcome Criteria: Father states he understands that the cause of leukemia is unknown.

Nursing Orders	*Rationale*
1. Review with father that the cause for leukemia is unknown but that stress alone could not be the cause.	1. Reducing a feeling of guilt can aid acceptance of illness.
2. Review importance of offering support to Beth at this time.	2. The diagnosis is also stressful to Beth.
3. Support father's capabilities.	3. Signs of leukemia are subtle and often are not detected immediately.
4. Stress that following an expected remission, Beth will again be able to play active games.	4. Support father in his interest in family activities.

Nursing Diagnosis: High risk for infection related to immunosuppression

Defining Characteristic: By definition, lack of functioning white blood cells are reduced with leukemia.

Goal: Beth will remain free of infection although white blood cell count is decreased during course of illness.

Outcome Criteria: Beth maintains a temperature below 99°F and has no body discharge or other signs of infection.

(continued)

records of the number and consistency of bowel movements in children receiving chemotherapy. If diarrhea is present, intravenous fluid will usually be administered to supplement fluid loss; an antidiarrheal agent may be prescribed for older children. Be certain to change diapers frequently in infants to prevent excoriation of the skin from the acid stool content. Diarrhea is frightening for children because of the loss of control they experience. Offer support and comfort for this annoying side effect of their primary therapy.

Nursing Diagnosis: High risk for diversional activity deficit related to neuropathy resulting from chemotherapy

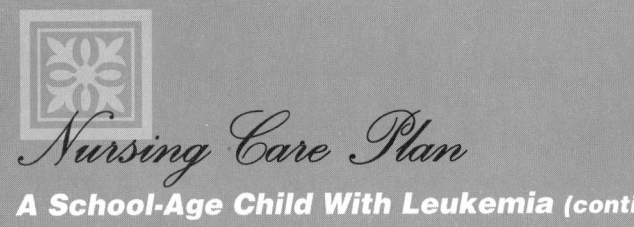
Nursing Orders	Rationale
1. Use good handwashing before giving care.	1. Most infection in health care facilities is spread by unclean hands of health care providers.
2. Screen visitors and staff for signs of infection and exclude them from contact as necessary.	2. Reduces exposure to infection.
3. Provide warm soaks to thumb (20 min) 4 times a day as prescribed. Assess site q 8 h for redness or possible infection.	3. Heat can reduce inflammation.
4. Administer gentamicin by intravenous infusion as prescribed.	4. An antibiotic can help cure infection.
5. Take oral temperature q 4 h.	5. Don't take rectal temperatures with children with leukemia because of possible rectal ulcerations.

Nursing Diagnosis: Fear related to painful procedures necessary for diagnosis and therapy

Defining Characteristic: Child screams at site of blood drawing needle.

Goal: Child demonstrates ability to control fear to a point of cooperation by 1 month's time.

Outcome Criteria: Beth uses a technique such as imagery to decrease fear.

Nursing Orders	Rationale
1. Prepare Beth thoroughly for painful procedures so she knows what to expect.	1. Reduces fear through knowledge of procedures.
2. Provide therapeutic play with syringes and needles.	2. Helps Beth work through feelings of fear.
3. Introduce Beth to concept of imagery and help her to use it for painful procedures.	3. Imagery is effective with children as they have good imaginations.
4. Encourage father to visit and serve as support person during painful procedures.	4. A support person can be instrumental in reducing stress.
5. Encourage Beth to verbalize her feelings about painful procedures.	5. Voicing feelings can help reduce fear.

Nursing Diagnosis: High risk for altered nutrition: less than body requirements, related to side effects of chemotherapy

Defining Characteristics: Side effects such as nausea and diarrhea can be expected with chemotherapy.

Goal: Child will ingest adequate nutrition for growth maintenance needs during chemotherapy period.

Outcome Criteria: Child ingests 1800-kcal diet daily.

(continued)

Goal: Child will maintain usual activity level during therapy.

Outcome Criteria: Child identifies activities he or she can participate in that do not require fine motor skills while neuropathy is present.

Vincristine therapy will result in neurologic symp-toms, such as weakness, tingling, and numbing of the extremities. These symptoms disappear when the medication is discontinued. Children may be unable to hold a pen or pencil or maneuver small parts of toys because their fingers are so affected. Use creative thinking to devise games they can accomplish until the numbness in the hands fades. Children on bedrest may develop

Nursing Orders	*Rationale*
1. Offer food early in day before chemotherapy when child is less apt to be nauseated. Support high caloric snacks such as malted milk and fortified breakfast foods.	1. Eating frequent small meals may be better accepted than large meals.
2. Allow child to select foods as much as possible. Praise for eating rather than scold for not eating or urging to eat more.	2. Make mealtime a positive experience.
3. Encourage parent to visit at mealtime or locate other children to make mealtime a social occasion.	3. Make mealtime a positive experience.
4. Weigh daily; maintain accurate intake and output measurements.	4. Assess for adequate fluid intake in presence of vomiting.
5. Encourage child to eat when she is hungry even if it is not mealtime.	5. Maintains adequate nutrition level.
6. Administer prescribed antiemetic 30 min before beginning of chemotherapy, regularly during chemotherapy.	6. Prevent nausea and vomiting rather than trying to correct it once it has occurred.
7. Assess skin turgor and moisture of mucous membrane every 8 h.	7. Vomiting can lead to dehydration.

Nursing Diagnosis: High risk for altered urinary elimination related to chemotherapy

Defining Characteristic: Some chemotherapeutic drugs cause toxicity in renal glomeruli.

Goal: Child will maintain renal function during chemotherapy period.

Outcome Criteria: Child voids 30 mL/h; specific gravity remains between 1.003 and 1.030.

Nursing Orders	*Rationale*
1. Maintain intravenous fluid infusion as prescribed or encourage oral fluid.	1. Encourages renal flow to reduce toxicity to glomeruli.
2. Encourage child to void frequently (every 4 h) during chemotherapy and before bedtime.	2. Reduces uric acid level in glomeruli and bladder.

(continued)

footdrop with vincristine and may need a footboard provided for them.

Nursing Diagnosis: High risk for infection related to depression of immune system with chemotherapy

Goal: Child will not develop an infection during treatment period.

Outcome Criteria: Child's temperature remains below 37.0°C; no areas of erythema or drainage are found on the skin.

Children with cancer are very susceptible to infection not only because their immune system is depressed by chemotherapy but also because they develop a degree of malnutrition that decreases the effectiveness of macrophage and phagocytosis function. The presence of a malignant process in the body may decrease the body's overall ability to recognize foreign invaders and respond with the usual efficient rejection process. Frequent intravenous insertion, the development of dry and cracking mucous membranes, and ulcer formation

Nursing Orders	**Rationale**
3. Assess urine samples for specific gravity and occult blood; monitor serum uric acid level.	3. Hemorrhagic cystitis can occur, especially with cyclophosphamide.
4. Administer allopurinol at prescribed dosage and time.	4. Helps reduce uric acid level.

Nursing Diagnosis: High risk for body image disturbance related to side effects of chemotherapy

Defining Characteristic: The physical changes that occur with chemotherapy can affect body image.

Goal: Child will demonstrate positive body image during chemotherapy period.

Outcome Criteria: Child continues in school and other age-appropriate activities; states that she is adjusting well to changes.

Nursing Orders	**Rationale**
1. Prepare both child and parent for effects of chemotherapy such as fatigue and alopecia. Help child select a cap to wear if desired.	1. Understanding and preparation can be the beginning of acceptance.
2. Introduce child to bald Cabbage Patch doll for a friend.	2. Helps child not to feel isolated with problem.
3. Stress that hair is lost because it breaks off at the skin surface; the root is not damaged so it will regrow.	3. Stresses that appearance change is temporary.
4. Stress that what people are inside is more important than what shows on the outside.	4. Helps child to understand that she is still loved for who she is as well as what she looks like during chemotherapy.

throughout the gastrointestinal tract provide ready sites for the entrance of microorganisms.

Although infection is occurring, it may be difficult to recognize because the usual response does not occur. Such common findings as local erythema, swelling, systemic fever, and swollen lymph glands may not be present or may be reduced in contrast to the degree of infection present.

Bacterial infections are common. Gram-negative bacteria, such as *Escherichia coli, Pseudomonas aerugi-*

nosa, and *Klebsiella pneumoniae,* and gram-positive bacteria, such as *Staphylococcus aureus* and streptococci, are common organisms involved in infections. Viral infections, such as varicella (chickenpox), varicella zoster (shingles), herpes simplex, viral hepatitis, and cytomegalovirus, are common invaders. Viral infections may occur because of the inability of children to produce interferon.

When bacterial infections are treated with antibiotics, overgrowth of fungal infections may occur. *Can-*

didiasis or *Aspergillosis* are common fungal invaders. When children are treated with immunosuppressive drugs, protozoal infections such as *Pneumocystis carinii* pneumonia (normally a very rare pneumonia) may occur.

When infection is discovered in children with cancer, the causative agent is identified by culture; specific antibiotics are then prescribed. The most important role in caring for children with cancer is not to assist with treatment after infection has occurred but to prevent infection. See the Focus on Nursing Care display that identifies interventions to reduce the possibility of infection in the child with neutropenia (lowered white blood cell count).

Chemotherapy Protocols

Chemotherapy is scheduled for children at set times and days and by different predetermined routes. At first, children remain in the hospital for treatment; later, they must be brought in on a specific day for therapy or parents administer it at home. Parents are shown the child's treatment protocol so that they know what drug the child will be receiving each day and on which days these must be administered. Knowing the protocol and specific drug therapy included helps parents begin to prepare the child for it, such as increasing fiber in the child's diet for a few days prior to the beginning of a constipation-causing drug like vincristine. An example of such a protocol is shown in Table 53-3.

Chemotherapy for acute lymphocytic leukemia (the most common cancer in children) is given first in a *remission* phase; next in a *sanctuary* phase; and finally, in a *maintenance* phase. In week 1 of this sample protocol, vincristine is given one time intravenously; oral prednisone is given daily. In week 2, another dose of vincristine is given, and oral prednisone is continued. In week 3, another dose of vincristine is given, and oral prednisone is continued; intrathecal (injection into the cerebrospinal fluid [CSF]) methotrexate is also given. In week 5, a course of L-asparaginase is begun, and prednisone is continued. Week 7 marks the beginning of the sanctuary phase; drug administration is further spaced during this period. A maintenance phase follows the sanctuary phase.

When a child who has received chemotherapy is discharged from the hospital, the parents may need to be reminded of some simple rules. They should not give the child aspirin, but acetaminophen can be used for headache or to reduce fever. Aspirin may interfere with blood coagulation, a problem already present due to lowered thrombocyte levels, and may increase the child's susceptibility to Reye's syndrome (see Chapter 49). A parent who wishes to give the child vitamins should be certain that the vitamin preparation does not contain folic acid. Administration of folic acid will interfere with the efficiency of methotrexate, a folic acid antagonist.

Live virus vaccines should not be given. The child's immune mechanism is so deficient that these vaccines could cause widespread viral disease. These children are particularly susceptible to infections and should be kept away from people with infections. They will need zoster immune globulin if they are exposed to chickenpox.

Bone Marrow Transplantation

Transplanting bone marrow that has been previously harvested from a child with cancer or transplanting marrow from a well person to a child with cancer has become a frequently used treatment for children. This can allow higher doses of chemotherapy and radiation to be used because, in the event of severe bone marrow depression, the child can have healthy marrow restored. Immune cells in the transplanted marrow may actually help to kill remaining cancer cells in the child's circulation.

If the child's own marrow is used, this is *autologous* transfusion. Bone marrow may be donated by someone who is histocompatible (immune compatible) with the child. This is an *allogeneic transplant*. A *synergeneic* transplant is one between twins (Geller, 1993).

Prior to transplant, the child receives a chemotherapy agent, such as cyclophosphamide, and total-body irradiation to kill as many marrow cells as possible, suppress the child's immune response to the transplanted tissue, and create space in the bone marrow to allow the newly transplanted cells a place to grow.

Bone marrow is removed from the child and treated

Table 53-3. *Sample Protocol for the Treatment of Acute Lymphocytic Leukemia*

Day	Remission Phase						Sanctuary Phase							
Day	1	8	15	22	29	36	43	50	57	64	71	78	85	92
Week	1	2	3	4	5	6	7	8	9	10	11	12	13	14
	V	V	V	V	L	L	M			M		V	M	
		M	M				M'+			M'+			M'+	
	P	P	P	P	P	P								

V = vincristine; P = prednisone; M = intrathecal methotrexate; L = L-asparaginase; M' = methotrexate IV; + = leucovorine.

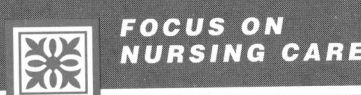

Guidelines for Care of the Child With Neutropenia

1. Admit the child with neutropenia to a private room that has been thoroughly cleaned before use. Begin reverse isolation.

2. To reduce the possibility of disease spread, do not care for children with infections such as bronchiolitis, diarrhea, or meningitis while also caring for a child with neutropenia.

3. The best safeguard against spreading infection is thorough and frequent handwashing. Wash hands before child care and after handling containers of potentially infected body secretions, such as tissues used for nasal discharge, diapers, or bedpans.

4. Screen visitors for signs of infection (e.g., nasal discharge, oral herpes, conjunctivitis, skin infections, rash). Prohibit people from visiting with the child who have infectious symptoms, who recently have been exposed to a communicable disease (e.g., chickenpox), or who have recently been immunized. Children who are exposed to varicella should receive zoster immune globulin.

5. Do not allow plants, fresh fruit and vegetables, or flowers in a child's room (they foster mold spores). Do not permit the child to have a goldfish (which fosters mold) or a pet turtle (a potential source of salmonella).

6. Provide for thorough body hygiene daily with mild soap and warm water. Encourage the child to brush the teeth with a soft toothbrush or cotton-tipped applicator to avoid breaking surface of mucous membrane.

7. Inspect the child's mouth daily for any bleeding sites or white patches that would indicate oral monilia (thrush). Keep the child's lips lubricated with Vaseline to avoid cracking and to prevent an entry site for microorganisms.

8. Assess temperature, pulse, and respiratory rate every 4 h. Avoid rectal temperature taking, which could puncture the rectal mucosa and provide an entry site for microorganisms. Administer acetaminophen as prescribed to maintain temperature within normal range (do not administer aspirin to the child with fever to prevent the possibility of Reye's syndrome).

9. Prevent dry skin by applying lotion. Use nonallergic tape on skin or cover skin with skin prep before applying adhesive tape to prevent excoriation on adhesive tape removal.

10. Inspect all skin surfaces daily for breaks in skin integrity or beginning areas of infection (erythema, pain, swelling, discharge). Primary sites where breaks may occur are elbows and heels. Potential sites for infection are intravenous or intramuscular injection sites, central venous sites, bone marrow aspiration sites, or diaper areas in infants. A stool softener may be necessary to prevent irritation of rectal mucosa from hard stool.

11. Provide a high-caloric, high-protein diet. Administer vitamin supplements as prescribed.

12. Prepare injection sites well with alcohol or povidone-iodine. Change intravenous tubing and solution sets and dressings on intravenous sites every 24–48 h.

13. Assess for signs of respiratory infection every 8 h (auscultate for chest sounds, cough, or "clearing throat"). Ask about throat pain or nasal discharge. Encourage the child to be mobile or to turn and reposition every 2 h; encourage deep breathing by games such as "Simon Says."

14. Assess for genitourinary health: cloudy, concentrated urine; pain; and frequency of urination. Encourage fluid to keep urine flow adequate. Test pH of urine samples (an alkaline finding suggests bacteria in urine). Teach the female child to wipe perineum front to back following voiding or a bowel movement. Encourage the female of menstrual age to change sanitary pads frequently (every 4 h) and to use sanitary pads (not tampons) to prevent toxic shock syndrome.

15. Avoid the use of urinary catheters; secure urine for culture by careful clean-catch technique.

16. Administer and monitor transfusions of granulocytes as prescribed.

17. Do not administer a live virus vaccine.

18. Explain the purpose of reverse isolation or care in laminar air-flow rooms. Provide sufficient supplies and activities so the child is not bored. Most articles can be sterilized by gas sterilization to be taken into the room. Encourage parents and other family members to visit, and be sure that you spend enough time in the child's room so that he or she does not feel abandoned.

to reduce the number of abnormal cells present (called purging) or removed from the donor in the operating room, under anesthesia, by the use of repeated punctures at the iliac crest (see Figure 44-3). It is then processed and transfused into the child intravenously. The new marrow migrates to the bone marrow in about 3 weeks. Until this time, the child is at extreme risk for infection. Everyone coming in contact with the child must wash their hands well; reverse isolation may be maintained. Transfusion of blood products may be necessary to maintain functional blood components until the transplanted marrow begins to function.

Not all medical centers perform bone marrow transplants, so a family may have to relocate for about 3 months for the therapy. Complications of bone marrow transplant are discussed in Chapter 44, as this technique is used with children with blood dyscrasias as well. Previously employed only with children with leukemia, it is now being used in children with solid tumors, particularly neuroblastoma and Hodgkin's disease (Bierman & Armitage, 1993).

Pain Assessment

Because growing tumors displace cells, causing anoxia to those cells, pain is a common symptom experienced by children with cancer. Methods to assess pain and interventions to help children deal with pain are discussed in Chapter 37 (see the Focus on Nursing Research box).

The Leukemias

Acute Lymphocytic Leukemia

Leukemia is the distorted and uncontrolled proliferation of white blood cells (leukocytes). It is the most frequently occurring type of cancer in children. Because the abnormally proliferating cells are so immature, they may be identifiable only at the immature, or "blast" or "stem," cell stage.

**FOCUS ON
NURSING RESEARCH**

Can Early-School-Age Children Accurately Locate Pain Using a Body Outline Drawing?

For this study, two nurse researchers asked 46 children aged 4 to 7 years who were hospitalized and experiencing pain to mark on a drawing of a body outline, using a felt-tip marker, where they felt pain. The child was then asked to indicate on his or her own body where pain was felt; medical charts were then examined to confirm points of discomfort. Twenty-four children in the study were male, 22 female, 31 white, and 15 of color. The mean number of pain marks made was 2.89 per child; although almost all body parts were marked by some child, the most frequently marked site was the abdomen (67%). The researchers concluded that asking children in this age group to locate pain by a body outline is an effective means of pain location, although they cautioned that some early-school-age children reverse right and left on a drawing.

Van Cleve, L. J., & Savedra, M. C. (1993). Pain location: Validity and reliability of body outline markings by 4- to 7-year-old children who are hospitalized. *Pediatric Nursing, 19,* 217.

Acute lymphocytic leukemia (ALL) is the most frequent type of leukemia in children, accounting for one third of all instances. The malignant cell involved is the immature lymphocyte, the lymphoblast. With the rapid proliferation of lymphocytes, the production of red blood cells and platelets falls, and invasion of body organs by the rapidly increasing white blood cell elements begins.

The highest incidence for ALL is in children between 3 and 5 years of age. The prognosis in children under 2 years or over 10 years at the time of first occurrence is not as good as in those between 2 and 10 years. The prognosis in children who have more than 20,000 white blood cells per millimeter or who have more than 10% L2 cells (see classification of cells below) in bone marrow at the time of diagnosis is not as good as in those with a lower white blood cell count and fewer L2 cells at first diagnosis. The incidence of ALL is slightly higher in males than females, and the disease is seen more often in white children than in children of other races (Mahoney, 1994c).

Although it can be shown that leukemia in mice and cats is of viral origin, the cause of leukemia in children is unknown. Radiation, exposure to chemicals, or genetic factors may have some influence on the occurrence of leukemia. Children with Down syndrome or Fanconi's syndrome are more likely to develop leukemia than are other children. It occurs more often in identical twins than in children who are only siblings (if one twin develops symptoms, the other is more likely to develop symptoms than is a nontwin sibling). Bone irradiation may be implicated, so children should be submitted to as few x-rays as possible, including x-rays while in utero.

Assessment

The first symptoms in children usually are pallor, low-grade fever, and lethargy (symptoms of anemia caused by the decreased red blood cell production). A child may have petechiae and bleeding from oral mucous membranes and may bruise easily because of the low thrombocyte count. As the spleen and liver begin to enlarge from infiltration, abdominal pain, vomiting, and anorexia will occur. As abnormal lymphocytes begin to invade the bone periosteum, the child experiences bone and joint pain. Central nervous system invasion will lead to symptoms such as headache or unsteady gait.

Physical assessment will reveal painless generalized adenopathy, especially of the submaxillary or cervical nodes. Laboratory studies will reveal a variable leukocyte count. In some children, the leukocyte count is normal or even slightly decreased but includes blast (very immature) cells; in other children, there is a marked leukocytosis of the blast cells. The platelet count and hematocrit will be low, but the red blood cells present will be normocytic and normochromic (of normal size and color).

A bone marrow aspiration is done to identify the type of white blood cell involved or the type of leukemia. If there are over 25% blast cells present, a leukemia diagnosis is established. In children, bone marrow is aspirated at the iliac crest rather than the sternum both because this is less frightening and because it yields more marrow. X-rays of the long bones may reveal lesions caused by the invasion of abnormal cells. A lumbar puncture may show evidence of blast cells in the CSF.

Therapeutic Management

About 90% of children with an initial good prognosis will have long-term survival. If a child experiences a relapse, the chances of long-term survival become greatly reduced. Although remission can be reinduced, the length of each subsequent remission tends to be shorter and less effective.

Leukemia is classified to define subgroups of cells and to predict the usual response to treatment. Lymphoblasts are classified as L1, L2, and L3, based on cell size, amount of cytoplasm present, shape of nucleus, and presence of nucleoli. A second classification system distinguishes cells as T cell or B cell. Blasts with T-cell characteristics clump or form rosettes when exposed to sheep erythrocytes and are described as being E positive. A third classification method includes the use of monoclonal antibodies that bind to antigens related to leukemic cells.

Blasts with B-cell characteristics can be recognized by the presence of immunoglobulin and antigen-antibody receptors on their surfaces. Most children with ALL have null-cell disease, or cells that are neither T or B cell. An antigen found with null-cell ALL has been named CALLA. Approximately 40% of children with ALL are CALLA positive. This finding is associated with a good prognosis. About 15% to 20% of children have T-cell involvement; prognosis with this type is poor. B-cell incidence is extremely rare (only a 5% incidence) and has a very poor prognosis. In contrast, a subtype termed *pre-B-cell ALL* has a good prognosis.

The goal of therapy for leukemia is complete cure, based on the use of chemotherapeutic agents. A chemotherapy program is aimed, first, at achieving a complete remission or absence of leukemia cells (induction phase); second, at preventing leukemia cells from invading or growing in the central nervous system (sanctuary phase); and third, at maintaining the original remission (maintenance phase). Chemotherapy in children is often administered by means of a Broviac (double-lumen catheter) into a subclavian vein. This can be clamped and "trapped" or kept open by a slow intravenous infusion to allow the child to be ambulatory between treatments.

Drugs frequently used to initiate a remission are vincristine, prednisone, and L-asparaginase. Doxorubicin or daunorubicin may be used. These are given over about a 1-month period. As many as 95% of children with ALL achieve remission with chemotherapy (a bone marrow aspiration shows less than 5% blasts in bone marrow). Because so many cells are destroyed by chemotherapy, a high level of uric acid is excreted during chemotherapy. This can lead to plugging of kidney glomeruli and loss of kidney function. To prevent this, a drug such as allopurinol to reduce formation of uric acid is administered with chemotherapy. Keeping a child well hydrated also helps maintain safe uric acid excretion.

Because many chemotherapy drugs do not cross the blood–brain barrier in effective concentrations, leukemic cells in the central nervous system continue to flourish even with chemotherapy. A combination of irradiation to the cranium and spinal column and intrathecal drug administration such as methotrexate, hydrocortisone, and ara-C (injection of drugs into the CSF by lumbar puncture) is next instituted to eradicate this source of leukemic cells (called a *sanctuary phase* because no "sanctuary" is given to malignant cells). Cranial radiation is less used today than previously because it may have a long-term side effect of causing minimal learning disorders.

The purpose of maintenance chemotherapy is to eliminate residual leukemic cells so that the child's immune system can complete the eradication. Standard maintenance therapy includes a combination of methotrexate and 6-mercaptopurine, vincristine, prednisone, and ara-C. This is given for up to 2 to 3 years. A drug such as leucovorin is usually given following systemic methotrexate to neutralize its action and protect normal cells from the effect of the drug. During the maintenance phase, the child must be monitored monthly for blood values. If there is serious bone marrow depression, medication levels may be lessened or a transfusion may be given.

If a bone marrow study done during the maintenance phase shows that leukemic cells are again evident, a new induction phase will be started, followed by a new sanctuary and maintenance phase. Children who are free of disease for 4 years are considered cured, and their maintenance therapy can then be stopped. Bone marrow transplantation or immunotherapy may be used with children who do not respond well to standard therapy (Geller, 1993).

Central Nervous System Involvement. If central nervous system involvement occurs, it can be severe and intense and can include blindness, hydrocephalus, and recurrent convulsions. The meninges and the sixth and seventh cranial nerves are the structures most often affected. With meningeal involvement, the child will have nuchal rigidity, headache, irritability, and perhaps vomiting and papilledema. A lumbar puncture will reveal the presence of blast cells in the CSF. Symptoms can be relieved by intrathecal injections of methotrexate, but check that children are not given oral or intravenous methotrexate at the same time, because some of the dose of intrathecal methotrexate is absorbed systemically and this could lead to a toxic reaction. Inserting Silicon tubing into a cerebral ventricle and threading it under the scalp (an Ommaya reservoir) provides easy access to the CSF for sampling or injection without the need for lumbar punctures (Figure 53-5). Radiation treatment of the skull and spine may also be effective in decreasing central nervous system symptoms.

Renal Involvement. Kidney involvement, resulting from invasion of leukemia cells, is a serious complication. The kidneys may enlarge, and their function will be impaired. Treatment is by radiation. Renal involvement may limit the use of chemotherapeutic agents, because they cannot be excreted effectively due to the kidney damage. If uric acid levels rise as a result of the breakdown of leukemic cells during chemotherapy, plugging of renal tubules with uric acid crystals and kidney failure may result. Oral administration of allopurinol will block the formation of uric acid. Keeping the child well hydrated and encouraging frequent voiding also help to prevent kidney damage.

Testicular Invasion. In boys, leukemic cells tend to invade the testes. Unless this problem is specifically addressed, these cells will not be destroyed by chemotherapy and so will grow and proliferate again once chemotherapy is halted. In most boys, therefore, the testes will be radiated to destroy this sanctuary site for cells. This will unfortunately lead to sterilization later in life. If a boy is past puberty and so is forming sperm, sperm banking might be suggested prior to chemotherapy and radiation so that he will have sperm for reproduction later in life.

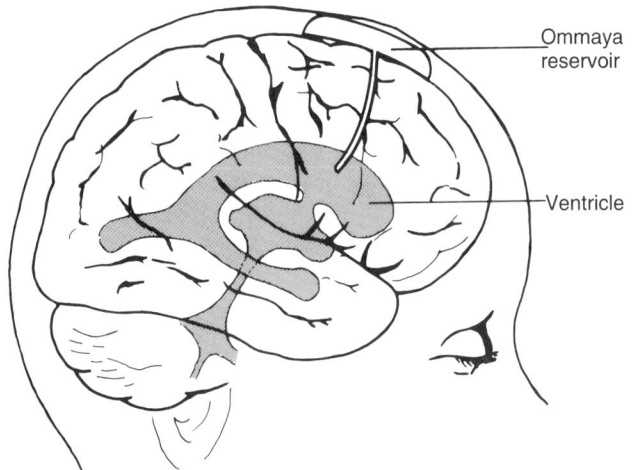

FIGURE 53-5
An Ommaya reservoir. Medication injected into the reservoir flows down to the ventricle and enters the cerebrospinal fluid.

Nursing Diagnoses and Related Interventions

Nursing Diagnosis: High risk for infection related to nonfunctioning white blood cells and immunosuppressive therapy

Goal: Child will not develop an infection during course of therapy.

Outcome Criteria: Child's temperature will remain below 37.0°C; no areas of erythema or drainage are present on skin.

Because the number of functioning white blood cells is reduced and the drugs used for treatment are immunosuppressive, children are extremely prone to infection during chemotherapy. Most deaths in children result from infections such as septicemia, pneumonia, or meningitis. *Pseudomonas* is frequently an invading organism.

While children are being cared for at home, parents must learn to observe them carefully and report any indication of infection promptly, such as low-grade fever or children being "just not themselves"; children can then receive prompt antibiotic therapy.

To increase the functioning leukocyte count, leukocytes may be transfused. Symptoms of increased temperature and chills from leukocyte transfusion tend to be more common than with red blood cell transfusion. This is not a true reaction and generally not a reason to stop the transfusion.

Children may be placed on prophylactic antibiotics to reduce the possibility of infection. Health care personnel and visitors entering their room must wash their hands well so that as few pathogens as possible are introduced into the room. Children who do not feel well have a low tolerance for waiting for their needs to be met. Having to wait for people to wash their hands or put on a gown and mask before they can enter a room may be more than children can tolerate. They need to know that you appreciate this. ("I know that it seems a long wait every time I come in, but handwashing is important.")

Nursing Diagnosis: High risk for fluid-volume deficit related to increased chance of hemorrhage from poor platelet production

Goal: Child will not develop a fluid-volume deficit during course of therapy.

Outcome Criteria: No evidence of hemorrhage is present (no epistaxis, hematuria, hematemesis); pulse and blood pressure remain normal for age group.

Because the platelet count is low due to poor platelet production and the effect of chemotherapy, children are extremely prone to massive hemorrhage. Epistaxis (nose bleed) is the most common source of bleeding; gastrointestinal, renal, or central nervous system bleeding also may occur.

Digital pressure is usually effective in stopping epistaxis. The application of Gelfoam soaked in topical thrombin may be necessary. In some children, postnasal packing is necessary. Children may need a transfusion to replace the lost blood volume. Platelet-rich plasma or a concentrated preparation of platelets will be ordered to improve the platelet count. Unfortunately, the life span of transfused platelets is short (1 to 3 days), so frequent platelet transfusion may be necessary.

Because children with leukemia have blood samples drawn frequently, receive transfusions, and have chemotherapeutic drugs given intravenously, they need the opportunity for therapeutic play with needles and syringe or intravenous tubing so that they can work through some feelings about these intrusive, hurtful procedures. Advocate for heparin traps or subclavian lines that minimize the number of venipunctures that must be done.

Following an intramuscular injection or the removal of an intravenous needle, compress the injection site securely to prevent bleeding. If the sites for intravenous infusion become obscured by large ecchymotic areas, the child's chances of remission through chemotherapy are reduced.

Nursing Diagnosis: Pain related to invasion of leukocytes

Goal: Child will experience a tolerable degree of pain during course of illness.

Outcome Criteria: Child states that pain is tolerable (if infant, not crying).

Children with acute leukemia experience pain because the vast number of white blood cells produced invades the periosteum of bones. They must be handled gently to keep pain to a minimum; assess pain using a standard scale for accuracy. They need to be repositioned in bed frequently because they tend to always assume a position of maximum comfort if they hurt. Placing a sheepskin underneath them helps to reduce the skin irritation caused by resting always in the same position.

Nursing Diagnosis: Altered health maintenance related to long-term therapy for leukemia

Goal: Child and parents demonstrate understanding of long-term health maintenance needs by hospital discharge.

Outcome Criteria: Parents and child state importance of regular health maintenance visits; child

continues chemotherapy regimen at home and keeps all ambulatory appointments.

During the maintenance phase of therapy, children can be allowed normal activity and should attend regular school. Parents need to report promptly any sign of infection so that antibiotic therapy can be started early. Because chickenpox can be fatal to a child who is immunosuppressed, the school should be asked to notify the child's parents if any other child in the school develops chickenpox so that appropriate immune protection can be given. Many children with leukemia are immunized by the experimental vaccine against chickenpox.

Evaluation of children at a follow-up visit should include not only the state of blood formation but also whether they are making forward-thinking plans or think of themselves as well children again.

Parents continue to need a great deal of support during the maintenance phase of therapy. They live from day to day, hoping that the remission will not end; they need a great deal of support if a relapse does occur. Parents who are told that their child has a heart defect that is not correctable know from the beginning that their child will die. In contrast, parents of the child with leukemia constantly hope that a remission is permanent, that their child will be one who is cured. In a sense, the child dies many times—at diagnosis and again if a relapse occurs. If death finally does occur, the reality of what has happened may be extremely difficult for the parents to accept. They may return to the hospital for visits weeks or months after the child's death, as though they must talk to some of the people who saw their child die to make it real for them. The Nursing Care Plan summarizes care.

Acute Myelogenous Leukemia

If leukemia is acute but does not involve a lymphocytic type, it is categorized as nonlymphoid leukemia (non-ALL, or ANLL). About 25% of childhood leukemia is of this type.

Acute myelogenous leukemia (AML) accounts for about 20% of all childhood leukemia. The frequency of the disorder increases in late adolescence, and it is the most common type of leukemia in adulthood.

Myelogenous leukemia is overproliferation of granulocytes. Granulocytes grow so rapidly that they often are forced out into the bloodstream still in the blast stage. The overproliferation of granulocytes limits the production of red blood cells and platelets.

Assessment

Children with AML will have the same symptoms as ALL or those related to anemia and easy bruising from the lack of red blood cells and platelets. Because they do not have mature granulocytes, they are susceptible to infection and may have had many recent upper respiratory infections. They tend to be tired and may have a low-grade fever. As the overproduction of cells in the bone marrow causes expansion of the bone marrow, periosteal pain is experienced. The liver and spleen enlarge from sequestration of abnormal cells. In addition, gingival (gumline) hypertrophy and perirectal necrotic lesions may be pronounced.

Therapeutic Management

The diagnosis of leukemia is established by bone marrow aspiration and biopsy. Cells are typed (M1 to M6) to establish prognosis. Following diagnosis, chemotherapy to effect remission will begin. Doxorubicin and cytosine arabinoside are two drugs commonly used for therapy. During their administration, children generally receive allopurinol to help the kidneys handle the amount of uric acid created by the great number of destroyed cells being evacuated from the blood. If children have extremely low leukocyte, erythrocyte, or platelet counts, they may receive transfusions of any of these products during this remission stage. It may take 1 to 2 months to reach a full remission state. A child is said to be in remission when bone marrow shows fewer than 5% blast cells.

Following the remission phase, a sanctuary phase is begun. The same drugs used for remission are continued. They are scheduled at spaced intervals to strike newly occurring cells at their most sensitive growth period to eradicate them most effectively. A sanctuary phase lasts about 12 weeks.

The third phase of therapy is maintenance. Additional chemotherapeutic agents commonly used are 2-azacitidine, cyclophosphamide, 6-thioguanine, and methyl-GAG. Maintenance therapy is continued indefinitely.

Remission is more difficult to achieve in children with ANLL than those with ALL; if one is achieved, it may be brief. Bone marrow transplantation may be attempted following the initial remission to assure new growth of normal granulocytes.

The Lymphomas

Hodgkin's Disease

Lymphomas are malignancies of the lymph or reticuloendothelial system; they are categorized as Hodgkin's or non-Hodgkin's lymphomas. Although Hodgkin's disease is better known, non-Hodgkin's lymphomas are more common in children (about 60% non-Hodgkin's to 40% Hodgkin's).

With Hodgkin's disease, there is a proliferation of lymphocytes and special *Reed-Sternberg cells* (large, multinucleated cells that are probably nonfunctioning monocyte-macrophage cells). Although Hodgkin's cells are capable of DNA synthesis and mitotic division, they are abnormal in that they lack both B- and T-lymphocyte surface markers and cannot produce immunoglobulins.

As with all neoplastic diseases, the etiology of Hodgkin's disease is unknown. It occurs more often in males than in females. It is rarely seen in children under 5 years of age. The incidence increases greatly during adolescence and young adulthood.

It occurs more frequently in children with rheumatoid arthritis or systemic lupus erythematosus, supporting the theory that the disease is associated with an abnormal immune response. Children who take phenytoin sodium (Dilantin) for long periods may develop a lymphoid hyperplasia that mimics Hodgkin's disease. In some children, there is an abnormal distribution of human leukocyte antigens to suggest that the disease may be inherited. Metastasis spread is through lymphatic channels. Late in the disease, spread to lung, liver, and bone marrow occurs.

Assessment

Symptoms of Hodgkin's disease usually begin with only one painless, enlarged, rubbery-feeling lymph node, usually a cervical node. Other nodes then become involved along with the liver, spleen, bone marrow, and eventually the central nervous system. The child usually has accompanying symptoms of anorexia, malaise, and loss of weight. Fever may be present. The sedimentation rate will be elevated; anemia is usually present from reduced red blood cell survival and poor iron utilization. Serum copper is elevated; the white blood cell count is usually normal.

Hodgkin's disease is confirmed by node biopsy and biopsy of the liver. Further studies (bone marrow, liver function, chest and abdominal computed tomography [CT] scan, lymphangiogram, and abdominal biopsy) are done to classify the clinical stage of the disorder. Chest x-ray reveals enlarged mediastinal nodes; the abdominal CT will reveal enlarged lymph nodes of the abdomen.

A lymphangiogram is begun by injection of dye into the hand or foot. This allows visualization of the lymphatic system. A catheter is inserted into a lymph vessel, and radiopaque dye is added as in angiography. Lymphatic channels can be visualized on x-ray. The lymph system does not eradicate opaque dye readily; in some children, lymph chains will still be outlined on x-ray for up to 1 year. The original dye injected into the skin to visualize the lymph vessels stains the skin a bluish green. This dye will remain as a skin stain for about a year. Nodes opacified from lymphangiogram dye can be used as markers of disease progress on plain, flat-plate x-ray films for 6 to 12 months.

Therapeutic Management

Four subcategories of Hodgkin's disease can be documented: lymphocyte predominant, nodular sclerosing, mixed cellularity, and lymphocyte depletion. The most frequently occurring types in children are nodular scle-rosing and lymphocyte predominant. The prognosis is best for the child with the lymphocyte-predominant type and worst for the child with the lymphocyte-depletion type.

The disease is staged according to regional involve-ment (Figure 53-6). Such staging may be determined by a laparotomy with partial or total splenectomy, and liver, multiple lymph node, and bone marrow biopsy. In girls, ovaries can be repositioned at the time of laparotomy to minimize the effect of radiation on them.

Treatment depends on the clinical stage at the time of diagnosis. Children in stages I or II receive radiation therapy to all lymph nodes above the diaphragm. Stages I and II are curable in about 90% of children. Children with stage III receive radiation therapy to the groin and retroperitoneum as well as to areas above the dia-phragm. Removal of the spleen at the time of laparo-tomy prevents the need for extensive radiation to this area. Chemotherapy may be begun. Children with stage IV disease are generally treated by a 6-month course of chemotherapy. Common agents used are mechloreth-amine (nitrogen mustard), vincristine (Oncovine), pro-carbazine, and prednisone; this is commonly referred to as MOPP therapy. Other drugs used are doxorubicin, bleomycin, vinblastine, and dacarbazine (Donaldson & Link, 1991). Children who have had their spleens re-moved generally are placed on prophylactic antibiotic therapy such as penicillin daily for 1 to 2 years to pre-vent them from contracting infections due to absence of the spleen. They should receive pneumococcal vaccine prior to spleen removal. If total splenectomy was done, the child will have a lifelong susceptibility to bacterial infection, most often *Pneumococcus*. Children should be followed conscientiously for symptoms of relapse during adult life.

A relapse is often retreatable, using a chemotherapy course different from that used initially. Adolescents with stages I and II who receive both radiation and chemotherapy have a 90% chance of a 5-year survival; this is as high as 80% in stage III. Those with stage IV and V disease, unfortunately, have a limited survival rate (25% to 50%).

Long-term effects of complete radiation may be re-tardation in bone growth, possibly scoliosis, hypothy-roidism, and nephritis. A secondary tumor may occur in as many as 10% to 12% of children from the extensive radiation. In males, aspermia may be a complication of MOPP therapy. Girls who have their ovaries reposi-tioned prior to radiation may have no detrimental effect on ovaries from the therapy. Newer regimens of an ABVD protocol (doxorubicin [Adriamycin], bleomycin, vinblastine, and dacarbazine) may be used to reduce these late toxicity problems.

Nursing Diagnoses and Related Interventions

The nursing diagnoses most often used with Hodgkin's disease address the child's impaired immune defenses, feelings about the diagnosis, or changed body image (particularly in the adolescent). Both the parents and the child need opportunities to express their feelings about the unfairness of this disease.

- High risk for infection related to impaired immune system
- Fear related to disease prognosis
- Body-image disturbance related to loss of hair following radiation

Nursing Diagnosis: High risk for powerlessness related to constant possibility of disease recurrence

Goal: Child will maintain positive attitude about self and ability of health care team to manage illness should a relapse occur.

Outcome Criteria: Child states that he or she feels healthy during remission; participates in school and

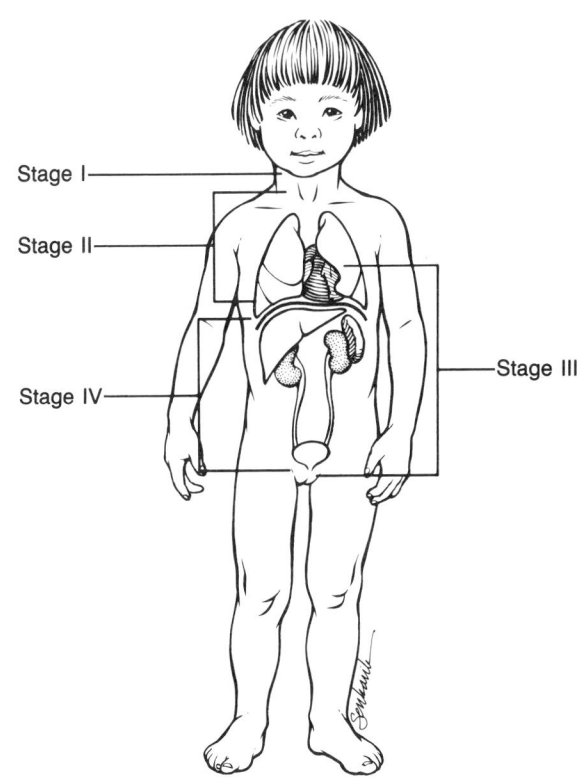

FIGURE 53-6
Staging of Hodgkin's disease. Stage I: Involvement of a single lymph node region or a single extralymphatic organ or site. Stage II: In-volvement of two or more lymph node regions on the same side of the diaphragm or localized involvement of an extralymphatic organ or site. Stage III: Involvement of lymph node regions on both sides of the diaphragm or localized involvement of an extralymphatic organ or site. Stage IV: Diffuse or disseminated involvement of extralym-phatic organs with or without associated lymph node involvement. An asymptomatic child is said to be in stage Ia, IIa, etc. A child with symptoms such as weight loss or fever is in stage Ib, IIb, etc.

extracurricular activities; and voices confidence in health care team to treat symptoms if they reappear.

The course of treatment for Hodgkin's disease is long. The adolescent lives from day to day, wondering when symptoms will reappear.

Adolescents should attend regular school during periods of remission so that they can lead as normal a life as possible. They should be told as much as they want to know about the disease. Some adolescents want to know exactly what stage they are in; others prefer not to be told so that they can continue to believe that a cure will be possible. Both adolescents and their parents need continued support from health care personnel during the long course of the disease.

Non-Hodgkin's Lymphoma

Non-Hodgkin's lymphomas are malignant disorders of the lymphocytes. They involve stem cells and lymphocytes in varying degrees of differentiation. In the pediatric population, diffuse lymphoblastic, undifferentiated, and large-cell lymphomas are commonly seen. Unlike Hodgkin's disease, spread is through the blood stream rather than directly by lymph flow, so it is unpredictable. Metastatic spread to the central nervous system tends to occur early in the disease. The most common age of occurrence is 5 to 15 years; non-Hodgkin's lymphomas occur slightly more often in males than in females (McClain, 1994).

The cause of non-Hodgkin's lymphomas may be an oncogenic virus. This occurs with increased frequency in children with agammaglobulinemia and acquired immunodeficiency syndrome or who are receiving long-term immunosuppressive therapy such as would be given following an organ transplant. Such states may reduce the body's ability to recognize and destroy oncologic viruses or malignant cells. These lymphomas can be divided into two groups: diffuse lymphoblastic lymphomas and diffuse, undifferentiated lymphomas. Cells can be classified as T-cell, B-cell, or non-T or non-B type; the prognosis for recovery is best if cells are non-T or non-B and worst if cells are B-cell type.

Assessment

Non-Hodgkin's lymphomas of the lymphoblastic type involve the lymph glands of the neck and chest most commonly, although axillary, abdominal, or inguinal nodes may be the first involved. If mediastinal lymph glands are swollen, the child may have a cough or chest "tightness." If mediastinal nodes press on the veins returning blood from the head, edema of the face may result. Diffuse, undifferentiated types present most commonly with an abdominal mass. If abdominal nodes are involved, the child notices abdominal pain; he or she may have diarrhea or constipation, and a mass may be palpable on examination. To establish the diagnosis, biopsy of the affected lymph nodes and bone marrow is performed. It is often difficult to distinguish between undifferentiated lymphoma cells and acute lymphoblastic leukemia. This can be established by bone marrow analysis (if a bone marrow biopsy shows over 25% blasts, the diagnosis is acute leukemia). Areas of metastases are identified by chest x-ray; lymphangiogram; gallium, liver-spleen, and CT scans; and bone marrow aspiration.

Therapeutic Management

Non-Hodgkin's lymphomas are treated by radiation of lymph nodes and by systemic chemotherapy. The initial phase of therapy is an induction phase (a time during which the child is put into remission, or no tumor can be detected by clinical means), followed by a maintenance phase up to 2 years long. Common drugs used are COMP therapy (cyclophosphamide, vincristine, methotrexate, and prednisone) and a multiple-agent program that includes cytosine arabinoside, cyclophosphamide, daunorubicin, vincristine, prednisone, BCNU, L-asparaginase, thioguanine, hydroxyurea, and methotrexate. Intrathecal chemotherapy may be included in the therapy because of the tendency for non-Hodgkin's lymphoma metastasis to the central nervous system. Because the breakdown of cells is so rapid with chemotherapy, careful assessment of hyperkalemia, hyperphosphate serum levels, and hypocalcemia must be done. A granulocyte-colony-stimulating factor may prevent neutropenia.

Autologous bone marrow transfusion (bone marrow removed at diagnosis before the disease has spread to the marrow and then replaced at a point that blood components are destroyed by chemotherapy) allows more aggressive chemotherapy to be used than formerly.

Eighty to ninety percent of children with non-Hodgkin's lymphoma with minimal symptoms will achieve remission (Kurtzberg & Graham, 1991). In a small percentage of children, the disorder may transform to ALL.

Burkitt's Lymphoma

Burkitt's lymphoma (a non-Hodgkin's lymphoma) is a specifically named but rare form of malignancy in the United States; it is generally seen in Africa. When this lymphoma does occur, however, it tends to affect children. Children 2 to 14 years of age have the highest incidence; the peak age of incidence is 7 years.

There is an association between Burkitt's lymphoma and Epstein-Barr virus, which causes infectious mononucleosis, in that the virus is present at the same time as Burkitt's lymphoma.

The first indication of disease is a detectable mass, which is usually painless unless it blocks some body system. Common primary sites are the submaxillary lymph nodes or those of the abdomen.

A Burkitt's lymphoma is a rapidly growing tumor; the cell mass may double in size in 24 hours. Surgery is used to remove the primary tumor. This is followed by chemotherapy; cyclophosphamide, methotrexate, doxorubicin, vincristine, and prednisone are commonly used agents. To prevent central nervous system involvement, intrathecal methotrexate may be given.

Because Burkitt's lymphomas are such rapidly growing tumors, they respond dramatically to chemotherapy (the cells are almost always in a susceptible state). Tissue breakdown may be so voluminous that the uric acid level of the urine may cause renal tubule plugging unless the child is kept very well hydrated and a drug such as allopurinol is administered concurrently.

Neoplasms of the Brain

Leukemia is the most common form of cancer in children. Brain tumor is the second most common form of cancer and the most common solid tumor form. Tumors tend to occur between 1 and 10 years of age, with 5 years being the peak incidence. In children, brain tumors tend to occur at the midline in the brain stem or cerebellum located beneath the tentorial membrane; in contrast, they usually are lateral and above the tentorial membrane in adults. This makes them particularly difficult to remove in children without damaging normal brain tissue (Friedman et al., 1991).

Assessment

Children with brain tumor will have symptoms of increased intracranial pressure: headache, vision changes, vomiting, and an enlarging head circumference from compression of cerebral fluid drainage. Lethargy, projectile vomiting, and coma are late signs.

The headache associated with brain tumor tends to be intermittent because of pressure changes related to position and the ability of the cranium to expand to some degree and temporarily relieve the associated pressure. Headache tends to occur on arising in the morning. It becomes intense on straining such as occurs with coughing or bowel movements. A parent may report these symptoms in the young child as an increasingly irritable child who is constipated because of reluctance to strain to pass stool. With some tumors, the pain is occipital. This is an important finding because this is an unusual location for a headache from any other cause.

Vomiting, like headache, tends to occur on arising. The child is not usually nauseated and so will eat immediately afterward, unlike the child who vomits because of gastrointestinal distress. The vomiting pattern occurs morning after morning. It will eventually become projectile after a long time, but projectile vomiting does not

present as an initial symptom. Vomiting in this pattern may be discounted by parents as school phobia (reluctance to attend school) as the children are able to eat again immediately and seem to recover about a half hour after they are out of bed (at the same time the school bus leaves).

Eye changes that occur are usually diplopia due to sixth cranial nerve involvement or strabismus due to suppression of vision in one eye. Children with strabismus may tend to tilt their head to the side or partially close one eye when viewing objects to compensate for the suppression and strabismus. The child may develop a torticollis (wry neck) or ptosis (lag of the eyelid). Papilledema (swelling of the optic nerve) may be evident on fundoscopic examination.

Apart from these generalized symptoms of increased intracranial pressure, a growing tumor will produce specific localized signs such as nystagmus (constant movement on horizontal movement of the eye), cranial nerve paralysis, or visual field defects. Tumors of the cerebellum tend to cause a definite head tilt due to vision suppression. As the tumor growth continues, symptoms of ataxia, personality change (emotional lability, irritability), and seizures may occur.

Four to six months may pass from the time of initial symptoms until symptoms become localized enough to arouse suspicion of a brain tumor. When this suspicion arises, the child needs a thorough neurologic examination; skull films, a bone scan, sonogram or magnetic resonance exam, cerebral angiography, or a CT scan will be done as needed. Myelography may be done to identify tumors that have seeded into the spinal column. Nuclear magnetic resonance scanning may detect small tumors even earlier than a CT scan reveals them. Lumbar puncture must be done cautiously or the release of CSF may cause the brain stem (under pressure from the tumor) to herniate into the spinal cord and interfere with respiratory and cardiac function.

Therapeutic Management

Therapy for brain tumors includes a combination of surgery, radiotherapy, and chemotherapy, depending on the location and extent of the tumor. Most tumors cannot be completely removed in children, so radiotherapy and chemotherapy measures become increasingly important. Radiation therapy may be intense because if tumor tissue is not rapidly proliferating, cells are not easily destroyed. Chemotherapy is limited in that many chemotherapeutic agents do not cross the blood-brain barrier. CCNU and vincristine are two drugs used. Administration of the drug directly into the ventricular system by a reservoir (Ommaya) may increase drug effectiveness.

The diagnosis of brain tumor is always a serious diagnosis in children. It is important to closely observe the child admitted for a possible diagnosis of brain tumor so that signs of increased intracranial pressure or new localizing signs are detected as they occur. Record pulse, blood pressure, and respiration rate accurately so that subtle changes become apparent. Note and document episodes of irritability, drowsiness, speech difficulty, and eye involvement. Statements such as "Child says he sees two forks when I show him one" or "Child is unable to see objects held in her left field of vision" are much more meaningful to a neurosurgeon than "Child has difficulty seeing." Describe completely any seizure activity observed, particularly the beginning movements of the seizure, because these may help to localize the point of maximum brain pressure. Side rails should be in place when a child is in bed for protection if a seizure occurs.

Preoperative Care

The child may receive a stool softener prior to surgery to prevent straining when moving bowels, which can cause increased intracranial pressure. Usually no preoperative enema is given, because expelling an enema will increase intracranial pressure.

Prior to surgery, a portion of the child's head is shaved. Prepare the child for this in a positive way. Emphasize that hair grows very fast again (Figure 53-7).

If the child will return to an intensive care unit for the first few days after surgery, a preoperative visit to the unit to meet the staff there should be made.

Postoperative Care

Following surgery, position the child as the surgeon prescribes. The position depends on the location of the tumor and the extent of surgery, but generally the child

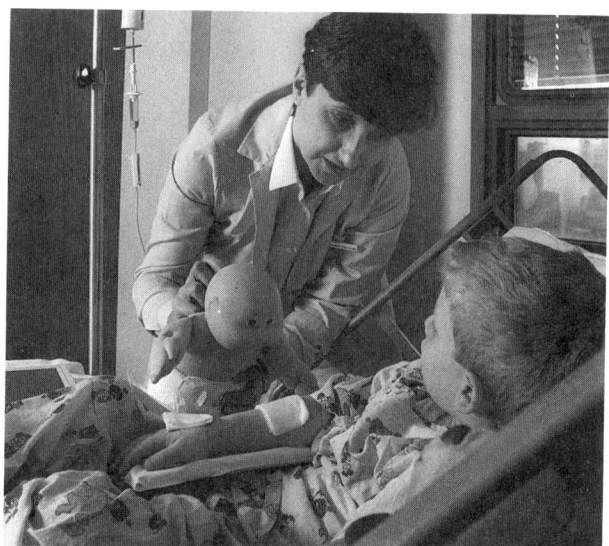

FIGURE 53-7
Preparing children for brain surgery is a major nursing responsibility. Here a nurse shows that hair loss can occur even in dolls. (Courtesy of the Department of Medical Photography, Children's Hospital, Buffalo, NY.)

is positioned on the unoperated side with the bed flat or only slightly elevated. Don't lower the head of the bed because this would tend to increase intracranial pressure from accumulation of increased blood in the area. Note carefully how much movement of the child's neck is allowed. If surgery was in the low occipital area, the surgeon may wish the child to be moved as though the head and neck were a single body part. A neck brace or cast can be applied to stabilize the head and neck.

The child can be expected to be comatose or extremely lethargic for a number of days after surgery due to brain irritation and edema. They may be placed on a ventilator. Unless ventilated, comatose children need to be positioned on their side so that oral secretions drain from the mouth to prevent aspiration. Many children have such extreme facial edema that their eyelids do not close completely or nasal breathing is impaired. Saline irrigation, eye drops, or eye dressings (with the eyes carefully closed under the dressings) may be ordered to keep the cornea from drying and ulcerating. Cool compresses over the eyes may help to reduce edema. Assess carefully the rate of pulse and respiration; pupillary size and ability to react to light; muscle strength (by asking the child to squeeze your hands); and level of consciousness (by asking the child his or her name or giving a simple instruction to follow).

Vital signs are taken frequently, about every 15 minutes, until they are stable and there is no apparent increase in intracranial pressure. The child's temperature may be either elevated or decreased because of the effect of the edema on the hypothalamus. Measures to reduce hyperthermia (sponging, antipyretics given by gavage or rectal administration because of lethargy or coma, or a hypothermia blanket) may be necessary to reduce the elevated temperature to below 101°F (38.4°C).

As the cerebral edema subsides and children begin to regain consciousness, they may need to be restrained to stop them from touching their head dressing or intravenous line. They should have as few restraints in place as possible, however, because if they fight restraints, intracranial pressure will increase.

The rate at which intravenous fluid is given must be regulated carefully; an increase in the infusion rate will increase intracranial pressure. Children may receive solutions of mannitol or hypertonic dextrose to aid in freeing the cerebral hemispheres of edematous fluid. As children regain consciousness, small amounts of oral fluid may be started. Make certain, when introducing fluid, that children are free of nausea from the anesthetic; vomiting increases intracranial pressure.

Observe head dressings carefully for drainage. A wet dressing is no longer a sterile dressing, because pathologic organisms may filter through its folds to reach the meninges and cause meningitis. Place a sterile towel under a wet dressing or reinforce the dressing with sterile compresses. Report signs of drainage and estimate the extent of the seepage so that you can tell later whether seepage has increased.

Children regaining consciousness after brain surgery generally are confused as to time and place; they may have difficulty performing simple tasks they could do easily before. Help the child gradually regain independence in self-care.

The child who will be receiving postoperative radiation therapy needs a good orientation about what to expect. Such children have had x-rays before, so the process and the machines involved are not new to them.

Following discharge from the hospital, the child should be allowed as near-normal activity as possible. A football helmet may be necessary to protect his or her head if a section of skull was removed or is not yet firmly knit. When the bulky head dressing is removed, the child may become aware of baldness for the first time. Children need support to return to school because some children will treat them differently now, having heard from their parents that they are dying or "had to have their head fixed." Parents should make the school administration aware of what has happened to the child; the school nurse should be encouraged to take an active role in helping the child readjust to school after a considerably long absence.

Late effects may occur in children who survive a malignant brain tumor. Long-term neurologic and pituitary dysfunction as well as intellectual retardation are not unusual in survivors of pediatric brain tumor, especially if they were treated with high doses of cranial radiation at a very young age.

Nursing Diagnoses and Related Interventions

Nursing Diagnosis: Fear related to diagnosis of brain tumor

Goal: Parents and child will demonstrate ability to cope with the level of fear present by 1 week.

Outcome Criteria: Parents and child continue to maintain function as a family, visit in hospital, and plan appropriately for discharge.

Parents of children with brain tumors generally are not prepared for their child's diagnosis. They bring the child to a health care facility because of insidious symptoms—vomiting, headache, strabismus. They may think that the child has a mild gastrointestinal upset or needs eyeglasses. They are shocked to learn that such benign symptoms are signs of a condition that may well kill their child. They are so upset at the time of the initial diagnosis that they cannot think of questions to ask. In the hours or days following the diagnosis, they have a great need to talk to people familiar with the care of children with brain tumors and to ask questions of the neurosurgeon.

Most parents want to hear a definite statement about prognosis: "All the tumor can be removed, your child will be as good as new"; "Your child's chances are one in four of surviving surgery . . . of having permanent effects," and so on. Because the type of tumor, its exact location, and its extent are not fully known until the time of surgery, these predictions cannot be made with more than an informed guess. Parents can be assured that it is normal in these instances for a surgeon not to make much of a guess. Otherwise, they may interpret a surgeon's unwillingness to give them definite figures as incompetence or lack of interest. Parents need to be assured that earlier diagnosis would not have made a difference in the outcome. This makes it possible for them to live with themselves afterward and not be overwhelmed by the guilt that would come if they thought they could have prevented a bad outcome. Symptoms of brain tumor *are* insidious, and the average parent cannot be expected to recognize them as important.

Parents must understand that because of the importance of brain tissue, brain surgery is never minor surgery. They must know how their child will appear following surgery: large, bulky head dressing; drowsy or unresponsive; possibly with facial edema. Even parents who are prepared are still shocked at the actual sight of their child. Following surgery, review with them once more that the child has a bulky dressing and is unconscious before you take them to the child's room.

Some parents may not "hear" the full extent of their child's diagnosis before surgery. They cannot believe that the surgeon will not be able to remove the entire tumor and cure their child. After surgery, when they are told that the entire tumor could not be removed, a very genuine grief reaction occurs. They are unable to sit and hold the child's hand, read to the child, and talk to him or her, because their minds have jumped ahead to the time when the child will die. The child may have difficulty relating to them because they are no longer acting like the parents he or she knew before but more like two strangers. Parents need a great deal of support from the time a child is first seen until the time the child has surgery, through discharge and readmissions, to the last hospital admission, when the child finally dies.

Children as young as 5 years of age are aware that the head and the brain are important parts of the body. They are very aware of the feeling tone they detect in parents and health care personnel. Because they undergo a number of diagnostic studies, followed by surgery and prolonged radiation therapy, they need opportunities to express their feelings about intrusive procedures through play with puppets or hospital equipment. Remember that when a patient becomes unconscious, hearing is often the last sense lost; although children do not appear to respond to you following surgery, they may be able to hear what is said over their head.

Types of Brain Tumors

Common sites for brain tumors in children are shown in Figure 53-8.

Cerebellar Astrocytomas

About one fourth of all brain tumors in children are cerebellar tumors, usually cerebellar astrocytomas. Astrocytomas are benign, slow-growing cystic tumors. They consist of overgrowths of glial cells, the cells that support the neurons of the brain. They are graded I to IV, I being the most benign, IV the most malignant. The peak age of incidence is 5 to 8 years.

Children with cerebellar tumors develop signs of increased intracranial pressure: ataxia, head tilt, and nystagmus. Papilledema is generally present. The onset of the growth is so insidious that the child may have symptoms for more than a year before the presence of the tumor becomes apparent. A skull x-ray will usually reveal separation of the cranial suture lines. A CT scan will reveal the location of the tumor.

The treatment is surgical removal. The recovery rate will depend on the nature of the tumor and its exact location. If the tumor is highly cystic and located in only one hemisphere, the chances of recovery are better than if it crosses the hemispheres or invades deeper structures such as the brain stem. The capsule of the tumor may be left to be dissolved by radiation. Overall, the survival rate for children with cerebellar astrocytomas is higher than in children with any other type of brain tumor (about 90%).

Because a portion of the cerebellum has been removed, ataxia and tremor may be more noticeable after surgery than before. After a few weeks, as operative edema subsides, these symptoms lessen and become barely noticeable. The child's head circumference should be measured daily following surgery, because hydrocephalus may occur from meningeal inflammation until edema subsides.

Medulloblastomas

Medulloblastomas are fast-growing malignant tumors, found most often in the cerebellum. The age of peak incidence in children is 3 to 5 years. These tumors tend to occur more frequently in boys than in girls. Metastasis occurs by spread through the CSF.

With such tumors, the signs of increased intracranial pressure become apparent after only about 2 months of growth. The major signs will be ataxia and fourth-ventricle compression, leading to hydrocephalus. A CT scan generally reveals the fourth-ventricle compression and the presence of the tumor. Because medulloblastomas grow rapidly, they usually are already large at the time of surgery; therefore, all portions of the tumor cannot be removed easily. The tumor, however, tends to be very sensitive to radiotherapy following surgery. Both the head and spinal cord areas of children are radiated to discourage CSF metastasis. Intrathecal chemotherapy with CCNU, vincristine, or methotrexate may be tried. An Ommaya reservoir (a collecting apparatus inserted under the scalp with a tube extending to the ventricles) may be inserted to allow for easy intrathecal injection without the need for lumbar puncture.

With the multiple approach of surgery and both chemotherapy and radiation, the survival rate of children following medulloblastoma is about 40%.

Ependymomas

Ependymomas are tumors that rise from the floor of the fourth ventricle and grow with intermediate speed. They tend to occur equally among boys and girls; the most common age of incidence is 2 to 6 years (Mahoney, 1990b). Because of the location of the tumor, obstructive hydrocephalus occurs; head tilt, ataxia, nystagmus, and vomiting also are evident. Vomiting occurs because the vomiting center of the brain is located just under the fourth ventricle.

A CT scan will reveal the obstruction in the ventricle. Surgery is difficult with ependymomas, because

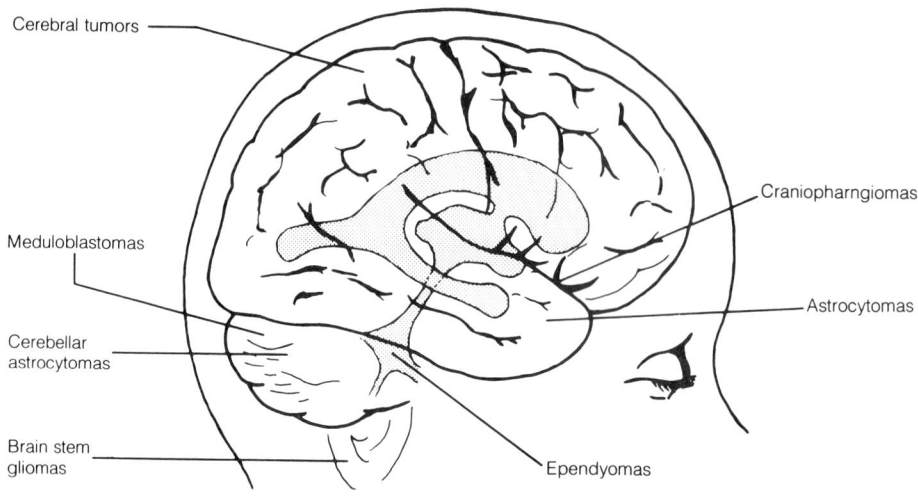

FIGURE 53-8

Common sites for brain tumors in children.

Cerebral tumors

Craniopharngiomas

Medulloblastomas

Astrocytomas

Cerebellar astrocytomas

Brain stem gliomas

Ependyomas

these tumors rarely can be separated completely from the structure of the ventricle. Ependymomas are highly radiosensitive, however, and so radiotherapy will be administered following surgery. The entire central nervous system may be radiated to discourage CSF metastasis. Chemotherapy with nitrosoureas may be attempted if symptoms recur. The prognosis for survival is increasing with ependymomas; the chances that there will be no recurrence of the tumor are about 50%.

Brain Stem Tumors

Gliomas, or tumors of the support tissue of the brain, are a form of tumor that occurs almost exclusively in children. This may occur as a brain stem tumor. The onset of symptoms of a growth in the brain stem is insidious; the first signs noted are generally those of cranial nerve involvement. Paralysis of the fifth, sixth, seventh, ninth, and tenth cranial nerves is typical. A symptom that is almost diagnostic is paralysis of conjugate gaze (inability of the eyes to work together).

Cerebellar pathway symptoms such as ataxia occur. Horizontal nystagmus is a frequent finding. Hemiparesis and a positive Babinski reflex (toes flaring upward on stimulation of the sole of the foot) are frequently present. Signs of increased intracranial pressure occur later than with tumors of the cerebellum, because the tumor is located so low in the brain. A CT scan will reveal upward displacement of the fourth ventricle because of the tumor growing beneath it.

Excision of brain stem tumors is generally not attempted because the brain stem contains the respiratory and cardiac centers. Radiotherapy is effective in temporarily reducing the size of the tumor. Intrathecal methotrexate may be helpful. Unfortunately, a relapse can be expected to occur in about 6 months. Survival following the initial diagnosis is limited.

Cerebral Tumors

Cerebral tumors tend to occur in school-age children. They present with headache and vomiting, motor weakness, or spasticity. In supratentorial tumors, the EEG is generally abnormal; therefore, the location of a cerebral tumor usually can be pinpointed by EEG. Brain scanning with radioactive isotopes is also an effective technique; echoencephalography will reveal space-occupying lesions in the cerebral hemispheres. Cerebral angiography or a CT scan may be helpful in localizing the tumor.

Most tumors of the cerebral hemisphere are astrocytomas. Removal of cerebral tumors is often difficult, because many essential brain parts, such as the motor and sensory areas, may be involved. The chance of full recovery following surgery and radiation is encouraging.

Optic Nerve Tumors

Tumors of the optic nerve occur almost exclusively in children. These tumors tend to be astrocytomas and to occur in very young children, around 2 years of age.

Exophthalmos is an early sign; nystagmus and strabismus (caused by diminished visual acuity) are common. On a fundoscopic examination, optic atrophy will be apparent.

The diagnosis is made by skull x-ray or CT scan. A mass will be seen encroaching on the third ventricle. Treatment is by surgical removal of the tumor, often followed by radiotherapy. Because the optic nerve is removed with the tumor, vision will be lost in the affected eye.

Craniopharyngiomas

Craniopharyngiomas are tumors located near the upper surface of the pituitary gland in the sella turcica. They tend to occur most frequently in children of school age. The tumor (although benign) compresses the foramen of Monro and so leads to signs of increased intracranial pressure from blocked CSF flow. The child notices visual field defects. Diminished pituitary activity may lead to growth retardation and sexual immaturity. Decreased secretion of antidiuretic hormone may lead to excessive urine output (diabetes insipidus). Diminished functioning of the hypothalamus may cause hypothermia or hyperthermia. Diagnosis is by skull x-ray, CT scan, or MRI.

Corticosteroids are administered before and after surgery to correct deficits in cortisone production that occur because of decreased pituitary stimulation to the adrenal glands. Symptoms of diabetes insipidus may be severe during the immediate postoperative period. As brain edema subsides, these symptoms diminish. In some children, corticosteroid and thyroid therapy and therapy for diabetes insipidus may have to be continued permanently. Hormonal therapy may be necessary at puberty to induce secondary sex changes. Human growth hormone may be necessary to achieve normal growth.

Sarcomas

Tumors derived from connective tissue such as bone and cartilage, muscle, blood vessels, or lymphoid tissue are called **sarcomas**. They are the second most frequently occurring neoplasms in adolescents (only lymphomas occur more frequently). Bone tumor may arise during adolescence because rapid bone growth is occurring at this time. Because girls have a puberty growth spurt earlier than boys, bone tumors tend to occur slightly earlier in girls than boys (13 compared with 14 to 15 years of age). The two most frequently occurring types are osteogenic sarcoma and Ewing's sarcoma (Figure 53-9).

Osteogenic Sarcoma

An **osteogenic sarcoma** is a malignant tumor of long bone involving rapidly growing bone tissue (mesenchymal-matrix forming cells). It tends to occur more com-

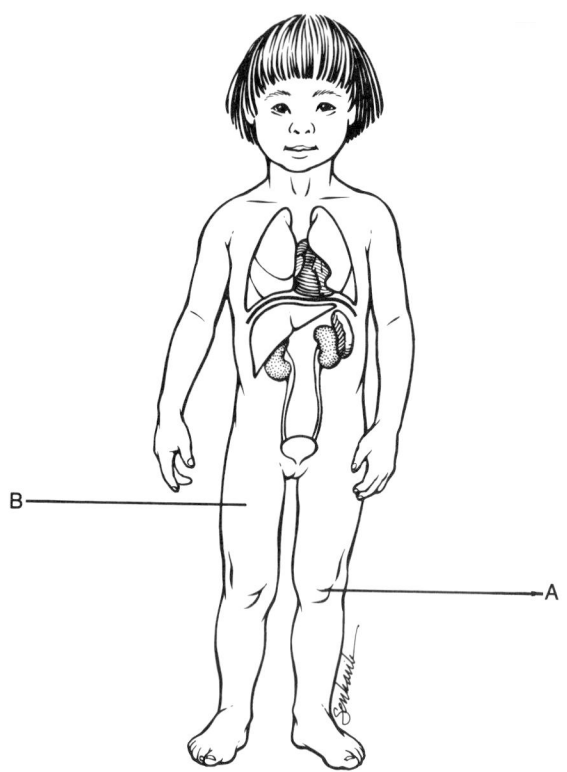

FIGURE 53-9

*Differing sites of occurrence of two bone neoplasms. (**A**) The epiphysis of bone is a common site of osteogenic sarcoma. (**B**) The diaphysis (midshaft) is one of the most frequent sites of Ewing's sarcoma.*

monly in boys than girls. The most common sites of occurrence are the distal femur (40% to 50%), proximal tibia (20%), and proximal humerus (10% to 15%) (see Figure 53-9). Osteogenic sarcoma can occur in children who have had radiation for other malignancies as a later life effect. Children with retinoblastoma have a higher incidence than normal of osteosarcoma, as if a hereditary influence may be present. Osteosarcomas can be induced by viruses in animals.

Metastasis occurs early because of the high vascularity present in bones. Metastasis to the lungs is the most common site; as many as 25% of adolescents have lung metastasis already at the time of initial diagnosis. If this is present, the adolescent usually has a chronic cough, dyspnea, and chest pain in addition to leg pain. Other common metastasis sites are brain and other bone tissue (Meyer & Malawer, 1991).

Assessment

Children with osteogenic sarcoma are often taller than average, indicating rapid bone growth. They notice pain and swelling at the tumor site. Often children report a history of recent trauma to the site (they fell playing basketball and bumped their knee) and attribute pain in the knee to this injury for some time. All adolescents with

extremity pain and swelling, particularly near the knee, should be referred for evaluation because of the possibility that a malignant process may be at work. It is important that both adolescents and their parents understand that trauma did not cause the process; it merely called attention to the knee where a malignant process was at work. This prevents adolescents from feeling they caused the tumor.

The area may be inflamed and feel warm, as tumors are highly vascular and therefore call increased blood into the area. As the tumor invades and weakens bone tissue, a pathologic fracture of the bone can occur.

For diagnosis, a biopsy is done of the area under suspicion. Because osteo cells produce alkaline phosphatase, rapidly growing bone cells will raise the serum level of this markedly, so serum analysis for alkaline phosphatase will be obtained. To see if metastasis is present, a complete blood count, urinalysis, chest x-ray, and chest CT and bone scans will be done. Caution children not to bear weight on an affected leg while waiting for tests or surgery. The bone may be so weakened by the growing tumor that weight bearing may cause a pathologic fracture at the tumor site.

Therapeutic Management

If the tumor is small at the time of diagnosis and the child has reached adult height, the single bone involved may be surgically removed and replaced with an internally placed bone or metal prosthesis. This will preserve the child's leg. If the tumor is extensive at the time of diagnosis, the leg may be amputated at the joint above the tumor (this usually therefore involves a total hip amputation). Lung metastasis sites can be removed by thoracotomy.

An adolescent may have chemotherapy to reduce the tumor size before surgery. Parents may be very concerned with the surgery delay and need an explanation that with bone tumor, this is an accepted and helpful intervention before surgery. Common drugs used are vincristine, methotrexate, cisplatin, cyclophosphamide, and doxorubicin.

Only a few years ago, a diagnosis of osteogenic sarcoma was very ominous; only a few children survived into adulthood. Today, 50% to 60% of adolescents in whom the diagnosis is made early and who are treated rigorously can be cured.

Nursing Diagnoses and Related Interventions

Diagnosis of malignant bone tumor is a shock to both parents and children. The symptoms begin so insidiously that the diagnosis seems unreal. Parents can be assured that any delay in seeking treatment would not have had a marked effect on the chances for a cure. Neither the adolescent nor the parents could have been expected to seek medical attention any earlier. This is important preparation because guilt-ridden parents cannot function effectively to help a child through this extensive an illness.

Be certain that goals established are realistic; it is not realistic, for example, for adolescents to accept amputation with understanding. The highest goal you might be able to achieve is that they realize amputation is necessary to save their life.

Nursing Diagnosis: Anticipatory grief related to scheduled tumor reduction or leg amputation surgery

Goal: Child will be able to accept necessity for surgery preoperatively.

Outcome Criteria: Child expresses feelings about loss of body part before and after surgery; states that he or she understands need for tumor reduction and implanted prosthesis even though this may mean that he or she will need to make some lifestyle changes.

If a decision for amputation is made, both the child and parents need a great deal of support. Adolescents concerned with body image may feel at first that they would rather die than undergo a mutilating operation such as amputation. They need time for discussion to be able to express their feelings. They may undergo a very real grief reaction for their old self, the football star, the former whole person that they were. Children pass through periods of denial (this can't be happening), to anger (it isn't fair this is happening), to bargaining (make this go away and I won't cheat on tests anymore), to acceptance (yes, this is happening to me and it's all right). Acceptance cannot be expected to be achieved for months. Talking to another adolescent who has had an amputation and is adjusting well can be a help, although not until children reach a point where they are interested in discussing what an amputation will mean to them. When having this great a crisis superimposed on the developmental crises of adolescents, it might be assumed that the suicide rate is above, average in these adolescents. This isn't true; the average adolescent is very interested in living and so will consent to surgery, chemotherapy, or radiation therapy (Perrone, 1993).

Hope is very high after surgery—the operation has been a success; surely all the tumor has been removed; the child will learn to walk with a prosthesis; everything will surely be all right. This aura of hope is therapeutic because it carries the family past the shock of the actual amputation procedure. Following amputation, children need visits from friends so they can see that true friends will accept them even with one leg. Hospital visiting rules may have to be broken or bent so that an adolescent's friends can visit. As long as visiting adolescents are free of symptoms of illness, their presence is vital in helping adolescents with amputations to accept their new body image. Tumor reduction surgery typically leaves a long leg scar. Some adolescents may have difficulty accepting this as it will be obvious when they wear a bathing suit or walking shorts.

Nursing Diagnosis: High risk for fluid-volume deficit related to postsurgical hemorrhage potential

Goal: Child does not experience hemorrhage from the amputation site during recovery period.

Outcome Criteria: Child's vital signs remain appropriate for age; no evidence of bleeding is present.

The greatest danger to the child after amputation is hemorrhage from the operative site. The stump is bandaged with a pressure or a rigid plastic dressing immediately following surgery to prevent edema. Observe the dressing every 15 minutes for the first 4 hours after surgery, then every hour for the first 24 hours. Take vital signs every 15 minutes until they are stable, and then every 1 to 4 hours thereafter until the danger of hemorrhage has passed (at least 48 hours after surgery). Each time you turn the child, check the bandage for the appearance of blood. You can usually control any bleeding present by direct pressure. A large tourniquet—large enough to wrap around the limb proximal to the surgical site—should be taped or tied to the foot of the bed to use to halt bleeding immediately, if hemorrhage begins, until healing is complete. The stump of the leg may be elevated for the first 24 hours to decrease vascular pressure on the incision so that pressure in blood vessels is decreased and edema is reduced; after that time, continuing to elevate the leg might lead to contraction of the leg at the hip. Helping children turn to lie on their abdomen also helps this forward-bending contraction from developing.

Nursing Diagnosis: Pain related to phantom limb phenomenon

Goal: Pain will be at a tolerable level following amputation.

Outcome Criteria: Child states that pain is tolerable. Child does not grimace or cry in pain.

Children who had pain in a leg before amputation may continue to feel this pain even though the leg has been amputated. This is "phantom limb pain"; it occurs because nerve tracts continue to report pain for a period after the pain has been relieved. Although you might think that phantom limb pain could be simply explained away, it cannot be. It is very real, and the child may need an analgesic to control it. In the immediate postoperative period, it helps children if you explain that their leg has been removed (so they can begin to adjust to the reality of the surgery) but acknowledge also that the pain is real and then get them medication to relieve it.

> *Nursing Diagnosis:* Health-seeking behaviors related to postamputation adjustment
>
> *Goal:* Child will demonstrate adjustment to prosthesis and return to former activities and friends.
>
> *Outcome Criteria:* Child identifies activities he or she can participate in and adjustments to routine he or she has made.

Before discharge from the health care facility, definite plans for follow-up care must be made. A temporary prosthesis (usually metal) is normally fitted immediately following surgery; plans for follow-up visits to fit a final lifelike prosthesis must be made. Adolescents should be encouraged to return to school and resume a near-normal routine as soon as possible. They may have to return later for refitting of a prosthesis after healing of the leg is complete. Unfortunately, as many as 50% of these adolescents will return later with metastatic lesions for additional chemotherapy, surgery, or terminal care.

Ewing's Sarcoma

Ewing's sarcoma is a malignant tumor occurring most often in the bone marrow of the diaphyseal area (midshaft) of long bones (Mahoney, 1994). It spreads longitudinally through the bone (see Figure 53-9). Ewing's sarcoma occurs primarily in young adolescents and older school-age children; it is slightly more common in males than females. It almost never occurs in blacks. Metastasis is usually present at the time of diagnosis; the lungs and bones are the most common sites for this. Eventually, central nervous system and lymph node sites become involved.

Assessment

Most children have had pain at the site of the tumor for some time before seeing a physician. At first, the pain is intermittent and the child attributes it to an injury (a friend punched her leg; she bumped it against a footstool). Finally, the pain becomes constant and so severe that the child cannot sleep at night. Because of this delay, at the time of the diagnosis multiple areas of involvement are often found.

X-ray will reveal an unusual "onion skin" reaction surrounding the invading tumor cells. A bone scan, bone marrow aspiration and biopsy, a CT scan of the lungs, and an intravenous pyelogram will probably be done to determine if metastasis to the lung, bone, kidney, or lymph nodes is present. A biopsy of the tumor site will be done for a definite diagnosis. During tests, the child may be out of bed but should not bear weight on the affected extremity. If the tumor has invaded a large area of bone, weight bearing may cause a pathologic fracture at the site.

Therapeutic Management

With Ewing's sarcoma, amputation is not likely unless the tumor is extensive at diagnosis. Therapy will be a combination of surgery to remove the primary tumor, radiation, and chemotherapy. Drugs often used are vincristine, actinomycin D, cyclophosphamide, and doxorubicin. High-dose radiation to the entire involved bone may be scheduled.

Fifty percent of children achieve a 5-year survival rate; older children have a better survival rate than younger children. Caution adolescents to continue to be careful about stress on a leg that has received extensive radiation (no football, no weight lifting with pressure on that leg) as it may not be as strong as normal.

Other Childhood Neoplasms

Neuroblastoma

Neuroblastomas are tumors that arise from the cells of the sympathetic nervous system; cells are very undifferentiated, highly invasive, and occur most frequently in the abdomen near the adrenal gland or spinal ganglia. They are the most common abdominal tumor in childhood. Neuroblastoma occurs primarily in infants and preschool children; it is slightly more common in boys than girls. There is an association between the development of neuroblastomas and fetal alcohol syndrome, Hirschsprung's disease, and neurofibromatosis. Common sites of metastasis are bone marrow, liver, and subcutaneous tissue.

Assessment

The growing tumor is most often discovered on abdominal palpation as an abdominal mass. Pressure on the adrenal gland from the tumor may cause excessive sweating, flushed face, and hypertension. Abdominal pain and constipation may be present. Compression on the spinal nerves or invasion into the intervertebral foramina may cause loss of motor function in lower extremities. The general symptoms of weight loss and anorexia may be present.

If the primary lesion is in the upper chest, children will have dyspnea; swallowing may be difficult, and neck and facial edema may occur from compression on the vena cava. If liver metastasis is present, children may have jaundice. If metastasis to the skin has occurred, blue or purplish-colored nodules (prominent raised areas) on arms or legs may be seen.

The extent of the tumor and any metastases present are identified by an intravenous pyelogram (a mass growing on the adrenal gland just above the kidney will demonstrate kidney compression); an arteriogram (neu-roblastomas are vascular tumors and incorporate veins and arteries into their structure as they grow); a sono-gram or CT scan of the chest, abdomen, and pelvis; gallium bone scan; and bone marrow aspiration and biopsy. If an adrenal tumor is present, it will stimulate production of adrenal gland hormones or catechol-amines. A urine for catecholamines or vanillyl-mandelic acid and homovanillic acid (the breakdown products of catecholamines) will be collected to demonstrate this. If children with stage IV disease have a high level of serum ferritin and the enzyme neuron-specific enolase, they have a poorer prognosis than those with low levels.

A biopsy of the tumor site will be planned so the tumor can be definitely identified and staged (Figure 53-10).

Therapeutic Management

If the tumor is localized, therapy will consist of surgical removal of the primary tumor, followed by radiation therapy. Chemotherapy has not shown any added bene-fit for children with stage I and stage II disease. With stage III involvement, both radiation and chemotherapy

are begun. A "second look" surgical procedure may be scheduled within several months to determine the effec-tiveness of treatment and to attempt the possible re-moval of further tumor (Fernbach, 1994). The use of aggressive chemotherapy followed by bone marrow transplantation to restore functioning bone marrow has promise in children with neuroblastoma (Shpall et al., 1993). Immunotherapy is also a possibility (Cheung, 1991).

Therapy for stage IV disease is combination chemo-therapy: cyclophosphamide, vincristine, cisplatin, and dacarbazine are used most frequently. Stage IV-s disease is a unique form because it has a very high rate of spon-taneous regression (about 80%). This occurs because the tumor either spontaneously degenerates or undergoes differentiation to normal tissue.

Children with stage I and stage II disease have a 5-year survival rate as high as 90%. Most children, unfortu-nately, are usually at a stage IV level at the time of diag-nosis, so prognosis is guarded (less than 10%). Although most children have a positive initial response to therapy, recurrence is common within the first year. The progno-sis in children under 2 years of age is better than that in children over 2 years.

Rhabdomyosarcoma

A **rhabdomyosarcoma** is a tumor of striated muscle. It arises from the embryonic mesenchyme tissue that forms muscle, connective, and vascular tissue. The peak age of incidence of these tumors is 2 to 6 years; a second peak occurrence is during puberty. Six different subtypes of tumors can be identified. Common sites of occurrence are the eye orbit, paranasal sinuses, uterus, prostate, bladder, retroperitoneum, arms, or legs. Central nervous system invasion occurs from direct tumor extension. This results in cranial nerve palsy, nuchal rigidity, brady-cardia, or bradypnea (due to brain stem compromise). Distant metastasis most commonly occurs in lungs, bone, or the bone marrow. The development of tumors is associated with a low socioeconomic level and breast cancer in family members (Hurwitz, 1990).

Assessment

The symptoms that occur relate to the site of the tumor (Table 53-4).

A biopsy specimen of the tumor is taken and exam-ined for tissue identification. Metastases is ruled out by bone scan, chest x-ray, CT scan, and bone marrow aspiration.

Therapeutic Management

The primary treatment is surgical removal of the tumor, followed by radiation and chemotherapy. Because a large area of the body may be irradiated, the white

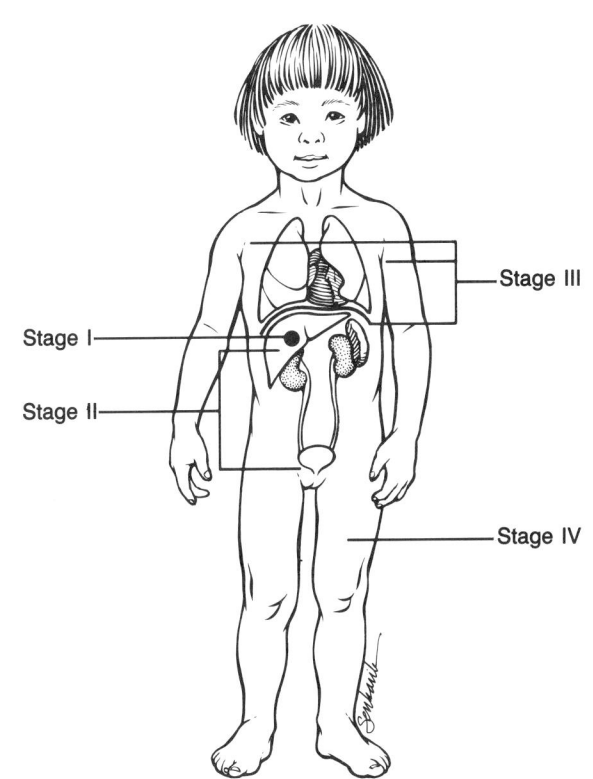

FIGURE 53-10

Staging of neuroblastoma. Stage I: Tumor is well encapsulated and is completely removed by surgery. Stage II: Tumor cannot be com-pletely removed by surgery, or there is lymph node involvement. Stage III: Tumor extends beyond the midline; regional lymph nodes may be involved bilaterally. Stage IV: Distant metastases are present at diagnosis, with involvement of bone, eyes, or liver.

Table 53-4. *Common Sites and Symptoms of Rhabdomyosarcoma*

Site of Tumor	Symptoms
Orbit	Proptosis (extruding eye); visible and palpable conjunctival or eye-lid mass
Neck	Hoarseness, dysphagia; visible and palpable mass in neck
Nasopharynx	Airway obstruction, epistaxis, dysphagia, visible mass in nasal or nasopharyngeal passages
Paranasal sinuses	Swelling, pain, nasal discharge, epistaxis
Middle ear	Pain, chronic otitis media, hearing loss, facial nerve palsy, mass protruding into external ear canal
Bladder and prostrate	Dysuria, urinary retention, hematuria, constipation, palpable lower abdominal mass
Vagina	Mass protruding from uterus or cervix into vagina, abnormal vaginal bleeding
Trunk, extremities	Visible and palpable soft-tissue mass
Testicles	Visible and palpable soft-tissue mass

blood cell count must be monitored closely during therapy. A number of chemotherapeutic drugs are effective, including vincristine, dactinomycin, cyclophosphamide, doxorubicin, and cisplatin. The child receives chemotherapy every 3 or 4 weeks for 18 to 24 months. If central nervous system extension has occurred, intrathecal chemotherapy may be included in the regimen.

A child's prognosis depends on the size of the tumor and whether metastasis was present at the time of initial diagnosis. If all the tumor can be removed and no lymph node metastasis has occurred, the chances are as high as 80% that the tumor will not recur. If some of the tumor has to be left because of its size or location, the chance of recurrence rises to about 50%. If metastasis to the lungs or bone was present at the time of the initial diagnosis, the prognosis is poor (about only 20% of children with this have long-term survival). In children who do survive, long-term complications, such as cataract formation, bone neoplasm, gastrointestinal stricture, and hemorrhagic cystitis, may occur from the extensive radiation used in the primary therapy.

Wilms' Tumor

Wilms' tumor (nephroblastoma) is a malignant tumor that rises from the metanephric mesoderm cells of the upper pole of the kidney (Steuber & Fernbach, 1994). It accounts for 20% of solid tumors in childhood; there is no increased incidence for sex or race. It occurs in association with congenital anomalies such as aniridia (lack of color in the iris), cryptorchidism, hypospadias, pseudohermaphroditism, cystic kidneys, hemangioma, and talipes disorders. There is a tendency for bilateral involvement to occur in siblings as if an autosomal dominant inheritance pattern may be present. Metastasis spread is most often to the lungs, regional lymph nodes,

liver, bone, and, eventually, brain by the blood stream. The maturity of cells (the more differentiated cells are) makes a difference in prognosis. If cells are mostly differentiated epithelial cells, the prognosis is best; if undifferentiated stromal cells, it is worst.

Assessment

A Wilms' tumor is usually discovered early in life (6 months to 5 years—peak at 3 to 4 years), although it apparently arises from an embryonic structure present in the child before birth. Wilms' tumors distort the kidney anteriorly so that the tumor is felt as a firm, nontender, abdominal mass. Parents sometimes are aware that their infant has a mass in the abdomen but bring him or her to a physician thinking that it is hard stool from chronic constipation. Fathers often discover the tumor when they toss a baby in the air, catch him or her by the abdomen, and feel the abdominal mass. Parents often report that the mass seemed to appear "overnight." This actually can happen as tumors can hemorrhage into themselves, doubling their size in a matter of hours. Wilms' tumor may present with hematuria, and a low-grade fever may be noted. Although hypertension may also occur from excessive renin production, blood pressure is not taken routinely in children of this age and so the tumor is rarely discovered by this method. The child may be anemic from lack of erythropoietin formation.

An intravenous pyelogram will reveal a mass displacing normal kidney structure. A CT scan or sonogram will reveal any points of metastasis. Kidney function studies, such as glomerular filtration rate or blood urea nitrogen, will be done to assess function of the kidneys prior to surgery. Little time, however, can be allotted for preoperative testing, because these tumors metastasize rapidly as a result of the large blood supply of kidneys and adrenal glands.

It is important that the child's abdomen not be palpated any more than is necessary for diagnosis, because handling appears to aid metastasis. Place a sign reading "No abdominal palpation" over the child's crib to prevent this.

Therapeutic Management

Wilms' tumors are staged according to the criteria of the National Wilms' Tumor Study Group (Table 53-5) to predict therapy and prognosis. The tumor will be removed by nephrectomy (excision of the affected kidney). This is generally followed immediately by radiation therapy (omitted in stage I tumors) and chemotherapy with dactinomycin, doxorubicin, or vincristine. The chemotherapy may be given at varying intervals for as long as 15 months. A second surgical procedure may be scheduled after 2 or 3 months to remove any remaining tumor.

If tumor involvement is bilateral, the operative decisions obviously become more complex. If tumors are small, they can both be removed, leaving functioning kidney cells intact. Only the kidney with the larger tumor may be removed. Tumors may be treated initially with radiation to shrink their size and then with surgery in about 3 months to remove any remaining tumor from kidneys.

Complications can occur from Wilms' tumor therapy. Both small bowel obstruction from fibrotic scarring and hepatic damage can occur from radiation to the lesion. Nephritis in the kidney can occur. In girls, radiation to ovaries may result in sterility. Radiation to lungs may result in interstitial pneumonia. Effects on bones can be scoliosis and hypoplasia of the ilium and lower rib cage, and epiphyseal radiation can lead to different growth rates in the two femurs. The extent of radiation may lead to the development of a second tumor. About 15% of children who survive Wilms' tumor develop a soft-tissue sarcoma, bone tumor, or leukemia in 5 to 25 years.

About 90% of children who had no metastatic spread survive for at least 5 years. In most protocols, if there is no recurrence in 2 years, the child is considered cured.

Table 53-5. Staging of Wilms' Tumor

Stage	Description
I	Tumor confined to the kidney and completely removed surgically
II	Tumor extending beyond the kidney but completely removed surgically
III	Regional spread of disease beyond the kidney with residual abdominal disease postoperatively
IV	Metastases to lung, liver, bone, distant lymph nodes, or other distant sites
V	Bilateral disease

Retinoblastoma

Retinoblastoma is a malignant tumor of the retina of the eye (Murphree & Cibis, 1993). A rare tumor, it accounts for only 1% to 3% of childhood malignancies. A small number (about 10%) develop because of an inherited autosomal dominant pattern. An alteration of chromosome 13 is present. Parents who have one child with retinoblastoma have about a 4% chance of having a second child with a similar tumor. If two or more children have the tumor, the parents are probably carriers, and it can be predicted that up to 50% of their children will be affected. Because of the dominant pattern of inheritance, a person who survives retinoblastoma has a 90% chance of having a child with a tumor. Parents who may be carriers, or the parent who has survived the disease, need genetic counseling so they are aware of the risk to their children. As the 5-year survival rate for children with retinoblastoma is good (at least 90%), this will become a very important counseling role in the future.

Retinoblastoma occurs most often, however, as spontaneous development, not the inherited type. Children with the inherited type tend to develop bilateral disease; those with the spontaneous type may or may not have the tumor in both eyes.

Assessment

Retinoblastoma occurs early in life, from about 6 weeks of age through the preschool period. It occurs equally in boys and girls, and there is no preference for either the right or left eye. One tumor or many individual tumors may be present. They are located on the retina or in the vitreous fluid or extend backward into the choroid, the optic nerve, and the subarachnoid space.

On examination, the child's pupil appears white (the red reflex is absent) or is described as a typical "cat's eye." The child will develop strabismus as the eye becomes nonfunctional. This tumor metastasizes readily along the course of the optic nerve to the subarachnoid space and brain; it quickly involves the second eye. Metastasis to distant body sites, such as the bone marrow and liver, occurs because of the rich blood supply to the brain.

Children with a family history should be examined at least three times yearly until they reach 5 years of age. When a tumor is suspected, an examination under general anesthesia is scheduled because children this age do not comply well with eye examinations. CT scanning and sonogram may be ordered to detect intraocular calcification or the presence of tumor. The possibility of distant metastasis is explored by lumbar puncture, liver and skeletal survey, and bone-marrow biopsy.

Therapeutic Management

Retinoblastomas are staged according to the Reese-Ellsworth system shown in Table 53-6. If the tumor is

Table 53-6. *Staging of Retinoblastoma (Reese-Ellsworth System)*

Group	Description
I	1. Solitary tumor, <4 disc diameters in size at or behind equator
	2. Multiple tumors, none >4 disc diameters in size at or behind equator
II	1. Solitary tumor, 4–10 disc diameters in size at or behind equator
	2. Multiple tumors, 4–10 diameters in size at or behind equator
III	1. Any lesion anterior to the equator
	2. Solitary tumor >10 disc diameters behind the equator
IV	1. Multiple tumors, some >10 disc diameters
	2. Any lesion extending anteriorly to ora serrata retinae
V	1. Massive tumors involving >50% of the retina

(Adapted from Reese, A. B. *Tumors of the eye* [3rd ed.]. Hagerstown, MD: Harper & Row; with permission.)

very small at the time of diagnosis, it may be treated with cryosurgery (freezing the tumor to destroy local cells). This will preserve partial vision in the eye. Photocoagulation to destroy the blood vessels supplying the tumor may be used. Localized radioactive applicators or plaques sutured to the sclera over the tumor may be used. Such plaques remain in place for 4 to 7 days. If the tumor is large, enucleation of the eye will be performed. This will distort the development of three-dimensional vision. If both eyes are involved, bilateral resection or enucleation may be scheduled, obviously resulting in blindness. The child may receive radiation treatment and chemotherapy (nitrogen mustard, vincristine, and cyclophosphamide are common drugs used) as well if metastasis of the tumor is demonstrated.

Following enucleation surgery, the child has a large pressure dressing applied to the empty socket. Observe for bleeding on the dressing and assess vital signs conscientiously. Young children may need to be restrained if someone cannot be with them constantly to keep them from tugging at the dressing and removing it. After about 48 hours, the pressure dressing is removed (usually by the operating surgeon) and a small eye patch is applied. Irrigation of the empty socket with normal saline or application of an antibiotic ointment may be prescribed with future dressing changes.

An eye prosthesis is fitted about 3 weeks after surgery. Prostheses in children do not need to be removed and cleaned daily, and in children this young, leaving the prosthesis in place prevents the child from playing with it (an interesting, colorful, round ball).

As discussed earlier, the long-term survival rate for children with retinoblastoma is as high as 90%. Evaluation of the child following retinoblastoma must include not only whether metastasis can be detected but whether the child is adjusting to the loss of sight in one or both eyes. Children who do not have binocular vision this early in life generally do not have difficulty adjusting to this. They notice it most as a school-ager when they are unable to compete in sports such as baseball that require three-dimensional sight. They may be restricted from obtaining a driver's license. If radiation was used for therapy, cataracts may develop several years later. Any radiation therapy has the risk of leading to the development of leukemia later in life. A high incidence of osteogenic and soft-tissue sarcomas that occurs may not be related to therapy as much as to a tendency for tumor growth.

Nursing Diagnoses and Related Interventions

Nursing Diagnosis: Decisional conflict related to approval of eye removal to save child's life

Goal: Parents and child will feel comfortable about decision regarding surgery postoperatively.

Outcome Criteria: Parents and child state they can accept removal of eye to save child's life.

With the diagnosis of retinoblastoma, parents are asked to make an almost impossible decision: to save their child's life, they must agree to the removal of an eye. Even following this procedure, the second eye may become involved or distant metastasis may occur.

Parents need support in the decision they make. If there is metastasis at a later date, they may feel guilty that they agreed to enucleation, thinking they have put the child through the pain of surgery for nothing. They may feel guilty that they did not notice that the child's eye was abnormal before metastasis occurred. They may have noticed that the eye was abnormal but thought nothing more than that the child needed glasses, and delayed coming for health care. Be certain that parents understand fully what surgery will entail (i.e., loss of the eye). Provide time for discussion to help them work through this very emotional time in their life.

Key Points

- Radiation is an important treatment modality in cancer therapy. Immediate side effects are anorexia, nausea, vomiting, and hair loss if radiation is to the head. Long-term effects may be growth retardation or learning disabilities.
- A chemotherapeutic agent is one capable of destroying malignant cells. Nursing diagnoses that may

apply to children receiving chemotherapy are High risk for altered nutrition, Fluid-volume deficit, Self-esteem disturbance, Altered oral mucous membrane status, Altered patterns of bowel elimination, Diversional activity deficit, and Infection.

- Help children to use time during chemotherapy in constructive ways, such as completing a project or writing a short story, in order to keep them mentally stimulated and advance emotional development.
- Be aware of the need to use gloves when preparing chemotherapy drugs to protect yourself from adverse effects of the medication.
- Leukemia is the distorted and uncontrolled proliferation of white blood cells and is the most frequently occurring type of cancer in children. About 90% of children with an initial good prognosis will now have long-term survival. Common nursing diagnoses identified with leukemia are High risk for infection, Fluid-volume deficit, Pain, and Altered health maintenance.
- Hodgkin's disease is a malignancy of the lymph system. It occurs most often in adolescents; the initial symptom is often one painless, enlarged lymph node. Therapy is with radiation and chemotherapy.
- Non-Hodgkin's lymphoma is a malignant disorder of the lymphocytes. Therapy is chemotherapy.
- Brain tumors are the most common solid tumors to occur in childhood. Beginning symptoms are usually those of increased intracranial pressure. Therapy is surgery followed by radiation and chemotherapy.
- Bone tumors occur in two main forms: osteogenic sarcoma and Ewing's sarcoma. These tumors tend to be fast growing because of the ready blood supply to bone. Nursing diagnoses identified for these are Anticipatory grief related to possible amputation, High risk for fluid-volume deficit, Pain, and Health-seeking behaviors related to life adjustments. Therapy is surgery followed by radiation and chemotherapy. Amputation is much less frequent today than formerly.
- Neuroblastomas are tumors that arise from the cells of the sympathetic nervous system. They are the most common abdominal tumor in childhood. Therapy is surgery, radiation, and chemotherapy.
- Rhabdomyosarcomas are tumors of striated muscle. The peak age of incidence is 2 to 6 years. Therapy is surgery and chemotherapy.
- Wilms' tumor (nephroblastoma) is a malignancy that arises from the metanephric mesoderm cells of the kidney. It is usually discovered early in life. Therapy is surgery followed by radiation and chemotherapy.
- Retinoblastoma is a malignant tumor of the retina of the eye. It may be inherited as an autosomal dominant pattern. Therapy is radiation, chemotherapy, and possibly enucleation.
- Following the diagnosis of cancer, help parents and

children to change their thinking from an older concept of cancer as being an always painful, fatal disease to a newer concept of it as a condition for which there is therapy and hope.
- Because the therapy for cancer involves so many return hospitalizations and so much parental concern, the siblings of children with cancer may begin to feel left out of family activities. Remind parents to incorporate the entire family in activities when possible to help them grow as a family during the course of therapy.
- Skin cancer is a type of malignancy that begins in childhood. Cautioning children about sensible sun exposure can be an important health promotion role for nurses.

Critical Thinking Exercises

1. Jose is a 6-year-old you see in a well-child setting. His mother tells you he wakes up every morning with a headache. He also vomits almost every morning just after he wakes up. She says this began just after he started school so she is certain it is related to this. The school nurse suggested Jose have his eyes examined. What additional questions would you want to ask to see if you should pursue this problem further?
2. Nancy is a 2-year-old who is going to be receiving chemotherapy following surgery for a neuroblastoma. How would you prepare her for this? What activities would you propose to keep Nancy occupied while an intravenous solution is infusing?
3. Salvatore is an adolescent who has been diagnosed as having Hodgkin's disease. How would you explain this disease to him? He is active in a school sports program and works part-time as a grocery store clerk. Will he need to halt these activities?

References

Bierman, P. J., & Armitage, J. O. (1993). Role of autologous transplantation in Hodgkin's disease. *Hematology/Oncology Clinics of North America, 7,* 591.

Cheung, N.V. (1991). Immunotherapy: Neuroblastoma as a model. *Pediatric Clinics of North America, 38,* 425.

Department of Health & Human Services. (1991). *Healthy people 2000.* Washington, DC: Public Health Service.

Donaldson, S. S., & Link, M. P. (1991). Hodgkin's disease: Treatment of the young child. *Pediatric Clinics of North America, 38,* 457.

Fernbach, D. J. (1994). Neuroblastoma. In F. A. Oski et al. (Eds.) *Principles and practice of pediatrics* (2nd ed.). Philadelphia: J.B. Lippincott.

Friedman, H. S., et al. (1991). Tumors of the central nervous system. *Pediatric Clinics of North America, 38,* 381.

Geller, R. B. (1993). Role of autologous bone marrow transplantation for patients with acute and chronic leukemia purged with cyclophosphamide. *Hematology/Oncology Clinics of North America, 7, 422.*

Gootenberg, J. E., & Pizzo, P. A. (1991). Optimal management of acute toxicities of therapy. *Pediatric Clinics of North America, 38, 269.*

Helman, L. J., & Thiele, C. J. (1991). New insights into the cause of cancer. *Pediatric Clinics of North America, 38, 201.*

Houghton, P. J., et al. (1991). Rhabdomyosarcoma: From the laboratory to the clinic. *Pediatric Clinics of North America, 38, 349.*

Hurwitz, R. L. (1994). Rhabdomyosarcoma. In F. A. Oski et al. (Eds.) *Principles and practice of pediatrics* (2nd ed.). Philadelphia: J.B. Lippincott.

Kurtzberg, J., & Graham, M. L. (1991). Non-Hodgkin's lymphoma. *Pediatric Clinics of North America, 38, 443.*

Mahoney, D. H. (1994a). Malignant bone tumors in children. In F. A. Oski et al. (Eds.) *Principles and practice of pediatrics* (2nd ed.). Philadelphia: J.B. Lippincott.

Mahoney, D. H. (1994b). Malignant brain tumor in children. In F. A. Oski et al. (Eds.) *Principles and practice of pediatrics* (2nd ed.). Philadelphia: J.B. Lippincott.

Mahoney, D. H. (1994c). Acute lymphoblastic leukemia in childhood. In F. A. Oski et al. (Eds.) *Principles and practice of pediatrics* (2nd ed.). Philadelphia: J. B. Lippincott.

McClain, K. L. (1994). Non-Hodgkin's lymphoma. In F. A. Oski et al. (Eds.) *Principles and practice of pediatrics* (2nd ed.). Philadelphia: J. B. Lippincott.

Meyer, W. H., & Malawer, M. M. (1991). Osteosarcoma. *Pediatric Clinics of North America, 38, 317.*

Murphree, A. L., & Cibis, G. W. (1993). Retinoblastoma. In G. W. Cibis et al., *Decision-making in ophthalmology.* St. Louis: B.C. Decker.

Perrone, J. (1993). Adolescents with cancer: Are they at risk for suicide? *Pediatric Nursing, 19, 22.*

Shpall, E. J., et al. (1993). Role of autotransplantation in neuroblastoma. *Hematology/Oncology Clinics of North America, 7, 647.*

Steuber, C. P., & Fernbach, D. J. (1994). Wilms' tumor. In F. A. Oski et al. (Eds.) *Principles and practice of pediatrics* (2nd ed.). Philadelphia: J. B. Lippincott.

Suggested Readings

Cohen, D. G. (1992). Retinoblastoma: A hereditary tumor in children. *Seminars in Oncology Nursing, 8, 235.*

Dallis, G. T., et al. (1993). "Right choices": Development and implementation of an American Cancer Society cancer prevention curriculum for secondary students. *Journal of Health Education, 24, 27.*

Davies, B. (1993). Sibling bereavement: Research-based guidelines for nurses. *Seminars in Oncology Nursing, 9, 107.*

Foote, A., et al. (1993). Orem's theory used as a guide for the nursing care of an 8-year-old child with leukemia. *Journal of Pediatric Oncology Nursing, 10, 69.*

Hollen, P. J., & Hobbie, W. L. (1993). Risk taking and decision-making of adolescent long term survivors of cancer. *Oncology Nursing Forum, 20, 769.*

Jessop, d. J., & Stein, R. E. (1994). Providing comprehensive health care to children with chronic illness. *Pediatrics, 93, 602.*

McGregor, S. E., et al. (1992). Attitudes about cancer and knowledge of cancer prevention among junior high students in Calgary, Alberta. *Canadian Journal of Public Health, 83, 256.*

Ritchie, M. A. (1992). Psychosocial functioning of adolescents with cancer: A developmental prospective. *Oncology Nursing Forum, 19, 1497.*

Ruccione, K. (1992). Wilms' tumor: A paradigm, a parallel and a puzzle. *Seminars in Oncology Nursing, 8, 241.*

Timmerman, P. R. (1993). Intravenous immunoglobulin in oncology nursing practice. *Oncology Nursing Forum, 20, 69.*

Walsh, B. A. (1992). Meeting the challenge of infection: A case study. *Journal of Pediatric Oncology Nursing, 9, 146.*

Unit

9

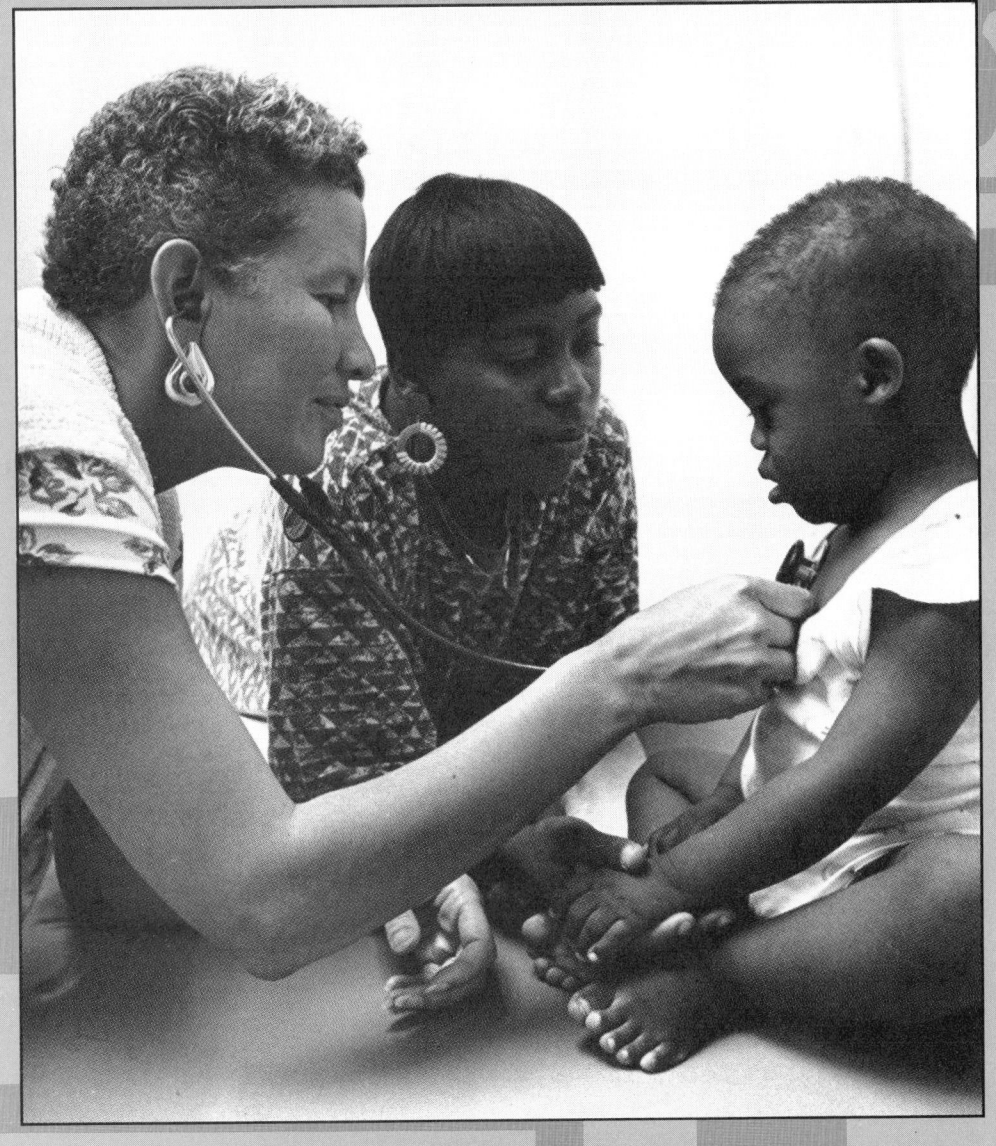

The Nursing Role in Restoring and Maintaining the Health of Children and Families With Mental Health Disorders

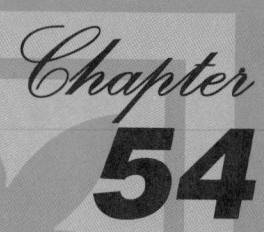

Chapter 54

Nursing Care of the Child With a Cognitive or Mental Health Disorder

Key Terms

- anhedonia
- catatonia
- choreiform movements
- complex vocal tics
- coprolalia
- echolalia
- expressed emotion
- flat affect
- graphesthesia
- hyperactivity
- labile mood
- motor tics
- palilalia
- stereognosis
- vocal tics

Objectives

After mastering the contents of this chapter, you should be able to:

1. Describe common cognitive and mental health disorders in children.

2. Assess a child for a cognitive or mental health disorder.

3. Formulate nursing diagnoses related to the cognitive or mental health disorders of childhood.

4. Plan nursing care for the child with a cognitive or mental health disorder such as helping parents plan a behavior modification program.

5. Implement nursing care for the child with a cognitive or mental health disorder such as teaching parents about the need for a safe environment.

6. Evaluate outcome criteria to be certain that nursing goals established for care were achieved.

7. Identify National Health Goals related to cognitive or mental health disorders that nurses can be instrumental in helping the nation to achieve.

8. Identify areas related to cognitive or mental health that could benefit from additional nursing research.

9. Analyze ways that care of the child with a cognitive or mental health disorder can be more family centered.

10. Synthesize knowledge of childhood cognitive and mental health disorders and nursing process to achieve quality maternal and child health nursing care.

Adele Pillitteri: MATERNAL AND CHILD HEALTH NURSING, 2nd Edition. © 1995 Adele Pillitteri.

A child who is mentally healthy has successfully mastered the tasks of each developmental phase, developed the ability to trust adults, and possesses a positive self-concept and sense of contentment. How is this state of health achieved and maintained? Perhaps the most important factor is a good emotional relationship with parents and a sense of safety and security in the home environment (Barthel & Herrman, 1991). Nurses who promote healthy family functioning during health care visits, who provide anticipatory guidance for parents about developmental milestones and needs, and who listen carefully to their clients—the children *and* the parents—can foster both the physical and mental health of children.

Mental health also implies that a child is able to meet the normal stressors of life with adaptive coping mechanisms. In fact, it is these stressors that provide the growth-producing challenges in life or help a child achieve the tasks of each developmental phase, for instance, establishing a sense of trust or independence. (This is one of the reasons why providing age-appropriate stimulation in the hospital environment is an essential nursing responsibility.) Some stressors in life, however, go beyond what is considered "the norm." Acute illness and hospitalization are examples of increased stress; chronic illness may provide an even greater stress, as the acute phase fades into recognition of long-term disability or an ultimately fatal prognosis. A nurse who is able to recognize the effects of illness and hospitalization on children and their families may also be able to provide interventions that can prevent maladaptive coping mechanisms from turning into emotional distress. Being aware of the potential emotional responses a child might have to a particular illness and implications for family functioning are essential to this ability.

Actual mental illness may develop during childhood as children suffer from the same mental illnesses that affect the adult population, such as depression or schizophrenia. In addition, a number of disorders exist that begin in childhood or adolescence and affect only children. Autism is an example of such a disorder. Some problems, such as separation anxiety, may consist of behavior that is considered normal at one stage of development (infancy) yet pathologic at another (adolescence). Current research attributes some of these disorders to genetic causes, others to disruption in family life or inadequate parent-child bonds. Children with mental illness, whatever the cause, must be evaluated and treated by specialists in the mental health field as early in their disease process as possible. It is often the child health nurse who is first aware of such problems, and as such, may be instrumental, through appropriate referrals, in helping the child and family adjust to the disorder. National Health Goals related to mental health are shown in the Focus on National Health Goals box.

NURSING PROCESS OVERVIEW
for the Care of the Child With Cognitive or Mental Illness

ASSESSMENT

Both a child's personality and mental growth potential are influenced by a number of factors, including genetic make-up, cultural background, family environment, and community resources. All of these things need to be taken into account when assessing a child's cognitive and mental health and well being. Assess children for emotional as well as physical problems at regular health maintenance visits. When an emotional problem has been identified or is suspected, a detailed history should be obtained of the presenting problem, presumed rea-

son for appearance of the problem, relevant past history, child's school and social history, child's developmental history, and family history and current pattern of family functioning (Barthel & Herrman, 1991).

Table 54-1 lists observational data to help in the assessment of a chief concern.

NURSING DIAGNOSIS

Nursing diagnoses established for ill children often address the response of children to their condition or treatment. Examples of these are:

- Anxiety related to surgical experience
- Diversional activity deficit related to lack of appropriate play materials for hospitalized child
- Fear related to potential loss of independence secondary to traumatic injury
- Self-esteem disturbance related to disfiguring scars following accident
- Impaired social interactions related to hearing deficit
- Powerlessness related to loss of independence and control in hospital environment
- Decisional conflict related to lack of relevant information
- Grieving related to loss of child in childbirth
- Hopelessness related to prolonged caretaking responsibilities for chronically ill child
- Ineffective family coping: compromised, related to overwhelming number of stressors placed on family at one time

Additional nursing diagnoses are appropriate when a problem of cognitive or mental health is present. Examples of these are:

- High risk for self-injury related to impulsivity
- Impaired social interaction related to short attention span and distractibility
- Impaired verbal communication related to verbal interruptions
- Altered family processes related to inability of child to follow instructions
- Altered thought processes related to schizophrenia
- Impaired verbal communication related to depression and withdrawn behavior
- Altered health maintenance related to inattention to food or hygiene needs
- Self-esteem disturbance related to lack of successful coping strategies
- Sleep pattern disturbance related to hallucinations
- Social isolation related to low self-esteem

FOCUS ON
National Health Goals

Cognitive and mental health disorders in children produce major costs to a nation, as well as to individual families, because they have the potential to reduce the earning power and contribution of future citizens. Two National Health Goals directly address this:

- Reduce to less than 10% the prevalence of mental disorders among children and adolescents from a baseline of 12%.
- Reduce the prevalence of serious mental retardation in school-aged children to no more than 2/1000 children from a baseline of 2.7/1000 (DHHS, 1991).

Nurses can be instrumental in helping the nation achieve these goals by educating parents to seek prenatal care so low birth weight can be reduced, educating about ways to reduce stress in families, and identifying children in school and health care agency settings who demonstrate a high level of stress as well as other symptoms of mental illness. Additional nursing research is needed for the following questions: What are the questions that best reveal mental stress at children's health maintenance visits? Can nurses identify adolescents who are high risk for eating disorders? What support measures are most helpful to families of a child with mental illness or mental retardation?

Table 54-1. *Guidelines for the Mental Health Interview of the Child*	
Observational Data	
General appearance	Height, weight, grooming and hygiene, nutrition, physical health, distinguishing features (deformities, tics), maturity level
Motor behaviors	Fine and gross, balance, bizarre motor activity
Speech and language	Receptive, expressive, content, tone, and articulation
Affect	Range of emotion, predominant emotion (depressed, angry, anxious, happy, irritable, labile), emotional reactions to process and/or content of interview (appropriate, inappropriate)
Thought process	Estimated intellectual level via language and knowledge base, orientation (to person, place, time), perceptual distortions (hallucinations, illusions, tangentiality, obsessions), attention span
Ability to relate to evaluator	Eye contact, attitude toward interviewer (negative, positive, shy, suspicious, withdrawn, friendly, self-centered)
Behaviors displayed during interview	Impulsivity, aggression, inhibition, low frustration tolerance, ability to have fun, sense of humor, creativity
Interactional Data	
Interpersonal relationships	Attitudes toward and perceptions of family and peers, transitional objects,* pets; social skills with peers, best friend
Self-concept and image	Self-appraisal (does child like self?), comparison of self with others (sibling, peers), what does child like most about self? what would he or she like to change about self? sense of pride in accomplishments, sex role, and gender identity
Conscience	Sense of right and wrong, acceptance of guilt, ability to accept limits in the evaluation

*Inanimate objects invested with ability to allay anxiety and tension in lieu of human relationships, especially the mother-child relationship.
(Gary, F., & Kavanagh, C. K. [1991]. *Psychiatric mental health nursing.* Philadelphia: J. B. Lippincott; with permission.)

- Ineffective family coping: compromised, related to chronic psychiatric illness in child

PLANNING

Although the diagnosis of an emotional disorder or a referral to a child guidance or psychiatric clinic does not carry the stigma it once did, many parents still believe such a referral is a mark of inadequacy or a sign of failure for themselves as parents. Helping parents to see that this type of referral is no different from one to a cardiologist or orthopedist can be an important nursing role.

Parents can be assured that everyone recognizes that there are many pressures and stresses on children today that parents cannot control or guard against completely. Many parents find it reassuring to be told that their contact with a child guidance clinic, psychologist, or psychiatrist will be kept confidential. They also feel reassured by knowing that the health care personnel making the referral will continue to offer episodic or health maintenance care—that they are not being "transferred out" but asked to seek additional help only in this one area.

Organizations that might be helpful for referral include the following:

Anorexia Nervosa and Related Eating Disorders
P.O. Box 5102
Eugene, OR 97405

Autism Society of America
8601 Georgia Avenue
Suite 503
Silver Spring, MD 20910

Tourette Syndrome Association
42-40 Bell Boulevard
Bayside, NY 11361

Table 54-2. Disorders Usually First Evident in Infancy, Childhood, or Adolescence

Developmental Disorders	Eating Disorders
Mental Retardation	Anorexia nervosa
Mild mental retardation	Bulimia nervosa
Moderate mental retardation	Pica
Severe mental retardation	Rumination disorder of infancy
Profound mental retardation	Eating disorder NOS
Unspecified mental retardation	*Gender Identity Disorders*
Pervasive Developmental Disorders	Gender identity disorder of childhood
Autistic disorder	Transsexualism
Specify if childhood onset	*Specify* sexual history: asexual, homosexual, heterosexual, unspecified
Pervasive developmental disorder NOS	Gender identity disorder of adolescence or adulthood, nontranssexual type
Specific Developmental Disorders	*Specify* sexual history: asexual, homosexual, heterosexual, unspecified
Academic skills disorders	Gender identity disorder NOS
Developmental arithmetic disorder	*Tic Disorders*
Developmental expressive writing disorder	Tourette's disorder
Developmental reading disorder	Chronic motor or vocal tic disorder
Language and speech disorders	Transient tic disorder
Developmental articulation disorder	*Specify*: single episode or recurrent Tic disorder NOS
Developmental expressive language disorder	*Elimination Disorders*
Developmental receptive language disorder	Functional encopresis
Motor skills disorder	*Specify*: primary or secondary type
Developmental coordination disorder	Functional enuresis
Specific developmental disorder NOS	*Specify*: primary or secondary type
Disruptive Behavior Disorders	*Specify*: nocturnal only, diurnal only, nocturnal and diurnal
Attention-deficit hyperactivity disorder	*Speech Disorders Not Elsewhere Classified*
Conduct disorder	Cluttering
Group type	Stuttering
Solitary aggressive type	*Other Disorders of Infancy, Childhood, or Adolescence*
Undifferentiated type	Elective mutism
Oppositional defiant disorder	Identity disorder
Anxiety Disorders of Childhood or Adolescence	Reactive attachment disorder of infancy or early childhood
Separation anxiety disorder	Stereotype/habit disorder
Avoidant disorder of childhood or adolescence	Undifferentiated attention-deficit disorder
Overanxious disorder	

NOS = Not otherwise specified.
(American Psychiatric Association. [1994]. *Diagnostic and statistical manual of mental disorders* [4th ed.]. Washington, DC: American Psychiatric Association; with permission.)

Parents of Down Syndrome Children
c/o Montgomery County Association for Retarded Citizens
11600 Nebel Street
Rockville, MD 20852

Toughlove International
P.O. Box 1069
Doylestown, PA 18901

IMPLEMENTATION

Often what parents and children need most when a cognitive or mental health disorder is present is a sympathetic but uninvolved person to hear out their story objectively and to provide support for them as they try to work through the situation to a satisfactory conclusion. Recognizing when you are the person best able to serve this function requires professional judgment. Serving in this capacity can be an important nursing role as well as a source of immense personal satisfaction.

EVALUATION

Children who have had an emotional concern at one point in life need ongoing evaluation by health care personnel at health care visits to see if the circumstances that led to the problem have truly been corrected or, because they were only superficially changed, are apt to resurface. On the whole, if the circumstances surrounding the child remain the same, the child's problem may return or will be manifested later in another way.

Examples of outcome criteria that might be established are:

- Child does not injure himself during the coming month.
- Parents state they are able to cope with child's dis-

Box 54-1
Common Causes of Mental Retardation

Chromosomal abnormalities such as Down syndrome and fragile X syndrome

Infection *in utero* such as rubella or cytomegalic inclusion disease

Anoxia at birth such as from umbilical cord compression

Fetal alcohol syndrome

Inherited metabolic disorders such as phenylketonuria

Lead poisoning

Hypothyroidism

Brain malformations such as anencephaly

Prematurity

Infection such as measles encephalitis

ruptive behavior since prescription of antipsychotic drug.
- Child ingests a minimum of 500 calories daily with no binge eating.

Classification of Mental Disorders

For many years, psychopathology in children was not classified according to a standard system, and, as a result, conditions were not clearly defined or described. Today, after several revisions, the American Psychiatric Association's *Diagnostic and Statistical Manual of Mental Disorders—Revised* (DSM-IV-R) (1994) provides a standardized classification system that can be used by all members of the mental health care team. Major cate-

gories of disorders that have been devised are given in Table 54-2.

Developmental Disorders

Mental Retardation

The DMS-IV defines mental retardation on the basis of two criteria: significantly subaverage general intellectual functioning—an intelligence quotient (IQ) of 70 or below—and concurrent deficits in adaptive functioning (APA, 1994). For infants, because available intelligence tests do not yield numerical values, a clinical judgment of significant subaverage intellectual function must be made.

Approximately 1% to 3% of children in the United States are mentally retarded. The incidence is twice as high in males as in females. A biologic cause for retardation can be documented in only about 25% of retarded children (Box 54-1). Fragile X syndrome is the most commonly inherited cause of mental retardation (Dooling, 1993).

Children with mental retardation are seen in health care settings for diagnosis, and they come to health settings throughout their lives for the same reasons as other children—for well-child care at ambulatory health maintenance visits; for treatment of lacerations or poisoning in emergency departments; or for treatment of illnesses such as pneumonia or appendicitis in in-service units. For these reasons, child health nurses need to be skilled in meeting the needs of mentally retarded children.

Classification

It is unfair to categorize children only according to results of intelligence tests, because children do not always perform well in testing situations. For discussion purposes, however, Table 54-3 lists a common method

Table 54-3. *Clinical Features of Mental Retardation*

	Mild	Moderate	Severe	Profound
IQ	50–55 to approx. 70	35–40 to 50–55	20–25 to 35–40	Below 20–25
Age of death (years)	50s	50s	40s	About 20
Percentage of population with mental retardation	85	10	4	1
Academic level achieved by adulthood	6th grade	2nd grade	Below first grade level in general	
Education	Educable	Trainable (self-care)		
Residence	Community	Sheltered	Mostly living in highly structured and closely supervised settings	
Economic capacity	Makes change; manages a job; income planning with effort or assistance	Makes small change; usually able to manage change well	Can use coin machines; can take notes to shopowner	Dependent on others for money management

(Adapted from Popper, C. W. [1988]. Disorders first evident in infancy, childhood or adolescence. In J. A. Talbott et al. [Eds.] *Textbook of psychiatry*. Washington, DC: The American Psychiatric Press; with permission.)

of classifying mental retardation as to subtype and IQ. The level of 70 was chosen as the upper limit of mental retardation because most children with IQs below this are so limited in their functioning that they require special services, protection, and schooling. IQ tests are considered to have an error of measurement of about five points. Many children with an IQ of 75 are therefore included in special schooling programs so that special help can be offered to them.

Mild Mental Retardation. About 80% of mentally retarded children fall into this category. In this group, a child's IQ is between 70 and 50. The category is equivalent to the educational category "educable." During early years, these children learn social and communication skills and are often not distinguishable from average children. They are able to learn academic skills up to about the sixth-grade level; as adults, they can usually achieve social and vocational skills adequate for minimum self-support. They need guidance and assistance when faced with new situations or unusual stress.

Moderate Mental Retardation. Children in this category have an IQ between 55 and 35. About 10% of mentally retarded children fall into this category. It is equivalent to the educational category of "trainable." During preschool years, these children learn to talk and communicate but they have only poor awareness of social conventions; they can learn some vocational skills during adolescence or young adulthood and to take care of themselves with moderate supervision. They are unlikely to progress beyond the second-grade level in academic subjects. As adults, they may be able to contribute to their own support by performing unskilled or semiskilled work under close supervision in a sheltered workshop setting. They may learn to travel alone to familiar places. They need supervision and guidance when in stressful settings.

Severe Mental Retardation. Children in this group have an IQ between 40 and 20. About 4% of mentally retarded children fall into this category. During the preschool period, these children develop only minimal speech and little or no communicative speech. They usually have accompanying poor motor development. During school years, they may learn to talk and can be trained in basic hygiene and dressing skills. As adults, they may be able to perform simple work tasks under close supervision but as a group do not profit from vocational training. They need constant supervision for safety.

Profound Mental Retardation. The IQ of this group of children is below 20. Less than 1% of mentally retarded children fall into this group. During the preschool period, these children show only minimal capacity for sensorimotor functioning. They need a highly structured environment and a constant level of help and supervision. Some children respond to training in minimal self-care, such as toothbrushing, but only very limited self-care is possible.

Assessment

Assessment for mental retardation is done by history taking and IQ testing. The assessment should be done as soon as parents become aware that their child is not developing normally so that they do not develop unrealistic expectations of the child or punish a child for doing things that he or she could not possibly understand not to do. This also allows parents to begin as early as possible to look at the things the child can do and to see where they can be of most help.

Intelligence is routinely measured with standardized tests, notably the Wechsler Intelligence Scale for Children (WISC) or Stanford-Binet. Adaptive behavioral functioning, which may vary in different environments, is judged according to a variety of means, including standardized instruments for assessing social maturity and adaptive skills. A composite picture of life functioning is drawn from multiple sources.

Parents may react to the diagnosis of mental retardation in the same way as parents who have been told that their child has a chronic or fatal illness—with a grief reaction. This may be manifested as disbelief, anger, or extreme sorrow. The grief may become a chronic sorrow, always present, always waiting to strike a parent especially hard at times when the child would have reached milestones in his or her life, such as the first day of school or high school graduation. Be certain that goals established for the family are realistic. You cannot make a child achieve more than an individual disability will allow, but you can help parents better accept the outcome (see the Focus on Cultural Awareness box).

Therapeutic Management

So that they can begin to plan, parents need a realistic prognosis for a child. This is difficult to offer in early life, because infant intelligence tests are not accurate and more sophisticated tests are difficult to administer until the preschool years. Prediction based on these early tests involves some subjective input so a child's potential may be over or under rated by them. Once parents have a realistic expectation based on the best judgement possible, however, they are ready, with guidance, to help children become all that they can be within their limitations.

Nursing Diagnoses and Related Interventions

Nursing Diagnosis: Health-seeking behaviors related to increasing knowledge of care needs of the mentally retarded child

Goal: Parents will demonstrate understanding of the

FOCUS ON CULTURAL AWARENESS

Mental illness disorders and mental retardation have always been perplexing to people, and so there is a history of poor acceptance of children with such disorders (Geissler, 1994). In ancient civilizations, physicians bored holes in children's heads to let out what they perceived to be evil spirits; modern television programs or movies still show distorted perceptions of how people with mental retardation or mental illness behave. These misperceptions make it difficult for parents to accept these diagnoses. Taking time to talk with them about modern management of mental illness disorders and the ways that children with mental retardation can be integrated into a family can be a major intervention in helping families adjust to and grow with these disorders.

needs of their child and care options before making any decisions.

Outcome Criteria: Parents identify their particular options and identify how each one will affect family functioning.

Parents of mentally retarded children have a number of important decisions to make concerning care of their child.

Institutional Care Versus Home Care. At one time, if a child was born with a syndrome such as Down syndrome, parents were advised to place the child in an institution immediately. Today, very few institutions of this type are available. Parents are encouraged to keep retarded children at home and maintain a home and school environment for them as near normal as possible. This plan has definite advantages for children who are mildly or moderately retarded. The give-and-take of a home environment improves their ability to relate to other people. Because a small group of people cares for them, their desire to achieve is increased. Children receive more stimulation in a normal home than they would in most institutions.

When children are severely retarded, keeping them at home becomes a more difficult task. If both parents work to earn an adequate family income, the responsibility for constant supervision of the child is on baby sitters or older children in the family. Obtaining baby sitters for severely retarded children is difficult and further compounds the problem. Day care and/or schooling outside the home may make home care more feasible.

Having a child who never grows up in terms of judgment puts a great deal of responsibility on parents

to provide constant watchful care; this responsibility grows greater as both the child and the parents grow older. Parent's freedom to go on vacation or have an adult life apart from the child is restricted. They may spend so much time with a retarded child that other children in the family feel unloved or a burden.

If parents are unable to care for a child at home, a suitable foster home placement may be possible to offer the child the advantage of a family setting. Halfway houses or group homes (6 to 12 retarded children living in a home with assigned counselors) provide a care setting in which a home atmosphere as well as community experiences are provided.

Before giving advice to any family about where a child should be raised, consider the individual circumstances of the family. Every family has its own coping mechanisms, and individual parents may be at different stages of coping, especially in the first year after the birth of a child with a severe disability. Be certain to consider the feelings of each family member and how adequately they are coping when planning with them.

Health Maintenance Needs. Mentally retarded children need the same health maintenance supervision as other children. At health care visits, parents may need a special review of precautions against accidents. Remind them to treat children according to their intellectual age, not their chronologic age. All 2-year-olds would turn on the burners of the stove to see the flame if they could reach them; most do not, however, because they cannot reach them. The mother who has a 6-year-old who thinks as a 2-year-old must be exceedingly careful. Her child can reach the same dangerous areas as any 6-year-old but, unfortunately, will explore and touch them with a 2-year-old's judgment.

Illness. It may be more difficult to detect illness in a mentally retarded child than in a child of normal intelligence. Such children cannot describe pain so may respond to pain by generalized crying like an infant. Parents must observe them closely for symptoms such as tugging at an ear, refusing to swallow food, rapid breathing, or limping, because these will help to localize discomfort. When they call health care personnel, parents may be apologetic about their lack of ability to judge the child. Assure them that you understand that this will always be a problem.

When mentally retarded children are seen in an emergency department or an ambulatory setting for care, they need simple explanations of what will happen. The average child aged 6 sees you with a thermometer in your hand and thinks, "She's going to take my temperature." Your explanation that you are going to do that only confirms what the child has already guessed. A mentally retarded child may be unable to make this association between the thermometer and what you are going to do. Your explanation, therefore, is the first introduction to the event. Make certain that it is adequate.

When retarded children are admitted to a hospital unit, nursing care planning must meet the needs of their intellectual age, not their chronologic one. For example, whether safety precautions such as restraints will be necessary must be judged according to intellectual age. The explanations and preparation for procedures also must be geared to intellectual age (see the Nursing Care Plan: A Hospitalized Adolescent With Mental Retardation).

When children are discharged from a hospital, parents need careful explanations of signs and symptoms to look for to ensure continued good health in the child. Remember that such signs are more difficult to elicit from the retarded child than from the average child. Parents must have a telephone number they can call to seek further information or advice if they are unsure of their own observations in the period immediately after discharge.

Education. Most mentally retarded children do well in preschool programs; this gives them a head start in learning to socialize with peers and to develop fine and gross motor coordination. These programs also offer parents some free time during the week to do things *they* wish to do.

The school chosen for the child will depend on the degree of retardation and on the school situations available in the community. Mentally retarded children should be included in regular classes, with average children, as much as possible (Sexson & Madan-Swain, 1993). This offers children a great deal of stimulation and helps them reach their best potential. It also helps them learn to work and socialize with people of average intelligence—something they will need to do the rest of their lives. You might need to advocate for school placement of a mentally retarded child in an inclusive program. By federal law, children have the right to the least restrictive environment possible. Retarded children need good instruction on bus safety and on locating the correct bus for the trip home from school. If they walk to school, they need appropriate supervision to ensure that they cross streets safely.

Nursing Diagnoses: Altered growth and development related to mental retardation.

Goal: Child will reach and maintain optimum level of functioning possible.

Outcome Criteria: Child is able to perform minimal self care; exhibits feelings of satisfaction with accomplishments.

Self-Care Activities. Children with mental retardation need to learn the maximum amount of self-care

possible as this can offer them a sense of control and accomplishment. Assess carefully if children need special aids to achieve such skills as brushing teeth, combing hair, taking a bath, and eating. Even after children learn how to perform these skills, they may need continued reminders to do them because they are unaware of the reason for or importance of the skill. If you do these skills for children, such as during a period of hospitalization, they can forget how to perform them and will need to be retaught after they return home (see the Focus on Family Teaching Box).

Play. Children with mental retardation enjoy play as much as children of normal intelligence. Guide parents to choose toys that are appropriate for their child's developmental, not chronologic, age. Some toys such as music boxes or record players that cover a wide age range are good choices for toys. Because mentally re-

FOCUS ON FAMILY TEACHING

Q. Sometimes I lose patience trying to teach my 4-year-old mentally retarded son the simplest task. What are guidelines I can use to be more successful?

A. Teaching mentally retarded children calls for extreme patience. Some general rules are:

- Short-term memory is often possible, whereas long-term memory is not. This means a child can only learn one step of a skill at a time (remembering three consecutive steps is long-term memory).

- Learning is not rewarding all by itself when intelligence is impaired. Introduce motivators for learning such as generous praise.

- Reduce the number of extra stimuli present. With too many stimuli present, a child cannot keep attention focused on the task to learn (or realize that the task is more important than surrounding stimuli).

- Seeing a skill performed is generally better than just hearing it explained.

- Mentally retarded children have difficulty with learning principles or abstractions. They may be able to learn to wash their hands, for example, but not why they should wash them (other than it pleases you).

- Remember that accomplishing even the most simple skill may be very difficult. Learning to tie shoes may take the same effort as a normal child spends learning algebra. Learning to cross streets safely may be equivalent to earning a high school diploma. Give praise accordingly.

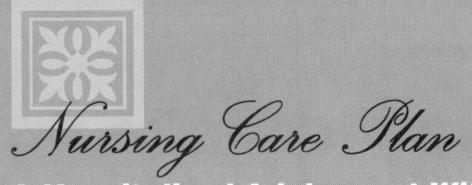

Nursing Care Plan

A Hospitalized Adolescent With Mental Retardation

Marsha is a 14-year-old girl admitted to your hospital unit for knee surgery. She will have a cast in place following the surgery. A nursing care plan you might design for her follows.

Assessment: 14-year-old, slightly obese, adolescent admitted for orthopedic surgery. Mother states she is "very retarded"; to treat her "like a 2-year-old." Has her favorite doll with her; often talks to doll about what she wants to do. Grows upset easily if daily routine is disturbed. Has a number of self-stimulation activities, such as head banging and hand biting. Likes to talk to people but doesn't know what to say, so often repeats questions like "What is your name? What car do you drive?" Can feed self and use bathroom independently. Can dress self and take shower with supervision. Attends ungraded program at Hoover School.

Nursing Diagnosis: High risk for self-care deficit related to change in routine and application of cast

Defining Characteristic: Parent states that Marsha can perform some self-care, but she relies heavily on routine. Hospitalization is a disruption in itself.

Goal: Marsha will maintain former self-care level during hospitalization.

Outcome Criteria: Marsha continues to dress and feed herself during hospitalization (cast will interfere with self-toileting, hygiene).

Nursing Orders	**Rationale**
1. Assess daily self-care routine at home so this is modified as little as possible.	1. Maintaining as nearly normal a routine as possible will help with adjustment to hospitalization.
2. Offer single explanations for all procedures (include doll in explanations to maintain interest).	2. Interacting at child's cognitive level is important for effective communication.
3. Teach new method of hygiene following surgery (bed bath) and use of bedpan (she will have large cast in place for 4 weeks) to both mother and child.	3. Child will need to carry out these self-care measures after return home. Teaching the mother as well helps insure cooperation.

Nursing Diagnosis: Diversional activity deficit related to hospitalization and change in routine

Defining Characteristic: Child displays self-stimulation activities.

Goal: Child will receive familiar stimulation and will not become upset during hospitalization beyond normal expectations.

Outcome Criteria: Marsha engages in few or no self-stimulation activities (head banging and hand biting) during hospitalization. Marsha shows interest in talking with health care providers.

Nursing Orders	**Rationale**
1. Place in room with school-age child if possible.	1. A roommate could provide social stimulation and role modeling.
2. Encourage parents to visit and assist with care.	2. Parental support is important for support and comfort.
3. Provide talk time at least twice daily.	3. Conversation provides social stimulation.
4. Protect as necessary against self-stimulation activities (pad side rails? provide mittens?) or distract to reduce such activities.	4. These measures protect against self-stimulation injury.

tarded children are older and stronger than the age of the children that toys were meant for, toys that are developmentally correct still may not be appropriate because they break too easily to be safe.

Social Relationships. The ability to communicate can be very delayed in mentally retarded children because ability to develop language is often so delayed. Speech therapy may be necessary to help them articulate correct sounds. Talking picture boards are boards with pictures on them (available commercially or made by parents) to which children can point if they want something, to speed communication.

Teaching early social behavior is important (saying "thank you," and "excuse me"; shaking hands; taking turns) in helping children relate with both other children and adults. As mentally retarded children imitate this type of behavior the same as other children, providing good role models is an effective way of teaching social behavior (Figure 54-1).

Encourage parents to enroll children in preschool programs to help them learn to be comfortable with other children at the earliest time possible. Many programs enroll children as early as 1 year of age to begin education. As a school-age child, participating in organized groups such as Girl Scouts or Special Olympics is an important way to learn to interact with others and feel successful (see the Focus on Nursing Research box).

Preparation for Adulthood. As mentally retarded children reach adolescence, they benefit from orienta-

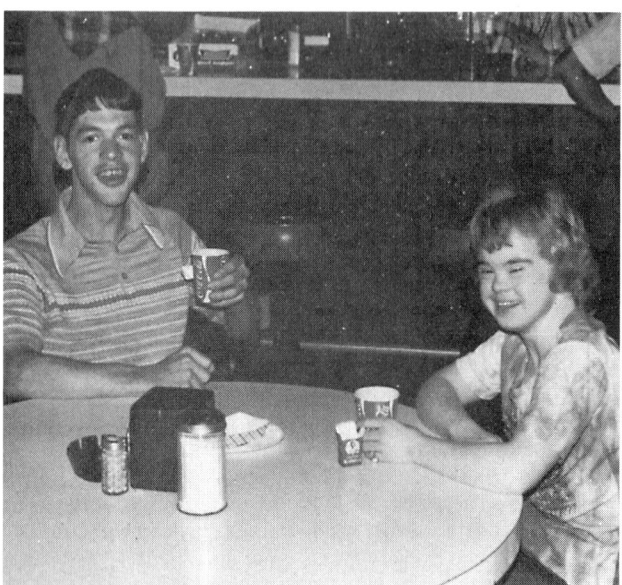

FIGURE 54-1
Children with mental retardation need as many near-normal experiences as possible to be prepared to adjust to the world. (From Blackwell, M. W. Care of the mentally retarded. Boston: Little, Brown, with permission.)

FOCUS ON NURSING RESEARCH

Are Children Aware That Unusual Behavior in Another Child Could Represent Mental Illness?

To find this answer, 168 children in grades 3 through 6 were asked to read vignettes that described behaviors of mentally ill children and adults, describe the probable motivation for the behaviors, and suggest solutions. Only 27% of the children who participated described vignette characters as mentally ill; only 11% suggested psychiatric therapy as a solution to changing the behavior. These findings are interesting because they suggest how little children know about mental illness; they probably reflect the difficulty parents have in discussing such problems as mental illness with children.

Poster, E. C. (1992). Children's concepts of the mentally ill. *Journal of Child and Adolescent Psychiatric and Mental Health Nursing, 5,* 28.

tion to sexual responsibility, the same as all children (David & Morgall, 1990). Girls can understand a simple explanation of menstruation and necessary menstrual hygiene. Both boys and girls need explanations of how pregnancy occurs and the measures they need to take to prevent this. Many adolescents rediscover masturbation as an enjoyable activity and, without the social awareness to recognize that other people do not find this a socially acceptable activity, practice it openly. As with all children, do not discourage this activity; just guide them to think of this as a "private activity" to do when they are alone.

If a girl is going to use a contraceptive and lives with a responsible adult, she can be given an oral contraceptive daily by that adult. Sterilization is not usually recommended because it is difficult for a mentally retarded adolescent to understand fully the implications of this (so consent is not fully informed) (AAP, 1990). If pregnancy should occur, a mentally retarded adolescent can be counseled to have an abortion but cannot be forced to have this done. Assisting the mentally retarded young adult through pregnancy is discussed in Chapter 17.

Pervasive Developmental Disorders: Infantile Autism

Infantile autism is a category of pervasive developmental disorders that is marked by serious distortions in psychologic functioning (Mays, 1993). There may be deficits in language, perceptual, and motor development; defective reality testing; and an inability to function in social settings. There is a lack of responsiveness to other people, gross impairment in communication skills, and bizarre responses to various aspects of the environment, all developing within the first 30 months of age (APA, 1994). It is a rare condition, occurring in only 2 to 4 children out of 10,000. It occurs about three times more often in boys than in girls.

The cause of the disorder is unknown, but it is linked with cerebellar and limbic system anomalies that probably occurred in utero (Lotspeich & Ciaranello, 1993). It has been associated with maternal rubella or phenylketonuria, meningitis, and encephalitis in the child. As many as 75% of children with the disorder are also mentally retarded.

Assessment

Common symptoms of autism are summarized in Box 54-2. Because of the lack of responsiveness to people that is part of the syndrome, normal attachment behavior does not develop. Infants fail to cuddle or make eye contact or exhibit facial unresponsiveness; they do not reach to be picked up as the average infant does. They are unable to play cooperatively or make friendships. Parents may first bring a child to a health care facility thinking he or she is deaf because of this.

The impairment in communication is shown in both verbal and nonverbal skills. Language may be totally absent. If a child does speak, grammatical structure may be impaired (the use of "you" when "I" is intended is common); there is inability to name objects (nominal aphasia) and abnormal speech melody, such as question-like rises at the end of statements.

Bizarre responses to the environment include intense reactions to minor changes in the environment (screaming if a toybox is moved across the room) and attachment to odd objects (always carrying a string or a shoe). Autistic children often persist in repetitive hand movements; rocking and rhythmic body movements are often observed. They are intensely preoccupied by moving objects such as a fan, the swirling water in the toilet bowl, or a spinning top. Music often holds a special interest for them. Hand biting may be so constant that they develop callouses on their hands.

In contrast to these bizarre mannerisms, long-term memory may be excellent and autistic children may be able to recall dates and spoken words from conversations that took place years before. This excellent memory previously led to the belief that most of these children have normal intelligence. Actually only about 25% of them have an IQ above 70 (APA, 1994). Intelligence testing is difficult, however, because they do not respond well to test situations and they score poorly on verbal parts of these tests. Tasks requiring manipulative or visual skills or immediate memory may be performed at above-normal levels.

Children with autism have a **labile mood** (crying occurs suddenly followed immediately by giggling or laughing). They may react with overresponsiveness to sensory stimuli, such as light or sound, but then be unaware of a major happening in the room, such as a fire alarm sounding.

Therapeutic Management

Autism is a perplexing condition. Parents need a great deal of support so that they do not reject the child because he or she seems to be rejecting them. Behavior modification therapy may be effective in controlling some of the bizarre mannerisms that accompany autism, but because the basic cause of the disorder is not known, therapy will not always succeed.

As children mature, they develop greater awareness of and attachment to parents and other familiar adults. A day care program can help to promote social awareness. Some children may eventually reach a point where they can become passively involved in loosely structured play groups. Some children are eventually able to lead independent lives, although social ineptness and awkwardness are apt to remain, especially if mental retardation accompanies the autism.

Box 54-2
Common Symptoms in the Child With Autism

Social isolation
Stereotyped behaviors
Resistance to any change in routine
Abnormal responses to sensory stimuli
Insensitivity to pain
Inappropriate emotional expressions
Disturbances of movement
Poor development of speech
Specific, limited intellectual problems

Disruptive Behavior Disorders

The disruptive behavior disorders include attention deficit with hyperactivity disorder (ADHD), undifferentiated attention-deficit disorder (without hyperactivity), and the conduct disorders. Because these disorders may begin with behavior problems not so different from what most families experience, parents may at first not believe that medical intervention is warranted. By the time they seek help, the parents may already be in a state of extreme distress about the unmanageability of their child.

It is important that these diseases be diagnosed as early as possible, before the child's behavior leads to a deteriorating level of self-esteem and compromised social skills and complications in family functioning develop. The home environment may be the most important factor in determining whether or not the energy of a child with an attention deficit disorder turns into a more complicated psychopathologic process or whether it can be channelled into purposeful, productive activity.

Attention Deficit With Hyperactivity Disorder (ADHD)

One of the most controversial of the childhood psychiatric disorders, attention deficit with hyperactivity disorder or ADHD, is estimated to occur in about 6% of U.S. school-age children (Leffert & Susman, 1993). Boys are affected more frequently than girls. The possible causes of ADHD as well as the reliability of symptoms for establishing its diagnosis and treatment methods have been under debate for the last 50 years. It may well be that ADHD serves as an umbrella diagnosis for a variety of behavioral-attention problems with a variety of causes. ADHD occurs more frequently among some families than in the general population, indicating a possible genetic etiologic component. ADHD has also been associated with situational anxiety, abuse, and neglect and may be one component in the development of a psychiatric illness such as schizophrenia. Both drug and behavior-modification treatment methods have been used with success, which may support the theory of varying causes.

Children with ADHD are unable to complete tasks effectively because of inattention or impulsivity. They are easily distracted and often may not seem to listen. Impulsivity is paramount—the child acts before he or she thinks, shifts excessively from one activity to another, and has difficulty with such tasks as awaiting turns in games. The child with ADHD exhibits excessive or exaggerated muscular activity, such as excessive climbing onto objects, constant fidgeting, and aimless or haphazard running.

Assessment

The disorder is diagnosable by 36 months of age, although it is often difficult to identify the disorder until later, when the child is asked to sit still in school for longer periods. Diagnosis is made on history and neurologic assessment. When the disorder is first suspected, a thorough initial history to reveal the extent of the problem should be recorded. Some children have enough control in a one-to-one situation for their behavior to be fairly normal in these settings. A child whom the parents report as hyperactive, therefore, may not be hyperactive in an ambulatory health care setting.

The history is especially important in evaluating the extent of the problem. The pregnancy and birth history, the child's ability to meet developmental milestones, and a typical day for the child should be reviewed carefully.

The term **hyperactivity**, or excess movement, is commonly carelessly used to describe any active child. Have the parent give an exact description of what the child is unable to do, such as sitting still long enough to finish a full meal, running to the window 10 times in 15 minutes, and so on, to document that hyperactivity truly exists.

Assess for activity that is not only excessive but also disorganized (Figure 54-2). Children with ADHD cannot sit still long enough to eat a meal or finish a school project. In school, they move from the back of the room to the front of the room, to the window, to the teacher's desk, to their own desk. They perform repetitive activities such as pencil tapping, arm swinging, and finger tapping. They will leave a project they are working on or a television program they are watching intently to run to the window or open the refrigerator door, unaware of why they are running. This is driven or compulsive behavior.

Variability is another important symptom. Everyone has good days and bad days, days when they perform at their peak, days when performance is less than optimum. In children with an attention deficit disorder, behavior is so variable that they have good and bad *moments.* This type of variability causes children to lose track of systems and methods, not just answers, so school performance falters. When asked to add, for example, a child might add 4 and 3 correctly and 5 and 4

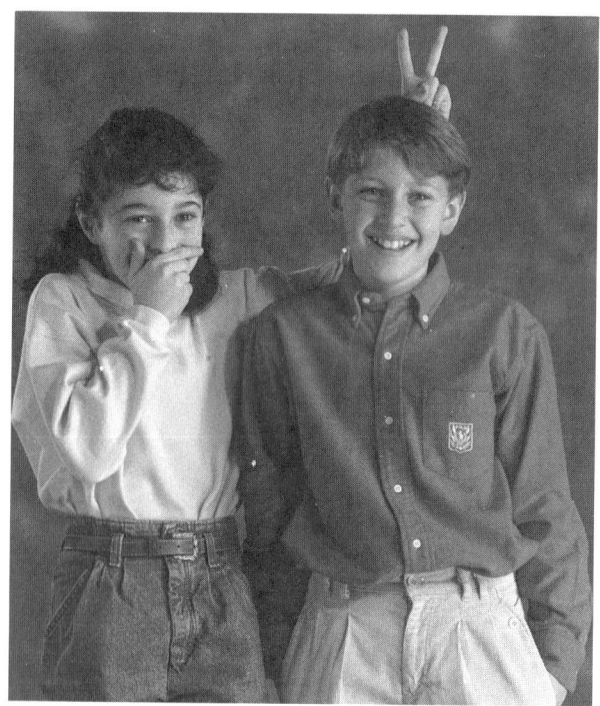

FIGURE 54-2
Observe children carefully to distinguish normal activity, as shown here, from the excessive activity of an attention-deficit disorder. (Courtesy of the Department of Medical Photography, Children's Hospital, Buffalo, NY.)

correctly, but then lose track of the system and add 2 and 3 as 23 or 32.

Such a high level of impulsiveness causes children to make statements without thinking, to touch objects they have just been told not to touch, or to speak or act before they have time to think about what they want to say or do. When they are angered, they shout or strike out before they can be offered an explanation. They cannot wait in line for a drink of water—their impulsiveness tells them that they must have their drink immediately.

Average children can filter out stimuli that are not important to them at that moment. Children with ADHD seem to have an "all-or-none" reaction to stimuli. They may block out all incoming stimuli and so do not hear their parents or a teacher calling them; they may be disciplined at school for something as extreme as not answering a fire drill (unaware that a bell was ringing and that children around them were moving toward the exit). At other times they cannot suppress any incoming stimuli. They mean to concentrate on a desk assignment in school, but outside the window they hear a bird singing; next to them they smell a girl's perfume; they feel their watch on their wrist—so cannot concentrate on the problem at hand. This may be reported by parents or teachers as an exceedingly short attention span.

Children with ADHD may also have difficulty with concepts such as *right* and *left, before* and *after, in front of, in back of, yesterday,* and *tomorrow,* as these concepts call for sequencing. If children cannot tell the difference between left and right, they can have difficulty forming common letters such as *b* and *d,* which vary only in the direction of the bottom loop. They can have difficulty with common tasks such as washing their hands, because they never know which way to turn a faucet. Turning door knobs and keys, tying shoe laces, and screwing on bottle caps are all complex tasks for a child who has difficulty with sequencing or space perception. They may show awkward motor movements and cannot work all muscles gracefully in proper sequence. These children may reach beyond an object and so spill a glass of milk at the table at every meal. They make strokes with a pencil longer than they meant them to be, so they rarely can hand in neat school assignments.

Long after the average child is speaking in fluent sentences, children with ADHD may have difficulty using conjunctions or prepositions correctly (sequencing of words). They may have difficulty learning to read, because to read words of more than one syllable, they must sound the first syllable, then retain that sound in their mind while they sound the second. If they have difficulty retaining the first syllable long enough to connect it with the second, they cannot construct the word. They can similarly have difficulty with arithmetic, because they may be unable to retain the sum of two numbers

long enough to add the sum of a third. Spelling will be equally difficult; not only are they unable to sequence the letters in a word correctly, but they cannot retain memory rules such as "i before e" to help them.

Children with ADHD do not have a deficit in intelligence, although they may seem to because of their impulsive behavior. They do not seem to be aware that their behavior is upsetting to family, friends, and teachers so are not anxious about their inability to conform to society's rules.

These children often show many "soft" neurologic signs, such as inability to use a pencil or scissors well. Testing them with a thorough neurologic examination is difficult because their attention span is so short. They often have difficulty performing tests such as a finger-to-nose test or rapid hand movements, such as touching one finger after another with their thumb. They tend to show "mirroring" with this movement (the second hand imitates what the first hand attempts to do). Cerebellar difficulty is evidenced further by inability to perform a tandem walk or a heel-to-shin test. They may be able to identify one touch but not two simultaneous touches on their body. They do not show the normal responses of **graphesthesia** (ability to recognize a shape that has been traced on the skin) or **stereognosis** (ability to recognize an object by touch). When asked to stand with arms outstretched, **choreiform movements** (aimless movements) and rising of the fingers are often present. More definite neurologic signs, such as a unilateral Babinski reflex or strabismus, may also be present. Tests must be made into a game so that their attention is maintained long enough to complete the assessment.

IQ testing is used to document the child's normal intelligence. The WISC, the test most often chosen for these children, consists of two portions: a verbal scale and a performance scale. The child is given three final scores: verbal IQ, performance IQ, and combination or full-scale IQ. The child with perceptual and motor deficits tends to do poorly on the performance scale but average or better on the verbal scale. Children with language difficulty do poorly on the verbal scale but average or above on the performance scale. Children with attention-deficit disorder show a "scatter" pattern on both performance and verbal portions: they do well on some portions, poorly on others.

Children who have difficulty filtering out stimuli do poorly on group-administered intelligence tests because they are too distracted by the children around them. These children, therefore, should take IQ tests individually. Neurologic examinations should be performed in rooms free of distractions such as attractive toys.

Children with an attention-deficit disorder are often referred to a health care facility because they have had difficulty in school. Parents may have been assured on previous occasions that although their child had difficulty settling down to tasks, this was because he was "all boy" or "every child is different." If the behavior problem was not handled well by school personnel, parents may be angry about the referral. They may want to establish that the school system is wrong and they are right rather than to obtain a true evaluation of the child. They may need time to accept that your role is not to be on anyone's side but to help establish whether or not their child has a condition that interferes with learning. As parents talk, they may find that they are relieved to describe the child's behavior to someone who is truly listening. They have been living with a difficult situation for a long time and may not be aware themselves of the strain this has produced until they start to describe it.

Therapeutic Management

A variety of treatment methods are used, often in combination, in the management of ADHD.

Environment. It is important that a stable learning environment be constructed for children with ADHD. This may include special instruction, free from the distractions of an entire class. Parents may have difficulty accepting the fact that their child needs special schooling (the intelligence test, after all, said that he or she was above average). They may need help in seeing that the condition interferes with intellectual functioning and that a special program must be constructed for the child to succeed (Campbell & Cohen, 1990).

Parents often have difficulty at home with discipline and management and appreciate some support and advice. Encourage them to be fair but firm. Children with a great deal of variability need rules to follow so that they do not constantly "run off the road." Although every child has a right to an opinion, many decisions that the average child enjoys making for himself or herself must be made for this child. "Do you want to wear your red or your blue shirt today?" is less effective than "Here is your blue shirt to wear today."

Children who are easily distracted have difficulty completing chores or picking up their toys. They can be assigned age-appropriate chores with the understanding that a parent must give many reminders to them to get the job completed. Teach parents to give instructions slowly and make certain that they have the child's attention before beginning instructions. Breaking down a chore into several steps may help (get the toybox is one step; pick up toys is a second). This avoids the confrontation that arises later if children do not hear or do not process what is said to them.

All children like to participate in dinner conversation or discussions about their day. These children often have difficulty telling a story or repeating a joke told to them (a sequencing problem). You can help them by asking questions such as "Why?" "Where?" or "Who?" to help them reach the point of the story. Encourage parents to be certain that when they correct behavior, their anger is about something the child has deliberately done

wrong, not about some incident that happened because of the child's inability to sequence, filter, or integrate concepts. Punishment should follow an offense quickly (it should not wait till Father gets home) because a child quickly forgets what he or she did. As with all children, parents should make certain the child understands that the parent is angry at the behavior, not the child. Children with attention-deficit disorders develop poor self-esteem, because although they are intelligent, they cannot succeed. Help parents to build, not hinder, the development of self-esteem at every stage possible.

Medication. A number of medications are helpful in controlling the excessive activity of the child with ADHD and lengthening the attention span or decreasing the distractibility so he or she can function in a normal classroom. Dextroamphetamine (Dexedrine) was the first drug used for this purpose.

More recently, methylphenidate hydro (Ritalin) or pemoline (Cylert) have been prescribed for this disorder. These drugs have side effects of insomnia and anorexia, so children on these medications must be observed to be certain these are not occurring. The insomnia may be relieved by administering the drug early in the day. Children receiving the drugs for long periods need careful height and weight assessment to see that long-term anorexia is not causing weight loss (Calis et al., 1990).

Diet. Dietary treatment of ADHD has been proposed but not substantiated in research. The Feingold diet (omitting salicylates and food dyes) became popular in the 1980s, but studies of this treatment have yielded contradictory findings. It has been found that food-dye restriction might be helpful for a small subgroup of children with ADHD. Megavitamin treatments have also proved ineffective and possibly dangerous.

Family Support. Parents of a child with ADHD often need frequent health care visits while their child is growing up; a responsive, listening ear is crucial to their ability to handle the challenge of raising a child with these symptoms. The best of parents grow short tempered and irritable at times with a child who does not seem to hear them or follow what they say. They may need reminders at intervals that their child does not act this way on purpose. Help them to understand that because of a very complex and as yet ill-understood syndrome of brain dysfunction, the behavior is the best their child can achieve.

Attention-deficit disorders are primarily a childhood condition. The symptoms of hyperactivity tend to "burn themselves out" with adolescence. The attention span lengthens, and the ability to filter improves. Children may have remaining motor difficulty, such as awkwardness, but most of the problems disappear. Perhaps the most significant aftereffect of ADHD is a persistent lowered self-esteem and/or reduction in social skills resulting from the time spent "not getting along" during childhood. If children can survive years of not fitting into an educational system and not meeting parent's expectations, they can eventually become intact, competent adults.

Conduct Disorders

Conduct disorders represent the most common psychiatric diagnosis of children and adolescents. The essential feature of these disorders is a repetitive and persistent pattern of violations of personal rights or societal rules, such as disobedience, stealing, fighting, destruction of property, fire setting, and early sexual behavior (APA, 1994).

Children may show aggressive behavior by purse snatching, mugging, or robbery with confrontation, or in less overt ways by persistent truancy, lying, or vandalism. Many teenage runaways (discussed in Chapter 33) may fall into this category.

Often these children fail to demonstrate a normal degree of affection, empathy, or ability to bond with others. They may have few meaningful peer relationships. Egocentrism is strong: they manipulate others for favors without any effort to return them. Feelings of guilt or remorse appear to be lacking. Unless there is an obvious immediate advantage, they do not extend themselves to others.

Conduct disorders are seen more frequently in males than in females, particularly when property or violent crimes are involved; however, the prevalence of conduct disorders in girls is increasing, which means that male predominance may be reduced over time. A number of etiologic factors have been described for this disorder, including genetic predisposition, neurologic deficit correlates, and sociologic factors related to poverty and cultural disadvantage. In addition, the home environment of aggressive children is frequently characterized by rejection, frustration, and harsh and inconsistent discipline; parents may have an unstable marital relationship; and children may have had a series of step or foster parents.

Therapy for children with conduct disorders is with drugs such as neuroleptics or lithium carbonate and to modify the home environment to one more consistent and less rejecting. This is difficult because parents are under stress already; learning better parenting to a child with acting-out behavior is difficult. Removing the child from the home to a structured day-care environment may be necessary. Unfortunately, this can be interpreted as more rejection by the child and compound the problem. Any new environment that is created must be consistent and loving, not institutional, to be effective. If hospitalized, such children can be very disruptive on a hospital unit.

Teaching parents behavior therapy (rewarding positive behavior) can also be effective. TOUGHLOVE is a national organization that can be helpful to some parents as a support group. The mainstay of the organization's philosophy is to set basic rules that children must follow or else move out of the parents' home. Critics of the method caution that although this approach may be effective in making children display acceptable behavior, it may not actually change the behavior (just drive it underground).

Anxiety Disorders of Childhood or Adolescence

Because anxiety is considered a normal part of certain phases of development (e.g., stranger anxiety of the 6- to 8-month old, separation anxiety in the toddler, fear of mutilation and the dark in the preschooler, and performance anxiety of the school-ager or adolescent), genuine anxiety disorders in children may often be overlooked. When left untreated, children may cope with fear by becoming overdependent on others for support or turning away from the problem and withdrawing into themselves. This can leave a child socially immature and unable to achieve in school. Three specific anxiety disorders have been defined in the DSM-III-R: separation anxiety disorder, overanxious disorder, and avoidant disorder of childhood or adolescence.

Separation Anxiety

Separation anxiety, a normal phase of development in the toddler (see Chapter 30), is considered a disorder when an older child shows excessive anxiety about separation or the possibility of separation from those to whom the child is attached. Children may worry when apart from parents that they will have an accident or become ill. They may have difficulty falling asleep at night or insist on sleeping with parents or just outside their parents' bedroom door. Such a degree of anxiety can be incapacitating to children as it prevents them from visiting at friend's houses, enjoying a camp experience, or enjoying school (Last & Strauss, 1990).

Separation anxiety tends to run in families and occurs slightly more frequently in girls than in boys. Unresolved internal conflicts, uncertainty about one's caregiver, and parent-induced anxious attachment are psychodynamic factors attributed to this disorder. Temperament is also considered a contributing factor. Treatment for separation anxiety includes individual counseling sessions combined with antidepressant medication. In addition, family therapy may be helpful in allowing the family to gain greater insight into the dynamics of the problem and the child to gain more confidence in his or her ability to function independently.

Separation anxiety is often associated with school phobia and school absenteeism. School phobia can be a transient phenomenon related to a particular situation at home (e.g., the arrival of a new baby) or at school (e.g., quarreling with friends), or it can be an ongoing syndrome with long-term effects. School phobia is discussed in Chapter 32.

Overanxious Disorder

Children who demonstrate generalized excessive worrying that is not limited to any particular object or event are diagnosed as having overanxious disorder (Popper, 1993). Future events, the possibility of injury or exclusion from peer groups, deadlines, or keeping appointments are examples of circumstances that worry such children. Physical signs such as gastrointestinal distress, duodenal ulcer, headache, or dizziness may be present. These children tend to be perfectionists and may appear overly mature because of their seriousness about many things other children take lightly. The child may be shy and self-deprecating and will often have habit disturbances, such as nail-biting, thumb-sucking, and enuresis. Like other anxiety disorders, an overanxious disorder can be incapacitating if the child spends more time worrying about being productive than in being productive. Family therapy may help a child and the child's family gain insight into the problem and begin focusing on real concerns. Antianxiety medicine may be helpful.

Avoidant Disorder of Childhood

An avoidant disorder is characterized by excessive drawing back from contact with strangers to such an extent that it interferes with normal social function or peer relationships. At the same time, the child expresses a desire for affection and acceptance from close family members. Although children do not have a basic communication disorder, they appear mute to strangers because of their inability to speak with them.

These children appear to lack confidence in themselves. This can occur in children as young as 2 years of age but generally manifests itself during adolescence. Family therapy is helpful in offering children insight into themselves and increased confidence in their ability to relate to others.

Eating Disorders

Pica

Children who eat nonfood substances such as dirt, clay, crayons, yarn, or paper are said to have pica (Lacey, 1990). *Pica* is the Latin word for magpie (a bird that will eat anything). Although this disorder is rarely diagnosed, it may be common. Its primary danger lies in the possibility of accidental or lead poisoning, but other complications include constipation and gastrointestinal malabsorption. Fecal impaction and intestinal obstruction can

also occur. In children, this disorder is seen predominantly between the ages of 1 and 6, although it may be present into adolescence (Figure 54-3). Often it is not diagnosed until the child presents with a pica-induced complication, particularly lead poisoning.

The condition may occur as a reaction to stress. Children with mental retardation tend to show more of the tendency than do those of average intelligence, probably because of their inability to distinguish edible from inedible substances. It is highly associated with iron deficiency anemia, so children with pica should be screened for this. With these children, correcting the anemia also corrects the pica (Bushnell, 1992).

Rumination Disorder of Infancy

The term *rumination* comes from the Latin word for "chewing the cud" (as cattle do). Rumination is the act of regurgitating and reswallowing previously ingested food. It is a rare disorder that generally affects infants between the ages of 3 and 12 months. It is seen most often in children with mental retardation. Both organic and environmental theories for the etiology of rumination have been explored. In some children, the existence of gastroesophageal reflux due to an esophageal sphincter disorder has been implicated. It has also been postulated that rumination is a form of self-stimulation by the infant, similar to head banging and body rocking. It may be related to an understimulating environment, but attempts to implicate the role of the primary caregiver in causing this disorder have failed. Most babies with rumination disorder seem happy and well cared for.

A parent may report that a child is constantly "spitting up" or vomiting or smells sour. Children can lose a great deal of fluid and electrolytes through this process

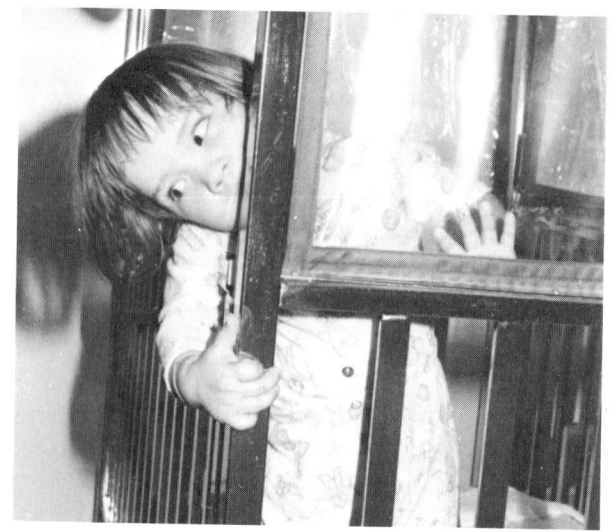

FIGURE 54-3
A hospitalized toddler chewing on a crib rail. Fortunately, the rail is harmless stainless steel. (Courtesy of Bruce Hill.)

and may show signs of failure to thrive. (Failure to thrive as a distinct problem is discussed in Chapter 55.) Distracting infants by holding, rocking, and talking to them tends to decrease rumination. Thickening formula with cereal occasionally is effective as this is more difficult to regurgitate. When the problem is severe, hospitalization may be necessary to provide an alternative feeding environment for the child and to give parents a needed break from feeding responsibilities. Attachment between the child and parent may be at risk because of the anxiety the parents suffer from their infant's constant regurgitation of food and lack of growth. Parents need support, reassurance, and education to help them re-establish this bond.

Anorexia Nervosa

Anorexia nervosa is a disorder characterized by preoccupation with food and body weight, creating a feeling of revulsion to food to the point of excessive weight loss (APA, 1994). It occurs most often in girls (95%), usually at puberty or during adolescence. As many as 1 in 250 girls between 12 and 18 years of age develop the disorder. It is more common among sisters and daughters of mothers who also had the disorder.

The specific cause of anorexia nervosa is unknown, but most theories have focused on psychodynamic views of the disorder as a phobic-avoidance response to food resulting from the sexual and social tensions generated by the physical changes associated with puberty (Meades, 1993). Anorexia nervosa tends to occur in girls who are described by their parents as perfectionist, "model children." They may be overvalued by both parents. Parents are fairly demanding and controlling. Girls who develop this disorder tend to have a poor self-image (they cannot live up to their parents' expectations). By excessive dieting, girls are able to feel a sense of control over their own body.

Anorexia nervosa often occurs in girls who were mildly overweight before the onset of the illness. Some girls with the phenomenon seem reluctant to grow up or mature physically. Lack of nutrition causes delayed psychosexual development. With a lean, nearly starved appearance, they do not appear as sexually developed or as old as they are. Some girls may be worried that they are pregnant, and the starvation may be an unconscious attempt to abort the pregnancy. In some girls, a period of stress or an unpleasant sexual encounter, such as a stranger making a pass at them on a bus, may have occurred prior to the anorexia nervosa. They may be attempting subconsciously to prevent further such sexual encounters.

Assessment

Girls with anorexia nervosa have an intense fear of becoming obese, perceive food as revolting and nauseat-ing, and refuse to eat or else vomit food immediately after eating. They often state they "feel fat" when they are actually as much as 25% less than normal weight. Refusal to eat may be accompanied by the use of laxatives or diuretics and extensive exercising to further lose weight. Girls may ingest ipecac to induce vomiting. These measures lead eventually to excessive weight loss, acidosis or alkalosis, dependent edema, hypotension, hypothermia, bradycardia, and lanugo formation (fine, neonatal-like hair). Compulsive mannerisms such as handwashing may develop. If the process is allowed to continue without therapy, it can lead to starvation and death. The use of ipecac can be exceptionally damaging. The mortality rate for the illness is between 1% and 15% (Palmer, 1990).

Therapeutic Management

By the time most children are seen at health care facilities, they are often already extremely underweight, pale, and lethargic. Menstruation is absent; this generally occurs when body weight falls below 95 lb. Often the child's parents have tried various methods of getting the child to eat, such as threatening, coaxing, and punishing, and so parent–child relationships are strained. Parents may feel guilty for insisting their child lose weight, if the girl was once overweight.

Be certain that goals established are realistic for the illness. A girl who grows nauseated just looking at food cannot quickly begin to take in a great deal of it. It is important to remember when caring for children with anorexia nervosa that although the condition began as a psychosocial problem, by the time a girl is seen for care a second important component is starvation. The girl generally must be removed from all oral foods and placed on intravenous fluid for at least 2 or 3 days. Total parenteral nutrition may be necessary to supply fat and protein. Girls generally accept total parenteral nutrition well because they view it as medicine, not as food. Enteral feedings may also be accepted and used to restore weight (Bufano et al., 1990).

As a girl's body image improves, the aversion to food diminishes. It is usually recommended that a girl gain enough to bring her weight up to 90 to 95 lb by an average gain of 3 lb weekly. Rapid gain of weight is not desirable because a girl may again begin dieting to reduce this weight gain. Weighing her once a week is better than every day to reduce her concentration on weight. Box 54-3 describes common strategies for care to be avoided because they interfere with helping the girl gain a positive self-image.

Children who have had anorexia nervosa need continued follow-up after weight is regained to be certain that they do not revert to their former dieting pattern. Counseling continues for 2 to 3 years to be certain that self-image is maintained. With counseling, most girls will achieve full recovery.

Lego, S. (1984). *The American handbook of psychiatric nursing.* Philadelphia: J. B. Lippincott, with permission.

Box 54-3
Nonproductive Approaches to Care of the Child With Anorexia Nervosa

1. Power struggles, such as insisting that the child eat, may make both the child and the staff feel angry, frustrated, helpless, and ineffective. Power struggles reenact familiar, pathologic family patterns.
2. An attempt to rebuild the anorexic's body in a hurry may terrify the child, who will then lose more weight. Overzealous nutritional restitution may be interpreted as a "cure" without psychological change within the client. Some clients have attempted suicide after weight gains.
3. Inconsistency in team approaches toward the client's deceitfulness about eating.
4. Aggressive interpretation of the unconscious meaning of symptoms in order to make the client change. These interpretations are alien to the client, who feels intruded upon by the all-knowing therapist (mother).
5. Impatience at the client's dawdling over food.
6. Use of trickery, bribery, cajoling, force, and threats to get the client to eat, stimulating more deceitfulness and power struggles.
7. Anxiety in staff, leading to excessive vigilance toward the client, similar to the intrusive mother's vigilance.
8. Arguing and excessive limit setting in response to the client's devaluation of nurses.
9. Intimidation by the very fragile anorexic who seems to be "running the show," leading staff to support the pathology instead of change.
10. Splitting among staff, especially disciplines and nursing shifts, leading to chaos.

---

crease the physical pain of abdominal distention and to improve self-concept (she feels more in control).

Children with bulimia may abuse purgatives or laxatives as well as diuretics to aid in weight control. The combination of frequent vomiting and the use of these drugs can result in serious physical complications, notably electrolyte abnormalities, which can ultimately lead to changes as severe as cardiac arrest. People with bulimia may also have severe erosion of their teeth because of the constant soaking in acidic gastrointestinal juices from vomiting. Esophageal tears may also result.

Like adolescents with anorexia nervosa, these girls exhibit great concern about their weight and overall body image and appearance. In contrast with anorexic girls, most girls with bulimia are only slightly underweight and so may be discounted as only slim unless a thorough history is obtained. As with anorexia nervosa, counseling is aimed at increasing the girl's self-esteem and sense of control (Giannini et al., 1990).

Tic Disorders

Tic disorders are abnormalities of semi-involuntary movement thought to result from dysfunction in the basal ganglia. *Tics* are rapid, repetitive muscle movements, such as rapid eye blinking or facial twitching. They generally become more pronounced in periods of stress and usually diminish in sleep. **Motor tics** include eye blinking, neck jerking, and facial grimacing. Simple **vocal tics** include coughing, throat clearing, snorting, and barking. Complex motor tics include facial gestures, grooming behaviors, jumping, touching, and smelling an object (Jankovic, 1994).

Children are most prone to these disorders between the ages of 9 and 13. They occur more frequently in boys than in girls and tend to be familial. The tic disorders are subclassified into Tourette's syndrome, chronic motor or vocal tic disorder, and transient tic disorder. Treatment generally focuses on reducing areas of stress in a child's life. Pointing out the mannerism to the child is not usually helpful and may intensify the manifestations, but behavior modification may be successful in curing a particular tic. If the stress is not removed, however, a child may substitute another nervous mechanism for the original tic.

Tourette's Syndrome

Tourette's syndrome is an inherited disorder in which the child suffers from a syndrome of facial and complex vocal tics (Scahill et al., 1993). **Complex vocal tics** include the repeated use of words or phrases out of context, specifically, **coprolalia** (use of socially unacceptable words, usually obscenities), **palilalia** (repeating

Bulimia Nervosa

Bulimia refers to episodic binge eating and purging (vomiting), accompanied by an awareness that the eating pattern is abnormal but not being able to stop. A period of depression usually follows the period of bingeing. Like anorexia nervosa, bulimia begins in adolescence or early adult life; it is seen predominantly in girls (Carlat & Camargo, 1991). The disorder may last for months or years; periods of normal eating may be interspersed, or the girl may constantly move from bingeing to fasting. Food consumed during a binge often has a high-caloric content and a texture that facilitates rapid eating. It may be eaten secretly, such as late at night or in the privacy of a bedroom. Following ingestion of this food, the girl notices abdominal pain; she vomits to de-one's own words), and **echolalia** (repeating the last sound heard or the phrase of another person) (APA, 1987). Some children with this syndrome have nonspecific electroencephalograph abnormalities and soft neurologic signs. The peak age of occurrence is before age 15; the syndrome lasts a lifetime. It occurs three times more frequently in boys than in girls. Often there is some other form of tic in other family members. Children with Tourette's syndrome can develop low self-esteem because of coprolalia before the syndrome is fully diagnosed. Fortunately, this syndrome responds to administration of dopamine receptor blockers such as haloperidol or fluphenazine (Scahill et al., 1993).

Elimination Disorders

Functional Encopresis

Encopresis is defined as repeated passage of feces in places not culturally appropriate for that purpose (APA, 1994). It is considered primary if a child was never fully toilet trained and secondary if the problem begins after effective training. Functional encopresis is said to exist only after medical causes such as fecal incontinence, lactase deficiency, thyroid disease, hypercalcemia, and Hirschsprung's disease have been ruled out. Isolated occurrences of encopresis may happen when a sibling is born (as part of an overall regression reaction) or if a child is visiting a strange house or new school and is too shy to ask for the bathroom. It can occur in school because a teacher will not allow children to use a bathroom when they wish or because some school bathrooms are occupied by children who tend to bully, so a quiet child may be afraid to go there. Encopresis is categorized as an emotional problem because it can be a manifestation of a poor parent–child relationship. In a few instances it occurs because of extreme constipation. Hard bowel movements cause anal fissures; because it hurts to move the bowels, children avoid bowel movements and their rectum becomes chronically distended. They are then no longer able to sense when they need to defecate, so involuntary defecation occurs. This is a distressing condition for children because other children in school can detect the odor of a bowel movement on their clothing.

Assessment

To document encopresis, take a careful history of the condition, including the number and times bowel accidents occur. Investigate any stress factors on the child. A physical examination that includes a rectal examination should be done to establish whether there is proper anal sphincter control. Therapy will then be based on the apparent cause (Sprague-McRae et al., 1993).

Therapeutic Management

The administration of 1 to 6 tbs of mineral oil daily for 2 or 3 months will often soften stools so that bowel movements are not painful. Children on long-term mineral oil therapy generally are given water-soluble vitamins A, D, and K, because these vitamins tend to be removed from the gastrointestinal tract with the mineral oil. Arranging to have children attempt to evacuate their bowels about two times daily (in the morning and after dinner) may create "habit" periods for them. If children evacuate their bowels before they leave for school in the morning, they are less likely to experience encopresis and embarrassment in school.

Emphasize to parents that children should not be punished for encopresis. Encourage them to pay as little attention as possible to bowel accidents and give praise for days when encopresis does not occur.

Functional Enuresis

Functional enuresis is defined as repeated involuntary or intentional urination during the day or at night after children have attained or are at an age at which they should have attained control over bladder function and when no organic cause for the problem can be found (APA, 1994). Although stress may be a factor in occurrences of functional enuresis, its primary cause is unknown; most children outgrow the problem by adolescence. Like functional encopresis, the most serious mental impairment associated with enuresis is related to the child's feelings of failure with each occurrence and associated rejection by peers or parents or other caregivers. All this contributes to a lowered sense of self-esteem. The problem and associated nursing diagnoses are described in more detail in Chapter 46. A similar problem is daytime urinary frequency or the need to void as many as ten or more times an hour. This also is associated with anxiety and fades with increased coping ability (Watemberg & Shaley, 1994).

Other Psychiatric Disorders Affecting Children

Childhood Depression

Children and adolescents both have depressive episodes similar to those experienced by adults. The incidence ranges from 0.3% for preschoolers to 14% in adolescents. Depression is becoming an increasing concern in our society because the escalating suicide rate among children and adolescents has become a major societal problem. A child is said to be depressed when five or more of the following symptoms exist for more than 2 weeks: loss of interest or pleasure, significant weight loss or gain, depressed mood, insomnia, psychomotor agitation, feelings of worthlessness or excessive or inappropriate guilt, diminished concentration, recurrent thoughts of death, or suicidal ideation (APA, 1994). Because these are symptoms easily missed, a history should be taken from the child as well as from the parents. Depression can be differentiated from "normal" sadness when children report they cannot remember the last time they felt happy or had a good time (**anhedonia**) (Figure 54-4).

Children who are depressed need treatment to prevent their depression from worsening to a point of school failure or suicide (Sadler, 1993). Counseling to discuss problems is necessary. Tricyclic antidepressants, monoamine oxidase inhibitors, second generation antidepressives, and lithium carbonate are all used in treatment. In addition to these pharmacologic approaches, family or individual counseling may be necessary to help the child regain self-esteem and the family to understand the level of depression that has occurred. Attempted suicide as a result of depression is discussed in Chapter 33.

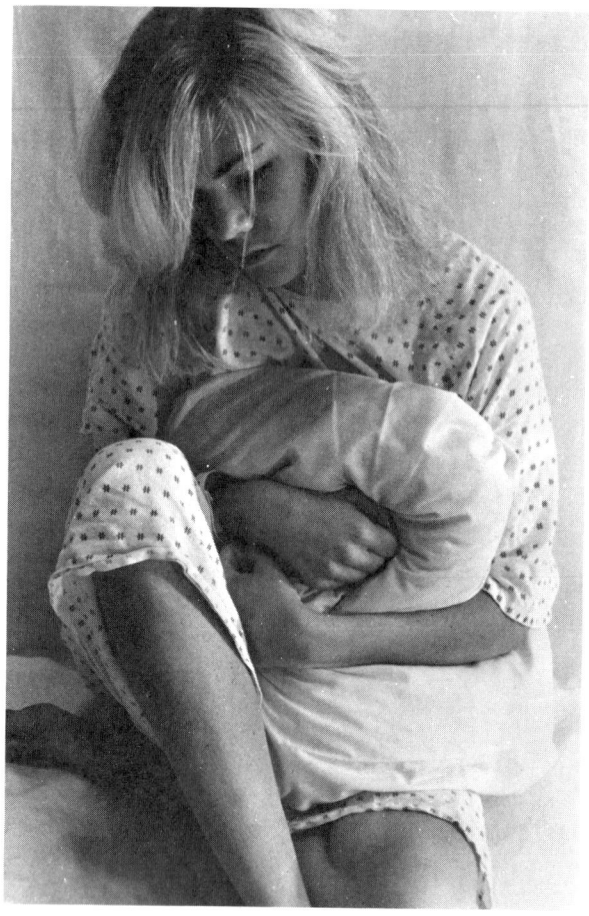

FIGURE 54-4
Observe children to detect depression or withdrawn behavior. Note this child's flat facial expression and the way the pillow is used for comfort. (Courtesy of Julie Golobic.)

Childhood Schizophrenia

Schizophrenia is actually a group of disorders of thought processes characterized by the gradual disintegration of mental functioning (APA, 1994). It is a devastating mental illness that usually strikes at a young age in adolescence or young adulthood. Symptoms during childhood are usually undifferentiated or ill defined.

Over the years there has been a great deal of debate about the cause of schizophrenia. For a long time, it was hypothesized that schizophrenia resulted solely from an impaired parent–child relationship. Current research, however, indicates that there is as much a genetic as an environmental basis for this disorder. It may well be that a combination of predisposing genetic factors in combination with poor parent–child communication is responsible for the development of the disorder. The influence of the family on the course of the illness has been the subject of intense research over the past 20 years. Some family environments—for example, those with high **expressed emotion**, or frequent, intense expression of emotion and a critical attitude—have been categorized as those most likely to cause relapse in children with schizophrenia discharged from hospitals. Neurologic studies have shown a linkage between schizophrenia and temporolimbic disease or frontal lesions.

Children with schizophrenia experience hallucinations (hear or see people or objects that other people cannot). They are not responsive (have a **flat affect**) and may withdraw so completely that they are stuporous (**catatonia**). Although schizophrenic manifestations may occur suddenly following a major stress in a child's life (such as rejection by a boyfriend or girlfriend), subtle signs of mental illness have usually been present for some time.

A diagnosis of a psychotic disorder of this extent is a shock to parents. Fortunately, therapy with modern antipsychotic drugs is effective in reducing children's hallucinations and bizarre thinking. Drugs that may be prescribed are trifluopromazine, chlorpromazine, and prochlorperazine (Spencer et al., 1993). Parents need help to support a child during a long period of therapy. Many children who are diagnosed as having schizophrenia in childhood will continue to have mental illness as adults, so they need continuing support.

Key Points

- Both mental retardation and mental illness pose long-term care concerns for children and their families.
- Mental retardation still carries a stigma in many communities; therefore, parents may have a more difficult time accepting this diagnosis in their child than they would a physical illness. Help parents to gain the insight that mental retardation occurs in a pro-

portion of infants in every population and having a child with this merely reflects a chance occurrence.

- Most children with mental retardation benefit from early schooling. Urge parents to enroll children in early education programs so the child has a "head start" on schooling.
- Mental illness often begins subtly in children and is first manifested as a behavior problem in school. Assess thoroughly any child referred for disruptive behavior in class for the possibility that he or she has a serious emotional problem.
- Infantile autism is a pervasive developmental disorder that has a syndrome of behaviors including fascination with movement, impairment of communication skills, and insensitivity to pain. Early identification is important so unreal expectations are not placed on the child.
- A number of disruptive behavior disorders such as attention deficit with hyperactivity disorder (ADHD) may occur in childhood. Such children may be treated with methylphenidate hydro (Ritalin) to reduce the hyperactivity and allow them to achieve better in school and interact better at home.
- Eating disorders seen in childhood are pica, rumination, anorexia nervosa, and bulimia. All these disorders can lead to loss of weight and electrolyte imbalances if left unrecognized and untreated.
- Children who are depressed are at high risk for committing suicide. They need thorough assessment and close observation to be certain this does not happen.
- Tic disorders are abnormalities of semi-involuntary movement thought to result from dysfunction of the basal ganglia. Tourette's syndrome is an example of this.
- Encopresis is the repeated passage of feces in places not culturally appropriate for that purpose. Therapy is both physiologic and psychological.
- Schizophrenia may occur in childhood. This usually presents as disorganized behavior. Long-term therapy is necessary.

Critical Thinking Exercises

1. Bethany is a 3-year-old with Down syndrome who is critically ill with pneumonia. It is difficult to believe that her mother did not recognize sooner how ill the child was becoming and bring her sooner for care. Why would a parent have reacted this way?
2. Todd is a second-grade student with attention deficit with hyperactivity disorder. His family feels "at its wits' end" because his attention span is so short and his behavior is so disruptive. What suggestions could you make to his mother to help him adjust better to the family routine?
3. Barry is an adolescent whose parents tell you

seems increasingly depressed, so much so that he sleeps almost all day on weekends. Does Barry need a referral or is he just demonstrating usual adolescent behavior? What questions would you want to ask to be able to tell?

References

American Academy of Pediatrics Committee on Bioethics. (1990). Sterilization of women who are mentally handicapped. *Pediatrics, 85,* 868.

American Psychiatric Association. (1994). *Diagnostic and statistical manual of mental disorders* (4th ed.). Washington, DC: American Psychiatric Association.

Barthel, R. D., & Herrman, C. (1991). Psychiatric mental health nursing with children. In F. Gary & C. K. Kavanagh (Eds.). *Psychiatric mental health nursing.* Philadelphia: J.B. Lippincott.

Bufano, G., et al. (1990). Enteral nutrition in anorexia nervosa. *Journal of Parenteral Enteral Nutrition, 14,* 404.

Bushnell, R. K. (1992). A guide to primary care of iron-deficiency anemia. *Nurse Practitioner, 17,* 68.

Calis, K. A., et al. (1990). Attention-deficit hyperactivity disorder. *Clinical Pharmacology, 9,* 632.

Campbell, L. R., & Cohen, M. (1990). Management of attention deficit hyperactivity disorder. *Clinical Pediatrics, 29,* 191.

Carlat, D. J., & Camargo, C. A. (1991). Review of bulimia in males. *American Journal of Psychiatry, 148,* 831.

David, H. P., & Morgall, J. M. (1990). Family planning for the mentally disordered and retarded. *Journal of Nervous and Mental Disease, 178,* 385.

Department of Health & Human Services. (1991). *Healthy people 2000.* Washington, DC: Public Health Service.

Dooling, E. C. (1993). Cognitive disorders in children. *Current Opinion in Pediatrics, 5,* 675.

Geissler, E. M. (1994). *Pocket guide to cultural assessment.* St. Louis: C. V. Mosby.

Giannini, A. J., et al. (1990). Anorexia and bulimia. *American Family Physician, 41,* 1169.

Jankovic, J. (1994). Basal ganglia and neurotransmitter disorders. In F. A. Oski et al. (Eds.). *Principles and practice of pediatrics* (2nd ed.). Philadelphia: J.B. Lippincott.

Lacey, E. P. (1990). Broadening the perspective of pica: Literature review. *Public Health Reports, 105,* 29.

Last, C. G., & Strauss, C. C. (1990). School refusal in anxiety-disordered children and adolescents. *Journal of the American Academy of Child and Adolescent Psychiatry, 29,* 31.

Leffert, N., & Susman, A. (1993). Attention deficit hyperactivity disorder in children. *Current Opinion in Pediatrics, 5,* 429.

Lotspeich, L. J., & Ciaranello, R. D. (1993). The neurobiology and genetics of infantile autism. *International Review of Neurobiology, 35,* 87.

Mays, R. M., et al. (1993). Autism in young children: An update. *Journal of Pediatric Health Care, 7,* 17.

Meades, S. (1993). Suggested community psychiatric nursing interventions with clients suffering from anorexia nervosa and bulimia nervosa. *Journal of Advanced Nursing, 18,* 364.

Palmer, T. A. (1990). Anorexia nervosa, bulimia nervosa: Causal theories and treatment. *Nurse Practitioner, 15,* 12.

Popper, C. W. (1993). Psychopharmacologic treatment of anxiety disorders in adolescents and children. *Journal of Clinical Psychiatry, 54,* 52.

Sadler, L. S. (1993). A review for school nursing professionals: Adolescent depression. *Journal of School Nursing, 9,* 12.

Scahill, L., et al. (1993). Tourette's syndrome. *Archives of Psychiatric Nursing, 7,* 209.

Sexson, S. B., & Madan-Swain, A. (1993). School reentry for the child with a chronic illness. *Journal of Learning Disabilities, 26,* 115.

Spencer, R. T., et al. (1993). *Clinical pharmacology and nursing management* (4th ed.). Philadelphia: J.B. Lippincott.

Sprague-McRae, J. M., et al. (1993). Encopresis: A study of treatment alternatives and historical and behavioral characteristics. *Nurse Practitioner, 18,* 52.

Watemberg, N., & Shaley, H. (1994). Daytime urinary frequency in children. *Clinical Pediatrics, 33,* 50.

Suggested Readings

Baker, M. H. (1990). Jennifer's life is a success story. *RN, 53,* 30.

Barry, A., & Lippmann, S. B. (1990). Anorexia nervosa in males. *Postgraduate Medicine, 87,* 161.

Edwards-Beckett, J. (1991). Caregiver attributions of success or failure of their mentally retarded dependent. *Journal of Pediatric Nursing, 6,* 121.

Finke, L. M., et al. (1993). National workshop: Implementation of practices with severely mentally and emotionally disturbed children and adolescents. *Journal of Child and Adolescent Psychiatric Mental Health Nursing, 6,* 31.

Fritsch, R. C., & Goodrich, W. (1990). Adolescent inpatient attachment as treatment process. *Adolescent Psychiatry, 17,* 246.

Griffin-Francell, C. (1993). Advocating for severely emotionally disturbed children and their families. *Journal of Child and Adolescent Psychiatric Mental Health Nursing, 6,* 33.

Hamburg, P., & Herzog, D. (1990). Supervising the therapy of patients with eating disorders. *American Journal of Psychotherapy, 44,* 369.

Kazdin, A. E. (1990). Premature termination from treatment among children referred for antisocial behavior. *Journal of Child Psychology and Psychiatry, 31,* 415.

Kennedy, P., et al. (1990). Use of the timeout procedure in a child psychiatry inpatient milieu: Combining dynamic and behavioral approaches. *Child Psychiatry and Human Development, 20,* 207.

Leung, A. K., et al. (1994). Attention-deficit hyperactivity disorder. *Postgraduate Medicine, 95,* 153.

Mansheim, P. (1990). Short-term psychiatric inpatient treatment of preschool children. *Hospital Community Psychiatry, 41,* 670.

Merlin, R. (1992). Understanding bulimia and its implications in pregnancy. *Journal of Obstetric, Gynecologic & Neonatal Nursing, 21,* 199.

Nehring, W. M. (1994). The nurse whose specialty is developmental disabilities. *Pediatric Nursing, 20,* 78.

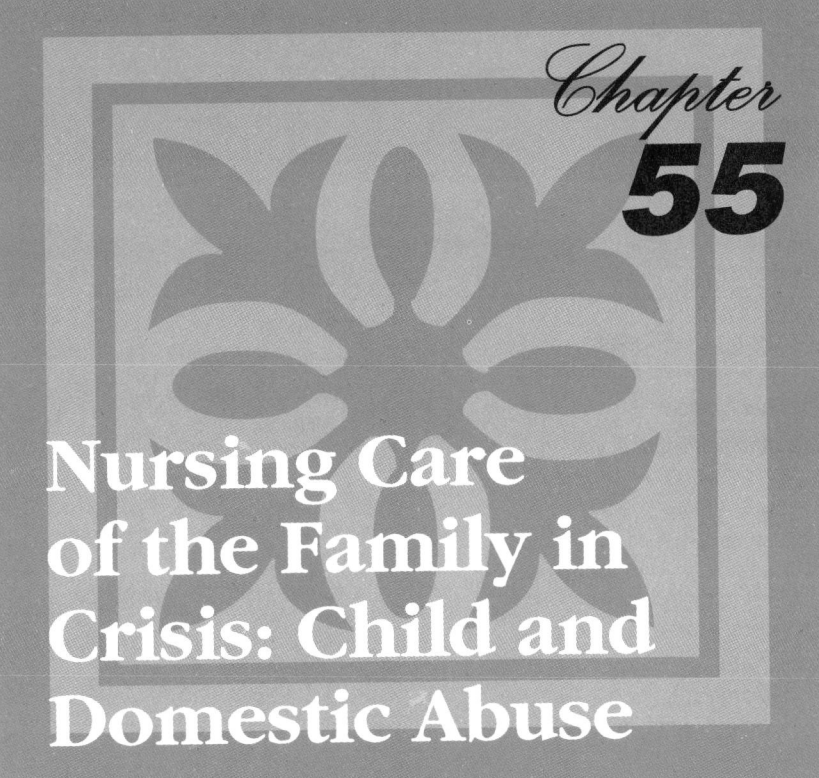

Chapter 55

Nursing Care of the Family in Crisis: Child and Domestic Abuse

Key Terms

- abuse
- battered child syndrome
- disorganization phase
- failure to thrive
- incest
- learned helplessness
- mandatory reporters
- molestation
- Munchausen syndrome by proxy
- pedophile
- permissive reporters
- rape trauma syndrome
- reorganization phase
- shaken baby syndrome
- silent rape syndrome

Objectives

After mastering the contents of this chapter, you should be able to:

1. Discuss the types of abuse seen in families and the theories explaining their occurrence.
2. Assess a physically or emotionally abused family.
3. Formulate nursing diagnoses related to the abused family.
4. Plan nursing care for the abused family such as ways to role model better parenting.
5. Implement nursing care for the family in which abuse occurred, for instance, assisting with immediate trauma care or counseling to prevent further abuse.
6. Evaluate outcome criteria to be certain that goals of nursing care were achieved.
7. Identify National Health Goals related to the abused family that nurses can be instrumental in helping the nation achieve.
8. Identify areas related to care of the abused child that could benefit from additional nursing research.
9. Use critical thinking to analyze ways that nurses can be instrumental in preventing child abuse.
10. Synthesize knowledge of family abuse with nursing process to achieve quality maternal and child health nursing care.

Adele Pillitteri: MATERNAL AND CHILD HEALTH NURSING, 2nd Edition. © 1995 Adele Pillitteri.

The increasing incidence of abuse in families is a growing concern in the United States. Abuse is associated with stress and has been linked to the inability of the family to handle external and internal stressors. Accordingly, abuse in the family is rarely an isolated event but rather an indication of how much the family needs care overall.

Abuse, which is defined as the "willful injury by one person of another" (Helfer & Kempe, 1987), takes many forms—child abuse, which can be physical or emotional and includes neglect and sexual abuse; wife battering or other forms of domestic violence; and maltreatment of the elderly. Maternity, child health, and family nurses need to be especially observant for signs of possible child abuse and prepared to handle this highly emotional and complex problem objectively. It is important, first and foremost, to ensure the safety of the victim, but this must be done with sensitivity to the importance of maintaining and improving overall family functioning.

Abuse has long-term consequences as children from abusive families may become abusive parents themselves (Lewis et al., 1991). It may lead to a posttraumatic stress disorder (Rowan et al., 1994). National Health Goals related to child abuse are shown in the Focus on National Health Goals box.

⊠ **NURSING PROCESS OVERVIEW**
for Care of the Family in Crisis

ASSESSMENT

Nurses are often the first persons to identify symptoms of possible child abuse because they are often the first to see a child undressed at a health care visit. When abuse in any form is suspected, it is essential to get as full a picture as possible. Talking with parents first, without the child, and then interviewing the child may help to uncover inconsistencies in the parents' explanation.

NURSING DIAGNOSIS

Nursing diagnoses associated with abuse should address both the physical and emotional results of abuse. Examples are:

- Pain related to burn on hand
- High risk for injury related to previous abuse
- High risk for violence directed at others related to admitted poor self-control
- Altered parenting related to high level of stress
- Ineffective family coping as manifested by child abuse related to alcohol use by father
- Self-esteem disturbance related to abuse

PLANNING

Planning must center first on ensuring the safety of the abused child and minimizing the effects of trauma. Long-term planning includes helping an abused family member find safe refuge and re-establishing self-esteem through a self-help or advocacy program. Teaching *empowerment,* or the ability to take charge of ones life, is particularly important for older children and women in abusing families. Organizations that are helpful for referral are:

Parents Anonymous
520 South Lafayette Park Place
Suite 316
Los Angeles, CA 90057

National Committee for Prevention of Child Abuse
332 South Michigan Avenue
Suite 1600
Chicago, IL 60604-4357

National Association of State Victims of Child Abuse
Laws (VOCAL)
P.O. Box 1314
Orangevale, CA 95662

Women Against Rape
P.O. Box 02084
Columbus, OH 43202

IMPLEMENTATION

The most important intervention related to family abuse is prevention. Nurses can do much in all settings to promote healthy ways of handling family stress. They can be particularly observant for families who seem to be at risk for abusive behavior. When instances of abuse are uncovered, role modeling is an intervention that can help parents who are ignorant about their children's needs and child behavior. Lecturing is not a useful intervention with any instance of abuse, but supportive education can be extremely valuable.

EVALUATION

Nurses are mandatory reporters of child abuse; identifying and reporting this problem is a legal responsibility as well as an important nursing action. Outcome criteria should focus on specific measures of improved parenting such as:

- Parent holds baby appropriately and maintains good eye contact.
- Parent admits to losing control with children at

home and voices desire to undergo counseling for problem.
- Parent states she has the Crisis Center telephone number by the telephone; will call for help if she realizes she may abuse child.
- Adolescent states she is able to continue to think of herself with high self-esteem in spite of sexual abuse by brother.
- Parent attends monthly meetings of Parents Anonymous.

Child Abuse

As many as 23 of every 1000 children are reported yearly as being victims of child abuse. As many as 1000 children die every year from abuse (Devlin & Reynolds, 1994). **Battered child syndrome**, a term used to de-

FOCUS ON
National Health Goals

Abuse of children is a national health disgrace as well as a national health concern. A number of National Health Goals address this issue:

- Increase to at least 30 the number of states in which at least 50% of children identified as neglected or physically or sexually abused receive physical and mental evaluation with appropriate follow-up as a means of breaking the intergenerational cycle of abuse.
- Reverse to less than 25.2/1000 the rising incidence of maltreatment of children younger than age 18, specifically, reduce physical abuse to 5.7/1000, sexual abuse to 2.5/1000, emotional abuse to 3.4/1000 and neglect to 15.9/1000 (DHHS, 1991).

Nurses can be instrumental in helping the nation achieve these goals by educating parents how to parent more effectively and identifying children in school or health care agency settings who have been abused or neglected. Additional nursing research would be helpful for the following questions: Can potentially abusing parents be identified on postpartal units and helped to avoid this? What counseling is necessary for adolescents who have been abused to help them be successful parents? What are the most helpful nursing interventions to use with parents when a child who has been abused is admitted to the hospital?

Table 55-1. *Incidence of Reported Child Abuse in the United States*

Type	Percentage of Total
Deprivation of necessities	54
Physical injury	25.5
Emotional maltreatment	7
Sexual maltreatment	8.5
Other	5

scribe victims of abuse (Helfer & Kempe, 1987), is one of the leading causes of childhood death and disability. About 10% of all children seen in hospital emergency departments for traumatic injuries (more than 1 million children annually) are victims of abuse. The incidence of various types of abuse is shown in Table 55-1.

To detect child abuse, the question of how an accident occurred must be asked whenever children are seen at a health care facility for injuries. Most childhood injuries are from accidents caused by the child's inability to distinguish safe situations from dangerous ones. A number of children are injured because parents overestimate their child's ability to do safely such things as lighting a fire to burn trash or using a saw in a wood project.

Because parenting is not an easy task, and good parenting is not an automatic or truly instinctive ability, there are children in every community who are injured because of abuse. Such abuse may be physical (the child is beaten, burned, or sexually molested) or neglect (the child is not fed, clothed, supervised properly, or offered medical care or educational opportunities). Abuse may also be psychological or emotional. A number of women who threatened the health of a fetus by drug abuse have been viewed by the courts as child abusers (Rhodes, 1990).

Child abuse is not limited to young children. A major reason that runaway youths leave home is that they have been abused (Powers et al., 1990).

Abuse not only places a child at immediate risk but can also lead to long-term effects. Physically abused children are found to be more angry, noncompliant, and hyperactive than others; they may demonstrate poor self-control and low self-esteem. Children whose parents do not interact with them (emotional abuse) are more withdrawn and have a flatter affect than others. Children who suffer sexual abuse have long-term effects of depression, guilt, and difficulty enjoying sexual relations at the same levels as others. As the abusive family is a disrupted one, children often have undiagnosed medical problems such as anemia, otitis media, lead poisoning, and sexually transmitted diseases (Flaherty & Weiss, 1990).

In addition, when children reach adulthood and begin parenting, they rear their children in basically the same way as they were reared. A concern is that parents who themselves received little love or were abused as children never form a basic sense of trust and so grow into nonloving and abusing parents unless there is effective intervention.

Reporting Suspected Child Abuse

State laws generally identify two types of responsibility in reporting child abuse: **mandatory reporters** and **permissive reporters**. Nurses are included in the mandatory category in most states; this means they *must* report suspected child abuse when they identify it. Failure to do so could result in a fine or possible loss of nursing licensure. The fact that the information was given in a confidential interview does not free the nurse from this responsibility.

All health care institutions and agencies have protocols on how the reporting should be handled. It is important to learn the protocol required in your particular agency, community, and state so you can effectively do this (see the Focus on Nursing Research box). Following

FOCUS ON NURSING RESEARCH

Does the Socioeconomic Status of Families Influence Reporting of Child Abuse?

In 1974, the Federal Child Abuse Prevention and Treatment Act required reporting of child abuse in all states. Although nurses have since this time been designated as mandated reporters of abuse, only recently have nurses begun to hold positions where they are directly responsible for abuse reporting.

This study investigated whether the gender and socioeconomic status of the victim influences the reporting of child abuse by nurses. Participants were registered nurses taking a 2-hour course in child abuse required by New York State for license renewal. Nurses were shown three vignettes of children being admitted to an emergency room with symptoms of possible abuse. When asked if they would or would not report the incident as child abuse, nurses indicated they were significantly less apt to report abuse when the victim was female rather than male and when the family was perceived as being from a middle rather than a low or high socioeconomic background. The implication of this finding is that female children from middle-class backgrounds may be left less protected than others as nurses become more actively involved in child abuse reporting.

Pillitteri, A., Seidl, A., Smith, C., & Stanton, M. (1992). Parent gender, victim gender, and family socioeconomic level influences on the potential reporting by nurses of physical child abuse. *Issues in Comprehensive Pediatric Nursing, 15,* 239.

official reporting of child abuse to an official child protection agency, a health care agency has the right, in most instances, to hold the child for 72 hours for protection to give an appointed caseworker time to investigate if abuse has occurred. Following the 72-hour time period, a court proceeding will determine whether a child should be returned to the parent's care. Because child abuse is a crime, the health care record of the child can be subpoenaed and displayed in court. Be certain when charting regarding child abuse that you make specific and factual notes (observations, not interpretations). Record conversation with parents in exact quotes when possible. Photographs of physical abuse aid the strength of the testimony of abuse, so these are usually ordered.

A second provision in most states is protection from having a lawsuit brought against a health care provider for reporting suspected abuse that is then proved false. This means it is better to err on the side of reporting suspected abuse rather than not reporting it, from both a child safety and a legal perspective. When abuse is officially reported, parents should be told that child abuse is suspected, as open lines of communication with parents are important both to protect the child and to arrange counseling help for the parents.

Theories of Child Abuse

The most commonly accepted theory as to why child abuse occurs is that a special triad of circumstances is present or that three factors are generally operating: a special parent, or one who has the potential to abuse a child; a special child, or a child who is seen as "different" in some way in the parent's eyes; and a special event or circumstance that brought about the abuse (Helfer & Kempe, 1987).

Special Parents

Only a small fraction of parents who abuse their children (probably less than 10%) have a history of mental illness. Many of these parents, however, do have a history of having been abused themselves as children. Such parents may have less self-control than other parents. They may be unfamiliar with the normal growth and development of children and so have unrealistic expectations of a child. These parents may be socially isolated, with no support persons readily available. The isolation may be by distance (a parent separated from other people in a farmhouse miles from neighbors), or it may be the type that exists in communities of apartment houses where neighbors do not routinely speak to one another. Abuse is strongly associated with excessive parental use of alcohol, a substance that removes inhibitions and self-control.

To prevent abuse, children may assume a role reversal with their parents or become the comforting, solacing persons. They recognize very early in life that when a parent is upset, they will be hurt. They learn to comfort the parent and reduce the parent's anxiety, thereby avoiding the hurt. This is a characteristic to look for in emergency departments—who is comforting whom?

In the emergency department, parents unable to deal with stress may not show the usual degree of compassion for children's degree of pain or offer to comfort. They may appear more concerned with how the injury affects them than how it affects the child: "This makes me look like a bad parent," not "I should have been more careful."

Special Children

Abused children are viewed as somehow "different" by parents. They may be more or less intelligent than other children in the family; they may have been unplanned. They may have a birth defect; they may have an attention span deficit. Because the child is perceived as somehow different, a good parent–child relationship does not develop. This is most likely to happen with children who are born prematurely or who have an illness at birth, because they are kept from parents or separated from them by special nurseries or equipment for the first weeks of life, when normal bonding occurs.

Special Circumstance: Stress

A third factor in child abuse is stress, which may be a response to an event that would not necessarily be stressful to an average parent. It might be something as common as a blocked toilet, an illness in the family, a lost job, a landlord asking for the rent, or a rainstorm that cancelled a planned activity. Child abuse crosses all socioeconomic levels because stress occurs at all levels. Stress generally has a greater impact when people do not have strong support people around them. Families whose internal support system is faulty or who have not formed outside support systems are apt to be families with a higher incidence of abuse.

Physical Abuse

Physical abuse is the action of a caregiver that causes injury to a child. It is commonly revealed by burns or head and hand injuries (see the Nursing Care Plan, p. 1746).

Assessment

Interview. Always ask parents to account for any injury to a child's body. It is important to remember, however, that most toddlers have a number of ecchymotic spots on their legs from bumping into tables or chairs. Some childhood diseases, such as leukemia or purpura, begin with easy bruising. Children with osteogenesis imperfecta will have frequent broken bones as a natural consequence of their disease. Because of inadequate fact finding in these instances, false reports lead to se-

Gerald is a 2-year-old boy admitted to your hospital unit for a diagnosis of physical child abuse. The following is a nursing care plan designed for him.

Assessment: Two-year-old child admitted to unit walking beside mother. Child dressed in wool coat and cap despite 80° heat outside. Circular lesions resembling cigarette burns on arms and legs; large 4-cm ecchymotic area on both buttocks and anterior thighs; sharp-pointed, blistered, and inflamed area on back of left hand resembling point of iron. Cast applied in emergency department present on right arm; fingers warm and pink; blanch readily on pressure.

Child lives with mother and mother's boyfriend (not child's father) in one-bedroom apartment; mother works as a cocktail waitress at night club. States that when she left to go to work last night, she left child in care of boyfriend. When she returned at 3:00 AM, child was crying in crib because "his arm hurt." States she thinks he "caught it in the side rail." States circular lesions are "mosquito bites"; mark on hand is a "birthmark."

Boyfriend accompanied mother and child to emergency department; was reluctant to allow nurses to remove child's clothing; stated, "It's too cold in here for that." Neither parent nor boyfriend were observed offering emotional support during examination. When physician suggested child may have been beaten and burned, mother said, "What can I do? I have to have someone watch him while I work."

Nursing Diagnosis: High risk for injury related to abusing parent

Defining Characteristic: Child has injuries characteristic of child abuse.

Goal: Child will sustain no further physical harm in the future.

Outcome Criteria: Child has no further ecchymotic or burned areas; states he has not been harmed.

Nursing Orders	*Rationale*
1. Obtain a pregnancy and birth history; be alert for description of undesired pregnancy, child hospitalized at birth, wrong sex of child, etc.	1. A pregnancy history is important to document characteristics associated with abuse.
2. Identify if triad of special parent, special child, special circumstance exists.	2. Triad characteristics are typical circumstances of abuse.
3. Obtain a history of child's physical symptoms; be alert to injury excessive for related cause.	3. A history inconsistent with physical symptoms is characteristic of abuse.
4. Undress child completely so total body can be examined; document abrasions, bruises, edematous or tender areas.	4. Physical assessment is important to document abuse.
5. Suspected child abuse reported to state capital by telephone; mother informed of official procedure.	5. Nurses are mandatory reporters of abuse.
6. Photographs to document child's physical appearance ordered.	6. Photographs can be important for documentation.
7. Encourage mother to visit during hospitalization; give care to child. Establish protective but welcoming atmosphere during parent's visits in hospital.	7. These are actions to encourage improved parenting.

(continued)

vere stress on the family that has been falsely accused and can interfere with the relationship between parents of an ill child and health care personnel who will then give care to the child (see the Focus on Cultural Awareness box).

When a child has been physically abused, the injury is usually out of proportion to the history of the injury given by the parent (Figure 55-1). The parent may report, for example, that the child was playing underneath the coffee table when he reared up quickly and hit

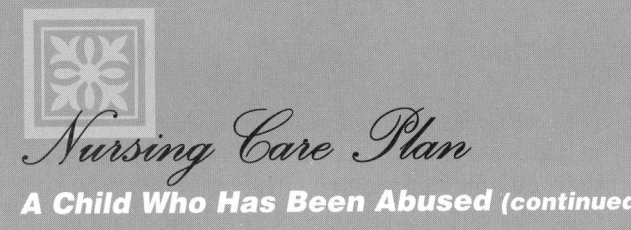

Nursing Care Plan
A Child Who Has Been Abused (continued)

Nursing Orders	**Rationale**
8. Use a primary assignment for nursing care to provide consistency in care.	8. Consistent nursing can help provide a sense of security.
9. Observe mother's parenting ability; document care level and child's response to parent; encourage mother to describe child care practices and expectations of child.	9. Assessing parenting ability is important to help determine if child will be safe with mother after hospital discharge.
10. Keep painful procedures to a minimum; provide stimulation and activities appropriate to age.	10. Providing comfort and support for child are important to help build self-esteem.

Nursing Diagnosis: Chronic low self-esteem of parent related to financial dependency

Defining Characteristic: Mother voices helplessness to improve her situation.

Goal: Mother will be able to be independent of boyfriend before hospital discharge.

Outcome Criteria: Mother has established a new living situation and means of support separate from boyfriend.

Nursing Orders	**Rationale**
1. Encourage mother to view self as responsible for her own and child's safety.	1. These are actions to help mother gain empowerment.
2. Ask mother if she is receptive to counseling.	2. A counselor could be helpful to mother to help her solve her child care problem.
3. Offer praise and reinforcement for sound decision-making or childrearing practice she demonstrates while child is hospitalized.	3. These are actions to help mother regain sense of self-esteem.
4. Empathize with difficulty of being a single parent, but do not condone abuse.	4. Being a single mother can be difficult; condoning child abuse would not be in either child's or mother's best interest.
5. Help mother locate source of emotional support, such as Parents Anonymous or a personal support person.	5. Helps mother find person to rely on other than present boyfriend.
6. Help mother secure competent child care while she is at work.	6. Child care arrangements could protect child from inadequate care while mother works.

his head, sustaining a large hematoma and temporary loss of consciousness, or that an infant "rolled off the couch" and now has two broken arms. In other instances, the parents may give conflicting stories or can give no reason for the injury ("He woke up from his nap and couldn't move his arm; I don't know what could be wrong.").

When questioned about the injury, abused children often repeat the parent's story; this loyalty to parents seems misplaced, but they may fear further beatings or

1747

1748 ▨ *Unit Nine: Children and Families With Mental Health Disorders*

FOCUS ON CULTURAL AWARENESS

There are some health practices that can be confused with child abuse. Coin-rolling, for example, a type of massage to draw illness out of the body used by Asians, leaves bruises on the back similar to those that would appear on a child who has been struck. Coin-rolling involves heating a coin and then vigorously rubbing it over the body, leaving red welts. Being aware of a practice such as coin-rolling aids understanding of the meaning of illness to parents and prevents false reports of child abuse (Geissler, 1994).

simply believe that living with such parents is better than not having anyone to live with. Ask about behavior problems in school or abnormal behavior, such as constant water drinking, as the constant stress these children live under can result in this type of manifestation.

It is often difficult to remain emotionally uninvolved and not grow angry when talking to the parents of an abused child. Emotional involvement is not constructive, however; it rarely helps the parents to change, and it may cause them to avoid seeking health care in the future, leaving the child totally unprotected.

Always assume that the parents have done the best they could under the circumstances in which they found themselves. The fact that they have brought the child for care means they are seeking help; this may be their way of saying, "Help me; I don't want this to happen again." Child abuse is rarely an isolated phenomenon. Often the mother is also a victim and needs as much help and protection as the child.

Physical Examination. When children are examined at both well child or ill child health care visits, be certain they are fully undressed so that their entire body can be observed during the course of the visit. Plot height and weight on a standard graph as these may be delayed in neglected children.

A number of injuries in children clearly signal child abuse. Children who are beaten with electrical cords, belts, or clotheslines have peculiar circular and linear lesions. Children beaten with a belt buckle have additional curved lacerations from the imprint of the buckle; few other weapons produce such contusions (Figure 55-2). Abrasions or ecchymotic areas on the wrists or ankles may be present from a child being tied to a bed or against a wall. Most parents protect their children's hands carefully, but children who are abused have a higher incidence of hand injury than others (Johnson et al., 1990).

Burns or scalds occur in about 10% of abused children. The peak age at which children accidentally burn themselves is 2 years; that of burns related to abuse is 3 years. When children burn their hand by accident, they usually burn the palm; burns from abuse are often on the dorsal surface. Scalding with hot water may be seen.

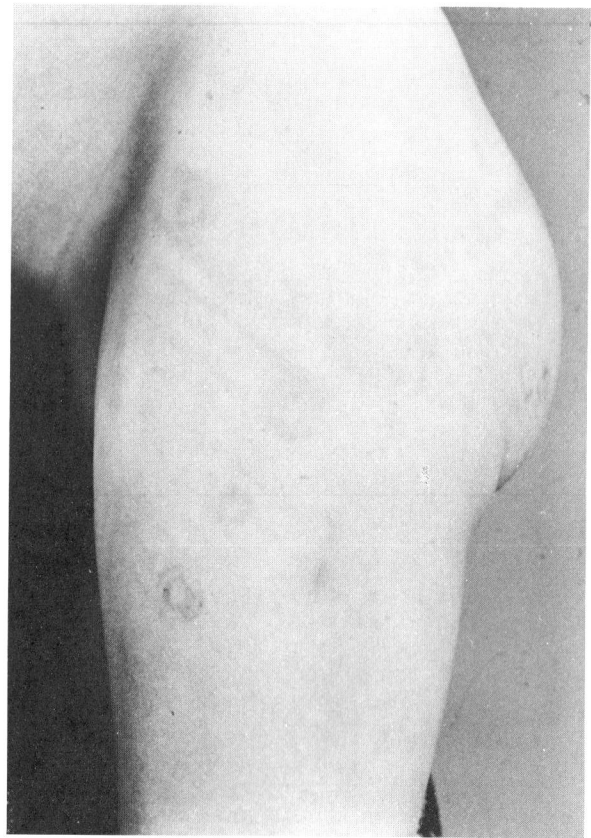

FIGURE 55-2
The leg of an abused child. Notice the peculiar diagnostic J-shaped marks from a beating with a belt. (Courtesy of the Department of Medical Photography, Children's Hospital, Buffalo, NY.)

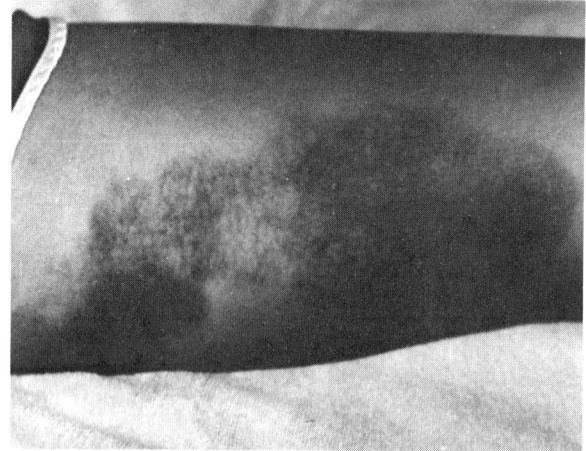

FIGURE 55-1
A large ecchymotic area on a child's leg. With this type of injury, carefully assessing the history of the accident would be appropriate.

A child placed in a tub of hot water, buttocks first, often has no burn in the center of his buttocks because they touched the tub; a ring of burns causing a "hole in the doughnut" effect appears around this. Young children do accidentally step into bathtubs containing water that is hot enough to burn. When this happens, however, the child usually falls forward and so also has burns on the hands and splash marks on the chest or face. When a child is lowered into scalding water as punishment, only the feet and the skin up to the knees are scalded.

Cigarette burns (Figure 55-3*A*) are a common finding on the bodies of physically abused children. A fresh cigarette burn causes a blister that resembles the scab of impetigo or pediculosis; differentiation at this stage is often difficult. Impetigo lesions, however, heal without scarring. Cigarette burns and pediculosis heal with a definite circular scar.

Human bites or chunks of hair pulled off the scalp may be present (Figure 55-3*B*). Head injury is common. Infants can suffer what has been termed **shaken baby syndrome**. Repetitive, violent shaking of a small infant by the arms or shoulders causes a whiplash injury to the neck, edema to the brain stem, retinal hemorrhages, and, potentially, a halt in respirations. In extreme instances, the infant may suffer brain hemorrhage and die. This is a particularly insidious form of child abuse because the damage inflicted on the infant is not readily apparent. Increased use of computed tomography scans and magnetic resonance imaging may help to detect these internal symptoms earlier (Spaide et al., 1990).

Broken bones are yet another frequent finding. Children who are preschool age and younger generally do not fall far enough in normal accidents to break bones; a broken bone at this age suggests the child was thrown or struck so hard that the bone broke. Common findings in connection with fractures include multiple fractures in different stages of healing, a single fracture with multiple bruises, rib or occipital fractures, and metaphyseal-

epiphyseal injuries. Bones are not always broken if a child is shaken roughly, but the periosteum is torn, and so the x-ray reveals a strange haziness along both sides of the bone shaft. Tibial torsion (twisting) is often seen (Mellick & Reesor, 1990). Deliberate poisoning is yet another form of child abuse. This usually occurs in a child younger than 2½ years.

Listen to children while they are being examined. If they did not hear the parent's explanation of the accident, while they are being examined they may say something that is not consistent with the parent's explanation of the accident. They may cry little in response to a painful procedure such as an injection, because they are not used to receiving comfort for pain. They may draw back from an examiner more than the average child would because they are afraid of adults. These are very subjective observations, however, because children react in different ways to the fear involved in a recent injury.

Nursing Diagnoses and Related Interventions

Nursing Diagnosis: High risk for injury related to documented abuse by parent

Goal: Child will not experience further abuse for lifetime.

Outcome Criteria: Child has no further physical injuries identifiable as being inflicted by abusing parent.

Prevent Further Abuse. Once child abuse has been discovered, the child can be removed from the home so that no more abuse occurs. It is impossible, however, to reverse the damage that has been done to the child's sense of trust and self-esteem. The goal of health providers with child abuse, therefore, must concentrate on prevention (see the Focus on Nursing Care display).

As many child abusers were abused themselves,

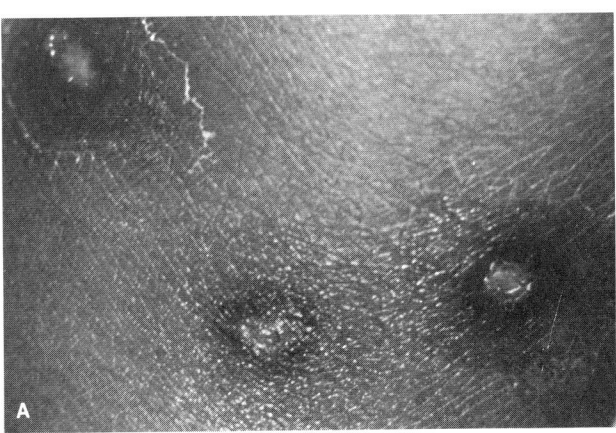
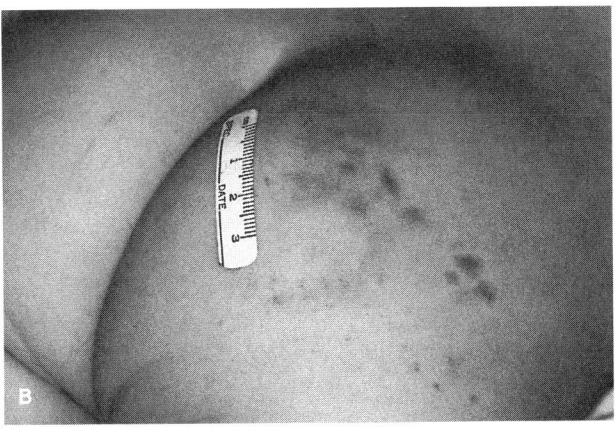

FIGURE 55-3
(**A**) *A cigarette burn on a child's arm.* (**B**) *A human bite mark on a child's buttock. (Courtesy of the Department of Medical Photography, Children's Hospital, Buffalo, NY.)*

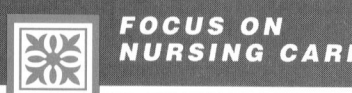

Measures to Prevent Child Abuse

1. Advocate courses in high school on parenting and growth and development of children.
2. Help children learn problem-solving techniques so they are not overwhelmed by mounting problems as adults.
3. Foster high self-esteem in children so they are not dependent on others but are self-assertive (they will not become a passive observer to battering).
4. Help parents with responsible reproductive life planning so children are desired.
5. Help parents locate support people in their community, such as Parents of Retarded Children or church or social contacts.
6. Teach children to verbalize their problems and to seek help for problems so they do not mount to overwhelming proportions.
7. Role model caring ways with children for parents.
8. Identify children who may be viewed as special in some way by parents (those separated at birth, premature, physically disabled).
9. Identify parents who were abused as children and offer specific help to them to break a chain of child abuse.
10. Advocate joining Parents Anonymous as an effective support group for parents who may be potential abusers.

stopping child abuse in any one generation helps prevent it in the next. Identifying parents who are potential abusers and helping them to seek assistance from adequate support people are necessary steps in prevention. Home visits and clubs of abusing parents, such as Parents Anonymous, can be highly effective in establishing crisis intervention lines so that parents can reach out for help in time of crisis. Interventions that appear promising are home visiting, family counseling, and therapy.

Some parents can be identified as potential child abusers during pregnancy. Listen carefully to the way pregnant women talk about the child they are expecting. The mother who is overly concerned about the physical appearance or sex of the child ("This had better be a girl" or "He'd better not have his father's nose") may have difficulty accepting a child who does not meet these predetermined expectations. Listen for a mother who is concerned about "not letting children get the upper hand" or who says a child "had better be good."

This mother may be telling you that she is worried about how she will act when the child is "bad."

Few mothers touch their newborns truly warmly the first time they see them. They may only touch the blanket at the first visit, touch them only with their fingertips at a second visit, and really pick them up and touch them on the second or third day of life. Be aware of a parent who, when she leaves the hospital with the infant, still does not touch him or her or makes disparaging remarks about the child's appearance.

By the time a baby is brought to a health care agency for an initial health maintenance visit, a good parent–child interaction should have begun. Listen for parents who say the baby is "nothing but trouble," "cries all the time," or "is bad." Ask new parents how it feels to be a new parent. "I'm enjoying it" is a different answer from "not what I expected" or "it's not much fun." Risk factors to look for during pregnancy and the early postpartal period are shown in Box 55-1. Specific observations to make during postpartum and pediatric health care checkups are summarized in Box 55-2.

Another nursing responsibility aimed at preventing child abuse is helping young parents learn more about normal growth and development of children and how to

Box 55-1

Women at High Risk for Potential Child Abuse or Neglect That Can Be Identified in the Pregnant or Postpartal Period

1. Mother has had frequent changes of address in the year before delivery (more than 2 changes of address in the previous 12 months).
2. Mother has had past or present psychiatric treatment.
3. Likely incompetence of mother as a parent is seen because of apparent emotional problems.
4. Likely incompetence of the mother as a parent is seen because of apparent lack of intellectual ability.
5. Mother has unrealistic expectations of the new child.
6. Mother refused (or dropped out of) prenatal classes.
7. Mother changed her decision regarding adoption of the child.
8. A previous child was abused or neglected.
9. Mother suffered parental violence or neglect as a child.

(Egan, T. G., et al. [1990]. Prenatal screening of pregnant mothers for parenting difficulties. *Social Science and Medicine, 30,* 289; with permission.)

1. Does the mother have fun with the baby?
2. Does the mother establish eye contact (direct *en face* position) with the baby?
3. How does the mother talk to the baby? Is everything she expresses a demand?
4. Are most of her verbalizations about the child negative?
5. Does she remain disappointed over the child's sex?
6. What is the child's name? Where did the name come from? When was the child named?
7. Are the mother's expectations for the child's development far beyond the child's capabilities?
8. Is the mother very bothered by the baby's crying? How does she feel about the crying?
9. Does the mother see the baby as too demanding during feedings? Is she repulsed by the messiness? Does she ignore the baby's demands to be fed?
10. What is the mother's reaction to the task of changing diapers?
11. When the baby cries, does she or can she comfort him or her?
12. What was (is) the husband's and/or family's reaction to the baby?
13. What kind of support is the mother receiving?
14. Are there sibling rivalry problems?
15. Is the husband jealous of the baby's drain on the mother's time and affection?
16. When the mother brings the child to the physician's office, does she become involved and take control over the baby's needs and what is going to happen (during the examination and while in the waiting room)? Or does she relinquish control to the physician or nurse (undressing the child, holding him or her, allowing the child to express fears, etc.)?
17. Can attention be focused on the child in the mother's presence? Can the mother see something positive for her in that?
18. Does the mother make nonexistent complaints about the baby? Does she describe to you a child that you do not see at all? Does she call with strange stories, such as the child has stopped breathing, changed color, or is doing something "on purpose" to aggravate the parent?
19. Does the mother make emergency calls for very small things, not major things?

(Kempe, C. N. [1976]. Approaches to preventing child abuse. *American Journal of Diseases of Children, 130,* 941, with permission.)

be better parents (Figure 55-4). Courses in high school that describe sound parenting and review normal growth and development of children and the responsibility involved in parenting are important measures in preventing child abuse. Classes conducted in high-risk prenatal settings might have an impact.

Provide Consistent Care and Support for the Abused Child. A major nursing role in caring for an abused child is supplying a consistent, caring, adult presence for the abused child or furnishing a relationship that the child has never enjoyed.

Use a primary or case management type of nursing care assignment with abused children to offer them consistency and the security of a one-to-one relationship (a type of in-depth relationship they have never enjoyed). Many abused children are not used to playing for their own enjoyment but only to the point that a parent wants to play a game; they watch you carefully for signs that you approve of their behavior. They are not used to such activities as sitting quietly and rocking or talking. Be careful when asking questions to imply that any answer is all right or they will supply what they think you want to hear rather than the truth (a question such as "That feels better, doesn't it?" will be followed by an instant "yes" even though the child feels no improvement in symptoms).

Evaluate and Promote Family Health. Nurses also can be instrumental in helping evaluate whether a child

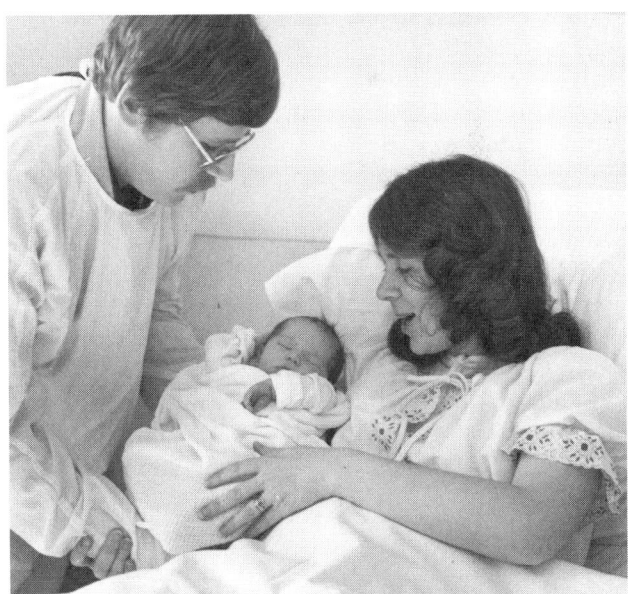

FIGURE 55-4
Teaching that all children have unique characteristics helps to prevent child abuse. Here, new parents explore the already noticeable unique aspects of their newborn. (Courtesy of the Department of Medical Photography, Children's Hospital, Buffalo, NY.)

would be safe in the parent's care in the future. When parents who are suspected child abusers visit in the hospital setting, be certain they are given the same welcome and orientation to the hospital unit and procedures as other parents. When caring for such a child, point out positive characteristics about the child or growth and development markers he or she has reached and realistic explanations of the age because lack of knowledge of normal growth and development may have contributed to the abuse.

For many parents, the response to a charge of child abuse is anger. For others, it is relief; now an unwanted child will be taken away from them. In some families, one of the parents is the abuser; the other is a victim also. The diagnosis of abuse may force the passive partner to make some important decisions about whether he or she wishes to continue a marriage or a relationship with the abusive partner. These are not easy decisions to make; if decision making of any kind were easy for this parent, the circumstances probably would never have reached the point where child abuse occurred.

Praise abusing parents for the things they do well; take time to talk to them away from the child so that your total attention is focused on them to meet their own childlike needs.

Sometimes a child is removed temporarily from a home following child abuse, then returned to the home later when the stress that led to abuse has been removed. Such children need careful follow-up, as parents may revert to an abuse pattern if stress should occur again.

If a child has to be removed permanently from a parent's care, the foster family should visit before discharge from the hospital to make the change less frightening for the child. Children being removed from their parents in this way can feel an acute sense of loss and may grieve for the nonabusing parent or siblings very much. An abused child may also grieve for the abusing parent, especially if the child convinced herself that she was responsible for the abuse, that the parent really was not to blame.

Evaluation of nursing goals for abused children must include not only whether they are physically safe but whether they are developing self-esteem, so that they can become adults who do not need role reversal with their children.

Physical Neglect

Physical neglect is a more subtle form of abuse than physical abuse but can be just as damaging to a child's welfare. A neglected child might appear unwashed, thin, and malnourished or be dressed without mittens or a coat or shoes in cold weather. There are some families in which no one has a warm coat to wear or receives enough food because there is no money for these

things; that is different from the family in which parents do have these things, but the children or this one particular child does not. This type of abuse may be missed by teachers because, never seeing the other members of the family, they believe that all are dressed poorly.

In a health care setting, the difference between one child's care and other family members may be more noticeable. Not bringing a child for immunizations or not seeking early medical care for an infection are other examples of neglect. Not requiring a child to attend school, deliberately keeping a child out of school without setting up a home school program, or allowing a child to go unsupervised after school may also be interpreted as neglect.

Neglect may be willful. Neglect may also occur if parents simply do not realize the normal needs of a child. Such parents need guidance from health care personnel.

Psychological Abuse

Psychological abuse includes constant belittling or threatening, rejecting, isolating, or exploiting the child. Psychological neglect is the absence of positive parenting (Brassard et al., 1993). Children who are psychologically abused are likely to have difficulty becoming emotionally confident adults. Emotional abuse is the most difficult form of abuse to detect as it may occur only in the home, and its effects, although severe, may be subtle; however, it can be every bit as damaging to the child as physical abuse.

The parent who uses only negative terms to describe a child may be psychologically abusing a child. Be sure to include enough growth and development questions during a health assessment to reveal this, and observe parent–child interaction to determine whether this interaction is positive and healthy or negative and potentially unhealthy.

Munchausen Syndrome by Proxy

Munchausen syndrome by proxy refers to a parent who repeatedly brings a child to a health care facility reporting symptoms of illness when, in fact, the child is well (Blouin, 1993). The parent might report a history of seizures, excessive sleepiness, or abdominal pain. The child undergoes extensive diagnostic procedures or therapeutic regimens needlessly. A mark of the syndrome is that the symptoms are those not easily detected by physical examination, only by history; the parent is someone with some degree of medical knowledge and tends to stay with the child in the hospital constantly, offering to give the majority of care. This can be very deceptive because wanting to stay and give care is also the hallmark of a very conscientious and caring parent. As this syndrome reveals distorted perceptions on the part of the parents, it is almost always necessary to remove the children from the home in order to protect them.

Failure to Thrive (Reactive Attachment Disorder)

Failure to thrive is a unique syndrome in which an infant falls below the third percentile for weight and height on a standard growth chart or is falling in percentiles on a growth chart. This condition can be divided into two categories: syndromes with organic causes, such as cardiac disease; and syndromes with nonorganic causes, which occur because of a disturbance in the parent–child relationship, resulting in maternal role insufficiency. Sometimes both physical and emotional factors play a role in failure to thrive.

The nonorganic and mixed types can be considered a form of child neglect although they represent a very complex interplay between parent and child. In many instances, the parent feels little emotional attachment to the child; she has a history of frequent moves and little family support (Lobo et al., 1993). Often a parent is not offering enough food (parents are not aware of the cues their infants are giving them when they need more food or else do not have enough concern for the children to feed them properly). Some infants are offered sufficient food, but the emotional deprivation they sense makes them so lethargic that they do not eat enough. A child may contribute to the poor-parenting interaction by being an irritable, fussy, colicky, or difficult-temperament child. In some instances, the child may have neurologic dysfunction from a birth injury and so may not respond as a normal child. The mother may have interpreted this lethargic behavior as lack of response to her and so did not carry out her half of the interaction adequately.

Assessment

All children should be weighed at routine health assessments, and their weight should be compared with standard growth curves so children who are failing to thrive can be identified. Because of little parent-child interaction, there may be accompanying motor and social developmental delays present.

Take a detailed pregnancy history. In many instances, a breakdown in the development of parenting began in the prenatal period. A pregnancy that was unplanned or not accepted, a boyfriend or husband who left during the pregnancy, the death of a close friend or parent, an economic catastrophe such as loss of a job, or a long distance move during pregnancy are all situations that can cause parenting to develop inadequately after pregnancy.

On physical examination, these infants generally demonstrate some typical behaviors. Overall, the infants may have poor muscle tone and appear lethargic. They

may not resist the examiner's manipulation as will the average infant. Many infants who are emotionally deprived rock on all fours excessively, as if seeking stimulation. They tend to be more reluctant to reach out for toys or initiate human contact than the average infant. They stare hungrily at people who approach them as if they are starved for human contact. Some health care personnel experience an uneasy feeling when caring for these infants, because this eye contact is so intense.

By the second month of life, the child demonstrates little cuddling or conforming to being held. By the third or fourth month, development in the prone position, such as lifting the head and chest and following an object with the eyes, is normal, but other behaviors that should appear in later months, such as sitting erect, pulling to a standing position, crawling, and walking, are delayed. This is because such behaviors depend, to some degree, on stimulation from a parent (the parent holds up the baby, and the baby practices bearing weight on his or her feet). Speech will be markedly delayed or absent because of the lack of interaction. Crying may be diminished or nonexistent.

By the time the infant with failure to thrive is seen in a health care facility, the baby's physical condition may be extremely poor. The child may be nearing acidosis from starvation. If an upper respiratory infection develops, the child's resistance to infection may be so low that it could result in death.

Therapeutic Management

With rare exceptions, children with failure to thrive need to be admitted to the hospital for evaluation and therapy. If the history and physical examination suggest that the cause for the extensive weight delay is nonorganic failure to thrive, studies other than routine admission blood work and urinalysis are delayed so as not to submit these understimulated children to needless pain.

Severe failure to thrive in the early months must be treated rigorously or it may lead to permanent neurologic damage or mental retardation because of protein deficits and interference with brain metabolism. Infants are placed on a diet appropriate for their ideal weight (the weight they would have been normally for the age). Gaining weight rapidly on this diet is diagnostic that their presenting illness was nonorganic failure to thrive.

Nursing Diagnoses and Related Interventions

A nursing diagnosis commonly used with children who fail to thrive is Altered nutrition: less than body requirements related to lack of desire to eat or parental neglect regarding nutritional needs. In addition, Altered parenting related to disturbance in parent–child bonding is often appropriate. A care plan designed for the family must be realistic. Parents cannot be made instantly to form a bond with their children, particularly if this lack of bonding has gone on for some time. On the other hand, one should never give up hope that this will happen. With the proper support and guidance over time, and when obstacles to bonding are removed, a healthy child–parent relationship could still develop.

> *Nursing Diagnosis:* Altered nutrition, less than body requirements, related to inadequate intake secondary to emotional deprivation
>
> *Goal:* Child will take in adequate nutrients for growth by 24 hours.
>
> *Outcome Criteria:* Child shows interest in bottle feedings; is able to establish a regular eating pattern; begins to increase in weight.

Ensure Adequate Nutrition. Keep a careful record of intake and output so the number of calories being taken in every day is accurate. Assess stools for pH and reducing substances (glucose) to be certain the child is absorbing nutrients. If a stool tests positive for glucose on a Clinistix test or has an acid pH (less than 5.5), it suggests that carbohydrates are not being absorbed.

Evaluate how well the infant sucks or is able to take food from the spoon and swallow. Record any symptoms such as pulling up the legs or crying after eating that would suggest gastrointestinal discomfort.

Nurture the Child. Because children with failure to thrive are suffering from emotional deprivation, they need effective "parenting" from nurses who care for them. This does not mean that everyone who passes the crib should stop and play with them for a few minutes. It means that a member of the nursing team should be chosen to be the child's "parent" during the hospital stay (a primary nursing or case management pattern of assignment). It is important that this person be able to spend time with the child, rocking him, giving him a leisurely bath, talking to him, exposing him to toys, and "parenting" him rather than just giving routine care. Be certain that the person chosen for this role accepts the role and understands that interaction with the child must be active. Passive rocking without talking to a child or paying attention to him or her, for instance, may be no different than the parents' care (Figure 55-5).

Support and Encourage the Parents. Encourage parents of children with failure to thrive to visit as much as possible—without encouragement, these parents may visit little or not at all. When they do visit, they should feed the child if they wish and interact with him or her as they choose. People cannot change their emotional feelings about other people overnight. Telling them that they ought to pick up the baby more or hold him or her more while feeding is ineffective and may only increase the parents' feelings of inadequacy. Giving some sug-

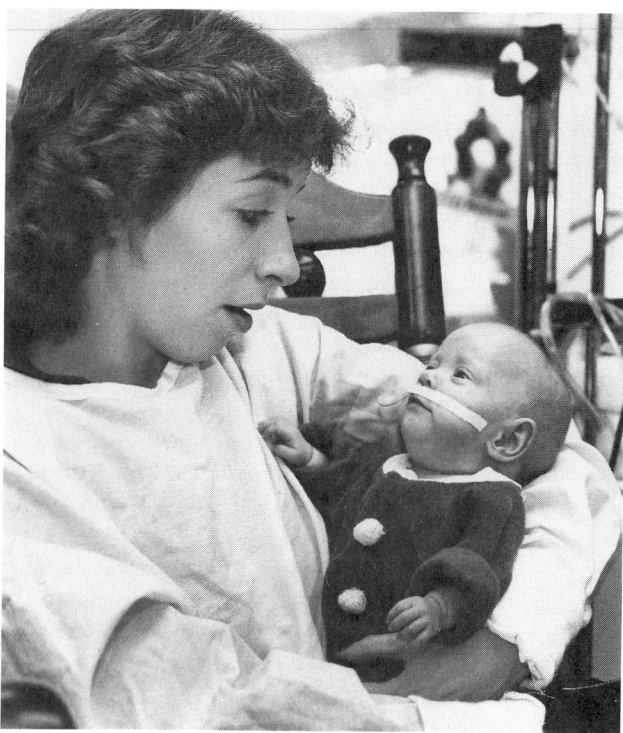

FIGURE 55-5
The child with failure to thrive should have a primary nurse assigned for care so that the child can enjoy a close attachment. (Courtesy of the Department of Medical Photography, Children's Hospital, Buffalo, NY.)

gestions about how the baby tries to communicate with them might be more effective. "Do you know what I think he's trying to say when he stops sucking like that? I think he's saying he's ready to be burped." Pointing out the infant's ability to respond to the parent may be helpful. "Look how he turns his head at the sound of your voice. He recognizes you."

Occasionally, a parent is so distraught by such factors as the illness or death of an older child or relative that they are simply unaware of how much of their energy and thought are being drained by these events. These parents quickly can become good parents to a deprived child as soon as they realize what has been happening. More often, however, the disturbance in a parent-child interaction began so long before or is so great that a parenting bond cannot be established at this point. If the infant is discharged with the parents, parents will need effective follow-up in the months to come to see that they maintain parenting at an acceptable level. There is a very thin line between the child who fails to thrive and one who is abused. Some of these children need to be placed in foster homes for their own safety and to ensure that they receive adequate care.

Evaluation and Follow-Up. Failure to thrive is easy to correct from a physiologic standpoint. When given proper food in a caring environment, the infant usually gains weight rapidly. Adequate follow-up to ensure that the emotional needs as well as the physical needs continue to be met is a much bigger problem—so big that the answer to the problem of infants who fail to thrive lies not in treatment but in prevention. Women who may be high risk for poor mothering need to be identified during pregnancy so they can have close follow-up in the postnatal period. At health maintenance visits, secure careful, thoughtful pregnancy histories to elicit information about the psychosocial events that could lead to mothering breakdown. Some mothers may need "respite" care for their children when they are overwhelmed by the task of mothering. They may need extended counseling to prevent mothering breakdown. Nurses can be instrumental persons in all phases of this care.

Sexual Abuse

Sexual abuse may be broadly defined as any sexual contact between children and adults. It involves the coercion of dependent, developmentally immature children and adolescents in sexual activities that they do not fully comprehend, to which they are unable to give informed consent, or that violate the social taboos of family roles (Helfer & Kempe, 1987). There may be as many as 360,000 cases of sexual abuse a year in the United States. Although the victim is usually female, the reporting of male abuse is increasing.

Sexual abuse is physically and emotionally destructive in that it leaves children unable to trust others, with a sense of ambivalence to intimacy and an overall sense of worthlessness. It should be suspected when a very young girl is pregnant (Boyer & Fine, 1992). Children should be taught at an early age that their bodies are their own and to report anyone who tries to touch them in a way they do not like (Figure 55-6; see the Focus on Family Teaching box).

Molestation

Molestation is sexual involvement such as oral–genital contact, genital fondling and viewing, or masturbation.

A **pedophile** is an adult who seeks out children for sexual gratification. In contrast to a rapist, whose crime is violent, the pedophile may be very gentle and limit the involvement to molestation. Such a person is usually a man who suffered sexual abuse himself as a child and repeatedly selects children who are of the same age at which his abuse occurred as victims (Greenberg et al., 1993). The relationship may involve people with either homosexual or heterosexual orientations. Many pedophiles take photos or videotapes of their activities with children to use for sexual gratification at a later date.

Rehabilitation of pedophiles is difficult because they are fixated emotionally at a childhood level (seeing themselves as children, they do not perceive relationships with children as wrong). Listen carefully to children who report that someone enjoys photographing

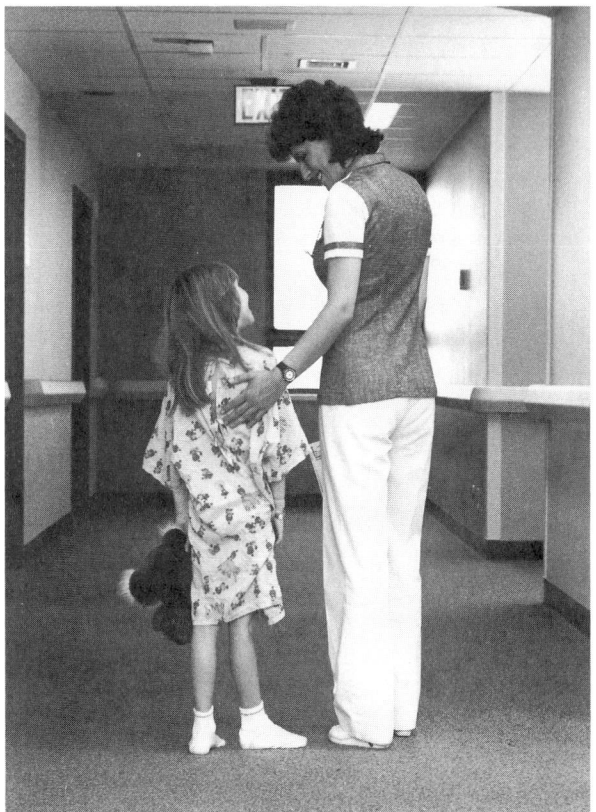

FIGURE 55-6
Teach children that their bodies are their own, and that they have to give permission before anyone can touch them. (Courtesy of the Department of Medical Photography, Children's Hospital, Buffalo, NY.)

them; ask children to describe what they mean by someone "touching" or "feeling" them to detect this type of abuse.

Incest

Incest is sexual activity between family members. It often involves an older male and a young girl, although it may involve an older female and younger male, brother or sister, or same-sex partners. It may involve foster, adopted, and stepchildren. Incest is a deviation from the norm and is so strongly viewed as such by most people that incest taboos are common to most cultures.

Incest usually occurs when a father dominates women in the family to such an extent that his wife finds condoning the incestuous relationship better than opposing him. Another situation is for a father to be submissive to a dominating wife. He then finds gratification in relating to a child (Crivillae, 1990). Although mothers in such instances often report that they knew nothing about the father–daughter relationship, it is highly unlikely that they did not suspect something was occurring. Some women even take themselves away from home in the evenings to allow the incest convenient time and space to happen.

Q. Every parent worries about the possibility of sexual abuse happening to his or her child. What are signs a parent should look for to detect if this is happening?

A. Signs of sexual abuse can be subtle. Common findings that it is occurring are:

- A child verbally reports sexual activity with an adult.
- A child has an awareness of sex that is beyond age expectations.
- A child engages in sexual expression with dolls.
- A child under 15 years old is pregnant.
- A child has perineal, vaginal, or anal inflammation or fissures.
- Symptoms of increased anxiety, such as sleep disturbance, development of tics, nail biting, or stuttering are present.
- A child has a change in school performance, develops a school phobia, or is truant.
- A child expresses fear of being left alone with a certain adult.
- A child develops vague abdominal pain or acting-out behavior.

Incest causes a great deal of guilt and loss of self-esteem in both the abusing and the abused persons—the abuser because he is aware that this act is not culturally approved yet he seems unable to end the relationship; the victim because she recognizes this act as wrong yet is unable to resist the older person's advances.

Assessment. The number of reported incidents of sexual abuse represents only a small portion of the actual number (Muram, 1993). Sexual abuse may be revealed on health history (e.g., a young girl worrying that she is pregnant); it may be revealed by a child's abnormal anxiety for a mother to return home from a hospitalization or anxiety on being left with a male in the family. Young girls who are submitted to this type of relationship often feel extremely low self-esteem and may envision that they are so "bad" that they deserve to be treated this way.

Allowing young children to play with anatomically correct dolls is a common way of determining whether or not sexual abuse is occurring (Everson & Boat, 1994). Use of such dolls is controversial as there is a concern that without a common protocol for their use, overinterpretation of the child's actions could result. The average reaction of a preschooler or young school-age child who has not been abused is to undress the dolls, giggle for a moment or two about how they look, and then redress or put them aside. The child who is involved in an incestuous relationship makes the dolls perform a sexual act, such as placing the male doll's penis in the female doll's mouth. Asking the child to draw a picture of what happened may also be an effective way of revealing abuse.

Abuse should be investigated in young girls who are seen for pubic lice or sexually transmitted diseases. Other physical indications are vaginal bleeding, urinary tract infection, and poor anal sphincter tone. Examining the girl in a knee–chest position may best reveal torn hymen fragments (Irons, 1993).

Therapeutic Management. Sexual abuse, like physical abuse, is required to be reported. The perpetrator will then be interviewed by the police as this is a criminal offense. It is important that this information be collected in such a way that the adult's rights are respected and the testimony is therefore admissible in court.

Both the adult and child involved in a sexual abuse relationship need psychological counseling—the child to improve self-esteem and the adult to channel sexual expression to less destructive outlets. Improvement is most apt to occur if parents can admit that the abuse has been occurring. To improve the child's self-esteem, it is important that the adult in the relationship admit the fault is all his. Follow-up care is best done by one of the people who sees the child initially so that he or she does not have to recount the incident to strangers again and again. Whether therapy for sexually transmitted diseases or protection against pregnancy needs to be initiated should be considered. Sexual abuse may be contributing to the spread of HIV infection (Zierler et al., 1991).

Parents may need as much counseling as the child, so that they can help the child to work through feelings about this situation. In many instances, the offender is a family member such as an uncle, stepfather, or older brother. Often the relationship has been going on for some time before it is reported. This is a particularly difficult situation to deal with, because the parents may feel guilty that they allowed the family member sufficiently easy access to the child or did not listen to the child's protestations that she did not like to be alone with this family member. If incest involves the father, it may be extremely difficult for the parents to continue to relate to each other effectively enough to help the child. All children should be taught some simple rules to help them avoid sexual abuse (see Box 32-1 in Chapter 32).

Rape

Rape is sexual activity that occurs under actual or threatened force of one person by another. *Forcible rape* is defined legally in most states as intercourse or penetration of a body orifice by a penis or other object. *Statutory rape* is sexual activity with a person under the age of consent (in most states, under 18 years of age) and is considered to have occurred in spite of the apparent willingness of the underage person. *Sexual assault* is used to refer to other forced sexual acts, such as oral–genital or anal–genital intrusion.

A growing phenomenon being reported today is "date rape," in which a man forces a date or casual friend into having coitus despite her voiced unwillingness. It may be very difficult for the victim of date rape to find a sympathetic ear as her companion insists he meant no harm: he simply didn't believe her (ACOG, 1993).

Both rape and sexual assault represent deviant behavior—acts of violence, not passion. They lack the components of privacy and mutual consent, which are elements of "normal" sexual behavior. Both rape and sexual assault are degrading and dehumanizing and leave the victim feeling completely helpless. Because adolescent girls are the most frequent victims of rape, they should be informed about ways to prevent rape (including date rape) (see Box 33-4 in Chapter 33).

Rape has become a crime of growing incidence over the last decade, although it is difficult to determine its actual incidence because so many rapes are unreported. It is believed, however, that the incidence of rape may be as high as one woman in five. Many women want to avoid the secondary, but no less severe, trauma associated with reporting rape, including social stigmatization and insensitive treatment by police. It is hoped that in the future more sensitive treatment, both socially and professionally, will help to narrow this gap so that more victims of rape can receive the immediate treatment and follow-up care so essential to a complete recovery.

The average rape victim is an adolescent girl, although victims can be any age, and they can be male. In more than half of reported rapes, the rapist is a stranger to the victim, although rapists frequently commit the act in the neighborhood in which they reside. Based on arrest data, the average rapist is a young adult male with a background of aggressive behavior. His motivation generally relates to expression of power or anger; sexual satisfaction does *not* appear to be a dominant motive. An excessive amount of alcohol intake often precedes rape. Rape tends to be a repetitive, planned activity rather than an isolated event.

Assessment

Many rape victims demonstrate immediate physical and emotional symptoms that can last for weeks. The symptoms describe what has been termed **rape trauma syndrome** and generally occur in two stages: disorganization and reorganization. In the immediate **disorganization phase**, the victim feels a combination of humiliation, shame and guilt, embarrassment, anger, and

vengefulness. She feels her life completely disrupted by the crisis and her inability to protect herself from the assault. She may tremble from fear and may be in great pain from perineal lacerations. She is apt to start visibly at the sound of anyone approaching or touching her. She needs gentle, sympathetic support people with her in the days following the event to allow her to feel safe. She may have nightmares of the attack occurring again. This immediate stage of disruption and disorganization generally lasts about 3 days.

The second stage of rape trauma syndrome, termed **reorganization**, may last for months or years. Many rape victims continue to report recurring nightmares, perhaps sexual dysfunction, and continuing inability to relate to men or face new and surprising situations. They may continue to have a great deal of difficulty discussing the rape. Many rape victims, trying to outlive this personal offense, change their residence at great sacrifice to finances and lifestyle. If not offered constructive counsel, victims may still feel guilt or shame when thinking about the rape as long as 20 to 30 years later.

When victims do not report rape and thus receive no counseling, symptoms indicative of **silent rape syndrome** can result. When the subject of rape is mentioned, people with silent rape syndrome may grow increasingly emotionally disturbed; it may be evident in their history that they altered their behavior toward men at a certain point in life and perhaps began to resist actions such as going outside or being alone in a house after that time. This can be devastating to their ability to maintain employment or remain independent. They need counseling as much as the person who reported a rape.

Emergency Care

Although most large city police forces have special officers assigned to investigate rape charges, a victim can be confused and further traumatized by police officers who imply that she provoked the attack or could have at least done more to resist or prevent it. This increases the victim's feeling of shame and degradation. It may be especially harmful to the adolescent as people she has been taught to respect have no concept of the degree of fright she has experienced or the strength of her attacker. Health care providers generally are the second group of people a victim sees following an attack, and they need to be extremely cautious that they do not show any of the same callous behavior.

Most health care agencies where many rape victims are seen have a rape trauma team with specially educated counselors to talk to the victim immediately following the rape and to offer long-term counseling as needed. Nurses serve as important members of such teams and may provide primary care following rape (Ledray & Arndt, 1994). Any nurse should be able to offer emergency support, as it might be a long time before a specifically designated staff member arrives, nor are such services available in every community.

Because rape is a crime, the hospital chart of a rape victim is often displayed as part of a court procedure. For the victim to bring charges against her attacker, she needs to have information concerning her appearance and her history detailed in the hospital chart, so it is important that statements in a chart are accurate and unbiased. In recording a history, quote the woman's exact words whenever possible. Describe her physical appearance carefully, including the presence and location of injuries such as bruises, lacerations, teeth marks, or abrasions and the condition of her clothing. Ask if she bathed or washed before coming for care as this can obscure evidence and obliterate the presence of sperm. Ask if she was menstruating or using a tampon. The force of penis penetration with rape can cause a tampon to tear through the posterior vaginal wall into the abdominal cavity, causing an extreme loss of blood. Photographs should be taken as necessary to document the extent of injuries. Any clothing that is ripped or stained should be considered to be evidence of violent assault and so not discarded.

Following this preliminary observation, a gynecologic examination will be done to evaluate the physical condition of the victim and to document that rape occurred. This is done by recording the existence of any vaginal or perineal lacerations and aspiration of sperm or acid phosphate from the vagina. Acid phosphate is a substance that is not normally present in vaginal secretions but is present in semen. The presence of acid phosphate is extremely important if the male is infertile or sterile, where sperm may not be present. Its presence is the best proof that rape occurred. A vaginal culture for gonorrhea and a Pap test are also taken. Blood will be drawn for a pregnancy test and a VDRL for syphilis. Prophylactic administration of antibiotics against gonorrhea and syphilis will be given. If the woman is not menstruating, she may be begun on oral contraceptives to avoid pregnancy. She may have a baseline blood sample drawn for HIV status.

Be certain during emergency care to offer privacy. There are many people who may want to ask the victim questions, including police officers or detectives, the victim's family, a rape trauma team, and the examining physician or nurse practitioner. Describing the experience is good, but lack of privacy during a perineal examination or when she is with her important support person demonstrates little more concern for her self-esteem than her attacker provided. Many victims are uncomfortable with a male physician examining them after rape as they are temporarily fearful of men. It is helpful if a female nurse remains with the victim during this time, although a male nurse can be equally supportive as it is not the male-female contrast that a victim is seeking as much as an aggression versus caring contrast. Table 55-2 summarizes common tests and procedures for emergency care of rape victims.

Table 55-2. *Common Specimen Procedures Following Rape**

Procedure	Purpose
Oral washing	Client rinses mouth with 5 mL sterile water; collected in test tube. Analyzed for blood group antigens or sperm of attacker.
Fingernail scraping	Scrape under all of client's fingernails and place scrapings in envelope. Analyzed for blood, skin, and clothing fibers of attacker.
Blood VDRL, HIV and HBsAg	Draw blood for antibody titer for syphilis, human immunodeficiency virus, and hepatitis B.
Blood typing	Client's blood is typed to differentiate it from attacker's type.
Pregnancy test	Either blood or a urine specimen may be obtained. Vaginal examination should be completed before woman voids.
Hair samples	Both scalp and pubic hairs of client (about 10) are removed for comparison with attacker's and placed in envelope.
Vaginal smear	Vagina is swabbed with dry applicator and smeared onto slide. Allow to dry for analysis of sperm.
Gonococcus smear	Cervix, vagina, rectum are cultured (also throat is cultured if oral coitus was attempted).
Vaginal washing	5 mL of sterile saline is placed in vagina and aspirated. Analyzed to detect sperm and acid phosphate.
Skin washings	Touch any dried stain of blood or semen on skin or clothing with a moistened cotton swab; drop into test tube. Analyzed for attacker's blood and semen.
Clothing care	Place any clothing stained or torn into a paper bag. Evidence of violent attack.

*Label all specimens carefully as to where they were obtained for medical therapy and legal evidence.

Legal Considerations

Nurses working in emergency departments may be asked to testify in court as to the victim's appearance following the assault, although the documentation in the chart is generally all that is necessary. Many victims, especially adolescents, do not press charges against their assailants because they were too frightened at the time to observe his appearance (or he was masked), so they are unable to identify him later or they are afraid that by naming him in court he will return and kill them. Whether the victim follows through with a legal action or not is her choice, but the incidence of rape might be reduced if rapists were aware that they are not apt to escape without a penalty for their crime. Taking the rapist to court may be the opportunity and appropriate time for the victim to "fight back" and so in the end not be as helpless as she was at the time of the actual attack.

Nursing Diagnoses and Related Interventions

Nursing Diagnosis: Rape trauma syndrome related to recent rape

Goal: Victim will demonstrate adequate coping behavior and, eventually, return to precrisis level of functioning.

Outcome Criteria: Victim is able to discuss what happened to her and her intense feelings about the crime; voices she can go forward with her life.

One of the major needs of any accident victim following a violent act is to talk about what happened. A person who can describe an incident begins to "put a fence around" or "contain" the event. This process brings the event down from "something terrible has happened to me," a situation that leaves a person with a continuing high anxiety level, to "this specific thing has happened to me," a situation that allows the traumatic event to be examined and dealt with. Something that is concrete and describable is rarely as frightening as "something out there." This also applies to rape.

Ask the victim to describe the incident to you with an introduction such as, "Most people find it helps to talk about what happened to them." Table 55-3 lists areas to explore with victims to help them reduce the incident to a size they can begin to work through.

Victims should be given the number of a counseling service to telephone before they leave the emergency department. As genital bruising may not be apparent until 24 hours after the rape, they may be asked to return for a reexamination the next day so this can be documented. Syphilis will not be apparent for up to 6 weeks

Table 55-3. *Areas to Explore in Rape Counseling*

Area	Considerations
The event	Where did the attack occur? What was happening at the time? This information is important for the victim to discuss and work through; otherwise, any time she is in similar circumstances again, she may have uncontrollable fears related to the attack. Walking home from school or waiting for an elevator in a public building are everyday actions that she will do often during her life. If she was raped in these circumstances, she can be assured that she was acting sensibly and that the rape was not her fault.
The assailant	Allowing an adolescent to review the description of the rapist may help her to realize that she may react in negative ways in the future to a man with the same build or description. The man may have approached her with a simple gesture, such as a hand on her shoulder. Others will perform this gesture again. She must work through her revulsion to handle it when it occurs in friendly circumstances.
The conversation	Describing the conversation with the rapist helps the adolescent to convince herself that she did not provoke the attack.
Details of the assault	Describing the actual assault is extremely difficult for most adolescents, but doing so allows them to work through it. Until they can describe the attack or the sexual act to which they had to submit, they may have difficulty in performing these same acts with persons of their choice.
Resistance to the assault	Many adolescents do not struggle during an assault because they realize that it could result in further harm to them. If someone asks them what they did to try to fight off the assailant, adolescents may feel again that they provoked or agreed to the attack. Reassure them that no action was probably the best action and the reason they are still alive. To improve self-esteem, counsel adolescents that rape is a violent crime and that usually the strength of an attacker is far too great for any female to resist effectively.

in serum, so they should return for a repeat VDRL at that time. They may be advised to return in 6 weeks for HIV testing. Be certain that victims have a support person to accompany them home and they are aware that if their distress becomes acute, they can return as needed to the health care facility for additional care or counseling. Inform them about any local support groups that may provide follow-up counseling for victims of rape. One such organization, Women Against Rape, is active in many communities.

> ***Nursing Diagnosis:*** Ineffective family coping, disabling, related to recent rape of family member
>
> ***Goal:*** Victim's partner and family will develop adequate coping mechanisms to be able to support victim.
>
> ***Outcome Criteria:*** Partner or other family members are able to express their feelings about the rape to health care provider; state confidence in their ability to support rape victim.

In many instances of rape of a woman, the victim's usual sexual partner has difficulty being a support person to her because he has as much difficulty dealing with the occurrence of rape as she does. Not too infrequently, a relationship that was meaningful before the rape will deteriorate as a result of a sexual partner seeing the victim as now "soiled" or mistakenly believing that the victim was somehow responsible for the trauma or actually enjoyed the experience. In other instances, a usual sexual partner may become so overprotective following the incident (not allowing the victim to go out alone any longer, checking on her constantly) that she is not free to maintain her identity. The man may be so filled with vengefulness and anger that he cannot effectively relate to her without his anger surfacing toward her as well as toward the attacker. Parents of a young adolescent may feel this same way. Counseling for the victim's partner or family may help them to be truly supportive (Box 55-3).

Domestic Abuse

As many as 30% of women seen in emergency departments for trauma have been battered. Like child abuse, this transcends all ethnic and social groups. If it appears to be more prevalent in the lower socioeconomic classes, it is because families at this level are more visible to service organizations and law enforcement officials. When wife battering occurs in middle or upper class houses, wives are often too embarrassed to let people know and keep the violence hidden longer.

Theories About Domestic Abuse

Violent marriages can be divided into two groups: those in which violence preceded the marriage and those in which the violence developed within the marriage. In the first and most frequently appearing group, violence is brought into the marriage by a man with a history of violence. His violence-prone characteristics usually erupt early in the courtship and grow progressively worse. He uses violence to handle any conflict and provokes a pervasive feeling of powerlessness in people around him. Such men usually have a history of early and prolonged exposure to family violence as children; alcohol is frequently associated with the expression of violence.

Women in this type of marriage react to their situation in three phases (Table 55-4). Wife abuse generally begins with a light level of abuse (stage I); during this first or *impact phase,* the woman uses denial as a defense mechanism. If the woman does not end the relationship at this point, abuse grows more frequent and more violent (by not stopping it, the woman is indirectly giving it permission to continue). During this second stage, she can no longer deny the violence is occurring. At the same time she cannot stop it because the violence is not provoked by her; she is only a convenient recipient of poorly controlled violent behavior. She is forced to use coping mechanisms such as becoming very obedient and cooperative, doing everything her husband wishes in a desperate effort to reduce the violence. This phase is termed *psychological infantilism* or **learned helplessness**. The level of abuse can continue until the woman is being almost constantly physically abused (stage III). A fetus is in danger if abuse of a pregnant woman is at stage II or III (Ribe et al., 1993). During this stage, the woman is forced to become more and more isolated; she sinks into hopelessness and depression; she has difficulty seeking help because she is unable to believe that outside people might want to help her.

For women in the second group of marriages, violence occurs as a last resort when all other attempts at communication have failed. In these marriages, the behavior of one partner threatens the psychological defenses of the other and each projects his or her feelings and shortcomings onto the other. Such a situation, however, is not typical of spouse abuse. In most instances, battered women marry husbands who bring violence into the marriage.

Assessment

Asking about the possibility of spouse abuse should be a priority with any woman seen for trauma and if child abuse has been identified in a family. Common injuries suffered by abused women are burns, lacerations, bruises, and head injury. Asking all women at physical

Box 55-3
Goals of Crisis Intervention for Families of Rape Victims

- Helping the family to openly express their immediate feelings in response to a rape as a shared life crisis
- Helping the family to be supportive of and reassuring to the victim
- Helping the family work through immediate practical matters and initiate problem-solving techniques
- Helping the family develop cognitive understanding of what the rape experience actually means to the victim and to the family
- Explaining the possibility of future psychologic and somatic symptoms that characterize a rape trauma syndrome and what the family can do to minimize these symptoms
- Activating qualities characteristic of healthy family functioning during the impact and resolution phases of the shared crisis
- Educating the family about rape as a *violent crime*, not a sexually motivated act, and eliminating focus on the victim's guilt or responsibility
- Eliminating the family's sense of guilt for not protecting the victim by assuring them that they could not have anticipated or prevented the rape
- Discouraging violent, destructive, or irrational retribution toward the rapist (under the guise of being on the victim's behalf) by encouraging a sharing of feelings of helplessness, sadness, hurt, and anger
- Encouraging discussion of the sexual relationship between partners; suggesting that the man let the victim know (a) that his feelings have not changed (when this is true) and that he still sexually desires her, (b) that he will wait for her to approach him, and (c) that sex therapy is available if they have difficulties that persist and want assistance in re-establishing normal sexual relations
- Explaining the possibility of sexually transmitted disease and pregnancy that may result from a rape, the preventive care necessary for the victim and spouse or boyfriend, and the follow-up care indicated

- Explaining that early crisis intervention often prevents long-term problems in resolving the crisis and that to seek counseling at this time does not imply mental illness (specify that crisis intervention usually lasts for 3 to 6 hours during the first few weeks post-rape)
- Referring the family for direct counseling when members' shared responses to the crisis interfere with their ability to cope adaptively
- Providing factual data, resource lists for counseling, and follow-up care *in writing* (because highly stressed persons do not hear or recall information verbally communicated)
- Letting families know that some decisions, such as whether to prosecute the rapist or move to a safer residence, can be postponed while more immediate needs, such as medical care, are taken care of. (This action helps the family (1) set priorities and organize decisions about what has to be done now, and (2) gain emotional distance from the urgency and confusion felt during a crisis state to permit sound decision making later.)
- Identifying how the family has handled crises in the past and encouraging members to use adaptive coping mechanisms for this crisis
- Encouraging contact with persons identified as supportive to the family and offering to contact such persons
- Assigning a primary nurse to spend time talking with the family in the emergency department waiting room while the victim receives medical care
- Allowing time for thoughts and feelings in a decision-making process
- Using empathic listening to convey understanding of the family's feelings and concerns
- Asking if the nurse can check back with the family the next day to see how they are getting along and answer any questions they may have

(Foley, T., & Davies, M. [1983]. *Rape: Nursing care of victims..* St. Louis: C. V. Mosby Company, p. 137; with permission.)

examinations to account for any bruise they have helps detect this (Furniss, 1993).

It is important that spouse abuse be identified because frequently, when a woman is abused, so are her children. Children raised in such a family learn that violence is an acceptable method of managing aggression and perpetuate it to the next generation. If abuse exists in a family, it may increase with pregnancy (Noel, 1992). Methods of assessing and caring for battered pregnant women are discussed in Chapter 14.

Therapeutic Management

An abused woman often feels that she is responsible for the abuse happening to her, that if she were a better person her partner would not resort to beating her. This sense of guilt helps to immobilize her. Because she may have no access to money and no skills to earn any, she needs a great deal of support to be able to leave the man. Even if she has a skill and has supported herself in the past, her self-esteem may be so low that she no

Table 55-4. *Levels of Wife Abuse*

Level	Description
I	Abuse is occasional; consists of slapping, punching, kicking, verbal abuse. Contusions occur
II	Abuse is becoming more frequent; beatings are sustained and cause fractures, such as a broken jaw or rib fracture
III	Abuse is even more frequent, perhaps daily. A weapon such as a gun, baseball bat, or broom handle may be used. Permanent disability or death from injuries such as intracranial hemorrhage or concussion may occur

longer believes she is able to put the skill to use. As the abuse becomes more violent, she may be afraid that the man will follow and kill her if she leaves. Other family members may be unwilling to shelter the woman for fear of being included in the man's violence.

It is important when caring for women who have been abused not to "blame the victim." Women are not beaten because of personality traits (hopelessness, powerlessness); instead, the dynamics of beatings have produced these traits in the woman (see the Focus on Nursing Care display). The fact that both spouse abuse and child abuse may exist in families strengthens the necessity for nursing care to be family-centered, so both these situations can be identified and halted.

Key Points

- At least 10% of children seen for traumatic injury received their injury from child abuse. A high suspicion for abuse should be present when burns, head injury, or rib fractures are present or when the history of the accident seems out of context for the injury.
- Child abuse may exist in many forms. It may be physical, emotional, or sexual, and may encompass neglect as well as abuse.
- In infants, a "shaken baby syndrome" results in retinal or intracranial hemorrhage. Babies with this syndrome may appear groggy or unresponsive in an emergency department.
- A triad of a "special parent, special child, special situation" is characteristic of the family in which child abuse occurs.
- Failure to thrive is a syndrome in which an infant falls below the third percentile for weight and height on a standard growth chart. It is associated with a disturbance in the parent–child relationship.
- Children who comfort parents in emergency settings may just be sensitive children or they may be

demonstrating "role reversal," a behavior characteristic of abused children.
- In families where a child is abused, the mother may also be a victim of abuse. Ask enough questions at health care visits to be certain that this problem does not exist as well.
- Child abuse is legally reportable. Nurses can initiate reporting as an independent action or through their health agency's referral network.
- Methods to prevent abuse that nurses can actively participate in include teaching about the expected growth and development of children, educating teenage parents for parenting roles, and teaching "empowerment," or a sense that children have control of their own lives.

FOCUS ON NURSING CARE

Promoting Health in the Abusive Family

1. At least 10% of children seen for trauma injury received their injury from child abuse. A high suspicion for abuse should be present when burns, head injury, or rib fractures are present or when the history of the accident seems out of context for the injury.

2. In infants, a "shaken baby syndrome" results in retinal or intracranial hemorrhage. Babies with this syndrome may appear groggy or unresponsive in an emergency department.

3. Children who comfort parents in emergency settings may just be abnormally sensitive children or they may be demonstrating "role reversal," a behavior characteristic of abused children.

4. In families where a child is abused, the mother may also be a victim of abuse. Ask enough questions at health care visits to be certain that this doesn't exist as well.

5. Child abuse is legally reportable. Nurses can initiate reporting as an independent action or through their health agency's referral network.

6. Methods to prevent abuse that nurses can actively participate in include teaching about the expected growth and development of children, educating teenage parents for parenting roles, and teaching "empowerment," or a sense that people have control of their own lives.

7. Sexual abuse of children can be prevented by teaching children to recognize abnormal advances and to know it is right to speak out about wrongs against them.

8. Abuse is a family, not an individual, problem. Therapy must include all family members to be effective.

- Sexual abuse of children can be prevented by teaching children to recognize abnormal advances and to know it is right to speak out about wrongs against them.
- Abuse is a family, not an individual, problem. Therapy must include all family members to be effective.

Critical Thinking Exercises

1. You weigh a baby at a well child conference and discover that the infant's weight is below the second percentile on a standardized growth chart. What questions would you want to ask the mother to see if you can account for this? What particular areas would you want to assess on a physical exam?
2. You are working in an emergency room and a father brings in a 2-year-old because he cannot move his arm. An x-ray shows the humerus to be broken. You notice in the chart that the child has been seen twice before, once for an ulnar fracture and once for a scald burn on his hand. The resident in charge of the emergency room dismisses the injuries as "typical of boys." What would be your action if you believe that there is suspicion of child abuse? What would be your legal responsibility?
3. Tanya is a 4-year-old who is seen in an ambulatory clinic for a purulent vulvovaginitis. A culture reveals this is from gonorrhea. What questions would you want to ask Tanya to determine how she contracted this? Suppose her parents are influential people in your community. Would this influence what questions you ask?

References

American College of Obstetricians and Gynecologists. (1993). Adolescent date rape. *International Journal of Gynaecology and Obstetrics, 42*, 209.

Blouin, A. M. (1993). Munchausen syndrome: A test of clinical reasoning. *Journal of Emergency Nursing, 19*, 513.

Boyer, D., & Fine, D. (1992). Sexual abuse as a factor in adolescent pregnancy and child maltreatment. *Family Planning Perspectives, 24*, 4.

Brassard, M. R. (1993). The psychological maltreatment rating scales. *Child Abuse and Neglect, 17*, 715.

Crivillae, A. (1990). Child physical and sexual abuse: The roles of sadism and sexuality. *Child Abuse and Neglect, 14*, 121.

Department of Health and Human Services. (1991). *Healthy people 2000.* Washington, DC: Public Health Service.

Devlin, B. K., & Reynolds, E. (1994). Child abuse: How to recognize it, how to intervene. *American Journal of Nursing, 94*, 26.

Everson, M. D., & Boat, B. W. (1994). Putting the anatomical doll controversy in perspective: An examination of the major uses and criticism of the dolls in child sexual abuse evaluations. *Child Abuse and Neglect, 18*, 113.

Flaherty, E. G., & Weiss, H. (1990). Medical evaluation of abused and neglected children. *American Journal of Diseases of Children, 144*, 330.

Furniss, K. K. (1993). Screening for abuse in the clinical setting. *AWHONNS Clinical Issues in Perinatal & Women's Health Nursing, 4*, 402.

Geissler, E. M. (1994). *Pocket guide to cultural assessment.* St. Louis: C. V. Mosby.

Greenberg, D. M., et al. (1993). A comparison of sexual victimization in the childhoods of pedophiles and hebephiles. *Journal of Forensic Sciences, 38*, 432.

Helfer, R. E., & Kempe, R. S. (1987). *The battered child.* Chicago: University of Chicago Press.

Irons, T. G. (1993). Documenting sexual abuse of a child. *Emergency Medicine, 25*, 56.

Johnson, C. F., et al. (1990). The hand as a target organ in child abuse. *Clinical Pediatrics, 29*, 66.

Ledray, L. E., & Arndt, S. (1994). Examining the sexual assault victim: A new model for nursing care. *Psychosocial Nursing and Mental Health, 32*, 7.

Lewis, D. O., et al. (1991). A follow-up of female delinquents: Maternal contributions to the perpetuation of deviance. *Journal of the American Academy of Child and Adolescent Psychiatry, 30*, 197.

Lobo, M. L., et al. (1993). Failure to thrive: A parent–infant interaction perspective. *Journal of Pediatric Nursing, 7*, 251.

Mellick, L. B., & Reesor, K. (1990). Spiral tibial fractures of children: A commonly accidental spiral long bone fracture. *American Journal of Emergency Medicine, 8*, 234.

Muram, D. (1993). Child sexual abuse. *Current Opinion in Obstetrics and Gynecology, 5*, 784.

Noel, N. L., et al. (1992). Domestic violence; the pregnant battered woman. *Nursing Clinics of North America, 27*, 871.

Powers, J. L., et al. (1990). Maltreatment among runaway and homeless youth. *Child Abuse and Neglect, 14*, 87.

Rhodes, A. M. (1990). Legal alternatives for fetal injury. *MCN: American Journal of Maternal Child Nursing, 15*, 111.

Ribe, J. K., et al. (1993). Blows to the maternal abdomen causing fetal demise: Report of three cases and a review of the literature. *Journal of Forensic Sciences, 38*, 1092.

Rowan, A. B., et al. (1994). Posttraumatic stress disorder in a clinical sample of adults sexually abused as children. *Child Abuse and Neglect, 18*, 51.

Spaide, R. F., et al. (1990). Shaken baby syndrome. *American Family Physician, 41*, 1145.

Zierler, S., et al. (1991). Adult survivors of childhood sexual abuse and subsequent risk of HIV infection. *American Journal of Public Health, 81*, 572.

Suggested Readings

Alexander, R., et al. (1990). Serial abuse in children who are shaken. *American Journal of Diseases of Children, 144*, 58.

Bourne, R., et al. (1993). When you suspect child abuse. *Patient Care, 27*, 22.

Else, L., et al. (1993). Personality characteristics of men who physically abuse women. *Hospital and Community Psychiatry, 44*, 54.

Hutchings, P. S., & Dutton, M. A. (1993). Sexual assault history in a community mental health center clinical population. *Community Mental Health Journal, 29*, 59.

Kitzinger, J. V. (1992). Counteracting, not reenacting, the violation of women's bodies: The challenge of perinatal caregivers. *Birth, 19*, 219.

Leonard, C. H., et al. (1990). Effect of medical and social risk factors on outcome of prematurity and very low birth weight. *Journal of Pediatrics, 116*, 620.

McCann, J. B., et al. (1994). Eating habits and attitudes of mothers of children with non-organic failure to thrive. *Archives of Disease in Childhood, 70*, 234.

Rhodes, A. M. (1993). Family violence. *MCN: American Journal of Maternal Child Nursing, 18*, 73.

Sadler, F., et al. (1992). Early identification of children at risk for child abuse and intervention. *Journal of Home Health Care Practice, 5*, 43.

Snyder, J. A. (1994). Emergency department protocols for domestic violence. *Journal of Emergency Nursing, 20*, 65.

Sullivan, C. A., et al. (1991). Munchausen syndrome by proxy: 1990. A portent for problems? *Clinical Pediatrics, 30*, 112.

Swett, C., et al. (1990). Sexual and physical abuse histories and psychiatric symptoms among male psychiatric outpatients. *American Journal of Psychiatry, 147*, 632.

Chapter 56

Nursing Care of the Family Coping With Long-Term or Fatal Illness

Key Terms

- anticipatory grief
- death
- grief process
- vulnerable children

Objectives

After mastering the contents of this chapter, you should be able to:

1. Describe common concerns of parents of children with a long-term or fatal illness.

2. Assess adjustment of the child and family with a long-term or fatal illness.

3. Formulate nursing diagnoses for the child with a long-term or fatal illness.

4. Plan nursing care for the child with a long-term or fatal illness such as planning for respite care.

5. Implement nursing care for the child with a long-term or fatal illness such as supporting a family through a period of acute grief.

6. Evaluate outcome criteria to be certain that nursing goals established for care were achieved.

7. Identify National Health Goals related to children with long-term or fatal illnesses that nurses could be instrumental in helping the nation achieve.

8. Identify areas related to care of the child with a long-term or fatal illness that could benefit from additional nursing research.

9. Use critical thinking to analyze ways that nursing care of the child with a long-term or fatal illness can be more family centered.

10. Synthesize knowledge of long-term and fatal illness in children with nursing process to achieve quality maternal and child health nursing care.

Adele Pillitteri: MATERNAL AND CHILD HEALTH NURSING, 2nd Edition. © 1995 Adele Pillitteri.

When children have acute illnesses, parents and the children themselves may be frightened by the sudden onset and severity of symptoms. Because human beings have a great capacity for coping with stress, however, they can usually adjust to the strain of disrupted daily routines, hospital visits, and caring for children as long as they are given adequate support.

When an illness becomes long term or is one that will ultimately have a fatal outcome, a family's capacity to cope can be stretched beyond its limits. Support is essential for the family to survive under this level of pressure and stress.

People cope with situations depending on their perception of the event, the type and kind of support they receive from people around them, and the ways that they have found successful in coping with stressful situations in the past. In working with parents of children with a long-term or fatal illness, discovering how the parents perceive the problem, what resources they have available to them, and how they plan to use these resources are crucial in planning nursing care.

Whether the medical diagnosis involves a permanent disability or impending death, a parent's first response will be a grief reaction: the parent has either lost the "perfect" child imagined during the pregnancy or the normal child he or she had up to the time of diagnosis. Depending on their age and maturity, children, too, may also respond with a grief response. National Health Goals related to care of the child with a long-term or

fatal illness are shown in the Focus on National Health Goals box.

⊠ **NURSING PROCESS OVERVIEW**
for Care of the Family Coping
With a Long-Term or Fatal Illness

ASSESSMENT

Because assessment of a family's coping abilities is best made not by a few quick contacts with a child and the family but gradually, over a period of many contacts, nurses' assessments of the degree of coping are often the most thorough and meaningful.

Observing children at home where they are most comfortable, or at school in a familiar atmosphere, often reveals a great deal more about their coping potential than a formal test situation does. Often a toy offered by a parent, sister, or brother will be grasped and manipulated by a child with a chronic disability; the same toy offered by a stranger will not be accepted. Children with a long-term illness, on the whole, have probably been through many tests and procedures in the diagnosis of their disorder; they may have reason to think of health care providers as hurting people, not people they achieve for. It may be possible to change their perception by maintaining a reassuring, gentle manner during assessment and subsequent care procedures.

NURSING DIAGNOSIS

Chronic illness takes many forms. A condition such as diabetes that requires daily attention (insulin injections) but that is stabilized may not be as stressful to parents as an illness such as muscular dystrophy, which slowly progresses in severity. In the former, although the child and family must adjust their lifestyle to incorporate the child's daily needs, they feel they have some control over the course of the illness and the child's overall health. In the latter, the child and family can feel powerless, lacking any ability to alter the course of the disease. They must simply wait for the next acute crisis to develop. Nursing diagnoses for both children with long-term and those with fatal illnesses should address both the child and the family as a whole. Some examples of nursing diagnoses when a long-term illness is present are:

- Altered family processes related to recent diagnosis of chronic illness in older child
- Ineffective family coping: compromised, related to child's disability
- Ineffective family coping: disabling, related to parents' inability to accept child's chronic illness
- Grieving related to child's chronic illness
- High risk for altered growth and development related to lack of age-appropriate stimulation because of disability

New issues develop when the child's disorder is considered terminal. The family must learn to accept not only the child's illness but also its fatal outcome. Some examples of nursing diagnoses when a fatal illness is present are:

- Hopelessness related to progression of child's disease
- Anticipatory grieving related to child's terminal illness
- Powerlessness related to inability to prolong child's life
- Decisional conflict related to treatment options and choice of setting for child's care

PLANNING

Be certain in planning care that goals established are realistic. You probably cannot alter the course of a child's illness, but you can help parents cope with the illness or impending death and aftermath.

Parents who have not yet accepted the seriousness of their child's illness may be inclined to make plans for a child that the child cannot possibly carry out. These parents are holding on to the hope that their child will eventually be cured or restored to full health. Sometimes this level of denial is essential to the parent's ability to cope with the child's daily needs and the needs of the rest of the family. Perhaps they feel they must shield the child or other family members from the truth. Focusing on goals that are hopeful but realistic, such as hope that the child will go through the day without experiencing pain or that their child will learn how to move about independently in a wheelchair, are the types of aims that

---

FOCUS ON
National Health Goals

Chronic illness in children is a major cost to the nation as well as individual families because it has the potential to reduce the earning power and contribution of future citizens. A number of National Health Goals address this. These are:

- Reduce to no more than 8% the proportion of people who experience a limitation in major activity due to chronic conditions from a baseline of 9.4%.
- Achieve for all disadvantaged children and children with disabilities access to high quality and developmentally appropriate preschool programs that help prepare children for school, thereby improving their prospects with regard to school performance, problem behaviors, and mental and physical health from a baseline of 47%.
- Reduce the death rate for children by 15% to no more than 28/100,000 children aged 1 to 14 and for infants by approximately 30% to no more than 7/1000 live births from baselines of 33/100,000 and 10.1/1000.
- Reduce the death rate for adolescents and young adults by 15% to no more than 85/100,000 people aged 15 through 24 from a baseline of 99.9/100,000 (DHHS, 1991).

Nurses can be instrumental in helping the nation achieve these goals by educating women to seek care for themselves during pregnancy so congenital anomalies are reduced and seeking immunizations for their children so diseases which can lead to long disability such as rubeola and meningitis can be prevented. Nursing research on the following areas would further these goals: What are special techniques for preparing children with multiple disabilities for surgery? How can children confined to wheelchairs maintain a high sense of self-esteem? What are the specific measures that are most helpful to parents at birth when they learn their child has been born with a disability?

move a family forward toward final, realistic acceptance of the child's illness.

Organizations that are helpful for referral are:

Candlelighters Childhood Cancer Foundation
7910 Woodmont Avenue
Suite 460
Bethesda, MD 20814

Helping Other Parents in Normal Grieving
Sparrow Hospital
1215 East Michigan Avenue
P.O. Box 30480
Lansing, MI 48909

IMPLEMENTATION

When children have a chronic or fatal illness, parents may begin to overprotect them so much that they neglect to encourage their growth. They may forget to provide play materials appropriate for their age or other forms of age-appropriate stimulation. Helping parents to look at their child's capabilities and arranging appropriate activities for him or her facilitates parents' acceptance of the diagnosis and the road ahead.

Helping parents to encourage their child's advancement toward developmental milestones is important. Suggestions for achieving developmental milestones are discussed with each age group in earlier chapters.

Teaching parents ways to remember to give medication over a number of years, ways to maintain quality care without becoming exhausted, and the importance of maintaining a lifestyle of their own are other important measures.

EVALUATION

Children with chronic or terminal illness need periodic follow-up care since plans made when children are newborns may no longer be suitable at 4 years of age. Plans made in the early school years may need to be modified by the time children are 12 years old. In addition to follow-up of their specific illnesses, children also need child health maintenance care. If a specialty clinic a child attends does not offer comprehensive health care, it must be obtained from an additional health care source. Otherwise, children are well protected from the complications of a special illness but unprotected from common childhood illnesses that could be even more devastating.

Evaluation of whether goals of care for the family of a child who died were met or not helps to strengthen your planning with the next dying child you care for, improve your self-esteem, and build confidence in your ability to care for dying children. Evaluation will reveal discrepancies between the wish and the reality of care, identifying areas you need to strengthen to grow as a health care provider. Some examples of outcome criteria that might be established are:

- Parents state realistic plans for their child regarding school placement.
- Parents state they have been able to deal with their grief over child's diagnosis to maintain normal family functioning.
- Child states she is aware illness is chronic but thinks of herself as a person able to accomplish many things in life.

The Child With a Disability or Chronic Illness

Family Adjustment

Because families have different resources and everyone reacts to situations differently, each family of a child with a long-term disability needs to be assessed as to its potential for providing necessary care (Figure 56-1). Through such assessment, appropriate interventions to help the family adapt can be started early in the course of the illness. Certain circumstances appear to increase parents' difficulty in adjusting to a disabling or long-term illness in their child. These are the degree and timing of the disability, the ages of the parents, and the availability of support people.

Degree of Disability

The seriousness of a disability obviously affects the ability of parents to adjust. A child who needs total care will require much more radical readjustment of parents' lives than will a child who only needs additional speech therapy for an hour a day. In most instances, parents' perception of the child's disability is as important as the child's condition itself. A parent who envisioned a son as someday being an Olympic runner, for example, may

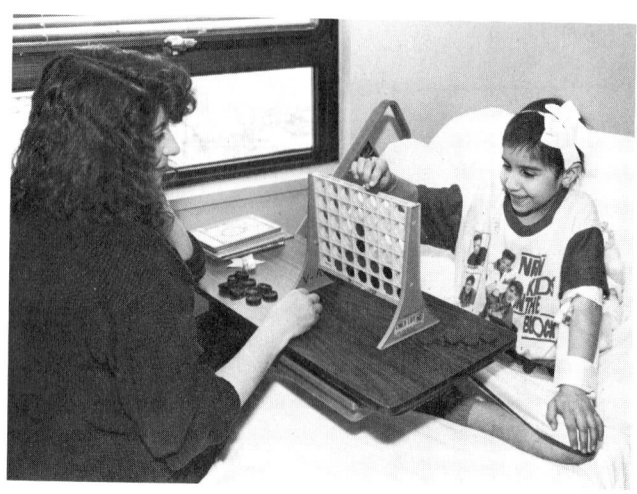

FIGURE 56-1
Urge parents to continue to care for children with long-term illnesses so that parent–child attachment is not broken. (Courtesy of the Department of Medical Photography, Children's Hospital, Buffalo, NY.)

perceive a son with subluxated hip as having a serious disability. A parent whose mental image of the child is that of a lawyer doing mainly desk work may not view the hip problem as a serious illness.

Many parents are not aware of the mental image that they carry of their child, an image that began to form the moment the woman realized she was pregnant. Hidden desires are often revealed if you ask parents, "If things could have been different, what kind of person would you have liked your child to be?" A parent who answers, "a kind person" can still have that wish fulfilled, no matter what the degree of disability. A parent who says "I always assumed my child would take over my business some day" may have some major mental adjusting to do.

Whether the disability is noticeable (spastic cerebral palsy) or not noticeable (controlled seizures) can make a difference in how parents adjust to the illness. A mother who takes her child with cerebral palsy shopping (a child who walks unsteadily and knocks over a display) may hear other shoppers say, "Wouldn't you think a mother would watch her child more carefully?" On days that her child wears long leg braces, however, shoppers' comments are more apt to be "Poor little thing. Isn't it wonderful that his mother brings him shopping with her?" She is happy to have signals (leg braces) that announce her child is different and cannot be held to standards for other children. Other parents might be more grateful that a child's disability is not a visible one—it makes the illness easier for them to accept.

Onset of the Illness

Whether a condition is apparent at birth (e.g., a myelomeningocele) or occurs at a later time (the child is struck by a car at 4 years of age) may make a difference in parents' ability to adjust. For most parents, never having had a well child makes the child's illness easier to accept.

Effect of Parental Age

Young parents may have more difficulty caring for a disabled child than older, more experienced parents because all phases of parenting are more difficult for them. Because of inexperience, young parents could have difficulty evaluating how much activity a child needs or what toys are appropriate. On the other hand, young parents may be more flexible than older parents. A young parent who has just this one child may have more time to spend in a daily exercise program than does a parent with five other children older than the affected child.

Availability of Support People

The family who has few close friends and lives some distance from relatives is apt to have more difficulty adjusting to illness in a child than will the family that has support people close by. People who have secondary support systems in the community, such as an organiza-

tion for parents of disabled children or a local church or synagogue, usually do better than parents without these resources. People who are able to use health care resources effectively adjust more easily than those who are not able to do so. Ability to use health care resources depends on a number of factors: the availability of transportation (you cannot take a child in a 50-lb cast on a bus); whether the parent speaks the same language as health care providers (it is frustrating to go for care and be unable to make your needs known); the financial situation and insurance coverage (it is frustrating to be told you need to see a specialist when you have no money to pay for one); and how helpful health care providers have been in the past. If the best advice that has been given the parents up to this point has been, "Take him home and treat him as near normally as possible," parents may not see health care providers as a source of useful information or help.

Life Events

A child's disability generally appears to be more acute at times the child would normally reach developmental milestones: at 12 months, when he should be taking his first step and is not (the baby book has a special page for a photograph of the child walking; the page in this child's book will remain blank); at 6 years, when she should begin school (she has already been going to a special preschool program for 4 years); first communion or Bar Mitzvah; time for a driving license; or voting age. When the child does not reach these milestones, parents are reminded of the disability in a particularly painful way.

Factors that indicate that a family will probably be able to adjust to caring for a disabled child are summarized in Table 56-1.

Grief Reaction

Parents can be expected to experience a **grief process** or regulated steps in grieving when they are told their child will be disabled or is fatally ill (Kübler-Ross, 1969). Table 56-2 summarizes the stages of a grief reaction. Most parents with a disabled child never arrive at a full stage of acceptance; for parents with a fatally ill child, this may come only with the child's death.

During the first period of grief (shock or denial), parents are unable to plan past short-term goals (learning to change a dressing or which pills to give each day). Trying to establish long-term goals at this point (what type of school the child will attend, the vocations that are open to him or her) is useless because it all must be done again when parents are truly ready to look this far ahead. During the stage of anger, parents may be unwilling to learn (the whole thing is so unfair; planning is asking too much of them; how can they trust you? If you were really helpful, you would cure their child). This is a time of waiting also, of holding back advice until par-

Table 56-1. *Factors That Make It Easier for Parents to Adjust to a Child's Handicap*

Factor	Rationale
Support persons are available.	Caring for a child is a series of crises during which support people become very important.
A strong marital bond exists between the parents.	A marriage partner can serve as the strongest support person.
A good relationship exists between the child's parents and their parents.	The parents (because they had good care) have a firm sense of trust and the ability to give care to another.
The handicapped child is other than the first-born.	The parents have had practice parenting.
The family lives close to shopping, schools, and transportation.	The family is not isolated.
The family has a strong religious faith.	Secondary support systems are important in times of stress.
The parents were told of the child's disability as soon as possible.	Handicap is easier to accept if parents never thought of the child as totally well.

(Modified from Battle, C. U. [1975]. Chronic physical disease: Behavioral aspects. *Pediatric Clinics of North America, 22*, 525.)

ents are more ready to accept it. During the bargaining stage of grief, parents are still not ready for planning. If their bargain is fulfilled (let their child be able to walk, and they will spend the rest of their life doing good), the plans they make now would have to be modified later.

During the next stage of grief—that is, depression—parents are ready to make plans but need a great deal of help in planning. Be careful in working with people who are depressed that you do not totally plan for them rather than with them. Many parents of disabled children have low self-esteem (they believe if they were really good people, they would have had a normal child). This makes them feel that your suggestions must be better than any they could make. After they return home, however, they are the people who must live with these plans and so should participate in making them. Young adults with disabilities show an above-average incidence of depression, probably from the chronic stress of the disability on their life, part of which occurs from poor planning (Turner & Beiser, 1990).

Some parents need guidance in making plans to prevent them from becoming so self-sacrificing that they ignore the needs and wishes of a marriage partner and other children (they will spend every waking moment with the ill child). Being a martyr is a way of easing guilt, a part of grief bargaining, a way of proving that

Table 56-2. *Stages of Grief*

Stage	Parents' Reaction	Description
1	Denial	Parents have difficulty realizing what has occurred. They ask, "How could this have happened?"
2	Anger	Parents react to the injustice of being singled out this way. They say, "It isn't fair this is happening."
3	Bargaining	Parents attempt to work out a "deal" to buy their way out of the situation. They say, "If my child gets well, I'll devote the rest of my life to doing good."
4	Depression	Parents begin to face what is happening. They feel sad and unprotected.
5	Acceptance	Acceptance is being able to say, "Yes, this is happening, and it is all right it is happening." With mental retardation or long-term illness, parents may never reach this stage but will always remain in the chronic sorrow of the depression stage.

(Modified from Kübler-Ross, E. [1969]. *On death and dying.* New York: Macmillan; with permission.)

they are equal to others—perhaps even the best parents in the entire world. These parents need time to talk about possible reasons why they feel they must push themselves in this manner. Perhaps this will help them find a middle-of-the-road approach to a child's care that allows time for all family members.

Siblings of disabled or fatally ill children need to be considered in plans as well (Williams et al., 1993). They almost automatically take second place (at least they feel that way) to the child who needs more care than they do; they are asked to assume more household chores than normally. Helping parents to reserve an hour a day that totally belongs to other children (playing a table game or walking in the park with them; teaching a child to sew) helps other children accept it better when parents must spend a great deal of time with the sick child. Parents may need a respite from the care of a sick child, such as an evening out while a baby sitter cares for the child. They may need to be reminded that siblings may need respite, too.

By the time a disabled child is of school age, parents should begin to make some concrete plans as to who will care for the child when they die. This is very difficult for parents; it asks them to contemplate their own death (something that people rarely want to do) and the vulnerability of children when it occurs. They might consult with family members about guardianship and with a lawyer to help them write a will that will provide future caretaking and economic support for the disabled child.

The Nurse and the Chronically Ill or Disabled Child

To help parents of children with a chronic illness, it is important to be familiar with the child's condition and the possible complications that could occur (Hutton, 1994). Over a period of years, parents become experts on the care of a child with a particular condition. This makes them apt to grow impatient with health care providers who appear to be unaware of things that they know. When children are admitted to a hospital for care, review with parents on admission their typical way of carrying out a procedure so that you can continue to care for their child in the same way the child is used to. On the other hand, be available to show a mother an easier way to do something if it seems appropriate. Frankly admitting to parents, "You're more familiar with the care of Jennifer than I am; you'll have to teach me some things," is a refreshing approach and not only allows parents to feel confidence in you (you are honest) but also increases their self-esteem (they are knowledgeable people).

It is also important to be familiar with community resources for disabled children in order to be of help to parents. Advising parents to see a dentist who special-

izes in caring for children with cerebral palsy when there is no one of that description less than 200 miles away not only is not helpful advice but is actually destructive. It raises expectations in parents that cannot be met—accentuating, not solving, a problem.

Sometimes parents of disabled children do not comply well with instructions or keep health care appointments consistently. This failure to comply usually is related to their adjustment to the illness. As long as denial, anger, bargaining, or depression is functioning (and there is rarely a parent who has successfully moved completely through these stages of grief to acceptance), coming for health care or evaluation is a major demand on parents. Each visit is more of a reminder of the child's illness than a time of reassuring health assessment.

Developmental Tasks

Children with disabilities often do not meet developmental milestones on schedule; achieving developmental tasks can be very difficult. When you are helping parents teach a child with a disability a developmental task, such as toilet training or using a spoon, it is good for them to break the task down into its component parts (reach for the spoon, grasp it, move it toward you, lift it, push it under the chosen food, lift it toward the mouth, etc.). This allows parents to appreciate that they are asking the child to do not a simple task but one that encompasses 20 or more coordinated motions. Helping them learn this technique allows them to be patient in teaching not only this task but all tasks in future years.

Caring for a chronically ill child is never easy. Support from interested health care personnel at all stages of the process is of great importance to the parents' acceptance of their child's illness. Ways to help children with disabilities achieve developmental tasks are discussed in Chapters 29 to 33. These include exposing them to normal events during a hospitalization (Figure 56-2).

Education

Children with a long-term disability often need provision for special education programs or at least for special hours of individualized instruction. Most of these children benefit from preschool programs, which may need adjustment to accommodate them (Crowley, 1990). They miss school more often than do their classmates in a normal school setting because of hospitalization or health supervision visits and so are likely to fall behind unless special plans to keep them with their school group are made. By federal law (Public Law 99-457, Education of the Handicapped Amendment), a school system must provide educational opportunities in the least structured setting possible beginning with preschool. You may have to be a strong child advocate to see that the best educational program available is being provided for a child (Sexson & Madan-Swain, 1993).

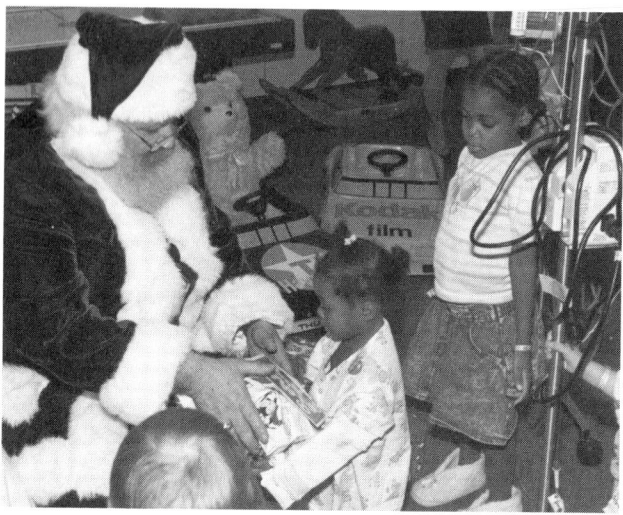

FIGURE 56-2

Helping children with long-term illnesses keep active and in touch with usual events during hospitalizations helps them meet developmental goals. (Courtesy of the Department of Medical Photography, Children's Hospital, Buffalo, NY.)

Home Care

Most children with a chronic illness are cared for at home today; planning for this care is discussed in Chapter 38. Caring not only for the disabled child but also for siblings must be discussed. Ways to involve the family in community activities are also important. Children as young as preschool age are aware that a disabled child is "different" and may not choose him or her as a playmate (see the Focus on Nursing Research box). Some chronically ill children are latchkey children (see Chapter 32) after school; assessing whether this poses problems for care is important (Holaday et al., 1993).

FOCUS ON NURSING RESEARCH

How Much Do Children With Cancer Know About Their Own Impending Death?

For this study, staff members who cared for children with progressive malignant disorders were asked to evaluate how much 31 children over 3 years of age and their families had discussed the child's pending death. In this small sample, the approach of death was mutually acknowledged in only 6 families (19%). Although it is generally suggested that the topic of death be mutually discussed by parents and children, in actual practice this occurs only rarely. Nurses could be helpful to families by broaching the subject with them and asking if they need help with the task.

Goldman, A., & Christie, D. (1993). Children with cancer talk about their own death with their families. *Pediatric Hematology and Oncology, 10,* 223.

The Child Who Is Terminally Ill

Caring for a dying child is one of the hardest tasks in nursing. Most people are raised to accept the fact that elderly people die—but they have also lived a long life. Most people can accept the death of middle-aged people with the same philosophy—they experienced at least a portion of their life. It is often more difficult to accept the death of children because they have had so little opportunity to live. It can be so difficult to work though your own feelings about a child's dying that you have difficulty caring for the child or supporting the parents.

Parental Grief Responses

Each parent reacts in a unique way to the diagnosis of terminal illness in a child (Brice, 1991). Being aware of the usual grief response that occurs in anticipation of the child's death helps in recognizing their response as grief and supporting them through this very difficult period.

Denial

A parent's usual reaction to a diagnosis of fatal illness in a child is denial, the first stage of grief (see Table 56-2). Although people are aware that children die, most proceed through life thinking, "it will not happen to my child." When it does, they respond with disbelief or denial. The likelihood of this response is enhanced by the fact that many fatal illnesses, such as brain tumor or leukemia, begin very insidiously. ("How can a few black-and-blue marks on a child's arms be the symptoms of a potentially fatal disease?")

How the parents handle this initial disbelief has a great deal to do with their relationship with health care personnel. If they have trusted health care personnel up to this point, they may be able to accept a diagnosis without questioning any further. If they do not have this relationship, they may feel the need to obtain a second diagnosis. This often involves considerable expense, but for many parents it is a necessary step in moving past this first reaction. Parents who feel a need for a third, fourth, or fifth opinion may be having an unusually difficult time resolving a "surely not me" response. They need a factual explanation of why it is certain their child has this disease, such as a copy of the blood report or the pathologist's biopsy report. They need time to talk about how they feel. Only when people can grasp that the illness is definitely present can they begin to accept that the child's disease will ultimately prove fatal.

During a stage of denial, parents' actions may be inappropriate to the child's condition. They may talk of an "upset stomach from the flu" when the child is vomiting blood or "his cold" when the child has cystic fibrosis. It is easy to view such denial as a step that should be hurried (parents cannot begin to deal with the problem as long as they deny that there is a problem). This is true, but neither can they deal with a problem when it hurts as much as this does. Denial is a temporary pain reliever and is a necessary step on the way to acceptance.

Anger

Parents can be expected to enter a stage of anger soon: a change from "Surely not me" to "It's not right that it's happening to me." When parents are angry about a diagnosis, they may be unable to direct their anger appropriately. They may find themselves angry with the child (scolding him or her for crying during a painful procedure). One parent may be angry with the other parent (criticizing him for reckless driving or for eating a fattening food for lunch). They may be angry with you (for not answering the child's light immediately). They may be angry with the medical, x-ray, laboratory, and dietary staff or with the entire health care delivery system. It can be difficult to react to this kind of angry attack because it seems unjustified (after all, you came as soon as you could). Be certain that your first reaction is not to be angry in return. This could result in your staying away from the child's room for the rest of the day, resisting being submitted to that kind of unfair criticism again, and therefore not meeting the child's basic need to have support people around him or her.

A more therapeutic reaction is to accept this angry response as the stage of grief that it is and respond accordingly: "I'm sorry it seemed to take me so long to answer your call bell, but you seem angry about more than just the light. Would it help to talk about it?"

Parents' reaction to the anticipated death of a child will depend to a great extent on their experience with death in the past and the meaning of this child to them. Because grandparents live longer and longer today, for some parents fatal illness in a child is their first contact with death. Another influencing factor is that different children mean different things to parents. A child born to them at a happy time in life can represent all that is good and happy in their life. Loss of this child could also mean loss of all the joy the child represents.

When you ask grieving parents to talk, therefore, they may talk not about the child at all but about how they felt when a parent died, how hard their job is for them, or how they feel their marriage is failing. This is part of grief: gathering resources, reworking stress from the past, arming themselves to face stress in the near future. Parents often receive support from other parents on the hospital unit whose children also are terminally ill in order to cope. They are helped by seeing parents of other children adjusting to approaching death—or if not adjusting, at least functioning in what passes for a normal manner.

Bargaining

Bargaining is an intermediate step in grief, a time when parents try to correct what is happening by making a bargain to be better persons (a change from "This isn't right" to "I can make it right.") They vow to be better people or function in a different way in exchange for their child's life. When parents realize that bargaining is ineffective, they are at a very low point: they have been let down not only by health care providers but also by the superior power with whom they tried to bargain. They may need more support when bargaining fails than at any other point.

Depression

When parents have passed through stages of denial, anger, and bargaining, a further step occurs: developing awareness of the true meaning of what is happening, with accompanying depression. This is a change from "I can make it happen" to "It is happening." An emotion such as crying is the most common sign that this stage has been reached. Parents may ask more questions about care, procedures, or medications than before. Be careful that you do not interpret this questioning as criticism. Parents are asking why a child must have a constant intravenous infusion in place not to criticize care but because this is the first time they are fully aware of its serious implication.

Parents may work through the expected loss of a child by talking about their plans for the child, the kind of child he or she was, or how the child was doing in school. They may suddenly shower him or her with expensive gifts or trips. They may have a great deal of difficulty leaving the child after visiting hours. On the surface, this reaction appears to be a step backward (they were accepting the diagnosis so well; now they seem demanding and overwhelmed by it). Actually, this is the first time they have actually begun to appreciate the diagnosis and what it means.

At about this stage, parents need to think about preparing other children in the family for the death of the sibling. Siblings may need to visit the dying child to be assured that death is not as frightening and horrible as they believed. If they are not allowed to visit, they may interpret this as proof that death is such a horrible sight that they are not allowed to be exposed to it rather than that visiting is against the hospital rules.

Some children feel responsible for the death of a sibling. They may have wished the child dead so that they could have a room all by themselves or so they could have her bicycle. They were told not to wrestle with him and they did anyway. These children need assurance that wishing for something does not make it come true and that the sibling's death is uncontrollable. It will happen no matter what they or their parents did or will do.

Acceptance

The acceptance stage of the grief process is resolution that the child will die (a change from "This is happening" to "It's all right this is happening"). Few parents reach this stage by the time of the child's death; grief work will need to continue for years past the time of the death.

Parental Coping Responses

Throughout the stages of grieving, parents will be developing important coping mechanisms to see them through this crisis. They may have already learned to cope positively with their child's illness and treatment measures, but the determination of death requires additional adjustments. Promoting the development of positive coping strategies while being sensitive to the unique needs of each family member is an important nursing responsibility. It may be difficult to determine when a coping strategy is truly helpful or when it has become maladaptive. For instance, seeking information is generally a very useful strategy of parents with ill children. Knowing what to expect reduces anxiety. Some parents, however, continue this procedure past the point at which information is helpful to them. They may believe that if they look hard enough, they'll discover a way to cure their child (prolonged denial), or they may "overintellectualize" their child's illness and impending death in an effort to block feelings of sadness.

Problem solving is always an effective coping strategy as long as parents are being realistic about which problems they can solve. Seeking and using the support of others, including health care providers and families with similar needs, is another positive strategy that the nurse can encourage by providing the names of support groups or individual families (with their permission) who have gone through similar experiences. The nurse may also need to help parents who are not comfortable accepting the help of others learn how to do so or simply learn how to feel comfortable expressing their feelings to others.

Parents may also be able to cope by searching for the meaning of their child's impending death in philosophical, spiritual, or religious terms. For these parents, body organ donation may be a meaningful way to give themselves some solace that their child will in some way live on.

Anticipatory Grief

If a child dies suddenly, the parents' grief response begins only with the actual death. Most parents, however, have some warning that death is expected and so begin a preparatory or **anticipatory grief** phase in which they gradually incorporate the reality of their child's fate into their thoughts. Such anticipatory mourning prepares parents for their child's death and saves them the abrupt, devastating, intolerable grief reaction that comes to parents whose child dies suddenly from trauma, such as a car accident, or from sudden infant death syndrome.

Although anticipatory grief does not shield the parents from experiencing renewed grief once their child has died, it can be a very useful process for them to work through. A danger of anticipatory grief is that a parent may reach the acceptance stage of the grief process too far in advance of the child's death. If this happens, parents may accept the child's death so thoroughly that they begin to treat the child as if he or she had already died. They stop visiting. When they do visit, they may spend most of their time visiting other children on the unit or sitting in the waiting room talking to other parents. When once they spent time comforting their child, now they may fail to rock or touch the child as much. They may "clean out" the child's room and throw or give away toys. Gradually they are drawing back from emotional attachment to shield themselves from the abrupt, stabbing pain that death will bring.

Children need a great deal of support if this happens, just as they did during the initial denial stage. Parents cannot help that the grief process did not time itself to coincide exactly with the child's death. They need understanding and not criticism for this reaction.

For some parents, when the child actually dies, the event may be anticlimactic. They have anticipated death so long that when it does occur, they cannot believe that it has actually happened. They may be so used to thinking constantly about their child's needs and having their child dependent on them that they do not know what to do. Some parents are reluctant to leave the hospital this final time. Leaving with the child's possessions is the step that will make the death real.

The Vulnerable Child Syndrome

When anticipatory grief proceeds so effectively that parents begin to think of a youngster as already dead and then the child does not die, parents may find that their grief reaction was so complete that they are unable to reverse it; they cannot view the child as they did before. They begin to treat him or her in a cold and unfeeling way—as if the child were not really there but did die. Such children are termed **vulnerable children** (Green & Solnit, 1964). They may develop behavior problems as they grow older (acting-out behavior such as temper tantrums, stealing in school, shoplifting as adolescents), as if to say, "Notice me: I am not dead." They require skilled counseling so that they can feel secure and learn to react effectively with others.

Children's Reactions to Death

When lifestyles were simpler and largely rural, death was accepted more commonly and comfortably than today because as children grew up on a farm they saw death as farm animals were slaughtered for food; they outlived cats, dogs, and chickens; they saw nests of field mice destroyed by plows or a dog. Families were often extended and so children watched family and friends gather to mourn when a family member died.

At the same time, children also saw new life: new crops, calves, and new chickens every spring. Birth, life, and death could be seen as cyclical changes that all would be experienced in their proper time.

Today, children reared in an inner city with no pets may have little or no exposure to death. Any family member who dies does so in a hospital; the rites of death are conducted at a funeral home from which the child is excluded. Death, therefore, can be a strange, frightening phenomenon to which they cannot relate or find comfort. Children's ability to understand death is shown in the Focus on Family Teaching box.

Infants and Toddlers

Infants and toddlers are certainly too young to appreciate death except as the loss of a person who cared for them and the presence of a void in their life. If such a loss interferes with the development of a sense of trust, its implications for the child's ability to achieve warm, close relationships could last a lifetime.

Preschoolers

Preschoolers learn about the concept of death when a pet dies or they discover a dead bird or mouse. They envision death as temporary, however, and appear to have little of the adult's fear of it. This casualness toward death is sometimes interpreted as callousness (the first response of a child who is told that his brother has just been killed in an automobile accident is to ask if he can have his brother's radio). This happens because he thinks of his brother as being gone only for a short time, making this a chance to take advantage of his property. This concept is strengthened by children's cartoons, in which characters frequently are killed and then immediately revive and go on with the story.

Because preschoolers fear separation greatly, they are stunned by the death of a parent. If a child grasps the concept that he himself is dying, his major worry might be that he will be alone and separated. He may need someone to stay with him constantly to assure him that he is not alone.

School-Agers

School-agers begin to have additional experience with death, so their knowledge of it as a final measure increases. They may think of it, however, as something that happens only to adults. Children's books deal only shallowly with the subject (Bowden, 1993). As children near the age of 8 or 9, they begin to appreciate that death is permanent. It is the same feeling they experienced when their parents left them at camp or went away for a weekend, but this time the separation will be permanent.

Most children of school age are aware of what is

FOCUS ON FAMILY TEACHING

Q. I'd like to talk to my child about the fact that he has a fatal illness. How old are children before they can grasp what death is?

A. Children's comprehension of death deepens as they grow older. Some general rules are:

• Infants undoubtedly have no understanding of their impending death. Important points for caring for an infant who is dying are to keep him or her comfortable and secure and to remain nearby to prevent loneliness and insecurity.

• Toddlers, likewise, do not understand death. Even though a close relative or friend may have died, they are unable to relate this with what is about to happen to them. Toddlers like routine, so allowing them opportunities to make choices and providing consistent care are the most important measures for them.

• Preschool children probably envision death as a long sleep. This makes them much more afraid of separation than of the thought of dying.

• Early school-age children understand death as separation but tend to view the separation as temporary. Over 9 years of age, children are able to realize that death is final. They still, however, are not as fearful of death as they are sad at the thought of being away from parents and frightened as to how they will manage without parents. Answer questions about death honestly (no one knows what it is really like but because it happens to everyone, it must not be anything to be fearful of). It is important to praise children for accomplishments to help them maintain their self-esteem so they can face this coming change.

• Adolescents have adult concerns and understanding of death. They may ask if it will be painful; they may feel angry over all that they will miss in life by dying. They may be concerned that they will need to answer for past ill deeds after death. Providing time and opportunities for them to ask and talk about death is important to help them work through a coming change. Allowing them to continue usual activities as much as possible helps them maintain self-esteem.

happening to them when their disorder has a fatal prognosis. They may learn from other children on the unit ("Are you the kid who's dying?"), from their parents' strange responses to questions, or from overhearing snatches of conversation about reports or physical findings. Most children are not as sad or afraid as adults are about facing death, however. Children, of necessity, meet new situations regularly—starting school, visiting a museum for the first time, boarding an airplane for the first time—and they cope with these experiences very well, as long as they know that someone they care about will be there to support them. Dying can be viewed in this same light as just another new experience for them. They are able to cope with it well if they know that there will be someone with them. If the parents become unable to relate to a child this age because of their grief, you will need to fill the gap (Figure 56-3).

Many children associate death with sleep (perhaps that was the explanation they were given for a grandparent's death) and so may be afraid to fall asleep without someone near them. They may need to have you sit with them while they fall asleep (if necessary, take patient charts to work on so you have the time to sit with them). The child may need the light left on (the better for you to work by) because he or she may associate death with darkness, not with naptime. Often the child who is dying is moved to the end of the hallway, away from the nurse's station. This frees the room for a child who needs frequent procedures (a justifiable move in terms of efficiency). Unfortunately, it may further isolate a child who needs support, as well as the child's parents, who also need your support and your presence nearby to face a hospital visit. Advocate as necessary for continued interaction with a child who is dying. Books about death to suggest for children to read are shown in Box 56-1.

Adolescents

Although adolescents have an adult concept of death, they also may feel immune to death. Driving at high

speeds and walking along the ledges of high cliffs reflect this judgment. They may deny symptoms for longer than usual because they believe it is impossible that anything serious could be happening to them. They appreciate time provided for discussion of how they view death and ways they contributed to their family even though they are dying young.

Environment for Death

The environment in which children die can influence their acceptance and their family's acceptance of death.

The Hospital

A few children who need a great deal of physical care (have a tracheotomy, require frequent blood gas determinations, need lung ventilation) may remain in a hospital for care because their family does not have the skill, energy, or money to care for them at home. In a hospital setting, be certain that visiting hours are extended to parents and other family members so that a child is not left alone when he or she needs people around the most. Be certain the child has opportunities to maintain contact with peers (see the Nursing Care Plan, p. 1778).

The Home

Most children today are not kept in the hospital past the time it is determined that therapy is no longer effective. Many families prefer that a child die at home surrounded by the family and familiar possessions rather than in a hospital. Time spent talking about arrangements—such as whom they should contact if the child suddenly becomes more ill than usual, how they will manage periodic check-ups, or how they will purchase medicine or supplies—is important preparation for home care. Assess how the family will schedule its time to have some leisure periods free so they can balance the care of the ill child in their lives.

Home care can be an extremely satisfying experience both for the child who is dying and for the family,

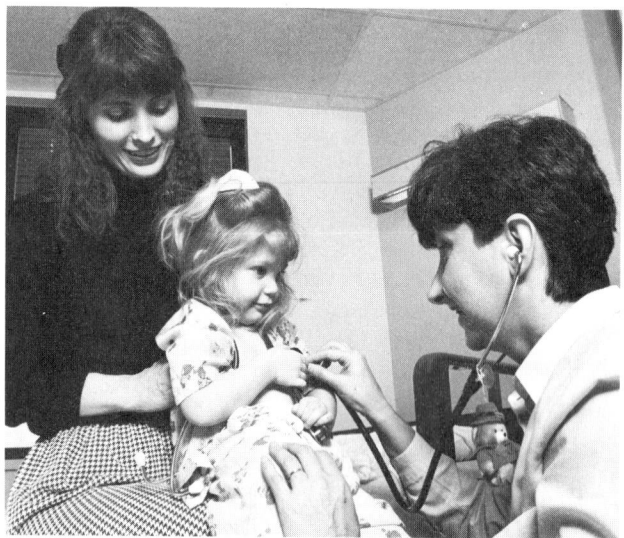

FIGURE 56-3
Primary nurse or one-to-one nursing relationships help children with long-term illnesses not to feel deserted. (Courtesy of the Department of Medical Photography, Children's Hospital, Buffalo, NY.)

as long as safeguards exist for protecting the caregivers' health as well as for providing good care for the child. This is discussed further in Chapter 38.

The Hospice

In 1967, St. Christopher's Hospice in London was opened as a facility for people who wanted to die in a homelike setting while still under skilled professional care. Most large communities today have similar hospice settings, although places for children are still not available in many communities. In a hospice, friends and family are allowed unlimited visiting; even younger children and pets can visit. Children are invited to bring those possessions that have importance to them. They are urged to choose the degree of pain relief they wish. Strong analgesia is often used to make a child pain free (a criticism of hospice care is that this level of analgesia slows respiratory rates and actually hurries death).

A basic philosophy of hospice care is that death is an extension or part of life, not a separate entity; thus, it can be dealt with—not with separate or awkward rituals but with the same warm concern as other situations in everyday life (Armstrong-Dailey, 1990).

Preparation for a Nursing Role With Dying Children and Their Families

Caring for dying clients can be an emotionally draining experience (Johnson, 1990). Although it is best that nursing assignments be consistent so a child has meaningful support, for everyone there is a point at which he or she may need a respite from caring for a certain child or help in offering support for the parents. This is not admitting weakness but recognizing humanness and a sense of compassion that interferes with client need. Humanness and compassion should be keystones of professional nursing; they are not qualities for which one needs to apologize.

Self-Awareness

Before you can offer support to children in any circumstance, you need to be aware of your own reactions and feelings. Thus, to offer support to a child who is dying, it is helpful to examine how you feel about caring for someone who is dying.

Fear. Fear is a natural response to death because the phenomenon is new and strange. To overcome this fear, put it into perspective. In nursing, you care for many people who have illnesses and experiences you will never have; thus, caring for people with experiences beyond your own is not really strange but almost routine in nursing.

People who have never seen someone die are often afraid that the moment of death will be terrifying to

watch. Death usually occurs gently, however, with body functioning just gradually lessening until it stops in a pain-free, quiet manner. People who have been declared dead and were then resuscitated by heroic measures report that death was not frightening but involved a feeling of exceptional calm and comfort; a number of people have said afterward that they wished they had been allowed to die rather than be called back to their body because death seemed so appealing (Dougherty, 1990).

Failure. Some health care professionals find themselves drawing back from care of dying children because death symbolizes failure to them. This can make children feel as if they have failed—they have not been able to keep their body from dying, despite everyone's best efforts.

Remind yourself that death is the ultimate outcome for everyone. At the point that death becomes unpreventable, the only failure that can exist is the failure of health care professionals to help a child achieve death with dignity and consideration and free of guilt that he or she has failed caregivers.

Grief

One of a person's greatest needs is intimacy and love, a feeling that someone cares and is concerned about him or her. In primitive times humans envisioned the heavens populated with many gods, probably from the need to be cared for and loved (if one god grew angry and ruined your grain crop, another would still love you). Nursing care is so intense that the relationship formed may be closer than you realize until the child is diagnosed as having a terminal illness or dies; only then do you feel the depth of the relationship (Whittam, 1993).

The grief that accompanies caring for dying children can be broken down into the same stages of grief experienced by the children themselves when they learn that they are dying.

Denial. There is a danger that a nurse who is in a stage of denial may care for children without mentioning that they have more than a simple illness. This includes omitting the use of such common expressions as "How are you this morning?" to avoid having to hear the answer. Denial may be so extensive that you avoid going into a child's room unless you have an important procedure to do. This is both confusing and lonely for children, because they miss the normal exchange of conversation and contact.

Nurses sometimes change professions following the loss of a child to whom they felt close because they are unwilling to submit themselves to that level of hurt again.

(*text continues on page 1780*)

Jennifer is an 8-year-old girl who is terminally ill with a diagnosis of brain tumor. The following is a nursing care plan devised for her.

Assessment: Frail-appearing 8-year-old, bald from the effects of radiation. Has vomiting if she sits upright. Weight plots at 10th percentile on growth scale. Child has periods of poor reactivity (Glasgow Coma Scale rating = 3). Is not able to get out of bed on her own. Is often found just staring into space. States she "knows she is dying" and is able to talk about it to grandmother. Parents cry at mention that child's condition is gradually deteriorating. Have not discussed possibility of Jennifer's death with younger siblings at home. Both parents openly critical of nursing care. Mother states that "poor care," both medical and nursing, is the reason child is not yet better.

Nursing Diagnosis: Altered nutrition, less than body requirements, related to malignant process

Defining Characteristic: Child's weight is at 10th percentile on standard growth chart.

Goal: Child will ingest by enteral tube an adequate caloric intake daily.

Outcome Criteria: Child maintains present weight; stomach residue remains under 10 mL before feedings; no diarrhea; urine output greater than 1 mL/kg/h; feedings of 1500 kcal daily absorbed.

Nursing Orders	Rationale
1. Administer enteral feedings by kangaroo pump of 500 mL in three feedings daily.	1. A pump allows for slow continual feedings to supply adequate calories daily.
2. Elevate head of bed to no more than 30 degrees during feeding.	2. Elevating head is important to prevent gastroesophageal reflux. Extreme elevation will initiate vomiting due to pressure changes in head; preventing vomiting is important to increase caloric intake and prevent aspiration.
3. Assess for stomach residue before feeding; return to stomach and reduce the amount of the feeding equal to the amount obtained.	3. Aspirating contents is an assessment for poor absorption; returning fluid prevents electrolyte loss through loss of stomach fluid.
4. Report stomach residual of over 20 mL to physician.	4. Stomach residual over 20 mL denotes poor absorption.
5. Assess intake and output; report urine output under 1/kg/h to physician.	5. This is assessment and documentation of normal urine output.
6. Make "mealtime" a social event by staying and talking to child during part of feeding.	6. Providing a pleasant atmosphere could increase intake and normalize feeding experience.

Nursing Diagnosis: High risk for altered skin integrity, related to sustained pressure on body parts secondary to limited ambulation

Defining Characteristic: Child is too weak to ambulate or move well on her own. Sustained pressure on body parts leads to loss of skin integrity.

Goal: Skin will remain intact during course of illness.

Outcome Criteria: No broken skin or erythema is present on body prominences.

(continued)

Nursing Orders	*Rationale*
1. Turn q2h.	1. Frequent turning is a method of decreasing continuous pressure on any one body part.
2. Massage body prominences following turning.	2. Massaging can increase circulation to body parts.
3. Lift out of bed to lounge chair daily; keep head of chair at less than 30-degree angle.	3. A change in position relieves consistent pressure; not elevating head prevents vomiting with position change.

Nursing Diagnosis: High risk for diversional activity deficit related to semiconscious state

Defining Characteristic: Child is often found doing nothing more than staring into space.

Goal: Child will demonstrate interest in herself and surroundings (including family) as long as physically possible.

Outcome Criteria: Child is oriented to time and place; completes at least one activity daily that offers stimulation; relates feelings of positive self-esteem.

Nursing Orders	*Rationale*
1. Speak to child to be certain she is awake and understands before touching.	1. Touching without warning is an uncomfortable type of stimulation.
2. Enjoys Simon and Garfunkel tape. Leave it playing for her during times she is alone. During times she doesn't respond well, play tape made by parents and siblings.	2. Listening to familiar sound provides stimulation.
3. Talk to Jennifer while giving care. When better, she liked to talk about "whale watching" she did last winter.	3. Conversation provides stimulation.
4. Turn bed toward window for optimal light.	4. Light can help with awareness of time of day.
5. Do not leave TV on in room as continuous background noise.	5. Continuous noise can result in overstimulation.
6. Read to child during AM and PM (favorite books: *Wizard of Oz* and *The Story of the Humpback Whale*).	6. Providing familiar activities can increase stimulation.

Nursing Diagnosis: Ineffective family coping: compromised, related to difficulty accepting daughter's diagnosis and expected outcome

Defining Characteristic: Parents state they are having difficulty preparing younger siblings; cannot discuss topic without crying.

Goal: Parents will demonstrate increased ability to cope with child's death by time of death.

Outcome Criteria: Parents state they are better prepared to face the expected outcome of their daughter's condition.

(continued)

Nursing Orders	*Rationale*
1. Encourage parents to discuss Jennifer's condition with medical staff.	1. Increasing parents' knowledge of child's condition can better help them focus on reality of situation.
2. Urge parents to attend a nursing staff meeting on Jennifer's care so they feel more a part of planning team.	2. Increasing parents' participation in care could increase self esteem and ability to cope with child's pending death.
3. Ask parents for suggestions on better positioning, stimulation activities, etc., at visits.	3. Increasing parent's participation in care could decrease sense of powerlessness in parents.
4. Ask parents if a secondary support group, such as the local chapter of Parents of Children with Cancer, or a minister would be helpful to them at this time.	4. Parents might benefit from additional spiritual and emotional support.
5. Urge parents to discuss feelings about child's condition. Be available to offer support as they begin to better grasp the meaning of the child's fatal prognosis.	5. Provides support to parents and helps them with acceptance of daughter's death.

Anger. Anger may be intense when a young child dies because the death seems so unfair. People who are angry have difficulty offering effective care. The person perceives himself or herself as giving thorough, comforting care, but you notice sharp, abrupt movements that are actually causing pain. Anger clouds judgment for decisions, such as which analgesic would be best to administer. Dying children cannot approach angry caregivers or ask questions; they are left alone and perhaps feel guilty that they have caused this anger. Anger is always destructive. Nurses may notice themselves making poor judgments in their personal lives (not following through on projects, spontaneous buying) because they carry this feeling of anger with them.

Bargaining. Caregivers begin to bargain for life the same as children themselves do. A statement such as "I hope that Tommy dies during the weekend while I'm off" is a bargaining statement. Statements of this kind are easy to overlook in your coworkers or yourself. Listening for them helps you to evaluate when a fellow worker is having difficulty caring for a particular patient and perhaps needs to change assignments. Hearing yourself say them should alert you that you are more involved with a child than you perhaps realize. You need to talk to someone about your feelings or ask for help. Remember that when bargaining fails, people reach their lowest point in grief. Recognizing bargaining statements in yourself helps you to be prepared for the depression that will follow.

Depression. Nurses who enter this phase may be ineffective caregivers, because depressed people are poor problem solvers (everything becomes a crisis). Nurses may make unwise decisions in their personal lives (drop out of a night school course, file for divorce, etc.) because they cannot effect good problem solving.

Depression is doubly destructive because when you are depressed, your reasoning processes are so slowed that you lose the ability to recognize that depression is the problem. When caring for a child who is expected to die, monitor your usual behavior to see if you are following your usual pattern. If irregularities occur (sleeping a great deal, not sleeping, loss of appetite), assess whether depression has overwhelmed you. When depressed, try to make no major decisions for at least a week to give your perspective time to change, or you may find later that you have made an irreversible decision.

Acceptance. The average person can reach a stage of acceptance in grief because he or she is subjected to few true losses in a lifetime. As a nurse on a unit where many terminally ill children come for care, you may find yourself facing loss or death over and over. Therefore, a stage of acceptance may never be reached. A caregiver who cannot reach a stage of acceptance is left in a stage of depression and cannot function.

To achieve a stage of acceptance, you may need to modify what it is you are accepting. You cannot accept the unfairness of death in children, but you can accept your ability to offer care that gives death dignity and compassion. Do not compensate for being unable to feel good by not feeling. This is a dangerous attitude because it also blocks your ability to feel happiness, love, and trust. You may need to ask for a temporary change of assignment to reestablish your perspective. You may need to concentrate on self-esteem therapy for yourself (doing something special for yourself, such as taking an evening for nothing but your own needs).

Caring for the Dying Child

A child may live for days, weeks, or even months in a "dying phase." Attentive physical and emotional care is essential to the child's maintaining a sense of security and positive self-esteem during this time. It is also essential to the grieving process for both the child and the child's family. Frequent and substantive communication is a major part of providing this care. Children, like their parents, need the opportunity to talk about their fears and feelings about death (Cohen, 1994). Practicing good communication skills when providing any care (e.g., when administering pain medication, starting intravenous lines, or providing basic comfort measures such as a bath) will help to establish a trusting relationship with a child, making her feel more comfortable about sharing her feelings with you (Figure 56-4). Box 56-2

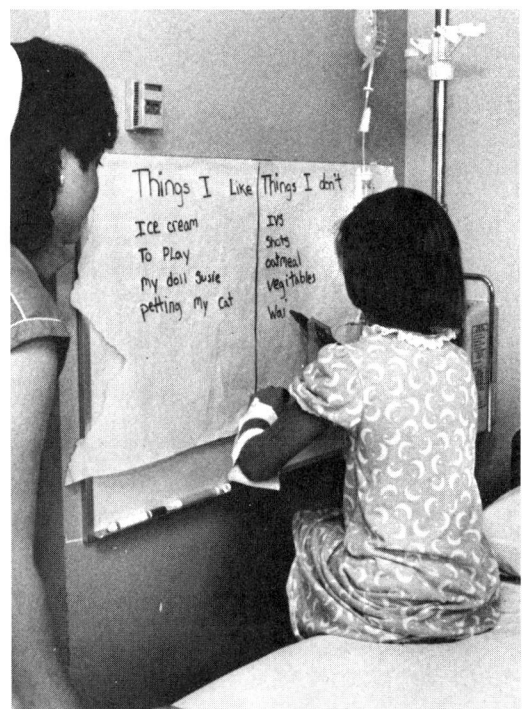

FIGURE 56-4
Helping children write out lists of what they like and don't like is a means of helping them express feelings. (Courtesy of the Department of Medical Photography, Children's Hospital, Buffalo, NY.)

1. Children who are dying need stimulation in as near normal a way as possible. Continue active conversation to provide this.

2. Use moments of silence therapeutically. Such moments occur normally just as speech occurs normally. Do not feel you have to chatter to fill quiet intervals.

3. Use the words *death* and *dying* as appropriate in conversation. Trying to avoid a word makes interchanges awkward. Statements such as "These flowers are dying," "That's a dead-end job," or "I'm dying to try that" may make it acceptable for the child you are caring for to voice for the first time what is happening to him or her—"I'm dying, too; let me tell you about dead-ending."

4. Preserve dying children's defenses. If they are using denial or bargaining, do not try to push them to the next step of grieving by confrontation. Children will move on to the next step when they are psychologically ready.

5. Many children assume that they will die at night. Therefore, night is "owned" by the dying. A child may talk more freely at night about fears or an unfulfilled life ambition than during the day. Children may also be more frightened at night and enjoy having someone sit beside them until they fall asleep.

6. Be supportive, not trite. A statement such as "All of us are dying" is true but not helpful. A supportive statement such as "This must be hard for you" is better.

7. Be aware that not all people's beliefs are the same as yours. A statement such as "God works in mysterious ways" may explain death for you but can be little comfort to a family who does not envision that as true. A statement such as "I believe God made some children die early to teach us to appreciate life" may evoke an angry response such as "Who could believe in a God like that?" rather than be comforting.

provides some specific guidelines on communicating with the child who is dying.

The Child's Family

For many children, hospitalization involves not one admission but a series of them, interspersed with ambulatory care. Parents need time during these ambulatory visits to talk about the problems they are having, not only with physical care (Should the child attend regular school? Could he come on vacation? How many times a day are they supposed to give the immunosuppressant?) but also about how it feels to live with a child who is dying (Are they having any difficulty answering the child's questions or siblings' questions?). Although many parents are reluctant to tell a child that he or she is dying, this is probably the soundest course once the child can see that his or her condition is deteriorating. There is often less anxiety in knowing what is happening than in hearing people whispering or spelling out words around you.

If the child is admitted to the hospital during an exacerbation of the disease, parents may again begin an anticipatory grief reaction: anger, bargaining, depression, acceptance. The process will be cut short by improvement and discharge, only to begin again at the next admission. Parents of a child being admitted for the 12th time for leukemia, therefore, may be in the same stage of grief as the parents whose child's leukemia is newly diagnosed.

When they are seen for health supervision visits, parents should be asked how other children in the family are managing. Often other children live with relatives so that the parents are free to spend a great deal of time visiting at the hospital. The parents may need reminding that although the dying child does need a lot of their time, other children find this illness in a sibling even more baffling than do the parents. When the ill child dies, siblings need active support to help them grieve (Davies, 1993).

The Onset of Death

As death nears in children, physiologic changes such as slowed metabolism, decreased cell oxygenation, and cell dysfunction begin to occur.

Stroke volume of the heart decreases, so the power to circulate blood becomes reduced. The child's skin feels cool and appears mottled or cyanotic because blood can no longer be pushed to distal sites. Just before death, blood will begin to pool in the dependent body parts, making them appear purple. As circulation fails, absorption of a drug from a muscle becomes virtually impossible; an emergency drug would need to be administered intravenously to have an effect.

As peripheral circulation fails, less heat is lost from the body and the temperature rises. The child's body may compensate for this by increased perspiration to increase heat loss through evaporation. This makes the child's skin feel not only cool but also damp. You may need to change linen frequently because of the increased moisture on the skin. Because perfusion of distal body parts is impaired, turn children slowly to allow their circulation system to accommodate to the change in position.

Slowed respiration leads to increased secretions in the lungs and the appearance of rales (the crackling sound of air being pulled through fluid in alveoli). To compensate for a few minutes of very slow respirations, a child may take a number of quick or extremely deep inhalations periodically. Be certain the child's chest is not compressed so he or she has optimal lung expansion to do this.

A decrease in muscular function leads to severe weakness and fatigue. More and more, a child maintains the exact position in which you placed him or her. As the throat muscles become lax, the possibility of aspiration increases. Assess children carefully for an intact gag reflex before offering oral fluid. If the gag or swallowing reflex is impaired, position children on their side to allow saliva to drain from the mouth and prevent aspiration. An often-noticed phenomenon is constant hand movement—picking at bedclothes, for example—that probably represents the loss of upper centers of voluntary muscular control. Neurologically, deep reflexes, such as the Achilles, begin to fade.

As children near death, they begin to demonstrate a lessened level of consciousness, although they may remain perfectly alert until seconds before death. Vision apparently blurs because children tend to turn toward a light. Touch seems to remain intact because children often quiet to a gentle stroking of the arm or shoulder; they grasp your hand meaningfully as if touch is appreciated and felt. Hearing remains intact. You may need to remind family members and, on occasion, other health care personnel of this. Continue to explain procedures to unconscious children as if they were conscious because they undoubtedly do hear you. Never make any comment in their presence that you would not make if they were alert. Continue to use the same gentle touch and nonverbal communication motions, such as holding a hand or brushing hair from the forehead, as if children were fully conscious. They may be fully aware of your actions even though they can give no indication of it.

Digestion slows as total body metabolism slows. Constipation due to poor bowel tone and decreased peristaltic action will occur (Huddleston et al., 1993). The abdomen may become distended from intestinal flatus. Dehydration with dry mucous membrane and conjunctivae will occur unless an intravenous supplement is begun. Mouth dryness will lead to cracking and secondary infection and pain; prevent this by frequent cleaning of the mucous membrane with clear water and applying Vaseline to the lips. If eye conjunctivae appear dry, ask a physician to prescribe moistening eye drops; keep any crusting at eyelids washed away so optimal vision is possible.

Keep skin surfaces from rubbing against one another by supporting pillows and good positioning. Keep skin dry from urine or feces from incontinence; this prevents painful decubitus ulcers from developing (normally not a major concern in children, but a concern here because of the lessened peripheral blood perfusion). Assess for pain (thrashing or moaning), and relieve this by administration of analgesics.

Documentation of Death

Defining when death occurs is controversial and involves both legal and ethical issues (Penticuff, 1990). Signs of death in a child not on ventilatory or mechanical assistance are the same as occur in adults: absence of respirations; no audible heart sounds by stethoscope; no pulse by palpation; no apparent blood pressure; absence of body movement or reflexes; and dilated, fixed pupils. **Death** is officially determined by unreceptivity and unresponsivity; no spontaneous muscular movement or breath; no reflex response; and a flat electroencephalogram—again, the same as in adults (AAP, 1987).

Organ Donation

Parents may be asked by their physician or a specifically designated transplant team before a child's death to grant permission for body organs to be transplanted following death. If parents make the decision to allow organ donation, mark this information on the child's care plan in a conspicuous place and alert the physician about the decision. When death does occur, the child's body will be maintained by a life-support system until a proper recipient for the body organ to be transplanted is located. The donation of body organs may help parents accept their child's death more easily, as they can feel their child has helped another person live (Wolf, 1990).

After Care

Before beginning any after care with a child following death, check with family members to see if they want to spend a few minutes with the child or if there are any religious rites they want to complete before the body is prepared for the morgue. This is necessary for some parents to be able to comprehend that death has really occurred. Some people have special prayers they want to say; others want to say a final, private goodbye. Check that the child's bed and room look neat and clean before you ask family if they would like to spend some time in the room, particularly if a final resuscitation attempt resulted in blood-soaked sponges or scattered equipment.

Remain in the room with the family in case they need your support, but be unobtrusive. Some parents fear touching a child's body after death, but touch is a strong and intimate communication technique that a family member may appreciate being shown how to use. Role model touching by holding the child's hand or brushing hair away from the forehead as if the child were still alive. Some parents may seem unable to leave the room or to let go of the child's hand. You may need gradually to separate their hands, saying something such as "I'll always remember Molly the way she was when I first met her—so full of life and always laughing. I'm sure that's how you'll always remember her, too." This helps parents begin to accept the fact that, in more than a physical sense, it is time to let go.

As a rule, crying is helpful for parents (Miles, 1990). You may need to tell them that it is all right to cry. On

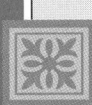

FOCUS ON CULTURAL AWARENESS

The way that death is viewed and the manner in which people express grief differ greatly across cultures. Some people are very expressive with grief; some are very restrained. The manner in which a child's body is handled after death also differs. Muslims, for example, forbid organ donations or transplants. Autopsies are not usually approved because it is important that children be buried quickly after death. Cremation is not permitted (Geissler, 1994). Being aware that grief is expressed differently by different cultures allows for better understanding of parents' concerns and reactions during a child's fatal illness.

the other hand, do not interpret a lack of tears as a lack of feeling. Crying is not everyone's response to death. It is not unprofessional for nurses to cry at a child's death. A parent's warmest memory of a hospital experience may be that a nurse cried as she said goodbye to his child—the implication being that the child made an impact on people other than family.

Autopsy Permission

If a child's death is a result of homicide, suicide, death within 24 hours after a hospital admission, suspected harmful death, or death in an institution or home where the child was not under a physician's care, an autopsy is required by law; parents have no input as to whether one is done. In other instances, it would be helpful to medical programs or research if an autopsy could be done (Vance, 1990) but parents must sign permission for this. Parents may refuse to allow autopsy permission for a child, thinking of their action as protecting the child from any more hurt or out of religious convictions (see the Focus on Cultural Awareness box). Autopsies advance medical science, so they should be done if at all possible; on the other hand, parents do have every right to refuse permission without being made to feel guilty for their actions.

Key Points

- Children with chronic illnesses need continual reassessment as, like all children, their needs change as they grow older. Larger doses of medicine will become necessary; such things as additional muscle strengthening exercises may be necessary.
- Factors that make it easier for parents to accept chronic illness in a child include the presence of support people and being told about the disability at as young an age as possible.
- Chronic illness in a child is often most difficult for parents to accept at what would have been the

child's "milestones" of development. Extra support for both the parents and child may be necessary at these times.

- Help children to do as much care for themselves as possible within the limits of a chronic illness. This empowers them to be as independent as possible.
- Children are about 9 years old before they are able to understand the meaning of death and that it is permanent.
- Children as well as parents are apt to need help to face a fatal diagnosis in the child. Urge parents and the child to ask for help to see them through this very difficult time in their lives.

Critical Thinking Exercises

1. Billy is a newborn with a myomeningocele. His parents are both 40 years old and live on a farm; finances are tight and they have no health insurance. Two grown children have expressed resentment at their parents being forced to spend so much time and money on a disabled child. How would you help this family? Do they have risk factors that might make adjusting to a disabled child more difficult than usual?

2. Tony is a 10-year-old who has an inoperable brain tumor. His parents have been told that he has only 6 more months to live. You notice Tony's parents in the waiting room of the hospital comforting a set of parents whose child was just hit by a car and killed instantly; you hear them say that losing a child suddenly is better than what they are experiencing. Why do you think Tony's parents feel this way? How could you help them with their feelings?

3. Adam is an adolescent with leukemia who wants to donate his corneas for transplant if he should die. His parents think this is totally wrong and say they will not allow it to happen. How would you counsel this family?

References

American Academy of Pediatrics, Task Force on Brain Death in Children. (1987). Guidelines for the determination of brain death in children. *Pediatrics, 80,* 298.

Armstrong-Dailey, A. (1990). Children's hospice care. *Pediatric Nursing, 16,* 337.

Bowden, V. R. (1993). Children's literature: The death experience. *Pediatric Nursing, 19,* 17.

Brice, C. W. (1991). Paradoxes of maternal mourning. *Psychiatry, 54,* 1.

Cohen, R., et al. (1994). Preschoolers' evaluations of physical disabilities: A consideration of attitudes. *Journal of Pediatric Psychology, 19,* 103.

Crowley, A. A. (1990). Integrating handicapped and chronically ill children into day care centers. *Pediatric Nursing, 16,* 39.

Davies, B. (1993). Sibling bereavement: Research-based guidelines for nurses. *Seminars in Oncology Nursing, 9,* 107.

Department of Health and Human Services. (1991). *Healthy people 2000.* Washington, DC: Public Health Service.

Dougherty, C. M. (1990). The near-death experience as a major life transition. *Holistic Nursing Practice, 4,* 84.

Geissler, E. M. (1994). *Pocket guide to cultural assessment.* St. Louis: C. V. Mosby.

Goldman, A., & Christie, D. (1993). Children with cancer talk about their own death with their families. *Pediatric Hematology and Oncology, 10,* 223.

Green, M., & Solnit, A. (1964). Reactions to the threatened loss of a child: A vulnerable child syndrome. *Pediatrics, 34,* 58.

Holaday, B., et al. (1993). Chronically ill children in self-care: Issues for pediatric nurses. *Journal of Pediatric Health Care, 7,* 256.

Huddleston, K. C., et al. (1993). Nutritional support of the critically ill child. *Critical Care Nursing Clinics of North America, 5,* 65.

Hutton, N. (1994). Special needs of children with chronic illness. In Oski, F. A., et al. (Eds.) *Principles and practice of pediatrics* (2nd ed.). Philadelphia: J. B. Lippincott.

Johnson, A. (1990). How paediatric nurses cope with child deaths. *Nursing Times, 86,* 53.

Kübler-Ross, E. (1969). *On death and dying.* New York: Macmillan.

Miles, A. (1990). Caring for families when a child dies. *Pediatric Nursing, 16,* 346.

Penticuff, J. H. (1990). Ethical issues in redefining death. *Journal of Neuroscience Nursing, 22,* 48.

Sexson, S. B., & Madan-Swain, A. (1993). School reentry for the child with chronic illness. *Journal of Learning Disabilities, 26,* 115.

Turner, R. J., & Beiser, M. (1990). Major depression and depressive symptomatology among the physically disabled. *Journal of Nervous and Mental Diseases, 178,* 343.

Vance, R. P. (1990). An unintentional irony: The autopsy in modern medicine and society. *Human Pathology, 21,* 136.

Whittam, E. H. (1993). Terminal care of the dying child. Psychosocial implications of care. *Cancer, 71,* 3450.

Williams, P. D., et al. (1993). Pediatric chronic illness: Effects on siblings and mothers. *Maternal-Child Nursing Journal, 21,* 111.

Wolf, Z. R. (1990). Nurses' experiences giving post-mortem care to patients who have donated organs: A phenomenological study. *Transplant Proceedings, 22,* 1019.

Suggested Readings

Birenbaum, L. K., & Robinson, M. A. (1991). Family relationships in two types of terminal care. *Social Science and Medicine, 32,* 95.

Burke, S. O., & Roberts, C. A. (1990). Nursing research and the care of chronically ill and disabled children. *Journal of Pediatric Nursing, 5,* 316.

Edwards, B. S. (1994). Ethical issues: When the family can't let go. *American Journal of Nursing, 94,* 52.

Jessop, D. J., & Stein, R. E. (1994). Providing comprehensive health care to children with chronic illness. *Pediatrics, 93,* 602.

Lawson, L. V. (1990). Culturally sensitive support for grieving parents. *MCN: American Journal of Maternal Child Nursing, 15,* 76.

Lynch, A. (1990). Respect for the dead human body: A question of body, mind, spirit, psyche. *Transplant Proceedings, 22,* 1016.

Parette, H. P., et al. (1990). The family physician's role with parents of young children with developmental disabilities. *Journal of Family Practice, 31,* 288.

Pharoah, P. O. (1990). Impairment, disability, and handicap. *Archives of Disease of Childhood, 65,* 819.

Rhymes, J. (1990). Hospice care in America. *Journal of the American Medical Association, 264,* 369.

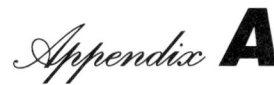

Rights of Pregnant Women and Children

The Pregnant Patient's Bill of Rights*

The Pregnant Patient has the right to participate in decisions involving her well-being and that of her unborn child, unless there is a clearcut medical emergency that prevents her participation. In addition to the rights set forth in the American Hospital Association's "Patient's Bill of Rights," the Pregnant Patient, because she represents TWO patients rather than one, should be recognized as having the additional rights listed below.

1. *The Pregnant Patient has the right,* prior to the administration of any drug or procedure, to be informed by the health professional caring for her of any potential direct or indirect effects, risks or hazards to herself or her unborn or newborn infant which may result from the use of a drug or procedure prescribed for or administered to her during pregnancy, labor, birth or lactation.

2. *The Pregnant Patient has the right,* prior to the proposed therapy, to be informed, not only of the benefits, risks and hazards of the proposed therapy but also of known alternative therapy, such as available childbirth education classes which could help to prepare the Pregnant Patient physically and mentally to cope with the discomfort or stress of pregnancy and the experience of childbirth, thereby reducing or eliminating her need for drugs and obstetric intervention. She should be offered such information early in her pregnancy in order that she may make a reasoned decision.

3. *The Pregnant Patient has the right,* prior to the administration of any drug, to be informed by the health professional who is prescribing or administering the drug to her that any drug which she receives during pregnancy, labor and birth, no matter how or when the drug is taken or administered, may adversely affect her unborn baby, directly or indirectly, and that there is no drug or chemical which has been proven safe for the unborn child.

4. *The Pregnant Patient has the right,* if cesarean birth is anticipated, to be informed prior to the administration of any drug, and preferably prior to her hospitalization, that minimizing her and, in turn, her baby's intake of nonessential preoperative medicine will benefit her baby.

5. *The Pregnant Patient has the right,* prior to the administration of a drug or procedure, to be informed of the areas of uncertainty if there is *no* properly controlled follow-up research which has established the safety of the drug or procedure with regard to its direct and/or indirect effects on the physiological, mental and neurological development of the child exposed, via the mother, to the drug or procedure during pregnancy, labor, birth or lactation—(this would apply to virtually all drugs and the vast majority of obstetric procedures).

6. *The Pregnant Patient has the right,* prior to the administration of any drug, to be informed on the brand name and generic name of the drug in order that she may advise the health professional of any past adverse reaction to the drug.

7. *The Pregnant Patient has the right* to determine for herself, without pressure from her attendant, whether she will accept the risks inherent in the proposed therapy or refuse a drug or procedure.

8. *The Pregnant Patient has the right* to know the name and qualifications of the individual administering a medication or procedure to her during labor or birth.

9. *The Pregnant Patient has the right* to be informed, prior to the administration of any procedure, whether that procedure is being administered to her for her or her baby's benefit (medically indicated) or as an elective procedure (for convenience, teaching purposes or research).

10. *The Pregnant Patient has the right* to be accompanied during the stress of labor and birth by someone she cares for, and to whom she looks for emotional comfort and encouragement.

11. *The Pregnant Patient has the right* after appropriate

*From Haire, D. B. (1975). The pregnant patient's bill of rights. *Journal of Nurse Midwifery, 20,* 29; from Committee on Patient's Rights, Box 1900, New York, NY 10001.

12. *The Obstetric Patient has the right* to have her baby cared for at her bedside if her baby is normal, and to feed her baby according to her baby's needs rather than according to the hospital regimen.

13. *The Obstetric Patient has the right* to be informed in writing of the name of the person who actually delivered her baby and the professional qualifications of that person. This information should also be on the birth certificate.

14. *The Obstetric Patient has the right* to be informed if there is any known or indicated aspect of her or her baby's care or condition which may cause her or her baby later difficulty or problems.

15. *The Obstetric Patient has the right* to have her and her baby's hospital medical records complete, accurate and legible and to have their records, including Nurses' Notes, retained by the hospital until the child reaches at least the age of majority, or to have the records offered to her before they are destroyed.

16. *The Obstetric Patient,* both during and after her hospital stay, *has the right* to have access to her complete hospital medical records, including Nurses' Notes, and to receive a copy upon payment of a reasonable fee and without incurring the expense of retaining an attorney.

It is the obstetric patient and her baby, not the health professional, who must sustain any trauma or injury resulting from the use of a drug or obstetric procedure. The observation of the rights listed above will not only permit the obstetric patient to participate in the decisions involving her and her baby's health care, but will help to protect the health professional and the hospital against litigation arising from resentment or misunderstanding on the part of the mother.

United Nations Declaration of the Rights of the Child*

Preamble

Whereas the peoples of the United Nations have in the Charter, reaffirmed their faith in fundamental human rights, and in the dignity and worth of the human person, and have determined to promote social progress and better standards of life in larger freedom,

Whereas the United Nations has, in the Universal Declaration of Human Rights, proclaimed that everyone

*United Nations. (1959). *Declarations of the rights of the child.* Geneva: The United Nations.

is entitled to all the rights and freedoms set forth therein, without distinction of any kind, such as race, color, sex, language, religion, political or other opinion, national or social origin, property, birth or other status,

Whereas the child by reason of his physical and mental immaturity, needs special safeguards and care, including appropriate legal protection, before as well as after birth,

Whereas the need for such special safeguards has been stated in the Geneva Declaration of the Rights of the Child of 1924, and recognized in the universal Declaration of Human Rights and in the statutes of specialized agencies and international organizations concerned with the welfare of children,

Whereas mankind owes to the child the best it has to give,

Now therefore the general assembly proclaims

This Declaration of the Rights of the Child to the end that he may have a happy childhood and enjoy for his own good and for the good of society and rights and freedoms herein set forth, and calls upon parents, upon men and women as individuals and upon voluntary organizations, local authorities and national governments to recognize these rights and strive for their observance by legislative and other measures progressively taken in accordance with the following principles:

Principle 1

The child shall enjoy all the rights set forth in this Declaration. All children, without any exception whatsoever, shall be entitled to these rights, without distinction or discrimination on account of race, color, sex, language, religion, political or other opinion, national or social origin, property, birth or other status, whether of himself or of his family.

Principle 2

The child shall enjoy special protection, and shall be given opportunities and facilities, by law and by other means, to enable him to develop physically, mentally, morally, spiritually and socially in a healthy and normal manner and in conditions of freedom and dignity. In the enactment of laws for this purpose the best interests of the child shall be the paramount consideration.

Principle 3

The child shall be entitled from his birth to a name and a nationality.

Principle 4

The child shall enjoy the benefits of social security. He shall be entitled to grow and develop in health; to this end special care and protection shall be provided both to him and to his mother, including adequate pre-natal care. The child shall have the right to adequate nutrition, housing, recreation and medical services.

Principle 5

The child who is physically, mentally or socially handicapped shall be given the special treatment, education and care required by his particular condition.

Principle 6

The child, for the full and harmonious development of his personality, needs love and understanding. He shall, wherever possible, grow up in the care and under the responsibility of his parents, and in any case in an atmosphere of affection and of moral and maternal security; a child of tender years shall not, save in exceptional circumstances, be separated from his mother. Society and the public authorities shall have the duty to extend particular care to children without a family and to those without adequate means of support. Payment of state and other assistance toward the maintenance of children of large families is desirable.

Principle 7

The child is entitled to receive education, which shall be free and compulsory, at least in the elementary stages. He shall be given an education which will promote his general culture, and enable him on a basis of equal opportunity to develop his abilities, his individual judgment and his sense of moral and social responsibility, and to become a useful member of society.

The best interests of the child shall be the guiding principle of those responsible for his education and guidance; that responsibility lies in the first place with his parents.

The child shall have full opportunity for play and recreation, which shall be directed to the same purposes as education; society and the public authorities shall endeavor to promote the employment of his right.

Principle 8

The child shall in all circumstances be among the first to receive protection and relief.

Principle 9

The child shall be protected against all forms of neglect, cruelty and exploitation. He shall not be the subject of traffic, in any form.

The child shall not be admitted to employment before an appropriate minimum age; he shall n no case be caused or permitted to engage in any occupation or employment which would prejudice his health or education, or interfere with his physical, mental or moral development.

Principle 10

The child shall be protected from practices which may foster racial, religious and any other form of discrimination. He shall be brought up in a spirit of understanding, tolerance, friendship among peoples, peace and universal brotherhood and in full consciousness that his energy and talents should be devoted to the service of his fellow men.

Composition and Ingredients of Infant Formulas

Adele Pillitteri: MATERNAL AND CHILD
HEALTH NURSING, 2nd Edition. © 1995
Adele Pillitteri.

Composition and Ingredients of Infant Formulas

Formula	Calories (Per oz)	(Per mL)	Percentage Weight Per Volume (g/100 mL) Protein	Fat	Carbohydrate	mEq/L Na	K	mg/L Ca	P	Ca/P Ratio	Fe	Approximate Solute Load Renal (mOsm/L)	GI (GI/L)	Protein	Fat	Carbohydrate	Comments
Cow's milk	20	.67	3.30 (21)*	3.30 (49)*	4.70 (30)*	21	39	1190	930	1.30/1	0.5	220	260	80% casein, 20% whey	Butterfat	Lactose	
Enfamil 20†	20	.67	1.50 (9)	3.80 (50)	6.98 (41)	8	18	465	317	1.47/1	1.1	100	270	40% casein, 60% whey	45% soy, 55% coconut oils	Lactose	
Enfamil premature	20	.67	2.00 (12)	3.40 (44)	7.40 (44)	11	19	793	402	2.00/1	1.7	180	220	40% casein, 60% whey	40% MCT oil, soy and coconut oil	Corn syrup solids, lactose	Premature infants
Human milk	21	.70	1.00 (6)	4.40 (55)	6.90 (39)	7	13	320	140	2.3/1	0.3	75	273	40% casein, 60% whey	Human milk, fat	Lactose	
Isomil	20	.67	1.80 (11)	3.69 (49)	6.80 (40)	14	24	700	500	1.40/1	12	122	230	Soy protein	Coconut and soy oils	Corn syrup solids and sucrose	For cow's milk protein or lactose intolerance
Isomil SF	20	.67	2.00 (12)	3.60 (48)	6.80 (40)	14	20	700	500	1.40/1	12	131	140	Soy protein	Coconut and soy oils	Corn syrup solids	For cow's milk protein, lactose, or sucrose intolerance
Lofenalac	20	.67	2.20 (13)	2.60 (35)	8.80 (52)	14	18	634	475	1.33/1	13	134	310	Processed casein hydrolysate to remove most of the phenylalanine	Corn oil	Corn syrup solids and modified tapioca starch	For phenylketonuria (PKU), low in phenylalanine
MJ 3232A‡	20	.67	1.90 (11)	2.80 (36)	9.10 (54)	12	19	634	423	1.50/1	13	124		Casein hydrolysate	MCT oil	Tapioca starch, mono- and disaccharide free	Management of disaccharidase deficiencies
MJ 80056 (per 100 g of diet powder)	20	.67	0.00 (0)	22.5 (41)	71.8 (59)	3	9	540	300	1.80/1	11		182	None	Corn oil	Corn syrup solids and modified tapioca starch	Protein-free formula for amino acid disorders

(continued)

490

Composition and Ingredients of Infant Formulas *Continued*

Formula	Calories (Per oz)	Calories (Per mL)	Percentage Weight Per Volume (g/100 mL) Protein	Percentage Weight Per Volume (g/100 mL) Fat	Percentage Weight Per Volume (g/100 mL) Carbohydrate	mEq/L Na	mEq/L K	mg/L Ca	mg/L P	Ca/P Ratio	Fe	Approximate Solute Load Renal (mOsm/L)	Approximate Solute Load GI (mOsm/L)	Protein	Fat	Carbohydrate	Comments
Nursoy	20	.67	2.10 (12)	3.60 (48)	6.90 (40)	9	19	630	440	1.40/1	12	122	266	Soy protein	Coconut, safflower, and soybean oils	Sucrose	For cow's protein or lactose intolerance
Nutramigen	20	.67	1.90 (11)	2.64 (35)	9.09 (54)	14	19	634	423	1.50/1	13	130	430	Casein hydrolysate	Corn oil	Corn syrup solids, modified corn starch	Use for sensitivity to intact milk protein, or for lactose intolerance
Portagen	20	.67	2.30 (14)	3.17 (41)	7.82 (45)	14	22	635	475	1.33/1	13	150	200	Sodium caseinate	88% MCT oil, 12% corn oil	Corn syrup sucrose	Use in fat malabsorption states, lactose intolerance (liver disease)
Pregestimil	20	.67	1.90 (11)	2.75 (35)	9.10 (54)	14	19	634	423	1.50/1	13	120	310	Casein hydrolysate with added l-cystine, l-tyrosine, l-tryptophan	60% corn oil, 40% MCT oil	Corn syrup solids, modified tapioca starch	Suitable for many malabsorption syndromes
Prosobee	20	.67	2.00 (12)	3.60 (48)	6.80 (40)	11	21	634	500	1.26/1	13	130	180	Soy protein isolate and methionine	Soy oil, coconut oil	100% corn syrup solids (glucose polymers)	Use for lactose and and cow's milk protein intolerance; sucrose intolerance; galactosemia
RCF			2.00 (20)	3.60 (80)	0 (0)	14	20	700	500	1.4/1	1.5	131§	60	Soy protein isolate	Coconut and soy oils	None	Contains no carbohydrates
Similac 20†	20§	.67	1.50 (9)	3.63 (48)	7.23 (43)	10	21	510	390	1.30/1	1.5	105	260	Nonfat cow's milk	Coconut and soy oils	Lactose	

Formula														Protein source	Fat source	Carbohydrate source	Comments
Similac 24LBW	24	.80	2.20 (11)	4.49 (42)	8.49 (42)	16	31	730	560	1.30/1	3.0	161	260	Nonfat cow's milk	MCT oil, coconut and soy oils	Lactose and corn syrup solids	Dilute initial feedings. For premature infants with fluid intolerance
Similac PM 60/40	20	.67	1.58 (9)	3.76 (50)	6.88 (41)	7	15	400	200	2.00/1	1.5	96	240	Casein and whey (60/40 ratio whey/casein)	Coconut and soy oils	Lactose	(Ca:P=2:1) For infants predisposed to hypocalcemia; low salt content
Similac special care	20	.67	1.83 (11)	3.67 (47)	7.17 (42)	13	24	1200	600	2.00/1	2.5	128	230	60% whey, 40% casein	MCT oil soy oil coconut oil	50% lactose 50% corn syrup solids	Premature infants Ca:P-2:1
Similac whey plus iron	20	.67	1.50 (9)	3.63 (48)	7.23 (43)	10	19	400	300	1.33/1	12	101	270	60% whey, 40% casein	Coconut, and soy oils	Lactose	
SMA 20	20	.67	1.59 (9)	3.60 (48)	7.20 (43)	6.5	14.3	440	330	1.33/1	12.7	126	271	Nonfat cow's milk, demineralized whey	Coconut safflower and soybean oils	Lactose	Low salt content
SMA Preemie	24	.80	2.00 (10)	4.40 (48)	8.60 (42)	14	19	750	400	1.88/1	3	175	300	60% whey, 40% casein	MCT oil, coconut and soy oils	Lactose and glucose polymers	Premature infants

*Percentage of calories supplied

†Also comes with iron (12 mg/L)

‡Mixed as 81 g diet powder plus 59 g added carbohydrate added

§Varies with amount carbohydrate added

||Ernst JA, et al. (1983). Vapor pressure method as determined by manufacturers method. *Pediatrics 72, 350.*

(Rowe P, (ed.) (1987). *The Harriet Lane handbook* (ed 11). Chicago: Year Book Medical Publishers, p. 338. Values listed were provided by manufacturers except where indicated otherwise.)

(Oski, F. A., et al., [1994]. *Principles and practice of pediatrics* [2nd ed]. Philadelphia: J. B. Lippincott, pg. 540–541.)

Excretion of Drugs in Breast Milk

Drugs that Appear to Pose Little or No Risk When Used During Lactation

Some Drugs Excreted in Human Milk but Without Apparent Clinical Significance		Some Drugs Not Excreted in Human Milk
Acetaminophen	Meperidine	Amitriptyline
Ampicillin	Mesoridazine	Cephalosporins, first and second generation
Antihistamines	Morphine	Chloroquine
β_2-Agonists	Nitrofurantoin	Desipramine
Caffeine	Novobiocin	Dextroamphetamine
Codeine	Propranolol	Heparin
Colchicine	Propantheline	Imipramine
Digoxin	Quinidine	Oxacillin
Diphenhydramine	Quinine	Pentazocine
Guanethidine	Scopolamine	Phenylbutazone
Hydroxyphenbutazone	Thyroid hormones	
Insulin	Tolmetin	
Lidocaine	Tranylcypromine	
Mefanimic acid		

(Swonger, A. K., & Matejski, M. P. [1991]. *Nursing pharmacology: An integrated approach to drug therapy and nursing practice* [2nd ed.] Philadelphia: J.B. Lippincott.).

Adele Pillitteri: MATERNAL AND CHILD HEALTH NURSING, 2nd Edition. © 1995 Adele Pillitteri.

Drugs Requiring Close Observation of Infant When Administered to Nursing Mothers

Drug	Comment
Alcohol	OK in small amounts; large amounts depress infant and inhibit lactation
Antimicrobials	
Cephalosporins, 3rd generation	Possible enterocolitis
Erythromycin	Concentrated in milk. Possible jaundice.
Isoniazid	Concentration is the same in milk as in serum; monitor child for possible toxicity
Kanamycin	Monitor child for toxicity
Nalidixic acid	Possible hemolytic anemia
Penicillin G or V	Possible hypersensitivity reactions
Barbiturates	Induce liver enzymes in infant
Benzodiazepines	Possible drowsiness
Carbamazepine	Possible tiredness, vomiting, or poor sucking
Chloral hydrate	Possible sedation in infant
Decongestants	May decrease milk volume
Diuretics (thiazides, spironolactone)	Avoid use during lactation; they decrease milk production and appear in milk
Glucocorticoids	Growth suppression; suppression of infant's production of glucocorticoids; retarded sexual development
Indomethacin	Convulsions reported in one breast-fed infant
Lithium	Monitor child for lithium toxicity
Meprobamate	Concentrated in milk 2 to 4× plasma level; monitor child for depressive effects
Methyldopa	Possible depression of respirations, blood pressure, and alertness
Minoxidil	Monitor for hypertrichosis
Neuroleptics	May cause galactorrhea in mother; not present in significant amounts in milk
Nicotine	Nicotine effects in infant occur if rate is greater than 20 cigarettes per day
Oral contraceptives	Gynecomastia in male infants
Phenytoin	One case of methemoglobinemia reported; induces liver enzymes
Primidone	Somnolence or drowsiness may occur in infant
Reserpine	Nasal stuffiness and lethargy in infant; galactorrhea in mother
Salicylates	Cause bleeding tendency; mother should take after feedings, not before. Possible skin rash
Vitamin D	Possible hypercalcemia in infant

(Swonger, A. K., & Matejski, M. P. [1991]. *Nursing pharmacology: An integrated approach to drug therapy and nursing practice* [2nd ed.]. Philadelphia: J.B. Lippincott.)

Drugs Contraindicated in Nursing Mothers

Drug Class	Comment
Antimicrobials (some)	
Amantadine	Possible vomiting, urinary retention, skin rash
Chloramphenicol	Infant's capacity to metabolize this drug is underdeveloped
Metronidazole	Avoid breastfeeding for 3 days after a single dose
Sulfonamides	Possible allergic skin reactions, jaundice, or hemolysis in G6PD-deficient infants
Streptomycin	Accumulates in liver of infant
Tetracyclines	Possible discoloration of teeth of infant
Antineoplastics	Nursing should be discontinued
Antithyroid drugs	May cause goiter or myxedema
Atropine	May cause atropine intoxication
Bromides	Cause rash and drowsiness
Cathartics	Diarrhea in infant
Cimetidine	Induces liver enzymes, suppresses gastric secretions, and stimulates the central nervous system in the infant
Ergot alkaloids	Vomiting, diarrhea, weak pulse, unstable blood pressure in the infant
Heavy metals	Mercury and lead poisoning can occur in infants if mother's milk is contaminated
Iodides	May cause thyroid impairment in infant
Narcotics	May cause addiction in infant
Oral anticoagulants (especially phenindione)	Cause hypocoagulation in the infant
Oral hypoglycemics	Tolbutamide achieves high concentration in milk; possible adverse effect on pancreas of infant
Radioactive drugs	Contraindicated in nursing mothers

(Swonger, A. K., & Matejski, M. P. [1991]. *Nursing pharmacology: An integrated approach to drug therapy and nursing practice* [2nd ed.]. Philadelphia: J.B. Lippincott.)

Temperature and Weight Conversion Charts

Conversion of Pounds to Kilograms

Pounds	0	1	2	3	4	5	6	7	8	9
0	—	0.45	0.90	1.36	1.81	2.26	2.72	3.17	3.62	4.08
10	4.53	4.98	5.44	5.89	6.35	6.80	7.25	7.71	8.16	8.61
20	9.07	9.52	9.97	10.43	10.88	11.34	11.79	12.24	12.70	13.15
30	13.60	14.06	14.51	14.96	15.42	15.87	16.32	16.78	17.23	17.69
40	18.14	18.59	19.05	19.50	19.95	20.41	20.86	21.31	21.77	22.22
50	22.68	23.13	23.58	24.04	24.49	24.94	25.40	25.85	26.30	26.76
60	27.21	27.66	28.12	28.57	29.03	29.48	29.93	30.39	30.84	31.29
70	31.75	32.20	32.65	33.11	33.56	34.02	34.47	34.92	35.38	35.83
80	36.28	36.74	37.19	37.64	38.10	38.55	39.00	39.46	39.91	40.37
90	40.82	41.27	41.73	42.18	42.63	43.09	43.54	43.99	44.45	44.90
100	45.36	45.81	46.26	46.72	47.17	47.62	48.08	48.53	48.98	49.44
110	49.89	50.34	50.80	51.25	51.71	52.16	52.61	53.07	53.52	53.97
120	54.43	54.88	55.33	55.79	56.24	56.70	57.15	57.60	58.06	58.51
130	58.96	59.42	59.87	60.32	60.78	61.23	61.68	62.14	62.59	63.05
140	63.50	63.95	64.41	64.86	65.31	65.77	66.22	66.67	67.13	67.58
150	68.04	68.49	68.94	69.40	69.85	70.30	70.76	71.21	71.66	72.12
160	72.57	73.02	73.48	73.93	74.39	74.84	75.29	75.75	76.20	76.65
170	77.11	77.56	78.01	78.47	78.92	79.38	79.83	80.28	80.74	81.19
180	81.64	82.10	82.55	83.00	83.46	83.91	84.36	84.82	85.27	85.73
190	86.18	86.68	87.09	87.54	87.99	88.45	88.90	89.35	89.81	90.26
200	90.72	91.17	91.62	92.08	92.53	92.98	93.44	93.89	94.34	94.80

Adele Pillitteri: MATERNAL AND CHILD
HEALTH NURSING, 2nd Edition. © 1995
Adele Pillitteri.

Conversion of Pounds and Ounces to Grams for Newborn Weights

Pounds	Ounces 0	1	2	3	4	5	6	7	8	9	10	11	12	13	14	15
0	—	28	57	85	113	142	170	198	227	255	283	312	430	369	397	425
1	454	482	510	539	567	595	624	652	680	709	737	765	794	822	850	879
2	907	936	964	992	1021	1049	1077	1106	1134	1162	1191	1219	1247	1276	1304	1332
3	1361	1389	1417	1446	1474	1503	1531	1559	1588	1616	1644	1673	1701	1729	1758	1786
4	1814	1843	1871	1899	1928	1956	1984	2013	2041	2070	2098	2126	2155	2183	2211	2240
5	2268	2296	2325	2353	2381	2410	2438	2466	2495	2523	2551	2580	2608	2637	2665	2693
6	2722	2750	2778	2807	2835	2863	2892	2920	2948	2977	3005	3033	3062	3090	3118	3147
7	3175	3203	3232	3260	3289	3317	3345	3374	3402	3430	3459	3487	3515	3544	3572	3600
8	3629	3657	3685	3714	3742	3770	3799	3827	3856	3884	3912	3941	3969	3997	4026	4054
9	4082	4111	4139	4167	4196	4224	4252	4281	4309	4337	4366	4394	4423	4451	4479	4508
10	4536	4564	4593	4621	4649	4678	4706	4734	4763	4791	4819	4848	4876	4904	4933	4961
11	4990	5018	5046	5075	5103	5131	5160	5188	5216	5245	5273	5301	5330	5358	5386	5415
12	5443	5471	5500	5528	5557	5585	5613	5642	5670	5698	5727	5755	5783	5812	5840	5868
13	5897	5925	5953	5982	6010	6038	6067	6095	6123	6152	6180	6209	6237	6265	6294	6322
14	6350	6379	6407	6435	6464	6492	6520	6549	6577	6605	6634	6662	6690	6719	6747	6776
15	6804	6832	6860	6889	6917	6945	6973	7002	7030	7059	7087	7115	7144	7172	7201	7228

Conversion of Fahrenheit to Celsius

Celsius	Fahrenheit	Celsius	Fahrenheit	Celsius	Fahrenheit
34.0	93.2	37.0	98.6	40.0	104.0
34.2	93.6	37.2	99.0	40.2	104.4
34.4	93.9	37.4	99.3	40.4	104.7
34.6	94.3	37.6	99.7	40.6	105.2
34.8	94.6	37.8	100.0	40.8	105.4
35.0	95.0	38.0	100.4	41.0	105.9
35.2	95.4	38.2	100.8	41.2	106.1
35.4	95.7	38.4	101.1	41.4	106.5
35.6	96.1	38.6	101.5	41.6	106.8
35.8	96.4	38.8	101.8	41.8	107.2
36.0	96.8	39.0	102.2	42.0	107.6
36.2	97.2	39.2	102.6	42.2	108.0
36.4	97.5	39.4	102.9	42.4	108.3
36.6	97.9	39.6	103.3	42.6	108.7
36.8	98.2	39.8	103.6	42.8	109.0

$(°C) \times (9/5) + 32 = °F$
$(°F - 32) \times (5/9) = °C$

Growth Charts

Nomogram for Estimating Surface Area of Infants and Young Children

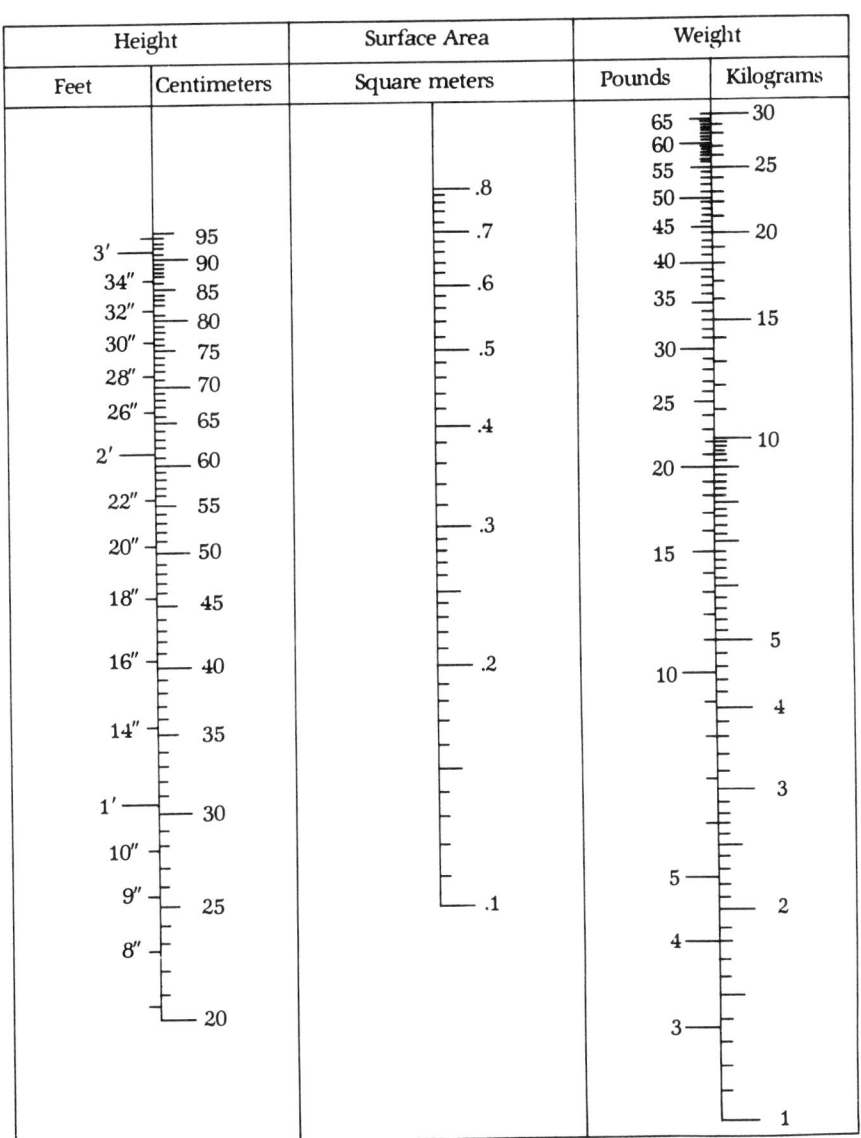

Height		Surface Area	Weight	
Feet	Centimeters	Square meters	Pounds	Kilograms

To determine the surface area of the child, draw a straight line between the point representing his or her height on the left vertical scale to the point representing his or her weight on the right vertical scale. The point at which this line intersects the middle vertical scale represents the child's surface area in square meters. (From Talbot, N. B., et al. [1980]. Functional endocrinology from birth to adolescence. Cambridge, MA: Harvard University Press. Copyright © 1952, 1980 by the President and Fellows of Harvard College. Reprinted by permission of the publisher.)

Adele Pillitteri: MATERNAL AND CHILD
HEALTH NURSING, 2nd Edition. © 1995
Adele Pillitteri.

BOYS: BIRTH TO 36 MONTHS
PHYSICAL GROWTH
NCHS PERCENTILES*

NAME _____ RECORD # _____

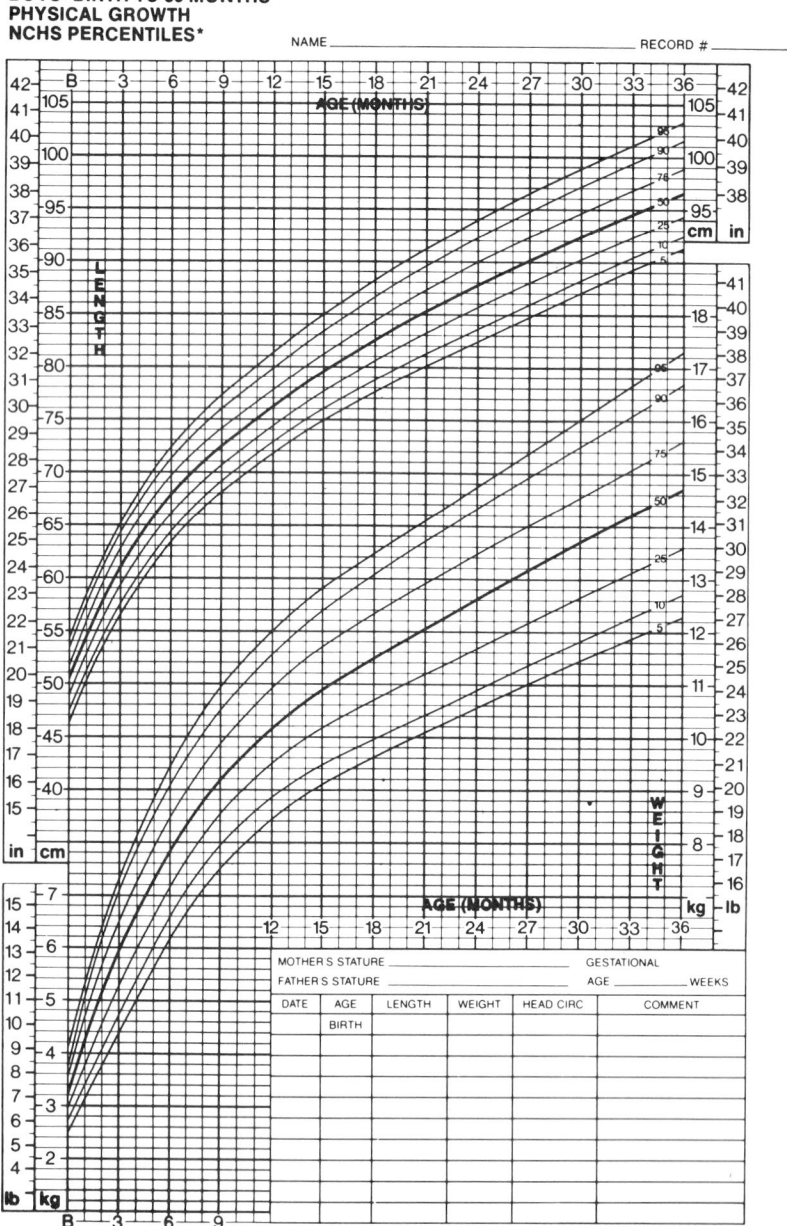

Source: *Adapted from Hamill, P. V. V., et al. (1979). Physical growth: National Center for Health Statistics percentiles.* American Journal of Clinical Nutrition, 32, *607. Data from the Fels Research Institute, Wright State University School of Medicine, Yellow Springs, OH. Courtesy of Ross Laboratories.*

GIRLS: BIRTH TO 36 MONTHS
PHYSICAL GROWTH
NCHS PERCENTILES*

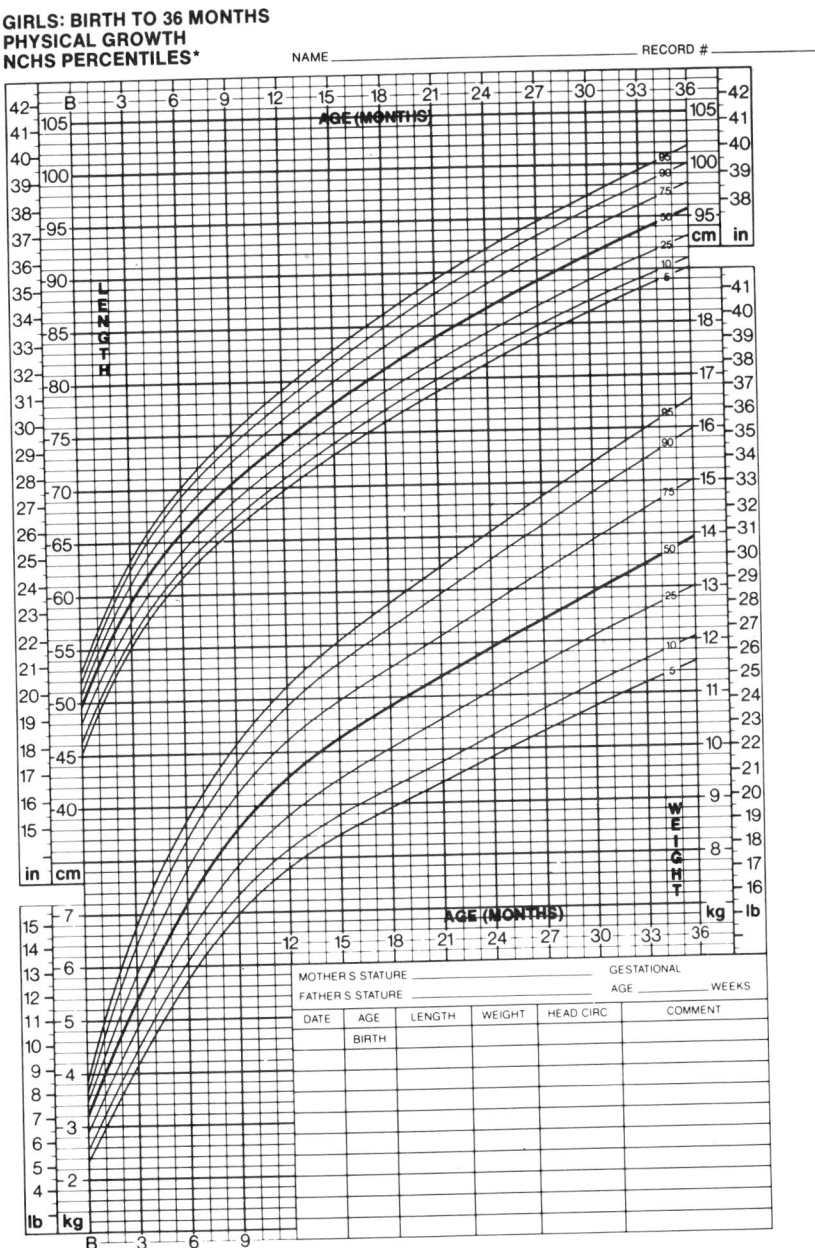

Source: *Adapted from Hamill, P. V. V., et al. (1979). Physical growth: National Center for Health Statistics percentiles.* American Journal of Clinical Nutrition, 32, 607. *Data from the Fels Research Institute, Wright State University School of Medicine, Yellow Springs, OH. Courtesy of Ross Laboratories.*

BOYS: 2 TO 18 YEARS
PHYSICAL GROWTH
NCHS PERCENTILES*

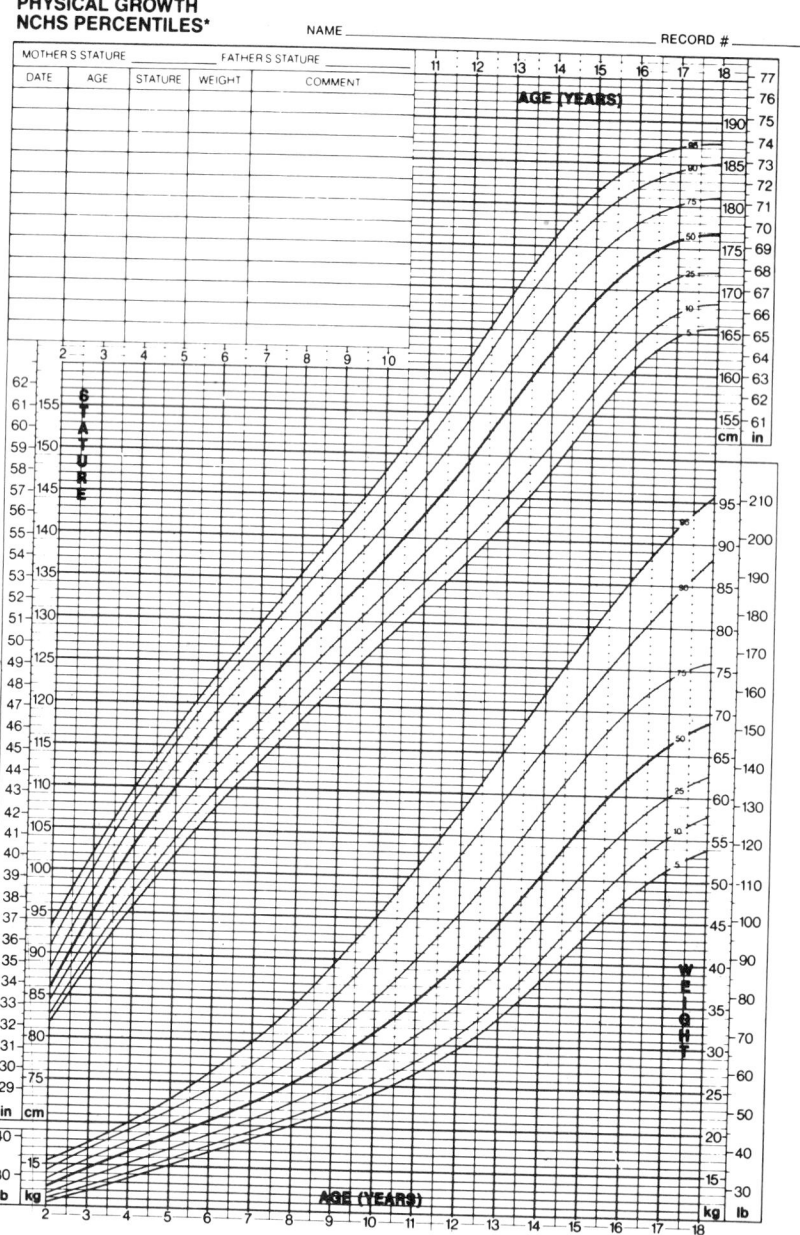

Source: *Adapted from Hamill, P. V. V., et al. (1979). Physical growth: National Center for Health Statistics percentiles.* American Journal of Clinical Nutrition, 32, 607. *Data from the Fels Research Institute, Wright State University School of Medicine, Yellow Springs, OH. Courtesy of Ross Laboratories.*

GIRLS: 2 TO 18 YEARS
PHYSICAL GROWTH
NCHS PERCENTILES*

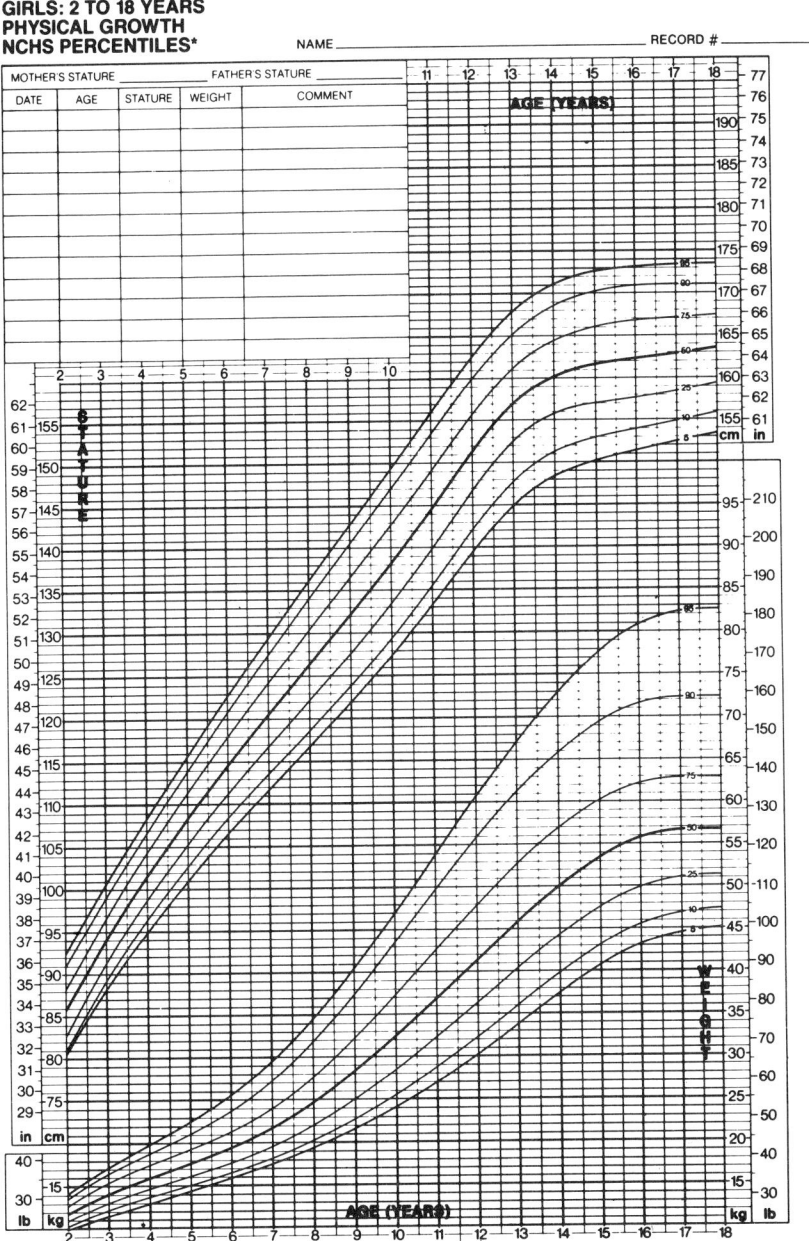

Source: *Adapted from Hamill, P. V. V., et al. (1979). Physical growth: National Center for Health Statistics percentiles.* American Journal of Clinical Nutrition, 32, 607. *Data from the Fels Research Institute, Wright State University School of Medicine, Yellow Springs, OH. Courtesy of Ross Laboratories.*

Head Circumference: Girls

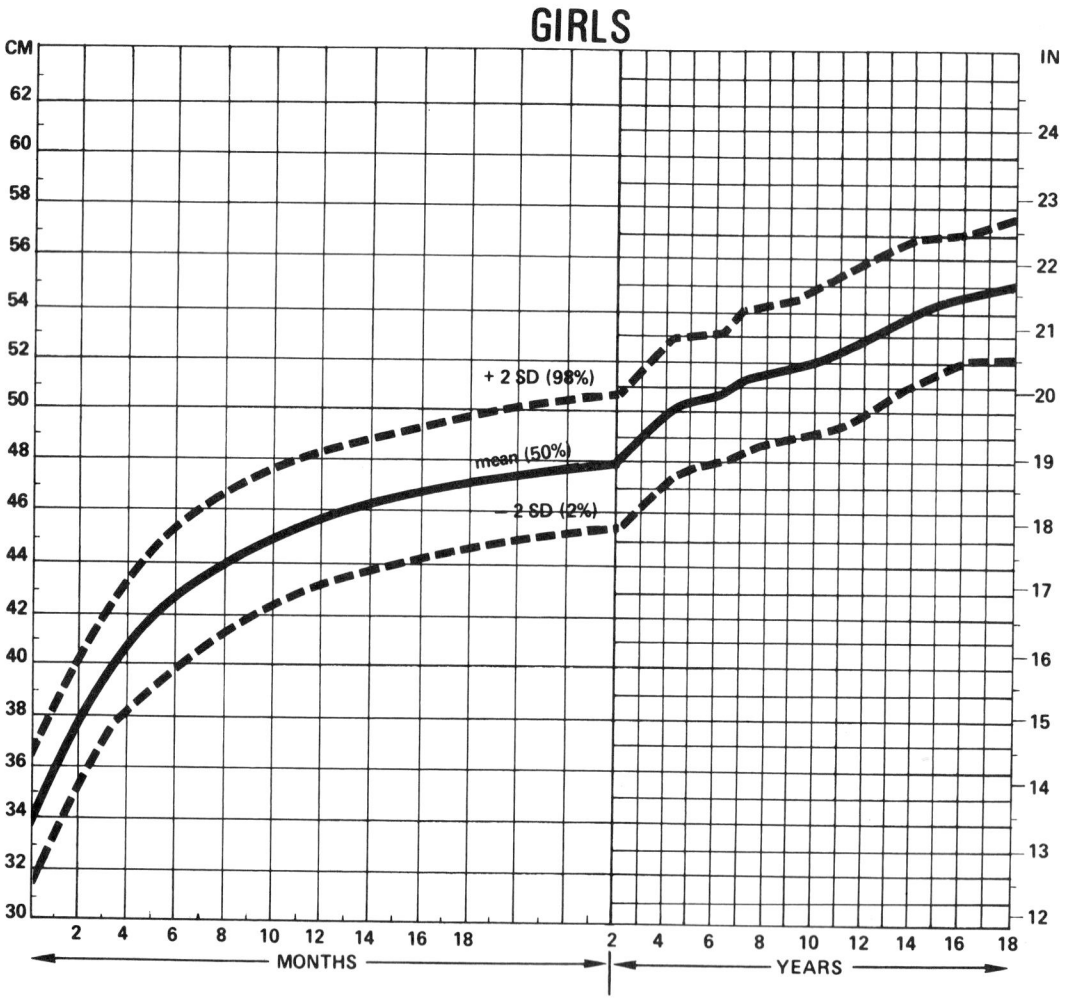

Source: *Nellhaus, G. (1968). Composite international and interracial graphs.* Pediatrics, 41, *106.* Copyright American Academy of Pediatrics 1968.

Head Circumference: Boys

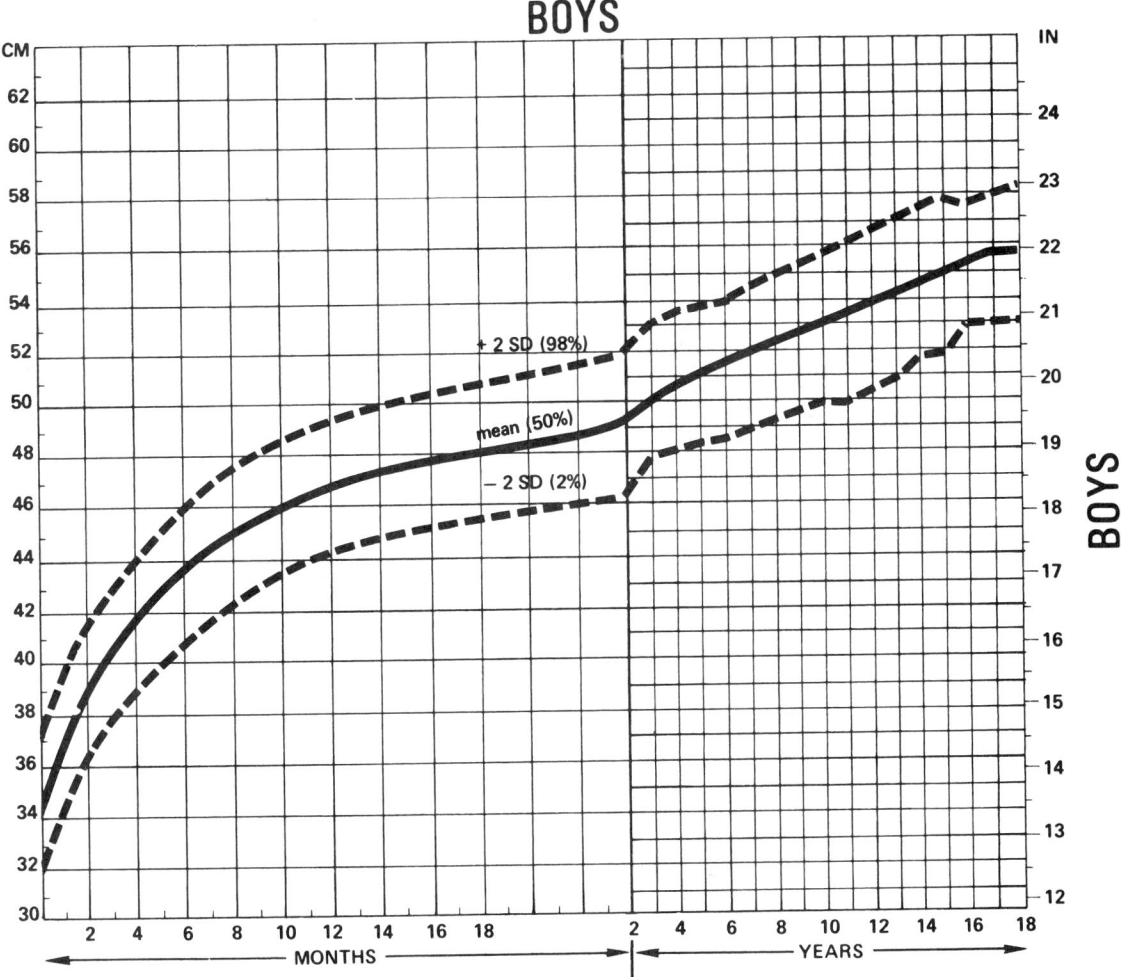

Source: *Nellhaus, G. (1968). Composite international and interracial graphs.* Pediatrics, 41, *106.* Copyright American Academy of Pediatrics 1968.

1983 Metropolitan Height and Weight Table for Women

Height		Weight*		
Feet	Inches	Small Frame (lb)	Medium Frame (lb)	Large Frame (lb)
4	10	102–111	109–121	118–131
4	11	103–113	111–123	120–134
5	0	104–115	113–126	122–137
5	1	106–118	115–129	125–140
5	2	108–121	118–132	128–143
5	3	111–124	121–135	131–147
5	4	114–127	124–138	134–151
5	5	117–130	127–141	137–155
5	6	120–133	130–144	140–159
5	7	123–136	133–147	143–163
5	8	126–139	136–150	146–167
5	9	129–142	139–153	149–170
5	10	132–145	142–156	152–173
5	11	135–148	145–159	155–176
6	0	138–151	148–162	158–179

*Weight in lb according to frame (in indoor clothing weighing 3 lbs, shoes with 1-in heels).

Source of basic data: Society of Actuaries and Association of Life Insurance Medical Directors of America (1990). *1979 build study.*

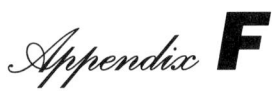

Standard Laboratory Values

Pregnant and Nonpregnant Women

Values	Nonpregnant	Pregnant
Hematologic		
Complete Blood Count (CBC)		
Hemoglobin, g/dL	12–16˙	11.5–14˙
Hematocrit, PCV, %	37–47	32–42
Red cell volume, mL	1600	1900
Plasma volume, mL	2400	3700
Red blood cell count, million/mm³	4–5.5	3.75–5.0
White blood cells, total per mm³	4500–10,000	5000–15,000
Polymorphonuclear cells, %	54–62	60–85
Lymphocytes, %	38–46	15–40
Erythrocyte sedimentation rate, mm/h	≤	30–90
MCHC, g/dL packed RBCs (mean corpuscular hemoglobin concentration)	30–36	No change
MCH (mean corpuscular hemoglobin per picogram)	29–32	No change
MCV/μm³ (mean corpuscular volume per cubic micrometer)	82–96	No change
Blood Coagulation and Fibrinolytic Activity†		
Factors VII, VIII, IX, X		Increase in pregnancy, return to normal in early puerperium; factor VIII increases during and immediately after delivery
Factors XI; XIII		Decrease in pregnancy
Prothrombin time (protime)	60–70 sec	Slight decrease in pregnancy
Partial thromboplastin time (PTT)	12–14 sec	Slight decrease in pregnancy and again decrease during second and third stage of labor (indicates clotting at placental site)
Bleeding time	1–3 min (Duke) 2–4 min (Ivy)	No appreciable change
Coagulation time	6–10 min (Lee/White)	No appreciable change
Platelets	150,000 to 350,000/mm³	No significant change until 3–5 days after delivery, then marked increase (may predispose woman to thrombosis) and gradual return to normal
Fibrinolytic activity		Decreases in pregnancy, then abrupt return to normal (protection against thromboembolism)
Fibrinogen	250 mg/dl	400 mg/dL
Mineral and Vitamin Concentrations		
Serum iron, μg	75–150	65–120
Total iron-binding capacity, μg	250–450	300–500
Iron saturation, %	30–40	15–30

(*continued*)

Adele Pillitteri: MATERNAL AND CHILD HEALTH NURSING, 2nd Edition. © 1995 Adele Pillitteri.

Pregnant and Nonpregnant Women Continued

Values	Nonpregnant	Pregnant
Vitamin B_{12}, folic acid, ascorbic acid	Normal	Moderate decrease
Serum proteins		
Total, g/dL	6.7–8.3	5.5–7.5
Albumin, g/dL	3.5–5.5	3.0–5.0
Globulin, total, g/dL	2.3–3.5	3.0–4.0
Blood sugar		
Fasting, mg/dL	70–80	65
2-hour postprandial, mg/dL	60–110	Under 140 after a 100-g carbohydrate meal is considered normal
Cardiovascular		
Blood pressure, mm Hg	120/80[‡]	114/65
Peripheral resistance, dyne/s · cm^{-5}	120	100
Venous pressure, cm H_2O		
Femoral	9	24
Antecubital	8	8
Pulse, rate/min	70	80
Stroke volume, mL	65	75
Cardiac output, L/min	4.5	6
Circulation time (arm-tongue), sec	15–16	12–14
Blood volume, mL		
Whole blood	4000	5600
Plasma	2400	3700
Red blood cells	1600	1900
Plasma renin, units/L	3–10	10–80
Chest x-ray studies		
Transverse diameter of heart	—	1–2 cm increase
Left border of heart	—	Straightened
Cardiac volume	—	70-mL increase
Electrocardiogram	—	15° left axis deviation
V_1 and V_2	—	Inverted T-wave
kV_4	—	Low T
III	—	Q + inverted T
aVr	—	Small Q
Hepatic		
Bilirubin total	Not more than 1 mg/dL	Unchanged
Cephalin flocculation	Up to 2+ in 48 h	Positive in 10%
Serum cholesterol	110–300 mg/dL	↑ 60% from 16–32 weeks of pregnancy; remains at this level until after delivery
Thymol turbidity	0–4 units	Positive in 15%
Serum alkaline phosphatase	2–4.5 units (Bodansky)	↑ from week 12 of pregnancy to 6 weeks after delivery
Serum lactate dehydrogenase		Unchanged
Serum glutamic-oxaloacetic transaminase		Unchanged
Serum globulin albumin	1.5–3.0 g/dL	↑ slight
	4.5–5.3 g/dL	↓ 3.0 g by late pregnancy
A/G ratio		Decreased
α_2-globulin		Increased
β-globulin		Increased
Serum cholinesterase		Decreased
Leucine aminopeptidase		Increased
Sulfobromophthalein (5 mg/kg)	5% dye or less in 45 min	Somewhat decreased

(continued)

Pregnant and Nonpregnant Women Continued

Values	Nonpregnant	Pregnant
Renal		
Bladder capacity	1300 mL	1500 mL
Renal plasma flow (RPF), mL/min	490–700	Increase by 25%, to 612–875
Glomerular filtration rate (GFR), mL/min	1C 32	Increase by 50%, to 160–198
Nonprotein nitrogen (NPN), mg/dL	2⁵	Decreases
Blood urea nitrogen (BUN), mg/dL	20 ⅝	Decreases
Serum creatinine, mg/kg/24 hr	20–22	Decreases
Serum uric acid, mg/kg/24 hr	257–750	Decreases
Urine glucose	Negative	Present in 20% of gravidas
Intravenous pyelogram (IVP)	Normal	Slight to moderate hydroureter and hydro-nephrosis; right kidney larger than left kidney
Miscellaneous		
Total thyroxine concentration	5–12 μg/dL thyroxine	↑ 9–16 μg/dL thyroxine (however, unbound thyroxine not greatly increased)
Ionized calcium		Relatively unchanged
Aldosterone		↑ 1 mg/24 hr by third trimester
Dehydroisoandrosterone	Plasma clearance 6–8 L/24 hr	↑ plasma clearance tenfold to twentyfold

* At sea level. Permanent residents of higher levels (e.g., Denver) require higher levels of hemoglobin.
From Bobak IM, et al. (1992). *Maternity and gynecologic care: The nurse and the family* (5th ed.). St Louis: C. V. Mosby.
† Pregnancy represents a hypercoagulable state.
‡ For the woman about 20 years of age.
   10 years of age: 103/70.
   30 years of age: 123/82.
   40 years of age: 126/84.

Infants and Children

The following reference values for laboratory tests represent guidelines only, since the reference range from one institution to the next will vary, depending on the laboratory method used. To simplify the interpretation of laboratory results reported in International System (SI) units, conversion factors (from SI to conventional units) are provided. SI base units are the gram (g), the liter (L), and the mole (mol). Other abbreviations used throughout this table are listed below.

SI Prefixes

Factor	Prefix	Symbol
10^3	kilo	k
10^{-1}	deci	d
10^{-2}	centi	c
10^{-3}	milli	m
10^{-6}	micro	μ
10^{-9}	nano	n
10^{-12}	pico	p
10^{-15}	femto	f

Abbreviations

Cl	confidence interval
d	day
F	female
h	hour
Hb	hemoglobin
M	male
MCHC	mean corpuscular hemoglobin concentration
MCV	mean corpuscular value
mEq	milliequivalent
min	minute
RBC	red blood cell
s	second
SD	standard deviation
U	unit
WBC	white blood cell
yr	year

Blood

Test	SI Reference Range	Conversion Factor	Conventional Units Reference Range

Adrenocorticotropic hormone (ACTH)	Cord: 130–160 ng/L
	1st week: 100–140
	Adult 0800 h: 25–100
	    1800 h: <50
			Cord: 130–160 pg/mL
			1st week: 100–140
			Adult 0800 h: 25–100
			    1800 h: <50

Alanine aminotransferase (ALT)	<1 yr: 5–28 U/L >1 yr: 8–20		Same as SI
Albumin	35–50 g/L		3.5–5.0 g/dL
Aldolase	Newborn: <32 U/L Child: <16 Adult: <8		Same as SI
Aldosterone	Newborn: 0.14–1.66 nmol/L 1 wk–1 yr: 0.03–4.43 1–3 yr: 0.14–1.66 3–5 yr: <0.14–2.22 5–7 yr: <0.14–1.39 7–11 yr: 0.14–1.94 11–15 yr: <0.14–1.39	nmol/L × 36.1 = ng/dL	Newborn: 5–60 ng/dL 1 wk–1 yr: 1–160 ng/dL 1–3 yr: 5–60 ng/dL 3–5 yr: <5–80 5–7 yr: <5–50 7–11 yr: 5–70 11–15 yr: <5–50
Alkaline phosphatase	Infant: 150–400 U/L 2–10 yr: 100–300 11–18 yr (M): 50–375 11–18 yr (F): 30–300 Adult: 30–100		Same as SI
α_1-antitrypsin	2–4 g/L		200–400 mg/dL
α-fetoprotein	Fetal: peak of 2–4 g/L Cord: <0.05 g/L >1 yr: <30 μg/L		Fetal: 200–400 mg/dL Cord: <5 >1 yr: <30
Ammonia nitrogen	9–34 μmol/L	μmol/L × 1.4 = μg/dL	13–48 μg/dL
Amylase	Newborn: 5–65 U/L >1 yr: 25–125		Same as SI
Androstenedione	Child: 0.17–1.7 nmol/L Adult (M): 2.4–5.2 Adult (F): 2.7–8.0	nmol/L × 28.7 = ng/dL	Child: 5–50 ng/dL Adult (M): 70–150 Adult (F): 76–228
Angiotensin-converting enzyme	<670 nmol · L^{-1} · S^{-1}	nmol · L^{-1} · S^{-1} × 0.06 = nmol/mL/min	<40 nmol/mL/min
Anion gap [Na − (Cl + HCO_3)]	7–14 mmol/L		7–14 mEq/L
Aspartate amino-transfer (AST)	<1 yr: 15–60 U/L >1 yr: ≤20 U/L		Same as SI
Bicarbonate	<2 yrs: 20–25 mmol/L >2 yrs: 22-26 mmol/L		<2 yrs: 20–25 mEq/L >2 yrs: 22–26
Bilirubin (total)	*Preterm* *Full term* Cord: <34 <34 μmol/L 0–1 d: <137 <103 1–2 d: <205 <137 3–5 d: <274 <205 Thereafter: <34 <17	μmol/L × 0.05848 = mg/dL	*Preterm* *Full term* Cord: <2 <2 mg/dL 0–1 d: <8 <6 1–2 d: <12 <8 3–5 d: <16 <12 Thereafter: <2 <1
Bilirubin (conjugated)	0–3.4 μmol/L	μmol/L × 0.05848 = mg/dL	0–0.2 mg/dL
Calcium (ionized)	1.12–1.23 mmol/L	mmol/L × 4 = mg/dL	4.48–4.92 mg/dL
Calcium (total)	Preterm < 1 wk: 1.5–2.5 mmol/L Term: <1 wk: 1.75–3 Child: 2–2.6 Adult: 2.1–2.6	mmol/L × 4 = mg/dL	6–10 mg/dL 7–12 8–10.5 8.5–10.5
Carbon dioxide (CO_2 content)	22–26 mmol/L		22–26 mEq/L

(*continued*)

Blood Continued

Test	SI Reference Range	Conversion Factor	Conventional Units Reference Range
Carbon monoxide (carboxyhemoglobin)	*% total HB* Nonsmokers: <0.02 Smokers: <0.01 Toxic: >0.20		*Fraction of HB sat* Nonsmokers: <2 Smokers: <10 Toxic: >20
Carotene	Infant: 0.37–1.30 μmol/L Child: 0.74–2.42 Adult: 1.12–3.72	μmol/L × 53.7 = μg/dL	Infant: 20–70 μg/dL Child: 40–130 Adult: 60–200
Ceruloplasmin	1–12 yr: 300–650 mg/L >12 yr: 150–600 mg/L		1–12 yr: 30–65 mg/dL >12 yr: 15–60
Chloride	94–106 mmol/L		94–106 mEq/L
Cholesterol	Infant: 1.81–4.53 mmol/L Child: 3.11–5.18 Adolescent: 3.11–5.44 Adult: 3.63–6.48	mmol/L × 38.61 = mg/dL	Infant: 53–135 mg/dL Child: 70–175 Adolescent: 140–250 Adult: 140–250
Complement, C_3	1 mo: 0.61–1.30 g/L 6 mo: 0.87–1.36 Adult: 1.11–1.71		1 mo: 61–130 mg/dL 6 mo: 87–136 Adult: 111–171
Complement, C_4	Newborn: 0.16–0.39 g/L Adult: 0.15–0.45 g/L		Newborn: 16–39 mg/dL Adult: 15–45
Complement, total hemolytic (CH 50)	75–160 U/mL		75–160 U/ml
Copper	0–6 mo: 3.1–11 μmol/L 6 yr: 14–30 12 yr: 12.5–25 Adult (M): 11–22 Adult (F): 12.6–24	μmol × 6.353 = μg/dL	0–6 mo: 20–70 μg/dL 6 yr: 90–190 12 yr: 80–160 Adult (M): 70–140 Adult (F): 80–155
Cortisol	0800 h (or pre-ACTH): 225–505 nmol/L Post-ACTH: twice pre-ACTH value	nmol/L × 0.0362 = μg/dL	0800 h (or pre-ACTH): 8–18 μg/dL Post-ACTH: twice pre-ACTH value
Creatine kinase	Newborn: 76–600 U/L Adult (M): 38–174 Adult (F): 96–140		Same as SI
Creatine kinase isoenzymes	*Fraction of total activity* CK-BB (CK-1): absent or trace CK-MB (CK-2): 0.04–0.06 CK-MM (CK-3): 0.94–0.96		*% Activity* CK-BB (CK-1): absent or trace CK-MB (CK-2): 4%–6% CK-MM (CK-3): 94%–96%
Creatinine	Newborn: 27–88 μmol/L Infant: 18–35 Child: 27–62 Adolescent: 44–88 Adult (M): 53–106 Adult (F): 44–97	μmol/L × 0.0113 = mg/dL	Newborn: 0.3–1.0 mg/dL Infant: 0.2–0.4 Child: 0.3–0.7 Adolescent: 0.5–1.0 Adult (M): 0.6–1.2 Adult (F): 0.5–1.1
Dehydroepiandrosterone (DHEA)	Child: 3–10 nmol/L Adult (M): 6–15 Adult (F): 7–18	nmol/L × 0.2884 = μg/L	Child: 1–3 μg/L Adult (M): 1.7–4.2 Adult (F): 2–5.2
Dehydroepiandrosterone sulfate (DHEA-S)	1–4 days: <52 μmol/L Child: 1.6–6.6	μmol/L × 0.37 = μg/mL	1–4 days: <20 μg/mL Child: 0.6–2.54
Estradiol	*Males* Pubertal stage I: 7–29 pmol/L II: 40 III: >73	pmol/L × 0.2723 = pg/mL	2–8 pg/mL 11 >20

(continued)

Blood *Continued*

Test	SI Reference Range	Conversion Factor	Conventional Units Reference Range
	Adult: 29–132		8–36
	Females		
	Pubertal stage I: 0–84 pmol/L		0–23 pg/mL
	II: 0–242		0–66
	III: 0–385		0–105
	IV: 73–1101		20–300
	Follicular: 37–330		10–90
	Midcycle: 367–1835		100–500
	Luteal: 184–881		50–240
Free fatty acids	Child: <1.10 mmol/L	mmol/L × 28.25 = mg/dL	Child: <31 mg/dL
	Adult: 0.3–0.9		Adult 8–25
Ferritin	Child: 7–144 µg/L		Child: 7–144 ng/mL
	Adult (M): 30–265		Adult (M): 30–265
	Adult (F): 10–110		Adult (F): 10–110
Fibrinogen	2–4 g/L		200–400 mg/dL
Folate	4–20 nmol/L	nmol/L × 0.4413 = ng/mL	1.8–9.0 ng/mL
Folate (RBCs)	340–1020 nmol/L packed cells	nmol/L × 0.4413 = ng/mL	150–450 ng/mL
Follicle-stimulating hormone (FSH)	Prepubertal: <5 IU/L		Prepubertal: <5 mIU/mL
	Adult (M): 1.5–16		Adult (M): 1.5–16
	Adult (F): 2–17.2		Adult (F): 2–17.2
Fructose	55–330 µmol/L	µmol/L × 0.018 = mg/dL	1–6 mg/dL
Galactose	Newborn: 0–1.11 mmol/L	mmol/L × 18.02 = mg/dL	Newborn: 0–20 mg/dL
	Thereafter: <0.28		Thereafter: <5
Gamma glutamyl transferase (GGT)	0–3 wk: 0–130 U/L		Same as SI
	3 wk–3 mo: 4–120		
	3 mo–1 yr (M): 5–65		
	3 mo–1 yr (F): 5–35		
	1–15 yr: 0–23		
	Adult: 0–35		
Gastrin	<100 ng/L		<100 pg/mL
Glucagon	50–100 ng/L		50–100 pg/mL
Glucose	Preterm: 1.1–3.6 mmol/L	mmol/L × 18.02 = mg/dL	Preterm: 20–65 mg/dL
	Full term: 1.1–6.1		Full term: 20–100
	1 wk–16 yr: 3.3–5.8		1 wk–16 yr: 60–105
	>16 yr: 3.9–6.4		>16 yr: 70–115
Haptoglobin	0.4–1.8 g/L		40–180 mg/dL
Hemoglobin A$_{1c}$	0.039–0.077 fraction of total Hb		3.9%–7.7% of total HB
β-Hydroxybutyrate	<100 µmol/L	µmol/L × 0.01041 = mg/dL	<1mg/dL
17-Hydroxyprogesterone	Prepubertal (M): 0.3–0.91 nmol/L	nmol/L × 0.33 = ng/mL	Prepubertal (M): 0.1–0.3 ng/mL
	Prepubertal (F): 0.61–1.52		
	Adult(M): 0.61–5.45		Prepubertal (F): 0.2–0.5
	Adult (F):		Adult(M): 0.2–1.8
	Follicular: 0.61–2.42		Adult (F):
	Luteal: 2.42–9.10		Follicular: 0.2–0.8
			Luteal: 0.8–3.0
Immunoglobulins A, G, M	*IgA*	*IgG*	*IgM*
	Newborn: 0–0.05 g/L	6.4–16 g/L	0.06–0.24 g/L
	1–3 mo: 0.03–0.66	3.0–10.0	0.15–1.50
	3–6 mo: 0.04–0.90	1.4–10.0	0.15–1.10
	6–12 mo: 0.45–2.25	4.0–11.5	0.43–2.25
	1–2 yr: 0.35–2.40	3.5–12.0	0.36–2.40

(continued)

Blood Continued

Test	SI Reference Range	Conversion Factor	Conventional Units Reference Range
	IgA	*IgG*	*IgM*
	2–6 yr: 0.40–1.90	5.0–13.0	0.50–1.99
	6–12 yr: 0.40–2.70	7.0–16.5	0.50–2.60
	12–16 yr: 0.50–2.32	7.0–15.5	0.45–2.40
	Adult: 0.70–3.90	6.5–15.0	0.40–3.4
Immunoglobulin E	Newborn: 0–24 µg/L		Newborn: 0–10 U/mL
	6–12 yr: 0–480		6–12 yr: 0–200
	Adult: 0–960		Adult: 0–400
Insulin, fasting	3–23 mU/L		3–23 µU/mL
Iron	Newborn: 20–48 µmol/L	µmol/L $\times$ 5.587 = µg/dL	Newborn: 110–270 µg/dL
	4–10 mo: 5.4–12.5		4–10 mo: 30–70
	3–19 yr: 9.5–27.0		3–10 yr: 53–119
	Adult: 13.0–33.0		Adult: 72–186
Iron-binding capacity	Newborn: 10.6–31.3 µmol/L	µmol/L $\times$ 5.587 = µg/dL	Newborn: 59–175 µg/dL
	Thereafter: 45–72		Thereafter: 250–400
Lactate	Venous: 0.5–2.0 mmol/L	mmol/L $\times$ 9.01 = mg/dL	Venous: 5–18 mg/dL
	Arterial: 0.3–0.8		Arterial: 3–7
Lactate dehydrogenase	Newborn: 160–1500 U/L		Same as SI units
	Infant: 150–360		
	Child: 150–300		
	Adult: 100–250		
Lactate dehydrogenase isoenzymes		*Fraction of total*	
		LD 1 (heart): 0.24–0.34	
		LD 2 (heart, RBCs): 0.35–0.45	
		LD 3 (muscle): 0.15–0.25	
		LD 4 (liver, muscle): 0.04–0.10	
		LD 5 (liver, muscle): 0.01–0.09	
Lead	<1.16 µmol/L	µmol/L $\times$ 20.7 = gmg/dL	<24 gmg/dL

Lipids	95th %ile values—mmol/L (mg/dL)			5th %ile values—mmol/L (mg/dL)	
	VLDL (Cholesterol)		*LDL (Cholesterol)*		*HDL (Cholesterol)*	
	M	F	M	F	M	F
	5–9 yr: 0.47 (18)	0.62 (24)	3.34 (129)	3.62 (140)	0.98 (38)	0.93 (36)
	10–14 yr: 0.57 (22)	0.59 (23)	3.41 (132)	3.52 (136)	0.96 (37)	0.91 (35)
	15–19 yr: 0.67 (26)	0.62 (24)	3.36 (130)	3.49 (135)	0.80 (31)	0.91 (35)
			mmol/L $\times$ 38.61 = mg/dL			

Test	SI Reference Range	Conversion Factor	Conventional Units Reference Range
Luteinizing hormone	Prepubertal: <5 IU/L		Prepubertal: <5 mIU/mL
	Adult (M): 3.9–18		Adult (M): 3.9–18
	Adult (F): 2.0–22.6		Adult (F): 2.0–22.6
Magnesium	0.75–1.0 mmol/L	mmol/L $\times$ 2 = mEq/L	1.5–2.0 mEq/L
Methemoglobin	<46 µmol/L	µmol/L $\times$ 0.0065 = g/dL	< 0.3 gdL
Osmolality	285–295 mmol/kg		285–295 mOsm/kg
Phosphorus	Newborn: 1.36–2.91 mmol/L	mmol/L $\times$ 3.097 = mg/dL	Newborn: 4.2–9.0 mg/dL
	1 yr: 1.23–2.00		1 yr: 3.8–6.2
	2–5 yr: 1.13–2.20		2–5 yr: 3.5–6.8
	Adult: 0.97–1.45		Adult: 3.0–4.5
Phytanic acid	<0.003 fraction of total serum fatty acids		<0.3% of total serum fatty acids
Potassium	<10 days: 3.5–6.0 mmol/L		<10 days: 3.5–6.0 mEq/L
	>10 days: 3.5–5.0		>10 days: 3.5–5.0
Progesterone	*Males*		
	Prepubertal: 0.35–0.83 nmol/L	nmol/L $\times$ 0.314 = ng/mL	0.11–0.26 ng/mL
	Adult: 0.38–0.95		0.12–0.30

(*continued*)

Blood Continued

Test	SI Reference Range	Conversion Factor	Conventional Units Reference Range
	Females		
	Prepubertal: <0.95		≤0.30
	Pubertal stage II: < 1.46		≤0.46
	III: <1.91		≤0.60
	IV: 0.16–41.34		0.05–13.0
	Follicular: 0.06–2.86		0.02–0.9
	Luteal: 19.08–95.40		6.0–30.0
Prolactin	Newborn: <200 μg/L		Newborn: <200 ng/mL
	Adult: <20 μg/L		Adult: <20 ng/mL
Protein, total	Preterm: 40–70 g/L		Preterm: 4.0–7.0 g/dL
	Term newborn: 50–71		Term newborn: 5.0–7.1
	1–3 mo: 47–74		1–3 mo: 4.7–7.4
	3–12 mo: 50–75		3–12 mo: 5.0–7.5
	1–15 yr: 65–86		1–15 yr: 6.5–8.6
Pyruvate	0.03–0.10 mmol/L	mmol/L × 8.81 = mg/dL	0.3–0.9 mg/dL
Renin	Adults: 0.30–1.14 ng · L^{-1} · S^{-1}	ng · L^{-1} · S^{-1} × 3.6 =	Adults: 1.1–4.1 ng/mL/h
Sodium	135–145 mmol/L	ng/mL/h	135–145 mEq/L
Somatomedin C	0–2 yr: 220–1000 IU/L		0–2 yr: 0.22–1.00 U/mL
	3–5 yr: 270–1600		3–5 yr: 0.27–1.60
	6–10 yr: 370–2100		6–10 yr: 0.37–2.10
	11–12 yr: 450–2800		11–12 yr: 0.45–2.80
	13–14 yr: 1100–4000		13–14 yr: 1.10–4.00
	15–17 yr: 1000–2900		15–17 yr: 1.00–2.90
	Thereafter: 460–1500		Thereafter: 0.46–1.50
Testosterone, free	Prepubertal: 2.08–13.19 pmol/L		Prepubertal: 0.06–0.38 ng/dL
	Adult (M): 48.6–201		Adult (M): 1.40–5.79
	Adult (F): 6.94–25		Adult (F): 0.20–0.73
Testosterone, total	Prepubertal: 0.35–0.70 nmol/L		Prepubertal: 10–20 ng/dL
	Adult (F): 0.8–2.6		Adult (F): 23–75
	Adult (M): 9.5–30		Adult (M): 275–875
Thyroid-stimulating hormone (TSH)	Cord 0–17.4 μU/L		Cord: 0–17.4 mIU/mL
	1–3 dyas: 0–13.3		1–3 days: 0–13.3
	Thereafter: 0–5.5		Thereafter: 0–5.5
Thyroxine (T$_4$), total	Cord: 95–168 nmol/L	nmol/L × 0.0775 = μg/dL	Cord: 7.4–13.0 μg/dL
	<1 mo: 90–292		<1 mo: 7.0–22.6
	1 mo–1 yr: 93–213		1 mo–1 yr: 7.2–16.5
	1–5 yr: 94–194		1–5 yr: 7.3–15.0
	5–10 yr: 83–172		5–10 yr: 6.4–13.3
	10–15 yr: 72–151		10–15 yr: 5.6–11.7
	Adult: 55–161		Adult: 4.3–12.5
Thyroxine (T$_4$), free	9–22 pmol/L	pmol/L × 0.0777 = ng/dL	0.7–1.7 ng/dL
Transferrin	Newborn: 1.30–2.75 g/L		Newborn: 130–275 mg/dL
	Adult: 2.20–4.00		Adult: 220–440

Triglycerides

Normal Upper Limits—mmol/L (mg/dL)	
Male	*Female*
0–4 yr: 1.12 (99)	1.26 (112)
5–9 yr: 1.14 (101)	1.19 (105)
10–15 yr: 1.41 (125)	1.48 (131)
15–19 yr: 1.67 (148)	1.40 (124)
	mmol/L × 88.55 = mg/dL

(continued)

Blood Continued

Test	SI Reference Range	Conversion Factor	Conventional Units Reference Range
Triiodothyronine (T$_3$)	Cord: 0.23–1.16 nmol/L	nmol/L × 65.1 = ng/dL	Cord: 15–75 ng/dL
	<1 mo: 0.49–3.70		<1 mo: 32–240
	1 mo–1 yr: 1.70–4.31		1 mo–1 yr: 110–280
	1–5 yr: 1.62–4.14		1–5 yr: 105–269
	5–10 yr: 1.45–3.71		5–10 yr: 94–241
	10–15 yr: 1.28–3.31		10–15 yr: 83–215
	Adult: 1.08–3.14		Adult: 70–204
Triiodothyronine resin uptake	0.25–0.35		25%–35%
Urea nitrogen	2–7 mmol/L	mmol/L × 2.8 = mg/dL	5–20 mg/dL
Uric acid	120–420 μmol/L	μmol/L × 0.0169 = mg/dL	2–7 mg/dL
Vitamin A	Newborn: 1.22–2.62 μmol/L	μmol/L × 28.65 = μg/dL	Newborn: 35–75 μg/dL
	Child: 1.05–2.79		Child: 30–80
	Adult: 1.05–2.27		Adult: 30–65
Vitamin B$_6$	14.6–72.8 nmol/L	nmol/L × 0.247 = ng/mL	3.6–18 ng/mL
Vitamin B$_{12}$	96–579 pmol/L	pmol/L × 1.355 = pg/mL	130–785 pg/mL
Vitamin C	11.4–113.6 μmol/L	μmol/L × 0.176 = mg/dL	0.2–2.0 mg/dL
Vitamin D$_3$ (1,25 dihydroxy)	60–108 pmol/L	pmol/L × 0.417 = pg/mL	25–45 pg/mL
Vitamin E	11.6–46.4 μmol/L	μmol × 0.043 = mg/dL	0.5–2.0 mg/dL
Zinc	10.7–22.9 μmol/L	μmol/L × 6.54 = μgdL	70–150 μg/dL

Hematology

Age	HB (g/dL) Mean	HB (g/dL) −2 SD	Hematocrit (%) Mean	Hematocrit (%) −2 SD	MCV (fL) Mean	MCV (fL) −2 SD	MCHC (g/dL RBC) Mean	MCHC (g/dL RBC) −2 SD	Reticulocyte (%)	WBC (1,000/mm^3) Mean	WBC (1,000/mm^3) 95% CI	Platelets (1,000/mm^3) Mean (Range)
Term												
(cord blood)	16.5	13.5	51	42	108	98	33.0	30.0	3.0–7.0	18.1	9.0–30.0	290
1–3 days	18.5	14.5	56	45	108	95	33.0	29.0	1.8–4.6	18.9	9.4–34.0	192
2 weeks	16.6	13.4	53	41	105	88	31.4	28.1		11.4	5.0–20.0	252
1 month	13.9	10.7	44	33	101	91	31.8	28.1	0.1–1.7	10.8	5.0–19.5	
2 months	11.2	9.4	35	28	95	84	31.8	28.3				
6 months	12.6	11.1	36	31	76	68	35.0	32.7	0.7–2.3	11.9	6.0–17.5	
6–24 months	12.0	10.5	36	33	78	70	33.0	30.0		10.6	6.0–17.0	(150–300)
2–6 years	12.5	11.5	37	34	81	75	34.0	31.0	0.5–1.0	8.5	5.0–15.5	(150–300)
6–12 years	13.5	11.5	50	35	86	77	34.0	31.0	0.5–1.0	8.1	4.5–13.5	(150–300)
12–18 years (M)	14.5	13.0	43	36	88	78	34.0	31.0	0.5–1.0	7.8	4.5–13.5	(150–300)
12–18 years (F)	14.0	12.0	41	37	90	78	34.0	31.0	0.5–1.0	7.8	4.5–13.5	150–300

Urine

Test	SI Reference Range	Conversion Factor	Conventional Units Reference Range
Aminolevulinic acid	8–53 μmol/d	μmol/d × 0.131 = mg/d	1–7 mg/d
Calcium	<0.1 mmol/kg/d	mmol/d × 40 = mg/d	<4 mg/kg/d
Copper	<0.6 μmol/d	μmol/d × 63.7 = gmg/d	<40 μg/d
Coproporphyrin	<300 nmol/d	nmol/d × 1.527 = μg/d	<200 μg/d
Cortisol, free	70–340 nmol/d	nmol/d × 0.362 = μgd	25–125 μg/d

(continued)

Urine Continued

Test	SI Reference Range	Conversion Factor	Conventional Units Reference Range
Creatinine	Infant: 71–177 μmol/kg/d Child: 71–194 Adolescent: 71–265	μmol/kg/d × 0.113 = mg/kg/d	Infant: 8–20 mg/kg/d Child: 8–22 Adolescent: 8–30
Cystine	40–260 μmol/d	μmol/d × 0.12 = mg/d	5–31 mg/d
Dehydroepiandrosterone (DHEA)	<5 yr: <0.3 μmol/d 6–9 yr: <0.7 10–15 yr: <1.4 Adult (M): <8.0 Adult (F): <4.2	μmol/d × 0.288 = mg/d	<5 yr: <0.1 mg/d 6–9 yr: <0.2 10–15 yr: <0.4 Adult (M): <2.3 Adult (F): <1.2
Epinephrine	<55 nmol/d	nmol/d × 0.183 < μg/d	<10 μg/d
Fluoride	<50 μmol/d	μmol/d × 0.019 = mg/d	<1 mg/d
Homovanillic acid (HVA)	*mmol/mol/creatinine* 1–12 mo: 0.75–21.7 1–2 yr: 2.5–14.3 2–5 yr: 0.43–8.4 5–10 yr: 0.31–5.6 10–15 yr: 0.15–7.4 15–18 yr: 0.31–1.24	mmol/mol creatinine × 1.61 = μg/mg creatinine	*μg/mg creatinine* 1–12 mo: 1.2–35.0 1–2 y r: 4.0–23.0 2–5 yr: 0.7–13.5 5–10 yr: 0.5–9.0 10–15 yr: 0.25–12.0 15–18 yr: 0.5–2.0
Metanephrines	*mmol/mol/creatinine* <1 yr: 0.001–2.64 1–2 yr: 0.15–3.09 2–5 yr: 0.20–1.72 5–10 yr: 0.25–1.55 10–15 yr: 0.001–0.38 15–18 yr: 0.03–0.69	mmol/mol creatinine × 1.74 = μg/mg creatinine	*μg/mg creatinine* <1 yr: 0.001–4.6 1–2 yr: 0.27–5.38 2–5 yr: 0.35–2.99 5–10 yr: 0.43–2.70 10–15 yr: 0.001–1.87 15–18 yr: 0.001–0.67
Norepinephrine	<590 nmol/d	nmol/d × 0.169 = μg/d	<100 μg/d
Osmolality	50–1200 μgmol/kg		50–1200 mOsm/kg
Oxalate	110–440 μmol/d	μmol/d × 0.088 = mg/d	10–40 mg/d
Porphobilinogen	0–8.8 μmol/d	μmol/d × 0.226 × mg/d	0–2 mg/d
Potassium	25–125 mmol/d (varies with diet)		25–125 mEq/d
Pregnanetriol	<7.4 μmol/d	μmol/d × 0.3365 = mg/d	<2.5 mg/d
Protein	10–140 mg/L		1–14 mg/dL
Steroids: 17-hydroxycorti-costeroid	Prepubertal: 2.76–15.5 μmol/d Adult (M): 11–33 Adult (F): 11–22	μmol/d × 0.3625 = mg/d	Prepubertal: 1–5.6 mg/d Adult (M): 4–12 Adult (F): 4–8
Steroids: 17-ketosteroids	<1 mo: ≤6.9 μmol/d 1 mo–5 yr: <1.73 6–8 yr: 3.47–6.9 Adult (M): 21–62 Adult (F): 14–45	μmol/d × 0.2884 = mg/d	< 1 mo: <2 mg/d 1 mo–5 yr: <0.5 6–8 yr: 1–2 Adult (M): 6–18 Adult (F): 4–13
Uric acid	1.48–4.43 mmol/d	mmol/d × 169 = mg/d	250–750 mg/d
Vanilylmandelic acid (VMA)	*mmol/mol creatinine* 1–6 mo: 1.71–9.71 6–12 mo: 1.14–8.57 1–5 yr: 1.14–5.71 5–10 yr: 0.86–4.00 10–15 yr: 0.57–3.43 >15 yr: 0.57–3.43	mmol/moil creatinine × 1.75 = μg/mg	*μg/mg creatinine* 1–6 mo: 3–7 6–12 mo: 2–15 1–5 yr: 2–10 5–10 yr: 1.5–7 10–15 yr: 1–6 >15 yr: 1–6

Cerebrospinal Fluid

Cell Count Range

Preterm: 0–25 WBC $\times$ 10^6 cells/L (57% polymorphonuclears)
Term: 0–22 WBC $\times$ 10^6 cells/L (61% polymorphonuclears)
Child: 0–7 WBC $\times$ 10^6 cells/L (0% polymorphonuclears)

Cell Count Percentiles

	Total WBC			Polymorphonuclears			Monocytes		
	25%	50%	75%	25%	50%	75%	25%	50%	75%
<6 wk	0.50	2.57	5.16	0	0	2.42	0	0.83	2.71
6 wk–3 mo	0.34	1.86	3.75	0	0	0.66	0	0.96	2.78
3–6 mo	0.00	1.11	2.31	0	0	0.40	0	0.43	1.64
6–12 mo	0.41	1.47	3.25	0	0	0.52	0.03	0.93	2.32
>12 mo	0.00	0.68	1.82	0	0	0	0	0.25	1.45

Test	SI Reference Range	Conventional Units Reference Range
Glucose	Preterm: 1.3–3.5 mmol/L	Preterm: 24–63 mg/dL
	Term: 1.9–6.6	Term 34–119
	Child: 2.2–4.4	Child: 40–80
Protein	Preterm: 0.65–1.50 g/L	Preterm: 65–150 mg/dL
	Term: 0.20–1.70	Term: 20–170
	Child: 0.05–0.40	Child: 5–40
Pressure	<200 mm H_2O	<200 mm H_2O

(Rowe, P. C. [1994]. Laboratory values. In F. A. Oski, et al. [Eds.] *Principles and practice of pediatrics* [2nd ed.]. Philadelphia: J. B. Lippincott.)

Pulse, Respiration, and Blood Pressure Values

Pulse Rate at Various Ages

Age	Range	Average
Newborn	70–170	120
1–11 months	80–160	120
2 years	80–130	110
4 years	80–120	100
6 years	75–115	100
8 years	70–110	90
10 years	70–100	90

	Girls		Boys	
	Range	Average	Range	Average
12 years	70–110	90	65–105	85
14 years	65–105	85	60–100	80
16 years	60–100	80	55–95	75
18 years	55–95	75	50–90	70

Variations in Respirations with Age

Age	Rate per Minute
Newborn	40–90
1 year	20–40
2 years	20–30
3 years	20–30
5 years	20–25
10 years	17–22
15 years	15–20
20 years	15–20

Normal Blood Pressure for Various Ages

Age	Systolic (Mean ± 2 SD)	Diastolic (Mean ± 2 SD)
Newborn	80 ± 16	46 ± 16
6 months–1 year	89 ± 29	60 ± 10*
1 year	96 ± 30	66 ± 25*
2 years	99 ± 25	64 ± 25*
3 years	100 ± 25	67 ± 23*
4 years	99 ± 20	65 ± 20*
5–6 years	94 ± 14	55 ± 9
6–7 years	100 ± 15	56 ± 8
8–9 years	105 ± 16	57 ± 9
9–10 years	107 ± 16	57 ± 9
10–11 years	111 ± 17	58 ± 10
11–12 years	113 ± 18	59 ± 10
12–13 years	115 ± 19	59 ± 10
13–14 years	118 ± 19	60 ± 10

* The point of muffling is shown as the diastolic pressure.

Average Blood Pressure in Adult American Females

	Age	White Women		Black Women	
		Average (mm Hg)	SD	Average (mm Hg)	SD
Systolic	Under 20	111.0	13.7	112.7	13.2
	20–29	116.9	13.8	119.1	14.7
	30–39	121.4	16.3	128.1	20.2
	40–49	129.3	19.6	138.3	22.8
Diastolic	Under 20	69.3	9.8	70.0	10.1
	20–29	73.7	7.2	75.4	9.7
	30–39	76.9	10.7	82.0	13.0
	40–49	80.6	11.6	86.9	13.9

SD = standard deviation.
(Adapted from Stamler, J, et al. [1976]. Hypertension screening of one million Americans. *Journal of the American Medical Association, 235*, 2299. Copyright ©1976, American Medical Association.)

Adele Pillitteri: MATERNAL AND CHILD HEALTH NURSING, 2nd Edition. © 1995 Adele Pillitteri.

NANDA Nursing Diagnoses

Pattern I: Exchanging

Altered Nutrition: More than body requirements
Altered Nutrition: Less than body requirements
Altered Nutrition: High risk for more than body requirements
Ineffective Infant Feeding Pattern
High Risk for Infection
High Risk for Altered Body Temperature
Hypothermia
Hyperthermia
Ineffective Thermoregulation
Ineffective Management of Self-Care Regimen
Dysreflexia
Constipation
Perceived Constipation
Colonic Constipation
Diarrhea
Bowel Incontinence
Altered Urinary Elimination
Stress Incontinence
Reflex Incontinence
Urge Incontinence
Functional Incontinence
Total Incontinence
Urinary Retention
Altered (Specify Type) Tissue Perfusion (Renal, cerebral, cardiopulmonary, gastrointestinal, peripheral)
Fluid Volume Excess
Fluid Volume Deficit
High Risk for Fluid Volume Deficit
Decreased Cardiac Output
Impaired Gas Exchange
Ineffective Airway Clearance
Ineffective Breathing Pattern
High Risk for Injury
High Risk for Suffocation
High Risk for Poisoning
High Risk for Trauma
High Risk for Aspiration
High Risk for Disuse Syndrome
High Risk for Peripheral Neurovascular Dysfunction
Altered Protection

Impaired Tissue Integrity
Altered Oral Mucous Membrane
Impaired Skin Integrity
High Risk for Impaired Skin Integrity

Pattern 2: Communicating

Impaired Verbal Communication

Pattern 3: Relating

Impaired Social Interaction
Social Isolation
Altered Role Performance
Altered Parenting
High Risk for Altered Parenting
Sexual Dysfunction
Altered Family Processes
Parental Role Conflict
Altered Sexuality Patterns

Pattern 4: Valuing

Spiritual Distress (distress of the human spirit)

Pattern 5: Choosing

Ineffective Individual Coping
Impaired Adjustment
Defensive Coping
Ineffective Denial
Ineffective Family Coping: Disabling
Ineffective Family Coping: Compromised
Family Coping: Potential for Growth
Noncompliance (Specify)
Decisional Conflict (Specify)
Health Seeking Behaviors (Specify)

Pattern 6: Moving

Impaired Physical Mobility
Activity Intolerance
Fatigue
High Risk for Activity Intolerance
Sleep Pattern Disturbance
Diversional Activity Deficit
Impaired Home Maintenance Management
Altered Health Maintenance

Adele Pillitteri: MATERNAL AND CHILD HEALTH NURSING, 2nd Edition. © 1995 Adele Pillitteri.

Feeding Self-Care Deficit
Impaired Swallowing
Ineffective Breastfeeding
Interrupted Breastfeeding
Effective Breastfeeding
Bathing/Hygiene Self-Care Deficit
Dressing/Grooming Self-Care Deficit
Toileting Self-Care Deficit
Altered Growth and Development

Pattern 7: Perceiving

Body Image Disturbance
Self-Esteem Disturbance
Chronic Low Self-Esteem
Situational Low Self-Esteem
Personal Identity Disturbance
Sensory/Perceptual Alterations (Specify) (Visual,
auditory, kinesthetic, gustatory, tactile, olfactory)
Unilateral Neglect
Hopelessness
Powerlessness
Relocation Stress Syndrome

Pattern 8: Knowing

Knowledge Deficit (Specific)
Altered Thought Processes

Pattern 9: Feeling

Pain
Chronic Pain
Caregiver Role Strain
Dysfunctional Grieving
Anticipatory Grieving
High Risk for Violence: Self-directed or directed at
others
High Risk for Self-Mutilation
Post-Trauma Response
Rape-Trauma Syndrome
Rape-Trauma Syndrome: Compound Reaction
Rape-Trauma Syndrome: Silent Reaction
Anxiety
Fear

Source: North American Nursing Diagnosis Association. *Taxonomy With Official Diagnostic Categories.* St. Louis, MO: NANDA.

Fractional Dose Calculations
for Pediatric Medication

Questions:

1. You have an order for aspirin gr XX. The bottle you have supplies tablets of 300 mg. How many tablets would you administer?

2. You have an order for gr 1/300 of atropine sulfate. It comes supplied as 0.4 mg/mL. How many milliliters would you administer?

3. You have an order for 1 tsp of liquid oral erythromycin. The bottle label tells you there are 250 mg in each 7 mL of solution. How many milligrams are you administering in each teaspoon?

4. You have an order for gr V of cough syrup. it is supplied as 120 mg in 10 mL. How many milliliters will you administer?

5. You have an order for liquid Tylenol of gr V. The bottle states there are 120 mg in each 5 mL. How many teaspoons should a mother administer?

Answers:

1. Using the formula $\dfrac{D}{H} \times \dfrac{QD}{QH}$ and the conversion factor gr 1 = 60

   mg:
   $$\begin{aligned} \text{gr } 1 &= 60 \text{ mg} \\ X &= 300 \text{ mg} \\ 60X &= 300 \text{ mg} \\ X &= 5 \text{ mg} \end{aligned}$$
   $$\begin{aligned} \text{gr } \dfrac{20}{5} &\times \dfrac{X}{1} \\ 5X &= 20 \\ X &= 4 \text{ tablets} \end{aligned}$$

2. Using the conversion factor gr $\dfrac{1}{60}$ = 1 mg:

$$\text{gr } \frac{1}{60} = 1 \text{ mg} \qquad 0.4 \text{ mg} = 1 \text{ mL}$$

$$\text{gr } \frac{1}{300} = X \qquad .2 \text{ mg} = x$$

$$\frac{1}{60} X = \frac{1}{300} \qquad X = 0.5 \text{ mL}$$

$$X = \frac{1}{5} \text{ or } 0.2 \text{ mg}$$

3. Using the conversion factor 1 tsp = 5 mL:

1 tsp = 5 mL	250 mg = 1.4 tsp
X tsp = 7 mL	X mg = 1 tsp
5X = 7	1.4X = 250 mg
X = 1.4 tsp	X = 178.5 mg

4. Using the conversion factor gr 1 = 60 mg:

gr 1 = 60 mg	120 mg = 10 mL
gr 5 = X	300 mg = X
gr V = 300 mg.	120 X = 3000
	X = 25 mL

5. Using the conversion factor, gr 1 = 60 mg:

gr 1 = 60 mg	120 mg = 5 mL
gr V = X	300 mg = X
X = 300 mg	120 X = 1500 mL
	X = 12.5 mL

   $$\begin{aligned} 1 \text{ tsp} &= 5 \text{ mL} \\ X \text{ tsp} &= 12.5 \text{ mL} \\ 5X &= 12.5 \\ X &= 2.5 \text{ tsp} \end{aligned}$$

Adele Pillitteri: MATERNAL AND CHILD HEALTH NURSING, 2nd Edition. © 1995 Adele Pillitteri.

Glossary

Abortion: The expulsion of products of conception before 20 weeks' gestation or before the age of viability.

Complete abortion: All the products of conception are expelled and no therapy is required.

Habitual abortion: An abortion that occurs following two previous consecutive pregnancy losses.

Incomplete abortion: An abortion in which not all of the products of conception are expelled. Further therapy is necessary to halt potential hemorrhage.

Imminent abortion: A situation where irreversible uterine evacuation has begun; the internal cervical os is dilated. At this point the pregnancy will inevitably be lost.

Missed abortion: A fetal death in which the products of conception have not yet been expelled.

Spontaneous abortion: A loss of pregnancy occurring before 12 weeks for unknown reasons.

Therapeutic abortion: An abortion that is performed to protect the woman's health. Often used interchangeably with induced or medical abortion.

Threatened abortion: Unexplained vaginal bleeding but without cramping or cervical os dilatation.

Abruptio placentae: A normally implanted placenta that separates prematurely between the 20th week of gestation and birth of the infant.

Abstinence: Refraining from sexual intercourse.

Abstract thought: The ability to think in terms of possibility rather than what really exists.

Abuse: To attack or injure.

Accessory heart sounds: Heart sounds other than a first and second sound.

Accommodation: The ability to adapt thought processes to fit what is perceived.

Acculturization: The process of losing cultural beliefs and values to those of another society.

Acute transplant rejection: An immediate reaction that occurs following organ transplantation indicating rejection.

Acrocentric: A chromosome with the "arms" crossing at a center point.

Acrocyanosis: Mottled cyanosis of hands and feet. Normal finding in newborns.

Active immunity: The condition of being unsusceptible to an organism through having developed the disease produced by the organism.

Acyanotic heart disease: Heart disease involving a left to right shunt or a stricture in blood flow.

Adaptability: Ability to change one's reaction to stimuli over time.

Adenocarcinoma: A malignancy in which the cells are arranged in the form of glands.

Adenology: The study of body glands, particularly male body health.

Adenosis: A disease of a gland.

Adipocyte: A fat cell.

Adolescence: The time period between 12 and 18 years.

Adrenarche: The physiologic changes that occur with puberty.

Adventitious sounds: Abnormal sounds heard on auscultation of the lungs.

Aerobic: Requiring oxygen for the maintenance of life.

Affective learning: The acquisition of behaviors involved in expressing feelings or attitudes.

Afterpains: Alternating contraction and relaxation of the uterine muscle following birth to accomplish involution. Most noticeable in women who are multigravida and nursing.

Aganglionic megacolon: The congenital absence of nerve innervation of a portion of the large bowel.

Agenesis: Congenital absence of an organ.

Age of viability: The age at which a fetus is likely to be able to live if born at that point: 20 to 24 weeks' gestation.

Agranulocyte: A white blood cell that does not contain cytoplasmic granules such as a monocyte.

Allele: Alternate forms of a gene found at the same chromosome locus.

Allergen: A substance that can produce a hypersensitivity reaction.

Allergic crease: An indentation across the nose frequently seen in children with allergies.

Allergic salute: A habit of rubbing the nose with the hand seen in children with allergies.

Allergic shiner: Dark circles often seen under the eyes of children with allergies.

Allogeneic transplantation: The grafting of tissue taken from the body of one person to another.

Allografting: Tissue grafting between two genetically dissimilar individuals.

Alternative birthing center: A free-standing facility for birth that encourages active maternal and family participation in labor and birth.

Amblyopia: Reduced vision in one eye.

Amelia: Absence of a limb.

Amenorrhea: Absence of menstrual flow.

Amniocentesis: Withdrawal of amniotic fluid from the uterus by means of introduction of a needle through the abdominal wall.

Amniotic cavity: The hollow space in the early embryo that forms the ectoderm.

Amniotic fluid embolism: A substance causing blockage in a maternal blood vessel caused by passage of amniotic fluid into the maternal blood stream.

Amniotic membrane: The innermost membrane surrounding the fetus that secretes amniotic fluid.

Amniotic sac: The sac formed by the amnion and chorion membranes that contains the fetus and amniotic fluid.

Anaerobic: Able to grow and function without oxygen.

Analgesic: Pharmacologic agent that relieves pain.

Anaphylaxis: An unusual or exaggerated reaction of the body to foreign protein that could result in death.

Anaerobic: Able to grow and function without oxygen.

Andrology: The branch of medicine that treats the man and diseases specific to the male sex.

Anencephaly: Absence of brain formation.

Angioedema: Temporary swelling of areas of the skin.

Anhedonia: The inability to feel pleasure or happiness from events normally experienced as such.

Ankyloglossia: Tongue-tie.

Anovulation: Absence of ovulation.

Anteflexion: A uterus that is bent forward just above the cervix.

Anteversion: A uterus that is tipped abnormally forward.

Anticipatory grief: Mourning that precedes actual loss.

Anticipatory guidance: Guidance given prior to expected use.

Adele Pillitteri: MATERNAL AND CHILD HEALTH NURSING, 2nd Edition. © 1995 Adele Pillitteri.

Antigen: A foreign body protein capable of evoking an antibody response.

Antitoxin: The antibody to the toxin of an antigen.

Aplastic anemia: A deficiency of blood components related to ineffective bone marrow production.

Apnea: Cessation of respirations.

Apparent life-threatening event: A phenomenon whereby an infant stops breathing; commonly called "near-miss" sudden infant death syndrome.

Appendicitis: Inflammation of the appendix.

Approach: A child's response to initial contact with a new stimulus.

Areola: The pigmented circle of epidermis that surrounds the nipple of the breast.

Arrhythmia: A deviation from the normal pattern of the heartbeat.

Artificial insemination: The artificial introduction of semen into the female vagina to initiate fertilization.

Aspermia: Absence of sperm.

Aspiration: The act of withdrawing a fluid by suction from the body; inhalation of a foreign object.

Aspiration studies: Diagnostic studies involving the withdrawal of a body fluid by suction.

Assimilation: The ability to change how a set is perceived to coincide with beliefs.

Astereognosis: The inability to identify objects by touch.

Astigmatism: An uneven cornea.

Atelectasis: Collapse of a lung.

Atopy: A hypersensitivity state.

Atresia: Absence or closure of a normal body passage.

Attention span: The length of time a child retains interest in an activity.

Attitude: A reference to the relationship of the fetal parts to each other or the degree of flexion of the fetal head.

Audiogram: A diagram showing the acuteness of an individual's hearing.

Augmentation of labor: Strengthening labor contractions by the use of a technique such as intravenous oxytocin.

Auscultation: Assessing through listening, either with an unassisted ear or with an instrument.

Autografting: Surgical transplantation of tissue from one part of the body to another part.

Autoimmunity: An immune response to one's own tissues.

Autologous transplantation: Grafting of tissue from one part of the body to the other.

Autonomic nervous system: The division of the nervous system that regulates involuntary body organs.

Autonomic dysreflexia: A syndrome that occurs as a result of impaired autonomic nervous system dysfunction. Simultaneous sympathetic and parasympathetic activity occurs leading to severe hypertension.

Autonomy: The ability to function independently.

Autonomy versus shame: The developmental task of the toddler period according to Erikson.

Autosome: A paired chromosome.

Azoospermia: Absence of spermatozoa.

Azotemia: The presence of excess nitrogenous waste in the blood stream.

Baby bottle syndrome: Severe tooth decay in infants caused by being put to bed with a bottle.

Balloon stenotomy: The technique of inserting a catheter with a deflated balloon attached through a narrow passageway, inflating the balloon and withdrawing the catheter to widen the constricted portion.

Ballottement: The sensation of an object rebounding after being pushed by an examining hand. Used for pregnancy diagnosis.

Bandl's ring: A pathologic retraction ring. Danger sign of labor.

Barium contrast studies: Diagnostic procedures carried out by instillation of a radiopaque substance and x-ray.

Battered child syndrome: A child who has been physically, sexually, or emotionally abused.

Barrier method: A method of reproductive life planning in which the sperm are prevented from entering the cervix.

Basal body temperature method: A method of natural family planning based on the use of body temperature on arising.

Battledore placenta: A placenta with the umbilical cord inserted on the periphery rather than the center.

Behavior modification: A form of therapy in which acceptable patterns of behavior are substituted for unacceptable patterns.

Beriberi: Polyneuritis caused by the deficiency of vitamin B_1 (thiamine).

Bicornate uterus: A uterus that has fundal horns; it may have an accompanying septum.

Bifidus factor: A growth producing factor that the bacteria *Lactobacillus bifidus* needs to grow.

Bilirubin: A breakdown product from the destruction of red blood cells. It is unconjugated or insoluble and toxic to body cells until it is conjugated and made soluble to water by the liver. Also referred to as indirect and direct.

Binocular vision: The use of both eyes simultaneously for vision.

Birthing bed: A bed designed for labor and birth.

Birthing chair: A chair designed for labor and birth in an upright position.

Birthing room: A room specially designed for labor and birth.

Blastocyst: A hollow sphere of cells that forms in very early fetal development.

Blood dyscrasias: Abnormal or pathologic conditions of the blood.

Blood plasma: The liquid portion of the blood.

B lymphocyte: The form of white blood cell responsible for producing antibodies.

Body mass index: Weight (in kg) divided by height (in meters^2).

Bougie: A cylindric flexible instrument for insertion into a body cavity to dilate it.

Braxton-Hicks contractions: Painless, erratic uterine contractions that occur toward the end of pregnancy. They ready the cervix for labor, but cervical dilatation does not occur with them.

Brazelton assessment: A scale for determining interactional behavior of the neonate.

Breech: Buttocks; used to denote a delivery presentation.

Broken fluency: The inability of the preschool child to speak with repeating sounds or words.

Bronchi: The two main air passages into the lungs.

Bronchial breathing: The sound heard over the trachea and main stem bronchus; the expiratory sound is longer than inspiratory.

Bronchoscopy: The visual examination of the respiratory tree by means of an endoscope.

Brown fat: Unique fat located between the scapula, around the neck, kidneys, adrenals and sternum that has a rich nerve and blood supply and generates heat in the neonate.

Bruit: The sound of irregular blood flow through a vessel or an organ.

Brushfield's spots: White spots on the iris in children with Down syndrome.

Bruxism: Grinding of the teeth.

Calendar method: A method of natural family planning based on the determination of fertile and nonfertile days each month.

Calorie counting: Calculation of calories ingested in 24 hours.

Caput succedaneum: A localized edematous area on the scalp of a newborn caused by pressure on the presenting part of the head against the cervix during labor.

Carcinoma: A malignant (cancerous) tumor.

Cardiac catheterization: A diagnostic procedure in which a catheter is introduced into a vein or artery and threaded into the heart.

Cardinal movements of labor: The typical sequence of positions assumed by the fetus as it descends through the pelvis during labor and delivery.

Caries: Destruction of the tooth enamel (dental cavities).

Carpal spasm: A convulsion or twitching of the wrist.

Cartilage: Connective tissue.

Case management nursing: A method of nursing which features total care and planning for an individual client.

Catatonia: A state manifested by immobility and inability to communicate.

Cavernous hemangioma: Dilated vascular spaces.

Celiac disease: A condition marked by malabsorption of the small bowel related to the intake of gluten.

Cell-mediated immunity: A delayed type IV hypersensitivity reaction initiated by T lymphocytes.

Central venous access devices: Devices which allow for blood sampling by insertion of a subdermal port.

Central venous pressure monitoring: The blood pressure in the vena cava; a measurement of the ability of the heart to handle the blood volume.

Centromere: The narrow junction point of a chromosome at which the two chromatids are joined.

Cephalic: Pertaining to the head; used to denote delivery presentation.

Cephalic presentation: A fetus positioned so the head will first contact the cervix at birth.

Cephalocaudal: Relating to the head and tail; progression of development in a fetus.

Cephalhematoma: An elevated area on the newborn's head caused by the extravasation of blood between the skull bone and its periosteum from the pressure of birth.

Cephalopelvic disproportion (CPD): A delivery condition in which the mother's pelvis is too small or too misshapen to allow the infant's head to pass through. The most common reason for which cesarean birth is performed.

Cerebrospinal fluid: The fluid surrounding the spinal cord.

Cervical cap: A latex barrier method of contraception that fits over the uterine cervix.

Cervical cerclage: A procedure in which a suture is placed in the uterine cervix to prevent it from dilating prematurely.

Cervical ripening. Softening of the cervix that occurs prior to labor.

Cesarean birth: Birth of an infant by surgical incision on the mother's abdomen and uterus.

Chadwick's sign: A change in color of the mucous membrane of the vagina from pink to deep violet because of increased vascularity due to pregnancy. A presumptive sign of pregnancy.

Chain of infection: The interrelated steps that allow infection to result.

Chalasia: Relaxation of the cardiac sphincter leading to regurgitation.

Chalazion: Inflammation of a meibomian gland of the eyelid.

Chancre: A painless ulcer that is a primary syphilitic lesion.

Chemotaxis: Movement of an organism from a region of high to low (or low to high) concentration.

Chemotherapeutic agent: A chemical used to treat disease that affects the causative organism of the illness but does not harm the host.

Chief concern: The reason stated by a person as to why he or she is visiting a health care facility.

Child health nursing: Nursing care of children.

Chloasma: Dark brown pigment causing discoloration of the face during pregnancy (the mask of pregnancy).

Choanal atresia: Obstruction of the posterior nares by membrane or bone.

Choreiform movements: Rapid uneven movements of the extremities.

Chorioamnionitis: Infection and inflammation of fetal membranes and amniotic fluid.

Choriocarcinoma: A malignant tumor that can occur following a hydatidiform mole.

Chorion: The outer of the two membranes that form the amniotic sac and contain the amniotic fluid and developing fetus during intrauterine life.

Chorionic gonadotropin, human (HCG): , A hormone produced by the trophoblast tissue. Used as the basis for pregnancy testing.

Chorionic membrane: The outermost fetal membrane.

Chorionic somatomammotropin, human (HCS): A hormone produced by the placenta in pregnancy; helps to regulate maternal glucose levels. Formerly termed human placental lactogen hormone.

Chorionic villi: Projections of the trophoblast that produce human chorionic gonadotropin and begin osmosis of nutrients to the embryo.

Chromosome: A rod-shaped structure composed of DNA and found within the nuclei of cells; carries genetic information.

Circumcision: The surgical removal of the foreskin of the penis.

Classic cesarean incision: A vertical midline incision of the upper segment of the uterus.

Class inclusion: The concept that objects can belong to more than one classification.

Clean-catch specimen: A urine that is as free of bacterial contamination as possible without the use of catheterization.

Cleansing breath: A deep breath taken at the beginning and end of breathing exercises to prevent hypoventilation.

Cleft lip and/or palate: Incomplete fusion of the lip or palate during intrauterine life.

Clinical nurse specialist: A nurse prepared at the master's level who has a special area of clinical expertise.

Clinodactyly: A congenital curvature of the little finger.

Clubbing of fingers: Abnormal enlargement of the distal fingers.

Coelocentesis: The transvaginal aspiration of fluid collected in the extraembryonic cavity early in pregnancy for analysis.

Cognitive learning: The acquisition of behaviors concerned with problem-solving ability.

Cognitive development: Intellectual growth; the ability to learn from experience.

Coitus: Sexual intercourse.

Coitus interruptus: A method of contraception in which the penis is withdrawn from the vagina before ejaculation.

Colostrum: The light yellow fluid secreted as the first milk following delivery.

Colposcopy: An examination of the vagina utilizing a colposcope.

Comedone: The lesion of acne arising from a plugged sebaceous gland.

Communicability: The ability to be transmitted from one person to another.

Communicable disease: Any disease transmitted from one person to another.

Community: A group of people who have a common interest and usually live in a common area.

Community ecogram: A diagram of the family's interactions with the community.

Complement: Enzymatic serum proteins arising from an antigen-antibody reaction.

Complete protein: Protein that contains all essential amino acids necessary for cell growth.

Complex vocal tics: The repeated spasmodic use of words or phrases out of context.

Computerized axial tomography: An x-ray technique that displays the appearance of a cross section of tissue.

Chalazion: Inflammation of a meibomian gland of the eyelid.

Conception: Impregnation of the female ovum by male spermatozoon.

Conceptus: The products of conception: the fetus, umbilical cord, fetal membranes , amniotic fluid, and placenta.

Concrete operational thought: Form of cognitive thought of the 7- to 12-year-old.

Conditioned response: A response that occurs when a secondary stimulant is substituted for an original stimulant.

Condom: A latex barrier method of contraception worn on the penis; provides some protection against STDs.

Conduction: The transfer of body heat to a cooler solid object in contact with a newborn.

Cones: The structures of the retina that allow for visualization of color.

Congestive heart failure: A condition characterized by inability of the heart to move blood received forward.

Conjugate vera: The pelvic measurement from the upper margin of the symphysis pubis to sacral promontory, a distance of about 10.5 to 11.5 cm.

Conjunctivitis: Inflammation of the mucous membrane lining the eyelid.

Consciously controlled breathing: Deliberately paced breathing.

Conscious relaxation: The deliberate relief of tenseness in muscle groups.

Consensual constriction: Constriction of the far pupil occurs when light is shown on the near pupil.

Conservation: The ability to discern that although substances change their shape they do not change their basic composition.

Contact dermatitis: Skin inflammation related to irritation by an object touching the skin.

Contraception: The prevention of conception.

Contraceptive: A device or method for preventing pregnancy.

Convection: The flow of heat from the body surface to cooler surrounding air.

Conventional development: The stage of moral development by Kohlberg from 7 to 12 years of age.

Convergence: The coordinated movement of the two eyes toward fixation of the same point.

Contractility: Ability of a muscle to tighten and produce tension.

Contrecoup injury: An injury to the opposite side of the brain from the side where a blow was struck.

Convalescent period: Time span until recovery from an illness is complete.

Coordination of secondary schema: The cognitive development stage of late infancy.

Coprolalia: Excess use of obscene language.

Cordocentesis: Analysis of fetal blood removed from the umbilical cord using amniocentesis technique.

Corona radiata: The crownlike grouping of cells that surrounds the ovum immediately after ovulation.

Cotyledon: A subdivision of the maternal surface of the placenta. Filled with maternal blood to allow for osmosis of nutrients to the fetal placental villi.

Couvade syndrome: Somatic symptoms experienced by the father during pregnancy simulating those of the pregnant mother.

Couvelaire uterus: Boardlike rigidity and discoloration of the uterus due to accumulation of blood in the myometrium from hemorrhage into the muscle wall; can occur with premature separation of the placenta.

Craniosynostosis: Premature closure of cranial sutures.

Crede treatment: The application of antibacterial therapy to a newborn's eyes.

Crowning: The appearance of the presenting part of the fetus at the vaginal orifice.

Cryptorchidism: Undescended testes.

Culdoscopy: The introduction of an endoscope through the posterior vaginal wall to view the pelvic organs.

Cultural norms: Customs generally accepted as right to follow by a community or society.

Cultural values: Beliefs generally held by the majority of people in a community or society.

Culture: The learned way of life of a community or society.

Cupping: A technique of postural drainage where the chest is struck with the curved palm.

Cutaneous stimulation: Massage of the skin to interfere with the transmission of painful sensations.

Cyanosis: Bluish discolorization of the skin and mucous membrane.

Cyanotic heart disease: Heart disease marked by a right to left shunt or unoxygenated blood entering the oxygenated circulation.

Cystocele: Pouching of the bladder into the anterior vaginal wall.

Cytomegalovirus: An organism representing a large herpes-type virus that causes serious neurological illnesses in newborns.

Cytotoxic response: A substance such as an antibody that has a specific harmful reaction against body cells.

Death: The state of being without brain wave response on an electroencephalogram.

Debridement: The removal of dirt, foreign bodies, or injured tissue from a wound or burn.

Deceleration: A decrease in the baseline reading of a fetal heart rate.

Decenter: The ability to focus on views other than your own.

Decerebrate posturing: A position with the arms extended, internal rotation of the wrists, and feet in plantar flexion.

Decidua basalis: The decidua portion under the implanted blastocyst.

Decidua capsularis: The portion of endometrium that covers the blastocyst.

Decidua vera: The portion of the decidua covering the nonimplanted portion of the uterus.

Deciduous teeth: "Baby" or first teeth.

Decorticate posturing: A position with the upper and lower extremities rigidly flexed.

Deep tendon reflexes: Contraction of muscles in response to a sharp stimulus; indicates spinal nerve integrity.

Deep vein thrombosis: A clot in an underlying vein such as the ovarian.

Dehydration: Excessive loss of fluid from body tissues.

Delayed hypersensitivity: Cell-mediated immunity.

Dermatoglyphics: The patterns of skin configurations on fingers and toes.

Demonstration: Performing an action to demonstrate the correct way for it to be done.

Development: An increase in the skill or ability to function: a qualitative change.

Developmental task: A skill responsibility arising at a particular time, the successful accomplishment of which will provide a foundation for the accomplishment of future tasks.

Diagonal conjugate: Distance from the sacral promontory to the lower posterior border of the symphysis pubis.

Dialysis: The removal of body waste products through the use of a semipermeable membrane.

Dialysis equilibrium syndrome: A phenomenon that occurs when electrolytes are being removed more rapidly from the blood stream than from the brain tissue during dialysis.

Diaphoresis: Profuse perspiration.

Diaphragm: A mechanical barrier contraceptive device fitted over the cervix in the woman.

Diaphragmatic excursion: The distance the diaphragm descends or rises on inspiration and expiration.

Diaphysis: The shaft of a long bone.

Diastasis recti: A separation of the rectus abdominis muscle.

Diastole: Contraction of the heart atria.

Diffusion: The state of being unsure of self-identity.

Dilatation: Stretching of the extenal os of the cervix large enough to allow the passage of the fetus.

Diplegia: Bilateral paralysis of any part of the body.

Diplopia: Double vision.

Direct care: Nursing care provided by the primary care nurse.

Discipline: To enforce a set of rules that govern behavior.

Dislocated hip: A congenital orthopedic condition in which a shallow acetabulum allows the femur head to slip from the socket.

Disorganization phase: A time period in which individuals are unable to organize thoughts clearly.

Distractibility: Ability to have interest diverted to a new object.

Distraction: A process that prevents or lessens the perception of pain by focusing attention to an object other than the pain.

Dominant trait: A characteristic that will be expressed in a heterozygous union.

Drowning: Asphyxiation because of submersion in water.

Drug dependence: Psychological craving for a drug.

Drug tolerance: The state in which cell adaptation to a drug occurs so increasingly larger doses are necessary to produce the usual effect.

Ductus arteriosus: A blood vessel joining the pulmonary artery and aorta in fetal life. Closes at birth.

Ductus venosus: A blood vessel joining the umbilical vein and the inferior vena cava in fetal life; closes at birth.

Dumping syndrome: The phenomenon in which the stomach empties too quickly into the duodenum.

Dysfunctional labor: Labor that progresses slower than usual due to ineffective contractions.

Dysmenorrhea: Painful menstruation.

Dyspareunia: Pain on sexual intercourse.

Dystocia: Difficult delivery.

Echocardiography: Ultrasonic examination of the heart.

Echolalia: A meaningless repetition of words.

Eclampsia: Severe pregnancy-induced hypertension after the point at which a woman has convulsed.

Ectoderm: Outermost of the three primary germ layers of the embryo.

Ectomorphic: A body build characterized by slenderness and fragility.

Ectopic pregnancy: A pregnancy implanted outside the uterine cavity; generally located in a fallopian tube.

Effacement: Thinning and shortening of the cervix that occurs just prior to dilatation.

Effleurage: Light, circular massage of the abdomen used as a distraction technique in prepared childbirth.

Egocentrism: Having all of one's ideas centered on oneself.

Eighth month anxiety: Separation anxiety that peaks at the eighth month of life.

Elderly primipara: A woman having her first pregnancy over age 35.

Electra complex: Freudian concept that preschool girls fall in love with their fathers.

Elective termination of pregancy: A therapeutic abortion.

Electrical impulse studies: Diagnostic studies that analyze the electrical activity of body cells.

Electrocardiogaphy: A study of the electrical activity of the heart.

Embryo: The intrauterine growth period from the time following implantation until organogenesis is complete (10th day to 5 to 8 weeks).

Enanthem: A rash on the mucous membrane.

Endocervix: The inner surface of the cervix.

Endometriosis: Abnormal implantation sites of the endometrial cells outside the uterus.

Endometritis: Inflammation of the inner uterine lining.

Endometrium: Inner layer of the uterus that is shed as menstruation.

Endomorphic: A body build characterized by a soft round physique.

Endorphin: A neuropeptide elaborated by the pituitary gland and acting on the central and peripheral nervous systems to reduce pain.

Endoscopy: Inspection of a body cavity by means of an endoscope.

En face: A position in which one person looks at another with his or her face in the same vertical plane as the other; typical position in which a mother holds her newborn.

Engagement: The entrance of the fetal presenting part into the superior pelvic strait.

Engorgement: Local congestion of the breast associated with lactation.

Entoderm: Innermost of the three primary germ layers of the embryo.

Enuresis: Involuntary discharge of urine.

Environmental control: The management of surroundings to lessen allergic responses.

Epidemic: A disease affecting a larger than usual number of people at one time.

Epidural anesthesia: Injection of a regional anesthetic outside the dura mater to reduce the pain of labor contractions.

Epiphyseal plate: The growth center of a long bone between the epiphysis and metaphysis.

Epiphysis: The head of a long bone.

Episiotomy: A surgical incision in the perineum to enlarge the vaginal opening for childbirth.

Epispadias: A urethral opening on the dorsal surface of the penis.

Erectile dysfunction: The inability to achieve erection in order to complete a sex act.

Erosion: Cell changes of the uterine cervix associated with irritation or infection.

Erythema toxicum neonatorum: Rash of the newborn marked by minute papules on an erythematous base caused from the first exposure to environmental contaminants.

Erythroblast: An immature red blood cell.

Erythrocyte: A red blood cell.

Erythroblastosis fetalis: Hemolytic disease of the newborn caused by isoimmunization resulting from Rh or ABO incompatibility.

Escharotomy: Surgical incision into the necrotic tissue formed after a burn.

Esophoria: Occasional medial deviation of an eye.

Esotropia: Consistent medial deviation of an eye.

Ethnicity: A person's nationality.

Ethnocentrism: The belief that one's own values or beliefs are superior to others.

Evaporation: The loss of heat through conversion of liquid to a vapor.

Ewing's sarcoma: A malignant tumor of the shaft of the long bone.

Exophoria: Occasional lateral deviation of an eye.

Exotropia: Consistent lateral deviation of an eye.

Exophthalmos: A marked protrusion of the eyeballs.

Expected date of birth (EDB): Calculated date on which birth will occur.

Expiration: Exhalation.

Expressed emotion: The outward showing of feelings.

Exstrophy of the bladder: A congenital disorder in which the bladder is exposed on the anterior surface of the abdomen.

External cephalic version: Rotating a fetus into a cephalic lie by external maneuvers against the mother's abdomen.

Extracorporeal membranous oxygenation: Oxygenation of the blood by a heart-lung machine.

Extremely very-low-birth-weight infant: A newborn weighing less than 1000 g or between 24 and 26 weeks' gestation age.

Extrusion reflex: A response that occurs when an object is placed on the newborn's tongue; fades at about 4 months of life.

Failure to achieve ejaculation: The failure to accomplish deposition of sperm with a sex act.

Failure to thrive: Retarded growth and development of a child for nonorganic reasons.

Family: Two or more people who live in the same household (usually), share a common emotional bond, and perform certain interrelated social tasks.

Family-centered nursing: A nursing philosophy in which the family is considered the unit of care.

Family nurse practitioner: A nurse prepared at the master's level who has expertise in the nursing care of families.

Family nursing: The concept that clients do not exist outside a family; the family rather than an individual is considered the client.

Family of orientation: One's birth family: oneself, mother, father, and siblings.

Family of procreation: One's marriage family: oneself, spouse, and children.

Family sculpture: A technique of family assessment that creates a live portrait of family members.

Family theory: Viewing situations or happenings from the family's point of view.

Fasciculation: A fine tremor.

Fertility awareness: A method of contraception based on body analyzing the consistency of vaginal secretions.

Fertility awareness: A method of contraception based on analyzing the consistency of vaginal secretions.

Fertilization: The union of the sperm and ovum.

Fetal alcohol syndrome: A fetus with growth retardation, mental deficiency, and facial, cardiac, and joint anomalies caused by the mother's consumption of alcohol during pregnancy.

Fetal descent: The maneuver of delivery in which the fetus passes beyond the ischial spines.

Fetoscope: A head stethoscope for listening to fetal heart sounds.

Fetoscopy: The visualization of the fetus by inspection through a fetoscope.

Fetus: The developing structure from the eighth week postfertilization until birth.

Fibrocystic breast disease: Benign fluid-filled cysts of the breast.

Fine motor development: Motor development concerned with small tasks such as writing.

Fistula: An abnormal passage or communication between two organs.

Flat affect: No outward sign of emotion.

Fluid shift: A change in compartments of body fluid.

Fluoroscopy: A radiology study that offers serial images.

Focusing: Attention on an alternative sensation to block out an incoming pain sensation.

Fomites: Nonliving materials such as combs that spread infection.

Foramen ovale: An opening between the atria of the heart during intrauterine life.

Forceps birth: Birth by the means of forceps to extract the fetus.

Foremilk: Breast milk formed prior to the let-down reflex.

Formal operational thought: A cognitive stage in which abstract thought is possible.

Fovea centralis: The location on the retina where cones are concentrated.

Frenulum: The attachment of the inferior surface of the tongue to the oral mucous membrane.

Funis: Umbilical cord.

Fusion: The ability of two eyes to see one image.

Gamma globulin: Antibodies.

Gating theory: A theory of pain control in which the person's perception of pain can be altered by interruption of the sensory input of pain.

Gavage: To feed by means of a tube passed into the stomach. Used with immature newborns.

Gene: A segment of DNA material that carries unit of heredity.

Genetics: The science of inheritance due to gene transmission.

Genogram: A diagram of family structure depicting essential family relationships; the interactive roles that exist in a family.

Genome: The total gene complement of an individual.

Genotype: The genetic composition of an individual.

General appearance: The overall appearance of a person prior to physical examination.

Genu valgus: Inward curving of the knees (knock knees).

Geographic tongue: A rough "maplike" appearance of the tongue from uneven papillae.

Gestational age: The number of weeks a fetus has been in utero.

Gestational trophoblastic disease: See Hydatidiform mole.

Gingiva: The gumline.

Glia cell: A supporting or connecting cell of the nervous system.

Globe: The shape of the eye.

Glomerular filtration rate: The rate at which body wastes are excreted by the kidney.

Glomerulonephritis: Inflammation of the glomeruli of the kidney.

Glucose tolerance test: A test of the body's ability to metabolize carbohydrate in reaction to a standardized dose of glucose.

Glycogen loading: Excessively decreasing and then increasing carbohydrate intake to better sustain energy for a sporting event.

Glycosuria: The presence of glucose in the urine.

Glycosylated hemoglobin: Hemoglobin that has absorbed glucose from circulating in a glucose-enriched serum.

Gonad: A gland that produces gametes (an ovary or testes).

Gonadostat: The unknown control mechanism that stimulates the hypothalamus to begin stimulation for puberty changes.

Goniotomy: An operation to increase the flow of aqueous humor from the anterior chamber of the eye.

Goodell's sign: Softening of the cervix during pregnancy because of the increased vascularity present. A probable sign of pregnancy.

Granulocyte: A white blood cell that contains cytoplasmic granules such as a neutrophil.

Graphesthesia: The inability to recognize a figure drawn on the skin.

Gravida: The number of pregnancies a woman has had; a pregnant woman.

Grief process: The predictable mourning response to loss.

Gross motor development: Motor development concerned with large tasks such as walking.

Growth: An increase in physical size; a quantitative change.

Gynecology: The study of reproductive diseases of women.

Gynecomastia: Excess development of male breast tissue; a transient occurence in normal adolescence.

Hand regard: The special fascination a 3-month-old has with his or her hands.

Hapten: A nonprotein substance that acts as an antigen by combining with particular bonding sites on an antibody.

Hawthorne effect: The phenomenon whereby people behave differently when they know they are being observed.

Heart murmur: An abnormal sound heard during auscultation caused by the flow of blood through an abnormal shunt or poorly functioning valve of the heart.

Hegar's sign: Softening of the lower uterine segment. A probable sign of pregnancy.

HELLP syndrome: A condition characterized by hemolysis, elevated liver enzymes, and a low platelet count.

Helper T cell: A type of white blood cell that stimulates B lymphocyte production.

Hemangioma: A collection of blood vessels.

Hematuria: Blood in urine.

Hemiplegia: Paralysis of one side of the body.

Hemochromatosis: Excess iron deposits in the body that have caused tissue destruction.

Hemoglobin: The iron-containing portion of red blood cells responsible for the transportation of oxygen to body cells. Expressed in mg/100 mL.

Hemoglobin A$_{1c}$: Glycosylated hemoglobin or hemoglobin with attached glucose.

Hemolysis: Destruction of red blood cells with release of hemoglobin.

Hemolytic disease of the newborn: Erythroblastosis fetalis; anemia caused by an incompatibility between mother and fetus.

Hemorrhagic disease of the newborn: Decreased clotting ability in a newborn caused by a deficiency of vitamin K.

Hemosiderosis: Increased body iron stores without associated tissue damage.

Hemosiderosis: Excess deposits of iron in the body without tissue damage.

Hepatitis: Inflammation of the liver.

Hermaphrodite: An individual with both testes and ovaries.

Heterografting: Tissue from another species used to temporarily cover a burned area.

Heterozygous: Possessing two different genes for a character trait.

Hiatal hernia: Projection of the stomach into the chest through the diaphragm.

High risk pregnancy: Any pregnancy in which some maternal or fetal factor is apt to result in the birth of a high-risk infant or in some way harm the mother.

Hind milk: Breast milk formed following the let-down reflex.

Hip dysplasia: A subluxated or dislocated hip.

Homans' sign: Pain in the calf of the leg on dorsiflexion of the foot; an indication of thrombophlebitis of a vein in the calf.

Home care: Nursing care conducted in a client's place of residence.

Homografting: Allografting.

Homologue: A structure similar in origin to another.

Homosexual: An individual whose sexual relations are with those of his or her own sex.

Homozygous: Possessing two like genes for a character trait.

Hordeolum: An infection at the margin of the eyelid occuring in a sebaceous gland of an eyelash.

Hormone: A chemical substance possessing a regulatory effect.

Hospice care: Care of a terminally ill individual in a facility designed to maintain a satisfactory life style until death.

Humoral immunity: Immunity created by antibody production.

Hydatidiform mole: Abnormal growth of proliferation of the trophoblast cells. No fetus forms and clear, fluid-filled, grapelike vesicles form in place of the placenta.

Hydramnios: An excessive amount of amniotic fluid (generally greater than 2000 mL).

Hydrocele: A collection of fluid in the sac surrounding the testis.

Hydrocephalus: An abnormally enlarged head size due to accumulated cerebrospinal fluid distending the cerebral ventricles.

Hydronephrosis: Distention of the pelvis of the kidney with urine as a result of obstruction of the ureter.

Hydrops fetalis: A fatal state caused by blood incompatibility evidenced by edema, anemia and congestive heart failure.

Hyperactivity: Excess driven behavior.

Hyperbilirubinemia: Excessive indirect bilirubin in serum.

Hypercholesterolemia: Elevated cholesterol levels in serum.

Hyperplasia: An increase in the number of cells.

Hyperptyalism: Excessive secretion of saliva.

Hypertrophia: An increase in size of body cells.

Hyperemesis gravidarum: Extreme vomiting during pregnancy or vomiting beyond the third month of pregnancy.

Hyperfunction: Excessive function.

Hyperglycemia: A greater than normal amount of glucose in the blood.

Hyperopia: Farsightedness.

Hyperphoria: Occasional upward deviation of an eye.

Hypertropia: Consistent upward deviation of an eye.

Hypersensitivity response: An immune response in which histamine is released.

Hypertension: Elevated blood pressure.

Hypertonic contractions: Contractions that maintain a high resting tone.

Hypertonic dehydration: Excessive loss of fluid from body tissues in which a greater proportion of fluid than electrolytes is lost.

Hypocalcemia: Lessened amount of calcium in the blood stream.

Hypofunction: Lessened function.

Hypoglycemia: A less than normal amount of glucose in the blood.

Hyposensitization: The process of lessening the response to an allergen.

Hypospadias: Opening of the urethra on the ventral surface of the penis.

Hypotonic contractions: Contractions that are infrequent and ineffective.

Hypotonic dehydration: Excessive loss of fluid from body tissues in which a greater proportion of electrolytes than fluid is lost.

Hypoxemia: Deficient oxygenation of the blood.

Hypoxia: Deficient oxygenation of body cells.

Id: A Freudian term for instinctive impulses.

Identity versus role confusion: The developmental task of the adolescent; learning what kind of person he or she is.

Immune response: The body's ability to combat outside invading organisms by leukocyte activity.

Immune serum: A solution of plasma that contains those antibodies normally present in adult human blood.

Immunity: The state of being nonsusceptible to an organism.

Immunocompetent: Capable of producing an effective immune response.

Immunogen: An antigen that produces an immune response.

Implantation: Contact between the blastocyst and the uterine endothelium that occurs 8 to 10 days after fertilization.

Impregnation: Fertilization.

Imprinting: The differential expression of genetic material that allows it to be possible to identify whether chromosomal material was inherited from the male or female parent.

Incest: Sexual relations between members of the same family.

Inclusion: The concept that children with disabilities should attend school classes with children without disabilities (formerly mainstreaming).

Incompetent cervix: A defect of the cervix that makes it unable to remain closed throughout pregnancy. Premature delivery occurs at about 20 weeks.

Incomplete protein: Protein that does not contain all the essential amino acids.

Incubation period: Time span for invasion of an organism until symptoms occur.

Indirect care: Nursing care that is completed by an auxillary person under the supervision of a nurse.

Induction of labor: Artificial stimulation of labor by a technique such as intravenous oxytocin.

Industry versus inferiority: The developmental task of the school-age child; learning how to do things well.

Infertility: The state of being unable to reproduce; sterile.

Inguinal hernia: Projection of intestine into the inguinal canal.

Initiative versus guilt: The developmental task of the preschooler according to Erikson.

Innocent heart murmur: An accessory heart sound that represents a benign origin.

Inspection: Observation.

Inspiration: Inhalation.

Insulin pump therapy: The subcutaneous administration of insulin by means of an automatic pump and syringe.

Interferon: A protein formed when cells are exposed to a virus that prohibits the growth of viruses.

Intermittent infusion devices: A device inserted in an intravenous line that allows for intermittent infusion of fluid or insertion of medicine (heparin trap).

Intrauterine device (IUD): A contraceptive device inserted into the uterine cavity.

Intrauterine growth retardation: A state in which a fetus's weight measures below the 10th percentile for gestational age.

Involution: The return of the uterus to its nonpregnant state.

Iron deficiency anemia: A microcytic, hypochromic anemia caused by an inadequate supply of iron.

Isoimmunization: The development of antibodies against antigens from the same species such as the development of anti-Rh antibodies.

Isotonic dehydration: An excessive loss of fluid from body tissues in which fluid and electrolytes are lost in proportion.

Intelligence: The ability to learn from experience.

Intensity of reaction: The degree of behavior exhibited by children in response to frustration.

Intercostal spaces: The hollow spaces between the ribs.

Intuitive thought: Spontaneous thought or thought without reasoning.

Intuitional thought: The cognitive develop period in which children are first able to view themselves as others see them.

Intussusception: Prolapse of a portion of intestine into an adjacent portion.

Involution: Reduction in size of the uterus after birth as it returns to its prepregnancy size and condition.

Irritable bowel syndrome: Inflammation of the bowel marked by diarrhea and pain.

Ischial tuberosity: The projections of the pelvic bone that mark the transverse diameter of the pelvic outlet.

Jaundice: A yellow color of the skin or mucous membrane. Caused by an increase in bilirubin.

Karyotype: A display of the number, size, and shape of chromosomes of a representative body cell.

Kegel's exercises: Periodic tightening and relaxation of the pubococcygeal muscles of the perineum to strengthen them.

Keratomalacia: Ulceration of the cornea resulting from vitamin A deficiency.

Kernicterus: Accumulation of indirect bilirubin in brain cells causing cell destruction.

Ketoacidosis: Acidosis accompanied by ketones in the body.

Killer T cell: A specialized lymphocyte that is able to bind to the surface of an antigen and destroy it.

Kinesthesia: The perception of one's own body parts, weight, and movement.

Koplik's spots: Peculiar blue- and white-centered red spots that occur on the mucous membrane in children with measles.

Kwashiorkor: A malnutrition syndrome caused by protein deficiency.

Labile mood: A rapidly changing mood.

Labor-delivery-recovery room: A room specially designed for a total birth experience and recovery period.

Labor-delivery-recovery-postpartum room: A room designed to accommodate a family during an entire birth experience hospital stay.

Lactase: The enzyme that breaks down lactose.

Lactiferous sinuses: The glands of the breasts where breast milk is stored.

Lactobacillus bifidus: A nonpathogenic organism that produces lactic acid from carbohydrates.

Lactoferrin: An iron-binding protein found in breast milk that interferes with the growth of bacteria.

Lacto-ovo-vegetarian: A diet mainly of fruits and vegetables but also dairy and egg products.

Lactose intolerance: The inability to digest lactose due to lactase deficiency.

Lactovegetarian: A diet mainly of fruits and vegetables but with some added dairy products.

Landau reflex: When held in a horizontal plane, an infant raises the head and flexes the arms and legs.

Lanugo: The fine, downy hair formed on the shoulders and back of the fetus.

Laparoscopy: Examination of the abdominal cavity and organs by insertion of a surgical instrument through the anterior abdominal wall.

Laparotomy: A surgical incision into the abdominal cavity.

Large-for-gestational-age (LGA) infant: A newborn who weighs above the 90th percentile for gestational age.

Latchkey child: A child who is without adult supervision for a part of each weekday.

Latent phase: A Freudian term for the development phase of the school-age child.

Latent tetany: Neuromuscular irritability as a result of a lowered calcium level.

Learned helplessness: A behavioral state of a person who believes he/she is ineffectual and unable to achieve.

Leboyer method: A method of birth that encourages subdued light and a welcoming bath for the baby at birth.

Left-to-right shunt: A passageway in the heart allowing oxygenated blood to pass into unoxygenated blood.

Leopold's maneuvers: A technique of manual palpation to discover the position and lie of the fetus.

Lesbian: A female homosexual.

Let-down reflex: A reflex initiated by an infant's suckling that releases oxytocin from the posterior pituitary, contract the myoepithelial cells surrounding milk glands and brings hindmilk forward to the nipple.

Letting-go phase: Rubin's last stage of postpartal adjustment during which the mother redefines her new role as a mother.

Leukocyte: A white blood cell.

Leukocytosis: An increase in the number of white blood cells.

Leukopenia: A decrease in the number of white blood cells.

Leukorrhea: A whitish vaginal discharge.

Libido: Sexual desire.

Lie: The relationship between the long axis of the fetus and the long axis of the mother.

Light refraction: The deviation that occurs when a ray of light strikes a fluid; allows light rays to fall on the retina for sight.

Lightening: Descent of the fetus into the pelvis at about 2 weeks prior to delivery. Also engagement.

Lithotomy position: An examining or delivery position with the patient lying supine; knees are flexed and heels are elevated in stirrups.

Liver transplantation: Grafting of the liver from one individual to another.

Lochia alba: A whitish vaginal discharge.

Lochia rubra: A vaginal discharge similar to a menstrual flow.

Lochia serosa: A pinkish or brown vaginal discharge.

Long bone: A bone of the arm or leg.

Lordosis: An increased anterior concavity of the spine.

Low-birth-weight infant: A newborn weighing 1500 to 2500 g and born between 30 and 36 weeks' gestation.

Low segment incision: A transverse incision in the supracervical portion of the uterus.

Lymphocyte production: The manufacture of white blood cells involved in immune responses.

Lymphokines: A substance secreted by killer cells to prevent migration of antigens.

Lymphoma: A tumor involving the lymphoid tissue.

Lysis: Dissolution.

Lysosome: A cytoplasmic particle capable of dissolving cells.

Macrobiotic: A diet in which protein is mainly derived from grains and seeds.

Macronutrient: A mineral needed by the body in an amount over 100 mg daily.

Macrophage: A phagocytic cell.

Macrosomia: Large body size.

Macula lutea: The location on the retina where central vision is perceived.

Magnetic resonance imaging: A diagnostic technique that uses magnetic and sound waves to reveal body composition and appearance.

Malignant: Cancerous.

Malocclusion: Abnormal alignment of the upper and lower jaw.

Mandatory reporters: Individuals designated as ones who must report child abuse.

Manifest tetany: Twitching of the muscles as a result of a lowered calcium level.

Mass: A collection of cells to form a tumor.

Mastitis: Inflammation of breast tissue.

Maternal and child health nursing: A conceptual approach to nursing care that views maternity and child health nursing as continuums, not separate entities.

Maternal-newborn nursing: Nursing that concentrates on the care of a family during pregnancy, labor and birth, and postpartum and of the infant immediately following birth.

Maturation: Coming of age or adulthood.

McDonald's rule: The fundus-to-symphysis distance in centimeters is equal to the week of gestation between the 20th to 31st weeks of pregnancy.

Means of transmission: The ways that communicable diseases can be spread.

Meconium: The first stool of the newborn, dark green or black in color.

Meconium plug: An unusually thickened portion of intestinal contents formed during fetal life that obstructs the intestine at birth. Associated with cystic fibrosis.

Meckel's diverticulum: Outpouching of the ilium related to yolk sac retention.

Megakaryocyte: An immature platelet.

Menarche: The first menstrual period or onset of menstruation.

Megaloblastic anemia: A hematologic disorder characterized by the production of immature, nonfunctional but large erythrocytes.

Meiosis: A process whereby a cell divides.

Melasma: Excessive body pigment that occurs during pregnancy.

Memory cell: A form of B lymphocyte that maintains the formula for producing antibodies.

Menorrhagia: An excessively profuse menstrual flow.

Mesoderm: One of the layers of primary germ cell tissue in the embryo.

Mesonephritic duct: The embryonic structure which allows the female reproductive organs to develop.

Metabolic acidosis: Excessive acid in the body resulting from a digestive or metabolic concern.

Metabolic alkalosis: Decreased acid or increased bicarbonate in the body resulting from a digestive or metabolic concern.

Metaphysis: The point in bone at which diaphysis and epiphysis meet.

Metastasis: The process by which tumor cells are spread to distant body parts.

Metrocentric: A chromosome with a central centromere.

Metrorrhagia: Vaginal bleeding between normal menstrual cycles.

Micronutrient: A mineral needed by the body in an amount under 100 mg daily.

Milia: Minute white papules commonly found on the nose and cheeks on neonates; unopened sebaceous glands.

Mittelschmerz: Pain in the middle of a menstrual cycle.

Molding: Overlapping of cranial bones or shaping of the fetal head that occurs to accommodate the head to the birth canal during labor.

Molestation: Unwelcome sexual involvement such as oral–genital contact, genital fondling, viewing, or masturbation.

Mongolian spot: A slate-gray area of pigment on the skin of the neonate.

Mood quality: The overall degree of happiness or sadness a child exhibits.

Morbidity: Illness.

Mores: Customs or beliefs commonly held.

Mortality (infant): The number of deaths per 1000 live births occurring at births or in the first 12 months of life.

Mortality (maternal): The number of maternal deaths per 100,000 live births that occur as a direct result of the reproductive process.

Morula: The developing blastomere structure as it multiplies rapidly and forms a bumpy surface.

Motor tics: A spasmodic action such as twitching of the face.

Multigravida: A woman who is having or has had more than one pregnancy.

Multipara: A woman who has delivered more than one child past the age of viability.

Mumps orchitis: Inflammation of the testis from invasion of the mumps virus.

Munchausen syndrome by proxy: A situation in which a parent repeatedly brings a child to a health care facility for care when the child is actually well.

Myometrium: The muscle layer of the uterus.

Myopathy: Abnormality of skeletal muscles other than that caused by nerve degeneration.

Myopia: Nearsightedness.

Myringotomy: An incision into the tympanic membrane.

Natal teeth: Erupted teeth in the newborn.

Natural family planning: Contraception involving no medical devices or chemicals.

Near drowning: The state of having inhaled water but a condition short of asphyxiation.

Neck-righting reflex: When the head of a newborn is turned right or left, the infant turns the shoulders as well.

Necrotizing enterocolitis: Death of intestinal tissue related to ischemia of the bowel.

Negative feedback: The regulatory process whereby hypofunction of a gland leads to increased production of a stimulating hormone.

Neonatal nurse practitioner: A nurse prepared at the master's level who has expertise with nursing care of the newborn infant.

Neonatal period: The first 28 days of life.

Neonatal teeth: Teeth present in a newborn.

Neonate: An infant during the first 28 days of life.

Neoplasm: An abnormal growth of new tissue.

Nephrosis: Degeneration of the renal tubules.

Neural plate: The embryonic structure from which the nervous system develops.

Neuroblastoma: A malignant tumor of nervous tissue.

Neurogenic bladder: A dysfunctional bladder caused by lack of nerve innervation.

Neuron: A nerve cell.

Nevus flammeus: A permanent port wine–colored birthmark.

Night grinding: Bruxism occurring at night.

Nocturnal enuresis: Involuntary release of urine at night (bedwetting).

Nondisjunction: Failure of two paired chromosomes to separate during cell division. Leads to the trisomy disorders.

Non-rapid-eye-movement (NREM) sleep: A type of sleep during which physiologic growth occurs.

Nonstress test: An assessment of fetal well-being determined from examination of the fetal heart rate in relationship to fetal activity.

Normoblast: An immature red blood cell.

Null cell: A lymphocyte that lacks the characteristic surface markers of either a B or T lymphocyte.

Nulligravida: A woman who has never been pregnant.

Nurse-midwife: A registered nurse with extended knowledge in care of the family during the prenatal, natal, and postnatal periods. Abbreviated as C.N.M. (Certified Nurse Midwife).

Nurse practitioner: A nurse prepared at the master's degree level with extensive skills in physical assessment, interviewing, and well-child counseling and care.

Nursing research: Scientific investigation of topics related to nursing.

Nutritional marasmus: Progressive wasting and emaciation from inadequate dietary intake.

Nystagmus: Rapid irregular eye movements.

Obesity: A body weight over 200 lbs or 50% above ideal body weight.

Object permanence: The awareness that an object continues to exist even when out of sight.

Obstetrics: The branch of medicine concerned with the care of women during pregnancy, childbirth and the postpartal period.

Oedipus complex: Freudian belief that preschool boys fall in love with their mother.

Oligohydramnios: Lessened amount of amniotic fluid.

Oligospermia: A sperm count less than normal.

Omphalocele: A congenital protrusion of intestine through a defect in the abdominal wall at the umbilicus.

Oncogenic virus: An organism capable of causing tumors.

Oocyte: An immature ovum.

Operculum: The mucous plug formed in the cervical canal during pregnancy.

Ophthalmia neonatorum: Infection of the conjunctivitis within the first 30 days of life; commonly used to describe gonorrheal infection of the conjunctiva.

Oral phase: The focus of the infant year according to Freud.

Orchiectomy: Excision of one or both testes.

Orchiopexy: Surgical fixation of an undescended testis into the scrotum.

Organic heart murmur: An accessory heart sound that signifies a structural heart defect.

Organogenesis period: The period of fetal life during which the major organs are forming; the 5th to 8th weeks.

Orientation: The ability to discern name, location, and time.

Orthopnea: The condition in which a person must sit upright in order to breathe comfortably.

Orthoptics: Eye exercises designed to correct visual control of binocular vision.

Osteosarcoma: A malignant tumor of the long bones usually involving mesenchyme cells.

Overhydration: Excessive fluid in body tissue.

Overweight: A weight greater than 20% above ideal weight or a body mass index over 26.1.

Ovo-vegetarian: A diet mainly of fruits and vegetables with some egg products allowed.

Oxytocin: A hormone secreted by the posterior pituitary. Acts to maintain and strengthen uterine contractions.

Pain: A subjective symptom of physical or mental suffering.

Palilalia: The rapid repetition of the same word or phrase.

Palpation: Use of the hand to determine manually the characteristics of tissue.

Pancytopenia: Deficiency of all cell elements of the blood.

Pandemic: Occurring throughout the population of a country.

Para: A term used to denote a woman who has produced a living child.

Parachute reaction: When an infant is held horizontally and lowered toward a surface, he or she pushes out the arms as if to break a fall.

Paralytic strabismus: Deviation of the eye from muscle dysfunction.

Paramesonephric (müllerian) ducts: The embryologic tissue that develops into the female reproductive organs.

Paraplegia: Motor or sensory loss of the lower extremities.

Paroxysmal coughing: A series of loud exhalations usually followed by a deep inspiration.

Paroxysmal nocturnal dyspnea: Sudden attacks of shortness of breath and tachycardia that awaken a person from sleep.

Parturition: The act of giving birth.

Passage: The internal pelvic rim through which a fetus must pass in order to be born.

Passenger: The fetus during labor and delivery.

Passive immunity: The condition being unsusceptible to an organism through antibodies crossing the placenta.

Patent urachus: An open connection between the bladder and umbilical cord.

Pathogen: Any microorganism capable of producing disease.

Pathologic retraction ring: An indentation horizontally across the uterus that denotes extreme stress on the divisions of the organ.

Patient-controlled analgesia: A medication delivery system whereby a client dispenses his or her own doses of IV narcotic analgesia.

Pedal spasm: Convulsion or twitching of the foot.

Pediatric nurse practitioner: A nurse prepared at the master's level who has expertise in the nursing care of children.

Pediatrics: The branch of medicine concerned with the development and care of children.

Pedophilia: An abnormal interest in children.

Pellagra: Inflammation, weakness, and disability related to deficiency of niacin.

Pelvic inflammatory disease: The inflammation of the internal female reproductive organs.

Peptic ulcer: An ulceration of the stomach or duodenum.

Percussion: Assessment by listening to the sound made by one finger striking another.

Perimetrium: The outer coat of the uterus.

Perinatal nursing: Nursing during the period surrounding birth.

Period of reactivity: Predictable stages of varying activity demonstrated by newborns in the first few hours following birth.

Periodic respirations: A respiratory pattern of immature infants in which short periods of apnea occur.

Periosteum: The fibrous, highly vascular covering of bone.

Peripartal cardiomyopathy: A unique form of heart disease that occurs only with pregnancy.

Peripheral nervous system: The division of the nervous system outside the central nervous system.

Peritoneal dialysis: The diffusion of fluid and electrolytes across the peritoneal membrane to simulate kidney function.

Peritonitis: Inflammation of the serous lining of the abdominal cavity.

Periventricular leukomalacia: Abnormal formation of the white matter of the brain caused by an ischemic episode in utero.

Permanence: The knowledge that an object exists even when it is out of sight.

Permissive reporters: Individuals who may report child abuse.

Pernicious vomiting: Another term for hyperemesis gravidarum.

Persistence: The degree to which a child will keep trying to perform an activity after failure.

Petechiae: Pinpoint nonraised, purplish spots on the skin caused by intradermal or submucosal hemorrhage.

Phagocytosis: Killings of cells.

Phallic phase: A Freudian term to describe the developmental phase of the preschooler.

Phenotype: The appearance of an individual in relation to his or her genetic makeup.

Phocomelia: Abnormal formation of arms or legs.

Phonocardiogram: A record of heart sounds recorded by microphone.

Photophobia: Sensitivity to light.

Phototherapy blanket: A commercial pad that emits ultraviolet rays; used in treatment of hyperbilirubinemia.

Physiologic jaundice: Yellowing of the skin that occurs from the normal breakdown of red blood cells at birth in the newborn.

Physiologic retraction ring: The junction of the upper and lower uterine segments during labor.

Physiologic splitting: A delayed second heart sound made by delayed closure of the aortic valve.

Pica: The indiscriminate eating of nonfood substances.

Pincer grasp: The ability to approximate the index finger and thumb to pick up an object.

Placenta accreta: Abnormal adherence of the placenta to the uterine wall making placental delivery very difficult.

Placenta circumvallata: A placenta with the fetal surface covered by chorion.

Placenta marginata: A placenta with the edge of the fetal surface covered by chorion.

Placenta previa: A placenta that is implanted in the lower uterine segment so that it touches or covers the internal os of the cervix.

Placenta succenturiata: A placenta with one or more accessory lobes.

Plasma cell: A form of B-lymphocyte that produces antibodies.

Play therapy: A form of psychotherapy in which children are helped to confront and gain insight into their fears.

Pneumothorax: Air in the chest cavity causing a lung to collapse.

Point of maximum impulse: The place on the chest where the impulse of the left ventricle can be felt.

Polycystic kidney: A condition in which normal kidney tissue is displaced by fluid-filled cysts.

Polycythemia: An excess of red blood cells.

Polydactyly: An extra digit on the hand or foot.

Polydipsia: Excessive thirst.

Polyuria: Excessive urine production.

Portal of entry: Site at which an infectious organism enters a body.

Portal of exit: Site at which an infectious organism leaves a body.

Position: Relationship of a chosen fetal reference point to its location in front, back, or sides of the maternal pelvis.

Positive reinforcement: Offering praise to motivate a child to learn.

Positive sign of pregnancy: A finding that definitely indicates a pregnancy is present.

Positron emission tomography (PET): A diagnostic technique involving a radioisotope and computed tomography.

Postcardiac surgery syndrome: A febrile episode occurring following extracorporeal membrane perfusion.

Postconventional development: The moral stage of development according to Kohlberg of the child older than 12 years.

Postmature syndrome: An infant born after 42 weeks of pregnancy with nutritional deficiencies.

Postpartal depression: A feeling of sadness following childbirth.

Postpartal neurosis: Faulty coping that occurs in the postpartal period.

Postpartal psychosis: A psychiatric disorder that occurs in the postpartal period.

Postperfusion syndrome: A febrile illness following extracorporeal perfusion; possibly caused by cytomegalovirus.

Post-term infant: An infant born after week 42 of pregnancy.

Post-term pregnancy: A pregnancy that has extended beyond 42 weeks.

Post-term syndrome: An infant of more than 42 weeks' gestation who has signs of dehydration and decreased growth such as dry skin, meconium staining, and intrauterine growth retardation.

Postural drainage: Positioning of a client in order to drain secretions from the pulmonary tree.

Postural proteinuria: Protein in urine present on standing in an upright posture.

Precipitous labor: Rapid or sudden labor of less than 3 hours' duration.

Preconventional reasoning: The type of moral reason according to Kohlberg that occurs in the young child.

Preeclampsia: The former name for pregnancy-induced hypertension.

Pregnancy-induced hypertension (PIH): Spasms of arterial vessels during pregnancy manifested by hypertension, edema, and albuminuria.

Prehensile ability: The ability to use the hands and fingers to grasp objects.

Preload: The volume of blood in the heart ventricles at the end of diastole.

Premature ejaculation: Deposition of sperm before vaginal penetration or the full enjoyment of the sexual partner.

Premature infant: An infant who weighs 2500 g or less at birth or is less than 38 weeks' gestational age.

Premature labor: Onset of labor before the 37th week of pregnancy or maturity of the fetus.

Premature rupture of the membranes: Spontaneous rupture of the membranes with loss of amniotic fluid prior to the onset of labor.

Premature separation of the placenta: Abruptio placentae.

Premenstrual syndrome: A cluster of symptoms such as irritability and headache experienced prior to menstrual flows.

Preoperational thought: Form of cognitive thought of children from 2 to 7 years of age.

Pre-religious stage: The infant period of moral reasoning.

Pressure anesthesia: Anesthesia achieved by pressure to nerve endings.

Presumptive signs of pregnancy: Findings that suggest but do not confirm that a pregnancy is present.

Preterm infant: An infant born before the 37th week of gestational age.

Preterm labor: Labor occurring before the 37th week of gestation.

Preterm premature rupture of membranes: Rupture of membranes before term.

Primary apnea: A state in which a newborn never breathed at birth.

Primary circular reaction: A stage of cognitive development in which an infant does not yet differentiate between those actions he or she causes and those that occur independently.

Primary dysfunctional labor: Labor that never effectively resulted in cervical dilatation and fetal descent.

Primary infertility: The state of never being able to conceive.

Primary nursing: A method of nursing in which the nurse assumes primary responsibility for planning care for an individual client.

Primigravida: A woman who is having her first pregnancy.

Primipara: A woman who has given birth to a viable child; common usage: a woman who is pregnant for the first time.

Probable signs of pregnancy: Findings that strongly suggest but do not confirm that a pregnancy is present.

Prodromal: Expectant period, or the period during which a disease is infectious before clinical symptoms appear.

Prolactin: A hormone produced by the anterior pituitary gland that stimulates milk production in the mammary glands.

Proteinuria: Protein in the urine.

Prune belly syndrome: A congenital disorder marked by kidney involvement and a flaccid abdominal wall.

Pseudoanemia: The apparent anemia that occurs early in pregnancy due to rapid expansion of blood volume.

Pseudocyesis: A psychological condition in which the woman believes she is pregnant when she is not.

Pseudohermaphrodite: An individual with external features of both sexes.

Psychomotor learning: The acquisition of motor skills.

Psychoprophylaxis: A method of prepared childbirth. Also the Lamaze method.

Ptosis: An abnormal condition in which an upper eyelid does not fully open.

Puberty: The stage of development at which the reproductive organs mature.

Pudendal block: Injection of an anesthetic agent into the perineum to achieve anesthesia of the pudendal nerve.

Puerperium: The first 6 weeks following childbirth.

Purpura: Confluent small blood spots under the skin.

Pyloric stenosis: Stricture of the valve between the stomach and duodenum.

Pyrosis: Heartburn.

Quadriplegia: Paralysis of the arms, legs, and trunk.

Quickening: The first movement of the fetus perceived by the mother.

Radiation: Loss of heat to a distant cold surface.

Rales: The sound of air moving through fluid in alveoli; a crackling sound.

Rape trauma syndrome: A series of predictable behaviors resulting from having been raped.

Rapid-eye-movement (REM) sleep: A pattern of sleep during which dreams and movement of the eyes under closed eyelids occur.

Radiopharmaceutical: A radioactive substance injected or swallowed for diagnostic procedures.

Reactive attachment disorder: Failure to thrive.

Reactivity pattern: The typical manner in which a child responds depending upon the child's temperament.

Recessive: A trait that will not be expressed unless two homozygous genes for the trait are present.

Rectocele: Herniation of the rectum into the posterior vaginal wall.

Redemonstration: Imitating an action that has just been demonstrated.

Reorganization phase: A time period in which a person reestablishes his or her ability to think clearly.

Reproductive life planning: Planning to space children or to prevent children from being conceived.

Reservoir: A container in which organisms grow.

Resonance: The sound produced by percussion over a hollow space.

Retinopathy of prematurity: The formation of fibrotic tissue behind the lens of the eye causing blindness; occurs primarily in premature infants from hyperoxemia.

Retraction: Inward movement of the chest wall on inspiration.

Reticulocytes: Immature red blood cells.

Retroflexion: A uterus that is bent backwards just above the cervix.

Retroversion: A uterus that is tipped abnormally backwards.

Reversibility: The cognitive ability to retrace steps.

Review of systems: A summary of body systems obtained at the end of a health interview.

Rhabdomyosarcoma: A malignant tumor arising from striated muscle cells.

Rh incompatibility: Sensitization to the Rh antigen by an Rh-negative woman; antibodies produced by the woman destroy the red blood cells of a Rh-positive fetus.

Rhythmicity: The degree to which a child maintains a regular or predictable pattern of behavior and response.

Rickets: Deficiency of vitamin D that leads to distortion of bones.

Right-to-left shunt: A passageway in the heart allowing unoxygenated blood to pass into oxygenated blood.

Ripe: A term used to describe the final softening of the cervix just prior to labor.

Rods: The retinal structures that perceive light.

Role fantasy: A type of thought in which the child is influenced by how he or she would like a situation to turn out.

Sadomasochism: A form of sexual expression marked by infliction of pain.

Salmonella: A gram-negative organism frequently responsible for food poisoning.

Sarcoma: A malignant tumor composed of tightly compacted cells.

Schema: A substage of cognitive development according to Piaget.

Secondary apnea: A state in which a newborn breathed at birth but respiratory activity halted.

Secondary dysfunctional labor: Labor that once was effective but becomes dysfunctional in terms of cervical dilatation and fetal descent.

Secondary circular reaction: The stage of cognitive development in which an infant learns that he or she can initiate pleasurable sensations.

Secondary infertility: The state of being unable to conceive although the ability was previously present.

Secondary schema: The Piagetian stage in which infants learn to control activities separate from their body.

Secondary stuttering: Difficulty with stammering that occurs after the child once spoke without the disorder.

Sensorimotor stage: The form of cognitive thought of children 1 month to 2 years of age.

Sensory overload: The overbombardment of stimuli to the senses.

Separation anxiety: Fear and apprehension caused by separation from the primary caregiver.

Septicemia: Infection of the blood.

Sequestrum: A portion of dead bone detached from healthy bone.

Sexually transmitted disease: An illness spread by sexual relations.

Shaken baby syndrome: An infant who has been repetitively, violently shaken.

Sheehan's syndrome: Pituitary necrosis and hypopituitarism occurring from circulatory collapse as a result of uterine hemorrhage.

Shoulder dystocia: Difficulty with delivery of a newborn's shoulder or shoulders.

Shoulder presentation: A fetal presentation in which the shoulder presents to the cervix.

Sickle cell crisis: An acute, episodic condition occurring with children with sickle cell anemia in which red blood cells cluster and cause circulatory obstruction and anoxia to tissue.

Sickle cell trait: The heterozygous form of sickle cell anemia; both hemoglobin S and hemoglobin A are present in red blood cells.

Silent rape syndrome: The predictable behaviors of an individual who was raped but allowed the rape to be unreported.

Sims' position: A resting position with the mother lying on her side, tipped slightly forward so the weight of the fetus rests on the bed surface.

Single proton emission computerized tomography (SPECT): A diagnostic procedure combining tomography and a radioisotope.

Sinus arrhythmia: Irregularity of the heartbeat influenced by inspiration and expiration.

Sitz bath: A bath in which only the hips and buttocks are submerged.

Skeletal traction: Application of tension to align bones by insertion of a pin through the bone.

Skilled home care: Nursing care that includes physician-prescribed procedures such as a dressing change.

Skin traction: Application of tension to align bone by wrapping the extremity in bandages.

Sleep deprivation: A state of confusion or depression caused by inadequate sleep.

Small for gestational age (SGA): A fetus whose weight is below the 10th percentile for number of weeks in utero.

Smooth muscle: Muscle not under voluntary control, such as that in the intestine.

Social smile: A smile in response to another's face; a developmental milestone of 2 months.

Somatic division: The division of the nervous system that acts to regulate voluntary skeletal muscles.

Somogyi phenomenon: The situation in which a child with diabetes mellitus needs less insulin but has symptoms suggestive of insulin lack.

Specificity: The concept that antibodies destroy only like antigens.

Speculum: An instrument with curved blades designed for examination of the vagina and cervix.

Spermatogenesis: The formation and maturation of spermatozoa.

Sperm count: The number of sperm present in a single ejaculation.

Sperm motility: The documented movement of sperm after ejaculation.

Spina bifida: Herniation of the spinal cord or meninges through a vertebral and skin defect; specifically, myomeningocele and meningocele.

Spina bifida occulta: A spinal defect in which a posterior vertebral surface is absent.

Station: Relationship of the presenting fetal part to an imaginary line drawn between the ischial spines of the pelvis.

Steatorrhea: Fat in stools.

Stenosis: A narrowing in a passageway.

Stereognosis: The ability to recognize an object by touch.

Stereopsis: Vision fusion.

Stereotyping: A fixed conception.

Strabismus: Deviation of an eye.

Strawberry hemangioma: A benign tumor of newly formed blood vessels.

Striated muscle: Skeletal muscle; muscle under voluntary control.

Stridor: A high-pitched inspiratory sound.

Stupor: Lethargy or unresponsiveness.

Stye: An infection of a sebaceous gland of the eyelid.

Subclinical disease: A disease so mild that it causes no symptoms.

Subconjunctival hemorrhage: Blood visible on the sclera from a ruptured conjunctival vessel.

Subluxated hip: A congenital orthopedic condition in which a shallow acetabulum allows the femur head freedom of movement.

Submetrocentric: A chromosome with the centromere below the midpoint so that "arms" of unequal length are created.

Substance abuse: The use of chemicals to improve the mental state or induce euphoria.

Superego: The part of the unconscious mind that acts as a monitor over the ego.

Superficial reflexes: A neural reflex initiated by stimulation of the skin.

Suppressor T cell: Specialized T-lymphocytes that reduce the production of immunoglobulins.

Surfactant: A lipoprotein secreted by the alveoli cells to reduce surface tension on expiration.

Susceptible host: A person vulnerable to contracting a disease.

Syncytiotrophoblast: The outer layer of the lining of the trophoblast villi.

Syndactyly: Webbing or joining of fingers or toes.

Synergeneic transplantation: The grafting of tissue from a genetically identical individual to another genetically identical.

Systole: Contraction of the ventricles.

Taboos: Actions that are prohibited in a specific culture.

Tachycardia: Rapid heart rate.

Tachypnea: Rapid respirations.

Taking-hold phase: The second phase of postpartal adjustment when the mother begins to take an active role in child care.

Taking-in phase: The first phase of postpartal adjustment when the mother is chiefly interested in her own care.

Talipes equinovarus: Congenital deformity of the foot.

Teaching plan: A prescription of goals and actions to ensure learning success.

Temperament: A person's innate emotional composition.

Teratogen: An agent capable of causing abnormality in a fetus.

Teratogenicity: The state of causing fetal harm.

Term infant: An infant born at 38 to 40 weeks' gestational age.

Tertiary circular reaction stage: The cognitive stage of development in which the child explores with trial and error to discover new properties of objects or events.

Thelarche: Breast development changes at puberty.

Therapeutic play: A technique useful to help children express fears or concerns.

Threshold of response: The point at which a child will exhibit evidence of frustration.

Thrombocyte: A platelet.

Thrombophlebitis: Inflammation of a vein with accompanying thrombus formation.

Thrush: Candidiasis of the mouth.

Thumb opposition: Ability to approximate the thumb and fingers in order to grasp.

Tic: A minor spasm; may be motor, such as blinking of an eye, or vocal, such as repeating a word or sound.

Tinea capitis: A fungal infection characterized by circular bald patches with erythema and scaling.

T-lymphocyte: A form of white blood cell involved in the immune response.

Tocolytic agent: A drug used to suppress preterm labor.

Tolerance: Progressive diminution of response to the effects of a substance introduced into the body.

Total parenteral nutrition: A method whereby total body nutritional needs are supplied intravenously.

Toxic shock syndrome: Infection occurring during the menstrual flow from organisms entering through the vagina.

Toxoid: A solution of toxins that still stimulates the formation of antitoxins.

Toxoplasmosis: An infection caused by a protozoan parasite and characterized by severe liver and brain involvement in the newborn; spread commonly by cat feces.

Transcultural nursing: A philosophy of nursing that focuses on the unique cultural beliefs of people.

Transition: The period just prior to full dilation in labor; the first few hours of life during which body systems stabilize.

Transcutaneous electrical nerve stimulation (TENS): A method of pain control by the application of electric impulses to nerve endings.

Transillumination: A diagnostic technique utilizing the phenomenon that a bright light shined on a body part will reveal whether the contents of the part are fluid.

Transsexual: A person of one sex whose perceived identity is of the opposite sex.

Transition: The last phase of the first stage of labor during which 8 to 10 cm of cervical dilation is achieved; the first few hours of life during which the newborn stabilizes body functions.

Transitional stool: Green-colored stool that occurs in newborns following meconium and prior to yellow breast-fed or formula-fed infant stools.

Transplant rejection: The immunologic response to the foreign tissue of a transplanted organ.

Transvestism: The practice of dressing in the clothes of the opposite sex.

Trauma: Physical injury caused by violent action.

Triage: The classification of injured persons as to degree of injury and priority for treatment.

Trophoblast: The outer layer of cells of the blastocyst that will become the placenta.

True conjugate: The distance between the interior surface of the symphysis pubis and sacral prominence.

Trust versus mistrust: The developmental task of the infant according to Erikson.

Tubal ligation: A method of contraception in which the fallopian tubes are cauterized, tied, or clamped to prevent migration of the fertilized oocyte to the uterus.

Tumor: An abnormal growth.

Tumor staging: A method to determine the extent of malignant involvement in order to determine and guide therapy.

Turgor: Elasticity of the skin implying adequate fluid content in subcutaneous tissue.

Tympanocentesis: An incision into the ear drum.

Ulcerative colitis: Inflammation of the bowel with shallow necrotic lesions.

Ultrasonography: A diagnostic study made by high frequency sound waves to reveal body organs.

Umbilical cord: The structure composed of two veins and one artery that connects the placenta to the fetus.

Umbilical cord prolapse: An umbilical cord that is presenting at the cervix prior to birth of the fetus.

Underweight: The state of being 10% to 20% less than ideal weight.

Uremia: Excessive urea or nitrogenous waste products in the body.

Uterine atony: Lack of uterus tone that leads to hemorrhage.

Uterine inertia: Dysfunctional labor.

Uterine inversion: Turning inside out of the uterus; could occur following childbirth from an action such as pulling on the umbilical cord before the placenta separates.

Uvea: The fibrous sheath under the sclera that includes the iris, ciliary body, and choroid of the eye.

Vaccine: A substance composed of microorganisms administered to create immunity.

Vacuum extraction: Assisting the birth of a baby by means of vacuum suction.

Vaginal birth after cesarean birth: A planned vaginal birth following a previous cesarean birth.

Vaginismus: Painful, involuntary spasms of the vagina.

Varicocele: Dilation of a blood vessel of the spermatic cord.

Vasectomy: A surgical ligating of the vas deferens that results in male sterility.

Vegan: A strict vegetarian.

Venipuncture: The entrance into a vein to withdraw blood or instill medication or fluid.

Ventral suspension: A position for examination; holding an infant lying in a prone position suspended horizontally.

Vernix caseosa: The cheesy covering of the fetus that protects it from water maceration.

Very-low-birth-weight: A newborn weighing between 1000 to 1500 g or between 26 and 30 weeks of gestation.

Vesicoureteral reflux: Back flow of urine from the bladder into the ureters on voiding.

Vesicular breathing: The type of breath sounds heard over lung periphery; inspiration is longer than expiration.

Viability: The ability to live after birth.

Vocal tics: A spasmodic action manifested by a verbal response.

Volvulus: A twisting of the intestine.

Voyeurism: The practice of obtaining sexual pleasure by looking at the nude body of another.

Vulnerable children: Children whose parents were told that they would die who then subsequently lived.

Vulvovaginitis: Inflammation of the external female reproductive organs.

Wharton's jelly: The gelatinous substance that gives bulk to the umbilical cord.

Wheezing: A whistling expiratory sound.

Yolk sac: The space in embryonic life from which the hemopoietic system develops.

Xerophthalmia: A deficiency of vitamin A resulting in reduction of eye fluid and diminished sight.

Zona pellucida: A layer of fluid that surrounds the ovum at ovulation.

Zygote: A fertilized ovum.

Index

Page numbers followed by f *indicate figures; those followed by* t *indicate tabular material; those in* italics *indicate terms defined in the Glossary.*

coexisting disease in, bleeding with, 400
complications of. *See also specific complication*
    in adolescent, 445–448
    high-risk pregnancy with, 379–422
    National Health Goals addressed to, 380–381
    nursing process with, 381–382
    in woman over 35, 451–452
constipation in, 260, 266*t*
    management of, 292–293
Crohn's disease and, 347–348
cystic fibrosis and, 344
danger signs of, 225*t*, 225–226
decreased decision-making in, 173
dental hygiene in, 182, 237, 255
diabetes mellitus and, 358–365. *See also* Diabetes mellitus
diagnosis of, 184–188, 205, 208*f*
    laboratory findings in, 184
    nursing care plan for, 186–187
domestic abuse in, 374–375
    nursing research on, 375
dressing in, 255
drug dependence and, 462–465
in drug-dependent client, 439–440
dyspnea in, 265
ectopic. *See* Ectopic pregnancy
edema in, 226
elective termination of, 110–113, *1825.* *See also* Abortion
emotional lability in, 173
emotional responses to, 171–173
endocrine changes in, 183
endocrine disorders and, 357–365
exercise in, 256–257
false, 415
fatigue in, 260–261, 266*t*
fetal health promotion during, 251–278
first trimester
    bleeding in, 383*t*, 385–393
    discomforts of, 260–264
    health promotion in, 260–264
    nursing diagnoses in, 260
    psychological tasks of, 167–168
flatulence in, 295
food cravings in, management of, 293–295
fourth trimester of, 603
fractures, 372–373
gastrointestinal changes in, 175*t*, 175, 176*f*, 181–182
gastrointestinal disorders and, 346–348
group B streptococcal infection in, 334
headache in, 265, 266*t*
health promotion during, 224
healthy adaptation to
    cultural influences on, 166
    family influences on, 166
    individual influences on, 166–167
    nursing process for, 164–165
    social influences on, 165–166
heart disease and, 350–357
heart valve prostheses and, 356
hematologic disorders in, 337–340
hemorrhoids in, 237–238, 262–263, 266*t*
hiatal hernia and, 346–347
high-risk. *See* High-risk pregnancy
human immunodeficiency virus infection and, 334–337
human papillomavirus infection in, 333–334
hypercholesterolemia in, 295
hyperthyroidism and, 358
hypotension in, 262

hypothyroidism and, 358
immune system in, 184
immunization in, 259–260
inadequate nutritional pattern in, nursing care plan for, 292–293
inflammatory bowel disease and, 347–348
influenza in, 343
integumentary changes in, 177–178
knee injury in, 373
late
    discomforts of, 264–266
    health promotion in, 264–266
    nursing diagnoses in, 264–265
length of, 205, 209
leukorrhea in, 264
maternal health promotion during, 251–278
methadone maintenance in, 464–465
middle
    discomforts of, 264–266
    health promotion in, 264–266
    nursing diagnoses in, 264–265
molar. *See* Hydatidiform mole
multiple, 411–414
    assessment in, 412
    incidence of, 411–413
    labor complications with, 582–583
    nursing diagnoses related to, 413–414
    nursing interventions related to, 413–414
    nutritional health promotion in, 298–299
    postpartal phase, problems in, 583
    therapeutic management of, 412–413
multiple sclerosis and, 349
muscle cramps in, 261*f*, 261–262, 266*t*
musculoskeletal changes in, 175*t*
musculoskeletal disorders and, 349–350
myasthenia gravis and, 349
nasal congestion in, 179
nasopharyngitis in, 342
nausea and vomiting in, 181
neurologic disorders and, 348–349
nutritional assessment in, 288–289
nutritional risk factors in, 288, 288*t*
nutrition in, components of, 282–287
obesity in, nutrition counseling with, 297–298
occupational hazards in, 258
orthopedic injuries in, 372–373
ovaries in, 175*t*, 177
perineal hygiene in, 255
physiologic changes in, 164, 173–184, 175*t*
pigmentation in, 175*t*, 178
pneumonia in, 343
postdate, 415
postmature, 415
post-term, 415
psychological changes of, 164–167
psychological tasks of, 167–173
pyrosis in, 181, 260, 295
renal changes in, 175*t*
renal disorders and, 340–342
reproductive tract in, 173–177
respiratory changes in, 178–179, 179*t*
respiratory disorders and, 342–344
resting in, 261
reworking of developmental tasks in, 169–170
rheumatic disorders and, 344–346
scoliosis and, 350
seat belt use in, 259
second trimester

bleeding in, 383*t*, 393–396
psychological tasks of, 168–169
seizure disorders and, 348–349
self-care needs in, 254–260
sexual activity in, 86, 256
    client concerns about, nursing care plan for, 87
sexual desire in, changes in, 173
sexually transmitted disease and, 330–337
sexual response in, 86
and sickle cell anemia, 338–340
signs of
    positive, 173, 185*t*, 185–188
    presumptive, 173, 184, 185*t*
    probable, 173, 184–185, 185*t*
skeletal changes in, 183
sleep in, 257–258
smoking cessation in, 272
spinal cord injury and, 454–456
sudden fluid discharge from vagina in, 226
syphilis in, 332–333
systemic changes in, 178–184
temperature in, 179
third trimester
    bleeding in, 383*t*, 396–400
    psychological tasks of, 169–170
trauma in, 366–375
travel in, 258–260
trichomoniasis in, 332
tubal. *See* Ectopic pregnancy
and tuberculosis, 1210
tuberculosis and, 343–344
ulcerative colitis and, 347–348
urinary disorders and, 340–342
urinary tract changes in, 182, 183*t*
urinary tract infection in, 340–341
uterine changes in, 173–176, 175*t*
vaginal bleeding in, 226
vaginal changes in, 175*t*, 177
varicosities in, 262, 262*f*, 266*t*
venous thromboembolic disease and, 356–357
viral hepatitis in, 347
vulvar pruritus in, 264
weight gain in, 282, 283*f*
in woman over 35, 449–453. *See also* Woman over 35, pregnancy in
in woman with cerebral palsy, 456–457
in woman with hearing impairment, 461–462
in woman with mental retardation, 457–458
in woman with special needs, 437–466
    National Health Goals addressed to, 439
    nursing process with, 439–441
in woman with visual impairment, 458–461
in women over 35, 438, 440
in women with disability, 438
work in, 258–259
Pregnancy counseling
    for woman with hearing impairment, 462
    for woman with mental retardation, 458
    for woman with visual impairment, 459–460
Pregnancy history, in child health assessment, 803–804
Pregnancy-induced hypertension, *1830.* *See* Hypertension, pregnancy-induced
    postpartal, 723–724

postictal state, 411
with pregnancy-induced hypertension, nursing interventions related to, 404–405
psychomotor, 1547
recurrent, 348
versus temper tantrums or breath holding, 895*t*
tonic-clonic, 1548
aura, 1548
convulsions of, 1548
in eclampsia, 410–411
injury prevention during, 1549
postictal state, 1548
in pregnancy, 348
prodromal period, 1548
safety measures during, 1549
types of, in children over 3 years old, 1547–1548
Seizure disorder(s), 1544–1551
child with, nursing care plan for, 1552–1553
diagnosis of, EEG in, 1529*f*, 1529–1530
family support measures with, 1549–1550
and pregnancy, 348–349
nursing diagnoses related to, 348–349
nursing interventions related to, 348–349
Self-awareness, of nurse caring for dying child, 1777
Self-care, in home care, 1111
Self-care needs, in pregnancy, 254–260
Self-catheterization, 1152
for bladder emptying, after spinal cord injury, 1559
Self-esteem
in adolescent, 956–957
strengthening, in woman with special needs, 440
Self-feeding, 993–994
Sella turcica, 1486
Semen, 63, 65
*p*H of, 65
Semen analysis, 124–125
Seminal vesicles, 64*f*, 65
functions of, 63
Seminiferous tubules, 64
obstruction, 120
Sensate focus, in labor, 313, 314*f*
Senses, in newborn, 650–651
Sensorimotor stage, 789, 792*t*, *1831*
Sensory deprivation, 1094–1095
Sensory development
in infant, stimulation of, 864–866
of infant, 857–858
Sensory function
assessment of, 829
tests of, 1526
Sensory overload, 1095–1096, *1831*
Sensory responses, in labor, 491
Separation
effect on children, 1016–1018
fear of, in preschooler, 911–912
Separation anxiety, 859, 1719, 1733–1734, *1831*
in hospitalization, 1023–1026
stages of, 1017*t*
in toddlers, 893–894
Septic abortion, 390–391
Septicemia, 1307, *1831*
Sequestrum, 1607, *1831*
Serous cystadenoma, ovarian, 232*t*
Serous otitis media, 1587–1588

Serum
electrolytes, preoperative assessment, 551
maternal, assays, in assessment of fetal well being, 216
osmolality, laboratory values, 1811*t*
*p*H, preoperative assessment, 551
Serum bilirubin test, 1393*t*
Serum glutamic oxaloacetic transaminase
in acetaminophen poisoning, 1647
laboratory values, in pregnant and non-pregnant women, 1806*t*
in Reye's syndrome, 1543
Serum glutamic oxaloacetic transaminase test, 1393*t*
Serum glutamic pyruvic transaminase
in acetaminophen poisoning, 1647
in Reye's syndrome, 1543
Serum glutamic pyruvic transaminase test, 1393*t*
Serum proteins test, 1393*t*
Serum sickness, 1284
Severe combined immunodeficiency syndrome, 1274
Sex
biologic, 1460
genetic, 1460
Sex chromosome(s), 77–78, 193
Sex education
for preschoolers, 915–917
for school-age child, 944
Sex preference, of mothers, for fetus, nursing research on, 168
Sex preselection, 131–132
Sex typing, 80
Sexual abuse, 1470–1471, 1755–1756
assessment for, 1756
incidence of, 1756
long-term effects of, 1744
prevention of, 935
signs of, 1756
therapeutic management of, 1756
Sexual activity
in adolescent, 966–968
after menopause, 83–84
age of initiation of, nursing research on, 944
in pregnancy, 86, 256
client concerns about, nursing care plan for, 87
Sexual assault, 1757
Sexual assessment, 60
Sexual concerns, of school-age children, 926–927
Sexual desire
changes in, in pregnancy, 173
inhibited, 89
Sexual differentiation, embryonic, 62, 193
Sexual dysfunction
biogenic, 88
primary, 88–89
psychogenic, 88
secondary, 89
Sexual expression, types of, 88
Sexual function
after childbirth, 630–631
after spinal cord injury, 1558
disorders of, 88–89
Sexual health, 58–91
promotion, nursing process and, 60–62
Sexual history, 60, 1460
in prenatal care, 232
Sexual identity, definition of, 80
Sexual Information and Education Council of the United States, 952

Sexuality, 80–85
in adolescent, 966–968
clients' concerns about, 58
client teaching about, 81
of individuals with physical disability, 84–85
of older adults, 84
Sexually transmitted disease, 1475–1479, *1831. See also specific disease*
National Health Goals addressed to, 1458
nursing diagnoses related to, 330
and pregnancy, 330–337
prevention of, 87, 330, 1475–1476
condoms in, 104
reportable, client anxiety related to, 1478
Sexual maturation, in school-age child, 926
Sexual orientation, types of, 86–88
Sexual physiology, 85
Sexual response cycle, 85–88
excitement stage of, 85
factors affecting, 84
menstrual cycle and, 86
orgasm, 85
plateau stage of, 85
in pregnancy, 86
resolution stage, 85
Shaken baby syndrome, 1749, *1831*
Sharing, by preschoolers, 913–914
Sheehan's syndrome, *1831*
postpartal, 712–713
Shigella, 1387
Shigellosis, 1387
Shock, with bleeding during pregnancy, 382–385, 384*f*
Shoes
for infant, 867
for toddler, 888–889
Short stature
assessment for, 1487–1488
self-esteem alteration and, 1488
Shoulder dystocia, 589–590, 741, *1831*
Shoulder presentation, *1831*
Show, 266, 485
in labor, 472
Sibling(s)
of children with congenital impairments, 1146
of disabled or fatally ill child, 1771
of infants, safety precautions with, 862
older, home birth and, 320–321
preparing for, 914–915
reactions to newborn, 679–680
Sibling education classes, 316
Sibling rivalry, in preschooler, 914
Sibling visitation, in postpartal period, 607–608, 608*f*
Sickle cell anemia, 1358–1360
child with
long-term health needs of, 1360
special precautions for, 1361
client education regarding, 1360
and pregnancy, 338–340
assessment in, 339
therapeutic management of, 339–340
tissue perfusion in, 1360
Sickle cell crisis, 1359, *1831*
nursing diagnoses related to, 1360
symptoms of, 1359*f*
Sickle cell disease, 144*t*
Sickle cell trait, 338–339, 1358, *1831*
testing, in first prenatal visit, 245
Side effects, 1293–1296
Silent rape syndrome, 1757, *1831*